THE GENETIC BASIS OF COMMON DISEASES

OXFORD MONOGRAPHS ON MEDICAL GENETICS

16. C. R. Scriver and B. Childs: *Garrod's inborn factors in disease*
18. M. Baraitser: *The genetics of neurological disorders*
19. R. J. Gorlin, M. M. Cohen, Jr., and L. S. Levin: *Syndromes of the head and neck, third edition*
21. D. Warburton, J. Byrne, and N. Canki: *Chromosome anomalies and prenatal development: an atlas*
22. J. J. Nora, K. Berg, and A. H. Nora: *Cardiovascular diseases: genetics, epidemiology, and prevention*
24. A. E. H. Emery: *Duchenne muscular dystrophy, second edition*
25. E. G. D. Tuddenham and D. N. Cooper: *The molecular genetics of haemostasis and its inherited disorders*
26. A. Boué: *Fetal medicine*
27. R. E. Stevenson, J. G. Hall, and R. M. Goodman: *Human malformations*
28. R. J. Gorlin, H. V. Toriello, and M. M. Cohen, Jr.: *Hereditary hearing loss and its syndromes*
29. R. J. M. Gardner and G. R. Sutherland: *Chromosome abnormalities and genetic counseling, second edition*
30. A. S. Teebi and T. I. Farag: *Genetic disorders among Arab populations*
31. M. M. Cohen, Jr.: *The child with multiple birth defects*
32. W. W. Weber: *Pharmacogenetics*
33. V. P. Sybert: *Genetic skin disorders*
34. M. Baraitser: *Genetics of neurological disorders, third edition*
35. H. Ostrer: *Non-mendelian genetics in humans*
36. E. Traboulsi: *Genetic diseases of the eye*
37. G. L. Semenza: *Transcription factors and human disease*
38. L. Pinsky, R. P. Erickson, and R. N. Schimke: *Genetic disorders of human sexual development*
39. R. E. Stevenson, C. E. Schwartz, and R. J. Schroer: *X-linked mental retardation*
40. M. J. Khoury, W. Burke, and E. Thomson: *Genetics and public health in the 21st century*
41. J. Weil: *Psychosocial genetic counseling*
42. R. J. Gorlin, M. M. Cohen, Jr., and R. C. M. Hennekam: *Syndromes of the head and neck, fourth edition*
43. M. M. Cohen, Jr., G. Neri, and R. Weksberg: *Overgrowth syndromes*
44. R. A. King, J. I. Rotter, and A. G. Motulsky: *The genetic basis of common diseases, second edition*

OXFORD MONOGRAPHS ON MEDICAL GENETICS NO. 44

The Genetic Basis of Common Diseases

Second Edition

Edited by

RICHARD A. KING
University of Minnesota

JEROME I. ROTTER
Cedars-Sinai Medical Center and UCLA

ARNO G. MOTULSKY
University of Washington

OXFORD
UNIVERSITY PRESS
2002

OXFORD
UNIVERSITY PRESS

Oxford New York
Auckland Bangkok Buenos Aires Cape Town Chennai
Dar es Salaam Delhi Hong Kong Istanbul Karachi Kolkata
Kuala Lumpur Madrid Melbourne Mexico City Mumbai Nairobi
São Paulo Shanghai Singapore Taipei Tokyo Toronto

and an associated company in Berlin

Published by Oxford University Press, Inc.,
198 Madison Avenue, New York, New York, 10016
http://www.oup-usa.org

Library of Congress Cataloging-in-Publication Data
The genetic basis of common diseases / edited by Richard A. King, Jerome I. Rotter, Arno G. Motulsky.—2nd ed.
p. ; cm.—(Oxford monographs on medical genetics ; no. 44)
Includes bibliographical references and index.
ISBN 0-19-512582-7
1. Medical genetics. 2. Genetic disorders. I. King, Richard A. (Richard Allen), 1939–
II. Rotter, Jerome I. III. Motulsky, Arno G., 1923– IV. Series.
[DNLM: I. Genetics, Medical. 2. Genetic Diseases, Inborn—genetics. 3. Genetic Predisposition to Disease. QZ 50 G3226 2002]
RB155 .G3593 2002
616'.042—dc21
2002018390

1 2 3 4 5 6 7 8 9

Printed in the United States of America
on acid-free paper

PREFACE TO THE SECOND EDITION

Ten years have elapsed since the first edition of this book appeared. At that time, the promise of better genetic understanding of common complex diseases had only recently emerged. The 1992 volume was a first attempt to describe genetic aspects of many of these diseases under one cover. The search for genes underlying common diseases has now become one of the most active areas of biomedical research and is supported by the government and nonprofit foundations as well as by the biotechnology and pharmaceutical industries.

The Human Genome Project has provided an almost complete sequence of the human genome and, together with novel methods of population genetics and statistics, is ready to be used for finding genes involved in complex multigenic diseases. New techniques involving the use of DNA markers such as single nucleotide polymorphisms (SNPs) are being applied more widely and include haplotypic combinations of SNPs in a given chromosomal region. Knowledge of the genetic basis of common disease is expanding and is increasingly brought to the clinic. Current excitement must be tempered, however, by the complexity of the problems: the difficulty in identifying susceptibility genes of modest effect, the large scale of the required family studies, the difficulty in proving that a provisionally identified gene is indeed responsible for susceptibility, and delineating the mechanisms by which implicated genes cause clinical disease. Thus, genetic elucidation of complex diseases has been slower than some observers had hoped for. While we are learning more about the role of various genes in complex diseases, the isolation of specific genes that were localized by linkage studies in complex diseases has been arduous and remains difficult. It is the goal of this second edition to convey current knowledge, excitement, and balance.

To accomplish this goal, the second edition of *The Genetic Basis of Common Diseases* has grown from 46 to 55 chapters. More importantly, it has been almost completely rewritten. There are 20 entirely new chapters, reflecting advances in diseases whose genetic knowledge was rudimentary at the time of the first edition. In a few cases, chapters have been combined, while other chapters have been divided. New chapters for specific diseases cover gallstones, hemochromatosis, osteoporosis, spondyloarthrophies, lupus erythematosis, mental retardation, common skin diseases and skin cancer, prostate cancer, hearing loss, and migraine. New general chapters address topics such as genetic counseling, evolution and disease, genetic effects of therapy, pharmacogenetics, and the role of mitochondrial variation. The authorship is virtually completely changed; close to 90% of the authors (103 out of 117) are new.

This second edition should be useful to readers with a clinical, genetic, or epidemiologic orientation who want to learn more about the genetics of common diseases or who can put this information to practical use in an increasing number of conditions. We hope that the presentation of current knowledge will lead to novel biomedical and genetic research that brings better understanding, prevention, and treatment of these diseases that constitute the majority of adult illnesses in the developed world.

Minneapolis, Minnesota R.A.K.
Los Angeles, California J.I.R.
Seattle, Washington A.G.M.
June 2002

CONTENTS

Part VI Genitourinary Disorders

Part VII Rheumatologic Diseases

Part VIII Cancer

Part IX Neuropsychiatric Disorders

Part X Other Common Problems

Part XI Therapy

CONTRIBUTORS

Dharam P. Agarwal, Ph.D., D.Sc.
Institute of Human Genetics
School of Medicine
University of Hamburg
Hamburg, Germany

Gregory J. Anderson, Ph.D.
Iron Metabolism Laboratory
Queensland Institute of Medical Research
Brisbane, Australia

Allen E. Bale, M.D.
Department of Genetics
Yale University
School of Medicine
New Haven, Connecticut

Robert Baloh, M.D.
Department of Neurology
University of California, Los Angeles
School of Medicine
Los Angeles, California

Michael A. Becker, M.D.
Rheumatology Section
Department of Medicine
The University of Chicago
Pritzker School of Medicine
Chicago, Illinois

Timothy W. Behrens, M.D.
Department of Medicine
University of Minnesota Medical School
Minneapolis, Minnesota

Thomas D. Bird, M.D.
Departments of Neurology and Medicine
University of Washington
School of Medicine
VA Medical Center
Seattle, Washington

Eugene R. Bleecker, M.D.
Center for Human Genomics
Department of Medicine
Wake Forest University School of Medicine
Winston-Salem, North Carolina

Claude Bouchard, Ph.D.
George A. Bray Professor
Executive Director
Pennington Biomedical Research Center
Louisiana State University
Baton Rouge, Louisiana

George Bray, M.D.
Boyd Professor
Pennington Biomedical Research Center
Louisiana State University
Baton Rouge, Louisiana

Suzanne J. Brown, M.D.
Department of Internal Medicine
Yale University
School of Medicine
New Haven, Connecticut

W. Ted Brown, M.D., Ph.D.
State University of New York
Downstate Medical Center
Brooklyn, New York

John D. Brunzell, M.D.
Department of Medicine
Division of Metabolism, Endocrinology, and Nutrition
University of Washington
School of Medicine
Seattle, Washington

Randall W. Burt, M.D.
Huntsman Cancer Institute
University of Utah
Salt Lake City, Utah

Ellen Buschman, Ph.D.
Department of Medicine
McGill University Health Centre
Montreal General Hospital
Montreal, Quebec
Canada

Frances Busfield, Ph.D.
Department of Diabetes and Endocrinology
Princess Alexandra Hospital
Brisbane, Australia

Martin C. Carey, M.D., D.Sc.
Department of Gastroenterology
Brigham and Women's Hospital
Harvard Medical School
Boston, Massachusetts

Suzanne B. Cassidy, M.D.
Department of Pediatrics
University of California, Irvine
School of Medicine
Irvine, California

Kay Chapman, Ph.D.
Institute of Molecular Medicine
University of Oxford
Oxford, United Kingdom

Ken C. Chiu, M.D.
Division of Endocrinology, Diabetes, and Hypertension
University of California, Los Angeles
School of Medicine
Los Angeles, California

Francis S. Collins, M.D., Ph.D.
National Human Genome Research Institute
National Institutes of Health
Bethesda, Maryland

Albert J. Czaja, M.D.
Division of Gastroenterology and Hepatology
Department of Medicine
Mayo Clinic and Mayo Foundation
Rochester, Minnesota

Richard C. Davis, Ph.D.
Department of Medicine
University of California, Los Angeles
School of Medicine
Los Angeles, California

Florence Demenais, M.D.
Department of Statistical Genetics and
Genetic Epidemiology of Multifactorial Diseases
INSERM EMI 00-06
Evry, France

Sevilla D. Detera-Wadleigh, Ph.D.
Genetics of Mood and Anxiety Unit
Mood and Anxiety Disorders Program
National Institute of Mental Health
National Institutes of Health
Bethesda, Maryland

Jared M. Diamond, Ph.D.
Department of Physiology
UCLA School of Medicine
Los Angeles, California

Michael J. Econs, M.D., F.A.C.P., F.A.C.E.
Departments of Medicine and Medical and Molecular Genetics
Indiana University School of Medicine
Indianapolis, Indiana

Steven C. Elbein, M.D.
Division of Endocrinology
University of Arkansas for Medical Sciences
John L. McClellan Veterans Hospital
Little Rock, Arkansas

Henry A. Erlich, Ph.D.
Human Genetics Department
Roche Molecular Systems
Alameda, California

David B. Everman, M.D.
Greenwood Genetic Center
Greenwood, South Carolina

Rena Ellen Falk, M.D.
Professor of Pediatrics
UCLA School of Medicine
Ahmanson Department of Pediatrics
Medical Genetics and Birth Defects Center
Cedar-Sinai Medical Center
Los Angeles, California

Magali Fernandez, M.D.
Department of Medicine
Ohio State University
College of Medicine
Columbus, Ohio

Nathan Fischel-Ghodsian, M.D.
Professor of Pediatrics
UCLA School of Medicine
Ahmanson Department of Pediatrics
Medical Genetics and Birth Defects Center
Cedar-Sinai Medical Center
Los Angeles, California

Tatiana Foroud, Ph.D.
Departments of Medical and Molecular Genetics and
Psychiatry
Indiana University School of Medicine
Indianapolis, Indiana

Patrick M. Gaffney, M.D.
Department of Medicine
University of Minnesota Medical School
Minneapolis, Minnesota

Thomas D. Gelehrter, M.D.
Department of Human Genetics
University of Michigan
Ann Arbor, Michigan

Lynn R. Goldin, Ph.D.
Genetic Epidemiology Branch
Division of Cancer Epidemiology and Genetics
National Cancer Institute
National Institutes of Health
Bethesda, Maryland

Stefan K.G. Grebe, Arzt, M.D., F.R.A.C.P.
Department of Pathology and Molecular Medicine
University of Otago
Wellington School of Medicine and Health Sciences
Wellington, New Zealand

Jonathan L. Haines, Ph.D.
Department of Molecular Physiology and Biophysics
Program in Human Genetics
Vanderbilt University Medical Center
Nashville, Tennessee

Edward J. Hollox, Ph.D.
Institute of Genetics
University of Nottingham
Nottingham, United Kingdom

Paul N. Hopkins, M.D., M.S.P.H.
Department of Internal Medicine
University of Utah
School of Medicine
Salt Lake City, Utah

Patrick H. Horn, B.S.
Department of Pediatrics
University of Oklahoma
College of Medicine
Oklahoma City, Oklahoma

Marshall Horwitz, M.D., Ph.D.
Division of Medical Genetics
Department of Medicine
University of Washington
School of Medicine
Seattle, Washington

Steven C. Hunt, Ph.D.
Department of Internal Medicine
University of Utah
School of Medicine
Salt Lake City, Utah

William B. Isaacs, Ph.D.
Department of Urology
Johns Hopkins University
School of Medicine
Baltimore, Maryland

C. Conrad Johnston, Jr., M.D.
Department of Medicine
Indiana University School of Medicine
Indianapolis, Indiana

Werner Kalow, M.D.
Department of Pharmacology
University of Toronto
Toronto, Ontario
Canada

Beth Y. Karlan, M.D.
Department of Obstetrics and Gynecology
University of California, Los Angeles
School of Medicine
Los Angeles, California

Francine Kauffman, M.D.
Department of Epidemiology and Biostatistics
INSERM U472
Villejuif, France

Richard A. King, M.D., Ph.D.
Department of Medicine
University of Minnesota Medical School
Minneapolis, Minnesota

Satu Kuokkanen, M.D., Ph.D.
Department of Obstetrics and Gynecology
Columbia University
College of Physicians and Surgeons
New York, New York

Jean-Marc Lalouel, M.D., D.Sc.
Department of Human Genetics
University of Utah
School of Medicine
Salt Lake City, Utah

Virginia K. Lasseter, B.A.
Department of Psychiatry
Johns Hopkins University
School of Medicine
Baltimore, Maryland

Bonnie S. LeRoy, M.S.
Department of Genetics, Cell Biology, and Development
The University of Minnesota
Minneapolis, Minnesota

Marie T. Lott, M.A.
Center for Molecular Medicine
Emory University
School of Medicine
Atlanta, Georgia

John Loughlin, Ph.D.
Institute of Molecular Medicine
University of Oxford
Oxford, United Kingdom

Aldons J. Lusis, Ph.D.
Departments of Medicine, of Microbiology, Immunology, and Molecular Genetics, and of Human Genetics
University of California, Los Angeles
School of Medicine
Los Angeles, California

George M. Martin, M.D.
Departments of Pathology and Genome Sciences
University of Washington
School of Medicine
Seattle, Washington

John A. McGrath, M.S.
Department of Psychiatry
Johns Hopkins University
School of Medicine
Baltimore, Maryland

Deborah A. Meyers, Ph.D.
Center for Human Genomics
Departments of Pediatrics and Public Health
Wake Forest University School of Medicine
Winston-Salem, North Carolina

Arno G. Motulsky, M.D.
Departments of Medicine (Division of Medical Genetics) and Genome Sciences
University of Washington
School of Medicine
Seattle, Washington

John J. Mulvihill, M.D.
Department of Pediatrics
University of Oklahoma
College of Medicine
Oklahoma City, Oklahoma

Katherine L. Nathanson, M.D.
Department of Medicine
University of Pennsylvania
School of Medicine
Philadelphia, Pennsylvania

Barbara Nepom, M.D.
Immunology Program
Virginia Mason Research Center
Seattle, Washington

Gerald T. Nepom, M.D., Ph.D.
Virginia Mason Research Center and
Department of Immunology
University of Washington School of Medicine
Seattle, Washington

Susan L. Neuhausen, Ph.D.
Department of Medical Informatics
University of Utah School of Medicine
Salt Lake City, Utah

Carole Ober, Ph.D.
Departments of Human Genetics
and Obstetrics and Gynecology
The University of Chicago
Chicago, Illinois

Beverly Paigen, Ph.D.
The Jackson Laboratory
Bar Harbor, Maine

Aarno Palotie, M.D., Ph.D.
Department of Pathology and Laboratory Medicine
University of California, Los Angeles
School of Medicine
Los Angeles, California

George Papadimitriou, M.D.
University Mental Health Research Institute
Eginition Hospital
Athens, Greece

Godfrey D. Pearlson, M.D.
Department of Psychiatry
Johns Hopkins University
School of Medicine
Baltimore, Maryland

Leena Peltonen, M.D., Ph.D.
Department of Human Genetics
University of California, Los Angeles
School of Medicine
Los Angeles, California
Biomedicum, University of Helsinki
National Public Health Institute
Helsinki, Finland

A.S. Peña, M.D., Ph.D., F.R.C.P.
Professor of Gastrointestinal Immunology
Head Laboratory of Immunogenetics
Department of Gastroenterology
Vrije Universiteit Medical Center
Amsterdam, The Netherlands

Margaret A. Pericak-Vance, Ph.D.
Center for Human Genetics
Department of Medicine
Duke University Medical Center
Durham, North Carolina

M. Alan Permutt, M.D.
Division of Endocrinology, Diabetes, and Metabolism
Washington University School of Medicine
St. Louis, Missouri

William D. Posten, M.D.
Department of Genetics
Yale University
School of Medicine
New Haven, Connecticut

Lawrie W. Powell, M.D., Ph.D.
Iron Metabolism Laboratory
Queensland Institute of Medical Research
Brisbane, Australia

Jon L. Pryor, M.D., Ph.D.
Department of Urologic Surgery
University of Minnesota Medical School
Minneapolis, Maryland

Ann E. Pulver, Sc.D.
Department of Psychiatry
Johns Hopkins University
School of Medicine
Baltimore, Maryland

Reed E. Pyeritz, M.D., Ph.D.
Division of Medical Genetics
Department of Medicine
University of Pennsylvania School of Medicine
Philadelphia, Pennsylvania

Leslie J. Raffel, M.D.
Medical Genetics—Birth Defects Center
Department of Pediatrics
Cedars-Sinai Medical Center
Department of Pediatrics
University of California, Los Angeles
School of Medicine
Los Angeles, California

Stephen S. Rich, Ph.D.
Department of Public Health Sciences
Wake Forest University
School of Medicine
Winston-Salem, North Carolina

Kenneth P. Roberts, Ph.D.
Departments of Urologic Surgery and Genetics, Cell Biology, and Development
University of Minnesota Medical School
Minneapolis, Minnesota

Jerome I. Rotter, M.D.
Director, Division of Medical Genetics
Cedars-Sinai Board of Governors' Chair in Medical Genetics
Departments of Medicine, Pediatrics, and Human Genetics
University of California, Los Angeles
Los Angeles, California

Janna Saarela, M.D., Ph.D.
Biomedicum, University of Helsinki
National Public Health Institute
Helsinki, Finland

Maren T. Scheuner, M.D., M.P.H.
Department of Medicine
University of California, Los Angeles
School of Medicine
Los Angeles, California

Harry W. Schroeder, Jr., M.D., Ph.D., F.A.C.M.G.
Division of Developmental and Clinical Immunology
Comprehensive Cancer Center
Departments of Medicine and Microbiology
University of Alabama at Birmingham
Birmingham, Alabama

Erwin Schurr, Ph.D.
Departments of Medicine and Human Genetics
McGill Centre for the Study of Host Resistance
Montreal General Hospital
Montreal, Quebec
Canada

R. Hal Scofield, M.D.
Department of Medicine
University of Oklahoma
College of Medicine
Arthritis and Immunology Program
Oklahoma Medical Research Foundation
Oklahoma City, Oklahoma

Thomas A. Sellers, Ph.D., M.P.H.
Department of Health Sciences Research
Mayo Clinic and Foundation
Rochester, Minnesota

Joe Leigh Simpson, M.D.
Department of Obstetrics and Gynecology
Baylor College of Medicine
Houston, Texas

Emil Skamene, M.D., Ph.D.
Departments of Medicine and Human Genetics
McGill University Health Centre
Montreal General Hospital
Montreal, Quebec
Canada

Jeffrey R. Smith, M.D., Ph.D.
Department of Medicine
Division of Genetic Medicine
Vanderbilt University Medical Center
Nashville, Tennessee

Dallas M. Swallow, Ph.D.
Department of Human Genetics
The Galton Laboratory
Department of Biology
University College London
London, United Kingdom

Karen L. Swartz, M.D.
Department of Psychiatry
Johns Hopkins University
School of Medicine
Baltimore, Maryland

Virginia P. Sybert, M.D.
Division of Dermatology
Department of Medicine
University of Washington
School of Medicine
Seattle, Washington

Kent D. Taylor, Ph.D.
Medical Genetics Birth Defects Center
Imflammatory Bowel Disease Center
Departments of Medicine and Pediatrics
Steven Spielberg Pediatric Research Center
Cedars-Sinai Research Institute
University of California, Los Angeles
School of Medicine
Los Angeles, California

Marian S. Verp, M.D.
Departments of Obstetrics and Gynecology
And Human Genetics
The University of Chicago
Chicago, Illinois

Ann P. Walker, M.A.
Department of Pediatrics
University of California, Irvine
Orange, California

Douglas C. Wallace, Ph.D.
Center for Molecular Medicine
Emory University
School of Medicine
Atlanta, Georgia

Barbara L. Weber, M.D.
Department of Medicine and Genetics
University of Pennsylvania
School of Medicine
Philadelphia, Pennsylvania

Maija Wessman, Ph.D.
Department of Biosciences
University of Helsinki
Helsinki, Finland

David West, Ph.D.
Xenogen
Alameda, California

Sarah F. Whitton
Department Pediatrics
University of Oklahoma
College of Medicine
Oklahoma City, Oklahoma

Denise G. Wiesch, Ph.D.
Division of Allergy, Immunology, and Transplantation
National Institute of Allergy and Infectious Diseases
National Institutes of Health
Bethesda, Maryland

Georgia L. Wiesner, M.D.
Departments of Genetics and Medicine
Case Western Reserve University
School of Medicine and
University Hospitals of Cleveland
Cleveland, Ohio

Jianfeng Xu, M.D., M.P.H.
Department of Public Health
Center for Human Genomics
Wake Forest University
School of Medicine
Winston-Salem, North Carolina

Huiying Yang, M.D., Ph.D.
Medical Genetics Birth Defects Center
Inflammatory Bowel Disease Center
Departments of Medicine and Pediatrics
Steven Spielberg Pediatric Research Center
Cedars-Sinai Research Institute
University of California, Los Angeles
School of Medicine
Los Angeles, California

Ping Yang, M.D., Ph.D.
Department of Health Sciences Research
Mayo Clinic
Rochester, Minnesota

John J. Zone, M.D.
Department of Dermatology
University of Utah School of Medicine
Salt Lake City, Utah

Part I

APPROACHES

1 Approach to Genetic Basis of Common Diseases

RICHARD A. KING, JEROME I. ROTTER, AND ARNO G. MOTULSKY

In broad terms, human genetics is the study of human biologic variation, and medical genetics is the study of how this variation can cause human disease. Individuals inherit copies of genes that produce disease or, more commonly, produce a susceptibility to a disease that becomes manifest with time and with environmental interaction. This book is devoted to common diseases in the adult population that have significant genetic susceptibility. Because individuals are not equally susceptible to the many disorders covered in this volume, the reasons for these differences are now being identified. Both the rapid increase in genetic knowledge stemming from the Human Genome Project and hard work in many laboratories throughout the world are providing critical information on gene mechanisms, pathways, and cellular processes that were unexplored and unknown when the first edition of this book was published. Appropriate disease classification, diagnosis, and management, along with the evaluation of patients' family members who may be at risk, will all benefit from genetic insights. Therefore, an understanding of genetic principles in common diseases should be part of every physician's and epidemiologist's armamentarium.

The generally accepted role of genetics in medicine has been the study of chromosomal and single-gene disorders that are clearly the result of specific changes within the genome of the affected individual (Rimoin et al., 1996; Vogel and Motulsky, 1997; Scriver et al., 2001). Many of these disorders are infrequent or rare, and they generally occur more frequently in children than in adults. Major aberrations in chromosome structure or number, or grossly abnormal gene function, account for such "classical" genetic disorders. Their recognition has played a major role in the advances of genetic knowledge. More complex problems such as diseases that "run in families" but do not follow the rules of Mendelian inheritance have been identified, but methods to assess their genetic components were lacking. This has changed in the last decade. Molecular techniques have gone beyond the mapping of genes to an understanding of their structure and regulation and to methods that may allow identification of individual copies (i.e., alleles) of genes that create susceptibility to disease either directly or indirectly by identifying DNA markers that segregate with the actual disease genes. The sequence of the entire human genome has become available. This has resulted in excitement, expansive predictions, and hope that genetics will solve the many medical problems of the population. Frequent stories about the "new genetics" are published in the popular press. We are concerned that the use of these new developments for prevention and treatment will require much more time than is often implied. There is no question that genetic susceptibility often will be critical in the pathogenesis of common diseases; however, our understanding of the complex problems of pathogenesis, prevention and treatment is yet in its infancy. What is exciting about the second edition of this book is that our understanding was just emerging when the first edition was published in 1992, but significant strides have been made in the ensuing years. Although this volume is large, it represents only the first steps in our understanding of human biology and variation as they provide a road map for the future of medicine.

COMMON DISEASES

What Are Common Diseases?

The subject of this volume is the genetic basis of common diseases.

Why common? Common disease means precisely what the term says, those diseases that are common in the population at large, such as coronary heart disease, diabetes, colon cancer, breast cancer, prostate cancer, depression, dementia, and osteoporosis, to name but a few (see contents listing for the others that are discussed here). These are the diseases that are responsible for the majority of morbidity, mortality, and health-care costs (both personal and societal) in the developed world. As such, they are responsible for the greatest burden to society and to the population at large. If we better understand the causes of these diseases, we hope to have a basis for developing more specific and more effective therapies, as well as means of prevention. If we can identify who is at risk, we will know to whom these means of prevention should be directed.

Why genetic? Because, as will be repeatedly demonstrated in this volume, all common diseases have a genetic component of susceptibility that plays a role in pathogenesis. Thus, the elucidation of genetic susceptibility will provide an overall understanding of etiology. Genetics has two major implications. One is that understanding the underlying genetics will lead to understanding the causes, which may lead to better and more specific therapies. The other is that with identification of the responsible genes, we will have developed tools to identify those who are at risk in families and in the population at large. This will allow the development of individualized health assessment and targeted prevention strategies.

As a practical definition of common diseases, we have set the frequency of 1 affected individual per 1000 for a given disease to be considered common and thus to be discussed in this volume. There are several reasons for using this criterion. Common diseases are those that most physicians will encounter in their practice, and the encounters will occur a number of times. At this frequency, these diseases contribute substantially to a society's health-care costs. Finally, they are sufficiently common that the frequency of the predisposing genes cannot be explained by recurrent mutation (see Chapter 4). Such genes therefore contribute substantially to the variation in the human genome and to the uniqueness of individuals. Occasionally, we include a subset of disease that is less frequent but which illustrates an important genetic principle applicable to common diseases.

HOW DO COMMON DISEASES DIFFER FROM TRADITIONAL SINGLE-GENE DISORDERS?

Currently, the best understood human genetic disorders are those single-gene disorders that present at birth or in childhood. Many of these follow Mendelian laws of inheritance and are either dominant or recessive and either autosomal or X-linked. For that reason, one can accurately predict the risk within families. Even more important, there often appears to be a clear predictive relationship between genotype and occurrence of the phenotype—that is, clinical disease. Thus, one abnormal allele at the fibrillin locus predicts Marfan syndrome, and two abnormal "sickle" alleles at the β-hemoglobin locus predict sickle cell anemia. For many Mendelian single-gene disorders the resulting diseases may vary in severity. Although many single-gene disorders exhibit variable expressivity of their phenotype, the problems of genotype–phenotype relationship are much greater for common complex diseases.

The relationship between genotype and phenotype in common diseases can appear at several levels. One is the number of basically different disease mechanisms that are included in a given disease category, and this is the concept of genetic *heterogeneity*. Thus both Type 1 and Type 2 diabetes are characterized by glucose intolerance (see Chapter 21 on Type 1 diabetes and Chapter 22 on Type 2 diabetes). But Type 1 diabetes is predominantly a disease of autoimmune destruction of the insulin-producing beta cells of the pancreatic islets, whereas Type 2 diabetes is most often a disease due to combined defects of insulin resistance and insulin secretion. Both result in hyperglycemia, but, for the most part, the underlying genetics and pathogenetic features are distinct. Many of the diseases reviewed in this volume have been demonstrated to exhibit, or are likely to exhibit, similar heterogeneity.

Even when we can accurately delineate heterogeneity, there is still enormous complexity. Often some forms of a common disease are due to single-gene mechanisms—for example, familial hypercholesterolemia due to low-density lipoprotein (*LDL*) receptor gene defects (see Chapter 7) and breast cancer due to abnormalities in the *BRCA1* and *BRCA2* genes (see Chapter 5). More frequently, however, the underlying susceptibility appears to be due to a number of genes acting in concert. A polygenic disease is one for which there are many such genes. If only a few genes (say two, three, or four) are required for susceptibility, the term *oligogenic* has been applied. Furthermore, the complexity not only relates to the number of genes but also may often reflect gene–gene interactions. Many questions arise with such interactions. Do the predisposing genes interact additively or independently, or multiplicatively and synergistically? Are certain genes necessary for disease susceptibility, while others only add to the susceptibility?

Environment often plays a major role in the pathogenesis of a common disease. The clearest example came from studies of migrant populations. For example, Japanese in Japan, compared to Western populations of European origin, have a relatively high frequency of stroke and gastric cancer and a relatively low frequency of coronary artery disease and colon cancer (Robertson et al., 1977; Flood et al., 2000). All of these diseases (stroke, coronary artery disease, gastric cancer, colon cancer) can be shown to have major genetic susceptibilities. Yet, when Japanese individuals migrate to the United States, their frequency of stroke and gastric cancer decreases and that of coronary artery disease and colon cancer increases. Since their genes have not changed, differences in the environment are clearly responsible. The implications of such observations are enormous for common diseases. Gene–environment interactions have to be considered in addition to gene–gene interactions. The responsible environmental factors are often yet to be defined, but they may range from diet, lifestyle (e.g., exercise), and smoking to infectious agents. It is quite clear that in many well-defined chronic infectious diseases (e.g., tuberculosis, hepatitis B, and malaria), genetic factors play a major role in both natural history and susceptibility (see Chapter 10). A recent example is *Helicobacter pylori*, the infectious cause of peptic ulcer. Yet in any population many more people are infected with *H. pylori* than ever develop ulcer, presumably for genetic reasons. Thus, in virtually all common diseases, we are facing interactions between genetic and environmental factors.

In addition to the terms *polygenic* and *oligogenic*, which refer to the number of genes involved, the designator *multifactorial inheritance* is applied, usually implying that one of the multiple etiologic factors is the environment. Another term commonly used is *complex diseases*, as cited earlier.

Risk and Burden of Common Diseases

The burden of common diseases such as cardiovascular, pulmonary, gastrointestinal, metabolic, neuropsychiatric, and oncologic diseases is great, since they are the leading causes of morbidity and mortality in the developed world. It is important to emphasize that the costs are not just borne by the patient and health-care system for medical-care expenses; costs to the individual and to society also include lost productivity and premature death, not to mention the suffering of the individual and their family. Examples of the magnitude of the costs are shown in Table 1–1. Besides the economic burden to a society and its individual citizens, another measure of the burden for an individual is the lifetime risk for mortality and morbidity of these diseases (Michaud et al., 2001). It is clear that since these diseases are common, virtually everyone in the population is at risk. Although such risks are often quoted as a single composite figure such as 1 in 50, the specific risk for an individual will be higher or lower than 1 in 50, depending on genetic makeup, environment, or other circumstances. What proportion is at risk for these common disorders? One study examined only common disorders such as heart disease, common cancers, and diabetes for

Table 1–1. Annual Cost of Common Diseases in the U.S. Population

Disease	No. of People Affected	Cost
Alzheimer's disease	4 million	$152 billion
Arthritis	43 million	$65 billion
Cancer	8.4 million	$107 billion
Cardiovascular disease	58 million	$287 billion
Diabetes	16 million	$98 billion
Multiple sclerosis	350,000	$5 billion
Osteoporosis	1.5 million fractures/year	$14 billion
Schizophrenia	2 million	$30 billion

Source: Data derived from National Center for Chronic Disease Prevention and Health Promotion, Centers for Disease Control (CDC) (*http://www.cdc.gov/nccdphp/majot.htm*) and Cowan and Kandel, 2001.

which beneficial intervention, such as early screening or treatment of an intermediate phenotype, was possible. Even for such a restricted group of common diseases, some 40% of young to middle-aged adults were at increased risk for these diseases, based on family history alone (Scheuner et al., 1997). The implication is that virtually every person is at increased risk to develop one or more common diseases.

Since these disorders appear in large measure to be due to the interaction of environmental factors with specific genetic susceptibilities, attempts have been made to quantify the relative role of genetics and environment by such statistical measures as the attributable risk for either genetic or environmental risk factors. Attributable risk is defined as the fraction of cases of a given disease caused by the specified risk factor. Such a measure is only useful if it is considered in relative terms. For example, the total effect on cholesterol levels in the U.S. population provided by the allele E4 of the apolipoprotein E (*APOE*) gene is approximately equivalent to that provided by mutations of the LDL receptor. An abnormal LDL receptor allele has a large effect on the individual by increasing cholesterol by 100 to 200 mg%, but the deleterious allele occurs only in 1 in 500 individuals. In contrast, apolipoprotein *E4* results in only 10 to 20 mg% elevation in cholesterol, but 3% to 4% of the population carry this allele (see Chapter 7). The effects are similar because they are spread over many more individuals.

Contrasting the burden of genes versus that of the environment is somewhat artificial. For example, if both a specific environmental factor and a specific gene are absolutely required for manifestation of a given disease, then the affected individual will always have both, and depending on their frequency in a given population, the attributable risk may be close to 1 (or 100%) when both risk factors are present. There is another way to approach this issue. If both a gene and an environmental factor are responsible for a disease, whether gene or environment appears to be the "predominant" factor will depend on their relative frequency. If the disease-predisposing allele is very common, and the environmental factor is somewhat rarer, the environmental factor will appear to be the predominant factor. If the environmental factor is ubiquitous, however, then genetic factors seem to be the principal determinants. Many common diseases of civilization such as Type 2 diabetes, obesity, coronary artery disease, and gallstones appear to fall in this category. Thus, the contributing environmental factors in the Western world are so ubiquitous that risk appears to be largely related to genetic differences. In such cases, the predominant environmental role can be inferred from the frequency changes of these diseases in migrant populations. Such observations and the response to preventive measures such as diet, exercise, and pharmaceutical interventions indicate that disease-predisposing genes interact with an appropriate environmental milieu. Thus, it is not either genes or environment but genes interacting with environment that leads to these diseases.

EFFECT OF COMMON DISEASE

Effect on an Individual: Disease Subsets, Diagnosis, and Therapy

In the practice of medicine, the physician wishes to come to an accurate diagnosis of the illness affecting a given patient ("What is it?"). This knowledge leads to two important classes of information for both patient and physician—prognosis ("What is going to happen?") and therapy ("What can be done about it?"). The diagnosis of most diseases is made phenotypically such as by a characteristic clinical picture or, more specifically, by evaluation of a tissue sample for breast or colon cancer, an angiography for coronary artery disease, elevated blood glucose for diabetes, or, for example, histology of a biopsy for inflammatory bowel disease. Each of these diseases has well-defined disease subsets—Crohn's disease vs. ulcerative colitis in inflammatory bowel disease and Type 1 diabetes (autoimmunity) vs. Type 2 diabetes (insulin resistance) in diabetes. These individual entities have different prognoses and different therapeutic strategies. Thus in Type 1 diabetes, where the process is ultimate destruction of pancreatic beta cells, there is virtually always a need for insulin injections as opposed to weight reduction, exercise, and oral agents as in Type 2 diabetes. The optimal surgery may be very different for a patient with ulcerative colitis than for one with Crohn's colitis, with the latter's tendency to fistula formation. This individualization of management and therapy will expand as more specific therapies are developed. Such disease categorizations can often be made clinically or by using other phenotypic measures. Often, differentiating phenotypic characteristics may not be available. Increasingly, genetic or molecular tests can aid in the distinction between disease subsets. Examples include breast cancer due to mutations in the *BRCA1* gene versus those in the *BRCA2* gene, and different mutator repair gene defects in hereditary nonpolyposis colorectal cancer. Establishing such distinctions is required because each specific entity may have a different prognosis and may require different approaches to treatment.

PRESYMPTOMATIC DIAGNOSIS AND SCREENING FOR COMMON DISEASES

The goal of diagnosis and screening for any disease is an accurate diagnosis so that the disease risk for an individual can be determined. While genetic screening has become the standard practice for a number of Mendelian single-gene disorders, such as Tay-Sachs disease, genetic screening for risk assessment for common disease is still in its infancy. There is general agreement that screening (other than for research purposes) should only be initiated if an abnormal test result provides useful information for the individual or for his or her family in the form of effective prevention or treatment. Unlike for rare genetic diseases where routine screening may not usually be cost-effective, screening for common diseases that can be prevented or treated can be justified for economic reasons.

Genetic screening for complex diseases can be approached at different levels. The first approach is the family history, a tool that is comprehensive and cost effective (Scheuner et al., 1997). Family history has a relatively high specificity, particularly with a family history of cancer. This approach continues to be the most effective method for identifying individuals at risk for the most common diseases.

A second approach for genetic screening is evaluation of the phenotype. Examples include measuring blood pressure, serum lipids, and fasting glucose; search by endoscopy for colonic polyps; and mammograms for breast cancer. This category of screening, depending on the condition, has sometimes been recommended for the population at large or for more restricted subgroups that are at an increased risk due to their medical history or findings on physical examination.

The third category of screening is at the gene (DNA) and gene product (enzymes or other proteins) level. While a more refined search by laboratory tests for a specific disease because of family history and other clues is a time-honored medical practice, DNA testing has engendered a great deal of discussion and even controversy. Biochemical tests for the diagnosis of genetic enzyme deficiency provide the same diagnostic information as DNA tests and have been standard practice for many years. The greatest current application is in risk assessment for breast and colon cancer. Usually, an individual is identified as being at high risk because of multiple affected family members. Ideally, the DNA of an affected family member is examined for a characteristic cancer mutation. Once such a mutation has become identified, this specific mutation in the person at risk can then be searched for. Absence of a mutation in those at risk usually means absence of the already discovered cancer gene.

Several examples will serve to make these points. Hemochromatosis is a disorder characterized by progressive iron overload by parenchymal tissue due to continuous increased absorption of iron by the intestines (see Chapter 18). In this disorder, screening can be accomplished with phenotypic markers of iron overload, with HLA-linked and associated markers, and with the direct predisposing mutations in the hemochromatosis gene. This disease appears to provide an excellent argument for family-based screening, since the available evidence strongly indicates that early intervention, which in this case is periodic phlebotomy before tissue damage occurs, minimizes morbidity and prevents excess mortality (Bacon, 2001). Some have even argued that screening for hemochromatosis should be applied to the population at large, or at least to individuals with associated diseases such as Type 2 diabetes, heart disease, and cirrhosis of the liver. In contrast, molecular genetic screening for schizophrenia (when such genes have been identified) would seem to be of little purpose, if no intervention has been developed. Screening for *BRCA1* and *BRCA2* mutations in families with dominant breast cancer can identify individuals who may elect to undergo intense screening with mammography and pelvis ultrasound, prophylactic mastectomy or oophorectomy, or chemoprevention with a drug like tamoxifen. Screening for Apo *E4* in Alzheimer's disease families would seem much more problematic unless specific intervention has been developed.

Prevention and Therapy

An important concept regarding common diseases is increasing success of specifically designed therapies and preventions. The fact that these diseases are due in significant measure to gene–environment interactions means that changes in the environment change the risk of occurrence of disease. In other words, it is almost certain that one can develop means to intervene in these diseases, either at the therapeutic (disease) stage or at the preventive (preclinical or initiating) stage. Such therapeutic and preventive successes are less striking for single-gene Mendelian disorders, many of which express similarly in virtually any environment. Thus, there is a great expectation that new therapies and preventive measures can be developed for common disorders. The inference is that these diseases are susceptible to environmental manipulations, and what else is a pharmaceutical but an introduced environmental agent? Second, if a given form of a disease is due to two or more genes (oligogenic to polygenic), some steps in which to prevent, halt, or reverse the pathogenetic process would be available for intervention. Hence, advances in understanding the genetics and pathophysiology of each of these diseases will often lead to advances in therapy and prevention.

MECHANISMS OF COMMON DISEASES: SUSCEPTIBILITY AND RESISTANCE

Genetic diseases are produced through single or complex mechanisms. A traditional view has been to consider a single mechanism for most genetic diseases. Categories of genetic diseases with single mechanisms include *(1)* chromosomal disorders, caused by an abnormality in chromosome number or structure; *(2)* Mendelian disorders caused by abnormalities of a single gene; and *(3)* non-Mendelian disorders caused by mitochondrial mutations or altered gene expression resulting from imprinting. This has led to historical emphasis on genetic diseases in children as well as acquisition of much new knowledge of gene identity and function. Common diseases in the adult population more frequently have complex mechanisms involving genetic susceptibility and environmental influences, but some may also be produced through single mechanisms.

Chromosomal Disorders

Chromosomal disorders are congenital or acquired. Acquired chromosomal abnormalities are important in the pathogenesis and evolution of hematologic (discussed in Chapter 43) and solid organ malignancies, but they are not generally part of the etiologic mechanisms for common diseases. They usually occur only in some cells in an organ but not in all of the cells of the body, and they usually develop later in life. Various congenital chromosomal disorders are common, occurring in approximately 1 in 150 live births (Jorde et al., 1999); they, with the exception of X and Y chromosomal disorders, usually present in the pediatric rather than the adult age group. Such chromosomal disorders are also known as constitutional or constitutive chromosomal disorders since they involve every cell in the body. The majority of congenital chromosomal disorders are sporadic and involve an extra chromosome because of nondisjunction in meiosis during formation of the egg or sperm. Less frequent are chromosomal rearrangements such as translocations that are sporadic and arise during meiosis or are inherited. A minority are chromosomal mosaic patterns in which there are two or more chromosomally distinct cell lines, such as 46,XX and 47,XX+21, in an affected individual. Mosaic chromosomal abnormalities are thought to arise most often from mitotic nondisjunction after conception. Recent technologic advances in the development of fluorescent in situ hybridization (FISH) have defined a large group of gene deletion syndromes, such as Williams and Wolf-Hirschhorn syndrome, that represent microscopically nonvisible chromosomal abnormalities (Strachan and Read, 1999). These syndromes are called *contiguous gene syndromes* because they are thought to result from the deletion of several genes linked together in a chromosomal region, with each gene contributing to some part of the observed phenotype.

Classic examples of chromosomal abnormalities that may be seen in the adult population are Down syndrome, caused by an extra chromsome 21 (trisomy 21); Turner syndrome, caused by the lack of a second sex chromosome in a female (45,X); and Klinefelter syndrome, caused by the presence of an extra X chromosome in a male (47,XXY). These are discussed in Chapter 53.

Abnormalities of chromosome number or structure produce an imbalance of genetic material and gene dose, resulting in a variety of structural and developmental defects. When an autosome is involved, the affected individual is almost always mentally retarded and has a number of physical abnormalities, including changes in the structure of the face, eyes, ears, mouth, heart, gastrointestinal tract, and extremities. The changes can be characteristic, as with Down syndrome, or they can be quite variable. Viable autosomal chromosomal abnormalities are apparent early in life and display little progression in severity over the lifespan of the individual. In fact, the majority are associated with a shortened lifespan and are not seen in the adult population. In contrast, abnormalities of the sex chromosomes, such as Turner and Klinefelter syndromes, are relatively common in the adult population. The spectrum of the phenotypes for these conditions is discussed in Chapter 53.

Mendelian Mechanisms

Mendelian disorders are due to a mutation in a single gene (Jorde et al., 1999). They are so named because they follow the well-delineated patterns of inheritance first described by Mendel in the nineteenth century.

Autosomal Dominant Inheritance

An autosomal dominant disorder is due to the mutation of a gene located on one of the autosomes (chromosome numbers 1 to 22). Normally, each individual has two copies (alleles) of each autosomal gene. A disorder is dominant if an alteration in one of the two alleles of a particular gene is sufficient to produce disease; the affected individual has one "abnormal" copy of a given gene and one "normal" copy of the same gene. In most cases, males and females are affected equally. Examples of common dominant disorders include familial breast cancer resulting from mutations of the *BRCA1* or *BRCA2* gene, familial polyposis resulting from mutations of the *APC* gene, and hypercholesterolemia resulting from mutations of the LDL receptor gene.

Each offspring of an affected individual has a 50% chance of receiving the dominant gene from the affected parent. Offspring who received the "normal" copy of the gene neither develop the disease nor pass it on. Thus, in an autosomal dominant disorder, one of the parents and, on average, 50% of the patient's siblings and 50% of their offspring are affected. This pattern of inheritance thus exhibits vertical transmission.

Autosomal dominant disorders exhibit several general features that are important in the adult population, such as *delayed age of onset*. Just because a disorder is genetic does not mean it is clinically evident at birth. For example, breast cancer can be an autosomal dominant disorder. In individuals with a mutation of *BRCA1* or *BRCA2*, the cancer usually does not develop until the third decade of life or later, and there is no evidence of disease in the first decade of life (see Chapter 35).

The second general feature is *pleiotropism*, which refers to multiple effects of a single gene. An example of pleiotropism is the Marfan syndrome in which a single abnormal gene can produce changes in the skeleton, eyes, heart, and great vessels by altering a structural protein common to these tissues (see Chapter 33). Pleiotropism may be an explanation for a number of common disease associations—for example, the increased occurrence of both insulin-dependent diabetes and autoimmune thyroid disease in the same individual and family suggests a common immunogenetic basis for these disorders.

The third general feature is *variable expression*, which describes the differences in the extent or severity of the manifestations of a disease among affected individuals. For example, in a single family with mitral valve prolapse, affected individuals may have significant mitral insufficiency or rhythm disturbances, while others have no symptoms and only an audible click on physical examination.

The fourth general feature, *penetrance*, is related to that of variable expressivity and is a statistical concept. When penetrance is 100%, all those who carry the gene will exhibit clinical findings; 50% penetrance means that only one-half of the gene carriers have clinical manifestations. Individuals known to carry the gene (proven by transmitting it to their offspring) who have no recognizable clinical manifestations of the disease (the far end of the spectrum of variable expressivity) are termed "nonpenetrant." Penetrance, like degree of expressivity, can be a function of the age of the patient; breast cancer is not present in the first decades of life. Penetrance should be expressed by careful definition of the disease phenotype under study. Thus, penetrance will be higher when abnormal laboratory findings in addition to clinical expression are used to determine penetrance.

Autosomal Recessive Inheritance

A disorder is inherited in an autosomal recessive pattern if two copies of an abnormal gene are needed for expression of the disease. Affected individuals are *homozygotes* (more formally, they are *homozygous for the disease gene*). Individuals with a single dose of the abnormal gene and a single dose of the normal gene are clinically normal but are carriers (*heterozygotes*) of the genes. Examples of relatively frequent autosomal recessive disorders include sickle cell disease, phenylketonuria, and cystic fibrosis. The parents usually are normal heterozygotes, and the risk to the siblings of the affected individual is 25%. One-half of all siblings carry one copy of the abnormal gene (heterozygotes), and one-fourth of the siblings are homozygous normal. This pattern of inheritance is horizontal aggregation. As in autosomal dominant disorders, both sexes are usually affected with the same frequency.

As with dominant disorders, recessive disorders can manifest at any time in life from the newborn period to middle age, but they are more frequently expressed in infancy or childhood. Because recessive disorders require two abnormal genes, they are more likely to occur if the parents have a common ancestor (consanguinity). The rarer the disorder (thus the rarer the abnormal gene), the higher the frequency of consanguinity among the parents of affected individuals. Conversely, if a disorder is quite common (e.g., hemochromatosis), no increased occurrence of consanguinity is observed.

The likelihood of a recessive disorder is increased if the frequency of the abnormal gene is high within some populations. This is the reason for the high frequency of a number of disorders in certain ethnic groups, including cystic fibrosis in U.S. and northern European populations (Mickle and Cutting, 2000; Grody et al., 2001), familial Mediterranean fever in Sephardic Jews and Armenians (Samuels et al., 1998), and Tay-Sachs disease in Ashkenazi Jews (Zerah et al., 1990).

At times a recessive disorder is so common that one may observe parent-to-offspring transmission because the affected homozygote has married a heterozygote. This has been termed *pseudodominant transmission*. For example, in the U.S. and European populations, heterozygosity for hemochromatosis occurs with a frequency of 10%, resulting in frequent matings between a homozygous affected and a heterozygous carrier (see Chapter

18). Since one-half of the offspring from this type of mating will be homozygous affected, 5% of the offspring of an affected individual would be expected to be homozygous affected. This has obvious important implications for disease screening for hemochromatosis.

X-Linked Inheritance

Males have one X and one Y chromosome, and females have two X chromosomes. The Y chromosome is small and appears to carry mainly male-determining genes. An abnormal gene located on an X chromosome may be dominant or recessive in expression in females. Because males have only one X chromosome, a mutant X chromosomal gene will always be expressed in males.

A male affected with an X-linked condition is *hemizygous*. A male affected with an X-linked disorder will pass the gene to none of his sons but to all of his daughters, who will then be carriers. Offspring of carrier (heterozygous) females and normal males can have four types of offspring, each with a 25% chance of occurrence: carrier females, normal females, normal males, and affected males.

Non-Mendelian Mechanisms

A variety of non-Mendelian mechanisms for human disease have been identified in the past few decades, including mitochondrial gene mutations, genetic imprinting and uniparental disomy, and gene methylation (Rimoin et al., 1996; Jorde et al., 1999; Scriver et al., 2001). Each of these mechanisms has the potential for being involved with the development of a common disease, and several have been shown to be part of a common disease process. Examples are the suggested association between the accumulation of mitochondrial mutations in cells in the central nervous system (CNS) and aging, and the association of altered gene expression in malignant cells with the loss of genetic imprinting. It is important to note, however, that most of these non-Mendelian mechanisms affect somatic tissue of an individual who already has a common disease, or they are not known to be involved with susceptibility to common diseases at this time. These mechanisms are clearly important with disease development and progression, but not with inherited susceptibility to the disease, and there are a few examples of their involvement in common disease, as discussed below.

Complex Mechanisms of Disease

Complex mechanisms of disease can involve the expression of a single gene, a few major genes, or a group of major genes and polygenes. In most cases, the effects of gene expression are also influenced by the environment. A brief discussion of these mechanisms follows.

Monogenic Mechanisms

Monogenic mechanisms that produce susceptibility to a common disease can result from inherited pathologic mutations in a single gene or from differences in expression of the gene because of inherited polymorphic differences or epigenetic effects. For example, pathologic mutations in a gene involved in DNA repair (*MSH2* or *MLH1*) produce increased susceptibility to colon cancer as part of the hereditary non-polyposis colon cancer (HNPCC) syndrome by allowing mutations in other colon cancer–related genes to develop (see Chapter 34). One of these other genes is the *APC* gene, mutations of which are responsible for familial polyposis coli and the development of multiple premalignant colon polyps. Mutations in *APC* are found in approximately 50% of sporadic colon cancer, indicating that alteration in this gene product plays a critical role in most colon cancers. To complicate matters, the expression of *APC* can also be altered by methylation of the gene (an epigenetic event), and this is a common mechanism for a noninherited increase in susceptibility to colon cancer through the development of a polyp. Another monogenetic example for a common disease is the suggestion that a frequent homozygous polymorphism in the gene for 5,10-methylene tetrahydrofolate reductase (MTHFR) influences homocysteine levels (see Chapter 7).

Oligogenic Mechanisms

Oligogenic inheritance is defined as the operation of a few different genes in a given case of the disease and not the action of a few genes in different cases of the disease. To date, the study of common diseases such as atherosclerosis, asthma, and cancer has led to the identification of several important genes, but the study of the interaction and cooperation between their effects is just beginning. An example of one type of oligogenic disease comes from atherosclerosis and coronary heart disease (CHD). Mutations in the LDL receptor gene are associated with hypercholesterolemia and an increased risk of CHD. The polymorphic variation of the MTHFR gene associated with elevated homocysteine levels together with the combination of a LDL receptor gene might increase the susceptibility to CHD above the level caused by either alone.

Multifactorial Mechanisms

Classic multifactorial inheritance includes susceptibility (liability) resulting from polygenes and the environment. Polygenes are defined as genes that have a small effect that often is additive. Current methods of gene mapping are not generally useful for identifying the location of polygenes, and association studies sometimes based on knowledge of the biology of the disease process, are frequently used in their identification. The availability of the human genome will help with the identification of polygenes, as will the development of better analytical tools for genetic-based association studies.

Gene–Environment Mechanisms

An important concept of gene–environment interactions is that they likely interact in different ways. It is not simply a matter of identifying the deleterious factors in the environment, from which all individuals need to be protected. A given environmental factor can be harmful to some and even helpful for others. Whether an environmental factor is good or bad can depend both on the individual's genes and even on different stages in an individual's life. Thus, for example, smoking is generally considered deleterious, but, in fact, it appears protective for ulcerative colitis (see Chapter 15). Sanitation of the water supply would appear to be a universal benefit to a society, minimizing infectious diseases. But such sanitations appear to be a risk factor for the inflammatory bowel diseases in those who are genetically predisposed (see Chapter 15). Thus, this realization of genetic individuality truly gives a scientific basis to the aphorism "what is one man's meat is another man's poison."

Interactive Mechanisms: Gene–Gene, Gene–Environment

The pathogenesis of common diseases must account for several characteristic aspects of their presentation, including adult onset, gender effects, parent-of-origin effects, lack of concordance in monozygotic twins, and changes in the disease process (i.e., fluctuations) over time. These characteristics are not easily explained with our current genetic models, and this has led to the hypothesis that epigenetic factors may play a significant role in the development and course of complex diseases (Petronis and Petroniene, 2000; Petronis, 2001). Epigenetic processes that are associated with the modification in gene expression involve gene-directed reversible changes in methylation of the DNA or the chromatin (Henikoff and Matzke, 1997; Martienssen and Henikoff, 1999). The resulting changes in gene expression could be important in sex or age differences, as well as the fluctuations in disease activity that are commonly observed.

A second potential mechanism that has been proposed to account for the variation in genetic susceptibility and clinical course of a common disease is the presence of modifier genes (Nadeau, 2001). These have been characterized best in mouse models of disease, but several human examples involving a variety of conditions have been suggested (Nadeau, 2001). The availability of the human genome sequence and the rapidly developing analytical tools for analysis of complex interactions is expected to lead to the identification of many alleles that have the ability to modify or change the genetic susceptibility of an individual to the development or course of a disease.

Interaction of the environment with heredity is obviously important. The concepts of "nature" and "nurture" are not mutually exclusive, and the involvement of environmental agents in disease causation does not rule out the operation of genetic factors. Thus in the twentieth century there was an increase and then a decline in the mortality of coronary heart disease. These fluctuations demonstrate the importance of environment, because gene frequencies do not change rapidly enough to account for such temporal alterations in incidence. Geneticists aim to show that different genotypes respond differently to a given environment. The demonstration that a specific environmental agent acts on well-defined genotypes will yield more rational preventive medicine. With better understanding, preventive measures could be directed at those subpopulations that are at high risk.

One of the most important areas of gene–environment interaction is pharmacogenetics, or how the genetic makeup of an individual influences how they respond to therapy or to environmental agents. Studies with identical and nonidentical twins have shown that the biotransformation of almost all drugs tested thus far is under some genetic control. Genetic variability presumably affects proteins involved in absorption, transport, metabolism, detoxification, and elimination of a drug or its components, but the specific proteins and pathways involved are often unknown. It can therefore be assumed that the metabolism of most foreign biochemical substances (xenobiotics) is also under genetic control. There is extensive evidence from animal work and to some extent from human data that carcinogenic chemicals often need to be activated before they exhibit their characteristic actions. Such activation of carcinogens shows genetic variability and therefore places some individuals at higher risk for cancer than others. Because a significant proportion of human cancer may be of environmental origin, genetic variation that affects metabolism of carcinogenic substances or activation of carcinogens is likely to determine why some, but not all individuals develop cancer when they are equally exposed to a given carcinogen. Genetic variability in DNA repair may also occur and may explain interindividual differences in cancer after exposure to carcinogens. The importance of the environment in many common cancers seems clear. The most common cancer of 40 years ago, cancer of the stomach, is sharply declining in frequency presumably because of better refrigeration in recent years with consequent removal of ingested natural carcinogens in contaminated foods. The most common cancer today, carcinoma of the lung, clearly is related to excessive cigarette smoking. In both cases, though, only a fraction of the population appears susceptible, possibly due to a genetic basis.

Mechanisms of Variation: Heterogeneity

The concept of *genetic heterogeneity* is important in understanding the genetic bases of common diseases. A single disorder, such as coronary artery disease, asthma, or diabetes mellitus, is in reality not one disease but a group of diseases, each with the same final common manifestation: respectively, a narrowed coronary artery, an inflamed airway that develops bronchospasm, or a high blood glucose level. Such a broadly defined disorder can have a number of different subtypes that are genetic or nongenetic in origin—that is, it may have a number of different genetic and nongenetic causes. A specific subtype may be caused by a single Mendelian gene, by two or three interacting major genes, by a set of genes acting in a polygenic pattern, or by an environmental agent. And it is possible that there will be subtypes that result from a complex combination of these causes, such as a major gene acting on a polygenic background. When the subtypes of a disease are indiscriminately combined, the overall familial aggregation may resemble the pattern expected in multifactorial inheritance.

It is useful to point out that delineating heterogeneity, or "splitting" disorders, has been common in medicine as knowledge of disease grows. Some 100 years ago, anemia, edema, and jaundice were disease categories, but it is now known that these are only clinical or laboratory signs, each with multiple causes. Identification of the different forms of anemia is obviously important for specific diagnosis and therapy. It must be recognized that many of the diseases that we deal with today, such as essential hypertension and coronary artery disease, are no more specific than the broad category of anemia.

Methods to Demonstrate Heterogeneity

The methods of demonstrating heterogeneity in a common disease are listed in Table 1–2. It is apparent that several of the findings that suggest a genetic component in a disease also provide evidence that such a component is genetically heterogeneous. Diabetes mellitus provides an excellent example of genetic heterogeneity for the following discussion, but it should be kept in mind that heterogeneity has been described for many common diseases such as asthma, colon cancer, and coronary artery disease.

Genetic Syndromes. The existence of several different monogenic syndromes that feature noninsulin-dependent diabetes, such as the various types of maturity-onset diabetes in the young (see Chapter 22) is proof that at least some forms of diabetes are genetically heterogeneous, because these syndromes are due to mutations at different loci. This also provides proof of pathogenetic heterogeneity, because different mechanisms lead to diabetes.

Epidemiologic and Ethnic Differences. Ethnic differences can suggest genetic or at least etiologic heterogeneity. The evidence is stronger if ethnic differences are observed not only in the frequency of a disorder but also in its clinical features. For exam-

Table 1–2. Criteria for Demonstrating Heterogeneity in Common Diseases

Criteria	Example
Rare genetic syndromes that feature a disease as part of a phenotype	*Peptic ulcer* Multiple endocrine neoplasia type 1 and gastrinomas; systemic mastocytosis; tremor-nystagmus ulcer syndrome
	Diabetes mellitus Hereditary pancreatitis; diabetes insipidus–optic atrophy syndrome; myotonic dystrophy
	Obesity Prader-Willi syndrome; Bardet-Biedl syndrome
	Colon cancer Familial polyposis coli
Animal models	*Diabetes mellitus* Mapping of different rodent diabetes genes to different chromosomes *Systemic lupus erythematosus* Mapping of different rodent SLE genes to different chromosomes
Ethnic variability in incidence and clinical features	*Diabetes mellitus* Ethnic groups differ in relative frequency of complications and ketoacidosis
Clinical manifestations	*Peptic ulcer* Gastric vs. duodenal ulcer, different age distribution; within duodenal ulcer, early and late ages of onset are associated with different clinical features and complications; association of ulcer with other diseases, e.g., chronic lung disease, renal stones (without hyperparathyroidism)
	Diabetes mellitus Insulin-dependent (Type 1) vs. noninsulin-dependent (Type 2) differ in frequency of obesity, age of onset, frequency of ketoacidosis
	Inflammatory bowel disease Crohn's vs. ulcerative colitis differ in frequency of strictures, fistulas, liver disease
Clinical genetic evidence	*Peptic ulcer* Gastric vs. duodenal ulcer, increased risk in families is site specific
	Diabetes mellitus Independent segregation of Type 1 and Type 2 in families; concordance rate in monozygotic twins much lower in Type 1
	Inflammatory bowel disease Complications and age of onset of Crohn's disease concordant in families
Physiologic differences	*Peptic ulcer* Within duodenal ulcer, abnormalities (acid hypersecretion, hyperpepsinogenemia I, increased gastrin response to a meal, increased rate of gastric emptying, acid stimulatory antibodies) present in some but not all families
	Diabetes mellitus Type 1 absolute insulin deficient, Type 2 variable insulin levels; Type 1 exhibits autoantibodies, that are not in Type 2
	Inflammatory bowel disease Ulcerative colitis, high frequency of antineutrophil cytoplasmic antibodies; Crohn's disease, high frequency of antibodies to *Saccharomyces cerevisiae*
Family studies with physiologic abnormalities as subclinical markers	*Coronary artery disease* Familial hypercholesterolemia, familial combined hyperlipidemia, familial hypertriglyceridemia
	Duodenal ulcer Hyperpepsinogenemia 1 families vs. normopepsinogenemia families
	Inflammatory bowel disease Presence or absence of familial antineutrophil cytoplasmic antibodies
Gene markers	*Peptic ulcer* Blood group O associated with duodenal, not gastric, ulcer
	Diabetes mellitus HLA antigens linked and associated with Type 1, not Type 2
	Cancer family syndromes Different families linked to different mutator DNA repair genes
	Breast cancer *BRCA1* vs. *BRCA2*

ple, both the frequency and the type of diabetes differ dramatically between some of the Southwest Amerindians, Mexican Americans, African Americans, and Causasians in the United States. These differences reflect both genetic and environmental heterogeneity. It is often difficult to disentangle genetics from environmental and socio-economic differences.

Clinical Differences. The finding of clinical differences within a population suggests heterogeneity of a disease. For example, the ages of onset for insulin-dependent Type 1 and insulin-independent Type 2 diabetes are generally different, although there has been a recent decrease of the age of onset for Type 2 diabetes that can approach that of Type 1. Family studies of clinical differences also provide evidence for separating disorders. With such studies it has been demonstrated that the increased risk for diabetes in a family is not for all diabetes but is specific for the type observed in the index case.

Physiologic Differences. As discussed previously, the study of the physiologic processes that lead to a disease can provide an understanding of the etiology of the disease. Type 1 diabetes is associated with loss of beta cells in the pancreas, anti-insulin antibodies, and loss of insulin, while Type 2 diabetes is associated with insulin resistance rather than the absolute loss of insulin.

Family Studies with Subclinical Markers. One of the most powerful methods both to demonstrate heterogeneity and to identify the specific genes involved in disease pathogenesis in a common disease involves family studies to demonstrate that physiologic heterogeneity is fundamental to disease pathogenesis. In many families of Type 1 diabetes patients, there is an increased aggregation of Type 1 diabetes, or other autoimmune diseases, but it is not consistent with a simple Mendelian mode of inheritance. In a number of these families, the diabetic patients have islet cell antibodies, as do a number of their clinically unaffected relatives. The unaffected relatives may develop anti-islet cell antibodies but do not always develop diabetes. The use of this *subclinical genetic marker*, the islet cell antibody, has been useful in identifying families with high or low risk for the development of Type 1 diabetes.

RECOGNITION OF GENETIC DETERMINANTS OF COMMON DISEASES

Diseases can be arranged on a continuum from those having a purely genetic cause (hemophilia) to those having a purely environmental cause (burns). The majority of common diseases lie between the two extremes and are the result of interaction between genetic and environmental factors. A number of methods are available to identify the genetic component of a common disease. It is particularly important to keep the distinction between genotype and phenotype in mind when considering common diseases because of the multicausality of most of these conditions. The *phenotype* of an individual is the clinical or measurable manifestation of the gene (or genes) that the individual possesses. The actual gene or genes are the *genotype*. The phenotype can range from a general list of clinical features to a specific description of polymorphic enzyme types. Consider an individual who is homozygous for the gene for hemochromatosis, a common autosomal recessive disorder that may lead to excessive iron storage in the liver, pancreas, testes, and heart. The genotype is the presence or absence of the hemochromatosis gene mutation in the individual. The clinical phenotype can be extremely variable; it may include hepatic cirrhosis, diabetes, hypogonadism, and congestive cardiomyopathy, all due to tissue damage from the excess iron.

Familial Aggregation and Ethnic Differences

A genetic component for a disease may be suspected from the finding of *(1)* familial aggregation (a higher frequency of the disease in first-degree relatives of patients with the disease than in the general population) or *(2)* marked variation of disease frequency among different ethnic groups. For example, breast cancer shows both familial aggregation and marked variation in frequency in different ethnic groups (see Chapter 35). The frequency of breast cancer is two- to threefold greater in relatives of breast cancer patients than in controls. Similar data are available for diabetes, atherosclerosis, rheumatoid arthritis, and colon cancer, among others. It should be noted that neither familial aggregation nor ethnic differences in disease *proves* a genetic component, since a shared or common familial environment or variable environments of different ethnic groups may produce these findings.

The demonstration of family aggregation for a number of common diseases has had a long evolution. Historically, the first reports were of one or more families with several cases of the disease of interest. This type of information does not allow conclusions regarding familial aggregation. In common diseases, the occurrence of multiple cases in a single family could easily be due to chance alone.

Often the next step in identifying a genetic component of a disease was a comparison of "the frequency of a positive family history" among cases with a disease to the frequency among a control group. For example, diabetics have an increased family history of diabetes, and patients with inflammatory bowel disease have an increased family history of inflammatory bowel disease. Such data are often reported as "positive"; however, this method of assessing familial aggregation has several problems. First, the proportion of affected relatives is not quantified, and their degree of relationship is sometimes not given. Second, there may be an important informational bias because affected individuals often know more about the family history of their disease than unaffected individuals do.

It is now recognized that the proportion of affected relatives of a specific class (e.g., first-degree relatives such as siblings and parents) must be compared with an appropriate control group to accurately assess familial aggregation. For example, siblings of an insulin-dependent diabetic are affected with insulin-dependent diabetes with a frequency of 5% to 10% compared to a 1 in 500 risk for the general population. Such empirically derived risks are important for genetic modeling to determine the actual mode of inheritance. They also become the initial basis for genetic counseling for these diseases. These risks are termed *empiric recurrence risks*, because they are based on the risk of recurrence actually observed, rather than on any theoretical genetic model (as in the case with Mendelian risks). Empiric risks must be used with caution, because they are not based on an underlying biologic model, and they may vary in different populations. They are often reassuring for genetic counseling, in that the risks are often smaller than those feared initially by an individual or family member.

Studies of different ethnic groups and migration patterns can show the importance of environmental factors and may suggest genetic factors that are involved in a disease. The frequency of noninsulin-dependent diabetes increased from practically zero to 5% to 10% in one generation when the Yemenite Jews migrated from Yemen to Israel, clearly illustrating an environmental effect (see Chapter 21). Although such evidence indicates the importance of environmental factors, it does not eliminate the potential importance of genetic factors—that is, Why did only a fraction of the population manifest disease? Differences in the clinical features of diseases between ethnic groups are also important because they suggest that the etiologic factors—be they genetic, environmental, or both—differ from one population to the next, indicating etiologic heterogeneity.

Animal Models

Animal models can provide indirect evidence for a genetic component. If a disease occurring in animals is analogous to a disease in humans, then the role of genetic factors among a species might be clarified by looking at differences among strains and by designing appropriate matings. Even if genetic factors are unequivocally demonstrated for the disease in animals, however, it is reasoning by analogy to make the same conclusion for the disease in humans. The genetic background of animals differs from that of humans, and genes that may be involved in a well-defined animal disease may play no role whatsoever in the human equivalent. Animal studies of common diseases therefore can only provide hints but never any definitive insights into the etiology of a common human disease. Such hints need to be then explored in studies in man.

Twin Studies

The classic method to determine whether familial aggregation is due to common genetic or to common environmental factors is to compare the concordance rates of disease (i.e., whether one or both members of a twin pair is affected) in monozygotic (MZ) and dizygotic (DZ) twin pairs. MZ twin pairs are genetically identical, whereas DZ twin pairs are no more genetically alike than are any pair of siblings. A higher concordance rate in MZ than in DZ twin pairs (especially like-sexed DZ pairs) indicates that a significant part of the familial aggregation is due to genetic factors, and equal rates of concordance indicate the familial aggregation is determined largely be environmental factors. A qualification is that it can sometimes be difficult to disentangle heredity from environment, because MZ twins, likely because of their genetic identity, tend to select similar environments. Coronary heart disease, celiac disease, inflammatory bowel disease, diabetes, and schizophrenia are examples of disorders in which the concordance rate is higher in MZ than in DZ twin pairs.

The MZ concordance is rarely 100%, suggesting environmental, genetic, epigenetic, or even random components to these diseases. The paramount importance of genetic factors is usually inferred if a disorder has a nearly 100% concordance rate in MZ twins (and less in DZ pairs), but even this deserves a cautionary note. The correct statement when 100% concordance in MZ twins is observed is that genetic factors are of great importance in the specific environment in which the individuals were studied. For example, noninsulin-dependent diabetes mellitus has virtually a 100% concordance rate in MZ twins in the Western world. On the other hand, the frequency of this disease varies severalfold in less than one generation in migrant populations. The migration data are evidence for the importance of environmental factors, while the MZ twin data suggest that the genetic factors are ubiquitous in the developed Western world and that individuals who develop the disease in the Western world are those with the appropriate genetic susceptibility.

Adoption Studies

Another approach for separating genetic from environmental effects is to compare the frequency of a disease in adopted versus biologic (related) relatives. The most common application of this method is with psychiatric conditions such as alcoholism, affective disorders, and schizophrenia. The concept is straightforward and takes advantage of the fact that adoption separates individuals from their biologic parents, with whom they share genes and environment, and moves them with their genes unchanged to a new family environment. Environmental factors are strongly implicated if an adopted individual's frequency of disease is more similar to that of the adopted parents, and the importance of genetic factors is established if the disease frequency is more similar to that of the biologic parents. It should be kept in mind that the selective placement of adoptees by adoption agencies into homes that are similar to those of the biologic parents may make the interpretation of adoption studies somewhat difficult.

Genetic Studies to Identify Genes

General Approach

Once it is decided that a disease process has a genetic basis, then the next step is to attempt to identify the gene. Before the advent of the Human Genome Project, a common intermediate step was to perform a *segregation analysis* to demonstrate the existence of the likely genetic model for the disease. In general, this was tedious and complex, and it often gave an unsatisfactory answer (i.e., it is genetic or not). The process of segregation analysis is less frequently used now, and direct gene mapping and identification methods are employed.

Linkage Analysis

Before we turn to strategies of gene finding based on prior hypotheses (e.g., candidate genes) or chromosomal locations (e.g., systematic genome scans), it is worthwhile to briefly review the analytic approaches that are used in all such studies. The goal of gene-finding efforts is to identify the specific gene(s) and the specific molecular variation(s) in that gene (known as alleles) that predispose to the disease. Classically, this problem was approached by finding a physiologic abnormality in a disease, then the responsible biochemical abnormality, then the abnormal protein responsible for the biochemical abnormality. One could then sequence the protein and infer the responsible DNA variation leading to the variant protein. Limitations to this approach included lack of understanding of the biochemical processes involved, thereby limiting the ability to examine for abnormal enzyme activity. Furthermore, the abnormal protein may not be abnormal per se but only be abnormal in the amount expressed. In addition, with modern molecular techniques, it is considerably easier to sequence DNA than it is to sequence a protein. Thus the more expeditious approach is to study some level of phenotype (e.g., disease, antibody) with variation defined at the DNA level. Gene-finding efforts take advantage of the fact that DNA is a linear structure—that is, a gene is a linear sequence of DNA base pairs and individual genes are arranged linearly along a chromosome.

Two basic study approaches are family-based linkage studies and population (usually case-control) association studies (Table 1–3). Linkage studies ask the question, Does the trait of interest (e.g., the presence of diabetes or inflammatory bowel disease) travel together in families with a particular chromosomal segment, identified by one or more genetic markers? Linkage studies take advantage of the fact that genes are arranged linearly along the 23 pairs (for 46 total chromosomes) of human chromosomes. During meiosis, the cellular division that produces the gametes, each chromosome pairs with its partner (known as the homologous chromosome, hence 22 autosomal pairs plus a pair of sex chromosomes), and exchanges genetic material. This exchange, termed *recombination*, is the basis for

Table 1–3. Contrasting Linkage and Association

Comparison	Linkage	Association
Theoretical basis	Predisposing gene located on chromosomal segment within range of genetic marker Depends on the fact that family members share entire chromosome segments transmitted as a unit	Testing specific variant allele of predisposing gene, or testing a marker that is extremely close to the allele
Type of sample	Family units: sib pairs, relative pairs, pedigrees	Case-control, nuclear families
Type of trait	Qualitative: e.g., presence of disease Quantitative	Qualitative Quantitative
Role to identify contribution of specific gene	Major genes: easy Genes of modest effect: difficult	Able to identify major, moderate, and minor genes
Ability to identify gene along a chromosome	Can be some genetic distance away, i.e., 5–20 cM (approximately 5–20 million bp)	Must be extremely close, either within the gene, or within several hundred kb of the gene (less than 1 cM)
Advantages	If linkage is observed, presence of a major gene likely Can look for genes without a prior hypotheses, e.g., systematic genome scan Can see the effect some distance from the disease gene Can identify an effect even if there are many different alleles	Can identify genes of minor effect For genes of effects smaller than major genes, has the greatest statistical power

detecting linkage. If two genes are close together on a chromosome, then the chance they would recombine is small. If they are far apart on the chromosome, then the chance that they would recombine is large. The frequency of recombination is reported in units termed centiMorgans (cMs), with 1 cM equivalent to a frequency of 1% recombination. The genetic distance of all the human chromosomes combined is somewhat greater than 3000 cMs. Since the 23 pairs of chromosomes are approximately 3 billion DNA base pairs (bp) long, the genetic distance of 1 cM is, on average, equivalent to a physical distance of 1 million bp.

Within one or two generations, there are only a few recombinant events per chromosome, and so large chromosomal segments are shared between parents and offspring and between siblings. Linkage asks whether a certain allele of a genetic marker is transmitted within a family (also referred to as *cosegregation*) with the disease or trait of interest. Because large chromosomal segments are shared in families, if the actual disease-predisposing gene is within 10 to 20 cMs (approximately equivalent to 10–20 million bp) of the genetic marker, then linkage will usually be observed. In performing a linkage analysis, one can have a prior hypothesis that a specific gene is involved. In that case, existence of linkage with a genetic marker at or near the gene of interest indicates that this is indeed the gene causing the disease, or that the disease gene is located in close physical proximity to that gene. Alternatively, one can perform a linkage analysis of the entire genome (the entire complement of human chromosomes), known as *systematic mapping* (also known as a *genome scan*). Here there is no prior hypothesis regarding the disease gene's location. Instead, one is taking advantage of the fact that 300 to 400 evenly spaced DNA markers will likely identify most linkages, because such a number of markers will on average be 10 cM apart and linkage usually extends over that distance. It is important to note that in conducting a linkage analysis, the form of the genetic marker, the allele, can differ between one family and another. The important question is whether the alleles at a marker locus travel together with the disease in families, but the measure is not allele-specific.

Linkage analysis is a statistical method to test whether a disease gene and a marker locus are located in the same chromosomal region (see Chapter 3). The LOD score method, also known as a model-based or parametric method, involves calculating the likelihood of obtaining the observed phenotypes in a sample of pedigrees, given that the recombination fraction between the relevant loci is a value theta (θ). This likelihood is compared to the likelihood of observing the same data, assuming no linkage between the two loci (recombination fraction = 0.5). The resulting value provides an estimate proportional to the odds in favor of linkage at recombination fraction θ compared to no linkage. In general, such linkage analyses have been applied primarily to disorders with "simple" inheritance patterns (that is, inheritance patterns due to a single, completely penetrant, Mendelian gene where the mode of inheritance and the allele frequencies are known). Misspecifying any of these parameters may lead to incorrect results that miss the real linkage or find false linkage when it does not exist.

However, optimally, statistical tools for gene mapping involving complex traits should be model free (also referred to as nonparametric), since one does not know a priori how many genes are involved in the disease, the mode of inheritance of each gene, and the penetrance or gene frequencies. Hence, model-free methods are the primary methods used in linkage analysis of complex traits, such as type 1 diabetes and inflammatory bowel disease. In the model-free approach, the concept is that if the disease gene is located very close to a marker locus, the siblings (or other relatives) who have similar phenotypes (i.e., affection status is concordant) will likely share the same marker alleles (i.e., identity-by-descent). Thus, it is important to determine whether the two siblings are truly sharing identical alleles from a common ancestor by studying not only affected siblings, but also parents and/or unaffected siblings from a nuclear family.

The power to detect linkage in complex traits depends on many factors, for some of which the relative effects are still unknown. The greater a gene contributes to a disorder, the easier it will be identified. A commonly used measurement for a genetic determination of a discrete trait is lambda (λ_S), as defined by Risch (1987): the risk to a relative of an affected individual, given that they share a particular allele, compared to the general population. For a quantitative trait, heritability can be used as a substitute. As will be discussed in the chapters on inflammatory bowel disease and Type 1 diabetes studies, some loci were identified with λ_s (risk to sibs) as low as 1.3.

Inflammatory bowel disease (IBD) is an excellent model to make this point (see Chapter 15). The single greatest risk factor for IBD is a positive family history (Yang and Rotter, 1995). The observed empirical risks of IBD in siblings of IBD patients ranges from 4% to 8%, depending on the type of the disease in probands and ethnicity (Yang et al., 1993). Familial risk in Crohn's disease (CD) is greater than that in ulcerative colitis (UC), and it is greater in Jewish individuals than in non-Jewish cases. If we take 5% as the average risk to siblings of CD probands and 1.5% as the risk to siblings of UC probands, and prevalence data for North America as summarized by Calkins and Mendeloff (1995)—0.04% to 0.1% for CD and 0.04% to 0.15% for UC—then the estimated relative risk to siblings (λ_S) is approximately 50 to 100 for CD and 10 to 30 for UC.

It is almost certain that there is genetic heterogeneity within IBD—for example, CD vs. UC, pANCA-positive UC/CD vs. pANCA-negative UC/CD. That is, these different forms of the disease may result from the expression of different genes. One way of reducing the analytic problem of heterogeneity is to divide the clinical phenotype into "subphenotypes." Thus, the families can be subdivided into families exhibiting only certain phenotypes such as CD only, UC only, pANCA-positive only, or some combinations of these traits to obtain more genetically homogeneous groups. Another way of obtaining etiologically homogenous families is to divide families by ethnicity. Because different ethnic groups may have different evolutionary histories, they may have different distributions of predisposing genes, different relative proportions of forms of the diseases, and different levels of linkage disequilibrium—all of which will affect the efficiency of a linkage study. While such phenotypic subdivision does not automatically translate into complete genetic homogeneity, it does tend to reduce the extent of genetic heterogeneity. The tradeoff for obtaining homogenous families is a decrease in the available sample size. Thus far, all available systematic linkage studies either analyzed CD alone or UC alone (with or without mixed families), or IBD all together.

Association Studies

In contrast to linkage, which asks whether chromosomal segments are shared between two family members with a disease, association tests whether a specific allele of a genetic marker is found with increased frequency in individuals with the disease compared to the frequency of that marker in individuals without the disease. If a disorder is found to be associated with a particular allele, this may suggest a causal relationship (i.e., the association may be due to one of the effects of the gene in which the marker allele lies). Or the disorder may be due to very nearby genes, a phenomenon known as *linkage disequilibrium* (see further discussion of linkage disequilibrium, below). Just as linkage takes advantage of recombination within current families, linkage disequilibrium takes advantage of the many more recombinant events that have occurred historically in a population. Thus, in contrast to linkage, which covers a chromosomal region of 10 to 20 cM (10–20 million bp), association due to linkage disequilibrium will usually occur over less than 1 cM (say 0.1–0.2 cM, or even much less), therefore over a distance of only a few hundred thousand or even a few thousand base pairs (Jorde et al., 1994; Kruglyak, 1997).

Association studies can be conducted in population-based case-control samples or family-based samples. The advantage of using a case-control sample is that it is relatively easy to recruit subjects, and each individual contributes one observation to the statistical test. In contrast, family-based association tests need to genotype at least three people in a family (affected and both parents) to obtain one case and one control. Although the population-based studies are more efficient in terms of time, money, and logistics, a drawback is their potential confounding due to ethnic stratification in an admixed population—that is, case-control data that are not genetically well matched may give us spurious associations. Therefore, family-based association studies are preferable or, at the minimum, are strongly complementary. The family-based transmission/disequilibrium test (TDT) (Spielman et al., 1993; Ewens and Spielman, 1995) can be used to test for linkage disequilibrium with the advantage that the controls are definitely and literally from the same genetic background since they are within the same family. Using families, we take genotypes transmitted to the affected child as "cases" and those from the same parents, but which were not transmitted to the affected children, as "controls." Since these cases and controls come from the same parents, they are genetically well matched for an association test. An additional importance of this method is that the samples collected for linkage studies (e.g., affected sib-pair families) will be suitable for linkage disequilibrium mapping as well, thus maximizing use of clinical epidemiologic resources.

Genome Scan

Systematic mapping, also referred to as the genome scan approach, has had a great success with Mendelian diseases. It is a much greater challenge to apply this approach to genetically complex disorders, since the strict one-to-one relationship between genotypes and phenotypes observed in monogenic disorders breaks down for complex diseases. For most complex diseases, it is likely that multiple genes influence the expression of the disease, which, in turn, makes it difficult to isolate and characterize the effects of each and every individual locus determining the disease. Such multiple genes may interact (epistasis) or induce susceptibility independently (locus heterogeneity). In addition, most complex diseases are influenced by environmental factors as well. As a consequence, genetic mapping in a complex disorder is considerably more difficult than for a Mendelian disorder. Despite advances in genotyping, statistical methodology and better phenotype definition, few replicable gene localizations have yet been obtained.

Experience has now shown that it has become possible to determine the approximate location of genes with only a moderate effect on complex disease expression. In this regard, work in diabetes, especially Type 1 insulin-dependent diabetes mellitus (IDDM) has served as a leading model. Since the initial recognition of the HLA region contribution to Type 1 diabetes (reviewed in Chapter 21), several other chromosome regions that may contain loci leading to susceptibility to IDDM have been detected by genome-wide linkage studies, although none of these loci appears to make a contribution to familial risk that is as strong as that of HLA. For example, the estimated sibling relative risks (λ_S) of IDDM2, the insulin gene (*INS*) minisatellite on chromosome 11p15, is only 1.3, as compared to 2.6 for HLA (Todd and Farrall, 1996). The effect of the non-HLA loci became more pronounced after stratified analysis on HLA. Once linkage has been established, it is possible to obtain additional evidence for the location of a putative susceptibility locus by linkage disequilibrium or association studies. The presence of association and linkage at INS demonstrated unambiguously its involvement in Type 1 diabetes susceptibility (see Chapter 21).

In the last few years it has become clear that highly polymorphic sequences such as microsatellites offer important advantages and are present at a sufficiently high density to allow construction of detailed linkage maps in both humans and animal models (see Chapter 2). The high degree of microsatellite polymorphism, combined with the relative ease of analysis by polymerase chain reaction (PCR), makes whole genome scanning an attractive method for genetic studies. Rapid genotyping of the human genome is now feasible and, indeed, becoming routine in many laboratories.

The primary advantage of whole genome mapping is that it can use PCR markers that can be typed by semiautomated, high-throughput methods. In particular, groups of markers can be simultaneously amplified from a single template (multiplex PCR) and combined on a single gel lane, where each marker is resolved from the others on the basis of size or fluorescent tag (multiplex electrophoresis). Moreover, analysis of the genotypes is now largely automated. A computer image of the fluorescent bands is transferred to disk by laser scanning the gel during electrophoresis. Imaging software identifies bands and computes their sizes from fluorescent size standards included with the samples. Database software can then associate the allele sizes with each individual's DNA on the basis of standardized lane positions. Although the computer-generated allele sizes need to be checked visually on the computer screen, most of the arduous lane-identification and allele-calling work is rapid and automatic.

Linkage Disequilibrium

Linkage disequilibrium (LD) is a population genetics phenomenon by which alleles (i.e., the various forms of a gene or marker) at different but close genetic loci on a chromosome remain together on chromosomes throughout generations within a population (also see Chapter 3). It has been demonstrated that linkage disequilibrium mapping (i.e., association) studies have greater power than linkage studies to identify genes with small effect (Risch and Merikangas, 1996). This assumes that the linkage disequilibrium exists between the genetic markers analyzed and the actual causative mutations (variations). However, two points should be kept in mind: *(1)* not all regions of the genome show a monotonic relationship between distance and extent of disequilibria between markers, *(2)* population history (age, size, migration, etc.) affects linkage disequilibrium and thus will affect gene mapping efforts of this nature. Therefore, assessing population genetic structure (e.g., amount of admixture or relative genetic distance between populations) may be important in study design and the interpretation of the results.

Once linkage to a DNA marker has been established, say in a genome scan, LD mapping can be applied to bring us closer to the disease locus (within 50–500 kb), to refine the location of a disease gene that is already mapped to a chromosomal region. Another use of LD mapping, which was proposed recently, is to map a disease gene de novo by performing whole genome association scans. New technologies have made the required dense markers at least theoretically in reach, for example, the development of a large number of well-characterized single nucleotide polymorphisms (SNPs). However, as of today, such markers are still in the process of being developed, and statistical issues regarding interpretation and significance of results from such studies remain under discussion.

Mouse–Human Homologies

Both linkage and association approaches are being actively utilized to find the genes underlying common diseases. Each of these approaches has its advantages and disadvantages in terms of the number of markers needed, length of the chromosomal region being examined, and magnitude of the genetic effect that can be identified. One additional approach to increase the power and potential of linkage studies in complex human diseases is to first identify regions of linkage in a mouse model, where genetics can be optimized by various breeding strategies and where the environment can be tightly controlled. If linkage is observed in the mouse, then the position of the homologous human locus is predicted using synteny maps of mouse and human genomes, and then linkage is tested in man for those specific homologous regions (see Chapter 3).

This approach is possible because many ancestral chromosomal segments have been conserved between mice and humans, although chromosomal rearrangements have scattered these syntenic regions on different chromosomes (Lander et al., 2001). This approach is becoming an increasingly active one in complex diseases, and a number of successes in disease gene localization have occurred using the mouse–human synteny paradigm for metabolic and autoimmune phenotypes. Examples of these successes have included apolipoprotein A-II and serum-free fatty acids related to atherosclerosis (Warden et al., 1993; Hedrick et al., 1993), multiple sclerosis (Kuokkanen et al., 1996), systemic lupus erythematosus (Tsao et al., 1997), obesity (Lembertas et al., 1997), and familial combined hyperlipidemia (Castellani et al., 1998; Pajukanta et al., 1998).

APPLICATION OF GENETICS IN COMMON DISEASES

Diagnosis

The physician who uses a genetic approach has the usual diagnostic skills available, including medical and family history, physical examination, laboratory tests, laboratory and imaging studies, and specialty consultations. Sometimes it is necessary to perform an evaluation on family members to make a correct diagnosis. As an example, a woman may present with breast cancer at the age of 55 years. If by taking a careful family history it is learned that she has a sister with breast cancer and an aunt with ovarian cancer, then a diagnosis of familial breast cancer associated with a mutation in *BRCA1* or *BRCA2* can be suspected. The physician taking a diagnostic genetic approach will not be satisfied with just obtaining a history of disease in relatives. Medical records documenting the type of cancer in the affected relatives should be obtained. Although this approach has been discussed with the example of a Mendelian disorder that accounts for a small but significant part of breast cancer, a similar approach can be used to arrive at a diagnosis of familial hypercholesterolemia with atherosclerosis, cirrhosis with hemochromatosis, or the autoimmune disorders that accompany insulin-dependent diabetes.

There are several lessons to be learned from genetics as regards clinical diagnosis. First, one can use the family as an additional investigative tool. This is done most effectively by actual examination of at-risk relatives. Relatives cannot be said to be unaffected unless they have been seen by a physician who was searching for the specific disorder segregating in the family.

Second, the family history can help focus the medical history and the physical and subsequent examinations. Time limitations and the high cost of medical care require that most physicians carry out a directed history and physical examination, asking questions and performing investigations that are specific to the patient's complaint and to the observations made during the examination rather than obtaining a "complete" history or perform a "complete" physical examination on a regular basis. Indeed, the examination itself is usually directed to the patient's complaints. In the same manner, a directed family history and directed examination of relatives can be very efficient and useful. A corollary of this lesson is that, when taking a history or performing a physical examination, the physician should ask directed questions and examine for specific findings that may indicate a syndromic form of what otherwise is a common disease.

Prognosis and Counseling

Genetic prognosis deals both with the prognosis for the individual affected with a specific disorder (rare or common) and with delineating disease risks for various relatives. Genetic counseling is the process by which such risks for a disease and the potential options for dealing with those risks are communicated to the individual and family at risk. As in genetic diagnosis, the entire family and not just the individual patient is properly considered.

The risk for a disease has two components. One is the numerical risk; the other is the burden or severity of the disorder. For example, lactose intolerance, cystic fibrosis, and hemochromatosis are autosomal recessive conditions, and when an individual is found to be affected with one of these disorders, the risk to a sibling is 25%. However, the burdens for the individual and family are very different. Lactose intolerance usually causes only modest symptoms and, in any case, is readily treated by limitation of the amount of lactose-containing food in the diet. In contrast, cystic fibrosis is a disorder that requires enormous medical attention and cost and still almost invariably leads to death by young adulthood. The consequences of the interventions are very different in terms of individual and family suffering and economic costs, and it is important that this information be conveyed to the family.

It is important also to delineate the quantitative risk for disease to family members as accurately as possible so they can make the best informed reproductive and health-care decisions. The ability to quantify a given relative's disease risk varies considerably. When a given disorder can be reliably diagnosed as a Mendelian disorder, accurate counseling can be given based on well-known Mendelian rules; for example, the genetic risk to siblings of an affected individual is 25% for an autosomal recessive disorder or 50% for an autosomal dominant disorder. There is a difference between clinical and genetic risk in that a disease can be expressed differently among individuals with the same genetic susceptibility. With hemochromatosis, for example, a male sibling of an affected individual has a greater chance of developing a complication of chronic iron overload than does a female sibling, even when both have the same genotype as that of their affected sibling. The actual clinical risk needs to be explained together with the genetic risk.

For the many non-Mendelian (multifactorial) disorders, however, well-defined rules predicting risk are not available. In these cases, physicians rely on empiric recurrence risks. While such empiric risk counseling is considerably less precise than that based on Mendelian risks, it is often reassuring in that the risks are often low, often ~5%. For example, the disease risk to siblings of an insulin-dependent diabetic is 5% to 10%, depending on the population studied.

For many common disorders, the only information that can be obtained is either the Mendelian or the empiric risk, but the patients and their families and physicians would prefer more helpful data. Instead of counseling a relative for hereditary nonpolyposis colon cancer (HNPCC), a dominant disorder, as having a 50% risk, it would be better to divide this risk group into those who actually have the disorder (100% risk) together with clinically apparent signs and those who do not carry the gene (0% risk). There are a number of methods that increasingly allow further refinement of a family member's disease risk. These are discussed in the next section.

Finally, an important component of genetic counseling is conveying to patients and their family the various options of dealing with the disorder and its risk of recurrence. We believe that for many of the disorders reviewed in this volume—those that are treatable and, especially, those for which early intervention improves the outcome (e.g., colon cancer and polyps)—preclinical screening is recommended to diagnose the disorder at a stage at which intervention will ameliorate or even prevent clinical disease. Prenatal diagnosis is rarely used in common diseases, since the genetic component is usually complex, the expression and penetrance of identified genes are variable, and the onset is later in life.

Presymptomatic Screening and Assessment

There are two major goals for presymptomatic genetic screening. One is research. Only by conducting such studies in families and in populations will we understand gene–gene and gene–environment interactions, the preclinical natural history of these diseases, the genotypic–phenotypic relationships, public health and resource evaluations, and accurate predictive ability of the various assessments (family history, phenotypic traits, molecular genotyping) of genetic risk. Another use of such information is in clinical trials (see below). It is these types of clinical genetic and genetic epidemiologic investigations that have generated the bulk of information provided in this volume.

The other goal for presymptomatic genetic screening is generally to prevent, delay, minimize, or reduce the risk and burden of clinical diseases. Thus, in general, clinical use of screening should be encouraged only when there is an intervention or interventions for which there is reasonable evidence that one can reduce the burden of clinical disease. Examples are decreasing cholesterol or homocysteine levels to reduce the risk of coronary artery disease, of polypectomy to reduce the risk of colon cancer, and of prophylactic oophorectomy for high ovarian cancer risks. It can be argued that reducing the burden of disease is not just reducing its occurrence but even its psychological consequences. Thus, one can make the argument that genetic screening to assess risk can reduce the anxiety of some individuals in the family who lack the segregating predisposing gene and thus are at the general population risk. For the individual found to be at risk and his family, there will be heightened anxiety and worry. At the same time, more meaningful personal, professional, family and financial planning becomes possible.

Therapy and Prevention

Obviously, the entire approach to understanding the genetic pathogenesis of common diseases is to produce effective forms of therapy and eventual prevention. The Human Genome Project now places this within the scope of biomedical research, but the advances are just beginning. There has been little application of the new genetic knowledge in the development of new therapies, and, essentially, no preventive strategies have developed. However, when the first edition of this book was published, there was little knowledge of the genetic basis of most of the diseases covered in the book, and that has changed. The ultimate full extent of the evolving new knowledge on prevention and therapy cannot yet be predicted. Medical practice, however, is likely to change.

REFERENCES

Bacon BR: Hemochromatosis: diagnosis and management. Gastroenterology 2001; 120:718–725.

Calkins BM, Mendeloff AI: The epidemiology of idiopathic inflammatory bowel disease. In: Kirsner JB, Shorter RG (eds). Inflammatory Bowel Disease. Baltimore: Williams and Wilkins, 1995:31–68.

Castellani LW, Weinreb A, Bodnar J, Goto AM, Doolittle M, Mehrabian M, Demant P, Lusis AJ: Mapping a gene for combined hyperlipidaemia in a mutant mouse strain. Nat Genet 1998; 18:374–377.

Cowan WM, Kandel ER: Prospects for neurology and psychiatry. JAMA 2001; 285:594–600.

Dreon DM, Fernstrom HA, Williams PT, Krauss RM: Reduced LDL particle size in children consuming a very-low-fat diet is related to parental LDL-subclass patterns. Am J Clin Nutr 2000; 71:1611–1616.

Dreon DM, Krauss RM: Diet–gene interactions in human lipoprotein metabolism. J Am Coll Nutr 1997; 16:313–324.

Ewens WJ, Spielman RS: The transmission/disequilibrium test: history, subdivision, and admixture. Am J Hum Genet 1995; 57:455–464.

Flood DM, Weiss NS, Cook LS, Emerson JC, Schwartz SM, Potter JD: Colorectal cancer incidence in Asian migrants to the United States and their descendants. Cancer Causes Control 2000; 11:403–411.

Grody WW, Cutting GR, Klinger KW, Richards CS, Watson MS, Desnick RJ: Laboratory standards and guidelines for population-based cystic fibrosis carrier screening. Genet Med 2001; 3:149–154.

Hedrick CC, Castellani LW, Warden CH, Puppione DL, Lusis AJ: Influence of mouse apolipoprotein A-II on plasma lipoproteins in transgenic mice. J Biol Chem 1993; 268:20676–20682.

Henikoff S, Matzke MA: Exploring and explaining epigenetic effects. Trends Genet 1997; 13:293–295.

Jorde LB, Carey JC, Bamshad MJ, White RL: Medical Genetics, 2d ed. St. Louis: Mosby, 1999.

Jorde LB, Watkins WS, Carlson M, Groden J, Albertsen H, Thliveris A, Leppert M: Linkage disequilibrium predicts physical distance in the adenomatous polyposis coli region. Am J Hum Genet 1994; 54:884–898.

Krauss RM, Dreon DM: Low-density-lipoprotein subclasses and response to a low-fat diet in healthy men. Am J Clin Nutr 1995; 62:478S–487S.

Kruglyak L: What is significant in whole-genome linkage disequilibrium studies? Am J Hum Genet 1997; 61:810–812.

Kuokkanen S, Sundvall M, Terwilliger JD, Tienari PJ, Wikstrom J, Holmdahl R, Pettersson U, Peltonen L: A putative vulnerability locus to multiple sclerosis maps to 5p14–p12 in a region syntenic to the murine locus Eae2. Nat Genet 1996; 13:477–480.

Lander ES, Linton LM, Birren B, Nusbaum C, Zody MC, Baldwin J, Devon K, Dewar K, Doyle M, FitzHugh W, et al.: Initial sequencing and analysis of the human genome. Nature 2001; 409:860–921.

Lembertas AV, Perusse L, Chagnon YC, Fisler JS, Warden CH, Purcell-Huynh DA, Dionne FT, Gagnon J, Nadeau A, Lusis AJ, Bouchard C: Identification of an obesity quantitative trait locus on mouse chromosome 2 and evidence of linkage to body fat and insulin on the human homologous region 20q. J Clin Invest 1997; 100:1240–1247.

Martienssen R, Henikoff S: The House and Garden guide to chromatin remodelling. Nat Genet 1999; 22:6–7.

Michaud CM, Murray CJ, Bloom BR: Burden of disease—implications for future research. JAMA 2001; 285:535–539.

Mickle JE, Cutting GR: Genotype–phenotype relationships in cystic fibrosis. Med Clin North Am 2000; 84:597–607.

Nadeau JH: Modifier genes in mice and humans. Nat Rev Genet 2001; 2:165–174.

Pajukanta P, Nuotio I, Terwilliger JD, Porkka KV, Ylitalo K, Pihlajamaki J, Suomalainen AJ, Syvanen AC, Lehtimaki T, Viikari JS, et al.: Linkage of familial combined hyperlipidaemia to chromosome 1q21–q23. Nat Genet 1998; 18:369–373.

Petronis A: Human morbid genetics revisited: relevance of epigenetics. Trends Genet 2001; 17:142–146.

Petronis A, Petroniene R: Epigenetics of inflammatory bowel disease. Gut 2000; 47:302–306.

Rimoin DL, Connor JM, Pyeritz, RE (eds): Principles and Practice of Medical Genetics, 3d ed. New York: Churchill Livingstone, 1996.

Risch N: Assessing the role of HLA-linked and unlinked determinants of disease. Am J Hum Genet 1987; 40:1–14.

Risch N, Merikangas K: The future of genetic studies of complex human diseases. Science 1996; 273:1516–1517.

Robertson TL, Kato H, Gordon T, Kagan A, Rhoads GG, Land CE, Worth RM, Belsky JL, Dock DS, Miyanishi M, Kawamoto S: Epidemiologic studies of coronary heart disease and stroke in Japanese men living in Japan, Hawaii and California: coronary heart disease risk factors in Japan and Hawaii. Am J Cardiol 1977; 39:244–249.

Samuels J, Aksentijevich I, Torosyan Y, Centola M, Deng Z, Sood R, Kastner DL: Familial Mediterranean fever at the millennium: clinical spectrum, ancient mutations, and a survey of 100 American referrals to the National Institutes of Health. Medicine (Baltimore) 1998; 77:268–297.

Scheuner MT, Wang SJ, Raffel LJ, Larabell SK, Rotter JI: Family history: a comprehensive genetic risk assessment method for the chronic conditions of adulthood. Am J Med Genet 1997; 71:315–324.

Scriver CR, Beaudet AL, Sly WS, Valle D (eds): The Metabolic and Molecular Bases of Inherited Disease, 8th ed. New York: McGraw-Hill, 2001.

Spielman RS, McGinnis RE, Ewens WJ: Transmission test for linkage disequilibrium: the insulin gene region and insulin-dependent diabetes mellitus (IDDM). Am J Hum Genet 1993; 52:506–516.

Strachan T, Read AP: Human Molecular Genetics. New York: Wiley-Liss, 1999.

Todd JA, Farrall M: Panning for gold: genome-wide scanning for linkage in type 1 diabetes. Hum Mol Genet 1996; 5(Spec No):1443–1448.

Tsao BP, Cantor RM, Kalunian KC, Chen CJ, Badsha H, Singh R, Wallace DJ, Kitridou RC, Chen SL, Shen N, et al.: Evidence for linkage of a candidate chromosome 1 region to human systemic lupus erythematosus. J Clin Invest 1997; 99:725–731.

Vogel F, Motulsky AG: Human Genetics: Problems and Approaches, 3d ed. Berlin: Springer, 1997.

Warden CH, Hedrick CC, Qiao JH, Castellani LW, Lusis AJ: Atherosclerosis in transgenic mice overexpressing apolipoprotein A-II. Science 1993; 261:469–472.

Yang H, McElree C, Roth MP, Shanahan F, Targan SR, Rotter JI: Familial empirical risks for inflammatory bowel disease: differences between Jews and non-Jews. Gut 1993; 34:517–524.

Yang H, Rotter JI: Genetic aspects of idiopathic inflammatory bowel disease. In: Kirsner JB, Shorter RG (eds). Inflammatory Bowel Disease. Baltimore: Williams and Wilkins, 1995:301–331.

Zerah M, Ueshiba H, Wood E, Speiser PW, Crawford C, McDonald T, Pareira J, Gruen D, New MI: Prevalence of nonclassical steroid 21-hydroxylase deficiency based on a morning salivary 17-hydroxyprogesterone screening test: a small sample study. J Clin Endocrinol Metab 1990; 70:1662–1667.

2 Molecular Genetics of Common Disease

JEFFREY R. SMITH, THOMAS D. GELEHRTER, AND FRANCIS S. COLLINS

Broadly stated, the subject of this volume is the role of hereditary factors in human disease. A few of the disorders discussed are inherited in classic Mendelian fashion, but in many others the nature of the genetic contribution cannot be explained by a single-gene hypothesis. In the former situation, the recent application of the powerful techniques of molecular genetics has led to rapid increases in our understanding with major therapeutic implications; in the latter, molecular genetic techniques offer the promise of detecting genetic heterogeneity and defining genetic factors more precisely than has previously been possible. The result of this new technology has been a shift in emphasis in the medical sciences from cellular metabolism to genetic information and its control. Thus, it is highly appropriate for a text such as this to include a chapter on molecular genetics, even though the widespread application of this approach to the solution of unique problems of the genetics of common disease is far from mature. Our goal in this chapter, therefore, is to present the basics of the molecular biology of information flow from DNA to RNA to protein, to describe some of the techniques of recombinant DNA that have allowed the molecular cloning of single genes, and to outline how these same strategies can be used to unravel the genetics of common disease.

PHYSICAL STRUCTURE OF THE HUMAN GENOME

DNA Structure

Though the existence of DNA was noted more than a century ago, it was not until 1944 that Avery and colleagues demonstrated, to the surprise of many, that DNA was capable of carrying genetic information. Less than a decade later, Watson and Crick (1953), in what is probably the most seminal one-page paper of the twentieth century, proposed the correct structure of DNA, consisting of an unbranched double helix composed of two intertwined chains with sugar-phosphate backbones (Fig. 2–1). A number of features of this structure are worthy of specific mention. *(1)* It is polar. There is a 5′ and a 3′ end to each strand, and the strands are arranged in antiparallel orientation. *(2)* The nucleotide bases are arranged inside the helix in a complementary fashion. A (adenine) on one strand always pairs with T (thymine) on the other, and C (cytosine) always pairs with G (guanine). Two hydrogen bonds stabilize the AT pairs, and three stabilize the GC pairs, accounting for the increased thermal stability of double-stranded GC-rich sequences. *(3)* It provides an elegant means of storing and coding vast amounts of information. The size of many genomes (N) in base pairs is fairly accurately known; because each position along the DNA strand can be A, C, G, or T, the number of possible combinations of information contained in such a genome is 4^N. For the human haploid genome, N is 3.2×10^9 (gigabases), so 4^N is approximately 10 to the two billionth power. *(4)* As suggested by Watson and Crick (1953) and confirmed through the experiments of Meselson and Stahl (1958), the complementary nature of DNA provides a mechanism for its replication in faithful fashion: each strand serves as the template for a new strand, a process referred to as *semi-conservative replication. (5)* The complementary nature also provides a means of error correction: if one strand is damaged, it can be repaired using the other as a template. *(6)* Complementarity of DNA strands also has enormous implications for experimental molecular biology because it allows separated complementary or near complementary strands to "find" each other in a complex mixture if slow annealing (hybridization) is allowed to occur after the strands have been thermally or chemically separated (denatured). As we shall see, the power of molecular hybridization to identify a particular nucleic acid sequence of low abundance in a mixture is at the heart of the success of molecular biology.

DNA Packaging: Nucleosomes and Chromatin

It is likely that each of the 46 human chromosomes is made up of a single molecule of double-stranded DNA. If stretched out, the DNA from a single cell would extend ~2 m in length: obviously, an efficient method of packaging must be utilized by cells to deal with a molecule of such complexity. An elaborate system of coiling, which also seems to be involved in the control of gene expression in as yet poorly understood ways, is present in mammalian cells (Felsenfeld, 1996; Wolffe and Guschin, 2000; Mello and Almouzni, 2001). Basic proteins, called *histones*, provide a core around which DNA is wound in a double loop comprising ~146 bp of DNA (Fig. 2–2). This unit is referred to as a *nucleosome*: the tight evolutionary conservation of histone structure implies an important functional role. The resulting "beads-on-a-string" DNA structure compacts the length by about a factor of 7: further organization occurs by arrangement of the nucleosomes in a solenoid fashion and by higher-order structural complexities.

The mechanism by which factors responsible for the regulation of gene expression interact with this monotonous histone–DNA complex represents an important area of investigation. There is evidence that regions of the DNA molecule that are involved in regulation may be locally free of histones. For example, certain areas (especially the 5′ ends) of actively expressed genes are unusually sensitive to cleavage by nonspecific nucleases such as DNase I, which do not efficiently cut histone-bound DNA (Gross and Garrard, 1988; Felsenfeld, 1996).

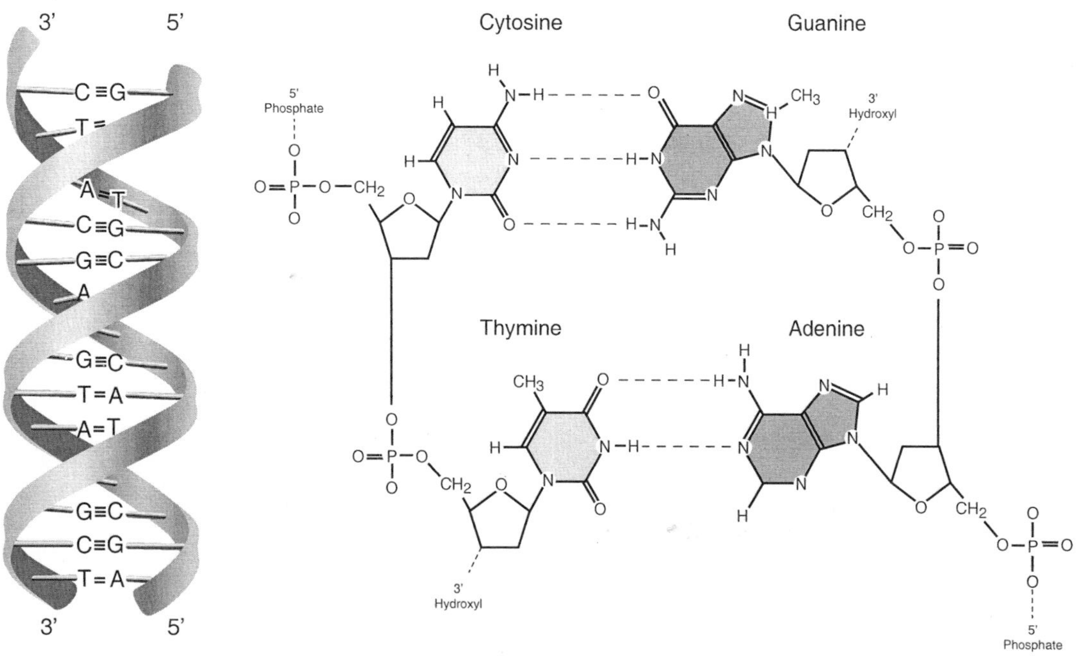

Fig. 2–1. Structure of double-stranded DNA. On the *right* are shown the hydrogen bonds that hold the double helix together.

Structure of Genes and Gene Families

One of the major surprises of eukaryotic genetics was the discovery that the DNA sequence of most eukaryotic genes does not code contiguously for its specific protein but is interrupted by regions of noncoding sequence, called *introns*, that have no clearly defined function and must be spliced out before a mature mRNA is produced. Two examples, shown in Figure 2–3, are the α- and β-*globin* genes of human hemoglobin (Stamatoyannopoulos et al., 1994). Both have three coding regions, called *exons*, interrupted by two noncoding introns of somewhat different lengths. Controversy exists regarding the role of introns and whether they were acquired in the evolution of eukaryotes or lost in the evolution of prokaryotes. Gilbert (1978) suggested that their presence might allow for more rapid evolution by a process of *exon shuffling*, which allows for blocks of coding regions to be combinatorially arranged to generate new proteins in a much more rapid fashion than would otherwise be possible. Multiple lines of evidence now support this hypothesis (Long et al., 1995; International Human Genome Sequencing Consortium, 2001; Venter et al., 2001). An example of such a protein is the low-density lipoprotein (LDL) receptor (Sudhof et al., 1985), which contains exon blocks separately homologous to the ninth component of complement and to the epidermal growth factor precursor; other exons are involved in discrete functions, such as membrane anchoring and recycling of the receptor.

The presence of introns also allows the generation of more than one protein molecule from a given gene by alternative splicing (Herbert and Rich, 1999). An example is the *Calcitonin* gene

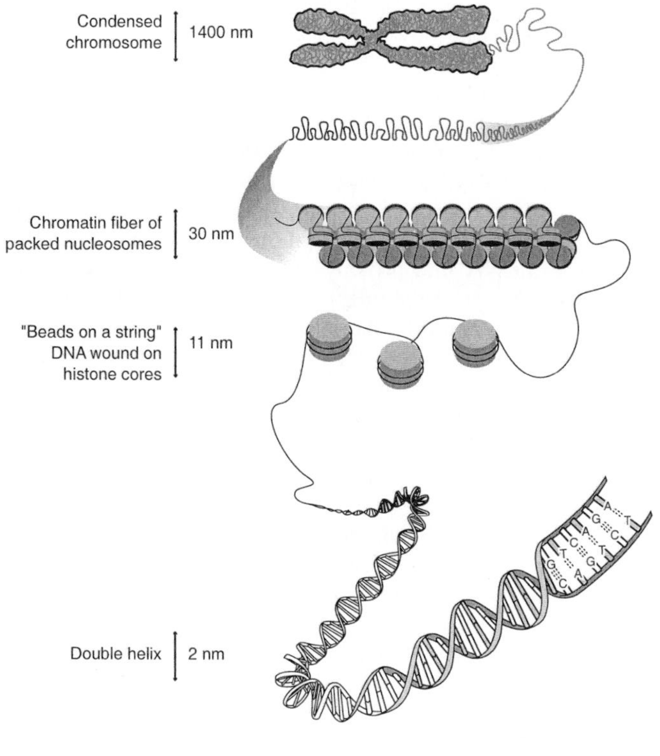

Fig. 2–2. Higher-order packaging of DNA by histones and other proteins.

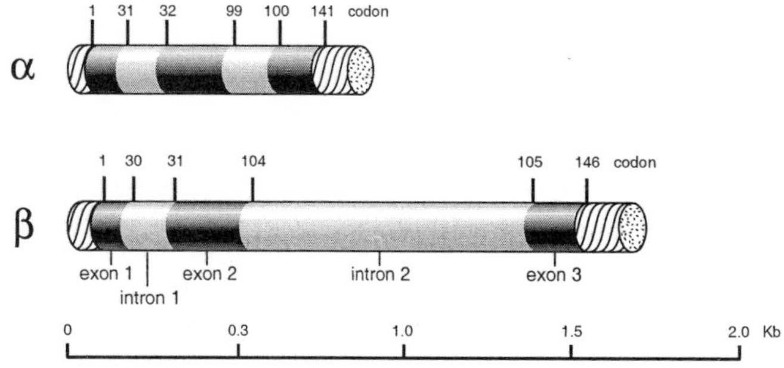

Fig. 2–3. Typical anatomy of the transcribed portion of a eukaryotic gene, as exemplified by the human α- and β-hemoglobin genes. *Hatched areas* are transcribed but not translated. *Darkly shaded areas* are exons; *lightly shaded segments* are introns.

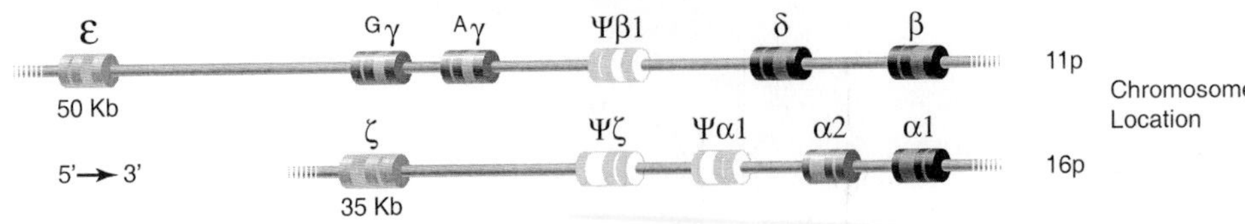

Fig. 2–4. Genomic structure of human hemoglobin genes on chromosomes 11 and 16. The beta cluster on chromosome 11 consists of five expressed genes (ε, G_γ, A_γ, δ, and β), and the α-globin cluster on chromosome 16 consists of three genes (ζ, α2, and α1). Interestingly, these genes are arranged on the chromosome in the order of their activation during development, such that ε and ζ code for embryonic hemoglobin and adult hemoglobin consists of δ, β, α1, and α2. Each cluster also contains at least one pseudogene, here designated ψβ1, ψζ, and ψα1. These represent genes which were once functional but have acquired inactivating mutations during the course of evolution. Also, the majority of the DNA in these clusters is intergenic and of mostly unknown function.

(Rosenfeld et al., 1983; Coleman and Roesser, 1998), which is spliced in one fashion in the thyroid and in another in the central nervous system, to yield protein products with quite different functions.

Genes of related function are sometimes, but not always, located near each other in the genome. Figure 2–4 shows the α- and β-globin clusters in humans (Stamatoyannopoulos et al., 1994). Adult hemoglobin is a tetrameric protein made of two α chains and two β chains. In embryonic life, human hemoglobin is primarily $\epsilon_2\zeta_2$ and in fetal life it is $\gamma_2\alpha_2$. All of the α-like chains are arranged within reasonable proximity on chromosome 16, and all of the β-like chains are arranged on chromosome 11, in both instances in the order of their developmental activation from 5′ to 3′. In both clusters, there are also *pseudogenes*, evolutionary remnants of once-functioning members of the cluster that have acquired inactivating mutations. Many other physically clustered gene families are known to exist in humans, including the class I and II major histocompatibility complex (MHC) genes (Steinmetz and Hood, 1983), the albumin–α-fetoprotein complex (Camper et al., 1989), and some of the apolipoprotein genes (Breslow, 1985). Furthermore, when entire families of genes share sequence homologies, implying a common evolutionary origin, these families are said to make up a *superfamily*; the best described superfamily (Hood et al., 1985) contains the immunoglobulin genes, the class I and II MHC genes, T-cell receptors, and certain other cell surface antigens.

It should be apparent from Figure 2–4 that only a small portion of the DNA in these gene complexes actually encodes protein. Only a third of the genome is transcribed, and ~98.8% of the genome does not encode proteins (International Human Genome Sequencing Consortium, 2001; Venter et al., 2001). In general, the sequence of noncoding DNA is evolutionarily less conserved and contains stretches that are repeated many times in the genome (Mazzarella and Schlessinger, 1997). An estimated 35% to 45% of the genome is comprised of these repetitive sequences; 11% is the so-called Alu sequence (because it contains an Alu I restriction site). While new Alu elements integrate preferentially in the gene-poor regions, over time they have accumulated predominantly in the gene-dense regions, suggesting some evolutionary benefit (International Human Genome Sequencing Consortium, 2001). The Alu sequence is roughly 300 bp in length and one member of a larger family of short interspersed nuclear elements found exclusively in primates. Long interspersed nuclear elements, such as the L1 element, comprise the other major repeat family (21% of the genome). Repetitive elements of both families can rarely migrate through the genome by a mechanism of retrotransposition: the sequence is transcribed into RNA, reverse-transcribed into cDNA, and integrated into a new genomic site. The genomic mutability conferred by this process may have major implications for evolution; repetitive elements provide "evolutionary grease" by promoting insertional mutagenesis, meiotic crossover events, and illegitimate recombination. Convincing evidence has been provided that germline short and long interspersed repetitive element retrotransposition can be a source of new mutations that cause medical illness (Moran et al., 1999). An additional 8% of the genome contains retrovirus-like repetitive DNA.

GENE EXPRESSION

All somatic cells contain the complete genome of the organism (there are an estimated 30,000–40,000 human genes) (International Human Genome Sequencing Consortium, 2001; Venter et al., 2001), with the exception of DNA rearrangements occurring in certain cells of the immune system. Yet in any given tissue, only a relatively small proportion of these genes are expressed. Understanding the control of gene expression is therefore fundamental to an understanding of virtually all aspects of human biology. Genes are expressed according to regulatory patterns of development, the cell cycle, tissue origin, hormonal influence, and metabolic pathway feedback. Networks of coordinately regulated genes have been termed *regulons* in prokaryotes. Complex networks in humans are being elucidated via new genome-scale systems that afford parallel assays of thousands of genes (Velculescu et al., 1995; Roth et al., 1998; Brown and Botstein, 1999), which will be discussed later in this chapter.

In general, it is the mature protein product of a gene that carries out its controlling influence. The level of this mature protein can be altered by *(1)* the rate of transcription of the gene into RNA, *(2)* the processing of this RNA, *(3)* the transport of the mRNA from nucleus to cytoplasm, *(4)* the rate of translation of the mRNA into protein on cellular ribosomes, *(5)* the rate of degradation of the mRNA, *(6)* posttranslational modification or sequestration of the protein, and *(7)* the rate of protein degradation. All of these control mechanisms have been implicated in specific instances. However, the most economic method is to control protein production at its earliest level: gene transcription.

There are three RNA polymerases in eukaryotic nuclei, each of which transcribes a different class of genes. RNA polymerase I transcribes the ribosomal DNA genes into 18S and 28S ribosomal RNA, and RNA polymerase III is involved in transcription of the transfer and 5S RNAs. RNA polymerase II is used for transcription of genes coding for proteins (Lee and Young, 2000). Our discussion here centers on the signals that target RNA polymerase II to a particular transcription-start site and control the quantity of mRNA produced from such a gene.

Figure 2–5 shows a schematic of the control elements of an idealized gene. *Cis*-acting sequence elements have been identi-

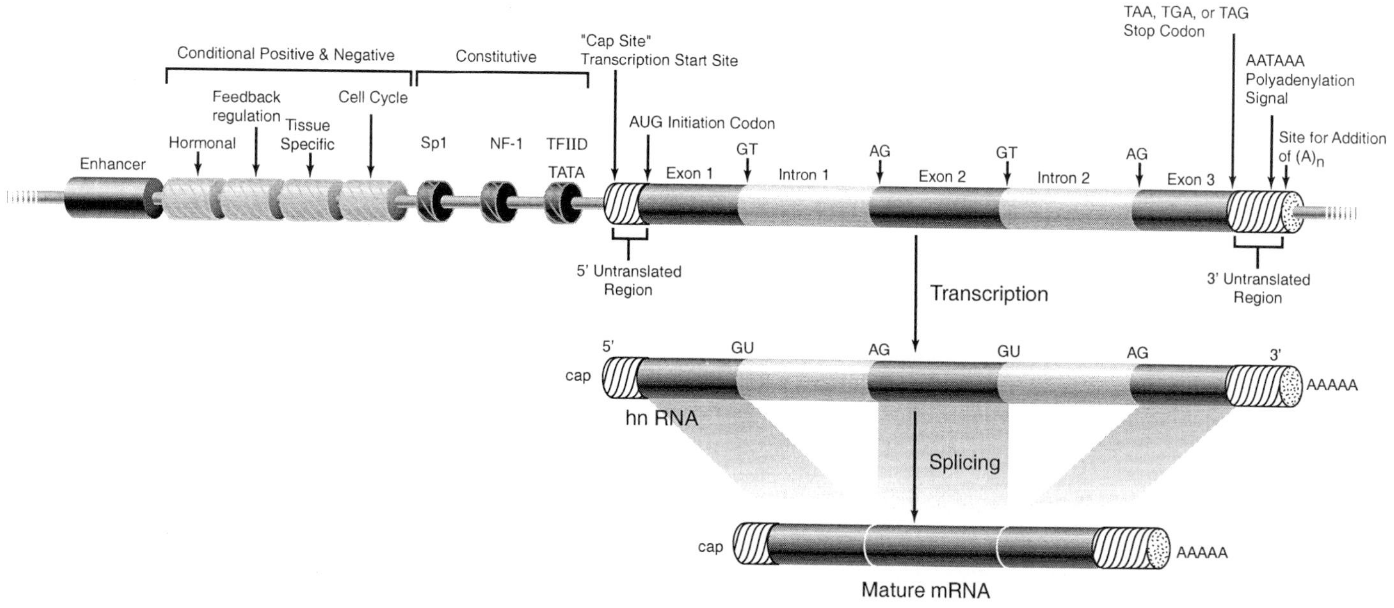

Fig. 2–5. Anatomy of a typical eukaryotic gene. *Top line* shows organization of the regulatory sequences, introns, and exons at the genomic level. *Center line* diagrams RNA transcript anatomy prior to splicing *(hnRNA)*. *Lower line* diagrams mature mRNA after splicing has been completed.

fied by a variety of methods, including functional assays using gene transfer into cultured cells, mutational analysis, and evolutionary comparison (Sudhof et al., 1987; Smith et al., 1990; Bishop, 1992). It is also possible to study physical interactions of DNA sequences and nuclear protein *trans*-acting factors in vitro (Wang et al., 1993; Briggs et al., 1993; Yokoyama et al., 1993), and successful in vitro transcription systems have been developed (Bennett et al., 1999). In vivo transcriptional control may also be evaluated by manipulation of test genes in mouse oocytes to create transgenic mice (Shimano et al., 1996).

The Promoter

The *promoter* is somewhat loosely defined as those sequence elements located 5′ to the gene that fix the site of transcription initiation and control gene expression in response to bound regulatory factors. While in some situations the promoter elements may extend for several kilobases, in many instances the important promoter elements are located within 400 bp of the 5′ end of the gene.

Many, but not all, genes contain a conserved TATA box sequence, which is located 25 to 30 bp 5′ to the start of transcription and seems to be involved in the precise localization of the start (Efstratiadis et al., 1980). It binds a transcription factor complex, TFIID, which interacts with RNA polymerase II and initiates transcription (Stargell and Struhl, 1996). However, many "housekeeping" genes, such as 3-hydroxy-3-methylglutaryl coenzyme A *reductase* (Osborne et al., 1985) and *Hypoxanthine-guanine phosphoribosyltransferase* (Melton et al., 1984), often lack such sequences. Auxiliary factors bind to specific sites within promoters to activate or repress transcription. Binding sites for transcription factors such as SP1 (the GC box) and NF-Y (the CCAAT box) (Maity and de Crombrugghe, 1998) are present in the promoter region of many of these genes. The frequency of such sites is relatively higher in "TATA-less" promoters (Mantovani, 1998). Interruption of the promoter by mutation can alter the normal pattern of expression with deleterious effects; one form of familial hypercholesterolemia observed within the founder French Canadian population results from deletion of the *LDL receptor* gene promoter (Hobbs et al., 1987).

Promoter elements also fix the start site of transcription to a particular location, though some degree of heterogeneity of start site in a 10 to 20 bp region is often seen, especially in genes lacking a TATA box. A particular modified nucleotide, 7-methylguanosine, called a *cap*, is added to the 5′ end of the growing mRNA chain (Varani, 1997). Thus, the site of initiation of transcription is also often called the *cap site*.

The pattern of expression of many genes is tightly regulated, and such regulation is often mediated by sequences in the gene promoter; e.g., expression may be guided by interaction of tissue-specific transcription factors with corresponding promoter binding sites. These binding sites would be expected to have similar sequences between genes co-expressed selectively in a given tissue; however, their identification by simple sequence comparison is difficult. The most successful approaches to this important issue have involved deletion or mutation of portions of a gene, followed by gene transfer into cultured cells or into transgenic mice so that the effects on tissue specificity can be observed. In the *Insulin* gene, e.g., Edlund et al. (1985) used this approach to define elements located 150 to 300 bp 5′ to the initiation site that are capable of conferring pancreatic islet-cell specificity (see also Dumonteil and Philippe, 1996). As further evidence of this tissue specificity, when the insulin promoter is placed in front of the transforming gene of simian virus 40 (SV40) (the *T-antigen* gene) and transgenic mice are generated, the mice develop pancreatic tumors at high frequency (Hanahan, 1985; Efrat et al., 1995). Also, using transgenic mice, sequences 5′ to the *Elastase* gene have been defined that confer pancreatic acinar-cell specificity (Ornitz et al., 1985; Kruse et al., 1995). A similar sequence is present in other acinar cell-specific genes, such as *Amylase* and *Chymotrypsin*. Not all tissue-specific elements are located in the promoter region though.

Enhancers

Enhancers are DNA sequences defined by the following properties: *(1)* they increase transcription from a nearby gene; *(2)* they operate over considerable distances and are relatively unaffected by altering this distance; and *(3)* they remain effective even if inverted (Blackwood and Kadonaga, 1998). The first enhancers described were those of certain DNA viruses, such as SV40, which bears a 72 bp twice-repeated sequence meeting these criteria and is capable of increasing transcription from a large number of genes and in almost any tissue tested. Tissue-specific enhancers have also been described. Perhaps the best example of the latter is the immunoglobulin heavy chain enhancer (Staudt and Lenardo, 1991). It appears to activate transcription from the rearranged immunoglobulin gene whose V-region promoter is brought into proximity to the enhancer by a DNA-rearrangement process responsible for combinatorial diversity at the locus. This particular enhancer has been shown to function selectively in beta cells.

Errant activation of transcription by an enhancer may be associated with disease. For example, somatic chromosomal rearrangements can approximate a tissue-specific enhancer adjacent to a normally quiescent oncogene to predispose malignancy. A reciprocal translocation, t(14;18)(q32;q21), positioning the immunoglobulin heavy chain enhancer adjacent to the *BCL2* gene in beta cells spurs development of non-Hodgkin's lymphoma (Pegoraro et al., 1984). A wide variety of mutations altering enhancer function have also been tied to disease. Sequence polymorphisms within enhancer transcription factor binding sites may alter expression levels to yield a phenotype. One salient example is of a single base change of an SP1 binding site within the first intron of the *COLIA1* gene (encoding a major collagen protein of bone), associated with osteoporosis and fracture risk (Grant et al., 1996).

Imprinting and X-Chromosome Inactivation

Two mechanisms have been identified that superimpose an additional level of transcriptional regulation by modulating the interaction of *cis*-acting promoter and enhancer sequences with *trans*-acting transcription factors. These epigenetic modes of regulation are termed *genomic imprinting* and *X-chromosome inactivation*.

Genomic imprinting is the phenomenon of differential expression of individual alleles of a gene according to the parent of origin. During gametogenesis, one allele is durably marked for suppression of expression throughout the life span of the organism. CG-rich direct repeats in regions of allele-specific differential methylation are hypothesized to signal regional imprinting, though this may be through a signal of secondary structure rather than of primary sequence (Constancia et al., 1998; Tilghman, 1999). Functional hemizygosity might result in disease from a single mutational event at the active allele, whereas in the absence of imprinting, mutational events at each of the two alleles would be required to abrogate the function of the locus.

X-chromosome inactivation operates in females to equalize X-linked gene dosage between males and females. Each cell of the female inactivates one of its two copies, resulting in mosaicism of X-chromosome gene expression in female tissues. X-chromosome inactivation is apparently maintained by the untranslated RNA *Xist* (X-inactivation-specific transcript) encoded by the *Xic* (X-inactivation center) locus (Heard et al., 1997). The transcript is expressed only from the allele on the inactive chromosome; DNA methylation silences the other copy. The exact mechanism by which *Xist* maintains X-chromosome inactivation remains unknown. Some X-linked genes escape the inactivation process, however, resulting in two active copies. Pseudoautosomal genes on the X chromosome with homologs on the Y chromosome escape X inactivation to yield equal dosage in females and males.

Splicing

As noted previously, most eukaryotic genes have their coding regions interrupted by introns that must be removed by a process called *splicing* to generate a mature mRNA that may be translated into a functional protein. While the function of introns remains unclear, the mechanism of splicing is better understood (Padgett et al., 1986; Maniatis and Reed, 1987; Sharp, 1994). At the beginning and end of an intron, certain nucleotide sequences are found (Fig. 2–5). The intron almost always begins with a GT (the splice donor) and ends with an AG (the splice acceptor); other adjacent bases tend to follow a certain consensus sequence. However, the necessary consensus sequences are not entirely sufficient for recognition by the splicing apparatus. One can find consensus sequences in transcribed genes that are not utilized. Inactivation of the normal splice signal by mutation occasionally activates one of these "cryptic" splice signals (Collins and Weissman, 1984).

A single gene can also use multiple potential splice junctions to generate a variety of transcripts and proteins, providing unique functions and enabling complex gene regulation. About 35% of human genes are subject to alternative splicing compared to 22% of *Caenorhabditis elegans* genes. Genes of human chromosomes 19 and 22 each produce an average of about three distinct alternatively spliced transcripts (compared to 1.34 splice variants per gene in *C. elegans*) (International Human Genome Sequencing Consortium, 2001). Polymorphisms associated with alternative splicing can have relevance for common disease. One such polymorphism is present in an alternatively spliced exon of *PPAR-*γ, a nuclear hormone receptor family transcription factor involved in adipocyte differentiation. One allele is associated with lower body mass index and improved insulin sensitivity; the other allele is associated with predisposition to Type 2 diabetes (Deeb et al., 1998). As with promoter and enhancer mutations, sequence alterations at conserved splice junctions can impair gene function and result in disease. Specific mutations at splice sites have been identified for a variety of common diseases, such as thalassemia (*β-globin*), hypercholesterolemia (*LDL receptor*), and breast cancer (*BRCA1*).

Polyadenylation

Messenger RNAs that code for protein are characterized by the addition of a string of ~200 adenosine residues at their 3′ end, which is involved in mRNA stability, transport out of the nucleus, and translational efficiency. A hexanucleotide signal, AATAAA, in the 3′-untranslated region is a consistent feature of such mRNAs, though other sequences in the vicinity of this site may also play a role in correct polyadenylation (Colgan and Manley, 1997). The A residues are added at a point 18 to 20 nt downstream from the AATAAA signal. Transcript cleavage and poly-A addition occur in a coupled reaction catalyzed by a large complex of multisubunit proteins that are additional targets for regulation. Polyadenylation site mutation can abrogate gene function (e.g., in specific forms of both α- and β-thalassemia) but can also play a more subtle role in common disease. A variant allele at the polyadenylation signal of *N-acetyltransferase-1* correlates with increased activity of the enzyme in metabolizing carcinogens and has been associated with increased risk for colon, bladder, and lung cancers (Bell et al., 1995; Bouchardy et al., 1998).

Translation

The capped, spliced, and polyadenylated mRNA is translocated from the nucleus to the cytoplasm. There, it complexes with ribosomes that "scan" the mRNA from its 5′ end until encountering the first AUG codon, at which point translation begins (Pestova et al., 2001). As shown in Figure 2–6, translation involves the sequential addition of amino acids, carried by transfer RNAs (tRNAs), whose "anticodon" sequences base pair with successive triplet codons of the mRNA as the strand is read. This process continues, according to the codon usage chart shown in Table 2–1, until a stop codon (UGA, UAA, or UAG) is encountered to signal chain termination. Unique codon usage tables are used by the mitochondrial genome. For example, the UGA stop codon of the nuclear genome encodes tryptophan in the mitochondrial genome.

Many polypeptides undergo further enzymatic posttranslational processing (Moldave, 1985; Han and Martinage, 1992), often involving cleavage of an amino-terminal leader sequence, addition of carbohydrate residues, phosphorylation, ubiquitination, prenylation, etc. These modifications are important mechanisms for regulating cellular functions. Study of the complete set of human proteins (*proteomics*) is now greatly facilitated through completion of the genome sequence. This important area is beyond the scope of this chapter.

Table 2–1. Genetic Code, Wherein Each Triplet RNA of Bases Specifies a Particular Amino Acid

First Position 5′ End	Second Position U	C	A	G	Third Position 3′ End
U	Phe	Ser	Tyr	Cys	U
	Phe	Ser	Tyr	Cys	C
	Leu	Ser	STOP	STOP	A
	Leu	Ser	STOP	Trp	G
C	Leu	Pro	His	Arg	U
	Leu	Pro	His	Arg	C
	Leu	Pro	Gln	Arg	A
	Leu	Pro	Gln	Arg	G
A	Ile	Thr	Asn	Ser	U
	Ile	Thr	Asn	Ser	C
	Ile	Thr	Lys	Arg	A
	Met	Thr	Lys	Arg	G
G	Val	Ala	Asp	Gly	U
	Val	Ala	Asp	Gly	C
	Val	Ala	Glu	Gly	A
	Val	Ala	Glu	Gly	G

The code is said to be "degenerate" since there are 64 possible triplets and only 20 amino acids. Note that three of the codons, UGA, UAG, and UAA, code for the termination of translation stop.

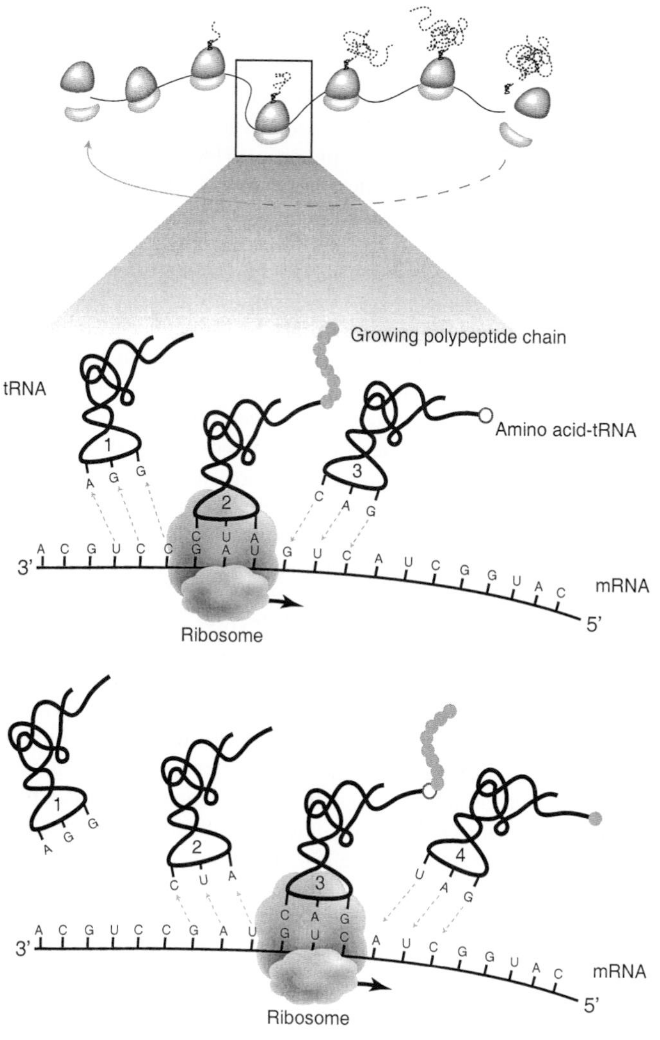

Fig. 2–6. The orderly process of protein translation, wherein a sequence of bases in mRNA is read by cytoplasmic ribosomes, using transfer RNAs (tRNAs) as the molecular adapters.

MUTATIONAL PATHOGENESIS

Mutations in any one of the transcriptional or translational elements of a gene may give rise to disease. They may diminish, augment, or change gene function altogether. An impressive example of the wide range of possible mutations is provided by the human *β-globin* gene (Olivieri, 1999). Over 200 mutant β chains have been described (Scriver et al., 2000). Mutant β-hemoglobin chains can result from mutations in the coding region that lead to an amino acid substitution; the most important of these is β^s (sickle β, where codon 6 is changed from GAG to GTG), causing sickle cell disease. In thalassemia disease there is a quantitative abnormality in α- or β-globin production. Over 60 mutations in the *β-globin* gene are known to diminish or abolish β-chain synthesis (Orkin and Kazazian, 1984; Kazazian, 1990). These include mutations in the promoter, the splicing signals, the coding regions (frameshifts or premature stops), and the polyadenylation signal. A rich pattern of genetic heterogeneity is found in other genetic diseases as well, though it may be particularly striking in the hemoglobinopathies because of positive selection pressures exerted by the malarial parasite (Weatherall and Clegg, 1981). Several online databases catalog gene mutations and genetic disease. Some of these are listed in Table 2–2. The vast and growing number of catalogued mutations makes such resources invaluable; e.g., there are more than 10,000 entries in the Online Mendelian Inheritance in Man database.

Like those in β-thalassemia, many mutations probably produce their phenotype by inactivating a gene and thereby reducing or eliminating its transcript, or by resulting in an altered pro-

Table 2–2. A Partial Listing of Important URLs for Major Sources of Information about Genetics and Genomics (Not Intended to Be Exhaustive)

General Links	
http://www.ncbi.nlm.nih.gov/	National Center for Biotechnology Information (NCBI)
http://www.nhgri.nih.gov/	National Human Genome Research Institute
Genome Maps	
http://cedar.genetics.soton.ac.uk/public_html/	Genetic Location Database
http://gdbwww.gdb.org/	Genome DataBase
http://www-genome.wi.mit.edu/	Whitehead Institute for Biomedical Research
http://www.genethon.fr/genethon_en.html	Genethon
http://cgap.nci.nih.gov/CHLC	Cooperative Human Linkage Center
http://www-shgc.stanford.edu/index.html	Stanford Human Genome Center
http://www.jax.org/	Jackson Laboratory
Sequence	
http://www.ncbi.nlm.nih.gov/genome/seq/	Human Genome Sequencing
http://www.sanger.ac.uk/	Sanger Centre
http://www.hgsc.bcm.tmc.edu/	Baylor College of Medicine
http://genome.wustl.edu/gsc/index.shtml	Washington University
Transcripts	
http://www.ncbi.nlm.nih.gov/genemap/	GeneMap
http://www.ncbi.nlm.nih.gov/UniGene/index.html	UniGene
http://www.ncbi.nlm.nih.gov/dbEST/index.html	dbEST: database of Expressed Sequence Tags
http://www.tigr.org/tigr_home/index.html	Institute for Genomic Research
Sequence Variants	
http://www3.ncbi.nlm.nih.gov/Omim/	Online Mendelian Inheritance in Man
http://www.ncbi.nlm.nih.gov/disease/	NCBI Genes and Disease Map
http://ariel.ucs.unimelb.edu.au:80/~cotton/mdi.htm	The Human Genome Organisation Mutation Database Initiative
http://www.uwcm.ac.uk/uwcm/mg/hgmd0.html	Human Gene Mutation Database, Cardif
http://www3.ncbi.nlm.nih.gov/SNP/index.html	dbSNP: single-nucleotide polymorphisms

tein product present in normal amounts but with reduced or absent function. The majority of recessive disorders are expected to fall into these categories, but other possible functional consequences of mutation exist. A mutation may result in a gene product that is not just lacking in function but actually damaging (a *dominant negative* mutation). An important example is that of the collagen genes (Prockop, 1984), mutations of which have been identified in the dominant condition osteogenesis imperfecta. Collagen is made up of a trimer of long helical protein subunits. If one or more of the three subunits is defective, the entire trimer is unstable and degraded. Thus, a defect in only one-half of the collagen chains results in degradation of seven-eighths of the associated trimers and is phenotypically worse than having one allele of the gene completely deleted. This observation illustrates one molecular mechanism for dominant genetic diseases.

It is also possible for mutation to increase the amount of a gene product or to affect tissue specificity or developmental timing. An example of the latter is a point mutation in the promoter of a human *Fetal hemoglobin* gene that results in persistent gross expression of fetal hemoglobin in adulthood (Collins et al., 1984; Karlsson and Nienhuis, 1985).

Finally, mutation may actually result in a new function. This process, which presumably is of great importance in evolution, can have dramatic consequences. A mutation in the α_1-*antitrypsin* gene, encoding an antiprotease, that generated a new anticoagulant factor similar to antithrombin III was observed: the patient suffered fatal bleeding diathesis (Owen et al., 1983).

Mechanism of Mutation

DNA mutation can occur at either the germline or somatic level to predispose to disease. In the latter case, expansion of the mutant cell population is ordinarily required for a phenotypic change and, thus, is seen primarily in malignancy. Mechanisms of genetic injury at both germline and somatic levels include *(1)* DNA replication error, *(2)* DNA repair error, *(3)* insertional mutagenesis, *(4)* chromosomal rearrangement, and *(5)* chromosome copy number error.

The error rate of DNA replication in *Escherichia coli* is about one error per 10^8 nucleotides incorporated, considerably lower than the rate of incorrect base insertion during polymerization, as a result of a proofreading activity associated with the polymerase. The polymerase can edit incorrectly added bases with 3′ to 5′ exonuclease activity. Rare, transient, tautomeric forms of bases (1 in 10^4) can base pair for incorporation but revert to the standard (and unpaired) base form after incorporation. Occasional unedited errors may still be corrected by a second mismatch repair system. As a result, the measured mutation rate can be as low as one mistake per 10^{11} nucleotides.

DNA-repair systems maintain surveillance for several additional mutational mechanisms as well (Fig. 2–7). The most frequent mutation in mammalian DNA involves the conversion of a C to a T in a CG dinucleotide. This occurs because methylation of cytosine is common and deamination of 5-methylcytosine results in the formation of thymine. Cytosine also suffers a low rate of deamination to form uracil, also ultimately converting a C-G to a T-A base pair in DNA replication if not repaired. Spontaneous deamination of adenine forms hypoxanthine, a base that can pair with cytosine in a subsequent round of replication to utimately alter an A-T to a G-C base pair. The change from one purine to another or one pyrimidine to another at a position is termed a *transition*; the interchange of a purine and pyrimidine is termed a *transversion*. In addition, slippage of DNA polymerase by looping out of the template strand or growing strand is believed to be a mechanism for deletion or insertion (respectively) of a single base pair. Other errors encountered for which specific repair mechanisms also exist include sugar-phosphate

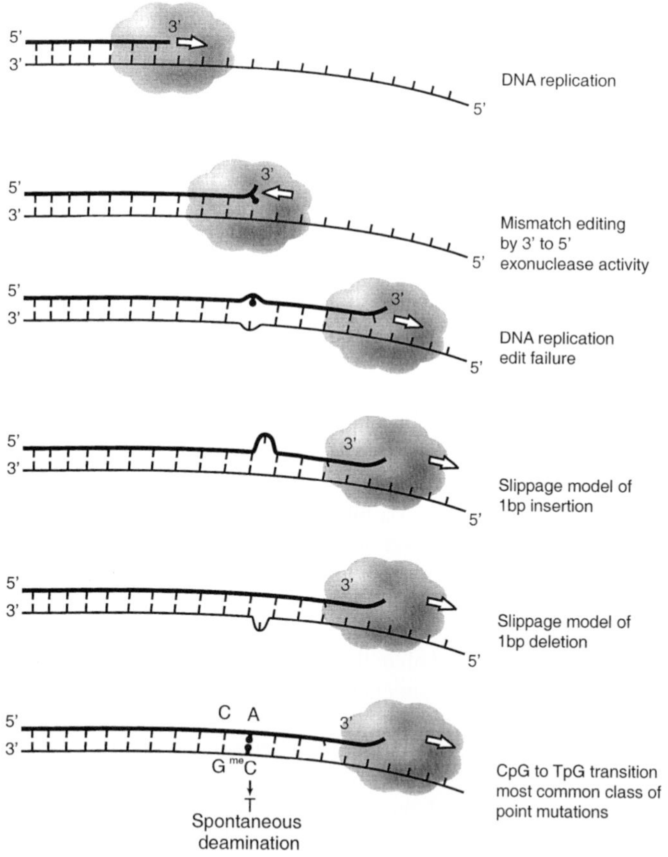

Fig. 2–7. Highly simplified diagram of the DNA-replication process, wherein DNA polymerase utilizes a template strand to synthesize double-stranded DNA using base pairing (Watson and Crick, 1953). Various types of replication error are indicated.

backbone breakage, pyrimidine dimer formation, base alkylation, and glycosidic bond breakage with base loss (leaving the sugar-phosphate backbone intact). Because information on one DNA strand is mirrored on the other, some repair pathways rely on the undamaged strand to guide replacement of the damaged one through a process termed *excision repair* (Krokan et al., 2000). Diploid cells may also utilize the second, unaltered copy of a region to repair double-stranded damage or missing duplex segments through recombination (*recombinational repair*).

The low rate of germline mutation escaping these repair mechanisms can give rise to polymorphisms in the population. (Strictly defined, a *polymorphism* is a sequence variant where the most common allele is found on fewer than 99% of chromosomes.) On average, any two individuals will differ at roughly one nucleotide every 1000 bp throughout the genome; these sites are termed single-nucleotide polymorphisms (SNPs). Some SNPs are detectable because they occur within sites recognized by specific bacterial restriction enzymes; these are termed *restriction fragment length polymorphisms* (RFLPs) since cleavage of genomic DNA by the enzyme can result in variable fragment sizes. Also scattered throughout the genome are tracts of simple sequence repeats (most commonly mono-, di-, tri-, and tetranucleotides) for which polymorphism in repeat length often develops by the slippage mechanism described above. Trinucleotide repeat expansions responsible for several diseases (such as Huntington's disease) have been identified; these are termed *triplet repeat diseases*. Polymorphisms can be associated with a phenotype if they occur in genes or regulatory regions, but most are silent. All polymorphisms may be used to distinguish genes and chromosomes in studies of inheritance and association of specific alleles with disease.

Mutations occurring within genes encoding DNA-repair enzymes predispose to the accumulation of somatic mutational events. These mutator genes include those responsible for ataxia-telangiectasia, hereditary nonpolyposis colon cancer, and Werner's syndrome of premature aging. A common phenotype is predisposition to malignancy, in some cases with sensitivity to DNA-damaging agents like ultraviolet or gamma irradiation (Lengauer et al., 1998).

Introduction of an ectopic DNA sequence into a gene can alter function by disrupting the coding sequence or expression, at either the germline or somatic level. Such mechanisms include transposition of repeat elements, viral integration, and gross chromosomal rearrangement (Fig. 2–8). With respect to repeat elements, insertion of a long interspersed repetitive element in

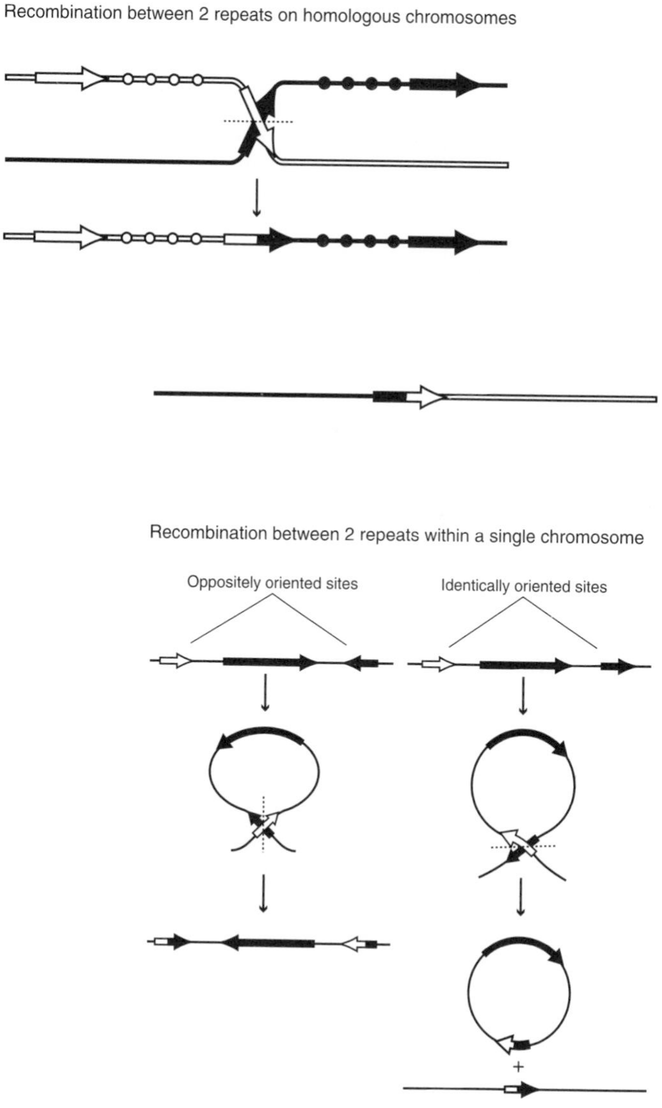

Fig. 2–8. Chromosomal rearrangements catalyzed by repeated sequences. Shown at the *top* is the consequence of unequal crossing over between two homologous chromosomes. One of the products has undergone a duplication, the other a deletion. In the *bottom panel*, the consequences of a rearrangement within a single chromosome are shown. When the sites are oriented in the same direction (as on the *right*), one of the products of the recombination event is an acentric circle, which is thus lost.

the *Factor VIII* gene has been noted as a heritable cause of hemophilia A (Kazazian et al., 1988). Moreover, illegitimate recombination at repeat elements can result in heritable deletions, such as an inter-Alu deletion at the *LDL receptor* gene resulting in familial hypercholesterolemia (Lehrman et al., 1986; Hobbs et al., 1986). Viral integration at the somatic level can introduce viral oncogenes or genes that inactivate cellular tumor suppressors, or it can activate nearby cellular oncogenes under the control of viral regulatory elements to disrupt the cell cycle. For example, integration of human papillomavirus types 16 and 18 is closely associated with development of cervical carcinoma (Park et al., 1995).

Some chromosomal rearrangements are present in germline DNA as a cause of heritable disease. For example, inversion of genomic sequence encoding the 5′ portion of the *Factor VIII* gene is the most common cause of hemophilia A; occurrence of a separate gene (the *A* gene) in two copies upstream of *Factor VIII* and one copy within an intron of *Factor VIII* facilitates the rearrangement (Fig. 2–8) (Antonarakis et al., 1995). Gross chromosomal rearrangements may be visible cytogenetically and guide identification of the genes responsible for disease. However, cytogenetics is rare as a mode for detecting genes predisposing to common diseases, with the notable exception of somatic changes in cancers.

Chromosomal copy number errors result in aberrant gene expression levels that cause disease, again at either the germline or somatic level. A mechanism for chromosomal loss or gain is diagrammed in Figure 2–9. Nondisjunction in meiosis I or II creates gametes with either absence of a chromosome or presence of an extra chromosome. Resultant trisomies, such as Down syndrome (trisomy 21), or nullisomies, such as Turner's syndrome (XO), are not rare causes of genetic disease by traditional standards but will not account for the heritable component of most common diseases. Mitotic nondisjunction is, however, a common somatic event, potentially leading to aneuploidy in malignancy. Growth advantage conferred by chromosomal rearrangements and aneuploidy results in relative expansion of a cell clone within a tumor and can provide a mechanism for evasion of therapeutic agents. Amplification or deletion of specific gene regions, rather than entire chromosomes, can also confer growth advantage within a tumor.

Selective loss of growth-controlling genes, often by gross deletion, may also predispose to transformation. The paradigm of "anti-oncogenes" or tumor-suppressor genes was developed for retinoblastoma and validated Knudson's (1971) two-hit hypothesis for tumor development (Fig. 2–10). The *Retinoblastoma* gene (*RB1*) product controls cell proliferation; loss of both copies is required for development of disease. Children inheriting a mutation in one copy (the first hit) require a single additional inactivating mutation in the second, wild-type copy (the second hit) to develop retinoblastoma. Their disease is of early onset and bilateral. In contrast, the sporadic form of the disease requires somatic mutation of both *RB1* genes in the same cell. Subsequent studies have revealed that the *RB1* pathway is inactivated in many additional sporadic cancer types as well. Figure 2–10 outlines potential mechanisms for the second somatic mutation. Inactivation of the wild-type copy of a tumor-suppressor gene by deletion creates loss of heterozygosity (LOH) at polymorphic markers in the deleted region. For the affected individual, only one allele at a polymorphic site is seen in the tumor compared to two alleles in normal tissues. LOH is more aptly termed *allelic imbalance*, however, because preferential amplification of

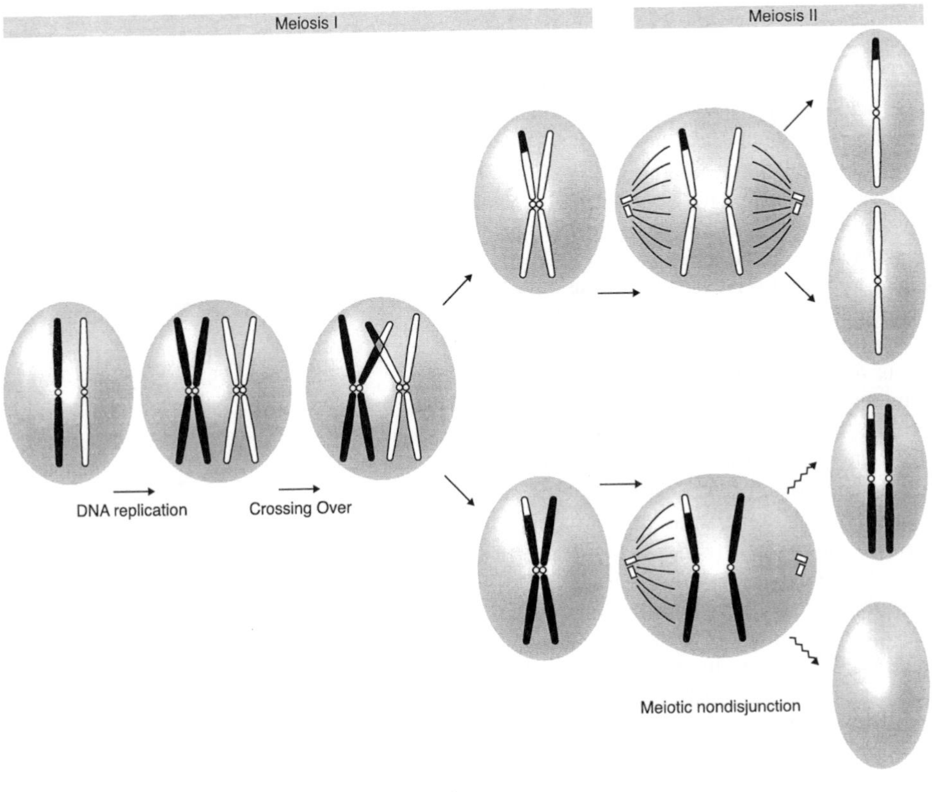

Fig. 2–9. Meiosis, crossing over, and an example of a nondisjunction in meiosis II.

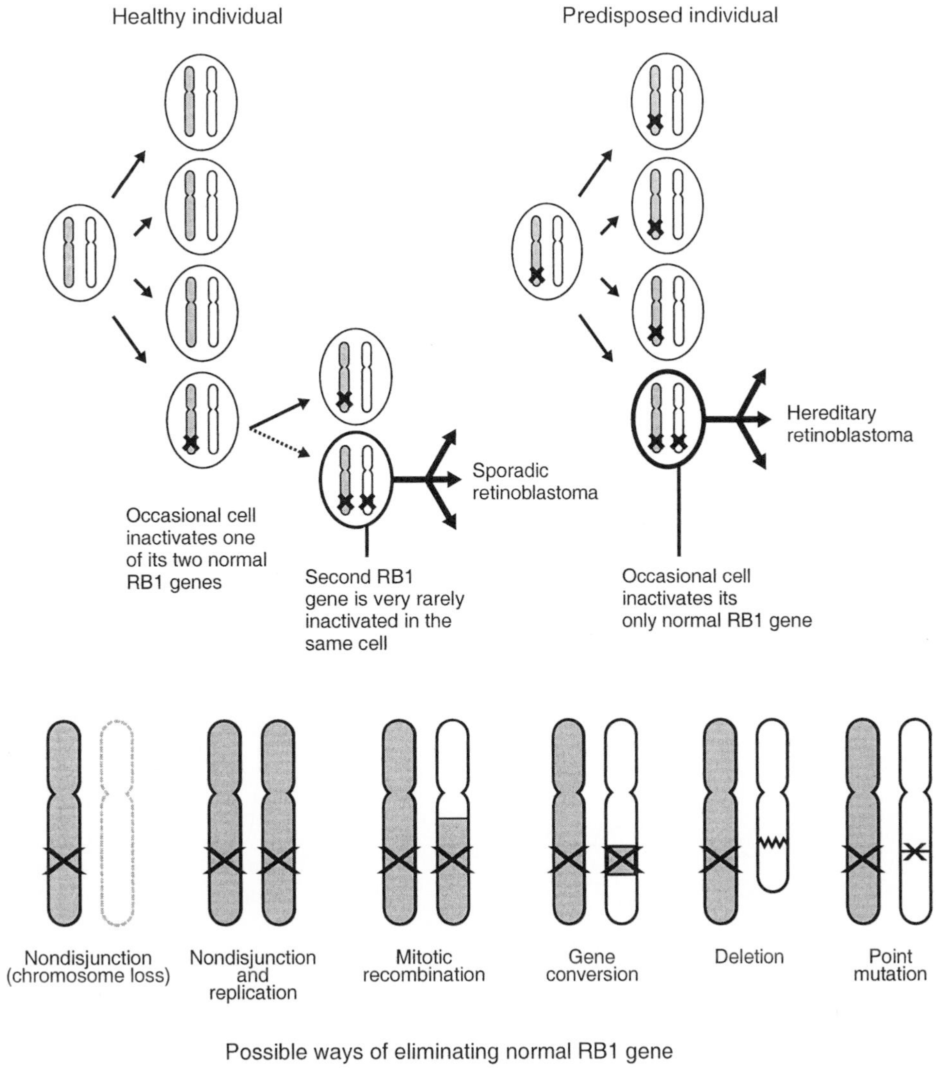

Fig. 2–10. The two-hit model of carcinogenesis, operative in retinoblastoma and a variety of other malignancies, in which tumor-suppressor genes are involved. At *top left* is shown the series of two "hits," or steps which must occur to result in loss of both copies of the *RB1* gene in an individual whose germline copies are normal. The consequence would be a sporadic retinoblastoma. At *top right* is shown the situation for an individual who has inherited one nonfunctional *RB1* gene. Loss of the second copy through only one additional somatic mutational event results in a retinoblastoma. *Lower panel* diagrams possible mechanisms that can result in inactivation of the wild-type *RB1* copy. All of these have been implicated in specific tumors.

one allele can appear similar to preferential loss of the other in typical assays (Fig. 2–11).

Classification of mutations by molecular mechanism does not always correspond clearly to disease phenotype. Traditional classification of Mendelian traits into recessive, dominant, codominant, or X-linked according to inheritance pattern is increasingly contrasted to molecular classification as disease genes are identified. Mutations causing loss of function can be recessive (cystic fibrosis), dominant (retinitis pigmentosa), or codominant (familial hypercholesterolemia). A subset of the loss-of-function mutations act in a dominant negative manner (*Collagen* and the oncogene *p53* are examples) and have a dominant phenotype. Most gain-of-function mutations are dominant (Huntington's disease). More complex patterns of disease–gene relationships may underlie many common diseases.

Genotype/Phenotype Correlation

A sequence variant may be functionally silent (a benign polymorphism), predispose to disease depending on additional environmental or genetic factors (a complex trait), or cause overt disease with a typical dominant, recessive, or X-linked pattern of inheritance (a simple Mendelian disease). In reality, even the most strongly Mendelian traits are modified by other genes and the environment, so the distinction between single-gene disorders and complex traits can be blurred. The probability of expressing a phenotype given a genotype is termed *penetrance*. Incomplete penetrance can be seen in Mendelian traits and is characteristic of complex traits.

The presence of both genetic and environmental components of disease predisposition may also confound understanding of disease etiology. Incomplete penetrance is a natural concomitant seen in complex traits; inheritance of a specific disease-predisposing allele may be neither necessary nor sufficient to cause disease. Modifier loci, which affect penetrance, severity, or associated phenotypic features, are also likely to complicate dissection of common diseases.

Molecular genetic techniques may be applied to both monogenic Mendelian disorders and the more common complex traits. Often, families with a monogenic trait are found among a much

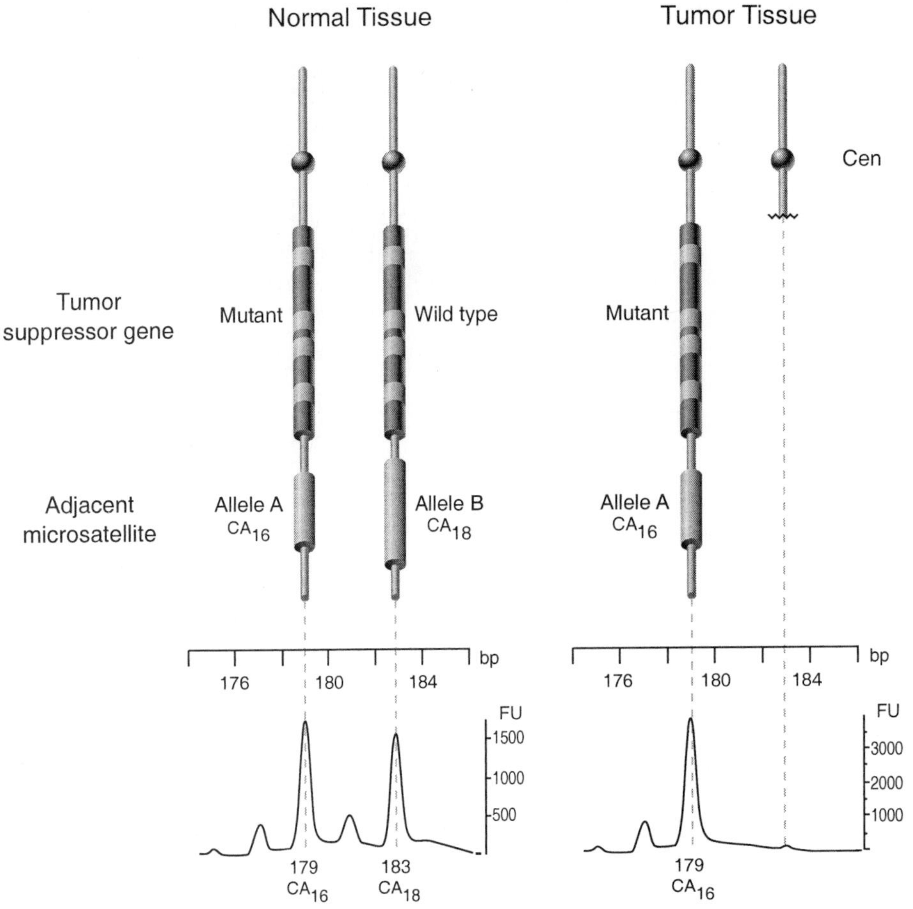

Fig. 2–11. Detection of the second hit for a tumor-suppressor gene, where the wild-type copy is lost by deletion. Also shown is a nearby microsatellite marker which is heterozygous in that individual's normal tissue. The genotype tracing below demonstrates major peaks at 179 and 183 bp. In the tumor tissue, however, the microsatellite locus has been deleted along with the nearby wild-type tumor-suppressor gene; thus, genotyping the tumor reveals only the 179 bp allele. This is the phenomenon of *loss of heterozygosity*.

larger group of individuals with a similar common, but not as strongly heritable, phenotype. The genes responsible for disease in the Mendelian families may also contribute more broadly to disease in the common cases; polygenic and environmental factors also likely play a role in common disease. Studies of those with a more severe phenotype and with familial disease may select cases more likely to have a monogenic form of the disease. Milder, less penetrant alleles of the same disease-predisposing genes identified for the simple Mendelian disorder may contribute to disease in the more common cases. In colon cancer, e.g., an array of mutated genes have been identified through the study of multiplex families. Among these genes is the *APC* tumor suppressor, which causes the highly penetrant autosomal dominant disorder familial adenomatous polyposis. A common variant (I1307K) of the *APC* gene, found in 6% of Ashkenazi Jews, doubles the risk of colon cancer, apparently because this sequence variant is susceptible to somatic mutation (Woodage et al., 1998).

DNA TECHNOLOGY

The revolution in molecular biology of recent years has been possible because of the development of a series of powerful laboratory techniques. Continued advances in automation and development of vast genomic database resources have brought the field to the forefront of medical science. These tools promise to uncover genetic predisposition to common disease and to enable tailored pharmacological therapy to suit individual patients according to their specific complement of alleles. Recombinant DNA technology has been of central importance in clinical genetics and promises to forever change the face of all of medicine. Broad understanding of the principles and terminology involved has become increasingly important to physicians.

Many of these techniques are directed at the need to detect very small changes, down to a single base pair, in the complex diploid human genome of 6.4 gigabases. Recombinant DNA allows the isolation and purification of relatively short, specific fragments of DNA from this highly complex mixture (referred to as *cloning*). The precise sequence of a cloned gene can be determined and its function studied in gene transfer systems. Furthermore, the cloned sequence can be used as a "probe" to identify similar sequences and to evaluate variability in the human genome.

Bacterial restriction enzymes can recognize and cleave specific DNA sequence sites. A cleaved fragment may be inserted into a *vector*, a DNA segment capable of autonomous replication, to prepare large quantities of the cloned fragment. The most

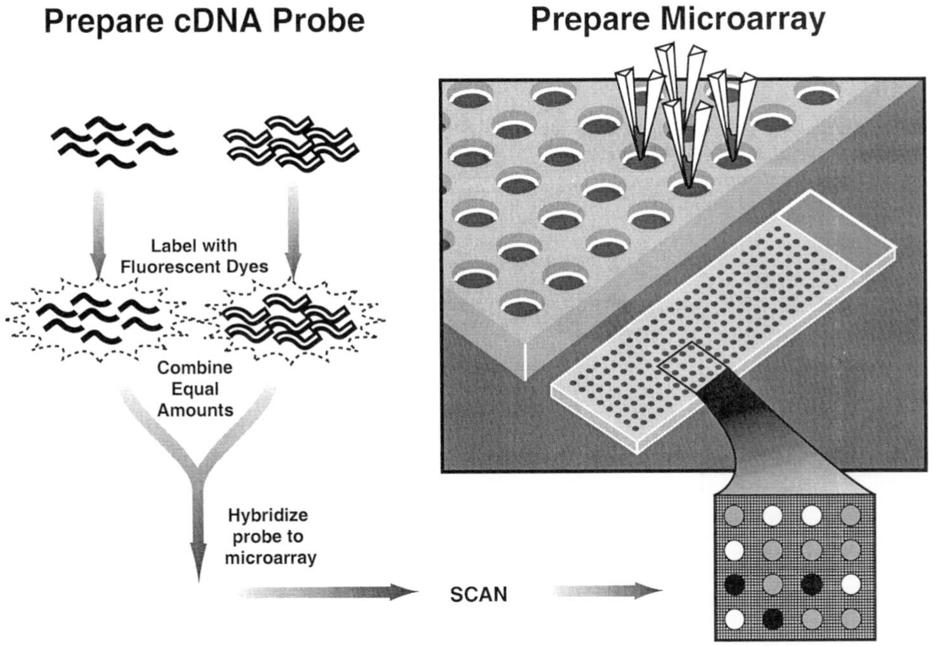

Fig. 2–12. Use of microarrays to assess gene expression. The high-density array is prepared by robotically spotting cloned DNA or polymerase chain reaction products from cDNAs of a large number of genes, each in a known address on the chip. Preparation of RNA from two different sources, labeling with two different fluorescent tags, and then hybridization to the chip allows assessment of the comparative abundance of mRNA expression from the two sources for each of the genes represented on the chip.

common vectors are *bacterial plasmids* (circular DNA molecules bearing antibiotic resistance genes) and *bacteriophages* (bacterial viruses). Replication of the vector containing the inserted fragment can allow milligram quantities of a given DNA fragment to be recovered. A transcribed sequence may also be cloned into a vector by starting with the mRNA transcript rather than genomic DNA. The single-stranded mRNA is first converted to double-stranded DNA using a retroviral enzyme called *reverse transcriptase*. The resulting cDNA may then be cloned into a vector. The collection of clones created from a genomic or RNA source is termed a *library*. Vast numbers of genomic sequences and expressed sequences have now been cloned and mapped to positions along each chromosome. The mapped genomic sequences are termed *sequence tagged sites* (STSs), and expressed sequences are termed *expressed sequence tags* (ESTs). Databases of the nucleotide sequence and map position for human STSs and ESTs have provided a framework for cloning and sequencing the entire human genome and for identifying its encoded genes. Increasingly, the map position of a gene of interest is being used as the primary mode for disease gene identification.

Detection of a specific desired sequence is facilitated by the unique ability of DNA to base pair, using selective hybridization of DNA strands. The selectivity derives from the ability of a single-stranded DNA to anneal to its complementary single strand while failing to anneal to unrelated sequences. A complex mixture of target clones may be separated (e.g., by plating bacterial colonies at low density, each containing a single clone of a library) and a replicate immobilized on a DNA-binding filter surface, followed by complementary target selection using a labeled probe. The identified clone may then be picked for further analysis. A related emerging technology employing microarrayed clones (Fig. 2–12) offers advantages in certain studies using selective hybridization (Duggan et al., 1999). The great density of clones that can be arrayed on a small surface translates into a powerfully parallel assay system. Thousands of cDNA clones from a specific tissue may be assayed concurrently for changes in mRNA levels in progression to malignancy. In addition, each clone has a specific "address" on an array, serving as an identifier in information databases of such things as clone sequence.

As an alternative to cloning, a complex DNA mixture (e.g., human genomic DNA prepared from blood) may be subjected to the polymerase chain reaction (PCR) to amplify a target sequence to high copy number for subsequent cloning or direct analysis (Fig. 2–13). It is first necessary to synthesize two short oligonucleotide primers based on known sequences. The two primers are synthetic single-stranded DNAs of about 17 to 35 nucleotides in length and are designed to bind complementary sequences on opposite strands of a denatured target DNA sequence, bracketing the region of interest. The DNA mixture is denatured to melt it into single-stranded DNA. The primers (in vast excess) are then annealed to the denatured target DNA at the two complementary sites. A DNA polymerase then extends the primers across the target sequence. The cycle is subsequently repeated to exponentially increase the number of copies of the target sequence. Thermostable DNA polymerases, such as *Taq*, withstand the high temperatures required for DNA denaturation to enable the process to continue without replenishment of polymerase. Thirty cycles of the PCR will amplify a single copy sequence about 1 billion-fold, adequate for assay by gel electrophoresis or other means. Practically, this allows investigation of genetic polymorphism (alleles), including gene mutations, without the need for cloning. Alleles can be detected in a matter of hours after receipt of a DNA sample.

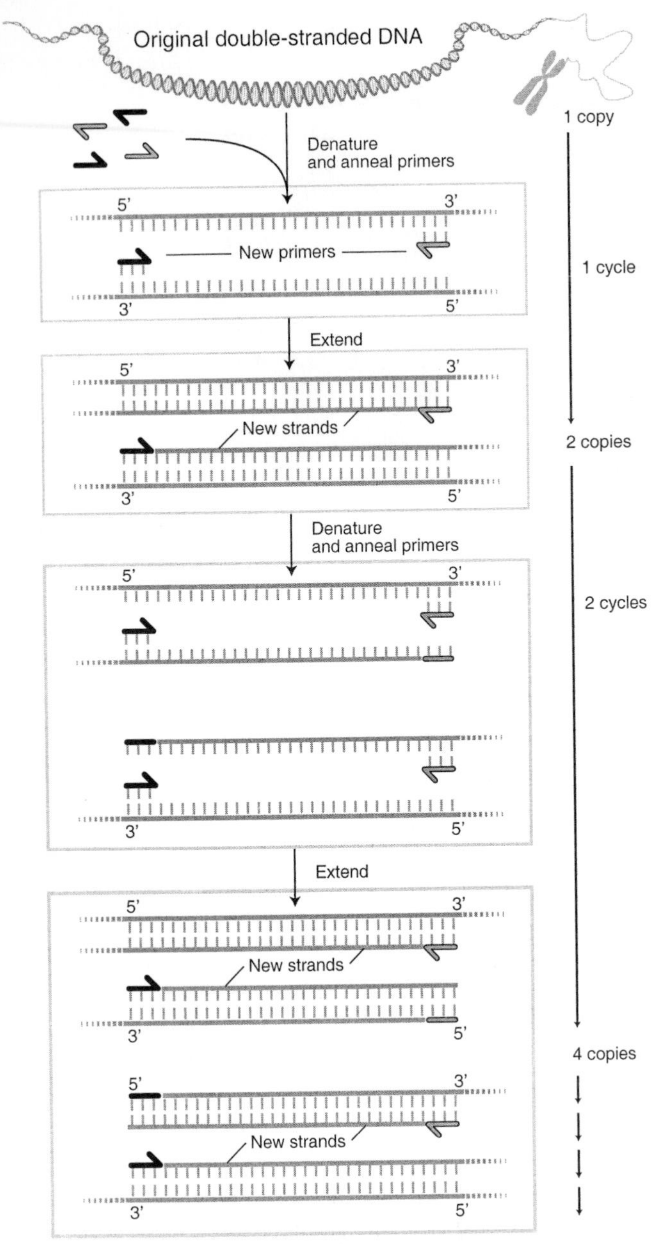

Fig. 2–13. Two polymerase chain reaction cycles are shown, but in practice one often proceeds for 25 to 30 cycles, resulting in roughly 1 billion-fold amplification of the DNA sequence that lies between the original primers. Note that the two primers delimit the region of amplification as cycles proceed.

TECHNIQUES TO STUDY COMMON DISEASE

The techniques described in this chapter and in Chapter 3 are suited to detailed characterization of specific mutations in single genes at the DNA level. While simple Mendelian disorders may be individually rare, they are not when considered in aggregate. Moreover, many common diseases have a genetic component; advances in genomics increasingly allow dissection of the complex genetics underlying these disorders. For some diseases, responsible genes have already been identified and the pathogenetic link between mutation and disease is understood (e.g., the *LDL receptor* and hypercholesterolemia). For many others, the availability of a complete human genome map, a draft sequence, and increasingly powerful techniques will facilitate chromosomal localization of the responsible genes. The complexities of underlying genetic factors in common disease (e.g., genetic heterogeneity, phenocopies, and incomplete penetrance) generally necessitate significantly increased study scale over that traditionally seen in the pursuit of simple Mendelian traits.

Genetic Mapping

Positional cloning is a strategy for identifying a disease-predisposing gene based on its location within the genome. This strategy can prevail even in the absence of knowledge about the underlying functional defect. The first gene identified by positional cloning was reported in 1986 (Monaco et al., 1986); the list of positionally cloned genes has grown dramatically since then as genomics tools have developed. Localization of a disease-predisposing gene to a chromosomal site allows screening of genes in this vicinity for identification of responsible mutations inherited by affected individuals. The original disease gene location is typically found by either of two methods: cytogenetic analysis or genetic mapping. The former method relies on identification of a cytologically recognizable chromosomal rearrangement. Methods for this include standard metaphase spreads with G-banding and hybridization to fluorescently labeled DNA probes to uniquely colorize individual chromosomes or chromosomal regions (chromosome painting, spectral karyotyping, fluorescent in situ hybridization). For tumor analysis, one can also use identification of regional LOH by PCR amplification of polymorphic markers or whole-genome copy number analysis by comparative genomic hybridization to evaluate relative amplification or loss of genomic sequences. The gene responsible for Peutz-Jeghers syndrome was narrowed to a specific chromosomal location with LOH and comparative genomic hybridization analysis of the tumors, which was then confirmed by pedigree linkage (Hemminki et al., 1997).

Genetic mapping is the more widely used method for delineating a genetic locus. Disease gene location is identified by statistically associating the inheritance of a particular region of the genome with the inheritance of disease in predisposed families (identification of *linkage*). The approach requires ascertainment of pedigrees or sibships segregating the disease and analysis of DNA to identify any shared genomic region(s) inherited by affecteds. Increasingly, this is done on a genome-wide basis; DNA of each individual is tested at regular intervals across each chromosome at polymorphic markers to distinguish the two copies of each chromosome within family members. This approach allows a region of sharing to be defined within which the disease-causing gene is located (Fig. 2–14). The closer a polymorphic marker is to the disease gene, the less likely a meiotic recombination event might occur to separate them and, consequently, the greater the statistical association between inheritance of the region's alleles and inheritance of disease. Figure 2–15 provides an example of the genome-wide survey done to localize genes predisposing to hereditary prostate cancer (Smith et al., 1996). Although genetic mapping is very labor-intensive and relies on statistical evidence, it is a powerful tool in genetic research. In contrast to genetic mapping for a simple Mendelian trait, mapping for a complex trait can require analysis of hundreds of pedigrees or sib pairs to build sufficient statistical power to identify a disease locus.

New mathematical methods of linkage analysis and increasingly dense genetic maps are being developed to accommodate the formidable difficulties posed by complex trait analysis. These are described in more detail in Chapter 3. *Association* studies

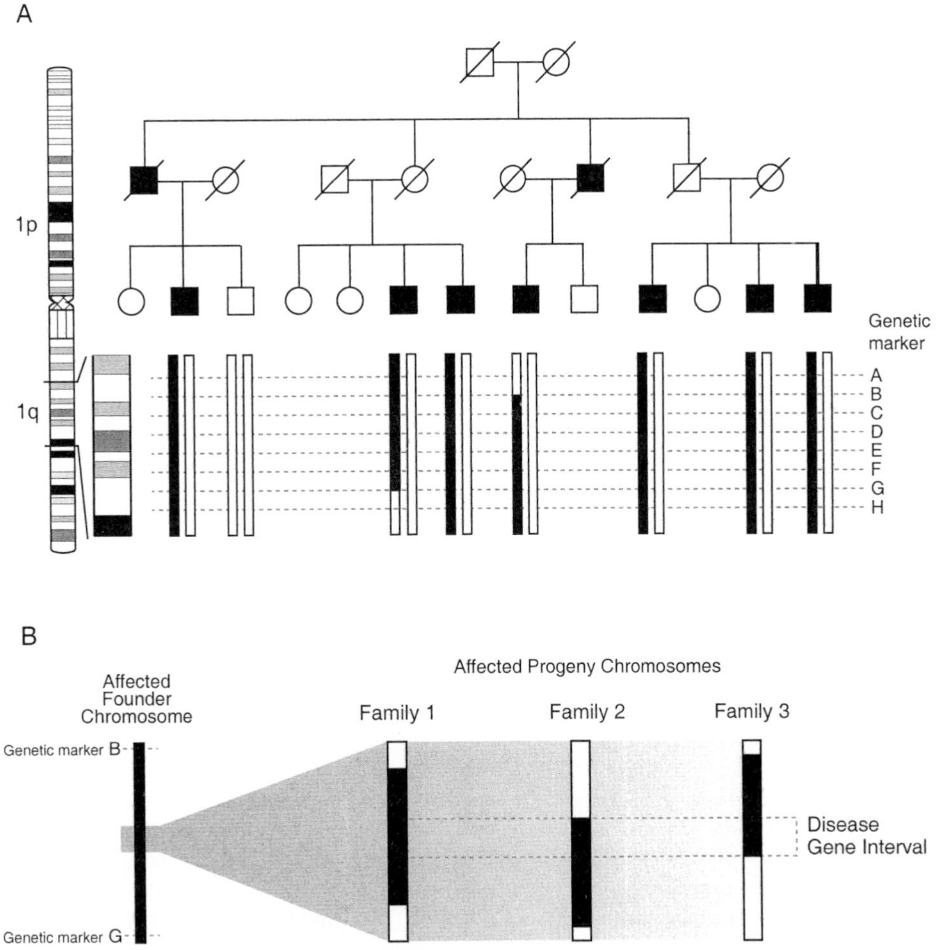

Fig. 2–14. Mapping of a disease locus by pedigree analysis. *A:* In this three-generation pedigree showing multiple males affected with prostate cancer, genetic markers A through H are used to track disease susceptibility. All of the affected males share a haplotype *(dark shading)* for markers B through G, which has presumably been inherited from a common founder in the first generation. Note the presence of a non-penetrant male in the second generation. *B:* If the disease allele is inherited from a common ancestor, then haplotypes may even be shared between different families. In this example, families 1, 2, and 3 represent different pedigrees with early-onset prostate cancer. By comparison of all three families, a small interval of haplotype identity can be perceived, which defines the boundaries of the disease-susceptibility gene.

can dramatically narrow a disease gene interval and are increasingly being used in the study of complex traits. Association studies do not require analysis of pedigrees but compare the prevalence of marker alleles in affected and unaffected individuals. A single disease-predisposing sequence variant introduced by a founding individual may be shared by present-day affected descendants. Ideally, one would like to score the causative variant directly as that confers the greatest statistical power. However, it is not necessary to score the functional variant directly as close neighboring polymorphisms that also mark the disease gene region will have been co-inherited. Specific alleles noted in the shared region will be statistically associated with inheritance of disease. The region's markers are said to be in *linkage disequilibrium* with the disease gene. These affected individuals will be distantly related to the founder and share a small DNA fragment: the greater the number of generations from the founder, the smaller the region of sharing (Fig. 2–14B). In a genome-wide association analysis, a potentially very high density of polymorphic markers might be required to detect an ancient shared segment. Typical simple sequence repeat polymorphic markers undergo a low rate of mutation that could obscure identification of very ancient shared alleles. SNP markers have a lower mutation rate and are present at higher density. Recent work has led to the identification and deposit in public databases of over 2 million SNPs (International SNP Map Working Group, 2001). Systematic surveys of more than 12 loci in the human genome suggest that linkage disequilibrium between adjacent SNPs operates over average distances of about 60 kb in northern European populations and somewhat less in African populations (Reich et al., 2001). Thus, sampling of a few hundred thousand well-chosen SNPs in a case-control association study may detect regions contributing to disease risk. SNPs are not individually as informative as repeat markers but may be amenable to high-throughput analysis to enable this emerging mode of gene discovery. SNP chips (Fodor et al., 1991), single-nucleotide primer extension (minisequencing) (Syvanen et al., 1990; Pastinen et al., 1997; Chen et al., 1999), matrix-assisted laser desorption ionization time-of-flight (MALDI-TOF) mass spectrometry (Ross et al., 1998), and the fluorogenic 5′ nuclease assay (Livak et al., 1995) show promise as new assays in SNP allelic detection.

Physical Mapping

An ordered map of genetic markers at the disease locus forms the basis for identification of a set of overlapping contiguous genomic clones, a *contig* or *physical map*, collectively representa-

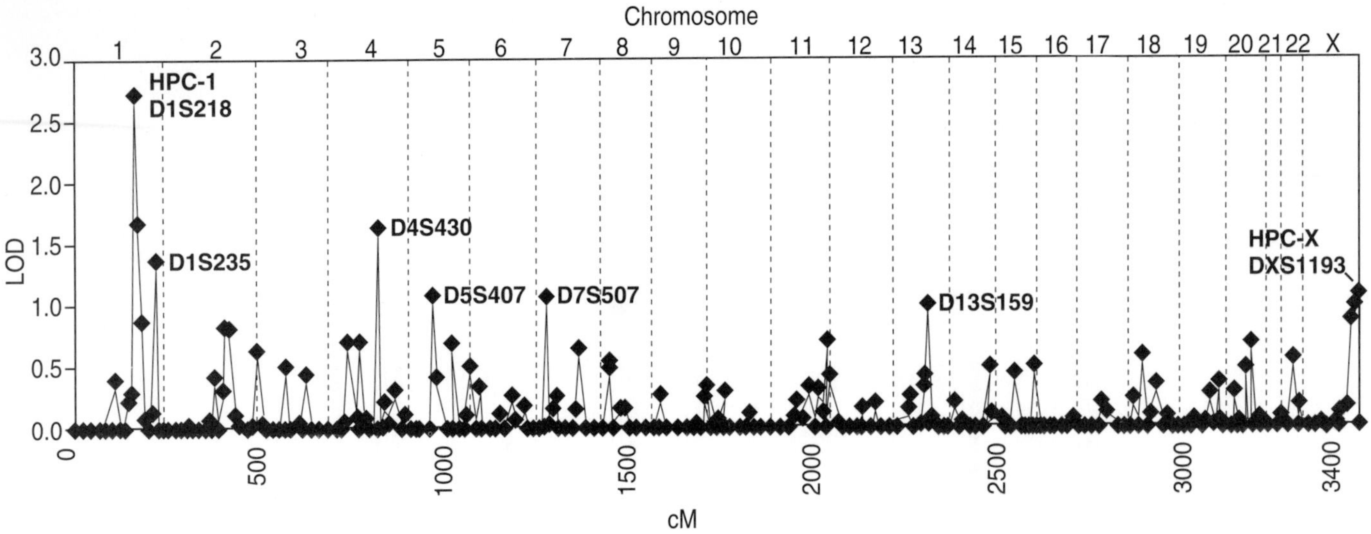

Fig. 2–15. Results of a genome-wide scan for prostate cancer susceptibility (Smith et al., 1996). Markers spaced on average 10 cM apart were tested against 66 families collected in the United States. Maximum single-point LOD scores for each marker are shown, beginning with chromosome 1 on the *left* and progressing all the way across the autosomes to the X chromosome. The strongest result, located on chromosome 1, was substantially refined with finer mapping and additional families to yield a LOD score >5 and has been denoted *HPC-1*. Other interesting LOD scores are apparent; the locus on the X chromosome has been confirmed by studying additional families.

tive of the region. Figure 2–16 illustrates the correlation of genetic and physical maps as a resource for positional cloning of disease genes. The Human Genome Project has constructed physical and genetic maps of the entire genome with an accompanying working draft sequence, about half of which is now in finished form. Public databases with maps of polymorphic genetic markers, STSs, ESTs, contigs, and draft and finished genomic sequences provide a framework for disease gene identification

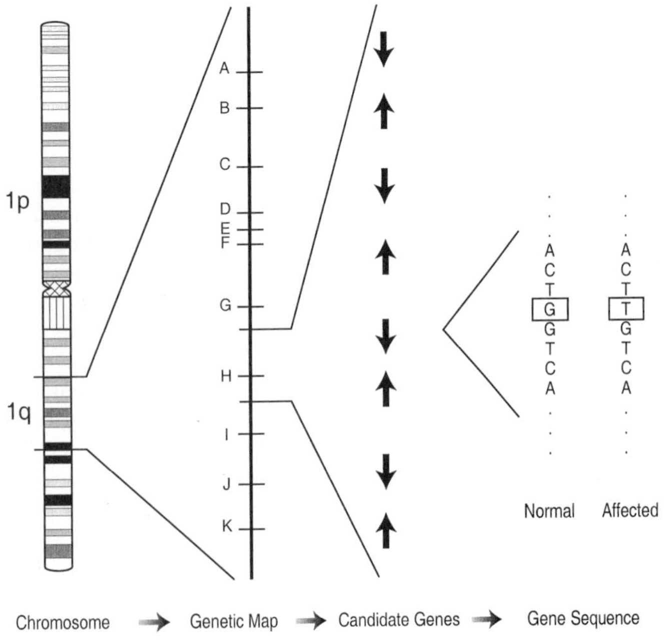

Fig. 2–16. Diagram of the steps involved in positional cloning, wherein one moves from mapping of the responsible locus using pedigree linkage methods to a physical map of the DNA in the interval to identification of candidate genes to analysis of their sequence, looking for differences between affecteds and unaffecteds.

once the locus is known. In addition, use of arrayed formats for samples is now employed to aid high-throughput screening and to enable resources to be shared between research groups. Pooling schemes allow arrayed libraries to be screened for a given sequence without individually assaying each address. For example, 10 96-well trays might require only 30 PCRs (rather than 960) to locate the well address of a clone: a positive reaction for a plate pool (10 reactions), column pool (12 reactions), and row pool (8 reactions). A specific clone can be associated with a unique address that serves as a reference for accessing it without the need for individual researchers to redundantly screen libraries. Increasingly, these public resources can be brought to bear for disease gene identification by positional cloning.

Candidate Gene Identification

Genes within the physical map of the region are candidates to be screened for a prediposing mutation. Genes may be found by several methods: *(1)* ESTs or full-length cDNAs may be mapped to the region, derived from expressed genes; *(2)* the completed sequence of genomic clones may be evaluated using gene-predicting software; and *(3)* molecular genetic techniques such as exon trapping can be applied to identify exons within genomic fragments. Genes of known or predicted function with biological relevance to the disease under study and those with appropriate tissue-specific expression are generally screened for causal mutations first.

The first two methods of transcript identification mine current public database resources. ESTs that map to clones within the contig may contain an overlapping sequence, often allowing a partial "virtual" transcript to be assembled. Increasingly, existing fully assembled sequences for genomic clones within the contig of interest may be found in public databases. These assembled sequences may already have been annotated for encoded genes. Sequences may also be generated in "sample sequencing" strategies designed to generate enough sequence to identify open

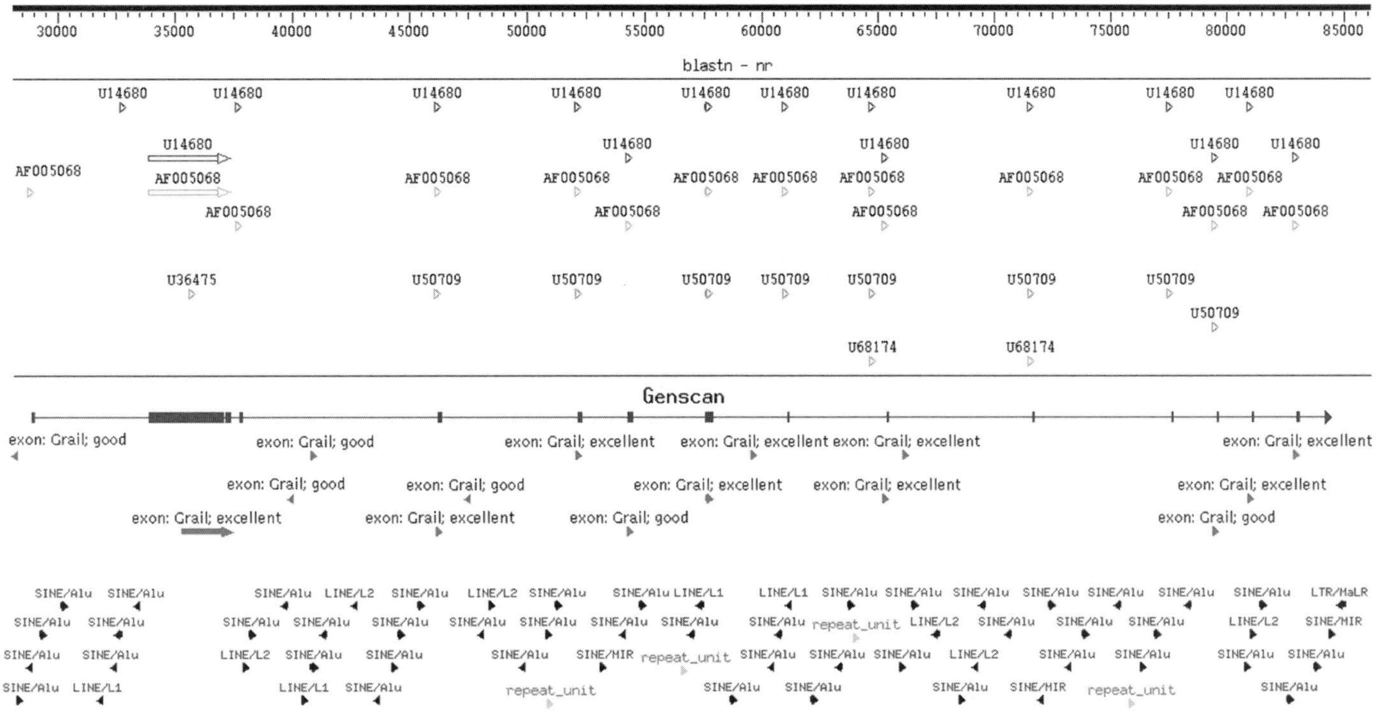

Fig. 2–17. Computational analysis of a 57 kb region of chromosome 17, which contains 12 exons of the *BRCA1* gene, including the unusually large exon 11 (located at 34000 to 38000 on the map.) The BLAST results *(top half)* show a large number of matches to ESTs, some of them (e.g., U14680) containing many exons. The purely computational Genscan *(continuous horizontal line at middle)* and Grail (individual exons just below, categorized as *good* or *excellent*) do a reasonably good job of finding the exons, but there are some false-positives and false-negatives. At *bottom*, the location of repetitive sequences is annotated.

reading frames but not to create an error-free finished sequence. Unannotated sequences may also be evaluated using software algorithms designed to identify homologies with known sequences and proteins and to predict promoters, transcription-start sites, exons, and poly-A sites. Figure 2–17 illustrates the output of several software tools available for evaluation of genomic sequences; in this example, the genomic clone contains part of the *BRCA1* coding sequence. Blast programs have identified numerous matches between the query genomic sequence and database EST sequences. The Grail and Genscan gene-predicting programs have identified numerous possible exons. Many repeat sequences are also noted. General agreement between these predictions correctly identifies most of the exons of the *BRCA1* gene within the genomic sequence, though not without some discrepancies.

Transcript identification can also be accomplished through molecular techniques such as exon trapping and direct selection. Exon trapping was first described in 1991 for selecting exons from cloned genomic fragments by virtue of functional 5′ and 3′ flanking splice sites (Fig. 2–18) (Buckler et al., 1991). A genomic library is created from a bacterial artificial chromosome clone within the contig, employing a vector that drives expression of an intron containing the cloning site and flanked by two vector-derived exons. If an insert of a genomic sequence at the cloning site contains an exon, functional 5′ and 3′ splice sites will allow it to be joined to the flanking exons during RNA processing in a cell. Introduction of the library into a cell line in which this processing occurs is followed by *(1)* RNA isolation, *(2)* cDNA synthesis, *(3)* PCR amplification of the spliced exon employing primer sites within the flanking vector-derived exons, and *(4)* subcloning of amplimers containing trapped exons for sequencing. The method will detect roughly 80% of internal exons within the clone (it will miss the first and the last), similar to the success rate for sequence-based software predictions. The second molecular technique, direct selection, is based on hybridization of cDNA fragments to immobilized DNA, followed by recovery of the selected cDNAs using PCR. The procedure permits cloning of cDNA fragments encoded by yeast and bacterial artificial chromosomes and can enrich cDNAs encoded in chromosome segments.

Often, these techniques for transcript identification yield only partial cloned or predicted sequences. After an exon or suspected transcript has been identified, transcript extension may be accomplished via PCR-based molecular techniques such as rapid amplification of cDNA ends (RACE) (Frohman et al., 1988) and interexon amplification, as well as via traditional cDNA cloning.

Among the candidate genes for a disease locus identified using these techniques, one is anticipated to have mutations or variants predisposing to the disease. Genes residing at the locus can sometimes be prioritized for mutation detection according to information that can be gleaned about each disease gene candidate. Homology between the candidate and known genes or between their predicted protein products can afford some insight about function. Quantitation of candidate gene expression levels in tissues and in patterns relevant to the disease process may also enable stratification of candidates.

Candidate genes suspected of predisposing to a disease may be identified through the positional cloning process but may also arise independently on consideration of disease-related molecular pathways. In contrast to the positional approach, the second approach (which has a much longer history) tests hypotheses of biological function through correlation of a candidate molecule variant with presence of disease and confirmation that the corresponding mutation plausibly alters function.

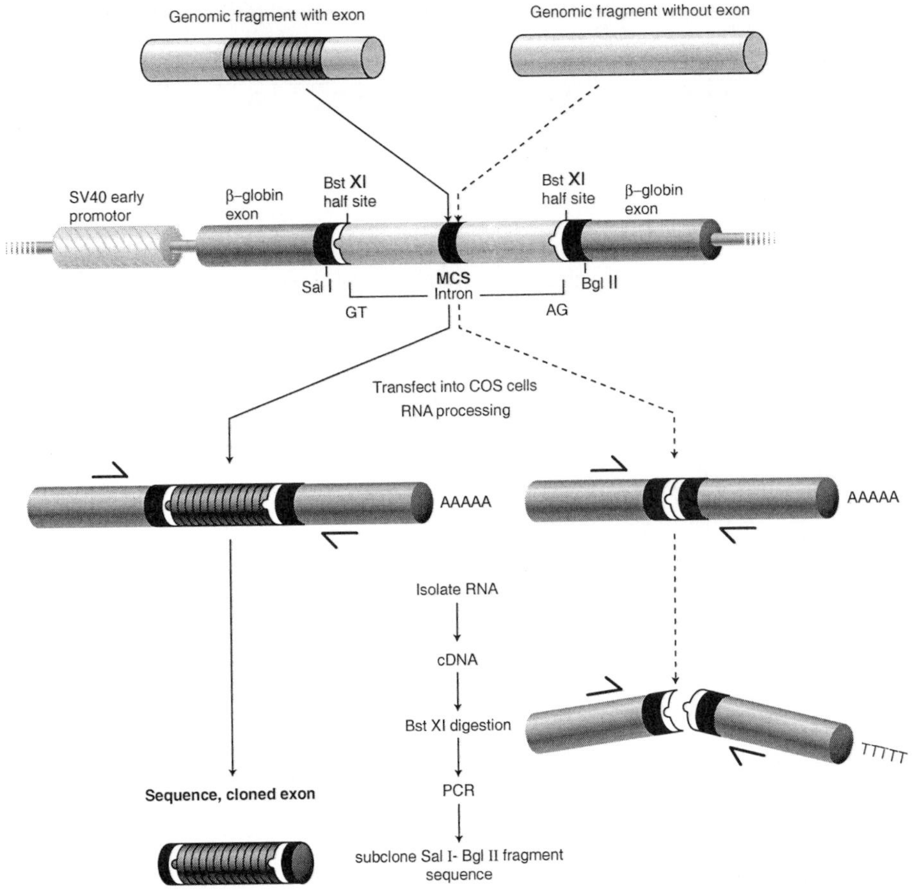

Fig. 2–18. The exon-trapping method of identifying the presence of exonic sequences within a genomic fragment. Cloned human genomic DNA (from a BAC or a cosmid) is digested with a restriction enzyme and then ligated into the multiple cloning site *(MCS)* of the exon-trapping vector, shown on the *second line* of the diagram. The vector provides a β-globin exon and a splice donor upstream of the MCS as well as a splice acceptor and an additional β-globin exon downstream. The vector is constructed so that BstXI half-sites are located at the splice donor and acceptor. If the genomic fragment cloned into this vector does not provide both a splice acceptor and a splice donor, then after transfection of the vector into COS cells and preparation of cDNA, the resulting construct will recreate the BstXI site. This can be readily digested prior to polymerase chain reaction *(PCR),* resulting in no product. If, however, the genomic fragment contains an exon, transfection into COS cells and RNA processing will result in splicing of that exon in between the β-globin flanking exons. In this case, BstXI will no longer digest the cDNA and, hence, the fragment can be amplified with the primers *(arrows),* resulting in rescue of the exon sequence. This method only traps exons that are flanked by introns on either side, so the first and last exons of a eukaryotic gene will not be recovered.

Candidate gene mutations or variants can be assayed by either molecular genetic techniques or biochemical or immunological assays. An example of the latter would be the early discovery of diminished LDL receptor quantity on monocytes of familial hypercholesterolemic patients (Bilheimer et al., 1978). Increasingly though, molecular genetic techniques have been applied for their ease and universality. A complete collection of full-length human cDNA clones would be of great advantage in this process of defining the anatomy of a candidate transcript. The Mammalian Gene Collection Project (Strausberg et al., 1999) aims to provide such a resource, both as sequence data and as actual clones. As of this writing (August 2001), 6190 full-length clones have been obtained and sequenced to high accuracy. That number should rise to 20,000 by mid-2002.

Mutation or Variant Detection

The techniques applicable for evaluation of candidate genes may be broadly grouped as *(1)* tests to identify novel sequence variants and *(2)* tests to genotype known sequence variants. In the former group, tests for gross genomic rearrangements at a candidate gene may be done through Southern blots (Southern, 1975). A Southern blot assays the sizes of genomic DNA restriction digest fragments containing the candidate gene. The digest is electrophoresed for size fractionation, then transferred to a membrane filter that can be hybridized with a labeled probe containing a portion of the candidate gene. A vast excess of unlabeled repetitive DNA is added to the hybridization to ensure that repeat elements present in the probe and target do not obscure the signal from unique sequences of the candidate gene. An altered banding pattern could result from any mutation changing the position of restriction sites, such as a deletion or an insertion. A Northern blot assays the size and quantity of an mRNA transcript from a candidate gene (Alwine et al., 1977). RNA prepared from a tissue in which the candidate gene is expressed is electrophoresed, then transferred to a filter for hybridization to a probe containing the gene sequence. Altered transcript size or quantity could reflect a culpable mutation. The RNA may also be analyzed by the protein truncation test (PTT) (Roest et al., 1993). This assay evaluates for premature translation termination in an in vitro translation system. A mutation resulting in a frameshift will typically create a premature termination codon that is readily detectable by this method. Over 80% of mutations

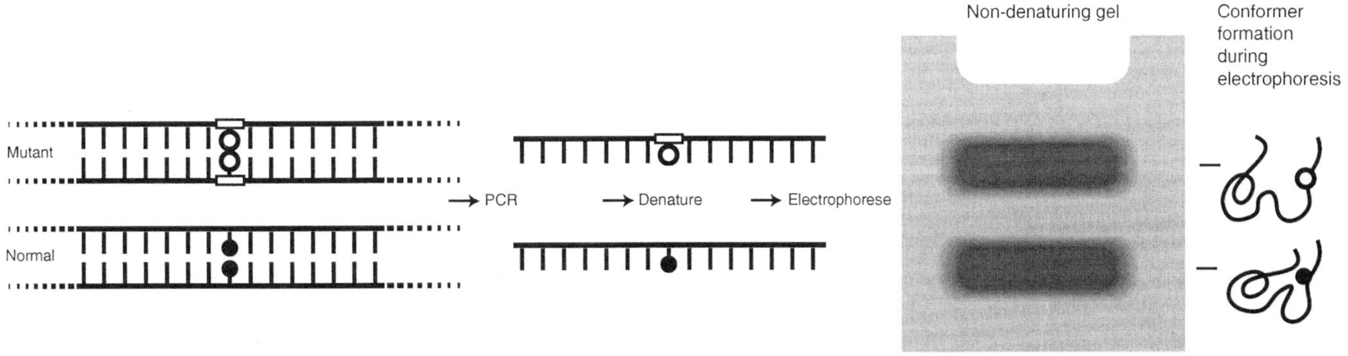

Fig. 2–19. The single-strand conformational polymorphism method of detecting a variant in a segment of genomic DNA. Polymerase chain reaction *(PCR)* primers are utilized to amplify a segment of DNA, commonly no greater than 200 to 300 bp in length. The PCR product is denatured and then electrophoresed on a nondenaturing gel. This allows secondary structure to form within the single-stranded DNA molecules. This secondary structure affects migration in an electrophoretic gel and is very sensitive to subtle changes in the DNA sequence, which affect the folding pattern. Hence, the presence of a variant frequently alters electrophoretic mobility. If such a shift is seen, it is possible to excise the aberrant band from the gel, reamplify it using the same PCR primers, and subject it to direct sequencing to determine the nature of the sequence variation.

catalogued for genes such as *APC* or *BRCA1* are detectable by PTT.

For most common diseases, however, one does not expect to find gross genomic rearrangements or loss-of-function mutations. To screen the sequence of a candidate gene for more subtle variations at the level of single-nucleotide changes, several methods can be applied. Dideoxy chain termination sequencing (Sanger et al., 1977) or pyrosequencing (Ronaghi, 2001) can be used to screen candidate genes for variation. Heterozygous affecteds can be detected, though this is potentially problematic. The large scale of the candidate gene screening effort in positional cloning projects with poorly refined disease gene intervals (often the case in complex traits) requires high-throughput sequencing facilities. Surrogate methods for detection of a single-nucleotide change in a candidate gene among affecteds are therefore often preferred. These methods include single-strand conformational polymorphism (SSCP), denaturing gradient gel electrophoresis (DGGE), and denaturing high-performance liquid chromatography (DHPLC). In SSCP, each exon of a candidate gene is assayed by PCR amplification, denaturation, and electrophoresis on a nondenaturing gel (Fig. 2–19). The single DNA strands assume conformations (*conformers*) of internal base pairing and homo- and heteroduplex formation that migrate through the gel with characteristic mobilities (Orita et al., 1989). In DGGE, the amplimers are not first denatured but electrophoresed through a gel containing a gradient of urea; variant duplex amplimers will denature more or less readily than the wild type and migrate differently (Fischer and Lerman, 1983).

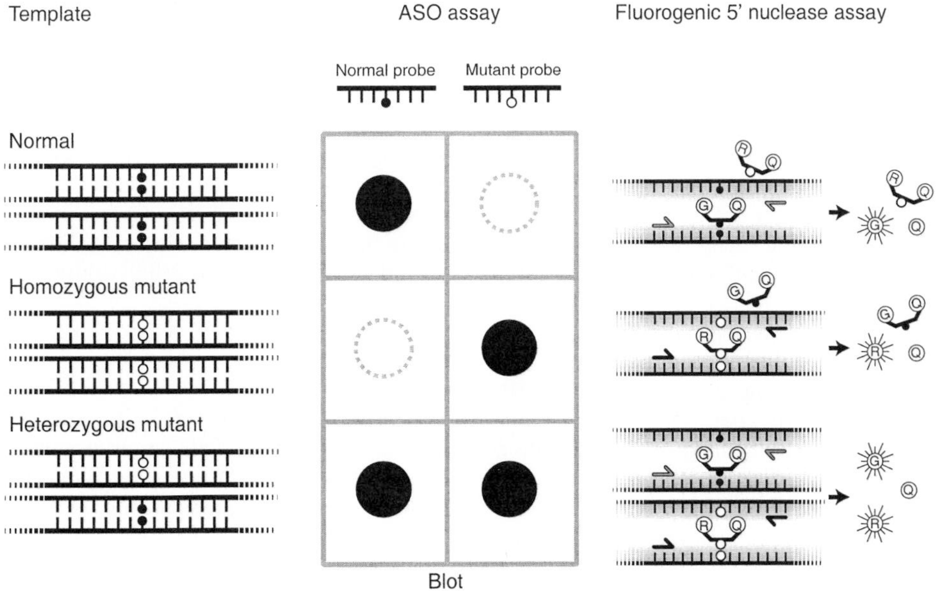

Fig. 2–20. Two methods to detect sequence variation in the heterozygous or homozygous state. In the *middle panel*, the allele-specific oligonucleotide *(ASO)* assay is shown. In this analysis, the polymerase chain reaction product from a DNA sample is spotted onto a filter and then probed with a radioactively labeled oligonucleotide (15–25 nucleotides) probe, which is specific for either the wild-type or the mutant sequence. Careful hybridization allows a perfect match of probe and target to remain annealed, whereas a mismatch is washed off. This allows distinction of heterozygous and homozygous genotypes. On the *right*, the fluorogenic 5′ nuclease assay (TaqMan®) is shown. This liquid-phase assay depends on the use of primers that contain both a fluorogenic tag (*G*, green; *R*, red) and a quencher *(Q)*. If the probe matches the target precisely, DNA polymerase will digest the probe as it marches through the region, releasing the fluorogenic marker and giving rise to a signal.

DHPLC separates homo- and heteroduplexes to identify variants (Oefner and Underhill, 1995). Polymorphisms noted as variants correlating with affected status by any of these methods are evaluated by subsequent sequencing.

In some cases, candidate genes with known mutations or polymorphisms are analyzed for associations with a new study population or disease. The methods outlined above can be used for this purpose, but a number of additional powerful techniques may also be applied. Single-nucleotide changes can be assayed by techniques relying on the discriminating power conferred by hybridization specificity or by incorporation of a chain-terminating dideoxynucleotide by DNA polymerase at a variant base position. Mutations associated with restriction sites may also enable use of an RFLP assay, but a more universal technique involves allele-specific oligonucleotide hybridization. Hybridization conditions may be tailored so that one labeled oligomer (probe) hybridizes selectively to the wild-type sequence and a second hybridizes selectively to the variant sequence. A PCR amplimer of the target gene region is immobilized by blotting onto a filter for subsequent hybridization to the labeled probes [a *dot blot* or *allele-specific oligohybridization* (ASO) assay]. Alternatively, a specially modified probe may be included in the initial PCR to enable direct detection during amplification without the need for blotting. The included probe is modified with both a fluorescent label and a quenching second dye; the fluorophore emits only after the probe hybridizes in the region between PCR primers and is degraded by the 5′ exonuclease activity of *Taq* to separate fluorescent and quenching dyes. Figure 2–20 illustrates both the ASO and fluorogenic 5′ nuclease assays (Livak et al., 1995).

Yet another common alternative is the single-nucleotide primer extension assay. Hybridization of an oligo primer immediately adjacent to the potential variant site is followed by primer extension employing a dideoxynucleotide triphosphate (ddNTP) anticipated to base pair with the variant. The identity of the terminating nucleotide may be distinguished through use of fluorescently labeled ddNTPs (a separate color for each), with detection by electrophoresis on an automated sequencer, or by fluorescence or fluorescence polarization on a microplate reader (Chen et al., 1999). Unlabeled terminating ddNTPs may also be used for detection with MALDI-TOF mass spectrometry (Ross et al., 1998). In the latter, the extended primer is pulsed from a surface by a laser, freeing it to accelerate in an electric field toward a detector. The time required for the product to reach the detector is determined by its charge-to-mass ratio and describes fragment molecular weight (and terminating nucleotide identity) extremely accurately.

A final technique for detecting sequence variation within candidate genes of known sequence is the gene chip, or SNP chip (Fodor et al., 1991). The assay has the potential to massively parallel assay large numbers of individual SNPs among thousands of candidate disease genes for a linkage or association study or to assay a single candidate disease gene at all positions in its sequence for an affected or at-risk individual. In Figure 2–21, the *BRCA1* gene is assayed for mutation on a gene chip (Hacia et al., 1996). Photolithographic techniques are used to synthesize unique oligonucleotides of defined sequence onto the chip surface. Each oligonucleotide is representative of a short region of the gene, the middle base of which is the site to be queried. Collectively, the oligonucleotides span the length of both strands of the gene. Potential sequence variants at each nucleotide position can also be represented. This essentially allows resequencing of the gene for individual patients. The technique can also be used for genome-wide linkage if a sufficient density of SNPs is tiled on the chip (Wang et al., 1998) and may in the future be useful for screening predefined polymorphisms within candidate genes for association with disease.

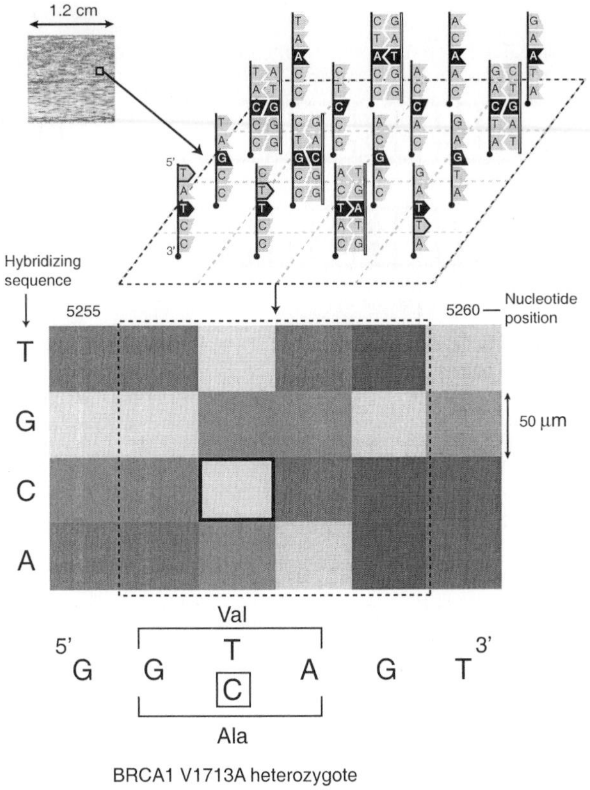

Fig. 2–21. Use of oligonucleotide chips for mutation detection. Based on light-mediated oligonucleotide synthesis, it is now possible to produce 250,000 or more probes on the surface of a 1.25 cm^2 silicon chip. The oligonucleotides, 15 to 25 nt in length, can be arrayed at high density in an addressable fashion. To query a biological sample for all possible substitutions in a particular gene sequence, the chip can be "tiled" not only for the wild-type sequence but also for nucleotide substitutions at every base. In the example, the normal sequence of GGTAGT has been tiled on the chip but so have all possible single-nucleotide substitutions. A wild-type biological sample would hybridize only to one feature in each column, but in this instance, an additional signal appears in the third base position due to the presence of a T-to-C substitution. This substitution results in a Val-to-Ala change in *BRCA1*. Oligonucleotides are shortened for purposes of clarifying the principle.

SUMMARY

Molecular genetics provides a framework for dissecting factors of common disease; delineation of genetic factors may also facilitate future study of interacting environmental factors. Identification of disease-predisposing genes is an entry point for studying relevant biological pathways and potential therapeutic approaches. Rapid advancements in the field have been made since the publication of the first edition of this volume. We have briefly reviewed the molecular basis of heredity, the molecular flow of information from DNA to RNA to protein, and the evolving genomics techniques that are driving a new era in medicine. Application of these techniques to complex traits is only beginning but carries great promise.

REFERENCES

Alwine JC, Kemp DJ, Stark GR: Method for detection of specific RNAs in agarose gels by transfer to diazobenzyloxymethyl-paper and hybridization with DNA probes. Proc Natl Acad Sci USA 1977; 74:5350.

Antonarakis SE, Kazazian HH, Tuddenham EG: Molecular etiology of factor VIII deficiency in hemophilia A. Hum Mutat 1995; 5:1–22.

Avery OT, Macleod CM, MacCarty M: Studies on the chemical nature of the substance inducing transformation of pneumococcal types. J Exp Med 1944; 79:137–158.

Bell DA, Badawi AF, Lang NP, Ilett KF, Kadlubar FF, Hirvonen A: Polymorphism in the *N-acetyltransferase 1* (*NAT1*) polyadenylation signal: association of *NAT1*10* allele with higher *N*-acetylation activity in bladder and colon tissue. Cancer Res 1995; 55:5226–5229.

Bennett MK, Ngo TT, Athanikar JN, Rosenfeld JM, Osborne TF: Co-stimulation of promoter for *Low density lipoprotein receptor* gene by sterol regulatory element-binding protein and Sp1 is specifically disrupted by the yin yang 1 protein. J Biol Chem 1999; 274:13025–13032.

Bilheimer DW, Ho YK, Brown MS, Anderson RG, Goldstein JL: Genetics of the low density lipoprotein receptor. Diminished receptor activity in lymphocytes from heterozygotes with familial hypercholesterolemia. J Clin Invest 1978; 61:678–696.

Bishop RW: Structure of the hamster *Low density lipoprotein receptor* gene. J Lipid Res 1992; 33:549–557.

Blackwood EM, Kadonaga JT: Going the distance: a current view of enhancer action. Science 1998; 281:61–63.

Bouchardy C, Mitrunen K, Wikman H, Husgafvel-Pursiainen K, Dayer P, Benhamou S, Hirvonen A: *N-Acetyltransferase NAT1* and *NAT2* genotypes and lung cancer risk. Pharmacogenetics 1998; 8:291–298.

Breslow JL: Human apolipoprotein molecular biology and genetic variation. Annu Rev Biochem 1985; 54:699–727.

Briggs MR, Yokoyama C, Wang X, Brown MS, Goldstein JL: Nuclear protein that binds sterol regulatory element of *Low density lipoprotein receptor* promoter. I. Identification of the protein and delineation of its target nucleotide sequence. J Biol Chem 1993; 268:14490–14496.

Brown PO, Botstein D: Exploring the new world of the genome with DNA microarrays. Nat Genet 1999; 21(Suppl 1):33–37.

Buckler AJ, Chang DD, Graw SL, Brook JD, Haber DA, Sharp PA, Housman DL: Exon amplification: a strategy to isolate mammalian genes based upon RNA splicing. Proc Natl Acad Sci USA 1991; 88:4005–4009.

Camper SA, Godbout R, Tilghman SM: The developmental regulation of *Albumin* and *Alpha-fetoprotein* gene expression. Prog Nucleic Acids Res Mol Biol 1989; 36:131–143.

Chen X, Levine L, Kwok PY: Fluorescence polarization in homogeneous nucleic acid analysis. Genome Res 1999; 9:492–498.

Coleman TP, Roesser JR: RNA secondary structure: an important *cis*-element in rat calcitonin/CGRP pre-messenger RNA splicing. Biochemistry 1998; 37:15941–15950.

Colgan DF, Manley JL: Mechanism and regulation of mRNA polyadenylation. Genes Dev 1997; 11:2755–2766.

Collins FS, Stoeckert CJ, Serjeant GR, Forget BG, Weissman SM: G gamma beta+ hereditary persistence of fetal hemoglobin: cosmid cloning and identification of a specific mutation 5′ to the *G gamma* gene. Proc Natl Acad Sci USA 1984; 81:4894–4898.

Collins FS, Weissman SM: The molecular genetics of human hemoglobin. Prog Nucleic Acids Res Mol Biol 1984; 31:315–462.

Constancia M, Pickard B, Kelsey G, Reik W: Imprinting mechanisms. Genome Res 1998; 8:881–900.

Deeb SS, Fajas L, Nemoto M, Pihlajamaki J, Mykkanen L, Kuusisto J, Laakso M, Fujimoto W, Auwerx J: A $Pro^{12}Ala$ substitution in PPAR-gamma-2 associated with decreased receptor activity, lower body mass index and improved insulin sensitivity. Nat Genet 1998; 20:284–287.

Duggan DJ, Bittner M, Chen Y, Meltzer P, Trent JM: Expression profiling using cDNA microarrays. Nat Genet 1999; 21(Suppl 1):10–14.

Dumonteil E, Philippe J: *Insulin* gene: organization, expression and regulation. Diabetes Metab 1996; 22:164–173.

Edlund T, Walker MD, Barr PJ, Rutter WJ: Cell-specific expression of the rat *Insulin* gene: evidence for role of two distinct 5′ flanking elements. Science 1985; 230:912–916.

Efrat S, Fusco-DeMane D, Lemberg H, al Emran O, Wang X: Conditional transformation of a pancreatic beta-cell line derived from transgenic mice expressing a tetracycline-regulated oncogene. Proc Natl Acad Sci USA 1995; 92:3576–3580.

Efstratiadis A, Posakony JW, Maniatis T, Lawn RM, O'Connell C, Spritz RA, DeRiel JK, Forget BG, Weissman SM, Slightom JL, et al.: The structure and evolution of the human beta-globin gene family. Cell 1980; 21:653–668.

Felsenfeld G: Chromatin unfolds. Cell 1996; 86:13–19.

Fischer SG, Lerman LS: DNA fragments differing by single base-pair substitutions are separated in denaturing gradient gels: correspondence with melting theory. Proc Natl Acad Sci USA 1983; 80:1579–1583.

Fodor SP, Read JL, Pirrung MC, Stryer L, Lu AT, Solas D: Light-directed, spatially addressable parallel chemical synthesis. Science 1991; 251:767–773.

Frohman MA, Dush MK, Martin GR: Rapid production of full-length cDNAs from rare transcripts: amplification using a single gene-specific oligonucleotide primer. Proc Natl Acad Sci USA 1988; 85:8998–9002.

Gilbert W: Why genes in pieces? Nature 1978; 271:501.

Grant SF, Reid DM, Blake G, Herd R, Fogelman I, Ralston SH: Reduced bone density and osteoporosis associated with a polymorphic Sp1 binding site in the *Collagen type I alpha 1* gene. Nat Genet 1996;14:203–205.

Gross DS, Garrard WT: Nuclease hypersensitivity sites in chromatin. Annu Rev Biochem 1988; 57:159–197.

Hacia JG, Brody LC, Chee MS, Fodor SP, Collins FS: Detection of heterozygous mutations in *BRCA1* using high density oligonucleotide arrays and two-colour fluorescence analysis. Nat Genet 1996; 14:441–447.

Han K, Martinage A: Post-translational chemical modification(s) of proteins. Int J Biochem 1992; 24:19–28.

Hanahan D: Heritable formation of pancreatic beta-cell tumours in transgenic mice expressing recombinant insulin/simian virus 40 oncogenes. Nature 1985; 315:115–122.

Heard E, Clerc P, Avner P: X-chromosome inactivation in mammals. Annu Rev Genet 1997; 31:571–610.

Hemminki A, Tomlinson I, Markie D, Jarvinen H, Sistonen P, Bjorkqvist AM, Knuutila S, Salovaara R, Bodmer W, Shibata D, et al.: Localization of a susceptibility locus for Peutz-Jeghers syndrome to 19p using comparative genomic hybridization and targeted linkage analysis. Nat Genet 1997; 15:87–90.

Herbert A, Rich A: RNA processing and the evolution of eukaryotes. Nat Genet 1999; 21:265–269.

Hobbs HH, Brown MS, Goldstein JL, Russell DW: Deletion of exon encoding cysteine-rich repeat of low density lipoprotein receptor alters its binding specificity in a subject with familial hypercholesterolemia. J Biol Chem 1986; 261:13114–13120.

Hobbs HH, Brown MS, Russell DW, Davignon J, Goldstein JL: Deletion in the gene for the low-density-lipoprotein receptor in a majority of French Canadians with familial hypercholesterolemia. N Engl J Med 1987; 317:734–737.

Hood L, Kronenberg M, Hunkapiller T: T cell antigen receptors and the immunoglobulin supergene family. Cell 1985; 40:225–229.

International Human Genome Sequencing Consortium: Initial sequencing and analysis of the human genome. Nature 2001; 409:860–921.

International SNP Map Working Group: A map of human genome sequence variation containing 1.42 million single nucleotide polymorphisms. Nature 2001; 409:928–933.

Karlsson S, Nienhuis AW: Developmental regulation of human globin genes. Annu Rev Biochem 1985; 54:1071–1108.

Kazazian HH Jr: The thalassemia syndromes: molecular basis and prenatal diagnosis in 1990. Semin Hematol 1990; 27:209–228.

Kazazian HH Jr, Wong C, Youssoufian H, Scott AF, Phillips DG, Antonarakis SE: Haemophilia A resulting from de novo insertion of L1 sequences represents a novel mechanism for mutation in man. Nature 1988; 332:164–166.

Knudson AG Jr: Mutation and cancer: statistical study of retinoblastoma. Proc Natl Acad Sci USA 1971; 68:820–823.

Krokan HE, Nilsen H, Skorpen F, Otterlei M, Slupphaug G: Base excision repair of DNA in mammalian cells. FEBS Lett 2000; 476:73–77.

Kruse F, Rose SD, Swift GH, Hammer RE, MacDonald RJ: Cooperation between elements of an organ-specific transcriptional enhancer in animals. Mol Cell Biol 1995; 15:4385–4394.

Lee T, Young R: Transcription of eukaryotic protein-coding genes. Annu Rev Genet 2000; 34:77–137.

Lehrman MA, Russell DW, Goldstein JL, Brown MS: Exon-Alu recombination deletes 5 kilobases from the *Low density lipoprotein receptor* gene, producing a null phenotype in familial hypercholesterolemia. Proc Natl Acad Sci USA 1986; 83:3679–3683.

Lengauer C, Kinzler KW, Vogelstein B: Genetic instabilities in human cancers. Nature 1998; 396:643–649.

Livak KJ, Flood SJ, Marmaro J, Giusti W, Deetz K: Oligonucleotides with fluorescent dyes at opposite ends provide a quenched probe system useful for detecting PCR product and nucleic acid hybridization. PCR Methods Appl 1995; 4:357–362.

Long M, de Souza SJ, Gilbert W: Evolution of the intron–exon structure of eukaryotic genes. Curr Opin Genet Dev 1995; 5:774–778.

Maity SN, de Crombrugghe B: Role of the CCAAT-binding protein CBF/NF-Y in transcription. Trends Biochem Sci 1998; 23:174–178.

Maniatis T, Reed R: The role of small nuclear ribonucleoprotein particles in pre-mRNA splicing. Nature 1987; 325:673–678.

Mantovani R: A survey of 178 NF-Y binding CCAAT boxes. Nucleic Acids Res 1998; 26:1135–1143.

Mazzarella R, Schlessinger D: Duplication and distribution of repetitive elements and non-unique regions in the human genome. Gene 1997; 205:29–38.

Mello J, Almouzni G: The ins and outs of nucleosome assembly. Curr Opin Genet Dev 2001; 11:136–141.

Melton DW, Konecki DS, Brennand J, Caskey CT: Structure, expression, and mutation of the *Hypoxanthine phosphoribosyltransferase* gene. Proc Natl Acad Sci USA 1984; 81:2147–2151.

Meselson M, Stahl FW: The replication of DNA in *Escherichia coli*. Proc Natl Acad Sci USA 1958; 44:671–682.

Moldave K: Eukaryotic protein synthesis. Annu Rev Biochem 1985; 54:1109–1149.

Monaco AP, Neve RL, Colletti-Feener C, Bertelson CJ, Kurnit DM, Kunkel LM: Isolation of candidate cDNAs for portions of the *Duchenne muscular dystrophy* gene. Nature 1986; 323:646–650.

Moran JV, DeBerardinis RJ, Kazazian HH Jr: Exon shuffling by L1 retrotransposition. Science 1999; 283:1530–1534.

Oefner PJ, Underhill PA: Comparative DNA sequencing by denaturing high-performance liquid chromatography (DHPLC). Am J Hum Genet 1995; 57:A266.

Olivieri NF: The beta-thalassemias. N Engl J Med 1999; 341:99–109.

Orita M, Iwahana H, Kanazawa H, Hayashi K, Sekiya T: Detection of polymorphisms of human DNA by gel electrophoresis as single-strand conformation polymorphisms. Proc Natl Acad Sci USA 1989; 86: 2766–2770.

Orkin SH, Kazazian HH Jr: The mutation and polymorphism of the human *Beta-globin* gene and its surrounding DNA. Annu Rev Genet 1984; 18:131–171.

Ornitz DM, Palmiter RD, Hammer RE, Brinster RL, Swift GH, MacDonald RJ: Specific expression of an elastase-human growth hormone fusion gene in pancreatic acinar cells of transgenic mice. Nature 1985; 313:600–602.

Osborne TF, Goldstein JL, Brown MS: 5′ end of *HMG CoA reductase* gene contains sequences responsible for cholesterol-mediated inhibition of transcription. Cell 1985; 42:203–212.

Owen MC, Brennan SO, Lewis JH, Carrell RW: Mutation of antitrypsin to antithrombin. Alpha 1-antitrypsin Pittsburgh (^{358}Met leads to Arg), a fatal bleeding disorder. N Engl J Med 1983; 309:694–698.

Padgett RA, Grabowski PJ, Konarska MM, Seiler S, Sharp PA: Splicing of messenger RNA precursors. Annu Rev Biochem 1986; 55:1119–1150.

Park TW, Fujiwara H, Wright TC: Molecular biology of cervical cancer and its precursors. Cancer 1995; 76(Suppl 10):1902–1913.

Pastinen T, Kurg A, Metspalu A, Peltonen L, Syvanen AC: Minisequencing: a specific tool for DNA analysis and diagnostics on oligonucleotide arrays. Genome Res 1997; 7:606–614.

Pegoraro L, Palumbo A, Erikson J, Falda M, Giovanazzo B, Emanuel BS, Rovera G, Nowell PC, Croce CM: A 14;18 and an 8;14 chromosome translocation in a cell line derived from an acute B-cell leukemia. Proc Natl Acad Sci USA 1984; 81:7166–7170.

Pestova T, Kolupaeva V, Lomakin I, Pilipenko E, Shatsky I, Agol V, Hellen C: Molecular mechanisms of translation initiation in eukaryotes. Proc Natl Acad Sci USA 2001; 98:7029–7036.

Prockop DJ: Osteogenesis imperfecta: phenotypic heterogeneity, protein suicide, short and long collagen. Am J Hum Genet 1984; 36:499–505.

Reich DE, Cargill M, Bolk S, Ireland J, Sabeti PC, Richter DJ, Lavery T, Kouyoumjian R, Farhadian SF, Ward R, et al.: Linkage disequilibrium in the human genome. Nature 2001; 411:199–204.

Roest PA, Roberts RG, Sugino S, van Ommen GJ, den Dunnen JT: Protein truncation test (PTT) for rapid detection of translation-terminating mutations. Hum Mol Genet 1993; 2:1719–1721.

Ronaghi M: Pyrosequencing sheds light on DNA sequencing. Genome Res 2001; 11:3–11.

Rosenfeld MG, Mermod JJ, Amara SG, Swanson LW, Sawchenko PE, Rivier J, Vale WW, Evans RM: Production of a novel neuropeptide encoded by the *Calcitonin* gene via tissue-specific RNA processing. Nature 1983; 304:129–135.

Ross P, Hall L, Smirnov I, Haff L: High level multiplex genotyping by MALDI-TOF mass spectrometry. Nat Biotechnol 1998; 16:1347–1351.

Roth FP, Hughes JD, Estep PW, Church GM: Finding DNA regulatory motifs within unaligned noncoding sequences clustered by whole-genome mRNA quantitation. Nat Biotechnol 1998; 16:939–945.

Sanger F, Nicklen S, Coulson AR: DNA-sequencing with chain-terminating inhibitors. Proc Natl Acad Sci USA 1977; 74:5463–5467.

Scriver CR, Sly WS, Childs B, Beaudet AL, Valle D, Kinzler K, Vogelstein B: The Metabolic and Molecular Bases of Inherited Disease, 8th ed. New York: McGraw-Hill, 2000.

Sharp PA: Split genes and RNA splicing. Cell 1994; 77:805–815.

Shimano H, Horton JD, Hammer RE, Shimomura I, Brown MS, Goldstein JL: Overproduction of cholesterol and fatty acids causes massive liver enlargement in transgenic mice expressing truncated SREBP-1a. J Clin Invest 1996; 98:1575–1584.

Smith JR, Freije D, Carpten JD, Gronberg H, Xu J, Isaacs SD, Brownstein MJ, Bova GS, Guo H, Bujnovszky P, et al.: Major susceptibility locus for prostate cancer on chromosome 1 suggested by a genome-wide search. Science 1996; 274:1371–1374.

Smith JR, Osborne TF, Goldstein JL, Brown MS: Identification of nucleotides responsible for enhancer activity of sterol regulatory element in *Low density lipoprotein receptor gene*. J Biol Chem 1990; 265:2306–2310.

Southern EM: Detection of specific sequences among DNA fragments separated by gel electrophoresis. J Mol Biol 1975; 98:503.

Stamatoyannopoulos G, Majerus PW, Perlmutter RM, Varmus H (eds): The Molecular Basis of Blood Diseases, 3rd ed. Philadelphia: Saunders, 2000. Stamatoyannopoulos G, and Grossveld F, Chapter 5: Hemoglobin Switching, 135–182.

Stargell LA, Struhl K: Mechanisms of transcriptional activation in vivo: two steps forward. Trends Genet 1996; 12:311–315.

Staudt LM, Lenardo MJ: Immunoglobulin gene transcription. Annu Rev Immunol 1991; 9:373–398.

Steinmetz M, Hood L: Genes of the major histocompatibility complex in mouse and man. Science 1983; 222:727–733.

Strausberg RL, Feingold EA, Klausner RD, Collins FS: The mammalian gene collection. Science 1999; 286:455–457

Sudhof TC, Goldstein JL, Brown MS, Russell DW: The *LDL receptor* gene: a mosaic of exons shared with different proteins. Science 1985; 228:815–822.

Sudhof TC, Van der Westhuyzen DR, Goldstein JL, Brown MS, Russell DW: Three direct repeats and a TATA-like sequence are required for regulated expression of the human *Low density lipoprotein receptor* gene. J Biol Chem 1987; 262:10773–10779.

Syvanen AC, Aalto-Setala L, Harju L, Kontula K, Soderlund H: A primer-guided nucleotide incorporation assay in the genotyping of *Apolipoprotein E*. Genomics 1990; 8: 684–692.

Tilghman SM: The sins of the fathers and mothers: genomic imprinting in mammalian development. Cell 1999; 96:185–193.

Varani G: A cap for all occasions. Structure 1997; 5:855–858.

Velculescu VE, Zhang L, Vogelstein B, Kinzler KW: Serial analysis of gene expression. Science 1995; 270:484–487.

Venter JC, Adams MD, Myers EW, Li PW, Mural RJ, Sutton GG, Smith HO, Yandell M, Evans CA, Holt RA, et al.: The sequence of the human genome. Science 2001; 291:1304–1351.

Wang DG, Fran JB, Siao CJ, Berno A, Young P, Sapolsky R, Ghandour G, Perkins N, Winchester E, Spencer J, et al.: Large-scale identification, mapping, and genotyping of single-nucleotide polymorphisms in the human genome. Science 1998; 280:1077–1082.

Wang X, Briggs MR, Hua X, Yokoyama C, Goldstein JL, Brown MS: Nuclear protein that binds sterol regulatory element of *Low density lipoprotein receptor* promoter. II. Purification and characterization. J Biol Chem 1993; 268:14497–14504.

Watson JD, Crick FHC: Molecular structure of nucleic acids: a structure for desoxyribose nucleic acid. Nature 1953; 171:737–738.

Weatherall DJ, Clegg JB: The Thalassemia Syndromes, 3rd ed. Oxford: Blackwell, 1981.

Wolffe AP, Guschin D: Chromatin structural features and targets that regulate transcription. J Struct Biol 2000; 129:102–122.

Woodage T, King SM, Wacholder S, Hartge P, Struewing JP, McAdams M, Laken SJ, Tucker MA, Brody LC: The APCI1307K allele and cancer risk in a community-based study of Ashkenazi Jews. Nat Genet 1998; 20:62–65.

Yokoyama C, Wang X, Briggs MR, Admon A, Wu J, Hua X, Goldstein JL, Brown MS: SREBP-1, a basic-helix-loop-helix-leucine zipper protein that controls transcription of the *Low density lipoprotein receptor* gene. Cell 1993; 75:187–197.

3 Genetic Epidemiologic Methods

STEPHEN S. RICH AND THOMAS A. SELLERS

The recognition that host factors influence risk of disease dates back at least to the time of the ancient Greeks. Around 200 CE Galen wrote, "But remember throughout that no cause is efficient without a predisposition of the body itself, otherwise, external factors which affect one would affect all." Despite this long-standing appreciation of variable response to the environment, the discovery of genetics (or Mendelian laws of inheritance) did not come for many centuries. Moreover, identifying the precise underlying basis for host susceptibility—namely, variation in genetic sequences—has not been possible until very recent times. This chapter provides a framework for one of the two general strategies for identifying genes: genetic epidemiology.

Genetic epidemiology strives to address four fundamental questions:

1. Does the disease, health condition, or phenotype cluster in families?
2. Is the familial aggregation a reflection of shared genes, shared environment, or a combination of genes and environment?
3. Is the pattern of disease consistent with Mendelian transmission of a single major gene?
4. Where are the chromosomal locations of these genes?

The positive answers to this series of questions are that, indeed, there is familial aggregation, the clustering appears to result (in part) from genetic factors, a gene with large effect does exist for the disease, and its location can be pinpointed to a region of about 1 million base pairs (bp) of DNA. From there, the work is passed to molecular geneticists and molecular biologists, who employ a variety of rapidly advancing techniques to further narrow the chromosomal position of the gene, and ultimately identify it. This latter phase of the scientific inquiry is known as *positional cloning*. Once called *reverse genetics*, this strategy does not require the study of families (Fig. 3–1). It is important to compare and contrast positional cloning with one that has yielded the identification of a far greater number of genes, namely, *functional cloning*. In the latter, proteins known to be involved in the disease process are identified, their protein sequence (and underlying genetic sequence) is determined, and the chromosomal location is then determined by finding where this particular sequence of DNA is found in the genome (Collins, 1995).

In this chapter, we provide an overview of the study design and analysis strategies and approaches that precede positional cloning and gene identification. In practice, the selection of design and analytic approach is based on a number of variables, such as the underlying genetic basis (e.g., monogenic, polygenic), the nature of the phenotype (simple dichotomy, quantitative trait), and the types of individuals sampled (unrelated individuals, sib pairs, nuclear families, extended pedigrees). Detailed coverage of all of these issues is not possible; the intent of this chapter is to provide familiarity with the key issues involved.

CAUSES OF FAMILIAL AGGREGATION

It is obvious to most people that the clustering of disease in a family is evidence that genetic factors may be operating. However, before reaching a final conclusion, several alternative explanations must first be considered. This is especially important for common diseases with known nongenetic influences. For example, given that there is a finite probability for the development of a particular disease in the population, even in the absence of any genetic contribution at all, the disease may afflict several members of the same family just by chance alone. This is especially true for the common diseases of major public health importance that are covered in other chapters in this book. If one in two Americans dies of some form of heart disease, and one in four dies of some form of cancer, it should probably be surprising for someone to *not* have a family history of these diseases.

The ability to determine whether a familial cluster of disease is greater than one would expect by chance alone requires data on the rates at which the disease occurs in the target population. If the rates of disease vary by age and sex, for example, then the expected occurrence of disease in a family must take this into consideration. The key point is that it is essential to consider the role of chance in the familial occurrence of disease and to use the known epidemiology of the disease to determine if the observed pattern of disease occurs at a frequency greater than that expected on the basis of population rates.

It is becoming commonplace in the practice of medicine to inquire if patients have a family history of specific diseases, often relating to the complaint for which the patient is being seen (family history of cancer if the patient had a high Prostate Specific Antigen (PSA) for example). Two additional factors that would affect the likelihood that someone reports a positive family history are age of the patient and family size. Although every person has at least two first-degree biological relatives (our parents), the person's number of siblings, aunts, uncles, cousins, and children are clearly random variables. For example, someone who has 15 close relatives at risk for a common chronic disease is almost certainly more likely to have a relative with the same disease than a person with only two relatives at risk. Similarly, because age is the single most important risk factor for many diseases of public health importance, an older person (with older relatives) is more likely to have a family history for nongenetic

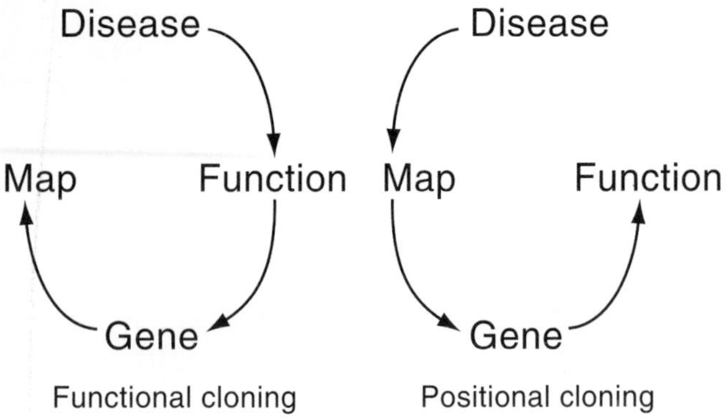

Fig. 3–1. Conceptual framework for positional cloning of a gene (*Source:* FS Collins, Nature Genetics 1993; 1:3.)

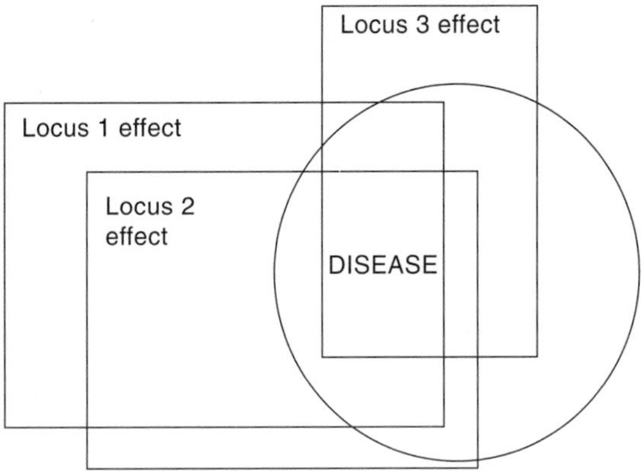

Fig. 3–3. Genetic (□) and environmental (○) influences on common human disease.

reasons than is a younger person (with corresponding younger relatives). It is generally held that if there are two forms of a disease, one genetic and the other not, the genetic form of the disease would tend to have an earlier age at onset. Therefore, cases of disease with an early age at onset and a family history tend to be those most likely to have a significant genetic influence (Fig. 3–2).

Most common diseases have at least some identified nongenetic factors that influence the risk of disease. This information on exposure–disease relationships must be considered as explanations for any observed clustering of disease in families (Fig. 3–3). For example, although roughly 95% of all lung cancer cases are smokers, fewer than 20% of heavy smokers ever develop the disease (Mattson et al., 1987). This observation has caused some to hypothesize that host factors might influence the response to environmental agents, such as tobacco. A complicating factor in the study of a disease with such a strong environmental risk factor is the extent to which family members also smoke cigarettes. Studies of twins conducted in the 1930s provided strong evidence that smoking habits clustered in families (Fisher, 1958). Therefore, if family members of cases are more likely to smoke than family members of controls, a greater proportion of cases would be expected to report a positive family history of lung cancer. In this case, however, clustering of cases in families would be due to shared lifestyle, rather than shared genes.

It is recognized that diet is related to disease risk in a variety of ways: high-fat diets, particularly saturated fat, are associated with coronary heart disease and cancer. Diets low in complex carbohydrates and fruits and vegetables are associated with diabetes and cancer. Several studies suggest that dietary intake patterns are familial in nature (Sellers et al., 1991b; Vachon et al., 1998). To the extent that family members share dietary habits that increase risk for a given disease, familial clustering of disease may occur. Similarly, behaviors and personality traits such as exercise habits, alcohol intake, and use of sunscreen may be learned within a family and indirectly relate to clustering of disease.

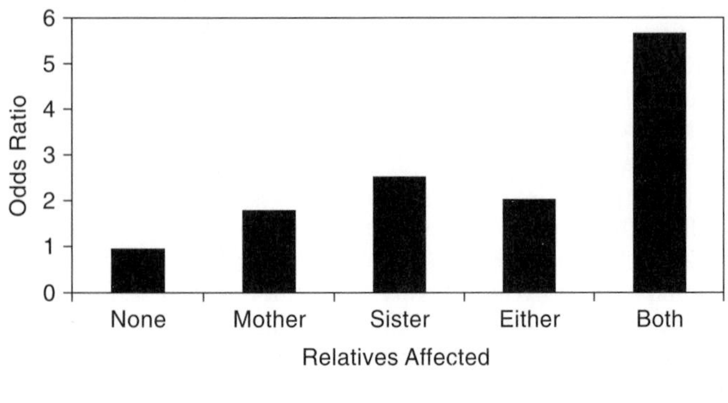

Fig. 3–2. Familial clustering of breast cancer.

Many risk factors shared by family members are a reflection of shared environment, such as water supply, radon from the soil, air quality, pesticides, lead paints—even occupation. A case report of a family with four members with mesothelioma, a rare cancer of the lining of the peritoneal cavity, was traced back to a common occupational exposure to asbestos (Krousel et al., 1986). Infectious diseases may also be included in this category, and there are a number of published examples where familial clustering of hepatitis or tuberculosis occurs from common exposures.

Before embarking on genetic analysis of the families, one should theoretically try to rule out shared environmental factors as the cause of the aggregation. This can be achieved with a study design known as a case-control family study. Because these studies are often costly and time-consuming, they are not frequently used and will not be discussed further in this chapter.

CASE-CONTROL AND ASSOCIATION STUDIES

Definitions and Contrasts

A case-control study is a popular epidemiologic method to determine if there is an association between an exposure and disease. They lend themselves nicely to studies of genetic factors, with genes being the relevant exposure of interest. A *case* is a person selected for study because he or she has the disease of interest. A *control* is a person with no history of the disease but is, nonetheless, at risk for the disease. The underlying hypothesis is that disease does not occur randomly, so that the cases differ in a systematic and identifiable way from the controls regarding the distribution of an *exposure* presumed to influence risk of the disease. When first exploring the hypothesis that a common disease has a genetic component, case-control studies comparing the frequency of reported family history are useful starting points.

The term *association study* can be used to describe case-control studies in which the exposure of interest is a gene that, based on knowledge of its presumed function, is a biologically plausible "candidate gene" for disease susceptibility. In this situation, the cases and controls would be expected to differ with respect to the frequency that the putative "high-risk" allele is found in the two groups. The most obvious situation would be one where every case carries the "defective" allele, and this allele appears in none of the controls. For some Mendelian traits, like Huntington disease, this is probably true, even though multiple mutations may occur within the gene. However, for common diseases with both genetic and environmental factors, this is less likely to occur.

Measure of Association

The strength of association between exposure and disease is quantified by the odds ratio. Translated literally, it means the odds of exposure given disease, relative to the odds of exposure given no disease. The interpretation of a study that finds a particular gene mutation to confer an odds ratio of 6.2 would be that cases were 6.2 times more likely than the controls to carry this particular genetic alteration. If a case-control study yields an odds ratio of 1.0, then the odds of exposure are the same among the cases and controls, implying no association. Odds ratios can also be less than 1, indicating that a particular exposure is protective against disease.

The odds ratio, as a measure of risk for an outcome when an antecedent factor is present, is particularly appealing to genetic studies, as the "antecedent factor" can be interpreted as the genotype (or risk allele). From the 2 × 2 table (Table 3–1), a series of cases (those with disease) and controls (those without disease) has been genotyped. The number in each cell is defined by n_{ij}, where the number with disease is $n_{.1} = n_{11} + n_{21}$, the number without disease is $n_{.2} = n_{12} + n_{22}$, and the total number of subjects is $n = n_{11} + n_{12} + n_{21} + n_{22} = n_{.1} + n_{.2} = n_{1.} + n_{2.}$.

Thus, the odds of "disease" is defined by $\Omega_D = \{P(D|G)/P(\text{not } D|G)\}$, and the odds of "no disease" is defined by $\Omega_{\text{not } D} = \{P(\text{not } D|G)/P(D|G)\}$, where Ω_D is the odds that the disease, D, will occur when the risk gene (genotype or allele) G is present. The measure of association based on Ω_D and $\Omega_{\text{not } D}$ is the ratio, $\omega = \Omega_D/\Omega_{\text{not } D}$. The sample odds ratio, o, is composed of two parts, with $O_D = n_{11}/n_{12}$ and $O_{\text{notD}} = n_{21}/n_{22}$. Thus, the sample odds ratio is estimated by $o = O_D/O_{\text{notD}} = (n_{11}/n_{12})/(n_{21}/n_{22}) = n_{11}n_{22}/n_{12}n_{21}$.

For many complex diseases, the role of selected candidate genes has been studied in the case-control format. For example, many autoimmune diseases (e.g., Type 1 diabetes, multiple sclerosis, autoimmune thyroid disease, systemic lupus erythematosus) have been evaluated in the context of the distribution of alleles (antigens) of the human major histocompatibility complex (HLA). Odds ratios (relative risks) of selected HLA antigens with autoimmune disease typically range from 2.5 to 4.5, but can be higher in selected subsets. For example, the well-known HLA–DR4 association with Type 1 diabetes has an odds ratio of nearly 4, yet 40% of cases and 10% of controls have the "risk allele" (Rich et al., 1984), demonstrating the "incomplete risk" associated with HLA and Type 1 diabetes. Even among hereditary cases of disease there may be different genes that contribute to the inherited risk. For example, hereditary colon cancer and hereditary breast cancer each have several different genes that confer increased risk. Therefore, one should expect to encounter a situation where there is a higher frequency of a disease allele among the cases than among the controls, but the concordance is less than perfect.

Table 3–1. The Model Fourfold Table to Test for Association

Genetic Factor	Disease: Present (D)	Disease: Absent (not D)	Total
Present (G)	n_{11}	n_{12}	$n_{1.}$
Absent (not G)	n_{21}	n_{22}	$n_{2.}$
Total	$n_{.1}$	$n_{.2}$	n

Ascertainment of Study Subjects

Of direct relation to the interpretation of the odds ratio is how the study groups were formulated. The internal and external validity of a case-control study is directly related to how the subjects were ascertained.

The ascertainment considerations might include the following:

1. Where will case probands be identified? A random sample of the population might be considered for a common condition (high prevalence), but this approach is inefficient for rare diseases. If the researcher is fortunate, there might be a disease registry that contains all incident cases in a defined geographic region. In many situations one is restricted to ascertainment of case probands from hospitals and clinics, which raises questions about their representativeness, especially if only specialized facilities are canvassed. Case probands may also be identified through death certificates (Ooi et al., 1986), although this selection method would prohibit the collection of biological samples from the index case. Careful definition of what constitutes a case is critical and should be agreed on before the start of the study. The critical issue in case ascertainment is trying to ensure that cases are representative of all cases (or a particular defined subset of cases).

2. Does the disease or trait require medical attention? It is not difficult to envision a number of important public health problems that may have a significant genetic component (e.g., alcohol or drug abuse), but the condition either does not require medical attention or required medical care is not sought. In those situations, it is virtually impossible to determine if all eligible case probands have been identified. Consequently, one cannot evaluate whether the cases are representative of all cases.

3. Is the prevalence of the disease known? When the incidence or prevalence of the condition under study is known, one has a much greater likelihood of evaluating whether or not the sampling frame of case probands includes all eligible cases with the disease.

4. Is there a survival effect of the disease? When the prevalence of the condition (Alzheimer's disease) is associated with a specific allele at a locus (ApoE) whose alleles also increase the risk of death from competing causes (cardiovascular events), then the distribution of genotypes will differ by age group. If so, careful matching on age is critical.

The purpose of control families derives from the need to be able to evaluate whether familial clustering among cases is greater than can be expected. This is especially important when there are no population-based rates to calculate the expected number of disease events in case families. Control families are also needed to be able to rule out common familial (measured) exposure as an explanation for any observed familial aggregation. Control families must be as similar as possible to the case families for all other (unmeasured) environmental exposures in order to determine properly whether a disease or trait truly has a genetic component.

Controls can be identified from several possible sources. One would be the same disease registry, clinic, or hospital from which the probands were drawn but with sampling based on a different disease. Another choice is random selection from the general population (e.g., neighborhood controls). Relatives of the proband's spouse have been used as controls since the turn of the twentieth century. This clever approach "matches" families on unmeasured lifestyle, economic, education, and even religious influences because likes tend to marry likes (Vandenberg, 1972).

TWIN STUDIES

When the question "Is it genetic?" arises, where "it" is a disease or other trait, the first thought often turns to twin studies and twin concordance rates. Studies of twins provide important information concerning the roles of genetic and environmental risk factors on disease risk (or on some other measurement). In the former, each member of a twin pair can be evaluated with respect to disease presence or absence of the disease in question. In the latter, each measurement is provided on each twin. Similarity in phenotype can then be correlated with similarity in "twin-ness." Monozygotic (MZ) twins are genetically identical, and dizygotic (DZ) twins are genetically half-identical (equivalent to a full sibling relationship, in which the twin pair shares one-half of their genes, on average). Thus, complete genetic determination of a trait would equate to MZ twins having 100% concordance and DZ twins having 50% concordance.

While a greater concordance in MZ twins versus DZ twins is expected for disorders with a genetic contribution, the presence of an MZ twin concordance less than 100% emphasizes the importance of environmental factors. For many common disorders of public health significance, the MZ twin concordance rates may be significantly less than 100%. One could hypothesize that as individuals age, the number of "random" environmental factors accumulate over time. This would increase the variation due to the environment and decrease the contribution due to genetic factors, thereby reducing the twin concordance rates for disorders that manifest in older ages (or increases the number of phenocopies). The effect of environment on genetic susceptibility needs to be considered for adult-onset disorders of public health importance. Common disorders of interest include Type 2 diabetes (Mayer et al., 1996; Hawkes, 1997), heart disease (Russell et al., 1998), stroke (Brass et al., 1996), hypertension (Busjahn et al., 1996; van den Bree et al., 1996), and Alzheimer's disease (Raiha et al., 1996; Meyer and Breitner, 1998).

Analysis of Twin Studies

Analysis of twin concordance data often uses linear model methods (such as analysis of variance) to estimate that portion of the total phenotypic variance that can be partitioned into "within-pair" and "between-pair" effects. These estimated variance components can be equated to genetic and environmental components of variance and, based on certain assumptions, the heritability of the phenotype can be estimated.

The heritability (h^2) of a trait can be defined as the ratio of the genetic variance to the phenotypic variance. When the genetic variance consists of additive, dominance, and epistatic effects, the heritability is said to be in the "broad sense" (h^2_B); this is the heritability that is often obtained from twin concordance studies. When the genetic variance is composed only of additive effects of genes (those effects that can be predicted from genes transmitted between parents and offspring), the estimated heritability is said to be in the "narrow sense" (h^2_N). Estimation of "narrow sense" heritability requires more extensive relationships than the classical twin design requires.

Table 3–2. Genetic Expectations for Relative Pairs

	Coefficient for		
Types of Relatives	σ^2_A	σ^2_C	σ^2_E
Spouse–spouse	0	1	1
MZ twins	1	1	1
DZ twins	1/2	1	1
Parent–offspring	1/2	1	1
Full sibs	1/2	1	1
Half sibs	1/4	1	1
Aunt–niece	1/4	0	1
First cousins	1/8	0	1

σ^2_A, additive genetic variance; σ^2_C, common (household) environmental variance; σ^2_E, random environmental variance.

Most analyses use twin pairs reared in the same family environment, although this necessarily confounds common genes with common environment. Using the relatively rare "twins reared apart" design, separation of common genes with common environment can be achieved (Tellegen et al., 1988; Hanson et al., 1989). Additional information can be obtained by extending the classical twin design to include additional relative types (Nance and Corey, 1976). For example, offspring of MZ twins are genetically half-siblings, while offspring of DZ twins are genetically first cousins. Models that incorporate these relationships have been shown to provide improved estimates of the role of genetic factors and can allow use of these data in efforts to map genes (Table 3–2).

Heritability estimates for specific traits, whether from twin or family designs, provide baseline information about the genetic architecture of the trait. High heritability, especially narrow sense heritability, suggests that the trait is a candidate for mapping. Low heritability suggests that the typical family-based design for mapping may be inefficient. What should be recognized, however, is that heritability does not provide information concerning the mode of inheritance, the number of loci, or the magnitude of individual locus effects on the trait. Further, the inference should be restricted to the population and the environment in which the trait is measured. Thus, heritability is a function of the trait measured at a point in time on a population in a specific environment. Changing any of these "parameters" may result in a different heritability.

SEGREGATION ANALYSIS

Definition and Utility

Although classical twin studies provide useful evidence for the influence of genetic factors on a given disease, they are less helpful in defining the mode of inheritance of a trait or for mapping the specific genes contributing to that trait. This section describes the basic approach for determination of the mechanism for understanding the inheritance of phenotypes and the approach to finding genes: segregation analysis.

Segregation analysis refers to the detection of Mendelian ratios in relatives. The historical basis is the experiments of Mendel, which showed that, for a simple discrete phenotype, it is possible to examine the proportion of offspring affected and compare them with expectations under Mendelian inheritance. Classical segregation analysis was primarily concerned with rare diseases. The questions regarding mode of inheritance concerned whether a single copy of the mutated gene was sufficient for disease (dominance) or whether two copies of the mutated gene (one from each parent) were required for disease (recessive). Therefore, one would expect to see one-half of the offspring of an affected parent in the case of autosomal dominant inheritance, and one-fourth of the offspring of unaffected parents in the case of autosomal recessive inheritance.

For complex human diseases the analysis is not quite so straightforward, for a number of reasons. For example, genetic susceptibility to a disease does not always express itself (incomplete penetrance) or does so with variable expressivity (gradations in severity or phenotypic features), often with a range in age at onset. These complicating factors make it difficult to infer the genetic influence on a disease or trait based on simple inspection of phenotypes in sibships. As a result, the "simple" segregation analysis, restricted to the calculation of proportions of affected children from parental mating types (affected × affected, affected × unaffected, unaffected × unaffected), no longer provided proportions that appeared Mendelian. Modern methods of segregation analysis (often termed *complex segregation analysis* due to its reliance on complicated statistical models) are based on more elaborate mathematical models of genetic transmission and liability (Elston, 1981), the concept of which is described next.

Analysis and Interpretation

Elucidation of the potential mode of inheritance of susceptibility to a disease is determined by comparing how well different hypotheses (genetic and nongenetic) fit the observed pattern of disease in a collection of families. A variety of computer software programs are available to perform this analysis, such as PAP (Hasstedt and Cartwright, 1981), POINTER (Lalouel and Morton, 1981), SAGE (1994), and MORGAN (Thompson, 1994). Coverage of these various options is beyond the scope of this chapter, as is discussion of the mathematical underpinnings of how the various hypotheses are constructed and tested. The concept, however, is basically as follows. In the traditional realm of science, hypotheses are generated and data are collected and analyzed to accept or refute the hypothesis. With segregation analysis, the outcome of the experiment (random mating and assortment of genes from parents to offspring) has already occurred (individuals who inherit the deleterious gene have an increased risk for disease). Thus, one is essentially asking the question, "Given the pattern of disease in these families, what is the likelihood that the underlying cause was transmission of an altered allele in a Mendelian fashion?"

Complex segregation analysis can be helpful in mapping genes by providing evidence that a single major gene might influence risk of the disease and by providing estimates of the parameters necessary for parametric (model-dependent) linkage analysis (providing estimates of allele frequency and penetrance). Certain assumptions are required, such as a single disease susceptibility locus with two alleles, random mating, and the trait locus in the population exhibiting Hardy-Weinberg equilibrium. Even with these simplifying assumptions, however, the analysis tends to be mathematically intensive and can be problematic even for powerful computers when the sample size is large and the sampling scheme is complex.

For most disease-related traits, the collection of families for segregation analysis begins with a proband. Correct specification of ascertainment of families is critical to the proper interpretation of segregation analysis because the likelihood of the data is dependent on the collection of the data (randomly ascertained, identified through a single proband, multiple affected relatives, etc.). Once families are identified, the data required for segregation analysis are relatively simple to collect, consisting of pedigree structure, disease state, current age, and age at diagnosis (for those affected). The basic format of data collection is the same whether a qualitative (disease) or a quantitative (continuous) trait is analyzed.

The basis for the computation intensity in segregation analysis is the large number of parameters that must be simultaneously estimated (in an iterative fashion) to fit a particular hypothesis. Such parameters include an estimate of the frequency of the disease allele, the transmission probabilities (of a hypothetical allele from a parent to a child), the genotype-specific means (for quantitative traits) or genotype-specific penetrance (for qualitative traits), the variance within genotypes, and any residual familial correlation not accounted for by the Mendelian locus (Fig. 3–4, Jarvik, 1998). The transmission probabilities denote the probability that a parent with a given genotype produces the high-risk allele. In the case of a single locus with two alleles, *A* and *a*, with *a* denoted as the high-risk allele, the transmission probabilities for parents with *AA*, *Aa*, and *aa* genotypes are 1.0, 0.5, and 0.0, respectively. Other mechanisms can produce non-Mendelian transmission probabilities (Weiss, 1995). For example, an environmental model can be constructed such that the transmission probabilities are all equal. Thus, the phenotype of the child is unrelated to the phenotype of the parents.

The analytical strategy is to compare how well various hypotheses (genetic and nongenetic) fit the observed family data using likelihood ratio tests. A general model is fit to the data with the fewest possible restrictions to the parameters. Models of Mendelian and non-Mendelian inheritance are constructed by restrictions placed on genetic parameters. For example, the Mendelian model would constrain the transmission probabilities to that expected under Mendelian transmission and have an absence of a polygenic effect, estimating those parameters relating to genotype-specific penetrance. The polygenic model would allow estimation of the heritability, in the absence of a single Mendelian locus (no transmission of a single susceptibility locus). Similarly, environmental models of susceptibility would

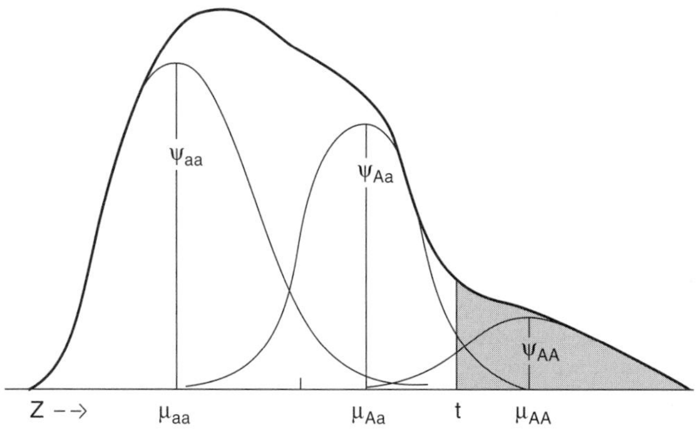

Fig. 3–4. Genetic liability model (*Source:* Modified from NE Morton, Outline of Genetic Epidemiology, Karger, 1982, p. 79.)

Table 3–3. Segregation Analysis of Human Lung Cancer

Parameter	Mendelian Dominant	Mendelian Recessive	Mendelian Codominant	No Major Type	Environmental Factors	General model
τ_{AA}	(1.0)	(1.0)	(1.0)	—	0.037	0.81
τ_{AB}	(0.5)	(0.5)	(0.5)	—	0.037	0.55
τ_{BB}	(0.0)	(0.0)	(0.0)	—	0.037	0.00
q_A	0.045	0.020	0.052	—	0.037	0.049
α	13.76	17.48	18.34	13.47	21.67	18.41
β_{AA}	−10.42	−9.87	−6.60	−10.80	−7.17	−6.57
β_{AB}	−10.42	−14.12	−15.03	−10.80	−11.56	−12.34
β_{BB}	−13.86	−14.12	−15.03	−10.80	−17.01	−15.03
γ	0.60	0.26	0.28	0.28	0.23	0.27
pk-yrs	0.61	0.82	0.87	0.66	1.09	0.88
pk-yrs^2	−0.071	−0.089	−0.10	−0.079	−0.12	−0.10
χ^2	8.48	9.77	0.21	19.44	12.41	—
df	3–4	3–4	2–3	5–6	2–3	—
p	<.075	<.044	>.90	<.004	<.006	—

Nos. in parentheses indicate parameters fixed at that value.
Source: Sellers et al., 1991a

have an absence of Mendelian locus parameters (allele frequency, transmission probabilities) and polygenic parameters (heritabilites). One then usually compares the goodness-of-fit of the general, Mendelian, environmental, and polygenic hypotheses. If the Mendelian model is favored, then further evaluation can be done to discriminate between Mendelian dominant, recessive, and codominant patterns of inheritance.

An example of segregation analysis is shown in Table 3–3) for lung cancer (Sellers et al., 1991a). Probands for the study were identified from a completely ascertained collection of lung cancer cases (over a 4-year period) in one of ten southern Louisiana parishes. The data for the analyses were based on three-generation pedigrees that were developed from interview and record review. The data on cancer status, age at onset, tobacco consumption, and employment history were obtained and verified. Using the regressive model implementation of complex segregation analysis, the pattern of lung cancer in these families was substantially explained by the Mendelian inheritance of a rare autosomal gene that produces an earlier age at onset. This is determined by the failure to reject the model with codominant inheritance ($p > .90$) as being significantly different from the general model. Using the parameters of the codominant model, the frequency of the risk allele is low (0.052), with nearly 28% of the population ($\gamma = 0.28$) ultimately expected to develop lung cancer. Using the estimated effects of the risk allele on age at onset (βs) and the pack-years of smoking (pk-yrs and pk-yrs^2), the cumulative risks of lung cancer to the putative gene and smoking could be obtained at specific ages.

A critical issue in complex segregation analysis is proper correction for ascertainment. Earlier in this chapter it was stressed that population-based sampling of cases should be performed. If it is determined that cases are more likely to have affected relatives than controls and the clustering is independent of measured risk factors, then the entire collection of cases (and their family members) should be subjected to segregation analysis, not just the subset of families with multiple affected members. Indeed, if one picks families because they "look genetic" and then performs a complex segregation analysis on the nonrandomly ascertained families, one is likely to prove the investigator's ability to recognize an autosomal form of transmission. The issue of correction for ascertainment represents a topic that is in need of additional research (Wijsman and Amos, 1997).

GENE MAPPING

Definition and Approaches

The ability to map disease susceptibility genes is a relatively recent development. The advances made in molecular genetics and human gene mapping have allowed a concerted effort to be made to map and identify genes that increase risk for diseases with significant public health impact. Until recently, only a small number of syndromes that focus on the extremes of common disease have been mapped, and fewer still have resulted in the relevant genes being identified. The ability to map and identify genes will contribute to our understanding of common disease in several ways:

1. Identification of specific chromosome loci confirms the hypothesis that specific mutations are involved in the etiology of common disease.
2. The diagnosis and recognition of subtypes of disease may be clarified.
3. Early stages of the disease may be detected, along with identification of those "at risk" who could be candidates for behavioral or medical intervention.
4. Knowledge of genetic risk may be incorporated to increase our ability to identify environmental risk factors and the manner in which they interact.

Data analysis for mapping disease susceptibility genes typically proceeds along two approaches: linkage studies and disequilibrium studies. Linkage studies can be separated into two methods: one uses maximum likelihood methods that are based on an assumed fully specified mode of inheritance (such as that obtained from complex segregation analyses); the other uses model-independent (no assumed mode of inheritance) methods. Disequilibrium studies are covered in the section on fine mapping.

Model-Based Linkage Studies

The maximum likelihood based LOD score approach has had tremendous historical success in mapping genes responsible for diseases determined by a single major locus. The fundamental approach is to track the inheritance of disease in families simultaneously with a specific genetic marker, using the expectation of disease status in family members that has been derived from the assumed genetic transmission model. Two statistics can be derived from the analysis of genetic data under the assumed model (Morton, 1955): the recombination fraction (θ), and the LOD score. The recombination fraction roughly equates crossing-over (in terms of proportion of recombinants) with genetic distance (in centiMorgan, cM, units) through a mapping function. The genetic distance can be roughly translated into physical distance (where 1 cM $\sim 10^6$ bp), although there are clearly "hot" and "cold" spots of recombination within even small chromosomal regions. Using the model-dependent approach and available protein polymorphisms, a number of important loci were mapped.

One complexity in identifying regions of the genome that may harbor disease susceptibility loci is that an apparently homogeneous disorder may, in fact, be due to different underlying genetic defects. The presence of phenotypic similarity in the presence of multiple genetic factors is considered "genetic heterogeneity." Application of model-based linkage approaches allow for the opportunity to discover heterogeneity as some families will appear "linked" to a candidate gene or genetic marker, while other families will appear "unlinked" to that same locus. Initially, methods were developed to determine the extent of genetic heterogeneity (independent loci contributing to the same phenotype) by using linkage admixture approaches (Morton, 1956; Smith, 1963).

The expansion of gene mapping began with the conceptualization of restriction fragment length polymorphisms (RFLPs) and their use in mapping disease susceptibility loci (Botstein et al., 1980). Using this technology, large numbers of highly polymorphic, anonymous DNA fragments that exhibit Mendelian inheritance could be followed in pedigrees. The fact that these DNA markers had many alleles (much more than typical protein polymorphisms) allowed each mating to be potentially informative for linkage. With identification of short tandem repeat polymorphisms (Weber and May, 1989), genetic marker number and polymorphic content further increased. The extent to which these genetic markers have proliferated, in parallel with technology development for laboratory procedures, has led to the development of protocols that allow the scanning of the entire human genome for linkage, with realistically high-quality, high-throughput genotyping. Using the additional information from tightly linked markers, multipoint methods emerged (Lathrop et al., 1984), which allowed even greater information content to be used in mapping disease susceptibility genes through model-dependent methods. Extensive coverage of linkage analysis—including biases, testing, evaluation, interpretation, and complexities (such as genetic heterogeneity)—is not possible in this chapter; however, these points have been well-described in the book by Ott (1991).

Model-Free Linkage Studies

Although traditional approaches to gene mapping have used families in which the trait (disease) is transmitted in a clear Mendelian fashion, common disease with late age at onset limits the usefulness of these methods. For complex traits, the inheritance pattern typically does not fit a simple single-gene model. The "parametric" method of assuming an underlying known genetic model for linkage therefore, may provide erroneous results (Risch et al., 1989; Risch and Guiffra, 1992). Further, many common diseases clearly exhibit familial aggregation, yet have no simple single gene model of transmission. In response to the failure to identify families with clear Mendelian transmission and in recognition of the need to develop methods for genetic analysis for adult disorders (often without parental data), research on affected relative (e.g., affected sibling) pair designs flourished. This method, originally attributed to Penrose (1953) and expanded by others (Haseman and Elston, 1972; Risch, 1990; Weeks and Lange, 1992; Kruglyak and Lander, 1995; Blangero and Almasy, 1997), is designed to detect linkage without the specification of an underlying genetic model (Fig. 3–5).

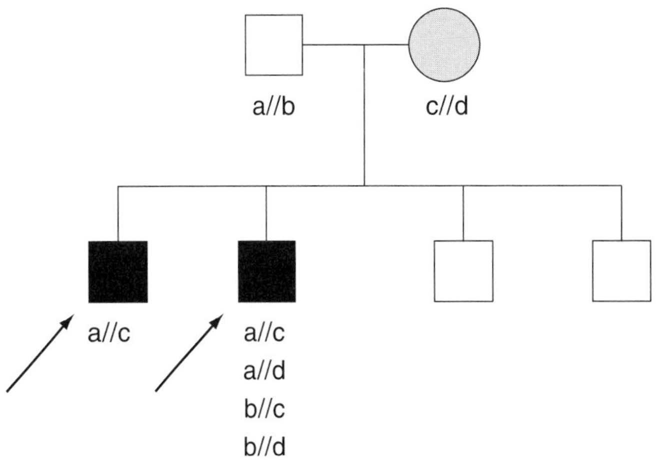

Fig. 3–5. Affected sib-pair family design. Filled boxes represent affected sibs, open symbols unaffected relatives, and arrows indicate probands.

In the context of linkage using relative pairs, the statistical test is essentially one of the deviations from expectation in relative pairs for individual genetic marker loci (or across the loci in a multipoint test). The probability (or the likelihood) for a collection of relative (e.g., sibling) pairs can be written as a function of the probability of relative pairs sharing alleles identical by descent at the marker locus. This probability is contrasted with the expectation under the null hypothesis of "no linkage"; the ratio of the maximized likelihood to the likelihood based on expectation of no linkage represents the test statistic, where large values of this statistic are indicative of linkage.

Deviations in sharing under linkage for concordant affected relative pairs are in the direction of an excess of sharing two alleles identical by descent. Deviations in sharing under linkage for discordant pairs (one affected, one unaffected) are in the direction of sharing no alleles. Thus, it has been noted that the collection of affected relative pairs with unaffected relatives may result in a complementary, and perhaps more powerful, analysis than the use of affected-only sib pairs (Rogus and Krolewski, 1996).

The robust model–independent methods have been implemented over the last decade with increasing success in the identification of regions of interest in the human genome. There is growing experience in using these methods, and while the effort to positionally clone genes for complex disease has yet to meet with widespread success, identification of candidate regions in which to search have been fruitful. These advances include the first major breakthrough—Type 1 diabetes (Davies et al., 1994)—and have extended to Type 2 diabetes (Hanis et al., 1996), prostate cancer (Smith et al., 1996), end-stage renal disease (Bowden et al., 1997), asthma (CSGA, 1997), febrile convulsions (Johnson et al., 1998), and systemic lupus erythematosus (Gaffney et al., 1998), and others.

FINE MAPPING/POSITIONAL CLONING

Barring the possibility that a candidate gene or a polymorphic marker will give dramatic and overwhelming evidence of linkage in a region, further evaluation of selected chromosomal regions that show evidence of linkage will be a necessary component of a mapping study. One of the weaknesses of the affected relative pair design appears to be the high number of "false positive" regions detected for linkage, either through sporadic cases or phenocopies that may be abundant for common disease. In this context, those chromosomal regions that show evidence of linkage need to be evaluated in two stages to reduce the region and reduce expense. In the initial phase of a study, an accepted (and perhaps the only practical) approach to further evaluate a region for linkage centers on genotyping and evaluating additional markers. Fortunately, genetic maps of highly polymorphic microsatellites are becoming increasingly dense and well characterized (Fig. 3–6). Thus, this process should be relatively easy either from existing linkage maps or from radiation hybrid maps. Although it has often been difficult to obtain precise relative orders of markers in the same map region with different (and poorly) integrated maps, the availability of physical map information should reduce this concern in the future.

Linkage Disequilibrium

An additional analytical approach that can be used consists of evaluating markers in a narrow region for linkage disequilibrium. This type of analysis assumes that a founder mutation that resulted in an allele at a marker locus almost completely segregates with the disease-causing allele. Over time, crossing-over should occur proportionally with genetic distance, so that strength of disequilibrium relates to the distance from the marker (with associated allele) to the disease locus. Thus, linkage disequilibrium could reflect population admixture, a recent disease-causing mutation, or natural selection. Each of these features could cause disequilibrium to be established (in the case of population admixture or recent mutation) or maintained (in the case of natural selection) in the population.

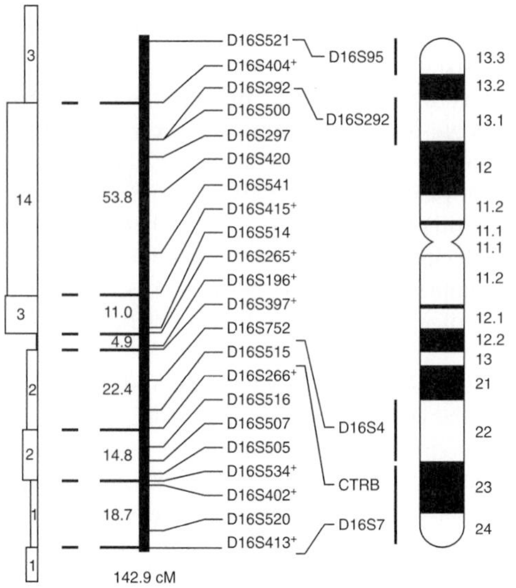

Fig. 3–6. Genetic map of human chromosome 16.

In the presence of true linkage, evidence for linkage disequilibrium would complement the results of nonparametric linkage analysis and could potentially narrow the region that contains a disease susceptibility gene. Association studies with genetic markers in regions of interest can be performed by implementing either a case-control or a family-based approach (Falk and Rubenstein, 1987; Spielman et al., 1993; Schaid, 1996). In these approaches, the genetic markers transmitted (and not transmitted) from parents to an offspring with disease (or a trait) are tabulated. Frequencies of transmitted and nontransmitted marker alleles are compared, with significant differences in transmission dependent upon both linkage and linkage disequilibrium.

Initial evaluation of regions with possible linkage can then be examined by detailed evaluation of the most promising regions based on disequilibrium studies. A number of outcomes are possible but, assuming the genome screen has been completed, there will likely be a number of candidate regions to focus on, some of which may still be false positive regions. In this case, multiple polymorphic markers or simple nucleotide polymorphisms (SNPs) in the candidate region can be evaluated in families, parent–child trios, or case-control sets.

Clearly, an advantage of the mapping approach by linkage disequilibrium is that limited family data are required for collection and analyses are performed under no assumptions of genetic transmission models. The ability to identify genes by linkage disequilibrium has yet to be fully explored. Further, the extent of disequilibrium over large genetic distances (over 1 cM) and resolving power (assuming current physical maps and possible genotyping errors) will likely vary by region in the genome and by the population studied.

Serendipity can play an important role in science. It is always possible that strong evidence for linkage will be identified with anonymous markers early in a study and a candidate region could quickly emerge. The next step in the mapping protocol would focus on efforts directed at identifying the gene involved. How exploitation of linkage is pursued at the physical mapping level would depend substantially on the nature of the linkage. Linkage to anonymous polymorphic loci would be a much more time-consuming and difficult positional cloning project. Once the candidate region has been reduced to a reasonable (approximately 1 Mb) size, the search for genes and their testing would follow what are, by now, relatively conventional paths with the same goals as enumerated for previously cloned candidate genes. There have been several encouraging reports that linkage disequilibrium can be seen even with complex diseases, so that, in addition to the increasingly comprehensive expressed sequence tag (EST) maps, disequilibrium would be a great asset in such a search. How difficult this would be to carry out an evaluation of a gene would depend on the size of the gene and its intron/exon organization, and could also potentially extend to evaluation of 5′ and 3′ noncoding regions.

COMPLICATIONS AND OPPORTUNITIES

The search for genes that form the basis of common disease will not be simple. There are advocates for both model-based and model-independent methods of linkage analysis, as well as for mapping by linkage disequilibrium methods. Proponents of the model-based methods correctly point out that this approach is more powerful than model-independent methods when the correct model is specified. Under incorrect specification of the genetic model, the model-based methods remain relatively robust, yet there remains concern that the estimates are biased and linkage results may be difficult to interpret; thus, for many investigators, model-independent methods are preferred.

For any method of analysis, several issues reduce the power of the study to identify disease-susceptibility genes. Many of these issues have been addressed by Ott (1991) but can be summarized in terms of misclassification—of the pedigree, the phenotype and the genotype—and the underlying disease etiology. Errors in pedigree structure (paternity and disease status) affect all methods, depending on the number and sizes of families ascertained. Paternity errors can often be detected using likelihood-based multipoint methods with highly polymorphic markers (Boehnke and Cox, 1997), while errors in phenotyping (disease status) can only be resolved by diligent review of records and clinical information. These errors in the phenotype increase misclassification rates and may increase recombination rates and reduce evidence for linkage. Variation in phenotype is another issue. In this case, affected status (asthma) could be defined by a threshold (on airways reactivity), in which the phenotype depends on seasonal exposure (high ragweed count in autumn increasing reactivity, low ragweed count in winter reducing reactivity). Genotyping errors also influence the power to detect genes for all methods.

Etiology of disease, and multiple means of disease causation, complicates attempts at mapping genes. The primary source of etiologic complexity is genetic heterogeneity. Genetic heterogeneity can be viewed as a geneticist's both bane and benefit. In the context of power to detect linkage for a common disease gene, heterogeneity at the genetic level will result in some families being viewed as linked, while others will be considered as not providing evidence for linkage (unlinked). These latter families may be "unlinked"—due either to a lack of polymorphism in the genetic marker locus for those families or to true heterogeneity. A statistical effect is that the result of heterogeneity increases the number of families (or relative pairs) that are required to detect linkage. In contrast, once linkage has been detected, the "linked" families can be contrasted with the "unlinked" families at the level of phenotype (clinical information). This latter investigation may shed light on the possible mechanism or target of the linked locus.

The use of relative pairs, rather than families, for tracking complex disease genes results in a small dilemma. Although they are easier to collect, relative pairs may no longer have sufficient information to allow for "family-by-family" detection of linkage (it is only as an aggregate that linkage to genetic markers can be made). Thus, if heterogeneity is important, possible subsets of loci could be missed (false negative effects). Recent developments for detecting linkage in the presence of heterogeneity are made difficult for complex disease, as both multiple genes and environmental interactions with genetic susceptibility may play important roles in susceptibility.

A second complication is replication of results. Given multiple loci that may contribute to disease, there is potential that the one (of ten) genes with large effect in population A is different from the one (of ten) genes of importance in population B. Even though both loci may contribute to common disease, the size of the effect in different populations may differ. One possible approach could be to evaluate the individual contributions at a locus, based on sharing alleles within specific regions, so that excess (but not significant) sharing at a locus would be consistent with significant excess sharing for a different population. Comparison of clinical characteristics in these groups may provide some insight into the basic mechanism underlying the form of disease under study.

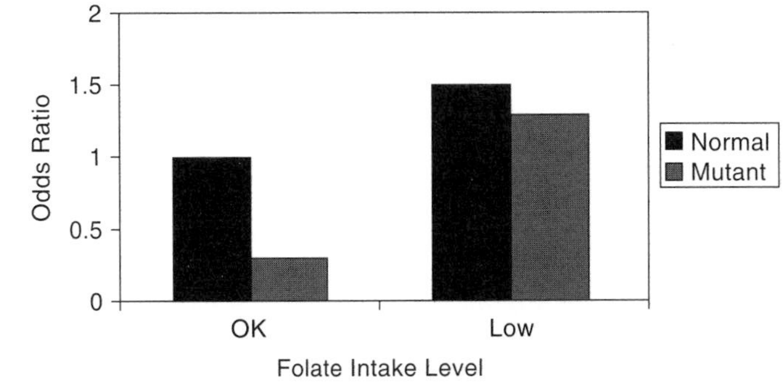

Fig. 3–7. MTHFR, diet, and colorectal cancer risk.

Finally, no discussion is complete without reference to interaction between genetic and environmental risk factors. The occurrence of a common disease in an individual is unlikely due to any one genetic factor or any one environmental factor. Rather, it is likely due to a complex interaction of genes and exposures that initiate a series of mutational events in target tissue that progresses to a clinically identifiable event (Fig. 3–7). Although the number of possible combinations of exposures and mutations in candidate genes are conceptually large, there may be a critical sequence of events that is required to progress from one "state" to another.

The approach to the study of interactions is statistical in concept, yet appreciation in genetic epidemiology is growing. Although one may consider evaluating gene–environment (or gene–gene) interaction in the context of a family study, most of the development of methods has been in the scope of a case-control study (Khoury and Flanders, 1996; Ottman, 1996; Beaty, 1998). In this approach, each candidate locus can be analyzed individually as a potential modifier of disease risk. In order to evaluate the relationships between inherited susceptibility (genotype) and environmental exposures (diet, physical activity, etc.), several strategies can be employed. One approach is stratification by genotype at each candidate locus, with analysis of "case" status with the second genetic (or environmental) exposure. For dichotomous exposures, this reduces to a comparison of contingency tables within genotype strata. Another approach uses logistic regression for continuous risk factors within genotype strata. Similarly, multivariate logistic regression can be used to predict group membership (case versus control status) based on age, sex, environmental risk factors that appear significant in univariate analyses, and genotype(s), with first-order interaction terms of genotype with environment and gene1 with gene2. Similar logistic regression methods will be used to address genotype–environment interaction effects on the continuous phenotypes. Recent efforts have been able to detect interactions between candidate genes and risk factors for common diseases (Hwang et al., 1995; Aragaki et al., 1997). Innovations in methodology and advances in molecular genetic technology illustrate the promise of the future in gene mapping.

FUTURE DIRECTIONS

What does the future hold? The future is full of mysteries and opportunities and, based on our biased view, may present a new approach to improving our public health and reducing disease risk. We can assume that the genetic map will be continually improved and genes will be continually discovered. Single nucleotide polymorphisms (SNPs) are rapidly becoming critical resources in gene mapping. It is estimated that the majority of genomic variation can be attributed to SNPs (Altshuler et al., 2000). A dense SNP map (including information on linkage disequilibrium across SNPs) could be used to scan the genome for disease-bearing haplotypes. This approach could greatly facilitate candidate region reduction. Improved high-throughput sequence analysis, coupled with the available public human DNA sequence of the human genome (Nierman et al., 2001; International Human Genome Sequencing Consortium, 2001), should facilitate the search for complex disease susceptibility genes.

We can assume that major epidemiologic risk factors will be identified. Thus, an obvious step will be the integration of the genetic and epidemiologic data (both as main effects and interaction effects) to form a "common disease clinic." This "clinic" will not only collect risk factor information, blood for DNA analysis, and behavioral data, but also will allow examination of an individual's risk for common disease. Using this approach, the "pre-patient" can be enrolled in intervention trials, behavior modification therapy sessions, or, if the risk is not amenable to environmental manipulation, gene therapy. This scenario, while futuristic, may be based on the work being conducted at this time in the examination of genes and environmental risk factors that predispose to disease.

REFERENCES

Altshuler D, Pollara VJ, Cowles CR, Van Etten WJ, Baldwin J, Linton L, Lander ES: An SNP map of the human genome generated by reduced representation shotgun sequencing. Nature 2000; 407:513–516.

Aragaki CC, Greenland S, Probst-Hensch N, Haile RW: Hierarchical modeling of gene–environment interactions: estimating NAT2 genotype-specific dietary effects on adenomatous polyps. Cancer Epidemiol Biomarkers Prev 1997; 6:307–314.

Beaty TH: Using association studies to test for gene–environment interaction in asthma and other complex diseases. Clin Exp Allergy 1998; 28(Suppl 1):68–73.

Blangero J, Almasy L: Multipoint oligogenic linkage analysis of quantitative traits. Genet Epidemiol 1997; 14:959–964.

Boehnke M, Cox NJ: Accurate inference of relationships in sib-pair linkage studies. Am J Hum Genet 1997; 61:423–429.

Botstein D, White RL, Skolnick M, Davis RW: Construction of a genetic linkage map in man using restriction fragment length polymorphisms. Am J Hum Genet 1980; 32:314–331.

Bowden DW, Sale M, Howard TD, Qadri A, Spray BJ, Rothschild CB, Akots G, Rich SS, Freedman BI: Linkage of genetic markers on human chromosomes 20 and 12 to NIDDM in Caucasian families with a history of diabetic nephropathy. Diabetes 1997; 46:882–886.

Brass LM, Hartigan PM, Page WF, Concato J: Importance of cerebrovascular disease in studies of myocardial infarction. Stroke 1996; 27:1173–1176.

Busjahn A, Faulhaber HD, Viken RJ, Rose RJ, Luft FC: Genetic influences on blood pressure with the cold-pressor test: a twin study. J Hypertens 1996; 14:1195–1199.

CSGA (Collaborative Study on the Genetics of Asthma): A genome-wide search for asthma susceptibility loci in ethnically diverse populations. Nat Genet 1997; 15:389–392.

Collins FS: Positional cloning moves from perditional to traditional. Nat Genet 1995; 9:347–350.

Davies JL, Kawaguchi Y, Bennett ST, Copeman JB, Cordell HJ, Pritchard LE, Reed PW, Gough SC, Jenkins SC, Palmer SM, et al: A genome-wide search for human type 1 diabetes susceptibility genes. Nature 1994; 371:130–136.

Elston RC: Segregation analysis. Adv Hum Genet 1981; 11:63–120.

Falk CT, Rubinstein P: Haplotype relative risks: an easy reliable way to construct a proper control sample for risk calculations. Ann Hum Genet 1987; 51:227–233.

Fisher RA: Lung cancer and cigarettes? Nature 1958; 182:108.

Friedlander Y, Austin MA, Newman B, Edwards K, Mayer-Davis EI, King MC: Heritability of longitudinal changes in coronary heart disease risk factors in women twins. Am J Hum Genet 1997; 60:1502–1512.

Gaffney PM, Kearns GM, Shark KB, Malmgren ML, Ortmann WA, Selby SA, Rohlf KE, Ockenden TC, Messner PR, King RA, et al.: A genome screen of systemic lupus erythematosus sib-pair families identifies potential susceptibility loci on chromosomes 6, 14, 16 and 20. Proc Natl Acad Sci USA 1998; 95:14875–14879.

Hanis CL, Boerwinkle E, Chakraborty R, Ellsworth DL, Concannon P, Stirling B, Morrison VA, Wapelhorst B, Spielman RS, Gogolin-Ewens KJ et al.: A genome-wide search for human non-insulin-dependent (type 2) diabetes genes reveals a major susceptibility locus on chromosome 2. Nat Genet 1996; 13:161–166.

Hanson B, Tuna N, Bouchard T, Heston L, Eckert E, Lykken D, Segal N, Rich SS: Genetic factors in the electrocardiogram and heart rate of twins reared apart and together. Am J Cardiol 1989; 63:606–609.

Haseman JK, Elston RC: The investigation of linkage between a quantitative trait and a marker locus. Behav Genet 1972; 2:3–19.

Hasstedt S, Cartwright P: PAP: Pedigree Analysis Package. Salt Lake City: Department of Medical Biophysics and Computing, University of Utah, 1981.

Hawkes CH: Twin studies in diabetes mellitus. Diabet Med 1997; 14:347–352.

Hwang SJ, Beaty TH, Panny SR, Street NA, Joseph JM, Gordon S, McIntosh I, Francomano CA: Association study of transforming growth factor alpha (TGF alpha) TaqI polymorphism and oral clefts: indication of gene–environment interaction in a population-based sample of infants with birth defects. Am J Epidemiol 1995; 141:629–636.

International Human Genome Sequencing Consortium: Initial sequencing and analysis of the human genome. Nature 2001; 409:860–901.

Jarvik GP: Complex segregation analyses: uses and limitations. Am J Hum Genet 1998; 63:942–946.

Johnson EW, Dubovsky J, Rich SS, O'Donovan CA, Orr HT, Anderson VE, Gil-Nagel A, Ahmann P, Dokken CG, Schneider DT, Weber JL: Evidence for a novel gene for familial febrile convulsions, FEB2, linked to chromosome 19p in an extended family from the Midwest. Hum Mol Genet 1998; 7:63–67.

Khoury MJ, Flanders WD: Nontraditional epidemiologic approaches in the analysis of gene–environment interaction: case-control studies with no controls. Am J Epidemiol 1996; 144:207–213.

Krousel T, Garcas N, Rothschild H: Familial clustering of mesothelioma: a report on three affected persons in one family. Am J Prev Med 1986; 2:186–188.

Kruglyak L, Lander ES: Complete multipoint sib-pair analysis of qualitative and quantitative traits. Am J Hum Genet 1995; 57:439–454.

Lalouel J-M, Morton NE: Complex segregation analysis with pointers. Hum Hered 1981; 31:312–321.

Lathrop GM, Laouel J-M, Julier C, Ott J: Strategies for multilocus linkage analysis in humans. Proc Natl Acad Sci USA 1984; 81:3443–3446.

Mattson ME, Pollack ES, Cullen JW: What are the odds that smoking will kill you? Am J Public Health 1987; 77:425–431.

Mayer EJ, Newman B, Austin MA, Zhang D, Quesenberry CP, Edwards K, Selby JV: Genetic and environmental influences on insulin levels and the insulin resistance syndrome: an analysis of women twins. Am J Epidemiol 1996; 143:323–332.

Meyer JM, Breitner JC: Multiple threshold model for the onset of Alzheimer's disease in the NAS-NRC twin panel. Am J Med Genet 1998; 81:92–97.

Morton NE: Sequential tests for the detection of linkage. Am J Hum Genet 1955; 7:277–318.

Morton NE: The detection and estimation of linkage between the genes for elliptocytosis and the Rh blood type. Am J Hum Genet 1956; 8:80–91.

Nance WA, Corey LA: Genetic models for the analysis of data from the families of identical twins. Genetics 1976; 83:811–826.

Ooi WL, Elston RC, Chen VW, et al.: Increased familial risk for lung cancer. J Natl Cancer Inst 1986; 76:217–222.

Ott J: Analysis of Human Genetic Linkage. Baltimore: Johns Hopkins University Press, 1991.

Ottman R: Gene–environment interaction: definitions and study designs. Prev Med 1996; 25:764–770.

Penrose LS: The general sib-pair linkage test. Ann Eugenics 1953; 18:120–144.

Raiha I, Kaprio J, Koskenvuo M, Rajala T, Sourander L: Alzheimer's disease in Finnish twins. Lancet 1996; 347:573–578.

Rich SS, Weitkamp LR, Barbosa J: Genetic heterogeneity of insulin-dependent (type 1) diabetes mellitus: evidence from a study of extended haplotypes. Am J Hum Genet 1984; 36:1015–1023.

Risch N: Linkage strategies for genetically complex traits: II. The power of affected relative pairs. Am J Hum Genet 1990; 46:229–241.

Risch N, Claus E, Guiffra L: Linkage and mode of inheritance in complex traits. Genet Epidemiol 1989; (Suppl):183–188.

Risch N, Guiffra L: Model misspecification and multipoint linkage analysis. Hum Hered 1992; 42:77–92.

Rogus JJ, Krolewski AS: Using discordant sib pairs to map loci for qualitative traits with high sibling recurrence risk. Am J Hum Genet 1996; 59:1376–1381.

Russell MW, Law I, Sholinsky P, Fabsitz RR: Heritability of ECG measurements in adult male twins. J Electrocardiol 1998; 30(Suppl):64–68.

SAGE (Statistical Analysis for Genetic Epidemiology). Cleveland: Department of Epidemiology and Biostatistics, Case Western Reserve University, 1994.

Schaid DJ: General score tests for associations of genetic markers with disease using cases and their parents. Genet Epidemiol 1996; 13:423–450.

Sellers TA, Bailey-Wilson JE, Elston RC, Wilson AF, Elston GZ, Ooi WL, Rothschild H: Evidence for Mendelian inheritance in the pathogenesis of lung cancer. JNCI 1990a; 82:1272–1279.

Sellers TA, Kushi LH, Potter JD: Can dietary intake patterns account for the familial aggregation of disease? Evidence from adult siblings living apart. Genet Epidemiol 1991b; 8:105–112.

Smith CAB: Testing for heterogeneity of the recombination fraction in human pedigrees. Ann Hum Genet 1963; 27:175–182.

Smith JR, Freije D, Carpten JD, Gronberg H, Xu J, Isaacs SD, Brownstein MJ, Bova GS, Guo Hm Bujnovszky P, Nusskern DR, et al.: Major susceptibility locus for prostate cancer on chromosome 1 suggested by a genome-wide search. Science 1996; 274:1371–1374.

Spielman RS, McGinnis RE, Ewens WJ: Transmission test for linkage disequilibrium: the insulin gene region and insulin dependent diabetes mellitus (IDDM). Am J Hum Genet 1993; 52:506–516.

Tellegen A, Lykken DT, Bouchard TJ, Wilcox KJ, Segal NL, Rich SS: Personality similarity in twins reared apart and together. J Pers Soc Psychol 1988; 54:1031–1039.

Thompson E: Monte Carlo programs for pedigree analysis: 1990–1993. Seattle: Department of Statistics, University of Washington, 1994.

Vachon CM, Sellers TA, Kushi LH, Folsom AR: Familial correlation of dietary intakes among postmenopausal women. Genet Epidemiol 1998; 15:553–563.

Vandenberg SG: Assortative mating, or who marries whom? Behav Genet 1972; 2:127–157.

van den Bree MB, Schieken RM, Moskowitz WB, Eaves LJ: Genetic regulation of hemodynamic variables during dynamic exercise: the MCV twin study. Circulation 1996; 94:1864–1869.

Venter JC, Adams MD, Myers EW, Li PW, Mural RJ, Sutton GG, Smith HO, Yandell M, Evans CA, Holt RA, et al.: The sequence of the human genome. Science 2001; 291:1304–1351.

Weber JL, May PE: Abundant class of human DNA polymorphisms which can be typed using the polymerase chain reaction. Am J Hum Genet 1989; 44:388–396.

Weeks DE, Lange K: A multilocus extension of the affected-pedigree-member method of linkage analysis. Am J Hum Genet 1992; 50:859–868.

Weiss KM: Genetic variation and human disease: principles and evolutionary approaches. Cambridge: Cambridge University Press, 1995: 69–115.

Wijsman EM, Amos CI: Genetic analysis of simulated oligogenic traits in unclear and extended pedigrees: summary of GAW10 contributions. Genet Epidemiol 1997; 14:719–735.

4 Evolution of Human Genetic Diseases

JARED DIAMOND AND JEROME I. ROTTER

What comfort is it to me that cause follows effect? I must have justice, or I'll destroy myself. All religions are based on this longing, and I'm a believer. But then there are the children: what am I to do about them? That's the question I can't answer. It's beyond all comprehension why children should suffer to pay for a divine system of justice. Justice isn't worth the tears of even a single tortured child. God demands too high an admission price for His divine system. And so, I respectfully give back to God my entrance ticket.

(Dostoevsky, *The Brothers Karamazov*)

Genetic diseases uniquely offend us. Of course we grieve when someone dies for other reasons, such as from an accident or a contracted illness. But we routinely try to understand such events by asking whether the victim did anything, or neglected to do anything, that led to his death. In genetic diseases that path to understanding is foreclosed. We cannot impute responsibility to the victim, because the cause of her death was present at the time of conception. Someone with a genetic disease or predisposition is a walking time bomb, programmed to explode (or at risk of exploding) at any time from infancy until late adulthood. We acknowledge that intervention, from treatment to prevention, is now possible for many genetic diseases and is certainly possible at some level for most of the diseases reviewed in this volume. However, in the case of many genetic diseases, there is still nothing that the victim can do to prevent the outcome. Why does God or fate play these supremely dirty tricks on us?

Our sense that the blow is undeserved becomes compounded by our sense of its meaninglessness. The death seems to be nothing more than the consequence of a purposeless genetic mistake, a mutation blindly passed on to a child who will be summarily disposed of by the implacable workings of natural selection. We can accept the notion of a mistake when we buy a pen that proves defective and that we have to discard in the trash. But we can't face saying, "My child was a mistake, so she ended up in the trash, and there's no more meaning to it than that."

At the root of this anguish lie difficult, controversial, still largely unresolved scientific questions. Given the overwhelming evidence that natural selection's filter tends to eliminate deleterious genes, then how is it that genetic diseases or harmful predispositions manage to persist? We often assume that many deleterious genes present at high frequency are sustained by counterbalancing natural selection, but very few such selective effects have been demonstrated convincingly in humans: are they really as widespread as we assume? Most of those likely selective effects are expected to be small: by what technique shall we succeed in demonstrating them convincingly? In many cases the founder effect has been proposed as an explanation alternative to counterbalancing selection: how can these two explanations be reliably distinguished? Even in the best-documented example of counterbalancing selection, that involving variant hemoglobins and malaria, why was hemoglobin S the variant that rose to high frequency in Africa, when hemoglobin E is instead the variant serving apparently the same function in tropical southeast Asia? Evolutionary biologists attribute many otherwise apparently deleterious traits of animal species to sexual selection, but this possible interpretation has been almost completely ignored in the medical genetic literature: what paradoxes of medical genetics might it resolve? Are effects of natural selection on old postreproductive people still very important? We believe so, but most medical geneticists (including many of our co-authors!) routinely dismiss this possibility, in the mistaken belief that genes acting after the age of reproduction cannot possibly have major selective consequences.

The evolution of human genetic diseases constitutes an important interface between the fields of evolutionary biology, medical genetics, and human history, but it has received much less attention than it deserves. The subject is important for several reasons, only one of which is for the understanding of the diseases themselves. In addition, an evolutionary perspective on human genes provides important insights into human history, as markers of prehistoric population expansions such as those of Bantu-speaking blacks over subequatorial Africa, of Polynesians into the Pacific, and of other expansions. Finally, just as evolutionary biology can illuminate medical genetics, so too can medical genetics illuminate evolutionary biology, because we know far more about humans than about any other animal or plant species. Except for a few endangered species with tiny remnant populations, such as the California condor, there is no other species of which all living individuals are named, for most of whose individuals the purported parentage is recorded, and for many of whose individuals the deep ancestry going back many generations is also known. Much is known about the human genome, and factors that are potentially of selective value have been intensively studied because of their medical importance. A dramatic example of the convergence of knowledge of human history and modern molecular biology is the recent demonstration that Jewish males who have the surname Cohen (and variants thereof), and who by biblical history are descended from Aaron (the brother of Moses) and constitute the hereditary priest class (termed the Cohanim), are indeed substantially more related at their Y chromosome to each other than they are to other Jewish males (Skorecki et al., 1997; Thomas et al., 1998). This distinction between Cohanim and other Jewish males occurs in both the Sephardi and Ashkenazi and is estimated to have originated some 3000 years ago, early in the first Temple period (Thomas et al., 1998).

We begin this chapter by discussing deleterious genes that became common locally and transiently as a result of either the founder effect or genetic drift. The rest of the chapter concerns genes for whose frequency the founder effect and drift do not provide adequate explanations and for which one must instead suspect operation of counterbalancing selective factors. We organize the discussion of counterbalancing selection in a series of categories, depending on who receives the selective benefit and who receives the penalty: genes that are bad for homozygotes but good for heterozygotes; genes that are bad for one sex but good for the opposite sex; genes that are bad for postnates but good for prenates; genes that are bad for the old but good for the young; and genes that are bad under one lifestyle but good under another lifestyle for the same individual. We then discuss the selective benefits that result from protection against infectious agents mediated by blood groups, and those that are not mediated by blood groups. Finally, we conclude by drawing attention to major unsolved questions.

Some readers may initially be put off by this chapter, regarding it as overly speculative. Yes, it is speculative: far more examples of counterbalancing selection probably remain to be identified than the few cases that have been convincingly established to date. Our motives in writing this chapter are to call attention to the treasure trove of unexplored problems that await those interested in the evolution of human genetic diseases.

FOUNDER EFFECT (AND GENETIC DRIFT)

In evolutionary biology the concept of the founder effect refers to "the establishment of a new population by a few original founders (in an extreme case, by a single fertilized female) which carry only a small fraction of the total genetic variation of the parental population" (Mayr, 1963). The resulting new population thereby instantly becomes genetically different from the parental population. A related phenomenon, genetic drift, has been defined as "random fluctuations in gene frequencies in effectively small populations" (Dobzhansky, 1951). That is, reduced genetic variation of the new population compared to the parental population is likely to arise not only at the moment of founding but also over succeeding generations, while the new population remains effectively small.

Although the founder effect is often thought to be important in speciation, it has rarely been observed directly in wild animal species, for the obvious reason that pedigrees of all individuals in an expanding animal population are generally unknown. In this respect, no other species can match the advantages of *Homo sapiens*, as already mentioned. Studies of human genetic disorders have documented the evolutionary significance of the founder effect in a way that would be impossible for other species.

As an example, consider the Afrikaner population of South Africa, which was founded by one shipload of immigrants from Holland in 1652 and subsequently augmented by modest additional numbers of immigrants over succeeding decades until immigration effectively ceased in the early 1700s. As documented by church registers, those early immigrants produced large families (often of 10 or more children), underwent a population explosion, and contributed disproportionately to the modern Afrikaner population, which now numbers in the millions. Some original settlers left tens of thousands of descendants alive today, and over 1 million living Afrikaners bear the names of one or another of only 20 original settlers (Botha and Beighton, 1983).

Among the founding immigrants on that first ship in the year 1652 were one carrier of the gene for Huntington's chorea and two carriers of lipoid proteinosis, while carriers of porphyria variegata and familial colonic polyposis arrived a few decades later (Dean, 1972; Botha and Beighton, 1983). In porphyria variegata, an autosomal dominant defect in the enzyme protoporphyrinogen oxidase, carriers develop a severe and sometimes lethal reaction to barbiturate anesthetics, but the condition was relatively benign and selectively neutral until the advent of modern medicine. All traceable Afrikaner carriers today prove to be descendants of one couple, Gerritt Jansz and Ariaantje Jacobs, who emigrated from Holland in 1685 and 1688, respectively (Dean, 1972). Now, more than 30,000 of their Afrikaner descendants carry the gene that they brought—resulting in a far higher incidence in South Africa than in Holland, due to this sampling accident. All South African cases of lipoid proteinosis, an autosomal recessive disorder that is more frequent in South Africa than anywhere else in the world, are traceable to one brother and sister who arrived in 1652 (Botha and Beighton, 1983). One of the brother's 5 children and 5 of the sister's 13 children carried the gene, as did 8 of the 17 offspring of the sister's eldest son, thereby propelling the gene toward its modern frequency. As for Huntington's chorea, a lethal autosomal dominant disease, most Afrikaner cases derived from a Dutch man who arrived in 1652 and his German wife who arrived in 1668.

Although the founder effect has been particularly easy to document among Afrikaners because of their church registers and interest in genealogy, there are many examples in other South African populations and in other parts of the world. In South Africa's Cape Colored population, the high frequency of an autosomal dominant bone disease (osteodental dysplasia) that causes complete loss of teeth by age 20 stems from one polygamous Chinese immigrant named Arnold who, aided by seven wives, transmitted the syndrome to at least 70 of 356 traceable descendants (Jackson, 1951). Hexadactyly has a high incidence (over 100 reported cases) among the Amish population of Lancaster County, Pennsylvania, because the few founders of that community included a certain Mr. Samuel King, and either Mr. King or his wife happened to carry the gene for hexadactyly (McKusick, 1979). Hereditary tyrosinemia is extremely rare in most of the world (less than 1 case in 100,000 newborns), but in the French Canadian population in the remote Chicoutimi area of Quebec Province it affects 1 in every 685 newborns, and an astonishingly high proportion of the population (estimated as 1 in 14) carries the gene as heterozygotes (Laberge, 1969; Bergeron et al., 1974; De Braekeleer and Larochelle, 1990; Mitchell et al., 1995). The historical background is that the Chicoutimi region was settled in the 1840s by a few dozen families who migrated north from Quebec's Charlevoix County, but few other settlers followed because of Chicoutimi's isolation, and most people living there today are descendants of those original families. The pedigrees of all of Chicoutimi's tyrosinemia patients have been traced back to just one couple, Louis Gagné and his wife Marie Michel, who emigrated to Quebec from France in the mid-seventeenth century. Evidently, either Louis or Marie carried the gene for tyrosinemia and passed it on to some of their nine children and uncounted grandchildren, at least two of whom moved to Charlevoix. Since only a small number of people from Charlevoix moved in turn to Chicoutimi, today's Chicoutimi population is rather inbred: the parents of the tyrosinemia patients share on the average as many genes as second cousins would. Hence it happens not infrequently that both a husband and wife are carriers of the Gagné/Michel curse, and both pass it on to their child, who is homozygous and consequently suffers from tyrosinemia.

These examples can be multiplied almost indefinitely. All known cases of Huntington's chorea on the island of Mauritius are descendants of a French nobleman's grandson, Pierre Dagnet d'Assigne de Bourbon (Hayden et al., 1981), while more than 500 cases in Australia are descended from one English widow called Ms. Cundick, who emigrated to Australia in 1858 with her 13 children by two marriages and passed the gene to offspring of both marriages (Hayden, 1981). The sixteenth-century population explosion that settled Central Finland as a result of small numbers of immigrants from the coast scattering over the interior bequeathed to modern Finns a characteristic legacy of several dozen genetic disorders, many of them still geographically concentrated in one or a few areas of central Finland (Norio et al., 1973; Sajantila et al., 1996; de la Chapelle and Wright, 1998; Peltonen et al., 1999; Peltonen, 2000). Achromatopsia (complete color blindness) is relatively common among inhabitants of Pingelap Island in Micronesia, much of whose population was "refounded" by the hereditary chief after the original population had been reduced to about 20 by a typhoon and subsequent starvation in the year 1775 (Sacks, 1996). At least some of the well-known genetic disorders of the Ashkenazi Jews may be attributable to the founder effect (Risch et al., 1995), although we doubt that this explanation applies to all or even most of the disorders in that population. Other small populations with characteristic genetic disorders likely to stem from founder effects include the Pitcairn Islanders descended from the HMS *Bounty* mutineers and their Polynesian wives, St. Helena islanders (Eickhoff and Beighton, 1985: e.g., familial genu valgum), and the inhabitants of remote Tristan de Cunha Island in the South Atlantic Ocean (Beighton, 1976; e.g., retinitis pigmentosa).

Still another example involves phenylketonuria (referred to as PKU) among the Yemenite Jews. This is an inborn error of metabolism caused by autosomal recessive mutations of the phenylalanine hydroxylase gene. The frequency of PKU varies dramatically between Ashkenazi and Sephardic Jews, with estimates from Israel of 1 in 180,000 for the former and 1 in 8500 for the latter, with a particularly high frequency in Jews of Yemenite origin (Thalhammer, 1975). One mutation, consisting of a deletion of the third exon, is apparently responsible for all the PKU cases among Yemenite Jews (Avigad et al., 1990). By use of family history and community documents, the origin of the mutation was traced to Yemen's capital city, San'a, before the eighteenth century.

An example of the founder effect that is particularly relevant to this volume is familial hypercholesterolemia, the autosomal dominant disorder predisposing to early coronary disease due to mutations in the LDL (low-density lipoprotein) receptor gene (Goldstein et al., 1995). The frequency of this disorder worldwide is 1 in 500, and with its high penetrance the disorder contributes significantly to coronary artery disease worldwide. At least four ethnic groups—Christian Lebanese, French Canadians, Afrikaners in South Africa, and Ashkenazi Jews in South Africa—have frequencies of the disorder 3- to 7-fold higher, in each case due to a founder effect. The greatest frequency worldwide (1 in 67) is in Ashkenazi South Africans, stemming from the emigration of a founder population of Lithuanian Jews to South Africa between 1880 and 1910 (Seftel et al., 1989; Goldstein et al., 1995).

When one observes some genetic order present at unusually high frequency in some small isolated population, how can one decide whether to attribute the high frequency to the founder effect or, instead, to effects of natural selection in response to distinctive local environmental conditions? A first clue is that deleterious genes tend eventually to be eliminated by natural selection. Hence one might suspect the founder effect as the explanation for high frequency of a deleterious gene in a population known to have been founded recently by a small number of founding individuals, but not in a long-established population thought to be descended from large numbers of initial colonists. For a second clue, one should ask whether the environment is sufficiently distinctive to have been likely to exert distinctive selective effects and whether the genetic condition might have any conceivable benefits in that environment. For example, no one has suggested a plausible reason why the South African environment should favor complete loss of teeth by age 20, or why a sixth finger is uniquely beneficial in Pennsylvania's Lancaster County; hence it seems likely that the high frequencies of osteodental dysplasia in South Africa's Cape Colored population and of hexadactyly in Lancaster County Amish stem from the founder effect rather than from natural selection. Conversely, until their modern diaspora, the Ashkenazi Jews lived for six centuries in a unique environment of Eastern Europe, being the sole population largely confined to urban ghettos (Motulsky, 1979). Furthermore, the urban history of the Ashkenazi extends back some 2000 years. Urban non-Jewish populations suffered high mortality from infectious diseases and unhygienic conditions and were not genetically self-sustaining or isolated but were continually subsidized by rural populations. Hence it is plausible that natural selection under conditions of urban ghettos might have been responsible for some genetic disorders of the Ashkenazim, a theme to which we shall return below.

Still a third clue to distinguishing between the founder effect and selection as explanations involves whether people affected by the disorder carry a single common mutation or several common mutations. If only a single mutation is involved, one might suspect the founder effect, but if several phenotypically similar mutants of the same gene have independently risen to high frequency in the same population, one should suspect natural selection. For instance, the occurrence of more than one frequent mutation in Tay-Sachs disease among Ashkenazi Jews argues for selection rather than the founder effect (Jorde, 1992), as does the occurrence of four frequent β-thalassemia alleles in the small Kurdistan Jewish population that originated in Northern Iraq (Rund et al., 1991; Motulsky, 1995).

Finally, natural selection can eliminate some deleterious genes more rapidly than others. Autosomal dominants that are expressed in all or many carriers and that kill or debilitate them before the age of reproduction are likely to be eliminated quickly. Autosomal dominant conditions with milder consequences, and autosomal recessive conditions whose heterozygotes are protected from effects of natural selection, are likely to be eliminated only slowly (compare A and B in Fig. 4–1). These considerations support the interpretation that the above-mentioned characteristic disorders of the Finns and Afrikaners are due largely to founder effects. Of the 19 earliest recognized genetic disorders of the modern Finns (Norio et al., 1973), 4 are autosomal dominants or sex-linked recessives that mainly lead just to visual impairment in adulthood and do not interfere with reproduction, while the other 15, despite including lethal diseases

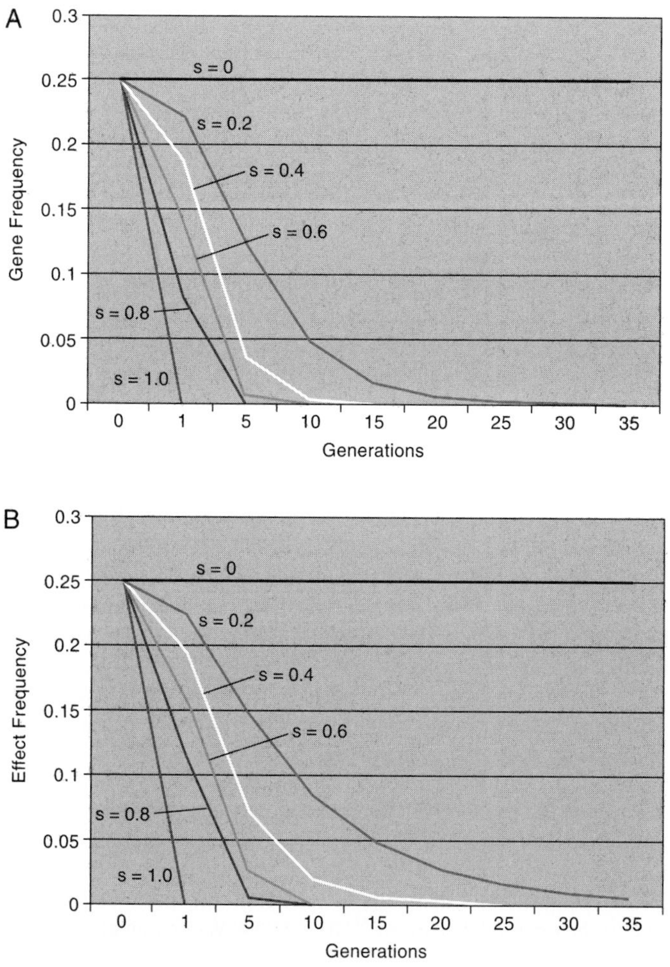

Fig. 4–1. Decrease with time (i.e., with number of generations) in the frequency of a deleterious gene, in the absence of new mutations to sustain it. The different curves depict selection coefficients of 0 (i.e., no selective disadvantage), 0.2, 0.4, 0.6, 0.8, and 1.0 against the gene. **A:** The disease gene is dominant; **B:** It is recessive. See Vogel and Motulsky (1997:510). Calculations kindly provided by Dr. Xiuqing Guo.

of childhood, are autosomal recessive conditions. Similarly, among the common genetic disorders of the Afrikaners, those that are lethal before adulthood or interfere with reproduction prove to be autosomal recessives (sclerosteosis, spondyloepimetaphyseal dysplasia), whereas the autosomal dominants are either benign (e.g., porphyria variegata before the advent of barbiturate anethestics) or else lethal only in the elderly (Huntington's chorea, familial colonic polyposis).

However, we do not wish to leave the impression that the role of founder effects can be dismissed in large human populations of ancient origins. Such populations stemming long ago from few founders may indefinitely retain nondeleterious or beneficial traits. Because many human populations must have gone through bottlenecks or must have radiated from only a few founders in the past, one must wonder whether founder effects have played a role in some familiar genetic differences between the world's largest populations today. For example, it is striking that the abnormal hemoglobin that conveys resistance to malaria is hemoglobin S in Africa but hemoglobin E in Southeast Asia. Given the evidence that population explosions within the last 6000 years in both Africa and Southeast Asia were associated with expansions of the first farmers, could this geographic difference in protective hemoglobins represent a legacy of the founder effect? We doubt it, for reasons that we shall mention below, but this is nevertheless a hypothesis that requires consideration. Other large populations in which the importance of founder effects should be seriously considered include Native Americans (Amerindians), most of whom are probably descended from a small number of immigrants across the Bering Straits region 13,000 years ago or earlier; Aboriginal Australians, similarly descended from a small number of immigrants around 55,000 years ago from Indonesia; the modern populations of the Philippines and Indonesia, derived from an expansion of Austronesian-speaking farmers out of Taiwan beginning around 6000 years ago; the Malagasy, descended from a mixture of colonists derived ultimately from Borneo and East Africa around A.D. 500; the modern Japanese, whose largest genetic component stems from immigrants from Korea into Kyushu around 400 B.C.; and western Europeans, among whom a major genetic component may go back to the first farmers who spread west into Europe from Anatolia beginning around 10,000 years ago (Cavalli-Sforza et al., 1994; Diamond, 1997).

BAD FOR HOMOZYGOTES, GOOD FOR HETEROZYGOTES

As mentioned, with time natural selection will tend to eliminate a deleterious gene that reached high frequency through the founder effect or genetic drift. As can be seen in Fig. 4–1, a gene introduced by the founder effect into a population at a frequency of 25% will rapidly decline in frequency (more rapidly for a dominant gene than for a recessive gene) if there is a significant selective disadvantage. Thus, a deleterious gene will tend to disappear with time if there is no counterbalancing advantage to maintain its frequency. If one nevertheless observes a gene with known deleterious effects to occur at high frequencies (far above those that could be sustained by mutation) in an old population, one should suspect that the gene may also carry some unknown positive selective value to offset the known negative selective value. In the remainder of this chapter we shall distinguish five types of such counterbalancing selection, depending on the relationship between the individuals who benefited from and the individuals who were penalized by the gene. This section will now consider the best-established cases, in which inheritance is autosomal recessive and in which individuals penalized are homozygotes while individuals benefited are heterozygotes.

Genetic Antimalarials

The best-established case of counterbalancing selection, discussed in all textbooks of genetics, involves a variant hemoglobin, hemoglobin S (Hb S) (sickle cell hemoglobin) (Allison 1954; Motulsky 1975; Fleming et al., 1979; Weatherall et al., 1995). In rural societies before modern medicine, the survival of homozygotes to reproductive age, or their successful reproduction, was very low. Nevertheless, in tropical Africa, heterozygotes constitute up to 40% of the population, a frequency far higher than could be attributed to recurrent mutations (Livingstone, 1985). Geographic and microgeographic variation in Hb S frequency in Africa and in the Mediterranean correlates with malaria's frequency, down to fine details: for example, Hb S frequency in South Africa declines from north to south down to negligible values among the Xhosa people, the only black African group who live south of the malaria zone. Field studies of differences between heterozygotes and homozygotes in malaria infection and mortality support the counterbalancing selection hypothesis.

As a human example of counterbalancing selection, Hb S is also almost unique in the availability of experimental evidence for selection, obtained several decades ago, before the rise of human subject protection committees and changes in ethical standards fortunately made such experiments impossible. Among 30 African subjects who were described as volunteers and who were deliberately exposed to malaria, only 2 out of 15 Hb S heterozygotes, but 14 out of 15 normal subjects (i.e., individuals who lack Hb S), developed malaria (Allison, 1954). The protection against malaria afforded by Hb S is such that heterozygotes enjoy a selective advantage of about 20% over normal individuals in malarial regions. This advantage proves sufficiently large to sustain the Hb S gene at its observed high frequencies in malarial regions of Africa. Given this degree of protection of the heterozygote, and assuming that the homozygote experienced 100% genetic lethality in that environment, one can calculate that it would take only 40 to 50 generations (equivalent to 1000–1200 years) to achieve the present equilibrium gene frequency in malarial regions (Weatherall et al., 1995; Vogel and Motulsky, 1997:525).

Other variant hemoglobins besides Hb S also occur at high frequencies in malarial regions: Hb C in West Africa, Hb D in India, Hb O in Arabia, and Hb E in Southeast Asia. The locally high frequencies of these hemoglobin variants are also likely to be due to counterbalancing selection that involves resistance to malaria, although the evidence is less abundant than in the case of Hb S. In addition to the variant hemoglobins, there are other well-known genetic antimalarials (Hill, 1998) whose postulated protective effect is supported by various strengths of evidence, which offer various magnitudes of protection and also of penalty, and which are transmitted by various patterns of inheritance besides autosomal recessive—such as G6PD deficiency (Ruwende et al., 1995), various HLA antigens (Hill et al., 1991, 1994), lack of the Duffy blood group, the thalassemias, and elliptocytosis. Most of these antimalarial traits give only relative resistance to falciparum malaria. The Duffy blood group is unique in that it gives absolute resistance to vivax malaria (Miller et al., 1976). Much of the supporting evidence is geographic, including evidence from micromapping, such as the altitudinal covariation of malaria incidence and of the frequency of the postulated antimalarial genes in Sardinia (G6PD deficiency) and New Guinea (thalassemia).

A related situation to the Duffy relationship in another disease is that of chemokine receptor CCR5 and HIV, in which homozygosity occuring in 1% of the population for a deletion allele apparently provides absolute protection to HIV infection; while heterozygosity of 18% of the population provides relative resistance (Dean et al., 1996; Carrington et al., 1997). This latter example illustrates that if we know the actual mechanism of resistance, we can start developing therapeutic approaches such as specifically designed drugs.

Hb S and the other genetic antimalarials offer important lessons and raise important questions. The same questions and possible lessons arise for other human genetic disorders that are likely to be sustained by counterbalancing selection, but much more abundant relevant evidence is available in the case of the antimalarials. We call attention here to six of these lessons or questions.

1. *Difficulties of proving counterbalancing selection.* It has been difficult to demonstrate convincingly the protective effects of the genetic antimalarials, even though they offer a protective selective advantage of up to 0.25. That means that it will be even more difficult to prove the selective advantages postulated or likely for other genetic disorders, in which benefits lower than 0.2 are likely to be the rule. Furthermore, the mode of inheritance must be taken into account. For example, G6PD deficiency, being X-linked, has five genotypes in the population (three in the female, two in the male), as opposed to the three genotypes in autosomal recessive disorders. As a consequence, selective advantages of somewhat smaller magnitude can be observed (Ruwende et al., 1995)

2. *Relation between selective advantage and disadvantage.* The higher the selective disadvantage borne by the homozygote, the higher must be the counterbalancing protective advantage to the heterozygote in order to sustain a gene at a given frequency. This point is already illustrated by available evidence for the genetic antimalarials: both the homozygote disadvantage and the heterozygote advantage apparently decrease in the sequence from Hb S to Hb C to Hb E, and in the sequence from Hb S to G6PD deficiency.

3. *Gene frequency changes with time in the absence of a counterbalancing advantage.* In cases of counterbalancing selection, one would predict that if the protective advantage for any reason were removed but the disadvantage remained, the gene should gradually decrease in frequency with time. Two examples appear to support this prediction for Hb S. Hb S was carried from Africa to the New World by African blacks who were originally transported as slaves, but the frequency of malaria in the New World varies greatly. In two New World areas with very low or zero incidence of malaria, the U.S. state of Georgia and the island of Curaçao, the frequency of the Hb S gene among the local black population is lower than in black populations from malarial regions of the New World and also lower than in African black populations still resident in Africa and more representative of the original condition (Jonxis 1959; Workman et al., 1963; Blumberg and Hesser, 1971). This suggests that, even within a mere few centuries of living in malaria-free regions of the New World, the Hb S gene decreased in frequency because there was no longer a counterbalancing benefit (protection against malaria) to sustain the gene's frequency in the face of selection tending to eliminate it because of its deleterious effect. This inference of decreasing Hb S frequency with time arose from genetic studies carried out for a different purpose: frequencies of various African gene markers were being measured in different New World black populations, and it was observed that a higher apparent frequency of white admixture was being calculated for black populations in nonmalarial regions. Of course, it is not the case that white admixture was especially high in Georgia and Curaçao; instead, Hb S frequency is low there because of the local absence of a counterbalancing advantage, and this low frequency was at first mistakenly attributed to high white admixture.

Another example is that the frequency of Hb S is below 1% in the Xhosa, the southernmost Bantu-speaking black population of Africa (Jenkins and Ramsay, 1986). All of the modern black populations of subequatorial Africa stem from an expansion of Bantu-speaking farmers that arose ultimately from north of the equator in Nigeria and Cameroon and reached the Cape of South Africa around 2000 years ago (Cavalli-Sforza et al., 1994; Diamond, 1997). One interpretation relates the near-absence of Hb S among the Xhosa to their having left Nigeria and Cameroon before the evolution of Hb S, but all linguistic and archaeological evidence suggests that the Xhosa are part of the same expansion wave that gave rise to all other black populations of subequatorial Africa. Instead, the likely explanation is that the Xhosa did carry the Hb S gene with them into South Africa beyond the range of malaria and that Hb S has been nearly eliminated among the Xhosa over the last 2000 years because it no longer provided any benefit to balance its penalties.

4. *Time depth.* How old are the mutations and high frequencies of Hb S and the other genetic antimalarials? Opinions vary: they could be recent innovations dating only from the rise of tropical agriculture and postulated associate rise of malaria within the past 8000 years; or they could be ancient, if malaria is an ancient affliction of humans, as it is of our closest relatives, the great apes. This interesting question awaits resolution. It may turn out that the answer varies geographically. For example, the mosquito vectors of human malaria differ between Africa and tropical Asia. Perhaps the genetic antimalarials are younger in Africa, where malarial mosquitos today are non-forest species associated with villages, than in tropical Asia, where mosquito vectors are forest species.

5. *Single or multiple mutations?* Hb S occurs at high frequency over a large area of the western Old World tropics and subtropics, from Africa and the Mediterranean east to Arabia and India. Does this wide distribution stem from a single mutation or from multiple independent mutations, each of which rose separately to high frequency because of selection by malaria? Linkage studies with DNA polymorphisms show that Hb S is associated with four different RFLP haplotypes, each of which is centered geographically: on the Atlantic coast of West Africa, on central West Africa, on Bantu-speaking African populations to the south and east, and on Arabia and India (Kan and Dozy, 1980; Pagnier et al., 1984). This has been interpreted to support four independent origins of Hb S in these four geographic regions, with all four mutants being pumped up independently to high frequencies by selection related to malaria. An alternative interpretation is that "ultimately all Hb S alleles derive from only one mutation, and that the present location of this allele in four RFLP haplotypes is explained by very rare recombination or by gene conversion" (Vogel and Motulsky, 1997:522). This question also awaits resolution.

6. *Different variant hemoglobins in different geographic regions.* The most obvious, but still infrequently asked, question arising from a distributional map of the genetic antimalarials is the following: why did Hb S and Hb E become widespread in Africa and tropical southeast Asia, respectively? (One could also ask why Hb C became common in West Africa, Hb D in India, and Hb O in Arabia.) At least six alternative interpretations suggest themselves:

1. The mutants may be extremely rare, and it may be pure chance that an Hb E mutant arose in Asia but an Hb S mutant arose in Africa. However, isolated mutants of both Hb S and Hb E are known from northern Europe, where the absence of malaria meant that they could not be pumped up to high frequency. Surely, then, Hb E mutants must also have arisen in Africa (as well as Hb S mutants in Asia), and each gene had its opportunity to take over in other regions but failed to profit from the opportunity.
2. Hb S may indeed have arisen first by chance in Africa, and Hb E in Asia. Each variant hemoglobin subsequently also arose in the other region, but by then one variant was already established and protecting the human population against malaria, so that variant hemoglobins came to exclude each other geographically by their competing protective effects.
3. The answer could involve interactions between variant hemoglobins and other proteins, coupled with the differing genetic backgrounds of Africans and Asians.
4. Each variant hemoglobin may interact with thalassemias and other genetic antimalarials, which differ between geographic areas and which may cause different variant hemoglobins to be advantageous in different areas.
5. Recalling that Hb S offers both stronger protection and more severe penalties than Hb E, one might wonder whether lower average severity of malaria in Asia than in Africa selected for genetic antimalarials of differing potency.
6. Different antimalarials may have been selected by different mosquito vectors and different malarial habitats in Asia and Africa.

Tay-Sachs Disease in Ashkenazi Jews

The high frequency of Tay-Sachs disease in Ashkenazi Jews has stimulated much discussion: should it be attributed to selection or to a founder effect (Jorde, 1992; Gravel et al., 1995; Motulsky, 1995)? Tay-Sachs also exists at high frequency in French Canadians and in a group of Pennsylvania Dutch; in each of those two populations only a single mutation is involved, no one has suggested what selective advantage might be involved, and a founder effect is assumed to be the explanation (Gravel et al., 1995). Many or most authors similarly assume that a founder effect, stemming from migrations of Jews from the Rhineland to eastern Europe around 600 to 700 years ago, accounts for their high Tay-Sachs frequency (Chase and McKusick, 1972; Chase, 1977; Risch et al., 1995).

An alternative interpretation (Myrianthopoulos and Aronsen, 1966; Myrianthopoulos and Melnick, 1977; Petersen et al., 1983) notes that eastern European Jews, because they were forced to concentrate in urban ghettos, were subjected to severe selection by a different suite of factors from those affecting the majority and primarily rural non-Jewish population of eastern Europe. A major selective agent in cities was tuberculosis (TB), accounting for up to 20% of all deaths. Several tantalizing correlations suggest that Tay-Sachs could have built up to high frequency as a "genetic antitubercular": comparisons of Jews and non-Jews within the same European city, class, and occupational group (for example, Warsaw garment workers) showed Jews to have only half the TB death rate of non-Jews, despite their being equally susceptible and equally exposed to infection; geographic variation within eastern Europe in frequency of the putative selective agent, TB, paralleled geographic variation in frequency of Tay-Sachs (cf. parallel geographic variation in malaria and the genetic antimalarials); and modern studies showed that grandparents of Ashkenazi Tay-Sachs children, half of whose grandparents were necessarily Tay-Sachs carriers, were reported to have an unexpectedly low risk of death from TB (Myrianthopoulos and Melnick, 1977). The presence of two common Tay-Sachs mutations, rather than just one, among Ashkenazim suggests that the gene was propelled by selection at least twice to high frequencies, weakening the hypothesis of a founder effect (Jorde, 1992). Finally, it has always seemed peculiar that the Ashkenazim should have high frequencies not only of Tay-Sachs but also of two other genetic disorders that resemble Tay-Sachs by resulting in lysosomal ganglioside accumulation: Gaucher disease and Niemann-Pick disease (Goodman and Motulsky, 1979; Rotter and Diamond, 1987). Unless this is really just a coincidence, it suggests some selective value of lysosomal ganglioside accumulation unique to the Ashkenazim. Could this be a group of genetic antituberculars (analogous to the genetic antimalarials) (Gravel et al., 1995)? Note, however, that the frequency of resistance to tuberculosis is much higher than the frequency of Tay-Sachs carriers, so that Tay-Sachs alone could at least provide only a fraction of the existing resistance to TB (see Chapter 10).

All these connections between Tay-Sachs and tuberculosis in the Ashkenazim remain speculative. How can this controversy be resolved?

Other Possible Cases of Heterozygote Advantage

Congenital adrenal hyperplasia appears to protect Yupik Eskimos against *Haemophilus influenzae* B infections (Petersen et al., 1984). The high frequency of cystic fibrosis (CF) in northern Europe has been speculatively attributed to protection against diarrheal infections because the CF defect involves the epithelial channel regulatory protein that controls gastrointestinal chloride secretion and that is harnessed by some bacterial toxins so as to cause diarrhea (Morral et al., 1994; Welsh et al., 1995). Familial Mediterranean fever (FMF) may protect against asthma: both affected homozygotes and obligate heterozygotes (parents of FMF cases) have been observed to have a reduced frequency of asthma (Danon and Zemer, 1992; Brenner-Ullman et al., 1994). This may be an example of "billiard," "downstream," or "secondary" selection, in that asthma itself has been proposed to result from selection against parasitic infections (see Chapter 11). Thus, FMF would be a secondary development, providing a selective advantage against the deleterious effects of the asthma genes that arose in the first place by protecting against parasitemia. These, and many other possible examples of human genetic disorders sustained at frequencies far above mutation rates by heterozygote advantage, await decisive tests.

BAD FOR MEN, GOOD FOR WOMEN

One can easily imagine how a gene that acts in both sexes might nevertheless produce more benefits for one sex than for the other sex. Currently the best candidate for involvement of such a gene in a disease is the gene for idiopathic hemochromatosis (IHC), a disorder of iron metabolism (see Chapter 18).

Throughout most of human history, and for most of the world's population today, the main problem in iron's metabolism is not getting enough of it. About one-third of the world's population today is considered iron-deficient, and the proportion must have been higher in the past, before the era of nutritional supplements and recognition of the role of parasites in contributing to anemia. Nevertheless, a few people, most of them elderly men, suffer from the opposite problem of too much iron.

IHC is an autosomal recessive disease with a heterozygote frequency of 10% in European populations, making it probably the commonest abnormal gene identified in the United States and Europe to date (see Chapter 18). One mutation accounts for 100% of IHC patients in Australia and for 85% in the United States and Europe. The symptoms arise from abnormally high rates of intestinal iron absorption, but buildup of body iron stores is still sufficiently slow that they do not reach toxic levels until middle age or later in life, and then mainly in people with a high dietary iron intake. Serious symptoms are 5 to 10 times less frequent in women than in men, because women routinely experience high iron losses through menstrual bleeding, pregnancy, and lactation. The principal symptoms are fibrosis, cirrhosis, and cancer of the liver, plus cardiomyopathy, diabetes, hypogonadism, and porphyria cutanea tarda. Only a fraction of elderly homozygous men develop symptoms. Heterozygotes rarely develop complications, although they do have slightly increased intestinal iron absorption; in fact, they have been observed to benefit slightly by having a lower frequency of iron deficiency anemia (Beutler et al., 2000)

Hemochromatosis and high intestinal iron absorption are considered diseases. This reflects a male-chauvinist evolutionary perspective (Diamond, 1989). Increased iron absorption is valuable for most women, and for most of our evolutionary history it has not harmed most men. From a liberated evolutionary perspective, the deaths of a few elderly men represent a small price to pay for protecting many women in the same population against the widespread dangers of anemia. One might similarly speculate how genes that promote high absorption, production, or storage of lipid might be branded as a genetic disorder when, in fact, such genes are actually beneficial for lactating women and are likely to produce hyperlipidemias mainly in men. For instance, the "atherogenetic lipoprotein phenotype" characterized by small LDL (low-density lipoprotein) particle size occurs in 10% to 20% of the population and triples the risk for coronary artery disease (Austin et al., 1988a, 1990; see Chapter 7). This is clearly a trait with major genetic contributions but with markedly reduced penetrance in young males (<20) and in premenopausal females (Austin et al., 1988b; Rotter et al., 1996). Thus, women are protected in large part until menopause. This lipid trait may well form one of the metabolic abnormalities consistent with Neel's thrifty gene hypothesis (Neel, 1962) (see below). More generally, for any given blood cholesterol level, women are more protected by their hormonal milieu, so women develop coronary disease on the average 10 years later than men (see Chapter 7). This is true even for such Mendelian disorders as familial hypercholesterolemia (Goldstein et al., 1995)

BAD FOR POSTNATES, GOOD FOR PRENATES

Today, when most of us survive to old age, "premature" death—that is, death before one's peak reproductive years—is considered an exceptional tragedy. In reality, that is true only if one defines "us" as "those of us who survive to be born." The combined risk of all postnatal "premature" human deaths pales before the risk of prenatal death through miscarriage. Of human pregnancies that the mother recognizes by a missed menstrual period, only about 15% end in miscarriage. But when introduction of modern hormonal tests permitted earlier detection of pregnancies that would otherwise have gone unrecognized, a higher fraction of those pregnancies was found to terminate without issue, yielding a total miscarriage rate of about 50%. Outcomes of attempted artificial fertilizations of ova within fallopian tubes point to further losses of embryos before implantation, suggesting overall miscarriage rates as high as 80%. This prenatal mortality means that each of our recognized children is actually the survivor of a set of phantoms, most of whom die before birth. Because, for an embryo, its entire reproductive career lies in the future, the selective value of mutations that would reduce the risk of miscarriage is large.

Type 1 diabetes may well exemplify a gene that is manifestly bad for postnates but that is maintained at high frequency because it is good for prenates. Evidence has been presented that suggests a potential selective advantage mechanism for Type 1 diabetes and at the same time provides at least a partial explanation of the recognition that the risk for Type 1 diabetes appears to be higher for offspring of males than females with Type

1, at least in the first 20 years of life (see Chapter 21). What has been observed in some, but not all, studies is preferential transmission of diabetogenic HLA haplotypes, not only to affected offspring but also to unaffected offspring (Vadheim et al., 1986; Thivolent et al., 1988). In addition, while this preferential transmission occurs for both high-risk diabetic alleles and haplotypes (both DR3 and DR4 associated) in fathers, it has been reported to occur for only the DR3-associated haplotypes in mothers, providing an explanation for the increased paternal risk. Furthermore, the available evidence suggests that this preferential transmission may occur via in utero selection, in that the history of miscarriages is a function of the parental DR3 and DR4 genotypes (Vadheim et al., 1985). These data may thus provide an explanation for the maintenance of the high frequency of this common genetic disease that used to be lethal. In addition, the suggestion that this prenatal selection could occur via immunologically mediated events raises the possibility that an additional consequence of these events, in fetuses that survive, might be immune changes presaging the eventual development of Type 1 diabetes (Vadheim et al., 1987) (see next section regarding pleiotropic effects).

GOOD FOR THE YOUNG, BAD FOR THE OLD

Senescence is an often-discussed puzzle of evolutionary biology. Why is it that any individual human or other animal, even if provided with unlimited food and complete protection from predators and the best possible medical care, nevertheless gradually "grows old," deteriorates in every biological function examined, and eventually dies? A leading theory of senescence by evolutionary biologists invokes postulated gene pleiotropy (Williams, 1957). That is, genes may have multiple effects, and in particular a gene that becomes deleterious late in life may be sustained in frequency by advantages that it brings early in life. Human medical science provides us with possible examples of such pleiotropic genes.

One such example is the polymorphism of *Apo E*, a gene with a modest effect on cholesterol levels (see Chapter 7 and Chapter 43). It has been speculated that lipids and lipoproteins could have a role as antiviral agents. If so, variation in a gene that affects cholesterol levels, such as *Apo E*, could have been selected for because of antiviral effects. It is now also clear that the specific *Apo E4* allele carries a severalfold increased risk for Alzheimer's disease (see Chapter 43). Hence a gene whose primary effect is on lipid metabolism may have a pleiotropic effect that results in accumulation of material in the brain.

Another possible example of such pleiotropy involves genes predisposing to inflammatory bowel diseases (IBD). It has been proposed that the genes predisposing to the various forms of IBD provided a selective advantage through mucosal immunoprotection in an unsanitary world (Rotter, 1994; see Chapter 15). Effective public sanitation, a development of modern civilization, has removed that selective advantage. But the mucosal immunoprotection is still primed genetically in those individuals with the IBD genes, which in effect are armed to defend the individual. When the IBD-predisposing genes are not adequately used in mucosal defense, as they would not be in the developed world, one of two events could then occur: *(1)* later exposure to an infectious agent could result in hyperstimulation of the immune response and subsequent chronic inflammation (analogous to paralytic polio, which occurs when infection develops after early infancy), or *(2)* even more likely, failure of exposure to a potentially injurious agent could leave the gut immunologic system in a continually primed state and thus set up the system for subsequent dysregulation—that is, a pleiotropic autoimmune reaction that leads to the diseases we recognize as ulcerative colitis and Crohn's disease (Rotter, 1994).

This hypothesis provides an explanation for the relatively high frequency of IBD in the Jewish population (see Chapter 15). The fact that those Jews with the highest frequency of IBD appear to be Ashkenazi Jews (i.e., those Jews whose origin is middle and eastern Europe) suggests that the selective factors had their greatest influence after the Ashkenazi split off from the Sephardic Jews (Rotter et al., 1992). That split arose historically when Europe and the Mediterranean became divided between Christian and Islamic kingdoms. However, the highest frequency of IBD appears to arise in those Ashkenazi Jews whose origin is in middle rather than eastern Europe (Roth et al., 1989; Zlotogora et al., 1990); the same finding applies to Tay-Sachs gene carriers (Petersen et al., 1983). But middle European countries, such as (modern) Austria, Hungary, and Czechoslovakia, are the ones that imposed on the Jews the greatest ghetto urbanization, hence presumably the greatest overcrowding and greatest defects in sanitation. This situation eased when Ashkenazi Jews from middle Europe were invited to settle in eastern Europe (i.e., Poland, Ukraine, and Russia). The frequency of both Tay-Sachs heterozygotes and IBD patients is higher in Jews of middle European than eastern European ancestry (Petersen et al., 1983; Roth et al., 1989; Zlotogora et al., 1990). Thus, the long-term urbanization that has been proposed as playing a selective role in the lysosomal diseases, such as Tay-Sachs, could have had a more general selection effect on other diseases as well.

BAD FOR ONE LIFESTYLE, GOOD FOR ANOTHER LIFESTYLE

Some genes are likely to be good under certain lifestyles (e.g., certain diets, salt intakes, or exercise levels) but bad under other lifestyles. There has been much discussion, in particular, about diseases associated with the shift from traditional lifestyles to a so-called Western lifestyle ("coca-colonization") in many parts of the world. Features associated with the Western lifestyle include high calorie intake, regular calorie intake, low levels of physical exercise, increased intake of carbohydrates (especially sugar) and saturated fat and salt, and decreased intake of complex carbohydrates and fiber. Since these lifestyle factors tend to be adopted together, it is usually uncertain which is most important in the resulting changes in disease patterns.

Coca-colonization tends to be accompanied by an explosion of common lifestyle-related diseases with a complex genetic basis, including Type 2 diabetes, hypertension, atherosclerosis, gallstones, and obesity. We shall discuss the first two of these five conditions in some detail and then mention the others more briefly. Explosions of similar health problems have also been noted in monkeys living on the equivalent of a Western lifestyle—affluent, overfed, underexercised monkeys in zoos. Our discussion will focus on the factors of human history and natural selection that may be involved.

Those of us committed to the Western lifestyle easily forget how different are the traditional lifestyles of non-Western peoples and, indeed, of almost all people throughout human evolution until recently. Instead of three predictable, unlimited, sugar-rich meals each day, frequent food shortages and rare gluts were the pattern of life. For example, one of us (J.D.) has experienced several times in the course of fieldwork in New Guinea that a group of New Guineans and I went virtually without food for several days, as a result of the failure of my arrangements for food delivery to our campsite. The first time this happened, when we reached a remote but empty campsite at sunset after a hard all-day climb, I expected to be lynched on the spot. Instead, my New Guinea companions were philosophical: "Orait, i no gat kaikai, yumi sleep nothing" (pidgin English for "Okay, so there's no food; we'll just sleep on empty stomachs"). Conversely, every year or two my New Guinea friends manage to have a gluttonous feast lasting several days, when food consumption shocks even me (rated by my friends as a bottomless pit) and when some people actually die of overeating.

Noninsulin-Dependent Diabetes Mellitus

The most plausible interpretation of the explosion of NIDDM (noninsulin-dependent diabetes, also known as Type 2 diabetes) accompanying westernization is Neel's (1962) "thrifty genotype" hypothesis. According to this view, under the conditions of fluctuating and usually meager food supply that prevailed throughout most of human history, those individuals with "thrifty" adaptations such as hair-triggered insulin release would thereby be enabled to convert more of their ingested calories into fat during occasional food gluts. They would thus be better able to survive bouts of starvation. Only under modern conditions of constantly available high-calorie food and little exercise would they develop NIDDM, as a result of excessively frequent insulin release and consequent development of insulin resistance.

The NIDDM epidemics involve two types of people (Bennett et al., 1997; de Courten et al., 1997; also Chapter 22). One type consists of people who moved from their homeland with a traditional lifestyle to a new land of residence with a Westernized lifestyle. Examples include the Yemenite Jews who were airlifted to Israel in 1949 and 1950 as an initially almost diabetes-free population and developed a 13% incidence of NIDDM within 20 years; Mexicans and Japanese who moved to the United States; Polynesian islanders who moved to New Zealand; Chinese who moved to Mauritius, Hong Kong, Singapore, and Taiwan; and Asian Indians who moved to Mauritius, Fiji, South Africa, and Great Britain. A role of genetic factors follows from the fact that the rise in NIDDM incidence remains significant even when the immigrant population is compared with members of the resident host population of the new homeland matched for obesity and other lifestyle risk factors.

The other type of peoples participating in the NIDDM explosion consists of peoples who rapidly adopted a Westernized lifestyle while remaining in their original homelands. These examples include Aboriginal Australians, many groups of Micronesians and Polynesians, and many groups of Native Americans, plus the two extreme examples to be described in the following paragraphs. A study comparing NIDDM incidence in several communities in the San Antonio area of Texas was instructive in demonstrating that the incidence of NIDDM increased with the population's estimated proportion of Native American genes, even after controlling for obesity (Chakraborty et al., 1986; Stern et al., 1992). This again suggests a role of genetic predisposing factors, in this case in the Native American population.

The two most striking examples consist of the two populations with the highest incidence of NIDDM in the world, the Pima Indians in Arizona and the Nauru Islanders in the Pacific Ocean, whose histories provide further insight into the evolution of genetic predisposing factors for NIDDM. The Pima Indians survived for more than 2000 years in the deserts of southern Arizona, using agricultural methods based on elaborate irrigation systems and supplemented by hunting and gathering (Bennett et al., 1997). Because rainfall in the desert varies greatly from year to year, crops failed about one year in every five, forcing the Pimas then to subsist entirely on wild foods, especially jackrabbits and mesquite beans. Many of their preferred wild plants were high in fiber and low in fat, and they released glucose slowly; thus they represent the ideal antidiabetic diet. After this long history of periodic but brief bouts of starvation, the Pimas experienced a more prolonged bout of starvation that began in the nineteenth century and ended in an intense famine for a decade late in the century, when white settlers diverted the water supply on which their agriculture depended. Today, the Pimas eat store-bought food.

Observers who visited the Pimas in the early 1900s reported obesity to be rare and diabetes almost nonexistent. Since the 1960s, obesity has become widespread among the Pimas, some of whom now weigh more than 150 kg. Half of them exceed the U.S. 90th percentile for weight in relation to height. Pima women consume about 3160 calories per day (50% above the U.S. average), 40% of which is fat. Associated with this obesity, Pimas have achieved notoriety in the diabetes literature by now having a frequency of NIDDM 19 times that of U.S. whites and matched in the world only by the Nauru Islanders. Half of all Pimas over age 35, and 70% of those still alive at age 55 to 64, are diabetic.

We interpret this history to suggest that the Pimas' traditional lifestyle, alternating between starvation and plenty, selected for a genetically thrifty metabolism shared with many other Native American groups and traditional peoples elsewhere. In the case of the Pimas, this genetic predisposition underwent further intense selection from the water diversions and crop failures of the nineteenth century, which left alive only those Pimas best able to accumulate fat in times of plenty. The result was an NIDDM explosion when supermarket food finally became constantly available.

The other extreme NIDDM epidemic has arisen on Nauru Island, a remote Pacific atoll occupied by 5000 Micronesians whose formerly energetic lifestyle depended on fishing and subsistence farming. Colonization by Great Britain, Australia, and New Zealand, and income from phosphate mining (Nauru rock has the world's highest concentration of phosphate, an essential ingredient to fertilizer), transformed Nauruans into one of the world's most sedentary peoples, with one of the world's highest per-capita incomes. Virtually all food is now imported and energy-dense; calorie intake is more than double the Australian-recommended norms; and obesity is rampant. NIDDM used to be nonexistent but within a few decades came to affect almost two-thirds of adults by age 55 to 64. The disease now contributes to most nonaccidental deaths on Nauru, with the paradoxical result that wealthy Nauru has one of the world's shortest human lifespans (Zimmet et al., 1990; Dowse et al., 1991; Zimmet, 1992).

Interestingly, the age-standardized prevalence of NIDDM and of impaired glucose tolerance actually declined from 1976 to 1987, despite no decline in environmental risk factors (Dowse et al., 1991). Evidently, NIDDM associated with the new lifestyle has already struck most of the genetically susceptible Nauruans, leaving the unaffected population to consist mostly of genetically resistant individuals. Nauru's epidemic of a genetic environmental disease thus resembles an infectious disease epidemic running its course, but the decline in disease frequency stems from an entirely different mechanism: interindividual variation in genetic susceptibility, rather than acquired immunity. Nauru illustrates natural selection operating on humans under our very eyes.

Selection for a thrifty genotype and for fat storage would have been especially intense on Nauru Islanders for three reasons. First, like other Micronesian and Polynesian populations of remote Pacific islands, the ancestors of the Nauruans reached their island by long canoe voyages on which many or most embarking colonists died by starvation, and only the initially fatter or metabolically more efficient people escaped death. Second, droughts and crop failures were common on Nauru in times past. Finally, just as mistreatment by American farmers imposed a final intense bout of starvation on the Pima Indians, mistreatment by the Japanese military similarly imposed a final bout on Nauruans: over one-quarter of the population of Nauru died of starvation during forcible deportment at the time of the Japanese occupation from 1942 to 1945. With this history, it is not surprising that only those Nauru Islanders with the greatest genetic predisposition to accumulate fat were still alive in 1945, thereafter to be undone by their rapid accumulation of wealth and their adoption of a hyper-Western lifestyle.

Hypertension

Compared with American whites of the same age and sex, on the average, American blacks have higher blood pressure, double the risk of developing hypertension, and nearly ten times the risk of dying from it. Around the world, only Japanese exceed U.S. blacks in their risk of dying from stroke. Of course, U.S. blacks and whites differ in lifestyle and environmental factors, both of which are known to contribute to the risk of hypertension. However, those factors do not appear to be the whole explanation: even after controlling for salt intake and other risk factors, American blacks are still at higher risk of hypertension than are American whites, which suggests additional genetic factors (Whelton et al., 1994; Burt et al., 1995; see Chapter 8).

In addition, hypertensive blacks are not merely similar to and proportionately more frequent than severely hypertensive whites. Instead, physiological differences seem to contribute as well. On consuming salt, blacks on the average retain it much longer before excreting it into the urine, and they experience a greater rise in blood pressure on a high-salt diet. Hypertension is more likely to be salt-sensitive in blacks than in whites. By the same token, black hypertension is more likely to be treated successfully by drugs that cause the kidneys to excrete salt (thiazide diuretics) and is less likely to respond to drugs that reduce heart rate and cardiac output (beta blockers, such as propanolol). These facts suggest qualitative and not just quantitative differences between the causes of black and white hypertension, with black hypertension more likely to involve renal salt handling.

To understand why U.S. blacks are now prone to die as a result of their kidneys' retaining salt, we need to ask under what conditions people might have benefited from kidneys that were especially efficient at retaining salt. That question is hard to understand from the perspective of modern Western society, where salt shakers are on every dining table, NaCl is cheap, and our bodies' main salt-related problem is how to get rid of it. Imagine, however, what the world used to be like before the ubiquitous salt shakers. Most plants contain very little sodium, yet animals require sodium at high concentrations in their extracellular fluids. As a result, carnivores readily obtain their needed sodium by eating herbivores, but herbivores themselves face problems in acquiring that sodium. That's why the animals that one sees coming to salt licks are deer and antelope, not lions and tigers. Similarly, some human hunter-gatherers obtained enough salt from the meat they ate. But when humans began to take up farming 10,000 years ago, we either had to evolve kidneys that were superefficient at conserving salt, learn to extract salt at great effort, or trade for salt at great expense.

Examples of these solutions abound in traditional societies. Brazil's Yanomamo Indians, whose staple food is low-sodium bananas, excrete on the average only 10 mg of salt daily, barely one-thousandth the salt excretion of the typical American. The New Guinea highlanders with whom one of us (J.D.) works, and whose diet consists up to 90% of low-sodium sweet potatoes, told me of the efforts to which they went to make salt a few decades ago, before Europeans brought it as trade goods. They gathered leaves of certain plant species, burned them, scraped up the ash, poured water through the ash to dissolve the solids, repeated the process many times over the course of several weeks, and finally evaporated the water to obtain small amounts of bitter but precious salt.

Thus, salt has been in very short supply for much of recent human evolutionary history. Those of us with efficient kidneys that are able to retain salt even on a low-sodium diet were better able to survive our inevitable episodes of sodium loss (of which more in a moment). Those kidneys proved to be detrimental only when salt became routinely available, leading to excessive salt retention and hypertension with its fatal consequences. That is why blood pressure and the frequency of hypertension have shot up recently in so many populations around the world, as they have made the transition from being self-sufficient subsistence farmers to patrons of supermarkets and purchasers of salt shakers.

Most American blacks originated via the slave trade from West African blacks, who must have faced the chronic problem of losing salt through sweating in their hot environment. Yet in West Africa, except on the coast and a few inland areas, salt was traditionally as scarce for farmers as it has been for Yanomamo and New Guinea farmers. By this argument, the genetic basis for hypertension in U.S. blacks was already widespread in many of their West African ancestors. In this view, American blacks would be no different from the many Polynesian, Melanesian, Kenyan, Zulu, and other populations that have recently developed high blood pressure under a Westernized lifestyle.

In addition, Wilson and Grim (1991) have proposed a historical interpretation that may have resulted in American blacks now being at even more risk for hypertension than were their African ancestors and other traditional farmers in low-salt environments. The scenario involves recent selection for superefficient kidneys, driven by massive mortality of black slaves from salt loss in the course of the slave trade. Slaves captured by raids in the interior of West Africa were chained together, given heavy loads, and marched to the coast for one or two months with little food and water, resulting in the deaths of about 25% of the captives en route. Another 12% died while awaiting purchase by slave traders and while being held on the coast in hot crowded buildings. Another 5% died as traders went up and down the coast buying and loading slaves for a few weeks or months until a ship's cargo was full. The dreaded Middle Passage across the Atlantic killed another 10%—as they were chained together in a hot, crowded, unventilated hold without sanitation. Of those who lived to land in the New World, 5% died while awaiting sale, 12% died while being marched or shipped from the sale yard to the plantation, and 10% to 40% of the survivors died during the first three years of plantation life, leaving only about 30% of the slaves initially captured still alive.

Salt loss was probably a major contributor to this chain of deaths during slave transport. One obvious cause of salt loss was sweating under hot conditions. A second was vomiting from seasickness during transport. Probably the biggest cause of salt loss at every stage, though, was from diarrhea due to crowding and lack of sanitation, constituting ideal conditions for the spread of gastrointestinal infections. (Please picture the toilet and handwashing arrangements for slaves chained in the hold of a ship.) All contemporary accounts of slave ships and plantation life emphasized diarrhea ("fluxes" in eighteenth-century terminology) as one of the leading killers of slaves.

Wilson and Grim reasoned, then, that slavery suddenly selected for superefficient kidneys surpassing the already efficient kidneys selected by thousands of years of West African history. Only those slaves who were best able to retain salt could survive the periodic risk of high salt loss to which they were exposed. Salt supersavers would have had the further advantage of building up, under normal conditions, more of a salt reserve in their body fluids and bones, thereby enabling them to survive longer or more frequent bouts of diarrhea. Those superefficient kidneys became a disadvantage only when modern medicine began to reduce diarrhea's lethal effect, thereby transforming a blessing into a curse. A test of this hypothesis will be to determine whether New World blacks, in addition to being more susceptible to hypertension than whites, are also more susceptible than the African black populations from which they were derived, when one controls for environmental risk factors.

Other Conditions

As examples of diseases of Westernization, we have discussed Type 2 diabetes and hypertension. Other such diseases include coronary atherosclerosis, obesity, gallstones, and inflammatory diseases such as Type 1 diabetes and the inflammatory bowel diseases (see individual chapters). In virtually all of these diseases, one can argue both for selective factors and for those selected genetic variations now contributing to disease in the Westernized world.

A final evolutionary question concerns why today's populations of white European ancestry have a relatively low frequency (compared to Native Americans, Pacific islanders, and other peoples) of genes predisposing to diabetes, hypertension, and other such lifestyle diseases. After all, until recently, most Europeans also lived under spartan conditions as peasant farmers until recently. The simplest answer may be that current developments among the Pimas and Nauru Islanders are telescoping into a single generation the lifestyle changes that developed over the course of many centuries in Europe. We refer to our indolent, obese, supermarket-based lifestyle as Western, precisely because it arose first among Europeans and white Americans and is only now spreading to other peoples. Perhaps genes related to diabetes and other such conditions have been undergoing elimination in Europe for centuries, as a result of many infants of diabetic mothers dying at birth, diabetic adults dying younger than other adults, and orphaned children and grandchildren of those diabetic adults dying of neglect. In addition, Europeans and Middle Easterners may have derived less advantage than other peoples from a thrifty genotype ever since the rise of Fertile Crescent agriculture 11,000 years ago, because that area's diversity of planted crops and domestic animals (the highest in the world) may have made starvation a less acute threat there than elsewhere in the world (Diamond, 1997).

SELECTION BY INFECTIOUS AGENTS ON BLOOD GROUPS

A model example of likely effects of natural selection on blood groups and other cell surface antigens is furnished by the Duffy blood group system and *Plasmodium vivax* malaria. The Duffy allele Fy^- is frequent among African blacks but is rare or absent elsewhere in the world. Blacks with this allele have complete resistance to the agent of *P. vivax* malaria, because the Duffy blood group is involved in receptor activity for *P. vivax*. This example illustrates the biological significance of a blood group polymorphism whose existence had been known previously but whose function was not known. Similarly, people lacking the P antigen of the blood group P system are naturally resistant to infection with parvovirus B19, because that antigen is the cellular receptor for the parvovirus.

A large and more controversial literature involves natural selection on the ABO blood group system (Vogel and Motulsky, 1997). One would expect these blood groups to be frequent targets of selection by infectious agents because the surfaces of many microbes bear proteins similar to the ABO antigens, with the result that the microbes may thereby escape recognition as foreign by the host's immune defenses. Various types of correlative evidence have been taken to suggest that individuals with blood group A are especially susceptible to several malignant tumors and to smallpox; that individuals with A, B, and AB are susceptible, and those with O resistant, to rheumatic fever and possibly to syphilis; and that individuals with O are susceptible to gastric and duodenal ulcers, and possibly to plague and cholera (Mourant et al., 1978). If these correlations are real and correctly interpreted, then one would expect selection on ABO frequencies to vary with time, depending on what epidemics have recently swept through an area. One would also expect that some selective effects that have been enormously important in human history, having caused a large proportion of human deaths, may be difficult to document convincingly now because the epidemics have been largely (plague) or completely (smallpox) eliminated.

An example of the available evidence and resultant controversies is a study by Vogel and Chakravartti (1966), carried out in rural areas of India where lack of resources for vaccination, limited access to modern medical care, and lack of understanding of hygiene and disease transmission combined to make smallpox epidemics virtually annual occurrences as recently as the 1960s. Realizing that a comparative study of survivors and victims might yield clues about genetic resistance to smallpox, Vogel and Chakravartti attempted to locate all cases of smallpox during severe epidemics in some Indian villages and small towns. They found a total of 415 unvaccinated smallpox patients, for all but 8 of whom they were also able to find a healthy brother or sister living in the same house and available as a control subject. ABO blood typing was carried out on patients and siblings.

It turned out that, although 52% of the patients (217 out of 415) died in this severe epidemic, risk varied greatly with ABO blood type. Among the 415 patients, 261 carried blood group A (i.e., were blood type A or AB), while 154 lacked A (i.e., blood type B or O). Among the 407 healthy controls, only 80 carried group A and 327 lacked it. The ratio of A to non-A among the patients (261:154), divided by the ratio among the controls (80:327), was 7, meaning that a person with group A blood type had a seven times higher risk of contracting smallpox than someone without it.

The 415 patients were then classified according to the severity of their symptoms. Among the 283 severe cases, most (201) had blood group A, but only 60 among the 132 mild cases had it. Hence, once patients had contracted smallpox, those with group A were three times more likely than those without it to develop a severe case.

Finally, when the 415 patients were classified as to whether they died or survived, most (155 of the 217) who died had group A, while the survivors consisted in nearly equal proportions of those with group A (106) and those without it (92). Hence, once a person had contracted smallpox, patients with group A had a double risk of dying. In short, people with group A are seven times more likely to contract smallpox, then three times more likely to develop a severe case, and finally twice as likely to die of it.

While the study by Vogel and Chakravartti seemingly yields a clear picture, it is considered controversial because two studies on hospital patients in Indian cities (Downie et al., 1966; Sukamaran et al., 1966) and one study in Brazil (Krieger and Vicente, 1969), comparing ABO frequencies between smallpox patients and controls, failed to confirm the conclusion by Vogel and Chakravartti. However, for many reasons, we find the study by Vogel and Chakravartti convincing and the contradictory studies unconvincing. Most of Vogel and Chakravartti's patients were unvaccinated children without medical care, exposed to an especially virulent epidemic, while many patients in the contradictory studies were apparently vaccinated adults who received medical care in large urban hospitals and possibly had been exposed to a less virulent epidemic. As a result, mortality in the other studies was only 0% to 16%, compared to 50% in Vogel and Chakravartti's study. The latter authors studied all patients that they could locate within a small area, and they compared the patients with siblings living in the same house. The other studies used the biased sample of patients who presented themselves at an urban hospital, and they compared the blood groups of those patients with those of so-called control subjects from other areas. However, the controls were inevitably poorly matched, especially within India, where blood group frequencies vary greatly with caste, religion, ethnic affiliation, and locality. In short, the study by Vogel and Chakravartti involved a much less biased set of "experimental" subjects, a set of control subjects far better matched to the experimental subjects, and a much greater selective effect of the smallpox epidemic.

The elimination of natural cases of smallpox in 1977 eliminated opportunities to convince skeptics by further studies. The study by Vogel and Chakravartti may thus serve not only as a model for the best evidence available of natural selection on ABO blood groups but also as a model for the reasons why even that best evidence has left skeptics unconvinced and why better evidence will be difficult to obtain. These uncertainties should not conceal the main conclusion: whatever the details, the ABO blood groups and other cell surface antigens are likely to play a major role in resistance to infectious disease, and infectious agents are likely to have been major determinants of ABO polymorphism.

SELECTION BY INFECTIOUS AGENTS ON GENES OTHER THAN THOSE FOR BLOOD GROUPS

Selection for genetic resistance to infectious agents presumably could involve genes expressed in any organ system affected by the pathogen (Hill and Motulsky, 1999). For example, it has been argued that acid hypersecretion may have been selected for as a protective factor for tuberculosis (Petersen and Rotter, 1983). (This is a further example of the pleiotropic mechanisms discussed here, since acid hypersecretion also predisposes to a disease, peptic ulcer.) Individuals with low acid production are exceptionally prone to infection (Gianella et al., 1972, 1973); hypochlorhydria precedes cholera infection (Nalin et al., 1978); and acid secretion and peptic activity of the stomach have a large genetic component (Rotter, 1980; see Chapter 13). In some cases, genetic susceptibility and resistance to a current agent may have resulted from selection in response to a prior agent. For instance, the CCR5 gene variants, which now provide protection against HIV, have a distribution similar to that of bubonic plague (Dean et al., 1996; Carrington et al., 1997), suggesting that plague could have selected for those CCR5 variants.

UNSOLVED QUESTIONS

The evolution of human genetic diseases offers more unsolved questions than established facts. The literature on genetic antimalarials demonstrates that even relatively large selective effects can be difficult to demonstrate. Most effects are likely to be of smaller selective strength and even more difficult to demonstrate. The literature on ABO blood groups demonstrates that some of the strongest selective effects in the past may no longer be operating in the present. As an indication of whole areas that are likely to be important but that have been ignored in the medical genetic literature, we mention two areas: sexual selection and the evolutionary significance of elderly people.

Sexual Selection

After Darwin (1859) had written his book *On the Origin of Species by Means of Natural Selection*, he went on to write an even longer book (Darwin 1871) entitled *The Descent of Man and Selection in Relation to Sex*. By sexual selection, Darwin meant increased success in transmitting genes affecting traits that enable the gene-bearer more successfully to attract mates of the opposite sex or to defeat rivals of the same sex, rather than genes affecting traits improving the individual's chances of surviving or of producing young. Darwin was impressed by many animal traits that would appear to interfere with survival and to be opposed by natural selection—such as bold color patterns of many nonpoisonous animals, or the exaggeratedly long plumes of some male birds. Darwin suggested that these traits became favored by sexual selection, which could act in opposition to natural selection. Evolutionary biologists studying animals now routinely take sexual selection into account when considering possible explanations for traits of animals.

It seems likely that sexual selection has also been important in the evolution of the human species, and indeed human biology was what brought Darwin to recognize the concept of sexual selection. In particular, Darwin noted that external and highly visible human characteristics, which tend to vary geographically and lack obvious interpretations in terms of natural selection, may have arisen through sexual selection. These traits include human geographic variation in hair color, hair form, eye color, and skin color. A zoologist from Outer Space visiting the Earth would quickly focus on the fact that black hair is fixed in many human populations, brown hair common in others, yellow hair common in a few, and red hair also common in a few. The extraterrestrial zoologist would also be impressed by our variously blue, green, or dark brown eyes. No one has suggested any remotely plausible reason why red hair should uniquely promote human survival only in Ireland and nowhere else in the world. Explanations in terms of natural selection for geographic variation in hair form and eye color are equally elusive. Even the explanations usually cited for geographic variation in human skin color dissolve under scrutiny (Diamond, 1992). Instead, as Darwin pointed out, skin and hair and eyes are among the main determinants of our esthetic preferences in selecting mates and sex partners and are likely targets of sexual selection.

Parts of the literature of medical genetics deserve re-examination from the perspective of sexual selection. For example, Zahavi and Zahavi (1997) have suggested that sexually selected traits and other animal signals tend to be traits that are expensive to synthesize and maintain and that thereby can be construed as honest signals of bearer quality: only an individual in good health and bearing good genes (hence, a good choice as mate) could afford to maintain the trait. Hamilton and Zuk (1982) have suggested that animals bearing expensive signals are thereby advertising to prospective mates that they are healthy, well nourished, free of parasites and sexually transmitted diseases, and therefore worthy of selection as mates. The literature on human infectious diseases and sexually transmitted diseases, and on their external manifestations, deserves reconsideration from the perspective on sexual selection developed by Zahavi and Zahavi, Hamilton and Zuk, and others.

Selective Value of the Elderly

The literature of medical genetics abounds with statements claiming that deleterious consequences of a gene emerging only late in life cannot be of selective value. The underlying assumption is that, once a man or woman has finished reproducing—that is, once the woman is postmenopausal or the man has fertilized his partner for the last time—the man's or woman's survival has no further consequences for the survival of offspring bearing his or her genes.

Even geneticists who make such statements would acknowledge that a child's survival in traditional societies is influenced by the survival of its parents at least until the child is a teenager or economically independent. However, it is evidently not obvious why parent survival is important past the age of offspring economic independence. This perspective would indeed be valid for tigers, rats, and most other mammalian species, in which parents have little or no significance for offspring after the latter's age of economic independence. For humans, however, we believe that this assumption is not only wrong but overlooks one of the most important features that distinguish human societies from those of most other mammals.

The death of an embryo, a fetus, or an infant forecloses no transmission of genes except through the foreclosed reproduction of the embryo/fetus/infant itself. Consider, however, the consequences of the death of an adult, especially of an elderly adult in a traditionally pre-literate society (Diamond, 2001). In the absence of books, elderly people are the repositories of knowledge. Their experience may mean the difference between life or death, not only for their children and grandchildren but also for their entire clan or tribe, many of whom are genetically related to them. For example, in quizzing New Guineans about local plant and animal species, one of us (J.D.) has regularly found that when his informants are stumped by a question, they turn to the oldest person in the village—often a man or woman over 80 years old, blind and crippled and toothless, but the repository of tribal knowledge. That person possesses the experience important to the tribe's survival, such as knowing which plants that are not normally considered edible were still found useful as famine foods at the time of the last big cyclone 70 years ago.

Thus, until the origins of writing around 3400 B.C. began to erode the value of the elderly to the low levels prevailing in modern Western society, natural selection operating on the elderly was far more important than their vanished capacity to sire or give birth to offspring would suggest. This is surely the genetic reason for the slowed senescence of humans, compared to our closest relatives the great apes, and for the otherwise baffling evolution of human female menopause. Even great apes in zoos, receiving far better medical care and nutrition than the vast majority of the world's humans, never survive past the age of 60, because without human language the social value of an old great ape (although much greater than that of an old tiger) is still less than that of an old human. Human female menopause evolved to preserve elderly women from the risk that death in pregnancy and childbirth and during lactation would jeopardize the mother's prior investment in other children and grandchildren. An important task for medical geneticists will be to identify traits whose positive selective value appears especially in the elderly, and which have therefore been responsible for the slowing of senescence in humans compared to our great ape relatives.

Identifying such traits may help us understand, and eventually delay, the aging process. This point illustrates, once again, that identifying the selective factors in human genetic diseases poses more than just an academic puzzle devoid of practical significance. Knowledge of those selective factors offers us a route to improving our lives in many ways, including by understanding the diseases themselves, intervening in them, and devising specific prevention strategies and therapies. Such gains in knowledge may partly compensate for the victimization of the innocent by genetic diseases—a victimization that, as we noted in the first paragraphs of this chapter, outrages our sense of justice. Geneticists can thereby fulfill the biblication admonition: "Justice, justice you shall pursue" (Deuteronomy 16:20).

REFERENCES

Allison AC: Protection afforded by sickle cell trait against subtertian malarial infection. Br Med J 1954; 1:290–294.
Andermann E, Scriver CR, Wolfe LS, Dansky L, Andermann F: Genetic variants of Tay-Sachs disease: Tay-Sachs disease and Sandhoff's disease in French Canadians, juvenile Tay-Sachs disease in Lebanese Canadians, and a Tay-Sachs screening program in the French-Canadian population. In: Kaback MM (ed), Tay-Sachs Disease: Screening and Prevention. New York: Alan R. Liss, 1977:161–188.
Austin MA, Breslow JL, Nennekens CH, Buring JE, Willett WC, Krauss RM: Low-density lipoprotein subclass patterns and risk of myocardial infarction. JAMA 1988a; 260:1917–1921.
Austin MA, King MC, Vranizan KM, Krauss RM: Atherogenic lipoprotein phenotype: a proposed genetic marker for coronary heart disease risk. Circulation 1990; 82:495–506.
Austin MA, King MC, Vranizan KM, Newman B, Krauss RM: Inheritance of low-density lipoprotein subclass patterns: results of complex segregation analysis. Am J Hum Genet 1988b; 43:838–846.
Avigad S, Cohen BE, Bauer S, Schwartz G, Frydman M, Woo SL, Niny Y, Shiloh Y: A single origin of phenylketonuria in Yemenite Jews. Nature 1990; 344:168–170.
Beighton P: Genetic disorders in Southern Africa. S Afr Med J; 1976; 50:1125–1128.
Bennett PH, Rewers M, Knowler W: Epidemiology of diabetes mellitus. In: Porte D, Sherwin R (eds), Diabetes Mellitus, 5th ed. Stamford, Connecticut: Appleton and Lange, 1997:373–400.
Bergeron P, Laberge C, Grenier A: Hereditary tyrosinemia in the province of Quebec: prevalence at birth and geographic distribution. Clin Genet 1974; 5:157–162.
Beutler E, Felitti V, Gelbart T, Ho N: The effect of HFE genotypes on measurements of iron overload in patients attending a health appraisal clinic. Ann Intern Med 2000; 133:329–337.
Blumberg BS, Hesser JE: Loci differently affected by selection in two American black populations. Proc Natl Acad Sci USA 1971; 68:2554–2558.
Botha MC, Beighton P: Inherited disorders in the Afrikaner population of Southern Africa: Part I. Historical and demographic background, cardiovascular, neurological, metabolic and intestinal conditions. S Afr Med J 1983; 64:609–612.
Brenner-Ullman A, Melzer-Ofir H, Daniels M, Shohat M: Possible protection against asthma in heterozygotes for familial Mediterranean fever. Am J Med Genet 1994; 53:172–175.
Burt VL, Whelton P, Roccella EJ, Brown C, Cutler JA, Higgins M, Horan MJ, Labarthe D: Prevalence of hypertension in the U.S. adult populations: results from the Third National Health and Nutrition Examination Survey, 1988–1991. Hypertension 1995; 25:305–313.

Carrington M, Kissner T, Gerrard B, Ivanov S, O'Brien SJ, Dean M: Novel alleles of the chemokine-receptor gene CCR5. Am J Hum Genet 1997; 61:1261–1267.

Cavalli-Sforza LL, Menozzi P, Piazza A: The History and Geography of Human Genes. Princeton, NJ: Princeton University Press, 1994.

Chakraborty R, Ferrell RE, Stern MP, Haffner SM, Hazuda HP, Rosenthal M: Relationship of prevalence of non-insulin dependent diabetes mellitus to Amerindian admixture in the Mexican Americans of San Antonio, Texas. Genet Epidemiol 1986; 3:435–454.

Chase GA: The Tay-Sachs disease gene among Ashkenazic Jews: founder effect and genetic drift. In: Kaback MM (ed), Tay-Sachs Disease: Screening and Prevention. New York: Alan R. Liss, 1977:107–110.

Chase GA, McKusick VA: Founder effect in Tay-Sachs disease. Am J Hum Genet 1972; 24:339–340.

Danon Y, Zemer D: Low asthma prevalence found in FMF. Immunol Allergy Pract 1992; 10:357–362.

Darwin C: On the Origin of Species by Means of Natural Selection or the Preservation of Favorite Races in the Struggle for Life. London: Murray, 1859.

Darwin C: The Descent of Man and Selection in Relation to Sex. London: Murray, 1871.

Dean G: The Porphyrias, 2nd ed. London: Pitman, 1972.

Dean M, Carrington M, Winkler C, Huttley GA, Smith MW, Allikmets R, Goedert JJ, Buchbinder SP, Vittinghoff E, Gomperts E, et al.: Genetic restriction of HIV-1 infection and progression to AIDS by a deletion allele of the CKR5 structural gene. Science 1996; 273:1856–1862.

De Braekeleer M, Larochelle J: Genetic epidemiology of hereditary tyrosinemia in Quebec and in Saguenay-Lac-St-Jean. Am J Hum Genet 1990; 47:302–307.

de Courten M, Bennett PH, Tuomilehto J, Zimmet P: Epidemiology of NIDDM in non-Europids. In: Alberti KGMM, DeFronzo RA, Keen H (eds), International Textbook of Diabetes Mellitus, 2nd ed. New York: Wiley, 1997:143–170.

de la Chapelle A, Wright FA: Linkage disequilibrium mapping in isolated populations: the example of Finland revisited. Proc Natl Acad Sci USA 1998; 95:12416–12423.

Deuteronomy. In Tanakh the Holy Scriptures, The New JPS Translation According to the Traditional Hebrew Text. Philadelphia: Jewish Publication Society, 1985.

Diamond JM: The cruel logic of our genes. Discover 10, 1989; 11:72–78.

Diamond JM: The Third Chimpanzee. New York: HarperCollins, York 1992.

Diamond JM: Guns, Germs, and Steel: The Fate of Human Societies. New York: Norton, 1997.

Diamond JM: Unwritten knowledge. Nature 2001; 410:521.

Dobzhansky T: Genetics and the Origin of Species, 3rd ed. New York: Columbia University Press, 1951.

Downie HW, Meiklejohn G, Vincent L, Rao AR, Sundara Babu BV, Kempe CH: Smallpox frequency and severity in relation to A, B and O blood groups. Bull WHO 1966; 33:623.

Dowse GK, Zimmet PZ, Finch CF, Collins V: Decline in incidence of epidemic glucose intolerance in Nauruans: implications for the "thrifty genotype." Am J Epidemiol 1991; 133:1093–1104.

Eickhoff S, Beighton P: Genetic disorders on the island of St. Helena. S Afr Med J 1985; 68:475–478.

Fleming AF, Storey J, Molineaux L, Iroko EA, Attai EDE: Abnormal haemoglobins in the Sudan savanna of Nigeria. I. Prevalence of haemoglobins and relationships between sickle cell trait, malaria and survival. Ann Trop Med Parasitol 1979; 73:161–172.

Giannella RA, Broitman SA, Zamcheck N: Gastric acid barrier to ingested microorganisms in man: studies in vivo and in vitro. Gut 1972; 13:251–256.

Giannella RA, Broitman SA, Zamcheck N: Influence of gastric acidity on bacterial and parasitic enteric infections. Ann Int Med 1973; 78:271–276.

Goldstein JL, Hobbs HH, Brown MS: Familial hypercholesterolemia. In: Scriver CR, Beaudet AL, Sly WS, Valle D (eds), The Metabolic and Molecular Bases of Inherited Disease, 7th ed. New York: McGraw-Hill, 1995:1981–2030.

Goodman RM, Motulsky AG (eds): Genetic Diseases among Ashkenazi Jews. New York: Raven Press, 1979.

Gravel RA, Clarke JTR, Kaback MM, Mahuran D, Sandhoff K, Suzuki K: The G_{M2} gangliosidoses. In: Scriver CR, Beaudet AL, Sly WS, Valle D (eds), The Metabolic and Molecular Bases of Inherited Disease, 7th ed. New York: McGraw-Hill, 1995:2839–2879.

Hamilton WD, Zuk M: Heritable true fitness and bright birds: a role for parasites? Science 1982; 156:1260–1262.

Hayden MR: Huntington's Chorea. New York: Springer, 1981.

Hayden MR, Berkowitz, AL, Beighton P, Yiptong C: Huntington's chorea on the island of Mauritius. S Afr Med J; 1981; 60:1001–1002.

Hill AVS: The immunogenetics of human infectious diseases. Annu Rev Immunol 1998; 16:593–617.

Hill AVS, Allsopp CEM, Kwiatkowski D, Anstey NM, Twumasi P, Rowe PA, Bennett S, Brewster D, McMichael AJ, Greenwood, BM: Common West African HLA antigens are associated with protection from severe malaria. Nature 1991; 352:595–600.

Hill AVS, Motulsky AG: Genetic variation and human disease: the role of natural selection. In: Stearns SC (ed). Evolution in Health and Disease. Oxford: Oxford University Press, 1999:50–61.

Hill AVS, Yates SN, Allsopp CEM, Gupta S, Gilbert SC, Lalvani A, Aidoo M, Davenport M, Plebanski M: Human leukocyte antigens and natural selection by malaria. Phil Trans R Soc Lond B 1994; 346:379–385.

Jackson WPU: Osteo-dental dysplasia (Cleido-cranial dysostosis). Acta Med Canad 1951; 139:292–303.

Jenkins T, Ramsay M: Malaria protective alleles in Southern Africa: relict alleles of no health significance? In: Roberts DF, De Stefano GF (eds). Genetic Variation and Its Maintenance. Cambridge: Cambridge University Press, 1986:135–147.

Jonxis JHP: The frequence of haemoglobin S and C carriers in Curacao and Surinam. Oxford: Blackwell, 1959.

Jorde LB: Genetic diseases in the Ashkenazi population: evolutionary considerations. In: Bonne-Tamir B, Adam A (eds). Genetic Diversity Among Jews. New York: Oxford University Press, 1992:305–318.

Kelly TE, Chase GA, Kaback MM, Kumor K, McKusick VA: Tay-Sachs disease: high gene frequency in a non-Jewish population. Am J Hum Genet 1975; 27:287–291.

Kan YW, Dozy AM: Evolution of the hemoglobin S and C genes in world populations. Science 1980; 209:388–391.

Krieger H, Vicente AT: Smallpox and the AB0 system in Southern Brazil. Hum Hered 1969; 19:654.

Laberge C: Hereditary tyrosinemia in a French Canadian isolate. Am J Hum Genet 1969; 21:36–45.

Livingstone FB: Frequencies of Hemoglobin Variants. New York: Oxford University Press, 1985.

Mayr E: Animal Species and Evolution. Cambridge: Harvard University Press, 1963.

McKusick, VA: Nonhomogeneous distribution of recessive diseases. In: Goodman RM, Motulsky AG (eds). Genetic Diseases among Ashkenazi Jews. New York: Raven Press, 1979:271–284.

Miller LH, Mason SJ, Clyde DF, McGinniss MH: The resistance factor to Plasmodium vivax in blacks: the Duffy-blood-group genotype, FyFy. N Engl J Med 1976; 294:302–304.

Mitchell GA, Lambert M, Tanguay RM: Hypertyrosinemia. In: Scriver CR, Beaudet AL, Sly WS, Valle D (eds). The Metabolic and Molecular Bases of Inherited Disease, 7th ed. New York: McGraw-Hill, 1995:1077–1106.

Morral N, Bertranpetit J, Estivill X, Nunes V, Casals T, Gimenez J, Reis A, Varon-Mateeva R, Macek M Jr, Kalaydjieva L, et al. The origin of the major cystic fibrosis mutation (ΔF508) in European populations. Nat Genet 1994; 7:169–175.

Motulsky AG: Glucose-6-phosphate dehydrogenase and abnormal hemoglobin polymorphisms—evidence regarding malarial selection. In: Salzano FM (ed). The Role of Natural Selection in Human Evolution. Amsterdam: North Holland, 1975:271–291.

Motulsky AG: Possible selective effects of urbanization on Ashkenazi Jews. In: Goodman RM, Motulsky AG (eds). Genetic Diseases among Ashkenazi Jews. New York: Raven Press, 1979:301–312.

Motulsky AG: Jewish diseases and origins. Nat Genet 1995; 9:99–101.

Mourant AE, Kopec AC, Domaniewska-Sobczak K: Blood Groups and Diseases: A Study of Associations of Diseases with Blood Groups and Other Polymorphisms. Oxford: Oxford University Press, 1978.

Myrianthopoulos NC, Aronson SM: Population dynamics of Tay-Sachs disease: I. Reproductive fitness and selection. Am J Hum Genet 1966; 18:313–327.

Myrianthopoulos NC, Melnick M: Tay-Sachs disease: a genetic-historical view of selective advantage. In: Kaback MM (ed). Tay-Sachs Disease: Screening and Prevention. New York: Alan R. Liss, 1977:95–106.

Nalin DR, Levin RJ, Levin MM, Hoover D, Bergquist E, McLaughlin J, Libonati J, Alam J, Hornick RB: Cholera, non-vibrio cholera and stomach acid. Lancet 1978; 2:856–859.

Neel JV: Diabetes mellitus: a thrifty genotype rendered detrimental by progress? Am J Hum Genet 1962; 14:353–362.

Norio R, Nevanlinna HR, Perheentupa J: Hereditary diseases in Finland. Ann Clin Res 1973; 5:109–141.

Pagnier J, Mears JG, Dunda-Belkhodja O, Schaefer-Rego KE, Beldjord C, Nagel RL, Labie D: Evidence for the multicentric origin of the sickle-cell hemoglobin gene in Africa. Proc Natl Acad Sci USA 1984; 81:1771–1773.

Peltonen L: Positional cloning of disease genes: advantages of genetic isolates. Hum Hered 2000; 50:66–75.

Peltonen L, Jalanko A, Varilo T: Molecular genetics of the Finnish disease heritage. Hum Mol Genet 1999; 8:1913–1923.

Petersen GM, Rotter JI: Genetic and evolutionary implications in peptic ulcer disease. Am J Phys Anthropol 1983; 62:71–79.

Petersen GM, Rotter JI, Cantor RM, Field LL, Greenwald S, Lim JS, Roy C, Schoenfeld V, Lowden JA, Kaback MM: The Tay-Sachs disease gene in North American Jewish populations: geographic variations and origin. Am J Hum Genet 1983; 35:1258–1269.

Petersen G, Rotter J, MacCraken J, Raelson J, New M, Terasaki P, Park M, Sparkes R, Ward J: Selective advantage of the 21-hydroxylase deficiency gene in Alaskan Eskimos: use of a linked marker to identify heterozygotes. Am J Hum Genet 1984; 36:177S.

Risch N, de Leon D, Ozelius L, Kramer P, Almasy L, Singer B, Fahn S, Breakefield X, Bressman S: Genetic analysis of idiopathic torsion dystonia in Ashkenazi Jews and their recent descent from a small founder population. Nat Genet 1995; 9:152–159.

Roth MP, Petersen GM, McElree C, Feldman E, Rotter JI. Geographic origins of Jewish patients with inflammatory bowel disease. Gastroenterology 1989; 97:900–904.

Rotter JI: The genetics of peptic ulcer disease—more than one gene, more than one disease. In: Steinberg AG, Bearn AG, Motulsky AG, Childs B (eds). Progress in Medical Genetics, No. 4 (New Series) 1980; 4:1–58.

Rotter JI: Inflammatory bowel disease. Lancet 1994; 343:1360.

Rotter JI, Bu X, Cantor RM, Warden CH, Brown J, Gray RJ, Blanche PJ, Krauss RM, Lusis AJ: Multilocus genetic determinants of LDL particle size in coronary artery disease families. Am J Hum Genet 1996; 58:585–594.

Rotter JI, Diamond JM: What maintains the frequencies of human genetic diseases? Nature 1987; 329:289–290.

Rotter JI, Yang H, Shohat T: Genetic complexities of inflammatory bowel disease and its distribution among the Jewish people. In: Bonne-Tamir B, Adam A (eds). Genetic Diversity among Jews: Diseases and Markers at the DNA Level. New York: Oxford University Press, 1992:395–411.

Rund D, Cohen T, Filon D, Dowling CE, Warren TC, Barak I, Rachmilewitz E, Kazazian HH Jr, Oppenheim A: Evolution of a genetic disease in an ethnic isolate: beta-thalassemia in the Jews of Kurdistan. Proc Natl Acad Sci USA 1991; 88:310–314.

Ruwende C, Khoo SC, Snow RW, Yates SNR, Kwiatkowski D, Gupta S, Warn P, Allsopp CEM, Gilbert SC, Peschu N, et al.: Natural selection of hemi- and heterozygotes for G6PD deficiency in Africa by resistance to severe malaria. Nature 1995; 376:246–249.

Sacks, O: The Island of the Colorblind. New York: Knopf, 1996.

Sajantila A, Abdel-Halim S, Savolainen P, Bauer K, Gierig C, Pääbo S: Paternal and maternal DNA linkages reveal a bottleneck in the founding of the Finnish population. Proc Natl Acad Sci USA 1996; 93:12035–12039.

Seftel HC, Baker SG, Jenkins T, Mendelsohn D: Prevalence of familial hypercholesterolemia in Johannesburg Jews. Am J Med Genet 1989; 34:545–547.

Skorecki K, Selig S, Blazer S, Bradman R, Bradman N, Waburton PJ, Ismajlowicz M, Hammer MF: Y chromosomes of Jewish priests. Nature 1997; 385:32.

Stern MP, Gonzalez C, Mitchell BD, Villalpando E, Haffner SM, Hazuda HP: Genetic and environmental determinants of type II diabetes in Mexico City and San Antonio, Texas. Diabetes 1992; 41:484–492.

Sukamaran PK, Master HR, Undesia JV, Balakrishnan B, Sanghvi LD: AB0 blood groups in active cases of smallpox. Indian J Med Sci 1966; 20:119.

Thalhammer O: Frequency of inborn errors of metabolism especially PKU, in some representative newborn screening centers around the world: a collaborative study. Hum Genet 1975; 30:273–286.

Thivolent CH, Beaufrere B, Betuel H, Gebuhrer, Chatelain P, Durand A, Tourniaire J, Francois R: Islet cell and insulin autoantibodies in subjects at high risk for development of Type I (insulin-dependent) diabetes mellitus: the Lyon family study. Diabetologia 1988; 31:741–746.

Thomas MG, Skorecki K, Ben-Ami H, Parfitt T, Bradman N, Goldstein DB: Origins of old testament priests. Nature 1998; 394:138–140.

Vadheim CM, Rotter JI, Maclaren NK, Riley WJ, Anderson CE: Preferential transmission of diabetic alleles within the HLA gene complex. New Engl J Med 1986; 315:1314–1318.

Vadheim CM, Rotter JI, Riley WJ, Akkina JE, Anderson CE: Prenatal selection for diabetes HLA genes and the onset of IDDM. Diabetes 1985; 34:21A.

Vadheim CM, Rotter JI, Riley WJ, Maclaren NK, Petersen GM, Cantor, RM: An interaction of genetic susceptibility and birth order in Type I diabetes. Clin Res 1987; 35:186A.

Vogel F, Chakravartti MR: AB0 blood groups and smallpox in a rural population of West Bengal and Bihar (India). Hum Genet 1966; 3:166–180.

Vogel F, Motulsky AG: Human Genetics, Problems and Approaches, 3rd ed. Berlin: Springer-Verlag, 1997.

Weatherall DJ, Clegg JB, Higgs DR, Wood WG: The hemoglobinopathies. In: Scriver CR, Beaudet AL, Sly WS, Valle D (eds). The Metabolic and Molecular Bases of Inherited Disease, 7th ed. New York: McGraw-Hill, 1995:3417–3484.

Welsh MJ, Tsui L-C, Boat TF, Beaudet AL: Cystic fibrosis. In: Scriver CR, Beaudet AL, Sly WS, Valle D (ed). The Metabolic and Molecular Bases of Inherited Disease, 7th ed. New York: McGraw-Hill, 1995:3799–3876.

Whelton PK, He J, Klag MJ: Blood pressure in Westernized populations. In: Swales JD (ed). Textbook of Hypertension. London: Blackwell Scientific, 1994:11–21.

Williams GC: Pleiotropy natural selection, and the evolution of senescence. Evolution 1957; 11:398–411.

Wilson TW, Grim CE: Biohistory of slavery and blood pressure differences in blacks today. Hypertension 17, 1991(Suppl 1):I122–I128.

Workman PL, Blumberg BS, Cooper AJ: Selection, gene migration and polymorphic stability in U.S. White and Negro population. Am J Hum Genet 1963; 15:429.

Zahavi A, Zahavi A: The Handicap Principle. New York: Oxford University Press, 1997.

Zimmet P: Challenges in diabetes epidemiology—from West to the rest. Diabetes Care 1992; 15:232–252.

Zimmet P, Dowse G, Finch C, Serjeantson S, King H: The epidemiology and natural history of NIDDM—lessons from the South Pacific. Diabetes Metab Rev 1990; 6:91–124.

Zlotogora J, Zimmerman J, Rachmilewitz D: Crohn's disease in Ashkenazi Jews. Gastroenterology 1990; 99:286–290.

5 Animal Models of Complex Genetic Disease

ALDONS J. LUSIS, DAVID WEST, AND RICHARD C. DAVIS

Animal models have been identified for most common genetic diseases. For example, Table 5–1 lists some disease models that occur among various inbred strains of mice. Even behavioral traits such as schizophrenia can be modeled in animals. Although "schizophrenic" mice have not been recognized, common genetic variations relevant to schizophrenia do occur among inbred strains of mice (Table 5–2). Animal models have a number of advantages for the dissection of complex diseases, and recent technical advances have further enhanced the use of these models for detailed analysis of molecular mechanisms and interactions in genetic diseases. The usefulness of planned genetic modifications in mice (transgenic and gene-targeted mice) for analysis of complex and Mendelian diseases is clear. Moreover, new applications of this technology, such as the use of transgenic mice to "sift" sequences for function, are being developed. The literature on the use of animal models to study complex genetic disease is large, and here we attempt only to summarize some of the approaches and to provide some examples. Some excellent reviews of the subject are available (Copeland et al., 1993; Frankel, 1995; Paigen, 1995; Silver, 1995; Bedell et al., 1997a, 1997b; Darvasi, 1998). Although the mapping and identification of the genes for complex diseases is greatly simplified in animal models (particularly mice), compared to studies in humans, a major question is: How relevant to human disease are these animal models? The available data suggest that some of the genetic factors and pathways will be shared between animal models and humans and that others will differ. Thus, through studies of animal models, we can expect to identify a subset of the genetic causes of complex human diseases. This should greatly aid the identification of the remaining factors.

STUDIES IN HUMANS AND ANIMAL MODELS ARE COMPLEMENTARY

Figure 5–1 shows a flowchart for the analysis of complex genetic traits in humans and rodent animal models. There are two approaches for identifying genes that contribute directly to complex traits in humans. The first is the candidate gene approach, involving either association or linkage analyses using known genes that are involved in pathways relevant to the trait. The second is a search of random parts of the genome to detect linkage to anonymous genes contributing to the trait. Currently, such linkage analyses usually involve whole genome scans using polymorphic markers. Once a locus contributing to the trait is identified, genes in the region are examined for possible involvement. In the case of Mendelian disorders, such a "positional cloning" strategy is straightforward (although laborious) given enough informative meioses. But for complex diseases, fine mapping (to within 1 cM or less) of the gene requires extremely large numbers of individuals. A fundamental problem with human studies is that genetic heterogeneity and environmental influences make it very difficult to detect the effects of moderate genetic influences, such as those likely to be involved in most common diseases (Lander and Schork, 1994). In addition, it can be difficult to extend such studies to the molecular level. Also, in the case of Mendelian disease, mutations with obvious consequences for gene expression (e.g., splice site or termination mutations) are usually involved, whereas with complex disorders, the genetic changes are likely to be subtle and difficult to distinguish from silent polymorphisms.

There are several important advantages in the use of animal models (particularly mice) for the dissection of complex traits (Fig. 5–1). First, mapping is much more straightforward in animal models: crosses can be planned, large numbers of progeny can be produced, and the environment can be controlled. Second, it is easier to move from a locus to a gene in rodent models. As in humans, candidate genes residing at a locus ("positional candidate genes") can be tested. But, in contrast to human studies, if none of the candidates are found to underlie the trait, it is still possible to isolate the chromosomal region on a common genetic background in rodents by constructing a "congenic strain" (see below). In turn, this makes possible biochemical and genetic studies, including positional cloning. Once the animal gene has been identified, the human homolog can be easily obtained by DNA hybridization or by reference to the human sequence, since most gene coding sequences are highly conserved between species. Finally, the mouse offers important advantages for functional studies. Over the last 10 years, transgenic mice and knockout mice have become essential tools for examining the role of specific genes in all areas of mammalian biology.

Genetic linkage groups are conserved between mouse and human chromosomes (DeBry and Seldin, 1996), a phenomenon that is sometimes called *conserved chromosomal synteny*. Thus, in some cases, knowledge of the location of a chromosomal region contributing to a complex trait in mice can allow one to predict where a particular locus is likely to reside in the human genome, even without knowledge of the underlying gene. For example, mouse multigenic obesity loci have been used to predict the locations of human obesity loci (Lembertas et al., 1997). Further examples of conserved chromosomal synteny for complex disease traits include loci for multiple sclerosis (Kuokkanen et al., 1996), Type 1 diabetes (Mein et al., 1998), and au-

Table 5–1. Naturally Occurring Mouse Models for Complex Human Genetic Diseases and Other Traits

Disorder	Strain
Alcoholism or drug addiction	C57BL/6
Asthma	A
Atherosclerosis	C57BL/6, DBA
Audiogenic seizures	DBA
Cleft palate	A
Deafness	LP
Dental disease	C57BL/6, BALB/c
Diabetes, Type 1	NOD
Diabetes, Type 2	C57BL/6
Epilepsy	EL, SWR
Granulosa cell tumors of the ovary	SWR
Germ cell tumors of the ovary	LT
Germ cell tumors of the testis	129
Hemolytic anemia	NZB
Hepatitis	BALB/c
Hodgkin's disease	SJL
Hypertension	MA/My
Kidney adenocarcinoma	BALB/c
Leprosy	BALB/c
Leukemia	AKR, C58, P
Lung tumors	A, MA
Measles	BALB/c
Osteoporosis	DBA
Polygenic obesity	NZB, NZW
Pulmonary tumors	A
Rheumatoid arthritis	MRL
Spina bifida	CT
Systemic lupus erythematosus	NZB, NZW
Trypanosomiasis A	BALB/c
Whooping cough (pertussis)	BALB/c

List complied in part from Copeland et al., 1993; Lusis, 1993; Crabbe et al., 1994; Frankel, 1995; Melo et al., 1996; Bedell et al., 1997a, 1997b; Lusis et al., 1998. See also references in Table 5–4.

toimmune disease (Tsao et al., 1997). Of course, the human and mouse genetic loci for complex traits will not always correspond since the genes that vary commonly in the population will often depend on chance rather than on selection.

ANIMAL MODELS

Naturally Occurring Models

Many complex diseases result from the effects of common quantitative genetic variations that can produce pathologic effects under particular environmental conditions or in old age. Frequently, quantitative variations with similar pathological effects arise among naturally occurring animal models. Table 5–1 lists common inbred strains of mice that exhibit susceptibility to aspects of complex human diseases. For example, genetic variation affecting the density of bones provide models for osteoporosis, and variations affecting the accumulation of body fat provide models for obesity and Type 2 diabetes.

Among animal models, the mouse is clearly the most useful mammal for genetic studies (Table 5–3). In particular, many genetic strains and variants with mutant genes are available (Doolittle et al., 1996), and the tools for genetic analysis, particularly a dense set of polymorphic markers, are most advanced in the mouse (Dietrich et al., 1995a; Mouse Genome Informatics Project, 1995). Therefore, this review will focus largely on studies with mice.

Of course, larger animals do have advantages for certain physiologic studies and may in some instances better reflect human pathology. Baboons and pigs, for example, develop atherosclerotic lesions that closely resemble those found in humans, while dogs exhibit a wide range of easily recognized behavioral patterns. The rat has been the classic mammal for physiologic studies and, for certain traits such as hypertension and diabetes, it continues to have advantages for genetic experimentation (Rapp and Dene, 1985; Hsu et al., 1994). The many similarities between mice and rats facilitate extrapolation of molecular and biologic information from one species to the other, and complete linkage maps with many highly polymorphic markers have been constructed in the rat (Jacob et al., 1995). Genetic studies in vertebrates such as the zebrafish, and even in invertebrates, will in many cases also be relevant to understanding complex human genetic disease.

Utility of Monogenic Models

A large number of mice with Mendelian mutations relevant to complex diseases have been identified. For example, there are Mendelian mouse models of obesity, autoimmune disease, behavioral disorders, and cancer. These resulted from rare spontaneous mutations during breeding. Because inbreeding tends to reveal recessive mutations; a mouse carrying a recessive mutation can pass on the mutation to multiple pups, which, if chosen for brother–sister mating, could produce progeny homozygous for the mutation. The concept that Mendelian diseases can provide valuable information about pathways contributing to complex disease is well established. For example, familial hypercholesterolemia demonstrated unequivocally that high-plasma cholesterol causes atherosclerosis, suggesting strongly that cholesterol contributes to the common, complex forms of atherosclerosis. Similarly, Mendelian forms of cancer, such as retinoblastoma, have revealed pathways that contribute to sporadic forms of the disease. An outstanding example of the importance of Mendelian mouse mutations are five mouse mutations that cause massive obesity: *obese* (*ob*), *diabetes* (*db*), *tubby*,

Table 5–2. Modeling of Behavioral Human Traits in Animals: Example of Schizophrenia

Human Trait	Animal Trait
Positive symptoms (hallucinations, delusions)	Increased responsivity to amphetamine (which exacerbate human symptoms)
Negative symptoms (social withdrawal, poverty of speech)	Decreased exploration (novel objects); decreased response to reward (sucrose drinking)
Cognitive impairment (memory deficit, impaired ability to make decisions)	Learning (maze)
Attention impairment (deficits in sustained attention and in filtering sensory information	Startle response, or prepulse inhibition of acoustic startle response

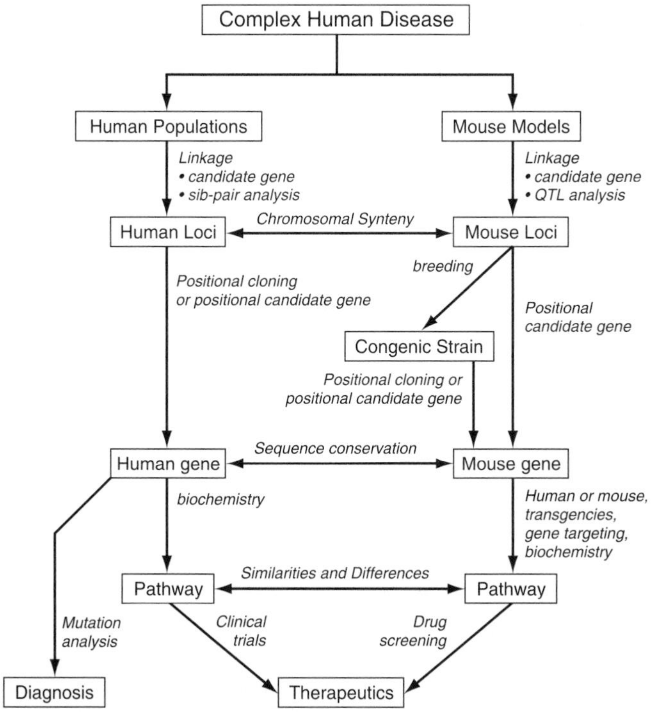

Fig. 5–1. Schematic diagram showing how mouse models can accelerate the identification of genes that contribute to complex genetic traits. The left side of the diagram indicates the steps involved in characterizing a gene for a complex trait directly in humans, and the right side indicates the steps used in mouse (or rat) models. The searches in humans and rodents are bridged by conserved chromosomal syntenies (allowing prediction of the chromosomal location of a gene in one species based on its location in the other species) and sequence conservation (allowing the identification of homologous genes by cross-hybridization). Animal models also facilitate dissection of pathways and the development of therapeutic procedures.

fat, and an allele of *agouti* (A^Y). All five of these genes have now been identified by using positional cloning or positional candidate gene strategies, and they have revealed a great deal about the mechanisms involved in body fat homeostasis and diabetes. None of these genes appears to be a factor in the common forms of human obesity, but studies of the genes have revealed novel pathways that are influenced by common variations. For example, linkage analysis has revealed loci that contribute to plasma leptin levels in human populations. An advantage of Mendelian over complex variations for gene discovery is that the former are more readily characterized at the molecular level.

Table 5–3. The Mouse Is the Most Useful Mammal for Genetic Studies

- Many different inbred mouse strains, encompassing great diversity
- Less expensive to maintain and breed than other mammals
- Short generation time.
- Genetic tools such as congenic strains, recombinant inbred strains, and recombinant congenic strains available
- A complete and detailed linkage map
- Mouse–human chromosomal homology relationships well understood
- Especially useful for gene manipulation and testing hypotheses (e.g., transgenic and gene-targeted mice)
- Well characterized in terms of biology (e.g., development, immune functions)

Engineered Animal Models of Complex Disease

A number of transgenic or gene-targeted mice exhibit dramatically increased susceptibility to various complex diseases. For example, mice with deficiencies of apolipoprotein E or the low-density lipoprotein (LDL) receptor as a result of gene targeting exhibit extreme hypercholesterolemia and tend to develop much more advanced atherosclerotic lesions than do naturally occurring susceptible inbred strains maintained on high-fat, high-cholesterol diets (Ishibashi et al., 1994; Breslow, 1996). Similarly, other transgenic or gene-targeted mice exhibit increased susceptibility to inflammatory disease, cancer, diabetes, and other common disorders. Very frequently, the phenotype will depend importantly on the genetic background. Among many known examples are the following: strain BALB/c mice with an interleukin 10 gene knockout tend to develop inflammatory bowel disease, whereas strain C57BL/6 with the same knockout are relatively resistant; strain MRL mice with a mutant *Fas* gene develop more severe autoimmune disease than do C3H mice with the mutation (Wang et al., 1997); strain C57BL/6 mice carrying a mutant adenomatous polyposis coli (*Apc*) gene develop more severe intestinal tumors than strain AKR mice with the mutation (Su et al., 1992; Dietrich et al., 1993); mice of the PL strain with a targeted deficiency in CD18 are much more likely to develop psoriasiform skin disease than are (C57BL × PL)F1 mice with the same deficiency (Bullard et al., 1996). As discussed below, this variable expression of phenotype on different genetic backgrounds offers the possibility of identifying "modifier genes" that contribute to complex traits.

Models Induced by Mutagenesis

New mutations can be generated in mice at relatively high frequencies using radiation, chemical mutagens, and transgene insertion (Rinchik, 1991; Russell and Russell, 1992; Justice et al., 1997). Mutagenesis screening has been particularly useful in identifying genes that cause developmental or specific biochemical defects, but it will also be useful in identifying genes that contribute to common diseases. The powerful germline mutagen *N*-ethyl-*N*-nitrosourea (ENU) appears to be particularly promising for large-scale studies of genetic functions in the mouse. ENU can induce mutations at a very high rate in mouse spermatogonia, equivalent to isolating a mutation in a single gene of choice in 1 of every 700 gametes screened. ENU is a point mutagen that is capable of inducing many different types of alleles, including both loss of function and gain of function mutations. Typical protocols involve the treatment of male mice with ENU, followed by mating to wild-type mice. The progeny are then tested or further bred to reveal the phenotype of interest (Rinchik, 1991). While the genome sequence is essentially complete in human and mouse, the function of many genes is unknown, even though most gene-coding sequences have been identified either by homology to expressed messenger RNA or by computer screening for likely exons. In an effort to identify disease-related effects of these genes, systematic, genome-wide mutagenesis screens are under way (Nadeau and Frankel, 2000; Nolan et al., 2000).

Justice and colleagues (1997) have proposed an ingenious method combining mutagenesis and targeted large deletions to obtain functional information about genes in a particular region. (See Fig. 5–2.) The method uses Cre/*loxP* engineering (see below) to generate specific deletions (up to several Mb) in regions

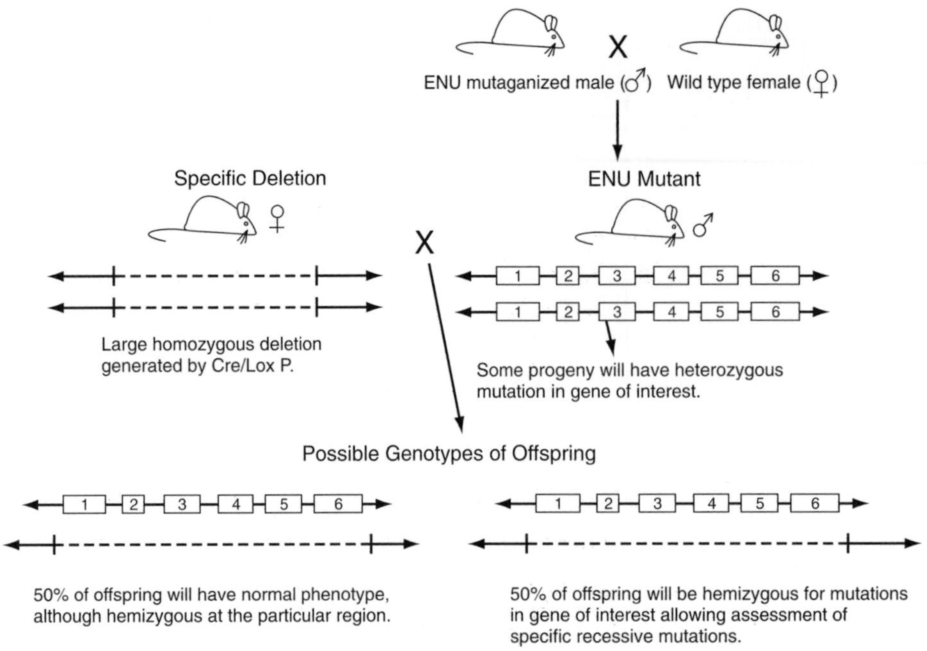

Fig. 5–2. Use of ENU (ethyl-nitrosourea) mutagenesis to explore the function of genes in large regions of the genome. ENU mutagenized male mice are mated to wild-type females to produce offspring hemizygous for random mutations in the gene of interest. These mice are mated with mice carrying homozygous deletions of the region created using *Cre/loxP* technology. Half of their offspring will carry the point mutation on one allele in combination with deletion of the other allele. This allows expression of the mutant phenotype, even if it is recessive in the hemizygous state.

thought to harbor genes-of-interest. Such regions could, for example, correspond to quantitative trait loci (QTLs) identified in genetic studies in mice. These haploid regions can then be further dissected with ENU mutagenesis in phenotype screens. ENU would induce mutations throughout the genome, but recessive mutations would be revealed by breeding to mice carrying deletions in the region of interest. According to the strategy of Justice et al. (1997), ENU-treated males would be bred to wild-type females, and their G1 progeny would then be mated to females carrying deletions. By incorporating genetic markers in the breeding scheme, mutant, carrier and noninformative offspring can be recognized. New phenotypes produced through mutagenesis would not themselves be complex, but, clearly, they could contribute to the dissection of complex traits, as discussed above.

GENETIC ANALYSIS

Traditional Crosses

Figure 5–3 summarizes various types of genetic crosses used to examine inheritance patterns and perform linkage analysis in rodents. Perhaps the most significant development in the history of mouse genetics was the production of "inbred strains," which were derived by brother–sister mating of stocks for 20 or more generations. Such inbred strains, being homozygous at all autosomal loci, greatly simplify genetic analysis and provide the same genetic material for studies in different laboratories. Most common inbred strains of mice are available from the Jackson Laboratories, Bar Harbor, Maine (home page: *http://www.jax.org/*). Many other suppliers and individual laboratories maintain other common or specialized strains. Silver's excellent book *Mouse Genetics* (1995) and other recent reviews such as Avner et al. (1998) provide detailed examination of the strengths and limitations of standard mouse crosses for genetic analysis of complex traits.

Inheritance is usually examined in backcrosses or in F2 crosses (Figure 5–3). Thus, two different parental inbred strains (designated A and B) can be crossed to generate F1 progeny (e.g., (A × B)F1). Such F1 progeny are genetically identical, with the exception of the sex chromosomes; one copy of an autosome is derived from parent A and the other from parent B. When such F1 mice are crossed to a parental strain, the backcross progeny—for example, (A × B)F1 × A—are all unique. Each derives one copy of each chromosome from parental strain A and one copy from the F1 animal. The latter are recombinant chromosomes generated during meiosis. Alternatively, one can cross two F1 progeny to generate F2 mice. Whereas the backcross mice will either be heterozygous or homozygous (for the A allele) at a particular locus, the F2 mice will exhibit various combinations of the parental genomes. The choice of F2 or backcross studies depends on the nature of the variation and the goals of the study (see Silver, 1995). The locations of genes contributing to the traits are determined by testing for cosegregation with "genetic markers" that differ between the parental strains. Complete linkage maps have been constructed for both mice and rats and, in the case of the mouse, thousands of polymerase chain reaction (PCR)-based microsatellite (or simple sequence repeat) markers are available. The mapping of genes for complex traits is discussed below.

Recombinant Inbred Strains

In addition to such traditional crosses, a number of special tools have been developed in rodents (Fig. 5–3B). *Recombinant inbred* (RI) strains are derived by inbreeding F2 progeny at random and then continuously brother–sister mating their progeny for 20 or more generations to generate a new set of inbred strains that are unique mixtures of the parental strains. Each RI strain in the set is a unique descendent of a specific F2 × F2 mating. Commercially maintained RI strain sets contain 2 to 26 differ-

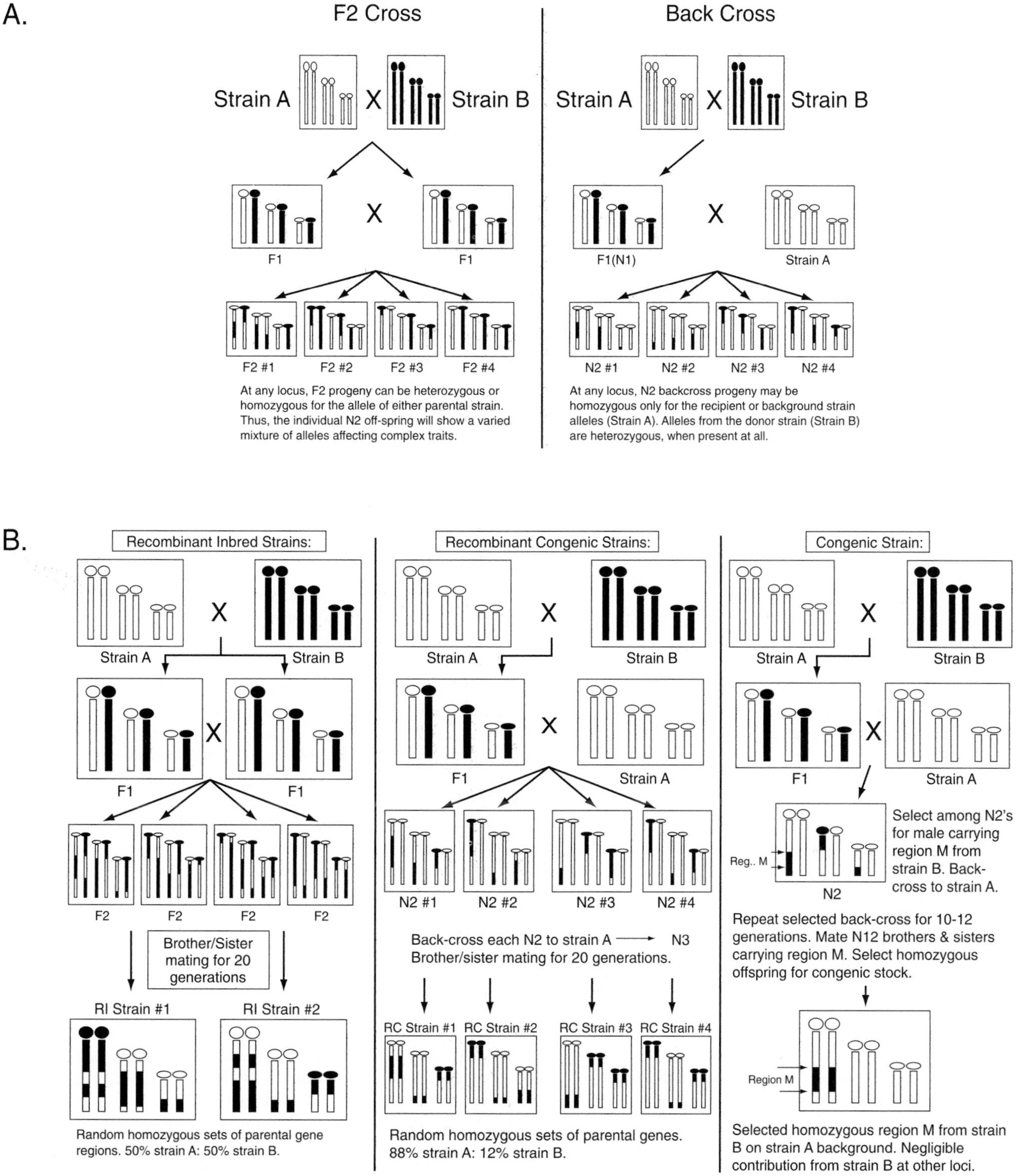

Fig. 5–3. Genetic crosses of animal models for studies of inheritance patterns and linkage. This figure summarizes various breeding strategies for analyzing genetic traits in animal models. Some of the strategies, such as the construction of recombinant inbred and congenic strains, are difficult with larger mammals and have been performed primarily with rodents. The figure shows three chromosomes in two different inbred strains, arbitrarily designated strain A (*open symbols*) and strain B (*closed symbols*). When these are crossed, the F1 mice inherit a copy of each chromosome from each parent. Thus, with the exception of the sex chromosomes, all of the F1 mice are genetically identical. **Top:** *Standard Crosses.* The inheritance of genetic traits can be analyzed by intercrossing the F1 mice to produce F2 progeny or by backcrossing the F1 mice to a parental strain to produce N2 progeny. F2 progeny contain recombinant chromosomes from each of their parents, whereas backcross (N2) mice contain recombinant chromosomes only from their F1 parents. The genetic distance between two polymorphic markers is estimated by determining the percentage of recombinant chromosomes in 100 progeny (100 tested chromosomes). Fifteen recombinants between two markers would signify a distance of 15 cM (although in some calculations distance is adjusted for the possibility of double recombinants). F2 animals have twice as many opportunities for inheriting recombinant chromosomes than N2 mice have, and the calculation of cM genetic distance is adjusted accordingly. **Bottom:** *Constructs for Analyzing Inheritance of Traits in Inbred Strains.* Recombinant inbred (RI) strains are derived by inbreeding random pairs of N2 progeny. Each RI strain has roughly 50% of its DNA from each of the parental strains A and B. However, different RI strains carry different regions from each parent. These strains are used to map genes that contribute to complex traits by associating inheritance of the trait with inheritance of specific parental alleles. Congenic strains are constructed by repeated backcrossing to one of the inbred parental strains (the recipient strain) while selecting for the presence of a particular locus from the other parental (donor) strain. After 10 or more generations, virtually all regions outside the selected donor region are homozygous for recipient DNA. Mice heterozygous at the locus of interest are intercrossed, and progeny homozygous for the donor region are selected to form a breeding stock (see text). Congenic strains allow assessment of genetic effects of a specific chromosomal region in the absence of variations induced by genetic heterogeneity at other loci.

ent RI strains derived from an initial cross between two established inbred mouse lines. At a particular locus, the RI strains in a set will be homozygous for either the parental allele of the A strain or the B strain. Thus, for a Mendelian trait, the RI strains would resemble one or the other parent. For complex (multigenic) traits, in contrast, the RI strains would be expected to exhibit unique phenotypes, depending on the combination of genes inherited.

RI strains are particularly valuable for genetic studies that require multiple animals of a particular recombinant genotype, such as toxicologic analyses. They have also proven useful for examining traits with large nongenetic variability. For example, atherosclerotic lesion development in mice challenged with a high-fat diet is clearly genetically determined but has a coefficient of variation (for lesion size) of about 50%. Thus, studies of RI strains, in which multiple animals of a particular recombinant genotype can be examined have greatly simplified linkage analysis of the trait (Paigen et al., 1987). Another important advantage of RI strains is that genotyping information is cumulative, avoiding the need to retype reference markers. The development of RI strains by Bailey and Taylor (Bailey, 1981) launched the first efforts to map complex traits such as alcohol preference, audiogenic seizures, cancer, atherosclerosis, and susceptibility to infections. The usefulness of RI strains is importantly limited by two factors, however. First, the relatively small number of RI strains in a particular set, usually less than 20, makes it difficult to analyze in detail traits that result from three or more genetic factors, necessitating confirmation of linkage by other means. Second, only a small fraction of the inbred strains are represented in the existing RI sets. Despite these limitations, RI strains have proved useful for examining a number of complex traits (Frankel, 1995).

Congenic and Recombinant Congenic Strains

A particularly important aspect of genetic analysis in rodents is the ability to isolate loci on common genetic backgrounds through the construction of *congenic* strains. Congenic strains were invented in the 1940s by G.D. Snell of The Jackson Laboratory for his systematic genetic analyses of histocompatibility. The process of constructing a congenic strain involves repeated backcrossing to a parental strain with selection at each generation for heterozygosity at the locus of interest (Fig. 5–3B). The use of congenic strains and other strategies for linkage analysis and fine-structure mapping is outlined in more detail below.

An approach that combines elements of both congenic strains and recombinant inbred strains is that of *recombinant congenic* (RC) strains. RC strains, pioneered by Peter Demant and colleagues (Fijneman et al., 1995), consist of various donor segments derived from one strain (about 12% of the genome) on the genetic background of a second strain (Fig. 5–3B). The strains are constructed by backcrossing F1 mice to the parental background strain and then, for a number of different N2 progeny, backcrossing to the same parental strain to generate N3 progeny. On average, these progeny will contain about 12.5% of the genome from the donor strain and 87.5% of the genome from the background or recipient strain. Pairs of such N3 mice are then repeatedly brother–sister mated to generate sets of 20 or more inbred RC strains. Several such panels of RC strains, in which the multiple donor regions cover the entire genome, have now been derived. Complex traits are dissected in these strains by testing the panel for a phenotype, followed by genetic crossing to define the relevant donor segments. Fine mapping is performed as with congenic strains (see below). An advantage of RC is that multigenic traits of interest have been partly dissected, avoiding the necessity to construct congenic strains from scratch. In addition, traits controlled by the interaction of multiple loci may be mapped using RC panels. A disadvantage, as with RI strains, is that only a limited number of RC strains are represented among existing panels (Fijneman et al., 1995; Frankel, 1995).

MAPPING COMPLEX TRAITS

Linkage Analysis

As previously discussed, inbred strains of mice (and rats) differ in numerous traits relevant to common diseases (Table 5–1). Some of these trait differences are due to major genes that can be dissected in a straightforward manner, but the vast majority are complex. Thus, when two inbred strains of mice differing in a complex trait of interest (for example, blood pressure or cholesterol level) are bred, the backcross or F2 mice will usually exhibit a continuum of values for the trait (from low to high blood pressure or cholesterol levels with no discrete groupings). (See Fig. 5–4.) This results from the fact that the progeny contain different combinations of the parental chromosomes. Nevertheless, because the mice can all be maintained under similar environmental conditions, and because they all differ for the same *set* of genetic factors, the chromosomal regions responsible can be defined much more easily than could those for the comparable human traits. Since the locations of the chromosomal regions harboring the genes of interest are unknown, genetic markers (such as highly polymorphic simple repeat sequences) must be typed along all parts of the genome (usually at intervals of about 10 cM in the 1500 cM mouse genome). Linkage maps for a number of mammalian species, including mice, rats, and pigs have been constructed (Dietrich et al., 1995a; Copeland et al., 1993; Jacob et al., 1995).

Linkage analyses of such data are usually relatively straightforward and are conveniently performed using programs such as MAPMAKER/EXP and MAPMAKER/QTL (Lander et al., 1987; Lander and Botstein, 1989; Lincoln et al., 1992a, 1992b) or Mapmanager (Manly, 1993). These programs use modifications of the classical method of a linear regression of phenotype on genotype, such as maximum likelihood methods for estimating the phenotype values between typed markers and the concept of "interval mapping" relating to the fact that intervals with no recombination between flanking markers can be treated as a "virtual" RFLP (restriction fragment length polymorphism) in which every gene is tightly linked. Thus, MAPMAKER/QTL uses genetic maps along with quantitative data from phenotypes to locate quantitative trait loci (QTLs) by an efficient interval mapping method that calculates LOD scores at 2 cM intervals between each marker. Examples of output from linkage analyses are shown in Fig. 5–5 with the peak LOD score corresponding to the most likely localization of the responsible gene. In this manner, genes contributing to numerous complex traits have now been mapped in mice or other mammals (Table 5–4).

One interesting recent suggestion is that genes for complex traits might be mapped in mice without carrying out genetic crosses between inbred strains. This method is based on measuring the association of known interstrain DNA polymorphisms

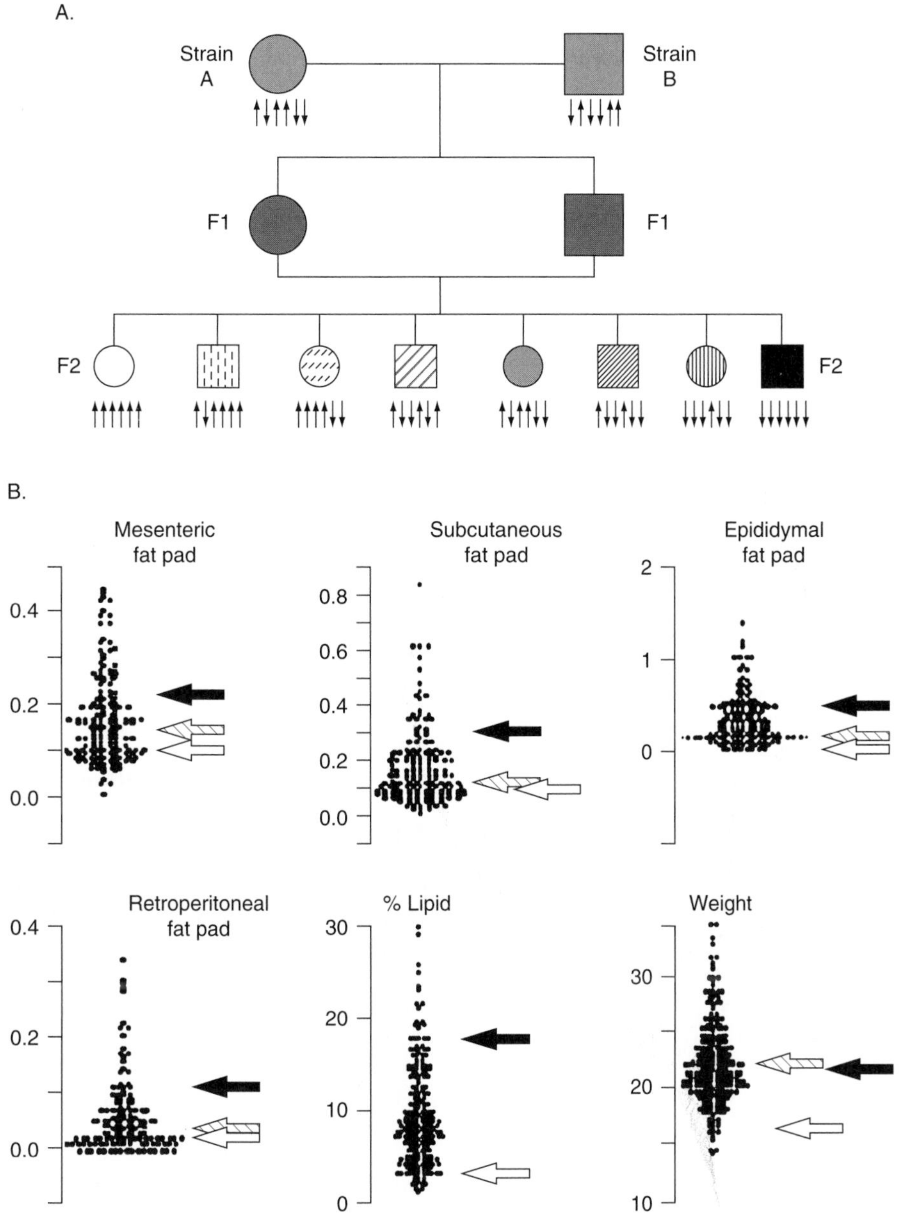

Fig. 5–4. Top: *Inheritance of a Quantitative Complex Phenotype in an F2 Cross between Two Inbred Strains.* The quantitative differences between strains are represented by shading of the symbols. The F1 progeny are genetically identical except for their sex chromosomes, since they inherit one copy of each autosome from each parent. When two F1 mice are crossed, F2 progeny are produced. Each F2 animal carries a unique combination of genes from their parental strains (See Fig. 5–3 Top). In the case of a Mendelian trait, the F2 progeny would exhibit a 1:3 ratio (for a recessive/dominant trait) or a 1:2:1 ratio (for a codominant trait). In contrast, in the case of a multigenic trait, the F2 progeny would exhibit a continuum for the trait due to the independent segregation of genes contributing to the trait. This is illustrated by the range of shading in the F2 progeny. Shown below each individual is a set of arrows representing genes that act to increase or decrease the trait. Most individuals exhibit an "average" phenotype because they inherit a mixture of genes that tend to enhance or suppress the trait. At the extremes, however, some individuals inherit a preponderance or enhancing or suppressing alleles. These individuals express the maximum or minimum of the trait. In between these extremes, the population shows a wide heterogeneity in expression of the trait. **Bottom:** *Wide Frequency Distribution.* Very wide frequency distribution of fat-pad weights, total body weights, and percentage of body fat in (B6 × CAST)F2 mice. Each point represents an individual mouse. *Filled arrow*, average values for B6 parental; *open arrow*, average value for the CAST mice; *hatched arrow*, average value for the (B6 × CAST)F1 mice. From Mehrabian et al. (1998) with permission.

with strain-specific phenotype differences. Grupe et al. (2001) tested the ability of this approach to detect loci for traits where previous QTLs had been identified using interstrain crosses. Using a single nucleotide polymorphism database and phenotype data for a set of about 15 inbred strains, they were able to successfully identify chromosomal regions for 19 of 26 previously mapped QTLs. An additional 19 loci were identified with no corresponding prior QTLs, presumably representing a mix of false positives and actual QTLs that had escaped previous detection. While this approach currently lacks the power of standard QTL mapping, it does offer a method to quickly screen the genome for strong QTLs and to focus more powerful mapping strategies on the most promising genomic regions. Moreover, the mouse phenome project, headquartered at Jackson Laboratories (*http://www.jax.org/phenome*), will attempt to provide comprehensive phenotype data for many complex disease–related traits in an extensive set of inbred strains. This data set, combined with strain-specific polymorphism data, should make it possible to routinely compute initial QTLs for relevant traits and to choose appropriate strains for further mapping and congenic studies.

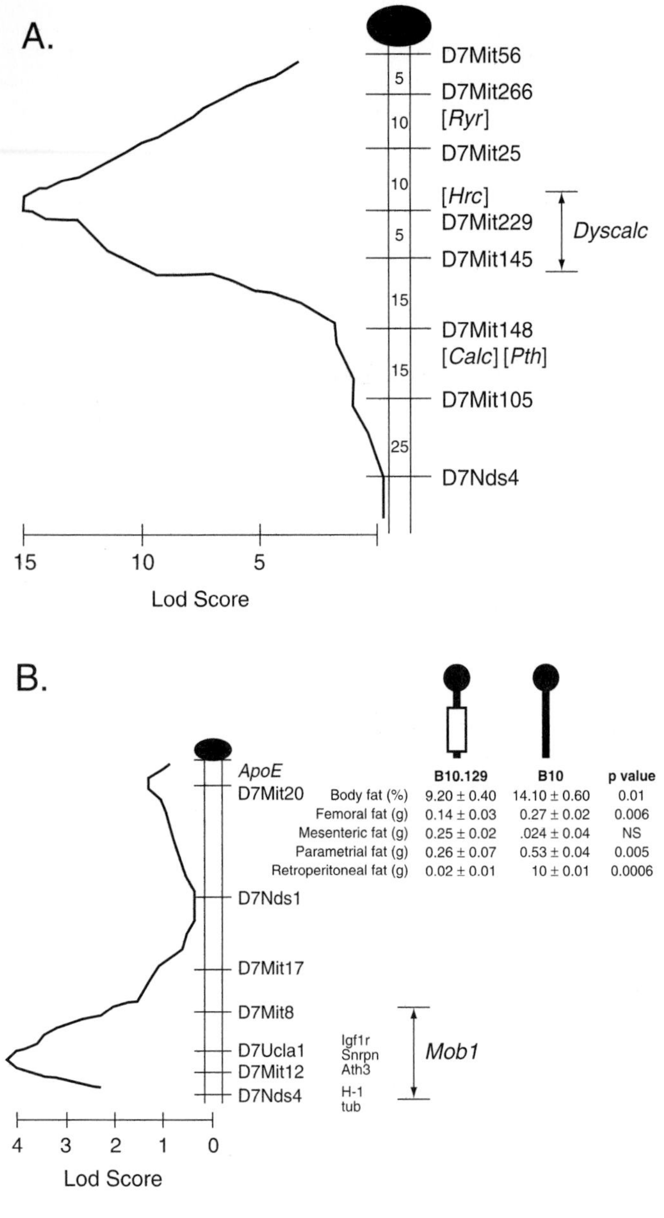

Fig. 5–5. (**A**) Chromosomal localization of a locus contributing to myocyte calcification (*Dyscalc*) on mouse Chr 7 using a (C57BL/6 × C3H/HeJ)F2 intercross. In this study, the inheritance of the semiquantitative trait of myocyte calcification was analyzed in a cross between inbred strains C3H (susceptible) and C57BL/6 (resistant). A total of 185 F2 progeny were analyzed for the trait, and each animal was typed for 50 genetic markers spanning the genome. Data were analyzed using the MAPMAKER/QTL, resulting in the output shown. An LOD score (the logarithm base ten of the odds ratio) is a measure of the likelihood that the data are explained by a gene in the region rather than by chance, and the peak LOD score corresponds to the most likely location of the gene. The chromosome is drawn with the centromere at the top. Microsatellite marker and gene symbols are given to the right of the chromosome, and the genetic distance (in cM between each marker or gene) is indicated between the bars of the chromosome. A plot of the LOD scores for linkage, calculated at two cM intervals along the chromosome, is shown on the left. The peak LOD score indicates the most likely position of the gene underlying the trait; the 95% confidence interval for the position of *Dyscalc* is indicated on the right. Candidate genes for *Dyscalc*, previously mapped to the same region of Chr 7, are indicated in brackets. From Ivandic et al. (1996) with permission. (**B**) Chromosomal localization of a locus contributing to multigenic obesity (*Mob1*) on mouse Chr 7 using a (C57BL/6 × *M. spretus*)F1 × C57BL/6 backcross. The chromosome is drawn with the centromere at the top. Microsatellite marker and gene symbols are given to the right of the chromosome. A plot of the LOD score, calculated at 2 cM intervals along the chromosome, is shown on the left. The peak LOD score indicates the most likely position of the gene underlying the trait; the 95% confidence interval for the position of *Mob 1* is indicated on the right. Candidate genes for *Mob 1*, previously mapped to the same region of Chr 7, are shown. Congenic strains whose donor strain regions overlap *Mob 1* have markedly different body fat profiles, confirming that a gene contributing to obesity is located in this region (*top right*). From Fisler et al. (1993) with permission.

Table 5–4. Mapping of Genes for Complex Traits in Rodents

Trait	Reference
Airway hyperresponsiveness	De Sanctis et al., 1995
Atherosclerosis	Paigen et al., 1987; Welch et al., 1996; Machleder et al., 1997
Blood pressure	Jacob et al., 1991; Schork et al., 1995, 1996; Zhang et al., 1997
Calcification (myocardial)	Ivandic et al., 1996
Diabetes, Type 1	She et al., 1994; Wicker et al., 1995
Diabetes, Type 2	Galli et al., 1996; Mehrabian et al., 1998
Epilepsy	Frankel et al., 1994, 1995a, 1995b
Lipid metabolism (plasma)	Mehrabian et al., 1993; Purcell-Huyhn et al., 1995; Machleder et al., 1997
Morphine preference	Berrettini et al., 1994
Neural tube defects	Neumann et al., 1994
Obesity	Warden et al., 1993; West et al., 1994; Taylor and Phillips, 1996, 1997
Renal disease	Brown et al., 1996
Susceptibility to infection (bacterial)	Dietrich et al., 1995
Systemic lupus erythematosus	Morel et al., 1994
Tail length	Alfred et al., 1997
Tumor suppressor genes	Dietrich et al., 1994
Tumor susceptibility (testicular)	Asada et al., 1994

Modifier Genes

A particularly important application of gene-targeted and transgenic mice is likely to be the identification of "modifier" genes that influence the phenotype resulting from mutations of specific genes. An outstanding example of the use of animals to identify modifier genes is in the area of cancer research. The adenomatous polyposis coli (*APC*) gene was first identified in human genetic studies. A single defective copy of the gene leads to the development of hundreds or thousands of polyps in the colon, which, unless they are removed, progress to become carcinomas. A mouse with the *Apc* mutation also exhibited intestinal polyps, and it was noted that the number of polyps was greatly influenced by the genetic background, suggesting the existence of modifier genes. Thus, strain C57BL/6 mice exhibited much larger numbers of polyps in the presence of the *Apc* mutation than did several other strains, including AKR. To map the modifier genes, backcrosses between C57BL/6 mice carrying the *Apc* mutation and various other strains were constructed, and the progeny with the *Apc* mutation were analyzed for polyp number, as well as for genetic markers that span the genome. When the results were statistically analyzed, a region on distal Chr 4 was found to be strongly associated with polyp number (Dietrich et al., 1993; Moser et al., 1995). Subsequently, MacPhee and colleagues (MacPhee et al., 1995; Gould et al., 1996) presented strong evidence that a secreted phospholipase A_2 (*Pla2g2a*) gene located within the distal Chr 4 QTL was the modifier gene. In addition to the location of the gene, the *Pla2g2a* gene was defective in C57BL/6 and certain other susceptible strains but not in relatively resistant strains, and the expression pattern of the gene was consistent with the phenotype, with high expression in the intestine. The identification of the *Pla2g2a* gene is an example of the "positional candidate gene approach," or "coincidence mapping," in which both positional and biochemical information are used to make conclusions about the role of a gene in a trait. Subsequently, *Pla2g2a* was expressed from a transgene and shown to suppress polyp formation, confirming its identity as the modifier gene (Cormier et al., 1997). It is hard to imagine how modifier genes such as *Pla2g2a* could be identified directly in humans since only family members carrying an *APC* mutation could be used for mapping purposes. In this situation, results would be importantly complicated by genetic heterogeneity (for example, the particular *APC* allele carried) and environmental factors (for example, diet clearly influences the disease). Once the gene was identified in mice, however, it became feasible to study its role in cancer in humans.

FINE MAPPING AND GENE IDENTIFICATION STRATEGIES

Positional Candidate Gene Approach

Once the chromosomal regions controlling the trait of interest have been mapped, the list of possible candidate genes for the trait is greatly reduced. Thus, biochemical and molecular studies can be focused on those genes that coincide with the identified chromosomal region. This approach, called the *positional candidate gene approach*, is proving useful in studies with humans as well as mice (Collins, 1995; Bedell et al., 1997b). The approach is nicely illustrated by the studies on arterial lipofuscin deposition (Qiao et al., 1993). Lipofuscin is a yellow-brown pigment consisting of oxidized lipids and protein, which frequently accumulates in macrophages in atherosclerotic lesions in humans. Its potential role in atherosclerosis has been unknown. Mehrabian et al. (1991) identified lipofuscin in heart valves and arteries in mice and showed that inbred strains of mice differ in the deposition of lipofuscin. Qiao et al. (1993) analyzed a genetic cross between a strain that develops lipofuscin (B6.C-*H25*^{c}) and a strain that is resistant (BALB/c); they observed that pigment deposition segregated as a recessive trait, mapping to mouse Chr 7. The region identified contained the gene for tyrosinase (*Tyr.*, Chr 7), which catalyzes the first step in melanin synthesis. At first, the tyrosinase gene seemed like a rather poor candidate, since lipofuscin is clearly distinct from melanin and tyrosinase was not known to be expressed in macrophages or the artery wall. But it was a rather straightforward candidate gene to examine, since many mutations of tyrosinase have been identified by virtue of their easily recognized consequence (albinism). When Qiao et al. (1993) studied a spontaneous point mutation of the tyrosinase gene on a susceptible genetic background, they observed an absence of lipofuscin, demonstrating a direct link between tyrosinase gene expression and lipofuscin. The nature of the link is as yet unclear, but it may be related to the pro-oxidant effects of tyrosinase. This study illustrates how defining chromosomal regions contributing to traits can help identify an underlying gene. In the absence of the knowledge of the chromosomal location of the lipofuscin gene, many more attractive candidate genes than tyrosinase would have been considered, and the testing of each candidate gene for a possible role would not have been feasible. Another good example of a positional candidate gene approach is the *Mom1* modifier of the *Apc* gene mutation, discussed above. Such a positional candidate gene approach has now been used to identify many genes for complex traits (Copeland et al., 1993; Bedell et al., 1997a, 1997b).

Isolating Individual Loci for Complex Traits Using Congenic Strains

Although most mammalian genes have now been partially sequenced, only a small fraction have been functionally characterized. Thus, the chances of finding the gene that underlies a complex trait from a list of candidate genes in the region of interest is small, even for relatively well characterized processes such as lipoprotein metabolism. One approach to identifying the critical gene in a quantitative trait locus is to make a congenic strain carrying that region (Flaherty, 1981; Silver, 1995). If a congenic region from a susceptible strain is isolated on a genetic background of another strain, the effects of the locus can be studied in isolation, using the background strain as control. Once the individual locus has been isolated, the trait becomes Mendelian in nature, since only a single genetic factor, differing between the congenic strain and background strain, now contributes to the trait. In effect, the congenic strategy removes genetic heterogeneity contributed by other loci. (See Fig. 5–6.) This greatly enhances the ability to distinguish affected and unaffected individuals and thus allows a much finer mapping of the responsible gene. By examining successively smaller congenic regions, the gene can be quickly localized in preparation for positional cloning.

Until recently, existing congenic strains covered only a very small fraction of the mouse genome, and, even for those regions, the donor and background strains may not differ in the trait of

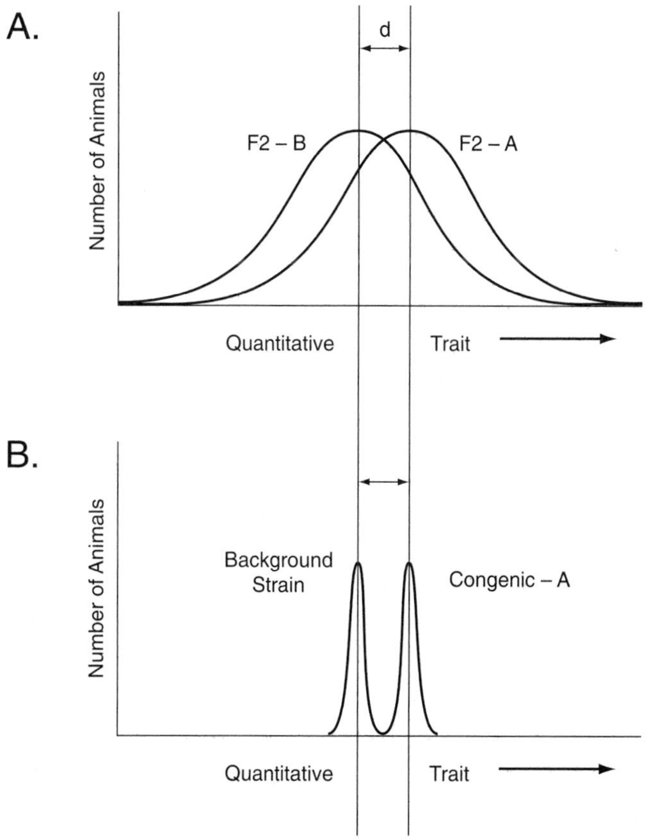

Fig. 5–6. Congenic mice assist in the identification of genes that contribute to complex diseases by eliminating genetic heterogeneity produced by other loci. Normally, the effect of a single gene in a complex trait is masked by other genes affecting that trait. **(A)** In an F2 cross between strains A and B, many genes affect a complex trait. The effect of a single locus shifts the value of a quantitative trait by the distance marked "d." However, the genetic heterogeneity at other loci broaden the population phenotype such that there is substantial phenotypic overlap between the population of F2 animals carrying the B allele (F2-B) at the locus and animals carrying the A allele (F2-A). **(B)** By contrast, when the A allele is isolated as a congenic on a background of strain B, genetic heterogeneity at other loci is lost, and the two classes of animals are much more easily resolved phenotypically. There is still some breadth to the phenotype peaks due to remaining environmental heterogeneity and experimental uncertainty.

interest. In such cases, recombinant congenic strains may be useful, although these also have been derived from a limited number of donor and background strains (Moen et al., 1996, 1997). Therefore, for most loci contributing to complex traits, it has been necessary to construct appropriate congenic strains. Classical construction of congenic strains involves selection at each generation for a particular phenotype. In the past, it was frequently not possible to distinguish the heterozygote from the background strain with respect to phenotype, and therefore congenic strains had to be created through complex breeding schemes. Today, the identification of a heterozygote is not a problem since one would know the map position of the locus of interest before undertaking production of the congenic strain, allowing the use of genetic markers to identify heterozygous and homozygous mice at the locus of interest.

The construction of a congenic strain is outlined in Fig. 5–3B. The first cross is between a recipient inbred strain and an animal that contains the donor allele. Progeny from this cross are repeatedly backcrossed to the recipient inbred strain, which provides the genetic background. At each generation, offspring heterozygous for the desired allele are selected for further breeding. The level of heterozygosity at other loci is reduced by an average of 50% in each backcross generation. Thus, the fraction of loci expected to be heterozygous at the Nth generation can be calculated as $[(1/2)^{N-1}]$. After 10 generations, the unselected portion of the genome is about 99.8% derived from the background strain. Typically, congenic strains are bred for about 10 generations, when they are usually intercrossed to obtain congenic stocks that are in the homozygous state. It is important to note that the rapid elimination of heterozygosity occurs only in regions of the genome that are not linked to the donor locus. It is possible to reduce the length of the chromosomal segment spanning the locus by screening backcross progeny for the occurrence of crossovers between the locus of interest and nearby DNA markers.

The availability of abundant genetic markers in the mouse and rat have made it possible to accelerate the construction of congenic strains using *marker-assisted selection protocols*. Basically, this involves the selection of progeny simultaneously for the presence of the desired target gene locus and the absence of undesired contaminating donor gene loci. The approach, also termed *speed congenics*, is relatively straightforward and allows the production of genetically defined congenic strains in less than half as many generations (Markel et al., 1997; Wakeland et al., 1997). This is of considerable importance since the time required for classical congenics, involving 10 or 12 generations of backcrossing, is several years.

In some cases, existing congenic strains, such as those constructed for studies of histocompatibility loci, have proven useful for studies of QTLs that, by chance, occur in the same regions. For example, four major loci contributing to multigenic obesity (termed *Mob1*, *Mob2*, *Mob3*, and *Mob4*) were mapped in a genetic cross between strains C57BL/6 and *Mus spretus* (Warden et al., 1995). Obesity in offspring of this cross was highly correlated with the specific combinations of parental alleles inherited for these four loci. (See Fig. 5–7.) Fortuitously, one of the loci (*Mob1*) on Chr 7 resides near a minor histocompatibility locus (*H-1*) for which congenic strains had been constructed a number of years ago. One congenic strain consisted of a C57BL/10 genetic background and a Chr 7 donor region derived from strain 129. Although the C57BL/10 background strain closely resembles the C57BL/6 strain used in the cross, the donor strain was very different from the *M. spretus* mice, which diverged from common laboratory strains (*Mus musculus*) several million years ago. Nevertheless, it was reasoned that the genetic variations influencing body fat in the C57BL/6 × *M. spretus* cross may be relatively common, since many inbred strains of laboratory mice vary in body fat and other obesity-related traits. Therefore, the congenic strain was examined for differences in body fat, as compared to the background strain. The results showed highly significant effects of the Chr 7 locus on body weight, retroperitoneal fat-pad weight, percentage of body water (inversely proportional to body fat), and plasma cholesterol. In fact, the congenic strain exhibited about 40% less overall body fat than the background C57BL/10 strain. These results strongly supported the linkage analysis (Warden et al., 1995).

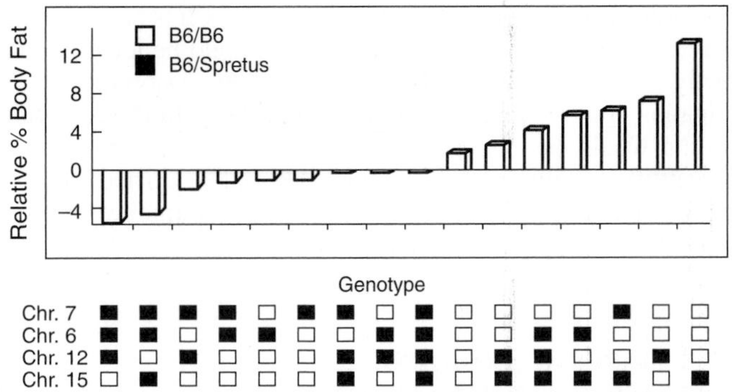

Fig. 5–7. Four loci important to the complex trait of obesity were observed in a backcross experiment between the mouse strain C57BL/6 and *M. spretus*. Obesity in the offspring of this cross was highly correlated with the specific combination of parental alleles inherited for these four loci. From Warden et al. (1993) with permission.

Increasingly, it will be possible to avoid the time and expense of constructing individual custom congenic strains for each QTL. In addition to congenics already developed by individual investigators, extensive sets of congenic strains that span the genome are becoming available. For instance, Iakoubova et al. (2001) have described two "libraries" of congenic animals with a set of introgressed segments covering all 19 autosomes and the X chromosome. Each of these libraries, referred to as *genome-tagged mice* (GTM), is comprised of more than 60 individual congenic strains. Both libraries use C57BL/6J as the background strain. The introgressed segments come either from DBA/2J (DBA-GTM library) or CAST/Ei (CAST-GTM library). Due to the small size of the introgressed chromosomal segment, GTMs allow direct initiation of positional cloning projects, as well as the resolution of multiple QTLs that may be present on a chromosome. They also greatly facilitate the direct mapping of QTLs and the analysis of gene–gene interactions.

Fine Mapping Using Large-Insert Transgenics and Engineered Deletions

Given sufficient family material, human genetic loci with relatively large effects on a complex trait can be mapped using existing nonparametric analyses. Generally, such a locus will be at least several cM in size. Depending on the nature of the population studied and the history of the underlying genetic variation, it may be possible to narrow the region using linkage disequilibrium. However, in most cases, such fine mapping would require a very high density of markers, perhaps 10 or more markers per cM. These are presently being developed, but it may be several years before such markers are available for the entire genome. An alternative approach for fine mapping is to "sift"

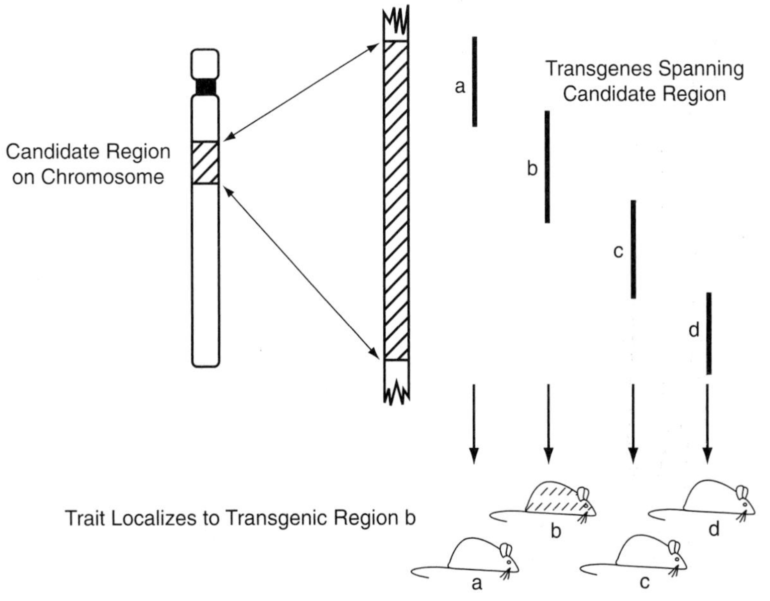

Fig. 5–8. Use of transgenics to map complex diseases. Once a candidate region has been identified and appropriate genomic clones spanning that region are available, then the creation of transgenic animals has the potential to more finely localize the responsible gene. As shown, the transgene must carry a dominant or codominant allele.

through that region of the human genome using transgenic mice or knockout mice.

Transgenic mice harboring large pieces of the human genome (up to about 1 million bp) can be created using YACs (yeast artificial chromosomes) or BACs (bacterial artificial chromosomes). Such transgenic mice can then be tested for the disease of interest, or, more likely, a trait related to the disease of interest (Peterson et al., 1993; Lamb and Gearhart, 1995; Perou et al., 1996). The ability to detect an effect in such cases requires that an extra copy of the underlying gene would influence the trait. Such a dose-dependent effect on the trait seems a likely possibility, although it would certainly not always be the case (for example, there may be a threshold level of a gene product, only below which an effect would occur). (See Fig. 5–8). An excellent example of this approach was the fine mapping of a region of human Chr 21, critical for certain Down syndrome phenotypes (Smith et al., 1997). Conceivably, a panel of transgenic mice (or embryonic stem cells) spanning the entire human genome could be created as a resource for screening regions affecting interesting traits (Edward Rubin, University of California at Berkeley, personal communication).

An alternative approach is to delete syntenic portions of the mouse genome (syntenic to the human disease gene loci) using homologous recombination. For example, large deletions can be created using the Cre/*loxP* system in which Cre sites are introduced by homologous recombination followed by expression of the Cre protein (see below). In the case of relatively large deletions, several hundred kb or more, it is unlikely that mice with homozygous deletions would be viable, and, thus, recognition of a gene would require the ability to observe an effect on the trait of interest in heterozygotes.

Positional Cloning in Animal Models

The basic principles of positional cloning in animal models are similar to those in humans: use genetic analysis to map the gene of interest to the smallest feasible interval; identify the genes that reside within that interval; examine the genes for possible involvement; identify the genetic variations underlying the trait. For the first steps in this process, animal models provide a number of important advantages over studies in humans. For the identification of genes involved in complex traits, rodents provide the ability to construct congenic strains, allowing fine structure mapping, as discussed above. In contrast, human fine-structure mapping for complex traits depends on linkage disequilibrium. Fine-structure mapping in rodents allows much greater resolution than in humans or other mammals because of the ability to construct large crosses. Since genetic mapping is generally much more efficient than molecular analysis, crosses of at least 1000 meioses are usually made. Such crosses allow the interval containing the gene to be narrowed to about a few tenths of a cM or less. In the mouse, this is equivalent to about one-half Mb or less, since, on average, 1 cM corresponds to about 2 Mb (Silver, 1995). An important problem for fine-structure mapping can be the lack of informative genetic markers of sufficient density. This problem is reduced by the use of interspecific genetic crosses, involving mouse species such as *M. spretus* and *M. castaneous*, which have diverged widely from common laboratory strains (Silver, 1995). Large-insert YACs, BACs, plasmid artificial chromosome (PAC), and phage P1 libraries are available for mice and rats (Haldi et al., 1996, 1997). A recent strategy for positional cloning that may prove increasingly important is complementation of mutations by construction of transgenics that contain large genomic inserts from the locus of interest (Hamilton et al., 1997). Another powerful tool in positional cloning has been to search for disease-specific changes in gene expression by screening expression libraries or using representational difference analysis (Lisitsyn et al., 1994). However, for complex diseases in a heterogeneous population, the expression of large numbers of genes are likely to be affected. Therefore, because of the ability to control genetic backgrounds, techniques such as representational difference analysis can be more readily applied in rodent models (for instance, for comparing expression differences between congenics and their background strains).

TRANSGENIC AND GENE-TARGETED MICE FOR EXAMINING GENE FUNCTIONS IN VIVO

Planned Genetic Modifications

The mouse offers advantages for elucidation of gene functions and pathways, not only because of the feasibility of experimental studies unethical in humans but also because of the ability to perform planned genetic modifications (Ramirez-Solis et al., 1995; Smithies and Maeda, 1995). The ability to generate transgenic and knockout mice has already had a major impact on research in many areas of mammalian biology, and the use of such genetically modified animals is rapidly expanding. Once a gene contributing to a complex trait has been identified, transgenic or gene-targeted mice can help define the molecular mechanisms involved. Genetically modified animals are also of great importance for the analysis of modifier genes, as discussed above. Below, we provide a very brief discussion of *(1)* transgenic animals, *(2)* gene-targeted animals, and *(3)* recent developments that have expanded the usefulness of genetically modified animal models.

Transgenic Animals

The experimental techniques for producing transgenic animals were first developed in mice (McLaren and Biggers, 1958; Gordon and Ruddle, 1981) and have been most extensively applied in mice (Silver, 1995), but they have also been extended to a number of other mammalian species, including large animals (Hammer et al., 1985). Transgenic technology is now used at virtually every major research facility throughout the world. The basic methodology is straightforward. The DNA construct of interest is microinjected into one of the pronuclei of fertilized single-cell eggs, and the eggs are transferred to the oviduct of appropriately synchronized pseudopregnant recipients. Of the animals that develop to term and are born and weaned, up to 30% will have incorporated the microinjected DNA into their genome, and the transgene will be heritable. Studies in transgenic animals allow one to ask questions pertaining to the overexpression of an endogenous gene product or the expression of a foreign gene product. Transgenic animals can also be used to examine the regulation of genes in vivo, and the occasional mutants that result from the insertion of a transgene into an endogenous gene can also be of value.

For studies in mice, an important consideration is the strain of females to be used as egg donors. In most cases, hybrid strains such as (C57BL/6 × SJL)F1 or (C57BL/6 × DBA)F1 have been used since they provide a higher yield of injectable eggs that withstand micromanipulation procedures better than eggs from inbred strains such as C57BL/6. This can lead to difficulties in the analysis of transgenic animals since they consist of a mixed genetic background. In such cases, if necessary, the transgene can be transferred onto a common genetic background by backcrossing, as described above for the construction of congenic strains. Alternatively, inbred strains such as C57BL/6 can be used for the construction of transgenic mice by harvesting and injecting significantly more eggs. The strain FVB/N is an exception to the rule that inbred strains are inefficient sources of embryos, and it is now being extensively used for transgenic studies (Taketo et al., 1991; Silver, 1995).

Animals carrying the transgene are usually identified and followed by DNA genotyping. Typically, a small segment of tail is removed, genomic DNA is isolated and analyzed by dot-blot analysis, polymerase chain reaction amplification, or Southern blotting. Transgenic animals will exhibit varying numbers of copies of the transgene, ranging from one to several hundreds. These copies are generally arranged as tandem head-to-tail repeats and are generally integrated into single random sites in the mouse genome. The level of expression of the transgene will depend on the nature of the construct, the promoter, the site of integration, and the number of copies that have been inserted. This is generally examined by determining the levels of expression of the gene product at the level of messenger RNA, protein, or activity.

In general, transgenes are designed with promoters that direct expression of the cDNA or genomic clones in specific tissues or cell types. Such tissue-specific expression can be achieved by using the gene's own regulatory sequences or by using heterologous regulatory sequences. Hundreds of different tissue-specific and cell type–specific regulatory sequences have been defined. Transgenic animal studies have been cataloged in a database that can be accessed via the Internet (*http://tbase.jax.org*). cDNA clones are frequently used for transgenic constructs because they are more available and more easily manipulated than are genomic clones. A problem with cDNA-based constructs is that they are frequently poorly expressed when integrated into a mouse chromosome, although heterologous introns placed between promoter sequences and cDNA coding sequences can enhance expression of some cDNAs (Palmiter and Brinster, 1986; Silver, 1995).

Transgenic animals, particularly mice, have been used for studies of virtually all of the major complex diseases. An outstanding recent example of the use of transgenic animals has been for studies of Alzheimer's disease (Higgins and Cordell, 1995). Naturally occurring inbred strains of mice do not exhibit any obvious Alzheimer's-related phenotypes, but transgenic mice expressing a mutant amyloid precursor protein (*App*) exhibit both amyloid plaques and memory deficits (Hsiao et al., 1996). Additionally, enhanced Alzheimer-type phenotypes occur in transgenic mice carrying both the mutant *App* and other genes known to be involved in Alzheimer's, such as presenilin 1 (Borchelt et al., 1997) and apolipoprotein E4 (Holcomb et al., 1998).

Gene-Targeted Mice

Whereas transgenic techniques permit the insertion of a cloned fragment of DNA into an animal's genome, thereby adding a new gene to the normal complement of genes, gene-targeted techniques can be used to disrupt a gene of interest to generate mice that are deficient in that gene product. Thus, gene-targeting techniques allow one to create "knockouts" of specific genes in the genome. This technology resulted from two separate biological advances. The first was the development of pluripotent mouse embryonic stem (ES) cells that could be microinjected into blastocysts to generate chimeric mice (Hogan et al., 1994). ES cells can contribute to the formation of all tissues of a developing mouse, including germ cells, and, therefore, they are capable of transmitting the ES genome to their progeny. The second advance was the ability to modify specific genes in cultured cell lines using homologous recombination with an appropriately modified and transfected "targeting" vector. In 1987, Thomas and Capecchi showed that ES cells had the machinery for homologous recombination by targeting the selectable gene for mouse hypoxanthine phosphoribosyl transferase (HPRT) gene (Thomas and Capecchi, 1987). Subsequently, nonselectable genes were targeted by a variety of laboratories (Mansour et al., 1988; Koller and Smithies, 1989). At the present time, these techniques have been used to create knockouts of hundreds of different genes, including many relevant to complex diseases.

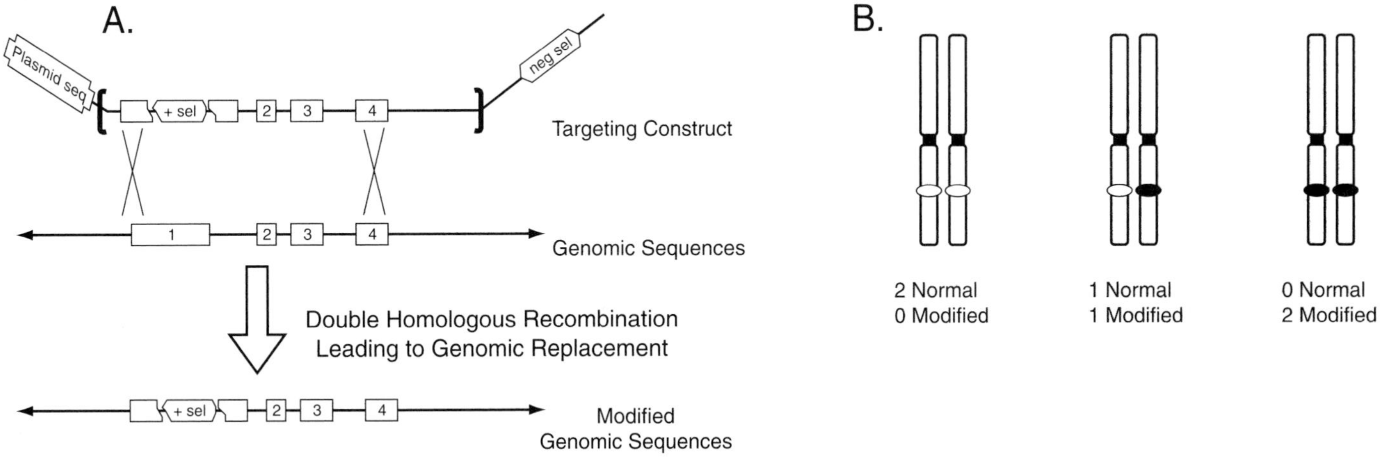

Fig. 5–9. Use of gene targeting to replace genomic sequences. **(A)** A large cloned genomic DNA segment is used as a targeting construct. In addition to the region with genomic homology (*shown between brackets at the top*) there are vector sequences and markers for negative selection (neg sel), usually herpesvirus thymidine kinase. A marker for positive selection (+ sel), usually neomycin resistance, is engineered into the homology region. Insertion of + sel into coding sequences as shown is likely to interrupt gene function, causing inactivation. As shown, the neomycin gene disrupts exon 1 of the gene. Insertion in intronic sequences often is not detrimental to gene function. In this case, additional specific functional mutations may be introduced in coding regions. Double homologous recombination between the targeting construct and genomic sequences in embryonic stem cells leads to replacement of the genomic sequences with the engineered sequences. **(B)** The normal gene sequence (*indicated by open ovals in homologous chromosomes at left and center*) is replaced hemizygously in the successfully targeted animal (*center*), and breeding may be used to produce animals homozygous for the modification (*right*). Gene dosage effects may be measured in animals carrying zero (*left*), one (*middle*), or two (*right*) copies of the modified DNA sequences.

The general strategy for inactivating a gene of interest in a mouse is as follows. (See Fig. 5–9.) A targeting vector containing flanking sequences homologous to the gene of interest but containing a mutation is constructed by routine molecular biology procedures. This targeting vector is then transfected into ES cells in culture, and cells that are appropriately targeted are selected. A variety of selection procedures, both positive and negative, are used since the frequency of targeting is generally extremely low in mammalian cells. The targeted cells are identified and confirmed by Southern analysis and then injected into the blastocyst cavity of developing mouse embryos to generate chimeric mice. The chimeric mice are subsequently bred to produce animals that are heterozygous for the targeted mutation, and these can then be bred to obtain homozygous mice. It should be noted that gene targeting of the mice is not a trivial undertaking. It requires skill in molecular cloning of DNA, cell-culture procedures, and expertise in microinjection and reimplantation of blastocysts. The latter is frequently performed in an experienced core facility. Generally, the successful implementation of gene targeting requires at least a 1-year full-time effort, and the characterization of the resulting mice frequently takes much longer than this. Thus, gene targeting is not advisable in the absence of a specific scientific hypothesis. A variety of reviews and papers addressing aspects of the technique are available (Thomas et al., 1992; Hasty and Bradley, 1993; Papaioannou and Johnson, 1993; Wurst & Joyner, 1993; Young et al., 1998). Smithies and Maeda (1995) have specifically discussed gene-targeted approaches to the analysis of complex genetic diseases.

There are two general types of gene-targeting vectors that have been used to disrupt genes: sequence-replacement vectors (Fig. 5–9) and sequence-insertion (Fig. 5–10). For both varieties of vectors, at least 5 kb of genomic DNA sequence homology to the gene of interest should be included in the vector to achieve reasonable targeting efficiencies. Most ES cell lines have been derived from mouse strain 129, and to maximize recombination efficiency, mouse strain 129 genomic clones should be used in the construction of targeting vectors. In designing a targeting vector, it is also important to consider the Southern blotting or PCR screening strategies that will be used to identify correctly targeted clones. The vast majority of gene-knockout experiments have used a sequence-replacement vector strategy.

Typically, a *neo* expression cassette, conferring resistance to the antibiotic G418, is used for both positive selection and for inactivation of the target gene. The *neo* gene is usually inserted into a critical 5′ exon of the target gene, leaving at least 1 kb of sequence homology on either side. Frequently, a negative selectable marker, usually the herpes simplex virus thymidine kinase (*HSVtk*), is attached outside the region of homology. Sequence-replacement vectors such as these are usually constructed simply by cloning the long and short arms of homology, often convenient restriction fragments in the gene, into plasmid vectors that already contain both the *neo* and the *HSVtk* genes. Before electroporation into ES cells, the sequence-replacement vectors are linearized at a unique site outside the segment of homology to increase targeting efficiency. Selectable markers are used to enrich correctly targeted cells since the efficiency of targeting is extremely low.

The *neo* gene provides a means of positive selection of ES cell clones in which the targeting vector has entered the cell and become integrated into the genome. Most such G418-resistant clones will have integrated the targeting vector randomly rather than by homologous recombination. The basis of the *HSVtk* negative selection strategy is that the HSVtk cassette is generally lost during the process of homologous recombination, since it lies outside the region of homology, but not during the process of random integration. Expression of the *HSVtk* gene renders the ES cells sensitive to the drug ganciclovir, and, therefore, treatment of the ES cells with ganciclovir will tend to remove clones that have integrated the targeting vector randomly. See Fig. 5–9 for a schematic of homologous recombination with both positive and negative selectable markers. Following selection, cell clones are grown briefly (extended culture risks the possibility that the cells will differentiate, such that they are no long pluripotent) and then stored as frozen stocks. To identify the correctly targeted ES clones, DNA is isolated from a portion of the cells to carry out confirmatory analysis.

The vast majority of gene-targeting experiments have been designed to produce mice with the null allele, allowing the ex-

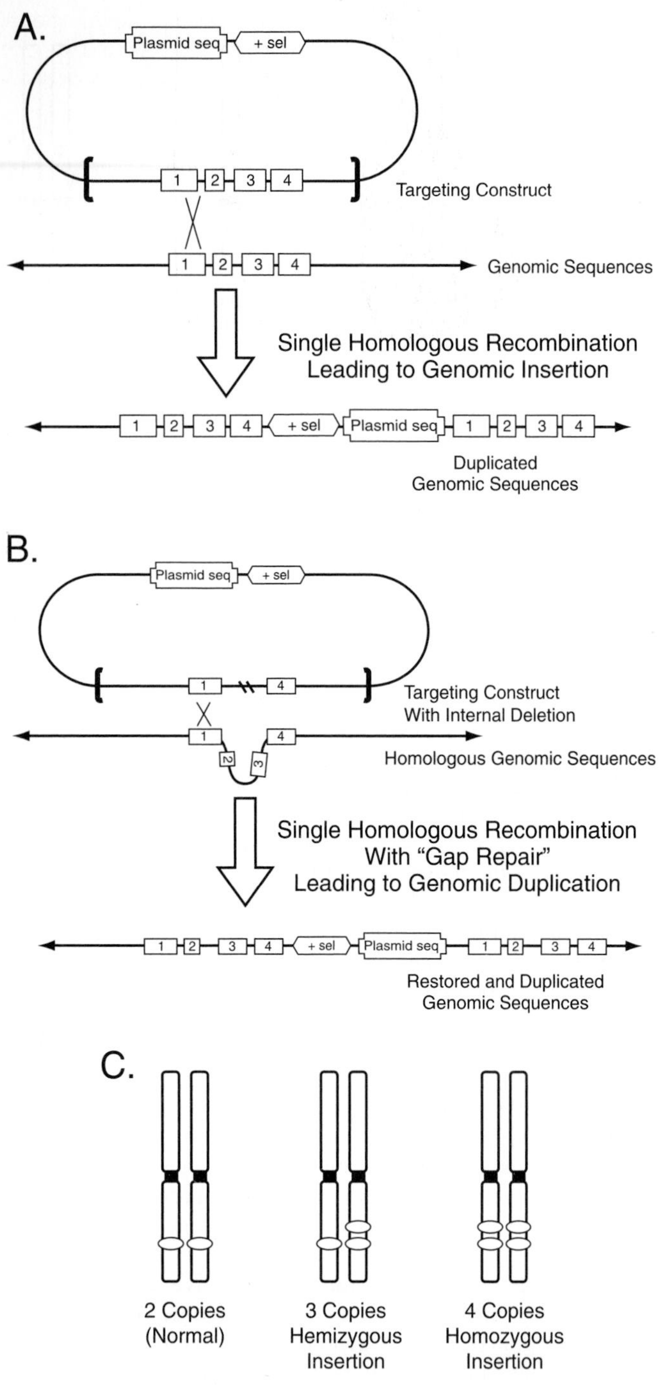

Fig. 5–10. Use of gene insertion to duplicate genomic sequences. **(A)** A large cloned genomic DNA segment is used as a targeting construct. In addition to the region with genomic homology (*shown between brackets at the top*), there are vector sequences and markers for positive selection (+ sel). A single homologous recombination leads to incorporation and duplication of the genomic sequences. **(B)** To duplicate very large genomic regions, it is possible to remove a substantial portion of the central homology region which, in some recombinants, will be replaced by "gap repair." **(C)** Successful targeting will produce an animal with three copies of the normal gene (*center*) that can be used to breed animals with four gene copies (*right*).

perimenter to ask what characteristics the animal exhibits in the absence of the gene product or in the presence of about half the normal amount of gene product. Generally, this is achieved by disrupting gene function with bacterial sequences inserted in the coding region of the gene. In addition, gene targeting can also be used to introduce subtle mutations into specific genes. A number of strategies have been described for this purpose. Probably the most widely used is the "hit-and-run" or "in-and-out" sequence-insertion vector strategy (Valancius and Smithies, 1991). In this strategy (see Fig. 5–11), a subtle mutation is usually inserted into a fragment of the gene of interest by site-directed mutagenesis. The mutated segment of homology is then cloned into a targeting vector that contains both *neo* and *HSVtk*. In the first step of the strategy, the linearized vector is incorporated into ES cells, and the cells are subjected to selection in G418. The resulting resistant ES cell clones, in which the gene-targeting vector has integrated into the cognate gene, are then identified by Southern blot analysis with a flanking probe. In the second step, the targeted ES cell clone is grown in the presence of ganciclovir or FIAU (1-(2-deoxy-2-fluoro-betaD-arabinofuranosyl)-5-iodouracil), which selects for the loss of the *HSVtk* gene. The loss of the *HSVtk* gene is expected to occur by spontaneous recombi-

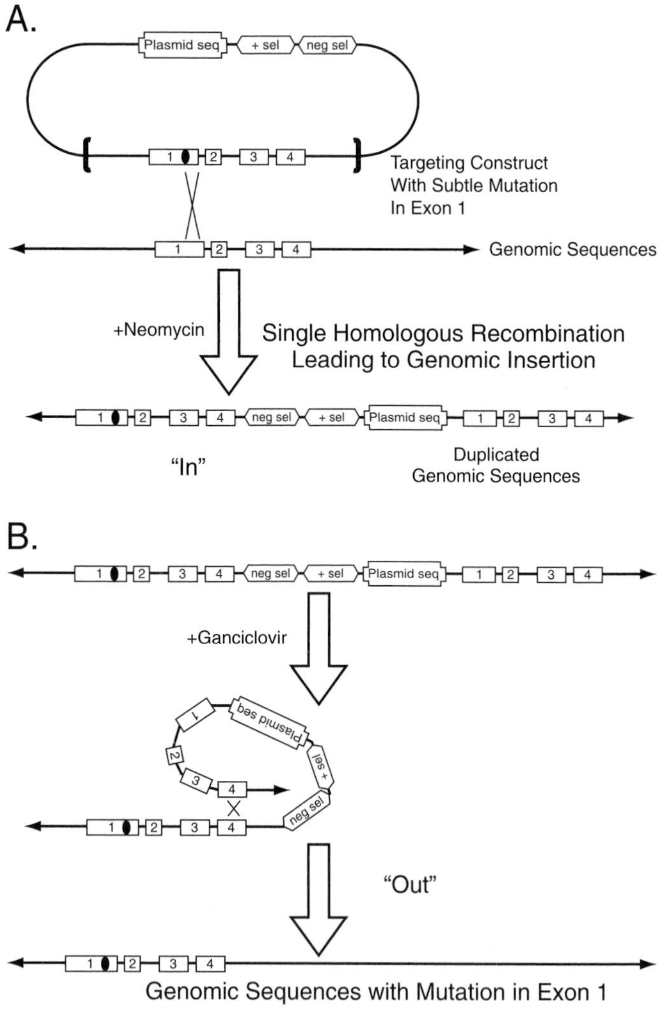

Fig. 5–11. Use of the "in and out" targeting procedure to introduce subtle mutations in the genome. **(A)** Gene modification is carried out by site-directed mutagenesis or other means in a plasmid construct. (The mutation is indicated by a solid oval in exon 1.) This insertion vector is used to incorporate the mutation into embryonic stem cells by homologous recombination. Cells that have incorporated the mutant construct are selected by neomycin resistance (+ sel) and then tested by PCR and/or restriction digest and Southern blot to identify clones incorporating the construct at the correct site. Correctly targeted constructs will duplicate the gene with one copy carrying the mutation. Plasmid sequences and selective markers (+ sel) and (neg sel) are also inserted in the genome. **(B)** Excision of the normal gene copy and plasmid sequences is accomplished by negative selection with ganciclovir or an equivalent drug that kills all cells carrying the negative selection (neg sel) marker. Some surviving cells will have escaped by excision of the marker. If the excision occurs by homologous intrachromosomal recombination, it is possible that the recombination event leaves the mutant copy of the gene while removing the normal gene along with selective markers and plasmid sequences.

nation between the normal endogenous sequences of the gene-of-interest and homologous gene segments supplied by the gene-targeting vector. The recombination event results in the deletion of the *HSVtk* gene, the *neo* gene, and plasmid sequences, while reduplicating the targeted gene sequences. If the intrachromosomal recombination occurred in the correct site, the gene of interest will contain the targeted subtle mutation.

After the targeting event has been identified, the appropriate ES cell clone is thawed and expanded, and the cells are microinjected into the cavity of 3.5-day mouse blastocysts, usually of C57BL/6 origin. Usually, about a dozen ES cells are injected into the blastocyst, which is held with a blunt-ended glass-holding pipet. The injected blastocysts are then implanted into the uterine horns of pseudopregnant females. Since the ES cells used for gene-targeting experiments are usually derived from strain 129 mice with coat color alleles distinct from those of the C57BL/6 blastocysts, the resulting chimeric pups can be identified by examining the coat color at about 1 week of age. Also, since ES cell lines are derived from male animals, microinjected ES cells can convert the sex of female blastocysts if sufficient numbers of the injected cells are incorporated into the developing embryo. Thus, male mice with chimeric coat color are selected to breed with females from an inbred strain such as C57BL/6. Transmission of the ES cell genome in the offspring can be detected by coat color, which is usually agouti fur (agouti is a dominant trait). Of the agouti pups, half should be heterozygous for the targeted allele. These heterozygotes can then be intercrossed to obtain homozygous animals.

Obviously, the targeted mice carry a mixture of genes from strain 129 and C57BL/6. To establish the targeted mutation on an inbred strain, the chimeric males (carrying targeted alleles from the 129 strain) should be bred with 129 strain females. However, strain 129 mice are not good breeders and are susceptible to infection. Alternatively, the targeted allele can be placed onto the genetic background of an inbred strain by repeated backcrossing, as discussed above for congenics. This can be performed in a relatively small number of generations using marker-assisted selection protocols (rapid congenics), as discussed above.

Recent Developments

A number of variations on transgenic and gene-targeting technologies have been developed over the years and have expanded the usefulness of genetically modified animal models. Below, we discuss some of the more widely used of these.

It has been difficult to express transgenes in a reversible or inducible manner, but recently a promising system for this has

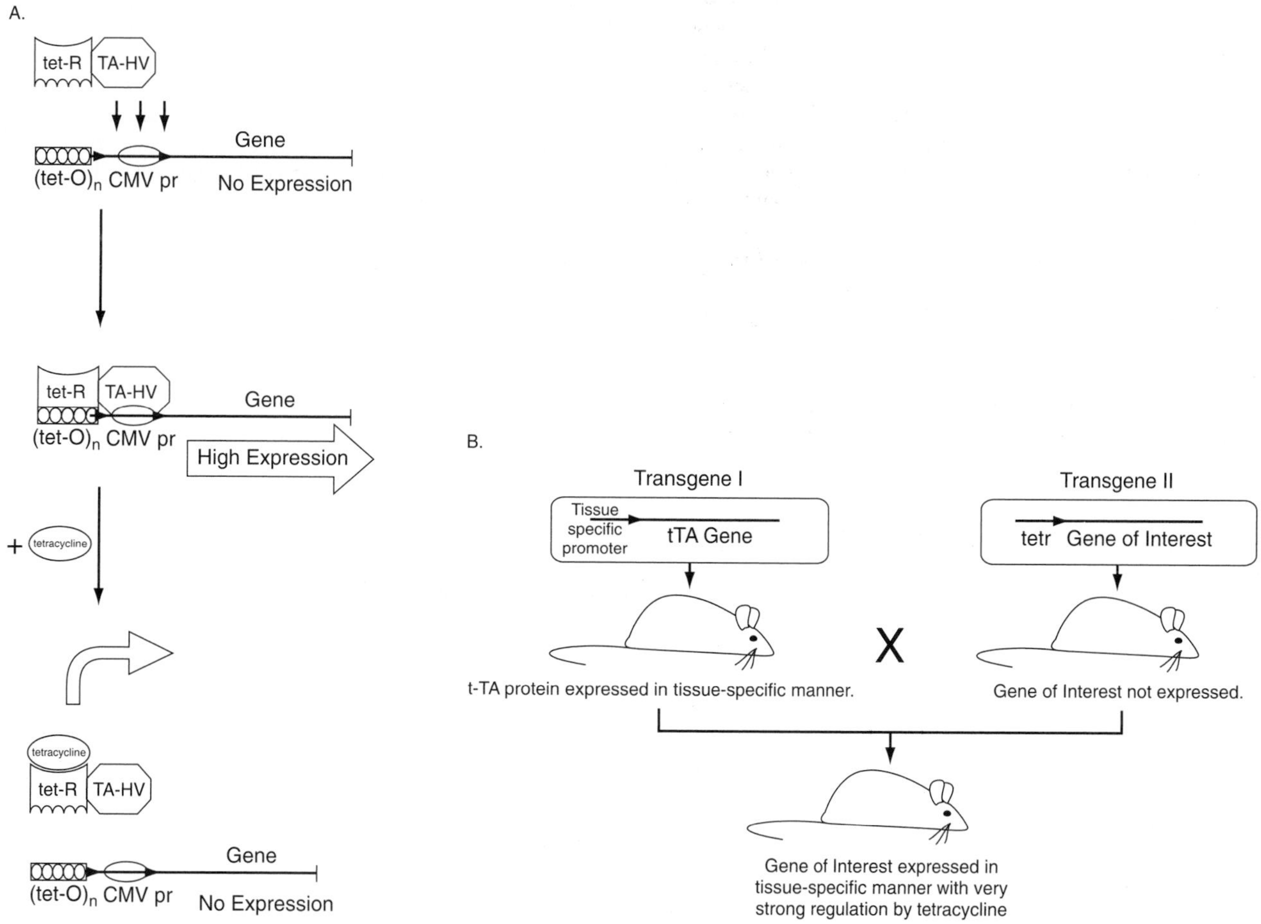

Fig. 5–12. Use of the tetracycline operon from E. coli to reversibly regulate transgene expression. **(A)** Coding sequences for the gene are placed downstream of a trans-activatable promoter such as the minimal promoter from cytomegalovirus IE. Immediately adjacent to the promoter are placed a tandem repeat of the bacterial tetracycline operon (tet-O_n) sequences that recognize and bind the tetracycline repressor (tet-R) protein. In the absence of a transactivator, no expression is seen. However, a fusion protein containing both tet-R and a transactivator such as that from herpesvirus (TA-HV) will bind to tet-O_n and transactivate high-level expression from the promoter. Tetracycline, when present, binds tet-R, releasing it from tet-O_n and interrupting transcription from the promoter. As a result, expression from the gene is reduced by 5 orders of magnitude. (Gossen and Bujard 1992). **(B)** Mice expressing the transgene for the tet-R/TA-HV fusion protein are mated with mice carrying the transgene for the tet-O_n/transactivable-promoter construct. In offspring carrying both transgenes, expression of the gene of interest is strongly regulated by tetracycline. Such expression can also be tissue-specific if the tet-R/TA-HV fusion protein is under the control of a tissue-specific promoter. (Passman and Fishman 1994).

been described (Gossen and Bujard, 1992; Passman and Fishman, 1994). The system takes advantage of a well-characterized regulatory system from *Escherichia coli*, the tetracycline-resistance operon (see Fig. 5–12). The system consists of the bacterial tetracycline repressor protein, which binds strongly to bacterial tetracycline operator sequences placed in the transcription unit. This binding can be displaced by low doses of tetracycline or its analogs. The repressor protein is converted in this system into a transactivator protein by fusion with the transcriptional activation domain from a viral protein. In tissue-culture cells, the fold induction of the system—that is, the ratio of promoter activity in the absence of tetracycline to activity in the presence of tetracycline—is several tens of thousands. This tetracycline-inducible system has been applied to transgenic animals where regulation is obtained by feeding tetracycline derivatives in a diet. Such derivatives are readily absorbed and have virtually no toxicity at the doses required to regulate the promoter elements. This system may be further refined by engineering animals that express the transactivator protein only in certain tissues (Fig. 5–12B), thus allowing tissue-specific regulation of expression of the target gene.

It seems likely that many of the variations contributing to complex traits will be quantitative, and Smithies and colleagues (Smithies and Kim, 1994) have developed specialized sequence-insertion vectors to duplicate a target gene in its endogenous chromosomal location for examining the effects of quantitative variations. The strategy is based on the fact that if a sequence-insertion vector contains an entire gene-of-interest, including the appropriate promoter and enhancer sequences, the targeted insertion of that vector would duplicate the entire locus (see Fig. 5–10A). For large genes, the construction of this type of vector would not be feasible. To circumvent this problem, Smithies and colleagues developed a "gap repair" duplication strategy (see Fig. 5–10B). In this strategy, vectors containing large gaps in the homologous sequences are used; such gaps are filled in during the homologous recombination event. Smithies and colleagues have used both duplications and null mutations to examine the effect of quantitative variations of the renin–angiotensin pathway on blood pressure in mouse models (Kim et al., 1995). For example, to duplicate the angiotensinogen gene, the targeting vector contained homology to the 5′ promoter region of the gene and the 3′ portion of the gene with a gap of about 8 kb in between. Very good targeting frequency was obtained, and Southern blot analysis confirmed that the gap was repaired and that the targeted chromosome contained two copies of the entire angiotensinogen gene. By breeding both mice with the duplicated gene and mice with the null mutation, animals containing no functional genes, one functional gene, two functional genes, three functional genes, and four functional genes were obtained (Figs. 5–9B and 5–10C). Angiotensinogen gene expression closely paralleled the number of copies of the gene. Blood pressure was found to be directly related to the number of angiotensinogen genes, with each gene, on average, increasing the blood pressure by 8 mm Hg. The beauty of this duplication strategy is that a precise number of copies of the duplicated gene is obtained, and the duplicated gene is expected to experience the same chromosomal environment as the native gene.

One of the most important technological advances for gene-targeting studies is the site-specific Cre/*loxP* recombination system. (See Fig. 5–13.) This system allows the development of mouse models in which a gene of interest is inactivated only in a tissue-specific or time-specific manner. It is based on a recombination system from bacteriophage P1 in which recombinase (*Cre*) catalyzes the recombination between two 36 bp sites called *lox*, for locus of crossing over. When two *loxP* sites are in the same orientation, *Cre* excises the intervening DNA sequences, and when the *loxP* sites are in the opposite orientation, *Cre* inverts the intervening DNA sequences. The Cre/*loxP* system was originally found to be sufficiently robust to function in mammalian tissue-culture cells, and subsequently it was found to also function in transgenic mice (Gu et al., 1994). The ability to knock out genes in selected tissues (see Fig. 5–14) has made it possible to study the role of genes for which traditional knockout experiments yielded lethal phenotypes. For example, Gu and coworkers (1994) wanted to determine the role of the DNA polymerase beta gene in T-lymphocyte function. However, the total knockout of this gene resulted in an embryonic lethal phenotype. To study the role of this gene in T-cells, they used a sequence-replacement vector to introduce *loxP* sequences flanking exon 1 of the DNA polymerase gene. In these studies, the introduction of the *loxP* sites in the 5′ flanking region and the first intron did not affect the expression of the gene. To knock

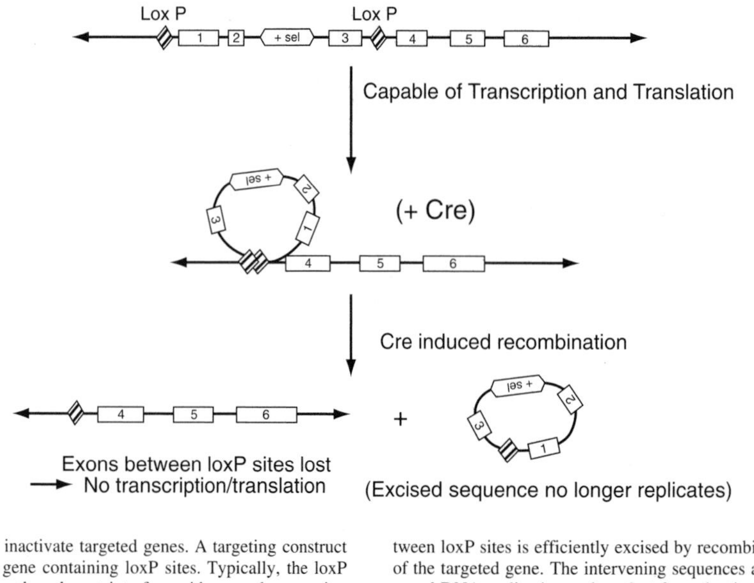

Fig. 5–13. Use of the Cre/*loxP* system to inactivate targeted genes. A targeting construct is used to replace the normal gene with a gene containing loxP sites. Typically, the loxP sites are placed in intronic sequences where they do not interfere with normal expression of the targeted gene. In tissues where the Cre recombinase is also expressed, the DNA between loxP sites is efficiently excised by recombination. This specifically disrupts function of the targeted gene. The intervening sequences are no longer included in normal chromosomal DNA replication and are lost from the tissue. ("+ sel" indicates the marker used for positive selection of the targeted gene construct.)

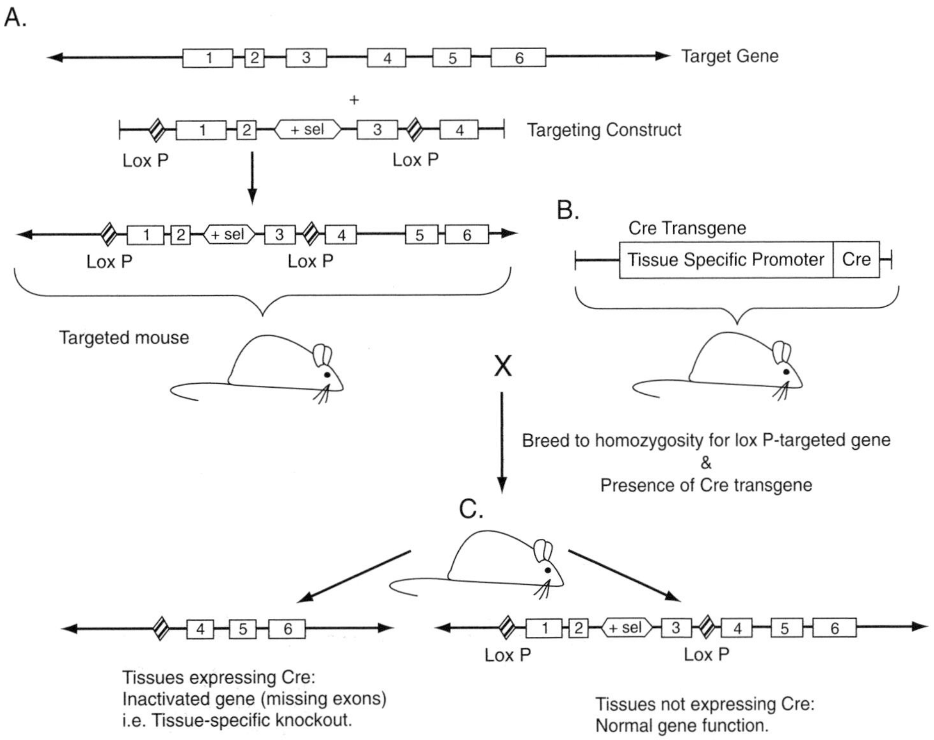

Fig. 5–14. Use of the Cre/*loxP* system to obtain tissue-specific inactivation of a target gene. **(A)** The targeting construct containing loxP sites is used to produce a mouse carrying a modified but functional gene in all tissues. **(B)** This targeted mouse is mated with a mouse carrying a Cre recombinase transgene regulated by a tissue-specific promoter. **(C)** Offspring carrying the Cre transgene and homozygous for the loxP-targeted gene are selected by DNA analysis. These mice experience inactivation of the targeted gene only in the specific tissue expressing Cre recombinase. Note that the same original targeted mouse can be mated to a panel of transgenic mice expressing Cre in different tissues. Moreover, the same panel of Cre transgenes with different tissue specificity can be used with any number of appropriately targeted genes. A useful variation of the procedure is to carry out tissue-specific activation of genes previously targeted for inactivation by insertion of DNA flanked by loxP sites. For example, tissue specificity of the Cre recombinase promoters can be monitored by using Cre to rescue inactivated transgenes for lac Z or green fluorescent protein.

out the polymerase gene in T-cells, but not in other tissues, mice with the *loxP* sites were mated with transgenic mice in which *Cre* was controlled by a promoter active only in T-cells. The progeny, containing both the *Cre* transgene and the modified polymerase gene, indicated that mature lymphocytes had undergone the *Cre*-mediated deletion of the polymerase gene but that the gene was normal in other tissues. Since these original studies, the *Cre/loxP* system has been used to create tissue-specific knockouts in many different systems. Many different variations of the original strategy have been devised. For example, it is possible to transiently express the *Cre* protein in ES cells to delete DNA fragments containing a drug resistance marker before generating mice (Araki et al., 1995). Also, transient expression of *Cre* with adenoviral vectors has been used for introducing gene knockouts both in vivo and in vitro (Anton and Graham, 1995).

FROM GENES TO PATHWAYS

Gene–Gene Interactions

Studies of interactions between genes contributing to complex diseases in humans are usually dependent on epidemiologic evidence, which is difficult to establish. Also, with the notable exception of cancer, where interactions can frequently be examined in tissue culture, it is usually not feasible to examine the molecular nature of the interactions. In contrast, gene–gene interactions can be studied in detail by using animal models, even if the identities of the underlying genes are unknown. For example, Fig. 5–7 shows the interactions of four separate loci contributing to body fat in a genetic cross between two strains of mice. The four loci, which together explain about 50% of the variance in body fat, exhibit clear nonadditive interactions (Warden et al., 1995).

Another outstanding example of the dissection of the analysis of gene–gene interactions involves noninsulin-dependent diabetes mellitus (NIDDM). The disease is characterized by insulin resistance in multiple tissues, followed by the failure of the pancreatic beta cells to adequately compensate. Reasoning that NIDDM involves multiple quantitative defects in the insulin-signaling pathway, Brüning and colleagues (Brüning et al., 1997) bred together gene-targeted mice for different components in the pathway. Thus, although neither mice heterozygous for a null mutation of the insulin receptor gene nor mice heterozygous for a null mutation of the insulin receptor substrate-1 gene exhibited dramatic insulin resistance or diabetes, mice in which both null mutations (in the heterozygous state) were combined exhibited dramatic insulin resistance (insulin levels elevated 5- to 50-fold) and significant diabetes. The analysis of other targeted mutations should allow examination of the steps in the pathway that have the potential to confer insulin resistance. Such mice are also likely to be useful for identification of modifier genes for the disease.

A particularly important advantage of studies in animal models is the ability to study interacting genes on a common genetic background. This same problem applies to gene–environment interactions and is discussed below. In addition, the ability to bring together specific alleles of interest by breeding and the ability to control the environment are crucial for studies where more than two genes are examined simultaneously and where the interactions are subtle.

Genetic–Environmental Interactions

Genetic–environmental interactions are clearly very difficult to study in detail in humans. In particular, it would be very difficult in humans to determine the relationship between a quantifiable phenotype, such as blood cholesterol, and various environments. One problem relates to our inability to carefully control the environment. But the major problem is that, in humans, a genotype cannot be replicated (except in identical twins), and, therefore, it is impossible to examine the effect of a number of different environments on a phenotype while holding the genotype constant. Consequently, the data available for humans represent average results over many different genotypes. An excellent potential model for detailed studies of genetic–environmental interactions is the mouse, because many different inbred strains, each representing a unique gene pool, have been derived by brother–sister mating. Numerous differences in dietary responsiveness have been observed among these strains, affecting traits such as atherosclerosis, obesity, diabetes, cancer, autoimmune disease, and inflammation. One particularly well characterized example involves changes in the levels of plasma lipoproteins and cholesterol levels in response to high-fat diets. Inbred strains of mice exhibit wide variations in response to high-fat diets (Kirk et al., 1995) and genes controlling responsiveness to dietary challenges have been mapped (Purcell-Huynh et al., 1995; Machleder et al., 1997).

Dissection of Multistep Pathways

Genetic approaches in mice, particularly the use of planned genetic modifications, have made feasible the detailed analysis of a number of pathways involved in complex disease processes. One good example concerns the development of early athero-

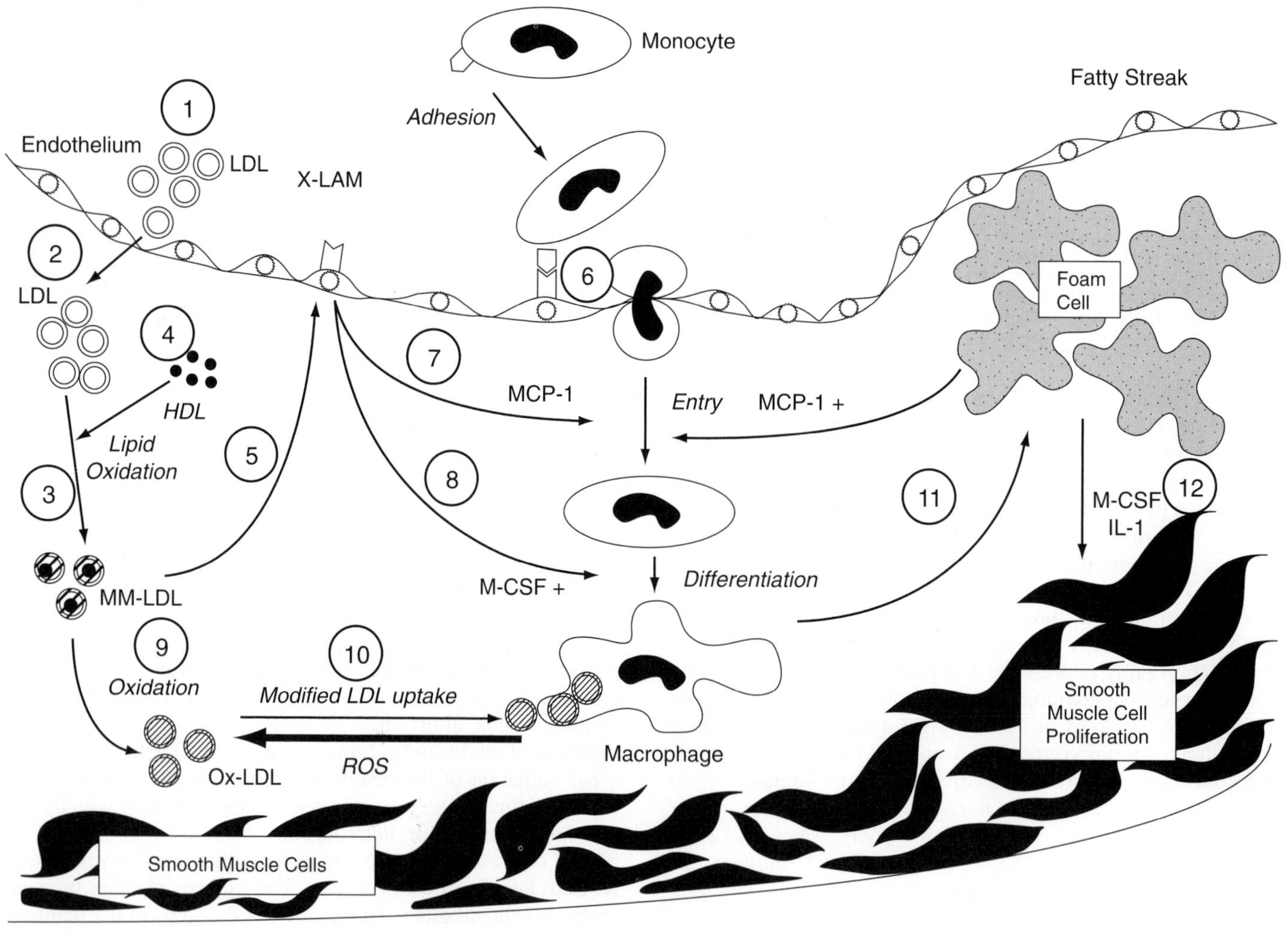

Fig. 5–15. A model for early steps in the development of the atherosclerotic lesion. Atherogenesis is clearly a complex disease involving the interaction of many genes. The detailed model shown here summarizes current thinking on early steps in lesion development. Most of these steps in the model have been tested in mouse model systems. **(1)** At high concentrations of LDL (or other atherogenic lipoproteins), the particles accumulate in the subendothelial space **(2)**. The trapped LDL particles become oxidized **(3)**, probably as a result of interactions with reactive oxygen species (ROS) produced by vascular cells. **(4)** The oxidation of LDL is inhibited by HDL, which carries an enzyme, paraoxonase, that is capable of destroying certain oxidized species. In vitro and in vivo studies suggest that such minimally modified LDL (MM-LDL) exhibits a potent biologic activity capable of inducing endothelial cells to express adhesion molecules for monocytes (X-LAM) **(5)**, monocyte chemotactic protein-1 (MCP-1) **(7)**, and macrophage-colony stimulating factor (M-CSF) **(8)**. The expression of these and other molecules results in the recruitment of blood monocytes to the artery wall **(6)**, where the monocytes differentiate into macrophages. With time, the LDL particles become highly oxidized (Ox-LDL) **(9)**, perhaps as a result of the high levels of ROS produced by macrophages. Such highly oxidized LDL particles are recognized by scavenger receptors on macrophages, resulting in rapid endocytosis **(10)**. Unlike the LDL receptor, the scavenger receptors are not downregulated by high levels of cellular cholesterol, and the macrophages continue to accumulate cholesterol until they give rise to cholesterol-engorged foam cells **(11)**. Such foam cells, the hallmark of fatty streaks, may contribute to the development of advanced lesions by the production of cytokines and growth factors such as M-CSF and interleukin-1 (IL-1) **(12)**. Reviewed in Lusis (2000). Table 5–4 summarizes how specific steps of the model have been tested using planned genetic modifications or naturally occurring mutations in mice.

Table 5–5. Dissection of Steps in Early Atherosclerosis Using Mouse Models

Hypothesis	Test
1. High levels of plasma LDL promote lipid infiltration of the artery wall.	1. Mice with extreme hypercholesterolemia (resulting from apolipoprotein E mutations) exhibit increased arterial lipid accumulation (Breslow, 1994).
2. LDL becomes trapped in the artery wall by interaction with proteoglycans and other matrix components.	2. Mice in which the heparin binding site of apolipoprotein B (the major protein of LDL) is deleted fail to accumulate lipids in the artery wall (Boren et al., 1998, and Innerarity, personal communication).
3. Lipids in LDL become oxidized and promote monocyte infiltration.	3. Deficiency of the antioxidant enzyme heme oxygenase promotes atherogenesis (Ishikawa and Lusis, personal communication).
4. HDL protects against atherosclerosis in part by reducing the accumulation of oxidized lipids.	4. Deficiency of paraoxonase, an esterase on HDL with the ability to destroy oxidized phospholipids, increases atherosclerosis (Shih et al., 1998).
7. Monocyte recruitment involves the chemotactic protein MCP-1.	7. MCP-1 receptor-deficient mice exhibit reduced atherosclerosis (Boring et al., 1998).
8. Macrophage growth and survival in artery wall is enhanced by M-CSF.	8. M-CSF-deficient mice exhibit dramatically reduced atherogenesis (Qiao et al., 1997; Rajavashisth et al. 1998).
10. The formation of foam cells involves receptors that recognize modified LDL.	10. Scavenger receptor–deficient mice exhibit reduced atherogenesis (Suzuki et al., 1997).
12. Foam cell accumulation is a prerequisite for later stages of atherosclerosis.	12. Mice deficient in M-CSF not only fail to accumulate foam cells but also do not exhibit smooth muscle cell proliferation (Qiao et al., 1997).

Numbers refer to steps diagrammed in Fig. 5–15.

sclerotic lesions. Tissue-culture studies and human epidemiological data suggested a multistep model for the disease (see Fig. 5–15). Since this model was proposed, in about 1990, many of the individual steps have been examined using transgenic and gene targeted mice as well as naturally occurring variations. As examples, Table 5–5 lists some of these steps (numbered according to Fig. 5–15), along with the specific model system used to investigate the pathway. A variety of other complex disease pathways have been successfully analyzed using animal model systems. These include the interactions of the Alzheimer's precursor protein with other genetic factors in Alzheimer's disease; homeostatic mechanisms, such as the leptin pathway in obesity; and interactions of the renin–angiotensin pathway in hypertension. None of these are readily amenable to investigation in humans, but the availability of animal models provides access to a detailed understanding of metabolic pathways that is otherwise unattainable. The success of these models and the continuing advancement of genetic strategies suggests that animal models will play a central role in our continued investigation of a variety of human afflictions.

Application of Animal Models in the Era of the Genome Project

With the advent of full genomic sequences for a number of species, particularly mouse and humans, it becomes possible to apply a variety of new techniques to investigate complex diseases in animal models (Rubin and Tall, 2000).

First, sequence data establish an absolute physical map and, within that map, provide numerous new polymorphisms whose positions are known precisely with respect to coding sequences. This combination greatly facilitates mapping of complex traits. In addition, sequence comparisons between species and between strains are likely to yield insights about the observed expression differences for the genes in question. Further, the availability of DNA microarrays, which contain probe sequences for large numbers of genes, makes it possible to simultaneously monitor shifts in expression for a full panel of disease-related genes in specific tissues of an animal model. Analysis of these data can follow two complementary approaches.

One approach is to assess the effect of the disease on candidate metabolic pathways or to reveal effects on pathways not previously considered. For example, hepatocyte nuclear factor 1a (HNF-1a) has been implicated in maturity onset diabetes of the young type 3 (MODY3) and, knockout mice exhibit hypercholesterolemia and have multiple defects in glucose and amino acid homeostasis. Shih et al. (2001) used expression arrays in knockout and control mice to show that HNF-1a is an essential regulator of bile acid and plasma cholesterol metabolism. Indeed, this transcription factor affects expression of multiple pathways, including bile acid synthesis, bile acid transport, plasma triglyceride hydrolysis, and reverse cholesterol transport. In a similar approach, Nadler et al. (2000) examined differences in gene expression between lean and obese mice and were able to identify 88 genes whose expression correlated with severity of diabetes. These included genes with known roles in signal transduction and energy metabolism, as well as genes not previously associated with diabetes. Interestingly, they found that genes normally involved in adipogenesis show decreased expression in obese mice. Finally, it was possible to identify novel genes whose expression is correlated with the transition from obese to diabetic. Thus, expression array analysis can greatly enhance the broader understanding of complex disease at the physiological level.

The second approach is to examine expression differences for all the genes underlying a QTL. For example, syndrome X, a complex of insulin resistance–related phenotypes is observed in the spontaneously hypertensive rat (SHR). QTLs for several of these traits have been mapped to distal Chr 4, and a congenic strain in which wild-type DNA replaces SHR DNA at this locus showed partial correction of the insulin-resistance phenotype. By profiling expression differences for genes within the congenic region, it was possible to identify CD-36 as a candidate gene responsible for the phenotypic changes (Aitman et al., 1999). Moreover, sequence comparisons between SHR and wild-type CD-36 genes revealed a rearrangement associated with suppression of CD-36 expression in SHR adipocytes. Thus, with a relatively complete physical map and an appropriate congenic construct, it was possible to identify CD-36 as a likely participant in the insulin-resistance QTL, and this conclusion was confirmed by inserting a wild-type CD-36 gene on the SHR genetic background (Pravenec et al., 2001).

In conclusion, studies in animal models are directly relevant to human disease in several ways. First, and foremost, they provide detailed mechanistic information about disease pathways, as exemplified by the studies of atherosclerosis discussed above. In particular, the advent of transgenic and knockout animals has greatly enhanced the ability to dissect metabolic pathways. As these constructs become refined (tissue-specific expression, regulated expression, etc.) they become ever more powerful tools to elucidate the corresponding human pathways. One example, among many, is investigation of the role of the renin–angiotensin system in hypertension (see Chapter 8). Furthermore, animal models, both naturally occurring variants and genetically modified strains, are increasingly useful in the development of new therapies, including gene therapy. Recent examples of such innovative therapies include treatment of the mdx mouse model for Duchenne's muscular dystrophy using normal stem-cell transplantation (Gussoni et al., 1999) and the prevention of diabetes in the NOD mouse with novel peptide vaccines (Berezhkovskiy et al., 1999). Finally, animal models provide one important avenue for gene identification. In a number of instances, studies in mice have lead directly to the identification of Mendelian disease genes. For example, in the case of deafness, studies in mice were important in the identification of several genes in non-syndromic hearing loss in humans (Liu et al., 1997; Verhoeven et al., 1998). For complex diseases, multiple contributing loci have been identified in animal models and, for some, such as familial combined hyperlipidemia (Castellani et al., 1998) and obesity (Lembertas et al., 1997) syntenic regions are associated with the similar disease in man. Clearly, such animal models will become ever more important for the discovery of human complex disease genes.

ACKNOWLEDGMENTS

We wish to acknowledge Arin Aboulilan for his valued assistance in preparation of the figures. Work in the authors' laboratories was supported by NIH grants HL30568, HL42488, HL28481, and HL58627.

REFERENCES

Aitman TJ, Glazier AM, Wallace CA, Cooper LD, Norsworthy PJ, Wahid FN, Al Majali KM, Trembling PM, Mann CJ, Shoulders CC, et al.: Identification of Cd36 (Fat) as an insulin-resistance gene causing defective fatty acid and glucose metabolism in hypertensive rats. Nat Genet 1999; 21:76–83.

Alfred JB, Rance K, Taylor BA, Phillips SJ, Abbott CM, Jackson IJ: Mapping in the region of Danforth's short tail and the localization of tail length modifiers. Genome Res. 1997; 7:108–117.

Anton M, Graham FL: Site-specific recombination mediated by an adenovirus vector expressing the Cre recombinase protein: a molecular switch for control of gene expression. J Virol 1995; 69:4600–4606.

Araki K, Araki M, Miyazaki J, Vassalli P: Site-specific recombination of a transgene in fertilized eggs by transient expression of Cre recombinase. Proc Natl Acad Sci USA 1995; 92:160–164.

Asada Y, Varnum DS, Frankel WN, Nadeau JH: A mutation in the Ter gene causing increased susceptibility to testicular teratomas maps to mouse chromosome 18. Nat Genet 1994; 6:363–368.

Avner P, Amar L, Dandolo L, Guenet JL: Genetic analysis of the mouse using interspecific crosses. Trends Genet 1998; 4:18–23.

Bailey DW: Recombinant inbred strains and bilineal congenic strains. In: Foster HL, Small JD, Fox JG (eds). The mouse in biomedical research: Vol 1. History, Genetics, and Wild Mice. New York: Academic Press, 1981:223–239.

Barsh GS: The genetics of pigmentation: from fancy genes to complex traits. Trends Genet 1996; 12:299–305.

Bedell MA, Jenkins NA, Copeland NG: Mouse models of human disease: Part 1. techniques and resources for genetic analysis in mice. Genes Dev 1997a; 11:1–10.

Bedell MA, Largaespada DA, Jenkins NA, Copeland NG: Mouse models of human disease: Part 2: Recent progress and future directions. Genes Dev 1997b; 11:11–43.

Berezhkovskiy L, Pham S, Reich EP, Deshpande S: Synthesis and kinetics of cyclization of MHC class II—derived cyclic peptide vaccine for diabetes. J Pep Res 1999; 54:112–119.

Berrettini WH, Ferraro TN, Alexander RC, Buchmerg AM, Vogel WH: Quantitative trait loci mapping of three loci controlling morphine preference using inbred mouse strains. Nat Genet 1994; 7:54–58.

Borchelt DR, Ratovitski T, van Lare J, Lee MK, Gonzales V, Jenkins NA, Copeland NG, Price DL, Sisodia SS: Accelerated amyloid deposition in the brains of transgenic mice coexpressing mutant presenilin 1 and amyloid precursor proteins. Neuron 1997; 19:939–945.

Boren J, Olin K, Lee I, Chait A, Wight TN, Innerarity T: Identification of the principal proteoglycan-binding site in LDL: a single-point mutation in apo-B100 severely affects proteoglycan interaction without affecting LDL receptor binding. J Clin Invest 1998; 101:2658–2664.

Boring L, Gosling J, Cleary M, Charo IF: Decreased lesion formation in CCR2$^{-/-}$ mice reveals a role for chemokines in the initiation of atherosclerosis. Nature 1998; 394:894–897.

Breslow JL: Insights into lipoprotein metabolism from studies in transgenic mice. Annu Rev Physiol 1994; 56:797–810.

Breslow JL: Mouse models of atherosclerosis. Science 1996; 272:685–688

Brown DM, Provoost AP, Daly MJ, Lander ES, Jacob HJ: Renal disease susceptibility and hypertension are under independent genetic control in the fawn-hooded rat. Nat Genet 1996; 12:44–51.

Brown RH, Jr: Amyotrophic lateral sclerosis: recent insights from genetics and transgenic mice. Cell 1995; 80:687–692.

Brüning JC, Winnay J, Bonner-Weir S, Taylor SI, Accili D, Kahn CR: Development of a novel polygenic model of NIDDM in mice heterozygous for IR and IRS-1 null alleles. Cell 1997; 88:561–572.

Bullard DC, Scharffetter-Kochanek K, McArthur MJ, Chosay JG, McBride ME, Montgomery CA, Beaudet AL: A polygenic mouse model of psoriasiform skin disease in CD-18-deficient mice. Proc Natl Acad Sci USA 1996; 93:2116–2121.

Castellani LW, Weinreb A, Bodnar J, Goto AM, Doolittle M, Mehrabian M, Demant P, Lusis AJ: Mapping a gene for combined hyperlipidaemia in a mutant mouse strain. Nat Genet 1998; 18:374–377.

Collins FS: Positional cloning moves from perditional to traditional. Nat Genet 1995; 9:347–350.

Copeland NG, Jenkins NA, Gilbert DJ, Eppig JT, Malltais LJ, Miller JC, Dietrich WF, Weaver A, Lincoln SE, Steen RG, et al.: A genetic linkage map of the mouse: current applications and future prospects. Science 1993; 262:57–66.

Cormier RT, Hong KH, Halberg RB, Hawkins TL, Richardson P, Mulherkar R, Dove WF, Lander ES: Secretory phospholipase Pla2g2a confers resistance to intestinal tumorigenesis. Nat Genet 1997; 17:88–91.

Crabbe JC, Belknap JK, Buck KJ: Genetic animal models of alcohol and drug abuse. Science 1994; 264:1715–1723.

Darvasi A: Experimental strategies for the genetic dissection of complex trait in animal models. Nat Genet 1998; 18:19–24.

DeBry RW, Seldin MF: Human–mouse homology relationships. Genomics 1996; 33:337–351.

De Sanctis GT, Merchant M, Beier DR, Dredge RD, Grobholz, JK, Martin TR, Lander ES, Drazen JM: Quantitative locus analysis of airway hyperresponsiveness in A/J and C57BL/6J mice. Nat Genet 1995; 11:150–154.

Dietrich WF, Copeland NG, Gilbert DJ, Miller JC, Jenkins NA, Lander ES: Mapping the mouse genome: current status and future prospects. Proc Natl Acad Sci USA 1995; 92:10849–10853.

Dietrich WF, Damron DM, Isberg RR, Lander ES, Swanson MS: Lgn1, a gene that determines susceptibility to *Legionella pneumophila*, maps to mouse chromosome 13. Genomics 1995; 26:443–450.

Dietrich WF, Lander ES, Smith JS, Moser AR, Gould KA, Luongo C, Borenstein N, Dove W: Genetic identification of Mom-1, a major modifier locus affecting min induced intestinal neoplasia in the mouse. Cell 1993; 75:631–639.

Dietrich WF, Radany EH, Smith JS, Bishop JM, Hanahan D, Lander ES: Genome-wide search for loss of heterozygosity in transgenic mouse tumors reveals candidate tumor suppressor genes on chromosomes 9 and 16. Proc Natl Acad Sci USA 1994; 91:9451–9455.

Doolittle DP, Davisson MT, Guidi JN, Green MC: Catalog of mutant genes and polymorphic loci. In: Lyon MF, Rastan S, Brown SDM (eds). Genetic Variants and Strains of the Laboratory Mouse, 3d ed. Oxford: Oxford University Press, 1996:17–854.

Fijneman RJ, Oomen LC, Snoek M, Demant P: A susceptibility gene for alveolar lung tumors in the mouse maps between Hsp 70.3 and G7 within the H2 complex. Immunogenetics 1995; 41:106–109.

Fisler JS, Warden CH, Pace HJ, Lusis AJ: BSB: a new mouse model of multigenic obesity. Obes Res 1993; 1:271–280.

Flaherty L: Congenic strains. In: Foster HL, Small JD, Fox JG (eds). The Mouse in Biomedical Research: Vol I. History, Genetics and Wild Mice. New York: Academic Press, 1981:215–222.

Frankel WN: Taking stock of complex trait genetics in mice. Trends Genet 1995; 11:471–477.

Frankel WN, Johnson EW, Lutz CM: Congenic strains reveal effects of the epilepsy quantitative trait locus, E12, separate from other E1 loci. Mamm Genome 1995b; 6:839–843.

Frankel WN, Taylor BA, Noebels JL, Lutz CM: Genetic epilepsy model derived from common inbred mouse strains. Genetics 1994; 138:481–489.

Frankel WN, Valenzuela A, Lutz CM, Johnson EW, Dietrich WF, Coffin JM: New seizure frequency QTL and the complex genetics of epilepsy in EL mice. Mamm Genome 1995a; 6:830–838.

Galli J, Li LS, Glaser A, Ostenson CG, Jiao H, Fakhrai-Rad H, Jacob HJ, Lander ES, Luthman H: Genetic analysis of non-insulin dependent diabetes mellitus in the GK rat. Nat Genet 1996; 12:31–37.

Gerlai R: Gene targeting studies of mammalian behavior: is it the mutation or the background genotype? Trends Neurosci 1996; 19:177–181.

Gordon JW, Ruddle FH: Integration and stable germ line transmission of genes injected into mouse pronuclei. Science 1981; 214:1244–1246.

Gossen M, Bujard H: Tight control of gene expression in mammalian cells by tetracycline-responsive promoters. Proc Natl Acad Sci USA 1992; 89:5547–5551.

Gould KA, Luongo C, Moser AR, McNeley MK, Borenstein N, Shedlovsky A, Dove WF, Hong K, Dietrich WF, Lander ES: Genetic evaluation of candidate genes for the *Mom1* modifier of intestinal neoplasia in mice. Genetics 1996; 144: 1777–1785.

Grupe A, Germer S, Usuka J, Aud D, Belknap JK, Klein RF, Ahluwalia MK, Higuchi R, Peltz G: In silico mapping of complex disease-related traits in mice. Science 2001; 292:1915–1918.

Gu H, Marth JD, Orban PC, Mossmann H, Rajewsky K: Deletion of a DNA polymerase beta gene segment in T cells using cell type–specific gene targeting. Science 1994; 265:103–106.

Gussoni E, Soneoka Y, Strickland CD, Buzney EA, Khan MK, Flint AF, Kunkel LM, Mulligan RC: Dystrophin expression in the mdx mouse restored by stem cell transplantation. Nature 1999; 401:390–394.

Haldi ML, Lim P, Kaphingst K, Akella U, Whang J, Lander ES: Construction of a large-insert yeast artificial chromosome library of the rat genome. Mamm Genome 1997; 8:284.

Haldi ML, Strickland C, Lim P, VanBerkel V, Chen X, Noya D, Korenberg JR, Husain Z, Miller J, Lander ES: A comprehensive large-insert yeast artificial chromosome library for physical mapping of the mouse genome. Mamm Genome 1996; 7:767–769.

Hamilton BA, Smith DJ, Mueller KL, Kerrebrock AW, Bronson RT, van Berkel V, Daly MJ, Kruglyak L, Reeve MP, Nemhauser JL, et al.: The vibrator mutations causes neurodegeneration via reduced expression of PITP alpha: positional complementation cloning and extragenic suppression. Neuron 1997; 18:711–722.

Hammer RE, Pursel VG, Rexroad CE Jr, Wall RJ, Bolt DJ, Ebert KM, Palmiter RD, Brinster RL: Production of transgenic rabbits, sheep, and pigs by microinjection. Nature 1985; 315:680–683.

Hasty P, Bradley A: Gene targeting vectors for mammalian cells. In: Joyner AL (ed). Gene Targeting: A Practical Approach. Oxford: Oxford University Press, 1993:1–31.

Higgins LS, Cordell B: Transgenic mice and modeling Alzheimer's disease. Rev Neurosci 1995; 6:87–96.

Hogan B, Beddington R, Costantini F, Lacy E: Manipulating the Mouse Embryo. Cold Spring Harbor, NY: Cold Spring Harbor Laboratory Press, 1994.

Holcomb L, Gordon MN, McGowan E, Yu X, Benkovic S, Jantzen P, Wright K, Saad I, Mueller R, Morgan D, et al.: Accelerated Alzheimer-type phenotype in transgenic mice carrying both mutant amyloid precursor protein and presenilin 1 transgenes. Nat Med 1998; 4:97–100.

Hsiao K, Chapman P, Nilsen S, Eckman C, Harigaya Y, Younkin S, Yang F, Cole G: Correlative memory deficits, Abeta elevation, and amyloid plaques in transgenic mice. Science 1996; 274:99–102.

Hsu LC, Kennan WS, Shepel LA, Jacob HJ, Szpirer C, Szpirer J, Lander ES, Gould MN: Genetic identification of Mcs-1, a rat mammary carcinoma suppressor gene. Cancer Res 1994; 54:2765–2770.

Hummler E: Implication of ENaC in salt-sensitive hypertension. J Steroid Biochem Mol Biol 1999; 69(1–6):385–390.

Iakoubova OA, Olsson CL, Dains KM, Ross D, Andalibi A, Lau K, Choi J, Kalcheva I, Cunanan M, Louie J, et al.: Genome tagged mice (GTM): two sets of genome wide congenic strains. Genomics 2001; 74:89–104.

Ishibashi S, Herz J, Maeda N, Goldstein JL, Brown MS: The two-receptor model of lipoprotein clearance: tests of the hypothesis in "knockout" mice lacking the low density lipoprotein receptor, apolipoprotein E or both proteins. Proc Natl Acad Sci USA 1994; 91:4431–4435.

Ivandic BT, Qiao J-H, Machleder D, Liao F, Drake TA, Lusis AJ: A locus on chromosome 7 determines myocardial cell necrosis and calcification (dystrophic cardiac calcinosis) in mice. Proc Natl Acad Sci USA 1996; 93:5483–5488.

Jacob HJ, Brown DM, Bunker RK, Daly MJ, Dzau VJ, Goodman A, Koike G, Kren V, Kurtz T, Lernmark Å, et al.: A genetic linkage map of the laboratory rat, *Rattus norvegicus*. Nat Genet 1995; 9:63–69.

Jacob HJ, Lindpaintner K, Lincoln SE, Kusumi K, Bunker RK, Mao YP, Ganten D, Dzau VJ, Lander ES: Genetic mapping of a gene causing hypertension in the stroke-prone spontaneously hypertensive rat. Cell 1991; 67:213–224.

Justice MJ, Zheng B, Woychik RP, Bradley A: Using targeted large deletions and high-efficiency *N*-ethyl-*N*-nitrosourea mutagenesis for functional analyses of the mammalian genome. Methods 1997; 13:423–436.

Kim HS, Krege JH, Kluckman KD, Hagaman JR, Hodgin JB, Best CF, Jennette JC, Coffman TM, Maeda N, Smithies O: Genetic control of blood pressure and the angiotensinogen locus. Proc Natl Acad Sci USA 1995; 92:2735–2739.

Kirk EA, Moe GL, Caldwell MT, Lernmark JA, Wilson DL, LeBoeuf RC: Hyper- and hypo-responsiveness to dietary fat and cholesterol among inbred mice: searching for level and variability genes. J Lipid Res 1995; 36:1522–1532.

Koller BH, Smithies O: Inactivating the β_2-microglobulin locus in mouse embryonic stem cells by homologous recombination. Proc Natl Acad Sci USA 1989; 86:8932–8935.

Kuokkanen S, Sundvall M, Terwilliger JD, Tienari PJ, Wikstrom J, Holmdahl R, Pettersson U, Peltonen L: A putative vulnerability locus to multiple sclerosis maps to 5p14–p12 in a region syntenic to the murine locus Eae2. Nat Genet 1996; 13:477–480.

Lamb BT, Gearhart JD: YAC transgenics and the study of genetics and human disease. Curr Opin Genet Dev 1995; 5:342–348.

Lander ES, Botstein D: Mapping Mendelian factors underlying quantitative traits using RFLP linkage maps. Genetics 1989; 121:185–199.

Lander ES, Green P, Abrahamson J, Barlow A, Daly MJ, Lincoln SE, Newburg L: MAPMAKER: an interactive computer package for constructing primary genetic linkage maps of experimental and natural populations. Genomics 1987; 1:174–181.

Lander ES, Schork NJ: Genetic dissection of complex traits. Science 1994; 265:2037–2048.

Lembertas AV, Perusse L, Chagnon YC, Fisler JS, Warden CH, Purcell-Huynh DA, Dionne FT, Gagnon J, Nadeau A, Lusis AJ, Bouchard C: Identification of an obesity quantitative trait locus on mouse chromosome 2 and evidence of linkage to body fat and insulin on the human homologous region 20q. J Clin Invest 1997; 100:1240–1247.

Lincoln S, Daly M, Lander E: Constructing genetic linkage maps with Mapmaker/Exp 3.0. Whitehead Institute Technical Report 3rd ed. 1992a. http://www-genome.wi.mit.edu/genome_software/other/mapmaker.html (as of 12/19/01).

Lincoln S, Daly M, Lander E: Mapping genes controlling quantitative traits with Mapmaker/QTL 1.1. Whitehead Institute Technical Report 3rd ed. 1992b. http://www-genome.wi.mit.edu/genome_software/other/qtl.html (as of 12/19/01)

Lisitsyn NA, Segre JA, Kusumi K, Lisitsyn NM, Nadeau JH, Frankel WN, Wigler MH, Lander ES: Direct isolation of polymorphic markers linked to a trait by genetically directed representational difference analysis. Nat Genet 1994; 6:57–63.

Liu XZ, Walsh J, Mburu P, Kendrick-Jones J, Cope MJ, Steel KP, Brown SD: Mutations in the myosin VIIA gene cause non-syndromic recessive deafness. Nat Genet 1997; 16:188–190.

Lusis AJ: The mouse model for atherosclerosis. Trends Cardiovasc Med 1993; 3:135–143.

Lusis AJ: Atherosclerosis. Nature 2000; 407:233–241.

Lusis AJ, Weinreb A, Drake TA: Genetics of atherosclerosis. In: Topol EJ (ed). Textbook of Cardiovascular Disease. Philadelphia: Lippincott-Raven, 1998:2389–2413.

Machleder D, Ivandic B, Welch C, Castellani LW, Reue K, Lusis AJ: Complex genetic control of HDL levels in mice in response to an atherogenic diet: coordinate genetic regulation of HDL levels and bile acid metabolism. J Clin Invest 1997; 99:1406–1419.

MacPhee M, Chepenik KP, Liddell RA, Nelson KK, Siracusa LD, Buchberg AM: The secretory phospholipase A2 gene is a candidate for the *Mom1* locus, a major modifier of Apc^{min}-induced intestinal neoplasia. Cell 1995; 81:957–966.

Manly K: A Macintosh program for storage and analysis of experimental genetic mapping data. Mamm Genome 1993; 4:303–313.

Mansour SL, Thomas KR, Capecchi MR: Disruption of the proto-oncogene *int-2* in mouse embryo-derived stem cells: a strategy for targeting mutations to non-selectable genes. Nature 1988; 336:348–352.

Markel P, Shu P, Ebeling C, Carlson GA, Nagle DL, Smutko JS, Moore KJ: Theoretical and empirical issues for marker-assisted breeding of congenic mouse strains. Nat Genet 1997; 17:280–284.

McLaren A, Biggers JD: Successful development and birth of mice cultivated in vitro as early embryos. Nature 1958; 182:877–878.

Mehrabian M, Demer LL, Lusis AJ: Differential accumulation of intimal monocyte-macrophages relative to lipoproteins and lipofuscin corresponds to hemodynamic forces on cardiac valves in mice. Arterioscler Thromb 1991; 11:947–957.

Mehrabian M, Qiao J-H, Hyman R, Ruddle D, Laughton C, Lusis AJ: Influence of the apoA-II gene locus on HDL levels and fatty streak development in mice. Arterioscler Thromb 1993; 13:1–10.

Mehrabian M, Wen P-Z, Fisler J, Davis RC, Lusis AJ: Genetic loci controlling body fat, lipoprotein metabolism, and insulin levels in a multifactorial mouse model. J Clin Invest 1998; 101:2485–2496.

Mein CA, Esposito L, Dunn MG, Johnson GCL, Timms AE, Goy JV, Smith AN, Sebag-Montefiore L, Merriman ME, Wilson AJ, et al.: A search for Type 1 diabetes susceptibility genes in families from the United Kingdom. Nat Genet 1998; 19:297–300.

Melo JA, Shendure J, Pociask K, Silver LM: Identification of sex-specific quantitative trait loci controlling alcohol preference in C57BL/6 mice. Nat Genet 1996; 13:147–153.

Moen CJ, Groot PC, Hart AA, Snoek M, Demant P: Fine mapping of colon tumor susceptibility (Scc) genes in the mouse, different from the genes known to be somatically mutated in colon cancer. Proc Natl Acad Sci USA 1996; 93:1082–1086.

Moen CJ, Stoffers HJ, Hart AA, Westerhoff HV, Demant P: Simulation of the distribution of parental strains genomes in RC strains of mice. Mamm Genome 1997; 8:884–889.

Morel L, Rudofsky UH, Longmate JA, Schiffenbauer J, Wakeland EK: Polygenic control of susceptibility to murine systemic lupus erythematosus. Immunity 1994; 1:219–229.

Moser AR, Luongo C, Gould KA, McNeley MK, Shoemaker AR, Dove WF: Apc^{Min}: a mouse model for intestinal and mammary tumorigenesis. Eur J Cancer 1995; 31A:1061–1064.

Mouse Genome Informatics Project: Mouse Genome Database (MGD): Jackson Laboratory, Bar Harbor, Maine. World Wide Web (http://www.informatics.jax.org/), 1998.

Nadeau JH, Frankel WN: The roads from phenotypic variation to gene discovery: mutagenesis versus QTLs. Nat Genet 2000; 25:381–384.

Nadler ST, Stoehr JP, Schueler KL, Tanimoto G, Yandell BS, Attie AD: (2000). The expression of adipogenic genes is decreased in obesity and diabetes mellitus. Proc Natl Acad Sci USA 2000; 97:11371–11376.

Neumann PE, Frankel WN, Letts VA, Coffin JM, Copp AJ, Bernfield M: Multifactorial inheritance of neural tube defects: localization of the major gene and recognition of modifiers in ct mutant mice. Nat Genet 1994; 6:357–362.

Nolan PM, Peters J, Strivens M, Rogers D, Hagan J, Spurr N, Gray IC, Vizor L, Brooker D, Whitehill E, et al.: A systematic, genome-wide, phenotype-driven mutagenesis programme for gene function studies in the mouse. Nat Genet 2000; 25:440–443.

Paigen K: A miracle enough: the power of mice. Nat Med 1995; 11:471–477.
Paigen B, Mitchell D, Reue K, Morrow A, Lusis AJ, LeBoeuf RC: *Ath-1*, a gene determining atherosclerosis susceptibility and high density lipoprotein levels in mice. Proc Natl Acad Sci USA 1987; 84:3763–3767.
Palmiter RD, Brinster RL: Germ-line transformation of mice. Annu Rev Genet 1986; 20:465–499.
Papaioannou V, Johnson R: Production of chimeras and genetically defined offspring from targeted ES cells. In: Joyner AL (ed). Gene Targeting: A Practical Approach. Oxford: Oxford University Press, 1993:107–146.
Passman RS, Fishman GI: Regulated expression of foreign genes in vivo after germline transfer. J Clin Invest 1994; 94:2421–2425.
Perou CM, Moore KJ, Nagle DL, Misumi DJ, Woolf EA, McGrail SH, Holmgren L, Brody TH, Dussault BJ, Jr., Monroe CA, et al.: Identification of the murine *beige* gene by YAC complementation and positional cloning. Nat Genet 1996; 13:303–308.
Peterson KR, Clegg CH, Huxley C, Josephson BM, Haugen HS, Furukawa T, Stamatoyannopoulos G: Transgenic mice containing a 248-kb yeast artificial chromosome carrying the human β-globin locus display proper developmental control of human globin genes. Proc Natl Acad Sci USA 1993; 90:7593–7597.
Pravenec M, Landa V, Zidek V, Musilova A, Kren V, Kazdova L, Aitman TJ, Glazier AM, Ibrahimi A, Abumrad NA, et al.: Transgenic rescue of defective Cd36 ameliorates insulin resistance in spontaneously hypertensive rats. Nat Genet 2001; 27:156–158.
Purcell-Huynh DA, Weinreb A, Castellani LW, Mehrabian M, Doolittle MH, Lusis AJ: Genetic factors in lipoprotein metabolism: analysis of a genetic cross between mouse strains NZB/BINJ and SM/J using a complete linkage map approach. J Clin Invest 1995; 96:1845–1858.
Qiao J-H, Tripathi J, Mishra NK, Cai Y, Tripathi S, Wang X, Imes S, Fishbein MC, Clinton SK, Libby P, et al.: Role of macrophage-colony stimulating factor in atherosclerosis: studies of osteopetrotic mice. Am J Pathol 1997; 150:1687–1699.
Qiao J-H, Welch CL, Xie P-Z, Fishbein MC, Lusis A: Involvement of the tyrosinase gene in the deposition of cardiac lipofuscin in mice: association with aortic fatty streak development. J Clin Invest 1993; 92:2386–2393.
Rajavashisth T, Qiao J-H, Tripathi S, Tripathi J, Mishra N, Hua M, Wang X, Loussararian A, Clinton S, Libby P, Lusis AJ: Heterozygous osteopetrotic (*op*) mutation reduces atherosclerosis in LDL receptor deficient mice. J Clin Invest 1998; 101:2702–2710.
Ramirez-Solis R, Liu P, Bradley A: Chromosome engineering in mice. Nature 1995; 378:720–724.
Rapp JP, Dene H: Development and characteristics of inbred strains of Dahl salt-sensitive and salt-resistant rats. Hypertension 1985; 7:340–349.
Rinchik EM: Chemical mutagenesis and fine-structure functional analysis of the mouse genome. Trends Genet 1991; 7:15–21.
Rubin EM, Tall A: Perspectives for vascular genomics. Nature 2000; 407:265–269.
Russell LB, Russell WL: Frequency and nature of specific-locus mutations induced in female mice by radiations and chemicals: a review. Mutat Res 1992; 296:107–127.
Schork NJ, Krieger JE, Trolliet MR, Franchini KG, Koike G, Krieger EM, Lander ES, Dzau VJ, Jacob HJ: A biometrical genome search in rats reveals the multigenic basis of blood pressure variation. Genome Res 1995; 5:164–172.
Schork NJ, Nath SP, Lindpaintner K, Jacob HJ: Extensions to quantitative trait locus mapping in experimental organisms. Hypertension 1996; 28:1104–1111.
She JX, Zhang LP, Scornik J, Wakeland EK: Additive susceptibility to insulin-dependent diabetes conferred by HLA-DQB1 and insulin genes. Autoimmunity 1994; 18:195–203.
Shih DM, Gu L, Hama S, Xia Y-R, Navab M, Fogelman AM, Lusis AJ: Genetic-dietary regulation of serum paraoxonase expression and its role in atherogenesis in a mouse model. J Clin Invest 1996; 97:1630–1639.
Shih DM, Gu L, Xia YR, Navab M, Li WF, Hama S, Castellani LW, Furlong CE, Costa LG, Fogelman AM, Lusis AJ: Mice lacking serum paraoxonase are susceptible to organophosphate toxicity and atherosclerosis. Nature 1998; 394:284–287.
Shih DM, Welch C, Lusis AJ: New insights into atherosclerosis from studies with mouse models. Mol Med Today 1995; 1:364–372.
Shih DQ, Bussen M, Sehayek E, Ananthanarayanan M, Shneider BL, Suchy FJ, Shefer S, Bollileni JS, Gonzalez FJ, Breslow JL, Stoffel M: Hepatocyte nuclear factor-1alpha is an essential regulator of bile acid and plasma cholesterol metabolism. Nature Genet 2001; 27:375–382.
Silver LM: Mouse Genetics: Concepts and Applications. New York: Oxford University Press, 1995.
Smith DJ, Stevens ME, Sudanagunta SP, Bronson RT, Makhinson M, Watabe AM, O'Dell TJ, Fung J, Weier HU, Cheng JF, Rubin EM: Functional screening of 2 Mb of human chromosome 21q22.2 in transgenic mice implicates minibrain in learning defects associated with Down syndrome. Nat Genet 1997; 16:28–36.
Smithies O, Kim H-S: Targeted gene duplication and disruption for analyzing quantitative genetics traits in mice. Proc Natl Acad Sci USA 1994; 91:3612–3615.
Smithies O, Maeda N: Gene targeting approaches to complex genetic diseases: atherosclerosis and essential hypertension. Proc Natl Acad Sci USA 1995; 92:5266–5272.
Su L-K, Kinzler KW, Vogelstein B, Preisinger AC, Moser AR, Luongo C, Gould KA, Dove WF: Multiple intestinal neoplasia caused by a mutation in the murine homolog of the APC gene. Science 1992; 269:13729–13732.
Suzuki H, Kurihara Y, Takeya M, Kamada N, Kataoka M, Jishage K, Ueda O, Sakaguchi H, Higashi T, Suzuki T, et al.: A role for macrophage scavenger receptors in atherosclerosis and susceptibility to infection. Nature 1997; 386:292–296.
Taketo M, Schroeder AC, Mobraaten LE, Gunning KB, Hanten G, Fox RR, Roderick TH, Stewart CL, Lilly F, Hansen CT: FVB/N: an inbred mouse strain preferable for transgenic analyses. Proc Natl Acad Sci USA 1991; 88:2065–2069.
Taylor BA, Phillips SJ: Detection of obesity QTLs on mouse chromosomes 1 and 7 by selective DNA pooling. Genomics 1996; 34:389–398.
Taylor BA, Phillips SJ: Obesity QTLs on mouse chromosomes 2 and 17. Genomics 1997; 43:249–257.
Thomas KR, Capecchi MR: Site-directed mutagenesis by gene targeting in mouse embryo–derived stem cells. Cell 1987; 51:503–512.
Thomas KR, Deng C, Capecchi MR: High-fidelity gene targeting in embryonic stem cells by using sequence replacement vectors. Mol Cell Biol 1992; 12:2919–2923.
Tsao BP, Cantor RM, Kalunian KC, Chen CJ, Badsha H, Singh R, Wallace DJ, Kitridou RC, Chen SL, Shen N, et al.: Evidence for linkage of a candidate chromosome 1 region to human systemic lupus erythematosus. J Clin Invest 1997; 99:725–731.
Valancius V, Smithies O: Testing an "in-out" targeting procedure for making subtle genomic modifications in mouse embryonic stem cells. Mol Cell Biol 1991; 11:1402–1408.
Verhoeven K, Van Laer L, Kirschhofer K, Legan PK, Hughes DC, Schatteman I, Verstreken M, Van Hauwe P, Coucke P, Chen A, et al.: Mutations in the human alpha-tectorin gene cause autosomal dominant non-syndromic hearing impairment. Nat Genet 1998; 19:60–62.
Wakeland E, Morel L, Achey K, Yui M, Longmate J: Speed congenics: a classic technique in the fast lane (relatively speaking). Immunol Today 1997; 18:472–477.
Wang Y, Nose M, Kamoto T, Nishimura M, Hiai H: Host modifier genes affect mouse autoimmunity induced by the lpr gene. Am J Pathol 1997; 151:1791–1798.
Warden CH, Fisler JS, Pace MJ, Svenson KL, Lusis AJ: Coincidence of genetic loci for plasma cholesterol levels and obesity in a multifactorial mouse model. J Clin Invest 1993; 92:773–779.
Warden CH, Fisler JS, Shoemaker SM, Wen P-Z, Svenson KL, Pace MJ, Lusis AJ: Identification of four chromosomal loci determining obesity in a multifactorial mouse model. J Clin Invest 1995; 95:1545–1552.
Warden CH, Hedrick CC, Qiao J-H, Castellani LW, Lusis AJ: Atherosclerosis in transgenic mice overexpressing apolipoprotein A-II. Science 1993; 261:469–472.
Welch CL, Xia Y-R, Schechter I, Farese R, Mehrabian M, Mehdizadeh S, Warden CH, Lusis AJ: Genetic regulation of cholesterol homeostasis: chromosomal organization of candidate genes. J Lipid Res 1996; 37:1406–1421.
West DB, Goudey-Lefevre J, York B, Truett GE: Dietary obesity linked to genetic loci on chromosomes 9 and 15 in a polygenic mouse model. J Clin Invest 1994; 94:1420–1416.
Wicker LS, Todd JA, Peterson LB: Genetic control of autoimmune diabetes in the NOD mouse. Annu Rev Cell Biol 1995; 6:679–714.
Wu H, Liu X, Jaenisch R: Double replacement: strategy for efficient introduction of subtle mutations into the murine *Col1a-1* gene by homologous recombination in embryonic stem cells. Proc Natl Acad Sci USA 1994; 91:2819–2823.
Wurst W, Joyner AL: Production of targeted embryonic stem cell clones. In: Joyner AL (ed). Gene Targeting: A Practical Approach. Oxford: Oxford University Press, 1993:33–61.
Young SG, Lusis AJ, Hammer RE: Genetically modified animals in cardiovascular research. In: Chein KR (ed). Molecular Basis of Cardiovascular Disease: A Companion to Brunwald's Heart Disease. Philadelphia: W.B. Saunders, 1999.
Zhang L, Xu D, West MJ, Summers KM: Association of the brain natriuretic peptide gene with blood pressure and heart weight in the rat. Clin Exp Pharmacol Physiol 1997; 24:442–444.

6 Genetic Counseling: History, Risk Assessment, Strategies, and Ethical Considerations

BONNIE S. LEROY AND ANN P. WALKER

In 1947, Sheldon Reed first used the term *genetic counseling* to describe the activities of geneticists at a handful of "heredity clinics" that had recently sprung up at a few universities and hospitals (Reed, 1955). Among the first of these were the Heredity Clinic at the University of Michigan, the Dight Institute at the University of Minnesota, and the Genetic Advisory Clinic at the Hospital for Sick Children in Great Ormond Street, London (Neel, 1994; Kevles, 1995). Then, as now, such clinics provided consultation for families with a history of genetic disease or for couples whose child had a birth defect or mental retardation. When possible, their geneticists established a diagnosis and pattern of inheritance, gave information about recurrence risk, and helped with reproductive decision making. It was this last exercise that was particularly sensitive since both the medical/scientific community and the public were still smarting from zealous mandatory eugenics programs that grew out of the early twentieth century's misguided attempts to apply Mendelian principles to complex traits and societal ills (Lubinsky, 1993). Reed (1974) hoped that introducing the idea of genetic counseling (which he viewed as "a kind of genetic social work without eugenic connotations") would divorce the emerging discipline of medical genetics from the eugenics movement.

In this chapter, we discuss the history of genetic counseling, its application to complex common diseases, factors that affect counseling strategies, and some of the ethical concerns inherent in providing this service. Examples of conditions for which genetic testing is presently available are used to demonstrate some points. We draw on our own experience, as well as the collective experience of others who provide care to families with these conditions and must make the difficult decisions concerning genetic testing and the test results. These examples provide some guidance about the possible approaches to genetic counseling and the difficulties expected when caring for families with complex diseases for which genetic testing is not yet available.

HISTORY, ORIGINS, AND PHILOSOPHY OF GENETIC COUNSELING

These early medical geneticists recognized that decisions about reproduction were complex and personal. Moreover, many were trained as research scientists rather than physicians and thus were unaccustomed to advising patients about health matters. Although many of them still held eugenic views (Resta, 1997), most were concerned that genetic counseling not be seen as coercive or eugenically motivated. In an article describing heredity clinics, Dice (1952) strongly made this point: "In no case, however, should the geneticist presume to tell a couple whether or not they should have a child." This reticence to give advice about reproductive decisions has since been central to the ethos of genetic counseling.

In the context of genetic counseling, the term *nondirective* has come to mean a particular approach in which the counselor does not render advice or encourage a particular course of action. He or she aims instead to promote autonomous decision making through genetic education and exploration of the client's values and beliefs. Development of this counseling approach was probably encouraged by the early involvement in human genetics of social workers and psychologists trained in Rogerian humanistic psychology (Wolff and Jung, 1995). While nondirectiveness, as used in genetic counseling, is distinct from the psychotherapeutic technique of the same name, both approaches have in common the goal of respecting and fostering the clients' capacity and ability to make and act on decisions, choices that often will have enormous impact on their lives.

Much has been said about the impossibility of achieving truly nondirective counseling and "value neutrality." Even when counselors avoid giving advice or making recommendations, they may convey covert messages by selecting or coloring the information that is discussed. Kessler (1992) makes the point that both directiveness and non-directiveness are both forms of persuasion, with the directive counselor trying to influence the client's behavior and the nondirective one, the client's way of thinking about the problem.

HOW GENETIC COUNSELING FOR COMMON DISEASES AND ADULT-ONSET CONDITIONS IS DIFFERENT: NEW CONTEXTS FOR GENETIC COUNSELING

While questions about reproductive risk will always comprise a major part of genetic counseling, new knowledge about the genes involved in adult-onset disorders and the genetic contributions to common diseases has meant that an increasing number of people are seeking genetic evaluations to answer questions about their *own* health. Genetic counseling now occurs in such diverse settings as infertility clinics, oncology units, and neurology services. In these sites, it may involve only a single geneticist rather than the more traditional team. In such situations, genetic testing might be done to see if an existing condition, such as congenital absence of the vas deferens, thyroid cancer, or early-onset Alzheimer's disease, has a genetic basis. In other cases, genetic counseling might be sought by a patient considering presymptomatic diagnosis for a later-onset condition, such as Huntington's disease (HD) or testing for predisposition to a familial disease, such as hereditary nonpolyposis colon cancer. Genetic counseling for common diseases in specialty clinics addressing disorders such as hypercholesterolemia and Alzheimer's disease has been reported (Bhatnagar et al., 2000; Liddell et al., 2001). In the near future, geneticists are likely to counsel people identified through population screening for relatively common genetic conditions in which morbidity may be reduced or prevented by simple medical interventions or lifestyle changes, as with hemochromatosis or alpha$_1$-antitrypsin deficiency. It is probable that pharmacogenetics will play an increasing role in identifying genetic factors that affect the response to drugs used for common ailments such as asthma or depression [e.g., albuterol, fluoxetine (Prozac)] (Begley, 1999). Those identified as being prone to react adversely may seek genetic counseling about the implications of these traits for themselves and other family members.

Differences in the Eugenic Implications of Testing for Common Diseases

When genetic evaluation is relevant to the patient's *own* health, rather than centered primarily on reproductive risk, concerns about eugenic motivations for testing become less important. One might argue, therefore, that a nondirective counseling stance is less necessary in the context of genetic evaluation for these disorders. In fact, as genetic tests move from academic centers to commercial laboratories and are ordered more frequently by nongeneticists who are used to a more prescriptive approach, they may occur with less deliberation and consideration than couples traditionally have given to prenatal diagnosis. However, the issues raised by genetic diagnosis in an adult, while different, are no less complex than those inherent in reproductive decision making. Furthermore, the far-reaching implications of diagnosing a genetic disorder in an adult or of predicting his or her risk for future disease make it especially important to promote patient autonomy with thorough education concerning the limitations of the test's utility and exploration of the impact that various test results would have.

Familial and Personal Implications of Genetic Diagnosis in Adulthood

At present, the very nature of presymptomatic or predisposition genetic testing usually implies that a disorder is present in the family. This means that the person considering testing is likely to have had direct experience with the condition, often in a parent. If a number of family members have been affected, the disease may comprise a significant aspect of the family's culture. Many at-risk individuals assume that they will ultimately develop the disease themselves and may even have made important life decisions based on this assumption. Thus, unlike the situation with prenatal diagnosis where a normal result usually represents unequivocal "good news," learning that one does *not* carry a familial mutation can require significant adjustments in beliefs, goals, and family dynamics (Sobel and Cowan, 2000). In contrast, a result predicting high risk of developing the disease may lead to feelings of despair, hopelessness, diminished self-worth, and, if the person has had children, guilt at having possibly transmitted the disorder to yet another generation. Looking into the near future, it is important to consider that presymptomatic or susceptibility genetic testing will be greatly expanded to include testing for diseases common in the population, including many of the disorders discussed in this book. This type of testing will provide a vast number of individuals more information about their risk for developing common diseases, but along with this knowledge will come information about other family members. The potential impact on other family members is one aspect of genetic testing that makes it so very complex.

The diagnosis of a genetic condition in adulthood, particularly in an asymptomatic individual, has numerous ramifications beyond the person's own health. Among these are the genetic implications for other family members, some of whom may not even have realized that they were at risk and may not have wanted this information. In unusual cases, an individual's test results may actually elucidate the mutation status of another family member, e.g., in a parent or identical twin. Testing sometimes stresses family relationships. This can happen when participation by key affected family members is needed to identify the causative mutation or for linkage studies or if at-risk individuals who are reluctant to be tested feel coerced. It can also occur when several family members learn their mutation status since those receiving normal results may no longer share the sibling bond of being at risk or may experience "survivor guilt" if they have been spared when a brother, sister, or parent has not.

Genetic evaluation for future disease risk can also have significant economic impact. Not the least of this is the expense of molecular diagnosis, which may be considered "experimental" by health maintenance organizations or third-party payors. Many people contemplating testing actually prefer not to involve their insurance carrier (assuming they *are* insured), fearing that billing for the evaluation or having test results in their medical record will call attention to the familial condition and potentially jeopardize future insurability or even employability. This limits access to many new diagnostic technologies to those who are well off or securely insured. Moreover, even when insurance will pay for testing, there is usually no mechanism to pay for studies on an affected family member whose mutation must be identified before testing the at-risk person can be fully informative.

Limitations and Ambiguities in Diagnosis

In most prenatal situations, a diagnosis can be fairly securely established on the basis of chromosome studies, DNA testing for a known mutation, biochemical analysis of amniotic fluid, or ultrasound findings. Genetic evaluation for common diseases and adult-onset disorders may be much less straightforward. Many common diseases are multifactorial, so even when major predisposing mutations or polymorphisms are known (e.g., with some diseases that have an autoimmune basis), the environmental or stochastic factors that trigger onset may be unclear. Certain other conditions, e.g., amyotrophic lateral sclerosis, are familial in only a small subset of cases. Even when a clearly dominant disease segregates in the family, it may be impossible to confirm the diagnosis if affected members in prior generations have died, records are unavailable, or diagnostic evaluations on these individuals were inadequate. Moreover, phenotypically similar diseases are often genetically heterogeneous. For instance, at least nine forms of dominant spinocerebellar ataxia are now known (Online Mendelian Inheritance in Man numbers 183090, 164400, 109150, 600223, 164500, 183086, 600224, 603516, and 603680; *www.ncbi.nlm.nih.gov*), and eight different genes contributing to hypertrophic cardiomyopathy have been identified (Yu et al., 1998; Bonne et al., 1998).

Absent proof of a causative mutation in a given family, genetic testing of an at-risk individual can raise more questions than it resolves. A negative test is completely reassuring only if it is clear that the disease in affected family members was related to a mutation in the gene studied. For example, failure to find a *BRCA1* or *BRCA2* mutation in an unaffected young woman is falsely reassuring if the patient's relatives who died with breast cancer actually had Cowden disease associated with a *PTEN* mutation. Furthermore, screening an entire gene often turns up mutations whose significance is unknown, either because they would have no obvious impact on protein function or because they have been seen in both affected individuals and controls.

Even when susceptibility or presymptomatic testing leads to identification of a mutation that clearly contributes to the familial disease, there may be limited information about penetrance and variability of the phenotype or about optimal preventive or surveillance strategies. This can present the client with a new set of uncertainties and dilemmas.

Thus, the issues raised by genetic evaluation for adult-onset and common diseases can be markedly more complex than the already difficult ones traditionally encountered in genetic counseling. Fortunately, this type of evaluation usually does not have the urgency of prenatal or pediatric diagnosis. Whenever possible, therefore, genetic counseling should strive to give patients ample opportunity to assimilate the complicated genetic information; to consider how making a diagnosis may affect them medically, psychologically, and economically; and to reflect on how this evaluation could affect family dynamics. This is best accomplished over a series of interactions, sometimes with input from other disciplines, e.g., psychology and social work.

For the purposes of this chapter, the term *genetic counselor* will be used to refer to the professional who performs genetic risk assessment, provides supportive counseling and help with decision making, and sometimes coordinates and interprets genetic testing. Usually, this will be a clinical or laboratory geneticist or a genetic counselor certified (at least in North America) by the American Board of Medical Genetics, the Canadian College of Medical Genetics, or the American Board of Genetic Counseling (Schneider and Kalkbrenner, 1998). However, other specialists who deal with common and adult-onset disorders with a genetic basis may also provide some elements of genetic counseling. Increasingly, primary care providers will need either to assume parts of the genetic counseling role themselves or to understand the complexities so that they can identify and refer patients appropriately and help their patients adjust to or act on the information they gain from a genetic evaluation. What follows then provides an overview of aspects of risk assessment, genetic testing, and psychosocial and ethical issues that are especially relevant to adult-onset common diseases.

RISK ASSESSMENT AND MODIFICATION: FAMILY HISTORY AND PEDIGREE

Pedigree Conventions

The earliest recorded use of a diagram with lines connecting individuals to their offspring to illustrate ancestry was in the fifteenth century. In the mid- to late 1800s, Pliny Earle and Francis Galton began to use pedigrees with symbols or names of family members to show inheritance of traits such as color blindness and "artistic ability" (Resta, 1993). Over the ensuing century and a quarter, numerous different conventions have been used for pedigree notation, sometimes leading to inconsistency and confusion. Moreover, the recent development and widespread utilization of assisted reproductive techniques has led to novel sorts of parent–child relationship that have often been creatively, but inconsistently, represented in pedigrees. To remedy these problems, the National Society of Genetic Counselors and the Pacific Northwest Regional Genetics Group constituted a committee to standardize pedigree nomenclature. This group did an extensive review of the genetics literature and surveyed geneticists about practices and preferences, to arrive at suggestions for standard ways of representing family relationships, reproductive histories, phenotypic features, genotypic information, results of medical evaluations, and current health status. These recommendations have been published with commentary (Bennett et al., 1995a–c; Marizita, 1995). Although seasoned geneticists may need to relearn some elements of pedigree notation, the new nomenclature, which actually makes it more straightforward to represent complex relationships and genetic information, is now widely accepted as the international standard for publication. The new conventions make it possible to denote, e.g., an asymptomatic individual who carries an HD mutation or a reproductive arrangement in which a pregnancy being carried by an infertile woman is the result of ovum donation by her sister followed by in vitro fertilization with her husband's sperm.

Targeting the Family History

Focusing questions about family members on history and symptoms potentially related to the disorder under consideration is an integral part of most genetic evaluations. Often, however, diseases with Mendelian inheritance are rare and their associated symptoms are distinctive. With common diseases, their very prevalence in the population makes the situation more complex since most cases do *not* result from the action of a single major gene but have a multifactorial or even entirely environmental basis. To differentiate the subset of disorders that have a primarily genetic etiology from those that occur in the general population, a number of additional pieces of evidence may be helpful.

With adult-onset diseases, the numbers and ages of not only affected but also unaffected family members become important. Often, individuals who are worried about their own risk will focus only on people in the family who have had the disease, ignoring those who never developed it. A history of a paternal grandmother and aunt with breast cancer would be of less concern, e.g., if both developed cancer in their seventies and each had five sisters who were cancer-free at the time of death in their eighties. Since the lifetime risk for breast cancer for any woman in the U.S. population is estimated to be about 1 in 9, this family does not really depart from what would be expected in the general population. With any late-onset disorder it is critical to record *all* family members' ages and causes of death because potential mutation carriers in the family may have died from other causes before developing the disease, making it difficult to determine if their offspring are at risk.

Sometimes information about the probable severity or natural history of a disease may need to be inferred from the family's own pedigree. This is particularly true if genotype-phenotype correlation is poorly understood, as is the case when many mutations have been described in the causative gene or when a family carries a "private" mutation that has not been seen before. In such cases, there will be no appropriate population-based data to give to asymptomatic individuals who are considering testing or who have received positive results. Since the most relevant information about penetrance, age at onset, disease course, etc. may come from the family's own pedigree, it is particularly important to document how the disease has behaved in other identified or obligate mutation carriers in the family. The sex of the parent who transmits the mutation may also be important, particularly in diseases that arise from unstable triplet repeats. In many neurogenetic disorders, e.g., HD, myotonic dystrophy, and certain of the spinocerebellar ataxias, greater expansion of the mutation (often roughly correlated with earlier onset or greater severity) occurs in either male or female meiosis. The sex of the affected parent may thus influence when symptoms begin to appear in the offspring.

With common later-onset diseases, nongenetic risk factors should also be taken into account. In assessing whether there is a significant genetic component to a familial disease, the potential effects of diet, exercise, and other aspects of lifestyle; gender; occupational exposures; and relevant medical history must be considered. Certain environmental factors can also affect the appearance of symptoms when a genetic disorder *is* present. For example, in evaluating a history for evidence of hemochromatosis, the fact that an at-risk woman is premenopausal or a frequent blood donor would make her less likely to be symptomatic (Burke et al., 2000). Similarly, personal and family history regarding obesity, diet, exercise, gestational diabetes, etc. can be helpful in estimating a particular individual's risk of developing Type 2 diabetes.

Attention to such details may be especially important in assessing cancer histories. For example, a melanoma might not be unusual if it occurred in a light-skinned person who worked outside all of his life. If, however, the melanoma arose in a part of the body *not* exposed to sun, at an unusually early age, or in an individual with numerous dysplastic nevi, it would be more significant. In Table 6–1, the case of hereditary cancer is used to illustrate the utility of directed questions to better target a family history for risk assessment.

Confirming Diagnoses and Medical History

With late-onset and common disorders, confirming diagnoses in multiple family members can be time-consuming and unsatisfying. However, it is also extremely important, given that affected individuals have often died and cannot be examined or tested. In some cases, disorders with similar symptoms may have been misdiagnosed (e.g., Friedreich's ataxia vs. a dominant spinocerebellar ataxia) or at least diagnosed before the heterogeneity of the disease was fully appreciated. It is also possible that people in the next generation may simply have confused conditions that sound similar (e.g., muscular dystrophy and multiple sclerosis, cystic fibrosis and fibrocystic disease). When such potential confusion exists, it can be helpful to elicit (using open-ended questions) particular things they and other family members remember about the affected relative(s). These would include where and by whom the person was diagnosed or treated, specific physical features, symptoms, and degree of disability including particular tasks that were difficult, onset and progression of the disease, changes in behavior or cognition, and medications or other treatments. While responses may be completely consistent with the disorder in question, they sometimes raise real doubts about the diagnosis. It is critical to impress upon concerned family members the importance of this information since negative results from presymptomatic or susceptibility testing for the wrong disease would not only be falsely reassuring to the person being tested but also have potentially disastrous implications for other at-risk individuals in the family.

Evaluating histories for the possibility of hereditary cancer predisposition presents a number of special challenges. Foremost among these is the accuracy of the available data. Because of the stigma attached to cancer, even in the recent past, younger members of a family may have only vague information about their relatives' cancers. They may not be clear on the specifics of tumor sites, ages at diagnosis, associated features, and relevant medical history (e.g., types of treatment, risk factors, and surgeries such as oopherectomy that might have precluded subsequent cancer occurrence). Young relatives may be uneasy about asking for records on affected individuals, particularly if cancer is a taboo subject in the family. In many cases, records no longer exist on deceased family members, and even when available, they may not be helpful; death certificates often list only the immediate cause of death, not alluding to the underlying disease process; primary cancers may not be differentiated from metastases or recurrences; pathology reports are of varying quality and specificity, etc. When the difference between uterine and ovarian cancer or between papillary and medullary thyroid carcinoma can be critical in differentiating between cancer syndromes, lack of accurate information can cloud the diagnosis. Practical experiences with genetic counseling for hereditary cancer clearly demonstrate the importance of confirming the diagnosis.

Table 6–1. Questions That Can Be Asked to Better Target a Family History for Risk Assessment: The Cancer Example

1. Are there multiple cases of the same or related cancers in the family (e.g., several individuals with medullary thyroid carcinoma or colon, endometrial, and ovarian cancers in different members of a hereditary nonpolyposis colon cancer family)?
2. Are there primary cancers arising in paired organs (e.g., bilateral breast cancer in a woman with a *BRCA1* mutation or bilateral renal cell carcinomas in Von Hippel-Lindau disease)?
3. Are there multifocal cancers or precursor lesions in the same organ or tissue (e.g., numerous adenomatous colon polyps in Gardner's syndrome; multiple dysplastic nevi in familial atypical moles and malignant melanoma syndrome; thyroid C-cell hyperplasia in a family with multiple endocrine neoplasia type IIA)?
4. Does this patient have a rare cancer (e.g., sarcomas and adrenocortical carcinomas in Li-Fraumeni syndrome, retinoblastomas, paragangliomas)?
5. Are there relatively common cancers occurring without the usual associated risk factors in the family (e.g., laryngeal cancer in individuals who have never smoked or pancreatic cancer in several family members with no history of alcohol abuse)?
6. Does this patient have an earlier age at onset than usually seen for the particular tumor (e.g., ovarian cancer in a 30-year-old)?

Assessing Risk: Using Pedigree Analysis to Establish A Priori Risks

When the diagnosis and mode of inheritance are clearly known, one can determine an at-risk individual's chance of carrying a disease-causing or predisposing mutation by applying familiar Mendelian principles. For dominant conditions, a priori risk is determined by the degree of relationship to the affected individual, i.e., 1/2 when a parent, sibling or child is affected, $(1/2)^2$ if the affected is a second-degree relative (e.g., aunt, nephew, or grandfather), or $(1/2)^3$ if the affected is a third-degree relative (e.g., first cousin, great uncle, or great grandparent). Unfortunately, however, in many adult-onset disorders, mutation carriers in the pedigree do not always make themselves known. Expression of the trait may be age-dependent, as is the case for many neurogenetic diseases; limited to one sex or the other (e.g., ovarian or prostate cancer); or influenced by environmental factors (diet and lifestyle, occupational exposures, etc.). This means that some mutation carriers in the family will have died before showing symptoms, and others will not be old enough for the trait to have appeared or will be of the "wrong" gender to have developed the disease. Furthermore, with common diseases such as breast cancer, even in a clearly dominant pedigree, an affected individual may not actually carry the familial predisposing mutation but instead represent a phenocopy who developed cancer for some unrelated and unknown reason. In such situations, risk assessment must often take additional empiric data into account, frequently using Bayesian calculations to modify a priori risks.

Evaluating, Synthesizing, and Incorporating Empiric Data about Risk and Penetrance

For many late-onset disorders, literature now exists on what proportion of mutation carriers will have developed a disease or manifested some specific symptoms by certain ages. The best example of such data is HD and *BRCA1*- and *BRCA2*-linked families (Brinkman et al., 1997; Offit, 1998). When such data exist, incorporating unaffected key family members' ages in the calculations can substantially alter the chance that an at-risk person carries the mutation. Although intuitively one would surmise that an asymptomatic 70-year-old individual whose parent was diagnosed at 37 years of age is less likely to develop the same condition, using empiric data may make it possible to generate a more specific modified risk figure. Caution must be exercised in using some of this information, however. In many cases, empiric data on age-dependent penetrance were gathered before the genetic basis of the condition was completely understood. Subsequent knowledge about disease-causing mutations may make the data less relevant.

For example, in the case of HD, the usual age at onset in people who carry the gene mutation is around 40 years. Therefore, if an at-risk individual lives to be 60 years old without symptoms, he or she has a statistical risk of less than 50% for having inherited the gene because some of the risk has been outlived. However, using age-dependent penetrance figures that were developed from a large study of HD patients prior to the knowledge of the mutation mechanism for this disease would not be appropriate in the case of an at-risk individual whose father developed symptoms in his late twenties. A child who inherited this father's mutation would probably have earlier onset of HD than empiric data would predict. This is due to a mechanism now known to be associated with the HD mutation, which is an expansion of a trinucleotide repeat region within the gene. In the above example, the father who developed symptoms in his twenties presumably had a large expansion mutation that was responsible for his early onset of symptoms; furthermore, we know that in HD the unstable repeat is likely to expand even further during male meiosis. This would place such a patient's children at risk for an earlier age at onset of symptoms than empiric data on age-dependent penetrance would predict.

Information on penetrance may have been developed from unrepresentative families. For example, initial data reflecting very high lifetime risks for cancer were generated from the breast–ovarian cancer families used for linkage studies that ultimately led to the mapping of *BRCA1* and *BRCA2*. These families were chosen precisely because the high penetrance of cancer made it easier to infer which members probably carried a predisposing mutation. A subsequent study showed that, at least among Jewish volunteers unselected for cancer history who were tested for three common Ashkenazi mutations, there was a much lower lifetime risk for breast or ovarian cancer in carriers (Struewing et al., 1997). Differences in penetrance estimates are presumably due not only to ascertainment but also to other modifying genes segregating in the families or to the fact that mutations in different parts of *BRCA1* and *BRCA2* may be associated with higher or lower cancer risks. Since it appears that most disorders are more likely to be characterized by such allelic heterogeneity than a single mutation, probable genotype–phenotype differences should be kept in mind when using penetrance data derived from affected families, who usually represent many different mutations. Whenever possible, mutation-specific figures should be used, although these are likely to be available only for very common mutations.

Disease Prevalence and Likelihood of Identifying a Predisposing Mutation

In some cases, the main question is not "What is the chance I have inherited the disease in my family?" but rather "What is the chance that the disease in my family is genetic?" For diseases that are common in the population, the answer may not be knowable. The vast majority of cancers are not clearly hereditary, and only subsets of conditions like Alzheimer's disease or amyotrophic lateral sclerosis are caused by a single major dominant gene. When only one or two members of a family are affected, differentiating between familial recurrences of a "sporadic" condition and a dominant disease with reduced penetrance is difficult. Moreover, for some conditions, there is a high rate of new mutations, so there may be no family history. This is true, e.g., in the instance of familial adenomatous polyposis, in which up to one-third of cases represent new mutations (Offit, 1998). Clues that increase the likelihood that a disease is due to a single dominant gene include earlier onset, more rapid progression, and sometimes greater severity. In the case of cancers, multifocal or bilateral malignancies or metachronous tumors affecting tissues or organs involved in a hereditary cancer syndrome are also likely to be hallmarks of a predisposing dominant gene.

As disease genes are cloned, it becomes possible to determine which affecteds carry a germline mutation, thereby giving an estimate of the proportion of cases in the population that are genetic and sometimes revealing phenotypic features that distinguish this group. There are limits to this strategy, however, since the testing method(s) may not detect all mutations in the known gene and additional causative genes may not have been found. For some diseases, estimates of the proportion of affected individuals whose disease is hereditary were made prior to the complete understanding of the condition's genetics. We now know, e.g., that many cases of neurogenetic disorders that apparently arose as "new mutations" were in fact due to a trinucleotide repeat expansion inherited from an asymptomatic parent with a premutation. Other nontraditional patterns of inheritance can also obscure the hereditary nature of some disorders. For instance, recognition that many paragangliomas are due to a dominant mutation in a maternally imprinted gene has increased the estimate of the proportion of cases that are inherited from about 10% to perhaps as high as 90% (W. S. Rubinstein, personal communication, 1999).

Many patients who come for genetic counseling about an adult-onset disease are considering genetic testing, often at considerable expense. When testing is available for a particular condition, another important question concerns the likelihood that such testing will reveal a causative mutation. Again, data are emerging using various parameters to estimate the chance that a mutation will be identified in the family. These are most widely available for breast cancer. There are now a number of published tables, graphs, and calculations to estimate the likelihood of finding a *BRCA1* and, in some cases, a *BRCA2* mutation (Shattuck-Eidens et al., 1995, 1997; Couch et al., 1997; Berry et al., 1997; Ford et al., 1998; Frank, et al., 1998). These take into account, variously, the age at breast cancer diagnosis in the proband, the average age at diagnosis in all affected family members, the presence or absence of ovarian cancer, the number of cases in the family, laterality, and ethnicity (Ashkenazi vs. non-Ashkenazi). No one method incorporates all of these parameters, however, and some use such strict criteria (e.g., requiring more than four affecteds) as to be useful in only a small proportion of cases. Additionally, these different techniques can produce widely differing estimates.

For example, in Fig. 6–1, five women in an Ashkenazi Jewish family have had breast cancer with or without ovarian cancer. If one takes Ruth to be the proband, estimates of identifying a *BRCA1* mutation in the family range from 86.7% (Frank et al., 1998) to 91% (Shattuck-Eidens et al., 1995) to 96.8% (Couch et al., 1997). A computer program, BRCAPRO, incorporates these models alone into those developed by Berry et al. (1997) and Parmagiani et al. (1998), making it possible to include unaffected individuals and their ages, using Bayesian analysis to further refine the risk. BRCAPRO gives a 99.6% chance that a *BRCA1* mutation is present in this family. In fact, Adele was found to carry the 185delAG *BRCA1*.

These models are actually more useful in intermediate-risk families, in which the likelihood of identifying a *BRCA1* or *BRCA2* mutation is much lower. Estimating the chance that a mutation will be identified given the family history can serve as a point of departure for discussion of the potential utility of testing, provided that the patient is aware of the limitations of the estimates.

The concerns discussed here will likely be similar in other common genetic diseases as mutations are identified and genetic testing becomes available.

Bayesian Modification of Risks

It is often helpful to use Bayesian analysis to modify an *a priori* risk based on pedigree analysis by incorporating additional information about penetrance, mutation likelihood, test sensitivity, etc. The following example demonstrates both the utility and the limitations of using such information. A much more extensive discussion of this topic was provided by Hodge (1998), who described a simple and straightforward technique for using Bayesian calculations in even more complex situations.

In the Figure 6–1 family, one could use published data on the age-dependent penetrance of breast and ovarian cancer in *BRCA1* carriers to modify the 25% a priori chance that Natalie, who has not had cancer at age 60, carries the mutation that was found in her cousin Adele. According to the data of Struewing and co-workers (1997), 50% of 185delAG carriers will have developed breast cancer by 60 and about 12% will have developed ovarian cancer. These authors found the penetrance rates of breast and ovarian cancer in noncarriers by age 60 to be about 8% and 1%, respectively. Using these figures, a Bayesian calculation lowers Natalie's chance of carrying 185delAG to about 13.9%. (The conditional probability that Natalie would be a carrier and not have breast cancer at 60 is 50%, while she would have a 92% chance of being unaffected if she were a noncarrier. The second conditional probability is the 88% chance that she would not have ovarian cancer at 60 if she were a carrier vs. a 99% chance of being unaffected if she were a noncarrier.) These

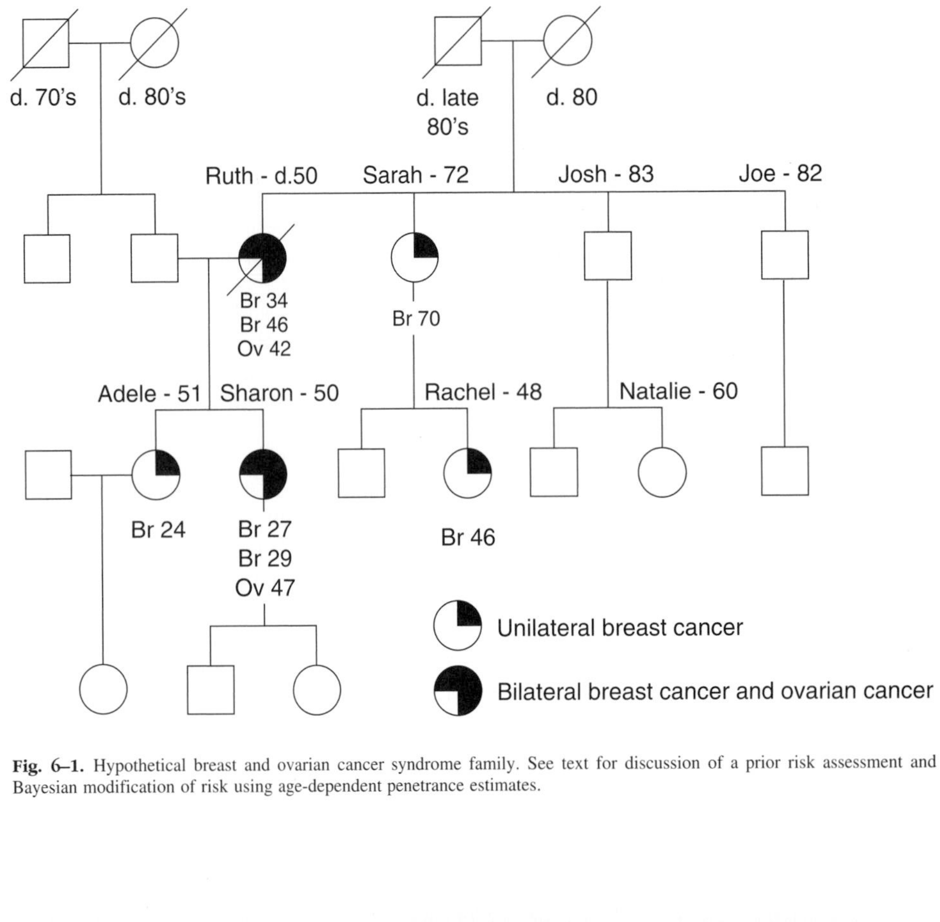

Fig. 6–1. Hypothetical breast and ovarian cancer syndrome family. See text for discussion of a prior risk assessment and Bayesian modification of risk using age-dependent penetrance estimates.

may not be the most appropriate figures to use, however. The data in this study were generated from 5318 Jewish volunteers who had been motivated to participate because they had more cancer in their families. Also, the family histories were not confirmed. Overreporting or ascertainment bias would have raised risk estimates for both carriers and noncarriers.

In Natalie's situation with a high-risk family, it might be better to use the data summarized by Offit (1998), which indicate that 77% of *BRCA1* heterozygotes from high-risk families will have developed breast cancer by 60 as opposed to 4% in the general population. Using these figures, Natalie's chance of being a carrier drops to about 7.4%. This demonstrates that caution should be exercised in using these types of estimate.

CONSIDERATIONS IN GENETIC TESTING FOR LATE-ONSET DISEASES: IDENTIFYING LABORATORY RESOURCES AND ASSESSING LABORATORY CAPABILITIES

Genetic testing is obviously only one component of a genetic evaluation. However, in many situations, it does provide the best means of clarifying genetic risk for a person who is concerned because of a family history of a common or late-onset disease that may or may not be hereditary. Identifying a mutation can differentiate a genetic disease from a nongenetic phenocopy or determine which of several genes that cause very similar conditions is responsible for the disease in that family. Molecular diagnosis will usually elucidate the pattern of inheritance, thus determining the a priori risk faced by various family members. It will also make it possible to describe the condition's natural history, variability, and penetrance more accurately and to identify mutation carriers long before they express symptoms or biomarkers of the disease. However, the success of using molecular diagnosis to inform genetic counseling is dependent not only on suspecting the correct disease or diseases to test for but also on the availability, sensitivity, and specificity of the test(s) and the quality of the laboratory analysis. For this reason, being able to identify and evaluate laboratory resources and tests is an important part of genetic counseling.

Research vs. Clinical Tests

Before molecular testing can be done, a disease gene must be at least closely mapped, so that the diagnosis can be inferred by linkage analysis, or cloned, so that causative mutations can be identified. Gene mapping usually takes place in a research setting, utilizing families in which the disease has been well characterized and confirmed by physical examination and/or other diagnostic procedures. In most cases such studies are done under protocols approved by the institutional review board, especially if samples or results can be linked to individuals. At this stage of research, it is rare for genotypes or other information to be reported back to patients or family members. Prior to sample collection, participants should sign an informed consent describing what, if anything, they will learn from their participation and how their samples may or may not be used in the future. In some cases, their disease gene may be found and characterized in a matter of weeks. In others, the gene may elude identification and complete characterization for years. Families should thus agree to participate in such research with the understanding that they themselves may never directly benefit from it.

The report of a gene's identification in the scientific and lay media often precedes by months or even years the availability of a diagnostic molecular test that is appropriate for clinical use. This is because the testing methodology must go through a process of internal and external validation wherein additional affecteds and normal controls are studied to determine the sensitivity, specificity, and replicability of the test. There is thus an investigational phase of test development, again conducted under institutional review board protocols, during which patients may or may not be able to get their test results. It has been suggested that a test not be used clinically until linkage studies are informative in 70% of matings and accurate within a 95% confidence interval (Lebo et al., 1990).

Any clinical testing in which results are reported to the referring provider or patient must be done in laboratories that meet federal standards for quality and proficiency established by the Clinical Laboratory Improvement Act/Amendment (CLIA 88, 1992). Laboratories providing research testing do not need to be CLIA-approved since they do not release results.

Even after a disease gene has been sequenced and causative mutations have been identified in research families, there may be very incomplete information about the frequency of polymorphisms in normal individuals or the clinical significance of different mutations. The availability of a clinical test does not, therefore, mean that the test will provide complete information. Furthermore, if a disease is rare, there may be limited commercial interest in developing a test even for clinical use.

Genetic Testing Directories

Since most genetic conditions are rare, finding a laboratory to do diagnostic or presymptomatic testing can be a daunting exercise. This task is now greatly simplified by an on-line database, GeneTests, funded by the National Library of Medicine and the Maternal and Child Health Bureau and maintained by geneticists at the University of Washington. This resource has up-to-date information on over 300 laboratories that collectively provide tests for over 550 disorders. Access for health-care professionals via the Internet (*http://www.genetests.org/about.html*) requires a one-time registration but is free. GeneTests lists both clinical and research tests but provides information on methodology only for clinical tests.

Evaluating Testing Methodology and Quality of Interpretation

In choosing a laboratory to do testing, it is important to consider both the quality of the laboratory and the methods of analysis that will be used. Indicators of laboratory quality include state licensure, CLIA approval, and the involvement of appropriately trained and experienced personnel who will be involved in interpreting results, including one or more who are certified in molecular genetics by the American Board of Medical Genetics.

The methodology that will be used for testing is also important as each method has its utilities and limitations. If a disease gene has been mapped, linkage analysis may identify mutation carriers within a family even before the gene has been cloned or completely characterized. Linkage studies are most useful for conditions in which only one causative gene has been identified, in families with several affected and unaffected individuals from which the mutation-bearing chromosome can be inferred, and when markers are either closely linked or actually located within the disease gene.

After a disease-causing gene has been cloned, there are several techniques that may make it possible to determine if a person has or will develop the condition. For some conditions, such as HD, there is a unique causative mutation. This means that an individual can have diagnostic or presymptomatic testing even if no one in the family has been conclusively diagnosed or is available to provide DNA. For other conditions, there are numerous mutations within a gene. Cystic fibrosis (CF) is a good example. In CF, over 800 mutations in *CFTR* have been described. Laboratories differ in how many of these are tested, thereby affecting the sensitivity of the test. The sensitivity of some tests may also differ according to the ethnic background of the person being tested since carrier frequencies and particular mutations are population-specific. For instance, testing for the most common CF mutations will detect 97% of Ashkenazi Jewish carriers but only 30% of those with Asian ancestry (National Institutes of Health Consensus, 1997). To provide the most appropriate testing and interpretation, the laboratory needs to know why the test is being ordered. CF testing in the context of male infertility, e.g., may appropriately include analysis of the 5T polymorphism found in intron 8 of *CFTR* (Chillon et al., 1995), which frequently is associated with congenital bilateral absence of the vas deferens.

Still, for some conditions, a high proportion of disease-causing mutations is rare or even unique to a particular family. For example, sequencing of the entire *BRCA1* and *BRCA2* genes is frequently done (ideally on DNA from an affected individual) when the pedigree suggests a dominant predisposition to breast or ovarian cancer. It is worth exploring if the laboratory will retest a sample as methodology improves or if issue amended reports when additional information becomes available about the significance of an identified mutation.

Diagnostic vs. Presymptomatic or Susceptibility Testing: Counseling Issues

Traditionally, genetic testing has been done to establish or confirm the diagnosis in a symptomatic individual in whom a specific disorder is suspected. In the context of genetic counseling for common or late-onset diseases, genetic testing can be done for some disorders in asymptomatic individuals who have a multitude of other reasons for wanting the information. Motivations may include any of the following: relief from uncertainty about the likelihood of developing a disease in the future; a need to inform important life decisions, such as education, career choice, marriage, reproduction, or medical interventions; a desire to know if one's children are at risk; or in some cases, coercion by a family member or health-care professional (Clark et al., 2000). The patient's motives should be extensively explored before a decision about this type of testing is made. In the course of this exploration, it may become evident that the test results will not provide the answers he or she is seeking.

Often, patients asking about presymptomatic testing are not fully aware of its complexity and potential impact on family dynamics. They may not know, e.g., that it may be necessary to test an affected family member who is not seeking genetic evaluation, to determine if presymptomatic or susceptibility testing will actually be informative. This can raise a number of problematic issues. It may be awkward or even impossible for them to ask a relative to be tested, especially if doing so would reveal that there might be a genetic basis to a health problem not thought (or at least acknowledged) to be familial. They will need to consider who should pay for a test that may not actually benefit the affected individual. They may not have thought about the fact that testing of one family member could reveal the genotype of another (e.g., a parent or identical twin) who does not want the information. They may not have considered the potential for test results to lead to insurance or employment discrimination. In some cases, patients are really asking the question "Do I have symptoms right now?" rather than "Do I have the gene?" A physical examination is more appropriate for these patients and will answer their questions better than a genetic test. After reflecting on all of these issues, some clients will decide that the information they stand to gain is not worth the risk.

Discussing Testing and Delivering Results

Because of the ramifications of diagnosing a genetic disorder or a predisposition for a genetic disease in an adult, genetic counseling needs to address certain issues that may be less prominent in other contexts. It is critical that sufficient time be allotted to discussing the implications of undergoing the process of diagnosis, in terms of what purpose the information will serve, who will be affected by it and how, and various courses of action that may be taken as a result. Educating the patient about the mechanics and limitations of testing is often complex. If laboratory analysis is involved, the waiting period between initiation of testing and results may be protracted, causing greater psychological distress than, e.g., cytogenetic testing. Lastly, both positive and negative results are likely to have far-reaching effects, mandating careful psychological evaluation and ongoing supportive counseling.

Assessing Patient Motivations and Readiness for Testing

It is important to explore the patient's reasons for seeking evaluation at this time. These may be as simple as following up on referral from the primary care physician or heightened awareness from a media report about potential genetic risks or the availability of testing. Other motivators may include a relative's or friend's recent diagnosis or death from the disease. There may be an important life event or decision pending, such as graduation, marriage, a career choice or change, or childbearing. Sometimes the patient or other family members have noticed symptoms that they fear may presage onset of the disorder, or the patient or physician may feel that a diagnosis is needed to inform decisions about medical or surgical interventions. Often, it is the patient's mounting anxiety that the condition is about to strike, perhaps because he or she is approaching an age when another close family member was diagnosed, that creates a need to know. In some cases, the patient has been pressured by other family members and really does not want to know (Grosfeld et al., 2000; Soldan et al., 2000).

An important part of prediagnostic counseling involves finding out about the patient's personal experience with the disease in question and determining how the patient feels about his or her own risk. Appropriate areas to explore with patients and their families who are interested in predictive or susceptibility genetic testing are listed in Table 6–2.

As with all genetic counseling, it is important to learn about the patient's family constellation and cultural background, educational level, degree of medical sophistication, and general approach to life. With presymptomatic evaluations, information about the patient's employment and insurance is especially relevant. By exploring the patient's support systems (family,

Table 6–2. Areas to Explore with Patients and Families Interested in Presymptomatic or Susceptibility Genetic Testing

1. How close is the patient to the affected people in the family biologically, generationally, geographically, and emotionally?
2. How old was the patient when key family members became affected (patient's developmental stage at this point may have had additional impact)?
3. What is the degree to which the patient identifies with affected family members ("I know I carry the gene because everyone says I take after my mother")?
4. What is the patient's perception of the disease's severity and natural history in people he or she has known, and how does he or she feel it affected the quality of life?
5. How burdensome does the patient feel the condition was for both the family and the affected individual (and was the patient involved in caretaking)?
6. What features of the condition worry the patient most or seem most distasteful (disfigurement, stigmatization, dying, being dependent, being undesirable)?
7. What are the family dynamics, attitudes about health issues (including secrecy in talking about them), and beliefs about causation and inheritance of the disorder?
8. How does the patient perceive his or her own risk (whether he or she will get the disease, how severely it will affect him or her, how he or she and others will cope)?
9. What is the emotional response to being at risk (vulnerability, loss of control, anger, poor self-esteem, guilt, isolation)?
10. How would learning his or her genetic status change his or her life or that of others?

friends, spiritual, occupational, etc.), the counselor acknowledges the stress that the evaluation may engender. Psychological assessment should include inquiries about the patient's current level of functioning: general level of stress and worry, ability to do daily tasks, appetite, sleeping patterns, drug or alcohol use, coping strategies, previous treatment for emotional problems, relationships, etc. It is often important to find out who the patient has told or plans to tell about considering a genetic evaluation or testing. The patient may wish to have a close friend or family member who is not at risk come with him or her for counseling sessions.

The Informed Consent Process

Patient education about the testing itself should review the inheritance of the condition as well as the risk assessment for the patient and other family members and how these were derived (pedigree analysis and Bayesian modifications). For some disorders, the family history and other data may also allow an estimate of the likelihood that a mutation will be identified. The testing methodology should be briefly reviewed so that the patient can understand the test's limitations (e.g., failure to find a mutation that is actually present in a different gene, missing a causative mutation when one is really present, identifying a change of unknown significance). Important discussion issues to consider with the patient during the informed consent process for genetic testing are listed in Table 6–3.

Once the issues around testing have been considered, both the patient and the genetic counselor need to reassess whether genetic testing and evaluation will provide the desired information and if this is the best time for the patient to undergo testing (in terms of coping ability, other stressors, utility of the information). In many cases, patients have not realized all of the ramifications of trying to learn their genetic status or have not contemplated the full impact of the information. They may come to the conclusion that evaluation should be deferred until a different point in their life or until advances in technology make the testing more helpful. However, those who decide to proceed should know that they still could opt to not learn or delay learning their results.

The Informing Interview

Much has been learned about genetic counseling for predictive and susceptibility genetic testing through the experiences with HD and cancer families. The genetic counselor should plan with the patient how they will get their results. It is nearly universally felt that these should be delivered face-to-face, unless there are extraordinary circumstances. Patients should be encouraged to identify a support person who will come with them, preferably someone who is not at risk or undergoing evaluation. It is worth "rehearsing" the informing day with patients so that they give thought to who will come with them, whom they will tell, what they will do afterward, how they will cope with either outcome, etc. Some counselors prefer not to know the results when they schedule the informing appointment and explain this to the patient when the specimen is obtained so that they will not be pressured into "tipping their hand" over the telephone. This also provides an out if the patient decides that he or she does not want to get the results. Many patients would be distressed by the thought that the counselor was privy to information they had chosen not to learn and are relieved that the envelope will remain sealed in their chart.

At the informing interview, patients should again be given an opportunity to consider if they are sure they want results and if they do or do not want the support person in the room when they get them. Delivery of the results should be empathetic but forthright. Genetic explanations should be limited to making sure that patients are comfortable with how the results were obtained and that they understand any attendant limitations or ambiguities. The counselor should be prepared for reactions ranging from stunned silence to severe distress. The patient and support per-

Table 6–3. Examples of Issues for Discussion During the Informed Consent Process for Genetic Testing

- Testing may not be truly informative or at least will provide limited reassurance if a specific mutation has not been identified in the family.
- Other people in the family will need to submit samples if the diagnosis is going to be inferred from linkage analysis.
- A positive test result does not necessarily mean that the disease is present or that it will develop in the future, and the test result cannot predict age at onset, severity, or disease course.
- Optimal preventive strategies or treatment for mutation carriers may be unknown.
- Testing positive may cause increased anxiety, depression, and stigmatization; lowered expectations and self-esteem; or altered family relationships.
- A positive test result can have financial implications, including the cost of increased surveillance or preventive surgery and potential loss of insurance or employment.
- A negative test may not guarantee that certain diseases (e.g., cancer) will not develop for some other reason.
- Testing negative can also have unexpected psychological effects, such as survivor guilt, the need to realign future plans, changes in family relationships, and more.

son should be afforded privacy, if they wish, and time to regain composure before they leave. Plans should be made for additional discussions or referrals. Many counselors ask permission to check in with the patient periodically by phone over the next few days or weeks.

Ongoing Support

One or more follow-up sessions or telephone calls should check for understanding of the test results, explore the patient's emotional state and the reactions of those with whom the patient has shared the news, and ask what (if any) actions the patient has taken as a result of the test results. Although most research has shown that even patients receiving positive test results return to their pretest state of psychological functioning within a few months of evaluation, the genetic counselor needs to be alert to depression and family dysfunction and to intervene when necessary. He or she should be prepared to provide appropriate referrals for medical, surgical, or psychological consultations and to offer information about available research protocols, support groups, and other community resources.

THE COUNSELING ASPECTS OF GENETIC COUNSELING: FACTORS INFLUENCING STRATEGY

The strategy of genetic counseling is best explained as a process that strives to empower patients through education and facilitate autonomous decision making utilizing the approach of client-centered counseling first described by Carl Rogers (Corey, 1996). The combination of respect for autonomy and the application of Rogers' theory and practice to decision making form the basis for the nondirective tenet of genetic counseling (Fine, 1993). The National Society of Genetic Counselors (1992) professional code of ethics illustrates the basis for this approach by emphasizing the "respect for client's beliefs, background and culture and the counselor's duty to enable clients to make autonomous decisions by providing all necessary information."

Kessler (1980) described the changes in emphasis in genetic counseling over the years as a "paradigm shift." Strategies in genetic counseling have involved multiple shifts in emphasis from, first, the communication of information counseling model to the preventive medicine model and, finally today, the psychosocial medicine approach. This strategy emphasizes patient self-determination and the genetic counselor's roles as a patient advocate, grief counselor, researcher, and health-care professional providing supportive care, education, resources, and referrals.

Over time, other counseling theories have been promoted in addition to the client-centered theoretical framework. These include the communication/psychological, cognitive/behavioral, and family systems approaches. In the communication/psychological approach, the genetic counselor facilitates individual and/or family decision making by providing unbiased information and promoting exploration of personal views and values regarding medical treatments and available options (Fine, 1993). The communication model, based on the tenets of nondirectiveness and client self-determination, includes principles from psychotherapy, family therapy, decision-making theory, and cross-cultural counseling. As such, the outcome of genetic counseling is not simply the acquisition of facts but the processing, assimilation, and personalization of this information that enable the individual to make an autonomous decision. Eunpu (1997) suggested applying family systems theory to genetic counseling because it addresses the individual, interactional, and intergenerational issues inherent in genetic conditions. Both genetic counseling and family systems therapists use family pedigrees or genograms for collecting and organizing information, assessing family patterns of disease and/or behaviors, developing hypotheses about how family dynamics are affected by the genetic diagnosis, and noting how these things in turn affect counseling and decision making.

Patient Expectations, Perceptions, and Needs

Paramount to effective genetic counseling is the clinician's attention to patient expectations, perceptions, and needs. Many studies have evaluated what patients expect from genetic counseling, how patients perceive their genetic risk, why they want genetic counseling and genetic testing, and what they need from this service. Once again, the majority of information available in this area of study comes from our experiences with genetic counseling for HD and cancer families.

Since genetic counseling is a relatively new medical service, patients often do not know what to expect or how to directly communicate their needs. This problem was clearly demonstrated by Hallowell and co-workers (1997), who assessed women's informational needs prior to cancer risk genetic counseling. Only 35% of the women in their study considered themselves adequately prepared for genetic counseling. All expected to discuss their family history and the risk of cancer, but 37% said they had no idea what else might be involved and therefore did not know what to expect. Although the majority reported that they were highly satisfied with the genetic counseling, uncertainty about what would occur in a consultation meant that they were unable to come to the session prepared to ask questions appropriate to their specific situation. The authors proposed that patients could benefit from precounseling education. One strategy suggested for dealing with this issue is to send patients written information about genetic counseling prior to the appointment. If patients and families know what to expect, they will come to the session more prepared to communicate their needs and help the clinician focus the genetic counseling.

What are the most important factors involved in the decision to seek genetic counseling and genetic testing? Hobus and colleagues (1995) reported their findings in a study that evaluated couples' decisions about whether or not to seek genetic counseling after the birth of a child with a major anomaly. The two most important factors in this decision were whether the couple was educated by their physician about the availability of genetic counseling and the couple's attitude toward genetic counseling. One of the factors affecting this attitude was the perception that genetic information would be an additional burden. Some couples who felt guilty about passing on "defective genes" to their child evidently thought that not knowing their risks would make reproductive decisions easier. The authors point out that such couples would benefit from understanding that the goals of genetic counseling include not only risk assessment and discussion of inheritance but also attention to their response and adaptation to the disease or risk.

Perception of risk is important in the decision to seek genetic counseling and testing, as is the perceived burden of the disease. Many people have a difficult time relating risk to their own situation. One study looked at people who had a 50% chance of inheriting the mutation for adult polycystic kidney disease, to see what they knew about their own risk. Only 32% knew their correct risk, while 41% knew that the condition was inherited but were unaware of their own risk (Ravine et al., 1991). People who are not aware of the fact that they may be at risk usually do not seek genetic services. This is of major concern in the case of adult polycystic kidney disease in that these individuals are probably unaware of recommendations for screening and treatment. However, if people believe that they are at high risk for a disease and that there is something they can do to *modify* that risk, they are more likely to seek genetic services. Those who do not think they are at risk and those at risk for a disease for which there is no cure or treatment are often less likely to seek genetic counseling.

Quaid et al. (2001) studied the perception of risk by patients affected with bipolar disorder. Patients were asked to estimate the genetic risk for bipolar disease in the general population as well as in their siblings, parents, and children. Patients more often than not overestimated the risk (Quaid et al., 2001). In another study of patients attending a familial cancer clinic, self-referred patients were often at lower risk than those referred by a physician or knowledgeable family members (Julian-Reynier et al., 1996). Patients came for genetic services because they perceived themselves to be at a high risk, but more importantly, 78% hoped to learn what they could do to prevent and screen for the cancer. An earlier study evaluating the anticipated uptake and impact of genetic testing for hereditary cancer found that most at-risk patients (79%) would want to be tested. The most common reasons for desiring testing were to learn if their children were at risk and to learn about prevention strategies (Struewing et al., 1995).

When patients with bipolar disorder and their spouses were asked if they would consider genetic testing for bipolar disorder if it became available, the majority said they would. Most felt that the benefits of knowing their genetic status outweighed any risks, although few would use the information to terminate an affected pregnancy or change their reproductive plans. They mostly hoped that the information would help them plan therapy (Trippitelli et al., 1998). These studies demonstrate that when patients are aware of their own risk and perceive that they can do something to modify it or the course of the disease, they will likely find genetic counseling and testing useful.

However, patients and clinicians do not always have the same perception about *how* the information will be useful. In a pilot study evaluating a method for assessing information recall in genetic counseling, researchers found that patients ranked information about implications for family members more highly than did genetic counselors (Michie et al., 1997a). Genetic counselors more frequently viewed information about testing, diagnosis, and prognosis as important compared to the patients. A follow-up study by the same researchers found that patients were able to correctly recall 76% of the key points in the counseling. Interestingly, recall was 100% for content involving family issues but only 68% to 78% for genetic or medical information (Michie et al., 1997b). Audrain and colleagues (1998) evaluated what women at risk for breast and ovarian cancer wanted from genetic counseling and testing. Almost all women in the study thought that genetic counseling "should include information about genetics; the benefits, risks, and limitations of testing; education about the meaning of the test result; and recommendations for surveillance and prevention". However, 50% to 60% of the women stated that genetic counseling should also involve discussion of their personal goals and values and the possible emotional impact of testing. They felt that these discussions were important in their decision about whether or not to be tested. Two-thirds wanted supportive counseling with disclosure of the results. The psychosocial needs of the women varied by age. More women who were under age 50 (73%–80%) felt that addressing psychosocial issues was vital than did women over 50 (50%).

Providing accurate and up-to-date information is essential, but it is only one component of effective genetic counseling. Identifying the patient's perception of risk, burden of disease, what they deem as important issues, and what they want from the genetic counselor are equally essential for meeting the patient's needs.

Family Dynamics

One of the distinctive aspects of genetic disorders is their impact on the family. When one individual is diagnosed with a genetic disease or found to carry a gene mutation, this information has implications for parents, brothers, sisters, children, and other family members. Lerman and Croyle (1996) described some of these issues in a publication based on their experiences in working with patients at risk for cancer. Different family members will have had different experiences with the disease, which shape how they perceive the disease and cope. At-risk family members fear for themselves but at the same time may feel guilty, angry, sad, and/or responsible for the condition. They may also want to place blame for the disease. Lerman and Croyle (1996) cite Kessler, a psychologist with vast experience in the field of genetic counseling, who has referred to the spouse as the "forgotten person." The spouse often receives little attention from the family or from care providers. This increases the strain on the marriage and affects family dynamics. In a study looking at the effects of predictive testing for HD on marital relationships, researchers found that partners of at-risk individuals demonstrated significantly higher levels of depression than those at risk (Quaid and Wesson, 1995). Partners face the possibility of significant changes in their marital relationship, increased risk to their children, and long-term caregiving responsibilities. A genetic condition affects multiple family members in a variety of ways and can have major psychological repercussions by disrupting relationships. Because of this, it is essential that a major component of genetic counseling should be to explore family issues.

Cultural Issues

Cultural differences often create barriers to medical care in general but can be especially challenging in genetic counseling. Not only language but also differences in communication styles can compromise the information exchange and exploration of psychosocial issues critical to effective genetic counseling. However, communication is only one of many hurdles. Different cultural beliefs about the causation, burden, and meaning of diseases can lead to misunderstandings. Genetic counseling's nondirective approach and preoccupation with patient autonomy may be unfamiliar to (and uncomfortable for) those from cultures in which people expect their healers to tell them what they should do to avoid or cure disease. Great disparities in education and economic status may also limit the usefulness of genetic counseling (Punales-Morejon and Penchaszadeh, 1992).

Greeson et al. (2001) used qualitative research methodology to understand the perception of disability in the Somali immigrant population in a city in the midwestern United States. The most consistent belief among participants was that disabilities and birth defects are considered a gift from God not to be questioned. They concluded that traditional genetic counseling would not be useful in this population; however, that does not mean that genetic medicine had nothing to offer. People were very interested in learning about anything that would improve the health of a person but not in anything that would predict or prevent what God had planned.

Rapp (1997) used the qualitative methodology of cultural anthropology to evaluate the impact of cultural issues among patients referred for prenatal genetic testing. She pointed out that not everyone sees mental retardation in the same way. Some families are less worried about mental retardation than about a physical handicap that would cause a child to be teased or not accepted. Risk is also relative, as is evident when Rapp (1997) quotes a genetic counselor's comment about her prenatal patient: "When she's got a 100% chance of running out of food stamps this month, a 50% chance she'll have to move before the year is over, and 25% chance that her brother will get caught up in street violence or drugs, one in a hundred for Down syndrome is the best odds she's facing." Religion also plays a large role in the perception of the burden of risk and in decision making. For many, it provides a belief system and support that may not appear to make sense to the medical community (Rapp, 1997).

Hughes and colleagues (1996) studied differences in perception of personal risk between white and African-American women who had one first-degree relative with breast cancer. They found that African-American women were significantly less likely to perceive themselves at risk than white women. The African-American women in the study also reported more daily psychological stress from worrying about their affected relative. The researchers suggested that "risk counseling for African American women should address not only personal risk factors and related concerns, but also aspects of the relative's breast cancer diagnosis." They also suggested that involving "other family members in risk counseling such as the index patient and/or siblings might facilitate the coping process." These studies emphasize the importance of cultural influences in providing genetic counseling.

Patient Decision Making

When providing complicated information to patients and families, it is important to think about how they hear and integrate this. Many studies have shown that people make medical decisions based on their perception of benefits vs. their perception of risk. These perceptions may have little to do with the actual genetic risk. Because of this, a patient's decision may seem totally illogical or not really based on fact. Wroe and co-workers (1998) compared a group of normal volunteers to a group of people at risk for a genetic condition to see why they would or would not pursue predictive testing if it were available. There was little difference between the two groups. Moreover, people who felt they were more at risk were more interested in genetic testing. In other words, people appeared to make decisions mostly based on reasons relevant to their own situation. Some of these reasons were grounded in emotion and had little to do with actual risk. The authors observed that "the decision maker appears to seek to maximise perceived gains relative to losses." They concluded that while the decision process is rational to the patient, it may not be clear to an outsider that the premises upon which the decision is based are sound.

Several studies have demonstrated the complex nature of patient decision making. Many have focused on patients' decisions about predictive testing for HD. This is an important population to learn from in that it was the first group with a genetic condition who faced the predictive testing decision. In this population, it is clear that the basis for decision making goes beyond the actual genetic risk for developing the disease. With current testing for HD, the results of predictive testing are usually definitive. To date, there is no available treatment or cure. Many people choose to be tested because it allows them to feel more in control of their future and reproductive decisions. Living with uncertainty is often agonizing. Reasons cited by those who choose not to have testing range from not wanting to know that their child will also face the risk to the lack of a cure for the disease to fear of losing health-care insurance to choosing uncertainty over certainty and to awareness that they will not be able to ignore the knowledge once it is known (Quaid and Morris, 1993; Decruyenaere et al., 1993). In one study, investigators found that nearly one-third of the patients who initially wanted testing withdrew from the testing program after counseling (Decruyenaere et al., 1997). The counseling in this testing program focused on helping people talk about what the information would mean in their own lives. This underscores the importance of counseling in helping patients understand the meaning of the genetic risk for themselves and in clarifying their perceptions of the possible benefits and losses inherent in testing.

Decision making about susceptibility testing for hereditary breast–ovarian cancer differs from HD predictive testing in that a positive result confers a high risk but not a virtual certainty of developing the disease. Furthermore, those at risk for breast–ovarian cancer have options such as screening or prophylactic surgery to reduce the risk of morbidity and mortality. Lerman and colleagues (1996) identified additional factors that went into decisions about testing for *BRCA1* and *BRCA2*. People wanting testing tended to come from a higher socioeconomic category and to have a greater number of relatives affected with breast cancer. Barriers to testing included lack of health-care insurance and concerns about insurance and employment discrimination. Some people also chose not to be tested because they did not perceive themselves to be at a high risk or were concerned over the possible negative psychological consequences of a positive result. Other patients seemed to perceive that the test did not provide enough conclusive information for them to alter decisions about reproduction or health-care behaviors. In another study, Lerman and co-workers (1995) found that women who received genetic counseling were much more likely to show improvement in their comprehension of personal risk (although they still overestimated their risk 3 months after counseling).

Lerman et al. (1997) pointed out the importance of enhancing the client's understanding of her own risk because those who perceive themselves at a very high risk sometimes choose not to participate in cancer screening, may overuse cancer screening, or may inappropriately decide to undergo prophylactic surgery. Again, interest in testing involves many outside factors beyond actual risk. The patient must feel that there are more personal advantages than disadvantages to the test (Jacobsen et al., 1997). Lerman et al. stated (1997) "it has been argued that optimal decision-making requires not only knowledge, but also a reasoned evaluation of the positive and negative consequences of alternate decisions." To help patients make good decisions, multiple factors must be considered and discussed. Patients should be helped to explore their personal risks, fears, and experience with the disease and their perception of the advantages vs. disadvantages of testing. Decision making is a process that takes time and optimally involves health-care professionals with special expertise.

Psychological Impact

Genetic information learned through genetic counseling and testing can be devastating and cause an emotional reaction that can interfere with complete understanding of the facts. Common reactions include denial, anger, fear, despair, guilt, shame, sadness, and grief (Djurdjinovic, 1998). Although these reactions are common when dealing with patients in many areas of medicine, guilt and shame play a particularly prominent role in genetics. It is not uncommon for patients to feel personally responsible for passing a gene on to a child or to be ashamed of their genetic family heritage. This is a particular problem when a diagnosis is newly made. The patient is shocked to learn not only that he or she has a disease but also that it is heritable. The diagnosis means an abrupt change in the patient's life and self-perception, which represents a transition from a familiar life to one that is full of unknowns (Delaporte, 1996). These are emotional rather than cognitive reactions, which can take years of counseling to resolve.

Taylor and Myers (1997) found that for patients who received the results of predictive linkage testing for HD, the long-term impact was significantly different in those found to be at low risk compared to those at high risk. The low-risk group was less anxious, less fearful, and less worried about the risk to their children. These patients also reported an increased sense of control and self-esteem. Lowered self-image was a common finding for those in the high-risk group. In addition, patients in the high-risk group did not usually find their stress and anxiety lowered by testing. Since many at-risk patients undergo testing to decrease their stress and anxiety, it is important for the counselor to realize that those with positive results will probably have as much stress as before, at least for a while.

Bloch and colleagues (1992) also studied the long-term effects of discovering an increased risk for HD on the basis of predictive linkage testing. After learning their results, patients initially showed shock and increased stress. However, after a year, most patients, especially those who openly communicated and reached out for support, were not more depressed or stressed. The authors emphasized the importance of pre- and post-test counseling for providing on-going support.

Lerman and colleagues (1996) reported similar findings for patients who had susceptibility testing for hereditary breast–ovarian cancer. In a follow-up study of patients who learned their gene status for *BRCA1*, those found *not* to carry the mutation demonstrated statistically significant reductions in symptoms of depression and functional impairment. This was not seen in those found to carry the mutation or in those who chose not to be tested. However, as with the HD patients, those found to carry the mutation had no *increase* in depression or functional impairment.

Genetic counseling plays an important role in helping patients deal with their emotional reactions. Berkenstadt and colleagues (1999) used the concept of *perceived personal control* as one aspect of measuring success in genetic counseling. Their work demonstrates a high association with perceived personal control among patients and families receiving genetic counseling services. They stated the following:

> Counselors aware of the concept of perceived control can emphasize specific issues that enhance counselee's sense of control. By focusing on how the information given enables more control of their future than before, the counselor can change the counselee's appraisal of the situation, even if only somewhat.

Addressing patient psychosocial issues, giving accurate genetic risk information, and providing ongoing support can help patients and families understand their risk, feel more in control of their lives, and better adjust to their situation. This is the essence of genetic counseling.

ETHICAL CONSIDERATIONS IN GENETIC COUNSELING

A myriad of ethical issues are inherent in the provision of genetic counseling services. Some are common to any medical service and others are more unique to genetic counseling (McCarthy Veach et al., 2001). Since a complete discussion of the ethical issues encountered by practitioners providing genetic counseling is beyond the scope of this chapter, we focus on a few that are the most common and troublesome.

Respect for Autonomy

Respect for patient autonomy is the guiding principle in contemporary genetic counseling. It is evident in the professional code of ethics for genetic counselors and in the nondirective approach embraced by the genetic counseling community (National Society of Genetic Counselors, 1992). However, there are occasions that challenge this principle. The most obvious examples involve a conflict in values that are either personal or professional in nature.

Respect for autonomy emphasizes the patient's freedom to make informed decisions without coercion from the counselor. It is the role of the counselor to provide accurate current medical and genetic information in a way that the patient can understand and find useful. Furthermore, the counselor should attempt to understand the patient's value system and facilitate decisions based on available options in relation to that particular patient and what is important to him or her at that point. In some cases, the values of the patient and the counselor conflict and dilemmas arise. In other cases, dilemmas arise when, in the process of trying to use technology to help, the potential for harm becomes apparent. Personal values can be challenged when a patient chooses a course of action that is considered immoral by the counselor. A good example of this is the case of a patient requesting prenatal testing for sex selection. With few exceptions, genetics professionals oppose the practice of sex selection (Wertz and Fletcher, 1993). Another common example of a counselor feeling conflicted is when a couple chooses to continue having children knowing that they are at a high risk for having a child with a severe or even a lethal disease. The counselor may feel that the couple is not considering what is in the best interest of the future child or of the other children in the family and therefore may have a difficult time providing unbiased counseling. Professional values can be challenged when a patient makes a request of the counselor that conflicts with the standards established by the profession. A case that illustrates this well is that of parents requesting genetic testing of their children when there is no obvious direct medical benefit. This practice is strongly discouraged by genetics professionals (ASHG and ACMG Report, 1995). Another example involves a difference in values that are cultural in nature. In some cultures, the patient expects the medical professional to make all decisions and the concept of autonomy is unfamiliar. Furthermore, diverse cultural views on disability and disease challenge the value system of traditional Western medicine. What may appear to be a minor physical disability to a genetics professional practicing in the United States may be unacceptable to someone from a different culture. Conversely, a condition involving mental retardation may not be considered a serious risk to patients from a different culture. Caplan (1993) argues that since no one can be value-neutral, it is important for the practitioner to know his or her own value system and to openly discus conflicts with the patient. Moreover, he asserts that not challenging the patient when these issues arise is not moral. In addition, he emphasizes that facilitating moral decision making is the role of the counselor.

Confidentiality

Confidentiality of medical information is a concern to all areas of medicine but is especially troublesome in the practice of genetics. In some cases, it is difficult to know who the primary patient is and therefore where the primary professional responsibility rests. This is because genetics involves families. The results of gene testing on one family member may have implications for another family member. Sometimes patients do not want to share information with others in the family even if the information may be medically significant to them. The American Society of Human Genetics Social Issues Subcommittee on Familial Disclosure (1998) published a statement suggesting that there are times when it may be considered ethical to breach patient confidentiality when the outcome may result in an individual avoiding a serious risk or when the individual may be in need of treatment. Maintaining confidentiality will become more of a challenge as the ability to test for more disease genes increases and the practice of genetics becomes more a part of primary care. It is easy to envision a situation where an entire family is seen in the same primary care setting and one family member wishes to be tested for a condition while others in the family either do not want testing pursued or are unaware of the risk.

Genetic Discrimination and Privacy

Concern over genetic discrimination and privacy of genetic information is growing. Cases of insurance and employment discrimination have been documented, and the public is becoming more aware of this concern. Lapham and colleagues (1996) in a survey study reported that members of genetic support groups could describe instances of being refused life and health insurance and being denied or fired from a job. For many patients, this is a great concern. Genetic testing is usually expensive, so patients want to use their insurance to cover the service. However, if an insurance company covers the service, then it has a right to the information. Moreover, insurance coverage, for most people, is tied to their employment. Because of this, patients need to be concerned about their genetic information finding its way back to their employer. To address this issue, many states have passed legislation in the attempt to protect patients. On a national level, this issue continues to receive vacillating attention. Bill Bradley, former U.S. senator, asserted that four elements are essential components to a national policy: balance, fairness, support, and public education (Bradley, 1999). In discussing balance, Bradley indicated that the individual's right to privacy and protection from discrimination needs to be balanced with the goals of science, the rights of the private sector and the public's need to equal access to new technology. He stated the following:

> America has always been about exploration, pushing back boundaries. Now, as the mysteries of our genetic make-up are explained, we have a new opportunity to blend compassion with enterprise and privacy with information. It is important to keep our eyes on the children, mothers and fathers, workers, healthy and ill who can be helped, or harmed, by the science and technology of genetics.

Justice

In the study of ethics, justice proposes fairness; i.e., everyone is treated in the same manner. This issue is of great concern in all areas of medicine but is especially challenging in the genetics arena. In a time when a great many people do not have access to basic medical care and basic medical care is not considered a right for everyone, medical genetics and genetic counseling may increasingly become services available only to the elite. This is an issue with which society as a whole must concern itself as our ability to provide more sophisticated genetic services advances. Since we all carry genes that are involved with the causation of complex common conditions, genetic counseling needs to be available to everyone. This will be more true as time goes on and genetic information can be better used to predict and prevent the problems associated with common diseases.

SUMMARY

Genetic counseling for common diseases, particularly those arising in previously healthy individuals later in life, will present challenges distinct from those encountered to date in other areas of genetic counseling. Among these will be the complexity of risk assessment since many such disorders will involve not just a single major gene but several genes. In addition, penetrance and expression will be influenced not only by the interaction between mutations and polymorphisms in these genes but by lifestyle and environmental factors as well. It is likely that many the genetic tests for a great number of these conditions will raise as many questions as they answer, with genotype–phenotype correlations being incompletely understood and optimal interventions and preventive strategies even less so. Genetic counselors will need to help patients and families cope with ambiguity and make decisions on the basis of imperfect information. They will have to guide patients in dealing with the psychological, social, and even economic impacts of learning that they or other family members are at risk, in some cases with resultant changes in family dynamics.

Geneticists and primary care providers will confront new and complex legal and ethical issues around privacy of genetic information, recontacting former patients about new developments, alerting other family members to possible risk or test availability, and experimental or expensive types of diagnosis and treatment. Unfortunately, all of this will have to be done with increasing economic and time constraints and inequities in access to health care. However, with appropriate genetic counseling, individuals at risk will have the opportunity to capitalize on a new understanding of the genetic basis of common ailments to improve their own health and quality of life. In this way, this book is a significant resource for any medical professional as we proceed into the era of genetic medicine.

REFERENCES

American Society of Human Genetics Social Issues Subcommittee on Familial Disclosure: Professional disclosure of familial genetic information. Am J Hum Genet 1998; 62:474–483.

ASHG and ACMG Report: Points to consider: ethical, legal and psychosocial implications of genetic testing in children and adolescents. Am J Hum Genet 1995; 57:1223–1224.

Audrain J, Rimer B, Cella D, Garber J, Peshkin BN, Ellis J, Schildkraut J, Stefanek M, Vogel V, Lerman C: Genetic counseling and testing for breast–ovarian cancer susceptibility: what do women want? J Clin Oncol 1998; 16:133–138.

Begley S: Screening for genes; matching medications to your genetic heritage. Newsweek 1999; Feb 8, 130(6):66.

Bennett RL, Steinhaus KA, Uhrich SB, O'Sullivan CK, Resta RG, Lochner-Doyle D, Markel DS, Vincent V, Hamanishi J: Recommendations for standardized human pedigree nomenclature. Am J Hum Genet 1995a; 56:745–752.

Bennett RL, Steinhaus KA, Uhrich SB, O'Sullivan CK, Resta RG, Lochner-Doyle D, Markel DS, Vincent V, Hamanishi J: Recommendations for standardized human pedigree nomenclature. J Genet Counsel 1995b; 4:267–279.

Bennett RL, Steinhaus KA, Uhrich SB, O'Sullivan CK, Resta RG, Lochner-Doyle D, Markel DS, Vincent V, Hamanishi J: Reply to Marizita and Curtis [letter to the editor]. Am J Hum Genet 1995c; 57:983–984.

Berkenstadt M, Shiloh S, Barkai G, Datznelson MB, Goldman B. Perceived personal control (PPC): a new concept in measuring outcome of genetic counseling. Am J Med Genet 1999; 82:53–59.

Berry DA, Parmigiani G, Sanchez J, Schildkraut J: Probability of carrying a mutation of breast–ovarian cancer gene *BRCA1* based on family history. J Natl Cancer Inst 1997; 89:227–238.

Bhatnagar D, Morgan J, Siddiq S, Mackness MI, Miller JP, Durrington PN: Outcome of case finding among relatives of patients with known heterozygous familial hypercholesterolemia. BMJ 2000; 321:1–5.

Bloch M, Adam S, Wiggins S, Huggins M, Hayden MR: Predictive testing for Huntington disease in Canada: the experience of those receiving an increased risk. Am J Med Genet 1992; 42:499–507.

Bonne G, Carrier L, Richard P, Hainque B, Schwartz K: Familial hypertrophic cardiomyopathy: from mutations to functional defects. Circ Res 1998; 83:580–593.

Bradley B: Privacy, safety, and genetics: finding the balance. Fam Syst Health 1999; 17:45–47.

Brinkman RR, Mezie MM, Theilmann J, Almqvist R, Hayden MR: The likelihood of being affected with Huntington disease by a particular age, for a specific CAG size. Am J Hum Genet 1997; 60:1202–1210.

Burke W, Imperatore G, McDonnell SM, Baron RC, Khoury MJ: Contribution of different HFE genotypes to iron overload disease: a pooled analysis. Genet Med 2000; 2:271–277.

Caplan AL: Neutrality is not morality: the ethics of genetic counseling. In: Bartels DM, LeRoy BS, Caplan A (eds). Prescribing Our Future: Ethical Challenges in Genetic Counseling. New York: Aldine de Gruyter, 1993:149–165.

Chillon M, Casals T, Mercier B, Bassas L, Lissens W, Silber S, Romey MC, Ruiz-Romero J, Verlingue C, Claustres M: Mutations in the cystic fibrosis gene in patients with congenital absence of the vas deferens. N Engl J Med 1995; 332:1475–1480.

Clark S, Bluman LG, Borstelmann N, Regan K, Winer EP, Rimer BK, Skinner CS: Patient motivation, satisfaction, and coping in genetic counseling and testing for BRCA1 and BRCA2. J Genet Counsel 2000; 9:219–235.

CLIA 88. Public Law 100–578 Clinical Laboratory Improvement Amendments of 1988, 42 USC 263a et seq. *Federal Register* 1992; 57:7001–7288.

Couch FJ, DeShano ML, Blackwood MA, Calzone K, Stopfer J, Campeau L, Ganguly A, Rebbeck T, Weber BL: *BRCA1* mutations in women attending clinics that evaluate the risk of breast cancer. N Engl J Med 1997; 336:1409–1415.

Corey G: Theory and Practice of Counseling and Psychotherapy, 5th edition. Pacific Grove, CA: Brooks/Cole Publishing 1996, p. 198–221.

Decruyenaere M, Evers-Kiebooms G, Boogaerts A, Cassiman JJ, Cloostermans T, Demyttenare K, Dom R, Fryns JP, Van den Berghe H: Predictive testing for Huntington's disease: risk perception, reasons for testing and psychological profile of test applicants. Genet Counsel 1995; 6:1–13.

Decruyenaere M, Evers-Kiebooms G, Boogaerts A, Cloostermans T, Cassiman JJ, Demyttenare K, Dom R, Fryns JP, Van den Berghe H: Non-participation in predictive testing for Huntington's disease: individual decision-making, personality and avoidant behaviour in the family. Eur J Hum Genet 1997; 5:351–363.

Decruyenaere M, Evers-Kiebooms G, Van den Berghe H: Perception of predictive testing for Huntington's disease by young women: preferring uncertainty to certainty? J Med Genet 1993; 30:557–561.

Delaporte C: Ways of announcing a late-onset, heritable, disabling disease and their psychological consequences. Genet Counsel 1996; 7:289–296.

Dice LR: Heredity clinics: their value for public service and research. Am J Hum Genet 1952; 4:1–13.

Djurdjinovic L: Psychosocial counseling. In: Baker DL, Schuette JL, Uhlmann WR (eds.) *A Guide to Genetic Counseling*. New York: Wiley-Liss, 1998:127–166.

Eunpu DL: Systemically-based psychotherapeutic techniques in genetic counseling. J Genet Counsel 1997; 6:1–20.

Fine BA: The evolution of nondirectiveness in genetic counseling and implications of the Human Genome Project. In: Bartels DM, LeRoy BS, Caplan A (eds). Prescribing Our Future: Ethical Challenges in Genetic Counseling. New York: Aldine de Gruyter, 1993:101–118.

Ford D, Easton EF, Stratton M, Narod S, Goldgar D, Devilee P, Bishop DT, Weber B, Lenoir G, Chang-Claude J, et al.: Genetic heterogeneity and penetrance analysis of the *BRCA1* and *BRCA2* genes in breast cancer families. Am J Hum Genet 1998; 62:676–689.

Frank TS, Manley SA, Olopade IO, Cummings S, Garber JE, Bernhardt B, Antman K, Russo D, Wood ME, Mullineau L, et al.: Sequence analysis of *BRCA2* and *BRCA2*: correlation of mutations with family history and ovarian cancer risk. J Clin Oncol 1998; 16:2417–2425.

Greeson CJ, McCarty Veach P, LeRoy BS: A qualitative investigation of Somali immigrant perceptions of disability: implications for genetic counseling. J Genet Counsel 2001; 10:359–378.

Grosfeld FJM, Lips CJM, Beemer FA, ten Kroode HFJ: Who is at risk for psychological distress in genetic testing programs for hereditary cancer disorders? J Genet Counsel 2000; 9:253–266.

Hallowell N, Murton F, Statham H, Green JM, Richards MPM: Women's need for information before attending genetic counselling for familial breast or ovarian cancer: a questionnaire, interview and observational study. BMJ 1997; 314:281–283.

Hobus I, Frets PG, Duivenvoorden HJ, Tibboel D, Niermeijer MF: Factors influencing whether or not couples seek genetic counselling: an explorative study in a paediatric surgical unit. Clin Genet 1995; 47:47–52.

Hodge SE: A simple, unified approach to Bayesian risk calculations. J Genet Counsel 1998; 7:235–261.

Hughes C, Lerman C, Lustbader E: Ethnic differences in risk perception among women at increased risk for breast cancer. Breast Cancer Res Treat 1996; 40:25–35.

Jacobsen PB, Valdimarsdottir HB, Brown KL, Offit K: Decision making about genetic testing among women at familial risk for breast cancer. Psychosom Med 1997; 5:459–466.

Julian-Reynier C, Eisinger F, Chabal F, Aurran Y, Nogues C, Vennin P, Gignon Y-J, Machelard-Roumagnac M, Maugard-Louboutin C, Serin D, et al.: Cancer genetics clinics: target populations and consultee's expectations. Eur J Cancer 1996; 32A:398–403.

Kessler S: The psychological paradigm shift in genetic counseling. Soc Biol 1980; 27:167–185.

Kessler S: Psychological aspects of genetic counseling. VII. Thoughts on directiveness. J Genet Counsel 1992;1:9–17.

Kevles DJ: In the Name of Eugenics. Cambridge, MA: Harvard University Press, 1995.

Lapham E, Kozma C, Weiss J: Genetic discrimination: perspectives of consumers. Science 1996; 274:621–624.

Lebo RV, Cunningham G, Simons MJ, Shapiro LJ: Defining DNA diagnostic tests appropriate for standard clinical care [letter to the editor]. Am J Hum Genet 1990; 47:583–590.

Lerman C, Biesecker B, Benkendorf JL, Kerner J, Gomez-Caminero A, Hughes C, Reed MM: Controlled trial of pretest education approaches to enhance informed decision-making for *BRCA1* gene testing. J Natl Cancer Inst 1997; 89:148–157.

Lerman C, Croyle RT: Emotional and behavioral responses to genetic testing for susceptibility to cancer. Oncology 1996; 10:191–199.

Lerman C, Lusbader E, Rimer B, Daly M, Miller S, Sands C, Balshem A: Effects of individualized breast cancer risk counseling: a randomized trial. J Natl Cancer Inst 1995; 87:286–292.

Lerman C, Narod S, Schulman K, Hughes C, Gomez-Caminero A, Bonney G, Gold K, Trock B, Main D, Lynch J, et al.: BRCA1 testing in families with hereditary breast–ovarian cancer. JAMA 1996; 275:1885–1892.

Liddell MB, Lovestone S, Owen MJ: Genetic risk of Alzheimer disease: advising relatives. Br J Psychiatry 2001; 178:7–11.

Lubinsky MS: Scientific aspects of early eugenics. J Genet Counsel 1993; 2:77–92.

Marizita M: Standardized pedigree nomenclature [letter to the editor]. Am J Hum Genet 1995; 57:982–983.

McCarthy Veach P, Bartels DM, LeRoy BS: Ethical and professional challenges posed by patients with genetic concerns: a report of focus group discussions with genetic counselors, physicians and nurses. J Genet Counsel 2001; 10:97–119.

Michie S, French D, Allanson A, Bobrow M, Marteau TM: Information recall in genetic counselling; a pilot study of its assessment. Patient Educ Counsel 1997a; 32:93–100.

Michie S, McDonald V, Marteau TM: Genetic counselling: information given, recall and satisfaction. Patient Educ Counsel 1997b; 32:101–106.

National Institutes of Health: NIH Consensus Statement on Genetic Testing for Cystic Fibrosis. Bethesda, MD: NIH, 1997.

National Society of Genetic Counselors: Code of ethics of the National Society of Genetic Counselors. J Genet Counsel 1992; 1:41–43.

Neel JV: *Physician to the Gene Pool, Genetic Lessons and Other Stories*. New York: Wiley, 1994:24.

Offit K: *Clinical Cancer Genetics*. New York: Wiley-Liss, 1998.

Parmigiani G, Berry DA, Aquilar O: Determining carrier probabilities for breast cancer susceptibility genes *BRCA1* and *BRCA2*. Am J Hum Genet 1998; 62:145–158.

Punales-Morejon D, Penchaszadeh VB: Psychosocial aspects of genetic counseling: cross-cultural issues. Birth Defects 1992; 28:11–15.

Quaid KA, Aschen SR, Smiles CL, Nurnberger JI: Perceived genetic risks for bipolar disorder in a patient population: an exploratory study. J Genet Counsel 2001; 10:41–51.

Quaid KA, Morris M: Reluctance to undergo predictive testing: the case of Huntington disease. Am J Med Genet 1993; 45:41–45.

Quaid KA, Wesson MK: Exploration of the effects of predictive testing for Huntington disease on intimate relationships. Am J Med Genet 1995; 57:46–51.

Rapp R: Communicating about chromosomes: patients, providers, and cultural assumptions. J Am Med Womens Assoc 1997; 52:28–32.

Ravine D, McGregor LR, Walker RG, Sheffield LJ: Perceptions of genetic risk in individuals with a one in two chance of developing autosomal dominant polycystic kidney disease. Med J Aust 1991; 154:689–691.

Reed S: Counseling in Medical Genetics. Philadelphia: W.B. Saunders, 1955.

Reed S: A short history of genetic counseling. Soc Biol 1974; 21:332–339.

Resta RG: The crane's foot: the rise of the pedigree in human genetics. J Genet Counsel 1993; 2:235–260.

Resta RG: Eugenics and nondirectiveness in genetic counseling. J Genet Counsel 1997; 6:255–258.

Schneider KA, Kalkbrenner KJ: National Society of Genetic Counselors Professional Status Survey. Perspect Genet Counsel 1998; 20:S1–S8.

Shattuck-Eidens D, McClure M, Simard J, Labrie F, Narod S, Couch F, Hoskins K, Weber B, Castilla L, Erdos M, et al.: A collaborative survye of 80 mutations in the *BRCA1* breast and ovarian cancer susceptibility gene: implications for presymptomatic testing and screening. JAMA 1995; 273:535–541.

Shattuck-Eidens D, Oliphant A, McClure M, McBride C, Gupte J, Rubano T, Pruss D, Tavtigian SV, Teng DH-F, Adey N, et al.: *BRCA1* sequence analysis in women at high risk for susceptibility mutations: risk factor analysis and implications for genetic testing. JAMA 1997; 278:1242–1250.

Sobel S, Cowan DB: The process of family reconstruction after DNA testing for Huntington disease. J Genet Counsel 2000; 9:237–251.

Soldan J, Street E, Gray J, Binedell J, Harper PS: Psychological model for presymptomatic test interviews: lessons learned from Huntington disease. J Genet Counsel 2000; 9:15–31.

Struewing JP, Hartge P, Wacholder S, Baker SM, Berlin M, McAdams M, Timmerman MM, Brody LC, Tucker MA: The risk of cancer associated with specific mutations of *BRCA1* and *BRCA2* among Ashkenazi Jews. N Engl J Med 1997;336:1401–1408.

Struewing JP, Lerman C, Kase RG, Giambarresi TR, Tucker MA: Anticipated uptake and impact of genetic testing in hereditary breast and ovarian cancer families. Cancer Epidemiol Biomarkers Prev 1995; 4:169–173.

Taylor CA, Myers RH: Long-term impact of Huntington disease linkage testing. Am J Med Genet 1997; 70:365–370.

Trippitelli CL, Jamison KR, Folstein MF, Bartko JJ, DePaulo JR: Pilot study on patients' and spouses' attitudes toward potential genetic testing for bipolar disorder. Am J Psychiatry 1998; 155:899–904.

Wertz DC, Fletcher JC: Prenatal diagnosis and sex selection in 19 nations. Soc Sci Med 1993; 37:1359–1336.

Wolff G, Jung C: Nondirectiveness and genetic counseling. J Genet Counsel 1995; 4:3–25.

Wroe AL, Salkovskis PM, Rimes KA: The prospect of predictive testing for personal risk: attitudes and decision making. Behav Res Ther 1998; 36:599–619.

Yu B, French JA, Jeremy RW, French P, McTaggart DR, Nicholson MR, Semsarian C, Richmond DR, Trent RJ: Counselling issues in familial hypertrophic cardiomyopathy. J Med Genet 1988; 35:183–188.

Part II

CARDIOPULMONARY DISEASES

7 Genetics of Coronary Atherosclerosis

ARNO G. MOTULSKY AND JOHN D. BRUNZELL

Coronary heart disease (CAD) is a common and well-studied disease that owes its origin to both genetic and environmental factors. It is emerging as a model for the elucidation of genetic factors in complex, common diseases. While the specific genes underlying the mechanisms of genetic susceptibility remain largely unknown in most other common diseases, a variety of genes predisposing to CAD have been identified. However, environmental factors are almost always also involved. Recent decades have seen many studies to demonstrate the role of hyperlipidemia as an important factor in the pathogenesis of CAD. Genetic variation and mutations affecting lipoproteins and their metabolism are increasingly clarified. The goal of the genetic approach is to elaborate a risk profile to identify those individuals who are most susceptible to develop CAD. Since prevention using diet or drugs is possible for various lipid abnormalities, appropriate measures can be directed at individuals who are at high risk. Since lipids play a major, but not the sole role, in this disease, ongoing and future research will need to identify non-lipid genetic and environmental factors that predispose to CAD so that better risk profiles will become available. In this chapter we will consider various common genetic factors that predispose to CAD.

THE ATHEROSCLEROTIC LESION

The cause of coronary heart disease is atherosclerosis of the coronary arteries. The term *atherosclerosis* refers to lipid-infiltrated lesions that thicken arterial intimal-media, narrow arteries, impair blood flow, and predispose to thrombosis. Atherosclerosis is generically defined as thickened and stiffened arteries. Clinical manifestations may occur with impairment of the coronary, cerebrovascular, and peripheral arterial circulation of the lower limbs. Aortic aneurysms may also occur.

Arteries consist of an outer shell of fibrous tissue and a few smooth muscle cells, plus an intermediate layer consisting of smooth muscle cells and an endothelial intimal lining. Two general types of atherosclerotic lesions are observed: the fatty streak and the fibrous plaque. Fatty streaks are largely confined to the inner lining of blood vessels and consist of lipid-laden macrophages derived from circulating monocytes. Fatty streaks are common and already may be seen in infants (Holman et al., 1958; McGill, 1968). It has been suggested by in vitro studies that oxidized, cholesterol-bearing, low-density lipoprotein (LDL) is more readily taken up by the early lesions than unmodified LDL (Steinberg and Witztum, 1990; Steinberg, 1997). The relevance of these observations for atherosclerosis is under intense study. Fatty streaks do not necessarily develop into fibrous plaques, and it is unknown what makes some of these lesions progress while others remain unchanged or regress.

Fibrous plaques are covered by a cap of dense connective tissue containing some smooth muscle cells. Beneath the fibrous cap, many smooth muscle cells (including cells with lipid droplets), as well as macrophages and some lymphocytes, can be seen. As the lesions progress, foam cells become necrotic and develop cholesterol deposits and calcification. Cracks, ulceration, intraplaque hemorrhage, fissures, and aneurysmal dilatation are often evident in such late lesions. Complete occlusion of a coronary vessel may occur when thrombosis develops. Any factors predisposing to clot formation or inhibiting clot lysis are therefore likely to predispose to CAD.

The details of the early pathogenesis of atherosclerosis have not been fully elucidated (Ross, 1986; Wissler, 1991; Ross, 1999—see also Havenith and Gotlieb, 1991; McGill et al., 2000). Endothelial injury has been suggested as the key event making for platelet adherence with release of platelets-derived growth factor (PDGF) to stimulate proliferation of the fibrous plaque. Endothelial injury, however, is not required, and release of a variety of other cytokine growth factors (such as fibroblast growth factor [FGF], epidermal growth factor [EGF], and transforming growth factor [TGF]) may be involved in fibrous plaque formation (Ross, 1986). Recent studies (Ross, 1999; Epstein et al., 2000) increasingly emphasize the role of inflammatory factors in pathogenesis and progression (Albert, 2000).

Future attention needs to be given to genetic and other variability in the mechanisms that lead to the fibrous plaque, such as the role of various inflammatory factors. Genetic differences in the various growth-promoting cytokines or in their receptors are also possible. Etiologic heterogeneity in CAD is likely. Since different pathophysiologic events appear involved, certain mechanisms may be more important than others in various subsets of patients.

Monoclonal Origin of Atherosclerosis

It has been demonstrated that the fibrous plaque often has a monoclonal origin. Testing cells from the atherosclerotic plaques of female heterozygotes for an X-linked genetic marker (such as G6PD variants), it was shown that all cells from a given atherosclerotic lesion exhibited an identical marker (Benditt and Benditt, 1973). In contrast, the surrounding unaffected tissue was a mosaic carrying either the normal or the variant G6PD marker, as expected from the normal phenomenon of X-inactivation in heterozygotes for an X-linked trait. It was therefore postulated that the early atherosclerotic lesion was monoclonal and had arisen by a mutational event in a *single* cell of a blood vessel. Since monoclonal origin of pathologic lesions has largely been observed in tumors that arise by somatic mutation, mutational origin from a single smooth-muscle cell was suggested. Since the monoclonal expansion in recent studies has also been found in nonatherosclerotic intima and media (Schwartz and Murry, 1998), it has been argued that the monoclonal nature of the plaque might have developed because of selective overgrowth of a small subpopulation of smooth muscle cells that all carried the identical genetic marker (Havenith and Gotlieb, 1991; Thomas and Kim, 1983). This mechanism appears most likely.

EPIDEMIOLOGIC STUDIES

Coronary heart disease accounted for about 27% of all deaths in the United States in the late 1980s and has remained the leading cause of death in recent years. Rates of CAD in the United States rose in the 1950s until more than 300 deaths per year per 100,000 population were observed in the mid-1960s. Since that time, the mortality has decreased with a lessened rate of decline in more recent years. In 1997, some 17.3% of all deaths were caused by CAD (Health Care Almanac and Yearbook, 2000). The mortality rates of CAD vary widely between different countries (Beaglehole, 1990). Rates in countries such as Finland, Northern Ireland, Ireland, Scotland, New Zealand, Australia, and England were higher than U.S. rates in the mid 1970s (Inter-Society Commission, 1984; Beaglehole, 1990). All other countries where statistics were kept showed lower rates. The lowest mortality was found in Japan and was one-sixth that of the United States. The recent decline in CAD mortality observed in the United States has also been noted in several other countries with high incidence. On the other hand, the frequency of CAD over the same time period has increased in several European countries, particularly those of Eastern Europe (Inter-Society Commission, 1984; Beaglehole, 1990). In general, the decline in coronary mortality in the United States has been concurrent with declines in cigarette smoking, the lessened amount of saturated fat consumed in the diet (Goldman and Cook, 1984), and in treatment of high blood pressure, as well as increased use of lipid-lowering therapy. The greatest mortality reduction has occurred among more educated and affluent groups, both in the United States and the United Kingdom. The low CAD mortality rate in France, which is $\frac{1}{3}$ that of the United States, is puzzling in view of French dietary practices (Tunstall-Pedoe, 1988) and has been explained by a higher consumption of red wine as a protective factor. Further work is needed.

Since mortality data are based on death certificates, possible vagaries in reporting, as well as international differences in the definition of CAD deaths, must be kept in mind when attempting to explain temporal and international differences. In general, however, most experts are convinced that the decrease of CAD in the United States (and increases in some other countries) is real. While morbidity data on the frequency of myocardial infarction are much harder to assess because of variable criteria for hospital admission, limited data suggest that CAD morbidity in the United States decreased along with mortality.

CAD death rates are about three times higher in middle-aged men than in premenopausal women, who tend to develop CAD 10 to 15 years later than men do. These sex differences diminish after menopause and in countries with a low incidence of CAD (Inter-Society Commission, 1984). When CAD mortality has declined in men, similar declines have also been seen in women. In those countries where there were increases, both sexes had analogous rates of change.

The important role of environmental factors was clearly shown in various migrant studies. When Japanese migrated from Japan to the Hawaiian Islands, their CAD rate doubled; with migration to the mainland United States, the rate tripled (Robertson et al., 1977). Similar increases were observed in Irish migrants in Boston, as compared with their brothers who stayed in Ireland (Kushi et al., 1985). CAD rates among various migrants became nearly similar to those observed in local populations of their adopted countries within 10 to 20 years after immigration.

Various studies on CAD differences in different racial and ethnic groups currently do not provide any insight into possible genetic differences between populations to explain variable rates. It may be significant, however, that Finns, who have the highest level of plasma cholesterol and the highest coronary heart disease rates, when compared with all other populations (Beaglehole, 1990), also have the highest gene frequency for the Apo E4 allele that raises cholesterol levels (see below) (Hallman et al., 1991).

Evidence for the Key Role of Cholesterol

The suggestion that lipids may be related to atherosclerosis was first made in nutritional studies on rabbits by Russian investigators before World War I (Ignatovski, 1908; Anitschkov and Chalatow, 1913). Cholesterol feeding produced arterial lesions resembling those of human atherosclerosis. A Dutch physician working in Java pointed out the higher level of serum cholesterol in premature CAD in Javanese ship stewards who ate typical Dutch food on Dutch ships (de Langen, 1916). Native Javanese living in Indonesia had lower cholesterol levels and a very low frequency of CAD. In the 1930s, Scandinavian investigators found families where familial hypercholesterolemia was accompanied by xanthomas and heart disease (Muller, 1939). Another Dutch physician working in China in 1941 related the low incidence of atherosclerosis in Beijing to the high unsaturated fatty acid and low cholesterol content of the Chinese diet (Snapper, 1941). The association of raised plasma cholesterol levels with coronary atherosclerosis in the United States was pointed out by Dock in 1946. By 1957, the Framingham Study (Dawber et al., 1957) had established the predictive nature of serum cholesterol for CAD. By that time, the association of autosomal dominant familial hypercholesterolemia with coronary heart disease had become generally accepted (Thannhauser and Magendantz, 1938; Adlersberg et al., 1949; Wilkinson, 1950).

Large-scale and extensive studies were carried out in many populations to buttress the cholesterol hypothesis. The degree of severity of coronary atherosclerosis, as well as the mortality rate of CAD, could be correlated with mean total cholesterol levels of a population (see Committee on Diet and Health, 1989, for extensive references). Thus, the correlation between CAD death rates for seven countries (Finland, Netherlands, Italy, Yugoslavia, Greece, United States, and Japan) and median cholesterol levels obtained 15 years earlier was .96. In another study of 19 different populations, those with cholesterol levels less than 180 mg/dl had very little atherosclerosis and CAD, while those with mean cholesterol levels above 220 mg/dl had high rates of CAD. The most impressive single study assessed the age-adjusted CAD death rate in 361,662 middle-aged U.S. men (ages 35–57) six years after a cholesterol determination (Martin et al., 1986). In this work the mortality rate doubled between a cholesterol level of 153 and 226 mg/dl (from 3.16 to 6.94 per 1000) and doubled again between 226 and 290 mg/dl (from 6.94 to 13.05 per 1000). The highest rates occurred with cholesterol levels above 300 mg/dl. These data indicated a definitive relationship of plasma cholesterol and CAD death rates over the *entire* range of normal and elevated cholesterol levels.

The key role of elevated cholesterol levels in the pathogenesis of CAD is clearly illustrated by familial hypercholesterolemia (Goldstein et al., 2001) (see below). Heterozygotes with cholesterol levels ranging between 280 and 450 mg/dl have a much increased frequency of coronary heart disease starting in young middle age. Homozygotes for this condition who have very high cholesterol levels (>500 mg/dl) often develop coronary heart disease in childhood with massive atherosclerosis. (In view of the rarity of this condition, homozygous familial hypercholesterolemia is not further discussed in this chapter.)

Various large-scale therapeutic trials such as the Helsinki Heart Study (Frick et al., 1987) and the U.S. Lipid Research Clinic Trial (Lipid Research Clinics Program, 1984a) have shown that reduction of cholesterol levels and an improvement of "lipid profile" by drugs is associated with a diminished morbidity from coronary heart disease. There was approximately a 2% reduction in morbidity for a 1% reduction in cholesterol levels in the United States (Lipid Research Clinics Program, 1984b). However, these therapeutic studies did not show a decreased CAD mortality. In large, more recent drug studies, improved CAD morbidity and mortality effects are established, both in primary prevention (Lipid Research Clinic Program 1984a,b; Shepherd et al., 1995) and secondary prevention studies (Brown et al., 1990; 4S Study, 1994; Sacks et al., 1998).

While a definitive relationship between plasma cholesterol and dietary intake of fat and cholesterol in population studies has been demonstrated, cholesterol levels among individuals have usually failed to show a clear association with diets (for references, see Committee on Diet and Health, 1989). These negative results have been ascribed to variable responses by individuals to cholesterol and fat intake. By analogy to animal studies, responses to lipid feeding are probably under genetic control (Katan and Beynen, 1987). Furthermore, statistical considerations make it difficult to demonstrate correlations within the relatively narrow range of cholesterol levels seen in most such studies.

The evidence coming from animal experimentation, epidemiologic studies, clinical correlations, genetic diseases, and therapeutic trials leaves little doubt about the role of cholesterol (Committee on Diet and Health, 1989), particularly of LDL cholesterol, in promoting atherosclerotic coronary heart disease.

Role of Triglycerides

The role of elevated triglycerides (TG) levels in risk for coronary heart disease is likely but less definite. Most, but not all, studies show an association of hypertriglyceridemia with CAD (Austin, 1991). Since cholesterol and triglyceride values are often correlated, this association might be mediated by the effects of elevated plasma cholesterol levels. However, even after triglyceride values are adjusted for cholesterol levels, the relation of hypertriglyceridemia to CAD remains in several studies. Because of inverse correlation of triglycerides with high-density lipoprotein (HDL) levels ($r = -.22$–$.65$, with higher inverse correlations in women), the predictive value of triglycerides for CAD often disappears when triglyceride values are adjusted for HDL (Havel, 1988). Furthermore, triglycerides seem to serve as a marker for many abnormalities, such as for increased very low density lipoprotein (VLDL), increased intermediate-density lipoprotein (ILDL), small dense LDL, and decreased HDL_2 (Brunzell and Hokanson, 1999).

A recent meta-analysis of prospective population studies examined the role of triglycerides as a CAD risk factor in 17 studies from 46,413 men and in 5 studies from 10,864 women (Hokanson and Austin, 1996). The relative risks (adjusted for HDL cholesterol) were 1.2 for men and 1.4 for women. Similar data were obtained from the Physicians Health Study (Stampfer et al., 1996) and a Danish investigation (Jeppsen et al., 1998; Agerholm-Larsen et al., 2000). In a 20-year follow-up of the Seattle study of families with familial combined hyperlipidemia and familial hypertriglyceridemia, elevated baseline triglyceride values were a predictor of subsequent cardiovascular mortality (Austin et al., 2000). Clinical trials specifically designed to study the role of decreasing triglyceride levels in reducing CAD-related events are necessary.

Role of HDL

While most individuals with low HDL cholesterol also have elevated triglyceride levels, a decrease in HDL cholesterol independently predicts risk for CAD in prospective trials (Gordon et al., 1989). Drug therapy to elevated HDL cholesterol has been repeatedly demonstrated to affect CAD independently from LDL cholesterol levels in primary (Lipid Research Clinics Program, 1984; Shepherd et al., 1995) and secondary (Brown et al., 1990; 4S Study, 1994; Sacks et al., 1998) intervention trials.

Decreases in both HDL_2 and HDL_3 cholesterol have been shown to predict risk of CAD (Stampfer et al., 1991). The decrease in HDL_2 cholesterol is related to increased hepatic lipase activity, which is in part related to a common promoter variant of the hepatic lipase gene. Decreases in hepatic lipase with intensive lipid lowering predicts regression of CAD by angiography (Zambon et al., 1999). A locus near the hepatic lipase gene has been linked to HDL cholesterol (Almasy et al., 1999). In part, the decrease in HDL_3 cholesterol is related to changes in cholesteryl ester transfer protein (CETP) activity and is mediated by variants in the CETP gene (Agerhom-Larsen et al., 2000; Barter, 2000; Inazu et al., 2000).

Role of Small Dense LDL

Small dense LDL can be measured by gradient gel electrophoresis or by density gradient ultracentrifugation in research laboratories, but this measurement is not readily available in routine laboratories. The association of small dense LDL with CAD was first demonstrated in several case-control studies of myocardial infarction (Austin et al., 1988a; Gardner et al., 1996). In the prospective Quebec Cardiovascular Study, small dense LDL particles were predictors of CAD in a large number of men who were initially free of CAD (Lamarche et al., 1997). Adjustment for triglyceride, LDL cholesterol, HDL cholesterol, Apo B levels had little effect on the relationship between small LDL and CAD. In a smaller study of 58-year-old men with the central obesity–insulin resistance syndrome, small dense LDL particles were associated with intimal-media thickness in the carotid and femoral arteries by ultrasound (Hulthe et al., 2000). Finally, the change in LDL peak particle density was the best predictor of coronary artery regression by angiography in middle-age men undergoing lipid-lowering therapy (Zambon et al., 1999). The combined changes in LDL density, LDL cholesterol level, and HDL_2 cholesterol level accounted for one-half of the change in coronary regression with intensive lipid-lowering therapy in this study.

There are several genetic mechanisms to account for small dense LDL particles (see also section on central obesity and insulin resistance below). Low lipoprotein lipase and high hepatic lipase activities are associated with decreased HDL cholesterol. Recently, mutations in the lipoprotein lipase gene, which cause LPL deficiency in the homozygous state, have been related to LDL particle size (Hokanson et al., 1999). This relationship may be mediated by modest hypertriglyceridemia via cholesteryl ester transfer protein (CETP) activity. Variation at the CETP locus also has been linked to LDL size (Talmud et al., 2000). Additionally, a variant in the hepatic lipase gene promoter, which affects heparin lipase activity, has been shown to be associated with LDL peak particle density (Zambon et al., 1998). These common gene variants affecting hepatic lipase and CETP, as well as other factors, such as gender and central obesity, interact to affect both LDL and HDL particle heterogeneity.

FAMILY STUDIES IN CORONARY ARTERY DISEASE

Familial Aggregation Studies

Familial aggregation of coronary artery disease has been known for many years. Osler (1897) pointed out that angina pectoris might occur in several generations; Fogge (1872) referred to multigenerational occurrence of fatty deposits in both skin and coronary arteries and thus presumably described familial hypercholesterolemia. Many later studies showed the marked familial aggregation of CAD in families who were affected with autosomal dominant familial hypercholesterolemia (see below) (Thannhauser and Magendantz, 1938; Muller, 1939; Adlersberg et al., 1949; Wilkinson, 1950).

Yater et al. (1948) and Gertler and White (1954) both described familial aggregation in men with premature coronary heart disease. Similar observations were made among graduates of the Johns Hopkins University Medical School (Thomas and Cohen, 1955) and in the Tecumseh epidemiologic study of CAD (Deutscher et al., 1966). Rose (1964) noted a three-fold excess mortality from coronary heart disease among parents of affected males as compared with controls. In another U.S. study (Rosenman et al., 1975), the occurrence of coronary heart disease was significantly associated with a history of parental CAD. Slack and Evans (1966) studied the first-degree relatives of 121 male and 96 female index cases with CAD for premature mortality (male deaths before 55 years and female deaths before 65 years), as compared with the general population. Male relatives of male index cases had a 5-fold increase of mortality while relatives of female index cases had a 7-fold increase. Female relatives of male patients had a 2.5-fold increased risk over control females. These data suggest that because of the lower population frequency of CAD among younger females, more CAD-determining genes need to be present among premenopausal women for CAD to become manifest. Consequently, first-degree relatives of female index cases with CAD would be expected to carry more of these genes, making for a stronger familial aggregation.

Extensive familial aggregation studies of premature CAD (defined as being younger than 56 years of age) in Finland (Rissanen, 1979a, 1979b; Rissanen and Nikkila, 1977, 1979) showed a 3.5-fold risk for CAD in brothers of male CAD cases, and a 2-fold risk in their sisters. There were resemblances in the severity and mortality of CAD among the brothers. The risk for the probands' brothers increased with decreasing age of onset among index cases (relative risks: 11.4, for index cases younger than 55 years of age; 8.3, for those 46 to 50 years of age; 1.3, for men 51 to 55 years of age). Heritability studies suggested very high heritability for CAD with onset before the age of 46 years.

Familial aggregation of CAD was also observed in two studies where index cases had angiocardiographically proven CAD (Hamby, 1981; Shea et al., 1984). Angiocardiographic indices of severity of CAD correlated with the degree of familial clustering. More extensive and severe lesions were seen among patients with the strongest family histories (Berg, 1991b). In a study of over 200 patients younger than 55 years with myocardial infarctions in Colorado (Nora et al., 1980), the highest risk in a study of 19 different risk factors was associated with a "positive family history" of ischemic heart disease.

Data from Seattle showed 2-fold increase of myocardial infarction among first-degree relatives of male index cases younger than 60 years (ten Kate et al., 1982). Surprisingly, however, the frequency of myocardial infarction among first-degree relatives of the spouses of these index cases was increased to a similar degree to that of the first-degree relatives of the male index cases (ten Kate et al., 1984). This finding was explained by "assortative mating" of CAD cases with spouses who came from families with a higher frequency of the various environmental factors (lifestyle, diet, cigarette smoking, etc.) that predispose to coronary heart disease. The finding of a higher frequency of coronary heart disease among the spouses of affected CAD patients (Kannel, 1976) fits this interpretation.

An important aspect of family studies of CAD was the question of whether familial aggregation could be fully accounted for by familial concentration of the known risk factors such as hyperlipidemia, diabetes, and hypertension. The Finnish data (Rissanen, 1979a, 1979b; Rissanen and Nikkila, 1977, 1979) suggested that no additional risk factors needed to be postulated and that hyperlipidemia and hypertension largely explained the observed familial aggregation. In contrast, data from Michigan (Snowden et al., 1982), the state of Washington (ten Kate et al., 1984), and Colorado (Nora et al., 1980) suggested that familial aggregation of coronary heart disease was not accounted for by familial clustering of the then known coronary risk factors, which at that time did not include Lp(a), Apo B levels, or lipoprotein heterogeneity. Additional genetic or environmental risk factors, or both, were required to explain familial aggregation.

Twin Studies

Twin studies in CAD may be difficult to interpret since the diagnostic end points under study such as myocardial infarction and sudden death may occur several years apart. While affected identical twins may have similar degrees of coronary narrowing from CAD, the thrombotic event that causes sudden death or myocardial infarction may be random so that significant twin discordance might be recorded at a given time.

Estimates of concordance of myocardial infarction among Danish monozygotic (MZ) and dizygotic (DZ) twins were 39% and 26% among males and 44% and 14% among females (Harvald and Hauge, 1963). The corresponding figures for Swedish MZ and DZ male twins were 48% and 28% (Lilliefors, 1970). In another Swedish study (de Faire, 1974) the frequency of death from CAD and other causes was determined in MZ and DZ twins aged 46 to 70 years. When one male MZ twin died of CAD, 90% of the male co-twins died of CAD, but only 36% of male co-twins died of CAD if the index case died of another cause. In further extensive Swedish studies (Marenberg et al., 1994), the relative risk for CAD in co-twins increased with younger ages of death from CAD in both male and female MZ and DZ twins. At older ages, genetic factors seemed less important since the MZ/DZ relative risk ratio for CAD approached 1. Among male

DZ twins, the CAD rate among co-twins of index cases with CAD mortality was 68%, as compared with 55% for those who died of other causes. In a smaller Norwegian study, the MZ concordance for coronary heart disease was 66% with a DZ concordance of 25% (Berg, 1983). A small angiocardiographic twin study failed to show differences in the dominance pattern of the coronary arterial supply and the location of coronary lesions between MZ and DZ twins. Thus, the observed higher concordance in CAD in MZ twins appears independent of the anatomical distribution of the coronary blood supply (Frings et al., 2000).

Familial Aggregation: General Principles

- Familial aggregation is strongest with decreasing age of affected patients—that is, in premature coronary heart disease. Genetic factors appear less important in coronary heart disease in older patients.
- The lack of Mendelian inheritance in most cases of coronary heart disease, a higher frequency in MZ twins compared with DZ twins, the 2 to 6 times increased familial aggregation among affected patients, and the definitive role of the environment such as smoking and diet in predisposing to coronary heart disease establish CAD as a multifactorial or complex disorder. An elucidation of various genetic factors requires a search for specific genes and their interaction with each other and the environment.
- Familial aggregation does not necessarily imply genetic determination. Families may share similar environments such as diets that are associated with a higher frequency of coronary heart disease in family members. A variety of dietary, epidemiologic, and genetic studies points out that a significant component of familial aggregation is mediated by environmental factors shared by families. Furthermore, there may be genetic–environmental interaction so that different genotypes may react differently to various environmental influences such as diet.
- A family history of premature coronary heart disease regardless of the nature of the various genetic and environmental factors that make for familial aggregation identifies high-risk individuals and families and should trigger further investigation.

GENETIC APPROACHES TO CORONARY ARTERY DISEASE

The origin of coronary atherosclerosis is multifactorial. The role of the different factors involved will vary between individuals and families. A definitive monogenic disorder such as familial hypercholesterolemia (FH) (see below) and a putative oligogenic condition such as familial combined hyperlipidemia (FCHL) accounted for 24% (FH 4%, FCHL 20%) of patients with premature myocardial infarction (younger than 60 years of age) (Goldstein et al., 1973). In such families, a characteristic family history of premature CAD can often be detected. However, in most cases of coronary heart disease, even though familial aggregation may occur, Mendelian transmission does not apply. The phenotype of CAD itself is far removed from gene action, which makes analysis difficult. A potentially useful approach for genetic analysis is not to use the diagnosis of CAD as the criterion but to investigate the possible genetic causes that underlie the various risk factors for CAD. The various lipid factors that cause hyperlipidemia are key candidates for such "intervening phenotypes." While a single genetic defect, as in familial hypercholesterolemia, may occasionally outweigh other etiologic factors, the participation of several genes interacting with environmental factors and with each other is more frequent.

Association Studies

Association studies of CAD with polymorphisms or genetic markers have often been done. This type of work was first carried out with a variety of blood groups and protein polymorphisms in a "blind" study for possible associations. Sing and Orr (1976) studied plasma cholesterol levels in 12 randomly selected blood group and protein markers. They found significant association for the ABO, nonsecretor, haptoglobin, and Gm genes. Carriers of the A allele, nonsecretors, Hp2, and Gm A, had higher cholesterol levels. On average, differences between high and low phenotypes ranged between 4 and 6 mg/dl. The causal relation between these polymorphisms and cholesterol is still unknown. A variety of other studies have identified a higher frequency of type A of the ABO blood group system in coronary thrombosis and myocardial infarction (rates of type A/O = 1.4) (Mourant et al., 1978).

More recently, monogenic DNA polymorphisms or markers have been studied in patients with hyperlipidemia or coronary heart disease, compared to matched controls (Deeb et al., 1986; Hegele and Breslow, 1987; Humphries, 1988; Fisher et al., 1989; Lusis, 2000). Such an approach has the highest chance of success in investigations of markers that are biologically related to the trait under study (Cooper and Clayton, 1988). A DNA variant of a lipid-related gene such as apolipoprotein B is more likely to show an association with hyperlipidemia than a randomly selected variant. The rationale in association studies for CAD is the existence of very close linkage of the marker gene to a mutation predisposing to CAD, such as that of an apolipoprotein gene. There must be linkage disequilibrium between the marker and the mutant gene on the same chromosome to allow cosegregation or "hitchhiking" of the pair. Linkage of the two genes must be very tight so that recombination in the patient's ancestors must not have separated the disease gene of interest from the linked marker. In association studies comparing affected and nonaffected individuals, controls must be carefully matched ethnically since variation in DNA marker frequency between populations is common—even in similar populations—and may give spurious results. The study of subjects with hyperlipidemia for association with markers of lipid-related genes is more likely to give meaningful results than such a search among patients with coronary heart disease since not all patients with CAD have hyperlipidemia and therefore any possible association with lipid-related markers would be weakened.

Because many statistical comparisons are often carried out in a search for possible associations with many different markers, appropriate allowance must be made for the possibility of "statistically significant" findings that have no biologic significance. Thus, very high levels of statistical significance should be demanded before accepting the results of an association study as being biologically real, and the level of significance should consider the number of observations made. However, this adjustment will lead to some loss of statistical power. Ideally, a repeat association study should be carried out on a new population sample to determine whether the association still holds. A frequent reason for ambiguous results is mutational heterogeneity: that is, different, independent mutations of the candidate gene (or even of an unlinked gene) have produced the same functional effects. Under such circumstances, the test population is, in fact, heterogeneous for the underlying mutation so that the association only applies to a subset of this population. If an association study shows a suggestive association of a marker with a disease, the transmission disequilibrium test (TDT) (Spielman et al., 1993) can be used for further substantiation. The test requires families with at least one affected child. Transmission of the associated marker allele from the heterozygous parent to an affected offspring is then assessed.

Association studies on unrelated individuals can be done more readily than family-based genetic investigations such as segregation or linkage studies. A large amount of work has been done with DNA variants of various lipoproteins and other markers. For the reasons explained, the results often were ambiguous and associations could frequently not be confirmed. Because of the disappointing results from a large volume of such case-controlled association studies, any conclusions must be viewed critically. See Risch and Merikangas (1996) and Risch (2000) for further discussion of various approaches.

Currently, much attention is being given to association studies of complex diseases with single nucleotide polymorphisms (SNPs) (Schork et al., 2000). SNP variants are very common, occur about every 1000 nucleotides in the genome, and can be readily detected. If a putative disease gene is located physically very close to a given SNP at a chromosomal location, the two genes will be transmitted together and the presence of the SNP could be used to signal the presence of the linked disease gene. Various disease genes in a given complex disease are hoped to be identified by constructing dense SNP maps and studying patterns of SNP association in patients and ethnically matched controls. Success with the technique will depend on distance of the SNP to the disease gene, evolutionary age of the SNP and of the disease gene, and the structure of the population under study. Very large numbers of SNPs in patients and controls may be required, and successful gene detection may vary for different diseases.

Segregation Analysis

Segregation analysis is the study of possible modes of inheritance of a trait in families. Ideally, a large number of families are studied. Investigation of large kindreds may be useful, but the results may not necessarily apply to other affected families if there is genetic heterogeneity. Again, investigations of an "intermediate phenotype," such as hyperlipidemia, are likely to be more fruitful in a search for major gene effects than is use of the more remote diagnostic end point such as coronary heart disease with its multiple genetic and environmental genetic factors. A variety of programs are available to allow search for the nature of the transmission of quantitative traits and complex diseases (Lalouel et al., 1983; MacCluer, 1989). In complex segregation analysis, the family data obtained are fitted to a variety of models that include entirely environmental causation, polygenic transmission, dominant inheritance, recessive inheritance, and "mixed" models that have a major locus with polygenic and environmental determinants. The genetic model that best fits statistically the observed family data is considered most likely to apply. Segregation analysis is a powerful statistical method but cannot be considered the "gold standard" to prove the exact mode of inheritance. The results from such an analysis show only that a certain mode of inheritance is likely. Once a major gene effect has been suggested, chromosomal mapping studies and molecular investigations need to be carried out. However, while relatively uncommon monogenic subtypes of complex diseases (such as familial hypercholesterolemia) have been found, no definite genes have been identified in various complex diseases by following this approach.

Linkage Studies

Linkage studies in families are powerful if there is unequivocal monogenic inheritance of the trait to be mapped (Ott, 1985). Recent years have seen remarkable success with this methodology by study of cosegregation of a disease gene and a marker gene in families. Mapping has often been achieved by a search for linkage of the disease gene with one of many anonymous DNA markers spread over all chromosomes (Botstein, 1991). Many monogenic diseases have been localized by this approach, and the mutant genes have been cloned (positional cloning). Application of linkage methodology to complex diseases has been less successful for a variety of reasons, including "fuzzy" phenotypes and genetic heterogeneity of the underlying mutations. These biological uncertainties raise statistical difficulties in the interpretation of linkage data. Many investigations on linkage for complex diseases in recent years have applied sib-pair techniques using affected sibs rather than carrying out complete family studies. Search for cosegregation of a DNA marker and the disease gene are then looked for in the affected sibs. Mapping of genes for major psychiatric diseases (such as schizophrenia and affective disorders) were claimed, but additional studies have failed to confirm the early findings. Relatively rare "Mendelizing" subtypes of a disease have frequently been identified by the linkage approach, but genes involved in complex disease have not yet been isolated by the various linkage studies even though gene localizations have often been reported.

Animal Studies

Gene mapping in rodent and other animal models of various human complex diseases has been suggested. Once relevant genes are identified, search for the analogous human gene can be undertaken, but there is no guarantee that the involved gene in the animal model is also operative in the human disease. A useful approach has been the creation of "knockout" and transgenic mice where a human candidate gene is removed or inserted into mice by appropriate techniques. The resultant molecular, biochemical, and pathophysiologic abnormalities are then studied.

GENETICS OF LIPOPROTEINS AND APOLIPOPROTEINS

The major classes of lipoproteins of particular interest for the etiology of CAD are VLDL (very low density lipoprotein), IDL (intermediate-density lipoprotein), LDL (low-density lipoprotein), and HDL (high-density lipoprotein) (Havel and Kane, 2001). These designations refer to the ultracentrifugal density of various lipid fractions (see Table 7–1). The major lipoprotein genes and many other genes relevant to the hyperlipidemias have been cloned, and their chromosomal location is known (Lusis 1988) (Table 7–2). The various apolipoproteins have many similarities of structure and sequence. Many apolipoprotein genes appear to be derived from a common ancestral gene and are therefore members of a multigenic family. Intensive molecular, biochemical, and genetic work now attempts to elucidate the role

Table 7–1. Major Classes of Lipoproteins

Type	Density	Electrophoretic Behavior	Associated Apolipoprotein
VLDL	0.93–1.006	Pre-β	B-100, C1, C2, C3, E
IDL	1.006–1.019	Broad-β	B-100, C1, C2, C3, E
LDL	1.0019–1.063	β	B-100
HDL	1.063–1.210	α_1-lipoprotein	A1, A2, C1, C2, C3, D, E

VLDL, very low density lipoprotein; IDL, intermediate-density lipoprotein; LDL, low-density lipoprotein; HDL, high-density lipoprotein.

of the various genes in the pathogenesis of the hyperlipidemias predisposing to atherosclerosis (Lusis, 1988).

Familial Aggregation of Plasma Cholesterol

Possible genetic control of plasma cholesterol was initially assessed by searching for correlation of plasma cholesterol values among family members. Significant correlations for first-degree relatives (sibs, parents, and their children) but not between spouses were obtained (Mayo et al., 1969; Berg, 1983). MZ twins had a higher correlation than DZ twins (Berg, 1983). The heritability of plasma cholesterol values in twin studies ranged between 0.8 and 0.34, with an average value of about 0.5 (Sing et al., 1990). Thus about one-half of the variability of plasma cholesterol values can be ascribed to genetic variation. However, the various family and twin studies cannot provide insight into the nature and number of the underlying genes. The role of specific genes has emerged from more recent work.

Genetics of Apo B

Since Apo B is the principal protein constituent of LDL, there are strong correlations between levels of total cholesterol, LDL cholesterol, and Apo B (Albers et al., 1989). Elevated levels of all of these factors lead to increased risks for coronary artery disease (Brunzell et al., 1984). Since there is intrafamilial correlation for plasma cholesterol levels, the findings of familial resemblance of Apo B levels is not surprising (Tiret et al., 1990). The association with CAD is stronger for Apo B levels than for total cholesterol levels in some studies. A small but significant number of individuals have elevated Apo B levels with normal cholesterol levels (LDL cholesterol below 200 mg/dl) and have been designated as having hyperapobetalipoproteinemia (Sniderman et al., 1980; Kwiterovich, 1991). The genetics of this condition has not been defined.

Several studies have been done to search for major gene effects on Apo B levels. Segregation analysis in several studies suggested that a single major gene with an allele frequency ranging between 0.15 and 0.21 existed and was associated with elevated Apo B levels (Hasstedt et al., 1987; Pairitz et al., 1988). The effects of this gene were codominant. For example, putative homozygotes with two copies of this gene had mean Apo B levels that were 55 mg/dl higher than those of heterozygotes whose Apo B levels were 35 mg/dl higher than levels in individuals not carrying this gene. This Apo B–elevating gene is unrelated to the apo E polymorphism (Pairitz et al., 1988) and to familial hypercholesterolemia (Hasstedt et al., 1987). The nature of this gene has not been identified, nor has it been mapped. It would be reasonable to suspect that a major gene that raised Apo B levels might be a regulatory or structural variant located at or around the Apo B gene or might be a gene that regulates hepatic Apo B degradation.

Population association studies have uncovered a few generally confirmed associations of DNA variants at the Apo B locus with Apo B levels. Thus, individuals who possess a common DNA variant of the Apo B XbaI polymorphism have a higher total cholesterol, Apo B, and LDL cholesterol levels in most but not all populations of European origin (Berg, 1986; Talmud et al., 1987; Alto-Setala et al., 1988; Deeb et al., 1992). In some studies, triglyceride elevations have also been observed. The association of this Apo B variant with hyperlipidemia was also noted in patients with CAD. In studies in Seattle (Deeb et al., 1992), allelic effects of the putative Apo B–enhancing DNA variant caused increases of about 3 mg/dl and decreases of 3 mg/dl for its normal allele at this locus. The difference for total cholesterol levels between the two respective homozygotes was on average 19 mg/dl. This Apo B XbaI polymorphism is located within the Apo B gene and does not alter the amino acid sequence. This marker is unlikely to affect Apo B levels directly, but presumably lies close to an as yet unidentified mutation of

Table 7–2. Apolipoproteins and Other Lipid-Related Genes: Location and Function

Gene	Chromosomal Location	Function
Apolipoprotein gene		
Apo A1	11q	HDL function
Apo A4	11q	Unknown
Apo C3	11q	Unknown
Apo B	2p	Chylomicrons VLDL, IDL, and LDL formation; ligand for LDL receptor
Apo D	2p	Unknown
Apo C1	19q	LCAT activation
Apo C2	19q	Lipoprotein lipase activation
Apo C3	11q	Modulates hepatic uptake of remnant
Apo E	19q	Ligand for LDL receptor
Apo A2	1p	Unknown
Other genes		
Lp(a)	6q	Lp(a) particle formation
LDL receptor	19p	Uptake of LDL particles
Lipoprotein lipase	8p	Hydrolysis of triglyceride lipoproteins
Hepatic lipase	15q	Hydrolysis of LDL and HDL lipids
LCAT	16q	Cholesteryl esterification
Cholesterol ester transfer protein and phospholipid transfer protein	16q	Facilities transfer of cholesteryl esters and phospholipids between lipoproteins

the Apo B gene that affects Apo B levels by an unknown mechanism. The presence of an immunologically detectable variant of Apo B linked to the Apo B locus is fairly common in normal sera and also suggests existence of yet unidentified Apo B variants (Gavish et al., 1989). The Apo B mutation at residue 3500 (Soria et al., 1989) interferes with binding of Apo B to the LDL receptor and is discussed below as a monogenic trait that causes familial hypercholesterolemia.

Genetics of Apolipoprotein E

Polymorphisms of apolipoprotein (Apo) E have been detected in all populations that have been examined (for further references, see Davignon et al., 1988; Hallman et al., 1991). The most common Apo E is known as Apo E3, with cysteine at site 112 and arginine at site 158. Apo E2 has cysteine at both sites, while Apo E4 has arginine at both these sites (Table 7–3). The various types of E lipoproteins are specified by corresponding $\epsilon 2$, $\epsilon 3$, and $\epsilon 4$ alleles on chromosome 19. Six genotypes with their corresponding apolipoproteins exist ($\epsilon 2$ $\epsilon 2$–E2 E2, $\epsilon 3$ $\epsilon 3$–E3 E3, $\epsilon 4$ $\epsilon 4$–E4 E4, $\epsilon 2$ $\epsilon 3$–E2 E3, $\epsilon 2$ $\epsilon 4$–E2 E4, $\epsilon 3$ $\epsilon 4$–E3 E4). The standard $\epsilon 3$ allele frequency ranges around 0.75 in populations of European origin, whereas $\epsilon 2$ and $\epsilon 4$ have average frequencies of 0.1 and 0.13, respectively. Apo E3 binds with high affinity to the LDL receptor, whereas Apo E2 had much reduced binding to the LDL receptor. A decrease in conversion of VLDL to LDL and a compensatory increase of LDL receptor activity in the liver leads to reduced levels of plasma LDL cholesterol, total cholesterol, and Apo B in E2 carriers. Apo E4 is associated with elevated levels of LDL, Apo B, and cholesterol. The resulting differences in cholesterol levels for a single ϵ allele are shown in Table 7–3. On average, the $\epsilon 4$ allele raises cholesterol levels by about 7 mg/dl, whereas the $\epsilon 2$ allele diminishes cholesterol levels about 14 mg/dl. The average effects on the plasma cholesterol level for any given individual (who has two Apo E alleles) can be roughly predicted from the genotype and may be considerable. Thus in a French study, the average cholesterol level of E2 E2 homozygotes was 199 mg/dl, and that of E4 E4 individuals was 240 mg/dl. The highest $\epsilon 4$ allele frequency (0.226) is observed in Finland, where the highest cholesterol levels and CAD rates in Europe have been observed. A small but definite proportion (6%–14%) of the genetic variability of cholesterol levels in different populations, therefore, can be ascribed to the Apo E polymorphism. These effects on cholesterol levels in a U.S. midwestern population (Sing et al., 1990) are noted in Table 7–4. Apo E–related differences in cholesterol levels could translate to significant variation in coronary heart disease frequencies. However, data relating Apo E phenotypes with its effects on plasma cholesterol levels did not always correlate perfectly with CAD rates (Sing et al., 1990). Determination of Apo E type in individual patients is not usually done in the workup of coronary heart disease.[1]

Table 7–3. Apo E Polymorphisms

Allele	Gene Product	Composition	Frequency	Average Allelic Effect on LDL Cholesterol (mg/dl)
ϵ_2	E2	pos. 112:cys pos. 158:cys	0.109	−14
ϵ_3	E3	pos. 223:cys pos. 158:arg	0.760	−0.16
ϵ_4	E4	pos. 112:arg pos. 158:arg	0.131	+7

Table 7–4. Effect of Apo E Genotypes on Plasma Cholesterol Levels in Minnesota

Genotype	Population Frequency (%)	Average Cholesterol Levels (mg/dl) in Normocholesterolemic Men
ϵ_2 ϵ_2	0.46	133
ϵ_2 ϵ_4	3.15	183
ϵ_3 ϵ_3	59.5	192
ϵ_3 ϵ_2	12.7	182
ϵ_3 ϵ_4	23.9	193
ϵ_4 ϵ_4	0.9	207
All genotypes	100.0	191

Allele frequencies: ϵ_2, .08; ϵ_3, 0.78; ϵ_4, 0.14.
Adapted from Sing and Orr (1990) with permission.

Lp(a) Polymorphism

Lp(a) (Loscalzo, 1990; Utermann, 1989, 2001) is a glycoprotein attached to Apo B and was discovered by Berg in 1963. It is entirely unrelated to the HDL apolipoprotein A. Lp(a) is highly homologous to plasminogen (McLean et al., 1987), and the genetic locus specifying Lp(a) is closely linked to the plasminogen gene on Chr 6 (Weitkamp et al., 1988). There is remarkable 1000-fold quantitative variation in Lp(a) levels in the population. Most individuals have very low levels. There is a high degree of allelic heterogeneity at the Lp(a) locus, with more than 20 common alleles having been identified (Kamboh et al., 1991; Lackner et al., 1991). Most persons are compound heterozygotes at this locus and carry two different alleles. Each allele determines a specific number of multiple tandem repeats of a unique coding sequence known as Kringle 4. The size of the Lp(a) gene correlates with the size of the Lp(a) protein. The smaller the size of the Lp(a) protein, the higher the Lp(a) levels. However, not all variation of Lp(a) levels can be accounted for by the Kringle size polymorphism.

High Lp(a) levels are associated with coronary heart disease. About 30% of Caucasian patients with premature heart disease have levels about the 95th percentile of the normal population. In men with CAD who are younger than 60 years of age, the excess or attributable risk for coronary heart disease of an Lp(a) level in the upper quartile was 28% (Rhoads et al., 1986). The corresponding figure for men 60 to 69 years of age was 13%. Lp(a) has also been used to predict the severity of coronary heart disease. It has been suggested that much of the familial aggregation of early CAD in the absence of monogenic hyperlipidemia may be caused by high Lp(a) levels (Durrington et al., 1988). The risk appears to be additive with other risk factors so that elevations of both LDL and Lp(a) confer a higher CAD risk.

Lp(a) levels are unrelated to variation in total cholesterol, HDL cholesterol, triglycerides, Apo A-I and A-II, and homocysteine, and they appear to be a genetic trait that is already expressed early in life (Berg, 1991). All studies of Lp(a) and CAD

[1]It should be noted that the e4 variant increases the risk of late-onset Alzhiemer disease in heterozygotes (2–4×) and homozygotes (~20×). Determination of E4 status therefore becomes a sensitive matter and should only be carried out with fully informed consent.

risk have been done on Caucasian and Japanese populations. Among African Americans, the distribution of Lp(a) levels is less skewed, and an association between Lp(a) levels and coronary heart disease has not been demonstrated (Scanu, 1991).

The mechanism by which Lp(a) predisposes to coronary heart disease is not fully understood. There is a direct association between Lp(a) serum concentration and amounts of Lp(a) deposited in the arterial wall (Rath et al., 1989). In vitro studies suggest that Lp(a), because of homology to plasminogen, may be the link between atherogenesis and thrombosis and may promote thrombosis or interfere with thrombolysis and fibrinolysis or both (Scanu, 1991).

Lp(a) determinations are optimally carried out with quantitative immunoelectrophoresis or in a simpler manner with enzyme-derived immunoelectrophoresis or with enzyme-derived immunoabsorbant assays (ELISA) if care is taken to prevent cross reactions with plasminogen (Berg, 1991).

Genetics of Apolipoprotein AI

Isolated reductions of HDL cholesterol are not common, but familial hypoalphalipoproteinemia does occur (Tall et al., 2001). Recent studies suggest that obligate heterozygote relatives of individuals with Tangier's disease are an important part of this group. Different allelic mutations in the ABC-1 gene have been found in Tangier's disease (Hayden et al., 2000). Such heterozygote defects are uncommon and may cause premature CAD (Hayden et al., 2000; Wang et al., 2000). However, in the presence of low LDL cholesterol levels, low HDL cholesterol has not been demonstrated to be associated with CAD. In familial hypercholesterolemia, low HDL cholesterol is associated with early CAD among affected family members as expected (NIH Consensus Panel, 1993).

COMMON HYPERLIPIDEMIAS

Familial Hypercholesterolemia

Familial hypercholesterolemia (FH) is the best understood type of hyperlipidemia (Goldstein et al., 2001). The classic form of the disease is caused by a variety of different mutations that interfere with normal LDL receptor function, thereby raising LDL cholesterol and apo B levels. Individuals with a single LDL receptor mutation are heterozygotes and carry a normal LDL receptor gene as well. The frequency of such heterozygotes ranges around 1 in 500 in most populations that have been studied (Goldstein et al., 2001). The rare mating between two heterozygotes can give rise to children with homozygous familial hypercholesterolemia who have a very high cholesterol level (more than 600 mg/dl) and may develop CAD as adolescents or even earlier. Since the homozygous condition is very rare (about 1 in 1,000,000), it will not be discussed here.

Heterozygote FH can be detected by cholesterol determinations early in life—even in cord blood. The condition may not be associated with any physical findings if hypercholesterolemia is only moderately severe. Nonvascular clinical findings include xanthomas of the Achilles tendon and of extensor tendons of the fingers. Achilles tendon involvement is common and appears somewhat characteristic of FH. Its extent can be assessed quantitatively by ultrasound testing. Corneal arcus and xanthelasmas are relatively common, but not specific. The various fat infiltrates are caused by deposits of LDL-derived cholesteryl esters in tissue macrophages. Self-limited polyarthritis and tenosynovitis occasionally occur and are unresponsive to anti-inflammatory drugs.

The principal risk of familial hypercholesterolemia is the increased formation of atheromas, particularly in the coronary vasculature. Premature coronary heart disease with its attendant morbidity and mortality often results. About 50% of affected heterozygotes develop clinically manifest coronary heart disease by age 50 years in males and 60 years in females. Thus a significant proportion of heterozygotes, particularly women, are symptom free in middle age. The combined data from three European studies indicate that 75% of male, but only 25% of female, heterozygotes will be dead by age 70 years (Goldstein et al., 2001). Other risk factors for CAD interact with FH and make for worse CAD risks (Hill et al., 1991). Cigarette smoking (Williams et al., 1975) and low HDL (Stone et al., 1974) predispose to earlier disease. Patients with higher Lp(a) levels have more frequent CAD (Seed et al., 1990). A significantly increased frequency of cerebrovascular accidents and of transient ischemic episodes has been reported (DeGennes et al., 1968). The risk of brain infarction is 20 times higher than in a control population (Kaste and Koivisto, 1988). Carotid atherosclerotic lesions assessed by Doppler techniques were three to six times more frequent among FH heterozygotes than in controls (Davignon et al., 1991). Peripheral vascular disease may also be more common. Most published data overestimate the morbidity and mortality of FH since heterozygotes without visible fat deposits and only moderate hypercholesterolemia may not be diagnosed as being gene carriers.

The pathology of the atherosclerotic lesion in the coronary vessels of heterozygotes for FH has not been specifically studied. No investigations of the distribution of atherosclerotic lesions in FH compared with a control population of CAD patients without FH are available.

Basic Defect

Heterozygote FH is caused by one of many mutations that interfere with normal function of the LDL receptor (Hobbs et al., 1990). The receptor is a ligand for Apo B and Apo E. Receptors are synthesized in the endoplasmic reticulum and are transported to the Golgi apparatus. They then move to the cell surface, where they cluster in coated pits and are recycled to the endosomes of the cell.

The LDL receptor gene (Russell et al., 1986; Hobbs et al., 1990) is located near the tip of the short arm of chromosome 19. The LDL receptor gene spans 45 kb and consists of 18 exons and 17 introns. Its mRNA is 5.6 kb long and specifies 860 amino acids. This gene is a cardinal example of "exon shuffling" in that it shares DNA coding blocks with other genes, including those for blood coagulation factors IX and X, protein C, C9 complement, and epidermal growth factor precursor. LDL receptor mutations can be categorized into five classes: *(1)* null mutations due to large deletions, insertions, and nonsense mutations; *(2)* transport defect mutations due to defective processing of the receptor; *(3)* binding defect mutations; *(4)* internalization defect mutations; and *(5)* recycling defective mutations. Affected heterozygotes only have 50% of the normal number of receptors. Such mutations interfere with LDL and IDL binding, and the reduced LDL and IDL clearance leads to elevated plasma LDL and cholesterol levels with their attendant clinical manifestations.

Many different FH mutations have been encountered in an outbred population of varying origin such as in the United States (Goldstein et al., 2001). A smaller number of mutations will be expected in countries whose inhabitants have a more restricted range of ancestry. In populations derived from a relatively small founder group, only a few mutations will occur, and the population frequency of FH may be higher than the 1 in 500 among Caucasians and Japanese. Thus in South Africans of Dutch origin (Afrikaners) the FH heterozygote frequency is 1:80 to 1:100 (Seftel et al., 1989), and 95% of mutations are accounted for by three different alleles (Kotze et al., 1991). The Afrikaner population is descended from about 2000 Dutch settlers who arrived in South Africa in the seventeenth and eighteenth centuries and have expanded to their current size of about 3 million individuals. Jews in South Africa are practically all of Lithuanian origin and arrived between 1880 and 1910. FH in this group has a high frequency (1 in 67) (Seftel et al., 1989) and can be largely ascribed to one mutation (Meiner et al., 1991). The current population of French Canadians of 5.8 million is descended from about 7000 French settlers who immigrated between 1608 and 1763. Five principal different FH mutations have been identified (Hobbs et al., 1990). One of these accounts for about 60% of all French Canadian mutations. However, only 80% of FH among French Canadians can be accounted for by the currently known five variants. In Finland, a characteristic deletion can be detected in over one-half of FH heterozygotes (Savolainen et al., 1991). In Lebanon, among Christians, FH appears to be common, and a single mutation has been identified several times. Its exact frequency remains unknown (Hobbs et al., 1990).

Familial Defective Apo B-100

A variant similar to familial hypercholesterolemia can sometimes be caused by a mutation that interferes with binding of apolipoprotein B to the LDL receptor (Innerarity et al., 1990). This is the "mirror image" condition of familial hypercholesterolemia due to LDL receptor mutations; the ligand Apo B itself is defective rather than its receptor. A CGG → CAG mutation at codon 3500 of Apo B affecting the receptor binding domain has changed a glutamine for an arginine residue and makes for markedly defective binding (3%–5% of normal) (Soria et al., 1989). This defect presumably is caused by severe distortion of the three-dimensional structure of the mutant Apo B. The condition is inherited as an autosomal dominant trait. Affected patients are heterozygotes. Several studies among U.S. and European whites suggest a frequency of around 1:500 to 1:1250, which is somewhat lower than that of FH (Innerarity et al., 1990; Tybjaerg-Hansen et al., 1998). The haplotype DNA pattern on which this mutation occurred was identical in eight unrelated individuals, suggesting common origin of all mutations for this defect (Ludwig and McCarthy, 1990). The average cholesterol level in heterozygotes was 269 mg/dl in the United States and 369 mg/dl in Europe (United Kingdom and Scandinavia) (Schuster et al., 1990; Tybjaerg-Hansen et al., 1990). The exact frequency of CAD remains unknown but probably is roughly related to cholesterol levels. Not unexpectedly, only European patients with the higher cholesterol levels had tendon xanthomas (Tybjaerg-Hansen et al., 1990). No physical findings were seen in the U.S. patients (Innerarity et al., 1990). No lipid abnormalities other than LDL cholesterol and cholesterol elevation are seen in patients with this defect. The phenotype of an adult man who was a compound heterozygote for both this defect and the LDL receptor defect of familial hypercholesterolemia was no different from that of other family members who had familial hypercholesterolemia alone (Rauh et al., 1991).

Polygenic Hypercholesterolemia

Familial correlations of cholesterol levels due to various genetic determinants suggest that some cases of hypercholesterolemia may be caused by the simultaneous presence of several cholesterol-raising genes. The Seattle study of myocardial infarct survivors classified individuals with an elevated cholesterol level and a distribution of cholesterol values among relatives that was shifted toward a higher mean level (Goldstein et al., 1973) to have *polygenic hypercholesterolemia*. Unlike in family members of patients with familial hypercholesterolemia who either were or were not affected, no bimodality was apparent. As various genes raising cholesterol levels are being elucidated, laboratory detection of their gene products is increasingly possibly. Polygenic hypercholesterolemia will become more clearly defined by the demonstration of specific alleles (such as the e4 allele of apo E and others) that are associated with higher cholesterol levels.

The frequency of polygenic hypercholesterolemia depends on the arbitrary cutoff (such as the upper 5th or 10th percentile) by which hypercholesterolemia is defined. The degree of cholesterol elevation will only be moderate, and no physical findings are expected. Environmental factors such as diet are likely to affect individuals with polygenic hypercholesterolemia more strongly, and the CAD risk probably is based on the severity of the hypercholesterolemia and on the presence of additional risk factors.

Familial Combined Hyperlipidemia

History and Definition

The genetic and biochemical defects in the common forms of hypertriglyceridemia—familial combined hyperlipidemia (FCHL) and familial hypertriglyceridemia (FHTG)—are unknown. FCHL was first described in the Seattle Myocardial Infarction Study in 1973 (Goldstein et al., 1973; see also Rose et al., 1973). In this study, patients under the age of 60 years who had survived for three months after a myocardial infarction (MI) and their families were investigated for lipid abnormalities. At least 11% of these MI survivors had a condition that was given the name of familial combined hyperlipidemia. This disease was characterized by increased triglyceride and/or cholesterol levels, which frequently varied within a single individual from time to time and could be detected in the proband and in some relatives. Apo B levels were found to be consistently elevated. Familial combined hyperlipidemia was also found in the Seattle Hypertriglyceridemia Study in families of individuals with hypertriglyceridemia, but no coronary artery disease, where relatives of probands with putative FCHL had twice the prevalence of MI than did relatives of individuals with FHTG or spouse controls (Brunzell et al., 1976). Note that the definite diagnosis of FCHL requires a family study among adult first-degree relatives. The prevalence of FCHL was also estimated in the Seattle Familial Atherosclerosis Treatment Study among males under the age of 60 with angiographically demonstrated coronary artery disease and elevated Apo B levels (Brown et al., 1990). Some 60% of these patients with Apo B levels above the 95th percentile of controls had FCHL, as shown by analysis of the lipid status in their families. About 15% of this study population had FH and 24% had elevations in Lp(a). Some elevation of Apo B occurs in one-third of patients with CAD. As much as 20% of premature CAD may be attributed to FCHL. The disorder has been reported in the United States, England, Canada, Finland, and Holland (Aro, 1973; Sniderman et al., 1980; Wojchechowski, 1991; Dallinga-Thie et al., 1997; De Graaf and Stalenhoef, 1998; Pajukanta et al., 1999).

Etiology and Pathogenesis

FCHL is typically characterized by an increase in triglyceride and cholesterol levels. The triglyceride is present in small VLDL and IDL, while the cholesterol is in small VLDL, in IDL, and in small dense LDL. All of these lipoproteins contain Apo B, the apolipoprotein consistently raised in FCHL. An individual's lipid pattern can shift from high triglycerides (TG) levels, to high TG and cholesterol levels, or to a high cholesterol level alone by shifting from one Apo B–containing lipoprotein to another cn a week to week basis.

The primary defect in FCHL appears to be caused by increased hepatic secretion of Apo B, presumably due to decreased hepatic degradation of Apo B (see Brunzell et al., 1995). In genetic linkage studies, the trait of increased Apo B levels in FCHL was not linked to the Apo B gene (Rauh et al., 1990). Insulin resistance with central obesity often has been found in FCHL (Hunt et al., 1989; Aitman et al., 1997; Bredie et al., 1997). Insulin resistance often is associated with hypertension, impaired glucose tolerance and dyslipidemia characterized by elevated triglycerides, increased amounts of small dense LDL, and a mild to moderate decrease in HDL_2 cholesterol. However, neither obesity nor insulin resistance accounts for the Apo B elevation in FCHL (Purnell et al., 2001). The genetic basis of central obesity and insulin resistance also is not known. However, central obesity and insulin resistance are major determinants of increased hepatic lipase activity, which leads to small dense LDL particles and decreased HDL_2 cholesterol (Brunzell and Hokanson, 1999).

A number of groups have performed linkage studies in families with familial combined hyperlipidemia. A locus on chromosome 1q21–q23 with a high LOD score was found in a genome-wide screen in Finnish families with FCHL and is convincing. This locus was linked to triglyceride and cholesterol levels in these families, but not to Apo B levels (Pajukanta et al., 1999). A homologous locus was found in a mouse model with hypertriglyceridemia (Castellani et al., 1998). However, the gene in both humans and mice is not yet known. Several candidate genes with modest LOD scores have been reported to be linked to small dense LDL particles in FCHL (see Aouizerat et al., 1999). Missense mutations in the LPL gene and in the AI, CIII, AIV cluster have been reported in a subgroup of individuals with one-half of normal postheparin plasma LPL activity (see Aouizerat et al., 1999).

The mode of inheritance of FCHL is best interpreted as an oligogenic or multigenic disorder. Additional genes are likely to be found to contribute to this phenotype.

Familial Hypertriglyceridemia

History and Definition

Familial hypertriglyceridemia (FHTG) was first clearly documented in the Seattle Myocardial Infarction Study. This common disorder appears to have autosomal dominant inheritance. Plasma triglyceride levels often are elevated in a parent and in half their offspring. LDL cholesterol levels often are low or normal, while HDL is triglyceride-enriched with depletion of HDL cholesterol (Brunzell et al., 1983).

Etiology and Pathogenesis

Individuals with FHTG have increased hepatic triglyceride synthesis with subsequent secretion of triglyceride-enriched, large VLDL. These individuals also have increased hepatic cholesterol and cholic acid synthesis (Angelin et al., 1987; Duane et al., 2000). Small bowel bile acid reabsorption is defective with decreased postprandial plasma bile acid levels. One of 26 probands was demonstrated to have a deletion in one allele for the ileal bile acid transporter gene (Love et al., 2001). Most individuals with FHTG have decreased message levels for this transporter gene in small intestinal absorptive cells (Duane et al., 2000). The decrease in plasma cholic acid appears to lead to the increase in hepatic triglyceride and cholic acid synthesis. LPL-related triglyceride removal and remnant lipoprotein catabolism are normal in most families with FHTG.

Comparisons of Genetic Hypertriglyceridemias

Both FHTG and FCHL are commonly expressed as dyslipidemia after late adolescence (Goldstein et al., 1973). However, children in some FCHL families may sometimes be affected with hyperlipidemia (Kwiterovich, 1991). Abnormal physical findings are uncommon in FHTG and FCHL. Occasionally, mild hepatomegaly is present and may be associated with hepatic fatty infiltration. Xanthomas of the skin are not seen with FHTG or FCHL unless other factors increasing triglyceride levels to over 2000 mg/dl are present. Individuals with FCHL tend to be centrally obese with its complications of insulin resistance, hypertension, and impaired glucose tolerance. Obesity seems not to be increased in FHTG (Brunzell and Bierman, 1977).

Premature atherosclerosis with onset of coronary disease in middle-aged men is common in FCHL. Coronary disease occurs prematurely in women as well, but about 10 years later than in men. Coronary disease occurs even earlier if an individual with FCHL is a smoker. In early studies, FHTG appeared to be associated with *premature* coronary disease (Goldstein et al., 1973), but recent long-term follow-up of families with FHTG has demonstrated increased CAD with hypertriglyceridemia in older patients (Austin et al., 2000).

Individuals with FHTG and FCHL have similar elevations in plasma triglyceride levels. Plasma total and LDL cholesterol and apolipoprotein B levels are higher in FCHL than in FHTG, but discrete cutpoints cannot be used to successfully distinguish these disorders. HDL cholesterol is only modestly reduced in FCHL. Paradoxically, HDL cholesterol can be much lower in FHTG, without an increase in premature coronary risk (Brunzell et al., 1983). This decrease is associated with a normal number of HDL particles. LDL particles are small and dense in FHTG and FCHL, but particle number is increased in FCHL. Hypertriglyceridemia is persistent in FHTG, while triglyceride-rich lipoprotein levels often change inversely with LDL levels in FCHL. A family history of premature coronary disease in a first- or second-degree relative suggests FCHL.

Many other conditions can lead to dyslipidemia similar to FCHL and FHTG. Central obesity with or without Type 2 diabetes is associated with dyslipidemia very similar to FCHL. Some antihypertensive agents (diuretics and beta blockers) can produce mild dyslipidemia. A phenotype, as seen in FHTG, can be found with oral estrogen replacement therapy, with alcohol intake, with Accutane or Zoloft therapy, and transiently on high-carbohydrate feeding (Chait and Brunzell, 1983).

Central Obesity and Insulin Resistance

The combination of central obesity, insulin resistance, hyperinsulinism, impaired glucose tolerance, hypertension, hypertriglyceridemia, low HDL cholesterol, and coronary artery disease has been noted to cluster in individuals and in families. This constellation has been called syndrome X (Reaven, 1988), the metabolic syndrome (Avogaro and Crepaldi, 1965), the insulin resistance syndrome (Haffner, 1996), the atherogenic lipoprotein phenotype (Austin et al., 1990), and the central obesity syndrome (Brunzell and Hokanson, 1999). This syndrome is thought to occur in 25% in normal men and premenopausal women (Austin 1988a,b; Reaven, 1988) in the Caucasian U.S. population. While the constellation of findings of "syndrome X" appears to be real, a genetic–epidemiologic analysis questioned the use of the term *syndrome*, which implies a non-random association of phenotypes related to a common genetic pathophysiology. The various findings in syndrome X did not meet this criterion and were ascribed to a combination of findings "attributable to first-order interactions" (Neel et al., 1998a, 1998b).

Computerized tomography demonstrates an accumulation of intra-abdominal, or visceral, fat in individuals with this syndrome (Despres et al., 1989; Fujimoto et al., 1994). Intra-abdominal fat appears to be the main adipose site accounting for insulin resistance and the resultant hyperinsulinism (Despres et al., 1989; Fujimoto et al., 1994; Tchernof et al., 1996). The amount of intra-abdominal fat accounts for a significant proportion of the gender dimorphism related to insulin resistance and dyslipidemia (Carr et al., 1999). Reduction of intra-abdominal fat by caloric restriction (Purnell et al., 2000) or exercise (Schwartz et al., 1992; Katzel et al., 1997) ameliorates insulin resistance and other components of the syndrome. The dyslipidemia of this syndrome consists of mild hypertriglycerdemia with reduced HDL_2 cholesterol in the presence of small dense LDL particles. Increased hepatic secretion of very low density lipoproteins leads to hypertriglyceridemia (Ginsberg, 2000). Central obesity and insulin resistance produce increased hepatic lipase activity (Brunzell and Hokanson, 1999), which causes LDL to be small and dense and HDL_2 to become HDL_3 by hydrolyzing lipids in these high-density lipoproteins.

Type 2 diabetes is often associated with central obesity and insulin resistance with resultant hyperinsulinemia. A defect in insulin secretion is present in those individuals who develop hyperglycemia (Kahn et al., 1994). First-degree relatives of individuals with Type 2 diabetes may have either decreased insulin secretion (as induced by glucose) or insulin resistance, or both. While the dyslipidemia in Type 2 diabetes is similar to that of the isolated central obesity syndrome, triglyceride levels tend to be higher.

CAD is related to the level of hyperglycemia in many cross-sectional studies. However, attempts to prevent CAD by lowering glucose have not been impressive (Seltzer, 1972; Abraira et al., 1995; Diabetes Control and Complications Trial Research Group, 1995; UKPDS, 1998). It is thought that components of the central obesity–insulin resistance syndrome other than glucose are the major predisposing factors for early CAD in diabetes (Brunzell and Hokanson, 1999).

Rare Genetic Hypertriglyceridemias

Rare genetic forms of hypertriglyceridemia have been classified by defects in specific proteins that regulate lipoprotein metabolism, such as lipoprotein lipase, apolipoprotein CII, hepatic lipase, and Apolipoprotein E. *Lipoprotein lipase deficiency* and *apolipoprotein CII deficiency* are autosomal recessive disorders that lead to severe hypertriglyceridemias due to the accumulation of dietary fat as chylomicrons in plasma (Brunzell and Deeb, 2001). Both disorders can present in childhood. Lipoprotein lipase deficiency has a prevalence of about 1 in 1 million; Apo CII deficiency is extremely rare. *Hepatic lipase deficiency* is also an extremely rare autosomal recessive cause with mild to moderate hypertriglyceridemia (Zambon et al., 2001). This disorder is unusual in that the elevation of triglycerides is due to triglyceride enrichment of particles in the intermediate-, low-, and high-density lipoprotein regions. Severe hypertriglyceridemia has been reported in some individuals with hepatic lipase deficiency. Premature coronary artery disease is common in this condition.

Chylomicronemia Syndrome

The chylomicronemia syndrome is the association of marked hypertriglyceridemia, including dietary fat as chylomicrons, with eruptive xanthomata, abdominal pain, paresthesias of the hands, and short-term memory loss (Brunzell and Deeb, 2001). This is a fairly common disorder in hospitalized patients. These findings all clear rapidly with reduction of plasma triglyceride levels. This syndrome is almost always due to the interaction of a common familial form of hypertriglyceridemia and an acquired form of hypertriglyceridemia. It is a much more common form of severe elevations in triglyceride than LPL or Apo CII deficiency. None of these severe hypertriglyceridemia seem to aggravate risk for CAD.

Remnant Removal Disease

Familial type III hyperlipoproteinemia (Mahley and Rall, 2001) is rarer (1:10,000) than the 1:1000 used as the definition of common disease and will only be discussed briefly. This adult type of hyperlipidemia is characterized by high cholesterol and high triglyceride levels caused by accumulation of remnant lipoprotein particles intermediate in characteristics between triglyceride-rich lipoproteins and LDL. There is an enrichment in apo E, and most patients have the homozygote ε2 ε2 genotype. Lipid infiltration of palms and soles is often seen, as are xanthomas of elbows and knees. Both CAD and peripheral vascular disease are common. The basis of the condition is usually due to coinheritance of homozygosity of the Apo ε2 allele, as well as the presence of any condition that causes hyperlipidemia, including familial combined hyperlipidemia and various acquired types of hyperlipidemia. About 1% of the population are ε2 ε2 homozygotes, but only about 1% of these individuals will carry the additional genetic or acquired factors that lead to full-blown type III disease.

OTHER ATHEROSCLEROTIC RISK FACTORS

Genetics of Risk Factors Other than Hyperlipidemia

Coronary heart disease is often seen in patients with normal cholesterol levels. While other lipids such as low HDL, high triglycerides, high Apo B, and elevated Lp(a) levels (see above) may occasionally be implicated, genetic factors affecting non-lipid mechanisms require attention.

How *hypertension* promotes atherosclerosis remains not fully understood, but there is agreement that hypertensives have about three times the frequency of atherosclerosis than normotensive controls (Doyle, 1995). Atherosclerotic changes are most notable in arterial sites exposed to high wall stress. While treatment of hypertension markedly reduces the frequency of cerebrovascular events, myocardial infarcts remain the principal cause of death in treated hypertensive patients. The combined presence of hypertension and hyperlipidemia occurs more frequently than by chance and is often accounted for by hypertension as a component of the central obesity–insulin resistance syndrome (see above). In elucidating the multifactorial pathogenesis of CAD, genetic determinants that predispose to hypertension may be operative and will interact with the various genetic and environmental factors predisposing to CAD. Similar considerations apply to *diabetes*, which is associated with a higher frequency of atherosclerosis (Manson et al., 1991). The genetic causation of Type 1 and Type 2 diabetes is polygenic. Apart from the genes involved in Type 2 diabetes associated with the central obesity–insulin resistance syndrome, the other genes predisposing to the common types of diabetes need yet to be identified.

Other pathophysiologic mechanisms involves in CAD that are potentially subject to genetic variation are various coagulation-related phenomena such as thrombogenesis, thrombolysis, and fibrinolysis, which affect thrombotic aspects of coronary disease as in myocardial infarction (Grant and Humphries, 1999). Elevated *fibrinogen* levels have been shown to be independent risk factors for CAD in several prospective studies (Ernst and Resch, 1993; Wang et al., 1997) and predict "all cause" and CAD mortality (Benderly et al., 1996). A polymorphism of the fibrinogen β-chain was found to be associated with increased fibrinogen levels and with familial myocardial infarction in an Italian study (Zito et al., 1997). Investigations with other fibrinogen polymorphisms have failed to show clear associations with fibrinogen levels and with CAD (Wang et al., 1997).

Two polymorphisms of coagulation *factor VII* (proconvertin) were claimed to reduce the risk of CAD in Italy in familial premature myocardial infarction patients (Iacoviello et al., 1998a,b). Another Italian study replicated these results (Girelli et al., 2000) and showed that these polymorphisms were major determinants of factor VII levels. Failure to replicate these results in other investigations (Lane et al., 1996; Doggen et al., 1998) has been ascribed to geographic variation in the frequency of these polymorphisms.

The *plasminogen activator inhibitor* (PAI-1) is the principal antagonist of fibrinolysis (see Kohler and Grant, 2000). A polymorphism (4G allele) of the PAI-1 gene is associated with ~30% increased levels of PAI-1 (Humphries et al., 1997) and was found to be associated more frequently with sudden cardiac death (77%) than with accidental deaths (68%) or mortality from other diseases (65%) (Mikkelsson et al., 2000). A meta-analysis of several other studies supported these findings (Iacoviello et al., 1998a).

Glycoprotein III (GP III a) is a cytokine that plays a key role in platelet aggregation and probably mediates intimal hyperplasia after endothelial injury. In a Finnish study, the presence of a polymorphism at the GP IIIa gene was associated with progression of CAD and with sudden death and myocardial infarction in middle-aged men (Mikkelson et al., 1999, 2000). Similar findings were noted in the United Kingdom (Carter et al., 1997) and in another Finnish study (Pastinen et al., 1998). In the Finnish investigation, the polymorphisms for both the 4G allele of the plasminogen inhibitor gene (*PAI-1*) and the *P1A2* allele of the glycoprotein III a gene were studied by array-based microsequencing. Concurrent carrier states of both gene variants caused a highly significant relative CAD risk of 4.5, which was higher than the individual risk for each of these polymorphisms. These data demonstrate that in complex diseases, analysis for several genetic variants is likely to be increasingly productive in elucidating the action of various genes in pathogenesis. Coagulation-related risk factors are unlikely to be found in CAD patients who do not have a thrombotic event, as in CAD without MI.

A variety of other polymorphic variants have been implicated in CAD. These include the insertion/deletion (I/D) variant of the angiotension-converting enzyme (ACE), the endothelial nitric synthase gene, the paraoxonase gene, and the heterozygote state for the C282Y gene that predisposes to hemochromatosis.

Most work has been done with the *angiotension-converting enzyme* (ACE) polymorphism. While suggestive results for association with various manifestations of coronary artery disease and an insertion/deletion polymorphism were frequently reported (Cambien et al., 1992; Mattu et al., 1995), large-scale population studies do not suggest any relationship (Lindpaintner et al., 1995). Absence of a relationship was further confirmed in mice that showed no effect on dietary-induced atherosclerosis with different ACE levels that were produced by manipulating ACE gene dosage (Knowles and Maeda, 2000). Analogous studies in model mice have been used successfully to demonstrate the role of other modifiers of atherosclerosis (Knowles and Maede, 2000).

Several polymorphisms of the *endothelial nitric synthase* (ENS) gene were reported to be associated with CAD in patients (Hibi et al., 1998; Hingorani et al., 1999; Stangl et al., 2000). Increased atherosclerosis (Knowles and Meade, 2000) in mice with ENS deficiency was consistent with the epidemiologic findings.

Paraxonase is an enzyme of unknown function that is a component of HDL. It has been postulated that paroxonase variants may alter the risk for coronary heart disease by clearing LDL of oxidized lipids in vivo (Heinecke and Lusis, 1998; Mackness et al., 1998). Several epidemiologic studies are consistent with this hypothesis, particularly in myocardial infarction with diabetes (Aubo et al., 2000; Imai et al., 2000), but other investigations did not confirm these findings (Cascorbi et al., 1999; Gardemann et al., 2000). However, knockout mice without paraoxonase activity were more susceptible to atherosclerosis than were their normal littermates (Shih et al., 1998).

It has been suggested that the heterozygote state for the typical C282Y polymorphism of the *HFE* gene that causes hemochromatosis in homozygotes occurs more frequently in patients with CAD (Roest et al., 1999; Tuomainen et al., 1999). Various data on the role of excess iron as a pathogenic factor in CAD have been invoked (Sullivan, 1999), but more data are required.

Homocysteine

Homocysteine has emerged as a risk factor for coronary artery disease as well as for cerebrovascular disease, peripheral artery disease, and venous thrombosis (Refsum et al., 1998; Robinson, 2000). It has been known for some time that homocystinuria—a rare inborn error of metabolism—is associated with thrombotic and atherosclerotic complications (see Mudd et al., 2001). Similar atherothrombotic disease was seen in several rare inborn errors of vitamin B12 metabolism and in severe methylene tetrahydrofolate reductase (MTHFR) deficiency (Mudd et al., 2001). All these conditions, despite different biochemical etiology, are characterized by very high levels of blood homocysteine. Based on these findings, it was suggested by McCully (1969) and later by Wilcken and Wilcken (1976) that lesser elevations of homocysteine—such as might be seen in heterozygotes for these conditions—would predispose to atherosclerosis. However, no definite association with vascular disease could be detected in a large family study of relatives of patients with homocystinuria (Mudd et al., 1981).

Many studies have been done in recent years to relate vascular disease (particularly CAD) to mild and moderate hyperhomocysteinemia (see Boushey et al., 1995). The combined data from a recent meta-analysis of 14 prospective studies show an odds ratio (OR) of 1.20 (95% confidence limits of 1.14–1.25) for CAD for 5 μmol/L homocysteine increments; the corresponding OR from retrospective data was 1.6 to 1.9 (Ueland et al., 2000). The difference between the prospective and retrospective data is explained because much of the homocysteine effect may be operative during short-term follow-up and less striking some years later.

A common polymorphism of the folic acid–related enzyme methylene tetrahydrofolate reductase (MTHFR) is found in the homozygote state (TT) in 10% to 15% of the Caucasian and Japanese populations and is associated with increased levels of homocysteine (~25%), particularly in individuals with suboptimal folate nutrition (see Rozen, 2000). However, a meta-analysis of 10 studies for CAD (Brattström et al., 1998) and 15 studies for venous thrombosis (Brattström and Wilcken, 2000) failed to show the expected correlation between the TT homozygote state for MTHFR and vascular disease. However, based on an odds ratio of 1.2 for homocysteine elevations in CAD (see above), it was argued that the known increase of homocysteine levels in homozygotes for the MTHFR polymorphism would give an odds ratio of 1.1 to 1.15, which could only be detectable with very large sample sizes that have not been achieved in most studies (Ueland et al., 2000). Furthermore, most investigations were carried out in European and American patients with good folate nutrition where increased homocysteine levels in MTHFR homozygotes are absent or less striking. Failure to exactly match the control population with patients by ethnicity may be another reason for the negative results since the frequency of the MTHFR polymorphism varies in populations (see Rozen, 2000).

While current data agree that increases of homocysteine levels are frequent in CAD, it has been suggested that homocysteine may not be a causal factor in vascular disease but might merely be a marker for atherosclerosis, possibly mediated by nephrosclerosis since kidney dysfunction raises homocystein levels (Brattström and Wilcken, 2000). Data including a relationship between homocysteine and preclinical atherosclerosis such as arterial intima-media thickness (IMT) (Malinow et al., 1993; Voutilainen et al., 1998; McQuillan et al., 1999), however, argue for a causal relationship. There is also excellent evidence that hyperhomocysteinemia interacts in a multiplicative manner with other CAD risk factors such as smoking, hypertension, and hypercholesterolemia (Graham et al., 1997), as well as with various thrombophilic polymorphisms (Green, 2000).

The homocysteine hypothesis is of potentially great medical and public health importance since folic acid supplementation (400 μg/day) reduces elevated homocysteine levels, regardless of origin (Clarke, 2000). Vitamin B6 (and vitamin B12 to a lesser extent) may also play a role. If homocysteine elevations per se are a causal factor in CAD, reduction of homocysteine levels might be expected to reduce CAD morbidity and mortality. Folate fortification of food (140 μg/100 g of food) was instituted in the United States in January 1998 to prevent neural tube defects during fetal development. If hyperhomocysteinemia is a true etiologic factor in vascular disease, a lower frequency of CAD in the United States might have occurred recently because of folate fortification but would be difficult to demonstrate. Clinical trials of CAD prevention by folate supplementation are needed and are largely being done in Europe where folate fortification of the food supply (which makes data interpretation difficult in the United States) has not been carried out. In the meantime, the potentially favorable effect of folate on cardiovascular health has been widely publicized in the United States, and folate supplementation with tablets (in addition to food fortification, which affects everyone) is increasingly practiced.

APPROACHES TO DIAGNOSIS

The diagnosis of CAD in its various manifestations uses many available diagnostic modalities, particularly coronary angiography. These cardiologic tests will not be discussed here. Since angiocardiography is associated with occasional morbidity and a rare death, a generally available noninvasive imaging test system to assess the presence or extent of CAD is desirable but does not yet exist.

The diagnosis of an underlying cause for CAD starts with the family history—particularly in patients with premature CAD. The various manifestations of early coronary heart disease (angina, sudden death, myocardial infarction) should be searched among family members and, if present, should lead to investigations for hyperlipidemia by initial testing for total and HDL cholesterol and triglyceride levels. If in the presence of familial CAD, cholesterol, triglyceride levels, and HDL are normal, testing of apo B and Lp(a) levels should be carried out to search for hyperlipidemias that may not be associated with hypercholesterolemia or hypertriglyceridemia. Determination of homocysteine levels may be useful. One might also consider evaluation of LDL heterogeneity as to size and density. HDL_2 cholesterol may contain the major antiatherosclerotic component of HDL, rather than HDL3. These measures are not routinely available in hospital laboratories, but reliable national laboratories now provide convenient services.

Diagnosis of Hyperlipidemic Conditions

Cholesterol elevations in *familial hypercholesterolemia* are often in the 99+ percentile (i.e., above 300 mg%) and are usually not associated with triglyceride elevation. LDL cholesterol and Apo B levels are increased, and Lp(a) levels are usually higher than in control populations (Seed et al., 1990), HDL usually is in the normal range. No practical biochemical tests exist to detect the LDL receptor defect, since all tests assaying for receptor activity show overlap with results of the normal population (Motulsky, 1989). In some populations with relatively few founders, such as French Canadians, Finns, Lebanese, South African Afrikaners, and Lithuanian Jews, only a few LDL receptor mutations are involved (see above), and search for the defect by direct DNA diagnosis is feasible using methodology that detects the specific mutation. The development of gene chips and of high-speed sequencing techniques in the future may make such testing possible. However, distinction between a benign polymorphic variant and a pathogenic mutation may be difficult.

Familial hypercholesterolemia can be readily diagnosed when a high cholesterol level, normal triglyceride level, tendon xanthomas, and a history of premature coronary heart disease are found in the patient and family members. With more moderate hypercholesterolemia, the diagnosis may be difficult; thus, differentiation from familial combined hyperlipidemia, familial cholesterol elevation due to defective Apo B-3500, and from polygenic hypercholesterolemias may not be readily possible. Hypercholesterolemia due to a defective Apo B-3500 lipoprotein can only be detected with DNA techniques that identify the characteristic mutation. It is likely that a certain number of patients with a diagnosis of familial hypercholesterolemia or polygenic hypercholesterolemia carry this defect.

Familial combined hyperlipidemia may present with hypercholesterolemia and hypertriglyceridemia, but hypertriglyceridemia or hypercholesterolemia alone is often seen, and the phenotype may vary from time to time. Apo B levels are elevated, and there are no LDL receptor abnormalities. A definite diagnosis cannot be made without family study. The diagnosis is usually suggested if there is either hypercholesterolemia or hypertriglyceridemia, or both, in at least two adult first-degree family members in addition to the dyslipidemia index case. Hypercholesterolemia is usually only moderate, and the high levels characteristic of FH are usually not seen. Tendon xanthomas are very unusual.

Familial hypertriglyceridemia is usually diagnosed when there are elevations of triglycerides in the absence of other lipid abnormalities, and a family study shows elevated triglyceride levels in other family members.

Assessment of CAD risk, regardless of diagnosis, is increasingly possible by testing for a risk profile including total, LDL, and HDL cholesterol; triglycerides; Lp(a) levels; and total homocysteine levels (Funke and Assmann, 1999). For large-scale screening, such a risk profile may be more useful and practical for CAD prediction than molecular tests, since data on *both* genetic and environmental factors are provided.

Population Screening

The testing scheme recommended by the U.S. National Cholesterol Education Program (National Cholesterol Education Program, 1988; Cleeman and Lenfant, 1998) urges massive cholesterol testing in the adult population, but no efforts are made to identify genetic factors affecting cholesterol levels. Such population-based surveys for lipid abnormalities raise many logistical and operational difficulties but have gained increasing acceptance. It has been suggested that identification of individuals at risk for CAD can be achieved by screening for cholesterol levels alone (National Cholesterol Education Program, 1988). Since cholesterol levels can be reduced by diet and drugs, the risk for CAD can be diminished and coronary heart disease can be avoided. According to the National Cholesterol Education Program in the United States, levels less than 200 mg/dl are considered desirable, values between 200 and 240 mg/dl are borderline, and levels above 240 mg/dl are considered abnormal. Follow-up is recommended for individuals with values above 200 mg/dl. Since a large fraction of the population would have to be followed, the practical consequences of instituting such schemes are considerable. Additional risk factors such as male gender, cigarette smoking, a family history of premature coronary heart disease, hypertension, diabetes, and central obesity must be considered before initiating cholesterol-lowering measures. Adults with borderline cholesterol results with two or more other risk factors, those with clinical premature arteriosclerotic heart disease, and individuals with cholesterol levels above 240 mg/dl are recommended for additional measurement of triglycerides, LDL, and HDL levels. Based on the LDL levels after such a work-up, initial dietary therapy is usually recommended. If there is no or little response to diet, therapy with an antihyperlipidemic drug can be considered.

The exact age at which testing should be started is somewhat arbitrary. Ideally, screening of men in their third decade or even earlier is appropriate since fatty streaks and occasional fibrous plaques can be observed in relatively young individuals. Since women develop coronary heart disease at a later age, testing might be considered about 10 years later.

Antihyperlipidemic therapy (similar to blood pressure–lowering treatment) requires that many people be treated to prevent a single coronary event (Cook and Sackett, 1995). Using various data on lipid-lowering treatment, it has been calculated that a large number of hyperlipidemics must be treated for 5 years to prevent a single myocardial infarction. However, treatment over longer periods would reduce these numbers to a more favorable ratio. Consideration of such data has made some observers question whether all-out population screening can be justified. The full assessment of population-wide cholesterol screening programs and their effect on morbidity and mortality will be awaited with interest.

Genetic Advice and Counseling

Family-oriented screening and counseling need encouragement and are recommended by all observers. The presence of premature coronary heart disease with hyperlipidemia should lead to a search for similar abnormalities among relatives who may require treatment. Identification of affected children, followed by dietary changes, may improve dietary compliance for the whole family.

Genetic advice in familial coronary heart disease is straightforward if a definite monogenic condition such as *familial hypercholesterolemia* is the underlying cause. Since affected patients are heterozygotes, the condition will have been inherited from one parent, and 50% of sibs of both sexes on the average will be affected. There is a 50% chance that children will carry the condition. Patients and their families should be advised about these risks, the natural history of FH, and the availability of effective treatment. Once a diagnosis of FH is suspected, it is mandatory to initiate testing among those most at risk to develop CAD in the near future—usually the patient's sibs. Because of an earlier age of onset in males, initial attention should be given to brothers, but sisters should not be neglected. Both parents should also be tested. Often the affected patient will have already exhibited some of the findings of coronary heart disease. Children in FH families need to be screened for cholesterol levels since early attention to reduction of hypercholesterolemia is likely to prevent coronary artery disease. Findings of elevated cholesterol and LDL cholesterol levels among affected relatives will usually make the diagnosis, and more complicated tests are not required.

Counseling for *familial combined hyperlipidemia* presents more difficulties. A search for abnormalities among adult sibs has the highest priority in view of the significant risk for coronary heart disease and the feasibility of treatment of the various lipid abnormalities. Since the condition or at least some of its components may be transmitted as an autosomal dominant trait, advice regarding a possible 50% risk among offspring should be given. Appropriate lipid testing needs to be carried out, keeping in mind that the detectable lipid abnormalities may not be apparent in children and young adults. *Familial hypertriglyceridemia* without other lipid abnormalities and in the absence of a family history for premature CAD appears to carry less CAD risk.

If a diagnosis of a specific hyperlipidemia cannot be made, family screening will still be worthwhile since relatives frequently will have lipid abnormalities. Most lipid abnormalities aggregate in families, even though the exact mode of inheritance is uncertain. Thus a search to identify other family members is helpful since treatment by diet and increasingly by drugs is often possible.

Lp(a) elevations are usually caused by the compound heterozygous state for two of many different Lp(a) variants that raise Lp(a) levels. A search for high Lp(a) levels in patients and relatives is useful for definition of the CAD risk profile of the tested individual. Some individuals may have high Lp(a) values in the absence of other kinds of hyperlipidemia. Lp(a) determination therefore should be part of the work-up in families with premature coronary heart disease. Members of the families with premature coronary heart disease in the absence of any lipid abnormalities are at significantly increased risk, but no definite risk figures can be quoted.

SOME PROBLEMS OF TREATMENT

A discussion of the treatment of coronary heart disease is beyond the scope of this chapter and is fully covered in textbooks of medicine and cardiology. However, management of a major risk factor for CAD that is best understood—hyperlipidemia—will be briefly considered. Therapy by a diet low in saturated fatty acids and low in cholesterol is initially recommended, and various dietary regimens are widely available (Krauss et al., 2000). There is considerable variability in response of individuals to such diets. The reasons are poorly understood since few human data exist. The mechanisms that govern such variability remain largely unknown, but it is likely that genetic factors are involved. Various studies suggest that a mean reduction of 10% to 15% in cholesterol levels may usually be achievable by diet (Krauss et al., 2000). However, dietary measures alone will not reduce cholesterol levels sufficiently in many patients with genetic hyperlipidemia, and drug therapy is often prescribed. Most patients with familial hypercholesterolemia will require medicinal therapy. Med Ped is an international program to detect and treat all individuals with FH through tracing of relatives. With this approach, some 5 to 15 new cases can often be detected, and effective lipid-lowering treatment that prevents CAD can be initiated (Williams et al., 1999, 2000). Treatment should be started at a relatively early age. There is no definite agreement whether children should be treated with drugs. Drug treatment (Schonfeld, 1991; Goldstein et al., 2001) starting in late adolescence presumably is appropriate.

Often the low-dose combination of a resin with a statin or niacin can be quite effective. Currently most drugs are used somewhat empirically (see Knopp, 1999), although the statins have become the accepted initial treatment for heterozygous FH. There is no accepted treatment for high Lp(a) levels, so that management of other existing lipid abnormalities (such as high cholesterol levels) becomes particularly important. The combined presence of high Lp(a) levels and cholesterol elevations increases the CAD risk and makes preventive measures important. The response to statin therapy in individuals with CAD is blunted in those who have at least one copy of the rare Taq 1B allele for the cholesteryl ester transfer protein (CETP) gene (Kuivenhoven et al., 1998). Similarly, individuals with the hepatic lipase promoter variant C-514 T on intensive lipid-lowering therapy have diminished CAD regression by coronary angiography (Zambon et al., 2001).

The need to consider *all* risk factors for CAD when initiating drug therapy against hyperlipidemia is important. Simplistic use of various algorithms for one risk factor such as hypercholesterolemia alone is not sufficient. Many other preventive measures—including weight reduction, cessation of smoking, careful attention to blood pressure control, and possible frequent use of small doses of aspirin—to prevent coronary thrombosis must be carried out. As the understanding of various hyperlipidemias and other CAD risk factors improves, it is likely that management will become less empirical and more specifically directed at the underlying basic defects.

One of the early attempts at *gene therapy* involved young individuals homozygous for the LDL receptor defect in familial hypercholesterolemia (Wilson and Chowdrory, 1990) by injecting autologous hepatocytes with normal LDL receptors. Although a transient decrease in LDL cholesterol was seen, an immunological response eliminated the new LDL receptors. The potential for gene therapy exists in the monogenic hyperlipidemias but awaits the development of better understanding of the underlying defects and of novel techniques to make this approach both safe and effective. However, gene therapy directed at reduction in size of the local lesions in coronary artery disease, regardless of etiology, is under active study.

CONCLUDING ASSESSMENT

- Coronary artery disease (CAD) is a common multifactorial disease. Males are more frequently affected, but sex differences diminish with advancing age. The disease occurs widely in many different populations and is a major cause of mortality. The mortality of CAD has declined in the United States in recent decades, partially because of nutritional (e.g., dietary fat) and lifestyle (e.g., less smoking) factors.
- The condition is caused by atherosclerotic obstruction of the coronary arteries. The underlying pathologic lesion is a fibrous plaque that becomes infiltrated by lipids. Coronary heart disease is a result of both environmental and genetic factors. Environmental factors can be shown by an increasing frequency of CAD among migrants who move to high-prevalence areas during a time period that is incompatible with genetic changes.
- Familial aggregation and twin data indicate that genetic factors play an important role in the pathogenesis of CAD. Familial aggregation is strongest with premature CAD (younger than 60 years) and cannot be fully accounted for by dyslipidemia, hypertension, or diabetes. Additional genetic and environmental factors including increased plasminogen activator inhibitor-1 and increased homocysteine levels contribute to familial aggregation. A positive "family history" for premature CAD is a strong risk factor by itself.
- Evidence from animal experimentation, epidemiologic studies, clinical correlations, genetic hyperlipidemias, and therapeutic trials indicate that lipids play a key role in the pathogenesis of CAD. Specifically, a high level of low-density lipoprotein (LDL) cholesterol and a low level of high-density lipoprotein (HDL) are strong risk factors.

- Approaches to the genetics of CAD include familial correlation studies with blood lipids, association studies with various genetic markers, segregation analysis searching for major genes, and linkage analysis to map the genes involved in pathogenesis. Most attention has been given to various hyperlipidemias and the underlying apolipoprotein defects.
- Cholesterol levels are correlated among family members but not in spouses. About 50% of the variability of plasma cholesterol is genetic in origin. A certain proportion of this variation can be accounted for by two alleles of the Apolipoprotein E locus that increase (E4) and decrease (E2) cholesterol levels, respectively. Polygenic hypercholesterolemia is the result of segregation of various genes raising cholesterol levels. It can be inferred that such genes contribute to the pathogenesis of CAD.
- HDL levels are genetically influenced, as shown by various family and twin studies. HDL levels are related to apolipoprotein A1 function, but only very rare mutations affecting this apolipoprotein and HDL levels have been reported. Polymorphisms at the apolipoprotein A1-C3 locus are often associated with hypertriglyceridemia. Mutations in a cell surface protein ABC-1 lead to lower HDL-C via a defect that decreases cellular cholesterol efflux.
- Apo(a) is an apoprotein attached to apolipoprotein B and forms Lp(a). High Lp(a) levels predispose to CAD and are an independent risk factor for CAD. Many Lp(a) alleles exist, and the structure of the Lp(a) gene can be related to Lp(a) plasma levels.
- Familial hypercholesterolemia is an autosomal dominant condition that strongly predisposes to CAD, particularly in men. Many different LDL receptor mutations can cause this condition. A specific mutation of apolipoprotein B (APO B-3500) leads to defective binding to the LDL receptor and also can cause familial hypercholesterolemia.
- Familial combined hyperlipidemia (FCHL) is a common condition (population frequency about 1%) manifesting with either hypercholesterolemia or hypertriglyceridemia, or with both conditions, in adults. Inheritance of elevated apolipoprotein levels appears to be autosomal dominant but has not definitely been proven by formal genetic analysis. The condition is associated with increased apolipoprotein B synthesis and is often accompanied by central obesity or diminished lipoprotein lipase activity. The basic defect or defects are unknown.
- Familial hypertriglyceridemia without other lipid abnormalities may occur, and autosomal dominant inheritance has been suggested but is not certain. Atherosclerosis is associated with this hypertriglyceridemia in older affected individuals. Most individuals have defects in the intestinal reabsorption of bile acids.
- Apolipoprotein B levels are usually correlated with total cholesterol and LDL cholesterol levels, but occasionally raised Apo B concentrations without an elevation in LDL cholesterol may be encountered. This condition has been called hyperapobetalipoproteinemia. The relation of this condition to a proposed major gene that raises Apo B levels and to familial combined hyperlipidemia (FHCL) needs further definition.
- A hyperlipidemic state should be suspected in premature CAD and is often associated with a family history of CAD. The specific diagnosis of autosomal dominant familial hypercholesterolemia may be difficult when hypercholesterolemia is only moderate and Achilles tendon xanthomas are lacking. Direct DNA methodology for the diagnosis of familial hypercholesterolemia is becoming available. The diagnosis of familial combined hyperlipidemia (FCHL) usually requires study of multiple family members. No pathognomonic diagnostic tests exist to be definitely certain about the diagnosis of FHCL in a single individual. Determinations of LDL, HDL, and Lp(a) are useful to define CAD risks and are recommended in the work-up of all patients with premature CAD and with hyperlipidemia, as well as in their family members. Apolipoprotein B determinations are emerging as a possible addition to LDL and HDL cholesterol testing.
- Wide-scale screening for hyperlipidemia in primary care settings using cholesterol determination has been proposed for adults. Since cholesterol levels above 200 mg/dl (the suggested cutoff for a desirable cholesterol level) are common, such programs raise major logistical problems regarding follow-up and appropriate management of identified hyperlipidemic persons. No attempts are usually made to distinguish genetic from environmental factors of hypercholesterolemia in such screening since a genetic classification is not required for lipid-lowering treatment.
- The search for hyperlipidemia in family members of patients with premature coronary heart disease has a high yield and is strongly recommended. Advice regarding risk can be given to affected relatives, and appropriate management can be started to prevent CAD.
- Management of hyperlipidemia uses low–saturated fat and low-cholesterol diets as the first step. In many of the genetic types of hyperlipidemia, additional drug therapy with antihyperlipidemic agents is indicated. Reduction of cholesterol levels and improvement of lipid profiles has been shown to decrease coronary atherosclerosis and to diminish the frequency of clinically manifest CAD. Currently, the various treatment regimens are used empirically—usually without attempts at genetic classification of the underlying condition.

REFERENCES

Abraira C, Colwell JA, Nuttall FQ, Sawin CT, Nagel NJ, Comstock JP: Veterans affairs cooperative study on glycemic control and complications in Type II diabetes (VA CSDM). Diabetes Care 1995; 18:1113–1123.

Adlersberg D, Parets AD, Boas EP: Genetics of atherosclerosis: studies of families with xanthoma and unselected patients with coronary artery disease under the age of fifty years. JAMA 1949; 141:246.

Agerholm-Larsen B, Nordestgaard BG, Steffensen R, Jensen G, Tybjaerg-Hansen A: Elevated HDL cholesterol is a risk factor for ischemic heart disease in white women when caused by a common mutation in the cholesteryl ester transfer protein gene. Circulation 2000; 101:1907–1912.

Aitman TJ, Godsland IF, Farren B, Crook D, Wong HJ, Scott J: Defects of insulin action on fatty acid and carbohydrate metabolism in familial combined hyperlipidemia. Arterioscler Thromb Vasc Biol 1997; 17:748–754.

Albers JJ, Brunzell JD, Knopp RH: Apoprotein measurements and their clinical application. Clin Lab Med 1989; 9:137–152.

Albert MA: The role of c-reactive protein in cardiovascular disease risk. Curr Cardiol Rep 2000; 2:274–279.

Almasy L, Hixson JE, Rainwater DL, Cole S, Williams JT, Mahaney MC, VandeBerg JL, Stern MP, MacCluer JW, Blangero J: Human pedigree-based quantitative-trait-locus mapping: localization of two genes influencing HDL-cholesterol metabolism. Am J Hum Genet 1999; 64:1686–1693.

Alto-Setala K, Tikkanen MJ, Taskinen MR, Nieminen M, Holmberg P, Kontula K: XbaI and c/g polymorphisms of the apolipoprotein B gene locus are associated with serum cholesterol and LDL-cholesterol levels in Finland. Atherosclerosis 1988; 74:65–74.

Angelin B, Hershon KD, Brunzell JD: Bile acid metabolism in hereditary forms of hypertriglyceridemia: evidence for an increased synthesis rate in monogenic familial hypertriglyceridemia. Proc Natl Acad Sci USA 1987; 84:5434–5438.

Anitschkow N, Chalatow S: Über experimentelle Cholesterinsteatose and ihre Bedeutung für die Entstehung einiger pathologischer Prozesse. Zentralbl Allg Pathol Pathol Anat 1913; 24:1–9.
Aouizerat BE, Allayee H, Bodnar J, Krass KL, Peltonen L, de Bruin TWA, Rotter JI, Lusis AJ: Novel genes for familial combined hyperlipidemia. Curr Opin Lipidol 1999; 10:113–122.
Aubo C, Senti M, Marrugat J, Tomas M, Vila J, Sala J, Masia R: Risk of myocardial infarction associated with Gln/Arg 192 polymorphism in the human paraoxonase gene and diabetes mellitus. The REGICOR Investigators. Eur Heart J 2000; 21:33–38.
Austin MA: Plasma triglyceride and coronary heart disease. Arterioscler Thromb 1991; 11:2–14.
Austin MA, Breslow JL, Hennekens CH, Buring JE, Willett WS, Krauss RM: Low-density lipoprotein subclass pattern and risk of myocardial infarction. JAMA 1988a; 260:1917–1921.
Austin MA, King M-C, Vranizan KM, Krauss RM: Atherogenic lipoprotein phenotype: a proposed genetic marker for coronary heart disease risk. Circulation 1990; 82:495–506.
Austin MA, King M-C, Vranzian KM, Newman B, Krauss RM: Inheritance of low-density lipoprotein subclass patterns: results of complex segregation analysis. Am J Hum Genet 1988b; 43:838–846.
Austin MA, McKnight B, Edwards KL, Bradley CM, McNeely MJ, Psaty BM, Brunzell JD, Motulsky AG: Cardiovascular disease mortality in familial forms of hypertriglyceridemia: a 20-year prospective study. Circulation 2000; 101:2777–2782.
Avogaro P, Crepaldi G: Essential hyperlipidemia, obesity and diabetes. Diabetologia 1965; 1:137.
Barter P: CETP and atherosclerosis. Arterioscler Thromb Vasc Biol 2000; 20:2029–2031.
Beaglehole R: International trends in coronary heart disease mortality, morbidity and risk factors. Epidemiol Rev 1990; 12:1–15.
Benderly M, Graff E, Reicher-Reiss H, Behar S, Brunner D, Goldbourt U: Fibrinogen is a predictor of mortality in coronary heart disease patients. The Bezafibrate Infarction Prevention (BIP) Study Group. Arterioscler Thromb Vasc Biol 1996; 16:351–356.
Benditt EP, Benditt JM: Evidence for a monoclonal origin of human atherosclerotic plaque. Proc Natl Acad Sci USA 1973; 70:1753.
Berg K: A new serum type system in man—the Lp system. Acta Pathol Microbiol Scand 1963; 59:369–382.
Berg K: Genetics of coronary heart disease. Prog Med Genet 1983; 5:35–90.
Berg K: DNA polymorphism at the apolipoprotein B locus is associated with lipoprotein level. Clin Genet 1986; 301:515–520.
Berg K: An overview of the genetics of coronary heart disease and its risk factors. In: Genetic Approaches to Coronary Heart Disease and Hypertension. Berlin: Springer-Verlag, 1991a:98–109.
Berg K: Atherosclerosis and coronary artery disease. In: Nora JJ, Berg K, Nora AH (eds). Cardiovascular Diseases: Genetics, Epidemiology and Prevention. New York: Oxford University Press, 1991b:3–40.
Botstein D: Linkage genetics in humans: origins and prospects. In: Lindsten J, Pettersson U (eds). Etiology of Human Disease at the DNA Level. New York: Raven Press, 1991:3–11.
Boushey CJ, Beresford SAA, Omenn GS, Motulsky AG: A quantitative assessment of plasma homocysteine as a risk factor for vascular disease: probable benefits of increasing folic acid intakes. JAMA 1995; 274:1049–1057.
Brattström L, Wilcken DEL: Homocysteine and cardiovascular disease: cause or effect? Am J Clin Nutr 2000; 72:315–323.
Brattström L, Wilcken DEL, Öhrvik J, Brudin L: Common methylenetetrahydrofolate reductase gene mutation leads to hyperhomocysteinemia but not to vascular disease: the result of a meta-analysis. Circulation 1998; 98:2520–2426.
Bredie SJ, Demacker PN, Stalenhoef AF: Metabolic and genetic aspects of familial combined hyperlipidaemia with emphasis on low-density lipoprotein heterogeneity. Eur J Clin Invest 1997; 27:802–811.
Brown G, Albers JJ, Fisher LD, Schaefer SM, Lin JT, Kaplan C, Zhao XQ, Bisson BD, Fitzpatrick VF, Dodge HT: Regression of coronary artery disease as a result of intensive lipid-lowering therapy in men with high levels of apolipoprotein B. N Eng J Med 1990; 323:1289–1298.
Brunzell JD, Albers JJ, Chait A, Grundy SM, Groszek E, McDonald GB: Plasma lipoproteins in familial combined hyperlipidemia and monogenic familial hypertriglyceridemia. J Lipid Res 1983; 24:147.
Brunzell JD, Austin MA, Deeb SS, Hokanson JE, Jarvik GP, Nevin DN, Wijsman E, Zambon A, Motulsky AG: Familial combined hyperlipidemia and genetic risk for atherosclerosis. In: Woodford FP, Davignon J, Sniderman A (eds). Atherosclerosis X. New York: Elsevier, 1995:624–627.
Brunzell JD, Bierman EL: Plasma triglyceride and insulin levels in familial hypertriglyceridemia. Ann Intern Med 1977; 87:198–199.
Brunzell JD, Deeb SS: Familial lipoprotein lipase deficiency, apo CII deficiency and hepatic lipase deficiency. In: Scriver CR, Beaudet AI, Sly WS, Valle D, Childs B, Kinzler KW, Vogelstein B (eds). The Metabolic and Molecular Basis of Inherited Disease, 8th ed. New York: McGraw-Hill, 2001:2789–2816.
Brunzell JD, Hokanson JE: Dyslipidemia of central obesity and insulin resistance. Diabetes Care 1999; 22(suppl. 3):C10.
Brunzell JD, Schrott HG, Motulsky AG, Bierman EL: Mycardial infarction in the familial forms of hypertriglyceridemia. Metabolism 1976; 25:313–320.
Brunzell JD, Sniderman AD, Albers JJ, Kwiterovich PO Jr: Apoproteins B and A-1 and coronary artery disease in humans. Atherosclerosis 1984; 4:79–83.
Cambien F, Poirier O, Lecerf L, Evans A, Cambou JP, Arveiler D, Luc G, Bard JM, Bara L, Ricard S, et al.: Detection polymorphism in the gene for angiotensin-converting enzyme is a potent risk factor for myocardial infarction [see comments]. Nature 1992; 359:641–644.
Carr MC, Hokanson JE, Deeb SS, Purnell JQ, Mitchell ES, Brunzell JD: A hepatic lipase gene promoter polymorphism attenuates the increase in hepatic lipase activity with increasing intra-abdominal fat in women. Arterioscler Thromb Vasc Biol 1999; 19:2701–2707.
Carter AM, Ossei-Gerning N, Wilson IJ, Grant PJ: Association of the platelet PI(A) polymorphism of glycoprotein IIb/IIIa and the fibrinogen Bbeta 448 polymorphism with myocardial infarction and extent of coronary artery disease. Circulation 1997; 96:1424–1431.
Cascorbi I, Laule M, Mrozikiewicz PM, Mrozikiewicz A, Andel C, Baumann G, Roots I, Stangl K: Mutations in the human paraoxonase 1 gene: frequencies, allelic linkages, and association with coronary artery disease. Pharmacogenetics 1999; 9:755–761.
Castellani LW, Weinreb A, Bodnar J, Goto AM, Doolittle M, Mehrabian M, Demant P, Lusis AJ: Mapping a gene for combined hyperlipidaemia in a mutant mouse strain. Nat Genet 1998; 18:374–377.
Chait A, Brunzell JD: Severe hypertriglyceridemia: the role of familial and acquired disorders. Metabolism 1983; 32:209–214.
Clarke R: An overview of the homocysteine lowering clinical trials. In: Robinson K (ed). Homocysteine and Vascular Disease. Dordrecht: Kluwer Academic, 2000:413–429.
Cleeman JI, Lenfant C: The National Cholesterol Education Program: progress and prospects. JAMA 1998; 280:2099–2104.
Committee on Diet and Health. Evidence of dietary components and increase: Fats and other lipids in diet and health. In: Implications of Reducing Chronic Disease Risk. Washington DC: National Academy Press, 1989:159–259.
Cook RJ, Sackett DL: The number needed to treat: a clinically useful measure of treatment effect. Brit Med J 1995; 310:452–454.
Cooper DN, Clayton JF: DNA polymorphism and the study of disease associations. Hum Genet 1988; 78:299–312.
Dallinga-Thie GM, van Linde-Sibenius Trip M, Rotter JI, Cantor RM, Bu XD, Lusis AJ, de Bruin TWA: Complex genetic contribution of the apoA1-CIII-AIV gene cluster to familial combined hyperlipidemia. J Clin Invest 1997; 99:953–961.
Davignon J, Gregg RE, Sing CF: Apolipoprotein E polymorphism and atherosclerosis. Atherosclerosis 1988; 8:1–21.
Davignon J, Roy M, Dufour R, Roederer G: Familial hypercholesterolemia. In: Steiner G, Shafrir E (eds). Primary Hyperlipoproteinemias. New York: McGraw-Hill, 1991:201–234.
Dawber TR, Moore FE, Mann GV: Coronary heart disease in the Framingham Study. Am J Public Health 1957; 47(Supp):4–24.
Deeb SS, Failor RA, Brown BG, Brunzell JD, Albers JJ, Motulsky AG, Wijsman E: Association of apolipoprotein B gene variants with plasma apoB and LDL cholesterol levels. Hum Genet 1992; 88:463–470.
Deeb S, Failor A, Brown BG, Brunzell JD, Albert JI, Motulsky AG: Molecular genetics of apolipoproteins and coronary heart disease. Cold Spring Harbor Symp Quant Biol 1986; LI:403–409.
de Faire U: Ischaemic heart disease in death discordant twins: a study on 205 male and female pairs. Acta Med Scand 1974; Suppl 568:1–109.
deGennes JL, Rouffy J, Chaer F: Complications vasculaires cerebrales des xanthomatoses tendineuses hypercholesterolemiques familiales. Bull Mem Soc Med Hosp Paris 1968; 119:569.
De Graaf J, Stalenhoef AFH: Defects of lipoprotein metabolism in familial combined hyperlipidaemia. Curr Opin Lipidol 1998; 9:189–196.
de Langen CD: Cholesterine-Stofwisseling en Rassen-pathologie. Geneeskd Tijdschr Ned Indie 1916; 56:1–34.
Despres JP, Moorjani S, Ferland M, Tremblay A, Lupien PJ, Nadeau A, Pinault S, Theriault G, Bouchard C: Adipose tissue distribution and plasma lipoprotein levels in obese women: importance of intra-abdominal fat. Atherosclerosis 1989; 9:203–210.
Deutscher S, Epstein FH, Kjelsberg MO: Familial aggregation of coronary heart disease. Circulation 1966; 33:911–934.
Diabetes Control and Complications Trial Research Group: Effect of intensive diabetes management on macrovascular events and risk factors in the Diabetes Control and Complications Trial. Am J Cardiol 1995; 75:894–903.
Dock W: The predilection of atherosclerosis for the coronary arteries. JAMA 1946; 131:875–878.
Doggen CJ, Manger Cats V, Bertina RM, Reitsma PH, Vandenbroucke JP, Rosendaal FR: A genetic propensity to high factor VII is not associated with the risk of myocardial infarction in men. Thromb Haemost 1998; 80:281–285.
Doyle AE: Does hypertension predispose to coronary disease? Conflicting epidemiological and experimental evidence. In: Laragh JH, Brenner BM (eds). Hypertension: Pathophysiology, Diagnosis and Management. New York: Raven Press, 1995:119–125.
Duane WC: Abnormal bile acid absorption in familial hypertriglyceridemia. J Lipid Res 1995; 36:96–107.
Duane WC, Hartich LA, Bartman AE, Ho SB: Diminished gene expression of ileal apical sodium bile acid transporter explains impaired absorption of bile acid in patients with hypertriglyceridemia. J Lipid Res 2000; 41:1384–1389.
Durrington PN, Hunt L, Ishola M, Arrol S, Bhatnagar D: Apolipoproteins(a), AI, and B and parental history in men with early onset ischaemic heart disease. Lancet 1988; i:1070–1073.
Epstein SE, Zhu J, Burnett MS, Zhou XF, Vercellotti G, Hajjar D: Infection and atherosclerosis: potential roles of pathogen burden and molecular mimicry. Arterioscler Thromb Vasc Biol 2000; 20:1417–1420.
Ernst E, Resch KL: Fibrinogen as a cardiovascular risk factor: a meta-analysis and review of the literature [see comments]. Ann Intern Med 1993; 118:956–963.

Fisher EA, Coates PM, Cortner JA: Gene polymorphisms and variability of human apoplipoproteins. Annu Rev Nutr 1989; 9:139–160.
Fogge CH: General xanthelasma or vitilogoidea. Trans Pathol Soc Lond 1872; 24:242.
4S Study. Randomised trial of cholesterol lowering in 4444 patients with coronary heart disease: the Scandinavian Simvastatin Survival Study (4S). Lancet 1994; 344:1383–1389.
Frick MKH, Elo O, Haapa K, Heinonen OP, Heinsalmi XX, Helo P, Huttunen JK, Kaitaniemi P, Koskinen P, Manninen V, et al.: Helsinki Heart Study: primary-prevention trial with gemfibrozil in middle-aged men with dyslipidemia. Safety of treatment, changes in risk factors, and incidence of coronary heart disease. N Eng J Med 1987; 317:1237–1245.
Frings AM, Mayer B, Bocker W, Hengstenberg C, Willemsen D, Riegger GA, Schunker H: Comparative coronary anatomy in six twin pairs with coronary artery disease. Heart 2000; 83:47–50.
Fujimoto WY, Abbate SL, Kahn SE, Brunzell J: The visceral adiposity syndrome in Japanese-American men. Obes Res 1994; 2:364–371.
Funke H, Assmann G: Strategies for the assessment of genetic coronary artery disease risk. Curr Opin Lipidol 1999; 10:285–291.
Gardemann A, Philipp M, Hess K, Katz N, Tillmanns H, Haberbosch W: The paraoxonase leu-Met54 and gln-Arg191 gene polymorphisms are not associated with the risk of coronary heart disease. Atherosclerosis 2000; 152:421–431.
Gardner CD, Fortmann SP, Krauss RM: Association of small low-density lipoprotein particles with the incidence of coronary artery disease in men and women. JAMA 1996; 276:875–881.
Gavish D, Brinton EZ, Breslow JL: Heritable allele-specific differences in amounts of apoB and low-density lipoproteins in plasma. Science 1989; 244:72–75.
Gertler MM, White PD: Coronary Heart Disease in Young Adults. Cambridge: Harvard University Press, 1954.
Ginsberg HN: Insulin resistance and cardiovascular disease. J Clin Invest 2000; 106:453–458.
Girelli D, Russo C, Ferraresi P, Olivieri O, Pinotti M, Friso S, Manzato F, Mazzucco A, Bernardi F, Corrocher R: Polymorphisms in the Factor VII gene and the risk of myocardial infarction in patients with coronary artery disease. N Engl J Med 2000; 343:774–780.
Goldman L, Cook EF: The decline in ischemic heart disease mortality rates: an analysis of the comparative effects of medical interventions and changes in lifestyle. Ann Intern Med 1984; 101:825–826.
Goldstein JL, Hazzard WR, Schrott HG, Bierman EI, Motulsky AG: Hyperlipidemia in coronary heart disease: II. Genetic analysis of lipid levels in 176 families and delineation of a new inherited disorder. J Clin Invest 1973; 51:1544–1568.
Goldstein JL, Hobbs HH, Brown MS: Familial hypercholesterolemia. In: Scriver CR, Beaudet AL, Sly WS, Valle D, Childs B, Kinzler KW, Vogelstein B (eds). The Metabolic and Molecular Basis of Inherited Disease, 8th ed. New York: McGraw-Hill, 2001:2863–2914.
Gordon DJ, Probstfield JL, Garrison RJ, Neaton JD, Castelli WP, Nobe JDK, Jacobs DR, Bangdiwala S, Tyroler HA: High density lipoprotein cholesterol and coronary heart disease: four prospective American studies. Circulation 1989; 79:8–15.
Graham IM, Daly LE, Refsum H, Robinson K, Brattstrom LE, Veland PM, Palma-Reis RJ, Boers GH, Shehan RG, Israelsson B, et al.: Plasma homocysteine as a risk factor for vascular disease: the European concerted action project. JAMA 1997; 277:1775–1781.
Grant PJ, Humphries SE: Genetic determinants of arterial thrombosis. Baillieres Best Pract Res Clin Haematol 1999; 12:505–532.
Green R: Homocysteine and coagulation factors: basic interactions and clinical studies. In: Robinson KL (ed). Homocysteine and Vascular Disease. Dordrecht: Kluwer Academic, 2000:349–370.
Haffner SM: The insulin resistance syndrome revisited. Diabetes Care 1996; 19:275–277.
Hallman DM, Boerwinkle E, Saha N, Sandholzer C, Menzel HJ, Csazar A, Utermann G: The apolipoprotein E polymorphism: a comparison of allele frequencies and effects in nine populations. Am J Hum Genet 1991; 49:338–349.
Hamby RI: Hereditary aspects of coronary artery disease. Am Heart J 1981; 101:639–649.
Harvald B, Hauge M: Hereditary Factors Elucidated by Twin Studies. Publication 1103, Genetics and Epidemiology of Chronic Disease. Washington DC: U.S. Public Health Service, 1963:61–67.
Hasstedt SJ, Wu L, Williams RR: Major locus inheritance of apolipoprotein B in Utah pedigrees. Genet Epidemiol 1987; 4:67–76.
Havel RJ: Lowering cholesterol 1988: rationale, mechanisms and means. J Clin Invest 1988; 81:1653–1660.
Havel RJ, Kane JP: Introduction: Structure and metabolism of plasma lipoproteins. In: Scriver CR, Beaudet AI, Sly WS, Valle D, Childs B, Kinzler KW, Vogelstein B (eds). The Metabolic and Molecular Basis of Inherited Disease, 8th ed. New York: McGraw-Hill, 2001:2705–2716.
Havenith MG, Gotlieb AI: Atherogenesis. In: Steiner G, Shafrir E (eds). Primary Hyperlipoproteinemias. New York: McGraw-Hill, 1991:75–107.
Hayden MR, Clee SM, Brooks-Wilson A, Genest Jr A, Attie A, Kastelein JJ: Cholesterol efflux regulatory protein, Tangier disease and familial high-density lipoprotein deficiency. Curr Opin Lipidol 2000; 11:117–122.
Health Care Almanac and Yearbook: USA health: an overview. Health Care Almanac and Yearbook, 2000.
Hegele RA, Breslow JL: Apolipoprotein genetic variation in the assessment of atherosclerosis susceptibility. Genet Epidemiol 1987; 4:163–184.
Heinecke J, Lusis A: Paraoxonase-gene polymorphisms associated with coronary heart disease: support for the oxidative damage hypothesis? Am J Hum Genet 1998; 62:20–24.
Hibi K, Ishigami T, Tamura K, Mizushima S, Nyui N, Fujita T, Ochiai H, Kosuge M, Watanabe Y, Yoshii Y, et al.: Endothelial nitric oxide synthase gene polymorphism and acute myocardial infarction. Hypertension 1998; 32:521–526.
Hill JS, Mayden MR, Frohlich J, Pritchard PH: Genetic and environmental factors affecting the incidence of coronary artery disease in heterozygous familial hypercholesterolemia. Arterioscler Throm 1991; 11:290–297.
Hingorani AD, Liang CF, Fatibene J, Lyon A, Monteith S, Parsons A, Haydock S, Hopper RV, Stephens NG, O'Shaughnessy KM, Brown MJ: A common variant of the endothelial nitric oxide synthase (Glu298 $\rightarrow$ Asp) is a major risk factor for coronary artery disease in the UK. Circulation 1999; 100:1515–1520.
Hobbs HH, Russel DW, Brown MS, Goldstein JL: The LDL receptor locus in familial hypercholesterolemia: mutational analysis of a membrane protein. Annu Rev Genet 1990; 24:133–170.
Hokanson JE, Austin MA: Triglyceride is a risk factor for cardiovascular disease independent of high-density lipoprotein cholesterol: a meta-analysis of population-based prospective studies. J Cardiovasc Risk 1996; 3:213–219.
Hokanson JE, Brunzell JD, Jarvik GP, Wijsman EM, Austin MA: Linkage of low-density lipoprotein size to the lipoprotein lipase gene in heterozygous lipoprotein lipase deficiency. Am J Hum Genet 1999; 64:608–618.
Holman RL, McGill JR HC, Strong JP, Geer JC: The natural history of atherosclerosis: the early aortic lesions as seen in New Orleans in the middle of the 20th century. Am J Pathol 1958; 34:209–235.
Hulthe J, Bokemark L, Wikstrand J, Fagerberg B: The metabolic syndrome, LDL particle size, and atherosclerosis: the Atherosclerosis and Insulin Resistance (AIR) Study. Arterioscler Thromb Vasc Biol 2000; 20:2140–2147.
Humphries SE: DNA polymorphisms of the apolipoprotein genes—their use in the investigation of the genetic component of hyperlipidaemia and atherosclerosis. Atherosclerosis 1988; 72:89–108.
Humphries SE, Panahloo A, Montgomery HE, Green F, Yudkin J: Gene–environment interaction in the determination of levels of haemostatic variables involved in thrombosis and fibrinolysis. Thromb Haemost 1997; 78:457–461.
Hunt SC, Wu LL, Hopkins PN, Stults BM, Kuida H, Ramire ME, Lalouel JM, Williams RR: Apolipoprotein, low density lipoprotein subfraction, and insulin associates with familial combined hyperlipidemia: study of Utah patients with familial dyslipidemic hypertension. Atherosclerosis 1989; 9:335–344.
Iacoviello L, Burrito F, Di Castelnuovo A, Zito F, Marially R, Donati MB: The 4G/5G polymorphism of PAI-1 promoter gene and the risk of myocardial infarction: a meta-analysis [letter]. Thromb Haemost 1998a; 80:1029–1030.
Iacoviello L, Di Castelnuovo A, De Knijff P, D'Orazio A, Amore C, Arboretti R, Kluft C, Benedetta Donati M: Polymorphisms in the coagulation factor VII gene and the risk of myocardial infarction. N Engl J Med 1998b; 338:79–85.
Ignatovski AI: Influence of animal food on the organism of rabbits. Izv Imp Voyenno-Med Akad Peter 1908; 16:154–176.
Imai Y, Morita H, Kurihara H, Sugiyama T, Kato N, Ebihara A, Hamada C, Kurihara Y, Shindo T, Oh-hashi Y, Yazaki Y: Evidence for association between paraoxonase gene polymorphisms and atherosclerotic diseases. Atherosclerosis 2000; 149:435–442.
Inazu A, Koizumi J, Mabuchi H: Cholesteryl ester transfer protein and atherosclerosis. Curr Opin Lipidol 2000; 11:389–396.
Innerarity TL, Mahley RW, Weisgraber KH, Bersot TP, Krauss RM, Vega GI, Grundy SM, Friedl W, Davignon J, McCarthy BJ: Familial defective apolipoprotein B-100: a mutation of apolipoprotein B that causes hypercholesterolemia. J Lipid Res 1990; 31:1337–1349.
Inter-Society Commission for Heart Disease Resources: Optimal resources for primary prevention of atherosclerotic diseases. Circulation 1984; 70:153A–205A.
Jeppsen J, Hein HO, Suadicani P, Gyntelberg F: Triglyceride concentration and ischemic heart disease: an eight-year follow-up in the Copenhagen Male Study. Circulation 1998; 97:1029–1036.
Kahn SE, Prigeon RL, McCulloch D, Boyko EJ, Bergman RN, Schwartz MW, Neifing JL, Ward WK, Beard JC, Palmer JP, et al.: The contribution of insulin-dependent and insulin-independent glucose uptake to intravenous glucose tolerance in healthy human subjects. Diabetes 1994; 43:587–592.
Kamboh MI, Ferrell RE, Kottke BA: Expressed hypervariable polymorphism of apolipoprotein (a). Am J Hum Genet 1991; 49:1063–1074.
Kane JP, Malloy MJ, Ports TA, Phillips NR, Diehl JC, Havel RJ: Regression of coronary atherosclerosis during treatment of familial hypercholesterolemia with combined drug regimens. JAMA 1990; 264:3007–3012.
Kannel WB: Some lessons in cardiovascular epidemiology from Framingham. Am J Cardiol 1976; 37:268–282.
Kaste M, Koivisto P: Risk of brain infarction in familial hypercholesterolemia. Stroke 1988; 19:1097.
Katan MB, Beynen AC: Characteristics of human hypo- and hyperresponders to dietary cholesterol. Am J Epidemiol 1987; 125:387–399.
Katzel LI, Bleecker ER, Rogus EM, Goldberg AP: Sequential effects of aerobic exercise training and weight loss on risk factors for coronary disease in healthy, obese middle-aged and older men. Metabolism 1997; 46:1441–1447.
Knopp RH: Drug treatment of lipid disorders. N Engl J Med 1999; 341:498–511.
Knowles JW, Maeda N: Genetic modifiers of atherosclerosis in mice. Arterioscler Thromb Vasc Biol 2000; 20:2336–2345.
Kohler HP, Grant PJ: Plasminogen-activator inhibitor type 1 and coronary artery disease. N Engl J Med 2000; 342:1792–1801.
Kotze MJ, Langenhoven E, Warnich L, du Plessis L, Retief AE: The molecular basis and diagnosis of familial hypercholesterolaemia in South African Afrikaners. Ann Hum Genet 1991; 55:115–121.
Krauss RM, Eckel RH, Howard B, Appel LJ, Daniels SR, Deckelbaum RJ, Erdman JW, Kris-Etherton P, Goldberg IJ, Kotchen TA, et al.: AHA dietary guidelines.

Revision 2000: a statement for healthcare professionals from the Nutrition Committee of the American Heart Association. Circulation 2000; 102:2284–2299.
Kuivenhoven JA, Jukema JW, Zwinderman AH, de Knijff P, McPherson R, Bruschke AV, Lie KI, Kastelein JJ: The role of a common variant of the cholesteryl ester transfer protein gene in the progression of coronary atherosclerosis: the Regression Growth Evaluation Statin Study Group. N Engl J Med 1998; 338:86–93.
Kushi LH, Lew RA, Stare FJ, Ellison CR, el Lozy M, Bourke G, Daly L, Graham I, Hickey N, Mulcahy R, Kevaney J: Diet and 20-year mortality from coronary heart disease: the Ireland-Boston Diet-Heart Study. N Eng J Med 1985; 312:811–818.
Kwiterovich PO Jr: Hyperapobetalipoproteinemia. In: Steiner G, Shafrir E (eds). Primary Hyperlipoproteinemias. New York: McGraw-Hill, 1991:235–248.
Lackner C, Boerwinkle E, Leffert CC, Rahmig T, Hobbs HH: Molecular basis of apolipoprotein(a) isoform size heterogeneity as revealed by pulsed-field gel electrophoresis. J Clin Invest 1991; 87:2077–2086.
Lalouel JM, Rao DC, Morton NE, Elston RC: A unified model for complex segregation analysis. Am J Hum Genet 1983; 35:816–826.
Lamarche B, Tchernof A, Moorjani S, Cantin B, Dagenais GR, Lupien PJ, Despres JP: Small, dense low-density lipoprotein particles as a predictor of the risk of ischemic heart disease in men: prospective results from the Quebec Cardiovascular Study. Circulation 1997; 95:69–75.
Lane A, Green F, Scarabin PY, Nicaud V, Bara L, Humphries S, Evans A, Lue G, Cambou JP, Arvailer D, et al.: Factor VII Arg/Gln353 polymorphism determines factor VII coagulant activity in patients with myocardial infarction (MI) and control subjects in Belfast and in France but is not a strong indicator of MI risk in the ECTIM study. Atherosclerosis 1996; 119:119–127.
Lilliefors I: Coronary heart disease in male twins: hereditary and environmental factors in concordant and discordant pairs. Acta Med Scand 1970;(Suppl):511:1–90.
Lindpaintner K, Pfeffer MA, Kreutz R, Stampfer MJ, Grodstein F, LaMotte F, Buring J, Hennekens CH: A prospective evaluation of an angiotensin-converting-enzyme gene polymorphism and the risk of ischemic heart disease. N Engl J Med 1995; 332:706–711.
Lipid Research Clinics Program: The Lipid Research Clinics Coronary Primary Prevention Trial results: I. Reduction in incidence of coronary heart disease. JAMA 1984a; 251:351–364.
Lipid Research Clinics Program: The Lipid Research Clinics Coronary Primary Prevention Trial results: II. The relationship of reduction in incidence of coronary heart disease to cholesterol lowering. JAMA 1984b; 251:365–374.
Loscalzo J: Lipoprotein(a): a unique risk factor of atherothrombotic disease. Atherosclerosis 1990; 10:672–679.
Love MW, Craddock AI, Angelin B, Brunzell JD, Duane WC, Dawson PA: Analysis of the ileal bile acid transporter gene (SLC10A2) in subjects with familial hypertriglyceridemia. Arterioscler Thromb Vasc Biol 2001; 21:XXX–XXX.
Ludwig EH, McCarthy BJ: Haplotype analysis of the human apolipoprotein B mutation associated with familial defective apolipoprotein B-100. Am J Hum Genet 1990; 47:712–720.
Lusis AJ: Genetic factors affecting blood lipoproteins: the candidate gene approach. J Lipid Res 1988; 29:397.
Lusis AJ: Atherosclerosis. Nature (Insight) 2000; 407:233–241.
MacCluer JW: Statistical approaches to identifying major locus effects on disease susceptibility. Monogr Hum Genet 1989; 12:50–78.
Mackness MI, Mackness B, Durrington PN, Fogelman AM, Berliner J, Lusis AJ, Navab M, Shih D, Fonarow GC: Paraoxonase and coronary heart disease. Curr Opin Lipidol 1998; 9:319–324.
Mahley RW, Rall Jr SC: Type III hyperlipoproteinemia (dysbetalipoproteinemia): the role of apolipoprotein E in normal and abnormal lipoprotein metabolism. In: Scriver CR, Beaudet AI, Sly WS, Valle D, Childs B, Kinzler KW, Vogelstein B (eds). The Metabolic and Molecular Basis of Inherited Diseases, 8th ed. New York: McGraw Hill, 2001:2835–2862.
Malinow MR, Nieto FJ, Szklo M, Chambless LE, Bond G: Carotid artery intimal-medial wall thickening and plasma homocyst(e)ine in asymptomatic adults: the Atherosclerosis Risk in Communities Study. Circulation 1993; 87:1107–1113.
Manson JE, Colditz GA, Stampfer MJ, Willett WC, Krolewski AS, Rosner B, Arky RA, Speizer FE, Hennekens CH: A prospective study of maturity-onset diabetes mellitus and risk of coronary heart disease and stroke in women. Arch Intern Med 1991; 151:1141–1147.
Marenberg ME, Risch N, Berkman LF, Floderus B, de Faire U: Genetic susceptibility to death from coronary heart disease in a study of twins. N Engl J Med 1994; 330:1041–1046.
Martin MJ, Hulley SB, Browner WS, Kuller GH, Wentworth D: Serum cholesterol, blood pressure, and mortality: implications from a cohort of 361,662 men. Lancet 1986; 2:933–936.
Mattu RK, Needham EW, Galton DJ, Frangos E, Clark AJ, Caulfield M: A DNA variants at the angiotensin-converting enzyme gene locus associates with coronary artery disease in the Caerphilly Heart Study [see comments]. Circulation 1995; 91:270–274.
Mayo O, Fraser GR, Stamatoyannopoulos G: Genetic influences on serum cholesterol in two Greek villages. Hum Hered 1969; 19:86–99.
McCully KS: Vascular pathology of homocysteinemia: implications for the pathogenesis of arteriosclerosis. Am J Pathol 1969; 56:111–128.
McGill HC Jr: Fatty streaks in the coronary arteries and aorta. Lab Invest 1968; 18:560–564.
McGill HC Jr, McMahan CA, Ziewske AW, Sloop GD, Walcott JV, Troxclair DA, Malcom GT, Tracy RE, Oalmann MC, Strong JP: Associations of coronary heart disease risk factors with the intermediate lesion of atherosclerosis in youth. Arterioscler Thromb Vasc Biol 2000; 20:1998–2004.
McLean JW, Tomlinson JE, Juang W-J, Eaton DL, Chen EY, Fless GM, Scanu AM, Lawn RM: cDNA sequence of human apolipoprotein(a) is homologous to plasminogen. Nature 1987; 330:132–137.
McQuilan BM, Beilby JP, Nidorf M, Thompson PL, Hung J: Hyperhomocysteinemia but not the C677T mutation of methylenetetrahydrofolate reductase is an independent risk determinant of carotid wall thickening: the Perth Carotid Ultrasound Disease Assessment Study (CUDAS). Circulation 1999; 99:2383–2388.
Meiner V, Landsberger D, Berkman N, Reshef A, Segal P, Seftel HC, van der Westhuyzen DR, Jeenah MS, Coetzee GA, Leitersdorf E: A common Lithuanian mutation causing familial hypercholesterolemia in Ashkenazi Jews. Am J Hum Genet 1991; 49:443–449.
Mikkelsson J, Perola M, Laippala P, Savolainen V, Pajarinen J, Lalu K, Penttila A, Karhunen PJ: Glycoprotein IIIa PI(A) polymorphism associates with progression of coronary artery disease and with myocardial infarction in an autopsy series of middle-aged men who died suddenly. Arterioscler Thromb Vasc Biol 1999; 19:2573–2578.
Mikkelson J, Perola M, Wartiovaara U, Peltonen L, Palotie A, Penttila A, Karhunen PJ: Plasminogen activator inhibitor-1 (PAI-1) 4G/5G polymorphism, coronary thrombosis, and myocardial infarction in middle-aged Finnish men who died suddenly. Thromb Haemost 2000; 84:78–82.
Motulsky AG: Genetic aspects of familial hypercholesterolemia and its diagnosis. Arteriosclerosis 1989; 9(Suppl I):1-3–1-7.
Mourant AE, Kopec AD, Domaniewska-Sobczak K: Blood groups and diseases: a study of associations of diseases with blood groups and polymorphisms. New York: Oxford University Press, 1978:34, 159–163.
Mudd SH, Havlik R, Levy HL, McKusick VL, Feinleib M: A study of cardiovascular risk in heterozygotes for homocystinuria. Am J Hum Genet 1981; 33:883–893.
Mudd SH, Levy HL, Kraus JP: Disorders of transsulfuration. In: Scriver CR, Beaudet AI, Sly WS, Valle D, Childs B, Kinzler KW, Vogelstein B (eds). The Metabolic and Molecular Basis of Inherited Diseases, 8th ed. New York: McGraw-Hill, 2001:2007–2056.
Muller C: Angina pectoris in hereditary xanthomatosis. Arch Intern Med 1939; 64:657–700.
National Cholesterol Education Program: Arch Intern Med 1988; 148:3.
Neel JV, Julius S, Weder A, et al.: Syndrome X: is it for real? Genet Epidemiol 1998a; 15:19–32.
Neel JV, Julius S, Weder AB, Yamada M, Viardia SLR, Haviland MB: Type II diabetes, essential hypertension, and obesity as "syndromes of impaired genetic homeostasis": the "thrifty genotype" hypothesis enters the 21st century. Pers Biol Med 1998b; 42:44–74.
NIH Consensus Development Panel on Triglyceride High-Density Lipoprotein and Coronary Heart Disease: Triglyceride, high-density lipoprotein, and coronary heart disease. JAMA 1993; 269:505–510.
Nikkila EA, Aro A: Family study of serum lipids and lipoproteins in coronary heart disease. Lancet 1973; 1:954–959.
Nora JJ, Lortscher RH, Spangler RD, Nora AH, Kimberling WJ: Genetic-epidemiologic study of early-onset ischemic heart disease. Circulation 1980; 61:503–508.
Osler W: Lectures on Angina Pectoris and Allied States. New York: Appleton & Co., 1897.
Ott J: Analysis of Human Genetic Linkage. Baltimore: Johns Hopkins University Press, 1985.
Pairitz G, Davignon J, Mailloux H, Sing CF: Sources of interindividual variation in the quantitative levels of apolipoprotein B in pedigrees ascertained through a lipid clinic. Am J Hum Genet 1988; 43:311–321.
Pajukanta P, Terwilliger JD, Perola M, Hiekkalinna T, Nuotio I, Ellonen P, Parkkonen M, Hartiala J, Ylitalo K, Pihajamäki J, et al.: Genomewide scan for familial combined hyperlipidemia genes in Finnish families, suggesting multiple susceptibility loci influencing triglyceride, cholesterol, and apolipoprotein B levels. Am J Hum Genet 1999; 64:1453–1463.
Pastinen T, Perola M, Niini P, Terwilliger J, Salomaa V, Vartianinen E, Peltonen L, Syvanen A: Array-based multiplex analysis of candidate genes reveals two independent and additive genetic risk factors for myocardial infarction in the Finnish population. Hum Mol Genet 1998; 7:1453–1462.
Purnell JQ, Kahn SE, Albers JJ, Nevin DN, Brunzell JD, Schwartz RS: Effect of weight loss with reduction of intra-abdominal fat on lipid metabolism in older men. J Clin Endocrinol Metab 2000; 85:977–982.
Purnell JQ, Kahn SE, Schwartz RS, Brunzell JD: Relationship of insulin sensitivity and apolipoprotein B levels to intra-abdominal fat in subjects with familial combined hyperlipidemia. Arterioscler Thromb Vasc Biol 2001; 21:567–572.
Rath M, Niendorf A, Reblin T, Dietel M, Krebberr HJ, Beisiegel U: Detection and quantitation of lipoprotein(a) in the arterial wall of 107 coronary bypass patients. Atherosclerosis 1989; 9:579–592.
Rauh G, Schuster H, Fischer J, Keller CH, Wolfram G, Zollner N: Identification of a heterozygous compound individual with familial hypercholesterolemia and familial defective apolipoprotein B-100. Klin Wochenschr 1991; 69:320–324.
Rauh G, Schuster H, Muller B, Schewe S, Keller C, Wolfram G, Zollner N: Genetic evidence from 7 families that the apolipoprotein B gene is not involved in familial combined hyperlipidemia. Atherosclerosis 1990; 83:81–87.
Reaven GM: Role of insulin resistance in human disease. Diabetes 1988;37:1595–1607.
Refsum H, Ueland PM, Nygard O, Vollset SE: Homocysteine and cardiovascular disease. Annu Rev Med 1998; 49:31–62.
Rhoads GG, Dahlen G, Berg K, Morton NE, Dannenberg AL: Lp(a) lipoprotein as a risk factor for mycardial infarction. JAMA 1986; 256:2540–2544.
Risch NJ: Searching for genetic determinants in the new millenium. Nature 2000; 405:847–856.
Risch NJ, Merikangas K: The future of genetic studies of complex human diseases. Science 1996; 273:1516–1517.

Rissanen AM: Familial aggregation of coronary heart disease in a high incidence area (North Karelia, Finland). Br Heart J 1979a; 42:294–303.
Rissanen AM: Familial occurrence of coronary heart disease: effect of age at diagnosis. Am J Cardiol 1979b; 44:60–66.
Rissanen AM, Nikkila EA: Coronary artery disease and its risk factors in families of young men with angina pectoris and in controls. Br Heart J 1977; 39:875–883.
Rissanen AM, Nikkila EA: Aggregation of coronary risk factors in families of men with fatal and non-fatal coronary heart disease. Br Heart J 1979; 42:373–380.
Robertson TL, Kato H, Rhodes GG, Kagan A, Marmot M, Syme SL, Gordon T, Worth RM, Belsky JL, Dock DS, et al.: Epidemiologic studies of coronary heart disease and stroke in Japanese men living in Japan, Hawaii and California: incidence of myocardial infarction and death from coronary heart disease. Am J Cardiol 1977; 39:239–243.
Robinson K (ed): Homocysteine and Vascular Disease. Dordrecht: Kluwer Academic, 2000.
Roest M, van der Schouw YT, de Valk B, Marx JJM, Tempelman MJ, de Groot PG, Sixma JJ, Banga JD: Heterozygosity for a hereditary hemochromatosis gene is associated with cardiovascular mortality in women. Circulation 1999; 100:1268–1273.
Rose G: The radiological patterns in ischaemic heart disease. Br J Prev Soc Med 1964; 18:75–80.
Rose HG, Krantz P, Weinstock M, Juliano J, Haft JI: Inheritance of combined hyperlipoproteinemia: evidence for a new lipoprotein phenotype. Am J Med 1973; 54:148.
Rosenman RH, Brand RJ, Jenkins CD, Friedman M, Straus R, Wurm M: Coronary heart disease in the Western Collaborative Study. JAMA 1975; 233:872–877.
Ross R: The pathogenesis of atherosclerosis—an update. N Engl J Med 1986; 314:488.
Ross R: Atherosclerosis—an inflammatory disease. N Engl J Med 1999; 340:115–126.
Rozen R: Molecular biology of methylenetetrahydrofolate reductase (MTHFR): interrelationships with folic acid, homocysteine, and vascular disease. In: Robinson K (ed). Homocysteine and Vascular Disease. Dordrecht: Kluwer Academic, 2000:271–289.
Russell DW, Lehrman MA, Sudhof TC, Yamamoto T, David CG, Hobbs HH, Brown MS, Goldstein JL: The LDL Receptor in Familial Hypercholesterolemia: Use of Human Mutations to Dissect a Membrane Protein. Cold Spring Harbor, New York: Cold Spring Harbor Laboratory, 1986:811–819.
Sacks FM, Moye LA, Davis BR, Cole TG, Rouleau JL, Nash DT, Pfeffer MA, Braunwald E: Relationship between plasma LDL concentrations during treatment with pravastatin and recurrent coronary events in the cholesterol and recurrent events trial. Circulation 1998; 97:1446–1452.
Savolainen MJ, Korhonen T, Aalto-Setala K, Kontula K, Kesaniemi A: Screening for a prevalent LDL receptor mutation in patients with severe hypercholesterolaemia. Hum Genet 1991; 87:125–128.
Scanu AM: Update on lipoprotein(a). Curr Opin Lipidol 1991; 2:253–258.
Schonfeld G: Drug treatment of hyperlipoproteinemias. In: Steiner G, Shafrir E (eds). Primary Hyperlipoproteinemias. New York: McGraw-Hill, 1991:321–335.
Schork NJ, Fallin D, Lanchbury S: Single nucleotide polymorphisms and the future of genetic epidemiology. Clin Genet 2000; 58:250–264.
Schuster H, Rauh G, Kormann B, Hepp T, Humphries S, Keller C, Wolfram G, Zollner N: Familial defective apolipoprotein B-100: comparison with familial hypercholesterolemia in 18 cases detected in Munich. Atherosclerosis 1990; 9:577–581.
Schwartz RS, Cain KC, Shuman WP, Larson V, Stratton JR, Beard JC, Kahn SE, Cerqueira MD, Abrass IB: Effect of intensive endurance training on lipoprotein profiles in young and older men. Metabolism 1992; 41:649–654.
Schwartz SM, Murry CE: Proliferation and the monoclonal origins of atherosclerotic lesions. Annu Rev Med 1998; 49:437–460.
Seed M, Hoppichler F, Reaveley D, McCarthy S, Thompson GR, Boerwinkle E, Utermann G: Relation of serum lipoprotein(a) concentration and apolipoprotein(a) phenotype to coronary heart disease in patients with familial hypercholesterolemia. N Eng J Med 1990; 332:1494–1499.
Seftel HC, Baker SG, Jenkins T, Mendelsohn D: Prevalence of familial hypercholesterolemia in Johannesburg Jews. Am J Med Genet 1989; 34:545–547.
Seltzer HS: A summary of criticisms of the findings and conclusions of the University Group Diabetes Program (UGDP). Diabetes 1972; 21:976–979.
Shea S, Ottman R, Gabrieli C, Stein Z, Nichols A: Family history as an independent risk factor for coronary artery disease. JACC 1984; 4:793–801.
Shepherd J, Cobbe SM, Ford I, Isles CG, Lorimer AR, MacFarlane PW, McKillop JH, Packard CJ: Prevention of coronary heart disease with ravastatin in men with hypercholesterolemia: West of Scotland Coronary Prevention Study Group. N Eng J Med 1995; 333:1301–1307.
Shih DM, Gu L, Xia Y-R, Navab M, Li W-F, Hama S, Castellani LW, Furlong CE, Costa LG, Fogelman AM, Lusis AJ: Mice lacking serum paraoxonase are susceptible to organophosphate toxicity and atherosclerosis. Nature 1998; 394:284–287.
Sing CF, Kaprio J, Perusse L, Moll PP: Genetic differences in risk of disease within and between populations. In: Simopoulos AP, Childs B (eds). Genetic Variation and Nutrition. Basel: Karger, 1990:220–235.
Sing CF, Orr JD: Analysis of genetic and environmental sources of variation in serum cholesterol Techumseh, Michigan: III. Identification of genetic effects using 12 polymorphic genetic marker systems. Am J Hum Genet 1976; 28:453–464.
Slack J, Evans KA: The increased risk of death from ischeaemic heart disease in first degree relatives of 121 men and 96 women with ischaemic heart disease. J Med Genet 1966; 3:239–257.
Snapper I: Chinese Lessons to Western Medicine. New York: Interscience Publishers, 1941.
Sniderman A, Shapiro S, Marpole D, Skinner B, Tend B, Kwiterovich PO, Jr.: Association of coronary atherosclerosis with hyperapobetalipoproteinemia (increased protein but normal cholesterol levels in human low density lipoproteins). Proc Natl Acad Sci USA 1980; 77:604–608.
Snowden CB, McNamara PM, Garrison RJ, Feinleib M, Kannel WB, Epstein FH: Predicting coronary heart disease in siblings—a multivariate assessment. Am J Epidemiol 1982; 115:217–222.
Soria LF, Ludwig EH, Clark HRG, Vega GL, Grundy SM, McCarthy BJ: Association between a specific apolipoprotein B mutation and familial defective apolipoprotein B-100. Proc Natl Acad Sci USA 1989; 86:587–589.
Spielman RS, McGinnis RE, Ewens WJ: Transmission test for linkage disequilibrium: the insulin gene region and insulin-dependent diabetes mellitus (IDDM). Am J Hum Genet 1993; 52:506–516.
Stampfer MJ, Krauss RM, Ma J, Blanche PJ, Holl LG, Sacks FM, Hennekens CH: A prospective study of triglyceride level, low-density lipoprotein particle diameter, and risk of myocardial infarction. JAMA 1996; 276:882–888.
Stampfer MJ, Sacks FM, Salvini S, Willett WC, Hennekens CH: A prospective study of cholesterol, apolipoproteins, and the risk of myocardial infarction. N Engl J Med 1991; 325:373–381.
Stangl K, Cascorbi I, Laule M, Klein T, Stangl V, Rost S, Wernecke KD, Felix SB, Bindereif A, Baumann G, Roots I: High CA repeat numbers in intron 13 of the endothelial nitric oxide synthase gene and increased risk of coronary artery disease. Pharmacogenetics 2000; 10:133–140.
Steinberg D: Low density lipoprotein oxidation and its pathobiological significance. J Biol Chem 1997; 272:20963–20966.
Steinberg D, Witztum JL: Lipoproteins and atherogenesis: current concepts. JAMA 1990; 264:3047–3052.
Stone NJ, Levy RI, Fredrickson DS, Verter J: Coronary artery disease in 116 kindreds with familial type II hyperlipoproteinemia. Circulation 1974; 49:476.
Sullivan JL: Iron and the genetics of cardiovascular disease. Circulation 1999; 100:1260–1263.
Tall AR, Breslow JL, Rubin EM: Genetic disorders affecting plasma high-density lipoproteins. In: Scriver CR, Beaudet AL, Sly WS, Valle D, Childs B, Kinzler KW, Vogelstein B (eds). The Metabolic and Molecular Basis of Inherited Disease, 8th ed. New York: McGraw-Hill, 2001:2915–2936.
Talmud PJ, Barni N, Kessling AM, Carlsson P, Darnfors C, Bjursell G, Galton D, Wynn V, Kirk H, Hayden MR, Humphries SE: Apolipoprotein gene variants are involved in the determination of serum cholesterol levels: a study in normo and hyperlipidemic individuals. Atherosclerosis 1987; 67:81–89.
Talmud PJ, Edwards KL, Turner CM, Newman B, Palmen JM, Humphries SE, Austin MA: Linkage of the cholesteryl ester transfer protein (CETP) gene to LDL particle size: use of a novel tetranucleotide repeat within the CETP promoter. Circulation 2000; 101:2461–2466.
Tchernof A, Lamarche B, Prud'homme D, Nadeau A, Moorjani S, Labrie F, Lupien PJ, Despres JP: The dense LDL phenotype: association with plasma lipoprotein levels, visceral obesity, and hyperinsulinemia in men. Diabetes Care 1996; 19:629–637.
ten Kate L, Boman H, Daiger SP, Motulsky AG: Familial aggregation of heart disease and its relation to known risk factors. Am J Cardiol 1982; 50:945–953.
ten Kate LP, Boman H, Daiger SP, Motulsky AG: Increased frequency of coronary heart disease in relatives of wives of myocardial infarct survivors: assortative mating for lifestyle and risk factors? Am J Cardiol 1984; 53:399–403.
Thannhauser SJ, Magendantz H: The different clinical groups of xanthomatous diseases: a clinical physiological study of 22 cases. Ann Intern Med 1938; 11:1662.
Thomas CB, Cohen BH: The familial occurrence of hypertension and coronary artery disease, with observations concerning obesity and diabetes. Ann Intern Med 1955; 42:90–127.
Thomas WA, Kim DN: Atherosclerosis as a hyperplastic and neoplastic process. Lab Invest 1983; 48:245.
Tiret L, Steinmetz J, Herbeth B, Visvikis S, Rakotovao R, Cudimetiere P, Cambien F: Familial resemblance of plasma apolipoprotein B: the Nancy Study. Genet Epidemiol 1990; 7:187–197.
Tunstall-Pedoe H: Theories on why the French have less heart disease: autres pays, autres moeurs. Br Med J 1988; 297:1557–1560.
Tuomainen T-P, Kontula K, Nyyssönen K, Lakka TA, Heliö T, Salonen JT: Increased risk of acute myocardial infarction in carriers of the hemochromatosis gene Cys282Tyr mutation: a prospective cohort study in men in eastern Finland. Circulation 1999; 100:1274–1279.
Tybjaerg-Hansen A, Gallagher J, Vincent J, Houlston R, Talmud PJ, Dunning AM, Seed M, Hamsten A, Humphries S, Myant NB: Familial defective apolipoprotein B-100: detection in the United Kingdom and Scandinavia, clinical characteristics of ten cases. Atherosclerosis 1990; 80:235–242.
Tybjaerg-Hansen A, Steffensen R, Meinertz H, Schnohr P, Nordestgaard BG: Association of mutations in the apolipoprotein B gene with hypercholesterolemia and the risk of ischemic heart disease. N Engl J Med 1998; 338:1577–1584.
Ueland PM, Refsum H, Beresford SAA, Vollset SE: The controversy over homocysteine and cardiovascular risk. Am J Clin Nutr 2000; 72:324–332.
UKPDS (UK Prospective Diabetes Study Group): Intensive blood-glucose control with sulphonylureas or insulin compared with conventional treatment and risk of complications in patients with Type 2 diabetes (UKPDS 33). Lancet 1998;352:837–852.
Utermann G: The mysteries of lipoprotein(a). Science 1989; 246:904–910.
Utermann G: Lipoprotein(a). In: Scriver CR, Beaudet AL, Sly WS, Valle D, Childs B, Kinzler KW, Vogelstein B (eds). The Metabolic and Molecular Basis of Inherited Disease, 8th ed. New York: McGraw-Hill, 2001:2753–2788.
Voutilainen S, Alfthan G, Nyyssonen K, Salonen R, Salonen JT: Association between elevated plasma total homocysteine and increased common carotid artery wall thickness. Ann Med 1998; 30:300–306.

Wang J, Burnett JR, Near S, Young K, Zinman B, Hanley AJ, Connelly PW, Harris SB, Hegele RA: Common and rare ABC1 variants affecting plasma HDL cholesterol. Arterioscler Thromb Vasc Biol 2000; 20:1983–1989.

Wang XL, Wang J, McCredie RM, Wilcken DE: Polymorphisms of factor V, factor VII, and fibrinogen genes: relevance to severity of coronary artery disease. Arterioscler Thromb Vasc Biol 1997; 17:246–251.

Weitkamp LR, Guttormsen SA, Schultz JS: Linkage between the loci for the Lp(a) lipoprotein (LP) and plasminogen (PLG). Hum Genet 1988; 79:80–82.

Wilcken DEL, Wilcken B: The pathogenesis of coronary artery disease: a possible role for methionine metabolism. J Clin Invest 1976; 57:1079–1082.

Wilkinson CF: Essential familial hypercholesterolemia: cutaneous metabolic and hereditary aspects. Bull NY Acad Med 1950; 26:670.

Williams RR, Hasstedt SJ, Wilson DE, Ash UO, Yanowitz FF, Reiber GE, Kuida IT: Evidence that men with familial hypercholesterolemia can avoid early coronary death. JAMA 1986; 255:219–224.

Williams RR, Hopkins PN, Stephenson S, Wu L, Hunt SC: Primordial prevention of cardiovascular disease through applied genetics. Prev Med 1999; 29(6 Pt 2):S41–S49.

Williams RR, Hopkins PN, Wu LL, Hunt SC: Applying genetic strategies to prevent atherosclerosis. In: Khoury MJ, Burke W, Thomson EJ (eds). Genetics and Public Health in the 21st Century. New York: Oxford University Press, 2000:463–485.

Wilson JM, Chowdhury JR: Prospects for gene therapy of familial hypercholesterolemia. Mol Biol Med 1990; 7:223–232.

Wissler RW: Update on the pathogenesis of atherosclerosis. Am J Med 1991; 91:3S–9S.

Wojchechowski AP, Farral M, Cullen P, Wilson TME, Bayliss JD, Farren B, Griffin BA, Caslake MJ, Packard CJ, Shepherd J, et al.: Familial combined hyperlipidemia linked to the apolipoprotein A1-CIII-AIV gene cluster on chromosome 11a23–q24. Nature 1991; 349:161–164.

Yater WM, Traum AH, Brown WG, Fitzgerald RP, Geisler MA, Wilcox BB: Coronary artery disease in men eighteen to thirty-nine years of age. Am Heart J 1948; 36:334–372.

Zambon A, Deeb SS, Bensadoun A, Foster KE, Brunzell JD: In vivo evidence of a role for hepatic lipase in human apoB-containing lipoprotein metabolism, independent of its lipolytic activity. J Lipid Res 2000; 41:1.

Zambon A, Deeb SS, Brown BG, Hokanson JE, Brunzell JD: A common hepatic lipase gene promoter variant determines clinical response to intensive lipid lowering treatment. Circulation 2001; 103:792–798.

Zambon A, Deeb SS, Hokanson JE, Brown BG, Brunzell JD: Common variants in the promoter of the hepatic lipase gene are associated with lower levels of hepatic lipase activity, buoyant LDL, and higher HDL_2 cholesterol. Arterioscler Thromb Vasc Biol 1998; 18:1723–1729.

Zambon A, Hokanson JE, Brown G, Brunzell JD: Evidence for a new pathophysiological mechanism for coronary artery disease regression: hepatic lipase—mediated changes in LDL density. Circulation 1999; 99:1959–1964.

Zito F, Di Castelnuovo A, Amore C, D'Orazio A, Donati MB, Iacoviello L: Bcl I polymorphism in the fibrinogen beta-chain gene is associate with the risk of familial myocardial infarction by increasing plasma fibrinogen levels: a case-control study in a sample of GISSI-2 patients. Arterioscler Thromb Vasc Biol 1997; 17:3489–3494.

8 Hypertension

STEVEN C. HUNT, PAUL N. HOPKINS, AND JEAN-MARC LALOUEL

The genetics of essential hypertension remains one of the most complex and daunting challenges facing human geneticists today. Apart from a few rare genetic syndromes, which may or may not be included under the rubric of essential hypertension, the underlying pathophysiology and etiology of hypertension in most individual cases cannot, by current methods, be ascertained. The protean mechanisms of blood pressure control, extensive compensatory mechanisms, and multiple interactions further obscure initiating factors. For example, initial volume expansion in controlled animal studies leads through compensatory mechanisms to hypertension perpetuated primarily by peripheral vasoconstriction with virtually normal vascular volume. Phenocopies and heterogeneity complicate the work of the genetic epidemiologist. Common forms of hypertension have relatively late onset and show marked interaction with environmental factors such as diet and exercise. Genes that are discovered will likely show incomplete penetrance since protective as well as susceptibility genes appear to be present. Nevertheless, there is now a large body of literature on the genetic association and linkage of various genes with blood pressure, hypertension, and intermediate phenotypes for blood pressure. Most of these studies have not found significant associations. There are some positive results, but only a subset of these have been replicated. Still fewer present pathophysiological data supporting a gene effect. This chapter reviews these findings and provides a perspective of how strong and consistent these results are and where these lines of research will eventually lead us in understanding the genetics of hypertension.

DISEASE DEFINITION

Diagnostic Criteria and Prevalence

Current diagnostic criteria for hypertension are given in Table 8–1. Since the 1993 report of the Joint National Committee on Detection, Evaluation, and Treatment of High Blood Pressure (JNC V, 1993), blood pressure has been classified into normal ranges and stages of hypertension. Blood pressure staging is based on the average of three separate readings taken one to several weeks apart. The reading at each visit should be the average of two or more measurements. Stage 4 pressures require immediate treatment after a single reading in that range. In the most recent report of the Joint National Committee (JNC VI, 1997), stages 3 and 4 were collapsed together because of the rarity of stage 4 (blood pressure ≥210/110 mm Hg). Nevertheless, treating persons with severe elevations remains urgent. A new recommendation in the JNC VI report is greater emphasis on whether other risk factors or target organ damage are present in considering when to initiate treatment and in determining the therapeutic goal (Table 8–2). Major risk factors are smoking, dyslipidemia, diabetes mellitus, age ≥60 years, being a male over age 45 or a postmenopausal female, and family history of cardiovascular disease (women ≤65 or men ≤55 years). Target organ damage is defined as left ventricular hypertrophy, angina or prior myocardial infarction, prior coronary revascularization, heart failure, stroke, transient ischemic attack, nephropathy, peripheral arterial disease, or retinopathy.

Sitting blood pressure measurements should be taken in a quiet room with the subject sitting in a chair that supports the back and allows the arm to be placed at the level of the heart. The first measurement should be taken after at least 5 minutes of rest, with 2 minutes of rest between subsequent measurements. Cuff size is critical for an accurate measurement and should be based on the circumference of the upper arm. It is recommended that the phase 5 Korotkoff sound be used for the diastolic blood pressure measurement.

The prevalence rates of hypertension in the United States are given in Table 8–3. As can be seen, the prevalence of hypertension is higher in blacks than whites and increases with age. Males have higher prevalence rates at younger ages, while females have equal or greater prevalence rates than males at older ages.

Clinical Presentation, Epidemiology, and Association with Other Diseases

Hypertension is generally asymptomatic. Headache may accompany moderate to severe elevations. However, the risk of atherosclerosis increases exponentially as blood pressure rises above optimal levels, defined as systolic and diastolic blood pressures under 120 and 80 mm Hg, respectively, in the Multiple Risk Factor Intervention Trial (MRFIT) 6-year follow-up of 356,222 middle-aged men (Fig. 8–1). Only 25% of the men had systolic blood pressures in this optimal range (Stamler, 1987). Importantly, the blood pressure strata where the attributable risk for coronary heart disease (CHD) was highest (a function of both prevalence and relative risk) were 85 to 89 mm Hg for diastolic blood pressure and 140 to 144 mm Hg for systolic blood pressure. Based on these MRFIT data, 32% of all CHD deaths can be attributed to diastolic blood pressure >80 mm Hg and 42% to systolic blood pressure >120 (Stamler, 1987). Systolic blood pressure is at least as predictive a risk factor as diastolic blood pressure, as shown in numerous prospective studies (Kannel et al., 1980; Garland et al., 1983; Harlan et al., 1984; Stamler, 1987; Neaton and Wentworth, 1992) and by the positive benefits realized by treating isolated systolic hypertension (SHEP Cooperative Research Group, 1991). In fact, coronary artery disease risk increases progressively with systolic pressure independently of

Table 8–1. Stages of Hypertension According to the Sixth Report of the Joint National Committee on Detection, Evaluation, and Treatment of Hypertension[a]

	Systolic (mm Hg)	Diastolic (mm Hg)
Optimal	<120	80
Normal	<130	<85
High normal	130–139	85–89
Stage 1 (mild)	140–159	90–99
Stage 2 (moderate)	160–179	100–109
Stage 3 (severe)	≥180	≥110

[a]For adults aged 18 and older not taking antihypertensive drugs and not acutely ill.
Source: JNC VI (1997).

diastolic pressure (Neaton et al., 1984). Including systolic blood pressure for the first time into the staging scheme for severity of hypertension in the JNC (1993) report was overdue and amply justified by epidemiological evidence.

How does hypertension promote atherosclerosis? Low-density lipoprotein (LDL) convection into the intima is highly dependent on the pressure gradient across the arterial wall, with up to 44 times more LDL collecting in the intima of test rabbit aorta at 160 mm Hg compared to 70 mm Hg (Curmi et al., 1990). The virtual exclusion of atherosclerosis from veins, even with homozygous familial hypercholesterolemia, further illustrates the importance of arterial pressure in the etiology of atherosclerotic disease (Buja et al., 1979). In some societies, where very low serum cholesterol levels predominate, hypertension does not appear to be a risk factor for coronary disease (Gordon et al., 1974; Kozarevic et al., 1976; Keys et al., 1984). In a nonhuman primate model, control of both hypertension and hyperlipidemia was necessary for atherosclerosis regression (Hollander et al., 1976). In a human multiple risk factor intervention study, substantial reductions in coronary risk occurred only in those who achieved a decrease in both cholesterol and blood pressure (Samuelsson et al., 1987). Thus, hypertension appears to interact with serum lipids to produce clinically relevant atherosclerosis.

Despite the overwhelming observational evidence for blood pressure as a risk factor for atherosclerosis in coronary as well as carotid arteries, not until 1990 had enough drug intervention experience accumulated to demonstrate not only a markedly reduced risk of stroke but also a modest reduction in coronary artery disease end points among patients treated for mild to moderate hypertension (Medical Research Council Working Party 1985; Collins et al., 1990; SHEP Cooperative Research Group, 1991; Dahlöf et al., 1991). Thus, drug treatment of mild to moderate hypertension resulted in reduction of coronary artery disease end points by 17% [95% confidence interval (CI) 10%–23%] and a decline in stroke incidence of 38% (95% CI 30%–44%) (Yusuf et al., 1993). An important recent meta-analysis showed significant benefit of low-dose diuretics and β-blockers in preventing coronary end points, while for higher-dose diuretics there was no significant benefit in coronary disease prevention (Psaty et al., 1997). In 1997, the first study of any of the newer antihypertensive agents (a calcium channel blocker in this case) showed a significant benefit on morbidity and mortality (Staessen et al., 1997a). In summary, the drug intervention studies have established even mild to moderate hypertension as a major causal risk factor for cardiovascular disease.

In addition to promoting atherosclerosis, hypertension can have direct adverse effects on arteries, arterioles, and the heart, resulting in potentially severe consequences beyond the more common manifestations of myocardial infarction and atherothrombotic stroke. Blood pressures in the range of stage 1 and stage 2 hypertension result in hypertrophy of the media in arteries and arterioles. Hypertrophy might be considered a physiological response which can protect the brain from breakdown of the blood–brain barrier in hypertensive individuals. Nevertheless, it also increases the response of arterioles to vasospastic stimuli, thus promoting and perpetuating increased peripheral vascular resistance and hypertension. In the heart, increasing afterload (from both higher blood pressures and alterations in elasticity of arteries) will lead to myocardial hypertrophy, itself a risk factor for cardiovascular disease, particularly sudden death, independently of blood pressure or other cardiovascular risk factors (Levy et al., 1990). When severe, left ventricular hypertrophy can lead to an imbalance between oxygen supply and demand and result in congestive heart failure. Even less-marked hypertension is a major risk factor for congestive heart failure, possibly through such a mechanism as well as through promotion of coronary atherosclerosis and ischemic myocardial damage (Levy et al., 1996; Aronow and Ahn, 1999).

As the arterial tree is exposed to stage 2 pressures for more prolonged periods or with stage 3 hypertension, pathological changes occur in both arteries and arterioles. Arteriosclerosis is an arterial change characterized by *myointimal hyperplasia*, a proliferation of smooth muscle cells in the intima. In addition, over time, collagen replaces much of the media. Arteries that have undergone these changes are stiff and do not accommodate the pulsatile changes in diameter that characterize systole in younger, more elastic arteries. The result is considerably increased stress on the heart (increased afterload) beyond that due to the increased blood pressure itself. In arterioles, a parallel process occurs, called *arteriolosclerosis*. Again, there is myointimal hyperplasia. Arterioles undergo a further change in the intima with excess pressure-driven insudation of fluids and protein from the plasma. There is initially an increase in glycoproteins and collagen and accumulation of some lipid. Even at this stage, swelling of the arteriolar wall can progress to the stage of lumen

Table 8–2. Treatment Recommendations According to Stage of Hypertension

Blood Pressure Stages (mm Hg)	Risk Group A (No Risk Factors, No TOD/CCD)	Risk Group B (At Least One Risk Factor, Not Including Diabetes; No TOD/CCD)	Risk Group C (TOD/CCD and/or Diabetes, with or without Other Risk Factors)
High normal (130–139/85–89)	Lifestyle modification	Lifestyle modification	Drug therapy
Stage 1 (140–159/90–99)	Lifestyle modification (up to 12 months)	Lifestyle modification (up to 6 months)	Drug therapy
Stages 2 and 3 (≥160/≥110)	Drug therapy	Drug therapy	Drug therapy

TOD, target organ damage; CCD, clinical cardiovascular disease.

Table 8–3. Prevalence Rates for Hypertension in the United States by Age, Race, and Gender. Data from the Third National Health and Nutrition Examination Survey, 1988–1991

	Prevalence of Hypertension (%)			
	Males		*Females*	
Age (years)	Black	White	Black	White
18–29	6.4	3.3	2.3	1.0
30–39	22.5	13.2	11.2	6.9
40–49	35.2	22.0	33.2	11.3
50–59	53.3	37.5	47.8	33.0
60–69	71.2	51.1	73.9	50.0
70+	60	60	80	70

Source: Burt et al. (1995).

compromise with adverse effects on several organs. With more severe hypertension, the endothelial barrier breaks down and plasma fluids and proteins flood the arteriole wall, causing vascular edema and fibrin deposition (fibrinoid change). As the process proceeds, necrosis of the arteriolar wall can occur (fibrinoid necrosis).

The consequences of arteriolosclerosis can be severe, especially when accompanied by the more advanced manifestations of fibrinoid change and fibrinoid necrosis. Even in the absence of any arterial compromise from atherosclerosis, characteristic end organ damage occurs. In the brain, lumen compromise of arterioles can lead to lacunar stroke. Clinical manifestations of such infarcts range from obvious, substantial motor deficits to subtle sensory or other neurological dysfunction, such as difficulty finding words. Dementia has also been associated with lacunae. In a 15-year longitudinal study, it was shown that elevated blood pressure precedes the onset of dementia and decreases only subsequent to the dementia (Skoog et al., 1996; Skoog, 1997). There are probably a number of potential causes of lacunar stroke besides hypertension, including emboli from atherosclerotic cerebral lesions. Weakening of brain arteriolar walls can result in *Charcot-Bouchard aneurysms*, small saccular defects that can burst and cause catastrophic cerebral hemorrhage. In the eye, microvascular changes can eventually lead to retinal ischemia and blindness. In the kidney, arteriolosclerosis is manifest as glomerulosclerosis and nephrosclerosis. When lumen compromise is sufficient, a vicious cycle of increasing ischemia, renin release, and further arteriolar damage leads to malignant hypertension. Untreated, malignant hypertension is associated with a 5-year mortality rate of 95%, with 65% dying from congestive heart failure, 14% from renal failure, 11% from myocardial infarction, and 5% from cerebral hemorrhage (Flaxman, 1936). Prevention of this kind of morbidity was clearly shown in early trials treating severely hypertensive patients (Veterans Administration Co-operative Study Group on Anti-Hypertensive Agents, 1967).

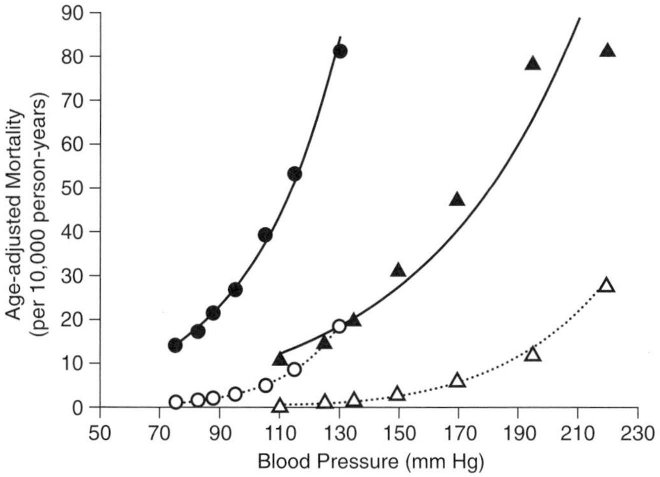

Fig. 8–1. Coronary heart disease (CHD) and stroke mortality vs. blood pressure after 6 years' follow-up of 347,978 men screened for the Multiple Risk Factor Intervention Trial (MRFIT). *Circles*, diastolic blood pressure; *triangles*, systolic blood pressure; *solid symbols*, CHD; *open symbols*, stroke. From Neaton et al. (1995).

Subtypes of Hypertension

Primary or essential hypertension comprises approximately 94% of all hypertension (Berglund et al., 1976; Rudnick et al., 1977). Secondary forms include hypertension resulting from renal parenchymal disease (glomerular and tubulointerstitial disease as well as vasculitis), renal vascular disease (atherosclerosis and fibromuscular dysplasia), urinary obstruction, and a variety of endocrine causes including Cushing's syndrome (with steroid medication use), primary hyperaldosteronism (adenomas and hyperplasia of adrenal glands), pheochromocytoma, acromegaly, juxtaglomerular tumors producing renin (very rare), hyperparathyroidism, hyperthyroidism, and oral contraceptive use (occasionally). Coarctation of the aorta and acute intermittent porphyria may also lead to hypertension.

Several rare, monogenic forms of hypertension are included in lists of secondary causes by some authors, though they are probably better considered as rare primary causes. These include glucocorticoid-remediable aldosteronism, Liddle's syndrome Gordon's syndrome (pseudohypoaldosteronism type II), apparent mineralocorticoid excess, and adrenogenital syndromes (with 11β-hydroxylase and 17α-hydroxylase deficiencies described) (Scheinman et al., 1999). Glucocorticoid-remediable aldosteronism is caused by crossover generation of a hybrid gene from two homologous genes on chromosome 8, 11β-hydroxylase and aldosterone synthase, resulting in increased 18-hydroxycortisol and 18-oxocortisol, increased aldosterone, and decreased renin activity (Lifton et al., 1992). This produces early-onset hypertension and stroke. Liddle's syndrome results in hypertension, hypokalemia, decreased renin activity, and decreased aldosterone secretion and is caused by mutations in both the β and γ subunits of the amiloride-sensitive epithelial sodium channel gene (Shimkets et al., 1994; Hansson et al., 1995a,b). Liddle's syndrome is responsive to triamterene or amiloride, which can inhibit the epithelial sodium channel. Mutations in two *WNK* kinase genes (chromosomes 12 and 17) lead to Gordon's syndrome, characterized by hypertension, increased salt reabsorption, and impaired hydrogen and potassium excretion (Wilson et al., 2001). A third, unknown locus on chromosome 1q has also been linked to this disorder (Mansfield et al., 1997).

Within the essential hypertension category, various attempts have been made to categorize subsets of hypertension. Some of these include low-renin hypertension, salt-sensitive hypertension, nonmodulation (inappropriate response of the renin–angiotensin–aldosterone system to angiotensin II infusion), and familial dyslipidemic hypertension. There is considerable overlap among these four groups, and they are especially common in African Americans. Each will be discussed in later sections.

GENERAL GENETIC AND EPIDEMIOLOGICAL EVIDENCE

Family Epidemiology

Family and Twin Studies

Blood pressure clearly correlates within families, as shown by nearly all large family studies from multiple countries, a few of which are listed in Table 8–4. Familial correlations generally range from 0.1 to 0.3, resulting in heritability estimates clustering around 20% (Miller et al., 1987; Hunt et al., 1989a; Tambs et al., 1992; Robinson et al., 1991). Brother-pair correlations are generally similar to sister-pair and brother–sister correlations. Parent–offspring correlations are usually slightly smaller than sib–sib correlations, possibly due to a generational effect that cannot be completely accounted for by age adjustment. A few studies have found lower father–offspring correlations than mother–offspring correlations (Miller et al., 1987; Koshechkin et al., 1991), which were attributed to the offspring sharing a more similar environment with the mothers than the fathers. However, other studies did not find a difference (Robinson et al., 1991; Tambs et al., 1992). If there is a maternal effect on blood pressure, it probably begins at very young ages. Blood pressure correlations have been shown to begin in infancy (6–12 months of age), with heritability estimates of 0.27 and 0.17 for systolic and diastolic blood pressure, respectively (Levine et al., 1982). Salt intake in the first 6 months after birth led to significantly higher blood pressures 15 years later, even though diet was not controlled after the study ended at 6 months (Geleijnse et al., 1997).

Heritability estimates are much higher when twins are used (Table 8–5). The high adult twin blood pressure heritabilities and the low infant twin heritabilities previously mentioned (Levine et al., 1982) suggest that heritability likely increases with age during the early years of life. A changing genetic variance over time is also supported by studies showing genotype by age interactions, the affected genotype having greater blood pressure increases with age than the normal genotype (Pérusse et al., 1991; Cheng et al., 1995). Environmental variance may remain more constant, however. Two studies have shown that spouse correlations do not increase the longer the spouses share a household environment and that sib correlations do not show large decreases years after they move out of the same home (Feinleib et al., 1979; Tambs et al., 1992).

Heritability estimates of blood pressure in a twin study were similar for supine measurements and 24-hour ambulatory measurements, suggesting that careful standard clinic measurements are valid for estimation of heritability despite the variability in blood pressure during the day (Fagard et al., 1995). Most of the difference in heritability estimates between twin and sibling data is probably due to different assumptions of the statistical models used to obtain the heritability estimates [e.g., same amount of shared environment for monozygotic (MZ) and dizygotic (DZ) twins] (Hunt et al., 1989a). This Utah study used a standardized clinic protocol on both family members and twin pairs ascertained from the same population and yet derived divergent estimates between the two samples. Adjustment for differences in environmental variables, including diet and physical activity, had little effect on the heritability estimates (Slattery et al., 1988). This suggests that either shared environment influences familial correlations in a more complicated way than can be adjusted for by simple regression techniques, that these particular environmental variables were not strongly correlated with blood pressure, or that model assumptions other than common environment are responsible for the differences. The existence of major genes for blood pressure also would violate the assumptions of both types of study. Averaging multiple measurements (four or more) of blood pressure over a period of at least 10 years, the Framingham Heart Study showed that heritabilities for systolic and diastolic blood pressure increased from 0.42 to 0.57 and 0.39 to 0.56, respectively (Levy et al., 2000). Thus, measurement error and daily fluctuations in blood pressure can have important effects on heritability estimates.

In a review of the literature using meta-analysis, the majority of 39 studies found increased blood pressure reactivity in hypertensive subjects, but the findings were not consistent across studies (Pickering et al., 1990). There are likely many factors involved in study variability, including heterogeneity of the underlying physiology. One study reported that mental stress was associated with vasoconstriction in obese subjects but with vasodilation in lean subjects, even though both groups increased mean arterial pressure (Rockstroh et al., 1992). Isometric stress was associated with exaggerated arterial pressure and resistance in both groups. In a 6.5-year prospective study, larger systolic and diastolic blood pressure responses to mental and physical stressors were associated with higher follow-up resting blood pressures (Matthews et al., 1993). Slightly lower heritability estimates than for resting blood pressure were found for changes in blood pressure in twins after participating in a mental arithmetic task of serial subtraction (Smith et al., 1987). Heritabilities for systolic and diastolic blood pressure changes during mental arithmetic were 0.46 and 0.54, respectively, after adjustment for baseline levels of blood pressure. Another study of mental stress found that stressed blood pressure heritabilities were higher than baseline heritabilities and that the shared environmental effects became smaller (Boomsma et al., 1998). The baseline and mental stress genetic effects were correlated with each other.

The cold pressor test, where blood pressure is measured while the hand is immersed in ice water, has been suggested to predict future hypertension (Wood et al., 1984). The response to this maneuver has also been shown to have a genetic component (McIlhany et al., 1975). The heritability estimates for change in systolic blood pressure were 0.72 in females and 0.36 in males and for change in diastolic blood pressure 0.68 in females and 0.53 in males. In a study looking at blood pressure and hemodynamic heritability (Bielen et al., 1991), heritabilities of resting systolic and diastolic blood pressures were 0.69 and 0.32 in 53 pairs of twins. Changes in blood pressure during a bicycle ergometer exercise test were not heritable, however, when either

Table 8–4. Sibling Blood Pressure Correlations

Location (References)	Systolic Blood Pressure	Diastolic Blood Pressure
Michigan, USA (Johnson et al., 1965)	0.17	0.12
Georgia, USA (Hayes et al., 1971)	0.20	0.17
Framingham, USA (Feinleib et al., 1975)	0.18	0.17
Utah, USA (Hunt et al., 1989a)	0.16	0.21
United Kingdom (Miall and Oldham, 1963)	0.33	0.20
Turkmenistan (Koshechkin et al., 1991)	0.27	0.11
Norway (Tambs et al., 1992)	0.22	0.23
Brazil (Robinson et al., 1991)	0.27	0.32
Tokelau (Ward et al., 1979)	0.17	0.13

Source: Hunt et al. (1994).

Table 8–5. Intraclass Blood Pressure Correlations and Heritability Estimates

Systolic Blood Pressure			Diastolic Blood Pressure			
rMZ	*rDZ*	h^2	*rMZ*	*rDZ*	h^2	Reference
0.85	0.50	0.70	0.80	0.54	0.52	McIlhany et al. (1975)
0.55	0.25	0.60	0.58	0.27	0.61	Feinleib et al. (1977)
0.87	0.59[a]	0.56	0.83	0.58[a]	0.50	Miller et al. (1987)
0.43	0.11	0.62	0.46	0.14	0.65	Hunt et al. (1989a)

r, intraclass or Pearson correlation between twins; h^2, heritability; MZ, monozygous; DZ, dizygous.
[a]Correlations from siblings rather than dizygous twins.
Source: Hunt et al. (1994).

work load or heart rate was fixed, with heritabilities of 0 for both systolic and diastolic blood pressure. Sizeable common environmental components were found for the change in blood pressure during exercise, ranging from 14% to 68%. However, two other studies have suggested a genetic component to a bicycle ergometer test (Hunt et al., 1989a; van den Bree et al., 1996). The second of these studies found both a genetic effect at baseline that continued throughout the exercise and an additional genetic component that appeared at the start of the exercise and remained until the end. These and other intervention tests have also been related to a positive family history of hypertension, e.g., the cold pressor test (Hines et al., 1936), mental arithmetic (Falkner et al., 1979), bicycle exercise and isometric handgrip (Ambrosioni et al., 1981), and standing blood pressure (Williams et al., 1984).

Adoption Studies

Adoption studies can also estimate heritability by comparing the adopted child's blood pressure to his or her natural and adopted parent's blood pressure and/or to the child's natural and adopted siblings. The genetic correlation estimates should be 0 when comparing the adopted child to the adopted parents or siblings. In the Montreal Adoption Survey, the intraclass correlation for systolic blood pressure between adopted siblings was 0.16 compared to the correlation of 0.38 between natural siblings (Mongeau et al., 1986). For diastolic blood pressure, the adoptee and natural sibling correlations were 0.29 and 0.53, respectively. Parent–adoptee correlations were not significantly different from 0 and much smaller than the significant parent–natural child correlations. Estimates of heritability were 61% and 58% for systolic and diastolic blood pressure, respectively. A study of twins reared together or reared apart yielded heritability estimates of 0.44 and 0.34 for systolic and diastolic blood pressure, respectively (Hong et al., 1994).

Family History

CHD, hypertension, and stroke aggregate within families, suggesting that genetic factors and/or common environmental factors make significant contributions to each of these end points (Hunt et al., 1986a). A family history of hypertension is an independent predictor of the development of hypertension (Hunt et al., 1986a, 1991; Friedman et al., 1988; Lauer et al., 1991). The prevalence of a positive family history of CHD (more than two affected) is increased threefold if the family has a positive family history of hypertension, stroke, or diabetes (Hunt et al., 1996a), suggesting, along with other data, that genetic components are common to the development of both hypertension and CHD.

Environmental Factors

Numerous environmental factors have been suggested to influence blood pressure, the incidence of hypertension, and the level of intermediate phenotypes for blood pressure. It is beyond the scope of this chapter to review this extensive literature. Therefore, some of the most important factors are mentioned here with references to more extensive reviews or meta-analyses. Reference works on hypertension should be consulted for detailed discussions (Swales, 1994; Laragh et al., 1995; Izzo and Black, 1999).

Dietary sodium is probably one of the most studied and controversial factors suggested to increase blood pressure. The Intersalt Study provided a wealth of data about population associations of salt intake and blood pressure and the increase with age (Elliott et al., 1996), but even this massive study is involved in controversy about whether it proved the salt hypothesis (Taubes, 1998). The Trials of Hypertension Prevention Collaborative Research Group (1997) found significantly reduced blood pressure after 36 months of reduced salt intake. The magnitude of the result was small, but extrapolating the result over 10 to 20 years becomes even more meaningful.

A meta-analysis of intervention trials suggested that a 21 to 70 mmol decrease in sodium intake produces reductions in systolic and diastolic blood pressure of 3.6/2.2 mm Hg (Grobbee and Hofman, 1986). Another meta-analysis showed that median 77 and 76 mmol decreases in sodium were associated with systolic and diastolic blood pressure decreases of 4.8/2.5 and 1.9/1.1 mm Hg in hypertensive and normotensive persons, respectively (Cutler et al., 1997). Infants who were randomized at birth to a low-sodium diet for the first 6 months after birth had lower blood pressures 15 years later (3.6/2.2 mm Hg) than infants assigned to a normal-sodium diet (Geleijnse et al., 1997). In addition, a study in chimpanzees showed that adding salt within the normal human dietetic range to a baseline low-salt diet increased systolic and diastolic blood pressure (33/10 mm Hg) over 20 months (Denton et al., 1995). The sodium-induced blood pressure changes were completely reversed within 6 months after removing the additional salt, and although most of the chimpanzees responded, there were clearly responders and nonresponders. In most human studies of salt sensitivity, there also has been a wide range of responses, even within the artificially defined subgroups of salt-sensitive and salt-resistant persons (Luft et al., 1977).

Other electrolytes are probably involved in various aspects of blood pressure control, such as calcium (Allender et al., 1996), potassium (Whelton et al., 1997), and magnesium (Whelton et al., 1989). Potassium may protect against cardiovascular disease, particularly stroke, even if blood pressure is not lowered (Tobian, 1988). The Dietary Approaches to Stop Hypertension study showed that fruits and vegetables reduced blood pressure even when dietary sodium intake was kept constant (Appel et al., 1997). Dietary fats have not been clearly linked to blood pressure (Ascherio et al., 1992). Lowering alcohol consumption helps to lower blood pressure, with an average of 1 mm Hg reduction for a reduction of one drink/day (Cushman et al., 1998).

Weight is clearly involved with blood pressure levels, if not as a cause at least as an aggravating factor (Landsberg, 1994; Hall, 1997; Hindmarsh and Brook, 1999; Jones, 1999). Obesity affects glucose metabolism, sympathetic activation, sodium excretion, and angiotensin production. It is considered to be the environmental factor for which intervention will have the greatest impact on blood pressure reduction. Unfortunately, long-term maintenance of weight loss is difficult. In the Trials of Hypertension Prevention study (1997), weight loss was maintained sufficiently over 36 months to significantly reduce blood pressure but required monitoring, training, and encouragement from study personnel.

Psychosocial factors, such as the degree of control one has over one's environment, can affect blood pressure, although other factors such as hostility are not as consistent from one study to another (Poulter et al., 1990; Pickering et al., 1990, 1996). Physical activity has a beneficial effect on multiple systems that control blood pressure (Fagard, 1995) and can reduce blood pressure even in the absence of weight loss.

PATHOPHYSIOLOGY: BIOLOGICAL BASIS OF GENETIC SUSCEPTIBILITY

Pathophysiology of Disease

In theory, every enzyme, hormone, cellular ion transporter, receptor, or structural component that is related to the control of blood pressure is a candidate gene for hypertension. As advances in each of the above areas are made, new candidate genes related to hypertension are suggested because they code for either the newly discovered gene product or the function of a known product that has some influence on some aspect of blood pressure control. Mutations in any of the genes controlling these variables could increase the susceptibility to hypertension. As the number of abnormalities increase, so does the susceptibility. Blood pressure physiology and possible abnormalities in the genes influencing that physiology will be discussed as each candidate gene is considered.

Because early studies showed that hypertension always followed transplantation of a kidney from hypertensive rats (Dahl et al., 1974), renal function and the renin–angiotensin system have received the most study for defects leading to hypertension. The kidney normally compensates for increased blood pressure by increasing fluid and sodium excretion. This response curve is very steep, so even small increases in blood pressure can return fluid and electrolyte balance to normal (Hall, 1994). Obesity shifts this curve to the right and may flatten the curve so that higher blood pressure levels are required to maintain fluid balance (Rocchini et al., 1989; Granger et al., 1994; Suzuki et al., 1996). A shift to the right without flattening, as seen in salt-insensitive subjects, means that blood pressure will be elevated but that natriuresis in response to blood pressure change will be nearly normal. A flattening of the response curve, as seen in more salt-sensitive individuals, requires a greater blood pressure increase to excrete a similar amount of sodium and fluid than in less salt-sensitive individuals.

One mechanism used to maintain normal pressure and electrolyte balance is the renin–angiotensin system. Renin is normally regulated by sodium loads sensed by the macula densa in the juxtaglomerular apparatus in the kidney or by reduced perfusion pressure. In the presence of decreased pressure or sodium loads, plasma renin is increased. Renin released from the kidney converts angiotensinogen of liver origin to angiotensin I, which is converted to angiotensin II by angiotensin-converting enzyme (ACE). Angiotensin II causes vasoconstriction and increases sodium reabsorption. Renin conversion of angiotensinogen to angiotensin I decreases the amount of angiotensinogen, but increased angiotensin II levels stimulate hepatic angiotensinogen production and release, returning angiotensinogen levels to normal. Higher angiotensin II levels also have a negative feedback on renin, decreasing renin levels (Sealey et al., 1990). Any genetic abnormality causing increased angiotensinogen production would increase angiotensinogen levels, resulting in higher amounts converted to angiotensin II. The higher angiotensinogen levels would also be maintained through higher feedback by angiotensin II. Increased angiotensin II directly increases sodium reabsorption in the proximal tubule and stimulates aldosterone release, increasing sodium and water retention, which increases blood pressure and should decrease renin. The importance of this positive and negative feedback system is illustrated in rats. If appropriate decreases in renin occur in the presence of high angiotensinogen levels, rats do not have increased blood pressure (Gahnem et al., 1994). However when renin does not appropriately decrease, blood pressure rises.

Genetic Studies of Pathophysiology

Low Renin

Hypertensive patients have been subdivided into three classes based on low, normal, and high plasma renin activity (Brunner et al., 1973). Persons with low renin are more likely to be salt-sensitive, female, older, responsive to diuretics, and African American (Drayer et al., 1981; Niarchos and Laragh, 1984). Low-renin hypertensive patients also appear to have abnormally low aldosterone responses to a low-salt diet or angiotensin II infusion compared to other hypertensive and normotensive patients (Fisher et al., 1999). While it appears that low-renin subjects may define a specific subset of hypertensive patients, there is no standard definition of low renin activity. A nomogram relating plasma renin activity to sodium excretion is often used for this definition (Laragh, 1992). The familiality of low renin activity is uncertain, although an abstract has reported significant familial concordance of low renin activity (Fisher et al., 2000).

Nonmodulation

Nonmodulation of the renin–angiotensin–aldosterone system has been suggested as an important intermediate phenotype, which is found in about 50% of hypertensive individuals with normal or high renin levels (Hollenberg and Williams, 1990). This phenotype is measured either as the change in renal blood flow after an infusion of angiotensin II while on a high-salt diet or as the change in aldosterone levels after an angiotensin II infusion while on a low-salt diet. Nonmodulators are persons who do not have normal changes in renal blood flow or aldosterone after these maneuvers. Classification as nonmodulators by the first method generally agrees with classification using the second method but is much less than 100% (Williams et al., 1992). Bimodality of the aldosterone response to angiotensin II was strong in the hypertensives ($p = 0.00009$) but borderline in the normotensives ($p = 0.05$). Trimodality in the hypertensives was also suggested ($p < 0.01$), with 8% of the sample in the highest mode. Multiple studies of the same patients have been done showing high stability of this phenotype.

Changes in renal blood flow in response to either angiotensin II infusion or change in sodium intake (10 to 200 meq/day) were significantly less in subjects with a positive family history of hypertension (Lifton et al., 1989). Concordance of the nonmodulation trait in hypertensive sib pairs was 3.5 times higher than expected, while that for modulating status in these hypertensive sib pairs was one-seventh of the expected value. Hopkins et al. (1996b) showed that variation at the angiotensinogen locus is associated with blunted renal plasma flow response to angiotensin II infusion. LDL cholesterol levels modify the blood pressure response to angiotensin II infusion, with higher lipid levels associated with greater increases of systolic and diastolic blood pressure (John et al., 1999; Vuagnat et al., 2001).

Salt Sensitivity

Approximately 30% of normotensive and 55% of hypertensive white subjects appear to have blood pressures that are sensitive to salt restriction (Luft et al., 1988). In black subjects, the percentages are 32% and 73%, respectively. These percentages change somewhat depending on the maneuver and cut points used to define salt sensitivity. Both low-renin subjects and African-American subjects (many of whom have low renin) are very salt-sensitive. The best studies analyze salt sensitivity as a continuous trait without trying to arbitrarily assign cut points. The changes in blood pressures after sodium restriction appear to be familial (Miller et al., 1987). Mother–offspring correlations were 0.26 ($p < 0.01$) and father–offspring correlations were 0.17 ($p < 0.10$) for mean arterial blood pressure change. Sibling correlations were 0.36 ($p < 0.01$), and MZ twin correlations were 0.68 ($p < 0.001$). However, in this study, spouse correlations for mean arterial change were greater ($r = 0.60$) than all other correlations but that for twins, even though baseline blood pressure correlations in the spouses were not significant. Watt et al. (1985) did not find differences in blood pressure reduction after sodium restriction between individuals with and without a parental history of hypertension.

Miller et al. (1987) showed that urinary sodium excretion changes were familial ($r = 0.42$ in siblings and $r = 0.73$ in twins), while there was no correlation between spouses for urinary sodium changes. The change in sodium excretion did not correlate with a change in blood pressure for any of the relationships. This may indicate that there is some component regulating sodium excretion that is genetic but not directly related to blood pressure responses because of the heterogeneity of that response within families (a gene–environment interaction) or the activation of other compensatory mechanisms in some family members. Thus, the heritability of blood pressure change or electrolyte change due to salt restriction is not resolved.

Dyslipidemia and Hypertension

Epidemiological studies have clearly shown consistent associations between hypertension and dyslipidemia, reported from the Framingham (Castelli et al., 1986) and the Lipid Research Clinic (Criqui et al., 1986) populations. Various names have been given to this syndrome, which is the most common syndrome associated with hypertension. Perhaps the most descriptive of these names is the *multiple metabolic syndrome*.

Twin and family studies suggest that genetic factors play an important role in the coaggregation of lipid abnormalities and hypertension, as shown from the National Heart, Lung, and Blood Institute (NHLBI) twin cohort (Selby et al., 1991) and in Utah families (Williams et al., 1988; Hunt et al., 1989b; Hopkins et al., 1996a). Sibling aggregation of both hypertension and lipid abnormalities occurred more often than expected by chance (Williams et al., 1988). In Utah sibling pairs ascertained only for the diagnosis of hypertension before age 60 in both siblings, high triglycerides and low high-density lipoprotein (HDL) cholesterol were found three times more often than expected ($p < 0.0001$). These abnormalities occurred in persons with normal weight as well as in the obese. This syndrome, descriptively labeled *familial dyslipidemic hypertension*, occurs in about 12% of persons with essential hypertension and 1% to 2% of the general population.

Siblings with this syndrome had increased fasting triglycerides, very low-density lipoprotein (VLDL) cholesterol, and apolipoprotein B and decreased HDL cholesterol (Hunt et al., 1989b). The syndrome itself appears heterogeneous. Results from the NHLBI twin study confirmed the Utah findings (Selby et al., 1991). In addition, this study showed that occurrence of CHD after 16 years of follow-up was much greater in persons with both hypertension and dyslipidemia than in persons with only hypertension or dyslipidemia (Fig. 8–2). LDL particles tend to be more dense and smaller in individuals with the multiple metabolic syndrome (Krauss, 1987; Hunt et al., 1989b).

Insulin Resistance

Similar to the salt hypothesis, it remains unclear whether hyperinsulinemia and insulin resistance cause hypertension. Most investigators agree that hyperinsulinemia does not cause hypertension, but there is less clarity about insulin resistance. Insulin resistance is hypothesized to promote hypertension in various ways: *(1)* stimulation of cation transport and Na reabsorption in the distal and proximal tubule, causing renal Na retention and hypertension (DeFronzo et al., 1975; Baum, 1987); *(2)* stimulation of norepinephrine secretion and increased blood pressure (Rowe et al., 1981); *(3)* stimulation of vascular endothelium and smooth muscle cells to hypertrophy, increasing peripheral vas-

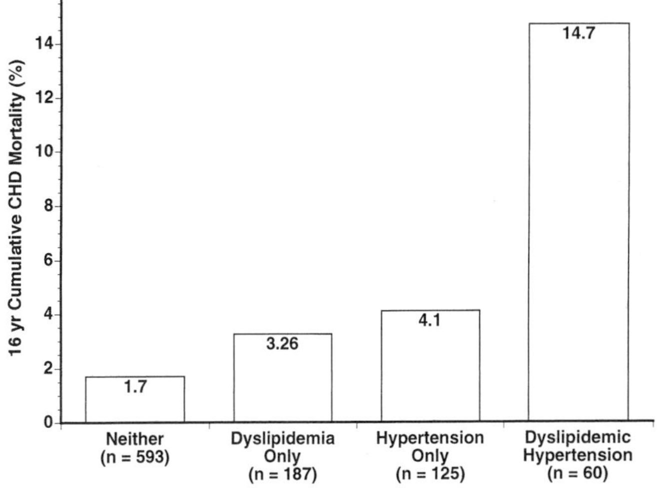

Fig. 8–2. Mortality rates for four subgroups of patients based on the presence or absence of hypertension and dyslipidemia.

cular resistance and blood pressure (i.e., growth factor-like effect of insulin) (King et al., 1985; Lever, 1986); *(4)* stimulation of intracellular calcium and increased smooth muscle contractility (Pershadsingh and McDonald, 1979; Draznin et al., 1987); and *(5)* obesity-related angiotensinogen production in adipose tissue associated with insulin resistance (Frederich et al., 1992).

Insulin resistance has been related to several metabolic and clinical conditions, including hyperinsulinemia, hypertension, CHD, diabetes, and obesity (Reaven, 1988). Insulin resistance has been included as part of the "deadly quartet" (Kaplan, 1989) and suggested to be the basis of syndrome X (Reaven and Hoffman, 1987; Fuh et al., 1987). Numerous examples of positive (Modan et al., 1985; Fuh et al., 1987; Ferrannini et al., 1987; Reaven, 1991) and negative (Mbanya et al., 1988; Asch et al., 1991; Schmidt et al., 1996; Neel et al., 1998) results are available relating insulin resistance to hypertension or blood pressure. A family-based study partially controlling for background genetic and environmental effects showed no association of insulin with isolated systolic blood pressure (Kronenberg et al., 2000). Further, evidence for associations of insulin with diastolic hypertension or with untreated blood pressure were not significant after further adjustment for body mass index (BMI). A few prospective studies have shown insulin to be related to the development of hypertension (Skarfors et al., 1991; Niskanen et al., 1991; Haffner et al., 1992; Lissner et al., 1992). Some studies on laboratory animals support the negative results in humans. Hypertensive and normotensive rats with acutely elevated insulin levels do not increase sodium reabsorption (Finch et al., 1990). Chronic insulin infusion (28 days) in normal dogs does not increase blood pressure or sympathetic stimulation (Hall et al., 1989, 1990). Further evidence is needed to determine whether hyperinsulinemia precedes lipid or lipoprotein abnormalities, or vice versa, or whether they occur simultaneously.

A gene for high insulin levels may contribute to the concordance of hypertension and diabetes. Between 30% and 50% of those with non-insulin-dependent diabetes mellitus (NIDDM) are hypertensive (Fuller, 1985). Approximately 40% of hypertensives have lipid abnormalities, and 46% of those with high cholesterol (>240 mg/dl) have hypertension (>140/90 mm Hg), indicating a strong clustering of these disorders. An analysis of the National Academy of Sciences twin registry showed that there was evidence for a common genetic determinant of hypertension, obesity, and diabetes (Carmelli et al., 1994). Fifty-nine percent of the variation in a common factor underlying the concordance of these three conditions was estimated to be explained by genetics. The genetic portion of the common factor explained 21% of the variance in hypertension, 11% for diabetes, and 6% for obesity. Each of the three conditions also had significant contributions from genes that were not common to the other conditions. The remaining variance was explained by environmental factors that were not shared by the twins. Another study showed genetic correlations of systolic blood pressure with the insulin resistance syndrome (Hong et al., 1997).

GENE IDENTIFICATION

Identifying Genetic Determinants of Hypertension

The advent of molecular techniques in the early 1980s held the promise that the genetic basis of human disorders would soon be understood in molecular terms. While such expectations have been met for a host of classic Mendelian disorders resulting from gain or loss of function at single loci, the same cannot be said of common human diseases, particularly hypertension. Nevertheless, the tools and resources made available by the Human Genome Project, the long history of epidemiological investigation of hypertension, advances in study design and analytical methods, and new technologies are cause for optimism that it will be possible to understand the genetic underpinnings of hypertension.

The implications of these findings for essential hypertension, a condition of unknown causes with a lifetime prevalence of 30% to 50% in affluent societies, have proven modest, however. Ambiguous phenotypic delineation, genetic heterogeneity, and various confounding factors have been appropriately cited to account for this sorry state, but such challenges have been encountered and handled adequately in classical genetics. The defining feature, then, of the genetics of common disease is that susceptibility imparted by genetic variation is modest and quantitative, results from differential response to environmental exposure, and achieves significance only through cumulative integration of lifetime experience.

Many investigators have suggested that intermediate phenotypes may help to reduce the problem of heterogeneity. Figure 8–3 suggests that many genes lead to the development of hypertension and that there are many confounding variables on these genetic effects. However, intermediate phenotypes should have both fewer genes influencing them and fewer confounding variables. Studying these phenotypes should make the genetic signal stronger and more easily detectable. Tables 8–6 and 8–7 show data suggesting that for many intermediate blood pressure phenotypes the genetic effects are larger, are less confounded, and may be more easily detected than simple measures of hypertension or blood pressure (Hasstedt et al., 1988a,b, 1989a,b; Hunt et al., 1993; Cheng et al., 1995, 1997).

If a person is to develop elevated blood pressure, some physiological mechanism must become abnormal prior to the elevation. While blood pressure may be resistant to the biochemical abnormality for many years, the intermediate phenotype must be abnormal for a sufficient time to cause the normal counterregulatory mechanisms to slowly fail. Because we know that hypertension develops over many years, it is expected that these abnormal physiological processes would be expressed for long periods of time before the onset of clinical hypertension.

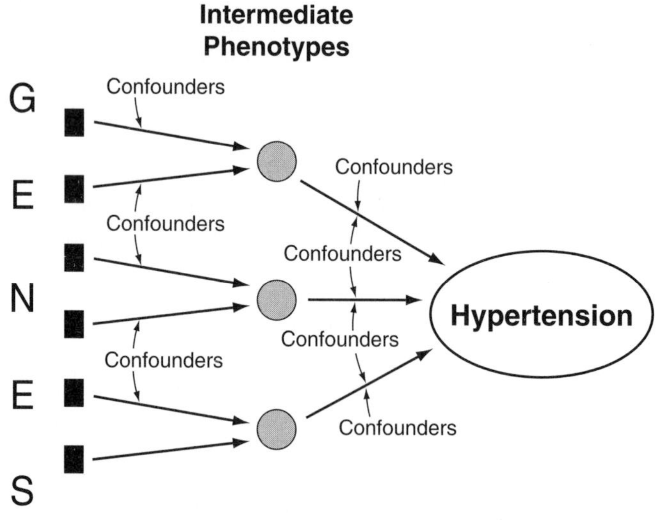

Fig. 8–3. Intermediate phenotypes may have fewer associated genes and less environmental confounding than blood pressure, hypertension, or cardiovascular end points.

Table 8–6. Major Gene and Total Heritabilities of Intermediate Phenotypes

Phenotype	Major Gene h^2	Polygenic h^2	Total h^2	Displacement
Na–Li countertransport	34%	46%	80%	2.8 SD
RBC Na	29	55	84	2.0
Ouabain binding site number	14	63	77	3.0
Kallikrein	51	27	78	2.3
Subscapular/suprailiac ratio	42	10	52	1.9
Math BP response	33	4	37	Depends on age
Exercise bike BP response	34	17	51	3.6
7-year DBP change	24	0	24	2.6

h^2, heritability; RBC, red blood cell; BP, blood pressure; DBP, diastolic blood pressure.

Many intermediate phenotypes have been shown to be elevated even in young children of hypertensive parents. For example, variation in the angiotensinogen gene (*AGT*) leads to elevated angiotensinogen levels in children (Bloem et al., 1995). Many lipid abnormalities are present in the twenties and thirties (Wilson et al., 1990, Kwiterovich 1995). Elevated sodium–lithium countertransport activities appear in childhood, as do low kallikrein levels (Zinner et al., 1976, 1978; Williams et al., 1983; Berry et al., 1989; Houtman et al., 1993). Obesity, a potent risk factor for cardiovascular disease, begins in many people at an early age (Freedman et al., 1987).

Heterogeneity and Confounding Effects on Gene Identification

Hypertension clearly has multiple causes and is heterogeneous even within defined populations. Clinical heterogeneity exists when different clinical manifestations of the same disease may be present (e.g., different blood pressures in patients with glucocorticoid-remediable aldosteronism). *Genetic heterogeneity* refers to a disorder with apparently different transmission patterns [e.g., pseudohypoaldosteronism, type I has both recessive and dominant forms (Kuhnle et al., 1995)]. *Locus heterogeneity* occurs when mutations at different loci lead to the same clinical phenotype, such as Liddle's and Gordon's syndromes and pseudohypoaldosteronism type I(Scheinman et al., 1999; Wilson et al., 2001). *Allelic heterogeneity* occurs when different mutations at the same locus can result in the same phenotype. As an example, over 600 mutations in the LDL receptor gene have been identified as causing familial hypercholesterolemia (Wilson et al., 1998).

Another cause of heterogeneity is the definition of hypertension. For example, clinicians do not start patients on antihypertensive medication in a uniform manner. Once a patient is treated for hypertension, any index of severity may be completely obscured or impossible to apply. Furthermore, hypertension can be self-perpetuating (as in salt-sensitive Dahl rats even after a high-salt diet is replaced with a low-salt diet) and can enter a rapidly escalating stage (malignant hypertension). In most cases, the investigator cannot determine with certainty whether a given patient's blood pressure is severely elevated because of a more powerful initiating stimulus or inadequate or delayed therapy.

One of the major research questions has been whether there are genes that have sufficiently large, identifiable effects on the variation in blood pressure between individuals or whether genetic control is a result of small effects from many genes. Heterogeneity masks the effects of any particular gene being studied due to variation in a phenotype that is independent of the genetic mechanism of interest. Unless the genetic effect is strong or the population subdivided to reduce heterogeneity, studies using blood pressure as a phenotype, or even using intermediate phenotypes associated with blood pressure, will be difficult.

Even though polygenes, by definition, each have a small effect on the phenotype or disease with which they are associated, the combination of polygenes can have a substantial effect. An example from two families with familial hypercholesterolemia illustrates this point (Fig. 8–4). The persons represented by black symbols have a specific mutation in the LDL receptor gene that leads to greatly elevated LDL cholesterol levels. There is clear

Table 8–7. Total Genetic Heritability (h^2, percent of total variance) and Common Environmental Effects (same household effect, c^2) Estimated in a Variance Components Analysis

Phenotype	h^2	c^2	Phenotype	h^2	c^2
Li–K cotransport	30	0	Math SBP	21	4
Na leak	43	0	Math DBP	23	8
Serum Mg	57	24	Grip SBP	16	0
Serum K	23	7	Grip DBP	17	0
Serum Ca	14	13	Sitting SBP	17	7
Uric acid	31	8	Sitting DBP	22	3
Creatinine	23	2	Standing SBP	16	10
Insulin	45	Not estimated	Standing DBP	21	3
Height	75	11	Cholesterol	42	8
BMI	24	0	TG	37	6
Scapular skinfold	32	3	HDL-C	45	15
Waist circumference	25	9	Urine aldosterone	30	Not estimated
Hip circumference	36	7	Urine PGE_2	40	Not estimated

BMI, body mass index; SBP, systolic blood pressure; DBP, diastolic blood pressure; TG, triglyceride; HDL-C, high-density lipoprotein cholesterol; PGE_2, prostaglandin E_2.
Source: Williams et al. (1991).

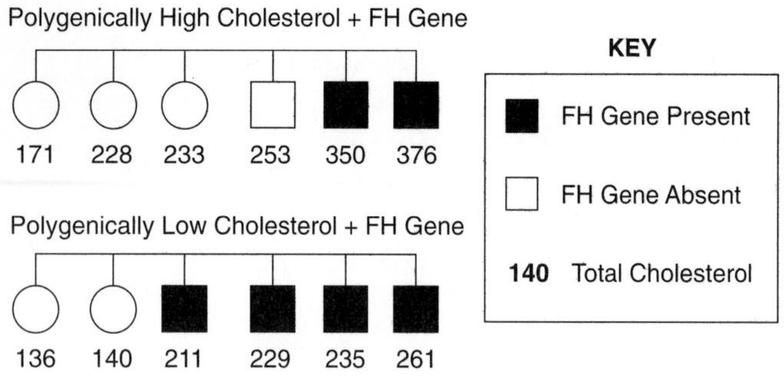

Fig. 8–4. Effect of different polygenic backgrounds on interpreting major gene segregation.

bimodality within each family, with an over 70 mg/dl difference in total cholesterol between mutation carriers and normal individuals. However, polygenic effects (possibly with some contribution from the environment) in the first family elevate the average cholesterol level in that family by 67 mg/dl. This causes an LDL receptor mutation carrier with polygenes for low cholesterol to have lower cholesterol than a normal person with polygenes for high cholesterol. The clear bimodality within individual families is masked by the polygenic effects when many of the two types of families are combined.

Polygenes also help to determine blood pressure levels. It appears that carriers of the gene for glucocorticoid-remediable aldosteronism within the same pedigree but in different branches have different average blood pressure levels (Lifton et al., 1992). If polygenes can confound segregation (bimodality) when superimposed over a gene with large effects, it is easy to see why finding segregation of blood pressure–related phenotypes may be so difficult when the genes are more common and have smaller effects.

This type of confounding is not limited to polygenes but also may be due to environmental factors. Obesity has a clear environmental component, in addition to a polygenic component, that could overwhelm any genetic signal of the trait being studied. A prime example of this type of confounding is the *AGT* gene. Persons on a normal-salt diet who are 235T homozygotes at the *AGT* locus have a blunted renal plasma flow response to a 3 $ng \cdot kg^{-1} \cdot min^{-1}$ angiotensin II infusion compared to the other two genotypes (Hopkins et al., 1996b). Greater BMI was associated with significantly lower renal plasma flow response in persons with the *TT* genotype ($r = -0.61$) than for the other two genotypes ($r = -0.38$). Therefore, weight loss may improve renal plasma flow response to a greater extent in the *TT* genotype, resulting in reduced blood pressure. Obesity could also easily confound the genetic relationships with renal blood flow.

In addition to confounding, obesity can mimic a genetic effect. Weight reduction results in loss of adipose tissue. Adipose tissue produces a significant amount of angiotensinogen, and angiotensinogen levels have been correlated with blood pressure reduction due to weight loss (Eggena et al., 1991). Loss of fat mass could directly reduce local angiotensinogen levels, local vasoconstriction, and possibly resistance changes of a more central nature. Differentiation of preadipocytes to adipocytes is related to activation of the angiotensinogen promoter (Tamura et al., 1994), suggesting that the greater the accrual of adipocytes during weight gain, the greater the activation of the *AGT* gene. Thus, a person with a gene for high angiotensinogen levels could appear to have normal levels after weight loss or a person gaining weight with a normal *AGT* gene could falsely appear to be a gene carrier.

The genetic segregation of urinary kallikrein provides another example of environmental confounding, this time by diet. Segregation analysis has found evidence for a major gene influencing urinary kallikrein excretion [produces vasodilation that counteracts the effects of angiotensin II (Fig. 8–5) (Hunt et al., 1993)]. There was also a significant interaction of genotype and dietary potassium intake on kallikrein levels. Those inferred to be homozygous for the high- or low-kallikrein genotype had a large separation of kallikrein means, and the separation did not vary by dietary potassium intake. However, those inferred to be heterozygotes had kallikrein levels similar to the high homozygotes when dietary potassium intake was high and had kallikrein levels similar to the low homozygotes when dietary potassium intake was low. Extrapolating these findings to various populations suggests that low urinary kallikrein excretion segregates as a dominant trait in populations or subgroups with low dietary potassium intake and as a recessive trait in subgroups with high potassium intake. In subgroups with intermediate potassium intake, there may be little evidence of bimodality or a major gene due to confounding by diet.

After fitting a major gene segregation model to blood pressure, Pérusse et al. (1991) found that persons assigned to the high blood pressure genotype had a significant rise in blood pressure with age; those in the other two genotypes had little or no increase in blood pressure with age. This indicates that the power to detect a major gene may depend on the age of the subjects being studied. The separation in blood pressure levels by genotype may increase with age, while environmental confounding may also increase.

These examples reinforce the complexity of blood pressure control and that genetic and environmental factors associated with blood pressure must be studied in the context of each other, rather than alone. These types of study necessitate large sample sizes to identify, estimate, and test for significant gene–environment interactions.

Linkage and Association

Anonymous Marker Genome Searches

Some investigators have attacked the problem of identifying genes related to hypertension using anonymous markers spread across each chromosome of the genome. Many monogenic trait genes have been identified after linking a marker to a particular

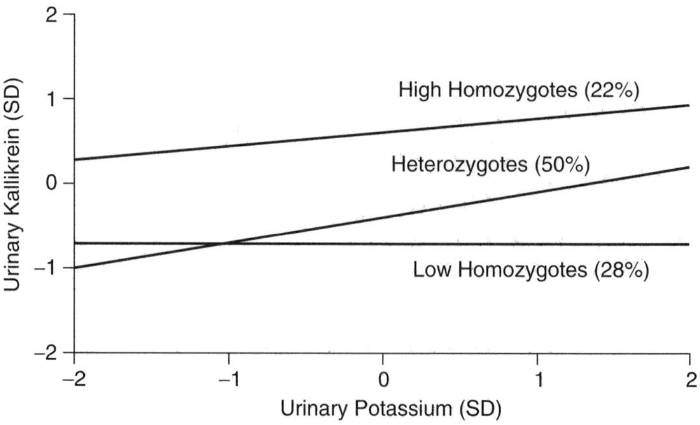

Fig. 8–5. Urinary kallikrein levels show interaction between urinary potassium excretion and the three kallikrein genotypes inferred from segregation analysis. Numbers in parentheses are the percent of persons estimated to be of each kallikrein genotype. Urinary potassium and kallikrein amounts are in standard deviation (SD) units.

region of a chromosome and determining what genes are nearby (positional candidate genes). If there are no obvious candidate genes or too many candidate genes, fine genetic mapping may be done (depending on the type of sample, e.g., pedigrees vs. sib pairs) to narrow the linked region so that one may proceed with physical mapping and cloning of the region. If the sample consists of sib pairs which have little power to resolve narrow locations, one can start sequencing known genes in the region for polymorphisms. It is difficult to know which of the genes in the region is responsible for the hypertension linkage, especially if the functional variant is in a regulatory region of the gene and does not cause a change in structure of a protein but changes the amount of protein or its activity.

Genome searches have been published using hypertension and blood pressure as phenotypes. A genome search using sib pairs that were discordant for blood pressure along with additional relatives found linkage to regions of chromosomes 2, 5, 6, and 15 (Krushkal et al., 1999). Five other chromosomes showed suggestive linkage. Follow-up of the region on 5q resulted in significant linkage and association of a region containing the α_{1B}- and β_2-adrenergic receptor genes and the dopamine receptor type 1A gene (Krushkal et al., 1998). A previous study had found evidence for linkage of salt sensitivity of diastolic blood pressure in African Americans to the β_2-adrenergic receptor, although baseline diastolic blood pressure was not significantly linked to this gene (Svetkey et al., 1997). Another study found no linkage of this receptor with systolic or diastolic blood pressure levels (Kamitani et al., 1998).

A number of genome scans for blood pressure, hypertension, and related phenotypes have been published (Kamitani et al., 1998; Krushkal et al., 1999; Xu et al., 1999; Sharma et al., 2000; Perola et al., 2000; Rice et al., 2000; Pankow et al., 2000; Levy et al., 2000; Hsueh et al., 2000; Atwood et al., 2001a; Rankinen et al., 2001; Zhu et al., 2001a; Cheng et al., 2001). While the initial scans showed little overlap in linked regions, there is now emerging concordance for some locations. For example, a number of scans have shown linkage on chromosome 1 around 192 cM. This is also within 20 cM of a familial combined hyperlipidemia locus (Pajukanta et al., 1998), which has been replicated by at least two different studies (Coon et al., 2000; Pei et al., 2000). Chromosome 2 has multiple locations suggesting linkage, with the two best regions around 40 to 80 cM (Rice et al., 2000; Levy et al., 2000; Hsueh et al., 2000) and around 100 to 120 cM (Rice et al., 2000; Atwood et al., 2001b).

Comparison of the results from genome scans is complicated by the use of different racial groups, which may have different underlying gene frequencies, changing the power of the analyses, or different environmental factors, increasing or decreasing the expression of a hypertension gene. Different family structures (concordant or discordant sib pairs, nuclear families, pedigrees) and treatment status (treated or untreated hypertension and normotension) also complicate study comparisons. Although not a genome scan, anonymous markers (based on homology to a rat linkage region) of hypertension were linked to a region approximately 18 cM proximal to the *ACE* gene on chromosome 17 (Julier et al., 1997). This result was replicated by the Framingham and Quebec Family Study genome searches (Levy et al., 2000; Rice et al., 2000) and by another study of this chromosome (Baima et al., 1999). Although it probably does not explain the strong linkage in the Framingham study (LOD score 4.7), the *WNK4* gene under linkage peak has been shown to cause Gordon's syndrome, a rare form of hypertension (Wilson et al., 2001).

Candidate Genes

Table 8–8 lists some of the classes of candidate genes that may be involved in hypertension. This list is necessarily incomplete because of rapid advances in this field and because one can usu-

Table 8–8. Suggested Candidate Gene Classes

Renin-angiotension-aldosterone system	Sympathetics
Angiotensinogen	α and β adrenoceptors
Angiotensin receptors	Dopamine β-hydroxylase
Renin	Dopamine receptors
Renin binding protein	Lipids and insulin
Angiotensin-converting enzyme	VLDL receptor
Glucocorticoid and mineralocorticoid receptors	LDL receptor
Kallikrein-kininogen system	apo A-I/C-III/A-IV
Kallikrein	Lipoprotein lipase
Kallikrein binding protein	Insulin and insulin receptor
Kininogen	TNF receptors
Bradykinin receptors	Coagulation factors
Prostaglandins	Fibrinogen
Cellular ion transport and concentration	Glycoprotein IIb/IIIa
Na-H antiporter isoforms	PAI-1
Anion exchange proteins	Homocysteine
Na,K-ATPase subunits	Others
Adducin	*SA* locus
Nitric oxide isoforms and natriuretic peptides	Neuropeptide Y and receptor
Nitric oxide synthase	Chromogranin A
Guanylyl cyclase A (receptors)	*MN*, haptoglobin
Natriuretic peptides	HLA
Natriuretic peptide receptors	Heat shock genes
Endothelin	
Endothelin	
Endothelin converting enzyme	
Endothelin receptors	

Table of genes suggested by molecular biology or by biochemical and physiological data to be related to hypertension. Some have been rejected as candidate genes. List is not exhaustive.
VLDL, very low-density lipoprotein; LDL, low-density lipoprotein; apo A-I, apolipoprotein A-I; TNF, tumor necrosis factor; PAI-1, plasminogen activator inhibitor 1; HLA, human leukocyte antigen.

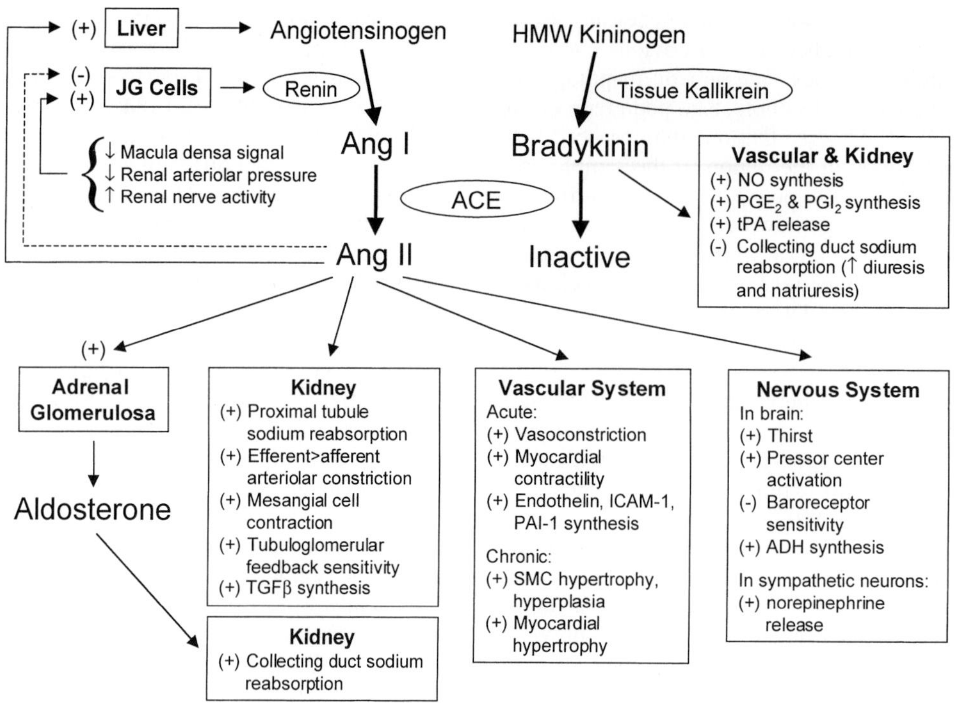

Fig. 8–6. Physiological pathways for the renin-angiotensin-aldosterone and kallikrein-kinin pathways and their connection through angiotensin-converting enzyme (*ACE*). *ANG*, angiotensin; *HMW*, high molecular weight; *JG*, juxtaglomerular; *NO*, nitric oxide; *PGE₂/I₂*, prostaglandin E_2/I_2; *TPA*, tissue plasminogen activator; *TGF*, transforming growth factor; *ICAM*, intracellular adhesion molecule; *PAI*, plasminogen activator inhibitor; *SMC*, smooth muscle cell; *ADH*, antidiuretic hormone.

ally find plausible mechanisms that relate a large number of other factors to blood pressure control.

Renin

Although tissue renin–angiotensin systems have also been identified, until recently the major emphasis has been on the global, circulating renin–angiotensin system (Fig. 8–6). Because of its strategic significance and its critical role in the acute regulation of angiotensin II formation, renin has been a leading candidate in genetic investigations of hypertension in both experimental models and human subjects. Linkage of a marker at the renin gene to blood pressure in rats (Rapp et al., 1989) stimulated further interest in the gene as a candidate in hypertension. Using congenic mice, it was later concluded that the linkage was not with the renin gene but with another unknown gene nearby (Zhang et al., 1997). In addition, the animal studies were not duplicated in humans. Pedigree studies and sib-pair studies provided no evidence of linkage to hypertension (Naftilan et al., 1989; Soubrier et al., 1990; Zee et al., 1991; Jeunemaitre et al., 1992b), while another study found no association of a marker at the renin locus with blood pressure in healthy subjects (Berge et al., 1994). While abnormalities in other genes may influence renin activity, the lack of linkage of a marker at the renin locus to hypertension does not make renin less important in blood pressure control per se. For example, patients with low renin activity have greater intracellular calcium-induced changes in membrane fluidity and abnormal membrane ion transport than other hypertensive or normotensive patients (Masuyama et al., 1988). Renin expression may also be reduced in the presence of elevated angiotensinogen levels (Danser et al., 1998), such as may be induced by a polymorphism in the *AGT* gene. In addition, in mice with only one *AGT* gene resulting in lower angiotensinogen levels, increased renin is produced in the absence of upregulation of the remaining *AGT* gene and any alteration in ACE production (Kim et al., 1999). The idea of interactions of various factors leading to hypertension and the difficulties in detecting and characterizing such interactions are what make hypertension research so challenging and interesting.

Angiotensin-Converting Enzyme

ACE was examined because of a dual role in blood pressure physiology. It converts angiotensin I to angiotensin II to increase vasoconstriction and release aldosterone for sodium retention. It also catabolizes active kinins, which are vasodilators. ACE is a more potent factor in the kallikrein–kinin system than in the renin–angiotensin system because of the lower K_m for bradykinin (Skidgel and Erdös, 1999). Bradykinin, a powerful vasodilator formed by the action of kallikrein on kininogen, stimulates prostaglandin formation. Higher ACE levels increase inactivation of bradykinin while increasing angiotensin II formation, leading to the hypothesis that abnormalities in the *ACE* gene are involved in hypertension. ACE blockers decrease angiotensin II formation and increase total bradykinin activity.

Associations exist between an insertion/deletion polymorphism of the *ACE* gene and both plasma ACE concentration and myocardial infarction (Staessen et al., 1997b). Despite a couple of early positive linkage studies, a large number of subsequent studies have suggested that mutations in the *ACE* gene were not involved in human hypertension (Jeunemaitre et al., 1992a; Schmidt et al., 1993; Ishigami et al., 1995; Castellano et al., 1995; Lachurié et al., 1995). The effects of the *ACE* gene may be context-dependent as linkage was found in men but not in women in two different studies (Fornage et al., 1998; O'Donnell et al., 1998). Additionally, other studies have found interactions between the *ACE* and *AGT* genes (Borecki et al., 1997; Vasku et al., 1998; Staessen et al., 2001) and between the *ACE* and α-

adducin genes (Barlassina et al., 2000) on blood pressure. Haplotype analyses of *ACE* variants also seem to increase the association of *ACE* with blood pressure (Zhu et al., 2001b).

Angiotensinogen

The *AGT* gene attracted less attention, in large part because of the perception that, due to its rather high and stable concentration in plasma, it was not an important determinant of the rate of angiotensin II formation. Indeed, early kinetic studies using partially purified preparations suggested that the plasma concentration of angiotensinogen was far in excess of the K_m of the reaction. Subsequent studies using highly purified substrate and enzyme revealed that the plasma concentration of angiotensinogen was near the K_m of the reaction (Gould and Green, 1971) and, as a consequence, could affect the rate of angiotensin II formation (Cain et al., 1971; Ménard and Catt, 1973). There is also a direct positive feedback mechanism of increasing angiotensin II levels on increased formation of angiotensinogen.

Plasma angiotensinogen was higher in hypertensive subjects and in the offspring of hypertensive parents than in normotensive controls (Fasola et al., 1968), and the correlation between angiotensinogen levels and blood pressure in another study was $r = 0.39$ (Walker et al., 1979). In the Four Corners Study (Watt et al., 1992), angiotensinogen concentrations were significantly associated with higher blood pressure in the subset most likely to show genetic predisposition, namely, the high blood pressure offspring of parents with high blood pressure. Antibodies raised against angiotensinogen lowered blood pressure, at least temporarily (Gardes et al., 1982), and injection of angiotensinogen increased blood pressure (Ménard et al., 1991).

Genetic support for *AGT* as a candidate gene in essential hypertension was first cited by Jeunemaitre et al. (1992c), who reported genetic linkage between a multiallelic marker of *AGT* and essential hypertension in hypertensive siblings. The evidence was more significant among siblings receiving a combination of two antihypertensive medications, and the linkage was stronger in males than females. Subsequent analysis revealed that a common variant in the gene, T235, which encodes a threonine instead of a methionine at codon 235 of the mature protein, occurred at higher frequencies in hypertensive patients than in normotensive controls and that this variant was associated with a modest (20%–40%) but significant increase in the plasma concentration of angiotensinogen. T235 occurred at a frequency of about 0.38, 15% of Caucasians being homozygous for the variant. A larger study confirmed that the 235T allele at the *AGT* locus was associated with higher angiotensinogen levels and increased blood pressure levels in French subjects (Jeunemaitre et al., 1993).

The work suggested that variants in the gene could predispose to essential hypertension. Admittedly, several important issues could not be resolved, including the proportion of subjects in whom this risk factor could be relevant and the relative magnitude of this genetic predisposition compared to environmental determinants of the disease. Jeunemaitre et al. (1992c) pointed out that the statistical inference of an association could not establish whether T235 was causally involved or simply a marker for one or more causal determinants to be identified.

No association was detected in populations of African descent, made more difficult because of the very high allelic frequency of the marker in such populations. Indicative of a possible functional effect in African Americans, however, a relationship between the *AGT* genotype and angiotensinogen levels was observed (Rotimi et al., 1994, 1997). Linkage between *AGT* and hypertension was quite significant in an African-Caribbean population from Saint-Vincent (Caulfield et al., 1995). In a prospective study of black and white children, *AGT* was associated with greater blood pressure increases over 5 years (Bloem et al., 1995). The correlation of serum angiotensinogen with the mean longitudinal diastolic blood pressure change was 0.24 for whites and 0.45 for blacks (both $p < 0.004$).

The situation in Caucasians was also confusing as a significant association was reported in only about half of the published studies. Caulfield and colleagues (1994) reported significant linkage but no association with T235. On the basis of linkage disequilibrium patterns of the multiallelic *AGT* marker, they suggested that there were distinct haplotypes of *AGT* for disease predisposition and disease protection, but this interpretation was not supported in an independent study (Jeunemaitre et al., 1997). So many studies were soon published, with such variation in phenotypic definition and recruitment of cases and controls, that they motivated comprehensive meta-analyses (Kunz et al., 1997; Staessen et al., 1999). These authors concluded that, overall, studies in Caucasians supported an association; that the evidence was greater when recruitment involved cases with a positive family history and ascertainment in referral centers, as in the original report of Jeunemaitre et al. (1992c); and that bias and confounding were present in many reports. In light of the very high prevalence of essential hypertension, its anticipated heterogeneity, and the fact that the majority of cases with mild hypertension may result from overweight and involve a number of environmental determinants, this apparent lack of replication in some reports should not come as a surprise.

A combined linkage analysis of multiple European populations did not find evidence for linkage, despite two of the subsamples having previously reported linkage (Brand et al., 1998a). Combining multiple groups with differing underlying population allele frequencies of the marker and using a pooled estimate of those frequencies could easily have removed evidence for linkage if it were present. Changing the pooled allele frequency estimates to estimate the effect on the linkage results will still not circumvent the problem of pooling heterogeneous data since inaccurate frequencies will always be used for a different subset of the data.

Another neglected factor in the evaluation of association studies was their relative lack of statistical power, i.e., their ability to identify as significant a modest difference in the frequency of T235 between cases and controls. The two reports commonly cited as evidence against an association (Bennett et al., 1993; Caulfield et al., 1994) had statistical power in the 50% range and, therefore, were essentially inconclusive. One study that had sufficient statistical power to detect an association of the *AGT* gene was negative using Chinese subjects (Niu et al., 1999), similar to most results in African Americans (Rotimi et al., 1994), both groups having high allele frequencies of T235. Also, no linkage was found in this population (Niu et al., 1998). A large study of the NHLBI Family Blood Pressure Program found little evidence for the association of *AGT* with blood pressure in large samples (Province et al., 2000b). Less than 1% of blood pressure variance was explained by the tested gene polymorphism. Another large study, from Denmark, showed a hypertension association of *AGT* and AGT levels only in females (Sethi et al., 2001).

Whether T235 was causal or a marker for another causal genetic variant required further examination. No differences in glycosylation, secretion, and stability were evident when *AGT* with either T235 or M235 was expressed in cultured cells; and these two substrates exhibited similar kinetics in their reaction with purified recombinant renin (Inoue et al., 1997). When haplotypes of T235 were generated through analysis of other *AGT* polymorphisms, no particular subset of haplotypes exhibited unambiguously greater association with hypertension than T235 as a whole (Jeunemaitre et al., 1997). Such reanalysis revealed that a common polymorphism in the proximal promoter of *AGT*, the presence of either guanine or adenine six residues upstream from the initiation site of transcription, was in complete linkage disequilibrium with T235 (Inoue et al., 1997). With few exceptions, all genes carrying T235 exhibited A at residue −6, while genes with M235 had a G at that site. Two implications of these findings were that all associations reported with T235 directly extended to A(−6) and that this polymorphism, as T235, could either be a marker or a causal determinant. In vitro binding studies with extract of nuclear proteins and transactivation experiments contrasting *AGT* promoters with either A or G at residue −6 supported the conclusion that the polymorphism affected both the binding of specific transacting factors and the transcriptional activity of the core promoter of *AGT* (Inoue et al., 1997). This suggested a molecular mechanism for *AGT*-mediated disease predisposition. These authors recognized that these *in vitro* experiments did not provide direct insight regarding the effect of this polymorphism on the function of the gene *in vivo* and that other haplotypes of the *AGT* gene may also be relevant. Additional polymorphisms have also been associated with angiotensinogen levels and hypertension, e.g., A-20C or C-18T variants (Ishigami et al., 1997; Sato et al., 1997; Zhao et al., 1999).

Through an innovative gene targeting strategy in mice, Kim et al. (1995) directly demonstrated that a modest increase in *AGT* expression *in vivo* leads to increased plasma levels of the protein and increased blood pressure. Table 8–9 shows that plasma AGT levels increased from 0% to 145% for mice with zero to four copies of the *AGT* gene. Mean arterial pressure correlated with *AGT* gene number ($r = 0.60$) and increased an average of 8 mm Hg with each additional copy of the *AGT* gene. Another direct demonstration that local angiotensinogen release in the kidney increases blood pressure used transgenic animals that overexpress angiotensinogen in the kidney (Ding et al., 1997). Blood pressure increased or remained constant depending on whether the transgenic system was activated.

The presence of T235 and A(-6) in all primate species examined suggests the hypothesis that the ancestral form of *AGT* is associated with disease predisposition. If so, the thrifty genotype hypothesis (Neel, 1999) would need to be considered. The ancestral form of the gene, advantageous for salt retention under the conditions of severe sodium restriction that prevailed during early primate and human evolution, may be disadvantageous relative to a new form under modern conditions of excess sodium intake.

Table 8–9. Serum Angiotensinogen Level and Mean Blood Pressure Level by Number of Angiotensinogen Genes in the Mouse

Number of *AGT* Genes	Angiotensinogen Level	Mean Blood Pressure (mm Hg)
1	35%	121
2	100%	130
3	124%	138
4	145%	146

Angiotensinogen level is relative to the two-gene mouse. Mean blood pressure estimated from Figure 2B of Kim et al. (1995).

Two longitudinal studies support the involvement of this gene in the development of hypertension (Bloem et al., 1995; Hunt et al., 1998). One was a clinical trial showing that after only a 3-year follow-up in the usual-care group, systolic and diastolic blood pressure and incidence of hypertension were higher but of borderline significance in persons with the *AA* genotype of the *AGT* gene than in those with the *GG* genotype (Hunt et al., 1998). Heterozygotes had intermediate blood pressure and a higher incidence of hypertension than persons with the *GG* genotype.

Despite higher blood pressures and an increased incidence of hypertension in the usual-care group with the *AA* genotype, there was a significant reduction in diastolic blood pressure and/or hypertension incidence in those assigned to the sodium-reduction or weight-loss intervention who had the *AA* and *AG* genotypes. The net blood pressure decrease with sodium reduction in those with the *AA* genotype was 2.5/3.3 mm Hg greater than the decrease in those with the *GG* genotype after 36 months. This mild effect is not surprising, given that the genetic effect of the *AA* genotype vs. the *GG* genotype raises angiotensinogen levels by only 10% to 30%. Only long-term elevation of angiotensinogen levels would be expected to slowly increase blood pressure as compensatory mechanisms reset or fail, the rate of that increase depending on other genetic and environmental factors. While persons with the *AA* genotype may develop hypertension to a greater degree than those with the other genotypes when there is no intervention, they also respond more favorably to salt-reduction or weight-loss intervention.

One mechanism proposed for the development of salt sensitivity is the failure to reduce angiotensin II to appropriate levels as sodium intake increases (Hall, 1986). Long-term administration of angiotensin II at subpressor doses has been shown to elevate blood pressure (Brown et al., 1981). The genetically determined higher angiotensinogen levels of the *AA* genotype on a normal (high)-salt diet would make it more difficult for these individuals to lower angiotensinogen when needed, making them more salt-sensitive. The resulting flattening of the pressure–natriuresis slope for the *AA* genotype would result in a greater blood pressure drop after sodium reduction than for the *GG* genotype, having a steeper response curve and a smaller blood pressure change (Suzuki et al., 1996).

The gene–environment interaction results of this large study have been replicated in another, smaller study in never-treated hypertensive subjects (Hunt et al., 1999a). The effects of this study were larger than those of the Trials of Hypertension Prevention Study (1997), possibly because the subjects were older and hypertensive and had potassium and magnesium supplementation in addition to sodium reduction. Mean systolic blood pressure reductions were 8.6 mm Hg for the M235T *TT* group (equivalent to the −6*AA* group), 9.0 mm Hg for the *MT* genotype group, and 5.3 mm Hg for the *MM* genotype group. Trends across genotypes were similar for diastolic blood pressure. These studies provided evidence that some of the variation in blood pressure response to a sodium intervention is explained by genetic factors, specifically the *AGT* gene. Preliminary results from the DASH study suggest that dietary factors, such as increased potassium and magnesium from a high fruit and vegetable diet and a reduced fat diet, may also interact with AGT and blood pressure even when dietary sodium is held constant (Svetkey et al., 2000).

Work on AGT illustrates the various challenges awaiting the geneticist in the search for an understanding of the genetic basis of common disease. The initial trial comes with the identification of a genetic hypothesis and its survival through replication attempts of varying significance and quality. The next hurdle is to develop a molecular hypothesis *in vivo*. For a trait such as blood pressure, the final test is that of elucidating the pathophysiological mechanism for disease predisposition, and there is little doubt that this final advance will also be the most daunting one.

Angiotensin Receptor Type 1 and Aldosterone

An association of the AT1 receptor for angiotensin II (causing vasoconstriction) has been reported, but there was no evidence for linkage (Bonnardeaux et al., 1994). Since association studies may be more powerful, these findings were interpreted as being compatible with a small genetic effect of the *AT1* receptor gene. Another study, in Caucasians, provided support for an association (Wang et al., 1997a), but no association was found in Germany (Schmidt et al., 1997) or Japan (Takami et al., 1998). A review of the evidence for association of the AT1 receptor is available (Duncan et al., 2001). A mild association of the 1166 polymorphism was found for infused angiotensin II blood pressure response, a response that is also aggravated by elevated LDL cholesterol levels (Vuagnat et al., 2001). Perhaps the strongest evidence for a genetic abnormality in this receptor comes from a Finnish study, which found both linkage and association with hypertension as well as, after controlling for disequilibrium in the linkage analysis, a LOD score of 5.13, a highly significant result (Kainulainen et al., 1999).

The aldosterone synthase gene did not show linkage with hypertension, but it did show association with hypertension in two studies (Brand et al., 1998b; Davies et al., 1999). Plasma aldosterone levels were lower in subjects with the allele associated with hypertension (Pojoga et al., 1998). Significant interactions were found with the aldosterone synthase gene, the α-adducin gene, and *ACE* on hypertension incidence (Staessen et al., 2001).

Kallikrein-Kinin System

Because of the reproducible physiological findings relating urinary kallikrein activity to blood pressure control and blood pressure differences between various patient groups, the components of the kallikrein–kinin system remain of great interest (Fig. 8–6). Kallikrein is an enzyme that converts kininogen to active kinin (bradykinin), which is a vasodilator. Urinary kallikrein activity is lower in blacks than whites (Horwitz et al., 1978) and lower in hypertensive than in normotensive patients (Keiser, 1980). It favorably responds (increases) to both sodium reduction and potassium supplementation (Margolius et al., 1974; Cappuccio and MacGregor, 1991). It segregates as a major gene, with the best genetic model suggesting that there is an interaction of this inferred gene with dietary potassium, as measured by urinary potassium excretion (Hunt et al., 1993). This model suggests that persons with the low kallikrein genotype do not modulate their kallikrein activity with changes in potassium excretion, while the heterozygotes may have kallikrein levels resembling either the high homozygous or low homozygous groups depending on whether their urinary potassium excretion is high or low (Fig. 8–5). If this genotype–potassium interaction can be substantiated in intervention trials, physicians would have an inexpensive and well-tolerated intervention to counteract the effects of low kallikrein on blood pressure that would be especially effective in heterozygotes (estimated to be 50% of the general population) but mostly ineffective in low homozygotes.

Susceptibility loci alone presumably do not account for hypertension in the absence of other risk factors. Defects in the renin–angiotensin vasoconstricting system and the kallikrein–kinin vasodilating system may act synergistically to promote hypertension. Long-term blockade of bradykinin B_2 receptors by Hoe-140 in WKY normotensive rats did not cause an increase in blood pressure (Madeddu et al., 1994). However, blockade of the B_2 receptors during a normally non-pressor infusion of angiotensin II caused significant blood pressure elevation. Infusion of low angiotensin II doses into Brown Norway normotensive rats with normal kallikrein levels did not increase blood pressure. If the same dose of angiotensin II is given to Brown Norway Katholiek rats, which have a complete lack of urinary kallikrein, blood pressure rises faster than in control rats (Majima et al., 1994). These two studies suggest that multiple defects may be necessary before normal compensatory mechanisms fail and blood pressure rises. Factors contributing to hypertension may also change as hypertension develops. In deoxycorticosterone acetate (DOCA) salt rats, it was suggested that mineralocorticoids increased kallikrein levels to compensate for elevated vasoconstriction (Nolly et al., 1994). As hypertension developed, kallikrein fell to low levels, no longer counteracting the vasoconstrictive effects of DOCA salt.

A polymorphic marker near the structural gene for tissue kallikrein (*KLK1*) was not linked to or associated with kallikrein levels or blood pressure (Friend et al., 1996; Berge et al., 1997). However, examining polymorphisms in the 5′ promoter of this gene suggested important associations in the regulatory region (Song et al., 1997). In addition, from presented but unpublished results (R. Slim et al. and S. Hunt et al), an amino acid change, R53H, in the kallikrein gene has been associated with dramatically reduced kallikrein activity in three different populations. Protein kinase C isoforms, particularly α, ε, and ζ, appear to be involved in post-receptor signal transduction following bradykinin binding to the B_2 receptors (Tippmer et al., 1994). There was no linkage of kininogen to hypertension (S. Hunt et al., unpublished results). Other than a negative association study of prostacyclin synthase and hypertension (Nakayama et al., 2001), no detailed genetic studies relating prostaglandins (which consist of both vasodilators and vasoconstrictors), cyclo-oxygenases, or protein kinase C to hypertension have yet appeared.

Ion-Transport Systems

Genetic defects have been sought that could explain the relationship of ion transport abnormalities to hypertension. Some of these systems include adducin, Na–Li countertransport, Na–K cotransport, Na,K-ATPase transport, Na–H antiporter, Na–Ca exchange, Ca-ATPase, Cl–HCO_3 transport, and the epithelial sodium channel (Fig. 8–7). Multiple mechanisms control the activity of these cellular transport systems and intracellular ion content, including genetic control of baseline or stimulated activity, ion concentration, the number of transporters, cellular pH, cellular membrane lipid composition, and local or systemic circulating factors.

The α-adducin gene is a candidate gene for human hypertension, which arose from studies in the Milan rat. Blood pressure cosegregated with the adducin gene in these rats, and the gene explained about 50% of the blood pressure difference between the normotensive and hypertensive strains (Bianchi et al., 1994). Similar cellular transport abnormalities were suggested in both Milan rats and hypertensive patients, with mutations in the α and β subunits of adducin being associated with changes in the membrane cytoskeleton, which affects Na,K-ATPase activity (Tripodi et al., 1996). Both linkage and association of α-adducin have been found in humans, with the linkage being sig-

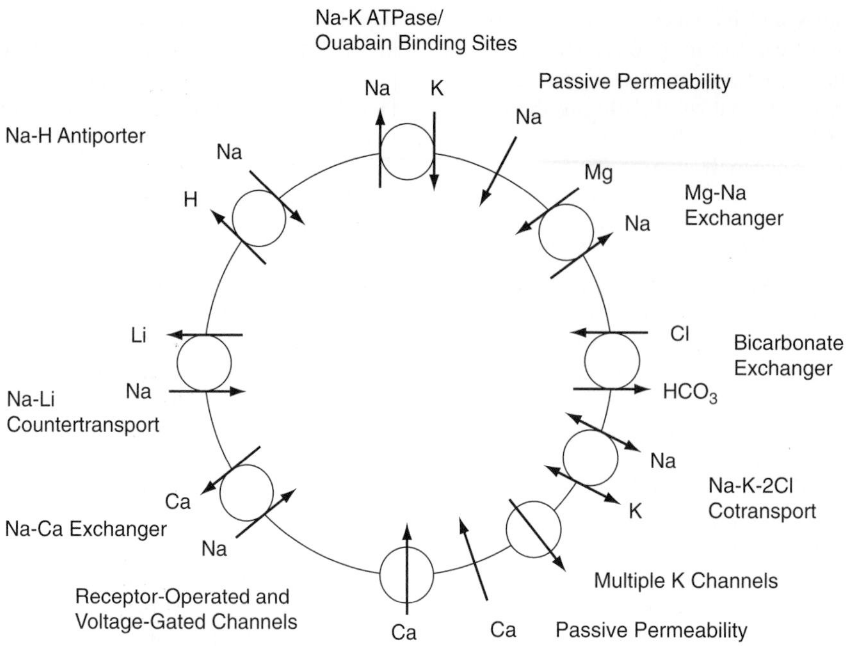

Fig. 8–7. Important cellular ion channels that regulate ion concentration, cell fluid volume, pH, electrical potential, and second-messenger systems.

nificant for three different polymorphic markers near the α-adducin locus (Cusi et al., 1997). Association was found in both French and Italian subjects in this study. In addition, the authors suggested that the defect was related to salt sensitivity, as shown by an acute salt loading and depletion protocol and by treatment with diuretics. Fractional excretion of lithium was measured to determine whether there were differences in renal function by adducin genotype. Those with the allele associated with hypertension had lower fractional lithium excretion, suggesting that they had increased sodium reabsorption (Manunta et al., 1999). It is possible that the reabsorption occurs as a result of abnormal Na,K-ATPase activity, although other abnormalities in Na–K–2Cl cotransport or the epithelial sodium channel could play a role (Cusi et al., 1993; Ferrandi et al., 1996).

Similar to angiotensinogen, however, there are some negative association studies. The α-adducin genotype was not associated with blood pressure, exchangeable sodium, intracellular sodium, or Na,K-ATPase sodium transport when comparing offspring of parents with high and low blood pressures (Kamitani et al., 1998). The frequency of the α-adducin allele associated with hypertension was much higher in the Japanese than in Caucasians, and no association was found comparing Japanese hypertensive and normotensive subjects (Kato et al., 1998). The Family Blood Pressure Program found the strongest association in Caucasians of the HyperGEN network (Province et al., 2000a). The SAPPHIRe network found a weak association only in a Chinese sample and not in the Japanese sample (Ranade et al., 2000). The other two networks of this program analyzed blood pressure, excluded medicated hypertensive subjects, and had negative results (Bray et al., 2000, Schork et al., 2000). A study in Australia also found no association (Wang et al., 1999). Negative results play an important role in assessing the relevance of a particular gene in the etiology of hypertension in the absence of pathophysiological data relating the gene to abnormalities associated with blood pressure. Large studies can assess the population impact on variation in a gene on a phenotype such as blood pressure. However, case-control studies become less important as the pathophysiological evidence increases and the number of positive findings increases. For example, even though α-adducin was associated with hypertension only in subjects from Milan and not Sardinia, the same physiological defects were seen in both groups (Glorioso et al., 1999). Most studies are powered to find a real effect only 80% of the time (with many having less power), while the positive studies require that fewer than 5% of subjects will show false-positive findings. The usual study design favors more false-negative than false-positive results. Therefore, the adducin gene joins angiotensinogen as a serious candidate for harboring common genetic mutations that contribute to the development of hypertension.

Genetic segregation models have suggested that Na–Li countertransport has recessive major gene effects that correlate with hypertension prevalence and incidence (Boerwinkle et al., 1986; Hasstedt et al., 1988b; Rebbeck et al., 1993). Na–H exchange (Aviv and Lasker, 1990) is closely related to, though not identical with, Na–Li countertransport and regulates cellular pH (Canessa et al., 1988; Semplicini, 1994). A heritability estimate of Na–H exchange was 54% in a twin study (Nowson et al., 1997). If alterations in ion transport found in blood cells are also present in kidney cells, increased Na reabsorption could occur. This may be followed by a compensating increased Na–Ca exchange to reduce cellular sodium, resulting in an increased intracellular calcium, increased smooth muscle contractility, and hypertension (Blaustein et al., 1984). Intracellular calcium may be a mediating factor between transport system abnormalities and vasoconstriction. Increased intracellular free Ca stimulates Na–H exchange across the plasma membrane, while increased cellular calcium in the juxtaglomerular cells in the kidney also has direct effects on renin release and enzyme activity (Fray et al., 1987).

The activity of the Na–H antiporter or Na–Li countertransport is modulated by other factors as well. Insulin increases activation of the antiporter, as it does with other transport systems (Moore, 1983). Metabolic cellular abnormalities reflected by cation and pH imbalances may stimulate insulin production to activate the Na–H exchange system (Resnick et al., 1987, 1990). In addition, catecholamines, which reduce the effectiveness of insulin on glucose uptake, increase intracellular levels of calcium (Roth et al., 1985; Landsberg and Young, 1985) and may be synergistic with the above mechanisms. Two linkage studies of the NHE-1 isoform of the Na–H antiporter with Na–Li countertransport activity and hypertension showed no evidence for linkage (Lifton et al., 1991; Dudley et al., 1991). Other isoforms are of interest, particularly NHE-3, but have not been studied. Na–K–2Cl cotransport has also been proposed to have a genetic basis of expression (Cusi et al., 1991). However, segregation analysis using large pedigrees has not been able to show evidence for a major gene controlling this phenotype. This transport system is responsible for nearly all NaCl reabsorption in the thick ascending limb of the loop of Henle (Garay et al., 1994, 1998). Salt loading increases a circulating factor that regulates the activity of this transporter, resulting in natriuresis.

Anion exchangers (AE) are cell membrane glycoproteins involved in chloride and bicarbonate exchange and have physiological relevance to blood pressure. AE-1 is the major glucose transporter of erythrocyte (and possibly other cell) membranes (Langdon and Holman, 1988). However, genetic studies of this class of ion exchangers have not been reported.

It has been suggested that alterations in cell membrane composition are related to ion transport rates and hypertension (Tsuda and Masuyama, 1990; Lijnen et al., 1994). For example, lipids and fatty acids, especially triglycerides, are correlated with transport activity (Corrocher et al., 1985; Hunt et al., 1986b, 1990). Membrane fluidity is decreased by cellular calcium loading (Sauerheber et al., 1980), and this decrease is greater in hypertensive than normotensive patients (Tsuda and Masuyama, 1990). Low dietary salt intake increases membrane fluidity (Masuyama et al., 1988). Epidemiological studies and cellular studies suggest that lipids or lipoproteins may affect blood pressure. Triglycerides predicted the development of hypertension in normotensive persons followed for 7 years (Hunt et al., 1991). After exposure to increasing doses of human LDL cholesterol (range 1–15 μg/ml), cultured smooth muscle cells and rat aortic ring contraction were increased in a dose-dependent fashion, apparently mediated by LDL-induced changes in intracellular pH and calcium concentration (Sachinidis et al., 1990). However, a cholesterol-lowering intervention study cast doubt on the importance of cholesterol levels *per se* on countertransport, even though membrane cholesterol was reduced (Lijnen et al., 1994).

Defects in the epithelial sodium channel cause Liddle's syndrome. However, many investigators hope to find other mutations in this transporter that may be associated with more common forms of hypertension with milder effects. There has been one positive linkage study to systolic blood pressure (Wong et al., 1999). After searching for polymorphisms in the β and γ subunits of the channel, no associations were found with hypertension (Persu et al., 1998, 1999). Another study tested for functional differences in the channel between hypertensive cases and controls and found no association (Baker et al., 1999). However, a large study in Japanese subjects found a low-frequency polymorphism in the γ subunit of the sodium channel gene that was associated with lower systolic blood pressure and hypotension (Iwai et al., 2001).

Ouabain Binding Sites, Na,K-ATPase Pump, and Intracellular Na

Natriuretic substances have been identified that inhibit the Na–K pump, including ouabain (Hamlyn et al., 1989), linoleic and oleic acids (Tamura et al., 1985), and lysophosphatidylcholine (Tamura et al., 1987). The last three substances have a common precursor, phosphatidylcholine, a phospholipid in the cell membrane. Population genetic analyses have not shown strong evidence for major gene determination of Na,K-ATPase pump activity, but a study in rats suggested that the α_1 Na,K-ATPase subunit may be involved with salt sensitivity (Herrera et al., 1998) and that there may be functional relevance of both the α_1 and α_2 subunits (Ruiz-Opazo et al., 1994, 1997). Segregation analysis of the number of ATPase sites, as measured by the amount of ouabain binding, has shown evidence for a recessive inheritance of an increased number of sites in about 2% of the population (Hasstedt et al., 1989b). High intraerythrocytic sodium levels appeared to segregate as a recessive trait, with a four-allele model fitting better than a two-allele model (Hasstedt et al., 1988a). Since we do not yet know cause-and-effect relationships, it is possible that higher numbers of pump sites are a response to increased intracellular sodium levels and vasoconstriction.

Principal Components Approach to Ion Transport

Genes involved with cellular ionic homeostasis do not act independently of other controls of cellular function. For example, a gene with large effects on the number of Na,K-ATPase exchange sites may also affect cellular concentrations of sodium, potassium, or calcium or changed activity of other associated transport systems. In addition to multiple effects of a single gene, each transport system likely reflects influences of multiple genetic variants. To separate multiple genetic influences on a single variable and allow for correlated secondary effects of other variables, the statistical technique of principal components was used to combine variables into independent linear equations. Variables that had the same genetic source of variance would most likely show high correlations with one of the newly defined equations, and variables that were not closely involved with a particular gene would show low correlations with that equation but might show high correlations with another equation that represented the greatest control over the expression of that variable. While somewhat complicated, this technique overcomes problems in genetic analysis of a syndrome, such as the multiple metabolic syndrome, which has multiple abnormal phenotypes. For example, it is not clear how insulin levels, lipid levels, glucose uptake, or obesity should be combined in a genetic analysis of the multiple metabolic syndrome. Using a principal components approach, however, allows these phenotypes to be combined into multiple equations, each representing a possible independent risk factor for this syndrome. Genetic analysis of these multivariate equations may proceed as though it were a single quantitative phenotype.

Using this methodology on multiple ion transport concentrations and transporters, 14 equations from 14 variables were formed. Segregation analysis showed evidence for five common and three rare major genes among these components (Hasstedt et al., 1994). Table 8–10 shows the four variables with the highest correlations on the five components suggested to have common major gene involvement. The first component segregates as a recessive major gene and appears to resemble the characteristics of familial dyslipidemic hypertension or the multiple metabolic syndrome. Inferred carriers are more obese with high triglyceride levels. In addition, their Na–Li countertransport levels are moderately elevated but not to the level predicted by the segregating major gene suggested for Na–Li countertransport. Urine creatinine, a correlate of weight, is also correlated with this component.

The second component with major gene effects is designated the ouabain binding component because there are higher in-

Table 8–10. Variables with the Strongest Correlations with Five Principal Components Inferred to Have Major Gene Inheritance

Principal Component	Familial Dyslipidemic HBP	Ouabain Binding Sites	Na–Li CNT	Na–Li CNT	BMI
Variable 1	BMI	RBC Na	Na–Li CNT	Na–Li CNT	BMI
Variable 2	Triglyceride	No. Sites	Urine K	Triglyceride	Urine K
Variable 3	Na–Li CNT	Plasma K	Plasma K	Urine K	Triglyceride
Variable 4	Urine creatinine	Plasma Na	Cell Na leak	Plasma Na	Urine creatinine
Inheritance	Recessive	Recessive	Dominant	Recessive	Recessive
Abnormal genotype	8.6%	7.6%	2.0%	3.1%	2.0%

HBP, high blood pressure; CNT, countertransport; BMI, body mass index; RBC, red blood cell.
Sources: Hasstedt et al. (1994), Hunt and Williams (1994).

traerythrocytic sodium levels in conjunction with a reduced number of ouabain binding sites. The activity of the Na,K-ATPase pump correlates poorly with this component. However, the reduced number of sites agrees with previous segregation analyses using only the number of sites as a univariate phenotype (Hasstedt et al., 1989b).

There may be two additional genes affecting Na–Li countertransport levels, one dominant (component 3) and one recessive (component 4). Each of these two independent components with major gene segregation had high correlations with Na–Li countertransport. The mean hourly countertransport levels in gene carriers were much higher (0.48 and 0.50 mmol/l red blood cells) than for gene carriers of component 1 (0.39 mmol/l red blood cells/hr). It appears that the two countertransport components have different biochemical profiles of the measured variables. If there are two genetic components to Na–Li countertransport, this would explain the suggested heterogeneity in other studies, where genetic transmission was not according to Mendelian expectations. The fifth genetic component appears to be a gene for moderate obesity but with normal triglyceride levels.

G-Protein β_3 Subunit

In functional studies of G proteins in hypertensive patients, increased signal transduction by pertussis toxin-sensitive G proteins was found. Association of the 825T allele in the gene encoding the β_3 subunit with hypertension was described, in which the polymorphism determines whether or not there is a splice variant. This splice variant was shown to be biologically active (Siffert et al., 1998). At least three additional studies have confirmed this association in other populations (Schunkert et al., 1998; Benjafield et al., 1998; Beige et al., 1999). One study found a significant association of the polymorphism in the Canadian Oji-Cree, but it was with the other allele (Hegele et al., 1998); another study found no association with hypertension or blood pressure in a large panel of French cases and controls (Brand et al., 1999b).

Subsequently, a study in German, Chinese, and South African subjects found consistent and significant increases in BMI with each additional T allele, suggesting that the association of the polymorphism with hypertension occurred through obesity-related mechanisms (Siffert et al., 1999). It is still not clear whether all of the hypertension association can be explained by obesity since diastolic blood pressure remained associated with 825T even after adjustment for BMI (Schunkert et al., 1998). Furthermore, this polymorphism appears to be associated with a differential blood pressure reduction among genotypes after 4 weeks of diuretic therapy. Systolic and diastolic blood pressure reductions were 6 and 5 mm Hg greater, respectively, in the 825TT subjects than in the 825CC subjects (Turner et al., 2001).

Nitric Oxide and Endothelin

Nitric oxide (NO) is a vasodilator in peripheral tissues and is equivalent to the endothelial relaxing factor. Nitric oxide synthase (NOS) has at least three isoforms, each with unique functions and tissue distributions (Salter et al., 1991). Neuronal NOS (NOS1) in the juxtaglomerular cells is involved with increased renin release, while endothelial NOS (NOS3) inhibits renin release and is found in the renal vasculature, not in the macula densa cells. Inducible NOS (NOS2) is expressed only after stimulation and inhibits sodium reabsorption in the thick ascending loop of Henle.

Constitutive endothelial NOS is calcium- and calmodulin-dependent and stimulated by a variety of hormones (acetylcholine, bradykinin, serotonin, norepinephrine, histamine, adenosine diphosphate), peptides (endothelin, vasopressin, substance P), and mechanical factors (flow or sheer stress), all of which mediate increased intracellular calcium concentrations. Among the effects of NO are increased permeability of potassium channels, increased Ca-ATPase, decreased phospholipase C activity with reduced concentration of inositol phosphatides, and decreased phosphorylation of myosin light chain. In smooth muscle, these effects lead directly and indirectly to relaxation. In platelets, NO leads to decreased aggregation and adherence. Interestingly, in endothelial and smooth muscle cells, increased cyclic guanosine monophosphate inhibits endothelin production, resulting in a negative feedback loop (since endothelin increases activity of constitutive NOS in endothelial cells).

Neuronal NOS produces NO in macula densa cells and is distinct from endothelial constitutive NOS. This macula densa NOS is induced by a high-salt diet and stimulated by perfusion of macula densa cells with a high-sodium solution. Production of NO by the macula densa counteracted the vasoconstriction observed in the afferent arterioles when the macula densa was perfused with a solution of higher salt concentration. Inhibition of NO production had no effect when the macula densa was perfused with a low-salt solution. The vasoconstrictor acting when NO synthesis was inhibited was not identified (Ito and Ren, 1993).

Several studies suggest impaired NO production in hypertensive individuals (Linder et al., 1990; Panza et al., 1990; Calver et al., 1992). At least part of the impaired NO production appears to be due to the high blood pressure itself, being in part reversible with lowered pressure (Lüscher et al., 1987). In kidneys, several mechanisms may contribute to the antihypertensive effects of NO. Renal blood flow appears to be controlled by the balance between angiotensin II and NO.

While the known peripheral and renal physiology of NO and NOS makes these very attractive candidate genes, three sib-pair studies failed to find linkage of endothelial NOS to hypertension (Bonnardeaux et al., 1995; Hunt et al., 1996b; Takami et al., 1999). A segregation analysis of basal endothelial NO levels in nuclear families found statistical evidence for a major gene and linkage to a marker at the *NOS3* locus (Wang et al., 1997b). Association studies have also shown conflicting results even within populations. One study in Japan of 1165 individuals showed no association of NOS3 with hypertension (Kato et al., 1999), while another Japanese study found association and replicated this association in a separate study group (Miyamoto et al., 1998). A third Japanese study also found significant association (Uwabo et al., 1998) but was followed by a study of two cities in Japan showing no association in either sample (Kajiyama et al., 2000). In Australian Caucasians, no association of NOS3 was found for hypertension (Friend et al., 1996). In Paris, an association was found for hypertension but not for blood pressure levels (Lacolley et al., 1998). Neuronal NOS was not associated with essential hypertension in a Japanese population (Takahashi et al., 1997). Inducible NOS was also not associated with hypertension in one study (Glenn et al., 1999) but was both linked to and associated with hypertension in an Australian sample (Rutherford et al., 2001). Thus, no clear pattern of results exists for these genes, and further physiological studies need to be performed to evaluate the functional significance of *NOS* gene polymorphisms. One such study of *NOS3* showed no endothelium-dependent vasodilation differences among $Glu^{298}Asp$ genotypes (Schneider et al., 2000).

Endothelins are a class of very potent vasoconstrictors, with endothelial cells producing only endothelin-1 (Lüscher et al., 1992). Endothelin-converting enzyme inhibitors and endothelin antagonists have shown some efficacy at reducing blood pressure in certain genetic animal models of hypertension (Nishikibe et al., 1993; McMahon et al., 1993). Serum and vascular concentrations of endothelin were increased in patients with atherosclerosis (Lerman et al., 1991). Endothelin may thus promote excess vasoconstriction, known to occur at diseased vascular sites, especially if unopposed by NO. Endothelin infusion causes renal afferent vasoconstriction, decreased glomerular filtration rate, salt retention, and hypertension (Kon and Badr, 1991). Salt-sensitive hypertension, which develops after endothelin infusion in animals, is prevented by captopril, implicating the renin–angiotensin system as a mediator of the hypertensive effects of endothelin (Mortensen and Fink, 1992). A dual endothelin-1/angiotensin II receptor or receptor group has been identified, which binds both hormones and may provide an important link between the coordination of these two systems (Ruiz-Opazo et al., 1998). These findings illustrate the intricate and sometimes unpredictable interplay between various systems that affect blood pressure. Whether endothelin levels play an important role in human essential hypertension remains enigmatic because plasma levels (which are variably elevated or normal in human hypertension) do not necessarily reflect endothelial production rates since most endothelin is probably not secreted luminally.

Linkage studies have not been reported for endothelin. One association study of hypertension suggests some genetic involvement of endothelin-1 but not its ET_A receptor (Stevens and Brown, 1995). The possibility of unknown variants in endothelin-1 and endothelin-2 being related to blood pressure, even though no association was found for the tested polymorphisms with hypertension, has been suggested (Brown et al., 2000). Another study also showed no evidence of association for either the ET_A or ET_B receptors with blood pressure (Nicaud et al., 1999). ET_A is selective for endothelin-1, while the ET_B receptor is nonselective for the endothelins. A study using a different marker at the endothelin locus found an association with blood pressure and a significant interaction with obesity and endothelin genotype on blood pressure in two different populations (Tiret et al., 1999). This again demonstrates the potential for important gene–environment interaction in the development of hypertension. Suggestive differences between normotensives with positive and negative family histories of hypertension for endothelin and sympathetic nerve activity responses to stress have been published (Noll et al., 1996). As with most candidate gene studies, there is at least one negative report of association, although with a different polymorphism (Berge and Berg, 1992).

Genetic defects could also occur in other links of the endothelin chain, such as endothelin-converting enzyme (ECE). Inhibition of this enzyme abolished increased forearm vasoconstriction induced by injected endothelin (Haynes et al., 1995). Genetic studies of endothelin-converting enzyme have not been published.

Sympathetic Nervous System

Physiological studies implicate the genes involved with catecholamine metabolism and receptors as important candidate genes. Normotensives with a positive family history of hypertension showed increased catecholamine levels in one study (Mo et al., 1995) but not in another (Yamakawa et al., 1992). Stress (behavioral but not physical) caused a greater catecholamine response in those with a positive family history of hypertension than in those without such a history (Fredrickson et al., 1991). Plasma epinephrine, norepinephrine, and dopamine showed high heritabilities (57%–74%) in twins (Williams et al., 1993). There is a growing body of evidence for the involvement of dopamine in blood pressure control (Jose et al., 1999). An association of the dopamine D_2 receptor gene has been found for systolic and diastolic blood pressure and hypertension (Rosmond et al., 2001). The dopamine D_1 receptor has also been associated with hypertension (Sato et al., 2000). Animals chronically infused with norepinephrine have increased smooth muscle cell DNA synthesis, which may occur through the α_1 adrenoceptor (deBlois et al., 1996). In humans, increases in insulin through a euglycemic clamp procedure are accompanied by increased sympathetic stimulation (Rowe et al., 1981). Renal catecholamine release also results in increased renal sodium reabsorption (DiBona, 1985). Linkage and association of the β_2-adrenergic receptor was described above in the genome search section. There was no association of α_2- or β_1-adrenergic receptor genes with hypertension (Zee et al., 1992; Baldwin et al., 1999).

Dyslipidemia and Hypertension

The atherogenic lipid profile, characterized by small and dense LDL, has been shown to segregate as a major gene trait in two studies. One study estimated dominant inheritance (Austin et al., 1988), while the other estimated recessive inheritance (de Graaf et al., 1992). The dense LDL phenotype was linked to the LDL receptor locus on chromosome 19 in two studies (Nishina et al., 1992; Rotter et al., 1996). However, it is not clear how the LDL receptor locus, which affects binding and removal of LDL cholesterol, could affect a syndrome such as familial dyslipidemic hypertension or familial combined hyperlipidemia, which more often have triglyceride and HDL abnormalities than the LDL cholesterol abnormality (Teng et al., 1986).

Other linkage studies have suggested that this syndrome is linked to the apo A-I/C-III/A-IV locus, which is involved in HDL, triglyceride, and insulin metabolism (Rotter et al., 1992, 1996). A locus for blood pressure, fasting insulin, and leptin was found on chromosome 7q (Cheng et al., 2001). It is likely that the heterogeneity of this syndrome results from multiple loci, as suggested by significant linkage results to four different genes in the latter study. It is also possible that the appearance of multiple lipid abnormalities defining this syndrome results from multiple common genetic abnormalities within a family and that individuals within this family who have only one genetic abnormality express only high triglyceride, high LDL, or low HDL.

A number of candidate genes have been proposed for familial combined hyperlipidemia, which phenotypically overlaps with familial dyslipidemic hypertension (Aouizerat et al., 1999a). Linkage of familial combined hyperlipidemia has been reported to the apo A-I/C-III/A-IV complex on chromosome 11 (Wojciechowski et al., 1991), following a previous positive association study (Hayden et al., 1987), but contradictory results exist. Using families selected for familial combined hyperlipidemia, linkage of dense LDL was found to markers for manganese-superoxide dismutase, cholesteryl-ester transfer protein, lecithin-cholesterol acyltransferase), and apo A-I/C-III/A-IV (Allayee et al., 1998). Other candidate genes have been considered for familial combined hyperlipidemia (Kwiterovich, 1993), and anonymous loci on chromosomes 1 and 11 have been suggested (Pajukanta et al., 1999; Aouizerat et al., 1999b). The locus on chromosome 1, near 170 to 180 cM, has been replicated in the NHLBI Family Heart Study (Coon et al., 2000), German and Chinese samples (Pei et al., 2000), and a study of diabetic pedigrees (Elbein et al., 1999). This locus is near the locus mildly linked to blood pressure in some genome scans (Krushkal et al., 1999; Levy et al., 2000; S. C. Hunt et al., unpublished results). A locus near the lipoprotein lipase gene on chromosome 8 showed linkage to systolic blood pressure in Taiwanese families with NIDDM (Wu et al., 1996) but not in Caucasians (Hunt et al., 1999b).

SA Gene

The *SA* gene was suggested as a candidate gene for hypertension based on comparisons of gene expression in the kidney between normotensive and hypertensive strains of rats and positive genetic association findings in humans (Iwai et al., 1994). However, subsequent human studies did not replicate the previous findings (Nabika et al., 1995; Harrap et al., 1995). Since the identification of this gene did not depend on statistical models and sample size considerations but only on actual gene expression and the association continues to be supported by animal studies, further study of this locus is warranted. However, a study in rats seems to exclude this locus from an association with elevated blood pressure (Hubner et al., 1999). The function of this gene is currently unknown.

Other Genes

Other genes have been tested for either association or linkage, including the β_3-adrenergic receptor (positive and negative associations) (Fujisawa et al., 1997; Tonolo et al., 1999), the glucagon receptor (positive and negative associations) (Morris and Chambers, 1996; Rutherford et al., 1998; Tonolo et al., 1999; Huang et al., 1999; Brand et al., 1999a), liver glucokinase (positive) (Chiang et al., 1997), and the protein phosphatase 1G subunit (negative) (Shen et al., 1997). Catalase, an antioxidant, has also shown positive and negative associations (Jiang et al., 2001; Ukkola et al., 2001). The 11β-hydroxysteroid dehydrogenase type 2 gene, which leads to apparent mineralocorticoid excess, did not contribute to essential hypertension in a linkage and association analysis (Brand et al., 1998c). This again shows that genes associated with severe monogenic forms of hypertension do not seem to contribute to common forms of essential hypertension.

CLINICAL APPLICATION AND RISK ASSESSMENT OF GENETIC INFORMATION

Because lipid abnormalities and Type 2 diabetes commonly co-occur with hypertension, patients with elevated blood pressure measurements during a clinical exam or blood pressure screen should always be followed up for these conditions. A family history of hypertension, dyslipidemia, or diabetes indicates that these patients should be more closely followed, especially if they already present near the upper limits of normal blood pressure, lipids, or glucose. A family history of CHD, stroke, or renal failure associated with hypertension may indicate the need for earlier onset of therapy and/or more aggressive therapy since these patients are likely to be more susceptible to the adverse effects of hypertension.

A physician should consider the presence of one of the known rare genetic hypertension syndromes if a patient (or relatives) has severe and early-onset hypertension. Also, the presence of early strokes accompanies glucocorticoid-remediable aldosteronism. Low renin and low potassium levels are present for both glucocorticoid-remediable aldosteronism and Liddle's syndrome, whereas aldosterone levels are high for glucocorticoid-remediable aldosteronism but low for Liddle's syndrome. Glucocorticoid-remediable aldosteronism is responsive to prednisone (suppresses hormone production), spironolactone (inhibits the aldosterone receptor), and amiloride (inhibits the distal renal epithelial sodium channel). Liddle's syndrome responds best to triamterene or amiloride, both of which inhibit the epithelial sodium channel. Future identification of specific defects of each newly defined essential hypertension syndrome may allow targeted drug treatment so that effective control of blood pressure is possible. For example, treatment with diuretics is contraindicated for glucocorticoid-remediable aldosteronism, whereas glucocorticoids provide effective treatment. Hypertension researchers hope that as the genetic defects are discovered in genes with more moderate effects a more targeted approach also will be possible. First-line medications may then be tailored to the genetic diagnosis, and the search for the best medication will be minimized. If early results can be confirmed, persons with the allele of either the *AGT* or the α-adducin gene, which increase blood pressure salt sensitivity, may need referral for specific dietary counsel to see if reduced sodium intake can reduce blood pressure levels without the need for medication.

While still in its infancy, there is hope that gene therapy can deliver functional genes to humans which will overcome the effects of dysfunctional genes or that antisense fragments can be delivered which will reduce the transcription of deleterious genes that lead to hypertension. Once perfected, it is believed that delivery of antisense oligodeoxynucleotides, perhaps from one to several times a year, can replace the need for daily antihypertensive medication and have few if any of the side effects now present with current drug treatment.

Gene therapy in rodents has shown successful temporary lowering of blood pressure for the angiotensinogen, kallikrein, endothelial NOS, angiotensin AT1 receptor, atrial natriuretic peptide, and adrenomedullin genes (Phillips, 1999). Therefore, if specific genes can be identified as imparting a measurable blood pressure change, persons with elevated blood pressure could have a panel of genes tested for mutations (gene chip technology) and be told which type of gene therapy will directly counteract the abnormality. There are a large number of obstacles to overcome, but many are optimistic of future success benefiting a large percentage of the world's population.

SUMMARY

The determination of blood pressure is a result of many genetically controlled factors interacting with each other and with the environment. The interlocking network of positive and negative feedback loops between physiological systems makes the study of hypertension very difficult.

As phenotypes are linked to specific genes, subdividing large samples of families into groups where specific genes segregate with hypertension or blood pressure elevations reduces the heterogeneity in the remaining families with unknown causes of hypertension. Since heterogeneity is reduced, epidemiological and genetic studies may have greater success at detecting differences in other variables that contribute to hypertension. Slowly, each factor will be pieced out of an exceedingly complex puzzle, which we hope will result in controlling the development of high blood pressure by targeting specific abnormalities to ultimately prevent its occurrence.

A sizeable number of reports show association and/or linkage of various markers at candidate genes with hypertension. These reports will continue to appear at an even greater rate. The key to maintaining a perspective of what the real genetic components are that lead to hypertension will be consistent replication by studies with sufficient power to test the hypothesis. Many reports of association or linkage studies have failed to be confirmed. Those that are confirmed may be studied in detail to discover how mutations at these loci change the function, amount, or activity of the gene product. The pathway of this product that leads to altered blood pressure may then be studied.

Previously identified epidemiological relationships with blood pressure and hypertension will need to be re-examined after subdivision by, or control for, genetic factors. The environmental contributions to the expression of these genes and the interaction of environmental factors with specific genotypes of multiple genes will greatly increase our understanding of blood pressure regulation.

ACKNOWLEDGMENTS

This book chapter is dedicated to the late Roger R. Williams, our friend and colleague, whose inspiration and scientific contributions to the genetic epidemiology of hypertension have been so valuable.

REFERENCES

Allayee H, Aouizerat BE, Cantor RM, Dallinga-Thie GM, Krauss RM, Lanning CD, Rotter JI, Lusis AJ, de Bruin TW: Families with familial combined hyperlipidemia and families enriched for coronary artery disease share genetic determinants for the atherogenic lipoprotein phenotype. Am J Hum Genet 1998; 63:577–585.

Allender PS, Cutler JA, Follmann D, Cappuccio FP, Pryer J, Elliott P: Dietary calcium and blood pressure: a meta-analysis of randomized clinical trials. Ann Intern Med 1996; 124:825–831.

Ambrosioni E, Costa FV, Montebugnoli L, Borghi C, Vasconi L, Tartagni F, Magnani B: Intralymphocytic sodium concentration. Clin Exp Hypertens 1981; A3:675–691.

Aouizerat BE, Allayee H, Bodnar J, Krass KL, Peltonen L, de Bruin TW, Rotter JI, Lusis AJ: Novel genes for familial combined hyperlipidemia. Curr Opin Lipidol 1999a; 10:113–122.

Aouizerat BE, Allayee H, Cantor RM, Davis RC, Lanning CD, Wen PZ, Dallinga-Thie GM, de Bruin TW, Rotter JI, Lusis AJ: A genome scan for familial combined hyperlipidemia reveals evidence of linkage with a locus on chromosome 11. Am J Hum Genet 1999b; 65:397–412.

Appel LJ, Moore TJ, Obarzanek E, Vollmer WM, Svetkey LP, Sacks FM, Bray GA, Vogt TM, Cutler JA, Windhauser MM, et al.: A clinical trial of the effects of dietary patterns on blood pressure. DASH Collaborative Research Group. N Engl J Med 1997; 336:1117–1124.

Aronow WS, Ahn C: Incidence of heart failure in 2,737 older persons with and without diabetes mellitus. Chest 1999; 115:867–868.

Asch S, Wingard DH, Barrett-Connor EL: Are insulin and hypertension independently related? Ann Epidemiol 1991; 1:23–44.

Ascherio A, Rimm EB, Giovannucci EL, Colditz GA, Rosner B, Willett WC, Sacks F, Stampfer MJ: A prospective study of nutritional factors and hypertension among US men. Circulation 1992; 86:1475–1484.

Atwood LD, Samollow PB, Hixson JE, Stern MP, MacCluer JW: Genome-wide linkage analysis of pulse pressure in Mexican Americans. Hypertension 2001a; 37:425–428.

Atwood LD, Samollow PB, Hixson JE, Stern MP, MacCluer JW: Genome-wide linkage analysis of blood pressure in Mexican Americans. Genet Epidemiol 2001b; 20:373–382.

Austin MA, King M-C, Vranizan KM, Newman B, Krauss RM: Inheritance of low-density lipoprotein subclass patterns: results of complex segregation analysis. Am J Hum Genet 1988; 43:838–846.

Aviv A, Lasker N: Proposed defects in membrane transport and intracellular ions as pathogenic factors in essential hypertension. In: Laragh JH, Brenner BM, eds. Hypertension: Pathophysiology, Diagnosis, and Management. New York: Raven, 1990:923–937.

Baima J, Nicolaou M, Schwartz F, DeStefano AL, Manolis A, Gavras I, Laffer C, Elijovich F, Farrer L, Baldwin CT, et al: Evidence for linkage between essential hypertension and a putative locus on human chromosome 17. Hypertension 1999; 34:4–7.

Baker EH, Portal AJ, McElvaney TA, Blackwood AM, Miller MA, Markandu ND, MacGregor GA: Epithelial sodium channel activity is not increased in hypertension in whites. Hypertension 1999; 33:1031–1035.

Baldwin CT, Schwartz F, Baima J, Burzstyn M, DeStefano AL, Gavras I, Handy DE, Joost O, Martel T, Manolis A, et al: Identification of a polymorphic glutamic acid stretch in the α2B-adrenergic receptor and lack of linkage with essential hypertension. Am J Hypertens 1999; 12:853–857.

Barlassina C, Schork NJ, Manunta P, Citterio L, Sciarrone M, Lanella G, Bianchi G, Cusi D: Synergistic effect of alpha-adducin and *ACE* genes causes blood pressure changes with body sodium and volume expansion. Kidney Int 2000; 57:1083–1090.

Baum M: Insulin stimulates volume absorption in the rabbit proximal convoluted tubule. J Clin Invest 1987; 79:1104–1109.

Beige J, Hohenbleicher H, Distler A, Sharma AM: G-protein beta3 subunit C825T variant and ambulatory blood pressure in essential hypertension. Hypertension 1999; 33:1049–1051.

Benjafield AV, Jeyasingam CL, Nyholt DR, Griffiths LR, Morris BJ: G-protein beta3 subunit gene (*GNB3*) variant in causation of essential hypertension. Hypertension 1998; 32:1094–1097.

Bennett CL, Schrader AP, Morris BJ: Cross-sectional analysis of Met235 $\rightarrow$ Thr variant of angiotensinogen gene in severe, familial hypertension. Biochem Biophys Res Commun 1993; 197:833–839.

Berge KE, Bakken A, Bohn M, Erikssen J, Berg K: Analyses of mutations in the human renal kallikrein (*hKLK1*) gene and their possible relevance to blood pressure regulation and risk of myocardial infarction. Clin Genet 1997; 52:86–95.

Berge KE, Berg K: No effect of a Taq1 polymorphism in DNA at the endothelin I (EDN1) locus on normal blood pressure level or variability. Clin Genet 1992; 41:90–95.

Berge KE, Berg K: No effect of a BglI polymorphism at the renin (REN) locus on blood pressure level or variability. Clin Genet 1994; 46:436–438.

Berglund G, Andersson O, Wilhelmsen L: Prevalence of primary and secondary hypertension: studies in a random population sample. BMJ 1976; 2:554–556.

Berry TD, Hasstedt SJ, Hunt SC, Wu LL, Smith JB, Ash KO, Kuida H, Williams RR: A gene for high urinary kallikrein may protect against hypertension in Utah kindreds. Hypertension 1989; 13:3–8.

Bianchi G, Tripodi G, Casari G, Salardi S, Barber B, Garcia R, Leoni P, Torielli L, Cusi D, Ferrandi M, et al.: Two point mutations within the adducin genes are involved in blood pressure variation. Proc Natl Acad Sci USA 1994; 91:3999–4003.

Bielen EC, Fagard RH, Amery AK: Inheritance of blood pressure and haemodynamic phenotypes measured at rest and during supine dynamic exercise. J Hypertens 1991; 9:655–663.

Blaustein MP, Hamlyn JM: Sodium transport inhibition, cell calcium, and hypertension. The natriuretic hormone/Na^+–Ca^{2+} exchange/hypertension hypothesis. Am J Med 1984:45–59.

Bloem LJ, Manatunga AK, Tewksbury DA, Pratt JH: The serum angiotensinogen concentration and variants of the angiotensinogen gene in white and black children. J Clin Invest 1995; 95:948–953.

Boerwinkle E, Turner ST, Weinshilboum R, Johnson M, Richelson E, Sing CF: Genetic analysis of the distribution of sodium lithium countertransport in a sample representative of the general population. Genet Epidemiol 1986; 3:365–378.

Bonnardeaux A, Davies E, Jeunemaitre X, Féry I, Charru A, Clauser E, Tiret L, Cambien F, Corvol P, Soubrier F: Angiotensin II type 1 receptor gene polymorphisms in human essential hypertension. Hypertension 1994; 24:63–69.

Bonnardeaux A, Nadaud S, Charru A, Jeunemaitre X, Corvol P, Soubrier F: Lack of evidence for linkage of the endothelial cell nitric oxide synthase gene to essential hypertension. Circulation 1995; 91:96–102.

Boomsma DI, Snieder H, de Geus EJ, van Doornen LJ: Heritability of blood pressure increases during mental stress. Twin Res 1998; 1:15–24.

Borecki IB, Province MA, Ludwig EH, Ellison RC, Folsom AR, Heiss G, Lalouel JM, Higgins M, Rao DC: Associations of candidate loci angiotensinogen and angiotensin-converting enzyme with severe hypertension: the NHLBI Family Heart Study. Ann Epidemiol 1997; 7:13–21.

Brand E, Bankir L, Plouin PF, Soubrier F: Glucagon receptor gene mutation (Gly^{40}Ser) in human essential hypertension : the PEGASE Study. Hypertension 1999a; 34:15–17.

Brand E, Chatelain N, Keavney B, Caulfield M, Citterio L, Connell J, Grobbee D, Schmidt S, Schunkert H, Schuster H, et al.: Evaluation of the angiotensinogen locus in human essential hypertension: a European study. Hypertension 1998a; 31:725–729.

Brand E, Chatelain N, Mulatero P, Fery I, Curnow K, Jeunemaitre X, Corvol P, Pascoe L, Soubrier F: Structural analysis and evaluation of the aldosterone synthase gene in hypertension. Hypertension 1998b; 32:198–204.

Brand E, Herrmann SM, Nicaud V, Ruidavets JB, Evans A, Arveiler D, Luc G, Plouin PF, Tiret L, Cambien F: The 825C/T polymorphism of the G-protein subunit beta3 is not related to hypertension. Hypertension 1999b; 33:1175–1178.

Brand E, Kato N, Chatelain N, Krozowski ZS, Jeunemaitre X, Corvol P, Plouin PF, Cambien F, Pascoe L, Soubrier F: Structural analysis and evaluation of the 11beta-hydroxysteroid dehydrogenase type 2 (*11beta-HSD2*) gene in human essential hypertension. J Hypertens 1998c; 16:1627–1633.

Bray MS, Li L, Turner ST, Kardia SL, Boerwinkle E: Association and linkage analysis of the alpha-adducin gene and blood pressure. Am J Hypertens 2000; 13:699–703.

Brown AJ, Casals-Stenzel J, Gofford S, Lever AF, Morton JJ: Comparison of fast and slow pressor effects of angiotensin II in the conscious rat. Am J Physiol 1981; 241:H381–H388.

Brown MJ, Sharma P, Stevens PA: Association between diastolic blood pressure and variants of the endothelin-1 and endothelin-2 genes. J Cardiovasc Pharmacol 2000; 35(Suppl 2):S41–S43.

Brunner HR, Sealey JE, Laragh JH: Renin as a risk factor in essential hypertension: more evidence. Am J Med 1973; 55:295–302.

Buja LM, Kovanen PT, Bilheimer DW: Cellular pathology of homozygous familial hypercholesterolemia. Am J Pathol 1979; 97:327–357.

Burt VL, Cutler JA, Higgins M, Horan MJ, Labarthe D, Whelton P, Brown C, Roccella EJ: Trends in the prevalence, awareness, treatment, and control of hypetension in the adult US population. Data from the Health Examination Surveys, 1960–1991. Hypertension 1995; 26:60–69.

Cain MD, Walters WA, Catt KJ: Effects of oral contraceptive therapy on the renin-angiotensin system. J Clin Endocrinol 1971; 33:671–676.

Calver A, Collier J, Moncada S, Vallance P: Effect of local intra-arterial N^G-monomethyl-L-arginine in patients with hypertension: the nitric oxide dilator mechanism appears abnormal. J Hypertens 1992; 10:1025–1031.

Canessa ML, Morgan K, Semplicini A: Genetic differences in lithium–sodium exchange and regulation of the sodium–hydrogen exchanger in essential hypertension. J Cardiovasc Pharmacol 1988; 12(Suppl 3):S92–S98.

Cappuccio RP, MacGregor GA: Does potassium supplementation lower blood pressure? A meta-analysis of published trials. J Hypertens 1991; 9:465–473.

Carmelli D, Cardon LR, Fabsitz R: Clustering of hypertension, diabetes, and obesity in adult male twins: same genes or same environments? Am J Hum Genet 1994; 55:566–573.

Castellano M, Muiesan ML, Rizzoni D, Beschi M, Pasini G, Salvetti M, Porteri E, Bettoni G, Kreutz R, Lindpaintner K, et al.: Angiotensin-converting enzyme I/D polymorphism and arterial wall thickness in a general population. The Vobarno Study. Circulation 1995; 91:2721–2724.

Castelli WP, Garrison RJ, Wilson PWF, Abbott RD, Kalousdian S, Kannel WB: Incidence of coronary heart disease and lipoprotein cholesterol levels. The Framingham Study. JAMA 1986; 256:2835–2838.

Caulfield M, Lavender P, Farrall M, Munroe P, Lawson M, Turner P, Clark AJL: Linkage of the angiotensinogen gene to essential hypertension. N Engl J Med 1994; 330:1629–1633.

Caulfield M, Lavender P, Newell-Price J, Farrall M, Kamdar S, Daniel H, Lawson M, De Freitas P, Fogarty P, Clark AJ: Linkage of the angiotensinogen gene locus to human essential hypertension in African Caribbeans. J Clin Invest 1995; 96:687–692.

Cheng LS, Carmelli D, Hunt SC, Williams RR: Segregation analysis of cardiovascular reactivity to laboratory stressors. Genet Epidemiol 1997; 14:35–49.

Cheng LS, Davis RC, Raffel LJ, Xiang AH, Wang N, Quinones M, Wen PZ, Toscano E, Diaz J, Pressman S, et al.: Coincident linkage of fasting plasma insulin and blood pressure to chromosome 7q in hypertensive hispanic families. Circulation 2001; 104:1255–1260.

Cheng LS-C, Carmelli D, Hunt SC, Williams RR: Evidence for a major gene influencing 7-year increases in diastolic blood pressure with age. Am J Hum Genet 1995; 57:1169–1177.

Chiang FT, Chiu KC, Tseng YZ, Lee KC, Chuang LM: Nucleotide(-258) G-to-A transition variant of the liver glucokinase gene is associated with essential hypertension. Am J Hypertens 1997; 10:1049–1052.

Collins R, Peto R, MacMahon S, Hebert P, Fiebach NH, Eberlein KA, Godwin J, Qizilbash N, Taylor JO, Hennekens CH: Blood pressure, stroke, and coronary heart disease. Part 2. Short-term reductions in blood pressure: overview of randomised drug trials in their epidemiological context. Lancet 1990; 335:827–838.

Coon H, Myers RH, Borecki IB, Arnett DK, Hunt SC, Province MA, Djousse L, Leppert MF: Replication of linkage of familial combined hyperlipidemia to chromosome 1q with additional heterogeneous effect of apolipoprotein A-I/C-III/A-IV locus. The NHLBI Family Heart Study. Arterioscler Thromb Vasc Biol 2000; 20:2275–2280.

Corrocher R, Steinmayr M, Ruzzenente O, Brugnara C, Bertinato L, Mazzi M, Furri C, Bonfanti F, De Sandr G: Elevation of red cell sodium–lithium countertransport in hyperlipidemias. Life Sci 1985; 36:649–655.

Criqui MH, Cowan LD, Heiss G, Haskell WL, Laskarzewski PM, Chambless LE: Frequency and clustering of nonlipid coronary risk factors in dyslipoproteinemia: the Lipid Research Clinic's program prevalence study. Circulation 1986; 73(Suppl 1):140–150.

Curmi PA, Juan L, Tedgui A: Effect of transmural pressure on low density lipoprotein and albumin transport and distribution across the intact arterial wall. Circ Res 1990; 66:1692–1702.

Cushman WC, Cutler JA, Hanna E, Bingham SF, Follmann D, Harford T, Dubbert P, Allender PS, Dufour M, Collins JF, et al.: Prevention and Treatment of Hypertension Study (PATHS): effects of an alcohol treatment program on blood pressure. Arch Intern Med 1998; 158:1197–1207.

Cusi D, Barlassina C, Azzani T, Casari G, Citterio L, Devoto M, Glorioso N, Lanzani C, Manunta P, Righetti M, et al.: Polymorphisms of alpha-adducin and salt sensitivity in patients with essential hypertension. Lancet 1997; 349:1353–1357.

Cusi D, Fossali E, Piazza A, Tripodi G, Barlassina C, Pozzoli E, Vezzoli G, Stella P, Soldati L, Bianchi G: Heritability estimate of erythrocyte Na–K–Cl cotransport in normotensive and hypertensive families. Am J Hypertens 1991; 4:725–734.

Cusi D, Melzi M, Barlassina C, Sereni F, Bianchi G: Genetic models of arterial hypertension—role of tubular ion transport. Pediatr Nephrol 1993; 7:865–870.

Cutler JA, Follmann D, Allender PS: Randomized trials of sodium reduction: an overview. Am J Clin Nutr 1997; 65(Suppl 2):643S–651S.

Dahl L, Heine M, Thompson K: Genetic influence of the kidneys on blood pressure. Evidence from chronic renal homografts in rats with opposite predispositions to hypertension. Circ Res 1974; 34:94–101.

Dahlöf B, Lindholm LH, Hansson L, Scherstén B, Ekmon T, Wester P-O: Morbidity and mortality in the Swedish Trial in Old Patients with Hypertension (STOP-Hypertension). Lancet 1991; 338:1281–1285.

Danser AH, Derkx FH, Hense HW, Jeunemaitre X, Riegger GA, Schunkert H: Angiotensinogen (M235T) and angiotensin-converting enzyme (I/D) polymorphisms in association with plasma renin and prorenin levels. J Hypertens 1998; 16:1879–1883.

Davies E, Holloway CD, Ingram MC, Inglis GC, Friel EC, Morrison C, Anderson NH, Fraser R, Connell JM: Aldosterone excretion rate and blood pressure in essential hypertension are related to polymorphic differences in the aldosterone synthase gene *CYP11B2*. Hypertension 1999; 33:703–707.

deBlois D, Schwartz SM, van Kleef EM, Su JE, Griffin KA, Bidani AK, Daemen MJAP, Lombardi DM: Chronic α_1-adrenoreceptor stimulation increases DNA synthesis in rat arterial wall. Modulation of responsiveness after vascular injury. Arterioscler Thromb Vasc Biol 1996; 16:1122–1129.

DeFronzo RA, Cooke CR, Andres R, Faloona GR, Davis PJ: The effect of insulin on renal handling of sodium, potassium, calcium, and phosphate in man. J Clin Invest 1975; 55:845–855.

de Graaf J, Swinkels DW, de Haan AFJ, Demacker PNM, Stalenhoef AFH: Both inherited susceptibility and environmental exposure determine the low-density lipoprotein-subfraction pattern distribution in healthy Dutch families. Am J Hum Genet 1992; 51:1295–1310.

Denton D, Weisinger R, Mundy NI, Wickings EJ, Dixson A, Moisson P, Pingard AM, Shade R, Carey D, Ardaillou R, et al.: The effect of increased salt intake on blood pressure of chimpanzees. Nat Med 1995; 1:1009–1014.

DiBona GF: Neural regulation of renal tubular sodium reabsorption and renin secretion. Fed Proc 1985; 44:2816–2822.

Ding Y, Davisson RL, Hardy DO, Zhu LJ, Merrill DC, Catterall JF, Sigmund CD: The kidney androgen-regulated protein promoter confers renal proximal tubule cell-specific and highly androgen-responsive expression on the human angiotensinogen gene in transgenic mice. J Biol Chem 1997; 272:28142–28148.

Drayer JI, Weber MA, Sealey JE, Laragh JH: Low and high renin essential hypertension: a comparison of clinical and biochemical characteristics. Am J Med Sci 1981; 281:135–142.

Draznin B, Kao M, Sussman KE: Insulin and glyburide increase cytosolic free-Ca^2 concentration in isolated rat adipocytes. Diabetes 1987; 36:174–178.

Dudley CR, Guiffra LA, Raine AE, Reeders ST: Assessing the role of *APNH*, a gene encoding for a human amiloride-sensitive Na^+/H^+ antiporter, on the interindividual variation in red cell Na^+/Li^+ countertransport. J Am Soc Nephrol 1991; 2:937–943.

Duncan JA, Scholey JW, Miller JA: Angiotensin II type 1 receptor gene polymorphisms in humans: physiology and pathophysiology of the genotypes. Curr Opin Nephrol Hypertens 2001; 10:111–116.

Eggena P, Sowers JR, Maxwell MH, Barrett JD, Golub MS: Hormonal correlates of weight loss associated with blood pressure reduction. Clin Exp Hypertens 1991; 13:1447–1456.

Elbein SC, Hoffman MD, Teng K, Leppert MF, Hasstedt SJ: A genome-wide search for type 2 diabetes susceptibility genes in Utah Caucasians. Diabetes 1999; 48:1175–1182.

Elliott P, Stamler J, Nichols R, Dyer AR, Stamler R, Kesteloot H, Marmot M: Intersalt revisited: further analyses of 24 hour sodium excretion and blood pressure

within and across populations. Intersalt Cooperative Research Group. BMJ 1996; 312:1249–1253.
Fagard R, Brguljan J, Staessen J, Thijs L, Derom C, Thomis M, Vlietinck R: Heritability of conventional and ambulatory blood pressures. A study in twins. Hypertension 1995; 26:919–924.
Fagard RH: Prescription and results of physical activity. J Cardiovasc Pharmacol 1995; 25(Suppl 1):S20–S27.
Falkner B, Onesti G, Angelakos ET, Fernandes M, Langman C: Cardiovascular response to mental stress in normal adolescents with hypertensive parents: hemodynamics and mental stress in adolescents. Hypertension 1979; 1:23–30.
Fasola AF, Martz BL, Helmer OM: Plasma renin activity during supine exercise in offspring of hypertensive parents. J Appl Physiol 1968; 25:410–415.
Feinleib M, Garrison R, Borhani N, Rosenman R, Christian J: Studies of hypertension in twins. In: Paul O, ed. Epidemiology and Control of Hypertension. New York: Grune and Stratton, 1975:3–17.
Feinleib M, Garrison RJ: The contribution of family studies to the partitioning of population variation of blood pressure. In: Sing CF, Skolnick M, eds. The Genetic Analysis of Common Diseases. New York: Alan R Liss, 1979:653–673.
Feinleib M, Garrison RJ, Fabsitz R, Christian JC, Hrubec Z, Borhani NO, Kannel WB, Rosenman R, Schwartz JT, Wagner JO: The NHLBI twin study of cardiovascular disease risk factors: methodology and summary of results. Am J Epidemiol 1977; 106:284–295.
Ferrandi M, Tripodi G, Salardi S, Florio M, Modica R, Barassi P, Parenti P, Shainskaya A, Karlish S, Bianchi G, et al.: Renal Na,K-ATPase in genetic hypertension. Hypertension 1996; 28:1018–1025.
Ferrannini E, Buzzigoli G, Bonadonna R, Giorico MA, Oleggini M, Graziadei L, Pedrinellia R, Brandi L, Bevilacqua S: Insulin resistance in essential hypertension. N Engl J Med 1987; 317:350–356.
Finch D, Davis G, Bower J, Kirchner K: Effect of insulin on renal sodium handling in hypertensive rats. Hypertension 1990; 14:514–518.
Fisher ND, Hurwitz S, Ferri C, Jeunemaitre X, Hollenberg NK, Williams GH: Altered adrenal sensitivity to angiotensin II in low-renin essential hypertension. Hypertension 1999; 34:388–394.
Fisher NDL, Hunt S, Hurwitz S, Jeunemaitre X, Hopkins P, Hollenberg NK, Williams GH: Heritability of low-renin hypertension. Am J Hypertens 2000; 13:2A.
Flaxman N: The course of hypertensive heart disease: 1. Age of onset, development of cardiac insufficiency, duration of life, and cause of death. Ann Intern Med 1936; 10:748–753.
Fornage M, Amos CI, Kardia S, Sing CF, Turner ST, Boerwinkle E: Variation in the region of the angiotensin-converting enzyme gene influences interindividual differences in blood pressure levels in young white males. Circulation 1998; 97:1773–1779.
Fray JCS, Park CS, Valentine AND: Calcium and control of renin secretion. Endocr Rev 1987; 8:53–93.
Frederich RC Jr, Kahn BB, Peach MJ, Flier JS: Tissue-specific nutritional regulation of angiotensinogen in adipose tissue. Hypertension 1992; 19:339–344.
Fredrickson M, Tuomisto M, Bergman-Losman B: Neuroendocrine and cardiovascular stress reactivity in middle-aged normotensive adults with parental history of cardiovascular disease. Psychophysiology 1991; 28:656–664.
Freedman DS, Shear CL, Burke GL, Srinivasan SR, Webber LS, Harsha DW, Berenson GS: Persistence of juvenile-onset obesity over eight years: the Bogalusa Heart Study. Am J Public Health 1987; 77:588–592.
Friedman GD, Selby JV, Quesenberry CP Jr, Armstrong MA, Klatsky AL: Precursors of essential hypertension: body weight, alcohol and salt use, and parental history of hypertension. Prev Med 1988; 17:387–402.
Friend LR, Morris BJ, Gaffney PT, Griffiths LR: Examination of the role of nitric oxide synthase and renal kallikrein as candidate genes for essential hypertension. Clin Exp Pharmacol Physiol 1996; 23:564–566.
Fuh MM-T, Shieh SM, Wu DA, Chen YDI, Reaven GM: Abnormalities of carbohydrate and lipid metabolism in patients with hypertension. Arch Intern Med 1987; 147:1035–1038.
Fujisawa T, Ikegami H, Yamato E, Hamada Y, Kamide K, Rakugi H, Higaki J, Murakami H, Shimamoto K, Ogihara T: Trp^{64}Arg mutation of beta3-adrenergic receptor in essential hypertension: insulin resistance and the adrenergic system. Am J Hypertens 1997; 10:101–105.
Fuller JH: Epidemiology of hypertension associated with diabetes mellitus. Hypertension 1985; 7(Suppl II):II-3–II-7.
Gahnem F, von Lutterotti N, Camargo MJ, Laragh JH, Sealey JE: Angiotensinogen dependency of blood pressure in two high-renin hypertensive rat models. Am J Hypertens 1994; 7:899–904.
Garay RP, Alvarez-Guerra M, Alda JO, Nazaret C, Soler A, Vargas F: Regulation of renal Na–K–Cl cotransporter *NKCC2* by humoral natriuretic factors: relevance in hypertension. Clin Exp Hypertens 1998; 20:675–682.
Garay RP, Cavalier S, Hannaert PA: The [Na^+,K^+,Cl^-] cotransport system: relevance in essential hypertension. In: Coca A, Garay RP, eds. Ionic Transport in Hypertension: New Perspectives. Boca Raton, FL: CRC Press, 1994:45–56.
Gardes J, Bouhnik J, Clauser E, Corvol P, Ménard J: Role of angiotensinogen in blood pressure homeostasis. Hypertension 1982; 4:185–189.
Garland C, Barrett-Connor E, Suarez L, Criqui MH: Isolated systolic hypertension and mortality after age 60 years: a prospective population-based study. Am J Epidemiol 1983; 118:365–376.
Geleijnse JM, Hofman A, Witteman JCM, Hazebroek AAJM, Valkenburg HA, Grobbee DE: Long-term effects of neonatal sodium restriction on blood pressure. Hypertension 1997; 29:913–917.
Glenn CL, Wang WY, Morris BJ: Different frequencies of inducible nitric oxide synthase genotypes in older hypertensives. Hypertension 1999; 33:927–932.
Glorioso N, Manunta P, Filigheddu F, Troffa C, Stella P, Barlassina C, Lombardi C, Soro A, Dettori F, Parpaglia PP, et al.: The role of alpha-adducin polymorphism in blood pressure and sodium handling regulation may not be excluded by a negative association study. Hypertension 1999; 34:649–654.
Gordon T, Garcia-Palmieri MR, Kapan A: Differences in coronary heart disease in Framingham, Honolulu and Puerto Rico: J Chron Dis 1974; 27:329–344.
Gould AB, Green B: Kinetics of the human renin and human renin substrate reaction. Cardiovasc Res 1971; 5:86–89.
Granger JP, West D, Scott J: Abnormal pressure natriuresis in the dog model of obesity-induced hypertension. Hypertension 1994; 23(Suppl 1):I-8–I-11.
Grobbee DE, Hofman A: Does sodium restriction lower blood pressure? BMJ 1986; 293:27–29.
Haffner SM, Valdez RA, Hazuda HP, Mitchell BD, Morales PA, Stern MP: Prospective analysis of the insulin-resistance syndrome (syndrome X). Diabetes 1992; 41:715–722.
Hall JE: Control of sodium excretion by angiotensin: intrarenal mechanisms and blood pressure regulation. Am J Physiol 1986; 250:R960–R972.
Hall JE: Renal and cardiovascular mechanisms of hypertension in obesity. Hypertension 1994; 23:381–394.
Hall JE: Mechanisms of abnormal renal sodium handling in obesity hypertension. Am J Hypertens 1997; 10:49S–55S.
Hall JE, Brands MW, Kivlighn SD, Mizelle HL, Hildebrandt DA, Gaillard CA: Chronic hyperinsulinemia and blood pressure. Interaction with catecholamines? Hypertension 1990; 15:519–527.
Hall JE, Coleman TG, Mizelle HL: Does chronic hyperinsulinemia cause hypertension? Am J Hypertens 1989; 2:171–173.
Hamlyn JM, Harris DW, Clark MA, Rogowski AC, White RJ, Ludens JH: Isolation and characterization of a sodium pump inhibitor from human plasma. Hypertension 1989; 13:681–689.
Hansson JH, Nelson-Williams C, Suzuki H, Schild L, Shimkets R, Lu Y, Canessa C, Iwasaki T, Rossier B, Lifton RP: Hypertension caused by a truncated epithelial sodium channel gamma subunit: genetic heterogeneity of Liddle syndrome. Nat Genet 1995a; 11:76–82.
Hansson JH, Schild L, Lu Y, Wilson TA, Gautschi I, Shimkets R, Nelson-Williams C, Rossier BC, Lifton RP: A de novo missense mutation of the beta subunit of the epithelial sodium channel causes hypertension and Liddle syndrome, identifying a proline-rich segment critical for regulation of channel activity. Proc Natl Acad Sci USA 1995b; 92:11495–11499.
Harlan WR, Hull AL, Schmouder RL, Landis JR, Larkin FA, Thompson FE: High blood pressure in older Americans. The first National Health Examination Survey. Hypertension 1984; 6:802–809.
Harrap SB, Samani NJ, Lodwick D, Connor JM, Fraser R, Davies DL, Lever AF, Foy CJ, Watt GC: The *SA* gene: predisposition to hypertension and renal function in man. Clin Sci (Colch) 1995; 88:665–670.
Hasstedt SJ, Hunt SC, Wu LL, Williams RR: The inheritance of intraerythrocytic sodium level. Am J Med Genet 1988a; 29:193–203.
Hasstedt SJ, Hunt SC, Wu LL, Williams RR: Evidence for multiple genes determining sodium transport. Genet Epidemiol 1994; 11:553–568.
Hasstedt SJ, Ramirez ME, Kuida H, Williams RR: Recessive inheritance of a relative fat pattern. Am J Hum Genet 1989a; 45:917–925.
Hasstedt SJ, Wu LL, Ash KO, Kuida H, Williams RR: Hypertension and sodium–lithium countertransport in Utah pedigrees: evidence for major locus inheritance. Am J Hum Genet 1988b; 43:14–22.
Hasstedt SJ, Wu LL, Kuida H, Williams RR: Recessive inheritance of a high number of sodium pump sites. Am J Med Genet 1989b; 34:332–337.
Hayden MR, Kirk H, Clark C, Frohlich J, Rabkin S, McLeod R, Hewitt J: DNA polymorphisms in and around the Apo-A1–CIII genes and genetic hyperlipidemias. Am J Hum Genet 1987; 40:421–430.
Hayes CG, Tyroler HA, Cassel JC: Family aggregation of blood pressure in Evans County, Georgia. Arch Intern Med 1971; 128:965–975.
Haynes WG, Ferro CE, Webb DJ: Physiologic role of endothelin in maintenance of vascular tone in humans. J Cardiovasc Pharmacol 1995; 26:S183–S185.
Hegele RA, Harris SB, Hanley AJ, Cao H, Zinman B: G protein beta3 subunit gene variant and blood pressure variation in Canadian Oji-Cree. Hypertension 1998; 32:688–692.
Herrera VL, Xie HX, Lopez LV, Schork NJ, Ruiz-Opazo N: The alpha1 Na,K-ATPase gene is a susceptibility hypertension gene in the Dahl salt-sensitive HSD rat. J Clin Invest 1998; 102:1102–1111.
Hindmarsh PC, Brook CG: Evidence for an association between birth weight and blood pressure. Acta Paediatr Suppl 1999; 88:66–69.
Hines EA Jr, Brown GE: The cold pressor test for measuring the reactibility of the blood pressure: data concerning 571 normal and hypertensive subjects. Am Heart J 1936; 11:1–9.
Hollander W, Madoff I, Paddock J: Aggravation of atherosclerosis by hypertension in a subhuman primate model with coarctation of the aorta. Circ Res 1976; 38(Suppl II):63–72.
Hollenberg NK, Williams GH: Abnormal renal function, sodium-volume homeostasis, and renin system behavior in normal-renin essential hypertension. In: Laragh JH, Brenner BM, eds. Hypertension: Pathophysiology, Diagnosis, and Management. New York: Raven Press, 1990:1349–1370.
Hong Y, de Faire U, Heller DA, McClearn GE, Pedersen N: Genetic and environmental influences on blood pressure in elderly twins. Hypertension 1994; 24:663–670.
Hong Y, Pedersen NL, Brismar K, de Faire U: Genetic and environmental architecture of the features of the insulin-resistance syndrome. Am J Hum Genet 1997; 60:143–152.
Hopkins PN, Hunt SC, Wu LL, Williams GH, Williams RR: Hypertension, dyslipidemia, and insulin resistance: links in a chain or spokes on a wheel? Curr Opin Lipidol 1996a; 7:241–253.

Hopkins PN, Lifton RP, Hollenberg NK, Jeunemaitre X, Hallouin MC, Skuppin J, Williams CS, Dluhy RG, Lalouel JM, Williams RR, et al.: Blunted renal vascular response to angiotensin II is associated with a common variant of the angiotensinogen gene and obesity. J Hypertens 1996b; 14:199–207.

Horwitz D, Margolius HS, Keiser HR: Effects of dietary potassium and race on urinary excretion of kallikrein and aldosterone in man. J Clin Endocrinol Metab 1978; 47:296–299.

Houtman PN, Shah V, Dillon MJ: Sodium–lithium countertransport and family history of hypertension in childhood. Acta Paediatr 1993; 82:1057–1060.

Hsueh WC, Mitchell BD, Schneider JL, Wagner MJ, Bell CJ, Nanthakumar E, Shuldiner AR: QTL influencing blood pressure maps to the region of PPH1 on chromosome 2q31–34 in Old Order Amish. Circulation 2000; 101:2810–2816.

Huang CN, Lee KC, Wu HP, Tai TY, Lin BJ, Chuang LM: Screening for the $Gly^{40}Ser$ mutation in the glucagon receptor gene among patients with type 2 diabetes or essential hypertension in Taiwan. Pancreas 1999; 18:151–155.

Hubner N, Lee YA, Lindpaintner K, Ganten D, Kreutz R: Congenic substitution mapping excludes *Sa* as a candidate gene locus for a blood pressure quantitative trait locus on rat chromosome 1. Hypertension 1999; 34:643–648.

Hunt SC, Cook NR, Oberman A, Cutler JA, Hennekens CH, Allender PS, Walker WG, Whelton PK, Williams RR: Angiotensinogen genotype, sodium reduction, weight loss, and prevention of hypertension: trials of hypertension prevention, phase II. Hypertension 1998; 32:393–401.

Hunt SC, Geleijnse JM, Wu LL, Witteman JCM, Williams RR, Grobbee DE: Enhanced blood pressure response to mild sodium reduction in subjects with the 235T variant of the angiotensinogen gene. Am J Hypertens 1999a; 12:460–466.

Hunt SC, Hasstedt SJ, Kuida H, Stults BM, Hopkins PH, Williams RR: Genetic heritability and common environmental components of resting and stressed blood pressures, lipids, and body mass index in Utah pedigrees and twins. Am J Epidemiol 1989a; 129:625–638.

Hunt SC, Hasstedt SJ, Wu LL, Williams RR: A gene–environment interaction between inferred kallikrein genotype and potassium. Hypertension 1993; 22:161–168.

Hunt SC, Hopkins PN, Williams RR: Hypertension: genetics and mechanisms. In: Fuster V, Ross R, Topol EJ, eds. Atherosclerosis and Coronary Artery Disease. Philadelphia: Lippincott-Raven, 1996a:209–235.

Hunt SC, Province MA, Atwood LD, Sholinsky P, Lalouel JM, Rao DC, Williams RR, Leppert MF: No linkage of the lipoprotein lipase locus to hypertension in Caucasians. J Hypertens 1999b; 17:39–43.

Hunt SC, Stephenson SH, Hopkins PN, Williams RR: Predictors of an increased risk of future hypertension in Utah pedigrees: a screening analysis. Hypertension 1991; 17:969–976.

Hunt SC, Williams RR: Genetic factors in human hypertension. In: Swales JD, ed. Textbook of Hypertension. Oxford: Blackwell, 1994:519–538.

Hunt SC, Williams RR, Ash KO: Changes in sodium–lithium countertransport correlate with changes in triglyceride levels and body mass index over two and one-half years of followup in Utah. Cardiovasc Drugs Ther 1990; 4:357–362.

Hunt SC, Williams RR, Barlow GK: A comparison of positive family history definitions for defining risk of future disease. J Chron Dis 1986a; 39:809–821.

Hunt SC, Williams CS, Sharma AM, Inoue I, Williams RR, Lalouel J-M: Lack of linkage between the endothelial nitric oxide synthase gene and hypertension. J Hum Hypertens 1996b; 10:27–30.

Hunt SC, Williams RR, Smith JB, Ash KO: Associations of three erythrocyte cation transport systems with plasma lipids in Utah subjects. Hypertension 1986b; 8:30–36.

Hunt SC, Wu LL, Hopkins PN, Stults BM, Kuida H, Ramirez ME, Lalouel J-M, Williams RR: Apolipoprotein, low density lipoprotein subfraction, and insulin associations with familial combined hyperlipidemia: study of Utah patients with familial dyslipidemic hypertension. Arteriosclerosis 1989b; 9:335–344.

Inoue I, Nakajima T, Williams CS, Quackenbush J, Puryear R, Powers M, Cheng T, Ludwig EH, Sharma AM, Hata A, et al.: A nucleotide substitution in the promoter of human angiotensinogen is associated with essential hypertension and affects basal transcription in vitro. J Clin Invest 1997; 99:1786–1797.

Ishigami T, Iwamoto T, Tamura K, Yamaguchi S, Iwasawa K, Uchino K, Umemura S, Ishii M: Angiotensin I converting enzyme (*ACE*) gene polymorphism and essential hypertension in Japan. Ethnic difference of *ACE* genotype. Am J Hypertens 1995; 8:95–97.

Ishigami T, Umemura S, Tamura K, Hibi K, Nyui N, Kihara M, Yabana M, Watanabe Y, Sumida Y, Nagahara T, et al.: Essential hypertension and 5′ upstream core promoter region of human angiotensinogen gene. Hypertension 1997; 30:1325–1330.

Ito S, Ren Y: Evidence for the role of nitric oxide in macula densa control of glomerular hemodynamics. J Clin Invest 1993; 92:1093–1098.

Iwai N, Baba S, Mannami T, Katsuya T, Higaki J, Ogihara T, Ogata J: Association of sodium channel gamma-subunit promoter variant with blood pressure. Hypertension 2001; 38(1):86–89.

Iwai N, Ohmichi N, Hanai K, Nakamura Y, Kinoshita M: Human *SA* gene locus as a candidate locus for essential hypertension. Hypertension 1994; 23:375–380.

Izzo JL, Black HR (eds.): Hypertension Primer: The Essentials of High Blood Pressure. Baltimore: Lippincott-Williams and Wilkins, 1999.

Jeunemaitre X, Charru A, Chatellier G, Dumont C, Sassano P, Soubrier F, Menard J, Corvol P: M235T variant of the human angiotensinogen gene in unselected hypertensive patients. J Hypertens 1993; 11(Suppl 5):S80–S81.

Jeunemaitre X, Inoue I, Williams C, Charru A, Tichet J, Powers M, Sharma AM, Gimenez-Roqueplo A-P, Hata A, Corvol P, et al.: Haplotypes of angiotensinogen in essential hypertension. Am J Hum Genet 1997; 60:1448–1460.

Jeunemaitre X, Lifton RP, Hunt SC, Williams RR, Lalouel J-M: Absence of linkage between the angiotensin converting enzyme locus and human essential hypertension. Nat Genet 1992a; 1:72–75.

Jeunemaitre X, Rigat B, Charru A, Houot AM, Soubrier F, Corvol P: Sib pair linkage analysis of renin gene haplotypes in human essential hypertension. Hum Genet 1992b; 88:301–306.

Jeunemaitre X, Soubrier F, Kotelevtsev Y, Lifton RP, Williams CS, Charru A, Hunt SC, Hopkins PN, Williams RR, Lalouel JM, et al.: Molecular basis of human hypertension: role of angiotensinogen. Cell 1992c; 71:169–180.

Jiang Z, Akey JM, Shi J, Xiong M, Wang Y, Shen Y, Xu X, Chen H, Wu H, Xiao J, et al.: A polymorphism in the promoter region of catalase is associated with blood pressure levels. Hum Genet 2001; 109:95–98.

John S, Delles C, Klingbeil AU, Jacobi J, Schlaich MP, Schmieder RE: Low-density lipoprotein-cholesterol determines vascular responsiveness to angiotensin II in normocholesterolaemic humans: J Hypertens 1999; 17:1933–1939.

Johnson BC, Epstein FH, Kjelsberg MO: Distributions and familial studies of blood pressure and serum cholesterol levels in a total community—Tecumseh, Michigan. J Chron Dis 1965; 18:147–160.

Jones DW: What is the role of obesity in hypertension and target organ injury in African Americans? Am J Med Sci 1999; 317:147–151.

Jose PA, Eisner GM, Felder RA: Role of dopamine in the pathogenesis of hypertension. Clin Exp Pharmacol Physiol Suppl 1999; 26:S10–S13.

Julier C, Delepine M, Keavney B, Terwilliger J, Davis S, Weeks DE, Bui T, Jeunemaitre X, Velho G, Froguel P, et al.: Genetic susceptibility for human familial essential hypertension in a region of homology with blood pressure linkage on rat chromosome 10. Hum Mol Genet 1997; 6:2077–2085.

Kainulainen K, Perola M, Terwilliger J, Kaprio J, Koskenvuo M, Syvanen AC, Vartiainen E, Peltonen L, Kontula K: Evidence for involvement of the type 1 angiotensin II receptor locus in essential hypertension. Hypertension 1999; 33:844–849.

Kajiyama N, Saito Y, Miyamoto Y, Yoshimura M, Nakayama M, Harada M, Kuwahara K, Kishimoto I, Yasue H, Nakao K: Lack of association between T-786 → C mutation in the 5′-flanking region of the endothelial nitric oxide synthase gene and essential hypertension. Hypertens Res 2000; 23:561–565.

Kamitani A, Wong ZY, Fraser R, Davies DL, Connor JM, Foy CJ, Watt GC, Harrap SB: Human alpha-adducin gene, blood pressure, and sodium metabolism. Hypertension 1998; 32:138–143.

Kannel W, Dawber T, McGee D: Perspectives on systolic hypertension. The Framingham Study. Circulation 1980; 61:1179–1182.

Kaplan NM: Upper-body obesity, glucose intolerance, hypertriglyceridemia, and hypertension. Arch Intern Med 1989; 149:1514–1520.

Kato N, Sugiyama T, Morita H, Nabika T, Kurihara H, Yamori Y, Yazaki Y: Lack of evidence for association between the endothelial nitric oxide synthase gene and hypertension. Hypertension 1999; 33:933–936.

Kato N, Sugiyama T, Nabika T, Morita H, Kurihara H, Yazaki Y, Yamori Y: Lack of association between the alpha-adducin locus and essential hypertension in the Japanese population. Hypertension 1998; 31:730–733.

Keiser HR: The kallikrein–kinin system in essential hypertension. Clin Exp Hypertens 1980; 2:675–691.

Keys A, Menotti A, Aravanis C, Blackburn H, Djordevic BS, Buzina R, Dontas AS, Fidanza F, Karvonen MJ, Kimura N, et al.: The Seven Countries Study: 2,289 deaths in 15 years. Prev Med 1984; 13:141–154.

Kim H-S, Krege JH, Kluckman KD, Hagaman JR, Hodgin JB, Best CF, Jennette JC, Coffman TM, Maeda N, Smithies O: Genetic control of blood pressure and the angiotensinogen locus. Proc Natl Acad Sci USA 1995; 92:2735–2739.

Kim HS, Maeda N, Oh GT, Fernandez LG, Gomez RA, Smithies O: Homeostasis in mice with genetically decreased angiotensinogen is primarily by an increased number of renin-producing cells. J Biol Chem 1999; 274:14210–14217.

King GL, Goodman AD, Buzney S, Moses A, Kahn CR: Receptors and growth-promoting effects of insulin and insulinlike growth factors on cells from bovine retinal capillaries and aorta. J Clin Invest 1985; 75:1028–1036.

Kon V, Badr KF: Biological actions and pathophysiologic significance of endothelin in the kidney. Kidney Int 1991; 40:1–12.

Koshechkin VA, Hudaiberdyev CB, Kabakova VA, Panin SV, Rozhkova TA, Solovjova EY: Genetic epidemiology of ischemic heart disease and arterial hypertension. In: Berg K, Bulyzhenkov V, Christen Y, Corvol P, eds: Genetic Approaches to Coronary Heart Disease and Hypertension. Berlin: Springer-Verlag, 1991:127–142.

Kozarevic D, Pirc B, Racic Z: The Yugoslavia cardiovascular disease study. II. Factors in the incidence of coronary heart disease. Am J Epidemiol 1976; 104:133–140.

Krauss RM: Relationship of intermediate and low-density lipoprotein subspecies to risk of coronary artery disease. Am Heart J 1987; 113:578–582.

Kronenberg F, Rich SS, Sholinsky P, Arnett DK, Province ME, Myers RH, Eckfeldt JH, Williams RR, Hunt SC: Insulin and hypertension in the NHLBI Family Heart Study: a sibpair approach to a controversial issue. Am J Hypertens 2000; 13:240–250.

Krushkal J, Ferrell R, Mockrin SC, Turner ST, Sing CF, Boerwinkle E: Genome-wide linkage analyses of systolic blood pressure using highly discordant siblings. Circulation 1999; 99:1407–1410.

Krushkal J, Xiong M, Ferrell R, Sing CF, Turner ST, Boerwinkle E: Linkage and association of adrenergic and dopamine receptor genes in the distal portion of the long arm of chromosome 5 with systolic blood pressure variation. Hum Mol Genet 1998; 7:1379–1383.

Kuhnle U, Hinkel GK, Akkurt HI, Krozowski Z: Familial pseudohypoaldosteronism: a review on the heterogeneity of the syndrome. Steroids 1995; 60:157–160.

Kunz R, Kreutz R, Beige J, Distler A, Sharma AM: Association between the an-

giotensinogen 235T-variant and essential hypertension in whites: a systematic review and methodological appraisal. Hypertension 1997; 30:1331–1337.
Kwiterovich PO Jr: Genetics and molecular biology of familial combined hyperlipidemia. Curr Opin Lipidol 1993; 4:133–143.
Kwiterovich PO Jr: Detection and treatment of elevated blood lipids and other risk factors for coronary artery disease in youth. Ann NY Acad Sci 1995; 748:313–332.
Lachurié M-L, Azizi M, Guyene T-T, Alhenc-Gelas F, Ménard J: Angiotensin-converting enzyme gene polymorphism has no influence on the circulating renin–angiotensin–aldosterone system or blood pressure in normotensive subjects. Circulation 1995; 91:2933–2942.
Lacolley P, Gautier S, Poirier O, Pannier B, Cambien F, Benetos A: Nitric oxide synthase gene polymorphisms, blood pressure and aortic stiffness in normotensive and hypertensive subjects. J Hypertens 1998; 16:31–35.
Landsberg L: Obesity-related hypertension and the insulin resistance syndrome. Trans Am Clin Climatol Assoc 1994; 106:69–75.
Landsberg L, Young JB: Catecholamines and the adrenal medulla. In: Wilson JD, Foster DW, eds. Williams Textbook of Endocrinology, 7th ed. Philadelphia: Saunders, 1985:891–965.
Langdon RG, Holman VP: Immunological evidence that band 3 is the major glucose transporter of the human erythrocyte membrane. Biochim Biophys Acta 1988; 945:23–32.
Laragh JH: The renin system and the renal regulation of blood pressure. In: Seldin DW, Giebisch G, eds. The Kidney: Physiology and Pathophysiology. New York: Raven, 1992:1411–1453.
Laragh JH, Brenner BM (eds): Hypertension: Pathophysiology, Diagnosis, and Management, 2d ed. New York: Raven, 1995.
Lauer RM, Burns TL, Clarke WR, Mahoney LT: Childhood predictors of future blood pressure. Hypertension 1991; 18(Suppl I):I-74–I-81.
Lerman A, Edwards BS, Hallet JW, Heublein DM, Sondberg SM, Burnett JCJ: Circulating and tissue endothelin immunoreactivity in advanced atherosclerosis. N Engl J Med 1991; 325:997–1001.
Lever AF: Slow pressor mechanisms in hypertension: a role for hypertrophy of resistance vessels? J Hypertens 1986; 4:515–524.
Levine RS, Hennekens CH, Perry A, Cassady J, Gelband H, Jesse MJ: Genetic variance of blood pressure levels in infant twins. Am J Epidemiol 1982; 116:759–764.
Levy D, DeStefano AL, Larson MG, O'Donnell CJ, Lifton RP, Gavras H, Cupples LA, Myers RH: Evidence for a gene influencing blood pressure on chromosome 17. Genome scan linkage results for longitudinal blood pressure phenotypes in subjects from the Framingham Heart Study. Hypertension 2000; 36:477–483.
Levy D, Garrison RJ, Savage DD, Kannel WB, Castelli WP: Prognostic implications of echocardiographically determined left ventricular mass in the Framingham Heart Study. N Engl J Med 1990; 322:1561–1566.
Levy D, Larson MG, Vasan RS, Kannel WB, Ho KKL: The progression from hypertension to congestive heart failure. JAMA 1996; 275:1557–1562.
Lifton RP, Dluhy RG, Powers M, Rich GM, Cook S, Ulick S, Lalouel J-M: A chimaeric 11β-hydroxylase/aldosterone synthase gene causes glucocorticoid-remediable aldosteronism and human hypertension. Nature 1992; 355:262–2625.
Lifton RP, Hopkins PN, Williams RR, Hollenberg NK, Williams GH, Dluhy RG: Evidence for heritability of non-modulation essential hypertension. Hypertension 1989; 13:884–889.
Lifton RP, Hunt SC, Williams RR, Lalouel JM: Exclusion of the Na^+/H^+ antiporter as a candidate gene in human essential hypertension by genetic linkage analysis. Hypertension 1991; 17:8–14.
Lijnen P, Celis H, Fagard R, Staessen J, Amery A: Influence of cholesterol lowering on plasma membrane lipids and cationic transport systems. J Hypertens 1994; 12:59–64.
Linder L, Kiowski W, Buhler FR, Luscher TF: Indirect evidence for release of endothelium-derived relaxing factor in human forearm circulation in vivo. Blunted response in essential hypertension. Circulation 1990; 81:1762–1767.
Lissner L, Bengtsson C, Lapidus L, Kristjansson K, Wedel H: Fasting insulin in relation to subsequent blood pressure changes and hypertension in women. Hypertension 1992; 20:797–801.
Luft FC, Grim CE, Higgins JT, Weinberger MH: Differences in response to sodium administration in normotensive white and black subjects. J Lab Clin Med 1977; 90:555–562.
Luft FC, Miller JZ, Cohen SJ, Fineberg NS, Weinberger MH: Heritable aspects of salt sensitivity. Am J Cardiol 1988; 61:1H–6H.
Lüscher TF, Boulanger CM, Dohi Y, Yang Z: Endothelium-derived contracting factors. Hypertension 1992; 19:117–130.
Lüscher TF, Vanhoutte PM, Raij L: Antihypertensive treatment normalizes decreased endothelium-dependent relaxations in rats with salt-induced hypertension. Hypertension 1987; 9:III193–III197.
Madeddu P, Parpaglia PP, Demontis MP, Varoni MV, Fattaccio MC, Glorioso N: Chronic inhibition of bradykinin B2-receptors enhances the slow vasopressor response to angiotensin II. Hypertension 1994; 23:646–652.
Majima M, Mizogami S, Kuribayashi Y, Katori M, Oh-ishi S: Hypertension induced by a nonpressor dose of angiotensin II in kininogen-deficient rats. Hypertension 1994; 24:111–119.
Mansfield TA, Simon DB, Farfel Z, Bia M, Tucci JR, Lebel M, Gutkin M, Vialettes B, Christofilis MA, Kauppinen-Makelin R, et al.: Multilocus linkage of familial hyperkalaemia and hypertension, pseudohypoaldosteronism type II, to chromosomes 1q31–42 and 17p11–q21. Nat Genet 1997; 16:202–205.
Manunta P, Burnier M, D'Amico M, Buzzi L, Maillard M, Barlassina C, Lanella G, Cusi D, Bianchi G: Adducin polymorphism affects renal proximal tubule reabsorption in hypertension. Hypertension 1999; 33:694–697.
Margolius HS, Horwitz D, Pisano JJ, Keiser HR: Urinary kallikrein excretion in hypertensive man: relationships to sodium intake and sodium-retaining steroids. Circ Res 1974; 35:820–825.
Masuyama Y, Tsuda K, Shima H, Ura M, Takeda J, Kimura K, Nishio I: Membrane abnormality of erythrocytes is highly dependent on salt intake and renin profile in essential hypertension: an electron spin resonance study. J Hypertens 1988; 6(Suppl 4):S266–S268.
Matthews KA, Woodall KL, Allen MT: Cardiovascular reactivity to stress predicts future blood pressure status. Hypertension 1993; 22:479–485.
Mbanya JC, Thomas TH, Wilkinson R, Alberti KG, Taylor R: Hypertension and hyperinsulinaemia: a relation in diabetes but not essential hypertension. Lancet 1988; 1:733–734.
McIlhany ML, Shaffer JW, Hines EA Jr: The heritability of blood pressure: an investigation of 200 pairs of twins using the cold pressor test. Johns Hopkins Med J 1975; 136:57–64.
McMahon EG, Palomo MA, Brown MA, Bertenshaw SR, Carter JS: Effect of phosphoramidon (endothelin converting enzyme inhibitor) and BQ-123 (endothelin receptor subtype A antagonist) on blood pressure in hypertensive rats. Am J Hypertens 1993; 6:667–673.
Medical Research Council Working Party: MRC trial of treatment of mild hypertension: principal results. BMJ 1985; 291:97–104.
Ménard J, Catt KJ: Effects of estrogen treatment on plasma renin parameters in the rat. Endocrinology 1973; 92:1382–1388.
Ménard J, El Amrani A-IK, Savoie F, Bouhnik J: Angiotensinogen: an attractive and underrated participant in hypertension and inflammation. Hypertension 1991; 18:705–706.
Miall WE, Oldham PD: The hereditary factor in arterial blood pressure. BMJ 1963; 1:75–80.
Miller JZ, Weinberger MH, Christian JC, Daugherty SA: Familial resemblance in the blood pressure response to sodium restriction. Am J Epidemiol 1987; 126:822–830.
Miyamoto Y, Saito Y, Kajiyama N, Yoshimura M, Shimasaki Y, Nakayama M, Kamitani S, Harada M, Ishikawa M, Kuwahara K, et al.: Endothelial nitric oxide synthase gene is positively associated with essential hypertension. Hypertension 1998; 32:3–8.
Mo R, Myking OL, Lund-Johansen P, Omvik P: The Bergen Blood Pressure Study: inappropriately low levels of circulating atrial natriuretic peptide in offspring of hypertensive families. Blood Press 1995; 3:223–230.
Modan M, Halkin H, Almog S, Lusky A, Eshkol A, Shefi M, Shitrit A, Fuchs Z: Hyperinsulinemia: a link between hypertension obesity and glucose intolerance. J Clin Invest 1985; 75:809–817.
Mongeau JG, Biron P, Sing CF: The influence of genetics and household environment upon the variability of normal blood pressure: the Montreal Adoption Survey. Clin Exp Hypertens 1986; 8:653–660.
Moore RD: Effects of insulin upon ion transport. Biochim Biophys Acta 1983; 737:1–49.
Morris BJ, Chambers SM: Hypothesis: glucagon receptor glycine to serine missense mutation contributes to one in 20 cases of essential hypertension. Clin Exp Pharmacol Physiol 1996; 23:1035–1037.
Mortensen LH, Fink GD: Captopril prevents chronic hypertension produced by infusion of endothelin-1 in rats. Hypertension 1992; 19:676–680.
Nabika T, Bonnardeaux A, James M, Julier C, Jeunemaitre X, Corvol P, Lathrop M, Soubrier F: Evaluation of the SA locus in human hypertension. Hypertension 1995; 25:6–13.
Naftilan AJ, Williams RR, Burt D, Paul M, Pratt RE, Hobart P, Chirgwin J, Dzau VJ: A lack of genetic linkage of renin gene restriction fragment length polymorphisms with human hypertension. Hypertension 1989; 14:614–618.
Nakayama T, Soma M, Takahashi Y, Rehemudula D, Tobe H, Sato M, Uwabo J, Kunimoto M, Izumi Y, Kanmatsuse K: Polymorphism of the promoter region of prostacyclin synthase gene is not related to essential hypertension. Am J Hypertens 2001; 14:409–411.
National Institutes of Health: Working group report on management of patients with hypertension and high blood cholesterol. Washington DC: NIH Publication 90-2361. US Department of Health and Human Services, 1990.
Neaton JD, Kuller L, Stamler J, Wentworth DN: Impact of systolic and diastolic blood pressure on cardiovascular mortality. In: Laragh JH, Brenner BM, eds. Hypertension: Pathophysiology, Diagnosis, and Management. New York: Raven, 1995:127–144.
Neaton JD, Kuller LH, Wentworth D, Borhani NO: Total and cardiovascular mortality in relation to cigarette smoking, serum cholesterol concentration, and diastolic blood pressure among black and white males followed up for five years. Am Heart J 1984; 108:759–769.
Neaton JD, Wentworth D: Serum cholesterol, blood pressure, cigarette smoking, and death from coronary heart disease. Arch Intern Med 1992; 152:56–64.
Neel JV: The "thrifty genotype" in 1998. Nutr Rev 1999; 57:S2–S9.
Neel JV, Julius S, Weder A, Yamada M, Kardia SLR, Haviland MB: Syndrome X: is it for real? Genet Epidemiol 1998; 15:19–32.
Niarchos AP, Laragh JH: Effects of diuretic therapy in low-, normal- and high-renin isolated systolic systemic hypertension. Am J Cardiol 1984; 53:797–801.
Nicaud V, Poirier O, Behague I, Herrmann SM, Mallet C, Troesch A, Bouyer J, Evans A, Luc G, Ruidavets JB, et al.: Polymorphisms of the endothelin-A and -B receptor genes in relation to blood pressure and myocardial infarction: the Etude Cas-Temoins sur l'Infarctus du Myocarde (ECTIM) Study. Am J Hypertens 1999; 12:304–310.
Nishikibe M, Tsuchida S, Okada M, Fukuroda T, Shimamoto K, Yano M, Ishikawa K, Ikemoto F: Antihypertensive effect of a newly synthesized endothelin antagonist, BQ-123, in a genetic hypertensive model. Life Sci 1993; 52:717–724.
Nishina PM, Johnson JP, Naggert JK, Krauss RM: Linkage of atherogenic lipopro-

tein phenotype to the low density lipoprotein receptor locus on the short arm of chromosome 19. Proc Natl Acad Sci USA 1992; 89:708–712.
Niskanen LK, Uusitupa MI, Pyorala K: The relationship of hyperinsulinemia to the development of hypertension in type 2 diabetic patients and in non-diabetic subjects. J Hum Hypertens 1991; 5:155–159.
Niu T, Chen C, Yang J, Wang B, Wang Z, Schork N, Fang Z, Xu X: Blood pressure and the T174M and M235T polymorphisms of the angiotensinogen gene. Ann Epidemiol 1999; 9:245–253.
Niu T, Xu X, Rogus J, Zhou Y, Chen C, Yang J, Fang Z, Schmitz C, Zhao J, Rao VS, et al.: Angiotensinogen gene and hypertension in Chinese. J Clin Invest 1998; 101:188–194.
Noll G, Wenzel RR, Schneider M, Oesch V, Binggeli C, Shaw S, Weidmann P, Lüscher TF: Increased activation of sympathetic nervous system and endothelin by mental stress in normotensive offspring of hypertensive parents. Circulation 1996; 93:866–869.
Nolly H, Carretero OA, Lama MC, Miatello R, Scicli AG: Vascular kallikrein in deoxycorticosterone acetate-salt hypertensive rats. Hypertension 1994; 23(Suppl 1):1185–1188.
Nowson CA, McMurchie EJ, Burnard SL, Head RJ, Boehm J, Hoang HN, Hopper JL, Wark JD: Genetic factors associated with altered sodium transport in human hypertension: a twin study. Clin Exp Pharmacol Physiol 1997; 24:424–426.
O'Donnell CJ, Lindpaintner K, Larson MG, Rao VS, Ordovas JM, Schaefer EJ, Myers RH, Levy D: Evidence for association and genetic linkage of the angiotensin-converting enzyme locus with hypertension and blood pressure in men but not women in the Framingham Heart Study. Circulation 1998; 97:1766–1772.
Pajukanta P, Nuotio I, Terwilliger JD, Porkka KV, Ylitalo K, Pihlajamaki J, Suomalainen AJ, Syvanen AC, Lehtimaki T, Viikari JS, et al.: Linkage of familial combined hyperlipidaemia to chromosome 1q21–q23. Nat Genet 1998; 18:369–373.
Pajukanta P, Terwilliger JD, Perola M, Hiekkalinna T, Nuotio I, Ellonen P, Parkkonen M, Hartiala J, Ylitalo K, Pihlajamaki J, et al.: Genomewide scan for familial combined hyperlipidemia genes in Finnish families, suggesting multiple susceptibility loci influencing triglyceride, cholesterol, and apolipoprotein B levels. Am J Hum Genet 1999; 64:1453–1463.
Pankow JS, Rose KM, Oberman A, Hunt SC, Atwood LD, Djousse L, Province MA, Rao DC: Possible locus on chromosome 18q influencing postural systolic blood pressure changes. Hypertension 2000; 36:471–476.
Panza JA, Quyyumi AA, Brush JE, Epstein SE: Abnormal endothelium-dependent vascular relaxation in patients with essential hypertension. N Engl J Med 1990; 323:22–27.
Pei W, Baron H, Muller-Myhsok B, Knoblauch H, Al-Yahyaee SA, Hui R, Wu X, Liu L, Busjahn A, Luft FC, et al.: Support for linkage of familial combined hyperlipidemia to chromosome 1q21–q23 in Chinese and German families. Clin Genet 2000; 57:29–34.
Perola M, Kainulainen K, Pajukanta P, Terwilliger JD, Hiekkalinna T, Ellonen P, Kaprio J, Koskenvuo M, Kontula K, Peltonen L: Genome-wide scan of predisposing loci for increased diastolic blood pressure in Finnish siblings. J Hypertens 2000; 18:1579–1585.
Pershadsingh HA, McDonald JM: Direct addition of insulin inhibits a high affinity Ca^2-ATPase in isolated adipocyte plasma membranes. 1979; 281:495–497.
Persu A, Barbry P, Bassilana F, Houot AM, Mengual R, Lazdunski M, Corvol P, Jeunemaitre X: Genetic analysis of the beta subunit of the epithelial Na^+ channel in essential hypertension. Hypertension 1998; 32:129–137.
Persu A, Coscoy S, Houot AM, Corvol P, Barbry P, Jeunemaitre X: Polymorphisms of the gamma subunit of the epithelial Na^+ channel in essential hypertension. J Hypertens 1999; 17:639–645.
Pérusse L, Moll PP, Sing CF: Evidence that a single gene with gender- and age-dependent effects influences systolic blood pressure determination in a population-based sample. Am J Hum Genet 1991; 49:94–105.
Phillips MI: Is gene therapy for hypertension possible? Hypertension 1999; 33:8–13.
Pickering TG, Devereux RB, James GD, Gerin W, Landsbergis P, Schnall PL, Schwartz JE: Environmental influences on blood pressure and the role of job strain. J Hypertens Suppl 1996; 14:S179–S185.
Pickering TG, Gerin W: Cardiovascular reactivity and the role of behavioral factors in hypertension: a critical review. Ann Behav Med 1990; 12:3–16.
Pojoga L, Gautier S, Blanc H, Guyene TT, Poirier O, Cambien F, Benetos A: Genetic determination of plasma aldosterone levels in essential hypertension. Am J Hypertens 1998; 11:856–860.
Poulter NR, Khaw KT, Hopwood BE, Mugambi M, Peart WS, Rose G, Sever PS: The Kenyan Luo migration study: observations on the initiation of a rise in blood pressure. BMJ 1990; 300:967–972.
Province MA, Arnett DK, Hunt SC, Leiendecker-Foster C, Eckfeldt JH, Oberman A, Ellison RC, Heiss G, Mockrin SC, Williams RR: Association between the alpha-adducin gene and hypertension in the HyperGEN Study. Am J Hypertens 2000a; 13:710–718.
Province MA, Boerwinkle E, Chakravarti A, Cooper R, Fornage M, Leppert M, Risch N, Ranade K: Lack of association of the angiotensinogen-6 polymorphism with blood pressure levels in the comprehensive NHLBI Family Blood Pressure Program. National Heart, Lung and Blood Institute. J Hypertens 2000b; 18:867–876.
Psaty BM, Smith NL, Siscovick DS, Koepsell TD, Weiss NS, Heckbert SR, Lemaitre RN, Wagner EH, Furberg CD: Health outcomes associated with antihypertensive therapies used as first-line agents. A systemic review and meta-analysis. JAMA 1997; 277:739–745.
Ranade K, Hsuing AC, Wu KD, Chang MS, Chen YT, Hebert J, Chen YI, Olshen R, Curb D, Dzau V, et al.: Lack of evidence for an association between alpha-adducin and blood pressure regulation in Asian populations. Am J Hypertens 2000; 13:704–709.
Rankinen T, An P, Rice T, Sun G, Chagnon YC, Gagnon J, Leon AS, Skinner JS, Wilmore JH, Rao DC, et al.: Genomic scan for exercise blood pressure in the Health, Risk Factors, Exercise Training and Genetics (HERITAGE) Family Study. Hypertension 2001; 38:30–37.
Rapp JP, Wang S-M, Dene H: A genetic polymorphism in the renin gene of Dahl rats cosegregates with blood pressure. Science 1989; 243:542–544.
Reaven G: Role of insulin resistance in human disease. Diabetes 1988; 37:1595–1607.
Reaven GM: Insulin resistance, hyperinsulinemia, and hypertriglyceridemia in the etiology and clinical course of hypertension. Am J Med 1991; 90(Suppl 2A):7S–12S.
Reaven GM, Hoffman BB: A role for insulin in the aetiology and course of hypertension? Lancet 1987; 2:435–436.
Rebbeck TR, Turner ST, Sing CF: Sodium–lithium countertransport genotype and the probability of hypertension in adults. Hypertension 1993; 22:560–568.
Resnick LM, Gupta RK, Gruenspan H, Alderman MH, Laragh JH: Hypertension and peripheral insulin resistance: possible mediating role of intracellular free magnesium. Am J Hypertens 1990; 3:373–379.
Resnick LM, Gupta RK, Soza RE, Corbett ML, Laragh JH: Intracellular pH in human and experimental hypertension. Proc Natl Acad Sci USA 1987; 84:7663–7667.
Rice T, Rankinen T, Province MA, Chagnon YC, Perusse L, Borecki IB, Bouchard C, Rao DC: Genome-wide linkage analysis of systolic and diastolic blood pressure: the Quebec Family Study. Circulation 2000; 102:1956–1963.
Robinson WM, Borges-Osório MR, Callegari-Jacques SM, Achutti AC, de Silveira LG, Klein CH, Costa EA: Genetic and nongenetic determinants of blood pressure in a southern Brazilian sample. Genet Epidemiol 1991; 8:55–67.
Rocchini AP, Key J, Bordie D, Chico R, Moorehead C, Katch V, Martin M: The effect of weight loss on the sensitivity of blood pressure to sodium in obese adolescents. N Engl J Med 1989; 321:580–585.
Rockstroh JK, Schmieder RE, Schächinger H, Messerli FH: Stress response pattern in obesity and systemic hypertension. Am J Cardiol 1992; 70:1035–1039.
Rosmond R, Rankinen T, Chagnon M, Perusse L, Chagnon YC, Bouchard C, Bjorntorp P: Polymorphism in exon 6 of the dopamine D(2) receptor gene (*DRD2*) is associated with elevated blood pressure and personality disorders in men. J Hum Hypertens 2001; 15:553–558.
Roth J, Grunfeld C: Mechanism of action of peptide hormones and catecholamines. In: Wilson JD, Foster DW, eds. Williams Textbook of Endocrinology, 7th ed. Philadelphia: Saunders, 1985:76–122.
Rotimi C, Cooper R, Ogunbiyi O, Morrison L, Ladipo M, Tewksbury D, Ward R: Hypertension, serum angiotensinogen, and molecular variants of the angiotensinogen gene among Nigerians. Circulation 1997; 95:2348–2350.
Rotimi C, Morrison L, Cooper R, Oyejide C, Effiong E, Ladipo M, Osotemihen B, Ward R: Angiotensinogen gene in human hypertension. Lack of an association of the 235T allele among African Americans. Hypertension 1994; 24:591–594.
Rotter JI, Bu X, Cantor RM, Warden CH, Brown J, Gray RJ, Blanche PJ, Krauss RM, Lusis AJ: Multilocus genetic determinants of LDL particle size in coronary artery disease families. Am J Hum Genet 1996; 58:585–594.
Rotter JI, Chen Y-DI, Bu X, Gray R, Brown J, Reaven GM, Krauss R, Lusis AJ: Quantitative fasting insulin levels in coronary artery disease families are linked to the apoA1-C3-A4 complex—identification of a major genetic locus for syndrome X? Am J Hum Genet 1992; 51:A26.
Rowe JW, Young JB, Minaker KL, Stevens AL, Pallotta J, Landsberg L: Effect of insulin and glucose infusions on sympathetic nervous system activity in normal man. Diabetes 1981; 30:219–225.
Rudnick KV, Sackett DL, Hirst S, Holmes C: Hypertension in a family practice. Can Med Assoc J 1977; 117:492–497.
Ruiz-Opazo N, Barany F, Hirayama K, Herrera VL: Confirmation of mutant $alpha_1$ Na,K-ATPase gene and transcript in Dahl salt-sensitive/JR rats. Hypertension 1994; 24:260–270.
Ruiz-Opazo N, Cloix JF, Melis MG, Xiang XH, Herrera VL: Characterization of a sodium-response transcriptional mechanism. Hypertension 1997; 30:191–198.
Ruiz-Opazo N, Hirayama K, Akimoto K, Herrera VL: Molecular characterization of a dual endothelin-1/angiotensin II receptor. Mol Med 1998; 4:96–108.
Rutherford S, Boatwright SD, Samwell GA, Morris BJ, Griffiths LR: A linkage and cross-sectional study of hypertension and obesity using a poly(A) Alu-repeat polymorphism at the glucagon receptor gene locus (17q25). Clin Exp Pharmacol Physiol 1998; 25:627–629.
Rutherford S, Johnson MP, Curtain RP, Griffiths LR: Chromosome 17 and the inducible nitric oxide synthase gene in human essential hypertension. Hum Genet 2001;109:408–415.
Sachinidis A, Mengden T, Locher R, Brunner C, Vetter W: Novel cellular activities for low density lipoprotein in vascular smooth muscle cells. Hypertension 1990; 15:704–711.
Salter M, Knowles RG, Moncada S: Widespread tissue distribution, species distribution and changes in activity of Ca^{2+}-dependent and Ca^{2+}-independent nitric oxide synthases. FEBS Lett 1991; 291:145–149.
Samuelsson O, Wilhelmsen L, Andersson OK, Pennert K, Berglund G: Cardiovascular morbidity in relation to change in blood pressure and serum cholesterol levels in treated hypertension. Results from the primary prevention trial in Goteborg, Sweden. JAMA 1987; 258:1768–1776.
Sato M, Soma M, Nakayama T, Kanmatsuse K: Dopamine D1 receptor gene polymorphism is associated with essential hypertension. Hypertension 2000; 36:183–186.
Sato N, Katsuya T, Rakugi H, Takami S, Nakata Y, Miki T, Higaki J, Ogihara T: Association of variants in critical core promoter element of angiotensinogen gene with increased risk of essential hypertension in Japanese. Hypertension 1997; 30:321–325.

Sauerheber RD, Lewis UJ, Esgate JA, Gordon LM: Effect of calcium, insulin and growth hormones on membrane fluidity: a spin label study of rat adipocytes and human erythrocyte ghosts. Biochim Biophys Acta 1980; 597:292–304.

Scheinman SJ, Guay-Woodford LM, Thakker RV, Warnock DG: Genetic disorders of renal electrolyte transport. N Engl J Med 1999; 340:1177–1187.

Schmidt MI, Watson RL, Duncan BB, Metcalf P, Brancati FL, Sharrett AR, Davis CE, Heiss G: Clustering of dyslipidemia, hyperuricemia, diabetes, and hypertension and its association with fasting insulin and central and overall obesity in a general population. Metabolism 1996; 45:699–706.

Schmidt S, Beige J, Walla-Friedel M, Michel MC, Sharma AM, Ritz E: A polymorphism in the gene for the angiotensin II type 1 receptor is not associated with hypertension. J Hypertens 1997; 15:1385–1388.

Schmidt S, van Hooft IMS, Grobbee DE, Ganten D, Ritz E: Polymorphism of the angiotensin I converting enzyme is apparently not related to high blood pressure: Dutch Hypertension and Offspring Study. J Hypertens 1993; 11:345–348.

Schneider MP, Erdmann J, Delles C, Fleck E, Regitz-Zagrosek V, Schmieder RE: Functional gene testing of the Glu^{298}Asp polymorphism of the endothelial NO synthase. J Hypertens 2000; 18:1767–1773.

Schork NJ, Chakravarti A, Thiel B, Fornage M, Jacob HJ, Cai R, Rotimi CN, Cooper RS, Weder AB: Lack of association between a biallelic polymorphism in the adducin gene and blood pressure in whites and African Americans. Am J Hypertens 2000; 13:693–698.

Schunkert H, Hense HW, Doring A, Riegger GA, Siffert W: Association between a polymorphism in the G protein beta3 subunit gene and lower renin and elevated diastolic blood pressure levels. Hypertension 1998; 32:510–513.

Sealey JE, Blumenfeld JD, Bell GM, Pecker MS, Sommers SC, Laragh JH: On the renal basis for essential hypertension: nephron heterogeneity with discordant renin secretion and sodium excretion causing a hypertensive vasoconstriction—volume relationship. In: Laragh JH, Brenner BM, eds. Hypertension: Pathophysiology, Diagnosis and Management. New York: Raven, 1990:1089–1103.

Selby JV, Newman B, Quiroga J, Christian JC, Austin MA, Fabsitz RR: Concordance for dyslipidemic hypertension in male twins. JAMA 1991; 265:2079–2084.

Semplicini A: The Li^+/Na^+ countertransport in hypertension. In: Coca A, Garay RP, eds. Ionic Transport in Hypertension: New Perspectives. Boca Raton, FL: CRC Press, 1994:89–117.

Sethi AA, Nordestgaard BG, Agerholm-Larsen B, Frandsen E, Jensen G, Tybjaerg-Hansen A: Angiotensinogen polymorphisms and elevated blood pressure in the general population: the Copenhagen City Heart Study. Hypertension 2001; 37:875–881.

Sharma P, Fatibene J, Ferraro F, Jia H, Monteith S, Brown C, Clayton D, O'Shaughnessy K, Brown MJ: A genome-wide search for susceptibility loci to human essential hypertension. Hypertension 2000; 35:1291–1296.

Shen GQ, Ikegami H, Fujisawa T, Hamada Y, Kamide K, Rakugi H, Higaki J, Murakami H, Shimamoto K, Ogihara T: Asp^{905}Tyr polymorphism of protein phosphatase 1 G subunit gene in hypertension. Hypertension 1997; 30:236–239.

SHEP Cooperative Research Group: Prevention of stroke by antihypertensive drug treatment in older persons with isolated systolic hypertension. Final results of the systolic hypertension in the elderly program (SHEP). JAMA 1991; 265:3255–3264.

Shimkets RA, Warnock DG, Bositis CM, Nelson-Williams C, Hansson JH, Schambelan M, Gill JR Jr, Ulick S, Milora RV, Findling JW, et al.: Liddle's syndrome: heritable human hypertension caused by mutations in the β subunit of the epithelial sodium channel. Cell 1994; 79:407–414.

Siffert W, Forster P, Jockel KH, Mvere DA, Brinkmann B, Naber C, Crookes R, Du PHA, Epplen JT, Fridey J, et al.: Worldwide ethnic distribution of the G protein beta3 subunit 825T allele and its association with obesity in Caucasian, Chinese, and Black African individuals. J Am Soc Nephrol 1999; 10:1921–1930.

Siffert W, Rosskopf D, Siffert G, Busch S, Moritz A, Erbel R, Sharma AM, Ritz E, Wichmann HE, Jakobs KH, et al.: Association of a human G-protein beta3 subunit variant with hypertension. Nat Genet 1998; 18:45–48.

Skarfors ET, Lithell HO, Selinus I: Risk factors for the development of hypertension: a 10-year longitudinal study in middle-aged men. J Hypertens 1991; 9:217–223.

Skidgel RA, Erdös EG: Angiotensin I-converting enzyme. In: Izzo JL Jr, Black HR, eds. Hypertension Primer. Dallas: American Heart Association, 1999:19–20.

Skoog I: The relationship between blood pressure and dementia: a review. Biomed Pharmacother 1997; 51:367–375.

Skoog I, Lernfelt B, Landahl S, Palmertz B, Andreasson LA, Nilsson L, Persson G, Oden A, Svanborg A: 15-year longitudinal study of blood pressure and dementia. Lancet 1996; 347:1141–1145.

Slattery ML, Bishop DT, French TK, Hunt SC, Meikle AW, Williams RR: Lifestyle and blood pressure levels in male twins in Utah. Genet Epidemiol 1988; 5:277–287.

Smith TW, Turner CW, Ford MH, Hunt SC, Barlow GK, Stults BM, Williams RR: Blood pressure reactivity in adult male twins. Health Psychol 1987; 6:209–220.

Song Q, Chao J, Chao L: DNA polymorphisms in the 5′-flanking region of the human tissue kallikrein gene. Hum Genet 1997; 99:727–734.

Soubrier F, Jeunemaitre X, Rigat B, Houot A-M, Cambien F, Corvol P: Similar frequencies of renin gene restriction fragment length polymorphisms in hypertensive and normotensive subjects. Hypertension 1990; 16:712–717.

Staessen JA, Fagard R, Thijs L, Celis H, Arabidze GG, Birkenhager WH, Bulpitt CJ, de Leeuw PW, Dollery CT, Fletcher AE, et al.: Randomised double-blind comparison of placebo and active treatment for older patients with isolated systolic hypertension. The Systolic Hypertension in Europe (Syst-Eur) Trial Investigators. Lancet 1997a; 350:757–764.

Staessen JA, Kuznetsova T, Wang JG, Emelianov D, Vlietinck R, Fagard R: M235T angiotensinogen gene polymorphism and cardiovascular renal risk. J Hypertens 1999; 17:9–17.

Staessen JA, Wang JG, Brand E, Barlassina C, Birkenhager WH, Herrmann SM, Fagard R, Tizzoni L, Bianchi G: Effects of three candidate genes on prevalence and incidence of hypertension in a Caucasian population. J Hypertens 2001; 19:1349–1358.

Staessen JA, Wang JG, Ginocchio G, Petrov V, Saavedra AP, Soubrier F, Vlietinck R, Fagard R: The deletion/insertion polymorphism of the angiotensin converting enzyme gene and cardiovascular-renal risk. J Hypertens 1997b; 15:1579–1592.

Stamler J: Epidemiology, established major risk factors, and the primary prevention of coronary heart disease. In: Parmley WW, Chatterjee K, eds. Cardiology. Philadephia: Lippincott, 1987:1:1–1:41.

Stevens PA, Brown MJ: Genetic variability of the ET-1 and the ETA receptor genes in essential hypertension. J Cardiovasc Pharmacol 1995; 26(Suppl 3):S9–S12.

Suzuki H, Ikenaga H, Hayashida T, Otsuka K, Kanno Y, Ohno Y, Ikeda H, Saruta T: Sodium balance and hypertension in obese and fatty rats. Kidney Int 1996; 55:S150–S153.

Svetkey LP, Chen YT, McKeown SP, Preis L, Wilson AF: Preliminary evidence of linkage of salt sensitivity in black Americans at the beta2-adrenergic receptor locus. Hypertension 1997; 29:918–922.

Svetkey LP, Moore TJ, Simons-Morton DG, Appel LJ, Bray GA, Sacks FM, Ard JD, Mortensen RM, Mitchell SR, Conlin PR, et al.: Angiotensinogen genotype and blood pressure response in the Dietary Approaches to Stop Hypertension (DASH) study. J Hypertens 2001; 19:1949–1956.

Swales JD (ed): Genetic Factors in Human Hypertension. Oxford: Blackwell, 1994.

Takahashi Y, Nakayama T, Soma M, Uwabo J, Izumi Y, Kanmatsuse K: Association analysis of TG repeat polymorphism of the neuronal nitric oxide synthase gene with essential hypertension. Clin Genet 1997; 52:83–85.

Takami S, Katsuya T, Rakugi H, Sato N, Nakata Y, Kamitani A, Miki T, Higaki J, Ogihara T: Angiotensin II type 1 receptor gene polymorphism is associated with increase of left ventricular mass but not with hypertension. Am J Hypertens 1998; 11:316–321.

Takami S, Wong ZY, Stebbing M, Harrap SB: Linkage analysis of endothelial nitric oxide synthase gene with human blood pressure. J Hypertens 1999; 17:1431–1436.

Tambs K, Moum T, Holmen J, Eaves LJ, Neale MC, Lund-Larsen G, Naess S: Genetic and environmental effects on blood pressure in a Norwegian sample. Genet Epidemiol 1992; 9:11–26.

Tamura K, Umemura S, Iwamoto T, Yamaguchi S, Kobayashi S, Takeda K, Tokita Y, Takagi N, Murakami K, Fukamizu A, et al.: Molecular mechanism of adipogenic activation of the angiotensinogen gene. Hypertension 1994; 23:364–368.

Tamura M, Inagami T, Kinoshita T, Kuwano H: A search for endogenous Na^+,K^+-ATPase inhibitor in acutely volume-expanded hog plasma led to lysophosphatidylcholine γ-stearoyl. J Hypertens 1987; 5:219–225.

Tamura M, Kuwano H, Kinoshita T, Inagami T: Identification of linoleic and oleic acids as endogenous Na+,K+,-ATPase inhibitors from acute volume-expanded hog plasma. J Biol Chem 1985; 260:9672–9677.

Taubes G: The (political) science of salt. Science 1998; 281:898–907.

Teng B, Sniderman AD, Soutar AK, Thompson GR: Metabolic basis of hyperapobetalipoproteinemia. Turnover of apolipoprotein B in low density lipoprotein and its precursors and subfractions compared with normal and familial hypercholesterolemia. J Clin Invest 1986; 77:663–672.

JNC V: The Fifth Report of the Joint National Committee on Detection, Evaluation, and Treatment of High Blood Pressure (JNC V). Arch Intern Med 1993; 153:154–183.

JNC VI: The Sixth Report of the Joint National Committee on Prevention, Detection, Evaluation, and Treatment of High Blood Pressure. Arch Intern Med 1997; 157:2413–2446.

Tippmer S, Quitterer U, Kolm V, Faussner A, Roscher A, Mosthaf L, Muller-Esterl W, Haring H: Bradykinin induces translocation of the protein kinase C isoforms alpha, epsilon, and zeta. Eur J Biochem 1994; 225:297–304.

Tiret L, Poirier O, Hallet V, McDonagh TA, Morrison C, McMurray JJ, Dargie HJ, Arveiler D, Ruidavets JB, Luc G, et al.: The Lys^{198}Asn polymorphism in the endothelin-1 gene is associated with blood pressure in overweight people. Hypertension 1999; 33:1169–1174.

Tobian L: The Volhard lecture. Potassium and sodium in hypertension. J Hypertens 1988; 4(Suppl 6):S12–S24.

Tonolo G, Melis MG, Secchi G, Atzeni MM, Angius MF, Carboni A, Ciccarese M, Malavasi A, Maioli M: Association of Trp^{64}Arg beta3-adrenergic-receptor gene polymorphism with essential hypertension in the Sardinian population. J Hypertens 1999; 17:33–38.

Trials of Hypertension Prevention Collaborative Research Group: Effects of weight loss and sodium reduction intervention on blood pressure and hypertension incidence in overweight people with high-normal blood pressure. Arch Intern Med 1997; 157:657–667.

Tripodi G, Valtorta F, Torielli L, Chieregatti E, Salardi S, Trusolino L, Menegon A, Ferrari P, Marchisio PC, Bianchi G: Hypertension-associated point mutations in the adducin alpha and beta subunits affect actin cytoskeleton and ion transport. J Clin Invest 1996; 97:2815–2822.

Tsuda K, Masuyama Y: Age-related changes in membrane fluidity of erythrocytes in essential hypertension. Am J Hypertens 1990; 3:714–716.

Turner ST, Schwartz GL, Chapman AB, Boerwinkle E: C825T polymorphism of the G protein beta(3)-subunit and antihypertensive response to a thiazide diuretic. Hypertension 2001; 37:739–743.

Ukkola O, Erkkila PH, Savolainen MJ, Kesaniemi YA: Lack of association between polymorphisms of catalase, copper-zinc superoxide dismutase (SOD), extracellular SOD and endothelial nitric oxide synthase genes and macroangiopathy in patients with type 2 diabetes mellitus. J Intern Med 2001; 249:451–459.

Uwabo J, Soma M, Nakayama T, Kanmatsuse K: Association of a variable number of tandem repeats in the endothelial constitutive nitric oxide synthase gene with essential hypertension in Japanese. Am J Hypertens 1998; 11:125–128.

van den Bree MB, Schieken RM, Moskowitz WB, Eaves LJ: Genetic regulation of hemodynamic variables during dynamic exercise. The MCV Twin Study. Circulation 1996; 94:1864–1869.

Vasku A, Soucek M, Znojil V, Rihacek I, Tschoplova S, Strelcova L, Cidl K, Blazkova M, Hajek D, Holla L, et al.: Angiotensin I-converting enzyme and angiotensinogen gene interaction and prediction of essential hypertension. Kidney Int 1998; 53:1479–1482.

Veterans Administration Co-operative Study Group on Anti-Hypertensive Agents: Effects of treatment on morbidity in hypertension. I. Results in patients with diastolic blood pressures averaging 115 through 129 mm Hg. JAMA 1967; 202: 1028–1034.

Vuagnat A, Giacche M, Hopkins PN, Azizi M, Hunt SC, Vedie B, Corvol P, Williams GH, Jeunemaitre X: Blood pressure response to angiotensin II, low-density lipoprotein cholesterol and polymorphisms of the angiotensin II type 1 receptor gene in hypertensive sibling pairs. J Mol Med 2001; 79:175–183.

Walker WG, Whelton PK, Saito H, Russell RP, Hermann J: Relation between blood pressure and renin, renin substrate, angiotensin II, aldosterone and urinary sodium and potassium in 574 ambulatory subjects. Hypertension 1979; 1:287–291.

Wang WY, Adams DJ, Glenn CL, Morris BJ: The Gly^{460}Trp variant of alpha-adducin is not associated with hypertension in white Anglo-Australians. Am J Hypertens 1999; 12:632–636.

Wang WY, Zee RY, Morris BJ: Association of angiotensin II type 1 receptor gene polymorphism with essential hypertension. Clin Genet 1997a; 51:31–34.

Wang XL, Mahaney MC, Sim AS, Wang J, Blangero J, Almasy L, Badenhop RB, Wilcken DE: Genetic contribution of the endothelial constitutive nitric oxide synthase gene to plasma nitric oxide levels. Arterioscler Thromb Vasc Biol 1997b; 17:3147–3153.

Ward RH, Chin PG, Prior IAM: Genetic epidemiology of blood pressure in a migrating isolate: prospectus. In: Sing CF, Skolnick MH, eds. Genetic Analysis of Common Diseases. New York: Alan R Liss, 1979:675–709.

Watt GCM, Foy CJW, Hart JT, Bingham G, Edwards C, Hart M, Thomas E, Walton P: Dietary sodium and arterial blood pressure: evidence against genetic susceptibility. BMJ 1985; 291:1525–1528.

Watt GCM, Harrap SB, Foy CJW, Holton DW, Edwards HV, Davidson HR, Connor JM, Lever A, Fraser R: Abnormalities of glucocorticoid metabolism and the renin—angiotensin system: a four-corners approach to the identification of genetic determinants of blood pressure. J Hypertens 1992; 10:473–482.

Whelton PK, He J, Cutler JA, Brancati FL, Appel LJ, Follmann D, Klag MJ: Effects of oral potassium on blood pressure. Meta-analysis of randomized controlled clinical trials: JAMA 1997; 277:1624–1632.

Whelton PK, Klag MJ: Magnesium and blood pressure: review of the epidemiologic and clinical trial experience. Am J Cardiol 1989; 63:26G–30G.

Williams GH, Dluhy RG, Lifton RP, Moore TJ, Gleason R, Williams R, Hunt SC, Hopkins PN, Hollenberg NK: Non-modulation as an intermediate phenotype in essential hypertension. Hypertension 1992; 20:788–796.

Williams PD, Puddey IB, Beilin LJ, Vandongen R: Genetic influences on plasma catecholamines in human twins. J Clin Endocrinol Metab 1993; 77:794–799.

Williams RR, Dadone MM, Hunt SC, Jorde LB, Hopkins PN, Smith JB, Ash KO, Kuida H: The genetic epidemiology of hypertension: a review of past studies and current results for 948 persons in 48 Utah pedigrees. In: Rao DC, Elston RC, Kuller LH, Feinleib M, Carter C, Havlik R, eds. Genetic Epidemiology of Coronary Heart Disease: Past, Pressent, and Future. New York: Alan R Liss, 1984: 419–442.

Williams RR, Hunt SC, Hopkins PN, Stults BM, Wu LL, Hasstedt SJ, Barlow GK, Stephenson SH, Lalouel JM, Kuida H: Familial dyslipidemic hypertension: evidence from 58 Utah families for a syndrome present in approximately 12% of patients with essential hypertension. JAMA 1988; 259:3579–3586.

Williams RR, Hasstedt SJ, Hunt SC, Wu LL, Hopkins PN, Berry TD, Stults BM, Barlow GK, Kuida H: Genetic traits related to hypertension and electrolyte metabolism. Hypertension 1991; 17(Suppl I):I-69–I-73.

Williams RR, Hunt SC, Kuida H, Smith JB, Ash KO: Sodium–lithium countertransport in erythrocytes of hypertension prone families in Utah. Am J Epidemiol 1983; 118:338.

Wilson DE, Emi M, Iverius PH, Hata A, Wu LL, Hillas E, Williams RR, Lalouel JM: Phenotypic expression of heterozygous LPL deficiency in the extended pedigree of a proband homozygous for a missense mutation. J Clin Invest 1990; 86:735–750.

Wilson DJ, Gahan M, Haddad L, Heath K, Whittall RA, Williams RR, Humphries SE, Day IN: A world wide web site for low-density lipoprotein receptor gene mutations in familial hypercholesterolemia: sequence-based, tabular, and direct submission data handling. Am J Cardiol 1998; 81:1509–1511.

Wilson FH, Disse-Nicodeme S, Choate KA, Ishikawa K, Nelson-Williams C, Desitter I, Gunel M, Milford DV, Lipkin GW, Achard JM, et al.: Human hypertension caused by mutations in WNK kinases. Science 2001; 293:1107–1112.

Wojciechowski AP, Farrall M, Cullen P, Wilson TME, Bayliss JD, Farren B, Griffin BA, Caslake MJ, Packard CJ, Shepherd J, et al.: Familial combined hyperlipidemia linked to the apolipoprotein AI-CIII-AIV gene cluster on chromosome 11q23–q24. Nature 1991; 349:161–164.

Wong ZY, Stebbing M, Ellis JA, Lamantia A, Harrap SB: Genetic linkage of beta and gamma subunits of epithelial sodium channel to systolic blood pressure. Lancet 1999; 353:1222–1225.

Wood DL, Sheps SG, Elveback LR, Schirger A: Cold pressor test as a predictor of hypertension. Hypertension 1984; 6:301–306.

Wu D-A, Bu X, Warden CH, Shen DDC, Jeng C-Y, Sheu WHH, Fuh MMT, Katsuya T, Dzau VJ, Reaven GM, et al.: Quantitative trait locus mapping of human blood pressure to a genetic region at or near the lipoprotein lipase gene on chromosome 8p22. J Clin Invest 1996; 97:2111–2118.

Xu X, Rogus JJ, Terwedow HA, Yang J, Wang Z, Chen C, Niu T, Wang B, Xu H, Weiss S, et al.: An extreme-sib-pair genome scan for genes regulating blood pressure. Am J Hum Genet 1999; 64:1694–1701.

Yamakawa H, Suzuki H, Nakamura M, Ohno Y, Saruta T: Disturbed calcium metabolism in offspring of hypertensive parents. Hypertension 1992; 19:528–534.

Yusuf S, Lessem J, Jha P, Lonn E: Primary and secondary prevention of myocardial infarction and strokes: an update of randomly allocated, controlled trials. J Hypertens 1993; 11(Suppl 4):S61–S73.

Zee RYL, Morris BJ, Griffiths LR: Association analyses of RFLPs for the α_2- and β_1-adrenoceptor genes in essential hypertension. Hypertens Res 1992; 15:57–60.

Zee RYL, Ying L-H, Morris BJ, Griffiths LR: Association and linkage analyses of restriction fragment length polymorphisms for the human renin and antithrombin III genes in essential hypertension. J Hypertens 1991; 9:825–830.

Zhang QY, Dene H, Deng AY, Garrett MR, Jacob HJ, Rapp JP: Interval mapping and congenic strains for a blood pressure QTL on rat chromosome 13. Mamm Genome 1997; 8:636–641.

Zhao YY, Zhou J, Narayanan CS, Cui Y, Kumar A: Role of C/A polymorphism at −20 on the expression of human angiotensinogen gene. Hypertension 1999; 33:108–115.

Zhu DL, Wang HY, Xiong MM, He X, Chu SL, Jin L, Wang GL, Yuan WT, Zhao GS, Boerwinkle E, et al.: Linkage of hypertension to chromosome 2q14–q23 in Chinese families. J Hypertens 2001a; 19:55–61.

Zhu X, Bouzekri N, Southam L, Cooper RS, Adeyemo A, McKenzie CA, Luke A, Chen G, Elston RC, Ward R: Linkage and association analysis of angiotensin I-converting enzyme (*ACE*)-gene polymorphisms with ACE concentration and blood pressure. Am J Hum Genet 2001b; 68:1139–1148.

Zinner SH, Margolius HS, Rosner B, Keiser HR, Kass EH: Familial aggregation of urinary kallikrein concentration in childhood: relation to blood pressure, race and urinary electrolytes. Am J Epidemiol 1976; 104:124–132.

Zinner SH, Margolius HS, Rosner B, Kass EH: Stability of blood pressure rank and urinary kallikrein concentration in childhood: an eight year follow-up. Circulation 1978; 58:908–915.

9 Chronic Obstructive Pulmonary Disease

FRANCINE KAUFFMANN AND FLORENCE DEMENAIS

By 2020, more than 3 million deaths from chronic obstructive pulmonary disease (COPD) could occur worldwide. This would represent an advance since 1990 from the sixth to the third cause of death, mostly because of the aging of the population and the effects of smoking (Murray and Lopez, 1997). In 1963, the protease inhibitor (*PI*) gene was discovered (Laurell and Eriksson, 1963); its deficient allele is a cause of early-onset emphysema, one rare subcategory of COPD. Other potential genetic markers, however, have been scarcely studied. The modern era of genetics is just starting for COPD, a complex set of diseases with a major environmental component. In recent years, several segregation analyses have been performed (Chen et al., 1996, 1999; Gilverber et al., 1998; Holberg et al., 1998; Rybicki et al., 1990; Chen et al., 1999; Wilk et al., 2000; Kurzius-Spencer et al., 2001). Published studies of genetic markers are exclusively association studies, although at least one genome-screening study to localize COPD genes is in progress (Silverman et al., 1998). In general, these studies have involved relatively small samples of subjects, with different inclusion criteria. Results of genetic studies obtained for asthma, the other obstructive disease presenting typically with reversible airflow limitation (see chapter 11) would likely be of interest for COPD, which is characterized by irreversible airflow limitation, as both asthma and COPD are related to pulmonary inflammation. Addressing the genetic–phenotypic heterogeneity, consideration of gene–environment interaction, and development of biological epidemiology would be useful approaches to develop the field, with the goals of understanding the pathophysiology, undertaking primary and secondary prevention of environmental risk factors, and finding new targets for drug treatment. Emphasis in this chapter is on the most recent data; complementary information may be found in reviews devoted to PI (Mittman, 1979; Fagerhol and Cox, 1981; Eriksson, 1996; WHO Memorandum, 1997) and on previous reviews on the genetics of COPD (Cohen and Chase, 1978; Kauffmann, 1984; Redline and Weiss, 1989; Kueppers, 1992; Luisetti and Pignatti, 1995; Sandford et al., 1997b; Barnes, 1999; Sandford and Paré, 2000).

DISEASE DEFINITION

Diagnostic Criteria

Chronic obstructive pulmonary disease is the most common term used clinically to include the functional aspect of chronic airflow limitation with the diagnoses of emphysema and chronic bronchitis (American Thoracic Society, 1995). The 1995 consensus statement of the European Respiratory Society includes chronic airflow limitation without chronic bronchitis or emphysema as COPD as well (Siafakas et al., 1995; Pride et al., 1998). Although asthma is generally excluded from that definition, its clinical presentation may be difficult to distinguish in numerous cases. Extensive literature has addressed the issue of definition for the various obstructive diseases (Samet, 1989; Snider 1995a, 1995b; Vermeire and Pride, 1991; Pride et al., 1998).

Figure 9–1 presents a nonproportional Venn diagram for patients with chronic bronchitis, emphysema, and asthma within the shaded area corresponding to COPD (American Thoracic Society, 1995; Snider, 1995b). *Chronic bronchitis* is defined by the presence of chronic or recurrent increases in bronchial secretions that are sufficient to cause expectoration. The secretions are present on most days for a minimum of 3 months a year for at least two successive years. *Emphysema* is defined anatomically by permanent, destructive enlargement of airspaces distal to the terminal bronchioles without obvious fibrosis. *Airflow limitation* is recognized by a reduction in the ratio of forced expiratory volume in 1 second (FEV_1) to vital capacity (VC). In moderate to severe disease, the severity of airflow is best assessed by FEV_1% predicted (Siafakas et al., 1995; Pauwels et al., 2001). *Chronic airflow limitation* is often defined by decrease in FEV_1% predicted and FEV_1/VC% predicted less than 1.64 residual SD (i.e., $FEV_1 < 70\%$ predicted and $FEV_1/VC < 11\%$ less than predicted (Rijcken and Britton, 1998)).

COPD has long been a diagnosis of exclusion—excluding specific causes of obstruction, as reflected by the term used in the Netherlands: CNSLD, or chronic nonspecific lung disease; this term includes asthma as well, but not α_1-antitrypsin deficiency (α_1ATD), which is considered to be a subcategory. At variance with the original diagram proposed by Snider are the representation of cystic fibrosis and fibrosis, as nonexcluding diagnoses if other features of COPD are fulfilled. Cystic fibrosis is not excluded because of the discovery in adulthood of minor forms of cystic fibrosis, and fibrosis is not excluded because airspace enlargment with fibrosis is less clearcut from emphysema than was thought earlier (Snider, 1995a). Emphysema is now considered to be a complex mix of fibrosis consequent on inflammation, as well as elastin degradation due to protease, antiprotease imbalance (Snider, 1992, 1995a; Cardoso and Thurlbeck, 1994). The importance of extracellular matrix remodeling in all obstructive diseases—including COPD (Paré and Bai, 1998) and asthma (Vignola et al., 1998)—is now recognized.

Brief Clinical Presentation

Most patients are males (although the sex ratio is decreasing), long-term smokers, and older than 50 years. COPD peak of onset is later than that of cardiovascular diseases. The usual symptoms are productive cough and dyspnea, first at exercise and then at rest. The intensity of shortness of breath impairs quality of

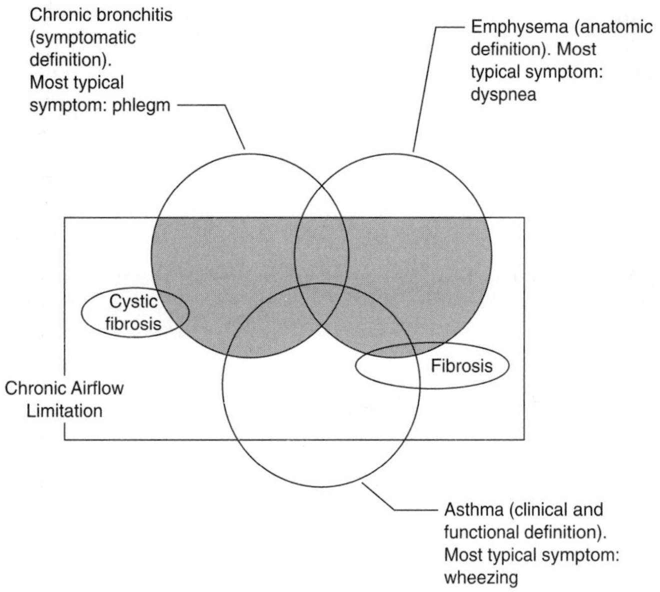

Fig. 9.1. Schema of chronic obstructive pulmonary disease. Shaded area represents COPD. Modified from Snider (1995b) with permission.

life and can end in total disability. Intermittent chest illnesses with increased cough, purulent sputum, wheezing, and dyspnea occur. Up to 30% of COPD patients may have a reversible component of airflow limitation. The history of wheezing and dyspnea may lead to an erroneous diagnosis of asthma. In advanced stages in some patients, low levels of oxygen in the arterial blood occur, resulting in increase in carbon dioxide in blood and tissues. Pulmonary hypertension may occur, and, at late stages, patients may have both respiratory and cardiac failure. Detailed clinical presentation may be found elsewhere (American Thoracic Society, 1995; Siafakas et al., 1995; Pauwels et al., 2001).

Defined Subtypes

COPD is phenotypically heterogeneous. The classic distinctions are between chronic bronchitis (COPD with productive cough, a disease of the airways) and emphysema (COPD with potential dyspnea as the sole symptom, a disease of the parenchyma). A functional diagnosis of emphysema is not possible, but it may be suggested by disorders of diffusing capacity. Criteria to define emphysema are based on anatomy—that is, postmortem or based on biopsies—but biopsies are not relevant for diagnostic purposes. Unless very late stages, X-rays are not precise enough for diagnosis, but in the last 10 years computed tomography scan has appeared to be a useful tool (Dirksen et al., 1997).

Two forms of emphysema are usually considered: the panacinar form, which involves the entire alveolus uniformly, predominating in the lower half of the lungs (usual type for PIZ (protease inhibitor Z) emphysema); the centriacinar type, which begins in the respiratory bronchioles and spreads peripherally (usual type in smoker emphysema, predominantly in the upper half of the lungs).

The classical description of advanced COPD (Burrows et al., 1964) of pink puffers (type A) and blue bloaters (type B) is still used (Calverley and Georgopousos, 1998). It is clear now (Thurlbeck, 1976) that type A does not represent the emphysematous type compared to the bronchitic type B. These two types are better described as the thin normocapnic (8%–10% of advanced COPD) and the fat hypercapnic (60%–80%). Blue bloaters benefit from long-term oxygen therapy. Mixed types occur. Staging based on either pulmonary function ($FEV_1 \geq 50\%$, 35%–49%, <35% predicted) (American Thoracic Society, 1995) or a combination of symptoms—in particular, degree of breathlessness, pulmonary function tests, and hypoxemia—have been proposed (Calverley and Georgopousos, 1998).

Distinguishing COPD from asthma is not always possible, as a reversible component is often observed in COPD and severe asthma has an irreversible airflow limitation. The issue of classification of COPD from the etiologic point of view is addressed later in this review.

GENERAL GENETIC AND EPIDEMIOLOGIC EVIDENCE

Clinical Epidemiology and Ethnic Differences

COPD is already one of the major causes of death in adults in most developed countries, as well as in developing countries (Murray and Lopez, 1997). The reliability and validity of COPD mortality data vary between countries and with time, according to clinical practice in diagnostic labeling and revisions of the international classification of diseases. Variations between countries have been reported (American Thoracic Society, 1995; Siafakas et al., 1995; Rijcken and Britton, 1998). In 1991, a death rate of 18.6 per 100,000 in relation to COPD and allied conditions occurred in the United States, which corresponded to more than 85,000 deaths (American Thoracic Society, 1995). Mortality rates of COPD and its allied conditions showed a quadrupling over 35 years from 1950 to 1985 in the United States, in men and women aged 55 to 84 (Feinleib et al., 1989). In England and Wales, where the epidemiology of smoking reached its mature phase earlier, mortality figures were relatively static between 1971 and 1990, with death rates in men and women older than 65 years in 1990 to 1992 around twice those reported in the United States (around 480 and 230 per 100,000, respectively (Rijcken and Britton, 1998). In France in 1992, respiratory disease represented the fourth cause of death after tumors, circulatory diseases, and external causes or 7% of deaths in both men and women. Obstructive respiratory diseases (chronic bronchitis, asthma, and emphysema) represented 34% of respiratory deaths in women and 44% in men. Projections mostly based on demographic data and trends in smoking habit (Murray and Lopez, 1997) show that COPD will be the third cause of death worldwide in 2020.

Mortality by COPD is relatively low compared to morbidity statistics. One of the reasons is the fact that numerous deaths are reported to be due to other causes (cardiac disease, acute pneumopathy, pulmonary embolism, acute respiratory insufficiency), since these diseases often occur in COPD patients. Secondary causes of death increase mortality approximately by 1.5-fold. Furthermore, the limits of death certificates as indicators of morbidity are shown by data from epidemiological surveys. For example, according to survey data in the Tecumseh study, COPD was mentioned as either the main or a secondary cause of death in death certificates of fewer than a fifth of those with COPD (Higgins and Keller, 1989). There are no reliable morbidity statistics for COPD over the world. Around 14 million persons in the United States suffer from COPD (American Thoracic Society, 1995). British data for 1982 to 1983 rank respiratory diseases as the third most common cause of days of certified incapacity (Siafakas et al., 1995). In 1991 in France, obstructive disease was ranked fifth of the costly long-term illnesses recognized by the social security after cardiovascular disease, tumors, psychiatric disorders, and diabetes (Kauffmann et al., 1996). In the United States in 1979, COPD cost $6.5 billion, with one-third for direct treatment costs, one-third for indirect morbidity costs, and one-third for indirect mortality costs. Projections for 2020 of disability-adjusted life years put COPD at 58 million (ranking after ischemic heart disease, unipolar major depression, traffic accidents, and cerebrovascular disease) with 5 million in developed regions and 53 million in developing regions (Murray and Lopez, 1997).

Therefore in terms of public health, COPD causes death, disability, reduction in quality of life, and cost in both genders and all regions of the world, and there has been a clear rising trend for all these in only a few decades. This rise suggests that, besides the already known major influence of smoking habits, we need to consider the effects of environmental factors (such as the interaction of childhood and adult environmental conditions of individuals) and of gene–environment interactions.

Gender and Ethnic Resemblance

The study of subjects who shared genes from the most remote to the closest degree of relationship are consistent with the hypothesis of the role of genetic factors in COPD. Gender, ethnic, family and twin resemblances have all been observed. Such resemblances may be due to genetic factors shared among these groups and shared environment through direct common environment (in utero, in family) or culturally transmitted (in ethnic groups, in genders, in families).

Genetic and environmental factors could explain the gender resemblance in COPD. The nature of environmental factors, their determinants, and their effects may be different (Becklake and Kauffmann, 1999; Kauffmann and Becklake, 2000). Exposure to factors common to both genders (such as active smoking and some occupational factors) is different. Although they are potentially common to both genders, some environmental factors may greatly differ between them (such as passive smoking, some occupational factors, domestic factors). Anatomic and hormonal factors, which have not yet undergone rigorous study for their relationship to COPD, are clearly under genetic control. The ratio of expiratory flow to pulmonary volume is higher in women than in men, for instance. The higher that ratio, the better is the pulmonary ventilation. A low ratio could be a consequence of dysanapsis (Mead, 1980), or the disproportionate growth of the primary structures of the lungs, the bronchi, and the alveoli. During all their life, women benefit from this anatomic advantage. The role of female hormones could be important or, on the contrary, it could negatively balance the families' anatomic advantage. Some data are already available for asthma, but information regarding COPD is lacking (Kauffmann et al., 1996). There is an increasing body of evidence that susceptibility to smoking may be greater in females than in males (Gold et al., 1996), suggesting the interaction of some gender-related factor (whether environmental or genetic) with the environmental factor of smoking.

The limitations of using geographical comparisons of ethnic distribution of morbidity and mortality due to differences in methods are illustrated above. Studies of migrants have been discussed elsewhere (Kauffmann, 1984). They are usually interpreted in terms of changing environment, but they could also suggest gene–environment interactions. Migrants often differ from those staying in their country of origin by environmental and sociocultural characteristics. Numerous studies have described classical functional parameters in different regions of the world, and the identification of important differences has led most authors to recommend the use of specific reference values according to sex, ethnic group, and region. The interpretation of the differences observed include anatomical and environmental factors. For example, the inadequate adjustment of total body size to compare ethnic groups has been shown (Ferris and Stoudt, 1971). The Cormic index (relation of sitting height, reflecting the size of the lung, to total height) is different among ethnic groups; because it is smaller in blacks than in Caucasians, the issue of proportional differences arose (Rossiter and Weill, 1974). These differences may be partially environmental (Mustafa, 1977), since malnutrition and repeated respiratory infections in childhood might influence both pulmonary and skeletal development. Altitude, social factors, mode of living, nutrition, and history of infections probably explain most geographical and ethnic differences. Studies taking these factors properly into consideration by samples at the same social level are difficult, if not impossible, and are of limited help in understanding the genetic determinants of COPD.

Family Epidemiology

Family Studies

Since the historical report by Pierre Louis (Figure 9–2; Louis, 1837), authors have reported isolated pedigrees of COPD, some of them corresponding to PIZ families. More than a century passed after Louis's report until a study included both cases and controls (Oswald et al., 1953). Table 9–1 presents the main studies ordered according to a decreasing selection bias toward familial resemblance. Type I describes studies in which diseased subjects and controls were interviewed for COPD in their first-degree relatives. Comparisons could be biased, as patients may be more prone to report familial antecedents than are nondiseased individuals. Type II describes studies based on health interviews of unselected individuals on their first-degree relatives. Type III describes studies with examinations of relatives of cases and controls. In type IV studies, examinations of different members of families from the general population were made. Among the studies conducted in the 1970s, important results came from two American studies: the Johns Hopkins University study (Cohen et al., 1975), based on families of COPD lung cancer patients and controls; and the Tecumseh Study conducted in the general population (Higgins et al., 1975). Both studies clearly showed familial resemblance in COPD.

Studies on familial resemblance have been described in detail elsewhere (Kauffmann, 1984; Redline and Weiss, 1989; Kueppers, 1992) and are summarized in Table 9–1. They showed an increased prevalence of COPD in relatives of cases over relatives of controls, higher correlations in lung function between parents and children and among siblings, and decreased similarity with decreased genetic relationship. Moreover, familial correlations of lung function measurements show little overlap with genetic determinants of asthma and atopic rhinitis (Palmer et al., 2001). More recently, segregation analyses have been performed to characterize the mode of transmission of pulmonary function indices (see below). As the relationships from a phenotypic and etiologic point of view between COPD and asthma are a matter of debate (see below), it is of interest to consider the recent studies that have assessed COPD in asthmatic families (Panhuysen et al., 1998) and asthma in COPD families (Silverman et al., 1998). In both cases, the prevalence of the other disease was low.

RECHERCHES

SUR

L'EMPHYSÈME DES POUMONS,

PAR M. LOUIS,

Médecin de la Pitié, membre de l'Académie royale de Médecine, etc., etc.

La question de l'hérédité a été étudiée par Jackson. Pour arriver à des résultats concluans à cet égard, il a pris des informations précises auprès d'un assez grand nombre de malades sur l'état de santé habituelle de leurs père et mère, frères ou sœurs, sur l'espèce de maladie qui les avait conduits au tombeau, et sur l'âge auquel ils avaient succombé. Ses questions ont principalement porté sur l'état de la respiration, sur la durée de l'oppression quand elle a eu lieu, sur l'état des membres, leur volume, etc. Il n'a considéré comme bien constatés que les faits attestés par des malades intelligens, doués d'une bonne mémoire, ayant toujours fait les mêmes réponses aux mêmes questions. En procédant avec cette réserve qui est commandée par la nature du sujet, il est arrivé aux résultats suivans :

1° Sur vingt-huit sujets atteints d'emphysème pulmonaire, dix-huit avaient leurs parens, père ou mère, atteints de la même affection, et plusieurs de ceux-ci avaient succombé dans son cours. Dans quelques cas, il en fut encore de même des frères et sœurs.

2° Sur cinquante individus non atteints d'emphysème, trois seulement avaient eu des parens affectés de cette maladie; d'où il suit, tout étant d'ailleurs égal de part et d'autre, que l'emphysème est fréquemment une affection héréditaire.

Fig. 9.2. Historical note: Pierre Charles Alexandre Louis. Translation modified from Louis (1838). The question as to its hereditary character was studied by J. Jackson. To obtain conclusive results in this respect, he [Jackson] took precise information in a large number of patients on the usual health of their father and mother, brothers or sisters, on the type of disease that brought them to the tomb and their age at which they succumbed. His questions mainly focused on the respiratory status, duration of breathlessness when it occurred. As well, he only considered observed facts attested by intelligent patients, with good memory and who always gave the same answers to the same questions. Proceeding with that reserve ordered by the nature of the topic, he arrived at the following results: *(1)* Of twenty-eight patients, affected with pulmonary emphysema, eighteen had their parents, father or mother with the same affection, and several of whom had died in the course of it. In some cases, the same was true of the brothers and sisters. *(2)* Of fifty individuals not affected with emphysema, three only were descended of parents, with the disease; whence, everything being equal from both, emphysema is frequently a hereditary affection.

This may be due to the extreme phenotype chosen for the probands by whom the families were ascertained, however. Considering very precise phenotypes is necessary for finding genetic factors in heterogeneous groups of diseases such as chronic obstructive pulmonary diseases and asthmas.

Twin Studies

Twin studies have confirmed the importance of genetic factors in COPD (Table 9–1). In one of the first studies in which the concordance of cough in monozygotic twins was compared to that in dizygotic twins (Cederlöf et al., 1967) it was concluded that the "constitutional factor" was more important than the smoking factor. Such conclusions are only valid under the classical twin model where any dissimilarity between monozygotic twins is attributed to environmental differences. However, the environment of monozygotic twins is closer than that of dizygotic ones (before and after birth), but is not identical. As more importance is now attributed to in utero and perinatal factors in the pathophysiology of obstructive diseases, these limitations may have more importance than previously thought (Weiss, 1995; Hoo et al., 1998; Rijcken and Britton, 1998). A strong concordance for ventilatory parameters has been shown in monozygotic twins (Feinleib et al., 1977; Hubert et al., 1978; Kauffmann, 1984; Redline et al., 1987; Kueppers, 1992; McClearn et al., 1994). In a large study of family members of adult twins, a direct relationship between shared genotype and the magnitude of the familial correlations for pulmonary function was evidenced; this conclusion was not altered by taking smoking habits into account (Redline et al., 1989). Finally, a study including twin pairs separated and reared apart confirms the high heritability of lung function parameters (McClearn et al., 1994). In that study, about one-half and two-thirds of the variance between VC and FEV_1 was due to genetic influence after the effects of age, sex, height, and pack years of smoking have been removed. That study, furthermore, conducted in aging twins shows that resemblance attributable to genetic factors persists throughout life.

Segregation Analyses of Pulmonary Function

The search for the major genes that influence pulmonary function has been carried out by segregation analysis, comparing different models to account for the familial transmission of lung function. Segregation analyses of pulmonary function were conducted in seven data sets from North America recruited in the following regions: Johns Hopkins Hospital, Baltimore (Rybicki et al., 1990); Humboldt town, Saskatchewan, Canada (Chen et al., 1996; Chen et al., 1999); Framingham town, Massachusetts (Givelber et al., 1998); Tucson, Arizona (Holberg et al., 1998; Kurzius-Spencer et al., 2001); and various U.S. centers as part of the NHLBI family heart study (Wilk et al., 2000). These analyses are summarized in Table 9–2. This table first presents a brief description of the family samples, which consisted of nuclear families or extended pedigrees and included only adults or adults and children. All seven samples were Caucasian subjects, plus other ethnic groups in two of them: African Americans in the John Hopkins study and Hispanics in the first Tucson study. The quantitative measures of the pulmonary function analyzed by these seven studies included the following: FEV_1 for six of the seven studies; FEV between 25% and 75% of the vital capacity ($FEF_{25-75\%}$); maximal expiratory flow rate at 50% of vital capacity (V_{max50}); the ratio of V_{max50} to forced vital capacity (V_{max50}/FVC) in the Canadian studies (Chen et al., 1996, 1999); the forced vital capacity (FVC) and the ratio of FEV_1/FVC in the NHLBI family heart study (Wilk et al., 2000). These measures were adjusted for covariates prior to segregation analysis. The covariates included, always, age, sex, and height (plus weight in four studies) and, as needed, ethnicity, ascertainment group or family position, history of respiratory symptoms or history of coronary heart disease. The smoking status was treated differently according to the seven analyses: the quantitative measures of pulmonary functions were adjusted for smoking before segregation analysis in most studies, except in two where it was included in the model of segregation analysis (Rybicki et al., 1990; Holberg et al., 1998).

All segregation analyses were carried out using regressive models (Bonney, 1984), which merge the goals of epidemiology and genetics by making it possible to estimate simultaneously the effects of genetic and environmental factors and their inter-

Table 9–1. Selected Familial and Twin Studies

Authors and Location	Population	Results
Case-control with interview of family members		
Louis (Paris, France) 1837	28 emphysema patients, 50 controls	Increase of emphysema in parents of patients
Oswald et al. (London, UK) 1953	300 chronic bronchitis patients, 300 controls matched for smoking	Relation with first-degree relatives' chronic bronchitis morbidity and mortality
General population with interview of family members		
Boudik et al. (Prague CSSR) 1970	8292 men, 52–67 yrs	Relation of chronic bronchitis in first-degree relatives
Deutscher and Higgins, (Tecumseh, MI) 1970	1487 men, 30+ yrs; 1 or 2 dead parents	Low FEV_1 score related to parental early death
Case-control with examination of family members		
Larson et al. (US), 1970	156 first-degree relatives, 86 spouses of 61 CAL	Resemblance in FEV_1, greater in nonsmokers
Cohen et al. (Baltimore, MD), 1975	290 relatives of CAL, 701 unrelated controls, all PiM	Resemblance in FEV_1/FVC, adjusted for age, sex, race, smoking; segregation analysis done in the same study
Kueppers et al. (Philadelphia, PA), 1977	1441 relatives of 114 CAL, 45–60; 114 controls, matched for smoking, occupation	Familial resemblance in FEV_1
Silverman et al. (US), 1998	44 families of severe (FEV_1% pred $< 40\%$) early onset with 249 relatives, 20 population-based family controls (83 subjects)	Familial resemblance of low FEV_1 in smokers; decreased similarity with increased genetic distance; genome screening in progress
General population with examination of family members		
Colley (Aylesburg, UK) 1974	2598 children 6–14 yrs with both parents	Familial resemblance for symptoms; adjusted for smoking and social class
Higgins and Keller (Tecumseh, MI), 1975	3817 children with both parents	Familial resemblance for FEV_1 and chronic bronchitis; FEV_1 correlations between parents and children decrease with age; no adjustment for smoking
Tager et al. (East Boston, MA), 1976	1st-, 2nd-, and 3rd-degree relatives of 430 subjects 45–54 yrs (68 COPD/362 controls)	Familial resemblance in COPD; decrease resemblance with increasing genetic distance; adjusted for smoking
Lebowitz et al. (Tucson, AZ), 1984	354 subjects ≥ 14 yr, both parents	No familial resemblance for FEV_1 after adjustment for age and height/weight^{-3}
Kauffmann et al. (France), 1989	945 population-based families with 2 parents and ≥ 1 child 6–10 yrs	Familial resemblance observed for lung function, between children and parents (stronger with mothers than fathers) and siblings; adjusted for parental smoking, education, body habitus; role of sex-specific lung growth pattern in familial resemblance
Xu et al. (China), 1999	203 population-based families in rural China and 2044 asthmatic families	Familial resemblance for FEV_1 (adjusted for age, sex, height, weight, education, smoking, asthma status) with parent–child and sibling correlations equal in random families but sib–sib correlations greater than parent–offspring correlations (with mother–child > father–child) in asthmatic families
Palmer et al. (Busselton, Australia), 2001	468 population-based families (family members 25–60 yrs of age)	Familial resemblance for FEV_1 and FVC adjusted for age, sex, height, smoking status (and possibly asthma and rhinitis) with mainly additive genetic effects for both FEV_1 (heritability = 38.9%) and FVC (heritability = 40.6%) and very little overlap with the genetic determinants of asthma and rhinitis
Twin studies		
Cederlöf et al. (Sweden), 1967	2793 MZ, 5008 DZ	Concordance for cough greater in MZ than DZ
Hubert et al. (Bethesda, MD), 1982	127 MZ, 141 DZ, 42–56 yrs	Greater resemblance in FEV_1 in MZ than DZ
Redline et al. (USA), 1987, 1989	256 MZ and 158 DZ twins 27–61 yrs; study of relatives of twins	Intrapair correlations for lung function adj for smoking greater in MZ than DZ; decrease in resemblance with decreasing genetic relatedness
McClearn et al. (Sweden), 1994	230 Swedish twin pairs (mean age 65 yrs) including 37MZ and 72 DZ reared apart	Resemblance for FEV_1 and VC; effect of rearing environment shown for VC. Adjusted for pack years

Table 9–2. Outcomes of Segregation Analyses of Pulmonary Function Measurements

Authors and Location	Family Sample	Phenotype Analyzed[a]	Analysis Model	Results and Best-Fitting Model
Rybicki et al. (Baltimore area, MD), 1990	85 American families ascertained through one COPD patient; 56 American families randomly selected	FEV_1 adjusted on usual covariates[a] except smoking	Class A regressive model with and without smoking as covariate	In COPD families, major gene, without residual correlations; in random families, no evidence for familial correlations
Chen et al. (Saskatchewan, Canada), 1996	214 Canadian nuclear families randomly selected	FEV_1 and $FEF_{25-75\%}$ adjusted on usual covariates plus smoking	Class D regressive model	Nontransmitted major factor for FEV_1 plus residual famililal correlations (Mendelian factor not rejected); familial correlations for $FEF_{25-75\%}$ without evidence for a major gene
Givelber et al. (Framingham, MA), 1998	1408 American pedigrees randomly selected	FEV_1 adjusted on usual covariates plus smoking	Class D regressive model	Nontransmitted major factor plus residual familial correlations (Mendelian factor rejected)
Holberg et al. (Tucson, AZ), 1998	222 American nuclear families without asthmatic family members; 87 American families with at least one asthmatic family member	FEV_1 adjusted on usual covariates	Class D regressive model with and without covariates (smoking and asthma)	In nonasthmatic families, familial correlations without evidence for a major gene (with and without smoking included); in asthmatic families, mother–child and sibling correlations and possible effect of a recessive gene (with and without inclusion of smoking)
Chen et al. (Saskatchewan, Canada), 1999	309 Canadian nuclear families randomly selected	V_{max50} V_{max50}/FVC, each adjusted on usual covariates, history of respiratory symptoms, smoking, and other environmental factors	Class D regressive model Class D regressive model	Nontransmitted major factor plus residual familial correlations Mendelian transmission of a codominant major gene without additional familial correlations
Wilk et al. (multi-center NHLBI family heart study, population-based), US, 2000	455 randomly selected Caucasian families	FEV_1, FVC, FEV_1/FVC each adjusted for usual covariates, smoking, history of coronary heart disease	Class D regressive model	FEV_1: Dominant major gene plus residual familial correlations FVC: Transmitted major factor plus residual familial correlations (transmission probabilities differing from Mendelian values, although not significantly) FEV_1/FVC: Non-Mendelian transmitted major factor plus residual familial correlations
Kurzius-Spencer et al. (Tucson, AZ), 2001	746 randomly selected Caucasian families	FEV_1 adjusted for usual covariates and either unadjusted for smoking or adjusted for smoking	Class D regressive model	Non-Mendelian transmitted major factor plus residual familial correlations (similar results with and without adjustment for smoking)

[a]Usual covariates include age, sex, height (weight), and eventually ethnicity, ascertainment group, and family position.

actions. The regressive models specify a regression relationship between each person's phenotype (measure of pulmonary function) and a set of explanatory variables, including a major gene effect, the phenotypes of preceding relatives to account for unspecified sources of familial correlations (due to other genes or to common environmental factors), and covariates that may interact with the major gene. Estimates of parameters and tests of hypotheses are based on maximum-likelihood theory. Several classes of regressive models have been described, which differ according to the patterns of familial correlations besides the major gene effect. The class A model, used in the Johns Hopkins study, assumes that, given parental phenotypes, the offspring phenotypes are not correlated (sibling correlation is a function of spouse and parent–offspring correlations), whereas the more general class D model, used in all other studies, allows for the sibling correlation not to be due only to common parentage. They both assume that correlations between any pair of sibs are equal.

As seen in table 9–2, all analyses show significant familial correlations, except one conducted in a small sample of 56 families (Rybicki et al., 1990). When considering FEV_1, there was some evidence for the transmission of a major gene in three family samples, two samples ascertained through either a COPD proband (Rybicki et al., 1990) or including an asthmatic subject (Holberg et al., 1998) and one randomly selected sample (Wilk et al., 2000). In the COPD families, the effect of a codominant major gene was highly significant ($p < .0001$) and accounted for all the observed familial correlation. However, the residual familial correlations were assumed to follow the class A model pattern, which may lead to false inference of a major gene, as shown by a simulation study (Demenais et al., 1990). Evidence for a recessive major gene effect in the asthmatic families was only of borderline significance ($p = .037$) and was detected when the nonsignificant father–offspring correlation was set to zero. In the NHLBI random sample (Wilk et al., 2000), a Mendelian dominant major gene model was not significantly different from the general transmission codominant model ($p = .058$), but the transmission probabilities under this general model were far from their Mendelian values and there was evidence for additional familial correlations. The patterns of familial correlations for FEV_1 estimated under the class D model differed by family samples. The spouse correlations were always not significantly different from zero. The sib–sib correlation was equal to the parent–offspring correlation, and both fit the polygenic mode of inheritance in the Humboldt Canadian and multicenter NHLBI data sets; in contrast, in all other samples the sib–sib correlation was greater than the parent–offspring correlation, suggesting effects of dominance variance or environmental factors shared by siblings. Interestingly, the mother–offspring correlation was higher then the father–offspring correlation in the Framingham pedigrees and even more in the Tucson asthmatic families, indicating a possible maternal effect as reported by other studies of pulmonary function in East Boston (Lewitter et al., 1984) and in the PAARC data (Kauffmann et al., 1989). The other measures of pulmonary function showed different patterns of familial transmission: evidence for a nontransmitted major factor, but residual familial correlations for V_{max50} (Chen et al., 1999) and presence of a transmitted major factor that did not follow a Mendelian pattern of inheritance plus additional familial correlations for FVC and FEV_1/FVC (Wilk et al., 2000). Moreover, there was significant evidence for the Mendelian transmission of a codominant major gene ($p < .001$), without any additional familial resemblance for the V_{max50}/FVC phenotype which represents airway-parenchymal dysanapsis (Chen et al., 1999).

Altogether, these seven studies show that familial aggregation of pulmonary function results from multiple genetic or common environmental factors when taking into account known risk factors such as smoking. Lung dysfunction may be controlled by one or a few genes, as suggested in the COPD and asthmatic families, and growth of airway relative to parenchyma (or airway–parenchymal dysanapsis) appears to be under major genetic control. These results clearly demonstrate heterogeneity of pulmonary function as outlined by the different patterns of familial correlations, which merits further investigation.

Associations with Other Diseases

The knowledge of associations with both other chronic diseases and rare genetic syndromes can suggest hypotheses regarding the etiology of COPD, including environmental factors, genetic factors, and physiopathological mechanisms.

The association of peptic ulcer to COPD was first described by Green and Dundee (1952). It has been reproduced in studies with cases and controls, when cases were either peptic ulcers or COPD patients (Rotter, 1980; Kauffmann and Brille, 1981). The relative risk is between two and three and is not explained by tobacco. Associations of peptic ulcer with antiprotease deficiency (André et al., 1974) and cystic fibrosis (Rotter, 1980) have been reported, but they could only explain a few cases. Hypotheses regarding salivary secretor gene, which is well known to be associated to peptic ulcer (see chapter 13) have been proposed for COPD (see below and Cohen et al., 1980).

Higher mortality and morbidity from COPD than expected has been observed in relatives of lung cancer patients (Tokuhata and Lilienfeld, 1963; Van der Wal et al., 1966), and this difference was apparent even in nonsmoking relatives of patients. Lung function tests have shown significantly lower FEV_1/FVC adjusted for age, sex, and smoking in lung cancer relatives than in controls (Cohen et al., 1977). The relationship of FEV_1 with 10-year lung cancer mortality adjusted for smoking was shown in a Danish population-based survey (Vestbo et al., 1991). Such association may suggest factors of interest for COPD from the literature on cancer genetics (see chapter 36). The role of genes controlling susceptibility to smoking, such as those with antioxidant properties, could be tested in both diseases. In contrast, designs in which emphysematous patients (precisely defined through lung biopsies) are compared to nonemphysematous patients, all with lung cancer (Schellenberg et al., 1998), are not appropriate to study factors common to both diseases.

Association of chronic airflow limitation with rheumatoid arthritis has been reported (Collins et al., 1976; Geddes et al., 1979). Pulmonary lesions observed in rheumatoid arthritis are particular forms of diseases of the small airways (Thurlbeck, 1982). Recent clinical results argue in favor of a specific obstructive disorder in rheumatoid arthritis (Vernegnègre et al., 1997), but there is no population-based study on this disease association. Genetic explanations have been proposed, but for now they are unconvincing. PIMZ has been implicated by some authors (Fagerhol et al., 1981). An explanation through the role of human leukocyte antigen (HLA) (HLA-DR4) has been proposed (Radoux et al., 1980) but not confirmed by further studies on larger data sets (Hassan et al., 1995) (see chapter 29).

Clinical studies have suggested that the lung could be a target organ for diabetes mellitus (Sandler, 1990). In population-based study, at its onset diabetes mellitus was associated with a significantly accelerated decline of ventilatory function in Denmark (Lange et al., 1990), but pulmonary function was unrelated to noninsulin dependent diabetes mellitus (NIDDM) in American older adults (Barrett-Connor and Frette, 1996). Negative correlation between FEV_1 and indirect measure of insulin resistance in nondiabetic men has also been observed (Lazarus et al., 1998). The authors raise the hypothesis that insulin could be one mechanism in the unexplained relationship of cardiovascular disease risk and decreased ventilatory function. As no familial or genetic data on the associations of lung function, diabetes mellitus, and cardiovascular diseases are available, it would be premature to raise a genetic explanation of the associations of intermediate phenotypes of COPD and diabetes, which needs first to be confirmed.

Asthma and COPD are both obstructive pulmonary diseases and share numerous phenotypic characteristics (Snider, 1995a). Although the two are usually considered under a common heading in the Netherlands, the discussion still continues about the Dutch hypothesis (Sluiter et al., 1991; Vermeire and Pride, 1991). Although wheezing is typical of asthma and bronchial hyperresponsiveness is one of its main features, they are also observed in COPD. Severe asthma is characterized by some degree of fixed chronic airflow limitation. Moreover, in addition to theories about common physiopathological mechanisms, a large group of patients are considered to have mixed forms of asthma and COPD, especially in smokers and in subjects aged 50 years or more. Although it is reasonable to design research protocols excluding such patients, in genetics studies (Panhuysen et al., 1998; Silverman et al., 1998) or clinical trials, the mixed forms do represent a fair number of individuals.

Associations of various genetic syndromes with COPD have been described. The first rare genetic syndrome in which COPD is an important manifestation is obviously α_1-antitrypsin (α1AT) deficiency of PIZ subjects (see below). The second one is cystic fibrosis (1 in 2500 live births in Caucasian populations). Adult patients with cystic fibrosis have a disease very similar to classical COPD (Boat and Petty, 1977). This has raised the question of the role of PIZ and cystic fibrosis heterozygotes (see below).

Young's syndrome, ciliary dyskinesia, immune deficiency syndromes, and connective tissue disorders share various features with COPD (Cohen and Chase, 1978; Kueppers, 1992). Kartagener's syndrome (triad of *situs inversus*, bronchitis, and sinusitis) is observed in 1 in 40,000); more generally, primary ciliary dyskinesia includes COPD (Mossberg et al., 1978). Primary ciliary dyskinesias suggest we should consider genetic determinants of mucociliary clearance in the pathophysiology of COPD, a hypothesis supported by strong twin resemblance (Camner et al., 1972). Several loci (19q13.3–qter, 9p21–p, 5p15–p14) have already been proposed for ciliary dyskinesia (Omran et al, 2000). Various immune deficiencies in which the main pulmonary manifestation is an increased susceptibility to infections have been associated with COPD (Kueppers 1992; Webb and Condemi, 1974; Luisetti and Pignatti, 1995). Genetically controlled collagen diseases are associated with some features of COPD. Marfan syndrome, Ehlers Danlos type V, and X-related cutis laxa present disorders similar to emphysema and parenchymal matrix remodeling (Kueppers 1992; Byers et al., 1980). Association of COPD with rare forms of genetically determined collagen disease and some animal models of emphysema (Snider et al., 1986)—both related to lysil oxidase activity—requires further investigations of the role of lysyl oxidase in common forms of human COPD.

Environmental Factors

Cigarette smoking and certain occupational exposures are established environmental risk factors for COPD. There is also good evidence that air pollution, poverty, nutritional factors such as antioxidants and polyunsaturated fatty acids, passive smoking, and childhood infections play a role in the etiology of COPD (Rijcken and Britton, 1998; Anto et al., 2000).

Mortality by COPD in smokers of 25 cigarettes per day is increased by 20 times that of nonsmokers (Doll et al., 1994). Smoking increased FEV_1 decline, as observed in many longitudinal surveys conducted in occupational cohorts and in general populations (Fletcher et al., 1976; Lange et al., 1998). Passive smoking at home (Kauffmann et al., 1983b) or at work and, more important, maternal smoking, in particular in utero exposure (Hoo et al., 1998), are also risk factors (Jaakkola, 2000). Therefore genetic factors explaining differential effects of smoking is an important issue. Moreover, part of the familial resemblance of COPD may be explained by familial resemblance in smoking habits. Occupational exposures to dust, gases, and fumes also accelerates FEV_1 decline (Kauffmann et al., 1982b; Becklake, 1989). There is conflicting evidence that indoor exposure to gas cooking relates to lower lung function (Jarvis et al., 1998). Outdoor particulate pollution aggravates COPD and is related to mortality (Dockery et al. 1993; Ackermann-Liebrich, 2000). Antioxidant defense is provided by dietary antioxidants and endogenous enzymes systems, which are under genetic control. There is increasing evidence that antioxidant vitamins C and E and fish oils may protect against the development of COPD (Schünemann et al., 2001; Tabak et al., 2001). The role of alcohol in COPD is not well understood. A deleterious effect of heavy drinking on FEV_1 decline has been shown (Lange et al., 1988), but there is some suggestion that alcohol consumption in smokers may have a protective effect on lung function (Lange et al., 1988; Garshick et al., 1989) and emphysema (Pratt and Vollmer, 1988). The anti-inflammatory effect of alcohol was suggested to explain these observations.

Besides the well-known role of infection with established COPD (Murphy and Sethi, 1992) during childhood (Samet et al., 1983; Shaheen et al., 1994; Johnston et al., 1998) or adulthood (for the British hypothesis, see below) (Fletcher et al., 1976; Krzyzanowski et al., 1990), its role as a risk factor in the natural history of COPD is a matter of debate. Childhood infections relate to adult decreased lung function. Whether childhood infections are a cause of low FEV_1 in adulthood or are a consequence of impaired lung function in early life is a question difficult to resolve (Johnston et al., 1998). Independent of clinical infections, the potential role of latent viral infections as an underlying factor of lung inflammation has been suggested (Hogg, 1997). The interrelationships of childhood infections with adult lung disease is further complicated by the current hypothesis that early childhood infections serve as a protective role toward asthma through a preferential lymphocyte maturation in Th1, instead of the pro-allergic Th2 (see chapter 11). All viral and bacterial respiratory infections potentially implicated may be modulated by genetic factors.

Of particular interest in the context of genetic studies is to distinguish environmental factors that are personal (active smoking, occupational exposures) from those shared by family members within the household such as smoking behavior, passive smoking (in utero, in childhood, in adulthood), dietary habits, indoor exposures like oxidants from gas cooking and allergens, and those common to several households, such as air pollution. Interactions between the various factors over time is not well understood. Accumulation of risks over the lifetime and pulmonary function tracking have pushed researchers to consider the whole life span, and an epidemiological model of COPD has been proposed in four life cycles: during pregnancy, during lung function growth (0–20 years), during the plateau phase (20–40 years), and during lung function decline (>40 years) (Rijcken and Britton, 1998).

PATHOPHYSIOLOGY: BIOLOGIC BASIS OF GENETIC SUSCEPTIBILITY

Pathophysiology of Disease

Three theories have dominated the debate on the etiology of COPD: the British hypothesis, the Dutch hypothesis and the protease–antiprotease theory (Fletcher et al., 1976; Speizer and Tager, 1979; Janoff, 1988; Burrows, 1990; Vestbo et al., 1998). Figure 9–3 shows these three hypotheses and how they have evolved. The British hypothesis proposed that acute respiratory infections (themselves strongly related to mucous hypersecretion) were a risk factor for impaired airway function. This hypothesis originated from clinical observation that infectious exacerbations in COPD patients led to continuing and permanent deterioration of FEV_1. It was reflected in the use of the term *obstructive chronic bronchitis* to indicate chronic bronchitis (i.e., mucous hypersecretion) complicated by obstruction of the airways.

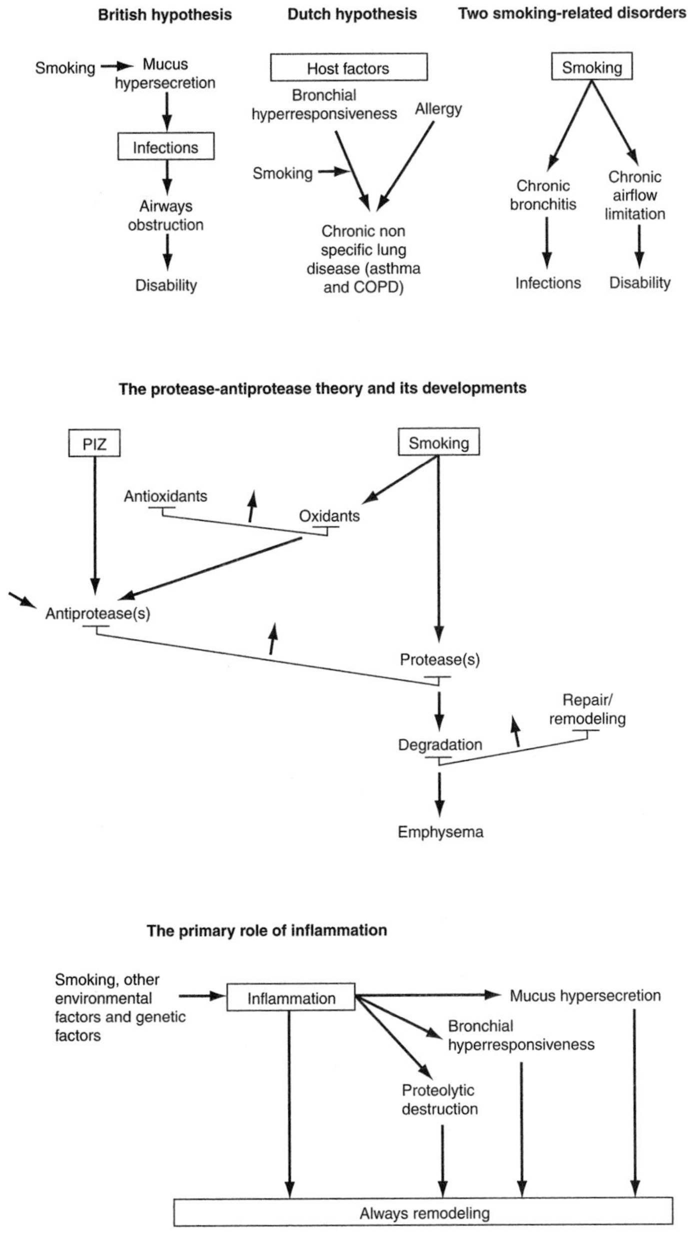

Fig. 9–3. Theories on the pathophysiology of COPD.

The Dutch hypothesis proposed that certain features observed in asthmatic patients, namely allergy and bronchial hyperresponsiveness, were risk factors for other obstructive airway diseases—that is, that there was some common host factor for asthma and COPD. It was typically reflected by use of the term *chronic nonspecific lung disease* (CNSLD) in the Netherlands to enable them to include asthma and COPD under a common heading. Thus, in some ways, the British hypothesis was an environmental hypothesis, and the Dutch hypothesis was a genetic hypothesis, although neither was phrased in those terms originally. Epidemiological studies were designed specifically to refute these hypotheses. Thus, the longitudinal study of Fletcher and colleagues addressed the question by examining the relationship between infections and mucous hypersecretion to FEV_1 decline.

The third hypothesis is the protease–antiprotease theory. It originates from two different types of observations: first, the observation of a genetic defect in the circulating level of α_1-antitrypsin (the main antiprotease in the serum) in emphysema with early onset and the demonstration of lung destruction (similar to human emphysema) in animal models after a single injection of protease; second, the fact that smoking, the major cause of emphysema, increased the number of circulating and lung neutrophils that contain elastase. It can therefore be considered as a genetic by environment hypothesis construct, and this is reflected in the term *destructive lung disease* (Gadek and Crystal, 1982). Most research on the subject has been done with the objective of supporting that hypothesis, not trying to refute it. The lack of any controlled trial on antielastase replacement therapy in PIZ individuals until 1998 (available since 1985) represents a missed occasion to support that causal theory.

The British hypothesis has been considered refuted since bronchial infections, or bronchial hypersecretion, were not a risk factor of FEV_1 decline after adjustment for smoking and FEV_1 level, in the 8-year study conducted by Fletcher et al. (1976) in an occupational cohort of London transport workers. Similar results have been observed in another 12-year occupational cohort in Paris area workers (Kauffmann et al., 1979). It was then considered that there were two disorders: the hypersecretory disorder (chronic bronchitis) and the obstructive disorder. As chronic bronchitis was not the factor leading to airway obstruction, the term *chronic airflow obstruction*, or, better, *chronic airflow limitation*, was proposed. This dichotomy fit with the difference in the site of chronic bronchitis (large airways) and of beginning of airflow limitation in small airways (Hogg et al., 1968). However, in two general populations surveys conducted later in Tucson, Arizona (Krzyzanowski et al., 1990) and Denmark (Vestbo et al., 1996), some effect of infections on FEV_1 decline was shown. Revisiting the original British hypothesis is worthwhile with this information on clinical infections, as well as in light of recent results about the potential role of early or latent viral infections (Hogg, 1997). Furthermore, the infectious hypothesis fits within a more general hypothesis on the role of airway inflammation as a major underlying factor of COPD (Rennard, 1998).

The Dutch hypothesis was not properly rebutted by the Fletcher study, as bronchial hyperresponsiveness was not directly measured. Since this report, several longitudinal epidemiological surveys have provided arguments supporting that hypothesis regarding the bronchial hyperresponsiveness part (Rijcken et al., 1995; Rijcken and Britton, 1988, Boezen et al., 2000). Allergy markers were also found to relate longitudinally to FEV_1 decline (Sherrill et al., 1995; Gottlieb et al., 1996), although it has not been observed in all studies. Bronchial hyperresponsiveness, a marked feature of asthma, is also considered to be an indicator of airway inflammation.

The protease–antiprotease theory is a seductive hypothesis in the mode of its formulation from different fields of research, its coherence, and its balance regarding a genetic factor (rare) and an environmental factor (frequent). However, overenthusiasm for the theory has overridden the observations which from the start suggested a more complex pattern (Gadek and Crystal, 1982; Janoff, 1988). Much research has been undertaken under the idea of the central role of $\alpha 1$AT and the importance of its inactivation by oxidants. The relative importance of small-airways inflammation and emphysema in the genesis of COPD has been debated (Burrows, 1990), and research has evolved in various directions. Besides the roles of $\alpha 1$AT and neutrophil elastase, studies have been conducted on several proteases and antiproteases. Besides the level of enzymes, studies have considered their activity, in particular, the oxidative inactivation of the antiprotease. Along with the destruction of parenchyma, consideration has been given to the possibility of level and quality of repair after elastolytic destruction. More generally, interest in the extracellular matrix in general, has increased, with the idea that excluding fibrosis associated with emphysema from COPD is inappropriate (Snider, 1995a). Insufficient repair after infections could play a role in the decrease in body weight that is observed in pink puffer patients. Animal models have suggested genetic factors in this broader context, where the whole lung matrix is considered. The blotchy mouse has progressive panlobular emphysema and is a genetic model of altered copper transport. In the blotchy mouse, lysyl oxidase (which cofactor is copper) activity is deficient and crosslinks of elastin and collagen are affected. The tight-skinned mouse has lungs with large airspaces and disorder in connective tissue (Snider et al., 1986).

Finally, the primary role of some inflammation (Rennard, 1998) with the remodeling consequences at the level of small airways, large airways, and parenchyma came through the various hypotheses, representing a more general model (see Figure 9–3). Inflammation may be modulated by genetic factors, and it is possible that insight into the genetic determinants of COPD may come from genetic studies on nonrespiratory inflammatory diseases, in addition to genetic studies of asthma. The lumping approach in analyzing the pathogenesis does not contradict the usefulness of trying to disentangle COPD for research purposes.

Genetic Studies of Pathophysiology

Studies of familial resemblance of intermediate phenotypes are particularly useful to approach the genetic determinants of common diseases. These phenotypes may be physiological or biological parameters. Physiological parameters are part of the studies of the familial resemblance of lung function tests, which have been reviewed above. Low lung function belongs to the definition of COPD and is not therefore an intermediate phenotype. Since the 1975 study of Higgins and Keller in the general population of Tecumseh, Michigan, it is known that familial resemblance of FEV_1 occurs for the whole distribution of the trait and is not restricted to familial resemblance of airflow limitation. Resemblance occurs also in families with median or high FEV_1 (Higgins and Keller, 1975). Therefore, understanding the genetic and environmental determinants of lung function values in their normal range is of great interest to elucidate the etiology of COPD. Twin studies have shown a genetic component in the response to hypoxia (Arkinstall et al., 1974; Kawakami et al., 1982), a phenotype of interest to understand potential genetic differences between type A and type B patients. Bronchial hyperresponsiveness, now recognized as a risk factor for COPD (Rijcken et al., 1995) has been studied for its familial resemblance because of its importance in asthma. These studies are reviewed in Chapter 11. More generally, studies conducted to understand the genetics of asthma will likely bring important information to understanding of familial resemblance of COPD.

The discovery of the implication of the $\alpha 1$AT level in emphysema and of its genetic determination was almost concomitant, and therefore there has been no need to study the familial resemblance of the $\alpha 1$AT serum level, which is a biological intermediate phenotype for emphysema. Clinical and a few epidemiological studies have considered elastin peptides and desmosine levels as markers of elastin metabolism and elastin degradation (Schriver et al., 1992; Stone et al., 1995; Frette et al. 1996). Problems in the measurement regarding the specificity, reproducibility, and cost of these biological markers have limited their use in epidemiological surveys, and no study of familial resemblance has been performed.

Total white blood cell count is a biomarker of exposure, response, and possibly susceptibility. In particular, it is an indicator of oxidative damage at the tissue level and thus a general biomarker of exposure to oxidant-generating stimuli (Crowell and Samet, 1995). However it is only an indirect marker of lung inflammation. Total white blood cell count has been the topic of numerous epidemiological surveys, but to our knowledge, no familial study has been performed. It might be of interest to study FEV_1 familial resemblance, taking into account smoking and leukocyte counts. Studies of familial resemblance for eosinophil counts have been performed in the context of asthma research (see Chapter 11), but none for total leukocyte or neutrophil counts.Overall, there is a paucity of studies of intermediate phenotypes, in particular of biological ones relevant to COPD.

In environmental epidemiology, the sequence of environment, internal dose, biologically effective dose, early biologic effect, altered structure or function, clinical disease, and prognostic significance is often used (Schulte, 1989). In Figure 9–4, genetic susceptibility is figured marginally as a potential modifying factor. In a parallel way, a sequence of gene(s), protein(s), functional changes, and disease is usually figured in the genetic literature with environmental factors, often not directly assessed, as modifiers. Figure 9–4 presents a synthesis of the two approaches with a balanced presentation of environment and genetics, figuring interactions. Low-level, intermediate-level, and high-level phenotypes between genes and clinical disease have been described (Schork, 1997). Figure 9–4 represents two levels of intermediate phenotypes. Both biological and physiological (already more complex) parameters are presented to illustrate intermediate phenotypes. More effort should be devoted to research on biological phenotypes through multidisciplinary research between biologists and epidemiologists, to find good markers in serum or induced sputum, which may be used in population-based studies (De Backer, 1998). Finding appropriate intermediate phenotypes for COPD in general and for specific

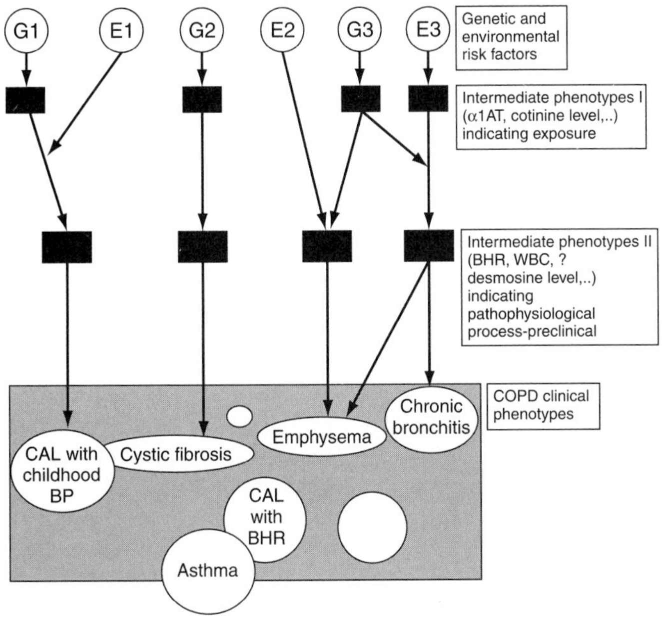

Fig. 9–4. Intermediate phenotypes: G1, G2, G3, genetic risk factors; E1, E2, E3, environmental risk factors; CAL, chronic airflow limitation; BP, bronchopneumopathies; BHR, bronchial hyperresponsiveness; $\alpha 1$ AT, α_1-antitrypsin.

forms of this heterogeneous disease would help in making progress in understanding of the mechanisms underlying COPD.

GENE IDENTIFICATION

Linkage and Association

With the recent advances in molecular genetics that have led to an increasing number of markers covering the whole genome, linkage analysis can be a powerful tool to detect genes involved in complex diseases. These analyses can be directed toward candidate regions or may be carried out in genome-wide searches, both being performed in asthma genetic studies (see Chapter 11). Model-free methods of linkage analyses are most often used since they do not require specification of a model for the disease, which is usually unknown (see Chapter 3). These methods search whether relatives who are similar with respect to the phenotype of interest (affected sib pairs) are also similar at the marker locus: that is, if they have inherited identical copies of the marker alleles, as will occur if a gene underlying the phenotype is linked to the marker. To our knowledge, only one genome-wide screen has been conducted for severe early-onset COPD (Silverman et al., 2001) Potential linkages were observed for moderate airflow obstruction ($FEV_1 < 60\%$ predicted, $FEV_1/FVC < 90\%$ predicted) to chromosomes 12 and 19, mild airflow obstruction ($FEV_1 < 80\%$ predicted, $FEV_1/FVC < 90\%$ predicted) to chromosomes 3 and 8 and chronic bronchitis to chromosomes 16, 19, and 22.

Another strategy is to search for associations of candidate genes with disease. Classically, marker allele frequencies are compared between cases and controls, which are matched for confounding factors, including ethnicity. An association occurs if the associated allele is the genetic variant causing the disease or is in linkage disequilibrium with the causal variant. Different mechanisms can cause a linkage disequilibrium: tight linkage between two loci and decreasing disequilibrium as the number of generations increases, but also admixture of populations with different frequencies of marker alleles and disease. Although cases and controls are matched for apparent ethnicity, the ethnic background of many populations is difficult to measure, and this may lead to spurious association. To circumvent this problem, family-based association studies have been proposed (Falk and Rubinstein, 1987) using the parents of a disease case as an alternative type of control: the two alleles of the parents that are not transmitted to their affected child are combined to create a pseudocontrol. The frequencies of marker allele among cases and pseudocontrols are used to derive an odds ratio (called the HHR: Haplotype Relative Risk). Another method has been then proposed, the transmission disequilibrium test (TDT), which tests for linkage in the presence of an association (Spielman et al., 1993; Schaid 1998) and has become a widely used tool to detect genes with small effects in multifactorial diseases. The TDT searches whether the proportion of marker alleles transmitted from heterozygous parents to their affected children differs from 50%, the expected value if there is no linkage and no association. Association studies for COPD were mainly done by comparing cases and controls and thus should be interpreted with caution.

Since the discovery of PI in 1963, an extensive literature has built up. Research on other genes potentially implicated in protease–antiprotease imbalance theory was then conducted. Some studies have looked at "classical" genetic markers available at the time (ABO, HLA, etc.). Some of them appeared to be reasonable candidate genes. It was only since 1995 that a few studies targeted specifically toward candidate genes emerged.

α_1-Antitrypsin (α_1AT)/α_1-Antiprotease (α_1AP) Deficiency

In 1963, Laurell and Eriksson, examining 1500 serum electrophoresis patterns done routinely, observed five subjects in which there was a missing band in the α_1 region (Laurell et al., 1963). They considered this dysproteinaemia to be due to an α1AT deficiency, a protein with a specific antitrypsin activity. They observed that three out of five subjects exhibited pulmonary disorders and evoked a genetic hypothesis to explain these observations. The major steps following that discovery until the availability of protein replacement therapy are summarized in Table 9–3, and a number of reviews describe them extensively (Fagerhol and Cox, 1981; Gadek and Crystal, 1982; Janoff, 1988; Kueppers, 1992; Eriksson, 1996; WHO memorandum 1997; Sandford et al., 1997a; Scwhaiblmair and Vogelmeier, 1998). The discovery of the protease inhibitor system has been a breakthrough. As often in such situations, the resulting new paradigm of the protease–antiprotease theory of destructive lung disease has for a while detracted attention from alternative and complementary hypotheses of the physiopathology of COPD.

The genetic system identified is called PI (protease inhibitor) to recognize that the activity of α1AT is to inhibit enzymes other than trypsin—in particular, elastase. It is therefore preferably called α_1-antiprotease (α1AP), but this term is not uniformly used. Some 49 alleles have been identified characterized by DNA sequencing and 100 by isoelectric focusing. Its nomenclature, based on the electrophoretic migration, was defined in Rouen in 1978. Sixteen alleles have been shown to be deficient in α1AT—in particular, PI null (0% activity of normal PIM), PIM_{malton} (12%), PIZ (15%: 5–6 μmol/l, or 30–40 mg/dl), PIP (30%), PIS (60%), and PII (68%). PIZ is present throughout all Caucasian populations (highest in Scandinavia at 2.6%, 1.4% in France,

Table 9–3. From PI Gene Discovery to the First Control Trial for Replacement Therapy (1963–1999)

1955	Protein found
1962	Protein named α_1-antitrypsin (α1AT)
1963	Deficiency of α1AT associated with emphysema
1964	Papain-induced animal emphysema
1967	Gene coding for α_1-antitrypsin named protease inhibitor (PI)
	Liver injury
1978	Rouen nomenclature of PI alleles
	NIH plan with four potential treatment steps
	Role of smoking in PIZ
	Debate on heterozygotes
	Oxidants and antioxidants
1982	Localization of PI on chromosome 14
1985	Availability of replacement therapy
	Discussion of prenatal diagnosis
1987	Discussion of proteases–antiproteases, extracellular matrix degradation and repair
1988	Setup of U.S. registry
1990	Gene therapy considered
1992	Secondary structure (loop) in PIZ explaining liver storage
1996	WHO meeting, published 1997
1997	Underdiagnosis by medical community noted
	Comparison of German (replacement) and Dutch (no replacement) registries of patients
1998	Data from the U.S. registry
1999	Results of the first Danish/Dutch controlled trial (n = 56)

1.2% in North American white population) and is absent from oriental and black populations without Caucasian admixture (Hutchison, 1998). PIS is rare in Northern Europe and concerns 7% of the French population. The other deficient alleles are very rare. Subtypes have been described among the M alleles. Normal α1AT serum levels in PIM are 20 to 53 μmol/l (150–350 mg/dl). The transmission of PI is autosomal codominant. In the absence of pedigree data, heterozygosity for PI null cannot be excluded when typing by isoelectric focusing technique; thus subjects are denoted by a monoallelic symbol, PIS and PIZ and not PISS and PIZZ. Except for rare variants, such as $PI_{Pittsburg}$, each α1AP has the same functional activity.

The PI gene locus is located on chromosome segment 14q32.1. It is part of a gene cluster that includes α_1-antichymotrypsin, protein C inhibitor, α_1-antitrypsin pseudogene/protease inhibitor-like gene, PI, and cortisol-binding globulin; it belongs to a supergene family (serine proteinase inhibitor, or serpin). The *PI* gene (SERPINA1) includes seven exons and six introns and is about 12 kb in length. Molecular genetics are described in the WHO report. IL-6 up regulates hepatocyte α1AT transcription. Translation of α1AT mRNA to the secretion of a globular protein of 418 aminoacids occurs (52,000 daltons) in fewer than 90 minutes. The principal site of synthesis is the liver parenchymal cells, but synthesis also occurs in mononuclear phagocytes, neutrophils, the intestinal epithelium, and the kidney parenchyma. In PIZ individuals, the synthesis is normal, but 85% of the α1AT produced is blocked in the terminal secretory pathway of the hepatocyte, resulting in liver dysfunction. Besides mutations of α1AT gene, which modifies the basal level of α1AT, mutations within the gene have been described that affect function, as a mutation in the 3′ flanking region that was related to COPD in some populations (Kalsheker et al., 1990), but not in others (Sandford et al., 1997a).

COPD in α_1-Antitrypsin Deficient Subjects

The typical characteristic is panlobular emphysema with basilar predominance. The severity of airflow limitation and the age of onset of symptoms are strongly related to smoking habits. Smoking may accelerate the onset of dyspnea up to 20 years. Detailed descriptions of patients from large series, such as the U.S. registry, which included 1129 patients (McElvaney et al., 1997) have been synthesized (Stoller, 1997). In the American series, 97% were PIZ, 1% were PISZ. FEV_1% predicted averaged 47%. A proportion of 79% reported a history of familial respiratory disease; 72% were ex-smokers, and 8% were current smokers. One-third of the patients reported a physician diagnosis of asthma. Data from the U.S. registry confirm that PISZ subjects are at lower risk of developing emphysema than are PIZZ subjects (Turino et al., 1996). Recent observations suggest that, besides underdiagnosis of PIZ, a substantial proportion of PIZ subjects may have only mild disease (Dahl et al., 2001b) and, besides smoking, other genes may modify the course of the disease in PIZ subjects, such as NOS3 (7q36), the constitutive endothelial nitric oxide synthase (Novoradovsky et al., 1999).

Heterozygotes PIMZ

Whether PIMZ heterozygotes were at risk of respiratory disease has been a matter of dispute. It is an important question as a large number of subjects are concerned. Table 9–4 summarizes results from two different types of studies: comparison of PIMZ prevalences in COPD cases and controls and comparison of respiratory characteristics, in particular lung function, between PIM and PIMZ subjects from the general population. The first series of studies is consistent and shows a relationship between COPD and PIMZ. The second series is also consistent but shows a lack of relationship between lung function and PIMZ. Potential self-selection against smoking may mask the association of PIMZ to lower lung function, when adjusting or matching for smoking (Kauffmann, 1985). Results from the general population of Copenhagen (Dahl et al., 2001), where the analysis was stratified according to clinically established COPD and was assessed by COPD hospitalization through the National Hospital register, reconciles these observations. PIMZ was associated with lower lung function, only in those with established COPD, suggesting that PIMZ acts as a modifying gene of the disease. A third type of design (reviewed in Kueppers, 1992) studied the prevalence of COPD in PIMZ heterozygotes who were identified as relatives of homozygous-deficient patients with lung disease. In this third series, most studies favor the association of the PIMZ phenotype with some degree of clinical or physiological abnormality. The discrepancy of the results according to the various designs (PIMZ from the general population or selected as a relative of a PIZ patient) may be explained by the presence of unknown familial factors (genetic or childhood shared environment) in PIMZ subjects belonging to families of PIZ patients (Kauffmann, 1984; Morse et al., 1977).

The hypothesis of additional familial factors to explain COPD in PIMZ was later supported. Comparison of the prevalence of airway obstruction and chronic bronchitis in first-degree relatives of COPD patients and first-degree relatives of controls showed that, in addition to α_1-antitrypsin deficiency (PIZ allele), personal cigarette smoking, and parental cigarette smoking, another component contributes to familial aggregation and it is likely to have a genetic basis (Khoury et al., 1985). Path and segregation analyses, conducted in families of PIZ subjects (Silverman et al., 1990), assessed whether factors other than the PI locus might contribute to familial resemblance of pulmonary function measures, FEV_1 and $FEF_{25-75\%}$ adjusted for the effects of PI type, age, and sex. Path analysis of the residual phenotypes indicated a highly significant cultural inheritance for both traits,

Table 9–4. Selected Studies on PIMZ Heterozygotes

Authors and Location	Population	Results
Case-control studies		
Talamo et al. (US), 1966	99 pulmonary clinic, 106 prisoners and employees	Nonsignificant increase
Kueppers and Dönhardt (US), 1974	89 hospital patients, 200 blood donors, 77 outpatients, 262 contestants in paternity suits	Significant association
Cox et al., 1976	163 outpatients, 209 blood donors, 512 schoolchildren	Significant association
Shigeoka et al., 1976	410 pulmonary function laboratory, 930 parents in community	Nonsignificant increase
Tarjan et al., (Hungary), 1994	Longitudinal 10 yrs; 28 PIMZ nonsmokers with dyspnea, 28 PIM controls	Significantly greater deterioration in lung function in PIMZ
Sandford et al. (Canada) 2001	Longitudinal 5 years; 283 smokers fast FEV_1 decliners (≥3% FEV_1% predicted/yr); 324 smokers no decline (≥0.4% gain/yr)	Significantly more MZ in fast than in slow decliners
Population-based studies		
Webb and Condemi (US), 1974	442 PIM, 18 PIMZ check-up center	No difference in lung function or symptoms
Eriksson et al. (Sweden, 1975)	100 PIM, 26 PIMZ unselected autopsies	Association with anatomic emphysema
Morse et al. (US), 1977	2637 PIM, 88 PIMZ general population 15–74 yrs old	No difference in lung function
Gulsvik and Fagerhol (Norway), 1979	1102 PIM, 55 PIMZ general population 15–70 yrs old	No association with $FEF_{25-75\%}$
Hamel and De Carrell, (N Zealand), 1981	499 PIM, 32 PIMZ, longitudinal, rural	No association with 3-yr FEV_1 slope
Bruce et al. (US), 1984	143 PIM, 143 PIMZ from six centers, matched for center and smoking	No association with lung function or symptoms
Dahl et al. (Denmark), 2001	8184 PIM, 498 PIMS, 12 PISS, 476 PIMZ, 10 PISZ, 6 PIZ, general population	MZ associated with reduced FEV_1 in those with clinically established COPD (hospitalization), but not among those without COPD

Source: Modified from Kueppers (1992) and Kauffmann (1984).

whereas a polygenic component was only demonstrated for $FEF_{25-75\%}$. However, additional adjustment of FEV_1 for significant interaction between PI type and pack-years of smoking increased the contribution of the polygenic component and decreased that of cultural inheritance. Segregation analysis, based on the mixed model (Lalouel and Morton, 1981), showed evidence that a major gene influences FEV_1 adjusted for age, sex, and PI type but presence of this major gene was not longer clearly demonstrated when adjusting also for the effect of pack-years and interaction between PI type and pack-years. This decrease in the evidence for a genetic factor might be explained if the role of the putative major gene is to enhance susceptibility to the effects of cigarette smoking. These different studies clearly indicate that other factors, genetic and environmental, contribute to familial aggregation of COPD besides the PI gene.

Other Antiproteases

Another serine protease inhibitor (SERPINA3), is α_1-antichymotrypsin, which inhibits neutrophil cathepsin G. The gene is located on chromosome 14 (14q32.11). The transmission is autosomal dominant. Twelve women out of 1872 Swedish middle-age women classified as heterozygotes were more often ex-smokers and had similar basal spirometry, but they had significantly higher residual volumes than the control subjects had (Lindmark et al., 1990). Mutations of the α_1-chymotrypsin gene were reported to be associated with COPD (Poller et al., 1993, Ishii et al., 2000), but not confirmed in another case control study (Sandford et al., 2001). It has been shown that the rare Leu-55–Pro variant associated with COPD (Poller et al, 1993) is due to an inactive conformation, explaining the loss of activity of the protein (Gooptu et al, 2000).

α_2-macroglobulin (A2M) is a serum protease inhibitor. The gene is located on chromosome 12p13.3–p12.3. Serum deficiency has been reported to be associated with COPD in a single patient (Poller et al., 1993; Sandford et al., 1998).

Salivary Secretor, Lewis, Red-Cell ABO Histo-Blood Groups

Lewis (*FUT3* gene located at 19p13.3), secretor (*FUT2* gene located at 19q13.3), and *ABO* (located at 9q34.2) loci control glycosyltransferases that act in concert on common precursor chains to build up oligosaccharide structures in exocrine secretions, such as the respiratory tract (Oriol, 1995). Studies on these systems are summarized in Table 9–5. In the 1960s when numerous reports searched for the associations of ABO, blood group with diseases (Mourant et al., 1978) and in particular COPD (Higgins et al., 1963), asthma (McConnell, 1959), and peptic ulcer (McConnell, 1959; Rotter, 1980), it was established that both blood group O and the salivary nonsecretor phenotype were independently related to peptic ulcers. In 1980, in the Johns Hopkins genetic epidemiologic study conducted in subjects related to COPD patients, lung cancer patients, and control subjects, Cohen et al. (1980) suggested an association of nonsecretor with lung function impairment and recalled the unexplained association of COPD with peptic ulcer and that the lung and the stomach shared the same embryologic origin. Furthermore, it was noticed from their data that salivary nonsecretor phenotype was significantly more prevalent in COPD-related subjects than in control subjects (Kauffmann, 1982a). Discordant results were observed in the various association studies between respiratory diseases and salivary secretor phenotype conducted later (Table 9–5). Longitudinal observations did not show associations of FEV_1 decline in adulthood with secretor (Higgins et al., 1982; Beaty et al., 1984). Lewis negative subjects were at increased risk of chronic airflow limitation, with an odds ratio of 7.2 in the general population of Humboldt in Canada (Horne et al., 1985).

A simultaneous analysis of the three preceding systems, based on their known biological interactions was conducted (Kauffmann et al., 1996). Very low lung function values were observed in the small group of Lewis-negative nonsecretors who lack both Le and Se controlled fucoses (1% of Caucasians). Lewis-positive, salivary ABH secretors who have these two fu-

Table 9–5. Studies on the Associations of Pulmonary Function with Histo-Blood Groups ABO/Secretor/Lewis

Author and Location	Population	Results
Cohen et al., (Baltimore, MD), 1980	1017 adults (129 COPD relatives, 31 lung cancer relatives, 857 controls)	FEV_1/FVC significantly lower in nonsecretors vs. secretors and in blood group A vs. others; adjusted for age, sex, smoking, social class, ascertainment
Abboud et al. (Canada), 1982	1422 pulp mill workers	No association of lung function with nonsecretor
Higgins et al. (Tecumseh, MI), 1982	General population; 15-yr incidence of low FEV_1	No association with ABO or secretor
Haines et al. (UK), 1982	2019 men, 766 women 18–64 yrs, at work	Significantly lower peak flow in nonsecretors
Kauffmann et al, (France), 1983	General population, 25–40 yrs: 43 never smokers with low FEV_1, 46 heavy smokers with high FEV_1	Increases of nonsecretor vs. secretor and Lewis negative vs. positive in low FEV_1, which were significant in blood group O subjects
Horne et al, (Humboldt, Canada), 1985	General population, rural, 893 subjects, 18–65 yrs	Significant increase of airflow limitation in Lewis negative (red cell typing); nonsignificant increase in nonsecretors.
Kauffmann et al. (France), 1996	228 coalminers	Significantly lower FEV_1 in subjects both Lewis negative and nonsecretors vs. others; in Lewis positive and secretors, significantly higher FEV_1 in blood group O vs. others; protective effect of alcohol consumption in Lewis negative

coses represent 79% of Caucasians. Among these subjects, lower lung function was observed in blood group A and to a lesser extent in blood group B than in blood group O subjects. Taking into account all the available information on the associations of the three genetic systems with COPD suggests that results are less discordant than previously thought (Kauffmann et al., 1996). Further studies of the combined effects of various histo-blood group genetic systems seem worthwhile, particularly for airflow limitation, wheezing, and asthma, possibly with reference to susceptibility to infectious agents.

Heterozygotes for Cystic Fibrosis

Cystic fibrosis (CF) is the most common autosomal recessive disease among Caucasian populations, with a prevalence very similar to PIZ. Mucus gland hypertrophy, inflammation, and fibrosis are observed in both CF and COPD patients. The early studies based on obligatory heterozygotes (Batten et al., 1963; Orzalesi et al., 1963; Hallett et al., 1965) have not shown clear results of an increase of airflow obstruction in parents of cystic fibrosis patients. However, parents of cystic fibrosis patients seem to be selected regarding smoking habits in these studies, which could mask the role of the genetic factor (Kauffmann, 1984). Associations of heterozygotes for cystic fibrosis and bronchial hyperresponsiveness were then suggested (Davis, 1989). Studies on obligate heterozygotes present some limitation as an association may result from the particular familial environment of cystic fibrosis patients.

In 1989, advances in the pathogenesis of the disease and determinations of heterozygotes became possible after cloning of the gene located on chromosome 7q31.2, the cystic fibrosis transmembane conductance regulator (CFTR) (Davidson and Porteous, 1998). The most common mutation is ΔF508. Clinical studies, based on case series, mostly do not support the view that common CFTR mutations predispose to chronic bronchitis (Dumur et al., 1990; Akai et al., 1992; Artlich et al., 1995). Some increase of ΔF508 was observed in one French study (6 out of 65 patients with chronic bronchitis; Dumur et al., 1990) but was not confirmed in another clinical series of 100 German patients with chronic bronchitis where only one was found ΔF508 (Artlich et al., 1995) and none in 21 chronic bronchitis with obstruction in Japan (Akai et al., 1992). None of these studies included a control group. Analyses of the various mutations in an Italian study showed an increase of the 5T variant for emphysema over a control group (Bombieri et al., 1998). Interesting findings come from a report of a population-based survey conducted in the general population of Copenhagen (Dahl et al., 1998). They found that ΔF508 carriers were significantly more often asthmatics than noncarriers and that among those with airflow limitation, FEV_1 was significantly lower in carriers than in noncarriers. Table 9–6 show that in these obstructed subjects, FEV_1 was independently related to environmental factors, social class, asthma, gender, and ΔF508. Their study was conducted in a representative sample of more than 10,000 individuals from the population of Copenhagen and concerned 250 carriers. A follow-up of that population showed that, in general, ΔF508 carriers did not have steeper 15-year FEV_1 decline than others (Dahl et al., 2001). However, whereas a history of asthma did not modifiy that relationship, ΔF508 heterozygosity was associated to steeper decline in those with a familial history of asthma (Dahl et al, 2001). Therefore, results suggest the role of various genes, among which CFTR mutations, and in particular ΔF508, may be involved in obstructive lung diseases (COPD and asthma).

Haptoglobin

Haptoglobin (Hp) is an α_2 sialoglycoprotein, an acute phase protein, with the primary role of binding with hemoglobin. It also

Table 9–6. Relation of Heterozygosity for ΔF508 to FEV_1 in 1009 Subjects with Airflow Obstruction from the General Population of Copenhagen[a]

Rank	Independent Variable	ΔR^{2b}	p	Change in FEV_1, ml (95% CI)
	Intercept		<.001	−228 (−954 to 498)
1	Height (cm)	.319	<.001	22 (18–25)
2	Age (years)	.113	<.001	−22 (−25 to −20)
3	Asthma	.068	<.001	−323 (−381 to −266)
4	Women	.022	<.001	−282 (−352 to −211)
5	Occupational dust	.012	<.001	−135 (−192 to −79)
6	ΔF508 heterozygosity	.004	.004	−217 (−385 to −60)
7	Household income	.005	<.001	
	Middle vs. high			−83 (−164 to −2)
	Low vs. high			−143 (−223 to −63)

[a]Airflow obstruction : predicted FEV_1 <80% and FEV_1/FVC ratio <0.7
[b]ΔR^2 = change in R^2 produced by adding independent covariate to model containing all previously ranked independent variables. F statistic: to approach normal distribution, FEV_1 was square-root transformed before analysis, but regression coefficients are shown for the untransformed values.
Source: After Dahl et al., (1998) with permission.

protects against free radicals and has an inhibitory effect on nitric oxide, cathepsin B, and prostaglandin synthesis, which confers to Hp an anti-inflammatory action (Langlois and Delanghe, 1996). The Hp_{α} gene is located on 16q22. There is a marked geographical difference with the lowest Hp_1 allele frequency in southeast Asia and the greatest in Africa and South America. A selective advantage seems to be provided by the Hp_2 allele. In the Northwestern European population, approximately 16% are Hp_1-1, 48% are Hp_2-1 and 36% are Hp_2-2. We observed a higher frequency of Hp_1 alleles in a group of subjects with high FEV_1 (although heavy smokers) than in a group of subjects with low FEV_1 (although nonsmokers), a difference only significant in subjects not belonging to group O (Kauffmann et al., 1983a). Indeed, a biological interaction between ABO and Hp is already known, since in families where parents have ABO incompatibility, there is a deficiency of Hp_2 children. Very few studies have considered Hp polymorphism. Hp_2-1 frequency was decreased in subjects with a family history of bronchial asthma (Fröhlander and Stjernberg, 1989).

Haptoglobin serum concentration rises markedly in infection or inflammation. Hp level has been shown in one epidemiological survey to be negatively related to FEV_1 but that hypohaptoglobinemia relates to wheezing (Kauffmann et al., 1991). Confirmation by other studies based on phenotype and haptoglobin concentrations data are needed before considering Hp gene as a risk factor. In this situation, as for histo-blood groups, interactions with current or past infections would be worthwhile to consider.

HLA, Gm, and Km

In the case of the HLA system, we have observed a significant increase in HLA-B7 antigen carriers and a deficiency of HLA-Bw16 antigen carriers in our groups with low FEV_1 (never smokers) compared to those with high FEV_1 (heavy smokers) (Kauffmann et al., 1983a). HLA-B16 also was shown as a protective factor for subjects with airway symptoms when working with laboratory animals (Sjöstedt et al., 1996). Although not statistically significant, these data are consistent with results of a case-control study, in which HLA-B16 was present in 11 of 200 controls but in none of 57 patients with chronic bronchitis (Anagnostopoulou et al., 1993). Another study showed an increased risk of bronchitis or pneumonia in HLA-B27 carriers (Hillderdal and Sapvenberg, 1983), an allele for which some trend was also observed in our study. A significant association of diffuse panbronchiolitis with HLA-Bw54 was also observed in an Asian population, a part of the world where only Bw54 and panbronchiolitis have been described (Sugiyama et al., 1990). No association was found with haplotypes of short (Km) and long (Gm) chains of immunoglobulins in one study (Kauffmann et al., 1983a).

Inflammatory Mediators

In the last years, several studies of candidate genes in the susceptibility to smoking—in particular, regarding the modulation of inflammation and antioxidant defense—have been conducted and showed interesting results (Table 9–7).

VitaminD–binding protein (or Gc) increases neutrophil chemotactic rates and is a macrophage-activating factor. The allele frequencies are 0.56 for 1S, 0.16 for 1F, and 0.28 for 2. Several case-control studies (Kueppers et al., 1977; Horne et al., 1990; Sandford et al., 1997; Schellenberg et al., 1998) observed a protective effect of allele 2 against COPD in smokers. The French study (Kauffmann et al., 1983a) did not refute the hypothesis of a protective role of this gene in smokers, as the two groups compared in that study (never smokers with low FEV_1 vs. heavy smokers with high FEV_1) did not let the authors study susceptibility factors to smoking. Therefore, the pattern regarding VitD-binding protein of allele 2 as a protective factor in smokers is consistent across published reports. The isoform Gc2 could help in maintaining the structural integrity of the lung that was chronically insulted by cigarette smoke (Schellenberg et al., 1998).

An increased TNFα expression could increase the inflammatory process. An association between chronic bronchitis and TNFα polymorphism has been reported (Table 9–7) (Huang et al., 1997), but it has not been confirmed in other studies (Higham et al., 2000; Patuzzo et al., 2000; Keatings et al., 2000; Sandford et al., 2001).

Preliminary results suggest that IL-10 polymorphism (gene located at 1q31–q32) may play a role in COPD (Küçükaycan et al., 2001), a result of interest if confirmed as IL-10 increases the tissue inhibitor of metalloprotease-1 (TIMP1) in cigarette smokers without modifying matrix metalloprotease-9 (MMP-9, gelatinase B) (Lim et al., 2000).

Genetic Polymorphisms in Xenobiotic Enzymes

Detoxification of xenobiotics, the components of tobacco smoke, is done in two phases: activation, usually governed by oxidation through cytochrome P-450, and detoxification by conjugation of the molecule with glutathione (through glutathionetransferase), sulfate (through sulfotransferase), or glycuronate (through glycuronyltransferase). Some of these aspects (which have been the topic of numerous reports on lung cancer, see Chapter 36) have been studied in COPD. Genetic susceptibility to oxidative stress in the development of COPD is receiving increasing interest (table 9–7; Cantlay et al., 1995; Harrison et al., 1997; Smith and Harrison, 1997; Koyama and Geddes, 1998; Schellenberg et al., 1998; Ishii et al., 1999; Patuzzo et al., 2000; Yamada et al., 2000; Yim et al., 2000; Sandford et al., 2001). It is biologically likely that interactions between these genetic systems occur to produce COPD. These recent studies have shown interesting associations of candidate genes with the susceptibility to tobacco components. Results are only partially consistent, however, and these association studies have been conducted on only small sample sizes.

Other Genetic Markers

A few studies have considered the potential role of several genetic markers, for which there were a priori no physiopathologic hypothesis and have been reviewed elsewhere (Kauffmann, 1984). Rhesus (located on 1p36.12–p34), MNS (located on 4q31), and complement C3 (located on 19p13.3) (Vestbo et al., 1993), Kell (located on 7q33) (Higgins et al., 1982), PTC (located on 5p15), and transferrin (located on 3q21) have been studied without conclusive results.

Genetic Control of Smoking Habits

As smoking is the major environmental factor for COPD, potential genetic influences on smoking habits are relevant to consider. Candidate genes for smoking behavior include the dopaminergic system and the activity and metabolism of nicotine (Rossing, 1998; Sandford and Paré, 2000). Twin studies sup-

Table 9–7. Other Association Studies (Oxidant/Antioxidant; Inflammation): Differential Susceptibility in Smokers

Authors and Locations	Gene	Localization	Population	Results
Cantlay et al. (UK), 1995	*CYP1A1*	15q22–q24	129 lung cancer smokers: 42 without emphysema, 87 with emphysema; 50 clinical lung disease; 281 blood donor controls	Val462carrier/IleIle OR cancer all 1.48 [0.83–2.61]; K no emphysema 0.52 [0.16–1.77]; K +emphysema 2.03 [1.10–3.73]; COPD 1.46 [0.66–3.25]
Huang et al., (Taiwan), 1997	*TNFα* (tumor necrosis factor)	6p21.3	42 men chronic bronchitis, FEV_1 <80%, FEV_1/FVC <69%; 42 local controls FEV_1 >80% (matched for smoking); 51 boys and 48 girls primary school	Genotype determination: TNF2 carriers vs. local controls 11.1 [2.90–42.6] and vs. pop controls 4.94 [2.09–11.7]
Smith and Harrison (UK), 1997	*EPHX1* (microsomal epoxide hydrolase)	1p11–qter	144 lung cancer patients: 94 with emphysema, 50 without emphysema; 68 COPD (all PIM); 57 chronic asthma; 203 blood donor controls	Two slow alleles (exon 3 and 4) vs. others; lung cancer alone 1.9 [0.6–5.9]; asthma 1.3 [0.4–4.3]; COPD 4.1 [1.8–9.7]; emphysema 5.0 [2.3–10.9]
Harrison et al. (UK), 1997	*GST M1* (glutathione *S* transferase M1	1p13.3	168 lung cancer patients: 57 without emphysema, 111 with emphysema; 384 blood donor controls	GSM1 deletion: cancer, 1.32 [0.91–1.90]; without emphysema 0.90 [0.52–1.58] and with emphysema 1.61 [1.04–2.49]
Schellenberg et al. (Canada), 1998	*VDBP* (GC) (vitamin D binding protein)	4q12–4q13	75 smoker lung cancer patients with COPD, 64 smoker lung cancer patients without COPD	Allele 2 carrier vs. 1–1 OR = 1.01 [0.49–2.1]; 2–2 vs. 1–1 OR = 0.17 [0.03–0.83]; no difference for neutrophil chemotaxis
Higham et al. (UK), 2000	*TNFα*	6p21.3	86 COPD, 63 eversmoker controls, 199 blood donors	No association of TNF2 carriers to COPD, nor to severity of airflow limitation/emphysema
Yoshigawa et al. (Japan), 2000	*EPHX1*	1p11–qter	71 lung cancer patients; 358 subjects, including 180 former workers of a poison gas factory	Variant allele exon 3 unrelated to COPD, but more prevalent in severe than in mild COPD
Yim et al. (Korea), 2000	*EPHX1, GSTM1*	1p11–qter	83 COPD, 73 healthy smokers	No association
Keatings et al. (UK), 2000	*TNFα*	6p21.3	106 COPD, 99 smoker controls	No difference between cases and controls, but in COPD patients, greater mortality associated to TNFα
Yamada et al. (Japan), 2000	*EPHX1*	1p11–qter	101 men with emphysema, 100 male smokers without emphysema	≥30 GT in the gene promoter associated to emphysema
Sandford et al., (Canada, 2001)	*VDBP (GC)* *EPHX1* *TNFα, LTA*	4q12–13 1p11–qter 6p21.3	Lung Health Study: Smokers followed 5 yrs. 283 fast FEV_1 decliners (≥3% FEV1% predicted/yr); 308 no decline (≥0.4% gain /yr)	No association of VDBP and TNF αG308A and LTA A252G polymorphisms; associations of haplotype frequencies of EPHX1 mutations, with His113/His139 associated (p = .03) with decline

port the hypothesis of genetic influences on smoking behavior. As noted by Rossing, the decline in smoking habits due to social pressures, may increase the genetic influence in remaining smokers. Genes coding for enzymes involved in dopamine receptors and transporters are of interest. The neural activity or metabolism of nicotine should also involve genes such as the cytochrome P-450 family and the nicotinic acetylcholine receptor. This area has not been addressed for now in studies of the genetics of COPD. Research in this area may be relevant for a pharmacogenetics approach in COPD, by identifying subjects for whom pharmacologic cessation aids may be most effective.

Gene–Environment Interactions

Various types of interactions may be considered (as shown in Figure 9–4) (Ottman, 1990): the genotype increases the expression of the risk factor and exacerbates its effect; the risk factor exacerbates the effect of the genotype; and both are required to raise the risk. Genetic factors may also modify exposure to the environment such as dopamin-genetic control intervening in nicotine addiction, and environmental mutagens may alter genetic structure. Some studies are designed to test gene–environment interaction (Yang and Khoury, 1997). Others cannot allow this type of analysis. A study of discordant monozygote twin pairs (Antti-Poika et al., 1992) is a powerful design, but only to evidence an environmental factor by removing genetic differences. A comparison of never smokers with low FEV_1 to heavy smokers with high FEV_1 (Kauffmann et al., 1983a) is a powerful design, but only to evidence a genetic factor by removing the smoking effect.

Little is known in COPD regarding gene–environment interactions. PIZ and smoking each influences alone the risk of COPD, and it is likely that PIMZ exacerbates the effect of smoking and other genetic factors (Silverman et al., 1990). The most recent studies have focused on the role of candidate genes in susceptibility to smoking.

Animal models suggest that there is a genetic control of airway inflammation related to oxidant exposure. Kleeberger et al (1993a, 1993b, 1997) have studied, in mouse models, the genetic control of response to acute and subacute exposure to ozone and concluded that airway inflammation, assessed by the number of polymorphonuclear leukocytes in bronchoalveolar lavage after acute (3 hr 2 ppm O_3) and subacute exposure (48 hr 0.3 ppm O_3) was controlled by different genes. A further study (Prows et al., 1997) suggested three major loci linked to acute lung injury related to ozone susceptibility. Kleeberger used mice to support linkage of O_3 susceptibility to a quantitative trait locus in the TNFα region, which was already implicated in pulmonary inflammatory disease. In the same region, other candidate genes include Mcpt6 and Mcpt7 which encode mast-cell proteases and histocompatibility genes and at a close location lies Sod2, which encodes MnSOD. This locus is also close to that related to hyperresponsiveness (DeSanctis et al., 1995). Drazen and Beier (1997) emphasized that respiratory responses to ozone represent a class of genotype–environment interaction, since these loci are in regions of conserved synteny in humans. Recent results from inbred strains of mice suggest that Toll-like recteor 4 (Tlr4) could play a role in ozone-induced lung hyperpermeability (Kleeberger et al, 2000). There is more generally a need for animal models of COPD, in relation in particular to susceptibility to cigarette smoke (March et al., 1999).

Stronger associations of nonsecretor gene with lung function in smokers (Haines et al., 1982) and of blood group A in heavy smokers (Khoury et al., 1986) than in nonsmokers have been reported. Some genetic factors could influence the physiologic deterioration of lung function in the normal aging process, and/or a greater susceptibility to smoking (Krzyzanowski et al., 1987). Further studies are needed to understand the potential modifying effect of genetic factors on factors related to lung growth (which may explain differences in adult FEV_1 levels), aging-related FEV_1 decline, and smoking-related FEV_1 decline. Differences in results from cross-sectional and longitudinal studies would provide information.

As for cardiovascular outcomes (Hein et al., 1993), a protective effect of alcohol consumption in Lewis-negative individuals (10% of Caucasians) was evidenced for FEV_1 in one study (Kauffmann et al., 1996). The potential protective role of alcohol consumption in smokers and in Lewis-negative subjects for both respiratory and cardiovascular outcomes needs to be further studied.

A reason for considering further histo blood groups is their known role in the adhesion of infectious agents. Facilitation of urinary, vaginal, gastric, and respiratory (Ramphal et al., 1991; Raza et al., 1991) infections has been related to the reaction of microorganism lectin receptors with specific host carbohydrates, such as the products of secretor, Lewis, or ABO genetic systems (Raza et al., 1991). Further studies of the combined effects of various glycosyltransferase genetic systems seem worthwhile, particularly for airflow limitation in asthma and respiratory childhood or old-age respiratory infections. In a different way, consideration of heterozygotes for cystic fibrosis goes with the same line as CFTR has been shown to interact with various infectious agents (Pier et al., 1998). The same genotype may either favor an infection or be a shield against it, depending on the specific agent concerned.

COPD HETEROGENEITY

COPD is a paradigm of complex diseases, for which there has not been enough work on phenotypes to address the heterogeneity. The issue of the disease phenotype to study is critical to maximize the ability to detect genes and more generally to understand the etiology. Considering the phenotypic heterogeneity is one means to understand genetic heterogeneity. Table 9–8 is an update of a classification proposed earlier (Kauffmann, 1984) to dissect the chronic obstructive pulmonary diseases, based on genetic, physiological (Evans and Green, 1998), and clinical knowledge to address the etiologic heterogeneity of these diseases, in particular regarding genetics. Such classification is proposed as an operational tool (which should evolve with knowledge) for etiologic research, not for clinical purposes. This table is an attempt to integrate classification based on our knowledge of genetic heterogeneity. When no specific cause is yet characterized, phenotype heterogeneity is also used as a starting point in disease classification. Environmental factors are not represented here, but groups such as COPD in nonsmokers may be studied. The study of physiological (bronchial hyperresponsiveness) or biological (measures of inflammation, lung destruction or repair) intermediate phenotypes should fit with such rationale. The interrelationships of COPD with asthma (here represented as a potential clinical mixed form) may change in the future, by considering following the so-called Dutch hypothesis that phenotypes associated with asthma, such as BHR and atopy are risk factors for COPD, and common inflammatory pathways may be less distinct than thought. The numerous recent results coming

Table 9–8. Classification of Chronic Obstructive Pulmonary Diseases According to Various Genetic, Physiological, and Clinical Criteria

1. PIZ emphysema
2. Chronic airflow limitation in PIMZ, PIMS
3. Chronic airflow limitation associated with rare genetic syndromes (cutis laxa, Ehlers Danlos, Marfan, cystic fibrosis, primary ciliary dyskinesia, IgA deficiency)
4. Chronic airflow limitation in homozygotes for CFTR mutations or in ΔF508 heterozygote carriers
5. Small airways disease
6. Emphysema
   - Panacinar
   - Centroacinar
7. Large airways disease
   - With or without bronchial hypersecretion (chronic bronchitis)
   - With or without bronchial hyperresponsiveness
8. According to childhood illness
   - with or without childhood respiratory diseases before 2 years
9. According to clinical form
   - Hypercapnia (type B blue bloaters)
   - Normocapnia (type A pink puffers)
10. According to other chronic diseases
    - Asthma
      - Allergic asthma
      - Intrinsic asthma
    - Peptic ulcer
    - Lung cancer

from the field of asthma genetics (see Chapter 11) would thus be of direct relevance to COPD genetics.

CLINICAL APPLICATION

Diagnosis, Screening, Counseling, and Prevention

α_1-antitrypsin deficiency is a paradigm of gene defects and explains a small proportion (1%) of a common disease. Understanding the etiologic heterogeneity of COPD could lead to the discovery of a few major genes, or oligogenes, but also of numerous genes with high relative risk for very restricted subgroups. The experience gained in diagnosis, screening, prevention, and treatment of α_1-antitrypsin deficiency could illustrate the success and the limitations of some current practices. Whereas it is demonstrated that removal from exposure to a modifiable environmental factor (smoking) markedly decreases the occurrence of emphysema in α1AT-deficient subjects, limited prevention programs have been undertaken, and research in that specific field is scarce. Whereas the availability of drug replacement therapy dates back to 1985 (table 9–3), only one small controlled clinical trial had been published by 1999 (Dirsken et al., 1999; Wencker et al., 2001).

Although of the same prevalence as cystic fibrosis in Caucasians, α1AT deficiency is markedly underdiagnosed. Detection is less than 10% in both the United States and the United Kingdom, and it reaches only 50% in Denmark, where active screening in the families of patients has been undertaken (WHO memorandum, 1997). Screening in unselected populations has permitted the assessment of prevalence of α1AT deficiency in various populations (Silverman et al., 1989; Thelin et al., 1996). Directed screening concerns subjects at higher than average risk of having α1AT deficiency: relatives of α1AT-deficient patients and subjects who are already suffering from respiratory disease. The former category also refers to counseling activities and the latter to case findings. The WHO report counsels that all patients with COPD and adults and adolescents with asthma should be screened once for α_1-antitrypsin deficiency using a quantitative test, followed by PI typing for those with abnormal results. In such a testing program in Salt Lake City (for individuals with chronic bronchitis, emphysema, and asthma and those with a family history of α1AT deficiency), 16,748 samples were tested in 5 years, with the detection of 515 subjects with α1AT < 11 μmol/l representing 15% of the known individuals with α1AT in the 5 years (WHO report). Although it has been done in the past (Wickle, 1998), direct information of family members of α1AT patients, is not appropriate. The initial approach to relatives should be made by the proband and be supported by information from a genetic counselor. Whereas the patient should obtain at his or her request the help needed to inform family members, he should not be taken out of the process for ethical reasons. Prenatal diagnosis may be relevant in the few families with a child with severe liver disease in early childhood, as intrafamilial resemblance for liver disease severity has been observed (α_1-Antitrypsin Deficiency, 1987; Cox and Mansfield, 1987).

Screening in unselected populations has been performed in Sweden and the United States. In Sweden, the neonatal screening performed in all 200,000 newborns in 1972–1974 was aimed at developing a primary prevention program, by decreasing exposure in the deficient subjects from air pollutants—in particular, tobacco smoke (Thelin et al., 1996). Regular somatic checkups at 6 months and 1, 2, and 4 years of age were proposed to the parents of 171 α1AT-deficient newborns that were detected. A specific effort to eliminate smoking habits was made. Decreasing parental smoking habits would have decreased exposure to passive smoking; moreover, because parental attitudes toward smoking have a strong effect on causing children to smoke or not, decreasing smoking by parents may result in decreasing smoking by their children. The neonatal screening was interrupted because negative psychological consequences for the parents and the parent–child relationship was reported by a number of pediatricians (McNeil et al., 1985). A research program was initiated when the children were 5 years of age to assess the psychological impact of the screening, and the cohort has been followed up through their twenties. Whereas the parents, in particular the mothers, did experience emotional reactions of shock and anxiety when they were first informed, their children later reported that identification of any such deficiency should be done as early as possible in life. Regarding smoking habits, there was no decrease in parental smoking for deficient children compared to controls (in fact, fathers were even more often smokers), but the children took up significantly less smoking by 18 years of age. This efficient measure suggests that screening is an effective preventive measure to change attitudes. Based on ethical standards, Thelin and colleagues (1996) concluded that they would now recommend a voluntary screening program offered to families sometime after the neonatal period. Voluntariness, confidentiality, and informed consent of the target family members to be screened have to be implemented. The appropriateness and necessary conditions for implementing screening in unselected populations is still a matter of debate. The recent WHO report recommends undertaking neonatal screening programs. Before the implementation of such programs, the WHO report recommends that laws and regulations must be in place to protect persons with severe α_1-antitrypsin deficiency from possible negative impacts; the permission of families must be obtained, and measures must be taken to provide appropriate counseling and support of persons and their families with α1AT deficiency.

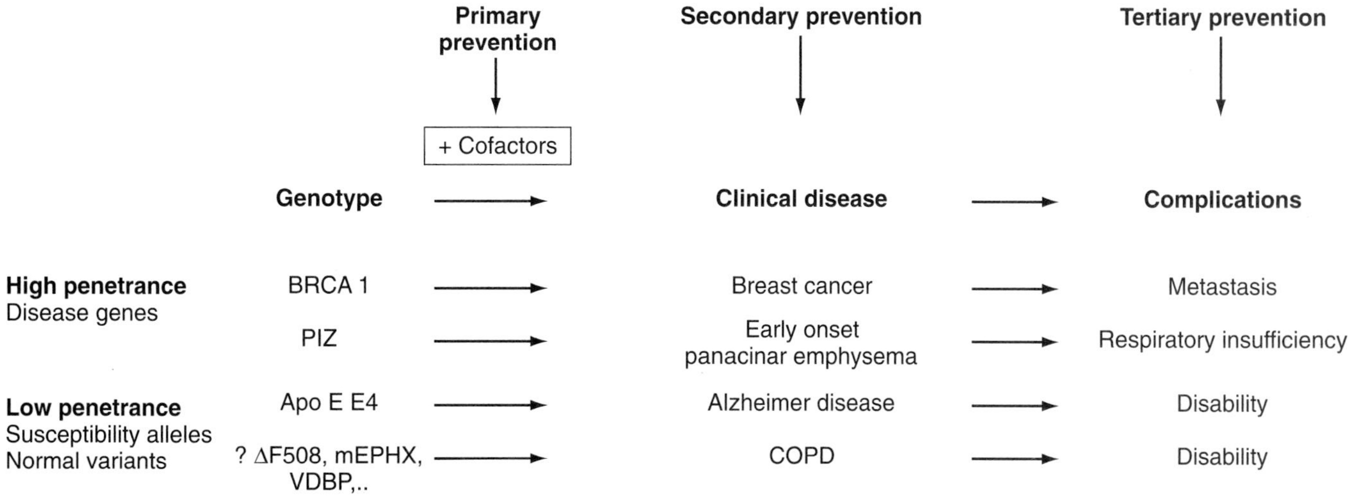

Fig. 9–5. Towards public health: the issue of prevention strategies in COPD, a moderate genetic disease. Modified from Khoury (1997) with permission.

An argument in favor of such screening is the efficiency to prevent a serious disease (emphysema) by modifying lifestyle habits (smoking), and that has been proven feasible (figure 9–5). α1AT deficiency has been qualified as a paradigm of an ecogenetic disorder, resulting from the interaction of exposure to smoking with a specific genetic predisposition to disease (Gelehrter et al., 1997). However, results from the general population of Copenhagen suggest that most PIZ, identified in a general population, have at most mild forms of the disease, which questions the usefulness of large-scale screening (Dahl et al., 2001). Besides α1AT deficiency, when discussing the interactions of genes with ozone-induced inflammation, Drazen and Beier (1997) concluded that when the genes responsible for this effect are identified in man, "these individuals unlucky enough to inherit alleles leading to enhanced susceptibility to ozone may be advised to refrain from strenuous outdoor activity on 'bad air' days." It is clearly one of the aims of genetic research to find genes which are shown to interact with modifiable environmental factors (Khoury, 1997) Figure 9–5 modified from Khoury shows the importance of such an approach for public health issues. It could be argued, however, that defining α1AT-deficient subjects as a specific target population for antismoking campaigns could be countereffective from a public health point of view by involuntarily reassuring the nondeficient subjects from stopping smoking, whereas the attributable risk of smoking habits in COPD is much greater than α1AT deficiency. Furthermore, the risk of shifting attention from the risk factor for the disease to potential discrimination against an individual's susceptibility to genotypes always has to be considered. Efficient preventive strategies on environmental exposure which interacts with genetic factors depend on the frequency of the genetic traits and environmental exposures, their relation to disease, and the nature of their interactions. Population-based epidemiological studies are needed before the results of basic genetic research can be translated into population-based interventions (Khoury and Wagener, 1995).

Therapy

Detailed discussion of treatment of COPD is beyond the scope of this review. The main treatment is discussed in specialized reviews (American Thoracic Society, 1995; Postma and Siafakas, 1998) concerns antismoking support, including nicotine replacement therapy, bronchodilators, anti-inflammatory drugs, antibiotics, antioxidants, mucolytics, vaccines, and oxygen therapy. Examples of potential applications of pharmacogenetics for COPD could be in relation to knowledge of the genetic control of nicotine addiction for the prescription of nicotine replacement therapy or of the genetic control of bronchial hyperresponsiveness (see chapter 11) for the prescription of bronchodilators.

Potential treatment options of α_1-antitrypsin deficiency (Schwaiblmair and Vogelmeier, 1998) are intravenous human plasma–derived augmentation therapy, aerosol augmentation therapy, recombinant α1AT augmentation therapy, gene therapy, augmentation of synthesis in the liver, synthetic inhibitors, lung volume reduction surgery, and lung transplantation. Under study are aerosol augmentation therapy to avoid the constraints of perfusion, synthetic inhibitors of low molecular weight. Gene therapy has been explored, but for now no stable expression of the α1AT gene has been obtained. The main discussion for now regards α_1-antitrypsin replacement therapy (Cohen, 1979; Hutchison and Hughes, 1997). This therapy is currently in a paradoxical phase. There is no doubt that the deficiency of the protein is a causal factor of emphysema in PIZ patients. Although replacement therapy has not been proven efficient clinically through a proper randomized control trial (Hutchison and Hughes, 1997; WHO report 1997; Dirksen et al., 1999; Seersholm et al., 1997), it has been approved by the American Food and Drug Administration and is currently on the market in very few countries. A multifactorial explanation seems likely. The feasibility of the trial was considered far from evident (Burrows, 1983), the disease was considered for a long time (Silverman et al., 1989) to be rare enough to qualify the drug as an orphan drug (Hay and Robin, 1991). The cost-effectiveness of the trial itself has been questioned on a basis that questions any trial for uncommon disorders (Hay and Robin, 1991). Demonstration of the causal link of protein deficiency to disease and demonstration that the administration of perfusion restores serum levels of α1AT to protective levels were major breakthroughs (Hubbard and Crystal, 1988). The demonstration of biochemical efficiency is only the first step to show clinical efficiency, however. Observational data of patients with and without replacement therapy from the American registry (McElvaney et al., 1997) and by the comparison of patients from the Danish (without replacement therapy) and German (with replacement therapy) registries (Seersholm et al., 1997) do not allow us to infer the clinical usefulness of the treatment. However, a better knowledge of the natural history of the α1AT-deficient patient has been gained through such registries, which should allow researchers to set up a feasible clinical trial in a near future. Besides mortality, changes in lung function and computed tomography can be used as endpoints. Preliminary results from a small Danish and Dutch-controlled trial suggests that efficiency could be shown in a larger set of patients, but it will probably be much smaller than was thought 15 years ago (Dirksen et al., 1999).

CONCLUSION

COPD is a common disease, with increasing prevalence worldwide and with both environmental (in particular, smoking) and genetic determinants. Although the PI gene was discovered 35 years ago, the genetic determinants of COPD are still largely unknown. PIZ explains 1% of COPD and there may be other rare genes involved with high penetrance. However, as in other common diseases, research in the genetic determinants of COPD may have to face the challenge of finding several frequent genes with low penetrance, each of which interacts with environmental factors. Different genes may be involved in the etiology of COPD and in its evolution toward severe forms and exacerbations. This would require combining family and case-control studies and applying different analytical methods, including segregation analyses, genome screening, linkage and association studies with candidate genes. Assessing the role of potential numerous candidate genes may be developed in larger scales through chip technology. Suggestions for new genes and proteins may come, besides several genome screens in progress, through mRNA differential display and proteomics (Barnes, 1999; Golpon et al., 2001). Addressing the heterogeneity of COPD, using current etiological and phenotypical knowledge, and searching through multidisciplinary research intermediate phenotypes either for COPD in general or for subcategories would be useful strategies.

REFERENCES

Abboud RJ, Yu P, Chan-Yeung M, Tan F: Lack of relationship between ABH secretor status and lung function in pulp mill workers. Am Rev Respir Dis 1982; 126:1089–1091.

Ackermann-Liebrich U: Outdoor air pollution. Eur Respir Mon 2000; 5(15):400–411.

Akai S, Okayama H, Shimura S, Tanno Y, Sasaki H, Takishima T: ΔF508 mutation of cystic fibrosis gene is not found in chronic bronchitis with severe obstruction in Japan. Am Rev Respir Dis 1992; 146:781–783.

American Thoracic Society: Standards for the diagnosis and care of patients with chronic obstructive pulmonary disease. Am J Respir Crit Care Med 1995; 152:S77–S120.

Anagnostopoulou U, Toumbis M, Konstanpopoulos K, Dostosovoulou-Fouskaki V, Zervas J: HLA-A and -B antigens in chronic bronchitis. J Clin Epidemiol 1993; 12:1413–1416.

André F, André C, Lambert R, Descos F: Prevalence of α_1 antitrypsin deficiency in patients with gastric or duodenal ulcer. Biomedicine 1974; 21:222–224.

α_1-Antitrypsin deficiency: Memorandum from a WHO meeting. Bull World Health Organ 1997; 75:395–415.

α_1-Antitrypsin deficiency and prenatal diagnosis. Lancet 1987; 1:421–422.

Anto JM, Vermeire P, Sunyer J: Chronic obstructive pulmonary disease. Eur Respir Mon 2000; 5(15):1–22.

Antti-Poika M, Nordman H, Koskenvuo M, Kaprio J, Jalava M. Role of occupational exposure to airway irritants in the development of asthma. Int Arch Occup Environ Health 1992; 64:195–200.

Arkinstall WW, Nirmal K, Klissouras V, Milic-Emili J: Genetic differences in the ventilatory response to inhaled CO_2. J Appl Physiol 1974; 36:6–11.

Artlich A, Boysen A, Bunge S, Entzian P, Schlaak M, Schwinger E: Common CFTR mutations are not likely to predispose to chronic bronchitis in Northern Germany. Hum Genet 1995; 95:226–228.

Barnes PJ: Molecular genetics of chronic obstructive pulmonary disease. Thorax 1999; 54:245–252.

Barrett-Connor E, Frette C: NIDDM, impaired glucose tolerance, and pulmonary function in older adults: the Rancho Bernardo study. Diabetes Care 1996; 19:1441–1444.

Batten J, Muir D, Simon G, Carter C: The prevalence of respiratory disease in heterozygotes for the gene for fibrocystic disease of the pancreas. Lancet 1963; i:1348–1350.

Beaty TH, Menkes HA, Cohen BH, Newill CA: Risk factors associated with longitudinal change in pulmonary function. Am Rev Respir Dis 1984; 129:660–667.

Becklake MR: Occupational exposures: evidence for a causal association with chronic obstructive pulmonary disease. Am Rev Respir Dis 1989; 140:S85–S91.

Becklake MR, Kauffmann F: Gender differences in airway behaviour over the human lifespan. Thorax 1999; 54:1119–1138.

Boat TF, Petty TL: Chronic bronchitis and cystic fibrosis: two chronic obstructive lung diseases of adults. Am Rev Respir Dis 1977; 116:1–2.

Boezen HM, Schouten JP, Weiss ST: The Dutch hypotheis on chronic nonspecific lung disease. Eur Respir Mon 2000; 5:37–47.

Bombieri C, Benetazzo M, Saccomani A, Belpinati F, Gilè LS, Luisetti M, Pignatti PF: Complete mutational screening of the CFTR gene in 120 patients with pulmonary disease. Hum Genet 1998; 103:718–722.

Bonney GE: On the statistical determination of major gene mechanisms in continuous human traits: regressive models. Am J Med Genet 1984; 18:731–749.

Boudik F, Goldsmith JR, Teichman V, Kauffmann PC: Epidemiology of chronic bronchitis in Prague. Bull WHO 1970; 42:711–722.

Bruce RM, Cohen BH, Diamond El, Fallat RJ, Knudson RJ, Lebowitz MD, Mittman C, Patterson CD, Tockman MS: Collaborative study to assess risk of lung disease in PIMZ phenotype subjects. Am Rev Respir Dis 1984; 130:386–390.

Burrows B: A clinical trial of efficacy of antiproteolytic therapy: can it be done? Am Rev Respir Dis 1983; 127:S42–S43.

Burrows B: Airways obstructive diseases: pathogenetic mechanisms and natural histories of the disorders. Med Clin N Am 1990; 74:547–559.

Burrows B, Niden AH, Fletcher CM, Jones NL: Clinical types of chronic obstructive lung disease in London and in Chicago. Am Rev Respir Dis 1964; 90:14–27.

Byers PH, Siegel RC, Holbrook KA, Narayanan AS, Bornstein P, Hall JG: X-linked cutis laxa: defective cross-linking formation in collagen due to decrease lysyl oxidase activity. N Engl J Med 1980; 303:61–65.

Calverley PMA, Georgopousos D: Chronic obstructive pulmonary disease: symptoms and signs. Eur Respir Mon 1998; 3(7):6–24.

Camner P, Philipson K, Friberg L: Tracheobronchial clearance in twins. Arch Environ Health 1972; 24:82–87.

Cantlay AM, Lamb D, Gillooly M: Association between the CYP1A1 gene polymorphism and susceptiblity to emphysema and lung cancer. J Clin Pathol: Mol Pathol 1995; 48:M210–M214.

Cardoso WV, Thurlbeck WM: Pathogenesis and terminology of emphysema. Am J Respir Crit Care Med 1994; 149:1383.

Cederlöf R, Edfors ML, Friberg L, Jonsson E: Hereditary factors, "spontaneous cough and smokers cough": a study on 7800 twin-pairs with the aid of mailed questionnaires. Arch Environ Health 1967; 14:401–406.

Chen Y: Genetic epidemiology of pulmonary function. Thorax 1999; 54:818–824.

Chen Y, Dosman JA, Rennie DC, Lockinger LA: Major genetic effects on airway–parenchymal dysanapsis of the lung: the Humboldt family study. Genet Epidemiol 1999; 16:95–110.

Chen Y, Horne SL, Rennie DC, Dosman JA: Segregation analysis of two lung function indices in a random sample of young families: the Humboldt family study. Genet Epidemiol 1996; 13:35–47.

Cohen AB: Opportunities for the development of specific therapeutic agents to treat emphysema. Am Rev Respir Dis 1979; 120:723–727.

Cohen BH, Ball WC, Bias WB, Brashears S, Chase GA, Diamond EL, Hsu SH, Kreiss P, Levy DA, Menkes HA, et al.: A genetic epidemiologic study of chronic obstructive pulmonary disease: I. Study design and preliminary observations. Johns Hopkins Med J 1975; 135:95–104.

Cohen BH, Bias WB, Chase GA, Diamond EL, Graves CG, Levy DA, Menkes H, Meyer MB, Permutt S, Tockman MS: Is ABH nonsecretor status a risk factor obstructive lung disease? Am J Epidemiol 1980; 111:285–291.

Cohen BH, Chase GA: Familial aggregation of chronic obstructive pulmonary disease: epidemiologic and genetic approaches. In: Litwin SD (ed). Genetic Determinants of Pulmonary Disease. New York: Dekker, 1978:201–371.

Cohen BH, Diamond EL, Graves CG, Kreiss P, Levy DA, Menkes HA, Permutt S, Quaskey S, Tockman MS: A common familial component in lung cancer and obstructive pulmonary disease. Lancet 1977; 2:523–526.

Colley JRT: Respiratory symptoms in children and parental smoking and phlegm production. Br Med J 1974; 2:201–204.

Collins RL, Turner RA, Johnson AM, Whitley NO, McLean RL: Obstructive pulmonary disease in rheumatoid arthritis. Arthritis Rheum 1976; 19:623–628.

Cox DW, Hoeppner VH, Levison H: Protease inhibitors in patients with chronic obstructive pulmonary disease: the alpha-1-antitrypsin heterozygote controversy. Am Rev Respir Dis 1976; 113:601–606.

Cox DW, Mansfield T: Prenatal diagnosis of α_1-antitrypsin deficiency and estimates of fetal risk for disease. J Med Genet 1987; 24:52–59.

Crowell RJ, Samet JM: Invited commentary: why does the white blood cell count predict mortality? Am J Epidemiol 1995; 142:499–501.

Dahl M, Nordestgaard BG, Lange P, Tybjaerg-Hansen A: Fifteen-year follow-up of pulmonary function in individuals heterozygous for the cystic fibrosis phenylalanine-508 deletion. J Allergy Clin Immunol 2001a; 107:818–823.

Dahl M, Nordestgaard BG, Lange P, Vestbo J, Tybjaerg-Hansen A: Molecular diagnosis of intermediate and severe α_1-antitrypsin deficiency: MZ individuals with chronic obstructive pulmonary disease may have lower lung function than MM individuals. Clin Chem 2001b; 47:56–62.

Dahl M, Tyaer-Hansen A, Lange P, Nordestgaard BG: ΔF508 heterozygosity in cystic fibrosis and susceptibility to asthma. Lancet 1998; 351:1911–1913.

Davidson DJ, Porteous DJ: The genetics of cystic fibrosis lung disease. Thorax 1998; 53:389–397.

Davis PB: Airway responsiveness and atopy in cystic fibrosis. In: Weiss S, Sparrow D (eds). Airway responsiveness and atopy in the development of chronic lung disease. New York: Raven Press, 1989:293–313.

De Backer W: Measures of inflammation in serum. Eur Respir Rev 1998; 8:1098–1102.

Demenais FM, Murigande C, Bonney GE: Search for faster methods of fitting the regressive models to quantitative traits. Genet Epidemiol 1990; 7:319–334.

DeSanctis GT, Merchant M, Beier DR, Dredge RD, Grobholz JK, Martin TR, Lander ES, Drazen JM: Quantitative locus analysis of airway hyperresponsiveness in A/J and C57BL/6J mice. Nat Genet 1995; 11:150–154.

Deutscher S, Higgins MW: The relationship of parental longevity to ventilatory function and prevalence of chronic nonspecific respiratory disease among sons. Am Rev Respir Dis 1970; 102:180–189.

Dirksen A, Dijkman JH, Madsen F, Stoel B, Hutchison DCS, Ulrik CS, Skovgaard LT, Kok-Jensen A, Rudophus A, Seersholm N, et al.: A randomized clinical trial of α_1-antitrypsin augmentation therapy. Am J Respir Crit Care Med 1999; 160:1468–1472.

Dirksen A, Friis M, Olesen KP, Skovgaard LT, Sorensen K: Progress of emphysema in severe alpha-1-antitrypsin deficiency as assessed by annual CT. Acta Radiol 1997; 38:826–832.

Dockery DW, Pope III A, Xu X, Spengler JD, Ware JH, Fay ME, Ferris BG, Speizer FE: An association between air pollution and mortality in six U.S. cities. N Engl J Med 1993; 329:1753–1759.

Doll R, Peto R, Wheatley K, Gray R, Sutherland I: Mortality in relation to smoking: 40 years' observations on male British doctors. Br Med J 1994; 309:901–911.

Drazen JM, Beier DR: The genetics of air pollution. Nat Genet 1997; 17:365–366.

Dumur V, Lafitte JJ, Gervais R, Debaecker D, Kestloot M, Lalau G, Roussel P: Abnormal distribution of cystic fibrosis ΔF508 allele in adults with chronic bronchial hypersecretion. Lancet 1990; 335:1340.

Eriksson S: A 30-year perspective on α_1-antitrypsin deficiency. Chest 1996; 110: 237S–242S.

Eriksson S, Moestrup T, Hagerstan I: Liver, lung and malignant disease in heterozygotes (PIMZ) α_1-antitrypsin deficiency. Acta Med Scand 1975; 198:243–247.

Evans DJ, Green M: Small airways: a time to revisit. Thorax 1998; 53:629–630.

Fagerhol MK, Cox DW: The Pi polymorphism genetic, biochemical and clinical aspects of human α_1-antitrypsin. Adv Hum Genet 1981; 11:1–62.

Falk CT, Rubinstein P: Haplotype relative risks: an easy reliable way to construct a proper control sample for risk calculations. Ann Hum Genet 1987; 51:227–33.

Feinleib M, Garrison RJ, Fabsitz R, Christian JC, Hrubec Z, Borhani NO, Kannel WB, Rosenman R, Schwartz JT, Wagner JO: The NHLBI twin study of cardiovascular disease risk factors: methodology and summary of results. Am J Epidemiol 1997; 106:284–295.

Feinleib M, Rosenberg HM, Collins JG, Delozier JG, Polenas R, Chevarley FM: Trends in COPD morbidity and mortality in the United States. Am Rev Respir Dis 1989; 140(3 Pt 2):S9–S18.

Ferris BG, Stoudt HW: Correlation of anthropometry and simple tests of pulmonary function. Arch Environ Health 1971; 22:672–676.

Fletcher CM, Peto R, Tinker CM, Speizer F: The Natural History of Chronic Bronchitis and Emphysema. Oxford: Oxford University Press, 1976.

Frette C, Jacob MP, Defouilloy C, Atassi C, Kauffmann F, Pham QT, Bignon J: Lack of a relationship of serum elastin peptide level to pulmonary emphysema assessed by high resolution computed tomography scans. Am J Respir Crit Care Med 1996; 153:1544–1547.

Frette C, Jacob MP, Wei SM, Bertrand JP, Laurent P, Kauffmann F, Pham QT: Relationship of serum elastin peptide level to single breath transfer factor for carbon monoxide in French coal miners. Thorax 1997; 52:1045–1050.

Fröhlander N, Stjernberg N: Association between haptoglobin groups and hereditary predisposition for bronchial asthma. Hum Hered 1989; 39:7–11.

Gadek JE, Crystal RG: α_1-antitrypsin deficiency. In: Stanbury JB, Wyngaarden JB, Fredrickson DS, Goldstein JL, Brown MS (eds). Metabolic Basis of Inherited Disease. New York: McGraw-Hill, 1982:1450–1467.

Garshick E, Segal MR, Worobec TG, Salekin CMS, Miller MJ: Alcohol consumption and chronic obstructive pulmonary disease. Am Rev Respir Dis 1989; 140:373–378.

Geddes DM, Webley M, Emerson PA: Airways obstruction in rheumatoid arthritis. Ann Rheum Dis 1979; 38:222–225.

Gelehrter TD, Collins FS, Ginsburg D: Principles of Medical Genetics. Baltimore: Williams and Wilkins, 1997:124–127.

Givelber RJ, Couropmitree NN, Gottlieb DJ, Evans JC, Levy D, Myers RH, O'Connor GT: Segregation analysis of pulmonary among families in the Framingham Study. Am J Respir Crit Care Med 1998; 157:1445–1451.

Gold DR, Wang X, Wypij D, Speizer FE, Ware JH, Dockery DW: Effects of cigarette smoking on lung function in adolescent boys and girls. N Engl J Med 1996; 335:931–937.

Golpon HA, Geraci MW, Moore MD, Miller HL, Miller GJ, Tuder RM, Voelkel NF: HOX genes in human lung: altered expression in primary pulmonary hypertension and emphysema. Am J Pathol 2001; 158:955–966.

Gooptu B, Hazes B, Chang WSW, Dafforn TR, Carrell RW, Read RJ, Lomas DA: Inactive conformation of the serpin α_1-antichymotrypsin indicates two-stage insertion of the reactive loop: implications for inhibitory function and conformational disease. Proc Natl Acad Sci USA 2000; 97:67–72.

Gottlieb DJ, Sparrow D, O'Connor GT, Weiss ST: Skin test reactivity to common aeroallergens and decline of lung function: the Normative Aging Study. Am J Respir Crit Care Med 1996; 153:561–566.

Green PT, Dundee JC: The association of chronic pulmonary emphysema with chronic peptic ulceration. Can Med Assoc J 1952; 67:438–439.

Gulsvik A, Fagerhol MK: α_1-antitrypsin phenotypes and obstructive lung disease in the city of Oslo. Scand J Respir Dis 1979; 60:267–274.

Haines AP, Imeson JD, Meade TW: ABH secretor status and pulmonary function. Am J Epidemiol 1982; 115:367–370.

Hallett WY, Knudson AG, Massey FJ: Absence of detrimental effect of the carrier state for the cystic fibrosis gene. Am Rev Respir Dis 1965; 92:714–724.

Hamel FA, De Carrell RW: Heterozygous α_1-antitrypsin deficiency: a longitudinal lung function study. NZ Med J 1981; 94:407–410.

Harrison DJ, Cantlay AM, Rae F, Lamb D, Smith CA: Frequency and glutathione *S*-transferase MI deletion in smokers with emphysema and lung cancer. Hum Exp Toxicol 1997; 16:356–360.

Hassan WU, Keaney NP, Holland CD, Kelly CA: Association of HLA-DR4 protease inhibitor phenotypes and keratoconjunctivitis sicca with pulmonary abnormalities in rheumatoid arthritis. Br J Rheumatol 1995; 34:37–40.

Hay JW, Robin ED: Cost-effectiveness of alpha-1-antitrypsin replacement therapy in treatment of congenital chronic obstructive pulmonary disease. Am J Public Health 1991; 81:427–433.

Hein HO, Sørensen H, Suadicani P, Gyntelberg F: Alcohol consumption, Lewis phenotypes and risk of ischaemic heart disease. Lancet 1993; 341:392–396.

Higgins ITT, Oldham PD, Kilpatrick GS, Drummond RJ, Bevan B: Blood groups of miners with coal-workers pneumoconiosis and bronchitis. Br J Ind Med 1963; 20:324–329.

Higgins MW, Keller JB: Familial occurrence of chronic respiratory disease and familial resemblance in ventilatory capacity. J Chronic Dis 1975; 28:239–251.

Higgins MW, Keller JB: Trends in COPD morbidity and mortality in Tecumseh, Michigan. Am Rev Respir Dis 1989; 140:S42–S48.

Higgins MW, Keller JB, Becker M, Howatt W, Landis JR, Rotman H, Weg JW, Higgins I: An index of risk for obstructive airway disease. Am Rev Respir Dis 1982; 125:144–151.

Higham MA, Pride NB, Alikhan A, Morrell NW: Tumour necrosis factor-α gene promoter polymorphism in chronic obstructive pulmonary disease. Eur Respir J 2000; 15:281–284.

Hillderdal G, Sapvenberg J: HLA B27: a risk factor for lung disease? Lancet 1983; 2:1195.

Hogg J: Latent adenoviral infections in the pathogenesis of COPD. Eur Respir Rev 1997; 7:216–220.

Hogg JC, Macklem PR, Thurlbeck WM: Site and nature of airway obstruction in chronic obstructive lung disease. N Engl J Med 1968; 278:1356–1360.

Holberg CJ, Morgan WJ, Wright AL, Martinez FD: Differences in familial segregation of FEV_1 between asthmatic and nonasthmatic families. Am J Respir Crit Care Med 1998; 158:162–169.

Hoo AF, Henschen M, Dezateux C, Costeloe K, Stocks J: Respiratory function among preterm infants whose mothers smoked during pregnancy. Am J Respir Crit Care Med 1998; 158:700–705.

Horne SL, Cockroft DW, Dosman JA: Possible protective effect against chronic obstructive airways disease by the GC2 allele. Hum Hered 1990; 40:173–176.

Horne SL, Cockroft DW, Lovegrove A, Dosman JA: ABO, Lewis and secretor status and relative incidence of airflow obstruction. Dis Markers 1985; 3:55–62.

Huang SL, Su CH, Chang SC: Tumor necrosis factor-α gene polymorphism in chronic bronchitis. Am J Respir Crit Care Med 1997; 156:1436–1439.

Hubbard RC, Crystal RG: Alpha-1-antitrypsin augmentation therapy for alpha-1-antitrypsin deficiency. J Am Med Assoc 1988; 84(suppl 6A):52–62.

Hubert HB, Fabsitz RR, Feinleib M, Gwinn C: Genetic and environmental influences on pulmonary function in adult twins. Am Rev Respir Dis 1982; 125:409–415.

Hutchison DCS: α-1-antitrypsin deficiency in Europe: geographical distribution of Pi types S and Z. Respir Med 1998; 92:367–377.

Hutchison DCS, Hughes MD: Alpha-1-antitrypsin replacement therapy: will its efficacy ever be proved? Eur Respir J 1997; 10:2191–2193.

Ishii T, Matsuse T, Teramoto S, Matsui H, Hosoi T, Fukuchi Y, Ouchi Y: Association between alpha-1-antichymotrypsin polymorphism and susceptibility to chronic obstructive pulmonary disease. Eur J Clin Invest 2000; 30:543–548.

Ishii T, Matsuse T, Teramoto S, Matsui H, Miyao M, Hosoi T, Takahashi H, Fukuchi Y, Ouchi Y: Glutathione S-transferase P1 (GSTP1) polymorphism in patients with chronic obstructive pulmonary disease. Thorax 1999; 54:693–696.

Jaakkola MS: Environmental tobacco smoke and respiratory disease. Eur Respir Mon 2000; 5(15):322–383.

Janoff A: Emphysema: proteinase-antiproteinase imbalance. In: Gallin JI, Goldstein IM, Snyderman R (eds). Inflammation: basic principles and clinical correlates. New York: Raven Press, 1988:803–814.

Jarvis D, Chinn S, Sterne J, Luczynska C, Burney on behalf of the European Community Respiratory Health Survey: the association of respiratory symptoms and lung function with the use of gas for cooking. Eur Respir J 1998; 11:651–658.

Johnston IDA, Strachan DP, Anderson HR: Effect of pneumonia and whooping cough in childhood on adult lung function. N Engl J Med 1998; 338:581–586.

Kalsheker NA, Watkings GL, Hill S, Morgan K, Stockley RA, Fick RB: Independent mutations in the flanking sequence of the alpha-1-antitrypsin gene are associated with chronic obstructive airways disease. Dis Markers 1990; 8:151–157.

Kauffmann F: Increase of ABH nonsecretor among relatives of COPD patients. Am J Epidemiol 1982; 115:298–300.

Kauffmann F: Genetics of chronic obstructive pulmonary diseases: searching for their heterogeneity. Bull Eur Physiopathol Respir 1984; 20:163–210.

Kauffmann F: Selection bias of PIMZ subjects. Am Rev Respir Dis 1985; 131:800.

Kauffmann F, Becklake MR: Sex and gender. Eur Respir Mon 2000; 5(15):288–304.

Kauffmann F, Brille D: Bronchial hypersecretion, chronic airflow limitation and peptic ulcer. Am Rev Respir Dis 1981; 124:646–649.

Kauffmann F, Drouet D, Lellouch J, Brille D: Twelve years spirometric changes among Paris area workers. Int J Epidemiol 1979; 8:201–212.

Kauffmann F, Drouet D, Lellouch J, Brille D: Occupational exposure and 12-year spirometric changes among Paris area workers. Br J Ind Med 1982; 39:221–232.

Kauffmann F, Frette C, Annesi I, Oryszczyn MP, Doré MF, Neukirch F: Relationships of haptoglobin level to FEV_1, wheezing, bronchial hyperresponsiveness and allergy. Clin Exp Allergy 1991; 21:669–674.

Kauffmann F, Frette C, Pham QT, Nafissi S, Bertrand JP, Oriol R: Associations of blood group-related antigens to FEV_1, wheezing, and asthma. Am J Respir Crit Care Med 1996; 153:76–82.

Kauffmann F, Kleisbauer JP, Cambon-de-Mouzon A, Mercier P, Constans J, Blanc M, Rouch Y, Feingold N: Genetic markers in chronic air-flow limitation. Am Rev Respir Dis 1983a; 127:263–269.

Kauffmann F, Tager IB, Muñoz A, Speizer FE. Familial factors related to lung function in children aged 6–10 years: results from the PAARC epidemiological study. Am J Epidemiol 1989; 129:1289–1299.

Kauffmann F, Tessier JF, Oriol P: Adult passive smoking in the home environment: a risk factor for chronic airflow limitation. Am J Epidemiol 1983b; 117:269–280.

Kawakami Y, Yamamoto H, Yoshikawa T, Shida A: Respiratory chemosensitivity in smokers: Studies on monozygote twins. Am Rev Respir Dis 1982; 126:986–990.

Keatings VM, Cave SJ, Henry MJ, Morgan K, O'Connor CM, Fitzgerald MX, Kalsheker N: A polymorphism in the tumor necrosis factor-α gene promoter region may predispose to a poor prognosis in COPD. Chest 2000; 118:971–975.

Khoury MJ: Relationship between medical genetics and public health: changing the paradigm of disease prevention and the definition of a genetic disease. Am J Med Genet 1997; 71:289–291.

Khoury MJ, Beaty TH, Newill S, Bryant S, Cohen BH: Genetic–environmental interactions in chronic airways obstruction. Int J Epidemiol 1986; 15:65–72.

Khoury MJ, Beaty TH, Tockman MS, Selj SG, Cohen BH: Familial aggregation in chronic obstructive pulmonary disease: use of the loglinear model to analyse intermediate environmental and genetic risk factors. Genet Epidemiol 1985; 2:155–166.

Khoury MJ, Wagener DK: Epidemiological evaluation of the use of genetics to improve the predictive value of disease risk factors. Am J Hum Genet 1995; 56:835–844.

Kleeberger SR, Levitt RC, Zhang LY: Susceptibility to ozone-induced inflammation: I. Genetic control of the response to subacute exposure. Am J Physiol 1993a; 264:L15–L20.

Kleeberger SR, Levitt RC, Zhang LY: Susceptibility to ozone-induced inflammation: II. Separate loci control responses to acute and subacute exposures. Am J Physiol 1993b; 264: L21–L26.

Kleeberger SR, Levitt RC, Zhang LY, Longphre M, Harkema J, Jedlicka A, Eleff SM, Disilvestre D, Holroyd KJ: Linkage analysis of susceptibility to ozone-induced lung inflammation in inbred mice. Nat Genet 1997; 17:475–478.

Kleeberger SR, Reddy S, Zhang LY, Jedlicka AE: Genetic susceptibility to ozone-induced lung hyperpermeability: role of toll-like receptor 4. Am J Respir Cell Biol 2000; 22:620–627.

Koyama H, Geddes DM: Genes, oxidative stress and the risk of chronic obstructive pulmonary disease. Thorax 1998; 53(suppl2):S10–S14.

Krzyzanowski M, Jedrychowski W, Wysocki M: ABO blood group system and cigarette smoking: interaction in chronic airways obstruction. Int J Epidemiol 1987; 16:293–294.

Krzyzanowski M, Sherrill DL, Lebowitz MD: Longitudinal analysis of the acute lower respiratory illnesses on pulmonary function in an adult population. Am J Epidemiol 1990; 131:412–422.

Küçükaycan M, Nicklin MJH, Buurman WA, Dentener MA, Wouters EFM: COPD is associated with IL-10 (−1117) polymorphism. Am J Respir Crit Care Med 2001; 163:A 693.

Kueppers F: Chronic obstructive pulmonary disease. In: King RA, Rotter JI, Motulsky AG (eds). The Genetic Basis of Common Diseases. New York: Oxford University Press, 1992:220–239.

Kueppers F, Dönhardt A: Obstructive lung disease in heterozygotes for alpha-1-antitrypsin deficiency. Ann Inten Med 1974; 80:209–212.

Kueppers F, Miller RD, Gordon H, Heppe NG, Offord K: Familial prevalence of chronic obstructive pulmonary disease in a matched pair study. Am J Med 1977; 63:1336–1342.

Kurzius-Spencer M, Holberg CJ, Martinez FD, Sherrill DL: Familial correlation and segregation analysis of forced expiratory volume in one second (FEV_1), with and without smoking adjustments, in a Tucson population. Ann Hum Biol 2001; 28:222–234.

Lalouel JM, Morton NE. Complex segregation analysis with pointers. Hum Hered 1981; 31:312–321.

Lange P, Groth S, Mortensen J, Appleyard M, Nyboe J, Jensen G, Schnohr P: Pulmonary function is influenced by heavy alcohol consumption. Am Rev Respir Dis 1988; 137:1119–1123.

Lange P, Groth S, Mortensen J, Appleyard M, Nyboe J, Schnohr P, Jensen G: Diabetes mellitus and ventilatory capacity: a five-year follow-up study. Eur Respir J 1990; 3:288–292.

Lange P, Parner J, Vestbo J, Schnohr P, Jensen G: A 15-year follow-up study of ventilatory function in adults with asthma. N Engl J Med 1998; 339:1194–1200.

Langlois MR, Delanghe JR: Biological and clinical significance of haptoglobin polymorphism in humans. Clin Chem 1996; 42:1589–1600.

Larson RK, Barman ML, Kueppers F, Fudenberg HH: Genetic and environmental determinants of chronic obstructive pulmonary disease. Ann Int Med 1970; 72:627–632.

Laurell CB, Eriksson S: The electrophoretic α_1-globulin pattern of serum in α_1-antitrypsin deficiency. Scand J Clin Lab Invest 1963; 15:132–140.

Lazarus R, Sparrow D, Weiss ST: Impaired ventilatory function and elevated insulin levels in nondiabetic males: the Normative Aging study. Eur Respir J 1998; 12:635–640.

Lebowitz MD, Knudson RJ, Burrows B: Familial concordance of pulmonary function measurements. Am Rev Respir Dis 1984; 129:8–11.

Lewitter FI, Tager IB, McGue M, Tishler PV, Speizer FE: Genetic and environmental determinants of level of pulmonary function. Am J Epidemiol 1984; 120:518–529.

Lim S, Roche N, Oliver BG, Mattos W, Barnes PJ, Fan Chung K: Balance of matrix metalloprotease-9 and tissue inhibitor of metalloprotease-1 from alveolar macrophages in cigarette smokers: regulation by interleukin-10. Am J Respir Crit Care Med 2000; 162(4 Pt 1):1355–1360.

Lindmark BE, Arborelus M, Erikson SG: Pulmonary function in middle-aged women with heterozygous deficiency of the serine protease inhibitor α_1-antichymotrypsin. Am Rev Respir Dis 1990; 141:884–888.

Louis PCA: Recherches sur l'emphysème des poumons. Mem Soc Med Obs 1837; 1:160–261.

Luisetti M, Pignatti PF: The search for susceptibility genes of COPD. Monaldi Arch Chest Dis 1995; 50:28–32.

March TH, Barr EB, Finch GL, Hahan FF, Hobbs CH, Ménache MG, Nikula KJ: Cigarette smoke exposure produces more evidence of emphysema in B6CF1 mice than in F344 rats. Toxicol Sci 1999; 51:289–299.

McClearn GE, Svartengren M, Pedersen NL, Heller DA, Plomin R: Genetic and environmental influences on pulmonary function in aging Swedish twins. J Gerontol 1994; 49:M264–M268.

McConnell RB: Secretion of blood group antigens in gastrointestinal disease. Gastroenterologia 1959; 92:103–113.

McElvaney NG, Stoller JK, Buist AS, Prakash UBS, Brantly ML, Schluchter MD, Crystal RD: α_1-antitrypsin deficiency registry: baseline characteristics of enrollees in the national heart, lung and blood institute registry of α_1-antitrypsin deficiency. Chest 1997; 111:394–403.

McNeil TF, Thelin T, Aspegren-Jansson E, Sveger T, Harty B: Psychological factors in cost–benefit analysis of somatic prevention: a study of the psychological effects of neonatal screening for α_1-antitrypsin deficiency. Acta Paediatr Scand 1985; 74:427–432.

Mead J: Dysanapsis in normal lungs assessed by the relationship between maximal flow, static recoil and vital capacity. Am Rev Respir Dis 1980; 121:339–342.

Mittman C: α_1-antitrypsin deficiency and other genetic factors in lung disease. In: P Macklem, S Permutt (eds). The Lung in the Transition between Health and Disease. New York: Dekker, 1979:245–269.

Morse JO, Lebowitz MD, Knudson TJ, Burrows B: Relation of protease inhibitor phenotypes to obstructive lung diseases in a community. N Engl J Med 1977; 296:1190–1194.

Mossberg B, Afzelius BA, Eliasson R, Camner P: On the pathogenesis of obstructive lung disease: a study on the immotile-cilia syndrome. Scand J Respir Dis 1978; 59:55–65.

Mourant AE, Kopec AC, Domaniewska-Sobczak K: Blood Groups and Diseases: A Study of Associations of Diseases with Blood Groups and Other Polymorphisms. Oxford: Oxford University Press, 1978.

Murphy TF, Sethi S: Bacterial infection in chronic obstructive pulmonary disease. Am Rev Respir 1992; 146:1067–1083.

Murray CJL, Lopez AD: Alternative projections of mortality and disability by cause 1990–2020: Global Burden of Disease study. Lancet 1997; 349:1498–1504.

Mustafa KY: Spirometric lung function tests in normal men of African ethnic origin. Am Rev Respir Dis 1977; 116:209–213.

Novoradovsky A, Brantly ML, Waclawiw MA, Chaudhary PP, Ihara H, Qi L, Eissa T, Barnes PM, Gabriele KM, Ehrmantraut ME, et al.: Endothelial nitric oxide synthase as a potential susceptiblity gene in the pathogenesis of emphysema in α_1-antitrypsin deificiency. Am J Respir Cell Mol Biol 1999; 20:441–447.

Omran H, Häffner K, Völkel A, Kuehr J, Ketelsen UP, Ross UH, Konietzko N, Wienker T, Brandis M, Hildebrandt F: Homozygosity mapping of a gene locus for primary ciliary dyskinesia on chromosome 5p and identification of the heavy dynein chain DNAH5 as a candidate gene. Am J Respir Cell Mol Biol 2000; 23:696–702.

Oriol R: ABO, Hl, Lewis and secretion: serology, genetics and tissue distribution. In: Cartron JP, Rouger P (eds). Blood Cell Biochemistry: Vol 6. Molecular Basis of Major Blood Group Antigens. New York: Plenum Press, 1995:37–73.

Orzalesi MM, Kohner D, Cook CD, Schwachman H: Anamnesis, sweat electrolyte and pulmonary function studies in parents of patients with cystic fibrosis of the pancreas. Acta Paediatr 1963; 52:267–276.

Oswald NC, Harold JT, Martin WJ: Clinical pattern of chronic bronchitis. Lancet 1953; 2:639–643.

Ottman R: An epidemiologic approach to gene–environment interaction. Genet Epidemiol 1990; 7:177–185.

Palmer LJ, Knuiman MW, Divitini ML, Burton PR, James AL, Bartholomew HC, Ryan G, Musk AW: Familial aggregation and heritability of adult lung function: results from the Busselton health study. Eur Respir J 2001; 17:696–702.

Panhuysen CIM, Bleecker E, Koeter GH, Meyers DA, Postma DS: Characterization of obstructive airway disease in family members of probands with asthma: an algorithm for the diagnosis of asthma. Am J Respir Crit Care Med 1998; 157:1734–1742.

Paré PD, Bai TR: Airway remodeling in chronic obstructive pulmonary disease. Eur Respir Rev 1998; 6:259–263.

Patuzzo C, Gilè LS, Zorzetto M, Trabetti E, Malerba G, Pignatti PF, Luisetti M: Tumor necrosis factor gene complex in COPD and disseminated bronchiectasis. Chest 2000; 117:1353–1358.

Pauwels RA, Buist AS, Calverley PM, Jenkins CR, Hurd SS: Global strategy for the diagnosis, management, and prevention of chronic obstructive pulmonary disease: NHLBI/WHO Global Initiative for Chronic Obstructive Lung Disease (GOLD) workshop summary. Am J Respir Crit Care Med 2001; 163:1256–1276.

Pier GB, Grout M, Zaidi T, Meluleni G, Mueschenborn SS, Banting G, Ratcliff R, Evans MJ, Colledge WH: Salmonella typhi uses CFTR to enter intestinal epithelial cells. Nature 1998; 393:79–82.

Poller W, Faber JP, Weidinger S, Tief K, Scholz S, Fischer M, Olek K, Kirchgesser M, Heidtmann HH: A leucine-to proline substitution causes a defective α_1-antichymotrypsin allele associated with familial obstructive lung disease. Genomics 1993; 17:640–743.

Postma DS, Siafakas NM: Management of Chronic Obstructive Pulmonary Disease. Eur Respir Mon 1998; 3(7):1–302.

Pratt PC, Vollmer RT: Effect of alcohol consumption on emphysema or pulmonary function. Am Rev Respir Dis 1988; 138:1358–1359.

Pride NB, Vermeire P: Definition and differential diagnosis. Eur Respir Mon 1998; 7:2–5.

Prows DR, Shertzer HG, Daly MJ, Sidman CL, Leikauf GD: Genetics analysis of ozone-induced acute lung injury in sensitive and resistant strains of mice. Nat Genet 1997; 17:471–474.

Radoux V, Cantin A, Bégin R, Masse S, Decarie F, Ménard HA: Airway disease in rheumatoid patients: a genetic predisposition. Am Rev Respir Dis 1980; 146:41–48.

Ramphal R, Carnoy C, Fievre S, Michalsky JC, Houdret N, Lamblin G, Strecker G, Roussel P: *Pseudomonas aeruginosa* recognizes carbohydrate chains containing type 1 (Galβ 1-3GlcNAc) or type 2 (Galβ 1-4GlcNAc) disaccharide units. Infect Immun 1991; 59:700–704.

Raza MW, Blackwell CC, Molyneaux P, James VS, Ogilvie MM, Inglis JM, Weir DM: Association between secretor status respiratory viral illness. Br Med J 1991; 303:815–818.

Redline S, Tishler PV, Lewitter FI, Tager IB, Muñoz A, Speizer FE: Assessment of genetic and nongenetic influences on pulmonary function: a twin study. Am Rev Respir Dis 1987; 135:217–222.

Redline S, Tishler PV, Rosner B, Lewitter FI, Vandenburgh M, Weiss ST, Speizer FE: Genotypic and phenotypic similarities in pulmonary function among family members of adult monozygotic and dizygotic twins. Am J Epidemiol 1989; 129:827–836.

Redline S, Weiss ST: Genetic and perinatal risk factors for the development of chronic obstructive pulmonary disease. In: Hensley MJ, Saunders NA (eds). Clinical Epidemiology of Chronic Obstructive Pulmonary Disease. New York: Dekker, 1989:139–168.

Rennard SI: COPD: overview of definitions, epidemiology, and factors influencing its development. Chest 1998; 113:235s–241s.

Rijcken B, Britton J: Epidemiology of chronic obstructive pulmonary disease. Eur Respir Mon 1998; 3(7):41–73.

Rijcken B, Schouten JP, Xu X, Rosner B, Weiss ST: Airway hyperresponsiveness to histamine is associated with accelerated decline of FEV_1. Am J Respir Crit Care Med 1995; 151:1377–1382.

Rossing MA: Genetic influences on smoking: candidate genes. Env Health Persp 1998; 106:231–238.

Rossiter CE, Weill H: Ethnic differences in lung function: evidence for proportional differences. Int J Epidemiol 1974; 3:55–61.

Rotter JI: The genetics of peptic ulcer: more than one gene, more than one disease. Prog Med Genet 1980; 4:1–58.

Rybicki BA, Beaty TH, Cohen BH: Major genetic mechanism in pulmonary function. J Clin Epidemiol 1990; 43:667–675.

Samet JM: Definitions and methodology in COPD research. In: Hensley MJ, Saunders NA (eds). Clinical Epidemiology of Chronic Obstructive Pulmonary Disease. New York: Dekker, 1989:1–23.

Samet JM, Tager IB, Speizer FE: The relationship between respiratory illness in childhood and chronic air-flow obstruction in adulthood. Am Rev Respir Dis 1983; 127:508–523.

Sandford AJ, Chagani T, Weir TD, Connett JE, Anthonisen NR, Paré PD: Susceptibility genes for rapid decline of lung function in the Lung Health Study. Am J Respir Crit Care Med 2001; 163:469–473.

Sandford AJ, Chagani T, Weir TD, Paré PD: α_1-antichymotrypsin mutations in patients with chronic obstructive pulmonary disease. Dis Markers 1998; 13:257–260.

Sandford AJ, Paré PD: Genetic risk factors for chronic obstructive pulmonary disease. Clin Chest Med 2000; 21:633–643.

Sandford AJ, Spinelli JJ, Weir TD, Paré PD: Mutation in the 3′ region of the α-1-antitrypsin gene and chronic obstructive pulmonary disease. J Med Genet 1997a; 34: 874–875.

Sandford AJ, Weir TD, Paré PD: Genetic risk factors for chronic obstructive pulmonary disease. Eur Respir J 1997b; 10:1380–1391.

Sandler M: Is the lung a "target organ" in diabetes mellitus? Arch Intern Med 1990; 150:1385–1388.

Schaid DJ: Transmission disequilibrium, family controls, and great expectations. Am J Hum Genet 1998; 63:935–941.

Schellenberg D, Paré PD, Weir TD, Spinelli JJ, Walker BAM, Sandford AJ: Vitamin D binding protein variants and the risk of COPD. Am J Respir Crit Care Med 1998; 157:957–961.

Schork NJ: Genetics of complex disease: approaches, problems, and solutions. Am J Respir Crit Care Med 1997; 156:S103–S109.

Schriver EE, Davidson JM, Sutcliffe MC, Swindell BB, Bernard GR: Comparison of elastin peptide concentrations in body fluids from healthy volunteers, smokers and patients with chronic obstructive pulmonary disease. Am Rev Respir Dis 1992; 145:762–766.

Schulte PA: A conceptual framework for the validation and use of biological markers. Env Res 1989; 48:129–144.

Schünemann HJ, Grant BJB, Frudenheim JL, Muti P, Browne RW, Drake JA, Klocke RA, Trevisan M: The relation of serum levels of antioxidant vitamins C and E, retinol and carotenoids with pulmonary function in the general population. Am J Respir Crit Care Med 2001; 163:1246–1255.

Schwaiblmair M, Vogelmeier C: α_1-antitrypsin: hope on the horizon for emphysema sufferers? Drug Aging 1998; 12:429–440.

Seersholm N, Wencker M, Banik N, Viskum K, Dirksen A, Kok-Jensen A, Konietzko N, WATL α_1-AT study group: Does α_1-antitrypsin augmentation therapy slow the annual decline in FEV_1 in patients with severe hereditary α_1-antitrypsin deficiency? Eur Respir J 1997; 10:2260–2263.

Shaheen SO, Barker DJP, Shiell AW, Crocker FJ, Wield GA, Holgate ST: The relationship between pneumonia in early childhood and impaired lung function in late adult life. Am J Respir Crit Care Med 1994; 149:616–619.

Sherrill DL, Lebowitz MD, Halonen M, Barbee RA, Burrows B: Longitudinal evaluation of the association between pulmonary function and total serum IgE. Am J Respir Crit Care Med 1995; 152:98–102.

Shigeoka JW, Hall WJ, Hyde RW, Schwartz RH, Mudholkar GS, Speers DM, Lin CC: The prevalence of alpha-1-antitrypsin heterozygotes (PIMZ) in patients with obstructive pulmonary disease. Am Rev Respir Dis 1976; 114:1077–1084.

Siafakas NM, Vermeire P, Pride NB, Paoletti P, Gibson J, Howard P, Yernault JC, Decrame M, Higenbottam T, Postma DS, Rees J, on Behalf of the Task Force: ERS consensus statement: optimal assessment and management of chronic obstructive pulmonary disease (COPD). Eur Respir J 1995; 8:1398–1420.

Silverman EK, Chapman HA, Drazen JM, Weiss ST, Rosner B, Campbell EJ, O'Donnell WJ, Reilly JJ, Ginns L, Mentzer S, et al.: Genetic epidemiology of severe, early-onset chronic obstructive pulmonary disease: risk to relatives for airflow obstruction and chronic bronchitis. Am J Respir Crit Care Med 1998; 157:1770–1778.

Silverman EK, Miletich JP, Pierce JA, Sherman LA, Endicott SK, Broze GJ, Campbell EJ: Alpha-1-antitrypsin deficiency: high prevalence in the St. Louis area determined by direct population screening. Am Rev Respir Dis 1989; 140:961–966.

Silverman EK, Mosley JD, Chapman HA, Drazen JM, Speizer FE, Campbell EJ, Reilly JJ, Ginns LC, Weiss ST: Genome screen linkage analysis of severe, early onset COPD. Am J Respir Crit Care Med 2001; 163:A909.

Silverman EK, Province MA, Campbell EJ, Pierce JA, Rao DC: Variability of pulmonary function in alpha-1-antitrypsin deficiency: residual family resemblance beyond the effect of the Pi locus. Hum Hered 1990; 40:340–355.

Sjöstedt L, Willers S, Ørbæk P: Human leukocyte antigens in occupational allergy: a possible protective effect of HLA-B16 in laboratory animal allergy. Am J Ind Med 1996; 30:415–420.

Sluiter HJ, Koeter GH, de Monchy JGR, Postma DS, de Vries K, Orie NGM: The Dutch hypothesis (chronic non-specific lung disease) revisited. Eur Respir J 1991; 4:479–489.

Smith CAD, Harrison DJ: Association between polymorphism in gene for microsomal epoxide hydrolase and susceptibility to emphysema. Lancet 1997; 350:630–633.

Snider GL: Emphysema: the first two centuries—and beyond—a historical overview with suggestions for future research: Part 2. Am Rev Respir Dis 1992; 146:1615–1622.

Snider GL: Defining chronic obstructive pulmonary disease. In: Calverley P, Pride N (eds). Chronic Obstructive Pulmonary Disease. London: Chapman and Hall, 1995a:1–8.

Snider GL: What's in a name? Names, definitions, descriptions, and diagnostic criteria of diseases, with emphasis on chronic obstructive pulmonary disease. Respiration 1995b; 62:297–301.

Snider GL, Lucey EC, Stone PJ: Animal models of emphysema. Am Rev Respir Dis 1986; 133:149–169.

Speizer FE, Tager IB: Epidemiology of chronic mucus hypersecretion and obstructive airways disease. Epidemiol Rev 1979; 1:124–142.

Spielman RS, McGinnis RE, Ewens WJ: Transmission test for linkage disequilibrium: the insulin gene region and insulin-dependent diabetes mellitus (IDDM). Am J Hum Genet 1993; 52:506–516.

Stoller JK: Clinical features and natural history of severe α_1-antitrypsin deficiency. Chest 1997; 111(suppl):123s–128s.

Stone PJ, Gottlieb DJ, O'Connor GT, Ciccolella DE, Breuer R, Bryan-Rhadfi J, Shaw HA, Franzblau C, Snider GL: Elastin and collagen degradation products in urine of smokers with and without chronic obstructive pulmonary disease. Am J Respir Crit Care Med 1995; 151:952–959.

Sugiyama Y, Kudoh S, Maeda H, Suzaki H, Takaku F: Analysis of HLA antigens in patients with diffuse panbronchiolitis. Am Rev Respir Dis 1990; 141:1459–1462.

Tabak C, Arts ICW, Smit HA, Heederik D, Kromhout D: Chronic obstructive pulmonary disease and intake of catechins, flavonols and flavones: the Morgen study. Am J Respir Crit Care Med 2001, 164:61–64.

Tager IB, Rosner B, Tishler PV, Speizer FE, Kars EH: Household aggregation of pulmonary function and chronic bronchitis. Am Rev Respir Dis 1976; 114:485–492.

Talamo RC, Blennerhasset JB, Austen KF: Familial emphysema and alpha-1-antitrypsin deficiency. N Engl J Med 1966: 275:1301–1304.

Tarjan E, Magyar P, Vaczi Z, Lantos A, Vaszar L: Longitudinal lung function study in heterozygous PIMZ phenotype subjects. Eur Respir J 1994; 7:2199–2204.

Thelin T, Sveger T, McNeil TF: Primary prevention in a high-risk group: smoking habits in adolescents with homozygous alpha-1-antitrypsin deficiency (ATD). Acta Paediatr 1996; 85:1207–1212.

Thurlbeck WM: Chronic Airflow Obstruction in Lung Disease. Philadephia: Saunders, 1976.

Thurlbeck WM: The pathology of small airways in chronic airflow limitation. Eur J Respir Dis 1982; 63:9–18.

Tokuhata GK, Lilienfeld AM: Familial aggregation of lung cancer in humans. J Natl Cancer Inst 1963; 30:289–312.

Turino GM, Barker AF, Brantly ML, Cohen AB, Connelly RP, Crystal RG, Eden E, Schluchter MD, Stoller JK: Clinical features of individuals with PI*SZ phenotype of α_1-antitrypsin deficiency. Am J Respir Crit Care Med 1996; 154:1718–1725.

Van der Wal AM, Huizinga E, Orie NGM, Sluiter JH, De Vries K: Cancer and chronic non specific lung disease (CNSLD). Scand J Respir Dis 1966; 47:161–172.

Vergnenègre A, Pugnere N, Antonini MT, Arnaud M, Melloni B, Treves R, Bonnaud F: Airway obstruction and rheumatoid arthritis. Eur Respir J 1997; 10:1072–1078.

Vermeire PA, Pride NB. A"splitting" look at chronic nonspecific lung disease (CNSLD): common features but diverse pathogenesis. Eur Respir J 1991; 4:490–496.

Vestbo J, Hein HO, Suaddicani P, Sørensen H, Gyntelberg F: Genetic markers for chronic bronchitis and peak expiratory flow in the Copenhagen Male Study. Dan Med Bull 1993; 40:378–380.

Vestbo J, Knudsen KM, Rasmussen FV: Are respiratory symptoms and chronic airflow limitation really associated with an increased risk of respiratory cancer? Int J Epidemiol 1991; 20:375–378.

Vestbo J, Prescott E: Update on the "Dutch hypothesis" for chronic respiratory disease. Thorax 1998; 53:S15–S19.

Vestbo J, Prescott E, Lange P, Jensen G, Schnohr P, Appleyard M, Nyboe J, Gronbaek M: Association of chronic mucus hypersecretion with FEV(1) decline and chronic obstructive pulmonary disease morbidity. Am J Respir Crit Care Med 1996; 153:1530–1535.

Vignola AM, Riccobono L, Mirabella A, Profita M, Chanez P, Bellia V, Mautino G, D'accardi P, Bousquet J, Bonsignore G: Sputum metalloproteinase-9/tissue inhibitor of metalloproteinase-1 ratio correlates with airflow obstruction in asthma and chronic bronchitis. Am J Respir Crit Care Med 1998; 158:1945–1950.

Webb DR, Condemi JJ: Selective immunoglobulin A deficiency and chronic obstructive lung disease: a family study. Ann Intern Med 1974; 125:158–162.

Weiss ST: Early life predictors of adult chronic obstructive lung disease. Eur Respir Rev 1995; 31:303–309.

Wencker M, Fuhrmann B, Banik N, Konietzko N: Longitudinal follow-up of patients with α_1-protease inhibitor deficiency before and during therapy with IV α_1-protease inhibitor. Chest 2001; 119:737–744.

Wickle JTR: Late onset genetic disease: where ignorance is bliss, is it folly to inform relatives? Br Med J 1998; 317:744–747.

Wilk JB, Djousse L, Arnett DK, Rich SS, Province MA, Hunt SC, Crapo RO, Higgins M, Myers RH: Evidence for major genes influencing pulmonary function in the NHLBI family heart study. Genet Epidemiol 2000; 19:81–94.

Xu X, Yang J, Chen C, Wang B, Jin Y, Fang Z, Wang X, Weiss ST: Familial aggregation of pulmonary function in a rural Chinese community. Am J Respir Crit Care Med 1999; 160:1928–1933.

Yamada N, Yamaya M, Okinaga S, Nakayama K, Sekizawa K, Shibahara S, Sasaki H: Microsatellite polymorphism in the heme oxygenase-1 gene promoter is associated with susceptibility to emphysema. Am J Hum Genet 2000; 66:187–195.

Yang Q, Khoury MJ: Evolving methods in genetic epidemiology: III. Gene–environment interaction in epidemiologic research. Am J Epidemiol 1997; 19:33–43.

Yim JJ, Park GY, Lee CT, Kim YW, Han SK, Shim YS, Yoo CG: Genetic susceptibility to chronic obstructive pulmonary disease in Koreans: combined analysis of polymorphic genotypes for microsomal epoxide hydrolase and glutathione S-tranferase M1 and T1. Thorax 2000; 55:121–125.

Yoshikawa M, Hiyama K, Ishioka S, Maeda H, Maeda A, Yamakido M: Microsomal epoxide hydrolase genotype and chronic obstructive pulmonary disease in Japanese. Int J Mol Med 2000; 5:49–53.

Part III

IMMUNOLOGIC AND INFECTIOUS DISEASES

10 Genetics of Human Susceptibility to Infectious Diseases: Progress and Prospects

ELLEN BUSCHMAN, EMIL SKAMENE, AND ERWIN SCHURR

In 1999, of a global total of 55.9 million deaths, 9.9 million were due to infectious and parasitic diseases (excluding respiratory infections). The leading killers among infectious diseases were human immunodeficiency virus/acquired immunodeficiency syndrome (HIV/AIDS, 2.6 million), diarrheal diseases (2.2 million), tuberculosis (1.6 million), and malaria (1 million) (WHO, 2000a). Why are these diseases such a public health threat, when most of them are either preventable or curable? Why are there no vaccines to prevent these diseases? Why do these diseases still frequently occur in epidemics? Answers to these questions can be found in the variable wealth of nations, the behavioral pattern of individuals, the state of our environment, the adaptive abilities of pathogens, and our own genetic constitution. Although in this chapter we focus exclusively on the role of genetics in infectious disease susceptibility, we first put the role of genetics in the context of overall susceptibility to infection.

A person's genetic constitution is one component of a complex interaction between external, environmental factors and genes that regulate resistance to infection. Certain infectious diseases have been endemic in developing nations for centuries, and the link between urban overcrowding, unsafe water, poor sanitation, inadequate nutrition, and the spread of infection is well known. From a public health perspective, it is obvious that these strong environmental factors of infection must be brought under control if any real gains in therapy are to be realized. Also, pathogens are continually expanding their habitat, through international travel of some 1.4 billion travelers per year (WHO, 2000b). Moreover, climatic changes, such as global warming and El Niño/southern oscillation, have been associated with changes in malaria and cholera incidence (Jan Bouma and Dye, 1997). Yet another variable in the formula for disease susceptibility comes from adaptive changes in pathogens and their carriers to infect populations with little established immunity. For example, the *Anopheles* mosquito, carrier of malaria, has become adapted to certain highland areas of Africa as well as urban centers, and the *Aedes* mosquito, carrier of dengue fever, has become established in the southwestern United States. Finally, certain pathogens have crossed species barriers, which explains the appearance of some of the 30 previously unknown human pathogens which have been identified since 1973 (WHO, 1999).

The correction of environmental problems and world poverty is likely to be a long struggle; thus, the identification of population-based genetic defenses in tandem with the availability of the draft human genome sequence has become a crucial link in the fight against infectious diseases. How do we know such genetic defenses exist, and how can genetics be used for disease control? Much of the older evidence is intuitive, but more solid evidence is continually emerging. The best evidence has come from the Δ32 bp mutation in the chemokine receptor gene *CCR5*, which is a human gene that can result in near total resistance to an infectious disease, HIV-1. Once a susceptibility gene is identified, the objective is to find the most widely applicable "exploitable targets" between host genes and infectious pathogens. The targets for therapy could be found in polymorphic variants of human genes that regulate specific antimicrobial mechanisms, rather than the microbes themselves. In traditional approaches, such genes may become the target for drug development or identify points for immuno-intervention such as cytokine therapy. Another set of attractive targets may be those host defenses which are strongly influenced by environmental factors, such as nutrition, as this link would represent a particularly useful and powerful mode of disease intervention in the developing world. One example of nutrition-based therapy is vitamin A, known to be useful in the prevention of measles. A similar reasoning has guided the recent search of vitamin D receptor polymorphisms in the susceptibility to tuberculosis and leprosy. In terms of vaccine development, the exploitable target may come from identification, in different ethnic populations, of specific antigens that efficiently interact with appropriate human leukocyte antigen (HLA) alleles. Even in the event that advances in genetic research do not lead to specific therapy against infectious diseases, advances should still provide valuable information concerning the control of epidemics and the ability to estimate vaccine efficacy. Most of all, it is improbable that universally protective vaccines against complex pathogens can be developed if fundamental, genetically controlled differences in the host response to infection are disregarded.

In February 2001, the working draft of the human genome sequence was completed (International Human Genome Sequence Consortium, 2001; Venter et al., 2001). In addition, many complete sequences are available for the genomes of pathogens such as *Mycobacterium tuberculosis*, *M. leprae*, and HIV-1. It is hoped that this sequence information can be transferred to DNA microarrays that will allow a new way to test the contribution of thousands of human loci to susceptibility to infection and to search for microbial antigenic peptides. However, even in this postgenome era, the effort to find the targets for therapy will still require three interactive disciplines: epidemiology, molecular genetics, and population genetics. Our objectives are simple, but our tools are becoming increasingly complex. In this chapter, we focus on advances from these three disciplines in the genetics of resistance to three of the most serious infectious disease threats that together account for over 5 million deaths per year (WHO, 2000a): tuberculosis (*M. tuberculosis*), HIV/AIDS (HIV-1), and malaria (*Plasmodium falciparum*).

WHY DO WE THINK THERE MAY BE A GENETIC COMPONENT FOR INFECTIOUS DISEASE SUSCEPTIBILITY?

It is widely believed that infectious diseases have been an important force of natural selection in human history (Haldane, 1948; O'Brien, 1998). This suggestion implies that alleles of certain genes decrease or increase the likelihood of survival during an infectious onslaught and, consequently, that only a proportion of a naive, i.e., previously unexposed, population will survive infection with a novel pathogenic agent. If this assumption is correct, the genetic make-up of a given population would be expected to differ before and after exposure to an infectious agent that causes serious morbidity or lethality among persons before they reach their full reproductive capacity.

Direct proof of a stated experimental hypothesis is not possible. However, there are several tragic events in recent human history that approximate such experimental verification. A widely quoted example that is thought to make a strong case for individual variability in the face of uniform infectious exposure is the contamination of one lot of bacille *Calmette-Guérin (BCG)* vaccine with a virulent strain of *M. tuberculosis* in Lübeck, Germany, in 1929. Of the 251 infants inoculated, 4 showed no signs of infection, 72 died of tuberculosis within 1 year of infection, and 175 overcame the infection (McKinney et al., 1998). Hence, an amazing 70% of immunologically naive babies survived infection with a massive dose of human-pathogenic *M. tuberculosis*. This high rate of survivors is in strong contrast to the extreme susceptibility of Native North Americans, for whom death rates of up to 90% were recorded following the introduction of *M. tuberculosis* into indigenous groups in the second half of the last century.

A second example is given by the study of survivors of a typhoid epidemic in Surinam, South America, that affected a group of Dutch settlers in 1845. For 367 individuals comprising 55 families, the overall mortality was 50%. However, six families had no deaths, while five families died out completely; the remaining 44 families lost a varying number of members (de Vries et al., 1979). When the gene frequencies of 64 direct descendants of the survivors were compared to the general Dutch population for allelic variants at 27 loci, it was found that HLA loci complement receptor 3 and heavy immunoglobulin G (IgG) chain allele frequencies differed significantly between epidemic survivors and the general population. Interestingly, no such difference was observed for immunologically nonrelevant genes, such as blood group antigens or serum enzymes (de Vries et al., 1979). These findings suggest that some selection of immune response "resistance" alleles had occurred during the epidemic.

A more recent example is given by the rates of HIV infection among the approximately 12,000 hemophiliacs who were infected with HIV from tainted blood products between 1978 and 1984, prior to the screening of blood donors for HIV. Despite the direct exposure to HIV, 10% to 25% of the recipients remained HIV-negative and about 1% of the HIV-positive recipients have remained in good health (O'Brien and Dean, 1997). In the ensuing 15 years, intensive research has revealed several host genes that can confer resistance to HIV infection and determine the rate of progression to AIDS. However, there are HIV-resistance mechanisms in highly exposed people which have yet to be identified.

Stronger evidence for the role of genetics in disease susceptibility, which will be discussed in more detail below, has also come from studies of family aggregation in leprosy (Shields et al., 1987), adoption studies (Sorensen et al., 1988), twin studies (Jepson, 1998), and several complex segregation analyses (Abel et al., 1995; Rodrigues et al., 1996; Alcais et al., 1997; Shaw et al., 1997). Several demonstrations of ethnic variability in disease susceptibility also point toward the role of genetic susceptibility factors (Stead et al., 1990; Stead, 1992). This evidence has been extensively reviewed (Schurr et al., 1990, 1991a; Hill, 1992, 1996a,b, 1997, 1998a,b; Blackwell et al., 1994, 1997; Davenport and Hill, 1996; Abel and Dessein, 1997, 1998; Bellamy and Hill, 1998a,b; Blackwell, 1998; Skamene et al., 1998).

Evidence also comes from genetic analysis of wild animal species, where genetic "footprints" and "fossils" have demonstrated selective gene adaptations of ancient epidemics or near extinction events (O'Brien, 1995). In cheetahs, genetic analysis has shown the entire species to have nearly identical major histocompatibility complex (MHC) genes and, therefore, to be greatly vulnerable to infection. Also, it is theorized that African monkeys are able to carry simian immunodeficiency virus (SIV) without disease due to the outcome of past genetic selection. To capitalize on these observations, researchers at the National Human Genome Research Institute (NHGRI) in Bethesda, Maryland, have embarked on "genetic prospecting," whereby nucleotide variants are being compared and dated between humans, chimpanzees, and gorillas to determine which genes may be most relevant to disease resistance (Hacia et al., 1999).

The other side of the same coin was pointed out by Neel (1962). If infectious agents have shaped the genetic makeup of populations in the past, is it possible that in the absence of such selective pressure, i.e., when infectious diseases are under control or eradicated, the selected genotypes may be detrimental to modern life? More specifically, could it be that the same genetic variants that protected against infectious diseases now predispose to common genetic disorders such as rheumatoid arthritis, atopy, hypertension, or even obesity? While intriguing, convincing experimental proof for such a suggestion is still missing. There is preliminary evidence that alleles of the human natural resistance–associated macrophage protein 1 (*NRAMP1*) gene that protect against tuberculosis may predispose to rheumatoid arthritis (Searle and Blackwell, 1999). It has also been speculated that protection from helminth infection, a condition where high IgE responsiveness is presumed to be beneficial, may be a risk factor for atopy (Palmer et al., 1997). Even when a clear association is made, caution is still advisable. For example, one allelic variant (235T) of the angiotensinogen gene, which is associated with hypertension, is found in high frequency among African Americans, Nigerians, and European Americans. However, the rates of hypertension are very different among these ethnic groups (Cooper et al., 1999). Studies such as these directly highlight the environmental and genetic complexity of disease development.

ANALYSIS OF GENETICALLY DETERMINED DISEASE SUSCEPTIBILITY

Phenotype Definition

Resistance or susceptibility to infectious disease is the result of the competitive biology of two species, the host and the infectious organism, in the context of a variable environment. The environmental stage on which the competition occurs has both biological, e.g., parasite reservoirs, vector biology, living habitats, and nonbiological, e.g., socioeconomic status, malnutrition, climatic changes, components. For genetic studies, researchers usually attempt to identify situations where the environment can be considered a constant parameter, at least over the short time that the study is conducted. Even in such situations, a comprehensive attempt at analyzing the genetic component of infectious disease susceptibility should take into account the competing genomes of both the host and the parasite. This ideal state of analysis has largely not been achieved, and parasitologists, virologists, microbiologists, and geneticists generally work independently on the biologies of parasite and host.

Due to a scarcity of experimental data, in this chapter we largely follow this unsatisfactory duality and essentially consider host phenotypes of susceptibility independently of the complex biology of the infectious organism. Similarly, we largely follow the now widely used convention of considering resistance and susceptibility as the opposite sides of the same coin, i.e., different alleles of the same gene. This usage implies that a "susceptibility" allele of a given gene increases the risk of infectious disease while an alternative "resistance" allele(s) of the same gene does not have such an effect (or vice versa). This does not necessarily imply that one allele increases and the other allele decreases risk of infectious disease relative to the general population. Clearly, it is important to keep *resistance* and *susceptibility* that act on the level of the individual apart from similar effects on the population level. It is now becoming increasingly clear that in many instances risk of infectious disease is under oligogenic control and that on the population level there are genes with specific alleles that increase such risk while alleles of other genes confer reduced risk of infectious disease. In this sense, it would be preferable to talk about *susceptibility* and *resistance* genes. However, since the allele effect on the population level is frequently not known, we prefer to use the terms to refer to the individual level as described above.

A far more serious problem that exceeds the challenge of using proper terminology is what to consider an appropriate definition for an infectious disease susceptibility phenotype. In Figure 10–1, the infectious process is simply divided into four stages: exposure to the pathogen, establishment of infection, progression of infection to disease, and clinical manifestation of the disease. As is immediately obvious, there is a multitude of resistance or susceptibility phenotypes that could be selected for further genetic analysis. If we assume that genetically controlled behavioral patterns that predispose to exposure are rare, the most likely points of possible genetic control are found during the innate and acquired phases of immunity.

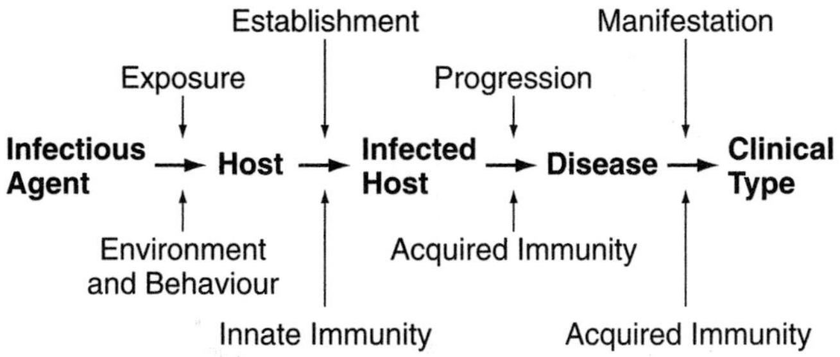

Fig. 10–1. The infectious process. The sequence of infection as it occurs in the human host is shown, separated by four *horizontal arrows*. The infectious process is divided into four stages, designated by the *vertical arrows pointing downward*: exposure to the pathogen, establishment of infection, progression of infection to disease, and clinical manifestation of disease. *Vertical arrows pointing upward* show the three main points of possible genetic control: environment and behaviour, innate immunity, and acquired immunity.

The phenotype selected for a study of infectious disease susceptibility can be very complex and represent the cumulative effect of many genes or the action of only one major gene. Intuitively, one would assume that early-stage phenotypes or well-defined clinical presentations are more likely to be under major gene control and less likely to show genetic heterogeneity. Conversely, phenotypes that occur later in the infectious process and are defined by more complex host–pathogen interaction are likely to be under multigenic control. While there are examples to support this intuition (e.g., total resistance to HIV controlled by the *CCR5* mutation vs. the several HLA and other genes controlling HIV disease progression), to what extent such intuition is correct is presently unclear; and it seems advisable to any prospective investigator to expect the possibility of genetic heterogeneity, oligogenic trait control, and possibly gene interaction in the genetic control of susceptibility to infectious diseases.

Evidence of Infection

An obvious phenotype in the study of infectious disease susceptibility is the onset of infection, i.e., the first detection of the disease-causing infectious agent in the host. For example, direct detection of viral RNA by reverse-transcription polymerase chain reaction or detection of antiviral envelope protein antibodies in a person's serum are two standard methods to establish HIV infection and, consequently, susceptibility to such infection. Several investigators have used the HIV infection phenotype, and genetic variants in several genes have been identified as risk modifiers for HIV infection (see below). However, there are other infectious diseases where susceptibility to infection does not appear to be a useful phenotype. For example, over 2 billion people are infected with *M. tuberculosis* worldwide, and in endemic regions the infection level can reach or exceed 80% of the general population if delayed-type hypersensitivity to purified protein derivative is used as a measure of *M. tuberculosis* infection. However, fewer than 10% of those infected advance to develop clinical tuberculosis by early adulthood. These numbers suggest that a possible *M. tuberculosis* infection susceptibility allele occurs at a very high population frequency and, hence, may be difficult to identify by genetic analysis. Conversely, genetic control of progression from infection to clinical disease may be easier to analyze.

Clinical Manifestations of Disease: Phenotype Designation According to Disease Severity

There are other examples of infectious diseases where a large proportion of the population in endemic areas is infected by the causative microorganism. Interestingly, for several medically important diseases, including malaria and schistosomiasis, the severity of infection, i.e., the number of parasites found in the host, varies dramatically from individual to individual (Abel and Dessein, 1998; Garcia et al., 1998a,b). In schistosomiasis, infection levels are under major gene control, and there is evidence that the same may hold true for malaria (Abel et al., 1991, 1992) (see below).

As mentioned above, extreme clinical manifestations of disease may provide good examples for genetic control of the infectious process. Consequently, stratification by disease severity may help to reveal the contribution of genes to the pathogenesis of the infectious process. For example, leprosy presents as a spectrum of clinical manifestations ranging from the benign paucibacillary tuberculoid to the disfiguring multibacillary lepromatous form. In several case-control association and family-based linkage studies, certain HLA class II alleles and *TNFA* promoter polymorphisms have been identified as risk modifiers for lepromatous leprosy (van Eden et al., 1982; Roy et al., 1997) or tuberculoid leprosy (van Eden et al., 1980; Weatherall et al., 1997). Such susceptibility alleles were not detected in studies of nonstratified populations that considered leprosy per se, i.e., leprosy irrespective of its specific clinical manifestations, as a susceptibility phenotype. Likewise, very significant associations between severe cerebral malaria and HLA and *TNFA* alleles have been observed in a large population-based case-control study in The Gambia (Hill et al., 1991; McGuire et al., 1994). These associations were not detected in cases with uncomplicated malaria, suggesting that certain HLA and *TNFA* alleles predispose or protect from severe malaria but not from simple infection with *Plasmodium* sp., the causative agents of malaria. A third example is the association of mucocutaneous, but not localized cutaneous, leishmaniasis with a *TNFA* promoter polymorphism (Cabrera et al., 1995). In addition to these well-documented examples, there is a substantial body of epidemiological evidence that uncommon clinical manifestations of common infectious diseases are clustered in certain ethnic or racial groups. For example, lymphoglandular tuberculosis is generally a rare manifestation of *M. tuberculosis* infection. However, in certain ethnic groups, the prevalence of lymphoglandular tuberculosis can exceed 50% of all tuberculosis cases (Sloane, 1996).

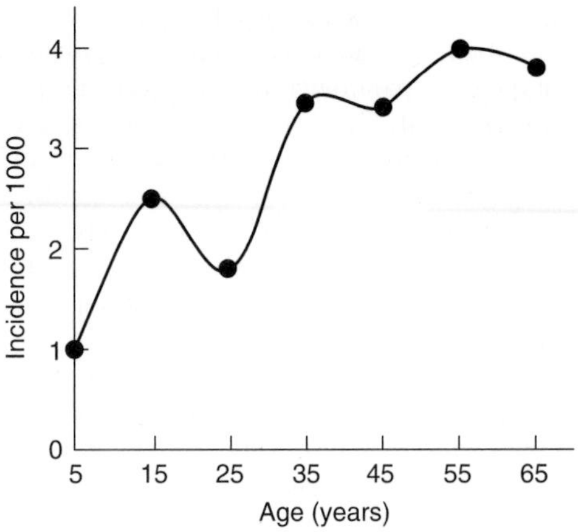

Fig. 10–2. Age and incidence of leprosy. Incidence of leprosy is plotted vs. age (in years). There is one peak before the age of 15 years, followed by a decline in incidence until age 25. Incidence then rises again to a maximum around age 55. The early peak may represent an interesting aspect for genetic studies of early–onset phenotypes in leprosy. From Nordeen (1985) with permission.

Designation According to Age at Onset

Many infectious diseases also display a very characteristic age at onset distribution. Frequently, there is a pronounced tendency for early onset among children. For example, the vast majority of deaths due to malaria occur in children under the age of 10 years, and one could be tempted to call malaria to some extent a pediatric disease. This pronounced age-dependent difference in mortality is also reflected in the age-dependent severity of infection, with children under age 10 displaying significantly higher infection levels than older age groups (Garcia et al., 1998a). Reduced infection levels in adults may reflect the development of antimalarial immunity and likely reflect constitutional age-related changes in the immune system of exposed individuals (Baird, 1995). Hence, genetic factors governing antimalarial immunity should be easier to detect and map among children (Garcia et al., 1998a).

Not all infectious diseases show an excess incidence among children. Nevertheless, even chronic diseases like tuberculosis and leprosy show a peak of cases before the age of 15 years (Fig. 10–2). Moreover, in chronic diseases, prevalence date and age at onset data may not be a good reflection of age-dependent risk factors since diagnosis of disease, which is often based on self-reporting, and onset of disease may differ significantly. A more interesting aspect for genetic studies of early-onset phenotypes in chronic diseases is the extent to which multiplex early-onset families are available for linkage studies. While there is good evidence that multiplex pediatric tuberculosis families are common, there appears to be little epidemiological evidence in favor of early-onset leprosy families. These observations suggest that stratification by age at onset may be a useful strategy in the genetic analysis of many, but not all, infectious diseases.

An additional observation that deserves further mention is that early-onset disease often results in extreme phenotypes. In tuberculosis, e.g., children who develop clinical disease are at high risk of developing miliary tuberculosis or tuberculous meningitis, two forms of tuberculosis with a very high fatality rate. Only in the young adult age group is there a significant shift to pulmonary tuberculosis as the most likely clinical form of the disease. The special status of pediatric forms of tuberculosis is also shown by the observation that the BCG vaccine, which is routinely given at birth in most tuberculosis-endemic countries, mainly reduces the frequency of miliary tuberculosis and tuberculous meningitis. In contrast, the effect of BCG vaccination in reducing pulmonary tuberculosis past puberty appears small. Taken together, the above considerations suggest that extreme disease manifestations in early-onset cases should offer a particularly good opportunity to tease apart the complex genetic system that governs susceptibility to infectious diseases.

Use of Biomarkers for Disease-Susceptibility Phenotypes

A final consideration for the choice of phenotype is to use surrogate markers of susceptibility, a widely employed strategy in genetic analysis. Certain parameters of the anti-parasitic immune response have been correlated with poor or good prognosis for infectious disease susceptibility, and it is possible to study the genetic control of such intermediate susceptibility markers in a stepwise effort to understand the presumably more complex genetic system for clinical disease susceptibility. Biomarkers are useful indicators of physiological and biochemical changes characteristic of the infection process. For example, for most intracellular parasitic infections, a T-helper 1 (Th1) type of response has been correlated with a good prognosis for the host to withstand the infectious onslaught by the parasite. Since the type of T-helper cell response is characterized by the production of certain cytokines, such as interferon-γ (IFN-γ) for Th1 and interleukin-4 (IL-4) for a Th-2 type response, it is possible to select the *in vitro* production of IFN-γ or IL-4 in response to parasite antigen as a quantitative trait for genetic analysis. Identification of genetic variants that control high or low cytokine production responsiveness would then provide candidate alleles for more focused analysis of susceptibility among patients. In addition to providing candidate genes for more detailed genetic analysis, this approach has the added advantage of distinguishing effective antiparasite host response mechanisms from physiological or immunological epiphenomena that are correlated with effective responses but have little impact *per se* on host susceptibility. One interesting example of this approach is the study of the genetic control of cytokine production and fatal meningococcal disease (Westendorp et al., 1997a,b).

STRATEGIES TO IDENTIFY CANDIDATE SUSCEPTIBILITY GENES

The advances of the Human Genome Project have spawned maps of the human genome of impressive resolution and accuracy (Hudson et al., 1995; Dib et al., 1996; Gyapay et al., 1996; Schuler et al., 1996; Wang et al., 1998). These maps are now being routinely used to search the entire genome for chromosomal regions that harbor genes involved in the control of disease phenotypes. However, present genome-wide searches cannot directly lead to the identification of specific genes controlling expression of the studied phenotypes, such as susceptibility to infection. Generally, chromosomal regions identified as likely harboring susceptibility genes are further analyzed by genetic and physical fine mapping and lists of candidate genes emerge from database searches or from direct experimental evidence, such as cDNA selection or exon trapping. Besides being located in a region of the genome that has been pinpointed as a likely location of a susceptibility gene, candidate genes identified by this strategy usually have a known or predicted function that makes biological sense, show a tissue expression pattern consistent with expression of the studied phenotype, and/or show allelic variants in affected individuals that may result in an abrogated function of the encoded protein.

Whole-genome scans are a tremendously powerful strategy to identify susceptibility loci that have a major effect on phenotype expression. Genome scans usually employ nonparametric methods of linkage analysis that evaluate the significance of excess allele sharing among affected pairs of offspring. Using this analytical approach, the numbers of sib pairs and families required to identify genes that have only a moderate effect on phenotype expression are too large to be practically feasible (Risch and Merikangas, 1996; Muller-Myhsok and Abel, 1997). Moreover, even when a major gene effect is being analyzed, the effort required to enroll a sufficient number of families can be excessive, especially in the context of infectious diseases. Likewise, the cost to genotype all family members with genetic markers spanning the entire genome may prove prohibitive for many laboratories, notably in developing countries where disease families are most readily available. For all of these reasons, it is a popular approach to identify candidate susceptibility genes by methods other than whole-genome scanning and then to evaluate the relative importance of such candidate genes in study designs that do not require enrollment of large numbers of sib pairs, such as population- or family-based case-control settings.

A popular approach to identifying candidate genes is the use of animal models, most commonly inbred strains of laboratory mice. The underlying assumption is that the mechanistic basis of disease resistance or susceptibility is the same in both the animal model and the human situation. Clearly, there is a large body of experimental evidence to support this claim. The main problem posed by the use of inbred strains of mice for genetic analysis is the paucity of genetic variability in such strains. In other words, only a very tiny proportion of genetic variability available in human populations is available for genetic analysis in inbred strains of mice. Hence, it is unlikely that the exact disease-causing genetic variants identified in mice will also be found in humans. What is likely, however, is that human orthologues of crucial genes identified in mice will be crucial in humans. Modern cellular immunology has amply proven this statement. By further extension, probably the most important application of mouse genetics to human disease will be the identification of biochemical and physiological pathways that are crucial for host resistance or susceptibility. Individual genes that encode proteins participating in the pinpointed pathway can then be further analyzed, possibly using genetically engineered strains of mice. Identification of the human orthologues encoding proteins participating in these pathways will provide a short list of human candidate genes that are now far less restricted by the lack of genetic variability in the mouse models.

Mouse models have been used to identify resistance/susceptibility loci for a large number of viral, bacterial, and eukaryotic pathogens (Buschman et al., 1995). However, only in a small number of these infectious disease susceptibility models has the causative gene been isolated and the molecular defect underlying the phenotype identified. The *Nramp1* gene is such an example, whereby through the use of transgenic animals it has been proven that a single G169D amino acid substitution is the cause of the susceptibility of certain inbred strains of mice to a large number of intracellular macrophage parasites (Vidal et al., 1993, 1995; Govoni et al., 1996). Since it is becoming increasingly clear that even among mice resistance/susceptibility to infectious disease is usually a multigenic trait, a number of recent studies have employed whole-genome scanning in the mouse in search of quantitative trait loci (QTL) that influence the expression of continuous susceptibility phenotypes. For example, in cutaneous leishmaniasis, two independent studies have localized QTLs to a total of eight different chromosomal regions (Beebe et al., 1997; Roberts et al., 1997). In one study, parasites were injected into the footpad and footpad swelling was used as the phenotype, leading to the identification of six QTL linkages (Beebe et al., 1997). In the other study, parasites were injected intradermally and the size of the developing cutaneous lesion was used as the phenotype, leading to the localization of two QTLs (Roberts et al., 1997). Interestingly, there was no overlap in the chromosomal regions identified in both studies, clearly demonstrating the importance of the phenotype for genetic analysis. In a similar set of experiments, mice were injected with *Plasmodium* parasites (the causative agents of malaria in humans) and the number of parasites at peak parasitemia was determined. In two studies (Fortin et al., 1997, 2001), loci on chromosomes 8 and 3 were detected, while a linkage on mouse chromosome 9 was detected in only one study (Foote et al., 1997). Although at first glance the phenotype analyzed was the same (peak parasitemia), the route of infection (intravenous vs. intraperitoneal) was different. Hence, it seems plausible that the locus on chromosome 9 may be related to the route of infection, thus providing another example of the importance of gene–environment interaction in infectious diseases. More examples of QTL mapping in mouse models are several recent scans to map loci influencing tuberculosis severity (Lavebratt et al., 1999; Mitsos et al., 2000; Kramnik et al., 2000). These analyses, conducted on mice of different genetic backgrounds, have identified several significant linkages: distal chromosome 1, proximal chromosome 7, proximal chromosome 9, and distal chromosome 3. Interestingly, the location of the chromosome 9 linkage exactly overlapped the one found in cutaneous leishmaniasis using lesion size as the phenotype (Roberts et al., 1997; Lavebratt et al., 1999).

Other investigators have pursued additional strategies to derive candidate genes for further genetic analysis, such as identifying the cause of hypersusceptibility to intracellular infections of children in families with parental consanguinity. This approach has so far identified deficiencies in the IFN-γ receptor *(INFGR1)* and IL-12 receptor *(IL12RB1)* genes as the cause of extreme susceptibility to mycobacteria that are only poorly pathogenic in humans (Jouanguy et al., 1996, 1999; Newport et al., 1996; Levin and Newport, 1997; Altare et al., 1998a,c; de Jong et al., 1998). Evidence is accumulating that different allelic variants of these receptor genes lead to varying degrees of susceptibility to mycobacterial infections (Jouanguy et al., 1997a,b, 1999) (see below). Two additional approaches for the identification of candidate susceptibility genes are the correlation of geographical distributions of known gene variants with infectious diseases and the "guessing" of candidate genes from the known pathology of the infectious disease. Both strategies have been used with remarkable success in the case of malaria and have resulted, e.g., in the identification of sickle hemoglobin and the thalassemias as important genetic factors influencing the risk of malaria in exposed populations (Weatherall et al., 1995; Weatherall, 1996a,b, 1997a).

The final aim of genetic studies of infectious diseases is the identification of molecular variants that modulate risk. In the mouse, such a proof can be provided in a straightforward fashion using transgenic animals expressing different forms of specific gene variants. In humans, this direct approach needs to be replaced with more indirect methods that are designed to test for linkage or association of a specific allelic variant with resistance or susceptibility to infectious disease. An excellent summary of different study designs has been provided (Abel and Dessein, 1998). It is important, however, to keep in mind that neither significant linkage nor association results provide proof of a causal relationship between genetic variant and studied phenotype. Especially in the context of complex genetic traits, reproducibility of observed linkages and associations lends credibility to the possible role of a genetic variant in influencing risk of disease. However, even in the event of a true linkage, reproducibility may not be easily achievable (Suarez et al., 1994), and linkage disequilibrium fine mapping is frequently used to provide further genetic evidence for or against the role of allelic variants in influencing expression of the phenotype. Such genetic studies need to be complemented by different functional assays that provide evidence consistent with the hypothesis that expression of allelic gene products can influence the underlying physiological events of resistance or susceptibility. In other words, the genetic evidence must be consistent with what is known about the biology of trait expression, supporting the claim that genetic analysis provides a swift way of identifying such physiological pathways that are particularly important for the pathogenesis of a studied trait.

CANDIDATE GENES FOR MAJOR INFECTIOUS DISEASES: AN OVERVIEW OF BASIC CONCEPTS

In Figure 10–3, we have presented our method of estimating the number of genes involved in the susceptibility to infection according to their timing of action in the immune response pathway. Basically, this concept is an extension of that shown in Figure 10–1 and theorizes that the number of host genes influencing disease susceptibility will increase as disease phenotypes appear later in the course of host defense. Thus, the most clear-cut disease phenotypes (i.e., resistance to HIV infection) will have

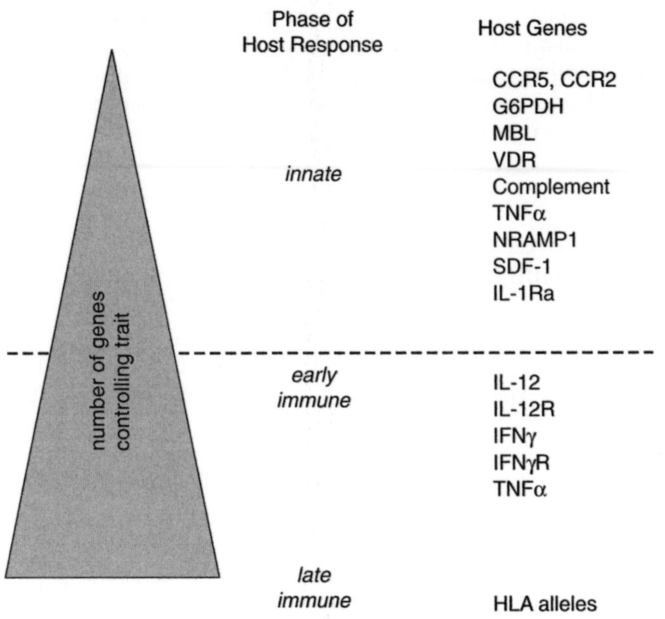

Fig. 10–3. Genetic susceptibility to infection. The number of genes controlling susceptibility to infection may be estimated according to their timing of action in the immune response pathway. The number of genes controlling the infection trait of interest decreases toward the point of the *gray triangle*. The phase of the host response (innate, early, and late immune) progresses toward the base of the triangle, along with the number of influencing genes. The host genes that act at the different phases are listed to the right and discussed in the text.

single-gene control (i.e., *CCR5* $\Delta 32$ mutation), which again is likely to act early in the infection process (i.e., viral entry/infection of macrophages). Likewise, the progression of AIDS is controlled at later stages of immunity by several genes, including the HLA alleles. Figure 10–3 also includes a list of genes that have been tested as candidate genes for susceptibility/resistance to tuberculosis/leprosy, HIV/AIDS, and malaria; the individual genes will be discussed throughout this chapter. Although certain of these genes are associated mainly with specific diseases, such as *CCR5* with HIV, it is worthwhile to consider a candidate's role in other infections as well, particularly in those infections found at the same time. There has also been increasing interest in examining the gene products that may be expressed at the route of entry of the infectious pathogen as these genes may present the first set of innate host genetic barriers.

In this chapter, we focus on the specific infectious diseases tuberculosis, leprosy, HIV, and malaria due to their importance and the abundance of recent genetics data. However, the principles presented, such as the strategies of analysis and investigation of candidate genes, are likely to be applicable to all major infectious and parasitic diseases.

Tuberculosis, Leprosy, and Genetics

There have been several major twin studies of tuberculosis and leprosy conducted over the last 70 years (Schurr and Skamene, 1996; reviewed in Jepson, 1998), which have suggested that genetic factors participate in host susceptibility. In leprosy, there is increased concordance of disease in monozygotic vs. dizygotic twins, and several complex segregation analyses have detected a strong genetic component of leprosy susceptibility (Abel and Dessein, 1997), while still other studies have reported a strong familial component of the disease (Shields et al., 1987). For tuberculosis, the results of most twin studies show that approximately 35% of susceptibility to tuberculosis is due to genetic factors, with the remaining influence due to environmental factors (Jepson et al., 1997; Jepson, 1998). In addition, several investigators have reported that certain racial or ethnic groups are more likely to develop leprosy and tuberculosis (reviewed in Schurr et al., 1991a). Regarding specific genes, a segregation analysis on Desirade Island showed that a single non-MHC gene controlled susceptibility to leprosy, while MHC genes have been shown to influence the type of acquired resistance or leprosy that develops. There is a dearth of segregation studies on tuberculosis; however, a segregation analysis in a northern Brazilian population concluded that tuberculosis susceptibility was under the control of two major loci (Shaw et al., 1997). Likewise, a genome scan for tuberculosis susceptibility loci detected suggestive evidence for the location of two candidate genes on human chromosome regions 15q and Xq (Bellamy and Hill, 1998a,b; Bellamy et al., 2000).

Genes Associated with Tuberculosis or Leprosy in Different Populations

NRAMP1. Since our group was the first to describe linkage of *NRAMP1* in a mycobacterial disease (Abel et al., 1998), we will emphasize our studies of testing *NRAMP1* for a possible role in leprosy and tuberculosis susceptibility as this chapter's first example of candidate gene testing. The key aspects of *NRAMP1* expression and function are outlined in Figures 10–4 and 10–5.

The mouse *Nramp1* gene, positionally cloned in 1993, is identical with the chromosome 1 mouse *Bcg/Ity/Lsh* locus, which controls murine susceptibility to BCG, *M. lepraemurium*, *M. avium*, *S. typhimurium*, and *L. donovani* (Vidal et al., 1993, 1995;

Tissue Expression of Nramp1 in Phagocytes

Mouse (spleen)	Human (lung)
• Mature monocytes/ macrophages	• polymorphonuclear leukocytes
• mature granulocytes	• monocytes

Genetic restriction (*Nramp1*) of resistance/susceptibility to infection

Under *Nramp1* control	NOT under *Nramp1* control
Mycobacterium bovis	*Pseudomonas aeruginosa*
Mycobacterium avium	*Listeria monocytogenes*
Salmonella typhimurium	*Legionella pneumophila*
Leishmania donovani	*Staphylococcus aureus*
Toxoplasma gondii	*Bacillus subtilus*

Fig. 10–4. Tissue expression and infections controlled by Nramp1. *Upper box* contrasts the different tissue expression of Nramp1 in mice and humans (Vidal et al., 1993; Cellier et al., 1997). *Lower box* lists the various pathogens which have been shown in the mouse to be under (or not under) the control of *Nramp1*.

Mouse Nramp1 - Structure

- Integral 12-transmembrane protein expressed in the macrophage phagosome
- Molecular weight of 100kDa; extensively glycosylated
- G169D mutation in TM4, *Bcg*[s] mice do not express Nramp1
- Consensus transport signature in TM8-9

Putative Function of NRAMP1 in lung macrophages

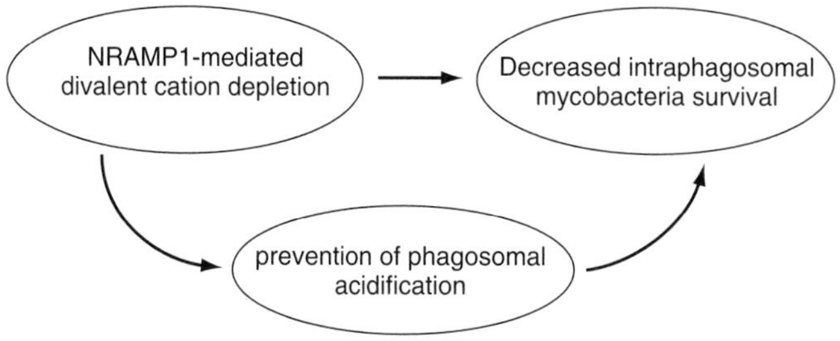

Fig. 10–5. Nramp1 structure and putative function. *Upper box* lists the biochemical properties of mouse Nramp1 (reviewed in Skamene et al., 1998), and the *lower diagram* shows the putative function of Nramp1 in controlling resistance to intracellular parasites (Hackam et al., 1998; Gruenheid et al., 1999).

Govoni et al., 1996). To what extent *Nramp1* is involved in murine susceptibility to *M. tuberculosis* is controversial (Medina and North, 1996). Sequencing of *Nramp1* cDNA from 27 inbred strains of mice identified a G169D substitution within predicted TM4 of the Nramp1 protein in all susceptible strains but in none of the resistant strains (Malo et al., 1994). Nramp1 is a transmembrane protein expressed in the phagosomes of mature macrophages of resistant mice; susceptible mice do not express the Nramp1 protein (Vidal et al., 1996).

The complete nucleotide sequence and genomic structure of the human *NRAMP1* gene region on chromosome region 2q35 have been determined (Marquet et al., 2000). Sequence analysis of human *NRAMP1*, located on chromosome 2q35, revealed extensive conservation of the primary nucleotide sequence with mouse *Nramp1*, suggesting that the protein is evolutionarily significant, and thus designated *NRAMP1* as a major candidate gene in host defense against mycobacterial infections. However, sequencing of homologous regions of human and bovine *NRAMP1* revealed a glycine at the position homologous to the G169D mouse *Nramp1* mutation, strongly suggesting that this mutation is unique to mouse *Nramp1*. *NRAMP1* expression studies revealed that the tissues with the highest expression of *NRAMP1* are peripheral blood leukocytes, followed by lung and spleen. In blood, polymorphonuclear leukocytes are the major site of *NRAMP1* expression, followed by monocytes (Cellier et al., 1997).

We have defined polymorphisms in the *NRAMP1* gene for linkage and association analysis of *NRAMP1* with mycobacterial disease (Buu et al., 1995; Liu et al., 1995; Abel et al., 1998). Using exon-specific primers, single-strand conformational polymorphism screening, direct sequencing of genomic DNA, and standard restriction fragment length polymorphism (RFLP) analyses, a total of 11 sequence variants within *NRAMP1* were identified in a screening panel of 15 unrelated individuals of mixed ethnic origin. The variants included a $(CA)_n$ microsatellite repeat in the immediate 5′ region of the gene, a single-nucleotide change in intron 4 (469+14G/C), a nonconservative single-base substitution at codon 543 that changes aspartic acid to asparagine (D543N), and a TGTG deletion in the 3′-untranslated region (UTR). The allele frequencies of these markers were determined among control panels of individuals of Caucasian, Asian, African, and Polynesian origin (Buu et al., 1995; Liu et al., 1995; Abel et al., 1998). In addition, a cluster of Alu repeats in the 5′ promoter region of *NRAMP1* was identified (Roger et al., 1998). These variants were tested in a case-control study of 410 adults with smear-positive pulmonary tuberculosis and 417 ethnically matched, healthy controls in The Gambia (Bellamy et al., 1998a,b). It was found that the 3′-UTR variant allele of *NRAMP1*, which is uncommon in Europeans, was present in 25% of Gambians. Heterozygotes for two *NRAMP1* polymorphisms in intron 4 and the 3′-UTR of the gene were significantly overrepresented among those with tuberculosis compared to those with the most common *NRAMP1* genotype. Thus, this allelic variant could partly explain the susceptibility to tuberculosis in The Gambia. The strongest evidence to date identifying *NRAMP1* as a major gene linked with tuberculosis susceptibility was detected in a tuberculosis outbreak in a community of aboriginal Canadians (Greenwood et al., 2000; Abel and Casanova, 2000). In this study, the *NRAMP1* gene (or a closely linked gene) seemed to control the progression from "infected" to "affected" status. The overall picture is that the influence of *NRAMP1* over susceptibility to tuberculosis and leprosy is genetically heterogeneous and dependent on the immunization status of the population.

Although far below tuberculosis in terms of mortality, leprosy has long been recognized as a serious mycobacterial infection on a global scale. We have been collecting DNA samples from multiplex leprosy families worldwide for several years (Schurr et al., 1991a,b). The first direct evidence of a role for *NRAMP1* in the susceptibility to leprosy came from families in southern Vietnam. A synopsis of how the analysis was performed and the results is given in Figure 10–6. Complex segregation analysis of this population revealed that Chinese families showed a strong implication for a complex genetic-epidemiological model of susceptibility, whereas Vietnamese families showed the presence of a major codominant gene with age-dependent penetrance controlling susceptibility to leprosy (Abel et al., 1995). In this population, 168 members of 20 multiplex leprosy families were genotyped for *NRAMP1* alleles and four closely linked polymorphic markers. Significant evidence for linkage was observed ($p < 0.005$–0.02), and the extent of allele sharing was strong (58%). Such a high degree of allele sharing is reminiscent of the *HLA* effect in insulin-dependent diabetes mellitus and suggests that *NRAMP1* may be a major leprosy susceptibility locus in this population. (Abel et al., 1998). Another study of *NRAMP1* in leprosy in this same Vietnamese population raised an important issue; significant linkage was observed between *NRAMP1* and the Mitsuda reaction, an in vivo diagnostic test for lepromatous leprosy that measures the specific immune response against lepromin (Alcais et al., 2000). These results imply that *NRAMP1* plays a regulatory role in the development of acquired antimycobacterial immune responses. Thus, although it is firmly accepted that mouse *Nramp1* is a determinant of natural resistance to infection and not acquired immunity, the human studies do not unequivocally show that this is the case for *NRAMP1*. It remains possible that, in humans, *NRAMP1* represents an immune response gene.

However, like the genetic analysis of other complex traits, the detection of specific leprosy susceptibility genes has been difficult. For example, a genome scan of leprosy susceptibility (Siddiqui et al., 2001) detected a susceptibility locus on chro-

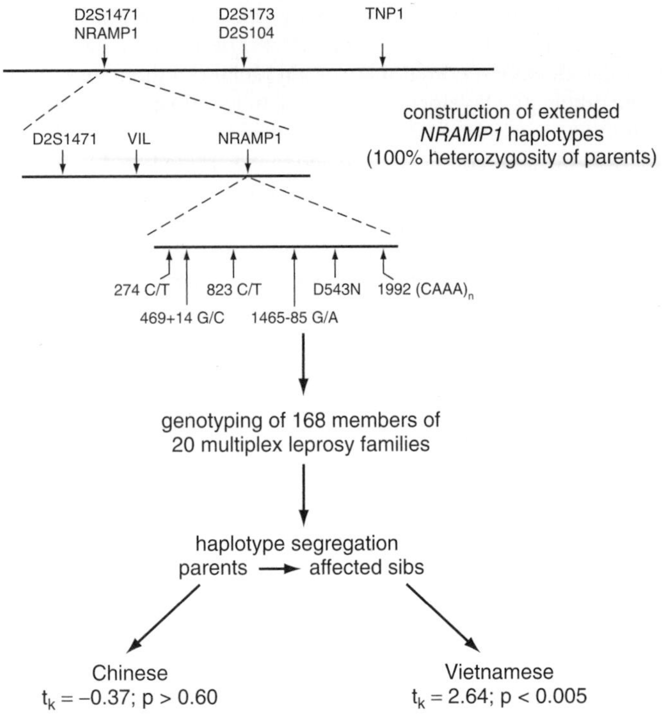

Fig. 10–6. Susceptibility to leprosy is linked to the human *NRAMP1* gene. Schematic diagram showing how linkage of *NRAMP1* with susceptibility to leprosy was detected in southern Vietnam. The markers used for the construction of extended *NRAMP1* haplotypes are shown at the *top*. Linkage analysis of extended *NRAMP1* haplotypes with leprosy susceptibility revealed that this Vietnamese family showed significant evidence of linkage ($p <$ 0.005). A high degree of haplotype sharing among affected sib pairs suggests that *NRAMP1* may be a major leprosy susceptibility locus in this population (Abel et al., 1998).

mosome 10p but failed to detect the *NRAMP1*, *VDR*, and *HLA* chromosomal regions detected in other studies. In a large study of multicase tuberculosis families in northern Brazil, no evidence for linkage of *NRAMP1* with the disease was found (Shaw et al., 1993, 1997). Two smaller studies of leprosy, one a case-control study in Calcutta, India (Roy et al., 1999), and the other a small analysis of seven families in French Polynesia (Levee et al., 1994; Roger et al., 1997), failed to detect any association or linkage of *NRAMP1* with leprosy. The study in Calcutta included seven ethnic groups, which may have contributed to a significant reduction in power (Roy et al., 1999). This lack of reproducibility is likely to result from genetic heterogeneity, very complex genetic trait control, as well as significant differences in the phenotypes studied.

Although the function of human NRAMP1 has yet to be identified, the function of mouse Nramp1 has been extensively studied. Nramp1 can prevent phagosome acidification, possibly through depletion of the phagosome of divalent cations such as Fe; both functions are required for microbial survival (Hackam et al., 1998; Gruenheid et al., 1999). Thus, it is conceivable that subtle variations of human NRAMP1 in lung alveolar macrophages may interfere with cation-dependent limitation of microbial growth. It may be that NRAMP1 has a main influence on mycobacteria that first contact the lung, which is the primary site of tuberculosis and possibly leprosy infection in humans as well as a primary site of NRAMP1 tissue expression in humans. In contrast, in *Leishmania* infection, which is contracted mainly through the skin, no association has been found with *NRAMP1* (Shaw et al., 1993; Blackwell et al., 1997; Maasho et al., 1998).

Vitamin D Receptor. The vitamin D receptor *(VDR)* gene is located on chromosome 12q12–q14 (Baker et al., 1988; Labuda et al., 1991) and encodes a 50 to 60 kDa nuclear receptor protein that belongs to the family of *trans*-activating transcriptional regulators. The VDR is homologous to steroid and thyroid hormone receptors. It binds to calcitriol, the active metabolite of vitamin D, a steroid hormone that regulates calcium metabolism and cell differentiation. Based on the observation that vitamin D metabolism is altered in patients with active tuberculosis (Gkonos et al., 1984), speculation arose that a defect in vitamin D metabolism predisposes to tuberculosis susceptibility (Barnes et al., 1989; Davies, 1989; Rook, 1989). This idea was supported by evidence that addition of vitamin D in vitro restricts growth of *M. tuberculosis* in macrophages (Crowle and Elkins, 1990). Generally, nonresponsiveness to vitamin D has been linked to a variety of mutations located in the *VDR*, and *VDR* polymorphisms have been described (Hustmeyer et al., 1993). These polymorphisms are biologically relevant because they are good predictors of bone density and the risk of osteoporosis (Morrison et al., 1994). The other impetus for investigating the *VDR* role in tuberculosis is that vitamin D–related intervention of tuberculosis would be an attractive therapy, much as vitamin A therapy is used for measles.

There are numerous *VDR* alleles, including six alleles (Aa, Bb, and Tt) of the *VDR* locus which are identified by three RFLPs (*Apa*1, *Bsm*1, and *Taq*1). The *Taq*1 RFLP distinguishes a T-C silent base change in the 3′ end of the *VDR* gene. The *tt* genotype has been associated with increased mRNA levels of *VDR* and a decrease in bone mineral density, primarily in females (Tao et al., 1998). In the same Gambian population which was used for the *NRAMP1* analysis, a weak association was found between VDR and tuberculosis (Bellamy et al., 1999). There was a slight underrepresentation of the relatively rare *tt* genotype in the tuberculosis group as opposed to the controls (6.6% vs. 12%), an effect which may have been influenced by a gender bias in this study. Also, serum vitamin D deficiency may contribute to the high occurrence of tuberculosis among Gujarati Asian subjects ($p = 0.008$) (Wilkinson et al., 2000). Moreover, the *VDR* genotypes of 91 untreated tuberculosis patients and 116 healthy people who had been sensitized to tuberculosis indicated that *VDR* polymorphisms are involved in tuberculosis susceptibility (Wilkinson et al., 2000).

A strong association was found between *VDR* genotypes and leprosy in a case-control study in Calcutta (Roy et al., 1999). In this population, the frequency of the *tt* genotype was 7.8%. In the tuberculoid form of leprosy, the *tt* genotype was significantly increased to 21.5%. The other striking association was a decrease of the *Tt* genotype in leprosy compared to controls. The authors suggested that the *tt* genotype may promote Th1-type immunity whereas the *TT* genotype may promote Th2-type immunity. However, given the very small population frequency of the *tt* compared to *TT VDR* genotype and the fact that most individuals are resistant to leprosy (and tuberculosis), it is unlikely that most individuals would resist these diseases with a Th2 immune response. It will be important to see if these *VDR* associations can be confirmed in other populations.

IL-1ra *and* TNFA. Identification of the tumor necrosis factor-α (*TNFA*) and the IL-1 receptor antagonist (*IL-1ra*) genes as potential mycobacterial susceptibility genes is interesting as both of these proteins had previously been identified as serum biomarkers of leprosy (Sampaio et al., 1993; Klausner et al., 1996) and tuberculosis (Bekker et al., 1998; Juffermans et al., 1998). *IL-1ra* has been identified as a susceptibility gene in a number of diseases, including systemic lupus erythematosus (Tjernstrom et al., 1999) and inflammatory bowel disease (Bioque et al., 1995). *IL-1ra* is located on chromosome 2q14–q21 in the same region as *IL1A* and *IL1B* and has five alleles that contain between two and six repeats of an 86 bp sequence (Nicklin). IL-1ra is a specific inhibitor of IL-1 activity on T cells and has been observed to be induced in peripheral blood monocytes by *M. tuberculosis* in vitro, possibly through a direct mechanism. In a case control study of modest size conducted on persons of Hindu origin in England, the production of IL-1Ra in response to *M. tuberculosis* in vitro was found to be influenced by an *IL-1ra* polymorphism: persons with the *IL-1ra* $A2^+$ allele produced approximately twofold more IL-1ra than persons with the *IL-1ra* $A2^-$ allele (Wilkinson et al., 1999). In addition, the *IL-1* (+3953) A1 allele was found in linkage disequilibrium with the *IL-1ra* $A2^-$ allele, and this haplotype was overrepresented in patients with tuberculous pleurisy. Although it is far from clear how the *IL-1ra* gene influences the host response to *M. tuberculosis*, it has been hypothesized that overproduction of IL-1ra may block the detrimental action of IL-1 early in the establishment of lung granulomas.

TNFA is located on chromosome 6p21.3–p21.1, within the HLA complex. TNF (also called cachectin) is produced primarily by activated macrophages and is clearly important for host protection against tumors and in several mouse models of parasitic and viral infection (Bermudez and Young, 1992; Karunaweera et al., 1992; Wilson et al., 1995). However, TNF has often been characterized by a more pathogenic role. Elevated serum levels of TNF have been associated with cachexia in cancer (Tisdale, 1999), with fatal cerebral malaria (McGuire et al., 1994), and with the lepromatous form of leprosy (Khanolkar-Young et al., 1995). The lowering of TNF levels, through anti-TNF antibodies or thalidomide treatment, has been linked with therapeutic effects in lepromatous leprosy (Sampaio et al., 1993; Klausner et al., 1996). A role for the *TNFA* polymorphic promoter variant at position −308 has been found in malaria and lepromatous leprosy (Roy et al., 1997). However, no role has been found for *TNFA* in the susceptibility to tuberculosis in a large pedigree analysis in Brazil (Shaw et al., 1997).

HLA, Tuberculosis, and Leprosy

Many studies have reported a role for HLA class I or II alleles in the susceptibility or resistance to *M. tuberculosis* and *M. leprae* (for reviews on this subject, see (Pauling et al., 1949; van Eden et al., 1980, 1982; Singh et al., 1983; van Eden and de Vries, 1984; Bodmer, 1996; Roy et al., 1997; Hill, 1998a). In most instances, these HLA studies have been characterized by weak linkage or association. Weak association may be in part due to the extreme polymorphism of the HLA complex, which gives low power in statistical analysis due to multiple corrections, the inability to detect HLA allelic specificities by the older method of serological typing, and the existence of genes in linkage disequilibrium with the HLA complex, such as the *TNFA* (Roy et al., 1997) and *TAP* genes (Rajalingam et al., 1997), which have been shown to independently modify the clinical type of leprosy. In addition, in our own hypothesis (Fig. 10–1), we suggested that it may be difficult to detect single *HLA* gene effects against the cumulative number of genes which regulate all events leading up to acquired immunity. Still, the importance of *HLA* genes in the immune response to mycobacteria cannot be disputed as multitudes of studies have shown that acquired immunity against *Mycobacteria* is mediated by class I and class II gene products. Class II gene products present antigens to cytotoxic T lymphocytes (CTLs), which lyse infected cells and produce IFN-γ. Class II gene products present antigen to $CD4^+$ T lymphocytes, which secrete cytokines that result in the activation of parasitized macrophages and promotion of the granulomatous response. In recent years, particularly with the use of molecular HLA typing by polymerase chain reaction, investigations have begun to reveal the existence of HLA class I and class II supertypes that may underlie the development of epitope-based vaccines for mycobacterial diseases (Sette and Sidney, 1998).

Three class I HLA supertypes have been identified (HLA-A2, HLA-A3, and HLA-B7), which are presumed to exist in up to 89% of the general population (Sette and Sidney, 1998). Other supertypes have also been reported (Bothamley, 1999). Each supertype encompasses several allelic specificities, which are distinguished by the peptide motifs and residue numbers recognized by their B and F binding pockets. The idea behind designing vaccines according to the supertypes is to define protective mycobacterial peptides that are recognized by class I and class II supertypes to afford maximum immunity. Since logic implies that those HLA types in association with disease should represent weak or otherwise inefficient binding pockets, the important issue here will be to assign the "direction of associations." There is evidence to suggest that certain HLA types occur more often in tuberculosis and leprosy (Pauling et al., 1949). For example, there have been several reports of class II HLA *DQB1*0503* and *DQB1*0501* associations with tuberculosis in Cambodians, Mexicans, and Indians, thus possibly representing a weak binding cleft (Teran-Escandon et al., 1999). In the Mexican study, the *DQB1*0402* allele was significantly decreased in patients; thus, one could hypothesize that this allele has a protective binding pocket. Molecular typing studies have revealed that *HLA-DRB1* alleles, where an arginine is usually conserved at two positions in the binding pocket, is increased in tuberculoid leprosy (Zerva et al., 1996).

Binding type cleft association has also been invoked in HLA class I association with tuberculosis (Bothamley, 1999). In a study of pulmonary tuberculosis in Indonesia, HLA-B60 was associated with tuberculosis and HLA-B44 with increased protection from tuberculosis. The authors suggested that this may reflect the ability of HLA-B44 over the HLA-B60 molecule to activate cytotoxic T cells. Accordingly, the authors then determined that among 14 secreted antigens of *M. tuberculosis*, HLA-B44 had 65 potential antigen binding sites while B60 had only seven predicted sites. Thus, the implication is that HLA-B44 could better stimulate cytotoxic and IFN-producing $CD8^+$ T cells than the HLA-B60 class I antigen (Bothamley, 1999). The hypothesis suggested by these studies is also supported by HLA associations with malaria.

Mycobacterial Infection and Genetic Immunodeficiency

It had long been suspected that children with rare, disseminated, nontuberculous mycobacterial infections might be associated with a recessive inherited immunodeficiency disorder. Over the last 4 years, Casanova and colleagues have been largely responsible for the description of genetically heterogeneous causes of this disorder (Jouanguy et al., 1997a,b; Altare et al., 1998b). The disorders are homozygous recessive and caused by mutations found in the *IFNGR1* or *IL12R* gene. In mice, IFN-γ has long been established as the major macrophage-activating cytokine secreted by T and natural killer (NK) cells and is required to form mature granulomas (Flynn et al., 1993). By virtue of these rare human mycobacterial susceptibility disorders, the crucial role of IFN-γ and IL-12 in the human immune response to mycobacteria has been brought into clear focus.

The first defined molecular basis of atypical mycobacteriosis, identified in 13 patients to date and the most severe deficiency, was a complete absence of the *IFNGR1* (ligand binding chain) (Jouanguy et al., 1996; Newport et al., 1996). The genetic mutation is a null mutation in which no receptor is expressed, and the affected patients had a complete absence of mature granulomas. A partial deficiency of *IFNGR1* studied in two patients, caused by a missense mutation in the extracellular domain, was associated with a milder course of disease and the presence of mature granulomas (Jouanguy et al., 1997a,b). Here, the receptor was partially expressed but did not function optimally. In the *IFNR2* gene, which encodes the signaling chain of the IFN receptor, a complete deficiency was linked to a frameshift mutation (Dorman and Holland, 1998). Although receptor expression was detected, there was a lack of response to IFN and no mature granulomas.

A patient with complete lack of the p40 *IL-12* gene subunit was detected, which resulted in complete lack of either the p40 molecule subunit or the IL-12 heterodimer (Altare et al., 1998d). A decreased response to IFN-γ was detected as a consequence of reduced levels of IL-12 since the response to IFN could be overcome by addition of exogenous IL-12 in vivo and in vitro. Finally, a complete deficiency in the *IL12RB1* gene, resulting in a null mutation, was detected in seven patients (de Jong et al., 1998). Although the receptor was not expressed, the deficiency was apparently much less severe than total *IFNR* deficiency and mature granulomas could be formed.

Although these immunodeficiency-associated mutations are rare, less severe, subtle mutations could conceivably exist in these genes on a more widespread, populational basis. It is possible that such subtle mutations in these important mycobacterial resistance genes would have a large effect in tuberculosis-endemic areas.

Mannose-Binding Protein or Lectin

Another immunodeficiency which has been associated with chronic recurrent infections, mainly in infants, is mannose-binding lectin (MBL) deficiency (Turner, 1996). Located on chromosome 10q11.2–q21, MBL encodes a 32 kDa protein. The MBL molecule in serum is composed of up to six 96 kDa subunits, where each subunit consists of three 32 kDa proteins assimilated in a "bunch of tulips" structure (Epstein et al., 1996). Serum MBL acts as an opsonin to promote phagocytosis of pathogens during the phase of innate immunity (Turner, 1996). A deficiency in serum MBL concentrations has been termed the world's commonest immune deficiency and is present in up to 30% of Africans. There are three known structural mutations in exon 1 of the MBL gene, which have been linked to reduced serum concentrations of MBL. Given the potential importance of this immunodeficiency in the susceptibility to infectious diseases such as HIV, tuberculosis, and malaria, studies have begun to examine MBL polymorphisms in different populations. However, in a study in The Gambia, MBL deficiency was not linked to susceptibility to malaria or tuberculosis (Bellamy et al., 1998b). Contrary to what was expected, a study in sub-Saharan Africa indicated that high levels of serum MBL may be involved in the pathogenesis of tuberculosis in immunocompetent individuals (Garred et al., 1997b).

Genetic Resistance to HIV/AIDS

The worldwide AIDS epidemic has been characterized by variation in the rate of AIDS disease progression as well as susceptibility to infectivity by HIV-1 (O'Brien and Dean, 1997; Mann and Tarantola, 1998). Two categories of host genes play clear roles in the outcome of HIV-1 exposure and subsequent disease progression: first, several chemokine receptor genes strongly modulate HIV-1 infectivity and infection; second, polymorphic variants of *HLA* genes alter the course of AIDS (O'Brien, 1998; Rowland-Jones, 1998). The overall effect of the host's genetic background on the outcome of HIV disease is convincing: it has been estimated that the combined genotypes of the chemokine receptor genes together with the *HLA* genes can predict the HIV status of 70% of long-term nonprogressors and 81% of progressors (Magierowska et al., 1999).

To date, three commonly found mutations in three chemokine genes have been shown to protect against HIV-1 infection or to decrease the rate of HIV-1 disease progression (Martin et al., 1998; O'Brien, 1998; Rowland-Jones, 1998). In the first stage of infection, the *CCR5* gene has been linked with resistance to contraction of HIV infection through the mechanism of viral entry (Dean et al., 1996; Liu et al., 1996). To infect macrophages, the macrophage-tropic (M-tropic) variant of HIV-1 (NSI strains) uses the CD4 molecule and the *CCR5* coreceptor for entry. Normally, the *CCR5* coreceptor serves as the receptor for the chemokines RANTES and macrophage inflammatory protein 1α (MIP-1α and MIP-1β; HIV has obviously usurped this cellular access (Smith et al., 1997). Approximately 10% of Caucasians carry a 32 bp deletion mutation in the *CCR5* gene on chromosome 3, which causes the *CCR5* receptor to not be expressed. Highly exposed Caucasians who carry the Δ32 mutation in homozygous recessive form were found to be protected from HIV infection, whereas persons heterozygous for the mutation were found to have a delayed form of disease progression (Dean et al., 1996; Liu et al., 1996). Homozygous individuals do not appear to have any immunological defects as a result of the lack of *CCR5*, which is interesting in terms of designing targeted therapy against the *CCR5* receptor. However, Δ32 homozygous individuals are not protected against (SIV) HIV strains that use the *CXCR4* coreceptor for entry. A second gene, *CCR2*, which is linked with decreased HIV-1 disease progression in Caucasians as well as African Americans, is also found near *CCR5* on chromosome 3 (Anzala et al., 1998). The *CCR2* mutation (*CCR2*-64I) causes a conservative amino acid change at position 64 of the CCR2 protein, so how this mutation delays HIV disease progression is not clear (O'Brien, 1998). The *CCR2* and *CCR5* mutations are never found in the same individual, due to the fact that the *CCR5* mutation has much more recently appeared (Martin et al., 1998). The *CCR2*-64I mutation has been linked with the resistance to HIV found in a cohort of Nairobi prostitutes (O'Brien, 1998). Lastly, a mutation in the stromal cell differentiation factor-1 (SDF-1) gene on chromosome 10, which encodes the ligand for the chemokine coreceptor *CXCR4*, has been found which delays progression to AIDS (Winkler et al., 1998). Again, as the mutation is found in the 3′-UTR of the gene, the protective function of the mutation is unknown. The striking fact is the high frequency of individuals possessing one or more protective *CCR5*, *CCR2*, or *SDF-1* genotypes: in Caucasians, the estimated frequency is 39.1% and in African Americans, 31.5% (Martin et al., 1998).

To date, one allelic form of *CCR5* has been associated with more rapid progression to AIDS in both Caucasians and African Americans (Martin et al., 1998). In this study, a total of nine mutations were identified in the promoter of *CCR5*. The most frequent of these, the *CCR5*-P1 promoter mutation, is a recessive mutation, which may account for as many as 10% to 17% of rapid AIDS progressors. The function of the promoter mutation is not yet known, but it may upregulate transcription or expression of the CCR5 receptor.

HLA-Mediated Resistance to HIV

The AIDS epidemic, which has now lasted some 20 years, has been an unprecedented situation to look for HLA resistance because this is a relatively new human infection. However, clear effects of *HLA* genes have been revealed on progression to AIDS and death. In a multicenter study in Caucasians, 28% to 40% of HIV-infected persons who had slower disease progression and extended survival (up to 10 years following infection) expressed maximal heterozygosity at HLA class I loci (Carrington et al., 1999). In contrast, 8% to 11% of persons who progressed to AIDS within 6 years were homozygous at one (or more) *HLA* class I locus (Carrington et al., 1999). Homozygous expression of the HLA alleles *B*35* and *Cw*04* was associated with more rapid progression to AIDS. Thus, the protective effect, or "heterozygote advantage," which has been invoked for other infectious diseases also operates against HIV-1. A more heterozygous range of class I HLA loci is thought to engender a wider spectrum of HIV-1-specific CTLs that more effectively keeps the emergence of new viral mutants in check. In contrast, HLA-B14 and -C8 are associated with nonprogression (Hendel et al., 1999). However, as the *B*35* and *Cw*04* alleles have been previously shown to efficiently present HIV epitopes (HLA-B35-restricted CTLs that exhibit cross-reactivity between the levels of virus throughout HIV infection), the effect of these alleles is not obvious. It was suggested that they may downmodulate the activity of NK cells. An effect of specific HLA class II alleles on HIV disease progression has also been suggested (Hendel et al., 1999).

Phenotypic and CTL-Mediated Resistance to HIV

There is general agreement that not all phenotypic highly exposed but persistently seronegative (HEPS) resistance to infection can be explained by the *CCR5* Δ32 deletion, other known chemokine factors, or HLA heterozygosity. The resistance mechanism in HEPS cases (described in three different high-risk cohorts, both African and Caucasian) appears to be one of "superimmune" resistance (Fowke et al., 1998; Bernard et al., 1999; Goh et al., 1999). These studies suggest that HIV resistance is likely the result of complex gene–environment interactions. However, one common phenotype appears to be superior CTL activity in that HEPS individuals are HIV-seronegative but demonstrate good anti-HIV T-cell immunity. Several HEPS groups demonstrated extensive CTL cross-reactivity between different HIV-1 viral sequences. It has also been suggested that highly resistant persons may have encountered a similar virus which conferred protection against HIV (O'Brien and Dean, 1997). By extension, one wonders if the HEPS phenotype is not caused by a mechanism similar to that found in the Lake Casitas mouse strain, which resist Friend virus 4 retrovirus because they have acquired, through evolution, chromosomal inserts of retroviral proteins which effectively block the murine receptor for this virus (O'Brien, 1995).

MBL/HIV

Three studies have investigated the role of MBL deficiency in the susceptibility to HIV/AIDS. The first analysis, of a Copenhagen cohort, indicated that homozygous carriers of variant MBL alleles are at increased risk of HIV infection and, following a diagnosis of AIDS, are associated with a shorter survival time (Garred et al., 1997a). The second study, conducted in Finland on 300 HIV-infected and control individuals, confirmed the Copenhagen results by showing that homozygosity for the MBL variant alleles was increased significantly in the HIV-1-infected group (Pastinen et al., 1998). However, a study in Amsterdam detected a weak protective effect of variant MBL alleles, causing slower progression to AIDS, in a cohort of 131 HIV-1 homosexual men (Maas et al., 1998). It will be important for investigators of HIV cohorts to further test the role of MBL in HIV infection.

Malaria

The modern concept of genetic susceptibility and resistance to infections began with J. B. S. Haldane, who proposed that the common occurrence of thalassemia in Mediterranean people arose as a specific defense mechanism against malaria (Haldane, 1948). Furthermore, over the last half-century, malaria-related investigations have provided extraordinary insight into host–pathogen co-adaptive responses. The so-called classical studies in malaria have revealed several common, population-specific disorders that involve the human erythrocyte, the host cell of *P. falciparum*. These disorders include the hemoglobinopathies, such as the α- and β-thalassemia mutations and sickle-cell anemia, as well as glucose-6-phosphate dehydrogenase (G6PD) deficiencies and the Duffy negative blood group, which provides complete protection against pl. vivax malaria (Nagel and Roth, 1989; Weatherall et al., 1995, 1997; Weatherall, 1996a, 1997a,b; Hill, 1996a).

It is now apparent that α- and β-thalassemia mutations arose independently in different malarious regions. The α^+-thalassemia condition, which confers approximately 25% protection against malaria, results from deletion of one α-globin gene on chromosome 16 and causes mild anemia with normal hemoglobin (Hb A) structure (Weatherall, 1996a). Children with α^+-thalassemia may develop better immunity to severe malaria through an increased early-life susceptibility to mild malaria (Allen et al., 1997). There exist numerous mutations in the *β-globin* gene, located on chromosome 11p12, which result in lowered production of β-globin subunits and a heterogeneous group of disorders known as the β-thalassemias. The mechanism of protection against malaria is presently unknown. The predominantly African trait of sickle-cell anemia, which was the first "genetic" disease identified, arises from a single substitution of valine for glutamic acid at position 6 in the β-globin chain (Pauling et al., 1949; Ingram, 1956). The deoxygenated form of sickle hemoglobin (Hb S) polymerizes and results in a more rigid red blood cell that blocks circulation. Sickle-cell anemia is less common than the thalassemias but considerably more protective against malaria in the heterozygous state, approximately 80% to 95% (Weatherall, 1996a).

The enzyme G6PD was identified and located to the X chromosome in the 1950s (Carson et al., 1956). The mechanism of protection of G6PD-deficient cells against malaria appears to be due to the role of G6PD as a housekeeping enzyme for the regeneration of NADPH, a coenzyme that protects against oxidative damage (Friedman and Trager, 1981). Red cells deficient in G6PD are more sensitive to hydrogen peroxide generated by the malaria parasite, resulting in death of the parasite. It was established in two large case-control studies of African children that the common form of G6PD deficiency is associated with a 46% to 58% reduction in risk of severe malaria for both female heterozygotes and male hemizygotes (Ruwende et al., 1995).

In addition to all of the disorders involving the erythrocyte, malaria is probably the best example of infectious disease–driven evolutionary adaptation that has resulted in the population- or ethnically unique HLA polymorphisms and variants seen today (Haldane, 1948; Gupta et al., 1994; Gupta and Hill, 1995; Bodmer, 1996; Gilbert et al., 1998). In our discussion below, we focus on three genes or genetic regions that have been associated with susceptibility/resistance to malaria infection: the *TNFA* gene, the HLA class I and class II genes, and the chromosome 5q31–q33 region.

Malaria and TNF

Malaria is a multifaceted disease, with symptoms ranging from mild fever to cerebral malaria, generalized convulsions, coma, severe anemia, and death. Although the disease is treatable and certain individuals can recover without treatment, malaria is always dangerous in children and is the major killer of African children under the age of 5 years (WHO, 1999). One of the major aims of research on malaria has been to determine if susceptibility to its various forms has a genetic cause. A relationship between TNF and malaria susceptibility was first reported by Grau et al. (1989), who found that children in The Gambia with severe cerebral malaria had very high serum concentrations of TNF. This finding was subsequently repeated, confirming that high circulating TNF levels in serum are a biomarker of malaria mortality (Kwiatkowski, 1990; Kwiatkowski et al., 1990). The suggestion was that TNF causes upregulation of intracellular adhesion molecule 1 (ICAM-1) on erythrocytes, which creates a fatal obstruction in the blood vessels (McGuire et al., 1996; Wahlgren, 1999). Incidentally, a common *ICAM-1* variant has been associated with increased risk of severe malaria in Kenya (Fernandez-Reyes et al., 1997). McGuire and co-workers (1994) documented a genetic cause for the high TNF levels, finding that a polymorphism in the promoter region of the *TNFA* gene, −308, called the *TNF2* allele, was significantly higher in Gambian children with cerebral malaria. The same variant has also been associated with malaria in Sri Lanka (Wattavidanage et al., 1999). Two more alleles predisposing to severe malaria have been described. In the Gambia, an allelic TNF variant, −238, was associated with severe anemia in children (McGuire et al., 1999). A variant at −376 was associated with cerebral malaria in both Kenya and The Gambia (McGuire et al., 1999). The −376 TNF variant was a G–A base pair change, which created a new transcriptional binding site that increased the production of TNF. The overall contribution of the *TNFA* alleles to the susceptibility to malaria is estimated to be approximately 18%, strongly suggesting a role for other host genes in susceptibility.

Malaria and HLA

P. falciparum has a complex life cycle, which includes erythrocytic stages as well as an intrahepatocytic liver stage (exoerythrocytic parasites), and expresses different antigens during each stage. Liver parasites are an important target of immune $CD8^+$ T cells, and one antigen, liver-stage antigen 1 (LSA-1), has been identified as possessing a protective class I HLA epitope. In Papua New Guinea, resistance to *P. falciparum* infection correlated with $CD8^+$ T-cell IFN-γ responses to an LSA-1 epitope that contained an HLA-A11-restricted sequence at a frequency of 40% (Hollingdale et al., 1998). Likewise, in The Gambia, HLA-B53 is found at 40% frequency and is associated with both protection against malaria and responses to LSA-1 (Hill et al., 1992). The opposite situation may operate for the class II HLA *P. falciparum* merozoite surface antigens (MSA-1, MSA-2), which are expressed during the parasite blood stage. A study in Gabon showed that the class II HLA alleles *DRB1*04* and *DPB1*1701* are associated with susceptibility to severe malaria and may be associated with certain MSA families (May et al., 1999). Thus, the overall effect of HLA alleles in the resistance and susceptibility to malaria appears to be stronger than that of the *TNFA* alleles.

Malaria and the Chromosome 5q31–q33 Region

An important aspect of the susceptibility to malaria is parasitemia of blood parasites. Several complex segregation analyses have tested for a possible major gene effect on the expression of this phenotype. While the first of these complex modeling analyses was consistent with a major gene effect (Abel et al., 1992), two additional studies were consistent with a major effect on blood infection levels, but this major effect did not follow simple Mendelian rules (Garcia et al., 1998a; Rihet et al., 1998a). All studies favored strong age–genotype interactions, suggesting that genetic studies in children may have higher power to detect the effect of individual genes on blood infection levels. To localize genes influencing blood parasitemia, two linkage studies have been conducted. In the first sib-pair linkage study performed on nine families from Cameroon, five candidate genome regions were analyzed for the presence of genes influencing blood infection. Borderline significant evidence for the presence of a locus on chromosome region 5q31–q33 was found (Garcia et al., 1998b). In the second study, 285 sib pairs belonging to 34 families from Burkina Faso were analyzed for linkage of the trait with chromosome region 5q31–q33 (Rihet et al., 1998b). In this extended family sample, highly significant evidence for the presence of a blood infection level–influencing gene on the studied chromosomal segment was obtained (Rihet et al., 1998b). Linkage of malaria to chromosome region 5q31–q33 is interesting for two reasons: first, this genome segment contains a large number of immunomodulatory genes, such as *IL-4*, *IL-12*, *IL-3*, and *CSF*, involved in Th1 vs. Th2 immune response regulation and possibly atopy; second, a major locus controlling the intensity of infection by *Schistosoma mansoni* had previously been located to the same genome region (Marquet et al., 1996). This opens the exciting possibility that allelic variants of a single major gene may influence susceptibility to at least two major infections and autoimmune disease.

CONCLUSION

The drive to understand the nature of genetics has always been powerful, yet more than a century after Mendel's (1865) paper, even in our postgenome era, we must realize that we may never arrive at the "true" function of a particular gene. Genetics alone will not conquer the present threat to public health by infectious diseases. However, understanding genetically controlled host responses in the host–parasite interplay will be crucial in efforts to control the most prevalent infections.

Here, we quote from Bateson (1900), perhaps somewhat out of context, where he had already outlined the neccessity of using clear phenotypes, which we have reiterated in this chapter. More than that, however, he displayed the optimism with which we would like to conclude our discussion.

> Enough has been said to show how necessary it is that the subjects of experiment should be chosen in such a way as to bring the laws of heredity to a real test. For this purpose the first essential is that the differentiating characters should be few, and that all avoidable complications should be got rid of. Each experiment should be reduced to its simplest possible limits. The results obtained by Galton, and also the new ones especially detailed in this paper have each been reached by restricting the range of observation to one character or group of characters, and there is every hope that by similar treatment our knowledge of heredity may be rapidly extended."

With those words in mind, we offer the following conclusions.

1. *How might identification of susceptibility genes help in infectious disease treatment?* The root of this question lies in the fact that the genetics of disease susceptibility is, in essence, just another method of identifying biochemical pathways important for the pathogenesis of the studied trait. That is to say, the identification of a gene which protects or predisposes to an infectious disease is a way to discover the role of a protein in the host biological defense against that pathogen. The hope of genetics is to find major gene effects because this should signify the most important proteins. Therapy may then not be based on the gene itself, i.e., gene therapy, but on strategies that can help or hinder the protein's activity. For example, a foreseeable approach could be the use of recombinant cytokines, the choice of which is dictated by our knowledge of genetically determined susceptibility traits. Likewise, identification of genetically controlled infection-resistance mechanisms would suggest therapeutic ways of intervention that are "approved by evolution."

2. *How can identification of susceptibility genes aid in identifying those at risk?* Genetic testing is, of course, presently a reality for many diseases. The question is how applicable will genetic testing be for infectious diseases, particularly in the developing world. Rather than to dismiss the possibility outright as too costly, there are several options. One is to identify populations at risk, a more-or-less approach that would target diagnostic services and medical personnel availability to populations at very high risk. Another is to appreciate that genetic testing of individuals, even in poor nations, could become a reality within the next decade if genomics technology continues at its present pace. Too expensive, many might say, but consider the following real scenario. There is presently an epidemic of multidrug-resistant tuberculosis raging in Russian prisons (estimated cost of treating one individual: $250,000). It is estimated that presently scores of thousands of individuals carry multidrug-resistance forms of the tubercle bacillus, and these numbers are increasing. As these individuals start developing tuberculosis (with a lifetime risk of 10%) and pass on their drug-resistant bacilli to other members of their communities, the cost of treatment becomes unimaginable. With a test to detect and target susceptible individuals most likely to advance from infection to clinically overt disease for preventive therapy, the threat of multidrug-resistant tuberculosis could be manageable. Tests that could be developed may be phenotypic tests that correlate with genetic susceptibility or resistance. The prototype of such tests is the purified protein derivative skin test, which has been used for decades to estimate *M. tuberculosis* infection rates in the developing world. The value of such a simple genetic skin test for tuberculosis susceptibility would be staggering.

3. *Will identification of susceptibility genes aid in the development of new vaccines?* Hard evidence for the influence of human genes in response to vaccines and antigens is restricted to the HLA. The discovery of HLA supertypes and HLA types that have co-evolved with pathogens such as malaria presents tangible possiblities for vaccine design. There is much evidence to show that HLA types have influenced the response to pathogens; there is also similar evidence for the MHC in mice. However, studies of human genetic susceptibility to infections have revealed that non-*HLA* genes are very strong modulators of the immune response; therefore, it is unlikely that immunity is influenced only by the HLA. While the genetic control of responses to vaccines is still in its infancy, there is every reason to expect that the discovery of human infectious disease susceptibility genes will have a major impact on future vaccine design. A good example of this is the present intense effort to develop an AIDS vaccine. One promising avenue of developing such a vaccine is the use of live attenuated forms of HIV-1 (Deacon et al., 1995). SIV infection in macaques is a close correlate of HIV. Experiments in macaques showed an astounding variety of individual responses to vaccination with live attenuated SIV strains, ranging from complete protection against reinfection with wild-type SIV to the development of AIDS due to the vaccination strain (Wyand et al., 1996; Baba et al., 1999). This variability in vaccine responses was unrelated to possible mutations within the virus genome and, hence, directly shows the importance of constitutive host factors in influencing vaccine efficacy (Baba et al., 1999).

It is our hope that the above prospects can become realities in the same way that a few years ago, the Human Genome Project was just a dim prospect on the horizon. Perhaps Robert H. Goddard put it best: "It is difficult to say what is impossible, for the dream of yesterday is the hope of today and the reality of tomorrow."

REFERENCES

Abel L, Casanova JL: Genetic predisposition to clinical tuberculosis: bridging the gap between simple and complex inheritance. Am J Hum Genet 2000; 67:274–277.

Abel L, Cot M, Mulder L, Carnevale P, Feingold J: Segregation analysis detects a major gene controlling blood infection levels in human malaria. Am J Hum Genet 1992; 50:1308–1317.

Abel L, Demenais F, Prata A, Souza AE, Dessein A: Evidence for the segregation of a major gene in human susceptibility/resistance to infection by *Schistosoma mansoni*. Am J Hum Genet 1991; 48:959–970.

Abel L, Dessein AJ: The impact of host genetics on susceptibility to human infectious diseases. Curr Opin Immunol 1997; 9:509–516.

Abel L, Dessein AJ: Genetic epidemiology of infectious diseases in humans: design of population-based studies. Emerg Infect Dis 1998; 4:593–603.

Abel L, Lap VD, Oberti J, Thuc NV, Cua VV, Guilloud-Bataille M, Schurr E, Lagrange PH: Complex segregation analysis of leprosy in southern Vietnam. Genet Epidemiol 1995; 12:63–85.

Abel L, Sanchez FO, Oberti J, Thuc NV, Hoa LV, Lap VD, Skamene E, Lagrange PH, Schurr E: Susceptibility to leprosy is linked to the human *NRAMP1* gene. J Infect Dis 1998; 177:133–145.

Alcais FO, Sanchez NV, Thuc VD, Lap J, Oberti PH, Lagrange E, Schurr L: Granulomatous reaction to intradermal injection of lepromin (Mitsuda Reaction) is linked to the human *NRAMP1* gene in Vietnamese leprosy sibships. J Infect Dis 2000; 181:302–308.

Alcais A, Abel L, David C, Torrez ME, Flandre P, Dedet JP: Evidence for a major gene controlling susceptibility to tegumentary leishmaniasis in a recently exposed Bolivian population. Am J Hum Genet 1997; 61:968–979.

Allen SJ, O'Donnell A, Alexander ND, Alpers MP, Peto TEA, Clegg JB, Weatherall DJ: α^+-Thalassemia protects children against disease caused by other infections as well as malaria. Proc Natl Acad Sci USA 1997; 94:14736–14741.

Altare F, Durandy A, Lammas D, Emile JF, Lamhamedi S, Le Deist F, Drysdale P, Jouanguy E, Doffinger R, Bernaudin F, et al.: Impairment of mycobacterial immunity in human interleukin-12 receptor deficiency. Science 1998a; 280:1432–1435.

Altare F, Jouanguy E, Lamhamedi S, Doffinger R, Fischer A, Casanova JL: Mendelian susceptibility to mycobacterial infection in man. Curr Opin Immunol 1998b; 10:413–417.

Altare F, Jouanguy E, Lamhamedi-Cherradi S, Fondaneche MC, Fizame C, Ribierre F, Merlin G, Dembic Z, Schreiber R, Lisowska-Grospierre B, et al.: A causative relationship between mutant *IFNγR1* alleles and impaired cellular response to IFNgamma in a compound heterozygous child. Am J Hum Genet 1998c; 62:723–726.

Altare F, Lammas D, Revy P, Jouanguy E, Doffinger R, Lamhamedi S, Drysdale P, Scheel-Toellner D, Girdlestone J, Darbyshire P, et al.: Inherited interleukin 12 deficiency in a child with bacille Calmette-Guerin and *Salmonella enteritidis* disseminated infection. J Clin Invest 1998d; 102:2035–2040.

Anzala AO, Ball TB, Rostron T, O'Brien SJ, Plummer FA, Rowland-Jones SL: *CCR2*-64I allele and genotype association with delayed AIDS progression in African women. University of Nairobi Collaboration for HIV Research. Lancet 1998; 351:1632–1633.

Baba TW, Liska V, Khimani AH, Ray NB, Dailey PJ, Penninck D, Bronson R, Greene MF, McClure HM, Martin LN, et al.: Live attenuated, multiply deleted simian immunodeficiency virus causes AIDS in infant and adult macaques. Nat Med 1999; 5:194–203.

Baird JK: Host age as a determinant of naturally acquired immunity to *Plasmodium falciparum*. Parasitol Today 1995; 11:105–111.

Baker AR, McDonell DP, Hughes M, Crisp TM, Mangelsdorf DJ, Haussler MR, Pike JW, Shine J, O'Malley BW: Cloning and expression of full length cDNA encoding human vitamin D receptor. Proc Natl Acad Sci USA 1988; 85:3294–3298.

Barnes PF, Modlin RL, Bikle DD, Adams JS: Transpleural gradients of 1,25-dihydroxyvitamin D in tuberculous pleuritis. J Clin Invest 1989; 83:1527–1533.

Bateson W: Problems of heredity as a subject for horticultural investigation. J R Horticult Soc 1900; 25:54–61.

Beebe AM, Mauze S, Schork NJ, Coffman RL: Serial backcross mapping of multiple loci associated with resistance to *Leishmania major* in mice. Immunity 1997; 6:551–557.

Bekker LG, Maartens G, Steyn L, Kaplan G: Selective increase in plasma tumor necrosis factor-alpha and concomitant clinical deterioration after initiating therapy in patients with severe tuberculosis. J Infect Dis 1998; 178:580–584.

Bellamy R, Beyers N, McAdam KP, Ruwende C, Gie R, Samaai P, Bester D, Meyer M, Corrah T, Collin M, et al.: Genetic susceptibility to tuberculosis in Africans: a genome-wide scan. Proc Natl Acad Sci USA 2000; 97:8005–8009.

Bellamy R, Hill AV: Genetic susceptibility to mycobacteria and other infectious pathogens in humans. Curr Opin Immunol 1998a; 10:483–487.

Bellamy R, Ruwende C, Corrah T, McAdam KP, Thursz M, Whittle HC, Hill AV: Tuberculosis and chronic hepatitis B virus infection in Africans and variation in the vitamin D receptor gene. J Infect Dis 1999; 179:721–724.

Bellamy R, Ruwende C, Corrah T, McAdam KP, Whittle HC, Hill AV: Variations in the *NRAMP1* gene and susceptibility to tuberculosis in West Africans. N Engl J Med 1998a; 338:640–644.

Bellamy R, Ruwende C, McAdam KP, Thursz M, Sumiya M, Summerfield J, Gilbert SC, Corrah T, Kwiatkowski D, Whittle HC, et al.: Mannose binding protein deficiency is not associated with malaria, hepatitis B carriage nor tuberculosis in Africans. QJM 1998b; 91:13–18.

Bellamy RJ, Hill AV: Host genetic susceptibility to human tuberculosis. Novartis Found Symp 1998b; 217:3–13.

Bermudez LE, Young LS: Tumour necrosis factor-α stimulates mycobactericidal–mycobacteriostatic activity in human macrophages by a protein kinase C–independent pathway. Cell Immunol 1992; 144:258–268.

Bernard NF, Yannakis CM, Lee JS, Tsoukas CM: Human immunodeficiency virus (HIV)–specific cytotoxic T lymphocyte activity in HIV-exposed seronegative persons. J Infect Dis 1999; 179:538–547.

Bioque G, Crusius JB, Koutroubakis I, Bouma G, Kostense PJ, Meuwissen SG, Pena AS: Allelic polymorphism in IL-1beta and IL-1 receptor antagonist (IL-1Ra) genes in inflammatory bowel disease. Clin Exp Immunol 1995; 102:379–383.

Blackwell JM: Genetics of host resistance and susceptibility to intramacrophage pathogens: a study of multicase families of tuberculosis, leprosy and leishmaniasis in north-eastern Brazil. Int J Parasitol 1998; 28:21–28.

Blackwell JM, Barton CH, White JK, Roach TI, Shaw MA, Whitehead SH, Mock BA, Searle S, Williams H, Baker AM: Genetic regulation of leishmanial and mycobacterial infections: the *Lsh/Ity/Bcg* gene story continues. Immunol Lett 1994; 43:99–107.

Blackwell JM, Black GF, Peacock CS, Miller EN, Sibthorpe D, Gnanandha D, Shaw JJ, Silveira F, Lins-Lainson Z, Ramos F, et al.: Immunogenetics of leishmanial and mycobacterial infections: the Belem Family Study. Philos Trans R Soc Lond B Biol Sci 1997; 352:1331–1345.

Bodmer J: World distribution of HLA alleles and implications for disease. In: Chadwick D, Cardew G (eds). Variation in the Human Genome. Ciba Foundation Symposium 197. Chichester: J. Wiley & Sons, 1996:233–258.

Bothamley GH: Differences between HLA-B44 and HLA-B60 in patients with smear-positive pulmonary tuberculosis and exposed controls. J Infect Dis 1999; 179: 1051–1052.

Buschman E, Schurr E, Skamene E: Constitutional resistance to mycobacterial onfections: role of genetic factors in resistance to infection. In: Verduin CM, Watson DA, van Dijk H, Verhoef J (eds). Constitutional Resistance to Infection. Austin: RG Landes, 1995:55–81.

Buu NT, Cellier M, Gros P, Schurr E: Identification of a highly polymorphic length variant in the 3′UTR of *NRAMP1*. Immunogenetics 1995; 42:428–429.

Cabrera M, Shaw M-A, Sharples C, Williams H, Castes M, Convit J, Blackwell JM: Polymorphism in tumour necrosis factor genes associated with mucocutaneous leishmaniasis. J Exp Med 1995; 182:1259–1264.

Carrington M, Nelson GW, Martin MP, Kissner T, Vlahov D, Goedert JJ, Kaslow R, Buchbinder S, Hoots K, O'Brien SJ: HLA and HIV-1: heterozygote advantage and B*35–Cw*04 disadvantage. Science 1999; 283:1748–1752.

Carson PE, Flanagan CL, Ickes CE, Alving AS: Enzymatic deficiency in primaquine-sensitive erythrocytes. Science 1956; 124:484–485.

Cellier M, Shustik C, Dalton W, Rich E, Hu J, Malo D, Schurr E, Gros P: Expression of the human *NRAMP1* gene in professional primary phagocytes: studies in blood cells and in HL-60 promyelocytic leukemia. J Leukoc Biol 1997; 61:96–105.

Cooper RS, Rotimi CN, Ward R: The puzzle of hypertension in African-Americans. Sci Am 1999; 280:56–63.

Crowle AJ, Elkins N: Relative permissiveness of macrophages from black and white people for virulent tubercle bacilli. Infect Immun 1990; 582:632–638.

Davenport MP, Hill AV: Reverse immunogenetics: from HLA–disease associations to vaccine candidates. Mol Med Today 1996; 2:38–45.

Davies PDO: The role of vitamin D in tuberculosis [letter]. Am Rev Respir Dis 1989; 139:1571.

Deacon NJ, Tsykin A, Solomon A, Smith K, Ludford-Menting M, Hooker DJ, McPhee DA, Greenway AL, Ellett A, Chatfield C, et al.: Genomic structure of an attenuated quasi species of HIV-1 from a blood transfusion donor and recipients. Science 1995; 270:988–991.

Dean M, Carrington M, Winkler C, Huttley GA, Smith MW, Allikmets R, Goedert JJ, Buchbinder SP, Vittinghoff E, Gomperts E, et al.: Genetic restriction of HIV-1 infection and progression to AIDS by a deletion allele of the *CKR5* structural gene. Hemophilia Growth and Development Study, Multicenter AIDS Cohort Study, Multicenter Hemophilia Cohort Study, San Francisco City Cohort, ALIVE Study [see comments] [published erratum appears in Science 1996; 274:1069]. Science 1996; 273:1856–1862.

de Jong R, Altare F, Haagen IA, Elferink DG, Boer T, van Breda Vriesman PJ, Kabel PJ, Draaisma JM, van Dissel JT, Kroon FP, et al.: Severe mycobacterial and *Salmonella* infections in interleukin-12 receptor–deficient patients. Science 1998; 280:1435–1438.

de Vries RR, Meera Khan P, Bernini LF, van Loghem E, van Rood JJ: Genetic control of survival in epidemics. J Immunogenet 1979; 6:271–287.

Dib C, Faure S, Fizames C, Samson D, Drouot N, Vignal A, Millasseau P, Marc S, Hazan J, Seboun E, et al.: A comprehensive genetic map of the human genome based on 5,264 microsatellites. Nature 1996; 380:152–154.

Dorman SE, Holland SM: Mutation in the signalling chain of the interferon gamma receptor is associated with severe mycobacterial infection. J Clin Invest 1998; 101:2364–2369.

Epstein J, Eichbaum Q, Sheriff S, Ezekowitz RA: The collectins in innate immunity. Curr Opin Immunol 1996; 8:29–35.

Fernandez-Reyes D, Craig AG, Kyes SA, Peshu N, Snow RW, Berendt AR, Marsh K, Newbold CI: A high frequency African coding polymorphism in the N-terminal domain of ICAM-1 predisposing to cerebral malaria in Kenya. Hum Mol Genet 1997; 6:1357–1360.

Flynn JL, Chan J, Triebold KJ, Dalton DK, Stewart TA, Bloom BR: An essential role for interferon gamma in resistance to *Mycobacterium tuberculosis* infection. J Exp Med 1993; 178:2249–2254.

Foote SJ, Burt RA, Baldwin TM, Presente A, Roberts AW, Laural YL, Lew AM, Marshall VM: Mouse loci for malaria-induced mortality and the control of parasitaemia. Nat Genet 1997; 17:380–381.

Fortin A, Belouchi A, Tam MF, Cardon L, Skamene E, Stevenson MM, Gros P: Genetic control of blood parasitaemia in mouse malaria maps to chromosome 8. Nat Genet 1997; 17:382–383.

Fortin A, Cardon LR, Tam M, Skamene E, Stevenson MM, Gros P: Identification of a new malaria susceptibility locus (Char4) in recombinant congenic strains of mice. Proc Natl Acad Sci USA 2001; 98:10793–10798.

Fowke KR, Nagelkerke NJD, Kimani J, Simonsen JN, Anzala AO, Bwayo JJ, MacDonald KS, Ngugi EN, Plummer FA: Resistance to HIV-1 infection among persistently seronegative prostitus in Nairobi, Kenya. Lancet 1998; 348:1347–1351.

Friedman MJ, Trager W: The biochemistry of resistance to malaria. Sci Am 1981; 244:158–164.

Garcia A, Cot M, Chippaux JP, Ranque S, Feingold J, Demenais F, Abel L: Genetic control of blood infection levels in human malaria: evidence for a complex genetic model. Am J Trop Med Hyg 1998a; 58:480–488.

Garcia A, Marquet S, Bucheton B, Hillaire D, Cot M, Fievet N, Dessein AJ, Abel L: Linkage analysis of blood *Plasmodium falciparum* levels: interest of the 5q31–q33 chromosome region. Am J Trop Med Hyg 1998b; 58:705–709.

Garred P, Madsen HO, Balslev U, Hofmann B, Pedersen C, Gerstoft J, Svejgaard A: Susceptibility to HIV infection and progression of AIDS in relation to variant alleles of mannose-binding lectin. Lancet 1997a; 349:236–240.

Garred P, Richter C, Andersen AB, Madsen HO, Mtoni I, Svejgaard A, Shao J: Mannan-binding lectin in the sub-Saharan HIV and tuberculosis epidemics. Scand J Immunol 1997b; 46:204–208.

Gilbert SC, Plebanski M, Gupta S, Morris J, Cox M, Aidoo M, Kwiatkowski D, Greenwood BM, Whittle HC, Hill AV: Association of malaria parasite population structure, HLA, and immunological antagonism. Science 1998; 279:1173–1177.

Gkonos PJ, London R, Hendler ED: Hypercalcemia and elevated 1,25-dihydroxyvitamin levels in a patient with end-stage renal disease and active tuberculosis. N Engl J Med 1984; 311:1683–1685.

Goh WC, Markee J, Akridge RE, Meldorf M, Musey L, Karchmer T, Krone M, Collier A, Corey L, Emerman M, et al.: Protection against human immunodeficiency virus type 1 infection in persons with repeated exposure: evidence for T cell immunity in the absence of inherited CCR5 coreceptor defects. J Infect Dis 1999; 179:548–557.

Govoni G, Vidal S, Gauthier S, Skamene E, Malo D, Gros P: The Bcg/Ity/Lsh locus: genetic transfer of resistance to infections in C57BL/6J mice transgenic for the $Nramp1^{Gly169}$ allele. Infect Immun 1996; 64:2923–2929.

Grau GE, Taylor TE, Molyneux ME, Wirima JJ, Vassalli P, Hommel M, Lambert PH: Tumor necrosis factor and disease severity in children with falciparum malaria. N Engl J Med 1989; 320:1586–1591.

Greenwood CMT, Fujiwara TM, Boothroyd LJ, Miller MA, Frappier D, Fanning EA, Schurr E, Morgan K: Linkage of tuberculosis to chromosome 2q35 loci, including NRAMP1, in a large aboriginal Canadian family. Am J Hum Genet 2000; 67:405–416.

Gruenheid S, Canonne-Hergaux F, Gauthier S, Hackam DJ, Grinstein S, Gros P: The iron transport protein NRAMP2 is an integral membrane glycoprotein that colocalizes with transferrin in recycling endosomes. J Exp Med 1999; 189:831–841.

Gupta S, Hill AV: Dynamic interactions in malaria: host heterogeneity meets parasite polymorphism. Proc R Soc Lond B Biol Sci 1995; 261:271–277.

Gupta S, Hill AV, Kwiatkowski D, Greenwood AM, Greenwood BM, Day KP: Parasite virulence and disease patterns in *Plasmodium falciparum* malaria. Proc Natl Acad Sci U S A 1994; 91:3715–3719.

Gyapay G, Schmitt K, Fizames C, Jones H, Vega-Czarny N, Spillett D, Muselet D, Prud'Homme JF, Dib C, Auffray C, et al.: A radiation hybrid map of the human genome. Hum Mol Genet 1996; 5:339–346.

Hacia JG, Fan JB, Ryder O, Jin L, Edgemon K, Ghandour G, Mayer RA, Sun B, Hsie L, Robbins CM, et al.: Determination of ancestral alleles for human single-nucleotide polymorphisms using high-density oligonucleotide arrays. Nat Genet 1999; 22:164–167.

Hackam DJ, Rotstein OD, Zhang W, Gruenheid S, Gros P, Grinstein S: Host resistance to intracellular infection: mutation of natural resistance-associated macrophage protein 1 (Nramp1) impairs phagosomal acidification. J Exp Med 1998; 188:351–364.

Haldane JBS: The rate of mutation of human genes. Hereditas 1948; 35:267–273.

Hendel H, Caillat-Zucman S, Lebuanec H, Carrington M, O'Brien S, Andrieu JM, Schachter F, Zagury D, Rappaport J, Winkler C, et al.: New class I and II HLA alleles strongly associated with opposite patterns of progression to AIDS. J Immunol 1999; 1993:6942–6946.

Hill AV: Malaria resistance genes: a natural selection. Trans R Soc Trop Med Hyg 1992; 86:225–226.

Hill AV: Genetic susceptibility to malaria and other infectious diseases: from the MHC to the whole genome. Parasitology 1996a; 112:S75–S84.

Hill AV: Genetics of infectious disease resistance. Curr Opin Genet Dev 1996b; 6:348–353.

Hill AV: Genetic susceptibility to multifactorial diseases. Trans R Soc Trop Med Hyg 1997; 91:369–371.

Hill AV: The immunogenetics of human infectious diseases. Annu Rev Immunol 1998a; 16:593–617.

Hill AV: Host genetics of infectious diseases: old and new approaches converge. Emerg Infec Dis 1998b; 4:695–697.

Hill AV, Allsopp CE, Kwiatkowski D, Anstey NM, Twumasi P, Rowe PA, Bennett S, Brewster D, McMichael AJ, Greenwood BM: Common west African HLA antigens are associated with protection from severe malaria. Nature 1991; 352:595–600.

Hill AV, Elvin J, Willis AC, Aidoo M, Allsopp CE, Gotch FM, Gao XM, Takiguchi M, Greenwood BM, Townsend AR, et al.: Molecular analysis of the association of HLA-B53 and resistance to severe malaria. Nature 1992; 360:434–439.

Hollingdale MR, McCormick CJ, Heal KG, Taylor-Robinson AW, Reeve P, Boykins R, Kazura JW: Biology of malarial liver stages: implications for vaccine design. Ann Trop Med Parasitol 1998; 92:411–417.

Hudson TJ, Stein LD, Gerety SS, Ma J, Castle AB, Silva J, Slonim DK, Baptista R, Kruglyak L, Xu SH, et al.: An STS-based map of the human genome. Science 1995; 270:1945–1954.

Hustmeyer FG, DeLuca HF, Peacock M: *ApaI*, *BsmI*, *EcoRV*, and *TaqI* polymorphisms at the human vitamin D receptor gene in Caucasians, blacks, and Asians. Hum Mol Genet 1993; 2:487.

Ingram VM: A specific chemical difference between the globins of normal human and sickle cell anemia hemoglobin. Nature 1956; 178:792–794.

International Human Genome Sequence Consortium: Initial sequence and analysis of the human genome. Nature 2001; 409:860–934.

Jan Bouma M, Dye C: Cycles of malaria associated with el Nino in Venezuela. JAMA 1997; 278:1772–1774.

Jepson A: Twin studies for the analysis of heritability of infectious diseases. Bull Inst Pasteur 1998; 96:71–81.

Jepson A, Banya W, Sisay-Joof F, Hassan-King M, Nunes C, Bennett S, Whittle H: Quantification of the relative contribution of major histocompatibility complex (MHC) and non-MHC genes to human immune responses to foreign antigens. Infect Immun 1997; 65:872–876.

Jouanguy E, Altare F, Lamhamedi S, Revy P, Emile JF, Newport M, Levin M, Blanche S, Seboun E, Fischer A, et al.: Interferon-gamma-receptor deficiency in an infant with fatal bacille Calmette-Guerin infection. N Engl J Med 1996; 335:1956–1961.

Jouanguy E, Altare F, Lamhamedi-Cherradi S, Casanova JL: Infections in IFNGR-1-deficient children. J Interferon Cytokine Res 1997a; 17:583–587.

Jouanguy E, Lamhamedi-Cherradi S, Altare F, Fondaneche MC, Tuerlinckx D, Blanche S, Emile JF, Gaillard JL, Schreiber R, Levin M, et al.: Partial interferon-gamma receptor 1 deficiency in a child with tuberculoid bacillus Calmette-Guerin infection and a sibling with clinical tuberculosis. J Clin Invest 1997b; 100:2658–2264.

Jouanguy E, Lamhamedi-Cherradi S, Lammas D, Dorman SE, Fondaneche MC, Dupuis S, Doffinger R, Altare F, Girdlestone J, Emile JF, et al.: A human IFNGR1 small deletion hotspot associated with dominant susceptibility to mycobacterial infection. Nat Genet 1999; 21:370–378.

Juffermans NP, Verbon A, van Deventer SJ, van Deutekom H, Speelman P, van der Poll T: Tumor necrosis factor and interleukin-1 inhibitors as markers of disease activity of tuberculosis. Am J Res Crit Care Med 1998; 157:1328–1331.

Karunaweera ND, Carter R, Grau GE, Kwiatkowski D, Del Giudice G, Mendis KN: Tumour necrosis factor–dependent parasite-killing effects during paroxysms in non-immune *Plasmodium vivax* malaria patients. Clin Exp Immunol 1992; 88:499–505.

Khanolkar-Young S, Rayment N, Brickell PM, Katz DR, Vinayakumar S, Colston MJ, Lockwood DN: Tumour necrosis factor-alpha (TNF-alpha) synthesis is asso-

ciated with the skin and peripheral nerve pathology of leprosy reversal reactions. Clin Exp Immunol 1995; 99:196–202.
Klausner JD, Freedman VH, Kaplan G: Thalidomide as an anti-TNF-alpha inhibitor: implications for clinical use. Clin Immunol Immunopathol 1996; 81:219–223.
Kramnik I, Dietrich WF, Demant P, Bloom BR: Genetic control of resistance to experimental infection with virulent *Mycobacterium tuberculosis*. Proc Natl Acad Sci USA 2000; 97:8560–8565.
Kwiatkowski D: Tumour necrosis factor, fever and fatality in falciparum malaria. Immunol Lett 1990; 25:213–216.
Kwiatkowski D, Hill AV, Sambou I, Twumasi P, Castracane J, Manogue KR, Cerami A, Brewster DR, Greenwood BM: TNF concentration in fatal cerebral, non-fatal cerebral, and uncomplicated *Plasmodium falciparum* malaria. Lancet 1990; 336:1201–1204.
Labuda M, Ross MV, Fujiwara TM, Morgan K, Ledbetter D, Hughes MR, Glorieux F: Two hereditary defects related to vitamin D metabolism map to same region of human chromosome 12q. Cytogenet Cell Genet 1991; 58:1978.
Lavebratt C, Apt A, Nikonenko BV, Schalling M, Schurr E: Severity of tuberculosis in mice is linked to distal chromosome 3 and proximal chromosome 9. J Infect Dis 1999; 180:150–155.
Levee G, Liu J, Gicquel B, Chanteau S, Schurr E: Genetic control of susceptibility to leprosy in French Polynesia; no evidence for linkage with markers on telomeric human chromosome 2. Int J Lepr Other Mycobact Dis 1994; 62:499–511.
Levin M, Newport M: Unravelling the genetic basis of susceptibility to mycobacterial infection. J Pathol 1997; 181:5–7.
Liu J, Fujiwara TM, Buu NT, Sanchez FO, Cellier M, Paradis AJ, Frappier D, Skamene E, Gros P, Morgan K, et al.: Identification of polymorphisms and sequence variants in the human homologue of the mouse natural resistance-associated macrophage protein gene. Am J Hum Genet 1995; 56:845–853.
Liu R, Paxton WA, Choe S, Ceradini D, Martin SR, Horuk R, MacDonald ME, Stuhlmann H, Koup RA, Landau NR: Homozygous defect in HIV-1 coreceptor accounts for resistance of some multiply-exposed individuals to HIV-1 infection. Cell 1996; 86:367–377.
Maas J, de Roda Husman AM, Brouwer M, Krol A, Coutinho R, Keet I, van Leeuwen R, Schuitemaker H: Presence of the variant mannose-binding lectin alleles associated with slower progression to AIDS. Amsterdam Cohort Study. AIDS 1998; 12:2275–2280.
Maasho K, Sanchez F, Schurr E, Hailu A, Akuffo H: Indications of the protective role of natural killer cells in human cutaneous leishmaniasis in an area of endemicity. Infect Immun 1998; 66:2698–2704.
Magierowska M, Theodorou I, Debre P, Sanson F, Autran B, Riviere Y, Charron D, Costagliola D: Combined genotypes of *CCR5, CCR2, SDF1*, and *HLA* genes can predict the long-term nonprogressor status in human immunodeficiency virus-1–infected individuals. Blood 1999; 93:936–941.
Malo D, Vogan K, Vidal S, Hu J, Cellier M, Schurr E, Fuks A, Bumstead N, Morgan K, Gros P: Haplotype mapping and sequence analysis of the mouse *Nramp* gene predict susceptibility to infection with intracellular parasites. Genomics 1994; 23:51–61.
Mann JM, Tarantola DJ: HIV 1998: the global picture. Sci Am 1998; 279:82–83.
Marquet S, Abel L, Hillaire D, Dessein H, Kalil J, Feingold J, Weissenbach J, Dessein AJ: Genetic localization of a locus controlling the intensity of infection by *Schistosoma mansoni* on chromosome 5q31–q33. Nat Genet 1996; 14:181–184.
Marquet S, Lepage P, Hudson TJ, Musser JM, Schurr E: Complete nucleotide sequence and genomic structure of the human *NRAMP1* gene region on chromosome region 2q35. Mamm Genome 2000; 11:755–762.
Martin MP, Dean M, Smith MW, Winkler C, Gerrard B, Michael NL, Lee B, Doms RW, Margolick J, Buchbinder S, et al.: Genetic acceleration of AIDS progression by a promoter variant of CCR5. Science 1998; 282:1907–1911.
May J, Meyer CG, Kun JF, Lell B, Luckner D, Dippmann AK, Bienzle U, Kremsner PG: HLA class II factors associated with *Plasmodium falciparum* merozoite surface antigen allele families. J Infect Dis 1999; 179:1042–1045.
McGuire W, Hill AV, Allsopp CE, Greenwood BM, Kwiatkowski D: Variation in the TNF-alpha promoter region associated with susceptibility to cerebral malaria. Nature 1994; 371:508–510.
McGuire W, Hill AV, Greenwood BM, Kwiatkowski D: Circulating ICAM-1 levels in falciparum malaria are high but unrelated to disease severity. Trans R Soc Trop Med Hyg 1996; 90:274–276.
McGuire W, Knight JC, Hill AV, Allsopp CE, Greenwood BM, Kwiatkowski D: Severe malarial anemia and cerebral malaria are associated with different tumor necrosis factor promoter alleles. J Infect Dis 1999; 179:287–290.
McKinney JD, Jacobs WR, Bloom B: Persisting problems in tuberculosis. In: Krause RM (ed). Emerging Infections. Biomedical Research Reports. New York: Academic Press, 1998:51–146.
Medina E, North RJ: Evidence inconsistent with a role for the *Bcg* gene (*Nramp1*) in resistance of mice to infection with virulent *Mycobacterium tuberculosis*. J Exp Med 1996; 183:1045–1051.
Mendel G: Experiments in plant hybridization [in German]. Verh Naturforsch Ver Brunn 1865; 4:3–47.
Mitsos LM, Cardon LR, Fortin A, Ryan L, LaCourse R, North RJ, Gros P: Genetic control of susceptibility to infection with *Mycobacterium tuberculosis* in mice. Genes Immun 2000, 1:467–477.
Morrison NA, Qi JC, Tokita A, Kelly PJ, Crofts L, Nguyen TV, Sambrook PN, Eisman JA: Prediction of bone density from vitamin D receptor alleles. Nature 1994; 367:284–287.
Muller-Myhsok B, Abel L: Genetic analysis of complex diseases. Science 1997; 275:1328–1329.
Nagel RL, Roth EF: Malaria and red cell genetic defects. Blood 1989; 74:1213–1221.
Neel JV: Diabetes mellitus: a thrifty genotype rendered detrimental by progress? Am J Hum Genet 1962; 14:353–362.
Newport MJ, Huxley CM, Huston S, Hawrylowicz CM, Oostra BA, Williamson R, Levin M: A mutation in the interferon-gamma-receptor gene and susceptibility to mycobacterial infection. N Engl J Med 1996; 335:1941–1949.
Nordeen SK: The epidemiology of leprosy. In: Hastings RC (ed). Leprosy. London: Churchill Livingstone, 1985:15–30.
O'Brien SJ: Genomic prospecting. Nat Med 1995; 1:742–744.
O'Brien SJ: AIDS: a role for host genes. Hosp Pract (Off Ed) 1998; 33:53–56.
O'Brien SJ, Dean M: In search of AIDS-resistance genes. Sci Am 1997; 277:44–51.
Palmer LJ, Pare PD, Faux JA, Moffatt MF, Daniels SE, LeSouef PN, Bremner PR, Mockford E, Gracey M, Spargo R, et al.: FcepsilonR1-beta polymorphism and total serum IgE levels in endemically parasitized Australian aborigines. Am J Hum Genet 1997; 61:182–188.
Pastinen T, Liitsola K, Niini P, Salminen M, Syvanen AC: Contribution of the *CCR5* and *MBL* genes to susceptibility to HIV type 1 infection in the Finnish population. AIDS Res Hum Retroviruses 1998; 14:695–698.
Pauling L, Itano HA, Singer SJ, Wells C: Sicke-cell anemia: a molecular disease. Science 1949; 110:543.
Rajalingam R, Singal DP, Mehra NK: Transporter associated with antigen-processing (*TAP*) genes and susceptibility to tuberculoid leprosy and pulmonary tuberculosis. Tissue Antigens 1997; 49:168–172.
Rihet P, Abel L, Traore Y, Aucan C, Fumoux F: Human malaria—segregation analysis of blood infection levels in a suburban area and a rural area in Burkina Faso. Genet Epidemiol 1998a; 15:435–450.
Rihet P, Traore Y, Abel L, Aucan C, Traore-Leroux T, Fumoux F: Malaria in humans: *Plasmodium falciparum* blood infection levels are linked to chromosome 5q31–q33. Am J Hum Genet 1998b; 63:498–505.
Risch N, Merikangas K: The future of genetic studies of complex human diseases. Science 1996; 273:1516–1517.
Roberts LJ, Baldwin TM, Curtis JM, Handman E, Foote SJ: Resistance to *Leishmania major* is linked to the H2 region on chromosome 17 and to chromosome 9. J Exp Med 1997; 185:1705–1710.
Rodrigues V, Abel L, Piper K, Dessein AJ: Segregation analysis indicates a major gene in the control of interleukin-5 production in humans infected with *Schistosoma mansoni*. Am J Hum Genet 1996; 59:453–461.
Roger M, Levee G, Chanteau S, Gicquel B, Schurr E: No evidence for linkage between leprosy susceptibility and the human natural resistance-associated macrophage protein 1 (*NRAMP1*) gene in French Polynesia. Int J Lepr Other Mycobact Dis 1997; 65:197–202.
Roger M, Sanchez FO, Schurr E: Comparative study of the genomic organization of DNA repeats within the 5′-flanking region of the natural resistance-associated macrophage protein gene (*NRAMP1*) between humans and great apes. Mamm Genome 1998; 9:435–439.
Rook GAW: The role of vitamin D in tuberculosis. Am Rev Respir Dis 1989; 138:768–770.
Rowland-Jones SL: Survival with HIV infection: good luck or good breeding? Trends Genet 1998; 14:343–345.
Roy S, Frodsham A, Saha B, Hazra SK, Mascie-Taylor CG, Hill AV: Association of vitamin D receptor genotype with leprosy type. J Infect Dis 1999; 179:187–191.
Roy S, McGuire W, Mascie-Taylor CG, Saha B, Hazra SK, Hill AV, Kwiatkowski D: Tumor necrosis factor promoter polymorphism and susceptibility to lepromatous leprosy. J Infect Dis 1997; 176:530–532.
Ruwende C, Khoo SC, Snow RW, Yates SN, Kwiatkowski D, Gupta S, Warn P, Allsopp CE, Gilbert SC, Peschu N, et al.: Natural selection of hemi- and heterozygotes for G6PD deficiency in Africa by resistance to severe malaria. Nature 1995; 376:246–249.
Sampaio EP, Kaplan G, Miranda A, Nery JA, Miguel CP, Viana SM, Sarno EN: The influence of thalidomide on the clinical and immunologic manifestation of erythema nodosum leprosum. J Infect Dis 1993; 168:408–414.
Schuler GD, Boguski MS, Stewart EA, Stein LD, Gyapay G, Rice K, White RE, Rodriguez-Tome P, Aggarwal A, Bajorek E, et al.: A gene map of the human genome. Science 1996; 274:540–546.
Schurr E, Buschman E, Malo D, Gros P, Skamene E: Immunogenetics of mycobacterial infections: mouse–human homologies. J Infect Dis 1990; 161:634–639.
Schurr E, Morgan K, Gros P, Skamene E: Genetics of leprosy. Am J Trop Med Hyg 1991a; 44:4–11.
Schurr E, Radzioch D, Malo D, Gros P, Skamene E: Molecular genetics of inherited susceptibility to intracellular parasites. Behring Inst Mitt 1991b; 88:1–12.
Schurr E, Skamene E: The Role of the *Bcg* Gene in Mycobacterial Infections. In: Rom W, Garay S (eds). Tuberculosis. Boston: Little, Brown, 1996:247–258.
Searle S, Blackwell JM: Evidence for a functional repeat polymorphism in the promoter of the human *NRAMP1* gene that correlates with autoimmune versus infectious disease susceptibility. J Med Genet 1999; 36:295–299.
Sette A, Sidney J: HLA supertypes and supermotifs: a functional perspective on HLA polymorphism. Curr Opin Immunol 1998; 10:478–482.
Shaw MA, Atkinson S, Dockrell H, Hussain R, Lins-Lainson Z, Shaw J, Ramos F, Silveira F, Mehdi SQ, Kaukab F, et al.: An RFLP map for 2q33–q37 from multicase mycobacterial and leishmanial disease families: no evidence for an *Lsh/Ity/Bcg* gene homologue influencing susceptibility to leprosy. Ann Hum Genet 1993; 57:251–271.
Shaw MA, Collins A, Peacock CS, Miller EN, Black GF, Sibthorpe D, Lins-Lainson Z, Shaw JJ, Ramos F, Silveira F, et al.: Evidence that genetic susceptibility to *Mycobacterium tuberculosis* in a Brazilian population is under oligogenic control: linkage study of the candidate genes *NRAMP1* and *TNFA*. Tuber Lung Dis 1997; 78:35–45.

Shields ED, Russell DA, Pericak-Vance MA: Genetic epidemiology of the susceptibility to leprosy. J Clin Invest 1987; 79:1139–1143.

Siddiqui MR, Meisner S, Tosh K, Balakrishnan K, Ghei S, Fisher SE, Golding M, Shanker NP Narayan, Sitaraman T, Sengupta U, et al.: A major susceptibility locus for leprosy in India maps to chromosome 10p13. Nat Genet 2001; 27:439–441.

Singh SP, Mehra NK, Dingley HB, Pande JN, Vaidya MC: Human leukocyte antigen (HLA)–linked control of susceptibility to pulmonary tuberculosis and association with HLA-DR types. J Infect Dis 1983; 148:676–681.

Skamene E, Schurr E, Gros P: Infection genomics: Nramp1 as a major determinant of natural resistance to intracellular infections. Annu Rev Med 1998; 49:275–287.

Sloane MF: Mycobacterial lymphadenitits. In: Rom W, Garay S (eds). Tuberculosis. Boston: Little, Brown, 1996:577–583.

Smith MW, Dean M, Carrington M, Huttley GA, O'Brien SJ: *CCR5-delta32* gene deletion in HIV-1 infected patients. Lancet 1997; 350:741.

Sorensen TI, Nielsen GG, Andersen PK, Teasdale TW: Genetic and environmental influences on premature death in adult adoptees. N Engl J Med 1988; 318:727–732.

Stead WW: Genetics and resistance to tuberculosis: could resistance be enhanced by genetic engineering? Ann Intern Med 1992; 116:937–941.

Stead WW, Senner JW, Reddick WT, Lofgren JP: Racial differences in susceptibility to infection by *Mycobacterium tuberculosis*. N Engl J Med 1990; 322:422–427.

Suarez BK, Hampe CL, Van Eerdewegh P: Problems of replicating linkage claims in psychiatry. In: Gershon ES, Cloninger CR (eds). Genetic Approaches to Mental Disorders. Washington DC: American Psychiatric Press, 1994:23–46.

Tao C, Yu T, Garnett S, Briody J, Knight J, Woodhead H, Cowell CT: Vitamin D receptor alleles predict growth and bone density in girls. Arch Dis Child 1998; 79:488–493.

Teran-Escandon D, Teran-Ortiz L, Camarena-Olvera A, Gonzalez-Avila G, Vaca-Marin MA, Granados J, Selman M: Human leukocyte antigen–associated susceptibility to pulmonary tuberculosis: molecular analysis of class II alleles by DNA amplification and oligonucleotide hybridization in Mexican patients. Chest 1999; 115:428–433.

Tisdale MJ: Wasting in cancer. J Nutr 1999; 129:243S–246S.

Tjernstrom F, Hellmer G, Nived O, Truedsson L, Sturfelt G: Synergetic effect between interleukin-1 receptor antagonist allele (IL1RN*2) and MHC class II (DR17,DQ2) in determining susceptibility to systemic lupus erythematosus. Lupus 1999; 8:103–108.

Turner MW: Mannose-binding lectin: the pluripotent molecule of the innate immune system. Immunol Today 1996; 17:532–540.

van Eden W, de Vries RR: HLA and leprosy: a re-evaluation. Lepr Rev 1984; 55:89–104.

van Eden W, de Vries RR, D'Amaro J, Schreuder I, Leiker DL, van Rood JJ: HLA-DR-associated genetic control of the type of leprosy in a population from Surinam. Hum Immunol 1982; 4:343–350.

van Eden W, de Vries RR, Mehra NK, Vaidya MC, D'Amaro J, van Rood JJ: HLA segregation of tuberculoid leprosy: confirmation of the DR2 marker. J Infect Dis 1980; 141:693–701.

Venter JC, Adams MD, Myers EW, Li PW, Mural RJ, Sutton GG, Smith HO, Yandell M, Evans CA, Holt RA: The sequence of the human genome. Science 2001; 291:1304–1351.

Vidal S, Tremblay ML, Govoni G, Gauthier S, Sebastiani G, Malo D, Skamene E, Olivier M, Jothy S, Gros P: The *Ity/Lsh/Bcg* locus: natural resistance to infection with intracellular parasites is abrogated by disruption of the *Nramp1* gene. J Exp Med 1995; 182:655–666.

Vidal SM, Malo D, Vogan K, Skamene E, Gros P: Natural resistance to infection with intracellular parasites: isolation of a candidate for Bcg. Cell 1993; 73:469–485.

Vidal SM, Pinner E, Lepage P, Gauthier S, Gros P: Natural resistance to intracellular infections: Nramp1 encodes a membrane phosphoglycoprotein absent in macrophages from susceptible (Nramp1 D169) mouse strains. J Immunol 1996; 157:3559–3568.

Wahlgren M: Creating deaths from malaria. Nat Genet 1999; 22:120–121.

Wang DG, Fan JB, Siao CJ, Berno A, Young P, Sapolsky R, Ghandour G, Perkins N, Winchester E, Spencer J, et al.: Large-scale identification, mapping, and genotyping of single-nucleotide polymorphisms in the human genome. Science 1998; 280:1077–1082.

Wattavidanage J, Carter R, Perera KL, Munasingha A, Bandara S, McGuinness D, Wickramasinghe AR, Alles HK, Mendis KN, Premawansa S.: TNFalpha*2 marks high risk of severe disease during *Plasmodium falciparum* malaria and other infections in Sri Lankans. Clin Exp Immunol 1999; 115:350–355.

Weatherall D, Clegg J, Kwiatkowski D: The role of genomics in studying genetic susceptibility to infectious disease. Genome Res 1997; 7:967–973.

Weatherall DJ: The genetics of common diseases: the implications of population variability. In: Variation in the Human Genome. Ciba Foundation Symposium 197. Chichester: Wiley, 1996a:300–308.

Weatherall DJ: Host genetics and infectious disease. Parasitology 1996b; 112:S23–S29.

Weatherall DJ: Thalassaemia and malaria, revisited. Ann Trop Med Parasitol 1997a; 91:885–890.

Weatherall DJ: The thalassaemias. BMJ 1997b; 314:1675–1678.

Weatherall DJ, Clegg JB, Higgs DR, Wood WG: The hemoglobinopathies. In: Scriver C, Beaudet AL, Sly WS, Valle D (eds). The Metabolic and Molecular Basis of Inherited Disease. New York: McGraw-Hill, 1995:3417–3484.

Westendorp RG, Langermans JA, Huizinga TW, Elouali AH, Verweij CL, Boomsma DI, Vandenbroucke JP, Vandenbroucke JP: Genetic influence on cytokine production and fatal meningococcal disease. Lancet 1997a; 349:170–173.

Westendorp RG, Langermans JA, Huizinga TW, Verweij CL, Sturk A: Genetic influence on cytokine production in meningococcal disease. Lancet 1997b; 349:1912–1913.

WHO: The World Health Report 1999. *http://www.who.int/whr/1999/en/disease.htm*, 1999.

WHO: The World Health Report 2000. *http://www.who.int/whr/2000/en/statistics.htm*, 2000a.

WHO: The World Health Report 2000. *http://www.who.int/infectious-disease-report/dlh-testimony*, 2000b.

Wilkinson RJ, Llewelyn M, Toossi Z, Patel P, Pasvol G, Lalvani A, Wright D, Latif M, Davidson RN: Influence of vitamin D deficiency and vitamin D receptor polymorphisms on tuberculosis among Gujarati Asians in west London: a case-control study. Lancet 2000; 355:618–621.

Wilkinson RJ, Patel P, Llewelyn M, Hirsch CS, Pasvol G, Snounou G, Davidson RN, Toossi Z: Influence of polymorphism in the genes for the interleukin (IL)-1 receptor anatagonist and IL-1beta on tuberculosis. J Exp Med 1999; 189:1863–1873.

Wilson AG, di Giovine FS, Duff GW: Genetics of tumour necrosis factor-α in autoimmune, infectious, and neoplastic diseases. J Inflamm 1995; 45:1–12.

Winkler C, Modi W, Smith MW, Nelson GW, Wu X, Carrington M, Dean M, Honjo T, Tashiro K, Yabe D, et al.: Genetic restriction of AIDS pathogenesis by an SDF-1 chemokine gene variant. ALIVE Study, Hemophilia Growth and Development Study (HGDS), Multicenter AIDS Cohort Study (MACS), Multicenter Hemophilia Cohort Study (MHCS), San Francisco City Cohort (SFCC). Science 1998; 279:389–393.

Wyand MS, Manson KH, Garcia-Moll M, Montefiori D, Desrosiers RC: Vaccine protection by a triple deletion mutant of simian immunodeficiency virus. J Virol 1996; 70:3724–3733.

Zerva L, Cizman B, Mehra NK, Alahari SK, Murali R, Zmijewski CM, Kamoun M, Monos DS: Arginine at positions 13 or 70–71 in pocket 4 of HLA-DRB1 alleles is associated with susceptibility to tuberculoid leprosy. J Exp Med 1996; 183:829–836.

11 Genetics of Asthma and Bronchial Hyperresponsiveness

DEBORAH A. MEYERS, DENISE G. WIESCH, AND EUGENE R. BLEECKER

DISEASE DEFINITION

Diagnostic Criteria

The diagnosis of asthma is based on the recurrence of a characteristic set of clinical symptoms (wheezing, intermittent dyspnea, cough, nocturnal cough, exercise-induced wheezing, and dyspnea) and physiologic manifestations of the disease (variable airflow obstruction and bronchial hyperresponsiveness, or BHR. There have been multiple consensus reports defining asthma, including those from the Ciba Foundation Guest Symposium (1971), the World Health Organization (1975), the American Thoracic Society (1987), and, more recently, several national panel reports on Guidelines for Treatment and Diagnosis of Asthma from the National Asthma Education Program (NHLBI, NIH) (National Heart, Lung and Blood Institute and National Institutes of Health, 1991, 1995; National Institutes of Health, 1991; National Heart, Lung and Blood Institute and World Health Organization, 1993, 1995; NIH Expert Panel, 1997). A brief summary of the NHLBI asthma definition is presented in Table 11–1. Since asthma is a chronic inflammatory disease of the airways and direct measurements of bronchial inflammation are not readily available, this definition does not provide exact criteria that can be applied in a standardized fashion across populations. There is heterogeneity in the clinical presentation of patients with asthma, with some individuals having a milder from of asthma while others have a much more severe and often progressive disease that is characterized by morphologic changes in the airways (airways remodeling). These differences in clinical asthma may reflect the stage and severity of inflammation in the airways. In some patients, asthma is characterized by recurrent acute episodes of inflammation, while other patients display structural changes in the bronchi or airways remodeling along with chronic inflammation. It is also possible that differences in disease expression (severity) may be influenced by polymorphisms in modifier genes.

No single physiologic test has sufficient sensitivity or validity for the diagnosis of asthma. Bronchial hyperresponsiveness—an increased bronchoconstrictor response to a variety of physical stimuli, chemical stimuli, or irritants—can be measured using pharmacologic, physical, or allergen challenge methods (Sparrow and Weiss, 1989). However, individuals without asthma may display airways hyperresponsiveness, especially individuals with aeroallergen sensitivity or allergic rhinitis and some chronic cigarette smokers (Pattemore et al., 1990; Woolcock et al., 1991; Sparrow et al., 1993). BHR is an associated phenotypic trait that can be studied in all family members and, thus, is useful for genetic studies. Response to a bronchodilator is another associated phenotype that is also not diagnostic of asthma since patients with normal lung function at the time of testing may not show bronchodilator reversibility. As yet, there are no easy to use or validated noninvasive measures of airways inflammation that can be used reliably to diagnose asthma (NIH Expert Panel, 1997). Thus, it is still necessary to rely on both the presence of symptoms and objective measures of pulmonary function in diagnosing asthma. Additional confounding variables include the effects of smoking and the presence of abnormal lung function due to premature birth (discussed below) or the presence of other obstructive lung diseases such as cystic fibrosis.

Asthma and COPD

There is also overlap of asthma with other diseases, particularly in adulthood. In childhood, diseases that may resemble asthma—for example, cystic fibrosis and bronchiectasis—can be excluded by using clinical criteria and diagnostic tests. In adults, the principal disease that overlaps with asthma in its manifestations is chronic obstructive pulmonary disease (COPD). COPD, a chronic disease of the airways, is characterized by progressive airflow obstruction that usually occurs in individuals with a long history of cigarette smoking and chronic bronchitis. This disease occurs almost exclusively in middle-aged or older individuals with at least a 20-year history of smoking one or more packages of cigarettes each day. The cardinal clinical feature is dyspnea, which results from impairment of ventilatory function due to airflow obstruction. Many patients also develop emphysema, a destructive process in the lung parenchyma in which there is both a reduction in lung elasticity and dilation and loss of the alveolar-capillary surface for exchange of O_2 and CO_2 in the lungs.

As smokers develop airflow obstruction, they may also have increased airways responsiveness, although not necessarily to the degree present in asthma (Woolcock et al., 1991; Tashkin et al., 1992). However, both symptoms and the presence of reversible airways disease may lead to a clinical picture consistent with asthma, and this is sometimes referred to as chronic obstructive bronchitis or chronic asthmatic bronchitis (American Thoracic Society 1987; Burrows 1990). Of course, some individuals with smoking-related lung disease may have first developed asthma earlier in life. This overlap between asthma and CPOD led to the "Dutch" hypothesis that these obstructive airways diseases are interrelated and require host susceptibility (genes), as well as environmental exposures, for their expression (Panhuysen et al., 1998). Interestingly, a relatively small proportion of chronic cigarette smokers (approximately 20%) develop either COPD or emphysema, or both, suggesting that there is also genetic susceptibility to the toxic effects of tobacco smoke in the lungs.

Table 11–1. Summary of NHLBI/NIH Definition of Asthma

A chronic inflammatory disorder of the airways in which many cells play a role—in particular, mast cells, eosinophils, and T lymphocytes.
In susceptible individuals this inflammation causes recurrent episodes of wheezing, breathlessness, chest tightness, and cough.
These symptoms are usually associated with widespread but variable airflow obstruction that is at least partly reversible, either spontaneously or with treatment.
Bronchial inflammation also causes an associated increase in airway responsiveness to a variety of stimuli.

National Heart, Lung and Blood Institute and National Institutes of Health, 1995.

Occupational Asthma

Several agents (including inorganic and organic dusts, gases, fumes, and irritants) have now been identified as causes of occupational asthma (Chan-Yeung and Malo, 1995). Exposure to these agents may be an important risk factor in triggering genetically susceptible individuals to develop respiratory symptoms and asthma. In addition, high levels of exposure may cause asthma in individuals with a lower degree of genetic susceptibility—perhaps due to polymorphisms or sequence variants in minor asthma-related genes.

Phenotype Definition in Genetic Studies

It is often useful to use associated phenotypes—especially those that represent objective or quantitative measures and can be assessed in all family members or the whole population sample—in genetic studies of common multigene disorders (Table 11–2). Asthma diagnosis based on clinical definitions may also be used; however, it is important that asthma is clearly defined and not open to variable interpretations, which may be a problem with using a reported physician's diagnosis or data derived from a questionnaire, both of which may be based on subjective data. The disease definition needs to be specific and reproducible so that results from different genetic studies may be compared. It is important to remember that in performing family studies, individuals will be present who are difficult to classify because of the presence of confounding factors such as smoking and individuals who have minimal symptoms of the disease. Thus, family units may be ascertained through a proband who meets both objective and subjective criteria for asthma, but other family members may be more difficult to classify.

With common disorders such as asthma, there will be a group of clearly affected individuals—for example, those defined by specific clinical criteria, including both objective pulmonary function and BHR testing, as well as subjective measures such as a clinical history of symptoms or treatment. Furthermore, using data from associated phenotypes, individuals can be categorized as either "affected" or "unaffected," providing either a dichotomous trait for genetic analysis or quantitative measures for QTL (quantitative trait loci) mapping. Some family members may meet some but not all of the criteria for disease status or may have intermediate values for an associated phenotype; therefore, it may not be appropriate to consider them unaffected, and, instead, an additional category of "uncertain" should be used. These individuals with intermediate phenotypes are important to follow over time, especially if they have the same genotype as their affected family members, to see if they develop the disorder after additional environmental exposures (for example, to allergens or respiratory infections). Family members with intermediate phenotypes represent a target population for studies on early disease identification and disease prevention, once the underlying genetic susceptibility is understood.

Table 11–2. Definition of Phenotype

Asthma
Clinical diagnosis (Symptoms and/or pulmonary function testing laboratory tests)
Associated phenotypes
Bronchial hyperresponsiveness (BHR), total serum IgE levels, specific allergic responses, blood eosinophil counts
Discrete or quantitative measures

When all individuals in families or extended pedigrees are studied clinically, it is useful to classify the phenotypes into one of a limited number of categories such as "asthma," "possible asthma," "uncertain airways disease," "COPD," or "unaffected," using a defined set of rules (Panhuysen et al., 1998) (Table 11–2). Since it will always be difficult to classify some family members, a category of "uncertain airways disease" is needed to avoid misdiagnosis. For example, a family member with a significant history of tobacco smoking who has airways hyperresponsiveness will be difficult to classify because of the known relationship between smoking, airways obstruction, and BHR (Tashkin et al., 1992). Family members who meet only some of the criteria for asthma may be classified as having "possible or probable asthma," and this group may be given less weight than the groups with definite asthma in the genetic analysis.

Assessment of bronchial inflammation should be considered in genetic studies of asthma and bronchial hyperresponsiveness. The usual methods include the use of bronchial biopsies and examination of respiratory fluids and cells obtained using bronchoalveolar lavage techniques (Djukanovic et al., 1990; Bleecker et al., 1992; Wenzel, 1999). Unfortunately, these measures rely on invasive techniques and cannot be performed in a large number of individuals. Other measures that may be more appropriate for family studies should be considered, such as analysis of induced sputum and total blood eosinophil counts (Fahy et al., 1993) and other forms of bronchial responsiveness testing, such as provocation with adenosine that may be more specific for asthmatic responses (Aalbers et al., 1991; Sporik et al., 1991). However, there may be considerable overlap between the allergic phenotype and inflammatory changes found in the airways of allergic non-asthmatics, asthmatics, and cigarette smokers (Brotherhood et al., 1989; Liu et al., 1990). Thus, even if they could be used in large population samples, invasive approaches may not provide ideal differentiation among subjects with different forms of obstructive pulmonary disease. Additional biomarkers and related measures of inflammation need to be developed to provide a sensitive and specific marker of inflammation and airways remodeling in asthma that can be routinely used in large sample studies.

GENERAL CLINICAL AND EPIDEMIOLOGIC EVIDENCE

Prevalence, Incidence, and Morbidity

In the United States in 1994, prevalence of asthma was estimated as 5.6 %, or 14.6 million persons based on the National Health Interview Survey (Adams et al., 1994). The disease was most prevalent in the youngest age groups, with 6.9%, or 4.8 million children under 18 years reporting asthma. Above 18 years of age, the prevalence was about 5% for all age groups. Geographically, asthma prevalence was slightly higher in the West and Northeast (5.9%) and slightly less in the South (5.5%) and Midwest (5.2%). These estimates are from the NHIS population-based interview survey (45,705 households randomly selected across the United States) where diagnostic testing was not performed. Prevalence rates have increased over all age and ethnic groups compared to an earlier NHIS survey in 1982 (Centers for Disease Control 1995). Over all groups, the prevalence rate increased by approximately 50% between the two surveys.

Studies on use of medical services such as rates of hospitalizations and use of ambulatory care clinics provide estimates of morbidity. In the United States in 1993, there were 198,000 hospitalizations for asthma for individuals under age 25 years. There has been a 28% increase in hospitalizations from 1980 to 1993 for this age group, mainly due to an increase in young children (under age 5). Rates were also consistently higher in African Americans than in Caucasians, with African Americans being 3.5 times more likely to be hospitalized for asthma than Caucasians (Centers for Disease Control, 1996).

For asthma as the principal diagnosis, there were approximately 13.7 million health-care visits annually in 1993 and 1994 in the United States. Approximately 80% of these were for physician office visits and 12% for emergency room visits (the rest were for outpatient department visits (Burt and Knapp, 1996). There were also ethnic differences, with African Americans having the highest rates for emergency room visits.

Ethnic and Geographic Differences

As described, estimates of prevalence and morbidity are higher in the United States for African Americans than for Caucasians. Asthma appears to be more prevalent in Hispanics in the United States than in either African Americans or Caucasians. Overall, asthma has been shown to be more prevalent in the more developed countries, with different frequencies in different racial and ethnic groups. Prevalence estimates for children who usually have the highest rates also differ considerably between countries, but although differences in prevalence estimates may occur between countries due to genetic and environmental differences, it is often very difficult to compare results across countries because different diagnostic criteria have been used. These rates may vary from as low as 0% to 46% (National Heart, Lung and Blood Institute and World Health Organization, 1995).

Gender and Size (Prematurity)

In general, epidemiologic studies have consistently found a higher prevalence rate for asthma in boys than in girls. Depending on the study, rates twice as high have been reported, and the degree of difference in observed rates tends to decrease with age (Schachter et al., 1984; Horwood et al., 1985). It has been hypothesized that these observed differences may be due to physical differences in airways anatomy. Lower flow rates and higher airways resistance have been observed in boys than in girls for ages 4 to 6 years (Doershuk et al., 1974; Taussig 1977). In general, for a given specific size, boys have smaller airways than girls have. It is possible that these observed differences may be related to the increased frequency of lower respiratory illnesses and wheezing observed in boys than in girls (Glezen and Denny, 1973; Monto and Ullman, 1974; Martinez et al., 1988). Thus, it is possible that boys may be more susceptible to developing asthma in childhood because of differences in bronchial anatomy (airways size).

Several studies have shown an association between premature birth and the development of symptoms consistent with asthma and other pulmonary disorders (Shepard et al., 1968; Outerbridge et al., 1972; Lamarre et al., 1973; Coates et al., 1977). However, this could be caused by one or a combination of several factors, such as pulmonary injury resulting from neonatal respiratory distress syndrome and mechanical ventilation, or from other factors associated with prematurity, including inadequate prenatal care or maternal smoking. In a cross-sectional study of 5000 German schoolchildren (aged 9–11 years), similar results were found for premature girls but not for premature boys. Premature girls had a significantly higher frequency of asthma and asthma symptoms (recurrent wheeze, shortness of breath, and cough) than full-term girls had, and the risk was highest in those who had been mechanically ventilated (Von Mutius et al., 1993).

However, it is important to consider confounding factors since premature birth is associated with race and socioeconomic status. In a study of African American children from a poverty area in Cleveland, Ohio, children with asthma had significantly lower birthweights and gestational age and were more likely to be placed on mechanical ventilation after birth (Oliveti et al., 1996). However, there was no evidence for an increased risk of asthma when other factors (such as lack of prenatal care, asthma in the mother, and mechanical ventilation of the infant) were considered. These studies suggest mechanical ventilation is a risk factor for asthma. It is not clear whether prematurity without mechanical ventilation also increases asthma risk.

Environmental Factors

Respiratory Infections

Asthma is a primary example of a complex genetic disease that is triggered by environmental exposures in genetically susceptible individuals. It is possible that variations in the level of genetic susceptibility plus differences in environmental exposures may determine whether an individual at risk for asthma develops mild, relatively asymptomatic asthma or a more progressive disease. Children may develop wheezing from viral infections of the lower respiratory tract which are frequent in childhood (Busse et al., 1992). Not all children who wheeze will develop asthma or bronchial hyperresponsiveness (Martinez et al., 1995), but it is clear that respiratory infections are an important risk factor for the development of asthma. For example, multiple studies have found a higher risk for asthma and related phenotypes such as bronchial hyperresponsiveness in children with a history of a hospitalization for a respiratory infection (Kattan et al., 1977; Sims et al., 1978; Gurwitz et al., 1981; Stokes et al., 1981; Henry et al., 1983). In addition, an increased risk of developing bronchial hyperresponsiveness was documented in children with a history of bronchiolitis or croup (Weiss et al., 1985). Therefore, respiratory infections in children are a risk factor for developing asthma and related phenotypes, whether or not the children were hospitalized because of the infection.

Several hypotheses may explain the observation of an increased risk of asthma or associated phenotypes following respiratory infections. One hypothesis is that viral infections enhance airway inflammation, which is an important factor in the development and progression of asthma (Busse et al., 1992). This is supported by observations that suggest a relationship between individuals who develop measurable virus-specific IgE levels and later develop asthma or a related phenotype (Welliver et al., 1981, 1986). However, whether virus-specific generation of IgE is a risk factor or a cause of asthma is not clear (Busse et al., 1992). In addition, viral infections may be a risk factor for the development of asthma symptoms since the increased degree of bronchial hyperresponsiveness that occurs after a viral respiratory infection makes the airways more responsive to a variety of nonspecific and allergic agents (Busse et al., 1992). Other studies have shown that viral respiratory infections may sensitize susceptible individuals (atopics and asthmatics) and increase the inflammatory response to allergen exposure (Busse et al., 1993).

However, the direct or indirect role of viral respiratory infections in the development of asthma is still not completely understood. It is also possible that the increased prevalence of asthma observed in industrial countries is due to a decrease in bacterial respiratory infections because of improvements in public health (Cookson and Moffatt, 1997; Holgate 1997; Shirakawa et al., 1997). Bacterial infections may promote activation of the TH1 lymphocyte phenotype, thus possibly inhibiting allergic TH2 lymphocytes responses in the lungs.

Diet and Breast Feeding

Diet—including breast feeding, food intolerance and sensitivity, and types of foods ingested—has been investigated as a potential risk factor for asthma. In general, there have been multiple studies evaluating these potential risk factors, with varying results. This is a complicated area of investigation, and it is difficult to obtain accurate data because of recall problems and difficulties in measuring specific food intake (Weiss, 1997). In addition, diets tend to be similar in that the same foods are eaten but in different amounts. Both positive and negative results have been obtained from studies on vitamin C intake (Troisi et al., 1995; Weiss, 1997); fatty acid composition of the diet (especially *n*-3 and *n*-6 polyunsaturated fatty acids found in fish oil) (Schwartz and Weiss, 1994; Troisi et al., 1995); and dietary sodium, potassium, and magnesium (Pistelli et al., 1993; Britton et al., 1994a, 1994b).

Studies on the role of breast-feeding influencing susceptibility to asthma have not given consistent results (Martin et al., 1981; Miskelly, 1988; Zeiger et al., 1989). A proposed advantage of breast-feeding to the infant is the acquisition of maternal antibodies and immune-competent cells, which should provide some protection against lower respiratory infections early in life. However, breast-feeding may also be a route of exposure to a variety of antigens from the mother, which may counteract some of the positive effects (Weiss, 1997).

Atopy

Atopy may be defined as a state of increased allergic response to environmental allergens, mediated by IgE (Shirakawa et al., 1997). The presence and degree of atopy may be determined by total serum IgE levels, allergen-specific IgE to the most common allergens, and positive skin-test responses to allergens. Questionnaire data are useful to evaluate symptoms and the presence of related diseases such as eczema, and allergic rhinitis (Coultas and Samet, 1993). A number of epidemiological studies have shown an association between clinical and laboratory measurements of atopy with the development of asthma. In a well-known study, Burrows et al. (1976) reported significant associations for various parameters in a random sample from Tucson, Arizona. Parameters of atopy included response to skin tests and total serum IgE levels, while parameters of asthma included wheezing, dyspnea, and diagnosed asthma. For example, in children (3–14 years), atopy (skin-test responsiveness) was strongly associated with attacks of wheezing and dyspnea, even if asthma had not been diagnosed. Other longitudinal studies performed on a birth cohort in New Zealand have shown that either total serum IgE levels or a combination of positive skin tests is closely related to the presence of airways hyperresponsiveness and the development of symptomatic asthma (Burrows et al., 1995).

Exposure to Allergens, Tobacco Smoking, and Pollution

Environmental factors are important in increasing the risk that a susceptible individual will develop asthma or BHR and can trigger disease exacerbations in an asthmatic. The major risk factors are exposure to allergens, both indoor and outdoor, and active and passive tobacco smoking. The role of pollutants, whether indoor or outdoor, is less clear, although some studies have shown an association with asthma exacerbations.

Since many asthmatics are also allergic, exposure to allergens is an important risk factor. However, many studies have focused on the risk of asthma exacerbations in individuals who already have the disease (Institute of Medicine, 1993). A prospective cohort study of 93 children at high risk for developing asthma (based on parental history) in the United Kingdom (Sporik et al., 1990) showed an association between levels of house dust mites and the development of wheezing and asthma. The children with higher levels of house dust mite antigen in their homes tended to wheeze at a younger age. A similar result was observed in a prevention trial where reduction of allergen exposure during early childhood appeared to delay the development of allergies and asthma (Hide et al., 1996).

Smoking is associated with an increased risk of asthma and asthma exacerbations in several different types of exposure, including active, passive, and maternal smoking. Active smoking has been shown to increase nonspecific airways responsiveness, perhaps by inducing airways inflammation (Floreani and Rennald, 1999; Weiss et al., 1999; Chalmers et al., 2001; Nolte et al., 2001; Wilson et al., 2001). Smokers report wheezing more frequently than do nonsmokers, and the frequency of wheezing and airways hyperresponsiveness decreases after individuals stop smoking (U.S. Department of Health and Human Services, 1986). However, long-term studies of individuals at risk for asthma have not been performed to show that cigarette smoking directly increases the risk of developing asthma (O'Connor et al., 1989; Weiss et al., 1999).

Passive smoking may increase risk for asthma through multiple pathways. One is by increasing risk and severity of respiratory infections in children exposed to smoke, especially early in life (U.S. Department of Health and Human Services, 1990). In addition, passive smoking may produce adverse effects in the lung and increase the degree of bronchial hyperresponsiveness. Moreover, some evidence suggests that in utero exposure to tobacco smoke has an effect on airways responsiveness after birth. For example, in a study of 63 normal infants, both parental smoking and a family history of asthma were associated with an increased level of airways responsiveness by histamine challenge (Young et al., 1991). It has also been shown that children whose mothers smoked during pregnancy had a lower level of airways function shortly after birth (Hanrahan et al., 1992). In summary, the California Environmental Protection Agency (1997) performed a meta-analysis showing an approximately 50% increase in risk for diagnosed asthma and a similar increase in risk for other wheezing syndromes associated with parental smoking. Exposure to tobacco smoke has also been shown to relate to asthma severity in children with asthma, as measured by an increase in medical care and degree of bronchial hyperresponsiveness (U.S. Department of Health and Human Services, 1986).

Outdoor air pollutants have been linked more to asthma exacerbations than seen as a risk factor for asthma (Molfino et al., 1991; Devalia et al., 1994; Committee on the Medical Effects of Air Pollution, 1995). Not all studies have shown an increase in exacerbations during times of heavy pollution, however. A few specific pollutants such as castor beans and soybeans have been associated with new outbreaks of asthma. For example, a very strong association was found between unloading of soybeans at the harbor in Barcelona, Spain, and the occurrence of an asthma epidemic (Anto et al., 1989); an antigen was later isolated from soybeans that was felt to be responsible for the outbreaks (Sunyer et al., 1989). Indoor air pollution including emissions from cooking stoves and heaters may also exacerbate asthma; however, it is unclear whether these exposures increase the likelihood of an individual developing the disease (Samet et al., 1993).

It is important to remember that it is difficult to study single risk factors for developing asthma or for asthma severity since children are likely to be exposed to multiple factors and may have a positive family history. Family history, certain types of indoor heating, and exposure to cigarette smoke all increased the risk of developing asthma in a case-control study of children seen in the emergency room with a new onset of asthma (Infante-Rivard, 1993).

Twin Studies

An increased frequency of asthma and related phenotypes in monozygotic (MZ) over dizygotic (DZ) twins provides evidence for a heritable component to these phenotypes. Several of the confounding factors such as gender, age, and exposure to environmental risk factors are avoided or minimized in twin studies. Twins of the same sex (and same age) are usually observed, and, especially in studies of children, both MZ and DZ twins share many of the same environmental exposures, including infections. Several large twin studies using questionnaire data on self-reported asthma have shown increased concordance in MZ versus DZ twins. In a large twin study with 7000 same-sex twins born between 1886 and 1925, the concordance rate for self-reported asthma in MZ twin pairs was 19.0%, while it was 4.8% in DZ twins (Edfors-Lubs, 1971). Although the frequency of asthma was higher, a similar difference was observed in a large study of several thousand twin pairs from the Australian twin register, with a concordance rate of 30% in MZ versus 12% in DZ pairs (Duffy et al., 1990). For BHR, similar results were observed in a smaller study where BHR was measured (Hopp et al., 1984, 1988). Assuming that like-sex twins, both MZ and DZ, tend to share a similar environment, especially in childhood, the increased concordance rate seen in MZ twins provides evidence for a significant genetic component in asthma.

Family Studies and Segregation Analysis

Another approach to estimating the genetic component for a common disease is familial aggregation studies where the risk to family members of different degrees of relationship is calculated. However, familial aggregation may be due to common genes, common environmental factors, or an interaction of genes and environment. The degree of familial aggregation can be estimated by calculating the increased risk to a family member (λ), which is the relative's risk compared to the prevalence in the population. These risk ratios can be used to postulate the number of loci involved in the disorder. However, these ratios are sensitive to the estimate of the population prevalence, which often differ between studies and depend on phenotype definition. In common disorders such as asthma, the estimates are usually quite small, in the range of 2 to 3, which reflects the complex nature of these multifactorial diseases and the expected difficulties in mapping genes that individually have a relatively small effect on the phenotype (Risch and Merikangas, 1996).

Significant familial aggregation asthma (often based on questionnaire data and associated phenotypes such as BHR and total serum IgE levels) has been described in numerous studies (Townley et al., 1986; Longo et al., 1987; Martinez et al., 1995; Holberg et al., 1996; Panhuysen et al., 1996). First-degree relatives of asthmatic individuals have a higher frequency of asthma and atopy than do control subjects and their families (Sibbald and Turner-Warwick, 1979; Hopp et al., 1984; Longo et al., 1987; Duffy et al., 1990). An increased incidence of another associated phenotype, BHR, has been described in parents of patients with asthma compared to controls (Hopp et al., 1984; Bruderman et al., 1987). While studies of relatives are helpful in determining whether a familial or genetic component is present, they do not generally provide insight into the mode of inheritance of the disorder or trait. It is also important to consider that a portion of the observed familial aggregation may be due to environmental factors, as well as to genetic influences.

It has been very useful to study familial aggregation in a set of Dutch families that were ascertained through a single proband, a parent who was originally studied approximately 20 years earlier (Figure 11–1). All of the probands had a diagnosis of asthma based on symptoms and objective testing (bronchial hyperresponsiveness to histamine and bronchodilator reversibility testing) (Panhuysen et al., 1998). In the first analysis of 320 offspring of a proband with asthma, 18% were classified as definite asthma and 8% as probable asthma. Thus, approximately one-quarter of the offspring (mean age = 23 years) in families selected because of one parent with asthma have an asthma phenotype. Another 21% had "unclassified" airway disease (asymptomatic BHR or cigarette smokers with some clinical asthmatic characteristics); 4% were classified as having COPD and 49% as unaffected (no lung disease). These results provide evidence for genetic susceptibility to asthma. Also, it is very interesting

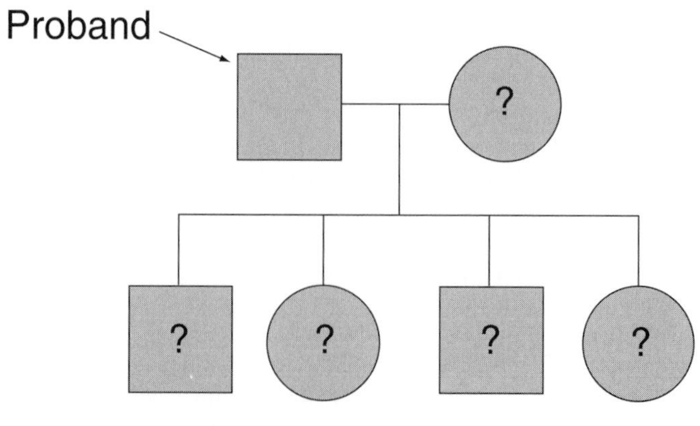

Fig. 11–1. Selection of Dutch families through a single proband. The Dutch families were ascertained through a parent with asthma who was previously studied approximately 25 years ago. The only criteria applied to the family was that there had to be at least two children and the spouse available for evaluation.

that approximately 40% of the offspring who were classified as having asthma based on questionnaire and laboratory studies did not have a prior physician's diagnosis, although their clinical findings were very similar to those with a diagnosis of asthma. These findings suggest underdiagnosis of this disease and that environmental exposures to immunologic or inflammatory agents may trigger clinical disease in "at-risk" individuals who share genetic susceptibility with their asthmatic siblings.

Segregation analysis may be performed on family data to determine whether the disease or trait is transmitted in the family and if it is consistent with a specific genetic model, such as a dominant or recessive major gene, or due to the equal effects of multiple genes (polygenic). The observed proportion of family members with a specific phenotype is compared to the expected number under various genetic models of inheritance. Segregation analysis has limited usefulness in common disorders for several reasons (Lander and Schork, 1994). Families must be ascertained in a pre-specified and appropriate manner that does not result in statistical bias favoring a specific mode of inheritance, which often results in a different type of ascertainment than that used for linkage studies (where families with multiple affected members are necessary). In addition, it is not possible to accurately model the complex nature of inheritance found in common disorders; segregation analysis is limited to testing for a single major gene (or two-locus) models. The possible models of inheritance usually do not even approximate the true situation in common disorders where both multiple genes and environmental factors determine genetic susceptibility (Landers and Schork, 1994).

There have been numerous segregation analyses for an asthma-related phenotype—total serum IgE levels (reviewed in Panhuysen et al., 1996) analyzed as a quantitative trait—but few studies of other measures of the allergic or asthmatic phenotype. These studies found evidence for a major gene, and this work was extended in the Dutch population to a two-locus epistatic model (Xu et al., 1995, 2000). The evidence for a major gene for BHR is less clear. In a family study of BHR to methacholine, evidence for a major gene was not found, and neither the genetic nor the environmental models could be excluded (Townley et al., 1986). In another study using response to inhaled carbachol in 80 non-asthmatic parents of asthma patients, suggestive evidence for autosomal dominant inheritance with incomplete penetrance was observed, but a formal segregation analysis was not performed (Longo et al., 1987). In a sample of Dutch families, segregation analysis was performed for bronchial hyperresponsiveness to histamine (Panhuysen et al., 1998). Some 92 families ascertained through a parent, the proband, with asthma diagnosed approximately 25 years ago were included in the analysis. Initially, no evidence for a major gene was observed; however, when IgE levels were included as a covariate, evidence for Mendelian inheritance of a susceptibility gene for BHR with high penetrance was found. Given the genetic complexity observed in common disorders, it is important to consider multiple related parameters in testing genetic models. They may be separate yet interacting genes for these correlated traits, BHR and serum IgE levels.

For the asthma phenotype, segregation analysis for asthma based on questionnaire data was performed and showed a strong familial polygenic component to asthma, suggesting the presence of multiple genes (Martinez and Holberg, 1995). This is not a surprising result but demonstrates the limitations of segregation analysis in common disorders since modeling three or four loci is not computationally feasible using currently available methods.

GENE IDENTIFICATION

Positional cloning has become easier to perform due to new technology developments that allow for rapid and accurate large-scale genotyping at a reasonable cost. However, cloning susceptibility genes for common disorders is still a major undertaking. Before beginning positional cloning studies for susceptibility genes for a common disorder such as asthma and allergy, it is important to determine the magnitude of the genetic component that underlies susceptibility and the number and types of families required for adequate statistical power. In addition, it is important to determine whether a family-based study or a case-control study is appropriate (Figure 11–2).

There are multiple sample designs that may be used in family studies for positional cloning ranging from studies of only affected siblings to studies of multigenerational pedigrees:

- Affected sib pairs
- Single affected proband
- Multiplex pedigrees
- Random populations
- Isolated and/or inbred populations

Families may be from a general heterogeneous population or a more genetically homogeneous population (possibly inbred) with a recent or more distant founder effect. As discussed previously, it is useful to study related phenotypes in the family members such as BHR and measurements of atopy, as well as the presence of clinical asthma. It is also important to consider the effect of age on the phenotype when performing studies on individuals from different generations. For example, it may not be possible to accurately phenotype a parent with a history of asthma as a child who is now a smoker with obstructive lung disease. This difficulty was avoided in the Dutch family study where clinical data were available on the probands from approximately 25 years previously when their asthma status was assessed.

In the Dutch study, families were ascertained through a single proband, an individual with asthma who was originally studied at a referral hospital approximately 25 years previously (Postma et al., 1995). The probands were studied a second time, along with their spouses, children, and grandchildren. The only criteria for study were that the proband had at least two offspring and a living spouse. This is an appropriate ascertainment scheme

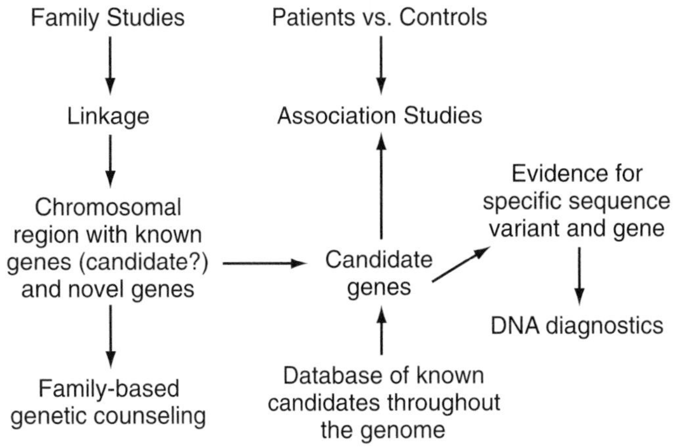

Fig. 11–2. Family vs. case-control studies. This flowchart shows the overall approach used in both linkage and association studies to delineate susceptibility genes. These results may then be useful in identifying individuals at high risk and early diagnosis.

to investigate the familial aggregation of asthma and to perform segregation analysis. However, since families will be studied that do not have additional members with asthma, some families will not be useful for asthma linkage studies but may be useful for mapping studies of closely associated phenotypes.

A commonly used approach for gene mapping studies is to ascertain and characterize affected siblings, although other pairs of relatives may also be used. In this study design, parents do not have to be phenotyped, and it is optional as to whether DNA samples are obtained from them. This design is often used for genome screening to identify chromosomal regions likely to contain susceptibility genes. A modified version of this approach has been used by the Collaborative Study of the Genetics of Asthma (CSGA) where families were ascertained through an affected sib pair (both with a doctor's diagnosis of asthma, symptoms, and BHR [or reversibility if it was not appropriate to perform hyperresponsiveness testing]). This was not strictly a sib-pair design since parents and other siblings were phenotyped and genotyped, and some families were extended to include additional relatives (CSGA, 1997; Xu et al., 2001).

Large multigenerational pedigrees may also be studied and ascertained through one or multiple probands. For common disorders, this design may encounter the problem of having the disease susceptibility genes entering the pedigree through multiple individuals (spouses, as well as the original founders). For example, a family with two affected siblings may be extended to include a first cousin with asthma; however, it is possible that the genetic susceptibility is different in the first cousin and is due to genes transmitted from the parent who married into the pedigree. In some studies, families where both parents have asthma are not included because of the increased likelihood of multiple susceptibility genes being transmitted in a family. However, if genetic susceptibility is due to the interaction of multiple genes, then bilineal families may be more representative, frequent in the population, and appropriate to include in the study.

Studies of isolated and inbred populations where the relationships between the nuclear families are known and may be traced back to a small number of founders are very useful; for example, the Old Order Amish in Pennsylvania and the Hutterites in South Dakota. One portion of the Hutterite community where everyone is descended from one pair of the original founders has been studied for asthma and related phenotypes by Carole Ober and her collaborators (1998). The family relationships are well documented, and, although individuals may leave the community, no one moves in, so the gene pool has remained restricted over multiple generations. However, even in a closed population, multiple genes may still be segregating for common diseases. The Pennsylvania Amish are a similar inbred population that has been studied for atopy and total serum IgE levels (Marsh et al., 1994).

It is also useful to study small families from more homogeneous populations with a known founder effect, even if the actual relationships between the families are not known. Homogenous populations have been studied in northern Holland (Postma et al., 1995). These populations are especially useful for fine-mapping studies since it may be possible to detect a shared haplotype of a small enough size that it limits the number of potential genes to be examined. Similar to studying inbred populations, the susceptibility genes that are present in a homogeneous population may be less common in the larger heterogeneous population. It is very useful to study different populations to replicate findings and to determine differences in gene frequencies.

Table 11–3. Linkage vs. Association

Type of Study	Definition
Linkage	Cosegregation of disease or trait with a specific chromosomal region in multiple families
Association	Presence of disease or trait in individuals with a specific allele in a relevant gene

Finally, it is important to distinguish between family-based linkage studies and association studies, using unrelated patients and appropriate controls (Table 11–3). Only subjects that meet the diagnostic criteria are included and not subjects with an unclear phenotype. A physician's diagnosis may be appropriate, since the genetic data should not be biased by underdiagnosis; however, if there is a significant degree of overdiagnosis, there would be a decrease in the statistical power to detect a difference between groups. It is important to include appropriate controls matched for important covariates such as age, gender, and ethnic group. Another approach is to study family "trios" by obtaining DNA samples from the proband's parents. In this case, the alleles not transmitted from the parent to the proband are then used to determine "control" allele frequencies (Spielman et al., 1993).

Genome-Wide Screens for Susceptibility Genes

Linkage analysis is performed to map the chromosomal location of susceptibility genes by demonstrating cosegregation of the phenotype and polymorphic DNA markers from a chromosomal region. Since the aim of a genome screen is to map susceptibility genes to chromosomal regions, markers are chosen for their ease of use in the laboratory and known polymorphic status and are not usually genes with known function. Genome-wide screens are especially useful in mapping genes with a relatively large phenotypic effect where the relevant polymorphisms are likely to be found in a large portion of the families. Multiple genome-wide screens have been performed for the asthma phenotype, and it is important in comparing results between studies to consider the population and type of family studied, definition of the phenotype, spacing of markers across the genome, and methods of genetic analysis. It has now become clear that there are multiple regions of the genome that are likely to contain susceptibility genes for asthma and BHR based on genome screens in different populations and on candidate gene studies.

In one of the first genome-wide screens, 80 Caucasian families were studied and genotyped for 253 autosomal markers. Analyses were performed for atopy and BHR as a quantitative trait (Daniels et al., 1996). Evidence for linkage to log of the slope of responsiveness to methacholine was seen for chromosomes 4 and 7 with p values $<.0005$ (D4S426, D7S484), and preliminary evidence was seen for linkage to chromosome 16 ($p < .05$ for D16S289). None of the measures of the atopic phenotype—including the associated phenotypes of total IgE levels, skin tests, or total eosinophil count—showed evidence for linkage to chromosome 4, but log of IgE levels was linked to chromosomes 7 and 16. The marker spacing used in this early study was broader than that used in later studies and may have decreased the power to detect genes of a lesser effect.

In the CSGA, a genome-wide screen using 360 markers at approximately 10 cM spacing was performed in families from different racial groups (African Americans, Caucasians, and Hispanics) ascertained through two siblings with asthma. All affected family members met the same criteria for asthma as the probands, which included a physician's prior diagnosis of asthma, the presence of asthma symptoms, and evidence of bronchial hyperresponsiveness or reversibility of airflow obstruction. Analyses were performed for the total sample and each racial group (Xu et al., 2001). The strongest evidence for linkage in the total sample was found on chromosome 14q32, 6p21 in Caucasians, 11q21 in African Americans, and 1p32 in the Hispanic population. Conditional analyses were performed by weighting the families based on the linkage results at these four regions. Both conditional analysis and affected sib-pair two-locus analysis provided further evidence for linkage at 5q31, 8p23, 12q22, and 15q13. These results were used to develop a gene–gene interactive model for asthma susceptibility loci, which will be useful for fine-mapping studies and gene identification. This may reflect a complex interaction between genes, which may occur in common diseases such as asthma, where there are likely to be more than two genes, as well as environmental factors, involved in susceptibility.

A genome screen for asthma and BHR was performed in a sample of 361 individuals as the primary sample and 292 individuals in a replication sample from the inbred Hutterite population (Ober et al., 1998). Across the genome, 292 autosomal and 3 X-Y pseudoautosomal DNA markers were genotyped. The analysis was performed using four phenotypes: "strict" asthma, BHR, asthma symptoms, and "loose" asthma (symptoms and/or BHR). Evidence for linkage was observed in both the initial sample and the replication sample for four chromosomal regions: 5q23–32q, 12q15–24q, 19q13, and 21q21 (p values from the pooled sample were $p = .001$ for D5S1480; .0025 for D12S375; .01 for D19S178; .03 for D21S1440). Evidence for linkage to chromosome 3p24.2–p22 was seen in the primary sample ($p = .01$ for D3S2432 and D3S1768) but was only marginally significant in the replication sample ($p = .035$ for D3S1768) and not significant in the pooled sample.

In a multicenter German study, 97 families with 156 affected sib pairs were genotyped for 351 markers across the genome. Four regions of the genome were detected for clinical asthma at the following markers: D2S2298 on 2pter ($p = .007$); D6S291 on 6p21.3 ($p = .008$); D9S1784 on 9q ($p = .007$); and D12S351 on 12q13 ($p = .01$). For BHR, similar results were seen for chromosomes 2 and 9 (Wjst et al., 1999).

A genome-wide screen was performed for BHR susceptibility genes using 348 DNA markers at approximately 10 cM intervals in 140 Dutch families ascertained through a proband with asthma originally studied approximately 25 years previously. The strongest evidence for linkage was seen on 5q in the same area reported previously using a candidate gene approach, and evidence was also seen for chromosome 3q (LOD = 2.8). Preliminary evidence was seen for three other chromosomes (1, 2, and 7) (Bleecker, 1998; Wiesch et al., 1999).

Several regions of the genome have been observed in at least two of the genome-wide screens, and some of these regions have also been seen in candidate gene studies. Other regions of the genome have only been observed in one study, and replication of these results is required. Interesting regions that have been observed in multiple genome-wide screens include 5q, 11, and 12q, all of which have also been found in candidate gene studies. Additional regions include 6p and multiple other chromosomal regions still to be delineated. For the larger chromosomes or regions of linkage, it is not clear that the same regions are being detected in the different studies. It is difficult to determine from genome-wide analysis whether multiple studies are detecting the exact same region; in some cases, the markers reported in different studies are at a significant distance from each other (for example, 30 cM). However, due to heterogeneity, it is difficult to accurately map the gene location in studies of common diseases, and additional markers need to be studied before such a comparison can be made (Table 11–4).

Table 11–4. Issues in Fine Mapping Complex Genetic Disorders

Multiple genes
Unknown mode of inheritance
Incomplete penetrance and phenocopies (not a 1:1 correspondence between phenotype and genotype)
Racial and population genetic differences

Chromosome 5

There are multiple biologic candidate genes on chromosome 5q that may be important in the regulation of IgE and the development or progression of inflammation associated with allergy and asthma. They include several cytokines (IL-3, IL-4, IL-5, IL-9, IL-13, granulocyte macrophage colony stimulating factor [GMCSF]), the β_2-adrenergic receptor, a glucocorticoid receptor, and multiple other candidates. Linkage to chromosome 5q has been seen in several populations for a range of phenotypes ranging from asthma and BHR to total serum IgE levels. In the inbred and genetically isolated Amish population, linkage to chromosome 5q in the region of several of the cytokines was observed for regulation of total serum IgE levels (Marsh et al., 1994). In the Dutch study, significant evidence for linkage was observed for several markers using both sib-pair analysis and the LOD score approach for two phenotypes: BHR and total serum IgE levels (Meyers et al., 1994; Postma et al., 1995). Additional analyses suggest that there may be separate loci on 5q for these two important components of the asthma phenotype (Panhuysen et al., 1996). Evidence for linkage of the asthma phenotype to this region has also been obtained in the same set of families (Panhuysen et al., 1998). A genome-wide screen has now been performed in these families for the BHR phenotype, and 5q is the strongest region. In the CSGA Caucasian families, preliminary evidence for linkage to this region of 5q was observed for the asthma phenotype (CSGA, 1997). Strong evidence for linkage to 5q (D5S1480) was observed in the Hutterites for the "loose" definition of asthma, which included subjects with asthma, BHR, or symptoms of athma (Ober et al., 1998).

Chromosome 6p

The HLA region and specific HLA haplotypes have been correlated with several measures of the allergic phenotype in a number of studies (Marsh et al., 1982; Blumenthal et al., 1992). Linkage to chromosome 6 has been found for several markers and eosinophil count in a genome screen of atopic families but not for BHR (Daniels et al., 1996). In the CSGA, there was evidence for increased allele sharing for markers on 6p21.3–p23 ($p = .01$) in the Caucasian sib pairs with asthma (CSGA, 1997). The German genome-wide screen also detected evidence for linkage to this region. Since many asthmatics are allergic, it is not yet possible to determine whether the evidence for this linkage is due to the major histocompatibility complex and its influence on the allergic response, or whether other susceptibility genes for asthma and BHR reside in this region.

Table 11–5. Genetic Approaches in Allergy and Asthma

Observations	Results
Several chromosomal regions with evidence for linkage have been identified for asthma and associated phenotypes	A few regions have been seen in multiple studies There is suggestive evidence for additional regions
Evaluation of candidate genes is ongoing	Functional candidates being evaluated Positional candidates being evaluated
Fine mapping and gene identification is under way at multiple centers	

Chromosome 11q

Evidence for linkage of a broadly defined allergic phenotype to markers on chromosome 11q was first described by Cookson et al. in 1989. In a later study, these investigators postulated that sequence variants in the FcϵRIβ gene may increase risk for developing allergy and possibly even asthma (Sandford et al., 1993). The postulated sequence variant (Leu181) has not been observed in several other studies, including the Dutch family studies (Amelung et al., 1998). This raises the issue of whether sequence variants in another gene on 11q confer susceptibility. There is continued evidence for linkage of the atopic phenotype to this region (Daniels et al., 1996). These studies illustrate the difficulty in finding sequence variants in a specific gene that may only confer a moderate increase in risk. Recently, a patent was released with a reported linkage to chromosome 11p (near the centromere) and the identification of a novel susceptibility gene found in an isolated inbred population of approximately 350 individuals living on an isolated south Atlantic island (Tristan du Cuhna). Until this finding is evaluated in more heterogenous populations, it is difficult to evaluate the importance of this result.

Chromosome 12q

There is a broad region on 12q with strong evidence for linkage from multiple studies and various phenotypes related to asthma, bronchial hyperresponsiveness, and allergy. Evidence for linkage for both asthma and total IgE levels was found in an Afro-Caribbean population and for total IgE levels in the Amish population (Barnes et al., 1996). In the CSGA, evidence for linkage was observed for the asthma phenotype in Caucasians (p = .004) and Hispanics (p = .026) but not in African Americans (CSGA, 1997). In a sample of randomly ascertained families and a sample of families ascertained for multiple members with asthma, evidence for linkage was seen for both asthma and allergic phenotypes (Dewar et al., 1997). Several candidate genes map to this region, including interferon γ (IFNγ), NOS1, and mast cell growth factor. As with the other chromosomal regions, evidence for linkage is found over a very wide region of the chromosome, and, until fine-mapping studies are complete, it is not possible to further localize this linkage.

Candidate Gene Associations

Association studies are performed to compare the frequency of a specific polymorphism (sequence variant) in a candidate gene in individuals with and without the disease phenotype. It is important to determine "a priori" the rationale for performing such a study since there are many candidate genes for most of the common disorders. Thus the criteria for choosing candidate genes include the following:

- Biologic plausibility
- Specific polymorphism in exon or regulatory region (functional change)
- Frequency of polymorphism high enough to detect in the population sample
- Candidate in chromosomal region showing evidence for linkage from previous study

For example, it is reasonable to test for an association with a sequence variant with a known function that is biologically important. It is also important to demonstrate significant evidence at an appropriate statistical level. For most candidate gene studies, there have been conflicting reports, which makes it difficult to determine the significance of the findings. Another explanation of an observed association is linkage disequilibrium: the observed polymorphism is physically close to the sequence variant important in the disorder, and there is co-inheritance of both polymorphisms due to linkage disequilibrium. Therefore, the polymorphism tested may not be the relevant functional polymorphism.

Another example of association studies are the recent studies of the IL-4 receptor and its multiple polymorphisms. In the first study, an association for the gln551arg polymorphism with atopy defined as an elevation in total serum IgE levels (with evidence for a gain of function mutation) was observed (Hershey et al., 1997). It has now become evident that there are multiple polymorphisms in this gene, several of which are in strong linkage disequilibrium with each other. From studies on the Hutterite population, the 406cyc allele was strongly associated with atopy based on skin-test responsiveness. Multiple pairwise haplotypes were strongly associated with asthma; but since this is an inbred founder population, there is strong linkage disequilibrium between many of the polymorphisms. Even in the families from the Collaborative Study on the Genetics of Asthma, there is strong linkage disequilibrium, and different haplotypes from those seen in the Hutterite population showed significant evidence for an association with asthma and atopy (Ober et al., 2000). Since it is not clear which polymorphism or combination of polymorphisms is responsible for the observed association, there may be additional important variants in the gene that are in linkage disequilibrium with those already studied. Since polymorphisms within a gene are often in linkage disequilibrium, this

Table 11–6. Relationship of Genotype to Phenotype

Frequency of polymorphism in the population
Functional effect
Inheritance in families: *susceptibility*
Relationship to clinical status: *disease expression*

example illustrates the difficulty in determining the role of a given polymorphism in a candidate gene that has a modest effect on risk.

Summary of Progress

Once linkage is confirmed in complex genetic disorders such as asthma or clinical allergic disease, finding the actual gene is a complex process (see Chapters 1 and 3). Fine-mapping studies include further clinical analyses and additional statistical analysis using techniques that include linkage disequilibrium and molecular and physical mapping with detection of mutations. It remains to be seen whether there will be single mutations that have a major effect on genetic susceptibility to asthma or whether, even within a major gene, there are multiple common sequence variants. Clearly, multiple genes influence the asthma phenotype, which is expected, given the frequency of the disease and the failure to detect a strong major gene effect from family studies. Significant progress has been made in the last decade. Several regions of the genome have been identified for susceptibility loci to asthma and BHR (Table 11–5). Future research will be focused in five major areas: completion of genome-wide searches in different populations; replication of previously reported linkages; development of multilocus models to investigate the role of multiple susceptibility loci; fine mapping of all the region(s) of interest; and candidate gene association studies. Determining the specific role of each gene in the development of asthma and BHR and correlations of phenotype to genotype will then become important areas of research (Table 11–6). These combined genetic, molecular, and clinical studies will lead to improved therapies and better techniques for early diagnosis of these disorders. By understanding the basic genetic mechanisms that lead to the development of allergy and asthma, new therapeutic interventions will be developed that will modify the development and clinical progression of these common disorders.

CLINICAL APPLICATIONS AND RISK ASSESSMENT

Since these disorders are usually common in the population and more prevalent than single-gene disorders, which are relatively rare, understanding the interaction between genes and the environment has major public health significance. Results of these studies will provide further insight into the pathophysiology of these disorders and should ultimately lead to new and more effective therapeutic interventions (Bleecker et al., 1992; Blecker and Meyers, 1995). In addition, these approaches may lead to new diagnostic methods for pre-symptomatic diagnosis, development of strategies for disease prevention in susceptible individuals, and delineation of the interaction between genotype and response to specific treatments (pharmacogenetics). Although positional cloning has not yet resulted in the identification of specific genes, these studies have already led to advances in our understanding of disease expression and characterization of the asthmatic phenotype (Bleecker et al., 1997). There is clearly an increased risk to developing asthma in family members of an asthmatic individual. However, because of population differences and the strong environmental influences, it is difficult to accurately estimate this risk in a manner appropriate for genetic counseling. Because there are probably multiple susceptibility genes for asthma, it may be reasonable to estimate risk to individuals based on the genes with the largest effect. Our ability to accurately assess risk for a given individual may vary in different populations and depend on the underlying genetic background (number of susceptibility genes and frequencies of the relevant polymorphisms).

Candidate gene studies may be performed to determine whether a polymorphism in a known gene is associated with the presence of disease (*susceptibility gene*) or with the phenotype expression of the disease (*dise*ase modifier/severity gene). An important example of the second type of study with clinical implications is the area of pharmocogenetics. Response to a given therapy varies among asthmatics, and part of this difference may be due to genetic differences in drug response. For example, there are differences in response to β-agonist therapy between asthmatics, which may be partially due to genotypic differences for polymorphisms in the β_2-adrenergic receptor gene (Drysdale et al., 2000; Israel et al, 2000).

There are several known functional polymorphisms of this gene on chromosome 5q, including those at codons 16, 27, and 164 (Reihsaus et al., 1993; Eason et al., 1995; Liggett, 1995). Because β-adrenergic therapy is the most common therapeutic agent used to treat asthma, it has been suggested that regular use of inhaled beta-agonists may be associated with adverse events in asthma (Sears et al., 1990). It is possible that differences in pharmacologic responses to β-agonist therapy between individuals with asthma may be affected by polymorphisms in this receptor. Israel and coworkers (2000) reported that individuals who are homozygous for arginine at position 16 (arg/arg) showed a decline in respiratory function when they underwent regular β_2-agonist therapy. This decline increased during a 4-week runout time period. Findings such as these are important because they may explain clinical observations related to adverse pharmacologic responses and may be used to identify a subgroup of individuals who are more likely not to respond as well as others to a specific therapy.

REFERENCES

Aalbers R, Kauffman HF, Koeter GH, Postma DS, De Vries K, de Monchy JG: Dissimilarity in methacholine and adenosine 5′-monophosphate responsiveness 3 and 24 h after allergen challenge. Am Rev Respir Dis 1991; 144:352–357.

Adams PF, Marano MA: Current estimates from the National Health Interview Survey, 1994. Vital Health Stat 1994; 10:193.

Amelung PJ, Postma DS, Xu J, Meyers DA, Bleecker ER: Exclusion of chromosome 11q and the FcϵR1β gene as aetiological factors in allergy and asthma in a population of Dutch asthmatic families [see comments]. Clin Exp Allergy 1998; 28:397–403.

American Thoracic Society: Standardization of spirometry. Am Rev Respir Dis 1987; 136:1285–1298.

American Thoracic Society: State of the Art Review: Health Effects of Outdoor Air Pollution. New York: ATS, 1995.

Anto JM, Sunyer J, Rodriguez-Roisin R, Suarez-Cervera M, Vazquez L: Community outbreaks of asthma associated with inhalation of soybean dust. N Engl J Med 1989; 320:1097–1102.

Barnes KC, Neely ND, Duffy DL, Freidhoff LR, Breazeale DR, Schou C, Naidu RP, Levett PN, Renault B, Kucherlapti R, et al.: Linkage of asthma and total serum IgE concentration to markers on chromosome 12q: evidence from Afro-Caribbean and Caucasian populations. Genomics 1996; 37:41–50.

Bleecker ER, McFadden ER Jr, Hurd SS, Goldstein RA, Ram JS: Investigative bronchoscopy in subjects with asthma and other obstructive pulmonary diseases: whether and when. Chest 1992; 101:297–298.

Bleecker ER, Meyers DA: Recent advances in the genetics of asthma. Clin Exp Allergy 25 (Suppl) 1995; 2:1–2.

Bleecker ER, Postma DS, Meyers DA: Genetic susceptibility to asthma in a changing environment. Ciba Found Symp 1997; 206:90–99.

Bleeker ER: Mapping susceptibility genes for asthma and allergy. Clin Exp Allergy 1998; 5:6–12.

Blumenthal M, Marcus-Bagley D, Awdeh Z, Johnson B, Yunis EJ, Alper CA: HLA-DR2, [HLA-B7, SC31, DR2], and [HLA-B8, SC01, DR3] haplotypes distinguish subjects with asthma from those with rhinitis only in ragweed pollen allergy. J Immunol 1992; 148:411–416.

Britton J, Pavord I, Richards K: Dietary sodium intake and the risk of airway hyperreactivity in a random adult population. Thorax 1994a; 49:875–880.

Britton J, Pavord I, Wisniewski A: Dietary magnesium, lung function, wheezing, and airway hyperreactivity in a random adult population. Lancet 1994b; 344:357–362.

Brotherhood JR, Budd GM, Hendrie AL, Jeffery SE, Beasley FA, Costin BP, Zhien W: Carbon monoxide unlikely to be a hazard to bushfire fighters [letter]. Med J Aust 1989; 151:719–720.

Bruderman I, Cohen R, Shachor J, Horowitz I: Bronchial response to methacholine in parents of asthmatic children. Chest 1987; 91:210–213.

Burrows B: Differential diagnosis of chronic obstructive pulmonary disease. Chest 1990; 97:16S–18S.

Burrows B, Lebowitz MD, Barbee RA: Respiratory disorders and allergy skin-test reactions. Ann Intern Med 1976; 84:134–139.

Burrows B, Sears MR, Flannery EM, Herbison GP, Holdaway MD: Relations of bronchial responsiveness to allergy skin test reactivity, lung function, respiratory symptoms, and diagnoses in thirteen-year-old New Zealand children. J Allergy Clin Immunol 1995; 95:548–556.

Burt CW, Knapp DE: Ambulatory care visits for asthma: United States, 1993–94. Adv Data 1996: 27:1–18.

Busse WW, Lemanske RFJ, Dick EC: The relationship of viral respiratory infections and asthma. Chest 1992; 101:385s–388s.

Busse WW, Lemanske RFJ, Stark JM, Calhoun WJ: The role of respiratory infections in asthma. In: Holgate ST, Kay AB (eds). Asthma. Physiology, Immunopharmacology, and Treatment. Fourth International Symposium. Boston: 1993:345–355.

California Environmental Protection Agency: Health effects of exposure to environmental tobacco smoke. CEPA, 1997.

Centers for Disease Control: Asthma—United States, 1982–1992. Morb Mortal Wkly Rep 1995; 43:952–955.

Centers for Disease Control: Asthma mortality and hospitalization among children and young adults—United States, 1980–1993. Morb Mortal Wkly Rep 1996; 45:350–353.

Chalmers GW, MacLeod KJ, Thomson L, Little SA, McSharry C, Thomson NC: Smoking and airway inflammation in patients with mild asthma. Chest 2001; 120:1917–1922.

Chan-Yeung M, Malo J-L: Occupational asthma. N Engl J Med 1995; 333:107–112.

Ciba Foundation Guest Symposium: Report of the Working Group on the Definition of Asthma. Edinburgh: Churchill Livingstone, 1971; 38:172–174.

Coates AL, Bergsteinsson H, Desmond K, Outerbridge EW, Beaudry PH: Long-term pulmonary sequelae of premature birth with and without idiopathic respiratory distress syndrome. J Pediatr 1977; 90:611–616.

Collaborative Study of the Genetics of Asthma (CSGA): A genome-wide search for asthma susceptibility loci in ethnically diverse populations. Nat Genet 1997; 15:389–397.

Committee on the Medical Effects of Air Pollutants: Asthma and Outdoor Air Pollution. London: Her Majesty's Stationary Office, 1995.

Cookson WOC, Moffatt MF: Asthma: an epidemic in the absence of infection? Science 1997; 275:41–43.

Cookson WOC, Sharp PA, Faux JA, Hopkin JM: Linkage between immunoglobulin E responses underlying asthma and rhinitis and chromosome 11q. Lancet 1989; 1:1292–1295.

Coultas DB, Samet JM: Epidemiology and natural history of asthma. In Tinkelman DG, Naspitz C (eds). Childhood Asthma. New York: 1993:71–114.

Daniels SE, Bhattacharrya S, James A, Leaves NI, Young A, Hill MR, Faux JA, Ryan GF, LeSouef PN, Lathrop GM, et al.: A genome-wide search for quantitative loci underlying asthma. Nature 1996; 383:247–250.

Devalia JL, Rusznak C, Herdman ML, Trigg CJ, Davies RJ: Effect of nitrogen dioxide and sulpher dioxide on airway response of mild asthmatic patients to allergen inhalation. Am J Respir Crit Care Med 1994; 344:1668–1671.

Dewar JC, Wilkinson J, Wheatley A, Thomas NS, Doull I, Morton NE, Lio P, Harvey JF, Liggett SB, Holgate ST, Hall IP: The glutamine 27 β_2-adrenoceptor polymorphism is associated with elevated IgE levels in asthmatic families. J Allergy Clin Immunol 1997; 100:261–265.

Djukanovic R, Wilson JW, Britten KM, Wilson SJ, Walls AF, Roche WR, Howarth PH, Holgate ST: Quantitation of mast cells and eosinophils in the bronchial mucosa of symptomatic atopic asthmatics and healthy control subjects using immunohistochemistry [see comments]. Am Rev Respir Dis 1990; 142:863–871.

Doershuk CF, Fisher BJ, Matthews LW: Specific airway resistannce from the perinatal period into adulthood: alterations in childhood pulmonary disease. Am Rev Respir Dis 1974; 109:452–457.

Drazen JM, Israel E, Boushey HA, Chinchilli VM, Fahy JV, Fish JE, Lazarus SC, Lemanske RF, Martin RJ, Peters SP, et al.: Comparison of regularly scheduled with as-needed use of albuterol in mild asthma. N Engl J Med 1996; 335:841–847.

Drysdale CM, McGraw DW, Stack CB, Stephens JC, Judson RS, Nandabalan K, Arnold K, Ruano G, Liggett SB: Complex promoter and coding region β_2-adrenergic receptor haplotypes alter receptor expression and predict in vivo responsiveness. Proc Amer Acad Sci USA 2000; 97:10483–10488.

Duffy DL, Nicholas MG, Battistutta D, Hopper JL, Mathews JD: Genetics of asthma and hay fever in australian twins. Am Rev Respir Dis 1990; 142:1351–1358.

Eason MG, Moreira SP, Liggett SB: Four consecutive serines in the third intracellular loop are the sites for β-adrenergic receptor kinase-mediated phosphorylation and desensitization of the α_{2A}-adrenergic receptor. J Biol Chem 1995; 270:4681–4688.

Edfors-Lubs M: Allergy in 7000 twin pairs. Acta Allergologica 1971; 26:249–285.

Eliasson O, Degraff A: The use of criteria for reversibility and obstruction to define patient groups for bronchodilator trials: influence of clinical diagnosis, spirometric, and anthropometric variables. Am Rev Respir Dis 1985; 132:858–864.

Fahy JV, Liu J, Wong H, Boushey HA: Cellular and biochemical analysis of induced sputum from asthmatic and from healthy subjects. Am Rev Respir Dis 1993; 147:1126–1131.

Floreani AA, Rennard SI: The role of cigarette smoke in the pathogenesis of asthma and as a trigger for acute symptoms. Curr Opin Pulm Med 1999; 5:38–46.

Glezen WP, Denny FW: Epidemiology of acute lower respiratory disease in children. N Engl J Med 1973; 288:498–505.

Gurwitz D, Mindorff C, Levison H: Increased incidence of bronchial reactivity in children with a history of bronchiolitis. J Pediatr 1981; 98:551–555.

Hall CB, Hall WJ, Gala CL, MaGill FB, Leddy JP: Long-term prospective study in children after respiratory syncytial virus infection. J Pediatr 1984; 105:358–364.

Hanrahan JP, Tager IB, Segal MR, Tosteson TD, Castile RG, Van Vunakis H, Weiss ST, Speizer FE: The effect of maternal smoking during pregnancy on early infant lung function. Am Rev Respir Dis 1992; 145:1129–1135.

Henry RL, Hodges IGC, Milner AD, Stokes GM: Respiratory problems 2 years after acute bronchiolitis in infancy. Arch Dis Child 1983; 58:713–716.

Hershey GK, Friedrich MF, Esswein LA, Thomas ML, Chatila TA: The association of atopy with a gain-of-function mutation in the a subunit of the interleukin-4 receptor. N Engl J Med 1997; 337:1720–1725.

Hide DW, Matthews S, Tariq S, Arshad SH: Allergen avoidance in infancy and allergy at 4 years of age. Allergy 1996; 51:89–93.

Holberg CJ, Elston RC, Halonen M, Wright AL, Taussig LM, Morgan WJ, Martinez FD: Segregation analysis of physician-diagnosed asthma in Hispanic and white families: a recessive component. Am J Respir Crit Care Med 1996; 154:144–150.

Holgate ST: Asthma genetics: waiting to exhale. Nat Genet 1997; 15:227–229.

Hopp RJ, Bewtra A, Biven R, Nair NM, Townley RG: Bronchial reactivity pattern in nonasthmatic parents of asthmatics. Ann Allergy 1988; 61:184–186.

Hopp RJ, Bewtra AK, Nair NM, Townley RG: Specificity and sensitivity of methacholine inhalation challenge in normal and asthmatic children. J Allergy Clin Immunol 1984; 74:154–158.

Horwood LJ, Fergusson DM, Shannon FT: Social and familial factors in the development of early childhood asthma. Pediatrics 1985; 75:859–868.

Infante-Rivard C: Childhood asthma and indoor environmental risk factors. Am J Epidemiol 1993; 137:834–844.

Institute of Medicine, Committee on the Health Effects of Indoor Allergens, Division of Health Promotion and Disease Prevention: Indoor Allergens: Assessing the Controlling Adverse Health Effects. Washington, D.C., National Academy Press, 1993.

Israel E, Drazen JM, Liggett SB, Boushey HA, Cherniack RM, Chinchilli VM, Cooper DM, Fahy JV, Fish JE, Ford JG, et al.: for the NHLBI's Asthma Clinical Research Network: The effect of polymorphisms of the β_2-adrenergic receptor on the response to regular use of albuterol in asthma. Am J Respir Crit Care Med 2000; 162:75–78.

Kattan M, Keens TG, Lapierre JG, Levison H, Bryan C, Reilly BJ: Pulmonary function abnormalities in symptom-free children after bronchiolitis. Pediatrics 1977; 59:683–688.

Lamarre A, Linsao L, Reilly BJ, Swyer PR, Levinson H: Residual pulmonary abnormalities in surviviors of idiopathic respiratory distress syndrome. Am Rev Respir Dis 1973; 108:56–61.

Lander ES, Schork NJ: Genetic dissection of complex traits. Science 1994; 265:2037–2048.

Liggett SB: Genetics of β_2-adrenergic receptor variants in asthma. Clin Exp Allergy 25(Suppl) 1995; 2:89–94.

Liu MC, Bleecker ER, Lichtenstein LM, Kagey-Sobotka A, Niv Y, McLemore TL, Permutt S, Proud D, Hubbard WC: Evidence for elevated levels of histamine, prostaglandin D2, and other bronchoconstricting prostaglandins in the airways of subjects with mild asthma. Am Rev Respir Dis 1990; 142:126–132.

Longo G, Strinati R, Poli F, Fumi F: Genetic factors in nonspecific bronchial hyperreactivity. Am J Dis Child 1987; 141:331–334.

Marsh DG, Meyers DA, Freidhoff LR, Ehrlich-Kautzky E, Roebber M, Norman PS, Hsu SH, Bias WB: HLA-Dw2: a genetic marker for human immune response to short ragweed pollen allergen Ra5. II. Response after ragweed immunotherapy. J Exp Med 1982; 155:1452–1463.

Marsh DG, Neely JD, Breazeale DR, Ghosh B, Friedhoff LR, Ehrlich-Kautzy E, Schou C, Krishnaswamy G, Beaty TH: Linkage analysis of IL-4 and other chromosome 5q31.1 markers and total serum IgE concentrations. Science 1994; 264:1152–1156.

Martin AJ, Landau LI, Phelan PD: Natural history of allergy in asthmatic children followed to adult life. Med J Aust 1981; 2:470–474.

Martinez FD, Holberg CJ: Segregation analysis of physician diagnosed asthma in Hispanic and non-Hispanic white families. Clin Exp Allergy 1995; 25:68–70.

Martinez FD, Morgan WJ, Wright AL, Holberg CJ, Taussig LM, Group Health Medical Associates: Diminished lung function as a predisposing factor for wheezing respiratory illness in infants. N Engl J Med 1988; 319:1112–1117.

Martinez FD, Wright AL, Taussig LM, Holberg CJ, Halonen M, Morgan WJ, Group Health Medical Associates: Asthma and wheezing in the first six years of life. N Engl J Med 1995; 332:133–138.

Meyers DA, Postma DS, Panhuysen CIM, Xu J, Amelung PJ, Levitt RC, Bleecker ER: Evidence for a locus regulating total serum IgE levels mapping to chromosome 5. Genomics 1994; 23:464–470.

Miskelly FG, Burr ML, Vaughan-Williams E, Fehily A, Butland BK, Merrett TG: Infant feeding and allergy. Arch Dis Child 1988; 63:388–393.

Molfino NA, Wright FC, Katz I, Tarlo S, Silverman F, McClean PA, Szalai JP, Raizenne M, Slutsky AS, Zamel N: Effect of low concentrations of ozone on inhaled allergen responses in asthmatic subjects. Lancet 1991; 338:199–203.

Monto AS, Ullman BM: Acute respiratory illness in an American community. JAMA 1974; 227:164–169.

National Heart, Lung and Blood Institute and National Institutes of Health: Guidelines for the diagnosis and management of asthma. Washington, DC: Printing Office, U.S. Government, 1991, 1995.
National Heart, Lung and Blood Institute and World Health Organization: Global initiative for asthma. Washington, DC: U.S. Government Printing Office, 1993, 1995.
National Institutes of Health: Workshop summary and guidelines: Investigative use of bronchoscopy, lavage and bronchial biopsies in asthma and other airways disease. J Allergy Clin Immunol 1991; 88:808–814.
NIH Expert Panel: Expert Panel Report II: Guidelines for the Diagnosis and Management of Asthma. Washington, DC: National Institutes of Health, National Asthma Education and Prevention Program, 1997.
Nolte H, Backer V, Porsbjerg C: Environmental factors as a cause for the increase in allergic disease. Ann Allergy Asthma Immunol 2001; 87:7–11.
Northway WH Jr, Moss RB, Carlisle KB, Parker BR, Popp RL, Pitlick PT, Eichler I, Lamm RL, Brown BW Jr: Late pulmonary sequelae of bronchopulmonary dysplasia. N Engl J Med 1990; 323:1793–1799.
Ober C, Cox N, Abney M, DiRienzo A, Lander ES, Changyaleket B, Gidley H, Durtz B, Lee J, Nance M, et al.: Genome-wide search for asthma susceptibility loci in a founder population. Hum Mol Genet 1998; 7:1393–1398.
Ober C, Leavitt SA, Tsalenko A, Howard TD, Hoki DM, Daniel R, Newman DL, Wu X, Parry R, Lester LA: for the CSGA: Variation in the IL4R gene confers susceptibility to asthma and atopy in ethnically diverse populations. Am J Hum Genet 2000; 66:517–520.
O'Connor GT, Sparrow D, Weiss ST: The role of allergy and nonspecific airway hyperresponsiveness in the pathogenesis of chronic obstructive pulmonary disease. Am Rev Respir Dis 1989; 140:225–252.
Oliveti JF, Kercsmar CM, Redline S: Pre- and perinatal risk factors for asthma in inner-city African-American children. Am J Epidemiol 1996; 143:570–577.
Outerbridge EW, Norgrady BM, Beaudry PH, Stern L: Idiopathic respiratory distress syndrome: recurrent respiratory illness in survivors. Am J Dis Child 1972; 123:99–104.
Panhuysen CI, Bleecker ER, Koeter GH, Meyers DA, Postma DS: Characterization of obstructive airway disease in family members of probands with asthma: an algorithm for the diagnosis of asthma. Am J Respir Crit Care Med 1998; 157:1734–1742.
Panhuysen CIM, Meyers DA: Genetic regulation of total serum IgE levels. In Liggett SB, Meyers DA (eds). The Genetics of Asthma. 1996:511–521.
Panhuysen CIM, Xu J, Postma DS, Bleecker ER, Meyers DA: Evidence for a major locus for bronchial hyperresponsiveness independent of the locus regulating total serum IgE levels. Am J Hum Genet 1996; 59:A231.
Pattemore PK, Asher MI, Harrison AC, Mitchell EA, Rea HH, Stewart AW: The interrelationship among bronchial hyperresponsiveness, the diagnosis of asthma, and asthma symptoms. Am Rev Respir Dis 1990; 142:549–554.
Pistelli R, Forastiere F, Corbo GM: Respiratory symptoms and bronchial responsivenss are related to dietary salt intake and urinary potassium excretion in male children. Eur Respir J 1993; 6:517–522.
Postma DS, Bleecker ER, Amelung PJ, Holroyd KJ, Xu J, Panhuysen CI, Meyers DA, Levitt RC: Genetic susceptibility to asthma: bronchial hyperresponsiveness coinherited with a major gene for atopy. N Engl J Med 1995; 333:894–900.
Reihsaus E, Innis M, MacIntyre N, Liggett SB: Mutations in the gene encoding for the β_2-adrenergic receptor in normal and asthmatic subjects. Am J Respir Cell Mol Biol 1993; 8:334–339.
Risch N, Merikangas K: The future of genetic studies of complex human diseases [see comments]. Science 1996; 273:1516–1517.
Samet JM, Lambert WE, Skipper BJ, Cushing AH, Hunt WC, Young SA, McLaren LC, Schwab M, Spengler JD: Nitrogen dioxide and respiratory illnesses in infants. Am Rev Respir Dis 1993; 148:1258–1265.
Sandford AJ, Shirakawa T, Moffatt MF, Daniels SE, Ra C, Faux JA, Young RP, Nakamura Y, Lathrop GM, Cookson WOC, Hopkin JM: Localisation of atopy and beta subunit of high-affinity IgE receptor on chromosome 11q. Lancet 1993; 341:332–334.
Schachter EN, Doyle CA, Beck GJ: A prospective study of asthma in a rural community. Chest 1984; 85:623–630.
Schwartz J, Weiss ST: The relationship of dietary fish intake to level of pulmonary function in the first National Health and Nutrition Examination Survey (NHANESI). Eur Respir J 1994; 7:1821–1824.
Sears MR, Taylor DR, Print CG, Lake DC, Li QQ, Flannery EM, Yates DM, Lucas MK, Herbison GP: Regular inhaled beta-agonist treatment in bronchial asthma. Lancet 1990; 336:1391–1396.
Shepard FM, Johnston RB, Klatte EC, Burko H, Stahlman M: Residual pulmonary findings in clinical hyaline-membrane disease. N Engl J Med 1968; 279:1063–1071.
Shirakawa T, Enomoto T, Shin-ichiro S, Hopkin JM: The inverse association between tuberculin responses and atopic disorder. Science 1997; 275:77–79.
Sibbald B, Turner-Warwick M: Factors influencing the prevalence of asthma among first-degree relatives of extrinxic and intrinsic asthmatics. Thorax 1979; 34:332–337.
Sims DG, Downham MAPS, Gardner PS, Webb JKG, Weightman D: Study of 8-year-old children with a history of respiratory syncytial virus bronchiolitis in infancy. Br Med J 1978; 1:11–14.
Sparrow D, O'Connor GT, Basner RC, Weiss ST: Predictors of the new onset of wheezing among middle-aged and older men: the normative aging study. Am Rev Respir Dis 1993; 147:367–371.
Sparrow D, Weiss ST: Methodological issues in airway responsiveness testing. In Weiss ST, Sparrow D (eds). Airway Responsiveness and Atopy in the Development of Chronic Lung Disease, New York: 1989:103–120.
Spielman RS, McGinnis RE, Ewens WJ: Transmission test for linkage disequilibrium: the insulin gene region and insulin-dependent diabetes mellitus (IDDM). Am J Hum Genet 1993; 52:506–516.
Sporik R, Holgate ST, Cogswell JJ: Natural history of asthma in childhood: a birth cohort study. Arch Dis Child 1991; 66:1050–1053.
Sporik R, Holgate ST, Platts-Mills TA, Cogswell JJ: Exposure to house-dust mite allergen (Der p I) and the development of asthma in childhood: a prospective study. N Engl J Med 1990; 323:502–507.
Stokes GM, Milner AD, Hodges IGC, Groggins RC: Lung function abnormalities after acute bronchiolitis. Pediatrics 1981; 98:871–874.
Tashkin DP, Altose MD, Bleecker ER, Connett JE, Kanner RE, Lee WW, Wise R: The lung health study: airway responsiveness to inhaled methacholine in smokers with mild to moderate airflow limitation. Am Rev Respir Dis 1992; 145:301–310.
Taussig LM: Maximal expiratory flow at functional residual capacity: a test of lung function for young children. Am Rev Respir Dis 1977; 116:1031–1038.
Townley RG, Bewtra A, Wilson AF, Hopp RJ, Elston RC, Nair N, Watt GD: Segregation analysis of bronchial response to methacholine inhalation challenge in families with and without asthma. J Allergy Clin Immunol 1986; 77:101–107.
Troisi RJ, Willett WC, Weiss ST, Trichopoulos D, Rosner B, Speizer FE: A prospective study of diet and adult-onset asthma. Am J Respir Crit Care Med 1995; 151:1401–1408.
U.S. Department of Health and Human Services: A Report of the Surgeon General: The Health Consequences of Involuntary Smoking. Washington, DC: U.S. Government Printing Office, 1986.
U.S. Department of Health and Human Services: A Report of the Surgeon General: The Health Benefits of Smoking Cessation. Washington, DC: U.S. Government Printing Office, 1990.
Von Mutius E, Nicolai T, Martinez FD: Prematurity as a risk factor for asthma in preadolescent children. J Pediatr 1993; 123:223–229.
Weiss ST, Utell MJ, Samet JM: Environmental tobacco smoke exposure and asthma in adults. Environ Health Perspect 1999; 6:891–895.
Weiss ST: Diet as a risk factor for asthma. In Chadwick DJ, Cardew G (eds). The rising trends in Asthma. Ciba Foundation Symposium 206. New York: Ciba Foundation, 1997:244–257.
Weiss ST, Tager IB, Munoz A, Speizer FE: The relationship of respiratory infections in early childhood to the occurrence of increased levels of bronchial responsiveness and atopy. Am Rev Respir Dis 1985; 131:573–578.
Welliver RC, Sun M, Rinaldo D: Predictive value of respiratory syncytial virus-specific IgE response for recurrent wheezing following bronchiolitis. J Pediatr 1986; 109:776–780.
Welliver RC, Wong DT, Sun M: The development of respiratory syncytial virus specific IgE and the release of histamine in nasopharyngeal secretions. N Engl J Med 1981; 305:841–846.
Wenzel SE: Inflammation, leukotrienes and the pathogenesis of the late asthmatic response [editorial; comment]. Clin Exp Allergy 1999; 29:1–3.
Wiesch DG, Meyers DA, Bleeker ER: Genetics of asthma. J Allergy Clin Immunol 1999; 104:895–901.
Wilson SR, Yamada EG, Sudhakar R, Roberto L, Mannino D, Mejia C, Huss N: A controlled trial of an environmental tobacco smoke reduction intervention in low-income children with asthma. Chest 2001; 120:1709–1722.
Wjst M, Fischer G, Immervoll T, Jung M, Saar K, Rueschendorf F, Reis A, Ulbrecht M, Gomolka M, Weiss EH, et al.: A genome-wide search for linkage to asthma. Genomics 1999; 58:1–8.
Woolcock AJ, Anderson SD, Peat JK, Du Toit JI, Guang Zhang Y, Smith CM, Salome CM: Characteristics of bronchial hyperresponsiveness in chronic obstructive pulmonary disease and in asthma. Am Rev Respir Dis 1991; 143:1438–1443.
World Health Organization: Epidemiology of chronic and non-specific respiratory diseases. Bull World Health Organ 1975; 52:251–260.
Xu J, Levitt RC, Panhuysen CI, Postma DS, Taylor EW, Amelung PJ, Holroyd KJ, Bleecker ER, Meyers DA: Evidence for two unlinked loci regulating total serum IgE levels. Am J Hum Genet 1995; 57:425–430.
Xu J, Meyers DA, Ober C, Blumenthal MN, Mellen B, Barnes KC, King RA, Lester LA, Howard TD, Solway J, et al.: Genomewide screen and identification of gene–gene interactions for asthma susceptibility loci in three U.S. populations. Am J Hum Genet 2001; 68:1437–1446.
Xu J, Postma DS, Howard TH, Koppelman GH, Zheng SL, Stine OC, Bleecker ER, Meyers DA: Major genes regulating total serum immunoglobulin E levels in families with asthma. Am J Hum Genet 2000; 67:1163–1173.
Young S, Le Souef PN, Geelhoed GC, Stick SM, Turner KJ, Landau LI: The influence of a family history of asthma and parental smoking on airway responsiveness in early infancy. N Engl J Med 1991; 324:1168–1173.
Zeiger RS, Heller S, Mellon MH, Forsythe AB, O'Connor RD, Hamburger RN, Schatz M: Effect of combined maternal and infant food-allergen avoidance on development of atopy in early infancy: a randomized study. J Allergy Clin Immunol 1989; 84:72–89.

12 IgA Deficiency and Common Variable Immunodeficiency

HARRY W. SCHROEDER, JR.

Among individuals of European ancestry, selective IgA deficiency (IgAD) is the most frequently recognized primary immunodeficiency (Rosen et al., 1997), but due to the severity of symptoms, common variable immunodeficiency (CVID) is the most common form of primary immune deficiency under the care of the clinical immunologist (Flori et al., 1997; Rosen et al., 1997). Individuals with CVID are typically panhypogammaglobulinemic, although some produce substantial amounts of IgM. Individuals with IgAD may also be deficient in IgG subclasses, especially IgG2 and IgG4 (Oxelius et al., 1981; French et al., 1995; Rosen et al., 1997). IgAD and CVID thus represent waystations along a range of humoral immunodeficiency that extends from a partial deficiency of serum IgA to the complete inability to produce antibodies of any isotype. The underlying defect is poorly understood, but it appears to result from a block in the ability of B cells, which are typically found in normal numbers in this disease, to differentiate into plasma cells of given isotypes (Cooper and Lawton, 1972; Rosen et al., 1997). The molecular basis of this developmental block remains unclear. B cells require the aid of other cells and organ systems to build and maintain serum antibody levels, and there is mounting evidence that T cell (Nordoy et al., 1998; Boncristiano et al., 2000; Di Renzo et al., 2000; Pozzi et al., 2001) or accessory cell (Cambronero et al., 2000) function may be abnormal. At present, however, in the absence of a molecular definition, IgAD and CVID remain diagnoses characterized by a clinical phenotype and represent diagnoses that encompass a heterogeneous group of disorders (Spickett et al., 1997).

DISEASE DEFINITION

Diagnostic Criteria

By definition, individuals with serum IgA concentrations that fall 2 SD below the mean for their age are considered to have partial IgA deficiency (Burgio et al., 1980). The diagnosis of complete IgA deficiency is reserved for those with undetectable levels of IgA in the serum and secretions (Rosen et al., 1992). Most clinical laboratories measure serum immunoglobulins by nephelometry, which cannot reliably measure serum IgA concentrations of less than 7 mg/dl (70 mg/L). IgA can be detected by the more sensitive hemmagglutination assay in approximately one-quarter of these patients (Vyas et al., 1975). Thus, diagnosis of complete IgA deficiency rests on the sensitivity of the assay for IgA.

Uncomplicated IgAD patients have normal serum concentrations of IgM, normal or elevated levels of IgG (Cunningham Rundles et al., 1983), and demonstrate normal cell-mediated immunity. A minority of patients may demonstrate additional evidence of immunological dysfunction, with inability to generate appropriate IgG2 anti-carbohydrate antibodies (Hammarstrom et al., 1985b; Lane and MacLennan, 1986), frank IgG subclass deficiencies (Oxelius et al., 1981; Ugazio et al., 1983; Preudhomme and Hanson, 1990), or evidence of impairment of T-cell function (Waldmann et al., 1976; Atwater and Tomasi, 1978; King et al., 1979).

Common variable immunodeficiency has long been considered a "wastebasket" category of primary immunodeficiencies that includes a number of immune disorders (Geha et al., 1974; Eibl et al., 1988). However, most CVID patients of northern European descent exhibit a distinctive phenotype that is characterized by a broad deficiency of Ig isotypes in spite of the presence of normal numbers of surface immunoglobulin bearing B-cell precursors in the peripheral blood (Cooper et al., 1971; Eibl et al., 1988). Almost all of these patients are IgA deficient and, by definition, exhibit total serum IgG levels of less than 500 mg/dl. Some IgG subclasses are more affected than others, with the sequential order of involvement being IgG4 > IgG2 > IgG1 > IgG3 (Wedgwood et al., 1986; Aucouturier et al., 1989). Many of these patients also have reductions of serum IgM and IgE (Stites et al., 1975). Most patients demonstrate normal cell-mediated immunity, but there is increasing evidence that abnormalities in T-cell function may contribute to the disease (Sneller et al., 1993; Fischer et al., 1996; Majolini et al., 1997; Thon et al., 1997; Nordoy et al., 1998; Boncristiano et al., 2000; Di Renzo et al., 2000; Pozzi et al., 2001). In a minority of cases, dysfunction of a broad array of other cell types of the hematopoietic system has been described (Belickova et al., 1994). In some cases, B-cell numbers are also reduced, although not to the same extent as that seen in X-linked agammaglobulinemia.

Brief Clinical Presentation

IgAD

The majority of individuals with IgAD have no obvious health problems, while others may suffer from chronic upper respiratory infections, as well as gastrointestinal disorders, autoimmune diseases, allergies, asthma, malignancies, and other genetic disorders (Ammann and Hong, 1971; Burgio et al., 1980; Fasth, 1982; Schaffer et al., 1991; Chee et al., 2001). The severity of clinical symptoms is likely related to factors such as the compensation by IgM or selected IgG subclasses in the secretions (Stobo and Tomasi, 1967; Brandtzaeg et al., 1968; Nilssen et al., 1993), associated deficits in selected IgG subclasses such as IgG2 and IgG4 (Oxelius et al., 1981; French and Harrison, 1986; Lane and MacLennan, 1986; Aucouturier et al., 1989; Preudhomme and Hanson, 1990), the level of IgE (Polmar et al., 1975), maintenance of intestinal secretory IgA in the absence of serum IgA

(Andre et al., 1978), whether the IgA deficiency is complete or partial (Morell et al., 1986), and the coexistance of other susceptibility factors.

The likelihood that an IgA-deficient individual who was identified serendipitously will require medical attention is difficult to assess because most studies in the literature reflect patients who were identified as a result of clinical symptoms (Seggev et al., 1988). Among IgAD patients referred to immunology clinics, more than 85% present with frequent, mild-to-moderate upper respiratory infections, including otitis media and sinusitis (West et al., 1962; Buckley, 1975; Ostergaard, 1980; Burks and Steele, 1986; Morell et al., 1986; Klemola, 1987; Schaffer et al., 1991). In children, symptoms often begin in the first year of life, although the physiologic lag in achieving serum IgA levels may delay the diagnosis until after the age of two (Burgio et al., 1980). The most common etiologic agents are encapsulated bacteria such as *H. influenzae* and *S. pneumoniae*. Respiratory infections begin early in childhood and may either disappear or persist throughout adult life (Ostergaard, 1980; Klemola, 1987; Hong and Ammann, 1989). In rare cases, patients with IgAD experience recurrent bronchitis, pneumonia, and even bronchiectasis (South et al., 1965). Many of these patients also have deficits in serum levels of IgG_2 and IgG_4 (Oxelius et al., 1981; Aucouturier et al., 1989; Preudhomme and Hanson, 1990). Chronic intermittent diarrhea is also a common complaint, and many patients are recurrently infested with the parasite *Giardia lamblia* (Amin, 1979). Systemic infections such as viral hepatitis, meningoencephalitis, and septicemia may also occur (Ammann and Hong, 1971; Ostergaard, 1980; Burks and Steele, 1986).

CVID

The clinical manifestations of CVID are similar but more severe than the ones seen in IgAD. A minority of patients with CVID present with no obvious health problems and are diagnosed serendipitously; most complain of mild to moderate upper respiratory tract infections (Watts et al., 1986; Chee et al., 2001). CVID patients are also at increased risk of developing gastrointestinal disorders, autoimmune diseases, and malignancies (Hausser et al., 1983; Couderc et al., 1987; Filipovich et al., 1994). Although allergic disorders are rare in CVID patients, there can be sufficient IgE to allow anaphylactic reactions to occur (Loria et al., 1987).

Respiratory symptoms often begin with recurrent sinusitis, otitis media, and mild bronchitis. The most common etiologic agents are encapsulated bacteria such as *H. influenzae* and *S. pneumoniae* (Sneller et al., 1993). The frequency and severity of infection appears to worsen in the second and third decades of life, and patients may present with recurrent pneumonia. Even when they are apparently asymptomatic, untreated patients can suffer recurrent subclinical pulmonary infections that can lead to irreversible chronic lung damage with bronchiectasis, unilateral hyperlucent lung, emphysema, and cor pulmonale (Watts et al., 1986). If after repeated infection the pulmonary mucosa becomes damaged, the spectrum of bacterial pathogens can broaden to include *Pseudomonas aeruginosa* and *Staphylococcus aureus* (Sneller et al., 1993).

Although most patients with CVID can clear viral infections normally, the lack of humoral immunity increases susceptibility to viral reactivation. For example, *Herpes zoster* (shingles) can occur in up to 20% of patients (Asherson, 1980), and frequent and severe recurrence of herpes simplex (Straus et al., 1984) and cytomegalovirus (Freeman et al., 1977) infections have also been reported. Antibody-deficient patients are at risk for severe enterovirus infections (Wilfert et al., 1977) and should never receive live viral vaccines (Kew et al., 1998). In rare cases, CVID patients have developed meningoencephalitis due to echovirus type 11 (Sneller et al., 1993). This latter infection has a progressive and usually fatal course that begins with fever, a dermatomyositis-like syndrome, edema, rashes, and hepatitis.

CVID patients often experience intermittent or chronic diarrhea, most commonly due to *Giardia lamblia*. Untreated patients may suffer for months or years. Affected individuals can undergo significant weight loss and develop a malabsorption syndrome that histologically may resemble celiac sprue (Sneller et al., 1993). There is an increased risk of infection from bacterial enteric pathogens such as *Salmonella*, *Shigella*, and *Campylobacter* (Sneller et al., 1993), as well as a fastidious gram-negative bacterium known as dysgonic fermenter-3 (Wagner et al., 1988). Patients with CVID are also at high risk for the development of hepatitis B and C, which can lead to chronic active hepatitis with fatal consequences (Hermans et al., 1976; Tong et al., 1977; Solley et al., 1979; Bjorkander et al., 1988).

Although it is not uncommon for CVID patients to be anergic, only a minority of patients develop infections characteristic of cell-mediated immune dysfunction, such as mycobacteria, *Pneumocystis carinii* (Bonagura et al., 1989), and fungi (Couch and Romyg, 1977; Gupta et al., 1987; Sneller et al., 1993). Some of these patients may demonstrate severe depression of the $CD8^+$ cytotoxic/suppressor T cell subset.

GENERAL GENETIC AND EPIDEMIOLOGIC EVIDENCE

Clinical Epidemiology and Ethnic Differences

IgAD

The prevalence of IgAD varies widely. It is the most frequently recognized primary immunodeficiency, having a prevalence of approximately 1 in 160 to 700 individuals of European ancestry (Bachman, 1965; Hobbs, 1968; Johansson et al., 1968; Pereira et al., 1997). Among individuals of African American descent, the prevalence is one-twentieth of that seen in European Americans (Lawton et al., 1972; Buckley, 1975) and appears even lower among Asians (Yadav and Iyngkaran, 1979; Kanoh et al., 1986). Among Israeli army recruits, the prevalence of IgAD is related to ethnicity, with more recruits of European descent affected than those of North African or Asian descent (Melamed et al., 1987). These differences support the view that genetic factors play a major role in the pathogenesis of the disease.

CVID

Common variable immunodeficiency has an estimated prevalence of 1:50,000 to 1:200,000 among northern Europeans (Fasth, 1982; McCluskey and Boyd, 1989). Men and women are equally affected. In our clinic population in the Southeastern United States, the prevalence among African Americans is one-twentieth that of Caucasians, markedly paralleling the relative prevalence of IgAD in the same populations. While patients with this disorder may present during childhood (Hosking and Roberton, 1983), most patients are diagnosed in the third decade of life, in which case the terms "late-" or "adult-onset" have been used (Hermans et al., 1976; Asherson, 1980; Cunningham-Rundles and Bodian, 1999). There are cases where a transition from normal serum immunoglobulin levels to an immunodeficiency state have been documented (Robbins, 1966; Johnson et al., 1997). Although CVID can thus be an "acquired" disease, the term *acquired immunodeficiency* has become synonymous with AIDS and should be reserved for patients in whom the diagnosis of HIV infection has been established.

Family Epidemiology

Family Studies

Individuals with either IgAD or CVID can be seen in multiplex families (Wollheim and Williams, 1965; Volanakis et al., 1992; Johnson et al., 1997). The mode of familial transmission is unclear since some pedigrees suggest a pattern of autosomal dominance and others autosomal recessive inheritance (Grundbacher, 1972; Oen et al., 1982; Cunningham Rundles, 1990). Coupled with the similarity in clinical phenotype, these observations support the hypothesis that IgAD and CVID reflect a common underlying genetic defect (Schaffer et al., 1989).

Twin Studies

Of the few studies of twins, three sets of identical twins have reported as discordant for IgAD (Hodgson, 1966; Leukonia et al., 1976; Skrede et al., 1977), one set of identical twins discordant for CVID has been reported (Cruchaud et al., 1965), and two sets of identical twins have been reported as concordant (Amarin and Grant, 1982; Schwaber and Roser, 1984). Among the more than 80 cases of CVID that this author has personally reviewed, there was one set of identical twins concordant for CVID.

Associations with Other Diseases

IgAD

Some symptomatic patients with IgAD have elevated IgE levels (Stites et al., 1975). The presence of IgE can introduce an allergic or asthmatic component to upper respiratory or pulmonary dysfunction (Buckley and Dees, 1969; Polmar et al., 1975). It has been proposed that the elevation of IgE serum concentrations is a compensatory response to the absence of IgA (Buckley, 1975). This appears to be a double-edged sword, because up to 20% of IgAD patients (Schaffer et al., 1991) may complain of allergic rhinitis, conjunctivitis, urticaria, and atopic eczema (Ostergaard, 1980; Oxelius et al., 1981; Burks and Steele, 1986; Schaffer et al., 1991). Allergic reactions may be enhanced due to the lack of IgA blocking antibodies in the serum (Turk et al., 1970), and unusually severe asthma has also been associated with IgAD (Horowitz and Hong, 1975).

Patients with IgAD are at higher risk for the development of a broad spectrum of autoimmune diseases (Ammann and Hong, 1971; Burks and Steele, 1986; Klemola, 1987). Juvenile rheumatoid arthritis and systemic lupus erythematosus have been reported in up to 7% of patients (Cassidy et al., 1969; Pelkonen et al., 1983; Rankin and Isenberg, 1997). Other autoimmune disorders reported in association with IgAD include Addison's disease, chronic nephritis, dermatomyositis, Evans syndrome, isolated hemolytic anemia, isolated idiopathic thrombocytopenic purpura, insulin-dependent diabetes mellitus (IDDM), pulmonary hemosiderosis, sarcoidosis, Sjögren's syndrome, and thyroiditis (Brouet and Seligmann, 1976; Hansen et al., 1982; Hoddinott et al., 1982; Cuesta et al., 1986; Schaffer et al., 1991). IgA deficiency appears to play a minimal role in the morbidity of these disorders. Henoch-Schönlein syndrome, or hemorrhagic purpura, has also been reported (Martini et al., 1985). Severe villous atrophy compatible with celiac disease can be found in up to 8% of children with IgAD (Meini et al., 1996), and approximately 2% to 3% of patients with celiac disease suffer from IgAD (Mulder et al., 1986; Quigley et al., 1986; Klemola et al., 1995; Heneghan et al., 1997; Cataldo et al., 1998). Most of these patients appear to have inherited the HLA-DR3, -B8, -A1 haplotype (Heneghan et al., 1997). Other gastrointestinal disorders include inflammatory bowel disease (Ammann and Hong, 1971), intestinal disaccharidase deficiency (Dubois et al., 1970), lactase deficiency (Dubois et al., 1970), pancreatic insufficiency (Penny et al., 1971), and pernicious anemia (Horowitz and Hong, 1975). Hepatobiliary disorders include chronic active hepatitis (Cuesta et al., 1986; Klemola, 1987), cholelithiasis (Danon et al., 1983), lupoid hepatitis, and primary biliary cirrhosis (James et al., 1986). Skin disorders reported in association with IgAD include pyoderma gangrenosum (Bundino and Zina, 1984), trachyonychia (Leong et al., 1982), and vitiligo (Wolf and Wolf, 1982). It is unclear whether these disorders are the end result of recurrent infections or the product of recurrent insult by antigens that would otherwise be cleared by IgA, or whether the underlying deficit that leads to IgAD also increases the risk of developing an autoimmune disorder. For example, autoimmune disorders such as IDDM and celiac disease are associated with the same HLA haplotypes as IgAD (see below) (French and Dawkins, 1990).

There are persistent reports in the literature associating IgAD with an increased risk for the development of gastrointestinal and lymphoid malignancies (Spector et al., 1978; Cunningham Rundles et al., 1980). Gastric and colonic adenocarcinoma have been frequently reported (Spector et al., 1978; Cunningham Rundles et al., 1980). IgAD patients have also been reported with acute lymphoblastic leukemia (Chevailler et al., 1990), hepatoma, lymphosarcoma, melanoma, multiple myeloma, ovarian carcinoma, squamous cell carcinoma, and malignant thymoma (Spector et al., 1978; Cunningham Rundles et al., 1980; Hong and Ammann, 1989). Cervical and bronchial lymphadenopathy can be found in IgAD patients who suffer from recurrent sinopulmonary infections (French, 1984). Patients with chronic gastrointestinal infections may demonstrate a nodular lymphoid hyperplasia of the small intestine that can lead to intestinal obstruction (Gryboski et al., 1968; Davis and Berk, 1977). Histologic evaluation reveals active B lymphocyte proliferation in the germinal centers of the Peyer's patches. These "constipated" lymph nodes have been mistaken for lymphoma. In some cases, it is possible to attribute the increased risk of malignancy to the lack of protection against ingested carcinogens (Borriello et al., 1985). In others, the simultaneous presence of IgAD and malignancy may simply reflect the high prevalence of IgAD in the Caucasian population.

CVID

Recurrent bacterial cellulitis is typically associated with disorders of the phagocytic cells of the blood. However, some patients with CVID can present with a history of skin infections (Loria et al., 1987). Patients may also present with erythroderma (White et al., 1985). The pathogenesis of these dermatologic manifestations remains unclear.

CVID patients appear to be at higher risk for the development of a broad spectrum of autoimmune diseases (Hermans et al., 1976; Asherson, 1980; Cunningham-Rundles and Bodian, 1999). The most common disorders are Coombs positive hemolytic anemia and idiopathic thrombocytopenic purpura (Hermans et al., 1976; Asherson, 1980; Cunningham-Rundles and Bodian, 1999), which in combination comprise Evans syndrome (Evans and Burn, 1979; Wang, 1988). Pernicious anemia can be found in up to 10% of patients (Twomey et al., 1969), and autoimmune neutropenia, Grave's disease, hypothyroidism, rheumatoid arthritis, systemic lupus erythematosus (SLE), and Sjögren syndrome have been reported (Hermans et al., 1976; Asherson, 1980; Webster et al., 1981; Cunningham-Rundles and Bodian, 1999). Given the pathogenic role of immunoglobulin in SLE, the concurrent presence of immune complexes and hypogammaglobulinemia in the same patient appears counterintuitive (Ashman et al., 1982; Stein et al., 1985; Goldstein et al., 1985). However, patients have been reported in which symptoms of lupus resolved as their serum levels of IgG declined (Sussman et al., 1983).

Untreated patients with CVID often complain of an asymmetrical, oligoarticular arthritis. In some cases, arthritis is the product of infection with encapsulated organisms (Sneller et al., 1993) or with *Mycoplasma* species (Johnston et al., 1983) and thus require antibiotic therapy. The etiology in other cases remains unclear. In the latter cases, the arthritis typically responds to therapy with intravenous gammaglobulin.

A sarcoid-like syndrome—characterized by non-caseating granulomas in the lung, lymph nodes, skin, bone marrow, and liver—can occur in patients with CVID (Edelstein et al., 1978; Keczkes et al., 1979; Friedman et al., 1983; Lee, 1984; Burmester et al., 1985; Sneller et al., 1993; Spickett et al., 1996b; Mechanic et al., 1997; Smith and Skelton, 2001), especially in African Americans (Fasano et al., 1996). In some cases, these granulomas may result from mycobacterial and fungal infections. For most patients, the cause remains unclear, and no treatment appears to be necessary. The granulomas can undergo spontaneous resolution without therapy.

CVID is associated with an increased risk for the development of gastrointestinal and lymphoid malignancies, especially non-Hodgkin's lymphomas (Gatti and Good, 1971; Gonzalez Vitale et al., 1982; Kinlin et al., 1985; Cunningham Rundles et al., 1987; Sander et al., 1992; Filipovich et al., 1994; Lai Ping and Mayer, 1997). Lymphomas in these patients are often of B cell origin and extra-nodal in location; they may be associated with Epstein-Barr infection and appear most commonly in females aged 50 or greater (Cunningham Rundles et al., 1991). A major difficulty in the diagnosis of lymphoma is the propensity of these patients to develop benign lymphoproliferative disorders. Up to 30% of patients with CVID will develop either diffuse lymphadenopathy or splenomegaly, or both (Sander et al., 1992). In most of these patients, the lymph node architecture is preserved, which is characteristic of reactive follicular lymphoid hyperplasia. In some patients, however, the lymph node architecture is disrupted by a polymorphic lymphocytic infiltrate.

CVID patients may also develop accumulations of lymphoid tissue in unusual sites (Hermans et al., 1966; Delamarre et al., 1976; De Smet et al., 1976). Up to 20% of patients may develop nodular lymphoid hyperplasia (Hermans et al., 1966; Delamarre et al., 1976; Bastlein et al., 1988). Nodules can also develop in the skin, bone marrow, or other tissues. Although these lesions may contain recognizable follicles, in CVID the nodules can also demonstrate abnormal architecture. This atypical lymphoid hyperplasia may be difficult to differentiate from a malignant lymphoma (Shackleford and McAlister, 1975; Ranchod et al., 1978; Gonzalez Vitale et al., 1982; Sander et al., 1992).

Environmental Factors

IgAD and CVID have been associated with congenital infection with rubella virus, cytomegalovirus, and *Toxoplasma gondii* (Soothill et al., 1966; Lawton et al., 1974) (Table 12–1). The ad-

Table 12–1. Humoral Immunodeficiency States

State or Disorder	Cause
Drug-induced state	Antimalarial agents (Schaffer et al., 1991)
	Captopril (Hammarstrom et al., 1991)
	Carbamazepine (Gilhus et al., 1982; Spickett et al., 1996a)
	Glucocorticoids (Butler and Rossen, 1973)
	Fenclofenac (Farr et al., 1985a)
	Gold salts (So et al., 1984; Guillemin et al., 1987)
	Penicillamine (Proesmans et al., 1976; Williams et al., 1988)
	Phenytoin (Sorrell et al., 1971; Seager et al., 1975; Aarli, 1976a, 1976b)
	Sulphasalazine (Farr et al., 1985b; Leickly and Buckley, 1986)
	Zonisamide (Maeoka et al., 1997)
	Thyroxine (Seager, 1984)[a]
Genetic disorders	Ataxia-telangiectasia
Monogenic diseases	Autosomal forms of SCID
	Hyper IgM immunodeficiency
	Transcobalamin II deficiency and hypogammaglobulinemia
	X-linked agammaglobulinemia
	X-linked agammaglobulinemia with growth hormone deficiency
	X-linked lymphoproliferative disorder (EBV associated)
	X-linked SCID
Chromosomal anomalies	Chromosome 18q-syndrome (Ogata et al., 1977; García Baez et al., 1980)
	Monosomy 22 (Taalman et al., 1987; Yamada et al., 1995)
	Trisomy 8 (Kurtyka et al., 1988)
	Trisomy 21 (Burgio et al., 1980)
Infectious diseases	Congenital rubella (Soothill et al., 1966)
	Congenital infection with CMV (Lawton et al., 1974; Magnan and Vervloet, 1995)
	Congenital infection with *Toxoplasma gondii* (Lawton et al., 1974; Magnan and Vervloet, 1995)
	Epstein-Barr virus (Saulsbury, 1989)
Malignancy	Chronic lymphocytic leukemia
	Immunodeficiency with thymoma
Systemic disorders	Hypercatabolism of immunoglobulins
	Excessive loss of immunoglobulins and lymphocytes

[a]Single report.

ministration of certain drugs has also been linked to a depression in serum immunoglobulin levels. Up to 20% of patients treated with phenytoin for idiopathic epilepsy suffer a mild decrease in serum IgA levels, and a few may develop complete IgA deficiency and CVID (De Gast et al., 1974; Bardana et al., 1983). Medications used for the treatment of rheumatoid arthritis and inflammatory bowel disease can also decrease production of antibody. Recovery of serum immunoglobulin levels can take months or years; persistence of antibody deficiency usually requires continued administration of the drug or continued infection with the virus or parasite.

PATHOPHYSIOLOGY OF DISEASE

IgAD

Although an association between IgAD and certain IgHγ haplotypes on chromosome 14 has been reported (Olsson et al., 1992; Oxelius et al., 1995), molecular and genetic analyses of the Cα gene locus in patients with IgAD have confirmed the integrity of the Cα genes and the basic genetic elements required for isotype switching (Hammarstrom et al., 1985a, 1987). IgAD individuals typically have normal numbers of IgA-bearing B-cell precursors in the peripheral blood (Conley and Cooper, 1981). However, in these cells a decrease in the switch frequency from IgM to IgA has been described (Islam et al., 1994; Wang et al., 1999), as well as a decrease in the expression of both secreted and membrane forms of Ca mRNA (Wang et al., 1999). Examination of the lymphoid organs reveals a profound deficit in IgA-producing plasma cells. Thus, the central feature in the pathogenesis of IgAD appears to be a selective arrest in the differentiation of the mature B cell into a plasma cell (Figure 12–1). The follicular hyperplasia that characterizes the lymphadenopathy seen in this disorder suggests that the ultimate block in differentiation may occur in the latter stages of the response to antigen.

Because the T cell aids the B-cell response to antigen, considerable effort has been devoted to the analysis of T-cell function in IgA-deficient individuals. In a few cases, evidence of selective IgA suppression by T cells has been reported (Waldmann et al., 1976; Atwater and Tomasi, 1978; King et al., 1979). However, when tested for their ability to support the differentiation of IgA B cells from normal individuals, T cells from IgAD patients typically drive development as well as T cells derived from normal individuals (Cassidy et al., 1979; de la Concha et al., 1982; Klemola et al., 1988). It should be noted that these in vitro results measure only the ability of T cells to drive relatively mature B cells to their final stage of differentiation. Thus, subtle dysfunction of the T cell, or of another component of the immune response to antigen, could block B-cell differentiation at an earlier stage than can be assessed with current techniques. Thus, the identities of the cell type, or types, that manifest the primary abnormality remain unclear.

CVID

Although some CVID patients have minimal numbers of circulating B cells (Preudhomme et al., 1973; Farrant et al., 1989), the majority have normal quantitites of IgA, IgG, and IgM-bearing B-cell precursors in the blood (Cooper et al., 1971). These cells appear unable to secrete normal amounts of immunoglobulin when stimulated in vitro by pokeweed mitogen in

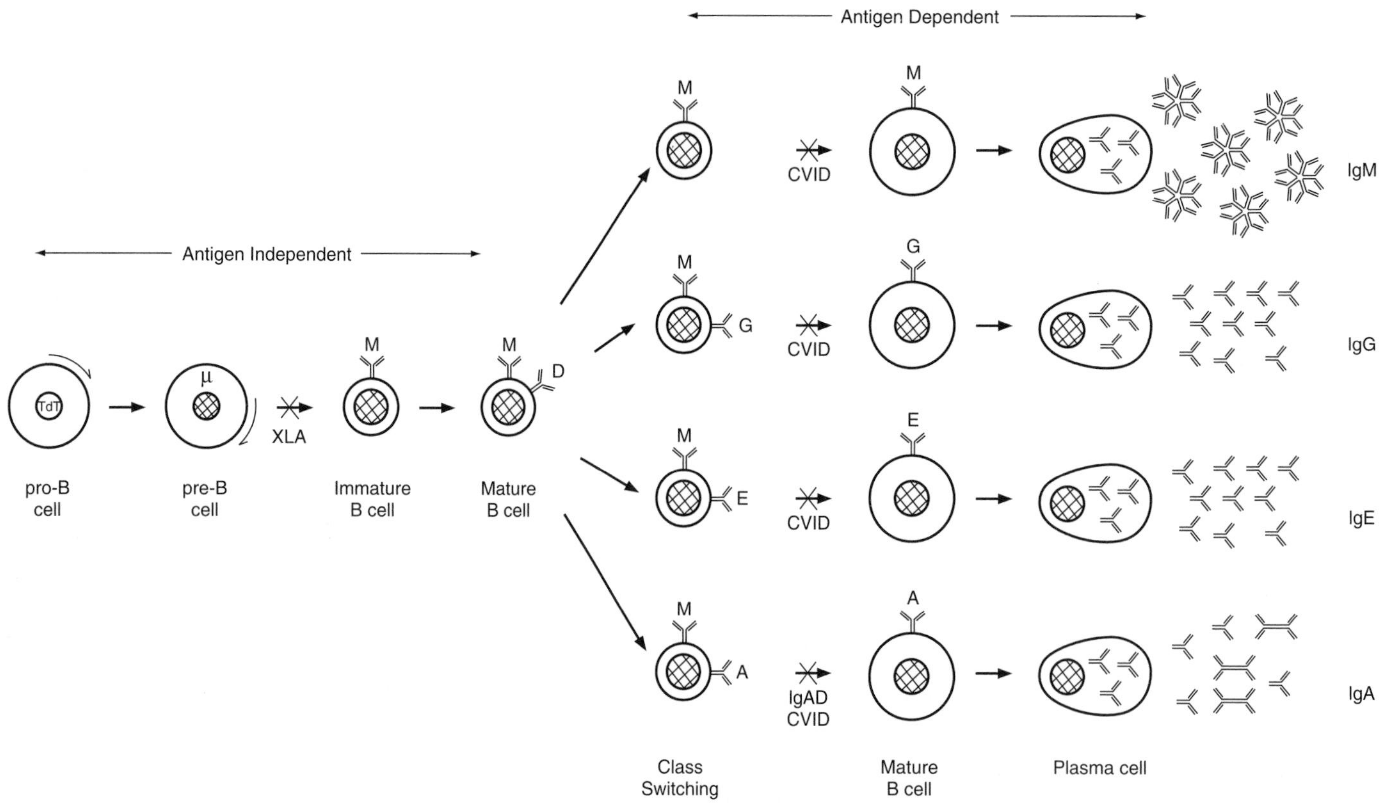

Fig. 12–1. A brief schematic of B-cell development illustrates the major stages traversed by the differentiating B lineage cell. Patients with X-linked agammaglobulinemia (XLA) have difficulty generating B cells. The B cells of patients with IgAD or CVID appear to be able to undergo class switching, but they have difficulty progressing to the plasma cell stage.

the presence of either endogenous T cells or exogenous allogeneic T cells from normal individuals (Choi et al., 1972; Wu et al., 1973; de la Concha et al., 1977; Ashman et al., 1980). To further define the B-cell defect, a number of increasingly sophisticated studies have been performed in which purified B cells from patients with CVID have been exposed to various stimuli in vitro. Stimuli used include T-dependent, T-independent, and T-cell-replacing conditions (Olerup et al., 1992; Saxon et al., 1992; Farrington et al., 1994; Iyer and Joshi, 1995). Attention has also been focused on B-cell stimulation in the presence of exogenous anti-CD40 and IL10 (Nonoyama et al., 1993; Eisenstein et al., 1994). These studies have the potential to allow sorting of CVID into individual disorders defined by mechanisms that underlie the pathogenesis of the defect, rather than the phenotype exhibited by the patient. For example, groups of CVID patients with defective expression of CD40 ligand, a key component of T-cell–B-cell comunication in class-switching (Farrington et al., 1994), reduced expression of CD28 and CD86, which are key components of T-cell—B-cell communication during antigen activation and apoptosis (Denz et al., 2000; Di Renzo et al., 2000), and abnormal expression of CD27, a marker of memory B cells (Brouet et al., 2000) have been identified. However, at present most of these studies have been limited to the descriptive grouping of patients into those in which there is little or no immunoglobulin production after stimulation; those in which there is some immunoglobulin production; and those in which there is near normal production of IgM, IgG, and IgA (De Gast et al., 1980; Saiki et al., 1982; Olerup et al., 1992; Spickett et al., 1992; Scott et al., 1994).

These studies emphasize the variability of the spectrum of immunodeficiency in this collection of patients. The ability of some patients to respond in vitro to various stimuli has raised the possibility that B cells from at least a subset of patients with CVID can be stimulated to respond normally to antigen if the factors necessary to drive B-cell differentiation could be provided (Spickett et al., 1992; Cunningham Rundles et al., 1994). These types of in vitro results measure only the ability of T cells to drive relatively mature B cells to their final stage of differentiation. Thus, although raising the possibility of novel therapeutic options, these studies have yet to elucidate the primary defect in CVID.

Although abnormal immunoglobulin production in CVID manifests as a B-cell defect, a number of studies have demonstrated that both T-cell numbers and function may also be abnormal in some patients (Pandolfi et al., 1993; Boncristiano et al., 2000), and cutaneous anergy is a frequent finding. The potential role of T-cell defects in CVID has been underscored by cases in which patients with CVID recovered serum antibody after infection with either HIV or hepatitis viruses (Osur et al., 1987; Wright et al., 1987; Antoniades et al., 1996; Wen et al., 1996).

A decrease in the relative numbers of $CD4^+$ to $CD8^+$ T cells is the most common laboratory finding in CVID patients who demonstrate alterations in their peripheral-blood T-cell profile (Pandolfi et al., 1993). In part, alteration of the CD4/CD8 ratio can reflect expansion of the $CD8^+$ natural killer cell population (Strannegard et al., 1982) or an increase in the subset of $CD8^+CD57^+$ T cells and NK cells (Baumert et al., 1992). However, in other patients, inversion of the ratio reflects a true decline in the absolute number of $CD4^+$ helper T cells (Pandolfi et al., 1993).

In vitro studies have shown that when T cells from some CVID patients are exposed to various T cell stimuli, they produce less IL-2, IL-4, IL-5, and IFNγ; express lower levels of the IL-2 receptor; and proliferate less well than normal T cells do (Kruger et al., 1984; Sneller and Strober, 1990; Baumert et al., 1992; Vukmanovic et al., 1992; Fischer et al., 1994). Defective recruitment and activation of ZAP-70 has also been observed in a subset of patients (Boncristiano et al., 2000). The contribution of these early blocks in T-cell-receptor-mediated T-cell activation to the pathogenesis of CVID remains unclear. However, these observations have led to novel therapeutic strategies for CVID (Cunningham Rundles et al., 1994).

IgA deficiency can be transmitted into a histocompatible sibling following the transplantation of bone marrow from an IgA-deficient donor into a recipient not previously deficient in IgA production (Hammarstrom et al., 1985b). A CVID patient with an acquired α-thalassemia, neutropenia, and thrombocytopenia proved to be heterozygous for a common allele of glucose-6-phosphate-dehydrogenase (G6PD). Through transcriptional analysis of the G6PD locus of the active X-chromosome in blood cells, it was determined that this female patient had clonal reticulocytes, platelets, granulocytes, and B and T lymphocytes (Belickova et al., 1994). These observations suggest that in some cases IgAD and CVID may result from an insult at the stem-cell level itself.

MOLECULAR GENETICS OF IGAD/CVID

Susceptiblity Gene for IgAD/CVID

A large array of genes that play important roles in the control of the immune response are located in the major histocompatibility complex (MHC) locus on chromosome 6 (Campbell and Trowsdale, 1997) (Fig. 12–2). There is a long history of an association between IgAD and some class I and class II alleles (Lewkonia et al., 1976; Ambrus et al., 1977; Hammarstrom et al., 1985b; Strothman et al., 1986; Vorechovsky et al., 1999). Among our clinic population in the Southeastern United States, for example, we have found that the majority of IgAD and CVID patients have one of two extended MHC haplotypes (Volanakis et al., 1992), which were initially defined by use polymorphic markers for 11 genes or their products between the HLA-DQB1 and the HLA-A genes (Fig. 12–2). In this population, haplotype I is characterized by the following alleles: HLA-DQB1*0201, HLA-DR3, C4B-Sf, C4A-0, G11–15, Bf-0.4, C2-a, HSP-7.5, TNFα-a2b3, HLA-B8, or HLA-A1; haplotype 2 includes all or a portion of HLA-DQB1*0201, HLA-DR7, C4B-S, C4A-L, G11–4.5, Bf-0.6, C2-b, HSP-9, TNFα-a7b4 or a11b4, HLA-B44, and HLA-A29. The combined results of three previous studies indicate prevalence of immunodeficiency of approximately one in eight in individuals randomly selected for homozygosity for haplotype 1 (Wilton et al., 1985; Volanakis et al., 1992; Alper et al., 2000).

A report from western Australia (French and Dawkins, 1990) provided the first indication that IgAD might be associated with a gene (or genes) located within the MHC class III cluster in linkage disequilibrium with these class I and/or class II alleles. The class III MHC region occupies about 1,100 kb of DNA between the class I and the class II gene clusters (Fig. 12–2) and contains at least 70 known genes (Campbell and Trowsdale, 1997). Many of these class III genes are expressed by cells of the lymphoid, myeloid, and monocyte lineages and have either a demonstrated or a potential role in innate or adaptive immune responses. Included are the genes encoding the complement pro-

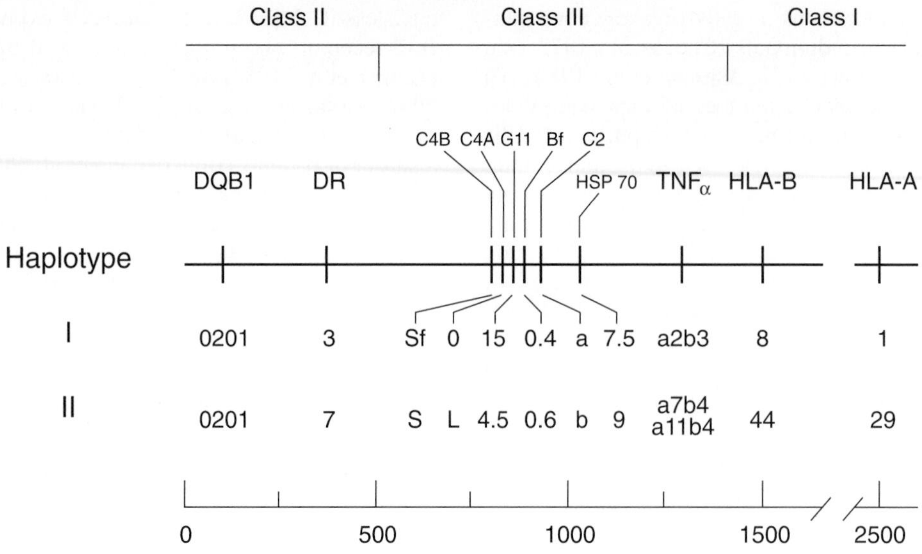

Fig. 12–2. Map of the MHC locus on chromosome 6 with the approximate location of 11 markers used to identify MHC haplotypes 1 and 2. Approximately two-thirds of patients with CVID or IgAD in our clinic population have inherited at least a portion of one of these two extended haplotypes.

teins C4A, C4B, C2, and factor B; the major heat-shock protein, HSP70; and the tumor necrosis factors α (TNFα) and β (TNFβ). The function of the products of most of the genes in the region is currently unknown.

The tight linkage disequilibrium between the class I, class II, and class III genes of both haplotypes I and II makes it difficult to determine which of these regions contains the gene or genes that provide susceptiblity for IgAD and CVID. There is a DR3$^+$ haplotype that is commonly found in individuals of Sardinian origin that is typically accompanied by HLA-B18 (Contu et al., 1992; Cucca et al., 1997). Finer analysis of the class III region indicated that this "Sardinian" haplotype was the product of an ancestral crossover event between HLA-DR and the C4 region of class III. Analysis of a large number of individuals homozygous for this Sardinian haplotype failed to reveal evidence of IgAD. Among our clinic population, two patients were identified who had all seven polymorphic markers tested in the class III region, including C4B and TNF, but lacked several of the class I and class II alleles characteristic of haplotype I (Volanakis et al., 1992). One individual had HLA-B8 but lacked HLA-DR3 and HLA-A1. The second had an even smaller fragment of haplotype 1 and lacked not only HLA-DR3 and HLA-A1 but also HLA-B8. Together, these studies suggested that the boundaries for the susceptibility locus for haplotype 1 lay between TNF and HLA-B on the telomeric class I end of the MHC, and between C4B and DR on the centromeric class II end, ruling out the class II region as the locus for susceptibility. Analysis of a large cohort of CVID patients afflicted with granulomas also demonstrated an association of polymorphisms in the TNF region with clinical disease (Mullighan et al., 1997).

Within our clinic population, a large family with eight affected members was identified, and family members underwent analysis of their extended MHC haplotypes and serum immunoglobulins (Schroeder et al., 1998). In this family, designated S12, 41 (56%) of 73 relatives by common descent were heterozygous and 9 (12%) were homozygous for a fragment or

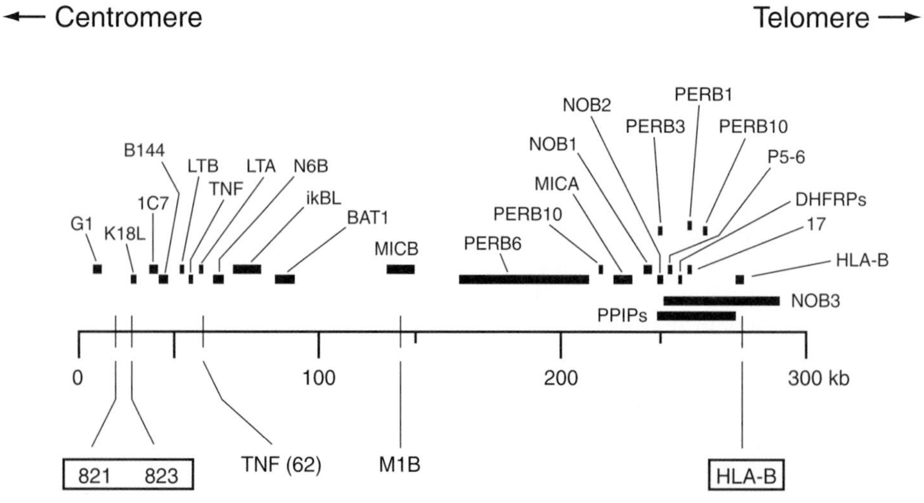

Fig. 12–3. A susceptibility locus for IgAD/CVID appears to lie within an interval delimited by microsatellite markers D821/D823 toward the class II terminus and HLA-B at the class I terminus of the MHC. Shown are the locations of 21 genes that have been mapped to this interval. From Campbell and Trowsdale (1997) and Schroeder et al. (1998) with permission.

the entire extended MHC in haplotype I. The remarkable prevalence of haplotype 1 proved to be due to the marital introduction into the family of 11 different copies of the haplotype, 8 sharing 20 identical genotype markers between HLA-DR3 and HLA-B8, and 3 that contained fragments of haplotype 1. In the analysis of the eight immunodeficient individuals and their unaffected relatives, crossover events suggest that the region between the class III markers D821/D823 and HLA-B8 contains a susceptibility locus for IgAD/CVID (Figure 12–3). This region contains 21 known genes, including TNFα and lymphotoxins α and β. Ongoing studies of additional families support the view that inheritance at this portion of the class III region derived from either haplotype I or II appears to be necessary for the development of IgAD/CVID in most cases of familial IgAD/CVID. It should be noted, however, that this view remains controversial, and other mapping studies place the class III locus for selective IgAD alone closer in proximity to class II than to class I (Vorechovsky et al., 2000).

Analysis of the patterns of inheritance of immunodeficiency among our clinic population suggests that neither IgAD nor CVID is attributable solely to a simple Mendelian trait. In the general population, individuals homozygous for the susceptibility locus are at high risk (7 of 54, or 13%) for immunodeficiency. In the study family of family S12 (Schroeder et al., 1998), the prevalence of immunodeficiency for haplotype 1 heterozygous individuals (4 of 41, or 10%) was equivalent to the risk for haplotype 1 homozygous individuals selected at random from the general population (Wilton et al., 1985; Volanakis et al., 1992; Kruskall et al., 1993). The risk for family members who are homozygous (four of nine, or 44%) was four-fold greater than homozygous individuals in the general population or heterozygous family members. Together, these data suggest an additive effect of the susceptibility locus. The increased prevalence of disease in family members, when compared with members of the general population, also suggests that factors in addition to MHC haplotype are contributing to immunodeficiency. Male-to-male transmission of immunodeficiency is well documented in this family; thus a second genetic factor could be transmitted as an autosomal dominant trait that requires the presence of the MHC susceptibility locus for development of the disease. Environmental factors could also be the source of the increased risk, and this view is supported by the fluctuations in serum immunoglobulins observed in affected individuals.

Role for Modifying Genes in IgAD/CVID

Mannose-binding lection (MBL) is an important component of the innate immune response. MBL alleles linked with low production of MBL are associated with an increased risk of infection, especially when adaptive immunity is already compromised. An association between low-production MBL alleles and infection in IgAD has yet to be demonstrated (Aittoniemi et al., 1999), but in CVID an association between these alleles and early age of disease onset has been reported (Mullighan et al., 2000).

CLINICAL APPLICATION AND RISK ASSESSMENT OF GENETIC INFORMATION

Diagnosis

It can be difficult to recognize IgAD and CVID in infants due to the physiologic delay in the acquisition of adult serum levels. Diagnosis of a humoral immunodeficiency is best achieved through a systematic evaluation of the patient's immunocompetence. The workup should begin with simple screening procedures, followed by appropriate tests of immune function. Due to the interdependence of the various components of the immune system, evaluation should include analysis of the humoral response (B-cell system), the cellular immune system (T cells), and agents that provide nonspecific resistance to infection (PMN's, complement, etc.).

History

Emphasis should be placed on the history of infections, including the age of onset of the patient's complaints, the frequency with which the infections occur, the location of the infections (e.g., the sinuses, the upper respiratory tract, the lungs, the gut, and the skin), the types of organisms involved (e.g., candida, herpes, *H. influenzae*, mycoplasmas, *G. lamblia*), and the response to therapy. In general, patients with B-cell deficiency will have an increased incidence of bacterial sinopulmonary infections; patients with T-cell defects and impaired cell-mediated immunity will experience recurrent viral, fungal, or protozoal infections; and patients with neutrophil disorders are susceptible to infections cause by high-grade bacterial pathogens, often outside mucosal sites. A history of previous immunization is useful, particularly a history of complications after vaccination with live organisms or a history of repeated infections in spite of vaccination with the appropriate vaccine. A history of neurologic abnormalities raises the possibility of therapy with phenytoin (an agent that can depress immunoglobulin production). A history of bleeding raises the possibility that the patient is suffering from idiopathic thrombocytopenic purpura (which is frequently found in patients with Wiskott-Aldrich syndrome and can be found in CVID). A history of autoimmune phenomena (e.g., autoimmune thyroiditis, SLE, skin rash, pernicious anemia) suggests the presence of HLA haplotypes that are also linked to IgAD and CVID. IgAD patients with anti-IgA antibodies in their serum may suffer anaphylaxis after transfusion with blood products that contain IgA. A history of surgical removal of the spleen, tonsils, or other lymphoid tissues, or a history of an unexplained lymphoproliferative process or malignancy, should be fully explored.

Physical Examination and Routine Laboratory and X-ray Studies

A complete physical examination should be performed with special emphasis on several important areas. The tympanic membranes should be inspected for evidence of acute or chronic otitis media, providing documentation for a history of recurrent infection. Tonsillar tissue is usually present in patients with common variable immunodeficiency, whereas patients lacking B cells due to a severe combined immunodeficiency (SCID) or to X-linked agammaglobulinemia will also lack tonsils. Patients with IgAD or CVID often have prominent peripheral and central lymphoid hyperplasia; thus the neck, axilla, and inguinal regions should be palpated for lymphadenopathy and the size of the spleen and liver should be evaluated. Auscultation of the chest may reveal wheezing, rales, or rhonchi, which is compatible with a history of chronic pulmonary disease. Congenital abnormalities of the face, neck, chest, limbs, heart, and other organs and neurologic abnormalities or behavioral disorders could suggest a multisystem abnormality such as a chromosomal disorder (e.g., $18q^-$ syndrome and DiGeorge syndrome). Examination of the skin may reveal scarring from previous viral or bacterial infections or may demonstrate eczema, petechiae, and purpura. Patients with abnormal immunoglobulin metabolism may demonstrate proteinuria on urinalysis, hypoalbuminemia and hypogammaglobulinemia, or dyscrasias of other components of the hematopoietic system, including thrombocytopenia, anemia, and leukopenia. X-rays of the chest should be evaluated for the thymic shadow, which is absent in DiGeorge syndrome and SCID and is potentially enlarged in patients with a thymoma. Silent and asymptomatic progression of pulmonary changes may occur in some patients, despite an adequate regimen of intravenous immunoglobulin-replacement therapy. For these patients, high-resolution computed tomography appears to be the method of choice for establishing and monitoring pulmonary changes (Kainulainen et al., 1999b).

Laboratory Evaluation of the Humoral Immune Response

Preliminary screening tests include quantitation of serum immunoglobulin levels, including IgG subclasses; a complete blood count with differential; and determination of serum isohemagglutinins. If these studies are normal, it is very unlikely that the patient is suffering from a humoral immune deficiency. A variety of methods are available for quantitation of serum immunoglobulins, but the most common are agarose gel electrophoresis and nephelometry. It is important to remember that the concentration of serum immunoglobulin in the sera of normal individuals increases with age and environment. Although no rigid values for the diagnosis of hypogammaglobulinemia exist, patients with a serum IgG of less than 500 mg/dl should be treated with replacement immunoglobulin therapy.

Although serum immunoglobulin levels are useful to detect gross abnormalities in immunoglobulin production, even normal immunoglobulin levels are not a guarantee that antibodies of the appropriate specificity are being generated (Williams, 1966). Isohemagglutinins are naturally occurring antibodies to the polysaccharides that distinguish group A and group B red blood cells. Due to natural immunization with enteric bacteria that cross-react with red cell antigens, all normal individuals over the age of three express titers greater than 1:8 against the A or B blood types (except, of course, for individuals who are of the AB blood type). Determination of anti-hemagglutinin levels is a routine procedure in hospital blood banks, and is thus an inexpensive screening test.

If these screening tests are abnormal, more sophisticated studies can be undertaken. At a minimum, assessment of the number of B cells (sIgM$^+$, or CD19$^+$), T cells (CD3$^+$), and T-cell subsets (CD4$^+$ and CD8$^+$) should be assessed through fluorescence-activated cell-sorting (FACS) analysis of the mononuclear cells present in the peripheral blood. Cell-mediated immunity can be assessed through subdermal injection with purified protein derivative (PPD) and appropriate controls (e.g., trichophyton, mumps, and candida). Finally, complement levels (CH50, C3, C4) should be determined to document adequate levels of mediators of innate resistance.

For those patients with borderline immunoglobulin levels, a normal profile of peripheral blood lymphocytes, and a history of recurrent infection, the best test of the patient's ability to mount a normal humoral response is to challenge his or her immune system with antigen. The patient should be tested with both T-cell-dependent (e.g., tetanus toxoid) and T-cell-unconjugated independent (e.g., pneumococcal polysaccharide) antigens (Mosier and Subbarrao, 1982). Postimmunization titers that exceed 800 ng antibody per ml are also considered normal (Zora et al., 1993), and a normal response requires a 4-fold increase in titer against the antigen in question. Almost all normal individuals develop a healthy response to pneumococcal polysaccharide type 3 and most respond to type 7, while a large proportion fail to develop "protective" titers to types 9 and 14. Hence, an inability to respond to type 7 or type 3 strongly suggests that the patient has a functional immunedeficiency (Herrod, 1993). Due to day-to-day variability in the measurement of antibody titers, it is advisable to submit matched sets of pre- and post-vaccination serum when the samples are sent to outside reference labs.

Counseling

A significant subset of young children diagnosed with partial IgA deficiency achieve normal serum levels by the second decade of life (Buckley, 1975; Joller et al., 1981; Blum et al., 1982; Plebani et al., 1986). Progression from IgAD to CVID may be a common pathway of disease acquisition, thus children who carry the diagnosis of IgAD should be re-tested during the teenage years, and young adults with a positive family history of immunodeficiency and recurrent sinopulmonary infection may require re-evaluation in spite of having demonstrated normal serum immunoglobulin levels earlier in life (Johnson et al., 1997).

The risk of immunodeficiency among the first-degree relatives of patients with asymptomatic IgAD is unknown. Among the CVID patients in our clinic who have inherited either all or a portion of the HLA-DR3, -B8, -A1 haplotype, the risk of IgAD and CVID appears to approach 40% in their children, but only 5% in their siblings (Schroeder, unpublished results). Because the manifestations of the disease can change over time, we currently recommend evaluation of the children of CVID probands at ages 5 and 10 and as young adults, or whenever there is evidence of repeated infection, autoimmunity, or lymphoid malignancies.

Therapy

IgAD

Most patients with IgAD are asymptomatic and do not require therapy. Due to the potential risk for anaphylaxis after exposure to exogenous IgA (Vyas et al., 1975; Branigan et al., 1983), patients with a complete absence of IgA should wear Medic Alert bracelets in case of accident or injury. They should only receive blood products from other IgA-deficient individuals or packed red blood cells from which the plasma has been removed by repeated washes (Vyas et al., 1975; Branigan et al., 1983).

Patients who experience recurrent upper respiratory infection should be treated with agents effective against encapsulated organisms such as *H. influenzae* and *S. pneumoniae*. Some patients with refractory sinusitis or otitis media benefit from continuous prophylactic therapy. Patients suffering from chronic diarrhea often are infested with *G. lamblia*, and because giardiasis may be difficult to document, patients may benefit from empiric therapy with metronidazole.

IgA-deficient patients can produce IgG or IgE anti-IgA antibodies (Vyas et al., 1975), placing them at risk for adverse reactions after transfusion with blood products or plasma from normal donors, and from some preparations of intramuscular or intravenous gammaglobulin therapy which, of course, contain IgA (Fudenberg et al., 1968; Vyas and Fudenberg, 1969; Schmidt et al., 1969). In one study, no difference was seen in the rate of adverse reactions between patients with or without detectable anti-IgA titers (Vyas et al., 1975); however, the severity of the reaction may differ. Patients with high anti-IgA levels (greater than 1:1,000) typically have potent antibodies directed against all IgAs. These patients are at risk for severe anaphylaxis. Patients with low anti-IgA antibody titers (less than 1:256) are often multiparous or multitransfused patients; they rarely demonstrate severe anaphylaxis after infusion with plasma or blood products but do present with hives and rashes. Serum complement typically falls as a result of this type of reaction. Transfusion reactions can be prevented through the use of blood products from other IgA-deficient individuals or through use of washed, packed red blood cells.

CVID

Therapy in CVID begins with the aggressive treatment of ongoing infections and the institution of prophylactic measures to prevent or ameliorate future infection. Patients with CVID tend to chronically harbor subclinical viral and bacterial infections (Kainulainen et al., 1999a). Thus, even patients that appear to be asymptomatic may benefit from empiric therapy with agents effective against encapsulated organisms such as *H. influenzae* and *S. pneumoniae* (Sneller et al., 1993). Patients with recurrent pneumonia and evidence of bronchiectasis may be infected with *Pseudomonas*, *S. aureus*, or other aggressive organisms, thus every effort should be made to identify the inciting agent. The course of treatment for immunodeficient patients is often prolonged, and intravenous administration of antibiotics may be required.

Immunoglobulin Therapy. The most effective therapy for hypogammaglobulinemic patients is the parenteral administration of donor immunoglobulin. Both historically and individually, there is a striking relationship between the quantity of immunoglobulin given and the patient's protection from infection and its sequelae. The initial recommendation from the World Health Organization called for the intramuscular administration of 100 mg/kg of gammaglobulin every 3 to 4 weeks. This dose increases the serum IgG level by 100 to 150 mg/dl, which is sufficient to reduce the likelihood of catastrophic infection (Janeway and Rosen, 1966). The introduction of intravenous preparations allowed for the administration of higher doses. Serum IgG levels typically increase by approximately 250 mg/dl for each 100 mg/kg infused intravenously (Sneller et al., 1993). A number of studies have demonstrated a steadily decreasing incidence of infection with increasing rates of intravenous gammaglobulin administration (up to 600 mg/kg) (Ammann et al., 1982; Cunningham Rundles et al., 1984; Roifman et al., 1985; Roifman and Gelfand, 1988; Buckley and Schiff, 1991). At higher doses, even patients with bronchiectasis demonstrate improvement in pulmonary function (Roifman et al., 1985). Currently, most clinical immunologists treat their patients with 400 mg/kg of intravenous gammaglobulin (1990). At this dose, the half-life for IgG and IgG subclasses is 30 to 40 days (Fischer et al., 1988). After reaching steady state levels approximately 6 months after starting therapy, patients should have achieved serum IgG levels of 500 mg/dl or greater 3 to 4 weeks after their last infusion. However, each patient demonstrates their own individual response to therapy, experiencing dramatic differences in the frequency and severity of infections with moderate changes in the dose of intravenous gammaglobulin. Moreover, patients suffering from serious infection often benefit from booster doses of intravenous gammaglobulin. Ultimately, dosage with intravenous immunoglobulin must be individualized based on the response of the patient. If the patient demonstrates no evidence of adverse reactions, infusions can be performed at home under appropriate supervision.

There are a number of different preparations of intravenous immunoglobulin licensed for use in the United States (Sneller et al., 1993). They differ by donor pool, by method of preparation, by carrier, and by IgA level. Although no patient has developed AIDS as a result of intravenous administration of immunoglobulin, hepatitis has been reported (Bjorkander et al., 1988; Schneider and Geha, 1994). Part of the difficulty lies in the consequences of screening donors for the presence of serum antibodies against infectious agents. Removing donors with past evidence of infection reduces the likelihood of transmission of that agent, while simultaneously eliminating neutralizing antibodies against that agent from the preparation. This leaves the patient somewhat defenseless against infection from that organism. A number of new preparations are currently undergoing testing, and the physician's armamentarium is likely to change over the next several years.

The potential for severe adverse reactions requires administration under the supervision of trained personnel. Initial administration should be performed in a hospital or clinic setting. When intravenous immunoglobulin is given slowly, most patients tolerate it well. The most frequent adverse reactions are nonanaphylactic and characterized by myalgias, back pain, abdominal pain, nausea, vomiting, chills, or fever (Sneller et al., 1993). Symptoms usually begin within the first 30 minutes of therapy and are not associated with dyspnea or hypotension. These symptoms can often be alleviated or prevented by reducing the rate of administration, pretreating with an antihistamine or a corticosteroid, or changing the preparation of intravenous gammaglobulin. Although most patients report mild euphoria after administration, some complain of headaches or fatigue that can last for several days. This type of reaction may occur in newly treated patients or in patients who are suffering from an active infection. In these cases, it can be beneficial to interrupt the infusion until the symptoms subside and then reinstitute therapy at a slower rate. Pretreatment with antihistamines or corticosteroids can also be helpful (Johansson et al., 1988).

Paradoxically, some patients with CVID can sustain severe anaphylaxis when they are given intravenous gammaglobulin or other blood products that contain serum or plasma (Benedict et al., 1977). These patients typically possess anti-IgA antibodies, including IgE anti-A antibodies (Ropars et al., 1979; Burks et al., 1986). Indeed, severe anaphylaxis characterized by flushing, urticaria, angioedema, dyspnea, anxiety, emesis, cyanosis, hypotension, and syncope (Buckley, 1988) can occur within 2 minutes after intravenous administration of less than 1 mg of IgA, which is the level present in less than 0.5 ml of human plasma (Benedict et al., 1977). One of the currently available preparations has been sufficiently depleted of IgA during manufacturing to allow its use in such patients (Buckley and Schiff, 1991). It should be noted, however, that the IgA level may vary by lot (R. Buckley, personal communication). For patients with a history of severe adverse reactions, it is advisable to try lots with the lowest IgA possible and to test the patient with the different lots in an intensive-care unit. Once having identified a lot that can be tolerated, the patient may receive therapy under more relaxed conditions.

Serum immunoglobulin concentrations in patients with CVID may change over time (Seligmann et al., 1991; Johnson et al., 1997), with some patients regaining normal serum IgG levels and no longer requiring immunoglobulin therapy. Careful review of the clinical history of these patients may reveal evidence of exposure to pharmacologic agents associated with the development of hypogammaglobulinemia (e.g., phenytoin). However, the majority of patients require intravenous gammaglobulin therapy for life.

Additional Supportive Therapy. Although IgG may be replaced, at present IgM and IgA cannot be provided to the patient. The absence of these multimeric proteins may help explain why even patients on high-dose replacement therapy may continue to suffer from chronic sinusitis or diarrhea. In such cases, patients often benefit from continued prophylactic therapy with antibiotics that are effective against encapsulated bacteria. Patients with CVID also are at risk from *G. lamblia*, as well as other enteric pathogens. Patients with chronic diarrhea often respond to treatment with empiric antibiotic therapy. Some patients develop hypogammaglobulinemic sprue or celiac disease, gluten-sensitive enteropathy, or lactose intolerance. These conditions may improve with avoidance of the inciting agent (Sperber and Mayer, 1988). Others develop a malabsorption syndrome that can lead to hypoalbuminemia, hypocalcemia (due to malabsorption of vitamin D), and decreased levels of vitamin A and carotene (Sneller et al., 1993). The cause of diarrhea and malabsorption in this latter patient subset remains unclear, and treatment is limited to supportive measures, with vitamin and mineral replacement as indicated.

Patients with bronchiectasis should be treated aggressively with intravenous gammaglobulin. In severe cases, aggressive pulmonary toilet will benefit the patient, including bronchodilator therapy, position, and postural drainage, or other physical therapies. The use of corticosteroids should be avoided.

Hypersplenism. Splenomegaly is common in untreated patients with CVID. Hypersplenism in most patients responds to aggressive therapy with antibiotics and intravenous immunoglobulin. The presumption is that the hypersplenism is secondary to reactive hyperplasia of lymphoid follicles within the spleen attempting to respond to infection (Prasad et al., 1957). However, development of esophageal varices, the other hematologic manifestations of hypersplenism (refractory thrombocytopenia, anemia, neutropenia, and lymphopenia), may require splenectomy as the therapy of last resort. The outcome for most such patients has been good (Cunningham-Rundles and Bodian, 1999), with resolution of symptoms. However, the risk of infection from encapsulated organisms increases in such patients, and they should be placed on penicillin prophylaxis (or an equivalent) (Lanzavecchia et al., 1978; Cunningham-Rundles and Bodian, 1999).

Immunodeficiency and Pregnancy. IgA-deficient mothers fail to secrete IgA in their colostrum (Barros et al., 1985). Although colostral IgM levels may be elevated in an attempt to compensate for the lack of maternal IgA, the newborn remains relatively unprotected against intestinal pathogens. Of greater concern are the children of mothers with untreated CVID who are born in a state of humoral immunodeficiency and are at great risk for life-threatening sinopulmonary infection (Hausser and Buriot, 1982; Smith and Hammarstrom, 1985; Madsen et al., 1986). To compensate for the loss of IgG across the placenta and to provide the infant with the passive immunity it will require, the level of intravenous gammaglobulin infusion should be increased to 600 mg/kg during the third trimester of pregnancy. In treated cases, the outcome of pregnancy has been favorable.

Malignancy. Although patients with CVID and, to a lesser extent, IgAD are at increased risk for developing a life-threatening lymphoproliferative disorders (Filipovich et al., 1994), it is essential to distinguish between a frank malignancy and the benign lymphoproliferative disorders that are so common in this patient population. For those patients unfortunate enough to develop a true lymphoid malignancy, the most common disorder is non-Hodgkin's lymphoma, specifically a B-lineage diffuse large-cell lymphoma (DLCL) lymphoma. These tumors typically harbor mutations in BCL-6 (Ariatti et al., 2000), which is a marker of transit through the germinal center and may reflect the prolonged, abortive B-cell stimulation that infected patients with this disease undergo. In these patients, the response to combination chemotherapy and/or radiation therapy protocols has been generally disappointing. Poor outcomes have been attributed to fewer tumor responses, excess toxicity from cancer therapy, and the exceptionally high risk of fatal infections in already immunodeficient patients. While complete and sustained remissions from non-Hodgkin's lymphomas have been achieved, the morbidity associated with cancer therapy has been higher than that seen in nonimmunodeficient patients. Epstein-Barr virus (EBV) has been associated with the development of B-cell lymphoproliferative disorders in these patients. There are no controlled trials regarding prophylactic therapy with acyclovir for patients with CVID or IgAD; however, the response in posttransplant patients suffering from EBV-associated lymphoproliferative disorders has been disappointing. Clinical remissions have been seen in a limited number of patients treated with α-interferon and weekly intravenous gammaglobulin infusions, but the efficacy of these treatments remains unclear (Filipovich et al., 1994).

Patients and their family members should be informed of the increased risk of gastrointestinal carcinomas in CVID and IgAD. Close attention should be paid to symptoms referable to the GI tract, and regular cancer screening should be encouraged.

Future Directions

Recent studies have demonstrated an increase in the level of endogenous serum antibody to antigenic challenge after stimulation with exogenous cytokines or other stimulators of the immune response (Cunningham Rundles et al., 1994). Serum TNFα production is noted to be high in CVID (Smith and Skelton, 2001), perhaps due to the association with the high-producing TNF alleles associated with the HLA-DR3, -B8, -A1 haplotype. Preliminary anecdotal reports suggest that use of anti-TNF reagents may ameliorate manifestations such as scarcoidal granulomas and hypogammaglobulinemic celiac disease. At present, however, such therapies are very much at the investigational stage. It is to be hoped that ongoing research into the genetics and biology of these intriguing diseases may yield new forms of therapy in the near future that may correct the deficit at its source and obviate the need for intravenous gammaglobulin infusions.

ACKNOWLEDGMENTS

The author thanks Drs. R. Duncan Campbell, Max D. Cooper, Sergei Nedospasov, and John E. Volanakis for their advice and participation in numerous collaborative studies of IgAD and CVID. This work was supported, in part, by NIH grant nos. AI33621, HD36292, and RR00032.

REFERENCES

Aarli JA: Changes in serum immunoglobulin levels during phenytoin treatment of epilepsy. Acta Neurol Scand 1976a; 54:423–430.

Aarli JA: Drug-induced IgA deficiency in epileptic patients. Arch Neurol 1976b; 33:296–299.

Aittoniemi J, Koskinen S, Laippala P, Laine S, Miettinen A: The significance of IgG subclasses and mannan-binding lectin (MBL) for susceptibility to infection in apparently healthy adults with IgA deficiency. Clin Exp Immunol 1999; 116:505–508.

Alper CA, Marcus-Bagley D, Awdeh Z, Kruskall MS, Eisenbarth GS, Brink, SJ, Katz AJ, Stein R, Bing DH, Yunis EJ, Schur PH: Prospective analysis suggests susceptibility genes for deficiencies of IgA and several other immunoglobulins on the [HLA-B8, SC01, DR3] conserved extended haplotype. Tissue Antigens 2000; 56:207–216.

Amarin ZO, Grant KA: Hypogammaglobulinemia during pregnancy in identical twin sisters. Int J Gynaecol Obstet 1982; 20:471–473.

Ambrus M, Hernadi E, Bajtai G: Prevalence of HLA-A1 and HLA-B8 antigens in selective IgA deficiency. Clin Immunol Immunopathol 1977; 7:311–314.

Amin N: Giardiasis: a common cause of diarrheal disease. Postgrad Med 1979; 66:151–156,158.

Ammann AJ, Ashman RF, Buckley RH, Hardie WR, Krantmann HJ, Nelson J, Ochs H, Stiehm ER, Tiller T, Wara DW, Wedgewood RW: Use of intravenous gamma globulin in antibody immunodeficiency: results of a multi-center controlled trial. Clin Immunol Immunopathol 1982; 22:60–67.

Ammann AJ, Hong R: Selective IgA deficiency: presentation of 30 cases and a review of the literature. Medicine 1971; 50:223–236.

Andre C, Andre F, Fargier C: Distribution of IgA 1 and IgA 2 plasma cells in various normal human tissues and in the jejunum of plasma IgA-deficient patients. Clin Exp Immunol 1978; 33:327–331.

Antoniades K, Hatzistilianou M, Pitsavas G, Agouridaki C, Athanassiadou F: Co-existence of Dubowitz and hyper-IgE syndromes: a case report. Eur J Pediatr 1996; 155:390–392.

Ariatti C, Vivenza D, Capello D, Migliazza A, Parvis G, Fassone L, Buonaiuto D, Savinelli F, Rossi D, Saglio G, Gaidano G: Common-variable immunodeficiency-related lymphomas associate with mutations and rearrangements of BCL-6: pathogenetic and histogenetic implications. Hum Pathol 2000; 31:871–873.

Asherson GL: Late-onset hypogammaglobulinemia. In: Asherson GL, Webster AD (eds). Diagnosis and Treatment of Immunodeficiency. London: Blackwell Scientific, 1980:37–60.

Ashman RF, Saxon A, Stevens RH: Profile of multiple lymphocyte functional defects in acquired hypogammaglobulinemia, derived from in vitro cell recombination analysis. J Allergy Clin Immunol 1980; 65:242–256.

Ashman RF, White RH, Wiesenhutter C, Cantor Y, Lasarow E, Liebling M, Talal N: Panhypogammaglobulinemia in systemic lupus erythematosus: in vitro demonstration of multiple cellular defects. J Allergy Clin Immunol 1982; 70:465–473.

Atwater JS, Tomasi TB, Jr.: Suppressor cells and IgA deficiency. Clin Immunol Immunopathol 1978; 9:379–384.

Aucouturier P, Lacombe C, Bremard C, Lebranchu Y, Seligmann M, Griscelli C, Preudhomme JL: Serum IgG subclass levels in patients with primary immunodeficiency syndromes or abnormal susceptibility to infections. Clin Immunol Immunopathol 1989; 51:22–37.

Bachman R: Studies on the serum γ_A-globulin level: III. The frequency of a-γ_A-globulinemia. Scand J Clin Lab Invest 1965; 17:316.

Bardana EJ, Gabourel JD, Davies GH, Craig S: Effects of phenytoin on man's immunity: evaluation of changes in serum immunoglobulins, complement, and antinuclear antibody. Am J Med 1983; 74:289–296.

Barros MD, Porto MH, Leser PG, Grumach AS, Carneiro Sampaio MM: Study of colostrum of a patient with selective IgA deficiency. Allergol Immunopathol (Madr.) 1985; 13:331–334.

Bastlein C, Burlefinger R, Holzberg E, Voeth C, Garbrecht M, Ottenjann R: Common variable immunodeficiency syndrome and nodular lymphoid hyperplasia in the small intestine. Endoscopy 1988; 20:272–275.

Baumert E, Wolff-Vorbeck G, Schlesier M, Peter HH: Immunophenotypical alterations in a subset of patients with common variable immunodeficiency (CVID). Clin Exp Immunol 1992; 90:25–30.

Belickova M, Schroeder HW, Jr., Guan YL, Brierre J, Berney S, Cooper MD, Prchal JT: Clonal hematopoiesis and acquired thalassemia in common variable immunodeficiency. Mol Med 1994; 1:56–61.

Benedict AA, Abplanalp HA, Pollard LW, Tam LQ: Inherited immunodeficiency in chickens: a model for common variable hypogammaglobulinemia in man? Adv Exp Med Biol 1977; 88P:197–205.

Bjorkander J, Cunningham Rundles C, Lundin P, Olsson R, Soderstrom R, Hanson LA: Intravenous immunoglobulin prophylaxis causing liver damage in 16 of 77 patients with hypogammaglobulinemia or IgG subclass deficiency. Am J Med 1988; 84:107–111.

Blum PM, Hong R, Stiehm ER: Spontaneous recovery of selective IgA deficiency: additional case reports and a review. Clin Pediatr 1982; 21:77–80.

Bonagura VR, Cunningham Rundles S, Edwards BL, Ilowite NT, Wedgwood JF, Valacer DJ: Common variable hypogammaglobulinemia, recurrent *Pneumocystis carinii* pneumonia on intravenous gamma-globulin therapy, and natural killer deficiency. Clin Immunol Immunopathol 1989; 51:216–231.

Boncristiano M, Majolini MB, D'Elios MM, Pacini S, Valensin S, Ulivieri, C, Amedei A, Falini B, Del Prete G, Telford JL, Baldari CT: Defective recruitment and activation of ZAP-70 in common variable immunodeficiency patients with T cell defects. Eur J Immunol 2000; 30:2632–2638.

Borriello SP, Reed PJ, Dolby JM, Barclay FE, Webster AD: Microbial and metabolic profile of achlorhydric stomach: comparison of pernicious anaemia and hypogammaglobulinaemia. J Clin Pathol 1985; 38:946–953.

Brandtzaeg P, Fjellander I, Gjeruldsen ST: Immunoglobulin M: local synthesis and selective secretion in patients with immunoglobulin A deficiency. Science 1968; 160:789–791.

Branigan EF, Stevenson MM, Charles D: Blood transfusion reaction in a patient with immunoglobulin A deficiency. Obstet Gynecol 1983; 61:47S–49S.

Brouet JC, Chedeville A, Fermand JP, Royer B: Study of the B cell memory compartment in common variable immunodeficiency. Eur J Immunol 2000; 30:2516–2520.

Brouet JC, Seligmann M: Letter: selective IgA deficiency and idiopathic thrombocytopenic purpura. Lancet 1976; 1:861–862.

Buckley RH: Clinical and immunologic features of selective IgA deficiency. Birth Defects 1975; 11:134–142.

Buckley RH: Common variable immunodeficiency. Curr Ther Allergy, Immunol Rheumatol 1988; 301–304.

Buckley RH, Dees SC: Correlation of milk precipitins with IgA deficiency. N Engl J Med 1969; 281:465–469.

Buckley RH, Schiff RI: The use of intravenous immune globulin in immunodeficiency disease. N Engl J Med 1991; 325:110–117.

Bundino S, Zina AM: Pyoderma gangrenosum associated with selective hereditary IgA deficiency. Dermatologica 1984; 168:230–232.

Burgio GR, Duse M, Monafo V, Ascione A, Nespoli L: Selective IgA deficiency: clinical and immunological evaluation of 50 pediatric patients. Eur J Pediatr 1980; 133:101–106.

Burks AW, Sampson HA, Buckley RH: Anaphylactic reactions after gammaglobulin administration in patients with hypogammaglobulinemia: detection of IgE antibodies to IgA. N Engl J Med 1986; 314:560–564.

Burks AW Jr., Steele RW: Selective IgA deficiency. Ann Allergy 1986; 57:3–13.

Burmester GR, Gramatzki M, von Gernler J, Bartels O, Kalden JR: Pulmonary sarcoidosis associated with acquired humoral and cellular immunodeficiency. Clin Immunol Immunopath 1985; 37:406–412.

Butler WT, Rossen RD: Effects of corticosteroids on immunity in man: I. Decreased serum IgG concentration caused by 3 or 5 days of high doses of methylprednisolone. J Clin Invest 1973; 52:2629–2640.

Cambronero R, Sewell WA, North ME, Webster AD, Farrant J: Up-regulation of IL-12 in monocytes: a fundamental defect in common variable immunodeficiency. J Immunol 2000; 164:488–494.

Campbell RD, Trowsdale J: A map of the human major histocompatibility complex. Immunol Today 1997; 18:Supplement.

Cassidy JT, Burt A, Petty R, Sullivan D: Selective IgA deficiency in connective tissue diseases. N Engl J Med 1969; 280:275.

Cassidy JT, Oldham G, Platts Mills TA: Functional assessment of a B cell defect in patients with selective IgA deficiency. Clin Exp Immunol 1979; 35:296–305.

Cataldo F, Marino V, Ventura A, Bottaro G, Corazza GR: Prevalence and clinical features of selective immunoglobulin A deficiency in coeliac disease: an Italian multicentre study. Gut 1998; 42:362–365.

Chee L, Graham SM, Carothers DG, Ballas ZK: Immune dysfunction in refractory sinusitis in a tertiary care setting. Laryngoscope 2001; 111:233–235.

Chevailler A, Ifrah N, Monteiro RC, Keyeux G, Renier G, Lefranc MP, Lesavre P, Hurez D: Association between acute lymphoblastic leukemia and partial IgA deficiency in a young man: a family study. Nouv Rev Fr Hematol 1990; 32:159–164.

Choi YS, Biggar WD, Good RA: Biosynthesis and secretion of immunoglobulins by peripheral-blood lymphocytes in severe hypogammaglobulinemia. Lancet 1972; 1:1149–1152.

Conley ME, Cooper MD: Immature IgA B cells in IgA-deficient patients. N Engl J Med 1981; 305:495–497.

Contu L, Arras M, Mulargia M, La Nasa G, Carcassi CXLA, Ledda A, Goddi F: Study of HLA segregation in 479 thalassemic families. Tissue Antigens 1992; 39:58–67.

Cooper MD, Lawton AR: Circulating B-cells in patients with immunodeficiency. Am J Pathol 1972; 69:513–528.

Cooper MD, Lawton AR, Bockman DE: Agammaglobulinemia with B lymphocytes: specific defect of plasma-cell differentiation. Lancet 1971; 2:791–795.

Couch JR, Romyg DA: Histoplasma meningitis with common variable hypogammaglobulinemia. Neurol Neurocir Psiquiatr 1977; 18:403–412.

Couderc LJ, Caubarrere I, Oksenlendler E, Clauvel JP: Vascular malformations and hypogammaglobulinaemia. Lancet 1987; 1:385.

Cruchaud A, Laperrouza C, Megevand R: Agammaglobulinemia in monozygous twins: therapeutic prospects. Birth Defects 1965; 315–327.

Cucca F, Zhu ZB, Khanna A, Cossu F, Congia M, Badiali M, Lampis R, Frau F, De Virgiliis S, Cao A, et al.: Evaluation of immunoglobulin A deficiency in Sardinians indicates a susceptibility gene encoded wtihin the HLA class III region. Clin Exp Immunol 1997; 111:76–80

Cuesta B, Fernandez J, Pardo J, Paramo JA, Gomez C, Rocha E: Evan's syndrome, chronic active hepatitis and focal glomerulonephritis in IgA deficiency. Acta Haematol 1986; 75:1–5.

Cunningham Rundles C: Genetic aspects of immunoglobulin A deficiency. Adv Hum Genet 1990; 19:235–266.

Cunningham-Rundles C, Bodian C: Common variable immunodeficiency: clinical and immunological features of 248 patients. Clin Immunol 1999; 92:34–48.

Cunningham Rundles C, Kazbay K, Hassett J, Zhhou Z, Mayer L: Brief report: enhanced humoral immunity in common variable immunodeficiency after long term treatment with polyethylene glycol-conjugated interleukin-2. N Engl J Med 1994; 331:918–921.

Cunningham Rundles C, Lieberman P, Hellman G, Chaganti RSK: Non-Hodgkin lymphoma in common variable immunodeficiency. Am J Hematol 1991; 37:69–74.

Cunningham Rundles C, Oxelius VA, Good RA: IgG2 and IgG3 subclass deficiencies in selective IgA deficiency in the United States. Birth Defects 1983; 19:173–175.

Cunningham Rundles C, Pudifin DJ, Armstrong D, Good RA: Selective IgA deficiency and neoplasia. Vox Sang 1980; 38:61–67.

Cunningham Rundles C, Siegal FP, Cunningham Rundles S, Lieberman P: Incidence of cancer in 98 patients with common variable immunodeficiency. J Clin Immunol 1987; 7:294–299.

Cunningham Rundles C, Siegal FP, Smithwick EM, Lion-Boule A, Cunningham Rundles S, O'Malley J, Barandum S, Good RA: Efficacy of intravenous gammaglobulin in primary humoral immunodeficiency disease. Ann Intern Med 1984; 101:435–439.

Danon YL, Dinari G, Garty BZ, Horodniceanu C, Nitzan M, Grunebaum M: Cholelithiasis in children with immunoglobulin A deficiency: a new gastroenterologic syndrome. J Pediatr Gastroenterol Nutr 1983; 2:663–666.

Davis TJ, Berk RN: Immunoglobulin deficiency diseases of the intestine. Gastrointest Radiol 1977; 2:7–11.

De Gast GC, The TH, Viersma JW, Marrink J, Arisz LA: Reversible hypogammaglobulinemia after diphenylhydantoin and hydroxyzine therapy. Neth J Med 1974; 17:261–269.

De Gast GC, Wilkins SR, Webster AD, Rickinson A, Platts Mills TA: Functional "immaturity" of isolated B cells from patients with hypogammaglobulinaemia. Clin Exp Immunol 1980; 42:535–544.

de la Concha EG, Oldham G, Webster AD, Asherson GL, Platts Mills TA: Quantitative measurements of T- and B-cell function in "variable" primary hypogammaglobulinemia: evidence for a consistent B-cell defect. Clin Exp Immunol 1977; 27:208–215.

de la Concha EG, Subiza JL, Fontan G, Pascual Salcedo D, Sequi J, Bootello A: Disorders of regulatory T cells in patients with selective IgA deficiency and its relationship to associated autoimmune phenomena. Clin Exp Immunol 1982; 49:410–418.

Delamarre J, Dupas JL, Chivrac D, Capron JP, Messerschmitt J: Hypogammaglobulinemia with lymphoid nodular hyperplasia of the small bowel: endoscopic diagnosis of one case. Endoscopy 1976; 8:214–216.

Denz A, Eibel H, Illges H, Kienzle G, Schlesier M, Peter HH: Impaired up-regulation of CD86 in B cells of "type A" common variable immunodeficiency patients. Eur J Immunol 2000; 30:1069–1077.

De Smet AA, Tubergen DG, Martel W: Nodular lymphoid hyperplasia of the colon associated with dysgammaglobulinemia. Am J Roentgenol 1976; 127:515–517.

Di Renzo M, Zhou Z, George I, Becker K, Cunningham-Rundles C: Enhanced apoptosis of T cells in common variable immunodeficiency (CVID): role of defective CD28 co-stimulation. Clin Exp Immunol 2000; 120:503–511.

Dubois RS, Roy CC, Fulginiti VA, Merrill DA, Murray RL: Disaccharidase deficiency in children with immunologic deficits. J Pediatr 1970; 76:377–385.

Edelstein AD, Miller A, Zimelman AP, Rocklin RE, Neiman RS: Adult severe combined immunodeficiency and sarcoid-like granulomas with hypersplenism. Am J Hematol 1978; 5:55–62.

Eibl MM, Griscelli C, Seligmann M, Aiuti F, Kishimoto T, Matsmoto S, Hanson LA, Hitzig WH, Thompson RA, Cooper MD, et al.: Primary immunodeficiency diseases. Immunol Rev 1988; 1:173–205.

Eisenstein EM, Chua K, Strober W: B cell differentiation defects in common variable immunodeficiency are ameliorated after stimulation with anti-CD40 antibody and IL-10. J Immunol 1994; 152:5957–5968.

Evans DI, Burn JL: Progressive hypogammaglobulinaemia in a child born to a mother with Hodgkin's disease. Arch Dis Child 1979; 54:313–315.

Farr M, Struthers GR, Scott DG, Bacon PA: Fenclofenac-induced selective IgA deficiency in rheumatoid arthritis. Br J Rheumatol 1985a; 24:367–369.

Farr M, Tunn E, Bacon PA, Smith DH: Hypogammaglobulinemia and thrombocytopenia associated with sulphasalazine therapy in rheumatoid arthritis. Ann Rheum Dis 1985b; 44:723–724.

Farrant J, Bryant A, Almandoz F, Spickett G, Evans SW, Webster AD: B cell function in acquired "common-variable" hypogammaglobulinemia: proliferative responses to lymphokines. Clin Immunol Immunopathol 1989; 51:196–204.

Farrington M, Grosmaire LS, Nonoyama S, Fischer SH, Hollenbaugh D, Ledbetter JA, Noelle RJ, Aruffo A, Ochs HD: CD40 ligand expression is defective in a subset of patients with common variable immunodeficiency. Proc Natl Acad Sci USA 1994; 91:1099–1103.

Fasano MB, Sullivan KE, Sarpong SB, Wood RA, Jones SM, Johns CJ, Lederman HM, Bykowsky MJ, Greene JM, Winkelstein JA: Sarcoidosis and common variable immunodeficiency: report of 8 cases and review of the literature. Medicine 1996; 75:251–261.

Fasth A: Primary immunodeficiency disorders in Sweden: cases among children, 1974–1979. J Clin Immunol 1982; 2:86–92.

Filipovich AH, Mathur A, Kamat D, Kersey JH, Shapiro RS: Lymphoproliferative disorders and other tumors complicating immunodeficiencies. Immunodeficiency 1994; 5:91–112.

Fischer MB, Hauber I, Eggenbauer H, Thon V, Vogel E, Schaffer E, Lokaj J, Litzman J, Wolf HM, Mannhalter JW, Eibl MM: A defect in the early phase of T-cell receptor-mediated T-cell activation in patients with common variable immunodeficiency. Blood 1994; 84:4234–4241.

Fischer MB, Wolf HM, Hauber I, Eggenbauer H, Thon V, Sasgary M, Eibl MM: Activation via the antigen receptor is impaired in T cells, but not in B cells from patients with common variable immunodeficiency. Eur J Immunol 1996; 26:231–237.

Fischer SH, Ochs HD, Wedgwood RJ, Skvaril F, Morell A, Hill HR, Schiffmann G, Corey L: Survival of antigen-specific antibody following administration of intravenous immunoglobulin in patients with primary immunodeficiency diseases. Monogr Allergy 1988; 23P:225–235.

Flori NM, Llambi JM, Boren TE, Borja SR, Casariego GF: Primary Immunodeficiency Syndrome in Spain: First Report of the National Registry in Children and Adults. J Clin Immunol 1997; 17:333–339.

Freeman HJ, Shnitka TK, Piercy JRA, Weinstein WM: Cytomegalovirus infection of the gastrointestinal tract in a patient with late onset immunodeficiency syndrome. Gastroenterology 1977; 73:1397–1403.

French MA: Lymphadenopathy and selective IgA deficiency. Br Med J 1984; 289:646–647.

French MA, Dawkins RL: Central MHC genes, IgA deficiency and autoimmune disease. Immunol Today 1990; 11:271–274.

French MA, Denis KA, Dawkins R, Peter JB: Severity of infections in IgA deficiency: correlation with decreased serum antibodies to pneumococcal polysaccharides and decreased serum IgG2 and/or IgG4. Clin Exp Immunol 1995; 100:47–53.

French MA, Harrison G: An investigation into the effect of the IgG antibody system on the susceptibility of IgA-deficient patients to respiratory tract infections. Clin Exp Immunol 1986; 66:640–647.

Friedman R, Ackerman M, Mallory G, Weng TR, Fireman P: Hypogammaglobulinemia with sarcoidlike granulomas. Am J Dis Child 1983; 137:774–776.

Fudenberg HH, Gold ER, Vyas GN, Mackenzie MR: Human antibodies to human IgA globulins. Immunochemistry 1968; 5:203–206.

García Baez M, González Espinosa C, Serna Alonso E, Mota Moraleda D: Delección de los brazos largos del cromosoma 18. An Esp Pediatr 1980; 13:1001–1006.

Gatti RA, Good RA: Occurrence of malignancy in immunodeficiency diseases. Cancer 1971; 28:89–98.

Geha RS, Schneeberger E, Merler E, Rosen FS: Heterogeneity of "acquired" or common variable agammaglobulinemia. N Engl J Med 1974; 291:1–6.

Gilhus NE, Aarli JA, Thorsby E: HLA antigens in epileptic patients with drug-induced immunodeficiency. Int J Immunopharmacol 1982; 4:517–520.

Goldstein R, Izaguirre C, Smith CD, Mierins E, Karsh J: Systemic lupus erythematosus and common variable panhypogammaglobulinemia: a patient with absence of circulating B cells. Arthritis Rheum 1985; 28:100–103.

Gonzalez Vitale JC, Gomez LG, Goldblum RM, Goldman AS, Patterson M: Immunoblastic lymphoma of small intestine complicating late-onset immunodeficiency. Cancer 1982; 49:445–449.

Grundbacher FJ: Genetic aspects of selective immunoglobulin A deficiency. J Med Genet 1972; 9:71.

Gryboski JD, Self TW, Clemett A, Herskovic T: Selective immunoglobulin A deficiency and intestinal nodular lymphoid hyperplasia: correction of diarrhea with antibiotics and plasma. Pediatrics 1968; 42:833.

Guillemin F, Bene MC, Aussedat R, Bannwarth B, Pourel J: Hypogammaglobulinemia associated with gold therapy: evidence for a partial maturation blockade of B cells. J Rheumatol 1987; 14:1034–1035.

Gupta S, Ellis M, Cesario T, Ruhling M, Vayuvegula B: Disseminated cryptococcal infection in a patient with hypogammaglobulinemia and normal T cell functions. Am J Med 1987; 82:129–131.

Hammarstrom L, Carlsson B, Smith CI, Wallin J, Wieslander L: Detection of IgA heavy chain constant region genes in IgA-deficient donors: evidence against gene deletions. Clin Exp Immunol 1985a; 60:661–664.

Hammarstrom L, de Lange GG, Smith CI: IgA2 allotypes determined by restriction fragment length polymorphism in IgA deficiency: re-expression of the silent A2m(2) allotype in the children of IgA-deficient patients. J Immunogenet 1987; 14:197–201.

Hammarstrom L, Lonnqvist B, Ringden O, Smith CI, Wiebe T: Transfer of IgA deficiency to a bone-marrow-grafted patient with aplastic anaemia. Lancet 1985b; 1:778–781.

Hammarstrom L, Smith CI, Berg CI: Captopril-induced IgA deficiency. Lancet 1991; 337–436.

Hansen OP, Sorensen CH, Astrup L: Evans' syndrome in IgA deficiency: episodic autoimmune haemolytic anaemia and thrombocytopenia during a 10-year observation period. Scand J Haematol 1982; 29:265–270.

Hausser C, Buriot D: Gamma globulin therapy during pregnancy in mother with hypogammaglobulinemia. Am J Obstet Gynecol 1982; 144:112.

Hausser C, Virelizier JL, Buriot D, Griscelli C: Common variable hypogammaglobulinemia in children: clinical and immunologic observations in 30 patients. Am J Dis Child 1983; 137:833–837.

Heneghan MA, Stevens FM, Cryan EM, Warner RH, McCarthy CF: Celiac sprue and immunodeficiency states: a 25-year review. J Clin Gastroenterol 1997; 25:421–425.

Hermans PE, Diax-Buxo JA, Stobo JD: Idiopathic late-onset immunoglobulin deficiency. Am J Med 1976; 61:221–236.

Hermans PE, Huizenga KA, Hoffman HN, Brown AL, Jr., Markowitz H: Dysgammaglobulinemia associated with nodular lymphoid hyperplasia of the small intestine. Am J Med 1966; 40:78–89.

Herrod HG: Management of the patient with IgG subclass deficiency and/or selective antibody deficiency. Ann Allergy 1993; 70:3–8.

Hobbs JR: Immune imbalance in dysgammaglobulinemia type IV. Lancet 1968; 1:110–114.

Hoddinott S, Dornan J, Bear JC, Farid NR: Immunoglobulin levels, immunodeficiency and HLA in Type 1 (insulin-dependent) diabetes mellitus. Diabetologia 1982; 23:326–329.

Hodgson G: Pyoderma and dysgammaglobulinaemia. Br J Dermatol 1966; 78:608.

Hong R, Ammann RJ: Disorders of the IgA system. In: Stiehm ER (ed). Immuno-

logic Disorders of Infants and Children. Philadelpha: W. B. Saunders, 1989:329–342.
Horowitz S, Hong R: Selective IgA deficiency—some perspectives. Birth Defects 1975; 11:129–133.
Hosking CS, Roberton DM: Epidemiology and treatment of hypogammaglobulinemia. Birth Defects 1983; 19:223–227.
Islam KB, Baskin B, Nilsson L, Hammarstrom L, Sideras P, Edvard-Smith CI: Molecular analysis of IgA deficiency: evidence for impaired switching to IgA. J Immunol 1994; 152:1442–1452.
Iyer RK, Joshi JM: Job's syndrome or hyperimmunoglobulin-E. J Assoc Physicians India 1995; 43:652.
James SP, Jones EA, Schafer DF, Hoofnagle JH, Varma RR, Strober W: Selective immunoglobulin A deficiency associated with primary biliary cirrhosis in a family with liver disease. Gastroenterology 1986; 90:283–288.
Janeway CA, Rosen FS: The gamma globulins: IV. Therapeutic uses of gamma globulin. N Engl J Med 1966; 275:826–831.
Johansson SG, Dannaeus A, Lilja G: Intravenous immunoglobulin treatment in the primary immunodeficiency diseases. Immunol Allergy Clin North Am 1988; 8:17–28.
Johansson SGO, Hogman CF, Killander J: Quantitative immunoglobulin determination. Acta Pathologica et Microbiologica Scandinavica 1968; 74:519.
Johnson ML, Keeton LG, Zhu Z-B, Volanakis JE, Cooper MD, Schroeder HW, Jr.: Age-related changes in serum immunoglobulins in patients with familial IgA deficiency and common variable immunodeficiency (CVID). Clin Exp Immunol 1997; 108:477–483.
Johnston CL, Webster AD, Taylor Robinson D, Rapaport G, Hughes GR: Primary late-onset hypogammaglobulinaemia associated with inflammatory polyarthritis and septic arthritis due to *Mycoplasma pneumoniae*. Ann Rheum Dis 1983; 42:108–110.
Joller PW, Buehler AK, Hitzig WH: Transitory and persistent IgA deficiency: reevaluation of 19 pediatric patients once found to be deficient in serum IGA. J Clin Lab Immunol 1981; 6:97–101.
Kainulainen L, Nikoskelainen J, Vuorinen T, Tevola K, Liippo K, Ruuskanen O: Viruses and bacteria in bronchial samples from patients with primary hypogammaglobulinemia. Am J Respir Crit Care Med 1999a; 159:1199–1204.
Kainulainen L, Varpula M, Liippo K, Svedstrom E, Nikoskelainen J, Ruuskanen O: Pulmonary abnormalities in patients with primary hypogammaglobulinemia. J Allergy Clin Immunol 1999b; 104:1031–1036.
Kanoh T, Mizumoto T, Yasuda N, Koya M, Ohno Y, Uchino H, Yoshimura K, Ohkubo Y, Yamaguchi H: Selective IgA deficiency in Japanese blood donors: frequency and statistical analysis. Vox Sang 1986; 50:81–86.
Keczkes K, Bilimoria S, Piercy DM: Pernicious anaemia and granulomatous skin lesions in a case of common variable hypogammaglobulinemia. Br J Dermatol 1979; 101:211–217.
Kew OM, Sutter RW, Nottay BK, McDonough MJ, Prevots DR, Quick L, Pallansch MA: Prolonged replication of a type 1 vaccine-derived poliovirus in an immunodeficient patient. J Clin Microbiol 1998; 36:2893–2899.
King MA, Wells JV, Nelson DS: IgA synthesis by peripheral blood mononuclear cells from normal and selectively IgA deficient subjects. Clin Exp Immunol 1979; 38:306–315.
Kinlen LJ, Webster ADB, Bird AG, Haile R, Peto J, Soothill JF, Thompson RA: Prospective study of cancer in patients with hypogammaglobulinemia. Lancet 1985; 1:263–266.
Klemola T: Deficiency of immunoglobulin A. Ann Clin Res 1987; 19:248–257.
Klemola T, Eskola J, Savilahti E: T- and B-cell functions in IgA-deficient patients. Scand J Immunol 1988; 28:301–306.
Klemola T, Savilahti E, Arato A, Ormala T, Partanen J, Eland C, Koskimies S: Immunohistochemical findings in jejunal specimens from patients with IgA deficiency. Gut 1995; 37:519–523.
Kruger G, Welte K, Ciobanu N, Cunningham Rundles C, Ralph P, Venuta S, Feldman S, Koziner B, Wang CY, Moore MA, et al.: Interleukin-2 correction of defective in vitro T-cell mitogenesis in patients with common varied immunodeficiency. J Clin Immunol 1984; 4:295–303.
Kruskall MS, Marcus-Bagley D, Awdeh Z, Eisenbarth GS, Brink SJ, Katz AJ, Hauser SL, Ahmed AR, Bing DH, Yunis EJ, et al.: Many individuals with the MHC conserved extended [HLA-B8, SC01, DR3] haplotype have immunoglobulin deficiencies. Clin Res 1993; 41:277A.
Kurtyka ZE, Krzykwa B, Piatkowska E, Radwan M, Pietrzyk JJ: Trisomy 8 mosaicism syndrome: two cases demonstrating variability in phenotype. Clin Pediatr 1988; 27:557–564.
Lai Ping SA, Mayer L: Gastrointestinal manifestations of primary immunodeficiency disorders. Semin Gastrointest Dis 1997; 8:22–32.
Lane PJ, MacLennan IC: Impaired IgG2 anti-pneumococcal antibody responses in patients with recurrent infection and normal IgG2 levels but no IgA. Clin Exp Immunol 1986; 65:427–433.
Lanzavecchia A, Frassoni F, Piovella F, Vitiello A, Maccario R, Ugazio AG: Common variable immunodeficiency: long-term clinical consequencies of splenectomy in a case of late-onset hypogammaglobulinaemia. Haematologica 1978; 63:326–332.
Lawton AR, Royal SA, Self KS, Cooper MD: IgA determinants on B lymphocytes in patients with deficiency of circulating IgA. J Lab Clin Med 1972; 80:26.
Lawton AR, Wu LY, Cooper MD: The cellular basis of IgA deficiency in humans. Adv Exp Med Biol 1974; 45:373–380.
Lee CA: Acquired hypogammaglobulinemia and sarcoidosis. Postgrad Med J 1984; 60:551–553.
Leickly FE, Buckley RH: Development of IgA and IgG2 subclass deficiency after sulfasalazine therapy. J Pediatr 1986; 108:481–482.
Leong AB, Gange RW, OConnor RD: Twenty-nail dystrophy (trachyonychia) associated with selective IgA deficiency. J Pediatr 1982; 100:418–420.
Lewkonia RM, Gairdner D, Doe WF: IgA deficiency in one of identical twins. Br Med J 1976; 1:311–313.
Loria RC, Jadidi S, Wedner HJ: Anaphylactic reaction to ampicillin in a patient with common variable immunodeficiency syndrome desensitized to penicillin. Ann Allergy 1987; 59:15–6,348.
Madsen DL, Catanzarite VA, Varela Gittings F: Common variable hypogammaglobulinemia in pregnancy: treatment with high-dose immunoglobulin infusions. Am J Hematol 1986; 21:327–329.
Maeoka Y, Hara T, Dejima S, Takeshita K: IgA and IgG2 deficiency associated with zonisamide therapy: a case report. Epilepsia 1997; 38:611–613.
Majolini MB, D'Elios MM, Boncristiano M, Galieni P, Del PG, Telford, JL, Baldari CT: Uncoupling of T-cell antigen receptor and downstream protein tyrosine kinases in common variable immunodeficiency. Clin Immunol Immunopathol 1997; 84:98–102.
Martini A, Ravelli A, Notarangelo LD, Burgio VL, Plebani A: Henoch-Schonlein syndrome and selective IgA deficiency. Arch Dis Child 1985; 60:160–162.
McCluskey DR, Boyd NAM: Prevalence of primary hypogammaglobulinemia in Northern Ireland. Proc R Coll Physicians Edinb 1989; 19:191–194.
Mechanic LJ, Dikman S, Cunningham Rundles C: Granulomatous disease in common variable immunodeficiency. Ann Intern Med 1997; 127:613–617.
Meini A, Pillan NM, Villanacci V, Monafo V, Ugazio AG, Plebani A: Prevalence and diagnosis of celiac disease in IgA-deficient children. Ann Allergy Asthma Immunol 1996; 77:333–336.
Melamed I, Kark JD, Zakuth V, Margalit G, Spirer Z: Serum immunoglobulin A levels and ethnicity in an Israeli population sample. Clin Immunol Immunopathol 1987; 42:259–264.
Morell A, Muehlheim E, Schaad U, Skvaril F, Rossi E: Susceptibility to infections in children with selective IgA- and IgA-IgG subclass deficiency. Eur J Pediatr 1986; 145:199–203.
Mosier DE, Subbarrao B: Thymus-independent antigens: complexity of B-lymphocyte activation revealed. Immunol Today 1982; 3:217–222.
Mulder CJ, Gratama JW, Trimbos Kemper GC, Willemze R, Pena AS: Thrombocytopenic purpura, coeliac disease and IgA deficiency. Neth J Med 1986; 29:165–166.
Mullighan CG, Fanning GC, Chapel HM, Welsh KI: TNF and lymphotoxin-α polymorphisms associated with common variable immunodeficiency: role in the pathogenesis of granulomatous disease. J Immunol 1997; 159:6236–6241.
Mullighan CG, Marshall SE, Welsh KI: Mannose binding lectin polymorphisms are associated with early age of disease onset and autoimmunity in common variable immunodeficiency. Scand J Immunol 2000; 51:111–122.
NIH Consensus Conference: Intravenous immunoglobulin: prevention and treatment of disease. JAMA 1990; 264:3189–3193.
Nilssen DE, Friman V, Theman K, Bjorkander J, Kilander A, Holmgren J, Hanson LA, Brandtzaeg P: Intestinal immunoglobulin production after oral cholera vaccination in patients with IgA deficiency with or without IgG subclass deficiency. Immunodeficiency 1993; 4:55–57.
Nonoyama S, Farrington M, Ishida H, Howard M, Ochs HD: Activated B cells from patients with common variable immunodeficiency proliferate and synthesize immunoglobulin. J Clin Invest 1993; 92:1282–1287.
Nordoy I, Muller F, Aukrust P, Froland SS: Adhesion molecules in common variable immunodeficiency (CVID)—a decrease in L-selectin-positive T lymphocytes. Clin Exp Immunol 1998; 114:258–263.
Oen K, Petty RE, Schroeder ML: Immunoglobulin A deficiency: genetic studies. Tissue Antigens 1982; 19:174–182.
Ogata K, Iinuma K, Kammura K, Morinaga R, Kato J: A case report of a presumptive +i(18p) associated with serum IgA deficiency. Clin Genet 1977; 11:184–188.
Olerup O, Smith CIE, Bjorkander J, Hammarstrom L: Shared HLA class II–associated genetic susceptibility and resistance, related to the HLA-DQB1 gene, in IgA deficiency and common variable immunodeficiency. Proc Natl Acad Sci USA 1992; 89:10653–10657.
Olsson PG, Hammarstrom L, Cox DW, Smith CIE: Involvement of both HLA and Ig heavy chain haplotypes in human IgA deficiency. Immunogenetics 1992; 36:389–395.
Ostergaard PA: Clinical and immunological features of transient IgA deficiency in children. Clin Exp Immunol 1980; 40:561–565.
Osur SL, Lillie MA, Chen PB, Ambrus JL Jr., Wilson ME: Elevation of serum IgG levels and normalization of T4/T8 ratio after hepatitis in a patient with common variable hypogammaglobulinemia. J Allergy Clin Immunol 1987; 79:969–975.
Oxelius VA, Carlsson AM, Hammarstrom L, Bjorkander J, Hanson LA: Linkage of IgA deficiency to Gm allotypes: the influence of Gm allotypes on IgA-IgG subclass deficiency. Clin Exp Immunol 1995; 99:211–215.
Oxelius VA, Laurell AB, Lindquist B, Golebiowska H, Axelsson U, Bjorkander J, Hanson LA: IgG subclasses in selective IgA deficiency: importance of IgG2–IgA deficiency. N Engl J Med 1981; 304:1476–1477.
Pandolfi F, Paganelli R, Cafaro A, Oliva A, Giovannetti A, Scala E, Quinti I, Aiuti F: Abnormalities of lymphocyte subpopulations in CVI do not correlate with increased production of IL-6. Immunodeficiency 1993; 4:19–23.
Pelkonen P, Savilahti E, Makela A-L: Persistent and transient IgA deficiency in juvenille rheumatoid arthritis. Scand J Immunol 1983; 12:273–279.
Penny R, Thompson RG, Polmar SH, Schultz RB: Pancreatitis malabsorption and IgA deficiency in a child with diabetes. J Pediatr 1971; 78:512–516.
Pereira LF, Sapina AM, Arroyo J, Vinuelas J, Bardaji RM, Prieto L: Prevalence of selective IgA deficiency in Spain: more than we thought (letter). Blood 1997; 90:893.

Plebani A, Ugazio AG, Monafo V, Burgio GR: Clinical heterogeneity and reversibility of selective immunoglobulin A deficiency in 80 children. Lancet 1986; 1:829–831.

Polmar SH, Waldmann TA, Terry WD: The relationship of IgA and IgE deficiency. Birth Defects 1975; 11:147–150.

Pozzi N, Gaetaniello L, Martire B, De Mattia D, Balestrieri B, Cosentini, E, Schlossman SF, Duke-Cohan JS, Pignata C: Defective surface expression of attractin on T cells in patients with common variable immunodeficiency (CVID). Clin Exp Immunol 2001; 123:99–104.

Prasad AS, Raeiner E, Watson DJ: Syndrome of hypogammaglobulinemia, splenomegaly, and hypersplenism. Blood 1957; 12:926–932.

Preudhomme JL, Griscelli C, Seligmann M: Immunoglobulins on the surface of lymphocytes in 50 patients with primary immunodeficiency diseases. Clin Immunol Immunopathol 1973; 1:241–256.

Preudhomme JL, Hanson LA: IgG subclass deficiency. Immunodeficiency Rev 1990; 2:129–149.

Proesmans W, Jaeken J, Eeckels R: D-penicillamine-induced IgA deficiency in Wilson's disease. Lancet 1976; 2:804–805.

Quigley EM, Carmichael HA, Watkinson G: Adult celiac disease (celiac sprue), pernicious anemia and IgA deficiency: case report and review of the relationships between vitamin B12 deficiency, small intestinal mucosal disease and immunoglobulin deficiency. J Clin Gastroenterol 1986; 8:277–281.

Ranchod M, Lewin KJ, Dorfman RF: Lymphoid hyperplasia of the gastrointestinal tract: a study of 26 cases and review of the literature. Am J Surg Pathol 1978; 2:383–400.

Rankin EC, Isenberg DA: IgA deficiency and SLE: prevalence in a clinic population and a review of the literature. Lupus 1997; 6:390–394.

Robbins JB: Immunochemical evidence for the development of an "acquired" hypogammaglobulinemic state. N Engl J Med 1966; 274:607–610.

Roifman CM, Gelfand EW: Replacement therapy with high dose intravenous gammaglobulin improves chronic sinopulmonary disease in patients with hypogammaglobulinemia. Pediatr Infect Dis J 1988; 7:S92–S96.

Roifman CM, Lederman HM, Lavi S, Stein LD, Levison H, Gelfand EW: Benefit of intravenous IgG replacement in hypogammaglobulinemic patients with chronic sinopulmonary disease. Am J Med 1985; 79:171–174.

Ropars C, Geay-Chicot D, Cartron JP, Doinel C, Salmon C: Human IgE response to the administration of blood components. Vox Sang 1979; 37:149–157.

Rosen FS, Wedgwood RJ, Eibl MM, Fischer A, Aiuti F, Notarangelo LD, Resnick IB, Hammarstrom L, Seger R, Chapel H, et al.: Primary immunodeficiency diseases: Report of a WHO scientific group. Clin Exp Immunol 1997; 109:S1–S28.

Rosen FS, Wedgwood RJ, Eibl MM, Griscelli C, Seligmann M, Aiuti F, Kishimoto T, Matsumoto S, Khakhalin LN, Hanson LA, et al.: Primary immunodeficiency diseases: Report of a WHO scientific group. Immunodeficiency Rev 1992; 3:195–236.

Saiki O, Ralph P, Cunningham Rundles C, Good RA: Three distinct stages of B-cell defects in common varied hypogammaglobulinemia. Proc Natl Acad Sci USA 1982; 79:6008–6012.

Sander CA, Medeiros LJ, Weiss LM, Yano T, Sneller MC, Jaffe ES: Lymphoproliferative lesions in patients with common variable immunodeficiency. Am J Surg Pathol 1992; 16:1170–1182.

Saulsbury FT: Selective IgA deficiency temporally associated with Epstein-Barr virus infection. J Pediatr 1989; 115:268–270.

Saxon A, Sidell N, Zhang K: B cells from subjects with CVI can be driven to Ig production in response to CD40 stimulation. Cell Immunol 1992; 144:169–181.

Schaffer FM, Monteiro RC, Volanakis JE, Cooper MD: IgA deficiency. Immunodeficiency Rev 1991; 3:15–44.

Schaffer FM, Palermos J, Zhu Z-B, Barger BO, Cooper MD, Volanakis JE: Individuals with IgA deficiency and common variable immunodeficiency share polymorphisms of major histocompatibility complex class III genes. Proc Natl Acad Sci USA 1989; 86:8015–8019.

Schmidt AP, Taswell HF, Gleich GJ: Anaphylactic transfusion reactions associated with anti-IgA antibody. N Engl J Med 1969; 280:188–193.

Schneider L, Geha R: Outbreak of hepatitis C associated with intravenous immunoglobulin administration—United States, October 1993–June 1994. Morb Mortal Wkly Rep 1994; 43:505–509.

Schroeder HWJ, Zhu ZB, March RE, Campbell RD, Berney, SM, Nedospasov SA, Turetskaya RL, Atkinson TP, Go RC, Cooper MD, Volanakis JE: Susceptibility locus for IgA deficiency and common variable immunodeficiency in the HLA-DR3, -B8, -A1 haplotypes. Mol Med 1998; 4:72–86.

Schwaber J, Roser FS: Lymphoid cell lines from patients with "non-secretory" agammaglobulinemia produce glycosylated heavy chains which are reduced in molecular weight. J Mol Cell Immunol 1984; 1:279–289.

Scott LJ, Bryant A, Webster DB, Farrant J: Failure in IgA secretion by surface IgA-positive B cells in common variable immunodeficiency. Clin Exp Immunol 1994; 95:10–13.

Seager J: IgA deficiency during treatment of infantile hypothyroidism with thyroxine. Br Med J 1984; 288:1562–1563.

Seager J, Jamison DL, Wilson J, Hayward AR, Soothill JF: IgA deficiency, epilepsy, and phenytoin treatment. Lancet 1975; 2:632–635.

Seggev JS, Ben Yosef N, Meytes D: Is selective IgA deficiency associated with morbidity? Review and reevaluation. Isr J Med Sci 1988; 24:65–69.

Seligmann M, Aucouturier P, Danon F, Preudhomme JL: Changes in serum immunoglobulin patterns in adults with common variable immunodeficiency. Clin Exp Immunol 1991; 84:23–27.

Shackleford MD, McAlister WH: Primary immunodeficiency diseases and malignancy. Am J Roentgenol Radium Ther Nucl Med 1975; 123:144–153.

Skrede S, Winther FO, Munthe E, Nordoy A: Transitory IgA-deficiency, persistent IgE deficiency and recurrent respiratory tract infectious disease after splenectomy. Arch Otorhinolaryngol 1977; 217:423–428.

Smith CI, Hammarstrom L: Intravenous immunoglobulin in pregnancy. Obstet Gynecol 1985; 66:39S–40S.

Smith KJ, Skelton H: Common variable immunodeficiency treated with a recombinant human IgG, tumour necrosis factor-α receptor fusion protein. Br J Dermatol 2001; 144:597–600.

Sneller MC, Strober W: Abnormalities of lymphokine gene expression in patients with common variable immunodeficiency. J Immunol 1990; 144:3762–3769.

Sneller MC, Strober W, Eisenstein E, Jaffe JS, Cunningham Rundles C: New insights into common variable immunodeficiency. Ann Int Med 1993; 118:720–730.

So AK, Peskett SA, Webster AD: Hypogammaglobulinemia associated with gold therapy. Ann Rheum Dis 1984; 43:581–582.

Solley GO, Dickson ER, Gleich GJ, Stobo JD: Chronic active liver disease with common variable hypogammaglobulinemia. Mayo Clin Proc 1979; 54:127–130.

Soothill JF, Hayes K, Dudgeon JA: The immunoglobulins in congenital rubella. Lancet 1966; i:1385.

Sorrell TC, Forbes IJ, Burness FR, Rischbieth RHC: Depression of immunological function in patients treated with phenytoin sodium (sodium diphenylhydantoin). Lancet 1971; 2:1233–1235.

South MA, Wolheim FA, Warwick WJ, Cooper MD, Good RA: Local deficiency aof immune globulin A in the saliva of patients with chronic sinopulmonary disease. J Pediatr 1965; 67:941.

Spector BD, Perry GSI, Kersey JH: Genetically determined immunodeficiency diseases and malignancy: report from the Immunodeficiency Cancer Registry. Clin Immunol Immunopathol 1978; 11:12–29.

Sperber KE, Mayer L: Gastrointestinal manifestations of common variable immunodeficiency. Immunol Allergy Clin North Am 1988; 8:423–434.

Spickett GP, Farrant J, North ME, Zhang JG, Morgan L, Webster AD: Common variable immunodeficiency: how many diseases? Immunol Today 1997; 18:325–328.

Spickett GP, Gompels MM, Saunders PW: Hypogammaglobulinemia with absent B lymphocytes and agranulocytosis after carbamazepine treatment. J Neurol, Neurosurg Psych 1996a; 60:459.

Spickett GP, Matamoros N, Farrant J: Lymphocyte surface phenotype in common variable immunodeficiency. Dis Markers 1992; 10:67–80.

Spickett GP, Zhang JG, Green T, Shrimankar J: Granulomatous disease in common variable immunodeficiency: effect on immunoglobulin replacement therapy and response to steroids and splenectomy. J Clin Pathol 1996b; 49:431–434.

Stein A, Winkelstein A, Agarwal A: Concurrent systemic lupus erythematosus and common variable hypogammaglobulinemia. Arthritis Rheum 1985; 28:462–465.

Stites DP, Ishizaka K, Fudenberg HH: The relationship of IgA and IgE deficiency. Birth Defects 1975; 11:151–153.

Stobo JD, Tomasi TB: A low molecular weight immunoglobulin antigenically related to 19S IgM. J Clin Invest 1967; 46:1397.

Strannegard O, Bjorkander J, Hanson LA, Hermodsson S: Natural killer cells in common variable immunodeficiency and selective IgA deficiency. Clin Immunol Immunopathol 1982; 25:325–334.

Straus SE, Seidlin M, Takiff H, Jacobs D, Bowen D, Smith HA: Oral acyclovir to suppress recurring herpes simplex virus infections in immunodeficient patients. Ann Intern Med 1984; 100:522–524.

Strothman R, White MB, Testin J, Chen SN, Ball MJ: HLA and IgA deficiency in blood donors. Hum Immunol 1986; 16:289–294.

Sussman GL, Rivera VJ, Kohler PF: Transition from systemic lupus erythematosus to common variable hypogammaglobulinemia. Ann Intern Med 1983; 99:32–35.

Taalman RD, Weemaes CM, Hustinx TW, Scheres JM, Clement JM, Stoelinga GB: Chromosome studies in IgA-deficient patients. Clin Genet 1987; 32:81–87.

Thon V, Wolf HM, Sasgary M, Litzman J, Samstag A, Hauber I, Lokaj J, Eibl MM: Defective integration of activating signals derived from the T cell receptor (TCR) and costimulatory molecules in both $CD4^+$ and $CD8^+$ T lymphocytes of common variable immunodeficiency (CVID) patients. Clin Exp Immunol 1997; 110:174–181.

Tong MJ, Nies KM, Redeker AG: Rapid progression of chronic active type B hepatitis in a patient with hypogammaglobulinemia. Gastroenterology 1977; 73:1418–1421.

Turk A, Lichtenstein LM, Norman PS: Nasal secretory antibody to inhalant allergens in allergic and nonallergic patients. Immunology 1970; 19:85–95.

Twomey JJ, Jordan PH, Jarrold T, Trubowitz S, Ritz ND, Conn HO: The syndrome of immunoglobulin deficiency and pernicious anemia: a study of 10 cases. Am J Med 1969; 47:340–349.

Ugazio AG, Out TA, Plebani A, Duse M, Monafo V, Nespoli L, Burgio GR: Recurrent infections in children with "selective" IgA deficiency: association with IgG2 and IgG4 deficiency. Birth Defects 1983; 19:169–171.

Volanakis JE, Zhu Z-B, Schaffer FM, Macon KJ, Palermos J, Barger BO, Go R, Campbell RD, Schroeder HW, Jr., Cooper MD: Major histocompatibility complex class III genes and susceptibility to immunoglobulin A deficiency and common variable immunodeficiency. J Clin Invest 1992; 89:1914–1922.

Vorechovsky I, Cullen M, Carrington M, Hammarstrom L, Webster AD: Fine mapping of IGAD1 in IgA deficiency and common variable immunodeficiency: identification and characterization of haplotypes shared by affected members of 101 multiple-case families. J Immunol 2000; 164:4408–4416.

Vorechovsky I, Webster AD, Plebani A, Hammarstrom L: Genetic linkage of IgA deficiency to the major histocompatibility complex: evidence for allele segregation distortion, parent-of-origin penetrance differences, and the role of anti-IgA antibodies in disease predisposition. Am J Hum Genet 1999; 64:1096–1109.

Vukmanovic S, Vuckovic S, Stosic-Grujicic S, Ramic Z, Abinun M: An unusual T-cell surface phenotype in vivo correlates with the failure to proliferate and produce IL-2 in vitro in a patient with common variable immunodeficiency. Clin Immunol Immunopathol 1992; 65:261–270.

Vyas GN, Fudenberg HH: Isoimmune anti-IgA causing anaphylactoid transfusion reactions. N Engl J Med 1969; 280:1073–1074.

Vyas GN, Perkins HA, Yang YM, Basantani GK: Healthy blood donors with selective absence of immunoglobulin A: prevention of anaphylactic transfusion reactions caused by antibodies to IgA. J Lab Clin Med 1975; 85:838–842.

Wagner DK, Wright JJ, Ansher AF, Gill VJ: Dysgonic fermenter 3–associated gastrointestinal disease in a patient with common variable hypogammaglobulinemia. Am J Med 1988; 84:315–318.

Waldmann TA, Broder S, Krakauer R, Durm M, Meade B, Goldman C: Defect in IgA secretion and in IgA specific suppressor cells in patients with selective IgA deficiency. Trans Assoc Am Physicians 1976; 89P215–24.:215–224.

Wang WC: Evans syndrome in childhood: pathophysiology, clinical course, and treatment. Am J Pediatr Hematol Oncol 1988; 10:330–338.

Wang Z, Yunis D, Irigoyen M, Kitchens B, Bottaro A, Alt FW, Alper CA: Discordance between IgA switching at the DNA level and IgA expression at the mRNA level in IgA-deficient patients. Clin Immunol 1999; 91:263–270.

Watts WJ, Watts MB, Dai W, Cassidy JT, Grum CM, Weg JG: Respiratory dysfunction in patients with common variable hypogammaglobulinemia. Am Rev Respir Dis 1986; 134:699–703.

Webster ADB, Platts-Mills TAE, Janossy G, Morgan M, Asherson GL: Autoimmune blood dyscrazias in five patients with hypogammaglobulinemia: response of neutropenia to vincristine. J Clin Immunol 1981; 1:113–118.

Wedgwood RJ, Ochs HD, Oxelius VA: IgG subclass levels in the serum of patients with primary immunodeficiency. In: Hanson LA, Soderstrom T, Oxelius VA (eds). Immunoglobulin Subclass Deficiencies. Vol. 20, Basel: Karger, 1986:80–89.

Wen L, Pao W, Wong FS, Peng Q, Craft J, Zheng B, Kelsoe G, Dianda LXOM, Hayday AC: Germinal center formation, immunoglobulin class switching, and autoantibody production driven by "non α/β" T cells. J Exp Med 1996; 183:2271–2282.

West CD, Hong R, Holland NH: Immunoglobulin levels from the newborn period to adulthood and in immunoglobulin deficiency states. J Clin Invest 1962; 41:2054–2064.

White WB, Shornick JK, Grant Kels JM, Ballow M: Erythroderma with spongiotic dermatitis: association with common variable hypogammaglobulinemia. Am J Med 1985; 78:523–528.

Wilfert CM, Buckley RH, Mohanakumar T, Griffith JF, Katz SL, Whisnant JK, Eggleston PA, Moore M, Treadwell E, Oxman MN, Rosen FS: Persistent and fatal central-nervous-system echovirus infections in patients with agammaglobulinemia. N Engl J Med 1977; 296:1485–1489.

Williams A, Scott DL, Greenwood A, Huskisson EC: The clinical value of measuring immunoglobulins when assessing penicillamine therapy in rheumatoid arthritis. Clin Rheumatol 1988; 7:347–353.

Williams RT: Acquired dysgammaglobulinaemia in a young man. Clin Exp Immunol 1966; 1:223–231.

Wilton AN, Cobain TJ, Dawkins RL: Family studies of IgA deficiency. Immunogenetics 1985; 21:333–342.

Wolf R, Wolf D: Vitiligo and selective IgA deficiency. Cutis 1982; 30:249–251.

Wollheim FA, Williams RC, Jr.: Immunoglobulin studies in six kindreds of patients with adult hypogammaglobulinemia. J Lab Clin Med 1965; 66:433–445.

Wright JJ, Birx DL, Wagner DK, Waldmann TA, Blaese RM, Fleisher TA: Normalization of antibody responsiveness in a patient with common variable hypogammaglobulinemia and HIV infection. N Engl J Med 1987; 317:1516–1520.

Wu LYF, Lawton AR, Cooper MD: Differentiation capacity of cultured B lymphocytes by peripheral blood lymphocytes in severe hypogammaglobulinemia. J Clin Invest 1973; 52:3180–3189.

Yadav M, Iyngkaran N: Low incidence of selective IgA deficiency in normal Malaysians. Med J Malaysia 1979; 34:145–148.

Yamada H, Nagaoka I, Takamori K, Ogawa H: Double filtration plasmapheresis enhances neutrophil chemotactic responses in hyperimmunoglobulin E syndrome. Artif Organs 1995; 19:98–102.

Zora JA, Silk HJ, Tinkelman DG: Evaluation of postimmunization pneumococcal titers in children with recurrent infections and normal levels of immunoglobulin. Ann Allergy 1993; 70:283–288.

Part IV

GASTROINTESTINAL DISORDERS

13 Peptic Ulcer and Gastritis

A. S. PEÑA

Evidence obtained under different experimental conditions cannot be comprehended within a single picture, but must be regarded as complementary in the sense that only the totality of the phenomena exhausts the possible information about the objects.

Niels Bohr, view of quantum theory (*http://www-groups.dcs.st-and.ac.uk/~history/Mathematicians/Bohr_Niels.html*)

The concept of peptic ulcer and gastritis has changed since Marshall and Warren (1984) demonstrated the presence of a gram-negative bacterium in the form of spiral bacteria, *Helicobacter pylori*, under the mucus of human gastric mucosa. It is now known that infection with these bacteria is the main cause of human gastritis and the major cause of peptic ulcer. *H. pylori* eradication is followed by significant long-term improvements in gastric histology (Forbes et al., 1996). In fact, it has been argued that we should consider *H. pylori* gastroduodenitis as a disease in its own right, with ulcer and cancer as its important complications (Axon and Forman, 1997). At present, most peptic ulcers are caused by *H. pylori* infection in people over the age of 60, and the second major cause of peptic ulcer is nonsteroidal anti-inflammatory drugs (NSAIDs) (Langman et al., 1994). It remains a matter of controversy and research as well as an appropriate question for this chapter in a book of human genetics as to why, when half of the world's population is infected by *H. pylori*, only a minority of people develop peptic ulcer or gastric cancer. Similarly, only a minority of the approximately 14 million patients in the United States who regularly take NSAIDs for various types of arthritis (Roth and Bennett, 1987) develop peptic ulcer. In these cases, the role of *H. pylori* appears to be independent of the effects of NSAIDs on the gastric mucosa, as will be discussed later. The strongest evidence that *H. pylori* infection is the cause of peptic ulcer is that treatment with antibiotics alone is effective not only for the clearance and eradication of the infection but also for the healing of the ulcer. Therefore, the pathogenesis of the ulcer is determined and probably follows the same principles of any infectious disease. The bacteria and the host form an interactive unit. The bacteria have to undergo evolutionary changes that are needed to survive the host response. Different strains are more virulent than others. In fact, *H. pylori* strains appear to be highly diverse (Logan and Berg, 1996), and new insights into the mechanisms that control the host response will determine the development of disease. Therefore, the pathogen and the host must be studied together; but in spite of significant advances in the fields of molecular genetics, cell biology, and molecular biology, this cannot and has not been done yet. Most of the information that we have is on the genetics of the bacteria. The lack of knowledge on the genetic host response to *H. pylori* gives us fragmentary knowledge that cannot be comprehended within a single picture. Blaser and Kirschner (1999) developed a mathematical model that incorporates the development of the host response concurrent with the establishment of *H. pylori*. They assumed that the major nutrient source for *H. pylori* results from inflammation and its exudates into the gastric lumen. Thus, the host response could include many possible factors, such as innate and adaptive immunity, as well as other mechanisms, such as iron sequestration. The capacity of the host to respond to the bacteria is critical to the colonization level and shows great heterogeneity, compatible with the heterogeneity of human response genes. Another factor is the growth rate of the host response, which affects the time to reach steady state and the size of the bacterial population. The model also assumes that if the bacteria cannot be eradicated by microbial evasion strategies, downregulation of the host response is beneficial to the host (Blaser, 1997). This is the situation in the majority of individuals infected by *H. pylori*. Host acid-secretory status and sensitivity to gastrin can be modulated by *H. pylori* infection, as will be discussed below. Once *H. pylori* has established itself in the stomach, virtually every patient develops gastritis, and variations in gastritis patterns have been associated with different gastric acid responses to *H. pylori* infection. The patterns of gastritis are important because they seem to determine disease outcome (Go, 1997; Sipponen and Hyvarinen, 1993). Also, the age at which the host acquires the infection appears to determine the outcome of the interaction between *H. pylori* and the host (Blaser, 1998). Figures 13–1 to 13–4 illustrate the different types of gastric mucosa found in the healthy human stomach (Figs. 13–1, 13–2) and some forms of gastritis (Figs. 13–3, 13–4).

GENERAL GENETIC AND EPIDEMIOLOGICAL EVIDENCE

Disease Definition

A peptic ulcer is a circumscribed inflammatory wound occurring in those parts of the gastrointestinal tract exposed to acid and pepsin, i.e., the lower esophagus, stomach, and upper intestine (duodenum). The vast majority of peptic ulcers are thus either

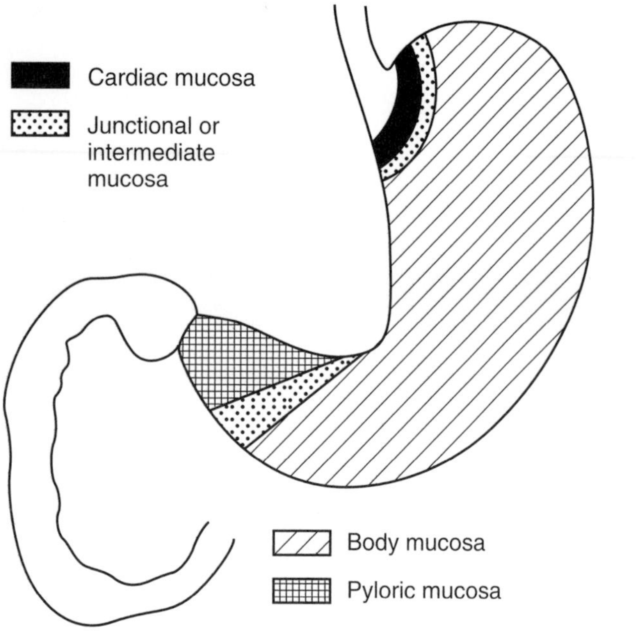

Fig. 13–1. Different types of gastric mucosa that occur in the healthy human stomach and their distribution. From Roca (1975) with permission.

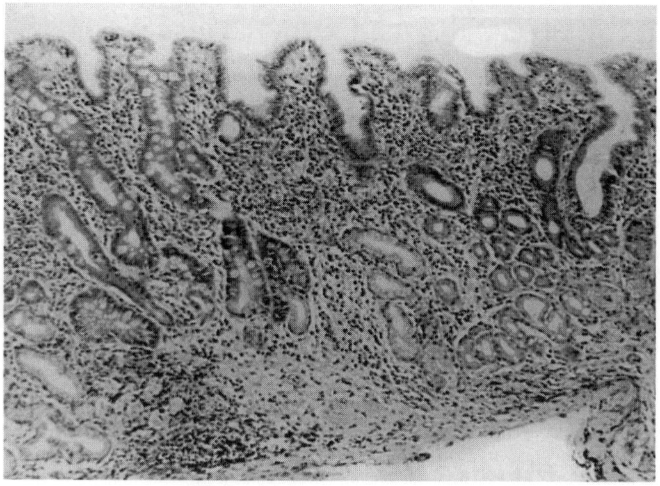

Fig. 13–3. Pyloric mucosa showing moderate atrophic gastritis. From Roca (1975) with permission.

gastric (occurring in the stomach) or *duodenal* (occurring in the first portion of the small intestine). Most duodenal ulcers occur within 1 to 2 cm of the pylorus. The concept that it is an inflammatory wound is important in understanding the pathogenesis. It invokes the inflammatory mechanisms not only of tissue destruction but also those of tissue repair.

The typical symptom of a peptic ulcer is epigastric abdominal pain that is worse at night and relieved by meals. This classic symptom occurs only in a portion of all ulcer patients. Many patients present with less classic abdominal pain but with the complications of ulcer, e.g., bleeding into the gastrointestinal tract. This can be in the form of chronic blood loss or occasionally a severe life-threatening hemorrhage. Another complication with a bad prognosis is *perforation*, penetration of the ulcer through the full thickness of the gastrointestinal tract wall. Occasionally, obstruction of gastric emptying is due to scarring, edema, and spasm of the pyloric channel. When this occurs, it may lead to obstruction and emaciation.

The diagnosis of a peptic ulcer is made by direct visualization using endoscopy and/or double-contrast barium. Giant duodenal ulcers are difficult to recognize and prone to perforation and massive hemorrhage. The radiologist plays an important role in making the correct diagnosis in these cases. Computed tomographic (CT) scanning has become an important tool in the diagnosis and management of diseases that affect the stomach and duodenum. By depicting the bowel lumen, wall, and extramural structures, CT can provide unique information that complements standard air contrast radiography and endoscopy. Proper scanning methods and knowledge of normal anatomy are necessary for optimal results. Some radiologists utilize the gas contrast technique for organ-specific examination in patients with known or suspected gastroduodenal disease. Gastric adenocarcinoma is an important indication for CT evaluation (Scatarige and DiSantis, 1989).

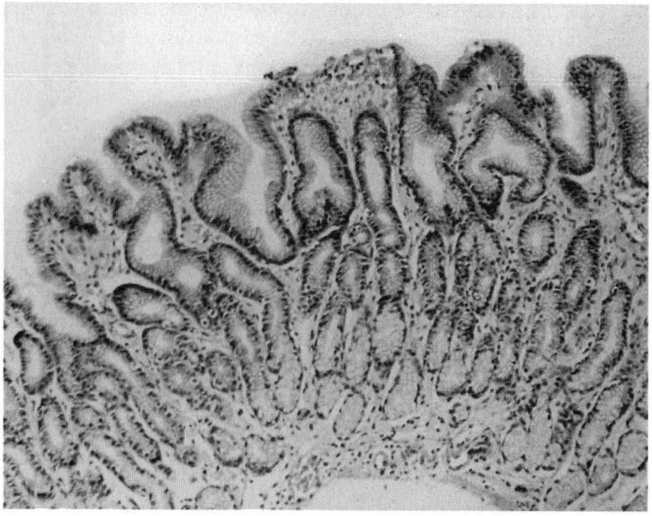

Fig. 13–2. Normal pyloric mucosa. The gastric pits are deeper and sometimes branched, while the glands are shorter and less tightly packed than in the body. From Roca (1975) with permission.

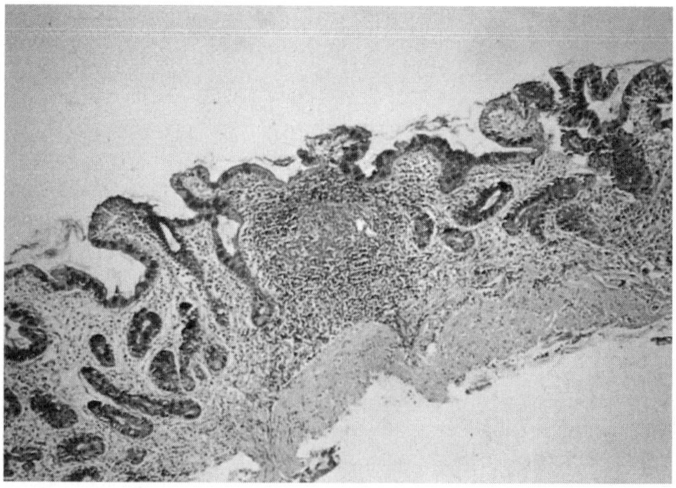

Fig. 13–4. Body mucosa showing atrophy and complete intestinalization. From Roca (1975) with permission.

The presence of *H. pylori* bacteria and the ingestion of NSAIDs have modified the concept of pathogenesis. The imbalance between the "aggressive" forces of acid and pepsin and the less well-defined "defensive" forces of mucosal resistance and regeneration is now seen as a secondary factor. Therefore, the goal of ulcer therapy is to eradicate the bacteria. The National Institutes of Health (1994) recommended antibiotic treatment of *H. pylori* for patients with gastroduodenal ulcers. In case of NSAID use, if these drugs cannot be stopped, the concomitant use of agents as gastroprotectives, misoprostol (Levine, 1995; Silverstein, 1998), H2 receptor antagonists for inhibition of acid secretion (Taha et al., 1996), or proton pump inhibitors (Hawkey et al., 1998; Yeomans et al., 1998) is indicated. When peptic ulcer has been induced by NSAIDs, eradication of *H. pylori* is not indicated; however, introduction of cyclo-oxygenase 2 antagonists may lead to modification of this advice (Hawkey, 1999).

Clinical Epidemiological and Ethnic Differences

Prevalence

Peptic ulcer is among the most common of the chronic diseases, occurring in 2% to 10% of the population (lifetime prevalence), depending on such factors as geography, the specific population, and level of health care (Kurata and Haile, 1984).

Rosenstock et al. (1996), in Denmark, examined the relationship between housing conditions, educational level, occupational factors, and serologically diagnosed acute and chronic *H. pylori* infection. They found an increased likelihood of chronic *H. pylori* infection in patients with a low socioeconomic level, a short duration of schooling, and lack of training/education; in unskilled workers; and in those with a high work-related energy expenditure. Some of the epidemiological factors found in peptic ulcer are due to these educational and occupational factors, which relate to the likelihood of chronic *H. pylori* infection. However, for the development of peptic ulcer, other permissive or associated cofactors are necessary. For example, peptic ulcer disease is twice as common in southern China compared with northern China; however, the overall *H. pylori* prevalence rate is similar in both populations (Ching and Lam, 1994; Wong et al., 1998).

The best available estimate of the point prevalence of peptic ulcer disease is based on an endoscopic survey of 358 subjects in Finland as part of a study of gastric carcinoma (Ihamaki et al., 1979). The prevalence of endoscopically verified peptic ulcer or ulcer scar was 5.9%. Active gastric ulcers were found in 0.28% and active duodenal ulcers in 1.4% of this population. This 5:1 ratio of duodenal to gastric ulcer is comparable to the ratio of 4:1 found in other studies (Pulvertaft, 1968). Similar prevalence figures were found in a nationwide population-based cohort of adult twins in Finland. The prevalence of peptic ulcer was 6.2% in men and 2.8% in women in 1975 (Räihä et al., 1998). The prevalence of ulcer disease in the western part of Scotland is about twice that in England and coincides with a high prevalence of *H. pylori* infection (Knill-Jones, 1991). Ulcer frequency is higher in the winter months, and this appears to be universal, being true in cold as well as in warm countries. Most places report a rise of ulcer rates among the elderly in recent decades. The male:female ratio also varies geographically: e.g., from 1:1 in the United States to 18:1 in India. In the last two decades in the United States, the male:female ratio has changed from 2:1 to 1:1. The duodenal ulcer:gastric ulcer ratio varies widely from place to place: e.g., from 0:8 in Japan to 19:1 in Africa and 32:1 in India. Placebo healing rates also differ geographically, ranging from 5% in the Philippines to 78% in Mexico (Lam, 1993). The time trends of gastric and duodenal ulcers during the past three decades are characterized by a notable decline in incidence and prevalence rates. This decline occurred in the United States, as well as in many European countries (Sonnenberg, 1995). Peptic ulcer has decreased continuously during the past 25 years in the United States. Figure 13–5 shows the time trends of death rates from gastric ulcer, duodenal ulcer, and erosive esophagitis for the period 1970 to 1995 (el-Serag and Sonnenberg, 1998). Similar trends have been observed in the United Kingdom (Bloom et al., 1990). In spite of these trends, increasing hospitalization and mortality rates from peptic ulcer complications have been reported from 1981 to 1993, particularly in elderly Danish people (Andersen et al., 1998). The incidence of *H. pylori* infection continues to be high (3%–10% per

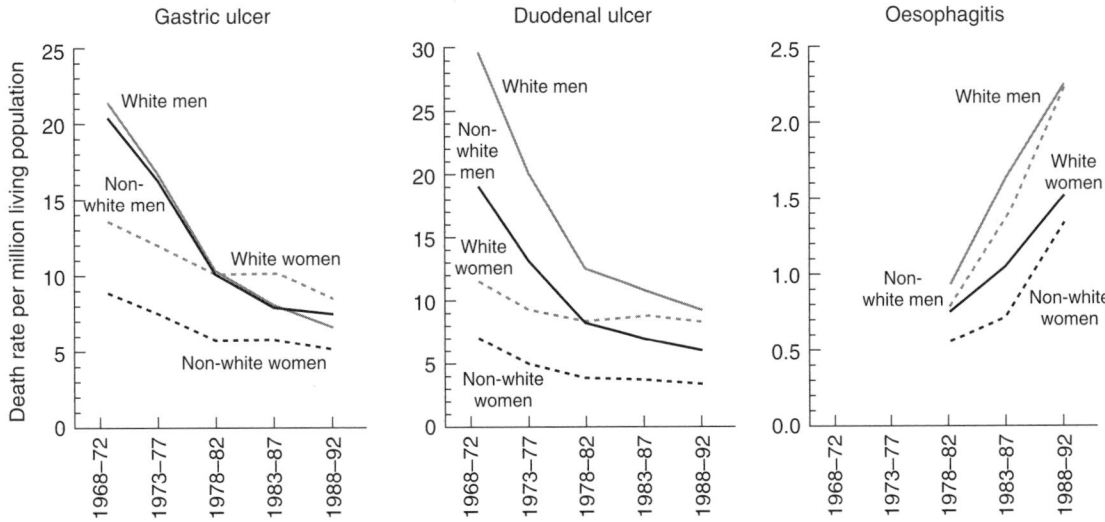

Fig. 13–5. Time trends of death rates from gastric ulcer, duodenal ulcer, and erosive esophagitis. From 1970 to 1995, hospitalization rates for gastric and duodenal ulcer as well as gastric cancer fell, while rates for gastroesophageal reflux disease rose significantly. Similar time trends were observed with respect to the death rates, as shown. Database of the U.S. Department of Veterans Affairs. Data points represent the average of consecutive time periods as shown on the *x* axis. From El-Serag and Sonnenberg (1998) with permission.

year) in developing countries. Throughout the world, the incidence of *H. pylori* infection appears to be higher in children than in adults, possibly due to lower standards of personal hygiene in younger populations (Parsonnet, 1995).

The findings obtained by prevalence studies strongly support multiple etiological factors. It is clear that, in addition to *H. pylori*, analgesics, work and social stress, cigarette smoking, dietary factors, and genetic factors have to be taken into account.

Incidence

Incidence rates obtained by Kurata and co-workers (1985a,b) in a large health maintenance organization in California were 0.024% for gastric ulcer and 0.062% for duodenal ulcer. A similar incidence of peptic ulcer diagnosed by X-ray, endoscopy, surgery, or necropsy in persons over 15 years of age living in Copenhagen County, Denmark, from 1963 to 1968 was reported in 1975; the annual incidence was 0.13% for duodenal ulcer, 0.03% for gastric ulcer, and 0.02% for combined duodenal and gastric ulcers (Bonnevie, 1975a,b). However, higher incidence rates have been reported in populations characterized by crowded housing and poor sanitation. For example, the average annual (1989–1993) age-adjusted incidence rate for hospitalization associated with a diagnosis of gastric and duodenal ulcer combined was 0.39% in the Indian population of Manitoba in Canada (Bernstein et al., 1999). *H. pylori* is consistently linked to conditions associated with residential crowding in childhood (Goodman and Correa, 1995).

Both gastric and duodenal ulcer rates increase with age (Kurata et al., 1985a,b). In the Danish studies, the incidence of duodenal ulcer increased almost linearly with age, reaching 0.3% in males over the age of 75. For gastric ulcer, the incidence was low before age 40 in males and reached its peak for those aged 60 to 64, while in women it increased with increasing age (Bonnevie, 1975a,b). Similar findings were reported from the United States: the age-specific incidence rates for duodenal ulcer increased from age 15, and the incidence rates for gastric ulcer increased until the fifth decade, leveled off, and then markedly increased at age 80 and above (Kurata et al., 1985a,b).

Results from a recent large, multicenter study in Britain suggest that about 40% of the 10,000 peptic ulcer bleeds that occurred in people over age 60 are related to drug treatment (Langman et al., 1994). In a high proportion, however, *H. pylori* infection probably also plays a part. A conservative estimate is that 65% of the mentioned 40% bleeding episodes are attributable to *H. pylori*.

The rate of *H. pylori* infection is inversely related to socioeconomic status. Childhood is the major acquisition period, as was demonstrated in a cross-sectional study of monozygotic and dizygotic twins who were reared apart or together in Sweden (Malaty et al., 1998). Among monozygotic twins reared apart and discordant for *H. pylori* status, infected twins were raised in homes under poorer socioeconomic conditions than those of their unaffected co-twins ($p = 0.02$). The density of the childhood home was consistently associated with acquisition of *H. pylori* infection ($p = 0.04$). This study confirmed the hypothesis that childhood acquisition of *H. pylori* infection is linked to hygiene practices. However, as will become clearer later, the incidence of peptic ulcer in families is greatly dependent on genetic factors that are independent of the presence of *H. pylori* infection.

Sex Differences

It has been repeatedly reported that twice as many men as women have peptic ulcers. In 1968, prevalence, hospitalization, and mortality measures in the United States showed a 2:1 ratio of men to women (Kurata et al., 1985a,b). Two decades later, changes in the rates for both males and females were reported. One-year prevalence data obtained through interviews showed that rates for males have decreased from 2.3% to 1.8% while rates for females have increased from 1.1% to 1.7%. Additionally, while for females there has been an increase in the reported period prevalence, hospitalizations and mortality data show small decreases. In males, however, all three measures of ulcer disease show a decrease. The data suggest that there may have been a real increase in peptic ulcer prevalence for women because of an increase in either incidence or disease duration. These changes are most likely caused by changes in various environmental exposures for females (Kurata et al., 1985b). Possibilities include increased smoking and a higher number of women entering the labor force. In favor of this hypothesis are the findings of a retrospective study of endoscopy in patients in northern Italy from 1981 to 1985: the number of confirmed duodenal ulcers exceeded that of gastric ulcers by a ratio of 6.6:1, and most of the confirmed duodenal ulcers were in males who smoked (Pelissero and Sategna-Guidetti, 1989). In Finland, however, the significant predictors of peptic ulcer were smoking and stress in men and the use of analgesics in women (Räihä et al., 1998).

Svanes et al. (1999) assessed the causes of death in patients treated for peptic ulcer perforation in western Norway during the period 1962–1990 and found that an excess mortality from lung cancer and from circulatory diseases that was higher in male than in female patients. This could be attributed mainly to smoking-related diseases. It is indirect evidence that smoking is an etiological factor of importance for ulcer perforation, which would explain the sex differences that have been recorded.

Ethnic Differences

For many years ethnic differences have been attributed to differences in the environment and changes in them have been attributed to the westernization of dietary habits. However, it was noted, e.g., that the increased incidence of duodenal ulcer in individuals whose origin is the Indian subcontinent is maintained in other countries (Robbs and Moshal, 1979). This observation may be explained by the presence of *H. pylori* in those individuals who usually emigrate with the entire family. A different situation appears to have occurred in European migrant workers in the 1970s since these were mainly males in the active part of life (20–40 years of age) who migrated from south to central and northern Europe to find work opportunities. Studies in Germany showed that chronic atrophic antral gastritis occurs in foreigners twice as often as in a comparative group of Germans, 77% of the duodenal ulcers and 88% of the gastric ulcers being found in the group of foreign workers examined aged 21 to 40 years (Horn and Herfarth, 1978; Quaquish et al., 1979). In those days, it was not possible to study the presence of *H. pylori* and to determine the specific strains that the immigrants carried, although the possible effects of other stressful environmental changes cannot be ruled out. Later a similar phenomenon was observed in black populations in South Africa (Moshal et al., 1981). Duodenal ulcer was not common in rural black South African communities. However, the number of Africans in the cities presenting with duodenal ulcer has steadily increased over the past 50 years. For example, in the Baragwanath Hospital in Johannesburg, the duodenal ulcer patients were primarily young men who were urbanized, more educated, and from higher socioeconomic classes compared with matched and unmatched samples of patients without gastrointestinal conditions in the same hospital (Segal et al., 1978).

Geographical Differences

Although peptic ulcer disease is declining in the developing world, it still occurs worldwide. In the Third World, there are areas where the incidence has always been high, e.g., certain parts of Africa and India, and areas where it is low. There are ethnic differences in the prevalence and clinical features of peptic ulcer in most Western countries. Duodenal ulcer is more prevalent than gastric ulcer. The opposite occurs in Japan, Korea (Watanabe et al., 1992), and certain isolated ethnic groups, such as inhabitants of the Faroe Islands (Kiaer et al., 1985).

The risk of developing peptic ulcer has risen in those generations born before the turn of the twentieth century and declined in all subsequent generations. The birth cohorts with the highest risk of developing gastric ulcer were born 10 to 20 years before those with the highest risk for duodenal ulcer. The birth-cohort pattern of peptic ulcer disease is similar in all European countries, the United States, Australia, and Japan. In gastric ulcer, the birth-related risk involves all ages over 5 years, while in duodenal ulcer it does not start before the age of 15 years. Gastric and duodenal ulcers are characterized by marked geographical variations that are similar for both types. Both sexes and all age groups older than 5 in the case of gastric ulcer and older than 15 in the case of duodenal ulcer share the similarity in geographical variation. The existence of a birth-cohort phenomenon implies that exogenous risk factors are responsible for the occurrence of peptic ulcer and that subjects are exposed to these risk factors during a limited period of childhood or early adulthood (Sonnenberg, 1995). A study in Britain found that absence of a fixed hot-water supply ($p = 0.0005$) and domestic crowding ($p = 0.0005$) in childhood were powerful independent risk factors for current infection with *H. pylori*. Among current living conditions, only the number of children living in the household was independently associated with *H. pylori* infection ($p = 0.004$) (Mendall et al., 1992).

According to epidemiological studies in Western countries during the second half of the nineteenth century, gastric ulcers were common and duodenal ulcers rare. Since the turn of the twentieth century, the prevalence of duodenal ulcer has increased sharply (Sonnenberg, 1993) and the frequency of gastric ulcer has decreased markedly. The same has been observed in Japan (Kawai et al., 1989). Patients with increased acid output have antral-predominant gastritis and are more likely to develop duodenal ulcers, whereas patients with low acid output have widespread inflammation involving the antrum and body of the stomach. Progression of *H. pylori*–induced body gastritis does not take place in individuals who are at the high end of the range of acid secretion. The bacterium is largely contained in the antrum by the high acid output of the corpus. These observations led to the proposal that the influence of *H. pylori* on production of gastric or peptic ulcer is dependent on local acid levels (Dixon, 1993; Lee et al., 1995). According to this hypothesis, *H. pylori*, although highly adapted for survival and growth in gastric acid, can flourish only on epithelium in which local acid levels are in the optimal range for the bacterium. A refinement of this hypothesis has been proposed (Veldhuyzen van Zanten et al., 1999). Both gastric and duodenal ulcers are located immediately adjacent to the transitional zones with a different type of mucosa, i.e., antral-body, body-cardia, and antrum-duodenum. As stated above, patients who are prone to develop duodenal ulcers have antral-predominant gastritis. The gastritis is confined to the antrum by high local acid levels at the antral-body transitional zone. Some bacterial colonization of body mucosa will occur, but any inflammation is generally superficial and does not progress. The existing high or high normal acid output may be increased further by the exaggerated gastrin response in the antrum. The net result is an increased acid load passing through the pylorus, which induces the formation of gastric metaplasia in the duodenum. Gastric metaplasia can be considered a distal extension of the antroduodenal transitional zone and will facilitate the spread of *H. pylori* infection from antrum to duodenum, thereby inducing a cascade of inflammation, duodenitis, and possibly ulceration. As a consequence, duodenal ulcers are located near the antroduodenal transitional zone (Veldhuyzen van Zanten et al., 1999).

Hypochlorhydria is markedly more frequent in Peru than in the United Kingdom (Recavarren-Arce et al., 1992). From an epidemiological review of the literature in Europe, it can be concluded that acquisition of *H. pylori* is the main cause of chronic gastritis in humans. In Europe, a small proportion (<1%) of gastritis cases are caused by *H. heilmannii* and somewhat more (5%) are of autoimmune origin. In the latter condition, *H. pylori* probably plays an indirect role.

Sipponen (1997) has summarized the epidemiological findings on chronic gastritis and *H. pylori* acquisition in developed countries: *(1)* *H. pylori* gastritis is acquired in childhood and adolescence (age >20) in more than 50% of the cases; *(2)* the risk and rate of acquisition are highest in early childhood, after which the rate exponentially declines; *(3)* new infections occur in adulthood but are quite rare (Kuipers et al., 1993); *(4)* *H. pylori* gastritis is a birth cohort–related phenomenon, i.e., rate and prevalence vary between cohorts; *(5)* the rate and risk of *H. pylori* infection are high in cohorts born at the beginning of the century but much lower in individuals born later; *(6)* this decline is due to a decrease in the rate and risk of *H. pylori* acquisition in childhood in particular. *H. pylori* gastritis–related complications, such as peptic ulcer diseases and gastric cancer, show epidemiological features similar to *H. pylori* gastritis. Both peptic ulcer and gastric cancer have declined in incidence over time. Sipponen (1997) has further suggested that gastric cancer is a birth-cohort phenomenon in the same way as *H. pylori* gastritis. The incidence of gastric cancer shows a positive but exponential relationship with the birth cohort-specific prevalence of gastritis in the general population. These observations explain the low prevalence of duodenal ulcer and gastric metaplasia in many developing countries despite a higher prevalence of *H. pylori*–associated gastritis. The age and geographical distributions of infection are changing with improvements in living conditions, particularly in the childhood period. More than one mode and route of transmission is possible, varying with local customs and practices. Infection may be acquired from environmental sources in certain parts of the developing world, but in most circumstances, it is probably acquired interpersonally (Mendall, 1997).

Family and Twin Studies

Family Studies

Several studies in the 1950s to the 1970s established that 20% to 50% of individuals with peptic ulcer have a positive family history in comparison with 5% to 15% of controls. Based on these studies, the prevalence of peptic ulcer, duodenal ulcer, and gastric ulcer in specific relatives compared to the prevalence among similar relatives of a control group gives a frequency of peptic ulcer two to three times greater in the first-degree relatives of peptic ulcer patients (Tarpila et al., 1982; Rotter et al., 1992). Later studies, using epidemiology, radiology, or endoscopy and histology, have confirmed these findings. In the northern part of Norway, statistically significant increased familial occurrences of peptic ulcer were found in relatives of patients with gastric or duodenal ulcer compared to the control group. The calculated relative risk (RR) of developing gastric or duodenal ulcer in patients with a positive family history was higher than in patients without a family history (Ostensen et al., 1985). In another study, the first-degree relatives of duodenal ulcer patients and of control probands were evaluated clinically and by gastroduodenal endoscopy for prevalence of duodenal ulcer. Endoscopic evidence of present or past duodenal or pyloric ulcer was found in 20 (13.0%) of the relatives of duodenal ulcer patients and in only 6 (3.9%) of the control relatives ($p <$ 0.01). The frequency of macroscopic duodenitis and gastric erosions was also significantly higher ($p < 0.05$) in relatives of patients than in those of controls. A history of epigastric pain was obtained in 54 (35.1%) endoscoped patient relatives and in 24 (15.6%) control relatives ($p < 0.01$). Thus, this study showed an increased prevalence of duodenal ulcer in the first-degree relatives of duodenal ulcer patients. The finding that duodenitis is also more prevalent in patient relatives than in controls supports the view that duodenitis is linked with duodenal ulcer (Tarpila et al., 1982).

Familiality of H. pylori and Relation to Ulcer

Several authors have demonstrated intrafamilial spread of *H. pylori* infection (Drumm et al., 1990; Valle et al., 1991; Graham et al., 1994). In a large family study in Finland of 59 duodenal ulcer probands (Valle et al., 1991), *H. pylori* was determined in 51 duodenal ulcer patients and 155 relatives and in 155 controls, matched by age and sex from a family sample representing the same geographical area. However, most of the children and parents remained without controls. The occurrence and score of *H. pylori* density showed an excellent correlation with the morphology of the mucosa, signs of acute inflammation, and the presence of gastric metaplasia in the duodenal bulb. The prevalence of *H. pylori* was 94% in probands with duodenal ulcer, which was significantly higher than in their relatives (56%) and controls (48%). The prevalence of *H. pylori* in their sibs was 64%, also significantly higher than in controls (51%). There was a subgroup of sibs with signs of active or past duodenal ulcer disease. These sibs had a higher than expected prevalence of *H. pylori.* Also, they had acid hypersecretion and high levels of serum pepsinogen I. This study clearly showed that the occurrence of *H. pylori* as well as of high-peak acid output and pepsinogen I levels should be considered as risk factors for duodenal ulcer in close relatives of probands with duodenal ulcer (Valle et al., 1991).

Among the close family members of a 12–year-old boy who developed a massive hemorrhage of a duodenal ulcer, two asymptomatic siblings were infected, as determined serologically, by C-13-urea breath test, and by histology. DNA fingerprinting using restriction endonucleases showed that all three children harbored an identical bacterial strain, indicating either cross-infection between the siblings or a common source. The authors suggested that the mother was the most likely source of this organism, considering that she had a history of peptic ulcer. The sister of the index patient had active and erosive gastritis, and his brother had nonactive gastritis only. This suggests that not only virulent strains of these bacteria but also host factors may be important for the ulcer pathogenesis (Dyrek et al., 1997). These observations are similar to those reported from studies in families when the probands are adults (van der Ende et al., 1996). These findings together with the increased familial clustering of *H. pylori* antibodies in families of *H. pylori*-positive children (Drumm et al., 1990) probably explain the well-established observations that the family history of a child with duodenal ulcer is frequently positive for ulcer disease in first-degree relatives. These results suggest that parent-to-child transmission and common infection sources are probable causes of intrafamilial clustering of *H. pylori* (Wang et al., 1993).

Spouses of patients with duodenal ulcer had a significantly higher seroprevalence of *H. pylori* infection than controls (71% vs. 58%, $p < 0.05$); at endoscopy, *H. pylori* infection was confirmed in 48 of 49 (98%) seropositive spouses. Endoscopic findings in these spouses showed active duodenal ulcer in 8 (17%), duodenal scar and cap deformity in 2 (4%), active gastric ulcer in 2 (4%), erosive duodenitis in 3 (6%), antral erosions in 2 (4%), antral erosions plus duodenitis in 1, and peptic esophagitis in 1. The prevalence of major endoscopic lesions was significantly higher in symptomatic spouses than in those who had never been symptomatic (Parente et al., 1996) (Table 13–1). These studies indicate that person-to-person spread of these bacteria may exist, and the fact that different members of the same family are infected by similar strains (Drumm et al., 1990; Bamford et al., 1993; Kalach et al., 1999) supports this possibility. Conjugal transmission has been demonstrated among 110 employees of a health insurance company and their partners. A very strong relation between partners' infection status persisted after control for age and other potential confounders: the adjusted odds ratio (OR) was 7.0 [95% confidence interval (CI) 1.8–26.7], and the risk of infection increased with the number of years lived with an infected partner (Brenner et al., 1999). These observations strongly point to the influence of environmental factors, including *H. pylori*, in disease pathogenesis. It is possible that peak acid output and pepsinogen I levels are a consequence of the infection or that other genetic and/or environmental factors contribute to regulate their levels. This will be discussed below.

Twin Studies

Comparison of monozygotic and dizygotic twins provides clues as to the magnitude of genetic factors (Koskenvuo et al., 1992). Several early studies established that the prevalence of peptic ul-

Table 13–1. Peptic Ulcer in Families and Familiality of *H. pylori* and Relation to Ulcer

	DU Relatives	Control Relatives	DU Sibs	Control Sibs	Spouse of DU	Spouse of Control	References
DU	13.0%	3.9%					Tarpila et al. (1982)
H. pylori	56%	48%	64%	51%			Valle et al. (1991)
H. pylori					71%	58%	Parente et al. (1996)
DU					21%		
GU					4%		

DU, present or past duodenal or pyloric ulcer; GU, gastric ulcer.

Table 13–2. Peptic Ulcer in an Unselected Nationwide Twin Population Study in Finland: Age-Adjusted Relative Risk (RR) and 95% Confidence Interval (CI) Compared with the General Population Risk

	Monozygotic Twins (n = 63) RR (95% CI)	Dizygotic Twins (n = 86) RR (95% CI)
Men	2.7 (2.0–3.6)	1.7 (1.4–2.2)
Women	2.7 (1.6–4.5)	1.2 (0.7–1.9)

Source: Räihä et al. (1998).

cer is higher in monozygotic twins than in dizygotic twins. Long-term clinical and radiological follow-up after initial diagnosis revealed that the ulcer site was usually concordant when both members of a twin pair were affected; i.e., both had either gastric or duodenal ulcer (Rotter et al., 1992). The concordance for monozygotic twins of the early studies based on X-rays varied between 14.3% and 52.6% vs. 6.3% and 35.7% for dizygotic twins, as summarized by Rotter et al. (1992).

Two studies have investigated the presence of environmental factors in twins in relation to peptic ulcers. The first consisted of 300 twins from a subregistry of the Swedish Twin Registry (Malaty et al., 1994). *H. pylori* status was evaluated using an enzyme-linked immunosorbent assay for anti-*H. pylori* immunoglobulin G (IgG). The probandwise concordance rate for *H. pylori* infection was higher in monozygotic twin pairs (81%) than in dizygotic twin pairs (63%) (p = 0.001) (Malaty et al., 1994). Probandwise concordance rates for *H. pylori* infection among 124 pairs of twins reared apart were 82% and 66% for monozygotic and dizygotic twins, respectively (p = 0.003). The heritability upon acquisition of *H. pylori* infection was approximately 0.66. The remaining variance was accounted for by shared rearing environmental factors (20%) and nonshared environmental factors (23%) (Malaty et al., 1994). The second study, based on a nationwide population-based cohort of adult twins in Finland born before 1958 with both twins alive in 1975, examined the concordance for peptic ulcer disease in monozygotic and dizygotic twins (Räihä et al., 1998). There were 63 monozygotic and 86 dizygotic pairs concordant for peptic ulcer disease. Table 13–2 shows the age-adjusted RR when one twin had peptic ulcer compared with the general population risk (Räihä et al., 1998). Thirty-nine percent (95% CI 32%–47%) of the liability to peptic ulcer disease was explained by genetic factors and 61% (95% CI 53%–68%) by individual environmental factors. In the incidence study (logistic regression analysis of the entire cohort initially free of peptic ulcer disease, with subjects diagnosed as having peptic ulcer after 1975), current smoking (RR = 2.2, 95% CI 1.5–3.2) and high stress levels (RR = 3.2, 95% CI 1.4–7.6) in men and regular use of analgesics (RR = 3.3, 95% CI 1.3–8.1) in women predicted peptic ulcer disease during the follow-up from 1976 to 1991. In the analysis of discordant pairs, smoking in men and regular use of analgesics in both sexes were predictors of peptic ulcer disease (Räihä et al., 1998). The higher concordance rate for peptic ulcer among monozygotic compared with dizygotic twins in this and previous studies indicates a genetic liability. This liability is not affected by sex, and it represents approximately 40% of the risk attributable to genetic factors according to the Finnish investigators.

How, then, can we understand the observations on genetic factors reviewed above in families and twins? The contribution of a family history of peptic ulcer and infection with *H. pylori* has been quantified in a cross-sectional study among 299 consecutive outpatients of a general practitioner in Germany. The adjusted ORs and 95% CIs for gastroscopically verified peptic ulcer were 3.8 (1.4–10.1) for persons with *H. pylori* infection, 8.4 (2.9–24.1) for persons with a family history of ulcer, and 29.5 (6.1–143.9) for persons with both risk factors compared to persons without these risk factors (Brenner et al., 1998a,b). In another large study of 863 children, German investigators found that the prevalence of infection was more than double among children whose mothers had a history of gastric or duodenal ulcer than among those whose mothers had no such history (OR = 2.4, 98% CI 0.9–6.4) (Brenner et al., 1998a,b). Table 13–3 shows

Table 13–3. Individual and Joint Relationships of Infection with *H. pylori* and Family History of Peptic Ulcer

H. pylori Infection	Family History	No.	Children Infected with *H. pylori* (%)	Peptic Ulcer (%)	Odds Ratio[a] (95% Confidence Interval)
No		22		4.1	1.0
		0			
Yes		79		12.7	3.8 (1.4–10.1)
	No	25		3.9	1.0
		8			
	Yes	41		22.0	8.4 (2.9–24.1)
No	No	19		2.6	1.0
		5			
Yes	No	63		7.9	3.7 (1.0–14.0)
No	Yes	25		16.0	8.4 (1.9–36.4)
Yes	Yes	16		31.3	29.5 (6.1–143.9)
	Mother No		13		1.0[b]
	Mother Yes		27		11.7 (3.8–36.2)[b]
	Father No		14		1.0[b]
	Father Yes		18		1.6 (0.4–5.5)[b]

[a]Adjusted for sex, age, and smoking by multiple logistic regression.
[b]Adjusted for nationality, mother's education, father's education, housing density, birth order, history of breast-feeding, attendance at nursery, antibiotic treatment, and history of ulcer in the other parent.
Source: Brenner et al. (1998a,b).

the individual and joint relationships of infection with *H. pylori* and of family history of peptic ulcer.

Another observation pointing to the importance of genetic susceptibility is the mutually exclusive presence of certain viruses and *H. pylori*. Peptic ulceration is rare in human immunodeficiency virus (HIV) infection and is frequently due to cytomegalovirus; of 497 HIV$^+$ patients with upper digestive tract symptoms, 23 (5%) had peptic ulcers at upper endoscopy with cytomegalovirus as the only organism significantly associated with peptic ulcer (Logan et al., 1990; Vaira et al., 1995; Varsky et al., 1998). Also, the prevalence of *H. pylori* with another member of the human retrovirus family, human T-cell leukemia virus type I (HTLV-I), in an endemic area of Japan has been found to be significantly low. The seroprevalence of *H. pylori* was 48% in 146 HTLV-I$^+$ individuals vs. 64% of 282 HTLV-I$^-$ controls ($p < 0.01$) (Isomoto et al., 1999).

Table 13–4. The Genetic Control of Inflammation

Innate immunity
LPS and Toll Like Receptors (TLRs)
Adherence molecules, Lewis antigens
Acquired immunity
Experimental animal models
"High" responders
"Low" responders
Proinflammatory response Th1
Host response in humans
Proinflammatory response Th1
Chemokines
Immunogenetics of response
Cytokine gene polymorphisms
Major histocompatibility complex
Genetics of adherence
ABO, secretor status, Lewis antigens

BIOLOGICAL BASIS OF GENETIC SUSCEPTIBILITY AND DISEASE SEVERITY

Three environmental factors have been identified as major risk factors for peptic ulcer in numerous clinical and epidemiological studies: *H. pylori*, NSAIDs, and cigarette smoking. The general population-attributable risks were 48% for *H. pylori*, 24% for NSAIDs, and 23% for cigarette smoking in a meta-analysis of English-language studies of risk for peptic ulcer–related gastrointestinal events (Kurata and Nogawa, 1997). What, then, is the biological basis of the susceptibility to acquire the infection and what determines the pattern of disease and its severity? Can the genetic factors of the host explain the heterogeneity of the response, and is this heterogeneity due to different strains of *H. pylori?* Observations reported in the last decade indicate that genetic host factors are important in determining the type and the severity of the disease.

Genetic Control of Inflammation

The host response is important for the immune defense against a variety of infections and to protect the organism against the invasion of foreign material. In the gastrointestinal tract, a fine balance exists between the microbial flora and the extraneous proteins that are meant to help the individual in its survival and its immune defense. It is probably survival that determines the genetic host response. Table 13–4 summarizes the different aspects relevant to the complex control of the immune response. It is important to recognize that immunity to infection is mediated by two systems, the innate and the acquired systems. Innate immunity provides a rapid antimicrobial host defense and probably determines to which antigens the acquired immune system will respond (Fearon and Locksley, 1996). The genes controlling these systems are different and probably work in a complementary fashion. Innate systems use germline-encoded proteins to identify microbial substances (Fearon, 1997).

Experimental animal models have provided evidence that the host response is an important determinant in the severity of gastritis and demonstrated the importance of the innate immune system. *H. felis* induces severe inflammation and gastric atrophy in certain strains of mice, such as C3H/He and SJL, whereas in other strains, such as C3H/HeJ and BALB/c, only mild gastritis results (Fox et al., 1996). Also, infection of CBA/Ca mice and the F_1 hybrids resulting from mating "high responder" strains with "low responders" induced little or no gastritis. Therefore, the non-responsiveness of CBA/Ca mice to *H. felis* infection is dominantly inherited. Analysis of the antibody responses in these mice revealed virtually undetectable anti-*Helicobacter* antibody levels despite colonization with high numbers of *H. felis*. It has been suggested that the lack of gastritis in CBA mice and their offspring may be due to active suppression of the immune response normally mounted against *H. felis* (Sutton et al., 1999). These observations probably apply to humans since the majority of people infected with *H. pylori* have mild gastritis with apparently no clinical consequences. The mechanisms of this suppression are probably different in mice and humans. In CBA mice, the host-dependent nature of these responses did not appear to be related to the major histocompatibility complex (MHC) haplotype of the strains as C3H/He mice, which have an inflammatory phenotype, and the non-responder CBA/Ca mice are MHC-identical but lack gastritis. In these cases, it appears that the mechanism is linked to the production of *Helicobacter* lipopolysaccharide (LPS). The LPS nonresponder C3H/HeJ strain failed to mount a significant inflammatory response to infection, in contrast to the closely related C3H/He strain, which has normal LPS responsiveness (Sakagami et al., 1996). LPS activates cells of the innate immune system so that host defense responses to the pathogen are mobilized to eliminate the infection. This includes induction of a multitude of new genes encoding proinflammatory cytokines, such as tumor necrosis factor-α (TNF-α), (LT-α, previously known as TNF-β), interleukin-1α (IL-1α), and IL-1β as well as other proteins with pro- or anti-inflammatory properties. Poltorak et al. (1998a,b) identified the LPS gene (*TLR4*) as being responsible for the failure of two mouse strains, C3H/HeJ and C57Bl/10ScCr, to respond to LPS. Mutations of the LPS gene selectively impede LPS signal transduction, rendering the mice resistant to endotoxin but highly susceptible to gram-negative infection. The C3H/HeJ strain contains a gene with a histidine-to-proline mutation at position 712, whereas the latter strain is homozygous for a *TLR4* null mutation. It is interesting that this gene encodes the Toll-4 receptor, a member of the IL-1 receptor family (Poltorak et al., 1998a,b).

These studies on genetic control of the innate immune response illustrate the complexity of the regulation. Through evolutionary selection, a series of innate immune defense mechanisms have evolved to protect the host against the constant threat of microbial injury and to direct the development of specific adaptive immune responses. How is this achieved?

Pathogens induce IL-12, which in turn elicits interferon-γ (INF-γ) production by natural killer cells. This contributes to early defense during certain bacterial, parasitic, and viral infections. During the induction of cell-mediated immunity, T lymphocytes expressing IFN-γ and TNF-α are generated within secondary lymphoid organs in an IL-12-dependent manner. Their extravasation into sites of infection results in the recruitment of macrophages, which become activated by these cytokines. IL-12 also facilitates the development of T-helper type 1 (Th1) lymphocytes, which are required for late protection against bacteria, parasites, and fungi. Therefore, the negative regulation of IL-12 during acute infections can be a key event in the establishment of chronic infection and protection against harmful excessive cellular immune responses (Orange and Biron, 1996a,b).

Whatever the exact mechanism, these experimental models clearly indicate that the intensity of nonspecific immune reactions and the host resistance to bacteria such as *H. pylori* and *H. felis*, as well as facultative intracellular pathogens, are associated in lines of mice selected for maximal or minimal acute inflammatory reactivity.

What is the relevance of these findings to the host response in *H. pylori* infection in humans? The proinflammatory cytokines IL-1β, IL-6, TNF-α, IL-8, IFN-γ, and IL-4 and the anti-inflammatory transforming growth factor (TGF-β) have been studied in antral biopsy specimens from *H. pylori*–infected duodenal ulcer patients and asymptomatic carriers with chronic gastritis only. For comparison, biopsy specimens from uninfected healthy individuals were also analyzed. An immunohistochemical technique was used to quantify the cytokine responses and identify the cell types associated with the cytokine expression. Compared to the levels in the healthy individuals, all of the studied cytokines, except IL-4, were increased in *H. pylori*–infected subjects. This demonstrated that the antral cytokine response is of the Th1 type since IFN-γ, but not IL-4, was upregulated in *H. pylori*–infected individuals. Furthermore, there were no significant differences in either proinflammatory or immunoregulatory cytokine levels when *H. pylori*–infected subjects with and without peptic ulcers were compared (Lindholm et al., 1998). Thus, like mice persistently infected with *H. felis*, which have a predominance of IFN-γ producing cells and an apparent Th1 response (Mohammadi et al., 1996), individuals with gastritis have a Th1 response (Bamford et al., 1998). Th1 cells also express Fas ligand and have the potential to enhance apoptosis in gastric epithelial cells expressing Fas. Should Th1 cells mediate these responses in the stomach, luminal acid and pepsin may have increased access to the underlying tissues, thereby increasing the chance of peptic ulcer formation (Ramsdell et al., 1994). Patients infected with strains expressing *cagA*, which may increase the risk of disease, produce higher levels of inflammatory cytokines (Peek et al., 1995; Yamaoka et al., 1999a,b). There is also evidence that TNF levels are increased in *H. pylori*–positive patients (Crabtree et al., 1991; Noach et al., 1994; Fan et al., 1995; Huseyinov et al., 1999). Urease produced by *H. pylori* stimulates dose-dependently the production of TNF (Harris et al., 1996). TNF-α had a direct inhibitory effect on isolated D cells, causing a reduction in both cellular content and, more markedly, release of somatostatin. It is possible that such products of inflammation are responsible for the deranged physiology (Beales and Calam, 1998a,b).

H. pylori infection associated with a predominant Th1 response by the host may lead to peptic ulcer through modulation of gastric secretion. This is in part due to TNF, which is able to induce functional alteration of gastric cells (Fiorucci et al., 1996; Weigert et al., 1996). In addition, TNF is a cytokine involved in *H. pylori*– and NSAID-induced gastroduodenal damage, ulcer repair (Tarnawski et al., 1997), and other mechanisms that regulate gastric function (Pasparakis et al., 1996; Beales and Calam, 1998a,b). After *H. pylori* eradication, duodenal ulcer patients showed a significantly decreased median level of TNF transcripts (Moss et al., 1994). TNF is also involved in NSAID-induced gastric damage, and agents that regulate TNF synthesis affect indomethacin-induced gastric damage (Santucci et al., 1995; Appleyard et al., 1996). The time course of resolution of the physiological abnormalities with anti-*H. pylori* treatment also favors inflammatory mediators rather than bacterially derived factors: hypergastrinemia persists in the early stages of antibacterial treatment despite severe depression of *H. pylori* and clearance of the polymorphonuclear cell infiltrate. Resolution of the physiology takes longer, as does clearance of the mononuclear cell infiltrate (Graham et al., 1993).

Chemokines, low molecular weight proteins that act as potent chemoattractants, are involved in the migration of inflammatory cells. They are divided according to the configuration of the first cysteine residues at the amino terminus of the proteins. Different subfamilies of chemokines attract different classes of inflammatory cells. C-C chemokines (the first two cysteines are adjacent to one another) predominantly attract monocytes and lymphocytes, while C-X-C chemokines (the first two cysteines (c) are separated by one amino acid (x)) attract polymorphonuclear neutrophils in addition to lymphocytes (Mackay, 1997), chemokines regulated on activation, normal T cell expressed and secreted (RANTES) is a member of the C-C chemokine family and a potent chemoattractant of T cells, natural killer cells, monocytes, eosinophils, basophils, and dendritic cells. Chemokines have been suggested to play an important role in *H. pylori*–associated gastritis (Moss et al., 1994; Noach et al., 1994; Fan et al., 1995; Beales and Calam, 1997; Ding et al., 1997; Lindholm et al., 1998; Yamaoka et al., 1998). *H. pylori* infection was associated with increased rates of expression of mRNA for the C-C chemokines: IL-8, neutrophil chemoattractants growth regulated α (GRO-α), and the C-X-C chemokines: RANTES, and macrophage inflammatory protein-1α. Increased levels of mucosal IL-8 and GRO-α correlated with the density of *H. pylori* in both the antrum and corpus. Interestingly, the levels of these chemokines correlated with cellular infiltration in the antrum but not in the corpus (Yamaoka et al., 1998). The interaction between proinflammatory cytokines and chemokines has not been fully studied, but it is likely that they interact in the modulation of the inflammatory response.

IMMUNOGENETICS OF THE CYTOKINE RESPONSE

There is also genetic control of the IL-1 family of cytokines and TNF. In healthy subjects, significant interindividual variations were found in in vitro production of IL-1 protein, which were interpreted as being inherited (Endres et al., 1989). In accordance with this finding are three biallelic base exchange polymorphisms described in the *IL-1B* gene: two in the promoter region, at position −31, −511 and the other in exon 5 at position +3953 from the transcriptional start site. The diallelic polymorphism at position −31 involves a *TATA* sequence which is involved in transcription of IL-1β. These polymorphisms were suggested to have an influence on IL-1β production (Pociot et al., 1992; Mochizuki et al., 1998; El-Omar et al., 2001; Santtila et al., 1998). Some authors have proposed that the inflammatory process produced by *H. pylori* infection is responsible for acid hyposecretion and have suggested the involvement of IL-1β

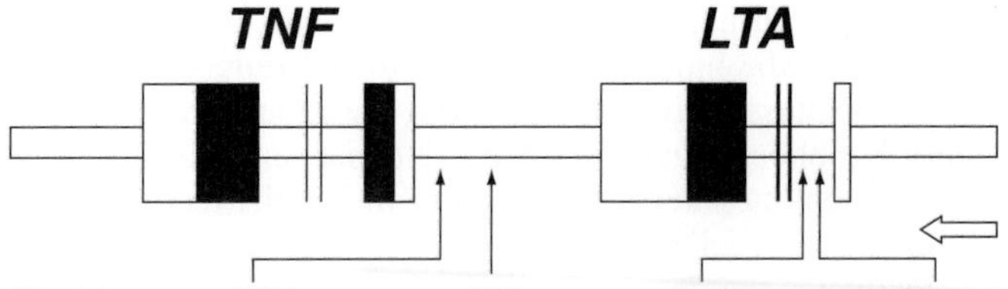

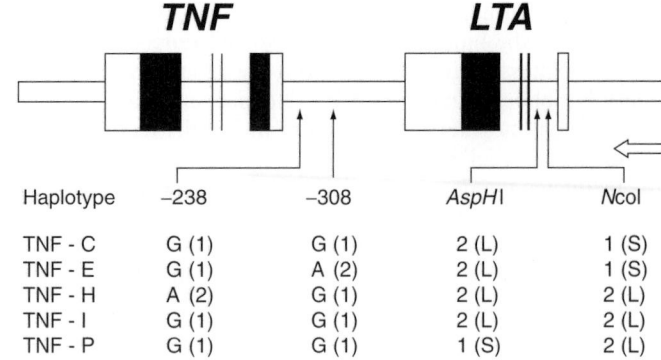

Haplotype	−238	−308	*AspHI*	*NcoI*
TNF - C	G (1)	G (1)	2 (L)	1 (S)
TNF - E	G (1)	A (2)	2 (L)	1 (S)
TNF - H	A (2)	G (1)	2 (L)	2 (L)
TNF - I	G (1)	G (1)	2 (L)	2 (L)
TNF - P	G (1)	G (1)	1 (S)	2 (L)

Fig. 13–6. Four restriction fragment length polymorphisms (RFLPs) in the *TNF* and *LTA* genes: five common haplotypes. RFLPs *NcoI* and *AspHI* in the first intron of the *LTA* gene and others at positions −238 and −308 in the promoter region of the *TNF* gene have been described. The *TNF-308* allele 2 may be responsible for the differences in secretion of TNF-[a]. This allele correlates strongly with haplotype TNF-E. This haplotype is in linkage disequilibrium with *HLA-DR3* in Caucasians.

(El-Omar et al., 1997). Preliminary results suggest that polymorphisms of the *IL-1B* gene are involved in the decreased production of gastric mucosal IL-1β in response to *H. pylori* and, therefore, are related to the pathogenesis of duodenal ulcer. An 86 bp variable number of tandem repeats (VNTR) in intron 2 of the *IL-1RA* gene has been described (Tarlow et al., 1993). TGF-β stimulates monocytes to produce several proinflammatory cytokines in a highly reproducible manner in vitro, but a less common allele of the 86 bp VNTR polymorphism (allele 2) of the *IL-1RA* gene was associated with increased production of IL-1Ra protein and reduced production of IL-1α protein (Danis et al., 1995). *H. pylori* stimulates granulocyte-macrophage colony-stimulating factor production from cultured antral biopsies and a human gastric epithelial cell line (Beales and Calam, 1997a–c), which also may have an indirect effect on IL-1 production. Furthermore, the production of IL-1β by mononuclear cells of blood donors is increased in individuals who carry allele 2 of the *IL-1RN* gene (Santtila et al., 1998). This strongly suggests that individuals who produce high amounts of IL-1β and lower amounts of IL-1ra have difficulty controlling inflammation. A study on the genetic control of these two cytokines showed no significant differences in carriage rate, genotype, and allele frequencies of *IL-1RN* and the *IL-1B+3954* gene polymorphisms between peptic ulcer patients and controls (García-Gonzalez et al., 2001). However, a strong allelic association between the *IL-1B* and *IL-1RN* genes was found in duodenal ulcer patients. Logistic regression analysis identified *H. pylori* infection and NSAIDs use as independent risk factors for peptic ulcer disease, whereas the simultaneous carriage of *IL-1B+3954* allele 2 and *IL-1RN* allele 2 was associated with reduced risk for duodenal ulcer disease (OR = 0.37, 95% CI 0.14–0.9). Thus, evidence exists that the *IL-1B* and *IL-1RN* genes in addition to bacterial and environmental factors play a key role in determining the final outcome of peptic ulcer disease.

The localization of the tandemly arranged *TNFA* and *LTA* genes in the central region of the MHC at the short arm of chromosome 6 has prompted special interest. The cytokines coded by these genes regulate diverse inflammatory processes. Stable interindividual differences in cytokine production are genetically determined, although it is not clear which genes control the cytokine production (Mølvig et al., 1988; Santamaria et al., 1989; Jacob et al., 1990). An AspHI restriction fragment length polymorphism, also in the first intron of the *LTA* gene (Ferencik et al., 1992), and others, at positions −238 and −308 in the promoter region of the *TNFA* gene, have been described (Wilson et al., 1992, 1993; D'Alfonso and Momigliano Richiardi, 1994) (Fig. 13–6). Variations at these positions might be important in the regulation of TNF-α and LT-α production (Bouma et al., 1996; Kroeger et al., 1997; Wilson et al., 1997; Allen, 1999). Some studies have shown that allele 2 of the *TNFA-308* gene polymorphism, which is related to increased TNF-α production, is associated with severe forms of different infections (McGuire et al., 1994; Cabrera et al., 1995; Nadel et al., 1996), suggesting that the excessive proinflammatory reaction may be detrimental for the individual.

TNF gene polymorphisms are good candidates to study further. Genes identified in the TNF-LT region are very important in the definition of ancestral MHC haplotypes since about 70% of these are ancestral haplotypes or recombinants of no more than two of them in the Caucasian population (Degli-Esposti et al., 1992; Abraham et al., 1993; Weissensteiner and Lanchbury, 1997). The frequency of *TNF-308* allele 2 is different among duodenal and gastric ulcers. This allele is in strong linkage disequilibrium with the HLA-A1-B8-DR3 ancestral haplotype in the Caucasian population (Wilson et al., 1993). The mean TNF secretion of individuals carrying HLA-DR3 was significantly higher compared to individuals without this haplotype (Jacob et al., 1990). The reason for the association between HLA-DR3 and high secretion of TNF has not been clarified, but evidence exists that the strongly linked *TNF-308* allele 2 may be responsible for the differences in secretion (Bouma et al., 1996; Wilson et al., 1997; Allen, 1999). This allele correlates strongly with haplotype TNF-E (Crusius et al., 1994). Therefore, in this case, this locus probably controls for the capacity of higher production of TNF. Preliminary studies from our laboratory have shown that more than one-fourth of patients with duodenal ulcer studied had the haplotype TNF-E. This haplotype carries allele 2 at position −308 in the promoter region of the *TNFA* gene. However, gastric ulcer patients have a low frequency of this haplotype and a strong positive association with haplotype TNF-I. Half of the patients studied with gastric ulcer were carriers of this haplotype. Being a carrier of haplotype TNF-I almost doubles the risk of developing peptic ulcer and increases the risk for gastric ulceration by a factor of 2.8 (Lanas et al., 2001). Carriers of haplotype TNF-I produced less LT-α than individuals who lacked this haplotype (Bouma et al., 1996). The differences in frequency of these haplotypes in duodenal and gastric ulcers support previous family and epidemiological data suggesting a difference in the genetic background for suffering from gastric or duodenal ulcers (Rotter et al., 1985; Hein et al., 1997; Räihä et al., 1998).

These data suggest that the normal physiological control of gastric secretory function and specifically of the pathogenesis of *H. pylori*–related diseases is determined to a certain extent by the inflammatory response (Beales and Calam, 1997a–c). It is clear that more work needs to be done to clarify the role of the genetic control in the inflammatory response. The interaction between virulent *H. pylori* strains and the genetic factors described above need to be addressed in future studies. The current working hypothesis is that genes that control the Th1 response interact with environmental factors to increase ulcer risk. These factors might help to determine the outcome of the type of ulcer, gastric or duodenal. The genetic control that determines whether an individual is a high responder or a low responder is also important to the other causes of peptic ulcer, such as NSAIDs and certain retroviruses. Knowledge in this area may explain the low prevalence of *H. pylori* in patients with HIV (Varsky et al., 1998) and in endemic areas of HTLV-I infection despite the high prevalence of *H. pylori* in the same population (Isomoto et al., 1999).

MHC and Peptic Ulcer

The association of the MHC antigens with peptic ulceration is weak (Rotter et al., 1977; Goedhard et al., 1983) and not confirmed in all studies. The negative and positive associations described between the *HLA-DQA1*0102* and *−DQA1*0301* alleles, respectively, and *H. pylori*–infected duodenal ulcer patients in a Japanese population remain to be confirmed in other studies (Azuma et al., 1995); and they are not present in patients from Spain (Santolaria et al., 1998). However, HLA-DQ5 was significantly higher in patients with *H. pylori* infection and evidence of atrophy or metaplasia than in those without atrophy or metaplasia in both infected and noninfected groups (Beales et al., 1995). However, the MHC has been suggested to be involved in the pathogenesis of this infection. The role of the MHC class I– and class II–restricted functions in *H. pylori* infection and immunity upon oral immunization has been examined in vivo during experimental challenges with *H. pylori SS1* in MHC class I and class II mutant mice compared with C57BL/6 wild-type mice (Pappo et al., 1999). The absence of these molecules resulted in significantly greater colonization of the bacteria. Oral immunization with *H. pylori* whole-cell lysates and cholera toxin adjuvant significantly reduced the magnitude of *H. pylori* infection in C57BL/6 wild-type and MHC class I knockout mice, but it had no effect on the *H. pylori* infection level in MHC class II-deficient mice. Interestingly, analysis of the anti-*H. pylori* antibody levels in serum showed a dominant serum IgG1 response in immunized C57BL/6 wild-type and MHC class I mutant mice but no detectable serum IgG response in MHC class II knockout mice. Populations of T-cell receptor $(TCR)^+CD4^+CD54^+$ cells localized to gastric tissue of immunized C57BL/6 wild-type and MHC class I knockout mice, but TCR^+CD8^+ cells predominated in the gastric tissue of immunized MHC class II-deficient mice. These observations show that $CD4^+$ T cells engaged after mucosal immunization may be important for the generation of a protective anti-*H. pylori* immune response and that $CD4^+CD8^+$ T cells regulate the extent of *H. pylori* infection in vivo (Pappo et al., 1999).

Class II MHC molecules are best known for their ability to bind and present antigens to $CD4^+$ T cells. However, engagement of class II MHC by T cells also has functional consequences for the antigen-presenting cell. For example, cross-linking class II MHC molecules with molecules such as microbial superantigens has been reported to induce apoptosis (Newell et al., 1993).

Fan et al. (1998) demonstrated that signaling through class II MHC molecules leading to induction of apoptosis can be induced by cross-linking IgM antibodies to surface class II MHC molecules. Antibodies recognizing class II MHC inhibited both the binding of *H. pylori* and the induction of apoptosis. However, IFN-γ increased the attachment of the bacteria as well as the induction of apoptosis in gastric epithelial cells in contrast to MHC II-negative cell lines. *H. pylori* induced apoptosis only in cells expressing class II MHC molecules constitutively or after gene transfection. These interesting results described novel receptors for *H. pylori* and provided a mechanism by which bacteria and the host response interact in the pathogenesis of gastric epithelial cell damage. They also give a glimpse into the molecular biological mechanisms that explain the described associations of the MHC with *H. pylori* infection and peptic ulcer.

Dissecting the fine regulation is going to be difficult. The presence of the TNF locus within the MHC may potentially complicate the interpretation of results in animal models in which the TNF locus is experimentally manipulated. The close genetic linkage between the TNF locus and other molecules within the MHC, many of which are plausible candidate genes in immunological disorders, undoubtedly complicates the study of these human diseases (Ruuls and Sedgwick, 1999).

ABO Blood Groups, Secretor Status, and Peptic Ulcer

The identification of *H. pylori* as a major cause of peptic ulcer has brought new light to the association of ABO blood groups and secretor status in these diseases. Most of the studies, since the early 1950s, have been directed to the ABO blood groups and later to the Lewis antigens (Clarke et al., 1956; Borén et al., 1993; Dickey et al., 1993; Niv et al., 1996). Nonsecretors and patients with *H. pylori* infection were significantly more likely to have gastroduodenal disease; however, no significant association was observed between secretor status and *H. pylori* infection (Dickey et al., 1993). Logistic regression analysis confirmed that these were independently associated with gastroduodenal disease. Overall, the RR of gastroduodenal disease for nonsecretors compared with secretors was 1.9 (95% CI 1.2–3.2). Nonsecretion of ABO blood group antigens is not related to *H. pylori* infection but is independently and significantly associated with endoscopic gastroduodenal disease (Dickey et al., 1993). It has been argued that knowledge of the genetic risk of peptic ulcer has predominantly been based on hospital materials. To minimize this selection bias, a large-scale epidemiological study was performed in Denmark (Hein et al., 1997). The lifetime prevalence of peptic ulcer in men with the Lewis phenotype Le(a+b−) and nonsecretors of ABH antigen was 15%, significantly higher than that in others, 11% ($p < 0.01$); the risk in phenotypes O and A was equally high, 12%, and that among other ABO groups, 7% ($p < 0.05$). Men with phenotype O had a significantly higher risk of hospitalization than others ($p < 0.01$). Compared with others, the attributable risk of peptic ulcer in men who were Le(a+b−) or nonsecretors, with the O or A phenotype, was 37%. No association was found with complement C3, MNS, or Rh blood groups. This study showed that the Le (a+b−) phenotype and the ABH non-secretor trait are relevant genetic markers of peptic ulcer and that the men in this population had increased susceptibility to *H. pylori* infection. The lifetime prevalence was equally high among men with the O or A phenotype, with more severe cases in men with phenotype O (Hein et al., 1997). Similar results have been reported in childhood duodenal ulcer disease (Nijevitch et al., 1999).

Lewis Antigens in Humans and *H. pylori*

Since bacterial attachment is a prerequisite for colonization of the gastric epithelial surface, it was first found that fucosylated epitopes in the glycoprotein(s) mediate the binding of *H. pylori* to the surface mucous cell. This was suggested by the fact that surface mucous cells of the stomach coexpress the adhesin receptor. Major fucosylated histo-blood group antigens, recognized by monoclonal antibodies specific for histo-blood group antigens H, B, and Le^b, block the binding. The lectin *Ulex europaeus* type 1 agglutinin, which is specific for α-L-fucose, also binds to the same cells that bind the bacteria (Falk et al., 1993). At the same time, Borén et al. (1993) found that gastric tissue lacking Le^b expression did not bind *H. pylori*. Bacteria did not bind to Le^b

antigen substituted with a terminal *N*-acetylgalactosamine α1–3 residue (blood group A determinant), suggesting that the availability of *H. pylori* receptors might be reduced in individuals of blood groups A and B compared with blood group O (Borén et al., 1993). Studies in Israel found that positivity for *H. pylori* was not associated with blood group O (Niv et al., 1996); in another study, patients with *H. pylori* infection and disease had a distribution of blood group antigens similar to a control population (Umlauft et al., 1996). Also, in an Indian community in northwestern Manitoba, Canada, no association between *H. pylori* seropositivity and age, sex, gastrointestinal complaints, medications, housing characteristics, and ABO or Lewis antigen status was found (Bernstein et al., 1999). However, a study in 523 subjects from Narino, Colombia, and 856 subjects from northern Spain found that Le(a+b−) and nonsecretor phenotypes showed a significant positive association with the expression of sulfomucins and gastric intestinal metaplasia (ORs = 2.4 and 2.6, respectively). Gastric metaplasia is a known marker of preneoplastic progression (Torrado et al., 1997).

It is now known that Lewis antigens occur in human gastric epithelium and in *H. pylori* LPS; their expression is polymorphic in both. Autoimmune mechanisms induced by bacterial Lewis expression have been proposed to cause gastritis (Appelmelk et al., 1996).

How can we reconcile the different findings? It has been found that *H. pylori* from patients with Lewis(a+b−) expressed Le^x more than Le^y, whereas isolates from patients with Lewis(a−b+) expressed Le^x less than Le^y, and isolates from Lewis(a−b−) patients expressed Le^x and Le^y approximately equally. The most significant finding is that *H. pylori* LPS can express type 1 Lewis blood group determinants, Le^a, H-1 (Le^d), and the type 1 chain precursor (Le^c), as well as the type 2 epitopes Le^x and Le^y. Both types are human oncofetal antigens. Figure 13–7 shows the structures of the Lewis carbohydrate structures according to Taylor et al. (1998). There is some evidence that the relative proportion of expression corresponds to the host Lewis phenotype, suggesting selection for host-adapted organisms (Wirth et al., 1997). Structural studies and additional serological experiments have shown that O chains from *H. pylori* LPS can also express fucosylated type 1 sequence, and that the LPS from a single *H. pylori* strain may carry O chains with type 1 and type 2 Lewis blood groups simultaneously. Therefore, these authors have concluded that *H. pylori* strain may have a different niche within the gastric mucosa and that each individual LPS blood group antigen may have a dissimilar role in *H. pylori* adaptation (Monteiro et al., 1998). Host-related microbial Lewis expression could help avoid host immune responses (Wirth et al., 1997) or be involved in autoimmunity by molecular mimicry between *H. pylori* LPS and the host, based on Lewis antigens (Appelmelk et al., 1996; Negrini et al., 1996; Monteiro et al., 1998). Clonal *H. pylori* populations from the primary culture of gastric biopsy specimens from 12 patients and 160 isolates from primary cultures from 16 experimentally infected rodents showed substantial differences in Lewis expression among the isolates from 9 of 12 (75%) patients (Wirth et al., 1999). These differences were unrelated to overall genetic diversity, as determined by polymerase chain reactions for randomly amplified polymorphic DNA or *cagA* status, and they persisted during subsequent in vitro passage. In contrast, Lewis expression was highly uniform in *H. pylori* isolates from different rodents infected for up to 20 weeks. Variation in *H. pylori* Lewis expression in genetically closely related organisms in human subjects may provide a pool of bacterial phenotypes for the continuous selection of optimally host-adapted populations suitable for persistence. However, no direct relationship has been found between Lewis antigen expression by *H. pylori* and gastric epithelial cells in infected patients (Fig. 13–8) (Taylor et al., 1998). Expression of Le^x and Le^y by *H. pylori* suggests their requirement for establishment and/or maintenance of infection. Therefore, as stated above the genetics of the host and of the bacteria should be studied together to comprehend within a single picture the totality of the phenomenon. It has been found that $\alpha(1,3)$-

Type 1 structures

Le^a: $\beta Gal1 \rightarrow 3\beta GlcNAc1 \rightarrow R$, with αFuc $\downarrow 1 \rightarrow 4$

Le^b: $\beta Gal1 \rightarrow 3\beta GlcNAc1 \rightarrow R$, with αFuc $\downarrow 1 \rightarrow 2$ and αFuc $\downarrow 1 \rightarrow 4$

Type 2 structures

Le^x: $\beta Gal1 \rightarrow 4\beta GlcNAc1 \rightarrow R$, with αFuc $\downarrow 1 \rightarrow 3$

Le^y: $\beta Gal1 \rightarrow 4\beta GlcNAc1 \rightarrow R$, with αFuc $\downarrow 1 \rightarrow 2$ and αFuc $\downarrow 1 \rightarrow 3$

Fig. 13–7. Le^a and Le^b determinants are blood group antigens: structures of type 1 and type 2 Lewis carbohydrate. The enzymes required for generation of these structures are shown next to the *arrows* and are 1,4-fucosyltransferase (Le^a and Le^b), 1,3-fucosyltransferase (Le^x and Le^y), and 1,2-fucosyltransferase (Le^b and Le^y). From Taylor et al. (1998) with permission.

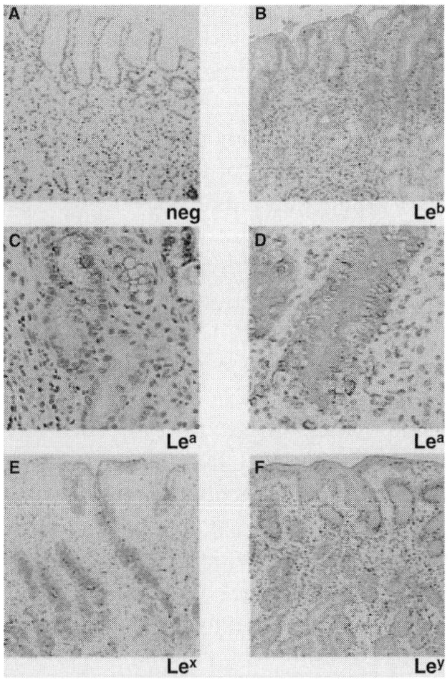

Fig. 13–8. Histological staining patterns of gastric biopsy specimens of Le^x and Le^y antigens. *A:* Negative control (*H. pylori*-negative) in which the primary antibody in the reaction was replaced by mouse serum. *B:* Anti-Le^b staining of gastric epithelium with *H. pylori*-associated gastritis. Positive staining in the superficial mucous cells, deep glands, and luminal secretions. In the stroma, mixed inflammatory cells are evident *(C)*. Anti-Le^a staining of gastric epithelium with *H. pylori*-associated gastritis. Positive staining in the superficial mucous cells and luminal secretions. In the stroma, mixed inflammatory cells are evident (original magnification ×275). *D:* Anti-Le^a staining of gastric epithelium with *H. pylori*-associated gastritis. Positive staining in the superficial mucous cells, deep glands, and luminal secretions. In the stroma, mixed inflammatory cells are evident (original magnification ×440). *E:* Anti-Le^x staining of gastric epithelium with *H. pylori*-associated gastritis. Positive staining in the superficial mucous cells, deep glands, and luminal secretions. In the stroma, mixed inflammatory cells are evident (original magnification ×110). *F:* Anti-Le^y staining of gastric epithelium with *H. pylori*-associated gastritis. Positive staining in the superficial mucous cells, deep glands, and luminal secretions. In the stroma, mixed inflammatory cells are evident (original magnification ×110). From Taylor et al. (1998) with permission.

and $\alpha(1,2)$-fucosyltransferases, which are present in several *H. pylori* strains, regulate the presence or absence of Le^y in the *H. pylori* LPS. Mutations in the fucosyltransferase gene and alterations in transcription and translation may be involved in this process (Wang et al., 1999). Biochemical studies have identified a 78 kDa protein from *H. pylori* strains (termed *BabA*) that allows binding to the blood group antigen Le^b, which is present on the surface of gastric epithelial cells (Covacci et al., 1993). Although two corresponding genes encoding *BABA* have been cloned (*BABA1* and *BABA2*), only the *BABA2* gene is transcribed. Bacteria harboring the *BABA2* gene express the adhesin and can thereby bind to Le^b antigens on gastric epithelial cells. Genotyping of *H. pylori* strains by the additional presence of the gene *BabA2* yielded a highly significant association with ulcer ($p = 2 \times 10^{-6}$) and distal gastric ($p = 0.014$) adenocarcinomas (Gerhard et al., 1999). These results indicate that the *BABA2* gene is of high clinical relevance and would be a useful marker to identify patients who are at higher risk for specific *H. pylori*–related diseases.

NSAIDS AND PEPTIC ULCER

The history of NSAID use is more common in duodenal and pyloric ulcer patients without infection than in patients in whom the ulcer is associated with *H. pylori* gastritis (Hyvarinen et al., 1996). Endoscopic evidence of gastric mucosal damage, such as erosions and submucosal hemorrhages, just 2 hours after aspirin administration was found. The mean serum salicylate concentration was approximately 12 mg/dl and gastric mucosal content of prostaglandin E_2 and $F_2\alpha$ was reduced by >95% in the fundus and antrum (Faust et al., 1990). NSAIDs cause peptic ulcer disease by mechanisms different from those of *H. pylori* infection. For example, NSAIDs inhibit the prostaglandin-dependent processes of blood flow and of mucus and bicarbonate secretion, which underlie mucosal protection, whereas *H. pylori* induces inflammation by activation of the cytokine network and, therefore, stimulates the production of prostaglandin synthesis, as discussed above. Gastric ulceration and bleeding are major complications of the chronic use of NSAIDs (Lanas and Hirschowitz, 1999). NSAIDs cause a topical irritant effect on the epithelium, impairment of the barrier properties of the mucosa, suppression of gastric prostaglandin synthesis, reduction of gastric mucosal blood flow, and interference with the repair of superficial injury. The presence of acid in the lumen of the stomach also contributes to the pathogenesis of NSAID-induced ulcers and bleeding in a number of ways. Acid impairs the restitution process, interferes with hemostasis, and can inactivate several growth factors that are important for mucosal integrity and repair. Profound suppression of gastric acid secretion has been shown to be effective in preventing NSAID-induced ulceration (Bastaki and Wallace, 1999). Concerning the interrelationship between the damaging effects of *H. pylori* and those of NSAIDs on the gastroduodenal mucosa, some pathogenic factors exert a damaging effect on the mucosa; therefore, an additive effect occurs, leading to aggravation of mucosal damage. However, mutual antagonism exists, leading to one of the pathogenic factors actually deriving some protection from the damaging potential of the other. Microscopically, *H. pylori*– and NSAID-associated gastritis are recognized as two separate entities. From two large, randomized, multicenter trials, it appears that antisecretory drugs are more effective in *H. pylori*-positive peptic ulcer patients taking NSAIDs than in *H. pylori*-negative patients taking these drugs (Chan and Sung, 1998; Hawkey et al., 1998a,b). These studies do not provide any evidence that *H. pylori* infection reduces the pathogenic effects of NSAIDs. Other studies, however, have shown protection against NSAID-associated gastroduodenal damage in *H. pylori*-negative patients. Thus, there are no firm conclusions on the role of *H. pylori* infection in patients with NSAID-associated peptic ulcers (Malfertheiner and Labenz, 1998; Hawkey, 1999).

In a study of female patients with rheumatoid arthritis of recent onset, a 24-hour gastric pH recording was performed both in basal conditions and after 1-month treatment with either indomethacin 150 mg/day or ketoprofen 300 mg/day. There was increased gastric acidity after 1 month of treatment with NSAIDs, supporting the use of antisecretory agents to prevent peptic ulcer in these patients (Savarino et al., 1998a,b). To achieve healing in these circumstances, it is necessary to augment the intragastric pH to around 4.0, a level necessary to inhibit peptic activity (Samloff, 1971); therefore, according to Hawkey (1999), the term *peptic ulcer* is more appropriate for an NSAID ulcer than for one caused by *H. pylori*.

HETEROGENEITY

It has been clear for a number of years that genetic factors predispose to peptic ulcer, but the mode of inheritance of this genetic predisposition has not been resolved. Originally, the hypothesis of polygenic or multifactorial inheritance was used to explain the genetics of peptic ulcer. *Polygenic inheritance* refers to the concept that the hereditary component of a given disorder is due to the contribution of many genes acting together, resulting in a continuum of genetic predisposition toward the disorder. Clinical disease would exist when the presence of a sufficient number of genes, in combination with environmental factors, exceeds a threshold level. The relatives of index patients would thus have genes in common with the patients in direct proportion to the closeness of their relationship. The multifactorial model predicts that the relatives will share some of the disease-predisposing genes and, hence, will be shifted toward the threshold for disease. The polygenic hypothesis basically assumed that peptic ulcer was the spectrum of one disease process. However, while there may be a polygenic contribution to peptic ulcer, the alternative mechanism of genetic heterogeneity is probably much more important.

Genetic heterogeneity was proposed as an alternative hypothesis that could explain both the familial aggregation of peptic ulcer disease and the lack of a simple Mendelian pattern of inheritance based on differences between ulcer patients in clinical and physiological studies (Lam and Sircus, 1975; Lam and Ong, 1976; Rotter and Rimoin, 1977; Lam and Lai, 1978; Rotter, 1981).

The existence of well-defined genetic and rare clinical syndromes that feature peptic ulceration is an important demonstration of genetic and etiological heterogeneity. The extensive ethnic variability, especially in clinical features, and the heterogeneity of genetic marker polymorphisms in the regulation of the inflammation are further proof of ulcer heterogeneity.

Clinical Studies

The separation of duodenal and gastric ulcers into two distinct disorders was confirmed by the classic clinical genetic study of Doll and Kellock (1951). Duodenal ulcer occurred no more frequently among relatives than in the general population. Likewise, the relatives of duodenal ulcer patients had three times as many duodenal ulcers compared with the control population but no increased risk of gastric ulcer.

The demonstration of clinical, physiological, or genetic differences within a disorder related to clinical features, such as ulcer location or age at onset, can also suggest genetic heterogeneity. In the case of gastric ulcer and duodenal ulcer, much of the evidence that indicates that these are separate and distinct disorders has been gathered in this fashion. Ulcer location is the dividing criterion, and then other features, such as age at onset, complications, male-to-female ratio, and acid secretion, are added.

Physiological Studies

A variety of studies among duodenal ulcer patients show that this entity by itself is clearly a heterogeneous group of disorders on physiological grounds alone (Lam, 1984). Some of the different physiological abnormalities among groups of duodenal ulcer patients may be a consequence of the infection by *H. pylori* or the use of NSAIDs, but many are likely to be due to genetic and etiological heterogeneity, including heterogeneity of interactions with environmental factors. It is obvious that many of the physiological abnormalities described previously are a consequence of *H. pylori* infection, the subsequent inflammatory response, or the use of aspirin or NSAIDs. However, abnormalities in acid secretion, pepsinogen-pepsin, and gastrin may also be independently controlled and genetic factors may be involved in their total output.

Abnormalities in Acid Secretion

Gastric acid secretion is necessary for the development of duodenal ulcers. Duodenal ulcers do not occur in persons who cannot secrete acid, and they are almost never seen in persons whose maximal acid secretion is <10 mmol/hour. The high parietal cell mass in duodenal ulcers is thought to be inherited because the *H. pylori* positivity and the consequent hypergastrinemia do not confer a consistent and equivalent increase of acid secretion in all populations with this infection. For instance, *H. pylori*-positive healthy volunteers have a significantly lower basal and stimulated acid output than patients with duodenal ulcer (El-Omar et al., 1995; Gillen et al., 1998). The maximal acid-secretory capacity in response to pentagastrin stimulation remains unchanged 1 year after *H. pylori* eradication (Gillen et al., 1998). If the increased parietal cell mass were caused by the trophic effect of bacteria-induced hypergastrinemia, it should resolve within 3 to 6 months, as shown in 45% of patients with gastrinoma after curative surgery (Pisegna et al., 1992). Therefore, the alterations of acid secretion in patients with duodenal ulcer have more to do with the genetic makeup of the host than the influence of the bacterium (Savarino et al., 1998a,b). Environmental factors such as tobacco are important since smoking has been associated with a 25% to 40% increase in maximal acid output (Feldman et al., 1996). The physiological response among *H. pylori*–infected patients with markedly different histology is probably different, and this should be taken into account (Graham, 1998).

Treatment of *H. pylori* infection results in recovery of acid secretion in patients with corpus gastritis (Yasunaga et al., 1994; Gutierrez et al., 1997). However, *H. pylori* eradication reduces the recurrence of duodenal ulcers. It is unclear why duodenal ulcers rarely recur in the absence of reinfection with *H. pylori*. The return to normality of several physiological abnormalities after eradication may explain the absence of recurrence. For example, pentagastrin-stimulated peak acid output was significantly higher in *H. pylori*-positive patients with duodenal ulcers than in *H. pylori*-negative controls and fell significantly after *H. pylori* eradication. In those few *H. pylori*-negative patients with recurrent duodenal ulcers, pentagastrin-stimulated peak acid output was significantly higher than in controls and similar to levels in *H. pylori*-positive patients with duodenal ulcers. Therefore, duodenal ulcer relapse after eradication of *H. pylori* may be related to high pentagastrin-stimulated peak acid output (Harris et al., 1997). The genetically determined high maximal acid output of patients with duodenal ulcer will result in an antral-predominant body-sparing type of *H. pylori* gastritis, producing increased antral gastrin release, which will in turn stimulate the healthy body of the stomach to secrete excess acid. In addition, dietary and environmental factors, such as intake of salt and antioxidants and smoking, together with differences in bacterial strains will influence both the gastritis and associated alterations in gastric secretory function and, thus, the disease outcome. Most chronic diseases are multifactorial in origin, and it would be a mistake to ignore the risk factors for peptic ulcer that were recognized in the pre-*H. pylori* era (Graham, 1998).

Abnormalities in Gastrin Secretion

Responses to cephalic stimulation in duodenal ulcer patients have been studied by modified sham feeding (food chewing followed by spitting and not swallowing), food teasing, and insulin hypoglycemia. Up to 30% of patients with duodenal ulcer have increased acid response to cephalic stimulation, independent of the size of the parietal mass (Lam, 1984). An increased cephalic acid response may be the result of increased vagal drive, increased sensitivity of the parietal cells to gastrin or cholinergic stimulation, increased parietal cell mass, and/or hyperfunction of the G cell.

Further heterogeneity in the sensitivity to gastrin stimulation has been demonstrated among different groups of duodenal ulcer patients. When patients were grouped by age at onset and maximal acid secretion, early-onset hypersecretors were more sensitive to pentagastrin than late-onset hypersecretors, while late-onset normosecretors were more sensitive than early-onset normosecretors (Lam, 1984; Lam and Koo, 1985). Furthermore, duodenal ulcer patients expressed increased sensitivity to their own endogenous gastrin (Lam et al., 1980; Lam, 1984).

In a small but unknown percentage of duodenal ulcer patients, G-cell hyperfunction occurs and is associated with acid hypersecretion (aggressive duodenal ulcer), and this phenotype can be familial (Lam, 1984). However, increased G-cell function appears to occur more frequently among duodenal ulcer patients with normal parietal cell mass and normal maximal acid output. Lam and Ong (1980) found an abnormal high meal-stimulated gastrin response in 35% of 144 patients with duodenal ulcer. They found evidence for two subgroups of patients. Patients with an early age at onset (<35 years) had higher postprandial gastrin than patients with later onset. Within the early-onset group, those with a positive family history of ulcer dyspepsia had higher gastrin levels than those without such a history. Gillen et al. (1998) suggested that acid response to gastrin distinguishes patients with duodenal ulcer from *H. pylori*–infected healthy subjects. They found that the sensitivity to gastrin was similar in duodenal ulcer patients and *H. pylori*-negative healthy volunteers but that *H. pylori*-positive healthy volunteers were less sensitive. However, the differences probably resulted from a comparison of *H. pylori* in patients without corpus gastritis, patients with duodenal ulcer, and those with different degrees of corpus gastritis (Graham, 1998).

Severe hypergastrinemia has been observed in some patients who had a longer duration of treatment with omeprazole for severe gastroesophageal reflux disease. These patients were characterized by a higher prevalence of *H. pylori* infection, corpus mucosal inflammation, and atrophic gastritis. This was reflected in lower serum pepsinogen A concentrations, pepsinogen A/C ratio, and mucosal somatostatin concentrations. This study clearly demonstrated that severe hypergastrinemia during omeprazole maintenance therapy for gastroesophageal reflux disease is associated with the duration of therapy and *H. pylori* infection but not with abnormalities of gastric emptying or vagal nerve integrity (Schenk et al., 1998).

Abnormalities in Pepsin and Pepsinogen Secretion

Pepsin appears to play a central role in the pathogenesis of peptic ulcers. It is difficult to distinguish between the role of acid alone and that of acid and pepsin together. Pepsinogen I (PG I), or pepsinogen A, and pepsinogen II (PG II), or pepsinogen C, are the pepsin precursors. PG I is derived exclusively from the peptic cells in the oxyntic glands of the stomach, while PG II is derived from the chief and mucous neck cells of the gastric fundus, the pyloric glands of the gastric antrum, and Brunner's gland of the proximal duodenum. Urine normally contains only PG 1, which reflects renal excretion of circulating PG 1. A high serum pepsinogen level was thought to reflect an increased secretory capacity of the gastric mucosa to secrete acid and pepsin, which was presumed to be a major factor in the pathogenesis of duodenal ulcer. When PG 1 and PG II were determined separately with radioimmunoassays, it was shown that one or both are higher than normal in some duodenal ulcer and in some gastric ulcer patients but that the ratio of PG I to PG II is lower in gastric ulcer patients than in duodenal ulcer patients due to different patterns of gastritis of the gastric body (Samloff et al., 1982, 1985).

Serum PG I levels also can be used to distinguish between appropriate and inappropriate hypergastrinemia. The combination of hypergastrinemia and a low serum PG I level is diagnostic of severe atrophic gastritis, or gastric atrophy, whereas the combination of hypergastrinemia and an elevated serum PG I level suggests Zollinger-Ellison syndrome (Samloff et al., 1982, 1985).

Of 120 duodenal ulcer cases in Liverpool, about one-half had hyperpepsinogenemia I (hyper-PG I). Family studies of patients with duodenal ulcers that are hyper-PG I or normo-PG I showed an independent segregation (Rotter et al., 1979a,b). Supporting the independence of hyper- and normo-PG I duodenal ulcers are observations made in clinically normal siblings of duodenal ulcer patients. The mean serum PG 1 of the normal siblings of hyper-PG I cases was significantly greater than that of the clinically normal siblings of the normo-PG I cases. In fact, the mean PG I level in the clinically normal siblings of the hyper-PG I cases was intermediate between the mean level in their siblings with duodenal ulcer and the mean level in healthy controls. In contrast, in the normo-PG I cases, the mean PG I values of the normal siblings and the duodenal ulcer patients were not different from those of healthy controls. Also, normal siblings of the hyper-PG I cases came from two separate distributions, one with an elevated PG I and one with a normal PG I. Habibullah et al. (1984) reported that healthy first-degree relatives of hyperpepsinogenemic duodenal ulcer patients had serum pepsinogen values intermediate between those of patients and controls. The segregation of hyperpepsinogenemia was consistent with an autosomal dominant inheritance, as was previously reported for PG I (Rotter et al., 1979a,b).

The association between the restriction fragment length polymorphism of the pepsinogen C (*PGC*) gene and peptic ulcer disease was investigated in 177 unrelated controls, 75 patients with gastric ulcer, and 70 patients with duodenal ulcer in Japan (Ohtaka et al., 1997). Four alleles were detected by polymerase chain reaction, 480 bp (allele 1), 450 bp (allele 2), 400 bp (allele 3), and 310 bp (allele 4). As shown in Table 13–5, the frequency of allele 4 was significantly higher in patients with gastric body ulcer than in controls ($p = 0.005$). Genotypes containing allele 4 were significantly more frequent in patients with gastric body ulcer than in patients with gastric angular, antral ulcer or healthy controls. The RR of gastric body ulcer associated with the presence of allele 4 was 4.63 and was statistically significant ($p = 0.005$). There were no significant differences in the allelic frequencies between the *H. pylori*-positive and *H. pylori*-negative groups in controls, patients with gastric body ulcer, or patients with gastric angular or antral ulcer. These results suggest a significant association between the genetic polymorphism at the *PGC* gene locus and gastric body ulcer. This association is independent from the presence of *H. pylori* infection (Konishi et al., 1994; Ohtaka et al., 1997). These interesting findings also indicate that the genetic etiology of gastric body ulcer is probably different from the one determining the development of an antral ulcer (Ohtaka et al., 1997).

Table 13–5. Associations between Genetic Polymorphisms at the *PGC* Gene Locus and Gastric Body Ulcer

		Allele Frequency of *PGC*-RFLP			
	No.	1	2	3	4
Controls	177	0.141	0.398	0.192	0.268
Gastric ulcer					
Body	40	0.113	0.350	0.088	0.450[a]
Angulus	25	0.140	0.400	0.180	0.280
Antrum	10	0.150	0.350	0.200	0.300
Duodenal ulcer	70	0.100	0.364	0.207	0.329

[a]Significantly different from controls, $\chi^2 = 9.92$ $p < 0.005$. The frequency of allele 4 in the PGC restriction fragment length polymorphism (RFLP) of patients with gastric body ulcer was significantly higher than that of controls. $\chi^2 = 14.84$ $p < 0.005$.
Source: Ohtaka et al. (1997).

PEPTIC ULCER IN CHILDREN

Peptic ulcer is an uncommon disorder in children (Rowland and Drumm, 1995). The fact that several ulcer risk factors, such as smoking, alcohol consumption, and the use of NSAIDs, are usually absent in children suggests that the etiology of peptic ulcer is more straightforward than in adults. For years it was debated whether childhood peptic ulcer is distinct from chronic adult duodenal ulcer. However, in children, as in adults, duodenal ulcer is more common than gastric ulcer (Tsang et al., 1990), although in older series antral ulcers were more frequent than duodenal ulcers (Nord et al., 1981). The natural course is similarly chronic (Azarow et al., 1996). As in adults, studies of children with primary duodenal ulcers have consistently demonstrated an increased male-to-female ratio in the range of 2:1 to 3:1; gastric ulcers tend to be more prevalent in girls, the male-to-female ratio being 1:2.25 (Nord et al., 1981). *H. pylori* is now recognized as the main cause of antral gastritis and ulceration in the child (Gryboski, 1991). Similar to the situation in adults, when *H. pylori* is eradicated, the gastritis improves (Mahony et al., 1992) and peptic ulcer is healed (Chan et al., 1997). Children develop the same physiological abnormalities in the presence of *H. pylori* infection as adults. In 71 children undergoing upper gastrointestinal endoscopy for investigation of upper abdominal pain, serum PGI and gastrin concentrations were measured. Before treatment there was a significant correlation between serum pepsinogen concentration, total inflammatory score, and *H. pylori* status, but no correlation between serum gastrin concentrations and *H. pylori* status. Similarly, the total inflammatory score and serum pepsinogen concentrations were significantly correlated. There was no such correlation in children negative for *H. pylori* (Oderda et al., 1990). *H. pylori* isolates from 32 children and adolescents were characterized with respect to putative virulence and colonization-associated properties. Only three of the subjects had duodenal ulcer. All but two of the remaining 29 had various degrees of chronic gastric inflammation. No significant correlation between degree of inflammation and presence of the cag-pathogenicity island was found. Neither was an association with cytotoxin production or the vacA alleles associated with cytotoxin expression or with the presence of Le^b observed, but children appeared to have lower expression of the Le^b oligosaccharide (Celik et al., 1998)

A SIMPLE CLASSIFICATION OF THE COMMON CAUSES OF PEPTIC ULCER

The accumulating evidence, reviewed above, suggests that two major causes of peptic ulcer exist, i.e., *H. pylori* and NSAIDs; but in both cases, the presence of a genetic predisposition is necessary to develop the disease. Multiple, additive predisposing genes, each with a small effect, determine the development of peptic ulcer. In the case of *H. pylori*, the genes that code for Lewis antigens, secretor status, and MHC are important in the susceptibility to acquire virulent strains. The genes involved in the regulation of the immune response determine the severity of the inflammatory reaction. Preliminary evidence suggests that these genes influence the site of lesion. Genes that code for PG I and PG II, and those determining total parietal cell mass also contribute to the determination of whether a gastric ulcer or a duodenal ulcer will develop. Age at onset of infection probably plays an important role in this respect as well.

Apart from the major role that *H. pylori* plays in the etiology of peptic ulcer and the regular use of aspirin and NSAIDs, especially in the elderly, other environmental factors, such as cigarette smoking and prolonged use of steroids in large doses, have been documented. Use of NSAIDs, *H. pylori*, and cigarette smoking have been identified as major risk factors for peptic ulcer in numerous clinical and epidemiological studies. As described above, these major environmental factors per se are insufficient and the presence of a family history also contributes to the development of a peptic ulcer. In summary, peptic ulcer is a polygenic and multifactorial disorder.

THERAPY

Peptic ulcer disease associated with *H. pylori* infection is curable. No optimal, simple antibiotic regimen has yet emerged. Simultaneous conventional ulcer therapy is recommended to facilitate symptom relief and healing. For refractory ulcers, only maximal acid inhibition offers an advantage over continued conventional therapy; cure of *H. pylori* infection is likely to facilitate healing of refractory ulcers. Only with complicated or refractory ulcers should conventional maintenance therapy be continued, at least until *H. pylori* is successfully eradicated. A search for NSAID use is indicated for all ulcer patients. Patients with peptic ulcer taking NSAIDs should discontinue use of these drugs whenever possible. *H. pylori*, if present, should be eradicated (Soll, 1996). Guidelines to assist the primary care physician, internist, and gastroenterologist with the diagnosis and treatment of new-onset dyspepsia have been published by the American Gastroenterological Association (Statement AGAMP, 1998). In younger patients with no alarming features who are *H. pylori*-negative, it is recommended that a trial of antisecretory therapy (e.g., H2 blocker or proton pump inhibitor) be prescribed for 1 month, and referral for early upper endoscopy is always indicated in older patients presenting with new-onset dyspepsia.

The important factors in selecting therapy are efficacy of eradication, prevention of resistance, avoidance or minimization of adverse effects, patient compliance, and cost. The most effective regimens include a bismuth preparation or an antisecretory drug (proton pump inhibitor or H2 receptor antagonist) plus two antibiotics administered for 14 days. Dual-drug therapies are no longer recommended. Triple-drug regimens are more likely to eradicate *H. pylori* and less likely to generate resistant strains among surviving organisms. In general, cure of the infection should be confirmed 4 weeks after completion of the treatment. Antibiotic resistance is an important consideration in choosing therapy, and patients should be made aware of the importance of compliance (Graham et al., 1999).

The result of the Canadian *H. pylori* Consensus Conferences recommend the testing and treatment of *H. pylori* infection in patients with known peptic ulcer disease and those with ulcer-like dyspepsia; it was decided that the urea breath test (not serology) should be used for routine diagnosis of *H. pylori* infection unless endoscopy is indicated for another reason. Recommended therapies were a twice daily, 7-day regimen of a proton pump inhibitor (omeprazole 20 mg, lansoprazole 30 mg, pantoprazole 40 mg) or ranitidine bismuth citrate 400 mg plus clarithromycin 500 mg and amoxicillin 1000 mg or plus clarithromycin 500 or 250 mg and metronidazole 500 mg. Regional centers should be established to monitor the prevalence of antibiotic-resistant *H.*

pylori infections (Hunt et al., 1999). The current attitudes to *H. pylori* infection in Switzerland among the members of the Swiss Society for Gastroenterology and Hepatology coincide with the Canadian guidelines. Peptic ulcer disease, mucosa-associated lymphoid tissue lymphoma, and therapy-resistant dyspepsia were clear indications for *H. pylori* eradication. Two antibiotics together with proton pump inhibitors constitute the most widely used eradication therapy (Binek et al., 1999).

Attention has been drawn to the high incidence of *H. pylori* in patients with bleeding peptic ulcer. This issue has been underestimated since many infected patients who present with bleeding do not receive eradication treatment. Rebleeding is largely preventable if more attention is given to diagnosis and treatment of *H. pylori.* Follow-up can be performed with a urea breath test (Garrigan et al., 1999). The combination of ranitidine bismuth citrate plus amoxicillin cures *H. pylori* infection in more than half of the patients treated. This treatment regimen is promising as a basis for future non-macrolide, non-imidazole triple-therapy regimens for eradicating *H. pylori*. Such regimens may be appropriate second-line treatments for patients who are resistant or unable to tolerate macrolide- or imidazole-containing therapies (Graham et al., 1998).

A 7-day triple therapy using lansoprazole (LAC15) is an efficient and economical regimen for the eradication of *H. pylori* (Sieg et al., 1999). The efficacy of 1-week bismuth triple therapy is adversely influenced by the presence of metronidazole resistance. In vitro studies suggest that ranitidine bismuth citrate plus metronidazole exhibit synergistic activity against metronidazole-resistant strains of *H. pylori.* One week of ranitidine bismuth citrate triple therapy with metronidazole and tetracycline is effective. This regimen is more appropriate in areas of high metronidazole resistance (Kung et al., 1999). In countries without the antibiotics used in western Europe and the United States, 1-week triple therapy consisting of tripotassium dicitrato bismuthate, low-dose furazolidone, and low-dose clarithromycin also achieves a high cure rate of *H. pylori* (Xiao et al., 1999). In a population of duodenal ulcer patients without predisposing risk factors for ulcer bleeding, antibiotic eradication or suppression of *H. pylori* infection prevented the occurrence of ulcer-related hemorrhage for up to 1 year after therapy (Sonnenberg et al., 1999).

In cases that require a surgical procedure, the treatment of choice for gastroduodenal ulcer is highly selective vagotomy. The laparoscopic approach shortens the hospital stay and improves the patient's comfort (Cadiere et al., 1999). However, laparoscopic repair of perforated peptic ulcer does not yield any additional benefits over open repair (Bergamaschi et al., 1999).

The empiric use of antibiotic therapy for patients with peptic ulcer without confirmation of the presence of *H. pylori* is not justified and cannot be recommended (Ciociola et al., 1999). NSAIDs are widely used for analgesic, anti-inflammatory, and antithrombotic indications. Such use carries the risk of gastrointestinal complications. NSAIDs promote ulcerous and nonulcerous lesions. Symptoms are poor predictors of serious lesions and complications, which may occur without previous symptoms. NSAIDs also delay the healing of peptic ulcers, even to the extent of intractability, and may cause recurrence after gastric surgery. Prophylactic therapy is indicated in high-risk patients (age >60 years, previous ulcer history, high-dose and concomitant use of corticosteroids or anticoagulants). Misoprostol, omeprazole, and high-dose famotidine have been shown to reduce the occurrence of both gastric and duodenal ulcers in NSAID users. As previously discussed, at present, the role of *H. pylori* in NSAID-induced gastroduodenal lesions is unclear, and there is no agreement in considering the organism as a risk factor and indicating its eradication in NSAID users (Lanas and Hirschowitz, 1999).

Since antibiotics can never be the ideal treatment of a condition, active research is concentrated on the development of vaccines to eradicate *H. pylori* and of safer drugs to replace the current NSAIDs.

Collection and interpretation of comprehensive family history data as an initial method for risk stratification for many preventable, chronic conditions has been shown to be feasible (Scheuner et al., 1997). Since such findings may have important implications for disease prevention and management, treatment of relatives of patients with peptic ulcer, gastric lymphoma, and gastric cancer must be considered. However, antimicrobial therapy for *H. pylori* infection remains an evolving area because of the search for simpler and more effective treatment regimens (Go and Fennerty, 1998). Also, although parent-to-child transmission and a common infection source are probable causes of intrafamilial clustering of *H. pylori*, DNA analysis of the gastric biopsy specimens of family members of *H. pylori*-positive patients has shown that only some of the children exhibited patterns identical to those of their siblings or to that of one of the parents (Wang et al., 1993). Therefore, at present, the guidelines to treat family members should be similar to those for patients with dyspepsia in primary care.

REFERENCES

Abraham LJ, Marley JV, Nedospasov SA, Cambon-Thomsen A, Crouau-Roy B, Dawkins RL, Giphart MJ: Microsatellite, restriction fragment-length polymorphism, and sequence-specific oligonucleotide typing of the tumor necrosis factor region. Comparisons of the 4AOHW cell panel. Hum Immunol 1993; 38:17–23.

Allen RD: Polymorphism of the human TNF-α promoter-random variation of functional diversity? Mol Immunol 1999; 36:1017–1027.

Andersen IB, Bonnevie O, Jorgensen T, Sorensen TI: Time trends for peptic ulcer disease in Denmark, 1981–1993. Analysis of hospitalization register and mortality data. Scand J Gastroenterol 1998; 33:260–266.

Appelmelk BJ, Simoons-Smit IM, Negrini R, Moran AP, Aspinall GO, Forte JG, Vries TD, Quan H, Verboom T, Maaskant JJ, et al.: Potential role of molecular mimicry between *Helicobacter pylori* lipopolysaccharide and host Lewis blood group antigens in autoimmunity. Infect Immun 1996; 64:2031–2040.

Appleyard CB, McCafferty DM, Tigley AW, Swain MG, Wallace JL: Tumor necrosis factor mediation of NSAID-induced gastric damage: role of leukocyte adherence. Am J Physiol 1996; 270:G42–G48.

Axon A, Forman D: *Helicobacter* gastroduodenitis: a serious infectious disease [editorial] [see comments]. BMJ 1997; 314:1430–1431.

Azarow K, Kim P, Shandling B, Ein S: A 45-year experience with surgical treatment of peptic ulcer disease in children. J Pediatr Surg 1996; 31:750–753.

Azuma T, Ito Y, Miyaji H, Dojyo M, Tanaka Y, Hirai M, Ito S, Kato T, Kohli Y: Immunogenetic analysis of the human leukocyte antigen DQA1 locus in patients with duodenal ulcer or chronic atrophic gastritis harbouring *Helicobacter pylori*. Eur J Gastroenterol Hepatol 1995; 7:S71–S73.

Bamford KB, Bickley J, Collins JS, Johnston BT, Potts S, Boston V, Owen RJ, Sloan JM: *Helicobacter pylori*: comparison of DNA fingerprints provides evidence for intrafamilial infection. Gut 1993; 34:1348–1350.

Bamford KB, Fan X, Crowe SE, Leary JF, Gourley WK, Luthra GK, Brooks EG, Graham DY, Reyes VE, Ernst PB: Lymphocytes in the human gastric mucosa during *Helicobacter pylori* have a T helper cell 1 phenotype. Gastroenterology 1998; 114:482–492.

Bastaki SM, Wallace JL: Pathogenesis of nonsteroidal anti-inflammatory drug gastropathy: Clues to preventative therapy. Can J Gastroenterol 1999; 13:123–127.

Beales ILP, Calam J: *Helicobacter pylori* infection and tumour necrosis factor-alpha increase gastrin release from human gastric antral fragments. Eur J Gastroenterol Hepatol 1997a; 9:773–777.

Beales ILP, Calam J: *Helicobacter pylori* stimulates granulocyte-macrophage colony-stimulating factor (GM-CSF) production from cultured antral biopsies and a human gastric epithelial cell line. Eur J Gastroenterol Hepatol 1997b; 9:451–455.

Beales ILP, Calam J: Stimulation of IL-8 production in human gastric epithelial cells by *Helicobacter pylori*, IL-1-beta and TNF-alpha requires tyrosine kinase activity, but not protein kinase C. Cytokine 1997c; 9:514–520.

Beales ILP, Calam J: Interleukin 1β and tumour necrosis factor α inhibit acid secretion in cultured rabbit parietal cells by multiple pathways. Gut 1998a; 42:227–234.

Beales ILP, Calam J: The histamine H3 receptor agonist $N\alpha$-methylhistamine produced by *Helicobacter pylori* does not alter somatostatin release from cultured rabbit fundic D-cells. Gut 1998b; 43:176–181.

Beales ILP, Davey NJ, Pusey CD, Lechler RI, Calam J: Long-term sequelae of *Helicobacter pylori* gastritis. Lancet 1995; 346:381–382.

Bergamaschi R, Marvik R, Johnsen G, Thoresen JE, Ystgaard B, Myrvold HE: Open vs laparoscopic repair of perforated peptic ulcer. Surg Endosc 1999; 13:679–682.

Bernstein CN, McKeown I, Embil JM, Blanchard JF, Dawood M, Kabani A, Kliewer E, Smart G, Coghlan G, MacDonald S, et al.: Seroprevalence of *Helicobacter pylori*, incidence of gastric cancer, and peptic ulcer–associated hospitalizations in a Canadian Indian population. Dig Dis Sci 1999; 44:668–674.

Binek J, Fantin AC, Meyenberger C: Attitude to *Helicobacter pylori* infection among Swiss gastroenterologists. Schweiz Med Wochenschr 1999; 129:441–445.

Blaser MJ: Ecology of *Helicobacter pylori* in the human stomach. J Clin Invest 1997; 100:759–762.

Blaser MJ: *Helicobacter pylori* and gastric diseases. BMJ 1998; 316:1507–1510.

Blaser MJ, Kirschner D: Dynamics of *Helicobacter pylori* colonization in relation to the host response. Proc Natl Acad Sci USA 1999; 96:8359–8364.

Bloom BS, Fendrick AM, Ramsey SD: Changes in peptic ulcer and gastritis/duodenitis in Great Britain, 1970–1985. J Clin Gastroenterol 1990; 12:100–108.

Bonnevie O: The incidence of gastric ulcer in Copenhagen County. Scand J Gastroenterol 1975a; 10:231–239.

Bonnevie O: The incidence of duodenal ulcer in Copenhagen County. Scand J Gastroenterol 1975b; 10:385–393.

Borén T, Falk P, Roth KA, Larson G, Normark S: Attachment of *Helicobacter pylori* to human gastric epithelium mediated by blood group antigens. Science 1993; 262:1892–1895.

Bouma G, Crusius JBA, Oudkerk Pool M, Kolkman JJ, von Blomberg BME, Kostense PJ, Giphart MJ, Schreuder GMT, Meuwissen SGM, Peña AS: Secretion of tumour necrosis factor alpha and lymphotoxin alpha in relation to polymorphisms in the TNF genes and HLA-DR alleles: relevance for inflammatory bowel disease. Scand J Immunol 1996; 43:456–463.

Brenner H, Rothenbacher D, Bode G, Adler G: The individual and joint contributions of *Helicobacter pylori* infection and family history to the risk for peptic ulcer disease. J Infect Dis 1998a; 177:1124–1127.

Brenner H, Rothenbacher D, Bode G, Adler G: Parental history of gastric or duodenal ulcer and prevalence of *Helicobacter pylori* infection in preschool children: population based study. BMJ 1998b; 316:665.

Brenner H, Rothenbacher D, Bode G, Dieudonne P, Adler G: Active infection with *Helicobacter pylori* in healthy couples. Epidemiol Infect 1999; 122:91–95.

Cabrera M, Shaw M-A, Sharples C, Williams H, Castes M, Convit J, Blackwell JM: Polymorphism in tumor necrosis factor genes associated with mucocutaneous leishmaniasis. J Exp Med 1995; 182:1259–1264.

Cadiere GB, Bruyns J, Himpens J, Van Alphen P, Verturyen M: Laparoscopic highly selective vagotomy. Hepatogastroenterology 1999; 46:1500–1506.

Celik J, Su B, Tiren U, Finkel Y, Thoresson AC, Engstrand L, Sandstedt B, Bernander S, Normark S: Virulence and colonization-associated properties of *Helicobacter pylori* isolated from children and adolescents. J Infect Dis 1998; 177:247–252.

Chan FK, Sung JJ: *Helicobacter pylori* eradication in long-term users of non-steroidal anti-inflammatory drugs [letter; comment]. Lancet 1998; 352:2016–2017.

Chan KL, Tam PK, Saing H: Long-term follow-up of childhood duodenal ulcers. J Pediatr Surg 1997; 32:1609–1611.

Ching CK, Lam SK: *Helicobacter pylori* epidemiology in relation to peptic ulcer and gastric cancer in south and north China. J Gastroenterol Hepatol 1994; 9:S4–S7.

Ciociola AA, McSorley DJ, Turner K, Sykes D, Palmer JB: *Helicobacter pylori* infection rates in duodenal ulcer patients in the United States may be lower than previously estimated. Am J Gastroenterol 1999; 94:1834–1840.

Clarke CA, Wyn Edwards J, Haddock RW, Howel-Evans AW, McConenell RB: ABO blood groups and secretor character in duodenal ulcer. Population and sibship studies. BMJ 1956; 3:725–731.

Covacci A, Censini S, Bugnoli M, Petracca R, Burroni D, Macchia G, Massone A, Papini E, Xiang Z, Figura N, et al: Molecular characterization of the 128-kDa immunodominant antigen of *Helicobacter pylori* associated with cytotoxicity and duodenal ulcer. Proc Natl Acad Sci USA 1993; 90:5791–5795.

Crabtree JE, Shallcross TM, Heatley RV, Wyatt JI: Mucosal tumour necrosis factor alpha and interleukin-6 in patients with *Helicobacter pylori* associated gastritis. Gut 1991; 32:1473–1477.

Crusius JBA, Bing X, Mulder CJJ, Mearin ML, Peña AS: Relevance of haplotypes in the TNF region in celiac disease. Eur Cytokine Netw 1994; 2:168.

D'Alfonso S, Momigliano Richiardi P: A polymorphic variation in a putative regulation box of the *TNFA* promoter region. Immunogenetics 1994; 39:150–154.

Danis VA, Millington M, Hyland VJ, Grennan D: Cytokine production by normal human monocytes: inter-subject variation and relationship to an IL-1 receptor antagonist (IL-1Ra) gene polymorphism. Clin Exp Immunol 1995; 99:303–310.

Degli-Esposti MA, Leaver AL, Christiansen FT, Witt CS, Abraham LJ, Dawkins RL: Ancestral haplotypes; conserved population MHC haplotypes. Hum Immunol 1992; 34:242–252.

Dickey W, Collins JSA, Watson RGP, Sloan JM, Porter KG: Secretor status and *Helicobacter pylori* infection are independent risk factors for gastroduodenal disease. Gut 1993; 34:351–353.

Ding SZ, Cho CH, Lam SK: *Helicobacter pylori* induces interleukin-8 expression in endothelial cells and the signal pathway is protein tyrosine kinase dependent. Biochem Biophys Res Commun 1997; 240:561–565.

Dixon M: Acid, ulcers, and *H. pylori*. Lancet 1993; 342:384–385.

Doll R, Kellock TD: The separate inheritance of gastric and duodenal ulcers. Ann Eugen 1951; 16:231–240.

Drumm B, Perez-Perez GI, Blaser MJ, Sherman PM: Intrafamilial clustering of *Helicobacter pylori* infection. N Engl J Med 1990; 322:359–363.

Dyrek I, Gaida G, Bock H, Mares A, Gaida H: Bleeding ulcus duodenum in a 12 year old boy as the first symptom of familial *Helicobacter pylori* infection. Monatsschr Kinderheilkunde 1997; 145:897–900.

El-Omar EM, Oien K, El-Nujumi A, Gillen D, Wirz A, Dahill S, Williams C, Ardill JE, McColl KE: *Helicobacter pylori* infection and chronic gastric acid hyposecretion. Gastroenterology 1997; 113:15–24.

El-Omar EM, Penman ID, Ardill JE, Chittajallu RS, Howie C, McColl KE: *Helicobacter pylori* infection and abnormalities of acid secretion in patients with duodenal ulcer disease. Gastroenterology 1995; 109:681–691.

El-Omar EM: The importance of interleukin 1β in *Helicobacter pylori* associated disease. Gut 2001; 48:743–747.

El-Serag HB, Sonnenberg A: Opposing time trends of peptic ulcer and reflux disease. Gut 1998; 43:327–333.

Endres S, Cannon JG, Ghorbani R, Dempsey RA, Sisson SD, Lonnemann G, Van der Meer JW, Wolff SM, Dinarello CA: In vitro production of IL 1beta, IL 1alpha, TNF and IL2 in healthy subjects: distribution, effect of cyclooxygenase inhibition and evidence of independent gene regulation. Eur J Immunol 1989; 19:2327–2333.

Falk P, Roth KA, Boren T, Westblom TU, Gordon JI, Normark S: An in vitro adherence assay reveals that *Helicobacter pylori* exhibits cell lineage-specific tropism in the human gastric epithelium. Proc Natl Acad Sci USA 1993; 90:2035–2039.

Fan X, Crowe SE, Behar S, Gunasena H, Ye G, Haeberle H, Van Houten N, Gourley WK, Ernst PB, Reyes VET: The effect of class II major histocompatibility complex expression on adherence of *Helicobacter pylori* and induction of apoptosis in gastric epithelial cells: a mechanism for T helper cell type 1–mediated damage. J Exp Med 1998; 187:1659–1669.

Fan XG, Chua A, Fan XJ, Keeling PW: Increased gastric production of interleukin-8 and tumour necrosis factor in patients with *Helicobacter pylori* infection. J Clin Pathol 1995; 48:133–136.

Faust TW, Redfern JS, Podolsky I, Lee E, Grundy SM, Feldman M: Effects of aspirin on gastric mucosal prostaglandin E_2 and F_2 alpha content and on gastric mucosal injury in humans receiving fish oil or olive oil. Gastroenterology 1990; 98:586–591.

Fearon DT: Seeking wisdom in innate immunity. Nature 1997; 388:323–324.

Fearon DT, Locksley RM: The instructive role of innate immunity in the acquired immune response. Science 1996; 272:50–53.

Feldman M, Cryer B, McArthur KE, Huet BA, Lee E: Effects of aging and gastritis on gastric acid and pepsin secretion in humans: a prospective study. Gastroenterology 1996; 110:1043–1052.

Ferencik S, Lindemann M, Horsthemke B, Grosse-Wilde H: A new restriction fragment length polymorphism of the human *TNF-B* gene detected by *AspHI* digest. Eur J Immunogenet 1992; 19:425–430.

Fiorucci S, Santucci L, Migliorati G, Riccardi C, Amorosi A, Mancini A, Roberti R, Morelli A: Isolated guinea pig gastric chief cells express tumour necrosis factor receptors coupled with the sphingomyelin pathway. Gut 1996; 38:182–189.

Forbes GM, Warren JR, Glaser ME, Cullen DJ, Marshall BJ, Collins BJ: Long-term follow-up of gastric histology after *Helicobacter pylori* eradication. J Gastroenterol Hepatol 1996; 11:670–673.

Fox JG, Li X, Cahill RJ, Andrutis K, Rustgi AK, Odze R, Wang TC: Hypertrophic gastropathy in *Helicobacter felis*–infected wild-type C57BL/6 mice and p53 hemizygous transgenic mice. Gastroenterology 1996; 110:55–166.

García-Gonzalez MA, Lanas A, Santolaria S, Crusius JBA, Serrano T, Peña AS: The polymorphic *IL-1β* and *IL-1RN* genes in the aetiopathogenesis of peptic ulcer. Clin Exp Immunol 2001; 125:368–375.

Garrigan K, McIntosh C, Fraser AG: Bleeding peptic ulcers: audit of eradication treatment for *H. pylori*. N Z Med J 1999; 112:178–180.

Gerhard M, Lehn N, Neumayer N, Born T, Rad R, Schepp W, Miehlke S, Classen M, Prinz C: Clinical relevance of the *Helicobacter pylori* gene for blood-group antigen-binding adhesin. Proc Natl Acad Sci USA 1999; 96:12778–12783.

Gillen D, el-Omar EM, Wirz AA, Ardill JE, McColl KE: The acid response to gastrin distinguishes duodenal ulcer patients from *Helicobacter pylori*–infected healthy subjects. Gastroenterology 1998; 114:50–57.

Go MF: What are the host factors that place an individual at risk for *Helicobacter pylori*–associated disease? Gastroenterology 1997; 113:S15–S20.

Go MF, Fennerty MB: Treatment of *Helicobacter pylori* infection. Curr Opin Gastroenterol 1998; 14:64–69.

Goedhard JG, Biemond I, Peña AS, Kreuning J, Schreuder GM, van Rood JJ: HLA and duodenal ulcer in the Netherlands. Tissue Antigens 1983; 22:213–218.

Goodman KJ, Correa P: The transmission of *Helicobacter pylori*. A critical review of the evidence. Int J Epidemiol 1995; 24:875–887.

Graham DY: Gastrin sensitivity and acid in *H. pylori*: revisited [letter]. Gastroenterology 1998; 115:509–510.

Graham DY, Breiter JR, Ciociola AA, Sykes DL, McSorley DJ: An alternative non-macrolide, non-imidazole treatment regimen for curing *Helicobacter pylori* and duodenal ulcers: ranitidine bismuth citrate plus amoxicillin. The RBC *H. pylori* Study Group. Helicobacter 1998; 3:125–131.

Graham DY, Go MF, Lew GM, Genta RM, Rehfeld JF: *Helicobacter pylori* infection and exaggerated gastrin release. Effects of inflammation and progastrin processing. Scand J Gastroenterol 1993; 28:690–694.

Graham DY, Malaty HM, Go MF: Are there susceptible hosts to *Helicobacter pylori* infection? Scand J Gastroenterol Suppl 1994; 205:6–10.

Graham DY, Rakel RE, Fendrick AM, Go MF, Marshall BJ, Peura DA, Scherger JE: Practical advice on eradicating *Helicobacter pylori* infection. Postgrad Med 1999; 105:137–140.

Gryboski JD: Peptic ulcer disease in children. Med Clin North Am 1991; 75:889–902.

Gutierrez O, Melo M, Segura AM, Angel A, Genta RM, Graham DY: Cure of *Helicobacter pylori* infection improves gastric acid secretion in patients with corpus gastritis. Scand J Gastroenterol 1997; 32:664–668.

Habibullah CM, Mujahid Ali M, Ishaq M, Prasad R, Pratap B, Saleem Y: Study of duodenal ulcer disease in 100 families using total serum pepsinogen as a genetic marker. Gut 1984; 25:1380–1383.

Harris AW, Gummett PA, Phull PS, Jacyna MR, Misiewicz JJ, Baron JH: Recurrence of duodenal ulcer after *Helicobacter pylori* eradication is related to high acid output. Aliment Pharmacol Ther 1997; 11:331–334.

Harris PR, Mobley HL, Perez-Perez GI, Blaser MJ, Smith PD: *Helicobacter pylori* urease is a potent stimulus of mononuclear phagocyte activation and inflammatory cytokine production. Gastroenterology 1996; 111:419–425.

Hawkey CJ: Personal review: *Helicobacter pylori*, NSAIDs and cognitive dissonance. Aliment Pharmacol Ther 1999; 13:695–702.

Hawkey CJ, Karrasch JA, Szczepanski L, Walker DG, Barkun A, Swannell AJ, Yeomans ND: Omeprazole compared with misoprostol for ulcers associated with nonsteroidal antiinflammatory drugs. Omeprazole versus Misoprostol for NSAID-induced Ulcer Management (OMNIUM) Study Group. N Engl J Med 1998a; 338:727–734.

Hawkey CJ, Tulassay Z, Szczepanski L, van Rensburg CJ, Filipowicz-Sosnowska A, Lanas A, Wason CM, Peacock RA, Gillon KR: Randomised controlled trial of *Helicobacter pylori* eradication in patients on non-steroidal anti-inflammatory drugs: HELP NSAIDs study. *Helicobacter* Eradication for Lesion Prevention [published erratum appears in Lancet 1998; 352:1634]. Lancet 1998b; 352:1016–1021.

Hein HO, Suadicani P, Gyntelberg F: Genetic markers for peptic ulcer. A study of 3387 men aged 54 to 74 years: the Copenhagen Male Study. Scand J Gastroenterol 1997; 32:16–21.

Horn J, Herfarth C: Duodenal ulcer of foreign workers. Med Klin 1978; 73:1417–1421.

Hunt RH, Fallone CA, Thomson AB: Canadian *Helicobacter pylori* Consensus Conference update: infections in adults. Canadian *Helicobacter* Study Group. Can J Gastroenterol 1999; 13:213–217.

Huseyinov A, Kutukculer N, Aydogdu S, Caglayan S, Coker I, Goksen D: Increased gastric production of platelet-activating factor, leukotriene-B_4, and tumor necrosis factor-alpha in children with *Helicobacter pylori* infection. Dig Dis Sci 1999; 44:675–679.

Hyvarinen H, Salmenkyla S, Sipponen P: *Helicobacter pylori*-negative duodenal and pyloric ulcer: role of NSAIDs. Digestion 1996; 57:305–309.

Ihamaki T, Varis K, Siurala M: Morphological, functional and immunological state of the gastric mucosa in gastric carcinoma families. Comparison with a computer-matched family sample. Scand J Gastroenterol 1979; 14:801–812.

Isomoto H, Mizuta Y, Fukushima K, Takeshima F, Miyazaki M, Murase K, Omagari K, Maeda T, Kamihira S, Shimokawa I, et al.: Low prevalence of *Helicobacter pylori* in individuals with HTLV-I infection. Eur J Gastroenterol Hepatol 1999; 11:497–502.

Jacob CO, Fronek Z, Lewis GD, Koo M, Hansen JA, McDevitt HO: Heritable major histocompatibility complex class II–associated differences in production of tumor necrosis factor alpha: relevance to genetic predisposition to systemic lupus erythematosus. Proc Natl Acad Sci USA 1990; 87:1233–1237.

Kalach N, Raymond J, Benhamou PH, Bergeret M, Dupont C: Managing intrafamilial dissemination of *Helicobacter pylori* gastric infection improves eradication rate in children [letter]. J Pediatr Gastroenterol Nutr 1999; 28:356.

Kawai K, Shirakawa K, Misaki F, Hayashi K, Watanabe Y: Natural history and epidemiologic studies of peptic ulcer disease in Japan. Gastroenterology 1989; 96:581–585.

Kiaer T, Roin J, Djurhuus J, Niclassen SD, Bonnevie O: Epidemiological aspects of peptic ulcer disease on the Faroe Islands. An interim report. Scand J Gastroenterol 1985; 20:1157–1162.

Knill-Jones RP: Geographical differences in the prevalence of dyspepsia. Scand J Gastroenterol Suppl 1991; 182:17–24.

Konishi J, Azuma T, Kohli Y, Fujiki N: Genetic heterogeneity of combined gastric and duodenal ulcers detected by pepsinogen C gene polymorphism. J Gastroenterol Hepatol 1994; 9:334–339.

Koskenvuo M, Kaprio J, Romanov K: Twin studies in metabolic diseases. Ann Med 1992; 24:379–381.

Kroeger KM, Carville KS, Abraham LJ: The −308 tumor necrosis factor-α promoter polymorphism effects transcription. Mol Immunol 1997; 34:391–399.

Kuipers EJ, Peña AS, van Kamp G, Uyterlinde AM, Pals G, Pels NF, Kurz-Pohlmann E, Meuwissen SGM: Seroconversion for *Helicobacter pylori*. Lancet 1993; 342: 328–331.

Kung NN, Sung JJ, Yuen NW, Li TH, Ng PW, Lai WM, Lui YH, Lam KN, Choi CH, Leung EM: One-week ranitidine bismuth citrate versus colloidal bismuth subcitrate-based anti-*Helicobacter* triple therapy: a prospective randomized controlled trial. Am J Gastroenterol 1999; 94:721–724.

Kurata JH, Haile BM: Epidemiology of peptic ulcer disease. Clin Gastroenterol 1984; 13:289–307.

Kurata JH, Honda GD, Frankl H: The incidence of duodenal and gastric ulcers in a large health maintenance organization. Am J Public Health 1985a; 75:625–629.

Kurata JH, Haile BM, Elashoff JD: Sex differences in peptic ulcer disease. Gastroenterology 1985b; 88:96–100.

Kurata JH, Nogawa AN: Meta-analysis of risk factors for peptic ulcer. Nonsteroidal antiinflammatory drugs, *Helicobacter pylori*, and smoking. J Clin Gastroenterol 1997; 24:2–17.

Lam SK: Pathogenesis and pathophysiology of duodenal ulcer. Clin Gastroenterol 1984; 13:447–472.

Lam SK: Epidemiology and genetics of peptic ulcer. Gastroenterol Jpn 1993; 28(Suppl 5):145–157.

Lam SK, Isenberg JI, Grossman MI, Lane WH, Walsh JH: Gastric acid secretion is abnormally sensitive to endogenous gastrin released after peptone test meals in duodenal ulcer patients. J Clin Invest 1980; 65:555–562.

Lam SK, Koo J: Gastrin sensitivity in duodenal ulcer. Gut 1985; 26:485–490.

Lam SK, Lai CL: Gastric ulcers with and without associated duodenal ulcer have different pathophysiology. Clin Sci Mol Med 1978; 55:97–102.

Lam SK, Ong GB: Duodenal ulcers: early and late onset. Gut 1976; 17:169–179.

Lam SK, Ong GB: Relationship of postprandial serum gastrin response to sex, body weight, blood group status, familial dyspepsia, duration, and age of onset of ulcer symptoms in duodenal ulcer. Gut 1980; 21:528–532.

Lam SK, Sircus W: Studies on duodenal ulcer. I. The clinical evidence for the existence of two populations. Q J Med 1975; 44:369–387.

Lanas A, García-González MA, Santolaria S, Crusius JBA, Serrano MT, Benito R, Peña AS: *TNF* and *LTA* gene polymorphisms reveal different risks in gastric and duodenal ulcer patients. Genes Immun 2001; 2:415–421.

Lanas A, Hirschowitz BI: Toxicity of NSAIDs in the stomach and duodenum. Eur J Gastroenterol Hepatol 1999; 11:375–381.

Langman MJ, Weil J, Wainwright P, Lawson DH, Rawlins MD, Logan RF, Murphy M, Vessey MP, Colin-Jones DG: Risks of bleeding peptic ulcer associated with individual non-steroidal anti-inflammatory drugs [published erratum appears in Lancet 1994; 343:1302]. Lancet 1994; 343:1075–1078.

Lee A, Dixon MF, Danon SJ, Kuipers E, Megraud F, Larsson H, Mellgard B: Local acid production and *Helicobacter pylori*: a unifying hypothesis of gastroduodenal disease. Eur J Gastroenterol Hepatol 1995; 7:461–465.

Levine JS: Misoprostol and nonsteroidal anti-inflammatory drugs: a tale of effects, outcomes, and costs. Ann Intern Med 1995; 123:309–310.

Lindholm C, Quiding-Jarbrink M, Lonroth H, Hamlet A, Svennerholm AM: Local cytokine response in *Helicobacter pylori*–infected subjects. Infect Immun 1998; 66:5964–5971.

Logan RP, Berg DE: Genetic diversity of *Helicobacter pylori* [published erratum appears in Lancet 1997; 349:64]. Lancet 1996; 348:1462–1463.

Logan RP, Polson RJ, Rao G, Walker MM, Pedley S, Harris JR, Pinching AJ, Baron JH: *Helicobacter pylori* and HIV infection. Lancet 1990; 335:1456.

Mackay CR: Chemokines: what chemokine is that? Curr Biol 1997; 7:R384–R386.

Mahony MJ, Wyatt JI, Littlewood JM: Management and response to treatment of *Helicobacter pylori* gastritis. Arch Dis Child 1992; 67:940–943.

Malaty HM, Engstrand L, Pedersen NL, Graham DY: *Helicobacter pylori* infection: genetic and environmental influences. A study of twins. Ann Intern Med 1994; 120:982–986.

Malaty HM, Graham DY, Isaksson I, Engstrand L, Pedersen NL: Co-twin study of the effect of environment and dietary elements on acquisition of *Helicobacter pylori* infection. Am J Epidemiol 1998; 148:793–797.

Malfertheiner P, Labenz J. Does *Helicobacter pylori* status affect nonsteroidal anti-inflammatory drug–associated gastroduodenal pathology? Am J Med 1998; 104:35S–42S.

Marshall BJ, Warren JR: Unidentified curved bacilli in the stomach of patients with gastritis and peptic ulceration. Lancet 1984; 1:1311–1315.

McGuire W, Hill AVS, Allsopp CEM, Greenwood BM, Kwiatkowski D: Variation in the TNF-alpha promoter region associated with susceptibility to cerebral malaria. Nature 1994; 371:508–510.

Mendall MA: Transmission of *Helicobacter pylori*. Semin Gastrointest Dis 1997; 8:113–123.

Mendall MA, Goggin PM, Molineaux N, Levy J, Toosy T, Strachan D, Northfield TC: Childhood living conditions and *Helicobacter pylori* seropositivity in adult life. Lancet 1992; 339:896–897.

Mochizuki T, Sugimura K, Sato Y, Ishizuka K, Honma T, Enomoto H, Matsuzawa J, Kobayashi M, Baba Y, Suriki A, et al.: *IL-1B* gene allele 2 involves the decreased production of gastric mucosal IL-1β in response to *Helicobacter pylori* of common genetic strain in Japan, and relates to the pathogenesis of duodenal ulcer. Gastroenterology 1998; 114:G947.

Mohammadi M, Czinn S, Redline R, Nedrud J: *Helicobacter*-specific cell-mediated immune responses display a predominant Th1 phenotype and promote a delayed-type hypersensitivity response in the stomachs of mice. J Immunol 1996; 156:4729–4738.

Mølvig J, Baek L, Christensen P, Manogue KR, Vlassara H, Platz P, Nielsen LS, Svejgaard A, Nerup J: Endotoxin-stimulated human monocyte secretion of interleukin-1, tumor necrosis factor-alpha, and prostaglandin-E_2 shows stable interindividual differences. Scand J Immunol 1988; 27:705–716.

Monteiro MA, Chan KH, Rasko DA, Taylor DE, Zheng PY, Appelmelk BJ, Wirth HP, Yang M, Blaser MJ, Hynes SO, et al.: Simultaneous expression of type 1 and type 2 Lewis blood group antigens by *Helicobacter pylori* lipopolysaccharides. Molecular mimicry between *H. pylori* lipopolysaccharides and human gastric epithelial cell surface glycoforms. J Biol Chem 1998; 273:11533–11543.

Moshal MG, Spitaels JM, Robbs JV, MacLeod IN, Good CJ: Eight-year experience with 3392 endoscopically proven duodenal ulcers in Durban, 1972–79. Rise and fall of duodenal ulcers and a theory of changing dietary and social factors. Gut 1981; 22:327–331.

Moss SF, Legon S, Davies J, Calam J: Cytokine gene expression in *Helicobacter pylori* associated antral gastritis. Gut 1994; 35:1567–1570.

Nadel S, Newport MJRB, Booy R, Levin M: Variation in the tumor necrosis factor-alpha gene promoter region may be associated with death from meningococcal disease. J Infect Dis 1996; 174:878–880.

National Institutes of Health: *Helicobacter pylori* in Peptic Ulcer disease. NIH Consensus Statement. Bethesda, MD: NIH, 1994:1–22.

Negrini R, Savio A, Poiesi C, Appelmelk BJ, Buffoli F, Paterlini A, Cesari P, Graffeo M, Vaira D, Franzin G: Antigenic mimicry between *Helicobacter pylori* and gastric mucosa in the pathogenesis of body atrophic gastritis. Gastroenterology 1996; 111:655–665.

Newell MK, Vanderwall J, Beard KS, Freed JK: Ligation of major histocompatibility complex class II molecules mediates apoptotic cell death in resting B lymphocytes. Proc Natl Acad Sci USA 1993; 90:10459–10463.

Nijevitch AA, Khamidullina SV, Khamidullina FM: Childhood duodenal ulcer associated with *Helicobacter pylori* and ABO blood groups [letter]. Am J Gastroenterol 1999; 94:1424–1425.

Niv Y, Fraser G, Delpre G, Neeman A, Leiser A, Samra Z, Scapa E, Gilon E, Bar-Shany S: *Helicobacter pylori* infection and blood groups. Am J Gastroenterol 1996; 91:101–104.

Noach LA, Bosma NB, Jansen J, Hoek FJ, van Deventer SJH, Tytgat GNJ: Mucosal tumor necrosis factor-alpha, interleukin-1 beta, and interleukin-8 production in patients with *Helicobacter pylori* infection. Scand J Gastroenterol 1994; 29:425–429.

Nord KS, Rossi TM, Lebenthal E: Peptic ulcer in children: the predominance of gastric ulcers. Am J Gastroenterol 1981; 75:153–157.

Oderda G, Vaira D, Dell'Olio D, Holton J, Forni M, Altare F, Ansaldi N: Serum pepsinogen I and gastrin concentrations in children positive for *Helicobacter pylori*. J Clin Pathol 1990; 43:762–765.

Ohtaka Y, Azuma T, Konishi J, Ito S, Kuriyama M: Association between genetic polymorphism of the pepsinogen C gene and gastric body ulcer: the genetic predisposition is not associated with *Helicobacter pylori* infection. Gut 1997; 41:469–474.

Orange JS, Biron CA: An absolute and restricted requirement for IL-12 in natural killer cell IFN-gamma production and antiviral defense. Studies of natural killer and T cell responses in contrasting viral infections. J Immunol 1996a; 156:1138–1142.

Orange JS, Biron CA: Characterization of early IL-12, IFN-alpha/beta, and TNF effects on antiviral state and NK cell responses during murine cytomegalovirus infection. J Immunol 1996b; 156:4746–4756.

Ostensen H, Gudmundsen TE, Ostensen M, Burhol PG, Bonnevie O: Smoking, alcohol, coffee, and familial factors: any associations with peptic ulcer disease? A clinically and radiologically prospective study. Scand J Gastroenterol 1985; 20:1227–1235.

Pappo J, Torrey D, Castriotta L, Savinainen A, Kabok Z, Ibraghimov A: *Helicobacter pylori* infection in immunized mice lacking major histocompatibility complex class I and class II functions. Infect Immun 1999; 67:337–341.

Parente F, Maconi G, Sangaletti O, Minguzzi M, Vago L, Rossi E, Bianchi Porro G: Prevalence of *Helicobacter pylori* infection and related gastroduodenal lesions in spouses of *Helicobacter pylori* positive patients with duodenal ulcer. Gut 1996; 39:629–633.

Parsonnet J: The incidence of *Helicobacter pylori* infection. Aliment Pharmacol Ther 1995; 9:45–51.

Pasparakis M, Alexopoulou L, Douni E, Kollias G: Tumour necrosis factors in immune regulation: everything that's interesting is . . . new. Cytokine Growth Factor Rev 1996; 7:223–229.

Peek RM Jr, Miller GG, Tham KT, Perez-Perez GI, Zhao X, Atherton JC, Blaser MJ: Heightened inflammatory response and cytokine expression in vivo to cagA$^+$ *Helicobacter pylori* strains. Lab Invest 1995; 73:760–770.

Pelissero A, Sategna-Guidetti C: Epidemiologic aspects of peptic ulcer disease in northern Italy. J Clin Gastroenterol 1989; 11:351–356.

Pisegna JR, Norton JA, Slimak GG, Metz DC, Maton PN, Gardner JD, Jensen RT: Effects of curative gastrinoma resection on gastric secretory function and antisecretory drug requirement in the Zollinger-Ellison syndrome. Gastroenterology 1992; 102:767–778.

Pociot F, Molvig J, Wogensen L, Worsaae HJN: A *TaqI* polymorphism in the human interleukin-1β (IL-1β) gene correlates with IL-1β secretion in vitro. Eur J Clin Invest 1992; 22:396–402.

Poltorak A, He X, Smirnova I, Liu MY, Huffel CV, Du X, Birdwell D, Alejos E, Silva M, Galanos C, et al.: Defective LPS signaling in C3H/HeJ and C57BL/10ScCr mice: mutations in *Tlr4* gene. Science 1998a; 282:2085–2088.

Poltorak A, Smirnova I, He X, Liu MY, Van Huffel C, Birdwell D, Alejos E, Silva M, Du X, Thompson P, et al.: Genetic and physical mapping of the Lps locus: identification of the Toll-4 receptor as a candidate gene in the critical region. Blood Cells Mol Dis 1998b; 24:340–355.

Pulvertaft CN: Comments on the incidence and natural history of gastric and duodenal ulcer. Postgrad Med J 1968; 44:597–602.

Quaquish I, Burkhardt HU, Heilmann KL: Gastric diseases in foreign workers in the German Federal Republic. MMW Munch Med Wochenschr 1979; 121:1563–1565.

Räihä I, Kemppainen H, Kaprio J, Koskenvuo M, Sourander L: Lifestyle, stress, and genes in peptic ulcer disease. A nationwide twin cohort study. Arch Intern Med 1998; 158:698–704.

Ramsdell F, Seaman MS, Miller RE, Picha KS, Kennedy MK, Lynch DH: Differential ability of Th1 and Th2 T cells to express Fas ligand and to undergo activation-induced cell death. Int Immunol 1994; 6:1545–1553.

Recavarren-Arce S, León-Barúa R, Cok J, Rodriguez C, Berendson R, Gilman RH, Ramírez-Ramos A, Watanabe J: Low prevalence of gastric metaplasia in the duodenal mucosa in Peru. J Clin Gastroenterol 1992; 15:296–301.

Robbs JV, Moshal MG. Duodenal ulceration in Indians and blacks in Durban. S Afr Med J 1979; 55:39–42.

Roca M: Gastritis, duodenitis and peptic activity of the human gastric and duodenal mucosa. D. Phil. Oxford, U.K., 1975.

Rosenstock SJ, Andersen LP, Rosenstock CV, Bonnevie O, Jorgensen T: Socioeconomic factors in *Helicobacter pylori* infection among Danish adults. Am J Public Health 1996; 86:1539–1544.

Roth SH, Bennett RE: Nonsteroidal anti-inflammatory drug gastropathy. Recognition and response. Arch Intern Med 1987; 147:2093–2100.

Rotter JI: Gastric and duodenal ulcer are each many different diseases. Dig Dis Sci 1981; 26:154–160.

Rotter JI, Petersen G, Samloff IM, McConnell RB, Ellis A, Spence MA, Rimoin DL: Genetic heterogeneity of hyperpepsinogenemic I and normopepsinogenemic I duodenal ulcer disease. Ann Intern Med 1979a; 91:372–377.

Rotter JI, Petersen GM, Samloff IM: Pepsinogens and other physiologic markers in genetic studies of peptic ulcer and related disorders. Prog Clin Biol Res 1985; 173:227–244.

Rotter JI, Rimoin DL: Peptic ulcer disease—a heterogeneous group of disorders? Gastroenterology 1977; 73:604–607.

Rotter JI, Rimoin DL, Gursky JM, Terasaki P, Sturdevant RA: HLA-B5 associated with duodenal ulcer. Gastroenterology 1977; 73:438–440.

Rotter JI, Shohat T, Petersen GM: Peptic ulcer disease. In: King RA, Rotter JI, Motulsky AG (eds). The Genetic Basis of Common Diseases. New York: Oxford University Press, 1992:240–278.

Rotter JI, Sones JQ, Samloff IM, Richardson CT, Gursky JM, Walsh JH, Rimoin DL: Duodenal-ulcer disease associated with elevated serum pepsinogen I: an inherited autosomal dominant disorder. N Engl J Med 1979b; 300:63–66.

Rowland M, Drumm B: *Helicobacter pylori* infection and peptic ulcer disease in children. Curr Opin Pediatr 1995; 7:553–559.

Ruuls SR, Sedgwick JD: Unlinking tumor necrosis factor biology from the major histocompatibility complex: lessons from human genetics and animal models. Am J Hum Genet 1999; 65:294–301.

Sakagami T, Dixon M, Orourke J, Howlett R, Alderuccio F, Vella J, Shimoyama T, Lee A: Atrophic gastric changes in both *Helicobacter felis* and *Helicobacter pylori* infected mice are host dependent and separate from antral gastritis. Gut 1996; 39:639–648.

Samloff IM: Pepsinogens, pepsins, and pepsin inhibitors. Gastroenterology 1971; 60:586–604.

Samloff IM, Varis K, Ihamaki T, Siurala M, Rotter JI: Relationships among serum pepsinogen I, serum pepsinogen II, and gastric mucosal histology. A study in relatives of patients with pernicious anemia. Gastroenterology 1982; 83:204–209.

Samloff IM, Varis K, Ihamaki T, Siurala M, Rotter JI: Serum pepsinogens I and II and gastric acid output: effect of gastritis. Prog Clin Biol Res 1985; 173:129–138.

Santamaria P, Gehrz RC, Bryan MK, Barbosa JJ: Involvement of class II MHC molecules in the LPS-induction of IL-1/TNF secretions by human monocytes. Quantitative differences at the polymorphic level. J Immunol 1989; 143:913–922.

Santolaria S, Barrios Y, Quintero E, Benito R, Lanas A: El gen HLADQA1 en la susceptibilidad a la infección por *Helicobacter pylori* en la úlcera péptica. Gastroenterol Hepatol 1998; 21:517A.

Santtila S, Savinainen K, Hurme M: Presence of the *IL-1RA* allele 2 (*IL1RN*2*) is associated with enhanced IL-1beta production in vitro. Scand J Immunol 1998; 47:195–198.

Santucci L, Fiorucci S, Di Matteo FM, Morelli A: Role of tumor necrosis factor alpha release and leukocyte margination in indomethacin-induced gastric injury in rats. Gastroenterology 1995; 108:393–401.

Savarino V, Celle G, Vigneri S: *Helicobacter pylori* and acid secretion. Gastroenterology 1998a; 115:510–511.

Savarino V, Mela GS, Zentilin P, Cimmino MA, Parisi M, Mele MR, Pivari M, Bisso G, Celle G: Effect of one-month treatment with nonsteroidal antiinflammatory drugs (NSAIDs) on gastric pH of rheumatoid arthritis patients. Dig Dis Sci 1998b; 43:459–463.

Scatarige JC, DiSantis DJ: CT of the stomach and duodenum. Radiol Clin North Am 1989; 27:687–706.

Schenk BE, Kuipers EJ, Klinkenberg-Knol EC, Bloemena E, Nelis GF, Festen HP, Jansen EH, Biemond I, Lamers CB, Meuwissen SG: Hypergastrinaemia during long-term omeprazole therapy: influences of vagal nerve function, gastric emptying and *Helicobacter pylori* infection. Aliment Pharmacol Ther 1998; 12:605–612.

Scheuner MT, Wang SJ, Raffel LJ, Larabell SK, Rotter JI: Family history: a comprehensive genetic risk assessment method for the chronic conditions of adulthood. Am J Med Genet 1997; 71:315–324.

Segal I, Dubb AA, Tim LO, Solomon A, Sottomayor MC, Zwane EM: Duodenal ulcer and working-class mobility in an African population in South Africa. BMJ 1978; 1:469–472.

Sieg A, Sellinger M, Schlauch D, Horner M, Fuchs W: Short-term triple therapy with lansoprazole 30 mg or 60 mg, amoxycillin and clarithromycin to eradicate *Helicobacter pylori*. Aliment Pharmacol Ther 1999; 13:865–868.

Silverstein FE: Improving the gastrointestinal safety of NSAIDs: the development of misoprostol-from hypothesis to clinical practice. Dig Dis Sci 1998; 43:447–458.

Sipponen P: *Helicobacter pylori* gastritis–epidemiology. J Gastroenterol 1997; 32:273–277.

Sipponen P, Hyvarinen H: Role of *Helicobacter pylori* in the pathogenesis of gastritis, peptic ulcer and gastric cancer. Scand J Gastroenterol Suppl 1993; 196:3–6.

Soll AH: Consensus conference. Medical treatment of peptic ulcer disease. Practice guidelines. Practice Parameters Committee of the American College of Gastroenterology [published erratum appears in JAMA 1996; 275:1314]. JAMA 1996; 275:622–629.

Sonnenberg A: The US temporal and geographic variations of diseases related to *Helicobacter pylori*. Am J Public Health 1993; 83:1006–1010.

Sonnenberg A: Temporal trends and geographical variations of peptic ulcer disease. Aliment Pharmacol Ther 1995; 9:3–12.

Sonnenberg A, Olson CA, Zhang J: The effect of antibiotic therapy on bleeding from duodenal ulcer. Am J Gastroenterol 1999; 94:950–954.

Statement AGAMP: Evaluation of dyspepsia. Gastroenterology 1998; 114:579–581.

Sutton P, Wilson J, Genta R, Torrey D, Savinainen A, Pappo A, Lee A: A genetic basis for atrophy: dominant non-responsiveness and helicobacter induced gastritis in F_1 hybrid mice. Gut 1999; 45:335–340.

Svanes C, Lie SA, Lie RT, Soreide O, Svanes K: Causes of death in patients with peptic ulcer perforation: a long-term follow-up study. Scand J Gastroenterol 1999; 34:18–24.

Taha AS, Hudson N, Hawkey CJ, Swannell AJ, Trye PN, Cottrell J, Mann SG, Simon TJ, Sturrock RD, Russell RI: Famotidine for the prevention of gastric and duodenal ulcers caused by nonsteroidal antiinflammatory drugs. N Engl J Med 1996; 334:1435–1439.

Tarlow JK, Blakemore AI, Lennard A, Solari R, Hughes HN, Steinkasserer A, Duff GW: Polymorphism in human IL-1 receptor antagonist gene intron 2 is caused by variable numbers of an 86-bp tandem repeat. Hum Genet 1993; 91:403–404.

Tarnawski A, Ohta M, Wahlstrom K, Itani R, Sarfeh IJ: Expression of cytokines: IL-1alpha, IL-6 and TNFalpha in normal and ulcerated duodenal mucosa. Effect of sucralfate treatment. Gastroenterology 1997; 112:309A.

Tarpila S, Samloff IM, Pikkarainen P, Vuoristo M, Ihamaki T: Endoscopic and clinical findings in first-degree relative of duodenal ulcer patients and control subjects. Scand J Gastroenterol 1982; 17:503–506.

Taylor DE, Rasko DA, Sherburne R, Ho C, Jewell LD: Lack of correlation between Lewis antigen expression by *Helicobacter pylori* and gastric epithelial cells in infected patients. Gastroenterology 1998; 115:1113–1122.

Torrado J, Ruiz B, Garay J, Cosme A, Arenas JI, Bravo JC, Fontham E, Correa P: Lewis, secretor, and ABO phenotypes, and sulfomucin expression in gastric intestinal metaplasia. Cancer Epidemiol Biomarkers Prev 1997; 6:287–289.

Tsang TM, Saing H, Yeung CK: Peptic ulcer in children. J Pediatr Surg 1990; 25:744–748.

Umlauft F, Keeffe EB, Offner F, Weiss G, Feichtinger H, Lehmann E, Kilganogler S, Schwab G, Propst A, Grunewald K, et al.: *Helicobacter pylori* infection and blood group antigens—lack of clinical association. Am J Gastroenterol 1996; 91:2135–2138.

Vaira D, Miglioli M, Menegatti M, Holton J, Boschini A, Vergura M, Ricci C, Azzarone P, Mule P, Barbara L, et al.: *Helicobacter pylori* status, endoscopic findings, and serology in HIV-1-positive patients. Dig Dis Sci 1995; 40:1622–1626.

Valle J, Pikkarainen P, Vuoristo M, Sipponen P, Kekki M, Siurala M: *Helicobacter pylori* and duodenal ulcer. A study of duodenal ulcer patients and their first-degree relatives. Scand J Gastroenterol Suppl 1991; 186:45–51.

van der Ende A, Rauws EA, Feller M, Mulder CJ, Tytgat GN, Dankert J: Heterogeneous *Helicobacter pylori* isolates from members of a family with a history of peptic ulcer disease. Gastroenterology 1996; 111:638–647.

Varsky CG, Correa MC, Sarmiento N, Bonfanti M, Peluffo G, Dutack A, Maciel O, Capece P, Valentinuzzi G, Weinstock D: Prevalence and etiology of gastroduodenal ulcer in HIV-positive patients: a comparative study of 497 symptomatic subjects evaluated by endoscopy. Am J Gastroenterol 1998; 93:935–940.

Veldhuyzen van Zanten SJ, Dixon MF, Lee A: The gastric transitional zones: neglected links between gastroduodenal pathology and *Helicobacter* ecology. Gastroenterology 1999; 116:1217–1229.

Wang G, Rasko DA, Sherburne R, Taylor DE: Molecular genetic basis for the variable expression of Lewis Y antigen in *Helicobacter pylori*: analysis of the $\alpha(1,2)$fucosyltransferase gene. Mol Microbiol 1999; 31:1265–1274.

Wang JT, Sheu JC, Lin JT, Wang TH, Wu MS: Direct DNA amplification and restriction pattern analysis of *Helicobacter pylori* in patients with duodenal ulcer and their families. J Infect Dis 1993; 168:1544–1548.

Watanabe Y, Kurata JH, Kawamoto K, Kawai K: Epidemiological study of peptic ulcer disease among Japanese and Koreans in Japan. J Clin Gastroenterol 1992; 15:68–74.

Weigert N, Schaffer K, Schusdziarra V, Classen M, Schepp W: Gastrin secretion from primary cultures of rabbit antral G cells: stimulation by inflammatory cytokines. Gastroenterology 1996; 110:147–154.

Weissensteiner T, Lanchbury JS: *TNFB* polymorphisms characterize three lineages of *TNF* region microsatellite haplotypes. Immunogenetics 1997; 47:6–16.

Wilson AG, de Vries N, Pociot F, di Giovine FS, van der Putte LBA, Duff GW: An allelic polymorphism within the human tumor necrosis factor alpha promoter region is strongly associated with *HLA A1*, *B8*, and *DR3* alleles. J Exp Med 1993; 177:557–560.

Wilson AG, di Giovine FS, Blakemore AIF, Duff GW: Single base polymorphism in the human tumour necrosis factor alpha (TNF alpha) gene detectable by *Nco*I restriction of PCR product. Hum Mol Genet 1992; 1:353.

Wilson AG, Symons JA, McDowell TL, McDevitt HO, Duff GW: Effects of a polymorphism in the human tumor necrosis factor α promoter on transcription activation. Proc Natl Acad Sci USA 1997; 94:3195–3199.

Wirth HP, Yang M, Peek RM Jr, Hook-Nikanne J, Fried M, Blaser MJ: Phenotypic diversity in Lewis expression of *Helicobacter pylori* isolates from the same host. J Lab Clin Med 1999; 133:488–500.

Wirth HP, Yang M, Peek RM Jr, Tham KT, Blaser MJ: *Helicobacter pylori* Lewis expression is related to the host Lewis phenotype. Gastroenterology 1997; 113:1091–1098.

Wong BC, Ching CK, Lam SK, Li ZL, Chen BW, Li YN, Liu HJ, Liu JB, Wang BE, Yuan SZ, et al.: Differential north to south gastric cancer–duodenal ulcer gradient in China. China Ulcer Study Group. J Gastroenterol Hepatol 1998; 13:1050–1057.

Xiao SD, Liu WZ, Hu PJ, Xia DH, Tytgat GN: High cure rate of *Helicobacter pylori* infection using tripotassium dicitrato bismuthate, furazolidone and clarithromycin triple therapy for 1 week. Aliment Pharmacol Ther 1999; 13:311–315.

Yamaoka Y, El-Zimaity HM, Gutierrez O, Figura N, Kim JK, Kodama T, Kashima K, Graham DY: Relationship between the cagA 3′ repeat region of *Helicobacter pylori*, gastric histology, and susceptibility to low pH. Gastroenterology 1999a; 117:342–349.

Yamaoka Y, Kita M, Kodama T, Sawai N, Tanahashi T, Kashima K, Imanishi J: Chemokines in the gastric mucosa in *Helicobacter pylori* infection. Gut 1998; 42:609–617.

Yamaoka Y, Kodama T, Gutierrez O, Kim JG, Kashima K, Graham DY: Relationship between *Helicobacter pylori* iceA, cagA, and vacA status and clinical outcome: studies in four different countries. J Clin Microbiol 1999b; 37:2274–2279.

Yasunaga Y, Shinomura Y, Kanayama S, Yabu M, Nakanishi T, Miyazaki Y, Murayama Y, Bonilla-Palacios JJ, Matsuzawa Y: Improved fold width and increased acid secretion after eradication of the organism in *Helicobacter pylori* associated enlarged fold gastritis. Gut 1994; 35:1571–1574.

Yeomans ND, Tulassay Z, Juhasz L, Racz I, Howard JM, van Rensburg CJ, Swannell AJ, Hawkey CJ: A comparison of omeprazole with ranitidine for ulcers associated with nonsteroidal antiinflammatory drugs. Acid Suppression Trial: Ranitidine versus Omeprazole for NSAID-Associated Ulcer Treatment (ASTRONAUT) Study Group. N Engl J Med 1998; 338:719–726.

14 Lactase Deficiency: Biological and Medical Aspects of the Adult Human Lactase Polymorphism

EDWARD J. HOLLOX AND DALLAS M. SWALLOW

Lactose, 4-*O*-β-D-galactopyranosyl-D-glucose, is a disaccharide that occurs widely in nature, but usually at low concentrations with other carbohydrates. Large amounts of the free molecule are present only in mammalian milks where it occurs at concentrations of between 4% and 8%. Lactose must first be hydrolyzed to the two constituent monosaccharides glucose and galactose to be transported across the intestinal epithelium. The digestion of dietary lactose is catalyzed by a β-galactosidase, lactase-phlorizin hydrolase (commonly called lactase, EC 3.2.1.23/3.2.1.62), which is located in the brush border membrane of small-intestinal epithelial cells. In most non-human lactose-producing mammals tested, a characteristic pattern of lactase activity has been observed: activity is high in the newborn and suckling period, declines after weaning, and remains low in adult animals (Rohmann and Nagano, 1903; Plimmer, 1906; Blaxter, 1961). The early research on lactose digestion in humans was carried out in countries where the population was mainly of European ancestry, so the high adult lactase activity that is common in Europeans was believed to be normal for all humans. Further research revealed that many humans show a postweaning decline of lactase activity similar to that in other mammals (Auricchio et al., 1963; Dahlqvist et al., 1963). The molecular basis of this variation has proved elusive, but the causal nucleotide change is believed to be within a regulatory element that controls developmental decline of lactase located near the lactase gene located at chromosome 2q21.

LACTASE DEFICIENCY AND LACTOSE INTOLERANCE

Physiological and Pathological Lactase Phenotypes

As early as 1906 it was shown that intestinal lactase activity in the mammalian small intestine does not depend on exposure to lactose in the diet (Plimmer, 1906). Since then it has been shown that in humans with low lactase levels, lactase cannot be induced to high levels by prolonged lactose administration (Cuatrecasas et al., 1965; Keusch et al., 1969b) or by milk consumption (Flatz and Rotthauwe, 1971; Gilat et al., 1972; Chua and Seah, 1973). Drinking cow's milk immediately after weaning does not prevent lactase downregulation (Keusch et al., 1969a; Flatz and Rotthauwe, 1971), and prolonged milk avoidance by lactase persistent subjects does not cause a decrease in lactase activity (Knudsen et al., 1968; Rosenweig and Herman, 1969). This, together with very good evidence summarized below (see Genetic and Epidemiological Evidence), indicates that low adult lactase activity is a genetic trait with variable frequencies throughout the world (see Distribution of the Lactase Phenotypes).

Although low adult lactase activity has often been called lactase deficiency, lactase is not physiologically required in adulthood and so should not be regarded as a deficiency but merely as one phenotype of a common polymorphism in which both phenotypes are physiologically normal. The phenotype of low lactase activity in adults is often termed adult-type hypolactasia, but may be more appropriately described as lactase restriction or lactase nonpersistence. The phenotype of high lactase activity in adults is usually called lactase persistence.

In addition to these two physiological phenotypes, two pathological conditions exist in which lactase deficiency is found. The first is an autosomal recessive condition, congenital lactase deficiency, or congenital alactasia, in which there are very low levels of lactase activity in infants (Savilahti et al., 1983). This is serious if undiagnosed, but extremely rare. The second is secondary lactase deficiency, which may develop as a result of gastrointestinal disease. Common causes of secondary lactase deficiency are acute and chronic enteritis, celiac disease, tropical sprue, severe protein malnutrition, and other enteropathies (Buller et al., 1991; Nichols et al., 1997). Secondary lactase deficiency is usually accompanied by gross morphological alterations of the intestinal epthelium. Although it may be difficult to distinguish between genetically determined lactase nonpersistence and secondary lactase deficiency, especially during the recovery phase of gastrointestinal disease, low activities of other disaccharidases such as sucrase-isomaltase indicate secondary lactase deficiency (Phillips et al., 1980).

Low Lactose Digestion Capacity and Lactose Intolerance

Low lactose digestion capacity implies that a dose of lactose is not quantitatively hydrolyzed and absorbed from the small intestine. This may occur in both lactase persistent and nonpersistent individuals, but there is a distinct dosage–dependent difference. Most individuals with lactase persistence can completely digest a single load of 50 to 100 g of lactose, which corresponds to 1 to 2 liters of cow's milk. In contrast, individuals with lactase nonpersistence digest much less lactose (Christopher and Bayless, 1971). With appropriate dosage, the two lactase phenotypes can be distinguished by lactose loading or tolerance tests, lactase-persistent individuals having high LDC and nonpersistent having low LDC (Table 14–1). The term *lactose intolerance* is used to imply the occurrence of gastrointestinal symptoms after ingestion of lactose or lactose-containing foods; it is a collective term for the symptoms that occur in some individuals with low LDC after lactose or milk consumption. Of course,

Table 14–1. Relationship of the Adult Lactase Phenotypes, the Lactose Digestion Capacity Phenotypes, and Putative Genotypes

Enzymatic Phenotype	Digestive Phenotype	Genotype
Lactase nonpersistence (or lactase restriction)	High LDC	*LCT–R/LCT–R (RR)*
		LCT–P/LCT–R (PR)
Lactase persistence	Low LDC	*LCT–P/LCT–P (PP)*

The designations *LCT–P* and *LCT–R* may represent groups of alleles with similar physiological action. LDC, lactose digestion capacity.

many individuals with low LDC tolerate substantial amounts of lactose (Johnson et al., 1993; Vesa et al., 1996; Suarez et al., 1997), and lactose intolerance depends on many environmental factors as discussed below (see Variables that Determine Lactose Intolerance). It is also important to note that lactose intolerance and milk intolerance are not synonymous. Only some of the patients reporting subjective milk intolerance have low LDC; other causes of milk intolerance, such as an allergy to certain milk proteins, are clinically important (Rosado and Solomons, 1983a).

Symptoms of Lactose Intolerance

In individuals with high LDC, dietary lactose is hydrolyzed, and the constituent monosaccharides are taken up by the glucose transporter SGLT1 (Martin et al., 1996).

In individuals with low LDC, the ingestion of relatively small amounts of lactose or lactose-containing foods may exceed the digestive capacity of the jejunum (Gudmand-Hoyer et al., 1970; Bedine and Bayless, 1973; Bayless et al., 1975; Lisker et al., 1978), but residual lactase hydrolyzes a variable portion of the disaccharide (Christopher and Bayless, 1971). Undigested lactose increases the osmotic pressure, causing water to diffuse into the small intestine (Launiala 1968; Christopher and Bayless 1971; Bond and Levitt 1976a). The increase in volume, up to 5-fold in some cases, stimulates peristalsis, and the unabsorbed lactose rapidly passes to the colon (Bond et al., 1975; Debognie et al., 1979). Colonic bacteria metabolize lactose to organic acids, including propionic, lactic, acetic, and formic acids (Bond and Levitt, 1976a; Hove et al., 1994). Formic acid is further metabolized by formic lyase to carbon dioxide and hydrogen, some of which is absorbed and excreted through the lungs (Calloway et al., 1966; Levitt, 1969; Perman et al., 1981; Klibanov et al., 1982). The amount of carbon dioxide and hydrogen may be reduced by methanogenesis, depending on the metabolic activity of the bacterial population, and this process may be so active that no hydrogen appears in the breath (Levitt and Ingelfinger, 1968; Bjorneklett and Jenssen, 1982). Increased peristalsis, gas formation, and colonic irritation are the main causes of symptoms of lactose intolerance, which are abdominal distension and pain, meteorism, borborygmi, flatulence, diarrhea, and, in some cases, heartburn, nausea, and vomiting. The incidence and severity of lactose intolerance depend on the amount and concentration of lactose and on other variables that regulate the individual tolerance threshold described next.

Variables That Determine the Symptoms of Lactose Intolerance

Some healthy individuals who are lactase nonpersistent may experience lactose intolerance after taking as little as 3 g of lactose, while others remain asymptomatic after the usual test dose of 50 g (corresponding to 1 liter of cow's milk) (Bedine and Bayless, 1973; Stephenson and Latham, 1974). The capacity of lactose digestion and the symptoms of lactose intolerance do not depend solely on residual lactase activity and the amount of ingested lactose. The following additional variables are thought to contribute to the regulation of the individual lactose tolerance threshold:

1. The velocity of gastric emptying is influenced by the preexisting tonicity of the gastric musculature, which shows a circadian variability (Heading, 1982). Consistency, temperature, osmolarity, and pH of food are additional determinants of gastric passage time (Welsh and Hall, 1977). In some tropical countries, it is customary to add molasses to milk to achieve better tolerance. Many subjects with low LDC report that they can induce diarrhea by drinking cold milk, whereas the same amount of warm milk produces no, or only slight, symptoms.
2. Small-intestinal passage time in individuals with low LDC ingesting a lactose-rich meal depends on the response of the small intestine to the osmotic challenge of undigested lactose. In addition to gastric and intestinal hormones, prostaglandins seem to be important stimulators of peristalsis, and individual differences in prostaglandin synthesis may partly explain the variable reaction to undigested carbohydrates (Buisseret et al., 1978; Alun Jones et al., 1982). The mouth-to-colon passage time, as determined by the breath hydrogen method (see Lactose Tolerance Test with Breath Hydrogen Determination), is related to symptoms. Subjects with a short passage time are prone to develop diarrhea after a load of undigestible carbohydrate, whereas subjects with a slow passage experience more symptoms caused by gas formation.
3. Colonic bacteria metabolize carbohydrates to short-chain organic acids and to gas. The balance between acid and gas production may be important in that short-chain organic acids but not sugars can be absorbed from the colon (Bond and Levitt, 1976a). When lactose-intolerant individuals ingest lactose over a 13-day period, fecal β-galactosidase activity rises, indicating that the colonic bacterial flora adapt to diet, including lactose (Briet et al., 1997).
4. Colonic irritability may depend on the action of prostaglandins formed in response to changes in consistency, pH, and volume of colonic contents. In animals, acidification of the colon increases persistaltic activity, and this may contribute to the diarrhea induced by lactose and unabsorbable carbohydrates (Bennet and Eley, 1976).
5. Low LDC may also be secondary to changes in either bowel transit time or inflammation that occurs in inflammatory bowel disease (Lisker et al., 1989; Mishkin, 1997; Mishkin et al., 1997), and symptoms of lactose intolerance are observed in patients undergoing chemotherapy treatment of a tumor because cytotoxic drugs lower individual LDC (Parnes et al., 1994).

Clinical Lactose Intolerance: Case Histories

Clinically important lactose intolerance is most likely to occur if individuals with low LDC suddenly alter their feeding habits. Two brief case histories from Flatz illustrate this point.

Case 1: A 53-year-old German male was reported to have been in good general health throughout his life. One of his sons, a nationally known football player, planned to change to a new team. Fans of the present team began to harass the father by telephone calls at odd hours, upsetting him and causing him to complain of upper abdominal pain. He consulted a physician and, in spite of normal results of an X-ray examination of the upper gastrointestinal tract, a high-milk diet was prescribed. The patient, who was not in the habit of consuming milk, changed abruptly to a diet containing the equivalent of 1 to 1.5 liters of cow's milk per day. Abdominal pain persisted, and he developed the additional symptoms of meteorism and flatulence, as well as passing two or three loose stools a day. Because of poor appetite and incipient weight loss, malignant bowel disease was suspected. He was referred to a gastroenterology department, where the personal history prompted the provisional diagnosis of lactose intolerance. Low LDC was demonstrated by lactose and sucrose tolerance tests. The symptoms abated after he returned to his previous almost milk-free diet. For several weeks, he received psychotherapy and an ataractic medication. After the son transferred teams, the father remained asymptomatic without medication.

Case 2: A 23-year-old Syrian male went to Germany to study at university. He was in good general health and nutrition when he arrived. In Syria, he seldom consumed milk, but in Germany he lived with students who drank large amounts of fresh milk. He tried to adjust to their dietary habits and began to drink between 0.5 and 0.75 liters of milk per day. He soon developed abdominal distension and pain, increased flatulence, and occasional diarrhea but did not connect these symptoms with the dietary change. He was very worried about his health and consulted the student medical service, from where he was referred to a gastroenterologist. After tests for occult blood in the stool and an X-ray examination of the colon were found to be normal, lactose intolerance was suspected. Selectively low lactase activity was proved by a small-intestinal biopsy, and lactose and glucose/galactose tolerance tests confirmed the diagnosis of low LDC. The patient remained asymptomatic after reducing his daily milk consumption to less than 0.2 liters.

A similar, more dramatic personal case history was published by a Sudanese physician (Ahmed, 1975). It is likely that many visitors from developing countries to Europe, North America, and Australia have similar experiences.

Clinical Importance of Low Lactose Digestion Capacity and Milk Rejection

Substantial consumption of fresh milk is limited to countries where most inhabitants are lactase persistent and so have high LDC (see Distribution of the Lactase Phenotypes). Conversely, populations who are predominantly lactase nonpersistent (and hence have low LDC) consume little or no fresh milk, so there is little chance of lactose intolerance. In these low-LDC individuals, the pharmacological action of lactose should be remembered: a glass of cold milk can be a convenient and cheap laxative. Even in populations with high milk consumption and a high frequency of lactase nonpersistence, clinically significant manifestations of low LDC are rare. Subjects with low LDC can digest considerable quantities of lactose as a result of residual lactase activity and adaptation of intestinal flora, and often milk intake is adjusted to their individual tolerance threshold (Bond and Levitt, 1976b; Briet et al., 1997).

Milk rejection because of lactose intolerance depends on the extent of milk consumption and on milk-drinking habits in families and other social groups within that population. In a study of children in the United States, black children with low LDC drank less milk than those with high LDC, but there was no difference in milk consumption between the two phenotypic groups in white children (Paige et al., 1971). Similarly, no significant difference in milk consumption between subjects with high and low LDC was observed in a Finnish Lapp population (Hasunen et al., 1977). These results suggested the influence of social factors on milk-drinking habits.

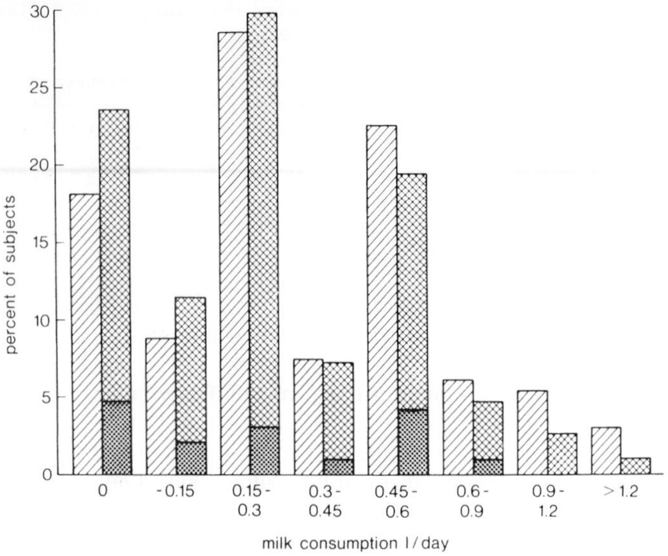

Fig. 14.1. Daily milk consumption and lactase phenotypes in 538 apparently healthy students, 18–25 years of age, from Germany and Austria. *Oblique hatching*, individuals with high lactose digestion capacity (high LDC); *cross hatching*, individuals with low LDC; *darkest parts of columns*, individuals with low LDC who reported an awareness of milk intolerance before the test. From Flatz (1982) with permission.

Lactase-persistent individuals in Germany and Austria consumed more milk (average 0.34 liters/day) than those with lactase restriction (0.27 liters/day), but the difference was not statistically significant (Fig. 14–1; Flatz, unpublished 1982). When three groups with no, moderate (<0.5 liters/day), and high (>0.5 liters/day) milk consumption were formed, the difference between the lactase phenotypic groups with high and low LDC was significant. Figure 14–1 also shows that only a few individuals with low LDC were aware of milk intolerance before the test, and, despite the high level of milk consumption in the population, milk consumption of more than half a liter per day by those aware of milk intolerance was very rare. Studies in the 1970s showed that in the United States awareness of milk intolerance among subjects with low LDC runs higher (55%–72%) than in Europe (Welsh, 1970; Bayless et al., 1975). Although milk intolerance may reduce milk consumption, awareness of milk intolerance did not always result in milk rejection (Bayless et al., 1975; Lisker et al., 1978). Moreover, milk intolerance is often reported by subjects with proven high LDC (Lisker et al., 1978; Rosado et al., 1987).

Low LDC, Irritable Bowel Syndrome, and Recurrent Abdominal Pain

Low LDC has been claimed to contribute to two clinical conditions: recurrent abdominal pain in children and irritable bowel syndrome in adults (Bayless and Huang, 1971; Pena and Truelove, 1972; Gudmand-Hoyer et al., 1973; Barr et al., 1979; Leibman, 1979; Porro et al., 1981; Lisker et al., 1989; Bohmer and Tuynmann, 1996). The validity of these studies is doubtful for two reasons:

1. The patient and control groups may not be comparable in terms of the frequency of lactase nonpersistence, due to differences within populations because of population stratification (see Table 14–2).
2. Many of the patients were aware of milk intolerance, and the exclusion of lactose from the diet may have had a placebo effect (MacLean, 1980).

Several studies do not support an important role for low LDC in the causation of irritable bowel syndrome or recurrent abdominal pain (Blumenthal et al., 1980; Christiensen, 1980; Lebenthal et al., 1981; Wald et al., 1982; Dearlove et al., 1983; Newcomer and McGill, 1983; Ferguson et al., 1984; Tolliver et al., 1996). A lactose-free diet does not always reduce abdominal symptoms in individuals with proven low LDC (Barr et al., 1979) but there is no doubt that individuals with lactase nonpersistence who drink milk beyond their tolerance threshold may get irritation of the bowel. Intolerance to various foods can elicit symptoms of irritable bowel syndrome in susceptible individuals, and it is possible that lactose intolerance occasionally may be responsible (Alun Jones et al., 1982).[1]

Disease Associations

The lactase phenotypes reflect a normal polymorphism rather than a disease. However, it is important to consider the effect,

[1]A recent more thorough 5-year follow-up study describes a subgroup of patients with irritable bowel disease who were clearly specifically lactose intolerant and in most cases their symptoms were improved on a lactose-free diet (Bohmer and Tuynman, 2001).

Table 14–2. Distribution of the Adult Lactase Phenotypes in Human Populations

Continent	Country	Population	*N*	% low LDC	% heterozygotes among those with High LDC	Frequency of Persistence Allele *LCT–P*
Americas	United States	**American white**	913	**22**	64	0.53
		American black	390	65	90	0.19
		American Mexican	305	52	84	0.28
		Pima Amerind	62	95	98	0.03
	Mexico	Mexican	401	83	95	0.09
	Greenland	Eskimo	119	85	96	0.08
		Eskimo-European	108	**38**	77	0.38
	Bolivia	Aymara Amerind	31	77	94	0.12
Europe	Estonia	**Estonian**	902	**27**	68	0.48
	Sweden	**Swedish**	400	**1**	18	0.9
	Germany	**German**	1872	**15**	56	0.61
	France	**North French**	62	**23**	65	0.52
		South French	71	**44**	80	0.34
	Russia	Russian	103	57	86	0.25
	Greece	Greek	800	52	84	0.28
	Italy	North Italian	383	50	83	0.29
		South Italian	197	67	90	0.18
	United Kingdom	**British white**	163	**5**	36	0.78
		British Afro-Carribean	50	82	95	0.09
	Poland	**Polish**	275	**37**	76	0.39
	Hungary	**Hungarian**	262	**41**	78	0.36
		Roma/Sinti	113	56	86	0.25
Africa	Egypt	**Sinai desert**	72	**11**	50	0.67
		Other	670	70	91	0.16
	Niger	**Tuareg**	118	**13**	53	0.64
	Sudan	**Beja**	281	**16**	57	0.60
		Dinka	213	76	93	0.13
	South Africa	Bantu-speaking	108	76	93	0.13
	Senegal	**Peuhle (Fuelbe)**	29	**0**	0	1.00
	Uganda/Rwanda	**Tutsi**	59	**7**	41	0.74
		Hutu	51	51	83	0.29
Middle East	Jordan	**Bedouin**	162	**24**	66	0.51
		Other Arab	204	75	93	0.13
	Israel	Jewish faith	276	68	91	0.17
Asia	India	**North Indian**	264	**27**	68	0.48
		Central Indian	125	63	88	0.21
		South Indian	60	67	90	0.18
	Russia	Khanty	115	72	92	0.15
	China	North (Han)	314	88	97	0.06
		Mongol	198	88	97	0.06
	Japan	Japanese	66	81	95	0.10
	Thailand	Thai	339	100	100	0
Australasia	Papua	Tribal groups	123	90	97	0.05
	Australia	Aborigine	45	84	96	0.08
		White	133	**5**	36	0.78
	New Zealand	Maori	30	64	89	0.20
		European	44	**9**	46	0.7

Most data were collected using lactose tolerance tests, and so the frequencies are shown as % low LDC. The percentage of persistent individuals that are heterozygous for the *LCT–P* allele and the frequency of the *LCT–P* allele are shown, and were calculated assuming the populations were in Hardy-Weinberg equilibrium. Numbers shown in bold are less than 50% low LDC. Data are from Swallow and Hollox (2000), where an extended version of this table is shown.

if any, of the lactase phenotypes on health and disease susceptibility. Studies on small groups of postmenopausal women suggested a role of low LDC in osteoporosis, but the difference between the control and patient groups may have been due in part to ethnic differences (Birge et al., 1967; Velebit et al., 1978). A larger study of women of northern European ancestry, however, gave similar results (Newcomer et al., 1978). In another examination of the influence of LDC on bone metabolism, cortical thickness of the clavicle was found to be significantly smaller in partially gastrectomized patients with low LDC than in those with high LDC (Kocian et al., 1973b). The etiological significance of these studies remains unknown, because osteoporosis does not seem to be unusually frequent in populations with low milk consumption and a high frequency of low LDC (Newcomer et al., 1978). In a study of healthy elderly people, no difference in bone mineral content between the two lactase phenotypes was noted, despite lower milk and calcium intake in the group with low LDC (Alhava et al., 1977). More recent studies give conflicting evidence about bone mineral density and low LDC (Horowitz et al., 1987; Honkanen et al., 1996, 1997). A great deal of evidence suggests that osteoporosis is primarily a defect of bone matrix formation and not of calcification, so an association with reduced calcium intake should not be expected.

It is even more difficult to decide whether prolonged milk intake by adult subjects with high LDC has any adverse effects. The hyperlipidemia of lactase-persistent subjects in one study (Sahi et al., 1977) was not correlated with individual milk consumption and does not establish an increased risk of coronary heart disease. Considering the present popularity and availability of skimmed and semi-skimmed milk, which both have reduced fat content, hyperlipidemia as a result of high milk consumption is less likely today. The geographic correlation between coronary heart disease, a high frequency of lactase persistence, and high milk consumption (Segall, 1980, 1994) may be coincidental, for various reasons. The correlation between presenile and senile cataracts and between high frequency of lactase persistence and high milk consumption is also controversial (Simoons, 1982; Bengtson et al., 1984). The etiological role of galactitol in cataract formation in hereditary disorders of galactose metabolism suggest a similar mechanism for the possible damage to the lens in individuals with high LDC consuming large amounts of milk. Healthy subjects with lactase persistence can rapidly convert the galactose from a dose of lactose equivalent to 1 liter of milk to glucose in the absence of hepatotoxic agents. In the presence of hepatotoxic agents, however, such as high alcohol intake, or where there is liver damage, it is conceivable that high milk intake may cause cataract formation in lactase-persistent people. In further studies of the correlation between lactase type and cataract, it may be advisable to determine the galactose tolerance of the test subjects in addition to the other variables.

A link between high LDC and ovarian cancer has been claimed (Cramer, 1989), but ethnic origin was not accounted for in the study and the results were not supported by other studies (Risch et al., 1994; Herrinton et al., 1995).

GENETIC AND EPIDEMIOLOGICAL EVIDENCE

Family Studies

The hypothesis of genetic determination of the lactase phenotypes was first derived from a population study and not from observations in families. Bayless and Rosensweig (1966) interpreted the difference in prevalence of low LDC between black Americans and white Americans as evidence for autosomal recessive inheritance of lactase nonpersistence. The early family studies were somewhat mixed in quality and conclusion, but the most convincing family data that suggested autosomal recessive inheritance of low LDC was achieved in a study of several large families from Finland (Sahi et al., 1973; Sahi 1974), reviewed in Swallow and Harvey (1993).

Twin Studies

Lactose tolerance tests with breath hydrogen determination were performed on 50 monozygotic and 52 dizygotic adult twin pairs in Budapest (Metneki et al., 1984). All monozygotic pairs were concordant with respect to breath hydrogen excretion after a load of lactose and with respect to the lactase phenotype. Among the dizygotic pairs, the distribution of concordance and discordance agreed with expectations, confirming the results of the family studies and corroborating the genetic etiology of the variability of lactose digestion capacity in healthy adults.

Lactase Phenotype–Genotype Correlation

Measurement of lactase activities in unrelated individuals provided further evidence of a genetic basis of the polymorphism. Because of the considerable variability in disaccharidase activity in intestinal material, the separation of subjects with lactase nonpersistence and lactase persistence on the basis of lactase activity alone is difficult. Disaccharidase activity ratios allow a more confident lactase phenotype diagnosis (Newcomer and McGill, 1967), and in jejunal specimens obtained at autopsy a trimodal distribution of sucrase/lactase ratios was reported in proportions compatible with Hardy-Weinberg equilibrium (Ho et al., 1982). A similar study using surgical biopsy material and a lactase/maltase ratio gave a separation of the three phenotypes corresponding to the putative genotypes *LCT–P/LCT–P*, *LCT–P/LCT–R*, and *LCT–R/LCT–R* (Flatz, 1984; see Fig. 14–2). The frequencies of the three phenotypes in both studies agree

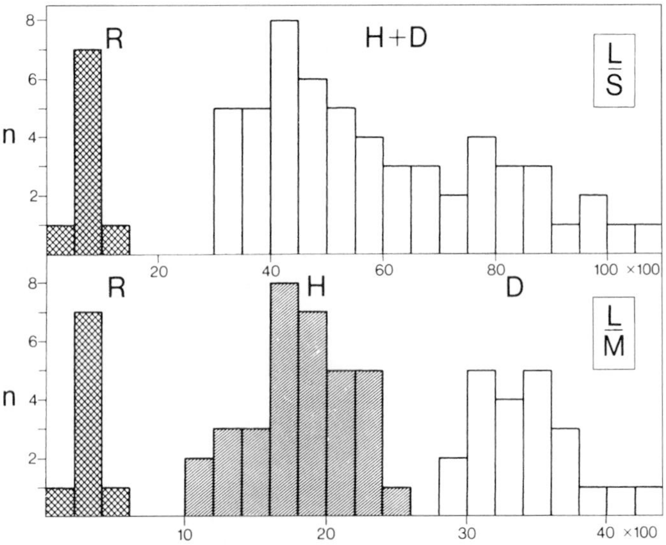

Fig. 14.2. Distribution of lactase/maltase (L/M) ratios determined in jejunal biopsy specimens from 65 healthy male German individuals. The three phenotypic groups (R, H, and D) correspond to the genotypes *LCT–R/LCT–R* (R), *LCT–P/LCT–R* (H), and *LCT–P/LAC–P* (D). From Flatz (1984) with permission.

with Hardy-Weinberg expectations and show a lactase gene dosage effect.

In summary, it is now generally accepted that lactase persistence or nonpersistence is determined by two alleles, *LCT–R* (lactase restriction or nonpersistence) and *LCT–P* (lactase persistence), as outlined in Table 14–1. Allele *LCT–P* is dominant over *LCT–R*, because *LCT–P/LCT–R* heterozygotes have sufficient lactase activity to digest 50 g of lactose, and hence register as lactase persistent in lactose tolerance tests.

Distribution of the Lactase Phenotypes

The distribution of the genetically determined adult lactase phenotypes in the world population is highly variable. A selection of the population data on this polymorphism is shown in Table 14–2; more complete versions can be found in Swallow and Hollox (2000). Both lactase alleles *LCT–P* and *LCT–R* are present in most populations, and the frequency of lactase restriction or low LDC ranges from 0% to 100%. Table 14–2 shows the absolute number of individuals and the frequency of low LDC, together with an estimate of the percentage of lactase-persistent individuals who are heterozygotes and a calculated value for the frequency of *LCT–P* in the population.

Low LDC (lactase nonpersistence) is the predominant phenotype in native populations of North and South America, sub-Saharan Africa, East and Southeast Asia, and Australia and the Pacific. The lactase-persistence phenotype is predominant in two distinct groups: central and northern Europeans (including Scandanavia, Germany, northern France, and the British Isles), and nomadic, milk-dependent populations in arid zones of North and Central Africa and Arabia. The two groups are separated by a peri-Mediterranean belt of people where lactase nonpersistence is the most common phenotype. There is a north–south gradient across Europe, with lactase persistence in the north and nonpersistence in the south. An east–west gradient also exists from persistent populations in Europe, stretching across the Ural region to the nonpersistent populations of the Far East (Kozlov et al., 1998).

Intermediate frequencies are found in populations originating from recent mixing of peoples with high and low LDC (compare the frequency of the persistence allele in Mexicans to American Mexicans, and of Eskimos to mixed European–Eskimo individuals in Table 14–2).

These data and the fact that nonpersistence is found in other mammals, show that, in fact, lactase persistence might be regarded as the "abnormal" condition, and there are several models that attempt to explain its high frequency in certain populations.

Natural Selection and Lactase Phenotype Distribution

Lactase persistence is the predominant allele only in populations with a tradition of production and consumption of milk. Dairying developed after the domestication of milking animals approximately 6000 to 9000 years ago, probably in the Near East (Simoons, 1971; Dudd and Evershed, 1998). It is generally assumed that the lactase persistence allele reached high frequency by natural selection, since milk provides a valuable source of nutrition for those who can digest it (Simoons, 1970, 1978). Another selective advantage of the ability to digest fresh milk may be that it provides an important source of water in arid regions (Cook, 1978). During the dry season, desert nomads are fully milk-dependent, and for the Beja people of Sudan, milk may be the only food for many months. Consumption of up to 3 liters of milk a day is not unusual (Habte et al., 1973), and considering the symptoms of lactose intolerance include diarrhea, which would cause water loss, selection in favor of tolerating lactose would be strong.

Additional selective forces may have acted on populations in northern Europe, where a tradition of mixed farming resulted in less dependence on milk (Ammermann and Cavalli-Sforza, 1971). Agriculture and dairying were introduced late into Scandanavia, probably not more than 4000 years ago, yet these countries have the highest frequencies of lactase persistence. Flatz and Rotthauwe (1973) suggested a "calcium absorption" hypothesis to explain the relatively rapid establishment of high persistence frequencies in northern Europe. This hypothesis is based on the assumption that rickets and osteomalacia were strong selective factors in areas with low solar irradiation. Milk is rich in calcium, lactose increases calcium absorption in humans (Greenwald et al., 1963; Pansu et al., 1979), and individuals with high LDC absorb more calcium than individuals with low LDC (Kocian et al., 1973a). The highly variable distribution of the persistence allele in the Mediterranean basin, Southwest Asia, and the Indian subcontinent could reflect differences in selective pressure or migrations from populations with high frequencies of lactase persistence.

A confounding effect when analyzing the environmental pressures that could have selected for lactase persistence is the genetic relatedness between the populations under study. Holden and Mace (1997) used a genetic and linguistic tree to control for this effect, and found that the results of a maximum likelihood analysis of environmental pressures against lactase persistence frequency supported selection of persistence due to increased nutrition, but did not support the calcium absorption hypothesis or the water requirement in arid zones hypothesis. However, when testing the calcium absorption hypothesis, solar irradiation on the ground was treated as proportional to geographical latitude, and this would result in an overestimation of solar irradiation in the unique climatic conditions of northwestern Europe. It may be that combinations of all three selective forces explain the current geographical distribution of lactase persistence.

Several attempts have been made to model these selective pressures mathematically to try to explain how the modern allele frequencies were reached in the 6000 to 9000 years since the development of agriculture. Most models assume coevolution of the milk-drinking cultural trait, high selection coefficients of around 5%, and a high initial allele frequency to reach a present-day frequency of 0.7 (Aoki 1986; Laland et al., 1995).

Nei and Saitou (1986) suggested that genetic drift and founder effects instead of selection resulted in high frequencies of the lactase persistence allele by chance in small groups who secondarily adopted dairying as their main economic activity and so became accustomed to high milk consumption. Further selection for the lactase persistence allele was possible but not essential to account for the present distribution of the lactase phenotypes.

Several populations with predominantly lactase nonpersistence (low LDC), such as the Mongols, Herero, and Dinka, consume significant quantities of milk. This is achieved by fermentation of fresh milk into products such as yoghurt, cheese, kefir, and kumiss. These products have lower amounts of lactose due to digestion by β-galactosidases supplied by the fermenting organisms, and they are also better tolerated by individuals with low LDC because of slower passage through the gastrointestinal tract (Kolars et al., 1984; Savaiano et al., 1984). Consumption of fermented milk is also common in Southern Europe and India.

In summary, it seems that the adoption of dairying allowed certain individuals a nutritional advantage if they were able to digest the lactose in milk satisfactorily. Three adaptations provided individuals with the means to harness this supply of food:

1. A symbiotic adaptation, which resulted in an increase in gut flora hydrolyzing lactose
2. A cultural adaptation, which provided lactose hydrolyzing flora by partial fermentation of the milk
3. A genetic adaptation, which allowed lactose to by hydrolyzed by persistence of childhood levels of the indigenous enzyme lactase

Origin of the Lactase Persistence Allele

Hypotheses concerning the evolution of the lactase phenotype distribution assume that lactase nonpersistence is the original phenotype. There is good evidence for this, in that most mammals that have been tested have the characteristic postweaning decline of lactase, except members of the Pinnepedia family (sea lions and walruses), which have no lactase in their digestive system or any lactose in their milk (Sunshine and Kretchmer, 1964). Unfortunately, there is little information concerning lactase in primates. A comprehensive study of baboons showed convincing down-regulation of lactase (Welsh et al., 1974), but in another study 9 out of 10 cebus monkeys (macaques, *Macaca fascicularis*) showed high LDC as adults (Wen et al., 1973). There are no published studies on the great apes, despite the interesting fact that weaning is very late in these species: 1640 days in the common chimpanzee and 1583 days in the gorilla, compared to 720 days in hunter-gatherer humans (Harvey et al., 1987). Adult gorillas and chimpanzees in the London Zoo are given occasional milkshakes without apparent adverse effects (A. Sainsbury, personal communication, 1997), but the lactose load may not be enough to cause symptoms of lactose intolerance.

All evolutionary models assume lactase nonpersistence is the original phenotype, but they also assume a reasonable lactase persistence allele starting frequency before the advent of agriculture. Since there was unlikely to be any milk consumption by adults before dairying (Simoons, 1971), other selective pressures may have been involved in the maintenance of a reasonable lactase persistence starting frequency. Maybe lactase persistence evolved as part of a social change, enabling higher primates to delay weaning, to space births, and to protect their offspring for longer. If the lactase persistence allele was already common in early humans, it is possible that selection by *falciparum* malaria against lactase persistence could account for the near absence of this allele in most African populations (Anderson and Vullo, 1994), although recent work does not support this (Meloni et al., 1998). The hypothesis was based on the fact that milk is rich in riboflavin and on evidence that cell multiplication of malarial parasites is inhibited in flavin-deficient erythrocytes, suggesting that mildly flavin-deficient individuals have increased resistance to malaria (Das et al., 1988).

Clinical Consequences of the Phenotypic Distribution in Populations

Unlike most autosomally inherited pathological enzyme deficiencies, adult lactase nonpersistence is a common trait. A large amount of skimmed milk powder, rich in lactose, is given as international aid to countries where the majority of the population are lactase nonpersistent: over 5000 metric tons were sent to Africa alone in 1997 (United Nations Food and Agriculture Organization, 1999). These individuals are often in poor nutritional condition and may suffer from acute or chronic gastrointestinal infections. If they also have genetically determined lactase nonpersistence, severe lactose intolerance may be expected after they ingest reconstituted milk. In 1971 the United Nations Food and Agriculture Organization summoned an advisory group to discuss this problem in relation to infant and adult nutrition. They concluded that "it would be highly inappropriate . . . to discourage producers to improve milk supplies and increase milk consumption among children because of the fear of milk intolerance" (quoted in Ransome-Kuti, 1977), yet as late as the early 1980s, according to the International Red Cross, uncontrolled distribution of powdered milk as aid "caused more health problems than it solved" (Perrin 1998) Modern aid agencies are more aware of the potential problems of milk, and the World Food Programme recommends following the United Nations policy for acceptance and use of milk products in refugee feeding program (United Nations High Commission for Refugees, 1989).

Even in populations with a high frequency of lactase persistence, many lactase-persistent individuals are heterozygous. Individuals who are heterozygous for lactase persistence have lower levels of lactase than homozygous persistent individuals due to the gene–dosage effect (Ho et al., 1982; Flatz, 1984). It is possible that heterozygotes are more likely than lactase-persistent homozygotes to suffer from lactose intolerance as a result of gastrointestinal disease. Table 14–2 shows the calculated percentage of lactase-persistent individuals likely to be heterozygous for the lactase-persistence allele, in a selection of populations, assuming the populations are in Hardy-Weinberg equilibrium.

The problem of lactose intolerance when an individual with low LDC drinks fresh milk in a culture which drinks a significant quantity of fresh milk is discussed above (see Clinical Lactose Intolerance: Case Histories). In addition, an individual from a population with a high prevalence of low LDC and whose culture does not involve drinking significant amounts of fresh milk may encounter problems due to lack of vitamin D. Since milk and milk products are rich in this vitamin, an individual may require vitamin D supplements when visiting or emigrating to countries with low solar irradiation due to the climate, such as those in northern Europe.

PHYSIOLOGICAL AND MOLECULAR BASIS OF THE LACTASE POLYMORPHISM

Description and Distribution of the Lactase-Phlorizin Hydrolase Protein

In the mammalian small-intestinal mucosa, dietary lactose is digested by lactase-phlorizin hydrolase (LPH), which is localized in the brush border where it exists as a dimer of two identical polypeptides with an apparent molecular mass of 160,000 each, both of which have lactase (β-galactosidase) and phlorizin hydrolase (β-glucosidase) activity (EC 3.2.1.23/62) (Semenza et al., 1975; Skovbjerg et al., 1981), and are highly glycosylated (Danielsen, 1990; Grunberg and Sterchi, 1995; Naim and Naim, 1996). The lactase polypeptide is synthesized as a precursor containing four domains—I, II, III, and IV—which resulted from ancient duplications of one subunit (Grabnitz et al., 1991). The cleavage of the signal sequence (which targets the polypeptide to the endoplasmic reticulum) occurs in the endoplasmic reticulum as expected (Mantei et al., 1988; Duluc et al., 1991). Domains I and II are removed by proteolytic cleavage to leave the mature lactase, with lactase-phlorizin hydolase activity in domains III and IV (Duluc et al., 1991; Wacker et al., 1992; Jost et al., 1997; Zecca et al., 1998). Most of the degradation of the cleaved protein containing domains I and II takes place intracellularly in the trans golgi network or a later compartment. The protein is then sorted to the brush border membrane (Buller et al., 1987; Naim et al., 1987; Witte et al., 1990; Lottaz et al., 1992; Rossi et al., 1992). As yet, there seems to be no enzymatic function for the cleaved protein containing domains I and II. It may be necessary, however, for this cleaved portion to exist in the endoplasmic reticulum, and it may act as a intramolecular chaperone (Oberholzer et al., 1993; Naim et al., 1994). Most of the protein molecule protudes into the intestinal lumen with a C-terminal anchor in the brush border membrane and a short cytoplasmic tail. Like other brush border proteins, lactase is thought to be mannosylated, glucosylated and trimmed in the endoplasmic reticulum, followed by complex glycosylation and other modifications in later compartments. Terminal glycosylation shows person-to-person variation, and this variation is controlled be the ABH and Lewis blood group glycosyltransferases (Green et al., 1988). The sugar moieties of lactase may have some effect on its enzymatic activity (Naim and Lentze, 1992).

Lactase expression varies along the crypt–villus axis in the mucosa: there is little or no lactase activity in the mucosal crypts, high lactase activity in the midvillus region, and a decrease in lactase activity toward the apex (Skovbjerg, 1981), Fig. 14–3. Studies of the distribution of lactase activity along the length of the small intestine, using enzyme assay or immunological methods, show that activity is lowest in the proximal duodenum and distal ileum and that activity is present at highest levels in the mid- to lower jejunum (Newcomer and McGill, 1966; Skovbjerg, 1981). No lactase activity is found in the stomach or in the colon. This distribution resembles that of sucrase-isomaltase activity, although there is more expression of sucrase-isomaltase in the colon (Newcomer and McGill, 1966; Skovbjerg, 1981; Wang et al., 1994). The distribution of lactase is similar in adults with lactase persistence and with lactase nonpersistence (Potter et al., 1985) but individuals with nonpersistence show generally less lactase protein (Skovbjerg et al., 1980, 1981; Potter et al., 1985). Several studies have shown evidence of mosiacism of lactase expression in nonpersistent individuals with clusters of a few lactase-producing cells in the jejunum (Maiuri et al., 1993, 1994) and duodenum (Lorenzsonn et al., 1993). This has been less evident in other studies (Harvey et al., 1994; Fig. 14–3), but it does suggest that the genetic switch is "leaky."

Localization and Cloning of the Lactase Gene

Human lactase-phlorizin hydrolase is encoded by a single gene consisting of 17 exons spanning approximately 70 kb on chromosome 2q21 (Mantei et al., 1988; Kruse et al., 1989; Boll et al., 1991; Harvey et al., 1993). Analysis of the exons in several persistent and nonpersistent individuals revealed polymorphism (including an exon 2 polymorphism, which changes valine to isoleucine, and an exon 13 polymorphism, which changes asparagine to serine), but none caused the phenotypic lactase persistence polymorphism (Boll et al., 1991).

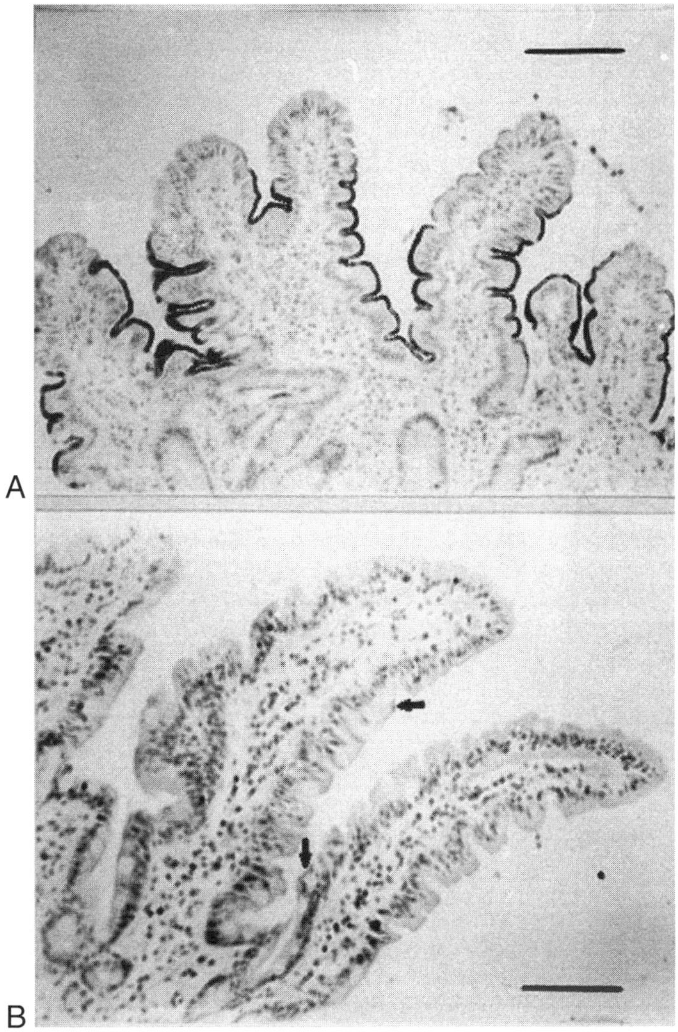

Fig. 14.3. Lactase expression in duodenal villi detected by immunohistology. (**A**) A lactase persistent individual. (**B**) A lactase-nonpersistent individual. The arrows indicate patches of cells with faint brush border staining. The scale bar represents 100 μm. From Harvey et al. (1994) with permission.

Analysis of Polymorphisms in the Lactase Gene

Seven polymorphic sites distributed across the lactase gene have been shown to be in linkage disequilibrium in Europeans and associate to form three common haplotypes, A, B, and C (Harvey et al., 1995), one of which is associated with lactase persistence (Harvey et al., 1998). Analysis of these and four other polymorphic sites in other populations showed similar lack of haplotype diversity in other non-Africans. In addition to the A, B, and C, a fourth common haplotype, U, was found, which was most common in Japanese and Chinese populations (Hollox et al., 2001). In the two sub-Saharan African populations studied, there was low linkage disequilibrium across the polymorphic sites and high haplotype diversity. Although the four common haplotypes were observed in the African populations, they accounted for a much lower proportion of the total diversity.

The four haplotypes that are common worldwide are only distantly related to each other, but the intermediate forms can be found in African populations, suggesting that these haplotypes evolved in Africa. Together, the evidence shows that non-African diversity is a subset of African diversity and supports the "out of Africa" theory for the origins of modern humans.

The A haplotype, which is associated with lactase persistence in northern Europeans, is at a much higher frequency (87%) than the lower frequencies of that haplotype in the other populations, which are mainly lactase nonpersistent. This suggests that recent directional selection for lactase persistence is reflected in the high frequency of the haplotype carrying lactase persistence due to a "genetic hitch-hiking" effect.

Transcriptional Control by a *cis*-Acting Element

In lactase nonpersistent individuals, the lactase gene down-regulates as in other mammals, but in persistent individuals the down-regulation does not occur. Several studies have attempted to find the mechanism of this down-regulation. An early study found poor correlation between lactase mRNA and enzyme levels (Sebastio et al., 1989), suggesting a control at the protein level, but the consensus is now that lactase mRNA levels reflect lactase protein levels. This suggests that reduced transcription is the primary level of control of down-regulation in humans (Montgomery et al., 1991; Escher et al., 1992; Fajardo et al., 1994; Harvey et al., 1994; Rossi et al., 1997), as well as rat (Sebastio et al., 1989; Buller et al., 1990; Duluc et al., 1993; Krasinski et al., 1994), sheep (Lacey et al., 1994) and pig (Torp et al., 1993), although in some studies regional differences and post-translational changes have also been suggested (Freund et al., 1989; Buller et al., 1990; Rossi et al., 1997).

The trimodal distribution of disaccharidase activity ratios (see Lactase Phenotype–Genotype Correlation) suggested a *cis*-acting element, and this was confirmed by analysis of marker polymorphisms in lactase mRNA from persistent heterozygotes that showed one allele expressed at high levels and the other allele expressed at low levels (Wang et al., 1995). This approach also showed that in children who are heterozygous for lactase persistence, one allele was progressively (though variably) down-regulated while the other allele was expressed at a high level (Wang et al., 1998; Figure 14–4).

The phenotypic polymorphism is due to this presence or absence of a genetic switch that controls the level of lactase mRNA, most probably at the level of transcription. However, there are a few unusual features, which suggest that the phenotype is sometimes dependent on more than control of transcription. Apart from the mosaicism of lactase in nonpersistent individuals, as mentioned above (Description and Distribution of the Lactase-Phlorizin Hydrolase Protein), studies in Italy showed poor correlation of steady state lactase enzyme activity and lactase mRNA (Rossi et al., 1997). There is also some evidence for abnormal processing and abnormal electroporetic mobility of the lactase protein (Sterchi et al., 1990; Witte et al., 1990; Harvey, 1994). These observations could reflect further genetic variation, such as variability in glycosylation of lactase or epigenetic and environmental differences.

Regulatory Elements Upstream of the Lactase Gene

Much of the work on lactase gene regulation has been done using the pig promoter as a model. Using the pig promoter in transgenic mice, it was shown that 1 kb of upstream sequence controlled lactase down-regulation, and a regulatory element within this region called CE-LPH1 was identified (Troelsen et al., 1994). This element binds a factor NF-LPH, which is much less abundant in the intestine of adult pigs when compared to suckling pigs (Troelsen et al., 1992). Rats have a homologous CE-LPH1 which interacts with several nuclear factors, but the developmental expression pattern of these factors is not clear (Boukamel and Freund, 1994; Hecht et al., 1997; Tanaka et al., 1997). Again using transgenic mice, the 2 kb of sequence upstream of rat lactase fused to a human growth hormone reporter gene shows correct cellular and tissue expression. This suggests that all the elements necessary for correct tissue and cell expression are within the 2 kb upstream of rat lactase (Krasinski et al., 1997).

Further work on pigs has shown that NF-LPH includes the intestine specific homeodomain transcription factor Cdx-2 and another homeodomain protein, HOXC-11. Activation by HOXC-11 depends on the presence of the transcription factor HNF-1α; and members of the subfamily of HNF-3/forkhead transcription factors are potential repressors of lactase transcription (Mitchelmore et al., 1998; Spodsberg et al., 1999). It is likely that the spatial pattern of expression of lactase depends on the tissue distribution of these transcription factors.

The human intestinal cell line Caco-2 was used to show that a 'GATA' sequence motif in an element 95 bp upstream of the transcription start site is required for full activity of the human lactase promoter and transcription from this transfected pro-

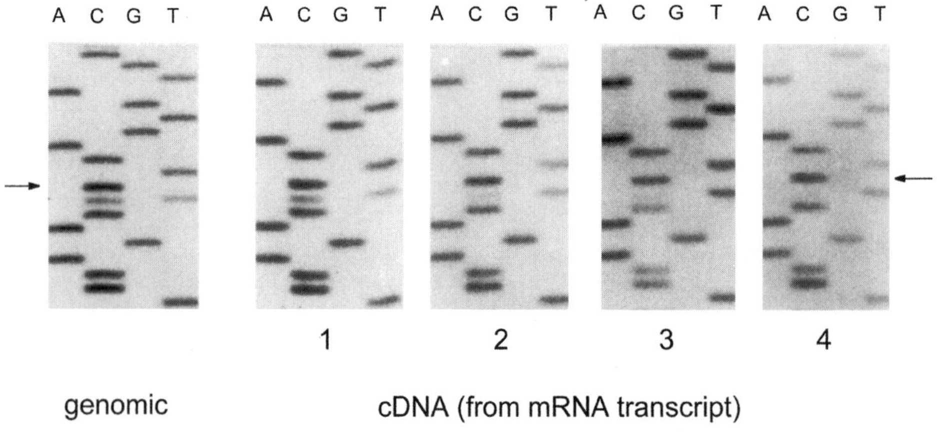

Fig. 14.4. Asymmetrical expression of lactase mRNA transcripts in children heterozygous for lactase persistence. These sequencing gels show genomic sequencing of a heterozygote for a C/T marker polymorphism in exon 1 (*left*), and four examples showing variable expression of the two mRNA transcripts detected by sequencing cDNA. All four individuals are heterozygous for this point (*arrows left and right*), but show variable expression of the C-containing allele. Individual 1 is 3 months old and shows equal expression of the C and T alleles (%C, 49, determined by phosphorimage analysis). Individual 2 is 42 months old (%C, 27), and individual 3 is 50 months old (%C, 20). In individual 4, who is 132 months (11 years) old, the C band is not visible, but trace amounts are detected by phosphorimaging (%C, 6). Both bands show equal intensity in genomic DNA from heterozygotes (%C, 51.25 ± 1.29, n = 4). From Wang et al. (1998) with permission.

moter, can be stimulated by co-expressing the zinc-finger transcription factor GATA-6 (Fitzgerald et al., 1998).

It would be surprising if the mechanism of down-regulation was not common to all mammals, but care must be taken in extrapolating the data on pigs and rats to humans. Substantial sequence analysis of over 9 kb upstream of the human lactase gene has revealed several polymorphisms, but none is causative of the phenotypic polymorphism (Harvey et al., 1998; Poulter unpublished, 1999). Interestingly, one of the polymorphisms 1 kb upstream of the gene is in a area conserved in pig and primates and greatly affects protein binding affinity of that DNA sequence, although the significance of this is not clear (Hollox et al., 1999).

The causative sequence change probably lies some way upstream of the lactase gene, and this has received support from a study describing the mapping of a locus for the congenital lactase deficiency found in Finns. The small Finnish founder population allowed an allelic association/identity by descent approach to position the locus at 2 cM (approximately 2 Mb) away from the lactase gene (Jarvela et al., 1998). This rare recessive congenital disease may involve the same complex *cis*-acting element as the common lactase-persistence polymorphism. The distances invoked for a potential *cis*-acting element are not entirely without precedent: elements have been identified as far away as 900 kb from the gene they control (for a review see Kleinjan and van Heyningen, 1998). Determination of the sequence change responsible for congenital lactase deficiency may help identify the sequence change responsible for the adult polymorphism.[2]

Timing of Lactase Down-Regulation

Lactase activity is low in fetuses, then rises postpartum to high levels in all healthy children in all populations (Auricchio et al., 1965; Antonowicz and Lebenthal, 1977; Villa et al., 1992; Wang et al., 1994, 1998). The timing of down-regulation appears to vary between and possibly within populations. In northern Thailand, for example, all 75 adults and 33 children above the age of 5 years studied had low LDC (Flatz et al., 1969; Figure 14–5), but a study in Finland demonstrated late conversion of lactase phenotype and an increase in the frequency of low LDC up to the age of 20 years (Sahi and Launiala, 1978; Sahi et al., 1983). Within an ethnically heterogenous group from London, down-regulation could be detected in mRNA levels from as early as 14 months, although one child of $4^1/_2$ years showed only slight down-regulation (Wang et al., 1998). It should be emphasized that these were all hospital patients. It is possible that environmental factors (other than milk consumption) influence the timing of lactase down-regulation, but it is also possible that it is controlled by some form of *cis*-acting or *trans*-acting allelic variation, perhaps in combination with epigenetic effects.

[2]It has recently been reported that a CT polymorphism at −14 kb is in complete association with lactase persistence in Finns (Enattah et al., 2002), the T allele being present in all persistent individuals and absent in nonpersistent individuals. These findings together with the fact that the T allele is present at appropriate frequency in other populations suggest that this nucleotide change may cause persistence.

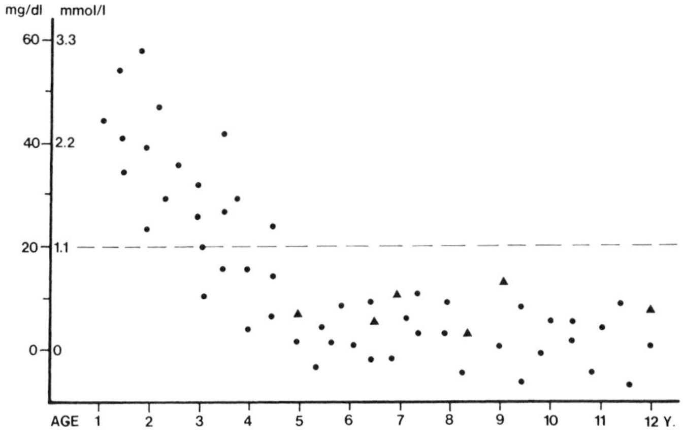

Fig. 14.5. Results of lactose tolerance tests (maximal increase in blood glucose concentration within 60 minutes after administration of 25 g lactose/m^2 calculated body surface) in 56 apparently healthy children from northern Thailand. All children over 5 years old have a low lactose digestion capacity (low LDC). Circles, children who drank no milk after weaning; triangles, children who regularly received cows' milk since the time of weaning. Based on data of Flatz (1977) with permission.

DIAGNOSIS OF LACTOSE INTOLERANCE AND CLINICAL APPLICATION

Disaccharidase Activity Determination

Direct diagnosis of the lactase phenotype is achieved by measuring disaccharidase activity in small-intestinal mucosal specimens obtained by endoscopy. The usual biopsy site was formerly the first jejunal loop, but more recent studies have shown that the distal duodenum is adequate (Escher et al., 1992; Harvey et al., 1994; Olsen et al., 1996; van Beers et al., 1998). The specimen is inspected and, if taken in a Crosby capsule, divided into three pieces for further analysis. If the enzyme assay is not carried out immediately after sampling, one piece (or one entire pinch biopsy) should be snap-frozen in liquid nitrogen and stored at −20°C. One piece of the specimen should be fixed and embedded in paraffin wax for morphological examination and immunohistology. The activity of disaccharidases is determined in tissue homogenates according to methods described by Dahlqvist (1964) and Phillips et al. (1980). A specific method for lactase eliminates the activity of acid β-galactosidase by inhibition with *p*-chloromercuribenzoate (Asp and Dahlqvist, 1972), but we have found this treatment is not necessary for human biopsy samples (Phillips et al., 1980; Harvey, 1994). Enzyme activity is expressed as micromoles of glucose liberated per minute. The usual reference parameters of protein, DNA, or tissue wet weight all have their merits and disadvantages, but tissue wet weight has the advantage that it does not use any of the sample. Disaccharidase activity varies considerably in biopsy specimens taken from a small area of mucosa in one person, and activity ratios give a more certain diagnosis of the lactase phenotypes then does lactase activity alone (see Lactase Phenotype–Genotype Correlation).

Tests for Lactose Digestion Capacity (Lactose Tolerance Tests)

Indirect methods for the diagnosis of the adult lactase phenotypes are more convenient and less invasive than intestinal biopsy. They are based on the principle that a large load of lactose will exceed the limited digestive capacity of individuals with lactase nonpersistence but not exceed the digestive capacity of those with lactase persistence. Lactose tolerance tests should be performed after a fast of at least 8 hours. The usual dose of lactose for adults is 50 g of lactose monohydrate dissolved in 400 ml of tap water, which is nearly an isotonic solution and so ensures rapid gastric passage. The solution should be at room temperature, and the proband should drink it in less than 3 minutes. One or more metabolites of lactose are determined in either the blood, or the breath, or both.

Blood Glucose Determination

Capillary blood samples are collected 5 minutes before and at regular intervals after the lactose administration (Dahlqvist, 1974). The blood glucose should be determined by an enzymatic method. In subjects with normal glucose metabolism, the maximum glucose concentration is usually observed 15 to 45 minutes after lactose administration. Subjects with high LDC show a marked increase in blood glucose concentration, and the maximum increase in glucose concentration after lactose is usually more than 1.4 mmol/liter (0.25 mg/ml). In subjects with low LDC, the blood glucose curve is flat, and the maximum increase is usually below 1.1 mmol/liter (0.2 mg/ml). If the result is in the diagnostically uncertain range between 1.1 and 1.4 mmol/liter, a repeat test is indicated. A few individuals with low LDC and delayed glucose metabolism may show a substantial increase in blood glucose concentration, so if this is suspected, a glucose tolerance test may clarify the diagnosis. A subsequent glucose-galactose test will exclude the rare monosaccharide malabsorption.

Many factors influence glucose metabolism, so the lactose tolerance test with blood glucose determination may be unreliable, especially in children (Krasilnikoff et al., 1975) and in subjects with delayed glucose metabolism (MacDonald et al., 1975).

Ethanol Administration and Blood or Urinary Galactose Determination

This test is based on the inhibition of conversion of galactose to glucose by ethanol in the liver (Jussila, 1969). The procedure is similar to the previously described glucose test, except that 0.3 g/kg body weight of ethanol is administered as a 40% solution 30 minutes before the lactose ingestion or together with the lactose, and both glucose and galactose levels are measured by enzymatic methods. The peak blood galactose concentration occurs approximately 40 minutes after lactose administration, and an increase in blood galactose concentration of more than 0.3 mmol/liter is diagnostic of high LDC. Methods measuring blood galactose determination once, 40 or 45 minutes after lactose ingestion, have been described (Kern and Heller, 1968; Isokoski et al., 1972), and measurement of galactose in the urine instead of blood is also reasonably accurate and very convenient (Arola et al., 1982; Grant et al., 1989).

The lactose tolerance test with blood and urinary galactose determination is more reliable than the glucose test (Jussila, 1969; Newcomer et al., 1975; Arola et al., 1988). In a twin study in Hungary several lactose metabolites were measured and the blood galactose test showed the highest intrapair correlation (Metneki et al., 1984). The disadvantage of this test is the necessity of administering alcohol, which limits its application to adults in societies permitting alcohol consumption.

^{14}C-Lactose or ^{13}C-Lactose

A small quantity of radioactively labeled lactose is added to the test dose, and the pulmonary excretion of $^{14}CO_2$ is determined (Salmon et al., 1969; Sasaki et al., 1970). Subjects with high LDC show an early excretion because of the metabolism of absorbed ^{14}C-glucose, whereas $^{14}CO_2$ appears late in the breath of subjects with low LDC because of bacterial fermentation in the colon. The ^{14}C-lactose test is no more reliable than the glucose test, probably because of overlapping of the $^{14}CO_2$ excretion periods in the two lactase phenotypes (Newcomer et al., 1975) and is not recommended because of unnecessary exposure to irradiation. Recently a more sophisticated approach has been used, in which a mixture of ^{13}C-lactose and ^{2}H-glucose is given, and it is claimed that lactase acitivity can be measured indirectly by determining the blood ratio of these two isotopes (Vonk et al., 2001).

Breath Hydrogen Determination

As mentioned (see Symptoms of Lactose Intolerance), unabsorbed carbohydrate is degraded by colonic bacteria, producing gas, mainly carbon dioxide and hydrogen. The gas chromatographic determination of hydrogen in breath samples is a convenient, noninvasive method of lactase phenotype diagnosis. Various breath-sampling techniques have been described: rebreathing methods require a complicated apparatus and are no more accurate than end-expiratory samples obtained with a simple device (Metz et al., 1976). For clinical studies, breath samples can be stored for several hours in plastic syringes without appreciable loss of hydrogen (Rosado and Solomons 1983b), and if longer storage is needed, vacutainers can be used, but retrieving the gas sample from them is complicated (Douwes et al., 1978). Normalization of the hydrogen concentrations to presumed alveolar carbon dioxide concentration largely eliminates the effects of individual sampling differences, especially in children (Niu et al., 1979; Skovbjerg et al., 1980). For population studies, collection of tidal air (multiple breath sampling by inflating a balloon) is suitable (Howell et al., 1981), and pressurized storage of breath in aluminium aerosol containers permits automated analysis of the samples (Howell et al., 1980).

In healthy individuals, maximum hydrogen excretion occurs between 90 and 210 minutes after a test dose of undigestible carbohydrate (Flatz et al., 1984). In clinical studies, breath sampling before and at intervals of 15 to 30 minutes for up to 3 to 4 hours after lactose administration is advisable. In field studies, at least two breath samples should be obtained after lactose load, preferably 110 to 120 and 150 to 160 minutes after ingestion (Flatz et al., 1984). In the case of low LDC, breath hydrogen concentration increases by at least 20 volumes per million (vpm) above the fasting concentration, whereas the increase is usually less than 15 vpm in subjects with igh LDC (Metz et al., 1976; Howell et al., 1980, 1981; Karcher et al., 1999). Breath hydrogen and carbon dioxide can be determined on a gas chromatograph fitted with a thermoconductivity detector. Simple electrochemical devices for the immediate determination of hydrogen in end-expiratory breath samples have been devised (Bartlett et al., 1981; Corbett et al., 1981). In a controlled study on biopsied individuals, the breath hydrogen test proved as reliable as the blood galactose test (Newcomer et al., 1975), but there are diagnostic problems such as:

1. Some individuals have high fasting hydrogen excretion, which may be caused by the ingestion of food containing undigestible oligosaccharides (e.g., beans) on the day before the test (Bayoumi et al., 1982).
2. Control of ventilation is important, and even moderate physical exercise, as well as breath holding, should be avoided during the test (Perman et al., 1985).
3. Smoking increases breath hydrogen concentration (Rosenthal and Solomons, 1983).
4. Not all individuals excrete hydrogen after a dose of unabsorbable carbohydrate because of methane production at the expense of hydrogen (Bjorneklett and Jenssen, 1982).

A recent study evaluated the use of a portable machine for measuring breath hydrogen (MicroH2), and it was found to be as reliable as the previously widely used machine, Quintron MicroLyzer (Peuhkuri et al., 1998). This makes this approach widely useable and avoids the need of storing breath samples.

Screening for Lactase Variability

Worldwide, newborn screening for lactase deficiency is performed regularly when infants receive the first feeding of mother's milk or other milk preparation. It is important that this is diagnosed rapidly, although in most cases the deficiency is transitory or secondary to other problems. Congenital lactase deficiency is exceptionally rare, except in Finland (Savilahti et al., 1983). Determination of the causal mutation(s) for this disease will provide, in the near future, a genetic test for Finnish individuals with a family history of the disease (Jarvela et al., 1998).

Screening for adult lactase nonpersistence and low LDC is mainly of interest to anthropologists and population geneticists at present. However, when the causal nucleotide differences are known, a DNA-based testing method will be possible and very valuable in distinguishing primary or secondary lactase deficiency in both adults and children with lactose malabsorption. This may help explain the poor recovery of lactase after inflammation has subsided.

Therapy of Lactose Intolerance

The best and only reasonable treatment of lactose intolerance in older children and adults is a reduction in the amount and a judicious diurnal spacing of the consumption of milk and lactose-rich milk products. Total milk avoidance is usually not necessary to relieve lactose intolerance. Low LDC can be a problem in infants with gastrointestinal disorders, and in adults it can be a result of gastrointestinal disease or a side effect of treatment, as mentioned (see Variables That Determine Lactose Intolerance), but low LDC is generally a rare cause of clinical problems. Relief of lactose intolerance by prostaglandin-synthesis inhibitors such as acetylsalicylic acid has been observed in one experiment (Leib, 1978). Even if the efficacy of this treatment were confirmed in a controlled study, it could not be recommended because of possible side effects of the medication. Enzymatic methods for diminishing the lactose content of milk are available (Rand, 1981) and exogenous β-D-galactosidase is available in pellet form for ingestion (Xenos et al., 1998). Lactose-free dairy products are available, especially in Finland and the United States, and these have a place in the nutrition of lactose-intolerant infants and small children, but most healthy adults and older children can tolerate the usual amounts of ordinary milk in the normal diet. There is a recent report of increasing lactose digestion in adults, albeit adult rats, by stable transfection of β-galactosidase into intestinal epithelial cells (During et al., 1998). The authors suggest that the research could be valuable in relation to humans, but this seems somewhat unlikely.

Milk Supplementation and Milk Avoidance in Disease Prevention

In most countries the proteins and carbohydrates in milk do not seem to offer special nutritional advantages in older children and adults, and milk is not an essential food in these age groups. The situation may be different for the dietary supply of calcium in human populations accustomed to a high intake of milk and milk products. If a large part of the daily calcium requirement is supplied by milk in the ordinary diet, people who abstain from milk consumption because of conscious or subconscious adaptation to lactose intolerance may have difficulties in maintaining calcium balance. However this effect is probably not important in causing calcium deficiency in modern times, and it is even more doubtful whether calcium alone can prevent osteoporosis. Bone formation and calcification depend on a multitude of independent variables, such as physical exercise, exposure to sunshine, hormonal status, exogenous and endogenous vitamin D, and the dietary calcium/phosphorous ratio. The World Health Organization recommends a daily intake of 400 mg calcium (Passmore et al., 1974), although a recent study suggests that the recommended amounts in some countries may be too low (Murray, 1996). Indeed, the recommended adult daily intake for calcium in the United Kingdom is 700 mg, and for men between 11 and 18 years of age it is as high as 1000 mg (United Kingdom Department of Health, 1998). Significant consumption of fresh milk, although an excellent source, is not necessary to achieve the recommended daily intake: calcium is present in other foods, such as cheese (approximately 700 mg in 100 g of cheddar cheese) and vegetables. The correction of hormonal deficiency, a healthy and active lifestyle, a sufficient supply of vitamin D, and the avoidance of excess phosphorus in the diet are as important as an adequate intake of calcium for preventing osteoporosis.

As with other food, excessive amounts of milk may have adverse effects, but milk consumption in moderate amounts below the individual tolerance threshold can be considered safe and nutritious.

ACKNOWLEDGMENT

This chapter was updated from the previous chapter in the first edition of this book written by Gebhard Flatz.

REFERENCES

Ahmed HF: Irritable bowel syndrome with lactose intolerance. Lancet 1975; 2:319–320.

Alhava EM, Jusilla J, Karjalainen P, Vuojolahti P: Lactose malabsorption and bone mineral content. Acta Med Scand 1977; 201:281–283.

Alun Jones V, McLaughlin P, Shorthouse N, Workman E, Hunter JO: Food intolerance: a major factor in the pathogenesis of irritable bowel syndrome. Lancet 1982; 2:1115–1117.

Ammermann A, Cavalli-Sforza L: Measuring the rate of spread of early farming in Europe. Man 1971; 6:674–688.

Anderson B, Vullo C: Did malaria select for primary adult lactase deficiency? Gut 1994; 35:1487–1489.

Antonowicz I, Lebenthal E: Developmental pattern of small intestinal enterokinase and disaccharidase activities in the human fetus. Gastroenterology 1977; 72:1299–1303.

Aoki K: A stochastic model of gene–culture coevolution suggested by the culture-historical hypothesis. Proc Natl Acad Sci USA 1986; 83:2929–2933.

Arola H, Koivula T, Jokela H, Isokoski M: Simple urinary test for lactose malabsorption. Lancet 1982; 2:524–525.

Arola H, Koivula T, Jokela H, Jauhiainen M, Keyrilainen O, Ahola T, Uusitalo A, Isokoski M: Comparision of indirect diagnostic methods for hypolactasia. Scand J Gastroent 1988; 23:351–357.

Asp N-G, Dahlqvist A: Human small intestine β-galactosidases: specific assay for three different enzymes. Analyt Biochem 1972; 47:527–538.

Auricchio S, Rubino A, Landholt M, Semenza G, Prader A: Isolated intestinal lactase deficiency in the adult. Lancet 1963; 2:324–326.

Auricchio S, Rubino A, Murset G: Intestinal glycosidase activities in the human embryo, fetus and newborn. Pediatrics 1965; 944–954.

Barr RG, Levine MD, Watkins JB: Recurrent abdominal pain of childhood due to lactose intolerance: a prospective study. N Engl J Med 1979; 300:1449–1452.

Bartlett K, Dobson JV, Eastham E: A new method for the detection of hydrogen in breath and its application to acquired and inborn sugar malabsorption. Clin Chim Acta 1981; 108:189–194.

Bayless T, Rosensweig N: A racial difference in the incidence of lactase deficiency: a survey of milk intolerance and lactase deficiency in healthy adult males. J Am Med Assoc 1966; 197:968–972.

Bayless TM, Huang SS: Recurrent abdominal pain due to milk and lactose intolerance in school-aged children. Pediatrics 1971; 47:1029–1032.
Bayless TM, Rothfeld B, Massa C, Wise L, Paige DM, Bedine M: Lactose and milk intolerance: clinical implications. N Engl J Med 1975; 292:1156–1159.
Bayoumi RAL, Flatz SD, Kuhau W, Flatz G: Deja and Nilotes: nomadic pastoralist groups with opposite distributions of the adult lactase phenotypes. Am J Phys Anthropol 1982; 58:173–178.
Bedine MS, Bayless TM: Intolerance of small amounts of lactose by individuals with low lactase levels. Gastroenterology 1973; 65:735–743.
Bengtson B, Steen B, Dahlqvist A, Jagerstad M: Does lactose intake induce cateract in man? Lancet 1984; 1:1293–1294.
Bennet A, Eley KG: Intestinal pH and propulsion: an explanation of diarrhoea in lactase deficiency and laxation by lactulose. J Pharm Pharmacol 1976; 28:192–195.
Birge SJ, Keutmann HT, Cuatrecasas P, Wheldon GD: Osteoporosis, intestinal lactase deficiency and low dietary calcium intake. N Engl J Med 1967; 276:445–448.
Bjorneklett A, Jenssen E: Relationship between hydrogen and methane production in man. Scand J Gastroenterol 1982; 17:885–892.
Blaxter K: Lactation and the growth of the young. In: Kow S, Cowie A (eds). Milk: The Mammary Gland and Its Secretion. New York: Academic Press, 1961:329–338.
Blumenthal I, Kelleher J, Littlewood JM: Recurrent abdominal pain and lactose intolerance in childhood. Br Med J 1980; 282:2013–2014.
Bohmer CJ, Tuynmann HA: The clinical relevance of lactose malabsorption in irritable bowel syndrome. Eur J Gastroenterol Hepatol 1996; 8:1013–1016.
Bohmer CJ, Tuynman HA: The effect of a lactose-restricted diet in patients with a positive lactose tolerance test, earlier diagnosed as irritable bowel syndrome: a 5-year follow-up study. Eur J Gastroenterol Hepatol 2001; 13:941–944.
Boll W, Wagner P, Mantei N: Structure of the chromosomal gene and cDNAs coding for lactase-phlorizin hydrolase in humans with adult-type hypolactasia or persistence of lactase. Am J Hum Genet 1991; 48:889–902.
Bond JH, Levitt MD: Fate of soluble carbohydrate in the colon of rats and man. J Clin Invest 1976a; 57:1158–1164.
Bond JH, Levitt MD: Quantitative measurement of lactose absorption. Gastroenterology 1976b; 70:1058–1062.
Bond JH, Levitt MD, Prentiss R: Investigation of small bowel transit time in man utilizing pulmonary hydrogen measurements. J Lab Clin Med 1975; 85:546–555.
Boukamel R, Freund J-N: The *cis*-element CE-LPH1 of the rat intestinal lactase gene promoter interacts in vitro with several nuclear factors present in endodermal tissues. FEBS Lett 1994; 353:108–112.
Briet F, Pochart P, Marteau M, Flourie B, Arrigoni E, Rambaud JC: Improved clinical tolerance to chronic lactose ingestion in subjects with lactose intolerance: a placebo effect? Gut 1997; 41:632–635.
Buisseret PD, Youlten LYF, Heinzelmann DI, Lassof MH: Prostaglandin synthesis inhibitors in prophylaxis of food intolerance. Lancet 1978; 1:906–909.
Buller HA, Kothe MJC, Goldman DA, Grubman SA, Sasak WV, Matsudaira PT, Montgomery RK, Grand RJ: Coordinate expression of lactase-phlorizin hydrolase mRNA and enzyme levels in rat intestine during development. J Biol Chem 1990; 265:6978–6983.
Buller HA, Montgomery RK, Sasak WV, Grand RJ: Biosynthesis, glycosylation and intracellular transport of intestinal lactase-phlorizin hydrolase in rat. J Biol Chem 1987; 262:17206–17211.
Buller HA, Rings EHHM, Montgomery RK, Grand RJ: Clinical aspects of lactose intolerance in children and adults. Scand J Gastroenterol 1991; 188(suppl):73–80.
Calloway DH, Colasito DJ, Mathews RD: Gases produced by human intestinal microflora. Nature 1966; 212:1238–1239.
Christiensen MF: Prevalence of lactose malabsorption in children with recurrent abdominal pain. Pediatrics 1980; 65:681–682.
Christopher NL, Bayless TM: Role of the small bowel and colon in lactose induced diarrhea. Gastroenterology 1971; 70:845–852.
Chua KL, Seah CS: Lactose intolerance: heriditary or acquired? Effect of prolonged milk feeding. Singapore Med J 1973; 14:29–33.
Cook GC: Did persistence of intestinal lactase into adult life originate in the Arabian peninsula? Man 1978; 13:418–427.
Corbett CL, Thomas S, Read NW, Hobson N, Bergman I, Holdsworth CD: Electrochemical detection for breath hydrogen determination: measurement of small bowel transit time in normal subjects and patients with the irritable bowel syndrome. Gut 1981; 22:836–840.
Cramer DW: Lactase persistence and milk consumption as determinants of ovarian cancer risk. Am J Epidemiol 1989; 130:904–910.
Cuatrecasas PD, Lockwood H, Caldwell J: Lactase deficiency in the adult: a common occurrence. Lancet 1965; 1:14–18.
Dahlqvist A: Method for assay of intestinal disaccharidases. Analyt Biochem 1964; 7:18–25.
Dahlqvist A: Enzyme deficiency and malabsorption of carbohydrates. In: Sipple HL, McNutt KW (eds). Sugars in Nutrition. New York: Academic Press, 1974:187–214.
Dahlqvist A, Hammond B, Crane R, Dunphy J, Littman A: Intestinal lactase deficiency and lactose intolerance in adults: preliminary report. Gastroenterology 1963; 45:488–491.
Danielsen EM: Biosynthesis of intestinal microvillar proteins: dimerization of aminopeptidase *N* and lactase-phlorizin hydrolase. Biochemistry 1990; 29:305–308.
Das BS, Das DB, Satpathy RN, Patnaik JK, Bose TK: Riboflavin deficiency and severity of malaria. Eur J Clin Nutr 1988; 42:277–283.
Dearlove J, Dearlove B, Pearl K, Primavesi R: Dietary lactose and the child with abdominal pain. Br Med J 1983; 2:1936.
Debognie JC, Newcomer AD, Millard JC, Hilbe A, Stainthorpe EM: Absorption of nutrients in lactase deficiency. Dig Dis Sci 1979; 24:225–231.
Douwes AC, Fernandes J, Rietveld W: Hydrogen breath test in infants and children: sampling and storing expired air. Clin Chim Acta 1978; 82:293–296.
Dudd SN, Evershed RP: Direct demonstration of milk as an element of archaelogical economies. Science 1998; 282:1478–1481.
Duluc I, Boukamel R, Mantei N, Semenza G, Raul F, Freund J-NF: Sequence of the precursor of intestinal lactase-phlorizin hydrolase from fetal rat. Gene 1991; 103:275–276.
Duluc I, Jost B, Freund J-N: Multiple levels of control of the stage- and region-specific expression of rat intestinal lactase. J Cell Biol 1993; 123:1577–1586.
During MJ, Xu R, Young D, Kaplitt MG, Sherwin RS, Leone P: Peroral gene therapy of lactose intolerance using an adeno-associated virus vector. Nat Med 1998; 4:1131–1135.
Enattah NS, Sahi T, Savilahti E, Terwilliger JD, Peltonen L, Jarvela I: Identification of a variant associated with adult-type hypolactasia. Nat Genet 2002; 30:233–237.
Escher JC, de Koning ND, van Engen CGJ, Arora S, Buller HA, Montgomery RK, Grand RJ: Molecular basis of lactase levels in adult humans. J Clin Invest 1992; 89:480–483.
Fajardo O, Naim HY, Lacey SW: The polymorphic expression of lactase in adults is regulated at the mRNA level. Gastroenterology 1994; 106:1233–1241.
Ferguson A, MacDonald DM, Brydon WG: Prevalence of lactase deficiency in British adults. Gut 1984; 25:163–167.
Fitzgerald K, Bazar L, Avigan MI: GATA-6 stimulates a cell-line specific activation element in the human lactase promoter. Am J Physiol 1998; 274:G314–G324.
Flatz G: Lactose tolerance: genetics, anthropology and natural selection. In: Armendares S, Lisker R (eds). Proceedings of the Fifth International Congress of Human Genetics. Mexico City: Excerpta Medica Amsterdam, 1977:386–396.
Flatz G: Gene dosage effect on intestinal lactase activity demonstrated in vivo. Am J Hum Genet 1984; 36:306–310.
Flatz G, Kunau W, Naftali D: Breath hydrogen test for lactose absorption capacity: importance of timing of hydrogen excretion and of high fasting hydrogen concentration. Am J Clin Nutr 1984; 39:752–755.
Flatz G, Rotthauwe HW: Evidence against nutritional adaption to tolerance to lactase. Humangenetik 1971; 13:118–125.
Flatz G, Rotthauwe HW: Lactose nutrition and natural selection. Lancet 1973; 2:76–77.
Flatz G, Saengudom C, Sanguanbhokai T: Lactose intolerance in Thailand. Nature 1969; 221:758–759.
Freund J-N, Duluc I, Raul F: Discrepancy between the intestinal lactase enzymatic activity and mRNA accumulation in sucklings and adults. FEBS Lett 1989; 248:39–42.
Gilat T, Russo S, Gelman-Malachi E, Aldor TAM: Lactase in man: a nonadaptable enzyme. Gastroenterology 1972; 62:1125–1127.
Grabnitz F, Seiss M, Rucknagel KP, Stauden Bauer W: Structure of the β-glucosidase gene bgl A of *Clostridium thermocellase*. Eur J Biochem 1991; 200:301–309.
Grant JD, Bezerra JA, Thompson SH, Lemen RJ, Kodolvsky O, Udall JN: Assessment of lactose absorption by measurement of urinary galactose. Gastroenterology 1989; 97:895.
Green FR, Greenwell P, Dickson L, Griffiths B, Noades J, Swallow DM: Expression of the ABH, Lewis and related antigens on the glycoproteins of the human jejunal brush border. In: Harris JR (ed). Subcellular Biochemistry. Vol. 12. New York: Plenum Press, 1988:119–153.
Greenwald E, Samachson S, Spencer H: Effect of lactose on calcium metabolism in man. J Nutr 1963; 79:531–538.
Grunberg J, Sterchi EE: Human lactase-phlorizin hydrolase: evidence of dimerization in the endoplasmic reticulum. Arch Biochem Biophys 1995; 323:367–372.
Gudmand-Hoyer E, Dahlqvist A, Jarnum S: The clinical significance of lactose malabsorption. Gastroenterology 1970; 53:460–473.
Gudmand-Hoyer E, Riis P, Wulff HR: The significance of lactose malabsorption in the irritable bowel syndrome. Scand J Gastroenterol 1973; 8:273–278.
Habte D, Sterky G, Hjaalmarsson B: Lactose malabsorption in Ethiopean children. Acta Paediatr Scand 1973; 62:649–654.
Harvey CB: The biochemical and genetical analysis of lactase phlorizin hydrolase: with specific reference to the lactase persistence/non-persistence polymorphism in man. PhD Thesis London: University of London, 1994:106–108.
Harvey CB, Fox MF, Jeggo PA, Mantei N, Povey S, Swallow DM: Regional localization of the lactase-phlorizin hydrolase gene, *LCT*, to chromosome 2q21. Ann Hum Genet 1993; 57:179–185.
Harvey CB, Hollox EJ, Poulter M, Wang Y, Rossi M, Auricchio S, Iqbal TH, Cooper BT, Barton R, Sarner M, Korpela R, Swallow DM: Lactase haplotype frequencies in Caucasians: association with the lactase persistence/non-persistence polymorphism. Ann Hum Genet 1998; 62:215–223.
Harvey CB, Pratt W, Islam I, Whitehouse DB, Swallow DM: DNA polymorphisms in the lactase gene: linkage disequilibrium across the 70kb region. Eur J Hum Genet 1995; 3:27–41.
Harvey CB, Wang Y, Hughes LA, Swallow DM, Thurrell WP, Sams VR, Barton R, Sarner M: Studies on the expression of intestinal lactase in different individuals. Gut 1994; 36:28–33.
Harvey PH, Martin RD, Clutton-Brock TH: Life histories in comparative perspective. In: Smuts BB, Cheney DL, Seyfarth RM, Wrangham RW, Struhsaker TT (eds). Primate Societies. Chicago: University of Chicago Press, 1987:181–196.
Hasunen K, Muhenon M, Sahi T, Kirjarinta M: Dietary intake in cases of lactose malabsorption in a Finnish Lapp population. Nordic Council Arctic Med Res 1977; 17:3–20.
Heading RC: Gastric emptying: a clinical perspective. Clin Sci 1982; 63:231–235.

Hecht A, Torbey CF, Korsmo HA, Olsen WA: Regulation of sucrase and lactase in developing rats: role of nuclear factors that bind to two gene regulatory elements. Gastroenterology 1997; 112:803–812.

Herrinton LJ, Weiss NS, Beresford SA, Stanford JL, Wolfla DM, Feng Z, Scott CR: Lactose and galactose intake and metabolism in relation to the risk of epithelial ovarian cancer. Am J Epidemiol 1995; 141:407–416.

Ho MW, Povey S, Swallow DM: Lactase polymorphism in adult British natives: estimating allele frequencies by enzyme assays in autopsy samples. Am J Hum Genet 1982; 34:650–657.

Holden C, Mace R: Phylogenetic analysis of the evolution of lactase digestion in adults. Hum Biol 1997; 69:605–628.

Hollox EJ, Poulter M, Wang Y, Krause A, Swallow DM: Common polymorphism in a highly variable region upstream of the human lactase gene affects DNA-protein interactions. Eur J Hum Genet 1999; 7:791–800.

Hollox EJ, Poulter M, Zvarik M, Ferak V, Krause A, Jenkins T, Saha N, Kozlov AI, Swallow DM: Lactase haplotype diversity in the Old World. Am J Hum Genet 2001; 68:160–172.

Honkanen R, Kroger H, Alhava E, Turpeinen P, Tuppurainen M, Saarkoski S: Lactose intolerance associated with fractures of weight-bearing bones. Bone 1997; 21:473–477.

Honkanen R, Pulkkinen P, Jarvinen R, Kroger H, Lindstedt K, Tupurainen M, Uusitupa M: Does lactose intolerance predispose to low bone density? A population based study of perimenopausal Finnish women. Bone 1996; 19:23–28.

Horowitz M, Wishart J, Mundy L, Nordin C: Lactose and calcium absorption in postmenopausal osteoporosis. Arch Intern Med 1987; 147:534–536.

Hove H, Nordgaard-Andersen I, Mortensen PB: Effect of lactic acid bacteria on the intestinal production of lactate and short-chain fatty acids, and the absorption of lactose. Am J Clin Nutr 1994; 59:74–79.

Howell JN, Schockenhoff T, Flatz G: Population screening for the adult lactase phenotypes with a multiple breaths version of the breath hydrogen test. Hum Genet 1981; 57:276–278.

Howell JN, Von der Fecht R, Flatz G: Hydrogen breath test for lactose tolerance adapted to population screening. Clin Chim Acta 1980; 103:229–231.

Isokoski M, Jusilla J, Sarna S: A simple screening method for lactose malabsorption. Gastroenterology 1972; 62:28–32.

Jarvela I, Enattah NS, Kokkonen J, Varilo T, Savilahti E, Peltonen L: Assignment of the locus for congenital lactase deficiency to 2q21, in the vicinity of but separate from the lactase-phlorizin hydrolase gene. Am J Hum Genet 1998; 63:1078–1085.

Johnson AO, Semenya JG, Buchowski MS, Enwonwu CO, Scrimshaw NS: Adaptation of lactose maldigesters to continued milk intakes. Am J Clin Nutr 1993; 58:879–881.

Jost B, Duluc I, Richardson M, Lathe R, Freund J-N: Functional diversity and interactions between the repeat domains of rat intestinal lactase. Biochem J 1997; 327:95–103.

Jussila J: Diagnosis of lactose malabsoption by the lactose tolerance test with peroral ethanol administration. Scand J Gastroenterol 1969; 4:361–368.

Karcher RE, Truding RM, Stawick LE: Using a cutoff of <10 ppm (less than 8 yr) ppm for breath hydrogen testing: a review of five years' experience. Ann Clin Lab Sci 1999; 29:1–8.

Kern F, Heller M: Blood galactose after lactose and ethanol: an accurate index of lactase deficiency. Gastroenterology 1968; 54:1250.

Keusch GT, Troncale FJ, Miller LH, Promadhat V, Anderson PR: Acquired lactose malabsorption in Thai children. Pediatrics 1969a; 43:540–545.

Keusch GT, Troncale FJ, Thavaramara B, Prinyanont P, Anderson PR, Bhamarapravathi N: Lactase deficiency in Thailand: effect of prolonged lactose feeding. Am J Clin Nutr 1969b; 22:638–641.

Kleinjan D-J, van Heyningen V: Position effect in human genetic disease. Hum Mol Genet 1998; 7:1611–1618.

Klibanov AM, Alberti BN, Zale SE: Enzymatic synthesis of formic acid from hydrogen and carbon dioxide and production of hydrogen from formic acid. Biotechnol Bioeng 1982; 24:25–36.

Knudsen K, Welsh M, Kronenberg R, Vanderveen J, Heidelbauch N: Effect of a nonlactose diet on human intestinal disaccharidase activity. Am J Dig Dis 1968; 13:593–597.

Kocian J, Skala I, Bakos K: Calcium absorption from milk and lactose free milk in healthy subjects and patients with lactase deficiency. Digestion 1973a; 9:317–324.

Kocian J, Vulterinova M, Beijblova O, Skala I: Influence of lactose intolerance on the bones of patients after partial gastrectomy. Digestion 1973b; 8:324–335.

Kolars JC, Levitt MD, Aouji M, Savaiano DA: Yogurt—an autodigestive source of lactase. N Engl J Med 1984; 310:1–3.

Kozlov AI, Balanovskaya EV, Nurbaev SD, Balanovsky OI: Gene geography of primary hypolactasia in populations of the Old World. Russian J Genet 1998; 34:445–454.

Krasilnikoff P, Gudmand-Hoyer E, Moltke H: Diagnostic value of disaccharidase tolerance in children. Acta Paediatr Scand 1975; 64:693–698.

Krasinski SD, Estrada G, Yeh KY, Yeh M, Traber PG, Rings EH, Buller HA, Verhave M, Montgomery RK, Grand RJ: Transcriptional regulation of intestinal hydrolase biosynthesis during postnatal development in rats. Am J Physiol 1994; 267:G584–G594.

Krasinski SD, Upchurch BH, Irons SJ, June RM, Mishra K, Grand RJ, Verhave M: Rat lactase-plorizin hydrolase/human growth hormone transgene is expressed on small intestinal villi in transgenic mice. Gastroenterology 1997; 113:844–855.

Kruse TA, Bolund L, Byskov A, Sjostrom H, Noren O, Mantei N, Semenza G: Mapping of the human lactase-phlorizin hydrolase gene to chromosome 2. Cytogenet Cell Genet 1989; 51:1026.

Lacey SW, Naim HY, Magness RR, Gething M-J, Sambrook JF: Expression of lactase-phlorizin hydrolase in sheep is regulated at the RNA level. Biochem J 1994; 302:929–935.

Laland KN, Kumm J, Feldman MW: Gene-culture coevolutionary theory: a test case. Curr Anthropol 1995; 36:131–156.

Launiala K: The mechanism of diarrhea in congenital disaccharidase malabsorption. Acta Paediatr Scand 1968; 57:425–430.

Lebenthal E, Rossi TM, Nord KS, Branski D: Recurrent abdominal pain and lactose malabsorption in children. Pediatrics 1981; 67:828–832.

Leib J: Prostaglandin-synthesis inhibitors in prophylaxis of food intolerance. Lancet 1978; 2:157.

Leibman WM: Recurrent abdominal pain in children: lactose and sucrose intolerance. Pediatrics 1979; 64:43–45.

Levitt MD: Production and excretion of hydrogen gas in man. N Engl J Med 1969; 282:122–127.

Levitt MD, Ingelfinger FJ: Hydrogen and methane production in man. Ann NY Acad Sci 1968; 150:75–81.

Lisker R, Aguilar L, Zavala C: Intestinal lactase deficiency and milk drinking capacity in the adult. Am J Clin Nutr 1978; 31:1499–1503.

Lisker R, Solomons NW, Perez Briceno R, Ramirez Mata M: Lactase and placebo in the management of the irritable bowel syndrome: a double-blind, cross-over study. Am J Gastroenterol 1989; 84:756–762.

Lorenzsonn V, Lloyd M, Olsen WA: Immunocytochemical heterogeneity of lactase-phlorizin hydrolase in adult lactase deficiency. Gastroenterology 1993; 105:51–59.

Lottaz D, Oberholzer T, Bahler P, Semenza G, Sterchi EE: Maturation of human lactase-phlorizin hydrolase: proteolytic cleavage of precursor occurs after passage through the Golgi complex. FEBS Lett 1992; 313:270–276.

MacDonald MJ, Horowitz R, Duncan TG: Use of the lactose ethanol tolerance test in diabetics. Am J Med Sci 1975; 269:193–199.

MacLean WC: Lactose intolerance. N Engl J Med 1980; 302:177.

Maiuri L, Raia V, Fiocca R, Solcia E, Cornaggia M, Noren O, Sjostrom H, Swallow D, Auricchio S, Dabelsteen E: Mosaic differentiation of human villus enterocytes: patchy expression of blood group A antigen in nonsecretors. Gastroenterology 1993; 104:21–30.

Maiuri L, Rossi M, Raia V, Garipoli V, Swallow D, Hughes L, Noren O, Auricchio S: Mosaic regulation of lactase in human adult-type hypolactasia. Gasteroenterology 1994; 107:54–60.

Mantei N, Villa M, Enzler T, Wacker H, Boll W, James P, Hunziker W, Semenza G: Complete primary structure of human and rabbit lactase-phlorizin hydrolase: implications for biosynthesis, membrane anchoring and evolution of the enzyme. EMBO J 1988; 7:2705–2713.

Martin MG, Turk E, Lostao MP, Kerner C, Wright EM: Defects in Na^+/glucose cotransporter (SGLT1) trafficking and function cause glucose–galactose malabsorption. Nat Genet 1996; 12:216–220.

Meloni T, Colombo C, Ruggiu G, Dessena M, Meloni GF: Primary lactase deficiency and past malarial endemicity in Sardinia. Ital J Gastroenterol Hepatol 1998; 30:490–493.

Metneki J, Cziezel A, Flatz SD, Flatz G: A study of lactose absorption capacity in twins. Hum Genet 1984; 67:296–300.

Metz G, Gassul MA, Leeds AR, Blendis LM, Jenkins DJA: A simple method for measuring breath hydrogen in carbohydrate malabsorption by end expiratory sampling. Clin Sci 1976; 50:237–240.

Mishkin B, Yalovsky M, Mishkin S: Increased prevalence of lactose malabsorption in Crohn's disease patients at low risk for lactose malabsorption based on ethnic origin. Am J Gastroenterol 1997; 92:1148–1153.

Mishkin S: Dairy sensitivity, lactose malabsorption and elimination diets in inflammatory bowel disease. Am J Clin Nutr 1997; 65:564–567.

Mitchelmore C, Troelsen JT, Sjostrom H, Noren O: The HOXC11 homeodomain protein interacts with the lactase-phlorizin hydrolase promoter and stimulates HNF1α-dependent transcription. J Biol Chem 1998; 273:13297–13306.

Montgomery RK, Buller HA, Rings EHHM, Grand RJ: Lactose intolerance and the genetic regulation of intestinal lactase-phlorizin hydrolase. FASEB J 1991; 5:2824–2832.

Murray TM: Prevention and management of osteoporosis: consensus statements from the Scientific Advisory Board of the Osteoporosis Society of Canada: 4. Calcium nutrition and osteoporosis. CMAJ 1996; 155:935–939.

Naim HY, Jacob R, Naim H, Sambrook JF, Gething M-JH: The pro-region of human intestinal lactase-phlorizin hydrolase. J Biol Chem 1994; 269:26933–26943.

Naim HY, Lentze MJ: Impact of *O*-glycosylation on the function of human intestinal lactase-phlorizin hydrolase: characterization of glycoforms varying in enzyme activity and localization of *O*-glycoside addition. J Biol Chem 1992; 267:25494–25504.

Naim HY, Naim H: Dimerization of lactase-phlorizin hydrolase occurs in the endoplasmic reticulum, involves the putative membrane spanning domain and is required for an effecient transport of the enzyme to the cell surface. Eur J Cell Biol 1996; 70:198–208.

Naim HY, Sterchi EE, Lentze MJ: Biosynthesis and maturation of lactase-phlorizin hydrolase in the human intestinal epithelial cells. Biochem J 1987; 241:427–434.

Nei M, Saitou N: Genetic relationship of human populations and ethnic differences in relation to drugs and food. In: Kalow W, Goedde HW, Agarwal DP (eds). Ethnic Differences in Reactions to Drugs and Other Xenobiotics. New York: Alan R Liss, 1986:21–37.

Newcomer AD, Hodgson SF, McGill DB, Thomas PJ: Lactase deficiency: prevalence in osteoporosis. Ann Intern Med 1978; 89:218–220.

Newcomer AD, McGill DB: Distribution of disaccharidase activity in the small bowel of normal and lactase deficient subjects. Gastroenterology 1966; 51:481–488.

Newcomer AD, McGill DB: Disaccharidase activity in the small intestine: prevalence of lactase deficiency in 100 subjects. Gastroenterology 1967; 53:881–889.

Newcomer AD, McGill DB: Irritable bowel syndrome: role of lactase deficiency. Mayo Clin Proc 1983; 58:339–341.

Newcomer AD, McGill DB, Thomas PJ, Hofmann AF: Prospective comparison of indirect methods for detecting lactase deficiency. N Engl J Med 1975; 293:1232–1236.

Nichols BL, Dudley MA, Nichols VN, Putnam M, Avery SE, Fraley JK, Quaroni A, Shiner M, Carrazza FR: Effects of malnutrition on expression and activity of lactase in children. Gastroenterology 1997; 112:742–751.

Niu HC, Schoeller DA, Klein PD: Improve gas chromatographic quantitation of breath hydrogen by normalization to respiratory carbon dioxide. J Lab Clin Med 1979; 94:755–763.

Oberholzer T, Mantei N, Semenza G: The pro sequence of lactase-phlorizin hydrolase is required for the enzyme to reach the plasma membrane: an intramolecular chaperone? FEBS Lett 1993; 333:127–131.

Olsen WA, Li BUK, Lloyd M, Korsmo H: Heterogeneity of intestinal lactase activity in children: relationship to lactase-phlorizin hydrolase messenger RNA abundance. Pediatr Res 1996; 39:877–881.

Paige DM, Bayless TM, Ferry GD, Graham GG: Lactose malabsorption and milk rejection in Negro children. Johns Hopkins Med J 1971; 129:163–169.

Pansu D, Bellaton C, Bronner F: Effect of lactose on duodenal calcium binding protein and calcium absorption. J Nutr 1979; 109:508–512.

Parnes HL, Fung E, Schiffer CA: Chemotherapy-induced lactose intolerance in adults. Cancer 1994; 74:1629–1633.

Passmore R, Nicol BM, Rac MN: Handbook on Human Nutritional Requirements. Geneva: World Health Organization, 1974.

Pena AS, Truelove SC: Hypolactasia and the irritable colon syndrome. Scand J Gastroenterol 1972; 7:433–438.

Perman JA, Modler S, Engel RR, Heldt G: Effect of ventilation on breath hydrogen measurements. J Lab Clin Med 1985; 105:436–439.

Perman JA, Modler S, Olson AC: Role of pH in production of hydrogen from carbohydrates by colonic bacterial flora. J Clin Invest 1981; 67:643–650.

Perrin P: The impact of humanitarian aid on conflict development. Int Rev Red Cross 1998; 323:319–333.

Peuhkuri K, Poussa T, Korpela R: Comparison of a portable breath hydrogen analyser (Micro H2) with a Quintron MicroLyzer in measuring lactose maldigestion, and the evaluation of a Micro H2 for diagnosing hypolactasia. Scand J Clin Lab Invest 1998; 58:217–224.

Phillips AD, Avigad S, Sacks J, Rice SJ, France NE, Walker-Smith JA: Microvillous surface area in secondary disaccharidase deficiency. Gut 1980; 21:44–48.

Plimmer RHA: On the presence of lactase in the intestines of animals and on the adaptation of the intestine to lactose. J Physiol (London) 1906; 35:20–31.

Porro GB, Petrillo M, Parente F, Sangaletti O, Della Vedova G: Recurrent abdominal pain and lactose intolerance. Br Med J 1981; 283:501.

Potter J, Ho M-W, Bolton H, Furth AJ, Swallow DM, Griffiths B: Human lactase and the molecular basis of lactase persistence. Biochem Genet 1985; 23:423–439.

Rand AG: Enzyme technology and the development of lactose hydrolyzed milk. In: Paige DM, Bayless TM (eds). Lactose Digestion: Clinical and Nutritional Implications. Baltimore: Johns Hopkins University Press, 1981:219–230.

Ransome-Kuti O: Lactose intolerance: a review. Post Grad Med J 1977; 53:73–87.

Risch HA, Jain M, Marrett LD, Howe GR: Dietary lactose intake, lactose intolerance, and the risk of ovarian cancer in southern Ontario (Canada). Cancer Causes Control 1994; 5:540–548.

Rohmann F, Nagano J: Über die Resorption und die fermentative Spaltung der Disaccharide im Dünndarm des aufgewachsenen Hundes. Arch Ges Physiol 1903; 95:533–605.

Rosado JL, Allen LH, Solomons NW: Milk consumption, symptom response, and lactose digestion in milk intolerance. Am J Clin Nutr 1987; 22:638–641.

Rosado JL, Solomons NW: Sensitivity and specificity of the breath hydrogen analysis test for detecting malabsorption of physiological doses of lactose. Clin Chem 1983a; 29:545–548.

Rosado JL, Solomons NW: Storage of hydrogen breath test samples in plastic syringes. Clin Chem 1983b; 29:583–584.

Rosenthal A, Solomons NW: Time-course of cigarette smoke contamination of clinical breath-analysis test. Clin Chem 1983; 29:1980–1981.

Rosensweig NS, Herman RH: Diet and disaccharidases. Am J Clin Nutr 1969; 22:99–102.

Rossi M, Maiuri L, Salvati VM, Russomanno C, Auricchio S: In vitro biosynthesis of lactase in preweaning and adult rabbit. FEBS Lett 1992; 313:260–264.

Rossi M, Mauiri L, Fusco MI, Salvati VM, Fuccio A, Auricchio S, Mantei N, Zecca L, Gloor SM, Semenza G: Lactase persistence versus decline in human adults: multifactorial events are involved in downregulation after weaning. Gastroenterology 1997; 112:1506–1514.

Sahi T: The inheritance of selective adult-type lactose malabsorption. Scand J Gastroenterol 1974; 9:1–73.

Sahi T, Isokoski M, Jussila J, Launiala K, Pyorala K: Recessive inheritance of adult-type lactose malabsorption. Lancet 1973; ii:823–826.

Sahi T, Jusilla J, Penttila I, Sarna S, Isokoski M: Serum lipids and proteins in lactose malabsorption. Am J Clin Nutr 1977; 30:476–481.

Sahi T, Launiala K: Manifestation and occurrence of selective adult-type lactose malabsorption in Finnish teenagers: a follow-up study. Dig Dis Sci 1978; 23:699–704.

Sahi T, Launiala K, Laitinen H: Hypolactasia in a fixed cohort of young Finnish adults: a follow-up study. Scand J Gastroenterol 1983; 18:865–870.

Salmon PR, Read AE, McCarthy CF: An isotope technique for measuring lactose absorption. Gut 1969; 10:685–689.

Sasaki Y, Ilo M, Kameda H, Ueda H, Aoyagi T, Christopher NL, Bayless TM, Wagner HM: Measurement of ^{14}C lactose absorption in the diagnosis of lactase deficiency. J Lab Clin Med 1970; 76:824–835.

Savaiano DA, Abou El Anouar A, Smith DE, Levitt MD: Lactose malabsorption from yogurt, pastuerized yogurt, sweet acidophilus milk, and cultured milk in lactase-deficient individuals. Am J Clin Nutr 1984; 40:1219–1223.

Savilahti E, Launiala K, Kuitunen P: Congenital lactase deficiency: a clinical study of 16 patients. Arch Dis Child 1983; 58:246–252.

Sebastio G, Villa M, Sartorio R, Guzzetta V, Poggi V, Auricchio S, Boll W, Mantei N, Semenza G: Control of lactase in human adult-type hypolactasia and in weaning rabbits and rats. Am J Hum Genet 1989; 45:489–497.

Segall JJ: Is lactose a dietary risk factor for ischaemic heart disease? Int J Epidemiol 1980; 9:271–276.

Segall JJ: Dietary lactose as a possible risk factor for ischaemic heart disease: review of epidemiology. Int J Cardiol 1994; 46:197–207.

Semenza G, Leese HJ, Colombo V, Lorenz-Meyer H: The small intestinal β-glycoside (lactase glucosylceramidase) complex. Mod Probl Paediatr 1975; 15:186–193.

Simoons FJ: Primary lactose intolerance and the milking habit: a problem in biological and cultural interrelations: II. A culture historical hypothesis. Am J Dig Dis 1970; 15:695–710.

Simoons FJ: The antiquity of dairying in Asia and Africa. Geograph Rev 1971; 61:431–439.

Simoons FJ: The geographic hypothesis and lactose malabsorption: a weighing of the evidence. Dig Dis 1978; 23:963–980.

Simoons FJ: A geographic approach to senile cataracts: possible links with milk consumption, lactase activity and galactose metabolism. Dig Dis Sci 1982; 27:257–264.

Skovbjerg H: Immunoelectrophoretic studies on human small intestinal brush border proteins: the longitudinal distribution of peptidases and disaccharidases. Clin Chem Acta 1981; 112:205–212.

Skovbjerg H, Gudmand-Hoyer E, Fenger H: Immunoelectrophoretic studies on human small intestinal brush border proteins: amount of lactase protein in adult-type hypolactasia. Gut 1980; 21:360–364.

Skovbjerg H, Sjostrom H, Noren O: Purification and characterisation of amphiphilic lactase-phlorizin hydrolase from human small intestine. Eur J Biochem 1981; 114:653–661.

Spodsberg N, Troelsen JT, Carlsson P, Enerback S, Sjostrom H, Noren O: Transcriptional regulation of pig lactase-phlorizin hydrolase: involvement of HNF-1 and FREACs. Gastroenterology 1999; 116:842–854.

Stephenson LS, Latham MC: Lactose intolerance and milk consumption: the relation of tolerance to symptoms. Am J Clin Nutr 1974; 28:86–88.

Sterchi E, Mills P, Fransen J, Hauri H, Lentze M, Naim H, Ginsel L, Bond J: Biogenesis of intestinal lactase-phlorizin hydrolase in adults with lactose intolerance: evidence for reduced biosynthesis and slowed-down maturation in enterocytes. J Clin Invest 1990; 86:1329–1337.

Suarez FL, Savaiano D, Arbisi P, Levitt MD: Tolerance to the daily ingestion of two cups of milk by individuals claiming lactose intolerance. Am J Clin Nutr 1997; 65:1502–1506.

Sunshine P, Kretchmer N: Intestinal disaccharidases: absence in two species of sea lions. Science 1964; 144:850–851.

Swallow DM, Harvey CB: Genetics of adult-type hypolactasia. Dyn Nutr Res 1993; 3:1–7.

Swallow DM, Hollox EJ: The genetic polymorphism of intestinal lactase activity in adult humans. In: Scriver CR, Beaudet AL, Sly WS, Valle D (eds). The Metabolic and Molecular Bases of Inherited Disease. New York: McGraw-Hill, 2000:1651–1663.

Tanaka T, Takase S, Goda T: A possible role of a nuclear factor NF-LPH1 in the regional expression of lactase-phlorizin hydrolase along the small intestine. J Nutr Sci Vitaminol (Tokyo) 1997; 43:565–573.

Tolliver BA, Jackson MS, Jackson KL, Barnett ED, Chastang JF, DiPalma JA: Does lactose maldigestion really play a role in the irritable bowel? J Clin Gastroenterol 1996; 23:15–17.

Torp N, Rossi M, Troelsen JT, Olsen J, Danielsen EM: Lactase-phlorizin hydrolase and aminopeptidase *N* are differentially regulated in the small intestine of the pig. Biochem J 1993; 295:177–182.

Troelsen J, Mehlum A, Olsen J, Spodsberg N, Hansen G, Prydz H, Noren O, Sjostrom H: 1 kb of the lactase-phlorizin hydrolase promoter directs post-weaning decline and small intestinal-specific expression in transgenic mice. FEBS Lett 1994; 342:291–296.

Troelsen J, Olsen J, Noren O, Sjostrom H: A novel intestinal *trans* factor (NF-LPH1) interacts with the lactase phlorizin hydrolase promotor and co-varies with the enzymic activity. J Biol Chem 1992; 267:20407–20411.

United Kingdom Department of Health: Quick reference primary care guide on the prevention and treatment of osteoporosis. Department of Health. London: 1998.

United Nations Food and Agriculture Organization: FAOSTAT Statistics Database (http://apps.fao.org), 1999.

United Nations High Commission for Refugees: Field Office Memorandum No. 76/89. Geneva: United Nations, 1989.

van Beers EH, Rings EHHM, Taminiau JAJM, Heymans HSA, Einerhand AWC, Dekker J, Buller HA: Regulation of lactase and sucrase-isomaltase gene expression in the duodenum during childhood. J Pediatr Gastroenterol Nutr 1998; 27:37–46.

Velebit L, Cochet B, Courvoisier B: Incidence de l'intolerance au lactose dans l'osteoporose postmenopausique. Schweiz Med Wochenschr 1978; 108:2061–2065.

Vesa TH, Korpela RA, Sahi T: Tolerance to small amounts of lactose in lactose maldigesters. Am J Clin Nutr 1996; 64:197–201.

Villa M, Menard D, Semenza G, Mantei N: The expression of lactase enzymatic activity and mRNA in human fetal jejunum: effect of organ culture and of treatment with hydrocortisone. FEBS Lett 1992; 301:202–206.

Vonk RJ, Stellaard F, Priebe MG, Koetse HA, Hagedoorn RE, De Bruijn S, Elzinga H, Lenoir-Wijnkoop I, Antoine JM: The 13C/2H-glucose test for determination of small intestinal lactase activity. Eur J Clin Invest 2001; 31:226–233.

Wacker H, Keller P, Falchetto R, Legler G, Semenza G: Location of the two catalytic sites in intestinal lactase phlorizin hydrolase: comparison with sucrase-isomaltase and other glycosidases, the membrane anchor of lactase phlorizin hydrolase. J Biol Chem 1992; 267:18744–18752.

Wald A, Chandra R, Fisher SE: Lactose malabsorption in recurrent abdominal pain in children. J Pediatr 1982; 100:65–68.

Wang Y, Harvey CB, Hollox EJ, Phillips AD, Poulter M, Clay P, Walker-Smith JA, Swallow DM: The genetically programmed down-regulation of lactase in children. Gastroenterology 1998; 114:1230–1236.

Wang Y, Harvey CB, Pratt WS, Sams VR, Sarner M, Rossi M, Auricchio S, Swallow DM: The lactase persistence/non-persistence polymorphism is controlled by a *cis*-acting element. Hum Mol Genet 1995; 4:657–662.

Wang Y, Harvey C, Rousset M, Swallow D: Expression of intestinal mRNA transcripts during development: analysis by a semi-quantitative RNA PCR method. Pediatr Res 1994; 36:514–521.

Welsh JD: Isolated lactase deficiency in humans: report on 100 patients. Medicine 1970; 49:257–277.

Welsh JD, Hall WH: Gastric emptying of lactose and milk in subjects with lactose malabsorption. Am J Dig Dis 1977; 22:1060–1063.

Welsh JD, Russell LC, Walker AW: Changes in intestinal lactase and alkaline phosphatase activity levels with age in the baboon (*Papio papio*). Gastroenterology 1974; 66:993–997.

Wen C-P, Antonowicz I, Tovar E, McGandy RB, Gershoff SN: Lactose feeding in lactose intolerant monkeys. Am J Clin Nutr 1973; 26:1224–1228.

Witte J, Lloyd M, Lorenzsonn V, Korsmo H, Olsen W: The biosynthetic basis of adult lactase deficiency. J Clin Invest 1990; 86:1338–1342.

Xenos K, Kyroudis S, Anagnostidis A, Papastathopoulos P: Treatment of lactose intolerance with exogenous β-D-galactosidase in pellet form. Eur J Drug Metab Pharmacokinet 1998; 23:350–355.

Zecca L, Mesonero JE, Stutz A, Poiree JC, Giudicelli J, Cursio R, Gloor SM, Semenza G: Intestinal lactase-phlorizin hydrolase (LPH): the two catalytic sites; the role of the pancreas in pro-LPH maturation. FEBS Lett 1998; 435:225–228.

15 Inflammatory Bowel Disease

HUIYING YANG, KENT D. TAYLOR, AND JEROME I. ROTTER

The inflammatory bowel diseases (IBD) consist principally of ulcerative colitis (UC) and Crohn's disease (CD)—two chronic idiopathic inflammatory diseases of the gastrointestinal tract. They are identified and diagnosed by the appearance of a set of clinical, radiologic, endoscopic, and histologic characteristics (Table 15–1). Ulcerative colitis and Crohn's disease are considered together because of their overlapping clinical, epidemiologic, and pathogenetic features and their shared complications and therapies. To some extent, however, they do, present distinct clinical, genetic, and pathologic characteristics, as shown in Table 15–1.

The common symptoms in UC and CD are diarrhea, abdominal pain, fever, and weight loss. Ulcerative colitis is a chronic inflammation of the colonic and rectal mucosa, characterized by relapses and remissions of rectal bleeding. The inflammation usually begins in the rectum and extends proximally in a continuous pattern without skipping areas of the colon. The inflammation is superficial—that is, it involves only the mucosal/submucosal layers, or the inner lining, of the gut. In contrast to UC, inflammation in Crohn's may occur anywhere in the gastrointestinal tract, from the mouth to the anus, both histologically and endoscopically, focally involved and skipped normal segments of the intestine are observed. The most common form of CD is *ileocolitis*, which affects both the small bowel and the colon (Lashner, 2000); when it affects the small bowel, the alternative term *regional ileitis* is used. In addition, inflammation in Crohn's involves all layers of the bowel wall—mucosa, submucosa, and muscular layer—and can even progress through the bowel wall. The chronic transmural inflammatory nature of CD can result in granulomas, abscesses, fistulae, and perianal complications. The term *indeterminate colitis* is used when one is not able to confidently assign the colitis to either UC or CD based on the clinical and pathological characteristics. In practice, this situation seldom arises and usually resolves itself with careful patient follow-up (Shanahan and Targan, 1994).

Traditionally the diagnosis of CD and of UC has been made on clinical, radiologic, endoscopic, and histologic findings. Recently, the use of disease-specific antibodies has begun to be explored for diagnostic purposes. A diagnostic role for the best established antibodies—anti-*Saccharomyces cerevisiae* antibody (ASCA) and perinuclear antineutrophil cytoplasmic antibodies (pANCA)—is being evaluated (Quinton et al., 1998). (These antibodies are discussed in more detail under disease pathophysiology, below.) It has been reported that the pANCA test has a sensitivity of 65% and specificity of 85% for UC and that the ASCA test has 61% sensitivity and 88% specificity for CD. The combination of a positive ASCA and negative pANCA yielded 49% sensitivity, 97% specificity, and 96% positive predictive value for CD. The combination of a positive pANCA and negative ASCA yielded 57% sensitivity, 97% specificity, and 92% positive predictive value for UC. Thus, because of their relatively low sensitivity, these markers cannot be used as screening tools. However, due to the high specificity of the combination of the two markers, in IBD patients with one of these two serological profiles, it appears that a rather definitive diagnosis of UC or CD can likely be made without further invasive testing, although this is not yet general practice. In addition, the use of these serological markers may play a role in the classification of individuals with indeterminate colitis.

Clinical subgroups have been defined, based on anatomic location of the disease to indicate disease extent, clinical course, and indication for surgery. Increasing evidence supports subgrouping Crohn's disease into perforating and nonperforating forms. Perforating CD is the more aggressive form, which often results in abscesses or free perforation and fistulae; it also has a higher reoperation rate. In contrast, the nonperforating form follows a more indolent clinical course and is associated with obstruction and bleeding (Greenstein et al., 1988). This clinical subgrouping has been further supported by cytokine mRNA profiles (Gilberts et al., 1994) and genetic marker studies (Esaki et al., 1999; Nemetz et al., 1999b) (see Disease Pathophysiology). Accurate disease subgrouping not only aids in clinical decision making and predicting prognosis but also is essential for studies of pathogenesis, genetic susceptibility, and response to therapy.

There is no etiologic-specific treatment for either form of IBD, although colectomy is a curative procedure for UC. Currently, initially supportive measures and anti-inflammatory agents (e.g., the sulfasalazines and corticorteroids) are commonly used, and immunosuppressive agents are added in the case of severe disease that is unresponsive to other agents.

In the past few years, immunotherapy directed against specific inflammatory molecules (cytokines, adhesion molecules) has become a promising approach to treating chronic IBD (Sands, 2000). Clinical trials have been conducted for anti-tumor necrosis factor (TNF) therapy, recombinant IL-10, and ICAM-1 antisense (Yacyshyn et al., 1998). Both short-term and long-term studies have demonstrated efficacy and safety of treatment with anti-TNF antibody (Infliximab) in bringing active disease to remission and maintaining remission in Crohn's disease (Targan et al., 1997b; Rutgeerts et al., 1999). However, even for these new agents, therapeutic response is not uniform. Only two-thirds of patients with moderate-to-severe, treatment-resistant Crohn's disease responded to this therapy (Targan et al., 1997). These responding and nonresponding groups may well have different underlying immunological and/or genetic backgrounds (see Clinical Application of Genetic Information).

The main reason for lack of specific treatments for these diseases is our continued lack of understanding of the etiology and

Table 15–1. Diagnostic Criteria and Clinical Characteristics of Ulcerative Colitis and Crohn's Disease

Method	Ulcerative Colitis (UC)	Crohn's Disease (CD)
Anatomic location	Colon and rectum	Any part of the alimentary tract; the most common form is ileocolitis.
Clinical	Diarrhea with or without rectal bleeding; abdominal pain and/or rectal cramping; weight loss and fatigue; fever	Symptoms vary with anatomic locations, but common symptoms are similar to those in UC. However, there are many complications; e.g., formation of strictures may lead to severe abdominal pain, nausea, and vomiting; fistulas and abscess may result in pain and fever
Radiologic	Fine granularity, small superficial erosions, and the symmetry and continuity of involvement	Thickening of mucosal folds, luminal narrowing, transmural disease tracts into the wall of the bowel, or fistula
Endoscopic	Disease almost always involves the rectum and extends proximally for varying distances; the inflammation is diffuse and continuous; ulceration in inflamed mucosa	Rectum often spared, asymmetric and skip areas of inflammation, discrete ulcers in normal mucosa, fissures, sinus and fistulous tracts, abscesses, strictures
Histologic	Disease principally involves mucosa: mucosa irregularity, ulceration, increased chronic inflammatory cells in lamina propria, Goblet cell mucin depletion, and glandular disarray	Disease is transmural, granulomas, fissures, serositis, and fistulas
Extraintestinal manifestations	Common extraintestinal manifestations include skin lesions, arthropathies, ophthalmologic problems, and hepatobiliary diseases and occur in about 21% of UC patients (Rankin, 1990).	Frequency (24%) and type of common extraintestinal disorders in CD are similar to those in UC (Monsen et al., 1990); thrombotic and thromboembolic vascular complications may occur in CD
Subgrouping	Proctitis; left-sided colitis; pancolitis	Based on anatomic location: ileocolonic, ileitis, jejunoileitis, colonic Crohn's disease. Based on nature of disease: perforating, nonperforating

pathogenesis of the various forms of IBD. Although exogenous or infectious agents might contribute to the pathogenesis or trigger the onset of disease, and the immune system almost certainly mediates the tissue damage, it is clear from available data that genetic factors determine the susceptibility of a given individual. Thus genetic studies are essential to delineate the basic etiologies of the various forms of IBD. It is only through understanding of these etiologies that we can develop radically new and specific therapies for these disorders. Such knowledge will also eventually provide the means to identify those at high risk for disease prevention.

In the remainder of this chapter the supporting evidence for genetic predisposition and progress in gene identification is reviewed. The evidence includes ethnic differences in disease frequency, familial aggregation, an increased monozygotic twin concordance rate compared with that in dizygotic twins, the existence of genetic syndromes that feature IBD, the important identification of genome scan loci for CD and UC, and, finally, associations between various forms of IBD and specific genetic markers.

GENERAL GENETIC AND EPIDEMIOLOGIC EVIDENCE

Clinical Epidemiology and Ethnic Differences

Because the etiology of IBD is unknown, descriptive epidemiological studies could play an important role in indicating the potential importance of genetic and environmental factors. Because of the difficulty of conducting population-based epidemiologic studies for these diseases, however, insufficient population-based studies have been done to estimate incidence and prevalence fully, especially in non-Caucasian populations. With the available data, the following can be generalized. Caucasians have a higher risk than non-Caucasian populations (Sonnenberg and Wasserman, 1991; Kurata et al., 1992; Probert et al., 1993). There seems to be a north to south gradient (Sonnenberg et al., 1991; Sonnenberg and Wasserman, 1991; Shivananda et al., 1996), and IBD appears to be less common in developing countries, but accurate data are lacking and the rate may increase with industrialization. In the Western world the most rapid increase of IBD occurred during the period 1960–1980 and reached a plateau in most countries (Trallori et al., 1996; Loftus et al., 1998). For the Caucasian population in North America, the annual incidence rate of IBD (per 100,000) during 1989–1994 in the central Canadian province of Manitoba was 14.6 for CD and 14.3 for UC. The prevalence (per 100,000) in 1994 was 198.5 for CD and 169.7 for UC (Bernstein et al., 1999). For a similar period (1983–1993), a lower incidence and prevalence was observed in Olmsted County, Minnesota (incidence: 6.9 and 8.3 per 100,000 for CD and UC, respectively) (Loftus et al., 1998, 2000). European countries have a similar population risk, as reported in the North American population (Russel and Stockbrugger, 1996; Shivananda et al., 1996; Trallori et al., 1996; Palli et al., 1998; Russel et al., 1998). In the United States, the Caucasian population has the highest risk among all racial groups, followed by blacks and Hispanics; the Asian population has the lowest risk (Sonnenberg and Wasserman, 1991; Kurata et al., 1992).

Although the differences in IBD frequency between various ethnic groups can have both environmental and genetic explanations, an important finding is the repeated observations that the Ashkenazi Jewish population has a consistently increased incidence or prevalence compared with other ethnic groups in the same geographic location. The fact that the Jewish and non-Jewish differences occur across different time periods as well as different geographic areas (Gilat et al., 1986; Rotter et al., 1992; Yang and Rotter, 1994), strongly suggest the existence of a ge-

Table 15–2. Inflammatory Bowel Disease Incidence/Prevalence Rates (per 100,000) among Jewish and Non-Jewish Populations by Area and Time Period

Area (Ref. No)	Disease	Period	Rate of Incidence: Jews	Non-Jews	Ratio[a]
Incidence comparisons					
North America					
Baltimore, MD (Monk et al., 1967)	Inflammatory bowel disease	1960–1963	16.7	5.4	3.1
	Ulcerative colitis	1960–1963	13.3	3.4	3.9
New York City (Korelitz, 1979)	Crohn's disease	1960–1963	3.4	1.72.0	
	Crohn's disease	?	12.6[b]	5.4	2.3
Scandinavia					
Malmo, Sweden (Brahme et al., 1975)	Crohn's disease	1965–1973	24.0[b]	6.0	4.0
Stockholm, Sweden (Hellers, 1979)	Crohn's disease	1960–1974	10.0	3.0	3.3
South Africa					
Western Cape (Novis et al., 1975)	Crohn's disease	1970–1974	2.8	0.8	3.5
Prevalence comparisons					
Edmonton, Canada (Pinchbeck et al., 1988)	Crohn's disease		309	143	2.2
	Ulcerative colitis		143	76	1.9
Southern Israel (Odes et al., 1991)	Crohn's disease	June 30, 1990	30	3.2[c]	9.4
	Ulcerative colitis		89	9.8[c]	9.1

[a]Ratio of Jewish to non-Jewish.
[b]As estimated in Krawiec et al. (1984).
[c]Israeli Arab.

netic predisposition as the most parsimonious explanation (see Table 15–2). Further support for such a hypothesis comes from studies of historical origins of Jewish subgroups and their relation to IBD frequency (Roth et al., 1989a; Zlotogora et al., 1990; Rotter et al., 1992).

Family Epidemiology

Family Studies

More than a dozen studies have demonstrated that familial aggregation is clearly increased in IBD, although the data fit no simple Mendelian pattern of inheritance (Yang and Rotter, 1994, 1995a; Russel et al., 1997). Several studies have shown there is an approximate 10- to 30-fold increase in disease prevalence among siblings compared to the community-wide prevalence (Mayberry et al., 1980; Fielding, 1986; Orholm et al., 1991, 1999; Binder, 1998). UC is increased among the relatives of UC patients, and CD is increased among the relatives of CD patients. However, the two diseases do exist in the same family with an increased frequency higher than just the co-occurrence by chance alone, suggesting an etiological relationship between UC and CD (Kirsner and Spencer, 1963; Yang et al., 1993a) (see Table 15–3). This may even identify a specific subset of IBD (mixed IBD), which currently would be defined by family history (Yang et al., 1993a). It has been observed that a positive family history is somewhat greater among CD patients than among UC patients (Kirsner and Spencer, 1963; McConnell and Vadheim, 1992; Yang et al., 1993a), and that the relatives of CD patients have a higher risk for IBD than those of UC patients (Roth et al., 1989b; Yang et al., 1993a). This suggests that to some degree CD is more often familial than UC, and it may indicate a more important role for genetic predisposition in this form of IBD. (As will be seen later in this chapter, this is supported by the twin data.) The authors' family data well represent the observations regarding familiality (Table 15–3) (Yang et al., 1993a). In that study, the age of relatives was also taken into account to estimate the lifetime risks for disease. The lifetime risks for the relatives of non-Jewish patients were consistently lower than the corresponding risks for relatives of Jewish patients from the same geographic area (Yang et al., 1993a) (Table 15–4). This has implications for the mode of inheritance of genetic susceptibility (see below).

Genetic Contributions Supported by Twin and Spouse Studies

Furthermore, while familial aggregation can be due to environmental factors alone, the increased monozygotic twin concordance rates, the rarity of IBD concordance in spouses, and the numerous instances of affected relatives whose disease onset is

Table 15–3. Positive Family History of Inflammatory Bowel Disease in Ulcerative Colitis and Crohn's Disease Probands: An Example

Disease in Proband[a]	No. of Probands	Disease in Relatives: Ulcerative colitis (%)	Crohn's Disease (%)	Mixed[b] (%)	Total (%)
Ulcerative colitis	269	37 (13.8)	6 (2.2)	4 (1.5)	47 (17.5)
Crohn's disease	258	19 (7.4)	32 (12.4)	9 (3.5)	60 (23.3)
Total	527	56 (10.6)	38 (7.2)	13 (2.5)	107 (20.3)

[a]Both Jews and non-Jews have the same trend.
[b]With several affected relatives, some are affected with UC and some with CD.
Source: Adapted from Yang et al. (1993a) with permission.

Table 15–4. Empiric Risks (%) for Inflammatory Bowel Disease in First-Degree Relatives of Patients with Inflammatory Bowel Disease

	Sibling	Parents	Offspring	Total
1. Uncorrected empiric risks for relatives of IBD probands				
Jewish probands affected with:				
Crohn's disease	8.0	3.0	1.8	4.5
Ulcerative colitis	2.4	3.2	1.9	2.6
Non-Jewish probands affected with:				
Crohn's disease	3.0	3.7	0	2.7
Ulcerative colitis	0.4	0.9	2.3	0.9
2. Corrected empiric lifetime risk for relatives of IBD probands[a]				
Jewish probands affected with:				
Crohn's disease	16.8	3.8	7.4	7.8
Ulcerative colitis	4.6	4.1	7.4	4.5
Non-Jewish probands affected with:				
Crohn's disease	7.0	4.8	0	5.2
Ulcerative colitis	0.9	1.2	11.0	1.6

[a]Corrected for age of at-risk relatives, using age-specific incidence data.
Source: Adapted from Yang et al. (1993a) with permission.

completely separated geographically and temporally from other affected family members (Kirsner, 1973), all provide support for a major genetic component to disease susceptibility.

A number of reports on twin data showed increased concordance rate of both CD and UC in monozygotic (MZ) twins as compared with dizygotic (DZ) twins (McConnell, 1983; Weterman and Pena, 1984). However, potential selection bias should be considered in reviewing these data since concordant pairs are more likely than discordant pairs to be reported. Nevertheless, in a population-based twin study, the same higher concordance rate for MZ twins than that for DZ twins, in both CD and UC (shown in Table 15–5) was also observed (Tysk et al., 1988). In addition, it seems that there is a greater concordance rate for CD than that for UC. The higher concordance rate in MZ twins than in DZ twins supports the argument that genetic factors are an important component in the development of IBD and that such genetic factors account for much of the familial aggregation. The observation that less than 100% of MZ twins are concordant indicates that there is reduced penetrance for the IBD genotype, presumably due to non-genetic factors. These non-genetic factors may be environmental, or they may be due to random stochastic variation such as occurs in development of B cells and T cells of the immune system (Hayward, 1989). The observation that the risk to dizygotic twins is not higher than the risk to siblings argues that environmental factors are ubiquitous throughout the population.

From the limited number of family studies investigating the risk in spouses, it seems that the incidence of reported spouse concordance does not appear to be increased over population risks and is dramatically less than the risk to siblings (Mayberry et al., 1980; Weterman and Pena, 1984; Yang and Rotter, 1995a). This would argue against any rapid acting environmental agents, although there are case reports of husband–wife couples both developing IBD after marriage (Comes et al., 1994; see also, Gene Environmental Interaction).

Rare Genetic Syndromes That Include IBD

IBD is clearly associated with three well-defined genetic syndromes (Yang and Rotter, 1997): Turner syndrome, also characterized by its association with autoimmunity (Hall, 1992); the autosomal recessive Hermansky-Pudlak syndrome (HPS; oculocutaneous albinism with a defect in the second phase of platelet aggregation leading to a bleeding diathesis and a ceroid-like pigment accumulation) (Schinella et al., 1980; Shanahan et al., 1989; Witkop et al., 1989; Mahadero et al., 1991); and glycogen storage disease type Ib in which there is neutropenia and abnormal neutrophil function (Couper et al., 1991; Roe et al., 1992). The gene for HPS, located on the long arm of chromosome 10, has recently been cloned (Wildenberg et al., 1995; Oh et al., 1996; Gardner et al., 1997). Mutations, as well as locus heterogeneity, have been identified (Hazelwood et al., 1997; Oh et al., 1998). Different mutations at the HPS locus have been shown to be associated with inflammatory bowel disease (Gahl et al., 1998). As regards glycogen storage disease, it seems likely that the neutropenia or the neutrophil dysfunction that occurs in this latter syndrome is the predisposing factor for the development of the Crohn's-like lesions in the bowel. Further circumstantial evidence implicating the neutrophil defect is the recognized occurrence of Crohn's-like lesions in other neutrophil or bone marrow stem-cell disorders such as chronic granulomatous disease (Ament and Ochs, 1973; Werlin et al., 1982; Sloan et al., 1996); congenital neutropenia (Vannier et al., 1982); autoimmune neutropenia (Stevens et al., 1991); leukocyte adhesion deficiency (D'Agata et al., 1996); and myelodysplastic syndromes (Eng et

Table 15–5. Ulcerative Colitis and Crohn's Disease in Monozygotic and Dizygotic Twins from Unselected Twin Registry

	Monozygotic Twins		Dizygotic Twins	
Disease	Concordant	Discordant	Concordant	Discordant
Crohn's disease	8 (44%)	10 (56%)	1 (4%)	25 (96%)
Ulcerative colitis	1 (6%)	15 (94%)	0 (0%)	20 (100%)

Source: Tysk et al. (1988) with permission.

al., 1992; Hebbar et al., 1997; Seymour, 1998). In addition, IBD has been less dramatically associated with several rare syndromes associated with immunodeficiency (Yang and Rotter, 1997). These studies of rare syndrome associations with IBD suggest that a variety of immunodeficiency states, autoimmune diseases, and miscellaneous genetic syndromes (Caruso et al., 1997; Compton et al., 1997), appear to increase the risk for IBD. These associations had suggested that studies of elements of the immune pathways may be useful in understanding the etiologies of at least some forms of IBD, and this hypothesis was subsequently supported by HLA and cytokine gene marker studies (see Genetic Marker Studies).

Inferences Regarding Mode of Inheritance

Although there is strong familial aggregation of IBD and although genetic susceptibility contributes to such familiality, there is no one simple genetic model that can explain the mode of inheritance of this disorder. The following observations have to be kept in mind when one attempts to explore potential genetic models.

1. From the monozygotic twin data, these are diseases with reduced penetrance—that is, genetic susceptibility does not appear to be the only determinant of disease.
2. The fact that dizygotic twins have a similar risk as that of siblings suggest that it is macro- not microenvironmental factors that determine the risk to IBD.
3. CD and UC are clearly genetically related, since they are found together with increased frequency in families; they are both increased in the Jewish population compared to the surrounding Caucasian population; moreover, the distinct distribution of countries of origin of U.S. Ashkenazi Jewish patients with IBD is true for both CD and UC (Yang et al., 1992).
4. Based on the stronger family history of IBD and greater MZ twin concordance for CD, genetic determinants appear to play a more deterministic role in CD than in UC. This does not mean UC is any less genetic, but it may be more influenced by stochastic variation, such as occurs in the development of the immune system.
5. There is now evidence for involvement of specific loci and genes (see Gene Identification).
6. Genetically modified animal models suggest that different genes can cause the same clinical phenotype.
7. Animal models also indicate the importance of gene and environmental interactions.

Simple Mendelian Model

It seems clear that the susceptibility to IBD as a whole is not inherited in any simple Mendelian mode of inheritance (Yang et al., 1993a; Kirsner, 1980). One approach is to ask whether the aggregation of disease within families is consistent with a specific mode of inheritance, an approach termed *segregation analysis*. Using a computerized genetic analytic technique termed *complex segregation analysis*, a recessive gene with incomplete penetrance was suggested for CD (Kuster et al., 1989; Orholm et al., 1993), while an additive major gene or a dominant major gene was proposed for UC (Monsen et al., 1989; Orholm et al., 1993). It is important to realize that the major gene effect concluded from complex segregation analysis is not equivalent to a major gene with simple Mendelian inheritance. While these analyses argue strongly against the multifactorial or polygenic model (discussed below), they cannot distinguish between simple Mendelian models and models with several major genes interacting (also known as multilocus or oligogenic model, see below), or models of genetic heterogeneity (i.e., several genetically distinct diseases with a similar phenotype). Nevertheless, keeping the genetic heterogeneity of IBD in mind, the possibility of simple Mendelian susceptibility may be true for a subset of IBD.

Multifactorial/Polygenic Models

A common explanation that used to be invoked frequently for diseases that demonstrate familial aggregation, but whose aggregation does not follow a Mendelian pattern of inheritance, is that they are due to multiple genes each of small effect (hence the term *polygenic*), acting together to provide the susceptibility to disease. Only when one has a sufficient number of these genes would an individual pass beyond a threshhold and clinical disease would result. If environmental factors were required as well, then the term *multifactorial* is applied. Since IBD does not fit a Mendelian pattern, the polygenic model was suggested.

McConnell had proposed a polygenic model as an explanation of the association between CD and UC: that there is one genotype, with perhaps 10 or 15 genes, which makes people liable to develop inflammatory bowel disease (McConnell, 1980; McConnell and Vadheim, 1992). Under this model, if a person has only a few of these genes, they are liable to develop UC; if they have many of these genes (a more complete genotype), the clinical and pathological picture that develops would more likely be CD. This would explain why the relatives of people with CD are much more likely to have inflammatory bowel disease than are relatives of people with UC. If a patient has a large number of these genes (and has CD), his or her relatives would be more likely to have a larger number of the genes compared to relatives of a patient with only a moderate number of the risk genes (i.e., a UC patient). Thus, CD patients would be more likely to have relatives with UC, and most of the relatives of UC patients would be likely to have too few of the high-risk genes to have any form of IBD.

However, the formal mathematical genetic analyses of large family data sets of both UC (Orholm et al., 1993; Monsen et al., 1989) and CD (Kuster et al., 1989; Orholm et al., 1993) have allowed the rejection of the simple polygenic model. Basically, what these formal genetic analyses have concluded is that the risk to relatives is too great to be explained by the polygenic model. In addition, genetically modified animal models (including knockouts) suggest that if one gene in the immunoregulatory pathway is sufficiently altered, it can lead to clinical disease; thus it may not require multiple genes with equal small effect to lead to disease.

Multilocus (Oligogenic) Models

There is increasing evidence that the genetic predisposition to a number of diseases is due to the interaction of two or more major genes, a form of inheritance termed *two locus* (if two major genes are involved) or *multilocus* or *oligogenic* (if more than two are involved) (Rotter, 1980, 1988; Greenberg and Rotter, 1981; Rotter and Landaw, 1984; Lin et al., 1985). This concept is important for IBD for several reasons. First, it is an etiologically attractive hypothesis that could explain more than one pathophysiologic defect being found in IBD patients. For example, in order to develop clinical Crohn's disease, one may need both a permeability defect that leads to increased exposure of the body's immune system to antigenic substances that ordinarily do not cross the gut mucosal barrier and a particular genetically determined immune response. An analogous hypothesis might include abnormal mucins and certain autoantibodies as the etiologic factors in UC. Second, the recurrence risks for multilocus disorders are very different from Mendelian disorders (Greenberg and Rotter, 1981; Rotter and Landaw, 1984; Lin et al., 1985). Third, a multilocus model could explain the relationship of UC and CD in families—that is, one gene may be insufficient by itself to lead to clinical disease yet predisposes to both diseases, but clinical disease occurs only when a second, more specific gene or genes interacts with the first, thus leading to the specific disease, CD or UC. Finally, if such a model for these diseases is indeed confirmed, it has important implications for genetic counseling and risk identification in relatives, since if even one locus is identified, family-based genetic-marker risk assessment begins to become feasible, as has been demonstrated for other autoimmune diseases (Lin et al., 1985).

There has been one intriguing study (as opposed to anecdotal case reports) of the risks to offspring for IBD when both parents themselves have IBD (Bennett et al., 1991). The results suggested that the risk was substantially greater than that of twice the empiric risk to offspring of couples when one parent has IBD, and was starting to approach the identical twin risks. This suggests another high-risk group, albeit somewhat rare. It also appears that there is a proclivity toward CD in these offspring, especially when the parents are concordant for CD. When the children were further divided into three groups—according to whether both parents, one parent, or neither parent had yet developed symptoms of IBD at the time of the children's conception—the risk for IBD were similar among these three groups. In addition, the concordance rate for the type of IBD (UC or CD) in those couples in whom both had onset of IBD after marriage was not greater than those in whom both or one was affected before marriage. These data argue for the position that some intrinsic (e.g., genetic) and not acquired factors are essential in the development of IBD and in the determination of the type of IBD. While strong environmental determinants limited to certain families could be an explanation, these data more likely argue for a limited number of genetically determined forms of IBD. In other words, such data are consistent with the assumption of a limited number of IBD-predisposing genes. The logic for such a conclusion is that if many different genes were required—if there were many different genetic forms of IBD—then the occurrence of genetic complementation would reduce the risks to offspring. But if, instead, there are a limited number of such genes, then the offspring of two affected parents are more likely to be homozygous at the loci for such genes and consequently affected. These data suggest that the actual number of genes predisposing is limited in number and thus are more consistent with the multilocus/oligogenic models, rather than polygenic, encouraging the search for the major genes that predispose to these diseases. The success of the genome scan efforts (reviewed below) also support the multilocus model.

Genetic Heterogeneity Models

The concept of genetic heterogeneity is that IBD is not a single disease but, rather, is several etiologically and genetically distinct diseases presenting a similar clinical picture. Each of the individual component diseases could conceivably be inherited in a Mendelian, polygenic, or multilocus mode of inheritance. Increasing evidence, from clinical differences, to subclinical markers, to genetic markers, supports this concept. The apparent physiologic and immunologic complexity of IBD argues that a heterogeneity model, while at first glance apparently more complex, may in the end be the most parsimonious. The etiology of specific subtypes of IBD may be more easily understood once these subgroups can be identified. Indeed, certain of these etiologically distinct IBD "diseases" may even be inherited in a Mendelian manner. The existence of the several genetic syndromes that feature IBD and several IBD knockout mice models is an immediate proof of at least some degree of genetic heterogeneity. In this context the interrelationship of CD and UC may mean that there is a form (or forms) of disease that result in UC alone, others that result in CD alone, and some that can present either as CD or UC. The different relative frequency of mixed disease (CD and UC) in the same family in Jewish versus non-Jewish families argues that the mixed form may be a distinct subgroup (Yang et al., 1993a). A major advantage of the heterogeneity model is that it can lead to directly testable etiologic hypotheses. For example, one possible corollary of such a model is that genetically determined physiologic abnormalities in the affected case are likely to be shared with their relatives, and these can differ in different groups of patients. Thus, clinically unaffected relatives of cases with a particular defect can be tested to see (1) if the defect is familial and (2) whether it is present before the disease. Along these lines, several different potential defects (reviewed below, Disease Pathophysiology) have been found in families with IBD (see Table 15–6). The available data on the familiality of antineutrophil cytoplasmic antibodies argue for genetic heterogeneity within UC, and, similarly, the data on ASCA argue for heterogeneity of CD. In addition, the genetic marker associations suggest heterogeneity within CD and within UC (see below). If the heterogeneity model is indeed the appropriate model, an understanding of the etiologies will only be possible by the subdivision of IBD on the basis of both physiologic defects and genetic marker associations into more etiologically homogeneous groups.

As will be seen, the available evidence argues that IBD is a heterogeneous group of disorders, with each subform an oligogenic disorder caused primarily by the interaction of a limited number of genes, although there may be more minor contributions from modifying genes.

Genetic Anticipation

Anticipation refers to the progressive increase in severity of an illness as it manifests in its transmission from parent to child, occurring in a more severe form and at an earlier age with succeeding generations. For a long time, the cause of anticipation had been attributed to artifact, due to ascertainment bias (McInnis, 1996). It was thought that when a more severe case of a disease presented clinically, milder clinical forms were identified among the parents, and this gave the appearance of anticipation. However, a prospective study of one paradigmatic disorder, myotonic dystrophy, clearly demonstrated the clinical phenomenon of anticipation (Howeler et al., 1989). Subsequently, the molecular basis of myotonic dystrophy, expansion of a trinucleotide (CTG) repeat (TNRs) at the 3′ end of a transcript encoding a protein kinase family member, was identified (Brook et al., 1992). Expansion of TNRs over subsequent generations are now known to be associated with a number of disorders, especially in the neuropsychiatric diseases. The significance and cause of anticipation is clear in those diseases that demonstrate both clinical anticipation and association with expansions in TNRs—for example, Huntington's disease (Huntington's Disease Collaborative Research Group, 1993), myotonic dystrophy, Fragile X syndrome (Verkerk et al., 1991), and spinocerebellar ataxia type 1 (Orr et al., 1993). If the phenomenon

Table 15–6. Subclinical Markers for Inflammatory Bowel Disease

Specific Disease	Marker	Type of Relatives Studied	Observations	Reference
Combined IBD	Autoantibodies to epithelial cell-associated component (ECAC) antigens	Family members	ECAC-C observed in 69.7% CD patients, 55.7% relatives, and only 8.0% control subjects	Fiocchi et al., 1989
	Antinuclear autoantibodies (ANA)	Family members	ANA observed in 18% CD patients, 43% UC patients, 13% relatives of CD, 24% relatives of UC, 2% control subjects	Folwaczny et al., 1997
	Goblet cell autoantibodies (GABs)	Family members	Positive GABs in 39% UC, 30% CD, 21% first-degree relatives of UC, 19% first-degree relatives of CD, 3% infectious enterocolitis, 2% healthy control subjects	Folwaczny et al., 1997
Crohn's disease	C3 dysfunction	Family members	Greater C3 dysfunction in CD (38%) and relatives (18%) than in control subjects	Elmgreen et al., 1985
	Intestinal permeability	Family members and twins	Increased in CD patients, conflicting results regarding relatives	Review in Hollander, 1993; Munkholm et al., 1994; Lindberg et al., 1995; Peeters et al., 1997
	Obligate anaerobic fecal flora	Family members	The flora of CD patients contained more anaerobic gram-positive coccoid rods and more gram-negative rods than that of healthy subjects; during 5 to 7 years follow-up, 3 of 9 children with a CD floral pattern showed CD symptoms and one such child was diagnosed as CD; none of 17 children with a normal flora showed CD symptoms	Van de Merwe et al., 1988
	Anti-*Saccharomyces cerevisiae* antibodies (ASCA)	Family members and twins	ASCA increased in CD patients, as compared with control subjects; ASCA positive in 50% CD, increased in healthy relatives	Lindberg et al., 1992; Sendid et al., 1997; Sutton et al., 2000; also see text
	Pancreatic autoantibodies	Family members	Positive pancreatic autoantibodies in 27% CD (14% type I, 13% type II), subtype showed familial cluster, 0.5% in first-degree relatives	Seibold et al., 1997
Ulcerative colitis	Antineutrophil cytoplasmic antibodies (ANCA)	Family members and twins	Specific for UC, increased in healthy relatives of UC patients, occur in a subset of CD patients	Shanahan et al., 1992; Seibold et al., 1994; Lee et al., 1995; Yang and Rotter, 1995b; also see text
	Colonic mucins	Twins	HCM species IV (mucin subtype) reduced in both UC and healthy co-twins, as compared with control subjects	Tysk et al., 1991
	Mucosal production of IgG subclass	Twins	UC patients and their healthy MZ co-twins showed a raised proportion of IgG1 (78%), as compared with control subjects (56%)	Helgeland et al., 1992
	IgA against gliadin	Twins	High IgA titers against gliadin in both UC patients and their healthy co-twins	Lindberg et al., 1992

of anticipation can be established for a disorder, then expansion of TNRs should be searched for, because at the moment that is the only biologic mechanism established for the etiology of anticipation. However, our understanding of the molecular events related to anticipation is far from complete (McInnis, 1996).

A number of studies have examined the possibility of anticipation in IBD. A lower age at diagnosis and a greater extent of disease in the younger member of two-generation pairs affected with CD was observed in a retrospective study (Polito et al., 1996). In another study, it was shown that children were younger than their parents at diagnosis in most but not all parent–offspring pairs, but in most pairs children did not have more severe disease than their parents (Grandbastien et al., 1998). In contrast, two large studies have found no evidence for genetic anticipation and have attributed the younger age of onset in the children to ascertainment bias (Lee et al., 1999; Hampe et al., 2000).

Anticipation is clearly an interesting hypothesis worth further pursuing in IBD. To date, the data have been inconclusive. It should be kept in mind that the expanding trinucleotide repeats are not the only cause of apparent anticipation (Fraser, 1997). Other molecular mechanisms, termed *epigenetic factors*, may also be involved in events similar to genetic anticipation, such as DNA methylation and chromatin conformation (Petronis et al., 1997). Furthermore, rapid changes in the environment could mimic the phenomenon of anticipation as well.

Associations with Other Diseases

It has been observed for many years that IBD is associated with several other disorders whose etiologies are unknown, but which appear to involve the immune system. The best-documented disease associations are with ankylosing spondylitis, primary sclerosing cholangitis, and psoriasis. All of these diseases occur more often than expected in IBD cases, and in their unaffected family members as well.

Ankylosing Spondylitis

Most disease association studies have shown that the frequency of UC patients with ankylosing spondylitis (AS) ranges from 1% to 6%, and the frequency of arthritis in UC patient series ranges from 2% to 15% (Moll, 1985). Among case series of CD patients, the frequency of peripheral arthropathies ranges from 5% to 10% (Moll, 1985; Purrmann et al., 1988). Approximately 90% of all AS patients are HLA-B27 positive, compared to a frequency of less than 10% in the general population. While the frequency of HLA-B27 in IBD patients reflects that of the general population, about 60% to 80% of IBD patients with spondylitis are HLA-B27 positive (Russell, 1975; Mallas et al., 1976; Huaux et al., 1977; Dekker-Saeys et al., 1978). There are also reports that the individuals with the phenotype B27,B44 are at especially high risk (estimated relative risk = 69) for the concurrent manifestation of CD and AS (Purrmann et al., 1988; Khan, 1989; Gilvarry et al., 1990). This strongly suggests that IBD is a potent initiating or potentiating factor in the development of AS. It is still not certain whether ankylosing spondylitis should be considered a complication of IBD or an associated disease. The accumulated data suggest that bowel disease may be present even when it is not manifested clinically (Jayson et al., 1970; Mielants and Veys, 1984a,b; De Keyser et al., 1998) and that patients with non-AS spondyloarthropathy and inflammatory gut lesions have greater risk of developing AS than do patients without gut inflammation (Mielants et al., 1995; De Vos et al., 1996). Of note is the increased risk for ankylosing spondylitis seen in the relatives of IBD patients even when the patients themselves have no evidence of ankylosing spondylitis (Russell, 1977). These data suggest that the intestinal inflammation may lead to joint disease in individuals who are genetically predisposed to these diseases, perhaps by allowing passage of potential antigens through the gut mucosa or by other mechanisms yet to be defined. It also suggests that there may well be subclinical, yet active, bowel disease in those patients in whom ankylosing spondylitis appears to develop before the bowel disease. Based on these data, the hypothesis should be actively considered that, etiologically, ankylosing spondylitis may often be secondary to a form of the idiopathic inflammatory bowel diseases, with the bowel disease being subclinical. It is conceivable that this spectrum of disease could occur in relatives of IBD patients, in whom clinical bowel disease is not apparent but in whom subclinical bowel disease leads to spondylitis. Thus, IBD is associated with factors that increase the risk for ankylosing spondylitis in persons genetically predisposed to this disease, and particularly in those with HLA-B27. The link between gut inflammation and arthropathy has also been demonstrated in animal models, notably the human leukocyte antigen B27 transgenic rats (see below, Animal Models) (Rath et al., 1996).

Psoriasis

The frequency of psoriasis, an inflammatory autoimmune disease of the skin, is increased in CD patients (7%–11%) as compared to that of the general population (1.1%–1.6%) (Yates et al., 1982; Lee et al., 1990). Of interest, the increased occurrence of psoriasis was also observed in the relatives of CD patients (Lee et al., 1990; Hammer et al., 1968). As with other IBD-associated diseases, the concurrence of psoriasis and CD at both the individual level and the family level suggests the possibility of a genetic link between the two disorders. In genome-wide scans for psoriasis susceptibility loci, the HLA region, along with several other novel loci, including loci on 16q (the long arm of chromosome 16), 20q, and 17q were identified (Matthews et al., 1996; Nair et al., 1997; Trembath et al., 1997; Bhalerao and Bowcock, 1998). The chromosome 16q region overlaps with a susceptibility locus of CD-*IBD1* (Hugot et al., 1996) (see Genome-Wide Linkage Studies). These data are consistent with the hypothesis that some genetic determinants are common for both disorders. Thus, recently identified NOD2 gene in 16q should be tested for association with psoriasis.

Primary Sclerosing Cholangitis

In the case of primary sclerosing cholangitis (PSC), the association is almost exclusively with ulcerative colitis (Chapman et al., 1980; Weisner and LaRusso, 1980). This association between PSC and UC has been recognized for several decades, and the most recent surveys of UC series have found the prevalence of PSC among UC patients to be approximately 5% overall, with a 10% to 15% prevalence among UC patients with hepatic abnormalities (Olsson et al., 1991; Wewer et al., 1991; Rasmussen et al., 1992). The converse association is much stronger. Approximately 50% to 70% of all PSC cases are affected with UC. This may be an underestimate, since IBD onset may have a substantial subclinical phase of IBD far longer than previously appreciated (Broome et al., 1995).

The significance of such association of PSC with UC has at least two aspects: the first is its obvious clinical importance; the second is pathogenetic and pertains to the possible immunologic mechanisms that link colitis and cholangitis. Although the pathogenesis of such association is still unknown, the following studies demonstrated the similarities between the two disorders in the immune response:

1. A higher proportion of patients with primary sclerosing cholangitis and UC have anti-colon antibodies (63%) and antibodies to portal tract antigens of the liver (compared to 17% of patients with UC alone) (Chapman et al., 1986).
2. A 40,000 molecular weight colonic epithelial protein has been identified with a unique epitope (or epitopes) that is shared by the skin and biliary tract epithelial cells (Das et al., 1990).
3. Antineutrophil cytoplasmic antibodies have been found in high frequency in both UC and PSC (Duerr et al., 1991; Lo et al., 1992; Seibold et al., 1992; Zauli et al., 1992).

If in fact there is a common antigenic target for immune-mediated attack on both colonic and biliary epithelial cells, identification of this antigen may facilitate understanding of the links between IBD and PSC, as well as the basic immunoregulatory disorder that underlies both diseases, and also allow development of an improved assay(s) for a disease marker or markers in UC and PSC.

Many diseases with either a suspected autoimmune etiology or pathogenesis, or both, have been found to be associated with genes of the HLA class II region (discussed in more detail in Gene Identification, Candidate genes). Primary sclerosing cholangitis is associated with the HLA antigens B8 and DR3 (Chapman et al., 1980; Shepherd, 1983). Although one study reported that of 29 patients with PSC, 100% had the HLA-DRw52a antigen, compared with 35% in the general population (Prochazka et al., 1990), such results could not be confirmed in Swedish patients with PSC (Olerup et al., 1991; Zetterquist et al., 1992). A dual association of both HLA-DR2 and -DR3 with PSC has been described (Donaldson, 1991). After all the DR3-positive individuals were removed, a significant secondary association with DR2 was noted (69% in PSC vs. 34% in controls). These data suggest that both DR2 and the HLA haplotype A1-B8-DR3 are independent factors that influence the development of PSC. This observation is particularly of interest because most HLA class II association studies with IBD observed a DR2-UC association (Sugimura et al., 1993; Toyoda et al., 1993; Hirv et al., 1999) (see below for details), and this was substituted by a DR3-UC association in a population in which the HLA DRB1*1502 (serologically DR2) is rare (Satsangi et al., 1998).

Although it is preliminary, it is worth noting that the degree of association between PSC and UC seems vary with race and sex. Turkish patients with IBD do not have an increased risk for PSC (Bayraktar et al., 1998), while Africans and Afro-Caribbeans, especially women, may be at increased risk for PSC (Kelly et al., 1997). Such difference suggests a different pathogenesis between PSC and IBD, although some aspects may be common for both diseases.

Pouchitis

Restorative proctocolectomy with ileal reservoir is a widely accepted procedure in the surgical treatment of UC. However, the most frequent long-term complication after ileal pouch–anal anastomosis (IPAA) for UC is a nonspecific inflammation of the ileal reservoir known as *pouchitis*. This complication seems to be related to the disease, not the operation, because the occurrence of pouchitis in patients after IPAA for familial adenomatous polyposis is significantly lower than those due to UC (Dozois et al., 1989). The cumulative risk of developing pouchitis varies between 15% and 46%, depending on the duration of follow-up (Sandborn, 1994).

The etiology and pathophysiology of pouchitis are not well understood. Many of the risk factors are similar to those for UC. Pouchitis has been found to be associated not only with UC but with the presence of extraintestinal manifestations of the disease (Lohmuller et al., 1990; Penna et al., 1996), with the presence of pANCA (Sandborn et al., 1995; P. Yang et al., 1996) and with the protective effect of smoking (Merrett et al., 1996). Therefore, it appears that pouchitis reflects the same underlying etiology and pathophysiology of UC, indicating the importance of host factors, such as genetic susceptibility and immunologic functions.

Other Immunologic Diseases

Multiple sclerosis is another disorder associated with IBD. Such an association has been demonstrated by the concurrence of multiple sclerosis and IBD both within families (Minuk and Lewkonia, 1986; Sadovnick et al., 1989) and within individuals (Rang et al., 1982; Kitchin et al., 1991; Purrmann et al., 1992). Of interest is the study of intestinal permeability in MS patients, which found that one-fourth of patients with MS also had increased intestinal permeability (Yacyshyn et al., 1996). An explanation for this, which could also be the explanation for several of the IBD-associated diseases, is that what is inherited is a generalized defect of the immune system that can predispose to several different autoimmune diseases. In support of this hypothesis for at least one form of IBD are studies of large series of IBD patients in which an increased frequency of a series of classic organ-specific autoimmune disorders are observed (e.g., autoimmune thyroid disease, insulin-dependent diabetes [IDDM], and systemic lupus erythematosus [SLE]) in UC patients, but not in those with Crohn's disease (Jarnerot et al., 1975; Snook et al., 1989; Snook, 1990). An increased co-occurrence of UC and celiac disease has been reported as well (Breen et al., 1987; Cottone et al., 1989). In addition, in this genome scan era, multiple putative susceptibility loci have been identified for a number of autoimmune disorders. Importantly, some of these loci are shared among many of the autoimmune diseases (Becker et al., 1997).

It is interesting to speculate whether other complications of IBD, whose etiology is currently unknown, and which affect only a portion of IBD patients, may have a similar etiologic relationship as the above-mentioned organ-specific autoimmune disorders and UC (i.e., an example of genetic pleiotropy). Complications that might be included in this etiologic model are uveitis, erythema nodosum, pyoderma gangrenosum, hepatitis, pancreatitis, and cirrhosis. In a large family with members affected with different autoimmune disorders, including rheumatoid arthritis, systemic lupus erythematosus, psoriasis, and IBD, it appears that family members with the same disease tend to share the same HLA haplotypes (Sels et al., 1997). If this holds true, it may raise a possibility that one set of genes, such as HLA, determine an individual's general autoimmunity and phenotypic specificity is governed by other genes.

Environmental Factors

The family and twin studies discussed above and the genetic linkage and association studies reviewed below are evidence that genetic factors play an essential role in the development of IBD. However, the following observations also argue for an environmental contribution to human IBD: (1) disease incidence has exhibited temporal trends and is correlated with industrialization; (2) there is much less than a 100% concordance rate in MZ twins; and (3) different disease risks have been observed for the same ethnic group residing in different geographical locations. Therefore, it is likely that both gene and environmental factors determine the risk of developing IBD. Evidence for specific environmental factors is enumerated below.

Infection

Two lines of evidence suggest that early infant and childhood infections may determine the risk of IBD later in life. The first line follows the hypothesis that delayed or reduced exposure to enteric infections may contribute to IBD etiology. It was reported that CD was more common in subjects whose first houses had a hot-water tap and separate bathroom than in controls without these facilities (Gent et al., 1994). A significant negative correlation between infant mortality and incidence of CD among 12 countries ($r = -.84$) was also consistent with this observation (Montgomery et al., 1997). Industrialization and improved domestic hygiene have resulted in reduced infant mortality. A possible consequence, however, is that low exposure of infants to enteric organisms may program the immune system of the gut at an early stage so that it is more susceptible to overreacting to a triggering agent later in life (Rotter, 1994). Such triggers could be an infectious agent, diet, or medication. The second line follows the intriguing, though still controversial, hypothesis that viral infection in early life has been reported to be associated with an increased risk for IBD. The possibility of an association between exposure to measles and the onset of IBD was described as early as 1950 (Sloan et al., 1950). Based on epidemiologic and basic scientific data for persistent measles virus in the intestine of patients with CD, it has been proposed that CD may be a chronic granulomatous vasculitis in reaction to a persistent infection with the measles virus within the vascular endothelium (Wakefield et al., 1995; Wakefield and Pounder, 1995). This proposal has stimulated a large number of investigations regarding measles infection, but the results have been controversial. Most studies have been confined to CD only. A recent large epidemiological study has assessed five childhood infections and diagnosis of IBD and IDDM in over 7000 British individuals in 1970 birth cohorts (Montgomery et al., 1999). This study observed that both measles and mumps infections during the same year, up to age 10, were associated with a substantially increased risk for both UC and CD, but not IDDM. Coinfection with chicken pox, pertussis, and meningitis with measles during the same year was not associated with increased risk for IBD. The authors concluded that an atypical paramyxovirus infection in childhood may increase the risk for later IBD. Data from Iceland support an association between a concurrent epidemic of mumps and measles, which are followed by an increased incidence of IBD (Montgomery et al., 1998). Although it is far from resolved, the role of viral infection in the development of IBD should be considered in genetic environmental studies.

Smoking

Smoking is almost the only environmental factor that consistently has been found to be associated with IBD. However, the relationship is quite complex in that cigarette smoking seems to be protective in UC and deleterious in CD. That smoking had a beneficial effect on UC patients was first reported in 1982 (Harries et al., 1982); this was followed by a demonstration of a dose–response relationship (Jick and Walker, 1983). Smoking was also found to be protective for pouchitis in patients with restorative proctocolectomy for UC (Merrett et al., 1996). In contrast, in a meta-analysis, smoking increased the risk of CD, with a summary odds ratio of 2.02 for current smokers, compared with lifetime nonsmokers (Calkins, 1989). The mechanism involved in this relationship is still unknown. However, nicotine may be one of the active compounds in cigarettes that is responsible for the relationship between smoking and IBD, based on the beneficial effect from a clinical trial of UC and a reversible deleterious effect in experimental models. In a randomized double-blind, placebo-controlled trial, transdermal nicotine administrations of the highest tolerated dosage for 4 weeks showed an effect in controlling the clinical presentation of mildly to moderately active UC (Sandborn et al., 1997). In an experimental model it was shown that exposure to cigarette smoke aggravates dinitrobenzene sulfonic acid–induced colitis in the rat, and this effect can be reversed by hexamethonium, which is a peripheral nicotine receptor antagonist (Galeazzi et al., 1999).

The Appendix and Appendectomy

The protective role of appendectomy in the development of UC was first reported in 1987 (Gilat et al., 1987) and was then followed by multiple confirmations (Rutgeerts et al., 1994; Smithson et al., 1995; Minocha and Raczkowski, 1997; Russel et al., 1997). The biological explanation is unclear, but results from T-cell receptor-α mutant mice and a histological study of the appendix in IBD patients have brought some light to understanding this relationship. Although the appendix has long been considered to be a redundant organ, the fact that this organ has a large blood supply and an abundance of lymphoid tissue indicates its potential important role in normal mucosal immune function. Since the mucosal lymphoid tissues of the appendix are predominantly composed of B cells and CD4 T-helper cells (Bjerke et al., 1986; Kawanishi, 1987), it was speculated that removing the appendix may alter the balance in favor of T-suppressor cells and thus protect against the development of UC (Rutgeerts et al., 1994). This hypothesis is supported by the observation that TCRα knockout mice spontaneously develop IBD similar to human UC (Mizoguchi et al., 1996). In this model, immunoglobulin was increased in the appendix of TCR$\alpha^{-/-}$ mice when compared with control TCR$\alpha^{+/-}$ mice, and cellular proliferation and number of B cells producing autoantibody to tropomyosin was higher in the appendix when compared with Peyer's patches in TCR$\alpha^{-/-}$ mice. Removal of the appendix in TCR$\alpha^{-/-}$ mice at a young age (<5 weeks) led to a marked reduction in mesenteric lymph node cells at 6 months and was associated with suppression of the development of IBD. Therefore, these investigators concluded that lymphoid tissue of the appendix is the priming site of cells involved in the development of IBD in TCR$\alpha^{-/-}$ mice. In a case-control study, a higher frequency of appendiceal inflammation was observed in UC patients (48%) than in cases of colonic carcinoma (Scott et al., 1998). In addition, the inflammatory changes seen within these appendices were more characteristic of the underlying IBD than were changes seen in acute appendicitis. Therefore, the appendix is involved in UC, either as a lesion or as a role in pathogenesis.

Other Environmental Factors

A meta-analysis of two cohort studies and seven case-control studies investigating the role of oral contraceptive agents in IBD revealed a modest association between the use of oral contraceptives and the development of CD (OR, 1.44) and UC (OR, 1.29) (Godet et al., 1995). Such a weak association indicates a minor and likely noncausal role of this risk factor.

Infection with *Mycobacterium paratuberculosis* has been suggested as a cause for CD. However, the results have been very conflicting (Brunello et al., 1991; Tanaka et al., 1991; Lisby et al., 1994; Rowbotham et al., 1995; Dumonceau et al., 1996). The absence of any benefit of a placebo-controlled trial with antituberculous chemotherapy in CD argues against the hypothesis that mycobacteria play an important role in the pathogenesis of CD (Thomas et al., 1998).

Gene and Environment Interaction

The importance of gene and environment interactions in the development of IBD are clearly demonstrated in animal models (Elson et al., 1995). For example, using recombinant DNA technology, transgenic rats expressing the human HLA-B27 and β_2 microglobulin genes have been produced. Certain transgenic rat lines developed a multiorgan disease manifested by colitis, arthritis, orchitis, and psoriasiform changes of the skin and nails (Hammer et al., 1990), features that resemble the human spondyloarthropathies. However, colitis and arthritis do not occur when B27 transgenic rats are raised under germ-free conditions, thus implicating the normal enteric bacterial flora as the source of the antigens driving these diseases (Taurog et al., 1994). Another model is that mice homozygous for the severe combined immunodeficiency (SCID) mutation develop IBD with adoptive transfer of CD4$^+$ T cells expressing high levels of CD45RB (see Animal Models). However, these mice do not develop IBD in germ-free conditions. Other studies have demonstrated that an abnormal immune response in the presence of a single murine pathogen, *Heliobacter hepaticus*, resulted in IBD (Cahill et al.,

1997). Similarly, IL-2 knockout mice do not develop colitis when they are raised in germ-free conditions (Elson et al., 1995). Although what genetic and environmental factors interact to cause human IBD is still unknown, such a model may explain at least some forms of IBD and may direct research efforts to study genes and environmental factors simultaneously in the etiologic studies of IBD.

In human studies, as reviewed above, environmental factors such as sanitation, measles virus infection and other perinatal or childhood infections, mycobacteria infection, appendectomy, oral contraceptive agents, and smoking have all been investigated, but none of these environmental studies has been evaluated taking genetic interactions into account.

If both environmental and genetic factors play an important role in the development of a disease, which factor will be identified as a predominant risk factor will depend on the relative distribution of these factors. For example, in Western societies, a common environment may have brought the majority of people to an equal footing in terms of good hygiene, better nutrition, and improved maternal and pediatric care. Those with susceptibility genes will be more likely to develop the disease than those who don't have such genes, given the same environment. In such cases, it will be difficult to evaluate environmental factors. In contrast, the increasing incidence in developing countries may provide a window of opportunity for researchers to study gene–environment interactions since the change in environmental factors (modernization) in a society is a progressive process and those who develop the disease will be the ones who are both genetically susceptible and environmentally vulnerable. Therefore, well-designed genetic epidemiological studies in developing countries are warranted.

AN EVOLUTIONARY PERSPECTIVE

One question that should be raised in the context of this broad discussion of the genetic susceptibility to IBD is why are these genes so frequent. One theoretical possibility is that this could be just due to new mutations. However, these genes clearly cause clinical disease—with major morbidity and even mortality. The mortality was certainly greater until modern supportive management became available. Thus if new mutations were the explanation, the mutation rate would have to equal both the mortality rate and the decreased reproduction due to the disease. For mutation to explain the IBD disease frequency in the modern world, the mutation rate clearly would have to be much greater than the estimated range of 1 in 100,000 to 1 in 1 million per gene locus that appears to be the mutation rate in man.

If new mutations are an inadequate explanation, there remain two other possible explanations—founder effect and genetic selection (see Chapter 4). Founder effect refers to the concept that a given gene appeared (presumably by mutation) in a small ancestral population (i.e., in a founder) and by random chance was transmitted to a large number of that founder's offspring. This would establish the gene in relatively high frequency in the original small population and its subsequent ancestors (Diamond and Rotter, 1987). Although this founder effect is a reasonable explanation for the high frequency of certain genes in certain ethnic groups, it is an inadequate explanation for a disease (or diseases) with as wide a distribution and as high a frequency as IBD.

This means we must turn to the consideration of selective advantage (Rotter and Diamond, 1987). The reason these genes are so relatively frequent, even though they are deleterious (cause disease) is that they also provide some compensating advantage to those individuals who have them (Rotter and Diamond, 1987). That is, these IBD-predisposing genes presumably provide some advantage in certain environments to which humans have been exposed. This advantage allows those humans with the gene (or genes) to better survive under these conditions, and thus the genes increase in frequency. A balance is achieved when the advantageous effect of the genes is matched by the frequency and severity of the diseases for which they predispose.

There are two reasons why it would be useful to understand how these IBD genes provide their selective advantage. One is that it would contribute to our understanding of human evolution and history. But there is an even more important reason. Understanding the actual mechanism of the selective advantage (or advantages) will provide an understanding of the underlying physiologic process at a very fundamental level; such understanding may allow us to identify the actual predisposing genes, provide a new understanding of disease pathogenesis, and thus suggest entirely new therapeutic approaches.

Is there any information that would allow us to speculate on the selective advantage provided by the IBD susceptibility genes? There are several basic observations that would underlie any such speculation. First, from the discussion throughout this chapter, it is apparent that IBD is indeed genetic, is clearly common, and occurs in many different ethnic groups throughout the world. Hence a selective advantage is likely necessary to account for its high frequency. Second, it is also apparent that IBD is genetically complex and is likely several different diseases. This means that there are likely several steps in the etiologic pathway that can contribute to any proposed selective advantage. Third, IBD appears to have increased dramatically in the developed world over the last century and is now appearing (or being recognized) with increasing frequency in the developing world. This indicates that some environmental factor or factors, still operating in historical times, provides the advantage in the developing world. It also raises the possibility that the disease is occurring because the selective advantage is no longer acting against the environmental factors that provided the selective advantage. Fourth, given the data reviewed above—that the DZ twin rate is no larger than the sibling recurrence risk—it seems whatever environmental factors are responsible are likely to affect the entire population. That is, the environmental factors are probably ubiquitous, rather than varying dramatically in frequency between families within a population or over a short time period (the few years of childhood). Fifth, IBD is an inflammatory and likely immunologic disease of the gut, so it is likely that environmental factors that provided the selective advantage operated at the level of the gut as well.

Putting this information together, the authors have proposed the following hypothesis: that the genes that predispose to the various forms of IBD provided a selective advantage in the form of mucosal immunoprotection in an unsanitary world (Rotter, 1994). Truly effective public sanitation is a development of modern civilization. The development of such sanitation then removes the selective advantage. But the mucosal immunoprotection is still primed genetically in those with the IBD genes, armed, if you will, to defend the organism. Thus, the authors have proposed that when the IBD-predisposing genes are not adequately used in mucosal defense, as they would not be in the developed world, one of two events could occur: (1) later exposure to an infectious agent could result in hyperstimulation of the immune response and subsequent chronic inflammation (analogous to paralytic polio, which occurs when infection occurs after early infancy); or (2) even more likely, failure of exposure to a potentially injurious agent conceivably leaves the gut immunologic system in a continually primed state and thus sets up the system for subsequent dysregulation—that is, an autoimmune reaction that eventuates in the diseases we recognize as ulcerative colitis and Crohn's disease (Rotter, 1994).

This hypothesis could provide a possible explanation for the relatively high frequency of IBD in the Jewish population (Rotter, 1994). It appears that IBD is highest in frequency in Ashkenazi Jews (i.e., those whose origin is middle and eastern Europe), suggesting that the selective factor or factors had their greatest influence after the Ashkenazi/Sephardic division (Rotter et al., 1992). This would correspond to the historical division of Europe and the Mediterranean between the Christian and Islamic kingdoms. However, the greatest frequency of IBD appears to arise in those Ashkenazi Jews whose origin is in middle Europe (Roth et al., 1989a; Zlotogora et al., 1990) and is similar to the distribution of Tay-Sachs gene carriers (Petersen et al., 1983). This is the region that imposed the greatest ghetto urbanization on the Jews and presumably had the greatest overcrowding and the consequent greatest defects in sanitation. This situation eased when the Ashkenazi Jews were invited to settle in eastern Europe, that is, in Poland, Ukraine, and Russia. The origin of both Tay-Sachs heterozygotes and IBD patients is highest in individuals from middle as opposed to eastern Europe (Zlotogora et al., 1990; Petersen et al., 1983). The lower frequency of IBD in Israel than in western Europe and in the United States would then be a possible consequence of the more developing nature of that society. Regardless, if the specific details of this hypothesis are correct, it will be important to determine if a genetically hyperresponding mucosal immune system is indeed responsible for the susceptibility to IBD.

PATHOPHYSIOLOGY: BIOLOGIC BASIS OF GENETIC SUSCEPTIBILITY

Recent parallel progress in the genetic and immunologic studies of human and rodent models has contributed great detail to our understanding of the pathophysiology of the inflammatory bowel diseases. Several genetic abnormalities have now been shown to affect the balance of T-cell responses to the antigens of bacteria commensal to the gut. Susceptibility to disease arises from an unfavorable genetic profile that creates an imbalance between antigen-specific effector and regulatory cells (e.g. TH-1, TH-2, TR-1/IL-10, or TH-3 /TGFβ cells). Disorders in T-cell responses have been associated with the presence of marker serum antibodies, each with a particular antigen specificity, as well as with distinct patterns of mucosal damage that together result in the broad spectrum of clinical manifestations of UC and CD. A clinical implication of this working hypothesis is that each distinct pattern will respond best to the specific therapy that addresses the specific imbalance at the foundation of that pattern. Future therapies may address these imbalances by altering cytokine profiles, by augmenting regulatory T-cell functions, or by changing the bacterial microenvironment in the gut.

Phenotypic Heterogeneity

Current evidence strongly supports the concepts that (1) IBD is not a single or even two diseases (e.g. Crohn's and UC) but, rather, is likely to be several distinct diseases presenting within the broad clinical picture of CD or UC; (2) these distinct diseases may have distinct etiologies and may require distinct therapies for successful treatment; and (3) close attention to clinical phenotype, to marker antibodies, and ultimately to polymorphisms of specific genes may identify these subgroups of CD and UC. These concepts are further supported by the fact that manipulation of many different genes in numerous rodent models of IBD (reviewed below) produces a wide spectrum of intestinal inflammation, broadly classifiable as CD-like or UC-like, yet each has specific characteristics that are unique to each model as well. Indeed, the wide spectrum of human intestinal inflammation seen in clinics is mimicked by the wide spectrum of intestinal inflammation seen in animal models.

The numerous rodent models further suggest that genetic heterogeneity—wherein defects in different genes or different combinations of genes lead to similar clinical manifestations—poses a major problem in elucidating the pathophysiology of IBD. Studies of the association of genetic variation with more homogeneous subgroups of disease, defined either by close attention to clinical detail or by subclinical markers, will therefore play an important role in sorting out the etiology of the different forms of IBD and ultimately will lead to the specific therapies needed for each subgroup.

Patients with either UC or CD show great variability in their disease phenotype for such characteristics as the following: age of onset; rate of relapse; fibrostenosis, perforating/fistulizing, internal or perianal "penetrating disease" (fistulae, abscesses, or perforations); presence of diarrhea, bleeding, or mucus discharge; duration of disease; location of disease (small bowel only, ileocolonic, colon only); number and types of surgery; development of chronic pouchitis after colectomy; and response to classes of medications such as corticosteroids, sulfasalazine or oral mesalamine, immunomodulatory agents (e.g., 6-mercaptopurine/azathioprine, methotrexate, cyclosporine), antibiotics, and topical therapies for distal colonic disease (Targan and Murphy, 1995; Vasiliauskas et al., 1996, 2000). Some patients can be clearly classified as having CD based on histological criteria, yet they have the UC-like features of left-sided colitis, more continuous and more shallow inflammation on endoscopy, and response to topical therapy (Vasiliauskas et al., 1996). As discussed above, some patients present with intermediate inflammation and cannot be classified as either CD or UC but are said to have indeterminate colitis.

Several lines of evidence suggest these phenotypic differences reflect underlying differences in immunological processes. IL-1β and IL-1 receptor antagonist mRNAs are increased in resected intestinal tissue from patients with nonperforating CD (the more benign form of CD) when compared with perforating CD (Gilberts et al., 1994). CD patients from families with multiple cases tend to have an early age at onset and more extensive disease than patients from families with no other cases (Colombel et al., 1996). Within families with multiply affected cases of CD, common familial patterns have been observed in the disease aggressiveness, age of onset (Bayless et al., 1996), disease location (Colombel et al., 1996; Cottone et al., 1997). Such familial distribution of clinical features suggests that certain genetic or environmental factors shared by family members may determine the clinical course of the disease. Thus, it may be beneficial to study a clinically homogenous group to understand the role of certain genetic and environmental factors.

Genetic Studies of Pathophysiology

Subclinical Markers

As commonly used, subclinical markers can be considered to be "intermediate phenotypes," or parameters that occur in the process of a disease's development and which, hopefully, are highly specific for that disease—for example, abnormal glucose tolerance and islet cell antibodies in diabetes, serum cholesterol in coronary artery disease, and adenomatous polyps in colon cancer. The study of subclinical markers promises to be a great aid to unravel the phenotypic heterogeneity of IBD. Markers with the greatest value in IBD research will be those that are closely related to the various underlying immunological processes that lead to the broad categories of intestinal inflammation.

As discussed above, the use of antineutrophil cytoplasmic antibodies with perinuclear immunofluorescent binding pattern (pANCA) in combination with antibodies to the cell-wall mannan of *S. cerevisiae* (ASCA) distinguish UC and CD. Several lines of evidence support the concept that the *serum* expression of these antibodies reflects *mucosal* processes. For pANCA, B cell clones taken from the mucosa of UC patients express pANCA (Targan et al., 1995), thus directly demonstrating pANCA in the intestinal mucosa. Further, pANCA is present in the sera of a high proportion of IL-10 knockout mice (Seibold et al., 1998). This reaction is eliminated by prior absorption of the pANCA$^+$ mouse sera with homogenized mouse cecal bacteria, suggesting that pANCA cross-reacts with enteric bacterial antigens. For ASCA, the specificity of the expression of anti-mannan antibodies, rather than anti-gliadin or anti-ovalbumin in CD patients (Lindberg et al., 1992), of antibodies to *Saccharomyces* and not to *Candida* (McKenzie et al., 1990), and of the expression of ASCA in patients with CD rather than with UC or other colitides, suggests that ASCA expression manifests a CD-related immune response rather than reflects a nonspecific intestinal insult resulting from the inflammation.

The expression of pANCA or ASCA also has been shown to extend the observed variability in IBD phenotype and provides further evidence for distinct subgroups within UC and CD. Within UC, the presence of pANCA has been associated with more severe forms of UC (treatment-resistant and left-sided UC; Vecchi et al., 1994), and the development of pouchitis following an ileal pouch–anal anastomosis procedure (Sandborn et al., 1995). Within CD, the presence of pANCA is associated with a more "UC-like" disease (more left-sided colitis; more distal, continuous, or shallow endoscopic appearance; more superficial histopathology—Vasiliauskas et al., 1996). Using pANCA as a phenotype, the authors have also provided evidence for heterogeneity within UC with family data (Shanahan et al., 1992), and this heterogeneity appears to have a genetic basis, as demonstrated by the use of HLA class II (Yang et al., 1993b) and the intercellular adhesion molecule-1 polymorphisms (H. Yang et al., 1995) (see Candidate Genes). High titers of ASCA in CD are associated with early age of disease onset, as well as both fibrostenosing and internal penetrating disease; in contrast, high ANCA levels are associated with a later age of onset and a different disease location (Vasiliauskas et al., 2000).

Recent studies support the hypothesis that genetic factors determine ANCA and ASCA expression, at least in part. First, ANCA and ASCA have been observed to be familial traits. For ANCA, an increased frequency of positive ANCAs has been observed in the clinically healthy relatives of UC patients, compared with environmental controls (Shanahan et al., 1992). Second-degree relatives, who did not share the same household with the probands, had an increased prevalence of ANCAs, and the household controls were not at an increased risk for ANCA. These results were further confirmed by an independent study (Seibold et al., 1994) but were not observed in another study (Lee et al., 1995). In a small twin study, 64% (9 of 14) of identical twins with UC had a positive ANCA, while of their 10 healthy monozygotic twins, 2 had ANCA (20%), which was greater than the frequency in healthy controls (5.8%) (P. Yang et al., 1995). These important epidemiologic observations suggest that the familial aggregation of ANCAs is due to shared genetic factors among the family members and not due to shared environmental factors. Further, in these family studies, there was a significant difference in the frequency of ANCAs in the relatives of probands whose sera were ANCA-positive compared with the relatives of probands whose sera were ANCA-negative (Shanahan et al., 1992; Seibold et al., 1994). This concordant familial distribution indicates heterogeneity within UC. Thus, ANCAs may be used as a marker of an underlying immunologic disturbance that is genetically determined (Shanahan, 1994).

For ASCA, the level of ASCA expression as a quantitative trait has been shown to be familial in both affected and unaffected relatives of CD patients, using intraclass correlation analysis (Sutton et al., 2000). A high percentage of CD patients (approximately half) and affected family members (also approximately half, but with a lower level of expression) were seropositive for anti-mannan Ig, compared to the normal control population (3.7%). Seropositivity or seronegativity was correlated among all affected relatives, and this association was stronger in affected first-degree relatives. Intraclass correlations revealed less variation in ASCA levels within rather than between families, and a significant familial aggregation was observed. There was no significant correlation among marital pairs. These findings demonstrated that ASCA in family members affected and unaffected with CD is a familial trait for both affected and unaffected relatives. The lack of correlation in marital pairs suggested that this familial aggregation is due in part to a genetic factor or childhood environmental exposure.

Second, preliminary observations suggest that genetic loci are associated with ANCA and ASCA expression. For ANCA, the intracellular adhesion molecule-1 ICAM1 G241R allele has been associated with ANCA expression (H. Yang et al., 1995). For ANCA and ASCA, an allele in the MHC Notch4 gene has been associated with high ASCA expression combined with absence of pANCA expression (Taylor et al., 2000). For ASCA, the TNF microsatellite "a" has been associated with ASCA seropositivity, regardless of whether the patient has CD or UC (Taylor et al., 1998), and that ASCA expression appears to be linked to markers near the MHC on chromosome 6 (IBD3) but not with the IBD1 locus on chromosome 16 (Yang et al., 2000).

When taken together, these observations suggest that ASCA and pANCA are serum markers for different mucosal inflammatory mechanisms that underlie distinct disease expression and that genetic variation may underlie these mechanisms. Use of clinical (fistulizing, perforating, fibrostenotic) and subclinical (ANCA, ASCA) characteristics may be useful in subdividing patient populations into more etiologically homogeneous groups for genetic studies and thus be the means for unraveling the genetic heterogeneity of these diseases in the future.

Other Subclinical Markers

Other potential subclinical markers are summarized in Table 15–6. Some of these, if confirmed, may lead to the understanding of host and environmental interactions, such as obligate anaerobic fecal flora.

The complement system plays a major role in the immune response and in the inflammatory process, thus making it a potential candidate in the etiology of IBD. Subnormal release of chemotactic activity for neutrophils (elicited by C5a2 from complement), increased in vivo C3 catabolism, increased levels of circulating C3c split products, and positive immunoconglutinin titers have all been reported in CD patients and suggest that complement may play a role in this disease (Hodgson et al., 1977; Lake et al., 1979; Potter et al., 1980; Amelio et al., 1981; Elmgreen et al., 1983, 1984, 1985). Complement levels are also known to vary with disease activity, supporting the possibility that the complement system could play a role in IBD etiology or pathophysiology (Ahrenstedt et al., 1990; Halstensen et al., 1989). Evidence supporting this concept includes the observation of enhanced local production of complement components in the small intestine of patients with Crohn's disease (Ahrenstedt et al., 1990; Ueki et al., 1996; Laufer et al., 2000). Furthermore, the proposal that the pathogenesis of Crohn's disease is mediated by multifocal gastrointestinal infarction is also consistent with a complement-mediated process (Wakefield et al., 1989, 1991; Hudson et al., 1992). A study of the protein polymorphism of the third component of complement (C3) was reported in a series of Danish patients with CD (Elmgreen et al., 1984). In this series, the F and FS phenotypes occurred significantly more often in the CD patients than in either UC patients or normal controls. The gene frequency of the F allele was 0.33 in CD with small bowel involvement only, 0.23 in all CD patients, 0.18 in UC patients and 0.17 in healthy volunteers. These data suggest that there may be etiologic differences not only between UC and CD but also between CD with and without colonic involvement. The molecular basis of polymorphisms between C3S and C3F has been suggested to be due to a single nucleotide change (Botto et al., 1990). The complement C3 gene is located within the peak linkage reported for IBD on chromosome 19 (see below).

One trait that has been investigated a number of times is that of intestinal permeability. Since the initial family study of intestinal permeability in CD (Hollander et al., 1986), there have been a number of several additional family studies. On first inspection, the results may appear somewhat inconsistent. It seems that a number of related factors may affect the results of an intestinal permeability study. These may include the type of probes, the method of administration of the probe—for example, fasting/nonfasting, with meals/without meals (Hollander, 1993); day urine collection/overnight urine collection, length of urine collection, and use of aspirin as a challenge (Bjarnason et al., 1991). It is important for this area of investigation to identify a sensitive and reproducible protocol for permeability testing that reliably separates Crohn's patients (or a subgroup of CD) from controls. In addition, it has been proposed that some of the statistical methods used to illustrate the increased permeability in the relatives of patients with CD may give misleading results (Hollander, 1993). Rather than comparing the means of permeability between the two groups—relatives and controls—one can examine the proportion of the asymptomatic relatives of patients with CD who have permeability values above the upper limits of the range of values in normal controls. The logic of this latter approach is that presumably only a proportion of CD relatives are genetically susceptible. Where this was done, the investigators found that approximately 10% of these relatives had a significant increase in intestinal permeability (May et al., 1993). When re-examining the published studies by this same approach (i.e., defining an increased level as greater than 2 SD above the mean in controls), the majority of such studies showed a significant increase in intestinal permeability in a fraction of the asymptomatic relatives of patients with CD (Hollander, 1993). Although there may be familiality of increased intestinal permeability, some family and twin studies do not support the hypothesis of a genetically determined intestinal leakiness in CD (Lindberg et al., 1995; Peeters et al., 1997). In addition, a variety of other disorders and relationships have shown increased permeability, including those with celiac disease, relatives of celiac disease patients (van Elburg et al., 1993), and even AIDS patients (Lim et al., 1993). These cumulative data would argue that these permeability abnormalities are likely not a fundamental inborn defect that predispose an individual to develop IBD but indicate early intestinal damage (preclinical expression). Natural history studies will be useful to resolve this "chicken and egg" issue and clarify the interpretation from cross sectional family studies. Genetic marker studies may also shed some light on this issue, especially those genes coding for structures in the permeability channels of the gut.

The potential importance of T cell receptor γ/δ genes in IBD has been suggested by a phenotypic study of γ/δ T lymphocytes in the intestinal mucosa of UC and CD (Fukushima, 1991). The different characterization and distribution of γ/δ_lymphocytes was found not only between patients with IBD and normal controls but also between patients with UC and those with CD. The T cell receptor α/δ complex lies in the chromosomal 14 linkage region (see below).

Immunoglobulin levels and subtypes have been investigated between IBD patients and controls and between CD and UC patients. One report observed a difference in immunoglobulin G (Gm allotype) markers in CD patients vs. controls, with a significant increase in frequency of the Gm (a,x,f;b,g) phenotype and Gm (a,x;g) haplotypes (Kagnoff et al., 1983). However, these results could not be replicated in later studies (Ockhuizen et al., 1985; Biemond et al., 1987; Gudjonsson et al., 1988; Field et al., 1989). No evidence for association or linkage with any specific immunoglobulin allotype was found in these latter studies. Given the studies of IgG subclass distribution in patients with UC or CD (Kett et al., 1987) and their family members (Helgeland et al., 1992) (see section on Subclinical Markers above for details), immunoglobulin genes still remain as potential candidate genes for IBD genetic studies.

Animal Models

Recognition and development of animal models of inflammatory bowel disease has progressed rapidly in recent years (Elson et al., 1995, 1998) (see Table 15–7). Chronic intestinal inflammation has been observed to occur in animals: (1) spontaneously (e.g., the rainforest cotton-top tamarin grown in the temperate climate of North America, or the C3H/HeJBir mouse strain); (2) after application or ingestion of chemicals (e.g., acetic acid instilled into the rectum or dextran sulfate sodium given in drinking water); (3) after genetic manipulation (e.g., rats expressing the human HLA-B27 molecule or various "knockout" strains of mice); and (4) after tissue transfer from one strain to another (e.g., transplantation of T-cell-depleted wild-type bone marrow into T cell–deficient (tgϵ 26) mice or transfer of $CD4^+$ $CD45RB^{hi}$ T cells into B- and T-cell-deficient–SCID mice). No single model completely reproduces the spectrum of human inflammatory bowel disease, but each model is useful, depending on the question being asked. Indeed, the wide spectrum of intestinal inflammation manifested by the sum total of these animal models is further evidence for the likely heterogeneity of the human inflammatory bowel diseases.

The basic lessons for IBD pathophysiology learned from these models are the following.

Table 15–7. Genetically Mediated Rodent Models of IBD

Model	Symbols	Inflammation	Bacteria Required	Comments	References
Induced by Agents					
Dextran sulfate sodium	DSS	Entire colon	Unknown	Identification of linkage to 5 genomic regions—multiple genes are required; this colitis is not T cell dependent	Mahler et al., 1998; 1999
Transgenic					
HLA-B27/β_2-microglobulin rat	HLAB27/β2m	Entire colon, small bowel, stomach	Yes	Increased colitis with *Bacterioides* spp.	Taurog et al., 1994; Rath et al., 1996, 1999
TNF knockin mouse, increased TNFproduction	TNFΔARE	Chronic ileitis	Unknown	No colitis in TNFΔARE + TNF receptor 1 double mutants;	Kontoyiannis et al., 1999; Cominelli et al., 1999
Targeted Disruption ("Knockouts")					
IL-2 knockout mouse	IL2$^{-/-}$	Entire colon	Colitis decreased, but not eliminated in germ-free environment	Increased transforming growth factor β, CD14, inducible nitric oxide synthase; IL-12 induces thymocytes to become colitis-inducing	Sadlack et al., 1993; Schultz et al., 1999; Meijssen et al., 1998; Harren et al., 1998; Ludviksson et al., 1997
IL-2 knockout mouse, raised pathogen-free, with colitis induced by keyhole limpet hemocyanin	IL2$^{-/-}$ with TNP-KLH induction	Entire colon	Mild colitis increased by induction with TNP-KLH in germ-free environment	Colitis reduced by anti-integrin αEβ7	Ehrhardt, 1997; Ludviksson et al., 1999
IL-10 knockout mouse	IL10$^{-/-}$	Colon, duodenum, jejunum	Yes; colitis can also be induced by *Helicobacter hepaticus* alone	Overproduction of Th1 cytokines; mediated by CD4$^+$ Th1 cells	Kuhn et al., 1993; Schultz et al., 1999; Davidson et al., 1996; Berg et al., 1996; Kullberg et al., 1998
Targeted Disruption ("Knockouts")					
Tumor necrosis factor knockout mouse	TNF$^{-/-}$	None	No	Defective antibacterial response; formation of B lymphocyte follicles; TNF receptor 1 also deficient in antibacterial response.	Pasparakis et al., 1996; 1997; Kaneko et al., 1999
T-cell receptor α knockout mouse	TCR$\alpha^{-/-}$	Entire colon	Unknown	No colitis in TCR$\alpha^{-/-}$ & IL4$^{-/-}$ double mutants (suggests Th2 pathway), but colitis in TCR$\alpha^{-/-}$ & IFN$\gamma^{-/-}$ double mutants; B-cells suppress colitis development but not required for initiation; initiation may require overproduction of IL1α and IL1β	Dianda et al., 1997; Mizoguchi et al., 1997; Mizoguchi et al., 1999
				IL-4 but not IFNγ required	Mizoguchi et al., 1999
Transplantation					
CD45RBhi cells to SCID mouse or to RAG minus mouse		Entire colon	Yes	Stat4/IL12 pathway involved; CD45RBlo cells from IL10$^{-/-}$ mouse no longer protect; TGFb is required for suppression of colitis by CD45RBlo; accelerated disease if T cells are depleted of natural killer cells	De Winter et al., 1999; Simpson et al., 1998; Powrie et al., 1996; Asseman et al., 1999; Fort et al., 1998
				Role of natural killer (NK) cells in down-regulation of Th1-mediated colitis	Fort et al., 1998

There are multiple paths to chronic intestinal inflammation. Chronic inflammation can be produced by creating transgenic animals in different genes: (1) targeted disruption ("knockout") of various genes in the mouse, interleukin-2 or its receptor, interleukin-10 (IL-10$^{-/-}$), T cell receptor α or β, transforming growth factor β, or G protein-α_{i2}, (2) enhancing expression of the tumor necrosis factor gene (TNF$^{\Delta ARE}$ "knockin"), or (3) adding of the human HLA-B27 and β_2-microglobulin genes to the rat (HLA-B27/β_2m). The involvement of different paths in these models is further supported by differences in cytokine profiles—for example, inflammation in the TNF$^{\Delta ARE}$ model is characterized by high levels of TNF (Kontoyiannis et al., 1999); inflammation in the IL-10$^{-/-}$ knockout model is characterized by high levels of IFNγ (Berg et al., 1996); and the inflammation in the T cell receptor $\alpha^{-/-}$ knockout model is characterized by high levels of IL-1α,β, and IL-4, but not IFNγ (Mizoguchi et al., 1997; Mizoguchi et al., 1999).

Intestinal inflammation is determined by multiple genes. In addition to the observations that several human genomic regions show linkage to IBD (see below) and that disruption of several different genes can lead to chronic intestinal inflammation (see previous section), breeding studies with mouse models also support the idea that many genes acting in concert predispose to IBD. For example, with the dextran sulfate sodium (DSS) mouse model, observed major differences in genetic susceptibility to DSS-induced colitis were observed (Mahler et al., 1998): strains C3H/HeJ and NOD/LtJ were particularly susceptible, strain C57BL/6J(B6) was partially resistant, and strain NON/LtJ was fully resistant to induction of inflammation. By crossing the susceptible C3H/HeJ strain to the partially resistant C57BL/6 strain and analyzing the colitis as a quantitative trait, these authors identified two loci with significant linkage to colitis (D5Mit216 and D2Mit94) and a further three loci with suggestive evidence for linkage (D18Mit119, D1Mit386, and D11Mit140) (Mahler et al., 1999). The linkage of DSS-induced colitis to the region on mouse chromosome 2 was confirmed using a NOD/LtJ × NON/LtJ cross. The D5Mit216 locus is syntenic with human linkage results on chromosome 5 (Ma et al., 1999). These results demonstrated that, similar to the human colitis, the rodent colitis in this model had more than one determining locus, and further work may lead to the identification of the specific genes determining colitis in this model.

Intestinal inflammation may require the presence of bacteria in the gut. When raised in bacteria-free conditions, inflammation does not occur with the IL-10 and TCRα knockouts (Dianda et al., 1997; Schultz et al., 1999). Using the HLA-B27/β_2m rat, it was observed that animals raised under germ-free conditions developed colitis only after gut colonization by bacterial mixtures containing *Bacteroides* species (Rath et al., 1996). When directly compared, inflammation induced by *B. vulgatus* was significantly more severe than that induced by *Escherichia coli* (Rath et al., 1999). This latter model raises the possibility that the HLA-B molecule may interact with bacterial antigens to produce IBD in humans. In contrast, inflammation is greatly reduced, but not eliminated, when the IL-2 knockout is raised in germ-free, compared with specific pathogen-free, conditions (Schultz et al., 1999). When taken together, these results suggest that live gut bacteria increase colonic inflammation in IBD and may be necessary for initiation of inflammation in some, but not all, models of disease.

Both pathogenic and protective CD4$^+$ cells are present in the normal animal. Intestinal inflammation occurs when a subpopulation of T cells from spleen or lymph node, CD4$^+$ CD45RB^{high}, are transferred into isogenic mice with severe combined immunodeficiency (SCID) or with a disruption of the recombination activating gene (RAG$^{-/-}$). In contrast, transfer of the entire CD4$^+$ population, or of the CD4$^+$ CD45RB^{low} subpopulation, does not induce inflammation. The CD4$^+$ CD45RB^{low} subset inhibits the CD4$^+$ CD45RB^{high} subset from inducing inflammation (Powrie et al., 1993).These observations suggested that normal mice have subsets of T cells that are capable of causing gut inflammation and that these subsets are kept in check by other subsets of T cells that protect the animal from inflammation. The induction by CD4$^+$ CD45RB^{high} cells can also be significantly reduced by treating the animal with anti-IFNγ, anti-IL-12, and IL-10, suggesting that pathogenesis in this model follows the Th1 pathway (Powrie et al., 1994; Simpson et al., 1998; De Winter et al., 1999). The suppression of inflammation by the CD4$^+$ CD45RB^{low} subset was inhibited by treatment with antitransforming growth factor beta (anti-TGBβ) but not anti-IL-4, suggesting a role for TGFβ in this suppression and that the inhibitory cells in the CD4$^+$ CD45RB^{low} subset may not be simply Th2 cells (Powrie et al., 1996).

IBD pathogenesis in this model can be dissected further by isolating the CD4$^+$ CD45RB^{high} cells from transgenics with alterations in various genes. Inflammation was greatly reduced, but not eliminated, when the CD4$^+$ CD45RB^{high} cells were isolated from knockouts in the signal transducer and activator of transcription-4 (STAT4$^{-/-}$) (Simpson et al., 1998), demonstrating that the IL-12/STAT-4 pathway plays the major role in the development of inflammation in this model. While this pathway controls IFNγ production and anti-IFNγ does reduce inflammation, conflicting results have been reported with CD4$^+$ CD45RB^{high} cells from IFNγ knockouts (Ito and Fathman, 1997; Simpson et al., 1998). These conflicts and the fact that some disease occurs with CD4$^+$ CD45RB^{high} cells from STAT-4 knockouts further reiterates the observations that there are multiple pathways to intestinal inflammation.

GENE IDENTIFICATION

Genome-Wide Linkage Studies

An intensive search for the susceptibility loci for IBD using the systematic mapping approach is currently under way by numerous laboratories worldwide. In this approach, no prior hypothesis is made as to the nature or location of the genetic susceptibility to disease. A *linkage panel,* or set of genetic markers equally spaced along the human genome, is systematically tested for linkage to the trait of interest using the appropriate statistical methods. A panel of 400 markers is necessary to give the 8 to 10 cM spacing over the entire human genome needed to detect a genetic effect in a complex trait. One of the problems with this approach is that it may be difficult to distinguish a true genetic effect in a complex trait from a random chance event that occurs because so many markers are tested in a sample (i.e., type 1 error) (see Chapter 1 and Chapter 3). This problem is potentially overcome when more than one laboratory observes linkage; therefore, the confirmation of linkage of a particular chromosomal region to IBD gives greater confidence that a susceptibility locus has in fact been identified.

Several genome scans have now been completed; these have examined linkage to CD, UC, or IBD combined. The putative regions identified by these scans have been further confirmed by yet more laboratories. This international effort is noteworthy within the study of the genetics of complex diseases in that several susceptibility loci for IBD have been identified by more than one laboratory. These results are summarized in Tables 15–8 to 15–12.

Table 15–8 shows the major IBD loci identified thus far. Consensus has been reached by the international IBD Genetics Consortium that the genome-wide approach provides evidence for susceptibility loci for IBD on chromosome 16 (IBD1) and on chromosome 12 (IBD2). Further agreement has been reached by some of the members of this consortium that this approach has also provided evidence for a third locus at or near the major histocompatibility complex (MHC) on chromosome 6 (IBD3), a fourth locus on chromosome 14, and a likely fifth locus on chromosome 5. More loci likely exist; some have prob-

Table 15–8. Susceptibility loci for IBD

Locus	Location (Chromosome)	Initial Report and Replications
IBD1	16q12	Hugot et al. 1996; Ohmen et al. 1996; Parkes et al. 1996; Mirza et al. 1998; Cho et al. 1998; Cavanaugh et al. 1998; Curran et al. 1998; Brant et al. 1998; Hugot et al. 1998
IBD2	12q13	Satsangi et al. 1996; Duerr et al. 1998; Curran et al. 1998; Yang et al. 1999a
IBD3	6p21 (MHC)	Yang et al. 1999b; Hampe et al. 1999a; Rioux et al. 2000;
IBD4	14q11	Ma et al. 1999; Duerr et al. 2000
IBD5	19p13	Cho et al. 1998; Duerr et al. 1998; Rioux et al. 2000
IBD6	5q31–q33	Ma et al. 1999; Rioux et al. 2000

ably already been detected by this effort. If a "cutoff" is arbitrarily set at LOD ≥ 2 or at $p < .001$ or at replication in two studies, then additional tentative loci may have also been identified on chromosomes 1, 3, 4, 5, 7, and 19.

Even though some of these results will represent false positives that are incurred during analysis of the genome screen data, clearly these results already support the following ideas: (1) there are multiple susceptibility loci for IBD; (2) CD and UC have some loci in common and do not share other loci; (3) some of these loci interact; (4) different loci play different roles in the IBD susceptibility of different populations.

Chromosome 16

The chromosome 16 locus (IBD1) was the first to be identified by a whole genome approach (Hugot et al., 1996), was quickly confirmed (Ohmen et al., 1996), and currently has the strongest support worldwide (Table 15–9). A two-point LOD score of 2.04 and an increased sharing of 0.67 between affected sib pairs was observed for marker D16S409 in an initial family panel with 25 sib pairs affected with CD with no known cases of UC (CD-only families) (Hugot et al., 1996). Significant linkage to this region was also observed in a second panel of 53 families. By further genotyping and multipoint analysis methods, linkage was localized to the region D16S409 and D16S419 with a significance of $p < 1.5 \times 10^{-5}$. This result was confirmed in an independent sample the same year (Ohmen et al., 1996). Subsequent genotyping to a 1cM resolution has resulted in a multipoint LOD score (MLS) of $Z = 2.81$ ($p = .0003$) at D16S416 to D16S3117 (Hugot et al., 1998). Linkage of this region was also observed in families with UC only (nonparametric linkage score (NPL) = 2.02, $p = .02$ at D16S3120) in only one study but, surprisingly, not in families with both CD and UC subjects (mixed families) (Mirza et al., 1998). Linkage of CD to this region of chromosome 16 has subsequently been observed by many but not all laboratories (summarized in Table 15–9).

In one study, linkage of IBD1 was strongest in families with an earlier age of onset of disease (Brant et al., 2000). Since an earlier age of disease onset is also associated with severity of CD, this observation suggests that IBD1 may play a role in determining the natural history of CD.

In an effort to combine the observations of the various laboratories worldwide in a single nonparametric analysis, members of the international IBD Genetics Consortium have combined genotype data for the same six markers broadly spanning the IBD1 region (The IBD International Genetics Consortium, 2001). A total of 613 families (386 CD only, 108 UC only, 119 mixed) had data available for both parents and at least two affected sib pairs. A multipoint LOD score of 5.8 for this locus was observed in CD but not in UC. This is among the highest LOD score observed in any complex trait and demonstrates the importance of the study of a large number of families in order to detect modest genetic effects by linkage. Approximately 10% to 15% of the susceptibility to CD was estimated to be accounted

Table 15–9. Linkage Studies on Chromosome 16 (IBD1)

Type of Family	Multipoint Linkage (LOD Score)	Two-point Linkage (*p* Value)	Association	Reference	Population	Comments
CD only	3.2	.0004	–	Hugot et al., 1996	France	Did not examine UC or mixed families
CD only	2.4	.02	–	Ohmen et al., 1996	North America	No linkage in UC and mixed families; linkage was observed in non-Jewish families only
CD only	2.4	.21	–	Cho et al., 1997	North America	No linkage in UC or mixed families and no Jewish and non-Jewish difference; interaction with locus on Chr 1
CD only	6.3	.000002	+	Cavanaugh et al., 1998	Australia	No linkage in mixed families
IBD		CD, .045 IBD, .058		Satsangi et al., 1996	United Kingdom	A marker 40 cM distal to this region, D16S407 gave a LOD 1.5 ($p = .004$) in CD families, zero in UC families
IBD	CD—1.5 UC—2 IBD—2.4			Curran et al., 1998	Northcentral Europe	
UC	2.2			Mirza et al., 1998	France	Did not report CD results
CD	2.8	.003		Hugot and Thomas, 1998	France	Families for this study were different from the families used in Hugot et al. 1996
CD	2.8			Brant et al., 1998	North America	This linkage was conducted in a large pedigree containing seven relatives affected with CD
IBD		.5	–	Vermeire et al., 1998	Belgium	
IBD				Rioux et al., 1998	Canada	Exclusion of $\lambda_s = 2.0$

for by this locus. The interval containing 1 LOD from the peak spans a less than 10 cM region.

After 5 years of intensive research, the IBD1 gene (CARD15/NOD2) was recently identified by Hugot et al. (2001) using positional cloning strategy, linkage followed by linkage disequilibrium mapping. They identified three independent variants of this gene associated with CD: a frameshift variant and two missense variants. NOD2 is a member of the Apaf-1/Ced-4 superfamily of apoptosis regulators, is expressed in monocytes, and acts as an intracellular receptor for components of microbial pathogens. These findings suggest that the chromosome 16 CD susceptibility locus alters components of the innate immunity system to create dysregulation of NF-kB in response to microbial lipopolysaccharides. The relative risks for simple heterozygous, homozygous, and compound heterozygous as compared with those no variant are 3, 38, and 44, respectively. The frequencies of the three variant alleles are 7%, 5%, and 29% in controls, UC, and CD patients, respectively. A candidate gene approach also demonstrated association between the NOD2 and CD (Ogura et al., 2001). Clearly, NOD2 is a susceptibility gene to CD, that is, it increases an individual's risk for CD, but it is neither sufficient nor necessary for the development of CD. As reviewed below, there are other loci to be identified. The identification of the NOD2 will shed light on the etiologic pathways of IBD and accelerate the discovery of additional susceptibility genes for IBD. A more severe, stricturing form of CD has also been associated with these mutations (Abreau et al., 2002; Lesage et al., 2002). The identification of the IBD1 gene is thus far one of a few successes in gene identification in complex diseases.

Chromosome 12

The chromosome 12 locus (IBD2) was the second region to be identified by a whole genome approach (Satsangi et al., 1996). A two-point LOD score of 5.47 ($p = 2.66 \times 10^{-7}$) was observed in their complete set of 186 sib pairs from CD only, UC only, and mixed families at the marker D12S83. An association between a "4-1-3" haplotype constructed with markers D12S83, D12S1662, and D12S1655 and UC was observed in further work using the transmission disequilibrium test (Parkes et al., 1998). Both the linkage and association findings have been replicated in North American studies: one observing an association to the same marker D12S83 in both CD and UC families using the transmission disequilibrium test (Duerr et al., 1998), and one to a marker 14 cM away at D12S85 in CD families (Yang et al., 1999a). Other linkage studies of this region are summarized in Table 15–10. The differences in the results for this interval have raised the possibility that there may be two loci in this region, one for CD and one for UC.

Thus far, a few candidate genes have been tested for association to either IBD, CD, or UC, based on their location within the IBD2 region, and negative results have been reported for interferon-γ (Hampe et al., 1998) and the natural resistance–associated macrophage protein (NRAMP2) (Stokkers et al., 2000).

Major Histocompatibility Complex

Based on the hypothesis that IBD pathogenesis may involve immunoregulatory factors, candidate genes within the major histocompatibility complex (MHC) on chromosome 6p21.3 IBD3 have long been tested for IBD susceptibility with conflicting results (see Candidate Gene Studies). In a recent study of the sharing of MHC haplotypes, which allowed the delineation of identity by descent of haplotypes (Yang et al., 1999b), linkage to the MHC was observed using several nonparametric methods: (1) an increased number of sib pairs sharing one or more haplotypes ($p = .004$); (2) an increased mean proportion of sharing between concordant affected ($p = .002$) and concordant unaffected ($p = .031$), pairs along with a decreased proportion in discordant pairs ($p = .007$); (3) a significant linear relation between the similarity of phenotype between members of a sib pair and the proportion of their shared haplotypes by regression analysis ($p = .00003$); (4) an increased sharing between pairs more distantly related than sib pairs ($p = .001$). Linkage was also observed in this region in a genome scan by the same investigators (Ma et al., 1999). Further support for linkage of the MHC region to IBD has been observed by two additional laboratories following the systematic mapping approach (summarized in Table 15–11): (1) a multipoint LOD score of 4.2 for D6S461 (Hampe et al., 1999b) and (2) a peak nonparametric LOD score of 2.3 ($p = .0026$) for D6S1017, with other NPL scores over 2 for nearby markers (Rioux et al., 2000). These observations suggest that the MHC is a third susceptibility region for IBD and is referred to as IBD3.

Table 15–10. Linkage and Association Studies on Chromosome 12 (IBD2)

Type of Family	Disease	Multipoint Linkage LOD Score	Two Point Linkage *p* Value	Association	Reference	Population	Comments
Chr. 12 ~80 cM[a]	IBD		CD-0.0073 UC-0.0025 IBD-2.7 × 10^{-7}	+	Satsangi et al., 1996 Parkes et al., 1998	United Kingdom	Linkage and association were reported in different papers
	IBD	CD-1.8 UC-1.8 IBD-2.8		+	Duerr et al., 1998	North America	
	CD	2.0	0.0004	+	Yang et al., 1998	North America	This peak is at D12S85, which is approximately 10–15 cM away from the peak observed in English families
	IBD	CD-1.8 UC-0.8			Curran et al., 1998		
	IBD	UC-0.8	0.24	–	Vermeire et al., 1998	Belgium	
IFNγ				–	Hampe et al., 1998	Europe	
VDR gene	Case-control			CD+ UC–	Simmons et al., 1998	United Kingdom	VDR gene maps to the region on Chr. 12 linked to IBD

[a]cM* distance from p telomere.

Table 15–11. Linkage Studies on Chromosome 6—MHC Region

Type of Family	Multipoint Linkage (LOD Score)	Two-point Linkage (p Value)	Association	Reference	Population	Comments
CD only		0.00003	+	Yang et al., 1999b	North America	Linkage observed using MHC haplotypes
IBD	4.2		+	Hampe et al., 1999b	Europe	D6S461 and D6S426 fine mapping peak outside of MHC, but nearby
UC	2.3		+	Rioux et al., 2000	Canada	Peak marker: D651017
UC		0.032		Satsangi et al., 1996		Peak marker: D6S276
CD				Hugot et al., 1994	Europe	Exclusion of MHC with parametric and nonparametric methods
IBD				Naom et al., 1996	United Kingdom	Exclusion of MHC with parametric methods
CD, UC, IBD				Cho et al., 1997		Evidence that MHC plays a minor role, if any

Chromosome 14

Evidence for linkage between CD and the marker D14S261 has been observed in two studies (Ma et al., 1999; Duerr et al., 2000) and to the general region of this marker in a third (Vermeire et al., 2000). This confirmation argues that this region constitutes the fourth IBD susceptibility locus, IBD4. Candidate genes in this region include the T-cell receptor α/δ complex.

Chromosome 19

Significant linkage of IBD to the marker D19S591 with a multipoint LOD of 4.6 has been observed in Canadian sib-pair families (Rioux et al., 2000). Some evidence for linkage to this same marker has also been reported by a second group (Duerr et al., 2000) (two-point LOD score 1.6, $p = .0067$) and to a neighboring region by a third group (Cho et al., 1998) (multipoint $p = .0059$). This region contains the genes for ICAM-1, complement component 3, thromboxane A2 receptor, leukotriene B4 hydroxylase, and the janus protein tyrosine kinases TYK2 and JAK3.

Chromosome 5

Evidence for linkage to the region D5S393–D5S673 has been observed in Jewish CD-only families (Ma et al., 1999) and in CD families with early onset disease (multipoint LOD 3.9) (Rioux et al., 2000). This region contains the genes for the cytokines interleukin 3, 4, 5, and 13 and CSF-2, and is syntenic to a mouse region implicated in the dextran sulfate-induced colitis model (Mahler et al., 1999). Completion of a dense genetic map of microsatellite markers and single-nucleotide polymorphisms of the cytokine gene cluster in this region has demonstrated a strong association between Crohn's disease and a specific haplotype spanning 250 kb (Rioux et al., 2001; Daly et al., 2001). However, the very strong linkage disequilibrium across this region thus far prevented any further identification of the causal mutation for CD because multiple single-nucleotide polymorphisms in the haplotype showed equal genetic evidence for susceptibility to CD.

Other Loci

The published genome scans have also proposed that other regions contain susceptibility loci for IBD (summarized in Table 15–12). The following evidence for linkage is worthy of note.

Chromosomes 3 and 7. A suggestion of linkage to the regions D3S1076–D3S1573 (mostly contributed by CD only families) and D7S484–D7S527 (contributed by both CD and UC families, depending on the marker in the region) was observed in the same study that reported the initial linkage to chromosome 12 (Satsangi et al., 1996). With further fine mapping, a peak single point linkage to CD has been observed by this group at marker D3S3521 (LOD = 3.5, $p = .00003$) with the support region (LOD within 1 of the peak) spanning D3S11–D3S3559 (Parkes et al., 1999). Evidence for linkage to these two regions has been observed in another study, with a multipoint $p = .014$ for CD only families to the chromosome 3 region, and a multipoint $p = .01$ for all IBD families to the chromosome 7 region (Cho et al., 1998). A mouse chromosome region containing a susceptibility locus for dextran sulfate-induced colitis, Dssc-1 (Mahler et al., 1999), is syntenic with this human chromosome 7 region.

For the chromosome 3 region, negative results have been reported for the G protein G-α-i-2 gene (GNAI2) (Zhang et al., 2000). A modest association between markers near the mutL homolog 1 gene (colon cancer, nonpolyposis type I; MLH1) and has been observed in a small sample of 45 CD, 36 UC, and 45 controls (Pokorny et al., 1997).

For chromosome 7, the mucin-3 (MUC3) gene has been tested for association to IBD; alleles of a 51 bp VNTR polymorphism are increased in UC patients from both Great Britain and Japan (Kyo et al., 1999). This observation of an association from two populations, combined with the observation of a reduction of altered mucin species IV in UC patients (Podolsky and Fournier, 1988), make this an attractive finding.

Chromosome 1. Two studies have observed evidence for linkage to the D1S2670–D1S2682 region (Cho et al., 1998; Hampe et al., 1999a). Families with linkage to this region also show greater linkage to IBD1, suggesting that this susceptibility locus interacts with IBD1 (Cho et al., 1998). Further narrowing of this region to 130 kb near D1S2697 and D1S3669 has been accomplished by homozygosity mapping in a collection of American Iraqi Chaldean families with IBD (Cho et al., 2000). Since both CD and UC are observed in these families, these authors have proposed that this locus determines a genetic susceptibility to IBD, with the concomitant inheritance of IBD1 then determining CD (Cho et al., 2000).

Table 15–12. "Other" Loci with Observed Linkage to IBD in Genome Screens

Chromosome	Locus	Location Broman (cM)	Interval	Interval Broman	Evidence: Single-Point LOD		Multipoint LOD		CD	UC	IBD	Reference
1	D1S1597	29.90			1.48							Duerr et al., 2000
	D1S552	45.33			2.03	3.14 IBD Non-Jewish	2.65	2.59 IBD Non-Jewish			0.00024	Cho et al., 1998
			D1S2670–D1S2682	262.96–288.29			Zmax = 2.08 IBD				0.0044	Hampe et al., 1999a
	D1S1609	274.53								mixed:	0.0023	Cho et al., 1998
2			D2S2952–D2S1400	17.88–27.6					0.0084m			Cho et al., 1998
			D2S305–D2S367	38.87–54.96			0.9	1.4 CD Jew	*			Ma et al., 1999
	D2S142	161.26							0.24	0.0071	0.0021	Satsangi et al., 1996
	D2Mit94	*180?*		*175–185?*							*0.0000178*	*Mahler et al., 1999*
	D2S117	194.50			1.30 CD		1.25					Duerr et al., 2000
3	D3S2432	57.92							0.014m			Cho et al., 1998
	D3S2432	57.92			2.24							Paavola et al., 2000
	D3S1076								0.0018	0.043	0.0026	Satsangi et al., 1996
	D3S3521	63.21	D3S11–D3S3559	61.52–67.94	CD 3.5; IBD 2.9				0.00003		0.0001	Parkes et al., 1999
	D3S1573	70.61			2.69				0.00029	0.011	0.00021	Satsangi et al., 1996
			D3S1766–D3S1285	78.64–91.18			2.4					Rioux et al., 2000
	D3S3045	124.16					1.31 CD					Duerr et al., 2000
	D3S2427		D3S3053–D3S2427	181.87–188.29	1.25		2.29 IBD	3.39 Non-Jew			0.00057	Cho et al., 1998
4	D4S1647	104.94			0.61	1.11 IBD Jew	1.15 IBD	2.11 IBD Jew			0.0025	Cho et al., 1998
	D4S2623	114.04			3.00	2.23 IBD Jew	2.76 IBD	2.76 IBD Jew				Cho et al., 1998
			D4S1575–D4S424	132.05–144.56			Zmax = 1.56 UC			0.009		Hampe et al., 1999a
5			D5S407–D5S647	64.67–74.07				1.2 CD	**			Ma et al., 1999
	D5S1462	105.29								0.0096		Cho et al., 1998
	D11Mit140		*D5S471–D5S393*	*129.83–140.93*							*0.004207*	*Mahler et al., 1999*
	D18Mit119	*140.70*									*0.000579*	*Mahler et al., 1999*
			D5S393–D5S673	140.7–155.9			0.7	2.2 Jew	***			Ma et al., 1999
			D5S816–D5S1480	139.33–147.49			3.0	3.9 early onset CD				Rioux et al., 2000
6			D6S262–D6S292	130.0–136.97	0.9	1.5 Non-Jew			*			Ma et al., 1999
7	D7S519	69.03			2.89				0.27	0.000056	0.00013	Satsangi et al., 1996
	D5Mit216		*(ELN at 84.52)*	*83.99–90.42*							*0.0000137*	*Mahler et al., 1999*
	D7S669	90.42			2.14				0.00018	0.014	0.000082	Satsangi et al., 1996
	D7S524	97.38							0.0011	0.042	0.00085	Satsangi et al., 1996
	D7S820	98.44								mixed:	0.01	Cho et al., 1998
	D7S648	128.41					0.91 CD					Duerr et al., 2000
8	D8S256	148.12							0.0044			Cho et al., 1998
9	D9S288	pter					0.1 CD	1.3 CD Jew				
	D9S1121	44.30			1.40				0.011			Duerr et al., 2000
	D9S2157	146.83							0.0054			Cho et al., 1998
	D9S164	147.90			1.01				0.031			Duerr et al., 2000
10			D10S548–D10S197	45.7–52.1			Zmax = 2.30 CD		0.0014			Hampe et al., 1999a
11	D11S1999	17.19							0.0028			Cho et al., 1998
14	D14S261	6.41			1.9 CD		1.9 CD	2.0 Jew CD	***			Ma et al., 1999
	D14S261	6.41	D14S261–D14S283		3.0 CD		3.6 CD	0.0002				Duerr et al., 2000
	D14S608	28.01								mixed:	0.004	Cho et al., 1998
17	D17S974	22.20			0.91				0.041			Duerr et al., 2000
			D17S925–D17S787	49.67–74.99			0.3	2.1 CD Jew	*			Ma et al., 1999
	D17S784	116.96					0	1.5 CD Jew	***			Ma et al., 1999
18	D18S474	71.32					1.1	1.9 CD Jew	* Jew			Ma et al., 1999
	(D1Mit386)		D18S60–D18S1091	91.62–107.4							0.00126	Mahler et al., 1999
	D18S61	105.00	D18S61–ATA82B02	105–106.8	1.34 CD		1.15 CD			0.013		Duerr et al., 2000
19			D19S591–D19S1034	9.84–20.75			4.6					Rioux et al., 2000
	D19S591	9.80			1.60 CD					0.0067		Duerr et al., 2000
			D19S1034–D19S586	20.75–32.94						0.0059		Cho et al., 1998
20			D20S95–D20S115	16.65–21.15			1.1	1.0 CD Jew	*			Ma et al., 1999
	D20S477	47.50			1.16 CD				0.021			Duerr et al., 2000
	D20S178	66.16					1.4		*			
21	D21S1253	20.45					1.1		**			
22	D22S315	21.47	D22S315–D22S421	21.47			Zmax = 1.52 IBD				0.0038	Hampe et al., 1999a
X			DXS1202–DXS1214	30.3–33.54			Zmax = 1.59 IBD				0.007	Hampe et al., 1999a
			DXS991	52.5					0.03			Satsangi et al., 1998
			DXS1001–DXS1047	75.79–82.07			Zmax = 1.71 UC			0.005		Hampe et al., 1999a

Locations of markers are from Broman et al., 1998 (http://research.marshfieldclinic.org/genetics). Shaded areas may represent the same locus due to "close" proximity or overlap of linkage results.
$^*0.01 < p < .05$; $^{**}0.001 < p < .01$; $^{***}p < .001$. "Dssc1-5" are mouse loci in the dextran sulfate–induced colitis model.
All p values are as reported by the authors, but different statistical methods were used. This table lists those loci as indicated to be important by each laboratory.
Lines in italics refer to mouse loci that are placed as close as possible to the given human regions by mouse-human synteny.

Candidate Gene Studies

In the candidate gene approach, genetic variants are tested based on a prior hypothesis regarding the role of that gene or gene product in the pathophysiology of the disease. Such a hypothesis may be based on evidence from clinical observation or physiological studies of affected individuals (in vivo studies), from studies of known disease-related processes (in vitro studies), from animal models of disease (transgenic construction or targeted disruption), and from the effects of drugs or chemicals on disease in either humans or animals (pharmacogenetic studies). For IBD, possible candidates could be selected from genes involved in the regulation of the balance between TH1 and TH2 cells, the response of humans to gut flora, and the release of cytokines during the immunological destruction and healing of the intestinal mucosa.

Major Histocompatibility Complex

The major histocompatibility complex (MHC) on chromosome 6p21.3 is the most gene-dense region of the human genome sequenced thus far, with 224 genes identified within 3.6 megabases (Mb) (MHC Sequencing Consortium, 1999). Since many of the genes in this cluster function in the regulation of the immune system and in antigen processing and presentation, the MHC is a candidate region for most, if not all, diseases with dysregulation of the immune system as the possible underlying pathophysiology. The MHC has therefore long been considered a candidate region for IBD. However, also among these genes are the most polymorphic human proteins known, the class I and class II molecules; and some of these proteins have over 100 allelic variants. This great variation and the high gene density of the MHC have contributed to the difficulty of assigning the specific role of a specific gene to the pathophysiology of IBD. General features of the immunogenetics of the various subregions of the MHC may be found in Chapter 28.

The MHC Class II Region. In general, the class II molecules are dimeric, with an α-chain and a β-chain that form a groove for presenting an extracellular antigenic peptide to $CD4^+$ T cells. The three class II molecules are HLA-DP, HLA-DQ, and HLA-DR. In each case the α- and β-chains are encoded by A and B genes, respectively. For HLA-DR, there is an invariant HLA-DRA gene and up to 3 distinct and highly polymorphic HLA-DRB genes. One of these HLA-DRB genes, HLA-DRB1, is present in all individuals and is the most polymorphic. The study of HLA-DRB1 genes has been an important tool in the study of the role of class II genes in IBD. Serological methods identify several HLA-DR types and subtypes and were used in the older studies, while molecular methods reveal even more subtypes at the nucleotide level and are the preferred techniques today. A meta-analysis of 29 studies reporting HLA-DR or HLA-DQ frequencies in CD and UC patients and in controls has been published (Stokkers et al., 1999). The results of this analysis and of recent association studies using molecular methods are summarized in Table 15–13.

The authors have identified an association between the combination of HLA-DR1/HLA-DQ w5 alleles and CD in Caucasians in the United States and HLA-DR2 and UC (Toyoda et al., 1993). The association between HLA-DR1 and CD has also been observed in France (Danze et al., 1996) and in the Netherlands (Bouma et al., 1997). Further molecular typing revealed that, of all the DR1 alleles, only the HLA-DRB1*0103 allele, and not other DR1 subtypes, was associated with both CD and UC (See Table 15–14) (Trachtenberg et al., 2000). This finding pointed to the importance of molecular typing over serological typing as the way to clarify the associations between class II alleles and IBD; an example of the associations between IBD and HLA alleles typed using molecular methods in one of the largest studies to date is given in Table 15–14. In Britain, HLA-DRB1*0103 has also been associated with UC (Satsangi et al., 1996) and with the extraintestinal manifestation of peripheral arthropathy in IBD patients but not in controls (Orchard et al., 2000). The authors have further observed that the association of DR2 with UC was due to the HLA-DRB1*1502 allele (Trachtenberg et al., 2000). In addition, a rare HLA-DRB1*0103–DQA1*0501–DQB1*0301 haplotype was dramatically associated with IBD with an odds ratio of 6.9, and a more common DR1 haplotype, HLADRB1*0103–DQA1*0101–DQB1*0501, was also assocated with IBD. This result suggested that an interaction between HLA-DR and HLA-DQ may determine the extent of disease risk.

A new association at another MHC class II locus, HLA-DP, has been recently observed; the common HLA-DPB1*0401 allele confers a modest risk for CD (Trachtenberg et al., 2000).

The results summarized in Tables 15–13 and 15–14 clearly point to a role for the MHC class II genes in the pathogenesis of IBD. HLA-DRB1*0103 differs from other HLA-DRB1 alleles by an LLEQR to ILEDE change at positions 67–71 in exon 2 (Trachtenberg et al., 2000). This change alters the peptide binding groove and may be involved in binding an IBD-related peptide to this antigen-presenting molecule. However, these results also suggest that there are interactions between multiple class II genes in the MHC and that further studies with larger sample sizes will be necessary to unravel the complex role of this region in the pathogenesis of IBD. Further, although great progress has been made in defining the association between IBD and MHC class II genes, three lines of evidence suggest that the contribution of the MHC to IBD is likely to consist of more than that provided by the class II region:

1. While some investigators have confirmed associations to the same class II alleles, others have observed associations to other class II alleles, particularly when studying other populations. This suggests that at least some MHC class II alleles are not the IBD susceptibility alleles but are in linkage disequilibrium with susceptibility alleles.
2. The results of two genome scans (Hampe et al., 1999b; Ma et al., 1999) suggest that the peak linkage to IBD in this region may be several centiMorgans telomeric from the MHC, and the result of a third (Rioux et al., 2000) suggests that the peak may be centromeric.
3. The magnitude of the linkage effect revealed above is not explained by the relatively modest associations of the MHC class II alleles heretofore observed. This evidence suggests that further linkage disequilibrium mapping of the MHC and IBD is also warranted.

Strategies to unravel the role of the potentially multiple MHC genes involved in the susceptibility to IBD are (1) to carry out this fine mapping using both case-control and family-based association tests (the TDT) and to follow leads that are positive with both methods, and (2) to examine the contribution of each locus in isolation from the others by methods that stratify the genotyping data at one locus with respect to another locus.

Notch4. A preliminary example of such a fine-mapping effort has revealed further susceptibility loci in the MHC class III re-

Table 15–13. Associations of CD and UC with HLA Class II Alleles

Serological	Genetic Allele	Frequency	Odds Ratio	p	Reference
DR					
DR1					
	DRB1*01	15% CD, 9% controls	1.75	.003 (corr*)	Danze et al., 1996
	DRB1*03	Not found in ANCA neg UC			Hirv et al., 1999
	DRB1*07	17% CD, 11% controls	1.58	.008 (corr)	Danze et al., 1996
	DRB1*07	18% CD, 10% controls	1.9	.0001	Reinshagen et al., 1996
	DRB1*0103	8.6% UC, 3.2% controls	2.9	.0074	Satsangi et al., 1996
		14%UC (16% extensive UC), 23% extraintestinal manifestations, 6% UC, 0.2% control	27.6	<.0001 .0002	Roussomoustakaki et al., 1997 Bouma et al., 1999
		Increased with extensive UC, colectomy	33, 84	<.0001	Bouma et al., 1999
		7.9% CD, 2.2% control	4.4	.002	Trachtenberg et al., 2000
		8.9% UC, 2.2% control	4.9	.001	Trachtenberg et al., 2000
		Meta-analysis, association with UC	*3.42*		Stokkers et al., 1999
DR2		70% UC, 31% controls	5.1	<.001	Asakura et al., 1982
		41% UC, 21% control	2.6	.008	Toyoda et al., 1993
		44% ANCA + UC, 21% ANCA − UC		.01	Yang et al., 1996
		Meta-analysis, association with UC	*2.0*		Stokkers et al., 1999
	DRB1*15	42% UC, 26% controls	2.1	.006	Bouma et al., 1999
		35% ANCA pos UC, 15% controls, 11% ANCA neg UC	2.9	.004	Hirv et al., 1999
		Meta-analysis, association with UC	*1.65*		Stokkers et al., 1999
	DRB1*1501 & DRB1*1502	Increased in ANCA pos UC			Hirv et al., 1999
	DRB1*1502	49% UC, 18% controls	2.8	<.0001	Futami et al., 1995
		12% UC, 5% controls	2.7	.005	Trachtenberg et al., 2000
		Meta-analysis, association with UC	*3.74*		Stokkers et al., 1999
		Negative for DR2 alleles			Duerr and Neigut, 1995
		Negative for DRB1*1502			Cariappa et al., 1998
DR4	DRB1*0410	13% CD, 3% controls	5.02	.001 (corr)	Nakajima et al., 1995
	DRB1*0410/DQA1*03/ DQB1*0402 haplotype	13% CD, 2.7% controls	5.6	.00011 (corr)	Nakajima et al., 1995
DR13	DRB1*1302/DRB3*030 1 haplotype	21% CD, 5.4% controls	4.6	.0066	Forcione et al., 1996 Cariappa et al., 1998
	DRB3*0301	*Meta-analysis, associated with CD*	1.18		Stokkers et al., 1999
DP					
	DPB1*0401	74% CD, 65% controls	1.6	.014	Trachtenberg et al., 2000
DQ					
	DQA1*03	88% CD, 68% control	3.36	.03 (corr)	Nakajima et al., 1995
	DQA1*0201	19% CD, 11% control	1.9	.0001	Reinshagen et al., 1996
	DQB1*0402	19% CD, 6% controls	3.89	.001 (corr)	Nakajima et al., 1995
	DQB1*0501	16% CD, 10% controls	1.61	.01 (corr)	Danze et al., 1996

corr*: *p* values adjusted for the number of tests performed.

gion around *Notch4*. The *Notch4* gene is located in the MHC class III region close to the border with the class II region. The function of the human *Notch4* gene is not currently known, but the family of Notch proteins are involved in the control of cell fate decisions during development (Artavanis-Tsakonas et al., 1999), including hematopoiesis (Milner and Bigas, 1999) and gut epithelium (Skipper and Lewis, 2000). Notch receptors and ligands are also expressed in the thymus, and the overexpression of *Notch1* in a mouse transgenic strain directs $CD4^+$ $CD8^+$ precursors to the CD8 lineage (Robey, 1999). The authors have observed that an allele of *Notch4* is associated with CD in Ashkenazi Jews in both a case-control study and a family-based study by TDT (Taylor et al., 1999). This genetic association was independent of the HLA-DRB1 associations discussed above, suggesting that multiple genes in the MHC may be determining IBD. In a study of well-characterized CD patients, this same allele was

Table 15–14. Summary of Class II Associations with CD, UC, or Both (IBD)

Disease	Class II Allele or Haplotype	% in Cases	% in Controls	p	OR
IBD	DRB1*0103	8.3	2.2	.001	4.6
CD		7.9	2.2	.002	4.4
UC		8.9	2.2	.001	4.9
IBD	DRB1*0103–DQA1*0501–DQB1*0301	2.8	0.4	.034	6.9
IBD	DRB1*0103–DQA1*0101–DQB1*0501	6.4	2.2	.007	3.5
UC	DRB1*1502	11.9	4.7	.006	2.6
CD	DPB1*0401	74.1	64.7	.014	1.6

Total subjects = 232 control, 304 CD, 270 UC.
Source: Trachtenberg et al. (2000) with permission.

also associated with a subset of CD patients characterized by an earlier age of onset of CD and no expression of pANCA combined with a high expression of ASCA (Taylor et al., 2000). These observations suggest that either the *Notch4* gene itself or a gene close by may also determine one of the subtypes of CD.

Tumor necrosis factor. Tumor necrosis factor (TNF) is involved in the regulation of inflammation at many levels; of particular interest for IBD is the role of TNF in the recruitment of circulating inflammatory cells to local tissue sites and in granuloma formation. An important role for TNF as a pro-inflammatory cytokine in CD has emerged in recent years (Van Deventer, 1997), and this pivotal role is prominent in the mouse models of intestinal inflammation that are the result of the alteration of the regulation of the TNF gene (reviewed above) and in the success of the use of anti-TNF antibody in the treatment of moderate to severe CD (Targan et al., 1997).

The genes for three members of the TNF superfamily—tumor necrosis factor (TNF), lymphotoxin-α (LTA) and lymphotoxin-β (LTB)—are located adjacent to each other at the border between the class III and class I region of the MHC (Bazzoni and Beutler, 1996; MHC Sequencing Consortium, 1999). Several studies have observed an association between polymorphisms in this region and (1) changes in TNF expression (Kroeger et al., 1997; Louis et al., 1998), (2) altered immune response to infectious diseases (McGuire et al., 1994, 1999; Wilson et al., 1995; Nadel et al., 1996; Hohler et al., 1998), and (3) increased joint damage in rheumatoid arthritis (Kaijzel et al., 1998). Five microsatellite markers, denoted as TNFa–e, broadly encompass this region (Nedospasov et al., 1991; Iris et al., 1993; Udalova et al., 1993; Kaijzel et al., 1998). The authors have observed an association between a haplotype of these microsatellite markers and CD (Plevy et al., 1996). TNF promoter polymorphisms have also been associated with CD (Kinouchi et al., 2000; Bonen et al., 2000). Two of the authors' recent observations suggest that genetic variation in the TNF region may determine the course of disease in subsets of IBD: (1) a haplotype in the LTA region may be associated with a lack of response to anti-TNF therapy in a group of patients with moderate to severe CD (Taylor et al., 2001); and (2) TNF microsatellite a is associated with the level of expression of ASCA antibody (Taylor et al., 1998).

Other Observed Associations

Interleukin 1-β and Interleukin 1 Receptor Antagonist. The interleukin 1 (IL1) family consists of three related proteins: interleukin 1-α (ILA), interleukin 1-β (IL1B), and interleukin 1 receptor antagonist (IL-1RA). The genes for all three proteins are located together on chromosome 2q14 but not within any region of linkage observed in genome scans (Table 15–14). IL-1A and IL-1B are cytokines with a wide spectrum of pro-inflammatory actions in many cell types, and IL-1RA inhibits the action of IL1A and IL1B by blocking the interleukin 1 receptor (Dinarello and Wolff, 1993). When these cytokines were measured in freshly isolated intestinal mucosal cells from IBD patients and controls, an imbalance in the ratio of IL-1 to IL-1RA was observed in both CD and UC patients, with the ratio correlating closely with the clinical severity of disease (Casini-Raggi et al., 1995). This observation was confirmed using biopsies from the inflamed mucosa of IBD patients (Andus et al., 1997). Further, removal of IL1RA by treating animals with anti-IL1RA or by gene knockout increases susceptibility to experimentally induced colitis (Ferretti et al., 1994). These observations support the hypothesis that an imbalance between IL-1 and IL-1 receptor antagonist is important in the etiology of IBD (Tountas et al., 1999; Dinarello, 2000).

The authors and others have observed an association between the IL1RA gene and UC, with an increased frequency of allele 2 of an 86 bp variable number of tandem repeats (VNTR) polymorphism in intron 2 of the IL1RA gene in UC (Mansfield et al., 1994; Tountas et al., 1999). The authors observed this increased frequency in patients from the Los Angeles area, particularly in a subset of UC patients from the Ashkenazi Jewish population, but not in patients from Milan. Biopsies from IBD patients with this genotype have a slight reduction of IL1-RA (Andus et al., 1997). These results suggest that genetic variation in the IL1RA gene may alter the ratio between interleukin 1 and its receptor antagonist and thus contribute to susceptibility to IBD. An association between polymorphisms in the IL1RA gene have been observed in some but not all subsequent studies (Louis et al., 1996; Heresbach et al., 1997; Stokkers et al., 1998; Nemetz et al., 1999a,b). Furthermore, some evidence supports the concept that IL1RA polymorphisms may also participate in determining the course and severity of IBD: for one, a significant association has been observed between two polymorphisms in the interleukin 1-β gene (IL1B; variants at -511 in the promoter and in exon 5) and nonperforating CD but not with perforating-fistulizing disease (Nemetz et al., 1999b), and for another, the IL1RA allele 2 has a higher frequency in surgically treated UC patients than in nonsurgically treated patients or controls (Heresbach et al., 1997). When taken together, the evidence supports an association between polymorphisms in the IL1RA gene and both CD and UC; the differences in these reports may be due to inadequate sample size and/or ethnic variation.

Intercellular Adhesion Molecule 1. Intercellular adhesion molecule 1 (ICAM1) is involved in one of the several steps of the normal capture and migration of leukocytes from the blood stream to the site of inflammation (Etzioni, 1996; Vainer, 1997). Several observations suggest that ICAM1 plays a direct role in IBD:

1. In mucosa taken from IBD patients and controls, a massive infiltration of ICAM1 positive cells has been correlated with the amount of inflammation in IBD (Nakamura et al., 1993), and the concentration of ICAM1 is significantly elevated in CD and UC patients and is also higher in active UC than in inactive UC (Vainer and Nielsen, 2000).
2. Plasma-soluble ICAM1 is also higher in patients with active UC, pouchitis, and CD (Patel et al., 1995).
3. Anti-ICAM treatment of rats reduces intestinal inflammation in the acetic acid–induced model of colitis (Wong et al., 1995).

The ICAM1 G241R polymorphism has been tested for association to IBD and the frequency of the mutant allele was higher for the ANCA-negative UC and for ANCA-positive CD subsets of disease, but not for CD or UC as a whole when compared with controls (H. Yang et al., 1995). This polymorphism may therefore play a role in determining the disease course of subsets of IBD. A negative result was reported for ANCA-negative UC (Hirv et al., 1999), but it should also be noted that the method of ANCA determination is not uniform worldwide. As discussed above, ICAM1 is located within the chromosome 19 linkage peak (see Table 15–14).

Interferon Gamma Receptor Subunit 1. Mutations in the interferon-γ receptor subunit 1 gene (IFNGR1) have been associated with impaired response to interferon-γ (Altare et al., 1998; Jouanguy et al., 2000) and susceptibility to mycobacterial infection (Newport et al., 1996; Jouanguy et al., 1997, 1999). The authors have observed an association between a polymorphism in this gene and the development of chronic pouchitis in UC patients who have undergone ileal-pouch anal anastomosis surgery (Fleshner et al., 2000). This observation raises the intriguing possibility that this receptor plays a role in determining the course of severe forms of UC. This gene is located in a peak of linkage to IBD (Ma et al., 1999).

Prothrombotic Gene Variants. Since IBD patients are also at a greater risk for thrombosis, the most frequent hereditary prothrombotic mutations have been tested for association with IBD. Currently, the results are contradictory, probably due to the small sample sizes of some of the studies and to geographic and ethnic differences. As in other diseases, the Factor V Leiden mutation seems to confer a higher relative risk for venous thrombosis in IBD patients. The thermolabile variant of the methylene tetrahydrofolate reductase gene (MTHFR C677T) was associated with IBD and probably accounts for a higher plasma homocysteine concentration in IBD patients than in controls (Mahmud et al., 1999). Negative results have been reported for the following genetic variants: Factor V Leiden (Helio et al., 1999; Vecchi et al., 2000). Factor XIII val34leu (Helio et al., 1999), the thermolabile variant of the methylene tetrahydrofolate reductase gene (MTHFR C677T), and prothrombin (Vecchi et al., 2000).

Natural Resistance-Associated Macrophage Protein 1 (NRAMP1). The NRAMP1 gene may be an important gene controlling response to infection by pathogens, particularly to *Mycobacteria* spp. (Govoni and Gros, 1998; Bellamy, 1999, 2000). An association has been observed between CD and a haplotype composed of two markers that flank NRAMP1—D2S434 and D2S1323 (Hofmeister et al., 1997). A negative result has also been reported (Stokkers et al., 2000).

In summary, the linkage data clearly identify specific genetic loci as contributing to the etiology of IBD. At least four, and likely more, loci can be identified from the current data. In moving from linkage to positional candidates, the best available data are for genes in both the MHC class II and in the border between the MHC class II and class III regions. Other candidate genes have been studied from function hypotheses (as has the MHC class II and TNF), and the best established of these is the interleukin receptor 1 family cluster.

CLINICAL APPLICATION OF GENETIC INFORMATION

In general, the genetic information described here is not yet used in clinical practice. Typing for ANCA and ASCA is on the verge of being used to diagnose CD vs. UC and in clarifying the cases of "indeterminate colitis." At the current time, genetic markers are not used diagnostically. As for the serum antibody markers pANCA and ASCA, they can be used in diagnosis. Even though they are found at increased risk in relatives, screening relatives clinically is not recommended as there is no recognized intervention. Counseling is based on empiric risks, which were reviewed in family epidemiology and are for the most part modest.

In the long term, genotyping patients for CD- and UC-associated genes will enable the determination of risk to relatives of IBD patients and of the optimal therapy for each individual; identifying the genes that predispose to each pathogenetic mechanism of IBD will point research into new directions to develop therapies and will enable the construction of mouse models for testing those therapies before starting clinical trials. The use of this genetic information in the nearest term is perhaps suggested by several preliminary IBD pharmacogenetic studies.

Since glucocorticoids are known substrates for a drug efflux pump protein (P-glycoprotein 170) expressed by the multidrug resistance gene (MDR), Farrell and coworkers (2000) compared the expression of this pump on the surface of lymphocytes obtained from IBD patients and controls, and observed that MDR expression was significantly elevated in CD and UC patients who required surgery because they failed medical therapy. This observation suggests that a genetic variation that affects the pharmacology of steroids may lead to the ineffectiveness of these drugs in some IBD patients. Inflammation of the large intestine has been observed in a mouse knockout of this gene, and this observation raises the possibility that MDR plays a more direct role in intestinal inflammation as well (Panwala et al., 1998).

Clinical response to 6-mercaptopurine (6-MP) depends on its conversion to 6-thioguanine (6-TG) and reaching a TG level greater than 235 (pmol/8 $\times 10^{-8}$ erythrocytes) (Dubinsky et al., 2000). Patients heterozygous for mutations that reduce the level of the enzyme thiopurine methyltransferase (TPMT) are able to attain this therapeutic level more readily on a given dose of 6-MP, because the drug is not converted into inactive nucleotides by this enzyme (e.g., 6-methylmercaptopurine or 6-MMP). These results suggest that TPMT genotyping may assist the clinician in optimizing the therapeutic response to 6-MP and in identifying individuals at increased risk for drug-induced toxicity.

Patients in the original clinical trial of the anti-TNF antibody were also typed for ANCA status and genotyped in the TNF region of the MHC. The response of pANCA patients was the lowest and not significantly different from placebo, and the response of sANCA patients (a different type of staining from pANCA) was the highest in this study. Homozygotes for the LTA NcoI-TNFc-aa13L-aa26 haplotype "1-1-1-1" did not respond to treatment. While these results must be interpreted with a great deal of caution because of the many comparisons made in this small study, these results raise the intriguing possibility that sANCA may identify a CD subgroup with a better response to Infliximab and that pANCA and homozygosity for the LTA "1-1-1-1" haplotype may identify CD subgroups with a poorer response.

While these studies are all recent, they each raise the possibility that the use of specific genetic markers, involved in either metabolism of the therapeutic agent or in the susceptibility to a form of IBD, may well guide therapy in the not too distant future.

GLOSSARY

ANCA	antineutrophil cytoplasmic antibody
AS	ankylosing spondylitis
ASCA	anti-*Saccharomyces cerevisiae* antibody
CD	Crohn's disease
cM	centiMorgan
HLA	human leukocyte antigen
HPS	Hermansky-Pudlak syndrome

IBD	inflammatory bowel disease
ICAM1	intracellular adhesion molecule 1
IFNG	interferon-γ
IL	interleukin
IL1RA	interleukin 1 receptor antagonist
IPAA	ileal pouch–anal anastomosis
LTA	lymphotoxin α
LTB	lymphotoxin β
MHC	major histocompatibility complex
MLS	multipoint LOD score
MTHFR	methylene tetrahydrofolate reductase
MUC3	mucin 3
NPL	nonparametric linkage score
NRAMP1	natural resistance–associated macrophage protein 1
pANCA	ANCA with perinuclear staining on indirect immunofluorescence
PSC	primary sclerosing cholangitis
SCID	severe combined immunodeficincy
TCR	T cell receptor
TGF	transforming growth factor
TNF	tumor necrosis factor
TNR	trinucleotide repeat
UC	ulcerative colitis
VNTR	variable number of tandem repeats

REFERENCES

Abreau MT, Taylor KD, Lin YC, Hang T, Gaiennie J, Vasiliauskas EA, Kam LY, Rojany M, Papadakis K, Rotter JI, Targan SR, Yang H: Mutations in NOD2 are associated with fibrostenosing disease in patients with Crohn's disease (CD). Gastroenterology 2002; 122:A108345.

Ahrenstedt O, Knutson L, Nisson B, Nilsson-Ekdahl K, Odlind B, Hallgren R: Enhanced local production of complement components in the small intestines of patients with Crohn's disease. N Engl J Med 1990; 322:1345–1349.

Altare F, Jouanguy E, Lamhamedi-Cherradi S, Fondaneche M C, Fizame C, Ribierre F, Merlin G, Dembic Z, Schreiber R, Lisowska-Grospierre B, et al.: A causative relationship between mutant IFNGR1 alleles and impaired cellular response to IFNG in a compound heterozygous child. Am J Hum Genet 1998; 62:723–726.

Amelio RD, Rossi P, Moli SLE, Ricci R, Montano S, Pallone F: In vitro studies on cellular and humoral chemotaxis in Crohn's disease using the under agarose gel technique. Gut 1981; 22:566–570.

Ament ME, Ochs HD: Gastrointestinal manifestations of chronic granulomatous disease. N Engl J Med 1973; 288:382–387.

Andus T, Daig R, Vogl D, Aschenbrenner E, Lock G, Hollerbach S, Kollinger M, Scholmerich J, Gross V: Imbalance of the interleukin 1 system in colonic mucosa: association with intestinal inflammation and interleukin 1 receptor antagonist genotype 2. Gut 1997; 41:651–657.

Artavanis-Tsakonas S, Rand MD, Lake RJ: Notch signaling: cell fate control and signal integration in development. Science 1999; 284:770–776.

Asakura H, Tsuchiya M, Aiso S, Watanabe M, Kobayashi K, Hibi T, Ando K, Takata H, Sekiguchi S: Association of the human lymphocyte-DR2 antigen with Japanese ulcerative colitis. Gastroenterology 1982; 82:413–418.

Asseman C, Mauze S, Leach MW, Coffman RL, Powrie F: An essential role for interleukin 10 in the function of regulatory T cells that inhibit intestinal inflammation. J Exp Med 1999; 190:995–1004.

Bayless TM, Tokayer AZ, Polito JM, Quaskey SA, Mellits ED, Harris ML: Crohn's disease: concordance for site and clinical type in affected family members—potential hereditary influences. Gastroenterology 1996; 111:573–579.

Bayraktar Y, Arslan S, Saglam F, Uzunalimoglu B, Kayhan B: What is the association of primary sclerosing cholangitis with sex and inflammatory bowel disease in Turkish patients? Hepato-Gastroenterol 1998; 45:2064–2072.

Bazzoni F, Beutler B: The tumor necrosis factor ligand and receptor families. N Engl J Med 1996; 334:1717–1725.

Becker KG, Simon RM, Biddison WE, Bailey-Wilson JE, McFarland HF, Trent JM: Clustering of non-MHC susceptibility candidate loci in human autoimmune diseases. Am J Hum Genet 1997; 61:A267.

Bellamy R: The natural resistance-associated macrophage protein and susceptibility to intracellular pathogens. Microbes Infect 1999; 1:23–27.

Bellamy R: Identifying genetic susceptibility factors for tuberculosis in Africans: a combined approach using a candidate gene study and a genome-wide screen. Clin Sci 2000; 98:245–250.

Bennett RA, Rubin PH, Present DH: Frequency of inflammatory bowel disease in offspring of couples both presenting with inflammatory bowel disease. Gastroenterology 1991; 100:1638–1643.

Berg DJ, Davidson N, Kuhn R, Muller W, Menon S, Holland G, Thompson-Snipes L, Leach MW, Rennick D: Enterocolitis and colon cancer in interleukin-10-deficient mice are associated with aberrant cytokine production and CD4(+) TH1-like responses. J Clin Invest 1996; 98:1010–1020.

Bernstein CN, Blanchard JF, Rawsthorne P, Wajda A: Epidemiology of Crohn's disease and ulcerative colitis in a central Canadian province: a population-based study. Am J Epidemiol 1999; 149:916–924.

Bhalerao J, Bowcock AM: The genetics of psoriasis: a complex disorder of the skin and immune system. Hum Mol Genet 1998; 7:1537–1545.

Biemond I, Delange GG, Weterman IT, Pena AS: Immunoglobulin allotypes in Crohn's disease in the Netherlands. Gut 1987; 28:610–612.

Binder V: Genetic epidemiology in inflammatory bowel disease. Dig Dis 1998; 16:351–355.

Bjarnason I, Smethurst P, Levi AJ, Menzies IS, Peters TJ: The effect of polyacrylic acid polymers on small-intestinal function and permeability changes caused by indomethacin. Scand J Gastroenterol 1991; 26:685–688.

Bjerke K, Brandtzaeg P, Rognum TO: Distribution of immunoglobulin producing cells is different in normal human appendix and colon mucosa. Gut 1986; 27:667–674.

Bonen DK, Ramos R, Lee S, Corradino S, Britton HM, Kirschner BS, Brant SR, Hanauer SB, Cho JH: Characterization of genomic and functional variation throughout the TNF gene in patients with IBD. Gastroenterology 2000; 118:A330–A331.

Botto M, Fong KY, So AK, Koch C, Walport MJ: Molecular basis of polymorphisms of human complement component C3. J Exp Med 1990; 172:1011–1017.

Bouma G, Crusius JB, Garcia-Gonzalez MA, Meijer BU, Hellemans HP, Hakvoort RJ, Schreuder GM, Kostense PJ, Meuwissen SG, Pena AS: Genetic markers in clinically well defined patients with ulcerative colitis (UC). Clin Exp Immunol 1999; 115:294–300.

Bouma G, Oudkerk Pool M, Crusius JB, Schreuder GM, Hellemans HP, Meijer BU, Kostense PJ, Giphart MJ, Meuwissen SG, Pena AS: Evidence for genetic heterogeneity in inflammatory bowel disease (IBD): HLA genes in the predisposition to suffer from ulcerative colitis (UC) and Crohn's disease (CD). Clin Exp Immunol 1997; 109:175–179.

Brahme F, Lindstrom G, Wenckert A: Crohn's disease in a defined population. Gastroenterology 1975; 69:342–351.

Brant SR, Fu Y, Fields CT, Baltazar R, Ravenhill G, Pickles M, Rohal P, Mann J, Kirschner BS, Jabs EW, et al.: American families with Crohn's disease have strong evidence for linkage to chromosome 16 but not chromosome 12. Gastroenterology 1998; 115:1056–1061.

Brant SR, Panhuysen C, Bailey-Wilson J, Lee S, Mann J, Rohal PM, Picco MF, Kirschner B, Hanauer SB, Cho JH, Bayless TM: Crohn's disease diagnosis before age 22 and with greater severity of disease identifies multiplex pedigrees at greater risk for locus IBD1. Gastroenterology 2000; 118:A708.

Breen EG, Coughlan G, Connolly CE, Stevens FM: Coeliac proctitis. Scand J Gastroenterol 1987; 22:471–477.

Broman KW, Murray JC, Shefield VC, White RL, Weber JL: Comprehensive human genetic maps: individual and sex-specific variation in recombination. Am J Hum Genet 1998; 63:861–869.

Brook JD, McCurrach ME, Harley HG, Buckler AJ, Church D, Aburantani H, Hunter K: Molecular basis of myotonic dystrophy: expansion of a trinucleotide (CTG) repeat at the 3′ end of a transcript encoding a protein kinase family member. Cell 1992; 68:799–808.

Broome U, Lofberg R, Lundqvist K, Veress B: Subclinical time span of inflammatory bowel disease in patients with primary sclerosing cholangitis. Dis Colon Rectum 1995; 38:1301–1305.

Brunello F, Pera A, Martini S, Marino L, Astegiano M, Barletti C, Gastaldi P, Verme G, Emanuelli G: Antibodies to *Mycobacterium paratuberculosis* in patients with Crohn's disease. Dig Dis Sci 1991; 36:1741–1745.

Cahill RJ, Foltz CJ, Fox JG, Dangler CA, Powrie F, Schauer DB: Inflammatory bowel disease: an immunity-mediated condition triggered by bacterial infection with *Helicobacter hepaticus*. Infect Immun 1997; 65:3126–3131.

Calkins BM: A meta-analysis of the role of smoking in inflammatory bowel disease. Dig Dis Sci 1989; 34:1841–1854.

Cariappa A, Sands B, Forcione D, Finkelstein D, Podolsky DK, Pillai S: Analysis of MHC class II DP, DQ and DR alleles in Crohn's disease. Gut 1998; 43:210–215.

Caruso ML, Cristofaro G, Lynch HT: HNPCC-Lynch syndrome and idiopathic inflammatory bowel disease: a hypothesis on sharing of genes. Anticancer Res 1997; 17:2647–2649.

Casini-Raggi V, Kam L, Chong YJ, Fiocchi C, Pizarro TT, Cominelli F: Mucosal imbalance of IL-1 and IL-1 receptor antagonist in inflammatory bowel disease: a novel mechanism of chronic intestinal inflammation. J Immunol 1995; 154:2434–2440.

Cavanaugh JA, Callen DF, Wilson SR, Stanford PM, Sraml ME, Gorska M, Crawford J, Whitmore SA, Shlegel C, Foote S, et al.: Analysis of Australian Crohn's disease pedigrees refines the localization for susceptibility to inflammatory bowel disease on chromosome 16. Ann Hum Genet 1998; 62:291–298.

Chapman RW, Arborgh BA, Rhodes JM, Summerfield JA, Dick R, Scheuer PJ, Sherlock S: Primary sclerosing cholangitis: a review of its clinical features, cholangiography, and hepatic histology. Gut 1980; 21:870–877.

Chapman RW, Cottone M, Selby WS, Shepherd HA, Sherlock S, Jewell DP: Serum autoantibodies, ulcerative colitis and primary sclerosing cholangitis. Gut 1986; 27:86–91.

Cho JH, Fu Y, Kirschner BS, Hanauer SB: Confirmation of a susceptibility locus for Crohn's disease on chromosome 16. Inflamm Bowel Dis 1997; 3:186–190.

Cho JH, Nicolae DL, Gold LH, Fields CT, LaBuda MC, Rohal PM, Pichles MR, Qin L, Fu Y, Mann JS, et al.: Identification of novel susceptibility loci for inflammatory bowel disease on chromosomes 1p, 3q, and 4q: evidence for epistasis between 1p and *IBD1*. Proc Natl Acad Sci USA 1998; 95:7502–7507.

Cho JH, Nicolae DL, Ramos R, Fields CT, Rabenau K, Corradino S, Brant SR, Espinosa R, LeBeau M, Hanauer SB, et al.: Linkage and linkage disequilibrium in chromosome band 1p36 in American Chaldeans with inflammatory bowel disease. Hum Mol Genet 2000; 9:1425–1432.

Colombel JF, Grandbastien B, Gower-Rousseau B, Plegat S, Evrard JP, Dupas JL, Gendre JP, Modigliani R, Belaiche J, Hostein J, et al.: Clinical characteristics of Crohn's disease in 72 families. Gastroenterology 1996; 111:604–607.

Comes MC, Gower-Rousseau C, Colombel JF, Belaiche J, Van Kruiningen HJ, Nuttens MC, Cortot A: Inflammatory bowel disease in married couples: 10 cases in Nord Pas de Calais region of France and Liege county of Belgium. Gut 1994; 35:1316–1318.

Cominelli F, Kontoyiannis D, Pizarro T, Kollias G: Contribution of TNF receptor (TNFR) types and T lymphocyte population to the pathogenesis of experimental Crohn's disease (CD) in TNF^{DARE} mutant mice. Gastroenterology 1999; 116:A690.

Compton RF, Sandborn WJ, Yang H, Lindor NM, Tremaine WJ, Davis MD, Khalil AA, Tountas NA, Tyan DB, Landers CJ, et al.: A new syndrome of Crohn's disease and pachydermoperiostosis in a family. Gastroenterology 1997; 112:241–249.

Cottone M, Brignola C, Rosselli M, Oliva L, Belloli C, Cipolla C, Orlando A, De Simone G, Aiala M, Di Mitri R, et al.: Relationship between site of disease and familial occurrence in Crohn's disease. Dig Dis Sci 1997; 42:129–132.

Cottone M, Cappello M, Puleo A, Cipolla C, Filippazzo MG: Familial association of Crohn's and coeliac diseases. Lancet 1989; 2:338.

Couper R, Kapelushnik J, Griffiths AM: Neutrophil dysfunction in glycogen storage disease IB: association with Crohn's-like colitis. Gastroenterology 1991; 100:549–554.

Curran ME, Lau KF, Hampe J, Schreiber S, Bridger S, Macpherson AJ, Cardon LR, Sakul H, Harris TJ, Stokkers P, et al.: Genetic analysis of inflammatory bowel disease in a large European cohort supports linkage to chromosomes 12 and 16. Gastroenterology 1998; 115:1066–1071.

D'Agata ID, Paradis K, Chad Z, Bonny Y, Seidman E: Leucocyte adhesion deficiency presenting as a chronic ileocolitis. Gut 1996; 39:5–8.

Daly MJ, Rioux JD, Scaffner SF, Hudson TJ, Lander ES: High-resolution haplotype structure in the human genome. Nat Genet 2001; 29:229–232.

Danze PM, Colombel JF, Jacquot S, Loste MN, Heresbach D, Ategbo S, Khamassi S, Perichon B, Semana G, Charron D, Cezard JP: Association of HLA class II genes with susceptibility to Crohn's disease. Gut 1996; 39:69–72.

Das KM, Vecchi M, Sakamaki S: A shared and unique epitope(s) on human colon, skin, and biliary epithelium detected by a monoclonal antibody. Gastroenterology 1990; 98:464–469.

Davidson NJ, Leach MW, Fort MM, Thompson-Snipes L, Kuhn R, Muller W, Berg DJ, Rennick DM: T helper cell 1-type $CD4^+$ T cells, but not B cells, mediate colitis in interleukin 10-deficient mice. J Exp Med 1996; 184:241–251.

De Keyser F, Elewaut D, De Vos M, De Vlam K, Cuvelier C, Mielants H, Veys EM: Bowel inflammation and the spondyloarthropathies. Rheum Dis Clin North Am 1998; 24:785–813.

Dekker-Saeys BJ, Meuwissen SG, Van Den Berg-Loonen EM, De Haas WH, Meijers KA, Tytgat GN: Ankylosing spondylitis and inflammatory bowel disease: III. Clinical characteristics and results of histocompatibility typing (HLA B27) in 50 patients with both ankylosing spondylitis and inflammatory bowel disease. Ann Rheum Dis 1978; 37:36–41.

De Vos M, Mielants H, Cuvelier C, Elewaut A, Veys E: Long-term evolution of gut inflammation in patients with spondyloarthropathy. Gastroenterology 1996; 110:1696–1703.

De Winter H, Cheroutre H, Kronenberg M: Mucosal immunity and inflammation: II. The yin and yang of T cells in intestinal inflammation: pathogenic and protective roles in a mouse colitis model. Am J Physiol 1999; 276:G1317–1321.

Diamond JM, Rotter JI: Observing the founder effect in human evolution. Nature 1987; 329:105–106.

Dianda L, Hanby AM, Wright NA, Sebesteny A, Hayday AC, Owen MJ: T cell receptor-α β-deficient mice fail to develop colitis in the absence of a microbial environment. Am J Pathol 1997; 150:91–97.

Dinarello CA: The role of the interleukin-1-receptor antagonist in blocking inflammation mediated by interleukin-1. N Engl J Med 2000; 343:732–734.

Dinarello CA, Wolff SM: The role of interleukin-1 in disease. N Engl J Med 1993; 328:106–113.

Donaldson PT: Dual association of HLA-DR2 and -DR3 with primary sclerosing cholangitis. Hepatology 1991; 13:129–133.

Dozois RR, Kelly KA, Welling DR, Gordon H, Beart RW Jr, Wolff BG, Pemberton JH, Ilstrup DM: Ileal pouch–anal anastomosis: comparison of results in familial adenomatous polyposis and chronic ulcerative colitis. Ann Surg 1989; 210:268–271.

Dubinsky MC, Lamothe S, Yang HY, Targan SR, Sinnett D, Theoret Y, Seidman EG: Pharmacogenomics and metabolite measurement for 6-mercaptopurine therapy in inflammatory bowel disease. Gastroenterology 2000; 118:705–713.

Duerr RH, Barmada MM, Zhang L, Davis S, Preston RA, Chensny LJ, Brown JL, Ehrlich GD, Weeks DE, Aston CE: Linkage and association between inflammatory bowel disease and a locus on chromosome 12. Am J Hum Genet 1998; 63:95–100.

Duerr RH, Barmada MM, Zhang L, Pfutzer R, Weeks DE: High-density genome scan in Crohn disease shows confirmed linkage to chromosome 14q11–12. Am J Hum Genet 2000; 66:1857–1862.

Duerr RH, Neigut DA: Molecularly defined HLA-DR2 alleles in ulcerative colitis and an antineutrophil cytoplasmic antibody-positive subgroup. Gastroenterology 1995; 108:423–427.

Duerr RH, Targan SR, Landers CJ, Sutherland LR, Shanahan F: Anti-neutrophil cytoplasmic-antibodies in ulcerative colitis: comparison with other colitides/diarrheal illnesses. Gastroenterology 1991; 100:1590–1596.

Dumonceau JM, Van Gossum A, Adler M, Fonteyne PA, Van Vooren JP, Deviere J, Portaels F: No *Mycobacterium paratuberculosis* found in Crohn's disease using polymerase chain reaction. Dig Dis Sci 1996; 41:421–426.

Ehrhardt RO, Ludviksson BR, Gray B, Neurath M, Strober W: Induction and prevention of colonic inflammation in IL-2 deficient mice. J Immunol 1997; 158:566–573.

Elmgreen J, Berkowicz A, Sorensen H: Hypercatabolism of complement in Crohn's disease. Acta Med Scand 1983; 214:403–407.

Elmgreen J, Both H, Binder V: Familal occurrence of complement dysfunction in Crohn's disease: correlation with intestinal symptoms and hypercatabolism of complement. Gut 1985; 26:151–157.

Elmgreen J, Sorensen H, Berkowicz A: Polymorphism of complement C3 in chronic inflammatory bowel disease: predominance of the C3F gene in Crohn's disease. Acta Med Scand 1984; 215:375–378.

Elson CO, Cong Y, Brandwein S, Weaver CT, McCabe RP, Mahler M, Sundberg JP, Leiter EH: Experimental models to study molecular mechanisms underlying intestinal inflammation. Ann NY Acad Sci 1998; 859:85–95.

Elson CO, Sartor RB, Tennyson GS, Riddell RH: Experimental models of inflammatory bowel disease. Gastroenterology 1995; 109:1344–1367.

Eng C, Farraye FA, Shulman LN, Peppercorn MA, Krauss CM, Connors JM, Stone RM: The association between the myelodysplastic syndromes and Crohn disease. Ann Intern Med 1992; 117:661–662.

Esaki M, Furuse M, Matsumoto T, Aoyagi K, Jo Y, Yamagata H, Nakano H, Fujishima M: Polymorphism of heat-shock protein gene HSP70-2 in Crohn disease: possible genetic marker for two forms of Crohn disease. Scand J Gastroenterol 1999; 34:703–707.

Etzioni A: Adhesion molecules: their role in health and disease. Pediatr Res 1996; 39:191–198.

Farrell RJ, Murphy A, Long A, Donnelly S, Cherikuri A, O'Toole D, Mahmud N, Keeling PW, Weir DG, Kelleher D: High multidrug resistance (P-glycoprotein 170) expression in inflammatory bowel disease patients who fail medical therapy. Gastroenterology 2000; 118:279–288.

Ferretti M, Casini-Raggi V, Pizarro TT, Eisenberg SP, Nast CC, Cominelli F: Neutralization of endogenous IL-1 receptor antagonist exacerbates and prolongs inflammation in rabbit immune colitis. J Clin Invest 1994; 94:449–453.

Field LL, Boyd N, Bowen TJ, Kelly JK, Sutherland LR: Genetic markers and inflammatory bowel disease: immunoglobulin allotypes (GM, KM) and protease inhibitor. Am J Gastroenterol 1989; 84:753–755.

Fielding JF: The relative risk of inflammatory bowel disease among parents and siblings of Crohn's disease patients. J Clin Gastroenterol 1986; 8:655–657.

Fiocchi C, Roche JK, Michener WM: High prevalence of antibodies to intestinal epithelial antigens in patients with inflammatory bowel disease and their relatives. Ann Intern Med 1989; 110:786–794.

Fleshner PR, Taylor KD, Yang H, Lin Y-C, Vasiliauskas EA, Targan SR, Rotter JI: Chronic pouchitis after ileal pouch–anal anastomosis for ulcerative colitis (UC) is associated with the interferon-γ receptor α-gene independent of perinuclear antineutrophil cytoplasmic antibody (pANCA) level. Gastroenterology 2000; 118:A338.

Folwaczny C, Noehl N, Endres SP, Heldwein W, Loeschke K, Fricke H: Antinuclear autoantibodies in patients with inflammatory bowel disease: high prevalence in first-degree relatives. Dig Dis Sci 1997; 42:1593–1597.

Forcione DG, Sands B, Isselbacher KJ, Rustgi A, Podolsky DK, Pillai S: An increased risk of Crohn's disease in individuals who inherit the HLA class II DRB3*0301 allele. Proc Natl Acad Sci USA 1996; 93:5094–5098.

Fort MM, Leach MW, Rennick DM: A role for NK cells as regulators of $CD4^+$ T cells in a transfer model of colitis. J Immunol 1998; 161:3256–3261.

Fraser FC: Trinucleotide repeats are not the only cause of genetic anticipation. Am J Med Genet 1997; 75:337.

Fukushima K: Immunohistochemical chracterization, distribution, and ultrastructure of lymphocytes bearing T-cell receptors in inflammatory bowel disease. Gastroenterology 1991; 101:670–678.

Futami S, Aoyama N, Honsako Y, Tamura T, Morimoto S, Nakashima T, Ohmoto A, Okano H, Miyamoto M, Inaba H, et al.: HLA-DRB1*1502 allele, subtype of DR15, is associated with susceptibility to ulcerative colitis and its progression. Dig Dis Sci 1995; 40:814–818.

Gahl WA, Brantly M, Kaiser-Kupfer MI, Iwata F, Hazelwood S, Shotelersuk V, Duffy LF, Kuehl EM, Troendle J, Bernardini I: Genetic defects and clinical characteristics of patients with a form of oculocutaneous albinism (Hermansky-Pudlak syndrome). N Engl J Med 1998; 338:1258–1264.

Galeazzi F, Blennerhassett PA, Qiu B, O'Byrne PM, Collins SM: Cigarette smoke aggravates experimental colitis in rats. Gastroenterology 1999; 117:877–883.

Gardner JM, Wildenberg SC, Keiper NM, Novak EK, Rusiniak ME, Swank RT, Puri N, Finger JN, Hagiwara N, Lehman AL, et al.: The mouse pale ear (ep) mutation is the homologue of human Hermansky-Pudlak syndrome. Proc Natl Acad Sci USA 1997; 94:9238–9243.

Gent AE, Hellier MD, Grace RH, Swarbrick ET, Coggon D: Inflammatory bowel disease and domestic hygiene in infancy. Lancet 1994; 343:766–767.

Gilat T, Grossman A, Fireman Z, Rozen P: Inflammatory bowel disease in Jews. In:

McConnell R, Rozen P, Langman M, Gilat T (eds). The Genetics and Epidemiology of Inflammatory Bowel Disease. New York: Krager, 1986:135–140.

Gilat T, Hacohen D, Lilos P, Langman MJ: Childhood factors in ulcerative colitis and Crohn's disease: an international cooperative study. Scand J Gastroenterol 1987; 22:1009–1024.

Gilberts EC, Greenstein AJ, Katsel P, Harpaz N, Greenstein RJ: Molecular evidence for two forms of Crohn disease. Proc Natl Acad Sci USA 1994; 91:12721–12724.

Gilvarry J, Keeling F, Fielding JF: Sibship Crohn's disease and ankylosing spondylitis. J Clin Gastroenterol 1990; 12:711–712.

Godet PG, May GR, Sutherland LR: Meta-analysis of the role of oral contraceptive agents in inflammatory bowel disease. Gut 1995; 37:668–673.

Govoni G, Gros P: Macrophage NRAMP1 and its role in resistance to microbial infections. Inflamm Res 1998; 47:277–284.

Grandbastien B, Peeters M, Franchimont D, Gower-Rousseau C, Speckel D, Rutgeerts P, Belaiche J, Cortot A, Vlietinck R, Colombel JF: Anticipation in familial Crohn's disease. Gut 1998; 42:170–174.

Greenberg DA, Rotter JI: Two locus models for gluten sensitive eneropathy: population genetic considerations. Am J Med Genet 1981; 8:205–214.

Greenstein AJ, Lachman P, Sachar DB, Springhorn J, Heimann T, Janowitz HD, Aufses AH Jr: Perforating and non-perforating indications for repeated operations in Crohn's disease: evidence for two clinical forms. Gut 1988; 29:588–592.

Gudjonsson H, Schanfield MS, Albertini RJ, McAuliffe TL, Beeken WL, Krawitt EL: Association and linkage studies of immunoglobulin heavy chain allotypes in inflammatory bowel disease. Tissue Antigens 1988; 31:243–249.

Hall JG: Turner syndrome. In: King RA, Rotter JI, Motulsky, AG (eds). The Genetic Basis of Common Diseases. New York: Oxford University Press, 1992:895–914.

Halstensen TS, Mollnes TE, Brandzaeg P: Persistent complement activation in submucosal blood vessels of active inflammatory bowel disease: Immunohistochemical evidence. Gastroenterology 1989; 97:10–19.

Hammer B, Ashurst P, Naish J: Diseases associated with ulcerative colitis and Crohn's disease. Gut 1968; 9:17–21.

Hammer RE, Maika SD, Richardson JA, Tang JP, Taurog JD: Spontaneous inflammatory disease in transgenic rats expressing HLA-B27 and human β_2m: an animal model of HLA-B27-associated human disorders. Cell 1990; 63:1099–1112.

Hampe J, Hermann B, Bridger S, MacPherson AJ, Mathew CG, Schreiber S: The interferon-γ gene as a positional and functional candidate gene for inflammatory bowel disease. Int J Colorectal Dis 1998; 13:260–263.

Hampe J, Heymann K, Kruis W, Raedler A, Folsch UR, Schreiber S: Anticipation in inflammatory bowel disease: a phenomenon caused by an accumulation of confounders. Am J Med Genet 2000; 92:178–183.

Hampe J, Schreiber S, Shaw SH, Lau KF, Bridger S, Macpherson AJ, Cardon LR, Sakul H, Harris TJ, Buckler A, et al.: A genomewide analysis provides evidence for novel linkages in inflammatory bowel disease in a large European cohort. Am J Hum Genet 1999a; 64:808–816.

Hampe J, Shaw SH, Saiz R, Leysens N, Lantermann A, Mascheretti S, Lynch NJ, MacPherson AJ, Bridger S, van Deventer S, et al.: Linkage of inflammatory bowel disease to human chromosome 6p. Am J Hum Genet 1999b; 65:1647–1655.

Harren M, Schonfelder G, Paul M, Horak I, Riecken EO, Wiedenmann B, John M: High expression of inducible nitric oxide synthase correlates with intestinal inflammation of interleukin-2-deficient mice. Ann NY Acad Sci 1998; 859:210–215.

Harries AD, Baird A, Rhodes J: Non-smoking: a feature of ulcerative colitis. Br Med J 1982; 284:706.

Hayward AR: Lymphoid cell development. In: Litwin SD, Scott DW, Reisfeld RA, Flaherty L, Marcus DM (eds). Human Immunogenetics. New York and Basel: Marcel Dekker, 1989:145–162.

Hazelwood S, Shotelersuk V, Wildenberg SC, Chen D, Iwata F, Kaiser-Kupfer MI, White JG, King RA, Gahl WA: Evidence for locus heterogeneity in Puerto Ricans with Hermansky-Pudlak syndrome. Am J Hum Genet 1997; 61:1088–1094.

Hebbar M, Kozlowski D, Wattel E, Mastrini S, Dievart M, Duclos B, Bonaz B, d'Almagne H, Belaiche J, Colombel JF, Fenaux P: Association between myelodysplastic syndromes and inflammatory bowel diseases: report of seven new cases and review of the literature. Leukemia 1997; 11:2188–2191.

Helgeland L, Tysk C, Jarnerot G: IgG subclass distribution in serum and rectal mucosa of monozygotic twins with or without inflammatory bowel disease. Gut 1992; 33:1358–1364.

Helio T, Wartiovaara U, Halme L, Turunen UM, Mikkola H, Palotie A, Farkkila M, Kontula K: Arg506Gln factor V mutation and Val34Leu factor XIII polymorphism in Finnish patients with inflammatory bowel disease. Scand J Gastroenterol 1999; 34:170–174.

Hellers G: Crohn's disease in Stockholm county, 1955–1974: a study of epidemiology, results of surgical treatment and long term prognosis. Acta Chir Scand 1979; 490(Suppl):1–84.

Heresbach D, Alizadeh M, Dabadie A, Le Berre N, Colombel JF, Yaouanq J, Bretagne JF, Semana G: Significance of interleukin-1β and interleukin-1 receptor antagonist genetic polymorphism in inflammatory bowel diseases. Am J Gastroenterol 1997; 92:1164–1169.

Hirv K, Seyfarth M, Uibo R, Kull K, Salupere R, Latza U, Rink L: Polymorphisms in tumour necrosis factor and adhesion molecule genes in patients with inflammatory bowel disease: associations with HLA-DR and -DQ alleles and subclinical markers. Scand J Gastroenterol 1999; 34:1025–1032.

Hodgson HJF, Potter BJ, Jewell DP: C3 metabolism in ulcerative colitis and Crohn's disease. Clin Exp Immunol 1977; 28:490–495.

Hofmeister A, Neibergs HL, Pokorny RM, Galandiuk S: The natural resistance-associated macrophage protein gene is associated with Crohn's disease. Surgery 1997; 122:173–179.

Hohler T, Kruger A, Gerken G, Schneider PM, Meyer zum Buschenfelde KH, Rittner C: Tumor necrosis factor alpha promoter polymorphism at position −238 is associated with chronic active hepatitis C infection. J Med Virol 1998; 54:173–177.

Hollander D: Permeability in Crohn's disease: altered barrier functions in health relatives? Gastroenterology 1993; 104:1848–1851.

Hollander D, Vadheim CM, Brettholtz E, Petersen GM, Delahunty T, Rotter JI: Increased intestinal permeability in Crohn's patients and their relatives: an etiological factor? Ann Intern Med 1986; 105:883–895.

Howeler CJ, Busch HFM, Geraedts JPM, Niermeijer MF, Staal A: Anticipation in myotonic dystrophy: fact or fiction? Brain 1989; 112:779–797.

Huaux JP, Fiasse R, de Bruyere M, Nigant de Deuxchaisnes C: HLA-B27 in sacroilitis. J Rheumatol 1977; 3:60–63.

Hudson M, Piasecki C, Sankey EA, Sim R, Wakefield AJ, More LJ, Sawyerr AFM, Dhillon AP, Pounder RE: A ferret model of acute multifocal gastrointestinal infarction. Gastroenterology 1992; 102:1591–1596.

Hugot JP, Laurent-Puig P, Gower-Rousseau C, Caillat-Zucman S, Beaugerie L, Dupas JL, Van Gossum A, Bonait-Pellie C, Cortot A, Thomas G: Linkage analyses of chromosome 6 loci, including HLA, in familial aggregations of Crohn disease. Am J Med Genet 1994; 52:207–213.

Hugot JP, Laurent-Puig P, Gower-Rousseau C, Olson JM, Lee JC, Beaugerie L, Naom I, Dupas JL, van Gossum A, Getaid T, et al.: Mapping of a susceptibility locus for Crohn's disease on chromosome 16 by a genome-wide nonparametric linkage analysis. Nature 1996; 379:821–823.

Hugot JP, Thomas G: Genome-wide scanning in inflammatory bowel diseases. Dig Dis 1998; 16:364–369.

Hugot JP, Zouali H, Colombel JF, Belaiche J, Cezard JP, Peeters M, Van Gossum A, Lofberg R, Pallone F, Gower-Rousseau C, et al.: Fine mapping of the inflammatory bowel disease susceptibility locus 1 (IBD1) in the pericentromeric region of chromosome 16. Gastroenterology 1998; 114:A999.

Hugot JP, Chamaillard M, Zouali H, Lesage S, Cesard JP, Belaiche J, Almer S, Tysk C, O'Morain CA, Gassull M, et al. Association of NOD2 leucine-rich repeat variants with susceptibility to Crohn's disease. Nature 2001; 411:599–603.

Huntington's Disease Collaborative Research Group: A novel gene containing a trinucleotide repeat that is expanded and unstable on Huntington's disease chromosomes. Cell 1993; 72:971–983.

The IBD International Genetics Consortium. International Collaboration Provides Convincing Linkage Replication in Complex Disease through Analysis of a Large Pooled Data Set: Crohn Disease and Chromosome 16. Am J Hum Genet 2001; 68:1165–1171.

Iris FJ, Bougueleret L, Prieur S, Caterina D, Primas G, Perrot V, Jurka J, Rodriguez-Tome P, Claverie JM, Dausset J, Cohen D: Dense Alu clustering and a potential new member of the NF-κ B family within a 90 kilobase HLA class III segment. Nat Genet 1993; 3:137–145.

Ito H, Fathman CG: CD45RBhigh CD4$^+$ T cells from IFN-γ knockout mice do not induce wasting disease. J Autoimmun 1997; 10:455–459.

Jarnerot G, Azad Khan AK, Truelove SC: The thyroid in ulcerative colitis and Crohn's disease II: thyroid enlargement and hyperthyroidism in ulcerative colitis. Acta Med Scand 1975; 197:83–87.

Jayson MIV, Salmon PR, Harrison WJ: Inflammatory bowel disease in ankylosing spondylitis. Gut 1970; 11:506–511.

Jick H, Walker AM: Cigarette smoking and ulcerative colitis. N Engl J Med 1983; 308:261–263.

Jouanguy E, Dupuis S, Pallier A, Doffinger R, Fondaneche MC, Fieschi C, Lamhamedi-Cherradi S, Altare F, Emile JF, Lutz P, et al.: In a novel form of IFN-γ receptor 1 deficiency, cell surface receptors fail to bind IFN-γ. J Clin Invest 2000; 105:1429–1436.

Jouanguy E, Lamhamedi-Cherradi S, Altare F, Fondaneche MC, Tuerlinckx D, Blanche S, Emile JF, Gaillard JL, Schreiber R, Levin M, et al.: Partial interferon-γ receptor 1 deficiency in a child with tuberculoid bacillus Calmette-Guerin infection and a sibling with clinical tuberculosis. J Clin Invest 1997; 100:2658–2664.

Jouanguy E, Lamhamedi-Cherradi S, Lammas D, Dorman SE, Fondaneche MC, Dupuis S, Doffinger R, Altare F, Girdlestone J, Emile JF, et al.: A human IFNGR1 small deletion hotspot associated with dominant susceptibility to mycobacterial infection. Nat Genet 1999; 21:370–378.

Kagnoff MF, Brown RJ, Schanfield MS: Association between Crohn's disease and immunoglobulin heavy chain (Gm) allotypes. Gastroenterology 1983; 85:1044–1047.

Kaijzel EL, van Krugten MV, Brinkman BM, Huizinga TW, van der Straaten T, Hazes JM, Ziegler-Heitbrock HW, Nedospasov SA, Breedveld FC, Verweij CL: Functional analysis of a human tumor necrosis factor-α (TNF-α) promoter polymorphism related to joint damage in rheumatoid arthritis. Mol Med 1998; 4:724–733.

Kaneko H, Yamada H, Mizuno S, Udagawa T, Kazumi Y, Sekikawa K, Sugawara I: Role of tumor necrosis factor-α in *Mycobacterium*-induced granuloma formation in tumor necrosis factor-α-deficient mice. Lab Invest 1999; 79:379–386.

Kawanishi H: Immunocompetence of normal human appendiceal lymphoid cells: in vitro studies. Immunology 1987; 60:19–28.

Kelly P, Patchett S, McCloskey D, Alstead E, Farthing M, Fairclough P: Sclerosing cholangitis, race and sex. Gut 1997; 41:688–689.

Kett K, Rognum TO, Brandtzaeg P: Mucosal subclass distribution of immunoglobulin G-producing cells is different in ulcerative colitis and Crohn's disease of the colon. Gastroenterology 1987; 93:919–924.

Khan MA: HLA-B27 and -B12 (B44) in Crohn's disease with ankylosing spondylitis. J Rheumatol 1989; 16:851–852.

King RA, Rotter JI, Motulsky AG (eds): The Genetic Basis of Common Diseases. New York: Oxford University Press, 1992.

Kinouchi Y, Simmon J, Van Heel D, Jewell DP: Polymorphism at position −1031 in the TNF gene confers susceptibility to Crohn's disease. Gastroenterology 2000; 118:A334.

Kirsner JB: Genetic aspects of inflammatory bowel disease. Clin Gastroenterol 1973; 2:557–576.

Kirsner JB: Inflammatory bowel disease: clinical, etiological and genetic aspects. In: Rotter JI, Samloff IM, Rimoin DL (eds). Genetics and Heterogeneity of Common Gastrointestinal Disorders. New York: Academic Press, 1980:261–280.

Kirsner JB, Spencer JA: Family occurrences of ulcerative colitis, regional enteritis and ileocolitis. Ann Intern Med 1963; 59:539–546.

Kitchin LI, Knobler RL, Friedman LS: Crohn's disease in a patient with multiple sclerosis. J Clin Gastroenterol 1991; 13:331–334.

Kontoyiannis D, Pasparakis M, Pizarro TT, Cominelli F, Kollias G: Impaired on/off regulation of TNF biosynthesis in mice lacking TNF AU-rich elements: implications for joint and gut-associated immunopathologies. Immunity 1999; 10:387–398.

Korelitz BI: From Crohn to Crohn's disease: An epidemiologic study in New York City. Mt Sinai J Med 1979; 46:533–540.

Krawiec J, Odes HSL, Krugliak P, Weitzman S: Aspects of the epidemiology of Crohn's disease in the Jewish population in Beer Sheva, Israel. Israel J Med Sci 1984; 20:16–21.

Kroeger KM, Carville KS, Abraham LJ: The −308 tumor necrosis factor-α promoter polymorphism effects transcription. Mol Immunol 1997; 34:391–399.

Kuhn R, Lohler J, Rennick D, Rajewsky K, Muller W: Interleukin-10-deficient mice develop chronic enterocolitis. Cell 1993; 75:263–274.

Kullberg MC, Ward JM, Gorelick PL, Caspar P, Hieny S, Cheever A, Jankovic D, Sher A: *Helicobacter hepaticus* triggers colitis in specific-pathogen-free interleukin-10 (IL-10)-deficient mice through an IL-12- and γ-interferon–dependent mechanism. Infect Immun 1998; 66:5157–5166.

Kurata JH, Kantor-Fish S, Frankl H, Godby P, Vadheim CM: Crohn's disease among ethnic groups in a large health maintenance organization. Gastroenterology 1992; 102:1940–1948.

Kuster W, Pascoe L, Purrmann J, Funk S, Majewski F: The genetics of Crohn disease: complex segregation analysis of a family study with 265 patients with Crohn disease and 5,387 relatives. Am J Med Genet 1989; 32:105–108.

Kyo K, Parkes M, Takei Y, Nishimori H, Vyas P, Satsangi J, Simmons J, Nagawa H, Baba S, Jewell D, et al.: Association of ulcerative colitis with rare VNTR alleles of the human intestinal mucin gene, MUC3. Hum Mol Genet 1999; 8:307–311.

Lake AM, Stitzel AE, Urmson RJ, Walker WA, Spitzer RE: Complement alterations in inflammatory bowel disease. Gastroenterology 1979; 76:374–379.

Lashner BA: Clinical features, laboratory findings, and course of Crohn's disease. In: Kirsner JB (ed). Inflammatory Bowel Disease. Philadephia: W.B. Saunders, 2000:305–314.

Laufer J, Oren R, Goldberg I, Horwitz A, Kopolovic J, Chowers Y, Passwell JH: Cellular localization of complement C3 and C4 transcripts in intestinal specimens from patients with Crohn's disease. Clin Exp Immunol 2000; 120:30–37.

Lee FI, Bellary SV, Francis C: Increased occurrence of psoriasis in patients with Crohn's disease and their relatives. Am J Gastroenterol 1990; 85:962–963.

Lee JC, Bridger S, McGregor C, Macpherson AJ, Jones JE: Why children with inflammatory bowel disease are diagnosed at a younger age than their affected parent. Gut 1999; 44:808–811.

Lee JC, Lennard-Jones JE, Cambridge G: Antineutrophil antibodies in familial inflammatory bowel disease. Gastroenterology 1995; 108:428–433.

Lesage S, Zouali H, Cezard JP, Colombel JF, Belaiche J, Almer S, Tysk C, O'Morain C, Gassull M, Binder V, et al. CARD15/NOD2 mutational analysis and genotype-phenotype correlation in 612 patients with inflammatory bowel disease. Am J Hum Genet 2002; 70:845–857.

Lim SG, Menzies IS, Lee CA, Johnson MA, Pounder RE: Intestinal permeability and function in patients infected with human immunodeficiency virus: a comparison with coeliac disease. Scand J Gastroenterol 1993; 28:573–580.

Lin HJ, Rotter JI, Conte WJ: Use of HLA marker associations and HLA haplotype linkage to estimate disease risks in families with gluten-sensitive enteropathy. Clin Genet 1985; 28:185–198.

Lindberg E, Magnusson K-E, Tysk C, Jarnerot G: Antibody (IgG,IgA,and IgM) to baker's yeast (*Saccharomyces cerevisiae*), yeast mannan, gliadin, ovalbumin and betalactoglobulin in monozygotic twins with inflammatory bowel disease. Gut 1992; 33:909–913.

Lindberg E, Soderholm JD, Olaison G, Tysk C, Jarnerot G: Intestinal permeability to polyethylene glycols in monozygotic twins with Crohn's disease. Scand J Gastroenterol 1995; 30:780–783.

Lisby G, Andersen J, Engaek K, Binder V: *Mycobacterium paratuberculosis* in intestinal tissue from patients with Crohn's disease demonstrated by a nested primer polymerase chain reaction. Scand J Gastroenterol 1994; 29:923–929.

Lo SK, Fleming KA, Chapman RW: Prevalence of anti-neutrophil antibody in primary sclerosing cholangitis and ulcerative colitis using an alkaline phoshatase technique. Gut 1992; 33:1370–1375.

Loftus EV Jr, Silverstein MD, Sandborn WJ, Tremaine WJ, Harmsen WS, Zinsmeister AR: Crohn's disease in Olmsted County, Minnesota, 1940–1993: incidence, prevalence, and survival. Gastroenterology 1998; 114:1161–1168.

Loftus EV Jr, Silverstein MD, Sandborn WJ, Tremaine WJ, Harmsen WS, Zinsmeister AR: Ulcerative colitis in Olmsted County, Minnesota, 1940–1993: incidence, prevalence, and survival. Gut 2000; 46:336–343.

Lohmuller JL, Pemberton JH, Dozois RR, Ilstrup D, van Heerden J: Pouchitis and extraintestinal manifestations of inflammatory bowel disease after ileal pouch-anal anastomosis. Ann Surg 1990; 211:622–667.

Louis E, Franchimont D, Piron A, Gevaert Y, Schaaf-Lafontaine N, Roland S, Mahieu P, Malaise M, De Groote D, Louis R, Belaiche J: Tumour necrosis factor (TNF) gene polymorphism influences TNF-α production in lipopolysaccharide (LPS)-stimulated whole blood cell culture in healthy humans. Clin Exp Immunol 1998; 113:401–406.

Louis E, Satsangi J, Roussomoustakaki M, Parkes M, Fanning G, Welsh K, Jewell D: Cytokine gene polymorphisms in inflammatory bowel disease. Gut 1996; 39:705–710.

Ludviksson BR, Gray B, Strober W, Ehrhardt RO: Dysregulated intrathymic development in the IL-2-deficient mouse leads to colitis-inducing thymocytes. J Immunol 1997; 158:104–111.

Ludviksson BR, Strober W, Nishikomori R, Hasan SK, Ehrhardt RO: Administration of mAb against alpha E beta 7 prevents and ameliorates immunization-induced colitis in IL2−/− mice. J Immunol 1999; 162:4975–4982.

Ma Y, Ohmen JD, Li Z, Bentley LG, McElree C, Pressman S, Targan SR, Fischel-Ghodsian N, Rotter JI, Yang H: A genome-wide search identifies potential new susceptibility loci for Crohn's disease. Inflamm Bowel Dis 1999; 5:271–278.

Mahadero R, Markowitz J, Fisher S, Daum F: Hermansky-Pudlak syndrome with granulosmatous colitis in children. J Pediatr 1991; 118:904–906.

Mahler M, Bristol IJ, Leiter EH, Workman AE, Birkenmeier EH, Elson CO, Sundberg JP: Differential susceptibility of inbred mouse strains to dextran sulfate sodium-induced colitis. Am J Physiol 1998; 274:G544–551.

Mahler M, Bristol IJ, Sundberg JP, Churchill GA, Birkenmeier EH, Elson CO, Leiter EH: Genetic analysis of susceptibility to dextran sulfate sodium-induced colitis in mice. Genomics 1999; 55:147–156.

Mahmud N, Molloy A, McPartlin J, Corbally R, Whitehead AS, Scott JM, Weir DG: Increased prevalence of methylenetetrahydrofolate reductase C677T variant in patients with inflammatory bowel disease, and its clinical implications. Gut 1999; 45:389–394.

Mallas EG, Mackintosh P, Asquith P, Cooke WT: Histocompatibility antigens in inflammatory bowel disease: their clinical significance and their association with arthropathy with special reference to HLA-B27 (w27). Gut 1976; 17:906–910.

Mansfield JC, Holden H, Tarlow JK, Di Giovine FS, McDowell TL, Wilson AG, Holdsworth CD: Novel genetic association between ulcerative colitis and the anti-inflammatory cytokine interleukin-1 receptor antagonist. Gastroenterology 1994; 106:637–642.

Matthews D, Fry L, Powles A, Weber J, McCarthy M, Fisher E, Davies K, Williamson R: Evidence that a locus for familial psoriasis maps to chromosome 4q. Nat Genet 1996; 14:231–233.

May GR, Sutherland LR, Meddings JB: Is small intestinal permeability really increased in relatives of patients with Crohn's disease? Gastroenterology 1993; 104:1627–1632.

Mayberry JF, Rhodes J, Newcombe RG: Familial prevalence of inflammatory bowel disease in relatives of patients with Crohn's disease. Br Med J 1980; 280:84.

McConnell RB: Inflammatory bowel disease: newer views of genetic influences. In: Berk JE (ed). Developments in Digestive Disease, Vol 3. Philadelphia: Lea and Febiger, 1980:129–137.

McConnell RB: Ulcerative colitis: genetic features. Scand J Gastroenterol 1983; 88(Supp):14–16.

McConnell RB, Vadheim CM: Inflammatory bowel disease. In: King RA, Rotter JI, Motulsky AG (eds). The Genetic Basis of Common Diseases. New York: Oxford University Press, 1992:326–348.

McGuire W, Hill AV, Allsopp CE, Greenwood BM, Kwiatkowski D: Variation in the TNF-α promoter region associated with susceptibility to cerebral malaria. Nature 1994; 371:508–510.

McGuire W, Knight JC, Hill AV, Allsopp CE, Greenwood BM, Kwiatkowski D: Severe malarial anemia and cerebral malaria are associated with different tumor necrosis factor promoter alleles. J Infect Dis 1999; 179:287–290.

McInnis MG: Anticipation: an old idea in new genes. Am J Hum Genet 1996; 59:973–979.

McKenzie H, Main J, Pennington CR, Parratt D: Antibody to selected strains of *Saccharomyces cerevisiae* (baker's and brewer's yeast) and *Candida albicans* in Crohn's disease. Gut 1990; 31:536–538.

Meijssen MA, Brandwein SL, Reinecker HC, Bhan AK, Podolsky DK: Alteration of gene expression by intestinal epithelial cells precedes colitis in interleukin-2-deficient mice. Am J Physiol 1998; 274:G472–479.

Merrett MN, Mortensen N, Kettlewell M, Jewell DO: Smoking may prevent pouchitis in patients with restorative proctocolectomy for ulcerative colitis. Gut 1996; 38:362–364.

MHC Sequencing Consortium. Complete sequence and gene map of a human major histocompatibility complex. Nature 1999; 401:921–923.

Mielants H, Veys EM: Ileal inflammation in B27-positive reactive arthritis. Lancet 1984a; 1:1072.

Mielants H, Veys EM: Inflammation of the ileum in patients with B27-positive reactive arthritis. Lancet 1984b; 1:288.

Mielants H, Veys EM, Cuvelier C, De Vos M, Goemaere S, De Clercq L, Schatteman L, Elewaut D: The evolution of spondyloarthropathies in relation to gut histology: II. Histological aspects. J Rheumatol 1995; 22:2273–2278.

Milner LA, Bigas A: Notch as a mediator of cell fate determination in hematopoiesis: evidence and speculation. Blood 1999; 93:2431–2448.

Minocha A, Raczkowski CA: Role of appendectomy and tonsillectomy in pathogenesis of ulcerative colitis. Dig Dis Sci 1997; 42:1567–1569.

Minuk GY, Lewkonia RM: Possible familial association of multiple sclerosis and inflammatory bowel disease. N Engl J Med 1986; 314:580–586.

Mirza MM, Lee J, Teare D, Hugot JP, Laurent-Puig P, Colombel JF, Hodgson SV, Thomas G, Easton DF, Lennard-Jones JE, Mathew CG: Evidence of linkage of the inflammatory bowel disease susceptibility locus on chromosome 16 (IBD1) to ulcerative colitis. J Med Genet 1998; 35:218–221.

Mizoguchi A, Mizoguchi E, Bhan AK: The critical role of interleukin 4 but not interferon-γ in the pathogenesis of colitis in T-cell receptor-α mutant mice. Gastroenterology 1999; 116:320–326.

Mizoguchi A, Mizoguchi E, Chiba C, Bhan AK: Role of appendix in the development of inflammatory bowel disease in TCR-α mutant mice. J Exp Med 1996; 184:707–715.

Mizoguchi E, Mizoguchi A, Bhan AK: Role of cytokines in the early stages of chronic colitis in TCRα-mutant mice. Lab Invest 1997; 76:385–397.

Moll JMH: Inflammatory bowel disease. Clin Rheum Dis 1985; 11:87–111.

Monk M, Mendeloff AI, Siegel CI, Lilienfeld A: An epidemiological study of ulcerative colitis and regional enteritis among adults in Baltimore: I. Hospital incidence and prevalence, 1960–1963. Gastroenterology 1967; 53:198–210.

Monsen U, Iselius L, Johansson C, Hellers G: Evidence for a major additive gene in ulcerative colitis. Clin Genet 1989; 36:411–414.

Monsen U, Sorstad J, Hellers G, Johansson C: Extracolonic diagnoses in ulcerative colitis: an epidemiological study. Am J Gastroenterol 1990; 85:711–716.

Montgomery SM, Bjornsson S, Johannsson JH, Thjodleifsson B, Pounder RE, Wakefield AJ: Concurrent viral epidemics in Iceland are a risk for inflammatory bowel disease. Gut 1998; 42:A41.

Montgomery SM, Morris DL, Pounder RE, Wakefield AJ: Paramyxovirus infections in childhood and subsequent inflammatory bowel disease. Gastroenterology 1999; 116:796–803.

Montgomery SM, Pounder RE, Wakefield AJ: Infant mortality and the incidence of inflammatory bowel disease. Lancet 1997; 349:472–473.

Munkholm P, Langholz E, Hollander D, Thornberg K, Orholm M, Katz KD, Binder V: Intestinal permeability in patients with Crohn's disease and ulcerative colitis and their first degree relatives. Gut 1994; 35:68–72.

Nadel S, Newport MJ, Booy R, Levin M: Variation in the tumor necrosis factor-α gene promoter region may be associated with death from meningococcal disease. J Infect Dis 1996; 174:878–880.

Nair RP, Henseler T, Jenisch S, Stuart P, Bichakjian CK, Lenk W, Westphal E, Guo SW, Christophers E, Voorhees JJ, Elder JT: Evidence for two psoriasis susceptibility loci (HLA and 17q) and two novel candidate regions (16q and 20p) by genome-wide scan. Hum Mol Genet 1997; 6:1349–1356.

Nakajima A, Matsuhashi N, Kodama T, Yazaki Y, Takazoe M, Kimura A: HLA-linked susceptibility and resistance genes in Crohn's disease. Gastroenterology 1995; 109:1462–1467.

Nakamura S, Ohtani H, Watanabe Y, Fukushima K, Matsumoto T, Kitano A, Kobayashi K, Nagura H: In situ expression of the cell adhesion molecules in inflammatory bowel disease: evidence of immunologic activation of vascular endothelial cells. Lab Invest 1993; 69:77–85.

Naom I, Lee J, Ford D, Bowman SJ, Lanchbury JS, Haris I, Hodgson SV, Easton D, Lennard-Jones J, Mathew CG: Analysis of the contribution of HLA genes to genetic predisposition in inflammatory bowel disease. Am J Hum Genet 1996; 59:226–233.

Nedospasov SA, Udalova IA, Kuprash DV, Turetskaya RL: DNA sequence polymorphism at the human tumor necrosis factor (TNF) locus: numerous TNF/lymphotoxin alleles tagged by two closely linked microsatellites in the upstream region of the lymphotoxin (TNFβ) gene. J Immunol 1991; 147:1053–1059.

Nemetz A, Kope A, Molnar T, Kovacs A, Feher J, Tulassay Z, Nagy F, Garcia-Gonzalez MA, Pena AS: Significant differences in the interleukin-1β and interleukin-1 receptor antagonist gene polymorphisms in a Hungarian population with inflammatory bowel disease. Scand J Gastroenterol 1999a; 34:175–179.

Nemetz A, Nosti-Escanilla MP, Molnar T, Kope A, Kovacs A, Feher J, Tulassay J, Nagy F, Garcia-Gonzalez MA, Pena AS: IL1B gene polymorphisms influence the course and severity of inflammatory bowel disease. Immunogenetics 1999b; 49:527–531.

Newport MJ, Huxley CM, Huston S, Hawrylowicz CM, Oostra BA, Williamson R, Levin M: A mutation in the interferon-γ receptor gene and susceptibility to mycobacterial infection. N Engl J Med 1996; 335:1941–1949.

Novis BH, Marks IN, Louw JH, Bank S: Incidence of Crohn's disease at Groote Schuur Hospital during 1970–1974. S Afr Med J 1975; 49:693–697.

Ockhuizen T, Westra H, Bijzet J, Post J, van Leeuwen M, van Rijswijk M: Immunoglobulin allotypes are not involved in systemic amyloidosis. J Rheumatol 1985; 12:742–746.

Odes HS, Fraser D, Krugliak P, Fenyves D, Fraser GM, Sperber AD: Inflammatory bowel disease in the Bedouin Arabs of southern Israel: rarity of diagnosis and clinical features. Gut 1991; 32:1024–1026.

Ogura Y, Bonen DK, Inohara N, Nicolae DL, Chen FF, Ramos R, Britton H, Moran T, Karaliuskas R, Duerr RH, et al. A frameshift mutation in NOD2 associated with susceptibility to Crohn's disease. Nature 2001; 411:603–606.

Oh J, Bailin T, Fukai K, Feng GH, Ho L, Mao JI, Frenk E, Tamura N, Spritz RA: Positional cloning of a gene for Hermansky-Pudlak syndrome, a disorder of cytoplasmic organelles. Nat Genet 1996; 14:300–306.

Oh J, Ho L, Ala-Mello S, Amato D, Armstrong L, Bellucci S, Carakushansky G, Ellis JP, Fong CT, Green JS, et al.: Mutation analysis of patients with Hermansky-Pudlak syndrome: a frameshift hot spot in the HPS gene and apparent locus heterogeneity. Am J Hum Genet 1998; 62:593–598.

Ohmen JD, Yang HY, Yamamoto KK, Zhao HY, Ma Y, Bentley LG, Huang Z, Gerwehr S, Pressman S, McElree C, et al.: Susceptibility locus for inflammatory bowel disease on chromosome 16 has a role in Crohn's disease, but not in ulcerative colitis. Hum Mol Genet 1996; 5:1679–1683.

Olerup O, Broome U, Einarsson K, Zetterquist H: Inability to attribute susceptibility to primary sclerosing cholangitis to specific amino acid positions of the HLA-DRw52 allele. N Engl J Med 1991; 325:1251–1252.

Olsson R, Danielsson A, Jarnerot G, Lindstrom E, Loof L, Rolny P, Ryden BO, Tysk C, Wallerstedt S: Prevalence of primary sclerosing cholangitis in patients with ulcerative colitis. Gastroenterology 1991; 100:1319–1323.

Orchard TR, Thiyagaraja S, Welsh KI, Wordsworth BP, Hill Gaston JS, Jewell DP: Clinical phenotype is related to HLA genotype in the peripheral arthropathies of inflammatory bowel disease. Gastroenterology 2000; 118:274–278.

Orholm M, Fonager K, Sorensen HT: Risk of ulcerative colitis and Crohn's disease among offspring of patients with chronic inflammatory bowel disease. Am J Gastroenterol 1999; 94:3236–3238.

Orholm M, Iselius L, Sorensen TIA, Munkholm P, Langholz E, Binder V: Investigation of inheritance of chronic inflammatory bowel disease by complex segregation anslysis. Br Med J 1993; 306:20–24.

Orholm M, Munkholm P, Langholz E, Nielsen OH, Sorensen IA, Binder V: Familial occurrence of inflammatory bowel disease. N Engl J Med 1991; 324:84–88.

Orr HT, Chung MY, Banfi S, Kwiatkowski YJ, Servadio A, Beaudet AL, McCall AE: Expansion of an unstable trinucleotide CAG repeat in spinocerebellar ataxia type 1. Nat Genet 1993; 4:221–226.

Paavola P, Helio T, Turunen U, Farkkila M, Kontula K: Suggestive evidence for linkage to chromosome 3p21 in Finnish inflammatory bowel disease families. Gastroenterology 2000; 118:A336.

Palli D, Masala G, Trallori G, Bardazzi G, Saieva C: A capture–recapture estimate of inflammatory bowel disease prevalence: the Florence population-based study. Ital J Gastroenterol Hepatol 1998; 30:50–53.

Panwala CM, Jones JC, Viney JL: A novel model of inflammatory bowel disease: mice deficient for the multiple drug resistance gene, mdr1a, spontaneously develop colitis. J Immunol 1998; 161:5733–5744.

Parkes M, Satsangi J, Lathrop GM, Bell JI, Jewell DP: Susceptibility loci in inflammatory bowel disease. Lancet 1996; 348:1588.

Parkes M, Satsangi J, Merriman A, Jewell DP: Precision mapping of chromosome 12 linkage in IBD: evidence for a haplotype association. Gastroenterology 1998; 114:A1058.

Parkes M, Vyas P, Satsangi J, Jewell DP: Fine mapping the IBD linkage on chromosome 3. Gastroenterology 1999; 116:A792.

Pasparakis M, Alexopoulou L, Episkopou V, Kollias G: Immune and inflammatory responses in TNFα-deficient mice: a critical requirement for TNFα in the formation of primary B cell follicles, follicular dendritic cell networks and germinal centers, and in the maturation of the humoral immune response. J Exp Med 1996; 184:1397–1411.

Pasparakis M, Alexopoulou L, Grell M, Pfizenmaier K, Bluethmann H, Kollias G: Peyer's patch organogenesis is intact yet formation of B lymphocyte follicles is defective in peripheral lymphoid organs of mice deficient for tumor necrosis factor and its 55-kDa receptor. Proc Natl Acad Sci USA 1997; 94:6319–6323.

Patel RT, Pall AA, Adu D, Keighley MR: Circulating soluble adhesion molecules in inflammatory bowel disease. Eur J Gastroenterol Hepatol 1995; 7:1037–1041.

Peeters M, Geypens B, Claus D, Nevens H, Ghoos Y, Verbeke G, Baert F, Vermeire S, Vlietinck R, Rutgeerts P: Clustering of increased small intestinal permeability in families with Crohn's disease. Gastroenterology 1997; 113:802–807.

Penna C, Dozois R, Tremaine W, Sandborn W, La Russo N, Schleck C, Ilstrup D: Pouchitis after ileal pouch–anal anastomosis for ulcerative colitis occurs with increased frequency in patients with associated primary sclerosing cholangitis. Gut 1996; 38:234–239.

Petersen GM, Rotter JI, Cantor RM, Field LL, Greenwald S, Lim JS, Roy C, Schoenfeld V, Lowden JA, Kaback MM: The Tay-Sachs disease gene in North American Jewish populations: geographic variations and origin. Am J Hum Genet 1983; 35:1258–1269.

Petronis A, Kennedy JL, Paterson AD: Genetic anticipation: fact or artifact, genetics or epigenetics? Lancet 1997; 350:1403–1404.

Pinchbeck BR, Kirdeikis J, Thomson ABR: Effect of religious affiliation and education status on the prevalence of inflammatory bowel disease in northern Alberta. Can J Gastroenterol 1988; 2(suppl A):95–100.

Plevy SE, Targan SR, Yang H, Fernandez D, Rotter JI, Toyoda H: Tumor necrosis factor microsatellites define a Crohn's disease–associated haplotype on chromosome 6. Gastroenterology 1996; 110:1053–1060.

Plevy SE, Taylor K, DeWoody KL, Schaible YF, Shealy D, Targan SR: Tumor necrosis factor (TNF) microsatellite haplotypes and perinuclear anti-neutrophil cytoplasmic antibody (pANCA) identify Crohn's disease (CD) patients with poor clinical responses to anti-TNF monoclonal antibody. Gastroenterology 1997; 112:A1062.

Podolsky DK, Fournier DA: Alterations in mucosal content of colonic glycoconjugates in inflammatory bowel disease defined by monoclonal antibodies. Gastroenterology 1988; 95:379–387.

Pokorny RM, Hofmeister A, Galandiuk S, Dietz AB, Cohen ND, Neibergs HL: Crohn's disease and ulcerative colitis are associated with the DNA repair gene MLH1. Ann Surg 1997; 225:718–725.

Polito JM, Rees RC, Childs B, Mendeloff AI, Harris ML, Bayless TM: Preliminary evidence for genetic anticipation in Crohn's disease. Lancet 1996; 347:798–800.

Potter BJ, Brown DJC, Watson A, Jewell DP: Complement inhibitors and immunoconglutinis in ulcerative colitis and Crohn's disease. Gut 1980; 2:1030–1034.

Powrie F, Carlino J, Leach MW, Mauze S, Coffman RL: A critical role for transforming growth factor-β but not interleukin 4 in the suppression of T helper type 1-mediated colitis by CD45RB(low) $CD4^+$ T cells. J Exp Med 1996; 183:2669–2674.

Powrie F, Leach MW, Mauze S, Caddle LB, Coffman RL: Phenotypically distinct subsets of $CD4^+$ T cells induce or protect from chronic intestinal inflammation in C. B-17 scid mice. Int Immunol 1993; 5:1461–1471.

Powrie F, Leach MW, Mauze S, Menon S, Caddle LB, Coffman RL: Inhibition of Th1 responses prevents inflammatory bowel disease in scid mice reconstituted with CD45RBhi CD4$^+$ T cells. Immunity 1994; 1:553–562.

Probert CS, Jayanthi V, Hughes AO, Thompson JR, Wicks AC, Mayberry JF: Prevalence and family risk of ulcerative colitis and Crohn's disease: an epidemiological study among Europeans and south Asians in Leicestershire. Gut 1993; 34:1547–1551.

Prochazka EJ, Terasaki PI, Park MS, Goldstein LI, Busuttil RW: Association of primary sclerosing cholangitis with HLA-DRw52a. N Engl J Med 1990; 322:1842–1844.

Purrmann J, Arendt G, Cleveland S, Borchard F, Furst W, Gemsa R, Bertrams J, Hengels K-J: Association of Crohn's disease and multiple sclerosis: is there a common background? J Clin Gastroenterol 1992; 14:43–46.

Purrmann J, Zeidler H, Bertrams J, Juli E, Cleveland S, Berges W, Gemsa R, Specker C, Reis HE: HLA antigens in ankylosing spondylitis associated with Crohn's disease: increased frequency of the HLA phenotype B27,B44. J Rheumatol 1988; 15:1658–1661.

Quinton JF, Sendid B, Reumaux D, Duthilleul P, Cortot A, Grandbastien B, Charrier G, Targan SR, Colombel JF, Poulain D: Anti-*Saccharomyces cerevisiae* mannan antibodies combined with antineutrophil cytoplasmic autoantibodies in inflammatory bowel disease: prevalence and diagnostic role. Gut 1998; 42:788–791.

Rang EH, Brooke BN, Hermon-Taylor J: Association of ulcerative colitis and multiple sclerosis. Lancet 1982; 2:555.

Rankin GB: Extraintestinal and systemic manifestations of inflammatory bowel disease. Med Clin North Am 1990; 74:39–50.

Rasmussen HH, Fallingborg J, Mortensen PB, Freund L, Tage-Jensen U, Kruse V, Rasmussen SN: Primary sclerosing cholangitis in patients with ulcerative colitis. Scand J Gastroenterol 1992; 27:732–736.

Rath HC, Herfarth HH, Ikeda JS, Grenther WB, Hamm TE Jr, Balish E, Taurog JD, Hammer RE, Wilson KH, Sartor RB: Normal luminal bacteria, especially *Bacteroides* species, mediate chronic colitis, gastritis, and arthritis in HLA-B27/human β_2-microglobulin transgenic rats. J Clin Invest 1996; 98:945–953.

Rath HC, Wilson KH, Sartor RB: Differential induction of colitis and gastritis in HLA-B27 transgenic rats selectively colonized with *Bacteroides vulgatus* or *Escherichia coli*. Infect Immun 1999; 67:2969–2974.

Reinshagen M, Loeliger C, Kuehnl P, Weiss U, Manfras BJ, Adler G, Boehm BO: HLA class II gene frequencies in Crohn's disease: a population based analysis in Germany. Gut 1996; 38:538–542.

Rioux JD, Daly MJ, Green T, Stone V, Lander ES, Hudson TJ, Steinhart AH, Bull S, Cohen Z, Greenberg G, et al.: Absence of linkage between inflammatory bowel disease and selected loci on chromosomes 3, 7, 12, and 16. Gastroenterology 1998; 115:1062–1065.

Rioux JD, Silverberg MS, Daly MJ, Steinhart AH, McLeod RS, Griffiths AM, Green T, Brettin TS, Stone V, Bull SB, et al.: Genomewide search in Canadian families with inflammatory bowel disease reveals two novel susceptibility loci. Am J Hum Genet 2000; 66:1863–1870.

Rioux JD, Daly MJ, Silverberg MS, Lindblad K, Steinhart H, Cohen Z, Delmonte T, Kocher K, Miller K, Guschwan S, et al. Genetic variation in the 5q31 cytokine gene cluster confers susceptibility to Crohn disease. Nat Genet 2001; 29:223–228.

Robey E: Regulation of T cell fate by Notch. Annu Rev Immunol 1999; 17:283–295.

Roe TF, Coates TD, Thomas DW, Miller JH, Gilsanz V: Brief report: treatment of chronic inflammatory bowel disease in glycogen storage disease type Ib with colony-stimulating factors. N Engl J Med 1992; 326:1666–1669.

Roth MP, Petersen GM, McElree C, Feldman E, Rotter JI: Geographic origins of Jewish patients with inflammatory bowel disease. Gastroenterology 1989a; 97:900–904.

Roth MP, Petersen GM, McElree C, Vadheim CM, Panish JF, Rotter JI: Familial empiric risk estimates of inflammatory bowel disease in Ashkenazi Jews. Gastroenterology 1989b; 96:1016–1020.

Rotter JI: The genetics of peptic ulcer disease: more than one gene, more than one disease. Prog Med Genet 1980; 4:1–58.

Rotter JI: Genetics in gastroenterology. In: Gitnick G, Hollander D, Kaplowitz N, Samloff IM, Schoenfield LJ (eds). Principles and Practices of Gastroenterology. New York: Elsevier, 1988:1501–1525.

Rotter JI: Inflammatory bowel disease. Lancet 1994; 343:1360.

Rotter JI, Diamond JM: What maintains the frequencies of human genetic diseases? Nature 1987; 329:289–290.

Rotter JI, Landaw EM: Measuing the genetic contribution of a single locus to a multilocus disease. Clin Genet 1984; 26:529–542.

Rotter JI, Yang H, Shohat T: Genetic complexities of inflammtory bowel disease and its distribution among the Jewish people. In: Bonne-Tamir B, Adam A (eds). Genetic Diversity among Jews: Diseases and Markers at the DNA Level. New York: Oxford University Press, 1992:395–411.

Roussomoustakaki M, Satsangi J, Welsh K, Louis E, Fanning G, Targan S, Landers C, Jewell DP: Genetic markers may predict disease behavior in patients with ulcerative colitis. Gastroenterology 1997; 112:1845–1853.

Rowbotham DS, Howdle PD, Trejdosiewicz LK: Peripheral cell-mediated immune response to mycobacterial antigens in inflammatory bowel disease. Clin Exp Immunol 1995; 102:456–461.

Russel MG, Dorant E, Volovics A, Brummer RJ, Pop P, Muris JW, Bos LP, Limonard CB, Stockbrugger RW: High incidence of inflammatory bowel disease in the Netherlands: results of a prospective study. Dis Colon Rectum 1998; 41:33–40.

Russel MG, Pastoor CJ, Janssen KM, Van Deursen CT, Muris JW, Van Wijlick EH, Stockbruuger RW, South Limburg IBD Study Group: Familial aggregation of inflammatory bowel disease: a population-based study in South Limburg, the Netherlands. Scand J Gastroenterol 1997; 32:88–91.

Russel MG, Stockbrugger RW: Epidemiology of inflammatory bowel disease: an update. Scand J Gastroenterol 1996; 31:417–427.

Russell AS: Transplantation antigens in Crohn's disease: linkage of associated ankylosing spondylistis with HL-Aw27. Am J Dig Dis 1975; 20:359–361.

Russell AS: Arthritis, inflammatory bowel disease, and histocompatibility antigens. Ann Intern Med 1977; 86:820–821.

Rutgeerts P, D'Haens G, Hiele M, Geboes K, Vantrappen G: Appendectomy protects against ulcerative colitis. Gastroenterology 1994; 106:1251–1253.

Sadlack B, Merz H, Schorle H, Schimpl A, Feller AC, Horak I: Ulcerative colitis-like disease in mice with a disrupted interleukin-2 gene. Cell 1993; 75:253–261.

Sadovnick AD, Paty DW, Yannakoulias G: Concurrence of multiple sclerosis and inflammatory bowel disease. N Engl J Med 1989; 321:762–763.

Sandborn WJ: Pouchitis following ileal pouch-anal anastomosis: definition, pathogenesis, and treatment. Gastroenterology 1994; 107:1856–1860.

Sandborn WJ, Landers CJ, Tremaine WJ, Targan SR: Antineutrophil cytoplasmic antibody correlates with chronic pouchitis after ileal pouch–anal anastomosis. Am J Gastroenterol 1995; 90:740–747.

Sandborn WJ, Tremaine WJ, Offord KP, Lawson GM, Petersen BT, Batts KP, Croghan IT, Dale LC, Schroeder DR, Hurt RD: Transdermal nicotine for mildly to moderately active ulcerative colitis: a randomized, double-blind, placebo-controlled trial. Ann Intern Med 1997; 126:364–371.

Sands BE: Therapy of inflammatory bowel disease. Gastroenterology 2000; 118:S68–82.

Satsangi J, Landers CJ, Welsh KI, Koss K, Targan S, Jewell DP: The presence of anti-neutrophil antibodies reflects clinical and genetic heterogeneity within inflammatory bowel disease. Inflamm Bowel Dis 1998; 4:18–26.

Satsangi J, Parkes M, Louis E, Hashimoto L, Kato N, Welsh K, Terwilliger JD, Lathrop GM, Bell JI, Jewell DP: Two stage genome-wide search in inflammatory bowel disease provides evidence for susceptibility loci on chromosomes 3, 7 and 12. Nat Genet 1996; 14:199–202.

Satsangi J, Welsh KI, Bunce M, Julier C, Farrant JM, Bell JI, Jewell DP: Contribution of genes of the major histocompatibility complex to susceptibility and disease phenotype in inflammatory bowel disease. Lancet 1996; 347:1212–1217.

Schinella RA, Grego A, Cobert BT, Denmark LW, Cox RP: Hermansky-Pudlak syndrome with granulomatous colitis. Ann Intern Med 1980; 92:20–23.

Schultz M, Tonkonogy SL, Sellon RK, Veltkamp C, Godfrey VL, Kwon J, Grenther WB, Balish E, Horak I, Sartor RB: IL-2-deficient mice raised under germfree conditions develop delayed mild focal intestinal inflammation. Am J Physiol 1999; 276:G1461–1472.

Scott IS, Sheaff M, Coumbe A, Feakins RM, Rampton DS: Appendiceal inflammation in ulcerative colitis. Histopathology 1998; 33:168–173.

Seibold F, Brandwein S, Simpson S, Terhorst C, Elson CO: pANCA represents a cross-reactivity to enteric bacterial antigens. J Clin Immunol 1998; 18:153–160.

Seibold F, Mork H, Tanza S, Muller A, Holzhuter C, Weber P, Scheurlen M: Pancreatic autoantibodies in Crohn's disease: a family study. Gut 1997; 40:481–484.

Seibold F, Slametschka D, Gregor M, Weber P: Neutrophil autoantibodies: a genetic marker in primary sclerosing cholangitis and ulcerative colitis. Gastroenterology 1994; 107:532–536.

Seibold F, Weber P, Klein R, Berg PA, Wiedmann KH: Clinical significance of antibodies against neutrophils in patients with inflammatory bowel disease and primary sclerosing cholangitis. Gut 1992; 33:657–662.

Sels F, Westhovens R, Emonds MP, Vandermeulen E, Dequeker J: HLA typing in a large family with multiple cases of different autoimmune diseases. J Rheumatol 1997; 24:856–859.

Sendid B, Quinton JF, Charrier G, Cortot A, Grandbastien B, Poulain D, Colombel JF: Anti-*Saccharomyces cerevisiae* mannan antibodies (ASCA) in healthy relatives of patients with Crohn's disease. Gut 1997; 41:A177.

Seymour JF: Association between myelodysplastic syndromes and inflammatory bowel diseases: report of seven new cases and review of the literature. Leukemia 1998; 12:1331–1332.

Shanahan F, Duerr RH, Rotter JI, Yang H, Sutherland LR, McElree C, Landers CJ, Targan SR: Neutrophil autoantibodies in ulcerative colitis: familial aggregation and genetic heterogeneity. Gastroenterology 1992; 103:456–461.

Shanahan F, Randolph LM, King R, Brogan M, Witkop C, Rotter JI, Targan SR, Oseas R: The Hermansky-Pudlak syndrome: an immunological assessment of 15 cases. Am J Med 1989; 85:823–828.

Shanahan F, Targan SR (eds): Inflammatory Bowel Disease: From Bench to Bedside. Baltimore: Williams & Wilkins, 1994.

Shepherd HA: Ulcerative colitis and persistent liver dysfunction. Quart J Med 1983; 52:503–513.

Shivananda S, Lennard-Jones J, Logan R, Fear N, Price A, Carpenter L, van Blankenstein M: Incidence of inflammatory bowel disease across Europe: is there a difference between north and south? Results of the European Collaborative Study on Inflammatory Bowel Disease (EC-IBD). Gut 1996; 39:690–697.

Simmons JD, Mullighan C, Welsh KI, Jewell DP: Vitamin D receptor gene polymorphism further evidence for an association with Crohn's disease. Gastroenterology 1998; 114:A1086.

Simpson SJ, Shah S, Comiskey M, de Jong YP, Wang B, Mizoguchi E, Bhan AK, Terhorst C: T cell–mediated pathology in two models of experimental colitis depends predominantly on the interleukin 12/Signal transducer and activator of transcription (Stat)-4 pathway, but is not conditional on interferon-γ expression by T cells. J Exp Med 1998; 187:1225–1234.

Skipper M, Lewis J: Getting to the guts of enteroendocrine differentiation. Nat Genet 2000; 24:3–4.

Sloan JM, Cameron CHS, Maxwell RJ, McClusky DR, Collins JSA: Colitis complicating chronic granulomatous disease: a clinicopathological case report. Gut 1996; 38:619–622.

Sloan WP, Bargen JA, Gage RP: Life histories of patients with chronic ulcerative colitis: a review of 2000 cases. Gastroenterology 1950; 16:25–38.

Smithson JE, Radford-Smith G, Jewell GP: Appendectomy and tonsillectomy in patients with inflammatory bowel disease. J Clin Gastroenterol 1995; 21:283–286.

Snook JA: Are the inflammatory bowel diseases autoimmune disorders? Gut 1990; 31:961–963.

Snook JA, de Silva HJ, Jewell DP: The association of autoimmune disorders with inflammatory bowel disease. Quart J Med 1989; 72:835–840.

Sonnenberg A, McCarty DJ, Jacobsen SJ: Geographic variation of inflammatory bowel disease within the United States. Gastroenterology 1991; 100:143–149.

Sonnenberg A, Wasserman IH: Epidemiology of inflammatory bowel disease among U.S. military veterans. Gastroenterology 1991; 101:122–130.

Stevens C, Peppercorn MA, Grand RJ: Crohn's disease associated with autoimmune neutropenia. J Clin Gastroenterol 1991; 13:328–330.

Stokkers PC, Huibregtse K Jr, Leegwater AC, Reitsma PH, Tytgat GN, van Deventer SJ: Analysis of a positional candidate gene for inflammatory bowel disease: NRAMP2. Inflamm Bowel Dis 2000; 6:92–98.

Stokkers PC, Reitsma PH, Tytgat GN, van Deventer SJ: HLA-DR and -DQ phenotypes in inflammatory bowel disease: a meta-analysis. Gut 1999; 45:395–401.

Stokkers PC, van Aken BE, Basoski N, Reitsma PH, Tytgat GN, van Deventer SJ: Five genetic markers in the interleukin 1 family in relation to inflammatory bowel disease. Gut 1998; 43:33–39.

Sugimura K, Asakura H, Mizuki N, Inoue M, Hibi T, Yagita A, Tsuji K, Inoko H: Analysis of genes within the HLA region affecting susceptibility to ulcerative colitis. Hum Immunol 1993; 36:112–118.

Sutton CL, Yang H, Li Z, Rotter JI, Targan SR, Braun J: Familial expression of anti-*Saccharomyces cerevisiae* mannan antibodies in affected and unaffected relatives of patients with Crohn's disease. Gut 2000; 46:58–63.

Tanaka K, Wilks M, Coates PJ, Farthing MJ, Walker-Smith JA, Tabaqchali S: *Mycobacterium paratuberculosis* and Crohn's disease. Gut 1991; 32:43–45.

Targan SR, Hanauer SB, van Deventer SJ, Mayer L, Present DH, Braakman T, DeWoody KL, Schaible TF, Rutgeerts PJ: A short-term study of chimeric monoclonal antibody cA2 to tumor necrosis factor-α for Crohn's disease. N Engl J Med 1997; 337:1029–1035.

Targan SR, Murphy LK: Clarifying the causes of Crohn's. Nat Med 1995; 1:1241–1243.

Taurog JD, Richardson JA, Croft JT, Simmons WA, Zhou M, Fernandez-Sueiro JL, Balish E, Hammer RE: The germfree state prevents development of gut and joint inflammatory disease in HLA-B27 transgenic rats. J Exp Med 1994; 180:2359–2364.

Taylor KD, Li Z, Barry M, Fischel-Ghodsian N, Plevy SE, Rotter JI, Targan SR, Yang H: Tumor necrosis factor microsatellite haplotype A11B4C1D3E3 is associated with anti-*Saccharomyces cerevisiae* antibody (ASCA) across clinical forms of inflammatory bowel disease. Gastroenterology 1998; 114:A1098.

Taylor KD, Vasiliauskas EA, Kam LY, Lin YC, Targan SR, Rotter JI, Yang H: Specific clinical and immunological features in Crohn's disease patients are associated with the MHC class III marker Notch4. Gastroenterology 2000; 118: A869.

Taylor KD, Yang H, Hang TD, Lin YC, Targan SR, Fischel-Ghodsian N, Rotter JI: Linkage disequilibrium mapping identifies a class III major histocompatibility complex (MHC) susceptibility haplotype to Crohn's disease in Ashkenazi Jews. Am J Hum Genet 1999; 65:A102.

Taylor KD, Plevy SE, Yang H, Landers CJ, DeWoody KL, Schaible TF, Shealy D, Barry MJ, Rotter JI, Targan SR, 2000. Factors associated with differential clinical responses to treatment with anti-TNF antibody (Infliximab): ANCA pattern and LTA haplotype. Gastroenterology 2001; 120:1347–1355.

Thomas GA, Swift GL, Green JT, Newcombe RG, Braniff-Mathews C, Rhodes J, Wilkinson S, Strohmeyer G, Kreuzpainter G: Controlled trial of antituberculous chemotherapy in Crohn's disease: a five-year follow-up study. Gut 1998; 42:497–500.

Tountas NA, Casini-Raggi V, Yang H, Di Giovine FS, Vecchi M, Kam L, Melani L, Pizarro TT, Rotter JI, Cominelli F: Functional and ethnic association of allele 2 of the interleukin-1 receptor antagonist gene in ulcerative colitis. Gastroenterology 1999; 117:806–813.

Toyoda H, Wang SJ, Yang HY, Redford A, Magalong D, Tyan D, McElree CK, Pressman SR, Shanahan F, Targan SR, Rotter JI: Distinct associations of HLA class II genes with inflammatory bowel disease. Gastroenterology 1993; 104:741–748.

Trachtenberg EA, Yang H, Hayes E, Vinson M, Lin C, Targan SR, Tyan D, Erlich H, Rotter JI: HLA class II haplotype associations with inflammatory bowel disease in Jewish (Ashkenazi) and non-Jewish Caucasian populations. Hum Immunol 2000; 61:326–333.

Trallori G, Palli D, Saieva C, Bardazzi G, Bonanomi AG, d'Albasio G, Galli M, Vannozzi G, Milla M, Tarantino O, et al.: A population-based study of inflammatory bowel disease in Florence over 15 years (1978–92). Scand J Gastroenterol 1996; 31:892–899.

Trembath RC, Clough RL, Rosbotham JL, Jones AB, Camp RD, Frodsham A, Browne J, Barber R, Terwilliger J, Lathrop GM, Barker JN: Identification of a major susceptibility locus on chromosome 6p and evidence for further disease loci revealed by a two stage genome-wide search in psoriasis. Hum Mol Genet 1997; 6:813–820.

Tysk C, Lindberg E, Jarnerot G, Floderus-Myrhed B: Ulcerative colitis and Crohn's disease in an unselected population of monozygotic and dizygotic twins: a study of heritability and the influence of smoking. Gut 1988; 29:990–996.

Tysk C, Riedesel H, Lindberg E, Panzini B, Podolsky D, Jarnerot G: Colonic glycoproteins in monozygotic twins with inflammatory bowel disease. Gastroenterology 1991; 100:419–423.

Udalova IA, Nedospasov SA, Webb GC, Chaplin DD, Turetskaya RL: Highly informative typing of the human TNF locus using six adjacent polymorphic markers. Genomics 1993; 16:180–186.

Ueki T, Mizuno M, Uesu T, Kiso T, Nasu J, Inaba T, Kihara Y, Matsuoka Y, Okada H, Fujita T, Tsuji T: Distribution of activated complement, C3b, and its degraded fragments, iC3b/C3dg, in the colonic mucosa of ulcerative colitis (UC). Clin Exp Immunol 1996; 104:286–292.

Vainer B: Role of cell adhesion molecules in inflammatory bowel diseases. Scand J Gastroenterol 1997; 32:401–410.

Vainer B, Nielsen OH: Changed colonic profile of P-selection, platelet-endothelial cell adhesion molecule-1 (PECAM-1), intercellular adhesion molecule-1 (ICAM-1), ICAM-2, and ICAM-3 in inflammatory bowel disease. Clin Exp Immunol 2000; 121:242–247.

Van de Merwe JP, Schroder AM, Wensinck F, Hazenberg MP: The obligate anaerobic faecal flora of patients with Crohn's disease and their first-degree relatives. Scand J Gastroenterol 1988; 23:1125–1131.

Van Deventer SJ: Tumour necrosis factor and Crohn's disease. Gut 1997; 40:443–448.

van Elburg RM, Uil JJ, Mulder CJ, Heymans HS: Intestinal permeability in patients with coeliac disease and relatives of patients with coeliac disease. Gut 1993; 34:354–357.

Vannier JP, Arnaud-Battandier F, Ricour C, Schmitz J, Buriot D, Griscelli C, Rey J: Chronic neutropenia and Crohn's disease in childhood: report of 2 cases. Arch Fr Pediatr 1982; 39:367–370.

Vasiliauskas EA, Kam LY, Karp LC, Gaiennie J, Yang H, Targan SR: Marker antibody expression stratifies Crohn's disease into immunologically homogeneous subgroups with clinical characteristics. Gut 2000; 47:487–496.

Vasiliauskas EA, Plevy SE, Landers CJ, Binder SW, Ferguson DM, Yang H, Rotter JI, Vidrich A, Targan SR: Perinuclear antineutrophil cytoplasmic antibodies in patients with Crohn's disease define a clinical subgroup. Gastroenterology 1996; 110:1810–1819.

Vecchi M, Gionchetti P, Bianchi MB, Belluzzi A, Meucci G, Campieri M, de Franchis R: p-ANCA and development of pouchitis in ulcerative colitis patients after proctocolectomy and ileoanal pouch anastomosis. Lancet 1994; 344:886–887.

Vecchi M, Sacchi E, Saibeni S, Meucci G, Tagliabue L, Duca F, De Franchis R: Inflammatory bowel diseases are not associated with major hereditary conditions predisposing to thrombosis. Dig Dis Sci 2000; 45:1465–1469.

Verkerk AJ, Pieretti M, Sutcliffe JS, Fu YH, Kuhl DP, Pizzuti A, Reiner O: Identification of a gene (*FMR*-1) containing a CGG repeat coincident with a breakpoint cluster region exhibiting length variation in Fragile X syndrome. Cell 1991; 65:905–914.

Vermeire S, Peeters M, Vlietinck R, Parkes M, Satsang J, Jewell D, Rutgeerts P: No evidence for linkage on chromsomes 16–12–7 and 3 in the Belgian population may reflect genetic heterogeneity of inflammatory bowel disease. Gastroenterology 1998; 114:A1109.

Vermeire S, Vlietinck R, Groenen P, Peeters M, Rutgeerts P: Replication of linkage on 14q11–12 in inflammatory bowel disease. Gastroenterology 2000; 118: A338.

Wakefield AJ, Ekbom A, Dhillon AP, Pittilo RM, Pounder RE: Crohn's disease: pathogenesis and persistent measles virus infection. Gastroenterology 1995; 108:911–916.

Wakefield AJ, Pounder RE: Measles virus in Crohn's disease. Lancet 1995; 345:660.

Wakefield AJ, Sankey EA, Dhillon AP, Sawyer AFM, More L, Sim R, Pittilo RM, Rowles PM, Hudson M, Lewis AMA, Pounder RE: Granulomatous vasculitis in Crohn's disease. Gastroenterology 1991; 100:1279–1287.

Wakefield AJ, Sawyer AM, Dhillon AP, Pittilo RM, Rowles PM, Lewis AAM, Pounder RE: Pathogenesis of Crohn's disease: multifocal gastrointestinal infarction. Lancet 1989; 2:1057–1062.

Weisner RH, LaRusso NF: Clinicopathologic features of the syndrome of primary sclerosing cholangitis. Gastroenterology 1980; 79:200–206.

Werlin SL, Chusid MJ, Caya J, Oechler HW: Colitis in chronic granulomatous disease. Gastroenterology 1982; 82:328–331.

Weterman IT, Pena AS: Familial incidence of Crohn's disease in the Netherlands and a review of the literature. Gastroenterology 1984; 86:449–452.

Wewer V, Gluud C, Schlichting P, Burcharth F, Binder V: Prevalence of hepatobiliary dysfunction in a regional group of patients with chronic inflammatory bowel disease. Scand J Gastroenterol 1991; 26:97–102.

Wildenberg SC, Oetting WS, Almodovar C, Krumwiede M, White JG, King RA: A gene causing Hermansky-Pudlak syndrome in a Puerto Rican population maps to chromosome 10q2. Am J Hum Genet 1995; 57:755–765.

Wilson AG, di Giovine FS, Duff GW: Genetics of tumour necrosis factor-α in autoimmune, infectious, and neoplastic diseases. J Inflamm 1995; 45:1–12.

Witkop CJ, Quevedo WC, Fitzpatrick TB, King RA: Albinism. In: Scriver C, Beaudet AL, Sly WS, Valle D (eds). The Metabolic Basic of Inherited Disease. New York: McGraw-Hill, 1989:2905–2948.

Wong PY, Yue G, Yin K, Miyasaka M, Lane CL, Manning AM, Anderson DC, Sun FF: Antibodies to intercellular adhesion molecule-1 ameliorate the inflammatory response in acetic acid–induced inflammatory bowel disease. J Pharmacol Exp Ther 1995; 274:475–480.

Yacyshyn B, Bowen-Yacyshyn M, Jewell L, Tami JA, Bennett CF, Kisner DL, Shanahan J: A placebo-controlled trial of ICAM-1 antisense oligonucleotide in the treatment of Crohn's disease. Gastroenterology 1998; 114:1133–1142.

Yacyshyn B, Meddings J, Sadowski D, Bowen-Yachyshyn M: Multiple sclerosis patients have peripheral blood CD45RO+ B cells and increased intestinal permeability. Dig Dis Sci 1996; 41:2493–2498.

Yang H, McElree C, Roth M-P, Shanahan F, Targan SR, Rotter JI: Familial empiric risks for inflammatory bowel disease: differences between Jews and non-Jews. Gut 1993a; 34:517–524.
Yang H, Ohmen JD, Ma R, Li Z, Bentley LG, Targan SR, Fischel-Ghodsian N, Rotter JI: Linkage and association between Crohn's disease and a putative locus on chromosome 12. Gastroenterology 1998; 114:A1119.
Yang H, Ohmen JD, Ma Y, Targan SR, Fischel-Ghodsian N, Rotter JI: Additional evidence of linkage between Crohn's disease and a putative locus on chromosome 12. Genet Med 1999a; 1:194–199.
Yang H, Plevy SE, Taylor K, Tyan D, Fischel-Ghodsian N, McElree C, Targan SR, Rotter JI: Linkage of Crohn's disease to the major histocompatibility complex region is detected by multiple non-parametric analyses. Gut 1999b; 44:519–526.
Yang H, Rotter JI: The genetics of inflammatory bowel disease. In: Targan SR, Shanahan F (eds). Inflammatory Bowel Disease: From Bench to Bedside. Baltimore: Williams & Wilkins, 1994:32–64.
Yang H, Rotter JI: Genetic aspects of idiopathic inflammatory bowel disease. In: Kirsner JB, Shorter RG (eds). Inflammatory Bowel Disease. Baltimore: Williams & Wilkins, 1995a:301–331.
Yang H, Rotter JI: Subclinical markers of human inflammatory bowel disease. Can J Gastroenterol 1995b; 9:161–167.
Yang H, Rotter JI: Inflammatory bowel disease. In: Rimoin DL, Connor JM, Pyeritz RE, Emery AEH (eds). Principles and Practice of Medical Genetics. London: Churchill Livingstone, 1997:1533–1553.
Yang H, Rotter JI, Toyoda H, Landers C, Tyan D, McElree CK, Targan SR: Ulcerative colitis: a genetically heterogeneous disorder defined by genetic (HLA class II) and subclinical (anti-neutrophil cytoplasmic antibodies) markers. J Clin Invest 1993b; 92:1080–1084.
Yang H, Shohat T, Rotter JI: The genetics of inflammatory bowel disease. In: McDermott RP, Stenson WF (eds). Inflammatory Bowel Disease. New York: Elsevier, 1992.
Yang H, Taylor KD, Lin YC, Targan SR, Rotter JI: Magnitude of anti-*Saccharomyces cerevisiae* antibody (ASCA) expression is linked in Crohn's disease families to the major histocompatibility complex (MHC) region. Gastroenterology 2000; 118:A339.
Yang H, Vora DK, Targan SR, Toyoda H, Beaudet AL, Rotter JI: Intercellular adhesion molecule 1 gene associations with immunologic subsets of inflammatory bowel disease. Gastroenterology 1995; 109:440–448.
Yang P, Jarnerot G, Danielsson D, Tysk C, Lindberg E: P-ANCA in monozygotic twins with inflammatory bowel disease. Gut 1995; 36:887–890.
Yang P, Oresland T, Jarnerot G, Hulten L, Danielsson D: Perinuclear antineutrophil cytoplasmic antibody in pouchitis after proctocolectomy with ileal pouch–anal anastomosis for ulcerative colitis. Scand J Gastroenterol 1996; 31:594–598.
Yates VM, Watkinson G, Kelman A: Further evidence for an association between psoriasis, Crohn's disease and ulcerative colitis. Br J Dermatol 1982; 106:323–330.
Zauli D, Baffoni L, Cassani F: Antineutrophil cytolasmic antibodies in primary sclerosing cholangitis, ulcerative colitis, and autoimmune diseases. Gastroenterology 1992; 102:1088–1095.
Zetterquist H, Broome U, Einarsson K, Olerup O: HLA class II genes in primary sclerosing cholangitis and chronic inflammatory bowel disease: No HLA-DRw52a association in Swedish patients with sclerosing cholangistis. Gut 1992; 33:942–946.
Zhang WJ, Koltun WA, Tilberg AF, Page MJ, Chorney MJ: Absence of GNAI2 codon 179 oncogene mutations in inflammatory bowel disease. Inflamm Bowel Dis 2000; 6:103–106.
Zlotogora J, Zimmerman J, Rachmilewitz D: Crohn's disease in Ashkenazi Jews. Gastroenterology 1990; 99:286–290.

16 Gallstones

BEVERLY PAIGEN AND MARTIN C. CAREY

Gallstones are calculi that form in bile within any part of the biliary tree, most frequently in the gallbladder (Nakayama 1997). As the exocrine secretion of the liver, bile is produced within spaces known as *canaliculi* that run between liver parenchymal cells. It constitutes an essential mechanism to facilitate lipid secretion by the liver and intestinal fat absorption (Crawford and Carey, 1998). Canaliculi are 1 to 2 μm canals formed between tight junctions surrounding canalicular membranes that are highly specialized but quantitatively minor (10%–15%) parts of the hepatocyte plasma membrane (Blovin, 1983). Bile is then conducted through an arborization of biliary passages of ever-increasing size (Fig. 16–1) into the upper part of the small intestine (Elias and Sherrick, 1969). Two large hepatic ducts exit from the liver (Fig. 16–1) and join together to form the common hepatic duct, which becomes the common bile duct. This large duct frequently shares its lumen with the major pancreatic duct (common channel), mixing bile and pancreatic juice prior to flowing into the duodenum, the first part of the small intestine (Last, 1963). The branching of the cystic duct distinguishes the transition between common hepatic and common bile ducts. The cystic duct acts as both the filling and emptying ducts of the gallbladder (Last, 1963). The gallbladder is a membranous, muscular sac adherent to the undersurface of the right lobe of the liver (Fig. 16–1), in which hepatic bile is concentrated and stored interdigestively (Rose, 1987; Reuss, 1991). Principally because of these functions, the majority of gallstones form in the gallbladder (Rains, 1964; Nakayama, 1997), often with no evidence of stones elsewhere in the biliary tree.

Gallstones are exceptionally common, occurring especially in Western populations. Several countries and even continents are notable exceptions, with gallstone prevalence rates approaching 0 (Burkitt and Tunstall, 1975). There is paleopathological evidence that the disease occurred but was not common in antiquity (Rains, 1964; Steinbock, 1991).

Gallstones would pass unnoticed in life were it not for the fact that they frequently produce pain and dangerous complications (Rains, 1964; Friedman, 1993; Nakayama, 1997). Since the disease can be treated definitively only by surgery and because surgery is commonly utilized, the total U.S. expense for the care of gallstone patients was $5 billion in 1985 (Brown and Everhart, 1994) and today is believed to approach $8 to $10 billion, or 1.3% to 1.5% of U.S. health-care costs (Everhart, 1994). In ancient Hippocratic and medieval Galenean physiology, bile constituted two of the four "bodily humors" determining a person's health and temperament (Rains, 1964; Heaton and Morris, 1971). Ever since the Greek physician Alexander of Tralle in the fifth century found "within the liver substance . . . dried up humors concreted like stones" (Thudichum, 1863; Rains, 1964), gallstones and bile have excited the interests of philosophers, apothecaries, embalmers, alchemists, artists, physicians, physiologists, chemists, pathologists, surgeons, epidemiologists, statisticians, economists, business administrators, and reviewers (see references in Thudichum, 1863; Sobotka, 1937; Rains, 1964; Heaton, 1973; Steinbock, 1991; Nakayama, 1997). The modern biophysical and pathophysiological era began with the understanding that gallstones are principally cholesterol calculi that phase-separate as crystals from supersaturated bile (Admirand and Small, 1968) and that bile constitutes a complex colloidal fluid of bile salt mixed micelles and phospholipid vesicles carrying large quantities of cholesterol (Carey and Cohen, 1987). Modern molecular biological and genetic approaches to bile, lipid secretion, enterohepatic circulation, and cholesterol gallstone formation have been productive in recent years (Russell and Setchell, 1992; Cohen et al., 1992; Higgins, 1992; Smit et al., 1993; Dawson and Oelkers, 1995; Khanuja et al., 1995; Müller and Jansen, 1997).

Here, we describe these recent discoveries and show how they pertain to gallstone disease, paying particular attention to cholesterol gallstones, which probably have a genetic basis. We will show how a preliminary understanding of cholesterol gallstones as a genetic disease is emerging from epidemiological, environmental, and pathophysiological studies in humans. Employing inbred mice as models (Khanuja et al., 1995), we discuss how the principal candidate proteins specified by a number of murine gallstone (*Lith*) genes may function and how they enter into the organism's biology. Extrapolating cautiously to humans, we demonstrate that a "thrifty" gallstone genotype (Neel, 1962; Weiss et al., 1984; Lowenfels, 1988) may have emerged during our pre-history because *LITH* genes conferred a pronounced survival advantage over individuals lacking the trait. They may have facilitated rapid absorption, assimilation, and storage of excess calories as fat while disposing of excess cholesterol by biliary secretion. Knowledge of the genes may not only provide a window on the kaleidoscopic past of the human race but also offer opportunities for prevention of cholesterol gallstone disease in the future (Carey, 1998).

DISEASE DEFINITION

Subtypes

Most gallstones form in the gallbladder through nucleation of sterile supersaturated bile (Carey, 1993a,b). They are composed chiefly of cholesterol monohydrate crystals (Rains, 1964) and/or precipitates of amorphous calcium bilirubinate often with cal-

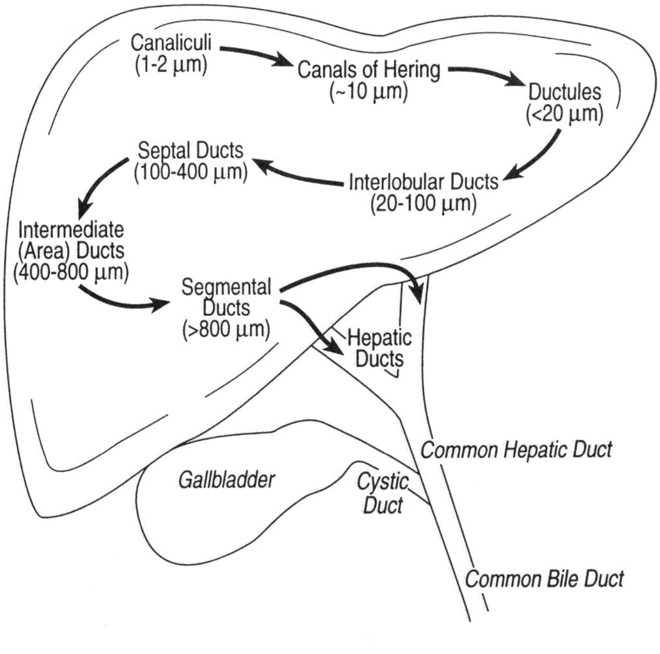

Fig. 16–1. Schematic depiction of the intrahepatic and extrahepatic biliary tree of humans, including the gallbladder. The purpose of the drawing is to display the sizes and nomenclature of the tunnel network within the liver beginning with canaliculi, which are tiny longitudinal tubes running between parenchymal liver cells (hepatocytes), and ending in the common bile duct, which conducts bile into the duodenum. The topology depicted within the liver has no relationship to reality and is employed here for convenience only.

cium carbonate or phosphate in one of the crystalline polymorphs (Cahalane et al., 1988). In typical Western populations, all gallstones from the same gallbladder are of similar composition (Park et al., 1982). Therefore, analysis of single gallstones from a number of gallbladders exhibits a bimodal distribution in terms of cholesterol contents (Sauerbruch et al., 1983). Figure 16–2 shows that the gallbladders of approximately one-quarter of a Boston cohort contained "black" pigment stones with less than 30% cholesterol by weight. Gallbladder pigment stones (Fig. 16–3A) are always small and multiple and generally black but can be dark brown, hard, brittle, lustrous, and sometimes spiculated. The nomogram (Fig. 16–2) indicates that the majority of gallstones are composed of at least 50% but generally more than 80% cholesterol. Cholesterol stones are much lighter in color than pigment stones and, when pure in composition, are white (Fig. 16–3B). They can be single (Fig. 16–3B) or multiple (Fig. 16–3C), round, oval, barrel-shaped, or faceted. Single stones (*cholesterol solitaire*) exhibit the highest cholesterol contents; it was from stones such as these that Michel Chevreul, the great French chemist, first obtained and identified the sterol, hence its common name (Chevreul, 1815). One of the curiosities of all cholesterol stones in humans (but not in laboratory animals) is that the nucleus is invariably pigmented with calcium bilirubinate (Rains, 1964). Stones with somewhat less cholesterol are generally multiple, often of similar size, and faceted (Fig. 16–3C), with colors varying from yellow to light brown depending on the calcium bilirubinate content. The calcium bilirubinate salts are invariably deposited in concentric rings and never tint the stones throughout (Hoppe-Seyler, 1903; Rains, 1964). Magnification of a fractured stone reveals cholesterol monohydrate crystals arrayed in radiating layers normal to the stone's surface. Calcium carbonate shells impart a considerable degree of hardness to stones and are frequent (Nakayama, 1997). Mucin glycoprotein (*mucus*) of gallbladder origin is a major component of both black pigment and cholesterol gallstones (Carey, 1993a,b). This sparingly soluble, high-molecular weight polymer acts not only as a heterogeneous nucleating agent (LaMont and Carey, 1992) but also as cement and scaffolding throughout the stones (Womack et al., 1963). Trace quantities of all other components of bile are found (Hoppe-Seyler, 1903; Rains, 1964), some of which may enter the stones by imbibition (Sanabria et al., 1996).

"Black" pigment and cholesterol gallstones are apparently caused by genetic, metabolic, and dietary factors (Carey, 1996, 1997). However, a less common type of pigment stone, known trivially as "brown," is infectious in origin (Cahalane et al., 1988). These pigment stones are putty-like in consistency, friable, and irregularly shaped, with a feculent odor from fermentation by entrapped anaerobic bacteria of colonic origin. They form in obstructed biliary passages and occasionally in the gallbladder. When brown stones occur intrahepatically, the disease is termed *hepatolithiasis*. This is primarily an Asian public health problem related to parasitic infestation from roundworms, particularly *Ascaris lumbricoides* or *Clonorchis sinensis*, and secondary bacterial infection of the biliary tree (Nakayama, 1997). The anaerobic bacteria produce a range of enzymes that hydrolyze ester and amide bonds of biliary lipids and conjugated bile pigments, leading to the intraductal precipitation of sparingly soluble lipids and their calcium salts (Cahalane et al., 1998). In the West, most cases of biliary tree obstruction are caused by a cholesterol or black pigment stone that has migrated from the gallbladder. The core and shell of such stones have distinct chemical compositions, consistent with the noninfectious gallbladder origin of the nucleus and the infectious origin of the mantle (Sauerbruch et al., 1983).

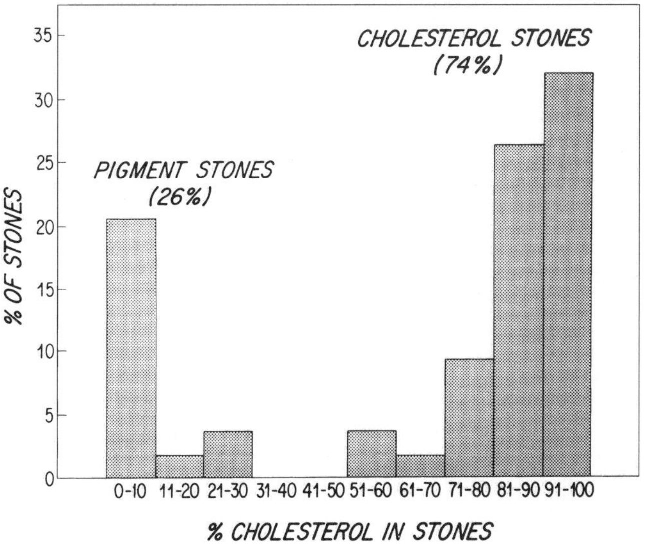

Fig. 16–2. Bimodal distribution of percent cholesterol in gallstones obtained from the gallbladders of different patients with sterile bile undergoing cholecystectomy at Brigham and Women's Hospital (Boston). The distribution of cholesterol by weight of each stone allows for a binary classification into ("black") pigment stones (<30% cholesterol) and cholesterol stones (>50% cholesterol) without a so-called mixed variety (stones courtesy of Dr. David C. Brooks, analysis by Michael J: Cahalane, Boston, MA).

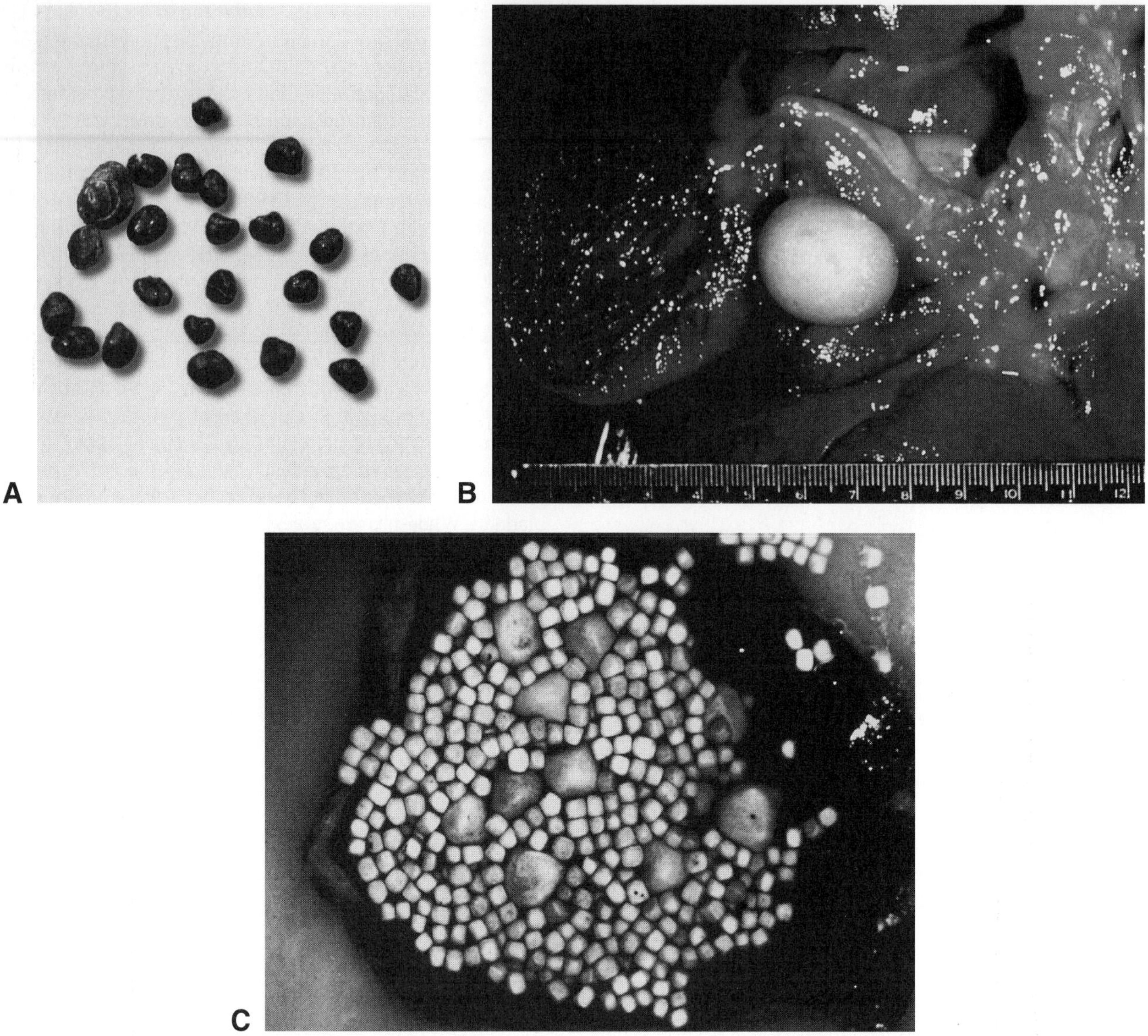

Fig. 16–3. *A:* "Black" pigment gallstones composed principally of the polymerized acid calcium salt of unconjugated bilirubin. *B:* A cholesterol gallstone of the round "solitaire" type lying at the infundibulum of an opened gallbladder. From Kamran Badizadegan as published in Cotran et al. (1989) with permission. *C:* Multiple-facet cholesterol gallstones with two size distributions (A and C courtesy of Drs. David C. Brooks).

Clinical Presentation

Silent Stones

Most (50%–90%) gallstones remain asymptomatic ("silent") throughout life. The likelihood of silent stones is influenced by gender (male > female), age (old > young), race (Caucasian > African American > Native American), presence of other metabolic disease (obesity, diabetes mellitus, alcoholism), stone type (cholesterol, especially solitaire > black pigment), latitude (tropics > temperate > Mediterranean > sub-Arctic), physical activity (regular exercise > sedentary), somatotype (slim > obese), cyesis (pregnancy > puerperium), and calorie intake (vegetarian diets > regular diet > low-calorie diet) (Apstein and Carey, 1994). Because gallstones become symptomatic in 10% to 50% of cases, *clinical* prevalence always underestimates *true* prevalence to a degree that depends on the population and the above factors (Carey and O'Donovan, 1984). It follows that the only reliable way to assess true gallstone prevalence rates is to screen all (or a scientifically chosen subset) of a population, stratified for age and gender, by ultrasonography or oral cholecystography (now obsolete for this purpose). These methods are highly specific and sensitive in making the diagnosis, and provided that all subjects with previous cholecystectomy are added to the numerator, accurate prevalence rates are obtained. Since 1970, when a true prevalence study was carried out by oral cholecystography on southwestern Native Americans (Sampliner et al., 1970), epidemiological studies have been carried out widely and rigorously and have proven most useful in tracking the genetic epidemiology of the disease.

Symptomatic Gallstones

When stones move or become temporarily or permanently impacted in the neck of the gallbladder, cystic duct, or biliary tree, they cause biliary pain, misnamed *colic* (Apstein, 1998). An attack of this severe, tearing, lacerating, and invariably constant pain usually begins, without a prodrome, in the epigastrium or right hypochondrium. Pain can radiate in any direction, including to sites such as the jaw, mammary gland, right shoulder, and genitals. It may occur only once or be daily in frequency. It is unremitting and therefore not a colic, lasts more than 30 minutes, and is characterized by frequent vomiting (Hoppe-Seyler, 1903). Most biliary pain is nocturnal (Rigas et al., 1990), occurring within 2 hours of retiring; however, in one-fourth of individuals, pain is postprandial or occurs during the late afternoon or both (Apstein, 1998). Invariably, the pain remits and a feeling of soreness over the gallbladder area persists for several hours. If the pain does not remit, a potentially life-threatening complication of gallstones, such as *cholecystitis* (inflammation of the gallbladder), *choledocolithiasis* (a stone impacted in the common duct), *cholangitis* (inflammation of the bile ducts), or *pancreatitis* (inflammation of the pancreas), secondary to an obstructing stone should be suspected.

Diagnostic Criteria

Because at least 85% of gallstones are radiolucent and do not show up on plain radiographs of the abdomen, ultrasonographic examination (Fig. 16–4A,B), with its resolution of approximately 3 mm, is key to the diagnosis for epidemiological purposes and family prevalence studies (Apstein, 1998). Mobile objects casting acoustic shadows (Fig. 16–4A) differentiate stones from adenomata or polyps of the gallbladder. Because both gallstone types (Fig. 16–3A,C) look alike upon ultrasound examination, the unanswered question for genetic epidemiologists is how frequently this might lead to diagnostic misclassification and therefore muddle genetic studies. This is a crucial issue when examining a family or subpopulation because, as inferred from pathophysiology, the genetic factors involved in cholesterol and black pigment gallstones are almost certainly different (Carey, 1993a,b). Therefore, it is critical to identify predisposing disorders for pigment stones, such as hemolysis, ineffective erythropoiesis, or ileal disease, by a careful medical history, physical examination, and laboratory tests. A cholecystectomized population at Brigham and Women's Hospital (Boston, MA) had a high percentage (26%) of pigment stones (Fig. 16–1), but clearly this ratio will differ in other countries and subpopulations. In some Native American tribes, pigment stone prevalence is vanishingly small (Ingelfinger, 1979); and in most of Africa, because of sickle cell disease, malaria, and a dearth of cholesterol stones, pigment stone disease may be the only type (Heaton, 1981). Although no precise methodology exists for differentiating cholesterol from pigment stones, computed tomographic (CT) scanning offers promise since there appears to be good correlation between stone CT density and cholesterol stone composition (Baron et al., 1988).

Biliary sludge is a radiological term for gelled gallbladder mucin containing entrapped crystals, liquid crystals, and/or calcium bilirubinate granules of sufficient size ($\geq 30\ \mu m$) to be visualized ultrasonographically (Fig. 16–4B) (Filly et al., 1980; Carey and Cahalane, 1988; Lee et al., 1988; Angelico et al., 1990). Sludge is certainly a transient stage in the formation of both cholesterol and pigment gallstones (Lee et al., 1985, 1988, 1994). Because stone formation is not inevitable (Carey and Cahalane, 1988), most epidemiologists do not include sludge as a criterion for the diagnosis of pre-stone disease. It is only when sludge is associated with inherited hemolytic anemias (Sarnaik et al., 1980) that one can be fairly certain that it is predestined to become black pigment gallstones (Bond et al., 1987).

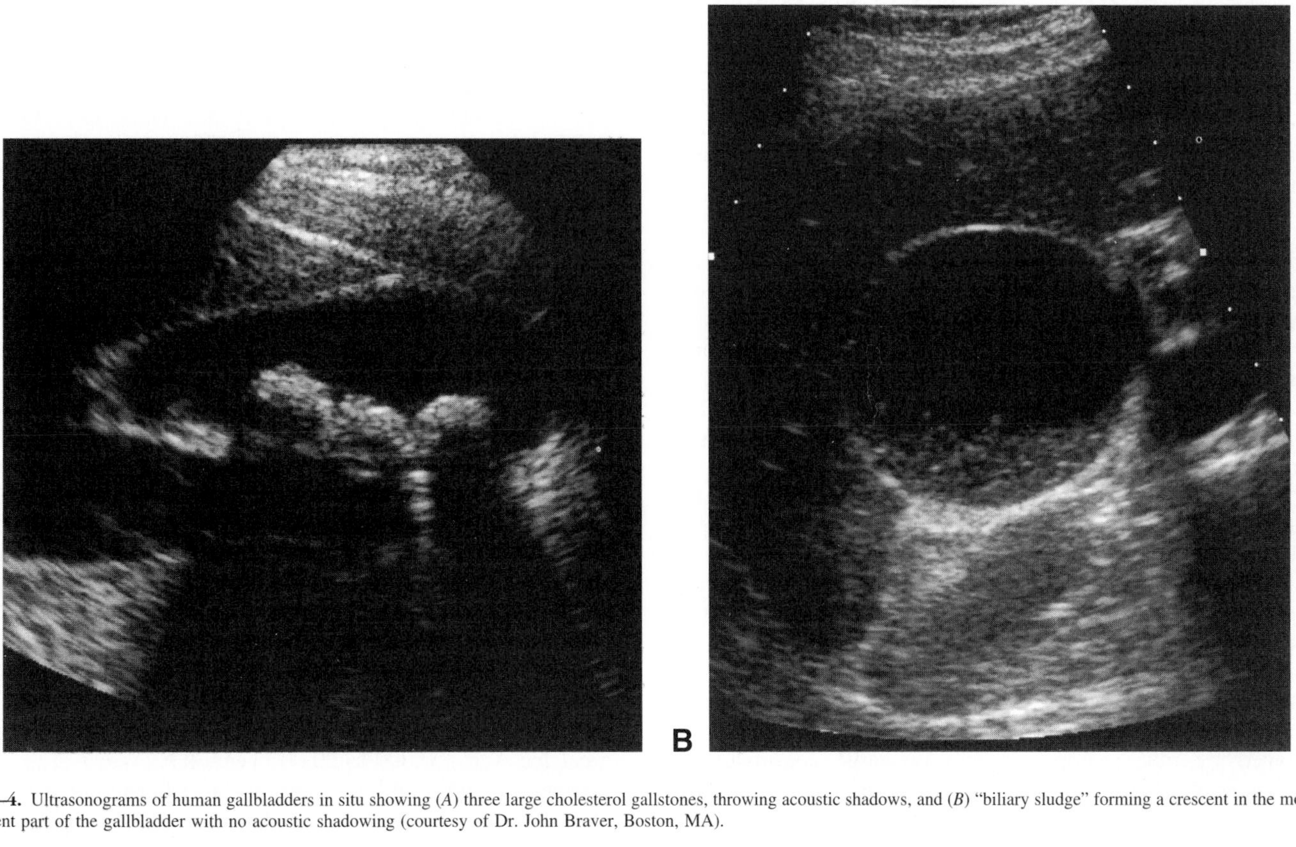

A B

Fig. 16–4. Ultrasonograms of human gallbladders in situ showing (*A*) three large cholesterol gallstones, throwing acoustic shadows, and (*B*) "biliary sludge" forming a crescent in the most dependent part of the gallbladder with no acoustic shadowing (courtesy of Dr. John Braver, Boston, MA).

GENERAL GENETIC AND EPIDEMIOLOGICAL EVIDENCE

Clinical Epidemiology and Ethnic Differences

General Considerations

The lack of accurate geographic information on gallstone prevalence worldwide typifies a common disease that is generally nonfatal and often asymptomatic. Until non-invasive imaging by ultrasonagraphy was introduced, only hospitalization/surgical data were available for clinically symptomatic disease and autopsy data for true (symptomatic plus asymptomatic) stone prevalence (Carey and O'Donovan, 1984). The biases in autopsy data are well known; the subjects are usually from urban populations and die in hospitals, often with multiple acute and chronic diseases. In all autopsy studies, stones were not chemically analyzed, so the true ratios of cholesterol to pigment cholelithiasis are not available. Similar biases can be associated with epidemiological surveys of free-living populations for gallstones in that stone type cannot be distinguished by ultrasonography or cholecystography. However, there is emerging evidence that in vivo attenuation values (Hounsfield units, HUs) by CT may provide excellent discrimination (Baron et al., 1988; Rambow et al., 1991) between cholesterol (<100 HU) and pigment stones (>100 HU), especially when taken together with radiographic features (Brink et al., 1994).

Comparisons of data in different cross-sectional or autopsy studies are fraught with difficulty because the crucial age and sex variables are often not considered (Heaton, 1981). Prevalence rates increase with age, and worldwide, cholesterol gallstones are at least twice as frequent in women compared with men. Cross-sectional studies conducted on a "convenience sample" of individuals are also problematic; e.g., the ultrasonographic screening of civil servants in Rome for gallstones (Rome Group for the Epidemiology and Prevention of Cholelithiasis, 1984, 1988a,b) was not representative of the Roman population.

Historically, G. B. Morgagni, the father of pathological anatomy, opined nearly a quarter of a millennium ago that gallstones favored women, increased in prevalence with advancing age, and often remained asymptomatic for life and that obesity was an important risk factor (Morgagni, 1769).

Geographic Variations

Geographic variations, when formally documented, provide a good estimate of the gallstone proneness of a population (Heaton, 1981). Autopsy prevalence rates (Fig. 16–5) in elderly women (aged 70–79 years, i.e., maximum prevalence rates) from 14 countries are based on reliable surveys published between 1951 and 1981 (Heaton, 1981). Gallstones are very common in Western countries (Cleland, 1953; Rodewald, 1957; Newman and Northup, 1959; Torvik and Høivik, 1960; Watkinson, 1967; Burnett, 1971; Marinovic et al., 1972; Douss and Castelden, 1973; Záhor et al., 1974; Kalos et al., 1977), with maximum rates that vary from 30% to 60%, especially in Chile, Sweden, and the Czech Republic (Fig. 16–5). In contrast, in developing countries, prevalence rates are low, from 0.1% in Ghana (Edington, 1957; Steinbock, 1991) to 4.4% in Thailand (Stitnimankarn, 1960); the 3% reported in Uganda (Owor, 1964) were mostly pigment stones, probably related to malaria or sickle cell disease. As evidenced by older autopsy studies on large cohorts, native Africans are strikingly free of cholesterol stone disease: Kenya, 0.1% (Vint, 1937); South Africa, 0.03% (Lopis, 1947) to 2% (Becker and Chatgidakis, 1952); Senegal, 0.1% (Edington, 1957;); Congo/Zaire, <0.01% (Trowell, 1960); Uganda, 0.9% with only 0.02% "cholesterol type" (Owor, 1964); Kenya, <0.01 (Trowell, 1981); south Kenya/Tanzania (the Masai tribe), 0% (Biss et al., 1971); and Ghana, 0% (Steinbock, 1991). The world-map projection (Fig. 16–6) shows approximate geographic distributions of gallstone disease categorized as rare (<5%), intermediate (5%–10%), common (10%–80%), and unknown (Grosse, 1966; Burkitt and Tunstall, 1975; Brett and Barker, 1976; Lowenfels, 1980; Heaton, 1981; Heaton et al., 1991a; Tsukanov et al., 1998). Although cholesterol gallstones are exceptionally rare in native populations of sub-Saharan Africa (Parnis, 1964; Shaper and Patel, 1964; Archampong, 1969; Onuigbo, 1977; Adedeji et al., 1986; Loefler, 1988), they are common in white populations of sub-Saharan Africa, particularly South Africa (Becker and Chatgidakis, 1952) and Zimbabwe, formerly Rhodesia (Burkitt and Tunstall, 1975). Gallstones are also rare in southern India (Malhotra, 1968), in Thailand (Stitnimankarn, 1960), and among the indigenous populations of New Guinea, Hawaii, Indonesia (Burkitt and Tunstall, 1975), and Siberia (Tsukanov et al., 1998). Intermediate prevalence rates have been reported from Spain, Greenland, the Balkans, north India, New Zealand and Easter Island (Maori population), Egypt, Arabia, South Korea, Japan, China, Singapore, and Israel (Heaton, 1973; Burkitt and Tunstall, 1975; Brett and Barker, 1976; Miquel et al., 1998). Prevalence rates are high throughout North, Central, and South America; most of Western Europe, especially Scandinavia and Finland; European Russia; Switzerland; Australia; New Zealand; and Hawaii (Brett and Barker, 1976; Heaton, 1981; Carey and O'Donovan, 1984; Nakayama, 1997). Overall, the worldwide distribution supports the theory that gallstones have a genetic basis and that gallstone (*LITH*) genes are "thrifty" genes (Neel, 1962; Shaheb, 1990) which emerged during inhospitable epochs involving the human race, e.g., during the last great Ice Age 100,000 to 20,000 years B.P. (Weiss et al., 1984; Lowenfels, 1988) and are likely to have been spread by small numbers of founder populations during several protracted human

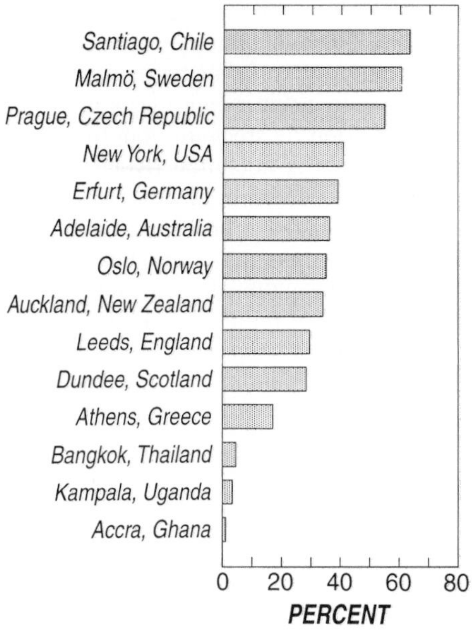

Fig. 16–5. Autopsy prevalence rates of gallstones in 70- to 79-year-old women in 14 countries based on reliable surveys published between 1951 and 1981. From Heaton (1981), with permission.

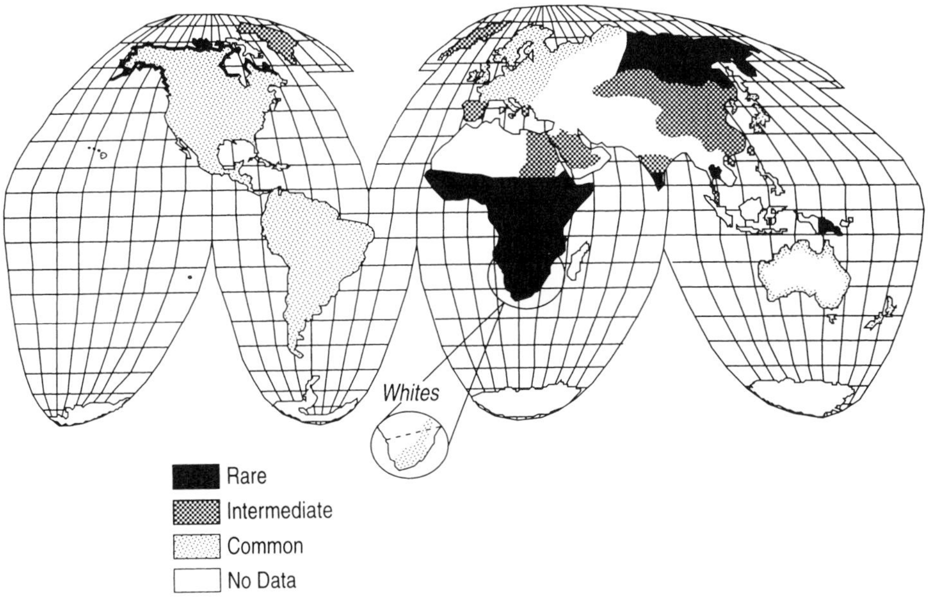

Fig. 16–6. World projection displaying countries and continents with rare, intermediate, common, and unknown prevalence rates of gallstones. Modified from Burkitt and Tunstall (1975), with up-to-date additions, see text and reference list.

migrations: *(1)* Native Americans from Beringia throughout the Americas c.12,000 years B.P. (Weiss et al., 1984), *(2)* Viking conquests of Europe 1200 to 800 years B.P. (Jones, 1984; Poser, 1995), and *(3)* Western European descendants of the Vikings to the Americas, Africa, Australia, and the Far East during the fifteenth to the twentieth centuries (Poser, 1995).

Population

The most reliable gallstone prevalence studies derive principally from defined populations of Scandinavia, Germany, Italy, American Hispanics, and Pima Indians of Arizona (summarized in Carey and O'Donovan, 1984; Knowler et al., 1984; Lowenfels et al., 1985; Diehl, 1991). Other good epidemiological studies, albeit clinical, have been carried out on Native American Chippewa (Thistle et al., 1971) and Micmac women (Williams et al., 1977a).

Native Americans. Many Native-American tribes demonstrate extraordinarily high prevalence rates of gallstones. These include the Micmac (eastern woodlands); Chippewa and Sioux (Great Plains); Shoshone and Arapaho (Great Basin); Navaho, Hopi, Papago, Apache, and Pima (southwest); and Seminoles (southeast) (Sievers and Marquis, 1962; Kravetz, 1964; Sievers and Fischer, 1981). The best studied tribes are the Micmac of Nova Scotia, Chippewa of Minnesota, and Pima of Arizona, which have the smallest European admixtures: Pima < Chippewa < Micmac (Geare, 1915; Hancock, 1933; Williams et al., 1986, 1992). Comess and colleagues (1967) highlighted the high prevalence of clinical gallstone disease, i.e., the sum of those with biliary pain, gallstone complications, and prior cholecystectomy, in Pima Indians compared to the population in the Framingham Study (Friedman et al., 1966). The age-adjusted clinical prevalence rates were 30% in 25- to 34-year-old and 45% in 35- to 44-year-old females, with males exhibiting much less clinical gallstone disease. Sampliner and colleagues (1970) published their classic epidemiological investigation of the true prevalence rate of gallstones in Pima Indians (Fig. 16–7). They examined a random sample of the population consisting of 50 males and 50 females in each of six age decades between 15 and 74 years. Oral cholecystography, the standard diagnostic tool at the time, was performed on those without previously documented gallstone disease, and nonvisualization of the gallbladder after ingestion of "iopanoic" acid was considered a positive result. True prevalence rates in Pima females ascended sharply from a few percent in adolescence to 70% and greater at age 25 to 34, remaining essentially constant thereafter into the seventh decade (Fig. 16–7). Gallstone prevalence in male Pimas showed a more gradual increase with advancing age until the sixth decade, thereafter equalling the rates for females (Fig. 16–7). The open sections of each histogram indicate prevalence rates of clinical (symptomatic) disease, including those cholecystectomized (Comess et al., 1967). Nearly half the females suffered from clinical disease compared to an appreciably lower percentages of

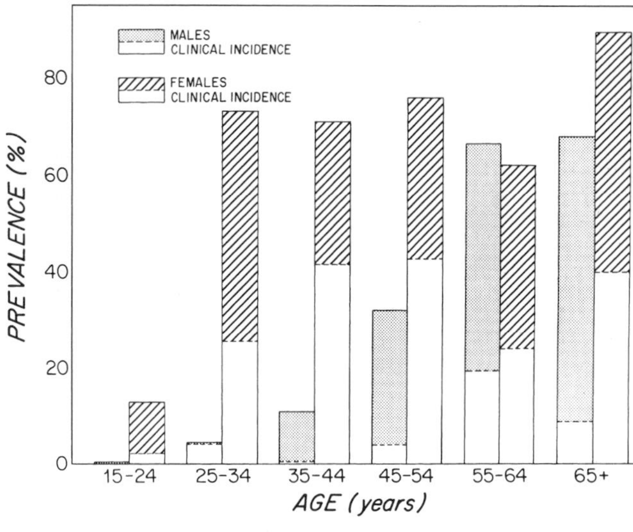

Fig. 16–7. True prevalence (*total bars*) and clinical prevalence (*open bars*) of gallstones in Pima Indians of Arizona, stratified for age decades and gender. From Carey and O'Donovan (1984) with permission.

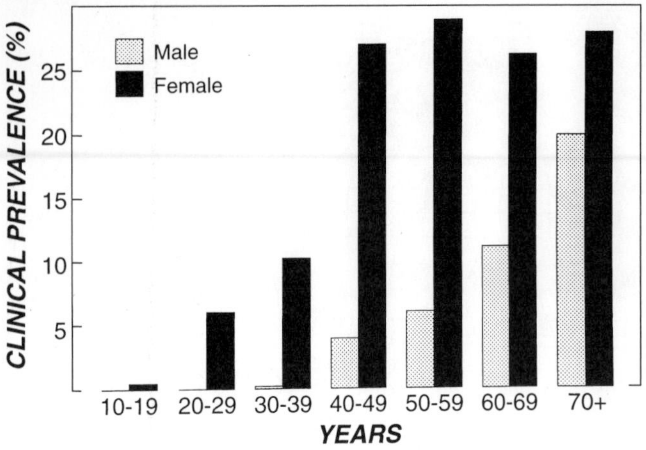

Fig. 16–8. Age- and gender-related prevalence rates of clinical (i.e., symptoms/cholecystectomy) gallbladder disease among Chippewa Indians of north Minnesota. Redrawn from data of Thistle et al. (1971).

males. Figure 16–8 displays clinical prevalence rates of gallstone disease among the Chippewa of Minnesota (Thistle et al., 1971), showing slightly higher rates of symptomatic disease, especially among males, than in the Pima. Other data, collected by Williams and colleagues (1977a) on Canadian Micmac women, corroborate these high prevalence rates among Native Americans. Nonetheless, since true prevalence rates of gallstones in the Chippewa and Micmac were not evaluated, the percentages of both populations remaining asymptomatic are not known.

Hispanic Populations. Hispanics have variable mixed Native American and Spanish ancestry (Long, 1991). Although past clinical data suggested high gallstone prevalence rates in Mexican Americans (Diehl and Stern, 1989), only two age- and gender-related true prevalence studies of Hispanics have been carried out by ultrasonography. Maurer and associates (1989) studied Puerto Ricans, Cuban Americans, and Mexican Americans in a gender- and age-stratified cross-sectional survey for gallstone disease from 1982 to 1984 as part of the Hispanic Health and Nutrition Examination Survey. Cases were defined as "subjects who had gallstones or who had their gallbladders surgically removed as indicated by ultrasound" (Tseng et al., 1998). Figure 16–9 reveals that gallstone prevalence rates increase markedly with advancing age and are more pronounced in females, with subgroup rates increasing in the rank order Puerto Ricans < Cuban Americans < Mexican Americans. Similar data were obtained by Miquel and colleagues (1998) in three Chilean subpopulations where prevalence rates varied in the rank order Native Americans > Hispanics > Easter Island Maoris (with no Native-American admixture as proven by mitochondrial DNA). Overall gallstone prevalence rates in Hispanics are much less than in Pima Indians and approximate those of northern Europeans, particularly Norwegians and Germans (Diehl, 1991). Developing information on the Mexican-American population of San Antonio, Texas, is consistent with the concept that variation in gallbladder disease in Hispanics is under strong genetic control (Duggirala et al., 1999).

African Americans. True prevalence data for African Americans are lacking; however, two older autopsy surveys, from Philadelphia, Pennsylvania (Lieber, 1952), and Birmingham, Alabama (Cunningham and Hardenbergh, 1956), suggest that prevalence rates in both genders increase with age, leveling off in the seventh to eighth decades to just below 20% (Fig. 16–10). In the younger age groups, females displayed slightly higher prevalence rates than males, and the gender ratio became equal in the seventh decade. This indicates that presumed cholesterol gallstone proneness is appreciably less, by one-fourth to one-sixth, in African Americans compared with U.S. Hispanics or Native Americans. This is in agreement with the documented low hospitalization incidence for gallbladder disease among African Americans (Sichieri et al., 1990). African-American populations are not pure-blooded Africans but are genetically admixed with Native Americans, particularly Cherokees, and with the descendents of northern European immigrants to the southern United States.

Western Europeans. Gallstones are exceptionally common throughout most of western Europe (Burkitt and Tunstall, 1975; Brett and Barker, 1976; Heaton, 1981; Carey and O'Donovan, 1984; Nakayama, 1997). As inferred from prevalence data in

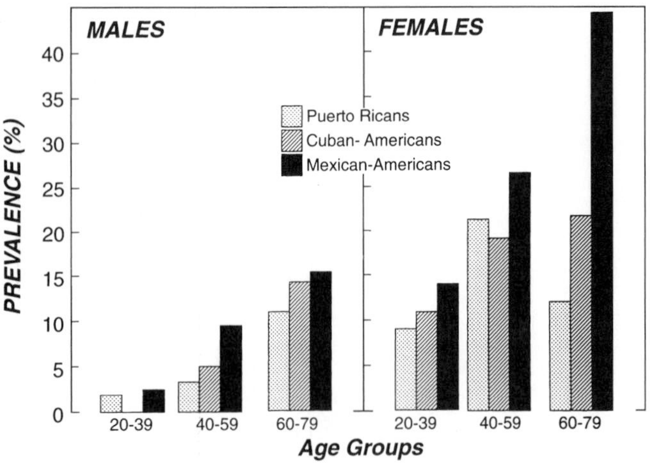

Fig. 16–9. Age- and gender-related prevalence rates of gallstones in Puerto Ricans, Cuban Americans, and Mexican Americans in the United States. Redrawn from Maurer et al. (1989).

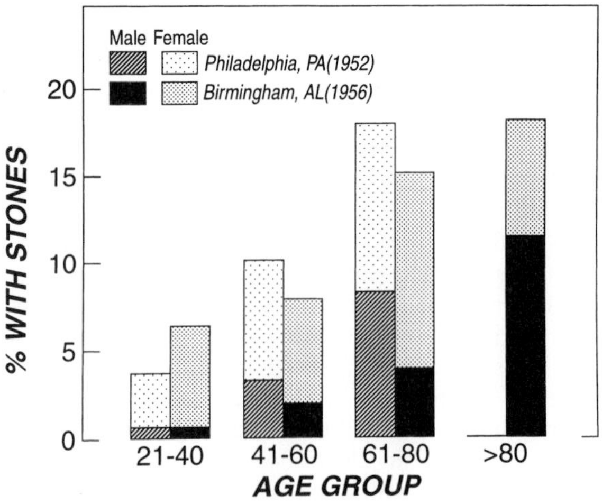

Fig. 16–10. Age- and gender-related prevalence rates of gallstones in African Americans based on 1952 and 1956 autopsy surveys in Philadelphia, PA, and Birmingham, AL. Plotted from data of Lieber (1952) and Cunningham and Hardenbergh (1956) with additions (sources in text).

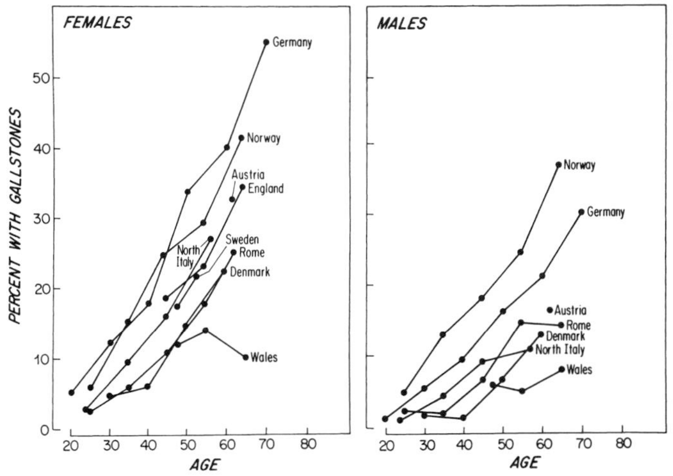

Fig. 16–11. Age- and gender-stratified prevalence rate of gallstones in countries of Western Europe by ultrasonography. Data from multiple sources (see text) and Heaton et al. (1991a,b).

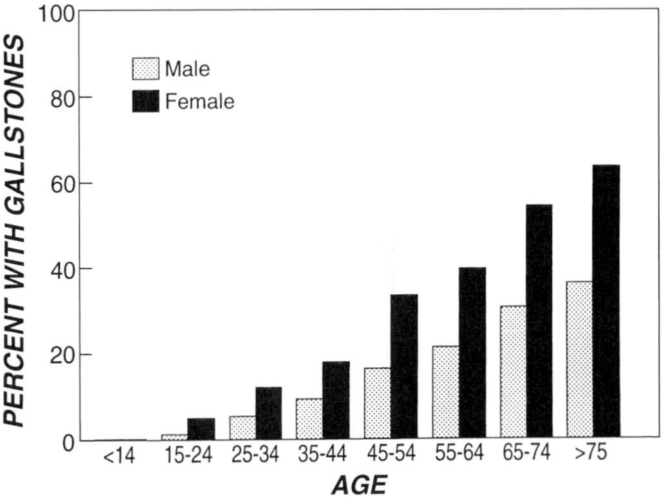

Fig. 16–12. Ultrasonographic mean prevalence rates of gallstones in two urban populations (Neuruppin, Schwedt) of northeast Germany stratified for age and gender. From Berndt et al. (1989) with permission.

Switzerland (Enderlin, 1958; Newman and Northup, 1959), the Czech Republic (Záhor et al., 1974), Romania (Acalovschi et al., 1995), Austria (Salzer et al., 1970), and Greece (Kalos et al., 1977), this appears to be the case also in central and eastern Europe. Figure 16–11 shows a compilation of the prevalence rates of gallstones documented by ultrasonography as functions of age in European females and males based on a number of reliable ultrasonographic studies (Heaton et al., 1991a). Gallstones are clearly endemic in Western Europe, with Scandinavia (Brett and Barker, 1976), Germany (Berndt et al., 1989), and Holland (Thijs et al., 1990b) predominating. In Scandinavia, prevalence rates decrease in the rank order of Norway (Glambek et al., 1987) > Sweden (Záhor et al., 1974) > Denmark (Jorgensen, 1987) > Finland (Brett and Barker, 1976) (not displayed), and the female-to-male ratio is ≈2:1 (Fig. 16–11). In Germany, prevalence rates appear to decrease as one travels southward (Brett and Barker, 1976; Massarratt et al., 1982; Balzer et al., 1986; Kratzer et al., 1998). The Sirmione, Italy, ultrasound study (Barbara et al., 1987) of 1930 subjects 18 to 65 years of age showed prevalence ranges of 1.1% to 11.0% in males and 2.9% to 27.0% in females (Fig. 16–11). Between 1985 and 1995, the Multicenter Italian Study on the Epidemiology of Cholelithiasis (MICOL) studied ultrasonographically two-thirds of 46,139 subjects aged 30 to 69 enrolled in 18 centers from 10 different regions (Attili et al., 1995). Gallstone prevalence rates displayed regional variations, with appreciably higher rates in northern than in central or southern Italy. As with all other studies on Caucasians, 70% to 90% of subjects were asymptomatic, a characteristic favoring males.

Age. As evidenced by data from two cities (Schwedt and Neuruppin) of northeastern Germany (Berndt et al., 1989), gallstone prevalence increases linearly with advancing age in both sexes (Fig. 16–12). Since gallstones do not disappear spontaneously, such data represent cumulative prevalence rates. There are two possible interpretations of these trends: *(1)* the incidence of gallstones, i.e., the percent of new cases appearing over a fixed time interval, remains the same in each decade, so if the ratio of cholesterol to pigment gallstone patients remained approximately 4:1 (Fig. 16–2), then age-related risk factors for both types of stone are identical throughout life; *(2)* assuming that cholesterol stones are a disease of youth and early middle age and that black pigment stones are a disease of late middle and old age, then these prevalence data (Fig. 16–12) might result from the integration of sigmoidal curves for each stone type (Trotman and Soloway, 1973). Because pigment gallstones are practically unknown in Pima Indians (Ingelfinger, 1979), the abrupt increase in stone prevalence in the second to fourth decades supports the suggestion of early onset of cholesterol stones (Fig. 16–7). One of the earliest autopsy studies, by von Recklinghausen and Schröder in 1892 (Moynihan, 1905) from Strasbourg (Fig. 16–13), showed a leveling off in prevalence rates in middle age but a sharp increase again in subjects 60 years and older. Heaton and colleagues (1991a) observed a similar trend in a prevalence study of gallstones in middle-aged females in Bristol, UK. In a clinical incidence study of 94 patients cholecystectomised over a 6-month period (Trotman and Soloway, 1975), there was a predominance of cholesterol stones in the younger age group and of pigment stones in the older age group, both being chemically verified (Fig. 16–14). Evidence against this subdivision derives from two unique populations, Chile (Valdiviesco et al., 1978) and Sweden (Einarsson et al., 1985), where aging was shown to augment the absolute as well as the relative biliary secretion rates of cholesterol.

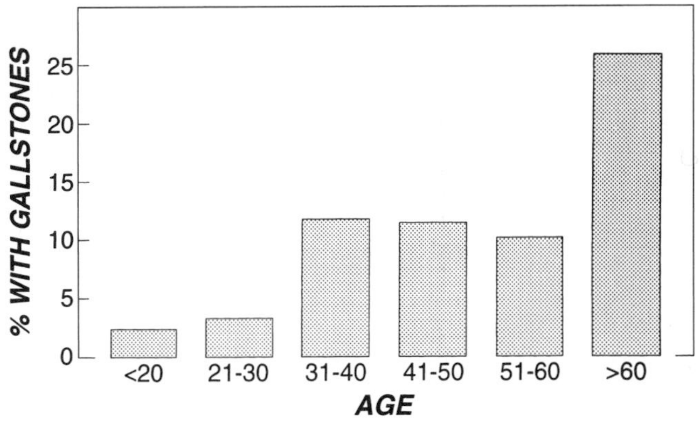

Fig. 16–13. Autopsy prevalence of gallstones in Strasbourg, France, during 1880–1887. Data of von Recklinghausen, collected by Schröder (1892) and cited by Moynihan (1905).

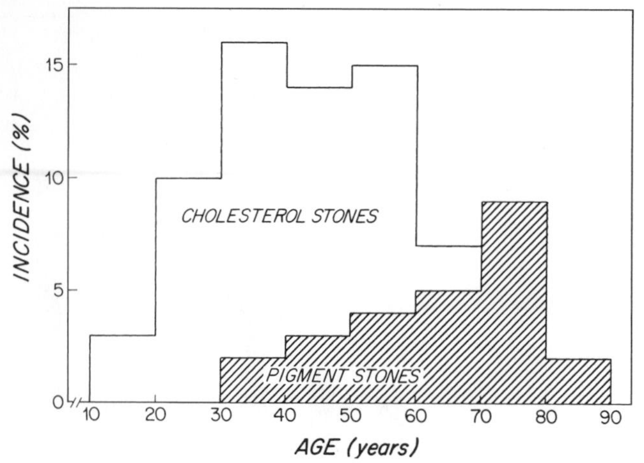

Fig. 16–14. Percent incidence of cholesterol and pigment gallstones in 94 consecutive cholecystectomies over a 6-month period in Philadelphia. Plotted from data of Trotman and Soloway (1975), published in Carey and O'Donovan (1984) with permission.

Gallstones are seldom found in prepubertal children and are rare in adolescent Caucasians. When they occur, they are mainly pigment stones associated with hemolytic anemia (Rains, 1964; Grosfeld et al., 1994). In the Sirmione study, only 1 of 135 in the 18- to 21-year-old subset had gallstones (Sama et al., 1990). However, in Mexican-American adolescents, cholesterol gallstones occur frequently, usually associated with obesity, family history, use of anovulatory steroids, and teenage pregnancy (Andrassy et al., 1976; Odom et al., 1976; Diehl, 1991). Both the Rome Group for the Epidemiology and Prevention of Cholelithiasis (1984, 1988a,b) and the Sirmione (Barbara et al., 1987) studies (Fig. 16–11) found gallstone prevalence rates that increased linearly with advancing age, typical of gallstone incidence in general. The 5-year rate of new stone formation in Sirmione was 3%, being higher in the 40- to 69-year age group (Sama et al., 1990), and in Chile the incidence was 6% in women under 31 years of age (Covarrubias et al., 1984).

Gender. Although in the Western world there is a 2:1 preponderance of cholesterol gallstones in females compared with males (Figs. 16–11, 16–12), a ratio of unity is observed in elderly Pimas (Sampliner et al., 1970). In some northern European populations (Bainton et al., 1976; Jorgensen, 1987), the gender ratio in the seventh decade of life also approaches unity (Fig. 16–7). Since ultrasonographic studies of patients with inherited hemolytic anemias (Sarnaik et al., 1980; Bond et al., 1987) reveal a female-to-male ratio of unity for black gallbladder stones, this again supports the probability that pigment stone disease predominates in old age (Trotman and Soloway, 1975). A female preponderance of cholesterol stones is observed in many animal models (Malet, 1985), but in certain inbred strains of mice, such as the gallstone-susceptible C57L/J strain, the gender ratio is reversed (Wang et al., 1997).

Family Epidemiology

Family Studies

For such a remarkably common disease, the literature concerning family inheritance is meager. Lord Moynihan of Leeds, a dominant voice in British surgery at the beginning of the last century, made the following fanciful statement (Moynihan, 1905):

> Ehret has found gall-stones in four generations, and some physicians are disposed to think that heredity must be considered playing a part. The number of suggestions that have been put forward are (*sic*) remarkable for their number and for their worthlessness. Much has been written, but little is known. It is in surgery as in finance—much poverty and much paper may coexist.

The anecdotal impression prevailed earlier in the last century that gallbladder disease (which is due to gallstones at least 98% of the time) is much more common in some families than in others (summarized in McConnell, 1966). In an age- and sex-controlled study of 74 family pedigrees of probands with gallbladder disease in Germany, Körner (1937) showed that gallstones were five times more common in families of affected individuals than in the control group. Jackson and Gay (1959) found that 72% of first-degree family members of 100 consecutive Caucasian patients undergoing gallbladder surgery had definite or suggestive evidence of gallbladder disease, utilizing oral cholecystography and history of cholecystectomy. Because of a higher female-to-male ratio in this study, Jackson and Gay (1959) suggested that gallstone disease may be inherited as a sex-linked dominant trait. In a cross-sectional ultrasonographic study of a large cohort ($n = 4581$) in Copenhagen, Jorgensen (1988a,b) found a positive 2:1 association between true gallstone disease in first-degree relatives of subjects with gallstones. In a paired subset ($n = 430$) of the Sirmione study (Barbara et al., 1987; Sama et al., 1990), the relative risk of gallstones was 3.3-fold higher in sons and daughters of parents with gallstones when controlled for age and other variables. In northern Germany, Nürnberg et al. (1989) found a threefold increased prevalence of gallstones in families of younger, asymptomatic female gallstone patients ($n = 1616$) compared with stone-free controls. In Ulm, Germany, a similar familial frequency of gallstones was found by Kratzer et al. (1998) among 1116 young to middle-aged healthy blood donors, most of whom were men. In the large Italian MICOL study (Attili et al., 1997), subjects with a history of gallstones in either parent had an increased risk of gallstones, with the risk being significantly higher when both parents had gallstone disease.

In northern Sweden during the 1960s and 1970s, very useful work on the familial occurrence of gallstones was done by van der Linden (1980). He attempted to sort out diagnostic and ascertainment bias with respect to control groups as well as to verify the presence of stones by oral cholecystography or cholecystectomy. van der Linden and Lindelöf (1965) restricted one investigation to proven gallstone patients who were married and who had siblings of the opposite sex. If the patient were a man, the occurrence of gallstones in his wife was compared with that in his sister nearest in age to his wife. If the patient were a woman, the occurrence of gallstones in her husband was compared with that in her brother nearest in age to her husband. Employing this approach, 263 individuals (87 males and 176 females, mean ages 49 and 51 years, respectively) were evaluated rigorously for gallstones. The data showed a clear 2:1 ratio in favor of familial occurrence, which was significant across the biometric criteria of Bross (1952) as well as the objection of Spiegel (1918) for the control group. Because familial occurrence does not necessarily reflect genetic factors, van der Linden and Westlin (1966) then studied the occurrence of gallstones in spouses who had lived together continuously and presumably shared the same environment, especially diet, during adult life. They employed a similar methodology and found that women married to patients with gallstone disease do not have a higher

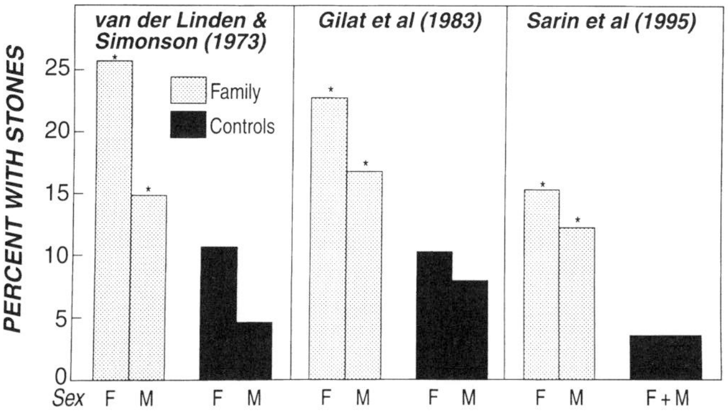

Fig. 16–15. Significant increases in true prevalence rates of gallstones by oral cholecystography, surgery, and/or ultrasonography in first-degree relatives of gallstone patients compared with controls. Data from van der Linden and Simonson (1973), Gilat et al. (1983), and Sarin et al. (1995).

prevalence of gallstones than other women. The impact of heredity has been corroborated (Fig. 16–15) in three carefully controlled true prevalence studies (by cholecystography, surgery, and ultrasonography) from Sweden (van der Linden and Simonson, 1973), Israel (Gilat et al., 1983), and north India (Sarin et al., 1995). For each cohort, the data showed significantly higher (≥2:1) prevalence rates of gallstones in the first-degree relatives of probands compared with controls. Furthermore, as McConnell (1966) suggested, the role of heredity should be particularly evident in family members of children with cholesterol stones. Such an effect was demonstrated (van der Linden and Simonson, 1973) by examining the first-degree relatives of gallstone patients under 22 years of age (Fig. 16–15). Another study examined the first-degree relatives of 27 children cholecystectomized before the age of 15 for cholesterol gallstone disease; 15 mothers, 2 fathers, and 7 of 10 siblings had gallstone disease (Hagberg et al., 1962). Hanis et al. (1985) also established that the probability of a Mexican American with gallbladder disease having a first-degree relative similarly affected was 1.8 times the random probability. Studies using index individuals have inherent biases since a certain amount of family aggregation would occur by chance, especially with high frequencies of the disease. Nowhere was this better exemplified than in a study of 316 adult Pima Indian women belonging to 144 sibships (Bennion and Knowler, 1980), where the investigators assessed 116 families with two sisters and 28 families with three sisters in the same age range (35–84 years) as controls. Table 16–1 shows that prevalence rates of gallstones in families with zero, one, two, or three sisters affected were identical to the expected frequencies. Since gallstones are most likely to be genetically determined in Pima Indians, this demonstrates the difficulty in assessing the impact of heredity on a disease when the putative genes are so prevalent.

Twin Studies

A natural boon to establishing the heritability of cholesterol gallstone disease would be twin studies. There are several anecdotal reports of concordance of cholesterol gallstones in small numbers of monozygous twins (summarized in McConnell, 1966). In a study by Doig (1957), 12 twin pairs were selected from a sample of 161 pairs by oral cholecystography because one twin was ill with gallstones. Concordance for gallstones was found in two pairs of monozygous males but not in two pairs of monozygous females; two of eight pairs of dizygotic twins were also concordant. In an important Danish study (Harvald and Hauge, 1956), 1900 unselected twin pairs born between 1870 and 1910 were sent a questionnaire by mail requesting that they describe “any and all admissions to hospital, where, when and for what condition.” No direct questions concerning cholelithiasis were asked. Gallstones were diagnosed from the chart descriptions of the hospitalized cases. In the entire cohort, the crude prevalence of cholelithiasis was 2.6%, clearly a minimal figure for adult Danes (Fig. 16–11). Of a total of 101 twin pairs with a diagnosis of cholelithiasis, concordance for gallstones was found among 14/25 monozygotic pairs compared with 6/40 (same sex) and 0/36 (different sex) dizygotic pairs. Kesäniemi et al. (1989) selected randomly adult male twins (17 monozygotic and 18 dizygotic pairs) from the Finnish Twin Cohort residing in the Helsinki area. Gallstones were ascertained by oral cholecystography and history of cholecystectomy in seven monozygotic and three dizygotic subjects. Two monozygotic and no dizygotic twin pairs were concordant for gallstones, giving 40% pairwise concordance for the former and 0% for the latter. All of these studies, albeit imperfect, constitute the best information we have on familial occurrence and concordance of gallstones in monozygotic twins. They add to the accumulating evidence for appreciable genetic control of hepatobiliary lipid metabolism and cholesterol secretion.

Associations with Other Diseases

Pigment Gallstones

The most obvious other disease association is the cause-and-effect relationship between congenital or acquired hemolytic anemias and black pigment gallstones (Trotman, 1983; Ostrow, 1984). By shortening the erythrocyte life span, hemolytic diseases increase production of bilirubin and augment conjugated bilirubin secretion into bile (Schull et al., 1977), and as a result of endogenous β-glucuronidase and perhaps nonenzymatic hydrolysis, the levels of biliary unconjugated bilirubin (UCB) become markedly elevated (Cahalane et al., 1988). Genetic hemolytic disorders that lead to high prevalence rates of pigment stones are hereditary spherocytosis (congenital hemolytic jaundice) (Bates and Brown, 1952), sickle cell disease (Rennels et al., 1984), thalassemia major (hereditary leptocytosis or Cooley’s

Table 16–1. Distribution of Numbers of Sisters with Gallstones in Pima Families with Two or Three Sisters 35 to 84 Years Old

	Families with Two Sisters				Families with Three Sisters				
Number Affected	0	1	2	Sum	0	1	2	3	Sum
Observed	35	57	24	116	6	11	6	5	28
Expected[a]	34.8	57.4	23.8	116	4.6	11.4	9.4	2.6	28

[a]Expected numbers were derived assuming a random distribution of the disease in the population.
Source: From Bennion and Knowler (1980) with permission.

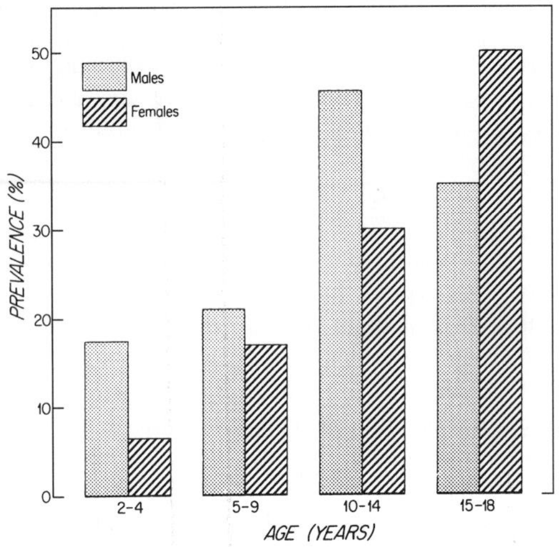

Fig. 16–16. True prevalence rates of "black" pigment gallstones (including pigment "biliary sludge") detected by ultrasonography in 224 young male and female patients with homozygous sickle cell disease. From Sarnaik et al. (1980), published in Carey and O'Donovan (1984) with permission.

anemia) (Goldfarb et al., 1990), and erythrocyte enzyme deficiencies (Grosfeld et al., 1994), all of which may elevate bilirubin levels in bile 10- to 20-fold (Fevery et al., 1980). Figure 16–16 displays the true prevalence of pigment gallstones (which includes biliary sludge) in 226 patients under age 18, evenly distributed between males and females with homozygous sickle cell disease (Sarnaik et al., 1980). Gallstone prevalence is high even in the youngest age group (2–4 years), and prevalence increases markedly within the first and second decades of life, reaching 35% for males and 50% for females. This and other studies of inherited hemolytic anemias (Rennels et al., 1984; Bond et al., 1987; Goldfarb et al., 1990) highlight *(1)* the early onset and high prevalence in the first and second decades of life and *(2)* the lack of a female preponderance, a feature uniformly present in cholesterol gallstone disease. Epidemiological information on patients reaching middle to old age suggest that pigment gallstone prevalence rates reach 60% to 80%, most marked in hereditary spherocytosis (Bates and Brown, 1952). As evidenced by an inbred mouse model [homozygous normoblastic (nb/nb) deer mice] of this condition (Trotman et al., 1980, 1981), not every subject with hemolytic anemia acquires pigment gallstones despite high UCB concentrations and ionized calcium levels in gallbladder bile. As in cholesterol gallstone disease, fewer than 25% of affected subjects become symptomatic from their stones (Sarnaik et al., 1980).

Cholesterol Stones

Obesity. Obesity dramatically increases cholesterol gallstone risk in proportion to the degree (Nakayama, 1997) and perhaps type (Diehl, 1991) of overweight, as well as female gender (Heaton, 1994). For example, in a large population study (Heaton et al., 1991a), a high waist:hip ratio predicted gallstones in men whereas a high body mass index and high weight gain since age 20 did not. In the Framingham Study, the risk for gallstones increased twofold in those 20% above the median weight (Friedman et al., 1966). In the large ultrasonographically surveyed Copenhagen cohort, gallstone prevalence correlated positively with body mass index in women but not in men (Jorgensen, 1989a–c), a feature also seen in the Rome Group for the Epidemiology and Prevention of Cholelithiasis (1988) study of Roman civil servants and in west Britain (Heaton et al., 1991a,b). In the Sirmione study (Sama et al., 1990), gallstone prevalence was significantly higher in obese subjects of younger age and, over 5 years of follow-up, incidence rates were three times higher in obese than in nonobese subjects. Most Mexican-American teenagers with cholesterol stones in Texas were markedly obese (Hanis et al., 1985). In the MICOL study of 29,584 males and females carried out on 14 cohorts between 1984 and 1987 in Italy (Attili et al., 1997), obesity proved to be one of the most consistent associations with gallstones.

The pathophysiological link between obesity and cholesterol gallstone disease is well established (Amaral and Thompson, 1985) and caused by markedly supersaturated bile from persistent hypersecretion of biliary cholesterol (Bennion and Grundy, 1975; Mabee et al., 1976; Shaffer and Small, 1977). Obese people overproduce total body cholesterol, most markedly in the liver, coincident with elevations in plasma very low-density lipoprotein (VLDL) cholesterol levels (Miettinen, 1971). Severe obesity is also associated with hepatic hypersecretion of bile salts and phospholipids (Shaffer and Small, 1977); however, the outputs are insufficient to counterbalance the massive increase in cholesterol secretion, so the bile becomes supersaturated (Carey and Small, 1978). Moderate to mild obesity in Caucasians or Pima Indians is coupled with normal secretion or hyposecretion of bile salts (Grundy et al., 1972, 1974; Northfield and Hofmann, 1975), further augmenting relative cholesterol supersaturation of bile. Obesity per se does not appear to alter gallbladder motor function (Vezina et al., 1990), but augmented stone nucleation, crystallization, and stone growth are apparently secondary to the effects of supersaturated cholesterol levels on gallbladder mucosa and muscle function (Shaffer, 1992).

Reduction of weight to ideal body mass causes a significant decrease of cholesterol secretion but not of bile salt and phospholipid outputs into bile (Bennion and Grundy, 1975). The end result is desaturation of bile when normal weight is regained (Bennion and Grundy, 1975). Prolonged starvation, nonetheless, has a profound effect, diminishing secretion rates of all biliary lipids (Reuben et al., 1985). Rapid weight reduction ($\geq$1.5 kg/week) in obese persons from bariatric surgery (Shiffman et al., 1991) or hypocaloric ($\approx$1000 kcal) diets (Broomfield et al., 1988; Liddle et al., 1989) is associated with 30% to 50% formation of new gallstones within a few weeks to months (Nakayama, 1997). This is linked pathophysiologically to hypersecretion of cholesterol into bile, decreased bile salt synthesis, induction of gallbladder mucin hypersecretion from elevated prostanoids, and elevated biliary calcium and gallbladder hypomotility (Marks et al., 1992; Shiffman et al., 1992). Deficient gallbladder contractility potentiates all risk factors and is caused by the subphysiological dietary stimulus (triglycerides $<$10 g/day) to cholecystokinin release from the proximal intestinal mucosa (Stone et al., 1992). The flux of cholesterol molecules into gallbladder smooth muscle cells from bile packs and stiffens the sarcolemmal membranes, decouples signal-transduction mechanisms (Yu et al., 1995, 1996), and paralyzes gallbladder muscle function (Behar et al., 1989). Gallbladder hypomotility and gallstone risk can be ameliorated, or even prevented, by adequate ($\geq$10–20 g/day) long-chain triglycerides in the diet (Stone et al., 1992; Gebhard et al., 1996); by large doses of oral ursodeoxycholic acid (Broomfield et al., 1988; Sugerman et al., 1995), which induces a phase change that prevents solid cholesterol crystallization in bile; and by "toxic" ($>$1 g/day) doses of acetylsalicylic acid (Broomfield et al., 1988), which suppress mucin hypersecretion (Sterling et al., 1995) and inhibit cholesterol crystal nucleation (Lee et al., 1981). When the gallbladder's contractile function recovers upon reestablishment of a normal diet, small stones often "disappear" (Liddle et al., 1989; Marks et al., 1994) from expulsion through the biliary tree into the duodenum. For this reason, new stones that form in the setting of rapid weight loss frequently cause biliary pain or a complication (Liddle et al., 1989; Marks et al., 1994). In the MICOL study in Italy (Attili et al., 1997), a history of dieting was associated with gallstone disease in both men and women.

Dyslipidemia. In comparing serum lipid profiles of Swedish gallstone patients, Ahlberg et al. (1980) found significantly higher serum triglyceride levels in gallstone patients over 40 years of age, a finding frequently confirmed in population-based case-control surveys (Nakayama, 1997). Several studies have documented a greater risk of cholesterol gallstones in subjects with low levels of high-density lipoprotein (HDL) cholesterol (Petitti et al., 1981; Scragg et al., 1984a; Jorgensen, 1989a). However, low HDL and high plasma triglycerides are generally inversely correlated and associated with upper body obesity. When body mass index was controlled by multivariate analysis in Japanese (Kono et al., 1988) and Danish (Jorgensen, 1989b) subjects, the relationship of serum triglycerides with cholesterol gallstone risk disappeared. In a case-control study from Holland, Thijs et al. (1990a,b) found the highest risk for gallstones in subjects with low HDL levels and high plasma triglyceride levels but body mass index was a confounding variable. By multivariate analysis, the Italian GREPCO (Rome Group for the Epidemiology and Prevention of Cholelithiasis, 1988a,b) and Sirmione (Barbara et al., 1987) studies supported the association between hypertriglyceridemia, low HDL cholesterol, and gallstone disease in both females and males. In view of these findings, especially in the large Italian studies, the evidence suggests that low plasma HDL and elevated triglycerides are statistically independent risk factors for cholesterol gallstone disease; but whether this relationship is totally independent of body mass index is questionable (Janson et al., 1985; Borch et al., 1998).

Emerging evidence suggests that an apolipoprotein E (apo E) polymorphsin may be an important genetic risk factor for cholesterol gallstones. The apo E4 isoform exhibits greater affinity for its hepatic receptor and correlates positively with cholesterol gallstone prevalence (Bertomeu et al., 1996), cholesterol content of stones (Juvonen et al., 1993), and speed of gallstone clearance as well as recurrence risk after extracorporeal shock-wave lithotripsy (Portincasa et al., 1996).

Diabetes Mellitus. The literature concerning diabetes as a gallstone risk factor is confusing. Essentially all autopsy studies in diabetics point to a statistically significant increase in cholesterol gallstone prevalence rates (Diehl, 1991; Nakayama 1997). This putative association caused much controversy in the older literature because of the potential biases involved (Nakayama, 1997). No association of diabetes and gallstones was found in a large retrospective case-control study of Canadian Caucasians (Honore, 1980) despite a considerable prevalence of obesity in the subjects. Likewise, two of the large Italian cross-sectional studies, Sirmione (Barbara et al., 1987) and GREPCO (Rome Group for the Epidemiology and Prevention of Cholelithiasis, 1988a,b), and the Danish studies (Jorgensen, 1989b) failed to observe an association of diabetes and gallstones. In contrast, a significant association of gallstones with diabetes was observed in the pan-Italian MICOL study (Attili et al., 1997). Furthermore, a rigorous case-control study of 336 middle-aged (30–69 years) gallstone patients matched with 336 controls (De Santis et al., 1997) showed by univariate analysis that diabetes mellitus was more frequent in the gallstone patients by a factor of 2 (18.3% vs. 9.9%) for men and of 4 (9.3% vs. 2.6%) for women.

The health of Native Americans is dominated by gallbladder disease and diabetes mellitus (Diehl, 1991; Grimaldi et al., 1993), and all Native-American populations exhibit significantly higher rates of both diseases than Caucasians (Nakayama, 1997). This is particularly exemplified by the Pima (Fig. 16–17), where prevalence rates of diabetes mellitus, gallstones, and obesity are as much as 10-fold higher than in the typical U.S. population (Carey and O'Donovan, 1984). Diabetes mellitus is a significant risk factor for clinical gallstone disease in Mexican Americans despite adjustment for confounding variables, including body mass index and body fat distribution (Hanis et al., 1985; Haffner et al., 1990), but then both diseases are very common in this population (Diehl and Stern 1989; Diehl 1991). Because the prevalence of these diseases in Mexican Americans parallels the degree of Native American admixture, they are likely to be caused by disease genes from the Native Americans (Hanis et al., 1986). Since the onset of Type 2 diabetes mellitus in Native Americans occurs many years later than that of gallstones (Diehl, 1991), a direct cause-and-effect relationship is unlikely. However, prediabetics are usually hyperinsulinemic for many years, and insulin upregulates *de novo* cholesterol synthesis appreciably (Bennion and Grundy, 1977; Scragg et al., 1984a,b). In fact, in one survey, obese males with gallstones (Heaton et al., 1991a) displayed significantly higher fasting plasma insulin levels compared to controls without gallstones. Moreover, biliary cholesterol saturation index is increased and gallbladder motility is decreased in diabetic subjects (Ponz de Leon et al., 1978; Stone et al., 1988).

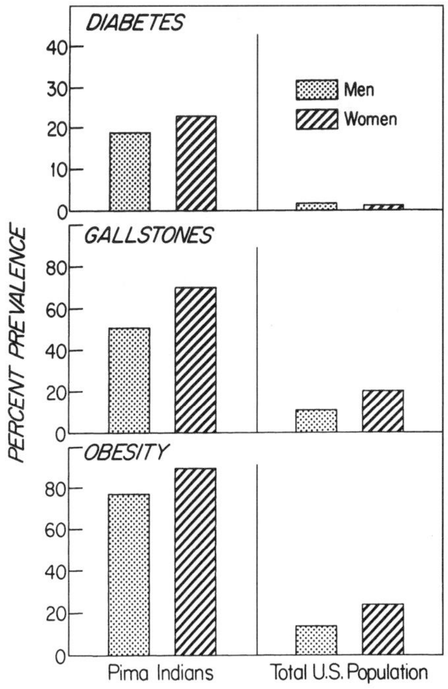

Fig. 16–17. The Native American burden: high age-adjusted prevalence rates of diabetes mellitus, gallstones, and obesity compared with U.S. national averages. From Carey and O'Donovan (1984) with permission.

Environmental Factors

As inferred from cross-sectional, case-control, and longitudinal studies, environmental factors impact upon cholesterol gallstone proneness, particularly diet, pregnancy, and certain medications (reviewed in Heaton, 1973, 1981; Sama et al., 1990; Diehl, 1991; Nakayama, 1997). Further, in each case, the pathophysiological basis is either known or can be speculated upon reasonably. Other imputed risk factors, such as migration, urban/rural residence, and economic/social status, and chronological changes will be discussed briefly since nutritional variations are probably responsible for most of these suggested associations and trends (Heaton, 1981; Diehl, 1991; Nakayama, 1997).

Diet

Conclusive data from large numbers of older and more recent studies (see references in Heaton, 1981; Low-Beer, 1985; Nakayama, 1997; Caroli-Bosc et al., 1998; Misciagna et al., 1999) implicate chronic overnutrition with refined nutrients, especially carbohydrates and depletion of dietary fiber, as crucial environmental triggers for cholesterol gallstone formation. On the basis of clinical evidence, gallstone disease was believed to be infrequent in Native Americans prior to World War II (Geare, 1915; Hancock, 1933; Salsbury, 1937; Weiss et al., 1984) but to increase markedly thereafter (Shaheb, 1990). The Tarahumara Indians of northeastern Mexico, who are closely related genetically to the southwestern U.S. Pima (Pennington, 1963; Shaheb, 1990), are not obese, do not acquire diabetes mellitus, are singularly free of hypertension, and apparently do not suffer from gallstones or atherosclerosis (Pennington, 1963; Connor et al., 1978). The Tarahumaran diet consists primarily of beans, corn, and squash; hence, it is high in complex carbohydrates, has no refined nutrients, and is low in fat and cholesterol and almost all dietary protein is derived from vegetable sources (Pennington, 1963; Connor et al., 1978; Cerqueira et al., 1979). When challenged with a hypercaloric Western diet, they display evidence of maladaptation with striking increases in plasma lipids, especially low-density lipoprotein (LDL) levels, and body weight (McMurry et al., 1991). Animals in the wild rarely form gallstones spontaneously, although the deer mouse (Schwab and Theis, 1989) and cotton rat (Pence et al., 1978) are notable exceptions in that they form cholesterol stones with annual cyclicity. Feeding an artificial diet containing high quantities of fat, carbohydrate, and/or cholesterol can produce cholesterol gallstones in several species, including mice, prairie dogs, rabbits, squirrel monkeys, and tupaias (Dam, 1969; DenBensten et al., 1974; van der Linden and Bergman, 1977; Schwaier, 1979; Holzbach, 1984; MacPherson et al., 1987; Liepa et al., 1988).

Total Calories. During and after World War I, autopsy studies in Rostock, Germany, (Mårtensson, 1937) indicated that gallstone prevalence rates decreased during the war years, especially in females; Taylor and Cotton (1973) reported similar findings during World War II in Holland. In a case-control study, Scragg et al. (1984a) found that young gallstone subjects in Adelaide, Australia, ate significantly more calories than controls, a finding that was not upheld in older gallstone patients in Melbourne, Australia (Wheeler et al., 1970). The U.S. nurses' study (Maclure et al., 1989; Stampfer et al., 1992) is notable not only for the size of the cohort (>60,000) but also for the strong positive correlation found between high energy intake and risk of clinical cholelithiasis. Studies on the habitual diet of gallstone patients in southern France over 21 years demonstrated an increased intake of total calories irrespective of dietary composition compared with age-matched controls (Sarles et al., 1969, 1970, 1978a,b). These findings were confirmed, also in southern France, in a multicenter cohort study (Caroli-Bosc et al., 1998). However, Micmac women in Shubenacadie, Canada, had the same total calorie and nutrient intake as female Caucasians from the same village (Johnston et al., 1977), even though the Micmacs were more obese and had more gallstones. Likewise, total calorie intake of Pima and Papago women in Arizona (Reid et al., 1971) did not differ from the U.S. average, even though they had more obesity and more gallstones. Pima women exceeded desirable weight by 157% compared to 116% for Caucasian females (Reid et al., 1971). Clearly, surveys of current dietary intake for a disease that putatively has genetic–metabolic expressions at puberty (Redinger and Small, 1972; Lowenfels et al., 1985) are fraught with lead-time errors. Perhaps also the long chronology involved in the natural history of the disease belies the results of the cross-sectional Italian MICOL study (Attili et al., 1998), which quantified the impact of diet on gallstone prevalence in 15,910 subjects of both sexes (14 Italian cohorts) that were controlled for the effects of obesity. These data failed to confirm that current high energy intake is associated with any increased risk of gallstones in either gender.

Cholesterol. Most cholesterol deposited in gallstones appears to be of dietary origin (Holzbach, 1984), and in the cholesterol-fed prairie dog, at least 80% of gallstone cholesterol is derived from the diet (Brenneman et al., 1972). The linkage between biliary cholesterol secretion in humans and cholesterol from the diet, that from lipoproteins, and that synthesized *de novo* is not well understood (Turley and Dietschy, 1982). Moreover, the contribution of *de novo* synthesized cholesterol to biliary cholesterol secretion is likely to be small, possibly <20% (Carey and LaMont, 1992). Mok et al. (1986) determined the $^{14}C/^{12}C$ cholesterol ratios in gallstones of Californians in the aftermath of 1960s Pacific atomic bomb testing and substantiated that a considerable amount of dietary cholesterol is deposited in human gallstones. This is consistent with the concept that a large fraction of cholesterol secreted into the bile may be derived from chylomicron remnants (Cooper, 1991). For example, ingestion of a high-cholesterol diet (5–10 eggs/day) increased biliary cholesterol secretion significantly over 15 to 21 days in gallstone subjects (Dam et al., 1971; Kern, 1994), and DenBesten et al. (1973) showed that ingestion of 750 mg (egg) cholesterol by 10 healthy men raised biliary cholesterol by 34%, with several subjects precipitating cholesterol monohydrate crystals (in duodenal bile). Similar findings were reported by Lee et al. (1985) in gallstone patients ingesting 500 to 1000 mg cholesterol/day, with the most marked increases in lithogenicity found in males. In an investigation of young male veterans, Duane (1994) determined that biliary cholesterol saturation did not increase significantly with consumption of cholesterol; however, cholesterol augmented bile salt loss from the small intestine, the so-called cholestyramine-like effect. Taken together, these and other data (summarized in Lee et al., 1985; Kern, 1994) suggest that individuals with supersaturated bile are easily tipped toward lithogenicity in response to a dietary cholesterol challenge. This phenomenon apparently does not occur in normal subjects, supporting a genetic predisposition in humans to eliminate excess dietary cholesterol in bile. The cholestyramine-like effect of cholesterol may result in enterohepatic cycling of bilirubin, increased conjugated bilirubin levels in bile, and precipitation of calcium bilirubinates following hydrolysis (Méndez-Sánchez et al., 1998), perhaps explaining why the nucleus of cholesterol gallstones is invariably pigmented.

Fat (Triglycerides). Dietary fat is mostly (>96%) long-chain triglyceride. The relative biliary lipid composition of volunteers (Dam et al., 1967) or of rhesus monkeys (Redinger et al., 1973) showed no consistent effects in response to ingestion of any natural triglyceride mixture. However, in an autopsy study (Sturdevant et al., 1973) of subjects who habitually ingested a low-saturated fat, low-cholesterol diet, gallstone prevalence was increased, yet a more recent case-control study did not substantiate this finding (Misciagna et al., 1999). In surveys of different populations, there are conflicting results, varying from no effect of fat intake (Sarles et al., 1969, 1978a,b; Pixley and Mann, 1988; Jorgensen and Jorgensen, 1989) to highly significant correlations between consumption of total fats (>125 g/day) (Caroli-Bosc et al., 1998; Scragg et al., 1984a) or saturated fats (Misciagna et al., 1999) and cholelithiasis.

A good example of a population with a negative association is the Masai of east Africa. These nomadic people have traditionally consumed dietary staples of cow's milk, ox blood, and fiber-enriched cereals. Despite the high intake of tryglycerides and cholesterol, they are remarkably free of Western diseases, including cholesterol gallstones and atherosclerosis (Biss et al., 1971). There are suggestions that blood and biliary cholesterol levels are kept low in the Masai by catabolism of dietary cholesterol into upregulated *de novo* bile salt synthesis (Biss et al., 1971). Although common in some animals, such as the domestic dog and rat, this positive regulatory phenomenon, which diverts neutral to acidic sterols, is not observed in most Caucasians, though unique exceptions have been reported (Kern, 1991).

In contrast, high intake of marine fish fat may protect against cholesterol gallstones, probably because of high contents of ω-3 polyunsaturated fatty acids in tissue triglycerides (Berr et al., 1992; Tierney et al., 1993; Nakayama, 1997). Canadian Inuit (Eskimo), who become acculturated to an urban environment, succumb rapidly to gallstone disease. For example, 47% of western urban young Inuit women acquire gallstones compared with 5% of nomadic eastern Inuit women of similar age, ≈30 years (Schaefer, 1981). Additional support for the protective effect of fish oils stems from a 1948–1949 study of north Greenland Inuit, who consumed very large quantities of fat but had a considerably lower prevalence of cholelithiasis than Caucasian residents (Ehrstrom, 1951). A hypocholesterolemic diet ingested by mental hospital inmates in Finland (Miettinen et al., 1976) was also protective against gallstone formation, possibly because of the level of fish meal in the diet. Animal studies also support the notion that triglycerides with ω-3 fatty acids are protective against gallstones. In the common cholesterol gallstone models, prairie dogs (Holzbach, 1984; Liepa et al., 1988), African green monkeys (Scobey et al., 1991), and hamsters (Holzbach, 1984), cholesterol gallstone formation can be inhibited markedly when fish oil is added isocalorically to the lithogenic diets (Magnuson et al., 1995; Scobey et al., 1991; Booker et al., 1990; Berr et al., 1993). The antilithogenic effects involve both reduction in cholesterol saturation of bile and inhibition of solid crystal nucleation, apparently because of stabilization of phase-separated liquid crystals (Magnuson et al., 1995). Nonetheless, in the Italian cross-sectional study of Roman civil servants, analysis of blood lipids as indices of prior dietary regimens revealed that erythrocyte ω-3 (or other) fatty acid compositions bore no relationship to gallstone risk (Arca et al., 1987).

Protein and Alcohol. High dietary levels of total protein, particularly animal protein, promote cholesterol cholelithiasis in rabbits (Borgman, 1965; Borgman and Haselden, 1968), hamsters (Kritchevsky and Klurfeld, 1983; Mahfouz-Cercone et al., 1984; Duffy et al., 1985), and monkeys (Jaskiewicz et al., 1987). Earlier human studies of protein intake and gallstone risk by Sarles et al. (1971) showed that healthy humans who habitually eat high-protein diets have elevated biliary cholesterol saturations. Smith and Gee (1979) showed that animal protein was an independent risk factor for cholelithiasis in humans. In the MICOL study (Attili et al., 1998), a positive association of high protein intake and risk of gallstones was found in males only; however, biochemical or biophysical mechanisms to explain this effect were not offered.

Moderate alcohol intake is associated with a diminution in risk of cholesterol gallstone disease (Nakayama, 1997). This was suggested in many earlier epidemiological and dietary studies (Sarles et al., 1969, 1978a,b; Coste et al., 1979), including the Framingham Study (Friedman et al., 1966). However, the first evidence for dose response in the protective effect of modest alcohol intake (<6 g/day) was the case-control study of Scragg et al. (1984a) in Adelaide, Australia. Biliary lipid alterations in duodenal bile were studied in 12 abstemious volunteers (Thornton et al., 1983a) before and after drinking a half-bottle of wine per day for several weeks. Biliary cholesterol saturations were reduced from 1.3 ± 0.1 to 1.1 ± 0.1, while plasma HDL cholesterol levels were elevated from 41.4 ± 1.9 mg/dl to 48.3 ± 3.1 mg/dl. In the Italian MICOL study, moderate alcohol consumption was also statistically significant in protecting against gallstone formation but in males only (Attili et al., 1998). Alcohol lowering of the cholesterol saturation of bile has also been documented in animal models (Topping et al., 1982; Schwesinger et al., 1988), but the mechanism is not known.

Nutrient intake may play a large role in the prevalence of pigment gallstone disease, especially in Asia (Nakayama, 1997). The prevalence of brown pigment stones caused by biliary infection and parasitic exposure correlates with low protein intake, especially in Japanese rural dwellers (Maki, 1961; Matsushiro et al., 1997). Consumption of diets enriched in carbohydrates causes pigment gallstones in the prairie dog and hamster (Prange et al., 1966; Conter et al., 1986; Malet et al., 1989; Strichartz et al., 1989a). It is likely that complex carbohydrates, by inducing enterohepatic cycling of bilirubin, may be a factor in black pigment gallstone formation in humans (Carey, 1993a,b, 1996). Clearly, when taken in excess for long periods, ethyl alcohol can cause alcoholic cirrhosis, a well-known risk factor for black pigment stone disease (Bouchier, 1969; Sheen and Liaw, 1989). There is also some evidence in animal models that high alcohol intake can increase biliary secretion rates of UCB (Schwesinger et al., 1985) and thereby provoke calcium bilirubinate precipitation directly.

Carbohydrate and Fiber. In his famous textbook *The Principles and Practice of Medicine*, William Osler (1892) described patients with gallstones as "often stout and usually very fond of starchy and saccharine food." Cleave and Campbell (1966) wrote a highly speculative but influential book proposing a "saccharine" hypothesis for many Western diseases. Sarles et al. (1969), on the basis of a large Mediterranean cohort, suggested that refined carbohydrates are conducive to elevating cholesterol saturation of bile and causing gallstones. Heaton (1973) proposed a refined carbohydrate hypothesis for cholesterol cholelithiasis independent of obesity, which implies a high-sucrose, white-flour diet that was fiber-depleted, results which were corroborated in a case-control study by Scragg et al. (1984a) from Australia. Nonetheless, in the first biochemical–physiological test of the hypothesis, Werner et al. (1984) failed to find a significant difference in biliary lipid secretion rates in 12 patients with cholesterol gallstones who ingested 120 g compared with 16 g/day sucrose for 6 weeks. However, in this study, the diets had only minor differences in rather low levels (<19 g/day) of dietary fiber. The Bristol group (Thornton et al., 1983b) found a significant (20%) diminution in cholesterol saturation of bile when refined sugar diets were compared with unrefined sugar diets, in which the differences (13 vs. 27 g/day) in dietary fiber were doubled. Interestingly, on the fiber-rich diet, there was a significant decrease in biliary deoxycholate conjugates, consistent with decreased bacterial catabolism of cholate in the large intestine (Marcus and Heaton, 1988). Supporting these concepts are results from the cross-sectional MICOL study (Attili et al., 1998) and a recent case-control study in Italy (Misciagna et al., 1999), where high levels of refined carbohydrates and low levels of dietary fiber were strongly associated with risk of gallstones in both males and females.

Impressed with the rarity of Western diseases in sub-Saharan Africa, Burkitt and Trowell (1975) emphasized that a deficiency of dietary fiber in the West may be an etiological factor in many common diseases, including gallstones. In several well-controlled studies on humans in Bristol, the influence on biliary cholesterol saturation of large doses of wheat bran (22–50 g/day) were studied. In the first study (Pomare et al., 1976), the cohort had radiolucent gallstones and cholesterol-supersaturated (duodenal) bile. In the other studies, the subjects had supersaturated (Watts et al., 1978) or unsaturated (McDougall et al., 1978; Watts et al., 1978; Huijbregts et al., 1980) bile but no gallstones. In individuals with supersaturated bile, moderate dietary levels of bran decreased cholesterol saturation significantly, but bran had no effect in those with unsaturated bile. In addition, bran uniformly decreased the biliary content of deoxycholate conjugates. Because of the suggested prolithogenic properties of secondary bile salts, two groups fed "physiological" doses of deoxycholic acid to volunteers and found that this hydrophobic bile acid induced cholesterol supersaturation of bile (Low-Beer and Pomare, 1975; Carulli et al., 1980). In addition, administration of antibiotics to humans to retard catabolism of cholate had a cholesterol-desaturating effect (Carulli et al., 1981). It is believed that dietary fiber prevents deoxycholate formation and/or its intestinal absorption by multiple mechanisms, including altering gut transit time, binding the bile acid, providing a substrate for bacterial fermentation and thereby luminal acidification, and inducing bile acid precipitation (Marcus and Heaton, 1988). Vegetarians, who have significantly higher intake of dietary fiber than nonvegetarians, may be protected from gallstone formation for similar reasons (Nakayama, 1997). Pixley et al. (1985) studied vegetarian women and controls and found a 50% diminution in gallstone occurrence, explained only in part by their slimness. Ahlberg et al. (1980) noted in Swedish vegetarians that there was a significant diminution in the deoxycholate pool, consistent with their resistance to cholesterol gallstone formation. The gallstone-protective effect of fiber has been substantiated in the Italian cross-sectional Sirmione (Sama et al., 1986) and MICOL (Attili et al., 1998) studies and a case-control study in southern Italy (Misciagna et al., 1999). However, the protective effect of dietary fiber (Smith and Gee, 1979) has not been substantiated in all studies (Scragg et al., 1984a; Caroli-Bosc et al., 1998). In a well-documented study, very high (120 g/day) dietary intake of legumes indigenous to Chile has been incriminated as posing an increased risk for gallstones (Nervi et al., 1989), apparently through a mechanism that lowers the phospholipid content of bile.

Fasting. Cholesterol saturation of human gallbladder bile varies diurnally, with higher levels following an overnight fast (Metzger et al., 1973). Upon varying the length (2–20 hours) of fasting in healthy human cholesterol saturation of the bile increased steadily (Williams et al., 1977a; Bloch et al., 1980). Paradoxically, prolonged fasting for up to 4 to 6 days reduced biliary cholesterol levels profoundly (Duane et al., 1976), most likely from cholesterol absorption by the gallbladder mucosa. Prolonged fasting also causes bile salt hyposecretion from a "sluggish" enterohepatic circulation of bile salts secondary to hypomotility of the gallbladder and small intestine (Vlahcevic et al., 1991; Carey and Duane, 1994). This not only may diminish endogenous cholesterol absorption (Duane et al., 1976) but in addition 3-hydroxy-3-methylglutaryl coenzyme A (HMG-CoA) reductase activity reaches a nadir after ≥14 hours of fasting. Although Jorgensen and Jorgensen (1989) failed to find a relationship between gallstone prevalence and the number of meals or snacks eaten in a 24-hour period in their large Copenhagen cohort, most human epidemiological and animal studies indicate prolonged fasting as a risk factor in cholesterol lithogenesis (Nakayama, 1997). In a prospective case-control study, Capron et al. (1981) found that young French women with gallstones had a longer duration of overnight fasting compared with matched controls and were frequent breakfast "skippers." In the Italian MICOL study (Attili et al., 1998), gallstone prevalence rate was significantly higher (relative risk 1.4) among subjects who had overnight fasts of 12 hours' duration or longer. The risk of prolonged fasting has been duplicated in the prairie dog gallstone model, and further, daily injections of a physiological dose of cholecystokinin octapeptide decreased gallstone incidence by 50% and reduced cholesterol saturation of bile to prelithogenic levels (Roslyn et al., 1981).

Pregnancy

In humans, cholesterol gallstone prevalence correlates directly with the number of full-term pregnancies (Rome Group for the Epidemiology and Prevention of Cholelithiasis, 1984; Scragg et al., 1984a; Barbara et al., 1987). Bennion and colleagues (1979) demonstrated that in Pima Indians bile becomes supersaturated at puberty, this being most pronounced in females and correlating positively with estrogen excretion. Caucasian females, but not males, at puberty develop supersaturated bile accompanied by sharp increases in conjugated deoxycholate levels in bile (von Bergman et al., 1986). Although the menstrual cycle appears to have no effect on biliary lipid secretion or composition or on the enterohepatic circulation, human pregnancy nevertheless has profound and progressive lithogenic effects on hepatobiliary and gallbladder function (Kern et al., 1981; Everson et al., 1982).

Kern et al. (1981) and Everson et al. (1982) examined pregnant women employing ultrasonography to document gallbladder function, analysis of duodenal bile to assess variations in biliary lipid composition, marker-perfusion techniques to measure biliary lipid secretion, and isotope dilution to measure bile salt pool size and kinetics by administering oral bile acids labeled with ^{13}C. They documented that in human pregnancy *(1)* cholesterol saturation of the bile increases monotonically, most markedly during the second and third trimesters; *(2)* the biliary cholesterol secretion rate increases relative to bile salt and phospholipid secretion rates; *(3)* proportions of chenodeoxycholate conjugates decrease with a decrease in synthesis; *(4)* following first-trimester increases in bile salt pool size, chenodeoxycholate and deoxycholate pool sizes decrease; and *(5)* fractional bile salt turnover rates decrease, which is consistent with a sluggish enterohepatic circulation (Kern et al., 1981). The second and third trimesters are associated with increased fasting and residual gallbladder volumes, as well as diminution in the rate and percentage of bile emptied with a meal (Braverman et al., 1980; Everson et al., 1982). The hyperestrogenism of pregnancy is believed to be responsible for the diminution in chenodeoxycholate synthesis and the stimulation of cholesterol hypersecretion into the bile, most likely from increased plasma LDL clearance via upregulation of hepatic B/E receptors (Brown and Goldstein, 1986). It appears that estrogen also activates HMG-CoA reductase, producing more total-body cholesterol (Kern et al., 1978; Reichen et al., 1987). Further, Everson et al. (1991) found that mixed conjugated estrogens (Premarin) given to anovulatory women enhanced chylomicron remnant clearance by two orders of magnitude, thereby diverting more dietary cholesterol into the bile. The increased levels of progesterone block G-protein function in gallbladder smooth muscle cells. In pregnancy, this effect is responsible for signal-transduction decoupling and impaired gallbladder contractility in response to cholecystokinin (Chen et al., 1998). Progesterone is also a potent inhibitor of hepatic acyl-coenzyme A:cholesterol acyltransferase (ACAT), thereby decreasing hepatic cholesteryl ester synthesis and presumably allowing more free cholesterol to enter an intrahepatic pool for biliary secretion (Nervi et al., 1983). Neither estrogen nor progesterone has any direct effect on hepatic bile salt secretion, but by inducing gallbladder dysmotility, progesterone causes a sluggish enterohepatic circulation and bile salt hyposecretion secondarily (Kern et al., 1981).

The lithogenic effects of supersaturated bile (estrogen) and gallbladder dysmotility (progestogen) in human pregnancy are hallmarked by the early appearance of biliary sludge, implying precipitated cholesterol crystals/microstones in gallbladder mucin gel (Carey and Cahalane, 1988). Maringhini and colleagues (1988) employed ultrasonography to follow a cohort of healthy pregnant women throughout the trimesters of pregnancy. There were progressive increases in the incidence of biliary sludge until parturition, when 42% of subjects had sludge with enlarged gallbladders and 10% had gallstones. The same investigators (Maringhini et al., 1987) followed a puerperal cohort of biliary sludge patients without gallstones and found that biliary sludge took 10 months to completely regress, at which time 7% of the patients had formed new gallstones. Valdivieso et al. (1993) obtained similar results in puerperal women in Chile; when followed for 40 weeks, 12% formed new gallstones compared with 1.3% in nulliparous controls. With puerperal recovery of gallbladder contractility, many women experience biliary pain for the first time and, in one-third, small stones disappear, presumably by migration through the biliary tree into the duodenum (Valdivieso et al., 1993).

Medications

Chronic intake of a number of widely used medications can increase cholesterol gallstone risk significantly. These drugs target the liver either to hypersecrete cholesterol or to hyposecrete bile salts, and some induce hypomotility of both the gallbladder and the gastrointestinal tract, all of which may pose an appreciable lithogenic risk.

Hormonal Steroids. Since the changes in levels of estrogenic and progestrogenic steroids of pregnancy influence biliary physiology in a prolithogenic fashion, it is anticipated that gallstone risk with anovulatory steroids would be similar. The large number of studies on this topic are beleaguered by contradictory outcomes, and it appears that the contemporary risk is small (summarized in Nakayama, 1997). The principal reasons for this are that *(1)* assessment in the early years was via clinical disease and not true prevalence of gallstones, e.g., in the Boston Collaborative Drug Surveillance Programme (1973) and in the Royal College of General Practitioners' Oral Contraceptive Study (1982), and *(2)* hormonal formulations, particularly the proportions of progestogens to estrogens, have decreased markedly since anovulatory steroids were introduced in 1961 (Djerassi, 1999). In the Rome Group for the Epidemiology and Prevention of Cholelithiasis (1988a,b), Sirmione (Barbara et al., 1987), and MICOL (Attili et al., 1995) studies, no differences in stone prevalence were found in those who used anovulatory steroids compared to those who did not. In fact, in the MICOL study (Attili et al., 1995) and in a recent Swedish study (Borch et al., 1998), the gallstone risk associated with anovulatory steroid use was appreciably negative. In contrast, the pharmacological use of large-dose estrogens in elderly men with metastatic prostate cancer results in strikingly increased prevalence rates of gallstones (Henriksson et al., 1989). In this Swedish investigation, bile lithogenicity increased 40% due to higher biliary cholesterol secretion rates and correlated positively with plasma LDL catabolism, as evidenced by lowered LDL cholesterol and increased expression of LDL receptors on the basolateral membranes of liver cells (Eriksson et al., 1989).

Fibrate Drugs. Clofibrate and its derivatives gemfibrozil, famfibrozil, and benzafibrate are powerful hypolipidemic agents in humans. By increasing biliary cholesterol secretion (Einarsson and Angelin, 1986), clofibrate, but apparently not the others, increases the relative risk for gallstones significantly, probably by a factor of 2 (Coronary Drug Project Research Group, 1977). In mice, these drugs stimulate biliary phospholipid secretion by increasing hepatocyte activity of multidrug resistance protein 2 (*Mdr2*) on the canalicular membrane responsible for transmembrane translocation of biliary lecithin (Chianale et al., 1996) and, thus, should be antilithogenic. However, in humans, biliary cholesterol secretion is also stimulated by a combination of upregulated HMG-CoA reductase activity and downregulated cholesterol 7α-hydroxylate activity (Einarsson, 1992; Ståhlberg et al., 1995). In contrast to their inhibitory effect on hepatic ACAT enzyme activity in laboratory animals (Ståhlberg et al., 1989), "fibrates" have no influence on ACAT in humans (Ståhlberg et al., 1989).

Octreotide/Somatostatin. Somatostatin is a natural gastrointestinal hormone, which inhibits the release into blood of other hormones, including cholecystokinin from the human gastrointestinal tract (Nakayama, 1997). In the rare somatostatinoma syndrome, wherein somatostatin is hyperproduced, cholesterol cholelithiasis occurs in all patients by the time of diagnosis (Krejs et al., 1979). Octreotide, the long-acting octapeptide analog of somatostatin, is employed to treat intractable secretory diarrhea (Lembcke et al., 1987) and, in acromegaly, to inhibit growth hormone and insulin-like growth factor release (Daughaday, 1990; Dowling et al., 1992). Six of seven patients treated with octreotide for acromegaly developed gallstones within 8 months of treatment and showed markedly reduced postprandial cholecystokinin release and gallbladder emptying (Moschetta et al., 2001). The pathogenesis of octreotide-induced gallstones is multifactorial and appears to involve *(1)* marked gallbladder stasis, *(2)* prolonged intestinal transit favoring transformation of cholate to deoxycholic acid (Hussaini et al., 1995), and *(3)* marked cholesterol supersaturation of bile most likely from the hypersecretory effects of deoxycholate (Marcus and Heaton, 1988) and probably augmented intestinal cholesterol absorption (Ponz de Leon et al., 1982).

Cyclosporin A and FK506. Cyclosporin A and FK506 are complex polypeptides that are powerful immunosuppressants employed principally to prevent organ rejection following successful human transplantation. As exemplified by heart transplantation, the agents are associated with a 40% to 60% risk of acquiring cholesterol gallstones within the first 2 postoperative years (Steck et al., 1991; Menegaux et al., 1998). As inferred principally from animal studies, the peptides have multiple effects on hepatocyte and enterocyte lipid transporters and lipid-synthesizing enzymes. They inhibit *(1)* sodium-dependent bile salt uptake across sinusoidal membranes of the liver (Kukongviriyapan and Stacey, 1991); *(2)* sterol 27-hydroxylase, a regulatory enzyme in the "acidic" pathway of bile salt synthesis (Dahlback-Sjoberg et al., 1993); *(3)* the bile salt export pump (BSEP) on the canalicular membrane (Kadmon et al., 1993); and *(4)* the apical sodium-coupled bile salt transporter (ASBT) of ileal enterocytes (Sauer et al., 1995). Although these drugs rarely cause overt cholestasis, they induce a relative bile salt deficiency without inhibiting biliary cholesterol secretion (Chan et al., 1998), thereby markedly supersaturating the bile with cholesterol. Gallstones formed as a result of these agents are composed of pure cholesterol monohydrate crystals, with very little of the drug's sparingly soluble biliary metabolites (Carey and Ko, unpublished observations, 1990).

Migration

Changes in gallstone prevalence rates with migration from underdeveloped to more developed countries are extremely poorly chronicled in terms of epidemiology and causality. These studies are frequently flawed by their anecdotal nature, small cohort size (Wheeler et al., 1970; Hills, 1971), clinical ascertainment criteria, and questionable controls (Maki, 1961; Wheeler et al., 1970; Hills, 1971; Yamase and McNamara, 1972; Burkitt and Tunstall, 1975; Nakayama, 1997). The trends, where real, are likely related to changes in dietary habits with acculturation.

Urban/Rural Residence

Profound urban/rural differences in gallstone prevalence rates (mainly estimated by autopsy and surgery) as well as stone composition have been documented from India (Malhotra, 1968; Sarin et al., 1986), Nigeria (Parnis, 1964), northwest Canada (Schaefer, 1981), South Africa (Bremner, 1971), Sudan (Osman, 1973), Sweden (Mårtensson, 1937), China (Wang and Yao, 1983), and Japan (Maki, 1961), especially pre- and post-World War II (reviewed in Nakayama, 1997). In each country, markedly lower prevalence rates of gallstones were observed in villages and rural communities compared with townships and big cities, and since rural stone type was mainly brown calcium bilirubinate stones, they were probably related to biliary parasites. In contrast, in urban dwellers, the principal stones were cholesterol stones and most likely related to genetic influences and diet. As exemplified by the large nationwide Chinese cohort study from 1984 through 1986, brown pigment stone prevalence throughout China correlated with rural residence and the presence of *A. lumbricoides* eggs in the stools of affected individuals (Nakayama, 1997).

Chronological Changes

In Westernized countries, cholecystectomy rates have increased 30% since the advent of laparoscopic cholecystectomy (1987), and this is due to hyperutilization (Nakayama, 1997), which contrasts with other abdominal operations performed laparoscopically. Several older autopsy studies have, nonetheless, suggested that true prevalence rates of gallstones have increased over the past 100 years, particularly in central and eastern Europe (Zschoch, 1965; Salzer et al., 1970; Brett and Barker, 1976; Kalos et al., 1977), Scandinavia (Mårtensson, 1937; Glambek et al., 1987), and Japan (Maki, 1961; Nakayama, 1997). Chronological increases in autopsy prevalence rates of gallstones during the twentieth century have been reported from Athens, Greece (Kalos et al., 1977), and Innsbruck, Austria (Salzer et al., 1970). The most remarkable autopsy reports are of gallstone prevalence rates at three time intervals over 110 years from the last quarter of the nineteenth until late into the twentieth century (1873–1882, 1973–1982, 1983–1992) from Cluj-Napoca, a Romanian city with a stable population of approximately 300,000 and necropsy rates of 17% to 21% (Acalovschi et al., 1987, 1995; Acalovschi, personal communication, 1998). Figure 16–18 summarizes the dramatic increases in gallstone prevalence rates, attaining those of other central European countries in both genders for all ages. The most notable environmental change in the population of Cluj-Napoca over the past century is a more "modern" lifestyle, with increased refined nutrients, especially sugars, low intake of dietary fiber, and increased prevalence of obesity (Acalovschi, personal communication, 1998). In this population, as in much of Europe, there is likely to be a *LITH* gene pool from the Vikings, who are known to have raided present-day Romania and to have reached the Black Sea during the tenth and eleventh centuries (Jones, 1984).

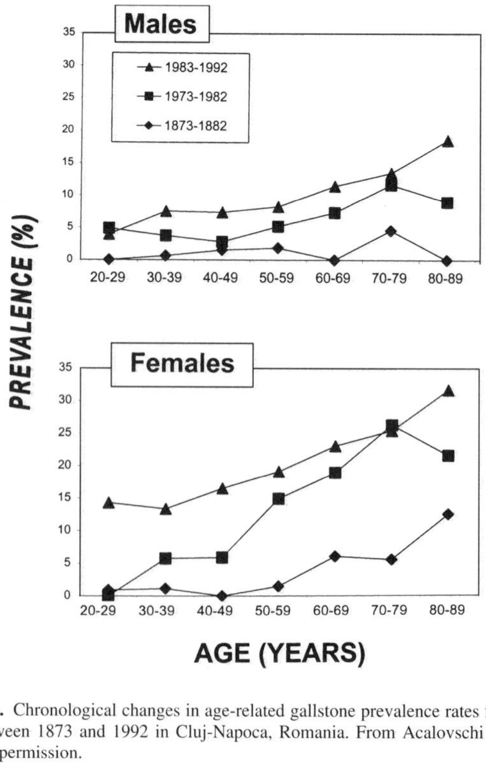

Fig. 16–18. Chronological changes in age-related gallstone prevalence rates from autopsy studies between 1873 and 1992 in Cluj-Napoca, Romania. From Acalovschi et al. (1987, 1995) with permission.

PATHOPHYSIOLOGY: BIOLOGICAL BASIS OF GENETIC SUSCEPTIBILITY

Pathophysiology of Disease

"Black" Pigment Gallstones

Gallbladder biles harboring black pigment gallstones contain an excess of conjugated bilirubins. The most obvious, but not the most common, cause is increased delivery of UCB to the liver from chronic hemolysis (Cahalane et al., 1988). Pigment gallstones are also associated with prolonged total parenteral nutrition and ileal disease, resection, or bypass (Carey, 1993a,b). The pathophysiology in these situations may be related to enterohepatic cycling of bilirubin from hypomotility of the gut and spillage of bile salts into the large intestine in ileal dysfunction syndromes (Brink et al., 1999). This results in solubilization of UCB and promotion of its absorption. Bile contains an endogenous β-glucuronidase which has a pH optimum of 4.0 to 5.0 (Cahalane et al., 1988), and at gallbladder pH of ~6.5, conjugated bilirubins are hydrolyzed slowly to form monoacid UCB (HUCB). This is the bilirubin species which precipitates with free biliary calcium. Most bile calcium is bound to bile salt/lecithin micelles and/or lecithin/cholesterol vesicles (Shiffman et al., 1992; Donovan et al., 1994). Biliary vesicles are absent in black pigment stone bile (Schriever and Jüngst, 1989) because sustained hypersecretion of bilirubin conjugates at the canalicular level uncouple lecithin and cholesterol from bile salt secretion rates (Apstein, 1984). When the ion product of $Ca(HUCB)_2$ exceeds its solubility product, nucleation and precipitation are thermodynamically possible (Ostrow, 1984). Because pigment stone bile is often supersaturated with inorganic calcium salts, this suggests that bile may also be more alkaline, possibly from buffering of secreted protons by the sialic acids of mucin glycoproteins (Cahalane et al., 1988; Carey, 1993a,b). Further, with elevated conjugated bilirubin and HUCB levels in bile, both free and bound calcium concentrations are increased because of Gibbs-Donnan forces (Brink et al., 1999). Once $Ca(HUCB)_2$ has precipitated, polymerization occurs slowly, apparently in biliary sludge and possibly triggered by free radicals of hepatic origin (Cahalane et al., 1988). A proposed scheme outlining the gallbladder pathophysiology of black pigment stone formation is shown in Figure 16–19.

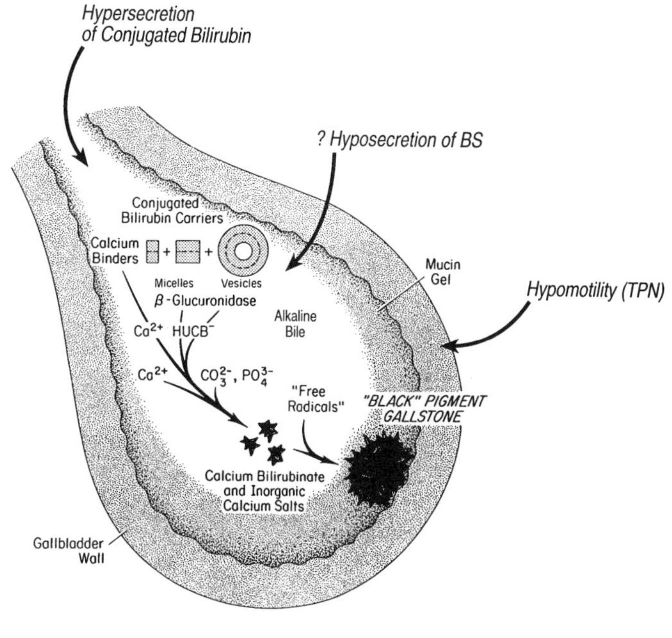

Fig. 16–19. Pathophysiology and physical–chemical pathogenesis of "black" pigment gallstones. Modified from Carey (1993a,b) with permission.

Cholesterol Gallstones

Cholesterol gallstones form only in the gallbladder from precipitation of cholesterol from supersaturated bile (Carey, 1993a,b; Apstein, 1998). Even in ideal-weight subjects, supersaturation is principally from hepatic hypersecretion of cholesterol (Nilsell et al., 1985) and, less commonly, from bile salt hyposecretion or both defects (Fig. 16–20). Cholesterol lithogenicity results in hypersecretion of mucin, presumably from upregulation of *MUC* genes, an early hallmark of lithogenic supersaturation (Carey, 1996). In addition, absorption of cholesterol molecules from bile induces gallbladder hypomotility from signal-transduction decoupling of gallbladder smooth muscle cells (Behar et al., 1989; Yu et al., 1995, 1996). Solid cholesterol crystals nucleate from a phase-separated liquid-crystalline phase, and subsequently cholesterol crystals grow and agglomerate in mucin gel to form macroscopic stones. Cholesterol absorption from the small intestine is within normal limits in cholesterol gallstone disease, but the rate of *de novo* cholesterol synthesis in the liver may be increased and bile salt synthesis decreased (Carey and Duane, 1994; Kern, 1994). Only in obese gallstone subjects are the secretion rates of all biliary lipids increased (Shaffer and Small, 1977). The cholesterol lithogenic state in humans is rather similar to that in C57L/J inbred mice with susceptible *Lith* alleles (Khanuja et al., 1995). With a high-fat diet plus 1% cholesterol and 0.5% cholic acid fed to the mice, five events occur rapidly: *(1)* conversion of the bile salt pool to mostly taurocholate, *(2)* increased intestinal cholesterol absorption, *(3)* increased hepatic cholesterol and phospholipid secretion rates, *(4)* markedly decreasesd *de novo* bile salt synthesis, and *(5)* a phase change in gallbladder bile that facilitates precipitation of cholesterol monohydrate crystals (Wang et al., 1999a,b). Assuming a genetic predisposition to cholesterol gallstones in many humans, the environmental trigger that promotes lithogenicity appears to be overnutrition typified by a diet enriched in refined carbohydrates, with high protein and fat, and deficient in fiber.

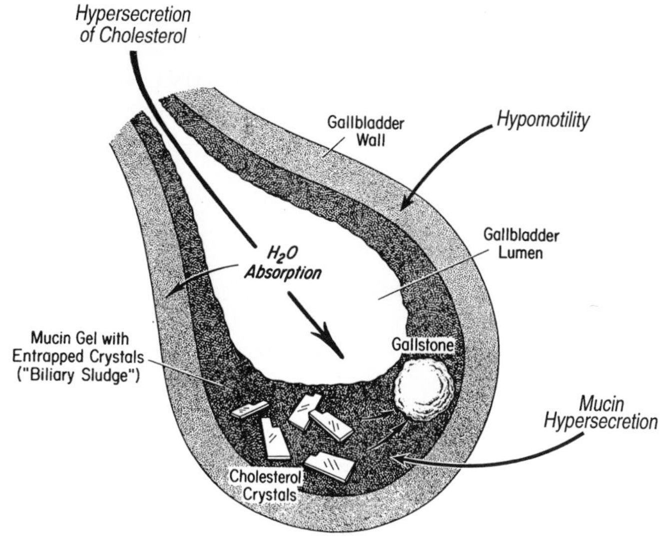

Fig. 16–20. Pathophysiology and physical-chemical pathogenesis of cholesterol gallstones. Modified from Carey (1993a,b) with permission.

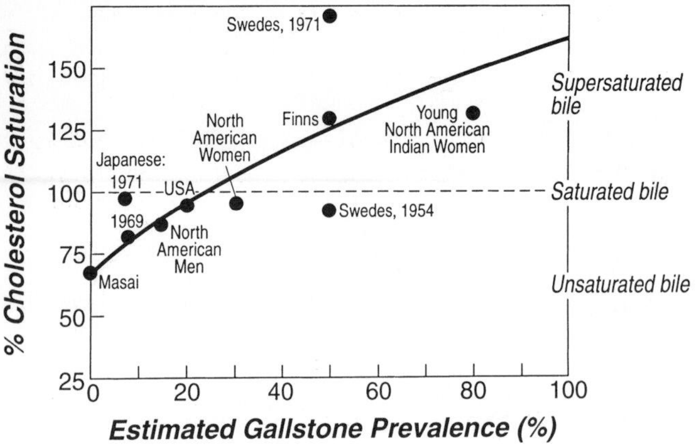

Fig. 16–21. Percent saturation of control gallbladder biles and estimated prevalence rates of gallstones in various populations. Replotted from Redinger and Small (1972), with adjustment for the equilibrium cholesterol saturation of (model) bile. From Carey and Small (1978) with permission.

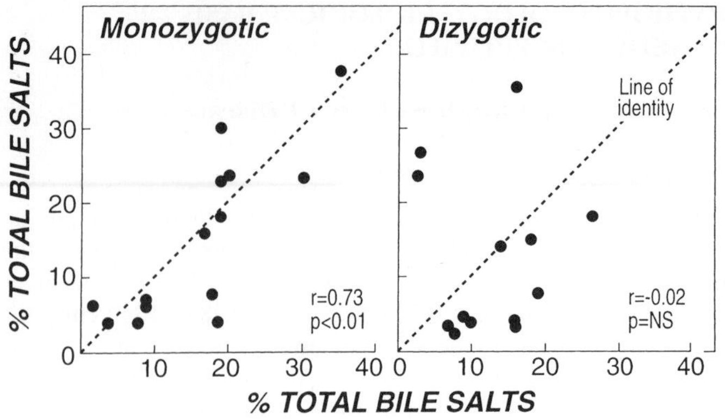

Fig. 16–23. Pairwise correlations of biliary deoxycholate levels as percent of total bile salts in monozygotic compared with dizygotic twins from Finland. Redrawn from Kesäniemi et al. (1989) with permission.

Genetic Studies of Pathophysiology of Cholesterol Gallstones

Based on autopsy, surgical, and cholecystographic studies, Redinger and Small (1972) pointed out that percent cholesterol saturation of control gallbladder biles was positively correlated with estimated prevalence rates of gallstones in the same population (Fig. 16–21). Very unsaturated bile was found in control populations with the lowest prevalence rates, whereas supersaturated bile in controls was derived from populations with very high prevalence rates. From a genetic perspective, these data suggest that if one does not have the *LITH* gene propensity to supersaturate bile, one develops gallstones only with difficulty in response to an environmental challenge. Clearly, in individuals who have susceptible *LITH* alleles, gallstones develop easily in the face of modest environmental challenges.

Figure 16–22 plots the relative lipid compositions of duodenal, i.e., stimulated, gallbladder bile of 39 young Chippewa women with cholesterol gallstones and their stone-free sisters (Danzinger et al., 1972). The relative lipid compositions of the gallstone biles plot above the micellar zone of the triangular phase diagram, implying supersaturated bile in all. In contrast, only half of the older sisters and none of the younger sisters displayed biliary cholesterol supersaturation. By duodenal bile microscopy, no cholesterol crystals were observed in the sisters with supersaturated bile. This unique study suggests that strong

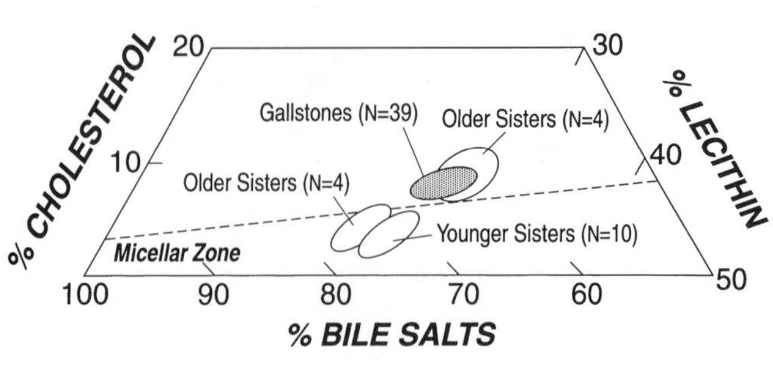

Fig. 16–22. Relative lipid compositions of bile plotted on a fragment of triangular coordinates, from older and younger sisters of Chippewa women with cholesterol cholelithiasis and supersaturated bile. Replotted from data of Danzinger et al. (1972).

age-dependent, genetic and environmental factors are involved in gallstone pathogenesis in this population.

In a Finnish study of male twins (Kesäniemi et al., 1989), the correlation coefficient for cholesterol saturation among 14 monozygotic twins was 0.46 (group mean 1.4 ± 0.5) compared to -0.01 in 13 dizygotic twins (group mean 1.4 ± 0.5). Biliary deoxycholate levels, which are excellent indices of bile lithogenicity in humans (Marcus and Heaton, 1988), were correlated pairwise with respect to each twin pair (Fig. 16–23). Percent deoxycholate showed a significant positive correlation in the monozygotic twins ($r = 0.73$) but no correlation in the dizygotic twins ($r = -0.02$). Likewise, the percent biliary cholesterol and biliary bile acids were more alike in monozygotic twins than in dizygotic twins, showing heritability of these traits as well. Taken together with the concordance for cholesterol gallstones in the monozygotic twins, this study suggests that at both the biochemical and biophysical levels percent biliary cholesterol, cholesterol saturation, and percent deoxycholate conjugates may be under significant genetic control.

GENE IDENTIFICATION

Human Linkage and Association Studies

So far, a limited number of studies linking genomic regions to gallstone disease have been carried out in humans. Among 232 Mexican Americans, a variant of the 5′ end of the cholesterol 7α-hydroxylase (*CYP7A1*) gene was associated with gallstones in men but not in women (Lin et al., 1994). *CYP7A1* is an attractive candidate gene because it is the rate-limiting step in the "neutral" pathway for formation of bile salts from cholesterol in the liver and because bile salts are crucial for bile production and keeping cholesterol molecules solubilized in mixed micelles in bile.

Because an inactive gallbladder favors stone formation, the genes for cholecystokinin and the cholecystokinin A receptor (*CCKAR*), which affect gallbladder motility, are attractive candidates. Genetic variation in *CCKAR* is associated with gallstone risk (Schneider et al., 1997), and an aberrant splicing of *CCKAR*, predicted to result in a nonfunctional receptor, was found in one obese patient with gallstones (Miller and Mitchell, 1995). In addition, certain polymorphisms of the apolipoprotein B and E genes and of the cholesterol ester transfer protein, all involved in carrying cholesterol in the plasma, are associated with gallstones (Juvonen et al., 1993, 1995; Bertomeu et al., 1996; Han et al., 2000). Missense mutations in the multidrug-resistant 3 gene (*ABCB4*), which encodes for the phosphatidylcholine transporter across the canalicular membrane of the hepatocyte, is the basis for one particular type of cholelithiasis and gallstone formation (Jacquemiu et al., 2001; Rosmorduc et al., 2001). This form is characterized by chronic cholestasis, recurrence of symptoms after cholecystectomy, and a high cholesterol/phospholipid ratio in bile.

In patients with hepatolithiasis, a common disorder in the Far East but rare in Western countries, low levels of MDR3 and phosphatidylcholine transfer protein occur together with markedly reduced phospholipid concentrations in bile (Shoda et al., 2001). Furthermore, HMG-CoA reductase activity was increased and *CYP7A1* activity was decreased in patients compared to controls. In this disorder, the formation of cholesterol-rich intrahepatic stones can be attributed to decreased biliary secretion of phospholipids in the setting of increased cholesterol synthesis and decreased bile salt synthesis.

Animal Studies

Strain Differences in Gallstone Formation

The major contribution to our understanding of genes associated with cholesterol gallstone disease comes from work using the mouse model. Evidence that genetic factors play an important role in the development of cholelithiasis has been provided by several studies comparing gallstone formation among different inbred strains of mice. Fujihara et al. (1978) reported that the prevalence of gallstones varied from 0% to 100% among six strains of laboratory mice. Alexander and Portman (1987) showed that C57BL/6 mice are susceptible to gallstone formation, whereas CBA mice are resistant; in both strains, bile was supersaturated with cholesterol but to different degrees. Studies on atherosclerosis in the mouse demonstrated that the high-fat and high-cholesterol diet (15% butter fat, 1% cholesterol, 0.5% cholic acid) used to produce atherosclerosis in female mice of inbred strains resulted in the formation of cholesterol gallstones in some strains but not in others after 18 weeks of diet consumption (Nishina et al., 1990; Paigen et al., 1990). This survey of gallstone susceptibility has been extended to both males and females of 48 inbred mouse strains fed the same diet for 8 weeks (Bouchard et al., data unpublished but posted at *www.jax.org/pub-cgi/phenome* in the Mouse Phenome Project). Gallstone-susceptible strains include the C57–C58 family of strains (C57BL/6, C57BL/10, C57L, C58) and PERA, CAST, and RIIIS.

Quantitative Trait Loci Mapping and the Gallstone Map

For analyzing quantitative polygenic traits, conventional genetic mapping methods, designed for single-gene traits, are inadequate. The technique of quantitative trait locus (QTL) analysis (Lander and Botstein, 1989) provided the approach for identifying, locating, and estimating the effects of genes in several chromosomal regions affecting gallstone formation. An additional advantage of QTL mapping is that it can be used to discover new loci, whereas transgenic and knockout mice usually provide information only on known genes.

In general, a QTL is assigned a name (in gallstones, *Lith1*, *Lith2*, etc.) if *(1)* statistical evidence shows that it is significant, which corresponds to $p < 0.0001$, a LOD score >3.3, or an F statistic that is significant after permutation testing, or *(2)* if the QTL has suggestive significance, which corresponds to $p < 0.003$ or a LOD score of at least 1.9 *and* is confirmed by constructing a congenic strain or is found a second time in an independent cross.

QTL analysis involves the following steps: *(1)* experimental crosses of inbred mice with different gallstone susceptibility, *(2)* measuring second-generation progeny (backcross or F_2) for the phenotype (weight of gallstones, extent of cholesterol monohydrate crystals, cholesterol supersaturation, or amount of mucin, an important intermediate phenotype in cholesterol gallstone formation), and *(3)* genotyping the progeny with polymorphic markers (simple sequence length polymorphisms, SSLPs) covering the whole genome. The progeny will have a distribution of the phenotype, such as total weight of gallstones in the gallbladder. In a QTL analysis, the distribution of alleles for each SSLP marker is compared between mice with no stones and mice with the largest stones. If the alleles at a single SSLP marker from the resistant strain are designated A and those from the susceptible strain are designated B, then a region of the chromosome that contains no gene affecting gallstone weight will have an equal distribution of A and B alleles in the mice with the smallest and largest stones. If a chromosomal region does contain a gene affecting gallstone weight, then mice with the smallest stones will have predominantly A alleles at the nearest SSLP and mice with the largest stones will have mostly B alleles. Several QTL regions can be found in a single cross since common complex diseases generally are polygenic. Table 16–2 lists all gallstone QTLs that have been identified to date; they are briefly summarized below.

The first study compared gallstone formation among resistant AKR/J mice, susceptible C57L/J mice, and their recombinant inbred strains, first filial (F_1) and backcross progeny (Khanuja et al., 1995). The data demonstrated that gallstone formation is a dominant trait, that gallstone susceptibility is determined by at least two unlinked genes, and that a major gene affects gallstone susceptibility, designated *Lith1* (for "lithogenic"). Subsequent QTL analysis of an extended 231 mouse backcross between these strains showed that *Lith1* mapped to chromosome 2 with a LOD score of 4.4, that *Lith2* mapped to chromosome 19, and that additional QTLs with LOD scores of 1.5 to 3 were found on chromosomes 6, 7, 8, 10, and X (Paigen et al., 2000). These QTLs and those described subsequently are depicted in Figure 16–24, which also shows the map positions of the candidate genes that may be involved in gallstone formation based on our current knowledge of the underlying pathophysiology.

To confirm the *Lith1* and *Lith2* genes, congenic strains that carry the C57L alleles only in the *Lith1* or *Lith2* regions on an AKR genetic background were constructed. The region of interest is introgressed into the genetic background of AKR by repeated backcrossing. At each backcross, about half of the alleles from the C57L parent are lost (except for the locus of interest). A congenic strain isolates the susceptibility alleles at one locus from all other QTLs in the same cross and thereby enables confirmation of the QTL and investigation of the pathophysiological changes that it causes. By convention, the nomenclature of a congenic strain follows this order: the symbol of the background strain, a period, the symbol of the donor strain of the introgressed locus, a dash, the name of the introgressed gene, and a superscript describing the allele (in this case, *s* for susceptible or *r* for resistant). *AK* is the symbol for AKR and *L* is the symbol for C57L. Thus, these congenic strains were named AK.L-$Lith1^s$ and AK.L-$Lith2^s$. Both congenics showed gallstone formation comparable to the C57L parent, confirming that both the

Table 16–2. Quantitative Trait Loci for Cholesterol Gallstones and Mucin in Inbred Mice[a]

Cross	Phenotype	Location		QTL Name[b]	Genetic Marker
		Chr.	cM		
(C57L × AKR)BC	Gallstone weight	2	0.23	*Lith1*	*D2Mit14*
(I/LN × PERA)F_2	Gallstone weight	4	50–70		*D4Mit204*
(C57BL/6 × C3H)F_2	Gallstone weight	5	25–55		*D5Mit205*
(AKR × SWR)BC	Mucin	5	70–90		*D5Mit46*
(C57L × AKR)BC	Gallstone weight	6	55–end		*D6Mit25*
(AKR × SWR)BC	Gallstone score	6	60–end		*D6Mit14*
(C57L × AKR) BC	Gallstone weight	7	15–45		*D7Mit85*
(C57L × AKR/BC	Gallstone weight	8	25–65		*D8Mit40*
(AKR × SWR)BC	Gallstone score	9	35–60	*Lith5*	*D9Mit307*
(C57L × AKR)BC	Gallstone weight	10	0–30		*D10Mit2*
(I/LN × PERA)F_2	Gallstone weight	10	25–60		*D10Mit12*
(C57BL/6 × C3H)F_2	Gallstone size	11	45–60		*D11Mit4*
(AKR × SWR)BC	Mucin	11	0–20		*D11Mit74*
(DBA/2 × CAST)F_2	Gallstone score	11	40–60		*D11Mit212*
(DBA/2 × CAST)F_2	Gallstone weight	13	15–35		*D13Mit19*
(I/LN × PERA)F_2	Gallstone weight	13	20–40		*D13Mit11*
(A × AKR)BC	Mucin	15	50–70		*D15Mit16*
(AKR × SWR)BC	Gallstone score	15	20–40		*D15Mit26*
(A × AKR)BC	Crystal and stone prevalence	17	0–15	*Lith3*	*D17Mit247*
(I/LN × PERA)F_2	Gallstone score	17	45–end		*D17Mit155*
(C57L × AKR)BC	Gallstone weight	19	0.4 cM	*Lith2*	*D19Mit58*
(C57L × AKR)BC	Gallstone weight	X	15–35	*Lith4*	*DXMit46*
(I/LN × PERA)F_2	Gallstone score	X	20–40		*DXMIT25*

[a]BC, backcross progeny; Chr, chromosome; F_2, intercross progeny; *Lith*, lithogenic gene; Mit, Massachusetts Institute of Technology; QTL, quantitative trait locus.
[b]QTL are named if significant or if confirmed by a congenic or presence in a second cross. Several QTL without names are significant but have not yet been named because the cross is not completely analyzed.

Lith1 and *Lith2* QTL regions contain genes that can cause gallstones.

Two additional crosses were carried out between the gallstone-resistant AKR strain and the gallstone-susceptible strains A/J and SWR/J. In the first cross, AKR mice were crossed to inbred strain A/J (A) and 227 male backcross progeny (A × AKR)F_1 × AKR were fed a lithogenic diet, examined for gallstone formation, and genotyped employing SSLP markers spanning the entire genome (Lammert et al., 1997). QTL analysis revealed a locus affecting gallstone formation with a LOD score >3.3 in the proximal region of chromosome 17 (Fig. 16–24) with the susceptibility allele contributed by the resistant strain AKR. This locus was designated *Lith3*. In this cross, another QTL was detected for mucin accumulation in the gallbladder on the distal end of chromosome 15, which co-localizes with the glycosylation-dependent cell adhesion molecule 1 (*Glycam1*), a glycoprotein like other mucins. GLYCAM1 was originally described as an endothelial adhesion molecule expressed in lymph nodes and subsequently located in different epithelial cells. By immunohistochemistry, we demonstrated that GLYCAM1 is expressed in gallbladder epithelial cells and secreted into the bile (Wittenburg et al., 2001). In the second cross, AKR was crossed to inbred strain SWR, and the F_1 progeny were backcrossed to AKR to obtain 330 progeny that were phenotyped for gallstones and for mucin accumulation in the gallbladder. Analysis of this cross led to the identification of a major QTL affecting gallstone formation on chromosome 9, named *Lith5*, and two interacting QTLs on chromosomes 6 and 15 (Wittenburg et al., unpublished data). In addition, a pair of interacting QTLs for mucin accumulation was found on chromosomes 5 (70–90 cM) and 11 (0–20 cM). The positional candidate gene for the mucin QTL on chromosome 5 QTL is *Muc3*, the mouse ortholog of the major human mucin gene in the gallbladder.

In a separate study, QTL analysis of 185 F_2 progeny of an intercross between the C57BL/6J and C3H/HeJ strains identified two loci, on chromosomes 5 and 11, associated with gallstone formation, HDL cholesterol concentration, and expression of CYP7A1 (Machleder et al., 1997). Gallstone formation was inversely correlated with plasma HDL cholesterol levels and CYP7A1 expression.

A set of eight additional QTL crosses for cholesterol gallstone formation are under way using four susceptible strains (C58/J, PERA/Ei, RIIIS/J, and CAST/Ei) and four resistant strains (LP/J, I/LnJ, DBA/2J, and 129SI/SclmJ), with each susceptible strain crossed to two resistant strains. Initial analyses of the first two crosses are available. In the cross between I/LnJ and PERA, gallstone QTL were found on chromosomes 4 (50–70 cM), 10 (25–60 cM), 13 (30–50 cM), 17 (distal end), and X (20–40 cM) (Wittenburg et al., unpublished data). In a cross between DBA/2J and CAST/Ei, gallstone QTL were found on chromosomes 11 (40–60 cM) and 13 (15–35 cM) (Lyons et al., unpublished data). When all of the crosses currently in progress are completed, 16 different inbred strains will have been examined for gallstone QTL. If the number of times each QTL has been discovered fits a Poisson distribution (for one, two, or three hits), then we should be able to estimate the total number of gallstone QTL among these strains, which represent a good sampling of the genetic diversity available in the mouse.

Table 16–2 and Figure 16–24 summarize the QTL found so far in mouse crosses. Three QTL have been identified for mucin and 15 for gallstone formation. The QTL on chromosomes 10, 11, 13, and X were each found in two separate crosses. Figure 16–24 depicts the QTL as well as the map locations of some of the key proteins involved in cholesterol and bile salt metabolism and transport (an earlier version of this map is in Lammert et al., 2001). The fact that a key protein maps to a QTL does not mean

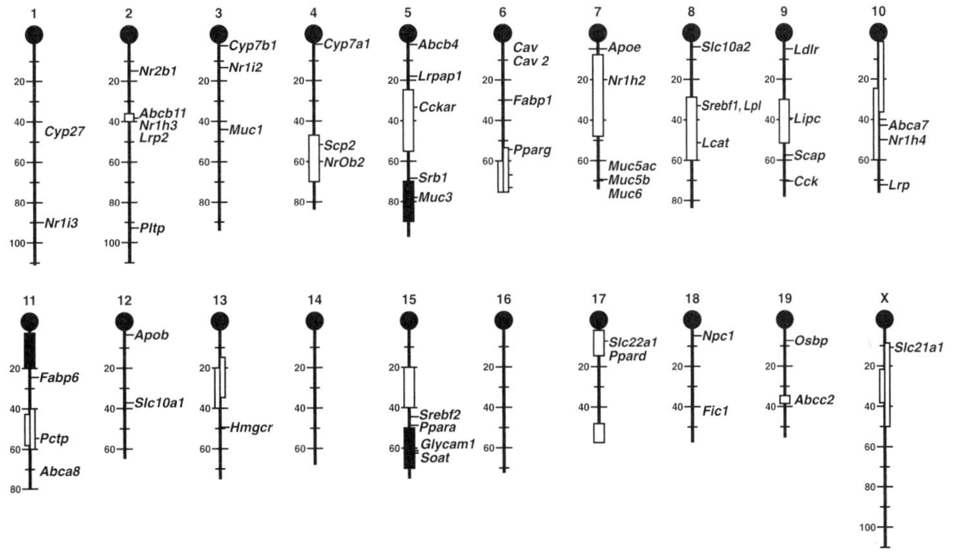

Fig. 16–24. Murine gallstone map: candidate genes and quantitative trait loci (QTL) on chromosomes of the mouse genome. *Open rectangular areas* represent QTL for cholesterol gallstones; *solid rectangles* represent QTL for mucin. The size of each QTL is 20 cM unless known to be more or less. *Vertical line* represents each chromosome, with the centromere at the proximal end, and genetic distances from the centromere are indicated to the left of the chromosomes (cM). *Light, long horizontal lines* on each chromosome represent 10 cM. *FIC1* has been mapped only in humans but is placed in the homologous region of chromosome 18 on the murine map. Gene symbols and names are as follows: *Abca7, Abcb4, Abcb11, Abcc2*, ATP-binding cassette subfamily A, B, or C, member 7, 4, 11, or 2; *Abcb4*, phosphatidylcholine translocator/multidrug resistant 3 (*Mdr2/MDR3*); *Abcb11*, bile salt export pump (*Bsep, Spgp*); *Abcc2*, multidrug resistance-associated protein 2/canalicular multispecific organic anion transporter (*Mrp2/Cmoat*); *Apob*, apolipoprotein B; *Apoe*, apolipoprotein E; *Cav*, caveolin; *Cav2*, caveolin 2; *Cck*, cholecystokinin; *Cckar*, cholecystokinin A receptor; *Cyp7a1*, cholesterol 7α-hydroxylase; *Cyp7b1*, oxysterol 7β-hydroxylase; *Cyp27*, sterol 27-hydroxylase; *Fabp1*, fatty acid binding protein 1, liver; *Fic1*, familial intrahepatic cholestasis 1; *Fabp6*, fatty acid binding protein 6, ileal; *Glycam1*, glycosylation-dependent cell adhesion molecule; *Hmgcr*, HMG-CoA reductase; *Lcat*, lecithin cholesterol acyltransferase *Ldlr*, low density lipoprotein receptor; *Lipc*, lipase, hepatic; *Lpl*, lipoprotein lipase; *Lrp*, Ldlr-related protein; *Lrpap1*, Lrp-associated protein 1; *Muc1, Muc3 Muc5ac, Muc5b, Muc6*, mucin genes; *Npc1*, Niemann-Pick type C1; *Nr1c1, Nr1c2, Nr1c3, Nr1h2, Nr1h3, Nr1h4, Nr1i2, Nr1i3, Nr2b1*, nuclear receptor subfamily 1 or 2, group C, H, or I, member 1–4; *Nr1c1, Nr1c2, Nr1c3*, peroxisomal proliferator activated receptor α, δ, γ (*Ppara, Ppard, Pparg*); *Nr1h2*, liver X receptor β (*Lxrb*); *Nr1h3*, liver X receptor α (*Lxra*); *Nr1h4*, farnesoid X receptor (*Fxr*); *Nr1i2*, pregnane X receptor (*Pxr*); *Nr1i3*, constitutive androstane receptor (*Car*); *Nr2b1*, retinoid X receptor α (*Rxra*); *Osbp*, oxysterol binding protein; *Pctp*, phosphatidylcholine transfer protein; *Pltp*, phospholipid transfer protein; Scap, *Srebf* cleavage activating protein; *Scp2*, sterol carrier protein 2; *Slc10a1*, sodium-dependent taurocholate (bile salt) cotransporting polypeptide (*Ntcp*); *Slc10a2*, apical sodium-dependent bile salt transporter/ileal bile acid transporter (*Asbt/Ibat*); *Slc21a1*, solute carrier family (organic anion transporter) member 1; *Slc22a1*, organic cation transporter; *Soat2*, acyl-CoA:cholesterol acyltransferase 2 (*Acat2*); *Srb1*, scavenger receptor class B, type 1; *Srebf1, Srebf2*, sterol regulatory element binding transcription factors 1 and 2.

that it is the gene determining gallstones, but such a map location does establish the gene as a positional candidate that deserves further testing. Thirteen of the 15 QTL co-localize with likely candidate genes in the same chromosomal region.

Studies of blood pressure demonstrate that hypertension QTL found in the mouse and rat models predict the location of hypertension QTL in humans (Sugiyama et al., 2001; Stoll et al., 2000). Thus, the location of these gallstone QTL in the mouse may be used to direct a search for gallstone QTL in humans. It may seem surprising that QTL found in rodent species can predict the location of QTL in humans. Since there may be more than 100 genes in the pathways for blood pressure regulation and since mutation is random, why do the same subset of genes appear as QTL in multiple species? It could result from an old mutation that occurred in the mammalian ancestor of mice, rats, and humans. We think this is a possible but unlikely reason. A more likely explanation is that only a subset of genes regulating a complex trait are rate-limiting and that only variation in this special subset causes a change in the trait. This makes sense with what we know from the large number of diseases inherited in a recessive fashion. Parents of the affected are normal even though they each carry only 50% of the responsible protein. Since many proteins are present in excess, a mutation affecting function to some degree will not affect the final phenotype. We suggest that primarily mutations in those proteins are rate-limiting or regulatory and affect the final phenotype. Since rate-limiting proteins are only a subset of all genes in a pathway, this could account for the concordance of disease QTL in different species. Variation in other genes may occur but may not result in a QTL because the protein is present in excess and small changes in concentration or activity will not affect the trait.

Candidate Genes

A consideration of the pathophysiology of gallstone disease indicates several major classes of candidate genes that encode proteins that may be important in cholesterol gallstone formation (Table 16–3). (Only the literature concerning their role in gallstone formation will be referenced; for references about their role in lipid metabolism, see the review by Lammert et al., 2001).

- Hepatic lipid-regulatory enzymes that could lead to excess cholesterol or decreased bile salt and/or phosphatidylcholine secretion into bile
- Lipoprotein receptors and related proteins that mediate cholesterol homeostasis
- Hepatic and intestinal membrane transporter proteins
- Hepatic and intestinal intracellular carriers of cholesterol, bile salts, or phosphatidylcholine
- Lipid- and bile salt-regulatory transcription factors
- Cholecystokinin and its receptors, which affect gallbladder motility
- Mucins, which promote cholesterol crystallization in bile

The nomenclature of these proteins is confusing because of changes to gene names due to their function and assignment to superfamilies. In general, human genes are capitalized and ital-

Table 16–3. Chromosomal Location of Candidate Gallstone and Mucin Genes in Mice and Humans

Gene Symbol (Former Symbol)	Gene Name (Former Gene Name)	Mouse Chromosome	cM	Human Ortholog
Hepatic lipid-regulatory enzymes				
Soat2	Sterol *O*-acyl transferase 2 (acyl-CoA:cholesterol acyltransferase)	15	62	12q13.3–q15
Cyp7a1	Cholesterol 7α-hydroxylase	4	0	8q11–q11.2
Cyp7b1	Oxysterol 7α-hydroxylase	3	1	8q12–22[b]
Cyp27	Sterol 27α-hydroxylase	1	nd	2q33–qter
Hmgcr	HMG-CoA reductase	13	49	5q13.3–14
Lipoprotein receptors and related genes				
Apob	Apolipoprotein B	12	2	2p24–p23
Apoe	Apolipoprotein E	7	4	19q13.2
Lrp2	Ldlr-related protein 2, megalin	2	39	2q31–q32.1
Ldlr	Low-density lipoprotein receptor	9	5	19p13.2
Lipc (Hpl)	Hepatic lipase	9	39	15q21–22
Lrp	Ldlr-related protein	10	72.5	12q13–q14
Lrpap1	Lrp-associated protein 1	5	18	4p16.3
Lcat	Lecithin cholesterol acyltransferase	8	53	16q22.1
Lpl	Lipoprotein lipase	8	33	8p22
Pltp	Phospolipid transfer protein	2	93	20q12–q13.1
Srb1	Scavenger receptor 1	5	68	12pter–qter
Hepatic and intestinal lipid membrane transporters				
Abca7	ATP-binding cassette, family A, member 7	10	44	19p13.3
Abcb11 (Bsep)	Bile salt export pump	2	38	2q24.3
Abcc2 (Cmoat)	Canalicular multispecific organic anion transporter	19	43	10q24
Abcb4 (Mdr2)	Multiple drug resistance 2 (phosphatidylcholine transmembrane transporter)	5	1	7q21
Fic1	Familial intrahepatic cholestasis type 1, ATPase class 1, type 8b1	18	nd	18q21–22
Slc2la1 (Oatp1)	Organic anion transporting polypeptide 1	X	nd	nd
Slc10a1 (Ntcp)	Sodium bile salt cotransporting polypeptide	12	37	14q21.1–21.2
Slc10a2 (Ibat)	Ileal bile salt cotransporter	8	2	13q33
Slc22a1 (Orct1)	Organic cation transporter 1	17	7	6q26
Hepatic and intestinal intracellular lipid carriers				
Akr1c3	3α-Hydroxysteroid dehydrogenase	2	nd	10p15
Cav	Caveolin	6	nd	7q31
Cav2	Caveolin 2	6	nd	7q31
Fabp1	Fatty acid binding protein 1 liver	6	30	2p11
Fabp6 (Illbp)	Fatty acid binding protein 6, ileal	11	24	5q23–35
Npc1	Niemann-Pick type C1	18	4	18q11
Osbp	Oxysterol binding protein	19	7	11q12–13
Pctp	Phosphatidylcholine transfer protein	11	52	17q21–24
Scp2	Sterol carrier protein 2	4	52	1p32
Lipid regulatory transcription factors				
Nr0b2 (Shp1)	Small heterodimer partner 1	4	61	nd
Nr1i3 (Car)	Constitutive androstane receptor	1	93	nd
Nr1h4 (Fxr)	Farnesoid × receptor	10	50	12q21–24[b]
Nr1h3 (Lxra)	Liver × receptor α	2	40	nd
Nr1h2 (Lxrb)	Liver × receptor β	7	20	nd
Nr1cl (Ppara)	Peroxisomal proliferator activated receptor α	15	48.8	22q12–13.1
Nr1c2 (Ppard)	Peroxisomal proliferator activated receptor δ	17	14	6p21.2–p21.1
Nr1c3 (Pparg)	Peroxisomal proliferator activated receptor γ	6	53	3p25
Nr1i2 (Pxr)	Pregnane X receptor	3	14	nd
Nr2b1 (Rxra)	Retinoid X receptor α	2	17	9q34
Scap	Srebf cleavage activating protein	9	58	nd
Srebf1	Sterol regulatory element binding transcription factor 1	8	33	17p11.2
Srebf2	Sterol regulatory element binding transcription factor 2	15	44.8	22q13
Gallbladder: cholecystokinin and mucins				
Cck	Cholecystokinin	9	71	3p22–21.3
Cckar	Cholecystokinin A receptor	5	34	4pter–qter
Glycam1	Glycosylation-dependent cell adhesion molecule 1	15	63	nd
Muc1	Mucin 1	3	44.8	1q21–23
Muc3	Mucin 3	5	78	7q22
Muc5ac	Mucin 5ac	7	69	11p15.5
Muc5b	Mucin 5b	7[b]	69	11p15.5
Muc6	Mucin 6	7[b]	69	11p15.5

[a]HMG-CoA, 3-hydroxy-3-methylglutaryl coenzyme A; nd, not determined; Ldlr, low-density lipoprotein receptor; Lrp, Ldlr-related protein; ATP, adenosine triphosphate; Srebf, sterol regulatory element binding transcription factor.

[b]Map position based on conserved homology between mouse and human genomes and assigned indirectly from localization in other species. Information on homologous regions was retrieved from the human/mouse homology databases maintained at the National Institutes of Health and The Jackson Laboratory. Map position of *Nr0b2* and *Scap* determined by Henning Wittenburg (personal communication).

icized and mouse genes begin with a capital letter and are italicized; when referring to the protein, the name is capitalized but not italicized for both species. Figure 16–24 shows the candidate gene map for cholesterol gallstone formation in the mouse. A QTL is given a descriptive name when it is first described, but when the protein is finally identified, the name changes to the name of the protein. For example, we named a major QTL for gallstones *Lith1*. We believe that the gene underlying this QTL is *sister to P-glycoprotein* (*Spgp*), the name given to the gene by the person who first cloned it (Childs et al., 1995). When the function of the protein was found to be the **b**ile **s**alt **e**xport **p**ump of mammalian liver (Gerloff et al., 1998), the gene name was changed to *Bsep*. Subsequently, it was shown that *Bsep* is a member of the **A**TP-**b**inding **c**assette (ABC) family of membrane transporters (Schriml and Dean, 2000), and finally, the nomenclature of the entire family of these transporters was changed to *Abc* followed by the class letter and subclass number; thus, *Bsep* became *Abcb11*.

Hepatic Lipid-Regulatory Enzymes. Hypersecretion of cholesterol from the liver into the bile is the primary cause of cholesterol gallstone formation in humans (Carey, 1993a,b) and in C57L mice (Wang et al., 1997). This excess cholesterol secretion can result from several processes in the liver: increased *de novo* cholesterol synthesis, decreased cholesterol catabolism to bile salts, or decreased cholesterol esterification. The following genes encode key regulatory enzymes of these processes: *Hmgcr*, *Cyp7a1*, sterol 27-hydroxylase (*Cyp27*), oxysterol 7α-hydroxylase (*Cyp7b1*), and acyl-CoA:cholesterol acyltransferase (*Acat2*), which has been renamed sterol *O*-acyltransferase (*Soat2*).

Hmgcr encodes the rate-limiting enzyme in cholesterol biosynthesis, and a QTL maps to the region containing this gene (Fig. 16–24). Comparison of HMG-CoA reductase activity in mice showed that the lithogenic diet downregulated the enzyme in gallstone-resistant mice but failed to downregulate it in gallstone-susceptible mice (Lammert et al., 1999a,b). Thus, susceptible mice continue to synthesize cholesterol in spite of its excess availability from the diet, indicating that something in the regulatory system of the enzyme is amiss.

Hepatic cholesterol can serve as a substrate for bile salt synthesis by two pathways. In the neutral pathway, *CYP7A1* catalyzes the first step and is rate-limiting. Polymorphisms in this gene have been associated with gallstones in humans (Lin et al., 1994). Although no murine gallstone QTL has been mapped in the region of the *Cyp7a1* structural gene on chromosome 4, in a cross between C57BL/6 and C3H strains, two QTL determining *CYP7A1* expression levels were found to be coincident on chromosomes 5 and 11 with QTL for gallstone formation (Machleder et al., 1997). In the alternative bile synthesis pathway, cholesterol side chain oxidation is initiated by *CYP27*. This is followed by hydroxylation on the fused-ring structure by the microsomal enzyme *CYP7B1*. No gallstone QTL so far mapped co-localizes with these genes.

Hepatic free cholesterol can be converted into cholesteryl ester by the rate-limiting enzyme ACAT2, encoded by *Soat2*. This enzyme catalyzes cholesterol esterification in the mouse liver and intestine (Farese, 1998). A knockout of this gene protected mice against hypercholesterolemia and gallstone formation when mice were fed a cholesterol-rich diet (Buhman et al., 2000; Zanlungo and Nervi, 2001). The mechanism appears to be the lack of cholesteryl ester synthesis and, hence, chylomicron assembly in the intestine, resulting in a reduced capacity to absorb cholesterol.

Lipoprotein Receptors or Related Proteins. The main type of cholesterol for biliary secretion is HDL cholesterol. Cholesterol is also delivered to the liver by LDL and chylomicron remnants, which are rich in cholesteryl esters. The genes encoding proteins that participate in this pathway are as follows: *Apob*, apolipoprotein B; *ApoE*, apolipoprotein E; *Ldlr*, LDL receptor; *Lrp2*, Ldlr-related protein 2; *Lipc*, hepatic lipase; *Lrp*, Ldlr-related protein; *Lrpap1*, Lrp-associated protein 1; *Lcat*, lecithin cholesterol acyltransferase; *Lpl*, lipoprotein lipase; *Pltp*, phospholipid transfer protein; and *Srb1*, scavenger receptor 1.

HDL cholesterol is taken up from blood by the scavenger receptor class BI (SR-BI) in liver and steroidogenic tissues. In mice, adenovirus-mediated overexpression of *Srb1* on both basolateral and canalicular membranes of hepatocytes has been shown to result in the disappearance of plasma HDL and to increase the amount of biliary cholesterol (Kozarsky et al., 1997). In turn, SR-BI-deficient mice had significantly reduced biliary cholesterol concentrations and secretion rates (Mardones et al., 2001).

LDLs are taken up by the LDL receptor (LDLR), which recognizes apolipoprotein E (apo E) and apolipoprotein B (apo B). Chylomicron remnants are taken up by LDLR or by the LDLR-related protein (LRP). LRP is associated with a 39 kDa protein, LRP-associated protein 1 (LRPAP1), which is necessary for the proper intracellular processing and membrane insertion of LRP.

In humans, a polymorphism of the *APOE* locus has been identified as a risk factor for cholesterol gallstones. *APOE* exists as three different alleles (E2, E3, and E4). The E4 genotype is associated with higher frequency of gallstones (Bertomeu et al., 1996), increased cholesterol content of stones (Juvonen et al., 1993), and higher risk of recurrence after clearance of gallstones by lithotropsy (Portincasa et al., 1996). In contrast, the E2 genotypes appear to protect against cholesterol gallstone formation (Niemi et al., 1999). The effects may be due in part to enhanced hepatic uptake of chylomicron remnants, increased intestinal cholesterol absorption and decreased bile salt synthesis (van Erpecum and Carey, 1996). Mice lacking *APOE* that were fed a high-cholesterol, lithogenic diet had decreased biliary cholesterol secretion and decreased gallstone formation compared to wild-type mice (Amigo et al., 2000).

Another member of the *Ldlr* gene family, called Ldlr-related protein 2 (*Lrp2*), also called *megalin*, is expressed on the apical surfaces of specialized epithelial cells, such as the distal small intestine, where it facilitates the uptake of vitamin B_{12}, and in the proximal renal tubules, where it facilitates the uptake of vitamin D_3. Because this receptor binds Apo E-containing lipoproteins, it might participate in cholesterol homeostasis. Even though *Lrp2* maps to the *Lith1* region, we consider it a less likely candidate gene because it is not expressed in hepatocytes.

Hepatic lipase (*Lipc*) increases chylomicron remnant and HDL cholesterol clearance in the liver. Outside the liver, lipoprotein lipase (*Lpl*) carries out hydrolysis of core triglycerides in chylomicrons and VLDL. Both of these lipases map to known gallstone QTL. Other genes that play a role in extrahepatic lipoprotein metabolism could affect the delivery of cholesterol to the liver. These include *Apob*, lecithin cholesterol acyltransferase (*Lcat*), phospholipid transfer protein (*Pltp*), and cholesterol ester transfer protein (*CETP*), which is absent in mice. Polymorphisms of the *APOB* gene in humans are associated with gallstone formation (Han et al., 2000). The map position for *Lcat* co-localizes with a gallstone QTL in the mouse. Since HDL is the main source of cholesterol for biliary excretion, proteins that affect HDL levels could affect gallstone formation. Increased

PLTP increases HDL and increased CETP lowers HDL. Polymorphisms of *CETP* in humans are associated with cholesterol gallstone formation (Juvonen et al., 1995); mice do not have CETP.

Hepatic and Intestinal Membrane Transporter Proteins

Transport of organic compounds from the liver into bile against a concentration gradient is accomplished by a set of ATP-binding cassette (ABC) transporters located in the canalicular membrane of the hepatocyte (Keppler and Arias, 1997). These export pumps belong to a large gene family of *P*-glycoproteins (Schriml and Dean, 2000) that includes *Mdr* genes and liver and blood–brain barrier genes. Alterations in the expression or function of these transport proteins may cause alterations in the composition of bile that contribute to cholesterol gallstones. At least four ABC transporters are involved in bile formation and probably gallstone susceptibility: *Abcb11*, also known as *Bsep*; *Abcc2*, the canalicular multispecific organic anion transporter also known as *Cmoat* or *Mrp2*; *Abcb4*, the phosphatidylcholine transmembrane transporter known as *Mdr2* in mice and *MDR3* in humans; and *Abca7*, the function of which is unknown but which maps to a gallstone QTL.

ABCB11 is a 170 kDa glycosylated plasma membrane protein that was first cloned from the pig (Childs et al., 1995) and then from the rat (Childs et al., 1998). It is related to the *P*-glycoprotein family by an ancient duplication that arose before the division of fish and mammals. It is localized exclusively to the canalicular membrane of the hepatocyte, and its function was shown in vitro to be the transport of monovalent bile salts (Gerloff et al., 1998). In humans, it was mapped to chromosome 2q31 (Childs et al., 1998). In the mouse, *Abcb11* was mapped using oligonucleotide primers designed to the 3′-untranslated region of the murine molecule and found to be nonrecombinant with *D2Mit56* in 188 mice from the Jackson Laboratory backcross panels between strains C57BL/6 and SPRET/Ei (Bouchard et al., 1999). This location is the same as that for the *Lith1* gene, as determined by backcrossing the *Lith1* congenic strain to AKR, collecting 423 progeny, and testing those with recombination events in the *Lith1* region for gallstone formation. *Lith1* was shown to be nonrecombinant with *D2Mit56* (Lammert et al., 1999a), suggesting *Abcb11* as a strong candidate gene. Its candidacy was further strengthened when C57L and the *Lith1* congenic were shown to have higher expression of Abcb11 protein and mRNA than AKR. Physiological studies of the AKR.L-*Lith1*^{s} congenic strain showed that the *Lith1* gene resulted in disproportionately high cholesterol secretion rates in the setting of elevated bile salt and phospholipid secretion rates, thus resembling the phenotype of obese human gallstone patients (Wang et al., 1999b). These data provide supporting evidence for the identity of *Abcb11* and *Lith1*. Since this is a gain of function, changes in the amino acid sequence of the protein are not expected; however, some alterations should be found in the regulatory sequences controlling gene expression. It is somewhat surprising that increased transport of bile acids should lead to a relative and absolute increase in cholesterol secretion (Carey and Duane, 1994). This may be related to increased cholesterol absorption from the intestine and high hepatic HMG-CoA reductase activity in susceptible strains. This effect may be most pronounced for the mixed bile salt pattern of intermediate hydrophobicity observed in mice on the lithogenic diet (Wang et al., 1997, 1999a,b) and in humans (Carey and Duane, 1994).

In humans, a lack of *ABCB11* is responsible for progressive familial intrahepatic cholestasis type 2 (PFIC2) (Strautnieks et al., 1998). In this disease, a near absence of bile salts leads to chronic cholestasis and liver cirrhosis before adulthood. These patients have subnormal biliary cholesterol levels; however, the bile is supersaturated, apparently from bile salt deficiency, and many patients develop gallstones (Bahar and Stolz, 1999).

Abcc2 (also known as *Cmoat* or *Mrp2*) is another member of the family of ABC transporters located on the canalicular membrane. It promotes biliary secretion of dianionic xeno- and endobiotics, including glutathione conjugates, bilirubin diglucuronide, and common bile salts conjugated with sulfate or glucuronide (Müller et al., 1996). ABCC2 is responsible to a large extent for the generation of bile salt-independent bile flow, apparently through glutathione secretion (Trauner et al., 1998). Oligonucleotide primers designed to the 3′-untranslated end of the molecule were used to map the gene to chromosome 19 (Lammert et al., 1998a), which is the *Lith2* region. To determine whether *Lith2* and *Abcc2* co-localize to a narrow region, a set of overlapping congenics on chromosome 19 was constructed. These congenic strains narrowed the gallstone-susceptibility locus to a 0.4 cM region containing *Abcc2*, suggesting that it is the candidate gene (Bouchard et al., 2000). The candidacy of *Abcc2* was further strengthened when a DNA change resulting in an amino acid difference was found in a putative binding site (Bouchard et al., 2000).

Abcb4 (alternate names for this gene are *Mdr2* (multiple drug resistance) in mice and *MDR3* in humans) maps to the top of chromosome 5 (Raymond et al., 1990; White et al., 1994). The exact function of this gene was unknown until ABCB4-deficient mice showed that the primary defect was a lack of phosphatidylcholine in bile; thus, the protein is a phosphatidylcholine transmembrane transporter, or "flippase" (Smit et al., 1993). Although the knockout mice had low absolute biliary cholesterol levels, bile was still supersaturated and cholesterol gallstones formed (Lammert et al., 1998b). These stones were composed mostly of anhydrous cholesterol crystals. *ABCB4* is mutated in some patients with progressive familiar cholestasis type 3 (de Vree et al., 1998).

Abca7, which maps to a gallstone QTL, is expressed in thymus, spleen, and bone marrow and induced when monocytes differentiate into macrophages (Kaminski et al., 2000a,b; Broccardo et al., 2001).

The gene named *FIC1* has been identified to be mutated in another form of familial progressive intrahepatic cholestasis (Byler's syndrome, PFIC1) (Bull et al., 1998; de Vree et al., 1998). *FIC1* maps to human chromosome 18. It is homologous to proteins that translocate aminophospholipids in plasma membranes, maintaining an asymmetrical lipid topology. Whether FIC1 has a role in gallstone formation is not known.

A second group of membrane transporters is located on the other side of the hepatocyte, the basolateral membrane; these transport biliary lipids or their precursors from blood into hepatocytes. These genes belong primarily to the family of solute carriers (*Slc*) and include *Slc22a1*, the organic cation tranporter (previously *Oct1*); *Slc21a1*, the organic anion transport protein 1 (previously *Oatp1*); *Slc10a1*, the sodium-dependant taurocholate cotransporting polypeptide (previously *Ntcp*); and *Slc10a2*, the ileal bile acid transporter (previously *Ibat*).

Slc22a1 transports a variety of cations, including choline (Koepsell, 1998; Green et al., 1998), which is essential for hepatic phosphatidylcholine synthesis. Its map position at the top of chromosome 17 places it within one of the gallstone QTL.

Slc21a1 is a member of the family of carriers that transport organic anions and prostaglandins into the liver (*Slc21*) and mediate hepatic uptake of unconjugated bile salts. It maps to the region of a gallstone QTL on chromosome X. *Slc10a1* is responsible for the sodium-dependant uptake of conjugated bile salts from the portal circulation (Hagenbuch and Meier, 1994). It maps to mouse chromosome 12. In the same gene family is *Slc10a2*, which is expressed in the ileum. Point mutations in this gene can produce primary bile salt malabsorption, diarrhea, failure to thrive, and reduced plasma levels of cholesterol and fat-soluble vitamins (Oelkers et al., 1997). The subsequent elevation of bilirubin in bile may increase the risk for black pigment gallstones (Brink et al., 1996, 1999). *Slc10a2* is also expressed in cholangiocytes and proximal renal tubular cells (Dawson, 1999) and may have a function in the cholehepatic shunting of conjugated bile salts. It does not appear to be an important candidate gene for cholesterol gallstone formation, although it may be a genetic factor predisposing to black pigment stones (see above, "Black" Pigment Gallstones). In the mouse, *Slc10a2* maps to chromosome 8 (Lammert et al., 1998b).

Hepatic and Intestinal Intracellular Lipid Carriers

Several intracellular proteins carry lipids in the cytosol of hepatocytes. These are coded for by *Scp2*, the sterol carrier protein 2; *Npc1*, Niemann-Pick type C1, which is involved in intracellular trafficking of LDL-derived cholesterol and is actually a membrane-bound protein; *Cav* and *Cav2*, which are caveolin 1 and caveolin 2; *Pctp*, the phosphatidylcholine transfer protein; *Osbp*, the oxysterol binding protein; and *Fabp1*, fatty acid binding protein 1. In the liver, bile salts are transported by the protein encoded by *Akr1c3*, a member of the aldo-ketoreductase supergene family. The intracellular bile salt transporter in the intestine is *Fabp6*, previously known as ILLBP (ileal lipid binding protein). The possible role of each of these genes in gallstone formation will be discussed.

SCP2 is a 13 kDa cytosolic protein that transports biliary cholesterol and phospholipids in liver (Puglielli et al., 1996; Leonard and Cohen, 1998). The source of the transported cholesterol appears to be HDL cholesterol (Kozarsky et al., 1997). Liver biopsies of gallstone patients showed elevated SCP2 concentrations (Ito et al., 1996), so expression of this protein was examined in gallstone-susceptible and -resistant mice. C57L, but not AKR, mice upregulated SCP2 about twofold when fed a lithogenic diet (Fuchs et al., 1998). The upregulation occurred early, prior to the appearance of cholesterol crystals in bile. This observation is consistent with the increased biliary cholesterol secretion following adenovirus-mediated overexpression of SCP2 in mouse liver (Zanlungo et al., 2000). *Scp2* maps to the gallstone QTL on chromosome 4, so it is an attractive candidate gene. However, *Scp2* knockout in gallstone-susceptible mice did not change biliary lipid secretion rates (Seedorf et al., 1998), and mice developed gallstones similar to the wild-type strain when fed the lithogenic diet (Fuchs et al., 1999a), suggesting that alternative pathways exist for transporting cholesterol in the liver.

NPC1 facilitates the intracellular trafficking of LDL-derived cholesterol by controlling the transfer of internalized LDL cholesterol out of endosomes and lysosomes (Loftus et al., 1997; Kobayashi et al., 1999). The recessive Niemann-Pick type C1 disease in humans results from mutations in this gene and is characterized by accumulation of unesterified cholesterol, nervous system degeneration, and hepatosplenomegaly (Carstea et al., 1997). In *Npc1* knockout mice, biliary cholesterol secretion is not increased when mice are fed a high-cholesterol diet, suggesting that NPC1 plays a regulatory role in delivering cholesterol to the canalicular membrane (Zanlungo et al., 2000). *Npc1* maps to mouse chromosome 18.

Caveolins are cholesterol binding proteins specific to the plasma membrane microdomains known as caveolae. They interact with several important signaling proteins (Sternberg and Schmid, 1999). Elevation of cellular cholesterol levels, as in Niemann-Pick disease, causes changes in the expression of caveolins (Murata et al., 1995; Engelman et al., 1998). In mice, caveolin 1 is overexpressed during cholesterol gallstone formation (Fuchs et al., 1999b) but caveolin 2 is upregulated in diosgenin-induced biliary cholesterol hypersecretion (Miquel et al., 1998). The caveolins do not map to a gallstone QTL.

PCTP is a very specific transporter of the molecular species of phosphatidylcholine typical of bile (Cohen, 1996; Cohen et al., 1999). However, mice do not express PCTP until 12 weeks of age and a *Pctp* knockout does not affect biliary phosphatidylcholine secretion (van Helvoort et al., 1999). *Pctp* maps to chromosome 11 and co-localizes with gallstone QTL from two different crosses. Current thinking is that OSBP acts as a cholesterol regulator or sensor in the Golgi apparatus. It binds oxysterols; may mediate sterol metabolism via HMGCR (HMG CoA reductase), the LDL receptor, and phospholipid synthesis; and induces bile salt synthesis (Lehto et al., 2001). FABP1 has been implicated in intracellular cholesterol trafficking, but it does not map to a gallstone QTL.

Intracellular movement of bile salts in the liver is mediated by bile salt binding proteins (Bahar and Stolz, 1999). One of these is 3α-hydroxysteroid dehydrogenase, AKR1C3, a membrane-bound protein which is required for bile salt synthesis (Khanna et al., 1995). Its exact map position is not known, but it is on chromosome 2.

FABP6 is a member of a family of fatty acid and bile acid binding proteins (reviewed in Banaszak et al., 1994). The 128-residue protein is expressed in the absorptive cells of the ileum and is the cytosolic receptor for bile acids that have undergone sodium-dependent active transport into the ileoctye by SLC10A2 (Wong et al., 1994). *Fabp6* maps to the edge of a gallstone QTL on chromosome 11, but it is not a very likely candidate gene. Mutations in *Fabp6* could interfere with intestinal bile salt absorption and perhaps contribute to pigment gallstone formation along with *Slc10a2*.

Lipid- or Bile Salt-Regulatory Transcription Factors

New insights have been provided into nuclear receptors that regulate cholesterol homeostasis and may play a role in cholesterol gallstone pathogenesis. Knowledge of key regulatory transcription factors is expanding rapidly, and the nomenclature is also in a state of flux. Nuclear receptors are ligand-activated transcription factors that specifically bind to their DNA response elements as dimers, often as heterodimers. Thus, they have two specificities: the ligands to which they bind and the DNA response elements. Three major groups will be discussed: nuclear receptors (*Nr*), peroxisome proliferator–activated receptors (*Ppar*), and sterol-regulatory element binding transcription factors (*Srebf*).

Dietary oxysterols are ligands of the liver X receptor α (LXRα) (Janowski et al., 1996; Peet et al., 1998), now renamed nuclear receptor NR1H3. Binding of oxysterols to OSBP might influence this signal-transduction pathway. Retinoid X receptor (NR2B1, RXR) is a common heterodimer partner of several nuclear receptors, including LXRα (Repa and Mangelsdorf, 1999). When bound to its ligand, the heterodimer NR1H3/NR2B1 induces the synthesis of CYP7A1. Both LXRα and RXR map to mouse chromosome 2. Bile acids, in particular chenodeoxycholic acid, and their conjugates are the physiological ligands for another nuclear receptor, the farnesoid X receptor (FXR) (Makishima et al., 1999; Parks et al., 1999; Wang H et al., 1999). FXR has been renamed *Nr1h4*. When bound to bile acids, the heterodimer NR1H4/NR2B1 represses transcription of CYP7A1 and activates the gene *Fabp6*. Bile acid synthesis is inhibited by an indirect mechanism: if bile acid levels increase, activated FXR induces transcription of the small heterodimer partner 1 (SHP-1), now renamed NROB2. Elevated NROB2 protein levels lead to transcriptional repression of CYP7A1 (Lu et al., 2000; Goodwin et al., 2000). FXR maps to mouse chromosome 10 within the region of a recently detected QTL. Another bile acid–activated nuclear receptor is the pregnane X receptor (PXR, NR1I2). This receptor seems to play an important role in protecting the liver from toxic bile acids by inducing *Cyp3a* expression and may have use in the treatment of cholestatic liver disease (Staudinger et al., 2001).

Another group of related nuclear receptors that are key regulators of lipid and carbohydrate metabolism are the peroxisome proliferator–activated receptors α, δ, and γ (*Ppara, Ppard, Pparg*). These have been renamed *Nr1c1, Nr1c2,* and *Nr1c3*, respectively. The hypolipidemic effects of the fibrate drugs are due to activation of PPARα and the antidiabetic effects of the glitazone drugs are due to activation of PPARγ. These three receptors have different tissue specificity and respond to different activators (Kliewer et al., 1994). PPARα is the main type in liver, PPARγ is the main type in adipose tissue, and PPARδ is expressed in many tissues (Kliewer et al., 1994). Peroxisomes catalyze β-oxidation of fatty acids as well as synthesis of cholesterol and specific steps in the oxidation of cholesterol to bile salts (Repa and Mangelsdorf, 1999).

The major role of PPARα is catabolism of fatty acids. It is activated by fatty acids and in turn activates transcription of the genes for fatty acid oxidation after formation of the heterodimer with RXR (i.e., NR1C1/NR2B1 heterodimer). The major role of PPARγ is adipogenesis, the making of fat cells, and lipid uptake and efflux from cells (Lowell, 1999). It also affects insulin resistance and is involved in reverse cholesterol transport, particularly from macrophages in partnership with LXRα (Chawla et al., 2001b). This effect is coupled to induction of ABCA1. Transplantation of *Nr1c3* knockout bone marrow into *Ldlr* knockout mice results in a significant increase in atherosclerosis, indicating that PPARγ is protective in vivo (Chawla et al., 2001b). No effect on gallstone formation was mentioned. PPARγ is highly expressed in macrophages and is an important regulator of the scavenger receptor CD36, which is genetically linked to oxidized lipid accumulation in macrophages (Chawla et al., 2001a). Finally, PPARδ is less well understood. PPARδ, which is distributed in many tissues, is involved in the upregulation of reverse cholesterol transport partly by increasing the expression of the reverse cholesterol transporter ABCA1 (Oliver et al., 2001). An agonist of PPARδ given to aging diabetic monkeys caused a rise in HDL cholesterol and a decrease in small, dense LDL, triglycerides, and insulin (Oliver et al., 2001).

Many proteins involved in cholesterol homeostasis are regulated by membrane-bound and ligand-activated transcription factors. Sterol regulatory element binding proteins (encoded by sterol regulatory element binding factor genes *SREBF1a, -1c* and *-2*), which have the characteristics of basic helix-loop-helix-leucine zipper transcription factors, upregulate transcription of *Hmgcr* and *Ldlr* (Brown and Goldstein, 1997). They are released from larger membrane-bound precursors by sterol-regulated proteolysis in the presence of **S**REBP **c**leavage **a**ctivation **p**rotein (SCAP), and metabolites of cholesterol, particularly oxysterols, block the proteolytic cleavage step and decrease SREBP production (Brown and Goldstein, 1997). SREBP1A and -1C are produced from a single gene. *Srebf1* maps to the gallstone QTL on mouse chromosome 8, and we have mapped *Scap* within the region of the gallstone QTL on chromosome 9. Furthermore, *Srebf2* maps within the region of the interacting QTL on chromosome 15 in the same cross (Wittenburg et al., unpublished data). Therefore, these transcription factors are attractive candidate genes for gallstone formation.

Cholecystokinin and Its Receptor

Stasis of bile in the gallbladder favors cholesterol crystallization and stone formation; as mentioned earlier, human studies implicate fasting with an increased risk of stones. Postprandial release of the hormone cholecystokinin causes the gallbladder to contract, so both this hormone and its receptor, cholecystokinin A (CCKAR), affect gallbladder motility and are attractive candidate genes. Polymorphisms of the *CCKAR* gene are associated with gallstones in humans (Schneider et al., 1997), and *Cckar* is a candidate gene for the QTL on mouse chromosome 5.

Mucins

Gallstone formation is also facilitated by mucin gel in the gallbladder, which promotes nucleation and holds the cholesterol crystals in place, thereby accelerating their growth into stones. Mucins are sparingly soluble, high-molecular weight glycoproteins. They are also the principal component of biliary sludge, a viscous gel of mucins, calcium bilirubinate granules, and cholesterol crystals. The formation of a thick mucin gel before stone formation in mice suggests that expression of *Muc* genes and mucin secretion by the gallbladder may be genetically determined. Human biliary epithelial cells strongly express *MUC3, MUC5b,* and *MUC6* and weakly express *MUC1, MUC2,* and *MUC5ab*. Also, GLYCAM1 is strongly expressed in mouse gallbladder. Of the three mucin QTL we have found, *Muc3* and *Glycam1* are candidate genes for two.

Contribution of the Mouse Model to Pathophysiology of Disease

Cholic acid, a primary bile acid, must be added to the diet for both gallstone formation and atherosclerosis in mice. It is clearly not required in humans since cholic acid conjugates are the major bile salts in healthy human bile (Carey and Duane, 1994). In fact, when a hydrophilic bile acid such as ursodeoxycholic acid is fed to humans, cholesterol is poorly absorbed, bile becomes unsaturated, gallstones dissolve, and LDL levels fall (Carey and Duane, 1994). This difference stems principally from a biochemical difference between mouse and human bile salts that affects cholesterol absorption from the small intestine. A major primary, i.e., synthesized intrahepatically from cholesterol, bile salt in mice is tauro-β-muricholate, a poor cholesterol solubilizer (Wang et al., 1997). In humans, with principally cholate and chenodeoxycholate conjugates (glycine as well as taurine amidates), cholesterol is more effectively solubilized, an essential step in cholesterol absorption from the gut. When mice are fed cholic acid, it is well absorbed by passive diffusion from all parts of the small intestine, efficiently extracted by the liver, conjugated intrahepatically, and converted to taurocholate, replacing a poor cholesterol solubilizer with an effective one and thus mimicking intestinal cholesterol solubilization and absorption in humans (Wang et al., 1997). Taurocholate aids cholesterol gallstone formation via two other mechanisms. In the first, taurocholate suppresses *de novo* bile salt synthesis, most likely by cholate's bacterial catabolic product deoxycholic acid, thereby making more intrahepatic cholesterol available for secretion into bile (Wang et al., 1999a). In the second, taurocholate allows a solid crystallization phase transition to occur in the gallbladder, whereas a mixture of equimolar taurocholate and tauro-β-muricholate, as occurs in the native bile salt pool of mice, would allow only a liquid crystalline phase transition to take place (Wang and Carey, 1996b).

The hepatic activities of the principal enzymes of cholesterol metabolism (HMGCR, CYP7A1, CYP27, ACAT) were measured in gallstone-susceptible C57L and SWR and -resistant AKR and SJL mice after consumption of chow or a lithogenic diet (Khanuja et al., 1995; Lammert et al., 1999c). Both susceptible and resistant strains exhibited large increases in ACAT activity and decreases in CYP7A1 and CYP27. CYP7A1 was repressed to a greater degree on the lithogenic diet in susceptible strains than in resistant strains. This is consistent with more catabolism of taurocholate to deoxycholate from gallbladder dysmotility, as evidenced by biliary bile salt molecular species analysis (Wang et al., 1997). The lithogenic diet downregulated HMGCR activity in the resistant strains but failed to do so in the susceptible strains (Wang et al., 1999b; Lammert et al., 1999c). This high synthetic rate of *de novo* cholesterol synthesis in the face of excess dietary cholesterol intake in C57L mice could be an important factor contributing to cholesterol hypersecretion. This experiment corroborated the results of previous human studies indicating an important role for HMGCR in gallstone formation, but this is not consistent across all human studies (Kern, 1994). Increased HMGCR activity has also been found in a gallstone-susceptible strain of hamster compared to a gallstone-resistant strain (Ferezou et al., 2000).

A powerful approach to determine the physiological effects of QTL such as *Lith1* and *Lith2* is to construct congenic strains of the loci. Congenic strains are mice that have been bred to have the same genome as a particular inbred strain except for a selected differential chromosomal segment, such as the QTL region containing one *Lith* gene (Silver, 1995). Two separate congenic strains for *Lith1* and *Lith2* were constructed; for each of the two loci, the C57L (susceptible) alleles of the locus were moved into strain AKR. To determine the physiological mechanisms affected by each locus, the process of gallstone formation in the congenics was compared to that in the parental strains by evaluating several phenotypes, including gallstone production, bile flow, and bile biochemistry. Both congenics had a prevalence of gallstones comparable to the susceptible C57L parent. The AK.L-*Lith1*^{s} congenic had biliary lipid hypersecretion similar to C57L but the AK.L-*Lith2*^{s} congenic did not. Furthermore, the increased bile flow typical of the C57L parent was found only in the AK.L-*Lith2*^{s} congenic but not in the AK.L-*Lith1*^{s} congenic. Thus, phenotyping of the congenic strains demonstrated that *Lith1* affects biliary lipid secretion and *Lith2* affects bile flow.

In a series of four related studies, additional physiological aspects of gallstone disease were identified by comparing the phenotypes of mice with gallstone-susceptible *Lith* alleles to those of mice with gallstone-resistant *Lith* alleles (Wang et al., 1997, 1999b; Lammert et al., 1999c; van Erpecum et al., 2001). Lammert et al. (1999c) conducted a further investigation into the role of regulatory enzymes by comparing the activities of HMGCR, CYP27, CYP7A1, and ACAT between the susceptible strains C57L, SWR, and AKXL-29 and the resistant strain AKR. Confirming the results of the previous study (Khanuja et al., 1995), HMGCR activity was downregulated in response to the lithogenic diet in the resistant AKR strain but failed to downregulate in all susceptible strains, resulting in continued cholesterol synthesis. Upon challenge with the lithogenic diet, activities of CYP27 and CYP7A1 were downregulated in all strains and lower in susceptible mice under all dietary conditions, resulting in a further increase in cholesterol saturation in susceptible mice. The study also found sharply increased levels of secondary bile salts in susceptible mice, probably because of a decrease in gallbladder motility and induced enterohepatic cycling. Since the mouse is a good hydroxylator of secondary bile salts (Wang et al., 1999a,b), levels in the bile represent only the "tip of the iceberg" of what is returned to the liver. The activity of ACAT, which converts cholesterol to cholesteryl ester, was increased in all strains on the lithogenic diet but higher in susceptible mice at intermediate and final time points compared to resistant mice. This was probably a consequence of the increased cholesterol availability in susceptible mice as cholesterol upregulates ACAT activity. Because of the lack of coordination in lipid-regulatory enzyme activity in susceptible mice, it was hypothesized that the principal effect of *Lith* genes is to cause hypersecretion of biliary cholesterol and that the various observed alterations of cholesterol metabolism are secondary feedback events on the lipid-regulatory enzymes. Inbred strains with susceptible *Lith* alleles exhibited not only alterations of hepatic lipid-regulatory enzymes but also decreased plasma HDL cholesterol and increased expression of the SRB1 receptor, the cytosolic SCP2, and CAV. These changes are indicative of high rates of cholesterol uptake and increased cytosolic trafficking (Fuchs et al., 1998, 2001). FABP1 was markedly increased in both susceptible and resistant strains. These data suggest a role of reverse cholesterol transport in gallstone susceptibility (Fuchs et al., 2001).

The pathophysiology of gallstone formation was further investigated in studies focusing on the gallbladder (Wang et al., 1997) and the hepatic secretion of biliary lipids (Wang et al., 1999a,b). The first study demonstrated the importance of cholesterol supersaturation and increased mucin secretion in gallstone formation (Wang et al., 1997). Gallstone-resistant AKR, susceptible C57L, and (C57L × AKR)F_1 mice of both genders were fed a lithogenic diet and examined for numerous factors involved in gallstone formation. Because the phenotype of the F_1 progeny mimicked that of the C57L parent, this study confirmed the previous finding that gallstone susceptibility is a dominant trait in the outcross (Khanuja et al., 1995). After mice consumed a lithogenic diet for 4 weeks, the cholesterol saturation index (CSI) of bile was under 100% in AKR mice and over 100% in C57L mice. After 21 days on the lithogenic diet, AKR mice formed a thin lining of mucin in the gallbladder, and this lining contained liquid crystals of cholesterol and phospholipid but no solid crystals of cholesterol monohydrate. In contrast, C57L mice formed a thick layer of mucin after 3 days on the lithogenic diet. After 14 days on the lithogenic diet, liquid crystals and cholesterol monohydrate crystals were observed in this mucin layer. Cholesterol crystals aggregated into small stones in the gallbladders of C57L mice by 28 days on the lithogenic diet. The gallbladders and gallstones were larger in C57L and F_1 mice than in AKR mice throughout the lithogenic feeding, and the number of gallstones after 56 days of lithogenic feeding was also greater in C57L and F_1 mice. This study provided information on other aspects of pathophysiology of cholelithiasis. A small percentage of AKR mice abruptly formed gallstones after 46 days on the lithogenic diet, suggesting that gallstone formation may be affected by an environmental factor such as severe hepatic steatosis. Three separate pathways of cholesterol monohydrate crystallization were identified in the gallbladder bile of C57, AKR, and F_1 mice: the well-known liquid crystal to solid cholesterol monohydrate crystallization pathway, the direct cholesterol monohydrate crystallization pathway, and an anhydrous cholesterol crystal to cholesterol monohydrate crystallization pathway. These pathways are identical to those found in human bile (Wang and Carey, 1996a,b).

The results of the study suggested several possible mechanisms for gallstone formation in susceptible mice. First, the more rapid supersaturation of bile in C57L and F_1 mice is likely to play a significant role. Second, the formation of a thick mucin layer prior to crystal formation suggests that the expression of *MUC* genes and mucin secretion in the gallbladder may be enhanced by components of supersaturated bile and/or the regulation of *Lith* genes. Third, the increase in hydrophobic bile salts of susceptible mice may enhance gallstone formation as hydrophobic bile salts induce cholesterol hypersecretion and rapid cholesterol crystal precipitation. Fourth, the somewhat lower total lipid concentration in the bile of susceptible mice may decrease the cholesterol-solubilizing capacity, thereby accelerating the formation of supersaturated bile. Finally, the larger gallbladders may reflect decreased gallbladder motility and greater mucin volumes of susceptible mice, and these factors may enhance gallstone formation by acting as a heterogeneous nucleating matrix.

Cholesterol saturation (Wang et al., 1997) and cholesterol and bile salt synthetic enzyme activities (Lammert et al., 1999c) differed between gallstone-susceptible and gallstone-resistant mouse strains. These differences appeared to be secondary to cholesterol hypersecretion. Therefore, a study was undertaken to examine the secretory rates of biliary lipids in susceptible and resistant strains (Wang et al., 1999a,b). The hepatic secretion of cholesterol, phospholipid, and bile salts was compared between C57L, AKR, and (AKR × C57L)F_1 mice fed a lithogenic diet. The CSI and relative lipid compositions of hepatic bile were also measured. This study produced several important findings indicating that the physiological basis of gallstone susceptibility is the development of lithogenic bile in the liver of susceptible mice. First, in susceptible mice, the development of cholesterol gallstones was preceded by the production of lithogenic hepatic bile; the lithogenic diet increased the CSI of hepatic bile in susceptible mice only. In addition, the lithogenic diet resulted in a change in the bile salt composition of hepatic bile in susceptible mice that paralleled the previously observed bile salt changes in gallstone bile (Wang et al., 1997), indicating that the liver, and not the gallbladder, is the primary cause of the changes in bile salt composition. Second, the lithogenic diet increased biliary cholesterol and phospholipid secretion only in susceptible mice and did not change bile salt secretion in any strains. Third, in response to the lithogenic diet, the cholesterol:phospholipid ratio of secreted lipids was increased only in susceptible mice and increased significantly over the entire time that mice were on the lithogenic diet, thereby priming the bile for the phase separation of cholesterol in the gallbladders of susceptible mice. Therefore, in the inbred mice, as in humans, the liver, and not the gallbladder, is the principal site for the production of abnormal bile associated with cholesterol gallstone formation.

The results of this study also indicated that the candidate gene for *Lith1* is a bile salt transporter on the canalicular membrane, ABCB11. Although its main function is bile salt secretion, ABCB11 upregulates phospholipid secretion by an indirect effect on ABCB4 gene expression. We speculate that cholesterol secretion is also increased as a secondary effect because the increased bile salts in the intestine cause increased cholesterol absorption, thereby increasing the amount of hepatic cholesterol available for secretion. Because the cholesterol:phospholipid ratio of hepatic bile indicates the cholesterol:phospholipid ratios of vesicles (Carey, 1993a,b) whose secretory activity is induced from the canalicular level (Crawford et al., 1995), the increased cholesterol:phospholipid ratios observed in susceptible mice suggest enhanced cholesterol secretion from the canalicular membrane. These results are similar to the elevated cholesterol:phospholipid ratios observed in human gallstone patients (Hofmann et al., 1982). Also, the increase in the cholesterol:phospholipid ratio in susceptible mice while consuming the lithogenic diet was correlated with an elevated CSI in the bile. Unexplored is the functionality of the SLC10A2 (ASBT) protein on the large cholangiocyte, which could induce cholehepatic shunting of canaliculus-secreted bile salts. Indeed, a bile salt hypersecretory state induced by knockout of the ferrochelatase gene in the mouse upregulated function and protein expression of SLC10A2 on the large cholangiocyte (Meerman et al., 1999), and it will be interesting to see whether this is also the case in cholesterol gallstone disease.

At various times during the past decade, it has been proposed that proteins in the bile promote crystallization of cholesterol. In vitro assays show that proteins isolated from human bile, such as immunoglobulins, α_1-acid glycoprotein, aminopeptidase-N, haptoglobin, and mucin, promote crystallization. The inbred mouse provides an excellent model to study the role of these proteins in gallstone formation. Using the susceptible C57L and resistant AKR inbred strains, the concentration of these pronucleating proteins as well as the biliary lipids and bile salt compositions in the early stages of gallstone formation were studied (van Erpecum et al., 2001). The in vitro crystallization-promoting immunoglobulins and aminopeptidase-N were not major factors in gallstone pathogenesis.

CLINICAL APPLICATION OF GENETICS INFORMATION

It is likely that many human populations are genetically predisposed to gallstones. It is possible that other individuals may have susceptibility alleles on the basis of genes for obesity and non-insulin-dependent diabetes mellitus. The consensus environmental factor is a diet comprising highly refined carbohydrates, too much cholesterol, too many calories, and too little dietary fiber. Although only a few genes affecting gallstone formation have been identified so far, much is known about the pathophysiology of their development. There are only a limited number of ways that hypersecretion of biliary cholesterol or hyposecretion of bile salt could occur. Based on our knowledge of the physical chemistry and pathophysiology of cholelithiasis today, a variety of nongenetic approaches (listed in Table 16–4) may be possible interventions to prevent gallstones. Clearly, stone prevention would be crucial for individuals at high risk of morbidity or mortality, not only from surgery, where the risks are slight but real, but from gallstone complications throughout an increasingly prolonged life span.

Table 16–4. Suggested Mechanisms and Targets for Gallstone Prevention

Mechanisms	Target
Keep gallbladder bile dilute	Na^+/N^+ exchanger (NHE-3)
Increase hydrophilicity of bile salts	Colonic bacteria with 7-epimerization: CDCA → UDCA
Antinucleating/antigrowth agents	*MUC* genes, COX2 immunoglobins
Increase biliary phospholipids	MDR-3 activity
Increase gallbladder emptying	CCKA receptor

CDCA, chenodeoxycholic acid; UDCA, ursodeoxycholic acid; COX2, cyclo-oxygenase 2; MUC, mucin; MDR, multidrug resistance; CCKA, cholecystokinin A.

Cholesterol Gallstone Prevention: Key Concepts

Three biophysical alterations in gallbladder bile are potential targets: *(1)* stabilization of cholesterol-supersaturated bile without altering cholesterol solubility, *(2)* shortening gallbladder residence time to inhibit or prolong nucleation time and prevent cholesterol injury to the mucosa and muscle, and *(3)* abolishing nucleation and crystallization kinetics by suppressing heterogeneous nucleation. Decreasing the rate of cholesterol secretion into bile at the hepatic level is not an attractive target since doing so will influence plasma LDL cholesterol levels deleteriously, as evidenced by experience with chenodeoxycholic acid therapy in the National Cooperative Gallstone Study (Grundy et al., 1984). Therefore, the main targets will be the factors influencing nucleation of cholesterol crystallization.

Mechanisms and Targets

A desirable aim would be to place the relative lipid composition of bile in region E of the bile phase diagram (Wang and Carey, 1996a,b), where liquid crystalline phase separation can occur but solid cholesterol crystallization is prevented. This is achievable by keeping gallbladder bile as dilute as hepatic bile (≈3g/dl); increasing the hydrophilicity of the bile salt pool with a novel bile acid, e.g, ursodeoxycholic or muricholic acids; and increasing the secretion rate of biliary phospholipid by upregulation of ABCB4 (MDR3). Approaches to modifiable targets might be *(1)* inhibition of the Na^+/H^+ exchanger (NHE-3) on the apical membranes of gallbladder absorptive cells to prevent absorption of biliary fluid; *(2)* quantitative conversion of chenodeoxycholic acid to urodeoxycholic acid by bioengineering a subpopulation of the colonic microflora with a 7-hydroxy epimerase to increase the bile salt pool hydrophilicity; *(3)* upregulation of ABCB4 (MDR3), the phosphatidylcholine "flippase" on the canalicular membrane, thereby increasing phospholipid secretion into bile, possibly achievable with hyodeoxycholate conjugates (common porcine bile salts) (Loria et al., 1997); *(4)* suppression of *MUC* genes to inhibit mucin secretion and thereby heterogeneous nucleation and crystal growth; and *(5)* promotion of gallbladder emptying with cholecystokinin receptor agonists.

Potential Strategies

Following the numerical order of the preceding section, *(1)* it may be possible to deliver to the gallbladder via the enterohepatic circulation an NHE-3 antagonist (Strichartz et al., 1989b). *(2)* Colonic microbes could be genetically bioengineered to quantitatively convert chenodeoxycholic acid into ursodeoxycholic acid. There appears to be a natural experiment in this regard. The bile of patients with Crohn's disease contains much higher levels of ursodeoxycholate conjugate than occurs in healthy people (Lapidus and Einarsson, 1991, 1998). It has been demonstrated that cecectomized rabbits quantitatively convert dietary chenodeoxycholic acid into ursodeoxycholate and not lithocholate (Yahiro et al., 1980). The increased biotransformation of chenodeoxycholic acid to ursodeoxycholic acid via 7-ketolithocholic acid (Miwa et al., 1986) in Crohn's patients may be related to altered gut flora induced by cecal disease. *(3)* Although in animal models "fibrates" induce *Abcb4* (*Mdr2*) gene expression and hypersecretion of biliary phospholipid (Chianale et al., 1996), they produce lithogenic bile in humans by increasing cholesterol secretion. However, the porcine bile salt hyodeoxycholate, which is available commercially as the taurine conjugate, is a potent inducer of biliary phospholipid hypersecretion in humans and other species and thereby desaturates bile (Loria et al., 1997). Perhaps this occurs by appreciable upregulation of *ABCB4* (*MDR3*), and if so, it would be interesting to discover whether other hydrophilic 6α-hydroxylated bile salts have similar action. *(4)* A potent cyclo-oxygenase inhibitor may prevent mucin hypersecretion by the gallbladder mucosa. It is not known presently how one might influence *MUC* gene expression selectively, but if gallbladder bile is kept dilute, this may prevent cholesterol-induced upregulation of *MUC* genes. *(5)* Gallbladder emptying could be accelerated with cholescytokinin agonists (Carey and Duane, 1994). This will depend on the development of safe, specific cholecystokinin agonists for limited use during periods of high gallstone risk, such as pregnancy and rapid weight reduction. However, once the repertoire of human *LITH* genes and their functions in gallstone pathogenesis become known and once the secondary gene responses involved are ascertained, multiple new targets for the prevention of gallstones should become feasible (Carey, 1998).

ACKNOWLEDGMENTS

We are most grateful to our colleagues and co-workers in Boston and Bar Harbor and our collaborators elsewhere, for their many contributions and support. We are particularly indebted to Drs. Kenneth W. Heaton (Bristol), Adolfo F. Attili (Rome), Frank Lammert (Aachen), Malcolm Lyons (Bar Harbor), and Henning Wittenburg (Boston) for their detailed, helpful, and constructive reviews of the manuscript. Supported in part by research grants DK 51568 (to B. P.), DK 36588, DK 52911, and DK 34854 (to M. C. C.) from the National Institutes of Health (U.S. Public Health Service).

REFERENCES

Acalovschi M, Dumitrascu D, Caluser I, Ban A: Comparative prevalence of gallstone disease at 100-year interval in a large Romanian town, a necropsy study. Dig Dis Sci 1987; 32:354–357.

Acalovschi M, Pascu M, Iobagiu S, Petrescu M, Olinici CD, Ban A, Dumitrascu D:

Increasing gallstone prevalence and cholecystectomy rate in a large Romanian town. A necropsy study. Dig Dis Sci 1995; 40:2582–2586.

Adedeji A, Akande B, Olumide F: The changing pattern of cholelithiasis in Lagos. Scand J Gastroenterol 1986; 21(Suppl 124):63–66.

Admirand WH, Small DM: The physicochemical basis of cholesterol gallstone formation in man. J Clin Invest 1968; 47:1043–1052.

Ahlberg J, Angelin B, Einarsson K, Hellstrom K, Leijd B: Biliary lipid composition in normo- and hyperlipoproteinemia. Gastroenterology 1980; 79:90–94.

Alexander M, Portman OW: Different susceptibilities to the formation of cholesterol gallstones in mice. Hepatology 1987; 7:257–265.

Amaral JF, Thompson WR: Gallbladder disease in the morbidly obese. Am J Surg 1985; 149:551–557.

Amigo L, Quinones V, Mardones P, Zanlungo S, Miquel JF, Nervi F, Rigotti A: Impaired biliary cholesterol secretion and decreased gallstone formation in apolipoprotein E-deficient mice fed a high-cholesterol diet. Gastroenterology 2000; 118:772–779.

Andrassy RJ, Treadwell TA, Ratner IA, Buckley CJ: Gallbladder disease in children and adolescents. Am J Surg 1976; 132:19–21.

Angelico M, De Santis A, Capocaccia L: Biliary sludge: a critical update. J Clin Gastroenterol 1990; 6:656–662.

Apstein MD: The inhibition of biliary phospholipid and cholesterol secretion by bilirubin in normal and Gunn rats. Gastroenterology 1984; 87:634–638.

Apstein MD: Biliary tract stone and associated diseases. In: Stein JM (ed). Internal Medicine, 5th ed. St. Louis: Mosby-Yearbook, 1998:2220–2231.

Apstein MD, Carey MC: Gallstones. In: Branch WT Jr (ed). Office Practice of Medicine, 3rd ed. Philadelphia: Saunders, 1994:277–295.

Arca M, Ciocca S, Montali A, Capocaccia R, Angelico F, Angelico M, Attili AF, Calvieri A, Capocaccia L, Conti R, et al.: Erythrocyte fatty acid composition and gallstone disease: results of an epidemiological survey. Am J Clin Nutr 1987; 46:110–114.

Archampong EQ: Cholelithiasis in Accra. Ghana Med J 1969; 8:134–139.

Attili AF, Capocaccia R, Carulli N, Festi D, Roda E, Barbara L, Capocaccia L, Menotti A, Okolicksanyi L, Ricci G, et al.: Factors associated with gallstone disease in the MICOL experience. Multicenter Italian Study on Epidemiology of Cholelithiasis. Hepatology 1997; 26:809–818.

Attili AF, Carulli N, Roda E, Barbara B, Capocaccia L, Menotti A, Okoliksanyi L, Ricci G, Capocaccia R, Festi D, et al.: Epidemiology of gallstone disease in Italy: prevalence data of the Multicenter Italian Study on Cholelithiasis (MICOL). Am J Epidemiol 1995; 141:158–162.

Attili AF, Scafato E, Marchioli R, Marfisi RM, Festi D: Diet and gallstones in Italy: the cross-sectional MICOL results. Hepatology 1998; 27:1492–1498.

Bahar RJ, Stolz A: Bile acid transport. Gastroenterol Clin North Am 1999; 28:27–58.

Bainton D, Davies GT, Evans KT, Gravelle IH: Gallbladder disease. Prevalence in a south Wales industrial town. N Engl J Med 1976; 294:1147–1149.

Balzer K, Goebell H, Breuer N, Rüping KW, Leder LD: Epidemiology of gallstones in a German industrial town (Essen) from 1940–1975. Digestion 1986; 33:189–197.

Banaszak L, Winter N, Xu Z, Bernlohr DA, Cowan S, Jones TA: Lipid-binding proteins: a family of fatty acid and retinoid transport proteins. Adv Protein Chem 1994; 45:89–151.

Barbara L, Sama C, Morselli-Labate AM, Taroni F, Rusticali AG, Festi D, Sapio C, Roda E, Banterle C, Puci A, et al.: A population study on the prevalence of gallstone disease: the Sirmione Study. Hepatology 1987; 7:913–917.

Baron RL, Rohrmann CA Jr, Lee SP, Shuman WP, Teefey SA: CT evaluation of gallstones in vitro: correlation with chemical analysis. AJR Am J Roentgenol 1988; 151:1123–1128.

Bates GC, Brown CH: Incidence of gallbladder disease in chronic hemolytic anemia (sperocytosis). Gastroenterology 1952; 21:104–109.

Becker JP, Chatgidakis CB: Carcinoma of the gall bladder and cholelithiasis on the Witwatersrand. An autopsy study of the racial incidence. S Afr J Clin Sci 1952; 3:13–22.

Behar J, Lee KY, Thompson WR, Biancani P: Gallbladder contraction in patients with pigment and cholesterol stones. Gastroenterology 1989; 97:1479–1484.

Bennion LJ, Grundy S: Effects of diabetes mellitus on cholesterol metabolism in man. N Engl J Med 1977; 296:1365–1371.

Bennion LJ, Grundy SM: Effects of obesity and caloric intake on biliary lipid metabolism in man. J Clin Invest 1975; 56:966–1011.

Bennion LJ, Knowler WC: Epidemiology of gallstones. In: Rotter JI, Samloff IM, Rimoin DC (eds). Genetics and Heterogeneity of Common Gastrointestinal Disorders. New York: Academic Press, 1980:297–312.

Bennion LJ, Knowler WC, Mott DM, Spagnola AM, Bennett PH: Development of lithogenic bile during puberty in Pima Indians. N Engl J Med 1979; 300:873–876.

Berndt H, Nürnberg D, Pannwitz H: Prävalenz der Cholelithiasis: Ergebnisse einer epidemiologischen Studie mittels sonographie in der DDR. Z Gastroenterol 1989; 27:662–666.

Berr F, Goetz A, Schreiber E, Paumgartner G: Effect of dietary n-3 versus n-6 polyunsaturated fatty acids on hepatic excretion of cholesterol in the hamster. J Lipid Res 1993; 34:1275–1284.

Berr F, Holl J, Jüngst D, Fischer S, Richter WO, Seifferth B, Paumgartner G: Dietary n-3 polyunsaturated fatty acids decrease biliary cholesterol saturation in gallstone disease. Hepatology 1992; 16:960–967.

Bertomeu A, Ros E, Zambon D, Vela M, Perez-Ayuso RM, Targarona E, Trias M, Sanlley C, Casals E, Ribo JM: Apolipoprotein E polymorphism and gallstones. Gastroenterology 1996; 111:1603–1610.

Biss K, Ho KJ, Mikkelson B, Lewis L, Taylor CB: Some unique biologic characteristics of the Masai of east Africa. N Engl J Med 1971; 284:649–699.

Bloch HM, Thornton JR, Heaton KW: Effect of fasting on the composition of gallbladder bile. Gut 1980; 21:1087–1089.

Blovin A: Anatomy, ultrastructure, and morphometry of the liver. In: Glaumenn H, Peters T Jr, Redman C (eds). Plasma Protein Secretion by the Liver. New York: Academic Press, 1983:31–53.

Bond LR, Hatty SR, Horn ME, Dick M, Meire HB, Bellingham AJ: Gallstones in sickle cell disease in the United Kingdom. BMJ 1987; 295:234–236.

Booker ML, Scott TE, LaMorte WW: Effects of dietary fish oil on biliary phospholipids and prostaglandin synthesis in the cholesterol-fed prairie dog. Lipids 1990; 25:27–32.

Borch K, Jönsson K-Å, Zdolsek JM, Halldestam I, Kullman E: Prevalence of gallstone disease in a Swedish population sample. Relations to occupations, childbirth, health status, life style, medications, and blood lipids. Scand J Gastroenterol 1998; 33:1219–1225.

Borgman RF: Gallstone formation in rabbits as affected by dietary fat and protein. Am J Vet Res 1965; 26:1167–1171.

Borgman RF, Haselden FH: Cholelithiasis in rabbits. Arch Pathol 1968; 88:598–601.

Boston Collaborative Drug Surveillance Programme. Oral contraceptives and venous thromboembolic disease, surgically confirmed gallbladder disease, and breast tumours. Lancet 1973; i:1399–1404.

Bouchard G, Nelson HM, Lammert F, Rowe LB, Carey MC, Paigen B: High-resolution maps of the murine chromosome 2 region containing the cholestrol gallstone locus, *Lith 1*. Mamm Genome 1999; 10:1070–1074.

Bouchard G, Paigen B, Carey MC: Functional and genetic studies of Abcc2 in inbred mice: evidence for a primary role of the canalicular conjugate organic anion transporter in Lith2 transmitted cholesterol gallstone susceptibility. In: Gerbes A, Beuers U, Jüngst D, Pape GR, Sachmann M, Sauerbruch T (eds). Hepatology 2000: Symposium in Honour of Gustav Paumgartner. Dordrecht: Kluwer, 2000:97–101.

Bouchier IAD: Postmortem study of the frequency of gallstones in patients with cirrhosis of the liver. Gut 1969; 10:705–710.

Braverman DZ, Johnson ML, Kern F Jr: Effects of pregnancy and contraceptive steroids on gallbladder function. N Engl J Med 1980; 302:362–364.

Bremner CG: The changing pattern of disease seen at Baraqwanath Hospital. S Afr J Surg 1971; 9:127–129.

Brenneman DE, Connor WE, Forker EL, DenBesten L: The formation of abnormal bile and cholesterol gallstones from dietary cholesterol in the prairie dog. J Clin Invest 1972; 51:1495–1502.

Brett M, Barker DJP: The world distribution of gallstones. Int J Epidemiol 1976; 5:335–341.

Brink JA, Kammer B, Mueller PR, Balfer DM, Prien EL, Ferrucci JT: Prediction of gallstone composition: synthesis of CT and radiographic features in vitro. Radiology 1994; 190:69–75.

Brink MA, Méndez-Sánchez N, Carey MC: Bilirubin cycles enterohepatically after ileal resection in the rat. Gastroenterology 1996; 110:1945–1957.

Brink MA, Slors JFM, Keulemans YCA, Mok KS, de Waart DR, Carey MC, Groen AK, Tytgat GNJ: Enterohepatic cycling of bilirubin: a putative mechanism for pigment gallstone formation in ileal Crohn's disease. Gastroenterology 1999; 116:1420–1427.

Broccardo C, Osorio J, Luciani MF, Schriml LM, Prades C, Shulenin S, Arnould I, Naudin L, Lafargue C, Rosier M, et al.: Comparative analysis of the promoter structure and genomic organization of the human and mouse *ABCA7* gene encoding a novel ABCA transporter. Cytogenet Cell Genet 2001; 92:264–270.

Broomfield PH, Chopra R, Sheinbaum RC, Bonorris GG, Silverman A, Schoenfield LJ: Effects of ursodeoxycholic acid and aspirin on the formation of lithogenic bile and gallstones during loss of weight. N Engl J Med 1988; 319:1567–1572.

Bross I: Sequential medical plans. Biometrics 1952; 8:180–205.

Brown DM, Everhart JE: Cost of digestive diseases in the United States. In: Everhart JE (ed). Digestive Diseases in the United States: Epidemiology and Impact. US Department of Health and Human Services, PHS NIDDK, NIH publication 94–1447. Washington DC: U.S. Government Printing Office, 1994:57–82.

Brown MS, Goldstein JL: A receptor-mediated pathway for cholesterol homeostasis. Science 1986; 232:32–47.

Brown MS, Goldstein JL: The SREBP pathway: regulation of cholesterol metabolism by proteolysis of a membrane-bound tnscription factor. Cell 1997; 89:331–340.

Buhman KK, Accad M, Novak S, Choi RS, Wong JS, Hamilton RL, Turley S, Farese RV Jr: Resistance to diet-induced hypercholesterolemia and gallstone formation in ACAT2-deficient mice. Nat Med 2000; 6:1341–1347.

Bull LN, van Eijk MJ, Pawlikowska L, DeYoung JA, Juijn JA, Liao M, Klomp LW, Lomri N, Berger R, Scharschmidt BF, et al.: A gene encoding a P-type ATPase mutated in two forms of hereditary cholestasis. Nat Genet 1998; 18:219–224.

Burkitt DP, Trowell HC: Refined Carbohydrate Foods and Disease. Some Implications of Dietary Fiber. London: Academic Press, 1975.

Burkitt DP, Tunstall M: Gallstones: geographical and chronological features. J Trop Med Hyg 1975; 78:140–144.

Burnett W: The epidemiology of gallstones. Tijdschr Gastroenterol 1971; 14:79–89.

Cahalane MJ, Neubrand MW, Carey MC: Physical–chemical pathogenesis of pigment gallstones. Semin Liver Dis 1988; 8:317–328.

Capron JP, Delamarre J, Herve MA, Dupas JL, Poulain P, Descombes P: Meal frequency and duration of overnight fast: a role in gallstone formation? BMJ 1981; 283:1435.

Carey MC: Pathogenesis of gallstones. Am J Surg 1993a; 165:410–419.

Carey MC: Pathogenesis of gallstones. Recent Prog Med 1993b; 83:379–391.

Carey MC: Formation and growth of cholesterol gallstones: the new synthesis. In: Fromm H, Leuschner U (eds). Bile Acids–Cholestasis–Gallstones. Dordrecht: Kluwer, 1996:147–175.

Carey MC: Pathogenesis of cholesterol and pigment gallstones: some radical new concepts. In: Gerok W, Loginov AS, Pokrowskij VI (eds). New Trends in Hepatology. Dordrecht: Kluwer, 1997:64–83.
Carey MC: Can cholesterol gallstones be prevented? In: Tytgat GNJ, Krejs GJ (eds). Gastroenterology and Hepatology: The Next Millennium. Paris: Lilly, 1998:37–44.
Carey MC, Cahalane MJ: Whither biliary sludge? Gastroenterology 1988; 95:508–523.
Carey MC, Cohen DE: Biliary transport of cholesterol in vesicles, micelles and liquid crystals. In: Paumgartner G, Stiehl A, Gerok W (eds). Bile Acids and the Liver. Lancaster, UK: MTP Press, 1987:287–300.
Carey MC, Duane WC: Enterohepatic circulation. In: The Liver: Biology and Pathobiology. Arias IM, Boyer JL, Fausto N, Jakoby WB, Schachter DA, Shafritz DA, (eds). Raven Press Ltd, New York. 1994:719–767.
Carey MC, LaMont JT: Cholesterol gallstone formation. 1. Physical-chemistry of bile and biliary lipid secretion. Prog Liver Dis 1992; 10:139–163.
Carey MC, O'Donovan MA: Gallstone disease: current concepts on the epidemiology, pathogenesis and management. In: Petersdorf RG, Adams RD, Braunwald E, Isselbacher KJ, Martin JB, Wilson JD (eds). Harrison's Principles of Internal Medicine. Update V. New York: McGraw-Hill, 1984:139–168.
Carey MC, Small DM: Physical-chemistry of cholesterol solubility in bile. Relationship to gallstone formation and dissolution in man. J Clin Invest 1978; 61:998–1026.
Caroli-Bosc FX, Deveau C, Peten EP, Delabre B, Zanaldi H, Hebuterne X, Hastier P, Viudes F, Belanger F, Caroli-Bosc C, et al.: Cholelithiasis and dietary risk factors: an epidemiologic investigation in Vidauban, southeast France. Dig Dis Sci 1998; 43:2131–2137.
Carstea ED, Morris JA, Coleman KG, Loftus SK, Zhang D, Cummings C, Gu J, Rosenfeld MA, Pavan WJ, Krizman DB, et al.: Niemann-Pick-C1 disease gene: homology to mediators of cholesterol homeostasis. Science 1997; 277:228–231.
Carulli N, Ponz de Leon M, Loria P, Iori R, Rosi A, Romani M: Effect of the selective expansion of the cholic acid pool on bile lipid composition: possible mechanisms of bile acid–induced biliary cholesterol desaturation. Gastroenterology 1981; 81:539–546.
Carulli N, Ponz ed Leon M, Zironi F, Iori R, Loria P: Bile acid feeding and hepatic sterol metabolism: effect of deoxycholic acid. Gastroenterology 1980; 79:637–641.
Cerqueira MT, McMurry-Fry M, Connor WE: The food and nutrient intakes of the Tarahumara Indians of Mexico. Am J Clin Nutr 1979; 32:905–915.
Chan FK, Zhang Y, Lee SS, Shaffer EA: The effect of liver transplantation and cyclosporin on bile formation and lipid composition in an experimental study in the rat. J Hepatol 1998; 28:329–336.
Chawla A, Barak Y, Nagy L, Liao D, Tontonoz P, Evans RM: PPAR-gamma dependent and independent effects on macrophage-gene expression in lipid metabolism and inflammation. Nat Med 2001a; 7:23–24.
Chawla A, Boisvert WA, Lee CH, Laffitte BA, Barak Y, Joseph SB, Liao D, Nagy L, Edwards PA, Curtiss LK, et al.: A PPAR gamma–LXR-ABCA1 pathway in macrophages is involved in cholesterol efflux and atherogenesis. Mol Cell 2001b; 7:161–171.
Chen Q, Chitinavis V, Xiao Z, Yu P, Oh S, Biancani P, Behar J: Impaired G protein function in gallbladder muscle from progesterone-treated guinea pigs. Am J Physiol 1998; 274:G283–G289.
Chevreul M: Recherches chimiques sur plusieurs corps gras et particulièrement sur leur combinaisons avec les alcalis. Ann Chim (Paris) 1815; 95:5–50.
Chianale J, Vollrath V, Wielandt AM, Amigo L, Rigotti A, Nervi F, Gonzalez S, Andrade L, Pizarro M, Accatino L: Fibrates induce *mdr2* gene expression and biliary phospholipid secretion in the mouse. Biochem J 1996; 314:781–786.
Childs S, Yeh RL, Georges E, Ling V: Identification of a sister gene to P-glycoprotein. Cancer Res 1995; 55:2029–2034.
Childs S, Yeh RL, Hui D, Ling V: Taxol resistance mediated by transfection of the liver-specific sister gene of P-glycoprotein. Cancer Res 1998; 58:4160–4167.
Cleave TL, Campbell GD: Diabetes, Coronary Thrombosis and the Saccharine Disease. Bristol: John Wright, 1966.
Cleland JB: Gallstones in seven thousand post-mortem examination. Med J Aust 1953; 2:488–489.
Cohen DE: Hepatocellular transport and secretion of biliary phospholipids. Semin Liver Dis 1996; 16:191–200.
Cohen DE, Green RM, Wu MK, Beier DR: Cloning, tissue-specific expression, gene structure and chromosomal localization of human phosphatidylcholine transfer protein. Biochim Biophys Acta 1999; 1447:265–270.
Cohen JC, Cali JJ, Jelinek DF, Mehrabian M, Sparkes RS, Lusis AJ, Russell DW, Hobbs HH: Cloning of the human cholesterol 7α-hydoxylase gene (*CYP7*) and localization to chromosome 8q11–q12. Genomics 1992; 14:153–161.
Comess J, Bennett PH, Burch TA: Clinical gallbladder disease in Pima Indians: the high prevalence in contrast to Framingham, Massachusetts. N Engl J Med 1967; 277:894–898.
Connor WE, Cerquerie MT, Connor RW, Wallace RB, Malinow MR, Casdorph HR: The plasma lipids, lipoproteins, and diet of the Tarahumara Indians of Mexico. Am J Clin Nutr 1978; 31:1131–1142.
Conter RL, Rosyln JJ, Pitt HA, DenBensten L: Carbohydrate diet-induced calcium bilirubinate sludge and pigment gallstones in the prairie dog. J Surg Res 1986; 40:580–587.
Cooper AD: Metabolic basis of cholesterol gallstone disease. Gastroenterol Clin North Am 1991; 20:21–46.
Coronary Drug Project Research Group. Gallbladder disease as a side effect of drugs influencing lipid metabolism. Experience in the Coronary Drug Project. N Engl J Med 1977; 296:1185–1190.
Coste T, Karsenti P, Berta JL, Cubeau J, Guilloud-Bataille M: Facteurs diétètiques de la lithiase biliare: comparaison de l'alimentation d'un groupe de lithiasiques à l'alimentation d'un group témoin. Gastroenterol Clin Biol 1979; 3:417–423.
Cotran RS, Kumar V, Robins SL: The liver and biliary tract. In: Cotran RS, Kumar V, Robins SL (eds). Pathological Basis of Disease, 4th ed. Philadelphia: Saunders, 1989:969.
Covarrubias C, Valdivieso V, Nervi F: Epidemiology of gallbladder disease in Chile. In: Capocaccia L, Ricci G, Angelico F, Angelico M, Attili AF (eds). Epidemiology and Prevention of Gallbladder Disease. Lancaster, UK: 1984:26–30.
Crawford JM, Carey MC: Bile production and secretion. In: Stein JM (ed). Internal Medicine, 5th ed. St. Louis: Mosby-Yearbook, 1998:2123–2229.
Crawford JM, Möckel G-M, Crawford AR, Hatch VC, Hagen SJ, Barnes S, Godleski JJ, Carey MC: Imaging biliary lipid secretion in the rat: ultrastructural evidence for vesiculation of the hepatocyte canalicular membrane. J Lipid Res 1995; 36:2147–2163.
Cunningham JA, Hardenbergh FE: Comparative incidence of cholelithiasis in the Negro and white races: a study of 6,185 autopsies. Arch Intern Med 1956; 1997:62–72.
Dahlback-Sjoberg H, Björkhem I, Princen HM: Selective inhibition of mitochondrial 27-hydroxylation of bile acid intermediates and 25-hydroxylation of vitamin D_3 by cyclosporin A: Biochem J 1993; 293:203–206.
Dam H: Nutritional aspects of gallstone formation with particular reference to alimentary production of gallstones in laboratory animals. World Rev Nutr Diet 1969; 11:199–239.
Dam H, Kruse I, Jensen HK, Kallehauge HE: Studies on human bile. II. Influence of two different fats on composition of human bile. Scand J Clin Lab Invest 1967; 19:367–378.
Dam H, Prange I, Jensen MK, Kallehauge HE, Fenger HJ: Studies on human bile. IV. Influence of ingestion of cholesterol in the form of eggs on the composition of bile in healthy subjects. Z Ernahrungswiss 1971; 10:178–187.
Danzinger RG, Gordon H, Schoenfield LJ, Thistle JL: Lithogenic bile in siblings of young women with cholelithiasis. Mayo Clin Proc 1972; 47:762–766.
Daughaday WH: Ocreotide is effective in acromegaly but often results in cholelithiasis. Ann Intern Med 1990; 112:159–160.
Dawson PA: Intestinal bile acid transport: molecules, mechanisms, and malabsorption. In: Paumgartner G, Stiehl A, Gerok W, Keppler D, Leuschner U (eds). Bile Acids and Cholestasis. Dordrecht: Kluwer, 1999:1–28.
Dawson PA, Oelkers P: Bile acid transporters. Curr Opin Lipidol 1995; 6:109–114.
DenBesten L, Connor WE, Bell S: The effect of dietary cholesterol on the composition of human bile. Surgery 1973; 73:266–273.
De Santis A, Attili AF, Ginanni Corradini S, Scafato E, Cantagalli A, De Luca C, Pinto G, Lisi D, Capocaccia L: Gallstones and diabetes: a case-control study in a free-living population sample. Hepatology 1997; 25:787–790.
de Vree JM, Jacquemin E, Sturm E, Cresteil D, Bosma PJ, Aten J, Deleuze JF, Desrochers M, Burdelski M, Bernard O, et al.: Mutations in the *MDR3* gene cause progressive familial intrahepatic cholestasis. Proc Natl Acad Sci USA 1998; 95:282–287.
Diehl AK: Epidemiology and natural history of gallstone disease. Gastroenterol Clin North Am 1991; 20:1–19.
Diehl AK, Stern MP: Special health problems of Mexican-Americans: obesity, gallbladder disease, diabetes mellitus and cardiovascular disease. Adv Intern Med 1989; 34:73–96.
Djerassi C: Review of the pill: a social history of oral contraceptives, 1950–1970, by ES Watkins. N Engl J Med 1999; 340:485–486.
Doig RK: Illness in twins III. Cholelithiasis. Med J Aust 1957; 11:716–717.
Donovan JM, Leonard MR, Batta AK, Carey MC: Calcium affinity for biliary lipid aggregates in model biles: complementary importance of bile salts and lecithin. Gastroenterology 1994; 107:831–846.
Douss TW, Castleden WM: Gallstones and carcinoma of the large bowel. N Z Med J 1973; 77:162–165.
Dowling RH, Hussaini SH, Murphy GM, Besser GM, Wass JAH: Gallstones during octreotide therapy. Metabolism 1992; 41:22–33.
Duane WC: Effect of lovastatin and dietary cholesterol on bile acid kinetics and bile lipid composition in healthy male subjects. J Lipid Res 1994; 35:501–509.
Duane WC, Ginsberg RL, Bennion LJ: Effects of fasting on bile acid metabolism and biliary lipid composition in man. J Lipid Res 1976; 17:211–219.
Duffy AM, Sullivan MS, DiMarco WM, Liepa GU: Effects of dietary protein on serum and biliary constituents and gallstone formation in hamsters. Nutr Rep Int 1985; 31:1319–1330.
Duggirala R, Mitchell BD, Blangero J, Stern MP: Genetic determinates of variation in gallbladder disease in the Mexican-American population. Genet Epidemiol 1999; 16:191–204.
Edington GM: Observations on hepatic disease in the Gold Coast: with special reference to cirrhosis. Trans R Soc Trop Med Hyg 1957; 51:48–55.
Ehrström MC: Medical studies in northern Greenland 1948–49, IV. Enlargement of the liver, biliary stone and peptic ulcer: incidence and etiology. Acta Med Scand 1951; 140:324–326.
Einarsson K: Abnormalities of biliary lipid secretion in cholesterol cholelithiasis. Presented at the 3rd World Congress on Biliary Lithotripsy, Orlando, FL.1992:19–20.
Einarsson K, Angelin B: Hyperlipoproteinemia, hypolipidemic treatment and gallstone disease. In: Grundy SM (ed). Bile Acids and Atherosclerosis. New York: Raven, 1986:67–97.
Einarsson K, Nilsell K, Leijd B, Angelin B: Influence of age on secretion of cholesterol and synthesis of bile acids by the liver. N Engl J Med 1985; 313:277–282.
Elias H, Sherrick JG: Morphology of the Liver. New York: Academic Press, 1969.
Enderlin N: Statistische Erhebungen über das Gallensteinleiden. Schweiz Med Wochenschr 1958; 88:855–858.
Engelman JA, Zhang XL, Galbiati F, Lisanti MP: Chromsomal localization, genomic organization, and developmental expression of the murine caveolin gene family

(*Cav-1, -2*, and *-3*). *Cav-1* and *Cav-2* genes map to a known tumor suppressor locus (6-A2/7q31). FEBS Lett 1998; 429:330–336.

Eriksson M, Berglund L, Rudling M, Henriksson P, Angelin B: Effects of estrogen on low density lipoprotein metabolism in males. Short-term and long-term studies during hormonal treatment of prostatic carcinoma. J Clin Invest 1989; 84:802–810.

Everhart JE: Gallstones. In: Everhart JE (ed). Digestive Diseases in the United States: Epidemiology and Impact. US Department of Health and Human Services, PHS NIDDK, NIH publication 94–1447. Washington DC: US Government Printing Office, 1994:647–692.

Everson GT, McKinley C, Kern F Jr: Mechanism of gallstone formation in women. Effect of exogenous estrogen (Premarin) and dietary cholesterol on hepatic lipid metabolism. J Clin Invest 1991; 87:237–246.

Everson GT, McKinley C, Lawson M, Johnson M, Kern F Jr: Gallbladder function in the human female: effects of the ovulatory cycle, pregnancy, and contraceptive steroids. Gastroenterology 1982; 82:711–719.

Farese RV Jr: Acyl CoA:cholesterol acyltransferase genes and knockout mice. Curr Opin Lipidol 1998; 9:119–123.

Ferezou J, Combettes-Souverain M, Souidi M, Smith JL, Boehler N, Milliat F, Eckhardt E, Blanchard G, Riottot M, Serougne C, et al.: Cholesterol, bile acid, and lipoprotein metabolism in two strains of hamster, one resistant, the other sensitive (LNP) to sucrose-induced cholelithiasis. J Lipid Res 2000; 41:2042–2054.

Fevery J, Verwilghen R, Tan TG, DeGroute J: Glucuronidation of bilirubin and the occurrence of pigment gallstones in patients with chronic hemolytic disease. Eur J Clin Invest 1980; 10:219–226.

Filly RA, Allen B, Minton MJ, Bernhoft R, Way LW: In vitro investigation of the origin of echoes with biliary sludge. J Clin Ultrasound 1980; 8:193–200.

Friedman GD: Natural history of asymptomatic and symptomatic gallstones. Am J Surg 1993; 165:399–404.

Friedman GD, Kannel WB, Dawber TR: The epidemiology of gallbladder disease: observations in the Framingham Study. J Chronic Dis 1966; 19:277–292.

Fuchs M, Ivandic B, Muller O, Schalla C, Scheibner J, Bartsch P, Stange EF: Biliary cholesterol hypersecretion in gallstone-susceptible mice is associated with hepatic up-regulation of the high-density lipoprotein receptor SRBI. Hepatology 2001; 33:1451–1459.

Fuchs M, Lammert F, Wang DQ-H, Paigen B, Carey MC, Cohen DE: Sterol carrier protein 2 participates in hypersecretion of biliary cholesterol during gallstone formation in genetically gallstone-susceptible mice. Biochem J 1998; 336:33–37.

Fuchs M, Muench C, Hafner A, Katzberg N, Seedorf U, Scheibner J, Stange EF: Disruption of the sterol carrier protein-2 gene does not prevent cholesterol gallstone formation [abstract]. Hepatology 1999a; 30:430A.

Fuchs M, Schalla C, Müller O, Stange EF: Caveolin-1 levels are up-regulated during biliary cholesterol (CHOL) hypersecretion: implications for bile formation [abstract]. Gastroenterology 1999b; 116:A1246.

Fujihara E, Kaneta S, Oshima T: Strain difference in mouse cholelithiasis and the effect of taurine on the gallstone formation in C57BL/C mice. Biochem Med 1978; 19:211–217.

Geare R: Some diseases prevalent among Indians of the southwest and their treatment. Med World 1915; 33:305–310.

Gebhard RL, Prigge WF, Ansel HJ, Schlasner L, Ketover SR, Sande D, Hotmeier K, Peterson FJ: The role of gallbladder emptying in gallstone formation during diet-induced rapid weight loss. Hepatology 1996; 24:544–548.

Gerloff T, Stieger B, Hagenbuch B, Madon J, Landmann L, Roth J, Hofmann AF, Meier PJ: The sister of P-glycoprotein represents the canalicular bile salt export pump of mammalian liver. J Biol Chem 1998; 273:10046–10050.

Gilat T, Feldman C, Halpern Z, Dan M, Bar-Meir S: An increased familial frequency of gallstones. Gastroenterology 1983; 84:242–246.

Glambek I, Kvaale G, Arnesjö B, Søreide O: Prevalence of gallstones in a Norwegian population. Scand J Gastroenterol 1987; 22:1089–1094.

Goldfarb A, Grisaru D, Gimmon Z, Okon E, Lebensart P, Rachmilewitz EA: High incidence of cholelithiasis in older patients with homozygous beta-thalassemia. Acta Haematol 1990; 83:120–122.

Goodwin B, Jones SA, Price RR, Watson MA, KcKee DD, Moore LB, Galardi C, Wilson JG, Lewis MC, Roth ME, et al.: A regulatory cascade of the nuclear receptors FXR, SHP-1, and LRH-1 represses bile acid biosynthesis. Mol Cells 2000; 6:517–526.

Green RM, Ananthanarayanan M, Suchy FJ, Beier DR: Genetic mapping of the Na^+-taurocholate cotransporting polypeptide to mouse chromosome 12. Mamm Genome 1998; 9:598–600.

Grimaldi CH, Nelson RG, Pettitt DJ, Sampliner RE, Bennett PK, Knowler WC: Increased mortality with gallstone disease: results of a 20-year population-based survey in Pima Indians. Ann Intern Med 1993; 118:185–190.

Grosfeld JL, Rescorla FJ, Skinner MA, West KW, Scherer LR 3rd: The spectrum of biliary tract disorders in infants and children. Experience with 300 cases. Arch Surg 1994; 129:513–518.

Grosse H: Die Cholelithiasis. Jena: Gustav Fischer, 1966.

Grundy SM, Duane WC, Adler RD, Aron JM, Metzger AL: Biliary lipid outputs in young women with cholesterol gallstones. Metabolism 1974; 23:67–73.

Grundy SM, Lan SP, Lachin J: The effects of chenodiol on biliary lipids and their association with gallstone dissolution in the National Cooperative Gallstone Study (NCGS). J Clin Invest 1984; 73:1156–1166.

Grundy SM, Metzger AL, Adler RD: Mechanism of lithogenic bile formation in American Indian women with cholesterol gallstones. J Clin Invest 1972; 51:3026–3043.

Haffner SM, Diehl AK, Mitchell BD, Stern MP, Hazuda HP: Increased prevalence of clinical gallbladder disease in subjects with non-insulin-dependent diabetes mellitus. Am J Epidemiol 1990; 132:327–335.

Hagberg B, Svennerholm L, Thorén L: Cholelithiasis in childhood. A follow-up study with special reference to heredity, constitutional factors and serum lipids. Acta Chir Scand 1962; 123:307–315.

Hagenbuch B, Meier PJ: Molecular cloning, chromosomal localization, and functional characterization of a human liver Na^+/bile acid cotransporter. J Clin Invest 1994; 93:1326–1331.

Han T, Jiang Z, Suo G, Zhang S: Apolipoprotein B-100 gene Xba I polymorphism and cholesterol gallstone disease. Clin Genet 2000; 57:304–308.

Hancock JC: Diseases among the Indians. Southwest Med 1933; 17:126–129.

Hanis CL, Chakraborty R, Ferrell RE, Schull WJ: Individual admixture estimates: disease associations and individual risk of diabetes and gallbladder disease among Mexican-Americans in Starr County, Texas. Am J Phys Anthropol 1986; 70:433–441.

Hanis CL, Ferrell RE, Tulloch BR, Schell WJ: Gallbladder disease epidemiology in Mexican Americans in Starr County, Texas. Am J Epidemiol 1985; 122:820–829.

Harvald B, Hauge M: A catamnestic investigation of Danish twins. A preliminary report. Danish Med Bull 1956; 3:150–158.

Heaton K: Gallstones. In: Trowell HC, Burkitt DP (eds). Western Diseases: Their Emergence and Prevention. Cambridge, MA: Harvard University Press, 1981:47–59.

Heaton KW: The epidemiology of gallstones and suggested etiology. Clin Gastroenterol 1973; 2:67–83.

Heaton KW: Epidemiology and prevention of gallstones, Eur J Gastroenterol Hepatol 1994; 6:852–856.

Heaton KW, Braddon FEM, Emmett PM, Mountford RA, Hughes AO, Bolton CH, Ghosh S: Why do men get gallstones? Roles of abdominal fat and hyperinsulinaemia. Eur J Gastroenterol Hepatol 1991a; 3:745–751.

Heaton KW, Braddon FEM, Mountford RA, Hughes AO, Emmett PM: Symptomatic and silent gallstones in the community. Gut 1991b; 32:316–320.

Heaton KW, Morris JS: Bitter humor: the development of ideas about bile salts. J R Coll Physicians Lond 1971; 6:83–87.

Henriksson P, Einarsson K, Eriksson A, Kelter U, Angelin B: Estrogen-induced gallstone formation in males. Relation to changes in serum and biliary lipids during hormonal treatment of prostatic carcinoma. J Clin Invest 1989; 84:811–816.

Higgins CF: ABC transporters: from microorganisms to man. Annu Rev Cell Biol 1992; 8:67–113.

Hills LL: Cholelithiasis and immigration. Med J Aust 1971; 2:94–95.

Hofmann AF, Grundy SM, Lachin JM, Lan S-P, Baum RA, Hanson RF, Hersh T, Hightower NC Jr, Marks JW, Mekhjian H, et al.: Pre-treatment biliary lipid composition in white patients wth radiolucent gallstones in the National Cooperative Gallstone Study. Gastroenterology 1982; 82:738–752.

Holzbach TR: Animal models of cholesterol gallstone disease. Hepatology 1984; 4:191S–198S.

Honore LH: The lack of a positive association between symptomatic cholesterol cholelithiasis and clinical diabetes mellitus: a retrospective study. J Chronic Dis 1980; 33:465–469.

Hoppe-Seyler G: Cholelithiasis. In: Nothnagel's Encyclopedia of Practical Medicine—American Edition. Baltimore: Saunders, 1903:525–607.

Huijbregts AWM, van Berg-Henegouwen GP, Hectors MPC, van Schaik, van der Werf SDJ: Effects of a standardized wheat bran preparation on biliary lipid composition and bile acid metabolism in young healthy males. Eur J Clin Invest 1980; 10:451–458.

Hussaini SH, Pereira SP, Murphy GM, Dowling RH: Deoxycholic acid influences cholesterol solubilization and microcrystal nucleation time in gallbladder bile. Hepatology 1995; 22:1735–1744.

Ingelfinger FJ: The chemistry of the American Indian's burden. N Engl J Med 1979; 300:917–918.

Ito T, Kawata S, Imai Y, Kakimoto H, Trzaskos JM, Matsuzawa Y: Hepatic cholesterol metabolism in patients with cholesterol gallstones: enhanced intracellular transport of cholesterol. Gastroenterology 1996; 110:1619–1627.

Jackson CE, Gay BC: Inheritance of gall-bladder disease. Surgery 1959; 40:853–857.

Jacquemin E, De Vree JM, Cresteil D, Sokal EM, Sturm E, Dumont M, Scheffer GL, Paul M, Burdelski M, Bosma PJ, et al.: The wide spectrum of multidrug resistance 3 deficiency: from neonatal cholestasis to cirrhosis of adulthood. Gastroenterology 2001; 120:1448–1458.

Janowski BA, Willy PJ, Devi TR, Falck JR, Mangelsdorf DJ: An oxysterol signalling pathway mediated by the nuclear receptor LXR alpha. Nature 1996; 383:728–731.

Janson L, Aspelin P, Eriksson S, Hildell J, Trall E, Östherg H: Ultrasonographic screening for gallstone disease in middle-aged women. Scand J Gastroenterol 1985; 20:706–710.

Jaskiewicz K, Weight MJ, Christopher KJ, Benade AJS, Kritchevsky D: A comparison of the effect of soya-bean protein and casein on bile composition, cholelithiasis and serum lipoprotein lipids in the vervet monkey (*Cercopithecus aethiops*). Br J Nutr 1987; 58:257–263.

Johnston JL, Williams CN, Weldon KLM: Nutrient intake and meal pattens of Micmac Indian and Caucasian women in Shubenacadie, NS: Can Med Assoc J 1977; 116:1356–1359.

Jones G: A History of the Vikings, 2nd ed. New York: Oxford University Press, 1984.

Jorgensen T: Prevalence of gallstones in a Danish population. Am J Epidemiol 1987; 126:912–921.

Jorgensen T: Gallstones in a Danish population: familial occurrence and social factors. J Biosoc Sci 1988a; 20:111–120.

Jorgensen T: Gallstones in a Danish population: fertility period, pregnancies and exogenous female sex hormones. Gut 1988b; 29:433–439.

Jorgensen T: Gallstones and plasma lipids in a Danish population. Scand J Gastroenterol 1989a; 24:916–922.

Jorgensen T: Gallstones in a Danish population. Relation to weight, physical activity, smoking, coffee consumption and diabetes mellitus. Gut 1989b; 30:528–534.

Jorgensen T, Jorgensen LM: Gallstones and diet in a Danish population. Scand J Gastroenterol 1989; 24:821–826.

Juvonen T, Kervinen K, Kairaluoma MI, Lajenen LH, Kesaniemi YA: Gallstone cholesterol content is related to apolipoprotein E polymorphism. Gastroenterology 1993; 104:1806–1813.

Juvonen T, Savolainen MJ, Kairaluoma MI, Lajunen LH, Humphries SE, Kesaniemi YA: Polymorphisms at the apoB, apoA-I, and cholesteryl ester transfer protein gene loci in patients with gallbladder disease. J Lipid Res 1995; 36:804–812.

Kadmon M, Klunemann C, Bohme M, Ishikawa T, Gorgas K, Otto G, Herfarth C, Keppler D: Inhibition by cyclosporin A of adenosine triphosphate-dependant transport from the hepatocyte into bile. Gastroenterology 1993; 104:1507–1514.

Kalos A, Delidou A, Kordosis T, Archimandritis A, Gananis A, Angelopoulos B: The incidence of gallstones in Greece: an autopsy study. Acta Hepatogastroenterol 1977; 24:20–23.

Kaminski WE, Orso E, Diederich W, Klucken J, Drobnik W, Schmitz G: Identification of a novel human sterol-sensitive ATP-binding cassette transporter (ABCA7). Biochem Biophys Res Commun 2000a; 273:532–538.

Kaminski WE, Piehler A, Schmitz G: Genomic organization of the human cholesterol-responsive ABC transporter ABCA7: tandem linkage with the minor histocompatibility antigen *HA-1* gene. Biochem Biophys Res Commun 2000b; 278:782–789.

Keppler D, Arias IM: Transport across the hepatocyte canalicular membrane. FASEB J 1997; 11:15–18.

Kern F Jr: Normal plasma cholesterol in an 88-year-old man who eats 25 eggs a day. Mechanism of adaptation. N Engl J Med 1991; 324:869–899.

Kern F Jr: Effects of dietary cholesterol on cholesterol and bile acid homeostasis in patients with cholesterol gallstones. J Clin Invest 1994; 93:1186–1194.

Kern F Jr, Erfling W, Simon FR, Dahl R, Mallory A, Starzl TE: Effect of estrogens on the liver. Gastroenterology 1978; 75:512–522.

Kern F Jr, Everson GT, DeMark B, McKinley C, Showalter R, Erfling W, Braverman DZ, Szczepanik-Van Leeuwen P, Klein PD: Biliary lipids, bile acids, and gallbladder function in the human female. Effects of pregnancy and the ovulatory cycle. J Clin Invest 1981; 68:1229–1242.

Kesäniemi YA, Koskenvuo M, Vuoristo M, Miettinen TA: Biliary lipid composition in monozygotic and dizygotic pairs of twins. Gut 1989; 30:1750–1756.

Khanna M, Qin KN, Wang RW, Cheng KC: Substrate specificity, gene structure, and tissue-specific distribution of multiple human 3 alpha-hydroxysteroid dehydrogenases. J Biol Chem 1995; 270:20162–20168.

Khanuja B, Cheah Y-C, Hunt M, Nishina PM, Chen HW, Billheimer JT, Carey MC, Paigen B: *Lith1*, a major gene affecting cholesterol gallstone formation among inbred strains of mice. Proc Natl Acad Sci USA 1995; 92:7729–7733.

Kliewer SA, Forman BM, Blumberg B, Ong ES, Borgmeyer U, Mangelsdorf DJ, Umesono K, Evans RM: Differential expression and activation of a family of murine peroxisome proliferator-activated receptors. Proc Natl Acad Sci USA 1994; 91:7355–7359.

Knowler WC, Carraher MJ, Pettitt DJ, Bennett PH: Epidemiology of cholelithiasis in the Pima Indians. In: Capocacia L, Ricci G, Angelico F, Angelico M, Attili AF (eds). Epidemiology and Prevention of Gallbladder Disease. Lancaster, UK: MTP Press, 1984:15–22.

Kobayashi T, Beuchat MH, Lindsay M, Frias S, Palmiter RD, Sakuraba H, Parton RG, Gruenberg J: Late endosomal membranes rich in lysobisphosphatidic acid regulate cholesterol transport. Nat Cell Biol 1999; 1:113–118.

Koepsell H: Organic cation transporters in intestine, kidney, liver, and brain. Annu Rev Physiol 1998; 60:243–266.

Kono S, Kochi S, Ohyama S, Wakisaka A: Gallstones, serum lipids, and glucose tolerance among male officials of self-defense forces in Japan. Dig Dis Sci 1988; 33:839–844.

Körner G: Über die familiare Härfung der Gallenblasenkrankheitern. Z Menschl Vererb. Konst 1937; 20:526–582.

Kozarsky KF, Donahee MH, Rigotti A, Iqbal SN, Edelman ER, Krieger M: Overexpression of the HDL receptor SR-BI alters plasma HDL and bile cholesterol levels. Nature 1997; 387:414–417.

Kratzer W, Kächele V, Mason RA, Hill V, Hay B, Haug C, Adler G, Beckh K, Muche R: Gallstone prevalence in Germany: the Ulm Gallbladder Stone Study. Dig Dis Sci 1998; 43:1285–1291.

Kravetz RE: Etiology of biliary tract disease in southwestern American Indians: analysis of 105 connective cholecystectomies. Gastroenterology 1964; 46:392–398.

Krejs GJ, Orci L, Conlon JM, Ravazzola M, Davis GR, Raskin P, Collins SM, McCarthy DM, Baetens D, Rubenstein A, et al.: Somatostatinoma syndrome. Biochemical, morphologic and clinical features. N Engl J Med 1979; 301:285–292.

Kritchevsky D, Klurfeld DM: Gallstone formation in hamsters: effect of varying animal and vegetable protein levels. Am J Clin Nutr 1983; 37:802–804.

Kukongviriyapan V, Stacey NH: Chemical-induced interference with hepatocellular transport. Role in cholestasis. Chem Biol Interact 1991; 77:245–261.

Lammert F, Carey MC, Paigen B: Chromosomal organization of candidate genes involved in cholesterol gallstone formation: a murine gallstone map. Gastroenterology 2001; 120:221–238.

Lammert F, Cohen DE, Paigen B, Carey MC, Beier DR: The gene encoding the multispecific organic anion transporter (*Cmoat*) of the hepatocyte canalicular membrane maps to mouse chromosome 19. Mamm Genome 1998a; 9:87–88.

Lammert F, Nelson HM, Wang DQ-H, Carey MC, Paigen B: Quantitative trait locus (QTL) mapping identifies a new murine gallstone gene on chromosome 17. Hepatology 1997; 26:401A.

Lammert F, Paigen B, Carey MC: Localization of the ileal sodium-bile salt cotransporter gene (*Slc10a2*) to mouse chromosome 8. Mamm Genome 1998b; 9:173–174.

Lammert F, Wang DQ-H, Cohen DE, Paigen B, Carey MC: Functional and genetic studies of biliary cholesterol secretion in inbred mice: evidence for a primary role of sister-P-glycoprotein, the canalicular bile salt export pump, in cholesterol gallstone pathogenesis. In: Paumgartner G, Stiehl A, Gerok W, Keppler D, Leuschner U (eds). Bile Acids and Cholestasis (Falk Symposium No. 108). Dordrecht: Kluwer, 1999a:224–228.

Lammert F, Wang DQ-H, Paigen B, Carey MC: Spontaneous cholesterol gallstone formation on normal diet characterizes mice with disrupted *mdr2* P-glycoprotein gene and provides new insights into cholesterol crystallization and bile formation. Gasterenterology 1998b; 114:A527.

Lammert F, Wang DQ-H, Paigen B, Carey MC: Phenotypic characterization of *Lith* genes that determine susceptibility to cholesterol cholelithiasis in inbred mice: integrated activities of hepatic lipid regulatory enzymes. J Lipid Res 1999c; 40:2080–2090.

LaMont JT, Carey MC: Cholesterol gallstone formation. 2. Pathobiology and pathomechanics. Prog Liver Dis 1992; 10:165–191.

Lander ES, Botstein D: Mapping Mendelian factors underlying quantitative traits using RFLP linkage maps. Genetics 1989; 121:185–199.

Lapidus A, Einarsson C: Bile composition in patients with ileal resection due to Crohn's disease. Inflamm Bowel Dis 1998; 4:89–94.

Lapidus A, Einarsson K: Effects of ileal resection on biliary lipids and bile acid composition in patients with Crohn's disease. Gut 1991; 32:1488–1491.

Last RJ: Anatomy, Regional and Applied, 3rd ed. London: Churchill, 1963:425–431.

Lee DTW, Gilmore CJ, Bonorris G, Cohen H, Marks JW, Cho-Sue M, Meiselman MS, Schoenfeld LJ: Effects of dietary cholesterol on biliary lipids in patients with gallstones and normal subjects. Am J Clin Nutr 1985; 42:414–420.

Lee SP, Carey MC, LaMont JF: Aspirin prevention of cholesterol gallstone formation in prairie dogs. Science 1981; 211:1429–1431.

Lee SP, Hayashi A, Kim YS: Biliary sludge: curiosity or culprit? Hepatology 1994; 2:523–525.

Lee SP, Maher K, Nicholls JF: Origin and fate of biliary sludge. Gastroenterology 1988; 1:170–176.

Lehto M, Laitinen S, Chinetti G, Johansson M, Ehnholm C, Staels B, Ikonen E, Olkkonen VM: The OSBP-related protein family in humans. J Lipid Res 2001; 42:1203–1213.

Lembcke B, Creutzfeldt W, Schleser S, Ebert R, Shaw C, Koop I: Effect of the somatostatin analogue sandostatin (SMS 201–995) on gastrointestinal, pancreatitic and biliary function and hormone release in normal men. Digestion 1987; 36:108–124.

Leonard AN, Cohen DE: Submicellar bile salts stimulate phosphatidylcholine transfer activity of sterol carrier protein 2. J Lipid Res 1998; 39:1981–1988.

Liddle RA, Goldstein RB, Saxton J: Gallstone formation during weight-reduction dieting. Arch Intern Med 1989; 149:1750–1753.

Lieber MM: The incidence of gallstones and their correlation with other diseases. Ann Surg 1952; 135:394–405.

Liepa GU, Gorman MA, Duffy AM: The use of animals in studying the effects of diet on gallstone formation. In: Breynen AC, West CE (eds). Use of Animal Models for Research in Human Nutrition, Vol 6. Basel: Karger, 1988:149–173.

Lin J-P, Hanis CL, Boerwinkle E: Genetic epidemiology of gallbladder disease in Mexican Americans and cholesterol 7α-hydroxylase gene variation. Am J Hum Genet 1994; 55:A48.

Loefler IJP: Gallstones and glaciers: hypothesis meeting at the equator. Lancet 1988; 2:683.

Loftus SK, Morris JA, Carstea ED, Gu JZ, Cummings C, Brown A, Ellison J, Ohno K, Rosenfeld MA, Tagle DA, et al.: Murine model of Niemann-Pick C disease: mutation in a cholesterol homeostasis gene. Science 1997; 227:232–235.

Long JC: The genetic structure of admixed populations. Genetics 1991; 127:417–428.

Lopis S: Incidence of cholelithiasis in Bantu. Clin Proc 1947; 6:338–347.

Loria P, Bozzoli M, Concari M, Guicciardi ME, Carubbi F, Bertolotti M, Piani D, Nistri A, Angelico M, Romani M, et al.: Effect of taurohyodeoxycholic acid on biliary lipid secretion in humans. Hepatology 1997; 6:1306–1314.

Low-Beer TS: Nutrition and cholesterol gallstones. Proc Nutr Soc 1985; 44:127–143.

Low-Beer TS, Pomare EW: Can colonic bacterial metabolism predispose to cholesterol gall stones? BMJ 1975; i:438–440.

Lowell BB: PPARγ: an essential rgulatory of adipogenesis and modulator of fat cell function. Cell 1999; 99:239–242.

Lowenfels AB: Gallstones and the risk of cancer. Gut 1980; 21:1090–1092.

Lowenfels AB: Gallstones and glaciers: the stone that came in from the cold. Lancet 1988; i:1385–1386.

Lowenfels AB, Lindstrom CG, Conway MJ, Hastings PR: Gallstones and risk of gallbladder cancer. J Natl Cancer Inst 1985; 75:77–80.

Lu TT, Makishima M, Repa JJ, Schoonjans K, Kerr TA, Auwerx J, Mangelsdorf DJ: Molecular basis for feedback regulation of bile acid synthesis by nuclear receptors. Mol Cell 2000; 6:507–515.

Mabee TM, Meyer P, DenBesten L, Mason EE: The mechanism of increased gallstone formation in obese human subjects. Surgery 1976; 79:460–468.

Machleder D, Ivandic B, Welch C, Castellani L, Reue K, Lusis AJ: Complex genetic control of HDL levels in mice in response to an atherogenic diet. Coordinate regulation of HDL levels and bile acid metabolism. J Clin Invest 1997; 99:1406–1419.

Maclure KM, Hayes KC, Colditz GA, Stampfer MJ, Speizer FE, Willett WC: Weight, diet, and the risk of symptomatic gallstones in middle-aged women. N Engl J Med 1989; 321:563–569.

MacPherson BR, Pemsingh RS, Scott GW: Experimental cholelithiasis in the ground squirrel. Lab Invest 1987; 56:138–145.

Magnuson TH, Lillemore KD, High RC, Pitt HA: Dietary fish oil inhibits cholesterol monohydrate crystal nucleation and gallstone formation in the prairie dog. Surgery 1995; 118:517–523.

Mahfouz-Cercone S, Johnson JE, Liepa GU: Effect of animal and vegetable protein on gallstone formation and biliary constituents in the hamster. Lipids 1984; 19:5–10.

Maki T: Cholelithiasis in the Japanese. Arch Surg 1961; 82:599–612.

Makishima M, Okamoto AY, Repa JJ, Tu H, Learned RM, Luk A, Hull MV, Lustig KD, Mangelsdorf DJ, Shan B: Identification of a nuclear receptor for bile acids. Science 1999; 284:1362–1365.

Malet PF: Animal models of gallstone formation. In: Cohen S, Soloway RD (eds). Gallstones, Vol 4. Contemporary Issues in Gastroenterology. New York: Churchill-Livingstone 1985:309–334.

Malet PF, Deng SQ, Soloway RD: Gallbladder mucin and cholesterol and pigment gallstone formation in hamsters. Scand J Gastroenterol 1989; 24:1055–1060.

Malhotra SL: Epidemiological study of cholelithiasis among railroad workers in India with a special reference to causation. Gut 1968; 9:290–295.

Marcus SN, Heaton KW: Deoxycholic acid and the pathogenesis of gallstones. Gut 1988; 29:522–533.

Mardones P, Quiñones V, Amigo L, Moreno M, Miquel JF, Schwarz M, Miettinen HE, Trigatti B, Krieger M, VanPatten S, et al.: Hepatic cholesterol and bile acid metabolism and intestinal cholesterol absorption in scavenger receptor class B type 1-deficient mice. J Lipid Res 2001; 42:170–180.

Maringhini A, Ciambra M, Baccelliere P, Raimondo M, Pagliaro L: Sludge, stones, and pregnancy. Gastroenterology 1988; 95:1160–1161.

Maringhini A, Marceno MP, Lanzarone F, Caltagirone M, Fusco G, Di Cuonzo G, Cittadini E, Pagliaro L: Sludge and stones in gallbladder after pregnancy. Prevalence and risk factors. J Hepatol 1987; 5:218–223.

Marinovic I, Guerra C, Larach G: Incidencia de litiasis biliar en material de autopsias y análisis de composición de los cálculos. Rev Med Chil 1972; 100:1320–1327.

Marks JW, Bonorris GG, Schoenfeld CJ: The sequence of biliary events preceding the formation of gallstones in humans. Gastroenterology 1992; 103:566–570.

Marks JW, Stein T, Schoenfield LJ: Natural history and treatment with ursodiol of gallstones formed during rapid weight loss in man. Dig Dis Sci 1994; 39:1981–1984.

Mårtensson KM: The incidence of gallstones in Sweden. The correlation of gallstones with various diseases and pathologic changes. Ann Surg 1937; 34:650–669.

Massarrat H, Klingemann, Kappert J: Die Häufigkeit der Cholelithiasis im autoptischen Material und ambulanten Krankengut aus Deutschland. Z Gastroenterol 1982; 20:341–345.

Matsushiro T, Suzuki N, Sato T, Maki T: Effect of diet on glucaric acid concentration in bile and the formation of calcium bilirubinate gallstones. Gastroenterology 1977; 72:630–633.

Maurer KR, Everhart JE, Ezzati TM, Johannes RS, Knowler WC, Larson DL, Sanders R, Shawker TH, Roth HP: Prevalence of gallbladder disease in Hispanic populations in the United States. Gastroenterology 1989; 96:487–492.

McConnell RB: The Genetics of Gastro-Intestinal Disorders. London: Oxford University Press, 1966:184–193.

McDougall RM, Yakymyshyn L, Walker K, Thurston OG: The effect of wheat bran on serum lipoproteins and biliary lipids. Can J Surg 1978; 21:433–435.

McMurry MP, Cerqueira MT, Connor SL, Connor WE: Changes in lipid and lipoprotein levels and body weight in Tarahumura Indians after consumption of an affluent diet. N Engl J Med 1991; 325:1704–1708.

Méndez-Sánchez N, Brink MA, Paigen B, Carey MC: Ursodeoxycholic acid and cholesterol induce enterohepatic cycling of bilirubin in rodents. Gastroenterology 1998; 115:722–732.

Menegaux F, Dorent R, Tabbi D, Pavie A, Chigot JP, Gandjbakhch I: Biliary surgery after heart transplantation. Am J Surg 1998; 175:320–321.

Meerman L, Koopen NR, Bloks V, Van Goor H, Havinga R, Wolthers BG, Kramer W, Stengelin S, Muller M, Kuipers F, et al.: Biliary fibrosis associated with altered bile composition in a mouse model of erythropoietic protoporphyria. Gastroenterology 1999; 117:696–705.

Metzger AL, Adler R, Heysfield S, Grundy SM: Diurnal variations in biliary lipid compositions. N Engl J Med 1973; 288:333–336.

Miettinen M, Turpeinen O, Karvonen MJ, Paavilainen E, Elosuo R: Prevalence of cholelithiasis in men and women ingesting a serum-cholesterol-lowering diet. Ann Clin Res 1976; 8:111–116.

Miettinen TA: Cholesterol production in obesity. Circulation 1971; 44:842–850.

Miquel JF, Covarrubias C, Villaroel L, Mingrone G, Greco AV, Puglielli L, Carvallo P, Marshall G, Del Pino G, Nervi F: Genetic epidemiology of cholesterol cholelithiasis among Chilean Hispanics, Amerindians, and Maoris. Gastroenterology 1998; 115:937–946.

Misciagna G, Centonze S, Leoci C, Guerra V, Cisternino AM, Ceo R, Trevisan M: Diet, physical activity and gallstones—a population-based case-control study in southern Italy. Am J Clin Nutr 1999; 69:120–126.

Miller LJ, Holicky EL, Ulrich CD, Wieben ED: Abnormal processing of the human cholecystokinin receptor gene in association with gallstones and obesity. Gastroenterology 1995; 109:1375–1380.

Miwa H, Yamomoto M, Nishida T, Yao T: Transformation of chenodeoxycholic acid to ursodeoxycholic acid in patients with Crohn's disease. Gastroenterology 1986; 90:718–723.

Mok HY, Druffel ER, Rampone WM: Chronology of cholelithiasis. Dating gallstones from atmospheric radiocarbon produced by nuclear bomb explosions. N Engl J Med 1986; 314:1075–1077.

Morgagni GB: Of the jaundice; and of bilious calculi. Letter XXXVII. In: Alexander B, Miller A, Cadell T (trans). The Seats and Causes of Diseases. Of Disorders of the Belly, Vol 2, Book III. London: Johnson and Payne, 1769.

Moschetta A, Stolk MF, Rehfeld JF, Portincasa P, Slee PH, Koppeschaar HP, Van Erpecum KJ, Vanberge-Henegouwen GP: Severe impairment of postprandial cholecystokinin release and gall-bladder emptying and high risk of gallstone formation in acromegalic patients during Sandostatin LAR. Aliment Pharmacol Ther 2001; 15:181–185.

Moynihan BGA: Gallstones and Their Surgical Treatment. Philadelphia: Saunders, 1905.

Müller M, Jansen PLM: Molecular aspects of hepatobiliary transport. Am J Physiol 1997; 292:G1285–G1303.

Müller M, Roelofsen H, Jansen PLM: Secretion of organic anions by hepatocytes: involvement of homologues of the multi-drug resistance protein. Semin Liver Dis 1996; 16:211–220.

Murata M, Peranen J, Schreiner R, Wieland F, Kurzchalia TV, Simons K: VIP21/caveolin is a cholesterol-binding protein. Proc Natl Acad Sci USA 1995; 92:10339–10343.

Nakayama F: Cholelithiasis: Causes and Treatment. New York: Igaku-Shoin, 1997.

Neel JV: Diabetes mellitus: a "thrifty" genotype rendered detrimental by "progress?" Am J Hum Genet 1962; 14:353–362.

Nervi F, Covarrubias C, Bravo P, Velasco N, Ulloa NC, Cruz F, Fava M, Severin C, Del Pozo R, Anetzana C, et al.: Influence of legume intake on biliary lipids and cholesterol saturation in young Chilean men. Gastroenterology 1989; 96:825–830.

Nervi FO, DelPozo R, Covarrubias CF, Ronco BO: The effect of progesterone on the regulatory mechanisms of biliary cholesterol secretion in the rat. Hepatology 1983; 3:360–367.

Newman HF, Northup JD: The autopsy incidence of gallstones. Int Abst Surg 1959; 109:1–13.

Niemi M, Kervinen K, Rantala A, Kauma H, Paivansalo M, Savolainen MJ, Lilja M, Kesaniemi YA: The role of apolipoprotein E and glucose intolerance in gallstone disease in middle aged subjects. Gut 1999; 44:557–562.

Nilsell K, Angelin B, Liljegvist L, Einarsson K: Biliary lipid output and bile acid kinetics in cholesterol gallstone disease: evidence for an increased hepatic secretion of cholesterol in Swedish patients. Gastroenterology 1985; 89:287–293.

Nishina PM, Verstuyft J, Paigen B: Synthetic low and high fat diets for the study of atherosclerosis in the mouse. J Lipid Res 1990; 31:859–869.

Northfield TC, Hofmann AF: Biliary lipid output during three meals and an overnight fast. I. Relationship to bile acid pool size and cholesterol saturation of bile in gallstone and control subjects. Gut 1975; 16:1–17.

Nurnberg D, Berndt H, Pannwitz H: Familial incidence of gallstones. Dtsch Med Wochenschr 1989; 114:1059–1063.

Odom FC, Oliver BB, Kline M, Rogers W: Gallbladder disease in patients 20 years of age and under. South Med J 1976; 69:1299–1300.

Oelkers P, Kirby LC, Heubi JE, Dawson PA: Primary bile acid malabsorption caused by mutations in the ileal sodium-dependent bile acid transporter gene (*SLC10A2*). J Clin Invest 1997; 99:1880–1887.

Oliver WR Jr, Shenk JL, Snaith MR, Russell CS, Plunket KD, Bodkin NL, Lewis MC, Winegar DA, Sznaidman ML, Lambert MH, et al.: A selective peroxisome proliferator-activated receptor delta agonist promotes reverse cholesterol transport. Proc Natl Acad Sci USA 2001; 98:5306–5311.

Onuigbo WIB: A necropsy study of gallstones in Nigerian Igbos. Digestion 1977; 15:353–355.

Osler W: The Principles and Practice of Medicine, 1st ed. New York: Appleton, 1892.

Osman AA: A Study of Dietary Factors in the Changing Pattern of Some Surgical Diseases in the Sudan. Khartoun, University of Sudan, 1973 Dissertation.

Ostrow JD: The etiology of pigment gallstones. Hepatology 1984; 4(Suppl):215S–222S.

Owor R: Gallstones in the autopsy population at Mulago Hospital, Kampala. East Afr Med J 1964; 41:251–253.

Paigen B, Ishida BY, Verstuyft J, Winters RB, Albee D: Atherosclerosis susceptibility differences among progenitors of recombinant inbred strains of mice. Arteriosclerosis 1990; 10:316–323.

Paigen B, Schork NJ, Svenson KL, Cheah YC, Mu JL, Lammert F, Wang DQ, Bouchard G, Carey MC: Quantitative trait loci mapping for cholesterol gallstones in AKR/J and C57L/J strains of mice. Physiol Genomics 2000; 4:59–65.

Park YH, Igimi H, Carey MC: The "mirroring" of gallstones: description of a novel silvering method for determining the surface area of an irregular object. In vitro demonstration that multiple gallstones from the same gallbladder dissolve in unsaturated "bile" at the same rate. Gastroenterology 1982; 83:1071–1078.

Parks DJ, Blanchard SG, Bledsoe RK, Chandra G, Consler TG, Kliewer SA, Stimmel JB, Willson TM, Zavacki AM, Moore DD, et al.: Bile acid: natural ligands for an orphan nuclear receptor. Science 1999; 284:1365–1368.

Parnis RO: Gallbladder disease in Nigeria. A five-year review. Trans R Soc Trop Med Hyg 1964; 58:437–440.

Peet DJ, Turley SD, Ma W, Janowski BA, Lobaccaro JM, Hammer RE, Mangelsdorf DJ: Cholesterol and bile acid metabolism are impaired in mice lacking the nuclear oxysterol receptor LXR alpha. Cell 1998; 93:693–704.

Pence DB, Mollhagen T, Swindle B: Cholelithiasis in the cotton rat, *Sigmodon hispidus*, from the high plains of Texas. J Wildlife Dis 1978; 14:208–211.

Pennington CW: The Tarahumara of Mexico. Salt Lake City: University of Utah Press, 1963.

Petitti DB, Friedman GD, Klatsky AL: Association of history of gallbladder disease with a reduced concentration of high-density-lipoprotein cholesterol. N Engl J Med 1981; 304:1369–1398.

Pixley F, Mann J: Dietary factors in the aetiology of gallstones: a case control study. Gut 1988; 29:1511–1515.

Pixley F, Wilson D, McPherson K, Mann J: Effect of vegetarianism on development of gallstones in women. BMJ 1985; 291:11–12.
Pomare EW, Heaton KW, Low-Beer TS, Espiner HJ: The effect of wheat bran upon bile salt metabolism and upon the lipid composition of bile in gallstone patients. Am J Dig Dis 1976; 21:521–526.
Ponz de Leon M, Ferenderes R, Carulli N: Bile composition and bile acid pool size in diabetes. Dig Dis Sci 1978; 23:710–715.
Ponz de Leon M, Iori R, Barbolini G, Pompei G, Zaniol P, Carulli N: Influence of small-bowel transit time on dietary cholesterol absorption in human beings. N Engl J Med 1982; 307:102–103.
Portincasa P, van Erpecum KJ, van de Meeberg PC, Dallinga-Thie GM, de Bruin TW, van Berge-Henegouwen GP: Apolipoprotein E4 genotype and gallbladder motility influence speed of gallstone clearance and risk of recurrence after extracorporeal shock-wave lithotripsy. Hepatology 1996; 24:580–587.
Poser CM: Viking voyages: the origins of multiple sclerosis? Acta Neurol Scand Suppl 1995; 161:11–22.
Prange I, Christensen F, Dam H: Alimentary production of gallstones in hamsters. 19. Composition of fistula bile from hamster on rice starch diet. Z Ernahrungswiss 1966; 7:59–64.
Puglielli L, Rigotti A, Amigo L, Nunez L, Greco AV, Santos MJ, Nervi F: Modulation of intrahepatic cholesterol trafficking: evidence by in vivo antisense treatment for the involvement of sterol carrier protein-2 in newly synthesized cholesterol transport into rat bile. Biochem J 1996; 317:681–687.
Rains AJH: Gallstones, Causes and Treatment. Springfield, IL: Thomas, 1964.
Rambow A, Staritz M, Wosiewitz U, Thelen M, Meyer zum Buschenfelde KH: Computerized tomography differentiation of pigment and cholesterol bile duct calculi. Z Gastronenterol 1991; 29:137–139.
Raymond M, Rose E, Housman DE, Gros P: Physical mapping, amplification, and overexpression of the mouse *mdr* gene family in multidrug-resistant cells. Mol Cell Biol 1990; 10:1642–1651.
Redinger RN, Hermann AH, Small DM: Primate biliary physiology X. Effects of diet and fasting on biliary lipid secretion and relative composition and bile salt metabolism in the rhesus monkey. Gastroenterology 1973; 64:610–621.
Redinger RN, Small DM: Bile composition, bile salt metabolism and gallstones. Arch Intern Med 1972; 130:618–630.
Reichen J, Karlaganis G, Kern F Jr: Cholesterol synthesis in the perfused liver of pregnant hamsters. J Lipid Res 1987; 28:1046–1052.
Reid JM, Fullmer SD, Pettigrew KD, Burch TA, Bennett PH, Miller M, Whedon GD: Nutrient intake of Pima Indian women: relationship to diabetes mellitus and gallbladder disease. Am J Clin Nutr 1971; 24:1281–1289.
Rennels MB, Dunne MG, Grossman NJ, Schwartz AD: Cholelithiasis in patients with major sickle hemoglobinopathies. Am J Dis Child 1984; 138:66–67.
Repa JJ, Mangelsdorf DJ: Nuclear receptor regulation of cholesterol and bile acid metabolism. Curr Opin Biotechnol 1999; 10:557–563.
Reuben A, Qureshi Y, Murphy GM, Dowling RH: Effect of obesity and weight reduction on biliary cholesterol saturation and the response to chenodeoxycholic acid. Eur J Clin Invest 1985; 16:133–142.
Reuss L: Salt and water transport by gallbladder epithelium. In: Schultz SG, Field M, Frizzell RA, Ranner BA (eds). Intestinal Absorption and Secretion. Handbook of Physiology. The Gastrointestinal System, Vol IV, Sect 6. Washington DC: American Physiological Society, 1991:303–322.
Rigas B, Torosis J, McDougall CJ, Vener KJ, Spiro HM: The circadian rhythm of biliary colic. J Clin Gastroenterol 1990; 12:409–414.
Rodewald H: Zur Pathologie der Gallenblase II. Mitteilung über die Häufigkeit der Gallensteine. Zentrabl Allgemein Pathol Pathol Anat 1957; 96:300–302.
Rome Group for the Epidemiology and Prevention of Cholelithiasis: The epidemiology of gallstone disease in Rome, Italy. Part I. Prevalence data in men. Hepatology 1988a; 8:904–906.
Rome Group for the Epidemiology and Prevention of Cholelithiasis: The epidemiology of gallstone disease in Rome, Italy. Part II. Factors associated with the disease. Hepatology 1988b; 8:907–913.
Rome Group for the Epidemiology and Prevention of Cholelithiasis: The prevalence of gallstone disease in an Italian adult female population. Am J Epidemiol 1984; 119:796–805.
Rose RC: Absorptive functions of the gallbladder. In: Johnson LR (ed). Physiology of the Gastrointestinal Tract, 2nd ed. New York: Raven, 1987:1455–1468.
Roslyn JJ, DenBensten L, Pitt HA, Kuchenbecker S, Polarek JW: Effects of cholecystokinin on gallbladder stasis and cholesterol gallstone formation. J Surg Res 1981; 30:200–204.
Rosmorduc O, Hermelin B, Poupon R: *MDR3* gene defect in adults with symptomatic intrahepatic and gallbladder cholesterol cholelithiasis. Gastroenterology 2001; 120:1549–1552.
Royal College of General Practitioners' Oral Contraceptive Study. Oral contraceptives and gallbladder disease. Lancet 1982; 2:957–959.
Russell DW, Setchell KDR: Bile acid biosynthesis. Biochemistry 1992; 31:4737–4739.
Salsbury C: Disease incidence among the Navajos. Southwest Med 1937; 21:230–233.
Salzer GM, Olbrich E, Kutschere H: Zur Epidemiologie der Cholelithiasis. Acta Hepatosplenol 1970; 17:65–74.
Sama C, Morselli-Labate AM, Cornia GL, Rusticali AG, Taroni F, Roda E, Barbara L: Diet and gallstones. A study on a general population. Dig Dis Sci 1986; 31:433S.
Sama C, Morselli-Labate AM, Taroni F, Barbara L: Epidemiology and natural history of gallstone disease. Semin Liver Dis 1990; 10:149–158.
Sampliner RE, Bennett PH, Comess LJ, Rose FA, Burch TA: Gallbladder disease in Pima Indians. Demonstration of high prevalence and early onset by cholecystography. N Engl J Med 1970; 283:1358–1364.
Sanabria JR, Gordon ER, Harvey PR, Goresky CA, Strasberg SM: Accumulation of unconjugated bilirubin in cholesterol pellets implanted in swine gallbladders. Gastroenterology 1996; 110:607–613.
Sarin SK, Kapur BML, Tandon RK: Cholesterol and pigment gallstones in northern India: a prospective analysis. Dig Dis Sci 1986; 31:1041–1045.
Sarin SK, Negi VS, Dewan R, Sasan S, Saraya A: High familial prevalence of gallstones in the first-degree relatives of gallstone patients. Hepatology 1995; 22:138–141.
Sarles H, Chabert C, Pommeau Y: Diet and cholesterol gallstones. A study of 101 patients with cholelithiasis compared to 101 matched controls. Am J Dig Dis 1969; 14:531–537.
Sarles H, Crotte C, Gerolami A, Mule A, Domingo N, Hauton J: The influence of caloric intake and of dietary protein on the bile lipids. Scand J Gastroenterol 1971; 6:189–191.
Sarles H, Gerolami A, Bord A: Diet and cholesterol gallstones. A further study. Digestion 1978a; 17:128–134.
Sarles H, Gerolami A, Cross RC: Diet and cholesterol gallstones. A multicenter study. Digestion 1978b; 17:121–127.
Sarles H, Hauton J, Planche NE, Lafont H, Gerolami A: Diet, cholesterol gallstones and composition of the bile. Am J Dig Dis 1970; 15:251–260.
Sarnaik S, Slovis TL, Corbett DP, Emami A, Whitten CF: Incidence of cholelithiasis in sickle cell anemia using the ultrasonic gray-scale technique. J Pediatr 1980; 96:1005–1008.
Sauer P, Kloters-Plachky P, Stiehl A: Inhibition of ileal bile acid transport by cyclosporin A in rat. Eur J Clin Invest 1995; 25:677–682.
Sauerbruch T, Stellard F, Soehendra N, Paumgartner G: Cholesteringehalt von Gallengangssteinen. Dtsch Med Wochenschr 1983; 108:1099–1102.
Schaefer O: Eskimos (Inuit). In: Trowell HC, Burkitt DP (eds). Western Diseases: Their Emergence and Prevention. Cambridge: Harvard University Press, 1981:113–128.
Schneider H, Sanger P, Hanisch E: In vitro effects of cholecystokinin fragments on human gallbladders. Evidence for an altered CCK-receptor structure in a subgroup of patients with gallstones. J Hepatol 1997; 26:1063–1068.
Schriever CE, Jüngst D: Association between cholesterol-phospholipid vesicles and cholesterol crystals in human gallbladder bile. Hepatology 1989; 9:541–546.
Schriml LM, Dean M: Identification of 18 mouse *ABC* genes and characterization of the *ABC* superfamily in *Mus musculus*. Genomics 2000; 64:24–31.
Schröder H: Beitrag zuss Aetiologie und Statistik der Cholelithiasis. Strassbourg: Goeller, 1892.
Schull DS, Wagner CI, Trotman BW, Soloway RD: Factors affecting bilirubin excretion in patients with cholesterol or pigment gallstones. Gastroenterology 1977; 72:625–629.
Schwab RG, Theis JH: Annual cyclicity of gallstone prevalence in deer mice (*Peromyscus maniculalus gambelii*). J Wildlife Dis 1989; 25:462–468.
Schwaier A: Tupaias (tree shrews)—a new animal model for gallstone research. Res Exp Med (Berl) 1979; 176:15–24.
Schwesinger WH, Kurtin WE, Johnson R: Alcohol protects against cholesterol gallstone formation. Ann Surg 1988; 207:641–647.
Schwesinger WH, Kurtin WE, Levine BA, Page CP: Cirrhosis and alcoholism as pathogenetic factors in pigment gallstone formation. Ann Surg 1985; 201:319–322.
Scobey MW, Johnson FL, Parks JS, Rudel LL: Dietary fish oil effects on biliary lipid secretion and cholesterol gallstone formation in the African green monkey. Hepatology 1991; 14:679–684.
Scragg RK, McMichael AJ, Baghurst PA: Diet, alcohol, and relative weight in gall stone disease: a case-control study. BMJ 1984a; 288:1113–1119.
Scragg RKR, Calvert GD, Oliver JR: Plasma lipids and insulin in gallstone disease: a case-control study. BMJ 1984b; 289:521–525.
Seedorf U, Raabe M, Ellinghaus P, Kannenberg F, Fobker M, Engel T, Denis S, Wouters F, Wirtz KW, Wanders RJ, et al.: Defective peroxisomal catabolism of branched fatty acyl coenzyme A in mice lacking the sterol carrier protein-2/sterol carrier protein-x gene function. Genes Dev 1998; 12:1189–1201.
Shaffer EA: Abnormalities of gallbladder function in cholesterol gallstone disease: bile and blood, mucosa and muscle—the list lengthens. Gastroenterology 1992; 102:1808–1812.
Shaffer EA, Small DM: Biliary lipid secretion in cholesterol gallstone disease: the effect of cholecystectomy and obesity. J Clin Invest 1977; 59:828–840.
Shaheb S: Cholelithiasis among American Indians. Gastroenterology 1990; 98:251–252.
Shaper AG, Patel KM: Diseases of the biliary tract in Africans in Uganda. East Afr Med J 1964; 41:246–250.
Sheen I-S, Liaw Y-F: The prevalence and incidence of cholelithiasis in patients with chronic liver disease: a prospective study. Hepatology 1989; 9:538–540.
Shiffman ML, Sugerman HJ, Kellum JM, Brewer WH, Moore EW: Gallstone formation after rapid weight loss: a prospective study in patients undergoing gastric bypass surgery for treatment of morbid obesity. Am J Gastroenterol 1991; 86:1000–1005.
Shiffman ML, Sugerman HJ, Kellum JM, Moore EW: Changes in gallbladder bile composition following gallstone formation and weight reduction. Gastroenterology 1992; 103:214–221.
Shoda J, Oda K, Suzuki H, Sugiyama Y, Ito K, Cohen DE, Feng L, Kamiya J, Nimura Y, Miyazai H, et al.: Etiologic significance of defects in cholesterol, phospholipid, and bile acid metabolism in the liver of patients with intrahepatic calculi. Hepatology 2001; 33:1194–1205.
Sichieri R, Everhart JE, Roth HP: Low incidence of hospitalization with gallblader disease among blacks in the United States. Am J Epidemiol 1990; 131:826–835.
Sievers ML, Fischer JR: Diseases of North American Indians. In: Rothschild VR (ed). Biocultural Aspects of Disease. San Diego: Academic Press, 1981.

Sievers ML, Marquis JR: The Southwestern American Indian's burden: biliary disease. JAMA 1962; 182:570–572.

Silver LM: Mouse Genetics. New York: Oxford University Press, 1995.

Smit JJ, Schinkel AH, Oude Elferinke RP, Groen AK, Wagenaar E, van Deemter L, Mol CA, Ottenhoff R, van der Lugt NM, van Roon MA, van der Valk MA, et al.: Homozygous disruption of the murine *mdr2* P-glycoprotein gene leads to a complete absence of phospholipid from bile and to liver disease. Cell 1993; 75:451–462.

Smith DA, Gee MI: A dietary survey to determine the relationship between diet and cholelithiasis. Am J Clin Nutr 1979; 32:1519–1526.

Sobotka H: Physiological Chemistry of the Bile. Baltimore: Williams and Wilkins, 1937.

Spiegel E: Beiträge zur klinischen Konstitutionspathologie. II. Organdisposition bei Ulcus pepticum. Dtsch Arch Klin Med 1918; 126:45–60.

Ståhlberg D, Angelin B, Einarsson K: Effects of treatment with clofibrate, bezafibrate, and ciprofibrate on the metabolism of cholesterol in rat liver microsomes. J Lipid Res 1989; 30:953–958.

Stahlberg D, Reihnér E, Rudling M, Berglund L, Einarsson K, Angelin B: Influence of bezafibrate on hepatic cholesterol metabolism in gallstone patients: reduced activity of cholesterol 7alpha-hydroxylase. Hepatology 1995; 21:1025–1030.

Stampfer MJ, Maclure KM, Colditz GA, Manson JE, Willett WC: Risk of symptomatic gallstones in women with severe obesity. Am J Clin Nutr 1992; 55:652–658.

Staudinger JL, Goodwin B, Jones SA, Hawkins-Brown D, MacKenzie KI, LaTour A, Liu Y, Klaassen CD, Brown KK, Reinhard J, et al.: The nuclear receptor PXR is a lithocholic acid sensor that protects against liver toxicity. Proc Natl Acad Sci USA 2001; 98:3369–3374.

Steck TB, Costanzo-Nordin MR, Keshavarzian A: Prevalence and management of cholelithiasis in heart transplant patients. J Heart Lung Transplant 1991; 10:1029–1032.

Steinbock RT: Studies in ancient calcified soft tissues and organic concretions. III: Gallstones (cholelithiasis). J Paleopathol 1991; 3:95–105.

Sterling RK, Shiffman MC, Sugerman HJ, Moore EW: Effect of NSAIDs on gallbladder bile composition. Dig Dis Sci 1995; 40:2220–2226.

Sternberg PW, Schmid SL: Caveolin, cholesterol and Ras signaling. Nat Cell Biol 1999; 2:E35–E37.

Stitnimankarn T: The necropsy incidence of gallstones in Thailand. Am J Med Sci 1960; 240:349–352.

Stoll M, Kwitek-Black AE, Cowley Jr AW, Harris EL, Harrap SB, Krieger JE, Printz MP, Provoost AP, Sassard J, Jacob HJ: New target regions for human hypertension via comparative genomics. Genome Res 2000; 10:473–482.

Stone BG, Ansel HJ, Peterson FJ, Gebhard RL: Gallbladder emptying stimuli in obese and normal-weight subjects. Hepatology 1992; 15:795–798.

Stone BG, Gavaler JS, Belle SH, Shreiner DP, Peleman RR, Sarva RP, Yingvorapant N, Van Thiel DH: Impairment of gallbladder emptying in diabetes mellitus. Gastroenterology 1988; 95:170–176.

Strautnieks SS, Bull LN, Knisely AS, Kocoshis SA, Dahl N, Arnell H, Sokal E, Dahan K, Childs S, Ling V, et al.: A gene encoding a liver-specific *ABC* transporter gene is mutated in progressive familial intrahepatic cholestasis. Nat Genet 1998; 20:233–238.

Strichartz SD, Abedin MZ, Abdou MS, Roslyn JJ: The effects of amiloride on biliary calcium and cholesterol gallstone formation. Ann Surg 1989a; 209:152–156.

Strichartz SD, Abedin MZ, Safairian EK, Roslyn JJ: Pigment gallstone formation and altered ion transport. Am J Surg 1989b; 157:163–167.

Sturdevant RAL, Pearce ML, Dayton S: Increased prevalence of cholelithiasis in men ingesting a serum-cholesterol-lowering diet. N Engl J Med 1973; 288:24–27.

Sugerman HJ, Brewer WH, Shiffman ML, Brollin RE, Fobi MAL, Linnier JH, MacDonald KG, MacGregor AM, Martin LF, Oram-Smith JL, et al.: Prophylactic ursodeoxycholic acid prevents gallstone formation following gastric bypass surgery–induced rapid weight loss: a multicenter, placebo controlled, randomized, double-blind prospective trial. Am J Surg 1995; 169:91–97.

Sugiyama F, Churchill GA, Higgins DC, Johns C, Makaritsis KP, Gavras H, Paigen B: Concordance of murine quantitative trait loci for salt-induced hypertension with rat and human loci. Genomics 2001; 71:70–77.

Taylor S, Cotton L: A Short Textbook of Surgery, 3rd ed. London: English Universities Press, 1973.

Thijs C, Knipschild P, Brombacher P: Serum lipids and gallstones: a case-control study. Gastroenterology 1990a; 99:843–849.

Thijs C, Knipschild P, van Engelshoven J: The prevalence of gallstone disease in a Dutch population. Scand J Gastroenterol 1990b; 25:155–160.

Thistle JL, Eckhart KL Jr, Nensel RE, Nobrega FT, Poehling GG, Reimer M, Schoenfield LJ: Prevalence of gallbladder disease among Chippewa Indians. Mayo Clin Proc 1971; 46:603–608.

Thornton J, Symes C, Heaton KW: Moderate alcohol intake reduces bile cholesterol saturation and raises HDL cholesterol. Lancet 1983a; ii:819–822.

Thornton JR, Emmett PM, Heaton KW: Diet and gall stones: effects of refined and unrefined carbohydrate diets on bile cholesterol saturation and bile acid metabolism. Gut 1983b; 24:2–6.

Thudichum JLW: A Treatise on Gallstones. London: Churchill, 1863.

Tierney S, Ahrendt SA, Fox-Talbot MK, Booker ML, Pitt HH, LaMorte WW, Lillemore KD: Fish oil reduces biliary cholesterol and prolongs nucleation of human gallbladder bile. Gastroenterology 1993; 104:A380.

Topping DL, Weller RA, Nader CJ, Calvert GD, Illman RJ: Adaptive effects of dietary ethanol in the pig: changes in plasma high-density lipoproteins and fecal steroid excretion and mutagenicity. Am J Clin Nutr 1982; 36:245–250.

Torvik A, Høivik B: Gallstones in an autopsy series. Incidence, complications and correlations with carcinoma of the gallbladder. Acta Chir Scand 1960; 120:168–174.

Trauner M, Meier PJ, Boyer JL: Molecular pathogenesis of cholestasis. N Engl J Med 1998; 339:1217–1227.

Trotman BW: Pigment gallstone disease. Semin Liver Dis 1983; 3:112–119.

Trotman BW, Bernstein SE, Balistreri WF, Wirt GD, Martin RA: Hemolysis-induced gallstones in mice: increased unconjugated bilirubin in hepatic bile predisposes to gallstone formation. Gastroenterology 1981; 81:232–236.

Trotman BW, Bernstein SE, Bove KE, Wirt GD: Studies on the pathogenesis of pigment gallstones in hemolytic anemia. Description and characterization of a mouse model. J Clin Invest 1980; 65:1301–1308.

Trotman BW, Soloway RD: Influence of age, race or sex on pigment and cholesterol gallstone incidence. Gastroenterology 1973; 65:573.

Trotman BW, Soloway RD: Pigment vs cholesterol cholelithiasis: clinical and epidemiological aspects. Am J Dig Dis 1975; 20:735–740.

Trowell HC: Non-infective Disease in Africa. London: Edward Arnold, 1960.

Trowell HC: Hypertension, obesity, diabetes mellitus and coronary heart disease. In: Trowell HC, Burkitt DP (eds). Western Diseases: Their Emergence and Prevention. Cambridge, MA: Harvard University Press 1981:3–32.

Tseng M, Williams RC, Maurer KR, Schonfield MS, Knowler WC, Everhart JE: Genetic admixture and gallbladder disease in Mexican Americans. Am J Phys Anthropol 1998; 106:361–371.

Tsukanov VV, Shtygasheva OV, Gorkovskaya IA, Tonkich DL, Zuev VV, Grichenko NN: Cholelithiasis epidemiology in a Siberian population. Digestion 1998; 59(Suppl 3):560.

Turley SD, Dietschy JM: Cholesterol metabolism and excretion. In: Arias IM, Popper H, Schacter D, Shafritz D (eds). The Liver: Biology and Pathobiology. New York: Raven, 1982:467–492.

Valdiviesco V, Covarrubias C, Siegel F, Cruz F: Pregnancy and cholelithiasis: pathogenesis and natural course of gallstones diagnosed in early puerperium. Hepatology 1993; 17:1–4.

Valdivieso V, Palma R, Wunkhaus R, Antezana C, Severin C, Contreras A: Effect of aging on biliary lipid composition and bile acid metabolism in normal Chilean women. Gastroenterology 1978; 74:871–874.

van der Linden W: Genetics of cholelithiasis. In: Rotter JT, Samloff IM, Rimoin DL (eds). Genetics and Heterogeneity of Common Gastrointestinal Disorders. New York: Academic Press, 1980:313–320.

van der Linden W, Bergman F: Formation and dissolution of gallstones in experimental animals. Int Rev Exp Pathol 1977; 17:173–233.

van der Linden W, Lindelöf G: The familial occurrence of gallstone disease. Acta Genet (Basel) 1965; 15:159–164.

van der Linden W, Simonson N: Familial occurrence of gallstone disease: incidence in parents of young patients. Hum Hered 1973; 23:123–127.

van der Linden W, Westlin N: The familial occurrence of gallstone disease II. Occurrence in husbands and wives. Acta Genet (Basel) 1966; 16:377–382.

van Erpecum KJ, Carey MC: Apolipoprotein E4: another risk factor for cholesterol gallstone formation? Gastroenterology 1996; 111:1764–1767.

van Erpecum KJ, Wang DQ-H, Lammert F, Paigen B, Groen AK, Carey MC: Phenotypic characterization of *Lith* genes that determine susceptibility to cholesterol cholelithiasis in inbred mice: soluble pronucleating proteins in gallbladder and hepatic biles. J Hepatology 2001; 35:444–451.

Van Helvoort A, de Brouwer A, Ottenhoff R, Brouwers JF, Wijnholds J, Beihnen JH, Rijneveld A, van der Poll T, van der Valk MA, Majoor D, Voorhout W, Wirtz KW, Elferink RP, Borst P: Mice without phosphatidyulcholine transfer protein have no defects in the secretion of phosphatidylcholine into bile or into lung airspaces. Proc Natl Acad Sci USA 1999; 28:11501–11506.

Vezina WC, Pardis RL, Grace DM, Zimmer RA, LaMont DD, Rycroft KM, King ME, Hutton LC, Chey WY: Increased volume and decreased emptying of the gallbladder in large (morbidly obese, tall normal and muscular normal) people. Gastroenterology 1990; 98:1000–1007.

Vint FW: Post-mortem findings in the natives of Kenya. East Afr Med J 1937; 37:337–340.

Vlahcevic ZR, Heuman DM, Hylemon PB: Regulation of bile acid synthesis. Hepatology 1991; 13:590–600.

von Bergman K, Becker M, Leiss O: Biliary cholesterol saturation in non-obese women and non-obese men before and after puberty. Eur J Clin Invest 1986; 16:531–535.

Wang DQ-H, Carey MC: Characterization of crystallization pathways during cholesterol precipitation from human gallbladder biles: identical pathways to corresponding model biles with three predominating sequences. J Lipid Res 1996a; 37:2539–2549.

Wang DQ-H, Carey MC: Complete mapping of crystallization pathways during cholesterol precipitation from model bile; influence of physical–chemical variables of pathophysiological relevance and identification of a stable liquid crystalline state in cold, dilute and hydrophilic bile salt-containing systems. J Lipid Res 1996b; 37:606–630.

Wang DQ-H, Lammert F, Cohen DE, Paigen B, Carey MC: Cholic acid aids absorption, biliary secretion and phase transitions of cholesterol in murine cholelithogenesis. Am J Physiol 1999a; 276:G751–G760.

Wang DQ-H, Lammert F, Paigen B, Carey MC: Phenotypic characterization of *Lith* genes that determine susceptibility to cholesterol cholelithiasis in inbred mice: pathophysiology of biliary lipid secretion. J Lipid Res 1999b; 40:2066–2079.

Wang DQ-H, Paigen B, Carey MC: Phenotypic characterization of *Lith* genes that determine susceptibility to cholesterol cholelithiasis in inbred mice. Physical-chemistry of gallbladder bile. J Lipid Res 1997; 38:1395–1411.

Wang DQ-H, Paigen B, Carey MC: Identification of cellular and biliary differences accounting for variations of intestinal cholesterol absorption efficiency in 12 strains of inbred mice. J Lipid Res 2001; 42:1820–1830.

Wang H, Chen J, Hollister K, Sowers LC, Forman BM: Endogenous bile acids are ligands for the nuclear receptor FXR/BAR. Mol Cells 1999; 3:543–553.
Wang HY, Yao BL: The characteristics of cholelithiasis of 166 cases in Xinjiang region. Bull Xinjiang Med Coll 1983; 6:314–326.
Watkinson G: The autopsy incidence of gallstones in England and Scotland. In: Proceedings of the 3rd World Congress of Gastroenterology, Tokyo. Basel: Karger, 1967:157–162.
Watts JM, Jablonski P, Toouli J: The effect of added bran to the diet on the saturation of bile in people without gallstones. Am J Surg 1978; 135:321–324.
Weiss KM, Ferrell RE, Hanis CL: A New World syndrome of metabolic diseases with a genetic and evolutionary basis. Yearbook Phys Anthropol 1984; 27:153–178.
Werner D, Emmett PM, Heaton KW: The effects of dietary sucrose on factors influencing cholesterol gallstone formation. Gut 1984; 25:269–274.
Wheeler M, Hills LL, Laby B: Cholelithiasis: a clinical and dietary survey. Gut 1970; 11:430–437.
White RA, Geissler EN, Adkison LR, Dowler LL, Alper SL, Lux SE: Chromosomal location of the murine anion exchanger genes encoding AE2 and AE3. Mamm Genome 1994; 5:827–829.
Williams CN, Johnston JL, Weldon KLM: Prevalence of gallstones and gallbladder disease in Canadian Micmac Indian women. Can Med Assoc J 1977a; 117:758–760.
Williams CN, Morse JWI, Macdonald IA, Kotoor R, Riding MD: Increased lithogenicity of bile on fasting in normal subjects. Am J Dig Dis 1977b; 22:189–194.
Williams RC, Knowler WC, Pettitt DJ, Long JC, Rokala DA, Polesky HF, Hackenberg RA, Steinberg AG, Bennett PM: The magnitude and origin of European-American admixtures in the Gila River Indian Community of Arizona: a union of genetics and demography. Am J Hum Genet 1992; 51:101–110.
Williams RC, Steinberg AG, Knowler WC, Pettitt DJ: Gm 3; 5, 13, 14 and stated admixture: independent estimates of admixture in American Indians. Am J Hum Genet 1986; 39:409–413.
Wittenburg HF, Lammert F, Wang D Q-H, Churchill GC, Carey MC, Paigen BJ: Genetic determinants of mucin accumulation in the murine gallbladder prior to gallstone formation: identification of susceptibility loci and candidate genes. Gastroenterology 2001; 120(Suppl 1):A-550.
Womack N, Zeppa R, Irvin G: The anatomy of gallstones. Ann Surg 1963; 157:670–686.
Wong MH, Oelkers P, Craddock AL, Dawson PA: Expression cloning and characterization of the hamster ileal sodium-dependent bile acid transporter. J Biol Chem 1994; 269:1340–1347.
Yahiro K, Setoguchi T, Katsuki T: Effect of cecum and appendix on 7α-dehydroxylation and 7β-epimerization of chenodeoxycholic acid in the rabbit. J Lipid Res 1980; 21:215–222.
Yamase H, McNamara JJ: Geographic differences in the incidence of gallbladder disease. Am J Surg 1972; 123:667–670.
Yu P, Chen Q, Biancani P, Behar J: Membrane cholesterol alters gallbladder muscle contractility in prairie dogs. Am J Physiol 1996; 271:G56–G61.
Yu P, Chen Q, Harnett KM, Amaral J, Biancani P, Behar J: Direct G protein activation reverses impaired CCK signaling in human gallbladders with cholesterol stones. Am J Physiol 1995; 269:G659–G665.
Záhor Z, Sternby NH, Kagan A, Uemera K, Vanecek R, Vichert AM: Frequency of cholelithiasis in Prague and Malmö. An autopsy study. Scand J Gastroenterol 1974; 9:3–7.
Zanlungo S, Amigo L, Mendoza H, Miquel JF, Vio C, Glick JM, Rodriguez A, Kozarsky K, Quinones V, Rigotti A, et al.: Sterol carrier protein 2 gene transfer changes lipid mtabolism and enterohepatic sterol circulation in mice. Gasteroenterology 2000; 119:1708–1719.
Zanlungo S, Nervi F: The *ACAT2* gene encodes a gatekeeper of intestinal cholesterol absorption that regulates cholesterolemia and gallstone disease. Hepatology 2001; 33:760–761.
Zschoch H: Die Häufigkeit von Gallensteinen und ihre Kombination mit anderen Befunden. Dtsch Z Verdau Stoffwechselkr 1965; 24:145–159.

17 Chronic Liver Disease

ALBERT J. CZAJA

Chronic liver disease reflects a sustained or self-perpetuating hepatic injury of a noxious, immunological, or infectious nature. Each cause of liver damage is associated with its own pathogenic mechanisms; and in each instance, multiple host-related, disease-specific, and environmental factors influence the clinical manifestations and outcome of the illness. The counterbalance of these various factors determines the clinical expression of the disease and distinguishes one patient from another with the same disorder and one disease from another.

As the pathogenic mechanisms of chronic liver disease have been unraveled, genetic bases for susceptibility and outcome have been described. These bases may reflect predispositions that are host-dependent but not disease-specific, such as female gender and human leukocyte antigen (HLA)-DR4 positivity in immune-predominant disorders, or they may reflect disease-specific gene polymorphisms that affect metabolic or detoxification pathways in a very selective fashion. The common forms of chronic liver disease are not dependent on genetic predisposition, and the genetic associations that have been defined are mainly modifying factors.

Alcoholic liver disease is an example of a noxious liver injury that is influenced by genetic determinants of patient behavior and ethanol metabolism. It may also be a model for the investigation of other forms of drug-related chronic hepatitis. Hepatocellular cancer is influenced by host predispositions, environmental factors, and disease-acquired deficits in genetic control. This complex interplay provides a template by which we can understand the bases of carcinogenesis in general. The immune-mediated chronic liver diseases, including primary biliary cirrhosis, primary sclerosing cholangitis, and autoimmune hepatitis, are associated with genetic predispositions that facilitate autoantigen presentation and immunocyte activation triggered by intrinsic and/or extrinsic factors. Perpetuation of the disease requires immune-mediated antigenic cross-reactivities, which are sustained by genetically encoded sites of antigen presentation and recognition. Virus-induced chronic liver disease illustrates the facilitatory effects of the host for clearance or tolerance of the etiological agent. It also underscores the variability of the pathogenic mechanisms associated with viral illness and the ethnic diversity of the host response. In this chapter, the genetic bases for each of these conditions are presented in the hope of improving diagnosis and therapy and stimulating future research.

ALCOHOLIC LIVER DISEASE

Alcoholic liver disease is the most common cause of cirrhosis in the Western world, accounting for 44% of deaths from cirrhosis in the United States (U.S. Department of Health and Human Services, 1993; Grant et al., 1994). It may also be the most frequent type of familial liver disease. The risk of liver injury increases with consumption, and the threshold for damage is 80 g of ethanol per day in men and 20 g per day in women (Lelback, 1975). Women are more susceptible to alcoholic liver injury than men, and blacks progress to cirrhosis more frequently than non-blacks (Frezza et al., 1990). Only 20% of men who consume alcohol beyond the risk threshold develop cirrhosis (Lelback, 1975). The effects of gender, race, and consumption on the risk for liver disease probably reflect genetic differences in alcohol metabolism. Nutritional factors and coexistent viral infections also impact on this risk.

The diagnosis of alcoholic liver disease requires a compatible clinical history and histological evidence of predominantly macrovesicular steatosis, hepatocyte necrosis, and lobular infiltration with polymorphonuclear leukocytes (Diehl et al., 1988). Condensations of cytoskeletal intermediary filaments may appear as eosinophilic fibrillar material within hepatocytes (Mallory bodies or alcoholic hyaline), and collagen deposition around the terminal hepatic venules and within sinusoids typifies the injury. Cirrhosis can develop without the intermediate stage of alcoholic hepatitis, and this progression probably relates to the fibrogenic properties of acetaldehyde. The histological pattern of alcoholic liver disease is not pathognomonic. Obesity-related or diabetes-associated steatohepatitis, drug-induced chronic liver disease, bacterial overgrowth syndromes, and jejunoileal bypass surgery for morbid obesity can produce similar changes (Sheth et al., 1997).

Genetic Aspects of Alcoholism

Multiple studies in monozygotic and dizygotic twins have demonstrated a genetic basis for alcoholism, and heritability estimates range from 0.3 to 0.6 for amount and frequency of alcohol consumed (Lumeng and Crabb, 1994). Adoption studies have supported the concept of an inheritable behavioral pattern that is alcohol-seeking. Indeed, 18% of adoptees with at least one alcoholic biological parent become alcoholic compared to only 5% of adoptees without this risk (Goodwin et al., 1973).

Gender also influences the risk for alcoholism, and studies in adopted women have indicated a higher frequency of alcoholism in the adoptees of alcoholic mothers than alcoholic fathers (Bohman et al., 1981). In contrast, severe alcohol abuse characterized by uninhibited behavior and/or criminality is limited to men, and it is nine times more common in sons of alcoholic fathers than sons of nonalcoholic fathers (Bohman et al., 1984).

Animal studies further support the hypothesis of a genetic influence on alcohol consumption (Lumeng and Crabb, 1994). Rats can be bred for high and low voluntary alcohol ingestion, and studies have demonstrated that the heavy drinkers seek ethanol mainly for its central nervous system effects (Lumeng et al., 1988). Alcohol-preferring lines have a deficiency in the neurotransmitters implicated in the reward areas of the brain (ventral tegmental area, lateral hypothalamus, nucleus accumbens, and medial prefrontal cortex), and lower than normal levels of serotonin and 5-hydroxyindoleacetic acid in these areas may affect alcohol preference (McBride et al., 1991). Indeed, ethanol stimulates the release of dopamine in the brain, and decreased dopaminergic signals or higher than normal densities of receptors responsive to γ-aminobutyric acid in the nucleus accumbens may influence the desire for alcohol. The genes regulating the sensitivities and densities of brain neurotransmitters and their receptors have not been defined.

Genetic Aspects of Alcoholic Liver Disease

Susceptibility to alcoholic liver disease has a genetic predisposition that is separate from the susceptibility to alcoholism. Concordance rates for alcoholic psychosis (21.1 vs. 6.0) and liver cirrhosis (14.6 vs. 5.4) are higher among male monozygotic twins than among male dizygotic twins (Hrubec et al., 1981). Concordance for alcoholism, however, is similar among twin pairs, and the greater concordance for a pathological outcome among monozygotic twins favors a genetic predisposition for the organ-specific complications of alcoholism. The low frequency of cirrhosis among heavy drinkers of alcohol (10%–20%) also suggests a separate genetic basis for a pathological outcome in some patients (Sorensen et al., 1984). This predilection does not refute a dose–response relationship between the amount of alcohol ingested and the risk of advanced liver disease (Lelback, 1975), but it does suggest that host-related factors modify individual susceptibility to alcohol injury.

Genes that regulate alcohol metabolism and tolerance, fibrogenesis, display of histocompatibility antigens, cytokine release, and lipid peroxidation have been implicated in the pathogenesis of alcoholic liver disease; and susceptibility to the biological disease is polygenic (Day and Bassendine, 1992; Bassendine and Day, 1998). The most actively investigated genes affecting this susceptibility are those that regulate ethanol metabolism in the liver.

Polymorphisms of Alcohol Dehydrogenase

The principal hepatic enzyme that oxidizes ethanol to aldehyde is alcohol dehydrogenase (ADH) (Fig. 17–1). Subunits of this enzyme are encoded at five different gene loci on chromosome 4, and polymorphisms can affect the rates of alcohol oxidation, aldehyde accumulation, and propensity for aldehyde-induced liver injury (Day and Bassendine, 1992). Two important polymorphisms of ADH have been described, and they have been designated *ADH2* and *ADH3*. The frequency of the *ADH3* allele is higher in English patients with cirrhosis than in normal English subjects (63% vs. 55%) (Day et al., 1991). This observation has justified speculation that the *ADH3*1* allele increases the risk of aldehyde-induced liver injury because of a faster conversion rate of ethanol to aldehyde. The association between *ADH3*1* and cirrhosis, however, has been weak, even after pooling the experiences of several studies (Day et al., 1993); and it has not been corroborated in other investigations among Caucasians (Couzigou et al., 1990; Poupon et al., 1992; Gilder et al., 1993). Furthermore, the *ADH3*1* allele is significantly decreased in Asian alcoholics compared to healthy subjects; and the rapid conversion of ethanol to aldehyde, which is mediated by *ADH3*1*, may actually have a protective effect against excess ethanol consumption in this population. Indeed, the side effects associated with rapid aldehyde accumulation may be a powerful deterrent against abusive drinking (Chao et al., 1994).

The *ADH2* alleles are common in Asians and rare in Caucasians (Chao et al., 1994). *ADH2*2* has been associated with alcohol abstinence in the Chinese (Chao et al., 1994), and *ADH2*1* has been associated with alcohol dependence and liver disease in the Japanese (Tanaka et al., 1996, 1997). The impact of these alleles in Asian alcoholics, however, may relate more to their association with other enzymes that catalyze ethanol oxidation than to their individual activity (Tanaka et al., 1996, 1997). Consequently, the true role of these polymorphisms in the modulation of alcohol tolerance and toxicity remains uncertain.

The ethnic variations in allelic expression, the rarity of certain polymorphisms in some populations, and the discrepant findings in studies of similar populations have weakened the candidacy of the *ADH* genes as important determinants of alcohol injury.

Polymorphisms of Aldehyde Dehydrogenase

The aldehyde produced by the oxidation of ethanol is catalyzed further to acetate by aldehyde dehydrogenase (ALDH) (Fig. 17–1). ALDH is encoded at four loci on four different chromosomes, and *ALDH2* on chromosome 12 encodes the major mitochondrial enzyme responsible for this conversion (Day et al., 1991). *ALDH2*1* and *ALDH2*2* are the two allelic forms of the *ALDH2* gene, and each encodes an enzyme with different catalytic activity. The *ALDH2*2* allele directs the synthesis of an inactive isoenzyme, and it is dominant over the *ALDH2*1* allele. Individuals homozygous or heterozygous for *ALDH2*2* are deficient in the oxidation of aldehyde, and this deficiency is protective against alcohol abuse. Facial flushing, nausea, and tachycardia are the unpleasant side effects of aldehyde toxicity that modulate alcohol consumption; and they are commonly experienced in Asians, who have a much higher frequency of *ALDH2*2* than Caucasians (Chao et al., 1994). Associations of *ALDH2*2* with the *ADH2*1*, *ADH2*2*, and *ADH3*1* alleles, which encode

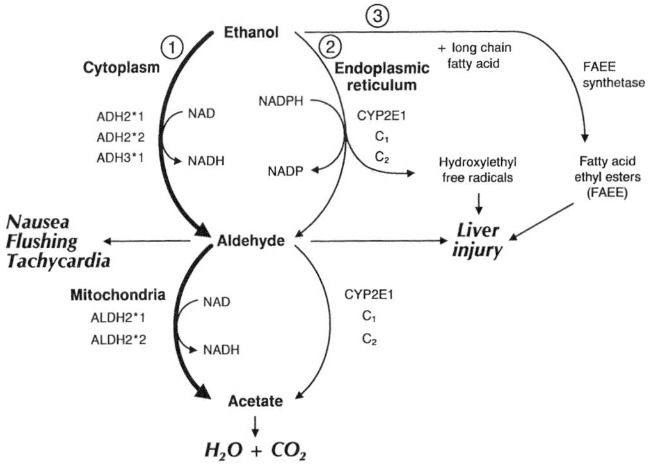

Fig. 17–1. Genetic factors influencing alcohol metabolism and toxicity. The principal metabolic pathway involving alcohol dehydrogenase (*ADH*) and aldehyde dehydrogenase (*ALDH*) polymorphisms is denoted by the *encircled number 1* and the *bold arrows*. Another metabolic pathway involving the microsomal ethanol oxidizing system is denoted by the *encircled number 2*, and it involves the c_1 and c_2 mutant alleles of cytochrome P-450 2E1 (*CYP2E1*). A nonoxidative pathway of ethanol metabolism is denoted by the *encircled number 3*, and it converts ethanol to fatty acid ethyl ester (*FAEE*) by FAEE synthetase. *NAD*, nicotinamide adenine dinucleotide; *NADH*, reduced form of NAD; *NADP*, NAD phosphate; *NADPH*, reduced form of NADP.

the more active ADH subunits for ethanol to aldehyde conversion, are particularly effective genetic deterrents against alcoholism (Chao et al., 1994; Tanaka et al., 1996).

Of Japanese patients with alcoholic liver disease, 15% are heterozygous for *ALDH2*2*, and 25% with the more severe forms of liver injury, including alcoholic hepatitis and cirrhosis, have this trait (Enomoto et al., 1991). A similar association between the *ALDH2*2* alleles and severe alcoholic liver disease has been described in the Chinese, but the difference in the frequencies of *ALDH2*2* in alcoholic patients with and without liver disease has not been statistically significant (19% vs. 12%, respectively) (Chao et al., 1994). These findings suggest that the *ALDH2*2* gene can protect against alcoholism among Asians but that individuals with this gene who drink alcohol are at a greater risk for developing cirrhosis (Chao et al., 1994). They also support the hypothesis that the rate of aldehyde accumulation rather than the rate of ethanol metabolism is important for end-organ damage (Day et al., 1991).

Different cell populations may also have varying thresholds of aldehyde injury and response patterns. Among alcoholic patients in China, the frequency of *ALDH2*2* is higher in patients with esophageal cancer than in those with cirrhosis or pancreatitis (Chao et al., 2000). Among alcoholic patients in Japan, the risk of cirrhosis, but not the risk of hepatocellular cancer, is associated with polymorphisms of the *ALDH2* gene (Takeshita et al., 2000).

ALDH2 polymorphisms cannot not be implicated in the pathogenesis of alcoholic liver disease in whites since the mutant *ALDH2*2* gene is nearly absent.

Polymorphisms of Cytochrome P450 2E1

The microsomal ethanol oxidation system is another pathway for the oxidation of ethanol, and cytochrome P-450 (CYP) 2E1 is its main enzyme (Fig. 17–1). The activity of CYP2E1 is inducible up to 20 times baseline by chronic alcohol consumption, and this volatility can stimulate the production of toxic metabolites and oxygen radicals (Savolainen et al., 1997). Messenger RNA for CYP2E1 is concentrated in perivenular hepatocytes, and this is where the first histological manifestations of alcohol injury appear in tissue (Takahashi et al., 1993). Polymorphisms in the 5′-flanking region of human *CYP2E1* have been described, and two mutations (*PstI* and *RsaI*) are in close linkage disequilibrium. These mutations can increase the transcriptional activity of the *CYP2E1* gene, which in turn can enhance ethanol metabolism, aldehyde concentration, and free radical production (Hayashi et al., 1991). The injurious effect of aldehyde on the liver is intrinsic to the hypothesis based on polymorphisms of *CYP2E1*, but in contrast to theories based on polymorphisms of the *ADH* and *ALDH* genes, the detrimental effects of free oxygen radicals and lipid peroxidation are also invoked.

The rare mutant allele that lacks the *RsaI* restriction site has been termed the c_2 allele, and it has higher transcriptional activity and enzyme activity than the more common wild-type allele, c_1 (Pirmohamed et al., 1995). Studies on American and British patients with alcoholic liver disease, patients with alcoholism without liver disease, patients with nonalcoholic liver disease, and healthy subjects have demonstrated a significantly higher frequency of the mutant c_2 allele in patients with alcoholic liver disease than in alcoholics without liver disease and normal subjects (Pirmohamed et al., 1995). This risk was especially increased in Caucasian individuals who carried the c_2 and *ADH3*2* alleles (Grove et al., 1998). These findings have supported the hypothesis that greater *CYP2E1* activity increases the conversion of ethanol to toxic intermediates and that these toxic metabolites are associated with end-organ damage (Pirmohamed et al., 1995). Similar findings have been reported in Japanese patients, the mutant c_2 allele being found in 84% of individuals with alcoholic liver disease and the wild type c_1 allele in heavy drinkers without liver disease (Tsutsumi et al., 1994; Tanaka et al., 1997).

The mutant c_2 allele of *CYP2E1* is rare in Caucasians, but it may synergize with other promoters of alcohol metabolism, such as *ADH3*2*, to enhance toxicity (Grove et al., 1998). Among healthy Mexican-Americans, the frequency of the *RsaI* polymorphism is significantly higher than in Caucasians, and this may indicate a greater likelihood of alcoholic liver disease in this ethnic group (Wan et al., 1998). A third, less common genetic polymorphism of *CYP2E1* (*TaqI*) has been associated with a reduced susceptibility to alcoholic liver disease. There is no evidence that *TaqI* alters alcohol metabolism, but it may be associated with other "protective" factors (Wong et al., 2000b).

Not all studies have corroborated the association between the polymorphisms of *CYP2E1* and alcoholic liver disease. Among Caucasian patients in the United States who had been screened and found negative for concurrent hepatitis C viral infection, the frequencies for the wild-type c_1 allele were 0.95 for alcoholics with severe liver disease, 0.95 for alcoholics without liver disease, and 0.98 for the general population. Only four of 53 patients with alcoholic liver disease had the mutant c_2 allele (Carr et al., 1995). Among Finnish patients, the allelic frequencies for *PstI* and *RsaI* were so low (0.01) that they did not have a major effect on the inherited susceptibility to alcoholic liver disease (Savolainen et al., 1997). Among Japanese patients, homozygosity for the wild-type c_1 allele was found to be an independent determinant of cirrhosis (Yamauchi et al., 1995) and the mutant c_2 allele was associated with nonfibrotic liver disease (Maezawa et al., 1994; Agarwal, 1997). Healthy Caucasians have higher frequencies of the *RsaI* and *PstI* alleles than healthy Japanese (0.98 vs. 0.81, respectively), and this difference may explain in part discrepancies between Caucasian and Asian studies. It does not, however, clarify the discrepancies between studies in similar ethnic groups (Maezawa et al., 1994; Carr et al., 1995; Yamauchi et al., 1995).

CYP2E1 metabolizes ethanol to aldehyde, but it also converts aldehyde to the less toxic acetate. The affinity of CYP2E1 for aldehyde is threefold greater than its affinity for ethanol. It should, therefore, preferentially metabolize aldehyde to acetate and thereby reduce the propensity for aldehyde-induced liver injury. Its ability to generate reactive oxygen species, however, may be its principal mode of liver toxicity. CYP2E1 is able to metabolize ethanol to a hydroxyethyl free radical, which may induce liver injury by alkylating hepatic proteins and inducing direct metabolic damage (Albano et al., 1991) or by modifying hepatic proteins and rendering them immunogenic (Clot et al., 1995). The factors that determine the balance between the aldehyde-metabolizing protective effects and the free radical–generating toxic effects of CYP2E1 are unknown. Their definition in the future, however, may explain differences in the observed pathological consequences of the c_2 allele in the same ethnic populations.

Acetylator status may also affect the transformation of compounds into toxic or nontoxic molecules, and polymorphisms of the N-*acetyltransferase-2 (NAT2)* gene have been associated with certain diseases. The *NAT2*5* allele, which is the most frequent slow acetylator allele, is decreased in patients with alcoholic cirrhosis compared to normal individuals; and it may be protective against alcoholic liver disease (Rodrigo et al., 1999). The basis for such protection is unknown, but the finding underscores the complexity of interactive and counterregulatory genetic factors that may be involved in modulating disease susceptibility and severity.

Free Radical Production

Free radical production has been implicated in the pathogenesis of alcoholic liver injury, and activated resident hepatic macrophages (Kupffer cells) contribute to this oxidative stress. Reduced nicotinamide-adenine dinucleotide phosphate (NADPH) oxidase is a major source of oxidants due to alcohol, and knockout mice that lack this subunit do not produce free radicals, activate nuclear factor (NF)-κB, generate tumor necrosis factor-α (TNF-α) mRNA, or demonstrate histological injury after chronic alcohol exposure (Kono et al., 2000). Furthermore, delivery of superoxide dismutase to alcohol-fed wild-type rats via recombinant adenovirus can blunt the manifestations of alcohol injury (Wheeler et al., 2001). These findings support the hypotheses that oxidant production is critical for liver damage and that gene delivery of antioxidant enzymes can prevent or treat the process. They also suggest other mechanisms whereby genetic differences in oxidant production and clearance may influence end-organ effects.

A genetic dimorphism encodes for either alanine or valine in the mitochondrial targeting sequence of manganese superoxide dismutase. Patients homozygous for alanine have a threefold increase in the risk of microvesicular steatosis and a 6- to 10-fold increase in the risk of alcoholic hepatitis and cirrhosis compared to patients with the valine genotype (Degoul et al., 2001). This finding suggests that genetic factors may influence functional differences in superoxide dismutase activity and thereby affect disease severity. Similarly, the release of proinflammatory cytokines from Kupffer cells that have been activated by gut-derived endotoxins may be affected by a polymorphism in the promoter region of the *CD14* gene, which encodes for endotoxin receptor. Patients with a thymine (T) for cytosine (C) substitution at position −159 in the promoter region of the *CD14* gene more commonly have advanced alcoholic liver disease and cirrhosis than patients with other genotypes. The risk for cirrhosis was especially high in individuals homozygous for the T allele (Jarvelainen et al., 2001). Other factors that influence oxidative stress may have a genetic basis, and they need to be defined before the interactive network causing liver injury is fully understood.

Polymorphisms of the Tumor Necrosis Factor Gene

TNF-α is cytotoxic to hepatocytes in experimental liver injury (McClain et al., 1993) and in humans with cancer (Schilling et al., 1992). Furthermore, it has been associated with liver injury during excessive alcohol consumption (McClain et al., 1993). Expression of mRNA for the TNF receptors p55 and p75 is significantly greater in patients with severe alcoholic cirrhosis than in healthy controls or patients with well-compensated cirrhosis (Hanck et al., 2000). Furthermore, knockout mice lacking TNF receptor-1 do not develop liver injury after long-term enteral feeding with ethanol, in contrast to wild-type mice and those lacking TNF receptor-2 (Yin et al., 1999). These findings have enhanced the candidacy of TNF-α as a mediator of alcoholic liver injury via the TNF receptor-1 pathway and its gene as a determinant of individual susceptibility to alcoholic liver disease (Grove et al., 1997; Yin et al., 1999).

Monocyte NF-κB is a potent transcription factor for the production of TNF-α, and endotoxin has been shown to increase its activity. Monocytes from patients with alcoholic hepatitis have significantly greater spontaneous NF-κB activity than monocytes from normal subjects and a greater response to endotoxin (Hill et al., 2000). These differences in constitutive and inducible NF-κB activity and TNF-α production in alcoholic liver disease may also reflect genetic factors.

Two polymorphisms have been described in the promoter region of the gene that encodes TNF-α (Wilson et al., 1993; D'Alfonso et al., 1994). Heterozygosity for the polymorphism, *TNFA-A*, has been associated more commonly with steatohepatitis than the wild-type allele (69% vs. 36%), and among patients with cirrhosis, heterozygosity for the *TNFA-A* allele is more frequent than heterozygosity for other alleles (92% vs. 77%) (Grove et al., 1997). The association between *TNFA-A* and alcoholic liver injury, however, has not been strong, and there have been no confirmatory studies.

The mechanisms of liver injury facilitated by *TNFA-A* are unknown, but they may involve increased transcription of TNF-α and induction of oxidative stress (Adamson et al., 1992) or apoptosis (Wright et al., 1992). Alternatively, *TNFA-A* may be in linkage disequilibrium with other genes that regulate more important cytotoxic mechanisms; and in this fashion, it may be a surrogate marker for these mechanisms rather than an effector of liver cell injury (Grove et al., 1997). Further study is warranted mainly because the polymorphism offers an alternative explanation for the genetic basis of alcoholic liver disease among Caucasians, in whom polymorphisms for genes that encode ADH, ALDH, and CYP2E1 are rare.

Cytokines

Interleukin (IL)-1β and IL-10 have been implicated in alcoholic liver injury, and the genes that encode these cytokines may modulate this effect (von Baehr et al., 2000). IL-1β is important in the inflammatory response, and serum levels are increased in alcoholic hepatitis and cirrhosis. The *IL-1β* gene has two polymorphisms, located at position −511 in the promoter region and +3953 in exon 5. Alcoholic patients in Japan who are carriers of the −511 allele have cirrhosis more commonly than alcoholic patients with liver disease but not cirrhosis, heavy drinkers without liver disease, and healthy individuals (Takamatsu et al., 2000). Furthermore, heterozygosity for a polymorphism of the *IL-1 receptor antagonist* gene (*IL-1RN*) has been associated with an increased frequency of fibrosis in Japanese alcoholics, despite a lower cumulative alcohol intake, than in alcoholics homozygous for the allele (Takamatsu et al., 1998). The same polymorphism is also overrepresented in Spanish alcoholics compared to nonalcoholics. Among the Spanish subjects, however, the polymorphism correlated with alcoholism in men rather than cirrhosis (Pastor et al., 2000).

IL-10 has anti-inflammatory, anti-immune, and antifibrotic actions; and polymorphisms that encode it may affect its secretion and actions. The polymorphism involving an adenine for cytosine substitution at position −627 in the promoter region is associated with low IL-10 expression, and its presence would be expected to enhance the inflammatory, immune-mediated, and/or profibrotic mechanisms of alcohol-induced liver injury. Among English patients, this expectation has been supported by a higher frequency of the adenine allele in drinkers with advanced liver disease compared to drinkers with no or mild disease and healthy controls (Grove et al., 2000).

The genetic effects on cytokine secretion and function in various disease states are being unraveled, and other associations are likely to be described in alcoholic liver disease. These effects can potentiate mechanisms of injury and characterize a host predisposition for a certain outcome, but they are not essential or specific for the disease.

Human Leukocyte Antigens

Associations have been made between the class I and class II HLAs and alcoholic liver disease, but these have been diverse and unsubstantiated. The class I HLA associations have included A1, A2, A9, A28, B5, B8, B13, B15, Bw35, and B40 and the class II HLA associations have included DR2, DR3, and DRw9 (Day et al., 1992). Theories that espouse an important immunological basis for alcoholic liver disease (Zetterman et al., 1981) have been strengthened by reports of an association between HLA-DR3 and alcoholic hepatitis and cirrhosis (Bron et al., 1982). These reports, however, have been contradicted by studies that have demonstrated other (Marbet et al., 1988) or no (List and Glund, 1994) HLA associations. Relationships to HLA in alcoholic liver disease may be fortuitous because of the large number of alleles that are assessed, or they may not be statistically significant when adjustments are made for the multiplicity of comparisons. Consequently, there is little firm evidence that the predilection for alcoholic liver disease is HLA-associated.

Other Candidate Genes

Polymorphisms of the genes encoding the enzymes that catalyze collagen production have also been implicated as genetic determinants of alcoholic liver disease. The restriction fragment length polymorphism of the *collagen* $\alpha 1$ gene on chromosome 17 and the *collagen* $\alpha 2$ gene on chromosome 7 each encode different polypeptide chains of type I collagen (Day and Bassendine, 1992). The restriction fragment length polymorphism of the *collagen* $\alpha 2$ locus has been associated with an increased risk for alcoholic cirrhosis (Weiner et al., 1988). This finding suggests that a polymorphism for the production of the predominant type of collagen in cirrhosis may be associated with increased transcriptional activity and an increased propensity for collagen deposition. This finding has not been confirmed in other studies using larger numbers of patients and controls (Day et al., 1990), but the concept of gene regulation of the mechanisms of collagen synthesis and degradation is an important area of future investigation.

Ethanol can also be metabolized in the liver by a nonoxidative pathway that forms fatty acid ethyl esters (FAEEs). These FAEEs are synthesized from ethanol and long-chain saturated or unsaturated fatty acids under the regulation of FAEE synthetase (Laposata and Lange, 1986) (Fig. 17–1). The pathway has been described in the myocardium, liver, pancreas, testes, and placenta. Its occurrence in different organs provides an explanation for tissue damage in areas that did not contain an oxidative pathway for ethanol metabolism (Lange et al., 1981; Hamamoto et al., 1990; Bearer et al., 1992; Werner et al., 1997). Subsequent studies have not only confirmed the toxicity of FAEE for intact human hepatoblastoma cells but also indicated that it could be synthesized in nonhepatic locations and transported to the liver as a component of low-density lipoproteins (Szczepiorkowski et al., 1995; Spector, 1995). The nonoxidative pathway is probably a minor route of ethanol degradation in the liver, but the FAEEs that are produced can incorporate into cell membranes and affect lipid metabolism (Lange et al., 1981; Lange and Sobel, 1983). The gene encoding for the activity of FAEE synthetase is another candidate for inclusion in the genotype of alcoholic liver disease.

HEPATOCELLULAR CARCINOMA

Hepatocellular carcinoma is a primary malignancy of the liver that typically develops on the background of pre-existent cirrhosis. It is the seventh most common malignancy in men and the ninth in women on a global scale (Parkin et al., 1988). Africa, especially central, eastern, and southern Africa, and Asia, especially China and Japan, have the highest annual incidence (>15 cases/100,000). North America and Europe have a relatively low annual incidence (<5 cases/100,000) (Parkin et al., 1988). In all instances, men have a greater predilection for the disease than women; and in high-risk regions, the male to female ratio averages 3.7:1 (Parkin et al., 1988).

Hepatocellular carcinoma is not an inherited disease, but the propensity for its occurrence and the mechanisms regulating its growth have a genetic basis. Certain types of chronic liver disease have a high risk for malignant transformation, such as genetic hemochromatosis (Niederau et al., 1996) and α_1-antitrypsin deficiency (Eriksson et al., 1989). These disorders are genetically acquired (Eriksson, 1964; Schroeder et al., 1985; Feder et al., 1996), and they carry with them the primary risk of cirrhosis and the secondary risk of neoplasm (Propst et al., 1994). Similarly, host-dependent predilections for chronic hepatitis and cirrhosis related to immunological mechanisms may enhance the susceptibility for primary liver neoplasm mainly because they promote the background liver disease that is requisite for the malignant transformation (Wang amd Czaja, 1988; Czaja et al., 1997b; Park et al., 2000). Emergence of a malignant clone also requires destabilization of the genome of the normal hepatocyte. Multiple alterations in suppressor and promoter genes facilitate this transformation and influence tumor invasion through loss of homeostatic functions and gain of oncogenic activity (Debruyne et al., 1999).

The pathogenic relationship between cirrhosis and hepatocellular cancer is unclear. All forms of cirrhosis have a propensity for malignant transformation (Kew and Popper, 1984), but the frequencies of its occurrence differ according to the etiology of the liver disease (Wang and Czaja, 1988; Park et al., 2000; Wong et al., 2000a). In some instances, the risk of neoplasm may be related to the etiological agent. In chronic hepatitis B viral (HBV) infection, the genome of the host hepatocyte may be integrated with portions of the viral genome that alter its stability (Shafritz et al., 1981). In genetic hemochromatosis, the hepatic iron accumulation may facilitate free radical production and lipid peroxidation (Dabbagh et al., 1994; Britton and Bacon, 1994; Houglum et al., 1997); and in α_1-antitrypsin deficiency, the inability to export the protein product may directly induce liver cell injury (Teckman and Perlmutter, 1996). In each of these instances, genetic factors that perpetuate viral infection or influence the occurrence and/or behavior of the liver disease may secondarily affect the propensity for liver neoplasm. In other instances, the cirrhosis itself may affect the clearance of carcinogens in a nonspecific fashion (Ohnishi et al., 1982) and the risk of primary liver tumor may be related to the duration of survival with cirrhosis (Wang and Czaja, 1988; Okuda, 2000). The low frequency of hepatocellular carcinoma in chronic hepatitis D (Rizzetto, 1983; Govindarajan et al., 1984; Kew et al., 1984) and its high frequency in chronic hepatitis C (Kiyosawa et al., 1990) are examples of how the relative aggressiveness of the liver disease affects the propensity for carcinogenesis.

Two primary genetic bases for hepatocellular carcinoma have been described, and they provide models for the further evaluation of host-dependent and disease-specific genetic propensities for tumor formation in individual liver diseases. Disturbances in the enzymatic detoxification of aflatoxin B_1 are host-derived genetic defects that enhance susceptibility to hepatocellular carcinoma in certain regions of the world (McGlynn et al., 1995). Alterations in tumor-suppressor genes are mainly environmental and/or disease-derived genetic defects that facilitate tumor formation by impairing growth regulation (Bressac et al., 1990; Ozturk, 1999; Buendia, 2000). In the former instance, the host susceptibility pre-exists and the risk of malignancy requires a particular trigger. In the latter instance, the host susceptibility is acquired and the risk of malignancy and tumor aggressiveness depends on the nature of the genetic alterations that are induced (Ozturk, 1999; Buendia, 2000). Both defects can coexist, and the host predisposition for a particular response to an environmental trigger may in turn affect the aberrations that develop subsequently in certain tumor-suppressor genes (Wong et al., 2000a).

De Novo Genetic Susceptibility

Genetic variations in metabolic pathways important in the elimination of carcinogens can affect tumor susceptibility in individual patients. The frequency of hepatocellular carcinoma is higher in certain regions of Asia than in areas of Africa where exposures to HBV and aflatoxin B_1 are similar (McGlynn et al., 1995). These observations suggest that primary population differences in the detoxification of aflatoxin 8,9-epoxide, which is the mutagenic metabolite of aflatoxin B_1, can affect the occurrence of hepatocellular cancer.

Polymorphisms Affecting Aflatoxin B_1 Detoxification

Detoxification of aflatoxin 8,9-epoxide requires glutathione *S*-transferase M1 and microsomal epoxide hydrolase (McGlynn et al., 1995). Deficiencies in the amount or activity of these enzymes can overload the hepatocyte with toxic metabolite, and DNA binding and alteration can occur. Mutations in the *p53* tumor-suppressor gene at codon 249 have been described after aflatoxin injury (Gerbes and Caselmann, 1993), and these genetic alterations may be consequences of a failure in epoxide detoxification (Fig. 17–2).

The isoenzyme glutathione *S*-transferase M1 is polymorphic in humans as a result of genetic deletion (Board et al., 1990), and DNA polymorphisms have also been described for microsomal epoxide hydrolase (Skoda et al., 1988). In each instance, mutation or absence of the gene for the individual enzyme impairs its activity (Brockmoller et al., 1993; Hassett et al., 1994), and this impairment may promote mutagenicity of the epoxide. A higher frequency of mutant alleles for both enzymes has been indicated in patients with DNA damage and hepatocellular carcinoma (McGlynn et al., 1995). Furthermore, the occurrence of hepatocellular cancer was greater in patients with HBV infection and the mutant allele for epoxide hydrolase than in patients with HBV infection or the mutant allele alone (McGlynn et al., 1995). These findings indicate a dynamic relationship between host predisposition, environmental toxins, viral infection, tumor-suppressor gene alterations, and tumor occurrence (Fig. 17–2).

Polymorphisms of CYP2A6 *and Carcinogen Clearance*

The inheritance of other genotypes that affect carcinogen clearance may have similar effects on mutations within tumor-suppressor genes, and their discovery promises to enhance the understanding of the genetic bases for liver tumor formation. In this regard, *CYP2A6* is not only abundant in liver tissue but important in the metabolic activation of liver-specific carcinogens such as aflatoxin B_1, nitrosamines, and 1,3-butadiene as well as various drugs, nicotine, and cotinine. Accordingly, it is another candidate enzyme under genetic control that may affect susceptibility to hepatocellular carcinoma (Raunio et al., 1998). The activity of *CYP2A6* is induced by chronic hepatocellular inflammation, including HBV infection, and this activation may initiate a cascade of events that translates chronic liver injury into tumor formation (Satarug et al., 1996; Kirby et al., 1996) (Fig. 17–2).

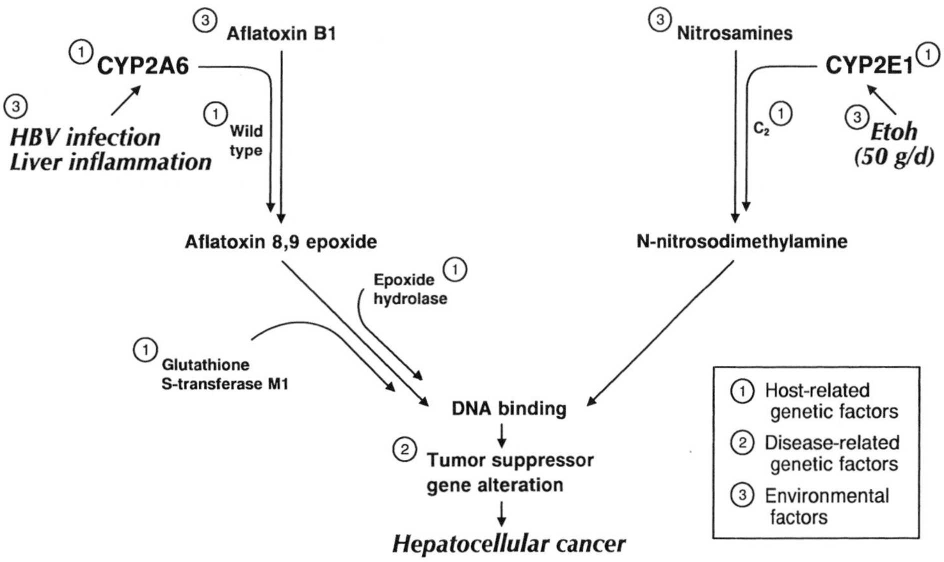

Fig. 17–2. Interactions between host-related, disease-related, and environmental factors in the development of hepatocellular carcinoma. Detoxification of aflatoxin B_1 depends on polymorphisms of cytochrome P-450 2A6 (*CYP2A6*) and the enzymes epoxide hydrolase and glutathione *S*-transferase M1. Homozygosity of the wild-type allele favors mutagenesis of aflatoxin B_1. The potential contribution of ethanol (*Etoh*)–inducible CYP2E1 in the activation of carcinogens is also shown. The c_2 allele has greater transcriptional activity than the c_1 allele, and it may activate carcinogens more readily. The various contributing factors and their interactions are denoted by *encircled numbers*, which indicate their nature. *HBV*, hepatitis B virus.

The *CYP2A6* gene is polymorphic, and two variant alleles have been described (Fernandez-Salguero et al., 1995). Initial studies indicated that individuals homozygous for functional *CYP2A6* were at greater risk of developing hepatocellular cancer than individuals with mutated alleles (Agundez et al., 1995). Subsequent studies, however, have not confirmed the protective effect of mutated alleles (Gullsten et al., 1997; Raunio et al., 1998). The low frequency of mutated *CYP2A6* alleles in Caucasians undoubtedly compromised the statistical power of the small early studies, and further investigations are warranted to better assess their importance.

Polymorphisms of CYP2E1

Ethanol-inducible *CYP2E1* expression has also been evaluated as a risk factor for hepatocellular carcinoma, and the c_2 allele associated with the *RsaI* polymorphism is overrepresented in patients with hepatocellular cancer and alcohol consumption of more than 50 g daily (Ladero et al., 1996) (Fig. 17–2). The c_2 allele has greater transcriptional activity than the c_1 allele, and individuals with this polymorphism may activate carcinogens such as *N*-nitrosodimethylamine more readily (Yang et al., 1990; Tsutsumi et al., 1993). The c_2 allele, however, is rare in Caucasians, and it is not primarily associated with liver malignancy in nonalcoholics. Accordingly, c_2 activity is best considered a genetically acquired but secondary risk factor for tumor formation in heavy drinkers.

Polymorphisms of Aldehyde Dehydrogenase

Polymorphisms of the *ALDH2* gene have also been assessed in alcohol-related hepatocellular carcinoma, and an overrepresentation of the inactive *ALDH2* genotype has not been found in patients with neoplastic disease. Consequently, a genetic disturbance in acetaldehyde metabolism cannot be implicated in tumor occurrence (Ohhira et al., 1996).

Human Leukocyte Antigens

Multiple studies have evaluated the association between HLAs and hepatocellular carcinoma, but no important or consistent relationships have been described in South African blacks (Kew et al., 1979) or in Chinese patients (Chan et al., 1980; Lin et al., 1987; Kam-Tao et al., 1995). However, studies have focused mainly on HBV infection in non-Caucasian patients, and the impact of HLA status on tumor propensity in Caucasian patients with other chronic liver diseases has not been defined.

Acquired Genetic Susceptibility

Primary inactivation of tumor-suppressor genes has been described, and the altered genes may have a germline source. The most common basis for their alteration, however, is chromosomal aberration resulting from exposures to environmental toxins or infectious agents (Fig. 17–2). Gene dysfunction alters the protein product that governs cell replication, and aberrant control of this process facilitates malignant transformation. Disturbances in tumor-suppressor gene function are typically acquired genetic defects (Fig. 17–2).

Aberrations of the p53 *Tumor-Suppressor Gene*

The tumor-suppressor gene product p53 is a common transcription factor that modulates cell-cycle activity, DNA repair, and apoptosis (Selivanova and Wiman, 1995); and 60% to 65% of all carcinomas have a mutation at the *p53* locus (Levine, 1993). The *p53* gene encodes a 53 kDa nuclear phosphoprotein that binds DNA and impairs progression from phase G_1 to phase S in cell division (Martinez et al., 1991). Typically, inactivation of *p53* results from a point mutation, which can have etiological specificity, such as the guanine-thymidine transversion in codon 249 following aflatoxin B_1 injury (Foster et al., 1983; Hsu et al., 1991). Other causes of *p53* inactivation include complexing with viral proteins (Yew and Berk, 1992) and binding to cell proteins, such as oncogene products (Momand et al., 1992). Point mutation at the *p53* locus results in accumulation of an abnormal protein product within cell nuclei, which can be detected by immunochemical staining (Collier et al., 1994).

As many as 67% of patients with cirrhosis and hepatocellular carcinoma may have increased p53 expression within cell nuclei. The *p53* gene product is also commonly overrepresented in nontumorous hepatocytes within regenerative nodules adjacent to malignant tissue. In contrast, increased p53 expression is infrequent in cirrhosis without detectable tumor (14%) and absent in patients without cirrhosis and normal subjects (Livni et al., 1995). These findings indicate a high frequency of the missense mutated *p53* gene in hepatocellular cancer and that a point mutation in the gene can occur in non-tumorous tissue before the development of malignancy. Additional studies in different ethnic groups are necessary to confirm these observations and to define the cause–effect relationship between the gene mutation and tumor occurrence.

The *p53* gene is on the short arm of chromosome 17, and alterations in it have been associated with aggressive tumor behavior (Jeng et al., 2000). The presence of *p53* mutations in hepatocellular carcinoma has been associated with poorly differentiated and anaplastic malignancies and a shortened tumor-free survival period after resection (Hayashi et al., 1995; Piao et al., 1997). Analyses of the patterns of mutation in the *p53* gene in tumor tissue have also been useful in distinguishing multifocal from single-source origins of tumor in individuals with multinodular disease. Furthermore, the basis for tumor recurrence (new vs. metastatic malignancy) can be assessed by determining the pattern of *p53* alteration and assuming that metastatic tumors derived from the same clone of tumor cells exhibit a constant mutation (Oda et al., 1992).

Associations between p53, Aflatoxin B_1, and Hepatitis B Virus

Mutations of *p53* have been most common in tumors of patients from Mozambique, Senegal, and Qidong, China, and they typically involve the guanine–thymidine transversion in codon 249 associated with aflatoxin B_1 toxicity (Unsal et al., 1994). The common association of HBV infection with hepatocellular cancer in these same geographical regions has been recognized, and it may be another cause of gene mutation. Integration of the HBV genome into chromosome 17p11.2–12 near the *p53* gene has been demonstrated (Slagle et al., 1991), and alteration of the *p53* gene in tumor tissue as a result of this integration is possible (Zhou et al., 1988; Goldblum et al., 1993). The overall frequency of *p53* mutations, however, outside of Africa and China has been low; and the importance of virus-induced structural changes in the *p53* gene is probably small, especially since the sites of genomic integration within the chromosome are variable. Indeed, the occurrence of *p53* mutations in other studies has been similar in tumors with and without HBV infection (Unsal et al., 1994). Furthermore, investigations of tumor tissue from geographic regions not endemic for aflatoxin B_1 exposure have failed to find high frequencies of *p53* mutations in patients with HBV or HCV infection (Shieh et al., 1993). Perhaps functional rather than structural changes in the *p53* gene are more common in virus-related hepatocellular carcinoma since gene products of HBV can bind p53 and block its entry into the cell nucleus (Ueda et al., 1995).

Aberrations of Other Tumor-Suppressor Genes

In geographical regions with low endemicity for aflatoxin B_1 exposure and HBV infection, *p53* alterations in hepatocellular carcinoma are unusual (0%–10% occurrence) (Kress et al., 1992; Vesey et al., 1994; Kubicka et al., 1995). Furthermore, the mutations that do occur are different from those in exon 7 at codon 249 (Diamantis et al., 1994; Kazachkov et al., 1996; Kubicka et al., 1997). Loss of heterozygosity for the tumor-suppressor genes *Rb-1 (retinoblastoma), EXT-1 (hereditary multiple exostosis),* and *APC (adenomatous polyposis coli)* have been described in hepatocellular carcinomas from Korea; and these alterations may also affect tumor cell growth. Indeed, multiple suppressor gene defects can accumulate during malignancy, and alterations other than those in *p53* can contribute to the malignant transformation. Accumulation of such defects during the course of malignancy has been associated with large tumors and poorly differentiated histological changes (Piao et al., 1997).

In Japan, hepatoma cell lines commonly have both *p53* and *Rb* alterations, whereas cell lines of pancreatic cancer have mainly *p53* alterations. These findings suggest that alterations in the tumor-suppressor gene *Rb* have tumor specificity and that they are important in liver carcinogenesis (Kaino, 1997). Other studies have supported this possibility by demonstrating loss of heterozygosity for the *Rb* gene in 86% of hepatocellular carcinomas with a *p53* mutation compared to none without a *p53* mutation. The tumors associated with aberrations in both genes were poorly or moderately undifferentiated and the observations suggested that the genetic alterations were interrelated and their effect additive (Tabor, 1994).

Inactivation of the tumor-suppressor gene $p16^{INK4A}$ by hypermethylation of its promoter region has been demonstrated in 73% of patients with hepatocellular cancer, 29% of patients with cirrhosis, and 24% of patients with chronic hepatitis B or C (Kaneto et al., 2001). These findings suggest that loss of p16 protein expression is an early event in tumor formation and that detection of this loss may identify high-risk individuals. The absence of p16 protein has been twice as common in metastatic hepatocellular cancers (74%) than in primary tumors (36%), and this finding has also suggested that inactivation of $p16^{INK4A}$ correlates with poor prognosis (Kaneto et al., 2001). Indeed, loss of p16 protein alone or with loss of Rb protein has been associated with decreased tumor differentiation, vascular invasion, and metastasis (Hui et al., 2000).

The $p16^{INK4A}$ gene encodes two cell-cycle regulators that inhibit cyclin-dependent kinase 4, and it is on chromosome 9p21. Alteration in $p16^{INK4A}$ by hypermethylation or homozygous deletion is more common in hepatocellular cancer than alterations in the other cell-cycle regulator gene, $p15^{INK4B}$, which encodes p15. This observation further strengthens the candidacy of $p16^{INK4A}$ as an important tumor-suppressor gene in hepatocellular cancer (Jin et al., 2000).

Aberrations have been found in chromosomes 1p, 4q, 5q, 6q, 8q, 11p, 13q, 16q, and 17p in hepatocellular carcinoma; and chromosomal gains as well as losses have been described that can affect activation of cellular oncogenes and the integrity of tumor-suppressor genes (Zimmermann et al., 1997). Aberrations of chromosomes 4q and 16q are particularly common in hepatocellular carcinomas (30%–60%) compared to other cancers, and these defects can affect the function of tumor-suppressor genes within these altered regions (Okuda, 1992). Among the Chinese, allelic loss of chromosomes 4q and 16q is not only common in hepatocellular cancer but also associated with increased serum α-fetoprotein levels. These observations suggest that chromosomal aberrations can influence not only tumor behavior but also phenotypic expression, possibly by affecting the gene for α-fetoprotein production (Yeh et al., 1996).

In Australia, allelic loss upstream from the tumor-suppressor gene *CDKN2A (MTS1/p16)*, located on chromosome 9p21–22, may inactivate regulatory sequences necessary for expression of *CDKN2A* or affect a second tumor-suppressor gene proximal to it (Biden et al., 1997). In Japan, frequent allelic losses at chromosome 13q may affect the tumor-suppressor function of the retinoblastoma gene (*Rb*) at 13q14 and the *BRCA2* gene (hereditary breast cancer gene) at 13q12–13 (Kuroki et al., 1995). These aberrations probably occur late in the course of the malignancy, and they have an uncertain composite effect on tumor behavior.

An interesting candidate as a tumor-suppressor gene in liver carcinogenesis is the *mannose 6-phosphate/insulin-like growth factor-II receptor gene* (*M6P/IGF2R*). This gene regulates cell growth by activating the growth inhibitor transforming growth factor-β (TGF-β) and inactivating the growth stimulator insulin-like growth factor-II (IGF-II). Alteration in this gene could increase cell proliferation and reduce apoptosis (Yamada et al., 1997). Dysplastic cirrhotic nodules characterized by enlarged pleomorphic nuclei commonly (63%) have aberrations at the *M6P/IGF2R* locus, and allelic loss is also frequent (90%) in cirrhotic nodules adjacent to tumor. In these latter instances, the same allele is inactivated in the cirrhotic nodule and the tumor tissue, suggesting that both have a clonal origin. These findings indicate that inactivation of the *M6P/IGF2R* allele occurs early in the development of liver cancer and that it may contribute to the formation of premalignant lesions that contain normal-appearing but genetically altered liver cells (Yamada et al., 1997).

β-Catenin

β-Catenin is an essential component of the cell-to-cell adhesion system that maintains normal tissue architecture, and it is also critical for the signal-transduction pathway mediated by Wnt proteins (Debruyne et al., 1999; Terris et al., 1999). The Wnt protein signaling pathway is critical for development and organogenesis, and its disruption has been described in several tumors (Satoh et al., 2000). Linkage of E-cadherin to actin microfilaments of the cytoskeleton requires complexing with β-catenin, and disturbances in this adhesion system can result in an invasive cell phenotype (Debruyne et al., 1999; Carruba et al., 1999). Mutations of the *β-catenin* gene in the region of the serine-threonine glycogen kinase-3β phosphorylation site are common in human and murine hepatocellular neoplasms. In chemical-induced carcinogenesis in mice, chemical-specific mutations are early events (Devereux et al., 1999).

Regulation of free cytoplasmic β-catenin depends on the actions of the *APC* suppressor gene, which downregulates the cytoplasmic level, and the *Wnt*-1 proto-oncogene, which stabilizes the level. Mutation of the *β-catenin* gene or its upregulation by inactivation of the *APC* gene results in oncogenic activity (Terris et al., 1999). Cytoplasmic accumulation of β-catenin upregulates Wnt signaling, which in turn stimulates cell proliferation and inhibition of apoptosis (Morin et al., 1997; Morin, 1999). Nineteen percent of hepatocellular carcinomas have alterations in the *β-catenin* gene, and nuclear accumulation of the protein can be demonstrated by immunohistochemical methods. Gene mutations have been demonstrated in the hepatocellular cancers of cirrhotic and noncirrhotic patients but not in fibrolamellar carcinomas, suggesting that they have tumor-type specificity (Terris et al., 1999).

Axin is a scaffolding protein which facilitates phosphorylation of β-catenin, and it is encoded by *AXIN1* (Clevers, 2000). *AXIN1* is mutated in hepatoma cell lines and primary hepatocellular cancer, and loss of functional axin leads to nuclear accumulation of β-catenin, which in turn upregulates downstream genes that stimulate cell proliferation. Transfer of *AXIN1* by adenovirus to mutated cells results in the destruction of β-catenin and apoptotic death of the cancer cells. These findings suggest that *AXIN1* may have tumor-suppressor function and that axin may be a treatment option (Satoh et al., 2000). The mutation frequency of *AXIN1* in hepatocellular cancer is low, and other genetic mutations may also affect the Wnt signaling pathway. Future therapies for cancers arising from disturbances in this pathway may include inhibitors of β-catenin activity (Clevers, 2000).

Oncogenes

The role of oncogenes in human hepatocellular cancer is unclear. Early studies failed to demonstrate activation of proto-oncogenes (Nagaya et al., 1987), and later studies evaluating the roles of *ras*, *myc*, and *fos* in liver carcinogenesis demonstrated overexpression in the absence of mutation (Tabor, 1994). Such overexpression may have reflected cell growth that was stimulated elsewhere in the regulatory pathway, including mutations in growth factor genes (*TGF-α* or *IGF-II*) or alterations in tumor-suppressor genes (Tabor, 1994).

Animal studies have been more successful in defining the role of oncogenes in hepatocellular carcinoma than human studies, and mutagenesis of *myc* proto-oncogenes by hepadnavirus insertion has been associated with liver cancer in the woodchuck (Hsu et al., 1988; Fourel et al., 1990). Overexpression of the c-*met* proto-oncogene product (c-*met*) in human carcinomas has refocused interest in this area, especially since it has been associated with an increased incidence of intrahepatic metastases (Ueki et al., 1997).

The c-*myc* promoter binding protein gene *MBP-1* is a eukayotic repressor that inhibits tumor formation by downregulating c-*myc* expression. It is located on chromosome 1p36, and it is ubiquitous in human tissues. Expression of MBP-1 protein is decreased in cirrhosis and, to a greater degree, in hepatocellular carcinoma (Fan et al., 2001). These observations have refocused attention on the possibility that mutations in the *MBP-1* gene may be a step in the cirrhosis–carcinoma sequence.

Undoubtedly, hepatocellular carcinoma is a product of multiple interactions, including environmental and infectious factors, host-dependent detoxification pathways, aberrations in tumor-suppressor gene function, overexpression of growth factors, and activation of oncogenes. The final product is probably a cumulative effect in which the number of interactions and their sequence is important.

PRIMARY BILIARY CIRRHOSIS

Primary biliary cirrhosis (PBC) is a chronic cholestatic liver disease of unknown cause that is characterized by inflammation and destruction of the interlobular bile ducts and the presence of antimitochondrial antibodies (AMAs) (Kaplan, 1987). Multiple AMAs (anti-M1 to anti-M9 antibodies) have been described based on the crude fractionation of mitochondrial proteins (Berg and Klein, 1989), but the major mitochondrial antigens specific for the disease are E2 subunits of the pyruvate dehydrogenase complex on the inner mitochondrial membrane (M2 antigens) (Van de Water et al., 1989a,b). AMAs are the immunoserological hallmarks of the disease, but they are not pathogenic (Krams et al., 1989; Berg and Klein, 1992). AMA-negative syndromes that are otherwise indistinguishable from PBC have been recognized and designated as autoimmune cholangitis or AMA-negative PBC (Brunner et al., 1987; Goodman et al., 1995; Czaja et al., 2000a).

The frequent concurrence of immunological diseases with PBC; its association with hypergammaglobulinema; the common occurrence of autoantibodies, including antinuclear antibodies (ANAs), smooth muscle antibodies (SMAs) and AMAs; the presence of autoreactive liver-infiltrating T cells (Lohr et al., 1993); the aberrant expression of class II HLAs on bile duct epithelium (Ballardini et al., 1984; Spengler et al., 1988); and the failure to define an etiological basis for the condition have justified its classification as an autoimmune liver disease (Kaplan, 1987). Women are afflicted with PBC nine times more commonly than men, and a genetically determined host predisposition for the condition has been established (Miller et al., 1983; James and Myszor, 1990). Alternative hypotheses of etiopathogenesis include *(1)* bacterial and viral infections that stimulate immunological cross-reactions between foreign and self-antigens (molecular mimicry) (Berg and Klein, 1992; Mason et al., 1998) or interfere directly with mechanisms of immune regulation (Talal et al., 1992); *(2)* somatic mutations in the genes responsible for the correct positioning of the M2 antigens on the mitochondrial membrane, resulting in their extrusion on the bile duct surface and presentation as autoantigens (Mackay and Gerschwin, 1989; 1990); and *(3)* disturbances in the sulfoxidation of certain compounds, resulting in the production of hepatotoxic substances of an endogenous (estrogens and monohydroxy bile acids) or exogeneous (chlorpromazine) origin (Olomu et al., 1988). In each instance, genetic determinants of autoantigen presentation and immunoreaction, viral clearance, and drug detoxification may be involved.

Epidemiology and Implications about Etiopathogenesis

The frequency of PBC has been assessed mainly in Europe, and the prevalence of symptomatic disease has been estimated to be 23 per million with an annual incidence of 4 per million (Triger et al., 1984). However, PBC is frequently an asymptomatic disease, and estimates of prevalence have varied greatly in different geographical regions and in accordance with detection methods. Estimated prevalences have ranged from 0 per million in Bilbao, Spain; 40 per million in eastern Scotland; 47 per million in northeast England; 75 per million in Pamplona, Spain; 92 per million in Malmo, Sweden; and 183 per million in Newcastle, England. Among English women over age 18, the point prevalence of definite disease is 302 per million. The mean annual incidence of PBC has also ranged widely from 4 per million to 15.2 per million (James and Myszor, 1990).

The apparent epidemic of PBC, especially in the United Kingdom and Scandinavia, undoubtedly reflects increased awareness and interest in the disease, broad application of biochemical screening techniques, and the relative longevity of asymptomatic patients with early-stage illness (James and Myszor, 1990). Indeed, PBC is still a rare condition only in Africa (Olubuyide et al., 1986). However, its variable prevalence and the regional differences in its occurrence suggest that genetic, environmental, and infectious causes may have contributing or interactive roles in its expression and behavior. Indeed, in one epidemiological study, the clustering of disease around a single water source emphasized these potential interrelationships (Triger, 1980).

Familial Occurrence and Implications About Etiopathogenesis

The presence of immune phenomena in relatives of patients with PBC and the occurrence of the disease in family members of an index case support a genetic basis. First-degree relatives have a high frequency of autoantibodies and hypergammaglobulinemia (up to 71%) (Feizi et al., 1972; Galbraith et al., 1974b; Salapuro et al., 1976; Shibasaki et al., 1990). They also commonly have a defect in suppressor T-cell function manifested as an inability to inhibit immunoglobulin G production (Miller et al., 1983) or undergo concanavalin A–induced transformation (Tsuji et al., 1992). These findings indicate an inheritable propensity for immune expression and susceptibility to PBC, but they do not predict disease occurrence or severity (Fig. 17–3).

The frequency of PBC among family members of cases is at least 4.3% in the United States (Bach and Schaffner, 1994) and 2.4% in northeast England (James and Myszor, 1990). Inclusion of family members with liver disease of an uncertain nature increases the frequency to 14.9% (Gregory and Bassendine, 1994). In each instance, the prevalence of PBC among family members exceeds that in the general population (22–25 per million in Canadian studies) (Villeneuve et al., 1991; Witt-Sullivan et al., 1990), and it further supports a genetic basis for the disease. Mothers, daughters, sisters, brothers, aunts, and cousins have been afflicted; and multiple case reports have confirmed familial clustering in different regions of the world (United States, United Kingdom, Sweden, and Japan) (Walker et al., 1972; Chohan, 1973; Brown et al., 1975; Tong et al., 1976; Fagan et al., 1977; Jaup and Zettergren, 1980; Kato et al., 1981; Bach and Schaffner, 1994).

Familial clustering of PBC can also implicate environmental or infectious factors, and epidemiological studies involving spouses and friends of index cases have suggested this possibility. PBC has been described in a mother, daughter, and unrelated close friend who nursed the daughter; in these cases, an environmental or infectious agent may have transmitted the disease (Douglas and Finlayson, 1979). Cluster patterns (Triger, 1980), AMA reactivity with human and bacterial mitochondria (Baum, 1989), homology between the E2 subunit of the pyruvate dehydrogenase complex of humans and that of *Escherichia coli* (Van de Water et al., 1989b), the high frequency of chronic bacterial infections especially with mutants of *E. coli* (Hopf et al., 1989), recurrence after liver transplantation (Van de Water et al., 1996), and the common (35%) occurrence of retroviral antibodies (Mason et al., 1998) have fostered speculations that an infection triggers antigenically misdirected immunopathic reactions (Fig. 17–3) (Van de Water et al., 1989b; Caldwell et al., 1992).

Antibodies against submitochondrial particles known to be devoid of M2 antigen have been described in 53% of healthy family members of patients with PBC, including husbands (40%) and husbands of healthy relatives (50%). Furthermore, these non-PBC-specific antibodies have been detected in 63% of technicians who have worked with PBC sera compared to 17% in other technicians and 15% in blood donors. The presence of these antibodies in patients with acute infectious diseases, their reaction to antigens in mitochondrial subfractions, and their predominant immunoglobulin M nature have justified their designation as "naturally occurring mitochondrial antibodies" (NOMAs). In the

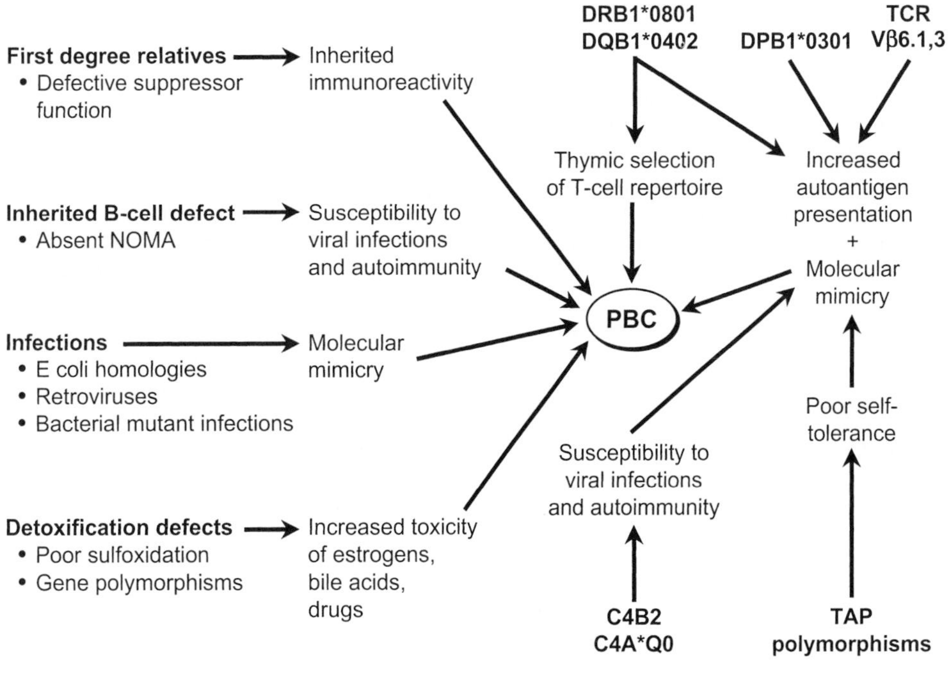

Fig. 17–3. Interactions between genetic, infectious, and metabolic factors in the development of primary biliary cirrhosis (*PBC*). *NOMA*, naturally occurring mitochondrial antibodies. The class II alleles of the major histocompatibility complex that have been implicated in susceptibility are shown, as well as the class III alleles that regulate components of the complement system. *TCR*, T-cell antigen receptor; *TAP*, transporter-associated-with-antigen-processing genes.

study of Klein and Berg (1990), NOMAs were present in only 6% of patients with PBC, and this low occurrence suggested a genetic defect for their expression in individuals with the disease.

Natural autoantibodies contribute to host defense against bacterial and viral infections (Holmberg and Coutinho, 1985; Cohen and Cooke, 1986; Czaja and Homburger, 2001a) and may be involved in the elimination of self-antigens and the maintenance of self-tolerance (Tomer and Shoenfeld, 1988). The high frequency of NOMAs in individuals in contact with PBC, either through direct (patient) or indirect (blood sample) exposure, suggests the transmission of an immunogenic or infectious agent from the PBC source to others. This agent could thereby stimulate B-cell clones to produce natural antibodies as a defense against infection and/or the loss of self-tolerance. In contrast, the absence of these antibodies in patients with PBC suggests an immune defect in the production of NOMAs and a susceptibility for infection and/or autoantigen expression that facilitates development of the disease (Fig. 17–3). This hypothesis for the emergence of PBC requires a somatic point mutation that alters the production of NOMAs in the host and the presence of a transmissible agent that induces NOMAs in relatives and disease in the propositus (Klein and Berg, 1990).

The frequency and significance of NOMAs in PBC cases and their kindred have not been established. NOMAs were not detected in any patients or relatives in a study from the United States, and an inherited deficiency in these naturally occurring antibodies could not be implicated as a basis for the disease. Furthermore, only 4% of blood relatives had AMAs, and these individuals either had PBC or sarcoidosis. The findings suggested a familial predisposition for PBC, but they also indicated that the expression of AMAs in relatives was a manifestation of disease rather than simply a genetic propensity (Caldwell et al., 1992).

Class I and Class II Human Leukocyte Antigens and Susceptibility

The class I and class II antigens of the major histocompatibility complex (MHC) are products of genes located on chromosome 6. Class I gene products are cell-surface molecules involved in cell recognition, and class II gene products facilitate the presentation of foreign and self-antigens to circulating immunocytes. Class II antigens affect immune expression and susceptibility to autoimmune disease, and they have been implicated as genetic risk factors for a variety of autoimmune disorders. As expected, class I antigens have not been associated with PBC (Galbraith et al., 1974a; Bassendine et al., 1985) and class II antigens have been incriminated (Gores et al., 1987).

HLA-DR8 occurs more commonly in patients with PBC than in control subjects (30% vs. 5%) (Gores et al., 1987; Czaja et al., 2001). This antigen is now recognized as a genetic risk factor for the disease not only in the United States but also in England (Mehal et al., 1994a), Germany (Manns et al., 1991), and Japan (Onishi et al., 1994) (Fig. 17–3). Not all ethnic groups exhibit the same HLA association with PBC: HLA-DR3 has been described in conjunction with the disease in Spain (Ercilla et al., 1979) and Denmark (Morling et al., 1992), and other (Miyamori et al., 1983; Seki et al., 1993) or no (Bassendine et al., 1985; Zhang et al., 1994) HLA associations have been reported in different regions of the same country. These inconsistencies have suggested a polygenic basis for PBC and/or a weak relationship with HLA. Indeed, only 20% of patients with PBC are HLA-DR8-positive.

Class III Human Leukocyte Antigens and Susceptibility

Genes of the MHC encode for three classes of protein on chromosome 6, and the HLA phenotype of PBC among Caucasian northern Europeans has been extended by assessment of class III gene products. Genes in the class III region of the chromosome encode the components of the complement system (C2, factor B, C4A, and C4B), and PBC has been associated with the *C4B2* allele in British patients (Briggs et al., 1987). Similar studies among unrelated German patients and two German families with PBC have confirmed the association of PBC with HLA-DR8 and indicated a high frequency of partial C4A deficiency in patients with PBC compared to control subjects (72% vs. 34%). The combined occurrence of the C4A null alleles (*C4A*Q0*) and HLA-DR8 denoted a high relative risk for PBC and suggested that the alleles were either in linkage disequilibrium or separate independent risk factors with an additive effect on susceptibility (Manns et al., 1991).

The C4 component of the complement system is involved in the elimination of viral infections and the clearance of immune complexes. Consequently, its deficiency could predispose to infections that might trigger a heightened immune response. The HLA-DR8 molecule might then be targeted by circulating immunocytes, present peptides that mimic infectious agents, or be linked to another susceptibility gene within the MHC that might affect other immune responses. The coexistence of these genetic determinants would predispose the host to a disease triggered by an infectious agent and perpetuated by an immune reaction (Manns et al., 1991) (Fig. 17–3).

Subsequent studies have weakened this hypothesis by demonstrating that HLA-DR8 and *C4B2* are in linkage disequilibrium and that the extended haplotype of HLA-DR8-*C4B2* does not confer greater susceptibility to PBC than HLA-DR8 alone. Currently, abnormalities in complement activation are not considered to be primary etiological mechanisms in the development of PBC (Mehal et al., 1994a).

Extended Haplotype

DNA-based molecular techniques have refined and extended the HLA haplotype for PBC in Caucasian patients of European extraction. The most frequent allele associated with PBC in this population is *DRB1*0801*, which is in strong linkage disequilibrium with *DQA1*0401/0601* and *DQB1*04* (Begovich et al., 1994) (Fig. 17–3). In British patients, the association of the haplotype DR8-*DQB1*0402* with PBC probably reflects the strong linkage disequilibrium between the HLA DR and DQ alleles (Underhill et al., 1992). These genes may affect susceptibility to PBC by interacting with T-lymphocyte precursors in the thymus and affecting the T-lymphocyte repertoire (Pullen et al., 1989). They may also affect the presentation of processed foreign or self-antigens to circulating immunocytes (Unanue and Allen, 1987) (Fig. 17–3). The strong linkage disequilibrium between the alleles has prevented further definition of the susceptibility locus, and it remains unclear if a single locus or multiple genes are involved (Begovich et al., 1994).

A negative association has been described between PBC and the *DRB1*1501-DQA1*0102-DQB1*0602* and the *DRB1*1302-DQA1*0102-DQB1*0604* haplotypes. These findings suggest a genetic basis for protection against the development of PBC. Since the *DQA1*0102* allele is common to both haplotypes, it may be the most important determinant (Begovich et al., 1994).

Protection may be genetically acquired if the class II allele fails to program T cells within the thymus against the autoantigen and/or impairs activation of CD4 lymphocytes by altering antigen display or recognition.

Similar molecular studies in Japan have also identified HLA-DR8 as a susceptibility factor, but the predominant allele among Japanese patients is *DRB1*0803* (Onishi et al., 1994). This allele is in strong disequilibrium with *DQA1*0103* and *DQB1*0601*, and the susceptibility phenotype *DRB1*0803-DQA1*0103-DQB1*0601* is different from that found in white Europeans. The *DQA1*0102* allele occurs infrequently in Japanese patients with PBC, and it may confer protection in this ethnic group. The HLA DQ locus of the MHC has been associated with antigenic non-responsiveness, and the *DQA1*0102* allele may modulate the immune response through effects on antigen-specific suppressor T-cell function (Hiryama et al., 1987). Clearly, the genes associated with PBC susceptibility are heterogeneous and can vary in different ethnic groups.

Other HLA associations with PBC have been described using molecular techniques, and the allele, *DPB1*0301* has been described in German patients (Mella et al., 1995) and the allele *DPB1*0501* in Japanese patients (Seki et al., 1993). The *DPB1* gene is located at the centromeric end of the HLA complex, and this location may affect its frequency of linkage disequilibrium with genes of the DR and DQ regions (Baish et al., 1993). Indeed, studies have not demonstrated linkage disequilibrium between *DRP1*0301* and HLA-DR8, and a similar lack of linkage may also exist between *DPB1*0501* and HLA-DR8 (Mella et al., 1995; Seki et al., 1993). The findings in the German and Japanese patients, therefore, may identify independent susceptibility alleles for PBC that can sensitize T cells against DPB epitopes, promote aberrant expression of HLA-DP molecules on bile duct epithelium, or associate with other susceptibility genes (Mella et al., 1995) (Fig. 17–3).

In the Japanese experience, 91% of patients with PBC had *DPB1*0501* (85%) or *DPB1*0202* (6%), and a comparison of the amino acid sequences of these two alleles with those of other *DPB1* alleles indicated that *DPB1*0501* and *DPB1*0202* shared a leucine at position 35 of the β1 domain of the DPB1 molecule that was not present at this location in the other *DPB1* alleles (Seki et al., 1993). This finding suggested that a single amino acid substitution could affect susceptibility to PBC, possibly by influencing configuration of the antigen-binding groove of the HLA molecule and the steric relationship between a presented antigen and a lymphocyte receptor (Brown et al., 1988).

Human Leukocyte Antigens and Disease Behavior

The susceptibility alleles for PBC do not have a strong influence on clinical expression or disease behavior (Czaja et al., 2001). Patients with HLA-DR8 have a higher serum bilirubin level than patients without this antigen, and this association may have a prognostic connotation (Gregory et al., 1993). The serum bilirubin level is an index of outcome in PBC, and it may be a surrogate marker for an underlying genetic predisposition, associated with HLA-DR8, that affects disease severity. This extrapolation has not been tested, and the association between HLA-DR8 and prognosis is hypothetical.

In the Japanese experience, all symptomatic patients with PBC had *DPB1*0501* and all asymptomatic patients did not. Furthermore, concurrent immune diseases, such as Sjögren's syndrome, occurred mainly in patients with HLA-DQ3. These observations suggest a genetic basis for disease expression and possibly disease severity (Seki et al., 1993).

Many diseases that occur in conjunction with autoimmune liver disease have HLA associations that exist outside the context of the liver disease (Czaja et al., 1993b). Their presence, therefore, does not necessarily imply an etiological relationship with the liver condition. Indeed, genetic predispositions for immune expression may facilitate the clustering of immune diseases that are host-dependent and not liver-specific (Czaja et al., 1996a). An immune phenotype consisting of female gender and HLA-DR4 positivity has been described in autoimmune liver disease, and it may influence the clinical manifestations of PBC without affecting disease occurrence (Czaja et al., 1998). Multiple extrinsic and instrinsic factors can affect the occurrence and clinical expression of PBC, and its manifestations and behavior may be variably affected by HLA associations.

Transporter Genes

Two interferon-γ–inducible genes within the class II (DR) region of the MHC are the *transporter-associated-with-antigen-processing* genes *TAP1* and *TAP2* (Monaco et al., 1990). Polymorphisms of these genes are few, but they encode membrane transporter molecules that are responsible for the movement of endogenous antigenic peptides across the endoplasmic reticulum. A heterodimer is formed that binds to class I heavy chains and β_2-microglobulin, and this interaction facilitates presentation of class I–restricted antigen to cytotoxic T cells (Monaco, 1992).

Aberrations in the *TAP* genes have been associated with defective antigen presentation in insulin-dependent diabetes (Faustman et al., 1991), and a similar dysfunction could impair the presentation of endogenous (self) antigens to immunocytes in other conditions. Since the development of self-tolerance requires presentation of self-antigens, an inability to do so may facilitate the emergence of autoimmune disease (Fig. 17–3).

Polymorphisms for the *TAP* genes have been sought in PBC, but a statistically significant association with the disease has not been found. HLA-DR8 is in linkage disequilibrium with *TAP1B* alleles in both PBC and normal subjects, but larger studies are needed to fully define the relevance of this association (Gregory et al., 1994).

Tumor Necrosis Factor-β

Transcription of TNF-β is regulated by genes located between the class I and class II regions of the MHC. The allele *TNFB*1* is in tight linkage disequilibrium with the HLA-B8-DR3 haplotype, and it may contribute to the propensity for immune expression (Pociot et al., 1991).

T lymphocytes from patients with PBC produce less TNF-β than T lymphocytes from normal subjects, and the amount of TNF-β mRNA is also less (Spengler et al., 1992). Polymorphisms of these genes may affect transcription of TNF and thereby alter individual susceptibility to autoimmune disease.

The low production of TNF-β mRNA in PBC has not been associated with a particular polymorphism (Messer et al., 1991), and it may be due to other factors, such as IL-2 production, which may affect transcription of the gene (Saxena et al., 1986). The genetic alterations affecting cytokine production and function in PBC are undefined, but variations in gene products at any point in the highly interactive immunoregulatory cascade may affect disease susceptibility and expression.

T-Cell Receptors

Antigen recognition by immunocytes requires an adequate repertoire of T-cell antigen receptors (TCRs), and these receptors are also under genetic control. The predominant cell type in the periportal infiltrate of PBC is the T lymphocyte, and almost all have α/β TCRs (Krams et al., 1990). Polymorphism of the *TCR* genes can alter immunoreactivity and disease expression (Zhao et al., 1994). In PBC, disease-specific alterations in the TCR repertoire have been demonstrated in blood and liver tissue (Mayo et al., 1996).

In the peripheral blood of patients with PBC, the mean level of Vβ6.1,3 expression is greater than in normal subjects, and in the liver tissue of these same patients, the mean level of Vβ6.1,3 expression is greater than in the blood (Mayo et al., 1996) (Fig. 17–3). These findings indicate that circulating T cells in PBC mainly express *Vβ* genes and that the liver-infiltrating T cells have a higher Vβ expression, possibly because of selective expansion and retention in response to the antigenic milieu (Mayo et al., 1996).

The biased pattern of Vβ expression in liver vs. blood is specific for PBC and suggests that a polymorphism in the *Vβ6.1* gene can affect T-lymphocyte receptors, which in turn react to certain antigens and predispose to the development of a particular disease (Mayo et al., 1996). Molecular analysis of the TCR repertoire in different regions of the liver has disclosed a relatively uniform distribution of TCR Vβ transcripts in PBC (Tsai et al., 1996) and oligoclonality of the liver-infiltrating T lymphocytes (Moebius et al., 1990). These findings are also consistent with selective recruitment of T lymphocytes to the liver by a particular antigen and expansion of the clone within the liver tissue (Tsai et al., 1996).

Molecular mimicry between self-antigens and foreign antigens may depend on the predominant TCR profile of circulating immunocytes, and polymorphisms of the *TCR* genes may influence the importance of this pathogenetic pathway in certain individuals (Fig. 17–3). Similarly, genetically determined and inappropriate regulation of T-helper 1 (Th1) and Th2 cytokine responses may affect immunoreactivity in certain patients. Th1 cells are now recognized as the predominant T-cell subset in PBC, and assessment for cytokine mRNA in the liver tissue of patients with PBC has disclosed the presence mainly of interferon-γ (Harada et al., 1997). The genetic bases for particular cytokine responses in PBC have not been determined, but this understanding in the future will undoubtedly add another aspect of genetic control to the evolving theory of pathogenesis.

Genetic Determinants of Liver Toxicity

Inherited defects in metabolic pathways that detoxify endogenous and exogenous compounds can render the liver susceptible to injury patterns that resemble PBC (Gregory and Bassendine, 1994). Eighty-four percent of patients with PBC are unable to efficiently conjugate compounds with sulfate compared to 24% of patients with other liver diseases and 22% of normal control subjects (Olomu et al., 1988). This metabolic aberration may impair the excretion of endogenous estrogens and monohydroxy bile acids (Vore, 1987), as well as certain drugs, including chlorpromazine (Walker and Combes, 1966). Diminished excretion of these compounds may in turn enhance their liver toxicity and induce a PBC-like picture (Fig. 17–3).

Deficiencies in sulfoxidation are not consequences of liver failure but probably reflect polymorphisms in genes regulating the pathway (Gregory and Bassendine, 1994). Additional studies are necessary to confirm these observations (Daly et al., 1993) and to explore the possibility that other polymorphisms similarly alter routes of detoxification and excretion and contribute to the development of PBC.

Polymorphisms of Cytotoxic T-Lymphocyte Antigen 4

Cytotoxic T-lymphocyte antigen 4 (CTLA-4) is a T-cell surface molecule that competes with the costimulatory molecule CD28 for the B7-1 and B7-2 ligands on antigen-presenting cells (McCoy and Le Gros, 1999). By interfering with the second signal of immunocyte activation, CLTA-4 modulates immune reactivity. The *CTLA-4* gene is on chromosome 2q33, and it has a single base exchange polymorphism in exon 1, where an adenine (A) for guanine (G) substitution at position 49 results in a threonine for alanine substitution in the expressed protein. The protein product of the polymorphism may have binding properties for the B7-1 and B7-2 ligands different from those of the protein encoded by genes without the base exchange. Consequently, it may be less effective at dampening immunocyte activation (Thompson and Allison, 1997).

Patients with PBC have overrepresentation of the G/A and G/G genotypes compared to normal individuals (Agarwal et al., 2000b), and these same genotypes distinguish patients with autoimmune hepatitis from normal control subjects (Agarwal et al., 2000a). These observations indicate that clinically distinct autoimmune diseases may be affected by a common set of susceptibility genes outside the MHC. These disease-nonspecific autoimmune promoters may synergize with other disease-specific genetic factors to influence disease occurrence and clinical expression. Other similarly nonspecific autoimmune promoters, such as polymorphisms for various cytokines or adhesion molecules, may also modulate the host response and disease behavior (Czaja and Donaldson, 2000b).

PRIMARY SCLEROSING CHOLANGITIS

Primary sclerosing cholangitis (PSC) is a chronic cholestatic liver disease of unknown cause that is associated with obliterative inflammatory fibrosis of the bile ducts (Chapman, 1990). The disease can be patchy or diffuse, and the bile ducts can be involved at any level of the biliary tree. The diagnosis is usually made by endoscopic retrograde cholangiopancreatography. A normal cholangiogram, however, does not exclude the disease as only the small intrahepatic bile ducts may be affected (Wee and Ludwig, 1985).

The disease is rare, with an estimated annual prevalence of 1 to 6 per 100,000 (Lee and Kaplan, 1995). A male predilection (2:1) is recognized, and 70% of individuals have concurrent chronic ulcerative colitis (CUC) (Chapman, 1991; van Milligen de Wit et al., 1995). PSC is present in 2% to 10% of patients with CUC (Chapman, 1991; Aitola et al., 1994), but it occurs infrequently in Crohn's disease, possibly because total colonic inflammation is rare in this condition (Chapman et al., 1980; Wiesner et al., 1980).

Multiple etiological mechanisms have been proposed; and infectious, environmental, toxic, vascular, and genetic factors may interact variably in different individuals. An immunological basis is suggested by the association of PSC with CUC (Wiesner and LaRusso, 1980), frequent concurrence with hypergammaglobulinemia and autoantibodies (SMAs and ANAs) (Chapman et al., 1980), detection of immunocytes reactive to biliary epithelial cells (McFarlane et al., 1979), association with HLA-B8 and -DR3 (Schrumpf et al., 1982), and aberrant expression of MHC class II antigens on bile duct cells (Chapman et al., 1988). Familial clustering of the disease implicates genetic factors in its pathogenesis (Quigley et al., 1983; Jorge et al., 1987; Isoyama et al., 1995), and the immunoregulatory mechanisms that orchestrate the individual host response and interweave the diverse etiological contributions undoubtedly have inheritable controls.

Familial Occurrence

The familial incidence of CUC is 2% to 29% (Kirsner and Spencer, 1963; Binder et al., 1966; Farmer et al., 1980), but familial PSC has rarely been documented. Many early reports of kinships with CUC described liver dysfunction, but assessments of the liver disease were inadequate for a confident diagnosis of PSC (Singer et al., 1971; Record et al., 1973; Waldram et al., 1975). Familial incidence of PSC is now recognized, but its occurrence is so low relative to the prevalence of CUC among the general population (40–100 cases/100,000) and among family members (2%–29%) that genetic bases alone are insufficient to explain its occurrence (Quigley et al., 1983; Jorge et al., 1987; Isoyama et al., 1995).

Perinuclear antineutrophil cytoplasmic antibodies (pANCAs) occur in 70% of patients with CUC and 82% of patients with PSC (Seibold et al., 1994). Among first-degree relatives of patients with CUC, 30% have pANCAs, as do 20% of first-degree relatives with PSC. In contrast, only 6% of relatives of patients with Crohn's disease have pANCAs. The occurrence of pANCAs is similar in the vertical and horizontal components of the pedigree, and it is comparable in relatives living with the proband and in those living separately (Seibold et al., 1994). Seronegativity for pANCAs in all relatives occurs in only 16% of families with CUC and in none of the families with PSC. Furthermore, seropositivity is present in relatives of seronegative patients and in individuals after transplantation. Titers of pANCAs are not affected by the activity of CUC, progression of the PSC, administration of corticosteroids, colectomy, or transplantation. Indeed, the autoantibody appears to be a genetic marker of PSC and CUC and not a consequence of the inflammatory process (Seibold et al., 1994). The familial occurrence of pANCAs and the independence of its behavior are stronger arguments for a genetic basis of PSC than the rare presence of the actual disease in family members. They suggest a genetically defined susceptibility for immunological expression which is common in family members and which might be expressed later as disease, after the interplay of other environmental, toxic, or infectious factors.

Human Leukocyte Antigens

PSC occurs commonly in conjunction with HLAs, which have been previously recognized as determinants of immune expression. HLA-B8 and -DR3 are present in at least 40% of individuals with PSC, and these same antigens have been described in insulin-dependent diabetes, autoimmune hepatitis, Grave's disease, dermatitis herpetiformis, celiac disease, and Sjögren's syndrome (Chapman et al., 1983; Schrumpf et al., 1982; Shepard et al., 1983). The common occurrence of HLA-B8 and -DR3 in diverse immune disorders suggests that each gene is linked to another gene that actually determines susceptibility to the particular disease. The same HLA phenotype among different autoimmune diseases may also promote similar clinical expressions, which can confound the diagnosis or create overlap syndromes (Czaja, 1998; Czaja et al., 2001).

Early studies in small numbers of patients awaiting liver transplantation indicated that HLA-DRw52a was present in all Caucasian patients with PSC and that the predominant haplotype of PSC was A1-B8-Cw7-DRw17-DRw52a-DQw2. They also demonstrated that PSC had a different HLA phenotype from PBC (Prochazka et al., 1990). Subsequent studies did not confirm the completeness of the association with HLA-DRw52a (Zetterquist et al., 1992), but they did indicate that PSC was associated with epitopes expressed on the DRβ3 molecule, which includes HLA-DRw52a (Noguchi et al., 1992).

Molecular DNA-based techniques have subsequently demonstrated that the DRB3 allele *DRB3*0101*, which encodes DRw52a, occurs in 55% of English patients with PSC compared to 22% of the normal population (Farrant et al., 1992) (Fig. 17–4). *DRB3*0101* is the most strongly associated susceptibility allele for PSC in Britain, and it occurs commonly in patients with a short median survival (9.3 years vs. 15.2 years) and requirement for liver transplantation (75%). These findings indicate that *DRB3*0101* affects not only susceptibility to the disease but also outcome (Farrant et al., 1992).

The absence of DRw52a in many patients with PSC suggests other risk factors for its occurrence. Exclusion of patients with *DRB3*0101* from the analysis of risk implicates *DRB5*0101* as another allele that can affect disease occurrence. Indeed, *DRB5*0101* is present in 53% of patients negative for *DRB3*0101*, and either *DRB3*0101* or *DRB5*0101* is present in 69% of patients with PSC compared to 47% of controls (Farrant et al., 1992).

*DRB3*0101* and *DRB5*0101* each encode a leucine residue at position 38 of the DRβ chain of the antigen binding groove of the HLA molecule (Fig. 17–4). The other *DRB* alleles commonly detected in PSC encode either a valine or an alanine residue at this position. Furthermore, patients with PSC more commonly have two DRβ molecules containing leucine at position 38 compared to normal subjects and a lower frequency of

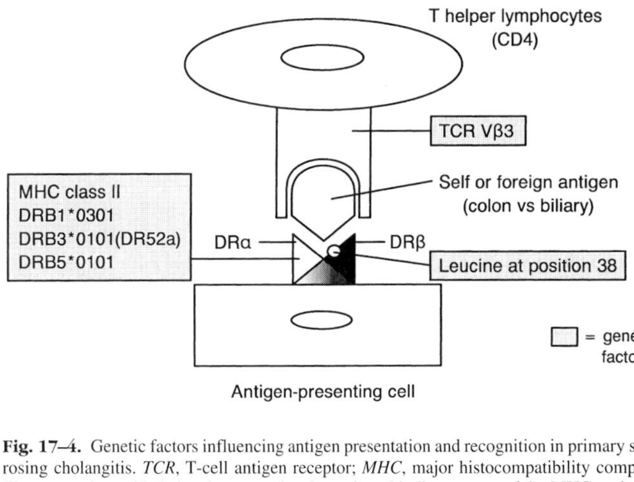

Fig. 17–4. Genetic factors influencing antigen presentation and recognition in primary sclerosing cholangitis. *TCR*, T-cell antigen receptor; *MHC*, major histocompatibility complex. The two amino acid chains that comprise the antigen-binding groove of the MHC molecule are shown as *DRα* and *DRβ*.

two DRβ molecules containing alanine at this position (Farrant et al., 1992). These findings suggest that susceptibility to PSC is affected by a single amino acid residue at position 38 of the DBβ chain. Since the hydrophobicity of leucine and alanine differs and position 38 of the DBβ chain is in the floor of the antigen binding groove of the HLA molecule, each amino acid may affect antigen presentation and/or recognition by affecting the steric configuration of the antigen binding complex. In this fashion, they may confer susceptibility (leucine residue) or protection (alanine residue) (Farrant et al., 1992) (Fig. 17–4).

The haplotype of PSC can be deduced, but it cannot be established without extensive family studies. Three different HLA haplotypes have been associated with susceptibility. *DRB1*0301-DRB3*0101-DQA1*0501-DQB1*0201* is the most common haplotype in patients compared to control subjects (39% vs. 19%) (Farrant et al., 1992). *DRB3*0101-DRB1*1301-DQA1*0103-DQB1*0603* and *DRB1*1501-DQB1*0602* have also been associated with susceptibility to PSC (Spurland et al., 1999; Norris et al., 2001). In contrast, *DRB1*0401-DRB4*0101-DQA1*0301-DQB1*0302* is the least common haplotype (0% vs. 16%), and it is associated with resistance to the disease (Farrant et al., 1992). *DRB1*0301*, which encodes for the serological determinant of DR3, and *DRB1*1301*, which encodes for one of the serological determinants of DRw6, are in linkage disequilibrium with *DRB3*0101*, which encodes for the serological determinant of DRw52a. Consequently, studies based on serological techniques that have found associations between PSC and DR3, DRw52a, and DR6 may have been identifying different aspects of the same genetic propensity. Similarly, serological studies that have identified an association between PSC and DR2 (Donaldson et al., 1991b) may have been recognizing the secondary association of the disease with *DRB5*0101*. Indeed, *DRB5*0101* encodes for one of the serological determinants of DR2.

The alleles encoding for DR4 are less common in PSC than in normal subjects (Czaja et al., 2001), as is the *DRB4*0101*, allele which encodes for DRw53 (Farrant et al., 1992). These negative associations with PSC may define a protective haplotype (Farrant et al., 1992; Czaja et al., 2001) or identify individuals with such an aggressive disease that early death eliminates them from inclusion in adult studies (Mehal et al., 1994b) (Fig. 17–4).

The HLA C antigens have been evaluated in PSC, and an association with *Cw*0701* has been described (Moloney et al., 1998). Amino acid substitutions at positions 77 and 80 of the HLA C heavy chain prevent natural killer (NK) cell–mediated lysis and may affect peripheral tolerance to autoantigens and surveillance mechanisms that clear virally infected or neoplastic cells. Furthermore, MHC class I antigens may alter the targeting activities of cytotoxic T lymphocytes by affecting their receptor function. In this fashion, they may limit the T-cell response to self- or foreign antigens and influence the propensity for an autoimmune reaction (Moloney et al., 1998). The associations of *Cw*0701* with PSC are weak, and they may reflect linkage disequilibrium with the HLA B8-*DRB3*0101-DRB1*0301* haplotype. Consequently, the *Cw*0701* allele may be only a surrogate marker for another prevailing genetic determinant. Since the associations of HLA-B8, *DRB1*0301*, and *DRB3*0101* with PSC are strong and the frequencies of each susceptibility allele, including *Cw*0701*, in PSC do not exceed 53%, it is unlikely that PSC is a single-gene disorder (Moloney et al., 1998). Environmental factors, genes of the MHC, and genes outside the MHC may each contribute to its pathogenesis.

Genetic Predispositions for Disease Expression and Behavior

Patients with and without *DRB3*0101* have similar clinical and laboratory features at presentation. Individuals with *DRB3*0101*, however, have a shorter survival and constitute a greater proportion of patients who undergo liver transplantation. These findings suggest that *DRB3*0101* is a determinant of prognosis (Farrant et al., 1992).

HLA-DR4 has also been implicated as a prognostic factor, and patients with HLA-DR4 have a more rapidly progressive disease than counterparts without HLA-DR4 (Fig. 17–4). The mean time from disease onset to end stage is 43 months in DR4-positive patients and 76 months in DR4-negative patients (Mehal et al., 1994b).

Gender and race are other inheritable risk factors that influence disease occurrence. Women and black Africans rarely have CUC (2% occurrence), but when CUC occurs in black African women, 75% develop PSC. In contrast, only 4 of 162 white Europeans with CUC develop PSC (2%) (Kelly et al., 1997). African origin rather than black race seems to be the principal determinant of susceptibility. Indeed, the frequency of PSC among black North American patients with CUC is only 12% (Simsek and Schuman, 1989). The lower prevalence of PSC in black Americans with CUC than in black Africans with CUC may reflect greater racial mixing in the former group and/or a higher incidence of unrecognized infectious cholangiopathies in the latter group (Forbes et al., 1993).

The specificity of the TCR for class II antigens that are aberrantly expressed on biliary epithelial cells can also affect susceptibility to PSC, and these receptors are genetically encoded (Broome et al., 1990). The TCR is an α/β heterodimer, which consists of a constant and a variable domain. The variable region is encoded by rearrangements of various gene segments that determine reactivity against certain peptide–MHC complexes, and it may be host-dependent (Davies and Metzger, 1983). In inflammatory and immune-mediated conditions, such as rheumatoid arthritis, Sjögren's syndrome and PBC, selected T-cell populations are expanded and have restricted TCR V (variable) gene segments, indicating reactivity to a particular antigen (Diu et al., 1993). Patients with PSC have a higher expression of Vβ3-positive lymphocytes in liver tissue than patients with PBC, and this difference is not evident in the peripheral blood (Fig. 17–4). This finding suggests that an antigen specific for PSC recruits certain types of T cell into the liver, which are encoded by the Vβ3 gene segment (Broome et al., 1997). Absence of the antigen, inadequate display of the antigen, and/or alterations in the TCR repertoire that recognizes the antigen may affect susceptibility to the disease and its clinical expression. Additional studies are necessary to fully define the genetic bases for certain TCR repertoires and their impact on disease occurrence and behavior.

Autoimmune Promoters

Fifty-eight percent of patients with PSC have the *TNF*2* allele compared to 29% of normal control subjects (Bernal et al., 1999). *TNF*2* is a polymorphism in the promoter region of the TNF-α gene (*TNF-A*) that involves a guanine (G) to adenine (A) substitution at position −308. The A variants of the −308 polymorphism may influence *TNF-A* transcription and result in high constitutive and inducible levels of TNF-α. The *TNF*2* allele was increased only in the presence of B8 and *DRB3*0101*, and it was independent of *DRB1*0301* in PSC. These findings indicate that polymorphisms within the HLA class III region may influence susceptibility to PSC in a disease-nonspecific fashion by favoring a type 1 cytokine response and a cell-mediated form of cytotoxicity based on the clonal expansion of cytotoxic T lymphocytes (Czaja, 2001). A similar polymorphism has been associated with type 1 autoimmune hepatitis (Cookson et al., 1999; Czaja et al., 1999).

The MHC class I chain-related (MIC) gene family includes *MICA* and *MICB*, which encode stress-induced antigens (Bauer et al., 1999). These self-antigens can evoke immune responses in T lymphocytes and NK cells, and they may impact on the development of inflammatory and autoimmune diseases. MIC genes map between *HLA-B* and *TNF-A*, and they may interact with other genes in the HLA region to affect susceptibility to PSC. The *MICA*002* allele has a strong dominant effect in reducing the risk of PSC, whereas the *MICA*008* allele has a recessive effect that increases risk (Norris et al., 2001). Only 4 of 112 (4%) British patients with PSC had *MICA*002* compared to 41 of 118 (35%) normal subjects. In contrast, *MICA*008* was more common in PSC than normal subjects (66% vs. 48%, $p = 0.002$), and the risk was highest in patients with homozygosity for the allele (58% vs. 22%, $p = 0.000006$). Stratification analysis demonstrated that the susceptibility associated with *MICA*008* was independent of HLA-B8 and other haplotypes associated with PSC (Norris et al., 2001).

Other polymorphisms of autoimmune promoter genes, including those of the *IL-1B* gene, the *IL-1 receptor antagonist* gene (*IL-1RN*), and the *IL-10 promoter* gene, have not been associated with susceptibility or resistance to PSC (Donaldson et al., 2000). Similarly, the alleles of the *DPB1* locus are not associated with disease occurrence in British patients (Underhill et al., 1995).

Genetic Associations with Cholangiocarcinoma

Cholangiocarcinoma is a major complication of PSC, and the pathogenic mechanisms for its occurrence are unknown. The *p53* tumor-suppressor gene regulates cell growth, and abnormalities in this gene have been associated with cancer. Seventy-nine percent of cholangiocarcinomas express p53 protein, and accumulation of the protein is also evident in neoplastic cells in biliary tissue separate from the main tumor (Rizzi et al., 1996). In contrast, p53 protein does not accumulate in biliary tissue involved with PSC but free of tumor. These findings support the hypothesis that the development of cholangiocarcinoma in PSC involves a defect in the *p53* gene.

Studies in Norway and the United States have strengthened and extended these observations by implicating K-*ras* mutations as an early event in the development of bile duct cancer. In Norway, K-*ras* mutations were found in 33% of tumors, especially in women (Boberg et al., 2000). In the United States, patients with tumors containing a K-*ras* mutation had shortened survival (Ahrendt et al., 2000). The overall frequency of K-*ras* mutations or p53 accumulation in the Norwegian population was 48% in tumor tissue compared to none of the control samples. K-*ras* mutations have also been detected in the bile of 30% of patients with PSC. Tumors or dysplasia have occurred only in the group with K-*ras* mutations in bile, though tumor occurrence has been infrequent and follow-up has been limited (Kubicka et al., 2001).

The tumor-suppressor gene *p16* has also been implicated in cholangiocarcinoma (Ahrendt et al., 1999). Allelic loss at chromosome 9p21 was present in 90% of tumors, and methylation of the *p16 promoter gene* was detected in 25%. These findings emphasize that multiple genetic abnormalities are common in different malignant transformations, the gene defects are similar in various tumors, and the final pathway of oncogenesis may be independent of the tumor type.

AUTOIMMUNE HEPATITIS

Autoimmune hepatitis is an inflammation of the liver of unknown cause that is characterized by interface hepatitis on histological examination, hypergammaglobulinemia, and autoantibodies (Czaja, 1984). The typical morphological changes include portal plasma cell infiltration, moderate to severe interface hepatitis, and panacinar hepatitis in the absence of steatosis, portal lymphoid aggregates, and cholestatic features (Czaja and Carpenter, 1993). Criteria for diagnosis have been codified by an international panel, and they require the exclusion of diseases such as Wilson disease, genetic hemochromatosis, α_1-antitrypsin deficiency, chronic viral hepatitis, and drug-induced hepatitis (Czaja, 1995; Alvarez et al., 1999).

An acute, even fulminant, presentation has been recognized, which can resemble an acute viral or toxic hepatitis (Nikias et al., 1994); and the requirement for 6 months of disease activity to establish chronicity has been waived (Czaja, 1995; Alvarez et al., 1999). The disease affects mainly women less than 40 years old (70%), and concurrent extrahepatic immune diseases are common (17%), including autoimmune thyroiditis, Graves' disease, synovitis, and ulcerative colitis (Czaja, 1995). An autoimmune basis is presumed mainly because immunoserological markers are present, autoreactive liver-infiltrating lymphocytes have been demonstrated, putative autoantigens have been described, corticosteroid therapy is effective at suppressing disease activity, and alternative etiological explanations have been elusive (Czaja and Manns, 1995b; Czaja, 2001). Three types of autoimmune hepatitis have been proposed based on immunoserological markers, but none has been endorsed by the International Autoimmune Hepatitis Group as a valid clinical entity (Czaja and Manns, 1995; Alvarez et al., 1999). Nevertheless, the designations have been useful as clinical descriptions and assimilated into the jargon.

Type 1 autoimmune hepatitis is characterized by the presence of SMAs and/or ANAs in serum, and it is the most common form among Caucasoid adults in the United States. *Type 2 autoimmune hepatitis* is characterized by the presence of antibodies to liver/kidney microsome type 1 (anti-LKM1) in serum, and it affects mainly children between the ages of 2 and 14 years (Homberg et al., 1987). Type 2 autoimmune hepatitis has been diagnosed in only 4% of American adults with autoimmune hepatitis (Czaja et al., 1992), whereas in Germany and France it is more common (Homberg et al., 1987). The autoantigen of type 1 disease is unknown, but the asialoglycoprotein receptor is a promising candidate (Vento et al., 1986). The autoantigen of type 2 disease is the cytochrome mono-oxygenase P-450 IID6 (CYP2D6) (Manns et al., 1989).

Type 3 autoimmune hepatitis is characterized by antibodies to soluble liver antigen/liver pancreas (anti-SLA/LP) (Manns et al., 1987; Stechemesser et al., 1993). The autoantigen is a 50 kDa cytosolic protein (Wies et al., 2000), and it has homology with a transfer ribonucleoprotein complex ($tRNP^{(Ser)Sec}$) that incorporates selenocysteine into peptide chains (Costa et al.,

2000). Type 3 autoimmune hepatitis shares clinical, laboratory, immunoserological, and prognostic features with type 1 disease; and it is unlikely to be a distinct entity (Czaja et al., 1993a; Kanzler et al., 1999).

Frequency and Familial Occurrence

The annual incidence of autoimmune hepatitis in Britain is 0.69/100,000 persons (Hodges et al., 1982), and its mean annual incidence and point prevalence in Norway are 1.9/100,000 and 16.9/100,000, respectively (Boberg et al., 1998). The Norwegian experience is based on a more homogeneous and closely screened population than the British study, and it is more likely to reflect disease occurrence among Caucasoid adults of North America. Prevalence decreases in regions near the Mediterranean, Africa, and the Middle East; and these changes may reflect alterations in the prevalence of certain HLA phenotypes (Ryder et al., 1978). The rarity of type 2 autoimmune hepatitis outside of Germany and France also suggests ethnic and/or regional variations in susceptibility.

Autoimmune hepatitis does occur in families, but its frequency is surprisingly low or underreported (Whittingham et al., 1970; Hilberg et al., 1971; Hodges et al., 1991). Autoantibodies, hypergammaglobulinemia, and/or the occurrence of extrahepatic immune-mediated diseases are more frequent in family members than liver disease (Galbraith et al., 1974b; Salapuro et al., 1976; Krawitt et al., 1987). This finding suggests that the genetic propensity for autoimmune hepatitis is difficult to trigger.

A variety of viral agents, including hepatitis A, hepatitis B, hepatitis C, and measles virus (Czaja, 1994), and drugs, including α-methyldopa, isoniazid, nitrofurantoin, diclofenac, and minocycline (Scully et al., 1993a; Herzog et al., 1997; Seeff, 1981), have been implicated as causes of the disease. These observations suggest that a common final pathway of pathogenesis can be initiated by various triggering factors, possibly through molecular mimicry, and that the process can be sustained in the absence of a trigger by genetic defects in self-tolerance (Czaja, 2001).

Defective Immune Suppression

Autoantibody production in autoimmune hepatitis is modulated by a type 2 cytokine response in which IL-10 is the principal mediator (Czaja et al., 2000b). The autoantibodies of the liver disease are not pathogenic, but they may be imprints of underlying immune mechanisms that can be characterized and monitored by the humoral manifestations (Czaja, 1999; Czaja and Homburger, 2001). The cytokine network is interactive and counterregulatory, and it modulates the activation and inhibition of immunocytes. Inhibitory actions may be manifested as suppression of T-lymphocyte functions. Suppressor T-cell dysfunction was initially described in patients with autoimmune hepatitis (Hodgson et al., 1978; Kashio et al., 1981; Vento et al., 1984) and in their first-degree relatives (Nouri-Aria et al., 1985; O'Brien et al., 1986; Krawitt et al., 1988). These observations suggested an inheritable basis for the suppressor defect.

Failures in suppressor T-cell function were suspected to cause inappropriate antibody production against normal hepatocyte membrane proteins. NK cells could then interact with the antigen–antibody complexes and induce liver cell injury through an antibody-dependent, cell-mediated form of cytotoxicity (Czaja, 1995a; Czaja, 2001). First-degree relatives with the suppressor T-cell defect commonly had the HLA-A1-B8-DR3 phenotype, and this association also indicated an inheritable risk factor for the disease (Nouri-Aria et al., 1985). Subsequent studies recognized associations between HLA-DR3 and polymorphisms of *CTLA-4* (Agarwal et al., 2000a) and of *TNF-A* (Cookson et al., 1999; Czaja et al., 1999). Consequently, early descriptions of inheritable defects in immune suppression may have reflected synergisms between a constellation of autoimmune promoters (Czaja, 2000).

The defect in immune suppression in autoimmune hepatitis is not antigen-specific, and it is present only in patients with active inflammation (Vento et al., 1984). Furthermore, the association of the suppressor T-cell defect with certain HLAs has not been demonstrated in all patients (Krawitt et al., 1987). A similar defect occurs in disease-free spouses, and this finding has suggested an environmental rather than a genetic trigger in some individuals (Krawitt et al., 1987). The nature and importance of defective humoral immunity in the development of autoimmune hepatitis remain unclear. A genetic basis for autoantibody expression cannot be discounted, but a primary pathogenetic role for suppressor T-cell dysfunction is unlikely (Czaja, 2000).

Class II Human Leukocyte Antigens

Cell-mediated cytodestruction involves a cascade of cellular and humoral interactions that are subject to multiple genetic influences, including autoantigen presentation, immunocyte activation, and cytokine signaling (Czaja, 2000). Immunoreactivity to autoantigens is determined by the configuration of the HLA antigen binding groove and the TCR of immunocytes. Genes encode these various structures and determine disease susceptibility and severity (Doherty et al., 1994a; Czaja and Donaldson, 2000).

HLA-DR3 and -DR4 are the inheritable risk factors for type 1 autoimmune hepatitis in Caucasoid individuals from northern Europe and North America (Donaldson et al., 1991a). Eighty-five percent of patients with the disease in the United States have one or both of these antigens (Czaja et al., 1993b). Susceptibility is polygenic, and it is carried by the *DRB1* gene. Molecular DNA-based techniques have indicated that *DRB1*0301* is the principal risk factor and that *DRB1*0401* is a secondary but independent risk factor (Fig. 17–5). In contrast, the

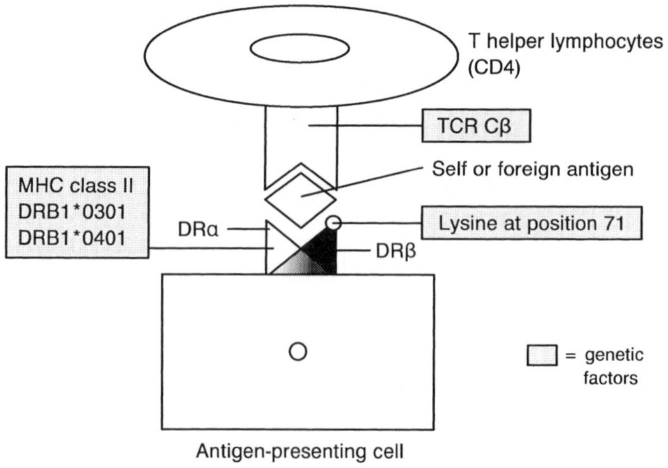

Fig. 17–5. Genetic factors influencing antigen presentation and recognition in white North Americans and British with type 1 autoimmune hepatitis. *TCR*, T-cell receptor; *MHC*, major histocompatibility complex. The two amino acid chains that comprise the antigen binding groove of the MHC molecule are shown as *DRα* and *DRβ*.

*DRB5*0101-DRB1*1501* haplotype confers protection (Strettell et al., 1997).

Analyses of amino acid sequence variations in the HLA antigen binding groove have indicated that the greatest risk for type 1 autoimmune hepatitis is associated with alleles that encode lysine at position DRβ71 (Strettell et al., 1997) (Fig. 17–5). *DRB1*0301* and *DRB1*0401* encode for lysine at this position and affect the steric configuration of the antigen binding groove in a similar fashion. *DRB1*0301* is in tight linkage disequilibrium with *DRB3*0101*, and *DRB1*0401* is in tight linkage disequilibrium with *DRB4*0103*. *DRB3*0101* also encodes for lysine at position DRβ71, whereas *DRB4*0103* encodes for arginine. Consequently, the *DRB1*0301-DRB3*0101* haplotype encodes two lysine residues at the critical DBβ71 position, and the *DRB1*0401-DRB4*0103* haplotype encodes only one. This difference of a single amino acid residue within the DBβ chain of the HLA molecule may account for the weaker association of *DRB1*0401* with disease susceptibility (Strettell et al., 1997) (Fig. 17–5).

The critical motif within the antigen binding groove of the HLA-DR molecule is represented by the sequence LLEQKR between positions DBβ67 and 72 (Doherty et al., 1994a; Strettell et al., 1997). In this sequence, lysine (K) is in position 71 and at the lip of the antigen binding groove. Position DBβ71 allows contact between the binding groove, antigenic peptide, and TCR of the immunocyte; it is a critical junction for immunocyte activation. Class II MHC molecules containing lysine at DBβ71 may be better able to orient antigenic peptides for immunocyte activation. They can also form dimers on the surface of antigen-presenting cells and thereby increase the intensity of antigen display and the vigor of immunocyte activation (Czaja and Donaldson, 2000).

*DRB1*1501* protects against type 1 autoimmune hepatitis and encodes an isoleucine (I) for a leucine (L) at position DRβ67. It encodes an alanine (A) for a lysine (K) at DRβ71 (Doherty et al., 1994a; Strettell et al., 1997). Alanine is a neutral, nonpolar, structurally different amino acid from the positively charged, polar lysine residue; and its substitution for lysine would affect the steric and electrostatic properties of the antigen-presenting complex. In this fashion, a single amino acid replacement at a critical location may protect against the disease.

Class III Human Leukocyte Antigens

The class III region of the MHC contains the genes that encode for the C4A and C4B isotypes of the complement pathway, and it been implicated in the development of autoimmune hepatitis. Low serum complement levels have been recognized in some patients with the disease (Munoz et al., 1982). C4 phenotyping has demonstrated null allotypes at the C4A or C4B locus in 90% of patients with autoimmune hepatitis of childhood onset and in healthy first-degree relatives (Vergani et al., 1985). The complement system clears immune complexes, neutralizes viruses, and eliminates micro-organisms; and a genetically determined deficiency in this system could enhance susceptibility to autoimmune hepatitis (Doherty et al., 1994b).

Molecular techniques using a complementary DNA probe for the *C4A* gene have demonstrated *C4A* gene deletion in over 50% of patients with autoimmune hepatitis, and these individuals have been distinguished by a younger age at disease onset (Scully et al., 1993b). Similar findings have been reported in English patients who also had a 21-hydroxylase A pseudogene. The C4 deletions in the British study were associated with increased mortality and frequency of relapse but not with age at onset (Doherty et al., 1994b). *C4* gene deletions are associated with the HLA-A1, -B8, and -DR3 antigens; and the *C4AQO* null allele has been included in the extended MHC haplotype of autoimmune hepatitis (Scully et al., 1993b).

Genetic Distinctions between Different Ethnic Groups

Not all ethnic groups have similar frequencies of HLA-DR3 and HLA-DR4, and there are regional variations in the occurrence of the disease and its clinical expression. The susceptibility alleles for type 1 autoimmune hepatitis are *DRB1*0405* in Japan (Seki et al., 1990, 1992), *DRB1*0405* in Argentine adults (Fainboim et al., 1994; Pando et al., 1999), *DRB1*1301* in Argentine children (Fainboim et al., 1994; Pando et al., 1999), *DRB1*1301* in Brazil (Bittencourt et al., 1999), and *DRB1*0404* in Mestizo Mexicans (Vazquez-Garcia et al., 1998). This multiplicity of race-dependent allelic risk factors for type 1 autoimmune hepatitis suggests that different alleles encode one or more common determinants that are critical for disease expression. Alternatively, there may be other genetic promoters of type 1 autoimmune hepatitis that are selected by region-specific etiological triggers and include both MHC-linked and MHC-independent loci.

The diversity of genetic risk factors for the same disease in different ethnic groups supports a *shared motif hypothesis* of pathogenesis (Czaja and Donaldson, 2000; Czaja, 2001). This hypothesis holds that the risk for type 1 autoimmune hepatitis relates to a short motif encoded in the antigen binding groove of the class II MHC molecule. The same or a similar motif can be encoded by several alleles, and each allele can thereby affect disease occurrence. *DRB1*0404* and *DRB1*0405* influence susceptibility in Mestizo Mexicans, Japanese, and Argentine adults; and they differ from the *DRB1*0401* allele in white northern Europeans and North Americans by encoding an arginine for a lysine at position DRβ71. Arginine is a positively charged, polar amino acid with structural and electrostatic similarities to lysine. It should not affect presentation of antigenic peptide or greatly alter susceptibility to the disease.

In contrast, *DRB1*1301* influences susceptibility in Argentine children and Brazilian patients, and it contradicts the shared motif hypothesis by encoding ILEDER at positions DRβ67–72. Glutamic acid (E), aspartic acid (D), and glutamic acid (E) are at DRβ positions 69, 70, and 71, respectively; and each of these amino acids is negatively charged and incongruous with the LLEQKR motif. The findings in South America are difficult to reconcile with those in North America and Britain unless the disease in South America is different, *DRB1*1301* is selected by environmental factors indigenous to South America, and/or *DRB1*1301* and *DRB1*0301* are linked to the *DRB3* gene. The *DRB3* gene encodes LLEQKR at DRβ67–72 (Czaja and Donaldson, 2000b).

Autoimmune Promoters

Not all patients with the same susceptibility alleles have the same clinical expression and behavior, and not all patients with type 1 autoimmune hepatitis have the same susceptibility alleles (Czaja and Donaldson, 2000; Czaja, 2001). Other factors must modify disease occurrence and outcome, and this likelihood has generated the *autoimmune promoter hypothesis*. This hypothesis purports that multiple autoimmune promoter genes inside and outside the MHC are drivers of the immune response. Immunoregulatory proteins can affect autoantigen presentation and processing, inflammation, fibrosis, apoptosis, immunocyte recruitment, and CD4 Th cell activation; and there may be synergy (epistasis) between primary and secondary susceptibility alleles of the MHC. These genes may promote the expression and clinical severity of type 1 autoimmune hepatitis by acting in concert as a permissive gene pool.

One such modifier in type 1 autoimmune hepatitis is a polymorphism of *TNF-A* involving an A for G substitution at position −308 (Cookson et al., 1999). Patients with the genotype TNF308 AA/AG have an earlier age at disease onset, higher frequency of *DRB1*0301*, and poorer response to corticosteroid therapy than patients with the TNF308 GG genotype (Czaja et al., 1999). Similarly, a polymorphism of *CTLA-4* may affect the immune response in a non-disease-specific fashion. Patients with a polymorphism involving a G for A substitution at position 49 in the first exon of *CTLA-4* have a CTLA-4 GG genotype that is associated with greater immunoreactivity and a higher frequency of *DRB1*0301* than patients with a CTLA-4 AA/AG genotype (Agarwal et al., 2000a). Other autoimmune promoters probably exist, and the full constellation of interactive immune modifiers remains to be described.

Genetic Distinctions between Types

HLA-B14, -DR3, and *-C4AQO* occur more commonly in patients with type 2 autoimmune hepatitis than in normal subjects (Manns and Kruger, 1994); but the genetic profiles of types 1 and 2 autoimmune hepatitis were not compared until recently. American patients with type 1 autoimmune hepatitis have the *DRB1*0301* allele more commonly than German patients with type 2 disease, and the frequency of *DRB1*04* alleles is also higher in American patients with type 1 disease after exclusion of individuals with the *DRB1*03* alleles (Czaja et al., 1997a). In contrast, German patients with type 2 autoimmune hepatitis have *DRB1*07*, *DRB1*15*, and *DQB1*06* more commonly than American patients with type 1 disease. They also have *DRB1*07*, *DRB4*01*, and *DQB1*06* more frequently than normal subjects from the United States (Czaja et al., 1997a). These findings suggest that regional variations in the prevalence of different types of autoimmune hepatitis reflect the genetic profiles of the populations at risk and that different types of autoimmune hepatitis have different susceptibility alleles. Similar findings have been reported in Brazil, where *DRB1*07* also characterizes type 2 autoimmune hepatitis (Bittencourt et al., 1999).

Human Leukocyte Antigens and Disease Expression and Behavior

The HLA phenotype determines susceptibility to autoimmune hepatitis and its behavior before and after corticosteroid therapy. These associations are stronger in autoimmune hepatitis than in other forms of chronic liver disease because the HLA associations are few and tight.

Patients with type 1 autoimmune hepatitis who are HLA-DR3-positive are younger at disease onset and have lower serum immunoglobulin G levels and fewer concurrent immune diseases than patients with HLA-DR4 (Czaja et al., 1993c). These patients also relapse more commonly after corticosteroid withdrawal (Czaja et al., 1990; Doherty et al., 1994a), require liver transplantation more often (Sanchez-Urdazpal et al., 1992), and deteriorate during corticosteroid therapy more frequently than patients with other HLA phenotypes (Czaja et al., 1993c). In contrast, patients with HLA-DR4 are older and more commonly women than patients with HLA-DR3. They also have concurrent extrahepatic immune diseases more often and respond better to corticosteroid therapy (Czaja et al., 1993c). DNA-based techniques have indicated that the *DRB1*0301* allele is associated with a poor treatment response and that the *DRB1*0401* allele is associated with a lower frequency of hepatic death or liver transplantation (Czaja et al., 1997b). *C4A* gene deletion has also been associated with an early age at onset (Scully et al., 1993b) and an adverse outcome after corticosteroid therapy (Doherty et al., 1994b). The *C4A* null allele is in linkage disequilibrium with HLA-DR3, and the poor prognoses associated with each genetic marker may be a polygenic effect (Scully et al., 1993b; Doherty et al., 1994b).

The reason that extrahepatic immune diseases occur more commonly in patients with HLA-DR4 is unclear. Many of the concurrent immune diseases have their own HLA associations outside the context of autoimmune hepatitis (Czaja et al., 1993b). The clustering of these diseases with HLA-DR4 may reflect another allele that is common to each disease or the existence of two linked loci that separately encode susceptibility for each condition (Payami et al., 1987). Studies from Argentina indicate that two HLA loci are involved in the extrahepatic manifestations of type 1 autoimmune hepatitis and that these loci are not linked (Marcos et al., 1994). HLA-A11 occurs more commonly in Argentine patients with type 1 autoimmune hepatitis and extrahepatic manifestations than in control subjects (31% vs. 6%), and joint expression of HLA-A11 and HLA-DR4 increases the odds ratio for concurrent immune features in a synergistic fashion. The implications are that autoreactive Th cells that have been sensitized by HLA-DR4 interact with the cytotoxic T cells sensitized by HLA-A11. Liver and nonliver tissues are then targeted by immunocytes in response to homologies between autoantigens in these different organs (Marcos et al., 1994).

Another explanation for the clustering of immune diseases with HLA-DR4 relates to the diversity of DR4 alleles that may present antigenic peptides. There are 26 possible alleles associated with HLA-DR4, in contrast to two alleles associated with HLA-DR3. Patients with HLA-DR4 may develop the disease by recognizing a more diverse range of autoantigens than patients with HLA-DR3, and some of these autoantigens may be gender-specific. Indeed, extrahepatic immune diseases are most common in women with HLA-DR4 (Czaja et al., 1998).

Female Gender

The reasons for the occurrence of autoimmune hepatitis mainly in women are unknown. The gender effect may be due to immunomodulatory mechanisms controlled by sex-linked genes or sex hormones that act on the immunocytes and/or the susceptibility alleles (Whitacre et al., 1999). An immunomodulatory gene on the X chromosome has been proposed, and the increased immune reactivity in women may reflect a "double dose" of this gene (Griffing et al., 1980; Chiovato et al., 1993). Alternatively, estrogens and other gender-related hormones may influence the vigor of the immune response by facilitating antigen processing and recognition (Van Griensven et al., 1997). The heightened immunoreactivity in women is manifested by higher serum levels of immunoglobulin after exposure to a fixed antigen load (Mackay et al., 1977), more common expression of natural autoantibodies (Tomer and Shoenfeld, 1988), and increased cell-mediated immunity after immunization (Whitacre et al., 1999).

Women are more likely to develop a type 1 cytokine response after exposure to an infectious agent or antigen than men

(Whitacre et al., 1999). During pregnancy, however, they have mainly a type 2 cytokine response. This shift may explain in part the differences in activity of certain autoimmune diseases observed during pregnancy. Changes in estrogen levels and the expression of estrogen receptors on immunocytes during pregnancy may contribute to these responses.

Estrogen has biphasic dose effects and two different receptors on immune cells. High estrogen levels, as in pregnancy, inhibit the proinflammatory type 1 cytokine response and promote a type 2 cytokine response, which favors antibody production and antibody-dependent pathogenic pathways (Whitacre et al., 1999). Conversely, low estrogen levels favor a type 1 cytokine response and promote cell-mediated pathogenic pathways. Pituitary hormones, such as prolactin and growth hormone, and sex hormones, such as progesterone and testosterone, counterregulate the immune response, probably by altering the cytokine milieu and/or estrogen receptor expression (Whitacre et al., 1999). Lastly, microchimerism can persist for years after pregnancy, and fetal cells in the maternal circulation have been associated with the initiation and exacerbation of autoimmune disease (Nelson, 1999; Lambert et al., 2000). Mechanisms by which microchimerism affects postpartum immunoreactivity are unknown, but it may compromise self-tolerance by promoting cross-reactivity.

Recognition that gender differences exist in the immune response does not translate into a coherent hypothesis of pathogenesis in autoimmune hepatitis. If there is a genetic basis for gender differences in this disease, it most likely relates to disparate modulations of the susceptibility genes by the sex hormones alone or in conjunction with secretions from the hypothalamic–pituitary–adrenal axis. Synergisms between the sex hormones, immunoregulatory cytokine profiles, and polymorphisms of various autoimmune promoters, such as Fas (CD95/APO-1), *CTLA-4*, and *TNF-A*, may enhance immunocyte activation by different complexes of antigenic peptide and class II molecules of the MHC.

T-Cell Antigen Receptors

T-cell antigen receptors recognize peptides presented by MHC class I or class II antigens, and this interaction triggers the activation of immunocytes. The TCR is comprised of α and β chains and γ and δ chains, which are encoded by genes from a germline pool. The diversity of the TCR in recognizing antigens relates to random interactions between these genes and the generation of chains with variable regions for antigen recognition and constant regions for attachment to the T-cell surface. Polymorphisms in the TCR repertoire could alter susceptibility to autoimmune hepatitis (Manabe et al., 1994). Studies in large families with HLA-identical siblings have demonstrated that HLA genes affect TCR variable segment frequencies and expression levels in peripheral blood lymphocytes. In this fashion, there can be a coordinated dual recognition of antigens by certain HLA and TCR molecules (Akolkar et al., 1993).

In an English study of autoimmune hepatitis, homozygosity for the TCR *C*β gene is more common in patients than in normal subjects, and this difference was greatest in individuals without HLA-DR3 and HLA-DR4 (Manabe et al., 1994) (Fig. 17–5). These findings indicate that susceptibility to autoimmune hepatitis involves the TCR β-chain genes and that particular combinations of TCR and HLA molecules can alter disease expression by affecting the TCR–antigen–HLA sandwich (Fig. 17–5). Heterozygosity for the TCR *C*β gene is significantly decreased in HLA-DR3-positive patients with early-onset disease. These observations imply that the TCR Cβ genotype can modify disease expression when associated with certain HLAs (Manabe et al., 1994).

CHRONIC VIRAL HEPATITIS

Chronic viral hepatitis is a hepatic inflammation of at least 6 months' duration that is due to a demonstrable viral agent. The infectious agent may be directly cytopathic or it may initiate immunopathic mechanisms that in turn cause liver cell injury. Host tolerance for the virus is necessary to perpetuate the viremia, and genetic predispositions may modulate immunoreactions to the virus that affect hepatocyte destruction and induce extrahepatic immune manifestations and/or diseases.

HBV and HCV are the prototypic viruses that cause chronic viral hepatitis, and each has a different predominant mechanism of cytodestruction. HBV is not directly cytopathic, and it accomplishes liver cell injury mainly through immunological mechanisms (Thomas et al., 1982). In contrast, HCV is a flavivirus that is cytopathic by nature. It can also evoke immunopathic mechanisms. In individuals with HCV, both cytopathic and immunopathic pathways can be present and one process may predominate over the other at different times in the illness (Gonzalez-Peralta et al., 1994).

Concurrent immune diseases in chronic viral hepatitis may be viral antigen-driven and associated with immune complex deposition (cryoglobulinemia, glomerulonephritis, cutaneous vasculitis and polyarteritis) or autoantigen-driven and associated with host-, rather than virus-, specific factors (autoimmune thyroiditis and Sjögren's syndrome). In the latter instance, viral antigens may resemble self-antigens and activate immunocytes through molecular mimicry. Antigen processing and immunocyte sensitization can also be enhanced by viral infection through the release of endogenous interferon (Czaja, 1997). Genetic predispositions may affect the persistence of viremia, severity of liver cell damage, extrahepatic manifestations, disease severity, risk of hepatocellular cancer, and responsiveness to antiviral agents. Studies defining these various genetic controls are still preliminary, but they already identify an exciting area of research.

Prevalence of Chronic Hepatitis B and Chronic Hepatitis C

The number of chronic infections with HBV in the United States is estimated as 1 million to 1.25 million, and the number of chronic infections with HCV is estimated as 3.5 million (Alter and Mast, 1994). Chronic hepatitis B accounts for 5000 deaths per year, and chronic hepatitis C accounts for 8000 to 10,000 deaths per year. The epidemiology of both diseases is changing as screening programs identify patients in the early asymptomatic stage more commonly, vaccination programs for HBV have been universalized, and public education efforts have emphasized transmission routes and prophylactic measures (Alter and Mast, 1994). Nevertheless, chronic hepatitis C is the most common cause of liver transplantation in the United States, and antiviral treatment remains inadequate for many individuals with the disease.

Human Leukocyte Antigens and Chronic Hepatitis B

Multiple studies have assessed the associations between HLA and chronic viral hepatitis, and the findings have been discrepant. The most secure conclusions are that genetic predispositions for disease susceptibility and behavior probably exist and that the importance of these predispositions remains uncertain.

Early reports suggested that HLA-Bw15, -Bw17, and -Bw35 were associated with transient or persistent hepatitis B surface antigenemia and that this relationship explained differences in disease prevalence among various geographic regions (Hillis et al., 1977). HLA-Bw15 was associated with transient antigenemia, HLA-Bw17 with persistent antigenemia, and HLA-Bw35 with either pattern of behavior. These findings implied that Bw35 was a marker of susceptibility and that the other HLA-B antigens were determinants of virus–host interaction (Hillis et al., 1977; Penner et al., 1977). The strongest association in these studies was between the HLA-B locus and the presence of hepatitis B surface antigen. Indeed, statistically significant associations between particular MHC class I antigens and certain patterns of disease behavior have not been demonstrated (Hillis et al., 1977).

Subsequent studies continued to suggest associations between the HLA-B locus and chronic HBV infection, but the results were variable and not compelling. HLA-B7 was ascribed a protective value in Caucasoid individuals (Sampliner et al., 1981). HLA-B35 occurred more commonly in Argentine patients with chronic hepatitis B than control subjects (45% vs. 16%) (Mota et al., 1987), and HLA-Bw15 was more frequent in Italian patients who were asymptomatic carriers of HBV than control subjects (33% vs. 8%) (Giani et al., 1979). These experiences were at variance with other studies, and the importance of class II HLA was not fully evaluated (van Hattum et al., 1987).

The first MHC class II antigens to be assessed in chronic hepatitis B were in Italian patients with and without superimposed hepatitis delta infection (Forzani et al., 1984). The frequency of HLA-DR3 was increased in patients without delta infection, whereas the frequency of HLA-DR4 was decreased (absent) in these same patients. These findings suggested that HLA-DR3 protected against delta infection by enhancing immune recognition or that it inhibited delta infection by promoting HBV replication and liver damage, possibly through autoimmune mechanisms. The absence of HLA-DR4 in these same patients implied that HLA-DR4 (or a gene in linkage disequilibrium with it) promoted clearance of the delta virus (Fig. 17–6). In contrast, persistence of delta virus was associated with HLA-DR2. HLA-DR2 could promote chronic delta infection by interfering with immune recognition of the viral antigen or by eliminating the thymus-derived lymphocytes that clear the virus (Forzani et al., 1984).

The Italian studies were not corroborated, but the roles of HLA-DR2, -DR3, and -DR4 in chronic hepatitis B could not be dismissed. Indeed, patients with chronic viral hepatitis (chronic hepatitis B or chronic hepatitis C) who were HLA-DR3-positive had higher serum γ-globulin and immunoglobulin G levels than patients with HLA-DR4 and a greater frequency of severe disease (Czaja et al., 1995). In contrast, patients with chronic viral hepatitis and HLA-DR4 had concurrent immune diseases more commonly than patients with other HLAs, and they had less severe disease (Fig. 17–6). These findings indicated that HLA-DR3 and HLA-DR4 could modify the clinical expression of chronic viral hepatitis, though the effects were often subtle.

Molecular DNA-based testing further clarified the MHC class II associations in HBV infection. Studies in children and adults in Gambia indicated a protective effect of *DRB1*1302* against the development of chronic hepatitis B, and *DRB1*1301* was recognized as a secondary protective factor (Thursz et al., 1995) (Fig. 17–6). *DRB1*1301* differs from *DRB1*1302* by a single amino acid substitution at position DRβ86 (valine for glycine), and HBV-infected patients with *DRB1*1301* or *DRB1*1302* are able to clear HBV infection more commonly than those with other alleles (Thursz et al., 1995) (Fig. 17–6). This protective effect against chronic HBV infection was also demonstrated in white Europeans, and the advantages against infection conferred by *DRB1*1301* and *DRB1*1302* were shown to span ethnic boundaries (Hohler et al., 1997b). *DRB1*1301* and *DRB1*1302* alleles may present the immunodominant epitopes of infectious agents to immunocytes more effectively than other alleles, or they may alter the thymic selection of T cells in favor of those active against the virus or antigenically similar agents.

Tumor Necrosis Factor and Chronic Hepatitis B

Cytokines have a modifying effect on HBV clearance, and genetically determined polymorphisms can alter this activity. Both TNF-α and interferon-γ inhibit transcription of the HBV core promoter (Romero and Lavine, 1996) and contribute to the elimination of HBV-infected cells to a greater degree than cytotoxic T cells (Guidotti et al., 1996). The TNF-α promoter polymorphism *TNF238.2* may be associated with the development of chronic hepatitis B (Hohler et al., 1998) (Fig. 17–6). The implication is that HBV interacts with *TNF238.2* and decreases transcription of *TNF-A* and/or that *TNF238.2* has impaired antiviral actions. Deficiencies in the production of TNF-α could then prevent viral clearance and promote chronic infection. *TNF238.2* is not in linkage disequilibrium with the HLA-B or -DR genes, and it must be considered an independent risk factor for chronic hepatitis B. Its effects must be balanced against those of *DRB1*1301* and *DRB1*1302* (Hohler et al., 1998) (Fig. 17–6).

Human Leukocyte Antigens and Chronic Hepatitis C

HLA associations with chronic hepatitis C have also been inconsistent, and this variability has challenged the legitimacy of any single study (Thio et al., 2000). Unlike HBV, HCV may induce liver cell injury by direct cytopathicity, immunoreaction, or both together or in sequence (Gonzalez-Peralta et al., 1994). These diverse mechanisms of liver cell damage may be important at different stages of the disease in the same individual, and each may be associated with different genetic controls at the time of its predominance. Similarly, disease severity against which

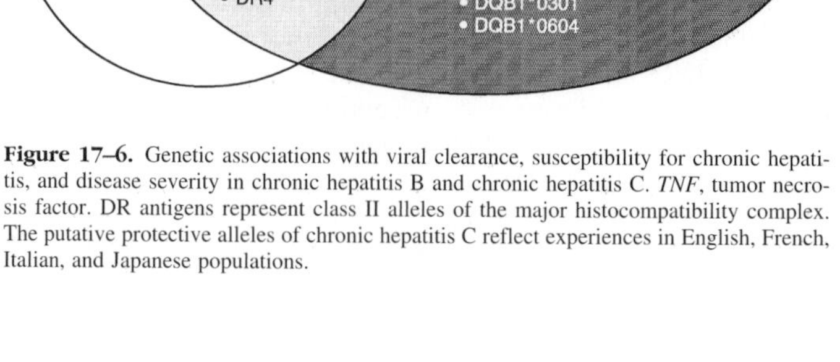

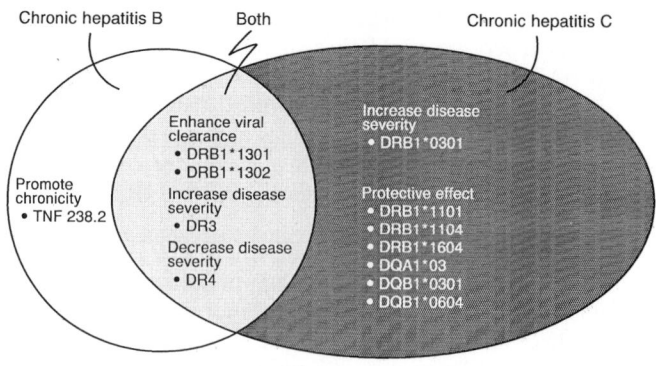

Figure 17–6. Genetic associations with viral clearance, susceptibility for chronic hepatitis, and disease severity in chronic hepatitis B and chronic hepatitis C. *TNF*, tumor necrosis factor. DR antigens represent class II alleles of the major histocompatibility complex. The putative protective alleles of chronic hepatitis C reflect experiences in English, French, Italian, and Japanese populations.

HLA associations are sought may also vary at different times in the same patient. Criteria based on laboratory indices of liver inflammation and/or histological features are limited by spontaneous fluctuations in disease activity and biases associated with patient selection and tissue sampling.

Studies from the United States which classified disease severity by clinical, laboratory, and histological criteria have failed to demonstrate a statistically significant association between the HLA-DR antigens and any clinical index of disease severity at presentation (Czaja et al., 1996b; Brandhagen et al., 2000). Furthermore, these studies have been unable to demonstrate a genetic propensity for chronic hepatitis C compared to an ethnically similar normal population (Czaja et al., 1996b).

In contrast, studies from Germany, comparing MHC class I and class II antigens in patients with chronic hepatitis C, have defined a higher frequency of *DRB1*0301* and a lower frequency of *DRB1*1301* in patients compared to controls (Hohler et al., 1997a) (Fig. 17–6). These findings are similar to those of earlier studies that had associated HLA-DR3 with chronic hepatitis B (Forzani et al., 1984) and severe inflammatory activity in chronic hepatitis B and C (Czaja et al., 1995; Czaja and Carpenter, 1997).

The autoimmune phenotype might define a host propensity for immune-dominant mechanisms of pathogenesis and/or more severe disease that is independent of the viral type. Furthermore, the protective effect that had been ascribed to *DRB1*1301* in chronic hepatitis B (Hohler et al., 1997b) was also found in chronic hepatitis C (Kuzushita et al., 1996; Hohler et al., 1997a). Indeed, HLA-DR13 may have a universal effect on the T-cell response to infectious agents (Hohler et al., 1997b) (Fig. 17–6).

The first HCV-specific association with class II HLA that was confirmed in other studies was with HLA-DR5. Patients with chronic hepatitis C and HLA-DR5 had milder disease and a lower frequency of cirrhosis than patients with other HLAs (Peano et al., 1994). Patients with chronic hepatitis C also had a lower occurrence of HLA-DR5 than normal subjects, suggesting that HLA-DR5 was protective against chronic infection (Zavaglia et al., 1996). Molecular DNA-based techniques subsequently indicated that HLA-DR11 was the most frequent split of HLA-DR5 in the Italian population and that this allele was protective against chronicity. Indeed, the protective haplotype was extended to *DRB1*1104-DQA1*0501-DQB1*0301* (Zavaglia et al., 1998). Subsequent studies in Germany indicated that *DRB1*11* and *DQB1*03* are associated with a reduced risk of end-stage liver disease in HCV-infected patients (Tillmann et al., 2001) (Fig. 17–6).

Studies in other Italian populations have indicated a lower frequency of HCV infection in transfusion-requiring patients with thalassemia major and the HLA-DR2 phenotype *DRB1*1601-DQB1*0502* (Conglia et al., 1996) (Fig. 17–6). *DQA1*03* has been described as protective against chronic HCV infection in Caucasian northern Europeans (Tibbs et al., 1996). *DRB1*1101* and *DQB1*0301* have been associated with viral clearance among the French (Alric et al., 1997), and *DRB1*1101*, *DRB1*1302*, and *DQB1*0604* have been associated with mild disease among the Japanese (Kuzushita et al., 1998) (Fig. 17–6). Self-limited HCV infection has been associated with *DRB1*1101* and *DQB1*0301* among the British, and *DRB1*0701* and *DRB4*0101* have been associated with persistent HCV infection (Thursz et al., 1999). The importance of host-dependent genetic factors in HCV clearance has been underscored by studies correlating the slope of change in the viral load of untreated patients of genotype 1b with diverse class II HLA (Fanning et al., 2001).

Table 17–1. Clinical Application of Genetic Factors in Chronic Liver Disease

Liver Disease	Genetic Factors	Clinical Application
Alcoholic liver disease	Neurotransmitters affect alcohol preference, *ADH3*1* affects rate of alcohol catabolism, *ALDH2*2* promotes aldehyde toxicities, *CYP2E1* c_2 generates toxic metabolites, *TNFA-A* affects apoptosis and steatosis, *Collagen* $\alpha 2$ associated with cirrhosis, fatty acid ethyl esters affect lipid metabolism	Risk assessment for alcoholism and liver disease, determining risk thresholds for liver disease in individuals
Hepatocellular cancer	Enzyme polymorphisms affect aflatoxin metabolism, *CYP2A6* affects activation of carcinogens, *CYP2E1* c_2 allele activates carcinogens, tumor-suppressor gene aberrations (*p53*, *Rb*) affect tumor risk and behavior, *myc*- and c-*met* proto-oncogenes affect tumor risk, *β-catenin* and *AXIN1* influence aggressiveness.	Cancer risk assessment, markers of tumor aggressiveness, determinants of tumor recurrence and origin
Primary biliary cirrhosis	HLA-DR8 associated with susceptibility, C4A null alleles (*C4A*Q0*) affect risk, *DQA1*0102* protective against disease, *DP1*0301* independent risk factor, T-cell receptor *Vβ6.1,3* affects antigen recognition, sulfoxidation deficiencies affect toxicities	Diagnostic aid, risk assessment, prognostic markers
Primary sclerosing cholangitis	HLA-DRw52a affects susceptibility, *DRB3*0101* affects risk and outcome, *DRB5*0101* is secondary risk factor, HLA-DR4 associated with aggressiveness	Diagnostic aid, risk assessment, prognostic markers
Autoimmune hepatitis	*DRB1*0301* is main risk factor, *DRB1*0401* is secondary risk factor, both affect prognosis, C4 null allotypes affect disease behavior, *DRB1*07* associated with type 2 disease	Diagnostic aid, prognostic factors, classification scheme
Chronic hepatitis B	HLA-DR3 associated with delta infection, HLA-DR4 protective against delta, *DRB1*1302* protective against chronicity, *DRB1*1301* secondary protective factor, *TNF238.2* promotes chronicity	Risk assessment for viral clearance, chronicity, superimposed delta infection
Chronic hepatitis C	*DRB1*0301* associated with risk; *DRB1*1301* affords protection; *DRB1*1104* affords protection; *DRB1*1302*, *DRB1*1601*, *DQA1*03*, *DQB1*0301*, *DQB1*0604*, *DRB1*1101* protective in various groups	Risk assessment for chronicity and severity

Among these diverse experiences, *DRB1*11* has been identified most commonly as protective, and it may be the most important genetic determinant of disease susceptibility and outcome in HCV infection. Class II MHC present viral antigens to CD4 Th cells, and the beneficial effect of the molecule encoded by *DRB1*1101* may reflect a superior ability to bind and present HCV antigens (Diepolder et al., 1999). Immunodominant CD4 T-cell clones from patients with self-limited HCV infection commonly recognize peptide presented by *DRB1*1101* (Diepolder et al., 1997) and by *DQB1*0301* (Lamonaca et el., 1999). This facility may enhance viral clearance.

Diverse autoimmune promoters may also affect disease outcome, and these are being unraveled in chronic hepatitis C. Angiotensin II, the main effector molecule of the renin–angiotensin system, has been shown to increase extracellular matrix; and it may be a mediator of fibrogenesis (Noble and Border, 1997). Polymorphisms of the *angiotensinogen promoter* gene and the *TGF-β1* gene are associated with high-producing genotypes, and these genotypes have been found more commonly in patients with chronic hepatitis C and progressive hepatic fibrosis than in patients with no or little hepatic fibrosis (Powell et al., 2000). The probability of other genetic effects on immunocyte activation, cytokine production, fibrogenesis, and malignant transformation is high.

CLINICAL APPLICATION AND RISK ASSESSMENT

The ultimate goals of defining the genetic bases for chronic liver disease are to prevent its occurrence and to improve therapy. The former objective is achieved by characterizing individuals and populations at risk and instituting protective measures. The latter objective is achieved in part by early diagnosis and accurate assessment of prognosis. None of the genetic associations with chronic liver disease has yet been incorporated into routine clinical practice, but each has the potential to achieve the ultimate objectives.

The recognition that alcohol-seeking behavior has a genetic basis that may relate to neurotransmitters and/or receptors in the gratification centers of the brain affords the opportunity to alter destructive behavior with targeted medication. By understanding the polymorphisms that affect ethanol catabolism and toxicity, individuals at risk for liver disease can be identified and counseled and alternative metabolic pathways can be promoted and/or destructive pathways suppressed by medication developed with highly selective actions. Risk thresholds for alcohol consumption can be estimated in the individual and safety limits proposed in a meaningful fashion. Families at high risk for alcoholism and alcoholic liver disease can be identified early and preventive measures instituted (Table 17–1).

The genetic polymorphisms that affect the detoxification of aflatoxin or activate carcinogens can be used in the assessment of populations at risk for hepatocellular carcinoma, and these estimates may stimulate improvements in specific environmental control measures. Knowledge about the aberrations in tumor-suppressor genes and the impact of proto-oncogenes on liver cancer can be applied to other malignant processes. The nature of the genetic aberrations can provide information about the individual carcinogen, the importance of co-morbid factors, the aggressiveness of the tumor, and the clonal origin of metastases or recurrences (Table 17–1).

The HLA class II determinants of PBC, PSC, and autoimmune hepatitis confirm the individuality of each entity and are useful in supporting a diagnosis, defining a variant syndrome or subtype, and justifying a treatment strategy. In PSC and autoimmune hepatitis, they influence disease expression and outcome and may be valuable prognostic indices. Subclassifications of autoimmune hepatitis that are now based on immunoserological markers may be founded in the future on the particular allele that determines presentation and behavior. In this fashion, the allele will define the disease like a virus or drug defines other liver conditions (Table 17–1).

Populations at risk for chronic hepatitis B and C may be identified by HLA screening, and individuals with infection may have specific HLA determinants of viral clearance and disease severity. Such insights could modify the vigor of a therapeutic action or identify individuals at risk for progression to cirrhosis, liver failure, and/or hepatocellular carcinoma. The requirement for special resources, such as liver transplantation, could then be better estimated and utilized. Characterization of the immunodominant epitopes presented by class II MHC molecules that facilitate viral clearance might result in T-cell vaccination programs that prevent chronic HCV infection (Table 17–1).

The genetic bases for chronic liver disease require further definition before clinical applications can burgeon. Studies have already indicated the importance of host factors in disparate liver conditions, and the complex interplay between the host, the disease, and the environment has become a recurrent theme whose variations must be learned in each condition. The promise of gene therapy can be realized only when all of the critical defects have been defined.

ACKNOWLEDGMENTS

Linda Grande is acknowledged for secretarial assistance.

REFERENCES

Adamson GM, Billings RE: Tumor necrosis factor induced oxidative stress in isolated mouse hepatocytes. Arch Biochem Biophys 1992; 294:223–229.

Agarwal DP: Molecular genetic aspects of alcohol metabolism and alcoholism. Pharmacopsychiatry 1997; 30:79–84.

Agarwal K, Czaja AJ, Jones DEJ, Donaldson PT: Cytotoxic lymphocyte antigen (*CTLA-4*) gene polymorphisms and susceptibility to type 1 autoimmune hepatitis. Hepatology 2000a; 31:49–53.

Agarwal K, Jones DE, Daly AK, James OF, Vaidya B, Pearce S, Bassendine MF: *CTLA-4* gene polymorphism confers susceptibility to primary biliary cirrhosis. J Hepatol 2000b; 32:538–541.

Agundez JAG, Ledesma MC, Benitez J, Ladero JM, Rodriguez-Lescure A, Diaz-Rubio E, Diaz-Rubio M: *CYP2A6* genes and risk of liver cancer. Lancet 1995; 345:830–831.

Ahrendt SA, Eisenberger CF, Yip L, Rashid A, Chow JT, Pitt HA, Sidransky D: Chromosome 9p21 loss and *p16* inactivation in primary sclerosing cholangitis-associated cholangiocarcinoma. J Surg Res 1999; 84:88–93.

Ahrendt SA, Rashid A, Chow JT, Eisenberger CF, Pitt HA, Sidransky D: *p53* overexpression and *K-ras* gene mutations in primary sclerosing cholangitis-associated biliary tract cancer. J Hepatobiliary Pancreat Surg 2000; 7:426–431.

Aitola P, Karvonen AL, Matikainen M: Prevalence of hepatobiliary dysfunction in patients with ulcerative colitis. Ann Chir Gynaecol 1994; 83:275–278.

Akolkar PN, Gulwani-Akolkar B, Pergolizzi R, Bigler RD, Silver J: Influence of HLA genes on T cell receptor V segment frequencies and expression levels in peripheral blood lymphocytes. J Immunol 1993; 150:2761–2773.

Albano E, Tomasi A, Persson J-O, Terelius Y, Goria-Gatti L, Ingelman-Sundberg M, Dianzani MU: Role of ethanol-inducible cytochrome P-450 (P-450IIE1) in catalysis of the free radical activation of aliphatic alcohols. Biochem Pharmacol 1991; 41:1895–1902.

Alric L, Fort M, Izopet J, Vinel J-P, Charlet J-P, Selves J, Puel J, Pascal J-P, Duffaut M, Abbal M: Genes of the major histocompatibility complex class II influence the outcome of hepatitis C virus infection. Gastroenterology 1997; 113:1675–1681.

Alter MJ, Mast EE: The epidemiology of viral hepatitis in the United States. Gastroenterol Clin North Am 1994; 23:437–455.

Alvarez F, Berg PA, Bianchi FB, Bianchi L, Burroughs AK, Cancado EL, Chapman RW, Cooksley WGE, Czaja AJ, Desmet VJ, et al.: International Autoimmune Hepatitis Group report. Review of criteria for diagnosis of autoimmune hepatitis. J Hepatol 1999; 31:929–938.

Bach N, Schaffner F: Familial primary biliary cirrhosis. J Hepatol 1994; 20:698–701.

Baish JM, Capra JD: Linkage disequilibrium within the HLA complex does not extend into HLA-DP. Scand J Immunol 1993; 37:499–503.

Ballardini G, Mirakian R, Bianchi FB, Pisi E, Doniach D, Bottazzo GF: Aberrant expression of HLA-DR antigens on bile duct epithelium in primary biliary cirrhosis: relevance to pathogenesis. Lancet 1984; 2:1009–1013.

Bassendine MF, Day CP: The inheritance of alcoholic liver disease. Baillieres Clin Gastroenterol 1998; 12:317–335.

Bassendine MF, Dewar PJ, James OFW: HLA-DR antigens in primary biliary cirrhosis: lack of association. Gut 1985; 26:625–628.

Bauer S, Groh V, Wu J, Steinle A, Phillips JH, Lanier LL, Spies T: Activation of NK cells and T cells by NKG2D, a receptor for stress-inducible MICA. Science 1999; 285:727–729.

Baum H: Nature of the mitochondrial antigens of primary biliary cirrhosis and their possible relationships to the etiology of the disease. Semin Liver Dis 1989; 9:117–123.

Bearer CF, Gould S, Emerson R, Kinnunen P, Cook CS: Fetal alcohol syndrome and fatty acid ethyl esters. Pediatr Res 1992; 31:492–495.

Begovich AB, Klitz W, Moonsamy PV, Van de Water J, Peltz G, Gershwin ME: Genes within the HLA class II region confer both predisposition and resistance to primary biliary cirrhosis. Tissue Antigens 1994; 43:71–77.

Berg PA, Klein R: Heterogeneity of antimitochondrial antibodies. Semin Liver Dis 1989; 9:103–138.

Berg PA, Klein R: Antimitochondrial antibodies in primary biliary cirrhosis. A clue to etiopathogenesis? J Hepatol 1992; 15:6–9.

Bernal W, Moloney M, Underhill J, Donaldson PT: Association of tumor necrosis factor polymorphism with primary sclerosing cholangitis. J Hepatol 1999; 30:237–241.

Biden K, Young J, Buttenshaw R, Searle J, Cooksley G, Xu D-B, Leggett B: Frequency of mutation and deletion of the tumor suppressor gene *CDKN2A (MTS1/p16)* in hepatocellular carcinoma from an Australian population. Hepatology 1997; 25:593–597.

Binder V, Weeke E, Olsen JH, Anthonisen P, Riis P: A genetic study of ulcerative colitis. Scand J Gastroenterol 1966; 1:49–56.

Bittencourt PL, Goldberg AC, Cancado ELR, Porta G, Carrilho FJ, Farias AQ, Palacios SA, Chiarella JM, Abrantes-Lemos CP, Baggio VL, et al.: Genetic heterogeneity in susceptibility to autoimmune hepatitis types 1 and 2. Am J Gastroenterol 1999; 94:1906–1913.

Board PG, Coggan M, Johnson P, Ross V, Suzuki T, Webb G: Genetic heterogeneity of the human glutathione transferases: a complex of gene families. Pharmacol Ther 1990; 48:357–369.

Boberg KM, Aadland E, Jahnsen J, Raknerud N, Stiris M, Bell H: Incidence and prevalence of primary biliary cirrhosis, primary sclerosing cholangitis, and autoimmune hepatitis in a Norwegian population. Scand J Gastroenterol 1998; 33:99–103.

Boberg KM, Schrumpf E, Berquist A, Broome U, Pares A, Remotti H, Schjolberg A, Spurkland A, Clausen OP: Cholangiocarcinoma in primary sclerosing cholangitis: K-*ras* mutations and *p53* dysfunction are implicated in the neoplastic development. J Hepatol 2000; 32:374–380.

Bohman M, Cloninger CR, von Knorring A-L, Sigvardsson S: An adoption study of somatoform disorders. III. Cross-fostering analysis and genetic relationship to alcoholism and criminality. Arch Gen Psychiatry 1984; 41:872–878.

Bohman M, Sigvardsson S, Cloninger CR: Maternal inheritance of alcohol abuse: cross-fostering analysis of adopted women. Arch Gen Psychiatry 1981; 38:965–969.

Brandhagen DJ, Gross JB Jr, Poterucha JJ, Germer JJ, Czaja AJ, Smith CI, Ribeiro AC, Guerrero RB, Therneau TM, Schiff E, et al.: Human leukocyte antigen DR markers as predictors of progression to liver transplantation in patients with chronic hepatitis C. Am J Gastroenterol 2000; 95:2056–2060.

Bressac B, Galvin KM, Liang T-J, Isselbacher KJ, Wands JR, Ozurk M: Abnormal structure and expression of *p53* gene in human hepatocellular carcinoma. Proc Natl Acad Sci USA 1990; 87:1973–1997.

Briggs DC, Donaldson PT, Hayes P, Welsh KI, Williams R, Neuberger JM: A major histocompatibility complex class III allotype (C4B2) associated with primary biliary cirrhosis (PBC). Tissue Antigens 1987; 29:141–145.

Britton RS, Bacon BR: Role of free radicals in liver diseases and hepatic fibrosis. Hepatogastroenterology 1994; 41:343–348.

Brockmoller J, Kerb R, Drakoulis N, Nitz M, Roots I: Genotype and phenotype of glutathione *S*-transferase class mu isoenzymes and psi in lung cancer patients and controls. Cancer Res 1993; 53:1004–1011.

Bron B, Kubski D, Widmann JJ, von Fliedner V, Jeannet M: Increased frequency of DR3 antigen in alcoholic hepatitis and cirrhosis. Hepatogastroenterology 1982; 29:183–186.

Broome U, Glaumann H, Hultcrantz R, Forsum U: Distribution of HLA-DR, HLA-DP, HLA-DQ antigens in liver tissue from patients with primary sclerosing cholangitis. Scand J Gastroenterol 1990; 25:54–58.

Broome U, Grunewald J, Scheynius A, Olerup O, Hultcrantz R: Preferential Vβ3 usage by hepatic T lymphocytes in patients with primary sclerosing cholangitis. J Hepatol 1997; 26:527–534.

Brown JH, Jardetzky T, Saper MA, Samraoui B, Bjorkman PJ, Wiley DC: A hypothetical model of the foreign antigen binding site of class II histocompatibility molecules. Nature 1988; 332:845–850.

Brown R, Clark MK, Doniach D: Primary biliary cirrhosis in brothers. Postgrad Med J 1975; 51:110–115.

Brunner G, Klinge O: A chronic destructive non-suppurative cholangitis-like disease picture with antibnuclear antibodies (immunocholangitis). Dtsch Med Wochenschr 1987; 112:1454–1458.

Buendia MA: Genetics of hepatocellular carcinoma. Semin Cancer Biol 2000; 10:185–200.

Caldwell SH, Leung PSC, Spivey JR, Prindiville T, De Medina M, Saicheur T, Rowley M, Reddy KR, Coppel R, Jeffers LJ, et al.: Antimitochondrial antibodies in kindreds of patients with primary biliary cirrhosis: antimitochondrial antibodies are unique to clinical disease and are absent in asymptomatic family members. Hepatology 1992; 16:899–905.

Carr LG, Hartleroad JY, Liang Y, Mendenhall C, Moritz T, Thomasson H: Polymorphism at the *P450IIE1* locus is not associated with alcoholic liver disease in Caucasian men. Alcohol Clin Exp Res 1995; 19:182–184.

Carruba G, Cervello M, Micelli MD, Farruggio R, Notarbartolo M, Virruso L, Giannitrapani L, Gambino R, Montalto G, Castagnetta L: Truncated form of β-catenin and reduced expression of wild-type catenins feature HepG2 human liver cancer cells. Ann NY Acad Sci 1999; 886:212–216.

Chan SH, Simons MJ, Oon CJ: HLA antigen in Chinese patients with hepatocellular carcinoma. J Natl Cancer Inst 1980; 65:21–23.

Chao Y-C, Liou S-R, Chung Y-Y, Tang H-S, Hsu C-T, Li T-K, Yin S-J: Polymorphism of alcohol and aldehyde dehydrogenase genes and alcoholic cirrhosis in Chinese patients. Hepatology 1994; 19:360–366.

Chao Y-C, Wang LS, Hsieh TY, Chu CW, Chang FY, Chu HC: Chinese alcoholic patients with esophageal cancer are genetically different from alcoholics with acute pancreatitis and liver cirrhosis. Am J Gastroenterol 2000; 95:2958–2964.

Chapman RW: The immunology of primary sclerosing cholangitis. Springer Semin Immunopathol 1990; 12:121–128.

Chapman RW: Aetiology and natural history of primary sclerosing cholangitis—a decade of progress? Gut 1991; 32:1433–1435.

Chapman RW, Arborgh BA, Rhodes JM, Summerfield JA, Dick R, Scheuer PJ, Sherlock S: Primary sclerosing cholangitis: a review of its clinical features, cholangiography and hepatic histology. Gut 1980; 21:870–877.

Chapman RW, Kelly P, Heryet A, Jewell DP, Fleming KA: Expression of the HLA-DR antigens on bile duct epithelium in primary sclerosing cholangitis. Gut 1988; 29:422–427.

Chapman RW, Varghese Z, Gaul R, Patel G, Kokinon N, Sherlock S: Association of primary sclerosing cholangitis with HLA-B8. Gut 1983; 24:38–41.

Chiovato L, Lapi P, Fiore E, Tonacchera M, Pinchera A: Thyroid autoimmunity and female gender. J Endocrinol Invest 1993; 16:384–391.

Chohan MR: Primary biliary cirrhosis in twin sisters. Gut 1973; 14:213–214.

Clevers H: Axin and hepatocellular carcinomas. Nat Genet 2000; 24:206–208.

Clot P, Bellomo G, Tabone M, Arico S, Albano E: Detection of antibodies against proteins modified by hydroxyethyl free-radicals in patients with alcoholic cirrhosis. Gastroenterology 1995; 108:201–207.

Cohen IR, Cooke A: Natural autoantibodies might prevent autoimmune disease. Immunol Today 1986; 7:363–364.

Collier JD, Carpenter M, Burt AD, Bassendine MF: Expression of mutant p53 protein in hepatocellular carcinoma. Gut 1994; 35:98–100.

Conglia M, Clemente MG, Dessi C, Cucca F, Mazzoleni AP, Frau F, Lampis R, Cao A, Lai ME, De Virgiliis S: HLA class II genes in chronic hepatitis C virus infection and associated immunological disorders. Hepatology 1996; 24:1338–1341.

Cookson S, Constantini PK, Clare M, Underhill JA, Bernal W, Czaja AJ, Donaldson PT: Frequency and nature of cytokine gene polymorphisms in type 1 autoimmune hepatitis. Hepatology 1999; 30:851–856.

Costa M, Rodriques-Sanchez JL, Czaja AJ, Gelpi C: Isolation and characterization of cDNA encoding the antigenic protein of the human tRNP$^{(Ser)Sec}$ complex recognized by autoantibodies from patients with type 1 autoimmune hepatitis. Clin Exp Immunol 2000; 121:364–374.

Couzigou P, Fleury B, Groppi A, Cassaigne A, Begueret J, Iron A: Genotyping study of alcohol dehydrogenase class I polymorphism in French patients with alcoholic cirrhosis. Alcohol Alcohol 1990; 25:623–626.

Czaja AJ: Natural history, clinical features, and treatment of autoimmune hepatitis. Semin Liver Dis 1984; 4:1–12.

Czaja AJ: Autoimmune hepatitis and viral infection. Gastroenterol Clin North Am 1994; 23:547–566.

Czaja AJ: Autoimmune hepatitis: evolving concepts and treatment strategies. Dig Dis Sci 1995; 40:435–456.

Czaja AJ: Extrahepatic immunologic features of chronic viral hepatitis. Dig Dis 1997; 15:125–144.

Czaja AJ: Frequency and nature of the variant syndromes of autoimmune liver disease. Hepatology 1998; 28:360–365.

Czaja AJ: Behavior and significance of autoantibodies in type 1 autoimmune hepatitis. J Hepatol 1999; 30:394–401.

Czaja AJ: Immunopathogenesis of autoimmune-mediated liver damage. In: Moreno-Otero R, Clemente-Ricote G, Garcia-Monzon C (eds). Immunology and the Liver: Autoimmunity. Madrid: Aran Ediciones, 2000:73–83.

Czaja AJ: Understanding the pathogenesis of autoimmune hepatitis. Am J Gastroenterol 2001; 96:1224–1231.

Czaja AJ, Carpenter HA: Sensitivity, specificity and predictability of biopsy interpretations in chronic hepatitis. Gastroenterology 1993; 105:1824–1832.

Czaja AJ, Carpenter HA: Histological findings in chronic hepatitis C with autoimmune features. Hepatology 1997; 26:459–466.
Czaja AJ, Carpenter HA, Manns MP: Antibodies to soluble liver antigen, P450 IID6 and mitochondrial complexes in chronic hepatitis. Gastroenterology 1993a; 105:1522–1528.
Czaja AJ, Carpenter HA, Santrach PJ, Moore SB: Genetic predispositions for the immunological features of chronic active hepatitis. Hepatology 1993b; 18:816–822.
Czaja AJ, Carpenter HA, Santrach PJ, Moore SB: Significance of HLA DR4 in type 1 autoimmune hepatitis. Gastroenterology 1993c; 105:1502–1507.
Czaja AJ, Carpenter HA, Santrach PJ, Moore SB: Significance of human leukocyte antigens DR3 and DR4 in chronic viral hepatitis. Dig Dis Sci 1995; 40:2098–2106.
Czaja AJ, Carpenter HA, Santrach PJ, Moore SB: Genetic predispositions for immunological features in chronic liver diseases other than autoimmune hepatitis. J Hepatol 1996a; 24:52–59.
Czaja AJ, Carpenter HA, Santrach PJ, Moore SB: DR human leukocyte antigens and disease severity in chronic hepatitis C. J Hepatol 1996b; 24:666–673.
Czaja AJ, Carpenter HA, Santrach PJ, Moore SB: Autoimmune cholangitis within the spectrum of autoimmune liver disease. Hepatology 2000a; 31:1231–1238.
Czaja AJ, Cookson S, Constantini PK, Clare M, Underhill JA, Donaldson PT: Cytokine polymorphisms associated with clinical features and treatment outcome in type 1 autoimmune hepatitis. Gastroenterology 1999; 117:645–652.
Czaja AJ, Donaldson PT: Genetic susceptibilities for immune expression and liver cell injury in autoimmune hepatitis. Immunol Rev 2000; 174:250–259.
Czaja AJ, Dos Santos RM, Porto A, Santrach PJ, Moore SB: Immune phenotype of chronic liver disease. Dig Dis Sci 1998; 43:2149–2155.
Czaja AJ, Homburger HA: Autoantibodies in liver disease. Gastroenterology 2001; 120:239–249.
Czaja AJ, Kruger M, Santrach PJ, Moore SB, Manns MP: Genetic distinctions between types 1 and 2 autoimmune hepatitis. Am J Gastroenterol 1997a; 92:2197–2200.
Czaja AJ, Manns MP: The validity and importance of subtypes in autoimmune hepatitis—a point of view. Am J Gastroenterol 1995; 90:1206–1211.
Czaja AJ, Manns MP, Homburger HA: Frequency and significance of antibodies to liver/kidney microsome type 1 in adults with chronic active hepatitis. Gastroenterology 1992; 103:1290–1295.
Czaja AJ, Rakela J, Hay JE, Moore SB: Clinical and prognostic implications of human leukocyte antigen B8 in corticosteroid-treated severe autoimmune chronic active hepatitis. Gastroenterology 1990; 98:1587–1593.
Czaja AJ, Santrach PJ, Moore SB: Shared genetic risk factors in autoimmune liver disease. Dig Dis Sci 2001; 46:140–147.
Czaja AJ, Sievers C, Zein NN: Nature and behavior of serum cytokines in type 1 autoimmune hepatitis. Dig Dis Sci 2000b; 45:1028–1035.
Czaja AJ, Strettell MDJ, Thomson LJ, Santrach PJ, Moore SB, Donaldson PT, Williams R: Associations between alleles of the major histocompatibility complex and type 1 autoimmune hepatitis. Hepatology 1997b; 25:317–323.
Dabbagh AJ, Mannion T, Lynch SM, Frei B: The effect of iron overload on rat plasma and liver oxidant status in vivo. Biochem J 1994; 300:799–803.
D'Alfonso S, Momigliano Richiardi P: A polymorphic variation in a putative regulation box of the TNFA promoter region. Immunogenetics 1994; 39:150–154.
Daly AK, Cholerton S, Gregory W, Idle JR: Metabolic polymorphisms. Pharmacol Ther 1993; 57:129–160.
Davies DR, Metzger H: Structural basis of antibody function. Annu Rev Immunol 1983; 1:87–117.
Day CP, Bashir R, James OFW, Bassendine MF, Crabb DW, Thomasson HR, Li T-K, Edenberg HJ: Investigation of the role of polymorphisms at the alcohol and aldehyde dehydrogenase loci in genetic predisposition to alcohol-related end-organ damage. Hepatology 1991; 14:797–801.
Day CP, Bashir R, Sykes B, Crabb D, Li T-K, Edenberg HJ, James OFW, Bassendine MF: Investigation of the role of five "candidate genes" in genetic susceptibility to alcoholic cirrhosis. Hepatology 1990; 12:923.
Day CP, Bassendine MF: Genetic predisposition to alcoholic liver disease. Gut 1992; 33:1444–1447.
Day CP, James OFW, Bassendine MF, Crabb DW, Li T-K: Alcohol dehydrogenase polymorphisms and predisposition to alcoholic cirrhosis [letter]. Hepatology 1993; 18:230–231.
Debruyne P, Vermeulen S, Mareel M: The role of the E-cadherin/catenin complex in gastrointestinal cancer. Acta Gastroenterol Belg 1999; 62:393–402.
Degoul F, Sutton A, Mansouri A, Cepanec C, Degott C, Fromenty B, Beaugrand M, Valla D, Pessayre D: Homozygosity for alanine in the mitochondrial targeting sequence of superoxide dismutase and risk for severe alcoholic liver disease. Gastroenterology 2001; 120:1468–1474.
Devereux TR, Anna CH, Foley JF, White CM, Sills RC, Barrett JC: Mutation of β-catenin is an early event in chemically induced mouse hepatocellular carcinogenesis. Oncogene 1999; 18:4726–4733.
Diamantis ID, McGandy C, Chen T-J, Liaw Y-F, Gudat F, Bianchi L: A new mutational hot-spot in the *p53* gene in human hepatocellular carcinoma. J Hepatol 1994; 20:553–556.
Diehl AM, Goodman Z, Ishak KG: Alcohollike liver disease in nonalcoholics. A clinical and histologic comparison with alcohol-induced liver injury. Gastroenterology 1988; 95:1056–1062.
Diepolder HM, Gerlach JT, Zachoval R, Hoffman RM, Jung MC, Wierenga EA, Scholz S, Santantonio T, Houghton M, Southwood S, et al.: Immunodominant $CD4^+$ T cell epitope within nonstructural protein 3 in acute hepatitis C virus infection. J Virol 1997; 71:6011–6019.
Diepolder HM, Scholz S, Pape GR: Influence of HLA alleles on outcome of hepatitis C virus infection. Lancet 1999; 354:2094–2095.
Diu A, Mobius U, Ferradini L, Genevee C, Roman S, Claudon M, Delorme D, Meuer S, Hercend T, Praz F: Limited T-cell receptor diversity in liver-infiltrating lymphocytes from patients with primary biliary cirrhosis. J Autoimmun 1993; 5:611–619.
Doherty DG, Donaldson PT, Underhill JA, Farrant JM, Duthie A, Mieli-Vergani G, McFarlane IG, Johnson PJ, Eddleston ALWF, Mowat AP, et al.: Allelic sequence variation in the HLA class II genes and proteins in patients with autoimmune hepatitis. Hepatology 1994a; 19:609–615.
Doherty DG, Underhill JA, Donaldson PT, Manabe K, Mieli-Vergani G, Eddleston ALWF, Vergani D, Demaine AG, Williams R: Polymorphisms in the human complement *C4* genes and genetic susceptibility to autoimmune hepatitis. Autoimmunity 1994b; 18:243–249.
Donaldson PT, Doherty DG, Hayllar KM, McFarlane IG, Johnson PJ, Williams R: Susceptibility to autoimmune chronic active hepatitis: human leukocyte antigens DR4 and A1-B8-DR3 are independent risk factors. Hepatology 1991a; 13:701–706.
Donaldson PT, Farrant JM, Wilkinson ML, Hayllar K, Portmann BC, Williams R: Dual association of HLA DR2 and DR3 with primary sclerosing cholangitis. Hepatology 1991b; 13:129–133.
Donaldson PT, Norris S, Constantini PK, Bernal W, Harrison P, Williams R: The interleukin-1 and interleukin-10 polymorphisms in primary sclerosing cholangitis: no associations with disease susceptibility/resistance. J Hepatol 2000; 32:882–886.
Douglas JG, Finlayson ND: Are increased individual susceptibility and environmental factors both necessary for the development of PBC? BMJ 1979; 2:419–420.
Enomoto N, Takase S, Takada N, Takada A: Alcoholic liver disease in heterozygotes of mutant and normal aldehyde dehydrogenase-2 genes. Hepatology 1991; 13:1071–1075.
Ercilla G, Pares A, Arriaga F, Bruguera M, Castillo R, Rodes J, Vives J: Primary biliary cirrhosis associated with HLA-DRw3. Tissue Antigens 1979; 14:449–452.
Eriksson S: Pulmonary emphysema and $alpha_1$-antitrypsin deficiency. Acta Med Scand 1964; 175:197–205.
Eriksson S, Carlson J, Velez R: Risk of cirrhosis and primary liver cancer in α_1-antitrypsin deficiency. N Engl J Med 1989; 314:736–739.
Fagan EA, Williams R, Cox S: Primary biliary cirrhosis in mother and daughter. BMJ 1977; 2:1195.
Fainboim L, Marcos Y, Pando M, Capucchio M, Reyes GB, Galoppo C, Badia I, Remondino G, Ciocca M, Ramonet M, Fainboim H, et al.: Chronic active autoimmune hepatitis in children. Strong association with a particular HLA-DR6 (DRB1*1301) haplotype. Hum Immunol 1994; 41:146–150.
Fan X, Solomon H, Schwarz K, Kew MC, Ray RB, Di Bisceglie AM: Expression of c-*myc* promoter binding protein (*MBP-1*), a novel eukayotic repressor gene, in cirrhosis and human hepatocellular carcinoma. Dig Dis Sci 2001; 46:563–566.
Fanning LJ, Levis J, Kenny-Walsh E, Whelton M, O'Sullivan K, Shanahan F: HLA class II genes determine the natural variance of hepatitis C viral load. Hepatology 2001; 33:224–230.
Farmer RG, Michener WM, Mortimer EA: Studies of family history among patients with inflammatory bowel disease. Clin Gastroenterol 1980; 9:271–278.
Farrant JM, Doherty DG, Donaldson PT, Vaughan RW, Hayllar KM, Welsh KI, Eddleston ALWF, Williams R: Amino acid substitutions at position 38 of the DRβ polypeptide confer susceptibility to and protection from primary sclerosing cholangitis. Hepatology 1992; 16:390–395.
Faustman D, Li X, Lin HY, Fu Y, Eisenbarth G, Avruch J, Guo J: Linkage of faulty major histocompatibility complex class I to autoimmune diabetes. Science 1991; 254:1756–1761.
Feder JN, Gnirke A, Thomas W, Tsuchihashi Z, Ruddy DA, Basava A, Dormishian F, Domingo R Jr, Ellis MC, Fullan A, et al.: A novel MHC class I-like gene is mutated in patients with hereditary haemochromatosis. Nat Genet 1996; 13:399–409.
Feizi T, Naccarato R, Sherlock S, Doniach D: Mitochondrial and other tissue antibodies in relatives of patients with primary biliary cirrhosis. Clin Exp Immunol 1972; 10:609–622.
Fernandez-Salguero P, Hoffman SMG, Cholerton S, Mohrenweiser H, Raunio H, Rautio A, Pelkonen O, Huang J, Evans WE, Idle JR, et al.: A genetic polymorphism in coumarin 7-hydroxylation: sequence of the human *CYP2A6* genes and identification of variant *CYP2A6* alleles. Am J Hum Genet 1995; 57:651–660.
Forbes A, Blanshard C, Gazzard B: Natural history of AIDS related sclerosing cholangitis—a study of 20 cases. Gut 1993; 34:116–121.
Forzani B, Actis GC, Verme G, Amoroso A, Borellia I, Curtoni ES, Rumi MG, Picciotto A, Marinucci G, Freni MA, et al.: HLA-DR antigens in HBsAg-positive chronic active liver disease with and without delta infection. Hepatology 1984; 4:1107–1110.
Foster PL, Eisenstadt E, Miller JH: Base substitutions induced by metabolically activated aflatoxin B_1. Proc Natl Acad Sci USA 1983; 80:2695–2698.
Fourel G, Trepo C, Bougueleret L, Henglein B, Ponzetto A, Tiollais P, Buendia MA: Frequent activation of N-*myc* genes by hepadnavirus insertion in woodchuck liver tumors. Nature 1990; 347:294–280.
Frezza M, Di Padova C, Pozzato G, Terpin M, Baraona E, Lieber CS: High blood alcohol levels in women: role of decreased gastric alcohol dehydrogenase activity and first pass metabolism. N Engl J Med 1990; 322:95–99.
Galbraith RM, Eddleston ALWF, Smith MGM, Williams R, McSween RN, Watkinson G, Dick H, Kennedy LA, Batchelor JR: Histocompatibility antigens in active chronic hepatitis and primary biliary cirrhosis. BMJ 1974a; 2:604–605.
Galbraith RM, Smith M, MacKenzie RM, Tee DE, Doniach D, Williams R: High prevalence of seroimmunologic abnormalities in relatives of patients with active chronic hepatitis or primary biliary cirrhosis. N Engl J Med 1974b; 290:63–69.
Gerbes AL, Caselmann WH: Point mutations of the *p53* gene, human hepatocellular carcinoma and aflatoxins. J Hepatol 1993; 19:312–315.

Giani G, Chiaramonte M, Pasini CV, Fagiolo U, Naccarato R: Hepatitis B surface antigenemia and HLA antigens [letter]. N Engl J Med 1979; 300:1056.
Gilder FJ, Hodgkinson S, Murray RM: ADH and ALDH genotype profiles in Caucasians with alcohol-related problems and controls. Addiction 1993; 88:383–388.
Goldblum JR, Bartos RE, Carr KA, Frank TS: Hepatitis B and alterations of the *p53* tumor suppressor gene in hepatocellular carcinoma. Am J Surg Pathol 1993; 17:1244–1251.
Gonzalez-Peralta RP, Davis GL, Lau JYN: Pathogenetic mechanisms of hepatocellular damage in chronic hepatitis C virus infection. J Hepatol 1994; 21:255–259.
Goodman ZD, McNally PR, Davis DR, Ishak KG: Autoimminue cholangitis: a variant of primary biliary cirrhosis. Clinicopathologic and serologic correlations in 200 cases. Dig Dis Sci 1995; 40:1232–1242.
Goodwin DW, Schulsinger F, Hermansen L, Guze SB, Winokur G: Alcohol problems in adoptees raised apart from alcoholic biological parents. Arch Gen Psychiatry 1973; 28:238–243.
Gores GJ, Moore SB, Fisher LD, Powell FC, Dickson ER: Primary biliary cirrhosis: associations with class II major histocompatibility complex antigens. Hepatology 1987; 7:889–892.
Govindarajan S, Hevia FJ, Peters RL: Prevalence of delta antigen/antibody in B-viral-associated hepatocellular carcinoma. Cancer 1984; 53:1692–1694.
Grant BF, Harford TC, Dawson DA, Chou P, Dufour M, Pickering R: Prevalence of DSM-IV alcohol abuse and dependence, United States, 1992. Alcohol Health and Research World 1994; 18:243–248.
Gregory WL, Bassendine MF: Genetic factors in primary biliary cirrhosis. J Hepatol 1994; 20:689–692.
Gregory WL, Daly AK, Dunn AN, Cavanagh G, Idle JR, James OFW, Bassendine MF: Analysis of HLA-classII–encoded antigen-processing genes *TAP1* and *TAP2* in primary biliary cirrhosis. Q J Med 1994; 87:237–244.
Gregory WL, Mehal W, Dunn AN, Cavanagh G, Chapman R, Fleming KA, Daly AK, Idle JR, James OFW, Bassendine MF: Primary biliary cirrhosis: contribution of HLA class II allele DR8. Q J Med 1993; 86:393–399.
Griffing WL, Moore SB, Luthra HS, McKenna CH, Fathman CG: Associations of antibodies to native DNA with HLA-DRw3: a possible major histocompatibility complex-linked human immune response gene. J Exp Med 1980; 152:319s-325s.
Grove J, Brown AS, Daly AK, Bassendine MF, James OF, Day CP: The RsaI polymorphism of *CYP2E1* and susceptibility to alcoholic liver disease in Caucasians: effect on age of presentation and dependence on alcohol dehydrogenase phenotype. Pharmacogenetics 1998; 8:335–342.
Grove J, Daly AK, Bassendine MF, Day CP: Association of a tumor necrosis factor promoter polymorphism with susceptibility to alcoholic steatohepatitis. Hepatology 1997; 26:143–146.
Grove J, Daly AK, Bassendine MF, Gilvarry E, Day CP: Interleukin 10 promoter region polymorphisms and susceptibility to advanced alcoholic liver disease. Gut 2000; 46:448–449.
Guidotti LG, Ishikawa T, Hobbs MV, Matzke B, Schreiber R, Chisari FV: Intracellular inactivation of the hepatitis B virus by cytotoxic T lymphocytes. Immunity 1996; 4:25–36.
Gullsten H, Agundez JAG, Benitez J, Laara E, Ladero JM, Diaz-Rubio M, Fernandez-Salguero P, Gonzalez F, Rautio A, Pelkonen O, et al.: *CYP2A6* gene polymorphism and risk of liver cancer and cirrhosis. Pharmacogenetics 1997; 7:247–250.
Hamamoto T, Yamada S, Hirayama C: Nonoxidative metabolism of ethanol in the pancreas: implication in alcoholic pancreatic damage. Biochem Pharmacol 1990; 39:241–245.
Hanck C, Glatzel M, Singer MV, Rossol S: Gene expression of TNF-receptors in peripheral blood mononuclear cells of patients with alcoholic cirrhosis. J Hepatol 2000; 32:51–57.
Harada K, Van de Water J, Leung PSC, Coppel RL, Ansari A, Nakanuma Y, Gershwin ME: In situ nucleic acid hybridization of cytokines in primary biliary cirrhosis: predominance of the Th1 subset. Hepatology 1997; 25:791–796.
Hassett C, Aicher L, Sidhu S, Omiecinski CJ: Human microsomal epoxide hydrolase: genetic polymorphism and functional expression in vitro of amino acid variants. Hum Mol Genet 1994; 3:421–428.
Hayashi H, Sugio K, Matsumata T, Adachi E, Takeneka K, Sugimachi K: The clinical significance of *p53* gene mutation in hepatocellular carcinomas from Japan. Hepatology 1995; 22:1702–1707.
Hayashi S, Watanabe J, Kaname K: Genetic polymorphism in the 5′-flanking region change transcriptional regulation of the human *cytochrome P4502E1* gene. J Biochem 1991; 110:559–565.
Herzog D, Hajoui O, Russo P, Alvarez F: Study of immune reactivity of minocycline-induced chronic active hepatitis. Dig Dis Sci 1997; 42:1100–1103.
Hilberg RW, Mulhern LM, Kenny JJ, Luparello FJ: Chronic active hepatitis: report of two sisters with positive lupus erythematosus preparations. Ann Intern Med 1971; 74:937–941.
Hill DB, Barve S, Joshi-Barve S, McClain C: Increased monocyte nuclear factor-kappa B activation and tumor necrosis factor production in alcoholic hepatitis. J Lab Clin Med 2000; 135:367–369.
Hillis WD, Hillis A, Bias WB, Walker WG: Associations of hepatitis B surface antigenemia with HLA locus B specificities. N Engl J Med 1977; 296; 1310–1314.
Hiryama K, Matsudhita S, Kikuchi I, Iuchi M, Ohta N, Sasazuki T: HLA-DQ is epistatic to HLA-DR in controlling the immune response to schistosomal antigen in humans. Nature 1987; 127:426–430.
Hodges JR, Millward-Sadler GH, Wright R: Chronic active hepatitis: the spectrum of disease. Lancet 1982; 1:550–552.
Hodges S, Lobo-Yeo A, Donaldson P, Tanner MS, Vergani D: Autoimmune chronic active hepatitis in a family. Gut 1991; 32:299–302.
Hodgson HJF, Wands JR, Isselbacher KJ: Alteration in suppressor cell activity in chronic active hepatitis. Proc Natl Acad Sci USA 1978; 75:1549–1553.
Hohler T, Gerken G, Notghi A, Knolle P, Lubjuhn R, Taheri H, Schneider PM, Meyer zum Buschenfelde K-H, Rittner C: MHC class II genes influence the susceptibility to chronic hepatitis C. J Hepatol 1997a; 27:259–264.
Hohler T, Gerken G, Notghi A, Lubjuhn R, Taheri H, Protzer U, Lohr HF, Schneider PM, Meyer zum Buschenfelde K-H, Rittner C: HLA-DRB1*1301 and *1302 protect against chronic hepatitis B J Hepatol 1997b; 26:503–507.
Hohler T, Kruger A, Gerken G, Schneider PM, Meyer zum Buschenfelde K-H, Rittner C: A tumour necrosis factor-alpha (TNF-α) promoter polymorphism is associated with chronic hepatitis B infection. Clin Exp Immunol 1998; 111:579–582.
Holmberg D, Coutinho A: Natural autoantibodies and autoimmunity. Immunol Today 1985; 6:356–357.
Homberg J-C, Abuaf N, Bernard O, Islam S, Alvarez F, Khalil SH, Poupon R, Darnis F, Levy V-G, Grippon P, et al.: Chronic active hepatitis associated with antiliver/kidney microsome antibody type 1: a second type of "autoimmune" hepatitis. Hepatology 1987; 7:1333–1339.
Hopf U, Stemerowicz R, Rodloff A, Galanos C, Moller B, Lobeck H, Freudenberg M, Galanos C, Huhn D: Relation between *Escherichia coli* R (rough)-forms in gut, lipid A in liver, and primary biliary cirrhosis. Lancet 1989; 2:1419–1422.
Houglum K, Ramm GA, Crawford DHG, Witztum JL, Powell LW, Chojkier M: Excess iron induces hepatic oxidative stress and transforming growth factor β1 in genetic hemochromatosis. Hepatology 1997; 26:605–610.
Hrubec Z, Omenn GS: Evidence of genetic predisposition to alcoholic cirrhosis and psychosis: twin concordances for alcoholism and its biological end points by zygosity among male veterans. Alcohol Clin Exp Res 1981; 5:207–215.
Hsu IC, Metcalf RA, Sun T, Welsh JA, Wang NJ, Harris CC: Mutational hotspot in the *p53* gene in human hepatocellular carcinomas. Nature 1991; 350:427–428.
Hsu TY, Moroy T, Etiemble J, Louise A, Trepo C, Tiollais P, Buedia MA: Activation of c-*myc* by woodchuck hepatitis virus insertion in hepatocellular carcinoma. Cell 1988; 55:627–635.
Hui AM, Shi YZ, Li X, Takayama T, Makuuchi M: Loss of $p16^{INK4}$ protein, alone and together with loss of retinoblastoma protein, correlate with hepatocellular carcinoma progression. Cancer Lett 2000; 154:93–99.
Isoyama K, Yamada K, Ishikawa K, Sanada Y: Coincidental cases of primary sclerosing cholangitis and biliary atresia in siblings? Acta Paediatr 1995; 84:1444–1446.
James OF, Myszor M: Epidemiology and genetics of primary biliary cirrhosis. Prog Liver Dis 1990; 9:523–536.
Jarvelainen HA, Orpana A, Perola M, Savolainen VT, Karhunen PJ, Lindros KO: Promoter polymorphism of the CD14 endotoxin receptor gene as a risk factor for alcoholic liver disease. Hepatology 2001; 33:1148–1153.
Jaup BH, Zettergren LSW: Familial occurrence of primary biliary cirrhosis associated with hypergammaglobulinemia in descendants: a family study. Gastroenterology 1980; 78:549–555.
Jeng KS, Sheen IS, Chen BF, Wu JY: Is the *p53* gene mutation of prognostic value in hepatocellular carcinoma after resection? Arch Surg 2000; 135:1329–1333.
Jin M, Piao Z, Kim NG, Park C, Shin EC, Park JH, Jung HJ, Kim CG, Kim H: p16 is a major inactivation target in hepatocellular carcinoma. Cancer 2000; 89:60–68.
Jorge AD, Esley C, Ahumada J: Family incidence of primary sclerosing cholangitis associated with immunological diseases. Endoscopy 1987; 19:114–117.
Kaino M: Alterations in tumor suppressor genes *p53*, *RB*, *p16/MTS1*, and *p15/MTS2* in human pancreatic cancer and hepatoma cell lines. J Gastroenterol 1997; 32:40–46.
Kam-Tao P, Leung NW-Y, Poon ASY, Wong KC, Chan TH, Lai KN: Molecular genetics of major histocompatibility complex class II genes in hepatocellular carcinoma. Dig Dis Sci 1995; 40:1542–1546.
Kaneto H, Sasaki S, Yamamoto H, Itoh F, Toyota M, Suzuki H, Ozeki I, Iwata N, Ohmura T, Satoh T, et al.: Detection of hypermethylation of the $p16^{INK4A}$ gene promoter in chronic hepatitis and cirrhosis associated with hepatitis B or C virus. Gut 2001; 48:372–377.
Kanzler S, Weidemann C, Gerken G, Lohr HF, Galle PR, Meyer zum Buschenfelde KH, Lohse AW: Clinical significance of autoantibodies to soluble liver antigen in autoimmune hepatitis. J Hepatol 1999; 31:635–640.
Kaplan MM: Primary biliary cirrhosis. N Engl J Med 1987; 316:521–528.
Kashio T, Hotta R, Kakumu S: Lymphocyte suppressor cell activity in acute and chronic liver disease. Clin Exp Immunol 1981; 44:459–466.
Kato Y, Suzuki K, Kumagai M, Nishimura N, Miyamori M, Kobayashi K, Hattori N, Nakanuma Y: Familial primary biliary cirrhosis. Am J Gastroenterol 1981; 75:188–191.
Kazachkov Y, Khaoustov V, Yoffe B, Solomon H, Klintmalm GB, Tabor E: p53 abnormalities in hepatocellular carcinoma from United States patients: analysis of all 11 exons. Carcinogenesis 1996; 17:2207–2212.
Kelly P, Patchett S, McCloskey D, Alstead E, Farthing M, Fairclough P: Sclerosing cholangitis, race and sex. Gut 1997; 41:688–689.
Kew MC, Dusheiko GM, Hadziyannis SJ, Patterson A: Does delta infection play a part in the pathogenesis of hepatitis B virus related hepatocellular carcinoma? BMJ 1984; 288:1727.
Kew MC, Gear AJ, Baumgarten I, Dusheiko GM, Maier G: Histocompatibility antigens in patients with hepatocellular carcinoma and their relationship to chronic hepatitis B virus infection in these patients. Gastroenterology 1979; 77:537–539.
Kew MC, Popper H: Relationship between hepatocellular carcinoma and cirrhosis. Semin Liver Dis 1984; 4:136–146.
Kirby GM, Batist G, Alpert L, Lamoureux E, Cameron RG, Alaoui-Jamali MA: Overexpression of cytochrome P-450 isoforms involved in aflatoxin B_1 bioactivation in human liver with cirrhosis and hepatitis. Toxicol Pathol 1996; 24:458–467.

Kirsner JB, Spencer JA: Family occurrence of ulcerative colitis, regional enteritis, and ileocolitis. Ann Intern Med 1963; 59:133–144.

Kiyosawa K, Sodeyama T, Tanaka E, Gibo Y, Yoshizawa K, Kakano Y, Furuta S, Akahane Y, Nishioka K, Purcell RH, et al.: Interrelationship of blood transfusion, non-A, non-B hepatitis and hepatocellular carcinoma: analysis by detection of antibody to hepatitis C. Hepatology 1990; 12:641–675.

Klein R, Berg PA: Demonstration of "naturally occurring mitochondrial antibodies" in family members of patients with primary biliary cirrhosis. Hepatology 1990; 12:335–341.

Kono H, Rusyn I, Yin M, Gabele E, Yamashina S, Dikalova A, Kadiiska MB, Connor HD, Mason RP, Segal BH, et al.: NADPH oxidase–derived free radicals are key oxidants in alcohol-induced liver disease. J Clin Invest 2000; 106:867–872.

Krams SM, Surh CD, Coppel RL, Ansari A, Ruebner B, Gershwin ME: Immunization of experimental animals with dihydrolipoamide acetyltransferase, as a purified recombinant polypeptide, generates mitochondrial antibodies but not primary biliary cirrhosis. Hepatology 1989; 9:411–416.

Krams SM, Van de Water J, Coppel RL, Esquivel C, Roberts J, Ansari A, Gershwin ME: Analysis of hepatic T lymphocyte and immunoglobulin deposits in patients with primary biliary cirrhosis. Hepatology 1990; 12:306–313.

Krawitt EL, Kilby AE, Albertini RJ, Schanfield MS, Chastenay BF, Harper PC, Mickey RM, McAuliffe TL: Immunogenetic studies of autoimmune chronic active hepatitis: HLA, immunoglobulin allotypes and autoantibodies. Hepatology 1987; 7:1305–1310.

Krawitt EL, Kilby AE, Albertini RJ, Schanfield MS, Chastenay BF, Harper PC, Mickey RM, McAuliffe TL: An immunogenetic study of suppressor cell activity in autoimmune chronic active hepatitis. Clin Immunol Immunopathol 1988; 46: 249–257.

Kress S, Jahn U-R, Buchmann A, Bannasch P, Schwarz M: *p53* mutations in human hepatocellular carcinomas from Germany. Cancer Res 1992; 52:3220–3223.

Kubicka S, Kuhnel F, Flemming P, Hain B, Kezmic N, Rudolph KL, Manns M, Meier PN: K-*ras* mutations in the bile of patients with primary sclerosing cholangitis. Gut 2001; 48:403–408.

Kubicka S, Trautwein C, Niehof M, Manns M: Target gene modulation in hepatocellular carcinomas by decreased DNA-binding of *p53* mutations. Hepatology 1997; 25:867–873.

Kubicka S, Trautwein C, Schrem H, Tillman H, Manns M: Low incidence of *p53* mutations in European hepatocellular carcinomas with heterogeneous mutation as a rare event. J Hepatol 1995; 23:412–419.

Kuroki T, Fujiwara Y, Nakamori S, Imaoka S, Kanematsu T, Nakamura Y: Evidence for the presence of two tumour-suppressor genes for hepatocellular carcinoma on chromosome 13q. Br J Cancer 1995; 72:383–385.

Kuzushita N, Hayashi N, Katayama K, Hiramatsu N, Yasumaru M, Murata H, Shimizu Y, Yamazaki T, Fushimi H, Kotoh K, et al.: Increased frequency of HLA DR13 in hepatitis C virus carriers with persistently normal ALT levels. J Med Virol 1996; 48:1–7.

Kuzushita N, Hayashi N, Moribe T, Katayama K, Kanto T, Nakatani S, Kaneshige T, Tatsumi T, Ito A, Mochizuki K, et al.: Influence of HLA haplotypes on the clinical courses of individuals infected with the hepatitis C virus. Hepatology 1998; 27:240–244.

Ladero JM, Agundez JAG, Rodriguez-Lescure A, Diaz-Rubio M, Benitez J: RsaI polymorphism at the cytochrome P4502E1 locus and risk of hepatocellular carcinoma. Gut 1996; 39:330–333.

Lambert NC, Evans PC, Hashizumi TL, Maloney S, Gooley T, Furst DE, Nelson JL: Cutting edge: persistent fetal microchimerism in T lymphocytes is associated with HLA-DQA1*0501: implications for autoimmunity. J Immunol 2000; 164:5545–5548.

Lamonaca V, Missale G, Urbani S, Pilli M, Boni C, Mori C, Sette A, Massari M, Southwood S, Bertoni R, et al.: Conserved hepatitis C virus sequences are highly immunogenic for CD4(+) T cells: implications for vaccine development. Hepatology 1999; 30:1088–1098.

Lange LG, Bergmann SR, Sobel BE: Identification of fatty acid ethyl esters as products of rabbit myocardial ethanol metabolism. J Biol Chem 1981; 256:12968–12973.

Lange LG, Sobel BE: Myocardial metabolites of ethanol. Circ Res 1983; 52:479–482.

Laposata EA, Lange LG: Presence of nonoxidative ethanol metabolism in human organs commonly deranged by ethanol abuse. Science 1986; 231:497–499.

Lee YM, Kaplan MM: Primary sclerosing cholangitis. N Engl J Med 1995; 332:924–933.

Lelback WK: Cirrhosis in the alcoholic and its relation to the volume of alcohol abuse. Ann NY Acad Sci 1975; 285:85–105.

Levine AJ: The tumor suppressor genes. Annu Rev Biochem 1993; 62:623–651.

Lin DY, Liaw YE, Huang CC: The distribution of HLA-A, B, C, DR antigens in Chinese patients with hepatocellular carcinoma in Taiwan. Tissue Antigens 1987; 29:110–114.

List S, Gluud C: A meta-analysis of HLA-antigen prevalences in alcoholics and alcoholic liver disease. Alcohol Alcohol 1994; 29:757–764.

Livni N, Eid A, Ilan Y, Rivkind A, Rosenmann E, Blendis LM, Shouval D, Galun E: p53 expression in patients with cirrhosis with and without hepatocellular carcinoma. Cancer 1995; 75:2420–2426.

Lohr H, Fleischer B, Gerken G, Yeaman SJ, Meyer zum Buschenfelde KH, Manns M: Autoreactive liver-infiltrating T cells in primary biliary cirrhosis recognize inner mitochondrial epitopes and the pyruvate dehydrogenase complex. J Hepatol 1993; 18:322–327.

Lumeng L, Crabb DW: Genetic aspects and risk factors in alcoholism and alcoholic liver disease. Gastroenterology 1994; 107:572–578.

Lumeng L, Murphy JM, McBride WJ, Li T-K: Basic neurochemical mechanisms of modulation of alcohol consumption in the P and NP rats. Pharmacol Excerpta Int Congr Ser 1988; 750:727–730.

Mackay IR, Gerschwin ME: Primary biliary cirrhosis: current knowledge, perspectives, and future directions. Semin Liver Dis 1989; 9:149–157.

Mackay IR, Gershwin ME: Primary biliary cirrhosis: considerations on pathogenesis based on identification of the M2 autoantigens. Springer Semin Immunopathol 1990; 12:101–109.

Mackay IR, Whittingham S, Tait B: Genetic control of immune responsiveness in man. Vox Sang 1977; 32:10–19.

Maezawa Y, Yamauchi M, Toda G: Association between restriction fragment length polmorphism of the human *cytochrome P450IIE1* gene and susceptibility to alcoholic liver cirrhosis. Am J Gastroenterol 1994; 89:561–565.

Manabe K, Hibberd ML, Donaldson PT, Underhill JA, Doherty DG, Demaine AG, Mieli-Vergani G, Eddleston ALWF, Williams R: T-cell receptor constant β germline gene polymorphisms and susceptibility to autoimmune hepatitis. Hepatology 1994; 106:1321–1325.

Manns M, Gerken G, Kyriatsoulis A, Staritz M, Meyer zum Buschenfelde KH: Characterization of a new subgroup of autoimmune chronic active hepatitis by autoantibodies against a soluble liver antigen. Lancet 1987; 1:292–294.

Manns MP, Bremm A, Schneider PM, Notghi A, Gerken G, Prager-Eberle M, Stradmann-Bellinghausen B, Meyer zum Buschenfelde K-H, Rittner C: HLA DRw8 and complement C4 deficiency as risk factors in primary biliary cirrhosis. Gastroenterology 1991; 101:1367–1373.

Manns MP, Johnson EF, Griffin KJ, Tan EM, Sullivan KF: Major antigen of liver kidney microsomal autoantibodies in idiopathic autoimmune hepatitis is cytochrome P450db1. J Clin Invest 1989; 83:1066–1072.

Manns MP, Kruger M: Immunogenetics of chronic liver diseases. Gastroenterology 1994; 106:1676–1697.

Marbet UA, Stalder GA, Thiel G, Bianchi L: The influence of HLA antigens on progression of alcoholic liver disease. Hepatogastroenterology 1988; 35:65–68.

Marcos Y, Fainboim HA, Capucchio M, Findor J, Daruich J, Reyes B, Pando M, Theiler GDC, Mendez N, Satz ML, et al.: Two-locus involvement in the association of human leukocyte antigen with the extrahepatic manifestations of autoimmune chronic active hepatitis. Hepatology 1994; 19:1371–1374.

Martinez J, Georgoff I, Levine AJ: Cellular localization and cell cycle regulation by a temperature-sensitive mutant of p53. Genes Dev 1991; 5:151–159.

Mason AL, Xu L, Guo L, Munox S, Jaspan JB, Bryer-Ash M, Cao Y, Sander DM, Shoenfeld Y, Ahmed A, et al.: Detection of retroviral antibodies in primary biliary cirrhosis and other idiopathic biliary disorders. Lancet 1998; 351:1620–1624.

Mayo MJ, Combes B, Jenkins RN: T-cell receptor VB gene utilization in primary biliary cirrhosis. Hepatology 1996; 24:1148–1155.

McBride WJ, Murphy JM, Gatto GJ, Levy AD, Lumeng L, Li T-K: Serotonin and dopamine systems regulating alcohol intake. Alcohol Alcohol Suppl 1991; 1:411–416.

McClain CJ, Hill D, Schmidt J, Diehl AM: Cytokines and alcoholic liver disease. Semin Liver Dis 1993; 13:170–182.

McCoy KD, Le Gros G: The role of CTLA-4 in the regulation of T cell immune responses. Immunol Cell Biol 1999; 77:1–10.

McFarlane IG, Wojcicka BM, Tsantoulas DC, Portmann BC, Eddleston ALWF, Williams R: Leukocyte migration inhibition in response to biliary antigens in primary biliary cirrhosis, sclerosing cholangitis and other chronic liver diseases. Gastroenterology 1979; 76:1333–1340.

McGlynn KA, Rosvold EA, Lustbader ED, Hu Y, Clapper ML, Zhou T, Wild CP, Xia X-L, Baffoe-Bonnie A, Ofori-Adjei D, et al.: Susceptibility to hepatocellular carcinoma is associated with genetic variation in the enzymatic detoxification of aflatoxin B_1. Proc Natl Acad Sci USA 1995; 92:2384–2387.

Mehal WZ, Gregory WL, Lo Y-MD, Cross SJ, Fleming KA, Bassendine MF, James OFW, Campbell RD, Chapman RW, Rosenberg WMC: Defining the immunogenetic susceptibility to primary biliary cirrhosis. Hepatology 1994a; 20:1213–1219.

Mehal WZ, Lo YMD, Wordsworth BP, Neuberger JM, Hubscher SC, Fleming KA, Chapman RW: HLA DR4 is a marker for rapid disease progression in primary sclerosing cholangitis. Gastroenterology 1994b; 106:160–167.

Mella JG, Roschmann E, Maier K-P, Volk BA: Association of primary biliary cirrhosis with the allele HLA-DPB1*0301 in a German population. Hepatology 1995; 21:398–402.

Messer G, Spengler U, Jung MC, Honold G, Eisenburg J, Scholz S, Albert ED, Pape GR, Riethmuller G, Weiss EH: Allelic variation in the TNF-β gene does not explain the low TNF-β response in patients with primary biliary cirrhosis. Scand J Immunol 1991; 34:735–740.

Miller KB, Sepersky RA, Brown KM, Goldberg MJ, Kaplan MM: Genetic abnormalities of immunoregulation in primary biliary cirrhosis. Am J Med 1983; 75:75–80.

Miyamori N, Kato Y, Kobayashi K, Hattori N: HLA antigens in Japanese patients with primary biliary cirrhosis and autoimmune hepatitis. Digestion 1983; 26:213–217.

Moebius U, Manns M, Hess G, Kober G, Meyer zum Buschenfelde KH, Meuer SC: T cell receptor gene arrangements of T lymphocytes infiltrating the liver in chronic active hepatitis B and primary biliary cirrhosis (PBC): oligoclonality of PBC-derived T cell clones. Eur J Immunol 1990; 20:889–896.

Moloney MM, Thomson LJ, Strettell MJ, Williams R, Donaldson PT: Human leukocyte antigen-C genes and susceptibility to primary sclerosing cholangitis. Hepatology 1998; 28:660–662.

Momand J, Zambetti GP, Olson DC, George D, Levine AJ: The *mdm*-2 oncogene product forms a complex with the p53 protein and inhibits p53 mediated transactivation. Cell 1992; 69:1237–1245.

Monaco JJ: A molecular model of MHC class-I–restricted antigen processing. Immunol Today 1992; 13:173–179.
Monaco JJ, Cho S, Attaya M: Transport protein genes in the murine MHC: possible implications for antigen processing. Science 1990; 250:1723–1726.
Morin PJ: β-catenin signaling and cancer. Bioessays 1999; 21:1021–1030.
Morin PJ, Sparks AB, Korinek V, Barker N, Clevers H, Vogelstein B, Kinzler KW: Activation of β-catenin–Tcf signaling in colon cancer by mutations in β-catenin or APC. Science 1997; 275:1787–1790.
Morling N, Dalhoff K, Fugger L, Georgsen J, Jakobsen B, Ranek L, Odum N, Svejgaard A: DNA polymorphism of HLA class II genes in primary biliary cirrhosis. Immunogenetics 1992; 35:112–116.
Mota A, Fainboim H, Terg R, Fainboim L: Association of chronic active hepatitis and HLA B35 in patients with hepatitis B virus. Tissue Antigens 1987; 30:238–240.
Munoz LE, DeVilliers D, Markham D, Whaley K, Thomas HC: Complement activation in chronic liver disease. Clin Exp Immunol 1982; 47:548–554.
Nagaya T, Nakamura T, Tokino T, Tsurimoto T, Mai M, Mayumi M, Kamino K, Yamamura K, Matsubara K: The mode of hepatitis B virus DNA integration in chromosomes of human hepatocellular carcinoma. Genes Dev 1987; 1:773–782.
Nelson JL: Microchimerism: implications for autoimmune disease. Lupus 1999; 8:370–374.
Niederau C, Fischer R, Purschel A, Stremmel W, Haussinger D, Strohmeyer G: Long-term survival in patients with hereditary hemochromatosis. Gastroenterology 1996; 110:1107–1119.
Nikias GA, Batts KP, Czaja AJ: The nature and prognostic implications of autoimmune hepatitis with an acute presentation. J Hepatol 1994; 21:866–871.
Noble NA, Border WA: Angiotensin II in renal fibrosis: should TGF-β rather than blood pressure be the therapeutic target? Semin Nephrol 1997; 17:455–466.
Noguchi K, Kobayashi M, Yagihashi A, Yoshida Y, Terasawa K, Konno A, Ichida F, Venek M, Iwatsuki S, Starzl TE, et al.: HLA antigens and primary sclerosing cholangitis. Transplant Proc 1992; 24:2775–2776.
Norris S, Kondeatis E, Collins R, Satsangi J, Clare M, Chapman R, Stephens H, Harrison P, Vaughan R, Donaldson P: Mapping the MHC-encoded susceptibility and resistance in primary sclerosing cholangitis: the role of MICA polymorphism. Gastroenterology 2001; 120:1475–1482.
Nouri-Aria KT, Donaldson PT, Hegarty JE, Eddleston AWLF, Williams R: HLA A1-B8-DR3 and suppressor cell function in first-degree relatives of patients with autoimmune chronic active hepatitis. J Hepatol 1985; 1:235–241.
O'Brien CJ, Vento S, Donaldson PT, McSorley CG, McFarlane IG, Williams R, Eddleston ALWF: Cell-mediated immunity and suppressor-T-cell defects to liver-derived antigens in families of patients with autoimmune chronic active hepatitis. Lancet 1986; 1:350–353.
Oda T, Tsuda H, Scarpa A, Sakamoto M, Hirohashi S: Mutation pattern of the *p53* gene as a diagnostic marker for multiple hepatocellular carcinoma. Cancer Res 1992; 52:3674–3678.
Ohhira M, Fujimoto Y, Matsumoto A, Ohtake T, Ono M, Kohgo Y: Hepatocellular carcinoma associated with alcoholic liver disease: a clinicopathological study and genetic polymorphism of aldehyde dehydrogenase 2. Alcohol Clin Exp Res 1996; 20:378A–382A.
Ohnishi K, Iida S, Iwana S, Goto N, Nomura F, Takashi M, Mishima A, Kono K, Kimura K, Musha H, et al.: The effect of chronic habitual alcohol intake on the development of liver cirrhosis and hepatocellular carcinoma: relationship to hepatitis B surface antigen carriage. Cancer 1982; 49:672–677.
Okuda K: Hepatocellular carcinoma: recent progress. Hepatology 1992; 15:948–963.
Okuda K: Hepatocellular carcinoma. J Hepatol 2000; 32(Suppl 1):225–237.
Olomu AB, Vickers CR, Waring RH, Clements D, Babbs C, Warnes TW, Elias E: High incidence of poor sulphoxidation in patients with PBC. N Engl J Med 1988; 318:1089–1092.
Olubuyide JO, Ayoola EA, Atoba MA: Hepatobiliary diseases in tropical Africa—the Ibadan experience. Trop Gastroenterol 1986; 7:54–61.
Onishi S, Sakamaki T, Maeda T, Iwamura S, Tomita A, Saibara T, Yamamoto Y: DNA typing of HLA class II genes: DRB1*0803 increases the susceptibility of Japanese to primary biliary cirrhosis. J Hepatol 1994; 21:1053–1060.
Ozturk M: Genetic aspects of hepatocellular carcinogenesis. Semin Liver Dis 1999; 19:235–242.
Pando M, Larriba J, Fernandez GC, Fainboim H, Ciocca M, Ramonet M, Badia I, Daruich J, Findor J, Tanno H, et al.: Pediatric and adult forms of type 1 autoimmune hepatitis in Argentina: evidence for differential genetic predisposition. Hepatology 1999; 30:1374–1380.
Park SZ, Nagorney DM, Czaja AJ: Hepatocellular carcinoma in autoimmune hepatitis. Dig Dis Sci 2000; 45:1944–1948.
Parkin DM, Laara E, Muir CS: Estimates of the worldwide frequency of 16 major cancers in 1980. Int J Cancer 1988; 41:184–197.
Pastor IJ, Laso FJ, Avila JJ, Rodriguez RE, Gonzalez-Sarmiento R: Polymorphism in the interleukin-1 receptor antagonist gene is associated with alcoholism in Spanish men. Alcohol Clin Exp Res 2000; 24:1479–1482.
Payami H, Khan MA, Grennan DM, Sanders PA, Dyer PA, Thomson G: Analysis of genetic interrelationship among HLA-associated diseases. Am J Hum Genet 1987; 41:331–349.
Peano G, Menardi G, Ponzetto A, Fenoglio LM: HLA-DR5 antigen—a genetic factor influencing the outcome of hepatitis C virus infection? Arch Intern Med 1994; 154:2733–2736.
Penner E, Grabner G, Dittrich H, Mayr WR: HLA antigens in HBs antigen positive chronic active hepatitis. Tissue Antigens 1977; 10:63–64.
Piao Z, Kim H, Jeon BK, Lee WJ, Park C: Relationship between loss of heterozygosity of tumor suppressor genes and histologic differentiation in hepatocellular carcinoma. Cancer 1997; 80:865–872.
Pirmohamed M, Kitteringham NR, Quest LJ, Allott RL, Green VJ, Gilmore IT, Park BK: Genetic polymorphism of *cytochrome P4502E1* and risk of alcoholic liver disease in Caucasians. Pharmacogenetics 1995; 5:351–357.
Pociot F, Molvig J, Wogensen L, Worsaae H, Dalboge H, Baek L, Nerup J: A tumour necrosis factor beta gene polymorphism in relation to monokine secretion and insulin-dependent diabetes mellitus. Scand J Immunol 1991; 33:37–49.
Poupon RE, Nalpas B, Coutelle C, Fleury B, Couzigou P, Higueret D: Polymorphism of alcohol dehydrogenase, alcohol and aldehyde dehydrogenase activities: implications in alcoholic cirrhosis in white patients. Hepatology 1992; 15:1017–1022.
Powell EE, Edwards-Smith CJ, Hay JL, Clouston AD, Crawford DH, Shorthouse C, Purdie DM, Jonsson JR: Host genetic factors influence disease progression in chronic hepatitis C. Hepatology 2000; 31:828–833.
Prochazka EJ, Terasaki PI, Park MS, Golstein LI, Busuttil RW: Association of primary sclerosing cholangitis with HLA-DRw52a. N Engl J Med 1990; 322:1842–1844.
Propst T, Propst A, Dietze O, Judmaier G, Braunsteiner H, Vogel W: Prevalence of hepatocellular carcinoma in alpha-1 antitrypsin deficiency. J Hepatol 1994; 21: 1006–1011.
Pullen AM, Kappler JW, Marrack P: Tolerance to self antigens shapes the T-cell repertoire. Immunol Rev 1989; 107:125–139.
Quigley EMM, LaRusso NF, Ludwig J, MacSween RNM, Birnie GG, Watkinson G: Familial occurrence of primary sclerosing cholangitis and ulcerative colitis. Gastroenterology 1983; 85:1160–1165.
Raunio H, Juvonen R, Pasanen M, Pelonen O, Paakko P, Soini Y: Cytochrome P4502A6 (CYP2A6) expression in human hepatocellular carcinoma. Hepatology 1998; 27:427–432.
Record CO, Eddleston ALWF, Shilkin KB, Williams R: Intrahepatic sclerosing cholangitis associated with a familial immunodeficiency syndrome. Lancet 1973; 2:18–22.
Rizzetto M: The delta agent. Hepatology 1983; 3:729–737.
Rizzi PM, Ryder SD, Portmann B, Ramage JK, Naoumov NV, Williams R: p53 protein overexpression in cholangiocarcinoma arising in primary sclerosing cholangitis. Gut 1996; 38:265–268.
Rodrigo L, Alvarez V, Rodriguez M, Perez R, Alvarez R, Coto E: *N*-Acetyltransferase-2, glutathione *S*-transferase M1, alcohol dehydrogenase, and cytochrome P450IIE1 genotypes in alcoholic liver cirrhosis: a case-controlled study. Scand J Gastroenterol 1999; 34:303–307.
Romero R, Lavine JE: Cytokine inhibition of the hepatitis B virus core promoter. Hepatology 1996; 23:17–23.
Ryder LP, Andersen E, Svejgaard A: An HLA map of Europe. Hum Hered 1978; 28:171–200.
Salapuro MP, Laitinen OI, Lehtola J: Immunological parameters, viral antibodies and biochemical and histological findings in relatives of patients with chronic active hepatitis and primary biliary cirrhosis. Scand J Gastroenterol 1976; 11:313–320.
Sampliner RE, Bias WB, Carney E, Hillis A, Hillis WD: HLA antigens and HBV infection: evaluation in the chronic carrier state and in a large family. Tissue Antigens 1981; 18:247–251.
Sanchez-Urdazpal L, Czaja AJ, van Hoek B, Krom RAF, Wiesner RH: Prognostic features and role of liver transplantation in severe corticosteroid-treated autoimmune chronic active hepatitis. Hepatology 1992; 15:215–221.
Satarug S, Lang MA, Yongvanit P, Sithithaworn P, Mairiang E, Mairiang P, Pelkonen P, Bartsch H, Haswell-Elkins MR: Induction of cytochrome P450 2A6 expression in humans by the carcinogenic parasite infection, *Opisthorchiasis viverrini*. Cancer Epidemiol Biomarkers Prev 1996; 5:795–800.
Satoh S, Daigo Y, Furukawa Y, Kato T, Miwa N, Nishiwaki T, Kawasoe T, Ishiguro H, Fujita M, Tokino T, et al.: *AXIN1* mutations in hepatocellular carcinomas, and growth suppression in cancer cells by virus mediated transfer of *AXIN1*. Nat Genet 2000; 24:245–250.
Savolainen VT, Pajarinen J, Perola M, Penttila A, Karhunen PJ: Polymorphism in the *cytochrome P450 2E1* gene and the risk of alcoholic liver disease. J Hepatol 1997; 26:55–61.
Saxena S, Nouri-Aria KT, Anderson MG: Interleukin 2 activity in chronic liver disease and the effect of in vitro α-interferon. Clin Exp Immunol 1986; 63:541–548.
Schilling PJ, Murray JL, Markowitz AB: Novel tumor necrosis factor toxic effects. Pulmonary hemorrhage and severe hepatic dysfunction. Cancer 1992; 69:256–260.
Schroeder WT, Miller MF, Woo SLC, Saunders GF: Chromosomal location of the human α_1-antitrypsin gene to 14q31–32. Am J Hum Genet 1985; 37:868–872.
Schrumpf E, Fensa O, Forre O, Doblong JH, Ritland S, Thorsby E: HLA antigens and immunoregulatory T cells in ulcerative colitis associated with hepatobiliary disease. Scand J Gastroenterol 1982; 17:187–191.
Scully LJ, Clarke D, Barr RJ: Diclofenac induced hepatitis. 3 cases with features of autoimmune chronic active hepatitis. Dig Dis Sci 1993a; 38:744–751.
Scully LJ, Toze C, Sengar DPS, Goldstein R: Early-onset autoimmune hepatitis is associated with a *C4A* gene deletion. Gastroenterology 1993b; 104:1478–1484.
Seeff LB: Drug-induced chronic liver disease, with emphasis on chronic active hepatitis. Semin Liver Dis 1981; 1:104–115.
Seibold F, Slametschka D, Gregor M, Weber P: Neutrophil autoantibodies: a genetic marker in primary sclerosing cholangitis and ulcerative colitis. Gastroenterology 1994; 107:532–536.
Seki T, Kiyosawa K, Inoko H, Ota M: Association of autoimmune hepatitis with HLA-Bw54 and DR4 in Japanese patients. Hepatology 1990; 12:1300–1304.
Seki T, Kiyosawa K, Ota M, Furuta S, Fukushima H, Tanaka E, Yoshizawa K, Kumagai T, Mizuki N, Ando A, et al.: Association of primary biliary cirrhosis with human leukocyte antigen DPB1*0501 in Japanese patients. Hepatology 1993; 18:73–78.
Seki T, Ota M, Furuta S, Fukushima H, Kondo T, Hino K, Mizuki N, Ando A, Tsuji

K, Inoko H, et al.: HLA class II molecules and autoimmune hepatitis susceptibility in Japanese patients. Gastroenterology 1992; 103:1041–1047.

Selivanova G, Wiman KG: p53: a cell cycle regulator activated by DNA damage. Adv Cancer Res 1995; 66:143–180.

Shafritz DA, Shouval D, Sherman HI, Hadziyannis SJ, Kew MC: Integration of hepatitis B virus DNA into the genome of liver cells in chronic liver disease and hepatocellular carcinoma. N Engl J Med 1981; 305:1067–1073.

Shepard HA, Selby WS, Chapman RWG, Nolan D, Barbatis C, McGee JOD, Jewell DP: Ulcerative colitis and persistent liver dysfunction. Q J Med 1983; 208:503–513.

Sheth SG, Gordon FD, Chopra S: Nonalcoholic steatohepatitis. Ann Intern Med 1997; 126:137–145.

Shibasaki T, Shimada T, Morita T, Sakai O: Immunogenetical penetrance in patients with primary biliary cirrhosis. Jpn J Med 1990; 29:533–536.

Shieh YSC, Nguyen C, Vocal MV, Chu H-W: Tumor-suppressor *p53* gene in hepatitis C and B virus-associated human hepatocellular carcinoma. Int J Cancer 1993; 54:558–562.

Simsek H, Schuman BM: Inflammatory bowel disease in 64 black patients: analysis of course, complications and surgery. J Clin Gastroenterol 1989; 11:294–298.

Singer MC, Anderson JGD, Frischer H, Kirsner JB: Familial aspects of inflammatory bowel disease. Gastroenterology 1971; 61:423–430.

Skoda RC, Demierre A, McBride OW, Gonzalez FJ, Meyer UA: Human microsomal xenobiotic epoxide hydrolase. Complementary DNA sequence, complementary DNA-directed expression in COS-1 cells, and chromosomal localization. J Biol Chem 1988; 263:1549–1554.

Slagle BL, Zhou YZ, Butel JS: Hepatitis B virus integration event in human chromosome 17p near the *p53* gene identifies the region of the chromosome commonly detected in virus-positive hepatocellular carcinomas. Cancer Res 1991; 51:49–54.

Sorensen TIA, Orholm M, Bentsen KD, Hoybye G, Eghoje K, Christoffersen P: Prospective evaluation of alcohol abuse and alcoholic liver injury in men as predictors of development of cirrhosis. Lancet 1984; 2:241–244.

Spector AA: Fatty acid ethyl esters: insight or intoxication [editorial]? Gastroenterology 1995; 108:605–607.

Spengler U, Moller A, Jung MC, Messer G, Zachoval R, Hoffmann RM, Eisenburg J, Paumgartner G, Riethmuller G, Weiss EH, et al.: T lymphocytes from patients with primary biliary cirrhosis produce reduced amounts of lymphotoxin, tumor necrosis factor and interferon gamma upon mitogen stimulation. J Hepatol 1992; 15:129–135.

Spengler U, Pape GR, Hoffmann RM: Differential expression of MHC class II subregion products in patients with primary biliary cirrhosis. Hepatology 1988; 8:459–462.

Spurland A, Saarinen S, Boberg KM, Mitchell S, Bromme U, Caballeria L, Ciusani E, Chapman R, Ercilla G, Fausa O, et al.: HLA class II haplotypes in primary sclerosing cholangitis patients from five European populations. Tissue Antigens 1999; 53:459–469.

Stechemesser E, Klein R, Berg PA: Characterization and clinical relevance of liver–pancreas antibodies in autoimmune hepatitis. Hepatology 1993; 18:1–9.

Strettell MDJ, Donaldson PT, Thomson LJ, Santrach PJ, Moore SB, Czaja AJ, Williams R: Allelic basis for HLA-encoded susceptibility to type 1 autoimmune hepatitis. Gastroenterology 1997; 112:2028–2035.

Szczepiorkowski ZM, Dickersin CR, Lopasata M: Fatty acid ethyl esters decrease human hepatoblastoma cell proliferation and protein synthesis. Gastroenterolgy 1995; 108:515–522.

Tabor E: Tumor suppressor genes, growth factor genes, and oncogenes in hepatitis B virus–associated hepatocellular carcinoma. J Med Virol 1994; 42:357–365.

Takahashi T, Lasker JM, Rosman AS, Lieber CS: Induction of P450IIE1 in human liver by ethanol is due to a corresponding increase in encoding mRNA. Hepatology 1993; 17:236–245.

Takamatsu M, Yamauchi M, Maezawa Y, Ohata M, Saito S, Toda G: Correlation of a polymorphism in the interleukin-1 receptor antagonist gene with hepatic fibrosis in Japanese alcoholics. Alcohol Clin Exp Res 1998; 22:141S-144S.

Takamatsu M, Yamauchi M, Maezawa Y, Saito S, Maeyama S, Uchikoshi T: Genetic polymorphisms of interleukin-1 beta in association with the development of alcoholic liver disease in Japanese patients. Am J Gastroenterol 2000; 95:1305–1311.

Takeshita T, Yang X, Inoue Y, Sato S, Morimoto K: Relationship between alcohol drinking, *ADH2* and *ALDH2* genotypes, and risk of hepatocellular carcinoma in Japan. Cancer Lett 2000; 149:69–76.

Talal N, Flescher E, Dang H: Are endogenous retroviruses involved in human autoimmune disease? J Autoimmun 1992; 5(Suppl A):61–66.

Tanaka F, Shiratori Y, Yokosuka O, Imazeki F, Tsukada Y, Omata M: High incidence of *ADH2*1/ALDH2*1* genes among Japanese alcohol dependents and patients with alcoholic liver disease. Hepatology 1996; 23:234–239.

Tanaka F, Shiratori Y, Yokosuka O, Imazeki F, Tsukada Y, Omata M: Polymorphism of alcohol-metabolizing genes affects drinking behavior and alcoholic liver disease in Japanese men. Alcohol Clin Exp Res 1997; 21:596–601.

Teckman JH, Perlmutter DH: Molecular pathogenesis of liver disease in α_1-antitrypsin deficiency. Hepatology 1996; 24:1504–1516.

Terris B, Pineau P, Bregeaud L, Valla D, Belghiti J, Tiollais P, Degott C, Dejean A: Close correlation between *β-catenin* gene alterations and nuclear accumulation of the protein in human hepatocellular carcinomas. Oncogene 1999; 18:6583–6588.

Thio CL, Thomas DL, Carrington M: Chronic viral hepatitis and the viral genome. Hepatology 2000; 31:819–827.

Thomas HC, Montano L, Goodall A, de Koning R, Oladapo J, Wiedman KH: Immunological mechanisms in chronic hepatitis B virus infection. Hepatology 1982; 2:116S-121S.

Thompson CB, Allison JP: The emerging role of CTLA-4 as an immune attenuator. Immunity 1997; 7:445–450.

Thursz M, Rhiannon Y, Goldin R, Trepo C, Thomas HC: Influence of class II genotype on outcome of infection with hepatitis C. Lancet 1999; 354; 2119–2124.

Thursz MR, Kwiatkowski D, Allsopp CEM, Greenwood BM, Thomas HC, Hill AVS. Association between an MHC class II allele and clearance of hepatitis B virus in the Gambia. N Engl J Med 1995; 332:1065–1069.

Tibbs C, Donaldson P, Underhill J, Thomson L, Manabe K, Williams R: Evidence that the HLA DQA1*03 allele confers protection from chronic HCV-infection in northern European Caucasoids. Hepatology 1996; 24:1342–1345.

Tillmann HL, Chen D-F, Trautwein C, Kliem V, Grundey A, Berning-Haag A, Boker K, Kubicka S, Pastucha L, Stangel W, et al.: Low frequency of HLA-DRB1*11 in hepatitis C virus induced end stage liver disease. Gut 2001; 48:714–718.

Tomer Y, Shoenfeld Y: The significance of natural autoantibodies. Immunol Invest 1988; 17:389–424.

Tong MJ, Nies KM, Reynolds TB, Quismorio FP: Immunological studies in familial primary biliary cirrhosis. Gastroenterology 1976; 71:305–307.

Triger DR: Primary biliary cirrhosis: an epidemiological study. BMJ 1980; 281:772–775.

Triger DR, Berg PA, Rodes J: Epidemiology of primary biliary cirrhosis. Liver 1984; 4:195–200.

Tsai SL, Lai MY, Chen DS: Analysis of rearranged T cell receptor (TCR) Vβ transcripts in livers of primary biliary cirrhosis: preferential Vβ usage suggests antigen-driven selection. Clin Exp Immunol 1996; 103:99–104.

Tsuji H, Mwai K, Akagi K, Fujishima M: Familial PBC association with impaired Con A–induced lymphocyte transformation in relatives. Dig Dis Sci 1992; 37:353–360.

Tsutsumi M, Matsuda Y, Takada A: Role of ethanol-inducible cytochrome P450 2E1 in the development of hepatocellular carcinoma by the chemical carcinogen, *N*-nitrosodimethylamine. Hepatology 1993; 18:1483–1489.

Tsutsumi M, Takada A, Wang J-S: Genetic polymorphisms of cytochrome P4502E1 related to the development of alcoholic liver disease. Gastroenterology 1994; 107:1430–1435.

Ueda H, Ullrich SJ, Gangemi JD, Kappel CA, Ngo L, Feitelson MA, Jay G: Functional inactivation but not structural mutation of p53 causes liver cancer. Nat Genet 1995; 9:41–47.

Ueki T, Fujimoto J, Suzuki T, Yamamoto H, Okamoto E: Expression of hepatocyte growth factor and its receptor c-*met* proto-oncogene in hepatocellular carcinoma. Hepatology 1997; 25:862–866.

Unanue ER, Allen PM: The basis for the immunoregulatory role of macrophages and other accesory cells. Science 1987; 236:551–557.

Underhill J, Donaldson P, Bray G, Doherty D, Portmann B, Williams R: Susceptibility to primary biliary cirrhosis is associated with the HLA-DR8-DQB1*0402 haplotype. Hepatology 1992; 16:1404–1408.

Underhill JA, Donaldson PT, Doherty DG, Manabe K, Williams R: HLA DRB polymorphism in primary sclerosing cholangitis and primary biliary cirrhosis. Hepatology 1995; 21:959–962.

U.S. Department of Health and Human Services, Eighth Special Report to the U.S. Congress on Alcohol and Health. National Clearinghouse for Alcohol and Drug Information. Washington, DC: 1993:1–35.

Unsal H, Yakicier C, Marcais C, Kew M, Volkmann M, Zentgraf H, Isselbacher KJ, Ozturk M: Genetic heterogeneity of hepatocellular carcinoma. Proc Natl Acad Sci USA 1994; 91:822–826.

Van de Water J, Cooper A, Surth CD, Coppel R, Danner D, Ansari A, Dickson R, Gershwin ME: Detection of autoantibodies to recombinant mitochondrial proteins in patients with primary biliary cirrhosis. N Engl J Med 1989a; 320:1377–1380.

Van de Water J, Gerson LB, Ferrell LD, Lake JR, Coppel RL, Batts KP, Wiesner RH, Gershwin ME: Immunohistochemical evidence of disease recurrence following liver transplantation for primary biliary cirrhosis. Hepatology 1996; 24:1079–1084.

Van de Water J, Surh CD, Leung PSC, Krams SM, Fregeau D, Davis P, Coppel R, Mackay IR, Gershwin ME: Molecular definitions, autoepitopes, and enzymatic reactivities of the mitochondrial autoantigens of primary biliary cirrhosis. Semin Liver Dis 1989b; 9:132–137.

Van Griensven M, Bergijk EC, Baelde JJ, De Heer E, Bruijn JA: Differential effects of sex hormones on autoantibody production and proteinuria in chronic graft-versus-host disease–induced experimental lupus nephritis. Clin Exp Immunol 1997; 107:254–260.

van Hattum J, Schreuder GMT, Schalm SW: HLA antigens in patients with various courses after hepatitis B virus infection. Hepatology 1987; 7:11–14.

van Milligen de Wit AWM, van Deventer SJH, Tytgat GNJ: Immunogenetic aspects of primary sclerosing cholangitis: implications for therapeutic strategies. Am J Gastroenterol 1995; 90:893–900.

Vazquez-Garcia MN, Alaez C, Olivo A, Debaz H, Perez-Luque E, Burguete A, Cano S, de la Rosa G, Bautista N, Hernandez A, et al.: MHC class II sequences of susceptibility and protection in Mexicans with autoimmune hepatitis. J Hepatol 1998; 28:985–990.

Vento S, Hegarty JE, Bottazzo G, Macchia E, Williams R, Eddleston ALWF: Antigen specific suppressor cell function in autoimmune chronic active hepatitis. Lancet 1984; 1:1200–1204.

Vento S, O'Brien CJ, McFarlane BM, McFarlane IG, Eddleston ALWF, Williams R: T-lymphocyte sensitization to hepatocyte antigens in autoimmune chronic active hepatitis and primary biliary cirrhosis. Gastroenterology 1986; 91:810–817.

Vergani D, Wells L, Larcher VF, Nasaruddin BA, Davies ET, Mieli-Vergani G, Mowat AP: Genetically determined low C4: a predisposing factor to autoimmune chronic active hepatitis. Lancet 1985; 2:294–297.

Vesey DA, Hayward NK, Cooksley WGE: *p53* gene in hepatocellular carcinomas from Australia. Cancer Detect Prevent 1994; 18:123–130.

Villeneuve J-P, Fenyves D, Infante-Rivard C: Descriptive epidemiology of primary biliary cirrhosis in the province of Quebec. Can J Gastroenterol 1991; 5:174–178.

von Baehr V, Docke WD, Plauth M, Liebenthal C, Kupferling S, Lochs H, Baumgarten R, Volk HD: Mechanisms of endotoxin tolerance in patients with alcoholic liver cirrhosis: role of interleukin 10, interleukin 1 receptor antagonist, and soluble tumour necrosis factors receptors as well as effector cell desensitization. Gut 2000; 47:281–287.

Vore M: Oestrogen cholestasis: membranes, metabolites or receptors. Gastroenterology 1987; 93:643–647.

Waldram R, Kopelman H, Tsantoulas D, Williams R: Chronic pancreatitis, sclerosing cholangitis and sicca complex in two siblings. Lancet 1975; 1:550–552.

Walker CO, Combes B: Biliary cirrhosis induced by chlorpromazine. Gastroenterology 1966; 51:631–640.

Walker JG, Bates D, Doniach D, Ball PAJ, Sherlock S: Chronic liver disease and mitochondrial antibodies. BMJ 1972; 1:146–148.

Wan YJ, Poland RE, Lin KM: Genetic polymorphism of *CYP2E1*, *ADH2*, and *ALDH2* in Mexican-Americans. Genet Test 1998; 2:79–83.

Wang KK, Czaja AJ: Hepatocellular cancer in corticosteroid-treated severe autoimmune chronic active hepatitis. Hepatology 1988; 8:1679–1683.

Wee A, Ludwig J: Pericholangitis in chronic ulcerative colitis: primary sclerosing cholangitis of the small bile ducts? Ann Intern Med 1985; 102:581–587.

Weiner FR, Eskries DS, Compton KV, Orrego H, Zern M: Haplotype analysis of a type I collagen gene and its association with alcoholic cirrhosis in man. Mol Aspects Med 1988; 10:159–168.

Werner J, Laposta M, Fernandez-Del Castillo C, Saghir M, Iozzo RV, Lewandrowski KB, Warshaw AL: Pancreatic injury in rats induced by fatty acid ethyl ester, a nonoxidative metabolite of alcohol. Gastroenterology 1997; 113; 286–294.

Wheeler MD, Kono H, Yin M, Rusyn I, Froh M, Connor HD, Mason RP, Samulski RJ, Thurman RG: Delivery of the Cu/Zn-superoxide dismutase gene with adenovirus reduces early alcohol-induced liver injury in rats. Gastroenterology 2001; 120:1241–1250.

Whitacre CC, Reingold SC, O'Looney PA: A gender gap in autoimmunity. Science 1999; 283:1277–1278.

Whittingham S, Mackay IR, Kiss ZS: An interplay of genetic and environmental factors in familial hepatitis and myasthenia gravis. Gut 1970; 11:811–816.

Wies I, Brunner S, Henninger J, Herkel J, Meyer zum Buschenfelde KH, Lohse AW: Identification of target antigen for SLA/LP autoantibodies in autoimmune hepatitis. Lancet 2000; 355:1510–1515.

Wiesner RH, LaRusso NF: Clinicopathologic features of the syndrome of primary sclerosing cholangitis. Gastroenterology 1980; 79:200–206.

Wilson AG, de Vries N, Pociot F, di Giovinr FS, van der Putte LBA, Duff GW: An allelic polymorphisms within the human tumor necrosis factor α promoter region is strongly associated with the HLA A1,B8 and DR3 alleles. J Exp Med 1993; 177:557–560.

Witt-Sullivan H, Heathcote J, Cauch K, Blendis L, Ghent C, Katz A, Milner R, Pappas SC, Rankin J, Wanless IR: The demography of primary biliary cirrhosis in Ontario, Canada. Hepatology 1990; 12:98–105.

Wong N, Lai P, Pang E, Fung LF, Sheng Z, Wong V, Wang W, Hayashi Y, Perlman E, Yuna S, et al.: Genomic aberrations in human hepatocellular carcinomas of differing etiologies. Clin Cancer Res 2000a; 6:4000–4009.

Wong NA, Rae F, Simpson KJ, Murray GD, Harrison DJ: Genetic polymorphisms of cytochrome p4502E1 and susceptibility to alcoholic liver disease and hepatocellular carcinoma in a white population: a study and literature review, including meta-analysis. Mol Pathol 2000b; 53:88–93.

Wright SC, Kumar P, Tam AW, Shen NP, Varma M, Larrick JW: Apoptosis and DNA fragmentation precede TNF-induced cytolysis in U937 cells. J Cell Biochem 1992; 29:249–260.

Yamada T, De Souza AT, Finkelstein S, Jirtle RL: Loss of the gene encoding mannose 6-phosphate/insulin-like growth factor II receptor is an early event in liver carcinogenesis. Proc Natl Acad Sci USA 1997; 94:10351–10355.

Yamauchi M, Maezawa Y, Mizuhara Y, Ohata M, Hirakawa J, Nakajima H, Toda G: Polymorphisms in alcohol metabolizing enzyme genes and alcoholic cirrhosis in Japanese patients: a multivariate analysis. Hepatology 1995; 22:1136–1142.

Yang CS, Yoo J-SH, Ishizaki H, Hong J: Cytochrome P450IIE1: roles in nitrosamine metabolism and mechanisms of regulation. Drug Metab Rev 1990; 22:147–159.

Yeh S-W, Chen P-J, Lai M-Y, Chin D-S: Allelic loss on chromosomes 4q and 16q in hepatocellular carcinoma: association with elevated α-fetoprotein production. Gastroenterology 1996; 110:184–192.

Yew PR, Berk AJ: Inhibition of p53 transactivation required for transformation by adenovirus early 1B protein. Nature 1992; 357:82–84.

Yin M, Wheeler MD, Kono H, Bradford BU, Gallucci RM, Luster MI, Thurman RG: Essential role of tumor necrosis factor alpha in alcohol-induced liver injury in mice. Gastroenterology 1999; 117:942–952.

Zavaglia C, Bortolon C, Ferrioli G, Rho A, Mondazzi L, Bottelli R, Ghessi A, Gelosa F, Iamoni G, Ideo G: HLA typing in chronic type B, D and C hepatitis. J Hepatol 1996; 24:658–665.

Zavaglia C, Martinetti M, Silini E, Bottelli R, Daielli C, Asti M, Airoldi A, Salvaneschi L, Mondelli MU, Ideo G: Association between class II alleles and protection from and susceptibility to chronic hepatitis C. J Hepatol 1998; 28:1–7.

Zetterman RK, Sorrell MF: Immunological aspects of alcoholic liver disease. Gastroenterology 1981; 81:616–624.

Zetterquist H, Broome U, Einarsson K, Olerup O: HLA class II genes in primary sclerosing cholangitis and chronic inflammatory bowel disease: no HLA DRw52a association in Swedish patients with sclerosing cholangitis. Gut 1992; 33:942–946.

Zhang L, Weetman AP, Bassendine M, Oliveira DBG: Major histocompatibility complex class-II alleles in primary biliary cirrhosis. Scand J Immunol 1994; 39:104–106.

Zhao TM, Whitaker SE, Robinson MA: A genetically determined insertion/deletion related polymorphism in human T cell receptor β chain (TCRB) includes functional variable gene segments. J Exp Med 1994; 180:1405–1414.

Zhou YZ, Slagle BL, Donehower LA, van Tuinen P, Ledbetter DH, Butel JS: Structural analysis of a hepatitis B virus genome integrated into chromosome 17p of a human hepatocellular carcinoma. J Virol 1988; 62:4224–4231.

Zimmermann U, Feneux D, Mathey G, Gayral F, Franco D, Bedossa P: Chromosomal aberrations in hepatocellular carcinomas: relationship with pathological features. Hepatology 1997; 26:1492–1498.

18 Hereditary Hemochromatosis

FRANCES BUSFIELD, G.J. ANDERSON, AND L.W. POWELL

In the late nineteenth century Trousseau (1865) recognized an association between cirrhosis with diabetes and pigmentation. The pigment was identified by von Recklinghausen (1889) as iron, and he coined the term *haemochromatose* since it was his belief that the iron originated from the blood. In 1935 Sheldon, a consultant physician at the University of Birmingham, reviewed 311 previously published cases of hemochromatosis and concluded that an inborn error of iron metabolism was responsible and that the disease was familial. Thus started a search for the genetic basis of hemochromatosis that was to last over 60 years. Due to the lack of information on the biochemical defect, it was not until the advent of contemporary positional cloning strategies that identification of the gene became possible. However, despite significant advances in our knowledge of iron transporters and iron metabolism, the biochemical basis of the defect leading to the inappropriate iron absorption in hemochromatosis is still uncertain.

DISEASE DEFINITION

Iron overload can be either acquired or inherited (Table 18–1). Hereditary hemochromatosis is an inherited disorder of iron metabolism that leads to inappropriately elevated iron absorption. If left untreated, hemochromatosis leads to the progressive accumulation of iron in the liver, heart, pancreas, and other tissues, resulting in cirrhosis, heart failure, and diabetes and contributing to early death. The iron overload is reflected in an elevation of biochemical markers of iron status, including the transferrin saturation and serum ferritin concentration. Clinical expression of the disease is exacerbated by a high dietary intake of iron.

Diagnosis and Differential Diagnosis

The diagnosis of hereditary hemochromatosis requires a high index of clinical suspicion and careful clinicopathological correlation—that is, the demonstration of excess stainable iron in parenchymal cells in the liver, elevated hepatic iron content, and a clinical history that excludes other causes of iron overload such as thalassemia. Careful history and appropriate laboratory investigations can identify most causes of secondary iron overload. Increasingly, however, the diagnosis of hereditary hemochromatosis is made less on the basis of the classical clinical features and more on the incidental finding of an elevated serum transferrin saturation and/or serum ferritin level. However, the diagnosis should be considered in any patient with unexplained hepatomegaly, abnormal skin pigmentation, cardiomyopathy, diabetes, arthritis, or hypogonadism.

The accepted criteria used for the diagnosis of expressed hemochromatosis (Bassett et al., 1986) are as follows:

1. Stainable hepatic iron grade 3 or 4 (of four grades) (Scheuer et al., 1962)
2. Hepatic iron concentration >80 μM/g dry weight (Bassett et al., 1986)
3. Hepatic iron index >1.9 (Bassett et al., 1986)
4. 5 grams or more of iron removed by phlebotomy therapy

A classification of the causes of hemochromatosis is given in Table 18–1. With the cloning of the hemochromatosis gene (*HFE*) in 1996 (Feder et al., 1996) more specific criteria for diagnosis and screening of HFE-associated hemochromatosis have been developed. These are discussed here under "Clinical Application and Risk Assessment of Genetic Information."

The degree of body iron overload is influenced by many factors, including age, sex, and blood loss, and these may result in delay in diagnosis in some subjects. Nevertheless, increased body iron stores with primarily parenchymal cell deposition of iron has been the hallmark of hereditary hemochromatosis for diagnostic and therapeutic purposes. This is clearly strengthened by a family history of the disease and evidence of mutations in the *HFE* gene.

Clinical Features of Hereditary Hemochromatosis

Hereditary hemochromatosis, a disorder that affects multiple organs, may be diagnosed in patients presenting with hepatic, cardiac, endocrine, rheumatologic, or dermatological symptoms or signs. Hemochromatosis is a progressive disorder, with clinical symptoms normally not becoming apparent until the 3rd to the 6th decades of life. The clinical expression of the disorder may be influenced by both genetic and environmental factors such as diet, blood donation, and menstruation. As a result of menstruation and parturition, fewer women than men show clinical signs of hemochromatosis by the age of 40. As hemochromatosis is being diagnosed at earlier stages than previously, the proportion of patients at initial presentation with cirrhosis or diabetes has decreased substantially from 84% and 55%, respectively (Milman, 1991), to 7% and 9% (Adams et al., 1997) over the last decade. In contrast, there has been little change in the percentage of patients presenting with arthropathy. Diagnosis is often difficult because of initial presentation with general complaints such as fatigue or abdominal pain. The main clinical features of the disorder are described below.

Hepatic Disease

The liver is normally the first organ affected in hemochromatosis, and hepatomegaly is very common in the symptomatic stage

Table 18–1. Classification of Iron Overload States

Familial or Hereditary Hemochromatosis	Acquired Iron Overload
1. HFE-related	1. Iron-loading anemias
a. C282Y homozygosity	a. Thalassemia major
b. C282Y/H63D compound heterozygosity	b. Sideroblastic anemia
c. Other rare *HFE* mutations	c. Chronic hemolytic anemias
2. Non-HFE-related	2. Dietary iron overload
a. Transferrin receptor 2 mutations	Eg. Sub-Saharan Africa
b. Ferroportin 1 mutations	3. Chronic liver disease
3. Juvenile hemochromatosis	a. Hepatitis C
4. Neonatal iron overload	b. Alcoholic liver disease
5. Autosomal dominant hemochromatosis (Solomon Islands)	c. Nonalcoholic steatohepatitis

(Milman, 1991; Niederau et al., 1996). One of the common features of iron overload is elevation of liver enzyme levels, in particular alanine aminotransferase and aspartate aminotransferase. With continued iron deposition cirrhosis may occur, this being the most common serious complication of hemochromatosis. There is also a 200-fold increase in risk for hepatocellular cancer in cirrhotic patients (Bradbear et al., 1985; Niederau et al., 1985). Niederau et al (1996) reported that this risk persists even after successful iron removal. Hepatic function is usually well preserved, and liver function tests may be normal despite substantial iron deposition and fibrosis.

Dermatologic Features

Excessive pigmentation is present in the majority of symptomatic patients but is absent in the early stages of iron accumulation. The "bronze" appearance is due to increased melanin in the epidermis and dermis with generalized atrophy of both.

Endocrine Disease

Diabetes mellitus develops in patients as tissue iron overload levels increase. Over the years a number of studies have been carried out to ascertain the prevalence of diabetes mellitus among hemochromatotic patients. The prevalence varies in these studies from 9% to 82% (Finch and Finch, 1955; Phelps et al., 1989; Adams et al., 1997). Iron deposition in the pancreas and development of insulin resistance (attributed to iron overload in hepatocytes) and/or cirrhosis probably contribute to the development of diabetes mellitus in hemochromatosis (Stocks and Powell, 1972). Insulin-dependent, non-insulin-dependent diabetes and associated diabetic complications such as retinopathy, nephropathy, and peripheral neuropathy may also be encountered.

Also relatively common is hypogonadotrophic hypogonadism, with up to 40% of patients suffering impotence (Niederau et al., 1996; Adams et al., 1997). Secondary amenorrhea in women is also well documented. In most instances of hypogonadism the evidence points toward hypothalamic or pituitary failure as the cause, with selective impairment of gonadotropin or gonadotropin-releasing hormone secretion (Stocks and Powell, 1972; Walton et al., 1983; Kelly et al., 1984).

Iron deposition is frequently seen in endocrine glands other than the pancreas and pituitary, but other endocrine manifestations such as Addison's disease, hypothyroidism, and hypoparathyroidism, although documented, are much less common.

Cardiac Disease

The most common cardiac complications in iron overload are cardiomyopathy and cardiac arrhythmias. Once a critical level of iron content is reached, cardiac failure with rapid deterioration can occur.

Arthropathy

In a study by Adams et al. (1997), arthritis was the most common finding after hyperpigmentation. The usual manifestations include metacarpophalangeal and proximal interphalangeal arthritis (Hamilton et al., 1981; Jones et al., 1992), and there may be progressive chondrocalcinosis due to calcium pyrophosphate dihydrate crystal deposition (Jones et al., 1992). The arthropathy is unrelated to the duration or the level of iron deposition, and, unlike most other manifestations of iron overload, removal of excess iron stores by phlebotomy does not reverse its progression (Hamilton et al., 1981).

Other Forms of Hereditary Iron Overload

Juvenile Hemochromatosis

While clinical symptoms of hereditary hemochromatosis normally manifest in the third to sixth decades of life, cases with onset of clinical symptoms before 30 years and as young as 17 years have been reported (Charlton et al., 1967; Felts et al., 1967; Lamon et al., 1979; Cazzola et al., 1983; Camaschella et al., 1997). In contrast to adult hereditary hemochromatosis, juvenile cases commonly present with hypogonadotrophic hypogonadism (Lamon et al., 1979) and die early if untreated, usually from cardiac dysfunction (Cazzola et al., 1983). The organs affected by the accumulation of iron are the same as in the adult disease, and the same periportal distribution of iron deposition is seen within the liver. Recent studies have shown that juvenile hemochromatosis is not due to mutations in the *HFE* gene but to a separate locus on chromosome 1 (Barton et al., 1997; Camaschella et al., 1997; Roetto et al., 1999).

Neonatal Hemochromatosis

Neonatal hemochromatosis is a generally fatal disease of infancy characterized by retardation of intrauterine growth, preterm birth, hepatic failure only hours after birth, and rapid progression to death (Knisely et al., 1987; Silver et al., 1987; Witzelbin and Uri, 1989; Knisely, 1994). Neonatal hemochromatosis has been successfully treated in a limited number of cases but the prognosis is usually fatal (Muller-Berghaus et al., 1997; Sigurdsson et al., 1998). Histopathologically abundant stainable iron in the liver and other tissues is typical. The etiology of neonatal hemochromatosis is unknown, but many consider it to be a recessive disorder with recurrence in siblings being reported in at least 24 sibships (listed in Verloes et al., 1996). However, neonatal hemochromatosis has been reported in maternal half sibs born to the same mother (Knisely, 1992; Jacknow et al., 1983; Verloes et al., 1996), which, together with the rarity of the disease making heterozygous pairings unlikely, would seem to argue against recessive inheritance. Hypotheses with respect to the cause have focused recently on intrauterine disturbances of iron metabolism (Jacknow et al., 1983; Rand et al., 1992; Verloes et al., 1996).

GENERAL GENETIC AND EPIDEMIOLOGIC EVIDENCE

Genetic Evidence

The genetic nature of hemochromatosis was for many years controversial. While most authors regarded it as an inborn error of iron metabolism (Sheldon, 1935), some considered it to be an acquired disease (MacDonald, 1964). A genetic etiology for hemochromatosis was firmly established in 1976, however, when Marcel Simon described the association between the disorder and HLA antigens A3 and B14 (Simon et al., 1976). Simon et al. found an increased frequency of HLA-A3 in unrelated hemochromatotic patients (78.4%) compared to controls (27%). Their findings were confirmed by numerous studies (Simon et al., 1977; Doran et al., 1981; Ritter et al., 1984; Summers et al., 1989). These studies all indicated that hemochromatosis was an inherited disease with the genetic defect located in close proximity to the class I major histocompatibility complex (MHC) on the short arm of chromosome 6, and that it was inherited as an autosomal recessive trait. Simon et al. (1977) observed that siblings sharing the same HLA-A and B-haplotypes as the proband are highly likely to be homozygous for hemochromatosis and develop iron overload, thus providing a useful diagnostic aid.

Direct evidence for the involvement of an MHC molecule in hemochromatosis was first provided from β_2-microglobulin knockout mice. These mice develop iron overload similar to that seen in hereditary hemochromatosis (Rothenberg and Voland, 1996; Santos et al., 1996). Since β_2-microglobulin binds to MHC class I molecules, it was postulated that the hemochromatosis gene would be an MHC molecule (Rothenberg and Voland, 1996). Subsequently, the *HFE* gene was identified by a large positional cloning effort 5 Mb telomeric to HLA-A and it encodes a nonclassical MHC class I molecule (Feder et al., 1996). In this initial study a common mutation was described in the *HFE* gene that leads to the substitution of a tyrosine for a cysteine at amino acid 282 (C282Y) of the HFE protein. Studies from a large number of countries have shown that homozygosity for the C282Y mutation accounts for 40% to 100% of hereditary hemochromatosis cases, depending on the population studied (Jazwinska et al., 1996; Jouanolle et al., 1996; Carella et al., 1997; UK Haemochromatosis Consortium, 1997; Piperno et al, 1998), with frequencies of 90% or more in most populations of northern European extraction. A second mutation in HFE (H63D) was also described, but its role in hereditary hemochromatosis is less clear. The frequency of C282Y/H63D compound heterozygotes is greater in hemochromatotics than in controls. With the frequency of compound heterozygotes twice that of C282Y homozygotes, complete penetrance of the compound heterozygous genotype would mean 50% of hemochromatosis cases should be compound heterozygotes. However, this genotype is only present in 2% to 7% of hereditary hemochromatosis cases, thus indicating low penetrance of iron overload with this genotype (Feder et al., 1996; Jouanolle et al., 1996; Barton et al., 1997; Carella et al., 1997; UK Haemochromatosis Consortium, 1997). More recently, another missense mutation in *HFE*, S65C, has been described, and some C282Y/S65C compound heterozygotes show evidence of iron loading (Pointon et al., 2000). In addition, several other rare mutations in the *HFE* gene have been described, but there is no clear evidence for their involvement in iron loading (summarized by Pointon et al., 2000).

Non-HFE Hemochromatosis

It is now clear that not all iron overload that is phenotypically similar to *HFE*-related hemochromatosis is caused by mutations in the *HFE* gene. This is particularly the case in populations in the Mediterranean region, where up to 60% of cases have no *HFE* mutations (Carella et al., 1997). Recently it has been shown that some of these cases can be accounted for by mutations in the transferrin receptor 2 gene (Camaschella et al., 2000; Roetto et al., 2001). In addition, an autosomal dominant form of iron overload has been reported in individuals with mutations in the ferroportin 1 gene (Njajou et al., 2001). Further investigation will no doubt implicate other genes in non-HFE-associated iron overload.

HFE Mutations in Juvenile and Neonatal Hemochromatosis

To date no cases of juvenile or neonatal hemochromatosis have been reported with the C282Y *HFE* mutation. Camaschella et al. (1997) describe the analysis of the *HFE* gene in seven Italian patients with juvenile hemochromatosis from five unrelated families (four with consanguineous parents). They reported that neither *HFE* mutation was present in any of the seven patients and that sequencing of the entire *HFE* gene in one patient revealed no other changes. Further to that, segregation analysis of markers closely associated with *HFE* in families with consanguineous parents showed that juvenile hemochromatosis was not linked to 6p but, rather, to 1q (Roetto et al, 1999), thus excluding *HFE* as the cause of hemochromatosis in these patients. It would appear that neonatal and juvenile hemochromatosis are genetically distinct from adult HFE-associated hemochromatosis and may result from mutations in other genes involved in iron homeostasis (Barton et al., 1997; Camaschella et al., 1997).

General Epidemiology

The controversy over the mode of transmission of hemochromatosis was settled in 1977 when Simon et al. demonstrated recessive transmission in 24 families by following the inheritance of HLA haplotypes. Due to the high carrier rate, occasional heterozygous–homozygous pairings occur, which give rise to a pseudodominant pattern of inheritance (Bassett et al., 1982). Hemochromatosis is a common inherited disorder in Caucasian populations where the incidence is 1 in 200 to 400 (Olynyk et al., 1999). In other populations the prevalence of hemochromatosis is very low (Merryweather-Clarke et al., 1997; Cullen et al., 1998). Incidence is highest in those populations with a Celtic origin, for example in Ireland, Wales, Australia, and regions of the United States with a high concentration of Irish immigrants (Smith et al., 1997).

Population Studies

With between 2 and 5 individuals per 1000 showing biochemical expression of iron overload, hemochromatosis is a very common disorder in Caucasian populations and one of the most common autosomal recessive disease traits (Edwards et al., 1988;

Leggett et al., 1990). The identification of HFE and the mutations responsible for hemochromatosis led to population studies to determine the frequency of these mutations in various ethnic populations. In one large study, Merryweather-Clarke et al. (1997) screened DNA samples from 2978 individuals from a variety of ethnic backgrounds for the C282Y and H63D mutations. The worldwide frequencies from this study were 1.9% for C282Y and 8.1% for H63D. The populations with the highest allele frequencies were 10% for C282Y in Irish chromosomes and 30.4% for H63D in Basque chromosomes. The C282Y mutation was most frequent in northern European populations and was rarely found in African, Asian, and indigenous Australasian populations, thus reflecting the geographic distribution of hemochromatosis (Merryweather-Clarke et al., 1997)—that is, in northern European populations—and consistent with the theory of Celtic or Nordic origin for the mutation. The finding of high H63D frequencies in populations not previously reported to suffer from hemochromatosis is consistent with the minor role of this mutation in causing iron overload (see below). A recent study by Cullen et al. (1998) looked at the frequency of the HFE mutations and the ancestry of chromosomes carrying these mutations in a number of non-Caucasian populations comprising Australian Aborigines, Chinese, and Pacific Islanders. The chromosomal ancestry was determined by HLA haplotyping. The C282Y mutation was found at very low frequency in Cape York Aborigines (1.07%), Melanesians (0.36%), and Polynesians 0.9%). Five of the six heterozygotes identified had HLA haplotypes common in Caucasians, and the sixth (Melanesian) had an HLA haplotype common in both Caucasian and Melanesian populations. This is consistent with the C282Y mutation being introduced into these populations by Caucasian admixture. The H63D mutation was present in the Aborigine and Chinese populations analyzed. All the Australian Aboriginal subjects with the H63D mutation also had a Caucasian HLA haplotype, which is consistent with the mutation being introduced by Caucasian admixture. The same was true for Chinese family subjects; however, in unrelated Chinese subjects, the H63D mutation was present on a wide variety of HLA haplotypes, several of which are rare in Caucasians. This makes it unlikely that the mutation was introduced into these southern and northern Chinese populations by Caucasian admixture. From this it would appear that, while the C282Y mutation is of Caucasian origin, the H63D mutation may have arisen independently in different populations.

Association of HFE Mutations with Other Diseases

Iron overload has been observed in association with a number of other disorders and in several of these the presence of either one or two copies of the C282Y mutation in the *HFE* gene has been shown to be responsible for increased hepatic iron content and increased severity of the disease.

Porphyria Cutanea Tarda

Sporadic porphyria cutanea tarda (PCT) is a disorder of porphyrin metabolism associated with hepatic siderosis. Liver damage of varying severity occurs and has been associated with alcohol abuse, iron overload, and infection with hepatitis C. Depletion of iron stores by phlebotomy induces clinical and biochemical remission, and a role for the hemochromatosis gene in PCT had been postulated. Since the identification of the HFE mutations, several studies have investigated the role of *HFE* as a genetic susceptibility factor in PCT (Roberts et al., 1997; Sampietro et al., 1998; Stuart et al., 1998). A significant increase in the frequency of the C282Y mutation in PCT patients compared to control populations was shown by two studies (Roberts et al., 1997; Stuart et al., 1998), with 44% of PCT patients having at least one copy of the C282Y mutation. The frequency of the H63D mutation in patients was not significantly different from that in controls, indicating that C282Y status but not H63D status is an important predisposing factor in the development of PCT.

In contrast to these two studies carried out in the United Kingdom and Australia, a study of Italian patients by Sampietro et al. (1998) reported a high prevalence of the H63D HFE mutation in patients with PCT. H63D was present in 50% of patients, compared to 24% of controls. The frequency of the C282Y mutation was not significantly different between patients and controls. This implicates H63D as the important predisposing factor in this Italian population. These findings, in conjunction with the work of Carella et al. (1997), implies that the HFE C282Y mutation is less important in iron overload disorders in Italy than elsewhere in Europe.

Familial porphyria cutanea tarda is associated with mutations in uroporphyrinogen decarboxylase (URO-D) and accounts for one-third of PCT patients (Bulaj et al., 2000). The phenotype is characterized by a photosensitive dermatosis accompanied by hepatic accumulation and urinary excretion of uroporphyrin and hepta-carboxylic porphyrins. In the absence of hepatic siderosis, individuals heterozygous for URO-D mutations do not usually express the porphyric phenotype. HFE mutations are frequently found in individuals heterozygous for URO-D mutations (Brady et al., 2000; Bulaj et al., 2000; Bonkovsky et al., 1998). A mouse model for familial PCT heterozygous for a URO-D null allele (URO-$D^{+/-}$) has been developed (Phillips et al., 2001). These mice only develop a porphyric phenotype when additional factors, such as injection with iron-dextran coupled with drinking water supplemented with δ-aminolevulinic acid were present. However, when these mice were crossbred with HFE knockout mice, a porphyric phenotype developed in the absence of any other factors (Phillips et al., 2001). This mouse model for familial PCT provides evidence for the role of *HFE* mutations in development of the porphyric phenotype. It is clear however, that the genetic background in which the iron overload occurs is important, as evidenced by the low incidence of PCT in humans with hemochromatosis and strain-dependent differences of mice in their susceptibility to iron loading (Lebouef et al., 1995; Fleming et al., 2001; Sproule et al., 2001).

Nonalcoholic Steatohepatitis

Nonalcoholic steatohepatitis (NASH) is a chronic liver disease, usually benign but occasionally progressing to cirrhosis. Mild hepatic iron overload is found in some NASH patients, and its association with HFE mutations has been investigated (George et al., 1998). The prevalence of the C282Y mutation in this Australian study was significantly greater in NASH patients (20%) than in controls (6%). No significant difference was found between the two groups for the frequency of the H63D mutation. It appears that the C282Y mutation has a predisposing effect for iron overload in NASH, although not all NASH patients with high iron stores had a C282Y mutation, indicating that other factors are involved.

Coronary Artery Disease

Coronary artery disease (CAD) has also aroused interest and debate with respect to iron and a possible role for HFE. It has been hypothesized that iron plays a causative role in the development of CAD based primarily on the disparity of CAD risk between males and premenopausal women (Sullivan, 1981). A study assessing the risk factors for CAD found the strongest correlation with cholesterol and liver iron levels combined (Lauffer, 1990). Interestingly, the highest rates of CAD mortality were found to occur in the United Kingdom, United States, Canada, and Australia where hemochromatosis is prevalent. In contrast, an autopsy study of hemochromatotics found a lower than normal incidence of CAD (Miller and Hutchins, 1994). In a recent study the prevalence of the C282Y mutation in CAD patients was shown to be similar to that in a control population (L. Coupland et al., personal communication), and the role of HFE mutations in CAD remains controversial.

Hepatitis C

Aggressive liver disease in chronic viral hepatitis C has been associated with increased levels of hepatic iron. A recent study that assessed the association of the HFE C282Y mutation with this more aggressive liver disease in chronic hepatitis sufferers found C282Y heterozygosity to be associated with an increased development of fibrosis (Smith et al., 1998). However, this has not been confirmed in other centers, and the topic remains controversial.

Arthritis

Arthritis is a clinical feature of hemochromatosis and it may be expected therefore that the prevalence of the HFE mutation in arthritic patients would be increased. In a study of 260 patients who attended the Royal Brisbane Hospital Rheumatolgy Clinic, the frequency of the C282Y mutation did not differ significantly from that of the control population (Devereaux et al., 1998).

Genotype–Phenotype Correlations

There is considerable variation in the phenotypic expression of hemochromatosis, some of which may be attributable to the gender of the individual and environmental factors such as alcohol intake and diet. Due to physiological blood loss in premenopausal women, the severity of iron loading is reduced and the onset of clinical and biochemical expression of the disorder delayed (Barton et al., 1996). Because there is greater concordance of both clinical manifestations and biochemical markers of iron within families than between families, it has been suggested that iron accumulation is primarily genetically determined (Muir et al., 1984; Crawford et al., 1993). Before the discovery of the *HFE* gene it had been established that homozygotes and heterozygotes for hemochromatosis assigned on the basis of HLA typing differed in the degree of iron loading, heterozygotes being intermediate in their levels of transferrin saturation, serum ferritin, hepatic parenchymal cell stainable iron, and hepatic iron concentration between normal individuals and homozygous subjects (Bassett et al., 1986; Adams, 1994; Bulaj et al., 1996). Since the discovery of the *HFE* gene and the mutations causing hemochromatosis, studies have been carried out to define more clearly the correlation between phenotype and *HFE* genotype.

In general, C282Y homozygotes make up the majority of subjects diagnosed with hereditary hemochromatosis, and they express more severe iron overload, as reflected in clinical manifestations and biochemical markers, than do individuals heterozygous or negative for this mutation (Crawford et al., 1998; Bacon et al., 1999). However, C282Y heterozygotes, compound heterozygotes, H63D homozygotes, and individuals without either mutation with raised biochemical markers and clinical expression have also been described (Barton et al., 1997; Martinez et al., 1997; Sham et al., 1997). Martinez et al. (1997) found compound heterozygotes to have a more severe phenotype than heterozygotes for C282Y alone. The variability of phenotype seen in conjunction with only two mutations further indicates that other factors, perhaps genetic, must be present to account for these differences. Additional evidence indicating this to be the case comes from significant variation in the iron parameters between hemochromatosis probands and obligate heterozygotes, all of whom are C282Y heterozygous and H63D negative (Barton et al., 1997). Strong evidence for the involvement of other genes in modifying the hemochromatosis phenotype comes from the two animal models of this disorder—HFE and β_2-microglobulin knockout mice. Each of these strains develops iron overload, but the degree of iron loading is very strongly influenced by the genetic background onto which the gene knockout is bred (Fleming et al., 2001; Sproule et al., 2001)

Finally, the presence of a genetic factor other than *HFE* is suggested by patients who are diagnosed with hemochromatosis and have significant iron overload in the absence of *HFE* mutations (Borot et al., 1997; Carella et al., 1997; Sham et al., 1997). These cases should only be considered as hereditary hemochromatosis if they have a family history of the disease and no other iron overload contributing factors such as iron-loading anemias, alcoholism, steatohepatitis, excessive dietary iron intake, or hepatitis C are present (Bacon et al., 1999). Clearly, hemochromatosis is a disease that reflects the interplay of genetic and environmental factors in its ultimate expression. In addition to the major effect of the C282Y mutation in the *HFE* gene, there is evidence for other genetic influences, both HLA related (Crawford et al., 1995) and non-HLA related (Carella et al., 1997). The obvious physiological and pathological factors affecting phenotypic expression include menstruation and pregnancy, as well as pathological blood loss. However, there is evidence that additional, as yet undetermined, factors are responsible for nonexpression or partial expression of the disease (Crawford et al., 1998).

PATHOPHYSIOLOGY

Normal Iron Metabolism

Iron is essential for life in most organisms; however, at high levels, it is toxic. For this reason and because there is no excretory mechanism for iron in humans, a system for the tight regulation of body iron levels is necessary. The major function of iron is in oxidation–reduction reactions that make use of its alternate oxidative states (de Silva et al., 1996). Iron is absorbed into the body from the diet through the small intestine. Of the total iron in the body, 60% to 70% is found in hemoglobin in red cells, with the remainder in myoglobin, iron-containing enzymes, transfer bound to transferrin, or storage bound to ferritin and hemosiderin.

Iron Absorption

The body has no mechanism for the active excretion of excess iron. Under normal circumstances the body loses around 1 mg of iron per day through nonmenstrual incidental losses. These losses are balanced by finely regulated uptake of iron from the diet. Regulation of total body iron content is achieved by controlling the level of absorption from the diet through the intestinal epithelial cells (de Silva et al., 1996). About 90% of dietary inorganic iron is non-absorbable due to its insolubility at neutral pH and its sequestration by dietary components. In contrast, iron in heme released from animal products during digestion is transported intact across the microvillus membrane and is absorbed more efficiently than non-heme iron (10%–30% vs. 1%–10%) (Morgan, 1996). It is likely that non-heme iron is only absorbed when it is in the ferrous (Fe^{2+}) form. The uptake of ferrous iron is mediated by the brush border membrane protein divalent metal transporter 1 (DMT1) (previously known as Nramp2 or DCT1) (Fleming et al., 1997; Gunshin et al., 1997). After uptake into the enterocyte, iron enters the cellular pool and may subsequently be either stored as ferritin or transported out of the cell across the basolateral membrane. Factors that are involved in the regulation of iron uptake include variations in body iron stores and the erythropoietic rate. When body iron stores become depleted, iron uptake rises and there is increased transfer across the basolateral membrane. In hemochromatosis there is an inappropriately high level of iron absorption and increased transfer of iron from intestinal cells into the body (McLaren et al., 1991), the intestinal cells acting as if they were iron depleted despite iron overload in the body (Powell et al., 1970; Cox and Peters, 1978; Raja et al., 1996).

Cellular Iron Metabolism

Absorbed iron becomes tightly bound to transferrin in the bloodstream and enters cells by receptor-mediated endocytosis of diferric transferrin after it is bound to transferrin receptors on the cell surface. The internalized endosome becomes acidified, and iron is released from transferrin. At this acid pH, apotransferrin remains bound to the receptor and is recycled to the cell surface where the neutral pH facilitates its release. The uptake of transferrin—and, hence, transferrin-bound iron—is controlled mainly by regulating the number of transferrin receptors on the plasma membrane. Transferrin receptor mRNA contains several iron responsive elements (IREs) in its 3′ untranslated region, and these IREs control the stability of the mRNA and thus the level of expression (Brittin and Ravel, 1971; Hentze and Kuhn, 1996). In iron deficiency, iron regulatory proteins (IRPs) are active and bind to the IREs in the transferrin receptor mRNA. This blocks the degradation of the mRNA, resulting in increased expression of the receptor. When iron is abundant, it binds to IRPs, making them inactive and incapable of binding IREs. This leaves the transferrin receptor mRNA susceptible to degradation by endonucleolytic cleavage, and reduced numbers of transferrin receptors are synthesized. Coordinately regulated along with the transferrin receptor is the synthesis of ferritin, the major protein for storing iron within cells. An IRE is also present at the 5′ end of ferritin mRNA. When IRPs bind in times of iron deficiency, translation of ferritin mRNA is blocked, thus reducing the levels of ferritin protein. Conversely, when iron is abundant, as is the case in hemochromatosis, ferritin translation proceeds and more apoferritin becomes available for iron storage (Harford and Klausner, 1990; Hentze and Kuhn, 1996; Addess et al., 1997; Rouault and Klausner, 1997).

In the normal cell, iron levels are regulated to ensure provision of sufficient iron for cellular function while avoiding the toxic effects of iron overload. While serum transferrin saturation and ferritin levels are increased in hemochromatosis, transferrin and ferritin appear to function normally, as do transferrin receptor and the IRPs (Sciot et al., 1987; Lombard et al., 1989; Pietrangelo et al., 1992; Flanagan et al., 1995). When the capacity of ferritin to store iron in a nontoxic form is exceeded, the amount of iron stored as hemosiderin increases, as does the amount of free iron which has the capacity to catalyze destructive oxidative reactions (Tavill et al., 1990).

The ferrous iron transporter DMT-1 not only plays an important role in iron uptake across the brush border membrane of intestinal epithelial cells (as noted above) but also is active in most cells and is likely to be the molecule that transports iron across the endosomal membrane after the receptor-mediated endocytosis of transferrin. DMT-1 is expressed ubiquitously with the highest levels on the villi of the duodenum (Fleming et al., 1997; Gunshin et al., 1997), and mutations in *DMT-1* are responsible for the abnormal intestinal and erythroid iron uptake that is observed in microcytic anemia mice and Belgrade rats (Fleming et al., 1997, 1998). *DMT-1* also has an IRE at the 3′ end of its mRNA, which makes its expression responsive to iron levels in the same way as does transferrin receptor mRNA. This responsiveness of DMT-1 to iron levels suggests it may play a role in the pathogenesis of hemochromatosis, and, indeed, elevated levels of this transporter have been found in the duodenum of hemochromatosis patients (Zoller et al., 1999, 2001) and HFE knockout mice (Fleming et al., 1999). This increase in DMT-1 expression is thought to be secondary to a dysregulation of iron absorption in hemochromatosis and not a primary abnormality of the disorder.

Several other molecules of iron homeostasis have been identified recently, although little is known of their biology at present. Of these, the most relevant to hemochromatosis are likely to be the iron export protein ferroportin 1 and transferrin receptor 2. Ferroportin 1 (also known as IREG1 or MTP1) is a membrane iron transporter that is expressed in most tissues (Abboud and Haile, 2000; Donovan et al., 2000; McKie et al., 2000). However, it is most highly expressed in those cells that actively export significant quantities of iron, such as the intestinal epithelial cells and reticuloendothelial cells. Its expression is also regulated by iron, and it possesses an IRE at the 5′ end of its mRNA. However, there is evidence that ferroportin 1 regulation is complex, with the IRE being utilized in some tissues, such as the liver, but not in others, such as the small intestine (Abboud and Haile, 2000). Recent data indicate that ferroportin 1 expression is increased in the duodenum of hemochromatosis patients (McKie et al., 2000; Zoller et al., 2001). Transferrin receptor 2 is a homolog of the "classical" transferrin receptor, but its expression is largely restricted to the liver (Kawabata et al., 1999). Unlike its much more extensively studied cousin, transferrin receptor 2 does not appear to be regulated by cellular iron levels. The high expression of this molecule in the liver led to the suggestion that it may play a role in the hepatic iron loading that is observed in hemochromatosis. Strong support for this has come from the description of an iron overload phenotype in patients with mutations in the transferrin receptor 2 gene (Camaschella et al., 2000; Roetto et al., 2001). These patients do not carry mutations in the *HFE* gene, but the possibility that variations in transferrin receptor 2 expression could modulate the phenotype in *HFE*-associate hemochromatosis is very real.

Pathogenesis of Hemochromatosis

The progressive accumulation of iron in the liver, pancreas, and heart in hemochromatosis eventually leads to cellular damage and results in fibrosis. The mechanism by which this damage is mediated is thought to be lipid peroxidation, which is brought about by the generation of reactive oxygen species (Britton et al., 1987). Iron has the capacity to initiate or propagate oxidation reactions through electron transfer (Tavill et al., 1990). Phospholipids in cell membranes are the most susceptible to oxidation, which leads to destruction of the membrane, release of hydrolytic enzymes within the cytosol, exposure of DNA to degrading enzymes, and loss of membrane potential in the mitochondria and culminates in cell death. Evidence supporting the theory of tissue damage via lipid peroxidation comes from the finding that hemochromatosis patients have higher levels of lipid peroxidation products and lower levels of vitamin E antioxidant than a control population (Young et al., 1994). Antioxidants such as vitamin E have the capacity to accept electrons, thus aiding in the prevention of oxidative damage (Stocker, 1994).

When the tissue iron content reaches a threshold of between 250 and 400 μmol/g dry weight, cirrhosis occurs; it is probably mediated by the activation and proliferation of hepatic stellate cells. Malondialdehyde, a product of lipid peroxidation, has been shown to activate hepatic stellate cells in vitro (Lee et al., 1995). Hepatic stellate cell activation is thought to be a critical step in formation of hepatic fibrosis and cirrhosis because of the high level of type I collagen produced by activated hepatic stellate cells (Friedman et al., 1985; Maher and McGuire, 1990). Increased collagen synthesis contributes to fibrous tissue formation within the liver, resulting in dysfunction of the organ (Tavill et al., 1990). The fibrogenic threshold is normally 400 μmol/g dry weight, but this may be reduced by factors such as alcohol intake and hepatic viral infections.

IDENTIFICATION OF A GENE FOR HEMOCHROMATOSIS

Positional Cloning of the Hemochromatosis Gene

Many years of biochemical studies and candidate gene analysis failed to lead to the identification of the basic defect underlying hemochromatosis. However, the localization of the affected gene to the short arm of chromosome 6 provided the basis for implementing a positional cloning strategy that was ultimately to meet with success. Positional cloning allows the isolation of disease genes on the basis of their chromosomal position without requiring knowledge of the function of the defective protein or its sequence.

Genetic Mapping: Linkage Disequilibrium and Haplotype Analyses

Following the localization of the hemochromatosis gene to chromosome 6, genetic mapping was employed to refine the candidate region by linkage disequilibrium and haplotype analyses. These studies follow highly polymorphic markers such as microsatellites in hemochromatosis families to determine their pattern of inheritance. Microsatellites in close proximity with the disease locus are seen to segregate with the disorder, and in this way a candidate region for the gene of interest can be identified. Identification of recombination between a marker and the disease allows the limits of the candidate region to be defined. In 1977 Simon et al. found an LOD score of 2.239 at a recombination fraction (θ) of 0.005 in six hemochromatotic families that supported linkage of hemochromatosis and the HLA locus. Stevens et al. (1977) concluded that a hemochromatosis gene might be on chromosome 6 close to the HLA locus and in linkage disequilibrium with *HLA-A3* in patients with hemochromatosis. LOD scores greater than +3.0, the score generally accepted as indicating linkage, were found by Cartwright et al. (1978). That this high LOD score was not due to A3, B7, B14 associations was supported by the finding of an LOD score of 4.14 at $\theta = 0.0$ in five pedigrees in which these antigens were not present in the probands (Dadone et al., 1982). In 1985 the first recombination between hemochromatosis and *HLA-A* was determined (Edwards et al., 1986), and it was proposed that the hemochromatosis locus lay between *HLA-A* and *HLA-B*. This, however, was disputed by the findings of David et al. (1986) and Powell et al. (1990), which placed the gene telomeric of *HLA-A*. David et al. (1986) studied a recombinant family with three HLA identical sibs; one (the proband) had hemochromatosis, while the other two were free from any clinical or biochemical signs of the disease. Restriction fragment length polymorphism (RFLP) analysis identified a 7.7 kb HindIII as being absent from the proband, and it was suggested that the hemochromatosis gene, or at least part of it, was located on this fragment.

By 1993 linkage analysis had identified a region between *HLA-A* and the microsatellite marker D6S105 with no recombinations for either marker (Jazwinska et al., 1993). Other markers were separated from the disease locus by recombination, and the centromeric and telomeric limits of the critical region were defined as *HLA-B* and D6S106, respectively. An allele association study of 82 unrelated hemochromatotics patients and 82 healthy unrelated controls found that allele 8 at D6S105 was present in 93% of patients and only 21% of controls, giving a relative risk for this allele of 48.4 (Jazwinska et al., 1993). HLA-A3 was present in 62% of patients and 26% of controls, giving a relative risk for A3 of 4.8. This association with D6S105 was confirmed in other population studies (Stone et al., 1994; Worwood et al., 1994). From this it was concluded that the hemochromatosis locus lay closer to D6S105 than to *HLA-A* and was in fact telomeric of *HLA-A*. The identification of a further recombinant in hemochromatosis families indicated that the gene was telomeric of *HLA-F* (Jazwinska et al., 1995). New microsatellite markers were identified, and further studies provided evidence that the gene was not only telomeric of *HLA-F* but also of D6S105 (Raha-Chowdhury et al., 1995). However, the search for the gene was hampered by the lack of highly polymorphic microsatellite markers telomeric of the class I MHC and an apparent suppression of recombination throughout the MHC region (Malfroy et al., 1997). This resulted in markers over a very large region showing linkage disequilibrium with the gene. So, 20 years after the first report of association with the MHC, the chromosomal region containing the gene remained greater than 4 Mb.

Ancestral Haplotypes

Haplotype analysis in unrelated patients can define the region most likely to contain the gene of interest in cases where the mutation occurred on a single ancestral chromosome. In such cases the ancestral haplotype is maintained at markers close to the gene, and unrelated patients will share this haplotype. Simon and Brissot (1988) suggested that a single mutation in a gene involved in iron homeostasis was responsible for hemochromatosis and that this mutation had occurred on a chromosome carrying the *HLA-A3, B7* haplotype. Over the years, recombination has led to the mutation appearing on chromosomes with haplotypes other than the ancestral haplotype. A haplotype study of 24 Australian families found strong linkage to *HLA* in 23 of the families, indicating that a single genetic locus was most likely to be the cause of hemochromatosis in Australia (Summers et al., 1989). A strong association was seen between the *A3* and *B7* haplotypes in Australia as reported in all other populations. In addition, *HLA-A2* and *HLA-B12* were in significant linkage disequilibrium in patients but not in controls, which indicated a new mutation or recent recombination between *HLA-A* and the hemochromatosis locus. Jazwinska et al. (1995) reported that hemochromatosis showed a very strong founder effect in Australia, with the majority of patients being of Celtic origin. They analyzed the chromosomes of 26 multiply affected hemochromatosis families for linkage disequilibrium and genetic heterogeneity and were able to assign the hemochromatosis status to 107 chromosomes—64 as affected and 43 as unaffected. One ancestral haplotype was predominant and was present in 33% of the affected chromosomes. This haplotype was exclusively associated with hemochromatosis with a haplotype relative risk of 903. The common ancestral haplotype identified, comprising markers spanning 2 Mb, was D6S248 allele 5, D6S265 allele 1, *HLA-A3*, *HLA-F2*, and D6S105 allele 8 (Jazwinska et al., 1995; Worwood et al., 1996).

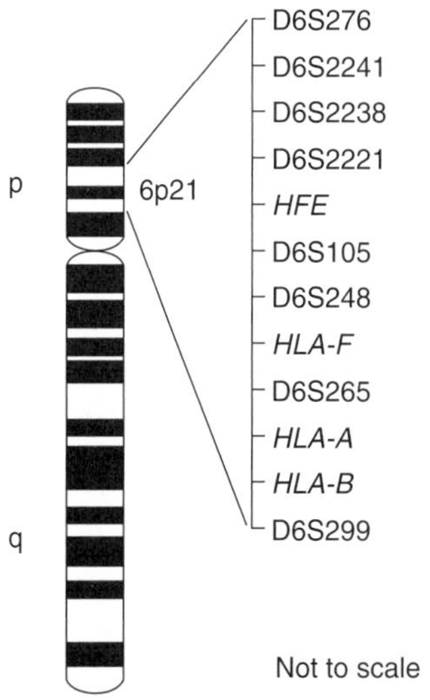

Fig. 18–1. Idiogram of chromosome 6 showing the order of markers in the HFE region.

Physical Mapping of the Candidate Region

Genetic mapping had identified a large candidate region between the markers HLA-F and D6S248 and stimulated the search for genes within this region. The proximal part of this candidate region containing the class I MHC had previously been extensively mapped (Campbell and Trowsdale, 1993; El Kalhoun et al., 1993; Abderrahim et al., 1994); however, the distal part of the region had been less well studied. Physical maps of this region were therefore constructed (Burt et al., 1996; Malaspina et al., 1996; Totaro et al., 1996). Using a combination of techniques, including cDNA selection and exon trapping, genes were identified from the region; however, none of the genes isolated in these studies proved to be the gene responsible for hemochromatosis (El Kalhoun et al., 1993; Totaro et al., 1996).

Identification of a Candidate Hemochromatosis Gene

In 1996 Feder et al. described the identification of a candidate hemochromatosis gene after an extensive positional cloning effort that exemplifies the stages involved in positional cloning. They first created a yeast artificial chromosome (YAC) contig consisting of nine YACs covering the 6 Mb region between D6S265 and D6S276 (Fig. 18–1). Using YAC-derived STSs and serial chromosome walking, they then assembled a set of smaller bacterial clones to cover the central 3 Mb region. New polymorphic markers, mainly CA repeats, were then isolated from both the YACs and the bacterial clones. These new polymorphic markers enabled them to identify a 600 kb region of maximum linkage disequilibrium in which the hemochromatosis gene was most likely to reside. Haplotype analysis of hemochromatosis chromosomes bearing eight ancestral alleles revealed a 400 kb region shared by all of them between markers D6S2221 and D6S2241 (Fig. 18–1). In addition, two hemochromatosis chromosomes bearing five contiguous ancestral alleles were recombinant and defined a minimal hemochromatosis candidate region of 250 kb between D6S2238 and D6S2241 (Fig. 18–1) common to all ancestral hemochromatosis chromosomes and 4.5 Mb telomeric of *HLA-A*.

Isolation of genes from within this 250 kb region was carried out using three independent methods: cDNA selection, exon trapping, and genomic DNA sequencing. These studies identified 15 genes from the region comprising 12 histone genes and 3 novel genes. The novel genes had sequence homologies to Ro/SSA ribonucleoprotein, a sodium phosphate transporter, and *HLA-A2*. The coding regions of all these genes were sequenced in two hemochromatotic patients and two controls. This sequencing identified only one mutation, which was consistent with the ancestral haplotype, a G to A transition at nucleotide 845 of the open reading frame of the class I like gene which they called *HLA-H*. This mutation resulted in a cysteine to tyrosine substitution at amino acid 282 (C282Y). Of 178 patients screened for this mutation, 148 (83%) were homozygous for the mutation, 9 (5%) were heterozygous, and 21 (12%) were homozygous for the wild-type allele, making this gene a strong candidate for the hemochromatosis gene. Several subsequent studies confirmed the high frequency of homozygosity for the C282Y mutation in hemochromatotic patients in various populations: 82% in another American series (Beutler et al., 1996), 92% in France (Jouanolle et al., 1996), 91% in the United Kingdom (UK Haemochromatosis Consortium, 1997), and 100% in a study of Australian muliplex families (Jazwinska et al., 1996). While the C282Y mutation appears to be the major disease causing mutation in these populations, Carella et al. (1997) reported that in Italy the disease appears to more heterogeneous than reported in northern Europe, with an overall C282Y homozygous frequency of 64%. This frequency is as low as 39% in southern Italy (Piperno et al., 1998).

The gene name *HLA-H* had previously been assigned to a pseudogene within the MHC class I region, and with the confirmation that the C282Y mutation in *HLA-H* was indeed causative of hemochromatosis, the gene was renamed *HFE* in accordance with the previously designated name for the hemochromatosis locus (Bodmer et al., 1997; Mercier et al., 1997).

A Second Mutation in HFE

Feder et al. (1996) described a second missense mutation within *HFE*, which resulted in a histidine to aspartic acid substitution at amino acid 63 (H63D) due to a C to G transition at nucleotide 187. This mutation was present in eight of the nine patients heterozygous for C282Y (compound heterozygotes), which represented a significant enrichment over the 17% frequency observed in control chromosomes. Subsequent studies have confirmed that a small percentage of H63D homozygotes and compound heterozygotes develop iron overload (Beutler, 1997;

Martinez et al., 1997; Risch, 1997; Sham et al., 1997). While H63D has been shown to play a role in hemochromatosis, the penetrance of this mutation appears to be low; healthy compound heterozygotes and H63D heterozygotes are described in the literature (Jouanolle et al., 1996; UK Haemochromatosis Consortium, 1997). Patients with non-C282Y-related iron overload tend to be older at presentation and have lower iron levels. Other factors often contribute to the iron overload in these patients, including anemias, hepatitis C, steatohepatitis, and alcohol intake (Sham et al., 1997; Bacon et al., 1999). At present, only C282Y homozygosity and compound heterozygosity are considered indicative of HFE-associated hereditary hemochromatosis (Bacon et al., 1999).

Other *HFE* Mutations?

While the two *HFE* mutations originally described can account for the majority of hereditary hemochromatosis, there are still cases of iron overload in 6p-linked families that have neither mutation and in which no other changes in the coding region or intron/exon boundaries of *HFE* could account for the disorder (Beutler et al., 1997; Carella et al., 1997). While the presence of abnormalities in the RNA untranslated regions and regulatory elements have yet to be explored, it is also possible that another tightly linked locus may be present on chromosome 6. However, a number of rare *HFE* mutations have been described in a limited number of individuals and may have a role to play in the etiology of hereditary hemochromatosis. Some of these mutations are mentioned below, and a detailed summary of rare coding and non-coding mutations in *HFE* can be found in Pointon et al. (2000).

There is a significant enrichment of the S65C mutation in hereditary hemochromatosis patients with one chromosome that does not carry either the C282Y or H63D mutations (Mura et al., 1999). In the hetrozygous state with C282Y, S65C appears to play a role in hereditary hemochromatosis (Barton et al., 1999). Two other mutations, G93R and I105T (Barton et al., 1999), were found to cause disease in the heterozygous state with either C282Y or H63D. In only one case has a mutation been described where it appears to be acting in a dominant manner. This is a frame shift mutation, P160ΔC, which deletes a single cysteine and introduces a premature termination codon 50 amino acids downstream of the deletion (Pointon et al., 2000). This is a rare mutation that appears to be private to the individual in which it was first described. Another deletion mutation V68ΔT leads to the creation of a premature termination codon 19 amino acids downstream of the deletion. The individual carrying this frameshift was also heterozygous for the C282Y mutation. (Liechti-Gallati et al., 1999). Both of these deletions cause a frameshift in the α_2 domain of HFE, leading to absence of the α_3 domain and, hence, the ability to interact with β_2-microglobulin. One splice site mutation IVS+1G to C has been described in a single family (Wallace et al., 1999). The mutation appears to cause hereditary hemochromatosis as a compound heterozygote with C282Y.

The HFE Protein

The *HFE* gene encodes for a 343 amino acid nonclassical MHC class I molecule. The HFE protein consists of a short cytoplasmic tail, a membrane-spanning domain, and three extracellular domains analogous to the α_1, α_2, and α_3 domains of MHC class I molecules (Fig. 18–2). Four cysteines which form structurally important disulfide bridges in the α_2 and α_3 domains of MHC

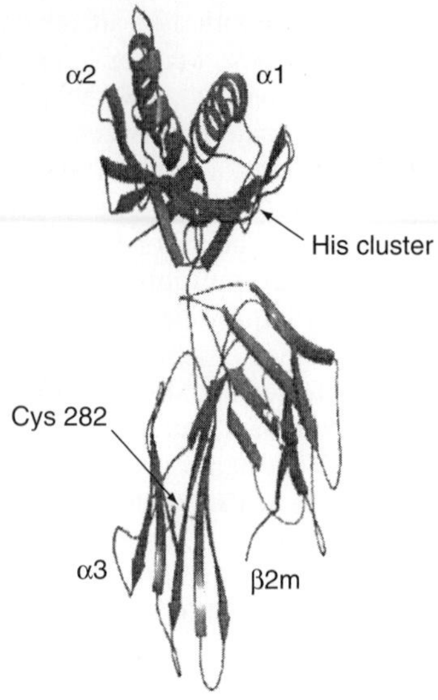

Fig. 18–2. Crystallographic structure of HFE protein. Modified from Lebrón et al. (1998) with permission.

class I molecules are conserved in HFE, indicating structural similarities to the MHC molecules. The α_1 and α_2 domains form the ligand-binding cleft in MHC class I molecules. Comparisons to the Fc receptor, another nonclassical class I MHC molecule, indicated that this cleft would be narrowed by the presence of a proline at amino acid 188 and so would not be able to bind a ligand. This prediction was confirmed recently with the determination of the crystal structure of HFE (Lebrón et al., 1998), which described the narrowing of this cleft so that peptide binding at this site becomes impossible. The α_3 domain is the most highly conserved within MHC class I molecules and interacts with β_2-microglobulin. The binding of β_2-microglobulin is essential for the correct cell surface presentation of the class I MHC molecules.

HFE mRNA is widely expressed in a variety of tissues, most notably the liver and small intestine (Feder et al., 1996). This would suggest a general role for HFE in cellular iron homeostasis rather than a specialized role in the regulation of iron absorption from the gut. Immunohistochemical analysis of the gastrointestinal tract has also shown that the HFE protein is present on the basolateral surfaces of some epithelial cells in the stomach, colon, and biliary tract and on the sinusoidal lining cells of the liver, but in the small intestine, the tissue most relevant to iron absorption, it shows a unique subcellular localization in the crypt cells (Parkkila et al., 1997b). Parkkila et al. (1997a) suggest that the different localization of HFE in the crypt cells of the small intestine indicates a different function for HFE at this site. However, the mechanism by which HFE contributes to the regulation of intestinal iron absorption remains obscure.

While many aspects of the biology of HFE have yet to be resolved, it is now clear that HFE is able to interact with the transferrin receptor (Parkkila et al., 1997a, 1997b; Lebrón et al., 1998; Waheed et al., 1999). Numerous studies conducted in cell lines transfected with HFE and the transferrin receptor suggest that wild-type HFE will interfere with the receptor-mediated uptake of transferrin and thus reduce the delivery of iron to cells (Feder et al., 1998; Gross et al., 1998; Roy et al., 1999, 2000). Overexpression of C282Y mutant HFE does not have this effect, however. The explanations for how the transferrin cycle is disrupted vary and include the following: an effect of HFE on the affinity of the transferrin receptor for transferrin (Feder et al., 1998); a direct competition between HFE and transferrin for binding to the receptor (Lebrón et al., 1999); interfering with iron delivery from transferrin in the endosome (Roy et al., 1999); and an altered rate of recycling of the transferrin receptor (Ikuta et al., 2000). Nevertheless, the relevance of these studies to the control of iron absorption has been questioned. In hemochromatosis, the delivery of plasma iron to the intestinal crypt cells appears to be reduced, whereas the in vitro studies suggest that cellular iron uptake should be increased in the presence of C282Y HFE. Further work is needed to resolve this discrepancy.

Kinetic analyses of iron uptake in duodenal biopsy specimens from patients with hemochromatosis suggested that the enhanced intestinal uptake in hemochromatosis is due to an increased affinity of the carrier for inorganic iron (Cox and Peters, 1978). Since transferrin is not expressed by cells of the small intestine and the transferrin receptor is localized predominantly to the basolateral plasma membrane (Banerjee et al., 1986; Anderson et al., 1990), as compared to the mainly subcellular localization of HFE, it appears that HFE plays a role in an as yet undefined pathway for iron uptake from the gut. One possibility is that HFE plays a role in recycling transferrin via the transferrin receptor in the enterocyte and that the C282Y mutation causes the recycling to be reduced; thus the enterocyte senses iron depletion and up-regulates DMT-1, ferroportin, and perhaps other molecules to increase iron absorption (Bacon et al., 1999). However, as noted above, there is as yet no experimental support for this attractive proposal.

Functional Significance of the Mutations

The C282Y mutation alters one of four cysteines which are highly conserved in both classical and nonclassical MHC class I molecules (Bjorkman and Parham, 1990). These four cysteine residues form intramolecular disulfide bridges that are essential for the stabilization of the molecule's tertiary conformation. Disruption of the disulfide bridge in the α_3 domain by the C282Y substitution prevents the binding of β_2-microglobulin, which is essential for correct intracellular processing and transport of HFE to the plasma membrane (Feder et al., 1997). The mutant protein is retained in the endothelial reticulum, fails to undergo late Golgi processing, and is not expressed on the cell surface. Over half of the newly synthesized C282Y mutant protein undergoes accelerated degradation before processing in the middle Golgi (Waheed et al., 1997). C282Y HFE is therefore not present on the cell surface and is unable to participate in its normal function.

The H63D mutation is located in the α_1 domain and, unlike the C282Y mutation, does not interfere with β_2-microglobulin binding. The intracellular processing, transport, and cell surface expression of H63D HFE does not differ from that of the wild-type protein (Waheed et al., 1997; Feder et al., 1998). The functional significance of this mutation was not therefore initially as clear as for the C282Y mutation. A clue to its significance was first indicated by Parkkila et al. (1997a), who, after noting the similar distribution of HFE and transferrin receptor on the syncytiotrophoblast membranes of the placenta, provided evidence via immunoprecipitation that these two molecules may interact. Further studies have confirmed this interaction and showed that it is pH dependent (Feder et al., 1998; Lebrón et al., 1998). Studies using transfected cell lines showed that wild-type HFE forms a stable complex with transferrin receptor, reducing its affinity for transferrin. While HFE H63D still complexes with transferrin receptor, it does not reduce its affinity for transferrin to the same extent as wild-type HFE (Feder et al., 1998; Lebrón et al., 1998). Whether this is the precise mechanism of action of HFE remains to be determined, but one can envisage that the binding of HFE to the transferrin receptor plays a key role in the regulation of cellular iron uptake, a role which is affected by both the C282Y and H63D mutations.

ANIMAL MODELS OF HEMOCHROMATOSIS

β_2-Microglobulin Knockout Mice

Before to the identification of HFE, evidence had been provided for involvement of an MHC class I molecule in hemochromatosis from β_2-microglobulin knockout mice (De Sousa et al., 1994; Rothenberg and Voland, 1996; Santos et al., 1996). These mice developed signs of iron overload similar to that observed in hemochromatosis. Iron overload was progressive with deposition in the liver having the same periportal distribution as seen in hemochromatosis. Irradiated β_2-microglobulin knockout mice reconstituted with normal hematopoietic cells redistribute the excess iron to Kupffer cells (Santos et al., 1996). This evidence for a defect in the iron storage ability of macrophages in β_2-microglobulin knockout mice is consistent with findings that macrophages from hemochromatotics have a reduced iron storage capacity. β_2-microglobulin mice are also at increased risk for spontaneous development of liver tumors (Rothenberg and Voland, 1996). These observations were extended by Santos et al. (1996), who described a 4-fold increase in serum iron concentration, elevated transferrin saturation ($>80\%$), and increased hepatic iron when compared to control mice with the same genetic background. Iron absorption in β_2-microglobulin knockout mice is excessively high in relation to the body iron stores, and the mice have an impaired ability to down-regulate iron absorption when iron loaded (Santos et al., 1998). Since β_2-microglobulin binding is essential for the normal functioning of class I MHC molecules, it was postulated by Rothenberg and Voland (1996) that the iron overloading observed was due to the disruption in function of an MHC class I molecule. While the actual role of an MHC class I molecule in iron metabolism was difficult to envisage, the tight linkage of hemochromatosis to the HLA region of chromosome 6 and the development of iron overload in β_2-microglobulin knockout mice clearly implicate a class I–like molecule in development of hemochromatosis. This model of hemochromatosis provided evidence that the nonclassical class I MHC molecule HFE could have a causative role in the development of hemochromatosis.

An interesting recent study has shown that β_2-microglobulin knockout mice crossed with *HFE* knockout mice develop more severe iron loading than mice lacking only the *HFE* gene (Levy et al., 2000). This finding suggests that, in addition to HFE, one or more β_2-microglobulin-dependent molecules are involved in body iron loading. Genetic studies of hemochromatosis patients have also provided evidence for the involvement of a second locus in the distal MHC region close to the microsatellite marker D6S105 (Pratiwi et al., 1999). The identity of these molecules is not known.

HFE Knockout Mice

The mouse homolog of *HFE* was cloned in 1997 by Hashimoto et al. (1997), and this enabled the production of *HFE* knockout mice (Zhou et al., 1998). The *HFE* knockout mice generated exhibited profound abnormalities in their control of iron metabolism. Knockout mice maintained on a standard diet exhibited an abnormally high transferrin saturation and showed excessive accumulation of iron in the liver. The iron deposition in the liver occurred predominantly in hepatocytes with a periportal distribution such as is seen in hemochromatosis. Iron deposition was also observed in the spleen and the small intestine but was absent from the pancreas, heart, lungs, and kidneys. Iron accumulation in these organs may occur at a later stage, or this difference in the pattern of iron accumulation may reflect a difference between murine and human iron homeostasis. Even on a standard diet, iron overload was evident in homozygous knockout mice by 10 weeks of age, while at the same age mice heterozygous for the knockout showed little evidence of abnormality. In addition to *HFE* knockout mice, mice bearing the C282Y mutation in HFE have been generated. Like the *HFE* knockouts, these animals accumulate iron in a pattern very similar to that found in hemochromatosis in humans. A surprising finding, however, is that the iron loading observed in C282Y knockin mice is less severe than that seen in *HFE* knockout mice (Levy et al., 1999). These data indicate that C282Y HFE has some residual function, even though current thoughts on the function of HFE suggest that C282Y HFE is tantamount to a functional knockout due to its inability to bind β_2-microglobulin.

It has been known for some time that mice show strain-dependent differences in their susceptibility to iron loading (Lebouef et al., 1995), indicating that at least one, and most likely multiple, genes are involved in determining iron status. Recent studies have shown that different genetic backgrounds also exert profound effects on iron loading in animal models of hemochromatosis. The ability of both *HFE* and β_2-microglobulin knockout mice to accumulate iron is highly dependent on the mouse strain onto which the gene deletion has been bred (Fleming et al., 2001; Sproule et al., 2001). This provides strong evidence for genetic modifiers of the hemochromatosis phenotype, and the genes responsible for these variations in mice may be the same as those responsible for the phenotypic variation observed between patients with the same *HFE* genotype in humans. Candidate genes could include any of the genes known to be involved in iron homeostasis described above, as well as those producing thalassaemia, heme oxygenase-1 deficiency and atransferrinemia (Craven et al., 1987; Yang et al., 1995; Poss and Tonegawa, 1997). The application of contemporary genetic methods to the analysis of these strain differences should lead to the identification of the genes responsible, and this will provide a major advance in understanding genotype–phenotype correlations in hemochromatosis. In addition, the various knockout mouse strains will provide models for testing putative prevention therapies and treatment strategies against iron overload.

CLINICAL APPLICATION AND RISK ASSESSMENT OF GENETIC INFORMATION

Diagnosis

It should be emphasized that hereditary hemochromatosis is now frequently recognized earlier in the natural history of the disease and before symptoms and physical signs develop. Once it is suspected on the basis of increased iron indices or family history of the disease, the performance of the C282Y mutation test can be helpful. Since the availability of a DNA diagnostic test based on this mutation, it has been possible to evaluate the expression of the disease in subjects diagnosed as homozygous or heterozygous for this mutation. The frequency of homozygosity for the C282Y mutation in patients with hemochromatosis varies throughout the world. However, in most populations of northern European extraction (notably Australia; Canada; and Brittany, France) over 90% of subjects are homozygous for the mutation. As stated above, in southern Italy and in some parts of the United States, only 60% or less of such subjects carry the mutation. Presumably other as yet unidentified HFE mutations or mutations in other genes are responsible for the iron overload, particularly in familial cases. In addition, a small proportion of subjects are compound heterozygotes—that is, have one copy each of the C282Y and H63D mutations.

It should also be emphasized that the expression of the disease is very variable. In one recent study (Crawford et al., 1998) of a series of patients referred for evaluation of iron overload, 33% of women and 6.7% of men homozygous for the C282Y mutation did not express iron overload to an extent that met the diagnostic criteria stated above. In addition, 8 of 171 subjects heterozygous for the mutation had modest iron overload in the range previously diagnosed as homozygous (hepatic iron index up to 3.7). However, there is no evidence that such subjects with partial expression of the disease had progressive iron overload with organ damage.

Role of Liver Biopsy in Diagnosis

The role of liver biopsy in the diagnosis of hereditary hemochromatosis has become controversial since the discovery of the *HFE* gene and its mutations. Before this, liver biopsy was an important means of establishing the definitive diagnosis. Now that the diagnosis can be confidently based on genetic testing for the C282Y mutation, however, particularly in the presence of elevated transferrin saturation of serum ferritin and a family history of hemochromatosis, liver biopsy is no longer essential for diagnosis in many cases. Nevertheless, it should be emphasized that liver biopsy is important for assessing whether liver injury, in particular cirrhosis, is present, and liver biopsy provides quantitative information on the amount of iron loading. Thus the use of liver biopsy in hereditary hemochromatosis might be restricted to those patients with a high probability of severe fibrosis or cirrhosis. Two recent studies have been helpful in this regard. First, in an analysis of a cohort of French patients homozygous for the C282Y mutation, noninvasive clinical and serum biochemical features were analyzed for their ability to predict the presence of significant liver fibrosis. Using mathematical modeling techniques, the authors devised an algorithm that would enable one to exclude confidently the presence of severe fibrosis on liver biopsy (Guyader et al., 1998). These authors found that in this cohort of 197 patients, none of 94 patients with a serum ferritin level less than 1000 μg/L, a normal serum aspartate aminotransferase level and absence of hepatomegaly had severe fibrosis on liver biopsy. A similar study from the Brisbane group (L.W. Powell, personal communication) showed similar findings, but in addition, concluded that with an alcohol intake in excess of 60 g per day and age over 45 years a significant proportion of subjects still had severe fibrosis or cirrhosis. They concluded that liver biopsy need not be performed if the serum ferritin level is $<$1000 μg/L and alcohol intake is $<$60 g per day. Both studies concluded that a serum ferritin level $>$1000 μg/L was the strongest independent predictor of fibrosis.

Role of HFE Mutation in Clinical Diagnosis

Testing for the mutations in *HFE* is indicated in all first-degree relatives of patients with hemochromatosis and also in patients with evidence of iron overload, such as elevated serum transferrin saturation, high serum ferritin levels, or excess iron staining or iron concentration on liver biopsy. It is particularly indicated in patients with known liver disease and evidence of iron overload, even if other causes of liver disease are present (such as hepatitis C or a history of alcohol abuse). *HFE* gene testing should include molecular analysis for both the C282Y and the H63D mutations. The finding of heterozygosity for C282Y is expected in 7% to 10% of subjects of northern European extraction. Heterozygosity for the H63D mutation is expected in approximately 15% to 20% of subjects and thus will be common in any Caucasian population studied. Heterozygosity may contribute to iron overload because of other conditions but should not be considered as the sole cause of iron overload or as diagnostic of hereditary hemochromatosis. At present, only homozygosity for C282Y and compound heterozygosity for C282Y/H63D should be considered indicative of hereditary hemochromatosis.

Screening

Screening for hemochromatosis should be considered in the context of:

1. Relatives of subjects known to have hemochromatosis
2. Individuals presenting for a standard medical check
3. The general population

With respect to relatives, screening for the C282Y mutation should be performed on all first-degree relatives (parents, siblings, children) of patients found to have hereditary hemochromatosis. HLA testing is no longer necessary. Family members identified as having C282Y homozygosity should be tested for transferrin saturation, serum ferritin, and elevated liver enzymes. Screening of young children of patients with hemochromatosis can be forgone if the spouse is tested and does not have the C282Y mutation (Adams, 1998). Subjects presenting for a routine medical examination should have the transferrin saturation measured because of the high prevalence of this disease in Caucasian populations (McLaren et al., 1998). If levels are above 45%, the estimation should be repeated on a fasting serum sample. If the fasting level is still above 45%, further investigation is warranted as outlined in Figure 18–3.

Screening for hemochromatosis in the general population is a more difficult and debatable question but would seem to be a reasonable and valuable public health measure. However, the problems raised by population screening are numerous, as has been discussed in detail elsewhere (Burke et al., 1998; Bacon et al., 1999).

The conclusion reached by two recent consensus conferences was that population screening using the C282Y mutation is premature until population studies currently in progress clarify unanswered questions, such as the degree of phenotypic expression, the logistics of documentation and counseling, and the effect of genetic discrimination. A more practical and feasible approach would seem to involve screening for evidence of iron overload using an inexpensive initial test, and recent studies from Canada and Australia would suggest that measurement of the unsaturated iron–binding capacity, which costs less than $1 per test, is the most cost-effective method (Adams and Chakrabarti, 1998; Hickman et al., 2000).

At present, testing of all newborns for C282Y homozygosity is not indicated (Burke et al., 1998). Tests for this mutation

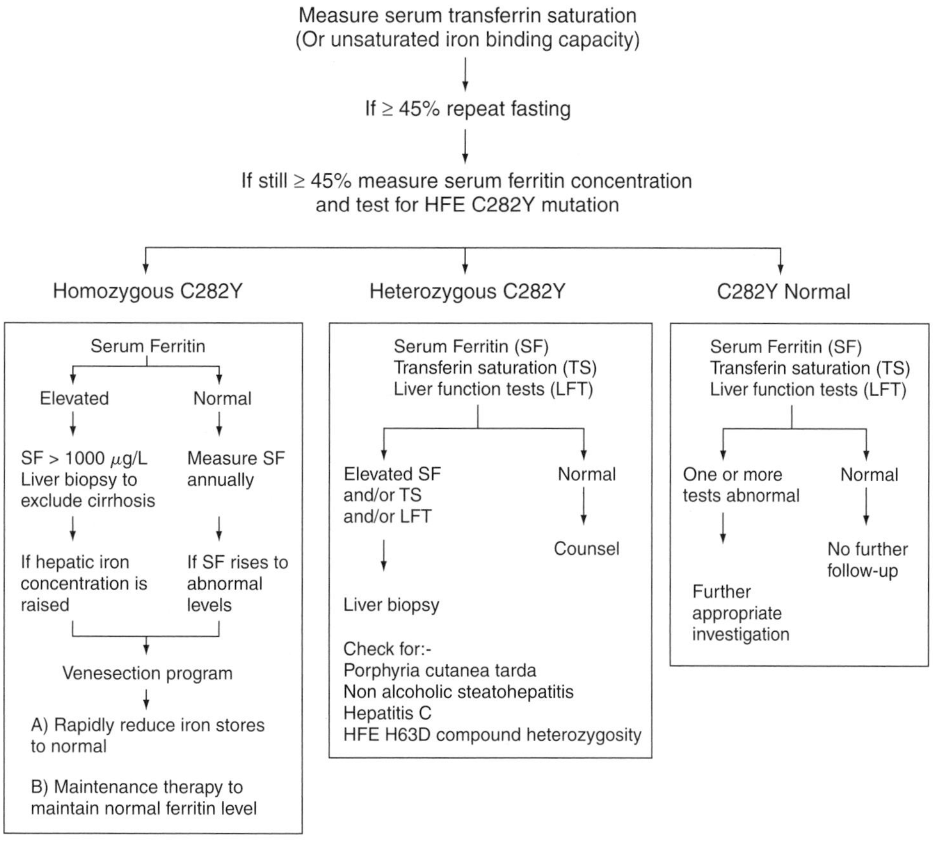

Fig. 18–3. Protocol for screening and management of hemochromatosis. Modified from Powell et al. (1998) in *Schiff's Diseases of the Liver*, eighth edition with permission.

are still comparatively expensive, and the implications for the child's health and medical care (insurability and compliance with therapy and monitoring) are complex. More appropriate would be the screening of all adults for iron overload using transferrin saturation, serum unsaturated iron–binding capacity, or serum ferritin, with confirmatory tests for the C282Y and H63D mutations in patients found to have an abnormality in the serum iron status tests. The optimal timing for such screening is uncertain but should probably be between the ages of 18 and 30 years, the time when the disease is likely to be evident from serum iron tests in most patients but before significant hepatic fibrosis or other serious organ damage has occurred. However, problems concerning how to capture young adults for such testing, how to keep records on results of such testing, and how to ensure accurate and reliable follow-up evaluation need to be addressed, as well as the sensitivity and specificity of screening tests. These issues hopefully will be resolved by population studies that are now being developed in several parts of the world.

Prevention and Counseling

Clearly, once the diagnosis of hereditary hemochromatosis has been made in an individual, first-degree relatives should be appropriately counseled and tested as outlined above. Hemochromatosis is an ideal disease for primary prevention since the disease can be detected well before serious complications develop and appropriate intervention (by phlebotomy therapy) has been shown to prevent all manifestations of the disease with the exception of arthropathy (Niederau et al., 1985). In addition, therapy is simple, through removal of blood on a regular basis, and increasingly blood transfusion services are now using such blood for transfusion if it meets the stringent criteria imposed for "normal" blood donations by blood transfusion services.

Subjects with established disease should also be counseled with respect to complications. This applies particularly to male cirrhotic patients who are at a high risk of developing primary liver cancer, particularly after the age of 55 years (Niederau et al., 1996). At present there is controversy concerning the cost-effectiveness of regular screening by ultrasound examination and alpha-feto protein levels. Preliminary analysis of a multinational prospective survey has shown that screening at intervals of six months can detect tumors as small as 1 cm in diameter, and resection or liver transplantation probably increases life expectancy (Dixon et al.,1998).

Therapy

Once the diagnosis of hereditary hemochromatosis is made, patients should be started on a course of iron depletion and monitoring. Initially patients with iron overload should undergo once or twice weekly therapeutic phlebotomy with regular monitoring of hemoglobin or hematocrit levels and testing of serum ferritin after each 1 to 2 grams of iron is removed (1 g = 4 donations) (Burke et al., 1998). In the typical disease some 8 to 25 units of blood must be removed before the serum ferritin level falls to 50 μg/L or less and serum transferrin saturation falls to 50% or less; these are the desirable end points for therapeutic phlebotomy.

Once primary iron depletion has been achieved, maintenance phlebotomy should be performed three to four times per year with repeat serum ferritin monitoring every year or so. The goal should be to keep the serum ferritin less than 50 μg/L. In all cases the patient should be aware that therapy of the disease is a lifelong commitment. Screening for primary liver cancer is discussed above. It should therefore be emphasized that patients diagnosed before the development of cirrhosis and treated appropriately have a normal life expectancy and should not be penalized for life-insurance purposes.

REFERENCES

Abboud S, Haile DJ: A novel mammalian iron-regulated protein involved in intracellular iron metabolism. J Biol Chem 2000; 275:19906–19912.

Abderrahim H, Sambucy JL, Iris F, Ougen P, Billault A, Chumakov IM, Dausset J, Cohen D, Le Paslier D: Cloning the human major histocompatibility complex in YACs. Genomics 1994; 23:520–527.

Adams PC: Prevalence of abnormal iron studies in heterozygotes for hereditary hemochromatosis: an analysis of 255 heterozygotes. Am J Hematol 1994; 45:146–149.

Adams PC: Implications of genotyping of spouses to limit investigation of children in genetic hemochromatosis. Clin Genet 1998; 53:176–178.

Adams PC, Chakrabarti S: Genotypic/phenotypic correlations in genetic hemochromatosis: evolution of diagnostic criteria. Gastroenterology 1998; 114:319–323.

Adams PC, Deugnier Y, Moirand R, Brissot P: The relationship between iron overload, clinical symptoms, and age in 410 patients with genetic hemochromatosis. Hepatology 1997; 25:162–166.

Addess KJ, Basilion JP, Klausner RD, Rouault TA, Pardi A: Structure and dynamics of the iron responsive element RNA: implications for the binding of the RNA by iron regulatory proteins. J Mol Biol 1997; 274:72–83.

Anderson GJ, Powell LW, Halliday JW: Transferrin receptor distribution and regulation in the rat small intestine: effect of iron stores and erythropoiesis. Gastroenterology 1990; 98:576–585.

Bacon BR, Powell LW, Adams PC, Kresina TF, Hoofnagle JH: Molecular medicine and hemochromatosis: at the crossroads. Gastroenterology 1999; 116:193–207.

Banerjee D, Flanagan PR, Cluett J, Valberg LS: Transferrin receptors in the human gastrointestinal tract: relationship to body iron stores. Gastroenterology 1986; 91:861–869.

Barton JC, Harmon L, Rivers C, Acton RT: Hemochromatosis: association of severity of iron overload with genetic markers. Blood Cells Mol Dis 1996; 22:195–204.

Barton JC, Sawada-Hirai R, Rothenberg BE, Acton R: Two novel missense mutations of the HFE gene (I105C and G93R) and identification of the S65C mutation in Alabama hemochromatosis probands. Blood Cells Mol Dis 1999; 25:146–154.

Barton JC, Shih WW, Sawada-Hirai R, Acton RT, Harmon L, Rivers C, Rothenberg BE. Genetic and clinical description of hemochromatosis probands and heterozygotes: evidence that multiple genes linked to the major histocompatibility complex are responsible for hemochromatosis. Blood Cells Mol Dis 1997; 23:135–145.

Bassett ML, Halliday JW, Powell LW: Value of hepatic iron measurements in early hemochromatosis and determination of the critical iron level associated with fibrosis. Hepatology 1986; 6:24–29.

Bassett ML, Doran TJ, Halliday JW, Bashir HV, Powell LW: Idiopathic hemochromatosis: demonstration of homozygous-heterozygous mating by HLA typing of families. Hum Genet 1982; 60(4):352–356.

Beutler E: The significance of the 187G (H63D) mutation in hemochromatosis. Am J Hum Genet 1997; 61:762–764.

Beutler E, Gelbart T, West C, Lee P, Adams M, Blackstone R, Pockros P, Kosty M, Venditti CP, Phatak PD, et al.: Mutation analysis in hereditary hemochromatosis. Blood Cells Mol Dis 1996; 22:187–194.

Bjorkman PJ, Parham P: Structure, function, and diversity of class I major histocompatibility complex molecules. Annu Rev Biochem 1990; 59:253–288.

Bodmer JG, Parham P, Ekkehard DA, Marsh SGE: Putting a hold on "HLA-H." Nat Genet 1997; 15:234–235.

Bonkovsky HL, Poh-Fitzpatrick M, Pimstone N, Obando J, Di Bisceglie A, Tattrie C, Tortorelli K, LeClair P, Mercurio MG, Lambrecht RW: Porphyria cutanea tarda, hepatitis C, and HFE gene mutations in North America. Hepatology 1998; 27:1661–1669.

Borot N, Roth M, Malfroy L, Demangel C, Vinel JP, Pascal JP, Coppin H: Mutations in the MHC class I-like candidate gene for hemochromatosis in French patients. Immunogenetics 1997; 45:320–324.

Bradbear RA, Bain C, Siskind V, Schofield FD, Webb S, Axelsen EM, Halliday JW, Bassett ML, Powell LW: Cohort study of internal malignancy in genetic hemochromatosis and other chronic nonalcoholic liver diseases. J Natl Cancer Inst 1985; 75:81–84.

Brady JJ, Jackson HA, Roberts AG, Morgan RR, Whatley SD, Rowlands GL, Darby C, Shudell E, Watson R, Paiker J, et al.: Co-inheritance of mutations in the uroporphyrinogen decarboxylase and hemochromatosis genes accelerates the onset of porphyria cutanea tarda. J Invest Dermatol 2000; 115:868–874.

Brittin GM, Raval D: Duodenal ferritin synthesis in iron-replete and iron-deficient rats: response to small doses of iron. J Lab Clin Med 1971; 77:54–58.

Britton RS, Bacon BR, Recknagel RO: Lipid peroxidation and associated hepatic organelle dysfunction in iron overload. Chem Phys Lipids 1987; 45:207–239.

Bulaj ZJ, Griffen BA, Jorde LB, Edwards CQ, Kushner JP: Clinical and biochemical abnormalities in people heterozygous for hemochromatosis. N Engl J Med 1996; 335:1799–1805.

Bulaj ZJ, Phillips JD, Ajioka RS, Franklin MR,Griffen LM, Guinee DJ, Edwards CQ, Kushner JP: Hemochromatosis genes and other factors contributing to the pathogenesis of porphyria cutanea tarda. Blood 2000; 95:1565–1571.

Burke W, Thomson E, Khoury MJ, McDonnell SM, Press N, Adams PC, Barton JC, Beutler E, Brittenham G, Buchanan A, et al.: Hereditary hemochromatosis: gene discovery and its implications for population-based screening. JAMA 1998; 280:172–178.

Burt MJ, Smit DJ, Pyper WR, Powell LW, Jazwinska EC: A 4.5 megabase YAC contig and physical map over the hemochromatosis gene region. Genomics 1996; 33:205–209.

Camaschella C, Cicilano M, Bosio S, Gubetta L, Di Vito F, Girelli D, Totaro A, Carella M, Grifa A, Gasparini P: Juvenile and adult hemochromatosis are distinct genetic disorders. Eur J Hum Genet 1997; 5:371–375.

Camaschella C, Roetto A, Cali A, De Gobbi M, Garozzo G, Carella M, Majorano N, Totaro A, Gasparini P: The gene *TFR2* is mutated in a new type of haemochromatosis mapping to 7q22. Nat Genet 2000; 25:14–15.

Campbell RD, Trowsdale J: Map of the human MHC. Immunol Today 1993; 14:349–352.

Carella M, D'Ambrosio L, Totaro A, Grifa A, Valentino MA, Piperno A, Girelli D, Roetto A, Franco B, Gasparini P, Camaschella C: Mutation analysis of the *HLA-H* gene in Italian hemochromatosis patients. Am J Hum Genet 1997; 60:828–832.

Cartwright GE, Skolnick M, Amos DB, Edwards CQ, Kravitz K, Johnson A: Inheritance of hemochromatosis: linkage to HLA. Trans Assoc Am Physicians 1978; 91:273–281.

Cazzola M, Ascari E, Claudiani G, Dacco M, Kaltwasser JP, Panaiotopoulos N, Schalk KP, Werner EE: Juvenile idiopathic haemochromatosis: a life-threatening disorder presenting as hypogonadotropic hypogonadism. Hum Genet 1983; 65:149–154.

Charlton RW, Abrahams C, Bothwell TH: Idiopathic hemochroamtosis in young subjects: clinical, pathological and chemical findings in four patients. Arch Pathol 1967; 83:132–140.

Cox TM, Peters T: Uptake of iron by duodenal biopsy specimens from patients with iron deficiency anaemia and primary haemochromatosis. Lancet 1978; 1:123–124.

Craven CM, Alexander J, Eldridge M, Kushner JP, Bernstein S, Kaplan J: Tissue distribution and clearance kinetics of non-transferrin-bound iron in the hypotransferrinemic mouse; a rodent model for hemochromatosis. Proc Natl Acad Sci USA 1987; 84:3457–3461.

Crawford DH, Halliday JW, Summers KM, Bourke MJ, Powell LW: Concordance of iron storage in siblings with genetic hemochromatosis: evidence for a predominantly genetic effect on iron storage. Hepatology 1993; 17:833–837.

Crawford DH, Jazwinska EC, Cullen LM, Powell LW: Expression of HLA-linked hemochromatosis in subjects homozygous or heterozygous for the C282Y mutation. Gastroenterology 1998; 114:1003–1008.

Crawford DH, Powell LW, Leggett BA, Francis JS, Fletcher LM, Webb SI, Halliday JW, Jazwinska EC: Evidence that the ancestral haplotype in Australian hemochromatosis patients may be associated with a common mutation in the gene. Am J Hum Genet 1995; 57:362–367.

Cullen LM, Gao X, Easteal S, Jazwinska EC: The hemochromatosis 845 G $\rightarrow$ A and 187 C $\rightarrow$ G mutations: prevalence in non-Caucasian populations. Am J Hum Genet 1998; 62:1403–1407.

Dadone MM, Kushner JP, Edwards CQ, Bishop DT, Skolnick MH: Hereditary hemochromatosis: analysis of laboratory expression of the disease by genotype in 18 pedigrees. Am J Clin Path 1982; 78:196–207.

David V, Paul P, Simon M, Le Gall JY, Fauchet R, Gicquel I, Dugast I, Le Mignon L, Yaouanq J, Cohen D, Bourel M: DNA polymorphism related to the idiopathic hemochromatosis gene: evidence in a recombinant family. Hum Genet 1986; 74:113–120.

de Silva DM, Askwith CC, Kaplan J: Molecular mechanisms of iron uptake in eukaryotes. Physiol Rev 1996; 76:31–47.

De Sousa M, Reimao R, Lacerda P, Hugo P, Kaufmann SHE, Porto G: Iron overload in β_2-microglobulin deficient mice. Immunol Lett 1994; 39:105–111.

Devereaux BM, Mortimore M, Coupland L, Klestov AC, Gunsberg M, Kevant S, Jazwinska EC, Powell LW: Screening for hereditary haemochromatosis (HHC) in a rheumatology clinic using genotypic markers. J Gastroenterol Hepatol 1998; 13(Suppl):A14.

Dixon JL, Do K-A, Fargion S, Conte D, Losowsky M, Powell L: Effectiveness of regular surveillance for hepatocellular carcinoma in haemochromatosis with cirrhosis. Hepatology 1998; 28(4, Pt. 2):1035.

Donovan A, Brownlie A, Zhou Y, Shepard J, Pratt SJ, Moynihan J, Paw BH, Drejer A, Barut B, Zapata A, et al.: Positional cloning of zebrafish *ferroportin1* identifies a conserved vertebrate iron exporter. Nature 2000; 403:776–781.

Doran T, Bashir HV, Trejaut J, Bassett ML, Halliday JW, Powell LW: Idiopathic hemochromatosis in the Australian population: HLA linkage and recessivity. Hum Immunol 1981; 2:191–200.

Edwards CQ, Griffen LM, Dadone MM, Skolnick MH, Kushner JP: Mapping the locus for hereditary hemochromatosis: localization between HLA-B and HLA-A. Am J Hum Genet 1986; 38:805–811.

Edwards CQ, Griffin LM, Goldgar D, Drummond C, Skolnick MH, Kushner JP: Prevalence of hemochromatosis among 11,065 presumably healthy blood donors. N Engl J Med 1988; 318:1355–1362.

El Kalhoun A, Chauvel B, Mauvieux N, Dorval I, Jouanolle A, Giequal I, Le Gall J, David V: Localization of seven new genes around the HLA-A locus. Hum Mol Genet 1993; 2:55–60.

Feder JN, Gnirke A, Thomas W, Tsuchibashi Z, Ruddy DA, Basava A, Dormishlan F, Domingo R, Ellis MC, Fullan A, et al.: A novel MHC class-I like gene is mutated in patients with hereditary haemochromatosis. Nat Genet 1996; 13:399–408.

Feder JN, Penny DM, Irrinki A, Lee VK, Lebrón JA, Watson N, Tsuchibashi Z, Sigal E, Bjorkman PJ, Schatzman RC: The hemochromatosis gene product complexes with the transferrin receptor and lowers its affinity for ligand binding. Proc Natl Acad Sci USA 1998; 1472–1477.

Feder JN, Tsuchihashi Z, Irrinki A, Lee VK, Mapa FA, Morikang E, Prass CE, Starnes SM, Wolff RK, Parkkila S, et al.: The hemochromatosis founder mutation in HLA-H disrupts β_2-microglobulin interaction and cell surface expression. J Biol Chem 1997; 272:14025–14028.

Felts JH, Nelson JR, Herndon CN, Spurr CL: Hemochromatosis in two young sisters. Case studies and a family survey. Ann Intern Med 1967; 67:117–123.

Finch SC, Finch CA: Idiopathic hemochromatosis, iron storage disease: iron metabolism in hemochromatosis. Medicine 1955; 34:381–430.

Flanagan PR, Hajdu A, Adams PC: Iron-responsive element-binding protein in hemochromatosis liver and intestine. Hepatology 1995; 22:828–832.

Fleming M, Trenor C, Su M, Foernzler D, Beier D, Dietrich W, Andrews N: Microcytic anaemia mice have a mutation in *Nramp2*, a candidate iron transporter gene. Nat Genet 1997; 16:383–386.

Fleming MD, Romano MA, Su MA, Garrick LM, Garrick MD, Andrews NC: *Nramp2* is mutated in the anemic Belgrade (b) rat: evidence of a role for Nramp2 in endosomal iron transport. Proc Natl Acad Sci USA 1998; 95:1148–1153.

Fleming RE, Holden CC, Tomatsu S, Waheed A, Brunt EM, Britton RS, Bacon BR, Roopenian DC, Sly WS: Mouse strain differences determine severity of iron accumulation in *Hfe* knockout model of hereditary hemochromatosis. Proc Natl Acad Sci USA 2001; 98:2707–2711.

Fleming RE, Migas MC, Zhou X, Jiang J, Britton RS, Brunt EM, Tomatsu S, Waheed A, Bacon BR, Sly WS: Mechanism of increased iron absorption in murine model of hereditary hemochromatosis: increased duodenal expression of the iron transporter DMT1. Proc Natl Acad Sci USA 1999; 96:3143–3148.

Friedman S, Roll F, Boyles J, Bissell D: Hepatic stellate cells: the principal collagen-producing cells of the liver. Proc Natl Acad Sci USA 1985; 82:8681–8685.

George DK, Goldwurm S, Macdonald GA, Cowley L, Walker NI, Ward PJ, Jazwinska EC, Powell LW: Increased hepatic iron stores on nonalcoholic steatohepatitis are associated with the hemochromatosis mutation and increased liver damage. Gastroenterology 1998; 114:311–318.

Gross CN, Irrinki A, Feder JN, Enns CA: Co-trafficking of HFE, a nonclassical major histocompatibility complex class I protein, with the transferrin receptor implies a role in intracellular iron regulation. J Biol Chem 1998; 273:22068–22074.

Gunshin H, Mackenzie B, Berger UV, Gunshin Y, Romero MF, Boron WF, Nussberger S, Gollan JL, Hediger MA: Cloning and characterization of a mammalian proton-coupled metal-ion transporter. Nature 1997; 388:482–488.

Guyader D, Jacquelinet C, Moirand R, Turlin B, Mendler M, Chaperon D, David V, Brissot P, Adams P, Deugnier Y: Noninvasive prediction of fibrosis in C282Y homozygous hemochromatosis. Gastroenterology 1998; 115:929–936.

Hamilton EB, Bomford AB, Laws JW, Williams R: The natural history of arthritis in idiopathic haemochromatosis: progression of the clinical and radiological features over 10 years. Q J Med 1981; 50:321–329.

Harford JB, Klausner R: Coordinate post-transcriptional regulation of ferritin and transferrin receptor expression: the role of regulated RNA-protein interaction. Enzyme 1990; 44:28–41.

Hashimoto K, Hirai M, Kurosawa Y: Identification of a mouse homolog for the human hereditary haemochromatosis candidate gene. Biochem Biophys Res Commun 1997; 230:35–39.

Hentze MW, Kuhn LC: Molecular control of vertebrate iron metabolism: mRNA-based regulatory circuits operated by iron, nitric-oxide and oxidative stress. Proc Natl Acad Sci USA 1996; 93:8175–8182.

Hickman PE, Hourigan LF, Powell LW, Cordingley F, Dimenski G, Ormiston B, Shaw J, Ferguson W, Johnson M, Ascough J, et al.: Automated measurement of unsaturated iron binding capacity provides an ongoing, cost effective, screening strategy for C282Y homozygous hemochromatosis. Gut 2000; 46:405–409.

Ikuta K, Fujimoto Y, Suzuki Y, Tanaka K, Saito H, Ohhira M, Sasaki K, Kohgo Y: Overexpression of hemochromatosis protein, HFE, alters transferrin recycling process in human hepatoma cells. Biochim Biophys Acta 2000; 1496:221–231.

Jacknow G, Johnson D, Freese D, Smith C, Burk B: Idiopathic neonatal iron storage disease. Lab Invest 1983; 48:7P.

Jazwinska EC, Cullen LM, Busfield F, Pyper WR, Webb SI, Powell LW, Morris CP, Walsh TP: Haemochromatosis and HLA-H [letter]. Nat Genet 1996; 14:249–251.

Jazwinska EC, Lee SC, Webb SI, Halliday JW, Powell LW: Localization of the hemochromatosis gene close to D6S105. Am J Hum Genet 1993; 53:347–352.

Jazwinska EC, Pyper WR, Burt MJ, Francis JL, Goldwurm S, Webb SI, Lee SC, Halliday JW, Powell LW: Haplotype analysis in Australian hemochromatosis patients: evidence for a predominant ancestral haplotype exclusively associated with hemochromatosis. Am J Hum Genet 1995; 56:428–433.

Jones AC, Chuck AJ, Arie EA, Green DJ, Doherty M: Disease associated with calcium pyrophosphate deposition disease. Semin Arthritis Rheum 1992; 22:188–202.

Jouanolle AM, Gandon G, Jezequel P, Blayau M, Campion ML, Yaouanq J, Mosser J, Fergelot P, Chauvel B, Bouric P, et al.: Haemochromatosis and HLA-H. Nat Genet 1996; 14:251–252.

Kawabata H, Yang R, Hirama T, Vuong PT, Kawano S, Gombart AF, Koeffler HP. Molecular cloning of transferrin receptor 2: a new member of the transferrin receptor-like family. J Biol Chem 1999; 274:20826–20832.

Kelly TM, Edwards CQ, Meikle AW, Kushner JP: Hypogonadism in hemochromatosis: reversal with iron depletion. Ann Intern Med 1984; 101:629–632.

Knisely AS: Neonatal hemochromatosis. Adv Pediatr 1992; 39:383–403.

Knisely AS: Iron and pediatric liver disease. Sem Liver Dis 1994; 14:229–235.

Knisely AS, Magid MS, Dische MR, Cutz E: Neonatal hemochromatosis. Birth Defects 1987; 23:75–102.

Lamon JM, Marynick SP, Roseblatt R, Donnelly S: Idiopathic hemochroamtosis in a young female: a case study and review of the syndrome in young people. Gastroenterology 1979; 76:178–183.

Lauffer RB: Iron stores and the international variation in mortality from coronary artery disease. Med Hypotheses 1990; 35:96–102.

Lebouef RC, Tolson D, Heinecke JW: Dissociation between tissue iron concentrations and transferrin saturation among inbred mouse strains. J Lab Clin Med 1995; 126:128–136.

Lebrón JA, Bennett MJ, Vaughn DE, Chirino AJ, Snow PM, Mintier GA, Feder JN, Bjorkman PJ: Crystal structure of the hemochromatosis protein HFE and characterization of its interaction with transferrin receptor. Cell 1998; 93:111–123.

Lebrón JA, West AP, Bjorkman PJ: The hemochromatosis protein HFE competes with transferrin for binding to the transferrin receptor. J Mol Biol 1999; 294:239–245.

Lee KS, Buck M, Houglum K, Chojkier M: Activation of hepatic stellate cells by TGFα and collagen type I is mediated by oxidative stress through *c*-myb expression. J Clin Invest 1995; 96:2461–2468.

Leggett BA, Halliday JW, Brown NN, Bryant S, Powell LW: Prevalence of haemochromatosis amongst asymptomatic Australians. Br J Haematol 1990; 74: 525–530.

Levy JE, Montross LK, Andrews NC: Genes that modify the hemochromatosis phenotype in mice. J Clin Invest 2000; 105:1209–1216.

Levy JE, Montross LK, Cohen DE, Fleming MD, Andrews NC: The C282Y mutation causing hereditary hemochromatosis does not produce a null allele. Blood 1999; 94:9–11.

Liechti-Gallati S, Varga D, Reichen J: Screening for haemochromatosis in Switzerland: detection of a new pathogenic mutation and two additional variants in exon 2 of the HFE gene. European Journal of Human Genetics. 1999; 7(Suppl 1):122.

Lombard M, Bomford A, Hynes M, Nauomov NV, Roberts S, Crowe J, Williams R: Regulation of the hepatic transferrin receptor in hereditary hemochromatosis. Hepatology 1989; 9:1–5.

MacDonald RA: Hemochromatosis and Hemosiderosis. Springfield, Illinois: Charles C. Thomas, 1964.

Maher JJ, McGuire RF: Extracellular matrix gene expression increases preferentially in rat stellate cells and sinusoidal endothelial cells during hepatic fibrosis in vivo. J Clin Invest 1990; 86:1641–1648.

Malaspina P, Roetto A, Trettel F, Jodice C, Blasi P, Frontali M, Carella M, Franco B, Camaschella C, Novelletto A: Construction of a YAC contig covering human chromosome 6p22. Genomics 1996; 36:399–407.

Malfroy L, Roth MP, Carrington M, Borot N, Volz A, Ziegler A, Coppin H: Heterogeneity in rates of recombination in the 6-Mb region telomeric to the human major histocompatibility complex. Genomics 1997; 43:226–231.

Martinez PA, Biron C, Blanc F, Masmejean C, Jeanjean P, Michel H, Schved J: Compound heterozygotes for hemochromatosis gene mutations: may they help to understand the pathophysiology of the disease? Blood Cells Mol Dis 1997; 23:269–276.

McKie AT, Marciani P, Rolfs A, Brennan K, Wehr K, Barrow D, Miret S, Bomford A, Peteres TJ, Farzaneh F, et al.: A novel duodenal iron-regulated transporter, Ireg1, implicated in the basolateral transfer of iron to the circulation. Mol Cell 2000; 5:299–309.

McLaren C, McLachlan G, Halliday J, Webb S, Leggett B, Jazwinska E, Crawford D, Gordeuk V, McLaren G, Powell L: The distribution of transferrin saturation in an asymptomatic Australian population: relevance to the early diagnosis of hemochromatosis. Gastroenterology 1998; 114:543–549.

McLaren GD, Nathanson MH, Jacobs A, Trevett D, Thomson W: Regulation of intestinal iron absorption and mucosal iron kinetics in hereditary hemochromatosis. J Lab Clin Med 1991; 117:390–401.

Mercier B, Mura C, Ferec C: Putting a hold on "HLA-H." Nat Genet 1997; 15:234–235.

Merryweather-Clarke AT, Pointon JJ, Shearman JD, Robson KJH: Global prevalence of putative haemochromatosis mutations. J Med Genet 1997; 34:275–278.

Miller M, Hutchins GM: Hemochromatosis, multiorgan hemosiderosis and coronary artery disease. JAMA 1994; 272:231–233.

Milman N: Hereditary haemochromatosis in Denmark 1950–1985: clinical, biochemical and histological features in 179 patients and 13 preclinical cases. Dan Med Bull 1991; 38:385–393.

Morgan EH: Cellular iron processing. J Gastroenterol Hepatol 1996; 11:1027–1030.

Muir WA, McLaren GD, Braun W, Askari A: Evidence for heterogeneity in hereditary hemochromatosis: evaluation of 174 persons in nine families. Am J Med 1984; 76:806–814.

Muller-Berghaus J, Knisely AS, Zaum R, Vierzig A, Kirn E, Michalk DV, Roth B: Neonatal haemochromatosis: report of a patient with favourable outcome. Eur J Ped 1997; 156:296–298.

Mura C, Raguenes O, Ferec C: HFE mutations analysis in 711 hemochromatosis probands: evidence for S65C implication in mild form of hemochromatosis. Blood 1999; 93:2502–2505.

Mura C, Nousbaum J-B, Verger P, Moalic M-T, Raguenes O, Mercier A-Y, Férec C: Phenotype–genotype corrolation in haemochromatosis subjects. Hum Genet 1997; 101:271–276.

Niederau C, Fischer R, Purschel A, Stremmel W, Haussinger D, Strohmeyer G: Long-term survival in patients with hereditary hemochromatosis. Gastroenterology 1996; 110:1107–1119.

Niederau C, Fischer R, Sonnenberg A, Stremmel W, Trampisch HJ, Strohmeyer G: Survival and causes of death in cirrhotic and in noncirrhotic patients with primary hemochromatosis. N Engl J Med 1985; 313:1256–1262.

Njajou OT, Vaessen N, Joosse M, Berghuis B, van Dongen JWF, Breuning MH, Snijders PJLM, Rutten WPF, Sandkuijl LA, Oostra BA, et al.: A mutation in *SLC11A3* is associated with autosomal dominant hemochromatosis. Nat Genet 2001; 28:213–214.

Olynyk JK, Cullen DJ, Aquilia S, Rossi E, Summerville L, Powell LW: A population-based study of the clinical expression of the hemochromatosis gene. N Engl J Med 1999; 341:718–724.

Parkkila S, Waheed A, Britton RS, Bacon BR, Zhou XY, Tomatsu S, Fleming RE, Sly WS: Association of the transferrin receptor in human placenta with HFE, the protein defective in hereditary hemochromatosis. Proc Natl Acad Sci USA 1997a; 94:13198–13202.

Parkkila S, Waheed A, Britton RS, Feder JN, Tsuchibashi Z, Schatzman RC, Bacon BR, Sly WS: Immunohistochemistry of HLA-H, the protein defective in patients with hereditary hemochromatosis, reveals unique pattern of expression in gastroentestinal tract. Proc Natl Acad Sci USA 1997b; 94:2534–2539.

Phelps G, Chapman I, Hall P, Braund W, MacKinnon M: Prevalence of genetic hemochromatosis among diabetic patients. Lancet 1989; 2:233–234.

Phillips JD, Jackson LK, Bunting M, Franklin MR, Thomas KR, Levy JE, Andrews NC, Kushner JP: A mouse model of familial porphyria cutanea tarda. Proc Natl Acad Sci USA 2001; 98:259–264.

Pietrangelo A, Rocchi E, Rigo G, Ferrari AL, Perini M, Ventura E, Cairo G: Regulation of transferrin, transferrin receptor and ferritin gene expression in the duodenum of normal anemic and siderotic subjects. Gastroenterology 1992; 102:802–809.

Piperno A, Sampietro M, Pietrangelo A, Arosio C, Lupica L, Montosi G, Vergani A, Fraquelli M, Girelli D, Pasquero P, et al.: Heterogeneity of hemochromatosis in Italy. Gastroenterology 1998; 11:996–1002.

Pointon JJ, Wallace D, Merryweather-Clarke AT, Robson KJH: Uncommon mutations and polymorphisms in the hemochromatosis gene. Genet Test 2000; 4:151–161.

Poss KD, Tonegawa S: Heme oxygenase 1 is required for mammalian iron reutilization. Proc Natl Acad Sci USA 1997; 94:10919–10924.

Powell LW, Campbell CB, Wilson E: Intestinal mucosal uptake of iron and iron retention in idiopathic hemochromatosis as evidence of a mucosal abnormality. Gut 1970; 11:727–731.

Powell LW, Summers KM, Board PG, Axelsen E, Webb S, Halliday JW: Expression of hemochromatosis in homozygous subjects: implications for early diagnosis and prevention. Gastroenterology 1990; 98:1625–1632.

Pratiwi R, Fletcher LM, Pyper WR, Do KA, Crawford DH, Powell LW, Jazwinska EC: Linkage disequilibrium analysis in Australian haemochromatosis patients indicates bipartite association with clinical expression. J Hepatol 1999; 31:39–46.

Raha-Chowdhury R, Bowen DJ, Stone C, Pointon JJ, Terwilliger JD, Shearman JD, Robson KJ, Bomford A, Worwood M: New polymorphic microsatellite markers place the haemochromatosis gene telomeric to D6S105. Hum Mol Genet 1995; 4:1869–1874.

Raja KB, Pountney D, Bomford A, Przemioslo R, Sherman D, Simpson RJ, Williams R, Peters TJ: A duodenal mucosal abnormality in the reduction of Fe(III) in patients with genetic haemochromatosis. Gut 1996; 38:765–769.

Rand EB, McClenathan DT, Whitington PF: Neonatal hemochromatosis: report of successful orthotopic liver transplantation. J Pediatr Gastroenterol Nutr 1992; 15:325–329.

Risch R: Haemochromatosis, HFE and genetic complexity. Nat Genet 1997; 17:375–376.

Ritter B, Safwenberg J, Olsson KS: HLA as a marker of the hemochromatosis gene in Sweden. Hum Genet 1984; 68:62–66.

Roberts AG, Whatley SD, Morgan RR, Worwood M, Elder GH: Increased frequency of the haemochromatosis Cys282Tyr mutation in sporadic porphyria cutanea tarda. Lancet 1997; 349:321–323.

Roetto A, Totaro A, Cazzola M, Cicilano M, Bosio S, D'Ascola G, Carella M, Zelante L, Kelly AL, Cox TM, et al.: Juvenile hemochromatosis locus maps to chromosome 1q. Am J Hum Genet 1999; 64:1388–1393.

Roetto A, Totaro A, Piperno A, Piga A, Longo F, Garozzo G, Cali A, De Gobbi M, Gasparini P, Camaschella C: New mutations inactivating transferrin receptor 2 in hemochromatosis type 3. Blood 2001; 97:2555–2560.

Rothenberg BE, Voland JR: β_2 knockout mice develop parenchymal iron overload: a putative role for class I genes of the major histocompatibility complex in iron metabolism. Proc Natl Acad Sci USA 1996; 93:1529–1534.

Rouault T, Klausner R: Regulation of iron metabolism in eukaryotes. Curr Topic Cell Reg 1997; 35:1–19.

Roy CN, Carlson EJ, Anderson EL, Basava A, Starnes SM, Feder JN, Enns CA: Interactions of the ectodomain of HFE with the transferrin receptor are critical for iron homeostasis in cells. FEBS Lett 2000; 484:271–274.

Roy CN, Penny DM, Feder JN, Enns CA: The hereditary hemochromatosis protein, HFE, specifically regulates transferrin-mediated iron uptake in HeLa cells. J Biol Chem 1999; 274:9022–9028.

Sampietro M, Piperno A, Lupica L, Arosio C, Vergani A, Corbetta N, Malosio I, Mattioli M, Fracanzani AL, Cappellini MD, et al.: High prevalence of the His63Asp HFE mutation in Italian patients with porphyria curtanea tarda. Hepatology 1998; 27:181–184.

Santos M, Clevers H, De Sousa M, Marx JJM: Adaptive response of iron absorption to anemia, increased erythropoiesis, iron deficiency and iron loading in β_2-microglobulin knockout mice. Blood 1998; 91:3059–3065.

Santos M, Schilham MW, Rademakers LPHM, Marx JJM, De Sousa M, Clevers H: Defective iron homeostasis in β_2-microglobulin knockout mice recapitulates hereditary hemochromatosis in man. J Exp Med 1996; 184:1975–1985.

Scheuer PJ, Williams R, Muir AR: Hepatic pathology in relatives of patients with haemochromatosis. J Pathol Bacteriol 1962; 84:53–64.

Sciot R, Paterson AC, Van Den Oord JJ, Desmet VJ: Lack of hepatic transferrin receptor expression in hemochromatosis. Hepatol 1987; 7:831–837.

Sham RL, Ou CY, Cappuccio J, Braggins C, Dunnigan K, Phatak PD: Correlation between genotype and phenotype in hereditary hemochromatosis: analysis of 61 cases. Blood Cells Mol Dis 1997; 23:314–320.

Sheldon JH: Haemochromatosis. Oxford: Oxford University Press, 1935.

Sigurdsson L, Reyes J, Kocoshis SA, Hansen TWR, Rosh J, Knisely AS: Neonatal hemochromatosis: outcomes of pharmacologic and surgical therapies. J Pediatr Gastroenterol Nutr 1998; 26:85–89.

Silver MM, Beverley DW, Valberg LS, Cutz E, Phillips MJ, Shaheed WA: Perinatal hemochromatosis: clinical morphologic and quantitative iron studies. Am J Pathol 1987; 128:538–554.

Simon M, Bourel M, Fauchet R, Genetet B: Association of HLA A3 and HLA B14 antigens with idiopathic hemochromatosis. Gut 1976; 17:332–334.

Simon M, Bourel M, Genetet B, Fauchet R: Idiopathic hemochromatosis: demonstration of recessive transmission and early detection by family HLA typing. N Engl J Med 1977; 297:1017–1021.

Simon M, Brissot P: The genetics of haemochromatosis. Hepatology 1988; 6:116–124.

Smith BC, Grove J, Guzail MA, Day CP, Daly AK, Burt AD, Bassendine MF: Heterozygosity for hereditary hemochromatosis is associated with more fibrosis in chronic hepatitis C. Hepatology 1998; 27:1695–1699.

Smith BN, Kantrowitz W, Grace ND, Greenberg MS, Patton TJ, Ookubo R, Sorger K, Semeraro JG, Doyle JE, Cooper AG, et al.: Prevalence of hereditary hemochromatosis in a Massachusetts corporation: is Celtic origin a risk factor? Hepatology 1997; 25:1439–1446.

Sproule TJ, Jazwinska EC, Britton RS, Bacon BR, Fleming RE, Sly WS, Roopenian DC: Naturally variant autosomal and sex-linked loci determine the severity of iron overload in β_2-microglobulin-deficient mice. Proc Natl Acad Sci USA 2001; 98:5170–5174.

Stevens FM, Walters JM, Watt DW, McCarthy CF: Inheritance of idiopathic haemochromatosis. Lancet 1977; 1:1107.

Stocker R: Lipoprotein oxidation: mechanistic aspects, methodological approaches and clinical relevance. Curr Opin Lipidol 1994; 5:422–433.

Stocks AE, Powell LW: Pituitary function in idiopathic haemochromatosis and cirrhosis of the liver. Lancet 1972; 2:298–300.

Stone C, Pointon JJ, Jazwinska EC, Halliday JW, Powell LW, Robson KJ, Monaco AP, Weatherall DJ: Isolation of CA dinucleotide repeats close to D6S105: linkage disequilibrium with haemochromatosis. Hum Mol Genet 1994; 3:2043–2046.

Stuart KA, Busfield F, Jazwinska EC, Gibson P, Butterworth LA, Cooksley WGE, Powell LW, Crawford DHG: The C282Y mutation in haemochromatosis (HFE) gene and hepatitis C virus infection are independent cofactors for porphyria cutanea tarda in Australian patients. J Hepatol 1998; 28:404–409.

Sullivan JL: Iron and the sex difference in heart disease risk. Lancet 1981; 1:1293–1294.

Summers KM, Tam KS, Halliday JW, Powell LW: HLA determinants in an Australian population of hemochromatosis patients and their families. Am J Hum Genet 1989; 45:41–48.

Tavill AS, Sharma BK, Bacon BR: Iron and the liver: genetic hemochromatosis and other hepatic iron overload disorders. Prog Liver Dis 1990; 9:281–305.

Totaro A, Rommens JM, Grifa A: Hereditary hemochromatosis: generation of a transcription map within a refined and extended map of the HLA class I region. Genomics 1996; 31:319–326.

Trousseau A: Glycosurie, diabete sucre. In: Clinique medicale de l'Hotel-Dieu de Paris. Vol 2, 2nd ed. Paris: Balliere, 1865:663.

UK Haemochromatosis Consortium: A simple genetic test identifies 90% of UK patients with haemochromatosis. Gut 1997; 41:841–844.

Verloes A, Temple IK, Hubert A, Hope P, Gould S, Debauche C, Verellen G, Deville J, Koulischer L, Sokal EM: Recurrence of neonatal haemochromatosis in half sibs born of unaffected mothers. J Med Genet 1996; 33:444–449.

von Recklinghausen FD: Über Hämochromatose. Tagebl Versamml Natur Ärzte (Heidelberg) 1889; 324–325.

Waheed A, Parkkila S, Saarnio J, Fleming RE, Zhou XY, Tomatsu S, Tsuchibashi Z, Britton RS, Bacon BR, Sly WS: Association of HFE protein with transferrin receptor in crypt enterocytes of human duodenum. Proc Natl Acad Sci USA 1999; 96:1579–1584.

Waheed A, Parkkila S, Zhou XY, Tomatsu S, Tsuchibashi Z, Feder JN, Schatzman RC, Britton RS, Bacon BR, Sly WS: Hereditary hemochromatosis: effects of C282Y and H63D mutations on association with β_2-microglobulin, intracellular processing and cell surface expression of the HFE protein in COS-7 cells. Proc Natl Acad Sci USA 1997; 94:12384–12389.

Wallace DF, Dooley JS, Walker AP: A novel mutation of *HFE* explains the classical phenotype of genetic hemochromatosis in a C282Y heterozygote. Gastroenterology 1999; 116:1409–1412.

Walters JM, Watt DW, Stevens FM, McCarthy CF: HLA antigens in haemochromatosis. Br Med J 1975; 4:520.

Walton C, Kelly WF, Laing I, Bullock DE: Endocrine abnormalities in idiopathic haemochroamtosis. Q J Med 1983; 52:99–110.

Witzelbin CL, Uri A: Perinatal hemochromatosis: entity or end result? Hum Pathol 1989; 20:335–340.

Worwood M, Dorak MT, Nicklin S: The frequency of the haemochromatosis-associated genotype D6S265-1:D6S105-8 in blood donors. Br J Haematol 1996; 93:838–840.

Worwood M, Raha-Chowdhury R, Dorak M, Darke C, Bowen D, Burnett A: Alleles at D6S265 and D6S105 define a haemochromatosis-specific genotype. Br J Haematol 1994; 86:863–866.

Yang B, Kirby S, Lewis J, Detloff PJ, Maeda N, Smithies O: A mouse model for β_0-thalassemia. Proc Natl Acad Sci USA 1995; 92:11608–11612.

Young IS, Trouton TG, Torney JJ, McMaster D, Callendar ME, Trimble ER: Genetic hemochromatosis and Wilson's Disease: role for oxidant stress? Free Radic Biol Med 1994; 16:393–397.

Zhou XY, Tomatsu S, Fleming RE, Parkkila S, Waheed A, Jiang J, Fei Y, Brunt EM, Ruddy DA, Prass CE, et al.: HFE gene knockout produces mouse model of hereditary hemochromatosis. Proc Natl Acad Sci USA 1998; 95:2492–2497.

Zoller H, Koch RO, Theurl I, Obrist P, Pietrangelo A, Montosi G, Haile DJ, Vogel W, Weiss G: Expression of the duodenal iron transporters divalent-metal transporter 1 and ferroportin 1 in iron deficiency and iron overload. Gastroenterology 2001; 120:1412–1419.

Zoller H, Pietrangelo A, Vogel W, Weiss G: Duodenal metal-transporter (*DMT-1, NRAMP-2*) expression in patients with hereditary haemochromatosis. Lancet 1999; 353:2120–2123.

19 Gluten-Sensitive Enteropathy

SUSAN L. NEUHAUSEN AND JOHN J. ZONE

Gluten-sensitive enteropathy (GSE, celiac disease, celiac sprue) is a common, under-diagnosed disease with significant morbidity and mortality if untreated. GSE refers to the histologic disorder of the small intestine, is characterized by intolerance to the dietary grain protein gluten, and ranges from minimal lymphocytic infiltration of the intestinal epithelium to severe atrophy of the villi (Trier, 1991). The histologic abnormality of the jejunum improves upon gluten withdrawal and recurs with reinstitution of a diet containing gluten (Trier, 1991). GSE is second only to cystic fibrosis as a cause of chronic malabsorption in children. Patients with GSE may have symptoms that include growth failure, abdominal pain, and diarrhea. Occult disease is frequently present with minimal symptoms or signs occurring in the presence of the histologic abnormality.

The terms *GSE* and *celiac disease* (*CD*) are often used interchangeably. In classical CD, there are clinical malabsorption symptoms. When individuals are asymptomatic, it is often referred to as *silent CD*. An extraintestinal manifestation is the gluten-sensitive skin disorder dermatitis herpetiformis (DH). Identification of non-human leukocyte antigen (HLA) genes for GSE would improve our understanding of the immunopathogenesis of the disease, which could lead to the development of preventive strategies and therapies directed at the molecular defect(s).

DISEASE DEFINITION

Brief Clinical Presentation

Symptoms of GSE frequently have their onset in the first 3 years of life, with the introduction of cereals into the diet. In infants less than 2 years of age, chronic diarrhea, failure to thrive, abdominal bloating, and vomiting can occur (Visakorpi, 1997). In children, the median age at onset is 4 to 5 years and common symptoms are loss of appetite and short stature (Greco, 1997). In young adults in their twenties to thirties, the presentation of GSE may be DH (Pruessner, 1998). There is a second peak of GSE incidence occurring in the third to fifth decades, with gastrointestinal symptoms or presentation with anemia, osteopenia, or other complications of the disease. These symptoms also present with other illnesses, so a clinical diagnosis is not sufficient. One of the criteria for a clinical diagnosis is a positive biopsy of the small intestine or skin. Individuals with GSE are then treated with a gluten-free diet; there may be frequent recurrence of symptoms after minor dietary indiscretions.

Subtypes

The GSE phenotype, like most genetic disorders, has a broad spectrum of expression. Three subtypes have been defined.

Clinical CD

Persons with classical symptoms can be diagnosed by the astute clinician and are termed *clinical CD*. Patients referred to as having CD are traditionally diagnosed on the basis of having symptomatic malabsorption in combination with severe mucosal flattening of the jejunum. Both the symptoms and the small intestinal inflammation improve with gluten restriction and recur with reintroduction of gluten into the diet.

Silent CD

Silent CD may represent a large proportion of GSE, including cases with minimal or no symptoms and signs who nonetheless have some degree of inflammation of the small intestinal mucosa.

DH

Last is the extraintestinal cutaneous manifestation of GSE, which involves a "direct disease process in another organ" (Visakorpi, 1997). The classical example of this is DH, which is characterized clinically by involvement of extensor surfaces with pruritic papulo-vesicles (Katz and Strober, 1978; Zone, 1991; Hall, 1992). Virtually all patients with DH demonstrate the pathognomonic deposition of granular immunoglobulin A (IgA) in the dermal papilla or along the basement membrane (Zone, 1991; Hall, 1992) and have some degree of histologic GSE (Fry et al., 1968; Leonard et al., 1983). However, only 15% to 20% of DH patients have overtly symptomatic CD. The prevalence of DH in patients with overt gastrointestinal symptoms of CD is unknown, but it is estimated at 5% to 10%. Abnormalities of the jejunal mucosa of patients with DH were first reported in 1966 (Marks et al., 1966). Subsequently, it was established that DH patients had an increased frequency of many of the clinical and laboratory abnormalities of GSE, including splenic atrophy and, on occasion, deficiencies of iron and folate (Fry et al., 1967; Pettit et al., 1972). The enteropathy was gluten-dependent, improving after withdrawal of gluten from the diet and recurring with challenge (Marks et al., 1968; Fry et al., 1968, 1969, 1982; Leonard et al., 1983; Reunala et al., 1984). Symptomatic malabsorption occurs in fewer than 15% of DH patients and predominantly in those with severe mucosal flattening. The degree of villous atrophy does not correlate with the severity of the skin disease and is not affected by treatment with dapsone (Marks et al., 1968; Shuster et al., 1968). DH is thus an independent marker of GSE.

Diagnostic Criteria

The first clinical report of GSE was published in 1888 by Samuel Gee (Gee, 1888). Since that time, various diagnostic criteria have been proposed. The European Society of Pediatric Gastroenterology and Nutrition (ESPGAN) criteria were first established in 1970 and revised in 1989 (Walker-Smith et al., 1990). The current criteria for diagnosis include a characteristic small intestinal mucosal abnormality on examination of a histological specimen from an intestinal biopsy and clinical remission of all symptoms on a strict gluten-free diet, which usually occurs within weeks to months. However, on occasion, histologic improvement and complete mucosal recovery may take years (Chartrand and Seidman, 1996). Previously, challenge with a gluten-containing diet with recurrence of symptoms was a criterion for diagnosis, but the 1989 revised criteria eliminated the requirement of gluten challenge. In minimally symptomatic or asymptomatic cases (e.g., first-degree relatives of GSE patients who are evaluated because of family history), a second biopsy is needed to prove recovery of the intestine on a gluten-free diet. In the past several years, serologic tests have been used to assist in the diagnosis of GSE, although, as discussed later, a small intestinal biopsy is still advisable.

Though the ESPGAN criteria have not undergone formal revision in more than a decade, there is increasing recognition that they need modification. Kaukinen et al. (2001) reviewed this topic, suggesting that the current diagnostic criteria involving small intestinal atrophy fail to account for minor mucosal lesions. They reported 10 adult patients suspected of having GSE on the basis of symptoms and positive serologic tests but with minimal histologic damage (Marsh grade I and grade II lesions). These patients showed clinical and serologic recovery on gluten-free diets. The authors proposed that serologic criteria may be more definitive in the diagnostic process than traditional biopsy.

Description of the Disease or Trait with Phenotypic Evaluation

The GSE phenotype, like most genetic disorders, has a broad spectrum of expression. It ranges from individuals with clinical symptoms and severe atrophy of the small intestinal microvilli to asymptomatic cases with minimal inflammation of the mucosal epithelium. Symptoms of clinical GSE may include diarrhea, steatorrhea, weight loss, dermatitis, and growth failure. Subtle malabsorptive symptoms include anemia, bleeding, abdominal pain, neuropathy, and bone pain (Visakorpi, 1997).

The current clinical standard for determination of GSE (the ESPGAN criteria) is a small intestinal biopsy and improvement of symptoms on a gluten-free diet. The morphology of the jejunum of individuals with no GSE and of patients with various expressions of the GSE phenotype has been established by a number of investigators (Demling et al., 1969; Marsh and Swift, 1969; Asquith et al., 1970; Halter et al., 1982). For evaluating the small intestinal biopsy for GSE, grading of overall morphology and determination of intraepithelial lymphocyte counts have been characterized (Kadunce et al., 1991; Marsh, 1992). There is an excellent correlation between intraepithelial lymphocyte counts and the severity of small intestinal damage (Kadunce et al., 1991). The GSE histologic lesion ranges from Marsh grade I, with normal villous height and increased intraepithelial lymphocytes, to Marsh grade III, with subtotal or total villous atrophy (Marsh, 1992; Oberhuber, 2000). Clinicians not aware of this spectrum of abnormality may make the diagnosis only in extreme cases. Traditionally, patients were diagnosed with GSE on the basis of having symptomatic malabsorption in combination with severe mucosal flattening of the jejunum.

The immune response to the dietary protein gliadin is thought to play an important part in the pathogenesis of GSE, as discussed below under Pathophysiology: Biologic Basis of Genetic Susceptibility. The antibody manifestations of this immune response are specific enough that they are of great diagnostic value in screening for GSE. In the 1980s, sensitive serologic tests for the screening of GSE first became available. These included IgA and IgG gliadin antibody (GA) and IgA endomysial antibody (EMA) tests (Savilahti et al., 1983; Chorzelski et al., 1984). The development of serologic testing in people with suggestive symptoms and in high-risk populations has greatly facilitated the evaluation for GSE (Catassi, 1997). GAs can be detected in sera using an enzyme-linked immunosorbent assay (ELISA). Although low levels of antibodies to many dietary proteins are frequently found in the serum of normals, patients with symptomatic GSE as a group have higher levels of IgA and IgG antibodies to gliadin compared to normals. IgG or IgA GAs were present in more than 75% of patients with symptomatic GSE, making them fairly sensitive markers of the disease. However, up to 10% to 15% of normals also had antibody levels above background for most normals, making the diagnostic value of this test less specific. Within the GA group, IgG GAs are regarded to be more sensitive but less specific markers for disease than IgA GAs (Ploski et al., 1993; Petronzelli et al., 1997). The IgG GA test is especially useful in screening for GSE in individuals with IgA deficiency. IgA deficiency is much more common in GSE patients for uncertain reasons (Collin et al., 1992). A sensitive screening strategy for at-risk populations includes testing for both IgG and IgA GAs. GA tests also correlate weakly with disease activity, as measured by adherence to a gluten-free diet (Burgin-Wolff et al., 1991).

Subsequent work showed that IgA antibodies to a tissue antigen in the endomysium were virtually never present in normals and present in more than 95% of patients with symptomatic GSE, giving a specificity >99% and a sensitivity >95% (Volta et al., 1991, 1992; Ferreira et al., 1992; Sategna-Guidetti et al., 1993; Grodzinsky et al., 1994; Unsworth, 1996; Valdimarsson et al., 1996). The IgA EMA test is less sensitive in children under 2 years of age (Burgin-Wolff et al., 1991). For adults, the quantity of IgA EMA correlates with the severity of the intestinal inflammatory process, but the exact point in the intestinal inflammation spectrum at which IgA EMA becomes negative is unknown (Rossi et al., 1988; Volta et al., 1992; Troncone et al., 1994). In a study by Volta et al. (1992), IgA EMA was correlated with the severity of the small intestinal abnormality. Only 1/9 (11%) patients with less severe intestinal involvement (partial villous atrophy or mild abnormalities) had positive tests for IgA EMA, whereas 19 of 22 (86%) patients with more severe flattening of the villi were positive (Volta et al., 1992). Rostami et al. (1999) reported that the sensitivity of the IgA EMA test was 100% for those with total villous atrophy, 70% for those with subtotal villous atrophy, and 31% for those with partial villous atrophy. Tursi et al. (2001), in a study of 92 patients with subclinical disease, found a higher sensitivity for the EMA test as it was positive in 97% of patients with total villous atrophy, 92% with subtotal villous atrophy, 89% with partial villous atrophy, and 40% with March grade II lesions.

Tissue transglutaminase (tTG) has been identified as the endomysial autoantigen involved in GSE (Dieterich et al., 1997). As a result, an ELISA was developed to measure IgA anti-tTG titers in serum samples (Dieterich et al., 1998a). Having a defined autoantigen should result in more accurate, reliable, and objective alternatives to the traditional immunofluorescence-based assays, which incorporate thin sections of primate esophagus or umbilical cord. The IgA tTG test, a quantitative assay, has a 95% concordance rate with the IgA EMA test (Troncone et al., 1999). Both tests enjoy an extremely high specificity, but the EMA test is somewhat more sensitive (Dieterich et al., 1998b; Sulkanen et al., 1998; Lock et al., 1999). The efficacy of testing tTG in GSE diagnosis has been demonstrated repeatedly. The sensitivity of tTG testing in diagnosing GSE has been reported to be between 84% and 100% (average 93%), and the specificity has varied from 91% to 100% (average 94%) in 13 studies (Dieterich et al., 1998b; Lampasona et al., 1998; Sulkanen et al., 1998; Amin et al., 1999; Bazzigaluppi et al., 1999; Biagi et al., 1999; Lock et al., 1999; Miller et al., 1999; Piaggio et al., 1999; Troncone et al., 1999; Vitoria et al., 1999, 2001; Hansson et al., 2000; Sblattero et al., 2000). Human recombinant tTG is now available (INOVA Diagnostics, San Diego, CA) and likely to improve the sensitivity of the tTG assay (Vitoria et al., 2001).

At the Eighth International Symposium on Celiac Disease in Naples, Italy, Porter et al. (1999) reviewed their experience with IgA EMA and IgA anti-tTG in a DH subset of GSE patients. They found that 15/27 (55.5%) had IgA EMA and 17/27 (62.9%) had IgA anti-tTG (Porter et al., 1999). Hall et al. (1999) reported that 20/27 (74%) DH patients had IgA anti-tTG using a human tTG antigen. Three of the IgA anti-tTG-negative cases had small intestinal biopsy, and all three demonstrated subtotal villous atrophy. They concluded that IgA anti-tTG was not sufficiently sensitive to be diagnostic for histologic GSE in DH patients (Hall et al., 1999). Dieterich et al. (1999) reported serologic results of IgA EMA and IgA anti-tTG in 61 DH patients. Forty-six of 61 (75%) patients were positive for IgA EMA and 43/61 (70%) were positive for IgA anti-tTG. No small intestinal biopsies were done in this study, but the percentage of patients with positive serology was clearly below the numbers reported for symptomatic GSE patients without DH. Because DH is an extraintestinal manifestation of GSE, these studies indicate that IgA anti-tTG does not define the true prevalence of histologic GSE. A proportion of cases with minimal GSE are likely to be missed with IgA EMA and IgA anti-tTG testing; therefore, the prevalence of GSE is likely underestimated in population studies using serologic screening methods.

The true specificity and sensitivity of antibody tests for the diagnosis of GSE are poorly understood. Most of the previous studies in the United States and Europe have focused on symptomatic cases; therefore, it is likely that they have overestimated the sensitivity of serologic testing. Specificity is also likely to have been misrepresented because control subjects were not evaluated by small intestinal biopsy, so it is unknown how many positive controls actually had histologic GSE with no symptoms.

In all likelihood, the current testing of high-risk groups by serology underestimates the true prevalence of GSE in these groups because of the potential for significant numbers of false-negatives when testing asymptomatic cases with minimal villous atrophy. Population studies using serologic screening with IgA EMA or IgA anti-tTG will miss all GSE cases that are negative for those antibodies. It would be necessary to perform intestinal biopsies on thousands of people to determine the percentage of subjects with histologic GSE who have negative serology. Methods to screen IgA EMA and IgA anti-tTG-negative GSE patients still need to be developed. The available serologic tests cannot substitute for a diagnostic biopsy. However, they can reduce the number of biopsies performed in a clinic by allowing the clinician to separate possibly affected from probably unaffected people.

GENERAL GENETIC AND EPIDEMIOLOGIC EVIDENCE

Clinical Epidemiology and Ethnic Differences

The epidemiology of GSE has been described as an iceberg (Maki et al., 1997). The visible tip is composed of patients with overt clinical manifestations, such as CD or DH. Underneath the sea level of the iceberg are the majority of cases, those with minimal or no symptoms and signs who nonetheless have inflammation of the small intestinal mucosa, so-called silent CD. Those in the middle of the iceberg are seropositive without classic symptoms, e.g., short stature, diarrhea. However, they may have occult anemia, osteopenia, osteoporosis, or minimal abdominal symptoms, including a feeling of bloating after eating. Those in the bottom of the iceberg are seronegative and presumably have no symptoms at all. Why some have significant small intestinal inflammation and are asymptomatic is unclear. There are people who will some day develop GSE but at the current time have a normal small intestinal biopsy. The amount of dietary gluten clearly can influence the spectrum of expression of this genetic disease, but the role of other precipitating factors, possibly including cross-reactive environmental proteins, is unclear (Kagnoff, 1988; Strober, 1992). The age at onset varies from infancy to late adulthood.

Distribution

Based on epidemiologic data, there appears to be a strong genetic component to the disease as the incidence is more prevalent in certain racial/ethnic groups, even in the same environment with similar diets. GSE occurs in most, if not all, Caucasian groups, including Europeans, Americans, Arabs, Indians, and Pakistanis (Misra et al., 1966; Strober, 1992). The prevalence of GSE has been reported to vary among countries. These differences may reflect different diets and/or differences in diagnoses. GSE has not been observed in Japanese and Chinese and rarely in African populations (Strober, 1992). There are rare reports of GSE in African Americans, although it is likely due to mixed ancestry with Caucasians.

Prevalence

The prevalence of the disease in Europe has shown marked regional variation (Greco et al., 1992), probably due to the relative mix of different ethnic groups in the population and to differences in diagnosis and population subsets (e.g., adult blood donors vs. children). In older studies, the prevalence of GSE ranged from 1/2000 to 1/3000 in areas of Scandinavia and Great Britain. However, with the advent of serologic testing, more reliable data on incidence and prevalence have been obtained than from previous data, which relied primarily on symptomatic cases and small intestinal biopsy. Prevalence rates are now estimated at 1/200 to 1/350 in the European population (Pruessner, 1998; Volta et al., 2001), 1/250 in Western Australia (Hovell et al.,

2001), and 1/680 in Brazil (Gandolfi et al., 2000). The ratio of symptomatic to asymptomatic cases is on the order of 1:5 to 1:7 (Greco, 1997). Therefore, many studies that have been performed in healthy blood donors likely have underestimated the frequency of disease. GSE in the United States was previously considered rare, but it now appears that U.S. rates are similar to those reported in Europe and Western Australia. Not et al. (1998) found that 8/2000 (1:250) blood donors in the Baltimore area tested positive serologically for GSE. Estimates in the United States will vary based on the genetic mix of the population. From a pilot study of serologic testing in children, 15/124 symptomatic and 2/35 asymptomatic children had positive serology. Of those positive children who had small intestinal biopsy, 5/8 had GSE (Fasano, 1996). In one study from Africa of Saharawi children in camps in Algeria, the prevalence of GSE based on positive EMA serology was 5.6%, much higher than that reported in European populations (Catassi et al., 1999).

Family Epidemiology

Familial aggregation of gluten sensitivity was first reported in 1935 (Thaysen, 1935). Multiple case families are common, with a risk to siblings ranging from <5% to >20% and most estimates between 10% and 12% (Trier, 1991; Houlston and Ford, 1996; Korponay-Szabo et al., 1998). DH and GSE are frequently seen within a family (Korponay-Szabo et al., 1998), and identical twins have been reported in which one has DH and the other GSE (Hervonen et al., 2000). The occurrence of GSE and DH in the same family supports DH being a manifestation of GSE rather than a separate disorder (Reunala et al., 1976). Why DH occurs in some GSE patients and families but not others is unknown.

Disorders of gluten sensitivity are both familial and HLA-linked. GSE has a marked familiality, with up to 70% of monozygotic twins concordant for the disease. Concordance in siblings is substantially lower than this, with HLA-identical sibs having a concordance of approximately 30% (Trier, 1991). This difference between concordance rates for monozygotic twins and HLA-identical siblings is a key piece of evidence that another gene(s), in addition to HLA, is involved in GSE. If HLA were the only genetic influence, rates would be similar for HLA-identical relatives. This is also reflected in segregation analysis of GSE, where familial aggregation was not explained by a single major locus and a gene in the HLA complex was insufficient to explain the familiality (Sherman et al., 1986).

Familial risks are suggestive that genes for GSE susceptibility interact multiplicatively rather than additively (Houlston and Ford, 1996). There is likely genetic heterogeneity so that more than one gene interacts with the HLA-linked locus. From calculations of sibling risk, Risch (1987) reported that a locus other than HLA might be the primary cause of familial aggregation of GSE, rather than an HLA-linked gene. Petronzelli et al. (1997) estimated that 36% of the sibling risk for GSE was due to HLA, Bevan et al. (1999) estimated 40%, and we estimated approximately 50% (Lewis et al., 2000). These estimates are sensitive to values assumed for sibling risk and prevalence.

Using family data, Pena et al. (1978) proposed that GSE results from interaction between HLA (or an HLA-linked gene) with dominant inheritance and a non-HLA gene with recessive inheritance. However, the model was inconsistent with the prevalence data on GSE. Greenberg et al. (1982) presented evidence both from segregation analysis and from HLA-typed sib pairs that supports a recessive model at HLA rather than a dominant model. The data from western Ireland of Hernandez et al. (1991) support a dominant model of the HLA-linked locus.

Associations with Other Diseases

GSE is associated with many other diseases as well as with complications from the disease (Visakorpi, 1997). Complications include a wide spectrum of metabolic effects, such as anemia, short stature, vitamin B_{12} deficiency, and osteoporosis, as well as seizures (Holmes, 1996; Trier, 1998; Murray, 1999; Dahele and Ghosh, 2001). In a case-control study of 458 cases with celiac sprue and 2692 controls, all treated at Veterans Administration hospitals, the comorbidity of other diseases with celiac sprue was examined. There were significant odds ratios associated with lymphoma, pulmonary eosinophilia, pancreatic insufficiency, Crohn's disease, functional bowel symptoms, chronic non-alcoholic hepatitis, and nutritional manifestations including vitamin B-complex deficiency, hypocalcemia, osteoporosis, iron-deficiency anemia, folate-deficiency anemia, and vitamin B_{12}-deficiency anemia (Delco et al., 1999).

Associations are identified as independent diseases in which the GSE phenotype occurs at an increased rate or in which the disease occurs more frequently in GSE patients. The reason for these associations is seldom clear, but GSE and the other disease may share a similar pathogenic mechanism, an underlying autoimmune mechanism, or genetic linkage of the responsible genes (Strober, 1992). Associated autoimmune disorders, primarily based on multiple case reports, include type 1 insulin-dependent diabetes (1.4%–16%), autoimmune thyroiditis (3.5%–14%), Sjögren's syndrome, Addison's disease, alopecia areata, IgA deficiency, inflammatory bowel disease (1.3%), as well as juvenile and adult rheumatoid arthritis (1%) (Cooper et al., 1978; Cronin and Shanahan, 1997; Kaukinen et al., 1999; Holmes, 2001; Not et al., 2001; Sategna-Guidetti et al., 2001). Kaukinen et al. (1999) examined 62 patients with more than one autoimmune endocrine disorder and reported that 14 (22.6%) had evidence of GSE ranging from minor mucosal changes to severe inflammation. All of them had the GSE-associated *HLA-DQ2* alleles. In a case-control study of GSE, there was a significantly higher proportion of autoimmune disorders in GSE cases than in controls (14.0% vs. 2.8%, respectively) (Ventura et al., 1999). There was also a significant trend for the association of later age at diagnosis of GSE with a number of autoimmune disorders, suggesting that length of exposure to gliadin may be important (Ventura et al., 1999).

There is evidence that some of the autoimmune associations are of the cause-and-effect type. GSE may cause autoimmune disorders through chronic autoimmune stimulation in the intestine, which then produces an increase in autoantibodies and, therefore, stimulates other autoimmune disorders (Strober, 1992; Reunala et al., 1997). In patients with arthritis, pericarditis, and autoimmune thyroiditis, symptoms diminish or disappear with adherence to a gluten-free diet (Laine and Holt, 1982; Pinals, 1986; Sategna-Guidetti et al., 2001). Alternatively, the association with autoimmune disease could be related to a GSE gene linked to HLA or a shared immunogenetic predisposition from HLA, which enables the autoimmune process. In one study, one-third of type 1 diabetic patients with HLA-DQ2 expressed IgA anti-tTG autoantibodies compared to fewer than 2% of patients lacking DQ2, suggesting a shared immunogenetic predisposition (Bao et al., 1999). In a prospective study of 90 patients with GSE, prevalence rates of diabetes and thyroid-related serum antibodies were 11.1% and 14.4%, respectively, and they tended to disappear with a gluten-free diet (Ventura et al., 2000). Holmes (2001) reviewed studies on the prevalence of GSE in type 1 diabetes and reported that it ranged from 1/6 to 1/103 in children and from 1/16 to 1/76 in adults.

In a study of 50 patients with GSE, the prevalence of autoimmune thyroid disease was increased over population levels (Cunningham and Zone, 1985). It was suggested that the association was due to a shared immunogenetic predisposition since more than 90% of patients with DH had the HLA-DR3 haplotype (Katz and Strober, 1978) and there is an increased prevalence of HLA-DR3 in thyroid disease. However, the association with autoimmune thyroid disease was subsequently shown to be much higher than that of HLA-DR3 controls (Gaspari et al., 1990), suggesting that it was not a shared predisposition due to HLA. In a study of autoimmune thyroid disease, 3.3% of patients were positive for IgA EMA and a diagnosis of GSE was confirmed with subsequent biopsy (Valentino et al., 1999). On a gluten-free diet, there was improvement of hypothyroidism and reduction of the thyroxine dosage.

The association between arthritis and GSE has been less well characterized. The studies have been varied, including cases with sacroiliitis, rheumatoid arthritis, and juvenile rheumatoid arthritis; but all have had positive serologic tests for GAs (Koot et al., 1989; Paimela et al., 1995; Usai et al., 1995; Mota Vargas et al., 1996; Miller, 1997). Arthritis in the GSE patients dramatically improved after gluten withdrawal, although the pathogenesis was unclear (Bourne et al., 1985; Pinals, 1986).

An increased prevalence of GSE has also been reported in Down syndrome (DS) patients. The reported prevalence of GSE in DS ranges from 4% to 17% (Castro et al., 1993; Zubillaga et al., 1993; Failla et al., 1996; George et al., 1996; Hansson et al., 1999; Csizmadia et al., 2000; Book et al., 2001), which is approximately 25 to 40 times that of the general Caucasian population rate of 0.4%. Gastrointestinal symptoms are commonly seen in DS patients, so it is unlikely that their presence would alert the clinician to a diagnosis of GSE. GSE therefore is not detected in most DS individuals on a clinical basis alone. In one report, IgA EMA was 100% specific for GSE in DS individuals (Failla et al., 1996). In another study, 7/43 DS children were IgA EMA-positive and all demonstrated villous atrophy (Carlsson et al., 1998). DS patients with GSE have the typical GSE HLA alleles, DR3, DR7, and DQ2 (Castro et al., 1993; Csizmadia et al., 2000; Book et al., 2001). Both GSE and DS have an association with autoimmune diseases, and the increased prevalence of GSE in DS suggests that a common link may be an altered immune system or genetic factors.

GSE is associated with gynecologic problems, including late menarche, early menopause, increased prevalence of secondary amenorrhea, increased infertility, higher miscarriage rates, and low-birth-weight babies (reviewed by Eliakim and Sherer, 2001). In a set of three studies of untreated GSE patients matched to controls, when the GSE patients adhered to a gluten-free diet, the gynecologic problems, miscarriage rates, and birth weights of babies were similar to those of controls (Sher and Mayberry, 1994; Ciacci et al., 1996; Smecuol et al., 1996). In a study of 845 pregnant women screened for GSE, 12 were identified as having the disease. Of those, five had small for gestational age newborns and three had preterm deliveries (of which one infant was small for gestational age) (Martinelli et al., 2000). Several of these researchers suggested that pregnant women should be routinely screened for GSE because of the high incidence of adverse outcomes that could be avoided through adherence to a gluten-free diet.

When compared to the general population, patients with GSE have an increased risk of developing esophageal and pharyngeal squamous carcinomas, small intestinal adenocarcinomas, and enteropathy-associated T-cell lymphoma (Wright, 1995; Ferguson and Kingstone, 1996; Green et al., 2001). The risk reported for enteropathy-associated T-cell lymphoma in individuals with GSE is 40- to 100-fold greater than in the general population (Hoggan, 1997). Lymphoma is of interest because in GSE patients the increased risk appears to be reversed with long-term adherence to a gluten-free diet (Egan et al., 1995; Collin et al., 1996). This implies that chronic stimulation of lymphocytes by gluten eventually produces malignant transformation of lymphocytes and that removal of that stimulation reverses the risk of malignant transformation.

Environmental Factors

The only known significant environmental factor that accentuates the disease is dietary exposure to gluten. The amount of gluten in the diet may affect age at diagnosis of GSE. In a study comparing the incidence of GSE in children suspected of having the disease, 6% of Danish children compared to 41% of Swedish children had GSE, with mean ages at diagnosis of 5.5 years and 1.5 years, respectively (Weile et al., 1995). The only clear difference was that the infant diet in Sweden contained more than 40 times the daily gliadin than the diet in Denmark.

Even given high exposure to gluten, not all individuals are susceptible to gluten sensitivity. There are clear genetic influences, yet they do not explain all of the susceptibility as only 60% to 70% of identical twins share the disease. There may be infectious agents or other environmental factors that are not yet identified. Kagnoff et al. (1984) looked for protein sequences that share amino acid sequence homology with α-gliadin, which had been shown to activate GSE. They found homology to the 54 kDa E1b protein of human adenovirus type 12 (Ad12), an adenovirus typically isolated from the intestinal tract. They suggested that antigens produced during intestinal viral infection could be important in the pathogenesis of GSE. In a study of sera from 41 children with untreated GSE, 16 children with DH, and 57 matched controls, serum antibodies to synthetic peptides from Ad12 and α-gliadin were measured. Antipeptide IgG antibodies to both Ad12 E1b and α-gliadin increased the risk of GSE and DH, suggesting that they may contribute to the development of the disease and that there may be a synergistic effect (Lahdeaho et al., 1993a,b).

PATHOPHYSIOLOGY: BIOLOGIC BASIS OF GENETIC SUSCEPTIBILITY

GSE is an immune-mediated inflammation of the small intestine characterized by both architectural and inflammatory changes of the mucosa, resulting in global malabsorption (Marsh, 1992). There is a spectrum of GSE observed from small intestinal biopsy specimens, illustrated in the scanning electron micrographs (Fig. 19–1). Briefly, normal specimens show predominantly finger-like villi (Fig. 19–1A) with lymphocyte counts of <200/1000 epithelial cells. Specimens with early GSE may have this same villous architecture in the presence of increased numbers of intraepithelial lymphocytes. The earliest abnormality of the villi consists of leaf- and tongue-like villi with cerebriform ridges (Fig. 19–1B). Next, the villi take on a cerebriform appearance

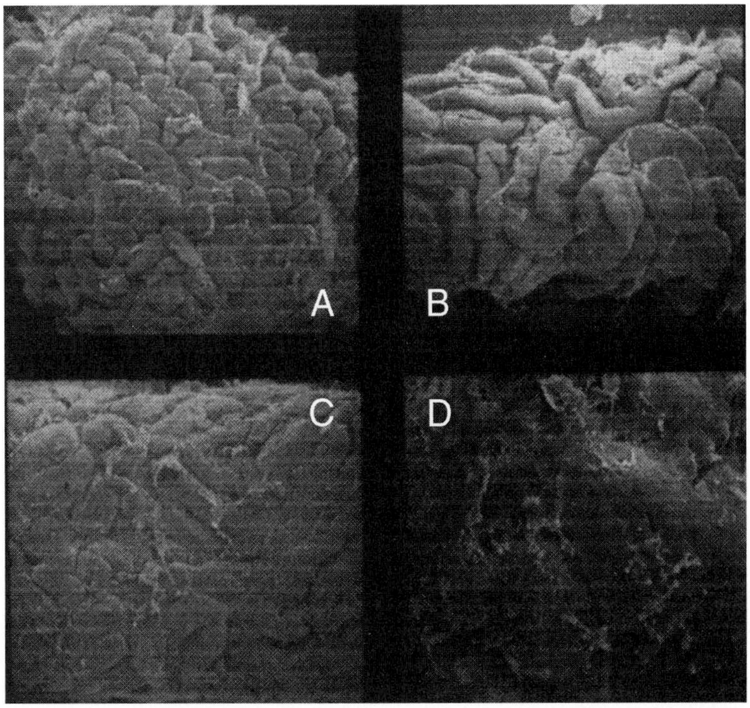

Fig. 19–1. Spectrum of villous architecture using electron microscopy. Mild stages of gluten-sensitive enteropathy may have fairly normal villous architecture and only infiltration of epithelium with lymphocytes. From Kadunce et al. (1991) with permission.

with an angular and convoluted morphology (Fig. 19–1C). In severe villous atrophy, which is seen in classical GSE, a flat or mosaic surface is seen with little evidence of villi (Fig. 19–1D). The loss of functional villi compromises absorption of nutrients by the small intestine, leading to nutrient deficiencies. The intraepithelial lymphocyte counts progressively increase to 400 to 500 lymphocytes/1000 epithelial cells in severe cases.

This pathologic picture is not specific for GSE since other inflammatory conditions of the intestine may show similar histology. However, there will be improvement of symptoms only with gluten restriction for those with GSE. Similar morphologic findings of the villous architecture have been reported in various immunodeficiency states, malabsorption syndromes associated with sensitivity to various food substances, and infections of the upper gastrointestinal tract (Strober, 1976; Walker-Smith et al., 1984; Trier, 1998). Infectious causes, such as giardia, can be evaluated by examination of stool for ova and parasites. Where there are other potential causes of villous atrophy, symptoms and/or the small intestinal morphology need to be re-evaluated after gluten restriction.

The specific immunologic mechanism that causes mucosal damage is unclear. However, current evidence suggests that environmental factors (including dietary gluten ingestion and adenoviral infection) as well as immune factors (intestinal T cell–mediated immunity and IgA antibody–mediated immunity) are important. No specific abnormality of a protein or enzyme has been identified in GSE, and no susceptibility gene other than the HLA association has been confirmed (Kagnoff, 1990; Howdle and Blair, 1992).

There is a strong humoral response. Increased numbers of plasma cells in the mucosa produce IgA, IgG, and IgM antibodies against grain peptides and connective tissue autoantigens. The humoral response appears to parallel the cellular injury. Secreted IgA directed against gliadin may target host antigens in the connective tissue of the jejunum, reticulin, and endomysium (Murray, 1999).

Immunohistochemical techniques have been used to further characterize changes in jejunal biopsies from patients with GSE. In the surface of the intestinal epithelium of GSE patients, the number of lymphocytes is markedly increased (Ferguson, 1977). The infiltrating cells are predominantly $CD3^{+}CD8^{+}$ α/β T-cell receptor-positive cells. The proportion and absolute density of γ/δ T cells are significantly increased. This constant increase in γ/δ T cells is the only permanent morphologic change in the jejunum and, as such, may be the most sensitive indicator of GSE (Savilahti et al., 1990). This has been identified in approximately 30% of family members of GSE patients, even in the absence of significant changes in villous morphology (Savilahti, 1997). Iltanen et al. (1999) also observed that in addition to an increased density of γ/δ^{+} cells, there are increases in α/β^{+} T cells, the ratio of γ/δ^{+} to $CD3^{+}$ T cells, and the ratio of γ/δ^{+} to α/β^{+} T cells. Activated T cells ($CD25^{+}$) were initially proposed as a marker for GSE but were found to be much less specific than the antibody tests (Savilahti, 1997).

Two autoantigens have been identified for GSE, the more frequently recognized tTG, identified in 1997, and a 55 kDa GSE-specific nuclear protein, reported in 2001 (Dieterich et al., 1997; Natter et al., 2001). tTG is the major autoantigen that reacts in the EMA test (Dieterich et al., 1997). The functions of tTG are to either cross-link or deamidate glutamine residues. Gliadin, which is approximately 35% glutamine residues, is a preferred substrate in vitro. Deamidation of gliadin by tTG uncovers epitopes that enhance binding to HLA-DQ2 on antigen-presenting cells, which are then recognized by intestinal T cells (Molberg et al., 1998). Molberg and colleagues (2001) demonstrated that deamidated gliadin epitopes are formed in situ by endogenous tTG, thus providing additional support that gliadin deamidation by tTG in vivo results in peptides that bind efficiently to DQ2 (or DQ8) molecules. Furthermore, tTG may become cross-linked to the gliadin peptide or its deamidated form, resulting in tTG–gliadin complexes. These complexes may then allow gliadin-specific T-helper cells to promote a specific antibody response to tTG by stimulated tTG-specific B cells (Dieterich et al., 1997).

Two possible explanations of how tTG is involved in lack of differentiation of the villous epithelium have been presented (Schuppan et al., 1998; Schuppan, 2000). tTG leads to activation in the lamina propria of $CD4^+$ T cells. As shown by in vitro studies, when gut fibroblasts are stimulated by activated $CD4^+$ T cells, they secrete matrix-degrading enzymes that are important in villous atrophy and crypt hyperplasia. Also, the humoral IgA response to tTG in GSE may be directly involved in the pathogenesis of villous atrophy. Differentiation of colon T84 cells into polarized epithelia is inhibited by IgA anti-tTG from GSE patients. Differentiation of intestinal epithelia may depend on activation of transforming growth factor-β, which requires tTG with plasmin. Thus, an excess of antibodies to tTG could prevent differentiation, resulting in the flat mucosa.

Suggestive candidate genes based on the pathophysiology of GSE are those that control T-cell immune responses. The classes of genes would include T-cell receptor genes; genes for protein antigen processing and peptide transport; the HLA genes that determine which peptides bind; and immune-modulating genes encoding for cytokines, cytokine receptors, and adhesion molecules (Sollid et al., 1997). The roles of several of these genes are discussed in the next section.

GENE IDENTIFICATION

Linkage and Association

Systematic/Random Markers with Clinical Disease and Physiologic Abnormalities

GSE is generally diagnosed through a small intestinal biopsy and antibody tests. Thus, the phenotype is generally considered to be the presence of an abnormal biopsy and/or positive serology rather than clinical symptoms. GSE with overt clinical symptoms accounts for only a small proportion of cases.

The first genome-wide search for linkage was published by Zhong et al. (1996), in which they studied 40 affected sib pairs from 11 families. They reported significant linkage approximately 30 cM from HLA on 6p23. Other suggestive regions were 11p11, 7q31.3, 22cen, 15q26, 5q33.3, 19p13.1, and 19q13.2. Houlston et al. (1997), studying 28 families, found no significant evidence for linkage to the regions suggested by Zhong et al. (1996), except for weak evidence at 15q26, where IDDM3 is localized (Field et al., 1994). This region was examined in a set of 99 Finnish families with at least one affected sib pair. There was no evidence for genetic linkage by nonparametric analysis; however, transmission disequilibrium testing gave evidence of linkage ($p = 0.03$) (Susi et al., 2001). Brett et al. (1998), in a study of 21 families with 60 affecteds and 125 unaffected family members, examined linkage to 6p23, 7q31.3, 11p11, 15q26, and 22cen and were unable to confirm linkage at any of these regions. In a genome-wide screen using the same families, there was evidence for linkage at D2S142 near CTLA-4 and at D7S515 as well as weaker hints at other regions (Yiannakou et al., 1999). Greco and co-workers (1998a) evaluated 39 sib pairs and their parents in a genome-wide screen of 281 markers. An additional 71 pairs in which one sib had symptomatic CD and the other had silent CD were used to further examine regions of interest. They were unable to confirm the candidate regions of Zhong et al. (1996) but did find weak evidence for linkage on 5qter and 11qter. In a replication set of 89 Italian sib pairs, they investigated previous linkage hints at 3q, 5q, 10q, 11q, 15q, and 19q and found nominal evidence at 5q (Greco et al., 2001). King et al. (2000) performed a genome-wide search with 16 GSE families and reported nominal evidence for linkage at 10q23.1 and 16q23.3. In a follow-up study of 17 regions, using 50 families, they found heterogeneity LOD scores >2.0 at 6p12, 11p11, 17q12, 18q23, and 22q13.3 (King et al., 2001).

It is surprising that little progress has been made in identifying the non-HLA genes responsible for GSE, especially given the high recurrence risk in siblings (approximately 30–60), compared to Type 1 diabetes mellitus (approximately 15) (Risch, 1987; Petronzelli et al., 1997; Bevan et al., 1999). From genome-wide screens, regions were identified in which there may be susceptibility genes (Zhong et al., 1996; Houlston et al., 1997; Greco et al., 1998a). However, regions showing linkage in one study have not been strongly replicated by other studies. Non-replication of linkage results in complex diseases is common and may be due to the low power of studies to detect genes of small effect and/or to a high degree of genetic heterogeneity among families. Larger data sets with more power likely are needed to find strong evidence for linkage.

Candidate Genes

In 1993, association and linkage studies of T-cell receptor genes (*TCRα*, *TCRγ*, and *TCRβ*) with GSE were carried out in a set of 49 cases and 70 controls (Roschmann et al., 1993). Relative risks were nonsignificant, ranging from 1.35 to 3.35 in the association studies, and no evidence for linkage was found in 23 families. In a second study, no evidence for linkage was found at *TCRα*, *TCRγ*, *TCRβ*, or *TCRδ* (Yiannakou et al., 1999).

Another region of interest is 2q33, where the *CD28* and *CTLA-4* genes, encoding receptors that regulate T-lymphocyte activation, are located. *CD28* promotes both T-cell proliferation and survival of activated T cells, whereas *CTLA-4* encodes a cell surface molecule that downregulates T-cell activation (Walunas et al., 1994; Noel et al., 1996). Holopainen et al. (1999) reported linkage to this region in a study of 100 Finnish families with GSE. They also observed allelic association with D2S116, which suggests a founder effect in these families. In a case-control study of 101 GSE cases and 130 healthy controls, a polymorphism in *CTLA-4* (49A → G) was significantly associated with GSE [$p = 0.002$, odds ratio (OR) = 2.36, 95% confidence interval (CI) 1.37–4.06] (Djilali-Saiah et al., 1998). Naluai et al. (2000) also reported an association of the 49A → G *CTLA-4* polymorphism with GSE in Swedish and Norwegian families, whereas Clot et al. (1999) found no evidence for linkage or association with this variant in Italian and Tunisian families with GSE. Interestingly, this polymorphism has been associated with autoimmune diseases such as Graves' disease (Yanagawa et al., 1995; Donner et al., 1997), multiple sclerosis (Harbo et al., 1999), rheumatoid arthritis in females (Gonzalez-Escribano et al., 1999), DR-4-associated rheumatoid arthritis (Seidl et al., 1998), and Type 1 diabetes (Donner et al., 1997; Marron et al., 1997).

Genes and Responsible Variation

Evidence of Association

There is a strong association of *HLA* with GSE. The strength of the *HLA* association with GSE has become stronger as more *HLA* genes have been examined. Initially, this association was described with the HLA class I alleles *A1* and *B8* (Falchuk et al., 1972). Stronger associations were subsequently described with the class II allele *DR3* (Park et al., 1983; Sachs et al., 1986; Hall et al., 1989; Sollid and Thorsby, 1993). In southern Europe, where the frequency of *DR3* is lower among the control population, significant class II associations were found with both *DR3* and *DR7* alleles (Sollid and Thorsby, 1993). Some groups have also shown an excess of *DR5/DR7* heterozygotes. A unifying hypothesis for the *HLA* associations came with the development of polymerase chain reaction–based *HLA* typing. *DR* and *DQ* are in strong linkage disequilibrium, and the *DR3/DQ2* haplotype carries the *DQA1*0501* and *DQB1*0201* alleles. As the strong association with *DR3* in all populations implies, the primary *HLA* susceptibility to GSE is the *DQ2* heterodimer formed by the *DQA1*0501* and *DQB1*0201* alleles. These alleles may be encoded in *cis* (on the same chromosome) with *DR3* or in *trans* (on different chromosomes) with the *DR5/DR7* haplotype (Sollid and Thorsby, 1993). The *DR7* allele exists in linkage disequilibrium with the *DQ* alleles *DQA1*0201* and *DQB1*0202*, while the *DR5* allele is found with the *DQ* alleles *DQA1*0501* and *DQB1*0301*. Fernandez-Arquero et al. (1998) identified a base pair change in the promoter region of *DQB*02*, which they believe is associated with the increased risk of GSE from the *DR7 DQA1*0201 DQB*0202* haplotype compared to those carrying *DQB1*0201* on the *DR3* haplotype.

New alleles (subtypes) of the *HLA* genes are still being identified, so the nomenclature of *HLA* genes is updated yearly (Bodmer et al., 1999) (sequences can be examined at *www.anthonynolan.com/HIG/data.html*). With knowledge of new subtypes, *HLA* allele designations in the literature have changed over time. For example, *DQB1*02* subtypes were not previously known, so the association was written as *DQA1*0501 DQB1*0201*. Based on current knowledge of subtypes, the appropriate nomenclature is *DQA1*05 DQB1*02* as the association of GSE with currently known subtypes has not been reported.

*DQ1*05 DQB1*02* is the most significant *HLA* association with the disease, with more than 90% of GSE and DH patients from northern and southern Europe carrying these alleles (Sollid and Thorsby, 1993; Tighe and Ciclitira, 1993; Houlston and Ford, 1996; Balas et al., 1997). The relative risk, to individuals who carry the *DQ2* heterodimer relative to the general population in the United States and Europe, is increased by 40- to 50-fold, and the absolute risk of developing GSE in individuals with those alleles is approximately 1% (Kagnoff, 1999). However, this calculation is not based on extensive sampling of *DQA1*05 DQB1*02*-positive individuals. Although this *HLA*-susceptibility haplotype occurs in a high proportion of GSE cases, it also occurs in approximately 18% of controls (Mazzilli et al., 1992). The frequency is similar across populations of northern Europeans, with haplotype frequencies of 0.127 in the United Kingdom and 0.149 in Switzerland (Doherty et al., 1992; Lango and Lindblum, 1993).

The remaining GSE cases are primarily *DR4-DQ8 (DQA1*03 DQB1*0302)* (Balas et al., 1997; Bouguerra et al., 1997; Polvi et al., 1998). Mantovani et al. (1993) reported that *DQB1*0302*, like *DQB1*02*, is missing aspartic acid at codon 57, and it could be that the substitution is a risk factor for GSE. Exon 2 of the *HLA*-associated alleles was sequenced to look for GSE-specific sequences, but none was identified (Kagnoff, 1988, 1990; Hall et al., 1991).

Lie et al. (1999) found that absence of an allele of marker D6S2223, telomeric to the HLA class I region, was associated with the presence of GSE (and Type 1 diabetes). It was independent of the *HLA-DQA1 DQB1* association as all controls and cases were homozygous for *DQA1*0501 DQB1*0201*. They suggested that a gene near D6S2223 may be involved in the pathogenesis of GSE and Type 1 diabetes.

Contribution to Pathophysiology

The strong association of *HLA* with GSE suggests primary involvement of *HLA* molecules and T cells in the pathogenesis. The primary *HLA* association in the majority of GSE cases is with the *DQ2* molecule and with *DQ8* in a minority of cases (Sollid et al., 2001). *HLA* molecules bind the peptide within a cleft in the tertiary structure of the receptor and present peptide fragments of antigens to T cells. The T cells then become activated, leading to the production of cytokines. Polymorphisms of the genes encoding these molecules are thought to alter the configuration of the cleft, thereby affecting individual antigen-binding affinities and influencing the T-cell response generated by these antigens. In GSE, the antigen is believed to be gliadin, the ethanol-soluble fraction of the wheat protein gluten. Class II alleles encode for cell surface antigens on the peptide receptor that are essential for the recognition of gliadin by $CD4^+$ T lymphocytes (Godkin and Jewell, 1998). The peptide-binding motif of the GSE-associated *HLA-DQ2* molecule is unique among HLA class II molecules (Sollid et al., 1997). T cells, isolated from $DQ2^+$ GSE patients, preferentially recognize the gliadin peptides presented by the *HLA DQ* molecules (Sollid et al., 1997). Polymorphisms in the genes encoding for both the α and β chains are important in the specificity of the disease-associated *HLA-DQ2* molecules, but the β-chain residue appears to be more important (Johansen et al., 1996). Gliadin-specific, *HLA-DQ2*-restricted T cells are often found in jejunal biopsies of celiac cases but not in controls (Molberg et al., 1997). This would explain the reports that individuals with two copies of *DQB1*201* have increased susceptibility to GSE (Ploski et al., 1993; Petronzelli et al., 1997). There is no evidence, however, that phenotypic differences in GSE patients (i.e., clinical features) are associated with different *HLA* genotypes (Greco et al., 1998b).

CLINICAL APPLICATION AND RISK ASSESSMENT OF GENETICS INFORMATION

Diagnosis

The standard diagnostic criteria for GSE were reviewed earlier (see Disease Definition). Diagnosis may be difficult because identification of the GSE phenotype can be confused by adherence to a gluten-free diet in high-risk groups. It is common in the United States for one family member to have a diagnosis of GSE made by biopsy. When a second family member develops gastrointestinal symptoms, he or she is put on a gluten-free diet without any evaluation. Gluten restriction would cause such people to have a normal small intestinal biopsy and negative IgA EMA, even if they actually do have GSE. Confirmation of the diagnosis requires reinstitution of gluten in the diet (a gluten challenge), but most individuals are unwilling to undergo a gluten challenge. With return to a normal diet, histologic changes in the small intestine may take 2 or more years to develop (Chartrand and Seidman, 1996). Lack of a confirmed diagnosis can be a significant problem because these people may actually have some other gastrointestinal ailment that should be treated and have no reason to adhere to a difficult diet of gluten restriction.

Screening

Biopsy requirements have been simplified to one or two duodenal biopsies rather than three jejunal biopsies (Walker-Smith et al., 1990). With the development of serologic tests, from IgA GA to IgA EMA to IgA anti-tTG, and with the increasing specificity and sensitivity of these tests, noninvasive screening procedures are now available. GSE screening possibly could be done for relatives of GSE cases and for patients with GSE-associated diseases such as diabetes mellitus, thyroid disease, and arthritis. Cronin and Shanahan (1997) suggested that because of the high incidence of GSE in Type 1 diabetes (1%–7.8%), all Type 1 diabetic patients should be screened for GSE by serology. They reported that individual patients with GSE on a gluten-free diet had improved glycemic control and posed the question of whether gluten restriction in diabetic patients with GSE would alter the rate and progression of diabetic complications.

Prevention

The only method to prevent GSE is to avoid gluten. Some researchers believe that delaying the introduction of wheat to infants may be helpful. Others believe that delayed introduction may cause occult disease, which then complicates diagnosis. Barley and rye should also be excluded. There is no evidence that oats are damaging (Janatuinen et al., 1995; Picarelli et al., 2001). There are many factors that affect compliance, including the limitations of the diet, inadequate labeling of foods, gluten in foods consumed outside the home, and use of gluten as an additive in food and pharmaceutical products.

Counseling

As this disease is not fatal, pretest counseling is not needed. Counseling to discuss risks of other diseases, nutritional needs, and diet is needed.

Therapy

There is no known therapy at this time other than dietary gluten restriction. Symptoms will subside with adherence to the diet. Even minor transgressions of the diet may result in recurrence of symptoms.

ACKNOWLEDGMENTS

The GSE work of S. L. N. and J. J. Z. is supported by the National Institutes of Health, grant NIH R01 DK50678.

REFERENCES

Amin M, Eckhardt T, Kapitza S, Fleckenstein B, Jung G, Seissler J, Weichert H, Richter T, Stern M, Mothes T: Correlation between tissue transglutaminase antibodies and endomysium antibodies as diagnostic markers of coeliac disease. Clin Chim Acta 1999; 282:219–225.

Asquith P, Johnson AG, Cooke WT: Scanning electron microscopy of normal and celiac jejunal mucosa. Am J Dig Dis 1970; 15:511–521.

Balas A, Vicario J, Zambrano A, Acuna D, Garcia-Novo D: Absolute linkage of celiac disease and dermatitis herpetiformis to HLA-DQ. Tissue Antigens 1997; 50:52–56.

Bao F, Yu L, Babu S, Wang T, Hoffenberg EJ, Rewers M, Eisenbarth GS: One third of HLA DQ2 homozygous patients with type 1 diabetes express celiac disease–associated transglutaminase autoantibodies. J Autoimmun 1999; 13:143–148.

Bazzigaluppi E, Lampasona V, Barera G, Venerando A, Bianchi C, Chiumello G, Bonifacio E, Bosi E: Comparison of tissue transglutaminase-specific antibody assays with established antibody measurements for coeliac disease. J Autoimmun 1999; 12:51–56.

Bevan S, Popat S, Braegger CP, Busch A, O'Donoghue D, Falth-Magnusson K, Ferguson A, Godkin A, Hogberg L, Holmes G, et al.: Contribution of the MHC region to the familial risk of coeliac disease. J Med Genet 1999; 36:687–690.

Biagi F, Ellis HJ, Yiannakou JY, Brusco G, Swift GL, Smith PM, Corazza GR, Ciclitira PJ: Tissue transglutaminase antibodies in celiac disease. Am J Gastroenterol 1999; 94:2187–2192.

Bodmer J, Marsh S, Albert E, Bodmer W, Bontrop R, Dupont B, Erlich H, Hansen J, Mach B, Mayr W, et al.: Nomenclature for factors of the HLA system, 1998. Tissue Antigens 1999; 53:407–446.

Book L, Hart A, Black J, Feolo M, Zone JJ, Neuhausen SL: Prevalence and clinical characteristics of celiac disease in Down syndrome in a US study. Am J Med Genet 2001; 98:70–74.

Bouguerra F, Babron MC, Eliaou JF, Debbabi A, Clot J, Khaldi F, Greco L, Clerget-Darpoux F: Synergistic effect of two HLA heterodimers in the susceptibility to celiac disease in Tunisia. Genet Epidemiol 1997; 14:413–422.

Bourne JT, Kumar P, Huskisson EC, Mageed R, Unsworth DJ, Wojtulewski JA: Arthritis and coeliac disease. Ann Rheum Dis 1985; 44:592–598.

Brett PM, Yiannakou JY, Morris MA, Rosen Bronson S, Mathew C, Curtis D, Ciclitira PJ: A pedigree-based linkage study of coeliac disease: failure to replicate previous positive findings. Ann Hum Genet 1998; 62:25–32.

Burgin-Wolff A, Gaze H, Hadziselimovic F, Huber H, Lentze MJ, Nussle D, Reymond-Berthet C: Antigliadin and antiendomysium antibody determination for coeliac disease. Arch Dis Child 1991; 66:941–947.

Carlsson A, Axelsson I, Borulf S, Forslund M, Lindberg B, Sjorberg K, Ivarsson S: Prevalence of IgA-antigliadin antibodies and IgA-antiendomysium antibodies related to celiac disease in children with Down syndrome. Pediatrics 1998; 101:272–275.

Castro M, Crino A, Papadatou B, Purpura M, Gainnotti A, Ferretti F, Colistro F, Mottola L, Digilio M, Lucidi V: Downs syndrome and celiac disease: the prevalence of high IgA antigliadin antibodies and HLA-DR and DQ antigens in trisomy 21. J Pediatr Gastroenterol Nutr 1993; 16:265–268.

Catassi C: Screening for coeliac disease. In: Maki M, Collin P, Visakorpi JK (eds). Coeliac Disease. Proceedings of the International Symposium on Coeliac Disease. Tampere, Finland: Institute of Medical Technology, University of Tampere, 1997:24–33.

Catassi C, Ratsch IM, Gandolfi L, Pratesi R, Fabiani E, El Asmar R, Frijia M, Bearzi I, Vizzoni L: Why is coeliac disease endemic in the people of the Sahara? Lancet 1999; 354:647–648.

Chartrand LJ, Seidman EG: Celiac disease is a lifelong disorder. Clin Invest Med 1996; 19:357–361.

Chorzelski TP, Beutner EH, Sulej J, Tchorzewska H, Jablonska S, Kumar V, Kapuscinska A: IgA anti-endomysium antibody. A new immunological marker of dermatitis herpetiformis and coeliac disease. Br J Dermatol 1984; 111:395–402.

Ciacci C, Cirillo M, Auriemma G, Di Dato G, Sabbatini F, Mazzacca G: Celiac disease and pregnancy outcome. Am J Gastroenterol 1996; 91:718–722.

Clot F, Fulchignoni-Lataud MC, Renoux C, Percopo S, Bouguerra F, Babron MC, Djilali-Saiah I, Caillat-Zucman S, Clerget-Darpoux F, Greco L, et al.: Linkage and association study of the *CTLA-4* region in coeliac disease for Italian and Tunisian populations. Tissue Antigens 1999; 54:527–530.

Collin P, Maki M, Keyrilainen O, Hallstrom O, Reunala T, Pasternack A: Selective IgA deficiency and coeliac disease. Scand J Gastroenterol 1992; 27:367–371.

Collin P, Pukkala E, Reunala T: Malignancy and survival in dermatitis herpetiformis: a comparison with coeliac disease. Gut 1996; 38:528–530.

Cooper BT, Holmes GKT, Cooke WT: Coeliac disease and immunologic disorders. BMJ 1978; 1:537–539.

Cronin CC, Shanahan F: Insulin-dependent diabetes mellitus and coeliac disease. Lancet 1997; 349:1096–1097.

Csizmadia CG, Mearin ML, Oren A, Kromhout A, Crusius JB, von Blomberg BM, Pena AS, Wiggers MN, Vandenbroucke JP: Accuracy and cost-effectiveness of a new strategy to screen for celiac disease in children with Down syndrome. J Pediatr 2000; 137:756–761.

Cunningham MJ, Zone JJ: Thyroid abnormalities in dermatitis herpetiformis: prevalence of clinical thyroid disease and thyroid antibodies. Ann Intern Med 1985; 102:194–196.

Dahele A, Ghosh S: Vitamin B_{12} deficiency in untreated celiac disease. Am J Gastroenterol 2001; 96:745–750.

Delco F, El-Serag HB, Sonnenberg A: Celiac sprue among US military veterans: associated disorders and clinical manifestations. Dig Dis Sci 1999; 44:966–972.

Demling L, Becker V, Classen M: Examinations of the mucosa of the small intestine with the scanning electron microscope. Digestion 1969; 2:51–60.

Dieterich W, Ehnis T, Bauer M, Donner P, Volta U, Riecken E, Schuppan D: Identification of tissue transglutaminase as the autoantigen of celiac disease. Nat Med 1997; 3:797–801.

Dieterich W, Laag E, Bruckner-Tuderman L, Reunala T, Karpati S, Zagoni T, Riecken E, Schuppan D: Antibodies to tissue transglutaminase as serologic markers in patients with dermatitis herpetiformis. J Invest Dermatol 1999; 113:133–136.

Dieterich W, Laag E, Schopper H, Volta U, Ferguson A, Gillett H, Riecken E, Schuppan D: Autoantibodies to tissue transglutaminase as predictors of celiac disease. Gastroenterology 1998a; 115:1317–1321.

Dieterich W, Laag E, Schopper H, Volta U, Ferguson A, Gillett H, Riecken EO, Schuppan D: Autoantibodies to tissue transglutaminase as predictors of celiac disease. Gastroenterology 1998b; 115:1317–1321.

Djilali-Saiah I, Schmitz J, Harfouch-Hammoud E, Mougenot JF, Bach JF, Caillat-Zucman S: *CTLA-4* gene polymorphism is associated with predisposition to coeliac disease. Gut 1998; 43:187–189.

Doherty D, Vaughan R, Donaldson P, Mowat A: *HLA*, *DQA*, *DQB* and *DRB* geno-

typing by oligonucleotide analysis: distribution of alleles and haplotypes in British Caucasoids. Hum Immunol 1992; 34:53–63.
Donner H, Rau H, Walfish PG, Braun J, Siegmund T, Finke R, Herwig J, Usadel KH, Badenhoop K: *CTLA4* alanine-17 confers genetic susceptibility to Graves' disease and to type 1 diabetes mellitus. J Clin Endocrinol Metab 1997; 82:143–146.
Egan LJ, Walsh SV, Stevens FM, Connolly CE, Egan EL, McCarthy CF: Celiac-associated lymphoma: a single institution experience of 30 cases in the combination chemotherapy era. J Clin Gastroenterol 1995; 21:123–129.
Eliakim R, Sherer DM: Celiac disease: fertility and pregnancy. Gynecol Obstet Invest 2001; 51:3–7.
Failla P, Ruperto C, Pagano A, Lombardo M, Bottaro G, Perichon B, Krishnamoorthy R, Romano C, Ragusa A: Celiac disease in Downs syndrome with HLA serological and molecular studies. J Pediatr Gastroenterol Nutr 1996; 23:303–306.
Falchuk ZM, Rogentine GN, Strober W: Predominance of histocompatibility antigen HLA-*A8* in patients with gluten-sensitive enteropathy. J Clin Invest 1972; 51:1602–1605.
Fasano A: Where have all the American celiacs gone? Acta Paediatr Suppl 1996; 412:20–24.
Ferguson A: Intraepithelial lymphocytes of the small intestine. Gut 1977; 18:921–937.
Ferguson A, Kingstone K: Coeliac disease and malignancies. Acta Paediatr Suppl 1996; 412:78–81.
Fernandez-Arquero M, Caldes T, Casado E, Maluenda C, Figueredo MA, De La Concha EG: Polymorphism within the HLA-*DQB1**02 promoter associated with susceptibility to coeliac disease. Eur J Immunogenet 1998; 25:1–3.
Ferreira M, Davies SL, Butler M, Scott D, Clark M, Kumar P: Endomysial antibody: is it the best screening test for coeliac disease? Gut 1992; 33:1633–1637.
Field LL, Tobias R, Magnus T: A locus on chromosome 15q26 (IDDM3) produces susceptibility to insulin-dependent diabetes mellitus. Nat Genet 1994; 8:189–194.
Fry L, Keir P, McMinn R, Cowan JD, Hoffbrand AV: Small-intestinal structure and function and haematological changes in dermatitis herpetiformis. Lancet 1967; 2:729–733.
Fry L, Leonard JN, Swain F, Tucker W, Haffenden G, Ring N, McMinn R: Long term follow-up of dermatitis herpetiformis with and without dietary gluten withdrawal. Br J Dermatol 1982; 107:631–640.
Fry L, McMinn RMH, Cowan JD, Hoffbrand AV: Effect of gluten-free diet on dermatological, intestinal, and haematological manifestations of dermatitis herpetiformis. Lancet 1968; 1:557–561.
Fry L, McMinn RMH, Cowan JD, Hoffbrand AV: Gluten-free diet and reintroduction of gluten in dermatitis herpetiformis. Arch Dermatol 1969; 100:129–135.
Gandolfi L, Pratesi R, Cordoba JC, Tauil PL, Gasparin M, Catassi C: Prevalence of celiac disease among blood donors in Brazil. Am J Gastroenterol 2000; 95:689–692.
Gaspari AA, Huang CM, Davey RJ, Bondy C, Lawley TJ, Katz SI: Prevalence of thyroid abnormalities in patients with dermatitis herpetiformis and in control subjects with HLA-B8/-*DR3*. Am J Med 1990; 88:145–150.
Gee S: On the celiac affection. St. Bartholomew's Hosp Rep 1888; 24:17–20.
George EK, Hertzberger-ten Cate R, van Suijlekom-Smit LW, von Blomberg BM, Stapel SO, van Elburg RM, Mearin ML: Juvenile chronic arthritis and coeliac disease in the Netherlands. Clin Exp Rheumatol 1996; 14:571–575.
Godkin A, Jewell D: The pathogenesis of celiac disease. Gastroenterology 1998; 115:206–210.
Gonzalez-Escribano MF, Rodriguez R, Valenzuela A, Garcia A, Garcia-Lozano JR, Nunez-Roldan A: *CTLA4* polymorphisms in Spanish patients with rheumatoid arthritis. Tissue Antigens 1999; 53:296–300.
Greco L: Epidemiology of coeliac disease. In: Maki M, Collin P, Visakorpi JK (eds). Coeliac Disease. Proceedings of the International Symposium on Coeliac Disease. Tampere, Finland: Institute of Medical Technology, University of Tampere, 1997:9–14.
Greco L, Babron MC, Corazza GR, Percopo S, Sica R, Clot F, Fulchignoni-Lataud MC, Zavattari P, Momigliano-Richiardi P, Casari G, et al.: Existence of a genetic risk factor on chromosome 5q in Italian coeliac disease families. Ann Hum Genet 2001; 65:35–41.
Greco L, Corazza G, Babron MC, Clot F, Fulchignoni-Lataud MC, Percopo S, Zavattari P, Bouguerra F, Dib C, Tosi R, et al.: Genome search in celiac disease. Am J Hum Genet 1998a; 62:669–675.
Greco L, Maki M, DiDonato F, Visakorpi JK: Epidemiology of coeliac disease in Europe and the Mediterranean area. A summary report on the multicentre study by the European Society for Paediatric Gastroenterology and Nutrition. Common food intolerances. I Epidemiology of coeliac disease. Dyn Nutr Res 1992; 2:25–44.
Greco L, Percopo S, Clot F, Bouguerra F, Babron M, Ellaou J, Franzeue C, Troneone R, Clerget-Darpoux F: Lack of correlation between genotype and phenotype in celiac disease. J Pediatr Gastroenterol Nutr 1998b; 26:286–290.
Green PHR, Stavropoulos SN, Panagi SG, Goldstein SL, McMahon DJ, Absan H, Neugut AI: Characteristics of adult celiac disease in the USA: results of a national survey. Am J Gastroenterol 2001; 96:126–131.
Greenberg DA, Hodge SE, Rotter JI: Evidence for recessive against dominant inheritance at the HLA-"linked" locus in coeliac disease. Am J Hum Genet 1982; 34:263–277.
Grodzinsky E, Hed J, Skogh T: IgA antiendomysium antibodies have a high predictive value for celiac disease in asymptomatic patients. Allergy 1994; 49:593–597.
Hall MA, Lanchbury JSS, Bolsover WJ, Welsh KI, Ciclitira PJ: HLA association with dermatitis herpetiformis is accounted for by a *cis* or *trans* associated DQ heterdimer. Gut 1991; 32:487–490.
Hall R, Bao F, Streilein R, Eisenbarth G, Smith A: IgA anti-transglutaminase antibodies in patients with dermatitis herpetiformis. J Invest Dermatol 1999; 112:616.
Hall RP, Sanders ME, Duqueisnoy RJ, Katz SI, Shaw S: Alterations in HLA-DP and HLA-DQ antigen frequency in patients with dermatitis herpetiformis. J Invest Dermatol 1989; 93:501–505.
Hall RPI: Dermatitis herpetiformis. Prog in Dermatol 1992; 26:1–12.
Halter SA, Greene HL, Helinek G: Gluten-sensitive enteropathy: sequence of villous regrowth as viewed by scanning electron microscopy. Hum Pathol 1982; 13:811–818.
Hansson T, Anneren G, Sjoberg O, Klareskog L, Dannaeus A: Celiac disease in relation to immunologic serum markers, trace elements, and HLA-DR and DQ antigens in Swedish children with Down syndrome. J Pediatr Gastroenterol Nutr 1999; 29:286–292.
Hansson T, Dahlbom I, Hall J, Holtz A, Elfman L, Dannaeus A, Klareskog L: Antibody reactivity against human and guinea pig tissue transglutaminase in children with celiac disease. J Pediatr Gastroenterol Nutr 2000; 30:379–384.
Harbo HF, Celius EG, Vartdal F, Spurkland A: *CTLA4* promoter and exon 1 dimorphisms in multiple sclerosis. Tissue Antigens 1999; 53:106–110.
Hernandez JL, Michalski JP, McCombs CC, McCarthy CF, Stevens FM, Elston RC: Evidence for a dominant gene mechanism underlying coeliac disease in the west of Ireland. Genet Epidemiol 1991; 8:13–27.
Hervonen K, Karell K, Holopainen P, Collin P, Partanen J, Reunala T: Concordance of dermatitis herpetiformis and celiac disease in monozygous twins. J Invest Dermatol 2000; 115:990–993.
Hoggan R: Considering wheat, rye, and barley proteins as aids to carcinogens. Med Hypotheses 1997; 49:285–288.
Holmes GK: Non-malignant complications of coeliac disease. Acta Paediatr Suppl 1996; 412:68–75.
Holmes GK: Coeliac disease and type 1 diabetes mellitus—the case for screening. Diabet Med 2001; 18:169–177.
Holopainen P, Arvas M, Sistonen P, Mustalahti K, Collin P, Maki M, Partanen J: *CD28/CTLA4* gene region on chromosome 2q33 confers genetic susceptibility to celiac disease. A linkage and family-based association study. Tissue Antigens 1999; 53:470–475.
Houlston R, Tomlinson I, Ford D, Seal S, Marossy A, Ferguson A, Holmes G, Hosie K, Howdle P, Jewell D, et al.: Linkage analysis of candidate regions for coeliac disease genes. Hum Mol Genet 1997; 6:1335–1339.
Houlston RS, Ford D: Genetics of coeliac disease. Q J Med 1996; 89:737–743.
Hovell CJ, Collett JA, Vautier G, Cheng AJ, Sutanto E, Mallon DF, Olynyk JK, Cullen DJ: High prevalence of coeliac disease in a population-based study from Western Australia: a case for screening? Med J Aust 2001; 175:247–250.
Howdle PD, Blair GE: Molecular biology and coeliac disease. Gut 1992; 33:573–575.
Iltanen S, Holm K, Ashorn M, Ruuska T, Laippala P, Maki M: Changing jejunal gamma delta T cell receptor (TCR)–bearing intraepithelial lymphocyte density in coeliac disease. Clin Exp Immunol 1999; 117:51–55.
Janatuinen EK, Pikkarainen PH, Kemppainen TA, Kosma VM, Jarvinen RM, Uusitupa MI, Julkunen RJ: A comparison of diets with and without oats in adults with celiac disease. N Engl J Med 1995; 333:1033–1037.
Johansen B, Jensen T, Thorpe C, Vartdal F, Thorsby E, Sollid L: Both alpha and beta chain polymorphisms determine the specificity of the disease-associated HLA-DQA molecules, with beta chain residues being most influential. Immunogenetics 1996; 42:142–150.
Kadunce DP, McMurry MP, Avots-Avotins A, Chandler JP, Meyer LJ, Zone JJ: The effect of an elemental diet with and without gluten on disease activity in dermatitis herpetiformis. J Invest Dermatol 1991; 97:175–182.
Kagnoff MF: Immunogenetic basis of celiac disease. In: Strober W, Lamm M, James SP, McGhee JR (eds). Mucosal Immunity and Infections at Mucosal Surfaces. New York: Oxford University Press, 1988:180–192.
Kagnoff MF: Understanding the molecular basis of coeliac disease. Gut 1990; 31:497–499.
Kagnoff MF: HLA genes and celiac disease. Presented at the Eighth International Symposium on Coeliac Disease, Naples, Italy, April, 1999.
Kagnoff MF, Austin RK, Hubert JJ, Bernardin JE, Kasarda DD: Possible role for a human adenovirus in the pathogenesis of celiac disease. J Exp Med 1984; 160:1544–1557.
Katz SI, Strober W: The pathogenesis of dermatitis herpetiformis. J Invest Dermatol 1978; 70:63–75.
Kaukinen K, Collin P, Mykkanen AH, Partanen J, Maki M, Salmi J: Celiac disease and autoimmune endocrinologic disorders. Dig Dis Sci 1999; 44:1428–1433.
Kaukinen K, Maki M, Partanen J, Sievanen H, Collin P: Celiac disease without villous atrophy: revision of criteria called for. Dig Dis Sci 2001; 46:879–887.
King AL, Fraser JS, Moodie SJ, Curtis D, Dearlove AM, Ellis HJ, Rosen-Bronson S, Ciclitira PJ: Coeliac disease: follow-up linkage study provides further support for existence of a susceptibility locus on chromosome 11p11. Ann Hum Genet 2001; 65:377–386.
King AL, Yiannakou JY, Brett PM, Curtis D, Morris MA, Dearlove AM, Rhodes M, Rosen-Bronson S, Mathew C, Ellis HJ, et al.: A genome-wide family-based linkage study of coeliac disease. Ann Hum Genet 2000; 64:479–490.
Koot VC, Van Straaten M, Hekkens WT, Collee G, Dijkmans BA: Elevated level of IgA gliadin antibodies in patients with rheumatoid arthritis. Clin Exp Rheumatol 1989; 7:623–626.
Korponay-Szabo I, Kovacs J, Lorincz M, Torok E, Goracz G: Families with multiple cases of gluten-sensitive enteropathy. Z Gastroenterol 1998; 36:553–558.
Lahdeaho ML, Lehtinen M, Rissa HR, Hyoty H, Reunala T, Maki M: Antipeptide antibodies to adenovirus E1b protein indicate enhanced risk of celiac disease and dermatitis herpetiformis. Int Arch Allergy Immunol 1993a; 101:272–276.
Lahdeaho ML, Parkkonen P, Reunala T, Maki M, Lehtinen M: Antibodies to E1b protein-derived peptides of enteric adenovirus type 40 are associated with celiac disease and dermatitis herpetiformis. Clin Immunol Immunopathol 1993b; 69:300–305.

Laine LA, Holt KM: Recurrent pericarditis and celiac disease. JAMA 1982; 252:3168.

Lampasona V, Bazzigaluppi E, Barera G, Bonifacio E: Tissue transglutaminase and combined screening for coeliac disease and type 1 diabetes–associated autoantibodies. Lancet 1998; 352:1192–1193.

Lango A, Lindblum B: HLA *DQA-DQB* haplotypes in a Swedish population. Eur J Immunogenet 1993; 20:453–460.

Leonard J, Haffenden G, Tucker W, Unsworth J, Swain F, McMinn R, Holdborow J, Fry L: Gluten challenge in dermatitis herpetiformis. N Engl J Med 1983; 308:816–819.

Lewis C, Book L, Black J, Sawitzke A, Cannon-Albright L, Zone J, Neuhausen S: Celiac disease and HLA genotype: accuracy of diagnosis in self-diagnosed individuals, dosage effect, and sibling risk. J Pediatr Gastroenterol Nutr 2000; 31:22–27.

Lie BA, Sollid LM, Ascher H, Ek J, Akselsen HE, Ronningen KS, Thorsby E, Undlien DE: A gene telomeric of the HLA class I region is involved in predisposition to both type 1 diabetes and coeliac disease. Tissue Antigens 1999; 54:162–168.

Lock RJ, Pitcher MC, Unsworth DJ: IgA anti-tissue transglutaminase as a diagnostic marker of gluten sensitive enteropathy. J Clin Pathol 1999; 52:274–277.

Maki M, Collin P, Visakorpi JK: Coeliac disease. Lancet 1997; 349:1755–1759.

Mantovani V, Corazza G, Bragliani M, Frisoni M, Zaniboni M, Gasbarrini G: Asp57-negative HLA DQ beta chain and *DQA1**0501 allele are essential for the onset of DQw2-postive and DQw2-negative coeliac disease. Clin Exp Immunol 1993; 91:153–156.

Marks J, Shuster S, Watson AJ: Small-bowel changes in dermatitis herpetiformis. Lancet 1966; 2:1280–1282.

Marks R, Whittle MW, Beard RJ, Robertson WB, Gold SC: Small bowel abnormalities in dermatitis herpetiformis. BMJ 1968; 1:552–555.

Marron MP, Raffel LJ, Garchon HJ, Jacob CO, Serrano-Rios M, Martinez Larrad MT, Teng WP, Park Y, Zhang ZX, Goldstein DR, et al.: Insulin-dependent diabetes mellitus (IDDM) is associated with *CTLA4* polymorphisms in multiple ethnic groups. Hum Mol Genet 1997; 6:1275–1282.

Marsh MN: Gluten, major histocompatibility complex, and the small intestine. Gastroenterology 1992; 102:330–354.

Marsh MN, Swift JA: A study of the small intestinal mucosa using the scanning electron microscope. Gut 1969; 10:940–949.

Martinelli P, Troncone R, Paparo F, Torre P, Trapanese E, Fasano C, Lamberti A, Budillon G, Nardone G, Greco L: Coeliac disease and unfavourable outcome of pregnancy. Gut 2000; 46:332–335.

Mazzilli M, Ferrante P, Mariani P, Martone E, Petronzelli F, Triglione P, Bonamico M: A study of Italian pediatric celiac disease patients confirms that the primary HLA association is to the DQ (alpha 1*0501, beta 1*0201) heterodimer. J Hum Immunol 1992; 33:133–139.

Miller A, Paspaliaris W, Elliott PR, d'Apice A: Anti-transglutaminase antibodies and coeliac disease. Aust N Z J Med 1999; 29:239–242.

Miller ML: Clinical aspects of juvenile rheumatoid arthritis. Curr Opin Rheumatol 1997; 9:423–427.

Misra RC, Kasthuri D, Chuttani HK: Adult coeliac disease in tropics. BMJ 1966; 2:1230–1232.

Molberg O, Kett K, Scott H, Throsby E, Sollid L, Lundin K: Gliadin specific, HLA DQ2-restricted T cells are commonly found in small intestinal biopsies from coeliac disease patients, but not from controls. Scand J Immunol 1997; 466:103–109.

Molberg O, Mcadam S, Korner R, Quarsten H, Kristiansen C, Madsen L, Fugger L, Scott H, Noren O, Roepstorff P, et al.: Tissue transglutaminase selectively modifies gliadin peptides that are recognized by gut derived T-cells in celiac disease. Nat Med 1998; 4:713–717.

Molberg O, Mcadam S, Lundin KE, Kristiansen C, Arentz-Hansen H, Kett K, Sollid LM: T cells from celiac disease lesions recognize gliadin epitopes deamidated in situ by endogenous tissue transglutaminase. Eur J Immunol 2001; 31:1317–1323.

Mota Vargas R, Nevado L, Pijierro Amador A, Bureo Dacal JC: Rheumatoid arthritis and celiac disease: a chance association? An Med Interna 1996; 13:252–253.

Murray JA: The widening spectrum of celiac disease. Am J Clin Nutr 1999; 69:354–365.

Naluai AT, Nilsson S, Samuelsson L, Gudjonsdottir AH, Ascher H, Ek J, Hallberg B, Kristiansson B, Martinsson T, Nerman O, et al.: The *CTLA4/CD28* gene region on chromosome 2q33 confers susceptibility to celiac disease in a way possibly distinct from that of type 1 diabetes and other chronic inflammatory disorders. Tissue Antigens 2000; 56:350–355.

Natter S, Granditsch G, Reichel GL, Baghestanian M, Valent P, Elfman L, Gronlund H, Kraft D, Valenta R: IgA cross-reactivity between a nuclear autoantigen and wheat proteins suggests molecular mimicry as a possible pathomechanism in celiac disease. Eur J Immunol 2001; 31:918–928.

Noel PJ, Boise LH, Thompson CB: Regulation of T cell activation by CD28 and CTLA4. Adv Exp Med Biol 1996; 406:209–217.

Not T, Horvath K, Hill I, Partanen J, Hammed A, Magazzu G, Fasano A: Celiac disease risk in the USA: high prevalence of antiendomysium antibodies in healthy blood donors. Scand J Gastroenterol 1998; 33:494–498.

Not T, Tommasini A, Tonini G, Buratti E, Pococco M, Tortul C, Valussi M, Crichiutti G, Berti I, Trevisiol C, et al.: Undiagnosed coeliac disease and risk of autoimmune disorders in subjects with type I diabetes mellitus. Diabetologia 2001; 44:151–155.

Oberhuber G: Histopathology of celiac disease. Biomed Pharmacother 2000; 54:368–372.

Paimela L, Kurki P, Leirisalo-Repo M, Piirainen H: Gliadin immune reactivity in patients with rheumatoid arthritis. Clin Exp Rheumatol 1995; 13:603–607.

Park MS, Terasaki PI, Razzaque A, Zone J: The 90% incidence of HLA antigen (Te24) in dermatitis herpetiformis. Tissue Antigens 1983; 22:263–266.

Pena AS, Mann DL, Hague NE, Heck JA, van Leeuwen HA, van Rood JJ, Strober W: Genetic basis of gluten-sentitive enteropathy. Gastroenterology 1978; 75:230–235.

Petronzelli F, Bonamico M, Ferrante P, Grillo R, Mora B, Mariani P, Apollonio I, Gemme G, Mazzilli MC: Genetic contribution of the HLA region to the familial clustering of coeliac disease. Ann Hum Genet 1997; 61:307–317.

Pettit JE, Hoffbrand AV, Seah PP, Fry L: Splenic atrophy in dermatitis herpetiformis. BMJ 1972; 2:438–440.

Piaggio MV, Demonte AM, Sihufe G, Garcilazo S, Esper MC, Wagener M, Aleanzi M: Serological diagnosis of celiac disease: anti-gliadin peptide antibodies and tissue anti-transglutaminase. Medicina 1999; 59:693–697.

Picarelli A, Di Tola M, Sabbatella L, Gabrielli F, Di Cello T, Anania MC, Mastracchio A, Silano M, De Vincenzi M: Immunologic evidence of no harmful effect of oats in celiac disease. Am J Clin Nutr 2001; 74:137–140.

Pinals RS: Arthritis associated with gluten-sensitive enteropathy. J Rheumatol 1986; 13:201–204.

Ploski R, Ek J, Thorsby E, Sollid L: On the HLA-DQ (alpha 1*0501, beta 1*0201)–associated susceptibility in celiac disease: a possible gene dosage effect of DQB1*0201. Tissue Antigens 1993; 41:173–177.

Polvi A, Arranz E, Fernandez-Arquero M, Collin P, Maki M, Sanz A, Calvo C, Maluenda C, Westman P, de la Concha EG, et al.: HLA-DQ2-negative celiac disease in Finland and Spain. Hum Immunol 1998; 59:169–175.

Porter WM, Lock RJ, Hardman CM, Unsworth JJ, Baker BS, Fry L: Tissue transglutaminase antibodies in dermatitis herpetiformis. Presented at the Eighth International Symposium on Coeliac Disease, Naples, Italy, April, 1999.

Pruessner HT: Detecting celiac disease in your patients. Am Fam Physician 1998; 57:1023–1041.

Reunala T, Collin P, Lewis HM, Fry L: Associated diseases and malignancy in dermatitis herpetiformis. In: Maki M, Collin P, Visakorpi JK (eds). Coeliac Disease. Proceedings of the International Symposium on Coeliac Disease. Tampere, Finland: Institute of Medical Technology, University of Tampere. 1997:75–79.

Reunala T, Kosnai I, Karpati S, Kuitunen P, Torok E, Savilahti E: Dermatitis herpetiformis: jejunal findings and skin response to a gluten free diet. Arch Dis Child 1984; 59:517–522.

Reunala T, Salo OP, Tiilikainen A, Selroos O, Kuitunen P: Family studies in dermatitis herpetiformis. Ann Clin Res 1976; 8:254–261.

Risch N: Assessing the role of HLA-linked and unlinked determinants of disease. Am J Hum Genet 1987; 40:1–14.

Roschmann E, Wienker TF, Gerok W, Volk BA: T-cell receptor variable genes and genetic susceptibility to celiac disease: an association and linkage study. Gastroenterology 1993; 105:1790–1796.

Rossi TM, Kumar V, Lerner A, Heitlinger L, Tucker N, Fisher J: Relationship of endomysial antibodies to jejunal mucosa pathology. Specificity towards both symptomatic and asymptomatic celiacs. J Pediatr Gastroenterol 1988; 7:858–863.

Rostami K, Kerckhaert J, Tiemessen R, von Blomberg BM, Meijer JW, Mulder CJ: Sensitivity of antiendomysium and antigliadin antibodies in untreated celiac disease: disappointing in clinical practice. Am J Gastroenterol 1999; 94:888–894.

Sachs J, Awad J, McCloskey D, Navarrete C, Festenstein H, Elliot E, Walker-Smith J, Griffiths C, Leonard J, Fry L: Different HLA associated gene combinations contribute susceptibility for coeliac disease and dermatitis herpetiformis. Gut 1986; 27:515–520.

Sategna-Guidetti C, Pulitano R, Grosso S, Ferfoglia G: Serum IgA antiendomysium antibody titers as a marker of intestinal involvement and diet compliance in adult celiac sprue. J Clin Gastroenterol 1993; 17:123–127.

Sategna-Guidetti C, Volta U, Ciacci C, Usai P, Carlino A, De Franceschi L, Camera A, Pelli A, Brossa C: Prevalence of thyroid disorders in untreated adult celiac disease patients and effect of gluten withdrawal: an Italian multicenter study. Am J Gastroenterol 2001; 96:751–757.

Savilahti E: Immunohistochemical markers of coeliac disease. In: Maki M, Collin P, Visakorpi JK (eds). Coeliac Disease. Proceedings of the International Symposium on Coeliac Disease. Tampere, Finland: Institute of Medical Technology, University of Tampere. 1997:139–152.

Savilahti E, Arato A, Verkasalo M: Intestinal gamma/delta bearing lymphocytes in coeliac disease and inflammatory bowel disease in children. Constant increase in celiac disease. Pediatr Res 1990; 28:579–581.

Savilahti E, Viander M, Perkkio M, Vainio E, Kalimo K, Reunala T: IgA anti-gliadin antibodies: a marker of mucosal damage in childhood coeliac disease. Lancet 1983; 1:320–322.

Sblattero D, Berti I, Trevisiol C, Marzari R, Tommasini A, Bradbury A, Fasano A, Ventura A, Not T: Human recombinant tissue transglutaminase ELISA: an innovative diagnostic assay for celiac disease. Am J Gastroenterol 2000; 95:1253–1257.

Schuppan D: Current concepts of celiac disease pathogenesis. Gastroenterology 2000; 119:234–242.

Schuppan D, Dieterich W, Riecken EO: Exposing gliadin as a tasty food for lymphocytes. Nat Med 1998; 4:666–667.

Seidl C, Donner H, Fischer B, Usadel KH, Seifried E, Kaltwasser JP, Badenhoop K: *CTLA4* codon 17 dimorphism in patients with rheumatoid arthritis. Tissue Antigens 1998; 51:62–66.

Sher KS, Mayberry JF: Female fertility, obstetric and gynaecological history in coeliac disease. A case control study. Digestion 1994; 55:243–246.

Sherman SL, Iselius L, Ellis A, Woodrow JC, MacLean CJ: Combined segregation and linkage analysis of coeliac disease. Genet Epidemiol Suppl 1986; 1:283–288.

Shuster S, Watson AJ, Marks J: Coeliac syndrome in dermatitis herpetiformis. Lancet 1968; 11:1101–1106.

Smecuol E, Maurino E, Vazquez H, Pedreira S, Niveloni S, Mazure R, Boerr L, Bai JC: Gynaecological and obstetric disorders in coeliac disease: frequent clinical onset during pregnancy or the puerperium. Eur J Gastroenterol Hepatol 1996; 8:63–89.

Sollid LM, Lundin KEA, Lundin HJS, Sjostrom H, Molberg O, Thorsby E: HLA-DQ molecules, peptides and T cells in coeliac disease. In: Maki M, Collin P, Visakorpi JK (eds). Coeliac Disease. Proceedings of the International Symposium on Coeliac Disease. Tampere, Finland: Institute of Medical Technology, University of Tampere, 1997:265–274.

Sollid LM, McAdam SN, Molberg O, Quarsten H, Arentz-Hansen H, Louka AS, Lundin KE: Genes and environment in celiac disease. Acta Odontol Scand 2001; 59:183–186.

Sollid LM, Thorsby E: HLA susceptibility genes in celiac disease: genetic mapping and role in pathogenesis. Gastroenterology 1993; 105:910–922.

Strober W: Gluten-sensitive enteropathy. Clin Gastroenterol 1976; 5:429–452.

Strober W: Gluten-sensitive enteropathy. In: King R, Rotter, JI, Motulsky AG (eds). Genetic Basis of Common Diseases. New York: Oxford University Press, 1992:279–304.

Sulkanen S, Halttunen T, Laurila K, Kolho KL, Korponay-Szabo IR, Sarnesto A, Savilahti E, Collin P, Maki M: Tissue transglutaminase autoantibody enzyme-linked immunosorbent assay in detecting celiac disease. Gastroenterology 1998; 115:1322–1328.

Susi M, Holopainen P, Mustalahti K, Maki M, Partanen J: Candidate gene region 15q26 and genetic susceptibility to coeliac disease in Finnish families. Scand J Gastroenterol 2001; 36:372–374.

Thaysen TEH: Ten cases of of ideopathic steatorrhea. Q J Med 1935; 4:359–395.

Tighe M, Ciclitira P: The implications of recent advances in coeliac disease. Acta Pediatr 1993; 82:805–810.

Trier JS: Celiac sprue. N Engl J Med 1991; 325:1709–1719.

Trier JS: Diagnosis of celiac sprue. Gastroenterology 1998; 115:211–216.

Troncone R, Caputo N, Micillo M, Maiuri L, Poggi V: Immunologic and intestinal permeability tests as predictors of relapse during gluten challenge in childhood celiac disease. Scand J Gastroenterol 1994; 29:144–147.

Troncone R, Maurano F, Rossi M, Micillo M, Greco L, Auricchio R, Salerno G, Salvatore F, Sacchetti L: IgA antibodies to tissue transglutaminase: an effective diagnostic test for celiac disease. J Pediatr 1999; 134:166–171.

Tursi A, Brandimarte G, Giorgetti G, Gigliobianco A, Lombardi D, Gasbarrini G: Low prevalence of antigliadin and anti-endomysium antibodies in subclinical/silent celiac disease. Am J Gastroenterol 2001; 96:1507–1510.

Unsworth F: Serologic diagnosis of gluten sensitive enteropathy. J Clin Pathol 1996; 49:704–711.

Usai P, Boi MF, Piga M, Cacace E, Lai MA, Beccaris A, Piras E, La Nasa G, Mulargia M, Balestrieri A: Adult celiac disease is frequently associated with sacroiliitis. Dig Dis Sci 1995; 40:1906–1908.

Valdimarsson T, Franzen L, Grodzinsky E, Skogh T, Strom M: Is small bowel biopsy necessary in adults with suspected celiac disease and IgA anti-endomysial antibodies? 100% positive predictive value for celiac disease in adults. Dig Dis Sci 1996; 41:83–87.

Valentino R, Savastano S, Tommaselli AP, Dorato M, Scarpitta MT, Gigante M, Micillo M, Paparo F, Petrone E, Lombardi G, et al.: Prevalence of coeliac disease in patients with thyroid autoimmunity. Horm Res 1999; 51:124–127.

Ventura A, Magazzu G, Greco L: Duration of exposure to gluten and risk for autoimmune disorders in patients with celiac disease. SIGEP Study Group for Autoimmune Disorders in Celiac Disease. Gastroenterology 1999; 117:297–303.

Ventura A, Neri E, Ughi C, Leopaldi A, Citta A, Not T: Gluten-dependent diabetes-related and thyroid-related autoantibodies in patients with celiac disease. J Pediatr 2000; 137:263–265.

Visakorpi JK: Changing features of coeliac disease. In: Maki M, Collin P, Visakorpi JK (eds). Coeliac Disease. Proceedings of the International Symposium on Coeliac Disease. Tampere, Finland: Institute of Medical Technology, University of Tampere, 1997:1–7.

Vitoria JC, Arrieta A, Arranz C, Ayesta A, Sojo A, Maruri N, Garcia-Masdevall MD: Antibodies to gliadin, endomysium, and tissue transglutaminase for the diagnosis of celiac disease. J Pediatr Gastroenterol Nutr 1999; 29:571–574.

Vitoria JC, Arrieta A, Ortiz L, Ayesta A: Antibodies to human tissue transglutaminase for the diagnosis of celiac disease. J Pediatr Gastroenterol Nutr 2001; 33:349–350.

Volta U, Bellentani S, Bianchi FB, Brandi G, De Franceschi L, Miglioli L, Granito A, Balli F, Tiribelli C: High prevalence of celiac disease in Italian general population. Dig Dis Sci 2001; 46:1500–1505.

Volta U, Molinaro M, Fusconi M, Cassani F, Bianchi F: IgA antiendomysial antibody test: a step forward in celiac disease screening. Dig Dis Sci 1991; 36:752–756.

Volta U, Molinaro N, De Franchis R, Forzenigo L, Landoni M, Fratangelo D, Bianchi FB: Correlation between IgA antiendomysial antibodies and subtotal villous atrophy in dermatitis herpetiformis. J Clin Gastroenterol 1992; 14:298–301.

Walker-Smith J, Guandalini S, Schmitz J, Shmerling D, Visakorpi J: Revised criteria for diagnosis of coeliac disease. Report of Working Group of European Society of Paediatric Gastroenterology and Nutrition. Arch Dis Child 1990; 65:909–911.

Walker-Smith JA, Ford RPK, Phillips AD: The spectrum of gastrointestinal allergies to food. Ann Allergy 1984; 53:629–636.

Walunas TL, Lenschow DJ, Bakker CY, Linsley PS, Freeman GJ, Green JM, Thompson CB, Bluestone JA: CTLA-4 can function as a negative regulator of T cell activation. Immunity 1994; 1:405–413.

Weile B, Cavell B, Nivenius K, Krasilnikoff PA: Striking differences in the incidence of childhood celiac disease between Denmark and Sweden: a plausible explanation. J Pediatr Gastroenterol Nutr 1995; 21:64–68.

Wright DH: The major complications of coeliac disease. Baillieres Clin Gastroenterol 1995; 9:351–369.

Yanagawa T, Hidaka Y, Guimaraes V, Soliman M, DeGroot LJ: *CTLA-4* gene polymorphism associated with Graves' disease in a Caucasian population. J Clin Endocrinol Metab 1995; 80:41–45.

Yiannakou JY, Brett PM, Morris MA, Curtis D, Mathew C, Vaughan R, Rosen-Bronson S, Ciclitira PJ: Family linkage study of the T-cell receptor genes in coeliac disease. Ital J Gastroenterol Hepatol 1999; 31:198–201.

Zhong F, McCombs CC, Olson JM, Elston RC, Stevens FM, McCarthy CF, Michalski JP: An autosomal screen for genes that predispose to celiac disease in the western counties of Ireland. Nat Genet 1996; 14:329–333.

Zone JJ: Dermatitis herpetiformis. In: Weston WL, Mackie RM, Provost TT (eds). Current Problems in Dermatology, Vol III. St Louis, MO: Mosby Year Book, 1991:1–41.

Zubillaga P, Vitoria J, A A, Echanzi P, Garcia-Masdevall M: Down syndrome and celiac disease. J Pediatr Gastroenterol Nutr 1993; 6:68–71.

Part V

ENDOCRINE DISORDERS

20 Thyroid Disease

STEFAN K. G. GREBE

The parenchymal component of the thyroid gland consists of two distinct cell populations: follicular cells, producing thyroid hormone, and C cells, producing calcitonin. Abnormalities of C cells are largely confined to hyperplasia and medullary carcinoma, both of which are rare. Nonetheless, they will be considered in this chapter, as they occur frequently in the context of genetically well-defined, inherited syndromes, and thus are showcases of hereditary neoplastic thyroid disease. The bulk of this chapter, however, will be devoted to the much more common, but in genetic terms generally much less well understood, diseases of the follicular cells of the thyroid gland.

Disorders of the thyroid gland, of which almost all affect the follicular portion, are extremely common. If minor or subclinical abnormalities of size, structure, and function are included, the majority of individuals in many human populations will suffer from some form of thyroid pathology during their lifetime. However, even when only clinically relevant structural and functional abnormalities are considered, diseases of the thyroid gland rival or surpass diabetes mellitus as the most common endocrine disorder. For example, in Western societies the combined lifetime risk of hypothyroidism or hyperthyroidism approaches 5% for men and 20% for women (Vanderpump and Tunbridge, 1996; Wang and Crapo, 1997), and the prevalence of clinically evident sporadic goiter is between 2% and 10% for men and 5% and 30% for women (Lamberg, 1991; Vanderpump and Tunbridge, 1996; Wang and Crapo, 1997; Bauch, 1998), while between 30% and 60% of the population may have ultrasonographic evidence of nodular thyroid disease (Bruneton et al., 1994; Wang and Crapo, 1997). Finally, in some developing countries, with persisting iodine deficiency, the prevalence of goiter, sometimes of extreme proportions, can approach 100% (Gaitan et al., 1991; Lamberg, 1991).

On a global scale, iodine deficiency and its associated conditions still account for the majority of thyroid disorders (Gaitan et al., 1991; Lamberg, 1991; Vanderpump et al., 1996), while in iodine-replete countries autoimmune hypo- and hyperthyroidism, sporadic goiter, and nodular thyroid disease (benign and malignant) make up the bulk of thyroid pathology (Vanderpump and Tunbridge, 1996; Wang and Crapo, 1997). Although there are few, if any, known genetic factors influencing the disease susceptibility to, or severity of, iodine deficiency, genetic makeup is increasingly being recognized as playing an important role in autoimmune and nodular thyroid disorders, as well as in sporadic goiter. In addition, there is a growing number of defined single-gene defect diseases of thyroid gland function. Almost every known step of thyroid hormone metabolism—from embryonic development of the gland, thyrotropin receptor function, iodine transport, thyroid hormone synthesis and metabolism, to serum thyroid hormone transport and end organ tissue action—may be affected by single-gene mutations. Although individually rare, these defects collectively make up a small, but significant, proportion of all thyroid disorders. In addition, they serve as prismatic cases highlighting the precise physiological role of the involved genes and the—sometimes unexpected—consequences of their alteration.

In this chapter I first review the normal thyroid anatomy and physiology and then briefly discuss the defined genetic syndromes of thyroid disease to highlight the role of various components of thyroid anatomy and physiology. This will serve as the foundation for the subsequent main portions of this chapter which discuss the genetic basis of autoimmune thyroid disease, goiter, and benign and malignant nodular thyroid disorders. C-cell hyperplasia and medullary carcinoma are included as a subsection of the discussion of nodular thyroid disease.

THE NORMAL THYROID GLAND

Gross Anatomy

The thyroid is the largest human endocrine gland. The physiological thyroid weight is about 20 g, although the average weight within a given human population may be considerably higher because of the high prevalence of pathological thyroid enlargement.

The gland is named for its close regional anatomical relationship to the laryngeal thyroid cartilage, which lies just superior and posterior to the gland and is often partly covered in its inferior lateral aspects by the upper poles of the thyroid gland. The thyroid gland is butterfly shaped, consisting of two roughly symmetrical lateral lobes on either side of the mid-line, a connecting isthmus and a variably present, and usually small, pyramidal lobe in the middle. The thyroid lobes are in close proximity to the great vessels of the neck laterally, and the recurrent laryngeal nerves traverse the gland. The gland has a thickish connective tissue capsule, with the parathyroid glands adherent to the back of the posterior portion of this capsule.

Embryogenesis

The follicular cell–containing portion of the thyroid gland develops from a median sprouting of thickened epithelium on the floor of the pharynx. As this tissue begins to migrate caudally along a central duct (thyroglossal duct) to its final position at the base of the neck, where it forms a left and a right lobe, it fuses with the mesodermal C-cell anlage, which has migrated medially from the two neural-crest-derived ultimobranchial bodies in the 4th pharyngeal pouch (Fisher and Polk, 1989; Mansberger and Wei, 1993).

The transcription factor TTF1 is crucial for the initial development of both types of thyroid precursor cells, with knockout mice lacking TTF1 showing total absence of both follicular cells and C cells (Kimura et al., 1996). The clonal expansion and differentiation of the follicular cells also has an obligatory requirement for the PAX8 transcription factor (Macchia et al., 1998; Mansouri et al., 1998) and a less stringent requirement for HOXA-3 (Manley and Capecchi, 1995). In addition, HOXA-3 influences the development and migration of the ultimobranchial bodies, thus regulating, in conjunction with other HOX-3-group paralogs such as HOXB-3 and HOXD-3, the orderly development and migration of thyroid C cells (Manley and Capecchi, 1995, 1998).

Once the thyroid gland has reached its final position, the thyroglossal duct usually regresses, although its caudal portion may form a small, central, pyramidal lobe. Thus, the initial structure of the gland resembles an exocrine gland, which is reflected in the loosely glandular structure of the mature gland with its left and right main lobes, each consisting of several ill-defined lobulae, which, in turn, are formed by the follicles that produce and store thyroid hormone. By contrast, the C cells are not obviously organized into glandular structures but remain interspersed throughout the gland.

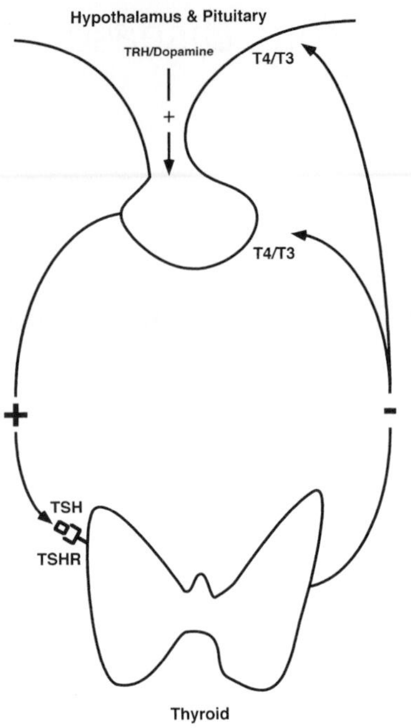

Fig. 20–1. Hypothalamic-pituitary-thyroid feedback regulation of thyroid hormone production. Pituitary-secreted thyrotropin (TSH) binds to TSH-receptors (TSHR) on thyrocytes and stimulates thyroid hormone production. Secreted thyroid hormones, thyroxine (T4) and triiodothyronine (T3), in turn, elicit negative feedback on TSH secretion. The negative feedback occurs on two levels: directly by down-regulating pituitary TSH secretion, and indirectly by diminishing hypothalamic thyrotropin-releasing hormone (TRH) and dopamine secretion.

Microscopic Anatomy

The thyroid follicle is the basic functional and organizational unit of the endodermally derived portion of the thyroid gland. It consists of a lumen filled with visible colloid, which is surrounded by a single layer of epithelial cells attached to a basement membrane. These thyrocytes are highly polar cells with a smooth outer surface attached to the basement membrane and a ragged apical surface with numerous pseudovillae on the follicular luminal aspect. A large Golgi apparatus is oriented toward the luminal side, and numerous vesicles, phagosomes, and lysosomes are present there, whereas the nucleus lies toward the basal side, and abundant endoplasmatic reticulum and mitochondria are more evenly distributed throughout the cells.

Between the follicles lies an extensive network of capillaries, so that each follicle is usually in contact with one or more capillaries and each capillary with several follicles. Scant connective tissue organizes the follicles into larger lobulae, which, in turn, form the lobes. C-cell nests are interspersed, being somewhat denser in distribution in the lateral regions of the gland. The C cells have the typical small, rounded appearance of neural crest–derived cells and contain calcitonin granules.

Follicular Cell Function and Regulation

The main function of follicular cells is to produce, store, and release thyroid hormone. This process is under pituitary feedback control, although a degree of thyroid autoregulation and autonomic control also exists (Grunditz and Sundler, 1996; Nagataki and Yokoyama, 1996). Pituitary thyrotropin (TSH) stimulates thyrocyte activity, hormone production, and secretion by binding to and transactivating thyrocyte cell-surface TSH receptors (TSHRs). In turn, secreted thyroid hormones exert negative feedback on pituitary TSH production, which is also subject to regulatory influences from hypothalamic centers via thyrotropin-releasing hormone and, to a lesser degree, dopamine and somatostatin. However, these hypothalamic influences play a minor role in regulating TSH secretion, compared with negative feedback regulation by circulating thyroid hormones (Grebe et al., 1995a) (Fig. 20–1).

Thyrocytes actively concentrate iodine via a sodium-iodide symporter (Dai et al., 1996; Smanik et al., 1996). Small amounts of iodine exist as inorganic intracellular iodine, but the major portion is coupled to tyrosine and thyronine residues of thyroglobulin (Tg), a 660 kDa dimeric protein (see below; J. Dunn, 1996; Taurog, 1996). Non-iodinated Tg is actively transported from cytosol to follicular lumen. Inorganic iodine may follow by diffusion but in the main is also actively transported to the follicular lumen, probably by the pendrin transmembrane anion transporter (Scott et al., 1999; Bidart et al., 2000). Iodination of Tg is a post-translational event occurring at the apical villae–luminae interface. It is catalyzed by thyroid peroxidase (TPO) and involves formation of activated iodine radicals, which react with tyrosine residues on Tg, followed by intramolecular coupling of pairs of mono- and diiodotyrosines to form predominately thyroxine (T4) or, to lesser degree, triiodothyronine (T3). The coupling step requires both thyroid peroxidase and H_2O_2 (Taurog, 1996). There are seven potential T4/T3 coupling sites in Tg, of which two are preferentially used (at amino acid residues 24 and 2572, accounting for greater than 50% of T4/T3 residues) (J. Dunn, 1996). Overall, approximately 27 atoms of iodine are bound per molecule of "mature" Tg: 3% to 4% in T3 residues, 30% to 35% in T4 residues, and the rest as iodotyrosines. The iodinated Tg is stored in the follicular lumen, forming the colloid. For thyroid hormone release, the colloid is reabsorbed at the apical membrane and proteolyzed. Iodinated tyrosine residues are deiodinated and recycled for synthesis of new Tg molecules, while the bulk of T3 and T4 residues are secreted from the basal membrane. Some T4 residues are partially

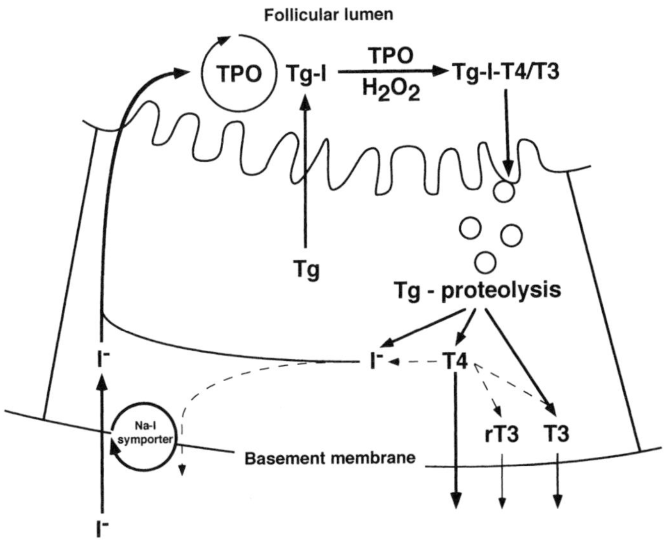

Fig. 20–2. Thyroid hormone synthesis. Iodide (I^-) is actively transported into thyrocytes through sodium-iodide symporters (Na-I symporters), passed to the apical membrane and excreted into the follicular lumen (probably largely through active transport by the Pendrin anion-transporter). Non-iodinated thyroglobulin (Tg) is also transported into the follicular lumen. In close proximity to the apical villae, thyroid peroxidase (TPO) catalyses the iodination of Tg tyrosine residues, followed (with H_2O_2 as a cofactor) by intramolecular coupling of some of the iodized tyrosine residues to thyroxine (T4) and triiodothyronine (T3). Fully processed Tg (Tg-I-T4/T3), containing mono- and diiodotyrosines, T3, and T4, reenters the thyrocytes via endocytosis and is proteolyzed in lysosomes. Free I^- is recycled, T3 is secreted, and T4 is mostly secreted and partly deiodinized to T3 and rT3, which are also secreted.

deiodinazed to rT3 or T3, which are then also secreted (A. Dunn, 1996; Taurog, 1996) (Fig. 20–2).

Thyroid Hormone Transport and Action

Following secretion, thyroid hormones are tightly bound by serum proteins, so that only about 1% circulate as free T4 or free T3. The major transporter is thyroxine-binding globulin (TBG), binding more than 70% of T4 and T3 with very high affinity, followed by transthyretin (TTR) and albumin, each of which binds 10% to 15% of the circulating T4 and T3. Binding to TTR and albumin is much weaker than to TBG; hence, these transporters are responsible for much of the delivery of T4 and T3 to cells, with hormone rapidly dissociating from them in the microcirculation. T4, which makes up the bulk of circulating thyroid hormones, is converted to T3 in the liver, kidney, and other peripheral organs. Biologically, T3 is three to five times more potent than T4; T4 serves as a storage form or "pro-hormone" (Robbins, 1996).

T3 (and to a lesser extent T4) enters cells by diffusion and combines with the nuclear thyroid hormone receptors. Thyroid hormone receptors (TRs) are a group of zinc finger transcription factors with high homology to steroid receptors. The main recognized subforms are α_1, β_1, and β_2, with the latter being expressed predominately in brain and pituitary tissues. Upon hormone binding, receptors undergo dimerization, either with other TRs or with related steroid superfamily-type receptors. Dimerized TRs can bind and transactivate thyroid hormone response elements (TREs) on DNA molecules. Monomeric TRs can also bind to TREs but can only transactivate them by recruiting other monomers to form dimers. TREs are typically six base pair palindromic, direct-repeat, or inverted-repeat nucleotide sequences with the consensus sequence of RGGTVA (IUB codes). They are primarily located in the promoter regions of genes, and their transactivation can result in either transcriptional activation or suppression. Many genes are thyroid hormone regulated and may contain several TREs, some of which may be positive transcriptional regulators, while other have negative regulatory effects on gene transcription. In addition, there are a large number of cofactors involved in thyroid hormone–mediated transcriptional control, as well as differences in tissue-specific responses. The result is a highly complex, partially tissue-specific, effect of thyroid hormones on gene expression.

INHERITED ABNORMALITIES OF THYROID DEVELOPMENT AND FUNCTION

For almost every step of thyroid development, thyroid hormone production, transport, and action there are recognized, well-defined inherited abnormalities. For most of these, the molecular basis is known. Individually each of these conditions is rare; however, in combination they account for a small, but significant, proportion of thyroid disorders. Following the outline used in the preceding section, these conditions include:

- Inherited developmental abnormalities of the hypothalamus or pituitary
- Primary developmental abnormalities of the thyroid gland
- TSH receptor abnormalities
- Abnormalities of iodide transport, with or without associated organification defects
- Abnormalities of thyroglobulin synthesis and function
- Organification defects
- Thyroid hormone transport abnormalities
- Thyroid hormone resistance

Table 20–1 briefly summarizes the salient aspects of the various conditions.

AUTOIMMUNE THYROID DISEASE

If trivial goiter and ultrasonographically (but not clinically) detectable nodular thyroid disease are excluded, autoimmune hypothyroidism and hyperthyroidism are the most common thyroid disorders in iodine-replete countries.

Autoimmune thyroid disease is characterized by the presence of autoantibodies against various thyroid components, namely the TSHR, TPO, and Tg, as well as by an inflammatory cellular infiltrate of variable severity within the gland. Among the autoantibodies found in autoimmune thyroid disease, TSHR autoantibodies are most closely associated with disease pathogenesis. Autoimmune thyrotoxicosis is virtually always caused by the production of TSHR-stimulating autoantibodies and at least 10% to 20% of patients with autoimmune hypothyroidism have evidence of TSHR-blocking antibodies (McIntosh et al., 1998; Rees Smith et al., 1988). The role of the Tg and TPO autoantibodies in relation to disease development is less well established; they may merely represent epiphenomena.

Patients with autoimmune thyroid disease are also more likely to suffer from other autoimmune conditions, in particular other organ-specific, endocrine autoimmune diseases, such as Type I diabetes and Addison's disease, suggesting a possible general predisposition to aberrant immune responses (Friedman

Table 20–1. Inherited Abnormalities of Thyroid Development and Function

Condition	Characteristics	Inheritance	References
Developmental abnormalities of hypothalamus and pituitary	Caused by a variety of different developmental abnormalities; variable loss of pituitary function; usually mild congenital (atrophic) hypothyroidism	Depends on underlying defect.	
Complete or partial thyroid agenesis	Atrophic congenital hypothyroidism; euthyroid family members may have minor structural or positional thyroid gland abnormalities; *TTF1*, *TTF2*, and *PAX8* implicated in some families	Most cases sporadic; inherited cases usually autosomal recessive	Acebron et al., 1995; Clifton-Bligh et al., 1998; Macchia et al., 1998
TSH resistance	Loss of function mutations of the TSH receptor; disease severity varies between severe and moderately severe congenital hypothyroidism	Usually autosomal recessive; heterozygote family members may have goiter or mild hypothyroidism	Takamatsu et al., 1993; Paschke et al., 1996; Mimouni et al., 1996; Krude et al., 1996; Abramowicz et al., 1997; Biebermann et al., 1997; Gagne et al., 1998
Familial non-autoimmune thyrotoxicosis	Gain of function mutations of the TSH receptor; highly variable severity and age of onset	Autosomal dominant	Thomas et al., 1982; Paschke, 1996; Schwab et al., 1996; Führer et al., 1997, 1998; Grüters et al., 1998
Iodide transport abnormalities	Loss of function mutations of the sodium iodide symporter. Severity of diseases dependent on mutation: congenital hypothyroidism, early onset hypothyroidism, or goiter.	Sporadic, autosomal dominant, and autosomal recessive	Wolff, 1983, 1997; Matsuda and Kosugi, 1997; Pohlenz et al., 1997, 1998
Iodide transport abnormalities with associated organification abnormalities	Also known as Pendred syndrome; caused by inactivating mutations/deletions of *PDS* (coding for a chloride-iodide transporter, with exclusive expression in thyroid tissue); goiterous hypothyroidism with abnormal organification/ thyroid dyshormonogenesis and deafness.	Autosomal recessive	Johnsen et al., 1989; Sheffield et al., 1996; Everett et al., 1997; Mustapha et al., 1998; Scott et al, 1999
Abnormalities of thyroglobulin synthesis or function	Mutations or deletions in the Tg gene lead to thyroid dyshormonogenesis, with goiterous hypothyroidism and (possible) predisposition to thyroid carcinoma	Autosomal dominant for most mutations and microdeletions (dominant negative effect of mutant in Tg dimer); autosomal recessive for defects leading to diminished Tg synthesis and for some mutations and microdeletions	Hasen and Bartalos, 1975; Wagar et al., 1982; Couch et al., 1986; Taylor and Rowe, 1987; Targovnik et al., 1989, 1991; Corral et al., 1993; Medeiros-Neto et al., 1993, 1997; Yoshida et al., 1996
Organification defects	Mainly TPO mutations, but also less well characterized defects in co-enzymes and factors involved in iodination and coupling, as well as Iodine transport into the follicular lumen; clinical disease spectrum similar to Tg abnormalities	Usually autosomal recessive	Tezuka et al., 1971; Niepomniszcze et al., 1977; Perez-Cuvit et al., 1977; Ismail-Beigi and Rahimifar, 1977; Medeiros-Neto et al., 1979, 1982; 1993; Niimi et al., 1985; Grüters et al., 1996; Bidart et al., 2000
Thyroid hormone transport abnormalities	May involve any of the thyroid hormone serum transport proteins; usually not associated with clinical disease; free hormone levels normal, but patients have abnormal total peripheral thyroid hormone levels, potentially leading to the erroneous diagnoses of hypo or (more commonly) hyperthyroidism	Usually autosomal dominant	Bratusch-Marrain et al., 1979; Frank et al., 1986; Trent et al., 1987; Young et al., 1987; Constans et al., 1992; Komatsu et al., 1994; Weiss et al., 1995; Sunthornthepvarakul et al., 1998
Thyroid hormone resistance	Mutations/deletions of thyroid hormone receptors; spectrum of disease severity ranges from few clinical signs to congenital hypothyroidism and ($\beta 2$ involvement) TSH-driven hyperthyroidism	Usually autosomal dominant (dominant negative effect of mutant in thyroid hormone receptor dimer)	Refetoff et al., 1993; Brucker-Davis et al., 1995

and Fialkow, 1978; Sasazuki et al., 1983; Torfs et al., 1986; Schleusener et al., 1991; Weetman, 1995; Heward and Gough, 1997). A minority of these patients simultaneously suffer from all three conditions plus (possibly) vitiligo and pernicious anemia, and these individuals are classified as suffering from autoimmune polyglandular syndrome type 2 or 3 (APS-2/3). Since the recent cloning of the *AIRE* gene, which when mutated results in another autoimmune polyglandular syndrome (APS-1) without thyroid involvement (Nagamine et al., 1997), there has been speculation whether some cases of APS-2 may be due to inherited single-gene defects. Thus far, the evidence supports only polygenic inheritance (Obermayer-Straub and Manns, 1998).

Familial clustering of autoimmune thyroid diseases has also long been recognized (Friedman and Fialkow, 1978; Schleusener et al., 1991; Weetman and McGregor, 1994; Heward and Gough, 1997; Tomer and Davies, 1997), and twin studies have suggested an inherited component of 50% or more (Schleusener et al., 1991; Heward and Gough, 1997; Tomer and Davies, 1997; Brix et al., 1998, 2000, 2001). Consequently, there has been considerable interest in the investigation of a possible association between polymorphisms of genes involved in immune responses and thyroid autoimmunity. This candidate gene approach has in recent times been supplemented by moves toward the use of more generalized, comprehensive genetic screens to identify thyroid autoimmunity susceptibility loci. Both approaches have their advantages and disadvantages (see chapters 3 and 4), but, despite all difficulties, association and linkage studies have already led to some significant advances in our understanding of autoimmune thyroid disease.

Autoimmune Hyperthyroidism (Graves' Disease)

Disease Definition

Diagnostic Criteria. Thyrotoxicosis is usually defined as symptoms or signs of thyroid hormone excess in conjunction with unequivocal biochemical evidence of elevated serum thyroid hormone levels and suppressed TSH levels, in the absence of pituitary disease. For the most part, autoimmune thyrotoxicosis is synonymous with Graves' disease, which the *International Statistical Classification of Diseases and Health Related Problems*, 10th edition (*ICD-10*), defines as "thyrotoxicosis with diffuse goiter, not due to chronic thyroiditis with transient thyrotoxicosis, or neonatal thyrotoxicosis" (WHO Collaborating Centres for Classification of Diseases, 1992). In clinical practice, this definition reflects the minimal set of diagnostic criteria, and additional clinical or radiological evidence is desirable for confirmation of diagnosis. In particular, one may also require evidence of either diffuse and uniformly increased radioisotope uptake on radioiodine or technetium scanning, typical extrathyroidal signs of Graves' disease (thyroid eye disease/exophthalmos, pre-tibial myxedema, or thyroid acropachy), or a positive result in a TSHR-stimulating autoantibody assay.

Clinical Features and Outcome. Patients may present with weight loss, irritability, insomnia, heat intolerance, loose bowel motions, tremor, and fatigue. However, numerous other symptoms may be present, or one of the main symptoms may predominate. On examination, the patient may be restless, tachycardic, sweaty, and tremulous. The tendon reflexes may be brisk, and there may be evidence of recent weight loss, signified by loose or poorly fitting clothing, and, occasionally, heart failure or psychotic behavior has been recorded. At presentation, in excess of one-half of the patients will have extrathyroidal signs of Graves' disease, most commonly thyroid eye disease, although this may be subtle. Virtually all patients will have at least a palpable goiter, and commonly the thyroid gland will be significantly enlarged. The goiter is usually smooth, although, given the high prevalence of nodular thyroid disease, coexisting nodules occasionally may be palpable. A vascular bruit over the goiter is considered pathognomonic.

The natural course of the disease is highly variable. Spontaneous remissions do occur, and some patients only develop minimal biochemical and clinical disease. However, in the majority of patients, Graves' thyrotoxicosis is at least initially progressive, and increasingly severe symptoms and signs tend to ensue over time. Since thyrotoxicosis will eventually affect virtually all organ systems, this results in considerable disease-related morbidity and, if the thyrotoxicosis is left untreated, between 10% and 50% mortality, mostly due to cardiac complications (White, 1886; McEwan, 1938; Sattler, 1952; Parker and Lawson, 1973). Given these facts, it is not surprising that Kocher was awarded the 1909 Nobel prize in medicine and physiology for his achievements in the development of thyroid surgery for treatment of Graves' disease. Today, with appropriate treatment, either in the form of antithyroid drug treatment or ablative treatment regimens such as surgery or radioiodine treatment, Graves' disease can be adequately managed in most patients, with little resultant morbidity and negligible mortality.

General Genetic and Epidemiological Evidence

Clinical Epidemiology. Although Graves' disease occurs in all ethnic groups, there are insufficient data to determine whether any particular races suffer from increased disease susceptibility. Published prevalence figures range from 0 in 1000 to 2.3 in 1000 for males and from 2 in 1000 to 27 in 1000 for females; the corresponding incidence figures are between 0 to 1000 per year and 0.9 to 1000 per year for males and between 0.3 to 1000 per year and 1.3 in 1000 per year for females (Vanderpump and Tunbridge, 1996). The condition is rare in the first decade of life and peaks in the fourth and fifth decades. Although new cases are rarely diagnosed after the age of 80, some studies suggest that Graves' disease is not uncommon in the sixth and seventh decade of life (Palmer, 1977). In all human populations studied to date, females are between 2 and 20 times more likely to suffer from Graves' disease than are males.

Family Epidemiology. It is established that Graves' disease aggregates in families. In 1937, Lehman from Germany reported identifying 38 individuals with thyrotoxicosis among first- and second-degree relatives of 15 index cases with "clinically typical" Basedow's/Graves' disease. Siblings of the index cases accounted for almost one-half of these cases, with 16 of 69 siblings affected. Bartels (1941) made similar observations in twin and family studies conducted in Denmark, finding evidence for a familial predisposition in approximately 60% of patients with thyrotoxicosis. Later Martin and Fisher (1945) reported that in a U.K. patient population, 17 relatives of 90 patients with Graves' disease had evidence of Graves' disease, while in a control group of 111 patients with nodular thyroid disease only 2 relatives were clinically affected by Graves' disease. More recently, other groups have confirmed these early observations (Friedman and Fialkow, 1978; Stenszky et al., 1985; Tomer and Davies, 1997).

Clinical studies have validated epidemiological observations of a female preponderance for Graves' disease, and it has been shown that 5.9% of daughters and 6.5% of sisters of thyrotoxic patients were also affected by autoimmune thyrotoxicosis, whereas none of the sons or brothers suffered from the condition (Stenszky et al., 1985). Finally, several investigators have reported a prevalence of up to 50% of thyroid autoantibodies in, mostly clinically unaffected, family members of patients with Graves' disease or Hashimoto's thyroiditis (Tomer and Davies, 1997).

Together these observations suggest strongly that either shared environmental or genetic factors play a significant role in determining the susceptibility to Graves' disease. Of these possibilities, the latter appears more likely, as a number of twin studies have shown concordance rates of 30% to 80% in monozygotic twins for Graves' disease, while in dizygotic twins the corresponding rates are only between 3% and 12% (Harvald and Hauge, 1956; Verschür, 1958; Brix et al., 1998, 2001). However, family and twin data also suggest that Graves' disease is not an entirely genetically determined condition; approximately half the risk can be ascribed to environmental factors. This is consistent with the now widely accepted concept that the development of autoimmune diseases in genetically susceptible individuals can be modified in permissive or protective environments.

Association with Other Diseases. In the combined genetic–environmental model, an abnormal immune response to thyroid autoantigens, and possibly to other autoantigens, is hypothesized, given permissive environmental circumstances. One might expect Graves' patients to also be at increased risk of other autoimmune disease, and, indeed, Graves' sufferers are at increased risk for non-organ-specific autoimmune diseases, such as rheumatoid arthritis, systemic lupus erythromatosis, psoriasis, and inflammatory bowel disease, and at even greater risk for other organ-specific autoimmune diseases, namely endocrine organ-specific disorders, such as Type I diabetes and Addison's disease. Organ-specific disorders of extraendocrine systems, such as celiac disease and multiple sclerosis, are also seen (Friedman and Fialkow, 1978; Sasazuki et al., 1983; Torfs et al., 1986; Schleusener et al., 1991; Weetman, 1995; Heward and Gough, 1997). Moreover, such associated diseases are overrepresented among Graves' disease relatives, regardless of whether they also suffer from autoimmune thyroid disease.

Environmental Factors. What constitutes the permissive or protective environmental factors that may determine whether a genetically predisposed individual will develop autoimmune disease in general, and Graves' disease in particular, remains unknown. Seasonal trends, significant regional variation in prevalence and occasional geographic clustering of Graves' disease cases have been reported (Tomer and Davies, 1993; Weetman and McGregor, 1994; McIver and Morris, 1998), suggesting the possibility that an infectious agent might be involved. This is further supported by the fact that a large proportion of recently diagnosed Graves' patients shows nonspecific serological evidence of recent infection and that the prevalence of ABO blood group nonsecretors, a condition associated with a slight predisposition to infection, is increased among Graves' disease patients (Tomer and Davies, 1993). All this constitutes circumstantial evidence for a potential role for infectious agents in precipitating Graves' disease.

Among possible pathogens *Yersinia enterocolitica* has received the most attention. *Yersinia enterocolitica* may cause gastroenteritis or intestinal lymphadenitis, but it has also been implicated in the pathogenesis of Reiter's syndrome and various other autoimmune phenomena. Patients who have evidence of past *Y. enterocolitica* infection display an increased rate of antithyroid autoantibodies, and Graves' disease patients are reported to frequently have detectable *Y. enterocolitica* antibodies (Arscott et al., 1992; Tomer and Davies, 1993; McIver and Morris, 1998). *Yersinia enterocolitica* can saturably bind human TSH and Graves' immunoglobulins at a specific binding site. Furthermore, human *TSHR* DNA probes hybridize with *Y. enterocolitica* DNA under relatively low stringency conditions, and *Y. enterocolitica* encoded proteins can elicit TSHR antibody production (Weiss et al., 1983; Heyma et al., 1986; Burman et al., 1991; Luo et al., 1994). Taken in conjunction, these data suggest that in some individuals, *Y. enterocolitica* infection may lead to the production of antibodies with cross-reactivity to the TSHR, resulting in Graves' disease or autoimmune thyroiditis. This hypothesis is further supported by the observation that rats and mice immunized with *Y. enterocolitica* proteins may develop a lymphocytic thyroiditis (Luo et al., 1993; Tomer and Davies, 1993). In these animal models, other autoimmune diseases may also occur after *Y. enterocolitica* immunization, suggesting this only reflects nonspecific immune hyperstimulation in rodents (Tomer and Davies, 1993). Because most individuals with *Y. enterocolitica* infection (including those with serological evidence of thyroid autoantibodies) do not develop clinical Graves' disease and because individuals with nonautoimmune thyroid diseases may also develop *Y. enterocolitica* antibodies, the role of *Y. enterocolitica* remains uncertain (Tomer and Davies, 1993; Resetkova et al., 1994). However, the balance of data is consistent with *Y. enterocolitica* infection being a permissive environmental factor in certain individuals with a genetic predisposition to abnormal immune responses and Graves' disease.

Similar conclusions can be reached for most other pathogens implicated in Graves' disease, in particular endogenous and exogenous retroviruses (Tomer and Davies, 1993). Interestingly, for this group of pathogens, an interaction with class II MHC genes conferring susceptibility to Graves' disease has been observed in one study, with only those individuals contracting Graves' disease who had both a "high-risk" HLA II haplotype and evidence of a particular retroviral infection (Jaspan et al., 1996).

Pathophysiological Basis of Genetic Susceptibility

General Pathophysiology. On the basis of the epidemiological information reviewed above, it seems plausible that on the background of polygenic susceptibility certain environmental factors, in conjunction with infections, can lead to Graves' disease. To understand precisely how this may occur, it is necessary to understand the pathophysiology of Graves' disease.

The sine qua non of Graves' disease in genetic terms is a predisposition to develop thyroid autoantibodies, which are capable of stimulating the TSHR. It is believed that these autoantibodies are produced either as a result of an immune reaction to some external trigger, possessing some similarity with the TSHR, or in response to aberrant autoantigen processing and presentation by thyrocytes, or by a combination of these factors. In addition, there needs to be an intrinsic ability of the patient's immune system to respond to such stimuli—that is, a failure of suppression of self-directed immune reactions.

The TSHR autoantibodies have the capability to transactivate the TSHR, thereby stimulating thyroid gland function and growth. As production of these TSHR-stimulating autoantibodies is not under normal pituitary feedback control, thyrotoxicosis ensues (Fig. 20–3). Simultaneously, there is lymphocytic infiltration of the gland, associated with some thyroid destruction, which may account for the spontaneous reversion of Graves' thyrotoxicosis to autoimmune hypothyroidism; this reversion occurs at a rate of approximately 3% per year. The active immune response in the gland may also serve to process and present further thyroid antigens, with resulting amplification of the autoimmune response, including further autoantibody production.

Finally, some aspects of the autoimmune response in Graves' disease also lead, in as yet unknown ways, to focal connective

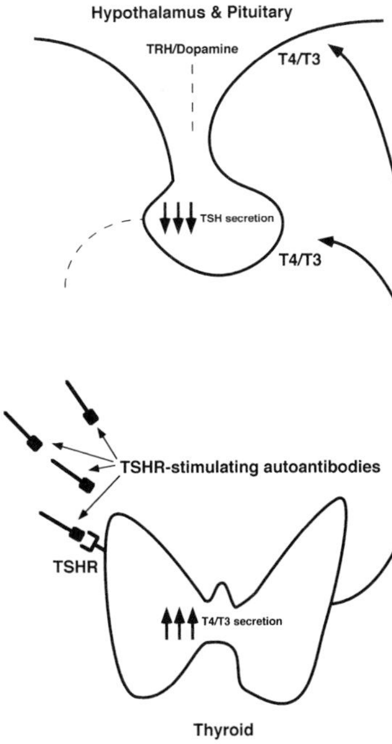

Fig. 20–3. Failure of hypothalamic-pituitary-thyroid feedback regulation of thyroid hormone production in Graves' disease. In Graves' disease, thyrotropin receptor autoantibodies (TSHR stimulating autoantibodies) bind to the TSHR and transactivate it, stimulating thyroid hormone production. With rising peripheral thyroid hormone levels, pituitary thyrotropin (TSH) secretion is appropriately diminished and eventually completely shut down. However, ongoing TSHR stimulation by autoantibodies continues to fuel thyroid hormone production, even in the absence of TSH.

tissue and muscle tissue changes, thereby initiating the various extrathyroidal manifestations of Graves' disease, in particular Graves' ophthalmopathy.

Possible Genetic Basis of Graves' Disease. Besides a predisposition to produce TSHR autoantibodies, genetic variability affecting several other aspects of the immune response in Graves' disease and the response of the thyroid gland itself to exposure to the TSHR-stimulating antibodies may predispose to Graves' disease or modulate its severity. Genetic factors may therefore influence the etiology, pathophysiology, and clinical course of Graves' disease by (1) predisposing an individual to an abnormal immune response, leading to TSHR-autoantibody production and lymphocytic infiltration of the thyroid gland; (2) influencing the magnitude and duration of TSHR-stimulating autoantibody production; (3) affecting the affinity of these antibodies to the TSHR and their ability to transactivate it; (4) altering the degree of thyroidal response to the stimulation; (5) changing the availability of substrate, mainly iodine, but also nutrients in general, for thyroid hormone production, to the thyrocytes, and (6) determining the relative proportion of inflammatory thyroid destruction to TSHR autoantibody–induced thyroid growth.

Any of these factors, possibly in conjunction with further, non-thyroid-related genes, may also influence the likelihood of disease remission and response to certain treatment modalities, including treatment side effects and the degree of extrathyroidal manifestations of Graves' disease.

Gene Identification

Based on the pathophysiological considerations elaborated above, it is clear that a large number of immune system–related and thyroid-related genes may influence the expression of the Graves' disease phenotype. The identification of disease genes under such circumstances is particularly difficult. If a candidate gene approach is used, many candidates may have to be examined. Any statistical calculations will require correction for multiple comparisons, and only a complex multivariate analysis will be able to determine the relative contributions of several different candidate genes to disease risk. Similarly, genome-wide screens will have to be designed to identify more than one disease gene, and, hence, greater numbers of markers will have to be screened in a larger number of subjects, thus greatly increasing the complexity of such an undertaking. Consequently, only a limited number of all possible candidate genes have thus far been examined, and as yet, no genome-wide screen has been completed.

Candidate Genes: Immune Response Genes. The basic elements of any immune reaction are presentation of antigens to immune cells, antigen recognition, and cellular or humoral immune response. A number of genes involved in several of these steps have been evaluated for their role in the development of Graves' disease.

Human Leukocyte Antigen Genes. At the level of antigen presentation, human leukocyte antigen (HLA) molecules have to present peptide fragments of antigens to immune competent cells. Human HLA genes are highly polymorphic; more than 120 different possible alleles for the HLA-A locus, over 250 for the HLA-B locus, more than 70 for the HLA-C locus, more than 260 known *DRB* alleles and about 20 *DQA*, 40 *DQB*, 15 *DPA*, and 85 *DPB* alleles (Mason and Parham, 1998; Marsh, 1998), giving rise to a staggering array of possible allelotypes. Some of these alleles may exhibit preferential binding of thyroid-related peptides or pathogen-derived peptides that mimic thyroid-related peptide fragments. This could be a mechanism by which an early Graves' disease autoimmune response is initiated.

In particular, HLA II molecules are strong candidates as disease-susceptibility genes for diseases that develop as a result of T-cell mediated autoimmunity. HLA II molecules are assembled in the endoplasmatic reticulum; are transported and modified through the Golgi; are released to the cytosol, where they take up degraded antigen; and are finally transported to the cell surface, where they present the antigen peptide fragments to $CD4^+$ T cells (Abbas et al., 1997; Thorsby, 1997). These $CD4^+$ T cells may then directly attack the presented foreign antigen, stimulate macrophages to attack the antigen, or stimulate antibody production by B lymphocytes. Thyrocytes and circulating T lymphocytes of Graves' patients show aberrant expression of HLA II molecules, making MHC class II genes obvious candidate genes to be involved in the first step of the autoimmune reaction in Graves' disease (Weetman and McGregor, 1984, 1994; McIver and Morris, 1998). Moreover, certain HLA class I and class II tissue types have been strongly linked to many other autoimmune diseases, as, for example, patients suffering from ankylosing spondylitis have more than a 150-fold increased likelihood of having the HLA I serotype B27, while the HLA II serotype DQ2 is more than 250-fold overrepresented in celiac disease patients (Thorsby, 1997).

A large number of studies have investigated the role of the MHC class I and II molecules in conveying susceptibility to Graves' disease; a review of the major papers (most cited or greater than 30 subjects) reveals 48 publications (Ofosu et al., 1996; Jaffiol et al., 1976; Barbesino et al., 1998a; Jaspan et al., 1996; Yanagawa et al., 1993, 1994; Yanagawa and DeGroot,

1996; Tamai et al., 1994, 1996; Shields et al., 1994; Cavan et al., 1994b; Uchigata et al., 1993; Hu et al., 1992; Roman et al., 1992; Mangklabruks et al., 1991; Weetman and McCorkle, 1990; Weetman et al., 1988; Boehm et al., 1988; Stenszky et al., 1985; Hawkins et al., 1985a; Dahlberg et al., 1981; Barlow et al., 1996; Onuma et al., 1994; Dong et al., 1992; Semana et al., 1990; Tandon et al., 1990; Payami et al., 1989; Yeo et al., 1989; Frecker et al., 1986, 1988; Kendall-Taylor et al., 1988; Sridama et al., 1987; Cho et al., 1987; Hawkins et al., 1985b; Allannic et al., 1980, 1983; McKenna et al., 1982; Uno et al., 1981; Farid et al., 1979, 1980a, 1980b; Badenhoop et al., 1992, 1996; Ratanachaiyavong et al., 1990, 1994; Omar et al., 1990; Philippou et al., 2001; Chen et al, 1999). The interpretation of these studies is somewhat difficult, as they have been conducted over more than two decades and HLA typing technology has changed considerably during this period. In particular, antibody panels for serotyping have become more sophisticated, with a much greater number of tissue types now being able to be resolved. This has led to changes in nomenclature and a significant amount of type reclassification. In addition, with the advent of genetic typing, it has been recognized that even the most advanced serological typing only detects a fraction of the expressed diversity. Thus, most of the recent studies on the relationship of HLA genes and Graves' disease have used some form of genetic typing. While this has increased the accuracy of typing and the likelihood that an observed association truly reflects certain genetic polymorphisms, it has also complicated comparison with the older literature. Finally, the profound linkage disequilibrium observed in the MHC region for some class I and class II marker combinations makes it difficult, regardless of typing method used, to unequivocally assign a permissive or protective relative risk to a single HLA marker.

Notwithstanding these methodological difficulties, it appears that a number of HLA markers are associated with an increased risk of Graves' disease. In Caucasian populations there is an association between A1, B8, and DR3 and various combinations of these three markers, and Graves' disease for both male and female patients. These observations are consistent across a large number of different association studies (Jaffiol et al., 1976; Badenhoop et al., 1992; Hu et al., 1992; Mangklabruks et al., 1991; Weetman and McCorkle, 1990; Stenszky et al., 1985; Dahlberg et al., 1981; Payami et al., 1989; Frecker et al., 1986, 1988; Kendall-Taylor et al., 1988; Allannic et al., 1980, 1983; McKenna et al., 1982; Farid et al., 1976, 1979, 1980b; Ratanachaiyavong et al., 1990, 1994; Mayr et al., 1976; Seignalet et al., 1975; Whittingham et al., 1975; Nelson and Pollet, 1975; Grumet et al., 1974). Since A1, B8, and DR3 are in strong linkage disequilibrium with each other, assignment of the HLA-related Graves' disease risk to a single one of these markers has been difficult. The strength of the observed association is generally greatest for DR3, suggesting that it might be the primary factor in determining Graves' risk in Caucasians. Multivariate logistic regression models using stepwise factor elimination have also suggested that A1 and B8 are only implicated through linkage disequilibrium with DR3 (Farid et al., 1980b; Payami et al., 1989). Linkage data further support a relationship between DR3 and Graves' disease in Caucasians (Uno et al., 1981; Stenszky et al., 1985; Shields et al., 1994). Although one study showed a lack of evidence for linkage between DR3 and Graves' disease (Roman et al., 1992), this study suffered from a lack of statistical power in that it only included 114 subjects from 27 families, 50 of which had Graves' disease. By a priori assumption of linkage equilibrium, when in fact the evidence from association studies supported a strong association of Graves' with DR3, the statistical power of this study was further weakened. By contrast, a subsequent study of a larger group of subjects, using a combination of segregation and linkage analysis, was free of these shortcomings and showed strong evidence of DR3 linkage to Graves' disease with a maximum LOD score of 6.6 (Shields et al., 1994).

DR3 (or rather its subtype, DR17) is a common HLA II serotype in Caucasians and is associated with unique patterns of immune responsiveness. Compared to $DR3^{-/-}$ individuals, normal $DR3^{+/-}$ or $DR3^{+/+}$ subjects display decreased interleukin 1 (IL-1) production and T-cell responsiveness to mitogens, diminished Fc receptor function, and increased immunoglobulin secretion after pokeweed mitogen stimulation, as well as different circulating CD4/CD8 cell ratios (Lawley et al., 1981; Ambinder et al., 1982; McCombs et al., 1986; Hashimoto et al., 1989, 1990). It is therefore biologically plausible that the DR3 haplotype predisposes to abnormal immune responses; however, the relative risks for Graves' disease conveyed by DR3 are relatively small, ranging from 2-fold to 7-fold. By contrast, much stronger associations have been observed for other HLA molecules in some other autoimmune diseases (also see above) (Thorsby, 1997). This suggests that the DR3 serotype either contributes to only a small degree of disease susceptibility or that another gene in linkage disequilibrium with DR3 accounts for the apparent disease–tissue type association. Based on the strong linkage data for a DR–Graves' linkage (Shields et al., 1994), this latter possibility seems more likely. It is further supported by the fact that, with the exception of Asian Indian populations, which are genetically close to Caucasians (Tandon et al., 1990), and South African Zulu (Omar et al., 1990), the DR3 serotype does not seem to be associated with Graves' disease in non-Caucasian populations (Uno et al., 1981; Hawkins et al., 1985a, 1985b; Cho et al., 1987; Sridama et al., 1987; Yeo et al., 1989; Dong et al., 1992; Uchigata et al., 1993; Cavan et al., 1994b; Onuma et al., 1994; Ofosu et al., 1996; Tamai et al., 1996; Yanagawa and DeGroot, 1996). In Chinese populations, B46 and DR9 show a mild to moderate degree of association with Graves' disease, which is comparable to B8 and DR3 in Caucasians (Hawkins et al., 1985a, 1985b; Yeo et al., 1989; Cavan et al., 1994b). DR9 has also been reported to be associated with Graves' disease in African Americans (Ofosu et al., 1996), while B46 is overrepresented in Japanese Graves' patients (Dong et al., 1992; Onuma et al., 1994). Japanese Graves' sufferers also have increased rates of DR8 (Uno et al., 1981), which, in turn, is also found at increased frequency in Korean Graves' subjects (Cho et al., 1987). Therefore, it appears that different populations show sometimes subtly and sometimes markedly different HLA type–Graves' disease risk associations, making it unlikely that any of the studied tissue types are uniquely associated with Graves' disease. Alternatively, many of the DR alleles are in linkage disequilibrium not only with HLA-A and HLA-B alleles but also with the other class II alleles, DP and DQ. Since different ethnic groups may display differing combinations of markers in linkage disequilibrium, this raises the possibility that a particular DP or DQ genotype might be the HLA-related factor that determines Graves' susceptibility. The variable A, B, and DR associations observed in different ethnic groups might then only reflect ethnic differences in marker combinations, which are in linkage disequilibrium with this hypothetical DP or DQ disease-associated haplotype.

Owing to difficulties in distinguishing DP and DQ alleles serologically, these have been studied less extensively in the early days of HLA typing. With the advent of improved monoclonal antibody panels and genetic typing, this situation has changed over the last 6 to 8 years, in particular for the DQ alleles. Consequently, many of the recent HLA–Graves' association studies have included DQ and, to a lesser degree, DP typing, and interesting results are beginning to emerge. The DR3 association in Caucasians now appears to be due to linkage disequilibrium between *DRB1*0301* (serologically DR3) and *DQA1*0501* (Yanagawa et al., 1993, 1994; Badenhoop et al., 1996; Barlow et al., 1996; Philippou et al., 2001), which seems to be the allele conferring the susceptibility, with relative risks as high as 10 being recorded. An important role for *DQA1* alleles in determining susceptibility to Graves' disease is further supported by the fact that certain other *DQA1* alleles (e.g., *DQA1*0201*) may be "protective" (Yanagawa et al., 1994, 1995). Similarly, some *DRB1*07* alleles may be protective (Chen et al., 1999). In the case of HLA molecules, the mechanisms of conveying disease susceptibility most likely involve preferential peptide binding and presentation. It is thought that HLA amino acid polymorphisms are the major factors determining antigen peptide fragment binding. While some amino acid polymorphisms will increase autoantigen binding and presentation, others may diminish it. Therefore, finding both protective and disease-associated alleles for a given HLA molecule increases the likelihood that it may be autoantigen presentation by this particular HLA molecule that influences disease risk.

Some DQ2 alleles (*DQB1*0201*) also seem to convey Graves' risk in Caucasians, although it is uncertain whether this is through linkage disequilibrium with *DQA1*0501*. Similarly, the DQ3 serotype, coded by the *DQB1* alleles **0301*, **0302*, and **0303*, seems to be associated with Graves' disease in African Americans (Ofosu et al., 1996). When analyzed on the genetic level, *DQB1*0301* and *DQB1*0303* have been found to convey an increased risk of Graves' disease in Caucasian and Chinese populations, respectively (Cavan et al., 1994b; Yanagawa et al., 1994b). As *DQB1*0501* has been found to have a "Graves' protective" effect (Tamai et al., 1994), it seems that certain DQA/B combinations might modulate Graves' disease susceptibility. Depending on the ethnic background, different A/B/DR combinations will be observed in linkage disequilibrium, accounting for the results of much of the earlier work. With ever increasing availability of molecular genetic HLA typing, it should soon be possible to confirm these hypotheses and to pinpoint more precisely which DQA/B combinations might convey the highest risks for the development of Graves' disease. Molecular modeling might then provide important insights into how such a hypothetical disease-associated HLA molecule may modify antigen binding and presentation.

Finally, DP alleles have thus far not been studied extensively, but they may also play a role. Among the known DP alleles, *DPB1*0501* has been found to be associated with Graves' disease in Japanese patients (Dong et al., 1992; Onuma et al., 1994), while *DPB1*0402* has been associated indirectly with Graves' susceptibility in Caucasians via linkage disequilibrium with DR17 (the Caucasian DR3 serotype; there is another DR3 serotype, DR18, which is found primarily in ethnic black Africans, including African Americans) and B8 (Ratanachaiyavong et al., 1994).

Clearly, there is the need for a large-scale, multi-ethnic association study using modern genetic HLA-typing approaches to determine definitively the roles of certain HLA allelotypes in conveying Graves' disease risk.

HLA Function Associated Genes. Genes encoding proteins that are involved in the regulation of transcription or translation of HLA molecules or in transport and degradation of either HLA molecules or antigenic peptides are potential candidate genes. Functional variation of these proteins may well affect HLA cell surface expression and antigen presentation. There are large numbers of transcription factors that regulate HLA expression, including cytokines (Abbas et al., 1997). Interferon-γ (InFγ) and tumor necrosis factor (TNF) are the best described cytokines in thyroid disease. They are known to up-regulate HLA-DR expression and adhesion molecule cell surface expression, and there is evidence of increased intrathyroidal InFγ and TNF production by infiltrating lymphocytes in Graves' disease (Buscema et al., 1989; Roura-Mir et al., 1997; Lahat et al., 1998). We are aware of only one study that has examined the relation of possible *InF*γ genetic polymorphisms to Graves' disease (Siegmund et al., 1998). The study examined the allele frequencies of a microsatellite repeat, located within the first intron of the *InF*γ gene, in 200 Graves' patients and 212 controls. They observed an excess of alleles *IFN-*γ**3* and *IFN-*γ**5* in Graves' patients, particularly in those who also carried the high-risk HLA allele *DQA1*0501*. However, the absolute frequency of these alleles was still low in the Graves' patients, suggesting the polymorphism probably does not contribute significantly to Graves' disease risk.

In contrast to the thus far limited research interest in *InF*γ, there have been five studies of *TNF*β gene polymorphisms in Graves' disease (Badenhoop et al., 1992; Cavan et al., 1994a; Kamizono et al., 2000; Maalej et al., 2000; Villanueva et al., 2000), with the increased interest in *TNF*β over *InF*γ probably partly because the *TNF*β gene is located in the MHC class III region, between class II and class I. The first study, in a Caucasian population, found a small increase in the frequency of the normally less frequent 5.5 kb *TNF*β gene NcoI restriction fragment polymorphism (RFLP) in Graves' patients (RR: 1.3); however, this polymorphism was in strong linkage disequilibrium with the Caucasian "high-risk" Graves' HLA haplotype A1/B8/DR3, and although the small increment in Graves' risk seemed to persist when the investigators controlled for DR3 status, the results do not support a major role for the *TNF*β gene as a possible Graves' disease susceptibility gene (Badenhoop et al., 1992). This is supported by the fact that subsequent studies in Chinese and North African populations failed to confirm the findings of the original study (Cavan et al., 1994a; Maalej et al., 2000). The remaining two studies examined the role of *TNF*β polymorphisms in the pathogenesis of Graves' ophthalmopathy, again with contradictory results. While Kamizono et al. (2000) found an association of a T 1031C polymorphism (located in the 5′ flanking region of the gene) with the presence and severity of Graves' ophthalmopathy in a Japanese patient population, no such associations were found by Villanueva et al.

Important proteins involved in intracellular processing and trafficking of antigens include the large multifunctional proteases (LMP2/7) and the transporters associated with antigen-processing proteins (TAP1/2), which, respectively, have a crucial role in antigen degradation into peptide fragments of suitable size for HLA binding and transport of the same to HLA complexes (Malnati et al., 1992; Momburg et al., 1992, 1994; Abbas et al., 1997; Thorsby, 1997). Both of these groups of molecules are encoded within the MHC class II region, between the HLA-DP and the HLA-DQ loci. This makes them particularly attractive Graves' disease susceptibility genes, given the established association between Graves' disease and this chromosomal region. There is also evidence that *LMP* and *TAP* genes are up-regulated in autoimmune thyroid disease (Sospedra et al., 1997; Vives-Pi et al., 1997). Thus far there have been no studies in Graves' disease patients examining *LMP* genes for genetic polymorphisms, but there has been a recent report examining a possible association between *TAP1/2* polymorphisms and Graves' disease risk. In a cohort of 235 Caucasian Graves' disease patients, alleles *TAP1*0301* (RR: 2.05) and *TAP2*0101* (RR: 2.2) were significantly overrepresented when compared with 218 healthy Caucasian controls, while the allele *TAP1*0401* showed a negative association with Graves' disease (RR: 0.25) (Rau et al., 1997). Moreover, in a subgroup of subjects selected for HLA *DQA1*0501* (127 patients, 70 controls), *TAP1*0301* (RR: 2.63) remained positively associated with Graves' disease, while the presence of *TAP1*0401* (RR: 0.22) continued to be inversely proportional to the presence of Graves' disease. This suggests that these two *TAP* alleles may convey HLA class II independent permissive or protective effects on Graves' disease risks. It will be interesting to see whether these promising early results will be reproduced in further studies, in particular in non-Caucasian populations.

T-cell Receptor Genes. Preferential peptide presentation to T cells will only result in an autoimmune response if T cells that recognize the autoantigen or pseudoautoantigen are present. The T-cell receptor determines antigen-HLA complex recognition and is therefore an obvious autoimmunity candidate gene. Normally, potentially autoreactive T cells are negatively selected in the infantile thymus; however, certain T-cell receptor polymorphisms may allow some enhanced degree of foreign–autoantigen cross-reactivity, and autoreactive T cells with certain T-cell receptor variants may also be less likely to be negatively selected.

A few studies have examined germline genetic T-cell receptor polymorphisms in relationship to Graves' disease. One early report suggested an overrepresentation of individuals heterozygous for a BglII RFLP at the T-cell receptor locus (RR: 3.01), which had additive increasing effects on disease risk with HLA-DR3 (combined RR: 8.31) (Demaine et al., 1987); thus far, this report not been confirmed. Subsequent studies have either found no association between Graves' disease and T-cell receptor polymorphisms (Demaine et al., 1989; Mangklabruks et al., 1991; Pickerill et al., 1993) or have suggested a relationship between T-cell receptor variants and autoimmune hypothyroidism rather than Graves' disease (Weetman et al., 1987).

Other Molecules Involved in Immune Response Regulation. Other molecules involved in thyrocyte–T cell interaction and in modulation of T-cell response are also of relevance and include CTLA4, cell-adhesion molecules, and various cytokines. The latter group of molecules, in particular the interleukins, are also important in the further steps of the autoimmune reaction, as they mediate many of the interactions between activated T cells and immune effector cells. Among this large group of potential Graves' susceptibility genes, the following have been studied: *CTLA4*, *IL-1α*, *IL-1β*, *IL-1*'s naturally occurring receptor antagonist *IL-1RN*, *IL-1* receptor, *IL-4*, *IL-4* receptor, *IL-6*, *IL-10* and *TGFβ*.

CTLA4 is a T-cell surface molecule that regulates T-cell response in ways that are not fully understood. Direct effects on T-cell receptor signaling may be involved in this process, as well as inhibition of CD28-dependent IL2-production. Overall, the net result of CTLA4 on T-cell function tends to be toward down-regulation.

Several studies have examined possible associations between Graves' disease and polymorphisms of the *CTLA4* gene on 2q33 (Yanagawa et al., 1995, 1997; Donner et al., 1997; Kotsa et al., 1997; Awata et al., 1998; Djilali-Saiah et al., 1998; Heward et al., 1998, 1999; Vaidya et al., 1999; Hunt et al., 2000; Park et al., 2000; Villanueva et al., 2000; Tomer et al., 2001), and it appears that *CTLA4* polymorphisms are associated with modest increases in autoimmune thyroid disease risk in general, and Graves' disease-risk in particular. It has been shown in a cohort of 133 Caucasian Graves' disease patients that the 106 base pair allele of an (AT)n microsatellite (*CTLA4.PCR1*), 642 nt upstream from the end of exon 3 in the 3′ UTR of the *CTLA4* gene, has been significantly overrepresented, compared to 85 control subjects (RR: 2.82) (Yanagawa et al., 1995). Interestingly, the observed increase in the frequency of the 106 bp allele was particularly pronounced among those Graves' disease individuals with "protective" HLA haplotypes (*DQA1*0201+/* DQA1*0501−). More recent work has corroborated these early observations, demonstrating an HLA-type independent significant increase in the 106 bp *CTLA4.PCR1* allele in 112 Caucasian Graves' disease patients compared to 91 control subjects (RR: 2.1) (Kotsa et al., 1997). In addition, this study found a similar relationship between frequency of the 106 bp *CTLA4.PCR1* allele in 44 patients with autoimmune thyroiditis and the 91 control subjects (RR: 2.2).

The 106 bp *CTLA4.PCR1* allele is in strong linkage disequilibrium with a nt 49 A to G polymorphism in exon 1 of the *CLTA4* gene. Not surprisingly, several studies have found very similar associations between this single-nucleotide polymorphism and Graves' disease or autoimmune thyroiditis, in Caucasian, Japanese, and Korean populations (Donner et al., 1997; Yanagawa et al., 1997; Awata et al., 1998; Djilali-Saiah et al., 1998; Heward et al., 1999; Hunt et al., 2000; Park et al., 2000). In addition, this polymorphism may predispose to IDDM (again with a more marked increase in risk for individuals with "non-permissive" HLA types), suggesting that *CTLA4* gene polymorphisms may convey some generalized increase in the risk of autoimmune endocrine disorders. This notion, of a *CTLA4* polymorphism-mediated generalized increase in autoimmune endocrine risk, is further supported by recent data that show genetic linkage of the *CTLA4* locus to thyroid autoantibody production, but not directly to Graves' disease or autoimmune hypothyroidism risk (Tomer et al., 2001). Finally, observations suggesting that *CTLA4* polymorphisms may, at least to a minor degree, also modulate Graves' ophthalmopathy risk again suggest a quite generalized role for genetic polymorphisms of *CTLA4* in autoimmune responses (Vaidya et al., 1999; Villanueva et al., 2000).

The autoimmune endocrine disease risk increase may be confined and specific to the 106 bp *CTLA4.PCR1* allele and the nt 49 A to G polymorphism, as most recently a nt −318 C to T change in the *CTLA4* promoter has been found to have no association with Graves' disease or autoimmune hypothyroidism in either Caucasians or Chinese individuals (Heward et al., 1998).

The mechanisms by which the 106 bp *CTLA4.PCR1* allele and the nt 49 A to G polymorphisms may affect CTLA4 function remain uncertain. The nt 49 A to G polymorphism results in a Thr to Ala change in the leader peptide of the expressed protein, which could affect protein targeting or trafficking. Alternatively, the length of the 3′ UTR *CTLA4.PCR1* microsatellite might affect *CTLA4* mRNA stability. Either mechanism could account for net changes in CTLA4-mediated T-cell down-regulation. It might be speculated that such effects could be particularly relevant in situations when antigen presentation is less permissive. The overwhelming effects of "high risk" HLA-type antigen presentation may overcome any down-regulation of T-cell response by CTLA4, while less-efficient presentation by "low-risk" HLA molecules may only elicit an autoimmune T-cell response if CTLA-4 mediated down-regulation is deficient.

Alternatively, both the nt 49 A–G polymorphism and the 3′ UTR 106 bp *CTLA4.PCR1* microsatellite polymorphism may simply be markers for as yet unidentified susceptibility genes located nearby and in linkage disequilibrium with these *CTLA4* polymorphisms. Most notably, such candidates include the homologous and adjacent *CD28* gene. However, genetic linkage studies have recently suggested that *CTLA4*, rather than *CD28*, is more likely to be the primary susceptibility gene (Tomer et al., 2001).

In contrast to the results for *CTLA4*, which suggest some possible general permissive role in Graves' disease etiology, neither *IL-1* nor *IL-1RN* genetic polymorphisms have been convincingly linked to Graves' disease. An initial report suggesting a weak association between the *IL-1RN*2* allele and Graves' disease (RR: 1.7) (Blakemore et al., 1995) has not been confirmed by a subsequent study (Cuddihy and Bahn, 1996). Similarly, specific *IL-1α* alleles do not seem to aggregate among Graves' patients (Cuddihy and Bahn, 1996). Other cytokines have only rarely been studied, but a recent report suggests that a *Il-4* gene promoter polymorphism may be overrepresented in patients with autoimmune thyroid disease, particularly those suffering from Graves' disease (Hunt et al., 2000).

Immune Effector Genes. TSHR-stimulating autoantibody production is the final pathogenetic link in the etiological chain of events leading to Graves' disease. The magnitude of autoantibody production and the characteristics of the antibodies produced are likely to be of importance in determining whether significant Graves' disease-causing TSHR stimulation occurs at all, and, if it does, whether it will be severe or mild. The diversity of antibodies results from both germline and somatic genetic recombination events. Some of the differences in the antibody repertoire between individuals may be detectable by the study of immunoglobulin gene polymorphisms relating to germline recombination events. IgG heavy-chain allotypes have been studied and linked to Graves' disease in one of the first linkage records describing HLA–Graves' disease associations (Uno et al., 1981). However, the results of several subsequent studies have been contradictory (Kozma et al., 1985; Rechavi et al., 1987; Shields et al., 1994; Tomer et al., 1997; Barbesino et al., 1998a), and at present it remains unclear what role inherited IgG heavy-chain polymorphisms may have in determining the susceptibility to, or the severity of, Graves' disease. In addition, a recent study examining the somatically expressed TSHR autoantibody repertoire in Graves' disease has failed to convincingly show significant repertoire restriction, further arguing against a genetically determined pre-selective effect on TSHR autoantibody diversity (McIntosh et al., 1998).

Candidate Genes: Genes Unrelated to Immune Responses. Based on the general considerations discussed in the section regarding the pathophysiological basis of Graves' disease genetic susceptibility, immune response–related genes are only one of the factors potentially contributing to the development of Graves' disease or modifying its severity. Another large group of candidate genes includes all those genes coding for thyrocyte-specific proteins. On the one hand, polymorphisms in any of these may lead to proteins with antigenic structures that have an increased likelihood of initiating an aberrant immune response, either directly or indirectly, by having greater resemblance to foreign antigens than less-permissive isoforms. On the other hand, polymorphisms of functional consequence in any of the genes involved in TSH signaling or thyroid hormone production could also increase the risk of Graves' disease. For example, TSHR polymorphisms may increase the receptors' affinity to TSHR autoantibodies or may increase the degree or duration of transactivation after TSHR stimulating autoantibody binding, thus leading to thyrotoxicosis in the face of relatively minor autoantibody production, as may well transiently occur in many individuals. Conversely, a polymorphism that leads to decreased TSHR autoantibody binding or decreased receptor transactivation on binding might mitigate the severity of an otherwise strong autoantibody attack on the gland. Similar considerations apply to the TSHR downstream signaling pathways, the enzymatic machinery involved in thyroid hormone synthesis, and iodide and hormone transporter proteins. Cell-cycle regulatory and apoptotic pathways may also be subject to functional variability due to genetic polymorphisms, thus influencing the glands' response to autoimmune attack and autoantibody-mediated TSHR stimulation. Finally, factors related directly to neither the immune response nor the thyrocytes may play a role. For example, the degree of angiogenesis in response to Graves' disease–initiated thyroid hyperplasia may be partly genetically determined. Differences in glandular blood flow stemming from such genetic variations in angiogenesis could result in differences in substrate availability to the Graves' gland, thus modifying disease severity.

Of all these nonimmune response–related factors, only the TSHR has thus far been studied. Shortly after the cloning of the *TSHR* gene, two studies examined the receptor for polymorphisms in Graves' disease, using relatively incomplete mutation screening in the form of RFLP (Cai et al., 1992; Monden et al., 1992). Both studies failed to find any genetic polymorphisms in the *TSHR* in Graves' patients. However, a later study sequenced the entire receptor cDNA in a Graves' patient and found a germline polymorphism at codon 52 (C to A, codon change Pro to Thr), which subsequently also was identified in 4 out of 50 normal controls (Bohr et al., 1993). One subsequent study found that this polymorphism was associated with Graves' disease in female patients (Cuddihy et al., 1995), but several subsequent studies in various Caucasian and Asian populations failed to confirm these observations (Watson et al., 1995; Allahabadia et al., 1998; Simanainen et al., 1999; Sunthornthepvarakul et al., 1999; Kaczur et al., 2000).

Most recently two linkage studies have suggested that the *TSHR* is not a major susceptibility gene for Graves' disease. De Roux et al. (1996) examined possible linkage of the *TSHR* to Graves' disease in 14 Welsh and English families with 223 members, 44 of which were affected. They found an LOD score of −4.53 for a dominant inheritance model, thus effectively rejecting the hypothesis that the *TSHR* is linked to Graves' disease under these assumptions. Further, detailed analysis also failed to find evidence for *TSHR* linkage under a variety of other genetic assumptions. The scenarios tested included combined segregation and linkage analysis, correction for HLA-DR3 status, allowances for thyroid autoantibodies in clinically unaffected family members, a recessive disease model, and possible linkage disequilibrium between disease and marker alleles. This suggests that the *TSHR* is unlikely to contribute more than 5% to 10% to the Graves' disease risk. Smaller contributions cannot be discounted as the study lacked sufficient size to exclude such small effects. Data by Tomer et al. (1997, 1998) have supported these findings in a linkage analysis. They studied eight candidate gene regions, including *HLA*, *Tg*, *TPO*, *IgH*, *CTLA4*, *TSHR*, *IDDM4*, and *IDDM5* in 19 Caucasian families with 107 members, 14 of which had Graves' disease and 32 autoimmune thyroiditis. With the exception of the *TSHR* locus, only one marker per locus was used, resulting—not unpredictably, for such a relatively small study using relatively few markers—in a lack of evidence for possible linkage of any of these loci to autoimmune thyroid disease. By contrast, in Graves' disease individuals, an LOD score of more than 2 was obtained for one of the *TSHR*-related markers, *D14S81*. Subsequent linkage analysis of the Graves' patients' DNA samples with additional markers suggested that a Graves' disease susceptibility gene may map between *D14S81* (LOD score > 2) and *D14S65* (LOD score > 1.7). This interval is in 25 to 35 cM distance to the *TSHR* gene locus, and markers closer to *TSHR* gave LOD scores close to 0. This again suggests that the *TSHR* is not a major susceptibility locus for Graves' disease. However, it also suggests that there may be a significant susceptibility gene in the vicinity of *TSHR* on chromosome 14, between *D14S81* and *D14S65*. Interestingly, *D14S81* maps immediately adjacent to *D14S1062*, which has been defined as the upper boundary for the interval containing a postulated familial nontoxic nodular thyroid goiter gene (*MNG1*), while *D14S65* falls within this region, close to its lower boundary at *D14S267* (Bignell et al., 1997). Subsequent fine-mapping studies have confirmed this close spatial relationship between *MNG1* and the hypothetical Graves' disease susceptibility gene (*GD1*), mapping the latter within approximately 2 cM telomeric to *D14S81*, within no more than 3 cM from the most likely location of *MNG1* (Tomer et al., 1998). It may be that this chromosomal region contains one or more genes involved in regulation of thyrocyte growth, or thyrocyte response to growth-promoting stimuli, such as TSH stimulation.

In addition to *GD1*, the same research group has identified two further potential Graves' disease susceptibility loci, *GD2* on chromosome 20 at 56 cM (Genethone map) and GD3 at 114 cM (Genethone map) on the X chromosome (Tomer et al., 1999). Further, a region in the vicinity of the HLA locus on chromosome 6 was linked to both autoimmune hypothyroidism and Graves' disease (Tomer et al., 1999). It must be said, though, that the LOD scores obtained for any of these loci were only in the range of 2.1 to 3.5. Until actual candidate genes are identified and tested, it thus remains possible that one or several of these susceptibility loci represent spurious linkage. Alternatively, as suggested by the authors, Graves' disease may be genetically heterogeneous or polygenic, with different susceptibility genes acting and interacting in different families. The now near complete (complete in draft form) human genome sequence should facilitate the identification of candidate genes, which will allow investigators to verify the obtained linkage results and to address the questions of heterogeneity and gene interactions.

The marked preponderance of female patients among individuals with autoimmune thyroid disease has prompted linkage studies of selected gender-related genes and the X chromosome (Barbesino et al., 1998b). These studies have effectively ruled out linkage to the estrogen receptor α and aromatase genes and have made linkage to the estrogen receptor β gene unlikely, although lack of precise mapping information about this gene's position precluded a conclusive result. By contrast, the analysis of the X-chromosome markers suggested the possible presence of a Graves' disease susceptibility locus at Xq21.33–2 within a 6 cM interval between *DX1196* and *DX1220*, with the maximum recorded LOD score being 2.5 at *DX8020*.

Finally, the known clustering of Graves' disease with other autoimmune endocrine diseases, in particular Type I diabetes, has prompted the investigation of known Type I diabetes susceptibility loci for linkage to Graves' disease (Vaidya et al., 2000). This has led to the identification of a potential Graves' disease susceptibility locus in the vicinity of the Type I diabetes susceptibility locus *IDDM6* on chromosome 18. Fine mapping yielded a maximum nonparametric linkage score of 3.46 (p = .0003) at *D18S487*. Since this region has been previously linked not only to Type I diabetes but also to a number of other autoimmune diseases, such as rheumatoid arthritis and systemic lupus erythematosus, it appears likely that it contains a gene(s) involved in general immune regulation, which, similar to *CTLA4* polymorphisms, may increase the overall susceptibility to autoimmune diseases.

Genome-Wide Screens. The International Consortium for the Genetics of Autoimmune Thyroid Disease has completed a genome-wide screen on 56 multigenerational families (354 individuals) with both Graves' disease and autoimmune hypothyroidism and is continuing their efforts. As outlined above, this has resulted in the identification of several candidate loci, which are awaiting verification and further study (Barbesino et al., 1998a, 1998b; Tomer et al., 1998, 1999).

Clinical Application of Genetic Information

To date, no definite strong Graves' disease susceptibility genes have been discovered. As described, the associations with various immune system–related genes, chiefly the HLA system, are relatively weak, and work on identifying other, nonimmune system–related susceptibility genes is recent and incomplete. Consequently, the effect of genetics on clinical management of Graves' disease has been small. Its major effect relates to the classical epidemiological–genetic observations of increased familial Graves' disease risk and increased personal and familial risk of other autoimmune, particularly endocrine system diseases. These epidemiological observations are applied daily by clinicians in patient counseling and planning of follow-up strategies. In this setting, occasionally HLA typing can be useful in identifying family members of index cases who are at particularly high risk or gauging an individual's risk for another autoimmune disease a little more precisely. Calculations based on available sib-pair data suggest that HLA-B8$^+$ females with an affected first-degree relative have a 11.44% chance of developing Graves' disease themselves, while those who are HLA-DR3$^+$ and have affected family members face a 14.91% risk. The corresponding percentages for B8 or DR3 positive males are 2.86% and 3.73%, respectively. By contrast, HLA-B8 and HLA-DR3 negative males or females with a family history of Graves' disease face only about one-third of the disease risk of their B8- or DR3-positive counterparts (Stenszky et al., 1985). However, links with permissive HLA histotypes are not of sufficient strength to allow more precise predictions, and the association of some HLA types with Graves disease is far to weak to be useful for any applications outside of personal or family counseling, such as population screening.

HLA typing may eventually find a larger role in predicting response to treatment or disease relapse. There have been a number of studies hinting at such relationships, but to date the results remain highly contradictory (Dahlberg et al., 1981; McKenna et al., 1982; Allannic et al., 1983; Schleusener et al., 1989; Ratanachaiyavong et al., 1990; Badenhoop et al., 1996; Tamai et al., 1996). The most interesting and clinically valuable finding among these studies may be the observation that in some populations the risk of serious, hematological side effects of antithyroid drug treatment are considerably higher in patients with certain HLA histotypes (Tamai et al., 1996). If confirmed, this observation could be of considerable clinical value.

Testing for other, non-HLA-related, possibly disease-linked, genetic polymorphisms remains of unproved value and at this point has to be considered as purely experimental, even in the limited setting of family counseling. *CTLA4* polymorphisms have emerged as the most promising candidates from this group, and pending further confirmation they may eventually find a place in identifying Graves'-susceptible individuals, in particular, those who may also be particularly predisposed to severe thyroid eye disease. Undoubtedly, over time, additional candidate genes will emerge. In the meantime, for those families who are participating in linkage studies, stronger predictions of disease risk for as yet clinically unaffected members are sometimes already possible, based on the linkage patterns observed over several generations.

Autoimmune Hypothyroidism (Autoimmune Thyroiditis)

Disease Definition

Diagnostic Criteria. Primary hypothyroidism is defined as symptoms or signs of thyroid hormone deficiency in the presence of lowered serum thyroid hormone levels and elevated serum TSH levels and in the absence of pituitary disease. Patients may or may not have a goiter. There is usually no history of thyroid or neck pain. On the basis of severity of biochemical and clinical abnormalities, hypothyroidism is subdivided into mild or subclinical hypothyroidism (no or minimal symptoms and normal or borderline low serum thyroid hormone levels and a TSH of no more than 2 or 3 time the upper limit of the normal reference range), and "frank" hypothyroidism (symptoms of hypothyroidism and clear reduction in serum thyroid hormone levels or elevation of the TSH level to more than 2 or 3 times the upper limit of the normal reference range).

While iodine deficiency is probably the most common cause of hypothyroidism on a global scale, in iodine-sufficient regions the majority of cases of hypothyroidism are due to autoimmune thyroiditis and iatrogenic hypothyroidism, the latter usually as a consequence of thyroid ablative therapy. A minority of patients will present with transient hypothyroidism due to subacute thyroiditis, and a very small minority of patients will suffer from congenital or hereditary forms of hypothyroidism, some of which are summarized in the section on inherited single-gene abnormalities of thyroid hormone metabolism. Consequently, in iodine-sufficient countries, patients with hypothyroidism are assumed to suffer from autoimmune thyroiditis, unless there is a history indicating previous thyroid ablation, subacute thyroiditis (prominent neck pain and transient thyrotoxicosis preceding the hypothyroidism), or congenital/hereditary hypothyroidism. The presence of autoantibodies to different thyrocyte components, chiefly Tg and TPO autoantibodies, is further supportive evidence.

Clinically, goiterous (often referred to as Hashimoto's thyroiditis) and nongoiterous (also called atrophic hypothyroidism) forms of autoimmune hypothyroidism are recognized. However, histologically, there are no significant differences between the two types: both feature variable degrees of fibrosis of the gland, inflammatory lymphocytic infiltrates, and loss of follicular epithelium.

Clinical Features and Outcome. As in thyrotoxicosis, the symptoms and signs of hypothyroidism can be highly variable between different patients with similar changes in thyroid hormone levels. Most patients will complain of some degree of fatigue, loss of energy, and sleepiness. Other common symptoms include depression, cold intolerance, hoarseness, constipation, dry skin, hair loss, weight gain, and menstrual disturbances. Muscle pain, compression neuropathies, and generalized neuropathy and anemia can occur. Occasionally pseudodementia or psychosis may be seen. Clinical signs include a general "puffy" appearance, non-pitting edema, dry skin, slow movements and speech, hoarseness, bradycardia, and hyporeflexia with delayed relaxation. A goiter may or may not be present; if present, it is usually painless and homogenous but can be nodular at times. Serum thyroid function tests confirm the diagnosis. In the absence of other causes for hypothyroidism, most cases are due to autoimmune thyroiditis, and the majority of patients will suffer permanent hypothyroidism. The exception are females with postpartum thyroiditis, which is transient in most, but not all, patients and individuals with silent, transient thyroiditis which is characterized by a small goiter and minimal lymphocytic infiltration. Transient thyroiditis may be asymptomatic and focal and is sometimes only discovered incidentally at thyroid biopsy or at autopsy.

Before the advent of thyroxine replacement therapy, hypothyroidism resulted in severe and usually lifelong disability and, sometimes, death by myxedema coma. Thyroxine treatment has radically altered this situation, with complete cure being the result in nearly all patients, although symptoms and signs of hypothyroidism may sometimes require several months of treatment for complete resolution. Despite this, the occasional patient will suffer some permanent damage; for example, pressure damage to a nerve, such as carpal tunnel syndrome, may no longer be reversible by the time treatment is initiated. For all but the transient cases, lifelong replacement therapy with thyroxine is indicated and will usually result in complete clinical and biochemical cure. Many patients with transient hypothyroidism may also benefit from some weeks or months of thyroxine treatment while thyroid function recovers.

General Genetic and Epidemiological Evidence

Clinical Epidemiology. As is the case for Graves' disease, hypothyroidism due to autoimmune thyroiditis occurs in all human populations, with no clear evidence for any ethno-specific disease risk. The incidence is between 0.6 in 1000 per year and 1 in 1000 per year for males and between 1 in 1000 per year and 11 in 1000 per year for females. The corresponding published prevalence rates are less than 1 in 1000 to 8 in 1000 for males and less than 1 in 1000 to more than 20 in 1000 for females (Vanderpump and Tunbridge, 1996). Autoimmune hypothyroidism is rare before the age of 25, but thereafter its incidence rises exponentially with age, reaching 15 to 20 in 1000 per year for females in the eighth and ninth decades of life (Vanderpump and Tunbridge, 1996). Again, females are far more likely than males to be affected at all ages, with the difference in risk comparable to the gender-specific risk difference observed in Graves' disease; however, the absolute numbers of patients are much larger than in Graves' disease, with females having as much as a 1 in 6 lifetime risk of developing autoimmune hypothyroidism.

Family Epidemiology. Similar to Graves' disease, autoimmune hypothyroidism clusters in families. Dunning (1959) first described the familial occurrence of Hashimoto's thyroiditis, and there have been many reports since, both for Hashimoto's thyroiditis and for atrophic autoimmune hypothyroidism (Hall et al., 1964; Lee et al., 1964; Assem et al., 1965; Hall, 1965; Foley et al., 1968; Hall et al., 1972; Gordin et al., 1979; McGregor et al., 1979). In addition to clinically evident cases within families, a high rate of thyroid autoantibody positivity among family members has been observed, further paralleling the experiences in Graves' disease (Hall et al., 1964, 1972; Assem et al., 1965; Gordin et al., 1979; Fenzi et al., 1986). Finally, again in concordance with the Graves' disease data, inheritance rather than shared environment seems to be the major factor in this familial clustering, as evidenced by substantially higher concordance rates in monozygotic twins versus dizygotic twins (Irvine et al., 1961; Brix et al., 2000)

The many parallels between Graves' disease and autoimmune hypothyroidism with regard to general and family epidemiology may reflect some shared underlying susceptibility mechanism. Families displaying clustering of either condition may also contain individuals who are affected by the other condition or have serological evidence of thyroid autoantibodies. For example, Doinach et al. showed in 1965 that among 195 relatives of patients with Hashimoto's thyroiditis, 21 suffered likewise, 2 were affected by atrophic hypothyroidism, 17 had Graves' disease, and a further 12 had either a goiter or positive serum thyroid autoantibody tests.

Association with Other Diseases. The susceptibility within individuals and families to other endocrine and non-endocrine autoimmune conditions is also shared between Graves' disease and autoimmune hypothyroidism. The spectrum of associated autoimmune conditions is virtually identical, again including, roughly in order of likelihood, Type 1 diabetes, Addison's disease, celiac disease, multiple sclerosis, rheumatoid arthritis, systemic lupus erythromatosis, psoriasis, and inflammatory bowel disease. In addition, there is a particularly strong association between autoimmune hypothyroidism and pernicious anemia (Lee et al., 1964; Doniach et al., 1965).

Environmental Factors. It appears that at least some of the genetic factors predisposing to the development of autoimmune hypothyroidism may be the same as those that predispose to Graves' disease. Given the appropriate environmental triggers, there may be a general genetic predisposition in some individuals to develop thyroid autoimmune disease. It even appears that some of this genetic predisposition may be of a very general nature, also increasing the risk of other autoimmune disease. Additional factors seem to determine whether individuals with such a generalized permissive genetic makeup will develop Graves' disease or autoimmune hypothyroidism and whether they will develop any of the associated autoimmune diseases. Some of these modifiers may also be genetic, but others are likely to be environmental. This hypothesis is supported by the fact that autoimmune hypothyroidism is associated with some environmental risk factors that are distinctly different from those observed in Graves' disease. Congenital rubella infection is associated with an increased prevalence of thyroid autoantibodies and autoimmune hypothyroidism, suggesting that under certain circumstances infectious agents may be involved in triggering autoimmune hypothyroidism. However, in general, there is much less evidence for infectious triggers in autoimmune hypothyroidism than in Graves' disease, and, in particular, neither *Yersinia enterocolitica* nor retroviruses seem to be important. By contrast, the general state of the immune system seems to be of particular importance, as evidenced by postpartum thyroiditis, which occurs during the immune reactivity rebound from the normal pregnancy-associated immunosuppressive state. Specifically, certain cytokines, in particular InFα, involved in immune system stimulation may play a prominent role in triggering autoimmune hypothyroidism in susceptible individuals (Weetman and McGregor, 1994; Amenomori et al., 1998; Fernandez-Soto et al., 1998). Other reasonably well supported environmental factors include iodine, in particular a sudden increase in environmental iodine exposure, and advancing patient age (Weetman and McGregor, 1994). Increases in iodine exposure are likely to trigger transient increased metabolic thyroid activity, while advancing age can be associated with increased clonal diversity within the thyroid on the basis of somatic mutations and clonal selection, resulting in foci of suboptimally controlled thyroid metabolic activity (Studer and Derwahl, 1995). In both cases there may be an increased likelihood of autoantigen presentation in susceptible individuals triggering autoimmune hypothyroidism; however, why this should not also lead to increased Graves' disease risk remains a mystery.

Pathophysiological Basis of Genetic Susceptibility

General Pathophysiology. The histopathology of autoimmune thyroiditis is not too dissimilar to Graves' disease, with a prominent cellular inflammatory infiltrate; however, nests of fibrosis and regions of clear loss of follicular cells are much more prominent than in Graves' disease. Increasing loss of follicular epithelium gradually leads to hypothyroidism. During this process, compensatory growth of intact follicles under the influence of rising TSH levels, in conjunction with the cellular inflammatory infiltrate, leads to the appearance of a goiter, typical for Hashimoto's thyroiditis. By contrast, if follicular destruction is particularly rapid or if significant titers of TSHR-blocking autoantibodies are present, no goiter will develop, leading to the clinical picture of atrophic autoimmune hypothyroidism (Fig. 20–4).

It is likely that presentation and abnormal processing of one or several thyroid autoantigens is one of the earliest steps in initiating the chain of events that lead to the final pathological picture. In contrast to Graves' disease, no likely causative or disease-initiating autoantigen has been identified, although the majority of patients with autoimmune thyroiditis will have measurable serum autoantibody levels to thyroid antigens, mainly Tg and TPO, but also TSHR autoantibodies. The latter are uncommonly found in the goiterous type of autoimmune hypothyroidism, but they probably occur in most instances of atrophic autoimmune hypothyroidism (Rees Smith et al., 1988; Tomer and Davies, 1993; Weetman and McGregor, 1994; McIntosh et al., 1998). In cases in which these TSHR autoantibodies have been functionally characterized, they are of the receptor blocking variety and thus probably contribute to the development of hypothyroidism when they are present (Fig. 20–4). They may also be partly responsible for the lack of a significant goiter in some patients (see above). By contrast, the TPO and Tg autoantibodies are probably epiphenomena rather than pathogenic, being secondary to thyrocyte destruction and exposure of hidden antigens. It does not appear that these antibodies mediate any significant thyrocyte destruction. For this reason, it was long assumed that T cell–mediated cytotoxicity is at the center of follicular destruction in autoimmune thyroiditis. However, evidence

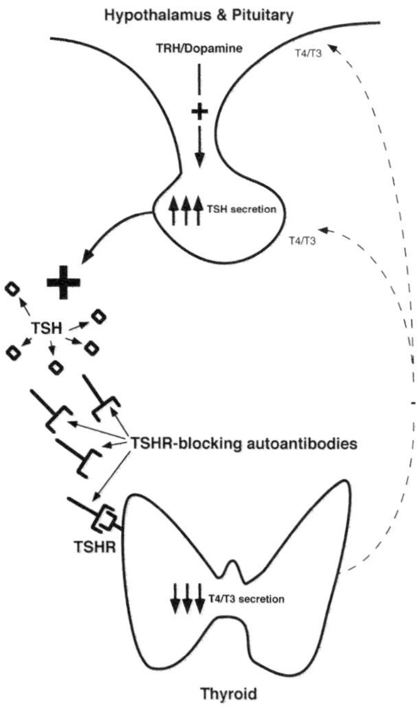

Fig. 20–4. Failure of hypothalamic-pituitary-thyroid feedback regulation of thyroid hormone production in autoimmune hypothyroidism with thyrotropin receptor-blocking autoantibodies. In atrophic autoimmune hypothyroidism, autoantibodies bind tightly to the thyrotropin receptor (TSHR), but fail to transactivate it. TSHRs blocked by these autoantibodies become inaccessible to thyrotropin (TSH) molecules. This results in diminished thyroid hormone production, which, in turn, leads to increased TSH secretion. However, in the presence of tightly bound TSHR-blocking autoantibodies, even high concentrations of TSH are unable to displace these autoantibodies from the TSHRs, and serum thyroid hormone levels fail to rise.

for a direct cytotoxic effect of T cells on thyrocytes has also been scant. Therefore, the last few years have seen a trend away from the study of T-cell cytotoxicity and toward other potential mechanisms of thyrocyte destruction.

There is now good evidence that apoptosis is the main mechanism of follicular cell death in autoimmune thyroiditis (Kotani et al., 1995; Tanimoto et al., 1995; Arscott and Baker, 1998; Giordano et al., 1997; Hammond et al., 1997; Ludgate and Jasani, 1997). IL-1β and Fas ligand (FasL) seem to be the mediators of the apoptotic response, with IL-1β regulating the level of Fas expression, and FasL cross-linking inducing apoptosis. Fas and FasL are constitutively expressed at low levels by normal thyrocyte; therefore, up-regulation of expression by IL-1β is probably at the center of the pathological apoptotic response in autoimmune thyroiditis (Giordano et al., 1997). Cytotoxic T cells seem to make a negligible contribution to either IL-1β or FasL production, so it seems unlikely they play any significant role in follicular cell death. It appears that infiltrating monocytes and macrophages are the main sites of IL-1β production and probably play a crucial role in the disease process (Giordano et al., 1997). However, recently CD4$^+$ T cells were shown to express FasL in response to MHC class II molecules presented by thyrocytes. Hence, in the context of aberrant HLA class II expression of thyrocytes, as it occurs in autoimmune hypothyroidism, CD$^+$ T-cell FasL expression may contribute to thyrocyte death (Kawakami et al, 2000). Further factors contributing to the increased thyrocyte apoptosis rate are yet to be determined, but BCL-2 down-regulation may be involved (Mitsiades et al., 1998), and it seems likely that other apoptosis-regulating pathways will be found to show abnormal activity in autoimmune thyroiditis.

Possible Genetic Basis of Autoimmune Thyroiditis. In summary, the steps involved in the development of autoimmune hypothyroidism are autoantigen recognition, followed by initiation of an abnormal immune response, which, in turn, leads to thyrocyte destruction. In this case, the abnormal immune response consists mainly in cellular inflammatory infiltration of the gland, with monocytes, macrophages, and CD4$^+$ cells initiating follicular cell apoptosis via IL-1β secretion and FasL expression. As thyrocytes are destroyed, further autoantigens are released, leading to a secondary humoral immune response. Most of the autoantibodies generated in this phase are of no pathogenetic significance, but if significant titers of TSHR-blocking autoantibodies are produced, they are likely to contribute to the disease, increasing its severity and limiting regenerative follicular growth due to TSH stimulation. Immune system–related genes that may be involved in the regulation of these events, as well as apoptosis-related genes and again the *TSHR* gene and other genes regulating TSH response in thyrocytes, are all potential disease candidate genes. The range of candidates to test is therefore very similar to Graves' disease, plus additionally apoptosis-related genes.

Gene Identification

Compared with Graves' disease, there is considerably less literature on candidate susceptibility genes for autoimmune hypothyroidism. Consequently, our knowledge about the genetic factors that influence the risk of autoimmune hypothyroidism is very incomplete. Efforts to find autoimmune thyroiditis susceptibility genes have largely mirrored similar efforts in Graves' disease. Often overlapping patient populations have been studied for similar candidate susceptibility genes, and often results of candidate gene studies of autoimmune thyroiditis and Graves' disease have been reported in combination. By contrast, the recent insights into the apoptotic basis of thyrocyte death have so far not been explored in any published genetic association or linkage studies of autoimmune hypothyroidism.

Candidate Genes: Immune Response Genes. Candidate immune response genes in autoimmune hypothyroidism include several genes that have also been studied in Graves' disease, most prominently the HLA genes.

Human Leukocyte Antigen (HLA) Genes. Association studies between HLA type and autoimmune hypothyroidism have yielded conflicting results. Unlike Graves' disease, where associations between certain HLA types and disease risk have at least been established within ethnic groups, and possible underlying common risk genes are beginning to emerge, no consistent association between HLA type and disease risk has been found for autoimmune thyroiditis.

Initial studies in Caucasian populations found no significant increase in DR3 in patients with autoimmune hypothyroidism (Weetman and McGregor, 1994). Subsequent studies, including a meta-analysis, have suggested a weak correlation between autoimmune hypothyroidism and HLA serotypes DR3 and DR4 (Jenkins et al., 1992; Weetman and McGregor, 1994). DR3 may be associated specifically with the atrophic variety of autoimmune thyroiditis (Farid et al., 1981), although other studies directly contradict these results, finding DR4 associated with goitrous hypothyroidism (Bogner et al., 1992). Overall, there is insufficient literature to draw any firm conclusions. In particular, DR4 may be associated with postpartum thyroiditis, one of the sometimes self-remitting subforms of autoimmune thyroiditis that occurs after pregnancy (Jansson et al., 1985). Caucasian subjects with any form of goiterous autoimmune hypothyroidism may also have increased frequencies of the DR5 serotype (Farid et al., 1981; Badenhoop et al., 1990; Tandon et al., 1991). In this group of patients, the combination of DR4 and DR5 seems to convey a particularly strong risk (RR: 15.3) (Badenhoop et al., 1990).

In non-Caucasian populations, even less data are available (Weetman and McGregor, 1994). Various HLA alleles have been implicated in these non-European populations (Weetman and McGregor, 1994), including a possible protective role of *DQA1*0102* and *DQB1*0602* in Japanese populations (Tamai et al., 1994). The relative paucity of studies makes these data difficult to interpret. However, one overall conclusion can be drawn from the comparison of the Caucasian and non-Caucasian data that, similar to Graves' disease, the risk haplotypes with regard to the DR locus are not the same in non-Caucasians as in Caucasians. This suggests that the primary susceptibility HLA locus for autoimmune hypothyroidism may be another HLA-II locus in linkage disequilibrium with DR in Caucasians and with other alleles in non-Caucasians. It also appears that HLA type is much less strongly associated with autoimmune hypothyroidism than with Graves' disease. Finally, some HLA subtypes may be selectively associated with autoimmune thyroid disease occurring in the context of cytokine treatment, in particular interferon-α treatment, with the HLA-A2 subtype conferring significantly increased susceptibility to the development of treatment-related autoimmune hypothyroidism (Kazikaki et al., 1999, 2000).

T-cell Receptor Genes. One of the studies examining T-cell receptor polymorphisms in Graves' disease also included a cohort of patients with autoimmune hypothyroidism. While this study failed to show any association between Graves' disease and T-cell receptor polymorphisms, it suggested a relationship between T-cell receptor variants and autoimmune hypothyroidism (Mangklabruks et al., 1991). Unfortunately, the study was relatively small, and limited information about the control population was provided. The role of T-cell receptor genetic polymorphisms in determining the risk of autoimmune hypothyroidism must therefore still be regarded as uncertain.

Other Molecules Involved in Immune Response Regulation. One of the studies reporting an association of the 106 bp *CTLA4.PCR1* microsatellite allele with Graves' disease found a similar association between autoimmune thyroiditis and the same *CTLA4.PCR1* microsatellite allele (Kotsa et al., 1997). These findings have been corroborated in Caucasian and Japanese populations for the *CTLA4* 49 A–G polymorphism, which is in linkage disequilibrium with the disease-associated 106 bp *CTLA4.PCR1* microsatellite allele (Awata et al., 1998; Djilali-Saiah et al., 1998). Interestingly, the homozygous 49 G–G genotype seems to be particularly strongly associated with atrophic autoimmune hypothyroidism, with an RR of almost 9 (Djilali-Saiah et al., 1998). As in Graves' disease, the known *CTLA4* promoter polymorphism does not seem to be overrepresented in patients with autoimmune hypothyroidism (Heward et al., 1998). Finally, once more paralleling the results in Graves' disease, limited linkage analysis has failed to show linkage of *CTLA4* to autoimmune hypothyroidism (Tomer et al., 1997; Barbesino et al., 1998a). This makes it unlikely that *CTLA4* polymorphisms contribute substantially more than 10% to the risk of autoimmune hypothyroidism or Graves' disease.

From the combination of these various findings, one can conclude that there is a high likelihood that *CTLA4*, or a nearby gene in linkage disequilibrium, exerts a minor permissive effect on autoimmune thyroid disease (Graves' disease and autoimmune hypothyroidism) in general, most likely through some changes in regulation of T-cell response. This is supported by the observation that thyroid autoantibody production seems to be linked genetically to the *CTLA4* locus (Tomer et al., 2001). However, further data need to be collected to confirm these preliminary conclusions and to refine risk estimates.

Candidate Genes: Genes Unrelated to Immune Responses. Work on candidate susceptibility genes unrelated to the immune system has been very limited in autoimmune hypothyroidism. There is some experimental evidence for TSHR expression down-regulation in autoimmune hypothyroidism, but there are few data as to the mechanisms behind this phenomenon (Schuppert et al., 1996), and the *TSHR* has not been subjected to mutation screening in patients with autoimmune hypothyroidism. Linkage data suggest that the *TSHR* gene locus is not a major autoimmune hypothyroidism susceptibility locus (Tomer et al., 1997, 1998), while data from the same linkage analysis project also exclude a major role of the X chromosome and 14 Graves' disease susceptibility loci in autoimmune hypothyroidism (Barbesino et al., 1998a, 1998b). The data from these studies also exclude a major role of several gender-specific genes in determining significant proportions of autoimmune hypothyroidism risk (Barbesino et al., 1998b).

Genome-Wide Screens. A whole genome screen for genes linked to autoimmune thyroid disease was recently completed in a modest-sized cohort of families. It has suggested a region close to the HLA locus as a site for a susceptibility gene for both Graves' disease and autoimmune hypothyroidism. It has also revealed two further candidate regions, *HT-1* at 96 cM on chromosome 13, and *HT-2* at 97 cM on chromosome 12 (both Genethone map). However, no candidate genes have been identified thus far, and the LOD score for *HT-1* was only 2.1 and *HT-2* appeared to be disease-linked in only a subgroup of families (Tomer et al., 1999). As in Graves' disease, identification and testing of the candidate genes must be awaited before firm conclusions can be drawn.

Clinical Application of Genetic Information

Since knowledge of genetic determinants of autoimmune hypothyroidism risks is much smaller than that for Graves' disease, it comes as no surprise that these limited findings have not affected clinical management. Possible exceptions include identifying individuals at particular risk of interferon-related hypothyroidism. For other patients, classical genetic epidemiology can assist in advising individual patients and their families about the risks of other autoimmune diseases and risks of autoimmune hypothyroidism or Graves' disease in other family members, but there are no known serological or genetic polymorphisms that might help refine such assessments. This is in contrast to Graves' disease, where at least HLA typing is starting to play a minor, but sometimes significant, role. One would hope that increasing genotype–phenotype knowledge will change this situation, although most benefits of increased genetic knowledge would be in the areas of counseling and risk assessment. The incentive for large studies is much less than for Graves' disease, where treatment is not always optimal and may have side effects, thus providing increased impetus for genotype–phenotype correlations, especially with regard to responses to treatment and risks of side effects. By contrast, hypothyroidism is usually so successfully and completely treated with thyroxine replacement that it is hard to imagine that increased genetic information would be able to improve such management, unless it would lead to disease prophylaxis.

NODULAR THYROID DISEASE AND GOITER

Traditionally, structural abnormalities of the thyroid gland have been subdivided into "simple" or "smooth" goiter, nodular goiter, and solitary thyroid nodules. This subdivision was largely based on gross clinical appearances, and it is now becoming clear that goiters without nodules are rare, as are solitary nodules, but that small nodules often exist in clinically not enlarged thyroid glands, and that overall nodularity and goiter size tend to go hand in hand.

If the presence of any thyroid nodularity, no matter how small, is regarded as abnormal, then between 30% and 60% of individuals in most populations suffer from nodular thyroid disease (Bruneton et al., 1994; Wang and Crapo, 1997). In iodine-deficient regions, these figures may approach 100% (Lamberg, 1991). Most of these nodules will only be detectable by ultrasonographic examination of the thyroid gland and will never cause any clinical disease. In contrast to such subclinical nodular thyroid disease, clinically relevant nodular thyroid disease can be defined as nodular thyroid disease which either leads to mechanical problems because of goiter or nodule size or causes functional thyroid abnormalities as a result of nodular autonomy or is associated with malignancy. Using such criteria, clinically relevant nodular thyroid disease affects a much smaller number of patients than thyroid nodularity per se, but is nonetheless common; in iodine-deficient countries, it is the most common form of thyroid disease, while in iodine-replete countries it is the second most common cause of thyroid disease behind autoimmune thyroid disease.

Traditionally, nodular thyroid disease is subdivided into multinodular goiter (MNG) and solitary thyroid nodules. MNG is the most common form of clinical nodular thyroid disease. In its pure form there is simply goiterous enlargement of the gland associated with glandular nodularity. Nodules may show cystic degeneration, and hemorrhage into such nodules can cause pain and swelling and occasionally serious compression of airways or vascular structures in the neck. Similar problems may also arise as a result of increasing goiter size, particularly if MNG has significant retrosternal components. In addition to the mechanical problems of MNGs, such goiters have a tendency to develop a degree of thyroid autonomy, sometimes resulting in a toxic nodular goiter, the second most common cause of thyrotoxicosis after Graves' disease. Finally, nodules within an MNG can be malignant, the risk being probably slightly less than for solitary nodules, between 1% and 10% of which are malignant (Grebe et al., 1997; Grebe and Hay, 1999). Solitary thyroid nodules are much less common than MNG, and the main concern with any solitary thyroid nodule, or any nodule within an MNG that has rapidly enlarged in size, is malignancy. Mechanical problems, similar to those observed in MNG nodules, may also occur, and a small percentage of solitary nodules may represent autonomous thyroid adenomas leading to thyrotoxicosis. Thus, the disease spectrum associated with MNG and solitary thyroid nodules shows considerable overlap, and, as high resolution ultrasonography is increasingly applied to the diagnosis of nodular thyroid disease, it is becoming clear that true solitary thyroid nodules are very rare. Many clinically diagnosed lesions show evidence of additional nodularity on ultrasound scanning, and in light of these observations the separation into MNG and solitary nodules appears artificial. It might be more appropriate to classify nodular thyroid disease on the basis of the major clinical pathology caused by the nodules into uncomplicated nodular thyroid disease, where mechanical problems predominate, nodular thyroid autonomy, and malignant nodular thyroid disease. Even with this reclassification, the boundaries between categories are fluent, with some uncomplicated goiters eventually developing autonomy or a toxic goiter harboring a thyroid carcinoma. However, some fundamental pathogenetic differences between "simple" goiter, thyroid autonomy, and thyroid malignancy are beginning to emerge, and in the following this classification scheme will be used to characterize the known data regarding genetic susceptibility factors in the pathogenesis of these forms of nodular thyroid disease. In addition, we will include a discussion of medullary thyroid carcinoma (MTC) in the section on malignant nodular thyroid disease.

Uncomplicated Nodular Thyroid Disease

Disease Definition

Diagnostic Criteria. Uncomplicated nodular thyroid disease encompasses MNG and solitary nodules of the thyroid gland, which show neither evidence of autonomous function nor of malignancy. The normal thyroid gland is not palpable, and, hence, any gland that is at least palpable is defined as a goiter. Goiters are loosely classified by size: grade I is palpable but not visible; grade II is visible; grade III is large; and grade IV has compression of airways or neck structures. Traditionally, goiters are also subdivided into "simple" or "smooth" goiters, without any palpable nodularity, and nodular goiters. However, increasing use of ultrasonography in goiter assessment has shown that almost all goiters will have some evidence of nodularity. Using high-resolution ultrasonography, nodularity can also be demonstrated in a number of normal-sized glands, and it seems that nodularity and glandular enlargement develop in tandem. True solitary nodules within a normal gland are rare; more commonly, a solitary nodule is found within a grade I or grade II goiter, and ultrasonographic examination most often reveals additional nodules, too small to be palpable.

Regardless of whether a prominent nodule is present clinically or whether there is palpable nodularity throughout the goiter, classification as uncomplicated nodular thyroid disease requires biochemical proof of euthyroidism and exclusion of malignancy; the latter is most commonly achieved by fine needle aspiration biopsy (FNAB). This examination has excellent sensitivity and specificity in diagnosing papillary thyroid carcinoma (PTC), undifferentiated thyroid carcinoma, and follicular neoplasms, although in the latter case it often fails to distinguish benign follicular adenomas (FA) from follicular thyroid carcinomas (FTC) (Grebe and Hay, 1999).

Clinical Features and Outcome. Patients usually present with a visible goiter or nodule. Often a small hemorrhage into a nodule has led to its sudden enlargement, precipitating the consultation. On detailed questioning and examination of old photographs, it is clear that a minor degree of thyroid enlargement has usually been notable for some time preceding the first presentation to a medical practitioner. Occasionally patients will present much later with a large goiter causing neck discomfort, significant cosmetic problems, or positional dyspnea. In the case of uncomplicated nodular thyroid disease, serum thyroid function tests will be normal and FNAB of palpable nodules will show no evidence of thyroid neoplasia.

Clinical problems relating to uncomplicated nodular thyroid disease are those of local pressure on neck structures, such as vessels, nerves, and airway. Such pressure can be elicited by a large nodular goiter per se, particularly if it contains retrosternal components, or can be caused by sudden enlargement of a nodule following a hemorrhage into cystic portions of the nodule. Significant mechanical problems are an indication for surgical nodule extirpation, partial thyroidectomy, or, sometimes, radioiodine treatment. Fortunately, such problems are rare, and more commonly minor neck discomfort or cosmetic considerations predominate. In these cases surgery may occasionally still be indicated, but more commonly observation alone is required in the first instance, as a sizable proportion of "simple" goiters and small nodules will disappear over time (Mack, 1995; Hurley and Gharib, 1996; Anders, 1998; Gharib and Mazzaferri, 1998). Thyroxine therapy in TSH-suppressive doses can lead to a modest decrease in nodule or goiter size, greater than the natural remission tendency, in some individuals. This regression is not significant in most patients and can be associated with cardiac side effects in some susceptible individuals (Gartner, 1994; Lima et al., 1997; Gharib and Mazzaferri, 1998), and, as a consequence, thyroxine treatment of nodular thyroid disease is not widely used or recommended. There is a tendency for some nodular goiters to become larger over time and to develop a degree of autonomy, thus necessitating therapeutic intervention; however, the majority of cases of uncomplicated nodular thyroid disease will not require any medical intervention other than follow-up.

General Genetic and Epidemiological Evidence

Clinical Epidemiology. The incidence and prevalence figures for uncomplicated nodular thyroid disease vary widely between studies. This is due, first, to the use of different definitions of goiter and, second, to the fact that most older studies have used palpation to identify goiters and nodules, whereas recent work uses ultrasound. In addition, goiter and nodule rates vary widely with environmental iodine content. Thus, published prevalence figures of uncomplicated nodular thyroid disease vary between 1% and more than 60%. Excluding data pertaining to only ultrasonographically detectable nodular thyroid disease, the prevalence is between 1% and 31%, with women under the age of 40 being most often affected and men over the age of 75 displaying the lowest goiter or nodule frequency (Vanderpump and Tunbridge, 1996). By contrast, ultrasonographic data indicate that thyroid gland nodularity increases with age in both sexes (Brander et al., 1991; Hintze et al., 1991; Hsiao and Chang, 1995), and it appears that larger nodules and goiters may become manifest at an earlier age, whereas overall glandular nodularity gradually increases with age.

Family Epidemiology. Traditionally, uncomplicated nodular thyroid disease has been regarded as sporadic. However, several defined inherited syndromes of abnormal thyroid metabolism can be associated with uncomplicated nodular thyroid disease or goiter; in particular, all syndromes of thyroid dyshormonogenesis are usually associated with smooth or nodular goiters (Table 20–1). In addition, there is accumulating evidence for strong genetic factors in the development of uncomplicated nodular thyroid disease. A Scottish twin study conducted during the 1960s suggested as much as a 40% contribution of inheritance to the development of nodular goiter in females (Greig et al., 1967). More recently, a Danish twin study has confirmed these observations, suggesting that in females as much as 82% of the risk to develop a simple goiter is inherited (Brix et al., 1999). Although these results may overestimate the importance of genetic components in the development of uncomplicated nodular thyroid disease, a number of reasonably well documented series of familial nontoxic goiter suggest a larger inherited component than is generally assumed (Murray et al., 1966; Couch et al., 1986; Bignell et al., 1997; Burgess et al., 1997).

Association with Other Diseases. Nodular goiters arising in young children in the context of severe environmental iodine deficiency can be associated with mental retardation or even syndromatic cretinism. The majority of cases of uncomplicated nodular thyroid disease that occur in iodine-replete countries are not statistically significantly associated with any other diseases. A minority of patients may suffer tracheomalazia or positional and sleep apnea as a consequence of their large nodular goiter, but this is a direct result of the thyroid pathology rather than a disease association.

Environmental Factors. Iodine deficiency, directly and indirectly through slightly elevated TSH levels, is the major known environmental factor that affects nodular goiter development.

Pathophysiological Basis of Genetic Susceptibility to Uncomplicated Nodular Thyroid Disease

General Pathophysiology. The underlying pathology of nodular goiter is a heterogeneous proliferation of follicular cells, with different thyroid regions displaying differing degrees of new follicle formation. In addition to the differences in proliferation, different regions of the gland may also show evidence of functional heterogeneity, with marked variation in follicular cell morphology, size, and colloid content (Studer and Derwahl, 1995). The different types of uncomplicated nodular thyroid disease all fall within this framework of basic pathological changes. Solitary nodules represent one end of this spectrum, where growth is confined to a single region of the gland; multinodular goiters, with heterogeneous proliferation of thyrocytes throughout the gland, are at the other end of the spectrum. The postulated underlying mechanism for these phenomena are somatic genetic follicular heterogeneity, resulting in differences in sensitivity of thyrocytes to goiterogenic stimulation and differences in duration of thyrocyte stimulation to such stimuli (Studer and Derwahl, 1995). Classically, the most proliferative regions of a MNG will display some degree of autonomy, and there will be a spectrum of growth potential and autonomy throughout the gland, reflecting the somatic genetic heterogeneity. Within these boundaries goiter growth will be promoted by any extrinsic or intrinsic growth and functional activity promoting factors.

Possible Genetic Basis of Uncomplicated Nodular Thyroid Disease. All those genetic factors that predispose thyrocytes to develop excessive somatic genetic variation in growth and function regulating genes could be candidate nodular thyroid disease susceptibility genes. This includes a wide range of genes coding for DNA repair systems, DNA damage checkpoint proteins, and apoptosis-related factors. In addition, genetic variability in genes coding for thyroid growth promoting factors or receptors can be expected to increase the overall background thyroid growth stimulation. This would have the effects of exaggerating any intrathyroidal variability in growth potential, leading to nodularity, and promoting overall growth, leading to goiter.

Gene Identification

Despite, or maybe because of, the wide array of potential candidate MNG susceptibility genes, until recently there have been very few efforts to identify candidate susceptibility genes. This lack of activity may be because it was believed that MNG was not a predominately inherited disorder. With the realization that MNG may have a much larger genetic component than previously thought, however, research efforts have increased. Because of the large number of potential candidate genes, classical linkage analysis has been chosen initially to identify susceptibility loci. This has resulted in the identification of a candidate locus, named *MNG1*, at 14q, mapping between *D14S1062* and *D14S267* (Bignell et al., 1997). The linkage of *MNG1* to familial euthyroid goiter has been confirmed in a second, independent study, which at the same time excluded linkage to the *Tg*, *TPO*, and the sodium-iodide symporter gene loci (Neumann et al., 1999). The MNG1 region overlaps a potential Graves' disease susceptibility locus, and it may harbor one or several genes involved in regulating thyrocyte response to growth promoting stimuli. Further work to refine the locus mapping and identification of candidate genes in this region is eagerly awaited. A second susceptibility locus for an autosomal-dominant form of multinodular goiter has been mapped to Xp22, to a presently still relatively large interval of 9.6 cM between *DXS1052* and *DXS8039*, with the maximum LOD score of 4.73 being obtained at *DXS8039* (Capon et al., 2000).

Clinical Application of Genetic Information

With the exception of those families involved in the familial MNG projects, there are no clinical applications of the scant genetic information available on uncomplicated nodular thyroid disease. Within the familial MNG syndrome, identification of the 14q and Xp susceptibility loci should facilitate risk assessment of clinically unaffected members by linkage analysis.

Toxic Nodular Goiter and Autonomous Adenoma

Disease Definition

Diagnostic Criteria. Nodular thyroid disease associated with clinical (symptoms or signs of hyperthyroidism) and biochemical (suppressed serum TSH with or without elevated peripheral serum thyroid hormone levels in the absence of pituitary disease) evidence of thyrotoxicosis is defined as toxic nodular thyroid disease. There must be evidence of autonomous function of one or more nodules and no evidence of other causes of thyrotoxicosis—in particular, Graves' disease. Autonomous thyroid nodules function independently of the normal negative pituitary–thyroidal feedback mechanisms, and for any given serum TSH level they produce inappropriately large amounts of thyroid hormone and will continue to produce thyroid hormone, even in the total absence of TSH stimulation. Toxic nodular thyroid disease caused by a single autonomous nodule is defined clinically as autonomous adenoma, although strictly the diagnosis of adenoma would require histopathological confirmation. If there is more than one toxic nodule present, toxic nodular thyroid disease is classified as toxic nodular goiter. In either case, confirmation of the suspected diagnosis can be achieved by scinti-scanning with iodine or technetium isotopes. In a typical case of autonomous adenoma, radionuclide uptake will be confined to one (usually the only) palpable nodule. Further confirmation of diagnosis can be achieved by T3 suppression and TSH stimulation testing. The former is particularly useful if there is some residual isotope uptake within the normal thyroid tissue. Following T3 administration any residual endogenous TSH secretion will be suppressed. On repeat scanning, residual uptake within normal thyroid tissue will diminish or disappear as a consequence of withdrawal of residual TSH stimulation. By contrast, there will be little or no change to the uptake within the autonomous nodule whose function is less, or not at all, dependent on TSH stimulation. TSH stimulation testing is based on the reverse principal that repeat scanning after TSH administration will show increased isotope uptake in the normal thyroid portions, as they appropriately resume hormone production upon TSH stimulation. Toxic nodular goiter displays a similar response to T3 suppression and TSH stimulation testing, but results are more difficult to interpret, as there will be multiple toxic nodules, which will also vary in their degree of TSH autonomy.

Clinical Features and Outcome. The onset of thyrotoxicosis in toxic nodular goiter and autonomous adenoma tends to be gradual, often over many years or, sometimes, even decades. Consequently, many patients have no or mild symptoms or signs of thyrotoxicosis at presentation. In the past, the diagnosis was most often suspected on the basis of a scintigram obtained in the course of the evaluation of nodular thyroid disease for malignancy. However, with the increasing use of FNAB as the initial assessment tool for diagnosing thyroid cancer, this route of serendipitous diagnosis of toxic nodular thyroid disease has become rare. Most patients today are diagnosed on the basis of suppressed serum TSH levels measured with a sensitive TSH assay. The test is rarely obtained because thyrotoxicosis is suspected, and more often it forms part of the routine evaluation of nodular thyroid disease or is ordered for "routine screening" reasons. Another sizable portion of patients are diagnosed during the evaluation of cardiac arrhythmias. The minority of patients who present with classical symptoms and signs of thyrotoxicosis have either large, relatively rapidly growing MNGs or autonomous adenomas, or they may have had a radiological procedure involving administration of iodine containing contrast medium. The considerable and sudden iodine load provides massive amounts of substrate for hormone production, sometimes triggering a sudden increase in hormone output by the autonomous nodules of a toxic MNG or an autonomous adenoma.

Untreated toxic nodular thyroid disease gradually worsens over time, and treatment on diagnosis is indicated in most cases. The exception to this may be the young patient with minimal biochemical thyrotoxicosis (suppressed TSH only), who might be safely observed for some time. Since there is no naturally occurring remission in toxic nodular thyroid disease, medical therapy would have to be lifelong, and therefore ablative forms of therapy are favored in toxic nodular thyroid disease. Toxic MNG is best treated by radioiodine ablation, while for autonomous adenoma percutaneous ethanol injection or surgery are viable alternatives. The latter is the treatment of choice for very large autonomous adenomas.

General Genetic and Epidemiological Evidence

Clinical Epidemiology. The incidence and prevalence rates of toxic nodular goiter and autonomous adenoma vary widely between countries, in line with the incidence and prevalence rates of endemic goiter. In regions of high iodine intake, all forms of toxic nodular thyroid disease account for no more than 5% to 10% of cases of thyrotoxicosis, whereas in low iodine-intake regions 30% to 50% of cases of thyrotoxicosis may be caused by toxic nodular goiter and autonomous adenoma (Vanderpump and Tunbridge, 1996; Bauch, 1998; Siegel and Lee, 1998). In most Western countries, which have intermediate to high levels of dietary iodine intake, between 4% and 30% of cases of thyrotoxicosis are due to toxic nodular thyroid disease, which translates into absolute incidence figures of 5 to 40 in 100,000 per year (Bauch, 1998). For each case presenting with thyrotoxicosis, there are several cases with clear evidence of autonomy that remain euthyroid (Bauch, 1998). On the present evidence, at least 30% of these will progress to thyrotoxicosis over time. Regardless of overall incidence and prevalence, cases of toxic MNG outnumber cases of autonomous adenomas by at least 2-fold (usually by a much greater margin) (Weetman and McGregor, 1994; Bauch, 1998; Siegel and Lee, 1998). The gender distribution of toxic nodular thyroid disease mimics that of Graves' disease, with females outnumbering males by at least 3 to 1. In both males and females, there are very few cases in the first two decades of life, but thereafter incidence rates continue to rise with age, particularly after the age of 50, so that the majority of patients with thyrotoxicosis who present in the sixth decade of life or later will be found to suffer from toxic nodular thyroid disease rather than Graves' disease (Bauch, 1998).

Family Epidemiology. Clustering of typical toxic nodular thyroid disease within families has not been reported, although familial thyrotoxicosis with diffuse thyroid autonomy, associated with uniform goiter with little nodularity does occur (Paschke, 1996; Führer et al., 1998). This was first reported by Thomas et al. (1982) in a French family, where 16 of 48 family members were affected. All affected individuals had hyperthyroidism with diffuse or mildly nodular goiter. There was no clinical or biochemical evidence of autoimmune thyroid disease. Histopathological examination showed absence of any inflammatory infiltration of the gland, and all individuals relapsed after initial anti-thyroid drug treatment. Several similar families have been described since this initial cohort (Schwab et al., 1996; Fuhrer et al., 1997, 1998; Grüters et al., 1998), but overall such clearly inherited cases of autonomous thyrotoxicosis are rare.

Association with Other Diseases. There are no known associations of toxic nodular thyroid disease with other medical conditions, other than those that may be precipitated or worsened by the thyrotoxicosis (e.g., cardiac arrythmias).

Environmental Factors. Paralleling the observations in uncomplicated nodular thyroid disease, iodine intake is the only known environmental factor implicated in the development of toxic nodular thyroid disease.

Pathophysiological Basis of Genetic Susceptibility

General Pathophysiology. Toxic nodular thyroid disease can be seen as a special case of uncomplicated nodular thyroid disease. The same basic pathophysiological factors are at work, but in addition there is a tendency of nodules, or in the case of an autonomous adenoma, *the* nodule, to develop a significant degree of autonomy. This is the cause of gradually developing thyrotoxicosis.

Possible Genetic Basis of Toxic Nodular Goiter and Autonomous Adenoma. Besides the genetic factors listed in the section on uncomplicated nodular thyroid disease, the TSH signaling pathway is of particular interest with regard to genetic susceptibility to toxic nodular thyroid disease. Indeed, a large proportion of autonomous nodules have been found to carry activating TSH receptor mutations (Siegel and Lee, 1998). These are generally somatic mutations, and any genetic factors favoring such mutations will have to be considered as potentially predisposing to autonomous nodules. It is conceivable that a number of toxic MNGs are equally affected, although in most cases, the germline-attributable risk seems to be low. The exception is the case of familial autonomous thyrotoxicosis, where TSH receptor mutations are high on the list of candidate disease genes.

Gene Identification

Somatic mutations of the TSHR have been identified in many autonomous nodules, but germline mutations seem to be rare (see above). Similarly, there is some recent evidence for somatic mutations or polymorphisms in the TSHR of patients with toxic MNGs. Interestingly, and despite a lack of convincing evidence for a strong heritable element in toxic MNG, there is also evidence for an overrepresentation of at least one ubiquitously occurring polymorphism of the TSH receptor in germline DNA of individuals with toxic MNG (Gabriel et al., 1999). Compared with a normal reference population, Gabriel et al. (1999) found a 3.5-fold increase in the frequency of the D727E polymorphism in germline DNA from U.S. patients with toxic MNG. They also found that this polymorphism induces increased cAMP responses to TSH stimulation, but not autonomous function. This polymorphism may therefore convey moderate growth advantages to thyrocytes and predispose to goiter formation or autonomy if additional factors are present. However, a second study in a European population failed to confirm an association of the germline D727E polymorphism with toxic nodular goiter (Muhlberg et al., 2000). Therefore, at present, the importance of this polymorphism in predisposing individuals to toxic MNG remains unclear.

It should also be noted that, as expected, many of the families with familial autonomous thyrotoxicosis show evidence of germline TSH receptor activating mutations (Paschke, 1996; Schwab et al., 1996; Führer et al., 1997, 1998; Grüters et al., 1998).

Clinical Application of Genetic Information

Individuals with familial toxic goiter can be clearly identified, even in the pre-symptomatic stage, by TSHR mutation screening, which will assist in guiding management. The much larger group of patients with apparent sporadic toxic nodular thyroid disease do not enjoy similar benefits, although longitudinal studies of individuals with TSHR D727E polymorphisms may eventually prove valuable in determining the risk of certain individuals of developing toxic MNG.

MALIGNANT NODULAR THYROID DISEASE

Malignant nodular thyroid disease encompasses malignant tumors of follicular epithelium, as well as malignant neoplasms that arise from C cells (medullary carcinoma). Follicular cell–derived thyroid carcinoma accounts for the vast majority of cases of thyroid malignancy, whereas the medullary carcinomas contribute fewer than 5% of the total cases.

Follicular Cell–Derived Thyroid Carcinoma

Disease Definition

Diagnostic Criteria. There are three main types of carcinomas derived from follicular thyroid epithelium: PTC, FTC, and anaplastic carcinomas. Initial presentation is usually as a thyroid nodule, which in most instances is clinically indistinguishable from a benign hyperplastic solitary nodule, a benign hyperplastic nodule within an MNG, or a benign functioning or nonfunctioning FA. Cytological or histological confirmation of diagnosis is always required.

PTCs show evidence of follicular cell differentiation, typically with papillary and follicular structures, as well as characteristic large, pale-staining nuclei with a "ground glass" appearance. These typical nuclear changes are the main defining feature of PTC and usually enable unequivocal identification of PTC cells on cytological examination. Papillary structures consist of complex branching papillae with a fibrovascular core covered by a single layer of tumor cells. Follicular elements, resembling FTC, are often interspersed (Hedinger, 1988; Rosai and Carcangiu, 1992).

FTC are characterized by varying degrees of resemblance to normal follicular architecture and function (including colloid formation), capsule formation with capsular invasion, local tissue and vascular invasiveness, and the absence of any features characteristic of PTC. Cytological features can vary considerably, with differing degrees of atypia and no clear distinction from FA. Major criteria for malignancy are unequivocal capsular or vascular invasion on histopathological examination (Hedinger, 1988; Rosai and Carcangiu, 1992).

Anaplastic carcinomas are poorly differentiated malignant thyroid tumors and often cannot be identified as arising from follicular epithelium. Cytologically, nuclear abnormalities and DNA aneuploidy are almost universal, and abundant mitotic figures are present. Cells are uniform and seldom form recognizable papillary or follicular structures. Not infrequently, only immunohistocytochemical staining for epithelial cell surface markers can unequivocally distinguish anaplastic thyroid carcinomas from thyroid lymphomas or sarcomas (Hedinger, 1988; Rosai and Carcangiu, 1992).

Clinical Features and Outcome. The major clinical challenge in thyroid carcinoma diagnosis is distinguishing malignant nodules from benign nodular thyroid disease. No more than 5% to 10% of thyroid nodules coming to medical attention will be malignant. Historical features that may suggest malignancy include prior exposure to ionizing radiation: a family history of thyroid and other malignancies; growth of a nodule over weeks or months rather than a much longer period; changes in speaking, breathing, or swallowing; and systemic symptoms of malignancy, such as weight loss, fatigue, and night sweats. Between 5% and 20% of patients with thyroid cancer may have distant metastases at presentation, and, in the absence of disturbances in thyroid function, systemic symptoms can be strong indicators of malignancy (Grebe et al., 1997; Grebe and Hay, 1999).

Typical signs of thyroid malignancy include firm consistency of the nodule, irregular shape, and fixation to underlying or overlying tissues. Evidence of suspicious regional lymphadenopathy may be present in up to one-third of patients with PTC but will be absent in most patients with hyperplastic nodules, FA, and FTC.

Thyroid function tests are rarely abnormal in patients with thyroid cancer. Even if biochemical evidence of hypo- or hyperthyroidism is found, malignancy is not excluded.

Ultrasonographic and scintigraphic appearance can occasionally be helpful in determining the diagnosis, but usually they are of little aid, and cytological or histological confirmation is always required. In the first instance, this is achieved by FNAB, which, if performed correctly, approaches 100% sensitivity and specificity for diagnosing PTC, benign hyperplastic lesion, and follicular tumors (FA and FTC) (Grebe et al., 1997; Grebe and Hay, 1999). However, it is of little assistance in distinguishing FA from FTC.

The primary treatment for all thyroid carcinomas is surgery, with complete tumor removal being the aim. As approximately 50% of tumor deaths in thyroid carcinoma are attributable to local airway and vascular complications, radical surgery is advised even for patients with distant metastasis. In patients without metastatic disease at presentation, complete surgical tumor removal will result in 10-year survival rates in excess of 80% for PTC and greater than 60% for FTC by the most conservative estimates. By contrast, most patients with anaplastic carcinomas will be dead within 1 year of diagnosis. In all types of thyroid carcinoma, younger patients tend to have a better prognosis than older patients (Grebe et al., 1997).

Patients with PTC or FTC are often offered adjuvant radioiodine therapy after surgery, based on the belief that this may eradicate minute residual tumor foci or "silent" metastasis, thus further improving outcome. However, it remains uncertain whether this results in a significantly improved prognosis for these patients, while the value of thyroxine treatment with TSH-suppressive doses following surgery also remains controversial (Grebe et al., 1997).

General Genetic and Epidemiological Evidence

Clinical Epidemiology. The annual incidence rate for thyroid cancer lies between 0.5 and 10 per 100,000 population in most countries (Franceschi and La Vecchia, 1994). Clinical thyroid malignancy is therefore relatively uncommon, comprising fewer than 1% of clinical human malignancies. Nonetheless, thyroid malignancies are more common and are associated with a higher number of fatal outcomes than are all other endocrine malignancies combined (Robbins et al., 1991). Incidence rates of PTC are greater than those for FTC, and both are far more common than anaplastic carcinomas (Grebe et al., 1997). However, the relative proportions of the three cancer types show wide geographic variation. Anaplastic carcinomas and FTC tend to be relatively more common in endemic goiter areas, and a number of case-control studies have strongly suggested that dietary iodine content is responsible for the increased rates of anaplastic cancer and FTC in these areas (Grebe and Hay, 1995).

Both PTC and FTC are more than twice as common in females than in males and tend to occur more commonly in middle age and later, although PTC patients are somewhat younger than FTC patients (Grebe and Hay, 1995; Grebe et al., 1997). Although thyroid cancer is more common in older patients and in women, the prevalence of benign nodular thyroid disease is also increased in these two groups, and the probability that a thyroid nodule is malignant is therefore actually greater in a young male patient than in an elderly female patient.

Family Epidemiology. Most thyroid cancers appear to be sporadic, although a generalized familial predisposition toward the development of various kinds of malignancy is sometimes observed in patients with thyroid cancer. In most instances such familial clustering of neoplasms is not significantly different from that of a random population sample, given the relative high prevalence of malignancies in most human populations. In some cases there may be a plausible genetic component, but evidence for this is usually weak and probably represents a mild, polygenic predisposition. However, there are also subgroups of patients with a definite family history, either of thyroid cancer alone (most commonly) or of thyroid cancer and other malignancies.

Overall, follicular cell–derived thyroid carcinomas occur in family members of patients with non-medullary thyroid cancer at standardized incidence rates of between 4.1 and 7.9, without any significant increase in risk of malignancy of other organs (Frich et al., 2001). This indicates that there is a familial predisposition to non-medullary thyroid carcinoma in a small but significant proportion of follicular cell–derived thyroid cancer patients. Several such families with apparent multigenerational inheritance of thyroid carcinoma, without any increased risk for the development of other malignancies, have been described (Lote et al., 1980; Cooper et al., 1981; Stoffer et al., 1986; Yashiro et al., 1987; Ozaki et al., 1988; Gorson, 1992; Kobayashi et al., 1995; Kwok and McDougall, 1995; Burgess et al., 1997; Loh, 1997; Medeiros-Neto et al., 1998; Kraimps et al., 1999; Lupoli et al., 1999; Malchoff et al., 2000).

Thyroid dyshormonogenesis—due to defects in thyroid hormone production, storage, or release—has been repeatedly linked to the occurrence of familial thyroid carcinoma (Cooper et al., 1981; Yashiro et al., 1987; Medeiros-Neto et al., 1998), and there is no evidence that individuals from these families suffer an increased risk of non-thyroidal malignancies. Occurrence of apparently familial thyroid carcinoma without thyroid dyshormonogenesis or a predisposition to develop tumors elsewhere has also been described in several families (Lote et al., 1980; Stoffer et al., 1986; Ozaki et al., 1988; Gorson, 1992; Kobayashi et al., 1995; Kwok and McDougall, 1995; Burgess et al., 1997; Loh, 1997; Lupoli et al., 1999). Although rare, these cases are more common than is familial thyroid malignancy associated with hormonal dysgenesis. Overall, the tumors in both groups do not seem to differ in biological behavior from ordinary, sporadic thyroid carcinomas, although there are some suggestions that they may have a less favorable prognosis (Lupoli et al., 1999).

A number of families display syndromatic occurrence of certain benign and malignant neoplasms, including thyroid cancer. Most prominent are individuals with Cowden's syndrome, who suffer from harmatomas in multiple organs and from benign and malignant tumors of breast, skin, and thyroid. The thyroid lesions run the full spectrum from MNG over FA to FTC (Liaw et al., 1997; Eng, 1998; Stratakis et al., 1998). Another group of patients are individuals with the Carney complex, who are susceptible to multiple lentigini, as well as benign and malignant neoplasms of endocrine glands, including the pituitary, adrenals, testes, and thyroid (Carney, 1995; Stratakis et al., 1996, 1997, 1998). Finally, individuals with the Gardner's syndrome variant of familial adenomatous polyposis coli display significantly increased rates of PTC (Haggitt and Reid, 1986; Giardiello et al., 1993; Kelly et al., 1993; Bülow et al., 1997; Soravia et al., 1998).

Some well-described generalized cancer-predisposing syndromes, such as Li-Fraumeni syndrome (inherited *TP53* mutations) and ataxia telangiectasia (AT) (inherited *ATM* mutations) can sometimes include thyroid carcinoma within their spectrum of malignancies, without thyroid tumors being a particular, specific, syndrome-characteristic feature.

Association with Other Diseases. With regards to benign disorders, many patients with follicular cell–derived thyroid carcinoma suffer from pre- or coexisting benign nodular thyroid disease. Other benign disorders do not seem to be associated with follicular cell–derived thyroid carcinoma; however, as mentioned above, thyroid carcinoma may be associated with various other human malignancies. In particular, breast cancer rates are significantly increased in individuals with thyroid carcinoma (Ron et al., 1984; McTiernan et al., 1987; Hall et al., 1991), much beyond what might be expected on the basis of the relatively small number of individuals with Cowden's syndrome. There is also a much lesser increase in the prevalence of many other malignancies in patients with thyroid carcinoma (Hall et al., 1991), suggesting a generalized "malignancy-permissive" genotype in many individuals.

Environmental Factors. The most firmly established environmental risk factor for thyroid cancer is previous exposure to ionizing radiation, particularly to the head and neck region during childhood (Grebe et al., 1997). This used to be a common problem in some exposed populations in Japan and the Pacific during the 1960s and 1970s, in the aftermath of atomic bomb use at the end of the World War II and atmospheric nuclear bomb tests during the 1950s and 1960s. In other countries, radiation treatment for benign medical conditions such as acne vulgaris, thymic enlargement, tinea capitis, and inflammatory connective tissue disorders contributed to rising numbers of thyroid cancer. More recently, significant and prolonged exposure to radioactive fallout in a number of countries in the southern part of the former Soviet Union in the wake of the Chernobyl nuclear reactor accident has led to increased rates of thyroid malignancies, often of an unexpectedly aggressive nature (Nikiforov et al., 1994).

The female preponderance of patients with follicular cell–derived thyroid cancer, and the association with breast cancer, has led to speculation about the role of estrogens as a risk factor for thyroid malignancy. The biological basis for these epidemiological observations could be that estrogen acts as a growth promoter on thyrocytes, and, indeed, some experimental evidence suggests that thyrocytes express estrogen receptors and further that estrogen may stimulate thyrocyte growth in cell culture systems (Grebe et al., 1997). It has also been shown that the partial estrogen antagonist tamoxifen inhibits growth of PTC cells both in vitro and in vivo (Hoelting et al., 1995). Nevertheless, risk factors for breast cancer that lead to increased estrogen exposure (such as low parity and absence of breast feeding) are, with the exception of increased body weight, not associated with an increased risk of thyroid cancer (Grebe et al., 1997). Therefore, on balance, the role of female sex hormones as a risk factor for the development of thyroid cancer in general must still be considered as unresolved.

Similarly, the issue whether iodine deficiency may increase overall thyroid cancer risk through providing a generalized goiterogenic thyroid growth promoting or permissive background remains contentious (Grebe and Hay, 1995; Grebe et al., 1997). It is accepted that environmental iodine content influences the relative number of PTC vs. FTC and anaplastic carcinomas, with iodine depletion increasing the proportion of FTC and anaplastic carcinomas, whereas a high environmental iodine content tends to increase the rates of PTC relative to FTC and anaplastic carcinomas (Grebe and Hay, 1995).

Pathophysiological Basis of Genetic Susceptibility to Follicular Cell–Derived Thyroid Carcinoma

General Pathophysiology. For FTC it is now becoming accepted that tumors, similar to most other human malignancies, develop in a multistep fashion. In this model of carcinogenesis, successive activation of various oncogenes and inactivation of various tumor suppressor genes leads to the phenotypic transformation of a normal follicular cell into a hyperplastic clone, with progression to an FA, then a well-differentiated FTC, and finally a poorly differentiated FTC or an anaplastic cancer. Damage to DNA repair systems might accelerate the various genetic events underlying this transformation, as may strong and prolonged external growth stimuli. There is a substantial and growing body of histopathological, cytogenetic, and molecular genetic evidence supporting such a model for FTC pathogenesis (Grebe et al., 1997).

By contrast, there is no firm evidence to suggest that PTC develops in the same multistep fashion. In particular, there are no known precursor lesions for PTC, and cytogenetic and molecular genetic changes and rearrangements are slight, most commonly involving genes coding for tyrosine kinase type receptors, in particular *RET* (Santoro et al., 1995; Grebe et al., 1997).

Possible Genetic Basis of Thyroid Carcinoma. The proposed multistep genetic model for FTC pathogenesis suggests that a number of known and novel oncogenes and TSGs, as well as DNA repair genes, might be involved in the disease etiology. Similarly, the family data on the link between dyshormonogenesis and carcinoma development suggest that constant TSH stimulation may act as a tumor promoting factor in FTC development. This is also consistent with the epidemiological data on geographical FTC prevalence, which suggests that environmental iodine deficiency increases the prevalence rates of FTC and anaplastic carcinoma. By contrast, there are no obvious candidate susceptibility genes for PTC, with the exception of genes coding for tyrosine kinase type receptors. Since activation of these genes in PTC usually involves genetic rearrangements, which have thus far not been detected in germline DNA of sufferers, rather than mutations, double-stranded DNA repair genes are the only obvious candidate susceptibility genes. Rearrangements that result in RET (or other tyrosine kinase type receptor) activation may then be selected for by conveying some thyroid-specific growth advantage to cells, which then eventually become malignant. It is known that several tyrosine kinase type receptors, when constitutively activated, can bring about cancerous transformation without additional genetic changes (Beug et al., 1995; Borrello et al., 1995; Santoro et al., 1995; Viglietto et al., 1995; Kitayama et al., 1996; Pasini et al., 1997). This may explain the transformation of PTC cells from benign to malignant without any obvious intermediate steps. However, DSB-repair gene defects in other human malignancies usually result in marked genetic disarray, not a common feature of PTC. Thus there are, to date, no clear candidate susceptibility genes for PTC, which would suggest themselves on the basis of the known pathophysiology.

Gene Identification

Gardner's Syndrome. The susceptibility gene for familial polyposis coli has been known for some time to be the *APC* gene. Patients with Gardner's syndrome who suffer from thyroid carcinoma, which affects about 20% of these individuals, do not differ in *APC* mutational spectrum from other familial polyposis coli patients. Almost all *APC* mutations are non-sense mutations and result in premature protein chain termination. The function of the APC protein is still a mystery, although several specific protein motifs have now been identified, including oligomerization domains, armadillo repeats, β-catenin binding sites, human-large-disk-protein binding sites, microtuble binding sites, and a number of potential binding sites for other as yet unidentified proteins. The polyposis phenotype seems to depend on the deletion of at least some of the several β-catenin sites, and it has been speculated that APC interaction with β-catenin is involved in its tumor suppressor function, probably by means of regulation of intracellular β-catenin levels or activity. β-catenin is involved in growth promoting signaling pathways, as well as in cell-to-cell signaling and cell adhesion/cell migration via interactions with cadherin and fascin (Polakis, 1997).

Cowden's Syndrome. The Cowden's syndrome disease gene has also been cloned. By 1996, linkage studies had mapped the site of the putative Cowden's syndrome gene to a 5 cM interval on 10q22–23 between markers *D10S541* and *D10S564*. The following year tumor genetic studies of somatic deletions in glioblastomas, breast, and prostate carcinomas identified a potential tumor suppressor gene, *PTEN/MMAC1*, which mapped to this interval (Li et al., 1997; Steck et al., 1997). Subsequently, mutation analysis of patients with Cowden's syndrome confirmed that *PTEN/MMAC1* was likely to be the Cowden's syndrome gene, with over 80% of affected individuals displaying germline mutations of *PTEN/MMAC1*(Liaw et al., 1997; Lynch et al., 1997; Marsh et al., 1998). *PTEN/MMAC1* codes for a dual-specificity protein tyrosine phosphatase, which can dephosphorylate serine, threonine, and tyrosine residues. It can therefore modulate or antagonize signals mediated by protein tyrosine kinases, many of which have been shown to be capable of acting as oncogenes. Studies of knockout mice have confirmed the role of *PTEN/MMAC1* as a tumor suppressor and have also confirmed its essential nature for embryonal development. Mutations have been observed in all exons of *PTEN/MMAC1*, but they cluster in exon 5, the putative phosphatase domain, and, to a lesser extent, in exons 7 and 8, the putative tyrosine kinase phosphorylation domains (Myers and Tonks, 1997; Di Cristofano et al., 1998). Within affected families, the family-specific germline mutations clearly segregate with the disease phenotype, and tumors of affected individuals show somatic loss of the *PTEN/MMAC1* wild-type allele, consistent with a classic inherited tumor suppressor model (Lynch et al., 1997; Marsh et al., 1998).

Carney Complex. Thyroid tumors were not initially recognized as a feature in Carney complex, but since the original description a significantly elevated rate of goiter, FA, and FTC in Carney complex patients has been noted. As the syndrome can involve pituitary hyperfunction, it is possible that this is the result of pituitary-driven continuous TSH stimulation, however, thyrotoxicosis should also ensue under these circumstances, and this has not been noted to date. It is therefore likely that the underlying genetic abnormality conveys a direct thyroid tumorigenic effect. Putative disease gene loci have been mapped to 2p16 and 17q22–24 by linkage analysis. Because of the similarities of Carney complex to the McCune-Albright syndrome, as well as other features, such as paradoxical responses to endocrine signals, genes involved in cyclic nucleotide-dependent signaling have been considered to be candidates for causing Carney complex

(Bertherat, 2001). Within the 17q22–24 region, such a gene, encoding a protein kinase A R1α regulatory subunit (*PRKAR1A*), was identified and subsequently proven to be inactivated through germline mutations, microdeletions, or deletions in patients with Carney complex who displayed linkage to 17q22–24, but not in those with linkage to 2p16 (Casey et al., 2000; Kirschner et al., 2000a, 2000b). Carney complex therefore seems to be caused by at least two distinct genetic alterations: inactivation of *PRKAR1A* and inactivation of an as yet unknown gene at 2p16, possibly another gene involved in cyclic nucleotide-dependent signaling. Candidate genes are currently being identified and examined. In addition, several known tumor suppressor genes mapping to the vicinity of 2p16, including one of the human mismatch repair genes, have been examined and excluded, while others are still being evaluated. It is likely that these studies will result in the cloning of the second Carney complex gene within the near future (Carney, 1995; Stratakis et al., 1996, 1997, 1998).

Thyroid Dyshormonogenesis. The genetic basis of tumors arising within the context of thyroid dyshormonogenesis syndromes mirrors the underlying genetic enzymatic defects, which include abnormalities in Tg, incomplete transport of Tg across the apical membrane, incomplete transport of iodine across the apical membrane (Pendred syndrome), and defects in any of the enzymes involved in Tg iodination and subsequent intra-thyrocyte thyroid hormone cleavage from iodinated Tg. The partial hormonogenesis block is overcome by increased mitogenic and metabolic stimuli to the thyrocytes, particularly TSH stimulation. This results in goiter formation and predisposes to tumor development by creating an environment that permits growth and transformation (Cooper et al., 1981; Niimi et al., 1985; Couch et al., 1986; Yashiro et al., 1987; Corral et al., 1993; Yoshida et al., 1996; Medeiros-Neto et al., 1998).

Familial PTC. Only a relatively small number of families of altogether less than 200 members with familial PTC have thus far been described (Lote et al., 1980; Stoffer et al., 1986; Ozaki et al., 1988; Gorson, 1992; Kobayashi et al., 1995; Kwok and McDougall, 1995; Burgess et al., 1997; Loh, 1997; Kraimps et al., 1999; Lupoli et al., 1999; Malchoff et al., 2000), although international efforts at linkage analysis are currently under way. These studies have thus far not produced any convincing results, other than excluding the *MNG1* locus as a thyroid carcinoma susceptibility locus (Bignell et al., 1997) and the relatively crude mapping of two new potential candidates in rare subforms of familial thyroid cancer. In familial PTC with oxyphilia, a possible disease-associated locus was identified in a single affected family in a relatively large region around D19S916 on 19p13.2 (LOD score 3.01) (Kraimps et al., 1999). In familial combined papillary thyroid and renal cell neoplasia, a rare syndrome, a possible disease locus was mapped in a large kindred at an LOD score of 3.58 to a 20 cM region on 1q21 (Malchoff et al., 2000). However, for the majority of familial PTC cases, no candidate regions or genes have as yet been identified. It is possible that the current disease families have too few members to allow successful linkage analysis or that the condition is heterogeneous, with different susceptibility genes involved in different families. These questions will only be resolved through continuing linkage analysis.

Clinical Application of Genetic Information

For individuals from one of the families with defined syndromes that include thyroid carcinoma susceptibility, the elucidation of the genetic basis of their family's condition has resulted in highly accurate disease prediction for presymptomatic individuals (Bülow et al., 1997). This predictive value is likely to result in reduced morbidity and mortality through targeted surveillance and early intervention. In individuals with dyshormonogenesis, thyroxine treatment may even prevent disease development altogether, provided commencement is sufficiently early. It is also possible that in some instances individuals with genetic evidence of Gardner's or Cowden's syndrome may opt for prophylactic thyroidectomy, and this is likely to result in complete abolition of any clinical thyroid carcinoma-related morbidity or mortality in these patients. For patients from familial PTC-only families, such advances are not yet available but are likely to become reality once the disease gene(s) is cloned.

Unfortunately, for the vast majority of follicular cell–derived thyroid carcinoma patients, who have sporadic tumors on the basis of some minor permissive genetic susceptibility, these developments have not resulted in significant clinical advances; however, the oncogenes and TSGs involved in hereditary tumor syndromes may also play a role in some sporadic tumors. Investigation of these candidate genes with regard to their role in the somatically acquired genomic changes in sporadic thyroid carcinoma should eventually result in greater understanding of sporadic thyroid carcinoma pathogenesis.

Medullary Thyroid Carcinoma

Disease Definition

Diagnostic Criteria. Medullary thyroid carcinoma (MTC) presents as a neck nodule, with confirmation of diagnosis by cytology or histology. Given a high level of suspicion, medullary carcinoma can be diagnosed with reasonable reliability from FNAB specimens, which will show highly cellular aspirates of heterogeneous, malignant-appearing cells that show no evidence of colloid and lack the typical features of papillary and follicular tumors. In these cases, confirmation of diagnosis is by histopathology of the operative specimen. MTC is a highly pleomorphic tumor with many variations in histological patterns, even within the same nodule. Typically, there are tumor nests of polygonal, oval, or spindle-shaped cells that exhibit the usual morphological features of malignant behavior. They show evidence of stromal, lymphatic, and vascular invasion, and many tumors show amyloid deposition. At the minimum, diagnosis requires evidence of well-demarcated collections of C cells that breach the follicular basement membranes. Simple C cell hyperplasia, although suspicious and often a precursor of MTC, is not sufficient, as this may occur in nonmalignant conditions such as autoimmune thyroiditis.

MTCs are hormonally active tumors that produce calcitonin and a variety of other neuropeptides. Elevated serum calcitonin levels are supportive evidence in the diagnosis of medullary carcinoma. In cases of highly de-differentiated tumors, elevated serum calcitonin levels or positive tumor-immunohistochemistry for calcitonin may be the only method of unequivocally diagnosing a medullary tumor.

Clinical Features and Outcome. Most patients with MTC present with a neck nodule or are identified in the course of screening of members of a family with MEN 2 or familial medullary thyroid carcinoma (FMTC). Some 80% of cases are sporadic tumors, with almost all presenting with thyroid nodules. Patients from MEN 2 or FMTC families are generally diagnosed at an earlier stage, or even when still asymptomatic, than are patients with sporadic tumors. Cervical lymph node metastasis at diagnosis is common, affecting about 40% of cases, as is recurrence in neck and mediastinal nodes, with cumulative nodal recurrence rates of 20% to 25%.

Most MTCs are hormonally active, producing calcitonin. In humans, calcitonin has no significant physiological role, and there are numerous compensatory mechanisms that maintain eucalcemia even in the face of massive hypercalcitoninemia. Consequently, MTC-induced hypercalcitoninemia is generally not noticed by patients. It can be accurately measured in serum samples, however, and this serves as a useful tumor marker, together with CEA, which is also often elevated (Normann et al., 1976; Saad et al., 1984; Schröder et al., 1988; Bergholm et al., 1989b; Gharib et al., 1992).

Disease stage at presentation is of paramount importance in determining outcome in MTC. Stage I and II patients generally have a favorable prognosis, whereas survival is poor in patients with stage III and IV disease. Radical, systematic lymph node dissection, either at primary surgery or as a secondary procedure, may improve outcome, but its effects are small in comparison to the benefits of early diagnosis (Normann et al., 1976; Saad et al., 1984; Schröder et al., 1988; Bergholm et al., 1989a, 1989b, 1997; Gharib et al., 1992).

General Genetic and Epidemiological Evidence

Clinical Epidemiology. MTC is a relatively rare tumor, accounting for less than 5% of all cases of thyroid malignancy. The traditional wisdom is that about 80% of affected individuals will have sporadic disease and 20% will be familial cases. However, in recent times it has become apparent that some of the sporadic cases may carry germline mutations in the *RET* proto-oncogene (see below), suggesting that they are either new, late-presenting, "founder" cases for new disease families or late-presenting familial cases from families which for one reason or another have not had any previous members formerly diagnosed. Most of the familial cases are from families with MEN2A, with FMTC and MEN2B following in order of frequency (Larsson and Nordenskjöld, 1990; Caruso et al., 1991; Marsh et al., 1995; Carney, 1998).

Among true sporadic cases of MTC there is a slight female preponderance of about 1.5:1. The mean age at diagnosis for these sporadic cases is between 50 and 60 years. There are no known risk factors for sporadic MTC and no evidence to suggest either geographic or ethnic clustering (Saad et al., 1984; Bergholm et al., 1989b; Larsson and Nordenskjöld, 1990; Caruso et al., 1991; Gharib et al., 1992; Marsh et al., 1995; Carney, 1998).

For patients with familial MTC, the sex ratio is essentially 1:1 and the lifetime penetrance of clinical disease for genetically affected individuals approaches 100%. Most subjects present between the age of 30 and 50, although some individuals will develop clinical MTC in their teens and first presentations above the age of 60 are recognized (Saad et al., 1984; Bergholm et al., 1989b; Larsson and Nordenskjöld, 1990; Caruso et al., 1991; Marsh et al., 1995; Carney, 1998; Gharib et al., 1992).

Family Epidemiology. MTC is one of the components of the multiple endocrine neoplasia syndrome, which is inherited in an autosomal dominant fashion. There are two subforms of MEN, designated MEN2A and MEN2B. MEN2A is characterized by MTC, with penetrance approaching 100%; usually bilateral pheochromocytomas, with a cumulative incidence of about 50%; and parathyroid tumors in 10% to 30% of cases. Patients with MEN2B usually lack parathyroid involvement, and affected individuals have a characteristic marfanoid habitus and suffer from mucosal neuromas. Occasional families appear to be affected exclusively by MTC. In a proportion of these cases there is underlying MEN2A, and the apparent lack of other organ involvement in family members is a chance event; however, the recent unraveling of the molecular pathogenesis of the MEN2 type syndromes suggests that there are also bonafide instances of FMTC (Larsson and Nordenskjöld, 1990; Caruso et al., 1991; Ponder, 1994; Borrello et al., 1995; Marsh et al., 1995; Pasini et al., 1997; Rossel et al., 1997; Carney, 1998; Santoro et al., 1998; Takahashi et al., 1998).

Association with Other Diseases. Familial MTC is often associated with the other endocrine neoplasias of the MEN2 type syndromes, as described above. There are no known specific disease associations for sporadic MTC, except a slight predisposition to malignancies in general, but this is a common observation in many human cancers.

Environmental Factors. The present theory of multistep genetic development of human malignancies predicts that carcinogenic environmental factors can hasten the manifestation of neoplasia in familial predisposed individuals. Such environmental influences may well account for some of the variability in age of onset of MTC in MEN and FMTC patients, and they may also play a role in determining whether a given individual will develop pheochromocytoma or parathyroid tumors. To date, the case numbers have been too small, potential environmental variables too numerous, the penetrance of MTC in this group of patients too high, and the genotype–phenotype correlations of some of the recognized underlying *RET* mutations too strong to allow identification of any specific environmental risk factors for inherited forms of MTC. Although more common than the tumors of familial origin, sporadic MTC has thus far not been linked to any specific environmental factors.

Gene Identification and Pathophysiological Basis of Genetic Susceptibility

Initial cytogenetic studies of tumors from MEN2 patients suggested frequent somatic deletions of chromosome band 20p12.2 (Grebe et al., 1997). While some subsequent molecular loss of heterozygosity (LOH) studies seemed to support the notion of statistically significant rates of loss of genetic material on chromosome 20 and also chromosome 22, linkage studies have disproved a role for chromosomes 20 and 22 in the development of MTC, suggesting instead linkage to chromosome 10 (Simpson et al., 1987; Grebe et al., 1997). This observation was confirmed by high-resolution linkage mapping studies of the paracentromeric region of chromosome 10 (Lichter et al., 1992). LOH studies failed to find evidence of somatic deletions in this region, suggesting that MEN2 was not caused by a mutation in a tumor suppressor gene but by oncogene activation (Nelkin et al., 1989). In inherited tumor suppressor gene defect syndromes, the inherited diseased allele generally carries inactivating point mutations or microdeletions, while the healthy allele is somatically deleted in tissues that are destined to become cancerous, thus leading to the required bi-allelic inactivation of the tumor suppressor. By contrast, oncogene activation may lead to disease by activation of only one of two oncogene alleles, thus fitting the observed lack of evidence of somatic genetic deletions in MTC from MEN2A patients. As the chromosomal region identified by linkage analysis in MEN patients was known to harbor a protooncogene, *RET*, coding for a tyrosine kinase type receptor, mutation screening in MEN2 patients focused on *RET*, subsequently confirming a high rate of *RET* mutations in MEN2 patients.

RET mutations can be demonstrated in more than 90% of individuals with inherited forms of MTC (Ponder, 1994; Ledger et al., 1995; Marsh et al., 1995; Robinson, 1998). As would be expected for gain of function mutations, a limited number of amino acid positions are involved. The known mutations are restricted to missense mutations of 14 of the over 1000 amino acids of the RET protein, and mutations of 6 of these 14 amino acids account for the vast majority of reported cases (amino acids 609, 611, 618, 620, 634, and 918). Within the framework of this limited number of mutation hotspots, extensive mutation analysis over recent years has revealed interesting genotype–phenotype relationships (Ponder, 1994; Ledger et al., 1995; Marsh et al., 1995; Robinson, 1998; Takahashi et al., 1998).

Some 98% of mutations in MEN2A are missense mutations of cysteine residues (within a large cysteine-rich domain), occurring on the extracellular receptor side within a 25 amino acid stretch immediately adjacent to the RET transmembrane domain (Ponder, 1994; Takahashi et al., 1998). Any of the six cysteine residues (Cys609, Cys611, Cys618, Cys620, Cys630, or Cys634) in this 25 amino acid segment of the extracellular cysteine-rich region may be affected, but over 50% of mutations will involve Cys634, while Cys630 is rarely mutated. Some of the 2% of individuals without germline mutations in any of these cysteine residues have mutations in codon 790, and very few MEN2A patients have no identifiable *RET* mutations (Marsh et al., 1995; Robinson, 1998; Takahashi et al., 1998). Within MEN2A families, the presence of any Cys634 mutation increases the likelihood of pheochromocytoma, and the C634R mutation may be linked to hyperparathyroidism.

Most families with FMTC will also show germline mutations of one of the cysteine residues most commonly affected in MEN2A, and most of the remainder will have mutations of codons 768, 791, 804 (in the proximal portion of the tyrosine kinase functional domain), and 891 (in the distal portion of the tyrosine kinase functional domain). Thus far it appears that these latter, less common, mutations are specific for FMTC, and it is also interesting to note that to date none of the FMTC families have shown a C634R mutation, which is distinctly common in MEN2A. In about 10% to 12% of FMTC families, there are no identifiable *RET* mutations (Robinson, 1998; Takahashi et al., 1998).

MEN2B families do not show mutations in the extracellular cysteine residue mutation hotspots affected in most MEN2A and FMTC families. Instead, about 95% of these families show a Met918Thr change, and some of the remainders have mutations in the close-by codons 883 or 912, also within the distal portion of the tyrosine kinase functional domain (Ledger et al., 1995; Marsh et al., 1995; Robinson, 1998; Takahashi et al., 1998). Somatic mutations of codon 918 also occur in many sporadic MTC, with published figures varying from about 30% to about 85% (Marsh et al., 1995). In sporadic MTC there is some evidence for an unfavorable prognostic impact of somatic codon 918 mutations, but MTC is diagnosed much earlier in MEN families due to the clinicians' anticipation of the likely development of the condition and resulting clinical, biochemical, and genetic screening. This earlier diagnosis reduces the proportion of patients dying of the disease. Because there are relatively few MEN2B families, no evidence has been found that relates adverse outcome of MTC specifically to MEN2B with codon 918 mutations.

Direct evidence linking the various *RET* mutations with tumor development comes in the form of ectopic and recombinant expression of the mutants in cell lines and from transgenic mouse experiments. Tyrosine kinase activity of the mutants is many fold increased over the wild type, and NIH 3T3 cells transfected with mutant *RET* show various degrees of malignant transformation (Asai et al., 1995; Borrello et al., 1995; Cirafici et al., 1997; Pasini et al., 1997; Rossel et al., 1997; Santoro et al., 1998; Takahashi et al., 1998). All known disease-associated *RET* mutants are capable of inducing malignant transformation, but the different mutants vary widely in their respective transforming activity. For all mutants, the long isoforms of *RET* are more potent in inducing transformation than the short isoforms. For the long RET isoform (1,114 aa) the M918T mutant displays the most potent transforming activity, while for the short RET isoform (1,072 aa) C634R is most active. The weakest transformants are the various Cys609 and Cys 611 mutants, which display about one-fifth of the transforming ability of C634R (Takahashi et al., 1998). When expressed in transgenic mice, the C634R mutant results in the development of MTC in these animals that is histologically similar to the human lesions (Michiels et al., 1997).

The molecular basis for the transforming ability and the carcinogenic potential of *RET* mutants lies in their ability to induce constitutive receptor activation in the absence of ligand. RET receptors are cell membrane receptors consisting of several distinct domains. The ligand, neurturin (NTN), is initially not bound to RET, but to a glycosyl-phosphatidylinositol (GPI)-linked coreceptor, neurturin receptor-α (NTNRα) (Durbec et al., 1996; Treanor et al., 1996; Buj-Bello et al., 1997; Klein et al., 1997). On binding, NTN, NTNRα, and RET receptors converge to form multimer receptor complexes (Buj-Bello et al., 1997; Klein et al., 1997). Formation of these multimer receptor complexes initiates dimerization of RET receptors through cadherin-like extracellular domains, and this activates the intracellular proximal and distal tyrosine kinase domains, resulting in tyrosine kinase activity (Santoro et al., 1998; Takahashi et al., 1998). The downstream intracellular transducers of RET signaling are still incompletely understood, but as in the case of many other tyrosine kinase type growth factor receptors, they probably involve the RAS pathways and result in growth promoting and mitogenic signals. The MEN2A and FMTC-associated *RET* mutations in the cysteine-rich extracellular domain induce constitutive RET dimerization in the absence of coreceptor or ligand through formation of disulfide bridges. The more potent Cys634 mutants result in formation of multiple disulfide bridges, leading to tight dimerization and continuous receptor activation, while most of the other mutants lead to weaker dimerization bonding, resulting in dimers that may eventually dissociate and will therefore not signal continuously (Santoro et al., 1998). These differences correlate with the clinical observations of a more severe disease spectrum in families with Cys634 mutations. Mutations in the distal tyrosine kinase domain, in particular the codon 918 mutations seen in MEN2B and sporadic MTC, also lead to constitutive RET activation (Cirafici et al., 1997; Rossel et al., 1997; Santoro et al., 1998). However, in this case this results from direct induction and activation of tyrosine kinase activity through the mutation, without the need for RET dimerization. Mutations in the proximal tyrosine kinase domain and other mutations in the distal domain have the same effect but show a lesser degree of tyrosine kinase activity in the absence of ligand or dimerization than do the 918 mutations (Ponder, 1994; Borrello et al., 1995; Cirafici et al., 1997; Pasini et al., 1997; Rossel et al., 1997; Santoro et al., 1998) (Fig. 20–5).

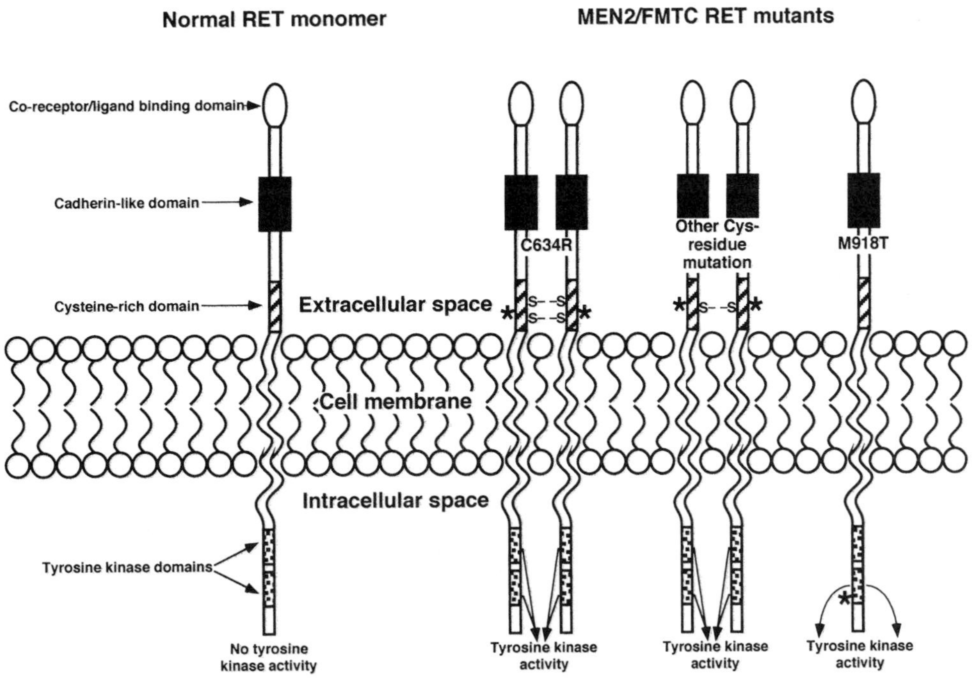

Fig. 20–5. Schematic depiction of some examples of RET activation by mutant RET-receptors (not drawn to scale). RET is a tyrosine kinase type cell-surface receptor that requires multimerization with a co-receptor, ligand, and a second RET receptor to initiate intracellular tyrosine kinase activity or signaling. *RET* gene mutations lead to aberrant RET tyrosine kinase activation by changing the amino-acid sequence of RET in such a way that either dimerization of RET receptors in the absence of co-receptor and ligand is induced, usually through the formation of disulfide bridges (S–S) between mutant RET molecules (C634R mutants and other extracellular cysteine residue mutations), or the tyrosine kinase region of the RET molecule is altered so that it no longer requires dimerization with other RET molecules to initiate tyrosine kinase activity (e.g., M918T mutant). The asterisks (*) indicate the approximate sites of the depicted examples of RET mutations.

Clinical Application of Genetic Information

MTC in its familial forms represents a classic example of a single-gene defect with well-established genotype–phenotype associations and well-researched molecular mechanisms of action. This may eventually result in highly specific therapies that could also benefit the larger group of sporadic MTC patients, many of whom share the codon 918 mutations at a somatic level with MEN2B patients (Marsh et al., 1995).

In addition, the unraveling of the molecular genetic basis of familial MTC has resulted in highly accurate diagnostic tests, which allow identification of asymptomatic family members. Since most deaths in MEN2 families and all deaths in FMTC families are due to MTC, such screening can have a dramatic impact on survival. Asymptomatic patients with genetic evidence of disease, who are generally very young, can be offered prophylactic thyroidectomy (Wells et al., 1994; Moley et al., 1998). In addition, affected individuals can be entered into regular biochemical screening programs that may permit early detection of hyperparathyroidism or pheochromocytoma, thus further reducing morbidity and mortality. These recent advances in determining the genetic basis of familial MTC have revolutionized the management of MEN2 and FMTC and have yielded substantial practical benefits for sufferers.

SUMMARY AND CONCLUSION

Diseases of the thyroid gland are the most common endocrine or metabolic diseases and cover a wide clinical spectrum, ranging from asymptomatic structural changes to debilitating or lethal functional and structural problems.

A thorough understanding of many of the steps involved in thyroid development, metabolic activity and regulation, thyroid hormone transport, and thyroid hormone action has been gained over the last four decades. These advances have resulted in an elucidation of the genetic basis and molecular mechanisms of a number of inherited single-gene defects that affect various facets of thyroid anatomy and function. Similarly, for some groups of patients with neoplastic diseases of the thyroid gland, most notably patients with familial forms of MTC, but also some individuals with familial follicular cell–derived thyroid carcinomas, predisposing single-gene defects have been identified. For most of these single-gene thyroid disorders, the unraveling of their genetic basis has resulted in tangible benefits for patients—in terms of both counseling and prevention and early intervention.

However, collectively, the well-described single-gene defect type disorders make up only a small proportion of all thyroid diseases. For the much larger group of patients suffering from autoimmune thyroid disease or various forms of benign or malignant nodular thyroid diseases and goiter, predisposing genetic factors remain yet to be determined. In particular, our knowledge of underlying genetic susceptibility is very poor for autoimmune hypothyroidism and most forms of nodular thyroid disease, while for Graves' disease some patterns of underlying genetic susceptibilities are beginning to emerge. Most notable are the copious data on HLA-disease relationships, which have allowed some limited improvements in family counseling of Graves' disease patients.

For the next decade it can be anticipated that this picture will change, as some large-scale susceptibility gene mapping projects in MNG, autoimmune hypothyroidism, and Graves' disease progress, and it is hoped that these studies will result in a more complete understanding of these diseases with resulting clinical benefits. With human single-nucleotide polymorphism databases growing in size, future linkage projects will be greatly facilitated. With the human genome sequencing project now almost complete (complete in draft form), identification and verification of candidate genes will be greatly facilitated. The next phase of the human genome project, functional genomics and expression profiling, will further advance our understanding of genotype–phenotype correlations and will result in the identification of several as yet unexpected relationships. Finally, cross-species correlations and transgenic animal models will allow yet more rapid and conclusive evaluation of the genetic basis of disease. Most of these advances will likely be brought to bear initially on cancer and cardiovascular disease, but eventually they will become so easily accessible and commonplace that they will be applied to the genetic basis of endocrine disease, particularly the common conditions such as diabetes and thyroid disease.

ACKNOWLEDGMENTS

This work was partly supported by a Health Research Council of New Zealand Repatriation Fellowship to Stefan Grebe. I am immensely grateful to Brett Delahunt for his kind advice, critique, and proofreading of the manuscript.

REFERENCES

Abbas AK, Lichtman AH, Pober JS: The major histocompatibility complex. In: Cellular and molecular immunology. 3rd ed. Philadelphia: W. B. Saunders, 1997:97–114.

Abramowicz MJ, Duprez L, Parma J, Vassart G, Heinrichs C: Familial congenital hypothyroidism due to inactivating mutation of the thyrotropin receptor causing profound hypoplasia of the thyroid gland. J Clin Investig 1997; 99:3018–3024.

Acebron A, Aza-Blanc P, Rossi DL, Lamas L, Santisteban P: Congenital human thyroglobulin defect due to low expression of the thyroid-specific transcription factor TTF-1. J Clin Investig 1995; 96:781–785.

Allahabadia A, Heward JM, Mijovic C, Carr-Smith J, Daykin J, Cockram C, Barnett AH, Sheppard MC, Franklyn JA, Gough SC: Lack of association between polymorphism of the thyrotropin receptor gene and Graves' disease in United Kingdom and Hong Kong Chinese patients: case control and family-based studies. Thyroid 1998; 8:777–780.

Allannic H, Fauchet R, Lorcy Y, Gueguen M, Le Guerrier AM, Genetet B: A prospective study of the relationship between relapse of hyperthyroid Graves' disease after antithyroid drugs and HLA haplotype. J Clin Endocrinol Metab 1983; 57:719–722.

Allannic H, Fauchet R, Lorcy Y, Heim J, Gueguen M, Leguerrier AM: HLA and Graves' disease: an association with HLA-DRw3. J Clin Endocrinol Metab 1980; 51:863–867.

Ambinder JN, Chiorazzi N, Gibofsky A, Fotino M, Kunkel HG: Special characteristics of cellular immune function in normal individuals of the HLA-DR3 type. Clin Immunol Immunopathol 1982; 23:269–274.

Amenomori M, Mori T, Fukuda Y, Sugawa H, Nishida N, Furukawa M, Kita R, Sando T, Komeda T, Nakao K: Incidence and characteristics of thyroid dysfunction following interferon therapy in patients with chronic hepatitis C. Intern Med 1998; 37:246–252.

Anders HJ: Compression syndromes caused by substernal goitres. Postgrad Med J 1998; 74:327–329.

Arscott PL, Baker JR Jr: Apoptosis and thyroiditis. Clin Immunol Immunopathol 1998; 87:207–217.

Arscott PL, Rosen ED, Koenig RJ, Kaplan MM, Ellis T, Thompson N Jr: Immunoreactivity to *Yersinia enterocolitica* antigens in patients with autoimmune thyroid disease. J Clin Endocrinol Metab 1992; 75:295–300.

Asai N, Iwashita T, Matsuyama M, Takahashi M: Mechanism of activation of the ret proto-oncogene by multiple endocrine neoplasia 2A mutations. Mol Cell Biol 1995; 15:1613–1619.

Assem ES, Trotter WR, Belyavin G: Thyroglobulin and thyroglobulin antibodies in the serum of normal adults. Immunology 1965; 9:21–29.

Awata T, Kurihara S, Iitaka M, Takei S-I, Inoue I, Ishii C, Negishi K, Izumida T, Yoshida Y, Hagura R, et al.: Association of CTLA-4 gene A–G polymorphism (IDDM12 locus) with acute-onset and insulin-depleted IDDM as well as autoimmune thyroid disease (Graves' disease and Hashimoto's thyroiditis) in the Japanese population. Diabetes 1998; 47:128–129.

Badenhoop K, Donner H, Braun J, Siegmund T, Rau H, Usadel KH: Genetic markers in diagnosis and prediction of relapse in Graves' disease. Exp Clin Endocrinol Diabetes 1996; 104(Suppl. 4):98–100.

Badenhoop K, Schwarz G, Schleusener H, Weetman AP, Recks S, Peters HB, Usadel KH: Tumor necrosis factor β gene polymorphisms in Graves' disease. J Clin Endocrinol Metab 1992; 74:287–291.

Badenhoop K, Schwarz G, Walfish PG, Drummond V, Usadel KH, Bottazzo GF: Susceptibility to thyroid autoimmune disease: molecular analysis of HLA-D region genes identifies new markers for goitrous Hashimoto's thyroiditis. J Clin Endocrinol Metab 1990; 71:1131–1137.

Barbesino G, Tomer Y, Concepcion E, Davies TF, Greenberg DA: Linkage analysis of candidate genes in autoimmune thyroid disease: 1. Selected immunoregulatory genes. J Clin Endocrinol Metab 1998a; 83:1580–1584.

Barbesino G, Tomer Y, Concepcion ES, Davies TF, Greenberg DA: Linkage analysis of candidate genes in autoimmune thyroid disease: 2. Selected gender-related genes and the X-chromosome. J Clin Endocrinol Metab 1998b; 83:3290–3295.

Barlow AB, Wheatcroft N, Watson P, Weetman AP: Association of HLA-DQA1*0501 with Graves' disease in English Caucasian men and women. Clin Endocrinol 1996; 44:73–77.

Bartels ED: Heredity in Graves' Disease. Copenhagen, Denmark: Munksgaard, 1941.

Bauch K: Epidemiology of functional autonomy. Exp Clin Endocrinol Diabetes 1998; 106(Suppl)4:S16–S22.

Bergholm U, Adami H-O, Bergström R, Bäckdahl M, Åkerström G, Swedish MTC Study Group: Long-term survival in sporadic and familial medullary thyroid carcinoma with special reference to clinical characteristics as prognostic factors. Acta Chir Scand 1989a; 156:37–46.

Bergholm U, Adami H-O, Bergström R, Johansson H, Lundell G, Telenius-Berg M, Åkerström G, Swedish MTC Study Group: Clinical characteristics in sporadic and familial medullary thyroid carcinoma. Cancer 1989b; 63:1196–1204.

Bergholm U, Bergström R, Ekborn A: Long-tern follow-up of patients with medullary carcinoma of the thyroid. Cancer 1997; 79:132–138.

Bertherat J: Protein kinase A in Carney complex: a new example of cAMP pathway alteration in endocrine tumors. Eur J Endocrinol 2001; 144:209–211.

Beug H, Schroeder C, Wessely O, Deiner E, Meyer S, Ischenko ID: Transformation of erythroid progenitors by viral and cellular tyrosine kinases. Cell Growth Differ 1995; 6:999–1008.

Bidart J-M, Mian C, Lazar V, Russo D, Filetti S, Caillou B, Schlumberger M: Expression of pendrin and the pendrin syndrome (PDS) gene in human thyroid tissues. J Clin Endocrinol Metab 2000; 85:2028–2033

Biebermann H, Schoneberg T, Krude H, Schultz G, Gudermann T, Gruters A: Mutations of the human thyrotropin receptor gene causing thyroid hypoplasia and persistent congenital hypothyroidism. J Clin Endocrinol Metab 1997; 82:3471–3480.

Bignell GR, Canzian F, Shayeghi M, Stark M, Shugart YY, Biggs P, Hamoudi R, Rosenblatt J, Buu P, Sun S, et al.: Familial nontoxic multinodular thyroid goiter locus maps to chromosome 14q but does not account for familial nonmedullary thyroid cancer. Am J Hum Genet 1997; 61:1123–1130.

Blakemore AI, Watson PF, Weetman AP, Duff GW: Association of Graves' disease with an allele of the interleukin-1 receptor antagonist gene. J Clin Endocrinol Metab 1995; 80:111–115.

Boehm BO, Schifferdecker E, Kuehnl P, Schoffling K: Linkage of HLA-DR β-specific restriction fragment length polymorphisms with Graves' disease. Acta Endocrinol 1988; 119:251–256.

Bogner U, Badenhoop K, Peters H, Schmieg D, Mayr WR, Usadel KH, Schleusener H: HLA-DR/DQ gene variation in nongoitrous autoimmune thyroiditis at the serological and molecular level. Autoimmunity 1992; 14:155–158.

Bohr UR, Behr M, Loos U: A heritable point mutation in an extracellular domain of the TSH receptor involved in the interaction with Graves' immunoglobulins. Biochim Biophys Acta 1993; 1216:504–508.

Borrello MG, Smith DP, Pasini B, Bongarzone I, Greco A, Lorenzo MJ, Arighi E, Miranda C, Eng C, Alberti L, et al.: RET activation by germline MEN2A and MEN2B mutations. Oncogene 1995; 11:2419–2427.

Brander A, Viikinkoski P, Nickels J, Kivisaari L: Thyroid gland: US screening in a random adult population. Radiology 1991; 181:683–687.

Bratusch-Marrain P, Haydl H, Waldhausl W, Dudczak R, Graninger W: Familial thyroxine-binding globulin deficiency in association with non-toxic goitre. Acta Endocrinol 1979; 91:70–76.

Brix TH, Christensen K, Holm NV, Harvald B, Hegedus L: A population-based study of Graves' disease in Danish twins. Clin Endocrinol 1998; 48:397–400.

Brix TH, Kyvik KO, Christensen K, Hegedus L: Evidence for a major role of heredity in Graves' disease: a population-based study of two Danish twin cohorts. J Clin Endocrinol Metab 2001; 86:930–934.

Brix TH, Kyvik KO, Hegedus L: Major role of genes in the etiology of simple goiter in females: a population-based twin study. J Clin Endocrinol Metab 1999; 84:3071–3075.

Brix TH, Kyvik KO, Hegedus L: A population-based study of chronic autoimmune hypothyroidism in Danish twins. J Clin Endocrinol Metab 2000; 85: 536–539.

Brucker-Davis F, Skarulis MC, Grace MB, Benichou J, Hauser P, Wiggs E, Weintraub BD: Genetic and clinical features of 42 kindreds with resistance to thyroid hormone: the National Institutes of Health Prospective Study. Ann Intern Med 1995; 123:572–583.

Bruneton JN, Balu-Maestro C, Marcy PY: Very high frequency (13 MHz) ultrasonographic examination of the normal neck: detection of normal lymph nodes and thyroid nodules. J Ultrasound Med 1994; 13:87–90.

Buj-Bello A, Adu J, Pinon LG, Horton A, Thompson J, Rosenthal A, Buchman VL, Davies AM: Neurturin responsiveness requires a GPI-linked receptor and the Ret receptor tyrosine kinase. Nature 1997; 387:721–724.

Bülow C, Bülow S, Group LCP: Is screening for thyroid carcinoma indicated in familial adenomatous polyposis? Int J Colorectal Dis 1997; 12:240–242.

Burgess JR, Duffield A, Wilkinson SJ, Ware R, Greenaway TM, Percival J, Hoffman L: Two families with an autosomal dominant inheritance pattern for papillary carcinoma of the thyroid. J Clin Endocrinol Metab 1997; 82:345–348.

Burman KD, Lukes YG, Gemiski P: Molecular homology between the human TSH receptor and Yersinia enterocolitica. Thyroid 1991; 1(Suppl.)1:S62.

Buscema M, Todd I, Deuss U, Hammond L, Mirakian R, Pujol-Borrell R, Bottazzo

GF: Influence of tumor necrosis factor-α on the modulation of interferon-γ of HLA class II molecules in human thyroid cells and its effect on interferon-γ binding. J Clin Endocrinol Metab 1989; 69:433–439.
Cai WY, Lukes YG, Burch HB, Djuh YY, Carr F, Wartofsky L, Rhooms P, Baker JR Jr, Burman KD: Analysis of human TSH receptor gene and RNA transcripts in patients with thyroid disorders. Autoimmunity 1992; 13:43–50.
Capon F, Tacconelli A, Giardina E, Sciacchitano S, Bruno R, Tassi V, Trischitta V, Filetti S, Dallapiccola B, Novelli G: Mapping a dominant form of multinodular goiter to chromosome Xp22. Am J Hum Genet 2000; 67:1004–1007.
Carney JA: The Carney complex (myxomas, spotty pigmentation, endocrine overactivity, and schwannomas). Dermatol Clin 1995; 13:19–26.
Carney JA: Familial multiple endocrine neoplasia syndromes: components, classification, and nomenclature. J Intern Med 1998; 243:425–432.
Caruso DR, O'Dorisio TM, Mazzaferri EL: Mulitple endocrine neoplasia. Curr Opin Oncol 1991; 3:103–108.
Casey M, Vaughan CJ, He J, Hatcher CJ, Winter JM, Weremowicz S, Montgomery K, Kucherlapati R, Morton CC, Basson CT: Mutations in the protein kinase A R1α regulatory subunit cause familial cardiac myxomas and Carney complex. J Clin Invest 2000; 106:R31–38.
Cavan DA, Penny MA, Jacobs KH, Kelly MA, Jenkins D, Mijovic CH, Chow CC, Cockram CS, Hawkins BR, Barnett AH: Analysis of a Chinese population suggests that the TNFB gene is not a susceptibility gene for Graves' disease. Hum Immunol 1994a; 40:135–137.
Cavan DA, Penny MA, Jacobs KH, Kelly MA, Jenkins D, Mijovic C, Chow C, Cockram CS, Hawkins BR, Barnett AH: The HLA association with Graves' disease is sex-specific in Hong Kong Chinese subjects. Clin Endocrinol 1994b; 40:63–66.
Chen Q-Y, Huang W, She J-X, Baxter F, Volpe R, MacLaren NK: HLA-*DRB1*03/DRB3*0101*, and *DRB3*0202* are susceptibility genes for Graves' disease in North American Caucasians, whereas *DRB1*07* is protective. J Clin Endocrinol Metab 1999; 84:3182–3186.
Cho BY, Rhee BD, Lee DS, Lee MS, Kim GY, Lee HK, Koh CS, Min HK: HLA and Graves' disease in Koreans. Tissue Antigens 1987; 30:119–121.
Cirafici AM, Salvatore G, de Vita G, Carlomagno F, Dathan NA, Melillo RM, Fusco A, Santoro M: Only the substitution of methionine 918 with a threonine and not with other residues activates RET transforming potential. Endocrinology 1997; 138:1450–1455.
Clifton-Bligh RJ, Wentworth JM, Heinz P, Crisp MS, John R, Lazarus JH, Ludgate M, Chatterjee VK: Mutation of the gene encoding human TTF-2 associated with thyroid agenesis, cleft palate and choanal atresia. Nat Genet 1998; 19:399–401.
Constans J, Ribouchon MT, Gouaillard C, Chaventre A, Clayton J: A new polymorphism of thyroxin-binding globulin in three African groups (Mali) with endemic nodular goitre. Hum Genet 1992; 89:199–203.
Cooper DS, Axelrod L, DeGroot LJ, Vickery AL Jr, Maloof F: Congenital goiter and the development of metastatic follicular carcinoma with evidence for a leak of nonhormonal iodide: clinical, pathological, kinetic, and biochemical studies and a review of the literature. J Clin Endocrinol Metab 1981; 52:294–306.
Corral J, Martin C, Perez R, Sanchez I, Mories MT, San Millan JL, Gonzalez-Sarmiento R: Thyroglobulin gene point mutation associated with non-endemic simple goitre. Lancet 1993; 341:462–464.
Couch RM, Hughes IA, DeSa DJ, Schiffrin A, Guyda H, Winter JS: An autosomal dominant form of adolescent multinodular goiter. Am J Hum Genet 1986; 39:811–816.
Cuddihy RM, Bahn RS: Lack of an association between alleles of interleukin-1α and interleukin-1 receptor antagonist genes and Graves' disease in a North American Caucasian population. J Clin Endocrinol Metab 1996; 81:4476–4478.
Cuddihy RM, Dutton CM, Bahn RS: A polymorphism in the extracellular domain of the thyrotropin receptor is highly associated with autoimmune thyroid disease in females. Thyroid 1995; 5:89–95.
Dahlberg PA, Holmlund G, Karlsson FA, Safwenberg J: HLA-A, -B, -C and -DR antigens in patients with Graves' disease and their correlation with signs and clinical course. Acta Endocrinol 1981; 97:42–47.
Dai G, Levy O, Carrasco N: Cloning and characterization of the thyroid iodide transporter. Nature 1996; 379:458–460.
Demaine A, Welsh KI, Hawe BS, Farid NR: Polymorphism of the T cell receptor β-chain in Graves' disease. J Clin Endocrinol Metab 1987; 65:643–646.
Demaine AG, Ratanachaiyavong S, Pope R, Ewins D, Millward BA, McGregor AM: Thyroglobulin antibodies in Graves' disease are associated with T-cell receptor β-chain and major histocompatibility complex loci. Clin Exp Immunol 1989; 77:21–24.
de Roux N, Shields DC, Misrahi M, Ratanachaiyavong S, McGregor AM: Analysis of the thyrotropin receptor as a candidate gene in familial Graves' disease. J Clin Endocrinol Metab 1996; 81:3483–3486.
Di Cristofano A, Pesce B, Cordon-Cardo C, Pandolfi PP: PTEN is essential for embryonic development and tumour suppression. Nat Genet 1998; 19:348–355.
Djilali-Saiah I, Larger E, Harfouch-Hammoud E, Timsit J, Clerc J, Bertin E, Assan R, Boitard C, Bach J-F, Caillat-Zucman S: No major role for the *CTLA-4* gene in the association of autoimmune thyroid disease with IDDM. Diabetes 1998; 47:125–127.
Dong RP, Kimura A, Okubo R, Shinagawa H, Tamai H, Nishimura Y: HLA-A and DPB1 loci confer susceptibility to Graves' disease. Hum Immunol 1992; 35:165–172.
Doniach D, Roitt IM, Taylor KB: Autoimmunity in pernicious anemia and thyroiditis: a family study. Ann NY Acad Sci 1965; 124:605–625.
Donner H, Rau H, Walfish PG, Braun J, Siegmund T, Finke R, Herwig JU, Badenhoop K: CTLA4 alanine-17 confers genetic susceptibility to Graves' disease and to Type 1 diabetes mellitus. J Clin Endocrinol Metab 1997; 82:143–146.
Dunn AD: Hormone synthesis: release and secretion of thyroid hormone. In: Braverman LE, Utiger RD (eds). Werner and Ingbar's The Thyroid. 7th Ed. Philadelphia: Lippincott-Raven, 1996:81–84.
Dunn JT: Thyroglobulin: chemistry and biosynthesis. In: Braverman LE, Utiger RD (eds). Werner and Ingbar's The Thyroid. 7th Ed. Philadelphia: Lippincott-Raven, 1996:85–95.
Dunning EJ: Struma lymphomatosa: a report of three cases in one family. J Clin Endocrinol Metab 1959; 19:1121–1125.
Durbec P, Marcos-Gutierrez CV, Kilkenny C, Grigoriou M, Wartiowaara KS, Suvanto P, Smith D, Ponder B, Costantini F, Saarma M, et al.: GDNF signalling through the Ret receptor tyrosine kinase. Nature 1996; 381:789–793.
Eng C: Genetics of Cowden syndrome: through the looking glass of oncology. Int J Oncol 1998; 12:701–710.
Everett LA, Glaser B, Beck JC, Idol JR, Buchs A, Heyman M, Adawi F, Nassir E, Baxevanis AD, Sheffield VC, Green ED: Pendred syndrome is caused by mutations in a putative sulphate transporter gene (PDS). Nat Genet 1997; 17:411–422.
Farid NR, Barnard JM, Marshall WH: The association of HLA with autoimmune thyroid disease in Newfoundland: the influence of HLA homozygosity in Graves' disease. Tissue Antigens 1976; 8:181–189.
Farid NR, Moens H, Larsen B, Payne R, Saltman K, Fifield F, Ingram DW: HLA haplotypes in familial Graves' disease. Tissue Antigens 1980a; 15:492–500.
Farid NR, Sampson L, Moens H, Barnard JM: The association of goitrous autoimmune thyroiditis with HLA-DR5. Tissue Antigens 1981; 17:265–268.
Farid NR, Sampson L, Noel EP, Barnard JM, Mandeville R, Larsen B, Carter ND: A study of human leukocyte D locus related antigens in Graves' disease. J Clin Invest 1979; 63:108–113.
Farid NR, Stone E, Johnson G: Graves' disease and HLA: clinical and epidemiologic associations. Clin Endocrinol 1980b; 13:535–544.
Fenzi GF, Giani C, Ceccarelli P, Bartalena L, Macchia E, Vitti P, Lari R, Ceccarelli C, Baschieri L, et al.: Role of autoimmune and familial factors in goiter prevalence: studies performed in a moderately endemic area. J Endocrinol Invest 1986; 9:161–164.
Fernandez-Soto L, Gonzalez A, Escobar-Jimenez F, Vazquez R, Ocete E, Salmeron J: Increased risk of autoimmune thyroid disease in hepatitis C vs hepatitis B before, during, and after discontinuing interferon therapy. Arch Intern Med 1998; 158:1445–1448.
Fisher DA, Polk DH: Development of the thyroid. Baillieres Best Prac Res Clin Endocrinol Metab 1989; 3:627–657.
Foley TP Jr, Schubert WK, Marnell RT, McAdams AJ: Chronic lymphocytic thyroiditis and juvenile myxedema in uniovular twins. J Pediatr 1968; 72:201–207.
Franceschi S, La Vecchia C: Thyroid cancer. Cancer Surv 1994; 19–20:393–422.
Frank K, Gartner R, Raue F, Ziegler R: Inherited thyroxine-binding globulin excess: study in a kindred. Exp Clin Endocrinol Diabetes 1986; 88:237–241.
Frecker M, Mercer G, Skanes VM, Farid NR: Major histocompatibility complex (MHC) factors predisposing to and protecting against Graves' eye disease. Autoimmunity 1988; 1:307–315.
Frecker M, Stenszky V, Balazs C, Kozma L, Kraszits E, Farid NR: Genetic factors in Graves' ophthalmopathy. Clin Endocrinol 1986; 25:479–485.
Frich L, Glattre E, Akslen LA: Familial occurrence of nonmedullary thyroid cancer: a population-based study of 5673 first-degree relatives of thyroid cancer patients in Norway. Cancer Epidemiol Biomarkers Prev 2001; 10:113–117.
Friedman JM, Fialkow PJ: The genetics of Graves' disease. Clin Endocrinol Metab 1978; 7:47–65.
Führer D, Mix M, Willgerodt H, Holzapfel HP, v. Petrykowski W, Wonerow P, Paschke R: Autosomal dominant nonautoimmune hyperthyroidism: clinical features, diagnosis, therapy. Exp Clin Endocrinol Diabetes 1998; 106(Suppl.)4:S10–S15.
Führer D, Wonerow P, Willgerodt H, Paschke R: Identification of a new thyrotropin receptor germline mutation (Leu629Phe) in a family with neonatal onset of autosomal dominant nonautoimmune hyperthyroidism. J Clin Endocrinol Metab 1997; 82:4234–4238.
Gabriel EM, Bergert ER, Grant CS, van Heerden JA, Thompson GB, Morris JC: Germline polymorphism of codon 727 of human thyroid-stimulating hormone receptor is associated with toxic multinodular goiter. J Clin Endocrinol Metab 1999; 84:3328–3335.
Gagne N, Parma J, Deal C, Vassart G, Van Vliet G: Apparent congenital athyreosis contrasting with normal plasma thyroglobulin levels and associated with inactivating mutations in the thyrotropin receptor gene: are athyreosis and ectopic thyroid distinct entities? J Clin Endocrinol Metab 1998; 83:1771–1775.
Gaitan E, Nelson NC, Poole GV: Endemic goiter and endemic thyroid disorders. World J Surg 1991; 15:205–215.
Gartner R: Thyroxine treatment of benign goiter. Acta Med Austriaca 1994; 21:44–47.
Gharib H, Mazzaferri EL: Thyroxine suppressive therapy in patients with nodular thyroid disease. Ann Intern Med 1998; 128:386–394.
Gharib H, McConahey WM, Tiegs RD, Bergstralh EJ, Goellner JR, Grant CS, van Heerden JA, Sizemore GW, Hay ID: Medullary thyroid carcinoma: clinicopathological features and long-term follow-up of 65 patients treated during 1946 through 1970. Mayo Clin Proc 1992; 67:934–940.
Giardiello FM, Offerhaus GJA, Lee DH, Krush AJ, Tersmette AC, Booker SV, Kelley NC, Hamilton SR: Increased risk of thyroid and pancreatic carcinoma in familial adenomatous polyposis. Gut 1993; 34:1394–1396.
Giordano C, Stassi G, De Maria R, Todaro M, Richiusa P, Papoff G, Bagnasco M, Testi R, Galluzzo A: Potential involvement of Fas and its ligand in the pathogenesis of Hashimoto's thyroiditis. Science 1997; 275:960–963.
Gordin A, Maenpaa J, Makinen T, Totterman TH, Tiilikainen A: Immunological and genetic markers in a family with Hashimoto's disease. Clin Endocrinol 1979; 11:425–435.

Gorson D: Familial papillary carcinoma of the thyroid. Thyroid 1992; 2:131–132.
Grebe SKG, Delahunt JW, Feek CM, Purdie G, Porter DJ: Lack of evidence for pituitary thyrotroph down-regulation after 1 week of oral thyrotrophin-releasing hormone and metoclopramide under conditions of constant peripheral thyroid hormone levels. Euro J Endocrinol 1995; 132:331–337.
Grebe SKG, Eberhardt NL, Jenkins RB: Cytogenetic abnormalities associated with endocrine neoplasia. In: Wolman SR, Sell S (eds). Human Cytogenetic Cancer Markers. Totowa, NJ: Humana Press, 1997:369–401.
Grebe SKG, Hay ID: Clinical evaluation of thyroid tumors. In: Thawley SE, Panje WR, Batsakis JG, Lindberg RD (eds). Comprehensive Management of Head and Neck Tumors. 2nd ed. Philadelphia: W. B. Saunders, 1999:1694–1709.
Grebe SKG, Hay ID: Follicular cell-derived thyroid carcinomas. Cancer Treat Res 1997; 89:91–140.
Grebe SKG, Hay ID: Follicular thyroid cancer. Endocrinol Metab Clin North Am 1995b; 24:761–801.
Greig WR, Boyle JA, Duncan A, Nicol J, Gray MJ, Buchanan WW, McGirr EM: Genetic factors in simple goitre formation: evidence from a twin study. Q J Med 1967; 36:175–188.
Grumet FC, Payne RO, Konishi J, Kriss JP: HL-A antigens as markers for disease susceptibility and autoimmunity in Graves' disease. J Clin Endocrinol Metab 1974; 39:1115–1119.
Grunditz T, Sundler F: Other factors regulating thyroid function: autonomic nervous control—adrenergic, cholinergic, and peptidergic regulation. In: Braverman LE, Utiger RD (eds). Werner and Ingbar's The Thyroid. 7th Ed. Philadelphia: Lippincott-Raven, 1996:247–253.
Grüters A, Köhler B, Wolf A, Söling A, de Vijlder L, Krude H, Biebermann H: Screening for mutations of the human thyroid peroxidase gene in patients with congenital hypothyroidism. Exp Clin Endocrinol Diabetes 1996; 104(Suppl.)4:121–123.
Grüters A, Schöneberg T, Biebermann H, Krude H, Krohn HP, Dralle H, Gudermann T: Severe congenital hyperthyroidism caused by a germline neo mutation in the extracellular portion of the thyrotropin receptor. J Clin Endocrinol Metab 1998; 83:1431–1436.
Haggitt RC, Reid BJ: Hereditary gastrointestinal polyposis syndromes. Am J Surg Pathol 1986; 10:871–887.
Hall P, Holm LE, Lundell G, Bjelkengren G, Larsson LG, Lindberg S, Wicklund H, Boice JD Jr: Cancer risks in thyroid cancer patients. Br J Cancer 1991; 64:159–163.
Hall PF: Familial occurrence of myxedema. J Med Genet 1965; 2:173–180.
Hall R, Dingle PR, Roberts DF: Thyroid antibodies: a study of first degree relatives. Clin Genet 1972; 3:319–324.
Hall R, Owen SG, Smart GA: Paternal transmission of thyroid autoimmunity. Lancet 1964; ii:115.
Hammond LJ, Lowdell MW, Cerrano PG, Goode AW, Bottazzo GF, Mirakian R: Analysis of apoptosis in relation to tissue destruction associated with Hashimoto's autoimmune thyroiditis. J Pathol 1997; 182:138–144.
Harvald B, Hauge M: A catamnestic investigation of Danish twins. Dan Med Bull 1956; 3:150–158.
Hasen J, Bartalos M: Dyshormonogenetic goitrous hypothyroidism in a patient with short arm deletion of E18 chromosome. Horm Res 1975; 6:28–35.
Hashimoto S, McCombs CC, Michalski JP: Mechanism of a lymphocyte abnormality associated with HLA-B8/DR3 in clinically healthy individuals. Clin Exp Immunol 1989; 76:317–323.
Hashimoto S, Michalski JP, Berman MA, McCombs C: Mechanism of a lymphocyte abnormality associated with HLA-B8/DR3: role of interleukin-1. Clin Exp Immunol 1990; 79:227–232.
Hawkins BR, Ma JT, Lam KS, Wang CC, Yeung RT: Analysis of linkage between HLA haplotype and susceptibility to Graves' disease in multiple-case Chinese families in Hong Kong. Acta Endocrinol 1985a; 110:66–69.
Hawkins BR, Ma JT, Lam KS, Wang CC, Yeung RT: Association of HLA antigens with thyrotoxic Graves' disease and periodic paralysis in Hong Kong Chinese. Clin Endocrinol 1985b; 23:245–252.
Hedinger CE: Histological typing of thyroid tumours. In: Hedinger CE (ed). International Histological Classification of Tumours, Vol. 11. Berlin: Springer, 1988:
Heward JM, Allahabadia A, Armitage M, Hattersley A, Dodson PM, MacLeod K, Carr-Smith J, Daykin J, Daly A, Sheppard MC, et al.: The development of Graves' disease and the CTLA-4 gene on chromosome 2q33. J Clin Endocrinol Metab 1999; 84:2398–2401.
Heward JM, Allahabadia A, Carr-Smith J, Daykin J, Cockram CS, Gordon C, Barnett AH, Franklyn JA, Gough SCL: No evidence for allelic association of a human CTLA-4 promoter polymorphism with autoimmune thyroid disease in either population-based case-control or family-based studies. Clin Endocrinol 1998; 49:331–334.
Heward JM, Gough SC: Genetic susceptibility to the development of autoimmune disease. Clin Sci 1997; 93:479–491.
Heyma P, Harrison LC, Robins-Browne R: Thyrotropin (TSH) binding sites on *Yersinia enterocolitica* recognized by immunoglobulins from humans with Graves' disease. Clin Exp Immunol 1986; 64:249–254.
Hintze G, Windeler J, Baumert J, Stein H, Kobberling J: Thyroid volume and goitre prevalence in the elderly as determined by ultrasound and their relationships to laboratory indices. Acta Endocrinol 1991; 124:12–18.
Hoelting T, Siperstein AE, Duh QY, Clark OH: Tamoxifen inhibits growth, migration, and invasion of human follicular and papillary thyroid cancer cells in vitro and in vivo. J Clin Endocrinol Metab 1995; 80:308–313.
Hsiao YL, Chang TC: Prevalence of goiter in Taiwanese adults: a preliminary study. J Formos Med Assoc 1995; 94:197–199.
Hu R, Beck C, Chang YB, DeGroot LJ: HLA class II genes in Graves' disease. Autoimmunity 1992; 12:103–106.
Hunt PJ, Marshall SE, Weetman AP, Bell JI, Wass JA, Welsh KI: Cytokine gene polymorphisms in autoimmune thyroid disease. J Clin Endocrinol Metab 2000; 85:1984–1988.
Hurley DL, Gharib H: Evaluation and management of multinodular goiter. Otolaryngol Clin North Am 1996; 29:527–540.
Irvine WJ, MacGregor A-G, Stuart AE, Hall GH: Hashimoto's disease in uniovular twins. Lancet 1961; ii:850–853.
Ismail-Beigi F, Rahimifar M: A variant of iodotyrosine-dehalogenase deficiency. J Clin Endocrinol Metab 1977; 44:499–506.
Jaffiol C, Seignalet J, Baldet L, Robin M, Lapinski H, Mirouze J: Systeme HLA et maladie de Basedow. Ann Endocrinol (Paris) 1976; 37:219–226.
Jansson R, Safwenberg J, Dahlberg PA: Influence of the HLA-DR4 antigen and iodine status on the development of autoimmune postpartum thyroiditis. J Clin Endocrinol Metab 1985; 60:168–173.
Jaspan JB, Sullivan K, Garry RF, Lopez M, Wolfe M, Clejan S, Yan C, Sander DM, Ahmed B, Bryer-Ash M: The interaction of a type A retroviral particle and class II human leukocyte antigen susceptibility genes in the pathogenesis of Graves' disease. J Clin Endocrinol Metab 1996; 81:2271–2279.
Jenkins D, Penny MA, Fletcher JA, Jacobs KH, Mijovic CH, Franklyn JA, Sheppard MC: HLA class II polymorphism contributes little to Hashimoto's thyroiditis. Clin Endocrinol 1992; 37:141–145.
Johnsen T, Sorensen MS, Feldt-Rasmussen U, Friis J: The variable intrafamiliar expressivity in Pendred's syndrome. Clin Otolaryngol 1989; 14:395–399.
Kaczur V, Takacs M, Szalai C, Falus A, Nagy Z, Berencsi G, Balazs C: Analysis of the genetic variability of the 1st (CCC/ACC, P52T) and the 10th exons (bp 1012–1704) of the TSH receptor gene in Graves' disease. Eur J Immunogenet 2000; 27:17–23.
Kakizaki S, Takagi H, Murakami M, Takayama H, Mori M: HLA antigens in patients with interferon-α-induced autoimmune thyroid disorders in chronic hepatitis C. J Hepatol 1999; 30:794–800.
Kakizaki S, Takagi H, Murakami M, Takayama H, Sato K, Mori M: HLA-A2 subtype in patients with interferon-α-induced autoimmune thyroid disorders in chronic hepatitis C. Liver 2000; 20:423–424.
Kamizono S, Hiromatsu Y, Seki N, Bednarczuk T, Matsumoto H, Kimura A, Itoh K: A polymorphism of the 5′ flanking region of tumour necrosis factor-α gene is associated with thyroid-associated ophthalmopathy in Japanese. Clin Endocrinol 2000; 52:759–764.
Kawakami A, Matsuoka N, Tsuboi M, Koji T, Urayama S, Sera N, Hida A, Usa T, Kimura H, Yokoyama N, et al.: $CD4^+$ T cell-mediated cytotoxicity toward thyrocytes: the importance of Fas/Fas ligand interaction inducing apoptosis of thyrocytes and the inhibitory effect of thyroid-stimulating hormone. Lab Invest 2000; 80:471–484.
Kelly MD, Hugh TB, Field AS, Fitzsimons R: Carcinoma of the thyroid gland and Gardner's syndrome. Aust N Z J Surg 1993; 63:505–509.
Kendall-Taylor P, Stephenson A, Stratton A, Papiha SS, Perros P: Differentiation of autoimmune ophthalmopathy from Graves' hyperthyroidism by analysis of genetic markers. Clin Endocrinol 1988; 28:601–610.
Kimura S, Hara Y, Pineau T, Fernandez-Salguero P, Fox CH, Ward JM: The T/ebp null mouse: thyroid-specific enhancer-binding protein is essential for the organogenesis of the thyroid, lung, ventral forebrain, and pituitary. Genes Devel 1996; 10:60–69.
Kirschner LS, Carney JA, Pack SD, Taymans SE, Giatzakis C, Cho YS, Cho-Chung YS, Stratakis CA: Mutations of the gene encoding the protein kinase A type I-α regulatory subunit in patients with the Carney complex. Nat Genet 2000a; 26:89–92.
Kirschner LS, Sandrini F, Monbo J, Lin JP, Carney JA, Stratakis CA: Genetic heterogeneity and spectrum of mutations of the PRKAR1A gene in patients with the Carney complex. Hum Mol Genet 2000b; 9:3037–3046.
Kitayama H, Tsujimura T, Matsumura I, Oritani K, Ikeda H, Ishikawa JO, Suzuki M, Yamamura K, Matsuzawa Y, Kitamura Y, Kanakura Y: Neoplastic transformation of normal hematopoetic cells by constitutively activating mutations of *c*-kit receptor tyrosine kinase. Blood 1996; 88:995–1004.
Klein RD, Sherman D, Ho WH, Stone D, Bennett GL, Moffat B, Vandlen R, Simmons L, Gu Q, Hongo JA, et al.: A GPI-linked protein that interacts with Ret to form a candidate neurturin receptor. Nature 1997; 387:717–721.
Kobayashi K, Tanaki Y, Ishiguro S, Mori T, Mitani Y, Shigemasa C: Family with nonmedullary thyroid neoplasms. J Surg Oncol 1995; 58:274–277.
Komatsu M, Hanamura N, Seki T, Narata M, Kuroda T: A family with hereditary high serum thyroxine-binding globulin. Endocrine J 1994; 41:467–470.
Kotani T, Aratake Y, Hirai K, Fukazawa Y, Sato H, Ohtaki S: Apoptosis in thyroid tissue from patients with Hashimoto's thyroiditis. Autoimmunity 1995; 20:231–236.
Kotsa K, Watson PF, Weetman AP: A CTLA-4 gene polymorphism is associated with both Graves' disease and autoimmune hypothyroidism. Clin Endocrinol 1997; 46:551–554.
Kozma L, Stenszky V, Kraszits E, Balazs C, Farid NR: The association of IgG heavy-chain allotypes (Gm) with Graves' disease in Hungary. Exp Clin Immunogenet 1985; 2:154–157.
Kraimps JL, Canzian F, Jost C, Menet E, Amati P, Levillian P, Harach R, Lesueur F, Barbier J, Romeo G, Bonneau D: Mapping of a gene predisposing to familial thyroid tumors with cell oxyphilia to chromosome 19 and exclusion of *JUN B* as a candidate gene. Surgery 1999; 126:188–194.
Krude H, Biebermann H, Göpel W, Grüters A: The gene for the thyrotropin receptor

(TSHR) as a candidate gene for congenital hypothyroidism with thyroid dysgenesis. Exp Clin Endocrinol Diabetes 1996; 104(Suppl.)4:117–120.

Kwok CG, McDougall IR: Familial differentiated carcinoma of the thyroid: report of five pairs of siblings. Thyroid 1995; 5:395–397.

Lahat N, Rahat MA, Sadeh O, Kinarty A, Kraiem Z: Regulation of HLA-DR and costimulatory B7 molecules in human thyroid carcinoma cells: differential binding of transcription factors to the HLA-DRα promoter. Thyroid 1998; 8:361–369.

Lamberg BA: Endemic goitre: iodine deficiency disorders. Ann Med 1991; 23:367–372.

Larsson C, Nordenskjöld M: Multiple endocrine neoplasia. Cancer Surv 1990; 9:703–723.

Lawley TJ, Hall RP, Fauci AS, Katz SI, Hamburger MI, Frank MM: Defective Fc-receptor functions associated with the HLA-B8/DRw3 haplotype: studies in patients with dermatitis herpetiformis and normal subjects. N Engl J Med 1981; 304:185–192.

Ledger GA, Khosla S, Lindor NM, Thibodeau SN, Gharib H: Genetic testing in the diagnosis and management of mulitple endocrine neoplasia type II. Ann Intern Med 1995; 122:118–124.

Lee FI, Jenkins GC, Hughes DT, Kazantizis G: Pernicious anemia myxedema and hypogammaglobulinemia: a family study. Br Med J 1964; 1:598–602.

Lehmann W: Zur Erbpathologie der Hyperthyrösen. Z induktive Abstammung Vererbung 1937; 73:531–535.

Li J, Yen C, Liaw D, Podsypanina K, Bose S, Wang SI, Puc J, Rodgers L, McCombie R, Bigner SH, et al.: PTEN, a putative protein tyrosine phosphatase gene mutated in human brain, breast, and prostate cancer. Science 1997; 275:1943–1947.

Liaw D, Marsh DJ, Li J, Dahia PL, Wang SI, Zheng Z, Bose S, Call KM, Tsou HC, Peacocke M, et al.: Germline mutations of the PTEN gene in Cowden disease, an inherited breast and thyroid cancer syndrome. Nat Genet 1997; 16:64–67.

Lichter JB, Wu J, Miller D, Goodfellow PJ, Kidd KK: A high-resolution meiotic mapping panel for the pericentromeric region of chromosome 10. Genomics 1992; 13:607–612.

Lima N, Knobel M, Cavaliere H, Sztejnsznajd C, Tomimori E: Levothyroxine suppressive therapy is partially effective in treating patients with benign, solid thyroid nodules and multinodular goiters. Thyroid 1997; 7:691–697.

Loh KC: Familial nonmedullary thyroid carcinoma: a meta-review of case series. Thyroid 1997; 7:107–113.

Lote K, Andersen K, Nordal E, Brennhvod IO: Familial occurrence of papillary thyroid carcinoma. Cancer 1980; 46:1291–1297.

Ludgate M, Jasani B: Apoptosis in autoimmune and non-autoimmune thyroid disease. J Pathol 1997; 182:123–124.

Luo G, Fan JL, Seetharamaiah GS, Desai RK, Dallas JS, Wagle N, Doan R, Niesel DW, Klimpel GR, Prabhakar BS: Immunization of mice with *Yersinia enterocolitica* leads to the induction of antithyrotropin receptor antibodies. J Immunol 1993; 151:922–928.

Luo G, Seetharamaiah GS, Niesel DW, Zhang H, Peterson JW, Prabhakar BS, Klimpel GR: Purification and characterization of *Yersinia enterocolitica* envelope proteins which induce antibodies that react with human thyrotropin receptor. J Immunol 1994; 152:2555–2561.

Lupoli G, Vitale G, Caraglia M, Fittipaldi MR, Abbruzzese A, Tagliaferri P, Bianco AR: Familial papillary thyroid microcarcinoma: a new clinical entity. Lancet 1999; 353:637–639.

Lynch ED, Ostermeyer EA, Lee MK, Arena JF, Ji H, Dann J, Swisshelm K, Suchard D, MacLeod PM, Kvinnsland S, et al.: Inherited mutations in PTEN that are associated with breast cancer, Cowden disease, and juvenile polyposis. Am J Hum Genet 1997; 61:1254–1260.

Maalej A, Kacem HH, Bellassoued M, Abid M, Makni H, Ayadi H: Polymorphisms of HLA DQB1 CAR1/CAR2 and TNFα IR2/IR4 microsatellite markers in patients affected with Graves disease. Clin Immunol 2000; 96: 91–93.

Macchia PE, Lapi P, Krude H, Pirro MT, Missero C, Chiovato L, Baserga M, Tassi V, Pinchera A, Fenzi G, et al.: PAX8 mutations associated with congenital hypothyroidism caused by thyroid dysgenesis. Nat Genet 1998; 19:83–86.

Mack E: Management of patients with substernal goiters. Surg Clin North Am 1995; 75:377–394.

Malchoff CD, Sarfarazi M, Tendler B, Forouhar F, Whalen G, Joshi V, Arnold A, Malchoff DM: Papillary thyroid carcinoma associated with papillary renal neoplasia: genetic linkage analysis of a distinct heritable tumor syndrome. J Clin Endocrinol Metab 2000; 85:1758–1764.

Malnati MS, Marti M, LaVaute T, Jaraquemada D, Biddison W, DeMars R: Processing pathways for presentation of cytosolic antigen to MHC class II-restricted T cells. Nature 1992; 357:702–704.

Mangklabruks A, Cox N, DeGroot LJ: Genetic factors in autoimmune thyroid disease analyzed by restriction fragment length polymorphisms of candidate genes. J Clin Endocrinol Metab 1991; 73:236–244.

Manley NR, Capecchi MR: The role of Hoxa-3 in mouse thymus and thyroid development. Development 1995; 121:1989–2003.

Manley NR, Capecchi MR: HOX group 3 paralogs regulate the development and migration of the thymus, thyroid, and parathyroid glands. Dev Biol 1998; 195:1–15.

Mansberger AR Jr, Wei JP: Surgical embryology and anatomy of the thyroid and parathyroid glands. Surg Clin North Am 1993; 73:727–746.

Mansouri A, Chowdhury K, Gruss P: Follicular cells of the thyroid gland require *Pax8* gene function. Nat Genet 1998; 19:87–90.

Marsh DJ, Coulon V, Lunetta KL, Rocca-Serra P, Dahia PL, Zheng Z, Liaw D, Caron S, Duboue B, Lin AY, et al.: Mutation spectrum and genotype–phenotype analyses in Cowden disease and Bannayan-Zonana syndrome, two hamartoma syndromes with germline *PTEN* mutation. Hum Mol Genet 1998; 7:507–515.

Marsh DJ, Learoyd DL, Robinson BG: Medullary thyroid carcinoma: recent advances and management update. Thyroid 1995; 5:407–424.

Marsh SGE: HLA class II region sequences. Tissue Antigens 1998; 51:467–507.

Martin L, Fisher RA: The hereditary and familial aspects of exophthalmic goitre and nodular goitre. Q J Med 1945; 14:207–219.

Mason PM, Parham P: HLA class I nucleotide sequences. Tissue Antigens 1998; 51:417–466.

Matsuda A, Kosugi S: A homozygous missense mutation of the sodium/iodide symporter gene causing iodide transport defect. J Clin Endocrinol Metab 1997; 82:3966–3971.

Mayr WR, Ludwig H, Schernthaner G, Hofer R: HLA CW3 in thyrotoxicosis patients with and without endocrine ophthalmopathy. Tissue Antigens 1976; 7:243–246.

McCombs CC, Michalski JP, deShazo R, Bozelka B, Lane JT: Immune abnormalities associated with HLA-B8: lymphocyte subsets and functional correlates. Clin Immunol Immunopathol 1986; 39:112–120.

McEwan P: Clinical problems in thyrotoxicosis. Br Med J 1938; i:1037–1042.

McGregor AM, Roberts DF, Hall R: A study of triplets with Hashimoto's thyroiditis. Postgrad Med J 1979; 55:894–896.

McIntosh R, Watson P, Weetman A: Somatic hypermutation in autoimmune thyroid disease. Immunol Rev 1998; 162:219–231.

McIver B, Morris JC: The pathogenesis of Graves' disease. Endocrinol Metab Clin North Am 1998; 27:73–89.

McKenna R, Kearns M, Sugrue D, Drury MI, McCarthy CF: HLA and hyperthyroidism in Ireland. Tissue Antigens 1982; 19:97–99.

McTiernan A, Weiss NS, Darling JR: Incidence of thyroid cancer in women in relation to known or suspected risk factors for breast cancer. Cancer Res 1987; 47:292–295.

Medeiros-Neto GA, Billerbeck AE, Wajchenberg BL, Targovnik HM: Defective organification of iodide causing hereditary goitrous hypothyroidism. Thyroid 1993a; 3:143–159.

Medeiros-Neto G, Bunduki V, Tomimori E, Gomes S, Knobel M, Martin RTZ, Zugaib M: Prenatal diagnosis and treatment of dyshormonogenetic fetal goiter due to defective thyroglobulin synthesis. J Clin Endocrinol Metab 1997; 82:4239–4242.

Medeiros-Neto G, Gil-DaCosta MJ, Santos CLS, Medina AM, Silva JCE, Tsou RM, Sobrinho-Simıes M: Metastatic thyroid carcinoma arising from congenital goiter due to mutation in the thyroperoxidase gene. J Clin Endocrinol Metab 1998; 83:4162–4166.

Medeiros-Neto GA, Nakashima T, Taurog A, Knobel M, Simonetti JP, Mattar E: Congenital goitre and hypothyroidism with impaired iodide organification and high thyroid peroxidase concentration. Clin Endocrinol 1979; 11:123–139.

Medeiros-Neto GA, Okamura K, Cavaliere H, Taurog A, Knobel M, Bisi HK, Mattar E: Familial thyroid peroxidase defect. Clin Endocrinol 1982; 17:1–14.

Medeiros-Neto G, Targovnik HM, Vassart G: Defective thyroglobulin synthesis and secretion causing goiter and hypothyroidism. Endocr Rev 1993b; 14:165–183.

Michiels FM, Chappuis S, Caillou B, Pasini A, Talbot M, Monier R, Feunteun J, Billaud M: Development of medullary thyroid carcinoma in transgenic mice expressing the RET protooncogene altered by a multiple endocrine neoplasia type 2A mutation. Proc Natl Acad Sci USA 1997; 94:3330–3335.

Mimouni M, Mimouni-Bloch A, Schachter J, Shohat M: Familial hypothyroidism with autosomal dominant inheritance. Arch Dis Child 1996; 75:245–246.

Mitsiades N, Poulaki V, Kotoula V, Mastorakos G, Tseleni-Balafouta S, Tsokos M: Fas/Fas ligand up-regulation and Bcl-2 down-regulation may be significant in the pathogenesis of Hashimoto's thyroiditis. J Clin Endocrinol Metab 1998; 83:2199–2203.

Moley JF, Debenedetti MK, Dilley WG, Tisell LE, Wells SA: Surgical management of patients with persistent or recurrent medullary thyroid cancer. J Intern Med 1998; 243:521–526.

Momburg F, Ortiz-Navarrete V, Neefjes J, Goulmy E, van de Wal Y, Spits H, Powis SJ, Butcher GW, Howard JC, Walden P, Hammerling GJ: Proteasome subunits encoded by the major histocompatibility complex are not essential for antigen presentation. Nature 1992; 360:174–177.

Momburg F, Roelse J, Howard JC, Butcher GW, Hammerling GJ, Neefjes JJ: Selectivity of MHC-encoded peptide transporters from human, mouse and rat. Nature 1994; 367:648–651.

Monden T, Yamada M, Satoh T, Iizuka M, Mori M: Analysis of the TSH receptor gene structure in various thyroid disorders: DNA from thyroid adenomas can have large insertions or deletions. Thyroid 1992; 2:189–192.

Muhlberg T, Herrmann K, Joba W, Kirchberger M, Heberling HJ, Heufelder AE: Lack of association of nonautoimmune hyperfunctioning thyroid disorders and a germline polymorphism of codon 727 of the human thyrotropin receptor in a European Caucasian population. J Clin Endocrinol Metab 2000; 85:2640–2643.

Murray IP, Thomson JA, McGirr EM, MacDonald EM, Kennedy JS, McLennan I: Unusual familial goiter associated with intrathyroidal calcification. J Clin Endocrinol Metab 1966; 26:1039–1049.

Mustapha M, Azar ST, Moglabey YB, Saouda M, Zeitoun G, Loiselet J: Further refinement of Pendred syndrome locus by homozygosity analysis to a 0.8 cM interval flanked by D7S496 and D7S2425. J Med Genet 1998; 35:202–204.

Myers MP, Tonks NK: PTEN: sometimes taking it off can be better than putting it on. Am J Hum Genet 1997; 61:1234–1238.

Nagamine K, Peterson P, Scott HS, Kudoh J, Minoshima S, Heino M, Krohn KJ, Lalioti MD, Mullis PE, Antonarakis SE, et al.: Positional cloning of the APECED gene. Nat Genet 1997; 17:393–398.

Nagataki S, Yokoyama N: Other factors regulating thyroid function: autoregulation—

effects of Iodine. In: Braverman LE, Utiger RD (eds). Werner and Ingbar's The Thyroid. 7th Ed. Philadelphia: Lippincott-Raven, 1996:241–247.

Nelkin BD, Nakamura Y, White RW, de Bustros AC, Herman J, Wells SAJ, Baylin SB: Low incidence of loss of chromosome 10 in sporadic and hereditary human medullary thyroid carcinoma. Cancer Res 1989; 49:4114–4119.

Nelson SD, Pollet JE: HL-A antigens and thyrotoxicosis. Tissue Antigens 1975; 5:38–40.

Neumann S, Willgerodt H, Ackermann F, Reske A, Jung M, Reis A, Paschke R: Linkage of familial euthyroid goiter to the multinodular goiter-1 locus and exclusion of the candidate genes thyroglobulin, thyroperoxidase, and Na^+/I^- symporter. J Clin Endocrinol Metab 1999; 84:3750–3756.

Niepomniszcze H, Medeiros-Neto GA, Refetoff S, DeGroot LJ, Fang VS: Familial goitre with partial iodine organification defect, lack of thyroglobulin, and high levels of thyroid peroxidase. Clin Endocrinol 1977; 6:27–39.

Niimi H, Sasaki N, Nakajima H: Congenital iodide organification defect accompanied by a large nodular goiter: a case report. Endocrinol Japonica 1985; 32:361–367.

Nikiforov Y, Gnepp DR: Pediatric thyroid cancer after the Chernobyl disaster: pathomorphological study of 84 cases (1991–1992) from the Republic of Belarus. Cancer 1994; 74:748–766.

Normann T, Gautvik KM, Johannessen JV, Brennhovd IO: Medullary carcinoma of the thyroid in Norway. Acta Endocrinol 1976; 83:71–85.

Obermayer-Straub P, Manns MP: Autoimmune polyglandular syndromes. Baillieres Clin Gastroenterol 1998; 12:293–315.

Ofosu MH, Dunston G, Henry L, Ware D, Cheatham W, Brembridge A, Alarif L: HLA-DQ3 is associated with Graves' disease in African-Americans. Immunol Invest 1996; 25:103–110.

Omar MA, Hammond MG, Desai RK, Motala AA, Aboo N, Seedat MA: HLA class I and II antigens in South African blacks with Graves' disease. Clin Immunol Immunopathol 1990; 54:98–102.

Onuma H, Ota M, Sugenoya A, Inoko H: Association of HLA-DPB1*0501 with early-onset Graves' disease in Japanese. Hum Immunology 1994; 39:195–201.

Ozaki O, Ito K, Suzuki A, Manabe Y, Honoda Y: Familial occurrence of differentiated, nonmedullary thyroid carcinoma. World J Surg 1988; 12:565–571.

Palmer KT: A prospective study into thyroid disease in a geriatric unit. N Z Med J 1977; 86:323–334.

Park YJ, Chung HK, Park DJ, Kim WB, Kim SW, Koh JJ, Cho BY: Polymorphism in the promoter and exon 1 of the cytotoxic T lymphocyte antigen-4 gene associated with autoimmune thyroid disease in Koreans. Thyroid 2000; 10:453–459.

Parker JLW, Lawson DH: Death from thyrotoxicosis. Lancet 1973; ii:894–897.

Paschke R: Constitutively activating TSH receptor mutations as the cause of toxic thyroid adenoma, multinodular goiter and autosomal dominant non autoimmune hyperthyroidism. Exp Clin Endocrinol Diabetes 1996; 104(Suppl)4:129–132.

Paschke R, Van Sande J, Parma J, Vassart G: The TSH receptor and thyroid diseases. Baillieres Clin Endocrinol Metab 1996; 10:9–27.

Pasini A, Geneste O, Legrand P, Schlumberger M, Rossel M, Fournier LR, Schuffenecker I, Lenoir GM, Billaud M: Oncogenic activation of RET by two distinct FMTC mutations affecting the tyrosine kinase domain. Oncogene 1997; 15:393–402.

Payami H, Joe S, Farid NR, Stenszky V, Chan SH, Yeo PP, Cheah JS: Relative predispositional effects (RPEs) of marker alleles with disease: HLA-DR alleles and Graves disease. Am J Hum Genet 1989; 45:541–546.

Perez-Cuvit E, Crigler JF Jr, Stanbury JB: Partial and total iodide organification defect in different sibships in a kindred. Am J Hum Genet 1977; 29:142–148.

Philippou G, Krimitzas A, Kaltsas G, Anastasiou E, Souvatzoglou A, Alevizaki M: HLA DQA1*0501 and DRB1*0301 antigens do not independently convey susceptibility to Graves' disease. J Endocrinol Invest 2001; 24:88–91.

Pickerill AP, Watson PF, Tandon N, Weetman AP: T cell receptor β-chain gene polymorphisms in Graves' disease. Acta Endocrinol 1993; 128:499–502.

Pohlenz J, Medeiros-Neto G, Gross JL, Silveiro SP, Knobel M, Refetoff S: Hypothyroidism in a Brazilian kindred due to iodide trapping defect caused by a homozygous mutation in the sodium/iodide symporter gene. Biochem Biophys Res Commun 1997; 240:488–491.

Pohlenz J, Rosenthal IM, Weiss RE, Jhiang SM, Burant C, Refetoff S: Congenital hypothyroidism due to mutations in the sodium/iodide symporter: identification of a nonsense mutation producing a downstream cryptic 3′ splice site. J Clin Invest 1998; 101:1028–1035.

Polakis P: The adenomatous polyposis coli (APC) tumor suppressor. Biochim Biophys Acta 1997; 1332:F127–F147.

Ponder BAJ: The gene causing multiple endocrine neoplasia type 2 (MEN 2). Ann Med 1994; 26:199–203.

Ratanachaiyavong S, Fleming D, Janer M, Demaine AG, Willcox N, McGregor AM: HLA-DPB1 polymorphisms in patients with hyperthyroid Graves' disease and early onset myasthenia gravis. Autoimmunity 1994; 17:99–104.

Ratanachaiyavong S, Gunn CA, Bidwell EA, Darke C, Hall R, McGregor AM: DQA2 U allele: a genetic marker for relapse of Graves' disease. Clin Endocrinol 1990; 32:241–251.

Rau H, Nicolay A, Usadel KH, Finke R, Donner H, Walfish PG: Polymorphisms of TAP1 and TAP2 genes in Graves' disease. Tissue Antigens 1997; 49:16–22.

Rechavi G, Givol D, Geltner D: Polymorphism of human immunoglobulin VH genes: a possible marker of autoimmune disease. Dis Markers 1987; 5:171–176.

Rees Smith B, McLachlan SM, Furmaniak J: Autoantibodies to the thyrotropin receptor. Endocr Rev 1988; 9:106–121.

Refetoff S, Weis RE, Usala SJ: The syndrome of resistance to thyroid hormone. Endocr Rev 1993; 14:348–399.

Resetkova E, Notenboom R, Arreaza G, Mukuta T, Yoshikawa N, Volpe R: Seroreactivity to bacterial antigens is not a unique phenomenon in patients with autoimmune thyroid diseases in Canada. Thyroid 1994; 4:269–274.

Robbins J: Thyroid hormone transport proteins and the physiology of hormone binding. In: Braverman LE, Utiger RD (eds). Werner and Ingbar's The Thyroid. 7th Ed. Philadelphia: Lippincott-Raven, 1996:96–110.

Robbins J, Merino MJ, Boice JD Jr, Ron E, Ain KB, Alexander R, Norton JA, Reynolds J: Thyroid cancer: a lethal endocrine neoplasm. Ann Intern Med 1991; 115:133–147.

Robinson BG: Multiple endocrine neoplasia syndromes. In: 80th Annual Meeting, Endocrine Society: Meet-the-Professor Handouts. The Endocrine Society Press, Bethesda, MA, USA. 1998:155–157.

Roman SH, Greenberg D, Rubinstein P, Wallenstein S, Davies TF: Genetics of autoimmune thyroid disease: lack of evidence for linkage to HLA within families. J Clin Endocrinol Metab 1992; 74:496–503.

Ron E, Curtis R, Hoffman DA, Flannery JT: Multiple primary breast and thyroid cancer. Br J Cancer 1984; 49:87–92.

Rosai J, Carcangiu ML: Atlas of tumor pathology: tumors of the thyroid gland. Washington, DC: Armed Forces Institute of Pathology, 1992.

Rossel M, Pasini A, Chappuis S, Geneste O, Fournier L, Schuffenecker I, Takahashi M, van Grunsven LA, Urdiales JL, Rudkin BB, Lenoir GM: Distinct biological properties of two RET isoforms activated by MEN 2A and MEN 2B mutations. Oncogene 1997; 14:265–275.

Roura-Mir C, Catalfamo M, Sospedra M, Alcalde L, Pujol-Borrell R: Single-cell analysis of intrathyroidal lymphocytes shows differential cytokine expression in Hashimoto's and Graves' disease. Eur J Immunol 1997; 27:3290–3302.

Saad MF, Ordonez NG, Rashid RK, Guido JJ, Stratton Hill C Jr, Hickey RC, Samaan NA: Medullary carcinoma of the thyroid. Medicine 1984; 63:319–342.

Santoro M, Grieco M, Melillo RM, Fusco A, Vecchio G: Molecular defects in thyroid carcinomas: role of the RET oncogene in thyroid neoplastic transformation. Eur J Endocrinol 1995; 133:513–522.

Santoro M, Melillo RM, Carlomagno F, Visvonti R, de Vita G, Salvatore G, Lupoli G, Fusco A, Vecchio G: Molecular biology of the *MEN2* gene. J Intern Med 1998; 243:505–508.

Sasazuki T, Nishimura Y, Muto M, Ohta N: HLA-linked genes controlling immune response and disease susceptibility. Immunol Rev 1983; 70:51–75.

Sattler H: Basedow's Disease. New York: Grune and Stratton, 1952.

Schleusener H, Bogner U, Peters H, Kotulla P, Schmieg D, Grüters A, Mayr WR: The relevance of genetic susceptibility in Graves' disease and immune thyroiditis. Exp Clin Endocrinol Diabetes 1991; 97:127–132.

Schleusener H, Schwander J, Fischer C, Holle R, Holl G, Badenhoop K, Hensen J, Finke R, Bogner U, Mayr WR, et al.: Prospective multicentre study on the prediction of relapse after antithyroid drug treatment in patients with Graves' disease. Acta Endocrinol 1989; 120:689–701.

Schröder S, Böcker W, Baisch H, Bürk CG, Arps H, Meiners I, Kastemdieck H, Heitz PU, Klöppel G: Prognostic factors in medullary thyroid carcinomas. Cancer 1988; 61:806–816.

Schuppert F, Deiters S, Rambusch E, Sierralta W, Dralle H, von zurMuhlen A: TSH-receptor expression and human thyroid disease: relation to clinical, endocrine, and molecular thyroid parameters. Thyroid 1996; 6:575–587.

Schwab KO, Söhlemann P, Gerlich M, Broecker M, v. Petrykowski W, Holzapfel HP, Paschke R, Grüters A, Derwahl M: Mutations of the TSH receptor as cause of congenital hyperthyroidism. Exp Clin Endocrinol Diabetes 1996; 104(Suppl)4:124–128.

Scott DA, Wang R, Kreman TM, Sheffield VC, Karniski LP: The Pendred syndrome gene encodes a chloride-iodide transport protein. Nat Genet 1999; 21:440–443.

Seignalet J, Mirouze J, Jaffiol C, Selam JL, Lapinski H: HL-A in Graves' disease and in insulin-dependent diabetes mellitus. Tissue Antigens 1975; 6:272–274.

Semana G, Allanic H, Quillivic F, Vallejo MT, Simon JP, Genetet B: Implication of the HLA-DRB3 gene in Graves' disease: predominance of allele Dw24. Hum Immunol 1990; 29:143–149.

Sheffield VC, Kraiem Z, Beck JC, Nishimura D, Stone EM, Salameh M, Glaser M: Pendred syndrome maps to chromosome 7q21–34 and is caused by an intrinsic defect in thyroid iodine organification. Nat Genet 1996; 12:424–426.

Shields DC, Ratanachaiyavong S, McGregor AM, Collins A, Morton NE: Combined segregation and linkage analysis of Graves disease with a thyroid autoantibody diathesis. Am J Hum Genet 1994; 55:540–554.

Siegel RD, Lee SL: Toxic nodular goiter: toxic adenoma and toxic multinodular goiter. Endocrinol Metab Clin North America 1998; 27:151–168.

Siegmund T, Usadel KH, Donner H, Braun J, Walfish PG, Badenhoop K: Interferon-γ gene microsatellite polymorphisms in patients with Graves' disease. Thyroid 1998; 8:1013–1017.

Simanainen J, Kinch A, Westermark K, Winsa B, Bengtsson M, Schuppert F, Westermark B, Heldin NE: Analysis of mutations in exon 1 of the human thyrotropin receptor gene: high frequency of the D36H and P52T polymorphic variants. Thyroid 1999; 9:7–11.

Simpson NE, Kidd KK, Goodfellow PJ, McDermid H, Myers S, Kidd JRJ, Duncan AM, Farrer LA, Brasch K: Assignment of multiple endocrine neoplasia type 2A to chromosome 10 by linkage. Nature 1987; 328:528–530.

Smanik PA, Liu Q, Furminger TL, Ryu K, Xing S, Mazzaferri EL, Jhiang SM: Cloning of the human sodium lodide symporter. Biochem Biophys Res Commun 1996; 226:339–345.

Soravia C, Sugg SL, Berk T, Mitri A, Cheng H, Gallinger S, Cohen Z, Asa SL, Bapat BV: Familial adenomatous polyposis-associated thyroid cancer. Am J Pathol 1998; 154:127–135.

Sospedra M, Tolosa E, Armengol P, Ashhab Y, Urlinger S, Lucas-Martin A, Foz-Sala M, Jaraquemada D, Pujol-Borrell R: Hyperexpression of transporter in antigen processing-1 (TAP-1) in thyroid glands affected by autoimmunity: a contributing factor to the breach of tolerance to thyroid antigens? Clin Exp Immunol 1997; 109:98–106.

Sridama V, Hara Y, Fauchet R, DeGroot LJ: HLA immunogenetic heterogeneity in black American patients with Graves' disease. Arch Intern Med 1987; 147:229–231.

Steck PA, Pershouse MA, Jasser SA, Yung WK, Lin H, Ligon AH, Baumgard ML, Hattier T, Davis T, Frye C, et al.: Identification of a candidate tumour suppressor gene, MMAC1, at chromosome 10q23.3 that is mutated in multiple advanced cancers. Nat Genet 1997; 15:356–362.

Stenszky V, Kozma L, Balazs C, Rochlitz S, Bear JC, Farid NR: The genetics of Graves' disease: HLA and disease susceptibility. J Clin Endocrinol Metab 1985; 61:735–740.

Stoffer SS, van Dyke DL, Vaden Bach J, Szpunar W, Weiss L: Familial papillary carcinoma of the thyroid. Am J Hum Genet 1986; 25:775–782.

Stratakis CA, Carney JA, Lin JP, Papanicolaou DA, Karl M, Kastner DLP, Chrousos GP: Carney complex, a familial multiple neoplasia and lentiginosis syndrome: analysis of 11 kindreds and linkage to the short arm of chromosome 2. J Clin Invest 1996; 97:699–705.

Stratakis CA, Courcoutsakis NA, Abati A, Filie A, Doppman JL, Carney JA, Shawker T: Thyroid gland abnormalities in patients with the syndrome of spotty skin pigmentation, myxomas, endocrine overactivity, and schwannomas (Carney complex). J Clin Endocrinol Metab 1997; 82:2037–2043.

Stratakis CA, Kirschner LS, Taymans SE, Tomlinson IP, Marsh DJ, Torpy DJ, Giatzakis C, Eccles DM, Theaker J, Houlston RS, et al.: Carney complex, Peutz-Jeghers syndrome, Cowden disease, and Bannayan-Zonana syndrome share cutaneous and endocrine manifestations, but not genetic loci. J Clin Endocrinol Metab 1998; 83:2972–2976.

Studer H, Derwahl M: Mechanisms of nonneoplastic endocrine hyperplasia—a changing concept: a review focused on the thyroid gland. Endocr Rev 1995; 16:411–426.

Sunthornthepvarakul T, Kitvitayasak S, Ngowngarmaratana S, Konthong P, Deerochanawong C, Sarinnapakorn V, Phongviratchai S: Lack of association between a polymorphism of human thyrotropin receptor gene and autoimmune thyroid disease. J Med Assoc Thailand 1999; 82:1214–1219.

Sunthornthepvarakul T, Likitmaskul S, Ngowngarmratana S, Angsusingha KK, Scherberg NH, Refetoff S: Familial dysalbuminemic hypertriiodothyroninemia: a new, dominantly inherited albumin defect. J Clin Endocrinol Metab 1998; 83:1448–1454.

Takahashi M, Iwashita AT, Murakami H, Ito S: Molecular mechanisms of development of multiple endocrine neoplasia 2 by *RET* mutations. J Intern Med 1998; 243:509–513.

Takamatsu J, Nishikawa M, Horimoto M, Ohsawa N: Familial unresponsiveness to thyrotropin by autosomal recessive inheritance. J Clin Endocrinol Metab 1993; 77:1569–1573.

Tamai H, Kimura A, Dong RP, Matsubayashi S, Kuma K, Nagataki S: Resistance to autoimmune thyroid disease is associated with HLA-DQ. J Clin Endocrinol Metab 1994; 78:94–97.

Tamai H, Sudo T, Kimura A, Mukuta T, Matsubayashi S, Kuma K, Sasazuki T: Association between the DRB1*08032 histocompatibility antigen and methimazole-induced agranulocytosis in Japanese patients with Graves disease. Ann Intern Med 1996; 124:490–494.

Tandon N, Mehra NK, Taneja V, Vaidya MC, Kochupillai N: HLA antigens in Asian Indian patients with Graves' disease. Clin Endocrinol 1990; 33:21–26.

Tandon N, Zhang L, Weetman AP: HLA associations with Hashimoto's thyroiditis. Clin Endocrinol 1991; 34:383–386.

Tanimoto C, Hirakawa S, Kawasaki H, Hayakawa N, Ota Z: Apoptosis in thyroid diseases: a histochemical study. Endocr J 1995; 42:193–201.

Targovnik H, Propato F, Varela V, Wajchenberg B, Knobel M, D'Abronzo HF, Medeiros-Neto G: Low levels of thyroglobulin messenger ribonucleic acid in congenital goitrous hypothyroidism with defective thyroglobulin synthesis. J Clin Endocrinol Metab 1989; 69:1137–1147.

Targovnik HM, Varela V, Abatangelo C, Wajchenberg BL, Medeiros-Neto G: Normal thyroglobulin and thyroperoxidase gene expression in thyroid congenital defective thyroglobulin synthesis. Thyroid 1991; 1:339–345.

Taurog A: Hormone synthesis: thyroid iodine metabolism. In: Braverman LE, Utiger RD (eds). Werner and Ingbar's The Thyroid. 7th Ed. Philadelphia: Lippincott-Raven, 1996:47–81.

Taylor BA, Rowe L: The congenital goiter mutation is linked to the thyroglobulin gene in the mouse. Proc Natl Acad Sci USA 1987; 84:1986–1990.

Tezuka U, Murakami T, Mishiro K, Fujino M, Takeichi O: Congenital goiter found in a district of Omuro, Kochi, Shikoku, Japan: familial goiter caused by possible defect of diiodotyrosine coupling to form thyroxine. Endocrinol Japonica 1971; 18:267–279.

Thomas JS, Leclere J, Hartemann P, Duheille J, Orgiazzi J, Petersen M, Janot C, Guedenet JC: Familial hyperthyroidism without evidence of autoimmunity. Acta Endocrinol 1982; 100:512–518.

Thorsby E: Invited anniversary review: HLA associated diseases. Hum Immunol 1997; 53:1–11.

Tomer Y, Barbesino G, Greenberg DA, Concepcion E, Davies TF: Linkage analysis of candidate genes in autoimmune thyroid disease: III. Detailed analysis of chromosome 14 localizes Graves' disease-1 (GD-1) close to multinodular goiter-1 (MNG-1). J Clin Endocrinol Metab 1998; 83:4321–4327.

Tomer Y, Barbesino G, Greenberg DA, Concepcion E, Davies TF: Mapping the major susceptibility loci for familial Graves' and Hashimoto's diseases: evidence for genetic heterogeneity and gene interactions. J Clin Endocrinol Metab 1999; 84:4656–4664.

Tomer Y, Barbesino G, Keddache M, Greenberg DA, Davies TF: Mapping of a major susceptibility locus for Graves' disease (GD-1) to chromosome 14q31. J Clin Endocrinol Metab 1997; 82:1645–1648.

Tomer Y, Davies TF: Infection, thyroid disease, and autoimmunity. Endocr Rev 1993; 14:107–120.

Tomer Y, Davies TF: The genetic susceptibility to Graves' disease. Baillieres Clin Endocrinol Metab 1997; 11:431–450.

Tomer Y, Greenberg DA, Barbesino G, Concepcion E, Davies TF: CTLA-4 and not CD28 is a susceptibility gene for thyroid autoantibody production. J Clin Endocrinol Metab 2001; 86:1687–1693.

Torfs CP, King MC, Huey B, Malmgren J, Grumet FC: Genetic interrelationship between insulin-dependent diabetes mellitus, the autoimmune thyroid diseases, and rheumatoid arthritis. Am J Hum Genet 1986; 38:170–187.

Treanor JJ, Goodman L, de Sauvage F, Stone DM, Poulsen KT, Beck CD, Armanini MP, Pollock RA, Hefti F, Phillips HS, et al.: Characterization of a multicomponent receptor for GDNF. Nature 1996; 382:80–83.

Trent JM, Flink IL, Morkin E, van Tuinen P, Ledbetter DH: Localization of the human thyroxine-binding globulin gene to the long arm of the X chromosome (Xq21–22). Am J Hum Genet 1987; 41:428–435.

Uchigata Y, Kuwata S, Tsushima T, Tokunaga K, Miyamoto M, Tsuchikawa K, Hirata Y, Juji T, Omori Y: Patients with Graves' disease who developed insulin autoimmune syndrome (Hirata disease) possess HLA-Bw62/Cw4/DR4 carrying DRB1*0406. J Clin Endocrinol Metab 1993; 77:249–254.

Uno H, Sasazuki T, Tamai H, Matsumoto H: Two major genes, linked to HLA and Gm, control susceptibility to Graves' disease. Nature 1981; 292:768–770.

Vaidya B, Imrie H, Perros P, Dickinson J, McCarthy MI, Kendall-Taylor P, Pearce SH: Cytotoxic T lymphocyte antigen-4 (CTLA-4) gene polymorphism confers susceptibility to thyroid associated orbitopathy. Lancet 1999; 354:743–744.

Vaidya B, Imrie H, Perros P, Young ET, Kelly WF, Carr D, Large DM, Toft AD, Kendall-Taylor P, Pearce SH: Evidence for a new Graves disease susceptibility locus at chromosome 18q21. Am J Hum Genet 2000; 66:1710–1714.

Vanderpump MPJ, Tunbridge WMG: The epidemiology of thyroid disease. In: Braverman LE, Utiger RD (eds). Werner and Ingbar's The Thyroid. 7th Ed. Philadelphia: Lippincott-Raven, 1996:474–482.

Verschür OV: Die Zwillingsforschung im Dienste der inneren Medizin. Verh Dtsch Ges innere Med 1958; 64:262–273.

Viglietto G, Chiappetta G, Martinez-Tello FJ, Fukunaga FH, Tallini G, Visconti R, Mastro A, Santoro M, Fusco A: RET/PTC oncogene activation is an early event in thyroid carcinogenesis. Oncogene 1995; 11:1207–1210.

Villanueva R, Inzerillo AM, Tomer Y, Barbesino G, Meltzer M, Concepcion ES, Greenberg DA, MacLaren N, Sun ZS, Zhang DM, et al.: Limited genetic susceptibility to severe Graves' ophthalmopathy: no role for CTLA-4 but evidence for an environmental etiology. Thyroid 2000; 10:791–798.

Vives-Pi M, Vargas F, James RF, Trowsdale J, Costa M, Sospedra M, Obiols G, Tampe R, Pujol-Borrell R: Proteasome subunits, low-molecular-mass polypeptides 2 and 7 are hyperexpressed by target cells in autoimmune thyroid disease but not in insulin-dependent diabetes mellitus: implications for autoimmunity. Tissue Antigens 1997; 50:153–163.

Wagar G, Lamberg BA, Sivula A, Saarinen P, Makinen T: Familial and sporadic thyroglobulin deficiency with goitre and hypothyroidism. Ann Clin Res 1982; 14:37–45.

Wang C, Crapo LM: The epidemiology of thyroid disease and implications for screening. Endocrinol Metab Clin North America 1997; 26:189–218.

Watson PF, French A, Pickerill AP, McIntosh RS, Weetman AP: Lack of association between a polymorphism in the coding region of the thyrotropin receptor gene and Graves' disease. J Clin Endocrinol Metab 1995; 80:1032–1035.

Weetman AP: Autoimmunity to steroid-producing cells and familial polyendocrine autoimmunity. Baillieres Clin Endocrinol Metab 1995; 9:157–174.

Weetman AP, McCorkle R: Evidence against extended DR3-related haplotypes in Graves' disease. J Immunogenet 1990; 17:403–407.

Weetman AP, McGregor AM: Autoimmune thyroid disease: developments in our understanding. Endocr Rev 1984; 5:309–355.

Weetman AP, McGregor AM: Autoimmune thyroid disease: further developments in our understanding. Endocr Rev 1994; 15:788–830.

Weetman AP, So AK, Roe C, Walport MJ, Foroni L: T-cell receptor α-chain V region polymorphism linked to primary autoimmune hypothyroidism but not Graves' disease. Hum Immunol 1987; 20:167–173.

Weetman AP, So AK, Warner CA, Foroni L, Fells P, Shine B: Immunogenetics of Graves' ophthalmopathy. Clin Endocrinol 1988; 28:619–628.

Weiss M, Ingbar SH, Winbald S, Kasper DL: Demonstration of a saturable binding site for thyrotropin in *Yersinia enterocolitica*. Science 1983; 219:1331–1333.

Weiss RE, Sunthornthepvarakul T, Angekow P, Marcus-Bagley D, Cox N, Alper CA, Refetoff S: Linkage of familial dysalbuminemic hyperthyroxinemia to the albumin gene in a large Amish kindred. J Clin Endocrinol Metab 1995; 80:116–121.

Wells SA, Chi DD, Toshima K, Dehner LP, Coffin CM, Dowton B, Ivanovich JL, Debenedetti MK, Dilley WG, Moley JF, et al.: Predictive DNA testing and prophylactic thyroidectomy in patients at risk for multiple endocrine neoplasia type 2A. Ann Surg 1994; 220:237–250.

White WH: On prognosis of secondary symptoms of exophthalmic goitre. Br Med J 1886; ii:151–152.

Whittingham S, Morris PJ, Martin FI: HL-A8: a genetic link with thyrotoxicosis. Tissue Antigens 1975; 6:23–27.

WHO Collaborating Centres for Classifiction of Diseases: Endocrine, nutritional and metabolic diseases (E00–E90): disorders of thyroid gland (E00–E07). In: WHO Collaborating Centres for Classifiction of Diseases (ed). International Statistical Classification of Diseases and Related Health Problems. 10th Ed. Geneva: World Health Organization, 1992:272–276.

Wolff J: Congenital goiter with defective iodide transport. Endocr Rev 1983; 4:240–254.

Yanagawa T, DeGroot LJ: HLA class II associations in African-American female patients with Graves' disease. Thyroid 1996; 6:37–39.

Yanagawa T, Hidaka Y, Guimaraes V, Soliman M, DeGroot LJ: CTLA-4 gene polymorphism associated with Graves' disease in a Caucasian population. J Clin Endocrinol Metab 1995; 80:41–45.

Yanagawa T, Mangklabruks A, Chang YB, Okamoto Y, Fisfalen ME, Curran PG, DeGroot LJ: Human histocompatibility leukocyte antigen-DQA1*0501 allele associated with genetic susceptibility to Graves' disease in a Caucasian population. J Clin Endocrinol Metab 1993; 76:1569–1574.

Yanagawa T, Mangklabruks A, DeGroot LJ: Strong association between HLA-DQA1*0501 and Graves' disease in a male Caucasian population. J Clin Endocrinol Metab 1994; 79:227–229.

Yanagawa T, Taniyama M, Enomoto S, Gomi K, Maruyama H, Ban Y, Saruta T: CTLA4 gene polymorphism confers susceptibility to Graves' disease in Japanese. Thyroid 1997; 7:843–846.

Yashiro T, Ito K, Akiba M, Kanaji Y, Obara T, Fujimoto Y, Hirayama A, Nakajima H: Papillary carcinoma of the thyroid arising from dyshormonogenetic goiter. Endocrinol Japonica 1987; 34:955–964.

Yeo PP, Chan SH, Thai AC, Ng WY, Lui KF, Wee GB, Tan SH, Lee BW, Cheah JS: HLA Bw46 and DR9 associations in Graves' disease of Chinese patients are age- and sex-related. Tissue Antigens 1989; 34:179–184.

Yoshida S, Takamatsu J, Kuma K, Murakami Y, Sakane S, Katayama S, Ohsawa N: A variant of adenomatous goiter with characteristic histology and possible hereditary thyroglobulin abnormality. J Clin Endocrinol Metab 1996; 81:1961–1966.

Young RA, Stoffer SS, Braverman LE: Familial dysalbuminemic hyperthyroxinemia associated with primary thyroid disease. Am J Med 1987; 82:221–223.

21 Type 1 Diabetes Mellitus

LESLIE J. RAFFEL AND JEROME I. ROTTER

INTRODUCTION AND HISTORICAL PERSPECTIVE: HOW DO WE KNOW THAT TYPE 1 DIABETES IS A GENETIC DISEASE AND SEPARATE FROM TYPE 2 DIABETES?

Diabetes mellitus is a diagnostic term for a group of disorders characterized by abnormal glucose homeostasis that results in elevated blood sugar. As a result of both physiological and genetic studies, it has become apparent over the past two decades that *diabetes* does not refer to a single entity but, like anemia, simply describes symptoms and/or laboratory abnormalities that can have a number of distinct etiologies. It is now clear that diabetes mellitus is not a single disease but a genetically heterogeneous group of disorders that have glucose intolerance in common (Rimoin and Schimke, 1971; Creutzfeldt et al., 1976; Rotter et al., 1978; Kobberling and Tattersall, 1982). While there has been controversy over the years as to how to best distinguish the genetically distinct forms of diabetes, it is generally accepted that Type 1, insulin-dependent diabetes mellitus (IDDM), should be considered separately from Type 2, non-insulin-dependent diabetes mellitus (NIDDM). This chapter describes what is currently known about the inheritance of Type 1 diabetes as well as the specific genes that are involved in causing this disorder and its complications. The genetic basis of Type 2 diabetes is discussed in Chapter 22.

Perhaps the earliest documentation of an appreciation of the genetic basis of diabetes, as well as acknowledgment of clinical heterogeneity within diabetes, dates back more than 2000 years. The Hindu physicians Charaka and Sushruta commented on "honey urine" of two causes: genetic, i.e., passed from one generation to another in "the seed," and environmental, i.e., injudicious diet. They also described two types of disease, one associated with emaciation, dehydration, polyuria, and lassitude and the other associated with stout build, gluttony, obesity, and sleepiness (Simpson, 1976; Cahill, 1979). The former description clearly refers to Type 1 diabetes, while the latter is an apt description of Type 2 diabetes.

In more modern times, the initial indications that Type 1 diabetes was genetically determined came as a result of family and twin studies, which also provided the first strong evidence that there was a genetic basis for all forms of diabetes. These studies were also key in the development of an appreciation that Type 1 and Type 2 diabetes were genetically distinct. The observation that clinical differences tended to run true in families constituted some of the first evidence (Cammidge, 1928, 1934; Harris, 1950; Simpson, 1962; Working Party, College of General Practitioners, 1965; Lestradet et al., 1972). These studies were followed by studies that estimated concordance rates for diabetes in twins. Using clinical diabetes as the criterion for being affected, most investigators have reported concordance rates between 45% and 96% for monozygotic (MZ) twins and between 3% and 37% for dizygotic (DZ) twins. Thus, the concordance of diabetes mellitus in MZ twins is significantly greater than that for DZ twins, suggesting an important genetic component in the etiology. As shown in Table 21–1, however, twin concordance rates vary greatly depending on the age at diagnosis. In late-onset diabetes (age ≥40 in the first affected twin), the MZ concordance rate was 90% or more, but in young-onset twin pairs (<40 years of age), the concordance rate was <50% (Pyke, 1979). Although not appreciated fully at the time, we now realize that these age-related differences reflect the fact that most cases of Type 1 diabetes present early in life, while the majority of Type 2 cases occur in later adulthood. Thus, while both forms demonstrate significantly increased concordance in MZ twins compared to DZ twins, the concordance is much lower in Type 1 diabetes, implying that environmental factors play a much greater role in its etiology. It is now generally accepted that the MZ twin concordance rate for Type 1 diabetes is in the range of 35% to 40% and that for Type 2 diabetes is close to 90%.

As summarized in Table 21–2, a number of lines of clinical and genetic evidence led to the eventual separation of Type 1 and Type 2 diabetes as clearly distinct groups of disorders. Physiological studies further supported the separation of the two types. The absolute insulinopenic response of juvenile-onset diabetics vs. the relative hyperinsulinemic response of maturity-onset diabetes parallels the therapeutic observation of the absolute insulin requirement of the juvenile (insulin dependent/Type 1) diabetic, which contrasts with the ability to manage most adult cases with oral hypoglycemics and/or diet (insulin independent/Type 2).

Immunological studies pinpointed the importance of immune mechanisms in the etiology of Type 1, but not Type 2, diabetes. Direct evidence for an autoimmune role in the pathogenesis of IDDM came from the discovery of organ-specific, cell-mediated immunity to pancreatic islets and then the successful demonstration of antibodies to the islet cells of the pancreas (Bottazzo et al., 1974). While these antibodies were first detected only in insulin-dependent diabetics with coexistent autoimmune endocrine disease, it soon became apparent that they were common (60%–80%) in most newly diagnosed juvenile diabetics. Islet-cell antibody studies supported the differentiation of IDDM from NIDDM as autoantibodies were present in 30% to 40% of the former group (even after onset) as opposed to 5% to 8% of the latter group. Many (possibly the majority) NIDDM patients who are antibody-positive appear to become insulin-dependent with time. They have flat insulin responses to a glucose load and the human leukocyte antigen (HLA)-associated DR3 and DR4 antigens (Groop et al., 1988). This suggested that etiologically these

Table 21–1. Concordance of Diabetes and Glucose Intolerance in Twins

Reference	Criteria	Age of Patients (Years)	Percent Concordant	
			Monozygotic	Dizygotic
White (1965)	Clinical		48.0	3.0
Werner (1936)	Clinical		75.0	10.0
Lemser (In Mimura and Miyao et al., 1962)	Clinical		85.5	29.2
Verschuer (In Mimura and Miyao et al., 1962)	Clinical		84.0	37.0
Steiner (1936)	Clinical		96.6	9.1
Harvald and Hauge (1963, 1965)	Clinical		47.0	9.5
Harvald and Hauge (1963, 1965)	Clinical	>70	73.0	32.0
Harvald and Hauge (1965)	GTT		57.0	9.0
Gottlieb and Root (1968)	Clinical	<40	10.0	3.1
Gottlieb and Root (1968)	Clinical	>40	70.0	3.5
Gottlieb and Root (1968)	GTT		14.0	35.0
Then Berg (1939)	GTT		65.0	22.0
Then Berg (1939)	GTT	>43	100.0	39.0
Pyke and Taylor (1967)	GTT		78.0	
Cerasi and Luft (1967)	Glucose infusion		92.0	
Mimura and Miyao (1962)	Combined data		80.5	28.0
Tattersal and Pyke (1972)	Clinical, GTT (96 pairs)	<40	52.5	
		>40	91.9	
Pyke and Nelson (1976)	Clinical, GTT (106 pairs)	<40	50.0	
		>40	92.9	
Pyke (1978)	Clinical, GTT (150 pairs)	<45	50.9	
		>45	88.6	
Pyke (1979)	Clinical, GTT (185 pairs)	Type 1 diabetes	55.3	
		Type 2 diabetes[a]	88.6	
Barnett et al. (1981)	Clinical, GTT (200 pairs)	Type 1 diabetes	54.4	
		Type 2 diabetes	90.6	
Matsuda and Kuzuya (1994)	Clinical (144 pairs)	Type 1 diabetes	47.0	8.0
		Type 2 diabetes	87.0	43.0
	GTT (glucose intolerance)	Type 1 diabetes	55.0	50.0
		Type 2 diabetes	98.0	92.0
Kaprio et al. (1992)	Clinical (614 pairs)	Type 1 diabetes	23.0	5.0
		Type 2 diabetes	34.0	16.0
Olmos et al. (1988)	Clinical (49 pairs)	Type 1 diabetes	34.0	
Japan Diabetes Society (1998)	Clinical (87 pairs)	Type 1 diabetes	45.0	0
		Type 2 diabetes	83.0	40.0
Kyvik et al. (1995)	Clinical, GTT (128 pairs)	Type 1 diabetes	53.0	11.0

[a]In the Type 2 diabetes discordant pairs, the index twin was ascertained only within 5 years of examination. GTT, glucose tolerance test.

Table 21–2. Separation of Type 1 from Type 2 Diabetes

Distinguishing Characteristics	Type 1 IDDM (Juvenile-Onset Type)	Type 2 NIDDM (Maturity-Onset Type)
Clinical	Thin, ketosis-prone, insulin required for survival, onset predominantly in childhood and early adulthood	Obese, ketosis-resistant, often treatable by diet or drugs, onset predominantly after age 40
Family studies	Increased prevalence of juvenile or Type 1	Increased prevalence of maturity or Type 2
Twin studies	<50% concordance in monozygotic twins	Close to 100% concordance in monozygotic twins
Insulin response to a glucose load	Flat	Variable
Associated with other autoimmune endocrine diseases and antibodies	Yes	No
Islet cell antibodies and pancreatic cell-mediated immunity	Yes	No
HLA associations and linkage	Yes	No

IDDM, insulin-dependent diabetes mellitus; NIDDM, non-insulin-dependent diabetes mellitus.

cases belong in the insulin-dependent category; i.e., they are just in a transitional state on the way to eventual insulin dependence and share the same underlying pathogenetic mechanisms as Type 1 diabetes. Thus immunological studies have served both to separate disorders (juvenile vs. adult) and to combine others (insulin-dependent and non-insulin-dependent yet antibody-positive).

Finally, the clear and consistent findings of HLA associations with juvenile insulin-dependent, but not maturity-onset non-insulin-dependent, diabetes became a major argument for etiological differences between these two disorders: approximately 95% of Type 1 diabetes patients have DR3 or DR4 or both (Platz et al., 1981; Rotter et al., 1983; Wolf et al., 1983; Maclaren et al., 1988).

There is, however, some evidence that families of either Type 1 or Type 2 diabetics have more of the other type of diabetes than do families in the general population (Gottlieb 1980; Dahlquist et al., 1989; Quatraro et al., 1990). Part of this overlap may be attributed to the insulin-independent phase of the insulin-dependent type (the frequency of which is still being defined), but it may also be the result of even further etiological heterogeneity (Irvine et al., 1979; Rich et al., 1991; Landin-Olsson et al., 1992).

GENERAL GENETIC AND EPIDEMIOLOGICAL EVIDENCE

What Is Type 1, Insulin-Dependent Diabetes Mellitus?

Type 1 diabetes mellitus is characterized by low or absent levels of endogenous insulin production (Table 21–2). This is secondary to destruction of the insulin-producing beta cells of the pancreas and is the single characteristic that most decisively separates Type 1 and Type 2 diabetes. It is estimated that 5% to 10% of all U.S. diabetic patients have Type 1 diabetes and that the incidence in U.S. children 0 to 14 years of age is in the range of 12 to 20/100,000 (Diabetes Epidemiology Research International Group, 1990). The incidence appears to vary dramatically worldwide, from an estimated low of 1/100,000 children in Asia to greater than 40/100,000 in some parts of Scandinavia (Diabetes Epidemiology Research International Group, 1988; Tuomilehto et al., 1999; EURODIAB ACE Study Group, 2000; Huen et al., 2000). In most regions of the world, the incidence appears to be increasing (Diabetes Epidemiology Research International Group, 1990; Dokheel, 1993; EURODIAB ACE Study Group, 2000; Huen et al., 2000; Kulaylat and Narchi, 2000). The increasing incidence suggests that some environmental risk factors for Type 1 diabetes are becoming more prevalent, but the nature of these environmental risks remains under investigation.

Natural History of Type 1 Diabetes

Patients with a new diagnosis of Type 1 diabetes typically present with acute illness, severe dehydration, ketoacidosis, and marked hyperglycemia. The history is generally that the individual was well until perhaps a week or two prior to presentation, when increased thirst and urination were noted. On occasion, an account is given of a viral upper respiratory tract infection or other mild infectious illness shortly before the increased thirst and urination began. As a result, until relatively recently, Type 1 diabetes was thought to be an acute-onset disorder. However, with the appreciation of the autoimmune nature of the beta-cell destruction, this assumption began to be questioned.

Several studies followed nondiabetic identical co-twins and triplets of Type 1 diabetic probands with serial testing for the presence of circulating autoantibodies (Verge et al., 1995; Redondo et al., 1999), and not surprisingly, many of these twins and triplets ultimately developed Type 1 diabetes. What was not anticipated, however, was that anti-islet-cell antibodies were often detectable months to many years prior to the time these co-twins became overtly diabetic. These studies demonstrated that Type 1 actually develops gradually. The autoimmune destruction of pancreatic beta cells progresses slowly over time, and it is not until the majority of these cells have been destroyed that diabetes becomes clinically apparent. It has been estimated that only 10% of the beta-cell mass remains at the time that overt diabetes is diagnosed (Wilson and Eisenbarth, 1990). Because of this residual insulin-secreting capacity, some patients go through a transient "honeymoon" phase in the early months after diagnosis, during which their requirement for exogenous insulin may decrease or even disappear. These remaining beta cells are lost within the first months to years following diagnosis, however, and all patients ultimately will require lifelong treatment with insulin.

With the recognition that there were functional beta cells still present at the time of diagnosis, treatment with immunosuppressants was attempted to see if Type 1 diabetes could be reversed. Although it was possible to produce a remission in some patients who were treated with cyclosporine within the first few months after diagnosis, the effect was short-lived in most and overt diabetes returned as soon as cyclosporine was discontinued (Assan et al., 1985; Vialettes et al., 1990; Martin et al., 1991; Robertson et al., 1992; Pozzilli et al., 1995). Thus, it appears that once beta-cell destruction has progressed to the point of overt diabetes, the process is too far along to effectively cure diabetes. Therefore, more recent attention has focused on attempts to intervene in high-risk individuals who have not yet progressed to clinical diabetes.

PATHOPHYSIOLOGY

Immunological Mechanisms

Type 1 diabetes is a chronic autoimmune disorder that gradually develops over many years. A variety of abnormalities in immune function and insulin release precede the "abrupt" development of the diabetic syndrome in patients genetically predisposed to diabetes (Atkinson et al., 1986; Eisenbarth 1986, Tarn et al., 1988). Eisenbarth (1986) proposed dividing the development of Type 1 diabetes into six stages: *(1)* genetic susceptibility, *(2)* triggering events, *(3)* active autoimmunity, *(4)* gradual loss of glucose-stimulated insulin secretion, *(5)* appearance of overt diabetes with some residual insulin secretion, and *(6)* complete beta-cell destruction. At the onset of Type 1 diabetes, as few as 10% of the beta cells remain, and within several years, essentially all beta cells are destroyed. The pace of these events may well relate to age at onset and the underlying genetic heterogeneity (Gorsuch et al., 1981). The implication of this natural history and the amount of beta-cell destruction present at clinical onset is that if interventional therapy is to be effective, it likely will have to be started well before the onset of the acute diabetic syndrome.

There remains substantial uncertainty as to what is the initiating event triggering the autoimmune destruction of beta cells. At the time of diagnosis, there are typically a variety of autoantibodies detectable, suggesting that the autoimmune process is directed at several different cellular components. As a group, the commonly occurring autoantibodies are referred to as *islet cell antibodies* (ICAs). Over the past decade, some of the specific components of ICAs have been identified, including antibodies reactive to glutamic acid decarboxylase (GAD65) and transmembrane tyrosine phosphatases (IA-2 and IA-2β) (Kukreja and Maclaren 1999). In addition to the ICAs, autoantibodies reactive against insulin (IAA) are frequently present at the time of diagnosis. In high-risk nondiabetic relatives of Type 1 diabetes patients, the number of detectable autoantibodies influences the overall risk of developing diabetes and the rate of beta-cell destruction in those who do become diabetic; individuals positive for only one antibody progress slowly, whereas those with autoantibodies to multiple antigens most often progress rapidly (Kukreja and Maclaren, 1999; Kimpimaki et al., 2000). Whether the autoantibodies are actually responsible for initiating beta-cell destruction or are merely a marker of the ongoing immune process remains unclear.

Nonobese diabetic (NOD) mice and BioBreeding (BB) rats are excellent models of the autoimmune form of Type 1 diabetes (Eisenbarth, 1986). Data from these animals indicate that T lymphocytes are important in the pathogenesis of islet T-cell destruction (Rossini et al., 1984; Mordes et al., 1987) as activated T lymphocytes from acute-diabetic BB rats can transfer diabetes to other animals (Koevary et al., 1985).

Similar evidence for the importance of T lymphocytes in human diabetes comes from studies of pancreatic transplantation between identical twins (Sutherland et al., 1984, 1989). When pancreata are transplanted from a nondiabetic twin to the diabetic MZ co-twin without immunosuppression, islet-cell destruction with massive T-cell infiltration and relapse of the diabetes occurs within weeks. Thus, the basic defect in Type 1 diabetes appears to be extrinsic to the pancreas and related to the activation of T lymphocytes, which then mediate destruction of the islets (Rimoin and Rotter, 1981).

The mechanisms resulting in the autoimmune destruction of the islets are complex, with both T cells and the cytokines they excrete involved (Almawi et al., 1999). Initially, it was thought that T-helper 1 (Th1) cells were responsible for the autoimmune damage and that Th2 cells afforded protection to the beta cells. However, it is now known that both Th1 and Th2 cells have roles in this destructive process (Mosmann and Coffman, 1989; Romagnani, 1995). Th1 cells produce interleukin-2 (IL-2), interferon-γ (IFN-γ), and tumor necrosis factor-α (TNF-α) and promote cell-mediated responses and delayed-type hypersensitivity, while Th2 cells produce IL-4, IL-5, IL-10, and IL-13 and stimulate humoral immunity. There is evidence of an alteration in the normal balance between these two pathways in Type 1 diabetes, as well as evidence that Th2 cells may be more important in the early initiation of the autoimmune process, whereas Th1 cells are implicated in the perpetuation of the destruction once the process has started (Anderson et al., 1993; Lee et al., 1996; Almawi et al., 1999).

Uncovering the basis of MZ twin discordance in Type 1 diabetes will be important in understanding the relationship of the basic underlying genetic defect in this disease to the subsequent immunological derangements and clinical disease. MZ twins, who are identical genotypically, can differ phenotypically by a variety of different mechanisms, including environmental exposure; lyonization, in the case of females; somatic mutation; activation of normally unexpressed genes; and gene rearrangement, as in the immunoglobulin and T-cell receptor genes (Rimoin and Rotter, 1985; Eisenbarth, 1987). T-cell activation through gene rearrangement may well be the proximal step in the development of Type 1 diabetes in an individual who is genetically predisposed to the disease. The various environmental agents discussed below may well operate in the triggering or selection of the appropriate T-cell receptor rearrangement, and the specific HLA type may be necessary for the interaction of these activated T cells and ICAs with the pancreas. In support of this concept are the tentative data for T-cell receptor associations (Millward et al., 1987; Ito et al., 1988; Hibberd et al., 1992).

Role of Environmental Factors

The MZ twin data, which show a Type 1 diabetes concordance of approximately 20% to 40%, raise the possibility that there are important environmental components to the etiology of Type 1 diabetes. As discussed above, the lack of 100% concordance in MZ twins, even though suggestive, does not absolutely require the involvement of environmental factors. Immunological gene rearrangements could also provide an explanation for such reduced penetrance (Rimoin and Rotter, 1985; Eisenbarth, 1987). However, the possibility of environmental factors having a significant role must be thoroughly investigated, especially regarding the implications for preventive strategies. As the pathogenetic processes which lead to Type 1 diabetes appear to be complex and may take years from initiation to completion, environmental agents could play one of several roles (Gamble 1980a,b). Environmental agents might function as initiating factors, i.e., factors which begin or continue the etiological processes that eventually terminate in Type 1 diabetes. If environmental factors function in this role, then more than one agent (e.g., several different viruses or viruses plus chemical agents) might be involved in the etiology. Alternatively, environmental factors could act mainly as precipitating factors, i.e., factors which convert preclinical diabetes into clinical disease. In either role (or both), what is clear is that environmental factors must act on genetically susceptible individuals for Type 1 diabetes to occur. Several classes of environmental agent have been implicated in the etiology of Type 1 diabetes.

Infectious Agents

A viral etiology for diabetes has been suggested for many years, with case reports of diabetes following an episode of an infectious disease dating back to the 1800s (Gunderson, 1927; Craighead, 1981). The current evidence for a role of viral agents comes from several sources, including case reports, epidemiological studies, clinical studies, and experimental animal and human models.

Anecdotally, a "viral-like illness" is known to precede the onset of many cases of Type 1 diabetes (Gamble, 1980b; Craighead, 1981). Several lines of epidemiological evidence are also consistent with an infectious etiology. For example, trends in age at onset of diabetes are consistent with a viral etiology (Gamble, 1980b). These data are most consistent with infectious agents playing a precipitating role in Type 1 diabetes, and the total number of infections during the preceding year has been shown to correlate with Type 1 diabetes risk (Blom et al., 1991). Another suggestion comes from studies on the time of clinical disease onset in pairs of siblings with Type 1 diabetes. At least one study suggested that sibling pairs are more likely to have onset of diabetes within a year of one another than would be expected by chance (Gamble, 1980b). Similarly, the period of discordance for Type 1 diabetes in MZ twins has been reported to be less than 3 years in 60% of twin pairs where both ultimately develop Type 1 diabetes (Kumar et al., 1993).

There is also limited evidence for a role of an infectious agent (e.g., mumps, coxsackievirus) from seroepidemiological studies, i.e., studies which compare viral and bacterial antibody titers in Type 1 diabetics and nondiabetic controls (King et al., 1983a,b; Schernthaner et al., 1985). Others have found no evidence of increased titers to coxsackievirus B in new-onset cases (Orchard et al., 1983; Frisk et al., 1992), while still others have suggested that titers of coxsackieviruses B3 and B4 are actually decreased in Type 1 diabetes (Palmer et al., 1982). Subsequent studies have utilized molecular techniques to determine the prevalence of viral DNA. In one series, Pak et al., (1988) detected the presence of cytomegalovirus (CMV) DNA in 22% of Type 1 diabetes patients compared to 2.6% of controls. There was a strong correlation between the CMV gene and ICAs in the diabetic patients, suggesting that persistent CMV infection may be relevant to pathogenesis in some cases. Additionally, Nairn et al. (1999) detected enterovirus RNA in 27% of children with new-onset Type 1 diabetes compared to only 4.9% of controls. Viral infection may also be important in adult-onset Type 1 diabetes as Andreoletti et al. (1998) detected coxsackievirus B3 or B4 genome in the blood of 5/14 (36%) newly diagnosed adults.

A study of the incidence of Type 1 diabetes in relation to the introduction of measles–mumps–rubella vaccination and the subsequent disappearance of mumps in Finland suggested that elimination of natural mumps infection has decreased the incidence of Type 1 diabetes (Hyöty et al., 1993). Measles vaccination itself was also correlated with a lower risk of Type 1 diabetes (Blom et al., 1991).

Evidence from clinical studies also suggests a role for infectious agents in Type 1 diabetes. The insulitis noted in early Type 1 diabetes could be consistent with viral infection of the pancreas, and autopsy studies have clearly documented pancreatic beta-cell damage in children dying from overwhelming viral infections (Jenson et al., 1980). Coxsackievirus B-specific antigens have specifically been found in the islets of Langerhans, and Coxsackievirus B4 itself has been isolated from the pancreas of a child dying of acute-onset Type 1 diabetes (Yoon et al., 1979). Several types of virus are capable of infecting human pancreatic beta cells in vitro, and data suggest that coxsackievirus B groups, rubella virus, and possibly CMV are capable of producing pathological beta-cell changes in vivo.

Molecular mimicry has been postulated to be a mechanism by which viral infection can impact the development of Type 1 diabetes (Atkinson et al., 1994). There are regions of sequence homology between GAD and the p2C protein of coxsackievirus B as well as between regions of both GAD and tyrosine phosphatase IA-2 and the VP7 protein of rotavirus (Kaufman et al., 1992; Honeyman et al., 1998). Tyrosine phosphatase IA-2 also demonstrates significant sequence homology with a variety of other viral genomes, including dengue, CMV, measles, and hepatitis C (Honeyman et al., 1998). Such observations raise the possibility that viral infection can trigger an anti-beta-cell autoimmune response by molecular mimicry. This possibility is further supported by the observation that the homologous peptides from both VP7 and IA-2 bind to HLA-DR4(*0401), while peptides from both p2C and GAD bind to DR3 (Honeyman et al., 1998; Vreugdenhil et al., 1998). Antibodies to GAD species and to the p2C protein have also been shown to cross-react in some, but not all, studies (Bach et al., 1997; Vreugdenhil et al., 1998; Vreugdenhil et al., 1999; Myers et al., 2000; Varela-Calvino et al., 2000; Schloot et al., 2001).

Evidence from experimental animal studies is strongly suggestive of a viral component to the etiology of Type 1 diabetes. Some of the first evidence came from the discovery that the M strain of the encephalomyocarditis (EMC) virus infects pancreatic beta cells and produces a diabetes-like disease in some strains of mice (Yoon and Notkins, 1976). This model has been widely studied, and it is now clear that the EMC-D variant (but not the EMC-B variant of the M strain) causes direct viral destruction of the beta cells in certain genetically susceptible mouse lines (SJL/JH, C3H/HeJ) (Boucher and Notkins, 1973; Craighead and Higgins, 1974; Hayashi et al., 1974; Onodera et al., 1978; Yoon et al., 1980, 1982, 1983; Iwo et al., 1983; Gould et al., 1984, 1985). In addition, in other mouse strains (e.g., Balb/cBy), EMC-M strains appear to initiate an immunologically mediated form of diabetes, suggesting that the same virus can have multiple effects, depending on the genetic predisposition of the host (Huber et al., 1985). Diabetes in SJL/J mice can be prevented by vaccination with live-attenuated EMC vaccine (Yoon and Ray, 1985). In BB/WOR diabetes-resistant rats, Kilham's rat virus (KRV) reproducibly induces Type 1 diabetes (Guberski et al., 1991). KRV does not produce diabetes in non-BB rats, however, clearly indicating that genetic factors are also necessary for Type 1 diabetes to develop.

That only some strains of mice are susceptible to virally induced diabetes strongly suggests a genetic component to disease susceptibility. The fact that only certain strains of virus are capable of inducing diabetes in specific animal models indicates that genetic factors in the agent are also important. The genetic/strain specificity of the agent may be particularly important in viruses which change their genetic characteristics rapidly in the population. This specificity may explain several puzzling aspects of Type 1 diabetes epidemiology, specifically, the changing incidence of Type 1 diabetes over time as well as the interesting observation that the proportion of complicated mumps cases who were ICA$^+$ decreased rapidly from the late 1970s to the mid-1980s (Helmke et al., 1986).

Experimental animal models suggest that infectious agents can cause diabetes or diabetes-like syndromes by at least four different mechanisms: *(1)* acute infection of the beta cell, leading to necrosis (EMC and reovirus models); *(2)* autoimmune mechanisms (rubella and KRV models); *(3)* persistent infection, leading to decreased growth and lifespan of the beta cell (lymphocytic choriomeningitis model); and *(4)* biochemical alterations in the cell or cell membrane, which lead to decreased insulin synthesis/release (Venezuelan encephalitis model) (Yoon, 1992). While our knowledge of infectious agents in human diabetes is less advanced, it is possible that all four mechanisms also occur in human disease.

Experimental animal models have also raised the hope that vaccination against promoting or initiating viral agents may protect genetically susceptible individuals against Type 1 diabetes. Vaccination against EMC virus in SJL/J mice and pertussis (whole-cell vaccine) in CD-1 mice with streptozotocin-induced diabetes suggests that beta-cell destruction can be either prevented or halted in at least some mouse models (Huang et al., 1984).

Viral infection can also prevent the development of Type 1 diabetes (Rabinovitch, 1996). Infection of NOD mice with lymphocytic choriomeningitis virus aborts the autoimmune reaction that produces Type 1 diabetes. The virus acts on a subset of

CD4$^+$ lymphocytes (Oldstone, 1990). Although most strains of the virus prevent Type 1 diabetes, at least one (Armstrong 53b variant, clone 13) does not, apparently due to alteration of the S RNA segment of the virus (Oldstone et al., 1990).

The best human models of infectious agents in Type 1 diabetes come from studies of individuals with the congenital rubella syndrome and from serial studies of children with viral infections who subsequently develop Type 1 diabetes. The incidence of Type 1 diabetes and other autoimmune diseases among children and young adults with the congenital rubella syndrome is markedly increased over that in the general population and may be as high as 15% to 40%. Cases of congenital rubella with Type 1 diabetes have an increased frequency of HLA-DR3 and -DR4 and a decreased frequency of HLA-DR2, much as in nonrubella Type 1 diabetes (Rubinstein et al., 1982). A significant proportion of patients with congenital rubella syndrome have T-cell subset abnormalities and a variety of autoimmune antibodies, including anti-thyroid microsomal, antithyroglobulin, anti-ICA, and anti-islet-cell surface antibodies, suggesting an autoimmune etiology (Rubinstein et al., 1982; Rabinowe et al., 1986). Rubella virus has been isolated from the pancreas of several cases with congenital rubella syndrome (De Prins et al., 1983), and at least one case is known of insulitis and beta-cell destruction in an infant with congenital rubella infection who died of acute diabetes (Patterson et al., 1981). This evidence suggests that rubella can indeed infect and damage the beta cell and that the diabetes seen in congenital rubella syndrome could be due either to initiation of an immune process by the rubella virus or to persistent pancreatic rubella infection.

Chemical Agents

Several chemical agents cause IDDM in experimental animals and humans. In the rat, streptozotocin and alloxan are classic diabetogenic agents, although the mechanism through which these beta-cell toxins cause diabetes is still not entirely understood. In humans, several agents cause diabetes upon ingestion, including the rodenticide *N*-3-pyridylmethl-*N′*-*p*-nitrophenylurea (RH-787, Vacor) and streptozotocin (Karam et al., 1980; Schulz et al., 1990). Some epidemiological studies have suggested a link between nitrate levels in drinking water and Type 1 diabetes risk (Kostraba et al., 1992; Virtanen et al., 1994), but other studies have failed to confirm this association (van Maanen et al., 2000).

Dietary Agents and Molecular Mimicry

The area of most recent interest as an environmental trigger for Type 1 diabetes has been dietary exposure. Several studies (Borch-Johnsen et al., 1984; Kostraba et al., 1993; Virtanen et al., 1993; Gerstein, 1994; Verge, 1994; Gimeno and de Souza, 1997) have reported an association of the introduction of cow's milk and cessation of breast-feeding with Type 1 diabetes risk. Elevated antibodies to several cow's milk proteins have also been found in children with Type 1 diabetes (Dahlquist et al., 1992; Virtanen et al., 1994). When it was reported that one epitope of bovine serum albumin, a 17–amino acid peptide (ABBOS), cross-reacts with p69, a beta-cell surface protein, the hypothesis was raised that early introduction of cow's milk into the infant diet could result in initiation of autoimmune injury to the beta cell via this molecular mimicry (Karjalainen et al., 1992; Robinson et al., 1993). Some studies of infant nutrition have not supported the association of autoimmunity to cow's milk and Type 1 diabetes risk; preliminary findings of the Diabetes Autoimmunity Study in the Young (DAISY) study actually suggested a protective effect of early cow's milk feeding (Atkinson et al., 1993; Bodington et al., 1994; Fava et al., 1994; Norris et al., 1995, 1996; Meloni et al., 1997; Couper et al., 1999). Therefore, while the possibility that cow's milk has some role in Type 1 diabetes remains, it appears unlikely that it is a major risk factor. This conclusion does not mean that dietary factors have no impact on diabetes risk, however, and the possible role of early infant and childhood diet requires further investigation (Kostraba, 1994).

GENE IDENTIFICATION

Difficulties in Genetic Analysis

With the discovery of HLA antigen associations with Type 1 diabetes, the genetic region that provides the major (but by no means only) genetic susceptibility to Type 1 diabetes was located. The genetics of Type 1 diabetes still remains an area of great complexity, however. There is no complete consensus as to which gene or combination of genes in the major histocompatibility complex (MHC) is responsible for the HLA-related susceptibility nor as to how many other genes outside of the HLA region (in most cases, on other chromosomes) are involved. There are several major difficulties that continue to confound attempts to analyze the genetics of Type 1 diabetes, including the reduced penetrance of the disorder, the confounding of linkage and association, and the heterogeneity within the disorder. However, even with all of these obstacles, major strides have been made in understanding the genetic complexities of this group of disorders.

One problem is the reduced penetrance of the Type 1 diabetes genotype. When the mode of inheritance is unknown, the only estimate we have for penetrance comes from identical twin concordance data. The largest twin data set (the British Diabetic Twin Study) reported concordance for Type 1 diabetes of some 50% (Pyke, 1979; Barnett et al., 1981). However, it is clear that this sample is not representative, with only a fraction of the twins in the British Isles identified and, thus, a presumed bias toward concordant pairs (Pyke, 1978). Studies on less biased, but much smaller, samples report concordances of approximately 20% (Gottlieb and Root, 1968). Finally, a prospective study of twins from the British group yielded a concordance estimate of about 36%, which is likely the best one available (Olmos et al., 1988). Thus, the best estimate is that perhaps only one-third of all persons with the genes for Type 1 diabetes actually develop clinical disease. The reduced penetrance indicates that what is inherited in Type 1 diabetes is disease susceptibility; other factors, presumably environmental, are required to convert genetic susceptibility into clinical disease. This view is supported by both the observations that the time of onset of Type 1 diabetes clusters in families and twin pairs (Gamble, 1980a; Olmos et al., 1988) and the epidemiological, experimental animal, and clinical evidence reviewed above for viral infections as a supervening factor in at least some cases (Craighead, 1981; Yoon, 1992; Smith et al., 1998; Nairn et al., 1999; Honeyman et al., 2000). However, it is not the only explanation as the somatic recombination that occurs within the immune system is also a potential explanation for the reduced penetrance (reviewed above).

A second problem in the genetics of Type 1 diabetes is that relationships between genes in the HLA region and Type 1 diabetes have been found in studies of both families and the population at large. The former observation connotes linkage and the latter, association. Linkage and association were classically characterized as being entirely distinct phenomena, although it is now appreciated that the two can occur together. Linkage is a reflection of the relative proximity of genetic loci on the chromosome map. Because of crossing over or recombination, specific alleles at the linked loci are not expected to be associated with the disease throughout a population. In contrast, disease association studies examine the prevalence of well-defined candidate gene polymorphisms among individuals with and without the disease of interest. Association usually implies that there is some etiological relationship between the gene marker allele and disease. Linkage is usually a phenomenon within families and not across populations, whereas association is a phenomenon across a population and not necessarily within families. For many years, most mathematical techniques for linkage detection included the assumption that there was no population association between the disease (phenotype) under study and the genetic marker alleles.

However, the genetics of the HLA region violate the cardinal rule of separation between linkage and association because alleles at various HLA loci are in "linkage disequilibrium." The HLA region has several well-defined loci: three serologically defined class I loci (A, B, and C); the class II genes (defined by serological methods, by mixed lymphocyte culture, and by molecular methods), which consist of at least three different subgroups (DP, DQ, and DR); and the class III loci, which include several components of the complement series. Each of these loci has multiple alleles or antigens (for further details, see chapter 28). These genes are located close to one another on chromosome 6 and thus are linked. However, certain pairs of HLA antigens also occur together in the population at a greater frequency than would be expected by chance (estimated by multiplying individual frequencies); i.e., they are associated. Since they are both linked and associated, certain pairs of HLA antigens are said to be in linkage disequilibrium.

Linkage disequilibrium may occur as a result of two different mechanisms. One is that selective forces exist that tend to favor and thus retain certain advantageous combinations of antigens. One of the major speculations regarding the etiology of various autoimmune diseases is that we are seeing today the residual of the selective advantage of these antigenic associations against the infectious diseases to which our species was exposed in the past. A second reason that linkage disequilibrium may be observed is simply because of the close physical proximity of two loci. If a given mutation associated with disease susceptibility has occurred relatively recently in human evolution, there may not have been enough time for multiple recombination events to have occurred between the disease gene and other nearby genetic regions. Linkage disequilibrium, which reflects the haplotype of the ancestral chromosomal region on which the disease-causing mutation occurred, may therefore be observed. This latter form of linkage disequilibrium is now recognized to occur commonly and is in fact exploited in the linkage disequilibrium single-nucleotide polymorphism (SNP) mapping being used in the wake of the Human Genome Project as a means of locating disease-causing genes (Collins, 1999). However, in a gene-dense region such as the HLA region, there may be such extensive linkage disequilibrium over long stretches of DNA that determining which gene is responsible for susceptibility to disease may be very difficult.

The HLA Region and Type 1 Diabetes

The earliest studies implicating the HLA region in Type 1 diabetes susceptibility demonstrated an increased frequency of the class I antigens B8 and B15 and then the class II HLA antigens DR3 and DR4 among Caucasian Type 1 diabetes patients (Singal and Blajchman, 1973; Nerup et al., 1974; Cudworth and Woodrow, 1975). Because of the linkage disequilibrium within the HLA region, the associations of B8 and B15 were thought to result from these alleles occurring with high frequency on DR3 (in the case of B8)– and DR4 (in the case of B15)–containing haplotypes. The Type 1 diabetes association was unusual among HLA disease associations because it involves two antigens, HLA-DR3 and -DR4. In addition, the relative risk for Type 1 diabetes in individuals who carry both DR3 and DR4 (compound heterozygotes) is greater than those homozygous for either DR3 or DR4 (Platz et al., 1981; Rotter et al., 1983; Wolf et al., 1983). This increased risk of the DR3/DR4 heterozygote was the first suggestion that more than one gene may predispose to Type 1 diabetes and, thus, was the first evidence for heterogeneity within Type 1 diabetes using HLA data (Svejgaard et al., 1975; Rotter and Rimoin, 1978).

Approximately 95% of all Type 1 diabetes cases (in Caucasian populations) have HLA-DR3, -DR4, or both compared to about 50% of individuals in the nondiabetic population (Platz et al., 1981; Rotter et al., 1983; Wolf et al., 1983; Maclaren et al., 1988). There are also more subtle relative increases in HLA-DR1 (especially among those who have only one copy of DR3 or DR4); conversely, DR2 and DR5 are decreased in individuals with Type 1 diabetes (Ilonen et al., 1978; Rubinstein et al., 1981; Anderson et al., 1983; Deschamps et al., 1984; Thomson, 1984; Thomson et al., 1988; Maclaren et al., 1988; Erlich et al., 1993a,b). HLA-DR3 and -DR4 (as defined serologically) are not pathognomonic of Type 1 diabetes; nearly half the U.S. population has either DR3 or DR4 (only 1%–3% have both), yet only a small percentage (about 0.5%) of these individuals will develop Type 1 diabetes. However, if one's sibling has Type 1 diabetes, the chance of a DR3 or DR4 individual developing Type 1 diabetes rises sharply (12%–24%). These observations suggested that DR3 and DR4, as defined serologically, could not adequately explain the risk for Type 1 diabetes present in the HLA region. Either the serological DR typing was not sensitive enough to detect the Type 1 diabetes-specific forms of DR3 and DR4 or other genes were responsible for at least some of the Type 1 diabetes susceptibility associated with the HLA region.

With the advent of molecular HLA typing, it became clear that both of these possible explanations are indeed important in understanding the role of the HLA region in Type 1 diabetes susceptibility. Initially, when the complexity of the HLA class II region was uncovered, attention focused on the hypothesis that another locus in tight linkage disequilibrium with DR was actually responsible for Type 1 diabetes susceptibility. Studies demonstrated that the HLA class II region is actually composed of at least three genetic loci, DR, DQ, and DP, each of which codes for a slightly different glycoprotein consisting of two peptide chains, α and β (Fig. 21–1). Because of this variability, there are differences at the DNA level between diabetics and nondiabetics, even when they share the same serological DR type.

Although studies in Caucasian populations initially implied that the primary locus for Type 1 diabetes susceptibility was the DQ β gene, the DQB1*0302 allele being associated with the highest risk, subsequent studies in other ethnic groups led to the realization that other genes within the class II region clearly are of importance as well. Thus, e.g., in Mexican-American Type 1 diabetes patients, DRB1*0402-DQB1*0302 and DRB1*0405-DQB1*0302 (European Caucasian haplotypes) are strongly associated with risk, whereas DRB1*0408-DQB1*0302 and

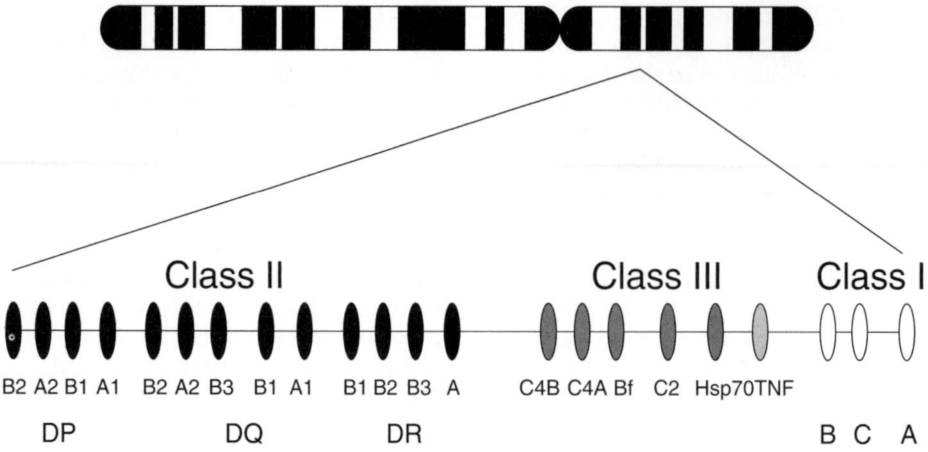

Fig. 21–1. The human leukocyte antigen (HLA) region on the short arm of chromosome 6. The class II region appears to be most directly involved in Type 1 diabetes.

DRB1*0411-DQB1*0302 (Native-American haplotypes) are actually protective against Type 1 diabetes, even though they all contain the DQB1*0302 allele (Erlich et al., 1993a,b). Additionally, the DPB1 locus has been shown to play a role in Type 1 diabetes susceptibility in both Caucasian and Mexican-American populations (Easteal et al., 1990; Erlich et al., 1993b; Noble et al., 1996, 2000; Cucca et al., 2001). There is now evidence that many of the class II loci are involved in Type 1 diabetes susceptibility, with associations reported with the DQ β region (DQBI*0302), the DQ α region (DQAI * 0301) and the DP β region (DPB1*0301), as well as with DR itself (Owerbach et al., 1983; Nepom et al., 1986; Horn et al., 1988; Vicario et al., 1992; Awata et al., 1992; Sanjeevi et al., 1993; Erlich et al., 1993b; Reijonen et al., 1997).

The HLA class II loci may not be the only portion of the HLA region conferring risk of Type 1 diabetes. Data have been reported that suggest that the class I region (HLA-B), class III region, and TNFA may also be involved in disease susceptibility (Thomson et al., 1988; Caplen et al., 1990; Fennessy et al., 1994; Nejentsev et al., 1997; Reijonen et al., 1997; Hanifi et al., 1998; Lie et al., 1999). Because of the extensive linkage disequilibrium across the HLA region, it may prove very difficult to determine exactly which of these loci actually contribute to Type 1 diabetes risk vs. loci that demonstrate associations only as a result of linkage disequilibrium.

Even with these difficulties, the observed increased risk for Type 1 diabetes in DR3/DR4 heterozygotes compared to either DR3/DR3 or DR4/DR4 homozygotes means that a single allele cannot explain the HLA region susceptibility to Type 1 diabetes. At a minimum, there must be two forms of Type 1 diabetes susceptibility, one associated with DR3 and another with DR4. Further evidence for at least two forms of Type 1 diabetes susceptibility comes from the observation that familial aggregation of Type 1 diabetes suggests that DR3 susceptibility acts in a recessive fashion, with most DR3-carrying Type 1 diabetes patients also having a second high-risk HLA haplotype (containing either DR3 or DR4). DR4-related Type 1 diabetes susceptibility, however, appears to act in a dominant fashion, as demonstrated by the observation of many DR4-carrying Type 1 diabetes patients who do not carry a second high-risk haplotype (MacDonald et al., 1986; Louis and Thomson, 1986; Thomson et al., 1988).

Phenotypic heterogeneity is also apparent between HLA-DR3- and DR4-associated Type 1 diabetes and further supports the concept that there is more than one form of genetic susceptibility encoded within the HLA region (Table 21–3) (Rotter, 1981; Schernthaner, 1982; Ludvigsson and Lindblom, 1984; Ludvigsson et al., 1986; Knip et al., 1986). The DR3 form of the disease (autoimmune form) is characterized by a greater persistence of pancreatic ICAs and antipancreatic cell-mediated im-

Table 21–3. Heterogeneity within Type 1 Diabetes

Evidence	DR3	DR4	Combined Form (DR3/DR4)
Linkage disequilibrium	A1, B8	B15, DQβ1*0302	Penetrance in monozygotic twins, risk to siblings
Insulin antibodies	Nonresponder (low antibody titers)	High responder (high antibody titers)	Occurrence in familial cases
Islet cell antibodies	Persistent	Transient	
Insulin autoantibodies	Less frequent	Increased frequency	Highest titers
Antipancreatic cell-mediated immunity	Increased	Not increased	
Thyroid autoimmunity	Yes	Less frequent	
Associated with other autoimmune endocrine diseases	Yes	No	
IgA deficiency	Increased	Not increased	
Age at onset	Any age	Younger age	Youngest
Ketoacidosis at clinical onset	Lesser frequency	Greater frequency	
Levels of C peptide	Preserved longer	Absent after shorter duration	Lowest

munity but a relative lack of antibody response to exogenous insulin. This form apparently has onset throughout life and probably accounts for a significant fraction of older-onset Type 1 diabetes. In the older age groups, this form of Type 1 diabetes may be treatable without insulin for a significant period of time, but the presence of ICAs presages eventual insulin dependence (Groop et al., 1988). The second form of Type 1 diabetes is associated with DR4. While not as strongly associated with autoimmune disease or ICAs, this form is accompanied by an increased antibody response to exogenous insulin (Rotter, 1981; Sklenar et al., 1982; Almer et al., 1985). For example, in this form of Type 1 diabetes, some individuals with the highest insulin antibody titers may have been treated with insulin for less than 5 years, thus indicating that prolonged duration of treatment is not the only explanation for an exaggerated immune response to insulin (Anderson et al., 1983). The relation between HLA-DR4 and insulin immunogenicity also can be seen before the initiation of exogenous insulin therapy, with the occurrence of insulin antibodies prior to disease onset (Karjalainen et al., 1986; Srikanta et al., 1986; Ziegler et al., 1991). DR4-associated Type 1 diabetes also appears to have an earlier age at onset, to exhibit seasonality, and to be related to viral infections.

The majority of investigators now believe that several different loci within the HLA region likely contribute to Type 1 diabetes susceptibility. With multiple genes participating, it is clear that the mechanisms by which the HLA region produces susceptibility must be complex. A more complete understanding of these mechanisms must await further clarification of both the number and identity of the HLA-linked genes that account for Type 1 diabetes risk.

Non-HLA Region Genes

Estimates of the proportion of genetic susceptibility to Type 1 diabetes for which the HLA region accounts vary, but even the highest estimates are in the range of 60% to 70%, clearly indicating that other, non-HLA loci must also play a role in Type 1 diabetes (Rotter and Landaw, 1984; Risch, 1987). Over the past 25 years, numerous other regions have been implicated in Type 1 diabetes susceptibility, but the data in support of most loci have remained fairly tentative.

The most substantiated locus is IDDM2, near the insulin gene on the short arm of chromosome 11. This region was first implicated in the early 1980s, when a polymorphic region 5′ to the insulin gene was discovered (Bell et al., 1984). The polymorphism results from the presence of a variable number tandem repeat (VNTR) region near the 5′-regulatory region. A number of population studies reported an association between Type I diabetes and class I alleles, which have smaller numbers of tandem repeats in this region compared to class III alleles (Bell et al., 1984; Hitman et al., 1985; Thomson et al., 1989; Raffel et al., 1991; Julier et al., 1991; Owerbach and Gabbay, 1993; Bennet et al., 1995). When these association studies were followed by family studies which failed to demonstrate linkage, however, there was some controversy as to whether the association was real. It is now appreciated that classical lod score linkage methods are rarely informative when analyzing loci contributing a comparatively small amount to disease susceptibility. As is true with the 5′ insulin VNTR, the high-risk alleles often occur very commonly in the general population, making it difficult to detect linkage without extremely large sample sizes. Thus, the failure to identify linkage between Type 1 diabetes and the insulin gene region was a consequence of the relatively small amount of genetic susceptibility to Type 1 diabetes afforded by this region. With the advent of family-based association methodologies, a role for IDDM2 in Type 1 diabetes susceptibility was better substantiated, and this locus is now well accepted (Raffel et al., 1992; Spielman et al., 1993; Owerbach and Gabbay, 1994). For many years, however, questions remained about exactly which gene is responsible for diabetes susceptibility in this region. Although it was proposed that loci upstream or downstream of the insulin gene might be involved, more recent studies make it fairly clear that the 5′ VNTR itself is responsible. The most attractive explanation is that this region affects expression of insulin mRNA in the fetal thymus and thus influences the development of tolerance to antigenic determinants of insulin (Vafiadis et al., 1997; Pugliese et al., 1997).

With the application of systematic chromosomal mapping to Type 1 diabetes, a variety of other candidate gene regions have been mapped (Table 21–4). As many as 14 loci have been implicated, with two or more distinct loci on chromosomes 2, 6, and 11. As these regions have been mapped using systematic approaches, the causative genes have by and large not yet been identified. Candidate genes within many of these regions have been investigated, but the majority have been excluded. The best data supporting a specific candidate gene suggest that *CTLA4* is

Table 21–4. Putative Type 1 Diabetes Loci in Humans

Locus	Chromosome Region	Candidate Genes in Region	References
IDDM1	6p21.3-6p21.3	Class II, class I *HLA* genes	See text
IDDM2	11p15.5–11p15.5	Insulin	See text
IDDM3	15q26–15q26		Field et al. (1994), Luo et al. (1995)
IDDM4	11q13–11q13	*LRP5*	Davies et al. (1994), Field et al. (1994), Hashimoto et al. (1994), Nakagawa et al. (1998)
IDDM5	6q25–6q25		Davies et al. (1994), Luo et al. (1996), Delepine et al. (1997)
IDDM6	18q21–18q21		Merriman et al. (1997, 1998), Cornelis et al. (1998)
IDDM7	2q31–2q31	*NeuroD/BETA2*	Copeman et al. (1995), Owerbach and Gabbay (1995), Kristiansen et al. (2000), Iwata et al. (1999)
IDDM8	6q27–6q27		Luo et al. (1995, 1996), Owerbach (2000)
IDDM10	10p11–10q11		Reed et al. (1997), Paterson and Petronis (2000)
IDDM11	14q24.3–14q31	*ENSA*	Field et al. (1996)
IDDM12	2q33–2q33	*CTLA-4*	Nistico et al. (1996), Marron et al. (1997, 2000)
IDDM13	2q34–2q34		Morahan et al. (1996), Fu et al. (1998), Larsen et al. (1999)
IDDM15	6q21–6q21		Delepine et al. (1997)
IDDM17	10q25–10q25		Verge et al. (1998)
IDDM18	5q31.1–q33.1	*IL12*	Adorini (2001), Morahan et al. (2001)
IDDMX	Xp11–Xp11		Davies et al. (1994), Cordell et al. (1995), Karvonen et al. (1997). Cucca et al. (1998)

likely IDDM12 on chromosome 2 (Marron et al., 1997, 2000; Larsen et al., 1999; Hill et al., 2000; Lowe et al., 2000). While proof that *CTLA4* is IDDM12, in the form of identification of the responsible mutations, has not yet been reported, there is compelling biological data supporting the linkage and association data implicating this gene. *CTLA4* has been shown to play a role in regulating apoptosis of activated T cells and to reduce proliferation of activated T cells by inhibiting production of IL-2 (Gribben et al., 1995; Krummel and Allison, 1996). Although candidate genes have been identified within some of the other chromosomal regions (Table 21–4), the data supporting them remain weak. Exactly how many of these regions will ultimately be proven to contain Type 1 diabetes susceptibility genes is unclear. While linkage of a number of the loci has been replicated in independent populations, several have been reported from only a single study population (IDDM11, IDDM15, IDDM17) and the linkages may ultimately turn out to be false-positives. While potentially interesting candidate genes have been localized within some of the linked regions (Table 21–4), recent successes in positional cloning for a variety of conditions have shown that the causative genes often are novel genes previously unsuspected to be involved in the disease process.

Understanding the ways in which the various loci interact to produce diabetes will be possible only after the actual susceptibility genes are cloned. It may well be that in any given individual only a portion of the Type 1 diabetes genes will be involved in disease causation. Whether all of the loci will be additive in their effects, as appears to be the case for HLA and the insulin gene region, or whether there will be synergistic interactions among some loci remains to be seen.

Support for the importance of non-HLA-region genes in the susceptibility to Type 1 diabetes also comes from experimental animal models. The NOD mouse, the best experimental animal model of Type 1 diabetes, has many similarities to human Type 1 diabetes. The disease is characterized by insulitis reminiscent of that seen in humans, and one susceptibility gene, *Idd-1*, has been shown to be tightly linked to the murine MHC (Prochazka et al., 1987; Miyazaki et al., 1990). Further supporting the idea of similarity in the disease process in NOD mice and humans is evidence suggesting sequence homology between the NOD I-A β gene (*Idd-1*) and the human allele HLA-DQB1*0302 (Miyazaki et al., 1990). Close to 20 other loci that are involved in the development of insulitis and Type 1 diabetes in the NOD mouse have been mapped (Ghosh et al., 1993; Miyazaki et al., 1994; Mouse Genome Database, 2001) (Table 21–5). These loci are scattered throughout the genome, although the mapping data suggest the presence of more than one Type 1 diabetes locus on a number of chromosomes, as in the case of mouse chromosomes 1, 3, 4, 6, 14, and 17 (Mouse Genome Database, 2001).

Initially, there was the hope that mouse Type 1 diabetes loci identification would aid in the localization of human Type 1 diabetes genes. Unfortunately, with the exception of the MHC in the mouse and the HLA in humans (and possibly the IL-12 gene, if recent studies hold up), no clear evidence exists that the same genes are responsible for Type 1 diabetes susceptibility in mice and humans. Although the existence of homologous susceptibility loci has not been excluded, it now appears that extension of the human mapping studies will be necessary to identify human Type 1 diabetes loci.

Given the growing data from both humans and experimental animal models that multiple genes participate in Type 1 diabetes susceptibility, the potential for genetic complexity is great. Not only can several loci provide susceptibility and/or protection, but there may be epistatic interactions among the various loci as well (Risch et al., 1993). Data collected thus far suggest that some loci act independently, while others display epistasis. Thus, e.g., although one study suggested that the 5′ insulin gene region provides risk preferentially to HLA-DR4-positive individuals (Julier et al., 1991), most studies of the Type 1 diabetes risk afforded by this region suggest that it acts independently of HLA (Raffel et al., 1991; Bain et al., 1992). In contrast, there does appear to be interaction between the HLA region and the

Table 21–5. Mouse Insulin-Dependent Diabetes Loci

Murine Locus	Murine Chromosome (cM)	Human Syntenic Region	References
Peri-insulitis	Chr. 1, distal	Chr. 1, 2, or 18	Garchon et al. (1991)
Idd5	1 (40.0)	Chr. 2q34-6	Cornall (1993), Ghosh et al. (1993), Yui et al. (1996)
Idd13	2 (71.0)	Chr. 2p or 15q	Serreze et al. (1994)
Idd3	3 (19.2)	Chr. 1 or 4	Cornall (1993), Denny et al. (1997), Encinas et al. (1999), Lord et al. (1995), Mcaleer et al. (1995), McDuffie (1998), Prochazka et al. (1987), Teuscher et al. (1996), Todd et al. (1991), Wicker et al. (1994), Yui et al. (1996)
Idd10	3 (48.5)	Chr. 1p13 or 1q21–22	Mcaleer et al. (1995), Podolin et al. (1997, 1998), Todd et al. (1991), Wicker et al. (1994), Yui et al. (1996)
Idd17	3 (39.0)		Podolin et al. (1997)
Idd18	3 (53.3)	Chr. 1p21	Podolin et al. (1997)
Idd9 (Idd9.1, Idd9.2, Idd9.3)	4 (82.0)	Chr. 1p36	Lyons et al. (2000), Mcaleer et al. (1995), Rodrigues et al. (1994)
Idd11	4 (64.6)	Chr. 1p35–36	Brodnicki et al. (2000), Morahan et al. (1994)
Idd15	5		Mcaleer et al. (1995)
Idd6	6	Chr. 12p12	Ghosh et al. (1993), Mcaleer et al. (1995), Yui et al. (1996)
Idd19	6 (60.5)	Chr. 12p12	Melanitou et al. (1998)
Idd7	7 (4.0)	Chr.19q13	Ghosh et al. (1993), Mcaleer et al. (1995)
Idd2	9 (22.0)	Chr. 11q	Mcaleer et al. (1995), Pearce et al. (1995), Prochazka et al. (1986, 1987, 1989)
Idd4	11 (44.0)	Chr. 17p13 or q11–12	Cornall (1993), Todd et al. (1991), Yui et al. (1996)
Idd14	13		Mcaleer et al. (1995)
Idd8	14 (3.5)	Chr. 10q24 or 3p	Ghosh et al. (1993)
Idd12	14 (12.0)		Morahan et al. (1994)
Idd1	17 (19.5)	Chr. 6p21, MHC	Ikegami et al. (1995), Prochazka et al. (1986, 1987, 1989), Yui et al. (1996)
Idd16	17 (18.0)	Chr. 6p21	Ikegami et al. (1995)

Gm locus; Field et al. (1984) reported that the immunoglobulin heavy chain allotype G1m(2) was associated with increased Type 1 diabetes risk in HLA-DR3 individuals, while G3m(5) resulted in increased risk in HLA-DR4 individuals. The interactions among loci may be even more complex; specific Gm allotypes have been reported to interact with a restriction fragment length polymorphism of the T-cell receptor β chain in Type 1 diabetes (Field et al., 1991), and interactions between HLD-DR and Gm have been reported to occur as a function of sex (Rich et al., 1986; Propert et al., 1991).

GENETICS OF DIABETIC COMPLICATIONS

Complications develop in most individuals with longstanding diabetes; most diabetics of 20 years' duration or more show evidence of at least one of these complications. Long-term diabetic complications affect the large blood vessels (coronary arteries, cerebral vasculature, and peripheral vasculature), also referred to as *macrovascular complications*; and microvascular complications include the eyes (diabetic retinopathy and cataract), the kidneys (diabetic glomerulosclerosis and renal failure), the nerves (distal neuropathy and autonomic neuropathy), and the skin and joints (Clements and Bell, 1985). These complications are the major causes of morbidity and early mortality in diabetes of all kinds (Pincus and White, 1933; Panzram and Zabel-Langhennig, 1981; Tunbridge, 1981; Dorman et al., 1985; Drury, 1985; Herman and Teutsch, 1985; Ulvenstam et al., 1985). As reviewed by Clements and Bell (1985), diabetics have at least a doubled risk for coronary heart disease, a risk for cataracts that is five times that of the general population, a 17-fold increased risk for kidney failure, a 25-fold increased risk for blindness, and a 50-fold increased risk for amputations.

Complications occur in all forms of diabetes, though not necessarily with the same frequency across the different types (Davidson and Smith, 1986; Nathan et al., 1986). While early studies suggested a disproportionate risk for complications in Type 1 diabetics, it now appears that complication rates may be more comparable across the various forms than was first recognized (Herman and Teutsch, 1985). Also, there still are difficulties in comparing studies across place and time, owing to differences in methods of detection and comparability of individuals screened.

The relative importance of various factors in the etiology of long-term diabetic complications has historically been controversial, it being unclear whether the duration of diabetes, the degree of metabolic control, or genetic predisposition has primacy. For Type 1 diabetes, duration of disease plays a significant role as it is highly unusual to see complications in patients with a disease duration of less than 5 to 10 years. The Diabetes Control and Complications Trial (DCCT), in the mid-1990s, clearly demonstrated that the risk of complications can be significantly reduced when glucose control is maximized (Diabetes Control and Complications Trial Research Group, 1995a–c). The DCCT also demonstrated, however, that genetic factors are important in the development of diabetic complications (Diabetes Control and Complications Trial Research Group, 1997).

Diabetic Nephropathy

Clinical nephropathy in the diabetic is defined as persistent proteinuria (>0.5 g/24 hours) in a diabetic of at least 10 years' duration with no other known renal disease, urinary tract infection, or cardiac failure (Viberti and Walker, 1988). It is estimated that 35% to 45% of long-term diabetics will develop clinical nephropathy (Oakley et al., 1974; Deckert et al., 1982; Anderson et al., 1983; Mogensen and Christensen, 1984; Viberti and Keen, 1984; Krolewski et al., 1985; Mathiesen et al., 1986; Viberti et al., 1987; Viberti and Walker, 1988). End-stage renal disease is currently an important cause of serious morbidity and premature mortality in diabetes (Herman and Teutsch, 1985; Winocour et al., 1987). Patients with nephropathy, proteinuria, or both are also significantly more likely to have clinically important macrovascular disease than are diabetics without nephropathy (Winocour et al., 1987; Borch-Johnsen and Kreiner, 1987; Jensen et al., 1987).

Clinical renal disease is rare prior to 10 years' duration of diabetes, although histological evidence of renal involvement is found earlier; close to 90% of diabetics with a disease duration of at least 10 years have evidence of glomerulosclerosis (Horey et al., 1962; Herman and Teutsch, 1985; Viberti and Walker, 1988). Surprisingly, only about 30% to 40% progress to clinical nephropathy, and the peak incidence of nephropathy occurs with a diabetes duration between 15 and about 20 years (Deckert and Poulsen, 1981; Mogensen, 1984; Nyberg et al., 1985; Kofoed-Enevoldsen et al., 1987). For those who do not have nephropathy 35 years after diagnosis, there is little risk of ever developing it (Andersen et al., 1983; Krolewski et al., 1985).

Hypertension has been demonstrated to be an independent risk factor for diabetic nephropathy (Mogensen et al., 1988; Noth et al., 1989). At first considered merely a secondary result of the kidney disease, several lines of evidence now strongly suggest that hypertension precedes clinical nephropathy and may play an important role in its genesis (Jensen et al., 1987). Elevated blood pressure at the onset of proteinuria is clearly associated with persistent proteinuria (Ishihara et al., 1984; Mathiesen et al., 1984; Hasslacher et al., 1985; Katzeff and Klein, 1987; Winocour et al., 1987). Even more important, small but significant increases in blood pressure have been reported in diabetics with low-level microproteinuria (Deckert et al., 1982; Mogensen and Christensen, 1984; Wiseman et al., 1984; Mathiesen et al., 1984; Viberti and Walker, 1988) and in diabetics who eventually progress to albuminuria or nephropathy prior to any evidence of kidney damage (Mogensen and Christensen, 1984; Hasslacher et al., 1985; Kofoed-Enevoldsen et al., 1987). Several studies have found decreased or reversed rates or kidney deterioration with improved control of hypertension (Mogensen, 1982; Bjorck et al., 1986; Christensen and Mogensen, 1987; Zander et al., 1987; Parving et al., 1987; Drury, 1985) and, conversely, an increased rate of deterioration in diabetics with higher blood pressure (Hasslacher et al., 1985).

Supporting a role for genetic susceptibility in the development of diabetic nephropathy is the demonstration of familial clustering of nephropathy (Seaquist et al., 1989; Quinn et al., 1996). In these two studies, 17% to 25% of Type 1 diabetes siblings of diabetic probands without nephropathy but 71% to 83% of Type 1 diabetes siblings of diabetic probands with nephropathy had evidence of nephropathy themselves. Fioretto et al. (1999) also demonstrated concordance in the severity and pattern of glomerular lesions in Type 1 diabetic siblings in the absence of concordance for glycemic control. Additionally, higher blood pressures have been observed in the siblings of Type 1 diabetic patients with hypertension compared to siblings of patients without hypertension, suggesting that genetic predisposition to hypertension may be one mechanism by which genetic factors impact risk for nephropathy. There is further evidence suggesting an interaction between cardiovascular risk and risk of nephropathy; overall, cardiovascular and stroke-related mortality has been reported to be increased in the parents of Type 1 diabetes subjects with nephropathy compared to normoalbuminuric subjects (Lindsay et al., 1999; Tarnow et al., 2000a).

Candidate gene studies have also been used to test for genetic influences on nephropathy in Type 1 diabetes. While early studies of nondiabetic nephropathy (both idiopathic membranous nephropathy and drug-induced nephropathy) suggested an association between HLA-DR3 and risk for kidney disease (Klouda et al., 1979; Wooley et al., 1980), studies of diabetic nephropathy have not suggested that HLA alleles play a role in this condition (Walton et al., 1984; Barbosa and Saner, 1984). A number of other candidate genes have been implicated in nephropathy risk, however. There are substantial data that the angiotensin-I-converting enzyme (*ACE*) gene is involved (Marre et al., 1994; Doria et al., 1994; Barnas et al., 1997; Jacobsen et al., 1998; Freire et al., 1998; Vleming et al., 1999; Gumprecht et al., 2000; Hadjadj et al., 2001). While most of these studies have looked directly at the risk for nephropathy, some investigators have also demonstrated associations between the *ACE* genotype and measures of renal blood flow, suggesting that the *ACE* gene may influence nephropathy risk by impacting blood pressure or some other aspect of renal hemodynamics (Fukumoto et al., 1996; Miller et al., 1997). This hypothesis is supported by the study of Jacobsen et al. (1998), who demonstrated an association between *ACE* genotype and response to ACE inhibitor therapy by changes in mean arterial blood pressure and reduction in albuminuria.

Further evidence that the renin–angiotensin pathway is important in nephropathy risk comes from studies demonstrating associations with the angiotensin receptor gene and the angiotensinogen gene (Marre et al., 1994; Doria et al., 1994; Fukumoto et al., 1996; Barnas et al., 1997; Miller et al., 1997; Jacobsen et al., 1998; Freire et al., 1998; Vleming et al., 1999; Gumprecht et al., 2000; Hadjadj et al., 2001). As with the *ACE* gene, blood pressure appears to be influenced by these candidate genes, suggesting that hypertension might be the pathway by which nephropathy risk is mediated.

Several studies have also implicated the aldose reductase gene in nephropathy (Shah et al., 1998; Moczulski et al., 2000; Hodgkinson et al., 2001). Aldose reductase is the rate-limiting step in the polyol pathway, and enzyme levels have been shown to be increased in Type 1 diabetes subjects with nephropathy compared to those without this complication (Shah et al., 1997). A variety of other candidate genes have been implicated in nephropathy risk (Table 21–6), but these associations are less well substantiated.

Diabetic Eye Complications

Eye complications associated with diabetes include an increased risk for cataracts and diabetic retinopathy. The retinopathy may be mild, consisting of background changes in the retina that have little impact on vision, or may develop into the vision-threatening proliferative neovascular changes seen in a proportion of diabetics of long duration.

Among Type 1 diabetics, an estimated 90% to 95% have background (nonproliferative) retinopathy after a diabetes duration of 15 years or more (Rosenstock and Raskin, 1988; Klein et al., 1988; Teuscher et al., 1988). Studies suggest that as many as 60% to 65% of all Type 1 diabetics will also have some proliferative eye changes 35 years after diagnosis (Klein et al., 1985a,b; Rosenstock and Raskin, 1988). Both background and proliferative retinopathy are strongly correlated with duration of diabetes (Ellis et al., 1983; Segal et al., 1983; Klein et al., 1985a,b; Nathan et al., 1986; Burger et al., 1986; Krolewski et al., 1987). In fact, diabetes duration is the strongest single predictor of diabetic retinopathy. With the development of more sensitive methods for detecting background retinopathy, it is now clear that some changes may be discernible within a few years in some Type 1 diabetics (Burger et al., 1986; Weber et al., 1986). However, clinically significant retinopathy is rare prior to 10 years' duration (Krolewski et al., 1987) and almost never occurs in childhood-onset diabetics prior to puberty (Knowles, 1971; Jackson et al., 1982; Weber et al., 1986). A number of studies have noted a slight male preponderance among diabetics with proliferative retinopathy (Deckert et al., 1979; Barbosa et al., 1980; Bodansky et al., 1982; Dornan et al., 1982; Klein and Klein, 1985).

Twin studies provide evidence that the risk for retinopathy in diabetics may have a genetic component. In the large British twin panel, MZ twins were found to have a high degree of concordance for complications such as diabetic retinopathy (Leslie and Pyke, 1982). Although the data were strongest for Type 2 diabetes, where concordance for complications was virtually complete, even in Type 1 pairs the investigators observed that 21 of 31 pairs of MZ twins were concordant for the level of retinopathy, either none, background, or proliferative retinopathy. This finding suggests that genetics factors, as opposed to shared environment alone, have a role in the development of retinopathy in these twins and presumably in all diabetic patients.

While a substantial body of data, as shown in Table 21–6, suggests an association between HLA and the risk for retinopathy (Barbosa et al., 1980; Johnston et al., 1981; Dornan et al., 1982; Gray et al., 1982; Baker et al., 1986; Cruickshanks et al., 1992; Agardh et al., 1996; Falck et al., 1997), there have also been many negative studies. In the more recent studies (when DR typing was available), DR4 has been the allele most often implicated in retinopathy risk. There has been a question as to whether this association is a result of the DR4-associated diabetes susceptibility locus, or if this might reflect the fact that HLA-DR4 is associated with more severe abnormalities in glycemic control, which then secondarily increase the risk for retinopathy. However, the work of Dornan and co-workers (1982), who reported that for each level of diabetic control (measured by HbA_{1c}), HLA-DR4-positive diabetics were more likely to have retinopathy than were DR4-negative diabetics, suggests that there is a primary role for DR4.

Genes in the renin–angiotensin and polyol pathways have also been implicated in retinopathy risk but not as convincingly as for nephropathy (Table 21–6).

Macrovascular Complications

The large-vessel (macrovascular) complications of diabetes include atherosclerotic disease of the coronary, cerebral, and peripheral arteries (Ledet et al., 1984). Macrovascular disease has been estimated to account for 50% or more of all deaths occurring in adult diabetics (Marks and Krall, 1971; Abadie et al., 1981; Tunbridge, 1981; Panzram and Zabel-Langhennig, 1981; Ledet et al., 1984; Drury, 1985; Herman and Teutsch, 1985; Ulvenstam et al., 1985; Davidson and Smith, 1986; Nathan et al., 1986; Dolan, 1986; Smith, 1986; Rosenstock and Raskin, 1988). In addition, there may be a specific diabetic cardiomyopathy (Ledet et al., 1984), as well as cardiac rhythm abnormalities sec-

Table 21–6. Candidate Genes Associated with Type 1 Diabetes Complications

Gene	Associated Trait	High-Risk Allele/Genotype	Reference
Nephropathy			
ACE	Nephropathy	D allele	Hadjadj et al. (2001)
ACE	Nephropathy	D allele	Barnas et al. (1997)
ACE	Nephropathy	D allele	Marre et al. (1994)
ACE	Chronic renal failure	D allele	Gumprecht et al. (2000)
ACE	Chronic renal failure	DD genotype	Vleming et al. (1999)
ACE	Glomerular filtration rate, renal plasma flow	D allele	Miller et al. (1997)
ACE	Arcuate artery resistance index	DD genotype	Fukumoto et al. (1996)
ACE	Response to *ACE* inhibitor therapy in subjects with nephropathy: reduction in mean arterial blood, pressure reduction in albuminuria	II genotype associated with improved response	Jacobsen et al. (1998)
ACE	Nephropathy	Intron 7 PstI polymorphism	Freire et al. (1998)
ACE	Nephropathy	XbaI minor allele	Doria et al. (1994)
AGT1R	Renal plasma flow, blood pressure response to hyperglycemia	CC genotype	Miller et al. (2000)
AGT1R	Hypertension	CC genotype	Van Ittersum et al. (2000)
AGT1R	Nephropathy in diabetics with poor glycemic control	C allele	Doria et al. (1997)
AGT	Urinary albumin excretion	235T allele (when interacting with *ACE* D allele)	Van Ittersum et al. (2000)
AGT	Chronic renal failure	235T allele	Gumprecht et al. (2000)
AGT	Nephropathy, chronic renal failure	235T allele	Rogus et al. (1998)
AGT	Nephropathy	235TT genotype	Fogarty et al. (1996)
AGT	Elevated blood pressure in patient with nephropathy	235TT genotype	Tarnow et al. (1996)
Aldose reductase	Nephropathy	Z-2, 106T alleles and Z-2/106T haplotype	Moczulski et al. (2000)
Aldose reductase	Nephropathy	Z-2 allele	Shah et al. (1998)
Aldose reducatase	Nephropathy	Z+2 allele is protective	Hodgkinson et al. (2001)
eNOS	Nephropathy	-786C/exon 4 a deletion haplotype	Zanchi et al. (2000)
MTHFR	Nephropathy	677 TT genotype	Shcherbak et al. (1999)
Pronatriodilatin	Nephropathy	T708 allele and ScaI A2 allele	Nannipieri et al. (1999)
Interleukin-1B	Nephropathy	IL1B*2 allele	Loughrey et al. (1998)
GLUT1	Nephropathy	Intron 2 XbaI 1.1kb allele	Hodgkinson et al. (2001)
Renin	Nephropathy	Intron 1 BglII bb genotype	Deinum et al. (1999)
Insulin gene VNTR	Nephropathy	II genotype	Raffel et al. (1991)
Retinopathy			
ACE	Retinopathy	DD genotype	Rabensteiner et al. (1999)
AGT	Retinopathy	235T allele	Van Ittersum et al. (2000)
Aldose reductase	Retinopathy	95A and CA repeat polymorphism	Kao et al. (1999a,b)
Aldose reductase	Retinopathy	Z-2 allele	Demaine et al. (2000)
HLA-DR/DQ	Retinopathy	DR3-DQ2/DR4-DQ8 haplotype	Agardh et al. (1996)
HLA-DR	Proliferative retinopathy	DR4	Cruickshanks et al. (1992)
HLA-DR	Retinopathy	DR1	Falck et al. (1997)
HLA-DR	Retinopathy	DR4/4, DR3/4, DRX/X	Baker et al. (1986)
HLA-DR	Retinopathy	DR4	Dornan et al. (1982)
HLA-B	Retinopathy	B7 protective	Gray et al. (1982)
HLA-A,B	Retinopathy	Ai-B8 combination	Johnston et al. (1981)
HLA-A,B	Proliferative retinopathy	B15; B7 protective	Barbosa et al. (1980)
Gm	Retinopathy	G2m(23)	Stewart et al. (1993)
Paraoxonase	Retinopathy	54L allele	Kao et al. (1998)
Coronary artery disease			
ACE	CAD in patients with nephropathy	D allele	Tarnow et al. (1995)
ApoE	CAD in patients with nephropathy	ApoE4 allele	Tarnow et al. (2000b)
ACE	Myocardial infarction in fathers of nephropathy probands	D allele	Tarnow et al. (2000a)
Neuropathy			
ATP1 A1	Neuropathy	Intron 1 BglII restriction site	Vague et al. (1997)
Aldose reductase	Neuropathy	Z+2 allele associated with reduced risk	Heesom et al. (1998)

ACE, angiotensin-converting enzyme; ApoE, apolipoprotein E; eNOS, endothelial nitric oxide synthase; MTHFR, methylenetetrahydrofolate reductase; AGT1R, angiotensin II type 1 receptor; GLUT1, glucose transporter 1; VNTR, variable number of tandem repeats.

ondary to autonomic neuropathy in diabetics (Blandford and Burden, 1984; Kereiakes et al., 1984).

Clearly, diabetes is associated with increased atherosclerosis and macrovascular complications at all ages. The increased risk associated with diabetes has been estimated to be between 1.5 and 2.5 times in men and between 1.7 and 4 times in women for coronary artery disease (Barrett-Connor and Orchard, 1985a,b), approximately twice for thromboembolic stroke (Abbott et al., 1987), and 50-fold for amputations secondary to peripheral vascular disease (Clements and Bell, 1985). The relative risk for coronary artery disease is particularly high in patients with Type 1 diabetes under the age of 40, owing to an increased risk for coronary artery disease at an age when the general population risk is very low (relative risk estimated to be around 28–35 times greater than for comparable nondiabetics) (Barrett-Connor and Orchard, 1985a,b).

As in the nondiabetic population, the risk for macrovascular disease rises with increasing age (Welborn et al., 1984). However, unlike nondiabetic women, premenopausal female diabetics do not appear to be afforded a relative protection against atherosclerotic cardiovascular disease (Garcia et al., 1974; Laakso et al., 1988). One finding in the World Health Organization Multinational Study was the slight but consistent increased prevalence of electrocardiographic abnormalities in female vs. male diabetics (Keen and Jarrett, 1979). Female diabetics are also at a relatively increased risk for cerebrovascular disease (Laakso et al., 1988). Relative risks for cardiovascular disease are particularly high for diabetics of both sexes prior to middle age, an age group that has low rates in the nondiabetic population (Tunbridge, 1981; Barrett-Connor and Orchard, 1985a,b). The relationship of diabetes duration (independent of attained age) and risk for macrovascular disease is less clear than for microvascular disease, and several studies have found no effect of duration (Pirart, 1977, 1978; Vigorita et al., 1980; Welborn et al., 1984; Barrett-Connor and Orchard, 1985; Jarrett and Shipley, 1988; Laakso et al., 1988).

Diabetics have an increased prevalence of several other known physiological risk factors for macrovascular disease, most notably hypertension and disordered lipid levels. These factors are often present for years prior to the development of overt cardiovascular disease. For example, Type 1 diabetics were found to have elevated systolic and diastolic blood pressures early in the course of diabetes when compared to closest-in-age siblings (Cruickshanks et al., 1985). Additional studies suggest that both Type I and Type 2 diabetics, as well as those with impaired glucose tolerance, are more likely to be hypertensive than are age- and sex-matched nondiabetic controls (Klein et al., 1985c).

Hypertension is another known risk factor for atherosclerosis. Most studies have found the prevalence of hypertension in Type 1 diabetes patients to be higher than in the general population. Klein and co-workers (1985c) found hypertension in 22% of Type 1 diabetes patients diagnosed before age 30. The duration of diabetes was significantly associated with higher systolic blood pressure. Furthermore, a specific association has been found between hypertension and the development of diabetic nephropathy. It has been suggested that the risk of kidney disease in Type 1 diabetes is associated with a genetic predisposition to hypertension (Krolewski et al., 1988; Seaquist et al., 1989; Nosadini et al., 1991).

Evidence suggesting that genetic factors may be involved in macrovascular complications comes from several sources. There are significant interpopulational differences in the frequency of macrovascular disease in diabetics as well as nondiabetics (Rimoin and Schimke, 1971; West, 1978; Keen, 1983; Uusitupa et al., 1985; Haffner et al., 1988, 1989; Lester and Keen, 1988; Pugh et al., 1988; Viberti, 1988). Additional evidence comes from clinical observations of cases with long-standing diabetes. For example, several studies from the Joslin Clinic suggest that some individuals with diabetes of 25 years' duration or more are complication-free, while others show evidence of microvascular and macrovascular disease even early in the course of their diabetes (Chazan et al., 1970; Ryan et al., 1970; Paz-Guevara et al., 1975; Lestradet et al., 1981). Other studies have noted that perhaps as many as one-quarter of diabetics of long duration do not show serious complications, including macrovascular disease (Ryan et al., 1970; Knowles, 1971; Oakley and Pyke, 1974; Pirart, 1978; Andersen et al., 1983; Nyberg et al., 1985). Even more interesting, there is evidence that some individuals remain relatively complication-free even with suboptimal control of their diabetes (Pirart, 1978; Deckert and Poulsen, 1981).

Several family studies suggest decreased longevity in the relatives of those Type 1 diabetes patients with early mortality and/or vascular complications. Chazan et al. (1970) found significantly decreased mean longevity in mothers and fathers of Type 1 diabetes patients with complications. Supporting this, Dorman and Drash (1986) reported increased familial mortality in parents and siblings of Type 1 diabetes probands who died young. Analogous results were seen in patients with early-onset ischemic heart disease by Nora et al. (1980), who reported that juvenile diabetes in a first-degree relative, although seen only at a relatively low frequency, was the third highest independent variable in increasing risk for coronary disease. Krolewski et al. (1981) found an increased frequency of coronary heart disease and hypertension in nondiabetic siblings of both Type 1 and Type 2 diabetes probands compared to control families, though the magnitude of risk was substantially greater among the sibs of the Type 2 diabetes patients. These studies suggest that the risks for vascular disease and diabetes are etiologically separate and that the risk for diabetic vascular disease is particularly high in individuals with both the genetic predisposition to vascular disease and metabolic derangements associated with diabetes.

Despite the epidemiological evidence for genetic control of macrovascular risk, surprisingly few studies have investigated candidate genes. The *ACE* and apolipoprotein E genes have been associated with coronary artery risk in patients with nephropathy and their families (Tarnow et al., 1995, 2000b), but confirmation of these findings is needed.

OTHER FORMS OF DIABETES MELLITUS

The separation of idiopathic diabetes into Type 1 and Type 2 diabetes by no means exhausts the potential heterogeneity within the diabetic phenotype. There could well be genetically distinct forms whose phenotypic presentation could include either Type 1 or Type 2 diabetes. The atypical forms of diabetes among African Americans (Winter et al., 1987; Banerji et al., 1994) may be examples. Evidence for "overlap" phenotypes includes suggestions of too high a frequency of either type in family members of the other type compared to the general population and reports that Type 2 diabetes in parents of Type 1 diabetes patients increased the risk to other siblings for Type 1 diabetes (Wagener et al., 1982; Chern et al., 1982). Some of this may be due to the occurrence of a Type 2 diabetes-like phase of Type 1 diabetes in patients with a more protracted natural history, but it quite possibly reflects further heterogeneity. In addition, it has been reported that in some non-Caucasian populations, i.e., South African Indian and black diabetics, regardless of the type of diabetes in the index case, there was an increase in Type 2 diabetes in first-degree relatives (Omar and Asmal, 1983). In addition, low order of magnitude HLA associations have been reported with HLA-Bw61 in diabetics of the Indian subcontinent (Serjeantson et al., 1981), and with HLA-A2 in Pima Indian diabetics (Williams et al., 1981). The genetic–etiological relation of these HLA associations with diabetes in these non-Caucasian populations appears to be fundamentally different from that of HLA and Type 1 diabetes in Caucasian populations. Since there is no evidence for a role of immunological factors in these types of diabetes, these HLA associations may have a polygenic background role more analogous to that of the mouse H2 locus and the effect of strain differences. Essentially, there are whole groups or classes of diabetes for which our knowledge of etiology, genetics, and nosology is minimal. This includes not only most forms of diabetes in the developing world but also gestational diabetes (National Diabetes Data Group, 1979).

EVOLUTIONARY SPECULATIONS

Heterogeneity within both the insulin-dependent and non-insulin dependent types appears extensive. An important question arises from the population genetic viewpoint. These diabetic disorders, whose susceptibility appears to be primarily genetically determined, are deleterious, and thus reproductive fitness should be impaired. As regards Type 2 diabetes, a possible explanation is the concept of a "thrifty" genotype, as first proposed by Neel (1962). He proposed that the diabetic genotype somehow allowed more efficient utilization of foodstuffs by the body in periods of famine, to which primitive humans were often exposed. Such a thrifty gene would therefore have a selective survival advantage and would tend to increase in frequency. However, in the modern Western world, with its continuous abundance of calories, such a gene would lead to diabetes and obesity. Neel's hypothesis has received support by observations in both humans and other species. The extremely high frequency of diabetes and obesity in populations such as the Pima Indians (Knowler et al., 1981) and Pacific Islanders (Zimmet, 1979) and its apparent increase with modernization and urbanization are entirely consistent with the thrifty-genotype hypothesis. Direct support comes from studies showing that heterozygotes for rodent diabetes–obesity genes exhibit a much better ability to survive fasting than normal rodents (Coleman, 1979).

What might be the selective advantage of the genes that predispose to Type 1 diabetes? Since Type 1 diabetes is a disorder in which autoimmunity and immune response genes seem implicated, a possible role in the resistance to infectious agents has been proposed. However, the problem of the selective advantage of Type 1 diabetes is much greater than for Type 2 diabetes. Before the onset of insulin therapy, Type 1 diabetes was usually a lethal disorder, at least in genetic terms (i.e., failure to reproduce). This was both because of its severity and because its onset was usually at such an age that reproduction would have been prevented altogether, or at least severely interrupted. Also, since susceptibility seems to be provided even by single HLA-linked genes, this negative selection is much greater than that for recessive genetic disorders such as sickle-cell anemia or Tay-Sachs disease, where negative selection operates only on those homozygous for the disease genes. Thus, the positive selective advantage would of necessity be dramatic and the positive selection should have continued into modern human history. Otherwise, the incidence of the disorder would have decreased dramatically prior to the advent of insulin therapy. However, no such positive selective advantage has been discerned, at least postnatally.

Evidence has accumulated that suggests a potential selective advantage mechanism for Type 1 diabetes and at the same time provides at least a partial explanation of the recognition that the risk for Type 1 diabetes appears to be higher to offspring of males with Type 1 diabetes than to offspring of females with Type 1 diabetes (at least in the first 20 years of life) (Degnbol and Green, 1978; Kobberling and Bruggeboes, 1980; Warram et al., 1984). What has been observed in some studies is preferential transmission of diabetogenic HLA haplotypes, not only to affected offspring but to unaffected offspring as well (Vadheim et al., 1986; Thivolent et al., 1988). In addition, while this occurs for both high-risk (DR3- and DR4-associated) diabetic alleles/haplotypes in fathers, it has been reported to occur for only the DR3-associated haplotypes in mothers, providing an explanation for the increased paternal risk. Furthermore, there is evidence that this may occur via in utero selection (Vadheim et al., 1986). These data may thus provide an explanation for the maintenance of the high population frequency for this previously frequent genetically lethal disease. In addition, the suggestion that this prenatal selection could occur via immunologically mediated events raises the theoretical possibility that an additional consequence of these events, in fetuses that survive, might be immune changes that presage the eventual development of Type 1 diabetes (Vadheim et al., 1987).

GENETIC COUNSELING IN TYPE 1 DIABETES

Risks for Type 1 Diabetes

Because the mode of inheritance in Type 1 diabetes is not straightforward, most genetic counseling is based on empiric risk estimates, which have been developed from both population-based and family-based epidemiological studies (Table 21–7). These recurrence risks are frequently reassuring to families as they are often less than the family has feared, particularly for siblings of the Type 1 diabetes patient. The empiric risk of recurrence for Type 1 diabetes is dependent on the relationship of the individual in question to the affected family member. For siblings, the empiric risk is approximately 5% to 10%. If the father is affected, the risk to his offspring is 4% to 6% compared to 2% to 3% if the mother is affected (Warram et al., 1984, 1988). For further refinement of sibling risks, HLA testing can be used to determine haplotype sharing with the diabetic sib (Gorsuch et al., 1982, Rotter et al., 1986). If two haplotypes are shared, the risk increases to 16% to 17% and is 20% to 25% if the haplotypes contain both DR3 and DR4 (Rotter and Rimoin, 1987). Siblings who share one haplotype have a risk in the range of 5% to 7%, while the risk is approximately 1% to 2% if no haplotypes are shared (Rotter and Rimoin, 1987). It is important to realize that the sibling of an individual with Type 1 diabetes still has a risk for Type 1 diabetes that is increased above that of the general population, even when the sib shares no HLA haplotypes with the diabetic in the family. Based on our understanding of the genetics of Type 1 diabetes as detailed above, there are at least three possible explanations for this persistent risk. Since the Type 1 diabetes gene(s) within the HLA region has not yet been absolutely identified, it is possible for siblings to have inherited the HLA-related Type 1 diabetes susceptibility gene but, due to recombination, different HLA types. Also, because the high-risk

Table 21–7. Risks for Type 1 Diabetes

Population risks	Overall 1/500
	HLA-DR related
	No high-risk allele 1/5000
	1 high-risk allele, i.e., DR3/x or DR4/x 1/400
	HLA-DR4 subset defined by molecular techniques 1/300
	HLA-DR3/3 or DR4/4 1/150
	HLA-DR3/4 1/40
Risks in relatives	
Siblings	Overall 1/14
	HLA haplotypes shared with diabetic sibling
	0 haplotypes shared 1/100
	1 haplotype shared 1/20
	2 haplotypes shared 1/6
	2 haplotypes shared and DR3/4 1/5 to 1/4
Offspring	Overall 1/25
	Offspring of affected female 1/50 to 1/40
	Offspring of affected male 1/20
Monozygotic twin of diabetic	1/3

HLA haplotypes (i.e., those containing DR3 or DR4) occur fairly commonly in the general population, it is possible that one or both parents of a child with Type 1 diabetes may actually carry two high-risk haplotypes. Thus, another child may inherit HLA-linked diabetes-susceptibility genes, even though he or she shares no HLA haplotypes with the index diabetic sibling. Lastly, it is possible that the increased risk is due to one or more of the non-HLA region susceptibility genes.

There is some question regarding the benefit of performing HLA typing (or any genetic marker) for the siblings of an individual with Type 1 diabetes when this information would not lead to any alteration in management. Particular attention must be paid to the potential negative effects of stigmatization and the risks of the child being treated as ill. The concept that HLA testing at best identifies someone more susceptible to developing Type 1 diabetes but in no way guarantees that he or she will become diabetic must be stressed. The potential for other negative effects, such as possibly being ruled ineligible for health, life, and/or disability insurance due to the presence of a "preexisting" condition, must also be discussed with every family contemplating more refined testing.

What is clear is that HLA testing is not appropriate as a screening tool for the general population. Approximately 50% of the nondiabetic population have the same HLA-DR types as patients with Type 1 diabetes. Thus, at least 98% of the people with DR3 or DR4 will never develop Type 1 diabetes. For every 1000 persons with HLA-DR3 or -DR4 in the population, only two to four will develop Type 1 diabetes (Table 21–7). Thus, population screening using HLA-DR serological typing will result in more false-positive results than true-positives in terms of genetic risk. Even molecular testing of the class II genes will result in many more false-positives than true-positives and will be fraught with the difficulties of different allelic associations depending on the ethnic and racial background of the individuals being tested, as described above. ICA or GAD antibody testing is also not yet specific enough to be effective for screening in the general population.

There may be situations in which HLA typing and/or autoantibody testing will be appropriate in the future. A variety of clinical trials are currently under way, testing various methods of intervention to prevent or delay the onset of Type 1 diabetes, including the Diabetes Prevention Trial (DPT-1, United States), the Type 1 Diabetes Prediction and Prevention Project (DIPP, Finland), the European Nicotinamide Diabetes Intervention Trial (ENDIT), the European Paediatric Prediabetes Subcutaneous Insulin Trial (EPP-SCIT), and the Finnish Trial to Reduce IDDM in the Genetically at Risk Study (TRIGR) (Carel and Bougneres, 1996; Coutant et al., 1997; Knip et al., 2000; Paronen et al., 2000). Should any of these prevention strategies prove effective, identifying those individuals at highest risk will be necessary to make appropriate interventions available to them.

Screening for Other Autoimmune Disorders

Diabetes is not the only autoimmune disorder for which relatives of an individual with Type 1 diabetes are at risk. Family members, as well as the patient, are at increased risk for autoimmune thyroid disease (Hashimoto's thyroiditis, Graves' disease), pernicious anemia secondary to autoimmune gastritis, autoimmune adrenal disease (Addison's disease), myasthenia gravis, vitiligo, and coeliac disease (Bottazzo et al., 1978; Raffel et al., 1996). A study looking at individuals with Type 1 diabetes and their relatives found that 21% of the diabetics and 22% of their first-degree relatives had evidence of autoimmune disease (Betterle et al., 1984). Of patients with persistent ICAs, 57% had other autoimmune conditions compared to 15% of those not found to have persistent ICAs (Betterle et al., 1984). Seventy-five percent of the autoimmune disease in relatives occurred in families in which there was a proband with autoimmune disease, indicating increased genetic susceptibility to other autoimmune disorders in certain Type 1 diabetes families.

The most common form of autoimmune disease in families with Type 1 diabetes is thyroid disease (Riley et al., 1981, Betterle et al., 1984). Although the proportion of Type 1 diabetes patients with clinical or subclinical thyroid disease has been reported to be as high as 35%, the actual proportion is thought to be closer to 15% to 20% (Fialkow et al., 1975; Betterle et al., 1984). In contrast, the prevalence of autoimmune thyroid disease in nondiabetic Caucasians is thought to be 4.5% (Riley et al., 1980). The prevalence of clinical or subclinical autoimmune thyroid disease in first-degree relatives of individuals with Type 1 diabetes is estimated to be 15% to 25% (Fialkow et al., 1975; Betterle et al., 1984). As is true with autoimmune thyroid disease in the general population, female family members have higher rates of thyroid and gastric autoimmunity than males.

Other autoimmune disorders are also seen with increased frequency in Type 1 diabetics and their relatives. Autoimmune gastritis, as evidenced by the detection of gastric parietal cell autoantibodies or pernicious anemia, is seen in 5% to 12% of individuals with Type 1 diabetes and in 2.5% to 6% of their first-degree relatives (Fialkow et al., 1975; Riley et al., 1982; Betterle et al., 1984; De Block et al., 1999). The prevalence of adrenal autoantibodies is 1% to 3% in individuals with Type 1 diabetes compared to up to 0.6% in nondiabetics (Riley et al., 1980; Betterle et al., 1984).

It is particularly important for the relatives of patients with Type 1 diabetes to be made aware of this increased risk for autoimmune disease since approximately 40% of all families which include an individual with Type 1 diabetes will have at least one other family member with latent or clinical autoimmune disease (Betterle et al., 1984). Although most physicians know of the association of Type 1 diabetes with other autoimmune diseases, the fact that close relatives are also at risk is not as well appreciated in the medical community. Since many of these autoimmune disorders can have relatively insidious onsets, with fairly nonspecific symptoms, making the relatives and their physicians aware of the increased risk may lead to earlier diagnosis.

Given this increased risk for autoimmune diseases, periodic screening of individuals with Type 1 diabetes and all of their first-degree relatives is warranted, particularly for thyroid dysfunction (via standard tests such as obtaining thyroxine and thyroid-stimulating hormone levels) and for vitamin B_{12} deficiency, which, if untreated, leads to pernicious anemia.

Pregnancy and Type 1 Diabetes

There is a markedly increased risk of congenital anomalies in the offspring of women with Type 1 diabetes (Kitzmiller et al., 1978; Mills, 1982). In the general population, the risk of having a child with a birth defect is 2% to 3%, whereas for women with Type 1 diabetes, the risk is increased threefold, to 6% to 10% (Gabbe, 1977; Kitzmiller et al., 1978; Cousins, 1983). The malformations seen in infants born to diabetic women tend to be more severe than those seen in infants of nondiabetic women and include abnormalities of the skeletal, renal, cardiac, and central nervous systems (Table 21–8) (Kucera, 1971; Soler et al.,

Table 21–8. Congenital Malformations in Infants of Diabetic Mothers

Malformation	Ratio of Incidences[a]
Caudal regression	200–600
Spina bifida, hydrocephalus, and other CNS defects	2
Cardiac defects (including transposition of the great vessels, ventricular septal defects, atrial septal defects)	4
Anal/rectal atresia	3
Renal malformations	5
Agenesis	6
Cystic kidney	4
Duplicated ureter	23
Situs inversus	84

[a]In diabetic vs. nondiabetic pregnancies.
Adapted from Mills et al. (1979) and Mills (1987).

1976; Gabbe, 1977; Mills, 1982; Neave, 1984). Virtually all anomalies occur with increased frequency in infants of diabetic mothers, but those which have the highest relative risk are caudal regression, renal agenesis, transposition of the great vessels, ventricular septal defects, atrial septal defects, situs inversus, focal femoral hypoplasia/unusual facies, and neural tube defects (anencephaly and meningomyelocele). Although these malformations are not specific for diabetes, caudal regression is seen much more often in infants of diabetic mothers than in the general population. The relative risk for caudal regression in the offspring of a diabetic woman has been estimated to be as high as 200 (Uusitupa et al., 1985). The relative risks for the other defects are not as high, due in large part to their higher incidence in the general population (Mills, 1982).

Disruption of embryogenesis leading to the abnormalities occurs prior to the eighth week of pregnancy, i.e., often before a woman realizes that she is pregnant (Mills et al., 1979). There is evidence that elevated glycosylated hemoglobin (HbA1c) levels may be associated with a high risk for malformations, and vigorous control of blood glucose levels prior to conception has been shown to significantly reduce the incidence of congenital malformations (Mills et al., 1979; Miller et al., 1981; Hanson et al., 1990; Kitzmiller et al., 1991; Nordstrom et al., 1998; McElvy et al., 2000). Although it is beneficial to optimize diabetes control even in women who present when they are already pregnant, postconceptional intervention is less likely to reduce the malformation risk (Suhonen et al., 2000). Beginning in early adolescence, diabetic women of childbearing age should be made aware of the risk of congenital malformations and counseled that planning their pregnancies is essential so that optimal metabolic control of their disease can be achieved prior to conception and continued throughout their pregnancy.

Because of the increased risk for major structural malformations, prenatal diagnostic tests should be recommended for all pregnant women who have Type 1 diabetes. These should be performed during the second trimester (usually between 16 and 20 weeks' gestation), providing women with abnormal results the opportunity to obtain genetic counseling regarding the anomaly (i.e., prognosis, treatment options) and to make informed decisions regarding pregnancy options. For women who have normal results, the information obtained via prenatal diagnosis can be very reassuring and help alleviate anxiety for the remainder of the pregnancy. Ultrasonography can be used to evaluate fetal growth and to rule out major fetal structural anomalies, such as renal agenesis, neural tube defects, and caudal regression. Fetal echocardiography, performed at 16 to 22 weeks following the first day of the last menstrual period, enables prenatal diagnosis of major structural cardiac malformations. Elevations of maternal serum alpha-fetoprotein are associated with open neural tube defects such as anencephaly and meningomyelocele (Brock and Sutcliffe, 1972; Wald and Cuckle, 1977); thus, maternal serum alpha-fetoprotein screening is recommended for all pregnant diabetics. Because maternal serum alpha-fetoprotein levels are altered in pregnant diabetics compared to nondiabetics, tables specific for diabetic women should be used when calculating these values, and it is therefore important that the laboratory performing the assay be made aware that the patient is diabetic (Milunsky et al., 1982; Reece et al., 1987; Baumgarten and Robinson, 1988). There is evidence that in the general population, folic acid supplementation, begun prior to conception, is helpful in decreasing the risk for neural tube defects (Czeizel and Dudas, 1992; Centers for Disease Control and Prevention, 2000; Czeizel, 2000; Stevenson et al., 2000). Although studies looking specifically at infants of diabetic mothers have not been reported, folic acid supplementation prior to conception should be strongly considered as the potential benefits (i.e., possibly reducing the risk for neural tube defects) outweigh any known risks.

Future Considerations and Counseling Summary

Given these recent advances in our knowledge of the genetics and heterogeneity of diabetes, what is the genetic counseling we can provide at this time to our diabetic patients? First, as in all genetic counseling, an accurate diagnosis must be made. On clinical grounds, one can distinguish between Type 1 (typically juvenile-onset), Type 2 (maturity-onset), and maturity-onset diabetes of youth. In distinguishing among these phenotypes, one already has important counseling information. In a given family, the increased risk for diabetes over the general population is in general only for the specific type of diabetes that has already occurred in the family, not for all types. Thus, if the index case presenting for counseling is a juvenile insulin-dependent diabetic, the increased risk for that patient's relatives is for Type 1 diabetes. If the index case is a non-insulin-dependent diabetic, the increased risk for the patient's relatives is, for the most part, for Type 2 diabetes only. Associated abnormalities or diseases may suggest one of the rare genetic syndromes that include diabetes, where the risk of recurrence is dependent on the specific diagnosis (Raffel et al., 1997; Raffel and Rotter, 2001).

Once we have accurately characterized the clinical phenotype of the patient, how do we proceed? At this stage, we must fall back on observed empirical recurrence risks, i.e., data concerning the observed recurrence of these disorders in a large number of families. Even these empiric recurrence risks have limitations since they have been reported mainly from Caucasian populations. Even with the reservation that these empirical risks can be safely applied only to the populations from which they were derived, the most reassuring aspect of the data is the overall low absolute risk for the development of clinical diabetes in first-degree relatives, especially for Type 1 diabetes.

The heterogeneity that has so far been discovered among typical diabetes mellitus probably represents just the tip of the iceberg, but even this demonstrable heterogeneity has immediate relevance to current research efforts into the pathogenesis and therapy of the diabetic state. The susceptibility to a given environmental agent may very well depend on the heterogeneity elucidated by these studies. There may also be heterogeneity in the complications associated with genetically distinct forms of diabetes, having implications for disease management. Only when each of the many disorders resulting in diabetes mellitus and/or glucose intolerance is delineated will specific prognostication and therapy be possible for all diabetic patients.

REFERENCES

Abadie E, Lombrail P, Passa P: Is sickle cell trait an additional risk factor for diabetic angiopathy. Diabetes Care 1981; 4:659.

Abbott RD, Donahue RP, MacMahon SW, Reed DM, Yano K: Diabetes and the risk of stroke: the Honolulu Heart Program. JAMA 1987; 257:949–952.

Adorini L: Interleukin 12 and autoimmune diabetes. Nat Genet 2001; 27:131–132.

Agardh D, Gaur LK, Agardh E, Landin-Olsson M, Agardh CD, Lernmark A: HLA-DQB1*0201/0302 is associated with severe retinopathy in patients with IDDM. Diabetologia 1996; 39:1313–1317.

Almawi WY, Melemedjian OK, Rieder MJ: An alternate mechanism of glucocorticoid anti-proliferative effect: promotion of a Th2 cytokine-secreting profile. Clin Transplant 1999; 13:365–374.

Almer LO, Ekberg G, Fankhauser S, Home PD, Worth R, Sailer S, Kurtz AB, Christy M: A prospective study of the immunogenicity of porcine insulin in HLA-typed new insulin-treated diabetics. Diabetes Res 1985; 2:221–224.

Andersen AR, Christiansen JS, Andersen JK, Kreiner S, Deckert T: Diabetic nephropathy in type 1 (insulin-dependent) diabetes: an epidemiological study. Diabetologia 1983; 25:496–501.

Anderson CE, Hodge SE, Rubin R, Rotter JL, Terasaki PI, Irvine WJ, Rimoin DL: A search for heterogeneity in insulin-dependent diabetes mellitus (IDDM): HLA and autoimmune studies in simplex, multiplex, and multigenerational families. Metabolism 1983; 32:471–477.

Anderson JT, Cornelius JG, Jarpe AJ, Winter WE, Peck AB: Insulin-dependent diabetes in the NOD mouse model. II. β-Cell destruction in autoimmune diabetes is a Th2- and not a Th1-mediated event. Autoimmunity 1993; 15:113–122.

Andreoletti L, Hober D, Hober-Vandenberghe C, Fajardy I, Belaich S, Lambert V, Vantyghem MC, Lefebvre J, Wattre P, Coxsackie B: Virus infection and beta cell autoantibodies in newly diagnosed IDDM adult patients. Clin Diagn Virol 1998; 9:125–133.

Assan R, Feutren G, Debray-Sachs M, Quiniou-Debrie MC, Laborie C, Thomas G, Chatenoud L, Bach JF: Metabolic and immunological effects of cyclosporin in recently diagnosed type 1 diabetes mellitus. Lancet 1985; 1:67–71.

Atkinson MA, Bowman MA, Campbell L, Darrow BL, Kaufman DL, Maclaren NK: Cellular immunity to a determinant common to glutamate decarboxylase and coxsackie virus in insulin-dependent diabetes. J Clin Invest 1994; 94:2125–2129.

Atkinson MA, Bowman MA, Kao KJ, Cambell L, Dush PJ, Shah SC, Simell O, Maclaren NK: Lack of immune responsiveness to bovine serum albumin in insulin-dependent diabetes. N Engl J Med 1993; 329:1853–1858.

Atkinson MA, Maclaren NK, Riley WJ, Winter WE, Fisk DD, Spillar RP: Are insulin autoantibodies markers for insulin-dependent diabetes mellitus? Diabetes 1986; 35:894–898.

Awata T, Kuzuya T, Matsuda A, Iwamoto Y, Kanazawa Y: Genetic analysis of HLA class II alleles and susceptibility to type 1 (insulin-dependent) diabetes mellitus in Japanese subjects. Diabetologia 1992; 35:419–424.

Bach JM, Otto H, Nepom GT, Jung G, Cohen H, Timsit J, Boitard C, van Endert PM: High affinity presentation of an autoantigenic peptide in type I diabetes by an HLA class II protein encoded in a haplotype protecting from disease. J Autoimmunity 1997; 10:375–386.

Bain SC, Prins JB, Hearne CM, Rodrigues NR, Rowe BR, Pritchard LE, Richie RJ, Hall JR, Undlien DE, Ronningen KS, et al.: Insulin gene region-encoded susceptibility to type 1 diabetes is not restricted to HLA-DR4 positive individuals. Nat Genet 1992; 2:212–215.

Baker RS, Rand LI, Krolewski AS, Maki T, Warram JH, Aiello LM: Influence of HLA-DR phenotype and myopia on the risk of nonproliferative and proliferative diabetic retinopathy. Am J Ophthalmol 1986; 102:693–700.

Banerji MA, Chaiken RL, Huey H, Tuomi T, Norin AJ, Mackay IR, Rowley MJ, Zimmet PZ, Lebovitz HE: GAD antibody negative NIDDM in adult black subjects with diabetic ketoacidosis and increased frequency of human leukocyte antigen DR3 and DR4: Flatbush diabetes. Diabetes 1994; 43:741–745.

Barbosa J, Ramsay RC, Knobloch WH, Cantrill HL, Noreen H, King R, Yunis E: Histocompatibility antigen frequencies in diabetic retinopathy. Am J Ophthalmol 1980; 90:148–153.

Barbosa J, Saner B: Do genetic factors play a role in the pathogenesis of diabetic microangiopathy? Diabetologia 1984; 27:487–492.

Barnas U, Schmidt A, Illievich A, Kiener HP, Rabensteiner D, Kaider A, Prager R, Abrahamian H, Irsigler K, Mayer G: Evaluation of risk factors for the development of nephropathy in patients with IDDM: insertion/deletion angiotensin converting enzyme gene polymorphism, hypertension and metabolic control. Diabetologia 1997; 40:327–331.

Barnett AH, Eff C, Leslie RDG, Pyke DA: Diabetes in identical twins: a study of 200 pairs. Diabetologia 1981; 20:87–93.

Barrett-Connor E, Orchard T: Diabetes and heart disease. In: National Diabetes Data Group. Diabetes in America: Diabetes Data Compiled 1984. NIH Publication 85-1468. Washington DC: US Department of Health and Human Services, 1985a:XVI-1–XVI-41.

Barrett-Connor E, Orchard TJ: Insulin-dependent diabetes mellitus and ischemic heart disease. Diabetes Care 1985b; 1:65–70.

Baumgarten A, Robinson J: Prospective study of an inverse relationship between maternal glycosylated hemoglobin and serum alpha-fetoprotein concentrations in pregnant women with diabetes. Am J Obstet Gynecol 1988; 159:77–81.

Bell GI, Horita S, Karam JH: A polymorphic locus near the human insulin gene is associated with insulin-dependent diabetes mellitus. Diabetes 1984; 33:176–183.

Bennett ST, Lucassen AM, Gough SC, Powell EE, Undlien DE, Pritchard LE, Merriman ME, Kawaguchi Y, Dronsfield MJ, Pociot F, et al.: Susceptibility to human type 1 diabetes at IDDM2 is determined by tandem repeat variation at the insulin gene minisatellite locus. Nat Genet 1995; 9:284–292.

Betterle C, Zanette F, Pedini B, Presotto F, Rapp LB, Monsciotti CM, Rigon F: Clinical and subclinical organ-specific autoimmune manifestations in type 1 (insulin-dependent) diabetic patients and their first degree relatives. Diabetologia 1984; 26:431–436.

Bjorck S, Nyberg G, Mulec H, Granerus G, Herlitz H, Aurell M: Beneficial effects of angiotensin converting enzyme inhibition on renal function in patients with diabetic nephropathy. BMJ 1986; 293:471–474.

Blandford RL, Burden AC: Abnormalities of cardiac conduction in diabetics. BMJ 1984; 289:1659.

Blom L, Nystrom L, Dahlquist G: The Swedish Childhood Diabetes Study: vaccinations and infections as risk determinants for diabetes in childhood. Diabetologia 1991; 34:176–181.

Bodansky HJ, Cudworth AG, Drury PL, Kohner EM: Risk factors associated with severe proliferative retinopathy in insulin-dependent diabetes mellitus. Diabetes Care 1982; 5:97–100.

Bodington MJ, McNally PG, Burden AC: Cow's milk and type 1 childhood diabetes: no increase in risk. Diabet Med 1994; 11:663–665.

Borch-Johnsen K, Joner G, Mandrup-Poulsen T, Christy M, Zachan-Christiansen B, Kastrup B, Nerup J: Relation between breast-feeding and incidence of insulin-dependent diabetes mellitus. Lancet 1984; 2:1083–1086.

Borch-Johnsen K, Kreiner S: Proteinuria: value as predictor of cardiovascular mortality in insulin dependent diabetes mellitus. BMJ 1987; 294:1651–1654.

Bottazzo GF, Florin-Christensen A, Doniach D: Islet-cell antibodies in diabetes mellitus with autoimmune polyendocrine deficiencies. Lancet 1974; ii:1279–1282.

Bottazzo GF, Mann JI, Thorogood M, Baum JD, Doniach D: Autoimmunity in juvenile diabetics and their families. BMJ 1978; 2:165–168.

Boucher DW, Notkins AL: Virus-induced diabetes mellitus. I: Hyperglycemia and hypoinsulinemia in mice infected with encephalomyocarditis virus. J Exp Med 1973; 137:1226–1239.

Brock DJH, Sutcliffe RG: Alpha-fetoprotein in the antenatal diagnosis of anencephaly and spina bifida. Lancet 1972; ii:197–199.

Brodnicki TC, McClive P, Couper S, Morahan G: Localization of *Idd11* using NOD congenic mouse strains: elimination of *Slc9a1* as a candidate gene. Immunogenetics 2000; 51:37–41.

Burger W, Hovener G, Dusterhus R, Hartmann R, Weber B: Prevalence and development of retinopathy in children and adolescents with type 1 (insulin-dependent) diabetes mellitus: a longitudinal study. Diabetologia 1986; 29:17–22.

Cahill GF Jr. Diabetes mellitus. In: Beeson PB, McDermott W, Wyngaarden JB (eds). Cecil Textbook of Medicine. Philadelphia: Saunders, 1979:1969–1989.

Cammidge PJ: Diabetes mellitus and heredity. BMJ 1928; ii:738–741.

Cammidge PJ: Heredity as a factor in the etiology of diabetes mellitus. Lancet 1934; i:393–395.

Caplen NJ, Patel A, Millward A, Campbell RD, Ratanachaiyavong S, Wong FS, Demaine AG: Complement C4 and heat shock protein 70 (HSP70) genotypes and type I diabetes mellitus. Immunogenetics 1990; 32:427–430.

Carel JC, Bougneres PF: Treatment of prediabetic patients with insulin: experience and future. European Prediabetes Study Group. Horm Res 1996; 45(Suppl 1):44–47.

Centers for Disease Control and Prevention: Neural tube defect surveillance and folic acid intervention—Texas–Mexico border 1993–1998. JAMA 2000; 283:2928–2930.

Cerasi E, Luft R: "What is inherited—what is added," hypothesis for the pathogenesis of diabetes mellitus. Diabetes 1967; 16:615–627.

Chazan BI, Balodimos MC, Ryan JR, Marble A: Twenty-five to forty-five years of diabetes with and without vascular complications. Diabetologia 1970; 6:565–569.

Chern MM, Anderson VE, Barbosa J: Empirical risk for insulin-dependent diabetes (IDD) in sibs: further definition of genetic heterogeneity. Diabetes 1982; 31:1115–1118.

Christensen CK, Mogensen CE: Antihypertensive treatment—long-term reversal of progression of albuminuria in incipient diabetic nephropathy: a longitudinal study of renal function. J Diabetes Complications 1987; 1:45–52.

Clements RS Jr, Bell DSH: Complications of diabetes: prevalence, detection, current treatment, and prognosis. Am J Med 1985; 79:2–7.

Coleman DL: Obesity genes: beneficial effects in heterozygous mice. Science 1979; 203:663–644.

Collins FS: Shattuck lecture. Medical and societal consequences of the Human Genome Project. N Engl J Med 1999; 341:28–37.

Copeman JB, Cucca F, Hearne CM, Cornall RJ, Reed PW, Ronningen KS, Undlien DE, Nistico L, Buzzetti R, Tosi R, et al.: Linkage disequilibrium mapping of a type 1 diabetes susceptibility gene (*IDDM7*) to chromosome 2q31–q33. Nat Genet 1995; 9:80–85.

Cordell HJ, Todd JA, Bennett ST, Kawaguchi Y, Farrall M: Two-locus maximum lod score analysis of a multifactorial trait: joint consideration of IDDM2 and IDDM4 with IDDM1 in type I diabetes. Am J Hum Genet 1995; 57:920–934.

Cornall RJ: Genetics of a multifactorial disease: autoimmune type 1 diabetes mellitus. Clin Sci (Colch) 1993; 84:257–262.

Cornélis F, Fauré S, Martinez M, Prud'homme JF, Fritz P, Dib C, Alves H, Barrera P, De Vries N, Balsa A, et al.: New susceptibility locus for rheumatoid arthritis suggested by a genome-wide linkage study. Proc Natl Acad Sci USA 1998; 95:10746–10750.

Couper JJ, Steele C, Beresford S, Powell T, McCaul K, Pollard A, Gellert S, Tait B, Harrison LC, Colman PG: Lack of association between duration of breast-feeding or introduction of cow's milk and development of islet autoimmunity. Diabetes 1999; 48:2145–2149.

Cousins L: Congenital anomalies among infants of diabetic mothers: etiology, prevention, prenatal diagnosis. Am J Obstet Gynecol 1983; 147:333–338.

Coutant R, Carel JC, Timsit J, Boitard C, Bougneres P: Insulin and the prevention of insulin-dependent diabetes mellitus. Diabetes Metab 1997; 23(Suppl 3):25–28.

Craighead JE: Viral diabetes mellitus in man and experimental animals. Am J Med 1981;70:127–133.

Craighead JE, Higgins DA: Genetic influences affecting the occurrence of a diabetes mellitus-like disease in mice infected with the encephalomyocarditis virus. J Exp Med 1974; 139:414–426.

Creutzfeldt W, Kobbeling J, Neel JV (eds): The Genetics of Diabetes Mellitus. Berlin: Springer-Verlag, 1976.

Cruickshanks KJ, Orchard TJ, Becker DJ: The cardiovascular risk profile of adolescents with insulin-dependent diabetes mellitus. Diabetes Care 1985; 8:118–124.

Cruickshanks KJ, Vadheim CM, Moss SE, Roth MP, Riley WJ, Maclaren NK, Langfield D, Sparkes RS, Klein R, Rotter JI: Genetic marker associations with proliferative retinopathy in persons diagnosed with diabetes before 30 yr of age. Diabetes 1992; 41:879–885.

Cucca F, Dudbridge F, Loddo M, Mulargia AP, Lampis R, Angius E, De Virgiliis S, Koeleman BPC, Bain SC, Barnett AH, et al.: The HLA-DPB1-associated component of the IDDM1 and its relationship to the major loci HLA-DQB1, -DQA1, and -DRB1. Diabetes 2001; 50:1200–1205.

Cucca F, Goy JV, Kawaguchi Y, Esposito L, Merriman ME, Wilson AJ, Cordell HJ, Bain SC, Todd JA: A male–female bias in type 1 diabetes and linkage to chromosome Xp in MHC HLA-DR3-positive patients. Nat Genet 1998; 19:301–302.

Cudworth AG, Woodrow JC: HL-A system and diabetes mellitus. Diabetes 1975; 24:345–349.

Czeizel AE: Primary prevention of neural-tube defects and some other major congenital abnormalities: recommendations for the appropriate use of folic acid during pregnancy. Pediatr Drugs 2000; 2:437–449.

Czeizel AE, Dudas I: Prevention of the first occurrence of neural tube defects by periconceptional vitamin supplementation. N Engl J Med 1992; 3227:1832–1835.

Dahlquist G, Blom L, Tuvemo T, Nystrom L, Sandstrom A, Wall S: The Swedish Childhood Diabetes Study: results from a nine year case register and a one year case-referent study indicating that type 1 (insulin-dependent) diabetes mellitus is associated with both type 2 (non-insulin-dependent) diabetes mellitus and autoimmune disorders. Diabetologia 1989; 32:2–6.

Dahlquist G, Savilahti E, Landin-Olsson M: An increased level of antibodies to β-lactoglobulin is a risk determinant for early-onset type 1 (insulin-dependent) diabetes mellitus independent of islet cell antibodies and early introduction of cow's milk. Diabetologia 1992; 35:980–984.

Davidson JC, Smith GW: Retinopathy in pancreatic diabetes in Qatar. Diabetes Care 1986; 9:432–433.

Davies JL, Kawaguchi Y, Bennett ST, Copeman JB, Cordell HJ, Pritchard LE, Reed PW, Gough SCL, Jenkins SC, Palmer SM, et al.: A genome wide search for human type 1 diabetes susceptibility genes. Nature 1994; 371:130–136.

De Block CE, De Leeuw IH, Van Gaal LF: High prevalence of manifestations of gastric autoimmunity in parietal cell antibody-positive type 1 (insulin-dependent) diabetic patients: the Belgian Diabetes Registry. J Clin Endocrinol Metab 1999; 84:4062–4067.

Deckert T, Egeberg J, Frimodt-Moller C, Sander E, Svejgaard A: Basement membrane thickness, insulin antibodies and HLA-antigens in longstanding insulin dependent diabetics with and without severe retinopathy. Diabetologia 1979; 17:91–96.

Deckert T, Parving HH, Andersen AR, et al. Diabetic nephropathy: a clinical morphometric study. In: Eschwege E (ed). Advances in Diabetes Epidemiology. Institut de la Sante et de la Recherche Medicale Symposium No. 22. New York: Elsevier, 1982:235–243.

Deckert T, Poulsen JE: Diabetic nephropathy: fault or destiny? Diabetologia 1981; 21:178–183.

Degnbol B, Green A: Diabetes mellitus among first and second-degree relatives of early onset diabetics. Ann Hum Genet 1978; 42:25–34.

Deinum J, Tarnow L, van Gool JM, de Bruin RA, Derkx FH, Schalekamp MA, Parving HH: Plasma renin and prorenin and renin gene variation in patients with insulin-dependent diabetes mellitus and nephropathy. Nephrol Dial Transplant 1999; 14:1904–1911.

Delepine M, Pociot F, Habita C, Hashimoto L, Froguel P, Rotter J, Cambon-Thomsen A, Deschamps I, Djoulah S, Weissenbach J, et al.: Evidence of a non-MHC susceptibility locus in type I diabetes linked to HLA on chromosome 6. Am J Hum Genet 1997; 60:174–187.

Demaine A, Cross D, Millward A: Polymorphisms of the aldose reductase gene and susceptibility to retinopathy in type 1 diabetes mellitus. Invest Ophthalmol Vis Sci 2000; 41:4064–4068.

Denny P, Lord CJ, Hill NJ, Goy JV, Levy ER, Podolin PL, Peterson LB, Wicker LS, Todd JA, Lyons PA: Mapping of the IDDM locus Idd3 to a 0.35-cM interval containing the interleukin-2 gene. Diabetes 1997; 46:695–700.

De Prins F, Van Assche FA, Desmyter J: Congenital rubella and diabetes mellitus. Lancet 1978; 1:439–440.

Deschamps I, Goderel I, Lestradet H, Schmid M, Busson M, Cohen D, Hors J: Segregation of HLA-DR2 among affected and non-affected offspring of 66 families with type 1 (insulin-dependent) diabetes. Diabetologia 1984; 27:80–82.

Diabetes Control and Complications Trial Research Group: Effect of intensive therapy on the development and progression of diabetic nephropathy in the Diabetes Control and Complications Trial. Kidney Int 1995a; 47:1703–1720.

Diabetes Control and Complications Trial Research Group: The relationship of glycemic exposure (HbA1c) to the risk of development and progression of retinopathy in the Diabetes Control and Complications Trial. Diabetes 1995b; 44:968–983.

Diabetes Control and Complications Trial Research Group: Progression of retinopathy with intensive versus conventional treatment in the Diabetes Control and Complications Trial. Ophthalmology 1995c; 102:647–661.

Diabetes Control and Complications Trial Research Group: Clustering of long-term complications in families with diabetes in the Diabetes Control and Complications Trial. Diabetes 1997; 46:1829–1839.

Diabetes Epidemiology Research International Group: Geographic patterns of childhood insulin-dependent diabetes mellitus. Diabetes 1988; 37:1113–1119.

Diabetes Epidemiology Research International Group: Trends in incidence of childhood IDDM in 10 countries. Diabetes 1990; 39:858–864.

Dokheel TM: An epidemic of childhood diabetes in the United States? Evidence from Allegheny County, Pennsylvania. Diabetologia 1993; 16:1606–1611.

Dolan TF Jr: Microangiopathy in a young adult with cystic fibrosis and diabetes mellitus. N Engl J Med 1986; 314:991–992.

Doria A, Onuma T, Warram JH, Krolewski AS: Synergistic effect of angiotensin II type 1 receptor genotype and poor glycaemic control on risk of nephropathy in IDDM. Diabetologia 1997; 40:1293–1299.

Doria A, Warram JH, Krolewski AS: Genetic predisposition to diabetic nephropathy: evidence for a role of the angiotensin I-converting enzyme gene. Diabetes 1994; 43:690–695.

Dorman JS, Drash AL: Concordance of diabetic complications in multiple sibling case families. Diabetes 1986; 35:48A.

Dorman JS, LaPorte RE: Mortality in insulin-dependent diabetes. In: National Diabetes Data Group. Diabetes in America: Diabetes Data Compiled 1984. NIH Publication 85-1468. Washington DC: US Department of Health and Human Services, 1985:XXX-1–XXX-9.

Dornan TL, Ting A, McPherson CK, Peckar CO, Mann JI, Turner RC, Morris PJ: Genetic susceptibility to the development of retinopathy in insulin-dependent diabetics. Diabetes 1982; 31:226–231.

Drury TF: Disability among adult diabetics. In: National Diabetes Data Group. Diabetes in America: Diabetes Data Compiled 1984. NIH Publication 85-1468. Washington DC: US Department of Health and Human Services, 1985:XXXVIII-10–XXXVIII-22.

Easteal S, Kohonen-Corish MRJ, Zimmet P, Serjeantson SW: HLA-DP variation as additional risk factor in IDDM. Diabetes 1990; 39:855–857.

Eisenbarth G: Type I diabetes mellitus: a chronic autoimmune disease. N Eng J Med 1986; 314:1360–1368.

Eisenbarth GS: Genes, generator of diversity, glycoconjugates, and auto-immune B cell insufficiency in type I diabetes. Diabetes 1987; 36:355–364.

Ellis D, Becker DJ, Daneman D, Lobes L Jr, Drash AL: Proteinuria in children with insulin-dependent diabetes: relationship to duration of disease, metabolic control, and retinal changes. J Pediatr 1983; 102:673–680.

Encinas JA, Wicker LS, Peterson LB, Mukasa A, Teuscher C, Sobel R, Weiner HL, Seidman CE, Seidman JG, Kuchroo VK: QTL influencing autoimmune diabetes and encephalomyelitis map to a 0.15-cM region containing IL2. Nat Genet 1999; 21:158–160.

Erlich HA, Rotter JI, Chang J, Shaw S, Raffel LJ, Klitz W, Bugawan T, Zeidler A: PCR/oligonucleotide probe typing of HLA class II loci in Mexican-American insulin dependent diabetes mellitus (IDDM) families reveals an association of HLA-DPB1*0301 with IDDM. Am J Hum Genet 1993a; 53:201A.

Erlich HA, Zeidler A, Chang J, Shaw S, Raffel LJ, Klitz W, Beshkov Y, Costin G, Pressman S, Bugawan T, et al.: HLA class II alleles and susceptibility and resistance to insulin dependent diabetes mellitus in Mexican-American families. Nat Genet 1993b; 3:358–364.

EURODIAB ACE Study Group: Variation and trends in incidence of childhood diabetes in Europe. Lancet 2000; 355:873–876.

Falck AA, Knip JM, Ilonen JS, Laatikainen LT: Genetic markers in early diabetic retinopathy of adolescents with type I diabetes. J Diabetes Complications 1997; 11:203–207.

Fava D, Leslie RD, Pozzilli P: Relationship between dairy product consumption and incidence of IDDM in childhood in Italy. Diabetes Care 1994; 17:1488–1490.

Fennessy M, Metcalfe K, Hitman GA, Niven M, Biro PA, Tuomilehto J, Tuomilehto-Wolf E: A gene in the HLA class I region contributes to susceptibility to IDDM in the Finnish population: Childhood Diabetes in Finland (DiMe) Study Group. Diabetologia 1994; 37:937–944.

Fialkow PJ, Zavala C, Nielson K: Thyroid autoimmunity: increased frequency in relatives of insulin dependent diabetes patients. Ann Intern Med 1975; 83:170–176.

Field LL, Anderson CE, Neiswanger K, Hodge SE, Spence MA, Rotter JI: Interaction of HLA and immunoglobulin antigens in type I (insulin-dependent) diabetes. Diabetologia 1984; 27:504–508.

Field LL, Stephure DK, McArthur RG: Interaction between T cell receptor beta chain and immunoglobulin heavy chain region genes in susceptibility to insulin-dependent diabetes mellitus. Am J Hum Genet 1991; 49:627–634.

Field LL, Tobias R, Magnus T: A locus on chromosome 15q26 (IDDM3) produces susceptibility to insulin-dependent diabetes mellitus. Nat Genet 1994; 8:189–194.

Field LL, Tobias R, Thomson G, Plon S: Susceptibility to insulin-dependent diabetes mellitus maps to a locus (IDDM11) on human chromosome 14q24.3–q31. Genomics 1996; 33:1–8.

Fioretto P, Steffes MW, Barbosa J, Rich SS, Miller ME, Mauer M: Is diabetic

nephropathy inherited? Studies of glomerular structure in type 1 diabetic sibling pairs. Diabetes 1999; 48:865–869.
Fogarty DG, Harron JC, Hughes AE, Nevin NC, Doherty CC, Maxwell AP: A molecular variant of angiotensinogen is associated with diabetic nephropathy in IDDM. Diabetes 1996; 45:1204–1208.
Freire MB, van Dijk DJ, Erman A, Boner G, Warram JH, Krolewski AS: DNA polymorphisms in the *ACE* gene, serum ACE activity and the risk of nephropathy in insulin-dependent diabetes mellitus. Nephrol Dial Transplant 1998; 13:2553–2558.
Frisk G, Friman G, Tuvemo T, Fohlman J, Diderhom H: Coxsackie B virus IgM in children at onset of type 1 (insulin-dependent) diabetes mellitus: evidence for IgM induction by a recent or current infection. Diabetologia 1992; 35:249–253.
Fu J, Ikegami H, Kawaguchi Y, Fujisawa T, Kawabata Y, Hamada Y, Ueda H, Shintani M, Nojima K, Babaya N, et al.: Association of distal chromosome 2q with IDDM in Japanese subjects. Diabetologia 1998; 41:228–232.
Fukumoto S, Ishimura E, Hosoi M, Kawagishi T, Kawamura T, Isshiki G, Nishizawa Y, Morii H: Angiotensin converting enzyme gene polymorphism and renal artery resistance in patients with insulin dependent diabetes mellitus. Life Sci 1996; 59:629–637.
Gabbe SG: Congenital malformations in infants of diabetic mothers. Obstet Gynecol 1977; 32:125–132.
Gamble DR: An epidemiological study of childhood diabetes affecting two or more siblings. Diabetologia 1980a; 19:341–344.
Gamble DR: The epidemiology of insulin-dependent diabetes, with particular reference to the relationship of viral infections to its etiology. Epidemiol Rev 1980b; 2:49–70.
Garchon HJ, Bedossa P, Eloy L, Bach JF: Identification and mapping to chromosome 1 of a susceptibility locus for periinsulitis in non-obese diabetic mice. Nature 1991; 353:260–262.
Garcia MJ, McNamara PM, Gordon T, Kannel WB: Morbidity and mortality in diabetics in the Framingham population: sixteen year follow-up study. Diabetes 1974; 23:105–111.
Gerstein HC: Cow's milk exposure and type 1 diabetes mellitus: a critical overview of the clinical literature. Diabetes Care 1994; 17:13–19.
Ghosh S, Palmer SM, Rodrigues NR, Cordell JH, Hearne CM, Cornall RJ, Prins JB, McShane P, Lathrop GM, Peterson LB, et al.: Polygenic control of autoimmune diabetes in nonobese diabetic mice. Nat Genet 1993; 4:404–409.
Gimeno SG, de Souza JM: IDDM and milk consumption: a case-control study in Sao Paulo, Brazil. Diabetes Care 1997; 20:1256–1260.
Gorsuch AN, Spencer KM, Lister J: Evidence for a long pre-diabetic period in type I (insulin-dependent) diabetes mellitus. Lancet 1981; 2:1363–1365.
Gorsuch AN, Spencer KM, Lister J, Wolf E, Bottazzo GF, Cudworth AG: Can future type I diabetes be predicted? A study in families of affected children. Diabetes 1982; 31:862–866.
Gottlieb MS: Diabetes in offspring and siblings of juvenile and maturity-onset type diabetes. J Chronic Dis 1980; 33:331–339.
Gottlieb MS, Root HF: Diabetes mellitus in twins. Diabetes 1968; 17:693–704.
Gould CL, McMannama KG, Bigley NJK, Giron DJ: Virus-induced murine diabetes: enhancement by immunosuppression. Diabetes 1985; 34:1217–1221.
Gould CL, Trombley ML, Bigley NJ, McMannama KG, Giron DJ: Replication of diabetogenic and non-diabetogenic variants of encephalomyocarditis (EMC) virus in ICR Swiss mice. Proc Soc Exp Biol Med 1984; 175:449–453.
Gray RS, Starkey IR, Rainbow S, Kurtz AB, Abdel-Khalik A, Urbaniak S, Eton RA, Duncan LJ, Clarke BF: HLA antigens and other risk factors in the development of retinopathy in type 1 diabetes. Br J Ophthalmol 1982; 66:280–285.
Gribben JG, Freeman GJ, Boussiotis VA, Rennert P, Jellis CL, Greenfield E, Barber M, Restivo J, Ke X, Gray GS, et al.: CTLA4 mediates antigen-specific apoptosis of human T cells. Proc Natl Acad Sci USA 1995; 92:811–815.
Groop L, Miettinen A, Groop PH, Meri S, Koskimies S, Bottazzo GF: Organ-specific autoimmunity and HLA-DR antigens as markers for beta-cell destruction in patients with type II diabetes. Diabetes 1988; 37:99–103.
Guberski KL, Thomas VA, Shek WR, Like AA, Handler ES, Rossini AA, Wallace JE, Welsh RM: Induction of type I diabetes by Kilham's rat virus in diabetes-resistant BB/Wor rats. Science 1991; 254:1010–1013.
Gumprecht J, Zychma MJ, Grzeszczak W, Zukowska-Szczechowska E: Angiotensin I-converting enzyme gene insertion/deletion and angiotensinogen M235T polymorphisms: risk of chronic renal failure: End-Stage Renal Disease Study Group. Kidney Int 2000; 58:513–519.
Gunderson E: Is diabetes of infectious origin? J Infect Dis 1927; 41:197–202.
Hadjadj S, Belloum R, Bouhanick B, Gallois Y, Guilloteau G, Chatellier G, Alhenc-Gelas F, Marre M: Prognostic value of angiotensin-I converting enzyme I/D polymorphism for nephropathy in type 1. Diabetes 2001; 12:541–549.
Haffner SM, Fong D, Stern MP, Pugh JA, Hazuda HP, Patterson JK, van Heuven WA, Klein R: Diabetic retinopathy in Mexican Americans and non-Hispanic whites. Diabetes 1988; 37:878–884.
Haffner SM, Hazuda HP, Stern MP, Patterson JK, Van Heuven WA, Fong D: Effects of socioeconomic status on hyperglycemia and retinopathy levels in Mexican Americans with NIDDM. Diabetes Care 1989; 12:128–134.
Hanifi Moghaddam P, de Knijf P, Roep BO, Van der Auwera B, Naipal A, Gorus F, Schuit F, Giphart MJ: Genetic structure of IDDM1: two separate regions in the major histocompatibility complex contribute to susceptibility or protection: Belgian Diabetes Registry. Diabetes 1998; 47:263–269.
Hanson U, Persson B, Thunell S: Relationship between hemoglobin A1c in early type 1 (insulin-dependent) diabetic pregnancy and the occurrence of spontaneous abortion and fetal malformations in Sweden. Diabetologia 1990; 33:100–104.
Harris H: The familial distribution of diabetes mellitus: a study of the relatives of 1,241 diabetic propositi. Ann Eugen 1950; 15:95–110.
Harvald B, Hauge M: Selection in diabete in modern society. Acta Med Scand 1963; 173:459–465.
Harvald B, Hauge M: Heredity factors elucidated by twin studies. In: Neel JV, Shaw MW, Schull WJ (eds). Genetics and the Epidemiology of Chronic Diseases. Public Health Service Publication 1163. Washington DC: Public Health Service, 1965:61–76.
Hashimoto L, Habita C, Beressi JP, Delepine M, Besse C, Cambon-Thomsen A, Deschamps I, Rotter JI, Djoulah S, James MR, et al.: Genetic mapping of a susceptibility locus for insulin-dependent diabetes on chromosome 11q. Nature 1994; 371:161–164.
Hasslacher C, Ritz E, Terpstra J, Gallasch G, Kunowski G, Rall C: Natural history of nephropathy in type I diabetes. Relationship to metabolic control and blood pressure. Hypertension 1985; 7:1174–1178.
Hayashi K, Boucher DW, Notkins AL: Virus-induced diabetes mellitus. II: Relationship between beta cell damage and hyperglycemia in mice infected with encephalomyocarditis virus. Am J Pathol 1974; 75:91–102.
Heesom AE, Millward A, Demaine AG: Susceptibility to diabetic neuropathy in patients with insulin dependent diabetes mellitus is associated with a polymorphism at the 5′ end of the aldose reductase gene. J Neurol Neurosurg Psychiatry 1998; 4:213–216.
Helmke K, Otten A, Willems WR, Brockhaus R, Mueller-Eckhardt G, Stief T, Bertrams J, Wolf H, Federlin K: Islet cell antibodies and the development of diabetes mellitus in relation to mumps infection and mumps vaccination. Diabetologia 1986; 29:30–33.
Herman WH, Teutsch SM: Kidney diseases associated with diabetes. In: National Diabetes Data Group. Diabetes in America: Diabetes Data Compiled 1984. NIH Publication 85-1468. Washington DC: US Department of Health and Human Services, 1985:XIV-1–XIV-31.
Hibberd ML, Millward BA, Wong FS, Demaine AG: T-cell receptor constant beta chain polymorphisms and susceptibility to type 1 diabetes. Diabet Med 1992; 9:929–933.
Hill NJ, Lyons PA, Armitage N, Todd JA, Wicker LS, Peterson LB: NOD Idd5 locus controls insulitis and diabetes and overlaps the orthologous CTLA4/IDDM12 and NRAMP1 loci in humans. Diabetes 2000; 49:1744–1747.
Hitman GA, Tarn AC, Winter RM, Drummond V, Williams LG, Jowett NI, Bottazzo GF, Galton DJ: Type 1 (insulin dependent) diabetes and a highly variable locus close to the insulin gene on chromosome 11. Diabetologia 1985; 28:218–222.
Hodgkinson AD, Millward BA, Demaine AG: Polymorphisms of the glucose transporter (*GLUT1*) gene are associated with diabetic nephropathy. Kidney Int 2001; 59:985–989.
Honeyman MC, Coulson BS, Stone NL, Gellert SA, Goldwater PN, Steele CE, Couper JJ, Tait BD, Colman PG, Harrison LC: Association between rotavirus infection and pancreatic islet autoimmunity in children at risk of developing type 1 diabetes. Diabetes 2000; 49:1319–1324.
Honeyman MC, Stone NL, Harrison LC: T-cell epitopes in type 1 diabetes autoantigen tyrosine phosphatase IA-2: potential for mimicry with rotavirus and other environmental agents. Mol Med 1998; 4:231–239.
Horey GE, Pryse-Davis J, Roberts DM: A survey of nephropathy in young diabetics. Q J Med 1962; 31:473–483.
Horn GT, Bugawan TL, Long CM, Erlich HA: Allelic sequence variation of the HLA-DQ loci: relationship to serology and to insulin-dependent diabetes susceptibility. Proc Natl Acad Sci USA 1988; 85:6012–6016.
Huang SW, Taylor G, Basid A: The effect of pertussis vaccine on the insulin-dependent diabetes induced by streptozotocin in mice. Pediatr Res 1984; 18:221–226.
Huber SA, Babu G, Craighead JE: Genetic influences on the immunologic pathogenesis of encephalomyocarditis (EMC) virus–induced diabetes mellitus. Diabetes 1985; 34:1186–1190.
Huen KF, Low LC, Wong GW, Tse WW, Yu AC, Lam YY, Cheung PC, Wong LM, Yeung WK, But BW, et al.: Epidemiology of diabetes mellitus in children in Hong Kong: the Hong Kong Childhood Diabetes Register. J Pediatr Endocrinol Metab 2000; 13:297–302.
Hyöty H, Hiltunen M, Reunanen A, Leinikki P, Vesikari T, Lounamaa R, Tuomilehto J, Akerblom HK: Decline of mumps antibodies in type 1 (insulin-dependent) diabetic children and a plateau in the rising incidence of type 1 diabetes after introduction of the mumps–measles–rubella vaccine in Finland: Childhood Diabetes in Finland Study Group. Diabetologia 1993; 36:1303–1308.
Ikegami H, Makino S, Yamato E, Kawaguchi Y, Ueda H, Sakamoto T, Takekawa K, Ogihara T: Identification of a new susceptibility locus for insulin-dependent diabetes mellitus by ancestral haplotype congenic mapping. J Clin Invest 1995; 96:1936–1942.
Ilonen J, Herva E, Tiilikainen A, Akerblom HK, Koivukangas T, Kouvalainen K: HLA-Dw2 as a marker of resistance against juvenile diabetes mellitus. Tissue Antigens 1978; 11:144–146.
Irvine WJ, Sawen JSA, Prescott RJ, Duncan LJP: The value of islet cell antibody in predicting secondary failure of oral hypoglycemic agent therapy in diabetes mellitus. J Clin Lab Immunol 1979; 2:23–26.
Ishihara M, Yukimura Y, Yamada T, Ohto K, Yoshizawa K: Diabetic complications and their relationships to risk factors in a Japanese population. Diabetes Care 1984; 7:533–538.
Ito M, Tanimoto M, Kamura H, Yoneda M, Morishima Y, Takatsuki K, Itatsu T, Saito H: Association of HLA-DR phenotypes and T-lymphocyte-receptor beta-chain-region RFLP with IDDM in Japanese. Diabetes 1988; 37:1633–1636.
Iwata I, Nagafuchi S, Nakashima H, Kondo S, Koga T, Yokogawa Y, Akashi T, Shibuya T, Umeno Y, Okeda T, et al.: Association of polymorphism in the *NeuroD/BETA2* gene with type 1 diabetes in the Japanese. Diabetes 1999; 48:416–419.
Iwo K, Bellomo SC, Mukai N, Craighead JE: Encephalomyocarditis virus–induced

diabetes mellitus in mice: long term changes in the structure and function of islets of Langerhans. Diabetologia 1983; 25:39–44.

Jackson RL, Ide CH, Guthrie RA, James RD: Retinopathy in adolescents and young adults with onset of insulin-dependent diabetes in childhood. Ophthalmology 1982; 89:7–13.

Jacobsen P, Rossing K, Rossing P, Tarnow L, Mallet C, Poirier O, Cambien F, Parving HH: Angiotensin converting enzyme gene polymorphism and ACE inhibition in diabetic nephropathy. Kidney Int 1998; 53:1002–1006.

Japan Diabetes Society: Diabetes mellitus in twins: a cooperative study in Japan: Committee on Diabetic Twins. Diabetes Res Clin Pract 1998; 5:271–280.

Jarrett RJ, Shipley MJ: Type 2 (non-insulin-dependent) diabetes mellitus and cardiovascular disease—putative association via common antecedents: further evidence from the Whitehall Study. Diabetologia 1988; 31:737–740.

Jensen T, Borch-Johnsen K, Deckert T: Changes in blood pressure and renal function in patients with type I (insulin-dependent) diabetes mellitus prior to clinical diabetic nephropathy. Diabetes Res 1987; 4:159–162.

Jenson AB, Rosenberg HS, Notkins AL: Pancreatic islet cell damage in children with fatal virus infections. Lancet 1980; ii:354–358.

Johnston PB, Middleton D, Archer DB, Hadden DR: HLA antigens in proliferative diabetic retinopathy. Int Ophthalmol 1981; 3:87–89.

Julier C, Hyer RN, Davies J, Merlin F, Soularue P, Briant L, Cathelineau G, Deschamps I, Rotter JI, Froguel P, et al.: The insulin-IGF2 region on chromosome 11p encodes a gene implicated in HLA-DR4 dependent diabetes susceptibility. Nature 1991; 354:155–159.

Kao YL, Donaghue K, Chan A, Knight J, Silink M: A variant of paraoxonase (*PON1*) gene is associated with diabetic retinopathy in IDDM. J Clin Endocrinol Metab 1998; 83:2589–2592.

Kao YL, Donaghue K, Chan A, Knight J, Silink M: A novel polymorphism in the aldose reductase gene promoter region is strongly associated with diabetic retinopathy in adolescents with type 1 diabetes. Diabetes 1999a; 48:1338–1340.

Kao YL, Donaghue K, Chan A, Knight J, Silink M: An aldose reductase intragenic polymorphism associated with diabetic retinopathy. Diabetes Res Clin Pract 1999b; 46:155–160.

Kaprio J, Tuomilehto J, Koskenvuo M, Romanov K, Reunanen A, Eriksson J, Stengard J, Kesaniemi YA: Concordance for type 1 (insulin-dependent) and type 2 (non-insulin-dependent) diabetes mellitus in a population-based cohort of twins in Finland. Diabetologia 1992; 35:1060–1067.

Karam JH, Lewitt PA, Young CW, Nowlain RE, Frankel BJ, Fujiya H, Freedman ZR, Grodsky GM: Insulinopenic diabetes after rodenticide (Vacor) ingestion. Diabetes 1980; 29:971–978.

Karjalainen J, Knip M, Mustonen A, Illonen J, Akerblom HK: Relation between insulin antibody and complement-fixing islet cell antibody at clinical diagnosis of IDDM. Diabetes 1986; 35:620–622.

Karjalainen J, Martin JM, Knip M, Ilonen J, Robinson BH, Savilahti E, Akerblom HK, Dosch H-M: A bovine albumin peptide as a possible trigger of insulin-dependent diabetes mellitus. N Engl J Med 1992; 327:302–307.

Karvonen M, Pitkaniemi M, Pitkaniemi J, Kohtamaki K, Tajima N, Tuomilehto J: Sex difference in the incidence of insulin-dependent diabetes mellitus: an analysis of the recent epidemiological data. Diabetes Metab Rev 1997; 13:275–291.

Katzeff HL, Klein I: Reversibility of diabetic nephropathy. Intern Med Specialist 1987; 8:69–74.

Kaufman DL, Erlander MG, Clare-Salzer M, Atkinson MA, Maclaren NK, Tobin AJ: Autoimmunity to two forms of glutamate decarboxylase in insulin-dependent diabetes mellitus. J Clin Invest 1992; 89:283–292.

Keen H, Jarrett RJ: The WHO multinational study of vascular disease in diabetes: 2. Macrovascular disease prevalence. Diabetes Care 1979; 2:187–195.

Keen H: Epidemiology and pathogenesis of vascular complications. Medicographia 1983; 5:2.

Kereiakes DJ, Naughton JL, Brundage B, Schiller NB: The heart in diabetes. West J Med 1984; 140:583–593.

Kimpimaki T, Kulmala P, Savola K, Vahasalo P, Reijonen H, Ilonen J, Akerblom HK, Knip M: Disease-associated autoantibodies as surrogate markers of type 1 diabetes in young children at increased genetic risk: Childhood Diabetes in Finland Study Group. J Clin Endocrinol Metab 2000; 85:1126–1132.

King ML, Bidwell D, Voller A, Bryant J, Banatvala JE: Coxsackie B viruses in insulin-dependent diabetes mellitus. Lancet 1983a; 2:915–916.

King ML, Shaikh A, Bidwell D, Voller A, Banatvala JE: Coxsackie B virus-specific IgM responses in children with insulin-dependent (juvenile-onset; type I) diabetes mellitus. Lancet 1983b; 1:1397–1399.

Kitzmiller JL, Cloherty JP, Younger MD: Diabetic pregnancy and perinatal morbidity. Am J Obstet Gynecol 1978; 131:560–580.

Kitzmiller JL, Gavin LA, Gin GD, Jovanovic-Peterson L, Main EK, Zigrang WD: Preconception care of diabetes: glycemic control prevents congenital anomalies. JAMA 1991; 265:731–736.

Klein R, Klein BE, Moss SE: A population-based study of diabetic retinopathy in insulin-using patients diagnosed before 30 years of age. Diabetes Care 1985a; 8(Suppl 1):71–76.

Klein R, Klein BE, Moss SE, Davis MD, DeMets DL: Retinopathy in young-onset diabetic patients. Diabetes Care 1985b; 8:311–315.

Klein R, Klein BE, Moss SE, Davis MD, DeMets DL: Glycosylated hemoglobin predicts the incidence and progression of diabetic retinopathy. JAMA 1988; 260: 2864–2871.

Klein R, Klein BE, Moss SE, DeMets DL: Blood pressure and hypertension in diabetes. Am J Epidemiol 1985c; 122:75–89.

Klein R, Klein BEK: Vision disorders in diabetes. In: National Diabetes Data Group. Diabetes in America: Diabetes Data Compiled 1984. NIH Publication 85-1468. Washington DC: US Department of Health and Human Services, 1985:XIII-1–XIII-36.

Klouda PT, Manos J, Acheson EJ, Dyer PA, Goldby FS, Harris R, Lawler W, Mallick NP, Williams G: Strong association between idiopathic membranous nephropathy and HLA-DRW3. Lancet 1979; 2:770–771.

Knip M, Douek IF, Moore WP, Gillmor HA, McLean AE, Bingley PJ, Gale EA: Safety of high-dose nicotinamide: a review. ENDIT Group: European Nicotinamide Diabetes Intervention Trial. Diabetologia 2000; 43:1337–1345.

Knip M, Illonen J, Mustonen A, Akerblom HK: Evidence of an accelerated β-cell destruction in HLA-Dw3,Dw4 heterozygous children with type 1 (insulin-dependent) diabetes. Diabetologia 1986; 29:347–351.

Knowler WC, Pettitt DJ, Savage PJ, Bennett PH: Diabetes incidence in Pima Indians: contributions of obesity and parental diabetes. Am J Epidemiol 1981; 113:144–156.

Knowles HC Jr: Long-term juvenile diabetes treated with unmeasured diet. Trans Assoc Am Physicians 1971; 84:95–101.

Kobberling J, Bruggeboes B: Prevalence of diabetes among children of insulin-dependent diabetic mothers. Diabetologia 1980; 18:459–462.

Kobberling J, Tattersall R: The Genetics of Diabetes Mellitus: London: Academic Press, 1982.

Koevary SB, Williams DE, Williams RM, Chick WL: Passive transfer of diabetes from BB/W to Wistar-Furth rats. J Clin Invest 75; 1985:1904–1907.

Kofoed-Enevoldsen A, Borch-Johnsen K, Kreiner S, Nerup J, Deckert T: Declining incidence of persistent proteinuria in type I (insulin-dependent) diabetic patients in Denmark. Diabetes 1987; 36:205–209.

Kostraba JN: What can epidemiology tell us about the role of infant diet in the etiology of IDDM? Diabetes Care 1994; 17:87–91.

Kostraba JN, Cruickshanks KJ, Lawler-Heavner J, Jobim LF, Rewers MJ, Gay EC, Chase HP, Klingensmith G, Hamman RF: Early exposure to cow's milk and solid foods in infancy, genetic predisposition and risk of IDDM. Diabetes 1993; 42:288–295.

Kostraba JN, Gay EC, Rewers M, Hamman RF: Nitrate levels in community drinking waters and risk of IDDM: an ecological analysis. Diabetes Care 1992; 15:1505–1508.

Kristiansen OP, Pociot F, Bennett EP, Clausen H, Johannesen J, Nerup J, Mandrup-Poulsen T: IDDM7 links to insulin-dependent diabetes mellitus in Danish multiplex families but linkage is not explained by novel polymorphisms in the candidate gene GALNT3: the Danish Study Group of Diabetes in Childhood and the Danish IDDM Epidemiology and Genetics Group. Hum Mutat 2000; 15:295–296.

Krolewski AS, Canessa M, Warram JH, Laffel LM, Christlieb AR, Knowler WC, Rand LI: Predisposition to hypertension and susceptibility to renal disease in insulin-dependent diabetes mellitus. N Engl J Med 1988; 318:140–145.

Krolewski AS, Czyzyk A, Kopczynski J, Rywik S: Prevalence of diabetes mellitus, coronary heart disease and hypertension in the families of insulin dependent and insulin independent diabetics. Diabetologia 1981; 21:520–524.

Krolewski AS, Warram JH, Christlieb AR, Busick EJ, Kahn CR: The changing natural history of nephropathy in type I diabetes. Am J Med 1985; 78:785–794.

Krolewski AS, Warram JH, Rand LI, Kahn CR: Epidemiologic approach to the etiology of type I diabetes mellitus and its complications. N Engl J Med 1987; 317:1390–1398.

Krummel MF, Allison JP: CTLA-4 engagement inhibits IL-2 accumulation and cell cycle progression upon activation of resting T cells. J Exp Med 1996; 183:2533–2540.

Kucera J: Rate and type of congenital anomalies among offspring of diabetic women. J Reprod Med 1971; 7:73–82.

Kukreja A, Maclaren NK: Autoimmunity and diabetes. J Clin Endocrinol Metab 1999; 84:4371–4378.

Kulaylat NA, Narchi H: A twelve year study of the incidence of childhood type 1 diabetes mellitus in the eastern province of Saudi Arabia. J Pediatr Endocrinol Metab 2000; 13:135–140.

Kumar D, Gemayel S, Deapen D, Kapadia D, Yamashita PH, Lee M, Dwyer JH, Roy-Burman P, Bray GA, Mack TM: North-American twins with IDDM genetic, etiological and clinical significance of disease concordance according to age, zygosity, and the interval after diagnosis in first twin. Diabetes 1993; 42:1351–1363.

Kyvik KO, Green A, Beck-Nielsen H: Concordance rates of insulin dependent diabetes mellitus: a population based study of young Danish twins. BMJ 1995; 311:913–917.

Laakso M, Ronnemaa T, Pyorala K, Kallio V, Puukka P, Penttila I: Atherosclerotic vascular disease and its risk factors in non-insulin-dependent diabetic and nondiabetic subjects in Finland. Diabetes Care 1988; 11:449–463.

Landin-Olsson M, Karlsson FA, Lernmark A, Sundkvist G, and the Diabetes Incidence Study in Sweden Group: Islet cell and thyrogastric antibodies in 633 consecutive 15- to 34-yr-old patients in the Diabetes Incidence Study in Sweden. Diabetes 1992; 41:1022–1027.

Larsen ZM, Kristiansen OP, Mato E, Johannesen J, Puig-Domingo M, de Leiva A, Nerup J, Pociot F: IDDM12 (CTLA4) on 2q33 and IDDM13 on 2q34 in genetic susceptibility to type 1 diabetes (insulin-dependent). Autoimmunity 1999; 31:35–42.

Ledet T, Gotzsche O, Hickendorff L: The pathology of diabetic cardiopathy: pathogenetic reflections. In: Jarret J (ed). Diabetes and Heart Disease: Metabolic Aspects of Cardiovascular Disease, Amsterdam: Elsevier, 1984:25–46.

Lee MS, Mueller R, Wicker LS, Peterson LB, Sarvetnick N: IL-10 is necessary and sufficient for autoimmune diabetes in conjunction with NOD MHC homozygosity. J Exp Med 1996; 183:2663–2668.

Leslie RD, Pyke DA: Diabetic retinopathy in identical twins. Diabetes 1982; 31:19–21.

Lester FT, Keen H: Macrovascular disease in middle-aged diabetic patients in Addis Ababa, Ethiopia. Diabetologia 1988; 31:361–367.

Lestradet H, Battiestelli J, Ledoux M: L'heredite dans le diabete infantile. Diabete 1972; 20:17–19.

Lestradet H, Papoz L, Hellouin de Menibus C, Levavasseur F, Besse J, Billaud L, Battistelli F, Tric P, Lestradet F: Long-term study of mortality and vascular complications in juvenile-onset (type I) diabetes. Diabetes 1981; 30:175–179.

Lie BA, Todd JA, Pociot F, Nerup J, Akselsen HE, Joner G, Dahl-Jørgensen K, Rønningen KS, Thorsby E: Undlien DE Undlien1: the predisposition to type 1 diabetes linked to the human leukocyte antigen complex includes at least one non-class II gene. Am J Hum Genet 1999; 64:793–800.

Lindsay RS, Little J, Jaap AJ, Padfield PL, Walker JD, Hardy KJ: Diabetic nephropathy is associated with an increased familial risk of stroke. Diabetes Care 1999; 22:422–425.

Lord CJ, Bohlander SK, Hopes EA, Montague CT, Hill NJ, Prins JB, Renjilian RJ, Peterson LB, Wicker LS, Todd JA, et al.: Mapping the diabetes polygene *Idd3* on mouse chromosome 3 by use of novel congenic strains. Mamm Genome 1995; 6:563–570.

Loughrey BV, Maxwell AP, Fogarty DG, Middleton D, Harron JC, Patterson CC, Darke C, Savage DA: An interleukin 1B allele, which correlates with a high secretor phenotype, is associated with diabetic nephropathy. Cytokine 1998; 10:984–988.

Louis EJ, Thomson G: Three-allele synergistic mixed model for insulin-dependent diabetes mellitus. Diabetes 1986; 35:958–963.

Lowe RM, Graham J, Sund G, Kockum I, Landin-Olsson M, Schaefer JB, Torn C, Lernmark A, Dahlquist G: The length of the CTLA-4 microsatellite (AT)N-repeat affects the risk for type 1 diabetes. Diabetes Incidence in Sweden Study Group. Autoimmunity 2000; 32:173–180.

Ludvigsson J, Lindblom B: Human lymphocyte antigen DR types in relation to early clinical manifestations in diabetic children. Pediatr Res 1984; 18:1239–1241.

Ludvigsson J, Samuelsson U, Beauforts C: HLA-DR3 is associated with a more slowly progressive form of type 1 (insulin-dependent) diabetes. Diabetologia 1986; 29:207–210.

Luo DF, Bui MM, Muir A, Maclaren NK, Thomson G, She JX: Affected sib-pair mapping of a novel susceptibility gene to insulin-dependent diabetes mellitus (IDDM8) on chromosome 6q25–q27. Am J Hum Genet 1995; 57:911–919.

Luo DF, Buzzetti R, Rotter JI, Maclaren NK, Raffel LJ, Nistico L, Giovannini C, Pozzilli P, Thomson G, She JX: Confirmation of three susceptibility genes to insulin-dependent diabetes mellitus: *IDDM4*, *IDDM5* and *IDDM8*. Hum Mol Genet 1996; 5:693–698.

Lyons PA, Hancock WW, Denny P, Lord CJ, Hill NJ, Armitage N, Siegmund T, Todd JA, Phillips MS, Hess JF, et al.: The NOD *Idd9* genetic interval influences the pathogenicity of insulitis and contains molecular variants of Cd30, Tnfr2, and Cd137. Immunity 2000; 13:107–115.

MacDonald MJ, Gottschall J, Hunter JB, Winter KL: HLA-DR4 in insulin-dependent diabetic parents and their diabetic offspring: a clue to dominant inheritance. Proc Natl Acad Sci USA 1986; 83:7049–7053.

Maclaren N, Riley W, Skordis N, Spillar R, Silverstein J, Klein R, Vadheim C, Rotter J: Inherited susceptibility to insulin-dependent diabetes is associated with HLA-DR1 (and DR3 and DR4) while DR5 (and DR2) are protective. Autoimmunity 1988; 1:197–205.

Marks HH, Krall LP: Onset, course, progression and mortality in diabetes mellitus. In: Marble A, White P, Bradley RF, Krasll L (eds). Joslin's Diabetes Mellitus, 11th ed. Philadelphia: Lea and Febiger, 1971:209–254.

Marre M, Bernadet P, Gallois Y, Savagner F, Guyene TT, Hallab M, Cambien F, Passa P, Alhenc-Gelas F: Relationships between angiotensin I converting enzyme gene polymorphism, plasma levels, and diabetic retinal and renal complications. Diabetes 1994; 43:384–388.

Marron MP, Raffel LJ, Garchon HJ, Jacob CO, Serrano-Rios M, Martinez Larrad MT, Teng WP, Park Y, Zhang ZX, Goldstein DR, et al.: Insulin-dependent diabetes mellitus (IDDM) is associated with CTLA4 polymorphisms in multiple ethnic groups. Hum Mol Genet 1997; 6:1275–1282.

Marron MP, Zeidler A, Raffel LJ, Eckenrode SE, Yang JJ, Hopkins DI, Garchon HJ, Jacob CO, Serrano-Rios M, Martinez Larrad MT, et al.: Genetic and physical mapping of a type 1 diabetes susceptibility gene (*IDDM12*) to a 100-kb phagemid artificial chromosome clone containing D2S72-CTLA4-D2S105 on chromosome 2q33. Diabetes 2000; 49:492–499.

Martin S, Schernthaner G, Nerup J, Gries FA, Koivisto VA, Dupre J, Standl E, Hamet P, McArthur R, Tan MH, et al.: Follow-up of cyclosporin A treatment in type 1 (insulin-dependent) diabetes mellitus: lack of long-term effects. Diabetologia 1991; 34:429–434.

Mathiesen ER, Oxenboll B, Johansen K, Svendsen PA, Deckert T: Incipient nephropathy in type 1 (insulin-dependent) diabetes. Diabetologia 1984; 26:406–410.

Mathiesen ER, Saurbrey N, Hommel E, Parving HH: Prevalence of microalbuminuria in children with type 1 (insulin-dependent) diabetes mellitus. Diabetologia 1986; 29:640–643.

Matsuda A, Kuzuya T: Diabetic twins in Japan. Diabetes Res Clin Pract 1994; 24(Suppl):63–67.

Mcaleer MA, Reifsnyder P, Palmer SM, Prochazka M, Love JM, Copeman JB, Powell EE, Rodrigues NR, Prins JB, Serreze DV, et al.: Crosses of NOD mice with the related NON strain: a polygenic model for IDDM. Diabetes 1995; 44:1186–1195.

McDuffie M: Genetics of autoimmune diabetes in animal models. Curr Opin Immunol 1998; 10:704–709.

McElvy SS, Miodovnik M, Rosenn B, Khoury JC, Siddiqi T, Dignan PS, Tsang RC: A focused preconceptional and early pregnancy program in women with type 1 diabetes reduces perinatal mortality and malformation rates to general population levels. J Matern Fet Med 2000; 9:14–20.

Melanitou E, Joly F, Lathrop M, Boitard C, Avner P: Evidence for the presence of insulin-dependent diabetes–associated alleles on the distal part of mouse chromosome 6. Genome Res 1998; 8:608–620.

Meloni T, Marinaro AM, Mannazzu MC, Ogana A, La Vecchia C, Negri E, Colombo C: IDDM and early infant feeding: Sardinian case-control study. Diabetes Care 1997; 20:340–342.

Merriman T, Twells R, Merriman M, Eaves I, Cox R, Cucca F, McKinney P, Shield J, Baum D, Bosi E, et al.: Evidence by allelic association-dependent methods for a type 1 diabetes polygene (*IDDM6*) on chromosome 18q21. Hum Mol Genet 1997; 6:1003–1010.

Merriman TR, Eaves IA, Twells RC, Merriman ME, Danoy PA, Muxworthy CE, Hunter KM, Cox RD, Cucca F, McKinney PA, et al.: Transmission of haplotypes of microsatellite markers rather than single marker alleles in the mapping of a putative type 1 diabetes susceptibility gene (*IDDM6*). Hum Mol Genet 1998; 7:517–524.

Miller E, Hare JW, Cloherty JP, Dunn PJ, Gleason RE, Soeldner JS, Kitzmiller JL: Elevated maternal hemoglobin A1c in early pregnancy and major congenital anomalies in infants of diabetic mothers. N Engl J Med 1981; 304:1331–1334.

Miller JA, Scholey JW, Thai K, Pei YP: Angiotensin converting enzyme gene polymorphism and renal hemodynamic function in early diabetes. Kidney Int 1997; 51:119–124.

Miller JA, Thai K, Scholey JW: Angiotensin II type 1 receptor gene polymorphism and the response to hyperglycemia in early type 1 diabetes. Diabetes 2000; 49:1585–1589.

Mills JL: Malformation in infants of diabetic mothers. Teratology 1982; 25:385–394.

Mills JL: Congenital malformations in diabetes. In: Infant of the Diabetic Mother Report of the 93rd Ross Conference on Pediatric Research. Columbus, OH: Ross Laboratories, 1987:12–19.

Mills JL, Baker L, Goldman AS: Malformations in infants of diabetic mothers occur before the seventh gestational week. Diabetes 1979; 28:292–293.

Millward BA, Welsh KI, Leslie RDG, Pyke DA, Demaine AG: T-cell receptor beta chain polymorphisms are associated with insulin-dependent diabetes. Clin Exp Immunol 1987; 70:152–157.

Milunsky A, Alpert E, Kitzmiller JL, Younger MD, Neff RK: Prenatal diagnosis of neural tube defects VIII: the importance of serum alpha-fetoprotein screening in diabetic pregnant women. Am J Obstet Gynecol 1982; 142:1030–1032.

Mimura G, Miyao S: Heredity and constitutions of diabetes mellitus. Bull Res Inst Diabet Med Kumamoto Univ 1962; 12:1–82.

Miyazaki J, Ishii M, Tashiro F: Current studies on the identification of susceptibility genes for IDDM in NOD mice: Nippon Rinsho 1994; 52:2772–2777.

Miyazaki T, Uno M, Uehira M, Kikutani H, Kishimoto T, Kimoto M, Nishimoto H, Miyazaki J, Yamamura K: Direct evidence for the contribution of the unique I-ANOD to the development of insulitis in non-obese diabetic mice. Nature 1990; 345:722–724.

Moczulski DK, Scott L, Antonellis A, Rogus JJ, Rich SS, Warram JH, Krolewski AS: Aldose reductase gene polymorphisms and susceptibility to diabetic nephropathy in type 1 diabetes mellitus. Diabet Med 2000; 17:111–118.

Mogensen CE: Long-term antihypertensive treatment inhibiting progression of diabetic nephropathy. BMJ 1982; 285:685–688.

Mogensen CE: Microalbuminuria predicts clinical proteinuria and early mortality in maturity-onset diabetes. N Engl J Med 1984; 310:356–360.

Mogensen CE, Christensen CK: Predicting diabetic nephropathy in insulin-dependent patients. N Engl J Med 1984; 311:89–93.

Mogensen CE, Schmitz A, Christensen CK: Comparative renal pathophysiology relevant to IDDM and NIDDM patients. Diabetes Metab Rev 1988; 4:453–483.

Morahan G, Huang D, Tait BD, Colman PG, Harrison LC: Markers on distal chromosome 2q linked to insulin-dependent diabetes mellitus. Science 1996; 272:1811–1813.

Morahan G, Huang D, Ymer SI, Cancilla MR, Stephen K, Dabadghao P, Werther G, Tait BD, Harrison LC, Colman PG: Linkage disequilibrium of a type 1 diabetes susceptibility locus with a regulatory IL12B allele. Nat Genet 2001; 27:218–221.

Morahan G, McClive P, Huang D, Little P, Baxter A: Genetic and physiological association of diabetes susceptibility with raised Na^+/H^+ exchange activity. Proc Natl Acad Sci USA 1994; 91:5898–5902.

Mordes JP, Desemone J, Rossini AA: The BB rat. Diabetes Metab Rev 1987; 3:725–750.

Mosmann TR, Coffman RL: Th1 and Th2 cells: different patterns of lymphokine secretion lead to different functional properties. Annu Rev Immunol 1989; 7:145–173.

Mouse Genome Database: Mouse Genome Informatics Web Site. Jackson Laboratory, Bar Harbor, ME, 2001: *http://www.informatics.jax.org/*.

Myers MA, Davies JM, Tong JC, Whisstock J, Scealy M, Mackay IR, Rowley MJ: Conformational epitopes on the diabetes autoantigen GAD65 identified by peptide phage display and molecular modeling. J Immunol 2000; 165:3830–3838.

Nairn C, Galbraith DN, Taylor KW, Clements GB: Enterovirus variants in the serum of children at the onset of type 1 diabetes mellitus. Diabet Med 1999; 16:509–513.

Nakagawa Y, Kawaguchi Y, Twells RCJ, Muxworthy C, Hunter KMD, Wilson A, Merriman ME, Cox RD, Merriman T, Cucca F, et al.: Fine mapping of the diabetes-susceptibility locus, *IDDM4*, on chromosome 11q13. Am J Hum Genet 1998; 63:547–556.

Nannipieri M, Penno G, Pucci L, Colhoun H, Motti C, Bertacca A, Rizzo L, De Giorgio L, Zerbini G, Mangili R, et al.: Pronatriodilatin gene polymorphisms, microvascular permeability, and diabetic nephropathy in type 1 diabetes mellitus. J Am Soc Nephrol 1999; 10:1530–1541.

Nathan DM, Singer DE, Godine JE, Harrington CH, Perlmuter LC: Retinopathy in older type II diabetics: association with glucose control. Diabetes 1986; 35:797–801.

National Diabetes Data Group: Classification and diagnosis of diabetes mellitus and other categories of glucose intolerance. Diabetes 1979; 28:1039–1057.

Neave C: Congenital malformations in offspring of diabetics. Perspect Pediatr Pathol 1984; 8:213–222.

Neel JV: Diabetes mellitus: a "thrifty" genotype rendered detrimental by "progress?" Am J Hum Genet 1962; 14:353–362.

Nejentsev S, Reijonen H, Adojaan B, Kovalchuk L, Sochnevs A, Schwartz EI, Akerblom HK, Ilonen J: The effect of HLA-B allele on the IDDM risk defined by DRB1*04 subtypes and DQB1*0302. Diabetes 1997; 46:1888–1892.

Nepom BD, Palmer J, Kim SJ, Hansen JA, Holbeck SL, Nepom GT: Specific genomic markers for the HLA-subregion discriminate between $DR4^+$ insulin-dependent diabetes mellitus and $DR4^+$ seropositive juvenile rheumatoid arthritis. J Exp Med 1986; 164:1–6.

Nerup J, Platz P, Ortved-Anderson O, Christy M, Lyngsoe J, Poulsen JE, Ryder LP, Staub-Nielsen L, Thomsen M, Svejgaard A: HLA antigens and diabetes mellitus. Lancet 1974; ii:864–866.

Nistico L, Buzzetti R, Pritchard LE, Van der Auwera B, Giovannini C, Bosi E, Martinez Larrad MT, Serrano Rios M, Chow CC, Cockram CS, et al.: The *CTLA-4* gene region of chromosome 2q33 is linked to, and associated with, type 1 diabetes. Hum Mol Genet 1996; 5:1075–1080.

Noble JA, Valdes AM, Cook M, Klitz W, Thomson G, Erlich HA: The role of HLA class II genes in insulin-dependent diabetes mellitus: molecular analysis of 180 Caucasian, multiplex families. Am J Hum Genet 1996; 59:1134–1148.

Noble JA, Valdes AM, Thomson G, Erlich HA: The HLA class II locus DPB1 can influence susceptibility to type 1 diabetes. Diabetes 2000; 49:121–125.

Nora JJ, Lortscher RH, Spangler RD, Nora AH, Kimberling WJ: Genetic—epidemiologic study of early-onset ischemic heart disease. Circulation 1980; 61:503–508.

Nordstrom L, Spetz E, Wallstrom K, Walinder O: Metabolic control and pregnancy outcome among women with insulin-dependent diabetes mellitus: a twelve-year follow-up in the county of Jamtland, Sweden. Acta Obstet Gynecol Scand 1998; 77:284–289.

Norris JM, Beaty B, Eisenbarth GS, Hamman RF, Rewers M: Lack of association between infant diet and prediabetic autoimmunity in high genetic risk children: the Diabetes Autoimmunity Study in the Young (DAISY). Diabetes 1995; 44(Suppl 1):6A.

Norris JM, Beaty B, Klingensmith G, Yu L, Hoffman M, Chase HP, Erlich HA, Hamman RF, Eisenbarth GS, Rewers M: Lack of association between early exposure to cow's milk protein and beta-cell autoimmunity: Diabetes Autoimmunity Study in the Young (DAISY). JAMA 1996;276:609–614.

Nosadini R, Fioretto P, Trevisan R, Crepaldi G: Insulin-dependent diabetes mellitus and hypertension. Diabetes Care 1991; 14:210–219.

Noth RH, Krolewski AS, Kaysen GA, Meyer TW, Schambelan M: Diabetic nephropathy: hemodynamic basis and implications for disease management. Ann Intern Med 1989; 110:795–813.

Nyberg G, Larsson O, Attman PO, Granerus G, Norden G: Time as a risk factor in diabetic nephropathy. Diabetes Care 1985; 8:590–593.

Oakley WG, Pyke DA, Tattersall RB, Watkins PJ: Long-term diabetes: a clinical study of 92 patients after 40 years. Q J Med 1974; 43:145–156.

Oldstone MB: Viruses as therapeutic agents. I: Treatment of nonobese insulin-dependent diabetic mice with virus prevents insulin-dependent diabetes mellitus while maintaining general immune competence. J Exp Med 1990; 171:2077–2089.

Oldstone MB, Ahmed R, Salvato M: Viruses as therapeutic agents. II: Viral reassortant map prevention of insulin-dependent diabetes mellitus to the small RNA of lymphocytic choriomeningitis virus. J Exp Med 1990; 171:2091–2100.

Olmos P, Hern RA, Heaton DA, Millward BA, Risley D, Pyke DA, Leslie RDG: The significance of the concordance rate for type 1 (insulin-dependent) diabetes in identical twins. Diabetologia 1988; 31:747–750.

Omar MAK, Asmal AC: Family histories of diabetes mellitus in young African and Indian diabetics. BMJ 1983; 286:1786.

Onodera T, Yoon J, Brown K, Notkins AL: Evidence for a single locus controlling susceptibility to virus-induced diabetes mellitus. Nature 1978; 276:693–696.

Orchard TJ, Atchison RW, Becker D, Rabin B, Eberhardt M, Kuller LH, LaPorte RE, Cavender D: Coxsackie infection and diabetes. Lancet 1983; 2:631.

Owerbach D: Physical and genetic mapping of *IDDM8* on chromosome 6q27. Diabetes 2000; 49:508–512.

Owerbach D, Gabbay KH: Localization of a type 1 diabetes susceptibility locus to the variable tandem repeat region flanking the insulin gene. Diabetes 1993; 42:1708–1714.

Owerbach D, Gabbay KH: Linkage of the VNTR/insulin-gene and type I diabetes mellitus: increased gene sharing in affected sibling pairs. Am J Hum Genet 1994; 54:909–912.

Owerbach D, Gabbay KH: The *HOXD8* locus (2q31) is linked to type I diabetes: Interaction with chromosome 6 and 11 disease susceptibility genes. Diabetes 1995; 4:132–136.

Owerbach D, Lernmark A, Platz P, Ryder LP, Rask L, Peterson PA, Ludvigsson J: HLA-DR beta chain DNA endonuclease fragments differ between health and insulin-dependent diabetic individuals. Nature 1983; 303:815–817.

Pak CY, Eun HM, McArthur RG, Yoon JW: Association of cytomegalovirus infection with autoimmune type 1 diabetes. Lancet 1988; ii:1–4.

Palmer JP, Cooney MK, Ward RH, Hansen JA, Brodsky JB, Ray CG, Crossley JR, Asplin CM, Williams RH: Reduced Coxsackie antibody titres in type 1 (insulin-dependent) diabetic patients presenting during an outbreak of coxsackie B3 and B4 infection. Diabetologia 1982; 22:426–429.

Panzram G, Zabel-Langhennig R: Prognosis of diabetes mellitus in a geographically defined population. Diabetologia 1981; 20:587–591.

Paronen J, Knip M, Savilahti E, Virtanen SM, Ilonen J, Akerblom HK, Vaarala O: Effect of cow's milk exposure and maternal type 1 diabetes on cellular and humoral immunization to dietary insulin in infants at genetic risk for type 1 diabetes: Finnish Trial to Reduce IDDM in the Genetically at Risk Study Group. Diabetes 2000; 49:1657–1665.

Parving HH, Andersen AR, Smidt UM, Hommel E, Mathiesen ER, Svendsen PA: Effect of antihypertensive treatment on kidney function in diabetic nephropathy. BMJ 1987; 294:1443–1447.

Paterson AD, Petronis A: Age of diagnosis-based linkage analysis in type 1 diabetes. Eur J Hum Genet 2000; 8:145–148.

Patterson K, Chandra RS, Jenson AB: Congenital rubella, inulitis and diabetes mellitus in an infant. Lancet 1981; 1:1048–1049.

Paz-Guevara AT, Hsu TH, White P: Juvenile diabetes mellitus after forty years. Diabetes 1975; 24:559–565.

Pearce RB, Formby B, Healy K, Peterson CM: Association of an androgen-responsive T cell phenotype with murine diabetes and *Idd2*. Autoimmunity 1995; 20:247–258.

Pincus G, White P: On the inheritance of diabetes mellitus. I. An analysis of 675 family histories. Amer J Medical Science 1933; 186:1–14.

Pirart J: Diabetes mellitus and its degenerative complications: a prospective study of 4,400 patients observed between 1947 and 1973 [in French]. Diabete et Metabolisme 1977; 3:97–107.

Pirart J: Diabetes mellitus and its degenertative complications: a prospective study of 4,400 patients observed between 1947 and 1973. Diabetes Care 1978; 1:168–188, 252–263.

Platz P, Jakobsen BD, Morling N, Ryder LP, Svejgaard A, Thomsen M, Christy M, Kromann H, Benn J, Nerup J, et al.: HLA-D and DR antigens in genetic analysis of insulin-dependent diabetes mellitus. Diabetologia 1981; 21:108–115.

Podolin PL, Denny P, Armitage N, Lord CJ, Hill NJ, Levy ER, Peterson LB, Todd JA, Wicker LS, Lyons PA: Localization of two insulin-dependent diabetes (*Idd*) genes to the *Idd10* region on mouse chromosome 3. Mamm Genome 1998; 9:283–286.

Podolin PL, Denny P, Lord CJ, Hill NJ, Todd JA, Peterson LB, Wicker LS, Lyons PA: Congenic mapping of the insulin-dependent diabetes (*Idd*) gene, *Idd10*, localizes two gene mediating the *Idd10* effect and eliminates the candidate *Fcgr1*. J Immunol 1997; 159:1835–1843.

Pozzilli P, Visalli N, Buzzetti R, Baroni MG, Boccuni ML, Fioriti E, Signore A, Mesturino C, Valente L, Cavallo MG, et al.: Adjuvant therapy in recent onset type 1 diabetes at diagnosis and insulin requirement after 2 years. Diabete et Metabolisme1995; 21:47–49.

Prochazka M, Le PH, Serreze D, Coleman D, Leiter EH: Genetic control of insulin-dependent diabetes in non-obese diabetic (NOD) mice. Mouse News Lett 1986; 75:32.

Prochazka M, Leiter EH, Serreze DV, Coleman DL: Three recessive loci required for insulin-dependent diabetes in nonobese diabetic mice. Science 1987; 237:286–289.

Prochazka M, Serreze DV, Worthen SM, Leiter EH: Genetic control of diabetogenesis in NOD/Lt mice: development and analysis of congenic stocks. Diabetes 1989; 38:1446–1455.

Propert DN, Tait BD, Harrison LC: Interaction of immunoglobulin allotypes (Gm and Km): HLA, and sex in insulin-dependent (type 1) diabetes. Dis Markers 1991; 9:43–45.

Pugh JA, Stern MP, Haffner SM, Eifler CW, Zapata M: Excess incidence of treatment of end-stage renal disease in Mexican Americans. Am J Epidemiol 1988; 127:135–144.

Pugliese A, Zeller M, Fernandez A Jr, Zalcberg LJ, Bartlett RJ, Ricordi C, Pietropaolo M, Eisenbarth GS, Bennett ST, Patel DD: The insulin gene is transcribed in the human thymus and transcription levels correlated with allelic variation at the INS VNTR-IDDM2 susceptibility locus for type 1 diabetes. Nat Genet 1997; 15:293–297.

Pyke DA: Twin studies in diabetes. In: Nance WE, Allen G, Parisi P (eds). Twin Research. Part C. Clinical Studies. New York: Alan R Liss, 1978:1–12.

Pyke DA: The genetic connections. Diabetologia 1979; 17:333–343.

Pyke DA, Nelson PG: Diabetes mellitus in identical twins. In: Creutzfeldt W, Kobberling J, Neel JV (eds). The Genetics of Diabetes Mellitus. Berlin: Springer-Verlag, 1976:194–205.

Pyke DA, Taylor KW: Glucose tolerance and serum insulin in unaffected identical twin of diabetics. BMJ 1967; ii:21–22.

Quatraro A, Consoli G, Magno M, Caretta F, Ceriello A, Giugliano D: Analysis of diabetic family connection in subjects with insulin-dependent diabetes mellitus (IDDM). Diabetes Metab 1990; 16:449–452.

Quinn M, Angelico MC, Warram JH, Krolewski AS: Familial factors determine the development of diabetic nephropathy in patients with IDDM. Diabetologia 1996; 39:940–945.

Rabensteiner D, Abrahamian H, Irsigler K, Hermann KM, Kiener HP, Mayer G, Kaider A, Prager R: *ACE* gene polymorphism and proliferative retinopathy in type 1 diabetes: results of a case-control study. Diabetes Care 1999; 22:1530–1535.

Rabinovitch A: Immunoregulatory and cytokine imbalances in the pathogenesis of IDDM: therapeutic intervention by immunostimulation? Diabetes 1996; 43:613–621.

Rabinowe SL, George KL, Loughlin R, Soeldner JS, Eisenbarth GS: Congenital rubella: monoclonal antibody–defined T-cell abnormalities in young adults. Am J Med 1986; 81:779–782.

Raffel LJ, Hitman GA, Toyoda H, Karam JH, Bell GI, Rotter JI: The aggregation of the 5′ insulin gene polymorphism in type I (insulin-dependent) diabetes mellitus families. J Med Genet 1992; 29:447–450.

Raffel LJ, Rotter JI: Diabetes mellitus. In: Rimoin DL, Connor JM, Pyeritz RE (eds). Principles and Practice of Medical Genetics, 4th ed. London: Churchill Livingstone, vol. 2, 2231–2276, 2001.

Raffel LJ, Vadheim CM, Klein R, Moss S, Riley WJ, Maclaren NK, Rotter JI: HLA-DR and the 5′ insulin gene polymorphism in insulin dependent diabetes. Metabolism 1991; 40:1244–1248.

Redondo MJ, Rewers M, Yu L, Garg S, Pilcher CC, Elliott RB, Eisenbarth GS: Genetic determination of islet cell autoimmunity in monozygotic twin, dizygotic twin, and non-twin siblings of patients with type 1 diabetes: prospective twin study. BMJ 1999; 318:698–702.

Reece AE, Davis N, Mahoney MJ, Baumgarten A: Maternal serum alpha-fetoprotein in diabetic pregnancy: correlation with blood glucose control. Lancet 1987; ii:275.

Reed P, Cucca F, Jenkins S, Merriman M, Wilson A, McKinney P, Bosi E, Joner G, Ronningen K, Thorsby E, et al.: Evidence for a type 1 diabetes susceptibility locus *(IDDM10)* on human chromosome 10p11–q11. Hum Mol Genet 1997; 6:1011–1016.

Reijonen H, Nejentsev S, Tuokko J, Koskinen S, Tuomilehto-Wolf E, Akerblom HK, Ilonen J: HLA-DR4 subtype and -B alleles in DQB1*0302-positive haplotypes associated with IDDM: the Childhood Diabetes in Finland Study Group. Eur J Immunogenet 1997; 24:357–363.

Rich SS, Panter SS, Goetz FC, Hedlund B, Barbosa J: Shared genetic susceptibility of type 1 (insulin-dependent) and type 2 (non-insulin-dependent) diabetes mellitus: contributions of HLA and haptoglobin. Diabetologia 1991; 34:350–355.

Rich SS, Weitkamp LR, Guttormsen S, Barbosa J: Gm, Km, and HLA in insulin-dependent type I diabetes mellitus: a log-linear analysis of association. Diabetes 1986; 35:927–932.

Riley WJ, Maclaren NK, Lezotte DC, Spillar RP, Rosenbloom AL: Thyroid autoimmunity in insulin-dependent diabetes mellitus: the case for routine screening. J Pediatr 1981; 98:350–354.

Riley WJ, Maclaren NK, Neufeld M: Adrenal autoantibodies and Addison's disease in insulin-dependent diabetes mellitus. J Pediatr 1980; 97:191–195.

Riley WJ, Toskes PP, Maclaren NK, Silverstein JH: Predictive value of gastric parietal cell autoantibodies as a marker for gastric and hematologic abnormalities associated with insulin dependent diabetes. Diabetes 1982; 31:1051–1055.

Rimoin D, Rotter JI: Genetic heterogeneity in diabetes mellitus and diabetic microangiopathy. Horm Metab Res 1981; 11:63–72.

Rimoin DL, Rotter JI: Progress in understanding the genetics of diabetes mellitus in genetic disorders. In: Berg K (ed). Medical Genetics: Past, Present and Future. New York: Alan R Liss, 1985:393–412.

Rimoin DL, Schimke RN: Endocrine pancreas. In: Genetic Disorders of the Endocrine Glands. St Louis: Mosby, 1971:150–216.

Risch N: Assessing the role of HLA-linked and unlinked determinants of disease. Am J Hum Genet 1987; 40:1–14.

Risch N, Ghosh S, Todd JA: Statistical evaluation of multiple-locus linkage data in experimental species and its relevance to human studies: application to nonobese diabetic (NOD) mouse and human insulin-dependent diabetes mellitus (IDDM). Am J Hum Genet 1993; 53:702–714.

Robertson RP, Klein DJ: Treatment of diabetes mellitus. Diabetologia 1992; 35(Suppl 2):S8–S17.

Robinson BH, Dosch H-M, Martin JM, Akerblom HK, Savilahti E, Knip M, Ilonen J: A model for the involvement of MHC class II proteins in the development of type 1 (insulin-dependent) diabetes mellitus in response to bovine serum albumin peptides. Diabetologia 1993; 36:364–368.

Rodrigues NR, Cornall RJ, Chandler P, Simpson E, Wicker LS, Peterson LB, Todd JA: Mapping of an insulin-dependent diabetes locus, *Idd9*, in NOD mice to chromosome 4. Mamm Genome 1994; 5:167–170.

Rogus JJ, Moczulski D, Freire MB, Yang Y, Warram JH, Krolewski AS: Diabetic nephropathy is associated with AGT polymorphism T235: results of a family-based study. Hypertension 1998; 31:627–631.

Romagnani S: Biology of human Th1 and Th2 cells. J Clin Immunol 1995; 15:121–129.

Rosenstock J, Raskin P: Diabetes and its complications: blood glucose control vs. genetic susceptibility. Diabetes Metab Rev 1988; 4:417–435.

Rossini AA, Slavin S, Woda BA, Geisberg M, Like AA, Mordes JP: Total lymphoid irradiation prevents diabetes mellitus in the biobreeding/Worcester (BB/W) rat. Diabetes 1984; 33:543–547.

Rotter JI: The modes of inheritance of insulin-dependent diabetes. Am J Hum Genet 1981; 33:835–851.

Rotter JI, Anderson CE, Rubin R, Congleton JE, Terasaki PI, Rimoin DL: HLA genotype study of insulin-dependent diabetes, the excess of DR3/DR4 heterozygotes allows rejection of the recessive hypothesis. Diabetes 1983; 32:169–174.

Rotter JI, Landaw EM: Measuring the genetic contribution of a single locus to a multilocus disease. Clin Genet 1984; 26:529–542.

Rotter JI, Rimoin DL: Heterogeneity in diabetes mellitus—update 1978: evidence for further genetic heterogeneity within juvenile onset insulin-dependent diabetes mellitus. Diabetes 1978; 27:599–608.

Rotter JI, Rimoin DL: The genetics of diabetes. Hosp Pract 1987; 22:79–88.

Rotter JI, Rimoin DL, Samloff IM: Genetic heterogeneity in diabetes mellitus and peptic ulcer. In: Morton NE, Chung CS (eds). Genetic Epidemiology. New York: Academic Press, 1978:381–414.

Rotter JI, Vadheim CM, Petersen GM, Cantor RM, Riley WJ, Maclaren NK: HLA haplotypes sharing and proband genotype in IDDM. Genet Epidemiol 1986; 3(Suppl 1):347–352.

Rubinstein P, Ginsberg-Fellner F, Falk C: Genetics of type I diabetes mellitus: a single, recessive predisposition gene mapping between HLA-B and GLO. Am J Hum Genet 1981; 33:865–882.

Rubinstein P, Walker ME, Fedun B, Witt ME, Cooper LZ, Ginsberg-Fellner F: The HLA system in congenital rubella patients with and without diabetes. Diabetes 1982; 31:1088–1091.

Ryan JR, Balodimos MC, Chazan BI, Root HF, Marble A, White P, Joslin AP, Quarter Century Victory Medal for Diabetes: A follow-up of patients one to 20 years later. Metabolism 1970; 19:493–501.

Sanjeevi CB, Zeidler A, Shaw S, Rotter J, Nepom GT, Costin G, Raffel L, Eastman S, Kockum I, Wassmuth R, et al.: Analysis of *HLA-DQA1* and *-DQB1* genes in Mexican Americans with insulin-dependent diabetes mellitus. Tissue Antigens 1993; 42:72–77.

Schernthaner G: The relation between clinical, immunological and genetic factors in insulin-dependent diabetes mellitus. In: Kobberling J, Tattersall RB (eds). The Genetics of Diabetes Mellitus. London: Academic Press, 1982:99–114.

Schernthaner G, Banatvala JE, Scherbaum W, Bryant J, Borkenstein M, Schober E, Mayer WR: Coxsackie B virus specific IgM responses, complement-fixing islet cell antibodies, HLA DR antigens and C-peptide secretion in insulin-dependent diabetes mellitus. Lancet 1985; 2:630–632.

Schloot NC, Willemen SJ, Duinkerken G, Drijfhout JW, de Vries RR, Roep BO: Molecular mimicry in type 1 diabetes mellitus revisited: T-cell clones to GAD65 peptides with sequence homology to Coxsackie or proinsulin peptides do not cross-react with homologous counterpart. Hum Immunol 2001; 62:299–309.

Schulz B, Hehmke B, Zander E, Ziegler B: Autoimmune reactions in a patient with malignant insulinoma treated by multiple low dose streptozotocin. Exp Clin Endocrinol 1990; 95:77–82.

Seaquist ER, Goetz FC, Rich S, Barbosa J: Familial clustering of diabetic kidney disease: evidence for genetic susceptibility to diabetic nephropathy. N Engl J Med 1989; 320:1161–1165.

Segal P, Treister G, Yalon M, Sandak R, Berezin M, Modan M: The prevalence of diabetic retinopathy: effect of sex, age, duration of disease and mode of therapy. Diabetes Care 1983; 6:149–151.

Serjeantson SW, Ryan DP, Zimmet P: HLA and non-insulin dependent diabetes in Fiji Indians. Med J Aust 1981; 1:462–464.

Serreze DV, Prochazka M, Reifsnyder PC, Bridgett MM, Leiter EH: Use of recombinant congenic and congenic strains of NOD mice to identify a new insulin-dependent diabetes resistance gene. J Exp Med 1994; 180:1553–1558.

Shah VO, Dorin RI, Sun Y, Braun M, Zager PG: Aldose reductase gene expression is increased in diabetic nephropathy. J Clin Endocrinol Metab 1997; 82:2294–2298.

Shah VO, Scavini M, Nikolic J, Sun Y, Vai S, Griffith JK, Dorin RI, Stidley C, Yacoub M, Vander Jagt DL, et al.: Z-2 microsatellite allele is linked to increased expression of the aldose reductase gene in diabetic nephropathy. J Clin Endocrinol Metab 1998; 83:2886–2891.

Shcherbak NS, Shutskaya ZV, Sheidina AM, Larionova VI, Schwartz EI: Methylenetetrahydrofolate reductase gene polymorphism as a risk factor for diabetic nephropathy in IDDM patients. Mol Genet Metab 1999; 68:375–378.

Simpson NE: The genetics of diabetes: a study of 233 families of juvenile diabetics. Ann Hum Genet 1962; 26:1–12.

Simpson NE: A review of family data. In: Creutzfeldt W, Kobberling J, Neel JV (eds). The Genetics of Diabetes Mellitus. Berlin: Springer-Verlag, 1976:12–20.

Singal DP, Blajchman MA: Histocompatibility (HL-A) antigens, lymphocytotoxic antibodies and tissue antibodies in patients with diabetes mellitus. Diabetes 1973; 22:429–432.

Sklenar I, Nerit M, Berger W: Association of specific immune responses to pork and beef insulin with certain HLA-DR antigens in type I diabetes. BMJ 1982; 285: 1451–1453.

Smith CP, Clements GB, Riding MH, Collins P, Bottazzo GF, Taylor KW: Simultaneous onset of type 1 diabetes mellitus in identical infant twins with enterovirus infection. Diabet Med 1998; 15:515–517.

Smith DA: Comparative approaches to risk reduction of coronary heart disease in Tecumseh non-insulin-dependent diabetic population. Diabetes Care 1986; 9:601–608.

Soler NG, Walsh CH, Malins JM: Congenital malformations in infants of diabetic mothers. Q J Med 1976; 45:303–313.

Spielman RS, McGinnis RE, Ewens WJ: Transmission test for linkage disequilibrium: the insulin gene region and insulin-dependent diabetes mellitus (IDDM). Am J Hum Genet 1993; 52:506–516.

Srikanta S, Ricker AT, McCulloch DR, Soeldner JS, Eisenbarth GS, Palmer JP: Autoimmunity to insulin, beta cell dysfunction and development of insulin-dependent diabetes mellitus. Diabetes 1986; 35:139–142.

Steiner F: Untersuchungen zur Frage der Erblichkeit des diabetes mellitus. Dtsch Arch Klin Med 1936; 178:497–510.

Stevenson RE, Allen WP, Pai GS, Best R, Seaver LH, Dean J, Thompson S: Decline in prevalence of neural tube defects in a high-risk region of the United States. Pediatrics 2000; 106:677–683.

Stewart LL, Field LL, Ross S, McArthur RG: Genetic risk factors in diabetic retinopathy. Diabetologia 1993; 36:1293–1298.

Suhonen L, Hiilesmaa V, Teramo K: Glycaemic control during early pregnancy and fetal malformations in women with type I diabetes mellitus. Diabetologia 2000; 43:79–82.

Sutherland DER, Goetz FC, Sibley RK: Recurrence of disease in pancreas transplants. Diabetes 1989; 38:85–87.

Sutherland DER, Sibley RK, Za XZ, Michael A, Srikanta S, Taub F, Najarian J, Goetz FC: Twin to twin pancrease transplantation reversal and reenactment of the pathogenesis of type I diabetes. Trans Assoc Am Physicians 1984; 97:80–87.

Svejgaard A, Platz P, Ryder LP, Staub-Nielsen L, Thomsen M: HLA and disease association—a survey. Transplant Rev 1975; 22:3–34.

Tarn AC, Thomas JM, Dean BM, Ingram D, Schwarz G, Bottazzo GF, Gale EAM: Predicting insulin-dependent diabetes. Lancet 1988; 1:845–850.

Tarnow L, Cambien F, Rossing P, Nielsen FS, Hansen BV, Lecerf L, Poirier O, Danilov S, Boelskifte S, Borch-Johnsen K: Insertion/deletion polymorphism in the angiotensin-I-converting enzyme gene is associated with coronary heart disease in IDDM patients with diabetic nephropathy. Diabetologia 1995; 38:798–803.

Tarnow L, Cambien F, Rossing P, Nielsen FS, Hansen BV, Ricard S, Poirer O, Parving HH: Angiotensin-II type 1 receptor gene polymorphism and diabetic microangiopathy. Nephrol Dial Transplant 1996; 11:1019–1023.

Tarnow L, Rossing P, Nielsen FS, Fagerudd JA, Poirier O, Parving HH: Cardiovascular morbidity and early mortality cluster in parents of type 1 diabetic patients with diabetic nephropathy. Diabetes Care 2000a; 23:30–33.

Tarnow L, Stehouwer CD, Emeis JJ, Poirier O, Cambien F, Hansen BV, Parving HH: Plasminogen activator inhibitor-1 and apolipoprotein E gene polymorphisms and diabetic angiopathy. Nephrol Dial Transplant 2000b; 15:625–630.

Tattersall RB, Pyke DA: Diabetes in identical twins. Lancet 1972; ii:1120–1124.

Teuscher A, Schnell H, Wilson PW: Incidence of diabetic retinopathy and relationship to baseline plasma glucose and blood pressure. Diabetes Care 1988; 11:246–251.

Teuscher C, Wardell BB, Lunceford JK, Michael SD, Tung KS: Aod2, the locus controlling development of atrophy in neonatal thymectomy-induced autoimmune ovarian dysgenesis, co-localizes with Il2, Fgfb, and Idd3. J Exp Med 1996; 183: 631–637.

Then Berg H: The genetic aspect of diabetes mellitus. JAMA 1939; 112:1091.

Thivolent CH, Beaufrere B, Betuel H, Gebuhrer, Chatelain P, Durand A, Tourniaire J, Francois R: Islet cell and insulin autoantibodies in subjects at high risk for development of type 1 (insulin-dependent) diabetes mellitus: the Lyon Family Study. Diabetologia 1988; 31:741–746.

Thomson G: HLA DR antigens and susceptibility to insulin-dependent diabetes mellitus. Am J Hum Genet 1984; 36:1309–1317.

Thomson G, Robinson WP, Kuhner MK, Joe S, Klitz W: HLA and insulin gene associations with IDDM. Genet Epidemiol 1989; 6:155–160.

Thomson G, Robinson WP, Kuhner MK, MacDonald JS, Gottschall JL, Barbosa J, Rich SS, Bertrams J, Baur MP, Partanen J, et al.: Genetic heterogeneity, modes of inheritance, and risk estimates for a joint study of Caucasians with insulin dependent diabetes mellitus. Am J Hum Genet 1988; 43:799–816.

Todd JA, Aitman TJ, Cornall RJ, Ghosh S, Hall JRS, Hearne CM, Knight AM, Love JM, McAleer MA, Prins J-B, et al.: Genetic analysis of autoimmune type 1 diabetes mellitus in mice. Nature 1991; 351:542–547.

Tunbridge WM: Factors contributing to deaths of diabetics under fifty years of age: on behalf of the Medical Services Study Group and British Diabetic Association. Lancet 1981; 2:569–572.

Tuomilehto J, Karvonen M, Pitkaniemi J, Virtala E, Kohtamaki K, Toivanen L, Tuomilehto-Wolf E: Record-high incidence of type I (insulin-dependent) diabetes mellitus in Finnish children, the Finnish Childhood Type I Diabetes Registry Group. Diabetologia 1999; 42:655–660.

Ulvenstam G, Aberg A, Bergstrand R, Johansson S, Pennert K, Vedin A, Wilhelmsen L, Wilhelmsson C: Long-term prognosis after myocardial infarction in men with diabetes. Diabetes 1985; 34:787–792.

Uusitupa M, Siitonen O, Pyorala K, Aro A, Hersio K, Penttila I, Voutilainen E: The relationship of cardiovascular risk factors to the prevalence of coronary heart disease in newly diagnosed type 2 (non-insulin-dependent) diabetes. Diabetologia 1985; 8:653–659.

Vadheim CM, Rotter JI, Maclaren NK, Riley WJ, Anderson CE: Preferential transmission of diabetic alleles within the *HLA* gene complex. N Engl J Med 1986; 315:1314–1318.

Vadheim CM, Rotter JI, Riley WJ, Maclaren NK, Petersen GM, Cantor RM: An interaction of genetic susceptibility and birth order in type I diabetes. Clin Res 1987; 35:186A.

Vafiadis P, Bennett ST, Todd JA, Nadeau J, Grabs R, Goodyer CG, Wickramasinghe S, Colle E, Polychronakos C: Insulin expression in human thymus is modulated by INS VNTR alleles at the IDDM2 locus. Nat Genet 1997; 15:289–292.

Vague P, Dufayet D, Coste T, Moriscot C, Jannot MF, Raccah D: Association of diabetic neuropathy with Na/K-ATPase gene polymorphism. Diabetologia 1997; 40:506–511.

Van Ittersum FJ, de Man AM, Thijssen S, de Knijff P, Slagboom E, Smulders Y, Tarnow L, Donker AJ, Bilo HJ, Stehouwer CD: Genetic polymorphisms of the renin–angiotensin system and complications of insulin-dependent diabetes mellitus. Nephrol Dial Transplant 2000; 15:1000–1007.

Van Maanen JM, Albering HJ, de Kok TM, van Breda SG, Curfs DM, Vermeer IT, Ambergen AW, Wolffenbuttel BH, Kleinjans JC, Reeser HM: Does the risk of childhood diabetes mellitus require revision of the guideline values for nitrate in drinking water? Environ Health Perspect 2000; 108:457–461.

Varela-Calvino R, Sgarbi G, Arif S, Peakman M: T-Cell reactivity to the P2C nonstructural protein of a diabetogenic strain of coxsackievirus B4. Virology 2000; 274:56–64.

Verge CF, Howard NJ, Irwig L, Simpson JM, Mackerras D, Silink M: Environmental factors in childhood IDDM: a population-based, case-control study. Diabetes Care 1994; 17:1381–1389.

Verge CF, Gianani R, Yu L, Pietropaolo M, Smith T, Jackson RA, Soeldner JS, Eisenbarth GS: Late progression to diabetes and evidence for chronic beta-cell autoimmunity in identical twins of patients with type I diabetes. Diabetes 1995; 44:1176–1179.

Verge CF, Vardi P, Babu S, Bao F, Erlich HA, Bugawan T, Tiosano D, Yu L, Eisenbarth GS, Fain PR: Evidence for oligogenic inheritance of type 1 diabetes in a large Bedouin Arab family. J Clin Invest 1998; 102:1569–1575.

Vialettes B, Picq R, du Rostu M, Charbonnel B, Rodier M, Mirouze J, Vexiau P, Passa P, Pehuet M, Elgrably F, et al.: A preliminary multicentre study of the treatment of recently diagnosed type 1 diabetes by combination nicotinamide–cyclosporin therapy. Diabet Med 1990; 7:731–735.

Viberti G: Recent advances in understanding mechanisms and natural history of diabetic renal disease. Diabetes Care 1988; 11(Suppl 1):3–9.

Viberti G, Keen H: The patterns of proteinuria in diabetes mellitus: relevance to pathogenesis and prevention of diabetic nephropathy. Diabetes 1984; 33:686–692.

Viberti GC, Keen H, Wiseman MJ: Raised arterial pressure in parents of proteinuric insulin dependent diabetics. BMJ 1987; 295:515–517.

Viberti GC, Walker JD: Diabetic nephropathy: etiology and prevention. Diabetes Metab Rev 1988; 4:147–162.

Vicario JL, Martinez-Laso J, Corell A, Martin-Villa JM, Morales P, Lledo G, Segurado OG, de Juan D, Arnaiz-Villena A: Comparison between HLA-DRB and DQ DNA sequences and classic serological markers as type 1 (insulin-dependent) diabetes mellitus predictive risk markers in the Spanish population. Diabetologia 1992; 35:475–481.

Vigorita VJ, Moore GW, Hutchins GM: Absence of correlation between coronary arterial atherosclerosis and severity or duration of diabetes mellitus of adult onset. Am J Cardiol 1980; 46:535–542.

Virtanen SM, Jaakkola L, Rasanen L, Ylonen K, Aro A, Lounamaa R, Akerblom HK, Tuomilehto J: Nitrate and nitrite intake and the risk for type 1 diabetes in Finnish children: Childhood Diabetes in Finland Study Group. Diabet Med 1994; 11:656–662.

Virtanen SM, Rasanen L, Ylonen K, Aro A, Clayton D, Langholz B, Pitkaniemi J, Savilahti E, Lounamaa R, Tuomilehto J, et al.: Childhood Diabetes in Finland Study Group: early introduction of dairy products associated with increased risk of IDDM in Finnish children. Diabetes 1993; 42:1786–1790.

Virtanen SM, Saukkonen T, Savilahti E, Ylonen K, Rasanen L, Aro A, Knip M, Tuomilehto J, Akerblom HK: Diet, cow's milk protein antibodies and the risk of IDDM in Finnish children: Childhood Diabetes in Finland Study Group. Diabetologia 1994; 37:381–387.

Vleming LJ, van der Pijl JW, Lemkes HH, Westendorp RG, Maassen JA, Daha MR, van Es LA, van Kooten C: The *DD* genotype of the *ACE* gene polymorphism is associated with progression of diabetic nephropathy to end stage renal failure in IDDM. Clin Nephrol 1999; 51:133–140.

Vreugdenhil GR, Geluk A, Ottenhoff TH, Melchers WJ, Roep BO, Galama JM: Molecular mimicry in diabetes mellitus: the homologous domain in coxsackie B virus protein 2C and islet autoantigen GAD65 is highly conserved in the coxsackie B-like enteroviruses and binds to the diabetes associated HLA-DR3 molecule. Diabetologia 1998; 41:40–46.

Vreugdenhil GR, Batstra MR, Aanstoot HJ, Melchers WJ, Galama JM: Analysis of antibody responses against coxsackie virus B4 protein 2C and the diabetes autoantigen GAD(65). J Medical Virol 1999; 59:256–261.

Wagener DK, Sacks JM, LaPorte RE, Macgregor JM: The Pittsburgh study of insulin-dependent diabetes mellitus. Risk for diabetes among relatives of IDDM. Diabetes 1982; 31:1115–1118.

Wald NJ, Cuckle H: Maternal serum alpha-fetoprotein measurement in antenatal screening for anencephaly and spina bifida in early pregnancy: United Kingdom Collaborative Study. Lancet 1977; i:1323–1332.

Walton C, Dyer PA, Davidson JA, Harris R, Mallick NP, Oleesky S: HLA antigens and risk factors for nephropathy in type 1 (insulin-dependent) diabetes mellitus. Diabetologia 1984; 27:3–7.

Warram JH, Krolewski AS, Gottlieb MS, Kahn RC: Differences in risk of insulin-dependent diabetes in offspring of diabetic mothers and fathers. N Engl J Med 1984; 311:149–152.

Warram JH, Krolewski AS, Kahn RC: Determinants of IDDM and perinatal mortality in children of diabetic mothers. Diabetes 1988; 37:1328–1334.

Weber B, Burger W, Hartmann R, Hovener G, Malchus R, Oberdisse U: Risk factors for the development of retinopathy in children and adolescents with type 1 (insulin-dependent) diabetes mellitus. Diabetologia 1986; 29:23–29.

Welborn TA, Knuiman M, McCann V, Stanton K, Constable IJ: Clinical macrovascular disease in Caucasoid diabetic subjects: logistic regression analysis of risk variables. Diabetologia 1984; 27:568–573.

Werner N: Blutzuckerregulation und Erbaniage. Dtsch Arch Klin Med 1936; 178:308.

West KM: Epidemiology of Diabetes and Vascular Lesions. New York: Elsevier, 1978.

White P: The inheritance of diabetes. Med Clin North Am 1965; 49:857–863.

Wicker LS, Todd JA, Prins JB, Podolin PL, Renjilian RJ, Peterson LB: Resistance alleles at two non-major histocompatibility complex-linked insulin-dependent diabetes loci on chromosome 3, *Idd3* and *Idd10*, protect nonobese diabetic mice from diabetes. J Exp Med 1994; 180:1705–1713.

Williams RC, Knowler WC, Butler WJ, Pettitt DJ, Lisse JR, Bennett PH, Mann DL, Johnson AH, Terasaki PI: HLA-A2 and type 2 (insulin-independent) diabetes mellitus in Pima Indians: an association of allele frequency with age. Diabetologia 1981; 21:460–463.

Wilson K, Eisenbarth GS: Immunopathogenesis and immunotherapy of type 1 diabetes. Annu Rev Med 1990; 41:497–508.

Winocour PH, Durrington PN, Ishola M, Anderson DC, Cohen H: Influence of proteinuria on vascular disease, blood pressure, and lipoproteins in insulin dependent diabetes mellitus. BMJ 1987; 294:1648–1651.

Winter WE, MacLaren NK, Riley WJ, Clarke DW, Kappy MS, Spillar RP: Maturity-onset diabetes of youth in black Americans. N Engl J Med 1987; 316:285–291.

Wiseman M, Viberti G, Mackintosh D, Jarrett RJ, Keen H: Glycaemia, arterial pressure and micro-albuminuria in type 1 (insulin-dependent) diabetes mellitus. Diabetologia 1984; 26:401–405.

Wolf E, Spencer KM, Cudworth AG: The genetic susceptiblity to type 1 (insulin-

dependent) diabetes: analysis of the HLA-DR association. Diabetologia 1983; 24:224–230.
Wooley PH, Griffin J, Panayi GS, Batchelor JR, Welsh KI, Gibson TJ: HLA-DR antigens and toxic reaction to sodium aurothiomalate and D-penicillamine in patients with rheumatoid arthritis. N Engl J Med 1980; 303:300–302.
Working Party, College of General Practitioners: Family history of diabetes. BMJ 1965; i:960–962.
Yoon JW: Induction and prevention of type 1 diabetes mellitus by viruses. Diabetes Metab 1992; 18:378–386.
Yoon JW, Austin M, Onodera T, Notkins AL: Virus-induced diabetes mellitus: isolation of a virus from the pancreas of a child with diabetic ketoacidosis. N Engl J Med 1979; 300:1173–1179.
Yoon JW, Cha CY, Jordan GW: The role of interferon in virus-induced diabetes. J Infect Dis 1983; 147:155–159.
Yoon JW, McClintock PR, Onodera T, Notkins AL: Virus-induced diabetes mellitus. XVIII: Inhibition by a non-diabetogenic variant of encephalomyocarditis virus. J Exp Med 1980; 152:878–882.
Yoon JW, Notkins AL: Virus-induced diabetes mellitus. VI: Genetically determined host differences in the replication of encephalomyocarditis virus in pancreatic beta cells. J Exp Med 1976; 143:1170–1185.
Yoon JW, Ray UR: Perspectives on the role of viruses in insulin-dependent diabetes. Diabetes 1985; 8:39–44.
Yoon JW, Rodriques MM, Currier C, Notkins AL: Long-term complications of virus-induced diabetes mellitus in mice. Nature 1982; 296:566–569.
Yui MA, Muralidharan K, Moreno-Altamirano B, Perrin G, Chestnut K, Wakeland EK: Production of congenic mouse strains carrying NOD-derived diabetogenic genetic intervals: an approach for the genetic dissection of complex traits. Mamm Genome 1996; 7:331–334.
Zanchi A, Moczulski DK, Hanna LS, Wantman M, Warram JH, Krolewski AS: Risk of advanced diabetic nephropathy in type 1 diabetes is associated with endothelial nitric oxide synthase gene polymorphism. Kidney Int 2000; 57:405–413.
Zander E, Schulz B, Mester J, Jutzi E, Templin R, Conde N: The progression of diabetic nephropathy in type I diabetics: relationship to metabolic control and blood pressure. J Diabetes Complications 1987; 1:53–57.
Ziegler AG, Standl E, Albert E, Mehnert H: HLA-associated insulin autoantibody formation in newly diagnosed type I diabetic patients. Diabetes 1991; 40:1146–1149.
Zimmet P: Epidemiology of diabetes and its macrovascular manifestations in Pacific population—the medical effects of social progress. Diabetes Care 1979; 2:144–153.

22 Type 2 Diabetes Mellitus

STEVEN C. ELBEIN, KEN C. CHIU, AND M. ALAN PERMUTT

Diabetes mellitus encompasses a number of metabolic diseases of diverse pathophysiology that result in hyperglycemia. As a consequence of this hyperglycemia, perhaps with modifying genetic factors, individuals with diabetes of any cause are at risk for microvascular complications (retinopathy, nephropathy, and neuropathy) and at markedly increased risk of macrovascular complications (cerebrovascular events and coronary heart disease). This chapter will review the definition, epidemiology, pathophysiology, and known genetic basis for the most common form of diabetes mellitus, Type 2 diabetes (T2DM). In contrast to Type 1 diabetes (T1DM), that involves autoimmune β-cell destruction, nearly complete or total absence of insulin secretion, and a tendency to ketoacidosis in the absence of insulin therapy, T2DM is itself a diverse disease with variable presentation, variable prevalence among different populations, and variable degrees of insulin deficiency and impaired insulin action. The genetic basis for this disease will show similar diversity—a prediction that is supported by growing data on T2DM susceptibility from multiple populations. However, as of this writing, available studies have only hinted at the full complexity of the genetic basis of typical T2DM.

DISEASE DEFINITION

From 1979 until 1997, the definition of diabetes rested on two similar sets of criteria: the National Diabetes Data Group (1979) and the World Health Organization (Harris et al., 1997). These criteria diagnosed diabetes based on a fasting glucose in excess of 140 mg/dl (6.1 mmol/l), or a glucose 2 hours following a 75 g oral glucose load in excess of 200 mg/dl (11.1 mmol/l). Both criteria also included an intermediate category with increased risk of cardiovascular disease and a high risk of future diabetes (progression at 5%/year) called impaired glucose tolerance (IGT). For the simpler World Health Organization criteria (Harris et al., 1985, 1997), IGT was characterized by normal fasting glucose but a 2-hour post-challenge glucose concentration between 140 mg/dl (6.1 mmol/l) and 200 mg/dl (11.1 mmol/l). Under National Diabetes Data Group criteria, IGT required an additional glucose in excess of 200 mg/dl (11.1 mmol/l), and those failing this additional criterion were designated as indeterminate.

In addition to IGT, the National Diabetes Data Group recognized five types of diabetes: insulin-dependent diabetes mellitus (IDDM), non-insulin-dependent diabetes mellitus (NIDDM), gestational diabetes mellitus (GDM), malnutrition-related diabetes mellitus, and all other types of diabetes. Although the terms insulin-dependent and non-insulin-dependent diabetes were not intended to refer to treatment, this was a constant source of confusion. Nonetheless, this classification recognized the broad separation between early-onset, autoimmune diabetes (IDDM) and later onset, far more common, and generally non-autoimmune diabetes (NIDDM). This classification is the basis for most ongoing studies. In 1997, an expert committee assembled by the American Diabetes Association proposed a new set of criteria and an updated classification (Expert Committee on the Diagnosis and Classification of Diabetes Mellitus, 1997). The new report recommends several changes. First, the old terminology is abandoned. The form of diabetes due primarily to β-cell failure and which results in ketoacidosis is now called Type 1 diabetes. The more prevalent, later-onset form of diabetes that results from a combination of insulin resistance and defective insulin secretion is now called T2DM. These terms will be used in this chapter. In addition, the new recommendations retain the categories of gestational diabetes mellitus (glucose intolerance first recognized during pregnancy, which brings a high risk of future T2DM) and IGT based on the oral glucose tolerance test.

Controversially, however, the new classification lowered the fasting glucose at which diabetes may be diagnosed from 140 mg/dl to 126 mg/dl. Thus, under the new criteria, only a glucose below 110 mg/dl (mmol/l) is considered normal. A fasting glucose between 110 mg/dl and 126 mg/dl is now called impaired fasting glucose (IFG), and a fasting glucose over 126 mg/dl and confirmed on a second day or by an independent test (such as a 75 g glucose tolerance test) is considered to be diabetes. This reclassification will have little effect on studies in most populations that used the oral glucose tolerance test to diagnose diabetes, but it will increase the number of diabetic subjects diagnosed by fasting glucose testing alone.

Clinical Presentation

T2DM often goes undetected, and diagnosis is made only by detecting hyperglycemia on fasting or random glucose. As much as 50% of T2DM may be undiagnosed (Harris, 1993), and onset may occur as much as 7 years before diagnosis (Harris et al., 1992). Most individuals with T2DM are obese. The onset is typically between the ages of 40 and 60 years. Those patients who are symptomatic present much like Type 1 diabetes, with polydipsia, polyuria, polyphagia, weight loss, and blurred vision. On occasion, particularly in elderly patients, the presentation may be in acute diabetic hyperosmolar coma with extremely high glucose levels and dehydration. Still more rarely, patients may present in diabetic ketoacidosis, although this presentation occurs almost exclusively among minority populations, particularly African American patients who have no evidence of autoimmunity. These subjects with atypical or "flatbush" diabetes present with an initial insulin secretory defect and insulin resistance, followed subsequently by improved insulin secretion; subsequent management and phenotype is typical of Type 2 diabetes, and patients are often managed with oral hypoglycemic agents (Banerji et al., 1994, 1995; Umpierrez et al., 1999). An additional atypical presentation of Type 2 diabetes has been seen in recent years. Increasingly, T2DM is observed in adolescent youth, often at or near the onset of puberty. Presentation is typical of Type 2 diabetes with obesity, often acanthosis nigricans, and generally in minority populations (Arslanian, 2000). Both the obesity and lack of autosomal dominant inheritance distinguish this form of diabetes from maturity onset diabetes of the young (see below); the etiology of this growing problem remains an enigma.

T2DM may be treated with oral sulfonylurea agents and other insulin secretagogues, which improve insulin secretion; oral "insulin sensitizers" such as biguanides (metformin), which act primarily to reduce hepatic glucose production (metformin); or most recently agonists of peroxisome proliferator activator receptor γ (PPARγ), such as the thiazolidinediones rosiglitazone and pioglitzaone, which primarily improve peripheral insulin action. Increasingly, combinations of these therapies are used to achieve synergistic effects. When oral treatments fail, insulin therapy is often instituted either alone or in combination with one or more oral therapies to achieve good glucose control. Both potential treatments and treatment regimens continue to proliferate. Importantly, insulin-treated individuals taken off insulin may experience very high glucoses, but typically do not develop diabetic ketoacidosis.

Subtypes of Diabetes

As we discuss above, two major classes of diabetes have been retained in recent recommendations of the Expert Committee on the Diagnosis and Classification of Diabetes Mellitus: type 1 diabetes (T1DM), marked by β-cell destruction of either autoimmune or idiopathic etiologies; and Type 2 diabetes (T2DM), the subject of this chapter. In previous classification schemes, maturity onset diabetes of the young (MODY) (Fajans, 1990) was considered to be a subtype of T2DM. In the most recent recommendations, subtypes with known genetic etiologies including MODY were not included under T2DM (Expert Committee on the Diagnosis and Classification of Diabetes Mellitus, 1997). Nonetheless, the physiology of these subtypes is often similar to more typical T2DM and will be included as such in this chapter. Although no other subgroups of T2DM have been suggested at this writing, other subgroups (mitochondrial diabetes; see below) clearly exist, and ongoing studies are likely to define additional genetic etiologies. A third major category is gestational diabetes mellitus (GDM), which appears to increase the risk of T2DM and may be an early manifestation of that disease (Peters et al., 1996). Diabetes fitting neither T1DM nor T2DM subgroups may be associated with a variety of other endocrine disorders, pharmacologic agents, infections, or a number of rare genetic diseases. Furthermore, as discussed above, diabetes may present with ketoacidosis but subsequently not reflect typical T2DM, or it may present in youth. The evolving recognition of these atypical presentations is not reflected in the current classification scheme, and no genetic studies of these entities have yet been performed. This chapter will cover only the pathophysiology and genetics of T2DM and subtypes that may be reasonably considered to fit under this broad umbrella.

TYPE 2 DIABETES AS A COMPLEX, INHERITED DISEASE

Evidence for Inheritance

Although environmental factors are usually required for the development of overt diabetes, genetic influence is clearly supported by three types of data: twin studies, familial aggregation of the disease, and different prevalence among various ethnic groups.

Twin Studies

Twin studies are an important approach of assessing the genetic influence in the etiology of a disease. Since monozygotic twins are genetically identical and dizygotic twins share no more genetic material than do siblings, a higher concordance rate in monozygotic twins than in dizygotic twins suggests that genetic influence plays an important role in the etiology of the disease. Several twin studies of T2DM have assessed its heritability. Pyke et al. (1976) reported a concordance rate of 100% in monozygotic twins whose diabetes was diagnosed after the age of 50. The concordance rate of T2DM in monozygotic twins increases with the number of years of follow-up (Tattersall and Pyke, 1972; Newman et al., 1987). In the National Heart, Lung, Blood Institute twin study (Newman et al., 1987), the concordance rate in monozygotic twins increased from 29% at the first examination (age of subjects: 42–55 years old) to 58% at the second examination (age of subjects: 52–65 years old). The Finnish Study (Kaprio et al., 1992) had the shortest period of follow-up and reported the lowest concordant rate of 34%. Almost all the twin studies reported a concordance rate of 50% or more in monozygotic twins with an average rate of 58.8%. In contrast, the concordance rate in dizygotic twins is 40% or less, with an average rate of 26.8% (Tattersall and Pyke, 1972; Pyke et al., 1976; Tattersall et al., 1980; Newman et al., 1987; Kaprio et al., 1992; Poulsen et al., 1999). A higher concordance rate in monozygotic twins than in dizygotic twins supports the role of inheritance in T2DM.

Prevalence among Different Ethnic Groups

The different prevalence of T2DM among various ethnic groups provides additional support for the genetic influence of the disease. The highest prevalence (50%) was noted in Pima Indians in Arizona (Knowler et al., 1990), followed by Nauruans in the South Pacific at 40%; in contrast, diabetes is almost absent among the non-Austronesian Melanesian people of Papua New Guinea (Zimmet et al., 1990). Similarly, the prevalence of diabetes varies among ethnic groups in the United States: 6.2% in whites, 9.3% in Cuban Americans, 10.2% in African Americans, 13% in Mexican Americans, 13.4% in Puerto Rican Americans (Harris, 1991), and 50% in certain Native Americans (Knowler et al., 1990).

Studies of genetically admixed populations also support the concept that diabetes is a genetic disease. The prevalence of T2DM among Mexican Americans parallels the proportion of Native American genetic admixture (Gardner et al., 1984; Hanis et al., 1991). Although non-Austronesian Melanesians are resistant to glucose intolerance (Zimmet and Baba, 1990), Melanesians with approximately 50% Austronesian and 50% non-Austronesian admixture have the second highest prevalence of glucose intolerance in the south Pacific region (King et al., 1984). Thus, moderate Austronesian admixture results in a significantly increased risk of T2DM.

Familial Aggregation

Family clustering is also observed in patients with T2DM. Although there is a wide range of variation in reports of the prevalence of positive family history of T2DM, it has been our experience that positive response rates increase as inquiry is made to investigate the family history of T2DM by specifying parents, grandparents, and siblings (S. Elbein, unpublished observations). A family history of diabetes has been shown to be a risk factor for T2DM within various ethnic groups (Knowler et al., 1990; Zimmet et al., 1990; Hanis et al., 1991). In African Americans, 83% of patients have a positive family history of diabetes, while only 37% of nondiabetic subjects report a positive family history (Chiu et al., 1992). The prevalence of T2DM in Pima Indians was as high as 80% in the subjects with both parents having early onset of diabetes (Knowler et al., 1990).

"Thrifty Genotype" Hypothesis

To explain the apparent increasing prevalence of T2DM worldwide, Neel (1999) proposed the "thrifty genotype" hypothesis. He suggested that the accumulation of diabetes gene(s) resulted from natural selection that favored energy storage as a defense against famine in the "hunter-gathering" era when food intake was irregular. The hypothesis suggested that with a constant food supply and an abundance of high-fat, energy-dense food sources, these genes have become a liability, resulting in obesity, insulin resistance, and T2DM.

"Thrifty Phenotype" Hypothesis

In contrast to the "thrifty genotype" hypothesis (Neel, 1999), Hales and Bankert (1992) proposed a "thrifty phenotype" hypothesis. They suggested a key role for nutritionally induced changes in fetal and infantile β-cell development. When nutrition becomes abundant and insulin resistance develops in later adult life, the increased demand for insulin exceeds the compromised β-cell capacity, resulting in impaired glucose tolerance or overt diabetes. Subsequently, "thrifty phenotype" was also applied to insulin resistance (Phillips et al., 1994) and the insulin resistance syndrome (Barker et al., 1993; Barker and Clark, 1997; Leon et al., 1996, 1998; Valdez et al., 1994).

Since birth records and weight at 1 year of age were available for those born in Hertfordshire, England, after 1911, Barker et al. (1989) were able to show a correlation of fetal and infantile growth retardation with increased prevalence of glucose intolerance and death rates from cardiovascular disease in adult life. A similar association was noted in Pima Indians (McCance et al., 1994), Mexican American and non-Hispanic white populations (Valdez et al., 1994), Swedish men (Leon et al., 1996; Lithell et al., 1996), schoolchildren in Jamaica (Forrester et al., 1996), health professionals in the United States (Curhan et al., 1996), and twins in Denmark (Poulsen et al., 1997).

In addition to compromised insulin secretory capacity, early nutritional deprivation may result in later insulin resistance. Phillips et al. (1994) examined 103 adult patients by insulin tolerance test, and showed an association of low ponderal index (birth weight/length^3) at birth with adult insulin resistance. Likewise, Martyn et al. (1998) showed that elevated fasting insulin levels in adults (a measure of insulin resistance) were inversely correlated with abdominal circumference at birth. Studies in rodents suggested a role for the liver in the effect of fetal nutrition on adult glucose tolerance. In laboratory rats, partial protein deprivation during pregnancy and lactation led to a 50% increase of hepatic glucokinase activity and 100% decrease of hepatic phosphenolpyruvate carboxykinase (Desai et al., 1997a). Protein restriction was associated with increased hepatic lobular volume, as well as with reduced perivenous concentration of glucokinase and decreased glucose uptake in the distal perivenous region. Consequently, hepatic glucose production was increased through decreased hepatic glucose uptake and increased gluconeogenesis (Burns et al., 1997). These mice exhibited hepatic insulin resistance to suppression of glucose output and hyperinsulinemia (Desai et al., 1997b). Maternal protein deprivation also caused altered islet structure (Berney et al., 1997) and reduced β-cell proliferation, islet size, and vascularization (Dahri et al., 1991). As might be anticipated, the offspring had reduced insulin secretion and reduced glucose tolerance. Whether these models of malnutrition explain the high prevalence of diabetes among various ethnic groups seems unlikely but remains to be determined by more careful studies.

Environmental Factors

The prevalence of T2DM differs with economic development in the world. While T2DM was absent or rare in traditional communities and in developing countries, the prevalence may increase over 2-fold in urban populations of similar genetic background (King and Rewers, 1993). The most dramatic example is the study of Aboriginal Australians, who developed diabetes while living in an urbanized environment: these individuals showed a marked improvement in carbohydrate and lipid metabolism after 7 weeks of a traditional hunter-gathering life style (O'Dea, 1984). Modernization has resulted in other changes, as outlined below.

Increased Longevity/Aging

The prevalence of diabetes increases with age (Harris, 1991). In underdeveloped regions, communicable diseases and natural disasters shorten life span, thus diminishing the development of diabetes. Modernization, with improved living conditions and the introduction of modern health care systems, prolongs life expectancy and permits later onset of diabetes.

Sedentary Lifestyle

In less-developed regions, most of the physical activity is derived from agricultural practices and food gathering. The developed economy is associated with a sedentary lifestyle and physical inactivity, which is a major risk factor for T2DM. This phenomena is seen in Mauritius, where the three major ethnic groups (Chinese, Indians, and Creoles) have a similar high prevalence of diabetes and where physical inactivity is an independent risk factor for all three groups (Dowse et al., 1991).

Dietary Change

Diet has long been implicated as a risk factor for diabetes. In agricultural regions, the traditional high-carbohydrate, high-fiber, low-fat diet consists largely of vegetable sources supplemented by a small quantity of wild game (Knowler et al., 1990; Zimmet and Baba, 1990). Financial rewards from modernization have resulted in a calorie-dense diet with refined carbohydrates, increased animal products, higher fat, and lower fiber. The resulting increased calories and increased dietary fat, along with the sedentary lifestyle, leads to obesity, particularly upper-body obesity, which is a strong risk factor for diabetes (Harris, 1990;

Knowler et al., 1990; Zimmet and Baba, 1990; Dowse et al., 1991; Bolton-Smith and Woodward, 1994).

The role of diet in glucose tolerance has been evaluated further in clinical trials. Brunzell and colleagues (1971) showed that a high-carbohydrate/low-fat diet improved glucose tolerance in mild diabetes. In non-diabetic elderly men (age 70–74 years), Chen et al. (1988) observed a 30% improvement in insulin sensitivity and a 150% improvement in the second-phase insulin response when dietary carbohydrate was increased from 49% (35% fat) to 85% (0% fat).

TYPE 2 DIABETES AS A COMPLEX GENETIC DISEASE

By definition, a complex disease results from the interaction of more than one gene and the environment. Although familial clustering has been noted, inheritance is non-Mendelian. Any single genetic defect may increase the susceptibility to the disease but may not be sufficient to cause the disease unless other genetic defects or environmental factors are present. For example, glucokinase mutations result in mild fasting hyperglycemia, but only 46% of carriers develop overt diabetes. This incomplete penetrance probably exemplifies most forms of T2DM.

Heterogeneity

Phenotypic (clinical) and genotypic (genetic) heterogeneity exist in T2DM. Both contribute to the complexity of the disease and provide challenges for genetic studies of T2DM. We discuss both, although a single major gene defect such as hepatocyte nuclear factor 1α (see below) may show a variable phenotype, depending on the precise mutation and perhaps other interactions. That phenotypic heterogeneity reflects an underlying genotypic heterogeneity in T2DM remains to be determined, but experience from both MODY and other complex diseases suggests that genotype–phenotype correlations will be incomplete at best.

Clinical Heterogeneity

The spectrum of clinical presentations may range from asymptomatic hyperglycemia to profound polyuria, polyphagia, polydipsia, and weight loss. The apparent decline of β-cell function in diabetic individuals is variable. In some patients the diabetes remains stable with diet alone, while other patients may require oral hypoglycemic agents to maintain normal blood glucose. About 50% of patients have progressive β-cell failure and eventually require insulin. A small subset of patients have a very rapid decline of β-cell function and require insulin treatment within a relatively short period of time. An unknown number of these patients with β-cell failure may have autoimmune diabetes (see below). Insulin sensitivity is also variable in patients with T2DM.

Diabetic complications develop in fewer than 50% of patients with T2DM, but some individuals develop diabetic retinopathy or nephropathy within a few years of diagnosis, despite excellent glycemic control. In contrast, some patients with poor glycemic control experience no microvascular complications. Family history is one determinant of diabetic nephropathy (see below).

Genetic Heterogeneity

Two forms of genetic heterogeneity may be distinguished: locus heterogeneity and allelic heterogeneity. Locus heterogeneity is the result of multiple loci, resulting in indistinguishable phenotypes. One example, MODY, in which at least five genes have been identified, is described below. Locus heterogeneity also appears to exist in late-onset T2DM, as described in detail below, although only one locus has been confirmed to date.

Allelic heterogeneity refers to multiple mutations at a single locus. For example, over 30 mutations have been described in the glucokinase gene (*MODY2*) on chromosome 7p, and even more variation has been observed in *HNF1*α (*MODY3*), as described below. Allelic heterogeneity may also involve different genes at the same genetic locus. Persistent hyperinsulinemic hypoglycemia of infancy (PHHI) was localized by linkage to chromosome 11p15.1 (Glaser et al., 1994). This locus encompasses both the sulfonylurea receptor (SUR) and the β-cell inward rectifier potassium channel (Kir6.2), and mutations in either gene result in the same phenotype familial hyperinsulinism.

Interactions between Genes

The interaction between genes can be characterized as epistatic, additive, or a combination of both. A possible epistatic model for diabetes might involve defects leading to both impaired insulin secretion and impaired insulin action (see below). While neither defect alone is likely to cause diabetes, the interaction between these defects could result in overt diabetes. Murine models reviewed below confirm the feasibility of this model. Under a pure additive model, each locus acts separately without interaction. For example, a defect in insulin secretion might explain one subset of diabetes, while a defect in insulin action might explain a second subset. A purely additive model appears to fit MODY, where multiple different genetic loci individually cause diabetes through a defect in insulin secretion (see below). For typical T2DM, a combination of different loci that in some cases interact (epistasis) is more likely than a simple model.

Degree of Genetic Influence

A widely used strategy to map the genes in a complex disease is the allele sharing among affected siblings, or "affected sib pair" (ASP) method. This method was used to map the susceptible loci for T1DM (Davies et al., 1994; Hashimoto et al., 1994). Advantages of the design are that model parameters need not be specified, penetrance does not complicate the analysis, and only affected siblings need to be recruited. On the other hand, allele sharing methods are less powerful than LOD score (parametric) methods in many settings, and the power depends on the underlying model even when no specific model is specified.

If one has an ideal map of genetic markers, key factors that determine power to detect linkage of a complex disease are λ_s (the ratio of the risk of diabetes for the sibling of a proband to the population risk), the number of genes involved, the type of interaction between genes and the sample size. As λ_s for any given gene decreases, the sample size required to map that gene increases. In contrast to T1DM (λ_s being 6%/0.4%, or about 15), the total λ_s of T2DM has been estimated at 2.5 to 3.5 (Rich, 1990).

Another way to estimate the genetic influence is to calculate the relative risk from the concordance rates between monozygotic and dizygotic twins (Newman et al., 1987; Kaprio et al., 1992; Poulsen et al., 1999). In contrast with T1DM, where the relative risk has been estimated at 4.93, the relative risk for T2DM ranges from 3.35 to 1.34, with an average of 2.10. Nevertheless, concordance in identical twins approaches 90% in

T2DM and is below 50% in T1DM, thus suggesting a smaller environmental component and higher penetrance in T2DM than in T1DM.

Pathogenesis of Type 2 Diabetes

The reader desiring a more extensive review of the pathogenesis of T2DM is advised to consult one of the several excellent reviews (e.g., DeFronzo et al., 1992). T2DM results from an imbalance between insulin sensitivity and insulin secretion, and either factor or both may be inherited (DeFronzo, 1997). Both tissue sensitivity to insulin and β-cell function are in a dynamic state of flux in T2DM. Insulin resistance may lead to the development of a defect in insulin secretion, and, similarly, impaired β-cell function can lead to a disturbance in insulin action (Moller and Flier, 1991; DeFronzo et al., 1992; Dinneen et al., 1992). Glucose itself may cause defects in insulin secretion and insulin action that may improve when hyperglycemia is treated (Gumbiner et al., 1990; Rossetti et al., 1990).

Insulin Resistance in the Pathogenesis of Type 2 Diabetes

Both longitudinal and cross-sectional studies have demonstrated that insulin resistance and hyperinsulinemia (Haffner et al., 1988; Gulli et al., 1992; Martin et al., 1992; Zimmet et al., 1999) are early detectable abnormalities in individuals at risk for T2DM. Furthermore, analyses of segregation and heritability in family studies have suggested that insulin resistance and hyperinsulinemia are inherited in a Mendelian fashion (Bogardus et al., 1989; Schumacher et al., 1992; Sakul et al., 1997). Martin et al. (1992) showed that insulin resistance preceded and predicted diabetes in offspring of two diabetic parents, and this conclusion has been supported in longitudinal studies of Pima Indians (Saad et al., 1988; Lillioja et al., 1993; Weyer et al., 1999).

Site(s) of Primary Insulin Resistance

Considerable evidence points to a target tissue defect in muscle insulin action as the major cause of insulin resistance in T2DM (Olefsky, 1995; DeFronzo, 1997). Glycolysis, glycogen synthesis, and glucose oxidation are all decreased (DeFronzo et al., 1992). Because hyperinsulinemia (258 pM) normalizes glycogen synthesis and total flux through glycolysis, but does not restore the normal distribution between oxidative and non-oxidative glycolysis (Del Prato et al., 1994), a defect in the partitioning of glycolytic flux between glucose oxidation and non-oxidative glycolysis has been suggested. The data are most consistent with a defect in the early stages of glucose metabolism such as glucose transport or glucose phosphorylation (DeFronzo et al., 1992; Rothman et al., 1995; DeFronzo, 1997). Studies of various candidate genes based on these hypotheses are described below.

In addition to the peripheral defect in insulin action that resides primarily in muscle, diabetes is characterized by diminished hepatic insulin action. Although diminished insulin suppression of hepatic glucose output is typical of the diabetic patient, systemic hyperinsulinemia and peripheral insulin resistance might be related to hepatic function. The liver normally extracts ~50% of insulin on its first pass. Hepatic bypass by way of pancreatic venous diversion in dogs leads to systemic hyperinsulinemia, which was shown to cause peripheral insulin resistance (decreased insulin-stimulated glucose deposition) (Miles et al., 1998), albeit with normal intravenous glucose tolerance. Glucose disposal in this model was decreased 30% due to post-receptor mechanisms.

β-Cell Compensation and Decompensation

Chiu and colleagues (2000) studied 26 glucose tolerant and normotensive subjects using a hyperglycemic clamp technique to assess both insulin sensitivity and β-cell function (first and second phase insulin responses). Both first- and second-phase insulin responses were tightly correlated with the insulin sensitivity index ($p = .001$ and $p < .001$, respectively). As insulin sensitivity index decreased (more insulin resistance), an increased β-cell response maintained glucose homeostasis. This relationship was also observed in a cross-sectional study by Kahn et al. (1993). However, in studies by Chiu et al. (2000), the insulin sensitivity index accounted for part but not all of the variance in β-cell function (36.3% for first phase and 51.2% for second-phase insulin responses). In studies of 126 members of 26 familial T2DM kindreds, Elbein et al. (2000b) observed a relationship between insulin sensitivity and first-phase insulin secretion that was similar to that observed by Kahn et al. (1993) in a normal population, but family members showed a markedly diminished compensation for decreased insulin sensitivity. Furthermore, the compensatory response of the β-cell to increase insulin secretion in response to the decreased insulin sensitivity of obesity failed in family members, whereas this response was normal in a control population without a family history of diabetes (Elbein et al., 2000b). Both genetic and environmental factors—and perhaps their interaction—are likely to account for these observations. Because of the compensatory increase in insulin secretion by the pancreas, insulin resistance alone is probably not sufficient to cause glucose intolerance, providing that pancreatic β-cells are able to respond with increased fasting and stimulated plasma insulin responses (Bergman, 1989). In cross-sectional studies, fasting insulin levels peak with a fasting glucose level of 140 mg/dl, but subsequently decline despite increasing plasma glucose (DeFronzo et al., 1992). Furthermore, in non-diabetic subjects (IGT and glucose tolerant), 30-minute insulin levels during oral glucose tolerance tests are inversely correlated with fasting glucose levels (Mitrakou et al., 1992). These results suggest that β-cell dysfunction is present in individuals with IGT as well as overt diabetes (Elbein et al., 2000b; Kahn, 2000). Furthermore, secondary insulin resistance and β-cell dysfunction may develop from hyperglycemia (Moller and Flier, 1991; DeFronzo et al., 1992; Dinneen et al., 1992; Del Prato et al., 1994). Thus, IGT and overt diabetes develop with β-cell failure, which, in turn, may result from glucose toxicity (Rossetti et al., 1990), an inherited genetic defect (Hattersley et al., 1992), or a combination of both.

Primary Defect in Type 2 Diabetes

Since fasting insulin concentration correlates well with the insulin sensitivity index, many epidemiological studies have used fasting insulin as a measure of insulin sensitivity. Based on such cross-sectional analyses, insulin resistance was detectable even before the development of overt diabetes, leading to the proposal that insulin resistance is the primary defect of T2DM.

Assessment of β-cell function is more difficult, and fewer investigators have examined β-cell function. Pimenta et al. (1995) showed a lower β-cell response in non-diabetic subjects with a diabetic first-degree relative than in individuals without a diabetic first-degree relative, but with no difference in insulin sensitivity. Their conclusions are supported by recent studies in Pima Indians (Sakul et al., 1997) and in Utah Caucasians (Elbein et al., 1999) that show strong heritability of insulin secretion when the response to insulin sensitivity is considered. A number of other studies support these conclusions (Dunaif and Finegood, 1996; Watanabe et al., 1999; Larsson and Ahren, 2000; Arslanian et al., 2001). Thus, while many studies support an early, inherited, and in some cases predictive role for insulin resistance in T2DM, many studies also support an early and inherited role for β-cell dysfunction. Genetic studies thus must determine whether the phenotypic defects result from a single genetic defect with pleiotropic effects on insulin sensitivity and secretion, a primary defect in insulin sensitivity that secondarily induces β-cell failure, a primary defect in β-cell function, or an oligogenic model in which both defects in insulin action and secretion are required to develop diabetes. Rodent models that begin to address these issues are discussed below.

Natural History of β-Cell Dysfunction and Insulin Sensitivity

The natural history of the β-cell function in T2DM has not been examined extensively until the United Kingdom Prospective Diabetes Study (1995; UKPDS), which recruited 5102 newly diagnosed T2DM subjects between 1977 and 1991. Fasting plasma glucose and insulin levels were assessed periodically, and insulin sensitivity and secretion were calculated from fasting plasma glucose and insulin levels using the homeostasis model assessment (HOMA) method (Matthews et al., 1985) during a 6-year follow-up period for those subjects who did not receive insulin treatment. These studies revealed that overt diabetes developed when β-cell function declined to about 50% of normal. β-cell function deteriorated significantly over 6 years in subjects who remained on diet therapy to 51%, 53%, and 28% at 0, 1, and 6 years, respectively. In subjects who initiated and remained on sulfonylurea therapy, insulin secretion increased from 46% to 78% in the first year after initiation of treatment but also declined subsequently to 52% at 6 years. A similar trend was seen in individuals treated with metformin, with an initial increase (51% to 66%) but eventual decline to 38% at 6 years. Regardless of the mode of treatment, β-cell function declined at a rate of 5% per year. Extrapolating from the 376 subjects in the diet-controlled group, β-cell function began to decline at -8.9 years before the diagnosis of overt diabetes and β-cell exhaustion would be predicted to occur at 11.9 years after the diagnosis of overt diabetes. These observations are consistent with the cross-sectional data that suggest an onset of T2DM at least 7 years before the clinical diagnosis of the disease, and that most patients will require pharmacologic therapy 8 to 10 years after diagnosis (Clauson et al., 1994). In contrast, insulin sensitivity in the UKPDS was relatively stable during the same time period (United Kingdom Prospective Diabetes Study, 1995). Whether treatment during the pre-diabetic period will diminish the rate of β-cell failure and, thus, overt diabetes is being evaluated by the NIH-sponsored Diabetes Prevention Program.

GENE IDENTIFICATION IN TYPE 2 DIABETES

Genetic studies of T2DM have been ongoing for nearly two decades. Until recently, most studies focused on candidate genes, as each gene in the pathway of insulin action or insulin secretion was cloned. Initially, these candidate gene studies were mostly association (case-control) studies (Rotwein et al., 1981) and may have been flawed because of admixture and spurious associations. In the last few years, linkage and molecular scanning techniques have become common; with the exception of glucokinase (see below), these techniques have had limited success. More recently, genome scanning methods have become a major focus in both academic and commercial laboratories. At least one susceptibility gene has been localized and cloned as a result of such studies (Hanis et al., 1996; Horikawa et al., 2000), and other regions appear promising (see below). Nonetheless, these studies have also demonstrated that the complexity of T2DM will make identification of susceptibility genes challenging. In contrast, major single-gene defects have been identified in the subset of diabetes with autosomal dominant inheritance (MODY). While such forms of diabetes are uncommon, they represent an unquestionable success of the genetic approach.

In this section, we review the single-gene causes of diabetes, candidate gene studies using association, linkage, and molecular scanning methods, and finally the current status of genome-wide scans. Because of the large number of negative studies and the growing number of candidate genes, a full review of all candidate gene studies is impossible. The reader is also cautioned that any textbook review is necessarily dated by the time of publication in this rapidly moving field. We concentrate on seminal studies of important candidates and studies that have at least appeared positive in some populations.

Single-Gene Causes of Type 2 Diabetes

Maturity Onset Diabetes of the Young (MODY)

The existence of large families with diabetes in multiple generations and with onset before age 25 was first noted by Fajans et al. (1996) and was denoted "maturity onset diabetes of the young." The disease was thought initially to represent mild diabetes, usually managed without insulin and with onset at an age that overlapped that of T1DM. In long-term prospective studies, many of these patients have indeed developed severe diabetes complications. The disease is characterized by autosomal dominant inheritance with high penetrance and early onset. Best studied is the large R–W kindred, carefully followed for several decades by Fajans. Studies of this family led to identification of the first diabetes locus, designated *MODY1*, by linkage to a region of chromosome 20q near the adenosine deaminase (ADA) locus (Bell et al., 1991; Bowden et al., 1992). However, few other families showed linkage to this region, and the identification of *hepatocyte nuclear factor 4α* (HNF4α) as the responsible gene (Yamagata et al., 1996a) awaited further clues.

The first MODY gene actually identified was based on candidate gene studies of glucokinase (Permutt et al., 1992), the rate-limiting step in β-cell glucose metabolism and the proposed glucose sensor for the β-cell (Matschinsky et al., 1993). Although this locus is known as *MODY2*, a more appropriate classification might be "diabetes due to glucokinase gene mutations." The glucokinase gene was first implicated by linkage in French families in which diabetes was defined as fasting hyperglycemia at 2 SD above normal, and MODY was defined as diabetes with onset before age 25 in one family member (Froguel et al., 1992, 1993). In subsequent studies, mutations were described throughout the glucokinase gene in French families (Froguel et al., 1993; Froguel, 1996), accounting for approximately 50% of French maturity onset diabetes of the young. No single mutation is common, which makes screening difficult. Although glucokinase mutations are unusual outside of France, they have been described also in British MODY families (Hattersley et al., 1992). As predicted by Matschinsky et al. (1993), the physiologic defect is an increase in fasting glucose, with a right shift of the glucose/insulin dose response curve (Froguel, 1996; Hattersley, 1998).

In careful physiologic studies (Byrne et al., 1994, 1995; Sturis et al., 1994), the glucokinase mutations caused an altered setpoint for insulin release in response to glucose. Although most studies have emphasized the effects on insulin secretion, Velho et al. (1996b) elegantly demonstrated impaired hepatic glycogen synthesis and augmented hepatic gluconeogenesis in seven glucokinase-deficient subjects. Clinically, glucokinase mutations result in mild diabetes that might easily go undiagnosed. Presentation with gestational diabetes may be common among those with mutations (Saker et al., 1996). Microvascular complications in this form of diabetes are unusual.

The third MODY locus (*MODY3*) was identified in French non-glucokinase MODY families by linkage to markers on chromosome 12q24 (Vaxillaire et al., 1995). This locus accounted for 33% of French MODY diabetes. In subsequent studies, families from Denmark, Germany, and the United States were also linked to a narrow interval near the anonymous marker D12S86 (Velho et al., 1996c). This defect was characterized clinically by severe hyperglycemia and a defect in insulin secretion at high glucose levels even in normoglycemic individuals (Byrne et al., 1996). Yamagata et al. (1996b) subsequently identified a novel pathway for diabetes pathogenesis with the discovery of hepatocyte nuclear factor 1α (*HNF1α*, or *TCF1*) as *MODY3*. This gene, a transcription factor expressed in both hepatocytes and β-cells, is a member of the steroid/thyroid hormone receptor superfamily (Yamagata et al., 1996b). In addition to the mutations originally described by Yamagata and colleagues, mutations have been identified in early onset, autosomal-dominant diabetic kindreds from Japan (Iwasaki et al., 1997), England, (Frayling et al., 1997), France (Vaxillaire et al., 1997), Finland (Glucksmann et al., 1997), Germany (Kaisaki et al., 1997), Denmark (Hansen et al., 1997e), and the United States (Glucksmann et al., 1997). Mutations have been identified in every exon and have included missense, frameshift, and promoter mutations (Ellard, 2000). Whereas each glucokinase mutation has appeared to arise independently (Froguel, 1996), a polycytidine tract in HNF1α exon 4 has lead to the same mutation—the insertion of an extra cytidine (Pro291fsinsC)—in multiple families from unrelated populations (Kaisaki et al., 1997). This region appears to be a mutational hotspot (Glucksmann et al., 1997; Kaisaki et al., 1997), and this mutation is the most common single mutation identified for MODY (Yamagata et al., 1998). Among English families, nine frameshift mutations accounted for 18% of all MODY, of which the single Pro291fsinsC mutation accounted for 13% (Frayling et al., 1997). The mechanism of diabetes pathogenesis from HNF1α mutations remains uncertain. In homozygous HNF1α knockout mice, insulin secretory responses to glucose and arginine were markedly reduced (<15%), but heterozygous mice were not hyperglycemic (Pontoglio et al., 1998). Yamagata et al. (1998) suggested that the common Pro291finsC mutation acted as a dominant negative by forming inactive heterodimers. More recently, promoter mutations were suggested as an additional cause of HNF1α dysfunction (Godart et al., 2000). Additionally, a mutation of the HNF4α binding site in the promoter clearly causes loss of function (Gragnoli et al., 1997).

Using the information from the identification of HNF1α as the *MODY3* gene, Yamagata and colleagues quickly identified the chromosome 20q, *MODY1* locus, as an upstream regulator of HNF1α, hepatocyte nuclear factor 4α (HNF4α, or TCF14). A single nonsense mutation in exon 7 (Gln to stop, Q268X) accounts for diabetes in the extensively studied, large, multigenerational R–W family (Yamagata et al., 1996a). Although this locus is a much less common cause of diabetes than is HNF1α, subsequent studies have identified several additional mutations in HNF4α (Lausen et al., 2000; Tripathy et al., 2000). Furuta et al. (1997) identified an arginine to tryptophan substitution in exon 4 in one of 57 Japanese MODY probands that segregated in three of five diabetics in the family, but with highly variable age of onset. Lindner et al. (1997a) identified a nonsense mutation at codon 154 (R154X) in a German family; Bulman et al. (1997) identified a missense mutation in exon 7 (E276Q) in a large English MODY family; and Hani et al. (1998) identified a missense mutation at codon 393 (V393I) in a single French family with onset before age 45. The nonsense mutation resulted in diminished insulin secretion to oral glucose, but no evidence for hepatic or renal dysfunction. Stoffel and Duncan (1997) showed widespread effects of the original *MODY1* mutation (Q268X) on genes of the glucose-dependent insulin secretion pathway.

Recently, additional rare mutations causing autosomal dominant diabetes have been identified. Using a candidate gene approach and the newly identified hepatocyte nuclear factor pathway, Horikawa and colleagues (1997) screened 57 Japanese MODY subjects for mutations of the gene *HNF1β* (TCF2). HNF1β is a homeodomain transcription factor closely related to HNF1α that appears to heterodimerize with HNF1β. A single nonsense mutation in the arginine at codon 177 in exon 2 (R177X) was identified. Subsequently, Nishigori et al. (1998a) identified a second frameshift mutation (A263fsinsGG) by screening 40 Japanese subjects with onset of T2DM before age 35, and additional variants were later identified by Cao and Hegele (2000) and Costa et al. (2000). Carriers had diabetes onset between ages 19 and 61 and appear to have renal dysfunction. Others have not identified mutations in this gene (Beards et al., 1998). Mutations of *HNF1β* are characterized by renal abnormalities in addition to T2DM (Horikawa et al., 1997; Bingham et al., 2000).

In a different pathway, Stoffers et al. (1997) evaluated the pancreatic homeodomain transcription factor *IPF1* (also known as *PDX1*). This factor regulates both pancreatic development and insulin gene expression. A deletion of a cytosine in exon 1 results in an inactivating mutation (Pro63fsdelC) that caused pancreatic agenesis in a homozygous individual and diabetes in heterozygous family members. As with other MODY mutations, both incomplete penetrance and the presence of phenocopies (diabetic individuals without this mutant allele) complicated the inheritance in this family. However, mutations of this gene appear to be rare in most populations (Chevre et al., 1998; Hara et al., 1998; Hansen et al., 2000b; Frayling et al., 2001). A sixth MODY gene was identified as *NeuroD1/BETA2* gene, in which both a missense and stop mutation were identified (Malecki et al., 1999), although mutations of *NeuroD1* also appear to be rare (Frayling et al., 2001). In a study of 101 Caucasian families from the United Kingdom, Frayling et al. (2001) reported that 63% were traced to mutations of *HNF1α*, 2% to *HNF4α*, 1% to *HNF1β*, and 20% to glucokinase. The other mutations were not detected in this study.

Insulin Gene Mutations

Arguably, the first dominant mutations associated with diabetes were identified in the insulin gene by HPLC before the availability of current molecular techniques (Steiner et al., 1990). Penetrance of insulin gene mutations with respect to diabetes has been variable, however, and most studies examined the intermediate phenotypes of hyperinsulinemia or hyperproinsulinemia. To date, three missense mutations have resulted in insulin with reduced activity: F24S, F25L, and H10D (Steiner et al., 1990). An additional four variants alter the normal cleavage of proinsulin into insulin and C-peptide, resulting in high levels of proinsulin with reduced insulin activity. While most variants alter the dibasic amino acid cleavage site for C-peptide, one mutation (His-B10-Asp) appears to result in secretion of intact proinsulin through the unregulated, constitutive pathway (Carroll et al., 1988). The most common defect is R65H, which has occurred in multiple families from multiple populations (Barbetti et al., 1990). However, such defects are rare and cannot account for a significant percentage of early-onset, dominant diabetes. Furthermore, Roder et al. (1996) later questioned whether the R65H variant was in fact responsible for impaired glucose tolerance, and suggested that the lower biological activity was compensated by the high levels of insulin secretion.

Insulin Receptor Mutations

The insulin receptor consists of a tetramer with two α-chain and two β-chain subunits encoded by a single gene. Taylor et al. (1992) suggested five classes of mutations: impaired receptor biosynthesis, impaired transport to the cell surface, decreased insulin binding, impaired tyrosine kinase activity, and accelerated receptor degradation. Mutations of the α-chain subunits tend to alter insulin binding, while mutations of the β-chain tyrosine kinase region tend to alter insulin action. Although a large number of mutations have been identified throughout the gene, recessive mutations of the α-chain generally result in leprechaunism, while Rabson-Mendenhall syndrome usually results from recessive β-chain defects rather than diabetes. Mutations causing insulin-resistant diabetes have more often been dominant and have impaired tyrosine kinase activity, although insulin-resistant diabetes has been linked to α-subunit mutations (Accili et al., 1989). Clinical features of insulin receptor mutations include hyperinsulinemia, acanthosis nigricans, and polycystic ovary syndrome. Glucose intolerance has been a variable feature of insulin receptor mutations, perhaps because robust pancreatic compensation often overcomes the insulin resistance in heterozygous subjects.

Mitochondrial DNA Mutations

The first mitochondrial mutation causing diabetes was described by Ballinger and colleagues in 1992 as a 10.4 kb deletion that resulted in maternal transmission of diabetes and sensorineural hearing loss. Subsequently, van den Ouweland et al. (1992) described in a Dutch family what is now the most prevalent mitochondrial mutation in most populations, an A to G transition at position 3243 that alters the leucine transfer RNA. Manifestations of this mutation vary widely, from normal glucose tolerance to insulin-deficient diabetes that is phenotypically indistinguishable from T1DM (Kadowaki et al., 1994; Velho et al., 1996a). The same variant causes hearing loss in over 50% of those affected and may result in cardiomyopathy, external ophthalmoplegia, vestibular dysfunction, and encephalopathy (Kadowaki et al., 1994). The highly variable presentation may stem from variable levels of mutant DNA in different tissues and in different family members (heteroplasmy) (Olsson et al., 1998). More recently, additional mutations with similar effects have been described at positions 3264 (Suzuki et al., 1997), 3271 (Tsukuda et al., 1997), 3256 (Hirai et al., 1998), 3426 (Shin et al., 1998), 8296 (Kameoka et al., 1998), 14709 (Vialettes et al., 1997), and 14577 (Tawata et al., 2000). Additionally, other deletions have been described (Nicolino et al., 1997), which may cause additional endocrinopathies. With the exception of the $tRNA^{Leu\ (UUR)}$ mutation, these variants are rare. Prevalence of the $tRNA^{Leu\ (UUR)}$ mutation ranges from 1% to 2% among unselected T2DM subjects to over 20% among subjects with maternally inherited diabetes and hearing loss (Kadowaki et al., 1994; Fukunaga et al., 1997; Tsukuda et al., 1997; Guillausseau et al., 2001). The prevalence among typical Caucasian T2DM subjects, even with a strong family history, appears to be much lower (Elbein and Hoffman, 1996; Newkirk et al., 1997). In a recent study of 54 French subjects with the 3243 $tRNA^{Leu}$ variant, Guillausseau and colleagues (2001) reported that 87% of subjects presented as T2DM, but all were lean; 73% had a maternal history of diabetes, and 46% progressed to insulin therapy within 10 years of diagnosis. All subjects had neurosensory hearing loss, 43% had myopathy, and 15% had cardiomyopathy. Finally, they reported a 28% frequency of renal disease after 12 years duration.

Genetic Susceptibility to Typical Type 2 Diabetes

Susceptibility to typical T2DM has been studied by two broad approaches: the analysis of candidate genes defined from the known physiologic defects and from genes identified in single-gene causes of diabetes, and the genome scan approach. Under the broader category of candidate gene studies, the primary approach until recently was the population association study. A smaller number of investigators have used linkage approaches to study the role of candidate genes in families and sib pairs with T2DM. Recently, many studies have attempted to identify mutations directly by either molecular scanning or sequencing of candidate genes in diabetic subjects. These approaches often generate genetic variants that may represent either biologically significant changes or simple nonfunctional polymorphisms. In the absence of rigorous biological tests of function of the variants, investigators have resorted to population association studies. The results of these studies have provided conflicting results that make interpretation of nearly all current candidate genes difficult. To date, no candidate qualifies as a major diabetes locus, but several variants appear to have some role in diabetes susceptibility. We will review candidate gene studies according to the broad categories of physiologic action: insulin secretion, insulin action, and other pathways including obesity.

Candidate Genes for Insulin Secretion

The insulin gene was the first candidate evaluated for diabetes. Initial association studies suggested an association of a variable number tandem repeat (VNTR) polymorphism 5′ to the insulin gene promoter with T2DM (Permutt and Rotwein, 1983). Although subsequent studies have identified this region as *IDDM2*, the role in T2DM has been uncertain (Permutt and Elbein, 1990). Recently the polymorphism was associated with the diabetes-susceptible polycystic ovary syndrome (Waterworth et al., 1997), and both overtransmission paternally derived alleles in sib trios (Huxtable et al., 2000) and altered insulin secretion were confirmed in T2DM (Ahmed et al., 1999). Another study associated the insulin gene VNTR region with juvenile obesity and hyperinsulinism (Le Stunff et al., 2000). Olansky et al. (1992) found a promoter variant that might contribute to diabetes in 5% to 6% of African American subjects. Linkage studies have not suggested a role for the insulin gene (Elbein et al., 1988). Insulin gene mutations are not a major susceptibility locus for T2DM, but the role of the VNTR will require further study.

Because hyperproinsulinemia is a common feature of T2DM and may be present before the development of hyperglycemia, defective conversion of proinsulin to insulin by prohormone convertases 2 and 3 has been examined. Yoshida et al. (1995) reported the association of a microsatellite polymorphism in prohormone convertase 2 with T2DM in Japanese subjects, but no SSCP (single-strand conformational polymorphism, a means of mutation screening) variant could explain this finding. Ohagi et al. (1996) found missense mutations of exons 2 and 14 in prohormone convertase 3 (PC3), but neither was associated with diabetes in 102 Japanese subjects. In a preliminary report, Kalidas et al. (1997) tested for PC3 involvement by linkage and SSCP in a mixed population and found no evidence for mutations causing diabetes or hyperproinsulinemia.

Amylin or islet amyloid polypeptide (IAPP) has been considered to be a strong candidate because IAPP-derived amyloid deposits are the most characteristic pathological feature of pancreases from Type 2 diabetic patients (Johnson et al., 1989). Cook et al. (1991) were unable to demonstrate linkage in a small study with a relatively uninformative polymorphism. Recent genome scans have also not reported linkage in this region. Nishi et al. (1990) failed to find any abnormalities upon sequencing of the coding regions from 25 individuals, including 13 African Americans and 10 Caucasians. However, Sakagashira and colleagues (1996) found a heterozygous missense mutation in exon 3 (S20G) by SSCP in 12 of 294 Japanese Type 2 diabetics. This mutation appeared to predispose to diabetes with early onset (<35 years), although one-third of patients with the same mutation had later onset of mild diabetes. In most populations, IAPP does not appear to be directly involved in susceptibility.

Glucokinase was suggested as a candidate, based on its role as a glucose sensor, a role that was confirmed in autosomal-dominant glucokinase mutations. Although microsatellite polymorphisms near the glucokinase gene were associated with T2DM in African American and Japanese populations (Chiu et al., 1992; Noda et al., 1993), neither linkage (Cook et al., 1992; Elbein et al., 1993a; Froguel et al., 1993; Janssen et al., 1994) nor direct screening suggest a role in typical T2DM (Chiu et al., 1993; Eto et al., 1993; Elbein et al., 1994a). Stone et al. (1994, 1996) reported a common variant in the β-cell promoter at position -30 that was associated with IGT and reduced insulin secretion in a Japanese-American population. Homozygosity for the -30 promoter variant was associated with IGT but not diabetes in a Japanese population (K. Yamada et al., 1997); however, several recent studies failed to find an association of this variant with diabetes or an impact on β-cell function (Rissanen et al., 1998; Urhammer et al., 1998; Elbein et al., 2001). Chiu and McCarthy (1996) reported a second promoter variant at -258 in the hepatic glucokinase promoter, which reduced activity 58% in in vivo studies and appeared to cause insulin resistance in homozygous glucose-tolerant African American subjects. Because both liver and pancreatic glucokinase are inhibited by a regulatory protein (GCKR), several groups also have studied the role of glucokinase regulatory protein. Vionnet et al. (1997) found no evidence for linkage in 751 French sib pairs, and no genome scan to date has found linkage in this region of chromosome 2p23. Hayward et al. (1998) recently described a common proline to leucine variant (P446L) in exon 15 in a highly conserved region. The role of this variant in diabetes is currently unknown.

Glucose enters the β-cell through the GLUT2 facilitative transporter. Additional support of a role for *GLUT2* in diabetes pathogenesis comes from the work of Unger (1991), who has reported decreased GLUT2 transporters in several murine forms of diabetes. Polymorphisms at this locus were not associated with T2DM in African Americans (Matsutani et al., 1990), and there was a lack of linkage to familial diabetes in Caucasians of northern European extraction (Elbein et al., 1992). Later, Lesage et al. (1997) found no evidence for linkage in 79 French diabetic families. Linkage was also rejected in Italian affected sib pairs (Baroni et al., 1992), and no reported genome scan has suggested linkage in this region. However, sib pair analysis in Pima Indians was suggestive of linkage with acute insulin response to glucose (Janssen et al., 1994). An amino acid variant (T110I) was found in exon 3 in 5% of Pima Indians, but this mutation was not associated with a low acute insulin response to glucose. Transfection experiments showed this variant has no effect on GLUT2 activity (Mueckler et al., 1994). Shimada et al. (1995) identified three mutations (V101I, T110I, G519E) in Japanese subjects, two of which were novel. An additional variant (P68L) was found by Matsubara et al. (1995). None of these variants were associated with diabetes, however, and any role of these mutations in insulin secretion is unclear. In contrast, Mueckler et al. (1994) showed that a fourth variant (V197I) abolished transport. GLUT2 mutations appear to be an extremely rare cause of diabetes. A recent analysis of the promoter region also failed to identify diabetes-susceptibility variants in Caucasian subjects (Moller et al., 2001).

A key component in glucose-stimulated insulin secretion is the sulfonylurea receptor gene (*SUR1* or *ABCC8*) and the associated ATP-sensitive K^+ channel subunit (Kir6.2), both of which have been mapped to chromosome 11p15.1 (Inoue et al., 1996). Using the map location, linkage of *SUR1* was rejected in Japanese sib pairs (Iwasaki et al., 1996), French sib pairs (Hani et al., 1997), Hispanic sib pairs (Stirling et al., 1995b), a white sib pair population from Dresden and Chicago (Lindner et al., 1997b), and multigenerational families from Utah (Elbein et al., 1996a). However, Stern et al. (1996a) found evidence for linkage to post-challenge glucose in this region of chromosome 11. Several sequence variants were found on SSCP screening of the gene, and a silent variant was associated with T2DM in several Caucasian populations (Hani et al., 1997; Inoue et al., 1996; 't Hart et al., 1999). A similar association was found with morbid obesity (Hani et al., 1997). This association cannot be explained by variants in the K^+ channel subunit (Inoue et al., 1997), although Hansen et al. (1997b) suggested higher insulin sensitivity in a few individuals with a combination of two amino acid variants. Elbein and colleagues (2001) recently showed that heterozygosity for silent *SUR1* variants (single-nucleotide polymorphisms) altered the ability of the β-cell to compensate for insulin resistance among members of Caucasian families with T2DM, and similar findings were reported by 't Hart and colleagues (2000). While lack of linkage in most studies suggests that *SUR1* does not play a major role in diabetes susceptibility, the finding of an association in several unrelated populations supports the possibility that there is a susceptibility gene in this region.

As discussed above, six genes have now been implicated in MODY. All have been evaluated in typical, late-onset T2DM. *HNF1α* was implicated by linkage of T2DM with an insulin secretion defect to the *MODY3* region of chromosome 12 in Botnian Finish diabetic families (Mahtani et al., 1996) and by suggestive evidence in a second set of Caucasian families (Bowden et al., 1997). Multiple investigators have screened for mutations by sequencing or molecular scanning methods, and most found few potentially diabetogenic mutations (Glucksmann et al., 1997; Iwasaki et al., 1997; Kaisaki et al., 1997; Urhammer et al., 1997b; S. Yamada et al., 1997; Elbein et al., 2000a). However, *HNF1α* mutations may be an important if unusual cause of familial T2DM with early onset (Kaisaki et al., 1997; Elbein et al., 1998). Although multiple linkage studies have implicated chromosome 20 (Bowden et al., 1997; Ji et al., 1997; Zouali et al., 1997; Ghosh et al., 1999b; Klupa et al., 2000; Permutt et al., 2001), mutations in *HNF4α* appear to be an unusual cause of late-onset T2DM (Hani et al., 1998). Available data do not support a significant role for *HNF1β* (Beards et al., 1998), insulin promoter factor 1 (*IPF1*) (Chevre et al., 1998; Hara et al., 1998; Frayling et al., 2001), or *NeuroD1/BETA2* (Frayling et al., 2001).

Candidate Genes for Insulin Action

Extensive studies of the insulin receptor gene do not support an important role for this gene in typical T2DM, based on both linkage and molecular scanning studies, although rare variants have been described (Taylor, 1992). A common variant (V985M) was found to influence glucose levels in members of one Utah family (Elbein et al., 1993b) and subsequently was associated with T2DM and elevated glucose in the Netherlands ('t Hart et al., 1996). Later studies did not replicate this finding (Hansen et al., 1997c) and did not find biological activity (Strack et al., 1997). Many investigators have examined the insulin substrate 1 (IRS1), a key protein in the insulin-signaling cascade. Although initial studies suggested an association of a common amino acid variant (G971Arg) with diabetes (Almind et al., 1993), subsequent results have been mixed (Laakso et al., 1994; Celi et al., 1995; Hitman et al., 1995; Mori et al., 1995; Sigal et al., 1996; Zhang et al., 1996). Although linkage has not been demonstrated to this region (see below) (Elbein et al., 1995), modest reductions (~40%) in phosphatidyinositol 3-kinase (PI-3 kinase) activity have been reported in some studies (Almind et al., 1996; Yoshimura et al., 1997) and decreased insulin action in vitro has been reported in others (Hribal et al., 2000). Impaired insulin secretion (Porzio et al., 1999; Stumvoll et al., 2001) has been reported also, and an interaction of the IRS1 variant with obesity is possible (Clausen et al., 1995). Other variants in IRS1 are uncommon and may predispose to diabetes in some cases, but deficiencies in PI-3 kinase activity are also modest in the heterozygous state (Imai et al., 1994, 1997; Armstrong et al., 1996; Ura et al., 1996; Celi et al., 2000).

Hansen et al. (1997d) found a common variant (M326I) in the p85α regulatory unit of PI-3 kinase, which, although not associated with T2DM, appeared to modestly reduce glucose effectiveness, glucose disappearance, and insulin sensitivity in the homozygous state. The real role of PI-3 kinase will require further evaluation. In the pathway of glucose transport, the insulin responsive (GLUT4) glucose transporter has been studied by linkage (Elbein et al., 1995; Lesage et al., 1997) and molecular scanning (Choi et al., 1991; Kusari et al., 1991; Buse et al., 1992). No linkage to T2DM has been demonstrated, and the single variant in exon 9 (*V383I*) (Kusari et al., 1991) was not associated with diabetes in several studies (Buse et al., 1992). *GLUT4* seems unlikely to contribute directly to T2DM. Similarly, hexokinase II, the peripheral equivalent of glucokinase in the pancreas, has not been implicated by linkage (Elbein et al., 1995; Hanis et al., 1996; Vionnet et al., 1997). Several groups have failed to find evidence that hexokinase variants were associated with diabetes, thus confirming the linkage studies (Echwald et al., 1995; Vidal-Puig et al., 1995; Taylor et al., 1996). Groop and colleagues (1993) initially reported an association of a restriction fragment polymorphism in muscle glycogen synthase (*GYS1*) with diabetes, hypertension, and insulin-stimulated glucose storage. Although subsequent studies suggested an association of this region with diabetes in Pima Indians (Majer et al., 1996), studies in other ethnic groups did not replicate the association (Kadowaki et al., 1993; Zouali et al., 1993; Zhang et al., 1996). Furthermore, linkage to the muscle glycogen synthase locus on 19q was rejected (Elbein et al., 1994b; Hanis et al., 1996; Mahtani et al., 1996; Vionnet et al., 2000), and no coding region mutations were identified in muscle mRNA (Vestergaard et al., 1991). Orho et al. (1995) identified a rare missense mutation (G464S, exon 11) in 2 of 228 Finnish Type 2 diabetic patients and no control subjects. Shimomura et al. (1997) found two variants (M416V, exon 10; P442A, exon 11); the former was also found in Finland but was not associated with diabetes or insulin resistance (Rissanen et al., 1997b). In contrast, Majer et al. (1996) found no variants in Pima Indians. While rare mutations may contribute to diabetes, glycogen synthase does not appear to play a major role (Rissanen et al., 1997b). Permana and Mott (1997) found no mutations in the type 1 protein phosphatase inhibitor, an enzyme in the phosphorylation cascade that activates glycogen synthase. Also in the phosphorylation cascade–controlling glycogen synthesis, Hansen et al. (1997a) found no significant mutations in glycogen synthase kinase isoforms 3α and 3β, and they mapped these genes to regions with no reported linkage to T2DM.

Recently, an additional candidate in the regulation of glycogen synthesis, the skeletal muscle regulatory G subunit of the glycogen-associated form of protein phosphatase 1 (*PPPIR3*) was implicated in the altered insulin-regulated glycogen synthesis of T2DM. Two common amino acid variants, Asp905Tyr (D905Y) and Arg883Ser (R883S), and a 5 bp 3′ untranslated region insertion/deletion variant have been identified (Hansen et al., 1995; Xia et al., 1998). Several studies have suggested an association of one or more of these variants with insulin sensitivity and T2DM (Hegele et al., 1998; Xia et al., 1998). As with other variants, this association is inconsistent (Shen et al., 1998; Maegawa et al., 1999; Hansen et al., 2000a). The three variants are in strong linkage disequilibrium. Xia and colleagues (1998) showed that the variable "ATTA" in the 3′ untranslated region alters mRNA levels by 10-fold, whereas the two amino acid variants had no effect on in vitro glycogen synthase activity (Permana et al., 2000).

A locus for insulin resistance was initially mapped by quantitative trait linkage to chromosome 4q near intestinal fatty acid binding protein (FABP2) (Prochazka et al., 1993). Subsequently, an amino acid variant (Ala54Thr; A54T) in *FABP2* was identified (Baier et al., 1995) and shown to alter intestinal fat binding and insulin sensitivity, and this finding was later confirmed in stably transformed cells (Baier et al., 1996). Unfortunately, as with many apparently functional variants, a role for this A54T in other populations has been inconsistent (Humphreys et al., 1994; Elbein et al., 1995; Mitchell et al., 1995; Stern et al., 1996b; Rissanen et al., 1997a; Vionnet et al., 1997; Hayakawa et al., 1999; Lei et al., 1999; Chiu et al., 2001), probably because the overall effect of this variant on glucose tolerance and insulin sensitivity is small.

A number of other loci have been examined, but they do not appear to play a role in T2DM. A potentially exciting novel gene, the RAS-related protein associated with diabetes, or *rad*, was overexpressed in the muscle of diabetic subjects (Reynet and Kahn, 1993; Caldwell et al., 1996), and initial reports suggested an association of *RAD* alleles with diabetes (Doria et al., 1995). Subsequent linkage and association studies have been negative (Elbein et al., 1995; Orho et al., 1996; Vionnet et al., 1997). An inhibitor of tyrosine kinase activity of the insulin receptor,

PC-1, was identified by Goldfine and colleagues (1998) and shown to be overexpressed in fibroblasts of insulin resistant subjects (Maddux et al., 1995). A common amino acid variant, Lys121Gln (K121Q) and variants in the 3′ untranslated region have been reported to alter PC-1 mRNA levels (Pizzuti et al., 1999; Costanzo et al., 2001; Frittitta et al., 2001), but association with diabetes and insulin resistance has been inconsistent (Pizzuti et al., 1999; Gu et al., 2000; Rasmussen et al., 2000).

Other Pathways, Other Candidate Genes

A number of candidate genes have been studied that alter energy metabolism or that affect glucose metabolism in ways not yet determined. A variant of the β_3-adrenergic receptor gene, Trp64Arg (W64R), was initially noted to influence insulin sensitivity, weight gain, and timing of diabetes onset (Clement et al., 1995; Kadowaki et al., 1995; Walston et al., 1995; Widen et al., 1995). As with other variants of small effect, subsequent studies have had variable results (Gagnon et al., 1996; Mauriege and Bouchard, 1996). Elbein et al. (1996b) found no effect on insulin levels, obesity, or diabetes in families ascertained for multiple diabetic siblings, and results have been inconsistent in a large number of other studies from various populations (Kadowaki et al., 1995; Fujisawa et al., 1996; Gagnon et al., 1996; Silver et al., 1996, 1997; Zhang et al., 1996; Arii et al., 1997; Keen et al., 1997; Kim-Motoyama et al., 1997; Moriarty et al., 1997; Nagase et al., 1997; Sakane et al., 1997; Yuan et al., 1997; Ghosh et al., 1999a; Benecke et al., 2000; Oeveren van-Dybicz et al., 2001). Mitchell et al. (1998) provided an intriguing explanation for the variable results. In a population from the San Antonio Heart Study, they found no association of the W64R variant with obesity until they conditioned on the major locus on chromosome 2 that controls leptin (Comuzzie et al., 1997). This study raises the general caution that failure to replicate a reported association may be the result of gene or environment interactions that obscure the effects of a relatively weak locus.

Hager and colleagues (1995) initially described the association of a missense variant (G40S) of the glucagon receptor with T2DM in French and Sardinian patients and suggested lower binding affinity for glucagon. They also found weak evidence for linkage. Gough et al. (1995) appeared to confirm the association in England. However, the distribution of the variant, even among Sardinians, and the association with T2DM have been highly variable (Fujisawa et al., 1995; Huang et al., 1995; Elbein and Hoffman, 1996; Hansen et al., 1996; Odawara et al., 1996; Ogata et al., 1996; Ristow et al., 1996; Urhammer et al., 1996; Tonolo et al., 1997a). Population stratification may be one explanation for the initially observed association. Furthermore, physiologic studies would suggest lower glucose response to glucagon (Tonolo et al., 1997b) and lower glucagon sensitivity (Hansen et al., 1996), which should be protective against diabetes.

Hegele et al. (1997) suggested that homozygosity for a variant of the paraoxonase-2 gene (*PON2*) was associated with elevated fasting glucose in subjects with T2DM, but not with diabetes or IGT itself. Following clues from a genome scan (see below), Baier and colleagues (1998) reported missense mutations of the vitamin D binding protein that were associated with differences in glucose tolerance in Pima Indians.

A number of investigators have examined loci for obesity as candidate genes for T2DM and obesity within Type 2 diabetic families. Multiple linkage studies have rejected these loci as major diabetes genes (Stirling et al., 1995a; Hasstedt et al., 1997; Otabe et al., 1998), despite some evidence for linkage of the leptin receptor locus to obesity (Clement et al., 1996). Comuzzie and colleagues (1997) reported a locus controlling leptin levels on chromosome 2, but this locus is not in a region with linkage to diabetes. Mutations of the leptin receptor gene seem unlikely to be an important cause of either obesity or T2DM (Maffei et al., 1996; Niki et al., 1996; Francke et al., 1997; Rolland et al., 1998; Chagnon et al., 1999, 2000; Clement et al., 1999; Lakka et al., 2000). In contrast, linkage and mutation screening studies have variably suggested a role for the uncoupling protein 2 (UCP2) in obesity and weight gain (Kubota et al., 1998; Otabe et al., 1998; Elbein et al., 1997; Urhammer et al., 1997a). A promoter variant, a 45 bp insertion in the 3′ untranslated region, and a common amino acid variant have all been associated with modest protection from obesity or with childhood obesity in some but not all studies (Urhammer et al., 1997a; Kubota et al., 1998; Dalgaard et al., 1999; Yanovski et al., 2000; Buemann et al., 2001; Esterbauer et al., 2001). Both the promoter and 3′ untranslated variants appear to alter RNA levels (Esterbauer et al., 2001). Although the effects of these variants are modest and the effects are not seen in all studies, the high prevalence of these variants in the population would imply a significant population-attributable risk (Esterbauer et al., 2001).

The recent development of pharmaceutical agents that act through the peroxisome activated receptor γ (PPARγ) has introduced a new pathway responsible for insulin sensitivity and obesity. A common amino acid change (Pro12Ala; P12A) in the PPARγ_2 gene was first described by Yen and colleagues (1997) and has now been studied carefully. Most studies have suggested that the common P12 allele results in decreased insulin sensitivity and increased risk of T2DM, along with more variably decreased body weight (Beamer et al., 1998; Koch et al., 1999; Altshuler et al., 2000; Clement et al., 2000; Cole et al., 2000; Hara et al., 2000; Jacob et al., 2000; Li et al., 2000; Meirhaeghe et al., 2000; Mori et al., 2001). The A12 allele has lower transactivation capacity (Deeb et al., 1998). The modest (1.25-fold increase) in diabetes risk and high frequency (0.85) of the P12 allele suggest a high population-attributable risk, accounting for up to 25% of T2DM. However, several paradoxes remain unresolved. Dominant negative mutations of the PPARγ gene cause diabetes, insulin resistance, and hypertension (Barroso et al., 1999), as might be expected given the pharmaceutical effects of activating PPARγ. Hasstedt et al. (2001) indeed showed an insulin-resistance-like phenotype among A12 carriers that was particularly prominent among A12 homozygotes, which is consistent with the reduced activity of this allele, rather than the improved insulin sensitivity seen in other studies (Deeb et al., 1998; Koch et al., 1999; Jacob et al., 2000). Interactions with obesity, glucose tolerance, and the environment may partially explain this paradox and the inconsistent directions of observed associations with insulin sensitivity and obesity (Ek et al., 1999; Koch et al., 1999).

Summary of Candidate Gene Studies

A large number of candidate genes have now been examined. The majority of studies support a role for the sulfonylurea receptor (ABCC8), although the causative variant is unknown, the P12A variant of the PPARγ_2 allele, the W64R variant of the β_3 adrenergic receptor gene, and the PPP1R3 3′ untranslated variant. The role of the UCP2 promoter and 3′ variant and the G972R variant of the IRS1 gene are less certain but likely. An additional variant in the calpain 10 gene (Baier et al., 2000; Horikawa et al., 2000) plays a similar role and is discussed below. None of these variants individually accounts for a large proportion of the diabetes risk in any single individual, but the population risk of these variants could be substantial because of their high frequency. Interactions between these variants and genes implicated in genome scans (see below) are likely and remain to be explored. The picture emerging from candidate gene studies and reinforced in the genome-wide scans discussed below is of common T2DM as a complex disease with many contributing factors that affect different individuals and all with small individual risk. Consequently, replication even in relatively large studies has been difficult to achieve. Lack of replication cannot be viewed as invalidating the initial observation until multiple studies have reported and confounding factors have been identified.

Genome Scans for Type 2 Diabetes

Because known candidate genes appear to play mostly minor, epistatic roles in diabetes susceptibility, the search for new loci using linkage analysis in sib pairs or families has been an important advance. These studies use regularly spaced microsatellite (simple tandem repeat) markers to map diabetes as either a dichotomous trait or a quantitative trait such as glucose or insulin that reflects diabetes risk. In the last few years many genome-wide scans have reported results, although reports are only in preliminary form and many studies are still in progress. Nearly all groups involved in exploring the genetics of T2DM have participated in the International Type 2 Diabetes Consortium, which has yet to formally report joint analyses but appears likely to identify regions that harbor susceptibility genes. To date, most studies have treated diabetes as a qualitative (dichotomous) trait, but several studies have attempted to examine glucose and insulin. The latter studies are reviewed first, then we review the current status (as of summer 2001) of the genome scans for T2DM.

Quantititive Trait Linkage Studies

In one of the first quantitative trait analyses, Prochazka and colleagues (1993) showed linkage of insulin action to chromosome 4q in a region that was later mapped to FABP2. This study was confirmed by Mitchell and colleagues (1995) in a Hispanic population. Subsequently, Stern and colleagues (1996a) used a multipoint variance components method to map quantitative trait loci controlling fasting and 2-hour post-challenge glucose in 32 Hispanic families from San Antonio to markers on chromosome 11p (LOD 3.77 with 2-hour glucose) in the general region of *ABCC8*, with less significant linkage in the same region with fasting glucose. They also found linkage near D6S290 in a region also proposed for Type 1 diabetes and near the membrane glycoprotein PC-1, although with much lower significance (LOD = 2.15). Using multiple methods to examine quantitative trait loci for fasting and 2-hour glucose, fasting and 2-hour insulin, measures of insulin secretion, and measures of insulin action, Pratley et al. (1998) studied 363 nondiabetic members of 109 Pima Indian families. They reported suggestive linkage of fasting insulin and in vivo insulin action to chromosome 3q21–q24, fasting insulin to 4p15–q12, 2-hour insulin to 9q21, and fasting glucose to 22q12–q13. No linkage exceeded a LOD score of 3.6, and most linkages were below a LOD score of 2.0. Based on the large number of tests performed, one would expect many of these scores to be false positives. Most intriguing is the evidence for linkage of 2-hour glucose during a glucose tolerance test to a region near *IDDM4* on chromosome 11q, thus confirming other suggestive data for a diabetes locus in this region (Elbein et al., 1996a). Watanabe and colleagues (2000) used data collected from the Finland–United States Investigation of Non-Insulin-Dependent Diabetes Mellitus Genetics (FUSION) Study to look at 14 traits related to diabetes in 580 families. Their best evidence for linkage in nondiabetic subjects was to chromosome 10 (acute insulin response), chromosome 13 (2-hour insulin), and chromosome 17p (insulin:glucose ratio). No logarithm of odds (LOD) score reached the threshold of 3.0, although the LOD score for insulin sensitivity in both diabetic and nondiabetic subjects exceeded 3.0 for 17p and for body mass index to chromosome 3p. In unpublished data from multi-generational Utah families, Elbein and Hasstedt (personal communication) examined 712 sib pairs from 111 sibships for fasting and post-challenge insulin and glucose, body mass index, and lipid levels. Triglyceride levels mapped to chromosome 19q near ApoE and ApoC2 genes with LOD 3.15, but no other trait met significance. The highest scores for insulin-related traits were 60 minute post-challenge glucose on chromosome 8p (LOD 2.25), fasting insulin on chromosome 7p (LOD 2.00), and insulin secretion from the oral glucose tolerance test on 19p (LOD 2.21). No other region overlapped with the quantitative trait studies of Pratley et al. (1998) or Watanabe et al. (2000). Mitchell and colleagues (2000) mapped a locus controlling insulin levels in Hispanic families to chromosome 3p14.2–p14.1. Other quantitative trait studies from the Amish Family Study (Hsueh et al., 2000) and the Hispanic study in San Antonio have been reported only in preliminary form. Surprisingly, most regions implicated in quantitative trait studies have not overlapped with regions implicated in genome-wide scans for T2DM.

Dichotomous Trait Linkage Studies of Type 2 Diabetes

In a genome-wide scan of 490 markers in 330 affected sib pairs from 170 sibships, Hanis et al. (1996) found evidence for a major locus at the telomere of chromosome 2q in Mexican Americans. This locus, which they called *NIDDM1*, accounted for 30% of familial clustering of T2DM and was replicated in a second set of 110 sib pairs from Starr County, Texas, but not in non-Hispanic whites or Japanese. Subsequent studies localized the susceptibility locus to an intronic single-nucleotide polymorphism (SNP) in the calpain 10 gene (*CAPN10*), a member of a cysteine-protease family that is ubiquitously expressed (Horikawa et al., 2000). A combination of two haplotypes conferred the highest risk and increased the risk of diabetes 2.8-fold. Homozygosity for the single SNP, SNP-43, resulted in insulin resistance, lower skeletal muscle mRNA levels, and higher fasting glucose in Pima Indians (Baier et al., 2000) but was not associated with diabetes. No other studies have demonstrated linkage to this region, and initial reports suggest that the high-risk haplotype is rare in Caucasians and may not explain much of the diabetes risk at all (Horikawa et al., 2000; Elbein et al., unpublished data). Among Utah families, association of neither CAPN10 SNPs nor haplotypes was found, but increased fasting glucose and post-challenge insulin levels were confirmed (Elbein et al., unpublished data). CAPN10 appears to explain only a small amount of diabetes risk in most populations, but a linkage signal in several studies proximal to *NIDDM1* might represent a second gene on echromosome 2q (Hanis et al., 1996; Hanson et al., 1998; Elbein et al., 1999b).

In a second genome scan, Mahtani et al. (1996) reported no region with significant linkage in an analysis of 26 families comprising 217 individuals. However, when families were ranked according to the insulin response to glucose at 30 minutes, the families in the lowest quartile (six families) showed linkage to

D12S366 on chromosome 12q near *MODY3*. Although this specific finding has not been replicated, and few investigators have measured insulin response to glucose in diabetic patients, several other studies have reported linkage on chromosome 12, some near the *HNF1α/MODY3* locus (Bowden et al., 1997; Shaw et al., 1998), including the large, multicenter Genetics of Type 2 Diabetes (GENNID) study (Ehm et al., 2000). The *HNF1α* gene is unlikely to account for this observation, since most linkage and screening studies have failed to implicate this locus (Kaisaki et al., 1997; S. Yamada et al., 1997b; Elbein et al., 1998; Nishigori et al., 1998b; Shaw et al., 1998). Recently, an additional region of chromosome 12q15 that is approximately 50 cM distant to the first observations was identified in Caucasian families (Bektas et al., 1999; Ehm et al., 2000). Work is in progress by Bektas et al. (2001) and others to pursue the apparent susceptibility loci on chromosome 12.

Multiple groups have reported linkage to different regions of chromosome 20, with some linkages reported in the general region of *MODY1*. Hani et al. (1996) reported evidence for linkage of T2DM to the phosphoenolpyruvate carboxykinase locus (*PCK1*) in French sib pairs, with the most important results in 25 sib pairs with diabetes onset before age 46. Subsequent analyses by this group have again suggested linkage ($p < .0004$) only in the 55 sib pairs with onset at or before age 45 (Zouali et al., 1997). Ji et al. (1997) also reported evidence for linkage (single locus significance $p < .005$) near the *MODY1* locus in 246 sib pairs from 29 Caucasian families with apparent autosomal-dominant transmission, and subsequent studies provided additional evidence for this locus (Klupa et al., 2000). The same region was implicated by Bowden et al. (1997) among Caucasian sib pairs with a history of diabetic nephropathy ($p = .005$), and more recently a chromosome 20q locus was implicated in 427 sib pairs of Ashkenazy Jewish ancestry (Permutt et al., 2001). However, the strongest evidence for a chromosome 20 locus derives from the large FUSION study of 716 Finnish T2DM sib pairs (Ghosh et al., 1999b), which implicated at least two regions on chromosome 20. Based on these data, the International Type 2 Diabetes Consortium re-examined this linkage with a uniform map in a large number of Caucasian and Hispanic populations, in Pima Indians, and a small African American population. While the most impressive findings were restricted to families from Finland, the combined data analysis of all data sets and Caucasian data sets confirms at least one significant locus on chromosome 20. Nonetheless, many data sets show no evidence for linkage anywhere on chromosome 20 (Frayling et al., 2000). Efforts are ongoing by multiple groups to identify these susceptibility genes, and the *MODY4/HNF4α* is probably not responsible for the observed linkage (Malecki et al., 1998).

Growing data support a third T2DM locus on chromosome 1q21–q24, roughly in the region of the apolipoprotein A2 gene. Hanson and colleagues (1998) found evidence for linkage in this region among Pima Indian siblings discordant for diabetes or when individuals with onset before age 45 were selected. In an independent analysis of 42 multigenerational Utah white families of northern European ancestry, Elbein et al. (1999b) identified the same locus under a recessive model (LOD = 4.29), with evidence also under nonparametric analyses. Subsequently, a large study of 637 members of 143 families from France showed suggestive linkage of lean (BMI under 27) diabetes to the same chromosome 1q21–q24 region (Vionnet et al., 2000), and most recently suggestive linkage in the same region was replicated in 743 sib pairs from the United Kingdom Warren 2 repository (Wiltshire et al., 2001). The same locus in the Amish population has been identified (St Jean et al., 2000). Furthermore, familial combined hyperlipidemia in Finland was linked to the same region (Pajukanta et al., 1998), and this finding was confirmed by linkage of the syntenic region to the murine familial combined hyperlipidemia (Castellani et al., 1998). As with all T2DM loci, heterogeneity is clearly evident in the failure of other large scans to find any locus on chromosome 1, and the failure of replication even among the same study population (Elbein et al., 1999b). As with other regions, a collaborative effort is under way to identify the susceptibility locus or loci responsible for these observations.

A large number of other loci have been implicated in other published genome scans, including additional loci among Caucasian and Hispanic individuals with T2DM that have not been replicated to date (Duggirala et al., 1999; Ehm et al., 2000; Vionnet et al., 2000). Among loci with some replication are two regions on chromosome 5q (Hager et al., 1998; Ehm et al., 2000; Vionnet et al., 2000; Wiltshire et al., 2001); chromosome 8p (Elbein et al., 1999b; Wiltshire et al., 2001) near the lipoprotein lipase gene; chromosome 10q23–q26 (Duggirala et al., 1999; Ghosh et al., 2000; Vionnet et al., 2000; Wiltshire et al., 2001) over a 50 cM region; chromosome 11q (Elbein et al., 1996a; Hanson et al., 1998); and chromosome 18p (Elbein et al., 1999b; Parker et al., 2001).

Summary of Genome-Wide Scans for T2DM Loci

As with candidate gene studies, genome-wide scans for T2DM have been frustratingly replete with lack of replication, even among the same populations ascertained in two or more phases (Ehm et al., 2000; Elbein et al., 1999b; Ghosh et al., 2000). The large number of regions implicated and the inconsistent linkage findings add to the confusing picture. What has emerged from the large amount of data now available is a picture of diabetes as a complex disease with multiple susceptibility loci, each of which contributes to different degrees in different populations. These loci individually do not appear to greatly increase the risk of T2DM in any single individual, and thus hopes of predicting diabetes risk from genetic susceptibility loci may require complex modeling. Subgroup analyses and analyses of epistatic interactions are in their infancy, but show some promise (Cox et al., 1999; Ghosh et al., 2000; Vionnet et al., 2000; Wiltshire et al., 2001). Collaborative efforts to identify these loci are encouraging. In addition to CAPN10 on chromosome 2, loci are likely to be identified on chromosomes 1q21–q24 and 20, with reasonable hope for loci also on chromosome 12q and possibly 5q and 10q. Perhaps one or more of these loci will identify specific genetic subgroups of diabetes that will drive future therapeutics.

Clues to Diabetes Loci from Animal Models

Appropriate review of the growing number of transgenic, knockout, and tissue-specific gene inactivation models would require at least a full chapter. Although the important insights from these models cannot be reviewed in any detail here, excellent reviews abound (Kahn et al., 2000; Mauvais-Jarvis and Kahn, 2000). Two types of studies offer insights into human disease: genome scans in rodent models of T2DM and knockout or transgenic mouse models of T2DM. Studies of the Goto-Kakizaki (GK) rat (Galli et al., 1996; Gauguier et al., 1996; Fakhrai-Rad et al., 2000) and the C57BL/6J (Seldin et al., 1994) diabetes-prone mouse suggest the future of animal models in identifying diabetogenic loci that may be important in humans. Seldin et al. (1994) mapped hyperglycemia by crossing the diabetes-susceptible C57BL/6J strain of mice with the diabetes-resistant A/J strain. Using a high-fat, high-sucrose diet to induce diabetes, they mapped hyperglycemia to a susceptibility locus near the glycogen synthase gene. As discussed above, the glycogen synthase gene seems unlikely to cause T2DM in humans, although some human data point to a similar location.

Galli et al. (1996) and Gauguier et al. (1996) mapped the quantitative traits of glycemia, hyperinsulinemia in response to glucose, and weight in the GK rat, a nonobese rodent model of T2DM. Different study designs, different crosses, and different marker maps make interpretation and comparison of these studies difficult. Galli et al. (1996) mapped three independent loci, the most significant of which on rat chromosome 1 controlled both post-challenge glucose and insulin response. Surprisingly, this locus showed no control over fasting glucose. Loci on chromosomes 2 and 10 controlled both fasting and post-challenge glucose levels, and a locus near insulin-like growth factor 1 (*IGF1*) (chromosome 7) controlled weight. Gauguier et al. (1996) used somewhat less stringent criteria for linkage but also reported loci on chromosomes 1 and 2 for post-challenge glucose and fasting insulin, respectively, and an obesity locus on chromosome 7. Whether the slightly different phenotypes between these studies are controlled by the same genes is unclear. Recently the syntenic regions in humans were examined and support for human loci on chromosomes 1q21 and 10q23.3 was noted (Fakhrai-Rad et al., 2000; Wiltshire et al., 2001). Other syntenic human regions are not yet certain.

Among studies of knockout animals, an insulin receptor substrate 2 (IRS2) knockout mouse demonstrated that a single gene could cause diabetes through defects in both peripheral insulin signaling and β-cell function (Withers et al., 1998). Specific defects in IRS2 do not appear to be important in people, however (Bernal et al., 1998; Kalidas et al., 1998). In another knockout model, Terauchi et al. (1997) used a double knockout of insulin receptor substrate 1 and glucokinase, neither of which cause hyperglycemia alone, to create a two-locus model of T2DM. While the specific defects in these models may not cause diabetes in humans, these experiments demonstrate the epistatic interactions that may cause human diabetes.

Genetics of Diabetes Complications

Microvascular complications of diabetes result from hyperglycemia, yet not all patients develop renal disease, for example, despite poor glycemic control. This fact and the familial aggregation and segregation of nephropathy and end-stage renal disease in diabetic subjects (Seaquest et al., 1989; Borch-Johnsen et al., 1992; Freedman et al., 1995; Trevisan and Viberti, 1995; Fogarty and Krolewski, 1997; Chowdhury et al., 1999; Adler et al., 2000; Imperatore et al., 2000; Covic et al., 2001) suggest that genetic predisposition plays a significant role. Several models of inheritance have been proposed, including a major dominant susceptibility gene that has support from several analyses (Rogus and Krolewski, 1996; Imperatore et al., 2000), an additive model in which poor glycemic control initiates diabetic nephropathy but genetic factors determine progression, or an interactive model in which only the subset of individuals with inherited susceptibility develop diabetic nephropathy in the presence of poor glycemic control. As with T2DM, studies of nephropathy have centered on candidate genes, including the renin–angiotensin axis (Parving et al., 1996; Chowdhury et al., 1995; Fogarty and Krolewski, 1997). Studies have included demonstrations of association and linkage of both M235T variant of the angiotensinogen gene and the insertion–deletion variant of the angiotensin-converting enzyme gene (Barnas et al., 1997; Jeffers et al., 1997; Marre et al., 1997; Rogus et al., 1998; Chowdhury et al., 1999; Sagnella et al., 1999; Solini et al., 1999), but the role of these genes remains controversial (Parving et al., 1996). Aldose reductase, which converts glucose to sorbitol, is the rate-limiting step in the polyol pathway. Aldose reductase expression is increased in the kidneys of individuals with poorly controlled diabetes (DeFronzo, 1995), and increased red cell and leukocyte aldose reductase activity have been reported with diabetic nephropathy and diabetic retinopathy (Heesom et al., 1997; Shah et al., 1997). A strong association of a microsatellite polymorphism with diabetic nephropathy was found in Type 1 diabetes (Heesom et al., 1997), and nephropathy linkage was reported in Pima Indians on chromosome 7q near the aldose reductase locus (Imperatore et al., 1998). An association of the 5′ microsatellite with both nephropathy and altered aldose reductase levels and gene expression in lymphocytes has been noted in other populations (Shah et al., 1997); however, not all studies have confirmed the association (Moczulski et al., 1997; Dyer et al., 1999; Maeda et al., 1999). Other studies have implicated the sorbitol pathway in the genetics of retinopathy or microvascular disease (Hasegawa et al., 1999; Kao et al., 1999; Olmos et al., 2000; Shimizu et al., 2000).

Using a discordant sib pair approach in nephropathy of type 1 diabetes, Moczulski et al. (1998) recently reported a locus near the human *AT1* gene on chromosome 3q. The importance of this gene in nephropathy associated with T2DM remains to be determined. Using a standard concordant sib approach in 98 Pima Indian sib pairs, Imperatore et al. (1998) found suggestive linkage to four regions, including a locus near the aldose reductase gene on chromosome 7; a locus on chromosome 20; and weaker evidence for linkage on chromosome 3, approximately 23 cM from the locus reported by Moczulski et al. (1998), and chromosome 9. Much additional work is required to define susceptibility loci for microvascular complications of diabetes.

GENETIC COUNSELING FOR DIABETES

For genetic counseling, the health care team ideally will require a number of items. These include knowledge of the gene defect responsible for the disease phenotype, a relatively simple and reliable means of detecting mutations in the gene; knowledge of the mode of inheritance and degree of penetrance; and knowledge of the clinical features of the disease, such as mean age of onset, and predisposing factors. Recently we mapped genes responsible for two disorders of carbohydrate metabolism, and through mutation analysis in families we encountered a number of problems that will highlight the complicating issues involved in counseling of families with even single-gene disorders. These issues will unquestionably be more complex when counseling families regarding a multifactorial disorder such as T2DM.

Wolfram Syndrome

Wolfram syndrome (WFS) (OMIM 222300) is a disorder characterized by a combination of familial juvenile-onset diabetes mellitus and optic atrophy (Barrett and Bundey, 1997). Other clinical features are commonly present, and it has also been referred to as the DIDMOAD syndrome for diabetes insipidus, diabetes mellitus, optic atrophy, and deafness. Most patients with this progressive, neurodegenerative disorder eventually develop all four cardinal manifestations and die prematurely with widespread atrophic changes throughout the brain (Rando et al., 1992). Insulin-dependent non-autoimmune diabetes mellitus occurs with mean age of onset at 6 to 8 years (Barrett and Bundey, 1997). The prevalence of the disease is low, and Wolfram has been estimated to account for 1 in 150 patients with insulin-dependent diabetes mellitus (Fraser and Gunn, 1977). The pathogenesis of Wolfram syndrome is unknown. Diagnosis is usually made in one or more offspring of unaffected often-related parents, suggesting autosomal recessive inheritance (Bretz et al., 1970; Cremers et al., 1977). In 1994, the Wolfram syndrome gene was shown to be linked to markers on the short arm of chromosome 4 (Polymeropoulos et al., 1994), and these results were later confirmed by another study (Collier et al., 1996). Then Inoue and colleagues (1998) confirmed linkage to chromosome 4p in 5 Wolfram pedigrees. Novel recombinants with markers that locate between previously identified markers allowed localization of the Wolfram syndrome gene to a critical region less than several hundred kilobases. A P1/BAC contig across the region was constructed, and genomic sequencing yielded several candidate genes. Among those identified, a novel gene encoding a putative transmembrane protein was cloned. Mutations in this gene, named WFS-1, were found in all affected individuals in six Wolfram syndrome families, and these mutations were strongly associated with the disease phenotype.

A Wolfram family was particularly gratifying for illustrating how genetic analysis and counseling can be effective when mutations in a single gene appear to be responsible for the disease phenotype. There was a child, age 10, with diabetes mellitus and diabetes insipidus. The parents were first cousins and sought confirmation of a preliminary diagnosis of Wolfram in their son. They also wanted to know whether the two younger sibs were affected. Direct sequencing of the *WFS-1* gene revealed that each parent was heterozygous for a 7 bp repeat insertion, resulting in a predicted frame shift and premature termination of the Wolfram protein. The affected child was homozygous for the mutation, while his unaffected sisters were heterozygous and homozygous normal, respectively. Thus in this monogenic disorder causing diabetes, physicians could be confident of their ability to give the family clinically useful information. As illustrated below, however, counseling for other monogenic disorders is not necessarily so straightforward.

Familial Hyperinsulinism

Familial hyperinsulinism (HI; OMIM:256450) is a disorder characterized by inadequate suppression of insulin secretion in the presence of severe, recurrent, fasting hypoglycemia (Dunne et al., 1997; Kane et al., 1997; Stanley, 1997; Stanley and Baker, 1999). In the majority of familial cases this disorder is inherited as an autosomal recessive trait. Clinical manifestations of HI, which occurs predominantly in neonates and infants under 1 year of age, are secondary to hypoglycemia and include seizures, coma, and large birth weight for gestational age. Most patients are treated with inhibitors of insulin secretion or subtotal pancreatectomy to prevent permanent neurologic damage.

Mutations in both the sulfonylurea receptor (*SUR1*) and *Kir6.2* genes on chromosome 11p15.1 have been involved in HI (Ashcroft et al., 1993; Aguilar-Bryan et al., 1995; Kane et al., 1996; Nestorowicz et al., 1996; Dunne et al., 1997; Ryan et al., 1998; Thornton et al., 1998; Glaser et al., 1999; Huopio et al., 2000; Grimberg et al., 2001). Evidence from electrophysiological and pharmacological studies of cells co-expressing both genes indicates that these molecules form subunits of the pancreatic β-cell ATP-sensitive potassium (K_{ATP}) channel. In islet β-cells, such channels function as regulators of glucose-induced insulin secretion by coupling the metabolic status of the cell to the membrane potential (Ashcroft et al., 1993; Dukes et al., 1994; Miki et al., 1999). Elevations in blood glucose concentration lead to increased rates of glucose metabolism in β-cells and consequent alterations in the intracellular ratio of ATP/ADP, resulting in K_{ATP} channel closure. The subsequent depolarization of the β-cell plasma membrane activates voltage-sensitive Ca^{2+} channels, and the ensuing influx of Ca^{2+} initiates insulin secretion. Evidence that HI is associated with molecular defects in SUR1 and pancreatic β-cell K_{ATP} channel function have been provided by the identification of eight different mutations in the *SUR1* gene that co-segregate with the disease phenotype (Nestorowicz et al., 1996; Nichols et al., 1996; Thomas et al., 1996; Dunne et al., 1997). Mutational analysis of *SUR1/Kir6.2* can be useful in certain ethnic groups with HI. Nestorowicz and colleagues (1966, 1998) demonstrated allelic homogeneity in HI patients of Ashkenazi Jewish descent, with two mutations in the *SUR1* gene accounting for 88% of HI chromosomes. The 3992–9G6A mutation accounts for 66% of the mutations, and most of the patients either are homozygous for this mutation or are compound heterozygotes with a delF1388 mutation. The 3992–9G6A mutation results in a new splice acceptor site, a frame shift, and a presumed premature truncation of the SUR1 protein. HI patients homozygous for this mutation have a severe phenotype. We have encountered two Ashkenazi Jewish families where the proband was homozygous 3992–9G6A and severely affected, yet there was another haploidentical sib who appeared to be clinically unaffected. We presume that this mutation results in variable aberrant splicing, accounting for some normal SUR1 protein and thus variable phenotypes. A similar situation has been encountered in cystic fibrosis where 10% normal CFTR channel protein is sufficient to yield a normal phenotype (Bienvenu et al., 1996).

Thus, Ashkenazi Jewish couples could be screened for mutations in SUR1/Kir6.2. We estimate the prevalence of the 3992–9G6A mutation at 0.01, while the delF1388 mutation is less frequent. But even if an unborn child is homozygous for the most common 3992–9G6A mutation, penetrance is certainly less than complete. Nevertheless, this information may have some clinical utility.

In the non-Ashkenazi Jewish families, genetic counseling for familial HI poses additional problems due to marked allelic heterogeneity in HI patients of various ethnic groups (Nestorowicz et al., 1998). A total of 20 different mutations in the SUR1 gene, including 17 novel mutations, were identified, bringing the total to 25. With one exception, each of these mutations was present on only 1% to 2% disease chromosomes. Mutations were successfully identified in only a fraction of the patients. The failure to detect mutations in *SUR1* in the majority of HI patients analyzed in this study may be due to mutations occurring outside the regions analyzed, including regions controlling gene expression, or because of locus heterogeneity. Recent evidence suggests that a locus for an autosomal dominant form of HI is not linked to *SUR1* (Kukuvitis et al., 1997) and that mutations in the *Kir6.2* locus are also associated with the HI phenotype (Thomas et al., 1996; Nestorowicz et al., 1997).

Together, these data have implications for the early diagnosis and genetic counseling of affected children and their families. While standard mutation screening may identify 88% HI alleles in the Ashkenazim, direct testing for specific mutations in non-Ashkenazi patients will be complicated by allelic and locus heterogeneity.

Maturity Onset Diabetes of the Young (MODY)

Because the MODY genes have only recently been discovered, little clinical data has been collected. There are few MODY1 families. We know that MODY 2 and 3 genes are highly penetrant, but genetic analysis will be difficult, as there is extensive allelic heterogeneity for glucokinase and HNF1α mutations. Only one family with a mutation in the *IPF1* gene (*PDX1*, an islet transcription factor; see MODY above) has been described. There are no commercial certified genetic diagnostic labs doing these analyses at present. Further, these families represent <1% of all diabetes. For T2DM we are dealing with a multifactorial disease, and genetic counseling, once we identify genes involved, will represent the next clinical challenge.

REFERENCES

Accili D, Frapier C, Mosthaf L, McKeon C, Elbein SC, Permutt MA, Ramos E, Lander E, Ullrich A, Taylor SI: A mutation in the insulin receptor gene that impairs transport of the receptor to the plasma membrane and causes insulin-resistant diabetes. EMBO J 1989; 8:2509–2517.

Adler SG, Pahl M, Seldin MF: Deciphering diabetic nephropathy: progress using genetic strategies [editorial]. Curr Opin Nephrol Hypertens 2000; 9:99–106.

Aguilar-Bryan L, Nichols CG, Wechsler SW, Clement JP, Boyd AE, Gonzalez G, Herrera-Sosa H, Nguy K, Bryan J, Nelson DA: Cloning of the β cell high-affinity sulfonylurea receptor: a regulator of insulin secretion. Science 1995; 268: 423–426.

Ahmed S, Bennett ST, Huxtable SJ, Todd JA, Matthews DR, Gough SC: INS VNTR allelic variation and dynamic insulin secretion in healthy adult non-diabetic Caucasian subjects. Diabet Med 1999; 16:910–917.

Almind K, Bjorbaek C, Vestergaard H, Hansen T, Echwald S, Pedersen O: Amino acid polymorphisms of insulin receptor substrate-1 in non-insulin-dependent diabetes mellitus. Lancet 1993; 342:828–832.

Almind K, Inoue G, Pedersen O, Kahn CR: A common amino acid polymorphism in insulin receptor substrate-1 causes impaired insulin signaling: evidence from transfection studies. J Clin Invest 1996; 97:2569–2575.

Altshuler D, Hirschhorn JN, Klannemark M, Lindgren CM, Vohl MC, Nemesh J, Lane CR, Schaffner SF, Bolk S, Brewer C, et al.: The common PPARγ Pro12Ala polymorphism is associated with decreased risk of Type 2 diabetes. Nat Genet 2000; 26:76–80.

Arii K, Suehiro T, Yamamoto M, Ito H, Ikeda Y, Nakauchi Y, Hashimoto K: Trp64Arg mutation of β_3-adrenergic receptor and insulin sensitivity in subjects with glucose intolerance. Intern Med 1997; 36:603–606.

Armstrong M, Haldane F, Taylor RW, Humphriss D, Berrish T, Stewart MW, Turnbull DM, Alberti KG, Walker M: Human insulin receptor substrate-1: variant sequences in familial non-insulin-dependent diabetes mellitus. Diabet Med 1996; 13:133–138.

Arslanian SA: Type 2 diabetes mellitus in children: pathophysiology and risk factors. J Pediatr Endocrinol Metab 2000; 13(Suppl)6:1385–1394.

Arslanian SA, Lewy VD, Danadian K: Glucose intolerance in obese adolescents with polycystic ovary syndrome: roles of insulin resistance and β-cell dysfunction and risk of cardiovascular disease. J Clin Endocrinol Metab 2001; 86:66–71.

Ashcroft SJ, Niki I, Kenna S, Weng L, Skeer J, Coles B, Ashcroft FM: The β-cell sulfonylurea receptor. Adv Exp Med Biol 1993; 334:47–61.

Baier LJ, Bogardus C, Sacchettini JC: A polymorphism in the human intestinal fatty acid binding protein alters fatty acid transport accross Caco-2 cells. J Biol Chem 1996; 271:10892–10896.

Baier LJ, Dobberfuhl AM, Pratley RE, Hanson RL, Bogardus C: Variations in the vitamin D–binding protein (Gc locus) are associated with oral glucose tolerance in nondiabetic Pima Indians. J Clin Endocrinol Metab 1998; 83:2993–2996.

Baier LJ, Permana PA, Yang X, Pratley RE, Hanson RL, Shen GQ, Mott D, Knowler WC, Cox NJ, Horikawa Y, et al.: A calpain-10 gene polymorphism is associated with reduced muscle mRNA levels and insulin resistance. J Clin Invest 2000; 106:R69–R73.

Baier LJ, Sacchettini JC, Knowler WC, Eads J, Paolisso G, Tatarahni PA, Mochizuki H, Bennett PH, Bogardus C, Prochazka M: An amino acid substitution in the human intestinal fatty acid binding protein is associated with increased fatty acid binding, increased fat oxidation, and insulin resistance. J Clin Invest 1995; 95:1281–1287.

Ballinger SW, Shoffner JM, Hedaya EV, Trounce I, Polak MA, Koontz DA, Wallace DC: Maternally transmitted diabetes and deafness associated with a 10.4 kb mitochondrial DNA deletion. Nat Genet 1992; 1:11–15.

Banerji MA, Chaiken RL, Huey H, Tuomi T, Norin AJ, Mackay IR, Rowley MJ, Zimmet PZ, Lebovitz HE: GAD antibody negative NIDDM in adult black subjects with diabetic ketoacidosis and increased frequency of human leukocyte antigen DR3 and DR4: flatbush diabetes. Diabetes 1994; 43:741–745.

Banerji MA, Chaiken RL, Lebovitz HE: Prolongation of near-normoglycemic remission in black NIDDM subjects with chronic low-dose sulfonylurea treatment. Diabetes 1995; 44:466–470.

Barbetti F, Raben N, Kadowaki T, Cama A, Accili D, Gabbay KH, Merenich JA, Taylor SI, Roth J: Two unrelated patients with familial hyperproinsulinemia due to a mutation substituting histidine for arginine at position 65 in the proinsulin molecule: identification of the mutation by direct sequencing of genomic deoxyribonucleic acid amplified by polymerase chain reaction. J Clin Endocrinol Metab 1990; 71:164–169.

Barker DJ, Clark PM: Fetal undernutrition and disease in later life. Rev Reprod 1997; 2:105–112.

Barker DJ, Hales CN, Fall CH, Osmond C, Phipps K, Clark PM: Type 2 (non-insulin-dependent) diabetes mellitus, hypertension and hyperlipidaemia (syndrome X): relation to reduced fetal growth. Diabetologia 1993; 36:62–67.

Barker DJ, Winter PD, Osmond C, Margetts B, Simmonds SJ: Weight in infancy and death from ischaemic heart disease. Lancet 1989; 2:577–580.

Barnas U, Schmidt A, Illievich A, Kiener HP, Rabensteiner D, Kaider A, Prager R, Abrahamian H, Irsigler K, Mayer G: Evaluation of risk factors for the development of nephropathy in patients with IDDM: insertion/deletion angiotensin converting enzyme gene polymorphism, hypertension and metabolic control. Diabetologia 1997; 40:327–331.

Baroni MG, Alcolado JC, Pozzilli P, Cavallo MG, Li SR, Galton DJ: Polymorphisms at the GLUT2 (β-cell/liver) glucose transporter gene and non-insulin-dependent diabetes mellitus (NIDDM): analysis in affected pedigree members. Clin Genet 1992; 41:229–234.

Barrett TG, Bundey SE: Wolfram (DIDMOAD) syndrome. J Med Genet 1997; 34:838–841.

Barroso I, Gurnell M, Crowley VE, Agostini M, Schwabe JW, Soos MA, Maslen GL, Williams TD, Lewis H, Schafer AJ, et al.: Dominant negative mutations in human PPARγ associated with severe insulin resistance, diabetes mellitus and hypertension. Nature 1999; 402:880–883.

Beamer BA, Yen CJ, Andersen RE, Muller D, Elahi D, Cheskin LJ, Andres R, Roth J, Shuldiner AR: Association of the Pro12Ala variant in the peroxisome proliferator-activated receptor-γ_2 gene with obesity in two Caucasian populations. Diabetes 1998; 47:1806–1808.

Beards F, Frayling T, Bulman M, Horikawa Y, Allen L, Appleton M, Bell GI, Ellard S, Hattersley AT: Mutations in hepatocyte nuclear factor 1β are not a common cause of maturity-onset diabetes of the young in the U.K. Diabetes 1998; 47:1152–1154.

Bektas A, Hughes JN, Warram JH, Krolewski AS, Doria A: Type 2 diabetes locus on 12q15: further mapping and mutation screening of two candidate genes. Diabetes 2001; 50:204–208.

Bektas A, Suprenant ME, Wogan LT, Plengvidhya N, Rich SS, Warram JH, Krolewski AS, Doria A: Evidence of a novel Type 2 diabetes locus 50 cM centromeric to NIDDM2 on chromosome 12q. Diabetes 1999; 48:2246–2251.

Bell GI, Xiang K, Newman MV, Xiang KS, Wu SH, Wright LG, Fajans SS, Spielman RS, Cox NJ: Gene for non-insulin-dependent diabetes mellitus (maturity-onset diabetes of the young subtype) is linked to DNA polymorphism on human chromosome 20q. Proc Natl Acad Sci USA 1991; 88:1884–1888.

Benecke H, Topak H, von zur MA, Schuppert F: A study on the genetics of obesity: influence of polymorphisms of the β_3-adrenergic receptor and insulin receptor substrate-1 in relation to weight loss, waist to hip ratio and frequencies of common cardiovascular risk factors. Exp Clin Endocrinol Diabetes 2000; 108:86–92.

Bergman RN: Toward physiological understanding of glucose tolerance: minimal model approach. Diabetes 1989; 39:1512–1527.

Bernal D, Almind K, Yenush L, Ayoub M, Zhang Y, Rosshani L, Larsson C, Pedersen O, White MF: Insulin receptor substrate-2 amino acid polymorphisms are not associated with random Type 2 diabetes among Caucasians. Diabetes 1998; 47:976–979.

Berney DM, Desai M, Palmer DJ, Greenwald S, Brown A, Hales CN, Berry CL: The effects of maternal protein deprivation on the fetal rat pancreas: major structural changes and their recuperation. J Pathol 1997; 183:109–115.

Bienvenu T, Beldjord C, Chelly J, Fonknechten N, Hubert D, Dusser D, Kaplan JC: Analysis of alternative splicing patterns in the cystic fibrosis transmembrane conductance regulator gene using mRNA derived from lymphoblastoid cells of cystic fibrosis patients. Eur J Hum Genet 1996; 4:127–134.

Bingham C, Ellard S, Allen L, Bulman M, Shepherd M, Frayling T, Berry PJ, Clark PM, Lindner T, Bell GI, et al.: Abnormal nephron development associated with a frameshift mutation in the transcription factor hepatocyte nuclear factor-1β. Kidney Int 2000; 57:898–907.

Bogardus C, Lillioja S, Nyomba BL, Zurlo F, Swinburn B, Puente E-D, Knowler WC, Ravussin E, Mott DM, Bennett PH, et al.: Distribution of in vivo insulin action in Pima Indians as a mixture of three normal distributions. Diabetes 1989; 38:1423–1432.

Bolton-Smith C, Woodward M: Dietary composition and fat to sugar ratios in relation to obesity. Int J Obes Relat Metab Disord 1994; 18:820–828.

Borch-Johnsen K, Norgaard K, Hommel E, Mathiesen ER, Jensen JS, Deckert T, Parving HH: Is diabetic nephropathy an inherited complication? Kidney Int 1992; 41:719–722.

Bowden DW, Gravius TC, Akots G, Fajans SS: Identification of genetic markers flanking the locus for maturity-onset diabetes of the young on human chromosome 20. Diabetes 1992; 41:88–92.

Bowden DW, Sale M, Howard TD, Qadri A, Spray BJ, Rothschild CB, Akots G, Rich SS, Freedman BI: Linkage of genetic markers on human chromosomes 20 and 12 to NIDDM in Caucasian sib pairs with a history of diabetic nephropathy. Diabetes 1997; 46:882–886.

Bretz GW, Baghdassarian A, Graber JD, Zacherle BJ, Norum RA, Blizzard RM: Coexistence of diabetes mellitus and insipidus and optic atrophy in two male siblings: studies and review of literature. Am J Med 1970; 48:398–403.

Brunzell JD, Lerner RL, Hazzard WR, Porte D Jr., Bierman EL: Improved glucose tolerance with high carbohydrate feeding in mild diabetes. N Engl J Med 1971; 284:521–524.

Buemann B, Schierning B, Toubro S, Bibby B, Sorensen T, Dalgaard L, Pedersen O, Astrup A: The association between the val/ala-55 polymorphism of the uncoupling protein 2 gene and exercise efficiency. Int J Obes Relat Metab Disord 2001; 25:467–471.

Bulman MP, Dronsfield MJ, Frayling T, Appleton M, Bain SC, Ellard S, Hattersley AT: A missense mutation in the hepatocyte nuclear factor 4α gene in a UK pedigree with maturity-onset diabetes of the young. Diabetologia 1997; 40:859–862.

Burns SP, Desai M, Cohen RD, Hales CN, Iles RA, Germain JP, Going TC, Bailey RA: Gluconeogenesis, glucose handling, and structural changes in livers of the adult offspring of rats partially deprived of protein during pregnancy and lactation. J Clin Invest 1997; 100:1768–1774.

Buse JB, Yasuda K, Lay TP, Seo TS, Olson AL, Pessin JE, Karam JH, Seino S, Bell GI: Human GLUT4/muscle-fat glucose-transporter gene: characterization and genetic variation. Diabetes 1992; 41:1436–1445.

Byrne MM, Sturis J, Clement K, Vionnet N, Pueyo ME, Stoffel M, Takeda J, Passa P, Cohen D, Bell GI, et al.: Insulin secretory abnormalities in subjects with hyperglycemia due to glucokinse mutations. J Clin Invest 1994; 93:1120–1130.

Byrne MM, Sturis J, Fajans SS, Ortiz FJ, Stoltz A, Stoffel M, Smith MJ, Bell GI, Halter JB, Polonsky KS, et al.: Altered insulin secretory responses to glucose in subjects with a mutation in the *MODY1* gene on chromosome 20. Diabetes 1995; 44:699–704.

Byrne MM, Sturis J, Menzel S, Yamagata K, Fajans SS, Dronsfield MJ, Bain SC, Hattersley AT, Velho G, Froguel P, et al.: Altered insulin secretory responses to glucose in diabetic and nondiabetic subjects with mutations in the diabetes susceptibility gene *MODY3* on chromosome 12. Diabetes 1996; 45:1503–1510.

Caldwell JS, Moyers JS, Doria A, Reynet C, Kahn RC: Molecular cloning of the human rad gene: gene structure and complete nucleotide sequence. Biochim Biophys Acta 1996; 1316:145–148.

Cao H, Hegele RA: Human hepatocyte nuclear factor 1β (HNF1B) 1968A/G polymorphism. J Hum Genet 2000; 45:98–99.

Carroll RJ, Hammer RE, Chan SJ, Swift HH, Rubenstein AH, Steiner DF: A mutant human proinsulin is secreted from islets of Langerhans in increased amounts via an unregulated pathway. Proc Natl Acad Sci USA 1988; 85:8943–8947.

Castellani LW, Weinreb A, Bodnar J, Goto AM, Doolittle M, Mehrabian M, Demant P, Lusis AJ: Mapping a gene for combined hyperlipidaemia in a mutant mouse strain. Nat Genet 1998; 18:374–377.

Celi FS, Negri C, Tanner K, Raben N, De Pablo F, Rovira A, Pallardo LF, Martin-Vaquero P, Stern MP, Mitchell BD, et al.: Molecular scanning for mutations in the insulin receptor substrate-1 (IRS-1) gene in Mexican Americans with Type 2 diabetes mellitus. Diabetes Metab Res Rev 2000; 16:370–377.

Celi FS, Silver K, Walston J, Knowler WC, Bogardus C, Shuldiner AR: Lack of IRS-1 codon 513 and 972 polymorphism in Pima Indians. J Clin Endocrinol Metab 1995; 80:2827–2829.

Chagnon YC, Chung WK, Perusse L, Chagnon M, Leibel RL, Bouchard C: Linkages and associations between the leptin receptor (LEPR) gene and human body composition in the Quebec Family Study. Int J Obes Relat Metab Disord 1999; 23:278–286.

Chagnon YC, Wilmore JH, Borecki IB, Gagnon J, Perusse L, Chagnon M, Collier GR, Leon AS, Skinner JS, Rao DC, et al.: Associations between the leptin receptor gene and adiposity in middle-aged Caucasian males from the HERITAGE family study. J Clin Endocrinol Metab 2000; 85:29–34.

Chen M, Bergman RN, Porte D Jr.: Insulin resistance and β-cell dysfunction in aging: the importance of dietary carbohydrate. J Clin Endocrinol Metab 1988; 67:951–957.

Chevre JC, Hani EH, Stoffers DA, Habener JF, Froguel P: Insulin promoter factor 1 gene is not a major cause of maturity-onset diabetes of the young in French Caucasians. Diabetes 1998; 47:843–844.

Chiu KC, Chuang LM, Yoon C: The A54T polymorphism at the intestinal fatty acid binding protein 2 is associated with insulin resistance in glucose tolerant Caucasians. Biomed Chromatogr Genet 2001; 2:7.

Chiu KC, Cohan P, Lee NP, Chuang LM: Insulin sensitivity differs among ethnic groups with a compensatory response in β-cell function. Diabetes Care 2000; 23:1353–1358.

Chiu KC, McCarthy JE: Promoter variation in liver glucokinase is a risk factor for non-insulin-dependent diabetes mellitus. Biochem Biophys Res Comm 1996; 221:614–618.

Chiu KC, Province MA, Permutt MA: Glucokinase gene is genetic marker for NIDDM in American blacks. Diabetes 1992; 41:843–849.

Chiu KC, Tanizawa Y, Permutt MA: Glucokinase gene variants in the common form of NIDDM. Diabetes 1993; 42:579–582.

Choi W-H, O'Rahilly S, Buse JB, Rees A, Morgan R, Flier JS, Moller DE: Molecular scanning of insulin-responsive glucose transporter (*GLUT4*) gene in NIDDM subjects. Diabetes 1991; 40:1712–1718.

Chowdhury TA, Dyer PH, Kumar S, Barnett AH, Bain SC: Genetic determinants of diabetic nephropathy. Clin Sci (Colch) 1999; 96:221–230.

Chowdhury TA, Kumar S, Barnett AH, Bain SC: Nephropathy in Type 1 diabetes: the role of genetic factors. Diabet Med 1995; 12:1059–1067.

Clausen JO, Hansen T, Bjorbaek C, Echwald SM, Urhammer SA, Rasmussen S, Andersen CB, Hansen L, Almind K, Winther K, et al.: Insulin resistance: interactions between obesity and a common variant of insulin receptor substrate-1. Lancet 1995; 346:397–402.

Clauson P, Linnarsson R, Gottsater A, Sundkvist G, Grill V: Relationships between diabetes duration, metabolic control and β-cell function in a representative population of Type 2 diabetic patients in Sweden. Diabet Med 1994; 11:794–801.

Clement K, Dina C, Basdevant A, Chastang N, Pelloux V, Lahlou N, Berlan M, Langin D, Guy-Grand B, Froguel P: A sib-pair analysis study of 15 candidate genes in French families with morbid obesity: indication for linkage with islet 1 locus on chromosome 5q. Diabetes 1999; 48:398–402.

Clement K, Garner C, Hager J, Philippi A, LeDuc C, Carey A, Harris TJ, Jury C, Cardon LR, Basdevant A, et al.: Indication for linkage of the human OB gene region with extreme obesity. Diabetes 1996; 45:687–690.

Clement K, Hercberg S, Passinge B, Galan P, Varroud-Vial M, Shuldiner AR, Beamer BA, Charpentier G, Guy-Grand B, Froguel P, et al.: The Pro115Gln and Pro12Ala PPAR γ gene mutations in obesity and Type 2 diabetes. Int J Obes Relat Metab Disord 2000; 24:391–393.

Clement K, Vaisse C, Manning BS, Basdevant A, Guy Grand B, Ruiz J, Silver KD, Shuldiner AR, Froguel P, Strosberg AD: Genetic variation in the β_3-adrenergic receptor and an increased capacity to gain weight in patients with morbid obesity. N Engl J Med 1995; 333:352–354.

Cole SA, Mitchell BD, Hsueh WC, Pineda P, Beamer BA, Shuldiner AR, Comuzzie AG, Blangero J, Hixson JE: The Pro12Ala variant of peroxisome proliferator-activated receptor-γ_2 (PPAR-γ_2) is associated with measures of obesity in Mexican Americans. Int J Obes Relat Metab Disord 2000; 24:522–524.

Collier DA, Barrett TG, Curtis D, Macleod A, Arranz MJ, Maassen JA, Bundey S: Linkage of Wolfram syndrome to chromosome 4p16.1 and evidence for heterogeneity. Am J Hum Genet 1996; 59:855–863.

Comuzzie AG, Hixson JE, Almasy L, Mitchell BD, Mahaney MC, Dyer TD, Stern MP, MacCluer JW, Blangero J: A major quantitative trait locus determining serum leptin levels and fat mass is located on human chromosome 2. Nat Genet 1997; 15:273–276.

Cook JT, Hattersley AT, Christopher P, Bown E, Barrow B, Patel P, Shaw JA, Cookson WO, Permutt MA, Turner RC: Linkage analysis of glucokinase gene with NIDDM in Caucasian pedigrees. Diabetes 1992; 41:1496–1500.

Cook JT, Patel PP, Clark A, Hoppener JW, Lips CJ, Mosselman S, O'Rahilly S, Page RC, Wainscoat JS, Turner RC: Non-linkage of the islet amyloid polypeptide gene with type 2 (non-insulin-dependent) diabetes mellitus. Diabetologia 1991; 34:103–108.

Costa A, Rodriguez C, Gomis R, Conget I, Casamitjana R, Bescos M: Follow up of a HNF-1α mutant carrier with a severely impaired β cell function. Diabetes Res Clin Pract 2000; 48:67–70.

Costanzo BV, Trischitta V, Di Paola R, Spampinato D, Pizzuti A, Vigneri R, Frittitta L: The Q allele variant (GLN121) of membrane glycoprotein PC-1 interacts with the insulin receptor and inhibits insulin signaling more effectively than the common K allele variant (LYS121). Diabetes 2001; 50:831–836.

Covic AM, Iyengar SK, Olson JM, Sehgal AR, Constantiner M, Jedrey C, Kara M, Sabbagh E, Sedor JR, Schelling JR: A family-based strategy to identify genes for diabetic nephropathy. Am J Kidney Dis 2001; 37:638–647.

Cox NJ, Frigge M, Nicolae DL, Concannon P, Hanis CL, Bell GI, Kong A: Loci on chromosomes 2 (NIDDM1) and 15 interact to increase susceptibility to diabetes in Mexican Americans. Nat Genet 1999; 21:213–215.

Cremers CW, Wijdeveld PG, Pinckers AJ: Juvenile diabetes mellitus, optic atrophy, hearing loss, diabetes insipidus, atonia of the urinary tract and bladder, and other abnormalities (Wolfram syndrome): a review of 88 cases from the literature with personal observations on 3 new patients. Acta Paediatr Scand Suppl 1977; 1–16.

Curhan GC, Willett WC, Rimm EB, Spiegelman D, Ascherio AL, Stampfer MJ: Birth weight and adult hypertension, diabetes mellitus, and obesity in U.S. men. Circulation 1996; 94:3246–3250.

Dahri S, Snoeck A, Reusens-Billen B, Remacle C, Hoet JJ: Islet function in offspring of mothers on low-protein diet during gestation. Diabetes 1991; 40(Suppl 2):115–120.

Dalgaard LT, Sorensen TI, Andersen T, Hansen T, Pedersen O: An untranslated insertion variant in the uncoupling protein 2 gene is not related to body mass index and changes in body weight during a 26-year follow-up in Danish Caucasian men. Diabetologia 1999; 42:1413–1416.

Davies JL, Yoshihiko K, Bennett S, Copeman JB, Cordell HJ, Pritchard LE, Reed PW, Gough SCL, Jenkins C, Palmer SM, et al.: A genome-wide search for human Type 1 diabetes susceptibility genes. Nature 1994; 371:130–136.

Deeb SS, Fajas L, Nemoto M, Pihlajamaki J, Mykkanen L, Kuusisto J, Laakso M, Fujimoto W, Auwerx J: A Pro12Ala substitution in PPARγ_2 associated with decreased receptor activity, lower body mass index and improved insulin sensitivity. Nat Genet 1998; 20:284–287.

DeFronzo RA: Diabetic nephropathy: etiologic and therapeutic considerations. Diabet Rev 1995; 3:510–550.

DeFronzo RA: Pathogenesis of Type 2 diabetes: metabolic and molecular implications for identifying diabetes genes. Diabet Rev 1997; 5:177–270.

DeFronzo RA, Bonadonna RC, Ferrannini E: Pathogenesis of NIDDM: a balanced overview. Diabetes Care 1992; 15:318–368.

Del Prato S, Leonetti F, Simonson DC, Sheehan P, Matsuda M, DeFronzo RA: Effect of sustained physiologic hyperinsulinaemia and hyperglycaemia on insulin secretion and insulin sensitivity in man. Diabetologia 1994; 37:1025–1035.

Desai M, Byrne CD, Meeran K, Martenz ND, Bloom SR, Hales CN: Regulation of hepatic enzymes and insulin levels in offspring of rat dams fed a reduced-protein diet. Am J Physiol 1997a; 273:G899–G904.

Desai M, Byrne CD, Zhang J, Petry CJ, Lucas A, Hales CN: Programming of hepatic insulin-sensitive enzymes in offspring of rat dams fed a protein-restricted diet. Am J Physiol 1997b; 272:G1083–G1090.

Dinneen S, Gerich J, Rizza R: Carbohydrate metabolism in non-insulin-dependent diabetes mellitus. N Engl J Med 1992; 327:707–713.

Doria A, Caldwell JS, Ji L, Reynet C, Rich SS, Weremowicz S, Morton CC, Warram JH, Kahn CR, Krolewski AS: Trinucleotide repeats at the rad locus: allele distributions in NIDDM and mapping to a 3-cM region on chromosome 16q. Diabetes 1995; 44:243–247.

Dowse GK, Zimmet PZ, Gareeboo H, George K, Alberti MM, Tuomilehto J, Finch

CF, Chitson P, Tulsidas H: Abdominal obesity and physical inactivity as risk factors for NIDDM and impaired glucose tolerance in Indian, Creole, and Chinese Mauritians. Diabetes Care 1991; 14:271–282.

Duggirala R, Blangero J, Almasy L, Dyer TD, Williams KL, Leach RJ, O'Connell P, Stern MP: Linkage of Type 2 diabetes mellitus and of age at onset to a genetic location on chromosome 10q in Mexican Americans. Am J Hum Genet 1999; 64:1127–1140.

Dukes ID, McIntyre MS, Mertz RJ, Philipson LH, Roe MW, Spencer B, Worley JF III: Dependence on NADH produced during glycolysis for beta-cell glucose signaling. J Biol Chem 1994; 269:10979–10982.

Dunaif A, Finegood DT: β-cell dysfunction independent of obesity and glucose intolerance in the polycystic ovary syndrome. J Clin Endocrinol Metab 1996; 81:942–947.

Dunne MJ, Kane C, Shepherd RM, Sanchez JA, James RF, Johnson PR, Aynsley-Green A, Lu S, Clement JP, Lindley KJ, et al.: Familial persistent hyperinsulinemic hypoglycemia of infancy and mutations in the sulfonylurea receptor. N Engl J Med 1997; 336:703–706.

Dyer PH, Chowdhury TA, Dronsfield MJ, Dunger D, Barnett AH, Bain SC: The 5′-end polymorphism of the aldose reductase gene is not associated with diabetic nephropathy in Caucasian Type I diabetic patients. Diabetologia 1999; 42:1030–1031.

Echwald SM, Bjorbaek C, Hansen T, Clausen JO, Vestergaard H, Zierath JR, Printz RL, Granner DK, Pedersen O: Identification of four amino acid substitutions in hexokinase II and studies of relationships to NIDDM, glucose effectiveness, and insulin sensitivity. Diabetes 1995; 44:347–353.

Ehm MG, Karnoub MC, Sakul H, Gottschalk K, Holt DC, Weber JL, Vaske D, Briley D, Briley L, Kopf J, et al.: Genomewide search for Type 2 diabetes susceptibility genes in four American populations. Am J Hum Genet 2000; 66:1871–1881.

Ek J, Urhammer SA, Sorensen TI, Andersen T, Auwerx J, Pedersen O: Homozygosity of the Pro12Ala variant of the peroxisome proliferation-activated receptor-γ_2 (PPAR-γ_2): divergent modulating effects on body mass index in obese and lean Caucasian men. Diabetologia 1999; 42:892–895.

Elbein SC, Bragg KL, Hoffman MD, Mayorga RA, Leppert MF: Linkage studies of NIDDM with 23 chromosome 11 markers in a sample of whites of northern European descent. Diabetes 1996a; 45:370–375.

Elbein SC, Chiu KC, Hoffman MD, Mayorga RA, Bragg KL, Leppert MF: Linkage analysis of 19 candidate regions for insulin resistance in familial NIDDM. Diabetes 1995; 44:1259–1265.

Elbein SC, Corsetti L, Goldgar D, Skolnick M, Permutt MA: Insulin gene in familial NIDDM: lack of linkage in Utah Mormon pedigrees. Diabetes 1988; 37:569–576.

Elbein SC, Hasstedt SJ, Wegner K, Kahn SE: Heritability of pancreatic β-cell function among nondiabetic members of Caucasian familial Type 2 diabetic kindreds. J Clin Endocrinol Metab 1999; 84:1398–1403.

Elbein SC, Hoffman M, Barrett K, Wegner K, Miles C, Bachman K, Berkowitz D, Shuldiner AR, Leppert MF, Hasstedt S: Role of the β_3-adrenergic receptor locus in obesity and noninsulin-dependent diabetes among members of Caucasian families with a diabetic sibling pair. J Clin Endocrinol Metab 1996b; 81:4422–4427.

Elbein SC, Hoffman M, Chiu K, Tanizawa Y, Permutt MA: Linkage analysis of the glucokinase locus in familial Type 2 (non-insulin-dependent) diabetic pedigrees. Diabetologia 1993a; 36:141–145.

Elbein SC, Hoffman M, Qin H, Chiu K, Tanizawa Y, Permutt MA: Molecular screening of the glucokinase gene in familial Type 2 (non-insulin-dependent) diabetes mellitus. Diabetologia 1994a; 37:182–187.

Elbein SC, Hoffman M, Ridinger D, Otterud B, Leppert M: Description of a second microsatellite marker and linkage analysis of the muscle glycogen synthase locus in familial NIDDM. Diabetes 1994b; 43:1061–1065.

Elbein SC, Hoffman MD: Role of mitochondrial DNA tRNA leucine and glucagon receptor missense mutations in Utah white diabetic patients. Diabetes Care 1996; 19:507–508.

Elbein SC, Hoffman MD, Matsutani A, Permutt MA: Linkage analysis of *GLUT1* (HepG2) and *GLUT2* (liver/islet) genes in familial NIDDM. Diabetes 1992; 41:1660–1667.

Elbein SC, Hoffman MD, Teng K, Leppert MF, Hasstedt SJ: A genome-wide search for Type 2 diabetes susceptibility genes in Utah Caucasians. Diabetes 1999b; 48: 1175–1182.

Elbein SC, Leppert M, Hasstedt S: Uncoupling protein 2 region on chromosome 11q13 is not linked to markers of obesity in familial Type 2 diabtetes. Diabetes 1997; 46:2105–2107.

Elbein SC, Sorensen LK, Schumacher MC: Methionine for valine substitution in exon 17 of the insulin receptor gene in a pedigree with familial NIDDM. Diabetes 1993b; 42:429–434.

Elbein SC, Sun J, Scroggin E, Teng K, Hasstedt SJ: Role of common sequence variants in insulin secretion in familial Type 2 diabetic kindreds: the sulfonylurea receptor, glucokinase, and hepatocyte nuclear factor 1α genes. Diabetes Care 2001; 24:472–478.

Elbein SC, Teng K, Eddings K, Hargrove D, Scroggin E: Molecular scanning analysis of hepatocyte nuclear factor 1α (TCF1) gene in typical familial Type 2 diabetes in African Americans. Metabolism 2000a; 49:280–284.

Elbein SC, Teng K, Yount P, Scroggin E: Linkage and molecular scanning analyses of MODY3/hepatocyte nuclear factor-1 α gene in typical familial Type 2 diabetes: evidence for novel mutations in exons 8 and 10. J Clin Endocrinol Metab 1998; 83:2059–2065.

Elbein SC, Wegner K, Kahn SE: Reduced β-cell compensation to the insulin resistance associated with obesity in members of caucasian familial Type 2 diabetic kindreds. Diabetes Care 2000b; 23:221–227.

Ellard S: Hepatocyte nuclear factor 1 α (HNF-1α) mutations in maturity-onset diabetes of the young. Hum Mutat 2000; 16:377–385.

Esterbauer H, Schneitler C, Oberkofler H, Ebenbichler C, Paulweber B, Sandhofer F, Ladurner G, Hell E, Strosberg AD, Patsch JR, et al.: A common polymorphism in the promoter of UCP2 is associated with decreased risk of obesity in middle-aged humans. Nat Genet 2001; 28:178–183.

Eto K, Sakura H, Shimokawa K, Kadowaki H, Hagura R, Akanuma Y, Yazaki Y, Kadowaki T: Sequence variations of the glucokinase gene in Japanese subjects with NIDDM. Diabetes 1993; 42:1133–1137.

Expert Committee on the Diagnosis and Classification of Diabetes Mellitus: Report of the expert committee on the diagnosis and classification of diabetes mellitus. Diabetes Care 1997; 20:1183–1197.

Fajans SS: Scope and heterogeneous nature of MODY [published errata appear in Diabetes Care 1990 (Mar); 13(3), following table of contents, and 1990 (Aug); 13(8):910]. Diabetes Care 1990; 13:49–64.

Fajans SS, Bell GI, Bowden DW, Halter JB, Polonsky KS: Maturity onset diabetes of the young (MODY). Diabet Med 1996; 13:S90–S95.

Fakhrai-Rad H, Nikoshkov A, Kamel A, Fernstrom M, Zierath JR, Norgren S, Luthman H, Galli J: Insulin-degrading enzyme identified as a candidate diabetes susceptibility gene in GK rats. Hum Mol Genet 2000; 9:2149–2158.

Fogarty DG, Krolewski AS: Genetic susceptibility and the role of hypertension in diabetic nephropathy. Curr Opin Nephrol Hypertens 1997; 6:184–191.

Forrester TE, Wilks RJ, Bennett FI, Simeon D, Osmond C, Allen M, Chung AP, Scott P: Fetal growth and cardiovascular risk factors in Jamaican schoolchildren. Br Med J 1996; 312:156–160.

Francke S, Clement K, Dina C, Inoue H, Behn P, Vatin V, Basdevant A, Guy-Grand B, Permutt MA, Froguel P, et al.: Genetic studies of the leptin receptor gene in morbidly obese French Caucasian families. Hum Genet 1997; 100:491–496.

Fraser FC, Gunn T: Diabetes mellitus, diabetes insipidus, and optic atrophy: an autosomal recessive syndrome? J Med Genet 1977; 14:190–193.

Frayling TM, Bulman MP, Ellard S, Appleton M, Dronsfield MJ, Mackie ADR, Baird JD, Kaisaki PJ, Yamagata K, Bell GI, et al.: Mutations in the hepatocyte nuclear factor-1α gene are a common cause of maturity onset diabetes of the young in the U.K. Diabetes 1997; 46:720–725.

Frayling TM, Evans JC, Bulman MP, Pearson E, Allen L, Owen K, Bingham C, Hannemann M, Shepherd M, Ellard S, et al.: β-cell genes and diabetes: molecular and clinical characterization of mutations in transcription factors. Diabetes 2001; 50(Suppl 1):S94–100.

Frayling TM, McCarthy MI, Walker M, Levy JC, O'Rahilly S, Hitman GA, Rao PV, Bennett AJ, Jones EC, Menzel S, et al.: No evidence for linkage at candidate Type 2 diabetes susceptibility loci on chromosomes 12 and 20 in United Kingdom Caucasians. J Clin Endocrinol Metab 2000; 85:853–857.

Freedman BI, Tuttle AB, Spray BJ: Familial predisposition to nephropathy in African-Americans with non-insulin-dependent diabetes mellitus. Am J Kidney Dis 1995; 25:710–713.

Frittitta L, Ercolino T, Bozzali M, Argiolas A, Graci S, Santagati MG, Spampinato D, Di Paola R, Cisternino C, Tassi V, et al.: A cluster of three single nucleotide polymorphisms in the 3′-untranslated region of human glycoprotein PC-1 gene stabilizes PC-1 mRNA and is associated with increased PC-1 protein content and insulin resistance–related abnormalities. Diabetes 2001; 50:1952–1955.

Froguel P: Glucokinase and *MODY*: from the gene to the disease. Diabet Med 1996; 13:S96–97.

Froguel P, Vaxillaire M, Sun F, Velho G, Zouali H, Butel MO, Lesage S, Vionnet N, Clement K, Fougerousse F, et al.: Close linkage of glucokinase locus on chromosome 7p to early-onset non-insulin-dependent diabetes mellitus. Nature 1992; 356:162–164.

Froguel P, Zouali H, Vionnet N, Velho G, Vaxillaire M, Sun F, Lesage S, Stoffel M, Takeda J, Passa P, et al.: Familial hyperglycemia due to mutations in glucokinase. definition of a subtype of diabetes mellitus. N Engl J Med 1993; 328:697–702.

Fujisawa T, Ikegami H, Yamato E, Takekawa K, Nakagawa Y, Hamada Y, Oga T, Ueda H, Shintani M, Fukuda M, et al.: Association of Trp64Arg mutation of the β_3-adrenergic receptor with NIDDM and body weight gain. Diabetologia 1996; 39:349–352.

Fujisawa T, Ikegami H, Yamato E, Takekawa K, Nakagawa Y, Hamada Y, Ueda H, Fukuda M, Ogihara T: A mutation in the glucagon receptor gene (Gly40Ser): heterogeneity in the association with diabetes mellitus. Diabetologia 1995; 38:983–985.

Fukunaga Y, Azuma N, Koshiyama H, Inoue D, Sato H, Yoshimasa Y, Nakao K: Mitochondrial DNA 3243 mutation is infrequent in Japanese diabetic patients with auditory disturbance [letter; comment]. Diabetes Care 1997; 20:1800–1803.

Furuta H, Iwasaki N, Oda N, Hinokio Y, Horikawa Y, Yamagata K, Yano H, Sugahiro J, Ogata M, Ohgawara H, et al.: Organization and partial sequence of the hepatocyte nuclear factor-4 α/*MODY1* gene and identification of a missense mutation, R127W, in a Japanese family with MODY. Diabetes 1997; 46:1652–1657.

Gagnon J, Mauriege P, Roy S, Sjostrom D, Chagnon YC, Dionne FT, Oppert JM, Perusse L, Sjostrom L, Bouchard C: The Trp64Arg mutation of the β_3-adrenergic receptor gene has no effect on obesity phenotypes in the Quebec Family Study and Swedish Obese Subjects cohorts. J Clin Invest 1996; 98:2086–2093.

Galli J, Li LS, Glaser A, Ostenson CG, Jiao H, Fakhrai Rad H, Jacob HJ, Lander ES, Luthman H: Genetic analysis of non-insulin dependent diabetes mellitus in the GK rat. Nat Genet 1996; 12:31–37.

Gardner LI Jr., Stern MP, Haffner SM, Gaskill SP, Hazuda HP, Relethford JH, Eifler CW: Prevalence of diabetes in Mexican Americans: relationship to percent of gene pool derived from Native American sources. Diabetes 1984; 33:86–92.

Gauguier D, Froguel P, Parent V, Bernard C, Bihoreau MT, Portha B, James MR, Penicaud L, Lathrop M, Ktorza A: Chromosomal mapping of genetic loci associated with non-insulin dependent diabetes in the GK rat. Nat Genet 1996; 12:38–43.

Ghosh S, Langefeld CD, Ally D, Watanabe RM, Hauser ER, Magnuson VL, Nylund SJ, Valle T, Eriksson J, Bergman RN, et al.: The W64R variant of the β_3-adrenergic receptor is not associated with Type II diabetes or obesity in a large Finnish sample. Diabetologia 1999a; 42:238–244.

Ghosh S, Watanabe RM, Hauser ER, Valle T, Magnuson VL, Erdos MR, Langefeld

CD, Balow J Jr, Ally DS, Kohtamaki K, et al.: Type 2 diabetes: evidence for linkage on chromosome 20 in 716 Finnish affected sib pairs. Proc Natl Acad Sci USA 1999b; 96:2198–2203.

Ghosh S, Watanabe RM, Valle TT, Hauser ER, Magnuson VL, Langefeld CD, Ally DS, Mohlke KL, Silander K, Kohtamaki K, et al.: The Finland–United States investigation of non-insulin-dependent diabetes mellitus genetics (FUSION) study: I. An autosomal genome scan for genes that predispose to Type 2 diabetes. Am J Hum Genet 2000; 67:1174–1185.

Glaser B, Chiu KC, Anker R, Nestorowicz A, Landau H, Ben Bassat H, Shlomai Z, Kaiser N, Thornton PS, Stanley CA, et al.: Familial hyperinsulinism maps to chromosome 11p14–15.1, 30 cM centromeric to the insulin gene. Nat Genet 1994; 7:185–188.

Glaser B, Furth J, Stanley CA, Baker L, Thornton PS, Landau H, Permutt MA: Intragenic single nucleotide polymorphism haplotype analysis of SUR1 mutations in familial hyperinsulinism. Hum Mutat 1999; 14:23–29.

Glucksmann MA, Lehto M, Tayber O, Scotti S, Berkemeier L, Pulido JC, Wu Y, Nir WJ, Fang L, Markel P, et al.: Novel mutations and a mutational hotspot in the *MODY3* gene. Diabetes 1997; 46:1081–1086.

Godart F, Bellanne-Chantelot C, Clauin S, Gragnoli C, Abderrahmani A, Blanche H, Boutin P, Chevre JC, Froguel P, Bailleul B: Identification of seven novel nucleotide variants in the hepatocyte nuclear factor-1α (TCF1) promoter region in MODY patients. Hum Mutat 2000; 15:173–180.

Goldfine ID, Maddux BA, Youngren JF, Frittitta L, Trischitta V, Dohm GL: Membrane glycoprotein PC-1 and insulin resistance. Mol Cell Biochem 1998; 182: 177–184.

Gough SC, Saker PJ, Pritchard LE, Merriman TR, Merriman ME, Rowe BR, Kumar S, Aitman T, Barnett AH, Turner RC: Mutation of the glucagon receptor gene and diabetes mellitus in the UK: association or founder effect? Hum Mol Genet 1995; 4:1609–1612.

Gragnoli C, Lindner T, Cockburn BN, Kaisaki PJ, Gragnoli F, Marozzi G, Bell GI: Maturity-onset diabetes of the young due to a mutation in the hepatocyte nuclear factor-4α binding site in the promoter of the hepatocyte nuclear factor-1α gene. Diabetes 1997; 46:1648–1651.

Grimberg A, Ferry RJ Jr., Kelly A, Koo-McCoy S, Polonsky K, Glaser B, Permutt MA, Aguilar-Bryan L, Stafford D, Thornton PS, et al.: Dysregulation of insulin secretion in children with congenital hyperinsulinism due to sulfonylurea receptor mutations. Diabetes 2001; 50:322–328.

Groop LC, Kankuri M, Schalin Jantti C, Ekstrand A, Nikula Ijas P, Widen E, Kuismanen E, Eriksson J, Franssila Kallunki A, Saloranta C, et al.: Association between polymorphism of the glycogen synthase gene and non-insulin-dependent diabetes mellitus. N Engl J Med 1993; 328:10–14.

Gu HF, Almgren P, Lindholm E, Frittitta L, Pizzuti A, Trischitta V, Groop LC: Association between the human glycoprotein PC-1 gene and elevated glucose and insulin levels in a paired-sibling analysis. Diabetes 2000; 49:1601–1603.

Guillausseau PJ, Massin P, Dubois-Laforgue D, Timsit J, Virally M, Gin H, Bertin E, Blickle JF, Bouhanick B, Cahen J, et al.: Maternally inherited diabetes and deafness: a multicenter study. Ann Intern Med 2001; 134:721–728.

Gulli G, Ferrannini E, Stern M, Haffner S, DeFronzo RA: The metabolic profile of NIDDM is fully established in glucose-tolerant offspring of two Mexican-American NIDDM parents. Diabetes 1992; 41:1575–1586.

Gumbiner B, Polonsky KS, Beltz WF, Griver K, Wallace P, Brechtel G, Henry RR: Effects of weight loss and reduced hyperglycemia on the kinetics of insulin secretion in obese non-insulin dependent diabetes mellitus. J Clin Endocrinol Metab 1990; 70:1594–1602.

Haffner SM, Stern MP, Hazuda HP, Mitchell BD, Patterson JK: Increased insulin concentrations in nondiabetic offspring of diabetic parents. N Engl J Med 1988; 319:1297–1301.

Hager J, Dina C, Francke S, Dubois S, Houari M, Vatin V, Vaillant E, Lorentz N, Basdevant A, Clement K, et al.: A genome-wide scan for human obesity genes reveals a major susceptibility locus on chromosome 10. Nat Genet 1998; 20:304–308.

Hager J, Hansen L, Vaisse C, Vionnet N, Philippi A, Poller W, Velho G, Carcassi C, Contu L, Julier C:. A missense mutation in the glucagon receptor gene is associated with non-insulin-dependent diabetes mellitus. Nat Genet 1995; 9:299–304.

Hales CN, Barker DJ: Type 2 (non-insulin-dependent) diabetes mellitus: the thrifty phenotype hypothesis. Diabetologia 1992; 35:595–601.

Hani E, Clement K, Velho G, Vionnet N, Hager J, Philippi A, Dina C, Inoue H, Permutt MA, Basdevant A, et al.: Genetic studies of the sulfonylurea receptor gene locus in NIDDM and in morbid obesity among French Caucasians. Diabetes 1997; 46:688–694.

Hani E, Suaud L, Boutin P, Chevre JC, Durand E, Philippi A, Demenais F, Vionnet N, Furuta H, Velho G, et al.: A missense mutation in hepatocyte nuclear factor-4 α, resulting in a reduced transactivation activity, in human late-onset non-insulin-dependent diabetes mellitus. J Clin Invest 1998; 101:521–526.

Hani E, Zouali H, Philippi A, Beaudoin J, Vionnet N, Passa P, Demenais F, Froguel P: Indication for genetic linkage of the phosphoenolpyruvate carboxykinase (PCK1) gene region on chromosome 20q to non-insulin-dependent diabetes mellitus. Diabetes Metab 1996; 22:451–454.

Hanis CL, Boerwinkle E, Chakraborty R, Ellsworth DL, Concannon P, Stirling B, Morrison VA, Wapelhorst B, Spielman RS, Gogolin-Ewens KJ, et al.: A genome-wide search for human non-insulin-dependent (Type 2) diabetes genes reveals a major susceptibility locus on chromosome 2. Nat Genet 1996; 13:161–166.

Hanis CL, Hewett-Emmett D, Bertin TK, Schull WJ: Origins of U.S. Hispanics: implications for diabetes. Diabetes Care 1991; 14:618–627.

Hansen L, Arden KC, Rasmussen SB, Viars CS, Vestergaard H, Hansen T, Moller AM, Woodgett JR, Pedersen O: Chromosomal mapping and mutational analysis of the coding region of the glycogen synthase kinase-3α and -β isoforms in patients with NIDDM. Diabetologia 1997a; 40:940–946.

Hansen L, Echwald SM, Hansen T, Urhammer SA, Clausen JO, Pedersen O: Amino acid polymorphisms in the ATP-regulatable inward rectifier Kir6.2 and their relationships to glucose- and tolbutamide-induced insulin secretion, the insulin sensitivity index, and NIDDM. Diabetes 1997b; 46:508–512.

Hansen L, Hansen T, Clausen JO, Echwald SM, Urhammer SA, Rasmussen SK, Pedersen O: The Val985Met insulin-receptor variant in the Danish Caucasian population: lack of associations with non-insulin-dependent diabetes mellitus or insulin resistance [letter]. Am J Hum Genet 1997c; 60:1532–1535.

Hansen L, Hansen T, Vestergaard H, Bjorbaek C, Echwald SM, Clausen JO, Chen YH, Chen MX, Cohen PT, Pedersen O: A widespread amino acid polymorphism at codon 905 of the glycogen-associated regulatory subunit of protein phosphatase-1 is associated with insulin resistance and hypersecretion of insulin. Hum Mol Genet 1995; 4:1313–1320.

Hansen L, Reneland R, Berglund L, Rasmussen SK, Hansen T, Lithell H, Pedersen O: Polymorphism in the glycogen-associated regulatory subunit of type 1 protein phosphatase (PPP1R3) gene and insulin sensitivity. Diabetes 2000a; 49:298–301.

Hansen L, Urioste S, Petersen HV, Jensen JN, Eiberg H, Barbetti F, Serup P, Hansen T, Pedersen O: Missense mutations in the human insulin promoter factor-1 gene and their relation to maturity-onset diabetes of the young and late-onset Type 2 diabetes mellitus in caucasians. J Clin Endocrinol Metab 2000b; 85:1323–1326.

Hansen LH, Abrahamsen N, Hager J, Jelinek L, Kindsvogel W, Froguel P, Nishimura E: The Gly40Ser mutation in the human glucagon receptor gene associated with NIDDM results in a receptor with reduced sensitivity to glucagon. Diabetes 1996; 45:725–730.

Hansen T, Andersen CB, Echwald SM, Urhammer SA, Clausen JO, Vestergaard H, Owens D, Hansen L, Pedersen O: Identification of a common amino acid polymorphism in the p85α regulatory subunit of phosphatidylinositol 3-kinase: effects of glucose disappearance constant, glucose effectiveness, and the insulin sensitivity index. Diabetes 1997d; 46:494–501.

Hansen T, Eiberg H, Rouard M, Vaxillaire M, Moller AM, Rasmussen SK, Fridberg M, Urhammer SA, Holst JJ, Almind K, et al.: Novel MODY3 mutations in the hepatocyte nuclear factor-1α gene: evidence for a hyperexcitability of pancreatic β-cells to intravenous secretagogues in a glucose-tolerant carrier of a P447L mutation. Diabetes 1997e; 46:726–730.

Hanson RL, Ehm MG, Pettit DJ, Prochazka M, Thompson DB, Timberlake D, Foroud T, Kobes S, Baier L, Burns DK, et al.: An autosomal genomic scan for loci linked to Type II diabetes mellitus and body-mass index in Pima Indians. Am J Hum Genet 1998; 63:1130–1138.

Hara K, Okada T, Tobe K, Yasuda K, Mori Y, Kadowaki H, Hagura R, Akanuma Y, Kimura S, Ito C, et al.: The Pro12Ala polymorphism in PPARγ_2 may confer resistance to Type 2 diabetes. Biochem Biophys Res Commun 2000; 271:212–216.

Hara M, Lindner TH, Paz VP, Wang X, Iwasaki N, Ogata M, Iwamoto Y, Bell GI: Mutations in the coding region of the insulin promoter factor 1 gene are not a common cause of maturity-onset diabetes of the young in Japanese subjects. Diabetes 1998; 47:845–846.

Harris MI: Noninsulin-dependent diabetes mellitus in black and white Americans. Diabetes Metab Rev 1990; 6:71–90.

Harris MI: Epidemiological correlates of NIDDM in Hispanics, whites, and blacks in the U.S. population. Diabetes Care 1991; 14:639–648.

Harris MI: Undiagnosed NIDDM: clinical and public health issues. Diabetes Care 1993; 16:642–652.

Harris MI, Eastman RC, Cowie CC, Flegal KM, Eberhardt MS: Comparison of diabetes diagnostic categories in the U.S. population according to the 1997 American Diabetes Association and 1980–1985 World Health Organization diagnostic criteria. Diabetes Care 1997; 20:1859–1862.

Harris MI, Klein R, Welborn TA, Knuiman MW: Onset of NIDDM occurs at least 4–7 yr before clinical diagnosis. Diabetes Care 1992; 15:815–819.

Harris MI, Hadden WC, Knowler WC, Bennett PH: International criteria for the diagnosis of diabetes and impaired glucose tolerance. Diabetes Care 1985; 8:562–567.

Hart LM, Dekker JM, van Haeften TW, Ruige JB, Stehouwer CD, Erkelens DW, Heine RJ, Maassen JA: Reduced second phase insulin secretion in carriers of a sulphonylurea receptor gene variant associating with Type II diabetes mellitus. Diabetologia 2000; 43:515–519.

Hasegawa G, Obayashi H, Kitamura A, Hashimoto M, Shigeta H, Nakamura N, Kondo M, Nishimura CY: Increased levels of aldose reductase in peripheral mononuclear cells from Type 2 diabetic patients with microangiopathy. Diabetes Res Clin Pract 1999; 45:9–14.

Hashimoto L, Habita C, Beressi JP, Delephine M, Besse C, Cambon-Thomsen A, Deschamps I, Rotter JI, Djoulah S, James MR, et al.: Genetic mapping of a susceptibility locus for insulin-dependent diabetes mellitus on chromosome 11q. Nature 1994; 371:161–164.

Hasstedt SJ, Hoffman M, Leppert MF, Elbein SC: Recessive inheritance of obesity in familial non-insulin-dependent diabetes mellitus, and lack of linkage to nine candidate genes. Am J Hum Genet 1997; 61:668–677.

Hasstedt SJ, Ren QF, Teng K, Elbein SC: Effect of the peroxisome proliferator-activated receptor-γ_2 Pro(12)Ala variant on obesity, glucose homeostasis, and blood pressure in members of familial Type 2 diabetic kindreds. J Clin Endocrinol Metab 2001; 86:536–541.

Hattersley AT: Maturity-onset diabetes of the young: clinical heterogeneity explained by genetic heterogeneity. Diabet Med 1998; 15:15–24.

Hattersley AT, Turner RC, Permutt MA, Patel P, Tanizawa Y, Chiu KC, O'Rahilly S, Watkins PJ, Wainscoat JS: Linkage of Type 2 diabetes to the glucokinase gene [see comments]. Lancet 1992; 339:1307–1310.

Hayakawa T, Nagai Y, Nohara E, Yamashita H, Takamura T, Abe T, Nomura G, Kobayashi K: Variation of the fatty acid binding protein 2 gene is not associated with obesity and insulin resistance in Japanese subjects. Metabolism 1999; 48:655–657.

Hayward BE, Dunlop N, Intody S, Leek JP, Markham AF, Warner JP, Bonthron DT:

Organization of the human glucokinase regulator gene *GCKR*. Genomics 1998; 49:137–142.

Heesom AE, Hibberd ML, Millward A, Demaine AG: Polymorphism in the 5′-end of the aldose reductase gene is strongly associated with the development of diabetic nephropathy in Type 1 diabetes. Diabetes 1997; 46:287–291.

Hegele RA, Connelly PW, Scherer SW, Hanley AJ, Harris SB, Tsui LC, Zinman B: Paraoxonase-2 gene (*PON2*) G148 variant associated with elevated fasting plasma glucose in noninsulin-dependent diabetes mellitus. J Clin Endocrinol Metab 1997; 82:3373–3377.

Hegele RA, Harris SB, Zinman B, Wang J, Cao H, Hanley AJ, Tsui LC, Scherer SW: Variation in the AU(AT)-rich element within the 3′-untranslated region of PPP1R3 is associated with variation in plasma glucose in aboriginal Canadians. J Clin Endocrinol Metab 1998; 83:3980–3983.

Hirai M, Suzuki S, Onoda M, Hinokio Y, Hirai A, Ohtomo M, Chiba M, Kasuga S, Hirai S, Satoh Y, et al.: Mitochondrial deoxyribonucleic acid 3256C-T mutation in a Japanese family with noninsulin-dependent diabetes mellitus. J Clin Endocrinol Metab 1998; 83:992–994.

Hitman GA, Hawrami K, McCarthy MI, Viswanathan M, Snehalatha C, Ramachandran A, Tuomilehto J, Tuomilehto-Wolf E, Nissinen A, Pedersen O: Insulin receptor substrate-1 gene mutations in NIDDM: implications for the study of polygenic disease. Diabetologia 1995; 38:481–486.

Horikawa Y, Iwasaki N, Hara M, Furuta H, Hinokio Y, Cockburn BN, Lindner T, Yamagata K, Ogata M, Tomonaga O, et al.: Mutation in hepatocyte nuclear factor-1β gene (TCF2) associated with MODY. Nat Genet 1997; 17:384–385.

Horikawa Y, Oda N, Cox NJ, Li X, Orho-Melander M, Hara M, Hinokio Y, Lindner TH, Mashima H, Schwarz PE, et al.: Genetic variation in the gene encoding calpain-10 is associated with Type 2 diabetes mellitus. Nat Genet 2000; 26:163–175.

Hribal ML, Federici M, Porzio O, Lauro D, Borboni P, Accili D, Lauro R, Sesti G: The Gly $\rightarrow$ Arg972 amino acid polymorphism in insulin receptor substrate-1 affects glucose metabolism in skeletal muscle cells. J Clin Endocrinol Metab 2000; 85:2004–2013.

Hsueh WC, Mitchell BD, Aburomia R, Pollin T, Sakul H, Gelder EM, Michelsen BK, Wagner MJ, St. Jean PL, Knowler WC, et al.: Diabetes in the Old Order Amish: characterization and heritability analysis of the Amish Family Diabetes Study. Diabetes Care 2000; 23:595–601.

Huang X, Orho M, Lehto M, Groop L: Lack of association between the Gly40Ser polymorphism in the glucagon receptor gene and NIDDM in Finland. Diabetologia 1995; 38:1246–1248.

Humphreys P, McCarthy M, Tuomilehto J, Tuomilehto Wolf E, Stratton I, Morgan R, Rees A, Owens D, Stengard J, Nissinen A, et al.: Chromosome 4q locus associated with insulin resistance in Pima Indians: studies in three European NIDDM populations. Diabetes 1994; 43:800–804.

Huopio H, Reimann F, Ashfield R, Komulainen J, Lenko HL, Rahier J, Vauhkonen I, Kere J, Laakso M, Ashcroft F, et al.: Dominantly inherited hyperinsulinism caused by a mutation in the sulfonylurea receptor type 1. J Clin Invest 2000; 106:897–906.

Huxtable SJ, Saker PJ, Haddad L, Walker M, Frayling TM, Levy JC, Hitman GA, O'Rahilly S, Hattersley AT, McCarthy MI: Analysis of parent–offspring trios provides evidence for linkage and association between the insulin gene and Type 2 diabetes mediated exclusively through paternally transmitted class III variable number tandem repeat alleles. Diabetes 2000; 49:126–130.

Imai Y, Fusco A, Suzuki Y, Lesniak MA, D'Alfonso R, Sesti G, Bertoli A, Lauro R, Accili D, Taylor SI: Variant sequences of insulin receptor substrate-1 in patients with noninsulin-dependent diabetes mellitus. J Clin Endocrinol Metab 1994; 79:1655–1658.

Imai Y, Philippe N, Sesti G, Accili D, Taylor SI: Expression of variant forms of insulin receptor substrate-1 identified in patients with noninsulin-dependent diabetes mellitus. J Clin Endocrinol Metab 1997; 82:4201–4207.

Imperatore G, Hanson RL, Pettitt DJ, Kobes S, Bennett PH, Knowler WC: Sib-pair linkage analysis for susceptibility genes for microvascular complications among Pima Indians with Type 2 diabetes. 1998; 47:821–830.

Imperatore G, Knowler WC, Pettitt DJ, Kobes S, Bennett PH, Hanson RL: Segregation analysis of diabetic nephropathy in Pima Indians. Diabetes 2000; 49:1049–1056.

Inoue H, Ferrer J, Warren-Perry M, Zhang Y, Millns H, Turner RC, Elbein SC, Hampe CL, Suarez BK, Inagaki N, et al.: Sequence variants in the pancreatic islet β-cell inwardly rectifying K+ channel Kir6.2 (Bir) gene: identification and lack of role in Caucasian patients with NIDDM. Diabetes 1997; 46:502–507.

Inoue H, Ferrer J, Welling CM, Elbein SC, Hoffman M, Mayorga R, Warren-Perry M, Zhang Y, Millns H, Turner R, et al.: Sequence variants in the sulfonylurea receptor (*SUR*) gene are associated with NIDDM in Caucasians. Diabetes 1996; 45:825–831.

Inoue H, Tanizawa Y, Wasson J, Behn P, Kalidas K, Bernal-Mizrachi E, Mueckler M, Marshall H, Domis-Keller H, Crock P, Rogers D, et al. A gene encoding a transmembrane protein is mutated in patients with diabetes mellitus and optic atrophy (Wolfram syndrome). Nat Genet 1998; 20:143–148.

Iwasaki N, Kawamura M, Yamagata K, Cox NJ, Karibe S, Ohgawara H, Inagaki N, Seino S, Bell GI, Omori Y: Identification of microsatellite markers near the human genes encoding the β-cell ATP-sensitive K+ channel and linkage studies with NIDDM in Japanese. Diabetes 1996; 45:267–269.

Iwasaki N, Oda N, Ogata M, Hara M, Hinokio Y, Oda Y, Yamagata K, Kanematsu S, Ohgawara H, Omori Y, et al.: Mutations in the hepatocyte nuclear factor-1α/*MODY3* gene in Japanese subjects with early- and late-onset NIDDM. Diabetes 1997; 46:1504–1508.

Jacob S, Stumvoll M, Becker R, Koch M, Nielsen M, Loblein K, Maerker E, Volk A, Renn W, Balletshofer B, et al.: The PPARγ_2 polymorphism pro12Ala is associated with better insulin sensitivity in the offspring of Type 2 diabetic patients. Horm Metab Res 2000; 32:413–416.

Janssen RC, Bogardus C, Takeda J, Knowler WC, Thompson DB: Linkage analysis of acute insulin secretion with *GLUT2* and glucokinase in Pima Indians and the identification of a missense mutation in *GLUT2*. Diabetes 1994; 43:558–563.

Jeffers BW, Estacio RO, Raynolds MV, Schrier RW: Angiotensin-converting enzyme gene polymorphism in non-insulin dependent diabetes mellitus and its relationship with diabetic nephropathy. Kidney Int 1997; 52:473–477.

Ji L, Malecki M, Warram JH, Yang Y, Rich SS, Krolewski AS: New susceptibility locus for NIDDM is localized to human chromosome 20q. Diabetes 1997; 46:876–881.

Johnson KH, O'Brien TD, Betsholtz C, Westermark P: Islet amyloid, islet-amyloid polypeptide, and diabetes mellitus. N Engl J Med 1989; 321:513–518.

Kadowaki H, Yasuda K, Iwamoto K, Otabe S, Shimokawa K, Silver K, Walston J, Yoshinaga H, Kosaka K, Yamada N, et al.: A mutation in the β_3-adrenergic receptor gene is associated with obesity and hyperinsulinemia in Japanese subjects. Biochem Biophys Res Commun 1995; 215:555–560.

Kadowaki T, Kadowaki H, Mori Y, Tobe K, Sakuta R, Suzuki Y, Tanabe Y, Sakura H, Awata T, Goto Y, et al.: A subtype of diabetes mellitus associated with a mutation of mitochondrial DNA: N Engl J Med 1994; 330:962–968.

Kadowaki T, Kadowaki H, Yazaki Y: Polymorphisms of the glycogen synthase gene and non-insulin-dependent diabtes mellitus. N Engl J Med 1993; 328:1568–1569.

Kahn CR, Bruning JC, Michael MD, Kulkarni RN: Knockout mice challenge our concepts of glucose homeostasis and the pathogenesis of diabetes mellitus. J Pediatr Endocrinol Metab 2000; 13(Suppl)6:1377–1384.

Kahn SE: The importance of the β-cell in the pathogenesis of Type 2 diabetes mellitus. Am J Med 2000; 108(Suppl)6a:2S–8S.

Kahn SE, Prigeon RL, McCulloch DK, Boyko EJ, Bergman RN, Schwartz MW, Neifing JL, Ward WK, Beard JC, Palmer JP, et al.: Quantification of the relationship between insulin sensitivity and β-cell function in human subjects: evidence for a hyperbolic function. Diabetes 1993; 42:1663–1672.

Kaisaki PJ, Menzel R, Linder T, Oda N, Rjasanowski I, Sahm J, Meincke G, Schulze J, Schmechel H, Petzold C, et al.: Mutations in the hepatocyte nuclear factor-1α gene in MODY and early-onset NIDDM: evidence for a mutational hotspot in exon 4. Diabetes 1997; 46:528–535.

Kalidas K, Dow E, Saker P, Walker M, Wareham N, Halsall D, O'Rahilly S, McCarthy M, Johnston D: Genetic analysis of PC3 gene in relation to hyperproinsulinemia and NIDDM. Diabetes 1997; 46(Suppl 1):178A.

Kalidas K, Wasson J, Glaser B, Meyer JM, Duprat LJ, White MF, Permutt MA: Mapping of the human insulin receptor substrate-2 gene, identification of a linked polymorphic marker and linkage analysis in families with Type II diabetes: no evidence for a major susceptibility role. Diabetologia 1998; 41:1389–1391.

Kameoka K, Isotani H, Tanaka K, Azukari K, Fujimura Y, Shiota Y, Sasaki E, Majima M, Furukawa K, Haginomori S, et al.: Novel mitochondrial DNA mutation in tRNA(Lys) (8296A $\rightarrow$ G) associated with diabetes. Biochem Biophys Res Commun 1998; 245:523–527.

Kane C, Lindley KJ, Johnson PR, James RF, Milla PJ, Aynsley-Green A, Dunne MJ: Therapy for persistent hyperinsulinemic hypoglycemia of infancy: understanding the responsiveness of β cells to diazoxide and somatostatin. J Clin Invest 1997; 100:1888–1893.

Kane C, Shepherd RM, Squires PE, Johnson PR, James RF, Milla PJ, Aynsley-Green A, Lindley KJ, Dunne MJ: Loss of functional KATP channels in pancreatic β-cells causes persistent hyperinsulinemic hypoglycemia of infancy. Nat Med 1996; 2:1344–1347.

Kao YL, Donaghue K, Chan A, Knight J, Silink M: An aldose reductase intragenic polymorphism associated with diabetic retinopathy. Diabetes Res Clin Pract 1999; 46:155–160.

Kaprio J, Tuomilehto J, Koskenvuo M, Romanov K, Reunanen A, Eriksson J, Stengard J, Kesaniemi YA: Concordance for Type 1 (insulin-dependent) and Type 2 (non-insulin-dependent) diabetes mellitus in a population-based cohort of twins in Finland. Diabetologia 1992; 35:1060–1067.

Keen RW, Samaras K, Richens KL, Spector TD, Campbell LV, Kelly PJ: β_3-adrenergic receptor gene polymorphisms and determination of adiposity and fat distribution in normal female twins [letter]. Diabetologia 1997; 40:122–123.

Kim-Motoyama H, Yasuda K, Yamaguchi T, Yamada N, Katakura T, Shuldiner AR, Akanuma Y, Ohashi Y, Yazaki Y, Kadowaki T: A mutation of the β_3-adrenergic receptor is associated with visceral obesity but decreased serum triglyceride. Diabetologia 1997; 40:469–472.

King H, Rewers M: Global estimates for prevalence of diabetes mellitus and impaired glucose tolerance in adults. Diabetes Care 1993; 16:157–177.

King H, Zimmet P, Bennett P, Taylor R, Raper LR: Glucose tolerance and ancestral genetic admixture in six semitraditional Pacific populations. Genet Epidemiol 1984; 1:315–328.

Klupa T, Malecki MT, Pezzolesi M, Ji L, Curtis S, Langefeld CD, Rich SS, Warram JH, Krolewski AS: Further evidence for a susceptibility locus for Type 2 diabetes on chromosome 20q13.1–q13.2. Diabetes 2000; 49:2212–2216.

Knowler WC, Pettitt DJ, Saad MF, Bennett PH: Diabetes mellitus in the Pima Indians: incidence, risk factors and pathogenesis. Diabetes Metab Rev 1990; 6:1–27.

Koch M, Rett K, Maerker E, Volk A, Haist K, Deninger M, Renn W, Haring HU: The PPARγ_2 amino acid polymorphism Pro12Ala is prevalent in offspring of Type II diabetic patients and is associated to increased insulin sensitivity in a subgroup of obese subjects. Diabetologia 1999; 42:758–762.

Kubota T, Mori H, Tamori Y, Okazawa H, Fukuda T, Miki M, Ito C, Fleury C, Bouillaud F, Kasuga M: Molecular screening of uncoupling protein 2 gene in patients with noninsulin-dependent diabetes mellitus or obesity. J Clin Endocrinol Metab 1998; 83:2800–2804.

Kukuvitis A, Deal C, Arbour L, Polychronakos C: An autosomal dominant form of familial persistent hyperinsulinemic hypoglycemia of infancy, not linked to the sulfonylurea receptor locus. J Clin Endocrinol Metab 1997; 82:1192–1194.

Kusari J, Verma US, Buse JB, Henry RR, Olefsky JM: Analysis of gene sequences of the insulin receptor and the insulin-sensitive glucose transporter (GLUT-4) in patients with common-type non-insulin dependent diabetes mellitus. J Clin Invest 1991; 88:1323–1330.

Laakso M, Malkki M, Kekalainen P, Kuusisto J, Deeb SS: Insulin receptor substrate-1 variants in non-insulin-dependent diabetes. J Clin Invest 1994; 94:1141–1146.

Lakka HM, Oksanen L, Tuomainen TP, Kontula K, Salonen JT: The common pentanucleotide polymorphism of the 3′-untranslated region of the leptin receptor gene is associated with serum insulin levels and the risk of Type 2 diabetes in non-diabetic men: a prospective case-control study. J Intern Med 2000; 248:77–83.

Larsson H, Ahren B: Islet dysfunction in insulin resistance involves impaired insulin secretion and increased glucagon secretion in postmenopausal women with impaired glucose tolerance. Diabetes Care 2000; 23:650–657.

Lausen J, Thomas H, Lemm I, Bulman M, Borgschulze M, Lingott A, Hattersley AT, Ryffel GU: Naturally occurring mutations in the human HNF4α gene impair the function of the transcription factor to a varying degree. Nucleic Acids Res 2000; 28:430–437.

Lei HH, Coresh J, Shuldiner AR, Boerwinkle E, Brancati FL: Variants of the insulin receptor substrate-1 and fatty acid binding protein 2 genes and the risk of Type 2 diabetes, obesity, and hyperinsulinemia in African-Americans: the Atherosclerosis Risk in Communities Study. Diabetes 1999; 48:1868–1872.

Leon DA, Koupilova I, Lithell HO, Berglund L, Mohsen R, Vagero D, Lithell UB, McKeigue PM: Failure to realise growth potential in utero and adult obesity in relation to blood pressure in 50 year old Swedish men. Br Med J 1996; 312:401–406.

Leon DA, Lithell HO, Vagero D, Koupilova I, Mohsen R, Berglund L, Lithell UB, McKeigue PM: Reduced fetal growth rate and increased risk of death from ischaemic heart disease: cohort study of 15,000 Swedish men and women born 1915–29. Br Med J 1998; 317:241–245.

Lesage S, Zouali H, Vionnet N, Philippi A, Velho G, Serradas P, Passa P, Demenais F, Froguel P: Genetic analyses of glucose transporter genes in French non-insulin-dependent diabetic families. Diabetes Metab 1997; 23:137–142.

Le Stunff C, Le Bihan C, Schork NJ, Bougneres P: A common promoter variant of the leptin gene is associated with changes in the relationship between serum leptin and fat mass in obese girls. Diabetes 2000; 49:2196–2200.

Li WD, Lee JH, Price RA: The peroxisome proliferator-activated receptor γ_2 Pro12Ala mutation is associated with early onset extreme obesity and reduced fasting glucose. Mol Genet Metab 2000; 70:159–161.

Lillioja S, Mott DM, Spraue M, Ferraro R, Foley JE, Ravussin E, Knowler WC, Bennett PH, Bogardus C: Insulin resistance and insulin secretory dysfunction as precursors of non-insulin-dependent diabetes mellitus; prospective studies of Pima Indians. N Engl J Med 1993; 329:1988–1992.

Lindner T, Gragnoli T, Furuta H, Cockburn BN, Petzold C, Rietzsch H, Weiss U, Schulze J, Bell GI: Hepatic function in a family with a nonsense mutation (R154X) in the hepatocyte nuclear factor-4α/*MODY1* gene. J Clin Invest 1997a; 100:1400–1405.

Lindner T, Gragnoli C, Schulze J, Rietzsch H, Petzold C, Schroeder HE, Cox NJ, Bell GI: The 31-cM region of chromosome 11 including the obesity gene Tubby and ATP-sensitive postassium channel genes, SUR1 and KIR6.2, does not contain a major susceptibility locus for NIDDM in 127 non-Hispanic white affected sibships. Diabetes 1997b; 46:1227–1229.

Lithell HO, McKeigue PM, Berglund L, Mohsen R, Lithell UB, Leon DA: Relation of size at birth to non-insulin dependent diabetes and insulin concentrations in men aged 50–60 years. Br Med J 1996; 312:406–410.

Maddux BA, Sbraccia P, Kumakura S, Sasson S, Youngren J, Fisher A, Spencer S, Grupe A, Henzel W, Stewart TA, et al.: Membrane glycoprotein PC-1 and insulin resistance in non-insulin-dependent diabetes mellitus. Nature 1995; 373:448–451.

Maeda S, Haneda M, Yasuda H, Tachikawa T, Isshiki K, Koya D, Terada M, Hidaka H, Kashiwagi A, Kikkawa R: Diabetic nephropathy is not associated with the dinucleotide repeat polymorphism upstream of the aldose reductase (*ALR2*) gene but with erythrocyte aldose reductase content in Japanese subjects with Type 2 diabetes. Diabetes 1999; 48:420–422.

Maegawa H, Shi K, Hidaka H, Iwai N, Nishio Y, Egawa K, Kojima H, Haneda M, Yasuda H, Nakamura Y, et al.: The 3′-untranslated region polymorphism of the gene for skeletal muscle-specific glycogen-targeting subunit of protein phosphatase 1 in the Type 2 diabetic Japanese population. Diabetes 1999; 48:1469–1472.

Maffei M, Stoffel M, Barone M, Moon B, Dammerman M, Ravussin E, Bogardus C, Ludwig DS, Flier JS, Talley M: Absence of mutations in the human OB gene in obese/diabetic subjects. Diabetes 1996; 45:679–682.

Mahtani MM, Widen E, Lehto M, Thomas J, McCarthy M, Brayer J, Bryant B, Chan G, Daly M, Forsblom C, et al.: Mapping of a gene for Type 2 diabetes associated with an insulin secretion defect by a genome scan in Finnish families. Nat Genet 1996; 14:90–94.

Majer M, Mott DM, Mochizuki H, Rowles JC, Pedersen O, Knowler WC, Bogardus C, Prochazka M: Association of the glycogen synthase locus on 19q13 with NIDDM in Pima Indians. Diabetologia 1996; 39:314–321.

Malecki MT, Antonellis A, Casey P, Ji L, Wantman M, Warram JH, Krolewski AS: Exclusion of the hepatocyte nuclear factor 4α as a candidate gene for late-onset NIDDM linked with chromosome 20q. Diabetes 1998; 47:970–972.

Malecki MT, Jhala US, Antonellis A, Fields L, Doria A, Orban T, Saad M, Warram JH, Montminy M, Krolewski AS: Mutations in NEUROD1 are associated with the development of Type 2 diabetes mellitus. Nat Genet 1999; 23:323–328.

Marre M, Jeunemaitre X, Gallois Y, Rodier M, Chatellier G, Sert C, Dusselier L, Kahal Z, Chaillous L, Halimi S, et al.: Contribution of genetic polymorphism in the renin-angiotensin system to the development of renal complications in insulin-dependent diabetes: Genetique de la Nephropathie Diabetique (GENEDIAB) study group. J Clin Invest 1997; 99:1585–1595.

Martin BC, Warram JH, Rosner B, Rich SS, Soeldner JS, Krolewski AS: Familial clustering of insulin sensitivity. Diabetes 1992; 41:850–854.

Martyn CN, Hales CN, Barker DJ, Jespersen S: Fetal growth and hyperinsulinaemia in adult life. Diabet Med 1998; 15:688–694.

Matschinsky F, Liang Y, Kesavan P, Wang L, Froguel P, Velho G, Cohen D, Permutt MA, Tanizawa Y, Jetton TL: Glucokinase as pancreatic β cell glucose sensor and diabetes gene. J Clin Invest 1993; 92:2092–2098.

Matsubara A, Tanizawa Y, Matsutani A, Kaneko T, Kaku K: Sequence variations of the pancreatic islet/liver glucose transporter (*GLUT2*) gene in Japanese subjects with noninsulin dependent diabetes mellitus. J Clin Endocrinol Metab 1995; 80:3131–3135.

Matsutani A, Koranyi L, Cox N, Permutt MA: Polymorphisms of *GLUT2* and *GLUT4* genes: use in evaluation of genetic susceptibility to NIDDM in blacks. Diabetes 1990; 39:1534–1542.

Matthews DR, Hosker JP, Rudenski AS, Naylor BA, Treacher DF, Turner RC: Homeostasis model assessment: insulin resistance and β-cell function from fasting plasma glucose and insulin concentrations in man. Diabetologia 1985; 28:412–419.

Mauriege P, Bouchard C: Trp64Arg mutation in β_3-adrenoceptor gene of doubtful significance for obesity and insulin resistance. Lancet 1996; 348:698–699.

Mauvais-Jarvis F, Kahn CR: Understanding the pathogenesis and treatment of insulin resistance and Type 2 diabetes mellitus: what can we learn from transgenic and knockout mice? Diabetes Metab 2000; 26:433–448.

McCance DR, Pettitt DJ, Hanson RL, Jacobsson LT, Knowler WC, Bennett PH: Birth weight and non-insulin dependent diabetes: thrifty genotype, thrifty phenotype, or surviving small baby genotype? Br Med J 1994; 308:942–945.

Meirhaeghe A, Fajas L, Helbecque N, Cottel D, Auwerx J, Deeb SS, Amouyel P: Impact of the peroxisome proliferator activated receptor γ_2 Pro12Ala polymorphism on adiposity, lipids and non-insulin-dependent diabetes mellitus. Int J Obes Relat Metab Disord 2000; 24:195–199.

Miki T, Nagashima K, Seino S: The structure and function of the ATP-sensitive K+ channel in insulin-secreting pancreatic β-cells. J Mol Endocrinol 1999; 22:113–123.

Miles PD, Li S, Hart M, Romeo O, Cheng J, Cohen A, Raafat K, Moossa AR, Olefsky JM: Mechanisms of insulin resistance in experimental hyperinsulinemic dogs. J Clin Invest 1998; 101:202–211.

Mitchell BD, Blangero J, Comuzzie AG, Almasy LA, Shuldiner AR, Silver K, Stern MP, MacCluer JW, Hixson JE: A paired sibling analysis of the β_3-adrenergic receptor and obesity in Mexican Americans. J Clin Invest 1998; 101:584–587.

Mitchell BD, Cole SA, Hsueh WC, Comuzzie AG, Blangero J, MacCluer JW, Hixson JE: Linkage of serum insulin concentrations to chromosome 3p in Mexican Americans. Diabetes 2000; 49:513–516.

Mitchell BD, Kammerer CM, O'Connell P, Harrison CR, Manire M, Shipman P, Moyer MP, Stern MP, Frazier ML: Evidence for linkage of postchallenge insulin levels with intestinal fatty acid-binding protein (FABP2) in Mexican-Americans. Diabetes 1995; 44:1046–1053.

Mitrakou A, Kelley D, Mokan M, Veneman T, Pangburn T, Reilly J, Gerich J: Role of reduced suppression of glucose production and diminished early insulin release in impaired glucose tolerance. N Engl J Med 1992; 326:22–29.

Moczulski DK, Rogus JJ, Antonellis A, Warram JH, Krolewski AS: Major susceptibility locus for nephropathy in Type 1 diabetes on chromosome 3q: results of novel discordant sib-pair analysis. Diabetes 1998; 47:1164–1169.

Moczulski D, Rogus JJ, Warram JH, Krolewski AS: Exclusion of aldose reductase gene as major locus for diabetic nephropathy in IDDM: results of family-based studies. Diabetes 1997; 46(Suppl 1):171A.

Moller AM, Jensen NM, Pildal J, Drivsholm T, Borch-Johnsen K, Urhammer SA, Hansen T, Pedersen O: Studies of genetic variability of the glucose transporter 2 promoter in patients with Type 2 diabetes mellitus. J Clin Endocrinol Metab 2001; 86:2181–2186.

Moller DE, Flier JS: Insulin resistance: mechanisms, syndromes, and implications. N Engl J Med 1991; 325:938–948.

Mori H, Hashiramoto M, Kishimoto M, Kasuga M: Amino acid polymorphisms of the insulin receptor substrate-1 in Japanese noninsulin-dependent diabetes mellitus. J Clin Endocrinol Metab 1995; 80:2822–2826.

Mori H, Ikegami H, Kawaguchi Y, Seino S, Yokoi N, Takeda J, Inoue I, Seino Y, Yasuda K, Hanafusa T, et al.: The Pro12 $\rightarrow$ Ala substitution in PPARγ is associated with resistance to development of diabetes in the general population: possible involvement in impairment of insulin secretion in individuals with Type 2 diabetes. Diabetes 2001; 50:891–894.

Moriarty M, Wing RR, Kuller LH, Ferrell RE: Trp64Arg substitution in the β_3-adrenergic receptor does not relate to body weight in healthy, premenopausal women. Int J Obes Relat Metab Disord 1997; 21:826–829.

Mueckler M, Kruse M, Strube M, Riggs AC, Chiu KC, Permutt MA: A mutation in the GLUT2 glucose transporter gene of a diabetic patient abolishes transport activity. J Biol Chem 1994; 269:17765–17767.

Nagase T, Aoki A, Yamamoto M, Yasuda H, Kado S, Nishikawa M, Kugai N, Akatsu T, Nagata N: Lack of association between the Trp64 Arg mutation in the β_3-adrenergic receptor gene and obesity in Japanese men: a longitudinal analysis. J Clin Endocrinol Metab 1997; 82:1284–1287.

National Diabetes Data Group. Classification and diagnosis of diabetes mellitus and other categories of glucose intolerance. Diabetes 1979; 28:1039–1057.

Neel JV: Diabetes mellitus: a "thrifty" genotype rendered detrimental by "progress"? Bull World Health Organ 1999; 77:694–703.

Nestorowicz A, Glaser B, Wilson BA, Shyng SL, Nichols CG, Stanley CA, Thornton PS, Permutt MA: Genetic heterogeneity in familial hyperinsulinism [published erratum appears in Hum Mol Genet 1998 (Sep); 7(9):1527]. Hum Mol Genet 1998; 7:1119–1128.

Nestorowicz A, Inagaki N, Gonoi T, Schoor KP, Wilson BA, Glaser B, Landau H, Stanley CA, Thornton PS, Seino S, et al.: A nonsense mutation in the inward rectifier potassium channel gene, Kir6.2, is associated with familial hyperinsulinism. Diabetes 1997; 46:1743–1748.

Nestorowicz A, Wilson BA, Schoor KP, Wilson BA, Glaser B, Landau H, Stanley CA, Thornton PS, Seino S, et al.: Mutations in the sulonylurea receptor gene are associated with familial hyperinsulinism in Ashkenazi Jews. Hum Mol Genet 1996; 5:1813–1822.

Newkirk JE, Taylor RW, Howell N, Bindoff LA, Chinnery PF, Alberti KGMM, Turnbull DM, Walker M: Maternally inherited diabetes and deafness: prevalence in a hospital diabetic population. Diabet Med 1997; 14:457–460.

Newman B, Selby JV, King MC, Slemenda C, Fabsitz R, Friedman GD: Concordance for Type 2 (non-insulin-dependent) diabetes mellitus in male twins. Diabetologia 1987; 30:763–768.

Nichols CG, Shyng SL, Nestorowicz A, Glaser B, Clement JP, Gonzalez G, Aguilar-Bryan L, Permutt MA, Bryan J: Adenosine diphosphate as an intracellular regulator of insulin secretion. Science 1996; 272:1785–1787.

Nicolino M, Ferlin T, Forest M, Godinot C, Carrier H, David M, Chatelain P, Mousson B: Identification of a large-scale mitochondrial deoxyribonucleic acid deletion in endocrinopathies and deafness: report of two unrelated cases with diabetes mellitus and adrenal insufficiency, respectively. J Clin Endocrinol Metab 1997; 82:3063–3067.

Niki T, Mori H, Tamori Y, Kishimoto-Hashirmoto M, Ueno H, Araki S, Masugi J, Sawant N, Majithia HR, Rais N: Human obese gene: molecular screening in Japanese and Asian Indian NIDDM patients associated with obesity. Diabetes 1996; 45:675–678.

Nishi M, Bell GI, Steiner DF: Islet amyloid polypeptide (amylin): no evidence of an abnormal precursor sequence in 25 Type 2 (non-insulin-dependent) diabetic patients. Diabetologia 1990; 33:628–630.

Nishigori H, Yamada S, Kohama T, Tomura H, Sho K, Horikawa Y, Bell GI, Takeuchi T, Takeda J: Frameshift mutation, A263fsinsGG, in the hepatocyte nuclear factor-1β gene associated with diabetes and renal dysfunction. Diabetes 1998a; 47:1354–1355.

Nishigori H, Yamada S, Kohama T, Utsugi T, Shimizu H, Takeuchi T, Takeda J: Mutations in the hepatocyte nuclear factor-1α gene (*MODY3*) are not a major cause of early-onset non-insulin-dependent (Type 2) diabetes mellitus in Japanese. J Hum Genet 1998b; 43:107–110.

Noda K, Matsutani A, Tanizawa Y, Neuman R, Kaneko T, Permutt MA, Kaku K: Polymorphic microsatellite repeat markers at the glucokinase gene locus are positively associated with NIDDM in Japanese. Diabetes 1993; 42:1147–1152.

Odawara M, Tachi Y, Yamashita K: Absence of association between the Gly40 → Ser mutation in the human glucagon receptor and Japanese patients with non-insulin-dependent diabetes mellitus or impaired glucose tolerance. Hum Genet 1996; 98:636–639.

O'Dea K: Marked improvement in carbohydrate and lipid metabolism in diabetic Australian aborigines after temporary reversion to traditional lifestyle. Diabetes 1984; 33:596–603.

Oeveren van-Dybicz AM, Vonkeman HE, Bon MA, van den Bergh FA, Vermes I: β_3-adrenergic receptor gene polymorphism and Type 2 diabetes in a Caucasian population. Diabetes Obes Metab 2001; 3:47–51.

Ogata M, Iwasaki N, Ohgawara H, Karibe S, Omori Y: Absence of the Gly40-ser mutation in the glucagon receptor gene in Japanese subjects with NIDDM: Diabetes Res Clin Pract 1996; 33:71–74.

Ohagi S, Sakaguchi H, Sanke T, Tatsuta H, Hanabusa T, Nanjo K: Human prohormone convertase 3 gene: exon-intron organization and molecular scanning for mutations in Japanese subjects with NIDDM: Diabetes 1996; 45:897–901.

Olansky L, Welling C, Giddings S, Adler S, Bourey R, Dowse G, Serjeantson S, Zimmet P, Permutt MA: A variant insulin promoter in non-insulin-dependent diabetes mellitus. J Clin Invest 1992; 89:1596–1602.

Olefsky JM: Diabetes Mellitus (Type II): Etiology and Pathogenesis. 3d ed.

Olmos P, Futers S, Acosta AM, Siegel S, Maiz A, Schiaffino R, Morales P, Diaz R, Arriagada P, Claro JC, et al.: (AC)23 [Z-2] polymorphism of the aldose reductase gene and fast progression of retinopathy in Chilean Type 2 diabetics. Diabetes Res Clin Pract 2000; 47:169–176.

Olsson C, Zethelius B, Lagerstrom-Fermer M, Asplund J, Berne C, Landegren U: Level of heteroplasmy for the mitochondrial mutation A3243G correlates with age at onset of diabetes and deafness. Hum Mutat 1998; 12:52–58.

Orho M, Carlsson M, Kanninen T, Groop LC: Polymorphism at the rad gene is not associated with NIDDM in Finns. Diabetes 1996; 45:429–433.

Orho M, Nikula Ijas P, Schalin Jantti C, Permutt MA, Groop LC: Isolated and characterization of the human muscle glycogen synthase gene. Diabetes 1995; 44: 1099–1105.

Otabe S, Clement K, Rich N, Warden C, Pecqueur C, Neverova M, Raimbault S, Guy-Grand B, Basdevant A, Ricquier D, et al.: Mutation screening of the human UCP2 gene in normoglycemic and NIDDM morbidly obese patients: lack of association between new UCP2 polymorphisms and obesity in French Caucasians. Diabetes 1998; 47:840–842.

Pajukanta P, Nuotio I, Terwilliger JD, Porkka KV, Ylitalo K, Pihlajamaki J, Suomalainen AJ, Syvanen AC, Lehtimaki T, Viikari JS, et al.: Linkage of familial combined hyperlipidaemia to chromosome 1q21–q23. Nat Genet 1998; 18:369–373.

Parker A, Meyer J, Lewitzky S, Rennich JS, Chan G, Thomas JD, Orho-Melander M, Lehtovirta M, Forsblom C, Hyrkko A, et al.: A gene conferring susceptibility to Type 2 diabetes in conjunction with obesity is located on chromosome 18p11. Diabetes 2001; 50:675–680.

Parving HH, Tarnow L, Rossing P: Genetics of diabetic nephropathy. J Am Soc Nephrol 1996; 7:2509–2517.

Permana PA, Kahn BB, Huppertz C, Mott DM: Functional analyses of amino acid substitutions Arg883Ser and Asp905Tyr of protein phosphatase-1 G-subunit. Mol Genet Metab 2000; 70:151–158.

Permana PA, Mott DM: Genetic analysis of human type 1 protein phosphatase inhibitor 2 in insulin-resistant Pima Indians. Genomics 1997; 41:110–114.

Permutt MA, Chiu KC, Tanizawa Y: Glucokinase and NIDDM: a candidate gene that paid off. Diabetes 1992; 41:1367–1372.

Permutt MA, Elbein SC: Insulin gene in diabetes: analysis through RFLP. Diabetes Care 1990; 13:364–374.

Permutt MA, Rotwein P: Analysis of the insulin gene in noninsulin-dependent diabetes. Am J Med 1983; 75:1–7.

Permutt MA, Wasson JC, Suarez BK, Lin J, Thomas J, Meyer J, Lewitzky S, Rennich JS, Parker A, Duprat L, et al.: A genome scan for Type 2 diabetes susceptibility loci in a genetically isolated population. Diabetes 2001; 50:681–685.

Peters RK, Kjos SL, Xiang A, Buchanan TA: Long-term diabetogenic effect of single pregnancy in women with previous gestational diabetes mellitus [see comments]. Lancet 1996; 347:227–230.

Phillips DI, Barker DJ, Hales CN, Hirst S, Osmond C: Thinness at birth and insulin resistance in adult life. Diabetologia 1994; 37:150–154.

Pimenta W, Korytkowski M, Mitrakou A, Jenssen T, Yki-Jarvinen H, Evron W, Dailey G, Gerich J: Pancreatic β-cell dysfunction as the primary genetic lesion in NIDDM: evidence from studies in normal glucose-tolerant individuals with a first-degree NIDDM relative. JAMA 1995; 273:1855–1861.

Pizzuti A, Frittitta L, Argiolas A, Baratta R, Goldfine ID, Bozzali M, Ercolino T, Scarlato G, Iacoviello L, Vigneri R, et al.: A polymorphism (K121Q) of the human glycoprotein PC-1 gene coding region is strongly associated with insulin resistance. Diabetes 1999; 48:1881–1884.

Polymeropoulos MH, Swift RG, Swift M: Linkage of the gene for Wolfram syndrome to markers on the short arm of chromosome 4. Nat Genet 1994; 8:95–97.

Pontoglio M, Sreenan S, Roe M, Pugh W, Ostrega D, Doyen A, Pick AJ, Baldwin A, Velho G, Froguel P, et al.: Defective insulin secretion in hepatocyte nuclear factor 1α-deficient mice. J Clin Invest 1998; 101:2215–2222.

Porzio O, Federici M, Hribal ML, Lauro D, Accili D, Lauro R, Borboni P, Sesti G: The Gly972 → Arg amino acid polymorphism in IRS-1 impairs insulin secretion in pancreatic β cells. J Clin Invest 1999; 104:357–364.

Poulsen P, Kyvik KO, Vaag A, Beck-Nielsen H: Heritability of Type II (non-insulin-dependent) diabetes mellitus and abnormal glucose tolerance: a population-based twin study. Diabetologia 1999; 42:139–145.

Poulsen P, Vaag AA, Kyvik KO, Moller JD, Beck-Nielsen H: Low birth weight is associated with NIDDM in discordant monozygotic and dizygotic twin pairs. Diabetologia 1997; 40:439–446.

Pratley RE, Thompson DB, Prochazka M, Baier L, Mott D, Ravussin E, Sakul E, Ehm MG, Burns D, Foroud T, et al.: An autosomal genomic scan for loci linked to prediabetic phenotypes in Pima Indians. J Clin Invest 1998; 101:1757–1764.

Prochazka M, Lillioja S, Tait JF, Knowler WC, Mott DM, Spraul M, Bennett PH, Bogardus C: Linkage of chromosomal markers on 4q with a putative gene determining maximal insulin action in Pima Indians. Diabetes 1993; 42:514–519.

Pyke DA, Theophanides CG, Tattersall RB: Genetic origin of diabetes: re-evaluation of twin data. Lancet 1976; 2:464.

Rando TA, Horton JC, Layzer RB: Wolfram syndrome: evidence of a diffuse neurodegenerative disease by magnetic resonance imaging. Neurology 1992; 42:1220–1224.

Rasmussen SK, Urhammer SA, Pizzuti A, Echwald SM, Ekstrom CT, Hansen L, Hansen T, Borch-Johnson K, Frittitta L, Trischitta V, et al.: The K121Q variant of the human PC-1 gene is not associated with insulin resistance or Type 2 diabetes among Danish Caucasians. Diabetes 2000; 49:1608–1611.

Reynet C, Kahn CR: Rad: a member of the Ras family overexpressed in muscle of Type II diabetic humans. Science 1993; 262:1441–1444.

Rich SS: Mapping genes in diabetes: genetic epidemiological perspective. Diabetes 1990; 39:1315–1319.

Rissanen J, Pihlajamaki J, Heikkinen S, Kekalainen P, Kuusisto J, Laakso M: The Ala54Thr polymorphism of fatty acid binding protein 2 gene does not influence insulin sensitivity in Finnish nondiabetic and NIDDM subjects. Diabetes 1997a; 46:711–712.

Rissanen J, Pihlajamaki J, Heikkinen S, Kekalainen P, Mykkanen L, Kuusisto J, Kolle A, Laakso M: New variants in the glycogen synthase gene (Gln71His, Met416Val) in patients with NIDDM from eastern Finland. Diabetologia 1997b; 40:1313–1319.

Rissanen J, Saarinen L, Heikkinen S, Kekalainen P, Mykkanen L, Kuusisto J, Deeb SS, Laakso M: Glucokinase gene islet promoter region variant (G to A) at nucleotide −30 is not associated with reduced insulin secretion in Finns. Diabetes Care 1998; 21:1194–1197.

Ristow M, Busch K, Schatz H, Pfeiffer A: Restricted geographical extension of the association of a glucagon receptor gene mutation (Gly40Ser) with non-insulin-dependent diabetes mellitus. Diabetes Res Clin Pract 1996; 32:183–185.

Roder ME, Vissing H, Nauck MA: Hyperproinsulinemia in a three-generation Caucasian family due to mutant proinsulin (Arg65–His) not associated with imparied glucose tolerance: the contribution of mutant proinsulin to insulin bioactivity. J Clin Endocrinol Metab 1996; 81:1634–1640.

Rogus JJ, Krolewski AS: Using discordant sib pairs to map loci for qualitative traits with high sibling recurrence risk. Am J Hum Genet 1996; 59:1376–1381.

Rogus JJ, Moczulski D, Freire MB, Yang Y, Warram JH, Krolewski AS: Diabetic nephropathy is associated with AGT polymorphism T235: results of a family-based study. Hypertension 1998; 31:627–631.

Rolland V, Clement K, Dugail I, Guy-Grand B, Basdevant A, Froguel P, Lavau M: Leptin receptor gene in a large cohort of massively obese subjects: no indication of the fa/fa rat mutation: detection of an intronic variant with no association with obesity. Obes Res 1998; 6:122–127.

Rossetti L, Giaccari A, DeFronzo RA: Glucose toxicity. Diabetes Care 1990; 13:610–630.

Rothman DL, Magnusson I, Cline G, Gerard D, Kahn CR, Shulman RG, Shulman GI: Decreased muscle glucose transport/phophorylation is an early defect in the pathogenesis of non-insulin-dependent diabetes mellitus. Proc Natl Acad Sci USA 1995; 92:983–987.

Rotwein P, Chyn R, Chirgwin J, Cordell B, Goodman HM, Permut MA: Polymor-

phism in the 5′-flanking region of the human insulin gene and its possible relation to Type 2 diabetes. Science 1981; 213:1117–1120.
Ryan F, Devaney D, Joyce C, Nestorowicz A, Permutt MA, Glaser B, Barton DE, Thornton PS: Hyperinsulinism: molecular aetiology of focal disease. Arch Dis Child 1998; 79:445–447.
Saad MF, Knowler WC, Pettitt DJ, Nelson RG, Mott DM, Bennett PH: The natural history of impaired glucose tolerance in the Pima Indians. N Engl J Med 1988; 319:1500–1506.
Sagnella GA, Rothwell MJ, Onipinla AK, Wicks PD, Cook DG, Cappuccio FP: A population study of ethnic variations in the angiotensin-converting enzyme I/D polymorphism: relationships with gender, hypertension and impaired glucose metabolism. J Hypertens 1999; 17:657–664.
Sakagashira S, Sanke T, Hanabusa T, Shimomura H, Ohagi S, Kumagaye KY, Nakajima K, Nanjo K: Missense mutation of amylin gene (S20G) in Japanese NIDDM patients. Diabetes 1996; 45:1279–1281.
Sakane N, Yoshida T, Umekawa T, Kondo M, Sakai Y, Takahashi T: β_3-adrenergic-receptor polymorphism: a genetic marker for visceral fat obesity and the insulin resistance syndrome. Diabetologia 1997; 40:200–204.
Saker PJ, Hattersley AT, Barrow B, Hammersley MS, McLellan JA, Lo YM, Olds RJ, Gillmer MD, Holman RR, Turner RC: High prevalence of a missense mutation of the glucokinase gene in gestational diabetic patients due to a founder-effect in a local population. Diabetologia 1996; 39:1325–1328.
Sakul H, Pratley R, Cardon L, Ravussin E, Mott D, Bogardus C: Familiality of physical and metabolic characteristics that predict the development of non-insulin-dependent diabetes mellitus in Pima Indians. Am J Hum Genet 1997; 60:651–656.
Schumacher MC, Maxwell TM, Wu LL, Hunt SC, Williams RR, Elbein SC: Dyslipidemias among normoglycemic members of familial NIDDM pedigrees. Diabetes Care 1992; 15:1285–1289.
Seaquest ER, Goetz FC, Rich S, Barbosa J: Familial clustering of diabetic kidney disease. N Engl J Med 1989; 320:1161–1165.
Seldin MF, Mott D, Bhat D, Petro A, Kuhn CM, Kingsmore SF, Bogardus C, Opara E, Feinglos MN, Surwit RS: Glycogen synthase: a putative locus for diet-induced hyperglycemia. J Clin Invest 1994; 94:269–276.
Shah VO, Dorin RI, Sun Y, Braun M, Zager PG: Aldose reductase gene expression is increased in diabetic nephropathy. J Clin Endocrinol Metab 1997; 82:2294–2298.
Shaw JT, Lovelock PK, Kesting JB, Cardinal J, Duffy D, Wainwright B, Cameron DP: Novel susceptibility gene for late-onset NIDDM is localized to human chromosome 12q. Diabetes 1998; 47:1793–1796.
Shen GQ, Ikegami H, Kawaguchi Y, Fujisawa T, Hamada Y, Ueda H, Shintani M, Nojima K, Kawabata Y, Yamada K, et al.: Asp905Tyr polymorphism of the gene for the skeletal muscle-specific glycogen-targeting subunit of protein phosphatase 1 in NIDDM. Diabetes Care 1998; 21:1086–1089.
Shimada F, Makino H, Iwaoka H, Miyamoto S, Hashimoto N, Kanatsuka A, Bell GI, Yoshida S: Identification of two novel amino acid polymorphisms in β-cell/liver (GLUT2) glucose transporter in Japanese subjects. Diabetologia 1995; 38:211–215.
Shimizu H, Ohtani KI, Tsuchiya T, Sato N, Tanaka Y, Takahashi H, Uehara Y, Inukai T, Mori M: Aldose reductase mRNA expression is associated with rapid development of diabetic microangiopathy in Japanese Type 2 diabetic (T2DM) patients. Diabetes Nutr Metab 2000; 13:75–79.
Shimomura H, Sanke T, Ueda K, Hanabusa T, Sakagashira S, Nanjo K: A missense mutation of the muscle glycogen synthase gene (M416V) is associated with insulin resistance in the Japanese population. Diabetologia 1997; 40:947–952.
Shin CS, Kim SK, Park KS, Kim WB, Kim SY, Cho BY, Lee HK, Koh CS, Shin CH, Lee JB: A new point mutation (3426, A to G) in mitochondrial NADH dehydrogenase gene in Korean diabetic patients which mimics 3243 mutation by restriction fragment length polymorphism pattern. Endocr J 1998; 45:105–110.
Sigal RJ, Doria A, Warram JH, Krolewski AS: Codon 972 polymorphism in the insulin receptor substrate-1 gene, obesity, and risk of noninsulin-dependent diabetes mellitus. J Clin Endocrinol Metab 1996; 81:1657–1659.
Silver K, Mitchell BD, Walston J, Sorkin JD, Stern MP, Roth J, Shuldiner AR: TRP64ARG β_3-adrenergic receptor and obesity in Mexican Americans. Hum Genet 1997; 101:306–311.
Silver K, Walston J, Wang Y, Dowse G, Zimmet P, Shuldiner AR: Molecular scanning for mutations in the β_3-adrenergic receptor gene in Nauruans with obesity and noninsulin-dependent diabetes mellitus. J Clin Endocrinol Metab 1996; 81:4155–4158.
Solini A, Giacchetti G, Sfriso A, Fioretto P, Sardu C, Saller A, Tonolo G, Maioli M, Mantero F, Nosadini R: Polymorphisms of angiotensin-converting enzyme and angiotensinogen genes in Type 2 diabetic sibships in relation to albumin excretion rate. Am J Kidney Dis 1999; 34:1002–1009.
Stanley CA: Hyperinsulinism in infants and children. Pediatr Clin North Am 1997; 44:363–374.
Stanley CA, Baker L: The causes of neonatal hypoglycemia. N Engl J Med 1999; 340:1200–1201.
Steiner DF, Tager HS, Chan SJ, Nanjo K, Sanke T, Rubenstein AH: Lessons learned from molecular biology of insulin-gene mutations. Diabetes Care 1990; 13:600–609.
Stern MP, Duggirala R, Mitchell BD, Reinhart LJ, Shivakumar S, Shipman PA, Uresandi OC, Benavides E, Blangero J, O'Connell P: Evidence for linkage of regions on chromosomes 6 and 11 to plasma glucose concentrations in Mexican Americans. Genome Res 1996a; 6:724–734.
Stern MP, Mitchell BD, Blangero J, Reinhart L, Krammerer CM, Harrison CR, Shipman PA, O'Connell P, Frazier ML, MacCluer JW, et al.: Evidence for a major gene for Type II diabetes and linkage analyses with selected candidate genes in Mexican-Americans. Diabetes 1996b; 45:563–568.
Stirling B, Cox NJ, Bell GI, Hanis CL, Spielman RS, Concannon P: Identification of microsatellite markers near the human OB gene and linkage studies in NIDDM-affected sib pairs. Diabetes 1995a; 44:999–1001.
Stirling B, Cox NJ, Bell GI, Hanis CL, Spielman RS, Concannon P: Linkage studies in NIDDM with markers near the sulphonylurea receptor gene. Diabetologia 1995b; 38:1479–1481.
St Jean P, Hsueh W-C, Mitchell BD, Ehm MG, Wagner M, Burns D, Shuldiner AR: Association between diabetes, obesity, glucose, and insulin levels in the Old Order Amish and SNPs on 1q21–q23. Am J Hum Genet 2000; 67:332 (Abstract).
Stoffel M, Duncan SA: The maturity-onset diabetes of the young (*MODY1*) transcription factor HNF4α regulates expression of genes required for glucose transport and metabolism. Proc Natl Acad Sci USA 1997; 94:13209–13214.
Stoffers DA, Ferrer J, Clarke WL, Habener JF: Early-onset Type-II diabetes mellitus (*MODY4*) linked to *IPF1*. Nat Genet 1997; 17:138–139.
Stone LM, Kahn SE, Deeb SS, Fujimoto WY, Porte Jr. D: Glucokinase gene variations in Japanese-Americans with a family history of NIDDM. Diabetes Care 1994; 17:1480–1483.
Stone LM, Kahn SE, Fujimoto WY, Deeb SS, Porte Jr. D: A variation at position −30 of the β-cell glucokinase gene promoter polymorphism is associated with reduced β-cell function in middle-aged Japanese-American men. Diabetes 1996; 45:422–428.
Strack V, Bossenmaier B, Stoyanov B, Mushack J, Haring HU: A 973 valine to methionine mutation of the human insulin receptor: interaction with insulin-receptor substrate-1 and Shc in HEK 293 cells. Diabetologia 1997; 40:1135–1140.
Stumvoll M, Fritsche A, Volk A, Stefan N, Madaus A, Maerker E, Teigeler A, Koch M, Machicao F, Haring H: The Gly972Arg polymorphism in the insulin receptor substrate-1 gene contributes to the variation in insulin secretion in normal glucose-tolerant humans. Diabetes 2001; 50:882–885.
Sturis J, Kurland IJ, Byrne MM, Mosekilde E, Froguel P, Pilkis SJ, Bell GI, Polonsky KS: Compensation in pancreatic β-cell function in subjects with glucokinase mutations. Diabetes 1994; 43:718–723.
Suzuki Y, Suzuki S, Hinokio Y, Chiba M, Atsumi Y, Hosokawa K, Shimada A, Asahina T, Matsuoka K: Diabetes associated with a novel 3264 mitochondrial tRNA(Leu)(UUR) mutation. Diabetes Care 1997; 20:1138–1140.
Tattersall RB, Pyke DA: Diabetes in identical twins. Lancet 1972; 2:1120–1125.
Tattersall RB, Pyke DA, Nerup J: Genetic patterns in diabetes mellitus. Hum Pathol 1980; 11:273–283.
Tawata M, Hayashi JI, Isobe K, Ohkubo E, Ohtaka M, Chen J, Aida K, Onaya T: A new mitochondrial DNA mutation at 14577 T/C is probably a major pathogenic mutation for maternally inherited Type 2 diabetes. Diabetes 2000; 49:1269–1272.
Taylor RW, Printz RL, Armstrong M, Granner DK, Alberti KGMM, Turnbull DM, Walker M: Variant sequences of the hexokinase II gene in familial NIDDM. Diabetologia 1996; 39:322–328.
Taylor SI: Lilly lecture: molecular mechanisms of insulin resistance—lessons from patients with mutations in the insulin-receptor gene. Diabetes 1992; 41:1473–1490.
Terauchi Y, Iwamoto K, Tamemoto H, Komeda K, Ishii C, Kanazawa Y, Asanuma N, Aizawa T, Akanuma Y, Yasuda K, et al.: Development of non-insulin-dependent diabetes mellitus in the double knockout mice with disruption of insulin receptor substrate-1 and β-cell glucokinase genes. Genetic reconstitution of diabetes as a polygenic disease. J Clin Invest 1997; 99:861–866.
't Hart LM, de Knijff P, Dekker JM, Stolk RP, Nijpels G, van der Does FE, Ruige JB, Grobbee DE, Heine RJ, Maassen JA: Variants in the sulphonylurea receptor gene: association of the exon 16-3t variant with Type II diabetes mellitus in Dutch Caucasians. Diabetologia 1999; 42:617–620.
't Hart LM, Stolk RP, Heine RJ, Grobbee DE, van der Does FEE, Maassen JA: Association of the insulin receptor variant Met-985 with hyperglycemia and non-insulin dependent diabetes mellitus in the Netherlands: a population-based study. Am J Hum Genet 1996; 59:1119–1125.
Thomas P, Ye Y, Lightner E: Mutation of the pancreatic islet inward rectifier Kir6.2 also leads to familial persistent hyperinsulinemic hypoglycemia of infancy. Hum Mol Genet 1996; 5:1809–1812.
Thornton PS, Satin-Smith MS, Herold K, Glaser B, Chiu KC, Nestorowicz A, Permutt MA, Baker L, Stanley CA: Familial hyperinsulinism with apparent autosomal dominant inheritance: clinical and genetic differences from the autosomal recessive variant. J Pediatr 1998; 132:9–14.
Tonolo G, Melis MG, Ciccarese M, Secchi G, Atzeni MM, Li LS, Luthman H, Maioli M: Glucagon receptor Gly40Ser amino acid variant in Sardinian hypertensive non-insulin-dependent diabetic patients. Sardinian Diabetic Genetic Study Group (SDGSG). Acta Diabetol 1997a; 34:75–76.
Tonolo G, Melis MG, Ciccarese M, Secchi G, Atzeni MM, Maioli M, Pala G, Massidda A, Manai M, Pilosu RM, et al.: Physiological and genetic characterization of the Gly40Ser mutation in the glucagon receptor gene in the Sardinian population. Sardinian Diabetes Genetic Study Group. Diabetologia 1997b; 40:89–94.
Trevisan R, Viberti G: Genetic factors in the development of diabetic nephropathy. J Lab Clin Med 1995; 126:342–349.
Tripathy D, Carlsson AL, Lehto M, Isomaa B, Tuomi T, Groop L: Insulin secretion and insulin sensitivity in diabetic subgroups: studies in the prediabetic and diabetic state. Diabetologia 2000; 43:1476–1483.
Tsukuda K, Suzuki Y, Kameoka K, Osawa N, Goto Y, Katagiri H, Asano T, Yazaki Y, Oka Y: Screening of patients with maternally transmitted diabetes for mitochondrial gene mutations in the tRNA[Leu(UUR)] region [see comments]. Diabet Med 1997; 14:1032–1037.
Umpierrez GE, Woo W, Hagopian WA, Isaacs SD, Palmer JP, Gaur LK, Nepom GT, Clark WS, Mixon PS, Kitabchi AE: Immunogenetic analysis suggests different pathogenesis for obese and lean African-Americans with diabetic ketoacidosis. Diabetes Care 1999; 22:1517–1523.
Unger RH: Diabetic hyperglycemia: link to impaired glucose transport in pancreatic β-cell. Science 1991; 251:1200–1205.

United Kingdom Prospective Diabetes Study: Relative efficacy of randomly allocated diet, sulphonylurea, insulin, or metformin in patients with newly diagnosed non-insulin dependent diabetes followed for three years. Br Med J 1995; 310: 83–88.

Ura S, Araki E, Kishikawa H, Shirotani T, Todaka M, Isami S, Shimoda S, Yoshimura R, Matsuda K, Motoyoshi S, et al.: Molecular scanning of the insulin receptor substrate-1 (IRS-1) gene in Japanese patients with NIDDM: identification of five novel polymorphisms. Diabetologia 1996; 39:600–608.

Urhammer SA, Clausen JO, Hansen T, Pedersen O: Insulin sensitivity and body weight changes in young white carriers of the codon 64 amino acid polymorphism of the β_3-adrenergic receptor gene. Diabetes 1996; 45:1115–1120.

Urhammer SA, Dalgaard LT, Sorensen TI, Moller AM, Andersen T, Tybjaerg-Hansen A, Hansen T, Clausen JO, Vestergaard H, Pedersen O: Mutational analysis of the coding region of the uncoupling protein 2 gene in obese NIDDM patients: impact of a common amino acid polymorphism on juvenile and maturity onset forms of obesity and insulin resistance. Diabetologia 1997a; 40:1227–1230.

Urhammer SA, Hansen T, Clausen JO, Eiberg H, Pedersen O: The g/a nucleotide variant at position −30 in the β-cell-specific glucokinase gene promoter has no impact on the β-cell function in Danish Caucasians. Diabetes 1998; 47:1359–1361.

Urhammer SA, Rasmussen SK, Kaisaki PJ, Oda N, Yamagata K, Moller AM, Fridberg M, Hansen L, Hansen T, Bell GI, et al.: Genetic variation in the hepatocyte nuclear factor-1α gene in Danish Caucasians with late-onset NIDDM. Diabetologia 1997b; 40:473–475.

Valdez R, Mitchell BD, Haffner SM, Hazuda HP, Morales PA, Monterrosa A, Stern MP: Predictors of weight change in a bi-ethnic population: the San Antonio Heart Study. Int J Obes Relat Metab Disord 1994; 18:85–91.

van den Ouweland JM, Lemkes HH, Ruitenbeek W, Sandkuijl LA, de Vijlder MF, Struyvenberg PA, van de Kamp JJ, Maassen JA: Mutation in mitochondrial tRNA(Leu)(UUR) gene in a large pedigree with maternally transmitted Type II diabetes mellitus and deafness. Nat Genet 1992; 1:368–371.

Vaxillaire M, Boccio V, Philippi A, Vigouroux C, Terwilliger J, Passa P, Beckmann JS, Velho G, Lathrop GM, Froguel P: A gene for maturity onset diabetes of the young (MODY) maps to chromosome 12q. Nat Genet 1995; 9:418–423.

Vaxillaire M, Rouard M, Yamagata K, Oda N, Kaisaki PJ, Borriraj VV, Chevre JC, Boccio V, Cox RD, Lathrop GM, et al.: Identification of nine novel mutations in the hepatocyte nuclear factor 1α alpha gene associated with maturity-onset diabetes of the young (MODY3). Hum Mol Genet 1997; 6:583–586.

Velho G, Byrne MM, Clement K, Sturis J, Pueyo ME, Blanche H, Vionnet N, Fiet J, Passa P, Robert JJ, et al.: Clinical phenotypes, insulin secretion, and insulin sensitivity in kindreds with maternally inherited diabetes and deafness due to mitochondrial tRNALeu(UUR) gene mutation. Diabetes 1996a; 45:478–487.

Velho G, Petersen KF, Perseghin G, Hwang JH, Rothman DL, Pueyo ME, Cline GW, Froguel P, Shulman GI: Impaired hepatic glycogen synthesis in glucokinase-deficient (MODY-2) subjects. J Clin Invest 1996b; 98:1755–1761.

Velho G, Vaxillaire M, Boccio V, Charpentier G, Froguel P: Diabetes complications in NIDDM kindreds linked to the MODY3 locus on chromosome 12q. Diabetes Care 1996c; 19:915–919.

Vestergaard H, Bjorbaek C, Andersen PH, Bak JF, Pedersen O: Impaired expression of glycogen synthase mRNA in skeletal muscle of NIDDM patients. Diabetes 1991; 40:1740–1745.

Vialettes BH, Paquis-Flucklinger V, Pelissier JF, Bendahan D, Narbonne H, Silvestre-Aillaud P, Montfort MF, Righini-Chossegros M, Pouget J, Cozzone PJ, et al.: Phenotypic expression of diabetes secondary to a T14709C mutation of mitochondrial DNA. Comparison with MIDD syndrome (A3243G mutation): a case report. Diabetes Care 1997; 20:1731–1737.

Vidal-Puig A, Printz RL, Stratton IM, Granner DK, Moller DE: Analysis of the hexokinase II gene in subjects with insulin resistance and NIDDM and detection of a Gln142-His substitution. Diabetes 1995; 44:340–346.

Vionnet N, Hani EH, Dupont S, Gallina S, Francke S, Dotte S, De Matos F, Durand E, Lepretre F, Lecoceur C, et al.: Genomewide search for Type 2 diabetes-susceptibility genes in French whites: evidence for a novel susceptibility locus for early-onset diabetes on chromosome 3q27–qter and independent replication of a Type 2-diabetes locus on chromosome 1q21–q24. Am J Hum Genet 2000; 67: 1470–1480.

Vionnet N, Hani EH, Lesage S, Philippi A, Hager J, Varret M, Stoffel M, Tanizawa Y, Chiu KC, Glaser B, et al.: Genetics of NIDDM in France: studies with 19 candidate genes in affected sib pairs. Diabetes 1997; 46:1062–1068.

Walston J, Silver K, Bogardus C, Knowler WC, Celi FS, Austin S, Manning B, Strosberg AD, Stern MP, Raben N, et al.: Time of onset of non-insulin-dependent diabetes mellitus and genetic variation in the β_3-adrenergic-receptor gene. N Engl J Med 1995; 333:343–347.

Watanabe RM, Ghosh S, Langefeld CD, Valle TT, Hauser ER, Magnuson VL, Mohlke KL, Silander K, Ally DS, Chines P, Blaschak-Harvan J, Douglas JA, Duren WL, Epstein MP, et al.: The Finland–United States investigation of non-insulin-dependent diabetes mellitus genetics (FUSION) study: II. An autosomal genome scan for diabetes-related quantitative-trait loci. Am J Hum Genet 2000; 67:1186–1200.

Watanabe RM, Valle T, Hauser ER, Ghosh S, Eriksson J, Kohtamaki K, Ehnholm C, Tuomilehto J, Collins FS, Bergman RN, et al.: Familiarity of quantitative metabolic traits in Finnish families with non-insulin-dependent diabetes mellitus: Finland–United States Investigation of NIDDM genetics (FUSION) study investigators. Hum Hered 1999; 49:159–168.

Waterworth DM, Bennett ST, Gharani N, McCarthy MI, Hague S, Batty S, Conway GS, White D, Todd JA, Franks S, et al.: Linkage and association of insulin gene VNTR regulatory polymorphism with polycystic ovary syndrome. Lancet 1997; 349:986–990.

Weyer C, Bogardus C, Mott DM, Pratley RE: The natural history of insulin secretory dysfunction and insulin resistance in the pathogenesis of Type 2 diabetes mellitus. J Clin Invest 1999; 104:787–794.

Widen E, Lehto M, Kanninen T, Walston J, Shuldiner AR, Groop LC: Association of a polymorphism in the β_3-adrenergic-receptor gene with features of the insulin resistance syndrome in Finns. N Engl J Med 1995; 333:348–351.

Wiltshire S, Hattersley AT, Hitman GA, Walker M, Levy JC, Sampson M, O'Rahilly S, Frayling TM, Bell JI, Lathrop GM, et al.: A genomewide scan for loci predisposing to Type 2 diabetes in a U.K. population (The Diabetes UK Warren 2 Repository): Analysis of 573 pedigrees provides independent Replication of a susceptibility locus on chromosome 1q. Am J Hum Genet 2001; 69:553–569.

Withers DJ, Gutierrez JS, Towery H, Burks DJ, Ren JM, Previs S, Zhang Y, Bernal D, Pons S, Shulman GI, et al.: Disruption of IRS-2 causes Type 2 diabetes in mice. Nature 1998; 391:900–904.

Xia J, Scherer SW, Cohen PT, Majer M, Xi T, Norman RA, Knowler WC, Bogardus C, Prochazka M: A common variant in PPP1R3 associated with insulin resistance and Type 2 diabetes. Diabetes 1998; 47:1519–1524.

Yamada K, Yuan X, Ishiyama S, Ichikawa F, Koyama KI, Koyanagi A, Koyama W, Nonaka K: Clinical characteristics of Japanese men with glucokinase gene β-cell promoter variant. Diabetes Care 1997; 20:1159–1161.

Yamada S, Nishigori H, Onda H, Takahashi K, Kitano N, Morikawa A, Takeuchi T, Takeda J: Mutations in the hepatocyte nuclear factor-1α gene (*MODY3*) are not a major cause of late-onset NIDDM in Japanese subjects. Diabetes 1997; 46:1512–1513.

Yamagata K, Furuta H, Oda N, Kaisaki PJ, Menzel S, Cox NJ, Fajans SS, Signorini S, Stoffel M, Bell GI: Mutations in the hepatocyte nuclear factor-4α gene in maturity-onset diabetes of the young (MODY1). Nature 1996a; 384:458–460.

Yamagata K, Oda N, Kaisaki PJ, Menzel S, Furuta H, Vaxillaire M, Southam L, Cox RD, Lathrop GM, Boriraj VV, et al.: Mutations in the hepatocyte nuclear factor-1α gene in maturity-onset diabetes of the young (MODY3). Nature 1996b; 384:455–458.

Yamagata K, Yang Q, Yamamoto K, Iwahashi H, Miyagawa J, Okita K, Yoshiuchi I, Miyazaki J, Noguchi T, Nakajima H, et al.: Mutation P291fsinsC in the transcription factor hepatocyte nuclear factor-1α is dominant negative [In Process Citation]. Diabetes 1998; 47:1231–1235.

Yanovski JA, Diament AL, Sovik KN, Nguyen TT, Li H, Sebring NG, Warden CH: Associations between uncoupling protein 2, body composition, and resting energy expenditure in lean and obese African American, white, and Asian children. Am J Clin Nutr 2000; 71:1405–1420.

Yen CJ, Beamer BA, Negri C, Silver K, Brown KA, Yarnall DP, Burns DK, Roth J, Shuldiner AR: Molecular scanning of the human peroxisome proliferator activated receptor γ (hPPARγ) gene in diabetic Caucasians: identification of a Pro12Ala PPARγ_2 missense mutation. Biochem Biophys Res Commun 1997; 241:270–274.

Yoshida H, Ohagi S, Sanke T, Furuta H, Furuta M, Nanjo K: Association of the prohormone convertase 2 gene (*PCSK2*) on chromosome 20 with NIDDM in Japanese subjects. Diabetes 1995; 44:389–393.

Yoshimura R, Araki E, Ura S, Todaka M, Tsuruzoe K, Furukawa N, Motoshima H, Yoshizato K, Kaneko K, Matsuda K, et al.: Impact of natural IRS-1 mutations on insulin signals: mutations of IRS-1 in the PTB domain and near SH2 protein bindings sites result in impaired function at different steps of IRS-1 signalling. Diabetes 1997; 46:929–936.

Yuan X, Yamada K, Koyama K, Ichikawa F, Ishiyama S, Koyanagi A, Koyama W, Nonaka K: β_3-adrenergic receptor gene polymorphism is not a major genetic determinant of obesity and diabetes in Japanese general population. Diabetes Res Clin Pract 1997; 37:1–7.

Zhang Y, Wat N, Stratton IM, Warren-Perry MG, Orho M, Groop L, Turner RC: UKPDS 19: Heterogeneity in NIDDM: separate contributions of IRS-1 and β_3-adrenergic-receptor mutations to insulin resistance and obesity respectively with no evidence for glycogen synthase gene mutations. Diabetologia 1996; 39:1505–1511.

Zimmet P, Baba S: Central obesity, glucose intolerance and other cardiovascular disease risk factors: an old syndrome rediscovered. Diabetes Res Clin Pract 1990; 10(Suppl 1):S167–S171.

Zimmet P, Boyko EJ, Collier GR, de Court: Etiology of the metabolic syndrome: potential role of insulin resistance, leptin resistance, and other players. Ann NY Acad Sci 1999; 892:25–44.

Zimmet P, Dowse G, Finch C: The epidemiology and natural history of NIDDM: lessons learned from the South Pacific. Diabetes Metab Rev 1990; 6:91–121.

Zouali H, Hani EH, Philippi A, Vionnet N, Beckmann JS, Demenais F, Froguel P: A susceptibility locus for early-onset non-insulin dependent (Type 2) diabetes mellitus maps to chromosome 20q, proximal to the phosphoenolpyruvate carboxykinase gene. Hum Mol Genet 1997; 6:1401–1408.

Zouali H, Velho G, Froguel P: Polymorphisms of the glycogen synthase gene and non-insulin-dependent diabetes mellitus. N Engl J Med 1993; 328:1568.

23 Obesity

GEORGE BRAY AND CLAUDE BOUCHARD

This chapter focuses on the genetic aspects of being overweight and relates them to the epidemiologic evidence that obesity is an epidemic and to the pathophysiologic consensus about causes of this epidemic. The location of body fat and the total amount of fat influence the health risks associated with obesity. The roles of increased food intake, reduced physical activity, and altered thermogenesis as physiologic mechanisms for the genetic development of excessive fat deposits are reviewed. Finally, a clinical approach to the use of this information is considered. For more detailed information about various facets of obesity, especially treatment, the reader is referred to several recent monographs (Bouchard et al., 1996; World Health Organization, 1998; National Heart, Lung and Blood Institute, 1998; Bray, 1998; Bray and Greenway, 1999).

Definition and Measurement of Body Fat and Its Distribution

Both overweight and fat distribution may be useful predictors of health risks associated with obesity and have genetic components that underlie their variance. We thus need to have a clear definition of these phenotypes. *Overweight* is an increase of body weight above a standard defined in relation to height. *Obesity* is an abnormally high percentage of body fat, which may be generalized or localized. To determine the degree of overweight and the amount of body fat, we need techniques and standards for quantitating body weight, body fat, and fat distribution. Several approaches are listed in Table 23–1.

Anthropometric Measurements

Anthropometric measurements include height and weight; circumferences of the chest, waist, hips, and extremities; and skinfold thickness (Heymsfield et al., 1998).

Height and weight can be related in several ways. Of these, the ratio termed the *body mass index* (BMI), or Quetelet index (kg/m^2), is most useful. The correlation of BMI with body fat as measured from body density is between 0.7 and 0.8. Table 23–2 is for determining BMI from pounds and inches or kilograms and centimeters.

The World Health Organization (1998) and the National Heart, Lung and Blood Institute (1998) have adopted a common classification of overweight and obesity. As BMI increases, risk to health increases. Obesity is defined as a BMI of 30 or more (Table 23–3).

The degree of body fat, or obesity, can be assessed from the thickness of skinfolds (Heymsfield et al., 1998). One difficulty with skinfold measurements is that the equations used to estimate body fat vary with age, sex, and ethnic background. Body fat increases with age even though the sum of the skinfold measurements remains constant. This finding implies that, with aging, fat accumulates at other than subcutaneous sites. The waist circumference alone or the ratio of waist or abdominal circumference to the hip circumference provides an index of central fatness and is an additional guide to health risks in epidemiologic studies. Men and women in the top quintile for waist circumference, i.e., the top 20%, have a substantially increased risk of heart disease and diabetes (Pouliot et al., 1994b).

Isotopic, Chemical, and Other Methods to Measure Body Composition

Both chemical and isotopic markers can be used to estimate body water, body fat, or potassium (Heymsfield et al., 1998; Bray, 1998). Measurement of body density provides a valuable quantitative technique for measuring body fat and fat-free mass (Table 23–1). Density is determined from the weight of the body when submerged in water compared to the weight of the body when out of water using the principle of Archimedes. The technique is relatively easy if appropriate facilities are available, but it remains primarily a research method.

Total body electrical conductivity also can be used to quantitate lean and fat tissue because of differences in the ability of these components to conduct electromagnetic waves (Heymsfield et al., 1998). However, the instrument used for this test is expensive. A relatively inexpensive instrument for measuring body fat uses electrical impedance. Electrodes are applied to one arm and leg, and the impedance is measured. Because impedance is related to the aqueous portion of the body, formulas can be used to estimate the percentage of fat in the body. There is concern, however, about the validity of this method (Bray et al., 2002). Dual-energy X-ray, or dual-photon absorptiometry, appears to be the best single method for estimating total body fat (Heymsfield et al., 1998). However, estimates of body fat using multicompartment models are the most reliable if they are available (Heymsfield et al., 1998; Bray et al., 2002).

Computerized tomographic (CT) scans and nuclear magnetic resonance imaging (MRI) (Table 23–1) can provide quantitative estimates of regional fat and give an intra-abdominal to extra-abdominal fat ratio. Ultrasonic waves applied to the skin are reflected by the fat, muscle, and other interfaces and can provide a measure of fat thickness in regional locations (Heymsfield et al., 1998). Finally, neutron activation of the whole body can be used to identify chemical components by their emission spectra (Heymsfield et al., 1998). This procedure is expensive and available in only a few centers.

Table 23–1. Methods for Body Measuring Composition[a]

	Cost	Ease of Use	Can Measure Regional Fat	External Radiation
Anthropometric				
Height and weight	$	E	No	
Diameters	$	E	+	
Circumferences	$	E	+	
Skinfolds	$	M	+	
Instrumental				
Hydrodensitometry	$$	E[b]	No	
Air displacement Plethysmography	$$$$	D[b]	No	
Dual X-ray absorptiometry	$$$	M[b]	+	tr
Isotope dilution	$$	M[b]	No	
Impedance (BIA)	$$	E[b]	+	
^{40}K counting	$$$$	D[b]	No	
Conductivity (TOBEC)	$$$	D[b]	±	
CT scan	$$$$	D[b]	++	++
MRI scan	$$$$	D[b]	++	
Neutron activation	$$$$+	D[b]	No	+++
Ultrasound	$$	M[b]	+	

[a]$, inexpensive; $$, some expense; $$$, expensive; $$$$, very expensive; tr, trace; E, easy; M, moderate experience needed; D, difficult; BIA, TOBEC, total-body electrical conductivity; CT, computed tomography; MRI, magnetic resonance imaging.
[b]Special equipment.
Source: Bray (1998).

In summary, overweight and obesity can be estimated in several ways. From a practical point of view, three methods are most useful. Measurements of height and weight, expressed as the BMI, provide an estimate of the degree of overweight. When available, dual-energy X-ray absorptiometry provides the easiest method of estimating total body fat. For estimating regional fat distribution, measurement of the waist circumference is practical. For accurate estimates of visceral fat, however, CT or MRI scans must be performed; and for accurate estimates of body fat, a four-compartment method is required.

The proportions of fat and nonfat components are depicted for a normal-weight (70 kg) and an obese (100 kg) male as well as for a normal-weight (55 kg) and an obese (85 kg) female; the extra 30 kg of weight adds ~50% to body weight but increases body energy stored as fat by 200% (Fig. 23–1).

Development and Anatomical Distribution of Adipose Tissue

Development of Body Fat

At birth, the human contains approximately 10% to 15% fat. This amount is higher than that for any other mammal except the whale. In the newborn period, body fat rises rapidly to reach a peak of about 25% by age 6 months and then declines to 15% to 18% in the prepubertal years.

Gender Differences

At puberty, there is a significant increase in the percentage of fat in females and a significant decrease in males. By age 18, males have approximately 15% body fat and females have about 25%. Fat increases in both sexes after puberty, and during adult life it rises to between 30% and 40% of body weight. Between ages 20 and 50, fat content in males approximately doubles and that in females increases by approximately 50%. Total body weight, however, rises by only 10% to 15%, indicating that there is a reduction in lean body mass (Bray, 1998).

Ethnic and Social Differences

In the United States, there is a lower percentage of overweight Caucasian women than either African-American or Hispanic women (Flegal et al., 1998). The nearly linear increase in prevalence with age is evident in all three groups, with peak values for overweight occurring between ages 40 and 70 years. For males, the percentage of overweight is lower for African Americans at all ages except the decade 40 to 49 years. Among males, the percentage of overweight becomes stable between the fourth and sixth decades of life.

Caucasian females at all ages are less obese (using a BMI of 30 or more) than African-American or Hispanic (Latino) females. The prevalence of obesity in African-American women is 37.4% and in Hispanic women, 34.2%. This contrasts with a figure of 22.4% for Caucasian women. The differences in obesity among males from different ethnic groups are much smaller. Caucasian males have a lower prevalence of obesity (BMI >30 kg/m^2) at all ages than African-American or Hispanic males, but these differences are small, with Caucasian males being 20% and African-American and Hispanic males being 21.3% and 23.1%, respectively.

Socioeconomic conditions play an important role in the development of obesity. Excess body weight is 7 to 12 times more frequent in women from lower social classes than in women from upper social classes. In men, social class and race have a much less pronounced relationship to overweight.

GENETIC AND EPIDEMIOLOGIC EVIDENCE

Epidemiology of Obesity

People in the United States and Canada are among the fattest people in the world. There are at least three possible explanations for the high prevalence of obesity in North America. First, the high proportion of automobiles, large amounts of time spent

Table 23–2. A Table of Body Mass Index Using Either Pounds and Inches or Kilograms and Centimeters

	Body Mass Index (kg/m^2)																					
Inches	19	20	21	22	23	24	25	26	27	28	29	30	31	32	33	34	35	36	37	38	39	40	Centimeters
58	*91*	*95*	*100*	*105*	*110*	*115*	*119*	*124*	*129*	*134*	*138*	*143*	*148*	*153*	*158*	*162*	*167*	*172*	*177*	*181*	*186*	*191*	
	41	**43**	**45**	**48**	**50**	**52**	**54**	**56**	**58**	**61**	**63**	**65**	**67**	**69**	**71**	**73**	**76**	**78**	**80**	**82**	**84**	**86**	**147**
59	*94*	*99*	*104*	*109*	*114*	*119*	*124*	*128*	*133*	*138*	*143*	*148*	*153*	*158*	*163*	*168*	*173*	*178*	*183*	*188*	*193*	*198*	
	43	**45**	**47**	**50**	**52**	**54**	**56**	**59**	**61**	**63**	**65**	**68**	**70**	**72**	**74**	**77**	**79**	**81**	**83**	**86**	**88**	**90**	**150**
60	*97*	*102*	*107*	*112*	*118*	*123*	*128*	*133*	*138*	*143*	*148*	*153*	*158*	*164*	*169*	*174*	*179*	*184*	*189*	*194*	*199*	*204*	
	44	**46**	**49**	**51**	**53**	**55**	**58**	**60**	**62**	**65**	**67**	**69**	**72**	**74**	**76**	**79**	**81**	**83**	**85**	**88**	**90**	**92**	**152**
61	*100*	*106*	*111*	*116*	*121*	*127*	*132*	*137*	*143*	*148*	*153*	*158*	*164*	*169*	*174*	*180*	*185*	*190*	*195*	*201*	*206*	*211*	
	46	**48**	**50**	**53**	**55**	**58**	**60**	**62**	**65**	**67**	**70**	**72**	**74**	**77**	**79**	**82**	**84**	**86**	**89**	**91**	**94**	**96**	**155**
62	*104*	*109*	*115*	*120*	*125*	*131*	*136*	*142*	*147*	*153*	*158*	*164*	*169*	*175*	*180*	*186*	*191*	*196*	*202*	*207*	*213*	*218*	
	47	**50**	**52**	**55**	**57**	**60**	**62**	**65**	**67**	**70**	**72**	**75**	**77**	**80**	**82**	**85**	**87**	**90**	**92**	**95**	**97**	**100**	**158**
63	*107*	*113*	*118*	*124*	*130*	*135*	*141*	*146*	*152*	*158*	*163*	*169*	*175*	*180*	*186*	*192*	*197*	*203*	*208*	*214*	*220*	*225*	
	49	**51**	**54**	**56**	**59**	**61**	**64**	**67**	**69**	**72**	**74**	**77**	**79**	**82**	**84**	**87**	**90**	**92**	**95**	**97**	**100**	**102**	**160**
64	*110*	*116*	*122*	*128*	*134*	*140*	*145*	*151*	*157*	*163*	*169*	*174*	*180*	*186*	*192*	*198*	*203*	*209*	*215*	*221*	*227*	*233*	
	50	**52**	**55**	**58**	**60**	**63**	**66**	**68**	**71**	**73**	**76**	**79**	**81**	**84**	**87**	**89**	**92**	**94**	**97**	**100**	**102**	**105**	**162**
65	*114*	*120*	*126*	*132*	*138*	*144*	*150*	*156*	*162*	*168*	*174*	*180*	*186*	*192*	*198*	*204*	*210*	*216*	*222*	*228*	*234*	*240*	
	52	**54**	**57**	**60**	**63**	**65**	**68**	**71**	**74**	**76**	**79**	**82**	**84**	**87**	**90**	**93**	**95**	**98**	**101**	**103**	**106**	**109**	**165**
66	*117*	*124*	*130*	*136*	*142*	*148*	*155*	*161*	*167*	*173*	*179*	*185*	*192*	*198*	*204*	*210*	*216*	*223*	*229*	*235*	*241*	*247*	
	54	**56**	**59**	**62**	**65**	**68**	**71**	**73**	**76**	**79**	**82**	**85**	**87**	**90**	**93**	**96**	**99**	**102**	**104**	**107**	**110**	**113**	**168**
67	*121*	*127*	*134*	*140*	*147*	*153*	*159*	*166*	*172*	*178*	*185*	*191*	*198*	*204*	*210*	*217*	*223*	*229*	*236*	*242*	*248*	*255*	
	55	**58**	**61**	**64**	**66**	**69**	**72**	**75**	**78**	**81**	**84**	**87**	**90**	**92**	**95**	**98**	**101**	**104**	**107**	**110**	**113**	**116**	**170**
68	*125*	*131*	*138*	*144*	*151*	*158*	*164*	*171*	*177*	*184*	*190*	*197*	*203*	*210*	*217*	*223*	*230*	*236*	*243*	*249*	*256*	*263*	
	57	**60**	**63**	**66**	**69**	**72**	**75**	**78**	**81**	**84**	**87**	**90**	**93**	**96**	**99**	**102**	**105**	**108**	**111**	**114**	**117**	**120**	**173**
69	*128*	*135*	*142*	*149*	*155*	*162*	*169*	*176*	*182*	*189*	*196*	*203*	*209*	*216*	*223*	*230*	*237*	*243*	*250*	*257*	*264*	*270*	
	58	**61**	**64**	**67**	**70**	**74**	**77**	**80**	**83**	**86**	**89**	**92**	**95**	**98**	**101**	**104**	**107**	**110**	**113**	**116**	**119**	**123**	**175**
70	*132*	*139*	*146*	*153*	*160*	*167*	*174*	*181*	*188*	*195*	*202*	*209*	*216*	*223*	*230*	*236*	*243*	*250*	*257*	*264*	*271*	*278*	
	60	**63**	**67**	**70**	**73**	**76**	**79**	**82**	**86**	**89**	**92**	**95**	**98**	**101**	**105**	**108**	**111**	**114**	**117**	**120**	**124**	**127**	**178**
71	*136*	*143*	*150*	*157*	*165*	*172*	*179*	*186*	*193*	*200*	*207*	*215*	*222*	*229*	*236*	*243*	*250*	*258*	*265*	*272*	*279*	*286*	
	62	**65**	**68**	**71**	**75**	**78**	**81**	**84**	**87**	**91**	**94**	**97**	**100**	**104**	**107**	**110**	**113**	**117**	**120**	**123**	**126**	**130**	**180**
72	*140*	*147*	*155*	*162*	*169*	*177*	*184*	*191*	*199*	*206*	*213*	*221*	*228*	*235*	*243*	*250*	*258*	*265*	*272*	*280*	*287*	*294*	
	64	**67**	**70**	**74**	**77**	**80**	**84**	**87**	**90**	**94**	**97**	**100**	**104**	**107**	**111**	**114**	**117**	**121**	**124**	**127**	**131**	**134**	**183**
73	*144*	*151*	*159*	*166*	*174*	*182*	*189*	*197*	*204*	*212*	*219*	*227*	*234*	*242*	*250*	*257*	*265*	*272*	*280*	*287*	*295*	*303*	
	65	**68**	**72**	**75**	**79**	**82**	**86**	**89**	**92**	**96**	**99**	**103**	**106**	**110**	**113**	**116**	**120**	**123**	**127**	**130**	**133**	**137**	**185**
74	*148*	*155*	*163*	*171*	*179*	*187*	*194*	*202*	*210*	*218*	*225*	*233*	*241*	*249*	*256*	*264*	*272*	*280*	*288*	*295*	*303*	*311*	
	67	**71**	**74**	**78**	**81**	**85**	**88**	**92**	**95**	**99**	**102**	**106**	**110**	**113**	**117**	**120**	**124**	**127**	**131**	**134**	**138**	**141**	**188**
75	*152*	*160*	*168*	*176*	*184*	*192*	*200*	*208*	*216*	*224*	*232*	*240*	*247*	*255*	*263*	*271*	*279*	*287*	*295*	*303*	*311*	*319*	
	69	**72**	**76**	**79**	**83**	**87**	**90**	**94**	**97**	**101**	**105**	**108**	**112**	**116**	**119**	**123**	**126**	**130**	**134**	**137**	**141**	**144**	**190**
76	*156*	*164*	*172*	*180*	*189*	*197*	*205*	*213*	*221*	*230*	*238*	*246*	*254*	*262*	*271*	*279*	*287*	*295*	*303*	*312*	*320*	*328*	
	71	**74**	**78**	**82**	**86**	**89**	**93**	**97**	**101**	**104**	**108**	**112**	**115**	**119**	**123**	**127**	**130**	**134**	**138**	**142**	**145**	**149**	**193**

To determine your body mass index, select your height in either inches or centimeters and move across the row until you find your weight in pounds or kilograms. Your body mass index can be read at the top. Italics are for pounds and inches; bold is for kilograms and centimeters.

Table 23–3. Classification of Overweight and Obesity[a] in Adults According to Body Mass Index (BMI)

Classification	BMI (kg/m^2)[b]	Risk of Comorbidities[c]
Underweight	<18.5	Low (but risk of other clinical problems increased)
Normal range	18.5–24.9	Average
Overweight	25.0–29.9	Mildly increased
Obese	≥30.0	
Class I	30.0–34.9	Moderate
Class II	35.0–39.9	Severe
Class III	≥40.0	Very severe

[a]Obesity is classified as BMI ≥30 kg/m^2.
[b]These values are age-independent and the same for both sexes. However, BMI may not correspond to the same degree of fatness across different populations.
[c]Both BMI and a measure of fat distribution (waist circumference or waist:hip ratio) are important in calculating the risk of obesity comorbidities. BMI <18.5 kg/m^2 signifies an increased risk of developing other clinical problems.
Source: World Health Organization (1998).

watching television, and the widespread availability of energy-saving devices may significantly reduce energy expenditure more than in other countries. Second, there may be differences in quantity or quality of dietary intake. Third, lower rates of smoking and smoking cessation may contribute to the higher rate of obesity in North America.

Time Trends within a Population

Several studies suggest that there has been a progressive increase in weight for height in the United States throughout the entire twentieth century. Data on inductees into the military service show that for men 5′ 8″ tall, weights rose from 147 lb in 1863 to 168 lb in 1991 (Bray, 1998). A similar increase has been observed in the Framingham cohort, with males showing a steady increase throughout the early part of this century and females showing a slight downward trend in average weight. Life insurance data and data from the National Center for Health Statistics also show a small increase in average weight for height. The National Center for Health Statistics data from surveys conducted in 1960–1962, 1970–1974, and 1976–1980 showed only a small change with time. Recent data from 1988–1994 show a marked increase for both men and women (Flegal et al., 1998) (Fig. 23–2).

Differences Between Populations

There are wide variations between populations in the prevalence of overweight. Among the fattest are some Polynesians, Melanesians, and Native Americans in the United States. In most developing countries, prevalence rates are much lower. The prevalence and time trends for several countries are shown in Fig. 23–3. The developed countries are highest in prevalence; the developing countries and those with a lower-fat diet are lowest but rising fast.

Family Epidemiology

It is well established that obesity runs in families (Bouchard et al., 1993). However, except for some rare Mendelian disorders, the vast majority of obese patients do not exhibit a clear pattern of Mendelian inheritance. Despite the difficulties associated with the study of the genetic basis of complex traits such as obesity, genetic epidemiologic studies are useful for addressing specific questions such as the extent of familial aggregation in obesity, the relative contribution of genetic and nongenetic factors, the role of maternal vs. paternal transmission, whether a trait is influenced by a major gene, and whether shared genetic and/or environmental factors contribute to the covariation among two or more phenotypes. Despite the large number of studies on the familial aggregation and heritability of the obesity phenotypes, there is no unanimity among researchers regarding the importance of genetic factors. A more complete review of these questions can be found elsewhere (Bouchard, 1994; Bouchard et al., 1998).

Family Studies

In traditional nuclear families, members share both genes and environments to some degree, and it is difficult to separate the genetic from the environmental components. Therefore, transmissibility or maximal heritability is usually reported, which includes both sources of shared variance. Several family studies have compared resemblance in pairs of spouses, parents and chil-

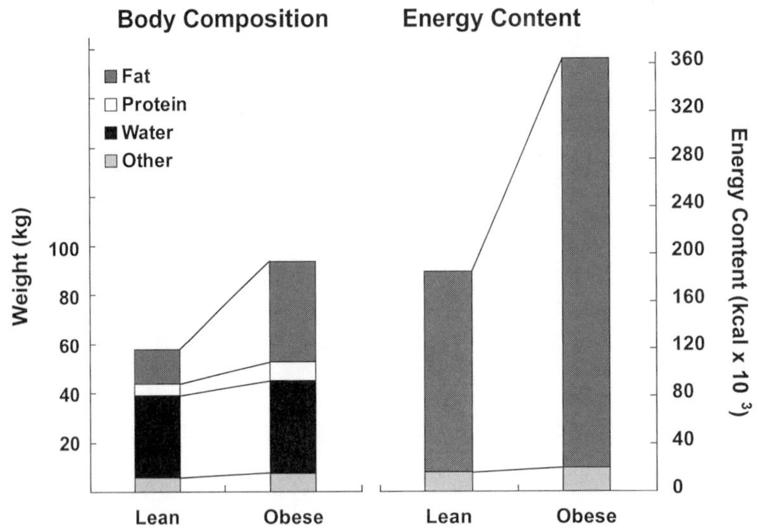

Fig. 23–1. Body composition in lean and obese individuals who differ by 30 kg. The measured components are on the *left*, and the calculated energy content on the *right* shows that most of the energy is stored in fat. Energy content nearly doubles with a 50% increase in body weight. From Bray (1998) with permission.

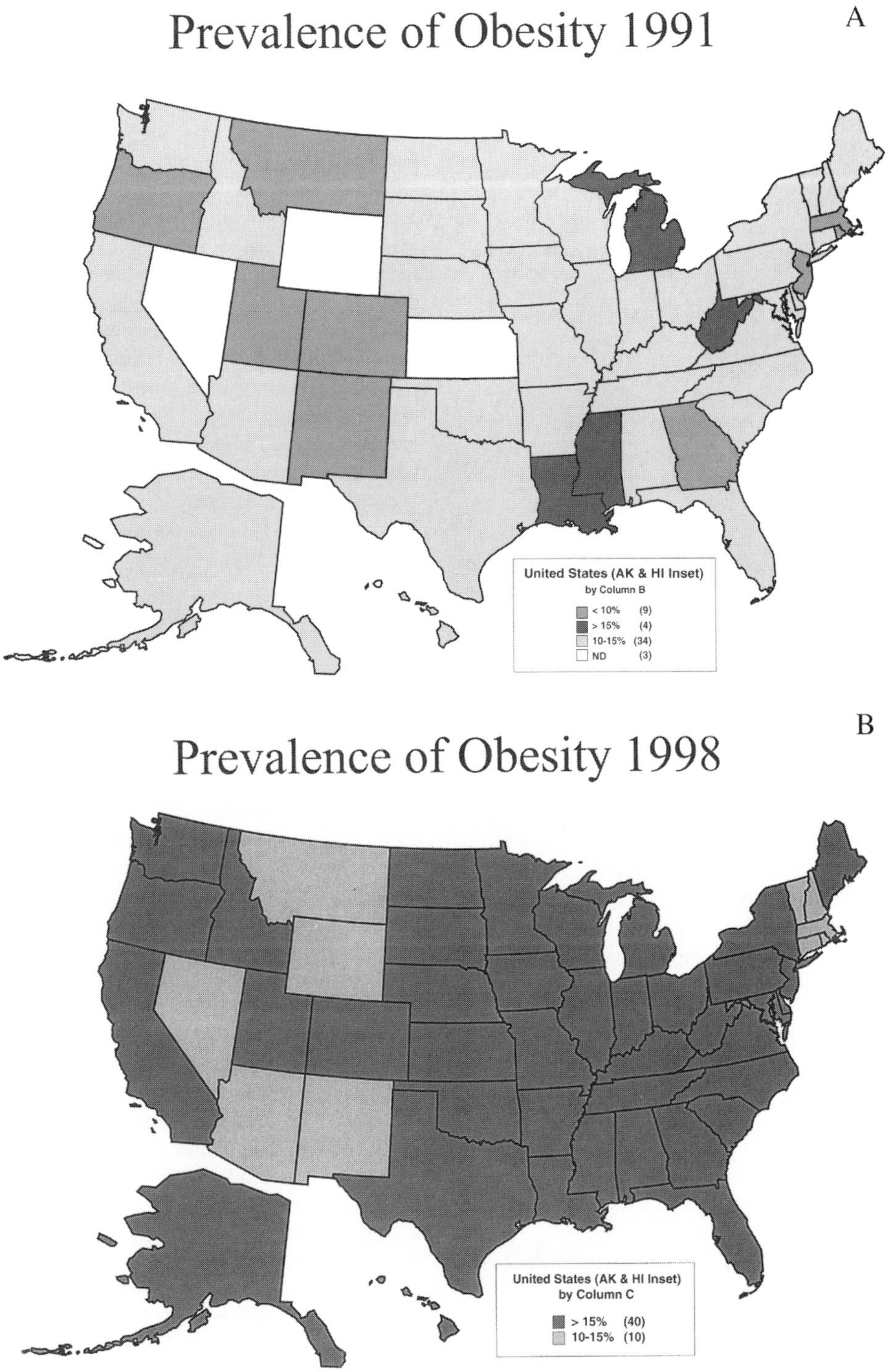

Fig. 23–2. Maps showing changing prevalence of obesity in the United States between 1991 *(A)* and 1998 *(B)*. Adapted from CDC.

dren, and brothers and sisters for body weight, BMI, and selected skinfold thicknesses (Mueller, 1983; Bouchard et al., 1988, 1993). Figure 23–4 presents the average correlations reported in four large family-based studies of BMI: the Framingham Heart Study (Heller et al., 1984), the Canada Fitness Survey (Perusse et al., 1988), the Quebec Family Study (Bouchard et al., 1988), and the Nord-Trøndelag Norwegian National Health Screening Service Family Study (Tambs et al., 1991).

The correlations among spouses are the lowest, reaching an average value of 0.13, whereas the correlations among monozygotic (MZ) twins are the highest, with an average value of 0.73. The parent–offspring, sibling, and dizygotic (DZ) twin correlations are 0.22, 0.28, and 0.27, respectively. These correlations suggest that individuals who share genes in addition to the familial environment tend to have more similar BMI values than those sharing only the environment, as with spouses. Doubling the average familial correlations (i.e., parent–offspring and sibling correlations) yields a transmissibility estimate of 50% to 55%. A study performed in families participating in the HERITAGE Family Study reported significant spouse, parent–

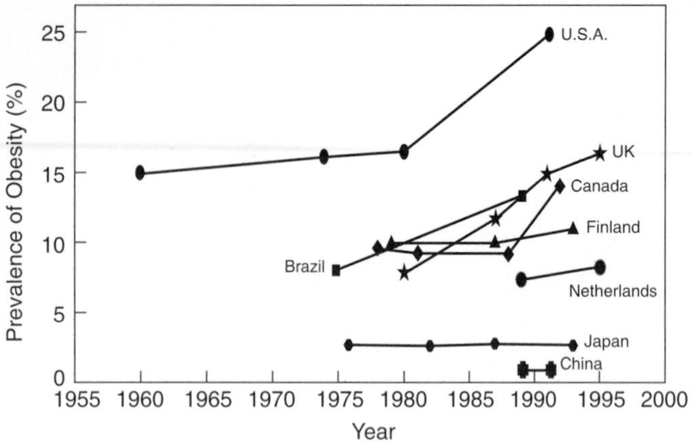

Fig. 23–3. Time trends in prevalence of obesity in women in several countries. Adapted from World Health Organization (1998) with permission.

offspring, and sibling correlations for subcutaneous fat based on eight skinfold measurements and percent body fat (derived from underwater weighing with maximal heritability estimates, including both genetic and environmental sources of variance) of 34% and 62%, respectively (Rice et al., 1997a). For fat-free mass, the maximal heritability reached 65% but was consistent with a genetic etiology as there was no significant spouse resemblance.

A sensible approach is to combine the information from all available types of relative and use maximum likelihood path analysis methods to obtain estimates of heritability. In a study of 74,994 persons from the population of Nord-Trøndelag, Norway, correlations in various kinds of relative were fitted to a path model to estimate genetic and environmental factors in the transmission of BMI, and a broad heritability coefficient of about 40% was obtained (Tambs et al., 1991). Similar estimates of familial variance were obtained for BMI in the Tecumseh, Michigan, study (Longini et al., 1984). In the Quebec Family Study, based on 1698 members of 409 families, including nine types of relative by descent or adoption, there was a total transmissible variance across generations for BMI of about 35%. For fat mass and percentage body fat estimated by densitometry, a genetic effect

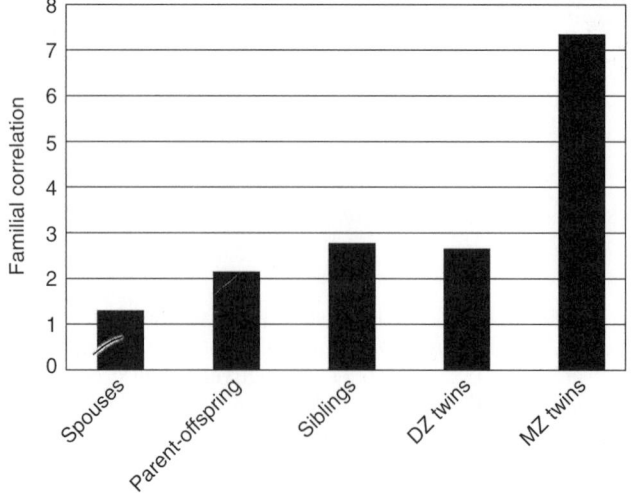

Fig. 23–4. Average familial correlations among various types of relative for body mass index derived from four large familial studies (Heller et al., 1984; Perusse et al., 1988; Bouchard et al., 1988; Tambs et al., 1991). *DZ*, dizygotic; *MZ*, monozygotic.

reaching 25% of the age- and sex-adjusted variance was reported (Bouchard et al., 1988).

The genetics of fat distribution has also been investigated in family studies. The evidence, mainly derived from skinfold measurements, reveals that, after adjusting for the total amount of body fat, about 30% to 50% of the variance in distribution of subcutaneous fat is accounted for by genetic factors (Bouchard et al., 1993). Instead of studying individual skinfolds or skinfold ratios, an alternative approach involves using principal components analysis to extract the factors underlying a set of skinfolds and investigate the familial aggregation basis of these factors. Based on six skinfold measures obtained in 1237 individuals from 308 nuclear families, Li et al. (1996) identified three principal components explaining 88% of the variance among the skinfold measurements. The first component represented a general measure of adiposity, whereas the second and third components contrasted the trunk-to-extremity and the upper-to-lower body skinfolds, respectively. The familial effects reached 46%, 52%, and 48% for each component, respectively, and were likely to be due to genetic factors since the spouse correlations were not significant (Li et al., 1996). The results support the previous findings and suggest a heritability of about 50% for the distribution of subcutaneous fat.

Heritability for waist circumference reached about 50% in two family studies (Katzmarzyk et al., 2000; Perusse et al., 2000) but dropped to about 30% after adjusting for BMI. The first heritability estimates of the abdominal visceral fat (AVF) depot, based on direct measurements, have been reported. In one study, AVF was measured by CT between vertebrae L4 and L5 in 366 adult subjects from the Quebec Family Study (Perusse et al., 1996). After adjustment for total body fat, the results were compatible with a genetic effect accounting for 56% of the variance in AVF. In another study, based on 437 subjects from the HERITAGE Family Study, a heritability estimate of 48% was reported for AVF after adjustment for total body fat (Rice et al., 1997b).

Leptin is involved in the regulation of food intake and energy expenditure (Campfield et al., 1996). Both expression of the leptin gene in adipose tissue and circulating levels of leptin are increased in most obese humans, suggesting that they are probably resistant to the action of leptin. However, in a fraction of the obese population, blood levels of leptin are low for the body mass or fat mass. The heritability of plasma leptin levels was estimated in a sample of 361 individuals from 118 African-American families (Rotimi et al., 1997). A heritability estimate of 39% was observed for age-adjusted leptin levels. In another study, the heritability of leptin was estimated to be 63% in Mexican-American families (Comuzzie et al., 1997).

Twin Studies

Twin studies allow for separation of the genetic component of variance. However, major problems with twin data are that MZ twins may share more environmental effects and dominance deviations than do DZ twins, thus inflating the genetic component. In fact, heritability estimates derived from twin data are usually higher than those derived from other family designs and, at times, are unrealistically high.

Heritability estimates of BMI derived from twin studies typically cluster between 50% and 80%. Comparison of MZ twins reared apart with MZ twins reared together is a useful design to assess the role of heredity with some control over the potentially confounding influences of a shared environment. Within-pair correlations for the BMI of MZ twins reared apart are generally similar to those of MZ twins reared together (Stunkard et al., 1990; MacDonald and Stunkard, 1990; Price and Gottesman, 1991), suggesting that shared familial environment did not contribute much to the variation in the BMI of MZ twins. Correlations of MZ twins reared apart provide a direct estimate of the genetic effect if it is assumed that members of the same pair were not placed in similar environments; that the twins were not, for some unspecified reasons, behaving similarly although they were living apart; and that intrauterine factors did not influence long-term variation in the BMI. According to these studies, the heritability of BMI would be in the range of 40% to 70%. Recent studies tend to corroborate these general trends. In a study of 53 pairs of MZ twins reared apart, Allison et al. (1996b) reported heritabilities between 0.50 and 0.70 for BMI. By combining these estimates with those previously reported in two other studies of MZ twins reared apart (Stunkard et al., 1990; Price and Gottesman, 1991), a heritability coefficient of 0.67 confidence interval [95% (CI) = 0.59–0.75] was obtained for BMI.

Total body fat, central abdominal fat, and nonabdominal fat were measured in 25 MZ and 18 DZ female twin pairs using dual-energy X-ray absorptiometry (Carey et al., 1996). Model fitting analysis of these data revealed that heritability of this central abdominal fat phenotype, adjusted for total amount of body fat, reached 73% and that common environmental effects were not significant (Carey et al., 1996).

Adoption Studies

Full adoption studies are useful for separating common environmental effects since adoptive parents and their adopted offspring (and adopted sibling pairs) share only environmental sources of variance, whereas the adoptees and their biologic parents share only genetic sources of variance.

Six adoption studies in which BMI data were available for both the biologic as well as adoptive relatives of the adoptees have been reported and generally found no significant contribution of shared family environment on BMI, suggesting that the familial resemblance could be attributed to genetic factors (Stunkard et al., 1986; Price et al., 1987; Sorensen et al., 1989, 1992a,b; Vogler et al., 1995). In the most recent of these studies, based on data from a Danish adoption registry, path analysis was used to estimate the heritability of BMI (Vogler et al., 1995). It was estimated to be 0.34, with all the remaining variance attributable to nonshared individual environmental factors.

In summary, the heritability of obesity phenotypes is highest with twin studies, intermediate with nuclear family data, and lowest when derived from adoption data. When several types of relatives are used jointly in the same design, heritability estimates typically cluster around 25% to 40% of the age- and gender-adjusted phenotype variance and tend to be slightly higher for fat-distribution phenotypes than for overall body fat, reaching a value of about 50% for abdominal visceral fat. There is no clear evidence for a specific maternal or paternal effect. In general, the common familial environmental effect appears to be marginal.

Genotype–Environment Interactions

Genotype–environment interaction arises when the response of a phenotype to environmental changes depends on the genotype of the individual. Although it is well known that there are interindividual differences in the responses to various dietary interventions, few attempts have been made to test whether these differences are genotype-dependent, particularly for obesity-related phenotypes.

It is generally recognized that there are some individuals prone to excessive accumulation of fat, some for whom losing weight represents a continuous battle, and others who seem relatively well protected against such a menace. Can such differences be accounted for by inherited differences? The results from a series of experiments performed with MZ twins revealed that the response to a positive or negative energy balance treatment is very heterogeneous among twin pairs but quite homogeneous within members of the same pair.

Twelve pairs of male MZ twins ate a 1000 kcal/day caloric surplus, 6 days a week, during a period of 100 days (Bouchard et al., 1990). Significant increases in body weight and fat mass were observed after the period of overfeeding. Data showed that there were considerable interindividual differences in the adaptation to excess calories and that the variation was not randomly distributed, as indicated by the significant within-pair resemblance in response. For instance, there was at least three times more variance in response between pairs than within pairs for the gains in body weight, fat mass, and fat-free mass (Fig. 23–5, left panel). These data demonstrate that some individuals are more at risk than others to gain fat when energy intake surplus is clamped at the same level for everyone and when all subjects are confined to a sedentary lifestyle. The within-identical-twin pair response

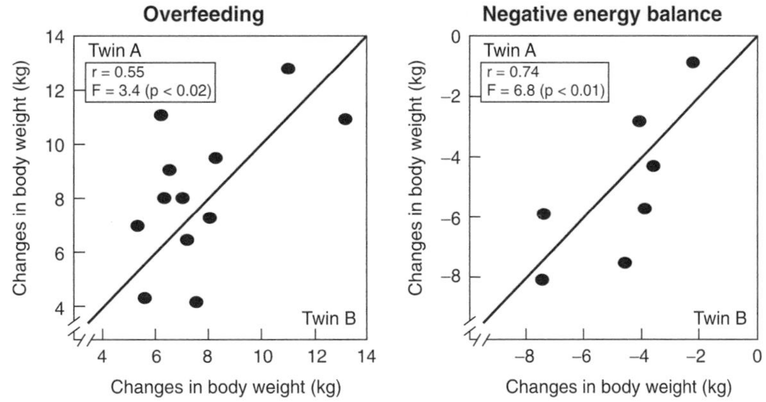

Fig. 23–5. Intrapair resemblance in the response of identical twins to long-term alterations in energy balance. *Left*: Changes in body weight in response to overfeeding (84,000 kcal surplus over 100 days) in 12 pairs of male identical twins (Bouchard et al., 1990). *Right*: Changes in body weight in response to a negative energy balance protocol induced by exercise (58,000 kcal deficit over 93 days) in seven pairs of male identical twins (Bouchard et al., 1994).

to the standardized caloric surplus suggests that the amount of fat stored is likely influenced by the genotype. This overfeeding study also revealed that there was six times more variance between pairs than within pairs for the changes in upper body fat and in CT-determined AVF when both were adjusted for the gain in total fat mass. These observations indicate that some individuals store fat predominantly in selected fat depots primarily as a result of undetermined genetic characteristics.

Seven pairs of young adult male identical twins completed a negative energy balance protocol during which they exercised on cycle ergometers twice a day, 9 of 10 days, over a period of 93 days, while being kept on a constant daily energy and nutrient intake (Bouchard et al., 1994). The mean total energy deficit caused by exercise above the estimated energy cost of body weight maintenance reached 244 MJ. Baseline energy intake was estimated over a period of 17 days preceding the negative energy balance protocol. Mean body weight loss was 5.0 kg, and it was entirely accounted for by the loss of fat mass. Body energy losses reached 191 MJ, which represented about 78% of the estimated energy deficit. Intrapair resemblance was observed in the changes in body weight (Fig. 23–5, right panel), fat mass, percent fat, sum of 10 skinfolds, and AVF level. Even though there were large individual differences in response to the negative energy balance and exercise protocol, subjects with the same genotype were more alike in responses than subjects with different genotypes. These results are remarkably similar to those for body-mass and body-fat gains in 12 pairs of twins subjected to the 100-day overfeeding protocol.

Genetic Effects on Temporal Trends

The prevalence of overweight and obesity increases with the age of the population up to about 65 years (Flegal et al., 1998). In genetic studies of obesity, the phenotypes are usually adjusted for age prior to analysis. This procedure corrects for age trends in the mean and variance, but temporal trends may still be evident in the covariances among family members. Correlation methods for tracking the familiarity estimates across time involve comparisons at different ages using either longitudinal measurements or cross-sectional data. It is, however, important to consider that with body-fat accretion up to a new body-mass level (e.g., a given obesity level), the causes of the positive energy balance that led to obesity become progressively masked. For instance, an apparent deficit in resting energy expenditure is compensated by an increase in the metabolic mass associated with weight gain (Ravussin et al., 1988). Similarly, an apparent deficit in lipid-oxidation rate is eliminated when the gain in fat mass has been large enough to ensure a greater reliance on lipid oxidation (Zurlo et al., 1990). This adds another dimension to the complexity of the task of understanding the causes of obesity and defining the role of genes.

Two studies using path analysis techniques (Province and Rao, 1985; Cardon, 1991) suggested that familial variance increased from birth to adulthood, which Cardon (1991), using adoptive and biologic families measured longitudinally, attributed to genetic (rather than environmental) factors. In adults (Korkeila et al., 1991; Fabsitz et al., 1980, 1992, 1994), there was a general decrease in the genetic heritability during adulthood. Fabsitz et al. (1992) suggested that there were two genetic effects, one increasing at or prior to age 20 years and the other decreasing after age 20 years. The presence of sex and age differences in the heritability of BMI was investigated in 1233 pairs of middle-aged (46–56 years) and elderly (60–76 years) MZ and DZ twins (Herskind et al., 1996). The heritability of BMI was higher in females compared to males in both middle-aged (0.77 vs. 0.46) and elderly (0.75 vs. 0.61) twins, and the age difference in the heritabilities was significant for males only. These results suggested the presence of age and sex differences in the heritability of BMI. In the aggregate, twin, family, and adoption studies suggest that the highest estimates of heritability are found during late adolescence and early adulthood, with decreases in the genetic effects at middle age and in the last decades of life (Pietiläinen et al., 1999; Rice et al., 1999; Huggins et al., 2000).

Evidence for Major Gene Effects

Heritability of the obesity phenotypes, as reviewed above, is thought to result primarily from the effects of several genes, each with small additive influences on the phenotypes. There are other types of genetic effect that are not necessarily additive in nature. For example, a major gene has a large impact on the phenotype. A common observation is that the obese proband in familial studies of obesity is, on the average, 10 to 15 BMI units heavier than his or her mother, father, brothers, or sisters (Reed et al., 1993; Adams et al., 1993; Lissner et al., 1994). Such a large difference between a proband and his or her first-degree relatives is suggestive of the contribution of a recessive gene having a large effect. This hypothesis can be tested by complex segregation analysis, in which the phenotype is assumed to be influenced by the independent and additive contributions from a major gene effect, a multifactorial background due to polygenes, and a unique environmental component (residual).

Several studies have tested the hypothesis of the segregation of a major gene for BMI or height-adjusted body mass, body-fat mass, subcutaneous fat distribution, or AVF (Table 23–4). Five of the 10 segregation studies of BMI, or some other measure of height-adjusted weight, provided evidence for the segregation of a recessive locus, with a frequency of about 0.2 and accounting for 35% to 45% of the variance, with a multifactorial component accounting for 40% to 45% of the variance. Four segrega-

Table 23–4. Overview of Segregation Analysis Studies for Obesity Phenotypes

Height-Adjusted Body Mass or Body Mass Index
- Two studies with no evidence of major gene effects (Karlin et al., 1981; Zonta et al., 1987)
- Three studies with evidence of major gene effects but with non-Mendelian transmission (Tiret et al., 1992; Rice et al., 1993a; Lecomte et al., 1997)
- Thirty-five studies with evidence for the segregation of a recessive locus with a frequency of about 0.20–0.30 and accounting for 35%–45% of the variance in addition to a multifactorial component accounting for 40%–45% of the variance (Price et al., 1990; Moll et al., 1991; Ness et al., 1991; Borecki et al., 1993; Borecki et al., 1998)

Fat Mass
- One study with evidence of a major gene effect but with non-Mendelian transmission (Lecomte et al., 1997)
- Three studies with evidence for the segregation of a recessive locus with frequencies between 0.35 and 0.47 and accounting for up to 65% of the variance in addition to a multifactorial component accounting for 20%–30% of the variance (Rice et al., 1993b, 1997b; Comuzzie et al., 1995)

Subcutaneous Fat Distribution
- Two studies with evidence for the segregation of a recessive locus with frequencies between 0.24 and 0.34 and a multifactorial component accounting for 30%–40% of the variance (Hasstedt et al., 1989; Borecki et al., 1995)

Abdominal Visceral Fat
- Two studies with evidence for the segregation of a recessive locus with frequencies around 0.30 and accounting for about 55% of the variance in addition to a multifactorial component accounting for about 20% of the variance (Bouchard et al., 1996; Rice et al., 1997c)

tion studies for fat mass and/or percent body fat have been reported. Two were conducted on the Quebec Family Study (Rice et al., 1993b) and the HERITAGE Family Study (Rice et al., 1997c) using underwater weighing techniques, and two were conducted in Mexican-American families (Comuzzie et al., 1995) and French Caucasian families (Lecomte et al., 1997) using bioelectrical impedance. In three of these studies (Rice et al., 1993b, 1997c; Comuzzie et al., 1995), the results were very similar and suggested the presence of a recessive locus accounting for about half of the variance, with an additional quarter of the phenotypic variance due to multifactorial effects. Two studies have also reported evidence of a recessive locus affecting the distribution of subcutaneous fat assessed from skinfold measurements (Hasstedt et al., 1989; Borecki et al., 1995).

A major gene hypothesis for AVF level was examined in the Quebec Family Study (Bouchard et al., 1996) and the HERITAGE Family Study (Rice et al., 1997c) cohorts. Very similar results were observed in both studies, with evidence of a putative recessive locus accounting for 51% and 57% of the variance of AVF and a multifactorial component accounting for an additional 21% and 17% of the variance. However, after adjusting AVF for fat mass, the transmission of the major gene was no longer Mendelian. It was suggested that the major gene previously noted for fat mass in the Quebec Family Study (Rice et al., 1993b) could also be responsible for the major gene detected for AVF. In other words, genetic pleiotropy was inferred, where the same major gene affected both fat mass and AVF. The hypothesis of a common genetic basis between fat mass and AVF was actually tested (Rice et al., 1996). The common familiality (shared genetic and familial environmental factors) between fat mass and AVF reached 29% to 50% (with sex differences), supporting the pleiotropy hypothesis and suggesting that there are genes affecting simultaneously fat mass and AVF.

These findings provide statistical evidence that there are subsets of obese families in which some genes appear to be more important than others in the etiology of obesity. Identification of these genes through linkage analyses is more likely to be successful in those families characterized by the strongest evidence for the segregation of major genes.

ENVIRONMENTAL FACTORS

Food Intake

Obesity is a problem of nutrient imbalance and results when the energy from excess foodstuffs is stored as fat rather than being used for metabolism (Bray and York, 1998). Do obese subjects ingest more food energy than they expend? The answer to this question is an unequivocal *yes*. Direct observations of food intake have shown that obese persons choose to eat larger meals than do lean persons. In a variety of studies on food choice, Stunkard and Kaplan (1977) found relative uniformity in the size of meals chosen in naturalistic settings. The energy content of the meals was strongly affected by eating site, and there was great variability in the amount of food chosen at each site. Thus, the major influence on how much people choose to eat is where they eat it. For instance, eating in a cafeteria leads to more food ingestion.

Based on both cross-sectional and longitudinal studies measuring food intake, obese people are often reported to eat less (National Research Council, Committee on Diet and Health, 1989). This apparent discrepancy has been resolved by the use of doubly labeled water to measure energy expenditure. This method shows that both obese and lean persons underreport their food intake (Bandini et al., 1990; Schoeller and Fjeld, 1991; Lichtman et al., 1992; Schutz and Jequier, 1998). As illustrated at the bottom of Figure 23–6, doubly labeled water ($^2H_2{}^{18}O$) is given to the subject. The top section of Figure 23–6 illustrates that deuterium ($^2H_2$) can leave the body only as water but ^{18}O can leave the body as both $C^{18}O_2$ and $H_2{}^{18}O$. Thus, ^{18}O is lost more rapidly than ^2H_2O, and the difference in rate of disappearance is proportional to CO_2 production (lower line in Fig. 23–6). The first measurement of $^2H_2$ and ^{18}O is within a few hours, and the second measurement is 7 to 14 days later (Fig. 23–6, lower panel). If one knows the respiratory quotient (RQ), it is possible to estimate reliably total energy expenditure. Data on a group of obese and lean subjects derived using this technique are shown in Figure 23–7 (Bandini et al., 1990; Welle et al., 1992; Prentice et al., 1996). In the three groups studied, obese subjects had higher total energy expenditure than lean ones. When compared with food intake, both obese and nonobese subjects underreported energy intake by 20% to 50% and 10% to 30%, respectively.

Energy requirements decline with age. Thus, to maintain body weight, food intake should show a corresponding decrease as a person ages. Values for energy intake from three surveys are presented in Figure 23–8 (Bray, 1989). Peak values occur in the second decade of life, followed by a gradual decline in successive decades for both sexes. Thus, the increase in body weight and body fat as a person ages cannot be attributed to increased nutrient intake but must be related to a relatively greater reduction in energy expenditure.

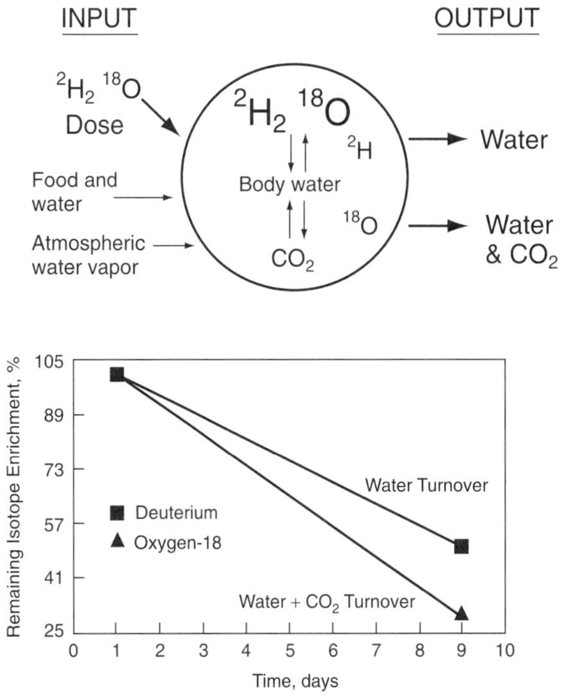

Fig. 23–6. Depiction of measurement of total body energy expenditure using doubly labeled water. A dose of water containing ^{18}O and ^2H is taken orally and allowed to mix with the body water. A baseline sample is then taken and the ratio of ^{18}O to ^2H determined. During metabolism, the ^{18}O can exit as water or CO_2, while the ^2H can only exit as water. Thus, the separation in the ratio of ^{18}O from ^2H is a measure of CO_2 production over the total time period. By estimating the respiratory quotient, the total energy expenditure can be calculated.

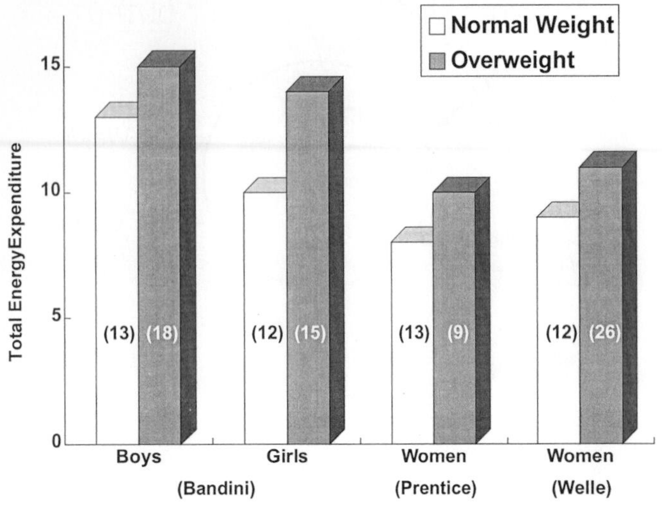

Fig. 23–7. Comparison of total energy expenditure in obese and lean subjects using doubly labeled water (Bandini et al., 1990; Prentice et al., 1996; Welle et al., 1992).

Fat Balance

To maintain normal body-fat stores requires that the nutrients present in the diet, especially fat, must be oxidized within the body in the proportion in which they occur in the diet. Figure 23–9 shows a typical distribution of macronutrients in a 2000 kcal diet and the fraction of body stores that these nutrients represent. Daily intake of carbohydrate nearly equals body stores of glucose. Thus, these stores are more vulnerable to changes in dietary carbohydrate than are either fat or protein, the other macronutrients. Oxidation of foodstuffs can be estimated from the RQ (the ratio of CO_2 produced to O_2 used). The corresponding ratio in food intake is referred to as the food quotient (FQ) (Flatt, 1995). As the FQ is reduced, i.e., as the percent of dietary fat increases, the RQ must also decline if weight is to remain stable. If it does not, the body continues to use carbohydrate stores and must replace these by eating more food to obtain carbohydrates or use back-up sources such as protein to provide a metabolic source of glucose. Whether this adjustment occurs efficiently and readily appears to have strong genetic determinants. Physiologically, adaptation to a high-fat, Western-type diet requires a decrease in carbohydrate oxidation to preserve carbohydrate stores. Schutz et al. (1992) and Astrup et al. (2000) have shown a strong relation between fat oxidation and body fat. If carbohydrate oxidation is reduced, the oxidation of fat will increase to provide for nutrient needs and lower the RQ. If the body is unable to reduce carbohydrate oxidation, one compensatory mechanism is to increase food intake to provide needed carbohydrates, increasing fat storage until a point is reached at which the oxidation of fatty acids increases to meet average daily fat intake. Recent studies have shown that this adaptation to a higher-fat diet is facilitated by exercise (Smith et al., 2000).

In summary, energy expenditure, and thus food intake, is higher in overweight than in lean subjects. Direct observation of obese subjects supports the conclusion that they choose to eat more food and often do so more rapidly than normal-weight subjects. Weight gain in adult life probably results from a decrease in energy expenditure rather than an increase in food intake, which actually seems to decline with age (Kromhout, 1983).

Energy Expenditure

Energy expenditure can be divided into several components, of which resting metabolic rate, thermic effect of food, and physical activity are the most important. Basal (resting) metabolic rate is defined as the total energy required by the body in the resting state and is influenced by age, sex, body weight, drugs, climate, and genetics. It represents approximately 70% of total energy expenditure. When corrected for body weight, the highest rate of energy expenditure occurs in infants. There is a gradual decline in this rate in childhood and a further, slower decline of approximately 2% per decade in adult life. Metabolic rates for women are usually lower than those for men of comparable height and weight, primarily because of the higher percentage of body fat in women (Schutz and Jequier, 1998). Basal metabolic rate has the strongest relationship to fat-free body mass (Ravussin et al., 1988), but it is also closely related to surface area and total body weight because heat loss is related to the surface area of the skin (Kleiber, 1961). In studies using both metabolic chamber (Garrow, 1981; Jequier and Schutz, 1983; deBoer et al., 1987; Bandini et al., 1990; Welle et al., 1992; Prentice et al., 1996) and doubly labeled water techniques, a higher body weight or greater lean body mass has been associated with a higher metabolic rate.

Metabolic rate clusters in families (Fontaine et al., 1985; Bogardus et al., 1986). If one individual is below the median for energy expenditure, other members of the family also tend to be below the median. A low resting metabolic rate in relation to lean body mass may also be a predictor for lower physical activity, higher body fat, and an increased likelihood of becoming obese (Ravussin et al., 1988).

Physical Activity

The relationship of physical activity to obesity can be studied by laboratory observations or by observation in the natural envi-

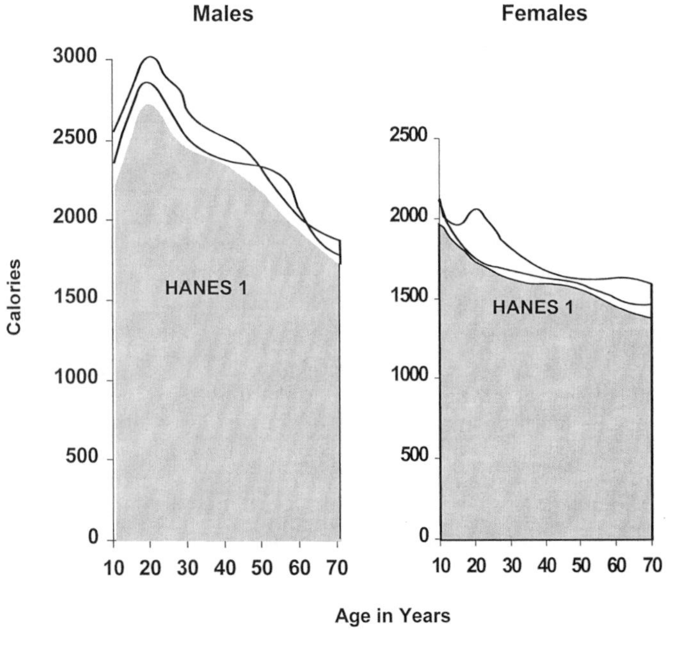

Fig. 23–8. Energy intake in relation to age in both males and females. NHANES1, National Health and Examination Survey I. Data from three national surveys. From Bray (1989) with permission.

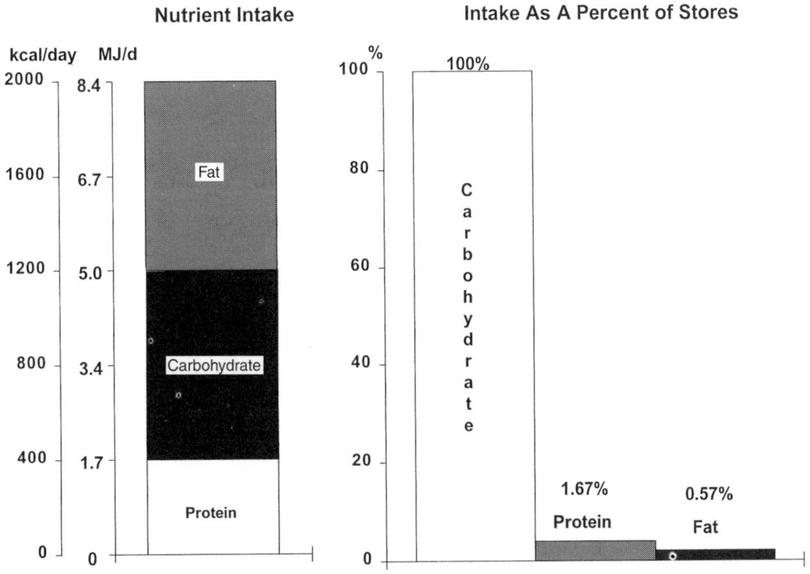

Fig. 23–9. Relationship of macronutrient intake to body stores of that macronutrient. A diet containing 40% fat, 40% carbohydrate, and 20% protein in terms of energy content is shown on the *left*. The relationship of each of these components to the body stores of the corresponding nutrient is shown on the *right* as a percent of nutrient stores.

ronment. In the laboratory, the treadmill and cycle ergometer have been the main tools used to examine the efficiency of exercising muscle in obese subjects. In both obese and lean individuals, the efficiency for coupling energy release to muscular contraction is approximately 30% (Bray, 1983); i.e., the work of turning the flywheel on a cycle ergometer accounts for 30% of the energy expended during cycling. Thus, there is no evidence to indicate an abnormality in the metabolic coupling of substrate metabolism to the contraction of muscular tissue in moderately or massively obese subjects (Bray, 1983).

The second approach to studying energy expenditure is observation. Obese individuals are often observed to be less active than normal-weight individuals. A lower level of spontaneous movement, however, does not necessarily imply reduced absolute energy expenditure because the overweight individual uses more energy for any given movement. In several prospective studies, the level of habitual physical activity or the level of sedentariness has been shown to be a strong predictor of weight gain over the follow-up period (Williamson et al., 1993). Thus, physically active adults have a reduced risk of becoming overweight or obese than do sedentary people. Also, maintaining a higher level of activity predicts greater success at maintaining weight loss (Williamson et al., 1993).

In normal-weight individuals, graded increases in physical activity have been reported to increase food intake (Woo et al., 1985a,b). In obese individuals, however, changing the level of physical activity has a much smaller effect on food intake (Woo et al., 1985a,b). Thus, the level of physical activity may modulate food intake and body fat in lean individuals. A disturbance in this system may play a key role in the development of obesity.

Thermic Effect of Food

When food is eaten, the metabolic rate initially rises and then returns toward normal. This process requires several hours, and during this time the increase in energy expenditure can approximate 10% of the total energy value of the ingested food. The thermic effect of food is highest with protein and lowest with fat (deJonge and Bray, 1997). One explanation for this thermogenic response to a meal is that it results from enhanced activity of the sympathetic nervous system, the effects of which are shown in activity of brown adipose tissue or muscle. If this is correct, a reduction in sympathetic activity of obese subjects compared with lean ones might provide a mechanism for enhanced metabolic efficiency that might allow energy to be stored rather than burned. A reduction in sympathetic nervous system activity to brown adipose tissue has been observed in many obese experimental species as well as humans (Bray et al., 1998) and might also explain why increasing physical activity does not significantly reduce food intake in obese subjects (Bray, 1991).

The concept that an altered thermic response to food may serve as a mechanism for the storage of extra calories, which causes human obesity, is intriguing and controversial (deJonge and Bray, 1997). Some studies have shown a difference between obese and lean subjects in energy produced after a meal, but other studies have not. The discrepancy may lie in the size of the meal eaten, the techniques of recording intake, the palatability of the food, and whether subjects had abnormal glucose tolerance. Golay et al. (1991) examined 55 subjects with varying degrees of obesity and impairment in glucose tolerance, including frank diabetes. The increment in energy expenditure was significantly lower in obese nondiabetic subjects and in those with impaired glucose tolerance than in normal volunteers. Obese diabetic subjects had a smaller response than normal-weight or obese nondiabetic subjects. There was a negative correlation between the degree of thermic response and circulating insulin. The thermic effect of glucose is partially blocked by propranolol, a drug that blocks β receptors (Acheson et al., 1988). This component of diet-induced thermogenesis is called *facultative thermogenesis*. These data suggest that there is an impairment in the thermic response to a meal in obese subjects and that one mechanism associated with this change is the anticipatory (cephalic phase) secretory response of the pancreatic system of releasing insulin. After weight loss, the thermic effect of a meal in obese subjects is reduced, providing additional evidence for this hypothesis.

In experimental animals, much of this effect is mediated through activation of uncoupling protein (UCP1) in brown adipose tissue. This thermogenic protein is a component of the inner mitochondrial membrane that enhances the leakage of protons through the mitochondrial membrane rather than coupling them to the generation of adenosine triphosphate (ATP). Using knowledge of the genetic structure of the brown adipose tissue UCP, at least two additional uncoupling proteins (UCP2 and UCP3) have been identified. UCP2 is widely distributed in fat and muscle, whereas UCP3 appears to be expressed only in muscle. Interest in these two uncoupling proteins as potential targets for drug treatment of obesity has stimulated a great deal of research on their function and control (Fleury et al., 1997; Vidal Puig et al., 1997; Kozak and Harper, 2000).

Age and Cold

Both energy expenditure and food intake decline with age. The rising prevalence of obesity with age implies that the matching of these two declining variables worsens with age. In a longitudinal study (Kromhout, 1983), body weight and food intake of middle-aged men were determined at two 5-year intervals. Food intake declined at each 5-year interval, whereas body weight increased, indicating that metabolic rate and/or physical activity had declined even faster than food intake.

Metabolic rate rises in cold environments. Under most circumstances, however, the availability of warm clothing and centrally heated housing mitigates this effect. No study has been able to provide evidence for a relationship between the prevalence of obesity and living in warm or cold climates across the range of human habitats.

Leptin Levels

Leptin was discovered in 1994 (Zhang et al., 1994) and is produced primarily in adipose tissue and placenta. Leptin is a member of the cytokine family and acts through the leptin receptor to modulate food intake, the sympathetic nervous system, and the hematopoietic system. Humans who lack either leptin (Montague et al., 1997) or the leptin receptor (Clement et al., 1998) are obese, as is the obese (*ob/ob*) mouse, which is leptin-deficient, and the diabetes (*db/db*) mouse, in which the leptin receptor is defective. When leptin is administered to either leptin-deficient humans or mice, food intake is reduced and the other defects of this deficiency are corrected. In mice that overexpress the leptin gene, essentially all body fat can be eliminated, indicating the potential value of this peptide as a treatment of obesity.

Familial Risk Levels

The risk of becoming obese when a biologic relative is obese is only partially understood (Perusse et al., 1998). The tendency for the risk of obesity to be higher in families of severely obese subjects was illustrated in a study where the prevalence of obesity (BMI >40 kg/m^2) was compared among 235 families of patients who were candidates for a surgical treatment of obesity and 152 families of normal-weight subjects matched for sex and age (MacLean and Rhode, 1996). Obese patients were 25 times more likely to have a first-degree relative with morbid obesity compared to control individuals [odds ratio (OR) = 24.5, 95% CI 10.4–57.7].

The familial aggregation of morbid obesity was also investigated in 221 families in Utah (n = 1560 subjects, ages 18 years and older) ascertained through a single morbidly obese proband (Adams et al., 1993). All probands had to be at least 45.5 kg over their ideal body weight. About 48% of the massively obese probands had one or more first-degree relatives who were also massively obese. When only probands with early onset of obesity were considered, i.e., probands who were massively obese before the age of 25, the prevalence of familial obesity reached 57%. Using data from 20,455 families from the general Utah population (more than 300,000 subjects), the authors estimated that the prevalence of massive obesity reached 6% in the Utah population, a value that was found to be significantly lower ($p <$ 0.00001) than in massively obese families (Adams et al., 1993). The risk of massive obesity was estimated to be about eight times higher (6% vs. 48%) in families segregating for morbid obesity than in the general population. The authors also calculated the risk of recurrence of obesity from parents to offspring and found that families with one or two obese parents had a 2.6 times increased risk ($p < 0.002$) of having one or more obese offspring (Adams et al., 1993). The results of this study suggest that obesity, and particularly early-onset obesity, strongly aggregates in families.

The prevalence of obesity in families of 729 obese women was also estimated by Reed et al. (1993). Obese probands were members of the National Association to Advance Fat Acceptance. The average age of the probands was 40 ± 9 years, and their average BMI was 47 ± 11 kg/m^2. The average BMI of the proband's first-degree relatives was also high, ranging from 28 kg/m^2 for adult children to 31 kg/m^2 for the proband's mother, and the majority of these probands (78%) had at least one other obese (BMI >30 kg/m^2) first-degree relative. Despite the high prevalence of obesity in these families, the familial correlations computed among first-degree relatives were similar to those observed in average-weight groups, which suggests that similar genetic factors could be involved in determining body mass in morbidly obese and nonobese subjects. The presence of one or two obese parents was associated with an increase of about 5 or 10 BMI units, respectively, in the BMI of the siblings of the probands. The familial aggregation of morbid obesity was also examined in a population-based sample of 1084 obese men (BMI ≥34 kg/m^2) and 1367 obese women (BMI ≥39 kg/m^2) of the Swedish Obese Subjects, an intervention trial aimed at determining the morbidity and mortality rates of obese individuals who underwent weight loss by surgical means (Lissner et al., 1994). Among the probands, 29% of the men and 34% of the women had one or more parent with a BMI >30 kg/m^2.

Familial risk can be quantified using the λ coefficient or standardized risk ratios, which are generally defined as the ratio of the risk of being obese when a biologic relative is obese compared to the risk in the population at large, i.e., the prevalence of obesity (Risch, 1990). Estimates of this risk based on BMI data have been reported (Allison et al., 1996a; Lee et al., 1997). Figure 23–10 depicts the age and gender-standardized risk ratios as computed from 2349 first-degree relatives of 840 obese probands and 5851 participants of the National Health and Nutrition Examination Survey III (Lee et al., 1997).

Figure 23–10 shows that the standardized risk ratio of obesity (BMI ≥30 kg/m^2) is about two times higher in families of obese individuals than in the population at large. Moreover, the risk increases with the severity of obesity in the proband as well as with the BMI threshold used to define obesity. Thus, the risk of extreme obesity (BMI ≥45 kg/m^2) is about seven to eight times higher in families of extremely obese subjects (Lee et al., 1997). These data illustrate that obesity aggregates in families, with a level that tends to increase with the severity of the condition.

However, the familial risk of obesity is only partially accounted for by genetic factors (Katzmarzyk et al., 1999). Indeed,

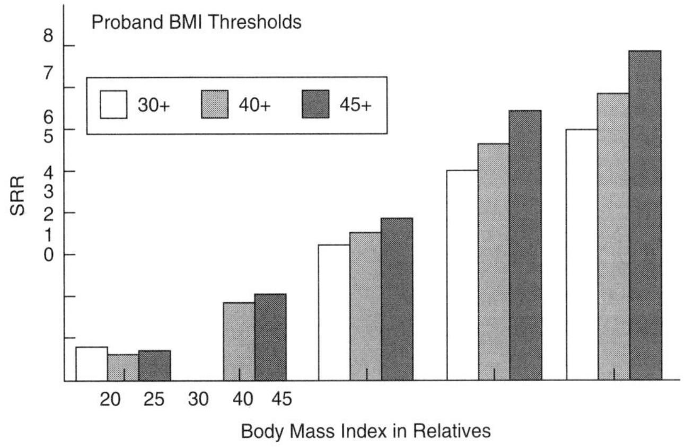

Fig. 23–10. Familial risk of obesity in relatives of obese probands in the University of Pennsylvania obesity studies. Values are age- and sex-standardized risk ratios (*SRR*) of the prevalence rate of obesity in relatives of probands to the population prevalence. *BMI*, body mass index. Adapted from Lee et al. (1997).

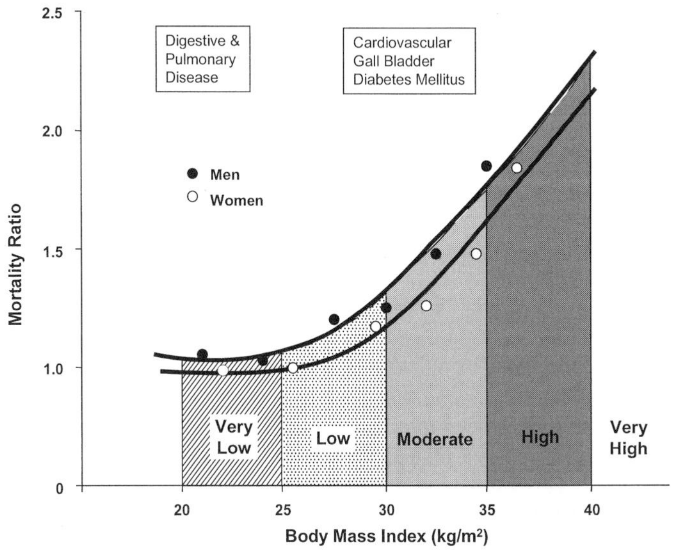

Fig. 23–11. Relationship between body mass index and mortality rates based on the American Cancer Society data. From Bray (1998) with permission.

a study was conducted in 1981 with 15,245 participants, ages 7 to 69 years, from a representative sample (6377 households) of the population of Canada. The standardized risk ratios for spouses and first-degree relatives of obese probands were generally only slightly higher in the case of the first-degree relatives. The data provided support for the hypothesis that the familial risk of obesity is only partially accounted for by genetic factors and may also depend on common environmental and other conditions.

Familial aggregation of massive obesity is stronger than for overweight or moderate obesity. The prevalence of obesity in families of markedly obese subjects is high, ranging from about 50% to 75% among various studies. The risk of severe obesity also appears to be higher for early-onset compared to late-onset obesity.

EFFECT OF OBESITY AND OVERWEIGHT ON MORTALITY AND MORBIDITY

It has been estimated that obesity causes 300,000 deaths per year in the United States (Allison et al., 1999). The detrimental effects of overweight on mortality have been demonstrated in a variety of prospective studies, e.g., those by the life insurance industry and the American Cancer Society (Stevens et al., 1998; Calle et al., 1999), the Norway study (Waaler, 1984), and the Nurses Health Study (Manson et al., 1995), which are consistent with many, but not all, smaller prospective studies (Society of Actuaries, 1980; Waaler, 1984). The overall relationship between BMI and excess mortality is shown in Figure 23–11, which plots relative mortality for various deviations of BMI using the American Cancer Society data (Bray, 1998). The data show a J-shaped curve, with the minimum mortality for both men and women occurring among individuals with a BMI of 22 to 25 kg/m^2. Deviations in BMI above this range are associated with an increase in mortality. Individuals with a BMI of 30 kg/m^2 clearly have increased mortality. As BMI approaches 40 kg/m^2, the curve becomes progressively steeper. In an examination of the relation of risk to BMI, Sjostrom (1992a,b) found that both studies with smaller numbers of subjects carried out over many years and studies with large numbers of subjects found a relationship of excess weight to mortality. Only studies with smaller numbers of subjects followed for short periods of time failed to find this relationship. The effect of excess weight on mortality applies to men and women (Manson et al., 1995) but may be less in women (Stevens et al., 1998), and particularly so in black women (Calle et al., 1999).

The curvilinear relationship between BMI and risk of mortality is similar to the relationship of rising blood pressure or increasing cholesterol to overall risk of mortality. These three risk factors and overall mortality are plotted in Figure 23–12. For each risk factor there are arbitrary cut-off points used to define risk. These have been aligned in the figure. The principal difference between the risk factors is the disease profile they predict. For a rising BMI, it is diabetes, gallbladder disease, cardiovascular disease, and some forms of cancer. It is interesting in this context that two reports, one from Japan and one from the Framingham Study, have defined relative morbidity using es-

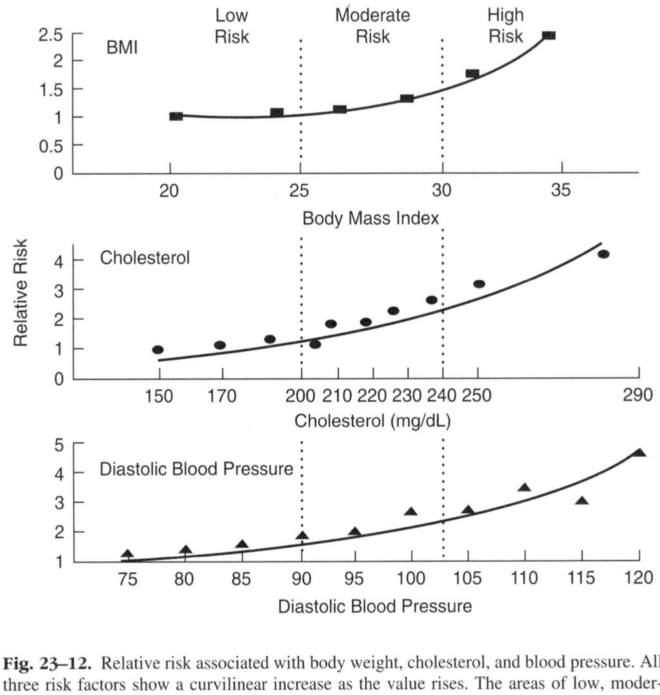

Fig. 23–12. Relative risk associated with body weight, cholesterol, and blood pressure. All three risk factors show a curvilinear increase as the value rises. The areas of low, moderate, and high have been identified by *vertical dashed lines*. *BMI*, body mass index. From Bray (1998) with permission.

timates of risk and found that the optimal BMI of 22 is very close to that from older estimates using mortality (Tokunaga et al., 1991; Garrison and Kannel, 1993).

Fat Distribution and Health Risks

One of the most important developments in understanding health risks associated with overweight has come from measurements of body fat distribution. There are two types of fat distribution: *(1)* the abdominal, android, upper-body, or male type and *(2)* the gynoid, lower-body, or female type. In the late 1940s, Vague (1956) suggested that a preponderance of upper-body fat might increase the risk for diabetes and cardiovascular disease. More than 30 years later, five prospective studies examining the relation of fat distribution to morbidity and mortality confirmed this hypothesis (Lapidus et al., 1984; Larsson et al., 1984; Stokes et al., 1985; Ducimetiere et al., 1986; Donahue et al., 1987; Kissebah and Krakower, 1994; Bjorntorp, 1997). Whether the distribution of fat was measured as the ratio of waist-to-hip circumference or a combination of skinfold thicknesses, all studies found a clear-cut and highly significant increase in the risk of death or an increased risk of diabetes, hypertension, heart attack, and stroke with increased upper-body obesity. Fat distribution was a more important risk factor for morbidity and mortality than overweight per se and had a relative risk ratio of ≥ 2.

In addition to the prospective data just described, cross-sectional studies have shown increased prevalence of glucose intolerance, insulin resistance, elevated blood pressure, and elevated blood lipids in both males and females with increased abdominal fat or upper-body obesity (Folsom et al., 1993; Pouliot et al., 1994b). Abdominal fatness also predicts the risk of breast cancer in women (Schapira et al., 1994). It has been suggested that the abdominal or android fat pattern may represent an increase in the size, number, or both of more metabolically active intra-abdominal fat cells. The current hypothesis is that these fat cells release free-fatty acids directly into the portal circulation, which might interfere with insulin clearance in the liver and thus affect various metabolic processes.

Comorbidity of Overweight and Obesity

With an increased BMI, there is an increased risk for diabetes mellitus, cardiovascular disease, and some types of cancer.

Diabetes Mellitus

The relationship between diabetes mellitus and obesity is strong (Colditz et al., 1995). Type 2 diabetes is almost nonexistent in individuals with a BMI below 20 kg/m^2. As BMI increases, the risk of diabetes increases dramatically (Colditz et al., 1995). Among the Pima Indians, the increased risk of diabetes in the obese has a strong familial tendency (Knowler et al., 1981). When one or both Pima Indian parents have diabetes, 100% of their offspring will develop diabetes if they become sufficiently obese. If neither parent has diabetes, fewer than 20% of their offspring develop diabetes. Recent studies show that modest weight loss can delay the onset of diabetes in humans with impaired glucose tolerance (Tuomilehto et al., 2001).

Hypertension

Increased blood pressure, like increased levels of insulin, is characteristic of obesity. Indeed, these two events may be related through the mechanism of insulin resistance (Ferrannini et al., 1991). The use of indirect sphygmomanometric methods to determine blood pressure in the obese requires an appropriately sized blood pressure cuff. When the blood pressure cuff is too short, greater differences are observed between systolic and diastolic pressures measured by direct intra-arterial methods than those obtained by indirect methods.

Hypertension has a striking correlation not only with body weight but also with lateral body build. The cardiac response to hypertension can include both concentric hypertrophy and dilatation (Messerli et al., 1987). Both central body fat distribution and increased total body fat appear to be related to the appearance of hypertension. During periods of severe caloric deprivation, such as occurred in World War I and World War II, hypertension was almost nonexistent. In clinical studies correlating changes in blood pressure with weight reduction, approximately 50% to 70% of those who lose weight have a fall in blood pressure (Davis et al., 1993; Stevens et al., 1993) and those who maintain the lower weight continue to have lower blood pressure (Stevens et al., 2001). One explanation might be reduced intake of salt, but careful studies have shown that blood pressure falls even if a fall in sodium intake is prevented by giving salt supplements (MacMahon et al., 1989). Weight reduction is more effective at lowering systolic blood pressure than diastolic blood pressure.

Cardiovascular System

In addition to the increased workload on the heart to pump larger volumes of blood, there is an increased risk of sudden death, probably due to cardiac arrhythmias associated with obesity. The increased risk of heart disease may be a reflection of an abnormal lipid pattern associated with obesity, decreased levels of high-density lipoprotein (HDL) cholesterol, and increased concentrations of low-density lipoprotein (LDL) cholesterol, particularly when these are the small and dense very-low-density lipoprotein (VLDL) particles (B pattern). In addition, obesity enhances C-reactive protein, a marker of inflammation. A higher C-reactive protein is a marker of risk for coronary heart disease. Obesity is viewed as a cardiac risk factor and a high BMI is associated with increased risk of coronary heart disease (Manson et al., 1995).

Cancer

Endometrial cancer, postmenopausal breast cancer, prostrate cancer, and colorectal cancer are related to the degree of obesity (Bray, 1998). One explanation for susceptibility to endometrial and breast cancer in obese women is the increased estrogen produced by the conversion of adrenal androgens (Δ^4-androstenedione) to estrone by aromatase in peripheral tissues. This factor is particularly important in the postmenopausal woman whose ovarian source of estrogen essentially disappears and where the predominant source of estrogen is peripheral conversion from adrenal androgens.

Gallbladder Disease

Gallbladder disease increases with obesity and age (Bray, 1998). One explanation for this association is the increased cholesterol excretion associated with obesity, independent of dietary intake. The quantity of cholesterol synthesized and excreted by the body per day increases by about 20 mg for each kilogram of adipose tissue. Thus, a 10 kg increase in adipose tissue mass increases cholesterol production and excretion by an amount comparable to that of the amount of cholesterol in one egg. Disturbances in nidation factors in the bile and alterations in the level of bile acids and phospholipids may lead to nidation and precipitation of cholesterol stones (Ko and Lee, 1998).

Pulmonary System and Sleep Apnea

Obesity itself, in the absence of underlying pulmonary disease, has little effect on respiratory function tests. However, sleep apnea is associated with obesity (Bray, 1998) in a linear fashion (Strohl et al., 1998). Sleep apnea poses a potentially serious problem. Recent data suggest that obstructive sleep apnea occurs because of local accumulation of fat in the tracheopharyngeal area. The obstructive episodes of sleep apnea produce interrupted sleep associated with hypoxia and hypercapnia. If not corrected, this condition can lead to right heart failure. Continuous positive airway pressure can be used at night to reduce or eliminate episodes of sleep apnea. Weight loss is of particular value in remediating this problem when even mild or moderate obesity is present.

Joint Disease and Skin Problems

Obesity is associated with an increase in osteoarthritis (Bray, 1998). Part of this is no doubt due to the added trauma of increased weight bearing, but the increased prevalence of osteoarthritis in non-weight-bearing joints suggests that additional factors may be involved. In addition to osteoarthritis, the prevalence of gouty arthritis is increased and may reflect alterations in urate clearance. Ketone bodies compete at the renal tubule for reabsorption of urate, and increased production of ketones from fat metabolism might account for the increased urate levels.

Among the skin problems associated with obesity are acanthosis nigricans, manifested by darkening of the skinfolds on the neck, elbows, and dorsal interphalangeal skin. Acanthosis nigricans is associated with increased insulin resistance and Type 2 diabetes. Skin turgor and friability may also be increased in obesity, enhancing the risk of fungal and yeast infections in skinfolds. Finally, venous circulatory disease is increased in obese subjects.

Endocrine System

Among the functional consequences of obesity are several alterations in the endocrine system. Hyperinsulinemia is a uniform finding and is directly related to the degree of obesity (Porte et al., 1998). Growth hormone secretion is reduced, but insulin-like growth factor I (IGF-I) is normal, suggesting that the lower level of growth hormone is sufficient to stimulate production of this important hormone. In both men and women, the level of sex hormone binding globulin is decreased, probably as a reflection of hyperinsulinemia. Testosterone levels are decreased in men, but free testosterone is normal until massive obesity appears, when it may also decline. The cyclic nature of the reproductive system in women makes it more susceptible to obesity. Obesity leads to an earlier onset of menarche, a greater frequency of irregular and anovulatory cycles, and earlier menopause. Distribution of body fat influences steroid metabolism in women. Women with central or visceral fat have a higher production of androgens, particularly testosterone, than women with less visceral fat and lower body obesity. Women with the gluteofemoral type of obesity have increased levels of estrone produced by peripheral aromatization of circulating adrenal Δ^4-androstenedione. Changes in thyroid hormone and its metabolism are predominantly a reflection of the level of nutrient intake. Triiodothyronine (T_3) can be increased by overfeeding and decreased by starvation. T_3 levels are also increased by high-carbohydrate diets and lowered by low-carbohydrate diets. In contrast, thyroxine (T_4) and thyrotropin are unaffected by these manipulations of the diet.

Obesity can sometimes be mistaken for Cushing's syndrome. The normal pattern of diurnal variation in plasma cortisol and the concentration of urinary free cortisol are normal in obesity but abnormal in Cushing's disease. If these differences are equivocal, suppression tests using exogenous dexamethasone may be needed.

Effects of Weight Loss

Does weight loss improve health? The insurance companies, the Framingham Study, and the Swedish Obese Subjects Study provide data suggesting that weight reduction may be beneficial (Ashley and Kannel, 1974; Goldstein, 1992; Sjostrom et al., 1997, 1999). In both men and women who intentionally lose and maintain a lower weight, the mortality rate is lower (Williamson et al., 1995). In a 2-year study, Sjostrom et al. (1997, 1999) found a graded effect of weight loss on a variety of cardiovascular and metabolic risk factors. Triglyceride and glucose declined, while HDL cholesterol increased. From the data obtained in the Framingham Study, a 10% reduction in relative weight for men was associated with a decrease in serum glucose of 0.14 mmol/l, a decrease in serum cholesterol of 0.292 mmol/l, a decrease in systolic blood pressure of 6.6 mm Hg, and a decrease in serum uric acid of 19.6 mmol/l (Ashley and Kannel, 1974). For each 10% reduction in the body weight of men, these data predict that there would be a 20% decrease in the incidence of coronary artery disease.

GENE IDENTIFICATION

Based on prevalence data from all continents (World Health Organization, 1998), there are an estimated 250,000,000 persons who are currently obese in the world, with a BMI of 30 and above, plus at least another 500,000,000 who are overweight, with BMI values ranging from 25 to <30 (Seidell, 2000). Efforts to identify the genes responsible for these obesity cases or the predisposition to obesity are still in an embryonic stage.

Several candidate genes for obesity have been identified. These candidate genes have been defined as such either because a mutation is known to influence the trait in one of the monogenic mouse models of obesity or because of their presumed functional implications in the physiopathology of the disease trait. In addition, positional candidate genes have been tested. In the case of obesity, these include those involved in the Mendelian syndromes exhibiting obesity as a clinical feature and quantitative trait loci (QTL) identified from human genome-wide searches or from polygenic animal models of obesity derived from crossbreeding experiments. A more complete discussion of the findings can be found in Perusse et al. (2001a).

Rare Mendelian Syndromes

Genetic syndromes characterized by the presence of obesity could potentially be useful in the identification of loci contributing to obesity. The current list of Mendelian disorders with obesity as one of their clinical features and that have also been mapped is presented in Table 23–5. The list was updated by searching the Online Mendelian Inheritance in Man (OMIM) computerized database. Only a small fraction of these disorders have been mapped and tested for potential association or link-

Table 23–5. Obesity-Related Mendelian Disorders with Known Map Location[a]

Mode of Inheritance	OMIM No.	Syndrome	Locus	Candidate Gene
Autosomal dominant	100800	Achondroplasia (ACH)	4p16.3	*FGFR3*
	103580	Albright hereditary osteodystrophy (AHO)	20q13.2–q13.3	*GNAS1*
	300800			
	103581	Albright hereditary osteodystrophy 2 (AHO2)	15q	N/A
	105830	Angelman syndrome with obesity (AGS)	15q11–q13	N/A
	147670	Insulin resistance syndromes (IRS)	19p13.3–p13.2	*INSR*
	122000	Posterior polymorphous corneal dystrophy (PPCD)	20q11	N/A
	151660	Familial partial lipodystrophy Dunnigan (FPLD)	1q21.2–q21.3	*LMNA*
	176270	Prader-Willi syndrome (PWS)	15q12	*SNRPN*
				NDN
	190160	Thyroid hormone resistance syndrome (THRS)	3p24.3	*THRB*
	181450	Ulnar-mammary syndrome or Schinzel syndrome (UMS)	12q24.1	*TBX3*
Autosomal recessive	203800	Alstrom syndrome (ALMS1)	2p13–p12	N/A
	209901	Bardet-Biedl syndrome 1 (BBS1)	11q13	N/A
	209900	Bardet-Biedl syndrome 2 (BBS2)	16q21	N/A
	600151	Bardet-Biedl syndrome 3 (BBS3)	3p13–p12	N/A
	600374	Bardet-Biedl syndrome 4 (BBS4)	15q22.3–q23	*MYO9A*
	603650	Bardet-Biedl syndrome 5 (BBS5)	2q31	N/A
	605231	Bardet-Biedl syndrome 6 (BBS6)	20p12	*MKKS*
	269700	Berardinelli-Seip congenital lipodystrophy (BSCL)	9q34	N/A
	216550	Cohen syndrome (COH1)	8q22–q23	N/A
	212065	Carbohydrate-deficient glycoprotein type 1a (CDGS1A)	16p13.3–p.13.2	*PMM2*
	227810	Fanconi-Bickel syndrome (FBS)	3q26.1–q26.2	*SLC2A2*
	139191	Isolated growth hormone deficiency (IGHD)	7p15–p14	*GHRH-R*
	601538	Combined pituitary hormone deficiency (CPHD)	5q	*PROP1*
X-linked	301900	Börjeson-Forssman-Lehmann syndrome (BFLS)	Xq26	*FGF13*
	303110	Choroideremia with deafness (CHOD)	Xq21.1–q21.2	N/A
	300148	Mehmo syndrome (MEHMO)	Xp22.13–p21.1	N/A
	300218	Mental retardation X-linked, syndromic 7 (MRXS7)	Xp11.3–q22	N/A
	300238	Shashi X-linked mental retardation syndrome (SMRXS)	Xq26–q27	N/A
	312870	Simpson-Golabi-Behmel 1 (SGBS1)	Xq26.1	*GPC3, GPC4*
		Simpson-Golabi-Behmel 2 (SGBS2)	Xp22	N/A
	309585	Wilson-Turner syndrome (WTS)	Xp21.2–q22	N/A

[a]Adapted from OMIM (Online Mendelian Inheritance in Man) computerized database. N/A, not available.

age relationships with obesity in the population at large. In one study, the chromosomal regions corresponding to several of these syndromes were tested for linkages with BMI using a total of 17 markers and data from 207 sibling pairs provided no significant evidence of linkage with any of the markers (Reed et al., 1995). These results suggest that the genes responsible for obesity in these genetic syndromes are probably not involved in determining obesity in otherwise clinically normal subjects. However, the prevalence of obesity was higher in subjects carrying one copy of the gene responsible for the Bardet-Biedl syndrome (BBS) (obligate heterozygote fathers of subjects affected by the syndrome) than in normal noncarrier subjects matched for age and sex, suggesting that this gene may affect the susceptibility to obesity in the general population (Croft et al., 1995).

There are now six loci that appear to be associated with BBS, all on different chromosomes. BBS6 has only recently been identified (Katsanis et al., 2001). Two BBS genes have been cloned, *BBS2*, which encodes a protein of unknown function (Nishimura et al., 2001), and BBS6, which encodes a chaperonin (Stone et al., 2000).

Two of these entries (OMIM 164160 and 600955) result from the first single-gene mutations ever reported in humans to be responsible for obesity. Montague et al. (1997) described two cases of severe obesity in children from a highly consanguineous pedigree. The two affected children, a boy 2 years of age with 54% body fat and his female 8-year-old cousin with 57% body fat, exhibited rapid development of obesity after birth, with hyperphagia and barely detectable serum leptin levels. Both children were homozygous for a frameshift mutation in the leptin gene leading to the introduction of 14 aberrant amino acids followed by a stop codon. A second consanguineous family with three leptin-deficient individuals has been reported (Strobel et al., 1998). In addition to hypogonadism and low leptin, this group reported reduced activity of the sympathetic nervous system using a cold pressor test, an orthostatic hypotension test, and absence of sympathetic skin responses with median nerve and auditory stimulation (Table 23–6).

Jackson et al. (1997) studied a 43-year-old woman, previously described by O'Rahilly et al. (1995), who exhibited high plasma levels of proinsulin, very low insulin levels, and a history of severe childhood obesity (body weight 36 kg at 3 years of age) but who was treated successfully with a diet. The clinical features of the patient were compatible with impaired prohormone processing and with the phenotype observed in the *fat* mouse, which is caused by a mutation in the carboxypeptidase E (*CPE*) gene (Naggert et al., 1995). Jackson et al. (1997) showed that the woman was a compound heterozygote for two mutations in the gene coding for prohormone convertase 1 (*PCSK1*). One mutation was a Gly^{483}Arg amino acid substitution leading to retention of the enzyme in the endoplasmic reticulum. The other was an A-to-C transversion in the donor splice site of intron 5, resulting in the loss of exon 5 and leading ultimately to a premature stop codon within the catalytic domain of the enzyme. Also, a splice mutation producing a skipping of exon 18, result-

Table 23–6. Cases of Human Obesity Caused by Single-Gene Mutations[a]

Gene	Mutation	Location	Case No.	Sex	Age	Weight (kg)	BMI (kg/m²)
PCSK1	Gly483Arg A → C+4 intron 5	5q15–q21	2	F	3	36	NA
LEP	Guanine deletion at codon 133,	7q31	3	F	8	86	45.8
			4	M	2	29	36.6
	C → T codon 105, exon 3		5	F	6		32.5
			6	M	22		55.8
			7	F	34		46.9
LEPR	G → A exon 16	1p31	8	F	19		65.5
			9	F	13		71.5
			10	F	19		52.5
POMC	G7013T and C deletion at nt 7133 exon 3,	2p23	11	F	3	30	NA
	C3804A exon 2		12	M	7	50	NA
PPARG	Pro115Gln	3p25	13	M	65		47.3
			14	F	32		38.5
			15	M	54		43.8
			16	M	74		37.9
MC4R	CTCT deletion at codon 211	18q21.3	17	M	4	32	28
			18	M	30	139	41
	GATT insertion at nt 732		19	F	78		37
			20	M[b]	73		35
			21	F	50		
			22	F	35		57
			23	F	34		50
			24	M	24		35
			25	F			33

[a]*LEP*, leptin; *LEPR*, leptin receptor; *MC4R*, melanocortin 4 receptor; *PCSK1*, protein convertase subtilisin/kexin type 1; *POMC*, proopiomelanocortin; *PPARG*, peroxisome proliferator–activated receptor γ; NA, not available; BMI, body mass index.
[b]Deceased individual not genotyped.
Adapted from Chagnon et al. (2000) and Perusse et al. (2001b).

ing in a truncated leptin receptor (LEPR) lacking both the transmembrane and the intracellular portions of the *LEPR* gene, has been reported in three sisters of a consanguineous family of Kabilian origin (Clement et al., 1998).

A rare syndrome with early onset of severe obesity, adrenal insufficiency, and reddish hair pigmentation resulting from two different mutations in exon 3 of proopiomelanocortin (POMC) was reported by Krude et al. (1998). A compound mutation was reported in one patient with the defect in exon 3 as well as a homozygous mutation in exon 2 within the untranslated 5′ end that would be expected to abolish translation of the wild-type POMC. The presence of severe early-onset obesity, low corticotropin, and red hair are consistent with predictions of the genetic defects.

In addition to these rare genetic forms of obesity is a more common form associated with a defect in the phosphorylation site of the peroxisome proliferator–activated receptor $\gamma 2$ (*PPAR*γ*2*). Among 121 unrelated obese individuals, defined as a BMI >29 kg/m^2, Ristow et al. (1998) identified four with a glutamine replacement for proline at position 115 (Pro^{115}Gln) of the PPARG2 molecule. In the control group of 237, there were no similar changes. The BMI of the affected individuals ranged from 37.9 to 47.3 kg/m^2 and was higher than the mean BMI of 33.6 kg/m^2 in the other 117 obese subjects. When the defective gene was transfected into fibroblasts, the phosphorylation at serine 114 was defective and the conversion of these fibroblasts to adipocytes was accelerated. It may well turn out to be a major defect in many massively overweight individuals.

Several carriers of mutations in the melanocortin-4 receptor (*MC4R*) gene have been reported (Chagnon et al., 2000; Perusse et al., 2001a). A German group reported on a total of 19 carriers of either a 4 bp deletion at codon 211 or a nonsense mutation at codon 35 (Hinney et al., 1999; Sina et al., 1999). However, the level of obesity was quite varied among carriers, suggesting variable penetrance. In a population of 209 severely obese (BMI >40 kg/m^2) French subjects, Vaisse et al. (2000) reported eight carriers of eight different mutations in the *MC4R* gene not found in 366 normal weight controls. Several of the mutations appeared to have a functional impact.

Single-Gene Rodent Models

Spontaneous mutations in five different genes have been found to be responsible for obesity in mouse models of obesity. These mutations are the *obese (ob)* mutation on mouse chromosome 6, the *diabetes (db)* mutation on mouse chromosome 4, the *agouti yellow* (A^y) mutation on mouse chromosome 2, the *fat* mutation on mouse chromosome 8, and the *tubby* mutation on mouse chromosome 7. Each of these genes has been cloned and its gene products identified (Perusse et al., 2001a). These mutations, their corresponding chromosomal regions in the human genome, and their gene products are shown in Table 23–7. Several studies

Table 23–7. Single-Gene Mutations in Mouse Models of Obesity and Their Role in Human Obesity

Mutation	Human Chromosome	Gene	Gene Product
Obese (*ob*)	7q31.1	*LEP*	Leptin
Diabetes (*db*)	1p31	*LEPR*	Leptin receptor
Agouti yellow (A^y)	20q11.2	*ASIP*	Agouti signaling protein
Fat (*fa*)	4q32	*CPE*	Carboxypeptidase E
Tubby (*tub*)	11p15.5	*TUB*	Insulin signaling protein

have investigated the role of these candidate genes in human obesity by linkage or association with markers targeted to cover the region of these genes. The results of these studies are also summarized in the last two columns of Table 23–7.

The Leptin (LEP) *and Leptin Receptor* (LEPR) *Genes*

The *obese* and *diabetes* mice are characterized by severe early-onset obesity. The genes responsible for obesity in these animals were found to encode a hormone secreted by the adipose tissue (leptin) and its receptor in the brain (leptin receptor). These genes (*LEP* and *LEPR*) are located on human chromosomes 7q31.3 and 1p31, respectively. Several studies have tested the linkage relationships between obesity and genetic markers flanking the *LEP* gene in humans with both positive and negative findings (Chagnon et al., 1998; Perusse et al., 1997, 2001a). Significant evidence of linkage with BMI, subcutaneous fat, and body-fat mass has been reported (Clement et al., 1996a; Reed et al., 1996; Duggirala et al., 1996). Despite numerous attempts to find association between specific mutations in the *LEP* gene and human obesity (Considine et al., 1995; Maffei et al., 1996; Niki et al., 1996; Carlsson et al., 1997), only two reports have shown human obesity to be due to a mutation in the *LEP* gene (Montague et al., 1997; Strobel et al., 1998). Other rare mutations in the *LEP* gene have been identified, but none was associated with obesity (Considine et al., 1995; Oksanen et al., 1997; Echwald et al., 1997a).

Several mutations in different exons and introns of the *LEPR* gene have been uncovered (Considine et al., 1996; Chung et al., 1996, 1997; Thompson et al., 1997; Gotoda et al., 1997; Echwald et al., 1997b; Francke et al., 1997; Matsuoka et al., 1997; Rolland et al., 1998), but only a few exhibited significant evidence of association with obesity (Perusse et al., 2001a). In a study based on 10 obese and 10 control subjects from the Pima Indian population, associations between percent body fat and three different mutations in the *LEPR* gene were observed (Thompson et al., 1997). A weak association with BMI was also observed in a British male population for another mutation ($Lys^{656}Asn$) but only in lean (BMI <28 kg/m^2) subjects (Gotoda et al., 1997). Three sisters with an early-onset severe form of obesity were homozygous for a splice mutation resulting in loss of exon 16 of *LEPR* (Clement et al., 1998). These results indicate a possible role of *LEPR* in the control of adiposity in humans, but the evidence is still weak. One study performed on 217 Pima Indian families provided no evidence of linkage between BMI or body fat and three markers surrounding the *LEPR* gene (Norman et al., 1996).

The Agouti Signaling Protein

The *agouti* gene is normally expressed in the skin of neonatal mice, where it controls the production of melanin pigments resulting in the wild-type coat color of mice. Mice carrying the dominant *agouti yellow* (A^y) mutation exhibit a complex syndrome that includes yellow fur, maturity-onset obesity, insulin resistance, hyperinsulinemia, and increased susceptibility to neoplasia (Miltenberger et al., 1997). The agouti protein antagonizes the binding of the α-melanocyte-stimulating hormone to the melanocortin receptors in hair follicles. Expression of the protein is normally restricted to the hair follicles, but the A^y mutation induces ectopic expression of the protein. The human equivalent of the mouse *agouti* gene is known as the agouti signaling protein (*ASIP*) and is located on chromosome 20q11–q12. No mutation in the *ASIP* gene has been found. Linkage between obesity phenotypes and markers flanking *ASIP* was tested in 45 obese families, and no significant evidence of linkage could be found (Xu et al., 1995). In contrast, weak evidence of linkage was observed in the Quebec Family Study (Lembertas et al., 1997) and other studies as well (Norman et al., 1998; Lee et al., 1999).

The Fat (Fat) *Gene*

The *Fat* mouse is characterized by early-onset (about 4 weeks) hyperproinsulinemia followed by obesity, apparent between 6 and 8 weeks of age (Chua, 1997). A mutation in the *CPE* gene, which codes for an enzyme involved in the processing of prohormones, is thought to be at the origin of the obesity phenotype in these mice. No evidence of linkage was reported between markers surrounding *CPE* at 4q32 and percent body fat in Pima Indians (Norman et al., 1996).

The Tubby (Tub) *Gene*

The *Tubby* mutation, like the *Fat* mutation, produces a late-onset and moderate form of obesity. The *Tub* gene appears to encode a protein involved in intracellular signaling by insulin (Kapeller et al., 1999). No mutation in the human equivalent of the gene has been reported. Negative linkage results have been observed in Pima Indians between five markers located in the corresponding human chromosomal region at 11p15.1, BMI, and percent body fat (Norman et al., 1996); but significant linkages with markers in the same area were observed in two studies (Hani et al., 1997; Clement et al., 1999).

In summary, most of the human linkage and association studies between obesity and the cloned genes from the mouse models have provided negative results. These results are not really surprising considering that genes with such a great impact on the phenotype are not expected to be responsible for a large number of obesity cases in humans. However, these candidate genes have provided new insights into the physiopathology of obesity. For instance, cloning of the *LEP* and *LEPR* genes has made it possible to describe another endocrine function of the adipocyte and has led to the identification of a new pathway in the regulation of food intake and energy expenditure.

QTL from Rodent Breeding Studies

Positional candidate genes of obesity can be identified from genomic scans with a set of evenly spaced genetic markers covering the entire genome of humans or rodents. The QTL correspond to regions of the genome containing markers showing significant evidence of linkage with the obesity phenotype. Synteny between the rodent and human genomes can be used to localize the human chromosomal region corresponding to the obesity QTL. The human chromosomal region defined in this manner can be further delineated by testing for linkage with a denser set of markers spanning the region. Candidate genes can then potentially be identified from maps of genes and sequenced transcripts (Schuler et al., 1996) and their putative functions anticipated based on sequence structure or homology with known genes. According to the latest version of the human obesity gene map, 115 QTL related to body weight or body fat have been identified from mouse and rat crosses (Perusse et al., 2001a). These QTL appear to identify about 30 unique sequences in the human genome (Chagnon et al., 1998). Only two studies have reported evidence of linkage between obesity and the human chromosomal regions syntenic to two of these QTL (Xu et al., 1995; Chagnon et al., 1997c).

QTL from Human Genomic Scans

The results from nine genome-wide scans for human obesity QTL have been reported to date. In Pima Indians, 660 markers were typed in 874 individuals, and linkages were observed with percent body fat and markers located at 11q21–q22 and 3p24.2–p22; however, no genes could be proposed as good candidates for these linkages (Norman et al., 1997). In a more recent report based on the same population, LOD scores of 2 and more were found at 11q21–q22 for percent body fat (LOD = 2.1), 11q23–q24 (LOD = 2.0) for 24-hour energy expenditure, and 18q21 (LOD = 2.3) for percent body fat (Norman et al., 1998). In another study, 169 markers were typed in 458 Mexican Americans and strong linkages with plasma leptin level and fat mass were observed on chromosome 2p21 (Comuzzie et al., 1997). The glucokinase regulatory protein and *POMC* genes have been suggested as candidates for these linkage relationships. In addition, a LOD score of 2.2 was obtained between a marker on 8p12 and fat mass in the same scan.

In the Paris-Lille Study, strong linkage (LOD = 4.9) was observed between markers on 10p12, with weaker ones on 5p11 (LOD = 2.9) and 2p21 (LOD = 2.4), and plasma leptin levels (Hager et al., 1998). Significant linkages were found on 20q13 (LOD = 1.5–3.2) in the University of Pennsylvania Family Study (Lee et al., 1999). In the Quebec Family Study, linkages were reported with fat-free mass for markers on 7p15.3 (LOD = 2.7), 15q25 (LOD = 3.6), and 18q12 (LOD = 3.6) (Chagnon et al., 2000). In the same study, several linkages were found with abdominal fat adjusted for total body fat with markers on 1p11, 4p15, 7q31, 9q22, 12q24, and 17q21 (Perusse et al., 2001b).

In the Finnish Family Study, linkages with obesity (BMI of 30 and above) were observed with markers on 18q21 (LOD = 2.4) and Xq24 (LOD = 3.5) (Ohman et al., 2000). Two regions were significantly linked with obesity phenotypes in the Take-Off Pounds Sensibly TOPS Family Study, one on 3q27 (LOD from 2.4 to 3.3) and the second on 17p12 (LOD = 5.0) (Kissebah et al., 2000). Several weak linkages were reported from a genomic scan performed on subjects from Caucasian families in the HERITAGE Family Study (Chagnon et al., 2001). These linkages were with markers on 8q23, 9q34, 10p15, 12p12, 14q11, and 19p13 and characterized by LOD scores of about 2. Finally, two linkages with LOD scores of 2 and above were found in the Old Order Amish Study, one on 10p12 with plasma leptin adjusted for BMI and the second on 14q for the same phenotype (Hsueh et al., 2001).

Linkage and Association with Candidate Genes

Candidate genes can also be defined on the basis of their roles in relevant biochemical and physiologic functions. One can conceive that a whole series of such candidate genes may be the target of study. For instance, there are likely to be candidate genes for body mass, body fat distribution, level of AVF, appetite and satiety signals, resting metabolic rate, diet-induced thermogenesis, physical activity level, nutrient partitioning, comorbidities of obesity, and others. Selected results of association and linkage studies conducted with candidate genes are reviewed here, and a listing of the positive findings is given in Table 23–8. A more detailed review can be found in Perusse et al. (2001a).

Lipoprotein lipase (LPL) is an enzyme involved in the hydrolysis of triglyceride-rich lipoproteins. LPL plays an important role in the regulation of plasma lipoprotein composition and concentrations and in the partitioning of exogenous triglycerides between the adipose tissue for storage and the skeletal muscle for oxidation. The activity of the adipose tissue LPL is increased in obese subjects. Despite evidence of association between polymorphisms in the LPL gene and levels of lipids and lipoproteins (Mattu et al., 1994; Gerdes et al., 1995; Georges et al., 1996), few studies have reported associations with obesity. In one study, a HindII restriction fragment length polymorphism (RFLP) of the *LPL* gene was related to a lower BMI (Jemaa et al., 1995). There is also evidence that the relationship between AVF and plasma triglyceride levels is modulated by genetic variation at the *LPL* gene (Vohl et al., 1995).

Besides their role as lipid-storage organs, adipocytes produce various factors that might serve as feedback signals to regulate fat cell size and adipose tissue metabolism (Fried and Russell, 1998). Among these factors are cytokines, such as tumor necrosis factor-α (TNF-α), the expression of which is increased with obesity in rodents and in humans. A study conducted on Pima Indians suggested a linkage between body fat and a marker near the TNF-α gene as well as significant evidence of association with BMI (Norman et al., 1995). A polymorphism in the promoter region of the TNFA gene was associated with increased percent body fat and serum leptin levels and decreased insulin sensitivity (Fernandez-Real et al., 1997).

Insulin resistance and hyperinsulinemia are commonly observed in obese individuals. Genes involved in insulin secretion and metabolism could be considered as strong candidate genes not only for Type 2 diabetes but also for obesity. Only one association has been reported so far (Weaver et al., 1992) between a polymorphism in the 5′ flanking region of the insulin gene (*INS*) and central obesity, assessed by the waist-to-hip ratio (p = 0.005) and fasting insulin (p = 0.012). Despite evidence that mutations in the insulin receptor gene (*INSR*) could be responsible for some rare insulin-related syndromes (Kahn et al., 1996), only one study reported that a mutation in intron 9 of *INSR* was associated with obesity (BMI >26) and only in hypertensive subjects (Zee et al., 1994). IGFs mediate the action of growth hormone under the control of insulin and, therefore, play a role in body mass development throughout the life span. In the spontaneous diabetic Goto-Kakizaki (GK) rat strain, a locus for impaired glucose tolerance and adiposity was identified near the *IGF2* gene (Gauguier et al., 1996). A polymorphism in the 3′-untranslated region of the *IGF2* gene was associated with BMI in 1474 middle-aged men (O'Dell et al., 1997). Insulin receptor substrate-1 (IRS-1) is the main substrate for the insulin and IGF-I receptors. A Gly^{972}Arg mutation in IRS-1 has shown significant interaction with obesity, which was associated with a 50% reduction in insulin sensitivity (Clausen et al., 1995). Moreover, the Gly^{972}Arg mutation may predispose to Type 2 diabetes in the presence of excess body weight (Sigal et al., 1996).

Unlike the agouti protein in the mouse, which is normally expressed only in the skin, human agouti is expressed, among

Table 23–8. Candidate Genes That Have Shown Evidence for the Presence of Association (A) or Linkage (L) with Body Mass Index (BMI) or Body Fat Phenotypes

Gene[a]	Location	Analysis	Phenotype	p value
LEPR	1p31	A	% Fat	0.003
ATP1A2	1q21–q23	A	% Fat	0.05
ACP1	2p25	A	BMI	0.02–0.002
		L	BMI	0.004
POMC	2p21	L[b]	Leptin, fat	LOD = 2.8–4.5
APOB	2p24–p23	A	BMI, % fat	0.05–0.005
APOD	3q27–qter	A	BMI	0.006
FABP2	4q28–q31	A	BMI, fat, % fat	0.01–0.008
GRL	5q31–q32	A	Fat	0.007–0.003
		L	BMI	0.009
TNFa	6p21.3	A	BMI, % fat	0.02–0.01
		L[b]	% Fat	0.05–0.002
LEP	7q31.3	A	Weight	0.05–0.006
		L[b]	BMI, fat, skinfolds	
LPL	8p22	A	BMI	0.05
ADRB3	8p12–p11.2	A	BMI, fat, weight	0.05–0.002
IGF2	11p15.5	A	BMI	0.02
SUR	11p15.1	A	Obesity	0.02
		L[b]	BMI	0.003
DRD2	11q22.2–q22.3	A	Weight	0.002
MC5R	18p11.2	A	BMI	0.003
		L	BMI, fat, % fat, skinfolds	0.02–0.001
MC4R	18q21.3	A	fat, % fat	0.002–0.004
INSR	19p13.3	A	Obesity	0.05
LDLR	19p13.2	A	BMI, obesity	0.02–0.004
ADA	20q12–q13.11	L	BMI, fat, % fat, skinfolds	0.04–0.001
MC3R	20q12–q13.11	L	BMI, fat, % fat, skinfolds	0.04–0.001

[a]*ACP1*, acid phosphatase; *ADA*, adenosine deaminase; *ADRB3*, β_3-adrenergic receptor; *APOB*, *APOD*, *APOA4*, apolipoproteins B, D, and A4; *ATP1A2*, sodium potassium adenosine triphosphatase α_2-subunit; *DRD2*, dopamine D_2 receptor; *FABP2*, fatty acid binding protein 2; *GRL*, glucocorticoid receptor; *HSD3B1*, 3β-hydroxysteroid dehydrogenase; *IGF2*, insulin-like growth factor II; *INSR*, insulin receptor; *LDLR*, low-density lipoprotein receptors; *LEP*, leptin; *LEPR*, leptin receptor; *LPL*, lipoprotein lipase; *MC3R*, *MC4R*, *MC5R*, melanocortin receptors 3–5; *POMC*, pro-opiomelanocortin; *SUR*, sulfonylurea receptor; *TNFa*, tumor necrosis factor α; *UCP1*, uncoupling protein 1.
[b]Linkages obtained using markers outside the gene.
Adapted from Chagnon et al. (1998).

other tissues, in the adipocytes (Wilson et al., 1996). The lack of known polymorphism in the *agouti* gene has precluded any association or linkage studies with this specific gene. However, because of the potential role of the melanocortin receptors in the expression of the agouti protein in the yellow mouse and the evidence that a knockout of the *MC4R* gene in mice reproduces the Agouti obesity phenotype (Huszar et al., 1997), melanocortin receptors were considered good candidate genes of obesity. Polymorphisms in the melanocortin receptor genes (*MC3R*, *MC4R*, and *MC5R*) were tested for linkage with obesity phenotypes in the Quebec Family Study. Evidence of linkage was observed between adiposity variables and *MC3R* (Lembertas et al., 1997) as well as between *MC5R* and BMI (p = 0.001), fat mass (p = 0.001), and resting metabolic rate (p = 0.002) (Chagnon et al., 1997a). Associations were observed for both *MC4R* and *MC5R* with adiposity but only in women (Chagnon et al., 1997a).

The fatty acid binding proteins (FABPs) are important regulators of the flux of free-fatty acids between the different compartments of the cell. The *FABP2* gene codes for the intestinal form of the protein, which is involved in the intracellular transport of long-chain fatty acids. An Ala^{54}Thr substitution in the *FABP2* gene has been associated with increased binding affinity and intracellular transport of fatty acids, lipid oxidation, and insulin resistance (Baier et al., 1996). The Ala^{54}Thr polymorphism has been associated with BMI and percent body fat (Hegele et al., 1996) as well as with abdominal fat (Yamada et al., 1997), while no evidence of association with obesity or insulin metabolism was observed in another study (Sipilainen et al., 1997).

Adrenergic receptors play an important role in the mobilization of lipids stored in the adipocytes through the regulation of catecholamine-induced lipolysis. Genetic variation in the α_2-, β_2-, and β_3-adrenergic receptors has been investigated for its role in obesity. The most studied polymorphism of the adrenergic receptors is a tryptophan-to-arginine mutation in codon 64 (Trp^{64}Arg) of the β_3-adrenergic receptor (*ADRB3*), which was associated with increased susceptibility to weight gain in a French group of massively obese subjects (Clement et al., 1995) and with a higher waist-to-hip circumference ratio and early onset of Type 2 diabetes in Finnish women (Widen et al., 1995). Following these reports, the *ADRB3* Trp^{64}Arg mutation was extensively studied in many different populations with respect to obesity, Type 2 diabetes, and hypertension. Negative results were reported in 21 of 28 studies with BMI, in 9 of 13 studies with waist-to-hip circumference ratio, and in 18 of 25 studies using other obesity phenotypes. Positive results, when found, were generally borderline (Mauriege and Bouchard, 1996; Chagnon et al., 1997b). This body of data suggests a marginal effect of the *ADRB3* Trp^{64}Arg mutation on obesity and its comorbidities. An additive effect of a *UCP1* mutation (Oppert et al., 1994) and the Trp^{64}Arg mutation in *ADRB3* has been reported in morbid obesity (Clement et al., 1996c). A study of 45 Mexican-American sib pairs concordant for a QTL on chromosome 2 previously shown to be linked to obesity in this population

(Comuzzie et al., 1997) but discordant for the *ADRB3* $Trp^{64}Arg$ mutation (i.e., the mutation present in one sibling but not in the other) revealed significant association of the variant with BMI and fat mass (Mitchell et al., 1998).

Polymorphisms of the α_2- and β_2-adrenergic receptor genes were tested for association with indicators of body fat and fat distribution in the Quebec Family Study with negative results, except for an association in women between a polymorphism in the α_2-adrenergic receptor and the tendency to accumulate more fat in the truncal-abdominal area compared to the limb (Oppert et al., 1995). Two polymorphisms in codons 16 ($Gly^{16}Arg$) and 27 ($Glu^{27}Gln$) of the β_2-adrenergic receptor gene were tested for association with obesity in 140 Swedish women exhibiting a large variation in body fat mass. The $Gln^{27}Glu$ polymorphism was markedly associated with obesity defined as a BMI value >27 kg/m^2 (Large et al., 1997). The fat mass of women homozygous for the mutation ($n = 22$) was on average 20 kg higher than those without the mutation ($n = 49$).

Adenosine deaminase (ADA) is an α-adrenergic agonist that regulates lipolysis and insulin sensitivity in human adipose tissue (Ohisalo et al., 1984; Kern et al., 1988). In an exploratory study of linkage with obesity phenotypes in the Quebec Family Study, significant evidence of linkage between ADA and BMI, as well as with subcutaneous fat, was observed (Borecki et al., 1994). This result was confirmed in a linkage study with markers on human chromosome 20 syntenic to the mouse multigenic obesity 5 (*Mob-5*) QTL (Lembertas et al., 1997).

One of the most consistent associations with obesity is with the apolipoprotein B gene (*APOB*), for which associations between a set of polymorphisms and BMI (Rajput-Williams et al., 1988) and total body fat and AVF (Pouliot et al., 1994a) have been reported. A weak association was also reported between a polymorphism in the gene coding for Apo D, a minor constituent of HDLs, and obesity (Vijayaraghavan et al., 1994). The LDL receptor (LDLR) is involved in serum cholesterol regulation. Two polymorphisms, located, respectively, in exons 12 and 18 of the *LDLR* gene, have shown association with obesity in hypertensive cases (Zee et al., 1992, 1995), while another microsatellite marker in exon 18 of the gene was associated with obesity in normotensive subjects (Griffiths et al., 1995).

Only a few studies have considered association and linkage relationships with fat distribution phenotypes. Glucocorticoids promote visceral fat accumulation (Pedersen et al., 1994), and omental fat cells have a higher glucocorticoid-binding capacity than do subcutaneous fat cells (Rebuffe-Scrive et al., 1985, 1990). A linkage between obesity (BMI >27) and a BclI RFLP at the glucocorticoid receptor gene (*GRL*) locus has been reported (Clement et al., 1996b), whereas an association has been observed with AVF level, particularly in normal-weight people (Buemann et al., 1997).

Uncoupling proteins are membrane mitochondrial proton transporters whose function is to "uncouple" mitochondrial respiration from the production of ATP, thereby consuming energy and generating heat, although this function is not fully established for UCP2 and UCP3. UCP1 is expressed exclusively in brown adipose tissue, while UCP2 has a wider range of tissular expression, including white adipose and skeletal muscle (Fleury et al., 1997; Gimeno et al., 1997). In a longitudinal study based on a 12-year follow-up period, Oppert et al. (1994) found that carriers of a BclI RFLP variant in the *UCP1* gene were more frequent among high fat gainers compared to low fat gainers. A strong linkage between markers encompassing the chromosomal region of the *UCP2* gene on chromosome 11q23 and resting metabolic rate was uncovered in the Quebec Family Study (Bouchard et al., 1997). A new uncoupling protein, UCP3, has been cloned and shown to be expressed only in skeletal muscle (Liu et al., 1998).

A GAIVS6 *UCP3* polymorphism was associated with adiposity (Lanouette et al., 2001). This was interpreted as supporting the hypothesis of a role of *UCP3* in fatty acid transport and metabolism. No other sequence variant in the *UCP3* gene was consistently associated with obesity phenotypes.

In summary, about 50 candidate genes and genomic positions have been associated or linked with human obesity phenotypes (Perusse et al., 2001a), only a few genes showing positive results in at least five studies. Several mutations have been identified and shown to be responsible for a handful of cases of human obesity. However, most obese individuals have developed this condition as a result of a genetic predisposition thought to arise from mutations at multiple genes. The field is, therefore, still at an embryonic stage when it comes to identifying the genes and mutations involved in the common forms of obesity. In addition, the complex task of defining gene–environment and gene–gene interactions at the molecular level has not even begun.

CLINICAL APPLICATION AND RISK ASSESSMENT OF GENETIC INFORMATION

Progress has been made in recent years concerning the diagnosis question as professional groups and national and international agencies have come closer together on the key features of body mass, body composition, and fat distribution that must be considered when it comes to the identification of obese and overweight patients at risk. However, these advances have not yet translated into the development of useful molecular tools. The advances of the last decade on the genetic and molecular basis of obesity and its comorbidities raised hope that innovative and preventive measures and new therapeutic approaches would soon become available. Unfortunately, these expectations have not materialized, and the difficulties to be overcome may have been underestimated.

Diagnosis

At the phenotypic level, diagnosis can be a simple matter for most patients. Using the classification scheme adopted by the World Health Organization (1998) and the National Heart, Lung and Blood Institute (1998), overweight in adults is defined as a BMI in the range from 25 to 29.9, while obesity is indicated at the BMI cut-off value of 30 (Table 23–2). Three classes of obesity are recognized: class I with a BMI from 30 to 34.9, class II from 35 to 39.9, and class III from 40 and higher (Table 23–3).

At the genetic level, little is known. Few of the 30 or so Mendelian diseases listed in OMIM that exhibit obesity as one of their clinical manifestations can be diagnosed at the molecular level. Mutations in a few candidate genes have been found to be the cause of an excessive level of fatness in a handful of patients (Table 23–6). Given the apparently extreme rarity of these genetic deficiencies, the diagnosis of these genetic obesity cases is not likely to become widespread in the near future. Further advances concerning the genes and mutations responsible for the predisposition to the most common forms of obesity are necessary before molecular diagnosis of the affected individual and perhaps of his or her family members, especially the youngest ones, becomes part of the typical diagnostic battery.

As with the comorbidities of obesity, there are differences in the susceptibility to hypertension, glucose intolerance, insulin resistance, and dyslipoproteinemia, to name but a few, in the presence of a persisting overweight or obese state. Thus far, several markers at key candidate genes, such as APOB, *LDLR*, *LPL*, *PPARγ2*, and other genes, have been associated with one or more comorbidities but only when people were heavier or fatter (Bouchard et al., 1998). The hope is that it will eventually be possible to identify at the molecular level those who are more at risk of developing these comorbidities if they become overweight or obese.

Screening

Since little can be done for the moment at the molecular level, screening individuals at risk must rely primarily on family history and age at onset of early signs of the disease. The risk of becoming obese and remaining obese is significantly increased in families in which one of the parents is obese and even more when both parents are affected. The worst-case scenario is observed when a child deviates strongly early on from the height and weight growth charts and exhibits early-onset obesity and parental obesity is also present. The risk for these children becoming obese adults is extremely high (Whitaker et al., 1997). Screening for these high-risk cases can be done in schools.

However, adult-onset obesity is a fast-growing segment of the affected population. One should remember that the maximal prevalence of obesity is reached around age 60 years. Effective screening of adult obesity cases must rely on public, private, and voluntary health settings, work sites, and physician's offices.

Prevention

Little has been done so far regarding prevention of obesity based on initial genetic risks. This is, however, a course of action that makes enormous sense, particularly in light of the limited success that is commonly achieved in the treatment of obesity. In the interim, for lack of strong molecular markers of risk, initiatives based on family-based screening programs would be very appropriate. Despite their merit, few examples of such programs can be found in the school and workplace environments or in health-care settings.

Counseling

Genetic counseling is of limited value at this time because so little is known about the genes and mutations predisposing individuals to obesity. Exceptions to this general rule include counseling opportunities if a parent has one of the rare mutations in the *LEP*, *LEPR*, *prohormone convertase 1*, or *POMC* gene (Montague et al., 1997; Jackson et al., 1997; Clement et al., 1998; Krude et al., 1998) or in *PPARG2* (Ristow et al., 1998) resulting in obesity. However, these cases are extremely rare and some of these patients do not undergo adequate sexual maturation. Genetic counseling to help future parents reach decisions with respect to the risk of having an obese child is therefore not truly useful at the moment. It may play a greater role when the genetic and molecular basis of the disease and its co-morbidities is better known.

Therapy

Several strategies can be used to treat overweight patients who meet the criteria for treatment. The discussion of these treatments has leaned heavily on two recent National Heart, Lung and Blood Institute reports (1998, 2000).

Behavior Therapy

Behavioral strategies to reinforce changes in diet and physical activity can produce a weight loss in obese adults in the range of 8% to 10% below baseline weight over 4 months to 1 year (Wing, 1998). Unless a patient acquires a new set of eating habits and physical activity skills, long-term maintenance of this weight reduction is unlikely to succeed. Most patients return to baseline weights in the absence of continued intervention. Thus, the physician or staff members must become familiar with techniques for modifying over the long term the life habits of overweight or obese patients.

The goal of behavior therapy is to alter the eating and activity habits of an obese patient. Techniques for behavior therapy have been developed to assist patients in modifying their life habits. The primary assumptions of behavior therapy are that by changing eating and physical activity habits it is possible to change body weight; that patterns of eating and physical activity are learned behaviors and can be modified; and that to change these patterns over the long term, the environment must be changed.

Behavior therapy, in combination with an energy deficit, provides additional benefits in assisting patients to lose weight over 1 year. Its effectiveness for long-term weight maintenance has not been shown in the absence of continued behavioral intervention (National Heart, Lung and Blood Institute, 1998). A recent report shows that the Internet can be used as a strategy for delivering behavioral therapy (Tate et al., 2001).

Changing eating and physical activity behaviors over the long term can be achieved either on an individual basis or in group settings. Group therapy has the advantage of lower cost. Following are some specific behavioral strategies as outlined in the National Heart, Lung and Blood Institute report (1998):

1. Self-monitor both eating habits and physical activity
2. Develop techniques to manage stressful situations
3. Control or modify stimuli that enhance eating
4. Learn techniques for problem solving in food-related situations
5. Develop cognitive strategies that restructure learning about food
6. Develop social support for weight loss progress and goals

Dietary Therapy

The majority of overweight and obese patients need to adjust their diet to reduce caloric intake and/or the percent of fat. Dietary therapy consists, in large part, of instructing patients on how to modify their diets to achieve a decrease in caloric as well as fat intake. A moderate reduction in caloric intake will produce slow but progressive weight loss. Ideally, caloric intake should be reduced by 500 kcal/day below the level required to maintain weight at the desired level (National Heart, Lung and Blood Institute, 1998). Alternatively, a patient may choose a diet of 1000 to 1200 kcal/day for women and 1200 to 1500 kcal/day for men. Very low-calorie diets with less than 800 kcal/day are not recommended for weight loss therapy because the deficits are too great and nutritional inadequacies will occur unless supplements of vitamins and minerals are taken. Moreover, clinical trials show that low-calorie diets are just as effective as very low-calorie diets in producing weight loss after 1 year. Although more weight is initially lost with very low-calorie diets, more is usually regained.

Following are some of the keys to successful modification of diet:

- Learn the energy value of different foods
- Know about food composition: fats, carbohydrates (including dietary fiber), and proteins
- Read nutrition labels to determine caloric content and food composition
- Develop new habits of purchasing, with a preference for low-calorie foods
- Avoid adding high-calorie ingredients during cooking (e.g., fats and oils)
- Avoid overconsumption of high-calorie foods (both high-fat and high-carbohydrate foods)
- Maintain adequate water intake
- Reduce portion sizes
- Limit alcohol consumption

Structured meal plans (Wing et al., 1996) or portion-controlled meals (Flechtner-Mors et al., 2000) can be valuable dietary tools to supplement behavioral therapy.

Physical Activity and Exercise

An increase in physical activity is an important strategy to help lose weight, to maintain weight loss, or to prevent weight gain with age (Bouchard and Blair, 1999). Physical activity increases energy expenditure and may inhibit food intake in overweight patients. Sustained levels of physical activity may also reduce overall cardiovascular risk (National Heart, Lung and Blood Institute, 1998). The effectiveness of programs to increase weight loss through increasing physical activity is disappointing, producing only an average 2% to 3% decrease in body weight as a result of only modest increases in physical activity in obese individuals (Ross and Janssen, 1999, 2001).

Many people live sedentary lives, have little training or skills in physical activity, and are difficult to motivate toward increasing their activity. Thus, starting a physical activity regimen may require supervision. The need to avoid injury during physical activity is high, particularly in obese subjects. The practitioner must decide whether exercise testing for cardiopulmonary disease is needed before embarking on a new physical activity regimen. This decision should be based on a patient's age, symptoms, and concomitant risk factors.

For most obese patients, physical activity should be initiated slowly and the intensity should be increased gradually. Table 23–9 provides a list of physical activities that can be performed to generate an energy expenditure of about 150 calories/day. Initial activities may be walking or swimming at a slow pace. With time, depending on progress, the amount of weight lost, and functional capacity, the patient may engage in more strenuous activities.

A regimen of daily walking is an attractive form of physical activity for most people, particularly those who are overweight or obese. The patient can start by walking for 10 minutes 3 days a week and build to 30 to 45 minutes of more intense walking at least 5 days a week. With this regimen, an additional 100 to 200 calories/day can be expended. Caloric expenditure will vary depending on the individual's body weight and intensity of the activity (Table 23–10). This regimen can be adapted to other forms of physical activity, but walking is particularly attractive because of its safety and accessibility. Some data suggest that making activity available at home may improve long-term adherence (Jakicic et al., 1999; Tate et al., 2001).

Table 23–9. Examples of Moderate Amounts of Activity[a]

Washing and waxing a car for 45–60 minutes	Less vigorous, more time[b] ↑
Washing windows or floors for 45–60 minutes	
Playing volleyball for 45 minutes	
Playing touch football for 30–45 minutes	
Gardening for 30–45 minutes	
Wheeling self in wheelchair for 30–40 minutes	
Walking 1.75 miles in 35 minutes (20 min/mile)	
Basketball (shooting baskets for 30 minutes)	
Bicycling 5 miles in 30 minutes	
Dancing fast (social) for 30 minutes	
Pushing a stroller 1.5 miles in 30 minutes	
Raking leaves for 30 minutes	↓ More vigorous, less time
Walking 2 miles in 30 minutes (15 min/mile)	
Water aerobics for 30 minutes	
Swimming laps for 20 minutes	
Wheelchair basketball for 20 minutes	
Basketball (playing a game) for 15–20 minutes	
Bicycling 4 miles in 15 minutes	
Jumping rope for 15 minutes	
Running 1.5 miles in 15 minutes (10 min/mile)	
Shoveling snow for 15 minutes	
Stair walking for 15 minutes	

[a]A moderate amount of physical activity is roughly equivalent to physical activity that uses approximately 150 calories of energy per day, or 1000 calories per week.
[b]Some activities can be performed at various intensities; the suggested durations correspond to expected intensity effort.

Pharmacotherapy

Weight-loss drugs can augment diet, physical activity, and behavior therapy in weight loss (Bray and Greenway, 1999). Because of the tendency to regain weight after weight loss, the use of long-term medication to aid in the treatment of obesity may be indicated.

The drugs currently approved as appetite suppressants work by increasing the secretion of dopamine, norepinephrine, or serotonin into the synaptic neural cleft, by inhibiting the reuptake of these neurotransmitters back into the neuron, or by both mechanisms. Sibutramine affects reuptake of both norepinephrine and

Table 23–10. Duration of Various Activities to Expend 150 kcal for an Average 70 kg (154 lb) Adult

Intensity	Activity	Approximate Duration in Minutes
Moderate	Volleyball, noncompetitve	43
Moderate	Walking, moderate pace (3 mph, 20 min/mile)	37
Moderate	Walking, brisk pace (4 mph, 15 min/mile)	32
Moderate	Table tennis	32
Moderate	Raking leaves	32
Moderate	Social dancing	29
Moderate	Lawn mowing (powered push mower)	29
Hard	Jogging (5 mph, 12 min/mile)	18
Hard	Field hockey	16
Very hard	Running (6 mph, 10 min/mile)	13

Source: Surgeon General's Report on Physical Activity and Health (1996).

Table 23–11. Drugs Approved by the Food and Drug Administration for Treatment of Obesity

Drug	Trade Name	Dosage	Drug Enforcement Agency Schedule	Cost per Day
Pancreatic lipase inhibitor approved for long-term use				
Orlistat	Xenical	120 mg tid before meals	—	$ 3.56
Norepinephrine–serotonin reuptake inhibitor approved for long-term use				
Sibutramine	Meridia, Reductil	5–15 mg/d	IV	$ 2.98–$ 3.68
Noradrenergic drugs approved for short-term use				
Diethylpropion	Tenuate	25 mg tid	IV	$ 1.27–$ 1.52
	Tepanil			
	Tenuate	75 mg q AM		
	Dospan			
Phentermine	Adipex	15–37.5 mg/d	IV	$ 0.67–$ 1.60
	Fastin			
	Oby-Cap			
	Ionamin slow release	15–30 mg/d		$ 1.75–$ 2.01
Benzphetamine	Didrex	25–50 mg tid	III	$ 1.19–$ 2.38
Phendimetrazine	Bontril	17.5–70 mg tid	III	$ 1.20–$ 5.25
	Plegine			
	Prelu-2			
	X-Trozine	105 mg qd		

serotonin. Orlistat, which blocks pancreatic lipase and decreases fat digestion, works by a different mechanism of action than other approved drugs (Table 23–11).

Clinical trials with sibutramine (Bray et al., 1999; Apfelbaum et al., 1999; James et al., 2000) and with orlistat (Sjostrom et al., 1998; Davidson et al., 1999; Rossner, 2000; Hauptman et al., 2000) show clinically significant weight loss. Net weight loss attributable to these drugs generally has been in the range of 10% below baseline (5% below placebo), although some patients lose significantly more weight. It is not possible to predict how much weight an individual will lose. Most of the weight loss usually occurs in the first 6 months.

Sibutramine increases blood pressure and pulse (Bray and Greenway, 1999). People with a history of high blood pressure, coronary heart disease, congestive heart failure, arrhythmias, or stroke should not take sibutramine; and all patients taking the medication should have their blood pressure monitored on a regular basis. Use of sibutramine in intermittent courses may achieve the benefits and minimize the side effects (Wirth and Krause, 2001). The risk for using appetite-suppressant drugs during pregnancy is unknown. With orlistat, there is a possible decrease in the absorption of fat-soluble vitamins and overcoming this may require vitamin supplementation.

Weight-loss drugs approved by the Food and Drug Administration for long-term use may be beneficial as an adjunct to diet and physical activity for patients with a BMI of ≥30 with no concomitant obesity-related risk factors or diseases and for patients with a BMI of ≥27 with concomitant obesity-related risk factors or diseases.

Not every patient responds to drug therapy. Tests with weight-loss drugs have shown that initial responders tend to continue to respond, while initial nonresponders are less likely to respond even with an increase in dosage. If a patient does not lose 2 kg (4.4 lb) in the first 4 weeks after initiating therapy, the likelihood of long-term response is low. This finding may be used as a guide to treatment, either continuing medication in the responders or stopping it in the nonresponders. If weight lost in the initial 6 months of therapy is more than 5% below baseline and is maintained after the initial weight-loss phase, this should be considered a success and the drug may be continued. It is important to remember that the major role of medications should be to help patients stay on a diet and physical activity plan while losing weight. Medications do not cure obesity, and weight loss or weight maintenance is unlikely to be maintained if the drug is stopped. Use of the drug may be continued as long as it is effective and the adverse effects are manageable and not serious. Since obesity is a chronic disorder, the short-term use of drugs is not helpful. The health professional should include drugs only in the context of a long-term treatment strategy and should consider intermittent therapy (Wirth and Krause, 2001).

Surgery for Weight Loss

Surgery is one option for weight reduction for some patients with severe and resistant obesity. The aim of surgery is to modify the gastrointestinal tract to reduce net food intake. Most authorities agree that weight loss surgery should be reserved for patients with severe obesity (BMI >35), in whom efforts at other therapy have failed and who are suffering from the complications of obesity. However, as laparascopic surgery improves, these criteria may need to be reassessed.

Surgical procedures in current use [gastric restriction (vertical gastric banding) and gastric bypass (Roux-en Y)] can induce substantial weight loss and reduce weight-associated risk factors and comorbidities (Sjostrom et al., 1997, 1999). Compared to other interventions available, surgery has produced the longest period of sustained weight loss. Assessing both perioperative risk and long-term complications is important and requires assessing the risk/benefit ratio in each case. Patients whose BMI equals or exceeds 40 kg/m^2 are potential candidates for surgery if they strongly desire substantial weight loss because obesity severely impairs the quality of their lives. Patients with a BMI between 35 and 39.9 kg/m^2 may also be considered for surgery if they have high-risk comorbid conditions (cardiovascular, sleep apnea, uncontrolled Type 2 diabetes) or weight-induced physical problems interfering with performance of daily life activities.

Since surgical procedures result in some loss of absorptive function, the long-term consequences of potential nutrient deficiencies must be recognized and adequate monitoring must be performed, particularly with regard to vitamin B_{12}, folate, and iron. Some patients may develop other gastrointestinal symptoms such as "dumping syndrome" or gallstones. Occasionally, patients may have postoperative mood changes or their presurgical depression symptoms may not be improved by the weight loss achieved. Thus, surveillance should include monitoring of indices of inadequate nutrition and modification of any preoperative disorders.

REFERENCES

Acheson KJ, Ravussin E, Schoeller DA, Christin L, Bourquin L, Baertschi P, Danforth E Jr, Jequier E: Two-week stimulation or blockade of the sympathetic nervous system in man: influence on body weight, body composition, and twenty-four hour energy expenditure. Metabolism 1988; 37:91–98.

Adams TD, Hunt SC, Mason LA, Ramirez ME, Fisher AG, Williams RR: Familial aggregation of morbid obesity. Obes Res 1993; 1:261–270.

Allison DB, Faith MS, Nathan JS: Risch's lambda values for human obesity. Int J Obes 1996a; 20:990–999.

Allison DB, Fontaine KR, Manson JE, Stevens J, VanItallie TB: Annual deaths attributable to obesity in the United States. JAMA 1999; 282:1530–1538.

Allison DB, Kaprio J, Korkeila M, Koskenvuo M, Neale MC, Hayakawa K: The heritability of body mass index among an international sample of monozygotic twins reared apart. Int J Obes 1996b; 20:501–506.

Apfelbaum M, Vague P, Ziegler O, Hanotin C, Thomas F, Leutenegger E: Long-term maintenance of weight loss after a very-low-calorie diet: a randomized blinded trial of the efficacy and tolerability of sibutramine. Am J Med 1999; 106:179–184.

Ashley FW, Kannel WB: Relation of weight change to changes in atherogenic traits: the Framingham Study. J Chronic Dis 1974; 27:103–114.

Astrup A, Grunwald GK, Melanson EL, Saris WH, Hill JO: The role of low-fat diets in body weight control: a meta-analysis of ad libitum dietary intervention studies. Int J Obes Relat Metab Disord 2000; 24:1545–1552.

Baier LJ, Bogardus C, Sacchettini JC: A polymorphism in the human intestinal fatty acid binding protein alters fatty acid transport across Caco-2 cells. J Biol Chem 1996; 271:10892–10896.

Bandini L, Schoeller DA, Dietz WH: Energy expenditure in obese and nonobese adolescents. Pediatr Res 1990; 27:198–203.

Bjorntorp P: Body fat distribution, insulin resistance, and metabolic diseases. Nutrition 1997; 13:795–803.

Bogardus C, Lillioja S, Ravussin E, Abbott W, Zawadzki JK, Young A, Knowler WC, Jacobowitz R, Moll PP: Familial dependence of the resting metabolic rate. N Engl J Med 1986; 315:96–100.

Borecki I, Rice T, Perusse L, Bouchard C, Rao DC: Major gene influence on the propensity to store fat in trunk versus extremity depots: evidence from the Quebec Family Study. Obes Res 1995; 3:1–8.

Borecki IB, Bonney GE, Rice T, Bouchard C, Rao DC: Influence of genotype-dependent effects of covariates on the outcome of segregation analysis of the body mass index. Am J Hum Genet 1993; 53:676–687.

Borecki IB, Higgins M, Schreiner PJ, Arnett DK, Meyer-Davis E, Hunt SC, Province MA: Evidence for multiple determinants of the body mass index: the National Heart, Lung, and Blood Institute Family Heart Study. Obes Res 1998; 6:107–114.

Borecki IB, Rice T, Perusse L, Bouchard C, Rao DC: An exploratory investigation of genetic linkage with obesity phenotypes: the Quebec Family Study. Obes Res 1994; 2:213–219.

Bouchard C (ed): The Genetics of Obesity. Boca Raton, FL: CRC Press, 1994.

Bouchard C, Blair SN: Introductory comments for the consensus on physical activity and obesity. Med Sci Sports Exerc 1999; 31(Suppl 11):S498–S501.

Bouchard C, Despres JP, Mauriege P: Genetic and nongenetic determinants of regional fat distribution. Endocr Rev 1993; 14:72–93.

Bouchard C, Perusse L, Chagnon YC, Warden C, Ricquier D: Linkage between markers in the vicinity of the uncoupling protein 2 gene and resting metabolic rate in humans. Hum Mol Genet 1997; 6:1887–1889.

Bouchard C, Perusse L, Leblanc C, Tremblay A, Theriault G: Inheritance of the amount and distribution of human body fat. Int J Obes 1988; 12:205–215.

Bouchard C, Perusse L, Rice T, Rao DC: The genetics of obesity. In: Bray GA, Bouchard C, James WPT (eds). Handbook of Obesity. New York: Marcel Dekker, 1998:157–190.

Bouchard C, Rice T, Lemieux S, Despres JP, Perusse L, Rao DC: Major gene for abdominal visceral fat area in the Quebec Family Study. Int J Obes 1996; 20:420–427.

Bouchard C, Tremblay A, Despres JP, Nadeau A, Lupien PJ, Theriault G, Dussault J, Moorjani S, Pineault S, Fournier G: The response to long-term overfeeding in identical twins. N Engl J Med 1990; 322:1477–1482.

Bouchard C, Tremblay A, Despres JP, Theriault G, Nadeau A, Lupien PJ, Moorjani S, Prudhomme D, Fournier G: The response to exercise with constant energy intake in identical twins. Obes Res 1994; 2:400–410.

Bray GA: The energetics of obesity. Med Sci Sports Exerc 1983; 15:32–40.

Bray GA: Overweight and fat distribution—basic consideration and clinical approaches. Dis Mon 1989; 7:451–537.

Bray GA: Obesity, a disorder of nutrient partitioning: the MONA LISA hypothesis. J Nutr 1991; 121:1146–1162.

Bray GA: Contemporary Diagnosis and Management of Obesity. Newtown, PA: Handbooks in Health Care Co, 1998.

Bray GA, Blackburn GL, Ferguson JM, Greenway FL, Jain AK, Mendel CM, Mendels J, Ryan DH, Schwartz SL, Scheinbaum ML, et al.: Sibutramine produces dose-related weight loss. Obes Res 1999; 7:189–198.

Bray GA, Bouchard C, James WPT (eds): Handbook of Obesity. New York: Marcel Dekker, 1998.

Bray GA, DeLany JP, Harsha DW, Volaufova J, Champagne CC: Evaluation of body fat in fatter and leaner 10-y-old African American and white children: the Baton Rouge Children's Study. Am J Clin Nutr 2001; 73:687–702.

Bray GA, Greenway FL: Current and potential drugs for treatment of obesity. Endocr Rev 1999; 20:805–875.

Bray GA, York DA: The Mona Lisa hypothesis in the time of leptin. Recent Prog Horm Res 1998; 53:95–118.

Buemann B, Vohl MC, Chagnon M, Chagnon YC, Gagnon J, Perusse L, Dionne F, Despres JP, Tremblay A, Nadeau A, et al.: Abdominal visceral fat is associated with a BclI restriction fragment length polymorphism at the glucocorticoid receptor gene locus. Obes Res 1997; 5:186–192.

Calle EE, Thun MJ, Petrelli JM, Rodriguez C, Heath CW Jr: Body-mass index and mortality in a prospective cohort of U.S. adults. N Engl J Med. 1999; 341:1097–1105.

Campfield LA, Smith FJ, Burn P: The OB protein (leptin) pathway. A link between adipose tissue mass and central neural networks. Horm Metab Res 1996; 28:619–632.

Cardon LR: Developmental analysis of the body mass index in the Colorado Adoption Project. Behav Genet 1991; 21:563–564.

Carey DGP, Nguyen TV, Campbell LV, Chisholm DJ, Kelly P: Genetic influences on central abdominal fat: a twin study. Int J Obes 1996; 20:722–726.

Carlsson B, Lindell K, Gabrielsson B, Karlsson C, Bjarnason R, Westphal O, Karlsson U, Sjostrom L, Carlsson LMS: Obese (*ob*) gene defects are rare in human obesity. Obes Res 1997; 5:30–35.

Chagnon YC, Chen WJ, Perusse L, Chagnon M, Nadeau A, Wilkison WO, Bouchard C: Linkage and association studies between the melanocortin receptors 4 and 5 genes and obesity-related phenotypes in the Quebec Family Study. Mol Med 1997a; 3:663–673.

Chagnon YC, Perusse L, Bouchard C: Familial aggregation of obesity, candidate genes and quantitative trait loci. Curr Opin Lipidol 1997b; 8:205–211.

Chagnon YC, Perusse L, Bouchard C: The human obesity gene map: the 1997 update. Obes Res 1998; 6:76–92.

Chagnon YC, Perusse L, Bouchard C: The molecular and epidemiological genetics of obesity. In: Lockwood D, Heffner T (eds). Obesity: Pathology and Therapy. New York: Springer-Verlag, 2001 (in press).

Chagnon YC, Perusse L, Lamothe M, Chagnon M, Nadeau A, Dionne FT, Gagnon J, Chung WK, Leibel RL, Bouchard C: Suggestive linkages between markers on human 1p32–p22 and body fat and insulin levels in the Quebec Family Study. Obes Res 1997c; 5:115–121.

Chagnon YC, Rice T, Perusse L, Borecki IB, Ho-Kim MA, Lacaille M, Pare C, Bouchard L, Gagnon J, Leon AS, et al.: Genomic scan for genes affecting body composition before and after training in Caucasians from HERITAGE. J Appl Physiol 2001; 90:1777–1787.

Chua SC Jr.: Monogenic models of obesity. Behav Genet 1997; 27:277–284.

Chung WK, Power-Kehoe L, Chua M, Chu F, Devoto M, Aronne L, Huma Z, Sothern M, Udall JN, Kahle B, et al.: Exonic and intronic sequence variation in the human leptin receptor (LEPR). Diabetes 1997; 46:1509–1511.

Chung WK, Power-Kehoe L, Chua M, Lee R, Leibel RL: Genomic structure of the human *OB* receptor and the identification of two novel intronic microsatellites. Genome Res 1996; 6:1192–1199.

Clausen JO, Hansen T, Bjorbaek C, Echwald SM, Urhammer SA, Rasmussen S, Andersen CB, Hansen L, Almind K, Winther K, et al.: Insulin resistance: interactions between obesity and a common variant of insulin substrate-1. Lancet 1995; 346:397–402.

Clement K, Dina C, Basdevant A, Chastang N, Pelloux V, Lahlou N, Berlan M, Langin D, Guy-Grand B, Froguel P: A sib-pair analysis study of 15 candidate genes in French families with morbid obesity: indication for linkage with islet 1 locus on chromosome 5q. Diabetes 1999; 48:398–402.

Clement K, Garner C, Hager J, Philippi A, LeDuc C, Carey A, Harris TJR, Jury C, Cardon LR, Basdevant A, et al.: Indication of linkage of the human *OB* gene region with extreme obesity. Diabetes 1996a; 45:687–690.

Clement K, Philipi A, Jury C, Pividal R, Hager J, Demenais F, Basdevant A, Guy-Grand B, Froguel P: Candidate gene approach of familial morbid obesity: linkage analysis of the glucocorticoid receptor gene. Int J Obes 1996b; 20:507–512.

Clement K, Ruiz J, Cassard-Doulcier AM, Bouillaud F, Ricquier D, Basdevant A, Guy-Grand B, Froguel P: Additive effect of A|G (−3826) variant of the uncoupling protein gene and the $Trp^{64}Arg$ mutation of the $beta_3$-adrenergic receptor gene on weight gain in morbid obesity. Int J Obes 1996c; 20:1062–1066.

Clement K, Vaisse C, Lahlou N, Cabrol S, Pelloux V, Cassuto D, Gourmelen M, Dina C, Chambaz J, Lacorte JM, et al.: A mutation in the human leptin receptor gene causes obesity and pituitary dysfunction. Nature 1998; 392:398–401.

Clement K, Vaisse C, Manning BSJ, Basdevant A, Guy-Grand B, Rinz J, Silver KD, Shuldiner AR, Froguel P, Strosberg D: Genetic variation in the beta 3-adrenergic receptor and an increased capacity to gain weight in patients with morbid obesity. N Engl J Med 1995; 333:352–354.

Colditz GA, Willett WC, Rotnitzky A, Manson JE: Weight gain as a risk factor for clinical diabetes mellitus in women. Ann Intern Med 1995; 122:481–486.

Comuzzie AG, Blangero J, Mahaney MC, Mitchell BD, Hixson JE, Samollow PB, Stern MP, MacCluer JW: Major gene with sex-specific effects influences fat mass in Mexican Americans. Genet Epidemiol 1995; 12:475–488.

Comuzzie AG, Hixson JE, Almasy L, Mitchell BD, Mahaney MC, Dyer TD, Stern MP, MacCluer JW, Blangero J: A major quantitative trait locus determining serum leptin levels and fat is located on human chromosome 2. Nat Genet 1997; 15:273–276.

Considine RV, Considine EL, Williams CJ, Hyde TM, Caro JF: The hypothalamus leptin receptor in humans: identification of incidental sequence polymorphisms and absence of the *db/db* mouse and *fa/fa* rat mutations. Diabetes 1996; 19:992–994.

Considine RV, Considine EL, Williams CJ, Nyce MR, Magosin SA, Bauer TL, Rosato

EL, Colberg J, Caro JF: Evidence against either a premature stop codon or the absence of *obese* gene mRNA in human obesity. J Clin Invest 1995; 95:2986–2988.

Croft JB, Morrell D, Chase CL, Swift M: Obesity in heterozygous carriers of the gene for the Bardet-Biedl syndrome. Am J Med Genet 1995; 55:12–15.

Davidson MH, Hauptman J, DiGirolamo M, Foreyt JP, Halsted CH, Heber D, Heimburger DC, Lucas CP, Robbins DC, Chung J, et al.: Weight control and risk factor reduction in obese subjects treated for 2 years with orlistat: a randomized controlled trial. JAMA 1999; 281:235–242.

Davis BR, Blaufox MD, Oberman A, Wassertheil-Smoller S, Zimbaldi N, Cutler JA, Kirchner K, Langford HG: Reduction in long-term antihypertensive medication requirements. Effects of weight reduction by dietary intervention in overweight persons with mild hypertension. Arch Intern Med 1993; 153:1773–1782.

deBoer JO, van Es AJ, van Raaij JM, Hautvast JG: Energy requirements and energy expenditure of lean and overweight women, measured by indirect calorimetry. Am J Clin Nutr 1987; 46:13–21.

deJonge L, Bray GA: The thermic effect of food and obesity: a critical review. Obes Res 1997; 5:622–631.

Donahue RP, Abbott RD, Bloom E, Reed DM, Yano K: Central obesity and coronary heart disease in men. Lancet 1987; 1:821–824.

Ducimetiere P, Richard J, Cambien F: The pattern of subcutaneous fat distribution in middle-aged men and the risk of coronary heart disease: the Paris Prospective Study. Int J Obes 1986; 10:229–240.

Duggirala R, Stern MP, Mitchell BD, Reinhart LJ, Shipman PA, Uresandi OC, Chung WK, Leibel RL, Hales CN, O'Connell P, et al.: Quantitative variation in obesity-related traits and insulin precursors linked to the *OB* gene region on human chromosome 7. Am J Hum Genet 1996; 59:694–703.

Echwald SM, Rasmussen SB, Sorensen TIA, Andersen T, Tybjaerg-Hansen A, Clausen JO, Hansen L, Hansen T, Pedersen O: Identification of two novel missense mutations in the human *OB* gene. Int J Obes 1997a; 21:321–326.

Echwald SM, Sorensen TD, Sorensen TI, Tybjaerg-Hansen A, Andersen T, Chung WK: Amino acid variants in the human leptin receptor: lack of association to juvenile onset obesity. Biochem Biophys Res Commun 1997b; 233:248–252.

Fabsitz RR, Carmelli D, Hewitt JK: Evidence for independent genetic influences on obesity in middle age. Int J Obes 1992; 16:657–666.

Fabsitz R, Feinleib M, Hrubec Z: Weight changes in adult twins. Acta Genet Med Gemellol (Roma) 1980; 29:273–279.

Fabsitz RR, Sholinsky P, Carmelli D: Genetic influences on adult weight gain maximum body mass index in male twins. Am J Epidemiol 1994; 140:711–720.

Fernandez-Real JM, Gutierrez C, Ricart W, Casamitjana R, Fernandez-Castaner M, Vendrell J, Richart C, Soler J: The TNF-alpha gene NcoI polymorphism influences the relationship among insulin resistance, percent body fat, and increased serum leptin levels. Diabetes 1997; 46:1468–1472.

Ferrannini E, Haffner SM, Mitchell BD, Stern MP: Hyperinsulinemia: the key feature of a cardiovascular and metabolic syndrome. Diabetologia 1991; 34:416–422.

Flatt J-P: McCollum Award Lecture, 1995. Diet, lifestyle, and weight maintenance. Am J Clin Nutr 1995; 62:820–836.

Flechtner-Mors M, Ditschuneit HH, Johnson TD, Suchard MA, Adler G: Metabolic and weight loss effects of long-term dietary intervention in obese patients: four-year results. Obes Res 2000; 8:399–402.

Flegal KM, Carroll MD, Kuczmarski RJ, Johnson CL: Overweight and obesity in the United States: prevalence and trends, 1960–1994. Int J Obes 1998; 22:39–47.

Fleury C, Neverova M, Collins S, Raimbault S, Champigny O, Levimeyrueis C, Bouillaud F, Seldin MF, Surwit RS, Ricquier C, et al.: Uncoupling protein-2: a novel gene linked to obesity and hyperinsulinemia. Nat Genet 1997; 15:269–272.

Folsom AR, Kaye SA, Sellers TA, Hong CP, Cerhan JR, Potter JD, Prineas RJ: Body fat distribution and 5-year risk of death in older women. JAMA 1993; 269:483–487.

Fontaine E, Savard R, Tremblay A, Després J-P, Poehlman E, Bouchard C: Resting metabolic rate in monozygotic and dizygotic twins. Acta Genet Med Gemellol (Roma) 1985; 34:41–47.

Francke S, Clement K, Dina C, Inoue H, Behn P, Vatin V, Basdevant A, Guy-Grand B, Permutt MA, Froguel P, et al.: Genetic studies of the leptin receptor gene in morbidly obese French Caucasian families. Hum Genet 1997; 100:491–496.

Fried SK, Russell CD: Diverse roles of adipose tissue in the regulation of systematic metabolism and energy balance. In: Bray GA, Bouchard C, James WPT (eds). Handbook of Obesity. New York: Marcel Dekker, 1998:397–413.

Garrison RJ, Kannel WB: A new approach to estimating healthy body weights. Int J Obes 1993; 17:417–423.

Garrow JS: Treat Obesity Seriously: A Clinical Manual. Edinburgh: Churchill Livingstone, 1981.

Gauguier D, Froguel P, Parent V, Bernard C, Bihoreau MT, Portha B, James MR, Penicaud L, Lathrop M, Ktorza A: Chromosomal mapping of genetic loci associated with non-insulin dependent diabetes in the GK rat. Nat Genet 1996; 12:38–43.

Georges JL, Regis-Bailly A, Salah D, Rakotovao R, Siest G, Visvikis S, Tiret L: Family study of lipoprotein lipase gene polymorphism and plasma triglyceride levels. Genet Epidemiol 1996; 13:179–192.

Gerdes C, Gerdes LU, Hansen PS, Faergeman O: Polymorphisms in the lipoprotein lipase gene and their associations with plasma lipid concentrations in 40-year-old Danish men. Circulation 1995; 92:1765–1769.

Gimeno RE, Dembski M, Weng X, Deng N, Shyjan AW, Gimeno CJ, Iris F, Ellis SJ, Woolf EA, Tartaglia LA: Cloning and characterization of an uncoupling protein homolog. A potential molecular mediator of human thermogenesis. Diabetes 1997; 46:900–906.

Golay A, Jallut D, Schutz Y, Felber JP, Jequier E: Evolution of glucose induced thermogenesis in obese subjects with and without diabetes: a six-year follow-up study. Int J Obes 1991; 15:601–607.

Goldstein DJ: Beneficial health effects of modest weight-loss. Int J Obes Relat Metab Disord 1992; 16:397–415.

Gotoda T, Manning BS, Goldstone AP, Imrie H, Evans AL, Strosberg AD, McKeigue PM, Scott J, Aitman TJ: Leptin receptor gene variation and obesity: lack of association in a white British male population. Hum Mol Genet 1997; 6:869–876.

Griffiths LR, Nyholt DR, Curtain RP, Gaffney PT, Morris BJ: Cross-sectional study of a microsatellite marker in the low density lipoprotein receptor gene in obese normotensives. Clin Exp J Pharmacol Physiol 1995; 22:496–498.

Hager J, Dina C, Francke S, Dubois S, Houari M, Vatin V, Vaillant E, Lorentz N, Basdevant A, Clément K, et al.: A genome-wide scan for human obesity genes reveals a major susceptibility locus on chromosome 10. Nat Genet 1998; 20:304–308.

Hani EH, Clement K, Velho G, Vionnet N, Hager J, Philippi A, Dina C, Inoue H, Permutt MA, Basdevant A, et al.: Genetic studies of the sulfonylurea receptor gene locus in NIDDM and in morbid obesity among French Caucasians. Diabetes 1997; 46:688–694.

Hasstedt SJ, Ramirez ME, Kuida H, Williams RR: Recessive inheritance of a relative fat pattern. Am J Hum Genet 1989; 45:917–925.

Hauptman J, Lucas C, Boldrin MN, Collins H, Segal KR: Orlistat in the long-term treatment of obesity in primary care settings. Arch Fam Med 2000; 9:160–167.

Hegele RA, Harris SB, Hanley AJG, Sadikian S, Connelly PW, Zinman B: Genetic variation of intestinal fatty acid binding protein associated with variation in body mass in aboriginal Canadians. J Clin Endocrinol Metab 1996; 81:4334–4337.

Heller R, Garrison RJ, Havlik RJ, Feinleib M, Padgett S: Family resemblances in height and relative weight in the Framingham Heart Study. Int J Obes 1984; 8:399–405.

Herskind AM, McGue M, Sorensen TIA, Harvald B: Sex and age specific assessment of genetic and environmental influences on body mass index in twins. Int J Obes 1996; 20:106–113.

Heymsfield SB, Allison DB, Wang ZM: Evaluation of total and regional body composition. In: Bray GA, Bouchard C, James WPT (eds). Handbook of Obesity, New York: Marcel Dekker, 1998:341–347.

Hinney A, Schmidt A, Nottebom K, Heibult O, Becker I, Ziegler A, Gerber G, Sina M, Gorg T, Mayer H, et al.: Several mutations in the melanocortin-4 receptor gene including a nonsense and a frameshift mutation associated with dominantly inherited obesity in humans. J Clin Endocrinol Metab 1999; 84:1483–1486.

Hsueh WC, Mitchell BD, Schneider JL, St Jean PL, Pollin TI, Ehm MG, Wagner MJ, Burns DK, Sakul H, Bell CJ, et al.: Genome-wide scan of obesity in the Old Order Amish. J Clin Endocrinol Metab 2001; 86:1199–1205.

Huggins RM, Hoang NH, Loesch DZ: Analysis of longitudinal data from twins. Genet Epidemiol 2000; 19:345–353.

Huszar D, Lynch CA, Fairchild-Huntress V, Dunmore JH, Fang Q, Berkemeier LR, Gu W, Kesterson RA, Boston BA, Cone RD, et al.: Targeted disruption of the melanocortin-4 receptor results in obesity in mice. Cell 1997; 88:131–141.

Jackson RS, Creemers JWM, Ohagi S, Raffin-Sanson ML, Sanders L, Montague CT, Hutton JC, O'Rahilly S: Obesity and impaired prohormone processing associated with mutations in the human prohormone convertase 1 gene. Nat Genet 1997; 16:303–306.

Jakicic JM, Winters C, Lang W, Wing RR: Effects of intermittent exercise and use of home exercise equipment on adherence, weight loss, and fitness in overweight women: a randomized trial. JAMA 1999; 282:1554–1560.

James WP, Astrup A, Finer N, Hilsted J, Kopelman P, Rossner S, Saris WH, Van Gaal LF: Effect of sibutramine on weight maintenance after weight loss: a randomised trial. STORM Study Group. Sibutramine Trial of Obesity Reduction and Maintenance. Lancet 2000; 356:2119–2125.

Jemaa R, Tuzet S, Portos C, Betoulle D, Apfelbaum M, Fumeron F: Lipoprotein lipase gene polymorphisms: associations with hypertriglyceridemia and body mass index in obese people. Int J Obes 1995; 19:270–274.

Jequier E, Schutz Y: Long-term measurements of energy expenditure in humans using a respiration chamber. Am J Clin Nutr 1983; 38:989–998.

Kahn RC, Vicent D, Doria A: Genetics of non-insulin-dependent (type-2) diabetes mellitus. Ann Rev Med 1996; 47:509–531.

Kapeller R, Moriarty A, Strauss A, Stubdal H, Theriault K, Siebert E, Chickering T, Morgenstern JP, Tartaglia LA, Lillie J: Tyrosine phosphorylation of *tub* and its association with Src homology 2 domain–containing proteins implicate *tub* in intracellular signaling by insulin. J Biol Chem 1999; 274:24980–24986.

Karlin S, Williams PT, Jensen S, Farquhar JW: Genetic analysis of the Stanford LRC Family Study data: I. Structured exploratory data analysis of height and weight measurements. Am J Epidemiol 1981; 113:307–324.

Katsanis N, Ansley S, Badano JL, Eichers ER, Lewis RA, Hoskins BE, Scambler PJ, Davidson WS, Beales PL, Lupski JR: Triallelic unheritance in Bardet-Biedl syndrome, a Mendelian recessive disorder. Science 2001; 293:2256–2259.

Katzmarzyk PT, Malina RM, Pérusse L, Rice T, Province MA, Rao DC, Bouchard C: Familial resemblance in fatness and fat distribution. Am J Hum Biol 2000; 12:395–404.

Katzmarzyk PT, Perusse L, Rao DC, Bouchard C: Familial risk of obesity and central adipose tissue distribution in the general Canadian population. Am J Epidemiol 1999; 149:933–942.

Kern PA, Ong JM, Goers JWF, Pedersen ME: Regulation of lipoprotein lipase immunoreactive mass in isolated human adipocytes. J Clin Invest 1988; 81:398–406.

Kissebah AH, Krakower GR: Regional adiposity and morbidity. Physiol Rev 1994; 74:761–811.

Kissebah A, Sonnenberg G, Myklebust J, Goldstein M, Broman K, James R, Marks J, Krakower G, Jacob H, Weber A, et al.: Quantitative trait loci on chromosomes 3 and 17 influence phenotypes of the metabolic syndrome. Proc Natl Acad Sci USA 2000; 97:14478–14483.

Kleiber M: Fire of Life: An Introduction to Animal Energetics. New York: John Wiley and Sons, 1961.
Knowler WC, Pettitt DJ, Savage PJ, Bennett PH: Diabetes incidence in PIMA Indians: contributions of obesity and parental diabetes. Am J Epidemiol 1981; 113:144–156.
Ko CW, Lee SP: Obesity and gallbladder disease. In: Bray GA, Bouchard C, James WPT (eds). Handbook of Obesity. New York: Marcel Dekker, 1998:709–724.
Korkeila M, Kaprio J, Rissanen A, Koskenvuo M: Effects of gender and age on the heritability of body mass index. Int J Obes 1991; 15:647–654.
Kozak LP, Harper M-E: Mitochondrial uncoupling proteins in energy expenditure. Ann Rev Nutr 2000; 20:339–363.
Kromhout D: Changes in energy and macronutrients in 871 middle-aged men during 10 years of follow-up (the Zutphen Study). Am J Clin Nutr 1983; 37:287–294.
Krude H, Biebermann H, Luck W, Horn R, Brabant G, Gruters A: Severe early-onset obesity, adrenal insufficiency and red hair pigmentation caused by *POMC* mutations in humans. Nat Genet 1998; 19:155–157.
Lanouette CM, Giacobino JP, Perusse L, Lacaille M, Yvon C, Chagnon M, Kuhne F, Bouchard C, Muzzin P, Chagnon YC: Association between uncoupling protein 3 gene and obesity-related phenotypes in the Quebec Family Study. Mol Med 2001; 7:433–441.
Lapidus L, Bengtsson C, Larsson B, Pennert K, Rybo E, Sjostrom L: Distribution of adipose tissue and risk of cardiovascular disease and death: a 12 year follow-up of participants in the population study of women in Gothenburg, Sweden. BMJ 1984; 289:1257–1261.
Large V, Hellstrom L, Reynisdottir S, Lonnqvist F, Eriksson P, Lannfelt L, Arner P: Human beta-2 adrenoreceptor gene polymorphism are highly frequent in obesity and associate with altered adipocyte beta-2 adrenoreceptor function. J Clin Invest 1997; 100:3005–3013.
Larsson B, Svardsudd K, Welin L, Wilhelmsen L, Bjorntorp P, Tibblin G: Abdominal adipose tissue distribution, obesity, and risk of cardiovascular disease and death: 13 year follow-up of participants in the study of men born in 1913. BMJ 1984; 288:1401–1404.
Lecomte E, Herbeth B, Nicaud V, Rakotovao R, Artur Y, Tiret L: Segregation analysis of fat mass and fat-free mass with age- and sex-dependent effects: the Stanislas Family Study. Genet Epidemiol 1997; 14:51–62.
Lee JH, Reed DR, Li WD, Xu W, Joo EJ, Kilker RL, Nanthakumar E, North M, Sakul H, Bell C, et al.: Genome scan for human obesity and linkage to markers in 20q13. Am J Hum Genet 1999; 64:196–209.
Lee JH, Reed DR, Price RA: Familial risk ratios for extreme obesity: implications for mapping human obesity genes. Int J Obes 1997; 21:935–940.
Lembertas A, Perusse L, Chagnon YC, Fisler JS, Warden CH, Purcell-Huynh DA, Dionne FT, Gagnon J, Nadeau A, Lusis AJ, et al.: Identification of an obesity quantitative trait locus on mouse chromosome 2 and evidence of linkage to body fat and insulin on the human homologous region 20q. J Clin Invest 1997; 100:1240–1247.
Li Z, Rice T, Perusse L, Bouchard C, Rao DC: Familial aggregation of subcutaneous fat patterning: principal components of skinfolds in the Quebec Family Study. Am J Hum Biol 1996; 8:535–542.
Lichtman SW, Pisarska K, Berman ER, Pestone M, Dowling H, Offenbacher E, Weisel H, Heshka S, Matthews DE, Heymsfield SB: Discrepancy between self-reported and actual caloric intake and exercise in obese subjects. N Engl J Med 1992; 327:1893–1898.
Lissner L, Sjostrom L, Bengtsson C, Bouchard C, Larsson B: The natural history of obesity in an obese population and associations with metabolic aberrations. Int J Obes 1994; 18:441–447.
Liu Q, Bai C, Chen F, Wang R, MacDonald T, Gu M, Zhang Q, Morsy MA, Caskey CT: Uncoupling protein-3: a muscle-specific gene upregulated by leptin in *ob/ob* mice. Gene 1998; 207:1–7.
Longini IM Jr, Higgins MW, Hinton PC, Moll PP, Keller JB: Genetic and environmental sources of familial aggregation of body mass in Tecumseh, Michigan. Hum Biol 1984; 56:733–757.
MacDonald A, Stunkard AJ: Body mass indexes of British separated twins. N Engl J Med 1990; 322:1530.
MacLean LD, Rhode BM: Does genetic predisposition influence surgical results of operations for obesity? Obes Surg 1996; 6:132–137.
MacMahon S, Cutler JA, Stamler J: Antihypertensive drug treatment. Potential, expected, and observed effects on stroke and on coronary heart disease. Hypertension 1989; 13(5 Suppl):I45–I50.
Maffei M, Stoffel M, Barone M, Moon B, Dammerman M, Ravussin E, Bogardus C, Ludwig DS, Flier JS, Talley M, et al.: Absence of mutations in the human *OB* gene in obese/diabetic subjects. Diabetes 1996; 45:679–682.
Manson JE, Willett WC, Stamfer MJ, Colditz GA, Hunter DJ, Hankinson SE, Hennekens CH, Speizer FE: Body weight and mortality among women. N Engl J Med 1995; 333:677–685.
Matsuoka N, Ogawa Y, Hosoda K, Matsuda J, Masuzaki H, Miyawaki T, Azuma N, Natsui K, Nishimura H, Yoshimasa Y, et al.: Human leptin receptor gene in obese Japanese subjects: evidence against either obesity-causing mutations or association of sequence variants with obesity. Diabetologia 1997; 40:1204–1210.
Mattu RK, Needham EW, Morgan R, Rees A, Hackshaw AK, Stocks J, Elwood PC, Galton DJ: DNA variants at the *LPL* gene locus associate with angiographical severity of atherosclerosis and serum lipoprotein levels in a Welsh population. Arterioscler Thromb 1994; 14:1090–1097.
Mauriege P, Bouchard C: $Trp^{64}Arg$ mutation in β_3-adrenoreceptor gene of doubtful significance for obesity and insulin resistance. Lancet 1996; 348:698–699.
Messerli FH, Nunez BD, Ventura HO, Snyder DW: Overweight and sudden death: increased ventricular ectopy in cardiomyopathy of obesity. Arch Intern Med 1987; 147:1725–1728.
Miltenberger RJ, Mynatt RL, Wilkinson JE, Woychik RP: The role of the *agouti* gene in the yellow obese syndrome. J Nutr 1997; 127:1902S–1907S.
Mitchell BD, Blangero J, Comuzzie AG, Almasy LA, Shuldiner AR, Silver K, Stern MP, MacCluer JW, Hixson JE: A paired sibling analysis of the beta-3 adrenergic receptor and obesity in Mexican Americans. J Clin Invest 1998; 101:584–587.
Moll PP, Burns TL, Lauer RM: The genetic and environmental sources of body mass index variability: the Muscatine Ponderosity Family Study. Am J Hum Genet 1991; 49:1243–1255.
Montague CT, Sadaf Farooqi I, Whitehead JP, Soos MA, Rau H, Wareham NJ, Sewter CP, Digby JE, Mohammed SN, Hust JA, et al.: Congenital leptin deficiency is associated with severe early-onset obesity in humans. Nature 1997; 387:903–908.
Mueller WH: The genetics of human fatness. Yearbook Phys Anthropol 1983; 26:215–230.
Naggert JK, Fricker LD, Varlamov O, Nishina PM, Rouille Y, Steiner DF, Carroll RJ, Paigen BJ, Leiter EH: Hyperproinsulinaemia in obese *fat/fat* mice associated with a carboxypeptidase E mutation which reduces enzyme activity. Nat Genet 1995; 10:135–142.
National Heart, Lung and Blood Institute: Clinical Guidelines on the Identification, Evaluation, and Treatment of Overweight and Obesity in Adults. Bethesda, MD: National Institutes of Health, 1998.
National Heart, Lung and Blood Institute, North American Association for the Study of Obesity: The Practical Guide. Identification, Evaluation, and Treatment of Overweight and Obesity in Adults. NIH Publication 00-4084. Bethesda, MD: National Institutes of Health, 2000.
National Research Council, Committee on Diet and Health: Calories: total macronutrient intake, energy expenditure, and net energy stores. In: Diet and Health: Implications for Reducing Chronic Disease Risk. Washington DC: National Academy Press, 1989:139–158.
Ness R, Laskarzewski P, Price RA: Inheritance of extreme overweight in black families. Hum Biol 1991; 63:39–52.
Niki T, Mori H, Tamori Y, Kishimotohashiramoto M, Ueno H, Araki S, Masugi J, Sawant N, Majithia HR, Rais N, et al.: Human *obese* gene: molecular screening in Japanese and Asian Indian NIDDM patients associated with obesity. Diabetes 1996; 45:675–678.
Nishimura DY, Searby CC, Carmi R, Elbedour K, Van Maldergem L, Fulton AB, Lam BL, Powell BR, Swiderski RE, Bugge KE, et al.: Positional cloning of a novel gene on chromosome 16q causing Bardet-Biedl syndrome (BBS2). Hum Mol Genet 2001; 10:865–874.
Norman RA, Bogardus C, Ravussin E: Linkage between obesity and a marker near the tumor necrosis factor-α locus in Pima Indians. J Clin Invest 1995; 96:158–162.
Norman RA, Leibel RL, Chung WK, Power-Kehoe L, Chua SC Jr, Knowler WC, Thompson DB, Bogardus C, Ravussin E: Absence of linkage of obesity and energy metabolism to markers flanking homologues of rodent obesity genes in Pima Indians. Diabetes 1996; 45:1229–1232.
Norman RA, Tataranni PA, Pratley R, Thompson DB, Hanson RL, Prochazka M, Baier L, Ehm MG, Sakul H, Foroud T, et al.: Autosomal genomic scan for loci linked to obesity and energy metabolism in Pima Indians. Am J Hum Genet 1998; 62:659–668.
Norman RA, Thompson DB, Foroud T, Garvey WT, Bennett PH, Bogardus C, Ravussin E: Genomewide search for genes influencing percent body fat in Pima Indians: suggestive linkage at chromosome 11q21–q22. Am J Hum Genet 1997; 60:166–173.
O'Dell SD, Miller GJ, Cooper JA, Hindmarsh PC, Pringle PJ, Ford H, Humphries SE, Day IN. ApoI polymorphism in insulin-like growth factor II (*IGF2*) gene and weight in middle-aged males. Int J Obes 1997; 21:822–825.
Ohisalo JJ, Ranta S, Huhtaniemi IT: Inhibition of adenosine 3′,5′-monophosphate accumulation and lipolysis by adenosine analogs in human subcutaneous adipocytes. J Clin Endocrinol Metab 1984; 58:32–35.
Ohman M, Oksanen L, Kaprio J, Koskenvuo M, Mustajoki P, Rissanen A, Salmi J, Kontula K, Peltonen L: Genome-wide scan of obesity in Finnish sibpairs reveals linkage to chromosome Xq24. J Clin Endocrinol Metab 2000; 85:3183–3190.
Oksanen L, Kainulainen K, Heiman M, Mustajoki P, Kauppinen-Makelin R, Kontula K: Novel polymorphism of the human ob gene promotor in lean and morbidly obese subjects. Int J Obes 1997; 21:489–494.
Oppert JM, Tourville J, Chagnon M, Mauriege P, Dionne FT, Perusse L, Bouchard C: DNA polymorphisms in alpha2- and beta2-adrenoceptor genes and regional fat distribution in humans: association and linkage studies. Obes Res 1995; 3:249–255.
Oppert JM, Vohl MC, Chagnon M, Dionne FT, Cassard-Doulcier AM, Ricquier D, Perusse L, Bouchard C: DNA polymorphism in the uncoupling protein (*UCP*) gene and human body fat. Int J Obes 1994; 18:526–531.
O'Rahilly S, Gray H, Humphreys PJ, Krook A, Polonsky KS, White A, Gibson S, Taylor K, Carr C: Impaired processing of prohormones associated with abnormalities of glucose homeostasis and adrenal function. N Engl J Med 1995; 333:1386–1390.
Pedersen SB, Jonler M, Richelsen B: Characterization of regional and gender differences in glucocorticoid receptors and lipoprotein lipase activity in human adipose tissue. J Clin Endocrinol Metab 1994; 78:1354–1359.
Perusse L, Chagnon YC, Bouchard C: Etiology of massive obesity: role of genetic factors. World J Surg 1998; 22:907–912.
Perusse L, Chagnon YC, Dionne FT, Bouchard C: The human obesity gene map: the 1996 update. Obes Res 1997; 5:49–61.
Perusse L, Chagnon YC, Weisnagel JS, Rankinen T, Snyder E, Sands J, Bouchard C: The human obesity gene map: the 2000 update. Obes Res 2001a; 9:135–168.
Perusse L, Despres JP, Lemieux S, Rice T, Rao DC, Bouchard C: Familial aggregation of abdominal visceral fat level: results from the Quebec Family Study. Metabolism 1996; 45:378–382.

Perusse L, Leblanc C, Bouchard C: Inter-generation transmission of physical fitness in the Canadian population. Can J Sport Sci 1988; 13:8–14.

Perusse L, Rice T, Chagnon Y, Després J, Lemieux S, Roy S, Lacaille M, Ho-Kim M, Chagnon M, Province M, et al.: A genome-wide scan for abdominal fat assessed by computed tomography in the Quebec Family Study. Diabetes 2001b; 50:614–621.

Perusse L, Rice T, Province MA, Gagnon J, Leon AS, Skinner JS, Wilmore JH, Rao DC, Bouchard C: Familial aggregation of amount and distribution of subcutaneous fat and their responses to exercise training in the HERITAGE Family Study. Obes Res 2000; 8:140–150.

Pietiläinen KH, Kaprio J, Rissanen A, Winter T, Rimpelä A, Viken RJ, Rose RJ: Distribution and heritability of BMI in Finnish adolescents aged 16y and 17y: a study of 4884 twins and 2509 singletons. Int J Obes 1999; 23:107–115.

Porte D Jr, Seeley RJ, Woods SC, Baskin DG, Figlewicz DP, Schwartz MW: Obesity, diabetes and the central nervous system. Diabetologia 1998; 41:863–881.

Pouliot MC, Despres JP, Dionne FT, Vohl MC, Moorjani S, Prudhomme D, Bouchard C, Lupien PJ: *ApoB-100* gene EcoRI polymorphism. Relations to plasma lipoprotein changes associated with abdominal visceral obesity. Arterioscler Thromb 1994a; 14:527–353.

Pouliot MC, Despres JP, Lemieux S, Moorjani S, Bouchard C, Tremblay A, Nadeau A, Lupien PJ: Waist circumference and abdominal sagittal diameter: best simple anthropometric indexes of abdominal visceral adipose tissue accumulation and related cardiovascular risk in men and women. Am J Cardiol 1994b; 73:460–468.

Prentice AM, Black AE, Coward WA, Cole TJ: Energy expenditure in overweight and obese adults: an analysis of 319 doubly-labelled water measurements. Eur J Clin Nutr 1996; 50:93–97.

Price RA, Cadoret RJ, Stunkard AJ, Troughton E: Genetic contributions to human fatness: an adoption study. Am J Psychiatry 1987; 144:1003–1008.

Price RA, Gottesman II: Body fat in identical twins reared apart: roles for genes and environment. Behav Genet 1991; 21:1–7.

Price RA, Ness R, Laskarzewski P: Common major gene inheritance of extreme overweight. Hum Biol 1990; 62:747–765.

Province MA, Rao DC: Path analysis of family resemblance with temporal trends: applications to height, weight and Quetelet index in northeastern Brazil. Am J Hum Genet 1985; 37:178–192.

Rajput-Williams J, Knott TJ, Wallis SC, Bell GI, Knott TJ, Sweetnam P, Cox N, Miller NE: Variation of apolipoprotein-B gene is associated with obesity, high blood cholesterol levels, and increased risk of coronary heart disease. Lancet 1988; ii:1442–1446.

Ravussin E, Lillioja S, Knowler WC, Christin L, Freymond D, Abbott WGH, Boyce V, Howard BV: Reduced rate of energy expenditure as a risk factor for body-weight gain. N Engl J Med 1988; 318:467–472.

Rebuffe-Scrive M, Bronnegard M, Nilsson A, Eldh J, Gustafsson J, Bjorntorp P: Steroid hormone receptors in human tissues. J Clin Endocrinol Metab 1990; 71:1215–1219.

Rebuffe-Scrive M, Lundholm K, Bjorntorp P: Glucocorticoid hormone binding to human adipose tissue. Eur J Clin Nutr 1985; 15:267–271.

Reed DR, Bradley EC, Price RA: Obesity in families of extremely obese women. Obes Res 1993; 1:167–172.

Reed DR, Ding Y, Xu W, Cather C, Green ED, Price RA: Extreme obesity may be linked to markers flanking the human *OB* gene. Diabetes 1996; 45:691–694.

Reed DR, Ding Y, Xu W, Cather C, Price RA: Human obesity does not segregate with the chromosomal regions of Prader-Willi, Bardet-Biedl, Cohen, Borjeson or Wilson-Turner syndromes. Int J Obes 1995; 19:599–603.

Rice T, Borecki I, Bouchard C, Rao DC: Segregation analysis of body mass index in an unselected French-Canadian sample: the Quebec Family Study. Obes Res 1993a; 2:288–294.

Rice T, Borecki IB, Bouchard C, Rao DC: Segregation analysis of fat mass and other body composition measures derived from underwater weighing. Am J Hum Genet 1993b; 52:967–973.

Rice T, Daw EW, Gagnon J, Bouchard C, Leon AS, Skinner JS, Wilmore JH, Rao DC: Familial resemblance for body composition measures: the HERITAGE Family Study. Obes Res 1997a; 5:557–562.

Rice T, Despres JP, Daw EW, Gagnon J, Borecki IB, Perusse L, Leon AS, Skinner JS, Wilmore JH, Rao DC: Familial resemblance for abdominal visceral fat: the HERITAGE Family Study. Int J Obes 1997b; 21:1024–1031.

Rice T, Despres JP, Perusse L, Gagnon J, Leon AS, Skinner JS, Wilmore JH, Rao DC, Bouchard C: Segregation analysis of abdominal visceral fat: the HERITAGE Family Study. Obes Res 1997c; 5:417–424.

Rice T, Perusse L, Bouchard C, Rao DC: Familial clustering of abdominal visceral fat and total fat mass: the Quebec Family Study. Obes Res 1996; 4:253–261.

Rice T, Pérusse L, Bouchard C, Rao DC: Familial aggregation of body mass index and subcutaneous fat measures in the longitudinal Québec Family Study. Genet Epidemiol 1999; 16:316–334.

Risch N: Linkage strategies for genetically complex traits. I. Multilocus models. Am J Hum Genet 1990; 46:222–228.

Ristow M, Muller-Wieland D, Pfeiffer A, Krone W, Kahn CR: Obesity associated with a mutation in a genetic regulator of adipocyte differentiation. N Engl J Med 1998; 339:953–959.

Rolland V, Clement K, Dugail I, Guy-Grand B, Basdevant A, Froguel P, Lavau M: Leptin receptor gene in a large cohort of massively obese subjects: no indication of the *fa/fa* rat mutation. Detection of an intronic variant with no association with obesity. Obes Res 1998; 6:122–127.

Ross R, Janssen I: Is abdominal fat preferentially reduced in response to exercise-induced weight loss? Med Sci Sports Exerc 1999; 31(Suppl 11):S568–S572.

Ross R, Janssen I: Physical activity, total and regional obesity: dose-response considerations. Med Sci Sports Exerc 2001; 33(Suppl 6):S521–S529.

Rossner S: Weight loss, weight maintenance, and improved cardiovascular risk factors after 2 years treatment with orlistat for obesity. European Orlistat Obesity Study Group. Obes Res 2000; 8:49–61.

Rotimi C, Luke A, Li Z, Compton J, Bowsher R, Cooper R: Heritability of plasma leptin in a population sample of African-American families. Genet Epidemiol 1997; 14:255–263.

Schapira DV, Clark RA, Wolff P, Jarrett A, Kumar NB, Aziz NM: Visceral obesity and breast cancer risk. Cancer 1994; 74:632–639.

Schoeller DA, Fjeld CR: Human energy metabolism: what have we learned from the doubly labeled water method? Annu Rev Nutr 1991; 11:355–373.

Schuler GD, Boguski MS, Stewart EA, Stein LD, Gyapay G, Rice K, White RE, Rodriguez-Tome P, Aggarwal A, Bajorek E, et al.: A gene map of the human genome. Science 1996; 274:540–546.

Schutz Y, Jequier E: Resting energy expenditure, thermic effect of food, and total energy expenditure. In: Bray GA, Bouchard C, James WPT (eds). Handbook of Obesity. New York: Marcel Dekker, 1998:443–455.

Schutz Y, Tremblay A, Weinsier RL, Nelson KM: Role of fat oxidation in the long-term stabilization of body weight in obese women. Am J Clin Nutr 1992; 55:670–674.

Seidell JC: The current epidemic of obesity. In: Bouchard C (ed). Physical Activity and Obesity. Champaign, IL: Human Kinetics, 2000 pp. 21–30.

Sigal RJ, Doria A, Warram JH, Krolewski AS: Codon 972 polymorphism in the insulin receptor substrate-1 gene, obesity, and risk of noinsulin-dependent diabetes mellitus. J Clin Endocrinol Metab 1996; 81:1657–1659.

Sina M, Hinney A, Ziegler A, Neupert T, Mayer H, Siegfried W, Blum WF, Remschmidt H, Hebebrand J, et al.: Phenotypes in three pedigrees with autosomal dominant obesity caused by haploinsufficiency mutations in the melanocortin-4 receptor gene. Am J Hum Genet 1999; 65:1501–1507.

Sipilainen R, Uusitupa M, Heikkinen S, Rissanen A, Laasko M: Variants in the human intestinal fatty acid binding protein 2 gene in obese subjects. J Clin Endocrinol Metab 1997; 82:2629–2632.

Sjostrom CD, Lissner L, Sjostrom L: Relationships between changes in body composition and changes in cardiovascular risk factors: the SOS Intervention Study. Swedish Obese Subjects. Obes Res 1997; 5:519–530.

Sjostrom CD, Lissner L, Wedel H, Sjostrom L: Reduction in incidence of diabetes, hypertension and lipid disturbances after intentional weight loss induced by bariatric surgery: the SOS Intervention Study. Obes Res 1999; 7:477–484.

Sjostrom L, Rissanen A, Andersen T, Boldrin M, Golay A, Koppeschaar HP, Krempf M: Randomised placebo-controlled trial of orlistat for weight loss and prevention of weight regain in obese patients. European Multicentre Orlistat Study Group. Lancet 1998; 352:167–172.

Sjostrom LV: Morbidity of severely obese subjects. Am J Clin Nutr 1992a; 55:508S–515S.

Sjostrom LV: Mortality of severely obese subjects. Am J Clin Nutr 1992b; 55:516S–523S.

Smith SR, deJonge L, Zachwieja JJ, Roy H, Nguyen T, Rood J, Windhauser M, Volaufova J, Bray GA: Concurrent physical activity increases fat oxidation during the shift to a high-fat diet. Am J Clin Nutr 2000; 72:131–138.

Society of Actuaries: Build Study of 1979. Chicago: Society of Actuaries/Association of Life Insurance Medical Directors of America, 1980.

Sorensen TIA, Holst C, Stunkard AJ: Childhood body mass index—genetic and familial environmental influences assessed in a longitudinal adoption study. Int J Obes 1992a; 16:705–714.

Sorensen TIA, Holst C, Stunkard AJ, Skovgaard LT: Correlations of body mass index of adult adoptees and their biological and adoptive relatives. Int J Obes 1992b; 16:227–236.

Sorensen TIA, Price RA, Stunkard AJ, Schulsinger F: Genetics of obesity in adult adoptees and their biological siblings. BMJ 1989; 298:87–90.

Stevens J, Cai J, Pamuk ER, Williamson DF, Thun MJ, Wood JL: The effect of age on the association between body-mass index and mortality. N Engl J Med 1998; 338:1–7.

Stevens VJ, Corrigan SA, Obarzanek E, Bernauer E, Cook NR, Hebert P, Mattfeldt-Beman M, Oberman A, Sugars C, Dalcin AT, et al.: Weight loss intervention in phase 1 of the Trials of Hypertension Prevention. The TOHP Collaborative Research Group. Arch Intern Med 1993; 153:849–858.

Stevens VJ, Obarzanek E, Cook NR, Lee IM, Appel LJ, Smith West D, Milas NC, Mattfeldt-Beman M, Belden L, Bragg C, et al.: Long-term weight loss and changes in blood pressure: results of the Trials of Hypertension Prevention, phase II. Ann Intern Med 2001; 134:1–11.

Stokes J III, Garrison RJ, Kannel WB: The independent contributions of various indices of obesity to the 22-year incidence of coronary heart disease: the Framingham Heart Study. In: Vague J, Bjorntorp P, Guy-Grand B, Rebuffe-Scrive M, Vague P (eds). Metabolic Complications of Human Obesities. Amsterdam: Excerpta Medica, 1985:49–57.

Stone DL, Slavotinek A, Bouffard GG, Banerjee-Basu S, Baxevanis AD, Barr M, Biesecker LG: Mutation of a gene encoding a putative chaperonin causes McKusick-Kaufman syndrome. Nat Genet 2000; 25:79–82.

Strobel A, Issad T, Camoin L, Ozata M, Strosberg AD: A leptin missense mutation associated with hypogonadism and morbid obesity. Nat Genet 1998; 18:213–215.

Strohl KP, Strobel RJ, Parisi RA: Obesity and pulmonary function. In: Bray GA, Bouchard C, James WPT (eds). Handbook of Obesity. New York: Marcel Dekker, 1998:725–739.

Stunkard AJ, Harris JR, Pedersen NL, McClearn GE: The body-mass index of twins who have been reared apart. N Engl J Med 1990; 322:1483–1487.

Stunkard AJ, Kaplan D: Eating in public places: a review of direct reports of eating behavior. Int J Obes 1977; 1:89–101.
Stunkard AJ, Sorensen TI, Hanis C, Teasdale TW, Chakraborty R, Schull WJ, Schulsinger F: An adoption study of human obesity. N Engl J Med 1986; 314:193–198.
Tambs K, Moum T, Eaves L, Neale M, Midthjell K, Lund-Larsen PG, Naess S, Holmen J: Genetic and environmental contributions to the variance of the body mass index in a Norwegian sample of first- and second-degree relatives. Am J Hum Biol 1991; 3:257–267.
Tate DF, Wing RR, Winett RA: Using Internet technology to deliver a behavioral weight loss program. JAMA 2001; 285:1172–1177.
Thompson DB, Ravussin E, Bennett PH, Bogardus C: Structure and sequence variation at the human leptin receptor gene in lean and obese Pima Indians. Hum Mol Genet 1997; 6:675–679.
Tiret L, Andre JL, Ducimetìre P, Herbeth B, Rakotovao R, Guegen R, Spyckerelle Y, Cambien F: Segregation analysis of height-adjusted weight with generation- and age-dependent effects: the Nancy Family Study. Genet Epidemiol 1992; 6:389–403.
Tokunaga K, Matsuzawa Y, Kotani K, Keno Y, Kobatake T, Fujioka S, Tarui S: Ideal body weight estimated from the body mass index with the lowest morbidity. Int J Obes 1991; 15:1–5.
Tuomilehto J, Lindstrom J, Eriksson JG, Valle TT, Hamalainen H, Ilanne-Parikka P, Keinanen-Kiukaanniemi S, Laakso M, Louheranta A, Rastas M, et al.: Prevention of type 2 diabetes mellitus by changes in lifestyle among subjects with impaired glucose tolerance. N Engl J Med 2001; 344:1343–1350.
U.S. Department of Health and Human Services. Physical activity and health: A report of the Surgeon General. Atlanta, GA: U.S. Department of Health and Human Services, Centers for Disease Control and Prevention, National Center for Chronic Disease Prevention and Health Promotion, 1996.
Vague J: Degree of masculine differentiation of obesities: factor determining predisposition to diabetes, atherosclerosis, gout, and uric calculous disease. Am J Clin Nutr 1956; 4:20–34.
Vaisse C, Clement K, Durand E, Hercberg S, Guy-Grand B, Froguel P: Melanocortin-4 receptor mutations are a frequent and heterogeneous cause of morbid obesity. J Clin Invest 2000; 106:253–262.
Vidal Puig A, Solanes G, Grujic D, Flier JS, Lowell BB: UCP3: an uncoupling protein homologue expressed preferentially and abundantly in skeletal muscle and brown adipose tissue. Biochem Biophys Res Commun 1997; 235:79–82.
Vijayaraghavan S, Hitman GA, Kopelman PG: Apolipoprotein-D polymorphism: a genetic marker for obesity and hyperinsulinemia. J Clin Endocrinol Metab 1994; 79:568–570.
Vogler GP, Sorensen TIA, Stunkard AJ, Srinivasan MR, Rao DC: Influences of genes and shared family environment on adult body mass index assessed in an adoption study by a comprehensive path model. Int J Obes 1995; 19:40–45.
Vohl MC, Lamarche B, Moorjani S, Prudhomme D, Nadeau A, Bouchard C, Lupien PJ, Despres JP: The lipoprotein lipase HindIII polymorphism modulates plasma triglyceride levels in visceral obesity. Arterioscler Thromb Vasc Biol 1995; 15:714–720.
Waaler HT: Height, weight and mortality: the Norwegian experience. Acta Med Scand 1984; 679:1–56.
Weaver JU, Kopelman PG, Hitman GA: Central obesity and hyperinsulinemia in women are associated with polymorphism in the 5′ flanking region of the human insulin gene. Eur J Clin Invest 1992; 22:265–270.
Welle S, Forbes GB, Statt M, Barnard RR, Amatruda JM: Energy expenditure under free-living conditions in normal-weight and overweight women. Am J Clin Nutr 1992; 55:14–21.
Whitaker RC, Wright JA, Pepe MS, Seidel KD, Dietz WH: Predicting obesity in young adulthood from childhood and parental obesity. N Engl J Med 1997; 337:869–873.
Widen E, Lehto M, Kanninen T, Walston J, Shuldiner AR, Groop LC: Association of a polymorphism in the $beta_3$-adrenergic-receptor gene with features of the insulin resistance syndrome in Finns. N Engl J Med 1995; 333:348–351.
Williamson DF, Madans J, Anda RF, Kleinman JC, Kahn HS, Byers T: Recreational physical activity and ten-year weight change in a US national cohort. Int J Obes Relat Metab Disord 1993; 17:279–286.
Williamson DF, Pamuk E, Thun M, Flanders D, Byers T, Heath C: Prospective study of intentional weight loss and mortality in never smoking overweight white women aged 40 to 64 years. Am J Epidemiol 1995; 141:1128–1141.
Wilson BD, Ollman MM, Kang L, Stoffel M, Bell GI, Barsh GS: Structure and function of ASP, the human homolog of the mouse agouti protein. Hum Mol Genet 1996; 4:223–230.
Wing R: Behavioral approaches to the treatment of obesity. In: Bray GA, Bouchard C, James WPT (eds). Handbook of Obesity. New York: Marcel Dekker, 1998:855–873.
Wing RR, Jeffery RW, Burton LR, Thorson C, Nissinoff KS, Baxter JE: Food provision vs structured meal plans in the behavioral treatment of obesity. Int J Obes Relat Metab Disord 1996; 20:56–62.
Wirth A, Krause J: Long-term weight loss with sibutramine: a randomized controlled trial. JAMA 2001; 286:1331–1339.
Woo R, Daniels-Kush R, Horton ES: Regulation of energy balance. Annu Rev Nutr 1985a; 5:411–433.
Woo R, Garrow JS, Pi-Sunyer FX: Effect of exercise on spontaneous calorie intake in obesity. Am J Clin Nutr 1985b; 36:470–477.
World Health Organization: Obesity—Preventing and Managing the Global Epidemic. Report of a WHO Consultation on Obesity. Geneva: World Health Organization, 1998.
Xu W, Reed DR, Ding Y, Price RA: Absence of linkage between human obesity and the mouse *Agouti* homologous region (20q11.2) or other markers spanning chromosome 20q. Obes Res 1995; 3:559–562.
Yamada K, Yuan X, Ishiyama S, Koyama K, Ichikawa F, Koyanagi A, Koyama W, Nonaka K: Association between $Ala^{54}Thr$ substitution of the fatty acid-binding protein 2 gene with insulin resistance and intra-abdominal fat thickness in Japanese men. Diabetologia 1997; 40:706–710.
Zee RYL, Griffiths LR, Moris BJ: Marked association of a RFLP for the low density lipoprotein receptor gene with obesity in essential hypertensives. Biochem Biophys Res Commun 1992; 189:965–971.
Zee RYL, Lou YK, Morris BJ: Insertion variant in intron 9, but not microsatellite in intron 2, of the insulin receptor gene is associated with essential hypertension. J Hypertens 1994; 12:S13–S22.
Zee RYL, Schrader AP, Robinson BG, Griffiths LR, Morris BJ: Association of HincII of low density lipoprotein receptor gene with obesity in essential hypertensives. Clin Genet 1995; 47:118–121.
Zhang Y, Proenca R, Maffei M, Barone M, Leopold L, Friedman M: Positional cloning of the mouse obese gene and its human homologue. Nature 1994; 372:425–432.
Zonta LA, Jayakar SD, Bosisio M, Galante A, Pennetti V: Genetic analysis of human obesity in an Italian sample. Hum Hered 1987; 37:129–139.
Zurlo F, Lillioja S, Esposito-Del Puente A, Nyomba BL, Raz I, Saad MF, Swinburn BA, Knowler WC, Bogardus C, Ravussin E: Low ratio of fat to carbohydrate oxidation as predictor of weight gain: study of 24-h RQ. Am J Physiol 1990; 259:E650–E657.

24 Genetics of Osteoporosis

TATIANA FOROUD, MICHAEL J. ECONS, AND C. CONRAD JOHNSTON, JR.

DISEASE DEFINITION

Osteoporosis is an important disorder, producing disability and excess mortality through the development of fractures. It has been defined as a disease characterized by low bone mass and microarchitectural deterioration of bone tissue, leading to enhanced bone fragility and a consequent increase in fracture risk (Consensus Development Conference, 1991). This definition is not quantitative, and it is thus difficult to use clinically. Since bone mass can be measured and it is an important determinant of fracture risk, the World Health Organization has defined the disorder related to measurement of bone mass. The diagnostic categories are as follows:

1. *Normal:* a value for bone mineral density (BMD) or bone mineral content (BMC) that is not more than 1 standard deviation (SD) below the young adult mean value.
2. *Low bone mass (or osteopenia):* a value for BMD or BMC that lies between 1 and 2.5 SD below the young adult mean value.
3. *Osteoporosis:* a value for BMD or BMC that is more than 2.5 SD below the young adult mean value.
4. *Severe osteoporosis (or established osteoporosis):* a value for BMD or BMC more than 2.5 SD below the young adult mean value in the presence of one or more fragility fractures (Kanis et al., 1994).

GENERAL GENETIC AND EPIDEMIOLOGIC EVIDENCE

Clinical Epidemiology

As noted above, osteoporosis is currently defined by low bone mass and the resulting increased risk of fracture. In the United States alone, up to 54% of postmenopausal white women, about 17 million women, have low bone mass and another 20% to 30%, or 6 to 9 million, have osteoporosis (Melton et al., 1992; Melton, 1995; Looker et al., 1997). The strongest predictors of low bone mass are age, gender, and race. Bone mass decreases with age, particularly among postmenopausal women. Blacks have the highest bone mass and whites the lowest (Liel et al., 1988; DiSimone et al., 1989). Men have a larger skeleton, and thus, greater bone mass than women (Geusens et al., 1986; Bevier et al., 1989). As a result, the risk of osteoporosis is greatest among elderly white women and less among white males and blacks of both genders.

Family Epidemiology

Family Studies

Numerous family studies have demonstrated significant familial correlation for BMD. An early study in a series of mother–daughter pairs estimated the heritability of radial BMC to be 72% (Lutz, 1986). Sowers et al. (1992), using a group of premenopausal sisters, estimated that genes account for 67% of the variability in femoral neck, 58% of the variability in Ward's triangle, and 45% of the variability in trochanter. A two-generation study of parents and their male and female offspring (Krall and Dawson-Hughes, 1993) reported heritability estimates of 45% to 60% for various bone sites. Consistent heritability estimates were obtained using both sibling and parent–offspring correlations. After adjusting for significant lifestyle variables, such as calcium intake, alcohol intake, and smoking, heritability estimates of 60% for total body, 47% for radius, 56% for os calcis, 62% for femoral neck, and 46% for spine were reported. Similar findings were reported by Jouanny and colleagues (1995), who found significant correlation between the BMD of children over 15 and their parents ($r = 0.27$, $p < 0.0001$). Offspring had a 4.3-fold higher risk of low BMD if one parent had low BMD and an 8.63-fold higher risk when both parents had low BMD.

Several studies have also documented lower BMD among individuals with a positive family history of osteoporosis (Evans et al., 1988; Seeman et al., 1989, 1994; Danielson et al., 1999; Rubin et al., 1999). A comparison of premenopausal daughters of women with and without osteoporosis compression fractures found that the daughters of women with osteoporosis had 7% (approximately 0.5–1 SD change) lower BMC at the lumbar spine ($p = 0.03$) compared to the daughters of women without postmenopausal osteoporosis (Seeman et al., 1989). There were also suggestive differences at the femoral neck (5% reduction, $p = 0.07$) and femoral midshaft (3% reduction, $p = 0.15$). In a second study, Seemen et al. (1994) compared the daughters of women with and without hip fractures and found that women whose mother had a hip fracture had lower BMD at the femoral neck ($p < 0.05$) and femoral shaft ($p < 0.001$) compared to women without a positive family history. However, they were unable to detect reduction at the lumbar spine (Seeman et al., 1994). Danielson et al. (1999) found higher heritability (h^2) estimates for BMD at the hip, spine, and calcaneus for premenopausal daughters ($0.50 < h^2 < 0.63$) compared to postmenopausal daughters (all $h^2 < 0.53$).

Lower BMD has also been found among elderly subjects with a positive family history of osteoporosis. A study in an elderly (60–89 years) population of both white men and women found that individuals with a positive family history of osteoporosis had lower BMD than those with a negative family history (Soroko et al., 1994). In particular, there was a stepwise decrease in BMD as the number of family members with a positive history of osteoporosis increased. Among men, a maternal history of osteoporosis was associated with lower hip BMD while positive paternal history was associated with lower spine BMD. Among women, only a positive paternal history of osteoporosis was associated with specific reductions in BMD levels at the spine and hip. These findings were confirmed in a large study of white women 65 years of age or older. In this sample, a maternal history of hip fracture doubled the risk of hip fracture, even after adjustment for bone density (Cummings et al., 1995).

Due to the strong effect of age on BMD, most studies have compared adult family members to establish the familiality of bone density measures. However, in a study of children between the ages of 5 and 20, significant correlation between parent and child BMD values was observed, with a father–child correlation of 83% and a mother–child correlation of 58% (Lonzer et al., 1996). Ferrari et al. (1998) estimated the heritability due to maternal descent only as one-half of the total heritability (0.5 h^2). In this sample of prepubertal girls, all under the age of 12, a series of BMC variables were measured. For the lumbar spine, femoral neck, and midfemoral diaphysis, estimates of heritability due to maternal descent (0.5 h^2) ranged from 18% to 37%. These significant parent–offspring correlations suggest that heredity influences bone density even in children who have not yet attained peak bone density.

Cardon et al. (2000) reported on eight families ascertained through a proband under the age of 35 years with a history of two or more fractures and spinal BMD at least 2.5 SD below the mean for age and gender. Formal segregation analysis performed for the spinal BMD phenotype in these families was consistent with a major gene having codominant inheritance.

Twin Studies

Bone Density. Twin studies have consistently demonstrated a significant genetic contribution to bone density. An early twin study examining a series of black and white, juvenile twins of both sexes identified significant heritability of both radial bone mass and bone width, with heritability estimates of 75% and 77%, respectively (Smith et al., 1973). A subsequent juvenile twin study (Dequeker et al., 1987) also found a significant, albeit lower, estimate of heritability (47%) for cortical bone (radius); however, the spine BMC heritability estimate was 88%.

The results of the early twin studies by Smith et al. (1973) were confirmed by Moller and colleagues (1978) in elderly male and female patients. In this sample, heritability for metacarpal total width was 77% and that for cortical width was 78%. Further evidence of significant BMD heritability was obtained in pre- and postmenopausal women as well as men (Pocock et al., 1987); significant heritability estimates were obtained for lumbar spine (92%), femoral neck (73%), Ward's triangle (85%), and trochanter (57%) BMD, with suggestive evidence of heritability from forearm BMC (42%).

Slemenda et al. (1991), in a sample of 171 female sibling pairs with a wide age range (25–80 years), found significant heritability estimates for radius BMC (52%) and BMD (70%) and for L2–L4 ($h^2 > 100\%$), femoral neck (88%), Ward's triangle (84%), and trochanter ($h^2 > 100\%$) BMD. The authors noted that the heritability estimates may be inflated due to failure of the assumption of no gene interactions. They suggested that the consistent evidence across several studies (Slemenda et al., 1991; Pocock et al., 1987) of extremely high heritability values may instead support interactions among a relatively small number of genes.

A large sample of 500 postmenopausal female twin pairs, aged 50 to 70 years, was used to confirm the heritability of numerous bone density measurements (Arden et al., 1996). Consistent significant heritability estimates were obtained over several sites, including the lumbar spine (78%), total hip (67%), femoral neck (84%), Ward's triangle (51%), distal forearm (61%), mid-forearm (46%), and whole body (76%).

Smith et al. (1973) also examined a series of adult male twins and found substantially lower heritability for bone mass (49%) and bone width (45%) compared to the juvenile sample. Higher heritability estimates were obtained in a second sample of adult male twins (Dequeker et al., 1987), in which the cortical bone BMC heritability estimate was 75%.

Bone Loss. Smith et al. (1973) utilized only white adult males and found a significant genetic contribution to midshaft bone mass and width. A follow-up study of a subset of this cohort continued to find strong genetic effects on midshaft radial width; however, there was no evidence of a genetic effect on bone loss over the 16-year interval between examinations, suggesting that environmental factors, rather than genes, have greater influence on the rate of bone loss with aging (Christian et al., 1989). A later study (Slemenda et al., 1992) in a large sample of older males (average age 63 years) confirmed the more prominent role of environment, rather than genetics, in bone loss. In that study, a statistically significant, but very similar, intraclass correlation for bone loss in both monozygotic and dizygotic twins was observed, suggesting a significant role of common environment, especially smoking and alcohol consumption, on bone loss. Contradictory evidence was obtained in a study of male and female twins with a wide age range (Kelly et al., 1993). In this sample, evidence of a genetic effect on rates of change in the lumbar spine and Ward's triangle was demonstrated, although there did not appear to be a significant genetic effect on changes in the femoral neck.

Summary of Genetic Studies

In summary, numerous studies have documented the substantial genetic contribution to BMD and peak BMD. However, genetic effects on the rate of bone loss have not been convincingly demonstrated. For these reasons, many studies seeking to identify genes underlying osteoporosis have relied primarily on BMD and, in many cases, on peak BMD, which appears to be the most heritable correlated phenotype.

PATHOPHYSIOLOGY: BIOLOGIC BASIS OF GENETIC SUSCEPTIBILITY

Few studies have evaluated the role of genetics on markers of bone formation and bone resorption. An initial study evaluated a sample of 140 pre- and post-menopausal female twin pairs for markers of bone formation (serum osteocalcin) and bone resorption (fasting urinary calcium:creatinine ratio and hydroxyproline:creatinine ratio). In this study, only the bone formation marker osteocalcin had a significant genetic contribution (80%) to trait variability (Kelly et al., 1991). These results were further examined using assays to detect circulating products of both type I collagen synthesis and degradation (Tokita et al., 1994). A significant correlation between serum osteocalcin and carboxy-terminal propeptide of type I procollagen (PICP) was found, and in concordance with the results of Kelly et al. (1991), genetic factors were estimated to account for 95% of the variance in serum PICP levels. PICP is cleaved extracellularly from the carboxyl terminus of procollagen, and its circulating levels are correlated with the bone collagen synthesis rate and osteoblast activity. Pyridinoline cross-linked carboxyl-terminal telopeptide of type I collagen, which is cleaved during the degradation of type I collagen, was not correlated with serum osteocalcin levels; however, the genetic contribution to the serum levels was estimated to be 64%.

In another sample of only postmenopausal twin pairs, markers of bone formation and resorption were examined to identify those with evidence of genetic effects (Garnero et al., 1996a). The three markers of bone formation, osteocalcin, PICP, and serum bone-specific alkaline phosphatase (BAP), had higher correlation among monozygotic compared to dizygotic twin pairs, although significant genetic effects were found only for PICP (99%) and BAP (64%). Among the four markers of bone resorption examined, free D-pyridinoline, total D-pyridinoline, urinary type I C-telopeptide breakdown products, and urinary type I collagen cross-linked N-telopeptide (NTX), the monozygotic twin correlation was significantly higher than the dizygotic twin correlation for free D-pyridinoline and NTX; however, significant heritability was found only for free D-pyridinoline (86%). Thus, the results of this second study do not confirm a significant genetic role for osteocalcin; however, serum PICP remained significantly heritable in both studies. Other findings found in one or the other study include significant heritability of BAP and free D-pyridinoline. The apparent inconsistency of findings from one study to the other may be due to the inherent technical difficulties and variability related to biochemical marker assays.

While twins have been examined most commonly to estimate the heritability of biochemical markers of bone turnover, Livshits et al. (2000) examined a sample of nuclear families from the Chuvasa region of the former Soviet Union and found that about 50% of the variation in PICP was attributable to genetic factors and about 40% of the variation in osteocalcin to genetic effects. Thus, a significant genetic contribution to PICP has been consistently reported; however, the apparent inconsistency of findings from one study to the other among the other biochemical measures may be due to the inherent technical difficulties and variability related to biochemical marker assays.

GENE IDENTIFICATION

Linkage and Association

High Bone Mass Family

One approach to identify genes for bone density is through families segregating apparently Mendelian forms of abnormal bone density. In one such family, extremely high bone density (the converse of osteoporosis) appeared to segregate as an autosomal dominant disorder (Johnson et al., 1997; Recker et al., 1998). Affected individuals in this family had spine BMD measurements greater than 3 SD above the mean without evidence of osteopetrosis or other osteosclerotic bone disorders. Affected individuals did not have clinical sequellae, and the proband was identified fortuitously when high bone mass was noted following X-rays related to a car accident. The family has been extended and now includes 22 individuals, 12 of whom have the high BMD phenotype. Using a genome screen approach, linkage to chromosome 11q12–13 was identified with a lod score of 5.74. Recently, these investigators have reported an amino acid change in the low density lipoprotein receptor-related protein 5 (LRP5) results in the high bone mass phenotype. The G-to-T transversion in exon 3 of the *LRP5* gene results in a glycine-to-valine amino acid change (G171V) (Little et al., 2002). This amino acid is evolutionarily conserved and appears to alter the local hydrophobic environment at the surface of the protein. This mutation was only observed in affected members of the high bone mass family and was not observed in over 1000 individuals from the general population who were screened. Interestingly, mutations in this same gene have also been found to produce the autosomal recessive disorder, osteoporosis pseudoglioma (Gong et al., 2001). A wide variety of mutations leading to LRP5 inactivation lead to this phenotype, which is characterized by very low bone mass and eye abnormalities. Carriers of mutations in *LRP5* also have reduced bone mass. LRP5 is believed to have its action on bone density through the Wnt signaling, which is a key pathway involved in various developmental processes, including skeletal differentiation. Thus, these two Mendelian disorders, with widely differing phenotypes, both are the result of changes in the same gene, with the osteoporosis pseudoglioma mutations resulting in protein inactivation while the high bone mass mutation is likely activating. A locus for autosomal recessive osteopetrosis (Heaney et al., 1997) has also been linked to this same region.

Low Bone Mass Families

A series of families with multiple members having osteopenia has been used to evaluate candidate genes for osteoporosis (Spotila et al., 1996) as well as to identify novel genetic linkage regions (Devoto et al., 1998). Ascertained through a proband with low bone density, seven families having a total of 37 members with osteopenia (corrected spinal Z-scores < -2.0) have been identified. Commingling analysis suggested that spinal BMD Z-scores had a bimodal distribution, consistent with an autosomal dominant mode of transmission. Parametric lod score linkage analysis was performed in these families to evaluate three candidate genes: *COL1A1*, *COL1A2*, and *vitamin D receptor* (*VDR*). Using an autosomal dominant model for the spine BMD inheritance, with the allele predisposing for low BMD having a frequency of 0.01, linkage to all three candidate genes was excluded, with lod scores below -2.0 (Spotila et al., 1996). Subsequently, parametric and nonparametric linkage analyses were performed in these seven families using data from a genome screen (Devoto et al., 1998). The maximum parametric lod score ($Z_{max} = 2.08, \theta = 0.05$) was obtained on chromosome 11q22–23 with the marker CD3D. Nonparametric sibling pair linkage analysis using 74 independent sibling pairs derived from these same seven families supported linkage to chromosome 1p36 with a maximum lod score of 3.51 at D1S450 (multipoint lod score = 2.29), chromosome 2p23–24 with a maximum lod score of 2.07 at D2S149 (multipoint lod score = 2.25), and chromosome 4qter with a maximum lod score of 2.95 at D4S1539. Extension of the study to include an additional 67 sibling pairs, each having at least one member with BMD values more than 2 SD below the norm, has increased the multipoint lod score on chromosome 1 to 3.01 (Spotila et al., 1998).

Sibling Pair Approach

Few large studies have been undertaken to identify novel genes underlying the risk for osteoporosis. Koller et al. (1998) reported linkage to chromosome 11q12–13, a region which was examined for linkage to peak BMD following the report of linkage of three Mendelian BMD-related phenotypes, autosomal dominant high bone mass (see above), autosomal recessive osteoporosis-pseudoglioma, and autosomal recessive osteopetrosis, to this chromosomal location. In the sample of 835 premenopausal Caucasian and African-American sisters, nonparametric linkage analysis supported a gene underlying peak BMD, with a maximum lod score of 3.5 for femoral neck BMD. When the two races were analyzed separately, the Caucasian sample (364 independent sibling pairs) obtained a maximum lod score of 2.78 while the African-American sisters (97 independent sibling pairs) had a maximum lod score of 1.52.

Subsequently, a 10 cM autosomal genome screen was completed in an initial sample of 429 Caucasian sister pairs (Koller et al., 2000). Multipoint nonparametric linkage analysis identified six chromosomal regions with lod scores above 1.85 in the genome screen sample; however, only the linkage findings on chromosomes 1, 5, 6, and 22 were at or near a marker locus and, therefore, pursued further in an expanded sample of 595 sister pairs (464 Caucasian, 131 African-American). The 11q region had already been pursued by genotyping an expanded sample of Caucasian and African-American sister pairs (Koller et al., 1998).

The results on chromosome 1q were the most promising of the genome screen. The initial genome screen resulted in a lod score of 3.11, which increased to 4.86 when additional Caucasian and African-American sister pairs were included in the analysis. Interestingly, this is not the same region of chromosome 1 reported by Devoto et al. (1998) in a genome screen employing pedigrees ascertained on the basis of an osteoporotic proband.

Evidence of linkage to chromosome 5p also increased with the inclusion of additional Caucasian and African-American sibling pairs, from a genome screen lod score of 1.9 to 2.2 after all available individuals were included in the analysis. Linkage to chromosome 6p was not substantially increased following the inclusion of additional Caucasian and African-American sibling pairs. However, when only Caucasian sister pairs were included in the analysis, the maximum lod score was 2.1. Finally, the initial evidence of linkage to chromosome 22 decreased substantially with the inclusion of additional sibling pairs, suggesting that the initial linkage result was likely spurious. These linkage findings provide substantial evidence that genetic loci influencing the highly heritable BMD phenotypes can be detected. These genetic studies have been completed in less than half of the final sample and suggest that samples of this size can be used to identify chromosomal regions in which to pursue high-density genotyping.

Niu et al. (1999) performed a genomewide screen for linkage to BMD in 153 sib pairs who were originally identified as extreme for blood pressure values. Using proximal forearm BMD, they obtained a peak lod score of 2.15 over a very large region (>50 cM) on chromosome 2. This large region of chromosome 2 appears to include the region previously identified by Spotila et al. (1998) using families ascertained through an individual with low BMD.

Animal Studies

The use of animal models with similar or related behaviors will likely provide important genetic clues that will improve the efficiency of identifying genes underlying peak bone density and osteoporosis. Genetic studies in a large baboon colony have identified a quantitative trait locus on chromosome 11 that influences BMD (Mahaney et al., 1997). This is the same chromosomal region identified in the high bone density family (Johnson et al., 1997) as well as in the sample of premenopausal sisters (Koller et al., 1998). In addition, the syntenic region on mouse chromosome 7 was identified in whole-body BMC studies of recombinant inbred mouse (Klein et al., 1998). The mouse studies identified additional quantitative trait loci that affect peak bone density on mouse chromosomes 1, 2, 7, 11, 14, 15, 16, 18, and 19.

Candidate Gene Studies

Vitamin D Receptor

Due to its important role in the regulation of calcium homeostasis, *VDR* was one of the first candidate genes evaluated for its role in peak bone density. Using twin pairs, Morrison et al. (1994) reported both linkage and association between a 3′-untranslated region (UTR) polymorphism in the *VDR* and spine BMD. Initial results suggested that the *B* allele, defined by absence of a Bsm-1 restriction site in the 3′-UTR, was associated with lower bone density and that the *VDR* locus might contribute as much as 75% to 80% of the variability in peak bone density, which would account for most, if not all, of the genetic contribution to BMD. In a series of over 300 unrelated healthy women, the majority of whom were postmenopausal, an association between *VDR* and lumbar spine and femoral neck BMD was observed. Among women with BMD values 2 SD below the mean, there was an overrepresentation of the *BB* genotype. Subsequently, the linkage data, although not the population association results, have been retracted (Morrison et al., 1997).

Prior to the recent partial retraction, numerous studies in a variety of age groups were undertaken to evaluate the role of this 3′-UTR *VDR* polymorphism on bone density and risk for osteoporosis. Work using an independent sample of premenopausal twin pairs (Hustmyer et al., 1994; Peacock et al., 1995) did not find any evidence to support the association between *VDR* and BMD. Conflicting results have been reported from a number of studies (Melhus et al., 1994; Yamagata et al., 1994; Looney et al., 1995; Spector et al., 1995; Krall et al., 1995; Fleet et al., 1995; Riggs et al., 1995; Garnero et al., 1995, 1996b; Harris et al., 1997; Gennari et al., 1998), although even those which were positive did not observe the magnitude of genetic effect reported initially by Morrison et al. (1994). In fact, three reports have found the reverse association to that initially reported (i.e., the *b* allele was associated with lower BMD). A recent meta-analysis (Cooper et al., 1996) of data from 16 studies found no significant association between the *VDR* locus and bone density when the twin data of Morrison et al. (1997), which was subsequently retracted (Morrison et al., 1997), were excluded from the analysis.

The *VDR* sequence, as originally reported by Baker et al. (1988), contains two ATG (methionine) sequences in the first four amino acids. A C/T polymorphism exists in the first potential ATG. Individuals with the T polymorphism start translation at the first methionine, while those with the C polymorphism start translation at the second site, resulting in a VDR protein that is three amino acids shorter. In light of the possibility that this polymorphism could lead to functional consequences (i.e., it is possible that one form of the VDR might be translated more easily or be more stable in vivo than the other form), Gross et al. (1996) performed an association study between this polymorphism and BMD in a population of Mexican-American women. They found that individuals homozygous for the longer VDR protein (genotype *ff*) had significantly lower spine BMD than individuals homozygous for the shorter VDR protein (genotype *FF*). Heterozygous individuals (genotype *Ff*) had intermediate spine BMD. A similar association was not observed in the same sample using femoral neck or forearm BMD. Association of BMD with the C/T polymorphism was not detected in a sample of premenopausal French women (Eccleshall et al., 1998). A large sample of 535 Caucasian and African-American sister pairs, which employed the start site polymorphism, did not find any evidence of linkage or association between *VDR* and BMD (Econs et al., 1998).

Collagen Type I αI Gene

Abnormalities in type I collagen have been shown to result in osteogenesis imperfecta, and mutations in the *COL1A1* and *COL1A2* genes, which encode the type I collagen proteins, have been documented in patients with osteogenesis imperfecta. As a result, more subtle polymorphisms in *COL1A1* and *COL1A2* were hypothesized to account, in part, for the genetic effects on BMD (Prockop et al., 1989; Spotila et al., 1991).

Some studies of the regulatory region of *COL1A1* have supported an association with bone mass (Grant et al., 1996; Uitterlinden et al., 1998). In two samples of white women, one from Aberdeen and the other from London, the majority of whom were postmenopausal, a common polymorphism was identified that results in a G → T substitution at the first base of a consensus site for the transcription factor Sp1 in the first intron of *COL1A1* (Grant et al., 1996). A subset of women from both samples having vertebral compression fracture was compared to age- and sex-matched control samples and those with fracture had a significant over-representation of the heterozygous and homozygous substitution genotypes. In both samples, spine BMD values were significantly higher in women homozygous for the wild-type allele (genotype *SS*) compared to women who were heterozygous (genotype *Ss*). However, in the Aberdeen sample only, there was significant evidence of a gene–dosage effect, with women homozygous for the substitution (genotype *ss*) having still lower spine BMD values. Results for hip BMD were not conclusive, although in the Aberdeen sample a similar trend was observed with an apparent association of higher BMD values with the *SS* genotype.

The association between *COL1A1* and BMD has been confirmed in another sample (Uitterlinden et al., 1998). A gene–dosage effect was observed at both the femoral neck and lumbar spine, with *SS* individuals having the highest BMD values, those with the *Ss* genotype having intermediate BMD values, and *ss* individuals having the lowest. Similar to the UK studies, incident nonvertebral fractures were also related in a dose-dependent fashion to the *COL1A1* genotype. Several other studies have reported similar findings (Langdahl et al., 1997c; Keen et al., 1997), while others have found much weaker evidence for association (Garnero et al., 1997; Haughton et al., 1998).

Similar to many reports of association between candidate genes and BMD, there have been a number of studies demonstrating no effect of the *COL1A1* Sp1 polymorphism on BMD (McLellan et al., 1997; Vandevyver et al., 1997; Hustmyer et al., 1997; Lim et al., 1997; Liden et al., 1998; Nogues et al., 1998; Heegaard et al., 1998; Jagger et al., 1998). Unfortunately, many of these negative reports have been published only in abstract form. However, they clearly demonstrate that there is not universal agreement among studies and that, in fact, the effect of the *COL1A1* Sp1 polymorphism, if present, is likely to be substantially less than originally estimated.

Estrogen Receptor

Decreased estrogen levels are associated with an increase in bone turnover and bone loss, while estrogen replacement therapy ameliorates loss of bone. Therefore, the estrogen receptor is a reasonable candidate gene for osteoporosis. Kobayashi et al. (1996), in a sample of postmenopausal Japanese women, found an association of a particular estrogen receptor haplotype with bone density. In particular, absence of a PvuII polymorphism (denoted P) and presence of an XbaI polymorphism (denoted x) on both chromosomes (denoted PPxx) was found to be associated with significantly lower lumbar spine and total-body BMD compared to all other observed genotypes at these two loci. Some studies appear to confirm an association of the estrogen receptor with BMD (Sowers et al., 1997; Huang et al., 1998), although the nature of the association is not consistent with the particular estrogen receptor haplotype initially reported nor with the absence or presence of the two initially reported polymorphisms (Nelson et al., 1997; Mahonen et al., 1997; Langdahl et al., 1997b; Sikic-Klisovic et al., 1998; Becherini et al., 1998; Zmuda et al., 1998). In a series of other studies, investigators have not replicated any association between the estrogen receptor and BMD (Jorgensen et al., 1997; Han et al., 1997a; Kindmark et al., 1998).

Other Candidate Genes

While several candidate genes have received the bulk of the attention of the osteoporosis research community, several other candidate genes have also been associated with BMD. For example, there has been a report of an association of an *interleukin-6* gene polymorphism with BMD (Murray et al., 1997). A 1-base deletion in the intron sequence eight bases prior to exon 5 (termed 713–8delC) has been associated with very low bone mass in osteoporotic women and with increased bone turnover in both osteoporotic and normal women (Langdahl et al., 1997a).

Clinical Application and Risk Assessment of Genetic Information

In light of the fact that specific genes that predispose to osteoporosis have yet to be identified, it is not currently possible to perform genetic testing for diagnosis or therapy of the disease. However, there are serious shortcomings in current strategies for the diagnosis and therapy of osteoporosis. Identification of genes that predispose to osteoporosis will provide numerous opportunities to influence screening, diagnosis, and therapy. How this will happen is, of course, dependent on the number of genes that influence the propensity to osteoporosis and their normal role in physiology. However, some benefits (and challenges) can already be anticipated from our current state of knowledge. Our discussion assumes that although many genes likely influence the predisposition to osteoporosis, only a limited number of genes play important roles in osteoporosis.

Diagnosis

Currently, diagnosis of osteoporosis is greatly dependent on assessing BMD and other risk factors for fracture. Discovery of genes that play important roles in determining peak bone mass, rates of bone loss, and bone microarchitecture (i.e., trabecular thickness, number) may allow clinicians to divide the currently large population of osteoporosis patients on the basis of pathophysiology. This may have important implications for therapy since patients who have osteoporosis based on different pathophysiologies may respond differently to various therapies. Additionally, genetic studies may allow early identification of patients at high risk for osteoporosis when preventive measures, such as optimizing intake of calcium and vitamin D, may be more effective than later in the course of the disease.

The prospect of early preventive strategies for this common disease raises the issue of genetic screening. In general, several conditions must be met for a screening test to be useful (Eddy, 1991): *(1)* the prevalence of the disease must be high in the screened population; *(2)* the test must be acceptable to the population screened; *(3)* there is an accepted therapeutic intervention, and early intervention improves outcome; *(4)* the cost of screening is acceptable; *(5)* the sensitivity and specificity of the test are sufficient to identify an acceptable percentage of affected individuals and to minimize the number of nondiseased individuals who are falsely identified and; *(6)* the risk of the test is acceptable. Clearly, osteoporosis is a common disease with a high prevalence, at least in postmenopausal Caucasian and Asian women. Conditions *2* through *5* are dependent on the type of genetic test employed. Although the physical risk of phlebotomy (or buccal smear) to obtain DNA is minimal, there is a risk of psychological harm in any genetic test. Patients need to be properly informed of all potential risks and benefits before screening is initiated.

For any genetic screening test for osteoporosis to be useful it must not only meet the above criteria but also be a better screening test than measurement of BMD. While current guidelines (Johnston et al., 1998) do not specifically use the term *screening*, BMD testing is recommended for all Caucasian women over the age of 65 and for all postmenopausal Caucasian women with additional risk factors regardless of age. Thus, densitometry is, in essence, already being used as a screening test. While the most cost-effective strategy has not been determined, BMD testing poses minimal risk but at a cost (approximately $30 for a peripheral measurement and $130 for a central measurement). For any potential genetic test to be useful it must outperform BMD testing on either a cost or a quality basis. Costs for genetic testing could be minimized if a limited number of functional polymorphisms could be tested in an automated fashion. However, it is unlikely that costs would be substantially below that of peripheral densitometry. Genetic tests might be more predictive of fracture than BMD if they provided information about risk factors other than BMD, such as trabecular microarchitecture, which is not available by other means. In any event, evidence that genetic tests are better than BMD testing would have to be obtained empirically.

Perhaps the most important application of the discovery of genes that influence predisposition to osteoporosis is the potential effects on therapy. There are two potential mechanisms by which identification of these genes could have major effects on therapy: pharmacogenetics and identification of molecular targets/pathways. While much of the current emphasis in pharmacogenetics is on using genotypic information to determine if the patient will have an adverse affect from a particular drug, pharmacogenetics will eventually allow clinicians to use genetic information to choose the best therapy for a particular individual. As noted above, patients who have osteoporosis based on different pathophysiologies may respond differently to various therapies. Currently, clinicians choose a therapy, use it for 2 years, and re-evaluate BMD to determine if the therapy increased BMD. If genetic testing allowed the clinician to determine which therapy would be most efficacious for a particular patient, therapy could be initiated with the most efficacious agent without delay or subjecting the patient to the side effects of a therapy that will not work.

In addition to pharmacogenetics, the discovery of genes that influence BMD and predisposition to osteoporosis will provide molecular targets for pharmacologic intervention. This is particularly important in osteoporosis since all currently approved therapies target osteoclastic bone resorption. Ideally, therapy should stimulate bone formation to replace lost bone, instead of simply preventing further loss. It is likely that some of the genes that influence predisposition to osteoporosis will have major effects on osteoblast regulation or function. Identification of these genes and the pathways that they regulate will provide opportunities to develop agents that increase osteoblast function. Discovery of a new class of pharmacologic agents that increase osteoblast activity and/or promote de novo bone formation could lead to curative therapy for osteoporosis.

ACKNOWLEDGMENTS

We gratefully acknowledge the support from Public Health Service grants P01 AG05793, P01 AG18397, K24AR02095, and K02AA00285.

REFERENCES

Arden NK, Baker J, Hogg C, Baan K, Spector TD: The heritability of bone mineral density, ultrasound of the calcaneus and hip axis length: a study of postmenopausal twins. J Bone Miner Res 1996; 11:530–534.

Baker AR, McDonnell DP, Hughes M, Crisp TM, Mangelsdorf DJ, Haussler MR, Pike JW, Shine J, O'Malley BW: Cloning and expression of full-length cDNA encoding human vitamin D receptor. Proc Natl Acad Sci USA 1988; 85:3294–3298.

Becherini L, Gennari L, Mansani R, Masi L, Gonneli S, Colli E, Falchetti A, Morelli AM: *Estrogen receptor-α* gene polymorphisms and osteoporosis: a large scale study on postmenopausal women. [abstract]. Bone 1998; 23(Suppl):SS269.

Bevier WC, Wiswell RA, Pyka G, Kozak KC, Newhall KM, Marcus R: Relationship of body composition, muscle strength, and aerobic capacity to bone mineral density in older men and women. J Bone Miner Res 1989; 4:421–432.

Cardon LR, Garner C, Bennett ST, Mackay IJ, Edwards RM, Cornish J, Hegde M, Murray MAF, Reid IR, Cundy T: Evidence for a major gene for bone mineral density in idiopathic osteoporotic families. J Bone Miner Res 2000; 15:1132–1137.

Christian JC, Yu P-L, Slemenda CW, Johnston CC Jr: Heritability of bone mass: a longitudinal study in aging male twins. Am J Hum Genet 1989; 44:429–433.

Consensus Development Conference: Prophylaxis and treatment of osteoporosis. Am J Med 1991; 90:107–110.

Cooper GS, Umbach DM: Are vitamin D receptor polymorphisms associated with bone mineral density? A meta-analysis. J Bone Miner Res 1996; 11:1841–1849.

Cummings SR, Nevitt MC, Browner WS, Stone K, Fox KM, Ensrud KE, Cauley J, Black D, Vogt TM, Study of Osteoporotic Fractures Research Group: Risk factors for hip fractures in white women. N Engl J Med 1995; 332:767–773.

Danielson ME, Cauley JA, Baker CE, Newman EB, Dorman JS, Towers JD, Kuller LH: Familial resemblance of bone mineral density (BMD) and calcaneal ultrasound attenuation: the BMD in Mothers and Daughters Study. J Bone Miner Res 1999; 14:102–110.

Dequeker J, Nijs J, Verstraeten A, Geusens P, Gevers G: Genetic determinants of bone mineral content at the spine and radius: a twin study. Bone 1987; 8:207–209.

Devoto M, Shimoya K, Caminis J, Ott J, Tenenhouse A, Whyte MP, Sereda L, Hall S, Considine E, Williams CJ, et al.: First-stage autosomal genome screen in extended pedigrees suggests genes predisposing to low bone mineral density on chromosomes 1p, 2p and 4q. Eur J Hum Genet 1998; 6:151–157.

DiSimone DP, Stevens J, Edwards J, Shary J, Gordon L, Bell NH: Influence of body habitus and race on bone mineral density of the radius, hip, and spine in premenopausal women. J Bone Miner Res 1989; 4:827–830.

Eccleshall TR, Garnero P, Gross C, Delmas PD, Feldman D: Lack of correlation between start codon polymorphism of the vitamin D receptor gene and bone mineral density in premenopausal French women: the OFELY Study. J Bone Miner Res 1998; 13:31–35.

Econs MJ, Koller DL, Considine EL, Takacs I, Christian JC, Conneally PM, Peacock M, Johnston CC, Foroud T: Association and sib pair linkage analysis studies between BMD and the vitamin D receptor (VDR) [abstract]. Bone 1998; 23(Suppl):S271.

Eddy DM (ed): Common Screening Tests. Philadelphia: American College of Physicians, 1991.

Evans RA, Marel GM, Lancaster EK, Kos S, Evans M, Wong SYP: Bone mass is low in relatives of osteoporotic patients. Ann Intern Med 1988; 109:870–873.

Ferrari S, Rizzoli R, Slosman D, Bonjour J-P: Familial resemblance for bone mineral mass is expressed before puberty. J Clin Endocrinol Metab 1998; 83:358–361.

Fleet JC, Harris SS, Wood RJ, Dawson-Hughes B: The BSM I vitamin D receptor restriction fragment length polymorphism (BB) predicts low bone density in premenopausal black and white women. J Bone Miner Res 1995; 10:985–990.

Garnero P, Arden NK, Griffiths G, Delmas PD, Spector TD: Genetic influences on bone turnover in postmenopausal twins. J Clin Endocrinol Metab 1996a; 81:140–146.

Garnero P, Borel O, Grant SFA, Ralston SH, Delmas PD: Sp1 binding site polymorphism in the *collagen type I α1* gene, peak bone mass, postmenopausal bone loss, and bone turnover: the OFELY Study [abstract]. J Bone Miner Res 1997; 12(Suppl):S490.

Garnero P, Borel O, Sornay-Rendu E, Delmas PD: Vitamin D receptor gene polymorphisms do not predict bone turnover and bone mass in healthy premenopausal women. J Bone Miner Res 1995; 10:1283–1288.

Garnero P, Borel P, Sornay-Rendu E, Arlot ME, Delmas PD: Vitamin D receptor gene polymorphisms are not related to bone turnover, rate of bone loss and bone mass in postmenopausal women: the OFELY Study. J Bone Miner Res 1996b; 11:827–834.

Gennari L, Becherini L, Masi L, Mansani R, Gonnelli S, Cepollaro C, Martini S, Montagnani A, Lentini G, Becorpi AM, et al.: Vitamin D and estrogen receptor allelic variants in Italian postmenopausal women: evidence of multiple gene contribution to bone mineral density. J Clin Endocrinol Metab 1998; 83:939–944.

Geusens P, Dequeker J, Verstraeten A, Nijs J: Age-, sex-, and menopause-related changes of vertebral and peripheral bone: population study using dual and single photon absorptiometry and radiogrammetry. J Nucleic Med 1986; 27:1540–1549.

Gong Y, Vikkula M, Boon L, Liu J, Beighton P, Ramesar R, Peltonen L, Somer H, Hirose T, Dallapaiccola B, et al.: Osteoporosis-pseudoglioma syndrome, a disorder affecting skeletal strength and vision, is assigned to chromosome region 11q12–13. Am J Hum Genet 1996; 59:146–151.

Gong Y, Slee RB, Fukai N, Rawadi G, Roman-Roman S, Reginato AM, Wang H, Cundy T, Glorieux FH, Lev D, et al.: LDL receptor-related protein 5 (LRP5) affected bone accrual and eye development. Cell 2001; 107:513–523.

Grant SF, Reid DM, Blake G, Herd R, Fogelman I, Ralston SH: Reduced bone density and osteoporosis associated with a polymorphic Sp1 binding site in the *collagen type I alpha 1* gene. Nat Genet 1996; 14:203–205.

Gross C, Eccleshall TR, Malloy PJ, Villa ML, Marcus R, Feldman D: The presence of a polymorphism at the translation initiation site of the vitamin D receptor gene is associated with low bone mineral density in postmenopausal Mexican-American women. J Bone Miner Res 1996; 11:1850–1855.

Han KO, Moon IG, Choi JT, Chung HY, Yoon HK, Min HK, Han IK: Nonassociation of estrogen bone density with estrogen receptor genotypes in Korean elderly women [abstract]. J Bone Miner Res 1997a; 12(Suppl):S256.

Han KO, Moon IG, Choi JT, Kim SW, Yoon HK, Min HK, Han IK: Nonassociation of estrogen receptor genotypes with bone mineral density and bone markers in Korean premenopausal women [abstract]. J Bone Miner Res 1997b; 12(Suppl): S256.

Harris SS, Eccleshall TR, Gross C, Dawson-Hughes B, Feldman D: The vitamin D receptor start codon polymorphism (FokI) and bone mineral density in premenopausal American black and white women. J Bone Miner Res 1997; 12:1043–1048.

Haughton MA, Gunnell AS, Grant SFA, Brown MA, Eisman JA: Linkage studies of the COL1A1 and VDR loci in the control of bone mineral density [abstract]. Bone 1998; 23(Suppl):S370.

Heaney C, Carmi R, Dushkin H, Sheffield V, Beier DR: Genetic mapping of recessive osteopetrosis to 11q12–13 [abstract]. Am J Hum Genet 1997; 61(Suppl):A12.

Heegaard A-MM, Jorgensen JL, Vestergaard AW, Hassager C, Grant SFA, Ralston SH: Lack of influence of Sp1 polymorphism in the collagen type Iα1 gene on the rate of bone loss in postmenopausal women followed for 18 years [abstract]. Bone 1998; 23(Suppl):S373.

Huang Q, Want Q, Zhang L, Zhou Q, Lu J: Relationship between bone mineral density and polymorphism of the estrogen receptor gene in Chinese postmenopausal women [abstract]. Bone 1998; 23(Suppl):S370.

Hustmyer FG, Liu G, Christian JC, Johnston CC, Peacock M: Is the polymorphism at the Sp1 binding site in the *COL1A1* gene associated with bone mineral density [abstract]. J Bone Miner Res 1997; 12(Suppl):S490.

Hustmyer FG, Peacock M, Hui S, Johnston CC, Christian J: Bone mineral density in relation to polymorphism at the vitamin D receptor gene locus. J Clin Invest 1994; 94:2130–2134.

Jagger C, Swan L, Harrison J, Rowan M, McColl J, Spooner R, Shapiro D, McLellan AR: Evidence that vitamin D receptor genotype, but not *COL1A1* genotype, may contribute to the heritability of bone mineral density: the Scottish Twin Study [abstract]. Bone 1998; 23(Suppl):S372.

Johnson ML, Gong G, Kimberling W, Recker SM, Kimmel DM, Recker RR: Linkage of a gene causing high bone mass to human chromosome 11 (11q12–13). Am J Hum Genet 1997; 60:1326–1332.

Johnston CC Jr, Cummings SR, Dawson-Hughes B, Lindsay R, Melton LJ, Slemenda CW: Physician's Guide to Prevention and Treatment of Osteoporosis. Washington DC: National Osteoporosis Foundation, 1998.

Jorgensen HL, Heegaard AM, Bayer L, Hansen L, Hassager C: PvuII and XbaI restriction fragment length polymorphism at the estrogen receptor (ER) locus and its relation to bone mineral density (BMD) and bone loss in postmenopausal Danish women [abstract]. J Bone Miner Res 1997; 12(Suppl):S254.

Jouanny P, Guillemin F, Kuntz C, Jeandel C, Pourel J: Environmental and genetic factors affecting bone mass. Similarity of bone density among members of healthy families. Arthritis Rheum 1995; 38:61–67.

Kanis JA, Melton LJ III, Christiansen C, Johnston CC, Khaltaev N: The diagnosis of osteoporosis. J Bone Miner Res 1994; 9:1137–1141.

Keen RW, Woodford-Richens KL, Grant SFA, Lanchbury JS, Ralston SH, Spector TD: Type I collagen gene polymorphism is associated with osteoporosis and fracture [abstract]. J Bone Miner Res 1997; 12(Suppl):S489.

Kelly PJ, Hopper JL, Macaskill GT, Pocock NA, Sambrook PN, Eisman JA: Genetic factors in bone turnover. J Clin Endocrinol Metab 1991; 72:808–813.

Kelly PJ, Nguyen T, Hopper J, Pocock N, Sambrook P, Eisman J: Changes in axial bone density with age: a twin study. J Bone Miner Res 1993; 8:11–17.

Kindmark A, Carling T, Melhus H, Ljunghall S: Estrogen receptors and osteoporosis: lack of association between disease and polymorphisms at three different loci [abstract]. Bone 1998; 23(Suppl):S369.

Klein RF, Mitchell SR, Phillips TJ, Belknap JK, Orwoll ES: Quantitative trait loci affecting peak bone mineral density in mice. J Bone Miner Res 1998; 13:1648–1656.

Kobayashi S, Inoue S, Hosoi T, Ouchi Y, Shiraki M, Orimo H: Association of bone mineral density with polymorphism of the estrogen receptor gene. J Bone Miner Res 1996; 11:306–311.

Koller DL, Econs MJ, Morin PA, Christian JC, Hui SL, Parry P, Curran ME, Rodriguez LA, Conneally PM, Joslyn G, et al.: Genome screen for QTLs contributing to normal variation in bone mineral density and osteoporosis. J Clin Endocrinol Metab 2000; 85:3116–3120.

Koller DL, Rodriguez LA, Christian JC, Slemenda CW, Econs MG, Hui SL, Morin P, Conneally PM, Joslyn G, Curran ME, et al.: Linkage of a QTL contributing to normal variation in bone mineral density to chromosome 11q12–13. J Bone Miner Res 1998; 13:1903–1908.

Krall EA, Dawson-Hughes B: Heritable and life-style determinants of bone mineral density. J Bone Miner Res 1993; 8:1–9.

Krall EA, Parry P, Lichter JB, Dawson-Hughes B: Vitamin D receptor alleles and rates of bone loss: influence of years since menopause and calcium intake. J Bone Miner Res 1995; 10:978–984.

Langdahl BL, Knudsen JY, Jensen HK, Gregersen N, Eriksen EF: A sequence variation: 713–8delC in the *transforming growth factor-beta1* gene has higher prevalence in osteoporotic women than in normal women and is associated with very low bone mass in osteoporotic women and increased bone turnover in both osteoporotic and normal women. Bone 1997a; 20:289–294.

Langdahl BL, Lokke E, Carstens M, Eriksen EF: Polymorphisms in the estrogen receptor gene show different distributions in osteoporotic patients and normal controls [abstract]. J Bone Miner Res 1997b; 12(Suppl):S255.

Langdahl BL, Ralston SH, Grant SFA, Eriksen EF: An Sp1 binding site polymorphism in the *COL1A1* gene predicts osteoporotic fractures in both men and women [abstract]. J Bone Miner Res 1997c; 12(Suppl):S489.

Liden M, Wilen B, Lunghall S, Melhus H: Polymorphism at the Sp1 binding site in the *collagen type I alpha 1* gene does not predict bone mineral density in postmenopausal women in Sweden. Calcif Tissue Int 1998; 63:293–295.

Liel Y, Edwards J, Shary J, Spicer KM, Gordon L, Bell NH: The effects of race and body habitus on bone mineral density of the radius, hip, and spine in premenopausal women. J Clin Endocrinol Metab 1988; 66:1247–1250.

Lim S-K, Li SZ, Won YJ, Shin W-Y, Lee HC, Huh KB: Lack of association between a polymorphic Sp1 binding site in *collagen type I alpha 1* gene and osteoporosis in Korea [abstract]. J Bone Miner Res 1997; 12(Suppl):S491.

Little RD, Carulli JP, Del Mastro RG, Dupuis J, Osborne M, Folz C, Manning SP, Swain PM, Zhao S-C, Eustace B, et al.: A mutation in the LDL receptor-related protein 5 gene results in the autosomal dominant high-bone-mass trait. Am J Hum Genet, in press (January, 2002).

Livshits G, Yakovenko C, Kobyliansky E: Quantitative genetic analysis of circulating levels of biochemical markers of bone formation. Am J Med Genet 2000; 94:324–331.

Lonzer MD, Imrie R, Rogers D, Worley D, Licata A, Secic M: Effects of heredity, age, weight, puberty, activity, and calcium intake on bone mineral density in children. Clin Pediatr 1996; 35:185–189.

Looker AC, Orwoll ES, Johnston CC Jr, Lindsay RL, Wahner HW, Dunn WL, Calvo MS, Harris TB, Heyse SP: Prevalence of low femoral bone density in older US adults from NHANES III. J Bone Miner Res 1997; 12:1761–1768.

Looney JE, Yoon HK, Fisher M, Farley SM, Farley JR, Wergedal JE, Baylink DJ: Lack of a high prevalence of the BB vitamin D receptor genotype in severely osteoporotic women. J Clin Endocrinol Metab 1995; 80:2158–2162.

Lutz J: Bone mineral, serum calcium, and dietary intakes of mother/daughter pairs. Am J Clin Nutr 1986; 44:99–106.

Mahaney MC, Morin P, Rodriguez LA, Newman DE, Rogers J: A quantitative trait locus on chromosome 11 may influence bone mineral density at several sites: linkage analyses in pedigreed baboons. J Bone Miner Res 1997; 12(Suppl 1):S118. Abstract nr 64.

Mahonen A, Turunen A-M, Kroger H, Maenpaa PH: Estrogen receptor gene polymorphism is associated with bone mineral density in perimenopausal Finnish women [abstract]. J Bone Miner Res 1997; 12(Suppl):S255.

McLellan AR, Jagger C, Spooner R, Sutcliffe R, Harrison J, Shaprio D: Are COL1A1 Sp1 polymorphisms important determinants of bone mineral density and osteoporosis in postmenopausal women in the UK [abstract]? J Bone Miner Res 1997; 12(Suppl):S119.

Melhus H, Kindmark A, Amer S, Wilen B, Lindh E, Ljungall S: Vitamin D receptor genotypes in osteoporosis. Lancet 1994; 344:949–950.

Melton L, Chrischilles E, Cooper C, Lane AW, Riggs BL: How many women have osteoporosis? J Bone Miner Res 1992; 7:1005–1010.

Melton LJ 3rd: How many women have osteoporosis now? J Bone Miner Res 1995; 10:175–177.

Moller M, Horsman A, Harvald B, Hauge M, Henningsen K, Nordin BEC: Metacarpal morphometry in monzygotic and dizygotic elderly twins. Calcif Tissue Res 1978; 25:197–201.

Morrison NA, Qi JC, Tokita A, Kelly PJ, Crofts L, Nguyen TV, Sambrook PN, Eisman JA: Prediction of bone density from vitamin D receptor alleles. Nature 1994; 367:284–287.

Morrison NA, Qi JC, Tokita A, Kelly PJ, Crofts L, Nguyen TV, Sambrook PN, Eisman JA: Prediction of bone density from vitamin D receptor alleles. Nature 1997; 387:106.

Murray RE, McGuigan F, Grant SF, Reid DM, Ralston SH: Polymorphisms of the interleukin-6 gene are associated with bone mineral density. Bone 1997; 21:89–92.

Nelson DA, Schlaen SE, Davis P, Wooley P: Estrogen receptor gene polymorphism and bone mass in black and white women [abstract]. J Bone Miner Res 1997; 12(Suppl):S255.

Niu T, Chen C, Cordell H, Yang J, Wang B, Wang Z, Fang Z, Schork NJ, Rosen CJ, Xu X: A genome-wide scan for loci linked to forearm bone mineral density. Hum Genet 1999; 104:226–233.

Nogues X, Garcia-Giralt N, Enjuanes A, Grinberg D, Mellibovsky L, Minguez S, Carbonell J, Serrano S, Diez A, Balcells S: Genetic study of bone mass determinants in perimenopausal Spanish women [abstract]. Bone 1998; 23 (Suppl):S371.

Peacock M, Hustmyer FG, Hui S, Johnston CC Jr, Christian JC: Vitamin D receptor genotype and bone mineral density—evidence conflicts on link. BMJ 1995; 311:874–875.

Pocock NA, Eisman JA, Hopper JL, Yeates MG, Sambrook PN, Ebert S: Genetic determinants of bone mass in adults: a twin study. J Clin Invest 1987; 80:706–710.

Prockop DJ, Constantinou CD, Dombrowski KE, Johima Y, Kadler KE, Kuivaniemi H, Tromp G, Vogel BE: Type I procollagen: the gene–protein system that harbors most of the mutations causing osteogenesis imperfecta and probably more common heritable disorders of connective tissue. Am J Med Genet 1989; 34:60–67.

Recker RR, Davies DK, Recker SM: Characterizing the phenotype in a kindred with autosomal dominant high bone mass [abstract]. Bone 1998; 23(Suppl):S274.

Riggs BL, Nguyen TV, Melton LJ 3rd, Morrison NA, O'Fallon WM, Kelly PJ, Egan KS,

Sambrook PN, Muhs JM, Eisman JA: The contribution of vitamin D receptor gene alleles to the determination of bone mineral density in normal and osteoporotic women. J Bone Miner Res 1995; 10:991–996.

Rubin LA, Hawker GA, Peltekova VD, Fielding LJ, Ridout R, Cole DEC: Determinants of peak bone mass: clinical and genetic analyses in a young female Canadian cohort. J Bone Miner Res 1999; 14:633–643.

Seeman E, Hopper JL, Back LA, Cooper ME, Parkinson E, McKay J, Jerums G: Reduced bone mass in daughters of women with osteoporosis. N Engl J Med 1989; 320:554–558.

Seeman E, Tsalamandris C, Formica C, Hopper JL, McKay J: Reduced femoral neck bone density in the daughters of women with hip fractures: the role of low peak bone density in the pathogenesis of osteoporosis. J Bone Miner Res 1994; 9:739–743.

Sikic-Klisovic E, Badenhop NE, Skugor M, Klisovic D, Ilich JZ, Landoll JD, Young AP, Matkovic V: Estrogen receptor gene polymorphism differentiates bone mass in adult males more than in females [abstract]. Bone 1998; 23(Suppl):S370.

Slemenda CW, Christian JC, Reed T, Reister TK, Williams CJ, Johnston CC Jr: Long-term bone loss in men: effects of genetic and environmental factors. Ann Intern Med 1992; 117:286–291.

Slemenda CW, Christian JC, Williams CJ, Norton JA, Johnston CC Jr: Genetic determinants of bone mass in adult women: a reevaluation of the twin model and the potential importance of gene interaction on heritability estimates. J Bone Miner Res 1991; 6:561–567.

Smith DM, Nance WE, Kang KW, Christian JC, Johnston CC Jr: Genetic factors in determining bone mass. J Clin Invest 1973; 52:2800–2808.

Soroko SB, Barrett-Connor E, Edelstein SL, Kritz-Silverstein D: Family history of osteoporosis and bone mineral density at the axial skeleton: the Rancho-Bernardo Study. J Bone Miner Res 1994; 9:761–769.

Sowers MF, Aron D, Burns T, Clark K, Willing M: Bone mineral density and its change in white women: estrogen and vitamin D receptor genotypes and their interaction [abstract]. J Bone Miner Res 1997; 12(Suppl):S175.

Sowers MFR, Boehnke M, Jannausch ML, Crutchfield M, Corton G, Burns TL: Familiality and partitioning the variability of femoral bone mineral density in women of child-bearing age. Calcif Tissue Int 1992; 50:110–114.

Spector TD, Keen RW, Arden NK, Morrison NA, Major PJ, Nguyen TV, Kelly PJ, Baker JR, Sambrook PN, Lanchbury JS, et al.: Influence of vitamin D receptor genotype on bone mineral density in postmenopausal women: a twin study in Britain. BMJ 1995; 310:1357–1360.

Spotila LD, Caminis J, Devoto M, Shimoya K, Sereda L, Ott J, Whyte MP, Tenehouse A, Prockop DJ: Osteopenia in 37 members of seven families: analysis based on a model of dominant inheritance. Mol Med 1996; 2:313–324.

Spotila LD, Constantinou CD, Sereda L, Ganguly A, Riggs BL, Prockop DJ: Mutation in a gene for type I procollagen (*COL1A2*) in a woman with postmenopausal osteoporosis: evidence for phenotypic and genotypic overlap with mild osteogenesis imperfecta. Proc Natl Acad Sci USA 1991; 88:5423–5427.

Spotila LD, Devota M, Caminis J, Kosich R, Korkko J, Ott J, Tenenhouse A, Prockop DJ: Suggested linkage of low bone density to chromosome 1p36 is extended to a second cohort of sib pairs [abstract]. Bone 1998; 23(Suppl):S277.

Tokita A, Kelly PJ, Nguyen TB, Qi J-C, Morrison NA, Risteli L, Rsteli J, Sambrook PN, Eisman JA: Genetic influences on type I collagen synthesis and degradation: further evidence for genetic regulation of bone turnover. J Clin Endocrinol Metab 1994; 78:1461–1466.

Uitterlinden AG, Burger H, Huang Q, Yue F, McGuigan FEA, Grant SFA, Hofman A, van Leeusen JPTM, Pols HAP, Ralston SH: Relation of alleles of the *collagen type Iα1* gene to bone density and the risk of osteoporotic fractures in postmenopausal women. N Engl J Med 1998; 338:1016–1021.

Vandevyver C, Philippaerts L, Cassiman J-J, Raus J, Geusens P: Bone mineral density in postmenopausal women is not associated with type I collagen (COL-1A1) dimorphisms [abstract]. J Bone Miner Res 1997; 12(Suppl):S490.

Yamagata Z, Miyamura T, Iijima S, Asaka A, Sasaki M, Kato J, Koizumi K: Vitamin D receptor gene polymorphism and bone mineral density in healthy Japanese women. Lancet 1994; 344:1027.

Zmuda JM, Cauley JA, Glynn NW, Lee M, Kuller LH, Ferrell RE: A common estrogen receptor gene variant is associated with hip bone density in older men [abstract]. Bone 1998; 23(Suppl):S269.

25 Hyperuricemia and Gout

MICHAEL A. BECKER

Gout (urate crystal deposition disease) is a clinical syndrome reflecting a heterogeneous group of genetic and acquired metabolic aberrations promoting *hyperuricemia* (supersaturation of serum with urate, the end product of purine metabolism) and deposition of monosodium urate and uric acid crystals in tissues (Wyngaarden and Kelley, 1976). Symptomatic manifestations of gout are direct consequences of crystal deposition and include recurrent attacks of a characteristic acute inflammatory arthritis (*acute gouty arthritis*); potentially destructive urate crystal aggregates (*tophi*), which favor connective tissue structures but may deposit in nearly any organ; uric acid urolithiasis, which may precede gouty arthritis or punctuate the course of gout; and renal impairment, which is usually due to comorbid states that are frequent among gout patients. Hyperuricemia is a proxy for extracellular fluid urate supersaturation and is present at some point in the course of nearly all patients with gout, but only a minority of hyperuricemic individuals ever experience clinical events resulting from urate deposition (Paulus et al., 1970; Fessel, 1979; Emmerson, 1996). Hyperuricemia is, thus, best considered a biochemical aberration that is the necessary pathogenetic common denominator predisposing to gout but is not itself sufficient to define a disease state.

Although asymptomatic hyperuricemia is not a disease state, it is a risk factor for development of gouty manifestations. The magnitude and duration of hyperuricemia, the sex and age of the individual, and prior clinical manifestations of crystal deposition appear to be major, but not absolute determinants of the level of risk (Hall et al., 1967; Wyngaarden and Kelley, 1976; Nishioka and Mikanagi, 1980; Zalokar et al., 1981; Campion et al., 1987). An acute attack of intensely inflammatory, disabling monoarticular arthritis is the most common initial gouty event, but in a substantial minority of patients, onset may involve an episode of uric acid urolithiasis or polyarticular gouty inflammation. A signature feature of gouty arthritis early in the disorder is a return to entirely normal joint and health status within days, if treated, or weeks, even if untreated. Also typical of gout is the distribution of inflammed joints early in the course, favoring the base of the great toe (first metatarsophalangeal joint, *podagra*); the instep, ankle, or knee joint; and the olecranon bursa at the elbow. The peak incidence of gout in men is in the fourth to sixth decade and in women, the sixth to eighth decade (Grahame and Scott, 1970; Wyngaarden and Kelley, 1976; Myers and Monteagudo, 1985; Macfarlane and Dieppe, 1985; Lally et al., 1986; Puig et al., 1991).

Recurrence of arthritis is the rule in untreated gout (nearly 80% of patients have recurrence within 2 years), though the duration of individual symptom-free (intercritical) periods varies widely. With multiple attacks, usually over years to decades, chronic and widespread joint pain and degeneration may result, often accompanied by tophaceous deposits, which rarely occur as the first manifestation of the disease. The combination of crystal-induced joint erosion and adjacent tophaceous deposits can lead to severe deformity and disability involving virtually any joint in the extremities or spine. Occasionally, the course of gout from the initial attack to the development of chronic tophaceous gout with joint deformity is truncated, evolving over months or a few years. This unfortunate path occurs more frequently in patients whose urate crystal deposition disease is secondary either to a disorder resulting in markedly excessive uric acid production (as in myeloproliferative or lymphoproliferative states) (Wyngaarden and Kelley, 1976) or to a drug or toxin that severely impairs renal uric acid excretion (e.g., cyclosporin A administration in organ transplant recipients or lead exposure in "moonshine" drinkers) (Reynolds et al., 1983; Burack et al., 1992; Baethge et al., 1993). Although many patients with hyperuricemia or gout develop chronic renal impairment and urate crystal deposition in the renal medullary interstitium is common in untreated gout, neither hyperuricemia nor gout is a major primary risk factor for chronic renal insufficiency (Liang and Fries, 1978; Fessel, 1979); rather, it is likely that the frequent association of gout with disorders such as hypertension, atherosclerosis, hyperlipidemia, obesity, and lead intoxication in men (Berger and Yu, 1975; Gibson et al., 1980; Langford et al., 1987) and with older age and diuretic use in women (Myers and Monteagudo, 1985; Macfarlane and Dieppe, 1985; Lally et al., 1986; Puig et al., 1991) introduces comorbidities that more directly account for impaired renal function in gout patients.

An additional renal risk for gout patients, however, is uric acid crystal deposition in the collecting system of the kidneys, most often manifested by one or more episodes of renal colic, dysuria, or excretion of gravel and blood in the urine (Yu and Gutman, 1967; Asplin, 1996). Uric acid crystals in the urinary tract also provide a nidus for calcium oxalate stone formation, and the result is a 20- to 30-fold increase in calcium stones among gout patients (Coe and Kavalach, 1974). Finally, patients with gout and hyperuricemia, particularly those with severe uric acid overproduction, are at risk for acute uric acid nephropathy, a form of oliguric or anuric renal failure due to uric acid crystal precipitation within the renal tubules (Cohen et al., 1980).

Prior to 1950, gout was a major clinical problem despite careful and accurate disease descriptions spanning two millennia and early recognition of the cause-and-effect relationship between urate deposition and gouty manifestations. In the past 50 years, advances in human purine biochemistry and physiology and identification of several inborn errors of purine metabolism have contributed to the development of effective therapies to reduce serum urate concentration, which have in turn resulted in successful management of most gouty patients. Nevertheless, the

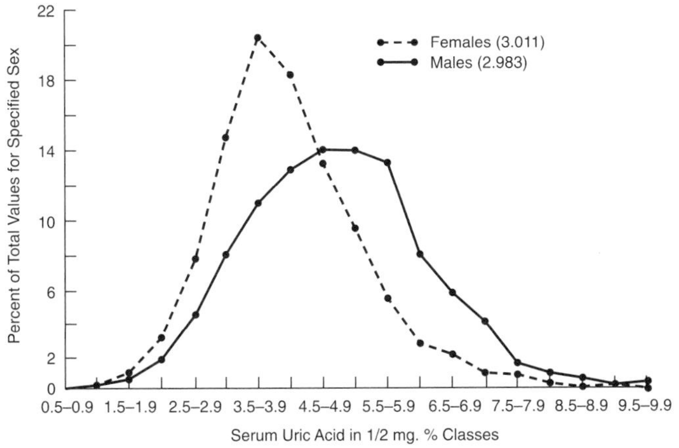

Fig. 25–1. Distribution of serum urate values in 0.5 mg/dl intervals among residents of Tecumseh, Michigan, 1959–1960. Among residents of the town, only hospitalized or severely ill persons were excluded from sampling. From Mikkelsen et al. (1965) with permission.

precise metabolic basis of gout remains uncertain in the majority of such individuals, and the recognition that urate metabolism, physiology, and crystal deposition are under multigenic control and are strongly affected by coexisting disease states, drug administration, and environmental exposures makes analysis of this problem very difficult.

GENERAL GENETIC AND EPIDEMIOLOGIC EVIDENCE

Clinical Epidemiology and Ethnic Differences

Automated enzymatic (uricase) methods measure production of H_2O_2 generated in the oxidation of urate (Price and James, 1988). They provide similar ease and greater accuracy and reproducibility in the clinical measurement of serum and urinary uric acid than prior colorimetric methods, although the uricase spectrophotometric assay remains preferable for research studies (Wyngaarden and Kelley, 1976). Most population studies utilizing the uricase spectrophotometric method have defined upper limits of normal serum urate [mean $\pm$ 2 standard deviations (SD)] at about 7.0 mg/dl in adult men and 6.0 mg/dl in premenopausal women. From physicochemical considerations, however, the theoretical limit of urate solubility in serum is about 6.5 mg/dl.

Serum urate values in both sexes are continuously distributed without any break suggesting that they represent a mixture of several distributions (Fig. 25–1). However, serum urate values are not normally distributed but skewed toward high values, a distribution observed in all studies of urate values in adult populations (Mikkelsen et al., 1965). In the Tecumseh, Michigan, population study, the 95th percentile for serum urate among men of all ages was 7.2 mg/dl, a supersaturating urate value. Overall, 7.4% of male subjects and 2.4% of female subjects were hyperuricemic by the clinical chemical criterion. Thus, hyperuricemia, which predisposes subjects to the risk of gout (Hall et al., 1967; Campion et al., 1987), is fairly common among adult Americans.

The magnitude of this risk is related to the degree and duration of hyperuricemia. In the Framingham Study (Hall et al., 1967), 16% to 17% of subjects, male or female, with serum urate of 7.0 to 7.9 mg/dl by the colorimetric method developed gouty arthritis. No women had higher values, but 25% of men with values of 8.0 to 8.9 mg/dl and 90% of those with values above 9 mg/dl on any single determination of serum urate developed gout over a span of two decades. Similarly, stone formation was correlated with daily urinary uric acid excretion, with a prevalence exceeding 50% when daily uric acid excretion exceeded 1100 mg.

Serum urate concentrations vary with age in patterns that are distinctive in men and women (Fig. 25–2). Childhood serum urate concentrations of 3 to 4 mg/dl rise during male puberty to adult levels before about age 20 and remain rather constant thereafter (Mikkelsen et al., 1965; Glynn et al., 1983). In contrast, women show only minor changes in urate concentrations until menopause, when values rise to more closely approximate those in adult men. The higher urinary fractional excretion of urate [defined as milligrams urinary urate per deciliter glomerular filtration rate (GFR)] in women of childbearing age appears to be due to diminished tubular uric acid postsecretory reabsorption (Mateos Anton et al., 1986). This is most likely related to the action of estrogenic compounds, but the precise mechanism is not well defined.

Many factors influence serum urate levels in adults: ethnic background (Gibson et al., 1984; Darmavan et al., 1992), anthropomorphic and social factors, and physiologic/pharmacologic determinants such as body weight, fat distribution (Takahashi et al., 1997), blood pressure (Hochberg et al., 1995), diet, drug and alcohol intake, and renal function (Wyngaarden and Kelley, 1976). In North America and Europe, the annual incidence of gout is estimated at 0.20 to 0.35/1000 persons, with an overall prevalence of 2 to 8/1000 (Wyngaarden and Kelley, 1976; Lawrence et al., 1998). Increasing age and serum urate concentration as well as male gender are associated with increased prevalence. For example, among French men aged 35 to 44 years, the prevalence of gout was 11/1000 previously asymptomatic men in the 35- to 39-year group and 20/1000 in those 40 to 44 years old (Zalokar et al., 1981).

In the New Zealand Maori population, with increased mean serum urate levels, the prevalence of gout in adult males and females is reported to exceed 10% and 4%, respectively (Gibson et al., 1984; Klemp et al., 1997). Additional studies in Maoris

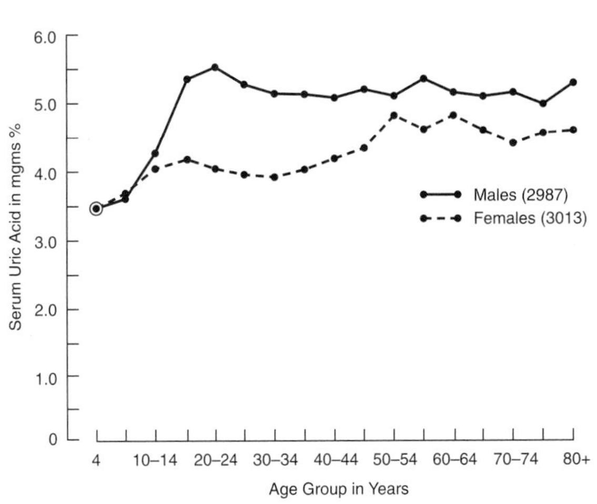

Fig. 25–2. Age- and sex-specific distribution of mean serum urate values in Tecumseh, Michigan, 1959–1960. From Mikkelsen et al. (1965) with permission.

have suggested the presence of a unique serum globulin that binds uric acid, resulting in increased serum urate levels and gout but low urate excretion (Klinenberg et al., 1977). The geographic concentration of hyperuricemic Pacific Islanders has led to speculation that they represent "one gouty family" or migration of a founding mutation across the Pacific. Filipinos residing in the Philippines have values similar to Caucasians, while those residing in Hawaii have higher values and those in the United States still higher. One study suggests that some Filipinos may have a diminished capacity for renal excretion of uric acid resulting in the development of hyperuricemia on a Western diet with its higher purine content (Healey and Bayani-Sioson, 1971).

Environmental Associations

Dietary Considerations

Studies of human volunteers maintained on purine-free diets have sought to determine baseline endogenous purine synthesis and degradation with attendant urate production. After 10 days on a purine-free formula diet, serum urate values declined from 4.9 to 3.1 ± 0.4 mg/dl and urinary excretion from 500 to 600 mg/day to 336 ± 39 mg/day in healthy young German men (Griebsch and Zollner, 1974). When purines were added to the diet, roughly 50% of yeast RNA or 25% of DNA was excreted in the urine, while plasma urate concentration and renal urate excretion increased linearly with increasing doses. These findings suggest that exogenous purines make a significant contribution to urate homeostasis in all subjects and that at least transient hyperuricemia can be induced in normal subjects by dietary excess alone. Foods rich in purines include organ meats and meat extracts, yeast, game birds, shellfish, legumes, fish and meat in general, and some vegetables.

Alcohol Consumption

The historic association of ethanol consumption with hyperuricemia and gout has been confirmed by physiologic studies. Acute ethanol infusion induces hyperuricemia, in part as a consequence of lactic acidemia sufficient to suppress renal uric acid excretion (Wyngaarden and Kelley, 1976) and in part as a result of adenine nucleotide degradation and increased uric acid production (Faller and Fox, 1982; Puig and Fox, 1984). Both binge drinking, possibly augmented by the ketonemia of fasting, and chronic alcohol ingestion induce hyperuricemia by altering excretion, probably with a substantial contribution of increased uric acid production as well.

Saturnine gout is a form of hyperuricemia/gout induced by lead poisoning, with lead nephropathy resulting in reduced urate excretion. It is historically associated with alcoholic hyperuricemia because of its occurrence in epidemic proportions among seventeenth and eighteenth century English port wine drinkers, whose fortified wine contained high levels of lead, and more recently among residents of the southeastern United States, where distillation of whiskey (moonshine) in automobile radiators also yields alcohol with a high lead content (Wyngaarden and Kelley, 1976; Batuman et al., 1981; Reynolds et al., 1983).

Obesity

Serum urate values show positive correlations with body size in almost every ethnic group or culture throughout the world (Mikkelsen et al., 1965; Acheson and O'Brien, 1966; Wyngaarden and Kelley, 1976). Measures of body weight, relative weight, ponderal index, or surface area detect the relationship, especially measures integrating height and weight. The relative contributions of dietary excess, augmented endogenous purine synthesis, and impaired renal excretion have not been well studied. Moreover, as discussed below, it is unclear whether obesity is independently associated with hyperuricemia or related through other disorders associated with each, such as hypertriglyceridemia, hypertension, and atherosclerosis.

The association of high serum uric acid values with obesity; diets rich in meats, seafood, and game; alcohol consumption; intelligence; achievement; and social status as well as higher hemoglobin and serum protein values led Acheson and O'Brien (1966) to comment that "the associates of a high uric acid are the associates of plenty."

Family Epidemiology

Family Studies of Serum Urate

All observers of large populations of hyperuricemic and gouty patients have noted a high frequency of family histories of gout, stones, or hyperuricemia. From earliest times, gout has been recognized as a familial disease (Garrod, 1931; Copeman, 1964; Wyngaarden and Kelley, 1976; Short, 1992; Porter, 1994). Thomas Sydenham remarked on early onset in patients with a parental history and, in 1823, Scudamore found a positive family history with direct inheritance from one or both parents in 60% of 522 patients. Garrod (1931) noted that 80% of his patients had a positive family history, Talbott reported 75%, and Grahame and Yu reported 40%. A number of studies have attempted to divine the mode of inheritance in gouty families. Early observations were confined to patients and family members with gout alone. However, beginning in the 1940s, investigators were able to detect not only overt gout but also asymptomatic hyperuricemia. Studies of the inheritance of common adult hyperuricemia have used three distinctly different proband sampling methodologies, and this has led to discrepant findings (reviewed in Short, 1992).

When normal subjects from populations with unimodal distribution curves for serum urate values, skewed toward higher values, are studied, a consistent answer emerges. Normal serum urate concentrations are polygenically determined or multifactorially determined with a polygenic component. This conclusion is reassuring because it makes good sense biologically. A phenotypic marker as complexly determined as serum urate is likely to be far removed from the sight of gene action. Each of the processes in uric acid production and disposal is under the control of multiple genes and subject to environmental modulators such as diet. Such a multidetermined marker should indeed fit a model of multifactorial (i.e., environmental and polygenic) influences on its expression.

These studies have been cited, however, to refute other studies that find evidence for major gene segregation in families with hyperuricemia ascertained through hyperuricemic or gouty probands. This conclusion is inappropriate because these two types of ascertainment sample different universes. What is clear is that "common" adult hyperuricemia, the focus of this chapter, may be sufficiently uncommon that one would not expect to ascertain many families in a limited random sampling of the population. Studies using hyperuricemic probands drawn from the tail of the urate distribution of normal populations make this point. In such studies, no cases of familial hyperuricemia were found among subjects above the 90th to 98th percentile of the normal population distribution for serum urate values. These studies suffer from sampling limited numbers of young nuclear families; thus, not surprisingly, they failed to detect affected relatives because, despite a substantial prevalence of hyperuricemia in adults (especially males), the majority (70% to 80%) of individuals are affected secondary to other disorders or acquired environmental circumstances. Thus, it appears that insufficient numbers of families of individuals with primary hyperuricemia have been studied to affirm or deny a major genetic hypothesis.

The results of a number of other studies on hyperuricemic or gouty probands, excluding persons with possible secondary hyperuricemia, have been remarkably consistent in documenting a strong family history of gout and hyperuricemia in the respective pedigrees (Smyth et al., 1948; Stecher et al., 1949; Hauge and Harvald, 1955; Rakic et al., 1964; Neel et al., 1965; Morton, 1979; Short, 1992). Primary hyperuricemia is more common in older subjects and decidedly more common in men than women. In families with more than one affected person, hyperuricemia appears in consecutive generations. Hyperuricemia within families shows father-to-son transmission. Within sibship and parent–child groups, correlation coefficients for urate values are poor, arguing that there are distinctly different groupings within these families, rather than a continuum of values characteristic of a polygenic trait. All attempts at simple threshold analysis of trait distribution, whether the threshold chosen is 7.0 mg/dl or the 95th percentile, have shown a pattern of segregation of hyperuricemia in adult first-degree relatives most consistent with autosomal dominant inheritance with late-onset, sex-dependent expression. The majority of studies using threshold analysis have also found pedigrees showing segregation ratios approaching 50% occurrence of hyperuricemia in older men, with a lesser percentage in older women (Smyth et al., 1948; Stecher et al., 1949; Hauge and Harvald, 1955; Rakic et al., 1964; Short, 1992).

In the late 1950s, it was argued that if a trait did not show bimodal distribution of values in families but rather a unimodal curve (albeit with dramatic skewing of the curve toward high values), inheritance of the trait could not result from expression of a single major gene. This view led investigators to conclude that, despite the threshold analyses, unimodal and rightward skewed urate distribution curves sufficed to define polygenic inheritance of hyperuricemia (Hauge and Harvald, 1955; Rakic et al., 1964; Neel et al., 1965). Because of such problems in interpretation, modern segregation analysis of quantitative traits using computer programs was devised and structured exploratory data analysis was invented to permit sophisticated modeling of the distribution of a quantitative trait within families (Carmelli et al., 1979).

Segregation analysis in a properly ascertained population, where the probands have common adult primary hyperuricemia, has been attempted only twice. Morton (1979) undertook a reexamination of data published in the 1940s (Smyth et al., 1948; Stecher et al., 1949). He analyzed 91 nuclear families with 326 members, 75 of whom were probands. Despite choosing to "use conservative methods to avoid asserting a nonexistent major locus," he found that a generalized major gene model fit the data surprisingly well. He, nonetheless, concluded that polygenic heritability accounted for nearly all of the genetic variance. Even in their simple threshold analysis of these same pedigrees, the earlier investigators had lamented the lack of enough older family members to prove the autosomal dominant hypothesis. The data set that Morton (1979) reanalyzed contained only 71 true probands, with 203 first-degree relatives, of whom only 141 were adults. This data set was probably too small to give a true test of the major gene hypothesis, especially when the model took no account of the late-onset, sex-dependent expression of the trait.

In the prior edition of this book, Short (1992) commented on analysis of serum urate in 65 probands with 304 adult first-degree relatives, including many older siblings and parents. When segregation analysis was performed with sex-specific means, the segregation pattern best fit the hypothesis of a codominant major gene segregating on a polygenic background. This analysis utilized the "mixed model" of the Pedigree Analysis Package (PAP) computer program (Hasstedt et al., 1979) and was likewise performed after age and sex adjustment and skewness correction (Cantor and Rotter, 1992). The mixed model tests the hypothesis that the observed segregation pattern is best explained by polygenic influence on the trait being analyzed as well as evidence of a megaphenic, or single major gene, influence. All 65 pedigrees were included, although by threshold analysis a second member with serum urate above the 95th percentile was present in only 42 of these families. Despite inclusion of possibly nontransmitting pedigrees, which should weaken evidence for a major gene hypothesis, the major gene model provided the best fit.

Family Studies of Renal Uric Acid Excretion

Disordered urate homeostasis is a physiologic disturbance often expressed in abnormal uric acid excretion, as well as, or in place of, altered serum urate concentration. In a brief examination of uric acid excretion in the relatives of patients with gout, Scott and Pollard (1970) concluded that there were strong correlations between probands and relatives for all measures of uric acid excretion. These correlations improved as measures of uric acid excretion that controlled for creatinine clearance were analyzed. Using the pedigrees mentioned above, Short (1992) employed segregation analysis of fractional excretion of uric acid, performed with sex-specific means, and found a best fit to the hypothesis of dominant inheritance of a major gene upon a polygenic background for common adult hyperuricemia and gout. Finally, when these pedigrees were analyzed for the combined traits of serum urate concentration and 24-hour urinary uric acid excretion corrected for creatinine clearance, the best fit hypothesis was a genetic, rather than an environmental or general, model and the segregation pattern fit a model of autosomal dominant gene segregation upon a polygenic background for common adult hyperuricemia and gout. In the absence, to date, of publications providing details of the studies carried out on these 65 families, interpretations (Short, 1992) must be regarded as provisional.

Twin Studies

There have been no adoption studies of primary adult hyperuricemia, but a few studies have compared serum urate concentrations in twin pairs. Rich et al. (1978) noted concordance rates of 84% for monozygotic twins and 43% for dizygotic twins of like sex. In twins, genetic effects appear more significant than environmental effects in determining serum uric acid concentrations. Whether based on half-sibling analysis or sib–sib correlations, there was evidence that some of the determining genetic factors were X-linked. These findings from twin pairs with serum uric acid values generally within the normal range are consistent with the polygenic determination of serum urate in most subjects. The possibility of X-linked genetic factors is also consistent with the higher degree of association of uric acid values in mothers and daughters compared with those of fathers and sons in the Tecumseh study (Mikkelsen et al., 1965).

Disease Associations

Obesity

Although there is a clear correlation, documented by many studies of widely divergent populations (Scott, 1977; Fessel and Barr, 1977; Brauer and Prior, 1978; Glynn et al., 1983; Seidell et al., 1986), between increasing body weight and increasing serum urate concentration, the basis for this relationship is complex and likely to be, at least in part, indirect. In the Tecumseh study, the proportion of subjects manifesting hyperuricemia ranged from 4.3%, when relative weight did not exceed the 20th percentile, to 11.4% among those whose relative weight was at or above the 80th percentile (Meyers et al., 1966). The correlation of body weight with uric acid levels was particularly prominent in the 35- to 44-year age group in the Framingham Study (Brand et al., 1985). Weight loss has been associated with modest reduction in serum urate in most, but not all, subjects studied (Nichols and Scott, 1972) and with decreased rates of purine nucleotide and uric acid synthesis (Emmerson, 1973). As would be expected from these observations, subjects with hyperuricemia alone or hyperuricemia and clinical gout (Grahame and Scott, 1970; Emmerson and Knowles, 1971; Wyngaarden and Kelley, 1976; Short, 1992) have higher incidences of obesity than control populations. In one study (Reynolds et al., 1983), 52% of gouty patients weighed greater than 20% over ideal body weight but 85% of these individuals were hypertensive and 48% had abnormal glucose tolerance and hyperlipidemia. Thus, the correlation of increasing weight with increasing serum urate concentration, which has also been observed in probands and first-degree relatives from pedigrees selected for the presence of common adult hyperuricemia (Short, 1992), may also reflect the other metabolic associations of obesity.

Diabetes

Hyperuricemia has been noted in varying numbers of adult diabetics; in part, the variation is related to the stringency of the criteria used to define diabetes. Hyperuricemia occurs in 2% to 50% of patients with overt diabetes, and abnormal glucose tolerance has been demonstrated in 7% to 74% of gouty subjects (Wyngaarden and Kelley, 1976). Since 80% to 90% of nonketotic adult diabetics are obese and as many as half of gouty subjects are overweight (Grahame and Scott, 1970), it is difficult to distinguish obesity from glucose intolerance as the primary association of hyperuricemia; in fact, an independent relationship between hyperuricemia/gout and diabetes has not been demonstrated in epidemiologic studies, such as the Israel Ischemic Heart Disease Study (Herman et al., 1967) or the Tecumseh study (Meyers et al., 1966). In a prospective component of the Israeli heart study, an increased risk for development of diabetes was noted in those with elevated serum urate but overt diabetics had lower uric acid levels owing to increased uric acid excretion (Medalie et al., 1974).

Hypertriglyceridemia

Although most published studies have not documented a significant association of hypercholesterolemia and hyperuricemia, hypertriglyceridemia is reported in up to 75% of individuals with gout and hyperuricemia (Wyngaarden and Kelley, 1976; Emmerson, 1998). This association is often confounded by the presence of obesity and increased alcohol consumption, both of which are known to increase plasma triglycerides (Grahame and Scott, 1970; Wiedemann et al., 1972; Ginsberg et al., 1974). Some observers have felt that a relationship between primary gout and hypertriglyceridemia persists even after allowance is made for greater weight and alcohol consumption (Collantes Estevez et al., 1990). Although one study of lean gouty subjects did not demonstrate an increase in hypertriglyceridemia, Emmerson (1998) has discussed impaired glucose tolerance and excessive insulin secretion as additional mediators of both metabolic aberrations. It appears that hyperuricemia resulting from impaired renal uric acid clearance is an integral part of the metabolic syndrome of hyperinsulinemia and resistance to insulin action (Reaven, 1988; Emmerson, 1998). Additional features of this syndrome include increased body mass index, abdominal obesity (Carey, 1998), hypertriglyceridemia, increased apolipoprotein B and very low-density lipoprotein cholesterol, reduced high-density lipoprotein cholesterol, hypertension, and coronary atherosclerosis (Reaven, 1988; Facchini et al., 1991; Vuorin-Markkola and Yki-Jarvinen, 1994; Lee et al., 1995).

Cardiovascular Disease

Associations between hyperuricemia and coronary heart disease, cardiovascular disease, and death have often been noted (Kagan et al., 1975; Wyngaarden and Kelley, 1976; Yano et al., 1977; Fessel, 1980; Reunanen et al., 1982; Brand et al., 1985; Bengtsson et al., 1988; Freedman et al., 1995; Lehto et al.,1998). Nevertheless, prospective studies of cardiac morbidity and mortality conducted since 1948 have most often concluded that the serum urate level is not an independent risk factor for the development of coronary artery disease (Rakic et al., 1964; Brand et al., 1985). The Tecumseh study found no association when urate values were adjusted for age, sex, and relative weight (Meyers et al., 1966). The Evans County, Georgia, study of 2530 subjects (Klein et al., 1973) and the Coronary Drug Research Group (1976) study of over 8000 men did not find an association between hyperuricemia and nonfatal myocardial infarction or death when the analysis was controlled for medication use. In the Israeli heart study, serum urate was unrelated to 5-year incidence of angina or myocardial infarction (Medalie et al., 1973a,b). A study of almost 5000 Finnish subjects failed to show hyperuricemia as an independent risk factor in multivariate analysis of a 5-year follow-up in persons without known heart disease (Reunanen et al., 1982). Significantly higher mortality in hyperuricemic men and women with known heart disease was attributable to an association with more advanced arterial disease and compromised renal function.

Several studies have renewed the concept that hyperuricemia may constitute an independent risk for cardiovascular disease and death (Freedman et al., 1995; Lehto et al., 1998; Ward, 1998). However, an extension of the Framingham Study (Culleton et al., 1999) supports the contention that other risk factors for both heart and vascular diseases are more important than hyperuricemia in atherosclerotic cardiovascular disease. In this study of 6763 subjects whose serum uric acid values were established in 1971–1976, hyperuricemia was not associated with increased risk for adverse outcomes (coronary heart disease, cardiovascular death, or death from all causes) in men or, after adjustment for other cardiovascular risks, in women.

There is, thus, at best weak evidence for hyperuricemia as an independent risk factor for coronary artery disease. The epidemiologic approach does not, however, resolve, and indeed may obscure, questions of the etiologic significance of hyperuricemia in conjunction with other known risk factors in the development or acceleration of coronary heart disease (Anker et al., 1997; Leyva et al., 1997). Etiologic data would speak to the question of whether asymptomatic hyperuricemia in the presence of other coronary risk factors should be treated. To date, the co-existence of coronary risk factors does not provide the basis for treating hyperuricemia any earlier or more vigorously than is recommended elsewhere in this chapter.

Hypertension

Hypertension is common in patients with primary gout, the prevalence ranging from 30% to 50% when confounding variables such as renal disease, age, or obesity are not included in the analysis (Rapado and Castrillo, 1977). Gout has been noted in 2% to 12% and hyperuricemia in 47% to 67% of untreated hypertensive subjects (Cannon et al., 1966; Wyngaarden and Kelley, 1976). When hypertension therapy and renal disease are excluded, the prevalence of hyperuricemia declines to 22% to 38%, still higher than would be expected in a normal population. In the Tecumseh study, no correlation was found between serum urate concentration and hypertension when values were age-, sex-, and relative weight-adjusted (Meyers et al., 1966). In the Israeli heart study, a simple correlation was observed between serum urate concentration and systolic blood pressure but the serum urate level had almost no power to predict blood pressure variation (Sive et al., 1971).

Renal urate excretion in normal individuals is efficient enough so that even a 50% loss of renal mass, as in transplant donors, does not result in hyperuricemia. Changes in renal vascular perfusion, however, impair uric acid excretion much more readily than loss of renal mass. Toxemia of pregnancy provides an excellent model of the early rise in serum urate as renal perfusion diminishes. Urate clearance has been shown to be inappropriately low for GFR in patients with renal and essential hypertension (Cannon et al., 1966). A critical study has shown an inverse correlation of serum urate concentration and renal blood flow and a direct correlation of serum urate with renal vascular and total peripheral resistance in untreated normotensive, mild, and established hypertensive subjects (Messerli et al., 1980). These physiologic findings were not accompanied by reduced GFR. The clinical observation that hyperuricemia may improve when antihypertensive therapy is initiated with agents that improve renal circulation, if diuretics are not employed, fits well with these findings. The significant hyperuricemia often seen in untreated hypertensives may be a marker for increased renal vascular resistance and early nephrosclerosis. Hyperuricemia and gout do not appear to cause hypertension, except perhaps in the rare instance of severe renal damage due to gouty nephropathy.

Renal Disease

Severe impairment of GFR results in urate retention and hyperuricemia, but gout is rather uncommon in this setting, perhaps because uric acid excretion and normouricemia are relatively well maintained in states of mildly or moderately impaired GFR. When, however, hyperuricemia is disproportionate to the degree of impaired GFR, as in renal vascular impairment with hypertension (Messerli et al., 1980), chronic lead nephropathy, polycystic renal disease, renal amyloidosis, analgesic nephropathy, medullary cystic disease, and obstructive uropathy with hydronephrosis, gout may emerge earlier in the renal disease. These forms of renal disease are characterized early by tubular, more than glomerular, impairment and often by early decrements in renal blood flow with interstitial renal damage (Emmerson, 1978).

Excess uric acid filtration and secretion can result in acute renal damage, as demonstrated by the syndrome of acute, potentially reversible uric acid nephropathy. The dramatically increased cell turnover of lymphoproliferative and myeloproliferative disorders is often accompanied by purine nucleotide and uric acid overproduction, sometimes manifested by severe hyperuricemia and hyperuricosuria leading to obstructive uropathy, especially during chemotherapy (Cohen et al., 1980). In acute uric acid nephropathy, the uric acid to creatinine concentration ratio in urine may exceed 1.0 (Tungsanga et al., 1984).

Chronic, longstanding, untreated tophaceous gout, frequently the outcome in an earlier era, was often associated with renal disease (Wyngaarden and Kelley, 1976). Renal failure was a serious complication of gout, and renal pathology revealed shrunken kidneys densely infiltrated with urate crystals and even tophi. Gouty kidney of this type is rarely seen in the modern era, when recurrent gout usually leads to antihyperuricemic treatment that successfully prevents tophus formation (Emmerson, 1996). Nevertheless, renal damage is detectable at autopsy in many untreated gouty subjects (Linnane et al., 1981), and such damage may occasionally result in renal insufficiency unrelated to other primary diagnoses. This occurrence appears to be very uncommon unless the degree of hyperuricemia is quite severe (>6 SD above the upper limit of normal for the respective gender) or daily urinary uric acid excretion exceeds at least 1000 mg.

Studies of serum creatinine in 113 subjects with asymptomatic hyperuricemia showed no increased incidence of azotemia over 8 years (Fessel, 1979). Evaluation of renal function by means of inulin and *p*-aminohippurate clearance in 112 gouty subjects followed for at least 12 years led to the conclusion that hyperuricemia alone had no deleterious effect on renal function (Berger and Yu, 1975). Even gout was in only a few cases related to diminished renal function not ascribable to aging, renal vascular disease, calculi, infection, or an independent nephropathy (Berger and Yu, 1975; Gibson et al., 1980). A study of 94 initially healthy men who became hyperuricemic over 14.9 years detected no deterioration in glomerular function attributable to hyperuricemia (Campion et al., 1987). These results support the concept that deterioration in glomerular function is minimal in mild to moderate hyperuricemia and gout. Changes in glomerular function are difficult to ascribe to hyperuricemia alone in an aging, often hypertensive population with many other renal risk factors. Tubular impairment, when measured by sensitive criteria, apparently occurs even in asymptomatic hyperuricemia; but the risk of morbidity from this defect would be small. The weight of evidence is that at the levels of hyperuricemia usually encountered, neither asymptomatic nor symptomatic hyperuricemia needs to be treated with the aim of preventing renal impairment (Berger and Yu, 1975; Wyngaarden and Kelley, 1976; Liang and Fries, 1978; Emmerson, 1996). The difficulty of establishing hyperuricemia or gout as a risk factor in chronic renal insufficiency is paralleled by a consequent inability to validate in a controlled fashion that antihyperuricemic treatment reduces the risk of renal impairment.

In recent years, interest has focused on an uncommon familial disease constellation in which early-onset hyperuricemia (with or without gout) occurs with hypertension and progressive renal impairment (Simmonds et al., 1980; Calabrese et al., 1990). Multiple family members of both sexes are affected in a generational pattern consistent with autosomal dominant inheritance. Genetic heterogeneity in the defects underlying the disorder among different affected families is suggested by differences in clinical course and by localization of two candidate 9 to 10 cM intervals for associated genes at 16p12 and 16p11.2 in Japanese (Kamatani et al., 2000) and Czech (Stiburkova et al., 2000) families, respectively. Affected patients can be modestly hyperuricemic in childhood; postpubertal subjects have more severe hyperuricemia; and gout occurs early, often becoming tophaceous without therapy. Progressive renal insufficiency leads to renal failure in the third or fourth decade of life. Metabolic studies suggest that reduced renal urate excretion leads to hyperuricemia (Simmonds et al., 1980; Puig et al., 1993). A primary role for a renal vascular defect manifested by impaired uric acid excretion prior to other renal functional or anatomic abnormalities has been suggested (Puig et al., 1993). These studies also suggest that disordered purine metabolism, urate crystal deposition, and gout are not the primary basis of the disorder, which may be better regarded as familial juvenile nephropathy with hyperuricemia (gout) rather than familial juvenile gouty nephropathy. As expected from this viewpoint, allopurinol administration has not proved consistent in retarding progression of the renal disease (Puig et al., 1993).

Renal Calculi

Hyperuricemia and hyperuricosuria constitute risk factors for urolithiasis. In the Framingham Study, 12.7% of males with serum uric acid above 7 mg/dl had stones, rising to 40% of those with serum uric acid above 9 mg/dl (Hall et al., 1967). When urate excretion was measured directly, the prevalence of urolithiasis ranged from 11% in those excreting less than 300 mg/day to 50% in those excreting more than 1100 mg/day (Yu and Gutman, 1967). The incidence of urolithiasis in Americans with gout has remained at about 20% since 1948 but is consistently higher in more arid climates (Asplin, 1996). In as many as 40% of hyperuricemic subjects, urate stone formation antedates attacks of arthritis, and the risk clearly rises with both duration and severity of hyperuricemia and hyperuricosuria (Yu and Gutman, 1967).

Recurrent uric acid stone-formers also include normouricemic patients with documented renal urate transport defects leading to hyperuricosuria. Both augmented tubular secretion and postsecretory reabsorptive defects have been described (Mateos Anton et al., 1984). A familial syndrome with recessive inheritance, in which defects in tubular urate reabsorption are severe enough to result in persistent hypouricemia, has also been described (Sperling et al., 1980). Hyperuricosuria also predisposes to formation of calcium stones (especially calcium oxalate stones) (Asplin, 1996). Idiopathic urolithiasis is common, most often resulting from reduced urine volume, increased urinary solute concentrations, and, in the case of uric acid stones, excessively acidic urinary pH. Thus, while patients with asymptomatic hyperuricemia, isolated hyperuricosuria, or gout are at significantly increased risk for urolithiasis, not all uric acid stone-formers have an identifiable disorder of urate homeostasis.

PATHOPHYSIOLOGY: BIOLOGIC BASIS OF GENETIC SUSCEPTIBILITY

Pathophysiology of Disease

Uric Acid Homeostasis

The end product of purine metabolism in most mammalian species is the highly soluble and readily excretable compound allantoin. Humans (and great apes), however, lack activity of the enzyme uricase, which catalyzes degradation of uric acid to allantoin, thus necessitating excretion of sparingly soluble uric acid as the end product of human purine metabolism (Hitchings, 1978). This situation conditions humans to the development of urate-supersaturated body fluids, with the attendant risks of urate crystal deposition and clinical sequelae. Uric acid is a weak organic acid, the un-ionized form of which predominates at acid pH and is soluble only to the extent of about 6.5 mg/dl in aqueous solution and about 15 mg/dl in normal urine at pH 5.0 (Wyngaarden and Kelley, 1976). Solubility of the ionized urate form that constitutes 98% of uric acid at the pH and sodium concentration of other extracellular fluids is also limited to about 6.5 mg/dl. Although mean serum urate concentrations in many normal adult male populations approach 6 mg/dl and most individuals excrete urine at supersaturating concentrations of uric acid, clinical manifestations of urate deposition are relatively uncommon. The factors determining in whom hyperuricemia and gout will develop are diverse and best understood in the context of the biochemical and physiologic mechanisms maintaining uric acid homeostasis in normal individuals and disrupting it in hyperuricemic individuals.

Purine Metabolism. Purines are compounds that contain the nine-member purine nucleus (Fig. 25–3), consisting of fused pyrimidine and imidazole rings. Purines are essential building blocks of DNA and RNA, act as molecular energy sources, and serve as coenzymes, neurotransmitters, and second messengers. Dietary intake of preformed purines and purines endogenously synthesized from nonpurine precursors (purine synthesis de novo) are the sole sources of new purines in the body. Interacting biochemical pathways comprise human purine metabolism, which culminates in the production of uric acid (Fig. 25–4). (A detailed description and display of the pathways and reactions of purine metabolism is found in Wyngaarden and Kelley, 1976.) Overall, purine metabolism involves three integrated and regulated processes: purine nucleotide synthesis, purine interconversions, and purine nucleotide catabolism through purine nucleosides and bases to uric acid. In the normal steady state, uric acid production (and excretion) balances in magnitude the sum of purine synthesis de novo and dietary intake.

Although net synthesis of purine nucleotides requires the multistep and energy-expensive pathway of purine synthesis de

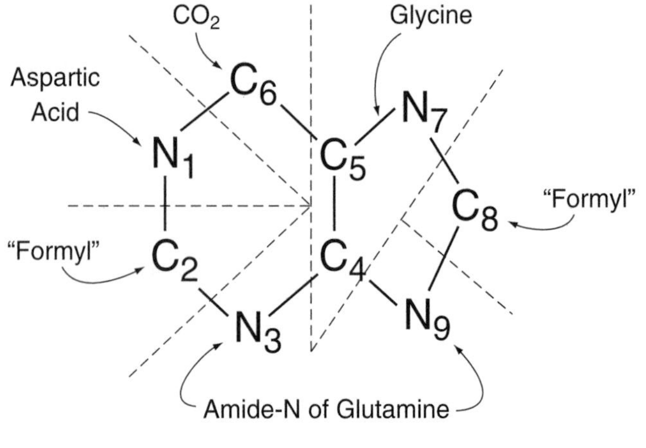

Fig. 25–3. Origins of the atoms of the purine ring. In the first reaction of the pathway of purine synthesis de novo, catalyzed by amidophosphoribosyltransferase, an amido group from glutamine is linked to the C1 of ribose-5-phosphate (donated by 5-phosphoribosyl 1-pyrophosphate) to form 5-phosphoribosylamine. In the subsequent nine reactions of the pathway, the purine ring is sequentially constructed on the ribose-5-phosphate backbone (not shown) by addition of the small molecule substituents indicated, with the N9 atom serving as the starting point. From Becker et al. (1997) with permission.

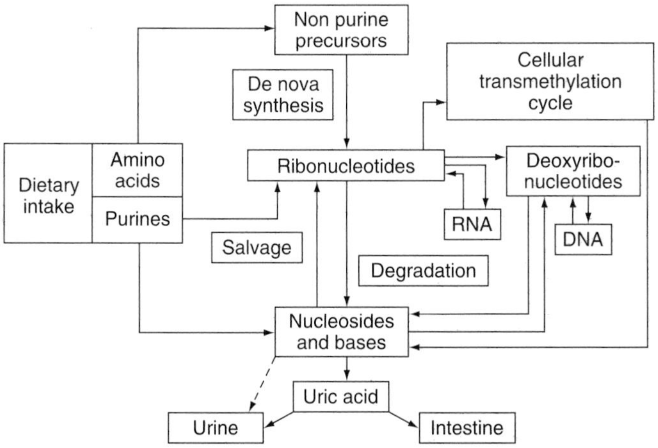

Fig. 25–4. Overview of human purine metabolism. There are two pathways leading to purine ribonucleotide synthesis. One is purine synthesis de novo (see Fig. 25–5), and the second is the purine salvage pathway by which purine bases, including those derived from purines contained in the diet, can be resynthesized to ribonucleotides. Purine ribonucleotides can be converted to the diphosphate and triphosphate forms as well as to cyclic nucleotides. Ribonucleoside diphosphate derivatives are converted to deoxyribonucleoside diphosphate derivatives, substrates for DNA synthesis. Adenosine triphosphate is a substrate for the cellular transmethylation cycle to form *S*-adenosylmethionine. During cellular transmethylation, *S*-adenosylhomocysteine and adenosine are formed and adenosine feeds into the pathway of purine nucleotide degradation. Purine ribonucleoside triphosphates are substrates for RNA synthesis, and nucleotides are products of RNA degradation. Purine ribonucleoside monophosphates are the main substrates for the pathway of purine nucleotide degradation, by which purine nucleotides are ultimately converted in humans to uric acid. From Fox (1986) with permission.

novo, the existence of alternative pathways of purine salvage provides efficient means for one-step reutilization of preformed purine rings, an important economy maintained by regulatory interactions between the pathways (Fig. 25–5). The compound 5-phosphoribosyl 1-pyrophosphate (PRPP), which is synthesized solely in a reaction catalyzed by PRPP synthetase (Becker, 2001), is a substrate in both de novo and salvage pathways of purine nucleotide synthesis; along with the purine nucleotide pathway products, it is an important regulator of the rate of purine synthesis de novo (Holmes et al., 1973a,b; Itakura et al., 1981; Becker et al., 1987a). A wealth of evidence (reviewed in Becker, 2001) supports the concept that the first reaction in purine synthesis de novo, catalyzed by amidophosphoribosyltransferase (AmidoPRT) (Holmes et al., 1973a), together with the preceding PRPP synthetase reaction comprise the dominant regulatory domain in which the interaction of PRPP and purine nucleotide products, acting as positive and negative allosteric effectors, respectively, of AmidoPRT adjust rates of purine synthesis (Fig. 25–5) (Holmes et al., 1973b; Bagnara et al., 1974; Itakura et al., 1981; Becker et al., 1987a). The structural bases for regulation of the activities of AmidoPRT (Smith et al., 1994) and PRPP synthetase (Eriksen et al., 2000) have been established.

Purine nucleotide and nucleoside interconversion reactions are integrated in a manner assuring adequate supplies of adenine and guanine nucleotides for nucleic acid synthesis and for the additional essential roles of purine compounds in differentiated cell activation, cellular energy metabolism, and nonpurine biosynthetic and catabolic pathways (Wyngaarden and Kelley, 1976; Fox, 1981). Similarly, purine catabolic reactions are regulated to assure a balance between purine reutilization in salvage reactions and irreversible degradation to uric acid (Fox, 1978). The final purine base oxidation reactions, through which hypoxanthine is converted to xanthine and xanthine to uric acid, are catalyzed by the enzyme xanthine oxidase, an important target of antihyperuricemic chemotherapy.

Uric Acid Physiology. Uric acid production and excretion are balanced processes in which, under normal circumstances, about two-thirds of the uric acid turned over daily is excreted by the kidneys and virtually all extrarenal urate disposal is accounted for by intestinal *uricolysis*, bacterial degradation of uric acid secreted into the gut (Wyngaarden and Kelley, 1976). Uric acid is synthesized mainly in the liver and released into the circulation, where only a small proportion (<4%) is protein-bound (Kovarsky et al., 1979). The vast majority of urate is thus available for filtration at the glomerulus and for mechanisms of renal uric acid handling that have been defined over a number of years as a result of pharmacologic and physiologic studies in experimental animals and humans.

Briefly, renal clearance of uric acid in normal subjects is only 7% to 10% that of creatinine or inulin clearance despite essentially free urate filtration at the glomerulus. This reflects net reabsorption of at least 90% to 93% of filtered urate (Roch-Ramel and Diezi, 1996) in a sequence of reactions initiated by a proximal tubular reabsorption process facilitated by active transport independent of non-ionic diffusion or passive forces (Roch-Ramel and Weiner, 1973). Study of an individual with marked hypouricemia and a urate clearance far exceeding that of inulin

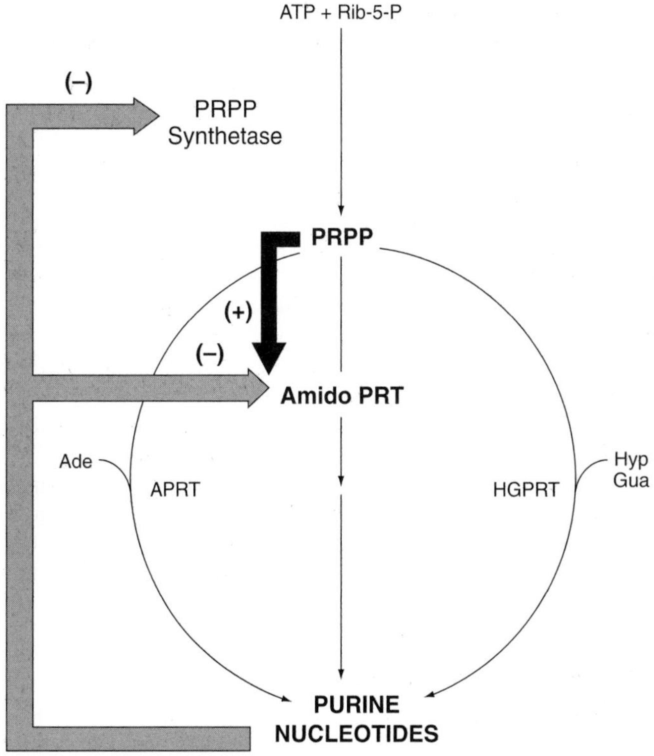

Fig. 25–5. Schematic representation of the pathways of 5-phosphoribosyl 1-pyrophosphate (*PRPP*) and purine nucleotide synthesis and the regulation of rates of purine synthesis de novo by PRPP and purine nucleotide end products. *Curved arrows* depict single-step purine base salvage pathways of purine nucleotide synthesis, requiring PRPP and catalyzed by the phosphoribosyltransferase (*PRT*) enzymes hypoxanthine-guanine PRT (*HGPRT*) and adenine PRT (*APRT*). Purine synthesis de novo is shown by a *thin solid arrow* representing the rate-limiting AmidoPRT reaction and a *dashed arrow* depicting the nine additional steps in this reaction sequence. Purine nucleotide inhibition (−) of PRPP synthetase and AmidoPRT is indicated by the *heavy hatched arrow*, and allosteric activation (+) of AmidoPRT by PRPP is shown by the *heavy dark arrow*. *Rib-5-P*, ribose-5-phosphate; *Ade*, adenine; *Hyp*, hypoxanthine; *Gua*, guanine. From Becker et al. (1997) with permission.

subsequently led to recognition of a third renal uric acid handling process, *proximal tubular urate secretion* (Praetorius and Kirk, 1950). Human tubular urate secretion is mediated by an energy-dependent transport system shared with a variety of endogenously generated and drug-derived organic acids, which potentially compete for the system.

Although tubular urate secretion may be of even greater importance than glomerular filtration in determining normal urinary uric acid excretion (Levinson and Sorensen, 1980; Puig et al., 1986), the relative contributions of reabsorption and secretion to this process in humans remain uncertain. In fact, a fourth component for human renal uric acid handling has been proposed, to reconcile the paradoxical drug effects on human uric acid excretion and the results of studies in Cebus monkeys and in families with apparent defects in renal uric acid handling (Diamond and Paolino, 1973; Levinson and Sorensen, 1980; Puig et al., 1983, 1986). This mechanism involves extensive post-secretory reabsorption of secreted urate at an anatomical site either coextensive with or distal to the secretory site. Resort to such a complicated scheme of physiologic mechanisms has been necessitated in part by the actions of drugs such as salicylates, probenecid, and pyrazinamide on uric acid excretion. For example, in low doses, salicylates decrease uric acid excretion, but increased doses result in uricosuria (Yu and Gutman, 1959). These effects remain best explained by hypothesizing inhibition of tubular secretion at low doses and inhibition of both secretion and reabsorption at higher doses. To date, however, confirmation of the four-component model of renal uric acid handling in humans and quantitation of the flux of uric acid through individual transport mechanisms have yet to be achieved (Roch-Ramel and Diezi, 1996).

Uric Acid Balance in Normal Humans. By means of sequential measurements of isotopic enrichment of urinary uric acid following intravenous administration of [^{15}N] or [^{14}C] urate, the size and dynamics of the miscible pool of uric acid and the contribution of renal excretion to uric acid disposal have been estimated at steady state in normal and hyperuricemic (gouty) individuals (Wyngaarden and Kelley, 1976). The miscible urate pool averages about 1200 mg in normal men with a mean rate of turnover of about 700 mg/day. The corresponding values in normal women are 600 mg and 0.6 pools/day, respectively. Untreated patients with gout invariably have enlarged uric acid pools, most often ranging from 2 to 4 g in the absence of tophaceous deposits but reaching as high as 30 g or more in tophaceous gout. Extrarenal uric acid disposal in hyperuricemic or gouty individuals is normal or increased, reaching as much as 50% of total daily excretion in patients with renal insufficiency. Thus, impaired intestinal uricolysis is not a mechanism of hyperuricemia (Sorensen, 1962).

Pathogenesis of Hyperuricemia in Humans

Although increased rates of turnover of the uric acid pool have been found in some patients with gout, most have turnover rates that overlap the normal range. Nevertheless, patients with excessive rates of purine synthesis de novo and uric acid overproduction, as manifested by increased incorporation of labeled precursors into urinary uric acid (Seegmiller et al., 1961; Wyngaarden and Kelley, 1976) and daily urinary uric acid excretion clearly exceeding that of normal individuals (Sorensen, 1962), invariably have accelerated uric acid pool turnover. Heterogeneity in the mechanisms accounting for uric acid accumulation, hyperuricemia, and predisposition to urate crystal deposition among gout patients is suggested by these findings. Subsequent study has confirmed that excessive production and diminished renal excretion of uric acid, acting singly or in combination, are the major abnormalities underlying uric acid accumulation in hyperuricemic individuals with or without gout (Wyngaarden and Kelley, 1976). Regardless of whether hyperuricemia occurs as a result of a hereditary metabolic disorder (primary hyperuricemia) or is a consequence of a coexisting acquired or inherited condition (secondary hyperuricemia), one or both of these mechanisms underlies the development of hyperuricemia. A mechanistic classification of hyperuricemia in humans is shown in Table 25–1.

Determination of the major mechanism responsible for hyperuricemia (i.e., uric acid overproduction or impaired renal uric

Table 25–1. Etiology of Hyperuricemia in Humans

Increased purine biosynthesis or urate production
Inherited enzymatic defects
Genetically undefined
HGPRT deficiency
PRPP synthetase overactivity
Glycogen storage disease (types I, III, V, VII)
Disease states leading to purine or urate overproduction
Myeloproliferative or lymphoproliferative disorders
Malignancies
Hemolysis
Psoriasis
Obesity
Tissue hypoxia
Down syndrome
Associated with drugs or dietary habits
Cytolytic agents
Vitamin B_{12} (pernicious anemia)
Warfarin
Nicotinic acid
4-Amino-5-imidazole carboxamide riboside
Pancreatic extract
Fructose
Ethanol
Excessive dietary purine intake
Decreased renal clearance of urate
Inherited defects of glomerular or tubular function (undefined)
Disease states leading to reduced urate clearance
Chronic renal insufficiency
Polycystic kidney disease
Familial juvenile nephropathy with hyperuricemia
Dehydration
Starvation
Diabetes insipidus
Lactic acidosis (tissue hypoxia)
Obesity
Hyperparathyroidism
Hypothyroidism
Sarcoidosis
Eclampsia
Bartter's syndrome
Lead poisoning (lead nephropathy)
Beryllium poisoning
Associated with drug administration
Diuretics
Ethanol
Salicylates (low dose)
Laxative abuse (alkalosis)
Cyclosporine
Pyrazinamide
Ethambutol
Levodopa
Methoxyflurane

HGPRT, hypoxanthine-guanine phosphoribosyltransferase; PRPP, 5-phosphoribosyl 1-pyrophosphate.

acid excretion) is of both therapeutic and investigative importance; in most instances, it can be made in individuals with normal renal function by measurement of daily urinary uric acid excretion, ideally with the patient at steady state with regard to dietary purine intake and excluding medications or other agents that affect uric acid production or excretion (Becker, 1988). When the determination is made after 3 to 5 days of an isocaloric, purine-free diet, mean values for uric acid excretion in adult white American males are about 425 mg/day, with 75 to 80 mg/day SD (Seegmiller et al., 1961; Wyngaarden and Kelley, 1976). Thus, values exceeding 600 mg/day are 2 SD above the mean and indicative of uric acid overproduction. When, as is frequently the case, such strict dietary control is impractical or impossible, daily uric acid excretion on a standard isocaloric diet is often measured. Although this is a less accurate and more often equivocal approach, uric acid excretion of more than 1000 mg/day is usually regarded as clearly excessive (Berger and Yu, 1975). For values between 800 and 1000 mg/day, retesting under closer dietary control is usually advisable. Standardized normal values are not available for women, children, and obese or very large individuals; but urinary uric acid excretion exceeding about 12 mg/kg body weight suggests uric acid overproduction.

Uric Acid Overproduction

In roughly 10% to 15% of patients with gout and primary hyperuricemia, as well as in most patients whose hyperuricemia reflects increased cell turnover (as in lymphoproliferative or myeloproliferative malignancy or psoriasis), a toxic state, or pharmacologic intervention resulting in increased uric acid production, excessive urinary uric acid excretion is demonstrable. In some patients with extensive tophaceous deposits or renal insufficiency or under circumstances in which there is increased extrarenal uric acid disposal, confirmation of suspected uric acid overproduction may require in vivo labeling studies (Seegmiller et al., 1961; Wyngaarden and Kelley, 1976) or direct measurement of rates of purine synthesis de novo in fibroblasts cultured from skin biopsy material (Becker et al., 1987b).

Sustained uric acid overproduction in patients with gout and primary hyperuricemia indicates excessive rates of purine synthesis de novo and, in our current understanding of the regulation of this pathway, likely reflects altered interaction between PRPP and purine nucleotides at the level of AmidoPRT activity (Holmes et al., 1973b; Becker et al., 1987a). Examples of circumstances in which inherited or acquired increases in PRPP availability or decreased purine nucleotide concentrations provide the apparent basis for excessive purine nucleotide and uric acid synthesis have been described. Although mutation in AmidoPRT leading to altered responsiveness to normal levels of allosteric effectors might be expected among at least some patients with inherited purine nucleotide and uric acid overproduction (Becker, 1976), defects in this key regulatory enzyme remain to be demonstrated.

Increased Phosphoribosyl Pyrophosphate Availability. Increased PRPP availability underlies excessive rates of purine synthesis de novo in two X chromosome–linked inborn errors of purine metabolism, PRPP synthetase superactivity (Sperling et al., 1972; Becker et al., 1973; Zoref et al., 1975) and hypoxanthine-guanine phosphoribosyltransferase (HGPRT) deficiency (Seegmiller et al., 1967; Kelley et al., 1967). Each of these disorders is characterized by uric acid overproduction, hyperuricemia, and hyperuricosuria; and in each, intracellular PRPP concentrations are increased (Rosenbloom et al., 1968; Kelley et al., 1969; Becker et al., 1973, 1987a,b). In PRPP synthetase superactivity, there is accelerated synthesis of this regulatory substrate (Becker et al., 1987b); in contrast, PRPP is synthesized at a normal rate in HGPRT deficiency but accumulates in excess as a result of underutilization of PRPP in purine base salvage (Becker et al., 1987b). Activation of AmidoPRT and acceleration of purine nucleotide and uric acid synthesis as a result of increased PRPP availability characterize both of these enzyme defects (Itakura et al., 1981). Although PRPP synthetase superactivity and HGPRT deficiency account for fewer than 10% of patients with primary uric acid overproduction, they provide the only confirmed instances in which increased PRPP availability in the absence of diminished intracellular purine nucleotide concentrations constitutes a unitary explanation for accelerated purine nucleotide and uric acid synthesis.

Abnormalities in carbohydrate metabolism may manifest themselves in hyperuricemia and gout, at least in part mediated by increased PRPP availability and uric acid overproduction. First, increased concentrations and rates of production of ribose-5-phosphate, the immediate precursor of PRPP, and PRPP were demonstrated in fibroblasts cultured from some patients with documented purine nucleotide and uric acid overproduction but no demonstrable enzyme defect (Becker, 1976). Second, it has been reported (but not confirmed) that an overactive electrophoretically variant form of the enzyme glutathione reductase is demonstrable at high frequency in erythrocyte extracts from patients with gout (Long, 1967). Third, a component of uric acid overproduction has been documented in the multifactoral hyperuricemia and gout that may appear as early as infancy in patients with autosomal recessive deficiency of glucose-6-phosphatase (glycogen storage disease type I) (Alepa et al., 1967). In all three of these circumstances, acceleration of the activity of the oxidative branch of the pentose phosphate pathway provides a tenable mechanism for excessive ribose-5-phosphate and PRPP availability and, ultimately, purine nucleotide and uric acid production. To date, however, no definitive experimental evidence has been provided to link rates of pentose phosphate generation to rates of PRPP and purine nucleotide synthesis under physiologic conditions (Becker, 2001). Nevertheless, hyperuricemia and gout are associated with such metabolic abnormalities as obesity, hypertriglyceridemia, and hyperinsulinemia/insulin resistance, raising the possibility that accelerated lipogenesis or carbohydrate excess might increase metabolic flux through the pentose phosphate pathway and consequently increase PRPP availability to account for these associations.

Decreased Purine Nucleotide Concentrations. Uric acid overproduction due to nucleotide depletion occurs in circumstances characterized by net degradation of adenosine triphosphate (ATP) as a consequence of either increased ATP consumption or impaired ATP regeneration (Fox et al., 1987). Under conditions of restricted inorganic phosphate, oxygen, glucose, or fatty acid supply, ATP synthesis may be impaired, leading to ATP depletion and hyperuricemia, particularly if the demands for ATP consumption are increased. Net ATP degradation results in accumulation of adenosine diphosphate (ADP) and adenosine monophosphate (AMP), which are rapidly converted to uric acid through the intermediates inosine, hypoxanthine, and xanthine. Increases in any or all of these intermediates accompanying excessive uric acid levels in serum or urine provide evidence to support activation of this mechanism of hyperuricemia (Fox and Kelley, 1972; Faller and Fox, 1982; Puig and Fox, 1984; Fox, 1985, 1986; Woolliscroft and Fox, 1986; Mineo et al., 1987; Yamanaka et al., 1992; Jinnai et al., 1993). In at least some instances of net ATP degradation, uric acid overproduction is supported by an increased rate of the pathway of purine synthesis de novo as a consequence of release of PRPP synthetase and AmidoPRT from purine nucleotide feedback inhibition (Raivio et al., 1975).

Physiologic and pathologic states associated with net ATP degradation and consequent hyperuricemia include strenuous training in otherwise normal individuals (Yamanaka et al., 1992), in which muscle hypoxia and adenylate depletion may ultimately contribute more to the hyperuricemia than the accompanying lactic acidemia and dehydration; glycogen storage disease type III (debrancher deficiency), type V (myophosphorylase deficiency), and type VII (muscle phosphofructokinase deficiency), in which mild exercise provokes myogenic hyperuricemia and hyperuricosuria as a consequence of impaired glucose availability for generation of ATP from ADP in muscle (Mineo et al., 1987); glucose-6-phosphatase deficiency (glycogen storage disease type I), in which hypoglycemia results in diminished ATP concentrations and purine catabolism (Greene et al., 1978); acute, severe illness, such as adult respiratory distress syndrome, myocardial infarction, or status epilepticus, in which tissue hypoxia may impair ATP synthesis from ADP in mitochondria, resulting in catabolism (Woolliscroft et al., 1986); and alcohol consumption in which this process plays a major role in the associated hyperuricemia (along with renal uric acid retention due to dehydration and metabolic acidosis) when the rate of ATP utilization in ethanol metabolism via acetate to form acetyl coenzyme A exceeds the capacity for ATP generation (Puig and Fox, 1984).

Decreased Uric Acid Excretion

A deficit in renal uric acid excretion is the major mechanism leading to hyperuricemia in 80% or more of individuals with gout (Wyngaarden and Kelley, 1976). Absolute underexcretion of uric acid, defined as daily excretion of less than about 275 mg of uric acid in a hyperuricemic person receiving a purine-free diet, is uncommon in primary gout. Even among the majority of gout patients, who excrete normal amounts of uric acid, however, these amounts are inappropriately low with respect to corresponding serum urate concentrations: gouty patients with primary underexcretion of uric acid have lower uric acid clearance rates than nongouty individuals (Wyngaarden and Kelley, 1976; Simkin, 1977; Levinson et al., 1982; Roch-Ramel and Diezi, 1996). When the urinary urate excretion rates of gouty and normal individuals are related to corresponding plasma urate concentrations, it appears that gouty persons must have a mean plasma urate value nearly 2 mg/dl greater on average than their nongouty counterparts in order to achieve equivalent excretion rates (Simkin, 1977). From these data, gouty patients are estimated to excrete an average of 41% less uric acid than normal subjects at any given plasma urate concentration. Similar findings are observed when the fractional excretion of urate (curate/cinulin or creatinine $\times$ 100) is studied (Simkin, 1977).

The complexity of renal uric acid handling provides for many potential sites of derangement among gouty patients. Decreased urate clearance in primary gout could be due to reduced urate filtration, enhanced tubular uric acid reabsorption, or diminished tubular urate secretion. Increased urate binding to plasma proteins has been reported in conjunction with the hyperuricemia of the Maoris of New Zealand (Gibson et al., 1984) and in a few other gouty subjects. Excessive plasma protein binding of urate could reduce the filtered load of urate, but these findings have not been accompanied by urate clearance data. Both increased reabsorption and decreased secretion of uric acid have also been proposed as the basis for the lower urate clearances observed in most patients with primary gout, but no compelling experimental evidence has been adduced to affirm enhanced proximal tubular reabsorption of uric acid as a common mechanism (Diamond and Paolino, 1973; Steele, 1973; Levinson and Sorensen, 1980). In contrast, diminished renal urate secretion per nephron has been implicated in the hyperuricemia of patients with primary gout unassociated with overproduction of uric acid (Rieselbach et al., 1970; Levinson and Sorensen, 1980; Puig et al., 1983, 1986). In a study employing benzbromarone, a drug that selectively inhibits reabsorption of secreted urate, to measure the minimum tubular secretory rate, such patients showed decreased secretion of uric acid in comparison to nongouty controls or gouty subjects with uric acid overproduction (Levinson and Sorensen, 1980). To date, no alteration in postsecretory reabsorption has been documented in conjunction with hyperuricemia.

In contrast to the limited insight into the individual contributions of uric acid handling mechanisms to renal urate retention in primary gout, mechanisms of secondary hyperuricemia and gout are better understood. For example, advanced chronic renal failure is commonly accompanied by hyperuricemia resulting from the progressive decline in GFR, which overcomes compensatory mechanisms that earlier in the course of the disease promote uric acid excretion through enhanced fractional excretion of filtered urate (Steele and Rieselbach, 1967). Similarly, conditions resulting in extracellular volume depletion are associated with hyperuricemia, in part due to reduced GFR. In such conditions as dehydration, diabetes insipidus, and diuretic therapy, however, enhanced reabsorption of uric acid plays an important, perhaps dominant, role in inducing hyperuricemia (Kahn, 1988). Diuretic treatment is an important and frequent cause of renal hyperuricemia (Myers and Monteagudo, 1985; Macfarlane and Dieppe, 1985; Lally et al., 1986; Puig et al., 1991). Finally, decreased tubular secretion as a mechanism for secondary renal hyperuricemia is exemplified by the effects of elevated blood levels of a wide array of endogenous and drug-derived organic acids (such as lactate, β-hydroxybutyrate, acetoacetate, and low-dose salicylates), which inhibit uric acid excretion by competing with urate at tubular secretory sites (Yu and Gutman, 1959; Goldfinger et al., 1965; Roch-Ramel and Diezi, 1996).

Genetic Expression in Common Primary Hyperuricemia

Urate production and excretion are influenced by a wide array of environmental and acquired factors and by multiple genetically determined physiologic and biochemical processes. Although most gout patients can be categorized with regard to the relative roles of uric acid production and renal excretion in their hyperuricemia (Becker, 1988), the more precise molecular bases of hyperuricemia within each category are unknown in the vast majority of affected individuals. In fact, given the comorbid associations of hyperuricemia, the prevalence and singularity of the designation *common adult primary hyperuricemia* remain in doubt. This situation is further complicated by the apparent differential expression of major environmental and even genetic influences on different members of the same pedigree, frequently resulting in inconsistencies in the biochemical and physiologic characteristics of the urate metabolic phenotype when the families of probands are analyzed (Short, 1992). Finally, the increase over the past several decades in secondary hyperuricemia and gout associated with drug agents, especially diuretics (Macfarlane and Dieppe, 1985; Scott, 1991), has skewed the balance be-

Table 25–2. Inherited Clinical Syndromes Associated with Gout

Disorder	Basis of Hyperuricemia	Clinical Features	Molecular Defect	Inheritance
HGPRT deficiency[a]	Purine and uric acid overproduction	Males affected *Severe:* infantile onset neurobehavioral disorder (Lesch-Nyhan syndrome) *Partial:* juvenile or early adult onset, variable neurological defects	Mutations in *HPRT* locus at Xq26–q27	X-linked
PRPP synthetase superactivity[b]	PRPP, purine, and uric acid overproduction	Adult-onset: Males only; rare neurological defects	Excessive PRPP synthetase isoform 1 expression due to accelerated *PRPS1* transcription	X-linked
		Infantile onset: Neurodevelopmental defects; carrier women affected	Mutations in *PRPS1* coding region (Xq22–q24)	
Glucose-6-phosphatase deficiency[c]	Purine and uric acid overproduction, impaired renal uric acid excretion	Type I glycogen storage disease and variants (GSD type I a–d)	Defects in components of hepatic microsomal glucose-6-phosphatase system	Autosomal recessive
Familial juvenile nephropathy with gout/hyperuricemia[d]	Impaired renal uric acid excretion	Juvenile to early adult onset; hypertension, progressive renal failure	Unknown, candidate affected intervals on chromosome 16p	Autosomal dominant

HGPRT, hypoxanthine-guanine phosphoribosyl transferase; PRPP, 5-phosphoribosyl 1-pyrophosphate.
Sources: [a]Lesch and Nyhan (1964), Seegmiller et al. (1967), Kelley et al. (1967), Jinnah and Friedman (2001); [b]Becker et al. (1995, 1996), Ahmed et al, (1999); [c]Chen (2001); [d]Simmonds et al. (1980), Calabrese et al. (1990), Puig et al. (1993), Kamatani et al. (2000), Stiburkova et al. (2000).

tween the prevalence of primary and secondary hyperuricemia sharply in favor of the latter (Short, 1992). As a consequence, identification of probands and families with unequivocal primary adult hyperuricemia has become even more difficult.

Success in breaking out specific subsets from the group of patients with primary hyperuricemia and gout has been achieved in some instances in which the genetic derangement has been strongly expressed (Table 25–2), usually in the form of extended clinical accompaniments, such as infantile-onset, symptomatic renal stone and/or neurologic disease in X-linked HGPRT deficiency (Lesch and Nyhan, 1964; Seegmiller et al., 1967); PRPP synthetase superactivity (Becker et al., 1995); or juvenile-onset hypertension, gout, and progressive renal failure in autosomal dominant familial nephropathy with hyperuricemia (Simmonds et al., 1980; Calabrese et al., 1990). Only the strong family histories identified among gout patients for centuries and a few pedigree studies (reviewed above and by Short, 1992), consistent with the view that an autosomal dominant gene defect is operative in many families showing adult-onset, male-predominant gout, lend credence to the major single-gene hypothesis in primary adult hyperuricemia. The identification and characterization of a candidate gene or genes remain dependent on future research initiatives. Perhaps detailed molecular and physiologic understanding of renal tubular urate transporters/ion channels (Leal-Pinto et al., 1997) will provide a start in this direction.

CLINICAL APPLICATIONS

Screening and Diagnosis of Disordered Urate Homeostasis

Aberrant urate homeostasis may come to light in a variety of settings. Most obvious and dramatic is the presentation of a 35- to 50-year-old man or a 60- to 80-year-old woman with acute gouty arthritis. More common is detection of asymptomatic hyperuricemia during a periodic health examination or in the course of evaluation or treatment for a common adult disorder such as hypertension. Occasionally, detection of hyperuricosuria or a uric acid urinary stone in the course of evaluation of renal calculi may unveil disordered urate homeostasis. Regardless of the context, all persistent hyperuricemia reflects extracellular fluid urate supersaturation and an expanded body urate pool. It is the deposition of urate or uric acid crystals from these fluids, however, that determines the clinical events defining gout.

The utility of a single random serum urate measurement as a screening marker for hyperuricemia is limited. For example, sequential measurements of serum urate in the relatives of gouty persons have revealed fluctuation in and out of the normal range in up to 30% of these subjects (Yu and Kaung, 1980). Furthermore, hyperuricemia has neither the specificity nor the sensitivity to permit its use as a primary criterion for the diagnosis of gout (Wallace et al.,1977). Serum urate values are normal in up to 40% of individuals suffering an acute attack of gouty arthritis (Logan et al., 1997), and, as discussed earlier, asymptomatic hyperuricemia is common in the adult male and postmenopausal female populations. The unequivocal diagnosis of gout requires demonstration of urate crystal deposition.

Given these considerations and recognizing their negative implications for establishing simplified means to distinguish affected from nonaffected members of the families of gouty/hyperuricemic propositi, it is perhaps best to discuss separate approaches to the evaluation of hyperuricemia and the diagnosis of gout.

Evaluation of Hyperuricemia

Asymptomatic hyperuricemia was formerly regarded as the preliminary stage in the classically defined progression of gout, preceding acute gouty arthritis, intercritical gout, and chronic tophaceous gout. Epidemiologic studies have established, however, that gouty manifestations are relatively infrequent among hyperuricemic persons and, on average, culminate one to two decades preceding hyperuricemia (Hall et al.,1967; Campion et al., 1987). Furthermore, despite the frequent disease associations of hyperuricemia, there is no compelling evidence that disordered uric acid metabolism is a causal factor in hypertension, hyperlipidemia, atherosclerosis, or, in most instances, chronic renal insufficiency (Berger and Yu, 1975; Fessel, 1979; Gibson et al., 1980; Campion et al., 1987; Langford et al., 1987). Finally, with the exception of acute uric nephropathy, the initial clinical manifestations of urate/uric acid crystal deposition are not life-threatening and are readily treatable. All of these points have led to a marked decline in the enthusiasm for routine prophylactic antihyperuricemic drug therapy in the vast majority of individuals with asymptomatic hyperuricemia (Liang and Fries, 1978).

The discovery of persistent asymptomatic hyperuricemia should prompt an appropriately limited and focused clinical and biochemical evaluation aimed at identifying persons at particularly high risk for gouty arthritis, tophi, or urolithiasis who thus might warrant antihyperuricemic treatment; individuals whose hyperuricemia signals an underlying disorder or environmental exposure requiring specific treatment; and hyperuricemia-inducing drugs or toxins, the removal of which can relieve or diminish the hyperuricemic state. The evaluation of hyperuricemia should start with a thorough history and physical examination, and laboratory work should be directed at discovering potential causes of hyperuricemia that may mandate treatment. For example, neoplastic disorders, psoriasis, and lead nephropathy may lead to hyperuricemia, as may any of the circumstances listed in Table 25–1.

If the above evaluation is unrewarding, hyperuricemia is regarded as a primary process. A 24-hour urine specimen should be collected for uric acid and creatinine while the individual is receiving a standard diet (excluding alcohol and drugs known to affect uric acid metabolism) in order to distinguish between uric acid overproduction (defined as urinary uric acid excretion >800 mg/day) and reduced urinary uric acid clearance as the major pathogenic mechanism underlying hyperuricemia. The distinction can guide further investigation of the underlying cause of hyperuricemia and, if treatment is necessary, will help direct the choice of antihyperuricemic medication.

About 80% to 90% of individuals with primary hyperuricemia (defined in this manner) demonstrate either excess dietary purine consumption or uric acid underexcretion or both. In the remainder, hyperuricemia reflects uric acid overproduction, in some instances as a consequence of inherited dysregulation of purine nucleotide synthesis de novo (HGPRT deficiency, PRPP synthetase overactivity), accelerated ATP catabolism, or increased rates of cell turnover. A means to distinguish among the three mechanisms is as follows: a uric acid to creatinine clearance ratio of <6% in the 24-hour urine specimen is indicative of underexcretion of uric acid; when hyperuricosuria is present in the 24-hour collection, a repeat collection should be obtained after the patient has received a purine-free diet for 5 days, with daily uric acid excretion exceeding 600 mg interpreted as uric acid overproduction; if serum urate and urinary uric acid excretion values decline to normal with the purine-free diet, excessive dietary purine consumption is implicated in hyperuricemia. Most patients who underexcrete uric acid and have a normal GFR show no other abnormality of renal function. The underlying defect, presumably in uric acid transport, may be acquired or intrinsic, possibly reflecting an inherited tubular transport defect(s).

Diagnosis of Gout

When on the basis of clinical history of physical examination gout is suspected, a definitive diagnosis should be sought. The reasons prompting this recommendation include exclusion of alternative possibilities (most commonly joint infection or pseudogout), avoidance of the use of potentially toxic medications for an improper indication, and validation of the diagnosis in members of families with a known gouty/hyperuricemic propositus.

The definitive diagnosis of gout requires demonstration of urate crystal deposition (or, in the case of uric acid urolithiasis, coexisting hyperuricemia) (Wallace et al., 1977). During an acute episode of gouty arthritis, aspiration of the affected joint and polarized compensated light microscopy of the synovial fluid permit detection of negatively birefringent, intracellular monosodium urate crystals in synovial fluid neutrophils in at least 85% of patients. Although specificity of urate crystal identification is absolute, an acute gout attack may occasionally be an accompaniment of a second acute intra-articular process, most notably septic arthritis or pseudogout.

The diagnosis of gout can also be established during the asymptomatic intercritical period by demonstration of urate crystals in the synovial fluid aspirated from a previously affected joint in 70% to 97% of gout patients who have not received antihyperuricemic treatment (Rouault et al., 1982; Pascual, 1991; Pascual et al., 1999). Despite occasional false-positive results in patients with asymptomatic hyperuricemia or renal failure, this provides a valuable means to establish diagnosis in most individuals for whom it was not made in the acute setting. The presence of urate crystals in joints previously affected only once supports the concept that, in general, the first clinical episode of gouty arthritis follows deposition of urate crystals in and around joints by a substantial period. In patients with suspected tophi, the diagnosis of gout can be confirmed by aspiration of a tophus and polarized microscopy, showing masses of urate crystals, usually without accompanying inflammatory cells.

When the presence of urate crystals cannot be established by polarized light microscopy, the diagnosis of gout must be regarded as, at best, provisional, relying on a typical history of episodic monoarticular arthritis separated by intercritical periods of complete wellness and, according to the traditional view, rapid clinical improvement after administration of oral colchicine (Wallace et al., 1977). Neither of these criteria, however, is specific; in fact, they can often be observed in pseudogout. Persistently normal serum urate levels, even during intercritical periods, would cast doubt on a diagnosis of gout, unless the history suggests an episode of acute hyperuricemia (as may occur with dehydration or an alcohol binge) or transient exposure to a medication causing hyperuricemia.

Prevention and Counseling

Given the high population prevalence of mild to modest asymptomatic hyperuricemia, the apparent chronicity and favorable outcome in the great majority of individuals, the readily treatable consequences of symptomatic urate or uric acid crystal deposition (gout), the strong likelihood that hyperuricemia is not causally related to the many associated disorders discussed above, and the occasional severely adverse responses to antihyperuricemic treatment (Hande et al., 1984; Singer and Wallace, 1986; Wallace et al., 1988a,b), several recommendations regarding this chemical aberration can be made. First, population-wide screening for hyperuricemia is unwarranted unless initiated in conjunction with a formal investigative aim. In this light, inclusion of serum urate determination in automated chemistry panels has probably not impacted favorably on the public health, and even when applied to hospitalized or otherwise ill patients, routine urate testing has had mixed consequences: the benefit of identifying hyperuricemia as a consequence of drug administration, for example, but the detriment of stimulating inappropriate antihyperuricemic treatment. Second, if for any reason persistent hyperuricemia nominally unrelated to an identifiable and/or correctable disorder or environmental cause is established, evaluation of uric acid excretion outlined in the preceding section should be undertaken with the aim of guiding a decision regarding further management (as outlined below, under Therapy of Primary Hyperuricemia and Gout). Third, if, as is the usual case, antihyperuricemic drug treatment is unwarranted, the nature of the chemical findings, the rationale for recommending only nondrug management (e.g., weight reduction, reduced ethanol intake, attention to hydration, and avoidance of high-purine, high-protein diets), and the range of possible clinical consequences should be discussed with the individual, planning for follow-up routinely appropriate to age and general medical status. Except in those instances in which the risk of gout, urolithiasis, or progressive renal insufficiency is high, pharmacologic prevention of urate crystal deposition is not currently advisable (Liang and Fries, 1978). Finally, unless the individual's clinical or family history or an investigative protocol mandates, screening of relatives is not recommended. Among salient historical data in patients with primary hyperuricemic gout that would prompt family screening would be identification of primary hyperuricemia/gout/uric acid urolithiasis in the patient or in a family member prior to age 20; a family history compatible with autosomal dominantly inherited hypertension, renal insufficiency, and hyperuricemia; multiple family members with otherwise unexplained hyperuricemia/gout or urolithiasis; membership in an ethnic group with particularly high prevalence of gout; and premenopausal female status. To date, insufficient information is available with regard to the genetic transmission of hyperuricemic states to provide more than general family risk assessment and counseling, except in specific subsets, such as X-linked HGPRT deficiency, PRPP synthetase overactivity, or autosomal dominant familial nephropathy with hyperuricemia. With regard to the immediate consequences of symptomatic urate crystal deposition, clinical manifestations appear to follow the severity and duration of hyperuricemia and are thus both more prevalent and earlier in onset among male family members.

Therapy of Primary Hyperuricemia and Gout

Asymptomatic Hyperuricemia

Primary hyperuricemia is urate supersaturation that is not explained by a coexisting disease process or environmental influence. The frequent but poorly understood associations of hyperuricemia with other prevalent disorders, such as obesity and hypertension, make the distinction between primary hyperuricemia and hyperuricemia secondary to these disorders less than clear. Nevertheless, once established, hyperuricemia usually persists indefinitely and warrants a decision regarding pharmacologic (antihyperuricemic) treatment.

The results of the evaluation of hyperuricemia suggested above should provide the means to estimate the risk in each individual for the development of gouty arthritis, tophi, uric acid or calcium oxalate stones, chronic renal insufficiency, or acute uric acid nephropathy. The estimated risk should then be balanced with the potential benefits and risks of life-long drug treatment, including the potentially severe and even life-threatening toxic reactions to such agents as allopurinol and colchicine (Hande et al., 1984; Singer and Wallace, 1986; Wallace and Singer, 1988a). For the great majority of persons with asymptomatic hyperuricemia, antihyperuricemic drug therapy is not justifiable by risk/benefit analysis (Liang and Fries, 1978; Emmerson, 1996). Gouty arthritis and tophi are readily treatable and reversible; prophylaxis against stone disease is not mandated in most individuals, but treatment should be initiated if a stone is discovered. Moreover, in the absence of a defined independent risk of asymptomatic hyperuricemia (or even of gout) for development of chronic renal insufficiency (Berger and Yu, 1975; Fessel, 1979; Gibson et al., 1980; Langford et al., 1987), a renal function-sparing role for antihyperuricemic drugs has been impossible to establish.

Table 28–3. Indications for Antihyperuricemic Drug Therapy in Patients with Gout and/or Hyperuricemia

Frequent and disabling attacks of acute gouty arthritis
Clinical or radiographic signs of chronic gouty joint disease
Presence of tophaceous deposits in soft tissues or subchondral bone
Gout with renal insufficiency
Recurrent urolithiasis
Serum urate levels persistently in excess of 13 mg/dl in men or 10 mg/dl in women
Urinary uric acid excretion exceeding 1100 mg/day
Impending cytotoxic chemotherapy or radiotherapy for lymphoma or leukemia

In three specific circumstances, however, the institution of antihyperuricemic treatment of asymptomatic persons is warranted, following the recommendations presented below (Table 25–3). First, data confirming the absence of a significant nephrotoxic risk of hyperuricemia are limited to urate values below 10 mg/dl in women and 13 mg/dl in men. Thus, persistent hyperuricemia with serum urate levels in excess of these unusually high values for the respective sex may carry some long-term renal risk, perhaps related to the likelihood of uric acid overproduction. Second, daily urinary uric acid excretion in excess of 1100 mg is associated with a 50% risk of uric acid calculi (Yu and Gutman, 1967; Hall et al., 1967). Finally, patients receiving radiotherapy or chemotherapy that is likely to result in extensive tumor cytolysis should be pretreated with allopurinol and fluid loading to prevent acute uric acid nephropathy (Cohen et al., 1980).

Gout

Gouty arthritis, tophus formation, and renal calculi associated with hyperuricemia are conditions for which specific treatment of gout is appropriate. Pharmacologic agents utilized in the treatment of gout can be classified as anti-inflammatory, prophylactic, and antihyperuricemic. These designations reflect different therapeutic aims. In the case of anti-inflammatory agents, the aim is prompt and safe termination of the acute arthritic attack. Prophylactic agents are given to prevent recurrences of acute gouty arthritis, in contrast to antihyperuricemic drugs, which are prescribed to prevent and reverse the consequences of urate crystal deposition in joints (gouty arthropathy), the urinary tract (nephrolithiasis), renal interstitium (urate nephropathy), connective tissues, and parenchymal organs (tophi).

Anti-inflammatory and prophylactic drugs effectively control and prevent attacks of gouty arthritis but do not reverse hyperuricemia or modify the natural history of gout. Achievement of this aim requires the long-term use of drugs to lower the serum urate concentration either by enhancing renal uric acid excretion (uricosuric agents) or by decreasing uric acid synthesis (xanthine oxidase inhibitors). By the same token, antihyperuricemic agents do not have anti-inflammatory properties and are not appropriate agents for treatment of acute gouty inflammation. It is critical for the physician to understand and convey to the patient the distinction between management directed at the acute inflammatory events of gout and that aimed at control of hyperuricemia in order to avoid prolongation of the symptomatic state in patients whose gout should be readily controlled (Nakayama et al., 1984; Lawry et al., 1988).

Antiinflammatory Therapy. Virtually any of the available nonsteroidal anti-inflammatory drugs (NSAIDs) or colchicine can be administered orally with the expectation of prompt and complete resolution of acute gouty arthritis, at least early in the disease. Aspirin is usually avoided because of the paradoxical effects of salicylates on serum urate concentrations (Yu and Gutman, 1959). NSAIDs and colchicine accelerate the natural resolution of acute gouty attacks, usually reversing the pain and disability within several days, rather than several weeks, as in untreated patients early in the course of their disease. Gastrointestinal intolerance associated with NSAID use dictates that the dose should be halved as soon as objective and subjective improvement is noted. Further dose reduction and withdrawal over several more days is most often safe and practical. Cyclooxygenase-2–selective anti-inflammatory agents are likely as efficacious as cyclooxygenase-nonselective NSAIDs and may ultimately prove to be significantly safer than the latter agents with regard to adverse gastrointestinal effects. Oral colchicine is a commonly used alternative and, when renal and hepatic function is normal, is given in a dose of 0.6 mg/hour until there is relief of the gouty inflammation, a total dose of 6 mg is reached, or nausea, vomiting, or especially diarrhea limits further use. Once the inflammation has been controlled, dosing can be reduced to 0.6 mg twice daily and continued, if gastrointestinal tolerance permits, until complete resolution of the attack. Oral prednisone (20 mg for 1 or 2 days and then reduced stepwise over 7 to 10 days) can also be employed to suppress acute gout, with, however, some risk of recurrence after withdrawal (Werlen et al., 1996).

Alternative anti-inflammatory regimens that may be equally effective and are especially useful in hospitalized (often postoperative) patients who are not receiving oral feedings include intra-articular steroid injection, parenteral corticosteroid, intramuscular corticotropin (40–80 USP units, twice daily for 2 days and then once daily for 2 to 3 days), and intravenous colchicine. The latter recourse should be taken only in patients with polyarticular gout or those unable to tolerate NSAIDs or oral medications. This approach should be limited to hospitalized patients, and supervision by a physician experienced in the use of colchicine by this route of administration is essential, as is adherence to published precautions (Wallace et al., 1988a,b), in order to avoid potentially life-threatening toxicity. Patients with leukopenia, hepatic disease, or renal insufficiency or who have recently used oral colchicine should not receive intravenous colchicine. The total intravenous dose should never exceed 4 mg during any 24-hour period or during any attack, and great care should be taken to avoid local infiltration of this highly sclerotic agent into the adjacent tissue.

Prophylactic Therapy. Oral colchicine (0.6 mg twice daily) is of value in reducing the frequency of recurrent acute gouty arthritis in at least some patients with a prior history of gout (Yu, 1982). Colchicine is an especially important adjunct early in the course of administration of antihyperuricemic drugs, when patients appear to be at increased risk for gouty attacks. In many patients, particularly elderly individuals, loose stools or diarrhea preclude use of the recommended dose. Satisfactory prophylaxis appears to be achievable, however, with 0.6 mg of colchicine daily or even every other day in such patients. Indomethacin (25 mg twice daily) and other NSAIDs are likely to be of prophylactic benefit in patients intolerant of low-dose colchicine.

Adverse reactions, such as colchicine neuromyopathy (Neuss et al., 1986; Kuncl et al., 1987) and NSAID-induced stomach ulceration, are potential complications of long-term administration of these prophylactic agents. Organ transplant recipients whose gout is associated with administration of cyclosporin A for immunosuppression may be particularly at risk for colchicine toxicity (Simkin and Gardner, 2000). Consequently, continued use of a prophylactic regimen after persistent normouricemia is achieved with antihyperuricemic drugs is not recommended. In patients without evident tophi, prophylaxis can be safely discontinued 6 to 12 months after normal serum urate values have been achieved, at which time tissue urate pools are presumably normalized. In patients with tophi, colchicine prophylaxis should be continued until resolution of tophi or until it becomes clear that tophaceous deposits will not resolve despite persistent normouricemia.

Antihyperuricemic Therapy. The general goal of antihyperuricemic therapy is to achieve a serum urate level substantially below that at which monosodium urate is saturated in extracellular fluids. In practice, concentrations of 5 to 6 mg/dl are satisfactory. Although concentrations in this range can sometimes be achieved by dietary modification, diets with restricted purine content are unpalatable and are neither practical nor effective in the management of hyperuricemia and gout in patients with normal dietary habits. A severely purine-restricted diet may reduce daily urinary uric acid excretion by 200 to 400 mg, but hyperuricemia often persists. With the availability of potent antihyperuricemic drugs, the dietary approach is rarely employed except in individuals with severe renal insufficiency or intolerance to pharmacologic therapy.

An antihyperuricemic drug is prescribed for an indefinite period, possibly for life, so great care is needed in establishing an indication for its use. Indications for antihyperuricemic drug therapy in patients with gout and/or hyperuricemia are listed in Table 25–3. Despite the high likelihood of recurrence after a single attack of acute gouty arthritis (Wyngaarden and Kelley, 1976), one or even several attacks does not provide an absolute indication for treatment of a reluctant individual; but clinical evidence of tophi or structural joint changes or radiologic evidence of tophi in bones constitutes such an indication. Probenecid and sulfinpyrazone are the uricosuric agents most commonly used in the United States, but losartan, an angiotensin II receptor blocker with uricosuric (Minghelli et al., 1998) as well as antihypertensive properties, is an attractive alternative in this patient population. Additional uricosuric drugs, such as benzbromarone (Perez-Ruiz et al.,1999), have gained use elsewhere. Allopurinol remains the only available xanthine oxidase inhibitor.

Allopurinol is likely to be effective in virtually all patients warranting therapy for gout, but safety considerations with allopurinol (Wallace et al., 1988a,b; Hande et al., 1984) and the demonstrated long-term efficacy of uricosuric drugs make the latter the drugs of choice in many patients with gout. The majority of patients with gout who excrete less than 800 mg of uric acid per day on a standard diet are potential candidates for uricosuric drug therapy in the absence of significant renal insufficiency (creatinine clearance <80 ml/min) or prior nephrolithiasis. Some consider older age (>60 years), uricoretentive diuretic therapy, and tophi as indications for use of allopurinol; but even so, a high proportion of gouty individuals remain candidates for uricosuric agents. In such patients, both uricosuric drugs and allopurinol have comparable efficacy at establishing normouricemia and ultimately decreasing or abolishing attacks of gout and preventing tophi and urolithiasis.

Uricosuric drugs are weak organic acids that promote renal clearance of uric acid by inhibiting renal tubular reabsorption of uric acid, predominantly at a postsecretory site (Wallace et al., 1988b). Enhanced uric acid excretion lasts for a relatively short period in patients whose uric acid production is not excessive because as the serum urate concentrations falls, uric acid excretion returns toward the baseline level. The patient returns to a steady state in which uric acid production and excretion are roughly equal. This occurs at a lower serum urate concentration, indicating the persistence of a relative uricosuric effect.

An acute fall in serum urate levels can precipitate acute gouty arthritis, especially if colchicine prophylaxis has been omitted. In addition, the transient increase in urinary uric acid excretion can promote stone formation. The likelihood of this complication can be minimized by starting with low doses of the uricosuric drug and by hydration (2 l of fluid daily); alkalinization of the urine is usually unnecessary.

Overall, probenecid and sulfinpyrazone are effective for most gouty patients, including 75% to 80% of those with tophaceous gout. Probenecid is started at 250 mg twice daily and dose increments are titrated according to the serum urate level. The usual maintenance dose is 500 to 1000 mg two or three times daily; the maximal effective dose is 3 g/day. Sulfinpyrazone is started at a dose of 50 mg twice daily, with increments over several weeks to 100 to 200 mg three or four times daily as needed. The maximum effective dose is 800 mg/day. Losartan, at an initial dose of 50 mg daily is usually titrated thereafter with the antihypertensive effect and appears to be safe when used in combination with thiazide diuretics (Shahinfar et al., 1999).

The major side effects of uricosuric drugs are rash, precipitation of acute gouty arthritis, gastrointestinal intolerance, and uric acid stone formation. Probenecid also increases urinary calcium excretion in gouty patients (Weinberger et al., 1983) and is contraindicated for use in patients with prior nephrolithiasis. Interference with the transport of other organic anions across cell membranes by uricosuric drugs is the basis of numerous drug interactions. For example, excretion of penicillin and ampicillin is decreased by probenecid, with prolongation of the half-lives of these antibiotics. Autoimmune hemolytic anemia has also been reported with probenecid therapy (Kickler et al., 1986).

Allopurinol is a hypoxanthine analog with multiple effects on human nucleotide metabolism (Elion, 1978). In addition to competitive inhibition of xanthine oxidase by allopurinol and pseudoirreversible inactivation of this enzyme by its major metabolite, oxipurinol, total urinary purine excretion is reduced during allopurinol administration, reflecting inhibition of purine synthesis de novo by drug-derived and endogenous nucleotide products of enhanced purine base reutilization. Both xanthine oxidase inhibition and deceleration of purine synthesis contribute to the promptly accompanying reduction in urate levels in serum and urine, but only the former (and more potent) mechanism is operative in individuals deficient in HGPRT. Allopurinol treatment also results in chemical states of xanthinuria, as a consequence of xanthine oxidase inhibition, and oroticaciduria and orotidinuria, as a result of inhibition of the pathway of pyrimidine nucleotide synthesis de novo by nucleotide derivatives of oxipurinol at the orotidylic acid decarboxylase step (Beardmore and Kelley, 1971).

Although the mean effective daily dose of allopurinol is 300 mg, there is considerable variation in the daily dose required to normalize the serum urate concentration (Rundles, 1985). The half-life of oxipurinol is prolonged in renal failure, necessitating a reduction in the allopurinol dose (Hande et al., 1984). Serum urate levels begin to fall within 2 days of allopurinol administration, reaching stable values within 2 weeks. The fall in serum urate levels early in the course of therapy of patients with extensive tophaceous deposits may lag substantially because of large pools of preformed urate. However, true refractoriness to the drug is rare and most commonly reflects a failure of patient compliance or of physician–patient communication (Wallace et al., 1988b).

The therapeutic effectiveness of allopurinol has been documented for more than 30 years. Side effects and adverse reactions, sometimes severe, have, however, been encountered. As with uricosuric agents, allopurinol administration can precipitate acute gouty arthritis, especially if colchicine prophylaxis has been omitted. Among adverse reactions in up to 3% to 5% of patients are rash, leukopenia, thrombocytopenia, diarrhea, and drug fever. Desensitization to allopurinol has been successfully accomplished in some patients with mild adverse reactions, such as skin rashes (Fam et al., 1992, 2001; Webster and Panush, 1985). However, desensitization protocols are cumbersome, and recurrence of hypersensitivity reactions has been reported (Unsworth et al., 1987).

The allopurinol-hypersensitive syndrome consisting of an erythematous skin rash, fever, hepatitis, eosinophilia, and renal failure, although unusual, is potentially life-threatening and more likely to occur in patients with mild renal insufficiency who are treated with standard doses of allopurinol and a diuretic (Hande et al., 1984; Singer and Wallace, 1986). The mortality rate in reported cases has approached 25%. Administration of allopurinol should thus be limited to the minimum dose necessary to achieve an adequate antihyperuricemic effect and to patients with appropriate indications for its use. Additional adverse reactions to allopurinol include gastrointestinal intolerance, severe skin rashes, vasculitis, interstitial nephritis, and urolithiasis composed of xanthine or oxipurinol crystals (especially in patients with florid purine overproduction). Among the important allopurinol drug interactions are potentiation of the cytolytic and immunosuppressive effects of 6-mercaptopurine and azathioprine, mandating at least 50% reductions in doses of these drugs in patients treated with allopurinol (Ragab et al., 1974); bone marrow suppression in patients treated with alkylating agents (Boston Collaborative Drug Surveillance Program, 1974); and an increase in the incidence of ampicillin-induced skin rashes (Boston Collaborative Drug Surveillance Program, 1972). Interactions between allopurinol and uricosuric drugs have also been demonstrated, but the combination has been safe in the unusual instances in which it has been undertaken.

ACKNOWLEDGMENT

Research discussed here from the author's laboratory was supported by United States Public Health Service grant DK-28554 from the National Institutes of Health.

REFERENCES

Acheson RM, O'Brien WM: The prediction of serum uric acid on haemoglobin and other factors in the general population. Lancet 1966; 2:777–778.

Ahmed M, Taylor W, Smith PR, Becker MA: Accelerated transcription of *PRPS1* in X-linked overactivity of normal human phosphoribosylpyrophosphate synthetase. J Biol Chem 1999; 274:7482–7488.

Alepa FP, Howell RR, Klinenberg JR, Seegmiller JE: Relationships between glycogen storage disease and tophaceous gout. Am J Med 1967; 42:58–66.

Anker SD, Leyva F, Poole-Wilson PA, Kox WJ, Stevenson JC, Coats AJ: Relation between serum uric acid and lower limb blood flow in patients with chronic heart failure. Heart 1997; 78:39–43.

Asplin JR: Uric acid stones. Semin Nephrol 1996; 16:412–424.

Baethge BA, Work J, Landreneau MD, McDonald JC: Tophaceous gout in patients with renal transplants treated with cyclosporine A. J Rheumatol 1993; 20:718–720.

Bagnara AS, Letter AA, Henderson JF: Multiple mechanisms of regulation of purine biosynthesis de novo in intact tumor cells. Biochim Biophys Acta 1974; 373:259–270.

Batuman V, Maesaka JK, Haddad B, Tepper E, Landy E, Wedeen RP: The role of lead in gout nephropathy. N Engl J Med 1981; 304:520–523.

Beardmore TD, Kelley WN: Mechanism of allopurinol-mediated inhibition of pyrimidine biosynthesis. J Lab Clin Med 1971; 78:696–704.

Becker MA: Patterns of phosphoribosylpyrophosphate and ribose-5-phosphate concentration and generation in fibroblasts from patients with gout and purine overproduction. J Clin Invest 1976; 57:308–318.

Becker MA: Clinical aspects of monosodium urate monohydrate crystal deposition disease (gout). Rheum Dis Clin North Am 1988; 14:377–394.

Becker MA: Phosphoribosylpyrophosphate synthetase and the regulation of phosphoribosylpyrophosphate production in human cells. Prog Nucleic Acid Res Mol Biol 2001; 69:115–148.

Becker MA, Kim M: Regulation of purine synthesis de novo in human fibroblasts by purine nucleotides and phosphoribosylpyrophosphate. J Biol Chem 1987a; 262: 14531–14537.

Becker MA, Levinson DJ: Gout and the pathogenesis of hyperuricemia. In: Koopman WJ (ed). Arthritis and Allied Conditions, 13th ed. Baltimore: Williams and Wilkins, 1997:2041–2071.

Becker MA, Losman MJ, Kim M: Mechanisms of accelerated purine nucleotide synthesis in human fibroblasts with superactive phosphoribosylpyrophosphate synthetases. J Biol Chem 1987b; 262:5596–5602.

Becker MA, Meyer LJ, Wood AW, Seegmiller JE: Purine overproduction in man associated with increased phosphoribosylpyrophosphate synthetase activity. Science 1973; 179:1123–1126.

Becker MA, Smith PR, Taylor W, Mustafi R, Switzer RL: The genetic and functional basis of purine nucleotide feedback-resistant phosphoribosylpyrophosphate synthetase superactivity. J Clin Invest 1995; 96:2133–2141.

Becker MA, Taylor W, Smith PR, Ahmed M: Overexpression of the normal phosphoribosylpyrophosphate synthetase 1 isoform underlies catalytic superactivity of human phosphoribosylpyrophosphate synthetase. J Biol Chem 1996; 271:19894–19899.

Bengtsson C, Lapidus L, Stendahl C, Waldenstrom J: Hyperuricaemia and risk of cardiovascular disease and overall death. A 12-year follow-up of participants in the population study of women in Gothenburg, Sweden. Acta Med Scand 1988; 224:549–555.

Berger L, Yu TF: Renal function in gout. IV. An analysis of 524 gouty subjects including long-term follow-up studies. Am J Med 1975; 59:605–613.

Boston Collaborative Drug Surveillance Program: Excess of ampicillin-rashes associated with allopurinol or hyperuricemia. N Engl J Med 1972; 286:505–507.

Boston Collaborative Drug Surveillance Program: Allopurinol and cytotoxic drugs. Interaction in relation to bone marrow suppression. JAMA 1974; 227:1036–1040.

Brand FN, McGee DL, Kannel WB, Stokes J, Castelli WP: Hyperuricemia as a risk factor of coronary heart disease: the Framingham Study. Am J Epidemiol 1985; 121:11–18.

Brauer GW, Prior IAM: A prospective study of gout in New Zealand Maoris. Ann Rheum Dis 1978; 37:466–472.

Burack DA, Griffith BP, Thompson ME, Kahl LE: Hyperuricemia and gout among heart transplant recipients receiving cyclosporine. Am J Med 1992; 92:141–146.

Calabrese G, Simmonds HA, Cameron JS, Davies PM: Precocious familial gout with reduced fractional urate clearance and normal purine enzymes. Q J Med 1990; 75:441–450.

Campion EW, Glynn RJ, DeLabry LO: Asymptomatic hyperuricemia. Risks and consequences in the Normative Aging Study. Am J Med 1987; 82:421–426.

Cannon PJ, Stason WB, Demartini FE, Sommers SC, Laragh JH: Hyperuricemia in primary and renal hypertension. N Engl J Med 1966; 275:457–464.

Cantor RM, Rotter JI: Analysis of genetic data: methods and interpretation. In: King RA, Rotter JI, Motulsky AG (eds). The Genetic Basis of Common Diseases. New York: Oxford University Press, 1992:49–70.

Carey DGP: Abdominal obesity. Curr Opin Lipidol 1998; 9:35–40.

Carmelli D, Karlin S, Williams R: A class of indices to assess major gene versus polygenic inheritance of distributed variables. Prog Clin Biol Res 1979; 32:711–729.

Chen Y-T: Glycogen storage diseases. In: Scriver CR, Beaudet AL, Valle D, Sly WS (eds). The Metabolic and Molecular Bases of Inherited Disease, 7th ed. New York: McGraw-Hill, 2001:1521–1551.

Coe FL, Kavalach AG: Hypercalciuria and hyperuricosuria in patients with calcium nephrolithiasis. N Engl J Med 1974; 291:1344–1350.

Cohen LF, Balow JE, Magrath IT, Poplack DG, Ziegler JL: Acute tumor lysis syndrome: a review of 37 patients with Burkitt's lymphoma. Am J Med 1980; 68:486–491.

Collantes Estevez E, Pineda Priego M, A-Non Barbudo J, Sanchez Guijo P: Hyperuricemia-hyperlipidemia–association in the absence of obesity and alcohol abuse. Clin Rheumatol 1990; 9:28–31.

Copeman WSC: A Short History of the Gout and the Rheumatic Diseases. Berkeley: University of California Press, 1964.

Coronary Drug Project Research Group: Serum uric acid: its asociation with other risk factors and with mortality in coronary heart disease. J Chronic Dis 1976; 29:557–569.

Culleton BF, Larson MG, Kannel WB, Levy D: Serum uric acid and risk for cardiovascular disease and death: the Framingham Heart Study. Ann Intern Med 1999; 131:7–13.

Darmavan J, Valkenburg HA, Muirden KD, Wigley RD: The epidemiology of gout and hyperuricemia in a rural population of Java. J Rheumatol 1992; 19:1595–1599.

Diamond HS, Paolino JS: Evidence for a postsecretory reabsorptive site for uric acid in man. J Clin Invest 1973; 52:1491–1499.

Elion GB: Allopurinol and other inhibitors of urate synthesis. In: Kelley WN, Weiner IM (eds). Uric Acid. Handbook of Experimental Pharmacology, Vol 51. New York: Springer-Verlag, 1978:485–514.

Emmerson BT: Alteration of urate metabolism by weight reduction. Aust N Z J Med 1973; 3:410–412.

Emmerson BT: Abnormal urate excretion associated with renal and systemic disorders, drugs and toxins. In: Kelley WN, Weiner IM (eds). Uric Acid. Handbook of Experimental Pharmacology, Vol 51. New York: Springer-Verlag, 1978:287–324.

Emmerson BT: The management of gout. N Engl J Med 1996; 334:445–451.

Emmerson BT: Hyperlipidaemia in hyperuricaemia and gout. Ann Rheum Dis 1998; 57:509–510.

Emmerson BT, Knowles BR: Triglyceride concentrations in primary gout and gout of chronic nephropathy. Metabolism 1971; 20:721–729.

Ericksen TA, Kadziola A, Bentsen A-K, Harlow KW, Larsen S: Structural basis for the function of *Bacillus subtilis* phosphoribosylpyrophosphate synthetase. Nat Struct Biol 2000; 7:303–308.

Facchini F, Chen Y-DI, Hollenbeck CB, Reaven GM: Relationship between resistance to insulin-mediated glucose uptake, urinary uric acid clearance, and plasma uric acid concentration. JAMA 1991; 266:3008–3011.

Faller J, Fox IH: Ethanol-induced hyperuricemia: evidence for increased urate production by activation of adenine nucleotide turnover. N Engl J Med 1982; 307:1598–1602.

Fam AG, Dunne SM, Iazzetta J, Paton TW: Efficacy and safety of desensitization to allopurinol following cutaneous reactions. Arthritis Rheum 2001; 44:231–238.

Fam AG, Lewtas J, Stein J, Paton TW: Desensitization to allopurinol in patients with gout and cutaneous reactions. Am J Med 1992; 93:299–302.

Fessel WJ: Renal outcomes of gout and hyperuricemia. Am J Med 1979; 67:74–82.

Fessel WJ: High uric acid as an indicator of cardiovascular disease: independence from obesity. Am J Med 1980; 68:40–44.

Fessel WJ, Bar GD: Uric acid, lean body weight and creatinine interactions: results from regression analysis of 78 variables. Semin Arthritis Rheum 1977; 7:115–121.

Fox IH: Degradation of purine nucleotides. In: Kelley WN, Weiner IM (eds). Uric Acid. Handbood of Experimental Pharmacology, Vol 51. New York: Springer-Verlag, 1978:93–124.

Fox IH: Metabolic basis for disorders of purine nucleotide degradation. Metabolism 1981; 30:616–634.

Fox IH: Adenosine triphosphate degradation in specific disease. J Lab Clin Med 1985; 106:101–110.

Fox IH: Disorders of purine and pyrimidine metabolism. In: Spittell JA (ed). Clinical Medicine, Vol 9. Philadelphia: Harper and Row, 1986:1–43.

Fox IH, Kelley WN: Studies on the mechanism of fructose-induced hyperuricemia in man. Metabolism 1972; 21:713–721.

Fox IH, Palella TD, Kelley WN: Hyperuricemia: a marker for cell energy crisis. N Engl J Med 1987; 317:111–112.

Freedman DS, Williamson DF, Gunter EW, Byers T: Relation of serum uric acid to mortality and ischemic heart disease. The NHANES I Epidemiologic Follow-Up Study. Am J Epidemiol 1995; 141:637–644.

Garrod AE: The Inborn Factors in Disease: An Essay. Oxford: Clarendon, 1931.

Gibson T, Highton J, Potter C, Simmonds HA: Renal impairment and gout. Ann Rheum Dis 1980; 39:417–423.

Gibson T, Waterworth R, Hatfield P, Robinson G, Bremner K: Hyperuricaemia, gout and kidney function in New Zealand Maori men. Br J Rheumatol 1984; 23:276–282.

Ginsberg H, Olefsky J, Farquhar JW, Reaven GM: Moderate ethanol ingestion and plasma triglyceride levels: a study in normal and hypertriglyceridemic persons. Ann Intern Med 1974; 80:143–149.

Glynn RJ, Campion EW, Silbert JE: Trends in serum uric acid levels 1961–1980. Arthritis Rheum 1983; 26:87–93.

Goldfinger S, Klinenberg JR, Seegmiller JE: Renal retention of uric acid induced by infusion of beta-hydroxybutyrate and acetoacetate. N Engl J Med 1965; 272:351–353.

Grahame R, Scott JT: Clinical survey of 354 patients with gout. Ann Rheum Dis 1970; 29:461–468.

Greene HL, Wilson FA, Hefferan P, Terry AB, Moran JR, Slonim AE, Claus TH, Burr IM: ATP depletion, a possible role in the pathogenesis of hyperuricemia in glycogen storage disease type I. J Clin Invest 1978; 62:321–328.

Griebsch A, Zollner N: Effect of ribonucleotides given orally on uric acid production in man. Adv Exp Med Biol 1974; 41B:443–449.

Hall AP, Barry PE, Dawber TR, McNamara PM: Epidemiology of gout and hyperuricemia. A long-term population study. Am J Med 1967; 42:27–37.
Hande KR, Noone RM, Stone WJ: Severe allopurinol toxicity. Description and guidelines for prevention in patients with renal insufficiency. Am J Med 1984; 76:47–56.
Hasstedt SJ, Cartwright PE, Skolnick MA, Bishop DT: PAP: a Fortran program for pedigree analysis. Am J Hum Genet 1979; 31:135A.
Hauge M, Harvald B: Heredity in gout and hyperuricemia. Acta Med Scand 1955; 152:247–257.
Healey LA, Bayani-Sioson PS: A defect in the renal excretion of uric acid in Filipinos. Arthritis Rheum 1971; 14:721–726.
Herman JB, Mount FW, Medalie JH, Groen JJ, Dublin TD, Neufeld HN, Riss E: Diabetes prevalence and serum uric acid: observations among 10,000 men in a survey of ischemic heart disease in Israel. Diabetes 1967; 16:858–868.
Hitchings GH: Uric acid: chemistry and synthesis. In: Kelley WN, Weiner IM (eds). Uric Acid. Handbook of Experimental Pharmacology, Vol 51. New York: Springer-Verlag, 1978:1–28.
Hochberg MC, Thomas J, Thomas DJ, Mead L, Levine DM, Klag MJ: Racial differences in the incidence of gout: the role of hypertension. Arthritis Rheum 1995; 38:628–632.
Holmes EW, McDonald JA, McCord JM, Wyngaarden JB, Kelley WN: Human glutamine phosphoribosylpyrophosphate amidotransferase. Kinetic and regulatory properties. J Biol Chem 1973a; 248:144–150.
Holmes EW, Wyngaarden JB, Kelley WN: Human glutamine phosphoribosylpyrophosphate amidotransferase. Two molecular forms interconvertible by purine ribonucleotides and phosphoribosylpyrophosphate. J Biol Chem 1973b; 248:6035–6040.
Itakura M, Sabina RL, Heald PW, Holmes EW: Basis for the control of purine biosynthesis by purine ribonucleotides. J Clin Invest 1981; 67:994–1002.
Jinnah HA, Friedmann T: Lesch-Nyhan disease and its variants. In: Scriver CR, Beaudet AL, Valle D, Sly WS (eds). The Metabolic and Molecular Bases of Inherited Disease, 8th ed. New York: McGraw-Hill, 2001:2537–2570.
Jinnai K, Kono N, Yamamoto Y, Kanda F, Ohno S, Tsutsumi M, Yamada Y, Kawachi M, Tarui S, Fujita T: Glycogenosis V (McArdle's disease) with hypeuricemia: a case report and clinical investigation. Eur Neurol 1993; 33:204–207.
Kagan A, Gordon I, Rhoads CG, Schiffman JC: Some factors related to coronary heart disease incidence in Honolulu Japanese men: the Honolulu Heart Study. Int J Epidemiol 1975; 4:271–279.
Kamatani N, Moritani M, Yamanaka, H, Takeuchi F, Hosoya T, Itakura M: Localization of a gene for familial juvenile hyperuricemic nephropathy causing underexcretion-type gout to 16p12 by genome-wide linkage analysis of a large family. Arthritis Rheum 2000; 43:925–929.
Kahn AM: Effect of diuretics on the renal handling of urate. Semin Nephrol 1988; 8:305–317.
Kelley WN, Greene ML, Rosenbloom FM, Henderson JF, Seegmiller JE: Hypoxanthine-guanine phosphoribosyltransferase deficiency in gout. Ann Intern Med 1969; 70:155–206.
Kelley WN, Rosenbloom FM, Henderson JF, Seegmiller JE: A specific enzyme defect in gout associated with overproduction of uric acid. Proc Natl Acad Sci USA 1967; 57:1735–1739.
Kickler TS, Buck S, Ness P, Shirey RS, Sholar PW: Probenecid induced immune hemolytic anemia. J Rheumatol 1986; 13:208–209.
Klein R, Klein BE, Cornoni JC, Maready J, Cassel JC, Tyroler HA: Serum uric acid. Its relationship to coronary heart disease risk factors and cardiovascular disease, Evans County, Georgia. Arch Intern Med 1973; 132:401–410.
Klemp P, Stansfield SA, Castle B, Robertson MC: Gout is on the increase in New Zealand. Ann Rheum Dis 1997; 56:22–26.
Klinenberg JR, Campion DS, Olsen RW: A relationship between free urate, protein-bound urate, hyperuricemia and gout in Caucasians and Maoris. Adv Exp Med Biol 1977; 76B:159–162.
Kovarsky J, Holmes EW, Kelley WN: Absence of significant urate binding to human serum proteins. J Lab Clin Med 1979; 93:85–91.
Kuncl RW, Duncan G, Watson D, Alderson K, Rogawski MA, Peper M: Colchicine myopathy and neuropathy. N Engl J Med 1987; 316:1562–1568.
Lally EV, Ho G Jr, Kaplan SR: The clinical spectrum of gouty arthritis in women. Arch Intern Med 1986; 146:2221–2225.
Langford HG, Blaufox MD, Borhani NO, Curb JD, Molteni A, Schneider KA, Pressel S: Is thiazide-produced uric acid elevation harmful? Analysis of data from the Hypertension Detection and Follow-up Program. Arch Intern Med 1987; 147:645–649.
Lawrence RC, Helmick CG, Arnett FC, Deyo RA, Felson DT, Giannini EH, Heyse SP, Hirsch R, Hochberg MC, Hunder GG, et al.: Estimates of the prevalence of arthritis and selected musculoskeletal disorders in the United States. Arthritis Rheum 1998; 41:778–799.
Lawry GV II, Fan PT, Bluestone R: Polyarticular versus monoarticular gout: a prospective comparative analysis of clinical features. Medicine 1988; 67:335–343.
Leal-Pinto E, Tao W, Rappaport J, Richardson M, Abramson RG: Molecular cloning and functional reconstitution of a urate transporter/channel. J Biol Chem 1997; 272:617–625.
Lee J, Sparrow D, Vokonas PS, Landsberg L, Weiss ST: Uric acid and coronary heart disease risk: evidence for a role of uric acid in the obesity-insulin resistance syndrome. Am J Epidemiol 1995; 142:288–294.
Lehto S, Niskanen L, Ronnemaa T, Laakso M: Serum uric acid is a strong predictor of stroke in patients with non-insulin-dependent diabetes mellitus. Stroke 1998; 29:635–639.
Lesch M, Nyhan WL: A familial disorder of uric acid metabolism and central nervous system function. Am J Med 1964; 36:561–570.
Levinson DJ, Decker DE, Sorensen LB: Renal handling of uric acid in man. Ann Clin Lab Sci 1982; 12:73–77.
Levinson DJ, Sorensen LB: Renal handling of uric acid in normal and gouty subjects: evidence for a 4-component system. Ann Rheum Dis 1980; 39:173–179.
Leyva F, Anker SD, Swan JW, Godsland IF, Wingrove CS, Chua TP: Serum uric acid as an index of impaired oxidative metabolism in chronic heart failure. Eur Heart J 1997; 18:858–865.
Liang MH, Fries JF: Asymptomatic hyperuricemia. The case for conservative management. Ann Intern Med 1978; 88:666–670.
Linnane JW, Burry AF, Emmerson BT: Urate deposits in the renal medulla. Nephron 1981; 29:216–222.
Logan JA, Morrison E, McGill PE: Serum uric acid in acute gout. Ann Rheum Dis 1997; 56:696–697.
Long WK: Glutathione reductase in red blood cells: variant associated with gout. Science 1967; 155:712–713.
Macfarlane DG, Dieppe PA: Diuretic-induced gout in elderly women. Br J Rheumatol 1985; 24:155–157.
Mateos Anton F, Garcia Puig J, Ramos T, Gonzalez P, Ordas J: Sex differences in uric acid metabolism in adults: evidence for a lack of influence of estradiol-17beta (E2) on the renal handling of urate. Metabolism 1986; 35:343–348.
Mateos Anton F, Puig JG, Gaspar G, Sanz AM, Herrero E, Ramos T, Martinez ME, Mantilla JM: Renal handling of uric acid in patients with recurrent calcium nephrolithiasis and hyperuricosuria. Nephron 1984; 37:123–127.
Medalie JH, Kahn HA, Neufeld HN, Riss E, Goldbourt U: Five year myocardial infarction incidence. II. Association of single variables to age and birthplace. J Chronic Dis 1973a; 26:329–349.
Medalie JH, Papier C, Herman JB, Goldbourt U, Tamir S, Neufeld HN, Riss E: Diabetes melllitus among 10,000 adult men. I. Five year incidence and associated variables. Isr J Med Sci 1974; 10:681–697.
Medalie JH, Snyder M, Groen JJ, Neufeld HN, Goldbourt U, Riss E: Angina pectoris among 10,000 men. Am J Med 1973b; 55:583–594.
Messerli FH, Frohlich ED, Dreslinski GR, Suarez DH, Aristmuno GG: Serum uric acid in essential hypertension: an indicator of renal vascular involvement. Ann Intern Med 1980; 93:817–821.
Meyers AR, Epstein FH, Dodge HJ, Mikkelsen WM: The relationship of serum uric acid to risk factors in coronary artery disease. Am J Med 1966; 45:520–528.
Mikkelsen WM, Dodge HJ, Valkenburg H: The distribution of serum uric acid values in a population unselected as to gout or hyperuricemia. Tecumseh, Michigan 1959–1960. Am J Med 1965; 39:242–251.
Mineo I, Kono N, Hara N, Shimizu T, Yamada Y, Kawachi M, Kiyokawa H, Wang YL, Tarui S: Myogenic hyperuricemia. A common pathophysiologic feature of glycogenosis types III, V, and VII. N Engl J Med 1987; 317:75–80.
Minghelli G, Seydoux C, Got JJ, Burnier M: Uricosuric effect of the angiotensin II receptor Antagonist losartan in heart transplant recipients. Transplantation 1998; 9:268–271.
Morton NE: Genetics of hyperuricemia in families with gout. Am J Hum Genet 1979; 4:103–106.
Myers OL, Monteagudo FSE: Gout in females: an analysis of 92 patients. Clin Exp Rheumatol 1985; 3:105–109.
Nakayama DA, Barthelemy C, Carrera G, Lightfoot RW Jr, Wortmann RL: Tophaceous gout: a clinical and radiographic assessment. Arthritis Rheum 1984; 7:468–471.
Neel JV, Rakic MT, Davidson RT, Valkenburg HA, Mikkelsen WM: Studies on hyperuricemia. II. A reconsideration of the distribution of serum uric acid values in the families of Smyth, Cotterman and Freyberg. Am J Hum Genet 1965; 17:14–22.
Neuss MN, McCallum RM, Brenckman WD, Silberman HR: Long-term colchicine administration leading to colchicine toxicity and death. Arthritis Rheum 1986; 29:448–449.
Nichols A, Scott JT: Effect of weight-loss on plasma and urinary levels of uric acid. Lancet 1972; 2:1223–1224.
Nishioka K, Mikanagi K: Hereditary and environmental factors influencing the serum uric acid throughout ten years population study in Japan. Adv Exp Med Biol 1980; 122A:155–159.
Pascual E: Persistance of monosodium urate crystals and low grade inflammation in the synovial fluid of patients with untreated gout. Arthritis Rheum 1991; 34:141–145.
Pascual E, Batlle-Gualda E, Martiez A, Rosas J, Vela P: Synovial fluid analysis for diagnosis of intercritical gout. Ann Intern Med 1999; 131:756–759.
Paulus HE, Coutts A, Calabro JJ, Klinenberg JR: Clinical significance of hyperuricemia in routinely screened hospitalized men. JAMA 1970; 211:277–281.
Perez-Ruiz F, Calabozo M, Fernandez-Lopez J, Herrero-Beites, Ruiz-Lucea E, Garcia-Erauskin G, Duruelo J, Alonso-Ruiz A: Treatment of chronic gout in patients with renal functional impairment. An open, randomized, actively controlled study. J Clin Rheumatol 1999; 5:49–55.
Porter R: Gout: framing and fantasizing disease. Bull Hist Med 1994; 68:1–28 and references therein.
Praetorius E, Kirk JE: Hypouricemia: with evidence for tubular elimination of uric acid. J Lab Clin Med 1950; 35:865–868.
Price CP, James DR: Analytical reviews in biochemistry: the measurement of urate. Ann Clin Biochem 1988; 25:484–498.
Puig JG, Fox IH: Ethanol-induced activation of adenine nucleotide turnover. Evidence for a role of acetate. J Clin Invest 1984; 74:936–941.
Puig JG, Mateos Anton F, Jimenez ML, Guitierrez PC: Renal handling of uric acid in gout: impaired tubular transport of urate not dependent on serum urate values. Metabolism 1986; 35:1147–1153.
Puig JG, Mateos Anton F, Sanz MA, Gaspar G, Lesmes A, Ramos T, Vazquez JO:

Renal handling of uric acid in normal subjects by means of the pyrazinamide and probenecid tests. Nephron 1983; 35:183–186.

Puig JG, Michan AD, Jimenez ML, Perez de Ayala C, Mateos FA, Capitan CF, de Miguel E, Gijon JB: Female gout: clinical spectrum and uric acid metabolism. Arch Intern Med 1991; 151:726–732.

Puig JG, Miranda ME, Mateos FA, Picazo ML, Jimenez ML, Calvin TS, Gil AA: Hereditary nephropathy associated with hyperuricemia and gout. Arch Intern Med 1993; 153:357–365.

Ragab AH, Gilkerson E, Myers M: The effect of 6-mercaptopurine and allopurinol on granulopoiesis. Cancer Res 1974; 34:2246–2249.

Raivio KO, Becker MA, Meyer LJ, Greene ML, Nuki G, Seegmiller JE: Stimulation of human purine synthesis de novo by fructose infusion. Metabolism 1975; 24:861–869.

Rakic MT, Valkenburg HA, Davidson RT, Engels JP, Mikkelsen WM, Neel JV, Duff IF: Observations on the natural history of hyperuricemia and gout. I. An eighteen year follow-up of nineteen gouty families. Am J Med 1964; 37:862–871.

Rapado A, Castrillo JM: Gout disease. Its natural history based on 1,000 observations. Adv Exp Med Biol 1977; 76B:223–230.

Reaven GM: Role of insulin-resistance in human disease. Diabetes 1988; 37:1595–1607.

Reunanen A, Takkunen H, Knebt P, Aromaa A: Hyperuricemia as a risk factor for cardiovascular mortality. Acta Med Scand (Suppl) 1982; 668:49–59.

Reynolds PP, Knapp MJ, Baraf HS, Holmes EW: Moonshine and lead. Relationship to the pathogenesis of hyperuricemia in gout. Arthritis Rheum 1983; 26:1057–1064.

Rich RL, Nance WE, Corey LA, Boughman JA: Evidence for genetic factors influencing serum uric acid levels in man. In: Nance WE (ed). Twin Research: Clinical Studies. New York: Alan R. Liss, 1978:187–192.

Rieselbach RE, Sorensen LB, Shelp WD, Steele TH: Diminished renal urate secretion per nephron as a basis for primary gout. Ann Intern Med 1970; 73:359–366.

Roch-Ramel F, Diezi J: Renal transport of organic ions and uric acid. In: Schrier RW, Gottschalk CW (eds). Diseases of the Kidney, 6th ed. Boston: Little, Brown, 1996: 231–249.

Roch-Ramel F, Weiner IM: Excretion of urate by the kidneys of Cebus monkeys: a micropuncture study. Am J Physiol 1973; 224:1369–1374.

Rosenbloom FM, Henderson JF, Caldwell IC, Kelley WN, Seegmiller JE: Biochemical bases of accelerated purine biosynthesis de novo in human fibroblasts lacking hypoxanthine-guanine phosphoribosyltransferase. J Biol Chem 1968; 243: 1166–1173.

Rouault T, Caldwell DS, Holmes EW: Aspiration of the asymptomatic metatarsophalangeal joint in gout patients and hyperuricemic controls. Arthritis Rheum 1982; 25:209–212.

Rundles RW: The development of allopurinol. Arch Intern Med 1985; 145:1492–1503.

Scott JT: Obesity and hyperuricemia. Clin Rheum Dis 1977; 3:25–35.

Scott JT: Drug-induced gout. Ballieres Clin Rheumatol 1991; 5:39–60.

Scott JT, Pollard AC: Uric acid excretion in the relatives of patients with gout. Ann Rheum Dis 1970; 29:397–400.

Seegmiller JE, Grayzel AI, Laster L, Liddle L: Uric acid production in gout. J Clin Invest 1961; 40:1304–1314.

Seegmiller JE, Rosenbloom FM, Kelley WN: Enzyme defect associated with a sex-linked human neurological disorder and excessive purine synthesis. Science 1967; 155:1682–1684.

Seidell JC, Bakx KC, Deurenberg P, van den Hoogen HJ, Hautvast JG, Stijnen T: Overweight and chronic illness: a retrospective cohort study with a follow-up of 6–17 years in men and women of initially 20–50 years of age. J Chronic Dis 1986; 39:585–593.

Shahinfar S, Simpson RL, Carides AD, Thijagarajan B, Nakagawa Y, Umans J, Parks JH, Coe FL: Safety of losartan in hypertensive patients with thiazide-induced hyperuricemia. Kidney Int 1999; 56:1879–1885.

Short EM: Hyperuricemia and gout. In: King RA, Rotter JI, Motulsky AG (eds). The Genetic Basis of Common Diseases. New York: Oxford University Press, 1992: 482–506.

Simkin PA: Urate excretion in normal and gouty men. Adv Exp Biol 1977; 76B:41–45.

Simkin PA, Gardner GC: Colchicine use in cyclosporine treated transplant recipients: how little is too much. J Rheumatol 2000; 27:1334–1337.

Simmonds HA, Cameron JS, Potter CF, Warren D, Gibson T, Farebrother D: Renal failure in young subjects with familial gout. Adv Exp Med Biol 1980; 122A:15–20.

Singer JZ, Wallace SL: The allopurinol hypersensitivity syndrome. Unnecessary morbidity and mortality. Arthritis Rheum 1986; 29:82–87.

Sive PH, Medalie JH, Kahn H, Neufeld HN, Riss E: Distribution and multiple regression analysis of blood pressure in 10,000 Israeli men. Am J Epidemiol 1971; 93:317–327.

Smith JL, Zaluzec EJ, Wery J-P, Niu L, Switzer RL, Zalkin H, Satow Y: Structure of the allosteric enzyme of purine biosynthesis. Science 1994; 264:1427–1431.

Smyth CJ, Cotterman CW, Freyberg RH: The genetics of gout and hyperuricemia—an analysis of 19 families. J Clin Invest 1948; 27:749–759.

Sorensen LB: The pathogenesis of gout. Arch Intern Med 1962; 109:379–390.

Sperling O, Boer P, Persky-Brosh S, Kanarek E, de Vries A: Altered kinetic property of erythrocyte phosphoribosylpyrophosphate synthetase in excessive purine production. Rev Eur Etud Clin Biol 1972; 17:703–706.

Sperling O, deVries A: Hereditary renal hypouricemia with hyperuricosuria and variably absorptive hypercalciuria and urolithiasis—a new syndrome. Adv Exp Med Biol 1980; 122A:149–153.

Stecher RM, Hersh AH, Solomon WH: The heredity of gout and its relationship to familial hyperuricemia. Ann Intern Med 1949; 31:595–614.

Steele TH: Urate secretion in man: the pyrazinamide suppression test. Ann Intern Med 1973; 79:734–737.

Steele TH, Rieselbach RE: The contribution of residual nephrons within the chronically diseased kidney to urate homeostasis in man. Am J Med 1967; 43:876–886.

Stiburkova B, Majewski J, Sebesta I, Zhang W, Ott J, Kmoch S: Familial juvenile hyperuricemic nephropathy: localization of the gene on chromosome 16p11.2 and evidence for genetic heterogeneity. Am J Hum Genet 2000: 66:1989–1994.

Takahashi S, Yamamoto T, Tsutsumi Z, Moriwaki Y, Yamakita J, Higashino K: Close correlation between visceral fat accumulation and uric acid metabolism in healthy men. Metabolism 1997; 46:1162–1165.

Tungsanga K, Boonwickit D, Lekhakula A, Sitprija V: Urine uric acid and urine creatinine ratio in acute renal failure. Arch Intern Med 1984; 144:934–937.

Unsworth J, Blake DR, D'Assis Fonseca AE, Baswick DT: Densensitization to allopurinol: a cautionary tale. Ann Rheum Dis 1987; 46:646.

Vuorin-Markkola H, Yki-Jarvinen H: Hyperuricemia and insulin-resistance. J Clin Endocrinol Metab 1994; 78:25–29.

Wallace SL, Robinson H, Masi AT, Decker JL, McCarty DJ, Yu T-F: Preliminary criteria for the classification of the acute arthritis of primary gout. Arthritis Rheum 1977; 20:895–900.

Wallace SL, Singer JZ: Systemic toxicity associated with intravenous administration of colchicine—guidelines for use. J Rheumatol 1988a; 15:495–499.

Wallace SL, Singer JZ: Therapy in gout. Rheum Dis Clin North Am 1988b; 14:441–457.

Ward HJ: Uric acid as an independent risk factor in the treatment of hypertension. Lancet 1998; 352:670–671.

Webster E, Panush RS: Allopurinol hypersensitivity in a patient with severe chronic tophaceous gout. Arthritis Rheum 1985; 28:707–709.

Weinberger A, Schindel B, Liberman UA, Pinkhas J, Sperling O: Calciuric effect of probenecid in gouty patients. Isr J Med Sci 1983; 19:377–379.

Werlen D, Gabay C, Vischer TL: Corticosteroid therapy for the treatment of acute attacks of crystal induced arthritis: an effective alternative to nonsteroidal antiinflammatory drugs. Rev Rhum Engl Ed 1996; 63:248–254.

Wiedemann E, Rose H, Schwartz E: Plasma lipoproteins, glucose tolerance and insulin response in primary gout. Am J Med 1972; 53:299–307.

Woolliscroft JO, Fox IH: Increased body fluid purine levels during hypotensive events: evidence for ATP degradation. Am J Med 1986; 81:472–478.

Wyngaarden JB, Kelley WN: Gout and Hyperuricemia. New York: Grune and Stratton, 1976.

Yamanaka H, Kawagoe Y, Taneguchi A: Accelerated purine nucleotide degradation by anaerobic but not by aerobic ergometer muscle exercise. Metabolism 1992; 41:364–369.

Yano K, Rhoads GG, Kagan A: Epidemiology of serum uric acid among 8,000 Japanese-American men in Hawaii. J Chronic Dis 1977; 30:171–184.

Yu T-F: The efficacy of colchicine prophylaxis in articular gout. A reappraisal after 20 years. Semin Arthritis Rheum 1982; 12:256–264.

Yu T-F, Gutman AB: Study of the paradoxical effects of salicylate in low, intermediate and high dosage on the renal mechanisms for excretion of urate in man. J Clin Invest 1959; 38:1298–1315.

Yu T-F, Gutman AB: Uric acid nephrolithiasis in gout. Predisposing factors. Ann Intern Med 1967; 67:1133–1148.

Yu T-F, Kaung C: The natural history of hyperuricemia among asymptomatic relatives of patients with gout. Adv Exp Med Biol 1980; 122A:1–7.

Zalokar J, Lellouch J, Claude JR: Serum urate and gout in 4663 young male workers. Semin Hop Paris 1981; 57:664–670.

Zoref E, de Vries A, Sperling O: Mutant feedback-resistant phosphoribosylpyrophosphate synthetase associated with purine overproduction and gout. Phosphoribosylpyrophosphate and purine metabolism in cultured fibroblasts. J Clin Invest 1975; 56:1093–1099.

Part VI

GENITOURINARY DISORDERS

26 Gynecologic Disorders

JOE LEIGH SIMPSON

The genetics of common gynecologic disorders have not been adequately investigated. This lack of knowledge has until recently contrasted strikingly with information about inherited tendencies in many other organ systems. There are several reasonable explanations. First, gynecologic disorders usually involve internal organ systems, making it more difficult to recognize genetic factors than in more readily accessible organ systems. Second, gynecologic disorders occur in members of only one sex (female); thus, fewer familial aggregates would be expected than if both sexes were affected. Third, there has been a relative paucity of gynecologists trained in genetics.

In this chapter we consider the genetics of common gynecologic disorders and the heritable tendencies in some common reproductive physiologic processes. Gynecologic cancers are discussed in chapter 35.

PELVIS CONTRACTURES AND UTERINE DYSTOCIA

Genetic Definitions

Familial tendencies influence the likelihood of undergoing Cesarean sections or operative vaginal deliveries. However, familial factors could reflect either heritable abnormalities of the bony pelvis or heritable abnormalities of uterine contractions. Thus, we shall consider both topics concurrently. Unfortunately, both lack crisp definitions.

Clinically, the term *pelvic contracture* is applied whenever a woman's bony pelvis is inadequate to permit birth of a normal size fetus. Standard texts (e.g., Gabbe et al., 1996) offer various definitions, such as area of pelvic inlet (123 cm^2 critical limit) or midplane (106 cm^2 critical limit) as discerned by X-ray pelvimetry. More practical are clinically derived (pelvic exam) estimates of the diagonal conjugate (distance between inferior border of symphysis pubis to sacral promontory), in turn usually 1.5 cm greater than the meaningful obstetric conjugate (distance between anterior posterior diameter of pelvic inlet). This should ordinarily be 10 cm or greater. However, diameters that may be adequate for a relatively small fetus may be inadequate for relatively larger fetuses. Also relevant is the classification of pelvic shapes into several subtypes. The most common subtype is gynecoid, which is the normal shape with an average posterior-sagittal diameter. An anthropid pelvis is long and oval-shaped with a long posterior-sagittal diameter. An android pelvis is heart-shaped with a short posterior-sagittal diameter.

Uterine dystocia is as ill-defined as bony contractions. The former is applied when uterine contractions are inadequate to expel the fetus yet the pelvis seems normal. Older criteria based on frequency and duration of contractions or the examiner's ability to indent the uterus are obsolete; current methods attempt to define inadequate contractions on the basis of intrauterine pressure transducer measurements. Contractions are considered inadequate if they are of less than 50 mm mg mercury every 3 minutes, or below 250 Montevideo units per 10 minutes.

General Genetic and Epidemiologic Evidence

Irrespective of imprecision of definitions, there is reason to believe heritable tendencies exist in pelvic contractions or uterine dystocia. Bone mass and shape are heritable in animals and presumably in humans as well. An anthropoid or android pelvis is more characteristic of blacks than whites. Naylor and Warburton (1974) formally showed that the length of the diagonal conjugate is heritable in whites, although not in blacks. Variation in bony structure surely accounts for some of the 20% to 25% U.S. births that necessitate Cesarean delivery.

Investigators in Utah studied women having been delivered by "Cesarean section, midforceps or high forceps"; matched controls were identified (Varner et al., 1996). Women born by Cesarean section showed an odds ratio (OR) of 1.41 for having a Cesarean section themselves (95% CI, 1.18–1.70). The OR for undergoing Cesarean section was increased when the index case had been delivered by mid or high forceps (OR 1.72; 95% CI, 1.20–2.47), had been born by Cesarean section for cephalopelvic disproportion (OR 1.83, 95% CI, 1.16–2.88) or had been born by Cesarean section because of dysfunction of labor (OR 5.97;95% CI, 1.5–23.6). The higher OR for the latter suggests that uterine factors are more likely to be heritable than are bony abnormalities. Despite the above, heritable factors play only a small role in Cesarean section in general. The attributable risk of heritable factors toward operative delivery was only 3.5%.

In a second study, a Swedish data base was used to verify that "dystocia" is familial (Berg-Lekas et al., 1998). The following International Classification of Disease (ICD) codes were used: (1) prolonged labor, uterine spasm, or rigid cervix (8th revision) or (2) uterine inertia, primary or secondary; hypertonic inordinate or prolonged uterine contractions; prolonged first- or second-stage labor or unspecific prolonged labor (9th revision). If a subject's mother had been delivered after dystocia, the OR was 1.7 (95% CI, 1.2–2.4) that her oldest daughter would also be delivered after dystocia. The OR was 1.8 for recurrence if an operative delivery occurred in the mother. The risk for an operative delivery among primiparous sisters was 3.5; the risk was 24.0 among twins. These studies indicate that familial tendencies affect labor and delivery. Presumably, to some extent these reflect genetic tendencies.

Biologic Basis of Genetic Susceptibility

The exact biologic basis of any existing genetic susceptibility is unclear because dysfunctional labor is multifaceted, as already shown by our concurrent discussion of both the bony pelvis and uterine contractions. Any of a variety of pathogenic factors could plausibly be responsible. In addition to bony abnormalities, potential mechanisms include perturbations of cervical collagen levels (Granstrom et al., 1989), oxytocin secretion or oxytocin receptors, and myometrial gap junction proteins like connexin 43. An initial attempt at detecting aberrant gene products contributing to dystocia has been made by Algovik et al. (1999). Using single-stranded conformational polymorphism (SSCP), blood from 23 women revealed no perturbations of endothelin 1 (END-1), prostaglandin F2α receptor, and 5α-reductase, type 1.

PELVIC RELAXATION

Disease Definition

In pelvic relaxation various pelvic organs—uterus, bladder, rectum—lose their integrity and often prolapse through the barrel of the vagina. There is no clear demarcation between normal variation and pathology. Moreover, levels of relaxation that are troublesome and symptomatic in some women seem asymptomatic in others.

General Genetic and Epidemiologic Evidence

There are no good prevalence data, but the common phenomenon of pelvic relaxation is clearly high in women of increased parity and advanced age. In fact, virtually all older parous women have some degree of pelvic relaxation. The only question is whether symptomatic problems are manifested. With the increasingly older U.S. and European population, pelvic relaxation is increasingly a major health care problem.

Factors specifically associated with pelvic organ prolapse include multiple prior vaginal births, especially given large (healthier) babies; preexisting nerve damage; estrogen deficiency; obesity; and increased intraabdominal pressure. Only one study has looked at familial tendencies in urinary incontinence. Mushkat et al. (1996) studied Israeli women diagnosed with urinary stress incontinence, which is typically defined as involuntary loss of urine due to anatomic displacement of the bladder neck. Diagnostic criteria include both clinical and urodynamic testing (cystometry; urethral pressure profiles). Controls consisted of women attending the same gynecology clinic "who desired treatment for any kind of micturition disorders." Information was gathered on relatives of 259 subjects with incontinence and compared to 165 women with no micturition disorder. Age and parity were similar, as was the presence of various medical conditions. Multivariate analysis was not performed. Questionnaire queries were made concerning leakage upon exertion, and symptoms that occurred at least twice weekly constituted the basis for diagnosis (affected relative). Prevalence of incontinence was 20.3% (158 of 780) among first-degree relatives of subjects, vs. 7.8% (37 of 474) in first-degree relatives of controls (Table 26–1). Diagnoses in relatives were probably accurate, but to confirm accuracy of cases ascertained by questionnaire urodynamic testing was offered to the 195 relatives said to be affected (158 being relatives of subjects and 37 relatives of controls). Of the 195, 48 were studied; all 48 had urinary stress incontinence by urodynamic testing, with 8 having combined stress incontinence and detrusor instability (dyssynergia, defined as loss of urine due to sudden and spontaneous detrusor muscle activity).

Duong and Korn (2001) stratified 415 San Francisco women by ethnic group, concluding that African American women (N = 59) had higher maximum urethral closure pressure than Hispanic (N = 195), white (N = 60), or Asian (N = 66) women. In the former, the mean was 58 ± 23 cm H_2O vs. 47 or 48 cm H_2O for other ethnic groups. Detrusor instability was diagnosed in more African Americans (29%) than in the other three ethnic groups (8%, 15%, 14%, respectively). Unfortunately, potential confounding variables were not adjusted by logistic regression.

The biologic basis of any genetic susceptibility is unclear, but a plausible hypothesis is the existence of defects or perturbations of connective tissue. The existence of many Mendelian disorders affecting connective tissue—for example, Erlers-Danlos Syndrome—reinforce the plausibility of hypothesizing connective tissue perturbation. It would be reasonable to expect that subtle abnormalities might exist in ostensibly normal women who experience bladder or uterine prolapse.

Some evidence supports differences in collagen or connective tissue between women who have and do not have pelvic relaxation. Women with both bladder neck collapse and urinary stress incontinence show cross-link modifications in their pubocervical fascia, compared to patients who have stress incontinence alone (Sayer et al., 1990). Collagen content in the vaginal cuff has been shown to be significantly reduced in premenopausal women who require vaginal hysterectomy for prolapse, compared to controls who did not. Significant increases in gelatinases (MMP2, MMP9) and cathepsin are further consistent with loss of collagen fiber strength. Intermolecular cross-links and advanced gylcation cross-links are increased in prolapsed tissue, without alteration. No change in the type I to type III collagen ratio was observed. Overall, this initial attempt comparing tissue in women with and without prolapse suggests collagen perturbation in the former.

A relationship exists between joint hypermobility and fascial relaxation (Norton et al., 1995). Given that hypermobile joint syndrome is more common in West African populations (Birrell et al., 1994), these populations might be predisposed toward urinary incontinence.

Table 26–1. Frequency of Women Who Do (Subjects) and Do Not (Control) Show Pelvic Relaxation in Relatives

		Affected Relatives			
Population	*N*	Mothers	Sisters	Daughters	All First-Degree Relatives
Subjects	259	71/203 (34.9%)	73/367 (19.9%)	14/210 (6.7%)	158/780 (20.3%)
Controls	165	19/149 (12.7%)	15/220 (6.8%)	3/105 (2.9%)	37/474 (7.8%)

Source: Data from Mushkat et al., 1996.

Table 26–2. Mean Differences (Months) in Age of Onset of First Menstruation

Population	Petri (1934)	Tisserant-Perrier (1953)	Fischbein (1977)
Identical twins	2.8 (N = 51)	2.2 (N = 46)	3.5 (N = 28)
Nonidentical twins	12.0 (N = 47)	8.2 (N = 39)	8.5 (N = 48)
Sibs	12.9 (N = 145)		
Mother–daughter	18.4 (N = 120)		
Unrelated	18.6 (N = 120)		

Clinical Application

Any woman known to be at increased risk for pelvic relaxation would be advised to be conscious of birth weight of her offspring; her physicians might be inclined to perform Cesarean delivery at relatively lower birth weight. More specific guidelines would be difficult to formulate. It might also be reasonable to consider different surgical approaches (e.g., sling operations) for patients who are predisposed to urinary stress incontinance prolapse.

AGE AT MENARCHE

General Genetic and Epidemiologic Evidence

In the United States the mean age of menarche is approximately 12 years. Age of menarche is clearly heritable, and this has been recognized by virtue of greater correlations for monozygotic (MZ) twins than for dizygotic (DZ) twins (Petri, 1934; Tisserant-Perrier, 1953; Fischbein, 1977) (Table 26–2). Age at menarche has differed less among sisters than among unrelated women, with the magnitude of the observed difference consistent with polygenic or multifactorial etiology.

Confounding social and environmental variables complicate human studies, but in the past decade additional intergenerational and familial studies concerning age of menarche have become available. The more recent studies (Table 26–3) differ from earlier studies by taking into account various confounding factors—for example, decreasing age at menarche in the general population. Familial tendencies still continue to prove substantive. Despite mothers showing higher mean ages of menarche than their daughters (4- to 12-month differences), correlations for age of menarche persist between mother–daughter and sister–sister pairs. Birth order and paternal occupation do not account for differences (Sanchez-Andres, 1997). These findings have been observed in Spanish women (Sanchez-Andres, 1997) and in South African Indians (Cameron and Nagdee, 1996), and they can be presumed applicable in all populations. Heritability also remains high, despite adjustments for weight, height, and skeletal maturation (Loesch et al., 1995). Malina et al. (1994) confirmed the familial correlation for age at menarche in a study of 44 MZ and 42 DZ twins. This correlation persisted even when comparing women who were university athletics to sisters and mothers who were not.

Using a Finnish twin registry, Kaprio et al. (1995) studied 468 MZ twin girls, 378 girls from like-sex DZ twin pairs, and 434 girls from unlike-sex DZ twin pairs; correlation(s) for age of menarche were .75, .34, and .32, respectively. Variance for age of menarche was estimated at 37% for additive genetic factors, 37% for dominance effects, and 26% for "unique environmental factors." Correlation between body mass and age at menarche was .57, suggesting that factors relating to mass could help explain the genetic correlation. Based on 1177 MZ and 711 DZ twins, Treloar and Martin (1990) concluded that the phenotypic variance in age of menarche due to genes was 65%. The most recent data (Sneider et al., 1998; Treolar et al., 1998) are consistent (Table 26–2).

One study has considered age at thelarche and pubache. In a longitudinal study of 74 pairs of sisters in Croatia, Jakic and Prebeg (1994) found that the onset of breast development showed greater correlation among sisters than among nonrelated individuals. The same held for age of onset of pubic hair development (pubarche).

Age of menarche does not necessarily correlate with age at menopause.

AGE AT MENOPAUSE

General Familial and Epidemiologic Evidence

In the United States, mean age at menopause is approximately 52 years. Menopause is defined as cessation of menstruation for at least six months. This variable is familial, predictably so because the germ cell number is normally distributed in nonhuman female mammals and presumably in humans. Different rodent strains show characteristic breeding durations, implying genetic control over either the rate of oocyte depletion or the number of oocytes initially present. It follows that some ostensibly normal (menstruating) women may have decreased oocyte reservoir or increased oocyte attrition on polygenic or stochastic grounds. In humans, assessing heritability of age of menopause is complicated because iatrogenic behavior (e.g., surgical hysterectomy) and other confounding factors (e.g, presence of leiomyomata) must be taken into account. Cramer et al. (1995) attempted to do so in a case-control study of 10,606 U.S. women between ages 45 and 54 years. Women with an early menopause (40–45 years) were age-matched with controls who were either still menstruating or had experienced menopause after 46 years of age. Of 129 early menopause cases, 37.5% had a similarly affected mother, sister, aunt, or grandmother. Only 9% of controls had a relative with early menopause (OR after adjustment 6.1, 95% CI, 3.9–9.4). The OR was greatest (9.1) for sisters and greater when menopause occurred before age 40. The findings of Cramer et

Table 26–3. Twin-Pair Correlation (r) and Heritability in Age of Menarche

Reference	Monozygotic (MZ) Twins	Dizygotic (DZ) Twins	Heritable (H^2)
Snieder et al. (1998)	0.61 (N = 275)	0.18 (N = 353)	45%
Treloar and Martin (1990)	0.65 (N = 1177)	0.18 (N = 711)	61–68% (youngest to oldest)
Kaprio (1995)	0.75 (N = 468)	0.31 (N = 378 like sex) (Sib-twin correlation 0.32)	37% (plus another 37% dominance, 26% environmental)

al. (1995) were confirmed by Torgerson et al., (1997), who studied women undergoing menopause during the five-year centile aged 45 to 49 years. The likelihood was increased that in their daughters menopause would occur in a similar five-year centile.

Twin studies also have confirmed heritability of age at menopause, and two such studies showed similar results (Treloar et al. (1998). Sneider et al. (1998) studied 275 MZ and 353 DZ United Kingdom twin pairs. For age at menopause, correlation (*r*) was .58 for MZ and .39 for DZ twins; heritability (h^2) was calculated to be 63%. Treloar et al. (1998) performed a similar study in 466 MZ and 262 DZ Australian twin pairs. For age at menopause the correlation (*r*) was .49 to .57 for MZ and .31 to .33 for DZ twin pairs. Differences between MZ and DZ held when iatrogenic causes of menopause were taken into account.

In 38 PCOS subjects Oksanen et al. (2000) found abnormalities in neither serum leptin nor leptin or leptin receptor genes. This is consistent with Urbanek et al.'s (1999) failure to find linkage. Takakura et al. (2001) found no inactivating mutations of FSHR (FSH receptor) in 38 PCOS cases. The search focused on exons 6, 7, 9, and 10.

Clinical Application

Anticipating an early age of menopause might be worthwhile in certain instances. In theory, women predisposed to early menopause might accelerate their childbearing options and not defer pregnancy. An exact age before which childbearing should be completed cannot be stated, perhaps by age 30 years. The age at which hormonal replacement therapy is begun should be advanced, but only after perimenopause or menopause has actually occurred.

INCOMPLETE MÜLLERIAN FUSION

Definitions

During early embryonic development, the Müllerian ducts are paired organs, later fusing and canalizing in the 150 to 200 mm embryo to form the upper vagina, uterus, and fallopian tubes (Simpson, 1976). Failure of fusion results in two hemiuteri, each associated with no more than one fallopian tube. Sometimes one Müllerian duct fails to contribute to the definitive uterus, leading to a rudimentary horn. Intrauterine septa may or may not persist. Renal anomalies coexist frequently. If one uterine horn is atretic, ipsilateral renal agenesis is common.

Specific terms are applied to the various uterine fusion defects (Fig. 26–1): *uterus unicornus* (absence of one uterine horn), with or without a coexisting contralateral rudimentary hemiuterus; *uterus arcuatus* (broadening and medial depression of the uterine fundus); *uterus subseptus* (persistence of complete uterine septum); *uterus bicornis unicollis* or *bicornuate uterus* (two separate uterine cavities, each leading to the same cervix; the fundus is deeply notched); *uterus bicornis bicollis* (two separate uterine cavities, each leading to a separate cervix); *uterus didelphys* (completely separated hemiuteri, each of which leads to a separate cervix and a separate vagina with the two vaginas separated by a septum); *completely separated hemiuteri* with not only separate cervices and separate vaginas but also separate perineal orifices.

General Genetic and Epidemiologic Evidence

Incomplete Müllerian fusion is relatively common, at least in its asymptomatic forms. Often the condition is detected only after an untoward reproductive event, specifically mid-trimester abortion or fetal malpresentation. Thus, the incidence of symptomatic cases is approximately 0.1% (Hay, 1958; Semmens, 1962), but frequency is much higher in asymptomatic form. As many as 2% to 3% of all postpartum uteri show minor structural changes (e.g., uterus arcuatus) (Hay, 1958; Greiss and Mauzy, 1961).

Familial aggregates of incomplete Müllerian fusion include multiple affected siblings, as well as affected mother and daughter (Nykiforuk, 1938; Tyler, 1939; Way, 1945; Holmes, 1956; Stevenson et al., 1959; Hay, 1961; Polishuk and Ron, 1974; Verp et al., 1983; Ergun et al., 1997). In some of these families affected relatives show different forms of incomplete Müllerian fusion (Ergun et al., 1997).

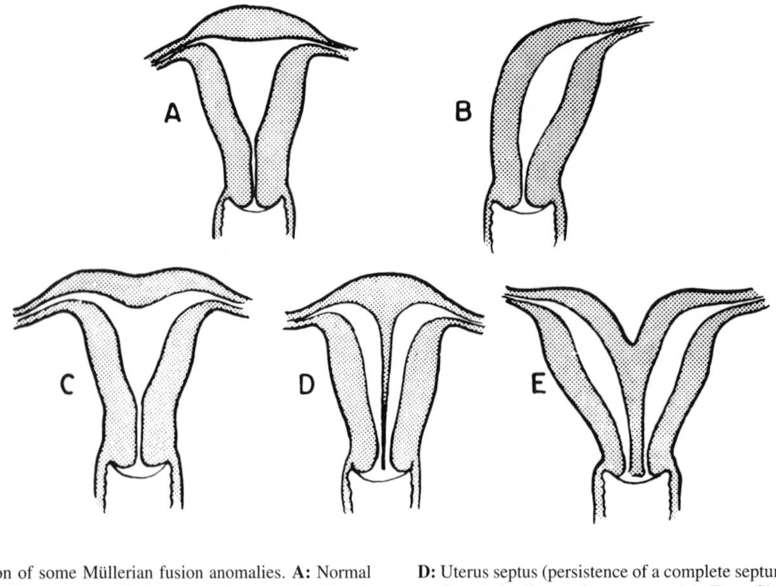

Fig. 26–1. Diagrammatic representation of some Müllerian fusion anomalies. **A:** Normal uterus, fallopian tubes, and vagina. **B:** Uterus unicornis (absence of one uterine horn). **C:** Uterus arcuatus (broadening and medical depression of a portion of the uterine fundus). **D:** Uterus septus (persistence of a complete septum). **E:** Uterus bicornis unicollis (two hemiuteri, each leading to the same cervix). From Simpson (1976) with permission.

One formal genetic study has been reported. Elias et al. (1984) found that 1 of 37 (2.7%) sisters of probands had a clinically symptomatic uterine anomaly; no (0 of 24) mothers, no (0 of 44) maternal aunts, and no (0 of 50) paternal aunts were affected. The 2.7% prevalence in siblings should be considered a minimum frequency because relatives could have had an undetected minor uterine anomaly. The opportunity to manifest symptoms that would suggest an anomaly would be limited if female relatives have not yet attempted pregnancy. Ideally one should thus perform hysteroscopy, hysterosalpingography ultrasound, or surgical exploration to exclude affected relatives. Even with these inherent limitations, the likelihood of first-degree female relatives being similarly affected with Müllerian fusion anomalies seems too low to be compatible with autosomal dominant or autosomal recessive etiology. That approximately 3% of clinically symptomatic female siblings were affected in the one formal study is consistent with predictions based on polygenic/multifactorial etiology, however.

Biologic Basis of Genetic Susceptibility

The pathogenesis of incomplete Müllerian fusion presumably involves perturbations of Müllerian fusion. No studies have investigated whether pathogenesis is different in familial cases than in nonfamilial cases. No HLA studies are reported.

Gene Identification

Studies into the molecular elucidation of isolated incomplete Müllerian fusion have not yet proved rewarding. Distinct from isolated Müllerian fusion defects are a variety of syndromes in which this malformation is only one component (Table 26–4). One of these is the hand-foot-genital (HFG) syndrome, an autosomal dominant disorder (Stern et al., 1970; Verp et al., 1983; Fryns et al., 1993). In HFG the etiology involves mutation of *HOXA13* (Mortlock and Innis, 1997). No mutations in *HOXA13* have been found in isolated incomplete Müllerian fusion (Stelling et al., 1998).

Clinical Application

An increased index of suspicion might facilitate early detection of a similar defect in a woman with an affected relative. A variety of clinical circumstances would suggest the possibility of Müllerian fusion defects. These reflect pregnancies in patients with incomplete Müllerian fusion being complicated by lack of space for the developing fetus (Jones and Rock, 1983). During labor, fetuses may be maintained in unusual positions (malpresentations). Thus, malpresentation or an unusual uterine contour suggests a uterine anomaly (Hay, 1958; Semmens, 1962). After delivery, the placenta may fail to separate from the uterus, resulting in hemorrhage (Blair, 1960; Wiebe, 1970). If a uterine

Table 26–4. Syndromes Associated with Incomplete Müllerian Fusion

Syndrome	Somatic Anomalies	Etiology
Bardet-Biedl	Retinal pigmentary degeneration (retinitis pigmentosa), polydactyly, obesity, mental deficiency	Autosomal recessive
Beckwith-Wiedemann	Macroglossia, omphalocele, macrosomia	Autosomal dominant, after uniparental disomy
Donohue (leprechaunism)	Elfin facies with thick lips; large, low-set ears; prominent breasts and external genitalia; hirsutism; abnormal carbohydrate metabolism; failure to thrive; motor and mental retardation	Autosomal recessive
Fraser	Cryptophthalmia, external ear and nose anomalies, laryngeal stenosis, syndactyly, skeletal defects, renal agenesis, large clitoris and labia majora, mental retardation	Autosomal recessive
Hand-foot-genital (HFG)	Metacarpal and metatarsal anomalies, malformed thumbs, displaced urethral meatus, urinary incontinence	Autosomal dominant
Johanson-Blizzard	Deafness, hypoplastic alae nasi, primary hypothyroidism, mental retardation	Autosomal recessive
Laryngeal atresia	Hydrocephaly, complete or partial laryngeal obstruction, tracheoesophageal fistula or atresia, renal hypoplasia, varus deformity of feet	Unknown
Meckel-Gruber	Microcephaly, posterior encephalocele, eye anomalies, cleft palate, polycystic kidneys, polydactyly	Autosomal recessive
Roberts	Sparse, silvery blond hair; midfacial hemangioma; cleft lip with or without cleft palate; limb reduction defect; intrauterine growth retardation	Autosomal recessive
Cavalcanti	Tibial aplasia, triphalangeal thumb, micratia, scaliosis, club foot; Müllerian aplasia also reported	Unknown
Rudiger	Bifid uvula, coarse facies, absent ear cartilage, hydronephrosis secondary to ureterovesical stenosis, short digits	Autosomal recessive
Thalidomide teratogenicity	Nasal hemangioma, neurosensory hearing loss, ear anomalies, limb reduction defects, visceral anomalies	Teratogen
Trisomy 18	Prominent occiput, malformed ears, micrognathia, short sternum, cardiac defects, horseshoe kidney, overlapping fingers, intrauterine growth retardation, severe development retardation	Chromosomal aneuploidy
Trisomy 13	Microcephaly, microphthalmia, malformed ears, cleft lip and palate, cardiac anomalies, polydactyly, intrauterine growth retardation, severe developmental retardation	Chromosomal aneuploidy
Urogenital adysplasia, hereditary (hereditary renal agenesis)	Oligohydramnios, flattened (Potter) facies, pulmonary hypoplasia, unilateral or bilateral absent kidneys, limb deformities	Autosomal dominant

horn is rudimentary, menstrual blood may be retained. Pregnancy in a rudimentary horn may terminate in uterine rupture or missed abortion, the latter of which can lead to lithopedian formation (Rolen et al., 1966). Frequency of second-trimester spontaneous abortion or premature labor is therefore increased (Blair, 1960). First-trimester abortions, usually genetic in etiology, are not necessarily increased.

Whether reconstructive surgery is warranted in women shown to have a fusion defect is sometimes arguable. However, surgery should ordinarily not be performed on asymptomatic women having no abnormal reproductive outcomes. This holds true whether the woman with such a defect does or does not have an affected relative.

LEIOMYOMAS

Disease Definition

Leiomyomas are common benign tumors of smooth muscle origin. They are dense, well-encapsulated, and usually multiple, and their locations may involve the uterine surface (serous), uterine wall (intramural), or uterine mucosa (submucous). Irregular bleeding is common. Large tumors may produce discomfort and obscure ovarian pathology, necessitating myomectomy or hysterectomy.

General Genetic and Epidemiology Evidence

Epidemiologic studies are difficult because leiomyomas are so common and because diagnosis of small tumors is often not appreciated. Valid prevalence figures would require dissecting uteri or performing high-quality pelvic ultrasound on a large asymptomatic sample. Otherwise, small intramural lesions would be missed. Presence or absence of leiomyomas also varies according to hormonal status, and pregnancy notably increases the size of the lesions.

Leiomyomas are two or three times more common in blacks than whites (Treloar et al., 1992; Kjerulff et al., 1993; Marshall et al., 1997). Differences in racial prevalence naturally suggest genetic factors. Black women undergoing hysterectomy are twice as likely as white women to have myomas as the major indication for their surgery (Meilahn et al., 1989; Kjerulff et al., 1993). Especially informative is a study of the Nurse's Health Study II Cohort (1989–present) that involved 116,678 registered nurses (Marshall et al., 1997). The age-standardized rate of ultrasound or hysterectomy-confirmed leiomyomas was 30.6 per 1000 woman-years in black women versus 8.9 per 1000 women years in white women. Confounding factors like parity, history of infertility, oral contraceptive usage, and body mass failed to account for this difference. Similarities in educational levels in the cohort makes it unlikely that the observed differences reflected biases of reporting or differences in health care use.

Familial Aggregates

Formal studies are limited. The first was a questionnaire study by Winkler and Hoffman (1938), who compared the prevalence of myomas in relatives of 356 subjects with that in relatives of 356 controls. Some 62 relatives of women with leiomyomas were said to be affected, compared with only 19 relatives of controls. Near relatives (defined by Winkler et al., 1938 as sibs, mothers, daughters, grandmothers, and granddaughters) were affected four times as often if the proband had leiomyomata; more distant relatives were affected twice as often. These data are consistent with polygenic/multifactorial etiology.

Two studies have been reported from Russia. Kurbanova et al. (1989) estimated risks for leiomyomata to be 9.7 ± 0.5% in the general population for women ages 20 to 60 years. Genetic data obtained from 1158 probands included 1173 first-degree relatives; clinical diagnoses were confirmed by contacting hospitals. Average risk was calculated per age. Risk until 60 years was 26.8% for daughters; risks until age 44 were 22.3% for sisters, 19.7% for daughters, and 15.8% for mothers. Heritability was 0.792 ± 0.018. The population risk of 9.7% hints at selection bias, but the 2- to 3-fold increase in first-degree relatives is meaningful.

In Russia, Vikhlyaeva and colleagues (1995) verified familial tendencies in Russian Caucasian women. The study was conducted in a sample of women in whom it was possible to obtain a family history and in whom it was also possible to perform a gynecologic examination on at least one first-degree relative. A total of 97 probands and 118 relatives (43 daughters, 33 sisters, 42 mothers) were studied through 457 pelvic ultrasounds and 51 laparoscopies or hysteroscopies. Leiomyomas were twice (2.2) as common among first-degree family members in which there were already two or more affected individuals. During the study leiomyomata were not infrequently (24.7%) found for the first time in a previously unaffected relative. Even accepting biases of ascertainment, the high prevalence of newly diagnosed cases must exceed the background prevalence.

Concordance for hysterectomy necessitated by leiomyomata is twice as high in monozygotic (MZ) twins than in dizygotic (DZ) twins (Treloar et al., 1992). In the context of an Australian twin study designed to compare age at menopause in MZ vs. DZ twins, it was noted that the higher correlations in MZ twins (r = .49–.57 vs. r = .31–.33) also reflected heritable correlations for leiomyomata (r = .66 MZ vs. r = .34 DZ) (Treloar et al., 1998).

Adenomyosis is a histologic phenomenon that is integrally related to leiomyomata. Familial adenomyosis has been reported (Arnold et al., 1994, 1995). There also exists an autosomal disorder (Reed syndrome) in which leiomyomata occur in both uterus and skin (Reed et al., 1973; Garcia Muret et al., 1988). This disorder (MCUL1, multiple cutaneous leiomyomata) is due to perturbation of genes on 1q42.3–q43 (Alam et al., 2001).

Finally, uterine leiomyomata are common in acromegaly. Of 12 cases studied by Cohen et al. (1998), 8 showed leiomyomata.

Gene Identifications

Leiomyomata have long been attractive for genetic analysis of disorders because it has been known since the 1960s that these tumors are monoclonal in origin. Perturbations of chromosomal regions 12q14–15q and 7q22 are most frequently observed (Mark et al., 1990; Nibert and Heim, 1990; Rein et al., 1991). On 7q a region is often deleted, whereas a region on 12q is involved in rearrangements. The most common single rearrangement is t(12;14), which is observed in 20% of cytogenetically abnormal leiomyomata (Meloni et al., 1992). Chromosomal region 12q is also perturbed in various other mesenchymal solid tumors, such as breast fibroadenoma (Calabrese et al., 1991; Ligon and Morton, 2000). That t(12;14) has been the only detectable aberration in some leiomyomas suggests that the clonal event leading to myomas involves this translocation and perturbations of genes near the break points. Xing et al. (1997) noted that del (7) (q22 → q32) is stable in vitro only if t(12;14) coexists; in the absence of the latter, del (7) becomes unstable. This suggests existence of a tumor-suppressor gene on 7q.

Perturbation of 12q14–15q in leiomyomata is thought to involve dysregulation of HMG1-C (high mobility group protein 1C) (Schoenberg-Fejzo et al., 1996). HMG1-C protein is disturbed in lipomas and other mesenchymal lesions (Ashar et al., 1995). Although HMG1-C is perturbed in t(12;14), the sequence of the gene itself seems undisturbed. In a search for complex rearrangements in t(12;14) myomas, the break point was 5′ to HMG1-C in 20 cases and 3′ to the gene in 4 other cases (Weremowicz, 1998).

One supporting argument for a role for HMG1-C is that leiomyomata not only express the related gene product HMG1Y, but also a 6p21.3 breakpoint in leiomyomata was found to span HMG1Y (Kazmierczak et al., 1996). Involvement of both HMG1C (chromosome 12) and HMG1Y (chromosome 6) suggests that HMG1 proteins in general could be pivotal. HMG proteins help remodel the double helix; thus, they are described as architectural factors. Perturbation of architectural proteins are usually hypothesized to alter binding of transcription factors. In turn, this could either interfere with tumor suppressor genes or facilitate growth promoting genes (oncogenes) (Ligon and Morton, 2000).

Other abnormalities in leiomyomata include trisomy 21, deletion of 3q, and rearrangements of 10q (Ligon and Morton, 2000).

Biologic Basis of Genetic Susceptibility

No studies have addressed the biologic differences between familial and nonfamilial leiomyomas. There are a few clinical correlations. In a case-control study, 301 black women undergoing hysterectomy for leiomyomas showed larger uteri with more myomas than did 281 matched white women undergoing the same procedure for the same indication (Kjerulff et al., 1996). Clinical correlations are, however, evolving between morphology of myomas and chromosomal status (Pandis et al., 1991). Submucous leiomyomas show fewer chromosomal abnormalities (12%) than either intramural (35%) or subserous (29%) leiomyomas show (Brosens et al., 1998).

Clinical Application

Clinical consequences of leiomyomas are discussed in standard gynecologic texts and need not be recounted here. Knowledge that her first-degree relative has leiomyomas plausibly should increase the index of suspicion for a given individual. Of course, large leiomyomas should be detected routinely whenever a pelvic examination is performed, especially if the patient presented for a symptom associated with leiomyomas (bleeding, pelvic discomfort, spontaneous abortion). Particularly useful to identify and difficult to detect is a submucous leiomyoma, which is not obvious on pelvic examination. Hysteroscopy, hysterosalpingography, or uterine curettage may be necessary.

Surgery is virtually never warranted on asymptomatic individuals, even if a leiomyoma is detected because a near relative was affected.

ENDOMETRIOSIS

Disease Definition

In endometriosis, endometrial tissue exists at sites outside the uterus, chiefly within the pelvic cavity. Ovaries, uterosacral ligaments, retrovaginal septum, and pelvic peritoneum are principal sites. Infertility is common in several cases, albeit for reasons not entirely understood. Dyspareunia and pelvic pain are common.

General Genetic and Epidemiology

Frequency of endometriosis among laparotomies at major hospitals has been estimated to be as high as 15% to 20% of gynecologic operations (Williams and Pratt, 1977; Ranney, 1978). This is probably an overestimate, and uncertainty as to representativeness of the samples render prevalence statements unwise. Probably the population prevalence in adult women is no more than 1% to 2%. However, a higher rate was reported by Treloar et al. (1999) in their large Australian twin sample.

It is frequently stated that affected women are white, upper socioeconomic, compulsive, mesomorphic, and perfectionistic (Kitchin, 1982; Kistner, 1986). In reality, all these traits reflect occurrence of the disease in women who delay childbearing. In turn, a relationship to delayed childbearing is consistent with observations that both pregnancy and progestogen therapy ameliorate the disease. Indeed, blacks are not infrequently affected (Chatman, 1976) and are said by some to have an incidence comparable to whites (Ridley, 1986). Epidemiologically verified risk factors are age, increased exposure to menstruation (shorter cycle interval or hypermenorrhea), reduced parity, and retrograde menstruation (Eszkenazi and Warner, 1997).

Familial Aggregates

Endometriosis has long been suspected of familial tendencies. Following an earlier questionnaire survey by Ranney (1971), Simpson et al. (1980) conducted the first formal genetic study in 1980. A total of 123 probands with histologically verified endometriosis were identified. Nine of 153 (5.9%) female sibs older than 18 years had endometriosis; 10 of the 123 (8.1%) mothers were affected. Only 1% of the patients' husband's first-degree

Table 26–5. Incidence of Endometriosis among Proband's First-Degree Relatives and Controls

	Proband's Relatives		
Study	Overall	Mothers and Sisters	Controls
Simpson et al., 1980	6.9% (19/276)	5.9% mothers 8.1% sisters	0.9% (2/211)*
Lamb et al., 1986	4.9%	6.2% mothers 3.8% sister	2.0%
Coxhead and Thomas, 1993	5.5% (7/127)		0.8% (2/258)*
Moen and Magnus, 1993	4.3% (45/1038)	3.9% mothers 4.8% sisters	0.6% (2/318)*

*Statistically significant

relatives (controls) had endometriosis (Table 26–5). Women with an affected sib or parent in the authors' sample were more likely to have severe than mild or moderate endometriosis (Malinak et al., 1980). Severe endometriosis was present in 11 of the 18 probands (61%) having an affected first-degree relative. Severe endometriosis was present in only 25 of 105 (23%) having no affected first-degree relative.

Other studies have been consistent with these initial observations (Table 26–5). Lamb et al. (1986) used questionnaires received from 491 members of the Endometriosis Association, based in the United States. A positive family history was reported by 18% of respondents. A total of 66 women were evaluated in greater detail, 43 returning a detailed questionnaire both they and a friend (control) completed. Endometriosis was present in 6.2% in mothers of probands and 3.8% in sisters; endometriosis was reported in fewer than 1% of first-degree relatives of friends. The frequency in second-degree relatives was 0.4% in grandmothers and 3.1% in aunts. In this study, most (93%) affected relatives were in the maternal lineage. A pitfall of this study is that no attempts were made to confirm the diagnosis in purportedly affected relatives said to be affected; however, members of the Endometriosis Association can be assumed to be knowledgeable concerning the disorder.

In Norway, Moen and colleagues (1993) conducted a study on 522 informative cases, of these, 3.9% mothers and 4.8% sisters had endometriosis; only 0.6% of sisters of women not having endometriosis (controls undergoing laparoscopy for other reasons) were affected. In this study either endometriosis or adenomyosis was considered grounds for diagnosis. Among relatives, affected mothers were far more likely to have adenomyosis than were affected sisters. This probably reflected ages. As in the U.S. cases of Simpson et al. (1980) and Malinak et al. (1980), familial cases in Norway were more likely to show severe endometriosis than were nonfamilial cases. In another report from the same Norwegian center, 8 monozygotic twins were observed among 515 endometriosis cases (Moen, 1994). Of the 8 sets, 6 were concordant and mothers were also affected in 3 cases.

Several groups are performing linkage studies, using sib pair analysis for DNA polymorphic variants. These studies have confirmed familial tendencies (Kennedy et al., 1995, 1997), but there are no control comparisons. The OXEGENE group recorded receipt of samples from 19 mother–daughter pairs and 56 sib pairs (Kennedy et al., 1995). In 18 families, 3 or more relatives in more than one generation were observed. All but 2 of 16 monozygotic twin pairs have been concordant for endometriosis (Hadfield et al., 1997). A similar study in Iceland has also yielded familial aggregates (Stefansson et al., 1998).

Higher concordance for MZ than DZ appears to exist (Simpson et al., 1980; Moen, 1994; Kennedy et al., 1995; Treloar et al., 1998). In addition, endometriosis detected in the context as a cause for surgical menopause shows greater correlation in MZ twins than in DZ twins ($r = 0.52$ vs. 0.19) (Treloar et al., 1998).

Although endometriosis is clearly heritable, the mode(s) of inheritance remains unclear. The magnitude of the increased risk (5%–8% of first-degree relatives) is more reminiscent of polygenic/multifactorial tendencies than is a single mutant gene. However, this recurrence risk is higher than the 2% to 5% expected for polygenic inheritance, and the frequency of affected relatives might be even higher if one could directly measure a gene product(s). Although Mendelian mechanisms cannot be excluded, quantative inheritance is more likely.

Another attractive etiologic possibility is genetic heterogeneity. One or more forms of endometriosis might be Mendelian, despite a larger proportion being nongenetic. At present the various forms would be clinically and histologically indistinguishable. HLA associations have often proved the first hint of genetic heterogeneity, different HLA associations connoting differing genotypes. However, HLA associations have not been observed with endometriosis (Moen et al., 1984; Simpson et al., 1984; Maxwell et al., 1989).

Gene Identification

Two general approaches are being pursued in identifying the major genes responsible for endometriosis. One approach is genome-wide analysis for linkage. Kennedy and colleagues (1995) are performing sib-pair analysis using polymorphic DNA markers; several regions of exclusion have been identified, but no linkage. Similar studies are being pursued in Icelandic women, where a "suggestive locus" was found on 9q. This was not in the region of the *GALT* gene (Stefansson et al., 1998).

The other approach is cytogenetic, using chromosome-specific probes to identify perturbed chromosomal regions. One vexing problem has been difficulty in obtaining and studying pure endometriosis tissue, in distinction from tissue samples admixed with contiguous (normal) endometrium or connective tissues. Techniques can be used that offer greater confidence that genetic information will truly reflect endometriosis tissue. Our group at Baylor College of Medicine uses touch preparations that allow histology or cytogenetic analysis of the mirror image micrograph. Using FISH with chromosome-specific probes, aneuploid cells were found in each of eight endometriotic samples (Kosugi et al., 1999). Monosomy 17 and trisomy 17 cells were also found in our earlier study (Shin et al., 1997). Various chromosome abnormalities, including tetrasomy 17, were also observed in a human endometriosis-derived established cell line (FbEM-1) (Bouquet de Joliniere et al., 1997). By comparative genome hybridization (CGH), a French team has found the following changes: 1q+, 4q−, 11p−, 13q−; loss of 9, 12, and 18; amplification of 6p (Gogusev et al., 1998).

The pattern of chromosomal aberrations in endometriosis, combined with the locally invasive nature of the disorder, suggests parallels between endometriosis and neoplasia. If the parallel holds, two "hits" (mutational events) would be necessary for development of endometriosis. Both hits may be somatic mutations, or one may be germline (genetic) and the other somatic (Bischoff and Simpson, 2000, 2001; Simpson and Bischoff, 2002). Consistent with this hypothesis are observations that monoclonal cell expansion occurs in endometriosis (Jimbo et al., 1997; Tamura et al., 1998). Overexpression of certain oncogenes (*c*-myc, *c*-erb, B1, and B2), as well as 6p DNA amplification, has been observed (Gogusev et al., 1998); however, no candidate genes on 6p have been overexpressed.

The third approach being pursued is to search for specific candidate genes. The first steps usually involved studies in which association was sought between endometriosis and normal individuals for selected genes (or polymorphisms at these loci).

One candidate gene is galactose-1-phosphate uridylyl transferase (*GALT*), specifically an adenine to guanine change (polymorphism) in exon 10 that results in substitution of aspartate for asparagine (N314D). An association was found with endometriosis by Cramer et al. (1996) but was not confirmed by Morland et al. (1998) or Hadfield et al. (1999). In the latter, frequencies of N314D were 15.8% (9 of 57) and 14.3% (13 of 91) in familial and sporadic endometriosis cases, respectively, vs. 11.3% (6 of 53) in female controls and 13.7% (13 of 95) in male controls.

An estrogen receptor gene polymorphism detectable by PvuII restriction endonucleose was reported by Georgiou et al. (1999):

homozygosity or heterozygosity was found in 72% (82 of 114) of endometriosis vs. 49% (56 of 114) controls.

Increased frequency for the null (deletion) allele of glutathione *S*-transferase M1 (GSTm1) was reported by Baranova et al. (1997): 86% (43 of 50) in endometriosis subjects vs. 46% (33 of 72) in controls. Baranova et al. (1997) also reported increased frequency of the slow acetylation allele of arylamine *N*-acetyltransferase 2 (NAT2). The potential significance of pharmacogenetic susceptibility involving this locus has been discussed elsewhere by Bischoff and Simpson (2001).

Oncogenes and Tumor Suppressor Genes in Endometriosis

The pattern of chromosomal aberrations combined with the invasive nature of endometriosis suggested parallels between the latter and neoplasia. Indeed, monoclonal expansion in endometriosis is accepted (Jimbo et al., 1997; Tamura et al., 1998), and overexpression of certain oncogenes (*c*-myc, *c*-erb B1 and B2) is recognized (Gogusev et al., 1998).

Candidates genes for those causing endometriosis could be found in the genes or chromosomal regions involved in ovarian endometrioid and endometrial cancer, even while realizing that less than 1% of endometriosis undergoes neoplastic transformation. Mutations in the tumor suppressor *PTEN* gene, located on 10q23, are reported in endometrioid but in neither serous nor mucinous epithelial ovarian tumours (Obata et al., 1998). Although Loss of Heterozygosity (LOH) was common among the endometrioid (43%) and serous (28%) tumors, somatic mutations involving *PTEN* in the remaining allele were observed only in the endometrioid (21%) tumors. These results demonstrate that the developmental pathways of the three epithelial ovarian cancer subtypes (serous, mucinous, endometrioid) appear to be different, and that somatic mutations in *PTEN* may represent early events in the transformation of benign endometriotic cells to malignancy. The PTEN protein is believed to function as a tyrosine phosphatase and play a part in signal transduction. Clearly, the role of *PTEN* in the pathogenesis of endometriosis should be pursued in the near future.

Using a two-colour FISH approach with probes specific to the p53 locus (17p13) and 17 centromere, we observed a significantly greater frequency of chromosome 17 aneuploidy in the endometriotic specimens ($n = 8$, mean 65%) than in the matched normal endometrial cells (mean 25%) (Kosugi et al., 1999; Simpson and Bischoff, 2002). Significant ($p < .0001$) differences were found between the distribution of FISH signals among various endometriosis samples, implying a high degree of heterogeneity involving chromosome 17 aneuploidy. We observed a high incidence of monosomy p53; 18% to 28% of cells scored in four of eight cases. In aggregate, these findings support a multistep pathway involving somatic genetic alterations in the development and progression of endometriosis, specifically, pointing to a role for *p53* in the pathogenesis of endometriosis. If so, *p53* would not be the initial perturbation (or Li-Fraumeni syndrome would exist). The first "hit" could be an oncogene or a matrix metalloproteinase (cell adhesion) gene, an antiadhesion gene like *muc-1*, a macrophage scavenger gene, or any of a host of other genes.

Clinical Application

Knowledge that a first-degree relative has endometriosis may influence both the timing of childbearing and the type of contraception. One logically might recommend early rather than delayed childbearing, at least in general terms. If an older sib has endometriosis, the age of onset would be expected to be similar. Use of oral contraceptives instead of intrauterine devices is recommended, and other recommendations for prophylaxis of endometriosis include avoiding gynecologic manipulation during menstruation, minimizing opportunities for reflux menstruations. Efficacy of these recommendations has not been tested formally.

POLYCYSTIC OVARIAN SYNDROME

Disease Definition

Polycystic ovarian (PCO) syndrome is characterized by clinically polycystic ovaries, hirsutism, anovulation, and often secondary amenorrhea. Ultrasound reveals many small ovarian cysts. Gonadotropin secretion is altered, as manifested by elevated luteinizing hormone/follicle-stimulating hormone (LH/FSH) ratios. Whether an alteration in the LH/FSH ratio is the primary defect is arguable. Despite agreement about the general description, no precise criteria for diagnosis are universally accepted. This has been a major hurdle in genetic elucidation (Simpson, 1992).

General Genetics and Epidemiology

Given the heterogeneous nature of PCOS (see below), even the scanty epidemiologic data available are not necessarily useful. For example, increased body fat alone could lead to increased estrone, as a result of an increased peripheral conversion from androstenedione. Increased estrone can lead to anovulation, then producing an elevated LH/FSH ratio. Yet the LH/FSH ratio can be elevated in nonobese women for other (central) reason. Epidemiologic studies that take heterogeneity like the above into account have not been conducted. HLA associations exist for DRW6 (Hague et al., 1990) and DQA1*0501 (Ober et al., 1992).

The exception is the 3% to 5% of all PCOS cases which are due to adult-onset errors of adrenal biosynthesis or other known etiologies (O'Driscoll et al., 1994; Talbot et al., 1996). The enzyme of greatest interest is 21-hydroxylase deficiency, but late-onset (nonclassical) 11-β hydroxylase deficiency, 3β-ol-dehydrogenase deficiency and 17α-hydroxylase deficiency are also associated with hirsutism and polycystic ovary phenotype (O'Driscoll et al., 1994). There are differences in the ethnic distribution of these various enzyme deficiencies, producing late-onset adrenal hypoplasia, PCOS, and hirsutism. Adult-onset 21-hydroxylase deficiency (nonclassical) is especially common in Ashkenazi Jews. A specific mutation in the CYP21 gene can be identified in perhaps 7% of Ashkenazim showing elevated 17α-hydroxyprogesterone. The most common mutations are Val282Leu and Pro454Ser, which are 68% and 7%, respectively, of cases in one series (Blanche et al., 1997). In the non-Ashkenazim, *CYP21* mutations represent a far less common a cause of hirsutism and PCOS. Adult onset 17α-hydroxylase deficiency is relatively more common in Japanese, whereas 11β-hydroxylase deficiency is more common in Arabic populations. Adult-onset deficiency for these enzymes is uncommon in other populations.

In nonadrenal hyperplasia, or "essential" PCOS, consensus exists that a dominant gene exists; however, such a gene cannot explain all cases. The first formal genetic study in PCOS was by Cooper et al. (1968), who in 1968 studied 18 patients with "Stein-Leventhal syndrome." (Like most studies to be cited, the uncommon adrenal enzyme deficiencies were not excluded.)

Oligomenorrhea was present in 4 mothers of 13 subjects, but in none of 13 control mothers. Oligomenorrhea was much more common in sisters of cases (9 of 19) than in sisters of controls (1 of 18). Hirsutism was also more common in both male and female relatives. When subjected to culdoscopy (a now obsolete method of pelvic visualization, used before laparoscopy), 8 cases of Stein-Leventhal syndrome were detected among 12 sisters of the affected probands. Male relatives also showed an increased prevalence of "pilosity." Overall, data suggested autosomal dominant inheritance. Given that autosomal dominant genes are characterized by variable expressivity and decreased penetrance, such inheritance would be consistent with the variable clinical findings in PCOS.

In the 1970s Givens, Cohen, Wilroy, Summitt, and others at the University of Tennessee, Memphis, published a series of reports concluding that PCOS was inherited in X-linked dominant fashion. Diagnostic criteria consisted of hirsutism and either polycystic or bilaterally enlarged ovaries. In their first report, Givens et al. (1971) described two families in which multiple individuals in more than two generations were affected. In one kindred affected females experienced myocardial infarction in their fifth decade; acanthosis nigricans, insulin resistance, and hypertension were present in many family members. Most subjects were African American. In a third kindred (Cohen et al., 1975) several males showed maturational arrest of spermatogenesis. Excluding index cases, Wilroy et al. (1975) tabulated that 47% of female offspring of affected females were affected. Among offspring of males having an elevated LH/FSH ratio, 89% of daughters were affected. That almost all daughters of affected males were affected is consistent with X-linked dominant inheritance.

In the United Kingdom there have been a number of studies. In 1979 Ferriman and Purdie (1979) studied 707 patients with "hirsutism and/or oligomenorrhea both with and without infertility." Of the 707, information on ovarian size was available in 467, as assessed by the now obsolete air contrast method of gynecography (ultrasound or, preferably, laparoscopy is recommended, if visualization is needed). Of the 467, 45 had "identifiable disorders" that included "adrenal, pituitary or hypothic disorders." Family history was available in 381 of the remaining 422 cases. Approximately 60% of the 381 showed enlarged and "presumed polycystic ovaries." Frequency of oligomenorrhea and infertility in first-degree relatives was compared to that in a control group of 179 normal women. Subjects were further stratified into those with or without hirsutism, as well as into those with or without enlarged ovaries. Familial tendencies were greatest among hirsute women with enlarged ovaries. Premature baldness was significantly increased in male relatives of hirsute women.

More recent British studies have also provided data supporting heritability of PCOS, specifically autosomal dominant inheritance. However, some of the conclusions have been challenged on the grounds of arguable ultrasound diagnostic criteria and high background prevalences. Clayton et al. (1992) randomly selected 1065 women, of whom 190 completed their study. In these ostensibly normal women the prevalence of polycystic ovaries by ultrasound was 22% (41/190) (Clayton et al., 1992), very similar to findings of Polson et al. (1988). By contrast, in hirsute women studied by O'Driscoll et al. (1994), the prevalence of PCOS on ultrasound was 52% in women with normal cycles and 81% in women with abnormal cycles.

Several related studies ostensibly show much higher prevalence rates for PCOS in normal and abnormal sample. Adams et al. (1986) performed ultrasound on 173 women presenting with anovulation or hirsutism. Polycystic ovarian disease was diagnosed in 87% of women with oligomenorrhea and in 92% with hirsutism (see below). The criteria of Adams et al. (1985, 1986) were 10 or more 2 to 8 mm ovarian cysts, plus one of the following: elevated LH, elevated androstenedione, elevated LH/FSH ratio. These criteria are reasonable, but the quality of ultrasound in the early 1980s was less than today's standard. Hague et al. (1988) used the criteria of Adams et al. (1985, 1986) to determine the frequency of PCOS in relatives of affected cases. Of 52 sisters of probands, 45 (87%) were affected; 24 of 36 (67%) mothers were affected. This high frequency of affected relatives is dramatically higher than the 50% predicted for either autosomal dominant or X-linked dominant inheritance. However, recall that the data of Wilroy et al. (1975) also showed an 87% recurrence rate for daughters of affected women. Non-Mendelian mechanisms would need to be invoked to account for such a distorted segregation ratio. More likely, nonspecific diagnostic criteria led to an overly sensitive diagnosis (false positives).

In other British studies, frequency of affected relatives was nearer the 50% expected for autosomal dominant inheritance. Carey et al. (1993) studied first-degree relatives of 10 probands. Of the 62 informative relatives, 58 could be fully screened by ultrasound. Of female first-degree relatives, 51% were affected. As in several other studies, male relatives showed premature balding.

The studies cited above were performed after ascertaining PCOS cases and relatives predominately on clinical or ultrasonographic criteria. Legro et al. (1998) studied 80 probands diagnosed on the bases of elevated testosterone associated with oligomenorrhea (<6 menses/year) or amenorrhea. Nonclassical 21-hydroxylase deficiency was excluded. Most in the sample were "non-Hispanic white" (87%); 10% were Hispanic, and 3% were African American. Of 134 sisters, 115 agreed to body mass index measurements and contributed a blood sample to determine serum testosterone, which was considered abnormal if it was greater than 2 SD above the control mean value. Excluding 36 sisters who were postmenopausal or could not be assessed because they were on oral contraception or other medicines that affect sex hormones, 46 of the remaining 81 were affected (46%) either on the basis of elevated T alone ($n = 19$) or both elevated T and oligomenorrhea ($n = 17$).

Kahsar-Miller et al. (2001) considered frequencies of both hirsutism alone and PCOS as defined clinically and biochemically (elevated T). Compared to a previously determined background of 4% in the Alabama population (Knochenhauer et al., 1998), frequency was increased 5- to 6-fold in first-degree relatives.

Concordantly affected twins have been observed (McDonough et al., 1972; Hutton and Clark, 1984), but discordance has been observed even for monozygotic twins. In an Australian study by Jahanfar et al. (1995), 19 MZ and 15 DZ twin pairs were identified. Using ultrasound criteria, 5 MZ and 6 DZ pairs were discordant.

Despite evidence of dominant tendencies, heritability due to a single dominant gene seems unlikely to explain all cases. Far fewer than 50% of symptomatic first-degree relatives seem clinically affected. The usual impression is that no more than 5% to 10% of first-degree relatives are symptomatic. When Mandel et al. (1982) studied 23 PCOS cases in Los Angeles, only 4 had a clinically affected relative; all 4 had an affected sister, and one also had an affected mother.

Lunde et al. (1989) studied 132 Norwegian women ascertained on the basis of ovarian wedge resection, multicystic ovaries, or other PCOS-like symptoms. Like other studies, female first-degree relatives showed hirsutism and menstrual irregularities more often than controls. Among sisters, the frequencies were 6% and 15%, respectively; among mothers, 12% and 13%. Male first-degree relatives showed early baldness.

In conclusion, formal explanations for the extant genetic data in essential (nonadrenal) PCOS include a single dominant gene of low penetrance and variable expressivity, along with polygenic/multifactorial inheritance or genetic heterogeneity. That HLA associations exist for DRW6 (Hague et al., 1990) and DQA1*O501 (Ober et al., 1992) are points in favor of genetic heterogeneity, given that HLA association are usually found in genetically heterogenous adult onset disorders having recurrence risks of 5% to 10%.

Gene Identification

This issue is muddied by lack of clarity concerning whether essential PCOS as defined above will involve any of the genes that cause nonclassical (adult-onset) adrenal hyperplasia and PCOS (*CYP21*, *CYP17*, *CYP11*). Of course, the few (5%) women with PCOS due to a demonstrable adrenal biosynthetic defect should have a mutation in the gene coding for these enzymes (21-hydroxylase, 17α-hydroxylase/17,20-lyase, or 11 β-hydroxylase). (Otherwise, the enzyme deficiency would be a secondary phenomenon.) The same principle applies to PCOS cases associated with insulin-resistance. Sorbara et al. (1994) sequenced the entire insulin receptor gene in 26 PCOS cases, finding mutations in 2. However, in 32 women studied by Talbot et al. (1996), no mutations were found in *INSR*. If insulin receptor perturbation is integral to PCOS, the mechanism of action must usually involve a more distant (downstream) step in insulin action (e.g., translation).

Whole-genome analysis to localize genes responsible for PCOS is under way, using sib-pair analysis with polymorphic DNA variants (Urbanek et al., 1998). A total of 150 families of European origin have been studied for linkage to 37 candidate genes, using affected sib-pair analysis and transmission/disequilibrium methods (Urbanek et al., 1999). Diagnostic criteria consisted of oligomenorrhea (<6 menses/year) and hyperandrogenism (>58 ng/dl total T or >15 ng/dl not bound to sex hormone–binding globulin). Of 134 sisters of index cases, 39 were affected, 46 were unaffected, and 49 were unknown. Polymorphic markers within 1 cM of each candidate gene were available for 28 candidate genes; for 9 candidate genes polymorphic markers were 1 to 4 cM distant. Analyzed were several regions previously stated to show association or linkage to PCOS: *INS*, *VNTR* (insulin variable number tandem repeats), *CYP11A*, *CYP1A*, *CYP17*, and *INSR* (insulin receptor). Strongest evidence for linkage was found between PCOS and follistation, which was 72% identity by descent. The nature of the perturbation in or near the follistation locus on chromosome was not determined, but a causative relationship is not implausible. Follistation neutralizes activin, a member of the TGFβ family that promotes ovarian folliculor development, inhibits these cell's androgen production, and increases both pituitary FSH and pancreatic β-cell insulin secretions. Inappropriately high follistation should inhibit follicular development, increase ovarian androgen production, and impair insulin release. These features are all characteristic of PCOS. Overexpression of follistation in transgenic mice results in a similar (PCOS-like) ovarian phenotype (Guo et al., 1998). Still, Calvo et al. (2001) found no mutations after sequencing exons 1, 2, 3, 4, and 6 of the follistation gene in 34 Spanish PCOS cases. Liao et al. (2000) similarly failed to find follistation perturbations in 64 Chinese cases.

Of the other candidate genes, only *CYP11A* showed nominally significant linkage (p = .02 before correction but $p > .05$ after correction). Among genes failing to show linkage and thus contradicting other studies were *INS*, *VNTR* (linkage shown by Waterworth et al., 1997, *CYP19*, *CYP17*, and *INSR*. Although Gharani et al. (1997) also showed association between CYP11A and PCOS, the specific allele they used (D15S520) was not shown to be linked to PCOS in the study of Urbanek et al. (1999).

Investigators at St. Mary's Hospital have long sought linkage and associations between PCOS and various cytochrome P450 genes involved in the adrenal biosynthetic pathways. The once promising association with CYP17 (17α-hydroxylase/17,20-lyase) is no longer accepted (Gharani et al., 1996; Techatraisak et al., 1997). Of current interest to this group is CYP11 (Gharani et al., 1997). There is also evidence (OR 8.20) for linkage between PCOS and the insulin gene on 11p15 (Waterworth et al., 1997), and between PCOS and the dopamine D3 receptor (Legro, 1995).

Clinical Application

Clinical management of nonadrenal PCO is a topic in all standard gynecologic texts. In the current context, an individual with familial PCO is managed no differently from an individual with PCO not having an affected relative. Hirsutism must be treated, and induction of ovulation may be necessary. Awareness of an affected relative naturally should heighten suspicion that a given individual has PCOS, especially if hirsutism or oligomenorrhea (infertility) coexists. However, PCOS and its symptoms are so pedestrian that clinicians will surely consider the diagnosis forthright in any symptomatic patient. That is, the diagnosis would be PCOS until proven otherwise (e.g., neoplasia). Asymptomatic patients rarely need treatment, even if FSH/LH ratios are altered and even if a relative is affected. An exception exists if an affected woman is asymptomatic but anovulatory, in which case periodic progestins are indicated.

PREMATURE OVARIAN FAILURE

Premature ovarian failure (POF) is generally defined as menopause at younger than 35 years of age. Some define POF as younger then 40 years of age. Causes of premature ovarian failure overlap with those responsible for complete ovarian failure and primary amenorrhea, a topic covered in more detail elsewhere (Simpson, 2000a). The many autosomal and X-linked genes causing ovarian failure may also be manifested as POF in some individuals. It is more profitable here to limit our comments to familial tendencies in POF, specifically when caused by other mechanisms. Detailed considerations are provided elsewhere (Simpson 2000a, 2000b; Simpson and Elias, in press).

To place familial POF as usually defined clinically in context, however, recall that these general causes exist: (1) X-chromosomal abnormalities, (2) autosomal recessive genes causing the various types of XX gonadal dysgenesis, and (3) autosomal dominant genes whose phenotype is restricted to POF.

X-Chromosomal Abnormalities

Premature rather than complete ovarian failure occurs to a varying extent with all X-abnormalities. At least 10% to 15% of 45,X/46,XX individuals menstruate, compared to fewer than 5% of 45,X individuals (Simpson, 1975). This percentage is surely a minimum because many mosaic individuals are so mildly affected that they are never detected clinically. Spontaneous menstruation occurs in about half of all 46,X,del(X)(p11) and in most 46,X,del(X)(p21 or 22) cases, albeit followed often by secondary amenorrhea and premature ovarian failure (Simpson, 2000a). Terminal deletions or X-autosomal translocations involving Xq21 to Xq26 are more likely to be associated with premature ovarian failure than with complete ovarian failure.

Increased frequency of premature ovarian failure occurs in women with the FRAXA premutation (FMR-1). FRAXA premutations accounts for some familial POF, for example 3 of 23 pedigrees studied by Conway et al. (1998). However, Kennevson et al. (1997) found FRAXA in 0 of 17 families, and Marozzi et al. (1999) found them in only 1 of 29. This phenomenon may or may not be independent of perturbations of terminal Xq ovarian maintenance genes.

Autosomal Recessive POF

The autosomal recessive mutations responsible for the various forms of XX gonadal dysgenesis may manifest as less severe ovarian pathology. The XX gonadal dysgenesis gene(s) are thus responsible for some aggregates of familial premature ovarian failure. In some families the propositus may have gonadal dysgenesis and streak gonads, but a sib may have ovarian hypoplasia with a few oocytes. These sibships indicate that the mutant gene responsible for XX gonadal dysgenesis shows variable expressivity. In Finland, Aittomaki (1994; Aittomaki et al., 1995), found that the FSH receptor mutation (C566T) that more commonly produced complete ovarian failure could also be manifested as POF, not infrequently coexisting in the same kindred as complete ovarian failure (COF).

Autosomal Dominant POF

The form(s) of POF that is most often associated with genetic tendencies is autosomal dominant. Coulam et al. (1983) reported POF in sibs who had an affected mother and aunt. Affected individuals in more than one generation were reported by Starup and Sele (1973) and by Austin et al. (1979). Mattison et al. (1984) reported five families in which POF segregated in autosomal or X-linked dominant fashion.

Of interest are studies being conducted in Italy (Testa et al., 1997; Vegetti et al., 1998). Women with POF recruited from a large northern Italian population base underwent pedigree studies to identify heritable POF. After excluding 10 cases with known etiologies (5 chromosomal, 3 prior ovarian surgery, 1 prior chemotherapy, 1 galactosemia), the remaining 71 probands were studied. In all, cessation of ovarian function (POF) occurred under age 40 years. Of the 71 probands, 22 (31%) had other affected relatives. Patterns of inheritance were consistent with autosomal or X-linked dominant inheritance because transmission through both maternal and paternal lineage was observed.

Blepharophimosis-Ptosis-Epicanthus

Blepharophimosis-ptosis-epicanthus (BPE) is an autosomal dominant multiple malformation syndrome long known to be associated with premature ovarian failure (Zlotogora et al., 1983; Panidis et al., 1994). Sib-pair analysis using polymorphic DNA variants (Harrar et al., 1995) localized the gene to chromosome 3 (3q22 → 24) (Amati et al., 1996). Positional cloning revealed mutation in the winged helix/forkhead transcription factor gene (*FOXL2*) yielding a truncated protein (Crisponi et al., 2001). The gene is expressed in the mesenchyma of mouse eyelids and in adult ovarian follicles. *FOXL2* cosegregated with that form of BPE associated with ovarian failure in four families and in one patient having a de novo mutation. Reported mutations produced stop codons or a 17bp duplication, causing a frameshift and truncated gene product.

Autosomal Chromosomal Rearrangements

Balanced autosomal chromosomal rearrangements can also lead to premature ovarian failure. The most common rearrangement is reciprocal translocation. The mechanism presumably involves meiotic breakdown. In men it is easier to study this relationship. Azoospermic or oligospermic men who are otherwise clinically normal may show balanced autosomal translocations and present for intracytoplasmic sperm injection (ICSI). Another 10% of ICSI candidates have sex chromosomal abnormalities, but these men usually show other systemic abnormalities (Klinefelter syndrome). A problem of similar magnitude probably exists in women, but difficulty in studying oocytes meiotically makes conclusive statements hazardous. Nevertheless, the pathogenesis presumably involves meiotic breakdown secondary to failure of synapsis.

Recognizing individuals with a chromosomal rearrangement is important because their offspring are at risk for unbalanced gametes; genetic counseling is obligatory.

Biologic Basis of Genetic Susceptibility

This issue is applicable here only for POF as traditionally defined—menopause occurring before age 30 or 40 in otherwise ostensibly normal women. In POF associated with X-chromosomal abnormality of XX gonadal dysgenesis, the issue is less genetic susceptibility than variable expression. Among the traditionally defined POF cases, the few familial aggregates show no identifying clinical characteristic. The biologic basis for familial cases could involve many genetic mechanisms, which are as yet undefined. Neither infectious nor immunologic factors have been identified, despite being sought in most studies cited. Logical hypotheses have centered on meiotic abnormalities, or, merely, the nearly untestable hypothesis that numbers of primordial follicles are decreased.

Clinical Application

The fact of familial aggregates of POF carries obvious clinical implications. First, endocrine status of younger sisters and daughters should be determined. Second, early childbearing should be encouraged. Individuals to whom this advice should be offered include those whose older sibling or parent has POF as traditionally designated. No precise age for childbearing can be stated, but as early as socially practical would be appropriate. The possibility of freezing oocytes or ovarian slices obtained early in life is now a genuine possibility. The rationale is that oocytes or tissue can be thawed and used for in vitro fertilization even if the patient is no longer spontaneously ovulating.

REFERENCES

Adams J, Franks S, Polson DW, Mason HD, Abdulwahid N, Tucker M, Morris DV, Price J, Jacobs HS: Multifollicular ovaries: clinical and endocrine features and response to pulsatile gonadotropin releasing hormone. Lancet 1985; 2:1375–1379.

Adams J, Polson DW, Franks S: Prevalence of polycystic ovaries in women with anovulation and idiopathic hirsutism. Br Med J 1986; 293:355–359.

Aittomaki K: The genetics of XX gonadal dysgenesis. Am J Hum Genet 1994; 54: 844–851.

Aittomaki K, Lucena JL, Pakarinen P, Sistonen P, Tapanainen J, Gromoll J, Kaskikari R, Sankila EM, Lehvaslaiho H, Engel AR: Mutation in the follicle-stimulating hormone receptor gene causes hereditary hypergonadotropic ovarian failure. Cell 1995; 82:959–968.

Alam NA, Bevan S, Churchman M, Barclay E, Barker K, Jaeger EE, Nelson HM, Healy E, Pembroke AC, Friedmann PS, et al.: Localization of a gene (*MCUL1*) for multiple cutaneous leiomyomata and uterine fibroids to chromosome 1q42.3–q43. Am J Hum Genet 2001; 68:1264–1269.

Algovik M, Lagercrantz J, Westgren M, Nordenskjöld: No mutations found in candidate genes for dystocia. Hum Reprod 1999; 14:2451–2454.

Amati P, Gasparini P, Zlotogora J, Zelante L, Chomel JC, Kitzis A, Kaplan J, Bonneau D: A gene for premature ovarian failure associated with eyelid malformation maps to chromosome 3q22–q23. Am J Hum Genet 1996; 58:1089–1092.

Arnold LL, Ascher SM, Simon JA: Familial adenomyosis: a case report. Fertil Steril 1994; 61:1165–1167.

Arnold LL, Meck JM, Simon JA: Adenomyosis: evidence for genetic cause. Am J Med Genet 1995; 55:505–506.

Ashar HR, Fejzo MS, Tkachenko A, Zhou X, Fletcher JA, Weremowicz S, Morton CC, Chada K: Disruption of the architectural factor MHGI-C: DNA-binding AT hook motifs fused in lipomas to distinct transcriptional regulatory domains. Cell 1995; 82:57–65.

Austin GE, Coulam CB, Ryan JR: A search for antibodies to luteinizing hormone receptors in premature ovarian failure. Mayo Clin Proc 1979; 54:394–400.

Baranova H, Bothorishvilli R, Canis M, Albuisson E, Perriot S, Glowaczower E, Bruhat MA, Baranov V, Malet P: Glutathione *S*-transferase M1 gene polymorphism and susceptibility to endometriosis in a French population. Mol Hum Reprod 1997; 3:775–780.

Berg-Lekas M-L, Hogberg U, Winkvist A: Familial occurrence of dystocia. Am J Obstet Gynecol 1998; 179:117–121.

Birrell FN, Adebajo AO, Hazleman BL, Silman AJ: High prevalence of joint laxity in West Africians. Br J Rheumatol 1994; 33:56–59.

Bischoff FZ, Simpson JL: Heritability and molecular genetic studies of endometriosis. Hum Reprod Update 2000; 6:37–44.

Bischoff FZ, Simpson JL: Genetics of endometriosis. In: Sciarra JJ (ed). Gynecology and Obstetrics, Vol. 5. Philadelphia: Lippincott, Williams and Wilkins, 2001; 1–7.

Blair RG: Pregnancy associated with congenital malformations of the reproductive tract. J Obstet Gynaecol Br Emp 1960; 67:36–42.

Bouquet de Joliniere J, Validire P, Canis M, Doussau M, Levardon M, Gogusev J: Human endometriosis-derived permanent cell line (FbEM-1): establishment and characterization. Hum Reprod Update 1997; 3:117–123.

Brosens I, Deprest J, Dal Cin P, Van den Berghe H: Clinical significance of cytogenetic abnormalities in uterine myomas. Fertil Steril 1998; 69:232–235.

Calabrese G, Di Virgilio C, Cianchetti E, Guanciali Franchi P, Stuppia L, Parruti G, Bianchi PG, Palka G: Chromosome abnormalities in breast fibroadenomas. Genes Chromosomes Cancer 1991; 3:202–204.

Calvo RM, Villuendas G, Sancho J, San Millan JL, Escobar-Morreale HF: Role of the follistatin gene in women with polycystic ovary syndrome. Fertil Steril 2001; 75:1020–1023.

Cameron N, Nagdee I: Menarcheal age in two generations of South African Indians. Ann Hum Biol 1996; 23:113–119.

Carey AH, Chan KL, Short F, White D, Williamson R, Franks S: Evidence for a single gene effect causing polycystic ovaries and male pattern baldness. Clin Endocrinol 1993; 38:653–658.

Chatman DL: Endometriosis in the black woman. Am J Obstet Gynecol 1976; 125:987–989.

Clayton RN, Ogden V, Hodgkinson J, Worswick L, Rodin DA, Dyer S, Meade TW: How common are polycystic ovaries in normal women and what is their significance for the fertility of the population? Clin Endocrinol (Oxf) 1992; 37:127–134.

Cohen O, Schindel B, Homburg R: Uterine leiomyomata: a feature of acromegaly. Hum Reprod 1998; 13:1945–1946.

Cohen PN, Givins JR, Wiser WL, Wilroy RS, Summitt RL, Coleman SA, Andersen RN: Polycystic ovarian disease, maturation arrest of spermiogenesis, and Klinefelter's syndrome in siblings of a family with familial hirsutism. Fertil Steril 1975; 26:1228–1238.

Conway GS, Payne NN, Webb J, Murray A, Jacobs PA: Fragile X premutation screening in women with premature ovarian failure. Hum Reprod 1998; 13:1184–1187.

Cooper HE, Spellacy WN, Prem KA, Cohen WD: Hereditary factors in the Stein-Leventhal syndrome. Am J Obstet Gynecol 1968; 100:371–387.

Coulam CB, Stringfellow S, Hoefnagel D: Evidence for a genetic factor in the etiology of premature ovarian failure. Fertil Steril 1983; 40:693–695.

Coxhead D, Thomas EJ: Familial inheritance of endometriosis in a British population: a case control study. J Obstet Gynaecol 1993; 13:42–44.

Cramer DW, Hornstein MD, Ng WG, Barbieri RL: Endometriosis associated with the N314D mutation of galactose-1-phosphate uridyltransferase (GALT). Mol Hum Reprod 1996; 2:149–152.

Cramer DW, Xu H, Harlow BL: Family history as a predictor of early menopause. Fertil Steril 1995; 64:740–745.

Crisponi L, Deiana M, Loi A, Chiappe F, Uda M, Amati P, Bisceglia L, Zelante L, Nagaraja R, Porcu S, et al.: The putative forkhead transcription factor FOXL2 is mutated in blepharophimosis/ptosis/epicanthus inversus syndrome. Nat Genet 2001; 27:157–166.

Duong TH, Korn AP: A comparison of urinary incontinence among African American, Asian, Hispanic, and white women. Am J Obstet Gynecol 2001; 184:1083–1086.

Elias S, Simpson JL, Carson SA, Malinak LR, Buttram VC Jr: Genetic studies in incomplete Müllerian fusion. Obstet Gynecol 1984; 63:276–279.

Ergun A, Pabuccu R, Atay V, Kucuk T, Duru NK, Gungor S: Three sisters with septate uteri: another reference to bidirectional theory. Hum Reprod 1997; 12:140–142.

Eskenazi B, Warner ML: Epidemiology of endometriosis. Obstet Gynecol Clin North Am 1997; 24:235–258.

Ferriman D, Purdie AW: The inheritance of polycystic ovarian disease and a possible relationship to premature balding. Clin Endocrinol 1979; 11:291–300.

Fischbein S: Onset of puberty in MZ and DZ twins. Acta Genet Med Gemellol (Roma) 1977; 26:151–158.

Fryns JP, Vogels A, Decock P, van den Berghe H: The hand-foot-genital syndrome: on the variable expression in affected males. Clin Genet 1993; 43:232–234.

Gabbe SG, Niebyl JR, Simpson JL (eds). Obstetrics: Normal and Problem Pregnancies, 3d ed. New York: Churchill Livingstone, 1996.

Garcia Muret MP, Pujol RM, Alomar A, Calaf J, de Moragas JM: Familial leiomyomatosis cutis et uteri (Reed's syndrome). Arch Dermatol Res 1998; 280(Suppl): S29–S32.

Georgiou I, Syrrou M, Bouba I, Dalkalitsis N, Paschopoulos M, Navrozoglou I, Lolis D: Association of estrogen receptor gene polymorphisms with endometriosis. Fertil Steril 1999; 72:164–166.

Gharani N, Waterworth DM, Batty S, White D, Gilling-Smith C, Conway GS, McCarthy M, Franks S, Williamson R: Association of the steroid synthesis gene *CYP11a* with polycystic ovary syndrome and hyperandrogenism. Hum Mol Genet 1997; 6:397–402.

Gharani N, Waterworth DM, Williamson R, Franks S: 5′ polymorphism of the *CYP17* gene is not associated with serum testosterone levels in women with polycystic ovaries. J Clin Endocrinol Metab 1996; 81:4174.

Givens JR, Wiser WL, Coleman SA, Wilroy RS, Andersen RN, Fish SA: Familial ovarian hyperthecosis: a study of two families. Am J Obstet Gynecol 1971; 110:959–972.

Gogusev J, Bouquet de Joliniere J, Doussau M, du Manoir S, Stojkoski A, Levardon M: Genetic abnormalities detected by comparative genomic hybridization in a human endometriosis-derived cell line. Mol Hum Reprod. 2000 Sep;6(9):821–827.

Granstrom L, Ekman G, Ulmsten U, Malmstrom A: Changes in the connective tissue of corpus and cervix uteri during ripening and labour in term pregnancy. Br J Obstet Gynaecol 1989; 96:1198–1202.

Greiss FC Jr, Mauzy CH: Genital anomalies in women: An evaluation of diagnosis, incidence, and obstetric performance. Am J Obstet Gynecol 1961; 82:330–339.

Guo Q, Kumar TR, Woodruff T, Hadsell LA, DeMayo FJ, Matzuk MM: Overexpression of mouse follistatin causes reproductive defects in transgenic mice. Mol Endocrinol 1998; 12:96–106.

Hadfield RM, Manek S, Nakago S, Mukherjee S, Weeks DE, Mardon HJ, Barlow DH, Kennedy SH: Absence of a relationship between endometriosis and the N314D polymorphism of galactose-1-phosphate uridyl transferase in a U.K. population. Mol Hum Reprod 1999; 5: 990–993.

Hadfield RM, Mardon HJ, Barlow DH, Kennedy SH: Endometriosis in monozygotic twins. Fertil Steril 1997; 68:941–942.

Hague WM, Adams J, Algar V, Drummond V, Schwarz G, Bottazzo GF, Jacobs HS: HLA associations in patients with polycystic ovaries and in patients with congenital adrenal hyperplasia caused by 21-hydroxylase deficiency. Clin Endocrinol (Oxf) 1990; 32:407–415.

Hague WH, Adams J, Reeders ST, Peto TE, Jacobs HS: Familial polycystic ovaries: a genetic disease. Clin Endocrinol 1988; 29:593–605.

Harrar HS, Jeffrey S, Patton MA: Linkage analysis in blepharophimosis-ptosis syndrome confirms localisation to 3q21–24. J Med Genet 1995; 32:774–777.

Hay D: The diagnosis and significance of minor degrees of uterine abnormality in relation to pregnancy. J Obstet Gynecol Br Emp 1958; 65:557–582.

Hay D: Uterus and unicollis and its relationship to pregnancy. J Obstet Gynaecol Br Emp 1961; 68:361–377.

Holmes JA: Congenital abnormalities of the uterus and pregnancy. Br Med J 1956; 1:1144–1147.

Hutton C, Clark F: Polycystic ovarian syndrome in identical twins. Postgrad Med J 1984; 60:64–65.

Jahanfar S, Eden JA, Warren P, Seppala M, Nguyen TV: A twin study of polycystic ovary syndrome. Fertil Steril 1995; 63:478–486.

Jakic M, Prebeg Z: Evaluation of genetic factors in the variability of menarche. Lijec Vjesn 1994; 116:123–127.

Jimbo H, Hitomi Y, Yoshikawa H, Yano T, Momoeda M, Sakamoto A, Tsutsumi O, Taketani Y, Esumi H: Evidence for monoclonal expansion of epithelial cells in ovarian endometrial cysts. Am J Pathol 1997; 150:1173–1178.

Jones HW Jr, Rock JA: Reparative and Constructive Surgery of the Female Generative Tract. Baltimore: Williams and Wilkins, 1983.

Kahsar-Miller MD, Nixon C, Boots LR, Go RC, Azziz R: Prevalence of polycystic ovary syndrome (PCOS) in first-degree relatives of patients with PCOS. Fertil Steril 2001; 75:53–58.

Kaprio J, Rimpela A, Winter T, Viken RJ, Rimpela M, Rose RJ: Common genetic influences on BMI and age at menarche. Hum Biol 1995; 67:739–753.

Kazmierczak B, Bol S, Wanschura S, Bartnitzke S, Bullerdiek J: PAC clone con-

taining the HMGI(Y) gene spans the breakpoint of a 6p21 translocation in a uterine leiomyoma cell line. Genes Chromosomes Cancer 1996; 17:191–193.
Kennedy S, Hadfield R, Barlow D, Weeks DE, Laird E, Golding S: Use of MRI in genetic studies of endometriosis. Am J Med Genet 1997; 71:371–372.
Kennedy S, Mardon H, Barlow D: Familial endometriosis. J Assist Reprod Genet 1995; 12:32–34.
Kennerson A, Cramer DW, Warren ST: Fragile X premutations are not a major cause of early menopause. Am J Hum Genet 1997; 61:1362–1369.
Kistner RW (ed): Gynecology, Principles and Practice, 4th ed. Chicago: Year Book, 1986.
Kitchin JD. Endometriosis. In: Sciarra JJ, Droegmuller W (eds). Gynecology and Obstetrics. Philadelphia: J.B. Lippincott, 1982; 1:1–25.
Kjerulff KH, Guzinski GM, Langenberg PW, Stolley PD, Moye NE, Kazandjian VA: Hysterectomy and race. Obstet Gynecol 1993; 82:757–764.
Kjerulff KH, Langenberg P, Seidman JD, Stolley PD, Guzinski GM: Uterine leiomyomas: racial differences in severity, symptoms and age at diagnosis. J Reprod Med 1996; 41:483–490.
Knochenhauer ES, Key TJ, Kahsar-Miller M, Waggoner W, Boots LR, Azziz R: Prevalence of the polycystic ovary syndrome in unselected black and white women of the southeastern United States: a prospective study. J Clin Endocrinol Metab 1998; 83:3078–3082.
Kosugi Y, Elias, S, Malinak RL, Nagata J, Isaka K, Takayama M, Simpson JL, Bischoff FZ: Increased heterogeneity of chromosome 17 aneuploidy in endometriosis. Am J Obstet Gynecol 1999; 180:792–797.
Kurbanova MK, Koroleva AG, Sergeev AS: Genetic-epidemiologic analysis of uterine myoma: assessment of repeated risk. S Genet 1989; 25:1896–1898. In Russian.
Lamb K, Hoffmann RG, Nichols TR: Family trait analysis: a case-control study of 43 women with endometriosis and their best friends. Am J Obstet Gynecol 1986; 154:596–601.
Legro RS: The genetics of polycystic ovary syndrome. Am J Med 1995; 98(1A): 9S–16S.
Legro RS, Driscoll D, Strauss JF III, Fox J, Dunaif A: Evidence for a genetic basis for hyperandrogenemia in polycystic ovary syndrome. Proc Natl Acad Sci USA 1998; 95:14956–14960.
Liao WX, Roy AC, Ng SC: Preliminary investigation of follistatin gene mutations in women with polycystic ovary syndrome. Mol Hum Reprod 2000; 6:587–590.
Ligon AH, Morton CC: Genetics of uterine leiomyomata. Genes Chromosomes Cancer 2000; 28:235–245.
Loesch DZ, Huggins R, Rogucka E, Hoang NH, Hopper JL: Genetic correlates of menarcheal age: a multivariate twin study. Ann Hum Biol 1995; 22:470–490.
Lunde O, Magnus P, Sandvik L, Hoglo S: Familial clustering in the polycystic ovarian syndrome. Gynecol Obstet Invest 1989; 28:23–30.
Malina RM, Ryan RC, Bonci CM: Age at menarche in athletes and their mothers and sisters. Ann Hum Biol 1994; 21:417–422.
Malinak LR, Buttram VC, Elias S, Simpson JL: Heritage aspects of endometriosis: II Clinical characteristics of familial endometriosis. Am J Obstet Gynecol 1980; 137:332–337.
Mandel FP, Chang RJ, Dupont B, Pollack MS, Levine LS, New MI, Lu JK, Judd HL: HLA genotyping of family members and patients with familial polycystic ovarian disease. J Clin Endocrinol Metab 1982; 56:862–864.
Mark J, Havel G, Grepp C, Dahlenfors R, Wedell B: Chromosomal patterns in human benign uterine leiomyomas. Cancer Genet Cytogenet 1990; 44:1–13.
Marozzi A, Dalpra L, Ginelli E, Tibiletti MG, Crosignani PG: FRAXA premutations are not a cause of familial premature ovarian failure. Hum Reprod 1999; 14: 573–575.
Marshall LM, Spiegelman D, Barbieri RL, Goldman MB, Manson JE, Colditz GA, Willett WC, Hunter DJ: Variation in the incidence of uterine leiomyoma among premenopausal women by age and race. Obstet Gynecol 1997; 90:967–973.
Mattison DR, Evans, MI, Schwimmer WB, White BJ, Jensen B, Schulman JD: Familial premature ovarian failure. Am J Hum Genet 1984; 36:1341–1348.
Maxwell C, Kilpatrick DC, Haining R, Smith SK: No HLA-DR specificity is associated with endometriosis. Tissue Antigens 1989; 34:145–147.
McDonough PG, Mahesh VB, Ellegood JO: Steroid, follicle-stimulating hormone, and luteinizing hormone profiles in identical twins with polycystic ovaries. Am J Obstet Gynecol 1972; 113:1072–1078.
Meilahn EN, Matthews KA, Egeland G, Kelsey SF: Characteristics of women with hysterectomy. Maturitas 1989; 11:319–329.
Meloni AM, Surti U, Contento AM, Davare J, Sandberg AA: Uterine leiomyomas: cytogenetic and histologic profile. Obstet Gynecol 1992; 80:209–217.
Moen M, Bratlie A, Moen T: Distribution of HLA-antigens among patients with endometriosis. Acta Obstet Gynecol Scand (Suppl) 1984; 123:25–27.
Moen MH: Endometriosis in monozygotic twins. Acta Obstet Gynecol Scand 1994; 73:59–62.
Moen MH, Magnus P: The familial risk of endometriosis. Acta Obstet Gynecol Scand 1993; 72:560–564.
Morland SJ, Jiang X, Hitchcock A, Thomas EJ, Campbell IG: Mutation of galactose-1-phosphate uridyl transferase and its association with ovarian cancer and endometriosis. Int J Cancer 1998; 77:825–827.
Mortlock DP, Innis JW: Mutation of *HOXA13* in hand-foot-genital syndrome. Nat Genet 1997; 15:179–180.
Mushkat Y, Bukovsky I, Langer R: Female urinary incontinence: does it have familial prevalence? Am J Obstet Gynecol 1996; 174:617–619.
Naylor AF, Warburton DA: Genetics of obstetrical variables: a study from the Collaborative Perinatal Project. Clin Genet 1974; 6:351–369.
Nibert M, Heim S: Uterine leiomyoma cytogenetics. Genes Chromosomes Cancer 1990; 2:3–13.
Norton PA, Baker JE, Sharp HC, Warenski, JC: Genitourinary prolapse and joint hypermobility in women. Obstet Gynecol 1995; 85:225–228.
Nykiforuk NE: Uterus didelphys. Can Med Assoc J 1938; 38:175–181.
Obata K, Morland SJ, Watson RH, Hitchcock A, Chenevix-Trench G, Thomas EJ, Campbell IG: Frequent *PTEN/MMAC* mutations in endometrioid but not serous or mucinous epithelial ovarian tumors. Cancer Res 1998; 58:2095–2097.
Ober C, Weil S, Steck T, Billstrand C, Levrant S, Barnes R: Increased risk for polycystic ovary syndrome associated with human leukocyte antigen DQA1*0501. Am J Obstet Gynecol 1992; 167:1803–1806.
O'Driscoll JB, Mamtora H, Higginson J, Pollock A, Kane J, Anderson DC: A prospective study of the prevalence of clear-cut endocrine disorders and polycystic ovaries in 350 patients presenting with hirsutism or androgenic alopecia. Clin Endocrinol (Oxf) 1994; 41:231–236.
Oksanen L, Tiitinen A, Kaprio J, Koistinen HA, Karonen S, Kontula K: No evidence for mutations of the leptin or leptin receptor genes in women with polycystic ovary syndrome. Mol Hum Reprod 2000; 6:873–876.
Pandis N, Heim S, Bardi G, Floderus UM, Willen H, Mandahl N, Mitelman F: Chromosome analysis of 96 uterine leiomyomas. Cancer Genet Cytogenet 1991; 55:11–18.
Panidis D, Rousso D, Vavilis D, Skiadopoulos S, Kalogeropoulos A: Familial blepharophimosis with ovarian failure. Hum Reprod 1994; 9:2034–2037.
Petri E: Untersuchungen zur Erbbedingtheit der Menarche. Z Morphol Anthropol 1934; 33:43–50.
Polishuk WZ, Ron MA: Familial bicornuate and double uterus. Am J Obstet Gynecol 1974; 119:982–987.
Polson DW, Adams J, Wadsworth J, Franks S: Polycystic ovaries: a common finding in normal women. Lancet 1988; 1:870–872.
Ranney B: Endometriosis: IV. Hereditary tendency. Obstet Gynecol 1971; 37:734–737.
Ranney B: Endometriosis. Obstet Gynecol Annu 1978; 7:219–244.
Reed WB, Walker R, Horowitz R: Cutaneous leiomyomata with uterine leiomyomata. Acta Dermatol Venereol 1973; 53:409–416.
Rein MS, Friedman AJ, Barbieri RL, Pavelka K, Flethcer JA, Morton CC: Cytogenetic abnormalities in uterine leiomyomata. Obstet Gynecol 1991; 77:923–926.
Ridley JH: The histogenesis of endometriosis. Obstet Gynecol Surv 1986; 23:1–35.
Rolen AC, Choquette AJ, Semmens JP: Rudimentary uterine horn: obstetric and gynecologic implications. Obstet Gynecol 1966; 27:806–813.
Sanchez-Andres A: Genetic and environmental factors affecting menarcheal age in Spanish women. Anthropol Anz 1997; 55:69–78. In German.
Sayer TR, Dixon JS, Hosker GL: A study of paraurethral connective tissue in women with stress incontinence of urine. Neurourol Urodynam 1990; 9:319.
Schoenberg-Fejzo M, Ashar HR, Krauter KS, Powell WL, Rein MS, Weremowicz S, Yoon SJ, Kucherlapati RS, Chada K, Morton CC: Translocation breakpoints upstream of the *HMGIC* gene in uterine leiomyomata suggest dysregulation of this gene by a mechanism different from that in lipomas. Genes Chromosomes Cancer 1996; 17:1–6.
Semmens JP: Congenital anomalies of female genital tract: functional classification based on review of 56 personal cases and 500 reported cases. Obstet Gynecol 1962; 19:328–350.
Shin JC, Ross HL, Elias S, Nguyen DD, Mitchell-Leef D, Simpson JL, Bischoff FZ: Detection of chromosomal aneuploidy in endometriosis by multi-color fluorescence in situ hybridization (FISH). Hum Genet 1997; 100:401–406.
Simpson JL: Gonadal dysgenesis and abnormalities of the human sex chromosomes: current status of the phenotypic–karyotypic correlations. Birth Defects 1975; 11(4):23–59.
Simpson JL (ed): Disorders of Sexual Differentiation: Etiology and Clinical Delineation. New York: Academic Press, 1976.
Simpson JL: Elucidating the genetics of polycystic ovary syndrome. In: Dunaif A, Givens JR, Haseltine FP, Merriam GR (eds). Polycystic Ovary Syndrome. Boston: Blackwell Scientific, 1992:59–69.
Simpson JL: Genetic programming in ovarian development and oogenesis. In: Lobo RA, Kelsey J, Marcus R (eds). Menopause Biology and Pathobiology. London: Academic Press, 2000a:77–94.
Simpson JL: Genetic factors in common disorders of female infertility. Reprod Med Rev 2000b; 8:173–202.
Simpson JL, Bischoff FZ: Heritability and molecular genetic studies of endometriosis. Bethesda, Maryland: National Institutes of Health (NIH), (In press).
Simpson JL, Bischoff, FZ: Heritability and molecular genetic studies of endometriosis. (In) Yoshinaga K, Parrott E.C. (Editors): *Endometriosis: Emerging Research and Intervention Strategies.* New York, Annuals of The New York Academy of Sciences Vol. 955, pp. 239–251, 2002.
Simpson JL, Elias S: Genetics in Obstetrics and Gynecology, 3d ed. Philadelphia: W.B. Saunders, (In press).
Simpson JL, Elias S, Malinak LR, Buttram VC Jr: Heritable aspects of endometriosis: I. Genetic studies. Am J Obstet Gynecol 1980; 137:327–331.
Simpson JL, Malinak LR, Elias S, Carson SA, Radvany RA: HLA association in endometriosis. Am J Obstet Gynecol 1984; 148:395–397.
Snieder H, MacGregor AJ, Spector TD: Genes control the cessation of a woman's reproductive life: a twin study of hysterectomy and age at menopause. J Clin Endocrinol Metab 1998; 83:1875–1880.
Sorbara LR, Tang Z, Cama A, Xia J, Schenker E, Kohanski RA, Poretsky L, Koller E, Taylor SI, Dunaif A: Absence of insulin receptor gene mutations in three insulin-resistant women with the polycystic ovary syndrome. Metabolism 1994; 43:1568–1574.
Starup J, Sele V: Premature ovarian failure. Acta Obstet Gynecol Scand 1973; 52:259–268.

Stefansson H, Geirsson RT, Guanason GA, Kong A, Frigge ML, Gulcher J, Stefansson K: A genome-wide search for endometriosis genes in Icelandic patients. Am J Hum Genet 1998; 63:A310.

Stelling JR, Bhagavath B, Gray MR, Reindollar RH: HOXA13 homeodomain mutation analysis in patients with Müllerian system anomalies. J Soc Gynecol Invest 1998; 5:140A.

Stern AM, Gall JC Jr, Perry BL, Stimson CW, Weitkamp LR, Poznanski AK: The hand-food-uterus syndrome: a new hereditary disorder characterized by hand and foot dysplasia, dermatoglyphic abnormalities, and partial duplication of the female genital tract. J Pediatr 1970; 77:109–116.

Stevenson AC, Dudgeon MY, McCluire HI: Observations on the results of pregnancies in women resident in Belfast: II. Abortions, hydatidiform males, and ectopic pregnancies. Ann Hum Genet 1959; 23:395–411.

Takakura K, Takebayashi K, Wang H-Q, Kimura F, Kasahara K, Noda Y: Follicle-stimulating hormone receptor gene mutations are rare in Japanese women with premature ovarian failure and polycystic ovary syndrome. Fertil Steril 2001; 75:207–209.

Talbot JA, Bicknell EJ, Rajkhowa M, Krook A, O'Rahilly S, Clayton RN: Molecular scanning of the insulin receptor gene in women with polycystic ovarian syndrome. J Clin Endocrinol Metab 1996; 81:1979–1983.

Tamura M, Fukaya T, Murakami T, Uehara S, Yajima A: Analysis of clonality in human endometriotic cysts based on evaluation of X chromosome inactivation in archival formalin-fixed, paraffin-embedded tissue. Lab Invest 1998; 78:213–218.

Tashiro H, Blazes MS, Wu R, Cho KR, Bose S, Wang SI, Li J, Parsons R, Ellenson LH: Mutations in *PTEN* are frequent in endometrial carcinoma, but rare in other common gynecological malignancies. Cancer Res 1997; 57:3935–3940.

Techatraisak K, Conway GS, Rumsby G: Frequency of a polymorphism in the regulatory region of the 17 α-hydroxylase-17,20-lyase (*CYP17*) gene in hyperandrogenic states. Clin Endocrinol (Oxf) 1997; 46:131–134.

Testa G, Vegetti W, Tibiletti MG, Dalpra L, De Lauretis L, Lalia M, Alagna F, Bolis PF, Crosignani PG: Pattern of inheritance in familial premature ovarian failure. Hum Reprod 1997; 12:202.

Tisserant-Perrier M: Etude comparative de certains processus de chroissance chez les jumeaux. J Genet Hum 1953; 2:87–103.

Torgerson DJ, Thomas RE, Reid DM: Mothers and daughters' menopausal ages: is there a link? Eur J Obstet Gynecol Reprod Biol 1997; 74:63–66.

Treloar SA, Do KA, Martin NG: Genetic influences on the age at menopause. Lancet 1998; 352:1084–1085.

Treloar SA, Martin NG: Age at menarche as a fitness trait: nonadditive genetic variance detected in a large twin sample. Am J Hum Genet 1990; 47:137–148.

Treloar SA, Martin NG, Dennerstein L, Raphael B, Heath AC: Pathways to hysterectomy: insights from longitudinal twin research. Am J Obstet Gynecol 1992; 167:82–88.

Treloar SA, O'Connor DT, O'Connor VM, Martin NG: Genetic influences on endometriosis in an Australian twin sample. Fertil Steril 1999; 71:701–710.

Tyler GT: Didelphys in sisters. Am J Surg 1939; 45:337–338.

Urbanek M, Driscoll DA, Legro RS, Dunaif A, Strauss DJ, Strauss JF, Spielman RS: Genetic analysis of candidate genes for polycystic ovary syndrome (PCOS). Am J Hum Genet 1998; 63:A313.

Urbanek M, Legro RS, Driscoll DA, Azziz R, Ehrmann DA, Norman RJ, Strauss JF III, Spielman RS, Dunaif A: Thirty-seven candidate genes for polycystic ovary syndrome: strongest evidence for linkage is with follistation. Proc Natl Acad Sci USA 1999; 96:8573–8578.

Varner MW, Fraser AM, Hunter CY, Corneli PS, Ward RH: The intergenerational predisposition to operative delivery. Obstet Gynecol 1996; 87:905–911.

Vegetti W, Grazia Tibiletti M, Testa G, de Lauretis Yankowski, Alagna F, Castoldi E, Taborelli M, Motta T, Bolis PF, Dalpra L, Crosignani PG: Inheritance in idiopathic premature ovarian failure: analysis of 71 cases. Hum Reprod 1998; 13:1796–1800.

Verp MS, Simpson JL, Elias S, Carson SA, Sarto GE, Feingold M: Heritable aspects of uterine anomalies: I. Three familial aggregates with Müllerian fusion anomalies. Fertil Steril 1983; 40:80–85.

Vikhlyaeva EM, Khodzhaeva ZS, Fantschenko ND: Familial predisposition to uterine leiomyomas. Int J Gynaecol Obstet 1995; 51:127–131.

Waterworth DM, Bennett ST, Gharani N, McCarthy MI, Hague S, Batty S, Conway GS, White D, Todd JA, Franks S, Williamson R: Linkage and association of insulin gene VNTR regulatory polymorphism with polycystic ovary syndrome. Lancet 1997; 349:986–990.

Way S: The influence of minor degrees of failure of fusion of the Müllerian ducts on pregnancy and labor. J Obstet Gynaecol Br Emp 1945; 52:325–333.

Weremowicz S, Somberger K, Dah Cin P, Vanni P, Morton CC: Characterization of *HMGIC* gene rearrangements in uterine leiomyomas by fluorescence in situ hybridization (FISH). Am J Hum Genetics 1998; 499:A91.

Wiebe D: Retained placenta of unusual type. Obstet Gynecol 1970; 35:153–154.

Williams TJ, Pratt JH: Endometriosis in 1,000 consecutive celiotomies: incidence and management. Am J Obstet Gynecol 1977; 129:245–250.

Wilroy RS Jr, Givens JR, Wiser WL, Coleman SA, Andersen RN, Summitt RL: Hyperthecosis: an inheritable form of polycystic ovarian disease. Birth Defects: 1975; 11(4):81–85.

Winkler H, Hoffman W: Zur Frage der Veriebbarket des Uterusmyom. Dtsch Med Wochenschr 1938; 64:253–256.

Xing YP, Powell WL, Morton CC: The del(7q) subgroup in uterine leiomyomata: genetic and biologic characteristics. Further evidence for the secondary nature of cytogenetic abnormalities in the pathobiology of uterine leiomyomata. Cancer Genet Cytogenet. 1997 Oct 1; 98(1):69–74.

Zlotogora J, Sagi M, Cohen, T: The blepharophimosis, ptosis, and epicanthus inversus syndrome: delineation of two types. Am J Hum Genet 1983; 35:1020–1027.

27 Infertility and Pregnancy Loss

CAROLE OBER, M. S. VERP, K. P. ROBERTS, AND J. L. PRYOR

Infertility and spontaneous abortion (SA) are common disorders. Because an early embryonic loss may present as a delayed menstrual period, some couples having very early pregnancy losses may mistakenly be thought to be infertile. In addition, some of the same factors may result in either failure to become pregnant (i.e., infertility), preclinical losses, or recognized pregnancy loss. Therefore, it is appropriate to consider both infertility and pregnancy loss in this chapter. In particular, we will focus on common genetic causes of male infertility (*CFTR* gene mutations, Y chromosome microdeletions, and Klinefelter syndrome), chromosome abnormality as the most common cause of pregnancy failure, and immunogenetic causes of infertility and spontaneous abortion.

CHROMOSOME ABNORMALITIES IN INFERTILE COUPLES

Infertility is the inability to conceive following one year of unprotected intercourse. Ten to 15% of U.S. couples are infertile. Although there are many nongenetic causes of infertility, chromosome abnormalities are present in a small number of infertile individuals. For example, infertile females or males with gonadal dysgenesis may have a 45,X or 47,XXY karyotype, and balanced chromosome rearrangements may occur at a higher than expected frequency in infertile individuals (Yoshida et al., 1997; Meschede et al., 1998; van der Ven et al., 1998) (Table 27–1). Interestingly, female partners of infertile males also have an increased frequency of karyotype abnormalities (Meschede et al., 1998; van der Ven et al., 1998; Yoshida et al., 1997), thus supporting the concept of infertility as a couple disorder with both partners subfertile.

GENETIC CAUSES OF MALE INFERTILITY

Among the 15% of couples with infertility (Mosher, 1985), male infertility is particularly problematic since it is estimated that the cause is unknown in up to 50% of cases (Dubin and Amelar, 1971; Hendry et al., 1973). However, it is becoming increasingly clear that many cases of idiopathic infertility may actually have a genetic etiology.

In the past there was little incentive for understanding the genetics of male infertility. It was generally accepted that genetic causes of infertility were rare and that there was relatively little that could be done for patients with infertility caused by a genetic abnormality. However, recent advances in our understanding of genetic causes of infertility and an increase in our ability to treat patients with severe oligospermia and azoospermia have made understanding the basics of reproductive genetics essential for the clinician treating infertility patients.

Y CHROMOSOME DELETIONS

Cytogenetic studies demonstrated that loss of the distal euchromatin of the Y chromosome was associated with severe infertility (Tiepolo and Zuffardi, 1976). This observation led to the proposal that a gene, or a set of genes, required for spermatogenesis resides on the long (q) arm of the Y chromosome. This region of the Y chromosome was designated AZF since it appeared to harbor an azoospermia factor gene or genes.

More recently, analysis of DNA from patients with Y chromosome deletions has led to mapping of the Y chromosome into a series of seven deletion intervals (Vollrath et al., 1992). Deletion intervals 1 through 4 reside on the p arm and include the centromere; deletion intervals 5 through 7 reside on the q arm. Sequence tagged sites (STS) have been aligned along the length of the Y chromosome (Vollrath et al., 1992), allowing fine mapping of small interstitial deletions (Nagafuchi et al., 1993; Kobayashi et al., 1994; Reijo et al., 1995, 1996b; Najmabadi et al., 1996; Nakahori et al., 1996; Qureshi et al., 1996; Stuppia et al., 1996; Vogt et al., 1996; Foresta et al., 1997; Girardi et al., 1997; Pryor et al., 1997; Simoni et al., 1997). Studies of Y deletions in infertile men demonstrate that most deletions occur in three regions in deletion intervals 5 and 6, designated AZFa, AZFb, and AZFc (Fig. 27–1) (Vogt et al., 1996). AZFc is the most common site of microdeletions. Although a correlation between deletions in these regions and specific phenotypes (hypospermatogenesis, spermatogenic arrest, etc.) has not been consistently demonstrated (Pryor et al., 1997), there appears to be a correlation between deletions in AZFb and a complete absence of advanced spermatids in the testis (Brandell et al., 1998). Therefore, testicular biopsy for sperm retrieval to be used in in vitro fertilization (IVF) with intracytoplasmic sperm injection (ICSI) may be contraindicated in patients with AZFb deletions.

Y chromosome microdeletions are found in approximately 10% to 15% of men with azoospermia or severe oligospermia (less than 5 million sperm per ml in the ejaculate), with values from different studies ranging from 3% to 29% (Najmabadi et al., 1996; Vogt et al., 1996; Foresta et al., 1997; Girardi et al., 1997; Pryor et al., 1997). In one study that examined the frequency of Y chromosome microdeletions in 200 infertile men, without selection for sperm count or other specific symptom, the frequency of deletions was 7% (Pryor et al., 1997). These data suggest that Y chromosome microdeletions constitute the second most common specific cause of male infertility, with varicocele being the most common cause. Furthermore, this same

Table 27–1. Chromosome Abnormalities in Infertile Patients and Their Partners

		Sex Chromosomes					Autosomes				
Reference	Sample	*N*	XXY	XYY	Yabn	XXX	Rcp t	Robert t	Inv	Other	Total (%)
Yoshida	Infertile males	1007	28	3	7		10	8	5	1	62 (6.2)
Meschede	Infertile males	432					2	2	2	1	7 (1.6)
van der Ven	Infertile males	305	1		1		5	1	1	1	10 (3.3)
Total	Infertile males	1744	29	3	8		17	11	8	3	79 (4.5)
van der Ven	Female partners	305				1	2	2	2	3	10 (3.3)
Meschede	Female partners	436				1	4	1			6 (1.4)
Total	Female partners	741				2	6	3	2	3	16 (2.2)

Data summarized from Meschede et al. (1998), van der Ven et al (1998), and Yoshida et al. (1997). Yabn, abnormal Y; Rcp t, reciprocal translocation; Robert t, Robertsonian translocation; Inv, inversion.

study showed that the frequency of Y chromosome microdeletions in patients with idiopathic infertility was 10%, indicating that Y chromosome deletions account for a substantial percentage of idiopathic infertility.

The Y chromosome microdeletions found in infertile men are absent in fertile men, indicating that these deletions are not simply correlated with infertility but actually cause the infertility (Reijo et al., 1995; Vogt et al., 1996; Pryor et al., 1997; Simoni et al., 1997). In addition, the near absence of deletions in the fathers of infertile men with Y chromosome deletions is strong evidence that these de novo deletions are responsible for the infertility (Reijo et al., 1995, 1996b; Vogt et al., 1996; Pryor et al., 1997; Girardi et al., 1997). However, not all microdeletions cause azoospermia—that is, some men with microdeletions of the Y chromosome can produce some sperm. This observation suggests that the deleted genes are not absolutely required for spermatogenesis but are necessary for optimal spermatogenesis, and it is consistent with the finding that deletions of the Y chromosome, in rare cases, can be transmitted by sexual intercourse (Nagafuchi et al., 1993; Kobayashi et al., 1994; Vogt et al., 1996; Pryor et al., 1997). More often, however, these deletions can be transmitted by assisted reproductive techniques such as intrauterine insemination (IUI), in vitro fertilization (IVF), and intracytoplasmic sperm injection (ICSI) (Kent-First et al., 1996a, 1996b; Mulhall et al., 1997; Pryor et al., 1997).

Gene Identification

The search for azoospermia factor genes led to the cloning of two candidate gene families from deletion interval 6 (Ma et al., 1993; Reijo et al., 1995; Affara et al., 1996; Najmabadi et al., 1996). The first such gene was predicted to encode a protein with an RNA binding motif and is referred to as *RBM* for RNA binding motif (originally named *YRRM* for Y-specific gene with RNA recognition motif) (Ma et al., 1993; Najmabadi et al., 1996). Two members of the *RBM* gene family have been cloned and characterized, but Southern analysis suggests that there are more than 15 copies of *RBM* genes scattered along both arms of the Y chromosome (Chandley and Cooke, 1994). Deletion of one or more of these genes in infertile men has been observed, qualifying these genes as AZF candidates (Ma et al., 1993; Najmabadi et al., 1996; Pryor et al., 1997). Consistent with a role in spermatogenesis, the *RBM* genes are expressed only in the testis (Elliott et al., 1996). Although the function of the *RBM* gene product is not known, these genes are related to the autosomal *hnRNPG* (heterogeneous nuclear ribonucleoprotein G) gene that encodes a protein involved in pre-mRNA processing and transport (Le Coniat et al., 1992; Weighardt et al., 1996).

The second AZF candidate gene cloned, from the distal portion of deletion interval 6, was named *DAZ* for deleted in azoospermia (Reijo et al., 1995). Although not related to the *RBM*

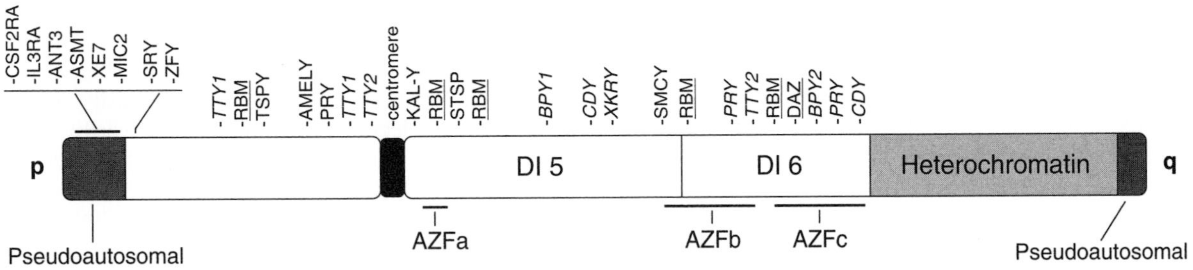

Fig. 27–1. Diagram of the Y chromosome with the relative locations of AZFa, AZFb, and AZFc—the three locations on the Y chromosome where deletions in infertile men preferentially occur. AZFa is found in the proximal portion of deletion interval 5; AZFb is located at the proximal end of deletion interval 6, extending into the distal part of deletion interval 5; and AZFc is found in the distal portion of deletion interval 6 (DI, deletion interval). Multiple copies of the *RBM* genes that have been localized to several regions on the Y chromosome and multiple copies of the DAZ gene are contained within AZFc (*underlined*). Also shown are the approximate locations of the Y-specific genes (*italics*) recently described by Lahn and Page (1997). Other well-characterized Y-chromosome genes are shown for reference. The heterochromatin varies in length between individuals and is noncoding. The pseudoautosomal region is that part of the Y chromosome which undergoes recombination with the X chromosome.

genes, the *DAZ* gene is also predicted to encode an RNA binding protein. The *DAZ* gene is also a member of a multigene family that has more than one copy on the Y chromosome. Another member of this family, *SPGY*, has also been cloned (Affara et al., 1995; Saxena et al., 1996). There is an autosomal homolog of *DAZ* on chromosome 3 in humans, termed *DAZH* or *DAZLA* (Saxena et al., 1996; Yen et al., 1996). In mice, the *DAZLA* ortholog is found on chromosome 17, while no ortholog is present on the Y chromosome (Reijo et al., 1996b). Both the Y-linked and autosomal *DAZ* genes are expressed in the testis, which is consistent with a functional role in spermatogenesis (Reijo et al., 1996b; Saxena et al., 1996; Yen et al., 1996). Mutation of the *DAZ* homolog in *Drosophila* causes meiotic arrest and infertility, adding additional evidence that *DAZ* is an AZF gene (Eberhart et al., 1996).

A comprehensive screen of expressed genes that reside in the nonrecombining region of the Y chromosome has resulted in the identification of 12 previously undescribed genes or gene families (Lahn and Page, 1997). Of these 12 new genes, 7 are found in multiple copy on the Y chromosome and are expressed in the testis, and these attributes are shared by *RBM* and *DAZ* (Fig. 27–1). Given the testicular expression of these genes and their location on the Y chromosome, these newly discovered genes are also candidate AZF genes. Infertility caused by microdeletions of Y chromatin could be attributed to the loss of any one or more of these genes.

Origin of Y Chromosome Deletions

The introduction of errors into the DNA sequence, such as mutations or deletions, normally occurs during DNA synthesis (i.e., DNA replication or repair) or during meiotic recombination. Errors occurring during recombination can be eliminated as a cause of these microdeletions as the deletions are found in the nonrecombining region of the Y chromosome. Therefore, it is most likely that Y chromosome deletions occur during DNA replication. Deletions that occur in the germline of the testis would result in sperm that carry the deletion and, if such a sperm fertilized an oocyte, would give rise to an individual who carried a Y chromosome deletion in all of his cells. Alternatively, a deletion occurring during DNA replication in the embryo would give rise to a mosaic individual with a possible deletion in the cells of the testicular germline. Because Y chromosome deletion analysis is normally performed on genomic DNA isolated from blood, mosaic individuals with a Y chromosome deletion confined to the germline would likely not be successfully diagnosed. It is likely that most individuals presenting with de novo Y chromosome microdeletions are not mosaics but, rather, inherited a Y chromosome that underwent a deletion event in their father's germline.

Indications for Y Chromosome Deletion Analysis

Y chromosome microdeletions occur with highest frequency in men with azoospermia and severe oligospermia (~15%) and are also prevalent in men with idiopathic infertility (~10%). Therefore, testing for Y chromosome microdeletions is a reasonable course of action for men with idiopathic infertility, as well as for those with azoospermia or severe oligospermia (<5 million sperm per ml). Couples considering in vitro fertilization with intracytoplasmic sperm injection, or other assisted reproduction options should also consider Y microdeletion analysis, since Y chromosome deletions have been passed on to male offspring using these techniques (Kent-First et al., 1996a, 1996b; Mulhall et al., 1997).

Clinical Implications of Y Chromosome Deletions

Although there is currently no treatment to improve fertility in men with Y chromosome deletions, knowledge of a Y chromosome microdeletion is useful for several reasons. First, detection of a deletion provides a diagnosis for infertility, and patients usually want to know why they are infertile. Second, a diagnosis of a Y chromosome microdeletion may influence the course of treatment for the patient. For instance, AZFb deletions may be a contraindication for testicular biopsy for sperm retrieval, or varicocele repair may not be beneficial in a patient with a Y chromosome deletion. Thus, with Y chromosome deletion information, the physician may be able to forego empirical treatments and direct the patient to assisted reproduction or adoption. Finally, knowledge of a Y chromosome microdeletion will allow couples who pursue assisted reproduction options to plan appropriately for the likelihood that a male child will eventually experience infertility. Although the male children of men with Y chromosome deletions conceived by assisted reproduction are not yet old enough to evaluate their fertility status, cases of inherited Y chromosome deletions suggests that infertility is passed on and may, in fact, be more severe in the offspring (Nagafuchi et al., 1993; Vogt et al., 1996; Pryor et al., 1997).

Klinefelter Syndrome

A male with one or more extra X chromosomes has Klinefelter syndrome, one of the most common causes of primary hypogonadism. This sex chromosomal anomaly has an incidence of around 1 in 500 male births (MacLean et al., 1964; Nielsen and Wohlert, 1991). Although the classic features of Klinefelter syndrome are often described as a triad of gynecomastia, small testes, and azoospermia, the clinical presentation can be quite variable. Therefore, a high degree of suspicion is appropriate when evaluating men presenting with severe oligo/azoospermia.

The pure form of Klinefelter syndrome, 47,XXY, occurs in 90% of cases, whereas the mosaic form 46,XY/47,XXY occurs in 10% of cases (Gordon et al., 1972). In half of the cases the extra X chromosome is of paternal origin, and in the other half it is of maternal origin (Lorda-Sanchez et al., 1992). If paternally derived, it results from non-disjunction in the first meiotic division; if maternally derived, it is the result of non-disjunction in either the first or second meiotic cycle (Lorda-Sanchez et al., 1992). Mosaic Kleinfelter syndrome results from mitotic nondisjunction in the embryo. Other variations of Klinefelter syndrome present with a single Y chromosome and 3, 4, or more X chromosomes. The clinical severity worsens as the number of X chromosomes increases.

As mentioned above, gynecomastia; small firm testes, and azoospermia are common features of Klinefelter syndrome. Other features include a eunuchoidal body habitus (long arms and legs due to a lack of testosterone at puberty, which delays epiphyseal closure of the long bones), obesity, varicose veins, diabetes, and learning disabilities (primarily verbal skills) (Money, 1993). Laboratory findings are consistent with hypogonadism and often include high follicle stimulating hormone (FSH), luteinizing hormone (LH), and estradiol levels, and low to normal testosterone levels. Despite these commonly described features, many men with Klinefelter syndrome lack gynecomastia or have soft rather than firm testes. Their body habitus may be completely normal, and many have no apparent learning disabilities. Therefore, the clinical presentation is highly variable and Klinefelter syndrome should be considered in the differential diagnosis of any male with significant hypogonadism.

The only consistent feature of Klinefelter syndrome is hypogonadism coincident with azoospermia and infertility. The typical histologic pattern in the testis is hylanized seminiferous tubules and Leydig cell hyperplasia (Gordon et al., 1972). In the classic form of Klinefelter syndrome there is a complete loss of germ cells, whereas in the mosaic form the findings are less severe. In one study, spermatids were found in 0.1% of seminiferous tubules in patients with 47,XXY vs. 16% of seminiferous tubules in patients with 46,XY/47,XXY (Gordon et al., 1972). Consistent with this is the description of fertility in those with 46,XY/47,XXY mosaicism (Warburg, 1963). However, no cases of fertility have been reported in men with classic Klinefelter syndrome until the recent advances in assisted reproductive techniques.

There are other health consequences associated with Klinefelter syndrome. Men with Klinefelter syndrome are estimated to have a 67-fold increased risk of developing an extragonadal tumor, primarily a germcell mediastinal tumor, compared to a male with a normal karyotype (Hasle et al., 1995). Men with Klinefelter syndrome also have an increased risk of developing breast cancer, although there is no uniform agreement on this association (Evans and Crichlow, 1987; Hasle et al., 1995; Hultborn et al., 1997). Men with Klinefelter syndrome are also at risk for bronchitis and diabetes. Thus, these men should undergo counseling and be aware of the possible health consequences of their diagnosis.

With the advent of intracytoplasmic sperm injection (ICSI), only a few sperm are needed for in vitro fertilization. Births have recently been described after ICSI using sperm obtained from the testicles of two men with Klinefelter syndrome (Palermo et al., 1998). One couple had a boy and the other had twins, a boy and a girl. All the children had normal karyotypes. However, men with mosaic or classic Klinefelter syndrome can produce sperm with 24 chromosomes (i.e., with an extra sex chromsosome) (Cozzi et al., 1994; Foresta et al., 1998). Therefore, ICSI confers a theoretical increased chance of passing on chromosomal errors to the progeny of men with Klinefelter syndrome. Genetic counseling and pre-implantation genetic screening of the embryo or amniocentesis needs to be discussed with the couple before to undertaking IVF and ICSI (In't Veld et al., 1997).

CFTR Gene Mutations and Male Infertility

Defects in the cystic fibrosis transmembrane conductance regulator (CFTR) protein are associated with an inability to properly transport chloride and sodium ions across epithelial cell layers. The resulting fluid imbalance across the epithelial cell lining of many different organs results in the classic symptoms of cystic fibrosis (Fick, 1990). Thick mucus forms in the lungs promoting bacterial infection, and the exocrine ducts of the pancreas become clogged, resulting in pancreatic insufficiency. A less appreciated but consistent symptom of CFTR defects is congenital bilateral absence of the vas deferens (CBAVD). It is thought that the fluid imbalance across the epithelial cell lining of the vas deferens, similar to that in the lungs, results in degeneration of the vas deferens in the neonate (Gaillard et al., 1997), although the exact cause of CBAVD in males with *CFTR* mutations is unknown. There are also clinical and genetic data to suggest that mild *CFTR* defects can result in obstruction of the vas deferens, without degeneration, resulting in obstructive azoospermia (Kanavakis et al., 1998).

Cystic fibrosis is the most common autosomal recessive disease in the Caucasian population, with a heterozygous carrier rate of 4% and a homozygous (or compound heterozygous) affected rate of 1 in 2500 live births (0.04%) (Welsh and Smith, 1995; Zielenski et al., 1995). The observation that obstructive azoospermia resulting from absence of the vas deferens is associated with CF led to the hypothesis that CBAVD in the absence of CF symptoms may be the result of *CFTR* mutations (Osborne et al., 1993; Culard et al., 1994; Oates and Amos, 1994; Casals et al., 1995; Chillon et al., 1995; Costes et al 1995; Jarvi et al., 1995; Jezequel et al., 1995; Le Lannou et al., 1995; Mercier et al., 1995; Rave-Harel et al., 1995; Zielenski et al., 1995; Dumur et al., 1996). Collectively, these studies showed that approximately 20% of men with CBAVD are homozygotes (or compound heterozygotes) for *CFTR* mutations, and nearly 50% are heterozygous for one of the tested mutations.

CBAVD in men who are heterozygous for *CFTR* mutations was unexpected. If a single *CFTR* mutation could cause CBAVD, one in every 25 Caucasian men would be expected to have this condition (i.e., the CBAVD frequency in men would equal the *CFTR* mutation carrier frequency). This is clearly not the case. The recent discovery of a set of allelic variants in intron 8 of the *CFTR* gene helps explain the expression of CBAVD in a large percentage of patients who are heterozygous for *CFTR* mutations. Intron 8 of the *CFTR* gene harbors a site with a variable number of thymidine (T) residues of 5, 7, or 9 T, each representing a variant form of this intron (Fig. 27–2). The 7T allele is the most common (c. 85%) in the normal population, with the 9T and 5T occurring at lower frequencies (c. 10% and 5%, respectively). While the 7T and 9T alleles produce normal CFTR mRNA, the 5T allele causes aberrant splicing of the *CFTR* hnRNA, resulting in the loss of exon 9 from 90% of the mRNA and with a consequent reduction in functional CFTR protein. The 5T allele is present in nearly 50% of men with CBAVD and in 60% to 80% of CBAVD patients who have a known *CFTR* mutation in their other allele. These statistics suggest that the reduction in functional CFTR mRNA caused by the 5T allele contributes to CBAVD. Both the 7T and 9T alleles are compatible with normal function of the *CFTR* gene, although the F508 mutation (the most common *CFTR* mutation in CF and CBAVD) appears to be preferentially associated with the 9T allele haplotype.

There are currently more than 700 known mutations of the *CFTR* gene. Therefore, it is not feasible to test for all, or even a majority, of the possible mutations in patients with CBAVD, and it is likely that some CF mutations in men with CBAVD are undetected. Even so, the frequency of *CFTR* mutations in the CBAVD population greatly exceeds the general population, which is consistent with a causative relationship. If the 5T allele is included as a *CFTR* mutation, then the majority of CBAVD patients are compound heterozygotes for *CFTR* mutations. When a mutation is present in both copies of the *CFTR* gene in a CBAVD patient without CF symptomology, at least one of the mutations is usually mild in nature (Chillon et al., 1995).

The frequency of the 5T allele in the general population, combined with the *CFTR* mutation carrier frequency, can potentially account for the 1 in 1000 frequency of CBAVD in the population (Lissens and Liebaers, 1997). The frequency of the 5T allele is about 5% (Chillon et al., 1995), and the frequency of *CFTR* mutations is 4%. Assuming that one *CFTR* mutation combined with the 5T allele always results in CBAVD, the expected frequency would be 0.2%, or 1 in 500. If the penetrance of the 5T allele is assumed to be 0.56 (Lissens and Liebaers, 1997), the frequency of CBAVD would be predicted to be 1 in 900, a value that is very close to the observed frequency.

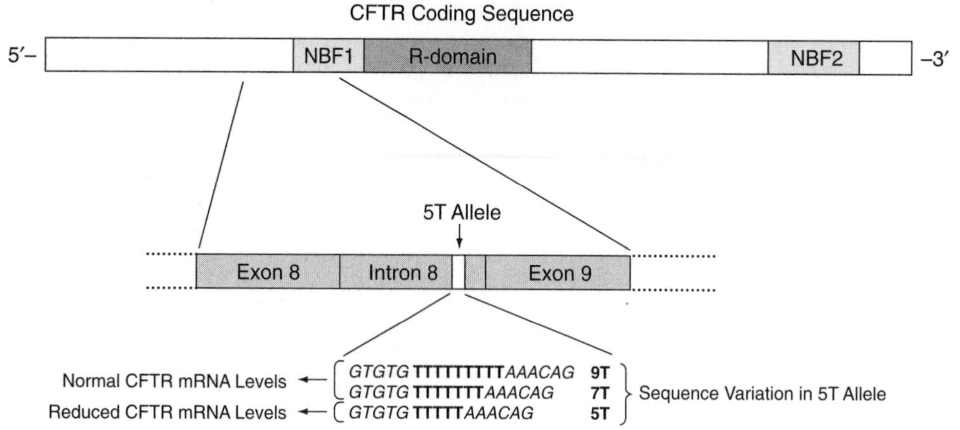

Fig. 27–2. Schematic representation of the 5T allele in the cystic fibrosis transmembrane conductance regulator (*CFTR*) gene. The 5T allele is a variable stretch of thymidine (T) residues of 5, 7, or 9 in intron 8. In the normal population, the 7T is the most common allele (c. 85%), with the 9T and 5T occurring with much less frequency (c. 10% and 5%, respectively). The 5T allele causes aberrant splicing of the *CFTR* hnRNA, resulting in the loss of exon 9 from 90% of the mRNA, with a consequent reduction in functional CFTR protein. Both the 7T and 9T alleles produce normal levels of functional *CFTR* mRNA.

CFTR mutations are not the only possible etiology of CBAVD. There is strong evidence to suggest that congenital abnormalities of the genitourinary system account for some cases. Several studies have demonstrated CBAVD in patients with renal anomalies such as renal agenesis (Casals et al., 1995; Dumur et al., 1996; Schlegel et al., 1996). In all of these reports, no *CFTR* mutations were found when CBAVD was associated with a renal abnormality.

CFTR Mutations and Non-CBAVD Infertility

Compared with the normal population, *CFTR* mutations are found at a high rate (17.5%–30%) in men with obstructive azoospermia but who have intact vas deferens bilaterally. This trend suggests that *CFTR* mutations can affect fertility without necessarily causing CBAVD (van der Ven et al., 1996; Kanavakis et al., 1998). In addition, Young's syndrome, which is manifested by obstructive azoospermia and chronic sinopulmonary disease, has been associated with an increased frequency of *CFTR* mutations, thus indicating another possible relationship between *CFTR* mutations and obstructive azoospermia (Hirsh et al., 1993). However, other studies have not found the same association (Friedman et al., 1995; Le Lannou et al., 1995).

The *CFTR* gene is expressed in the testis, and therefore it is possible that *CFTR* mutations may affect spermatogenesis (Larriba et al., 1998). Very few studies have addressed this question. In one study of 80 men with low semen quality, the *CFTR* mutation rate was 17.5% (van der Van et al., 1996). This study tested for only 13 *CFTR* mutations and did not include the 5T allele. A qualitative effect of the 5T allele on spermatogenesis has been suggested by Larriba et al. (1998), who correlated expression of CFTR mRNA splice variants in testis biopsy tissue to testicular histology.

Clinical Implications of CBAVD

Mutations in the cystic fibrosis transmembrane conductance regulator gene are the most common cause of congenital absence of the vas deferens. Therefore, men who present with infertility and CBAVD have a very high likelihood of harboring at least one CF mutation. Before proceeding with IVF and ICSI on such couples, CF mutation screens should be performed on both partners to determine the risk of having a CF child. The couple should then receive appropriate genetic counseling. In addition, if the patient with CBAVD has at least one *CFTR* mutation, he should be worked up for possible mild CF.

Other Genetic Causes of Male Infertility

There are many genetic causes for infertility that have a low incidence in both the general and infertile male population. Several of these genetic causes were recently reviewed and categorized into pre-testicular, testicular, and post-testicular causes (Mak and Jarvi, 1996). Although these causes of male infertility are rare, some of them illustrate basic concepts in reproductive physiology and are presented in Table 27–2.

Genetic Considerations for the Infertile Male

Although the birth of Louise Brown by IVF in 1978 heralded a great advance in treating the infertile couple, it had little effect on the infertile male with severe oligospermia or azoospermia because more than 1 million motile sperm (approximately 100,000 per egg) are typically required for IVF. However, with the advent of ICSI in 1995, only one viable sperm per egg is necessary for a chance of conception. This is a major advance for men with severe infertility, but it has also introduced the possibility of transmitting to the offspring a genetic cause of infertility or a congenital abnormality in which infertility is part of the disease spectrum. This increases the responsibility of the clinician to detect genetic causes of infertility before proceeding with IVF and ICSI so that the couple can make informed decisions.

Men with CBAVD should undergo testing for *CFTR* gene mutations. In addition, some clinicians feel that even if a *CFTR* gene mutation is not detected in these men, it is likely that they are heterozygous, and possibly homozygous (compound heterozygous), for an unidentified *CFTR* mutation. If true, then all female partners of men with CBAVD should also undergo genetic testing, regardless of the result from screening the male patient.

Finally, men with severe oligospermia (defined as less than 5 million sperm per ml) or azoospermia should have a karyotype to evaluate for Klinefelter syndrome and testing for microdeletions of the Y chromosome. As has been discussed, it is possible to have a conception by harvesting sperm in a man with Klinefelter syndrome, but there is an increased risk for a child

Table 27–2. Classic Genetic Causes of Male Infertility

Disorder	Features	Genetics	Reference
Kallman syndrome	Anosmia or hyposmia, midline defects such as cleft lip, renal anomalies, cryptorchidism, eunuchoidal skeletal proportions, low gonadotropins (FSH and LH), low testosterone	X-linked recessive	Franco et al., 1991
Young syndrome	Azoospermia, thick inspissated material within the epididymis, pulmonary infections	Autosomal recessive	Handelsman et al., 1984
Immotile-cilia syndrome	Bronchiectasis, chronic sinusitis, chronic cough, agenesis of frontal sinuses, immotile sperm; Kartagener syndrome is a subset of this group (50%) and has the classic triad situs inversus, bronchiectasis, and chronic siusitus.	Autosomal recessive	Elliasson et al., 1977
5-Reductase deficiency	Decreased or absent dihydrotestosterone causes abnormal development of external genitalia with micropenis, perineoscrotal hypospadius, and a blind vaginal pouch; there is a variable degree of masculinization at puberty	Autosomal recessive	Imperato-McGinley and Peterson, 1976; Schweikert, 1993
Androgen insensitivity syndrome	Variable from normal-appearing female external genitalia; abdominal or inguinal testes and an absent uterus (called testicular feminization syndrome) to incomplete pseudohermaphroditism	X-linked recessive	Aiman et al., 1979; Brown, 1995

with a sex chromosomal abnormality. Therefore, these couples should undergo genetic counseling prior to IVF and ICSI. Men with microdeletions of the Y chromosome will most assuredly pass them on to any male progeny, and these children may ultimately have similar reproductive potential. Although the majority of couples are unlikely to abandon IVF given the diagnosis of a microdeletion of the Y chromosome, informed consent is necessary. Finally, our understanding of genetic causes of infertility is still very limited. There are probably hundreds of genes on the sex chromosomes and autosomes that are involved in reproduction and have not been identified. It is likely that many men with idiopathic infertility have a genetic etiology for their infertility and are passing genetic infertility to their progeny when able to conceive through assisted reproductive techniques. In this situation IVF with ICSI is truly a double-edged sword: it can create fertility where none existed before, yet can pass on genetic abnormalities at the same time. Patients need to be made aware of these issues.

CYTOGENETIC CAUSES OF INFERTILITY AND FETAL LOSS

Cytogenetic Studies in Gametes and Early Embryos

Extrapolating from studies of pre-clinical losses and pre- and postimplantation abnormalities, approximately 70% of fertilized ova are lost before the first missed period. Although the causes of these preclinical pregnancy failures are not known, recent studies of oocytes, sperm, and early embryos fertilized in vitro (IVF) reveal a high frequency of chromosome abnormalities. Thus, it is likely that a majority of fertilization failures and preclinical losses are due to chromosomal abnormalities.

Unfertilized oocytes obtained from stimulated cycles of patients in IVF programs have shown a 37% incidence of hyperhaploidy, hypohaploidy, and diploidy (Kamiguchi et al., 1993). The few studies performed on unstimulated oocytes show lower but still significant aneuploidy rates (approximately 10%) (Hassold et al., 1993). An increase in oocyte aneuploidy with advanced maternal age has been demonstrated in some but not all, studies (Plachot, 1997). Chromosome abnormalities in sperm are also common. Approximately 10% of sperm from fertile men show either aneuploidy or, more commonly, structural chromosome rearrangements (Martin et al., 1991). Paternal age has little effect on the frequency of aneuploidy, although an age effect is seen for structural chromosome abnormalities (Guttenbach et al., 1997). Studies of infertile men have shown a significantly higher rate of sperm disomy than control donors show (Martin, 1997).

Studies in European IVF patients demonstrated chromosome abnormalities in 23% to 40% of early preimplantation embryos (Zenses and Casper, 1992). The high frequency of chromosome abnormalities is not unexpected, given the high incidence of chromosome abnormalities in oocytes and sperm and the fact that chromosome abnormalities for the most part do not seem to prevent fertilization and zygote formation. In addition to trisomies and structural chromosome aberrations, triploidy due to polyspermy is common. Embryonic chromosome abnormalities are especially common in certain patient populations. In one study of 32 infertile couples (mean age 32.0 ± 3.8 years) with two or more IVF failures, more than 50% of embryos with normal morphology had chromosome abnormalities, thus perhaps explaining the implantation failure and infertility of these couples (Magli et al., 1998). In another study of IVF patients with recurrent spontaneous abortions, 17 of 39 embryos tested for chromosomes 13, 16, 18, 21, 22, X and Y had numerical chromosome abnormalities (Vidal et al., 1997).

Chromosome Abnormalities in Clinically Recognized Sporadic Pregnancy Losses

Among pregnancies that survive the preclinical period, 12% to 15% end as first trimester spontaneous abortions, with a decreasing incidence per week as gestation continues. Embryonic death usually precedes spontaneous loss by several weeks, and ultrasound studies show a high continuation rate (i.e., 96.7% continue to 16 weeks) when an intact pregnancy with fetal heart beat is seen prior to 10 weeks gestation (Christians and Stoutenbeek, 1984). The general mechanism of spontaneous abortion may be abnormal fetal–maternal villus circulation, leading to declining hormonal production by villus tissue and decidual necrosis. Increased cell death (apoptosis) and decreased cell proliferation in muscularized blood vessels have been found in chromosomally abnormal placentas (Qumsiyeh et al., 1998), suggesting that trophoblast failure rather than embryonic death itself may be the impetus to uterine irritability, contraction, and subsequent pregnancy failure (Rushton, 1981). This hypothesis is consistent with studies of confined placental mosaicism (CPM). CPM is the presence of a cytogenetically abnormal cell line in the placenta but not in the fetus. CPM usually arises from a trisomic conceptus that loses one of the trisomic chromosomes in an early cell division, leading to trisomic/diploid mosaicism. The inner cell mass, which develops into the embryo, may by chance or by selection include only diploid cells. CPM has been associated with spontaneous abortion (Johnson et al., 1990; Wapner et al., 1992), but not all studies have confirmed this finding (Roland et al., 1994; Wolstenholme et al., 1994).

Numerical and Structural Abnormalities

Studies of first trimester pregnancy losses demonstrate cytogenetic abnormalities in approximately 50%, with a frequency of 66% in spontaneous abortions of less than 8 weeks developmental age. In contrast, the rate of chromosome abnormalities in induced abortuses is 4.7% in the seventh and eighth weeks of gestation (Burgoyne et al., 1991) and 3.2% at 5 to 15 weeks gestation (Kajii et al., 1978). Loss rates also increase with maternal age, with rates at 35 to 39 years almost twice those at 30 to 34 years (Wilson et al., 1984; Hoesli et al., 2001). Both chromosomally normal and chromosomally abnormal pregnancy losses increase with maternal age (Fig. 27–3), although not all chromosomes show the same degree of maternal age effect. Mean maternal age is most significantly correlated with trisomies 15, 16, 18, 20, 21, and 22 and X polysomies (Hassold et al., 1984). Most autosomal trisomies and X polysomies are maternal in origin (over 75% due to maternal meiosis I non-disjunction), but 45,X, 47,XYY, triploidy, and most de novo structural abnormalities primarily occur as male gametic errors; reduced (or absent) meiotic recombination between homologous chromosomes has been associated with non-disjunction in both male and female gametes (Hassold et al., 1993).

The most common findings in chromosomally abnormal first trimester abortuses are autosomal trisomies (53%), monosomy X (19%), and polyploidy (22%); additional sex chromosomes (0.4%), monosomy (0.2%), and structural rearrangements (3.3%) are infrequent (Warburton et al., 1991). The most common autosomal trisomy in first trimester abortuses is trisomy 16, a chromosome constitution virtually never seen in liveborns. Therefore, for the most part, the chromosome abnormalities found in first trimester losses are so deleterious that they prevent embryonic development and pregnancy advancement beyond the earliest stages.

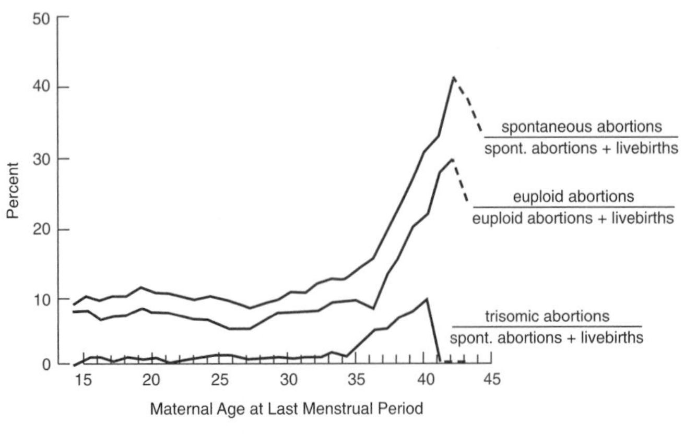

Fig. 27–3. Estimated rates of spontaneous abortion, euploid abortion, and trisomic abortion by maternal age. From Stein et al. (1980) with permission.

Table 27–3. Regression-Smoothed Rates of Chromosome Abnormality at Different Gestational Ages

Maternal Age	CVS	Amniocentesis	Live Births
35	1/109	1/140	1/212
36	1/83	1/111	1/169
37	1/64	1/88	1/131
38	1/48	1/70	1/103
39	1/37	1/56	1/81
40	1/28	1/44	1/64
41	1/21	1/35	1/50
42	1/16	1/28	1/39
43	1/12	1/22	1/31
44	1/9	1/18	1/24
45	1/7	1/14	1/19

Source: Modified from Hook et al. (1983) with permission.

In the second trimester of pregnancy, losses are less common (2%) and the proportion due to chromosome abnormality decreases to 10% to 40% (Ruzicska and Czeizel, 1970; Warburton et al., 1986; Craver and Kalousek, 1987). Only 5% to 10% of fetuses lost at more than 20 weeks gestation have chromosome abnormalities (Bauld et al., 1974; Machin and Crolla, 1974; Warburton et al., 1986). Among second trimester losses and perinatal deaths, trisomies 13, 18, and 21, monosomy X, and sex chromosome polysomies predominate (Warburton et al., 1991). Therefore, as pregnancy progresses, chromosome abnormalities in fetal losses become more similar to those found in liveborns. Further evidence that chromosomally abnormal conceptuses are disproportionately lost early in pregnancy is the difference in the rate of chromosome abnormalities found in prenatal diagnosis specimens obtained at 9 to 11 weeks, at 16 to 18 weeks, and at livebirth (Hook et al., 1983) (Table 27–3).

Uniparental Disomy

Uniparental disomy (UPD) is the inheritance of both homologous chromosomes of a pair from the same parent. Androgenesis, the presence of two paternal haploid chromosomes sets and no maternal chromosomes, results in hydatidiform mole in at least some cases. Gynogenesis is the combination of two maternally derived pronuclei and no paternal pronucleus. The discovery of each of these abnormalities in human or mice embryos has suggested that some pregnancy losses may be due to inheritance of all 46 embryonic chromosomes, or one homologous pair, from one parent (Henderson et al., 1991). However, in two studies that examined a total of 89 early losses, both maternal and paternal genomic contributions were found in all cases, excluding androgenesis or gynogenesis as a cause of the losses (Henderson et al., 1991; Hsu et al., 1994). UPD for a single chromosome could not be excluded in these studies, but only two cases of UPD (of chromosome 21) in embryonic abortuses have been reported (Henderson et al., 1994).

Recurrent Spontaneous Abortion

Although sporadic pregnancy loss is common, recurrent spontaneous abortion (RSA; ≥3 consecutive spontaneous abortions) occurs in only $^{1}/_{2}$% to 1% of pregnant women (Stray-Pederson and Stray-Pederson, 1984; Alberman, 1988). RSA can be further categorized into primary RSA (when a couple has no liveborn children) and secondary RSA (when couples with three or more losses also have one or more liveborn children). In the majority of couples with RSA, genetic, endocrinologic, anatomic, autoimmunologic, or infectious causes for the pregnancy losses cannot be identified (Tho et al., 1979; Harger et al., 1983; Hill et al., 1992), suggesting that in some of these couples the losses may not have been due to a fixed systemic factor. Thus, it is not surprising that in couples with idiopathic RSA, the likelihood of a successful pregnancy after three or more spontaneous abortions can be as high as 65% (Ober et al., 1995b).

Inherited Thrombophilias

Recently, mutations in two coagulation factor genes, factor V and prothrombin, have been implicated in recurrent pregnancy loss, particularly in losses that occur after 20 weeks gestation (Martinelli et al., 2000; Seligsohn and Lubetsky, 2001). The precise role of these common mutations in early pregnancy losses, as well as mutations in other genes in coagulation pathways (deficiencies of antithrombin, protein C or protein S, methylenetetrahydrofolate reductase gene mutation), remains to be elucidated.

Sporadic vs. Recurrent Aneuploidy

Because cytogenetic abnormalities are found in more than half of sporadic miscarriages, and the frequency of aneuploid conceptuses increases with maternal age, it is not surprising that couples with idiopathic RSA may have one or more chromosomally abnormal abortuses. However, it is still not known if there is a subgroup of couples with genetically controlled recurrent nondisjunction as a cause of their RSA, or whether the occurrence of aneuploid fetuses among couples with recurrent miscarriage is sporadic and a function of maternal age. A large study by Boue et al. (1975) suggests that genetically controlled recurrent aneuploidy is not likely to be a common cause of RSA and that the occurrence of more than one chromosomally abnormal abortuses among couples with recurrent miscarriage is likely due to chance factors. In their study, the frequency of recurring abortion was 16.5% among 286 women with a karyotyped abnormal abortus and 23.0% among 134 women with a karyotyped normal abortus. This relationship was consistent across maternal age groups and prior reproductive histories. Furthermore, couples with a chromosomally abnormal abortus do not appear to be at increased risk for a subsequent chromosomally abnormal abortus after maternal age is taken into account (Warburton et al., 1987). Therefore, a genetic predisposition to recurrent aneuploidy remains only a theoretical possibility and a potential (infrequent) cause of RSA.

Structural Chromosome Abnormalities

On the other hand, *structural* chromosome abnormalities are not infrequently associated with RSA. In 2% to 5% of couples with recurrent pregnancy losses, one of the partners will have a balanced chromosome rearrangement—a translocation. Females are more likely to carry a translocation than are males, and reciprocal translocations are slightly more common than Robertsonian translocations. Although balanced in the parent, a chromosome rearrangement may result in unbalanced gametes with duplications or deficiencies of genetic material. If a conception results from such a gamete, the embryo will be chromosomally unbalanced. These embryos are more likely to spontaneously abort than are embryos with normal chromosomes.

X Chromosome Abnormalities

Other cytogenetic mechanisms that have been implicated in RSA involve the sex chromosomes. A low frequency of 45,X cells (or 45X/46,XX) has been reported in a number of studies of women with RSA. However, the association between the presence of 45,X cells in women and RSA is equivocal because 45,X cells are frequently found with advancing maternal age. Therefore, unless the proportion of such cells is substantial (>10%), this finding is unlikely to be of significance. Skewed X-inactivation has also been associated with RSA. For example, Lanasa et al. (1999) showed that 7 of 48 (14.6%) women with unexplained RSA had skewed X-inactivation, compared with only 1.5% of 67 control females. In this study, skewed X-inactivation was defined as preferential activation of the same X chromosome in 90% or more of peripheral leukocytes. The same group had previously reported a family ascertained through a female with Duchenne muscular dystrophy in which the trait for skewed X-inactivation was maternally inherited. Among women carrying this trait, there was a statistically significant increase in spontaneous abortions. This trait co-segregated with a locus on Xq28 (Z_{max} = 6.92), suggesting the presence of a specific locus for RSA on the X chromosome (Pegoraro et al., 1997).

It is tempting to speculate that both skewed X-inactivation and 45,X/46,XX mosaicism could contribute to a common mechanism in women experiencing RSA. For example, the expression of both alleles at a locus on Xq28 may be necessary for maintenance of pregnancy. Pregnancy failure may result if there is not balanced expression of both alleles, either through skewed X-inactivation or the preferential loss of an X chromosome.

Recently, another explanation for pregnancy failure secondary to skewed X-inactivation has been advanced. Sangha et al. (1999) also have found skewed X-inactivation in 18% (14 of 76) of patients with RSA and only 5% (6 of 111) of controls. These authors suggest that skewed X-inactivation may result from selection against trisomic cells in a mosaic trisomic embryo. The embryo subsequently develops into a woman who retains trisomic cells in her gonadal (germline) tissue. She is then likely to produce trisomic conceptuses herself and have RSA. The skewed X-inactivation in this scenario is not the etiology of the losses but merely a marker for the mosaic aneuploidy in the woman.

Genetic Counseling in Couples with RSA

Cytogenetic studies in both partners should be performed in couples with three spontaneous abortions, couples with a combination of spontaneous abortions and abnormal liveborn children, and couples with two spontaneous abortions and a family history of spontaneous abortions or abnormal liveborn children. Individuals with balanced structural rearrangements are at increased risk for both recurrent abortions and abnormal liveborns. Counseling for parents with balanced rearrangements should be specific for their rearrangement if empiric data exist. If other family members are known to have the balanced rearrangement, the extended family history of spontaneous abortions, abnormal liveborns, and normal liveborns is relevant to the estimation of risk for pregnancy loss or abnormal liveborns. Chromosome diagnosis should be offered to appropriate relatives of an individual with a structural rearrangement to avoid the tragedy of another member of the family having an infant with unbalanced chromosomes. Most balanced chromosome rearrangements do not preclude the birth of normal children, but may result in multiple losses with unbalanced chromosomes. A few rare translocations (eg., t21q;21q) will result in only losses or abnormal liveborns.

Recommendations for cytogenetic studies in tissues from aborted fetuses are less straightforward. Among couples with unexplained RSA there is still a fairly high likelihood (>30%) that an aborted fetus is aneuploid. Although determining that an abortus is chromosomally abnormal will usually not reveal the cause for prior miscarriages (unless a familial structural rearrangement is found), it will offer an explanation for that particular miscarriage. This information is often psychologically comforting to couples with RSA. Furthermore, knowing that a particular abortus is abnormal may allow the couple to refrain from empirical treatments devised for couples with nongenetic pregnancy loss.

Women with more than one pregnancy loss, particularly at 20 or more weeks of gestation, should be offered testing for the factor V Leiden mutation (American College of Medical Genetics, 2000). If the results are positive, testing for the prothrombin 20210A mutation should be considered, as well as measurement of plasma homocysteine levels to detect homozygotes for mutations in the methylenetetrahydrofolate reductase (MTFHR) gene, which result in high homocysteine levels. Testing for other thrombophilias should depend on the family history, such as presence of venous thrombosis.

IMMUNOGENETIC CAUSES OF INFERTILITY AND FETAL LOSS

The survival of allografts in mammals is influenced by genes of the major histocompatibility complex (MHC). Humans rapidly reject foreign tissues that have human leukocyte antigens (HLA) different from their own (van Rood and Claas, 1990; Ratner et al., 1991). A notable exception is fetal tissue. Maternal tolerance of the allogeneic fetus remains a paradox and is the subject of continuing investigation in immunogenetics and reproductive immunology (Ober, 1998). At the center of this research are the HLA genes and the role that these genes play in normal and abnormal pregnancy.

Three key observations made over the years provide a framework for evaluating the role of HLA in pregnancy. First, the classical HLA genes (*HLA-A*, *HLA-B*, *HLA-DR*, *HLA-DQ*) that are responsible for the rapid rejection of allografts in humans are *not* expressed in tissues at the maternal–fetal interface (Sunderland et al., 1981b; Faulk et al., 1982; Johnson and Stern, 1986). Instead, a nonclassical gene, *HLA-G* (Geraghty et al., 1987), is primarily expressed in these tissues (Sunderland et al., 1981a; Ellis et al., 1990; Kovats et al., 1990; Yelavarthi et al., 1991; Chumbley et al., 1994). Although *HLA-G* has very limited polymorphisms (reviewed in Ober and Aldrich, 1997), variation in this gene has been associated with recurrent miscarriage (Aldrich et al., 2001; Pfeiffer et al., 2001), as discussed below. Another nonclassical gene with very low levels of polymorphism, *HLA-E*, is expressed in all tissues that express other class I HLA genes (including *HLA-G*) (Braud et al., 1997; Lee et al., 1998). Lastly, the classical gene, *HLA-C*, is transiently expressed in tissues at the maternal–fetal interface (King et al., 1996). *HLA-C* also shows reduced polymorphism relative to other classical HLA, and variation in *HLA-C* has not been associated with adverse reproductive outcomes. Therefore, the absence of expression of the highly polymorphic HLA loci at the maternal–fetal interface may facilitate maternal tolerance of the fetal allograft (Hunt and Orr, 1992; Le Bouteiller, 1994; Loke et al., 1994; Ober and Aldrich, 1997; Hunt et al., 2000).

The second important observation is that 20% of primigravidae and 40% of multigravidae women have detectable levels of antibodies directed against paternally derived HLA that have been inherited by the fetus (Payne and Rolfs, 1958; van Rood et al., 1958). Despite the fact that the classical HLA are not expressed at the maternal–fetal interface, these antibodies are directed against the polymorphic epitopes of the classical HLA loci. Presumably, sensitization occurs when fetal nucleated cells enter the maternal circulation, either during pregnancy or at parturition. Regardless of their origin, the presence of anti-HLA antibodies in 20% to 40% of healthy pregnancies indicates that the maternal immune system does recognize fetal HLA and that sensitization to paternal HLA during pregnancy is not harmful. In fact, it has been suggested that these antibodies may be beneficial (Beer and Billingham, 1976).

The third set of observations suggests that maternal–fetal *in*compatibility with respect to MHC antigens may be advantageous in mammalian pregnancy. That is, only fetuses with MHC genes that differ from maternal MHC genes (i.e., histo*in*compatible fetuses) can elicit the production of maternal antibodies against paternal MHC or other alloimmune responses that may be beneficial in pregnancy. Empiric evidence that maternal–fetal histo*in*compatibility may be beneficial came first from animal studies. For example, placental sizes were larger and implantation rates higher in histo*in*compatible murine pregnancies than in histocompatible murine pregnancies (Billington, 1964; James, 1965; Kirby, 1970). If human fetuses with paternally derived HLA that are identical to maternal HLA (i.e., histocompatible fetuses) are at a selective disadvantage during pregnancy, then couples who match for some HLA should have poorer reproductive outcomes than couples who do not match for any HLA, because some of the fetuses of couples who match for HLA will be histocompatible with the mother. Although this hypothesis was proposed over 20 years ago (see, for example, Beer and Billingham, 1976, and Kirby, 1970), the role of HLA matching in pregnancy failure and success remains controversial. However, because the relationship between HLA and pregnancy outcome has potential diagnostic and therapeutic implications, the remainder of this chapter will focus on this topic.

HLA-G

HLA-G Is a Unique HLA Gene

The fetal cells that come into direct contact with maternal tissues in the pregnant uterus uniquely express a nonclassical, class I HLA protein, called HLA-G. Although another nonclassical HLA protein, HLA-E, and the classical HLA-C are also expressed in these tissues, expression of the highly polymorphic HLA class I (HLA-A and HLA-B) and class II (HLA-DR, -DQ, and -DP) proteins are suppressed in these tissues. Further, whereas HLA-E and HLA-C are ubiquitously expressed in all nucleated cells, HLA-G protein expression is restricted to fetal tissues, with the highest expression in the extravillous cytotrophoblast, the placental cells that invade deeply into the maternal deciduas (Hunt et al., 2000).

HLA-G and Recurrent Miscarriage

Although many studies have described HLA-G allele frequencies in worldwide population samples (reviewed in Ober and Aldrich, 1997), surprisingly few studies have examined the relationship between polymorphisms in HLA-G and miscarriage. Three small studies, each in fewer than 40 couples with recurrent miscarriage, examined a subset of HLA-G polymorphisms that did not include the HLA-G*0104 and *0105N alleles (Karhukorpi et al., 1997; Penzes et al., 1999; Yamashita et al., 1999). None of these small and incomplete studies found an association between the *HLA-G* alleles and recurrent miscarriage. More recently, two studies in larger samples and with complete genotyping reported significant associations between the *HLA-G* genotype and recurrent miscarriage (Aldrich et al., 2001; Pfeiffer et al., 2001). One study of 78 couples with recurrent miscarriage and 52 fertile controls reported an increased frequency of the *01013 and *0105N allele in aborters compared with controls ($p = .007$) (Pfeiffer et al., 2001). Furthermore, they showed that woman carrying either of these "high-risk" alleles were less likely to give birth to a living child in their next pregnancy than women not carrying these alleles ($p = .06$). Curiously, the *01013 allele differs from other *0101 alleles only at silent sites, yet no *0101 allele other than *01013 was associated with increased miscarriage rates. In a previous study these investigators showed low levels of soluble G1 protein in plasma from nonpregnant subjects carrying the *01013 and *0105N alleles (Rebmann et al., 2001). They suggested that this might be due to differences in the transcriptional regulation of these different alleles (Pfeiffer et al., 2001).

A second study (Aldrich et al., 2001) examined the relationship between *HLA-G* genotypes and pregnancy outcome in couples participating in the REMIS study (described below; Ober et al., 1999b). In this study both partners in 113 couples with a history of unexplained recurrent miscarriage were genotyped for 12 HLA-G alleles, including the four major alleles and the *01013 allele. The presence of an HLA-G*0104 or an HLA-G*0105N allele in either parent was significantly associated with an increased risk of miscarriage, after adjusting for maternal age, number of previous miscarriages, presence of a previous liveborn child, and treatment group assignment ($p = .006$, odds ratio = 3.62, 95% CI, 1.45–9.03). There was no association in this study with the *01013 allele as in the Pfeiffer study described above, but both studies reported an association with the null, *0105N allele. Because both the *0104 and *0105N polymorphisms are present in exon 3 and therefore affect only the full-length HLA-G1 isoforms, but not the shorter HLA-G2 isoforms, the investigators interpreted these results as evidence for a critical role of the G1 isoform in maintaining pregnancy. The mechanism is still unknown, but it could mediate effects in pregnancy through one of the many ascribed functions of HLA-G, including antigen presentation (Lee et al., 1995), inhibition of T-cell proliferation (Kapasi et al., 2000; Le Gal et al., 1999), interactions with natural killer cells (Colonna et al., 1998), or other as yet unknown mechanisms.

In summary, although the many roles of HLA-G during pregnancy are not fully elucidated, the studies discussed above suggest that it plays an important role in establishing and maintaining pregnancy, and that certain *HLA-G* alleles are associated with miscarriage. The HLA-G*0105N allele, which is a null allele for the full-length HLA-G1 isoforms, was associated with increased risk for miscarriage in two independent studies (Aldrich et al., 2001; Pfeiffer et al., 2001), indicating that low levels of the G1 protein is a risk factor for miscarriage. Other alleles, such as the HLA-G*01013 and HLA-G*0104 alleles, may also be associated with miscarriage in different population samples, but these associations need to be confirmed in additional studies. At the present time, HLA-G genotyping in couples with recurrent miscarriage is not recommended because this information would not provide any useful information regarding management. In particular, the presence of high-risk alleles was unrelated to the efficacy of treatment with paternal mononuclear cell immunization (Aldrich et al., 2001). Therefore, the *HLA-G* genotype of couples with a history of recurrent miscarriage would not identify a subgroup of patients who would benefit from this treatment.

HLA Matching and Pregnancy Failure

HLA Matching and Unexplained Infertility

Some couples with unexplained infertility may be experiencing recurrent loss of blastocysts during the peri-implantation period. If histo*in*compatible embryos are more likely to implant successfully compared with histocompatible embryos, then HLA matching could account for infertility in some couples. A small number of studies have tested this hypothesis by HLA typing couples with unexplained infertility.

Three early studies did not reveal increased matching of HLA-A, HLA-B, or HLA-DR locus antigens in couples with unexplained infertility compared either to fertile controls (Nordlander et al., 1983; Persitz et al., 1985) or to theoretically derived expectations of matching (Jeannet et al., 1985); however, the sample sizes in these studies were small ($N = 14$, 18, and 16, respectively). By contrast, one larger study of 79 unexplained infertility subjects reported that couples with primary infertility ($N = 48$) but not secondary infertility ($N = 31$) were less likely to produce HLA-DQ heterozygous offspring (i.e., they shared more HLA-DQ antigens) than were fertile controls ($p = .014$) (Coulam et al., 1987). Differences with respect to matching antigens at the HLA-A, HLA-B, or HLA-DR loci were not observed in primary or secondary unexplained infertility couples (Coulam et al., 1987).

Other studies of HLA matching in unexplained infertility focused on infertile couples who failed to achieve a successful pregnancy with assisted reproductive technology (ART). Because failure to achieve a clinical pregnancy following ART would result from implantation failure, these subjects may be less heterogeneous than all couples with unexplained infertility. Weckstein and colleagues (1991) first reported increased HLA matching among couples with a failure after ART compared with couples with a subsequent success ($p < .01$). Balasch and colleagues (1993) reported similar results. In the Balasch study, the frequency of HLA matching was higher in the ART failures than in the infertile controls ($p < .005$) and the fertile control group ($p = .01$). A third, larger study of couples with unexplained infertility showed significantly more HLA matching among the women who failed to become pregnant after ART than among women with successful pregnancies: 44.4% of couples with failures and 21.5% of successful couples shared three antigens ($p = .015$; comparison between couples with failures and fertile controls, $p = .021$; comparison between successful couples and normal fertile controls, $p = .44$) (Ho et al., 1994). Further, among the individual loci, there was an excess of matching at the HLA-DQ locus among the couples with failures, but this difference was not statistically significant after adjusting for multiple comparisons (empiric $p = .001$) (Jin et al., 1995).

These studies (Weckstein et al., 1991; Balasch et al., 1993; Ho et al., 1994) suggest that a subgroup of couples presenting as "infertile" may in fact be experiencing recurrent implantation failures. Increased HLA matching among couples who fail ART further suggests that *in*compatibility for HLA genes may enhance the likelihood of implantation, supporting the hypothesis suggested by Kirby in 1970.

HLA Matching and Recurrent Miscarriage

The first two studies to examine HLA matching in couples with recurrent miscarriage reported significantly increased matching among aborters compared with control couples (Komlos et al., 1977; Schacter et al., 1979). At least 30 additional studies of

HLA matching in recurrent miscarriage have been reported (Reviewed in Ober and van der Ven, 1998), with about half showing increased matching of HLA in couples with recurrent miscarriage. However, even among studies reporting an association, there is little agreement with regard to the MHC gene or region associated with spontaneous abortion. For example, some investigators reported associations between recurrent miscarriage and matching antigens at the class I loci, HLA-A or HLA-B; others reported associations with matching antigens at the class II loci, HLA-DR or HLA-DQ; and yet others reported increased matching over all loci.

These conflicting data may be due to chance findings in small samples, differences between centers with regard to tissue typing methodology, the numbers of antigens identified by the laboratory or present in the particular population, the choice and number of control couples, and the selection and stratification of couples with recurrent abortion. However, even considering these factors, discrepancies between studies are difficult to explain, and the role of HLA matching in recurrent miscarriage remains controversial. Nonetheless, it is clear that HLA matching neither predicts pregnancy outcome nor identifies a subgroup of couples that would benefit from specific treatments (Cowchock et al., 1990; Cowchock and Smith, 1992; Mowbray et al., 1983; Smith and Cowchock, 1988; Christiansen et al., 1994). Therefore, HLA typing should not be included as part of the clinical evaluation of couples with recurrent miscarriage.

HLA Matching and Sporadic Miscarriage

To elucidate the reproductive effects of HLA matching, Ober and colleagues have been conducting prospective, population-based studies in the Hutterites for over 15 years (Ober et al., 1983, 1985, 1988, 1992, 1998b, 1997, 1999c; Robertson et al., 1999; Weitkamp and Ober, 1998). This population is very appropriate for such studies for the following reasons. First, the Hutterites are descendants of fewer than 90 founders (Martin, 1970). This results in a limited repertoire of HLA haplotypes in the population (Weitkamp and Ober, 1999) and the increased likelihood of marrying someone with the same haplotype that was inherited identical-by-descent from a common ancestor (Ober et al., 1997). As a result, many Hutterite couples will match for all or part of an HLA haplotype. Second, the Hutterites are among the most fertile human populations. For example, only 2% of Hutterite couples are childless (Sheps, 1965) and the median completed sibship size was 10 among married women born between 1901 and 1940, during which time contraceptive use was rare (Mange, 1964; Ober et al., 1999a). Third, the Hutterites practice a communal lifestyle. As a result, environmental and social factors that either influence fertility or attitudes toward pregnancy are relatively uniform across the population.

These studies have consistently shown decreased fertility among Hutterite couples matching for HLA compared with Hutterite couples not matching for HLA. These differences have been observed with respect to interbirth intervals (Ober et al., 1983, 1988), the length of the interval to a positive pregnancy test (Ober et al., 1992), and clinically recognized sporadic miscarriage rates (Ober et al., 1998b). Of note is that none of the approximately 500 Hutterite couples in these studies would meet the definition for recurrent miscarriage; that is, none have had three *consecutive* miscarriages and all couples with three miscarriages have at least two liveborn children (Ober et al., 1998b).

Results of a 10-year prospective study in Hutterite women were recently reported (Ober et al., 1998b). Women enrolled in this study conducted a home pregnancy test within two days of a missed period. All participants maintained a diary with their

Table 27–4. Fetal Loss Rates by HLA Matching in the Hutterites

	No. of Alleles/Haplotypes Shared		
HLA Locus/Haplotype	0	1	Value
A	0.12 (13/106)	0.17 (25/145)	.537
C	0.12 (19/156)	0.20 (19/95)	.033
B	0.10 (16/157)	0.23 (22/94)	.019
DRB1	0.15 (20/136)	0.16 (18/115)	.649
DQA1	0.14 (14/97)	0.16 (24/154)	.757
DQB1	0.13 (19/145)	0.18 (18/101)	.344
DPB1	0.13 (12/93)	0.16 (26/158)	.444
Haplotype	0.13 (28/221)	0.33 (10/30)	.002

The numbers in parentheses are the number of losses to the number of pregnancies. All p values were adjusted for wife's age, wife's inbreeding coefficient, and multiple pregnancies per couple.
Source: Modified from Ober et al. (1998b) with permission.

menstrual dates, results of pregnancy tests, and pregnancy outcomes after a positive pregnancy test. Information regarding breast feeding, contraceptive use, and other factors that might influence pregnancy rates (such as travel away from spouse) were also recorded in the diaries. Data were obtained for 251 pregnancies in 111 couples. Fetal loss rates by HLA matching are shown in Table 27–4. Loss rates were highest among couples matching for HLA-B antigens (0.23 vs. 0.10, $p = .019$) or for the entire 16-locus haplotype (0.33 vs. 0.13, $p = .002$). At the time of the study, HLA-B typing was determined by serology rather than DNA-based typing, which might have revealed molecular heterogeneity. Thus, it is possible that HLA-B matching per se accounts for the association with the whole haplotype, but molecular typing of HLA-B alleles will have to be performed to test this hypothesis. Furthermore, these data do not exclude the possibility that alleles at an as yet unknown locus linked to HLA-B underlies the observed association. Regardless, these studies demonstrate that matching for HLA-B alleles or alleles at an HLA-B-linked locus, or matching for alleles at all loci on the haplotype, is associated with an increased sporadic fetal loss rate in the Hutterites. These results are similar to results of a study in captive pigtailed macaques that demonstrated significantly increased sporadic fetal loss in pairs matching for class I MHC antigens.

The restricted number of HLA haplotypes in the Hutterites increases both the proportion of couples that match for HLA and the likelihood of matching for alleles at an unknown locus that is in linkage disequilibrium with the matched locus. Therefore, it is much easier to detect the effects of unknown loci in the Hutterites than in outbred couples. This may explain the consistent associations between HLA matching and fertility in the Hutterites and the very discrepant and controversial results in outbred couples with recurrent miscarriage. Additionally, the effects of HLA sharing on miscarriage rates in the Hutterites may not be an important cause of *recurrent* miscarriage, which has been the focus of studies in outbred couples. Consistent with this is the observation that HLA matching is not a significant predictor of pregnancy outcome in outbred couples with recurrent miscarriage (Cowchock et al., 1990; Cowchock and Smith, 1992; Mowbray et al., 1983; Smith and Cowchock, 1988; Christiansen et al., 1994).

Immunotherapy for Recurrent Pregnancy Loss

Based on the premise that maternal–fetal histo*in*compatibility enhances pregnancy outcome, mononuclear cell immunization was suggested as a treatment for recurrent spontaneous abortion (Beer et al., 1981; Taylor and Faulk, 1981). The purpose of immunotherapy is to artificially stimulate "normal" maternal immunologic responses in women who do not, on their own, respond in an immunologically appropriate manner in pregnancy (Beer et al., 1988; Scott et al., 1987). These responses presumably protect the feto-placental unit and promote successful pregnancy. This model is analogous to the reduced rate of rejection after kidney transplantation in patients who have previously had blood transfusions (Opelz and Terasaki, 1978) and to the decreased murine fetal resorption rates after immunization with allogeneic cells (Bobe et al., 1987; Chaouat et al., 1987).

Four approaches to immunotherapy in couples with RSA have been used: (1) intravenous transfusion with individual or pooled third-party (non-husband) leukocytes (Taylor and Faulk, 1981; Unander and Lindholm, 1986; Christiansen et al., 1994); (2) intravenous transfusion, intradermal injection, and/or subcutaneous injections of husbands' mononuclear cells (Beer et al., 1981; Mowbray et al., 1983; Smith and Cowchock, 1988; Carp et al., 1990; Cauchi et al., 1991; Ho and Gill, 1991; Gatenby et al., 1993); (3) intravenous transfusion with pooled trophoblast membrane extracts (Johnson et al., 1991); and (4) immunization with pooled seminal plasma vaginal suppositories (Stern and Coulam, 1992). Because of the potential risks associated with exposure to unrelated (non-husband) donor cells and fluids, immunization with husbands' mononuclear cells is now the most common immunotherapy protocol used in couples with RSA.

Several small trials were conducted evaluating the efficacy of immunotherapy using husbands' cells. In the first randomized, controlled trial, Mowbray and colleagues (1985) reported significantly better outcomes in women immunized with husband's compared to wife's (placebo) cells. Among 53 couples who became pregnant, 77% of women immunized with husbands' cells had a successful outcome (defined as pregnancy at ≥28 weeks of gestation) compared with 37% of women immunized with their own cells (placebo) (p = .01). In a second (non-blinded) study of 99 women with RSA, success rates were higher among immunized women than among women immunized with autologous cells (controls), but the differences did not reach statistical significance (p = .680) (Ho and Gill, 1991). A third (blinded) study of 46 women with RSA reported higher success rates in women treated with saline (control) than among women immunized with husbands' cells (p = .30) (Cauchi et al., 1991).

Several meta-analyses of the results of randomized controlled trials have been presented (Fraser et al., 1993; Recurrent Miscarriage Immunotherapy Trialist Group, 1994; Jeng et al., 1995). In one analysis of both published and unpublished results (Recurrent Miscarriage Immunotherapy Trialist Group, 1994), a small but statistically significant effect in favor of leukocyte immunotherapy was found. Results were reported on a relative risk scale—that is, as the ratio of live birth rates in treated and control groups. In that paper, two analysis teams worked independently and arrived at estimated ratios of 1.16 (95% CI, 1.01–1.34) and 1.21 (95%, CI 1.04–1.37), respectively. In a more recent meta-analysis including updated data from these trials (Jeng et al., 1995), the effect of immunotherapy did not reach statistical significance (livebirth rate ratio of 1.12; 95% CI, 0.97–1.31). Taken together, the published trials and meta-analyses of published and unpublished studies yielded conflicting results, indicating the need for large randomized trials (Jeng et al., 1995).

An NICHD-funded multicenter, randomized trial evaluating the efficacy of immunotherapy for preventing recurrent miscarriage has recently been completed (Ober et al., 1999b). Following an immunization protocol nearly identical to Mowbray's (Mowbray et al., 1985), 179 women were randomized into a treatment (husband's cells) or control (saline) group. All women were followed for one year after immunization, and couples not achieving pregnancy within 6 months were reimmunized with the same treatment they received initially. Success was defined as a pregnancy that continued to 28 or more weeks of gestation. In the intent-to-treat analysis of all randomized subjects, failures included (1) women who failed to become pregnant within 12 months of randomization, and (2) women who experienced a pregnancy loss before 28 weeks of gestation. A secondary analysis was performed, including only women who became pregnant within 12 months of randomization, with failure defined as a pregnancy loss before 28 weeks of gestation. A subgroup analysis limited to women with no previous livebirths (primary aborters) was also performed.

After the last subject was enrolled, an independent data monitoring and safety board recommended that no further immunizations be given because the miscarriage rate was higher in the treatment group than in the control group (Ober et al., 1999b). In the intent-to-treat analysis, the success rates were 36% (31 of 86) in the treatment group and 48% (41 of 85) in the control group (odds ratio 0.54; 95% CI, 0.28–1.02; p = .056). In the analysis of pregnant subjects only, the success rates were 46% (31 of 68) in the treatment group and 65% (41 of 63) in the control group (odds ratio 0.40; 95% CI, 0.19–0.84; p = .015). The results were nearly identical in the analysis of primary aborters, with a statistically significant increase in loss rates in the women in the treatment group who achieved pregnancy (success rates 39% vs. 63%; odds ratio 0.37; 95% CI, 0.16–0.86; p = .021). When the data from this trial were added to the data from the previous meta-analyses (discussed above), the estimated livebirth ratio was 1.04 (95% CI, 0.97–1.20), indicating that immunotherapy does not improve the livebirth rate (Ober et al., 1999b). Based on these results, the authors recommended that immunotherapy with the husband's mononuclear cells not be used as a treatment for recurrent miscarriage.

SUMMARY

In sum, both infertility and early pregnancy loss are common human conditions. Manifestations of these conditions can include a normal adult phenotype with reproductive failure, anomalous embryonic development, or recurrent loss of apparently normal concepti. Genetic abnormalities, both single-gene disruptions and numerical and structural chromosome disorders, account for a large proportion of these conditions. Each family with reproductive failure deserves a thorough and thoughtful evaluation. Accurate estimates of recurrence risk and likelihood of successful reproduction, as well as plans for appropriate intervention, will follow the evaluation.

REFERENCES

Affara N, Bishop C, Brown W, Cooke H, Davey P, Ellis N, Graves JM, Jones M, Mitchell M, Rappold G, et al.: Report of the Second International Workshop on Y Chromosome Mapping 1995. Cytogenet Cell Genet 1996; 73:33–76.

Aiman J, Griffin JE, Gazak JM, Wilson JD, MacDonald PC: Androgen insensitivity as a cause of infertility in otherwise normal men. N Engl J Med 1979; 300:223–227.

Alberman E: The epidemiology of repeated abortions. In: Beard RW, Sharp F (eds). Early Pregnancy Loss: Mechanisms of Treatment. London: Springer-Verlag, 1988:9–17.

Aldrich CL, Stephenson MD, Karrison T, Odem RR, Branch DW, Scott JR, Schreiber JR, Ober C: *HLA-G* genotypes and pregnancy outcome in couples with unexplained recurrent miscarriage. Mol Hum Reprod 2001; 7:1167–1172.

American College of Medical Genetics: Consensus Statement on Factor V Leiden Mutation Testing, October 31, 2000. Genet in Med 2001; 3:139–148.

Balasch J, Inmaculada J, Martorell J, Gayá A, Vanrell JA: Histocompatibility in in vitro fertilization couples. Fertil Steril 1993; 59:456–458.

Bauld R, Sutherland GR, Bain AD: Chromosome studies in investigation of stillbirths and neonatal deaths. Arch Dis Child 1974; 49:782–788.

Beer AE, Billingham RE: The Immunobiology of Reproduction. Upper Saddle River, NJ: Prentice Hall, 1976.

Beer AE, Quebbeman JF, Ayers JWT, Haines RF: Major histocompatibility complex antigens, maternal and paternal immune responses, and chronic habitual abortions in humans. Am J Obstet Gynecol 1981; 141:987–997.

Beer AE, Quebbeman JF, Zhu X: Nonpaternal leukocyte immunization in women previously immunized with paternal leukocytes: immune responses and subsequent pregnancy outcome. In: Clark DA, Croy BA (eds). Reproductive Immunology. New York: Elsevier Science Publishers, 1988:261–268.

Billington WD: Influence of immunologic dissimilarity of mother and foetus on size of placenta in mice. Nature 1964; 202:317–318.

Bobe P, Stanislawski M, Kiger N: Immunogenetic studies of spontaneous abortion in mice. In: Gill TJ, Wegmann TG (eds). Immunoregulation and Fetal Survival. New York: Oxford University Press, 1987:252–262.

Boue J, Boue A, Lazar P: Retrospective and prospective epidemiological studies of 1500 karyotyped spontaneous abortions. Teratology 1975; 12:11–26.

Bourrouillou G, Colombies P, Dastugue N: Chromosome studies in 2136 couples with spontaneous abortions. Hum Genet 1987; 74:399–401.

Brandell RA, Mielnik A, Liotta D, Ye Z, Veeck LL, Palermo GD, Schlegel PN: AZFb deletions predict the absence of spermatozoa with testicular sperm extraction: preliminary report of a prognostic genetic test. Hum Reprod 1998; 13:2812–2815.

Braud V, Jones Y, McMichael A: The human major histocompatibility complex class Ib molecule binds signal sequence-derived peptides with primary anchor residues at positions 2 and 9. Eur J Immunol 1997; 27:1164–1169.

Brown TR: Human androgen insensitivity syndrome. J Androl 1995; 16:299–303.

Burgoyne PS, Holland K, Stephens R: Incidence of numerical chromosome anomalies in human pregnancy estimation from induced and spontaneous abortion data. Hum Reprod 1991; 6:555–565.

Carp HJ, Toder V, Gazit E: Immunization by paternal leukocytes for prevention of primary habitual abortion: results of a matched control trial. Gynecol Obstet Invest 1990; 29:16–21.

Casals T, Bassas L, Ruiz-Romero J, Chillon M, Gimenez J, Ramos MD, Tapia G, Narvaez H, Nunes V, Estivill X: Extensive analysis of 40 infertile patients with congenital absence of the vas deferens: in 50% of cases only one CFTR allele could be detected. Hum Genet 1995; 95:205–211.

Cauchi MN, Lim D, Kloss YM, Pepperell RJ: Treatment of recurrent aborters by immunization with paternal cells: controlled trial. Am J Reprod Immunol 1991; 25:16–17.

Chandley AC, Cooke HJ: Human male fertility: Y-linked genes and spermatogenesis. Hum Mol Genet 1994; 3:1449–1452.

Chaouat G, Kolb J-P, Chaffaux S, Riviere M, Lankar D, Athanassakis I, Green D, Wegmann TG: The placenta and survival of the fetal allograft. In: Gill TJ, Wegmann TG (eds). Immunoregulation and Fetal Survival. New York: Oxford University Press, 1987:239–251.

Chillon M, Casals T, Mercier B, Bassas L, Lissens W, Silber S, Romey M-C, Ruiz-Romero J, Verlingue C, Claustres M, et al.: Mutations in the cystic fibrosis gene in patients with congenital absence of the vas deferens. N Engl J Med 1995; 332:1475–1480.

Christians GCML, Stoutenbeek P: Spontaneous abortion in proven intact pregnancies. Lancet 1984; 2:571–572.

Christiansen OB, Mathiesen O, Husth M, Lauritsen JG, Grunnet N: Placebo-controlled trial of active immunization with third party leukocytes in recurrent miscarriage. Acta Obstet Gynecol Scand 1994; 73:261–268.

Chumbley G, King A, Gardner L, Lowlett S, Holmes N, Loke YW: Generation of an antibody to HLA-G in transgenic mice and demonstration of the tissue reactivity of this antibody. J Reprod Immunol 1994; 27:173–186.

Colonna M, Samaridis J, Cella M, Angman L, Allen RL, O'Callaghan CA, Dunbar R, Ogg GS, Cerundolo V, Rolink A: Human myelomonocytic cells express an inhibitory receptor for classical and nonclassical MHC class I molecules. J Immunol 1998; 160:3096–3100.

Costes B, Girodon E, Ghanem N, Flori E, Jardin A, Soufir JC, Goossens M: Frequent occurrence of the CFTR intron 8 $(TG)_n$ 5T allele in men with congenital bilateral absence of the vas deferens. Eur J Hum Genet 1995; 3:285–293.

Coulam CB, Moore SB, O'Fallon WM: Association between major histocompatibility antigen and reproductive performance. Am J Reprod Immunol Microb 1987; 14:54–58.

Cowchock FS, Smith JB: Predictors for livebirth after unexplained spontaneous abortion: correlations between immunologic test results, obstetric histories, and outcome of next pregnancy without treatment. Am J Obstet Gynecol 1992; 167:1208–1212.

Cowchock FS, Smith JB, David S, Scher J, Batzer F, Corson S: Paternal mononuclear cell immunization therapy for repeated miscarriage: predictive variables for success. Am J Reprod Immunol 1990; 22:12–17.

Cozzi J, Chevret E, Rousseaux S, Pelletier R, Benitz V, Jalbert H, Sele B: Achievement of meiosis in XXY germ cells: study of 543 sperm karyotypes from an XY/XXY mosaic patient. Hum Genet 1994; 93:32–34.

Craver RD, Kalousek DK: Cytogenetic abnormalities among spontaneously aborted previable fetuses. Am J Med Genet Suppl 1987; 3:113–119.

Culard JF, Desgeorges M, Costa P, Laussel M, Razakatzara G, Navratil H, Demaille J, Claustres M: Analysis of the whole CFTR coding regions and splice junctions in azoospermic men with congenital bilateral aplasia of epididymis or vas deferens. Hum Genet 1994; 93:467–470.

Dubin L, Amelar RD: Etiologic factors in 1294 consecutive cases of male infertility. Fertil Steril 1971; 22:469–474.

Dumur V, Gervais R, Rigot JM, Delomel-Vinner E, Decaestecker B, Lafitte JJ, Roussel P: Congenital bilateral absence of the vas deferens (CBAVD) and cystic fibrosis transmembrane regulator (CFTR): correlation between genotype and phenotype. Hum Genet 1996; 97:7–10.

Eberhart CG, Maines JZ, Wasserman SA: Meiotic cell cycle requirement for a fly homologue of human Deleted in Azoospermia. Nature 1996; 381:783–785.

Elliasson R, Mossberg B, Camner P, Afzelius BA: The immotile-cilia syndrome: a congenital ciliary abnormality as an etiologic factor in chronic airway infections and male sterility. N Engl J Med 1977; 297:1–6.

Elliott DJ, Ma K, Kerr SM, Thakrar R, Speed R, Chandley AC, Cooke H: An RBM homologue maps to the mouse Y chromosome and is expressed in germ cells. Hum Mol Genet 1996; 5:869–874.

Ellis SA, Palmer MS, McMichael AJ: Human trophoblast and the choriocarcinoma cell line BeWo express a truncated HLA class I molecule. J Immunol 1990; 144:731–735.

Evans DB, Crichlow RW: Carcinoma of the male breast and Klinefelter's syndrome: is there an association? CA Cancer J Clin 1987; 37:246–251.

Faulk WP, Hsi BL, McIntyre JA, Yeh CJG, Mucchielli A: Antigens of the human extra-embryonic membranes. J Reprod Fertil (Suppl) 1982; 31:181–189.

Fick RB Jr: Cystic fibrosis and bronchiectasis. In: Stein JH (ed). Internal Medicine. Boston: Little, Brown, 1990:711–717.

Foresta C, Ferlin A, Garolla A, Rossato M, Barbaux S, Debortoli A: Y-chromosome deletions in idiopathic severe testiculopathies. J Clin Endocr Metab 1997; 82:1075–1080.

Foresta C, Galeazzi C, Bettella A, Stella M, Scandellari C: High incidence of sperm sex chromosomes aneuploidies in two patients with Klinefelter's syndrome. J Clin Endocr Metab 1998; 83:203–205.

Franco B, Guioli S, Pragliola A, Incerti B, Bardoni B, Tonlorenzi R, Carrozzo R, Maestrini E, Pieretti M, Taillon-Miller P, et al.: A gene deleted in Kallmann's syndrome shares homology with neural cell adhesion and axonal path-finding molecules. Nature 1991; 353:529–536.

Fraser EJ, Grimes DA, Schulz KF: Immunization as a therapy for recurrent spontaneous abortion: a review and meta-analysis. Obstet Gynecol 1993; 82:854–859.

Friedman KJ, Teichtahl H, De Kretser DM, Temple-Smith P, Southwick GJ, Silverman LM, Highsmith WE Jr, Boucher RC, Knowles MR: Screening Young syndrome patients for CFTR mutations. Am J Respir Crit Care Med 1995; 152:1353–1357.

Gaillard DA, Carre-Pigeon F, Lallemand A: Normal vas deferens in fetuses with cystic fibrosis. J Urol 1997; 158:1549–1552.

Gatenby PA, Cameron K, Simes RJ, Adelstein S, Bennett MJ, Jansen RPS, Shearman RP, Stewart GJ, Whittle M, Doran TJ: Treatment of recurrent spontaneous abortion by immunization with paternal lymphocytes: results of a controlled trial. Am J Reprod Immunol 1993; 29:88–94.

Geraghty DE, Koller BH, Orr HT: A human major histocompatibility complex class I gene that encodes a protein with a shortened cytoplasmic segment. Proc Natl Acad Sci USA 1987; 84:9145–9149.

Girardi SK, Mielnik A, Schlegel PN: Submicroscopic deletions in the Y chromosome of infertile men. Hum Reprod 1997; 12:1635–1641.

Gordon DL, Krmpotic E, Thomas W, Gandy HM, Paulsen A: Pathologic testicular findings in Klinefelter's syndrome. Arch Intern Med 1972; 130:726–729.

Guttenbach M, Engle W, Schmid M: Analysis of structural and numerical chromosome abnormalities in sperm of normal men and carriers of constitutional chromosome aberrations: a review. Hum Genet 1997; 100:1–21.

Handelsman DJ, Conway AJ, Boylan LM, Turtle JR: Young's syndrome: obstructive azoospermia and chronic sinopulmonary infections. N Engl J Med 1984; 310:3–9.

Harger JH, Archer DF, Marchese SG, Muracca-Clemens M, Garver KL: Etiology of recurrent pregnancy losses and outcome of subsequent pregnancies. Obstet Gynecol 1983; 62:574–581.

Hasle H, Mellemgaard A, Nielsen J, Hansen J: Cancer incidence in men with Klinefelter syndrome. Br J Cancer 1995; 71:416–420.

Hassold T, Hunt PA, Sherman S: Trisomy in humans: incidence, origin and etiology. Curr Opin Genet Dev 1993; 3:398–403.

Hassold T, Warburton D, Kline J, Stein Z: The relationship of maternal age and trisomy among trisomic spontaneous abortions. Am J Hum Genet 1984; 36:1349–1356.

Henderson DJ, Bennett PR, Rodeck CH, Gau GS, Blunt S, Moore GE: Trophoblast from anembryonic pregnancy has both a maternal and a paternal contribution to its genome. Am J Obstet Gynecol 1991; 165:98–102.

Henderson DJ, Sherman LS, Loughna SC, Bennett PR, Moore GE: Early embryonic failure associated with uniparental disomy for human chromosome 21. Hum Mol Genet 1994; 3:1373–1376.

Hendry WF, Sommerville IF, Hall RR, Pugh RC: Investigation and treatment of the subfertile male. Br J Urol 1973; 45:684–692.

Hertig AT, Rock J: On the development of the early human ovum with special reference to the trophoblast of the previllous stage: a description of seven normal and five pathologic ova. Am J Obstet Gynecol 1944; 47:149–184.

Hill JA, Polgar K, Harlow BL, Anderson DJ: Evidence of embryo and trophoblast toxic cellular immune respone(s) in women with recurrent spontaneous abortion. Am J Obstet Gynecol 1992; 166:1044–1052.

Hirsh A, Williams C, Williamson B: Young's syndrome and cystic fibrosis mutation delta F508. Lancet 1993; 342:118.

Ho HN, Gill TJ: Immunotherapy for recurrent spontaneous abortion in a Chinese population. Am J Reprod Immunol 1991; 25:10–15.

Ho H-N, Yang Y-S, Hsieh R-P, Lin H-R, Chen S-U, Chen HF, Huang SC, Lee T-Y, Gill TJ III: Sharing of human leukocyte antigens in couples with unexplained infertility affects the success of in vitro fertilization and tubal embryo transfer. Am J Obstet Gynecol 1994; 170:63–71.

Hoesli IM, Walter-Gobel I, Tercanli S, Holzgreve W: Spontaneous fetal loss rates in a non-selected population. Am J Med Genet 2001; 100:106–109.
Hook EB, Cross PK, Jackson L, Pergament E, Brambati B: Maternal age-specific rates of 47,+21 and other cytogenetic abnormalities diagnosed in the first trimester of pregnancy in chorionic villus biopsy specimens: comparison with rates expected from observations at amniocentesis. Am J Hum Genet 1988; 42:797–807.
Hook EB, Cross PK, Schreinemachers DM: Chromosomal abnormality rates at amniocentesis and in live-born infants. JAMA 1983; 249:2034–2038.
Horsman DE, Dill FJ, McGillivray BC, Kalousek DK: X chromosome aneuploidy in lymphcyte cultures from women with recurrent spontaneous abortions. Am J Med Genet 1987; 28:981–987.
Hsu CC, McConnell J, Doe B, Braude P: Androgenesis and gynogenesis are not causative in early pregnancy loss in humans. Am J Obstet Gynecol 1994; 170:1351–1358.
Hultborn R, Hanson C, Kopf I, Verbiene I, Warnhammar E, Weimarck A: Prevalence of Klinefelter's syndrome in male breast cancer patients. Anticancer Res 1997; 17:4293–4297.
Hunt JS, Orr HT: HLA and maternal-fetal recognition. FASEB J 1992; 6:2344–2348.
Hunt JS, Petroff MG, Morales P, Sedlmayr P, Geraghty DE, Ober C: HLA-G in reproduction: studies on the maternal-fetal interface. Hum Immunol 2000; 61:1113–1117.
Imperato-McGinley J, Peterson RE: Male pseudohermaphroditism: the complexities of male phenotypic development. Am J Med 1976; 61:251–272.
In't Veld PA, Halley DJJ, van Hemel JO, Niermeijer MF, Dohle G, Weber RFA: Genetic counselling before intracytoplasmic sperm injection. Lancet 1997; 350:490.
James DA: Effects of antigenic dissimilarity between mother and foetus on placental size in mice. Nature 1965; 205:613–614.
Jarvi K, Zielenski J, Wilschanski M, Durie P, Buckspan M, Tullis E, Markiewicz D, Tsui LC: Cystic fibrosis transmembrane conductance regulator and obstructive azoospermia. Lancet 1995; 345:1578.
Jeannet M, Bischof P, Bourrit B, Vuagnat P: Sharing of HLA antigens in fertile, subfertile, and infertile couples. Transplant Proc 1985; 17:903–904.
Jeng GT, Scott JR, Burmeister LF: A comparison of meta-analytic results using literature vs individual patient data. JAMA 1995; 274:830–836.
Jezequel P, Dorval I, Fergelot P, Chauvel B, Le Treut A, Le Gall JY, Le Lannou D, Blayau M: Structural analysis of *CFTR* gene in congenital bilateral absence of vas deferens. Clin Chem 1995; 41:833–835.
Jin K, Ho H-N, Speed TP, Gill TJ III: Reproductive failure and the major histocompatibility complex. Am J Hum Genet 1995; 56:1456–1467.
Johnson A, Wapner RJ, Davis GH, Jackson LG: Mosaicism in chorionic villus sampling: an association with poor perinatal outcome. Obstet Gynecol 1990; 75:573–577.
Johnson PM, Ramsden GH, Chia KV, Hart CA, Farquharson RG, Francis WJA: A combined randomized double-blind and open study of trophoblast membrane infusion (TMI) in unexplained recurrent miscarriage. In: Chaouat G, Mowbray J (eds). Cellular and Molecular Biology of the Materno-Fetal Relationship. Paris:, INSERM/John Libbey Eurotext, 1991:277–284.
Johnson PM, Stern PL: Antigen expression at human materno-fetal interfaces. Prog Immunol 1986; 6:1056–1069.
Kajii T, Ohama K, Mikamo K: Anatomic and chromosomal anomalies in 944 induced abortuses. Hum Genet 1978; 43:247–258.
Kamiguchi Y, Rosenbusch B, Sterzik K, Mikamo K: Chromosomal analysis of unfertilized human oocytes prepared by a gradual fixation air-drying method. Hum Genet 1993; 90:533–541.
Kanavakis E, Tzetis M, Antoniadi T, Pistofidis G, Milligos S, Kattamis C: Cystic fibrosis mutation screening in CBAVD patients and men with obstructive azoospermia or severe oligozoospermia. Mol Hum Reprod 1998; 4:333–337.
Kan-ming T, Wa-lun Y, Fai-man L, Tak-sum L: A cytogenetic study of 514 Chinese couples with recurrent spontaneous abortions. Chin Med J 1996; 109:635–638.
Kapasi K, Albert SE, Yie S, Zavazava N, Librach CL: HLA-G has a concentration-dependent effect on the generation of an allo-CTL response. Immunol 2000; 101:191–200.
Karhukorpi J, Laitinen T, Tiilikainen AS: HLA-G polymorphism in Finnish couples with recurrent spontaneous miscarriage. Br J Obstet Gynaecol 1997; 104:1212–1214.
Kent-First MG, Kol S, Muallem A, Blazer S, Itskovitz-Eldor J: Infertility in intracytoplasmic-sperm-injection-derived sons. Lancet 1996a; 348:332.
Kent-First MG, Kol S, Muallem A, Ofir R, Manor D, Blazer S, First N, Itskovitz-Eldor J: The incidence and possible relevance of Y-linked microdeletions in babies born after intracytoplasmic sperm injection and their infertile fathers. Mol Hum Reprod 1996b; 2:943–950.
King A, Boocock C, Sharkey AM, Gardner L, Beretta A, Siccardi AG, Loke YW: Evidence for expression of HLA-C class I mRNA and protein by human first trimester trophoblast. J Immunol 1996; 156:2068–2076.
Kirby DR: The egg and immunology. Proc R Soc Med 1970; 63:59–61.
Knapp LA, Ha JC, Sackett GP: Parental MHC antigen sharing and pregnancy wastage in captive pigtailed macaques. J Reprod Immunol 1996; 32:73–88.
Kobayashi K, Mizuno K, Hida A, Komaki R, Tomita K, Matsushita I, Namiki M, Iwamoto T, Tamura S, Minowada S, et al.: PCR analysis of the Y chromosome long arm in azoospermic patients: evidence for a second locus required for spermatogenesis. Hum Mol Genet 1994; 3:1965–1967.
Komlos L, Zamir R, Joshua H, Halbrecht I: Common HLA antigens in couples with repeated abortions. Clin Immunol Immunopath 1977; 7:330–335.
Kovats S, Main EK, Librach C, Stubblebine M, Fisher SJ, Demars R: A class I antigen, HLA-G, expressed in human trophoblasts. Science 1990; 248:220–223.
Lahn BT, Page DC: Functional coherence of the human Y chromosome. Science 1997; 278:675–680.
Lanasa MC, Hogge WA, Kubik CJ, Blancato J, Hoffman EP: Highly skewed X-chromosome inactivation is associated with idiopathic recurrent spontaneous abortion. Am J Hum Genet 1999; 65:252–254.
Larriba S, Bassas L, Gimenez J, Ramos MD, Segura A, Nunes V, Estivill X, Casals T: Testicular CFTR splice variants in patients with congenital absence of the vas deferens. Hum Mol Genet 1998; 7:1739–1743.
Le Bouteiller P: HLA class I chromosomal region, genes, and products: facts and questions. Crit Rev Immunol 1994; 14:89–129.
Le Coniat M, Soulard M, Della Valle V, Larsen CJ, Berger R: Localization of the human gene encoding heterogeneous nuclear RNA ribonucleoprotein G (*hnRNP-G*) to chromosome 6p12. Hum Genet 1992; 88:593–595.
Lee N, Goodlett DR, Ishitani A, Marquardt H, Geraghty DE: HLA-E surface expression depends on binding of TAP-dependent peptides derived from certain HLA class I signal sequences. J Immunol 1998; 160:4951–4960.
Lee N, Malacko AR, Ishitani A, Chen MC, Bajorath J, Marquardt H, Geraghty DE: The membrane-bound and soluble forms of HLA-G bind identical sets of endogenous peptides but differ with respect to TAP association. Immunity 1995; 3:591–600
Le Gal FA, Riteau B, Sedlik C, Khalil-Daher I, Menier C, Dausset J, Guillet JG, Carosella ED, Rouas-Freiss: HLA-G-mediated inhibition of antigen-specific cytotoxic T lymphocytes. Int Immunol 1999; 11:1351–1356.
Le Lannou D, Jezequel P, Blayau M, Dorval I, Lemoine P, Dabadie A, Roussey M, Le Marec B, Legall JY: Obstructive azoospermia with agenesis of vas deferens or with bronchiectasia (Young's syndrome): a genetic approach. Hum Reprod 1995; 10:338–341.
Lissens W, Liebaers, I: The genetics of male infertility in relation to cystic fibrosis. Bailliere's Best Pract Res Clin Obst Gynaecol 1997; 11:797–817.
Loke YW, King A, Chumbley G: Human trophoblast cell surface molecules: HLA-G and reproduction. Trophoblast Research 1994; 8:331–337.
Lorda-Sanchez I, Binkert F, Maechler M, Robinson WP, Schinzel AA: Reduced recombination and paternal age effect in Kleinfelter syndrome. Hum Genet 1992; 89:524–530.
Ma K, Inglis JD, Sharkey A, Bickmore WA, Hill RE, Prosser EJ, Speed RM, Thomson EJ, Jobling M, Taylor K, et al.: A Y-chromosome gene family with RNA-binding protein homology: candidates for the azoospermia factor AZF controlling human spermatogenesis. Cell 1993; 75:1287–1295.
Machin GA, Crolla JA: Chromosome constitution of 500 infants dying during the perinatal period. Humangenetik 1974; 23:183–198.
MacLean N, Harnden DG, Brown WM, Mantel DJ: Sex-chromosome abnormalities in newborn babies. Lancet 1964; 1:286–290.
Magli MC, Ferraretti AP, Munne S, Gianaroli L: Incidence of chromosomal abnormalities from a morphologically-normal cohort of embryos in poor prognosis patients. J Assist Reprod Genet 1998; 15:297–301.
Mak V, Jarvi KA: The genetics of male infetility. J Urol 1996; 156:1245–1257.
Mange AP: Growth and inbreeding of a human isolate. Hum Biol 1964; 36:104–133.
Martin AO: The founder effect in a human isolate: evolutionary implications. Am J Phys Anthropol 1970; 32:351–368.
Martin RH: Genetics of human sperm. J Assist Reprod Genet 1997; 14:453–454.
Martin RH, Ko E, Rademaker A: Distribution of aneuploidy in human gametes: comparison between human sperm and oocytes. Am J Med Genet 1991; 39:321–331.
Martinelli I, Taioli E, Cetin I, Marinoni A, Gerosa S, Villa MV, Bozzo M, Mannucci PM: Mutations in coagulation factors in women with unexplained late fetal loss. N Engl J Med 2000; 343:1015–1018.
Mercier B, Verlingue C, Lissens W, Silber SJ, Novelli G, Bonduelle M, Audrezet MP, Ferec C: Is congenital bilateral absence of vas deferens a primary form of cystic fibrosis? Analyses of the *CFTR* gene in 67 patients. Am J Hum Genet 1995; 56:272–277.
Meschede D, Lemcke B, Exeler JR, DeGeyter C, Behre HM, Nieschlag E, Horst J: Chromosome abnormalities in 447 couples undergoing intracytoplasmic sperm injection-prevalance, types, sex distribution and reproductive relevance. Hum Reprod 1998; 13:576–582.
Money J: Specific neuro-cognitive impairments associated with Turner (45,X) and Klinefelter (47,XXY) syndromes: a review. Soc Biol 1993; 40:147–151.
Mosher WD: Reproductive impairments in the United States, 1965–1982. Demography 1985; 22:415–430.
Mowbray JF, Gibbings CR, Sidgwick AS, Ruszkiewicz M, Beard RW: Effects of transfusion in women with recurrent spontaneous abortion. Transplant Proc 1983; 15:896–899.
Mowbray JF, Liddell H, Underwood JL, Gibbings C, Reginald PW, Beard RW: Controlled trial of treatment of recurrent spontaneous abortion by immunisation with paternal cells. Lancet 1985; 1:941–943.
Mulhall JP, Reijo R, Alagappan R, Brown L, Page D, Carson R, Oates RD: Azoospermic men with deletion of the DAZ gene cluster are capable of completing spermatogenesis: fertilization, normal embryonic development and pregnancy occur when retrieved testicular spermatozoa are used for intracytoplasmic sperm injection. Hum Reprod 1997; 12:503–508.
Nagafuchi S, Namiki M, Nakahori Y, Kondoh N, Okuyama A, Nakagome Y: A minute deletion of the Y chromosome in men with azoospermia. J Urol 1993; 150:1155–1157.
Najmabadi H, Chai NN, Kapali A, Subbarao MN, Bhasin D, Woodhouse E, Yen P, Bhasin S: Genomic structure of a Y-specific ribonucleic acid binding motif-containing gene: a putative candidate for a subset of male infertility. J Clin Endocrinol Metab 1996; 81:2159–2164.
Nakahori Y, Kuroki Y, Komaki R, Kondoh N, Namiki M, Iwamoto T, Toda T, Kobayashi K: The Y chromosome region essential for spermatogenesis. Horm Res 1996; 46:20–23.

Nielsen J, Wohlert M: Sex chromosome abnormalities found among 34,910 newborn children: results from a 13-year incidence study in Arhus, Denmark. Birth Defects Orig Artic Ser 1991; 26:209–223.
Nordlander C, Fuchs T, Hammarström L, Smith CIE: Human leukocyte antigens group A in couples with unexplained infertility. Fertil Steril 1983; 40:60–65.
Oates RD, Amos JA: The genetic basis of congenital bilateral absence of the vas deferens and cystic fibrosis. J Androl 1994; 15:1–8.
Ober C: HLA and pregnancy: the paradox of the fetal allograft. Am J Hum Genet 1998; 62:1–5.
Ober C, Aldrich A: HLA-G polymorphisms: neutral evolution or novel function? J Reprod Immunol 1997; 36:1–21.
Ober C, Aldrich C, Rosinsky B, Robertson A, Walker MA, Willadsen S, Verp MS, Geraghty DE, Hunt JS: HLA-G1 protein expression is not essential for fetal survival. Placenta 1998a; 19:127–132.
Ober C, Elias S, Kostyu DD, Hauck WW: Decreased fecundability in Hutterite couples sharing HLA-DR. Am J Hum Genet 1992; 50:6–14.
Ober C, Elias S, O'Brien E, Kostyu DD, Hauck WW, Bombard A: HLA sharing and fertility in Hutterite couples: evidence for prenatal selection against compatible fetuses. Am J Reprod Immunol Microbiol 1988; 18:111–115.
Ober C, Hauck WW, Kostyu DD, O'Brien E, Elias S, Simpson JL, Martin AO: Adverse effects of HLA-DR sharing on fertility: a cohort study in a human isolate. Fertil Steril 1985; 44:227–232.
Ober C, Hyslop T, Elias S, Weitkamp LR, Hauck WW: Human leukocyte antigen matching and fetal loss: results of a 10-year prospective study. Hum Reprod 1998b; 13:33–38.
Ober C, Hyslop T, Hauck WW: Inbreeding effects on fertility in humans: evidence for reproductive compensation. Am J Hum Genet 1999a; 64:225–231.
Ober C, Karrison T, Odem RR, Barnes RB, Branch DW, Stephenson MD, Baron B, Walker MA, Scott JB, Schreiber JR: The Recurrent Miscarriage (REMIS) Study: a randomized clinical trial to evaluate the efficacy of mononuclear cell immunization in the prevention of recurrent miscarriages. Lancet 1999b; 354:365–369.
Ober C, Martin AO, Simpson JL, Hauck WW, Amos DB, Kostyu DD, Fotino M, Allen FH: Shared HLA antigens and reproductive performance in the Hutterites. Am J Hum Genet 1983; 35:990–1004.
Ober C, van der Ven K: Immunogenetics of reproduction: an overview. In: Olding LB (ed). Current Topics in Microbiology and Immunology. Vol. 222. Berlin: Springer-Verlag, 1997:1–23.
Ober C, Weitkamp LR, Cox N: HLA and mate choice. In: Johnston R, Müller-Schwarz D, Sorensen P (eds). Chemical Signals in Vertebrates 8. New York: Plenum Press, 1999c: pp. 189–200.
Ober C, Weitkamp LR, Cox N, Dytch H, Kostyu D, Elias S: HLA and mate choice in humans. Am J Hum Genet 1997; 61:497–504.
Opelz G, Terasaki PI: Improvement of kidney-graft survival with increased numbers of blood transfusions. N Engl J Med 1978; 299:799–803.
Osborne LR, Lynch M, Middleton PG, Alton EW, Geddes DM, Pryor JP, Hodson ME, Santis GK: Nasal epithelial ion transport and genetic analysis of infertile men with congenital bilateral absence of the vas deferens. Hum Mol Genet 1993; 2:1605–1609.
Palermo GD, Schlegel PN, Sills ES, Veeck LL, Zaninovic N, Menendez M, Rosenwaks Z: Births after intracytoplasmic injection of sperm obtained by testicular extraction from men with Klinefelter's syndrome. N Engl J Med 1998; 338:588–590.
Payne R, Rolfs MR: Fetomaternal leucocyte incompatibility. J Clin Invest 1958; 37:1756–1763.
Pegoraro E, Whitaker J, Mowery-Rushton P, Surti U, Lanasa M, Hoffman EP: Familial skewed X inactivation: a molecular trait associated with high spontaneous-abortion rate maps to Xq28. Am J Hum Genet 1997; 61:160–170.
Penzes M, Rajczy K, Gyodi E, Reti M, Feher E, Petranyi G: HLA-G gene polymorphism in the normal population and in recurrent spontaneous abortion in Hungary. Transplant Proc 1999; 31:1832–1833.
Persitz E, Oksenberg JR, Margalioth EH, Hacohen S, Schenker J, Brautbar C: Histoincompatibility in couples with unexplained infertility. Fertil Steril 1985; 43:733–738.
Pfeiffer KA, Fimmers R, Engels G, van der Ven H, van der Ven K: The HLA-G genotype is potentially associated with idiopathic recurrent spontaneous abortion. Mol Hum Reprod 2001; 7:373–378.
Plachot M: The human oocyte: genetic aspects. Ann Genet 1997; 40:115–120.
Portnoi M-F, Joye N, Van Den Akker J, Morlier G, Taillemite J-L: Karyotypes of 1142 couples with recurrent abortion. Obstet Gynecol 1988; 72:31–34.
Pryor JL, Kent-First M, Muallem A, Van Bergen A, Nolten WE, Meisner L, Roberts KP: Microdeletions in the Y chromosome of infertile men. N Engl J Med 1997; 336:534–539.
Qumsiyeh MB, Ahmed MN, Kim K-R, Bradford W: Towards an understanding of the etiology of spontaneous abortion (SAB): increased apoptosis and decreased cell proliferation of chromosomally abnormal versus normal chorionic villi. Am J Hum Genet 1998; 63:A171.
Qureshi SJ, Ross AR, Ma K, Cooke HJ, McIntyre MA, Chandley AC, Hargreave TB: Polymerase chain reaction screening for Y chromosome microdeletions: a first step towards the diagnosis of genetically determined spermatogenic failure in men. Mol Hum Reprod 1996; 2:775–779.
Ratner LE, Hadley GA, Hanto DW, Mohanakumar T: Immunology of renal allograft rejection. Arch Pathol Lab Med 1991; 115:283–287.
Rave-Harel N, Madgar I, Goshen R, Nissim-Rafinia M, Ziadni A, Rahat A, Chiba O, Kalman YM, Brautbar C, Levinson D, et al.: CFTR haplotype analysis reveals genetic heterogeneity in the etiology of congenital bilateral aplasia of the vas deferens. Am J Hum Genet 1995; 56:1359–1366.
Rebmann V, van der Ven K, Päßler M, Pfeiffer K, Krebs D, Grosse-Wilde H: Association of soluble HLA-G plasma levels with HLA-G alleles. Tissue Antigens 2001; 57:15–21.
Recurrent Miscarriage Immunotherapy Trialist Group: Worldwide collaborative observational study and meta-analysis on allogenic leukocyte immunotherapy for recurrent spontaneous abortion. Am J Reprod Immunol 1994; 32:55–72.
Reijo R, Alagappan RK, Patrizio P, Page DC: Severe oligozoospermia resulting from deletions of azoospermia factor gene on Y chromosome. Lancet 1996a; 347:1290–1293.
Reijo R, Lee TY, Salo P, Alagappan R, Brown LG, Rosenberg M, Rozen S, Jaffe T, Straus D, Hovatta O, et al.: Diverse spermatogenic defects in humans caused by Y chromosome deletions encompassing a novel RNA-binding protein gene. Nat Genet 1995; 10:383–393.
Reijo R, Seligman J, Dinulos MB, Jaffe T, Brown LG, Disteche CM, Page DC: Mouse autosomal homolog of DAZ, a candidate male sterility gene in humans, is expressed in male germ cells before and after puberty. Genomics 1996b; 35:346–352.
Robertson A, Charlesworth D, Ober C: The effect of inbreeding avoidance on Hardy-Weinberg equilibrium: examples of neutral and selected loci. Genet Epidemiol 1999; 17:165–173.
Roland B, Lynch L, Berkowitz G, Zinberg R: Confined placental mosaicism in CVS and pregnancy outcome. Prenat Diagn 1994; 14:589–593.
Rushton DI: Examination of products of conception from previable human pregnancies. J Clin Pathol 1981; 34:819–835.
Ruzicska P, Czeizel A: Cytogenetic studies on mid-trimester abortuses. Humangenetik 1970; 10:273–297.
Sangha KK, Stephenson MD, Brown CJ, Robinson WP: Extremely skewed X-chromosome inactivation is increased in women with recurrent spontaneous abortion. Am J Hum Genet 1999; 65:913–917.
Saxena R, Brown LG, Hawkins T, Alagappan RK, Skaletsky H, Reeve MP, Reijo R, Rozen S, Dinulos MB, Disteche CM, Page DC: The DAZ gene cluster on the human Y chromosome arose from an autosomal gene that was transposed, repeatedly amplified and pruned. Nat Genet 1996; 14:292–299.
Schacter B, Muir A, Gyves M, Tasin M: HLA-A,B compatibility in parents of offspring with neural-tube defects or couples experiencing involuntary fetal wastage. Lancet 1979; 1:796–799.
Schlegel PN, Shin D, Goldstein M: Urogenital anomalies in men with congenital absence of the vas deferens. J Urol 1996; 155:1644–1648.
Schweikert H-U: The androgen resistance syndromes: clinical and biochemical aspects. Eur J Pediatr 1993; 152:S50–57.
Scott JR, Rote NS, Branch WR: Immunologic aspects of recurrent abortion and fetal death. Obstet Gynecol 1987; 70:645–656.
Seligsohn U, Lubetsky A: Genetic susceptibility to venous thrombosis. N Engl J Med 2001; 344:1222–1231.
Sheps MC: An analysis of reproductive patterns in an American isolate. Popul Stud 1965; 19:65–80.
Simoni M, Gromoll J, Dworniczak B, Rolf C, Abshagen K, Kamischke A, Carani C, Meschede D, Behre HM, Horst J, Nieschlag E: Screening for deletions of the Y chromosome involving the *DAZ* (deleted in azoospermia) gene in azoospermia and severe oligozoospermia. Fertil Steril 1997; 67:542–547.
Smith JB, Cowchock FS: Immunological studies in recurrent spontaneous abortion: effects of immunization of women with paternal mononuclear cells on lymphocytotoxic and mixed lymphocyte reaction blocking antibodies and correlation with sharing of HLA and pregnancy outcome. J Reprod Immunol 1988; 14:99–113.
Stein Z, Kline J, Susser E, Shrout P, Warburton D, Susser M: Maternal age and spontaneous abortions. In: Porter IH, Hook EB (eds). Human Embryonic and Fetal Death. New York: Academic Press, 1980:107–127.
Stern JJ, Coulam CB: Seminal plasma treatment of recurrent spontaneous abortion. Am J Reprod Immunol 1992; 27:50.
Stray-Pederson B, Stray-Pederson S: Etiologic factors and subsequent reproductive performance in 195 couples with a prior history of habitual abortion. Am J Obstet Gynecol 1984; 148:140–146.
Stuppia L, Mastroprimiano G, Calabrese G, Peila R, Tenaglia R, Palka G: Microdeletions in interval 6 of the Y chromosome detected by STS-PCR in 6 of 33 patients with idiopathic oligo- or azoospermia. Cytogenet Cell Genet 1996; 72:155–158.
Sunderland CA, Naiem M, Mason DY, Redman CWG, Stirrat GM: The expression of major histocompatibility antigens by human chorionic villi. J Reprod Immunol 1981a; 3:323–331.
Sunderland CA, Redman VWG, Stirrat GM: HLA-A, -B, -C antigens are expressed on nonvillous trophoblasts of the early human placenta. J Immunol 1981b; 127:2614–2615.
Taylor C, Faulk WP: Prevention of recurrent abortions with leucocyte transfusions. Lancet 1981; 2:68–69.
Tho TP, Byrd JR, McDonough PG: Etiologies and subsequent reproductive performance of 100 couples with recurrent abortion. Fertil Steril 1979; 32:389–395.
Tiepolo L, Zuffardi O: Localization of factors controlling spermatogenesis in the nonfluorescent portion of the human Y chromosome long arm. Hum Genet 1976; 34:119–124.
Unander AM, Lindholm A: Transfusions of leukocyte-rich erythrocyte concentrates: a successful treatment in selected cases of habitual abortion. Am J Obstet Gynecol 1986; 154:516–519.
van der Ven K, Messer L, van der Ven H, Jeyendran RS, Ober C: Cystic fibrosis mutation screening in healthy men with reduced sperm quality. Hum Reprod 1996; 11:513–517.
van der Ven K, Peschka B, Montag M, Lange R, Schwanitz G, van der Ven H: In-

creased frequency of congenital chromosomal aberrations in female partners of couples undergoing intracytoplasmic sperm injection. Hum Reprod 1998; 13:48–54.

van Rood JJ, Claas FHJ: The influence of allogeneic cells on the human T and B cell repertoire. Science 1990; 248:1388–1393.

van Rood JJ, van Leeuwen A, Eernisse JG: Leucocyte antibodies in sera from pregnant women. Nature 1958; 181:1735–1736.

Vogt PH, Edelmann A, Kirsch S, Henegariu O, Hirschmann P, Kiesewetter F, Kohn FM, Schill WB, Farah S, Ramos C, et al.: Human Y chromosome azoospermia factors (AZF) mapped to different subregions in Yq11. Hum Mol Genet 1996; 5:933–943.

Vollrath D, Foote S, Hilton A, Brown LG, Beer-Romero P, Bogan JS, Page DC: The human Y chromosome: a 43-interval map based on naturally occurring deletions. Science 1992; 258:52–59.

Wapner RJ, Simpson JL, Golbus MS, Zachary JM, Ledbetter DH, Desnick RJ, Fowler SE, Jackson LG, Lubs H, Mahony RJ, et al.: Chorionic mosaicism: association with fetal loss but not with adverse perinatal outcome. Prenat Diagn 1992; 12:347–355.

Warburg E: A fertile patient with Klinefelter's syndrome. Acta Endocr 1963; 43:12–26.

Warburton D, Byrne J, Canki N: Chromosome Anomalies and Prenatal Development: An Atlas Oxford Monographs on Medical Genetics No. 21. New York: Oxford University Press, 1991.

Warburton D, Kline J, Stein Z, Hutzler M, Chin A, Hassold T: Does the karyotype of a spontaneous abortion predict the karyotype of a subsequent abortion? Evidence from 273 women with two karyotyped spontaneous abortions. Am J Hum Genet 1987; 41:465–483.

Warburton D, Kline J, Stein Z, Strobino B: Cytogenetic abnormalities in spontaneous abortions of recognized conceptions. In: Porter IH, Hatcher NH, Willey AM (eds). Perinatal Genetics: Diagnosis and Treatment. Orlando: Academic Press, 1986:23–40.

Weckstein LN, Patrizio P, Balmaceda JP, Asch RH, Branch DW: Human leukocyte antigen compatibility and failure to achieve a viable pregnancy with assisted reproductive technology. Acta Eur Fertil 1991; 22:103–107.

Weighardt F, Biamonti G, Riva S: The roles of heterogeneous nuclear ribonucleoproteins (hnRNP) in RNA metabolism. Bioessays 1996; 18:747–756.

Weitkamp LR, Ober C: HLA and mate choice. Am J Hum Genet 1998; 62:986–987.

Weitkamp LR, Ober C: Ancestral and recombinant 16-locus HLA haplotypes in the Hutterites. Immunogenetics 1999; 49:491–497.

Welsh MJ, Smith AE: Cystic fibrosis. Sci Am 1995; 273:52–59.

Wilcox AJ, Weinberg CR, O'Connor JF, Baird DD, Schlatterer JP, Canfield RE, Armstrong EG, Nisula BC: Incidence of early loss of pregnancy. N Engl J Med 1985; 319:189–194.

Wilson RD, Kendrick V, Wittmann BK, McGillivray BC: Risk of spontaneous abortion in ultrasonically normal pregnancies. Lancet 1984; 2:920–921.

Wolstenholme J, Rooney DE, Davison EV: Confined placental mosaicism, IUGR, and adverse pregnancy outcome: a controlled retrospective U.K. collaborative survey. Prenat Diagn 1994; 14:345–361.

Yamashita T, Fujii T, Tokunaga K, Tadokoro K, Hamai Y, Miki A, Kozuma S, Juji T, Taketani Y: Analysis of human leukocyte antigen-G polymorphism including intron 4 in Japanese couples with habitual abortion. Am J Reprod Immunol 1999; 41:159–163.

Yelavarthi K, Fishback JI, Hunt JA: Analysis of *HLA-G* mRNA in human placental and extraplacental membrane cells by in situ hybridization. J Immunol 1991; 146:2847–2854.

Yen PH, Chai NN, Salido EC: The human autosomal gene DAZLA—testis specificity and a candidate for male infertility. Hum Mol Genet 1996; 5:2013–2017.

Yoshida A, Miura K, Shirai M: Cytogenetic survey of 1,007 infertile males. Urol Int 1997; 58:166–176.

Zenses MT, Casper RF: Cytogenetics of human oocytes, zygotes, and embryos after in vitro fertilization. Hum Genet 1992; 88:367–375.

Zielenski J, Patrizio P, Corey M, Handelin B, Markiewicz D, Asch R, Tsui LC: *CFTR* gene variant for patients with congenital absence of vas deferens [letter]. Am J Hum Genet 1995; 57:958–960.

Part VII

RHEUMATOLOGIC DISEASES

28 Immunology and Immunogenetics

GERALD T. NEPOM AND HENRY A. ERLICH

Genetic control of the immune response involves a complex set of cellular and molecular interactions. Hundreds of genes are involved in immune recognition, activation and function, with distinct patterns of expression and regulation. Genetic polymorphisms at some of these loci are a key determinant of the immune response, accounting for variation within the population. For autoimmune- and immune-mediated diseases, our understanding of disease mechanisms, phenotypic heterogeneity, and disease susceptibility is being rapidly advanced by a thorough understanding of the key genetic participants in immune response pathways. This chapter introduces the key elements of the human immune response and summarizes the crucial role of the major histocompatibility complex (MHC, 6p21) in this process.

ELEMENTS OF THE IMMUNE RESPONSE

The immune system consists of interacting molecules and cells which are designed to *(1)* recognize intracellular and extracellular threats (primarily pathogens); *(2)* alert and activate lymphocytes and monocytes suitable for response to these threats; *(3)* instruct and commit the responding cells to an appropriately regulated response to the threat; *(4)* amplify the response if necessary by recruitment of additional cells, including polymorphonuclear leukocytes and macrophages, as well as additional lymphocytes and monocytes; and *(5)* ultimately complete and terminate the immune response after the threat has resolved. A general outline of this pathway is illustrated in Figure 28–1. Each step involves an interaction between two or more cells, mediated by specific intramolecular interactions. In the sections which follow, the key molecules in these interactions are discussed in the context of their functional hierarchy in this pathway.

Role of Antigen-Presenting Cells in Antigen Recognition

Antigens are molecular constituents (peptides, lipids, carbohydrates) that alert the immune system to the presence of a new exposure or threat. Antigens, whether derived from infectious pathogens or from altered self-proteins, make their entry into the immune pathway through the surveillance system established by bone marrow–derived monocytes, macrophages, and especially dendritic cells, which are distributed throughout the body. For example, viral infection is followed by intracellular proteolysis of some of the virus-encoded proteins, and peptides generated in this way become the key antigens that signal a specific viral threat. In the absence of intracellular infections, dendritic cells actively survey their surroundings by endocytosis and thereby incorporate proteins, which are subsequently proteolyzed and presented as potential antigens.

Antigen presentation is an engineering marvel of structural biology. Peptides generated by proteolysis within an antigen-presenting cell (APC) are loaded onto specialized molecules, encoded by the human leukocyte antigen (HLA) loci, through an intricate and very specific binding interaction. Depending on the size and shape of each specific peptide antigen, it has the potential to bind some, but not all, HLA molecules. HLA molecules, in turn, differ widely between individuals. This individual variation is due to the extensive genetic polymorphisms of the HLA genes themselves, discussed below. Thus, it is the specific combination of an antigen–HLA complex which provides the first genetically controlled determinant of antigen-specific recognition. In the presence of a successful binding interaction between peptide and HLA molecule within an APC, this complex is then arrayed on the APC membrane, where the surfaces of both the antigen and the HLA molecule are presented to the extracellular environment (Braciale and Braciale, 1991).

As described in Table 28–1, there are two general categories of HLA molecules that perform this antigen presentation function. MHC class I molecules generally bind short peptides in the endoplasmic reticulum, predominantly representing an array of proteins actively being synthesized intracellularly (e.g., viral proteins). HLA class II molecules generally bind peptides present in endosomal compartments, due to the presence of a chaperone molecule, called the *invariant chain*, which binds to class II molecules in the endoplasmic reticulum and blocks the peptide-binding site until it is removed by a separate catalyst (HLA-DM) present in the endosome. After removal of the invariant chain, HLA class II molecules bind peptides, which are degraded in endosomal compartments, representing both endogenously and exogenously derived proteins (Pieters, 1997).

The specificity of the peptide–HLA interaction relies on structural complementarity between the antigenic peptides and the binding groove of the HLA molecules. As illustrated in Figure 28–2, the binding groove of HLA molecules contains a series of pockets, which are bordered by combinations of different amino acids. Different HLA alleles encode different HLA molecules with similar overall structural homology but key differences in these amino acids that line the exterior of the peptide binding pockets. Thus, unique peptide-binding profiles are generated for different HLA molecules. For this reason, individuals with different HLA genes will bind different peptides, creating a very straightforward link between genetic polymorphisms and variable responses (Engelhard, 1994; Rammensee, 1995; Strominger and Wiley, 1995; Young et al., 1995).

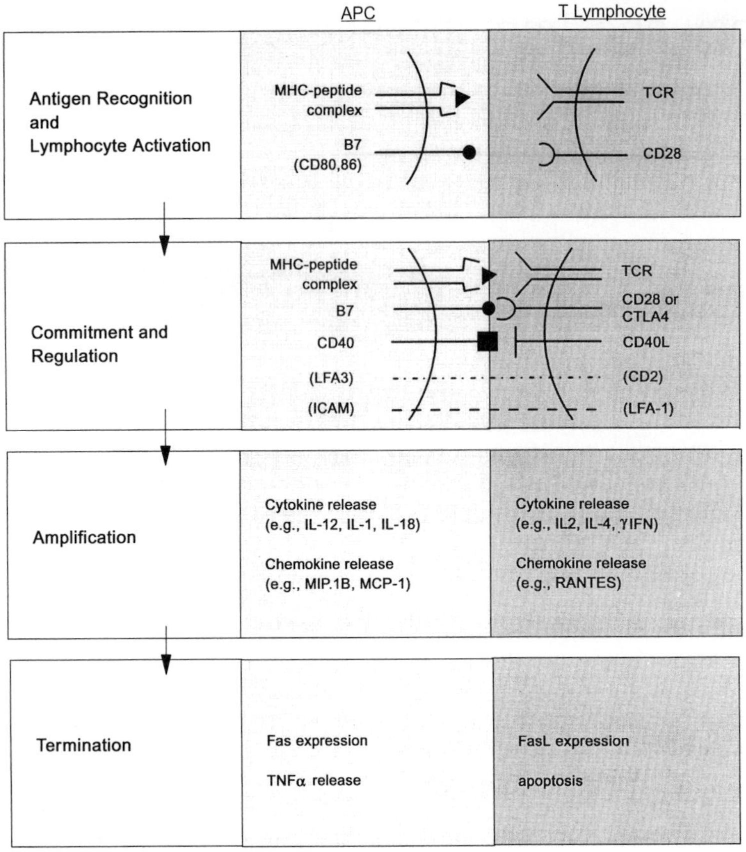

Fig. 28–1. The antigen recognition pathway. *MHC*, major histocompatibility complex; *TCR*, T-cell receptor; *IL*, interleukin; *IFN*, interferon; *TNF*, tumor necrosis factor.

Genetic Basis for T-Cell Specificity during Antigen Recognition and Activation

When the peptide–MHC complex is present on the surface of APCs, it serves as a beacon for transmitting information about the antigen to the T lymphocytes. The T cell accomplishes this recognition through expression of a molecular complex called the *T-cell receptor* (TCR). The TCR consists of an α and a β chain, which are unique to each individual T cell, complexed with the γ, δ, and ϵ chains of the CD3 molecule, along with a homodimer of ζ chains, which are important in transmitting activation signals to the interior of the T cell. When this TCR complex contacts the peptide–MHC complex, the TCR α and β chains bind to the exposed portions of the peptide and HLA molecules on the APC surface. If there is sufficient structural complementarity in this interaction and if there are enough identical peptide–MHC complexes on the APC to serially bind TCR molecules for sufficient duration, then signal transduction events occur, mediated by phosphorylation of the ζ-chain components (Valitutti et al., 1995; van Oers et al., 1998; Boniface et al., 1998; Itoh et al., 1999). Subsequent interactions with tyrosine kinases, adaptor proteins, and other intracellular effector pathways translate the TCR interaction signal into a cascade of intracellular events and transcription factor activation (Robey and Allison, 1995; Peterson et al., 1998; Peterson and Koretzky, 1999).

One key aspect of the genetic control of this TCR recognition event lies in the specificity of the TCR α- and β-chain structures. Both the α and the β chains of the TCR consist of variable regions and constant regions, separately encoded by V segments and C segments analogous to immunoglobulin variable and constant domains, respectively. As with immunoglobulin genes, the genome contains a large number of TCR V-region

Table 28–1. Cellular and Molecular Components of Antigen-Specific Immune Recognition

Molecule	Distribution	Function
T-cell receptor	T lymphocytes	Binds to MHC–peptide complexes and triggers T-cell activation
CD4	Subset of T lymphocytes	Directs recognition toward peptides complexed with class II MHC molecules
CD8	Subset of T lymphocytes	Directs recognition toward peptides complexed with class I MHC molecules
Costimulators	T lymphocytes	Augment, amplify, or regulate the activation (e.g., CD28, CTLA4, CD2) signal transduced by the T-cell receptor
MHC (HLA) class I	All cells	Binds peptides for presentation to lymphocytes ($CD8^+$ T cells and NK cells)
MHC (HLA) class II	Antigen-presenting cells	Binds peptides for presentation to $CD4^+$ T lymphocytes

MHC, major histocompatibility complex; NK, natural killer.

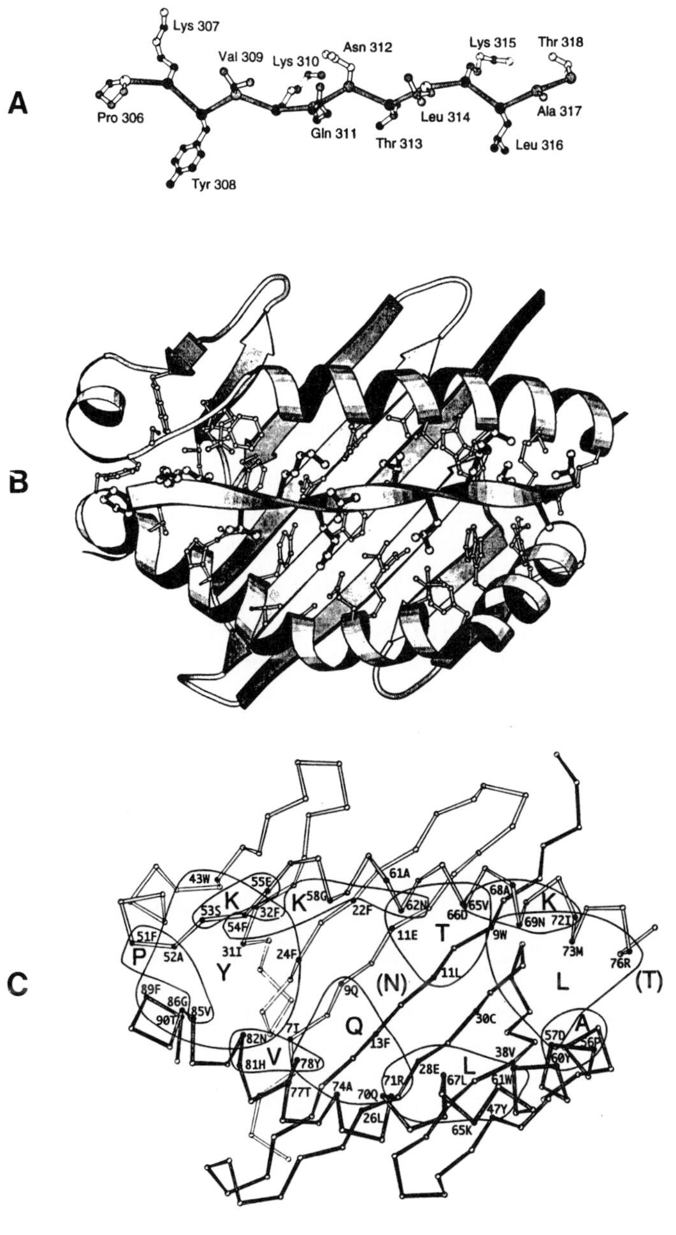

Fig. 28–2. Structual interactions between antigenic peptides and HLA class II molecules. Peptides *(A)* are bound in extended conformation with the central groove of class II molecules *(B)* where specific side chain interactions and hydrogen bond interactions determine binding avidity. *C:* Sites within the MHC molecule, with peptide removed, which determine specific binding interactions. These sites vary between different individuals and are the basis for HLA genetic variation influencing antigenic peptide binding. Adapted from Stern et al. (1994).

segments. Genomic rearrangement events during the maturation of the T lymphocyte juxtapose individual V segments with C segments, resulting in transcription of intact α- and β-chain mRNA. A huge potential repertoire of TCR specificities is generated in this way, with the formation of different combinations of V segments, joining segments, and C-region combinations, with additional junctional diversity introduced during genomic rearrangement. It has been estimated that the potential repertoire contains as many as 10^{16} possible unique TCR α and β structures, a number comparable to estimates of the total diversity of immunoglobulins (Mak et al., 1986; Wilson et al., 1988; Weiss, 1991).

The interaction between the α–β TCR and the peptide–MHC complex involves intermolecular, and therefore intercellular, contacts in which the specificity of TCR binding is controlled both by peptide contact sites and by MHC contact sites. Both the peptide and the MHC molecules contribute to the overall avidity of trimolecular interaction and, therefore, to activation of the T cell through the TCR. In this way, the specific type of HLA molecule involved in the peptide–MHC complex controls the binding not only of its specific peptides but also of its corresponding TCR. This MHC-controlled TCR recognition is known as *MHC restriction* and represents a key checkpoint for genetic control of the T-cell immune response, based on the genetics of the HLA component expressed by the APC (Zinkernagel and Doherty, 1979). HLA genetic polymorphism thus controls this interaction through three structural mechanisms: directly through binding the antigenic peptide, directly through binding to the TCR, and indirectly by altering the conformation of the bound peptide and influencing the interaction between peptide and TCR.

In addition to the TCR complex, the interaction between T lymphocytes and APCs involves a number of coactivator and costimulator molecules. CD4 and CD8 molecules are expressed on mature T lymphocytes, where they associate with the TCR complex and bind to MHC molecules. CD4 molecules bind to MHC class II molecules, and CD8 molecules bind to HLA class I molecules, providing the molecular basis for identifying subsets of T lymphocytes which are MHC-restricted for MHC class II or class I molecules, respectively. Table 28–1 summarizes these key elements of MHC-restricted antigen-specific recognition.

The immune system has several fail-safe mechanisms to prevent aberrant or unregulated TCR activation as well as several feedback mechanisms designed to guide pathways of T-cell commitment to specific effector functions. These secondary signals are provided by a set of costimulator molecules on the APC and T-cell surfaces, some of which are illustrated in Figure 28–1. After TCR engagement of the peptide–MHC complex, co-ligation of the B7-CD28 molecules pushes the T lymphocyte toward a differentiation and commitment pathway, which is subject to further regulation by additional pairs of costimulatory molecules, such as CD40–CD40 ligand, lymphocyte function associated molecule–CD2, and intracellular adhesion molecule–LFA1. Alternative regulatory interactions, such as that between B7 and CTLA4, are also potential modulators during the early events in this pathway (Chen et al., 1992; Jenkins and Johnson, 1993; Lenschow et al., 1996; Croft and Dubey, 1997).

Thymic Education: Positive and Negative Selection

The diversity of TCR specificities creates a broad functional potential for antigenic recognition, an essential component of the adaptive immune response. Of necessity, TCR specificities which are potentially reactive with self-antigens are also created during random TCR gene rearrangement, creating the potential for autoreactive T cells. In the normal course of T-cell maturation, however, several TCR selection steps are designed to protect the individual from expression of such T cells. This pathway of T-cell development is called *thymic education* since it occurs predominantly in the thymus, the site of T-cell maturation.

After expression of rearranged TCR genes, immature T lymphocytes in the thymus are capable of receiving antigen-specific signals from HLA–peptide complexes expressed on APCs. Early in the maturation process, such T cells encounter HLA–peptide complexes presented by thymic epithelial cells arrayed in the thymic cortex. In a process known as *positive selection,* T cells at this immature stage receive growth and differentiation signals as a result of TCR ligation. T cells with rearranged TCR capable of reacting with self-HLA and self-peptide complexes continue to develop and mature (Kisielow et al., 1988; Marrack et al., 1988; Benoist and Mathis, 1989; Bevan, 1997). T cells with TCR that do not recognize self-HLA–peptide complexes die within the thymus. This positive selection of T cells based on HLA–peptide recognition is responsible for MHC restriction, wherein T-cell specificity is directed toward particular HLA specificities. Thus, following TCR α and β gene rearrangement, $CD4^+$, $CD8^+$ immature T cells are positively selected to be restricted to either specific class I molecules ($CD8^+$ T cells) or specific class II molecules ($CD4^+$ cells).

After positive selection, the T cells traffic to the thymic medullary areas, where they encounter HLA–peptide complexes expressed on a different type of APC, hematopoietically derived monocytes and dendritic cells similar to the mature APCs used by the peripheral immune system to respond to antigenic challenge. In the thymic medulla, however, T cells are in an immature stage of development; and when they encounter very strong antigenic signals from the HLA–peptide complex, they trigger a programmed death response, which results in the deletion, or *negative selection*, of autoreactive cells. This remarkable developmental step is an immunologic fail-safe mechanism programmed to protect an individual from the maturation of self-reactive T lymphocytes (Kisielow and von Boehmer, 1995). Experimental animal models of immune maturation have demonstrated that failure of this negative selection maturation step results in several types of systemic and organ-specific autoimmunity. A complex set of poorly characterized developmental regulatory genes controls this T-cell maturation pathway, some of which are likely to contribute to human autoimmunity and aberrant immune responses (Alberola-Ila et al., 1996; Anderson et al., 1997).

Cytokines and Chemokines Amplify and Regulate the Immune Response

The intracellular activation cascades set in motion by binding through the TCR result in mobilization of transcription factors, which act on genes controlling various lymphocyte effector functions. Cytokine gene expression is among the most important of these early activation functions. Cytokine expression provides an important means for immune cells to communicate with each other during the course of an immune response, thereby providing a flexible language for increasing, decreasing, or changing the recruitment of a specific effector function. For example, interferon-γ (IFN-γ) release is an early cytokine response by T lymphocytes following TCR activation, which results in activation of APC macrophages and monocytes, causing the release of monocyte-derived cytokines such as interleukin-12 (IL-12) and tumor necrosis factor (TNF). These in turn are potent proinflammatory cytokines that accelerate local inflammatory responses and release of mediators such as nitric oxide and superoxides. Other cytokines, such as IL-2 and IL-3, are growth factors produced by T cells which stimulate expansion of lymphocytes and other hematopoietic cells. Several cytokines have multiple functions; e.g., IL-4 is an activation and growth factor that recruits B lymphocytes while at the same time augmenting the growth and differentiation of T lymphocytes.

Structurally distinct molecules, termed *chemokines*, are also made by activated lymphocytes and APCs and function as chemoattractants for migrating leukocytes. Dozens of such chemokines have been described, with overlapping specificities and cellular profiles (Baggiolini et al., 1997; Zlotnik et al., 1999) (Table 28–2). It is likely that multiple chemoattractants released at sites of immune activation establish chemotactic gradients, which determine the amplitude and type of immune cell recruitment.

Functional Distinction between Th1 and Th2 Cells

Following T-cell activation, commitment, and amplification steps, a typical immune response involves T cells with a broad variety of effector function and cytokine profiles. Within this heterogeneity, however, two specific subsets of T lymphocytes have been described with interesting, somewhat reciprocal phenotypes (Mosmann and Coffman, 1989; Romagnani et al., 1998).

Table 28–2. Some Principal Cytokines and Chemokines Involved in Cellular Immune Responses

Cytokines	Cell Source	Function
IL-1	mϕ, monocyte	Activates lymphocytes, endothelium
IL-2	T cell	Lymphocyte growth factor
IL-3	T cell	Hematopoietic growth factor
IL-4	T cell	Activation, growth and differentiation factor
IL-5	T cell	B-cell and eosinophilic growth and differentiation
IL-10	T cell	Hematopoietic cell regulator
IL-12	Activated mϕ, monocyte	T and NK cell activator, differentiation factor
IL-18	Activated mϕ, monocyte	T and NK cell activator
Interferon-γ	T cell	Activation and differentiation factor
TNF-α	T cell, monocyte, and mϕ	Activation and effector factor for multiple cells
Chemokines Family	**Example**	**Cell Source**
CXC (12 members)	IL-8	mϕ, monocytes, fibroblasts
CC (20 members)	MIP-1β	Monocytes, endothelium, mϕ
	MCP-1	Monocytes, fibroblasts, mϕ
	Rantes	T cells

TNF, tumor necrosis factor; NK, natural killer.

T-helper 1 (Th1) cells are T lymphocytes that are committed to release proinflammatory cytokines such as IFN-γ and IL-2, which amplify the cellular immune response, but that do not produce cytokines such as IL-4 or IL-5. Th2 cells, however, produce IL-4, IL-5, IL-13, and sometimes IL-10, which amplify the humoral immune response and modulate lymphocyte function but do not produce IFN-γ. The development of Th1 cells is induced in vivo and in vitro by IL-12, whereas Th2 cells are induced by IL-4. The Th1 and Th2 dichotomy may reflect a functionally important classification since experimental studies of Th1 and Th2 lymphocytes have shown that they not only produce reciprocal sets of cytokines but also appear to counterregulate each other. In other words, cytokines produced by Th1 cells tend to block the further differentiation of additional Th2 lymphocytes, and production of cytokines by Th2 cells tends to block the commitment of additional Th1 lymphocytes. Expression of this kind of reciprocal feedback loop leads in vivo to highly polarized types of immune response, often dominated by either the Th1 or the Th2 phenotype at the expense of the other. This functional dichotomy also has potential implications for immunotherapy in that immune-mediated diseases dominated by Th1 responses may potentially be modulated by therapies which enhance expression of a Th2-type response. Similarly, diseases such as allergic asthma, mediated primarily by a Th2 response, may respond to therapies designed to shift the immune system toward a Th1 response (Constant and Bottomly, 1997; Maggi 1998; Morel and Oriss, 1998; De Vries et al., 1999).

Downregulation and Termination of T-Cell Responses

As a counterbalance to immune activation, the immune system has several mechanisms for downregulating lymphocytes and terminating an ongoing immune response. When these terminator pathways go awry, uncontrolled immune amplification and autoimmune disease may ensue. Some mechanisms for lymphocyte regulation are mediated through cell-surface intermolecular interactions, analogous to pathways used for activation. One of the most important of these pathways is the interaction between CTLA-4 molecules, expressed on T lymphocytes, and CD80/CD86 molecules (B7), expressed on APCs. The CTLA-4–B7 recognition system acts as a counterbalance to the CD28–B7 recognition system, important in T-cell activation. When the CTLA-4 protein is expressed on T lymphocytes and activated by contact with the B7 molecule on APCs, it recruits phosphatases to the site of TCR activation complexes, which intersect and interrupt the kinase-mediated activation pathways, resulting in a negative signaling pathway (Lee et al., 1998).

A less subtle form of immune downregulation is mediated by the TNF cytokine family and by the fas–fas ligand set of cell-surface ligands. These terminator effector pathways induce death of the target cells, known as *apoptosis*, by triggering signaling cascades that activate death-mediating molecules, e.g., caspases, and inhibit protective molecules, e.g., BCL-2 (Vaux, 1998).

B Lymphocytes Participate in the Proliferative, Differentiation, and Effector Functions of the Immune Response

B lymphocytes lack the TCR complex and therefore do not recognize MHC-restricted antigen. However, these cells have a functionally analogous receptor, the B-cell receptor, which contains a membrane-bound immunoglobulin molecule. This surface immunoglobulin binds to antigens found in the extracellular compartment, and B-cell activation is accomplished by simultaneous receipt of a signal through the B-cell receptor and a cooperating signal provided by the activated T lymphocytes. In this way, B lymphocytes become immune effector cells, recruited and activated in parallel with T-cell responses (Monroe, 1998; Benschop and Cambier, 1999). There are many functional interactions between the B lymphocyte and the T lymphocyte in such cognate recognition. Interaction between specific costimulatory molecules encourages the T lymphocyte to secrete IL-4, biasing it toward a Th2 pattern of cytokine release. Some of the same cytokines act on B cells to drive production of antibodies and lead to isotype switching, the maturation step in which antibody molecules switch from immunoglobulin M (IgM) to IgG molecules. TCR activation and co-ligation of accessory molecules also lead to B-cell division and differentiation to antibody-producing plasma cells, a process facilitated by the Th2 cytokine release of mediators such as IL-4, IL-5, and IL-6.

Release of soluble antibodies by plasma cells forms the effector arm of the humoral immune response. Diversity of the antibody specificity is determined by a combinatorial set of genomic rearrangements between variable segments, constant segments, and diversity and joining segments. In addition to the huge diversity of antibody repertoire generated by such genomic combinatorial flexibility, antibody molecules undergo a process of affinity maturation, in which the immunoglobulin genes in mature B cells are mutated in a fashion leading to production of antibodies with higher antigen-binding affinity. Genetic defects in these B-cell maturation pathways generally lead to either hyper- or hypoproduction of immunoglobulin; genomic variation within the population of V segments is hypothesized to influence the B-cell repertoire for antigen specificity and to lead to more subtle phenotypic variation (McIntosh et al., 1998; Wiens et al., 1998; Kelsoe, 1999).

Immunologic Effectors beyond the T-Cell/B-Cell Sphere of Influence

Because of the broad distribution, circulatory patterns, and surveillance functions of the immune system, essentially all cells of the body are capable of some form of immune interaction. Most endothelial and epithelial cells can be induced by cytokines such as IFN-γ to acquire APC properties, e.g., and many secrete chemokines following activation. Complement components are serum proteins that bind to immunoglobulin molecules following antigen interaction and mediate additional forms of lytic effector functions. Additional hematopoietic lineages, such as natural killer (NK) cells, form a primitive form of lymphocyte, and neutrophils perform important surveillance and effector functions as well. NK cells are capable of killing cells that lack HLA class I molecules, a counterinsurgency immune response to loss of HLA expression in virus-infected cells and some tumors. NK cells express cell-surface receptors that transmit an inhibitory signal when occupied by a paired HLA class I molecule; thus, cells which have lost HLA expression, and therefore have avoided recognition by $CD8^+$ cytotoxic lymphocytes, release this inhibitory signal and are vulnerable to immune surveillance by NK cells (Raulet et al., 1997; Raulet, 1999). Together, all of these elements of the immune response provide broad and sometimes chaotic accompaniment to the more direct and specific form of immune activation directed by the MHC-restricted, antigen-specific T lymphocyte.

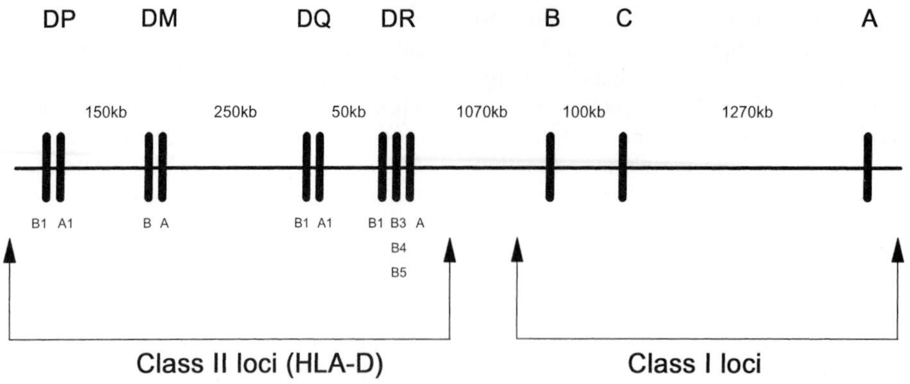

Fig. 28–3. Simplified map of the expressed genes of the HLA class I and class II regions.

Because of the central role for the T-cell response in terms of antigen recognition and genetic determinism, much attention has been focused on the specific nature of the MHC elements that restrict TCR recognition. As discussed in the next section, this focus on MHC elements underlying the genetic control of the immune response is validated and reinforced by the observation that only specific MHC genotypes are associated with particular autoimmune responses in clinical disease.

GENETIC CONTROL OF THE IMMUNE RESPONSE

The HLA region, also known as the human MHC, contains several multigene families located on the short arm of chromosome 6 (6p21.3). A simplified map for the HLA region is shown in Figure 28–3. Both the HLA class I and class II genes encode highly polymorphic cell-surface molecules that bind and present processed antigens in the form of peptides to T lymphocytes; recognition by the T cell of the HLA–peptide complex along with a costimulatory signal results in T-cell activation. Class I molecules, HLA-A, -B, and -C, are found on most nucleated cells. They are cell-surface proteins that present peptides derived primarily from endogenously synthesized proteins (e.g., viral and tumor peptides) to $CD8^+$ T cells. These heterodimers consist of an HLA-encoded α chain associated with a non-MHC-encoded, monomorphic polypeptide, β_2-microglobulin.

The HLA class II molecules consist of HLA-encoded α and β chains associated as heterodimers on the surface of APCs such as B cells, macrophages, and dendritic cells. Class II molecules, HLA-DR, -DQ, and -DP, serve as receptors for processed peptides, derived predominantly from membrane and extracellular proteins (e.g., bacterial peptides), and are presented to $CD4^+$ T cells. Both the HLA-DQ and -DP regions contain one functional gene for each of their α (*DQA1* and *DPA1*) and β (*DQB1* and *DPB1*) chains as well as the pseudogenes *DQA2*, *DQB2*, *DPA2*, and *DPB2*. The HLA-DR region, however, contains one functional gene for the α chain (*DRA*) but either one or two functional genes for the β chain, depending on the haplotype. All individuals express a DRB1-encoded polymorphic polypeptide, which is found on the cell surface in association with the monomorphic α chain, forming the main HLA-DR molecule. The other functional class II *DRB* genes, *DRB3*, *DRB4*, and *DRB5*, encode a β chain that forms a second cell-surface heterodimer with the *DRA*-encoded α chain. In general, the *DRB3* locus is found on haplotypes where *DRB1* is **03*, **11*, **12*, **13*, or **14*; the *DRB4* locus is found on haplotypes where *DRB1* is **04*, **07*, and **09*; and the *DRB5* locus is found on haplotypes where *DRB1* is **15* or **16* (previously *02). *DRB1*01*, **08*, and **10* haplotypes typically have only the *DRB1* locus (see Box 28–1).

Many other genes with important immune functions are found within the MHC. In the class III region, between the HLA-DR region (class II) and the HLA-B locus (class I), are found the complement genes encoding C2 and C4 as well as the TNF-α and -β loci. The MHC class I–associated chain A (MICA) and MICB loci (see below) are located just centromeric of HLA-B. The TAP1 and TAP2 loci are located between the DQ and DM loci. The TAP loci encode the peptide transporter molecules involved in loading the newly synthesized class I molecules in the endoplasmic reticulum with peptides derived from proteolysis of proteins in the cytoplasm by the proteosome. The LMP2 and LMP7 genes, located near the TAP loci, encode the IFN-γ-interferon inducible subunits of the proteosome. HLA-E and HLA-G are class I loci, whose polymorphism and tissue distribution are both much more limited than those of the classical HLA-A, -B, and -C genes. There are many other genes within the MHC whose function has not been elucidated. In general, these loci are much less polymorphic than the HLA class I and class II loci.

X-ray crystallographic structural studies have revealed that the outer domain of both class I molecules and the class II α–β heterodimers forms a peptide-binding groove, consisting of a β-

Box 28–1. HLA Nomenclature

The nomenclature for HLA polymorphism is complex and has, to some extent, proved something of a barrier to investigators outside the HLA field. Let us consider the DRB1 locus as an illustrative example. Serologically defined antigens (also known as serotypes or specificities) are designated as DR1, 2, 3, 4, 5, 6, 7, 8, 9, and 10. The DR2 serotype can be split into DR15 and DR16; DR3 can be split into DR17 and DR18; DR5 can be split into DR11 and DR12; and DR6 can be split into DR13 and DR14. In the WHO nomenclature for DNA sequence-defined alleles, the locus (e.g., DRB1) is followed by an asterisk (*) and two digits that identify the allele group (e.g., DRB1*04, which in this case corresponds to the DR4 serotype) and two digits that identify the allele or DR4 subtype (e.g., *DRB1*0401*, *DRB1*0402*, *DRB1*0403*). An additional digit is used to designate silent variants, ie., different nucleotide sequences that encode the same amino acid sequence (e.g., *DRB1*08041* and *08042*). For some loci, all alleles within a single allele group designation (e.g., HLA-B*15) do not necessarily encode the same serological type.

sheet floor and two α-helical walls (Stern et al., 1994; Jardetzky et al., 1996). Typically, the peptides bound in class I clefts are octamers or nonamers, with the ends of the peptide buried in pockets of the cleft (Bjorkman et al., 1987; Madden et al., 1991). Peptides bound in the class II groove are somewhat longer, usually 12 to 14 mer, with the ends protruding from the cleft. Based on the sequences of peptides eluted from purified HLA molecules, specific peptide-binding sequence motifs have been inferred for different class I and class II molecules (Falk et al., 1994; Barouch et al., 1995), allowing modeling of the interaction between these residues and the polymorphic residues within the pockets of the binding groove. Some polymorphic residues within the binding groove bind to the peptide, while others bind to the TCR (Garboczi et al., 1996). It is the complex of specific peptide bound within a given HLA antigen that is recognized by the TCR of $CD4^+$ cells for class II molecules and of $CD8^+$ cells for class I molecules.

ALLELIC DIVERSITY AND POPULATION GENETICS

HLA class I and class II genes are the most polymorphic coding sequences in the human genome. The number of alleles at these loci is listed in Table 28–3. Virtually all of this extensive sequence diversity is localized, for the class II loci, to the second exon and, for the class I loci, to the second and third exons. The HLA class II polymorphic second exon codes for the outer domain of the α and β chains, which together form the peptide-binding groove with its characteristic β-sheet floor and two α-helical walls. The first part of the second exon encodes the β-sheet floor and the second part encodes the α-helical wall of the groove (Fig. 28–2). For the class I molecule, the peptide-binding groove is formed by a single chain; the β-sheet floor and two α-helical walls are encoded by the second and third exons.

The patterns of allelic sequence diversity for both the class I and class II loci are highly unusual; some alleles differ in the second and third exons by as much as 15%, and the sequence variation is distributed as a patchwork of localized polymorphic sequence motifs. The allelic diversity at these loci is thought to have been generated by recombinational mechanisms such as gene conversion-like events or, to a lesser extent, by reciprocal recombination (Erlich and Gyllensten, 1991). Thus, new alleles appear to have been created by shuffling these polymorphic motifs. In addition, point mutation has contributed to sequence diversity at the HLA loci.

Although a very large number of alleles (e.g., >200 for HLA-DRB1) can be found in the global human population, a much smaller number (e.g., 30–50 for HLA-DRB1) is present in most individual populations, and many populations that have gone through bottlenecks or founding events (e.g., Native Americans) show more limited allelic diversity. In general, different populations tend to have different distributions of alleles as well as different patterns of linkage disequilibrium (Table 28–4).

Strong linkage disequilibrium is a striking feature of the population genetics of the HLA region. In all populations, particular haplotypes consisting of specific alleles at the linked HLA loci are found much more frequently than would be expected at random. For example, the *HLA-A*0101-HLA-B*0801-DRB1*0301* haplotype is common among Caucasians but not other groups. The linkage disequilibrium for this haplotype extends to the DPB locus (with the *DPB1*0101* allele), about 3 Mb telomeric of HLA-A. Although a variety of evolutionary forces can create linkage disequilibrium, selection for particular combinations of HLA alleles has been suggested as the primary cause for these extended haplotypes. This strong linkage disequilibrium makes it difficult to assess which allele or which combination of alleles on a disease-associated HLA haplotype is responsible for the observed correlations with disease. Because the patterns of linkage disequilibrium differ among various populations, disease association studies in many different ethnic groups can prove valuable in identifying the contributions of individual alleles. For example, the distribution of DR-DQ haplotypes bearing the *DRB1*0405* allele is strikingly different (Table 28–4) and, hence, informative with respect to discriminating between HLA-DR– and HLA-DQ–associated susceptibility to disease. Among Europeans, the haplotype *DRB*0405-DQB1*0302* is strongly associated with type I diabetes; among Africans, *DRB1*0405* can be coupled to *DQA1*0301* and *DQB1*0201*; in the Japanese and other Asian populations, it is coupled to *DQA1*0301* and *DQB1*0401*; and in the Philippines, it is coupled to *DQA1*0101* and *DQB1*0503*.

Table 28–3. Allelic Diversity at the Human Leukocyte Antigen (HLA) Class I and Class II Loci

Locus	No. of Alleles
HLA-A	120
HLA-B	250
HLA-C	70
DRA	2
DRB1	260
DRB3	11
DRB4	8
DRB5	12
DQA1	19
DQB1	36
DPA1	15
DPB1	84

HLA alleles based on the 1998 WHO Nomenclature Report (Bodmer et al., 1999). Alleles listed include silent variants, which represent a small minority of alleles at these loci.

Table 28–4. Different Populations Have Different Patterns of Linkage Disequilibrium: Global Distribution of HLA-DRB1*0405 Haplotypes

DRB1/DQA1/DQB1	Area
*0405/*0301/*0302	Europe
*0405/*0301/*0401/2	Asia
*0405/*0301/*0201	Africa
*0405/*0101/*0503	Philippines

HLA AND DISEASE

Linkage of genes within the HLA region to several different diseases has been demonstrated by cosegregation studies in families or with nonparametric approaches such as haplotype sharing among affected sib pairs. The genetic region identified by linkage studies can be large, on the order of 5 cM (5% recombination). Higher-resolution mapping of disease genes can be provided by disease association studies because these depend on strong linkage disequilibrium between the genetic marker and

Table 28–5. A Selected List of HLA-Associated Diseases

	HLA Antigen	Allele or Haplotype	Putative Autoantigen
		Class II	
Autoimmune/inflammatory			
IDDM[a]	DR3	DRB1*0301-DQB1*0201	Insulin
(Type I diabetes)	DR4	DRB1*04-DBQ1*0302	Glutamic acid decarboxylase-65, IA-2
	DR2 (protective)	DRB1*1501-DQB1*0602	
Multiple sclerosis	DR2	DRB1*1501-DQB1*0602	Unknown
Pemphigus vulgaris	DR4	DRB1*0402-DQB1*0302	Pe V antigen complex
	DR6	DRB1*1401-DQB1*0503	
Celiac disease	DR3	DRB1*0301-DQB1*0201	α-Gliaden
	DR7	DRB1*0701-DQB1*0201	
Rheumatoid arthritis (RA)	DR4	DRB1*0401, DRB1*0404, DRB1*0405	Unknown
Pauciarticular juvenile RA	DR8	DRB1*0801	Unknown
	DPw2	DRB1*0201	
Myasthenia gravis	DR3	DRB1*0301-DQB1*0201	Acetylcholine receptor
Stiffman's syndrome	DR3	DRB1*0301-DQB1*0201	Glutamic acid decarboxylase
		Class I	
Psoriasis	HLA-Cw6	HLA-C*06	Unknown
Ankylosing spondylitis	HLA-B27	HLA-B*27	Unknown
Behçets disease	HLA-Bw51	HLA-B*51	Unknown
Unknown etiology			
Narcolepsy	DR2	DRB1*1501-DQB1*0602	—

[a]The highest-risk DR4 alleles are *DRB1*0405*, **0402*, and **0401*; and the highest-risk genotype is the *DR3/DR4-DQB1*0302* heterozygote. IDDM, insulin-dependent diabetes mellitus.

the disease allele. In general, the association of a marker with a given disease implies that the genetic marker is significantly less than 1 cM away from the disease gene. In case-control association studies, the frequency of a given genetic marker among unrelated patients is compared with the frequency in matched controls. Although many parameters influence linkage disequilibrium, e.g., population history, age of the marker, and age of the disease alleles, in general, the strength of linkage disequilibrium is inversely related to physical distance. Thus, a strong association with a given disease suggests either that the associated marker locus is very close to the disease locus or that it may itself confer susceptibility to the disease.

For autoimmune diseases where the function of the HLA molecules is directly implicated in immune pathogenesis, it is likely that the HLA genes are not simply markers in linkage disequilibrium with some other disease locus but causally related to disease (see Potential Immunologic Mechanisms Underlying Disease Associations, below). HLA alleles that are positively associated with disease are referred to as *susceptible*, while negatively associated alleles are termed *protective*. Table 28–5 lists some of the most thoroughly studied diseases and their associated HLA alleles.

Most of these diseases are autoimmune disorders and the associations with specific HLA alleles have been demonstrated in numerous case-control studies in a variety of populations (reviewed by Tiwari and Terasaki, 1985). Most of these diseases are associated with alleles in the HLA class II region, but several, such as the well-known correlation of ankylosing spondylitis and HLA-B27, are associated with specific class I alleles. For some diseases, the associated HLA alleles confer a very high risk. The relative risk (RR) or odds ratio (OR, see below) for ankylosing spondylitis and B27 is well over 100. For other disease associations, such as multiple sclerosis and DR2, the RR is more modest, on the order of 3. For some diseases, there is a hierarchy of risk associated with different alleles and genotypes rather than a single predisposing allele. For type I diabetes, the RR for the heterozygous genotype *DR3/DR4-DQB1*0302* is about 30 to 40 while the RR for *DR3/DR3* and *DR4/DR4-DQB1*0302* homozygotes is around 5 to 8 and *DR1/DR4-DQB1*0302* and *DR4-DQB1*0302/DR8* heterozygotes confer a lesser but significant risk. The DR4-associated susceptibility to type I diabetes reflects contributions both from the DQB1 locus, where **0302* but not **0301* is associated with disease, as well as from the DRB1 locus, where **0401*, **0402*, and **0405* are disease-associated. The *DRB*0403-DQB1*0302* haplotype is negatively associated with type I diabetes. This pattern of disease association, involving specific combinations of HLA alleles, found either in *cis* in haplotypes or in *trans* in genotypes, has been observed in other diseases as well.

Some associations are negative, suggesting a protective role for the associated alleles or haplotypes, such as DR2 and Type 1 diabetes. The RR for the DR2 haplotype common among Caucasians, *DRB1*1501-DQB1*0602*, is around 0.05. Other DR2 haplotypes are not negatively associated with Type 1 diabetes; based on the disease association observed with various DR2 haplotypes, the dominant protection conferred by the *DRB1*1501-DQB1*0602* haplotype appears to be attributable to the *DQB1*0602* allele.

With the advent of DNA-based typing methods, it has become possible to evaluate the role of individual polymorphic amino acid residues in HLA disease associations. Comparing a sequence that is disease-associated with closely related sequences that are not can point to specific polymorphic sequence motifs and, given the known structure, to specific pockets in the peptide-binding groove as functionally important in disease susceptibility or resistance. For example, comparing *DRB1*0402* (associated with pemphigus vulgaris) to the other DR4 alleles or *DRB1*0103* (associated with inflammatory bowel disease) to the other DR1 alleles implicates the motif I-DE in the third hypervariable region (codons 67–71), which is common to both alleles (Scharf et al., 1989; Trachtenberg et al., 1999). The role of DQB1 position 57 in Type 1 diabetes susceptibility based on the negative association of Asp^{57} with disease is well known (Todd et al., 1987), but the susceptibility of a given haplotype cannot be predicted by the presence of an individual amino acid residue. Clearly, there are some haplotypes that contain DQB1 Asp^{57}

Table 28–6. Definition of Risk Estimates

	Marker +	Marker −
Disease +	*a*	*b*
Disease −	*c*	*d*

Odds ratio (relative risk[a]) $= \dfrac{ad}{cb}$

Absolute risk $= \dfrac{a/(a+b)}{c/(c+d)} \times$ disease incidence

Etiologic fraction (population attributable risk) $= \dfrac{[a/(a+b) - c/(c+d)]}{1 - [c/(c+d)]}$

a, number of patients with marker; *b*, number of patients without marker; *c*, number of controls with marker; *d*, number of controls without marker.

[a]The relative risk used by epidemiologists for prospective studies differs slightly from the odds ratio used in case-control studies and is defined as $a/(a+c)/b(b+d)$. For rare diseases where *a* and *b* are small relative to *c* and *d*, this expression approximates the odds ratio.

(e.g., *DRB1*0801-DQB1*0402* in Caucasians or *DRB1*0405-DQB1*0402* in Asians) and are positively associated with type I diabetes (Nepom and Erlich, 1991).

Risk Estimates

As noted above, a variety of diseases have been associated with specific HLA class I or class II alleles. Risk estimates for the disease-associated marker can be calculated based on the distribution of the marker in patients and controls. The mathematical definitions of various parameters used to estimate genetic risk are shown in Table 28–6. The OR (or RR) gives the probability that someone with the specific marker will get a given disease relative to someone without the marker. *Absolute risk* refers to the probability that someone with the marker will get the disease; this estimate is related to the disease incidence. The *etiologic fraction* (or *population attributable risk*) measures what proportion of the disease risk can be attributed to this gene.

Studies of multiplex families or of affected sib pairs also allow one to estimate the proportion of the total genetic risk attributable to a given genetic region defined by a specific marker; this approach involves calculating a value (λ) from the ratio of expected to observed affected sib pairs that share zero haplotypes (Risch, 1987). For insulin-dependent diabetes mellitus (IDDM), e.g., the observed proportion of affected sib pairs sharing zero HLA haplotypes is about 0.06 and the expected proportion is 0.25, yielding a λ for HLA of about 4.1. For IDDM, the familial clustering or sibling risk ratio (total λ), the ratio of sibling risk to population prevalence, is about 15. This familial clustering ratio may include components of both genetic risk and shared environmental factors. A value of about 50% for the proportion of familial clustering attributable to the HLA region (Noble et al., 1996) can be calculated, making certain assumptions from these estimates of λ.

Potential Immunologic Mechanisms Underlying Disease Associations

Although most diseases associated with HLA are autoimmune or inflammatory in nature, HLA polymorphism may also influence certain infectious diseases and cancers. HLA associations have been reported for cervical cancer, Hodgkin's disease, and nasopharyngeal carcinoma (Apple et al., 1994; Klitz et al., 1994; Liebowitz, 1994), which have a viral etiology as well. Cervical carcinoma and precancerous cervical lesions are caused by human papillomavirus, while Hodgkin's disease and nasopharyngeal carcinoma are associated with Epstein-Barr virus. Relatively few studies of infectious diseases have revealed strong HLA associations, although specific HLA-B and HLA-DRB1 alleles have been associated with resistance to severe malaria in African populations (Hill et al., 1992) and other HLA alleles have been associated with leprosy, tuberculosis, and hepatitis (Hill, 1998). In general, the fundamental mechanisms underlying these HLA disease associations are not fully understood.

Some diseases are clearly associated with specific HLA alleles because these alleles are in linkage disequilibrium with disease-causing mutations or polymorphic variants at a nearby locus (see Role of Non-HLA Genes within the MHC in Disease, below). For systemic lupus erythematosus (SLE), complement deficiencies appear to play a role in pathogenesis; the *C4A* null allele in linkage disequilibrium with the B8-DR3 haplotype may account for the DR3 association with SLE observed in Caucasians (Arnett and Reveille, 1992). For many of the HLA-associated diseases, however, the observed association is likely due to variation in the amino acid sequence of the HLA molecules themselves.

The primary function of the HLA class I and class II molecules is to bind antigenic peptides and present them to $CD8^+$ and $CD4^+$ T cells, respectively. The differential predisposition for some autoimmune diseases associated with certain HLA alleles could simply reflect the ability of a particular HLA molecule to bind and present a specific peptide derived from an autoantigen. For example, the autoimmune dermatologic disease pemphigus vulgaris is associated with the DR4 subtypes, *DRB1*0402-DQB1*0302*, as well as the *DRB1*1401-DQB1*0503* haplotype (Scharf et al., 1988, 1989). Peptides derived from the putative autoantigen PeV antigen complex have been shown to bind to the *DRB1*0402*-encoded molecule but not to other DR4 molecules. Presumably, the *DRB1*1401-DQB1*0503* association reflects either other peptides or other mechanisms (see below).

In addition to their role in antigen presentation, class I and class II molecules shape the developing T-cell repertoire in the thymus. As noted above, T cells that react strongly with self-peptides and self-MHC are clonally deleted. Thus, another potential explanation for HLA disease association is that certain allelic polymorphisms in HLA molecules might influence positive or negative selection such that certain V_{beta} TCR-expressing T cells are eliminated from the periphery or the repertoire of T cells available for antigen reactivity is altered. A potential mechanism of thymic elimination of particular T-cell clones is, in principle, consistent with the dominant protection observed for DR2 and Type 1 diabetes (see above).

Another model for HLA disease associations involves differential stimulation of the class II–restricted $CD4^+$ helper subsets Th1 and Th2. As noted above, each of these distinct subpopulations produces its own set of cytokines and mediates separate effector functions. Preferential simulation of the Th1 subset appears to play a role in several autoimmune diseases. Thus, while susceptible and resistant HLA alleles may encode molecules that present peptides from the same autoantigen, they may bind different subsets of peptides or bind peptides with different affinities and thereby stimulate different subsets of T cells. An additional model for a class II protective role has been proposed, suggesting that susceptible and protective alleles compete with peptides during the processing of autoantigens, resulting in reduced levels of susceptible class II–autoantigen complexes for T-cell activation (Nepom, 1990).

Yet another proposed mechanism suggests that it is the genetic variation in regulatory regions affecting gene expression, such as promoter sequences, rather than the coding sequence polymorphism that is responsible for the observed HLA disease associations. While regulatory sequence polymorphism remains a plausible model for many candidate gene (e.g., cytokine and cytokine receptor loci) disease associations, this hypothesis requires linkage disequilibrium with the coding sequence variation identified by serologic or DNA-based typing to account for the HLA association. Several alternative mechanisms have also been proposed. Different disease associations may reflect different mechanisms.

Role of Non-HLA Genes within the MHC in Disease

There are a variety of non-HLA genes within or near the MHC that may be responsible for several HLA-associated diseases. Some of these diseases have no obvious immunopathology. For example, hereditary hemochromatosis, an autosomal recessive disease of excessive iron storage associated with HLA-A3, is now known to result from a mutation in the *HFE* locus, a class I-like gene, whose product associates with β_2-microglobulin and is involved in iron transport (Feder et al., 1996). The *HFE* locus is about 3 Mb telomeric of HLA-A, and the C282Y mutation, present in homozygous form in the vast majority of Caucasian patients, is in strong linkage disequilibrium with HLA-A3. Mutations in the *21-OH* locus, located between the DR region and HLA-B, give rise to congenital adrenal hyperplasia. A puzzling and intriguing example of an HLA-associated disease is narcolepsy, a condition with no evidence of immunopathology yet strongly associated with the DQB1 allele *0602, with no evidence for another nearby disease gene (Ellis et al., 1997).

There are also several non-HLA genes within the MHC with an immunologic function that have been implicated in disease susceptibility. Polymorphisms in the promoter of the TNF-α locus have been associated with several autoimmune as well as infectious diseases (Hill, 1998; Knight et al., 1999). These polymorphisms are thought to affect the level of TNF-α produced in response to certain stimuli. Null alleles at the *C4* locus (a component in the complement cascade) appear to contribute to several diseases, including SLE.

The role of the MICA and MICB loci, about 45 kB centromeric of HLA-B, remains unclear. These genes encode a class I-like glycoprotein that may serve as a ligand/restriction element for the TCR of γ–δ T cells. There are over 25 alleles at each of these loci (Ando et al., 1997). It has been suggested that certain alleles of MICA and/or MICB may predispose to certain HLA-associated diseases, such as Behçet's disease or celiac disease. This latter disease is an interesting candidate because it appears to involve the action of γ–δ T cells in the gut. However, the issue of linkage disequilibrium with disease-associated B locus alleles (e.g., B51), in the case of Behçet's disease, or DR-DQ haplotypes (e.g., DR3-DQ2), in the case of celiac disease, will have to be examined carefully to assess the true role of polymorphism at these loci in disease susceptibility.

Non-MHC Disease Genes

Although the HLA loci and, possibly, other genes within the MHC play a critical role in many autoimmune and inflammatory diseases, other genes also contribute significantly to disease risk. Linkage studies using segregation analyses (parametric) and haplotype sharing among affected sib pairs (nonparametric, see above) have been carried out for a variety of diseases, notably Type 1 diabetes, multiple sclerosis, and inflammatory bowel disease, using genome-wide scans with microsatellite markers (Todd and Farrall, 1996; Ohmen et al., 1996; Kuokkanen et al., 1997). These studies have identified several regions of significant linkage, including the MHC, for all of these diseases, although not all studies of the same disease have implicated the same chromosomal locations (Becker et al., 1998). In general, the genes responsible for the disease linkage to a chromosomal region have not been identified, and extensive association studies with candidate genes and anonymous genetic markers mapping in these regions are under way in many laboratories. For example, association studies carried out in several populations suggest that the insulin (chromosome 11p15) and the CTLA4 (chromosome 2q33) loci may be involved in susceptibility to type I diabetes (reviewed by Todd and Farrall, 1996).

Celiac Disease: An Informative Example

Celiac disease (CD) is an inflammatory autoimmune disease of the intestinal mucosa, elicited by ingestion of wheat gluten or gliadin. In terms of elucidating immunologic mechanisms, CD is one of the most informative of the HLA-associated diseases because the pathogenic antigen is known and antigen-specific T cells can be recovered from the gut and analyzed in vitro. In terms of identifying the molecule responsible for the observed disease association with the DRB1*0301-DQA1*0501-DQB1*0201 and DRB1*0701-DQA1*0201-DQB1*0201 haplotypes, the genetics of CD is also instructive. The strongest associations with CD are with the DR3 haplotype (DRB1*0301-DQA1*0501-DQB1*0201) and the genotype DR11/DR7 (DRB1*11-DQA1*0501-DQB1*0301/DRB1*0701-DQA1*0201-DQB1*0201). A unifying interpretation of this association pattern is that the molecule responsible for the disease association is the DQ heterodimeric molecule with the α chain encoded by DQA1*0501 and the β chain encoded by DQB1*0201 (Sollid et al., 1989). This molecule is encoded in *cis* by the DR3 haplotype and formed as a *trans*-complementing heterodimer in a DR11/DR7 heterozygote. This model represents strong evidence that the HLA polymorphism associated with CD is not simply a genetic marker in linkage disequilibrium with some other disease gene but is causally related to disease susceptibility.

T cells have been isolated from the gut of CD patients that recognize specific peptides in the context of the DQ2 molecule. The sequence analysis of peptides bound to the molecule encoded by DQA1*0501 and -0201 has been determined and the binding motif identified (Vartdal et al., 1996). Surprisingly, this motif, which contains glutamic acid, is not found in gliadin and other components of wheat gluten. The resolution to this apparent paradox was the discovery of an enzyme, tissue transglutaminase, present in the gut. This enzyme converts glutamine to glutamic acid in gliadin, creating peptides that are bound by the DQ2 molecule and presented to T cells. Increased levels of tissue transglutaminase have been observed in jejunal biopsies of patients, and antibodies to this enzyme are a hallmark of CD (van de Wal et al., 1998). Thus, the genetics of CD can be best explained by preferential binding and presentation of a modified gliadin peptide by the DQ molecule encoded by the disease-associated alleles DQA*0501 and DQB1*0201. Demonstration of the role of this DQ molecule in CD does not mean, however, that other genes within (see above) and outside the MHC do not also contribute to genetic susceptibility for this disease. As noted above, multiple genes as well as environmental factors are likely to be involved in all of the many diseases associated with specific HLA alleles.

Serologic and Cellular HLA Typing Methods

Historically, HLA typing has been performed using a combination of the serologic microcytotoxity and, in special cases, the mixed lymphocyte reaction assays. In the microcytotoxicity assay, which can be used to type both class I and II antigens, an antiserum (or monoclonal antibody) is mixed with live lymphocytes and allowed to bind to the cell-surface molecules. Specific binding is then detected with the addition of complement, which lyses the cells and allows the uptake of a dye. The microcytotoxicity assay requires viable cells and uses antisera obtained primarily from individuals who have been sensitized to HLA differences, such as multiparous women or individuals who have received multiple transfusions. Consequently, these reagents are limiting in quantity and difficult to standardize. Although, as noted above, about 200 DRB1 alleles (different amino acid sequences) have been identified, serologic reagents can distinguish only 15 different groups of DR molecules encoded by these alleles.

DNA-Based Techniques

Over the last two decades, molecular genetic techniques have been used to isolate the genes encoding the HLA class I and class II molecules and to characterize their genomic organization. Development of the polymerase chain reaction (PCR) in the mid-1980s greatly facilitated the analysis of sequence polymorphism at both the class I and II loci. Based on the available database of class II allelic sequence diversity, a variety of relatively simple and rapid PCR-based methods have been developed to carry out HLA class II typing at the DNA level. The first approaches utilized labeled sequence-specific oligonucleotide (SSO) probes to hybridize to PCR products amplified from the sample and immobilized on a nylon or nitrocellulose filter, the dot blot method (Saiki et al., 1989). Under appropriate hybridization and wash conditions, these SSO probes would bind only to the complementary sequence in the amplified DNA and were able to distinguish single-nucleotide differences. Given enough primers and probes, the SSO method is, in principle, capable of distinguishing all of the alleles at a given HLA locus.

Another approach, based on the specificity of primer extension rather than probe hybridization, has also been applied to HLA typing. This method is known variously as allele-specific amplification, sequence-specific priming, and the amplification refractory mutation system (Newton et al., 1989). Here, a specific primer pair is designed for each polymorphic sequence motif or pair of motifs, and the presence of the targeted polymorphic sequence in a sample is defined as a positive PCR, typically identified as a band on a gel. If the PCR is negative, the sample is assumed to lack one or both of the specific motifs. Allele-specific amplification can be used in conjunction with SSO probe typing for high-resolution typing. Other PCR-based methods, such as restriction fragment length polymorphism, single-strand conformation polymorphism, and directed heteroduplex analysis, have also been developed but are not widely used.

A new approach to SSO probe analysis of HLA polymorphism has been developed that facilitates DNA-based HLA typing. The conventional dot blot involved an immobilized PCR product hybridized to each of many labeled SSO probes. The reverse blot (or immobilized probe) method is based on hybridization of the PCR product, labeled with biotinylated primers during amplification, to an array of immobilized probes on a membrane (Saiki et al., 1989). This procedure requires only a single PCR and a single hybridization reaction to obtain information from the entire SSO probe panel; all of the probe reactivity information is contained on a single membrane, making it amenable to automated data interpretation.

Chain termination DNA sequencing using electrophoresis on a slab gel or capillary electrophoresis is also used for high-resolution HLA typing. In general, different DNA typing methods are appropriate for different uses, depending on the cost and the level of resolution and throughput required.

CLINICAL APPLICATIONS

Transplantation

In the transplantation of solid organs and bone marrow stem cells, differences in the HLA class I and class II molecules (sometimes referred to as antigens due to the serologic typing methods used in the past) between donor and recipient can elicit alloreactive T-cell responses in the host and result in either acute or chronic donor graft rejection. For bone marrow transplantation, however, the most critical clinical issue is graft-vs.-host disease, the attack of the host tissue by activated alloreactive donor T cells in the graft. (For patients with leukemia, this alloreactivity has some beneficial consequences and is referred to as the *graft-vs.-leukemia effect.*) For most solid organ transplants, HLA matching for donor and recipient is only one of many issues to be considered and, given current immunosuppressive protocols, even transplants using mismatched organs can have a good outcome. However, HLA matching of donor and recipients is particularly important for bone marrow stem cell transplantation, and matching at 6/6 or 5/6 antigens (both alleles at the HLA-A, -B, and -DR loci) is typically required for a bone marrow transplant. An HLA-matched sibling is the best-matched donor since he or she has inherited the same HLA haplotypes as the recipient, but for most patients, such a donor is not available. Registries for unrelated bone marrow donors have been established in many parts of the world; the U.S. National Marrow Donor Program now has well over three million donors, making the identification of a matched unrelated donor much more likely for those patients who do not have a matched sibling. In general, the move from serologic typing to DNA-based typing has resulted in much more precise matching and, consequently, a reduction in graft-vs.-host disease and improved survival in bone marrow transplantation (Petersdorf et al., 1998). Transplants involving stem cells from umbilical cord blood have been performed with considerable success (Kurtzberg et al., 1996; Hurley et al., 1999). These initial studies have suggested that, because there appear to be fewer activated T cells in the cord blood than in the bone marrow of adults, it may be possible to successfully transplant patients with 4/6 antigen matches. If true, this property of cord blood stem cell transplants would be very important for patients with rare HLA types who fail to find a 5/6 or 6/6 match in the bone marrow donor registries.

HLA-DR Genotyping for Clinical Utility in Rheumatoid Arthritis

As noted above, specific HLA class II alleles are associated with rheumatoid arthritis (RA), with risk in Caucasoid populations increased 5- to 10-fold for individuals with specific *HLA-DR4* genes, such as *DRB1*0401* and *DRB1*0404*. However, these same alleles are prevalent in the normal population, so screening for disease susceptibility based on the presence of these alleles is not highly predictive and not clinically indicated. The absolute risk to an individual positive for one of these specific *DR4* susceptibility alleles is, on average, only 8% (range 5% to 12%) compared to a population prevalence of approximately 1% (Nepom and Nepom, 1992). In addition, there is marked clinical heterogeneity in the spectrum of RA associated with these HLA genes. While 80% to 90% of patients with longstanding erosive forms of RA are positive for the *DR4* susceptibility alleles, only 55% to 65% of newly diagnosed RA patients carry these same alleles. This observation has been the subject of considerable clinical interest as it appears to indicate that patients diagnosed with RA represent a spectrum of clinical heterogeneity which is caused in part by an underlying genetic heterogeneity. Indeed, further studies have shown that the *DR4* susceptibility genes are most prevalent in patients with rheumatoid factor and severe erosive RA and that other class II susceptibility genes, such as *DRB1*0101*, are markers for a broader clinical spectrum, which includes seronegative and nonerosive forms of RA (Nepom and Nepom, 1998).

This genetic distinction between severe erosive RA and other forms of polyarthritis has potential clinical utility for prognosis. When individuals newly diagnosed with RA are analyzed, the presence of *DR4* RA susceptibility alleles (e.g., *DRB1*0401* or **0404*) is predictive of progression to erosive disease. For example, in studies of patients who met clinical criteria for RA but did not yet have erosive disease (X-ray evidence of joint erosions), there was excellent correlation between the presence of *DR4* susceptibility alleles and the likelihood of onset of erosive disease within 2 years (Gough et al., 1994; Wagner et al., 1997; Valenzuela et al., 1999). Patients who lacked these *DR4* susceptibility genes had a high frequency of nonerosive polyarthritis and a low frequency of erosive and progressive RA. In other studies using unselected RA patients, there was little additional prognostic value shown for use of these genetic tests in patients who already had erosive disease, indicating that the positive predictive value of *DR4* analysis is limited to use in early patients who do not yet have severe disease (Seidl et al., 1999).

Therefore, while the association between *HLA-DR* genes and RA suggests a role for HLA molecules in disease susceptibility, the current practical clinical utility lies in the association between specific RA-susceptibility alleles and prognosis for progressive erosive forms of disease. *HLA-DR4* genetic analysis is potentially useful in this regard as a means to select patients for alternative forms of therapy. In a randomized clinical trial comparing an aggressive form of multidrug therapy for RA with a single-drug regimen, there was a marked distinction in clinical outcome that corresponded to the *HLA-DR4* genetic analysis (O'Dell et al., 1998). The *DR4*-negative patients, as expected, had overall a milder disease course over the 2-year clinical trial and they responded well to both arms of the clinical trial; i.e., patients treated with the single-drug regimen responded to therapy with an excellent clinical outcome (83% response). In contrast, the *DR4*-positive patients who were randomized to the single-drug regimen did very poorly, with a marginal (32%) clinical response. The *DR4*-positive patients who received the multidrug treatment, however, had a 94% response rate, which was comparable to the *DR4*-negative groups (88%). Thus, use of *HLA-DR4* genetic typing to influence the selection of aggressive vs. standard therapies in RA for newly diagnosed Caucasoid patients, i.e., those who do not yet have joint erosions, may be a valuable adjunct to medical management in this disease.

HLA Genotyping for Prediction of IDDM Susceptibility

Autoimmune diabetes (juvenile diabetes, Type 1 diabetes) is a complex immunologic cascade in which genetic susceptibility underlies the immune activation events that lead to disease. The immunologic consequence of this genetically controlled activation is chronic progressive destruction of insulin-producing islet cells, which may occur for months or years before identification of insulin deficiency and clinical diabetes. This long prediabetic interval provides an opportunity to use genetic typing for identification of at-risk individuals, with the hope of future intervention and disease prevention.

A number of different screening strategies for identifying diabetes risk have been suggested. In the United States, screening programs are currently designated as research protocols and utilize HLA class II genotyping as a means to select initial individuals of interest. As noted above, the HLA genes most closely associated with IDDM in the United States are the *HLA-DQB1*0302* and *DQB1*0201* alleles at the *DQ* locus on haplotypes containing the linked *HLA-DRB1*04* and **03* alleles, respectively. Relatively simple genotyping for these alleles identifies haplotypes associated with increased risk of IDDM. The highest-risk genotype for IDDM is the *DR3-DQB1*0201,DR4-DQB1*0302* heterozygote; this genotype is present in 30% to 40% of Caucasian patients but only 2% to 3% of the general population. However, there are also notable genetic modifiers in IDDM, including other genes within the HLA class II complex (Nepom and Erlich, 1991; Noble et al., 1996). Thus, the *DQB1*0602* allele is associated with protection from IDDM, even in individuals heterozygous for one of the IDDM-susceptibility haplotypes. Moreover, not all *DR4* subtypes confer equal risk. At the *DRB1* locus, the presence of alleles such as *DRB1*0403* indicates a lower disease risk, even on haplotypes containing *DQB1*0302*. Other genes both within and outside the MHC also appear to contribute to genetic risk. Thus, HLA testing to assess genetic risk is complex, and interpretation of risk associated with inheritance of known susceptibility genes will benefit from additional genotype analysis. This is a particular consideration also for non-Caucasoid populations, where the information about susceptibility and resistance genes in IDDM is less complete.

Estimates for the risk of IDDM vary according to HLA genotype, family history, ethnicity, and age. Since the association between high-risk HLA alleles and IDDM is highest in the youngest age groups, current genetic screening strategies based on HLA genes are intended for use in children and newborn populations. The highest HLA risk group, individuals heterozygous for the *DR3-DQB1*0201* and *DR4-DQB1*0302* haplotypes in Caucasian populations, is estimated to have an absolute risk of IDDM of about 10% compared to a population prevalence of 0.4%. Risks for individuals who carry only one of these HLA-susceptibility haplotypes are, of course, lower, and risks for individuals with the protective *HLA DQB1*0602* gene are <0.1%. Since these HLA-susceptibility genes are also prevalent in the nondiabetic population, efforts have been made to improve the predictive value of genetic screening by addition of immunologic tests that measure autoantibodies to several islet cell autoantigens, such as GAD65 and insulin (Gottlieb and Eisenbarth, 1998). This strategy is based on the rationale that genetic susceptibility is an underlying risk factor that permits the immune system to initiate an activation pathway directed against the insulin-producing islet cell. After such immune activation has occurred but before the clinical onset of diabetes, plasma antibodies that serve as a second tier to the IDDM risk-assessment process are detectable. Thus, HLA genetic testing can identify a subset of high-risk individuals for periodic monitoring for the appearance of islet cell autoantibodies.

SUMMARY

The immune system is a complex network of interacting molecules and cells. Many of the genes specifying components of the immune system are polymorphic and likely to lead to variation in specific immune responses to foreign and self-antigens (autoimmunity). In fact, the HLA class I and class II loci are the most polymorphic coding sequences in the human genome. Susceptibility and protection to a variety of diseases, many of which are common human disorders, are associated with specific alleles at HLA class I and class II loci. Other loci within the MHC as well as those in the rest of the genome, such as cytokine and cytokine receptor genes, are also likely to influence disease susceptibility and progression. Recent developments in the genetic analysis of complex diseases are likely to have a significant clinical impact on the ability to predict disease predisposition as well as disease severity.

REFERENCES

Alberola-Ila J, Hogquist KA, Swan KA, Bevan MJ, Perlmutter RM: Positive and negative selection invoke distinct signaling pathways. J Exp Med 1996; 184:9–18.

Anderson G, Hare KJ, Platt N, Jenkinson EJ: Discrimination between maintenance and differentiation-inducing signals during initial and intermediate stages of positive selection. Eur J Immunol 1997; 27:1838–1842.

Ando H, Mizuki N, Ota M, Yamazaki M, Ohno S, Goto K, Miyata Y, Wakisaka K, Bahram S, Inoko H: Allelic variants of the human MHC class I chain–related B gene (*MICB*). Immunogenetics 1997; 46:499–508.

Apple RJ, Erlich HA, Klitz W, Manos MM, Becker TM, Wheeler CM: HLA DR-DQ associations with cervical carcinoma show papillomavirus-type specificity. Nat Genet 1994; 6:157–162.

Arnett F, Reveille JD: Genetics of systemic lupus erythematosus. In: Nepom GT (ed). Rheumatic Disease Clinics of North America. Philadelphia: WB Saunders, 1992:865–892.

Baggiolini M, Dewald B, Moser B: Human chemokines: an update. Annu Rev Immunol 1997; 15:675–705.

Barouch D, Friede T, Stevanovic S, Tussey L, Smith K, Rowland J, Braud V, McMichael A, Rammensee HG: HLA-A2 subtypes are functionally distinct in peptide binding and presentation. J Exp Med 1995; 182:1847–1856.

Becker KG, Simon RM, Bailey-Wilson JE, Freidlin B, Biddison WE, McFarland HF, Trent JM: Clustering of non-major histocompatibility complex susceptibility candidate loci in human autoimmune diseases. Proc Natl Acad Sci USA 1998; 95:9979–9984.

Benoist C, Mathis D: Positive selection of the T cell repertoire: where and when does it occur? Cell 1989; 58:1027–1033.

Benschop RJ, Cambier JC: B cell development: signal transduction by antigen receptors and their surrogates. Curr Opin Immunol 1999; 11:143–151.

Bevan MJ: In thymic selection, peptide diversity gives and takes away. Immunity 1997; 7:175–178.

Bjorkman PJ, Saper MA, Samraoui B, Bennett WS, Strominger JL, Wiley DC: The foreign antigen binding site and T cell recognition regions of class I histocompatibility antigens. Nature 1987; 329:512–518.

Bodmer JG, Marsh SGE, Albert ED, Bodmer WF, Bontrop RE, Erlich HA, Hansen JA, Mach B, Mayr WR, Parham P, et al.: Nomenclature for factors of the HLA system, 1998. Tissue Antigens 1999; 53:407–446.

Boniface JJ, Rabinowitz JD, Wulfing C, Hampl J, Reich Z, Altman JD, Kantor RM, Beeson C, McConnell HM, Davis MM: Initiation of signal transduction through the T cell receptor requires the multivalent engagement of peptide/MHC ligands. Immunity 1998; 9:459–466.

Braciale TJ, Braciale VL: Antigen presentation: structural themes and functional variations. Immunol Today 1991; 12:124–129.

Chen L, Ashe S, Brady WA, Hellstrom I, Hellstrom KE, Ledbetter JA, McGowan P, Linsley PS: Costimulation of antitumor immunity by the B7 counterreceptor for the T lymphocyte molecules CD28 and CTLA-4. Cell 1992; 71:1093–1102.

Constant SL, Bottomly K: Induction of Th1 and Th2 $CD4^+$ T cell responses: the alternative approaches. Annu Rev Immunol 1997; 15:297–322.

Croft M, Dubey C: Accessory molecule and costimulation requirements for CD4 T cell response. Crit Rev Immunol 1997; 17:89–118.

De Vries JE, Carballido JM, Aversa G: Receptors and cytokines involved in allergic TH2 cell responses. J Allergy Clin Immunol 1999; 103:S492–S496.

Ellis MC, Hetisimer AH, Ruddy DA, Hansen SL, Kronmal GS, McClelland, Quintana L, Drayna DT, Aldrich MS, Mignot E: HLA class II haplotype and sequence analysis support a role for DQ in narcolepsy. Immunogenetics 1997; 46:410–417.

Engelhard VH: Structure of peptides associated with class I and class II MHC molecules. Annu Rev Immunol 1994; 12:181–207.

Erlich HA, Gyllensten UB: Shared epitopes among HLA class II alleles: gene conversion, common ancestry and balancing selection. Immunol Today 1991; 12:411–414.

Falk K, Rötzschke O, Stevanovic S, Jung G, Rammensee HG: Pool sequencing of natural HLA-DR, DQ, and DP ligands reveals detailed peptide motifs, constraints of processing, and general rules. Immunogenetics 1994; 39:230–242.

Feder JN, Gnirke A, Thomas W, Tsuchihashi Z, Ruddy DA, Basava A, Dormishian F, Domingo RJ, Ellis MC, Fullan A, et al.: A novel MHC class I-like gene is mutated in patients with hereditary haemochromatosis. Nat Genet 1996; 13:399–408.

Garboczi DN, Ghosh P, Utz U, Fan QR, Biddison WE, Wiley DC: Structure of the complex between human T-cell receptor, viral peptide and HLA-A2. Nature 1996; 384:134–141.

Gottlieb PA, Eisenbarth GS: Diagnosis and treatment of pre-insulin dependent diabetes. Annu Rev Med 1998; 49:391–405.

Gough A, Faint J, Salmon M, Hassell A, Wordsworth P, Pilling D, Birley A, Emery P: Genetic typing of patients with inflammatory arthritis at presentation can be used to predict outcome. Arthritis Rheum 1994; 37:1166–1170.

Hill AV: The immunogenetics of human infectious diseases. Annu Rev Immunol 1998; 16:593–617.

Hill AV, Elvin J, Willis AC, Aidoo M, Allsopp CE, Gotch FM, Gao XM, Takiguchi M, Greenwood BM, Townsend AR: Molecular analysis of the association of HLA-B53 and resistance to severe malaria. Nature 1992; 360:434–439.

Hurley CK, Wade JA, Oudshoorn M, Middleton D, Kukuruga D, Navarrete C, Christiansen F, Hegland J, Ren E-C, Andersen I, et al.: A special report: histocompatibility testing guidelines for hematopoietic stem cell transplantation using volunteer donors. Tissue Antigens 1999; 53:394–406.

Itoh Y, Hemmer B, Martin R, Germain RN: Serial TCR engagement and down-modulation by peptide:MHC molecule ligands: relationship to the quality of individual TCR signaling events. J Immunol 1999; 162:2073–2080.

Jardetzky TS, Brown JH, Gorga JC, Stern LJ, Urban RG, Strominger JL, Wiley DC: Crystallographic analysis of endogenous peptide associated with HLA-DR1 suggests a common, polyproline II-like conformation for bound peptides. Proc Natl Acad Sci USA 1996; 93:734–738.

Jenkins MK, Johnson JG: Molecules involved in T-cell costimulation. Curr Opin Immunol 1993; 5:361–367.

Kelsoe G: V(D)J hypermutation and receptor revision: coloring outside the lines. Curr Opin Immunol 1999; 11:70–75.

Kisielow P, Teh HS, Blüthmann H, von Boehmer H: Positive selection of antigen-specific T cells in thymus by restricting MHC molecules. Nature 1988; 335:730–733.

Kisielow P, von Boehmer H: Development and selection of T cells: facts and puzzles. Adv Immunol 1995; 58:87–209.

Klitz W, Aldrich CL, Fildes N, Horning SJ, Begovich AB: Localization of predisposition to Hodgkin disease in the HLA class II region. Am J Hum Genet 1994; 54:497–505.

Knight JC, Udalova I, Hill AVS, Greenwood BM, Peshu N, Marsh K, Kwiatowski D: A polymorphism that affects OCT-1 binding to the TNF promoter region is associated with severe malaria. Nat Genet 1999; 22:145–150.

Kurtzberg J, Laughlin M, Graham ML, Smith C, Olson JF, Halperin EC, Ciocci G, Carrier C, Stevens CE, Rubinstein P: Placental blood as a source of hematopoietic stem cells for transplantation into unrelated recipients. N Engl J Med 1996; 335:157–166.

Kuokkanen S, Gschwend M, Rioux JD, Daly MJ, Terwilliger JD, Tienari PJ, Wikstrom J, Palo J, Stein LD, Hudson TJ, et al.: Genome-wide scan of multiple sclerosis in Finnish multiplex families. Am J Hum Genet 1997; 61:1379–1387.

Lee KM, Chuang E, Griffin M, Khattri R, Hong DK, Zhang W, Straus D, Samelson LE, Thompson CB, Bluestone JA: Molecular basis of T cell inactivation by CTLA-4. Science 1998; 282:2263–2266.

Lenschow DJ, Walunas TL, Bluestone JA: CD28/B7 system of T cell costimulation. Annu Rev Immunol 1996; 14:233–258.

Liebowitz D: Nasopharyngeal carcinoma: the Epstein-Barr virus association. Semin Oncol 1994; 21:376–381.

Madden DR, Gorga JC, Strominger JL, Wiley DC: The structure of HLA-B27 reveals nonamer self-peptides bound in an extended conformation. Nature 1991; 353:321–325.

Maggi E: The TH1/TH2 paradigm in allergy. Immunotechnology 1998; 3:233–244.

Mak TW, Caccia N, Kimura N, Spolski R, Iwamoto A, Ohashi P, Reis MD, Toyonaga B: Structures and evolution of the T-cell antigen receptor genes. Cold Spring Harb Symp Quant Biol 1986; 51(Pt 2):797–802.

Marrack P, Lo D, Brinster R, Palmiter R, Burkly L, Flavell RH, Kappler J: The effect of thymus environment on T cell development and tolerance. Cell 1988; 53:627–634.

McIntosh R, Watson P, Weetman A: Somatic hypermutation in autoimmune thyroid disease. Immunol Rev 1998; 162:219–231.

Monroe JG: Antigen receptor-initiated signals for B cell development and selection. Immunol Res 1998; 17:155–162.

Morel PA, Oriss TB: Crossregulation between Th1 and Th2 cells. Crit Rev Immunol 1998; 18:275–303.

Mosmann TR, Coffman RL: TH1 and TH2 cells: different patterns of lymphokine secretion lead to different functional properties. Annu Rev Immunol 1989; 7:145–173.

Nepom GT: A unified hypothesis for the complex genetics of HLA associations with IDDM I diabetes. Diabetes 1990; 39:1153–1157.

Nepom GT, Erlich H: MHC class II molecules and autoimmunity. Annu Rev Immunol 1991; 9:493–525.

Nepom GT, Nepom B: Genetics of the major histocompatibility complex in rheumatoid arthritis. In: Klippel JH, Dieppe PA (eds). Rheumatology. London: Mosby, 1998:5.7.1–5.7.12.

Nepom GT, Nepom BS: Prediction of susceptibility to rheumatoid arthritis by human leukocyte antigen genotyping. In: Nepom GT (ed). Rheumatic Disease Clinics of North America. Philadelphia: WB Saunders, 1992: 785–792.

Newton CR, Graham A, Heptinstall LE, Powell SJ, Summers C, Kalsheker, Smith JC, Markham AF: Analysis of any point mutation in DNA. The amplification refractory mutation system (ARMS). Nucleic Acids Res 1989; 17:2503–2516.

Noble JA, Valdes AM, Cook M, Klitz W, Thomson G, Erlich HA: The role of HLA class II genes in insulin-dependent diabetes mellitus: molecular analysis of 180 Caucasian, multiplex families. Am J Hum Genet 1996; 59:1134–1148.

O'Dell J, Nepom BS, Haire C, Gersuk VH, Gaur L, Moore GF, Drymalski W, Palmer W, Eckhoff PJ, Klassen LW, et al.: HLA-DRB1 typing in rheumatoid arthritis: predicting response to specific treatments. Ann Rheum Dis 1998; 57:209–213.

Ohmen JD, Yang HY, Yamamoto KK, Zhao HY, Ma Y, Bentley LG, Huang Z, Gerwehr S, Pressman S, McElree C, et al.: Susceptibility locus for inflammatory bowel disease on chromosome 16 has a role in Crohn's disease, but not in ulcerative colitis. Hum Mol Genet 1996; 5:1679–1683.

Petersdorf EW, Gooley TA, Anasetti C, Martin PJ, Smith AG, Mickelson, EM, Woolfrey AE, Hansen JA: Optimizing outcome after unrelated marrow transplantation by comprehensive matching of HLA class I and II alleles in the donor and recipient. Blood 1998; 92:3515–3520.

Peterson EJ, Clements JL, Fang N, Koretzky GA: Adaptor proteins in lymphocyte antigen-receptor signaling. Curr Opin Immunol 1998; 10:337–344.

Peterson EJ, Koretzky GA: Signal transduction in T lymphocytes. Clin Exp Rheumatol 1999; 17:107–114.

Pieters J: MHC class II restricted antigen presentation. Curr Opin Immunol 1997; 9:89–96.

Rammensee HG: Chemistry of peptides associated with MHC class I and class II molecules. Curr Opin Immunol 1995; 7:85–96.

Raulet DH: Development and tolerance of natural killer cells. Curr Opin Immunol 1999; 11:129–134.

Raulet DH, Held W, Correa I, Dorfman JR, Wu MF, Corral L: Specificity, tolerance and developmental regulation of natural killer cells defined by expression of class I-specific Ly49 receptors. Immunol Rev 1997; 155:41–52.

Risch N: Assessing the role of HLA-linked and unlinked determinants of disease. Am J Hum Genet 1987; 40:1–14.

Robey E, Allison JP: T-cell activation: integration of signals from the antigen receptor and costimulatory molecules. Immunol Today 1995; 16:306–310.

Romagnani S, Kapsenberg M, Radbruch A, Adorini L: Th1 and Th2 cells. Res Immunol 1998; 149:871–873.

Saiki RK, Walsh PS, Levenson CH, Erlich HA: Genetic analysis of amplified DNA with immobilized sequence-specific oligonucleotide probes. Proc Natl Acad Sci USA 1989; 86:6230–6234.

Scharf SJ, Friedman A, Brautbar C, Szafer F, Steinman L, Horn G, Gyllensten U, Erlich HA: HLA class II allelic variation and susceptibility to pemphigus vulgaris. Proc Natl Acad Sci USA 1988; 85:3504–3508.

Scharf SJ, Freidmann A, Steinman L, Brautbar C, Erlich HA: Specific HLA-DQB and HLA-DRB1 alleles confer susceptibility to pemphigus vulgaris. Proc Natl Acad Sci USA 1989; 86:6215–6219.

Seidl C, Koch U, Buhleier T, Moller B, Wigand R, Markert E, Koller-Wagner G, Seifried E, Kaltwasser JP: Association of (Q)R/KRAA positive HLA-DRB1 alleles with disease progression in early active and severe rheumatoid arthritis. J Rheumatol 1999; 26:773–776.

Sollid LM, Markussen G, Ek J, Gjerde H, Vartdal F, Thorsby E: Evidence for a primary association of celiac disease to a particular HLA-DQ α/β heterodimer. J Exp Med 1989; 169:345–350.

Stern LJ, Brown JH, Jardetzky TS, Gorga JC, Urban RG, Strominger JL, Wiley DC: Crystal structure of the human class II MHC protein HLA-DR1 complexed with an influenza virus peptide. Nature 1994; 368:215–221.

Strominger JL, Wiley DC: The 1995 Albert Lasker Medical Research Award. The class I and class II proteins of the human major histocompatibility complex. JAMA 1995; 274:1074–1076.

Tiwari J, Terasaki P: HLA and Disease Associations. New York: Springer-Verlag, 1985.

Todd JA, Bell JI, McDevitt HO: *HLA-DQβ* gene contributes to susceptibility and resistance to insulin-dependent diabetes mellitus. Nature 1987; 329:599–604.

Todd JA, Farrall M: Panning for gold: genome-wide scanning for linkage in type 1 diabetes. Hum Mol Genet 1996; 5(Suppl):1443–1448.

Trachtenberg E, Yang H, Hayes E, Vinson M, Li S, Targan S, Tyan D, Erlich H, Rotter J: HLA class II haplotype associations with inflammatory bowel disease. Hum Immunol 2000; 61:326–333.

Valenzuela A, Gonzalez-Escribano MF, Rodriguez R, Moreno I, Garcia A, Nunez-Roldan A: Association of HLA shared epitope with joint damage progression in rheumatoid arthritis. Hum Immunol 1999; 60:250–254.

Valitutti S, Muller S, Cella M, Padovan E, Lanzavecchia A: Serial triggering of many T-cell receptors by a few peptide–MHC complexes. Nature 1995; 375:148–151.

van de Wal Y, Kooy YM, van Veelen PA, Pena SA, Mearin LM, Molberg O, Lundin KE, Sollid LM, Mutis T, Benckhuijsen WE, et al.: Small intestinal T cells of celiac disease patients recognize a natural pepsin fragment of gliadin. Proc Natl Acad Sci USA 1998; 95:10050–10054.

van Oers NS, Love PE, Shores EW, Weiss A: Regulation of TCR signal transduction in murine thymocytes by multiple TCR zeta-chain signaling motifs. J Immunol 1998; 160:163–170.

Vartdal F, Johansen BH, Friede T, Thorpe CJ, Stevanovic S, Eriksen JE, Sletten K, Thorsby E, Rammensee HG, Sollid LM: The peptide binding motif of the disease associated HLA-DQ (alpha1*0501, beta1*0201) molecule. Eur J Immunol 1996; 26:2764–2772.

Vaux DL: Immunopathology of apoptosis—introduction and overview. Springer Semin Immunopathol 1998; 19:271–278.

Wagner U, Kaltenhauser S, Sauer H, Arnold S, Seidel W, Hantzschel H, Kalden JR, Wassmuth R: HLA markers and prediction of clinical course and outcome in rheumatoid arthritis. Arthritis Rheum 1997; 40:341–351.

Weiss A: Molecular and genetic insights into T cell antigen receptor structure and function. Annu Rev Genet 1991; 25:487–510.

Wiens GD, Roberts VA, Whitcomb EA, O'Hare T, Stenzel-Poore MP, Rittenberg MB: Harmful somatic mutations: lessons from the dark side. Immunol Rev 1998; 162:197–209.

Wilson RK, Lai E, Concannon P, Barth RK, Hood LE: Structure, organization and polymorphism of murine and human T-cell receptor alpha and beta chain gene families. Immunol Rev 1988; 101:149–172.

Young AC, Nathenson SG, Sacchettini JC: Structural studies of class I major histocompatibility complex proteins: insights into antigen presentation. FASEB J 1995; 9:26–36.

Zinkernagel RM, Doherty PC: MHC-restricted cytotoxic T cells: studies on the biological role of polymorphic major transplantation antigens determining T-cell restriction-specificity, function, and responsiveness. Adv Immunol 1979; 27:151–177.

Zlotnik A, Morales J, Hedrick JA: Recent advances in chemokines and chemokine receptors. Crit Rev Immunol 1999; 19:1–47.

29 Rheumatoid Arthritis

BARBARA NEPOM AND RICHARD A. KING

Many diseases are thought to date to antiquity, but the record is most convincing for arthritis. Bony fossils have preserved a history of bone and joint diseases spanning 600 million years, which includes the time of dinosaurs, the forebears of common domestic animals, and early humans (Pemberton and Osgood, 1934; Hormell, 1940; Benedek and Rodnan, 1982; Thould and Thould, 1983). Rheumatic disease has been of interest since the time of Hippocrates, with more recognized patterns and classifications being recent developments (Short, 1974; Benedek and Rodnan, 1982; Thould and Thould, 1983). Guillaume de Baillou first used the term *rheumatism* in reference to joint disease in 1642. Laudie-Beavais, 1772–1840, provided the first specific description of rheumatoid arthritis (RA) in 1800, and A. B. Garrod proposed the term *rheumatoid arthritis* in 1892 (Hormell, 1940; Short, 1974; Benedek and Rodnan, 1982; Abdel-Nasser et al., 1997). The historical evidence supports the hypothesis that RA is a disease of the New World of relatively recent origin (Abdel-Nasser et al., 1997). No clear written or paleopathologic evidence of RA before the eighteenth century has been found. The complexity and diverse nature of arthritis and related disease are recognized, as seen by the American Rheumatism Association classification, which includes over 100 entities. This chapter reviews the genetic basis of RA.

DISEASE DEFINITION

RA is a chronic systemic inflammatory disease with the cardinal feature of persistent and progressive arthritis involving the synovial (diarthrodial) joints (Goronzy et al., 1987; Anderson, 1987; Lee and Weinblatt, 2001). The surrounding tendons, ligaments, fascia, muscle, and bone may also be involved. Any synovial joint may be affected, but there is a predilection for the small joints of the hand and foot (Wollheim, 1998). The articular manifestations of RA include morning stiffness, synovial inflammation, and eventual structural damage of the cartilage and bone of the joint. Extra-articular manifestations involving the skin, eyes, lungs and respiratory tract, heart, gastrointestinal tract, kidneys, neurologic system, and blood occur and are an integral component of the systemic nature of RA. The clinical spectrum of RA is wide, with unpredictable disease progression, joint involvement, and extra-articular involvement.

The diagnosis of RA is usually made by evaluation of the clinical, serologic, and radiologic features of joint involvement and inflammation. Symmetrical synovitis with serologic changes is present in the early phase of the disease, with radiologic evidence of bony erosions developing later. RA is an autoimmune disease, and the major autoantibodies are the rheumatoid factor (RF), an autoantibody directed against antigenic determinants on the Fc (constant) portion of the heavy chain of immunoglobulin G (Dorner and Alexander, 1987; Sutton et al., 2000). Polyclonal RFs are not specific for RA, however, and are found, usually in less abundance, in acute and chronic inflammatory and infectious diseases such as bacterial endocarditis and sarcoidosis, as well as with advancing age (Jonsson et al., 2000; Radstake et al., 2000; Witte et al., 2000; Heliovaara et al., 2000). Furthermore, RFs are not found in all patients with RA, and this disease can develop in the absence of RFs (Gonzalez-Gay et al., 2001; Kaltenhauser et al., 2001; Papadopoulos et al., 2001). Given these diagnostic limitations, however, RF remains one of the laboratory hallmarks of RA (Goronzy and Weyand, 1987).

Diagnosing RA is often a challenging problem in clinical practice and in the genetic evaluation of this disease. The individual with classic, well-established chronic RA is obvious but represents an unknown portion of all individuals with RA. RA is a progressive disease with insidious onset in which mild cases are common and remissions occur, and these factors make specific diagnosis difficult. Furthermore, RA may be present in the absence of arthritis. The remittent nature and the usual slow progression of mild RA have been well documented, and it appears that individuals with RA can be symptom-free for long periods of time. These considerations have led to the speculation that many cases do not develop the complete syndrome of classic RA and that the majority of mild cases are never seen by a physician and go undiagnosed.

To overcome these difficulties, broadly accepted diagnostic criteria for RA have been established for use in research and clinical practice as a mechanism for a uniform approach to diagnosis. The American Rheumatism Association established classification criteria in 1958, and these were revised in 1987 (Table 29–1) (Arnett et al., 1988). An individual is diagnosed with RA if he or she has satisfied at least four of the seven criteria. Criteria 1 through 4 must be present for at least 6 weeks. Individuals with two clinical diagnoses are not excluded. Terms such as *classic*, *definite*, and *probable* RA, as used in many population studies in the past, are not to be used with the current classification. Other diagnostic criteria, such as the New York criteria, have been used in the past, but the ARA criteria are now those most widely used (Bennett and Burch, 1967; Fries et al., 1994).

GENERAL GENETIC AND EPIDEMIOLOGIC EVIDENCE

Clinical Epidemiology and Ethnic Differences

RA is found in all parts of the world and in all ethnic groups, with an overall prevalence estimated to be approximately 1% and incidence estimated to be approximately 0.03% (reviewed in Abdel-Nasser et al., 1997; Lawrence et al., 1989, 1998; Harris, 1990; Hazes et al., 1990; Gabriel, 2001). The distribution is

Table 29–1. American Rheumatism Association 1987 Revised Criteria for Rheumatoid Arthritis[a]

1. Morning stiffness
2. Arthritis of three of more joints
3. Arthritis of the hand joints
4. Symmetrical arthritis
5. Rheumatoid nodules
6. Serum rheumatoid factor
7. Radiologic changes

[a]For classification purposes, a patient shall be said to have rheumatoid arthritis if he or she has satisfied at least four of these seven criteria. Criteria 1 through 4 must be present for at least 6 weeks. Patients with two clinical diagnoses are not excluded. The designations *classic*, *definite*, and *probable* rheumatoid arthritis are not to be made (Arnett et al., 1988).

not uniform, however; and there are populations with higher and lower rates of disease (Table 29–2). Some of the variation is related to the different diagnostic criteria used in the various studies, but a significant part appears to represent true population differences (MacGregor et al., 1994). The prevalence of RA in the Caucasian populations of North America and Europe is approximately 1% (Table 29–2), and some studies have suggested that the incidence and severity of disease may be declining in these populations (Spector, 1990). The highest prevalence of RA has been reported in Native Americans (O'Brien et al., 1967; Beasley et al., 1973b; Harvey et al., 1981; Boyer et al., 1991). It has been estimated that RA is twice as prevalent in Native Americans than in the general North American Caucasian population, and these data have been used to provide further support for the New World origin of the disease (Rubin and Voorneveld, 1991; Abdel-Nasser et al., 1997). A similar increase in prevalence is not found in the Alaskan and Canadian Eskimo populations (Beasley et al., 1973a; Oen et al., 1986; Boyer et al., 1991). The prevalence in Asian populations is estimated to be approximately one-third to one-half that in the North American and European Caucasian populations (Mijiyawa, 1995; Abdel-Nasser et al., 1997). Low rates of RA are also reported in the sub-Saharan populations of Africa, and the rates may be lowest in these populations. Prevalence also declines with age in Caucasian populations (Laiho et al., 2001).

Table 29–2. Prevalence of Rheumatoid Arthritis in Different Populations

	Prevalence (%)			
Population	Female	Male	Total	Reference
Europe				
Denmark	1.2	0.3	0.9	Sorensen (1973)
Netherlands	1.8	0.5	1.1	Lawrence (1977)
Sweden			0.9	Hellgren (1970)
North America				
Pima Indians	7	3	5.3	Del Puente et al. (1989)
United States	1.6	0.7	1.0	Engel et al. (1966)
Tecumseh, MI	0.7	0.3	0.5	Mikkelsen et al. (1967)
Caribbean				
Jamaica	2.2	1.5	1.9	Lawrence et al. (1966)
Asia				
China (rural island)	0.4	0.2	0.3	Beasley et al. (1983)
China (mainland)	0.6	0.04	0.3	Wigley et al. (1994)
Taiwan	0.5	0.2	0.34	Chou et al. (1994)
Africa				
Lesotho	0.4	0.0	0.3	Moolenburgh et al. (1986)
South Africa (urban)	1.4	0.0	0.9	Solomon et al. (1975)

Source: Abdel-Nasser et al. (1997).

RA is more common in females than males, as shown in Table 29–2, and the reason for this is unknown. Some insight into this comes from the observation that there is often an amelioration of active disease during pregnancy, followed by a postpartum relapse (Hazes et al., 1990b; Da Silva and Spector, 1992; van der Horst-Bruinsma et al., 1998). Several potential explanations include differences in hormone levels and/or differences in immunity and immunosuppression (Da Silva, 1995; Da Silva and Spector, 1992). That hormone levels are directly or indirectly involved can be seen from studies showing a reduced risk of developing RA with the use of oral contraception (Kay and Wingrave, 1983; Spector and Hochberg, 1989; Hazes and van Zeben, 1991). Gender may also influence the clinical course and pattern of extra-articular manifestations (Weyand et al., 1998). At this time, these observations are interesting but not helpful in understanding the basic genetic susceptibility or pathogenetic mechanisms of RA, and further work will be necessary to place these observations in the proper context.

Population Differences in Disease

The clinical variability of RA is great, making comparisons between populations difficult. This is further compounded by the difficulties in diagnosis and an incomplete understanding of the etiology. Some studies, however, suggest that there are population differences in the clinical manifestations of disease (reviewed in Abdel-Nasser et al., 1997). For example, an Israeli study of patients of Sephardic origin and Ashkenazi origin showed a greater severity of disease, as defined by pain and disability, in the former group, although there also were socioeconomic differences between the two (Amit et al., 1996). Several studies have found greater severity of disease in British patients compared to Greek (Drosos et al., 1992, 1995) or black Zimbabwean (Chikanza et al., 1994) patients. Differences in articular and extra-articular manifestations have been found when Asian population samples have been compared to British (Veerapen et al., 1993) or Australian (Moran et al., 1986, 1987) population samples. Taken together, these and other studies only suggest population differences in disease severity and articular and extra-articular manifestations, but there are no data to support a strong genetic role in these differences.

Family Epidemiology

Family, twin, and human leukocyte antigen (HLA) studies have provided evidence for a genetic component to the susceptibility to RA. The basic autoimmune nature of the disease and its association with the HLA system obviously point to an immunogenetic basis, but the specific mechanisms that provoke or disregulate the immune system are unknown.

Family Studies

A genetic or a familial component of RA has been considered since the early description of the disease, and impressive pedigrees with affected members in three and four generations and large family surveys are available. The true familial aggregation has been difficult to document, however; and there are several reasons for this, the first being the problem of diagnosis. Many useful studies have been published since establishment of the ARA classification, but documentation of RA by historical evidence in distant dead relatives is not exact and can easily be biased. Second, RA is a common disease and families with more than one affected member may occur by chance alone rather than representing a familial genetic expression of disease. Third, the etiology of RA is unknown. Even with these shortcomings, a review of family studies provides useful information.

Until the advent of HLA studies, the most commonly used method for the genetic analysis of RA was the family study. Probands with RA were selected, and the occurrence of RA in relatives was determined in families or compared to that in a control population. The results of these studies have often been conflicting, and a true familial occurrence of RA has not always been obvious (Wordsworth and Bell, 1991; Deighton and Walker, 1991; Kwoh et al., 1996). In the previous edition of this book, data were presented from 16 reports published over the period 1950 through 1970, which showed a frequency between 1.1% and 15% in first-degree relatives of a proband with RA and a frequency of 0.6% and 9.0% in controls (King, 1992). All studies showed a higher incidence of RA in first-degree relatives of a proband with RA than in relatives of controls.

More recent studies have continued to find the analysis of familial expression problematic when conducted without consideration of HLA status. These studies indicate that approximately 10% to 13% of probands with RA have one or more first-degree relatives with RA compared to rates of 3% to 9% in control relatives, and the risk of RA in first-degree relatives is only a modest 1.6- to 1.7-fold higher than in the control population (Deighton et al., 1992b; Rigby et al., 1991; Jones et al., 1996; Barrera et al., 1999; Kwoh et al., 1996; Koumantaki et al., 1997). The sex of the proband as well as the characteristics of the disease can influence familial risk, with siblings of probands with severe RA at greater risk that those of probands with mild disease; and RA clustering is more likely to be found in large rather than small sibships or in sibships of females rather than males (Lawrence, 1970; Deighton et al., 1992a,b; Barrera et al., 1999). Risk to relatives is also higher for female probands with RA than for male probands with RA (Kwoh et al., 1996). An interesting finding that may help explain some of the conflicting results is that the false-positive status for family members is high (62%) when clinical status is verified by examination (Kwoh et al., 1996). Without careful examination of all family members, using established classification criteria to verify reported cases of RA in a family, it may not be possible to determine an accurate familial incidence of RA.

Twin Studies

Twin studies can be helpful in defining a genetic component of a common disease, but they must be critically assessed because problems of study design and ascertainment can bias their interpretation (reviewed in Chapter 3). Available twin studies include case reports and population surveys. Case reports of limited size, published in the period 1936 through 1969, showed greater concordance for RA in monozygous (MZ) twin pairs (32%, $n = 18/57$) vs. dizygous (DZ) twin pairs (13%, $n = 5/38$) (King, 1992). Lawrence (1970) studied 428 twins chosen from patients attending 23 arthritis clinics in the United Kingdom and the Netherlands. Concordance for seropositive RA was 32% for MZ and 6% for DZ twin pairs. As this was the first large twin study that approached a population-based study, these results were widely accepted and the general literature on RA soon reflected an approximate 30% concordance for MZ twin pairs (Jarvinen and Aho, 1994). Subsequent population-based studies have not found the same high level of concordance.

The nationwide Finnish Twin Cohort consisted of 4137 MZ and 9162 DZ same-sex twin pairs born before 1958 and alive in 1975 (Aho et al., 1986). Based on insurance records for medication, there were 261 cases of RA in the cohort, and the RA concordance rates were 12.3% for MZ twin pairs and 3.5% for DZ twin pairs. The U.K. nationwide study of 91 MZ and 112 DZ twin pairs found concordance rates of 15.4% for MZ twins and 3.6% for DZ twins (Silman et al., 1993). Finally, the Australian Twin Registry study of 3808 pairs of twins found 258 with self-reported RA in one or both members of the pair (Bellamy et al., 1992). MZ concordance for RA was 21% (3/14), while no DZ twin pairs (0/9) were concordant.

Taken together, most of the earlier, smaller twin studies and the more recent larger studies demonstrate increased MZ twin concordance for RA compared to that in DZ twins, suggesting a genetic component to RA susceptibility. Based on the twin data, the strength of the genetic component of susceptibility is not great, and this correlates well with the modest relative risks associated with the family studies discussed above.

There are some additional interesting aspects of twin studies in RA. The above studies did not take HLA status into account. When HLA typing is included in the analysis (see Gene Identification below), disease concordance is greatly increased in MZ twins, who are also concordant for HLA type, and this is most marked for MZ twins who share the RA-susceptible epitope of *HLA-DRB1* (see Gene Identification below) (Jawaheer et al., 1994). Jawaheer et al. (1994) suggested that RA concordance in MZ twin pairs is rare in the absence of the shared epitope. The clinical course of disease in MZ twins does not usually follow a concordant pattern, except for similar ages at onset (MacGregor et al., 1995a).

BIOLOGIC BASIS OF GENETIC SUSCEPTIBILITY

RA is a chronic autoimmune inflammatory disease involving primarily the synovial tissue of the joints (Thomas, 1998; Maini and Feldmann, 1998). The immunopathology is complex, involving many components of the immune system, and a clear description of the pathogenesis is difficult because there is no animal model and the etiologic agent that starts the process is unknown.

Family and twin studies have indicated that genetic and environmental factors are involved in the development of RA. Identification of infectious agents in RA has been the goal of many studies, but no single agent or group of agents has been identified. Several potential candidates are Epstein-Barr virus (EBV) (Bluestein and Hasler, 1984; Venables, 1988), *Mycobacterium tuberculosis* (van Eden et al., 1985, 1988; Holoshitz et al., 1986, 1989) and *Proteus mirabilis* (Tiwana et al., 1999; Ebringer and Wilson, 2000). EBV capsid protein has an amino acid motif (QKRAA) that matches closely the amino acid sequence of the *HLA-DRβ1* susceptibility sequence (see below), and this has suggested a possible link between RA and persistent EBV infection through cross-reactivity (Roudier et al., 1988, 1989; Auger and Roudier, 1997). A major problem with this hypothesis is that EBV is nearly ubiquitous, with evidence of high infection rates in the general population, and there is no explanation for the small proportion that do develop RA, as well as those with RA who do not have evidence of EBV infection (Maini and Feldmann, 1998). The interest in *M. tuberculosis* comes from animal models that show mycobacterium protein with immunologic cross-reactivity with cartilage proteins. One mycobacterial protein is a member of a family of heat-shock proteins (hsp65) and is expressed in diseased joints, where it could be a target for T-cell autoreactivity (van Eden et al., 1985, 1988; Holoshitz et al., 1986). Sequence differences between bacterial and human heat-shock proteins (Gaston et al., 1989) and the inability to identify organisms in the joints of patients with RA argue against *M. tuberculosis* being a major etiologic factor in RA.

The classic immunologic disregulation in RA is activation of T cells (see Chapter 28) (Maini and Feldmann, 1998; Thomas, 1998; Miossec, 2000; Aarvak et al., 2000; Lee and Weinblatt, 2001; Panayi et al., 2001; Nepom, 2001). The T cell is the major infiltrating cell of the synovium; most are $CD4^+$ and located in perivascular nodules, while fewer numbers of $CD8^+$ T cells are found diffusely in the diseased tissue. Recognition of antigen by $CD4^+$ T cells is HLA-DR-restricted, and the association of specific HLA-DR molecules with RA (see below) is consistent with a central role of T cells in the pathogenesis of RA. The disregulation is thought to arise from the development of antigen-presenting cells that activate the T cells through the presentation of self-antigen (Thomas, 1998). One model places the antigen-presenting cell at the center of the self-perpetuating process of joint inflammation by priming T cells to endogenous or joint-derived self-antigen and then maintaining a pool of autoreactive memory T cells capable of localizing to the joint (Thomas, 1998). As noted above, the origin of the initial stimulating antigen remains unknown.

Altered cytokine expression is prominent in RA (Maini and Feldmann, 1998; Brennan et al., 1998; Feldmann and Maini, 1999; Arend, 2001; Klimiuk et al., 2001; Jain et al., 2001; Smith et al., 2001). The rheumatoid synovium expresses many cytokines, some of which are important for cell growth or for expression of class II HLA molecules; but it is not clear which, if any, cytokine is involved in disease pathogenesis rather than in inflammation and progression. It seems that there is some level of genetic control of cytokine expression and that polymorphic variation influencing the degree and timing of expression of different genes may play a role in disease variability; but the genetic analysis of this type of variability has only begun, and little data are available.

More recent ideas on the pathogenesis of RA have involved fibroblasts and other cells found in the joint (Sen et al., 2000; Volin and Koch, 2000). Synovial fibroblasts undergo an alteration of phenotype, associated with the synthesis of inflammatory cytokines and cell-surface adhesion molecules (Case et al., 1989; Harada et al., 1999; Miyazawa et al., 1999; Sarkissian and LaFyatis, 1999). One suggestion is that synovial tissue fibroblasts change phenotype, clonally expand, aggregate, and form nodules. Expression of cell cycle-regulatory genes and the processes of proliferation and apoptosis are altered, resulting in synovial hyperplasia and eventual joint destruction (Volin and Koch, 2000). Another potential explanation involving the fibroblasts derives from their expression of embryonic growth factors of the wingless (*wnt*) and frizzled (*fz*) families (Sen et al., 2000). These growth factors could signal their replacement by immature and more destructive mesenchymal and bone marrow cells, which are associated with perpetuation of disease and destruction of the joint tissue. Further studies of fibroblast behavior may provide new insight into the chronic process of RA.

GENE IDENTIFICATION

HLA-DR Genes

DR4 Association with RA

By far the best-studied and most reproducible genetic association in RA is with the *HLA-DR* genes of the major histocompatibility complex (MHC) (Andersson et al., 2000; Roudier, 2000; Weyand and Goronzy, 2000; Zanelli et al., 2000). Association of RA with HLA-DR4 was first noted over 20 years ago (McMichael et al., 1977; Stastny, 1978). Since then a plethora of studies have confirmed this association with a striking degree of reproducibility such that the genetic contribution of *DR4* is generally accepted. Early studies were based on detection of *DR* alleles through serologic or cellular techniques, and the nomenclature used was sometimes confusing or imprecise, reflecting the level of understanding of *HLA* genes at the time. In brief, *DR4* is a serologically defined entity present on a number of different *DR4*-positive molecules. These can be discriminated further on the basis of cellular recognition in mixed lymphocyte reactions into different subtypes of DR4, such as Dw4, Dw14, etc. Nucleotide sequence information now allows definition of specific unique alleles. For example, Dw4 is now called *DRB1*0401*, designating it as allele 1 among the homologous DR4-positive alleles, while Dw14 is called *DRB1*0404*, another allele within the DR4 family.

Most early studies, performed predominantly in North American or northern European populations, demonstrated a 65% to 80% prevalence of DR4 among patients with RA (Stastny, 1978; Panayi et al., 1978; Jaraquemada et al., 1979; Karr et al., 1980; Gran et al., 1983; Legrand et al., 1984; Ollier et al., 1984; Zoschke and Segall, 1986). When cellularly defined subtypes were investigated, Dw4 (**0401*) was the most highly associated among DR4-positive haplotypes, being in the range of 35% to 60% of the total patient population typed as positive for Dw4 (McMichael et al., 1977; Stastny, 1978; Thomsen et al., 1979; Jaraquemada et al., 1979; Young et al., 1984; Zoschke and Segall, 1986). As DNA-based techniques became available, an increase in the frequency of the **0404* allele (previously called Dw14) was noted in addition to the increase in **0401* (Nepom et al., 1986, 1989; Wordsworth et al., 1989; Ronningen et al., 1990; Wallin et al., 1991). In contrast, some DR4-positive alleles were not associated with disease, like **0402* (Dw10) and **0407* (Dw13), indicating that all DR4 alleles are not proportionately increased among patients (Mattey et al, 2001a,b; Seidl et al., 2001; Snijders et al., 2001). When populations are stratified by age, the association between RA and *DR4* genes is strongest for younger patients and may be less important in elderly patients (Hellier et al., 2001).

Other DR Genes

Some non-*DR4* genes, such as *DR1*, have also been associated with RA, although more weakly than *DR4*. For example, *DR1* is often not significantly increased among patient groups as a whole, but if all *DR4*-positive patients and controls are removed from the analysis, it becomes highly significant, accounting for the majority of non-*DR4* patients (Thomsen et al., 1979; Woodrow et al., 1981; Khan and Khan, 1986; Nepom et al., 1989; Gao et al., 1990; Wallin et al., 1991; van Zeben et al., 1991; Kim et al., 1995). Figure 29–1 compares the frequencies of the most commonly associated alleles in a series of studies encompassing northern European and North American Caucasian populations, all using DNA-based typing methods. This demonstrates the remarkable similarity of results when comparable populations and techniques are utilized.

In some studies, a negative association of certain *DR* alleles has been observed. Both British (Ollier et al., 1984; Jaraquemada et al., 1986) and Canadian (Gladman and Anhorn, 1986; Panayi et al., 1987) studies found a decrease of *DR2* and *DR7* alleles among RA patients. Other groups found only a decrease of *DR2* (Panayi et al., 1978; Young et al., 1984), and most other studies

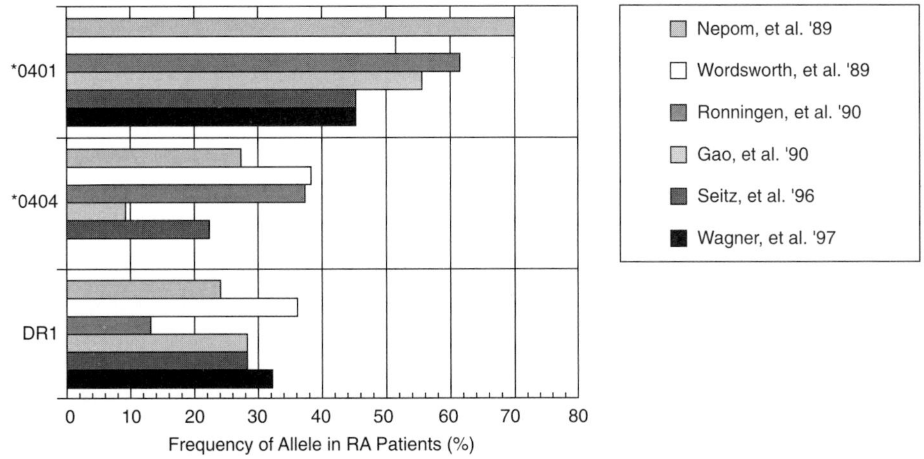

Fig. 29–1. Comparison of frequencies of the most commonly associated *HLA-DR* alleles among representative studies. Results are remarkably similar when comparable populations and HLA typing techniques are used; in this case, all reports studied northern European or North American Caucasian populations and utilized DNA-based typing methods.

have reported no significant negative associations. The extent of any protective effect is not clear.

The Shared Epitope Hypothesis

With the advent of DNA sequencing of individual *DRB1* alleles, Gregersen and colleagues (1987) observed that the alleles associated with RA share a similar sequence at amino acids 70–74 in the third hypervariable region of the *DRB1* molecule (QKRAA, represented by the **0401* allele, or *QRRAA*, seen in the **0404* and **0101* alleles). From this emerged the shared epitope hypothesis, which suggests that risk for RA is conferred by the structural element encoded by this small region of sequence homology, even though other polymorphic regions of the genes can be quite divergent. The concept was further strengthened when it was demonstrated that within certain populations where *DR4* genes are uncommon, such as the Yakima Indians of eastern Washington State, RA is associated with the presence of another *DRB1* allele, **1402*, that is quite dissimilar to *DR4* genes except for an exact match in the region of the shared epitope (Willkens et al., 1991). Similarly, a gene called **1001* (formerly *DR10*) was shown to be increased in frequency in RA patients in other populations where the *DR4* susceptibility alleles are uncommon (Blanar et al., 1989; Gao et al., 1991); this gene has an RRRAA sequence at amino acids 70–74, similar to the shared epitope. Figure 29–2 demonstrates these sequence homologies among genes both associated and not associated with RA.

How the shared epitope fragment confers susceptibility to RA is unknown. A number of models are currently being investigated, all variations on the fact that the polymorphic amino acids in an HLA molecule govern which antigenic peptides may bind to it and that the conformation of the resulting unique HLA/peptide complex determines recognition by a T-cell receptor (Snijders et al., 2001). In one model, a shared epitope-containing HLA molecule bound to a self-peptide influences T-cell selection in the thymus, allowing development of self-reactive T cells, which are subsequently activated in the periph-

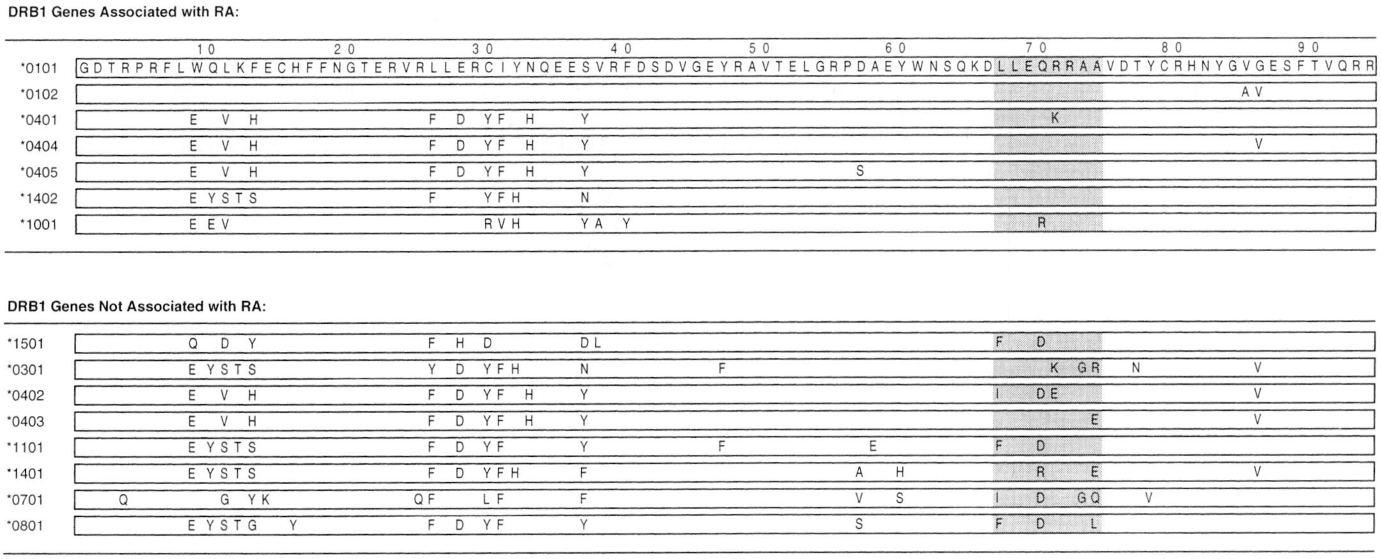
DRB1 Genes Associated with RA:
10 20 30 40 50 60 70 80 90
*0101 GDTRPRFLWQLKFECHFFNGTERVRLLERCIYNQEESVRFDSDVGEYRAVTELGRPDAEYWNSQKDLLEQRRAAVDTYCRHNYGVGESFTVQRR
*0102 A V
*0401 E V H F D YF H Y K
*0404 E V H F D YF H Y V
*0405 E V H F D YF H Y S
*1402 E YSTS F YFH N
*1001 E EV RVH YA Y R
DRB1 Genes Not Associated with RA:
*1501 Q D Y F H D DL F D
*0301 E YSTS Y D YFH N F K GR N V
*0402 E V H F D YF H Y I DE V
*0403 E V H F D YF H Y E V
*1101 E YSTS F D YF Y F E F D
*1401 E YSTS F D YFH F A H R E V
*0701 Q G YK QF LF F V S I D GQ V
*0801 E YSTG Y F D YF Y S F D L

Fig. 29–2. Amino acid sequences of *HLA-DRB1* genes associated with rheumatoid arthritis (*RA*) demonstrating the shared epitope. Amino acid sequences, using the single-letter code, of representative DRB1 genes are aligned. *Upper panel* lists genes associated with RA, with the shared epitope region shaded, showing the striking degree of homology in this sequence stretch. *Lower panel* lists common genes not associated with RA, demonstrating very little sequence homology within the shared epitope region.

ery. In a second model, the structure of the susceptible HLA molecule allows binding of a particular arthritogenic peptide in the periphery, which leads to an aberrant immune response in the joint. A third model suggests that the shared epitope itself is processed and presented as the relevant antigen, bound by another HLA molecule. Still another possibility is that there is direct T-cell recognition of the shared epitope on the class II molecule, which dominates over peptide-specific recognition. Molecular mimicry mechanisms may play a role in several of these models.

HLA Association Studies in Different Ethnic Populations

One area that has undergone extensive investigation in recent years is the extension of HLA association studies into different geographic and ethnic populations. Table 29–3 summarizes some of these studies. The overriding impression is the striking reproducibility of HLA alleles conferring risk for RA in diverse population groups. For example, *DRB1*0401* is elevated in RA patients from Scandinavia (Thomsen et al., 1979; Ronningen et al., 1990), Greece (Stavropoulos et al., 1997), Italy (Angelini et al., 1992), and India (Taneja et al., 1996), as well as in U.S. (Stastny 1978; Nepom et al., 1989) and British (Jaraquemada et al., 1986; Wordsworth et al., 1989) Caucasians. However, the presence and strength of association of particular alleles depends on their background frequency in that population. For example, among Caucasians of northern European ancestry, the *DRB1* alleles **0401*, **0404*, and **0101* are the most highly associated with RA (Thomsen et al., 1979; Wordsworth et al., 1989; Ronningen et al., 1990; Seitz et al., 1996). In many Asian countries, however, including Japan and China, the most frequent *DR4* allele in the general population is **0405*, another shared epitope-containing allele, and that is the gene with the highest RA association in those groups (Chan et al., 1994; Yen et al., 1995; Kim et al., 1995; Zhao et al., 1996; Takeuchi et al., 1996; Wakitani et al., 1997).

Other populations have a low background frequency of all shared epitope-positive *DR4* alleles, and in those cases non-*DR4* genes are most highly associated with disease. For example, among Israeli Jews the most common *DR4* allele is **0402*, which does not contain the shared epitope. In that population, the highest association is with the shared epitope-containing alleles *DR1* and **1001* (Schiff et al., 1982; Gao et al., 1991). Similarly, the Spanish have a relatively low frequency of *DR4* alleles, and studies reveal *DR10* to be most highly associated with disease (Yelamos et al., 1993). The association of the **1402* allele with RA in the Yakima population has already been mentioned; in fact, studies in a number of Native American populations have shown the same association, including the Tlingit of Alaska (Nelson et al., 1992) and the Pima of Arizona (Williams et al., 1995).

Among populations with a low background frequency of all shared epitope-positive *DR* alleles, the overall percentage of RA patients carrying such an allele may be quite low. Some studies of African Americans, e.g., report that fewer than half of RA patients carry the shared epitope (Alarcon et al., 1983; McDaniel et al., 1995). Even in populations with a strong association of shared epitope-positive alleles among RA patients, some patients will be negative for these alleles; carrying one of these alleles is neither necessary nor sufficient for disease expression. This may indicate that a different mechanistic pathway leads to the phenotype of RA in these individuals and/or that a different constellation of other genetic and environmental factors has pushed the individual over the threshold of disease expression.

Disease Severity and the Effect of Gene Dose

Another area of complexity concerns disease heterogeneity. RA includes a spectrum of clinical features of disease, including variation in severity, age at onset, and extra-articular disease manifestations. Most of the early studies of HLA and RA utilized patient groups drawn from university or tertiary care centers and tended to include patients with well-established, severe disease. When community-based populations were studied, the results were sometimes less clear. Thomson et al. (1993) reported in a British study that *DR4* alleles were not significantly elevated in a series of newly diagnosed cases of RA from the community (42% of patients compared to 37% of controls). At the other extreme, 96% of a group of RA patients positive for RF who were followed at the Mayo Clinic, a tertiary care center, expressed the shared epitope (Weyand et al., 1992a). These variations led to the suggestion that HLA genetic risk factors might contribute to disease severity as well as to susceptibility. A number of other studies agree that among patients initially diagnosed with polyarthritis or probable RA, follow-up reveals a higher frequency of the shared epitope, particularly in the context of a *DR4* allele, in those individuals with a more severe disease course (Salmon et al., 1993; Combe et al., 1995; Wagner et al., 1997; Mattey et al., 2001a,b; Seidle et al., 2001). Patients carrying only a *DR1* allele, in contrast, have milder disease (McCusker et al., 1991; Nepom et al., 1992; Wakitani et al., 1997; Seidl et al., 2001). A few studies report an association of shared epitope-positive alleles with RA susceptibility but not severity (Mottonen, 1988; Suarez-Almazor et al., 1995). Finally, a study of gene dose and age at onset in families with affected parents and offspring has suggested anticipation with earlier disease onset but not disease outcome in the offspring of an affected parent (Radstake et al., 2001).

Evaluation of radiographically determined bony erosions as a measure of disease severity seems to confirm a correlation of RA-associated alleles with worse disease. Young et al. (1984) first reported that *DR4* expression was associated with more erosive disease, while *DR2* negatively correlated with erosions. Olsen et al. (1988) confirmed the association of *DR4* with erosive disease and found that *DR1* was not correlated with erosions. Other studies corroborated these findings, including groups from Europe (van Zeben et al., 1991; McMahon et al., 1993; Combe et al., 1995; Moreno et al., 1996; Salvarani et al., 1998; Plant et al., 1998; Kaltenhauser et al., 2001), Japan (Doita et al., 1990; Wakitani et al., 1997), China (Chan et al., 1994; Zhao et al., 1996), Taiwan (Yen et al., 2001), and Korea (Kim et al., 1997).

Furthermore, gene dosage appears to play a role in determining risk for disease. In an early report, we demonstrated a synergistic risk for disease in patients with RF-positive (adult-like) juvenile RA carrying what is now called the **0401/*0404* genotype (Nepom et al., 1984); such individuals had a relative risk for disease of 116. We and others subsequently confirmed this in adult RA, showing that individuals with two shared epitope-positive alleles, in particular the **0401/*0404* combination, were at increased risk for disease (Nepom et al., 1986; Wordsworth et al., 1992; Gough et al., 1994; MacGregor et al., 1995a). MacGregor et al. (1995a) reported that the risk of RA in individuals carrying a single shared epitope allele was four times that of shared epitope-negative individuals; the risk in those with two shared epitope-positive alleles was eight times higher; and the risk of individuals with the **0401/*0404* combination was 26 times higher. In all patients, this genotype was associ-

Table 29–3. Relative Risk for Rheumatoid Arthritis (RA) in Different Populations

Population	References	No. RA Patients	Associated Specificity or Gene	% Positive in Patients	% Positive in Controls	Relative Risk
North America						
Canada	Gladman and Anhorn (1986)	48	*DR4*	63	28	4.3
	Suarez-Almazor et al. (1995)	103	*DR4*	54	35	2.3
United States						
Caucasians	McMichael et al. (1977)	39	*Dw4*	36	12	3.0
	Stastny (1978)	80	*DR4*	70	28	6.0
			Dw4	54	16	6.1
	Karr et al. (1980)	35	*DR4*	71	40	3.8
	Zoschke and Segall (1986)	42	*DR4*	86	30	14.3
			Dw4	57	14	8.2
	Olsen et al. (1988)	151	*DR4*	65		
	Nepom et al. (1989)	41	*DR4*	63	32	3.7
			**0401*	51	15	6.1
			**0404*	27	7	4.6
			DR1	24	22	1.1
	Gao et al. (1990)	88	*DR4	63	33	3.5
			**0401*	55	19	5.3
			DR1	28	19	1.7
Blacks	Karr et al. (1980)	35	*DR4*	46	14	5.1
	Ueno et al. (1981)	18	*DR4*	39		
	Alarcón et al. (1983)	85	*DR4*	22	7.4	3.6
	Alarif et al. (1983)	50	*DR4*	58	18	4.3
	McDaniel et al. (1995)	86	*04	27	13	2.4
Native Americans						
Chippewa	Harvey et al. (1983)	12	*DR4*	100	68	13.4
Yakima	Willkens et al. (1991)	18	**1402*	83	60	3.3
Tlingits	Nelson et al. (1992)	32	*1402	91	80	2.3
Pimans	Williams et al. (1995)	47	*1402	98	95	2.3
Hispanics	Ueno et al. (1981)	17	*DR4*	77	38	5.2
	Teller et al. (1996)	67	*DR4*	43	24	2.4
Mexico	Debaz et al. (1998)	83	**0404*	29	7	5.4
			**0401*	7	1	9.8
			**1001*	8	1	6.8
South America						
Chile	Massardo et al. (1990)	64	*DR4*	48	32	2.0
			DR9	16	4	4.5
	Gonzalez et al. (1997)	129	**0404*	19	6	3.0
Europe						
Norway	Gran et al. (1983)	122	*DR4*	65	27	5.0
	Rønningen et al. (1990)	54	**0401*	61	25	4.8
			**0404*	37	9	6.1
Denmark	Thomsen et al. (1979)	36	*Dw4*	44	17	
Britain	Jaraquemeda et al. (1979)	107	DR4	69	24	8.9
			Dw4	39	20	2.5
	Young et al. (1984)	95	*DR4*	55	36	2.1
	Ollier et al. (1984)	77	*DR4*	74		
	Jaraquemada et al. (1986)	440	*DR4*	65	31	4.1
			Dw4	49	25	2.8
	Panayi et al. (1987)	50	*DR4*			
	Wordsworth et al. (1989)	139	*DR4*	95	17	10.5
			*0401	70	12	11.0
			**0404*	38	5	14.3
			DR1	36	33	1.2
Netherlands	van Zeben et al. (1991)	134				
			DR4	50	27	2.7
			DR1	25	17	1.7
Germany	Wagner et al. (1997)	66				
			DR4	56	25	3.8
			**0401*	45	20	3.4
			DR1	32	21	1.5
Austria	Scherak et al. (1980)	40				
			DR4	55	23	4.1
Switzerland	Seitz et al. (1996)	83	**04*	82	31	10.1
			**0401*	45	14	3.8
			**0404*	22	11	6.0
			**0405*	7	1	2.0
			**0101/0102*	28	13	2.3

(*continued*)

Table 29–3. Relative Risk for Rheumatoid Arthritis (RA) in Different Populations (*Continued*)

Population	References	No. RA Patients	Associated Specificity or Gene	% Positive in Patients	% Positive in Controls	Relative Risk
Europe (*continued*)						
France	Legrand et al. (1984)	77				
			DR4	31	10	8.5
	Benazet et al. (1995)	73	**0101*	44	13	5.2
			**0401*	25	7	4.7
			**0404*	18	5	4.5
			**0405*	7	1	8.2
Spain	Yelamos et al. (1993)	70	*DR4*	41	23	2.4
			**0405*	13	2	4.3
			DR10	13	4	3.8
Basques	de Juan et al. (1994)	62	*DR1*	35	25	2.2
			DR10	15	1	16.8
	Sanchez et al. (1990)	90	*DRw10*			5.3
			DR4			1.8
Portugal	Queiros et al. (1982)	80	*DR4*	49	12	8.5
Italy	Angelini et al. (1992)	48	**0401*	19	6	4.0
			**0404*	15	3	5.2
Greece	Boki et al. (1992)	92	**DR4*	23	12	2.1
			DRw10	6.5	0	12.7
	Carthy et al. (1993)		**0101*	23	7	4.0
			**1001*	21	6	4.3
			**0405*	14	4	4.5
	Drosos et al. (1995)	92				
	Stavropoulos et al. (1997)	86	*0101*			
			0401			
			0405			
			**1001*			
Yugoslavia	Jajic et al. (1990)	127	*DR1*	45	22.3	2.8
			DR4	34	21	1.9
Russia	Konenkov et al. (1994)		**0404*/0408			
			(0401)			
Middle East						
Israel	Schiff et al. (1982)	49	*DR1*	31	11	3.5
	Gao et al. (1991)	49	*DR1*	18	8	2.8
			**0404*	10	0	10.0
			**0405*	10	0	10.0
			**1001*	16	0	16.6
Kuwait	Sattar et al. (1990)	85	*DR3*	34	2	23.6
Asia and India						
India	Woodrow et al. (1981)	35	*DR1*	60	17	7.0
	Ollier et al. (1991)	44	*DR1*	18	6	3.5
			DR4	21	12	1.9
			DRw10	27	9	3.8
	Agrawal et al. (1995)	74	*DR1*	28	10	3.6
			DR4	72	24	8.0
	Taneja et al. (1996)	75	**0405*	20	5	5.1
			**0401*	11	2	5.0
			**1001*	28	11	3.3
Pakistan	Hameed et al. (1997)	86	DR10	15	5	3.9
			**0401/4/5/8*	12	2	5.7
China	Seglias et al. (1992)	66	*DR4*	42	18	3.4
	Molkentin et al. (1993)	23	*DR4*	43	14	4.6
	Zhao et al. (1996)	86	*DR4*	49	18	4.4
			**0405*	30	4	6.1
Taiwan	Yen et al. (1995)	144	*DR4*	47	26	2.5
			**0405*	39	13	5.1
Singapore	Chan et al. (1994)	70	**0405*	40	13	4.7
			**1001*	14	1	13.2
Korea	Kim et al. (1995)	95	*DR4*	60	31	3.3
			**0405*	44	12	7.2
	Hong et al. (1996)	61	*DR4*	61	29	3.7
			**0405*	43	7	9.4
			**0401*	10	1	8.8
Japan	Maeda et al. (1981)	88	*DR4*	71	46	2.8
	Nakai et al. (1981)	63	*DR4*	71	42	3.5
	Ohta et al. (1982)	148	*DR4*	67	41	3.0
	Takeuchi et al. (1996)		*DR4*	57		
			**0405*	47		

(*continued*)

Table 29–3. Relative Risk for Rheumatoid Arthritis (RA) in Different Populations (*Continued*)

Population	References	No. RA Patients	Associated Specificity or Gene	% Positive in Patients	% Positive in Controls	Relative Risk
Asia and India (*continued*)						
	Wakitani et al. (1997)	852	**0405*	50	29	2.4
			**0101*	14	8	1.8
Australia	Sherritt et al. (1996)	114	*DR4*	54	39	1.9
			DR1	33	13	3.3
New Zealand Polynesians	Tan et al. (1993)	30	*DR4*	67	26	5.6
			**0405*	37	5	11
Africa						
Zimbabwe	Martell et al. (1990)	26	*DR4*			
	Cutbush et al. (1993)	69	**0405*	22	4	7.3
			**1001*	19	2	9.3
South African blacks	Mody et al. (1989)	100	*DR4*	44	10	7.4
	Martell et al. (1989)	33	*DR4*			3.9

ated with a more severe disease course. A Greek study calculated the relative risk for RA of an individual carrying a single shared epitope-positive allele as 2.85, which increased to 8.57 for those with two susceptibility alleles (Stavropoulos et al., 1997). In that population, **0401* conferred the highest risk, followed by **0405*, **0101*, and **1001*.

Numerous additional studies have confirmed that gene dosage also affects disease severity. Eberhardt et al. (1996) found that progressive large joint damage was significantly more prevalent among patients homozygous for *DR4* alleles. Similarly, Toda et al. (1994) demonstrated a more rapid progression of bone destruction in the wrists and fingers among Japanese patients carrying two susceptibility alleles. Combe et al. (1995) divided patients into those with severe articular damage and those with limited radiologic abnormalities; 34.1% of the former group had two susceptibility alleles compared to 8.5% in the latter group (and 7.9% in normal controls). In a group of patients with erosive disease, Seitz and colleagues (1996) showed that patients with two susceptibility alleles had a significantly earlier onset of disease than those with a single dose.

Weyand et al. (1992a,b, 1995) and Weyand and Goronzy (2000) reported several elegant studies leading to a model of a hierarchy of *DR* genotypes determining disease severity and extra-articular manifestations. Their first report analyzed a series of 102 RF-positive RA patients with erosive disease (Weyand et al., 1992a). All but four individuals expressed at least one shared epitope-positive allele, and nearly half had two such alleles. Nodular disease, extra-articular major organ system disease, and the need for joint surgery were significantly higher in patients with two susceptibility alleles. Furthermore, among patients with two shared epitope-positive alleles, those with two *DR4* alleles had worse disease than those with at least one non-*DR4* allele.

Subsequent reports by the same group extended their observations and suggested the following hierarchy. Among individuals with RA, those with no shared epitope-positive alleles are likely to have nonerosive, RF-negative, mild disease. The presence of a *DR4*-negative, shared epitope-positive allele (such as *DR1* or *DR10*) moves them slightly along the spectrum toward more severe disease, while having a single shared epitope-positive *DR4* allele implies a greater chance of RF-positive, erosive disease. A double dose of shared epitope-positive alleles increases the likelihood of extra-articular disease in addition to erosive articular disease. If only one susceptibility allele is *DR4*-positive, nodular disease is likely, while the presence of two *DR4* alleles suggests major organ involvement (e.g., **0401/*0404*). Finally, in this population, vasculitis was particularly common among patients with the **0401/*0401* genotype (Weyand et al., 1992b). Other groups have similarly suggested a continuum of disease severity and *HLA* gene dose (Mattey et al., 2001a,b). Although not all investigators have reproduced this continuum precisely and there is undoubtedly a great deal of overlap among the clinical groups, it is likely that this type of hierarchy does exist, with individual shared epitope-positive alleles contributing differing degrees of risk and certain combinations providing synergism.

Disease Heterogeneity

In addition to the spectrum of disease severity as discussed above, some clinical and/or laboratory constellations of findings are considered to be subsets of RA, and these too have been investigated for possible immunogenetic associations. One of the most common delineations is between RF-positive (seropositive) and RF-negative (seronegative) disease (Goronzy et al., 1987; Anderson, 1987; Lee and Weinblatt, 2001). This has clinical significance in that seronegative patients generally have a milder, less erosive disease course and require less aggressive treatment.

Whether these represent two diseases or variations of the same disease is unknown, and immunogenetic associations may help to resolve this question. One difficulty is with patient selection. Seronegative RA can be difficult to distinguish from other polyarthritis syndromes. One study beginning with 50 seronegative RA patients found that at least 37 actually had other diseases (Kaarela et al., 1990). In addition, patients negative for RF at one time can be positive at other times or when the test is performed by a different method. When these factors are taken into account, most studies of seronegative RA find an excess of the same shared epitope-positive *DRB1* alleles as those seen in seropositive RA. Several studies report an association of *DR4* alleles with seronegative RA (Panayi et al., 1987; Calin et al., 1989; al Jarallah et al., 1994). Furthermore, *DR4* correlates with more severe disease among these patients: Calin et al. (1989) found more destructive disease radiographically in both seropositive and seronegative patients who carried *DR4*.

Other studies agree that shared epitope-positive alleles are associated with seronegative RA but demonstrate an interesting twist: whereas *DR4* alleles are most highly associated with seropositive RA and *DR1* alleles are more weakly associated, the

DR1 association is relatively stronger in seronegative RA (Bardin et al., 1985; Ploski et al., 1994; Vehe et al., 1994; Weyand et al., 1995). In our small study of persistently seronegative RA patients with erosive disease, 81% carried the shared epitope, 50% were positive for *DR4* alleles, and 38% had a *DR1* allele (Vehe et al., 1994). This compares to 85%, 63%, and 24%, respectively, among our seropositive population (Nepom et al., 1989). Weyand et al. (1995) reported a similar trend when comparing seronegative vs. seropositive RA: 35% vs. 91% carried a *DR4* allele, and 42% vs. 23% carried a *DR1* allele, respectively. More recent studies have suggested that the *HLA* shared epitope and the presence or absence of RF may be independently associated with disease severity (Mattey et al., 2001b). In patients with longstanding disease who were RF-positive, there was no apparent association between the presence of the shared epitope and the severity of disease as judged by the bony erosions present, while RF-negative patients showed an association between disease severity and the presence of the shared epitope.

The overall conclusion from these studies, all of which were performed in Caucasian populations, seems to be that seronegative RA is associated with alleles carrying the shared epitope, although the association is somewhat stronger with the *DR1* alleles and less strong with the *DR4* alleles compared to seropositive disease. In addition, many authors have demonstrated that RF production is closely associated with *DR4* alleles (Dobloug et al., 1980; Nelson et al., 1994; Olsen et al., 1988; Queiros et al., 1982). These findings are consistent with the continuum of disease severity and specific alleles described above.

Felty's syndrome is a rare variant of RA characterized by neutropenia and splenomegaly in addition to arthritis. It is highly associated with *HLA-DR4* alleles; in fact, many groups report a near 100% frequency of *DR4* in this patient group (Friman et al., 1985; Westedt et al., 1986; Campion et al., 1990). The *DRB1*0401* gene (*Dw4*) appears to be particularly elevated in these patients (Lanchbury et al., 1991; Wallin et al., 1991; Coakley et al., 2000), but **0404* is also seen often, especially in the **0401/*0404* combination as described in RA above (Wordsworth et al., 1992; Bowman et al., 1994). More recently, a syndrome of chronic proliferation of large granular lymphocytes has been described (Loughran and Starkebaum, 1987). These patients often also have neutropenia and splenomegaly, and up to one-quarter have RA; the relationship among RA, Felty's syndrome, and large granular lymphocyte syndrome is unclear. We and others have investigated the immunogenetic bases of these conditions and come to the same conclusion, i.e., that individuals with large granular lymphocyte syndrome who also have arthritis share the extreme excess of *DR4* alleles seen with Felty's patients, while large granular lymphocyte syndrome patients without arthritis are similar to controls (Bowman et al., 1994; Starkebaum et al., 1997).

Other Genes in the MHC

A large number of genes in the MHC are in disequilibrium, such that when one polymorphic allele is inherited, alleles at other loci are usually inherited too. For example, in Caucasians who carry the *DRB1* allele **0301*, often the entire extended haplotype *A1*, *B8*, *DQA1*0501*, *DQB1*0201* will also be present (see Chapter 28). Linkage disequilibrium is strongest between the *DR* and *DQ* alleles. Class I alleles (*HLA-A*, *-B*, etc.) are less strongly linked, and the *DP* locus is generally not linked. Inserted between the class I and class II regions is the class III region, containing other non-*HLA* genes, such as the genes for tumor necrosis factor (TNF), 21-hydroxylase, heat-shock proteins (HSP), and certain complement components. Also included in the MHC are some genes functioning in antigen-processing pathways, like *TAP-1* and *TAP-2* (transporters associated with antigen processing). Thus, when association studies report correlations between a particular gene and a disease, the question arises whether that gene or a linked gene actually confers susceptibility. Additive or synergistic risk contributed by multiple genes could also be envisioned since many of these gene products act along similar pathways in the immune response. A variety of studies have therefore evaluated other genes in the MHC besides those at the *DR* locus for association with RA, either as primary disease-associated candidate genes or as modulators of such genes.

Other HLA Class II Genes

Among Caucasian populations, *DR4* alleles are usually linked with one of two *DQB1* genes, either **0301* or **0302*. Some early studies reported an increase in what is now called the **0301* allele among RA patients (Baum, 1983; Sansom et al., 1987; Stephens et al., 1989), and one reported an increase in the **0302* allele (Wallin et al., 1988). Subsequent authors have generally agreed, however, that the *DR* association is primary, although the possibility that *DQ* alleles may somehow modulate disease expression has not been ruled out (Fugger and Svejgaard, 1997; Seidl et al., 1997; Mattey et al., 2001a,b). Similarly, several reports have claimed an increase in the *DQB1*0301* allele in RA patients with Felty's syndrome (Sansom et al., 1987; So et al., 1988; Clarkson et al., 1990), while other reports suggest that this is secondary to the *DR* association (Lanchbury et al., 1991; Coakley et al., 2000).

The question of an association of *HLA-DP* alleles with RA is even more confusing. An approximately equal number of studies have reported either no association of any *DP* allele with RA (Pawelec et al., 1988; Begovich et al., 1989; Sage et al., 1991; Hutchings et al., 1993) or an association of RA with the *DPB1* allele **0401* (Stephens et al., 1989; Perdriger et al., 1992; Seidl et al., 1997). Although all of these studies were performed on Caucasian patients, differences in ethnic background may play a role in the varying outcomes. In any case, the degree of any positive *DP* associations is weak at best, and none of the authors suggests that the effect of DP is as important as that of *DR*.

The more recently described HLA class II gene *HLA-DM* has also been investigated for possible relevance to RA. The DM heterodimer is a "nonclassical" HLA molecule with homologies to both class I and class II genes; it is involved in the intracellular processing and presentation of antigens by class II molecules. Although much more conserved than other *HLA* genes, several alleles have been described based on limited nucleotide polymorphisms in the third exon of the *DMA* and *DMB* genes. Analysis of RA patients, normals, and *DR*-matched controls in a French study revealed an increase in the *DMA*0103* allele among patients with *DRB1*01* as well as in patients negative for shared epitope-containing *DR* alleles, although only 13% of the patients had this *DM* allele (Pinet et al., 1997). Three other studies, from Taiwan (Yen et al., 1997), Japan (Takeuchi et al., 1997), and Canada (Singal and Ye, 1998), showed no association of *DM* alleles independent of *DR*.

Non-HLA Genes in the MHC

In addition to the *HLA* class II genes, several other genes located in the MHC have been investigated for their possible contribution to RA. TNF-α has been the focus of intense interest recently since the cytokine has been shown to be central in the inflammatory cascades operating within affected synovia. The response of some refractory patients to treatment with anti-TNF biologic agents has been gratifying and may provide a clue to pathogenesis (Elliott et al., 1994). Thus, it was logical to evaluate the presence of particular TNF alleles as potential contributors to RA susceptibility.

The TNF locus lies in the MHC between the class III and *HLA-B* genes and includes the TNF-α and TNF-β (lymphotoxin) genes. A series of microsatellite markers and single-base polymorphisms (including two in the TNF-α promoter region) define over 40 haplotypes (Udalova et al., 1993; D'Alfonso and Richiardi, 1994; Mulcahy et al., 1996). The results of association studies among RA patients are conflicting. Danis et al. (1995) found an increase in a promoter region polymorphism among RA patients compared to normals, but were unable to demonstrate a corresponding functional difference in TNF-α protein production in vitro. Mulcahy et al. (1996) reported an increase in RA patients of a particular haplotype defined by five microsatellite markers in the TNF-α and TNF-β regions, as well as with two of these markers individually. Wilson et al. (1995) found no differences in TNF-α alleles between patients and normals, nor did Vinasco et al. (1997a) find an association of either TNF-α promoter region polymorphisms or TNF-β markers with disease.

Still other groups report an association of particular TNF alleles with RA, but find that these correlations are due to linkage with the DR alleles. Hajeer and colleagues (1996) reported an increase in a TNF allele called *TNFa6* with RA, but concluded this increase was secondary to linkage with DRB1*0401. Similarly, Field et al. (1997) found an increase in the *TNFa2* allele among patients, but when they were segregated into DR4-positive and DR4-negative groups, the increase was only present in the former population, and the authors determined that the DR association was primary. Interestingly, a *DRB1*0401*-containing haplotype has been associated with a relatively high level of TNF alpha production (Pociot et al., 1993), suggesting that the combination of certain DR and TNF-α alleles may be functionally relevant in RA. The significance of such potential interactions remains to be clarified.

The *TAP* genes, also located within the MHC, encode proteins that function in transporting cytoplasmic antigenic peptides into the endoplasmic reticulum for binding to HLA class I molecules. Limited polymorphisms discovered within these genes prompted a search for association with RA. Most reports attribute any skewing of *TAP-2* alleles in RA to linkage with *DR* (Marsal et al., 1994; Vandevyver et al., 1995; Vinasco et al., 1998), although two reports suggest an increased frequency of a *TAP-2* allele among *DR4*-positive RA patients compared to HLA haplotype-matched controls (Singal et al., 1994; Hillarby et al., 1996).

Other polymorphic genes within the class III region have also been studied for possible association with RA, such as the complement component *C4B* (Clarkson et al., 1990) and *HSP-70* (Quadri et al., 1996; Vinasco et al., 1997b). No convincing associations with particular alleles that could not be accounted for by linkage with *DR* susceptibility genes have been reported.

Genes Outside the MHC

Since MHC genes do not account for all of the susceptibility for RA, investigators have searched for associations with candidate genes outside of this region, without striking success to date. As T lymphocytes are felt to be important in disease pathogenesis, it was logical to investigate the polymorphic T-cell receptor (TCR) genes for association with disease. Germline polymorphisms have not shown reproducible associations (reviewed in Wordsworth, 1998). Many studies have subsequently looked for similarities in usage of TCR families and genes; however, very little consensus has emerged, so the role of TCR genetics in RA remains unclear.

Associations with polymorphic immunoglobulin genes have been sought in RA as well. Many studies showed no association, and most of those observing an increase in particular allotypic markers found that they were enriched among patients who were *DR4*-positive. The possible role of these polymorphisms remains to be clarified.

Cytokine genes are another category of candidate genes that may be relevant to the pathogenesis of RA. In addition to the TNF genes discussed above, other cytokine loci have been evaluated for possible skewing in RA. Weak linkage has been suggested in preliminary studies for several genes, including the interleukin-5 (IL-5) receptor, interferon-γ, IL-2 (John et al., 1998), and the IL-1 gene cluster (Cox et al., 1998). In other reports, no evidence for linkage was seen for the IL-10 promoter (Hajeer et al., 1998), interferon-α and -β, IL-1 and the IL-1 receptor, IL-6, the IL-8 receptor, CD40L (John et al., 1998), or the cytokine gene cluster on chromosome 5q23–31, which includes IL-3, IL-4, IL-5, granulocyte-macrophage colony-stimulating factor, and IL-9 (Barrett et al., 1998).

As there is such a strong female preponderance in RA, one other area of investigation relates to hormone-related genes. Preliminary evidence of possible linkage to RA has been found by one group for markers near the genes for corticotropin-releasing hormone and estrogen synthetase (Barrett et al., 1998) as well as prolactin (Brennan et al., 1997).

Genome-Wide Screening

Much effort has gone into collecting large series of patients and family members for comprehensive genome-wide linkage studies. Information from these studies should be available in the near future. A few preliminary results have already been presented as of this writing. Hardwick and colleagues (1997) confirmed linkage to the HLA region, along with another possible locus on chromosome 6 outside of the HLA region, using 315 microsatellite markers in 293 individuals from a set of 89 multicase families. Shunichi et al. (1997) studied 41 Japanese families with at least two affected sibs with 358 microsatellite markers and found preliminary evidence of linkage near markers on chromosome 1 (*D1S214*), chromosome 8 (*D8S556*), and the X chromosome (*DXS1047* and *DXS1227*). The authors suggested the genes for TNF receptor 2 and CD40L as candidate genes in these regions.

The European Consortium on RA Families (ECRAF) reported data from a genome scan on 114 sib pairs from 97 families, using 309 microsatellite markers (Cornelis et al., 1998). As in the previous study, linkage was significant only for the HLA region ($p < 2.5 \times 10^{-5}$). However, 19 other markers in 14 regions showed nominal linkage, with significance values of $p < 0.05$. Two of these regions were studied in a second set of 194 sib pairs from 164 families, and one of them, defined by marker *D3S1267* at chromosome 3q13, resulted in significantly improved linkage ($p < 0.002$). Of interest, this region overlaps one previously implicated in IDDM susceptibility (called insulin-dependent diabetes mellitus (IDDM9). Candidate genes in the region include those encoding CD80 and CD86, costimulatory molecules important in T-cell activation. ECRAF has subsequently reported an RA susceptibility locus on chromosome 1 (Cornelis, 1998). This was also tested on a second set of affected sib-pair families. Marker *D1S228* reached a significance of $p =$

0.04. Furthermore, they demonstrated an effect of HLA on sharing at this locus, suggesting an interaction between the two regions. One candidate gene in this area is *TNFR2*, which encodes a TNF receptor, a gene also suggested by the Japanese group. A recent study of *TNFR2* has also suggested an association between an allele of this gene, defined by a single-nucleotide polymorphism, and RA (Barton et al., 2001b).

A group of collaborators in the United States formed the North American Rheumatoid Arthritis Consortium with the goal of collecting 1000 families containing affected sib pairs (Gregersen, 1998). This type of extremely large sample collection will be required in many cases to confirm in a statistically robust manner the linkage of particular genetic regions with RA and should allow the degree of confidence that makes the subsequent work of finding the individual gene linked to disease worthwhile. While the challenge of determining the identity and function of individual genes linked to disease should not be minimized, with the techniques available we are likely on the threshold of a much greater understanding of the genetic basis of complex diseases like RA.

The availability of high-throughput methods has led to an increased number of linkage studies (Myerscough et al., 2000; Jawaheer et al., 2001; Merriman et al., 2001; Barton et al., 2001a). These studies attempt to replicate the findings from the first set of studies, to identify candidate genes in regions that are critical to other autoimmune diseases, and to develop correlations between laboratory animal models and human disease. This is an exciting area of ongoing research. No specific gene has been identified to date that explains familial RA, but this work is providing insight into potential pathways of disease that collectively are responsible for the genetic susceptibility to this common disease.

CLINICAL APPLICATION AND RISK ASSESSMENT

Diagnosis and Screening

As discussed above, certain *HLA* alleles, such as *DRB1*0401* and **0404*, are highly associated with RA. In particular, they are strongly correlated with more severe, erosive disease, and gene dosage appears to play a role, with a "double dose" of susceptibility alleles correlating with extra-articular disease manifestations. This has raised the issue of whether these alleles confer susceptibility or are markers only of disease severity; perhaps a more useful way to think of it is that they confer susceptibility for severe disease. In any event, this raises the question of the clinical utility of knowing these genotypes. Is knowledge of *HLA* genotypes useful in screening the general population for those at risk of RA? Is it useful in making the diagnosis of RA in a patient with early, undifferentiated arthritis? Is it useful in predicting disease severity in an individual patient and, thus, potentially guiding therapy?

To address these issues, one can calculate risk estimates for specific genes in particular populations, as exemplified in Table 29–4. These numbers are based on a Caucasian, North American population, with the prevalence of RA assumed to be approximately 1% (which is an upper-limit estimate, particularly for severe disease). Thus, this represents the high end of predictive value. For *DRB1*0401*, the most prevalent allele among patients in this population, the estimated risk is 1 in 35. Consequently, 97% of individuals carrying the **0401* allele will not develop RA. Even in the case of the highest risk, 1 in 7 for an **0401/*0404* heterozygote, over 85% of individuals will not get

Table 29–4. Estimated Risk Ratios for *HLA-DRB1* Genes Associated with Rheumatoid Arthritis (RA)

Gene	Estimates per 10,000 Population		Approximate Risk Ratio
	RA-Positive	Normals	
**0401*	50	1800	1 in 35
**0404*	25	500	1 in 20
**0101*	25	2000	1 in 80
**0401* or **0404*	65	2300	1 in 35
**0401*, **0404*, or **0101*	90	4200	1 in 46
**0401* and **0404*	15	100	1 in 7
Other	10	5800	1 in 580

disease, making this uninformative for screening the general population. Furthermore, there is currently no known intervention for delaying or preventing RA. For similar reasons, *HLA* genotyping helps little in the diagnosis of RA, which remains a clinical diagnosis. While the association of these susceptibility alleles with RA is quite strong and reproducible, as many as 40% of the normal population will have at least one of these alleles, so it is not helpful in making the diagnosis of RA in an individual patient.

Relationship to Therapy

Once the diagnosis of RA is made, knowing the patient's *HLA* genotype may be helpful in predicting disease course and guiding therapy. As discussed above, disease severity is correlated with the presence and number of specific alleles. Several studies have assessed this issue prospectively. Wagner et al. (1997) followed 55 patients with recent-onset RA for a median observation time of 2 years and found that those individuals carrying a shared epitope in the context of a *DR4*-positive allele had a significantly increased risk (relative risk = 13.75) of developing bony erosions, while there was no increased risk of developing erosions in those expressing the shared epitope on DR1 only or not expressing it at all.

In another prospective study, Gough and colleagues (1994) evaluated 120 RA patients for the development of erosions after 1 year. Although the authors did not distinguish between the shared epitope expressed on a *DR4* as opposed to a *DR1* allele, they found a strikingly similar relative risk of 13.5 for the development of erosions among patients positive for either the shared epitope or RF.

If *HLA* genotyping is useful in predicting which patients will develop erosive disease, does this have clinical utility in guiding therapy? One study suggested that it does, at least within the Caucasian population. Eighty-four RA patients enrolled in a treatment trial comparing methotrexate alone, hydroxychloroquine plus sulfasalazine, and all three drugs together were genotyped for *HLA-DR* (O'Dell et al., 1998). A marked difference was seen in the frequency of successful outcomes among patients stratified by shared epitope status. Among patients receiving methotrexate alone, only 32% of those positive for the shared epitope met criteria for "successful completion," while 94% of shared epitope-positive patients in the group treated with all three drugs were successful completers. Those in the hydroxychloroquine plus sulfasalazine group were intermediate in outcome. In addition, in the methotrexate-only group, gene dosage appeared to play a role: 83% of patients negative for the shared epitope, 36% of patients with a single dose of the shared epitope, and only 25% of patients with a double dose of the shared epitope had successful outcomes with this less aggressive treatment. These data are consistent with the concept that RA patients carrying one or, especially, two doses of the shared epitope may require earlier, more aggressive treatment to control disease and prevent erosions. Prospective studies with longer follow-up are needed to clarify the ultimate clinical usefulness of these markers. As more treatment options become available, especially biologic agents such as anti-TNF-α reagents, the need for determining which patients require more aggressive treatment will become more acute.

In the past, a number of studies reported associations between HLA class II specificities and toxic reactions to certain therapeutic agents. The most reproducible correlation seemed to be between *HLA-DR3* and toxic reactions, particularly proteinuria, to either gold salts or D-penicillamine (Panayi et al., 1978; Wooley et al., 1980; Speerstra et al., 1983; Bensen et al., 1984; Legrand et al., 1984). As the use of these drugs has waned in favor of newer therapies, this issue has become less pertinent. It remains to be seen whether *HLA* genotyping is helpful in predicting which patients will respond to the newer drugs or biologic agents and/or which will have significant side effects.

A current issue is the availability and cost of testing for these markers. *HLA* genotyping is generally performed only in centralized tissue typing laboratories or in research protocols, often at prohibitive cost. However, technological advances should make rapid, accurate, and automated typing feasible and available to most clinical laboratories. One such method has been described (Nepom et al., 1996), and this and/or similar techniques will likely become available in the near future.

REFERENCES

Aarvak T, Chabaud M, Thoen J, Miossec P, Natvig JB: Changes in the Th1 or Th2 cytokine dominance in the synovium of rheumatoid arthritis (RA): a kinetic study of the Th subsets in one unusual RA patient. Rheumatology (Oxford) 2000; 39:513–522.

Abdel-Nasser AM, Rasker JJ, Valkenburg HA: Epidemiological and clinical aspects relating to the variability of rheumatoid arthritis. Semin Arthritis Rheum 1997; 27:123–140.

Agrawal S, Aggarwal A, Dabadghao S, Naik S, Misra R: Compound heterozygosity of HLA-DR4 and DR1 antigens in Asian Indians increases the risk of extra-articular features in rheumatoid arthritis. Br J Rheumatol 1995; 34:41–44.

Aho K, Koskenvuo M, Tuominen J, Kaprio J: Occurrence of rheumatoid arthritis in a nationwide series of twins. J Rheumatol 1986; 13:899–902.

Alarcon GS, Koopman WJ, Acton RT, Barger BO: DR antigen distribution in blacks with rheumatoid arthritis. J Rheumatol 1983; 10:579–583.

Alarif LI, Ruppert GB, Wilson R Jr, Barth WF: HLA-DR antigens in blacks with rheumatoid arthritis and systemic lupus erythematosus. J Rheumatol 1983; 10:297–300.

al Jarallah KF, Buchanan WW, Sastry A, Singal DP: Seronegative rheumatoid arthritis and HLA-DR4. J Rheumatol 1994; 21:190–193.

Amit M, Guedj D, Wysenbeek AJ: Expression of rheumatoid arthritis in two ethnic Jewish Israeli groups. Ann Rheum Dis 1996; 55:69–72.

Anderson RJ: Rheumatoid arthritis. B. Clinical and laboratory features. In: Klippel JH (ed). Primer on the Rheumatic Diseases. Atlanta: Arthritis Foundation, 1987:161–167.

Andersson EC, Svendsen P, Svejgaard A, Holmdahl R, Fugger L: A molecule basis for the *HLA* association in rheumatoid arthritis. Rev Immunogenet 2000; 2:81–87.

Angelini G, Morozzi G, Delfino L, Pera C, Falco M, Marcolongo R, Giannelli S, Ratti G, Ricci S, Fanetti G: Analysis of *HLA DP*, *DQ*, and *DR* alleles in adult Italian rheumatoid arthritis patients. Hum Immunol 1992; 34:135–141.

Arend WP: Physiology of cytokine pathways in rheumatoid arthritis. Arthritis Rheum 2001; 45:101–106.

Arnett FC, Edworthy SM, Bloch DA, McShane DJ, Fries JF, Cooper NS, Healey LA: The American Rheumatism Association 1987 revised criteria of rheumatoid arthritis. Arthritis Rheum 1988; 31:315–324.

Auger I, Roudier J: A function for the QKRAA amino acid motif: mediating binding of DnaJ to DnaK. Implications for the association of rheumatoid arthritis with HLA-DR4. J Clin Invest 1997; 99:1818–1822.

Bardin T, Legrand L, Naveau B, Marcelli-Barge A, Debeyre N, Lathrop GM, Poirier JC, Schmid M, Ryckewaert A, Dryll A: *HLA* antigens and seronegative rheumatoid arthritis. Ann Rheum Dis 1985; 44:50–53.

Barrera P, Radstake TR, Albers JM, van Riel PL, van de Putte LB: Familial aggregation of rheumatoid arthritis in the Netherlands: a cross-sectional hospital-based survey. European Consortium on Rheumatoid Arthritis Families (ECRAF). Rheumatology (Oxford) 1999; 38:415–422.

Barrett JH, Worthington J, John S, Myerscough A, Hajeer A, Panayi GS, Lanchbury JS, Silman AJ, Ollier WER: Linkage analysis of candidate gene loci in rheumatoid arthritis: evidence suggestive of linkage to corticotropin releasing hormone (CRH) and estrogen synthetase (CYP19). Am J Hum Genet 1998; 63:A281.

Barton A, Eyre S, Myerscough A, Brintnell B, Ward D, Ollier WER, Lorentzen JC, Klareskog L, Silman A, John S, et al.: High resolution linkage and association mapping identifies a novel rheumatoid arthritis susceptibility locus homologous to one linked to two rat models of inflammatory arthritis. Hum Mol Genet 2001a; 10:1901–1906.

Barton A, John S, Ollier WE, Silman A, Worthington J: Association between rheumatoid arthritis and polymorphism of tumor necrosis factor receptor II but not tumor necrosis factor receptor I, in Caucasians. Arthritis Rheum 2001b; 44:61–65.

Baum J: Treatment of juvenile arthritis. Hosp Pract 1983; 18:121–126.

Beasley RP, Bennett PH, Lin CC: Low prevalence of rheumatoid arthritis in Chinese. Prevalence survey in a rural community. J Rheumatol Suppl 1983; 10:11–15.

Beasley RP, Retailliau H, Healey LA: Prevalence of rheumatoid arthritis in Alaskan Eskimos. Arthritis Rheum 1973a; 16:737–742.

Beasley RP, Willkens RF, Bennett PH: High prevalence of rheumatoid arthritis in Yakima Indians. Arthritis Rheum 1973b; 16:743–748.

Begovich AB, Bugawan TL, Nepom BS, Klitz W, Nepom GT, Erlich HA: A specific *HLA-DP* β allele is associated with pauciarticular juvenile rheumatoid arthritis but not adult rheumatoid arthritis. Proc Natl Acad Sci USA 1989; 86:9489–9493.

Bellamy N, Duffy D, Martin N, Mathews J: Rheumatoid arthritis in twins: a study of aetiopathogenesis based on the Australian Twin Registry. Ann Rheum Dis 1992; 51:588–593.

Benazet JF, Reviron D, Mercier P, Roux H, Roudier J: *HLA-DRB1* alleles associated with rheumatoid arthritis in southern France. Absence of extraarticular disease despite expression of the shared epitope. J Rheumatol 1995; 22:607–610.

Benedek TG, Rodnan GP: A brief history of the rheumatic diseases. Bull Rheum Dis 1982; 32:59–68.

Bennett AH, Burch TA: New York symposium on population studies in the rheumatic diseases. Bull Rheum Dis 1967; 17:453–458.

Bensen WG, Moore N, Tugwell P, D'Souza M, Singal DP: *HLA* antigens and toxic reactions to sodium aurothiomalate in patients with rheumatoid arthritis. J Rheumatol 1984; 11:358–361.

Blanar MA, Burkly LC, Flavell RA: NF-kappaB binds within a region required for B-cell-specific expression of major histocompatibility complex class II gene Eαd. Mol Cell Biol 1989; 9:844–846.

Bluestein HG, Hasler F: Epstein-Barr virus and rheumatoid arthritis. Surv Immunol Res 1984; 3:70–77.

Boki KA, Panayi GS, Vaughan RW, Drosos AA, Moutsopoulos HM, Lanchbury JS: HLA class II sequence polymorphisms and susceptibility to rheumatoid arthritis in Greeks. The HLA-DR β shared-epitope hypothesis accounts for the disease in only a minority of Greek patients. Arthritis Rheum 1992; 35:749–755.

Bowman SJ, Sivakumaran M, Snowden N, Bhavnani M, Hall MA, Panayi GS, Lanchbury JS: The large granular lymphocyte syndrome with rheumatoid arthritis. Immunogenetic evidence for a broader definition of Felty's syndrome. Arthritis Rheum 1994; 37:1326–1330.

Boyer GS, Templin DW, Lanier AP: Rheumatic diseases in Alaskan Indians of the southeast coast: high prevalence of rheumatoid arthritis and systemic lupus erythematosus. J Rheumatol 1991; 18:1477–1484.

Brennan FM, Maini RN, Feldmann M: Role of pro-inflammatory cytokines in rheumatoid arthritis. Springer Semin Immunopathol 1998; 20:133–147.

Brennan P, Hajeer A, Ong KR, Worthington J, John S, Thomson W, Silman A, Ollier B: Allelic markers close to prolactin are associated with *HLA-DRB1* susceptibility alleles among women with rheumatoid arthritis and systemic lupus erythematosus. Arthritis Rheum 1997; 40:1383–1386.

Calin A, Elswood J, Klouda PT: Destructive arthritis, rheumatoid factor, and HLA-DR4. Susceptibility versus severity, a case-control study. Arthritis Rheum 1989; 32:1221–1225.

Campion G, Maddison PJ, Goulding N, James I, Ahern MJ, Watt I, Sansom D: The Felty syndrome: a case-matched study of clinical manifestations and outcome, serologic features, and immunogenetic associations. Medicine (Baltimore) 1990; 69:69–80.

Carthy D, Ollier W, Papasteriades C, Pappas H, Thomson W: A shared *HLA-DRB1* sequence confers RA susceptibility in Greeks. Eur J Immunogenet 1993; 20:391–398.

Case JP, Lafyatis R, Remmers EF, Kumkumian GK, Wilder RL: Transin/stromelysin expression in rheumatoid synovium. A transformation-associated metalloproteinase secreted by phenotypically invasive synoviocytes. Am J Pathol 1989; 135:1055–1064.

Chan SH, Lin YN, Wee GB, Koh WH, Boey ML: HLA class 2 genes in Singaporean Chinese rheumatoid arthritis. Br J Rheumatol 1994; 33:713–717.

Chikanza IC, Stein M, Lutalo S, Gibson T: The clinical, serologic and radiologic features of rheumatoid arthritis in ethnic black Zimbabwean and British Caucasian patients. J Rheumatol 1994; 21:2011–2015.

Chou CT, Pei L, Chang DM, Lee CF, Schumacher HR, Liang MH: Prevalence of rheumatic diseases in Taiwan: a population study of urban, suburban, rural differences. J Rheumatol 1994; 21:302–306.

Clarkson R, Bate AS, Grennan DM, Chattopadhyay C, Sanders P, Davis M, Kelly C: *DQw7* and the *C4B* null allele in rheumatoid arthritis and Felty's syndrome. Ann Rheum Dis 1990; 49:976–979.

Coakley G, Brooks D, Iqbal M, Kondeatis E, Vaughan R, Loughran TP Jr, Panayi GS, Lanchbury JS: Major histocompatibility complex haplotype associations in Felty's syndrome and large granular lymphocyte syndrome are secondary to allelic association with *HLA-DRB1*0401*. Rheumatology 2000; 39:393–398.

Combe B, Eliaou JF, Daures JP, Meyer O, Clot J, Sany J: Prognostic factors in rheumatoid arthritis. Comparative study of two subsets of patients according to severity of articular damage. Br J Rheumatol 1995; 34:529–534.

Cornelis F: New susceptibility locus on chromosome 1 for rheumatoid arthritis (RA). Arthritis Rheum 1998; 41(Suppl):S242.

Cornelis F, Faure S, Martinez M, Prud'Homme JF, Fritz P, Dib C, Alves H, Barrera P, de Vries N, Balsa A, et al.: New susceptibility locus for rheumatoid arthritis suggested by a genome-wide linkage study. Proc Natl Acad Sci USA 1998; 95:10746–10750.

Cox A, Camp NJ, Dale M, di Giovine FS, Silman AJ, Ollier WER, Worthington J, Duff GW: Linkage disequilibrium mapping of rheumatoid arthritis severity/susceptibility loci in the interleukin-1 gene cluster using TDT and sib-TDT. Am J Hum Genet 1998; 63:A286.

Cutbush S, Chikanza IC, Biro PA, Bekker C, Stein M, Lutalo S, Garcia-Pacheco JM, McCloskey DS, Lanchbury JS, Sachs JA: Sequence-specific oligonucleotide typing in Shona patients with rheumatoid arthritis and healthy controls from Zimbabwe. Tissue Antigens 1993; 41:169–172.

D'Alfonso S, Richiardi PM: A polymorphic variation in a putative regulation box of the *TNFA* promoter region. Immunogenetics 1994; 39:150–154.

Danis VA, Millington M, Hyland V, Lawford R, Huang Q, Grennan D: Increased frequency of the uncommon allele of a tumour necrosis factor alpha gene polymorphism in rheumatoid arthritis and systemic lupus erythematosus. Dis Markers 1995; 12:127–133.

Da Silva JA: Sex hormones, glucocorticoids and autoimmunity: facts and hypotheses. Ann Rheum Dis 1995; 54:6–16.

Da Silva JA, Spector TD: The role of pregnancy in the course and aetiology of rheumatoid arthritis. Clin Rheumatol 1992; 11:189–194.

Debaz H, Olivo A, Vazquez Garcia MN, de la RG, Hernandez A, Lino L, Burgos R, Fernandez-Vina M, Stastny P, Gorodezky C: Relevant residues of DRβ1 third hypervariable region contributing to the expression and to severity of rheumatoid arthritis (RA) in Mexicans. Hum Immunol 1998; 59:287–294.

Deighton CM, Roberts DF, Walker DJ: Effect of disease severity on rheumatoid arthritis concordance in same sexed siblings. Ann Rheum Dis 1992a; 51:943–945.

Deighton CM, Walker DJ: The familial nature of rheumatoid arthritis. Ann Rheum Dis 1991; 50:62–65.

Deighton CM, Wentzel J, Cavanagh G, Roberts DF, Walker DJ: Contribution of inherited factors to rheumatoid arthritis. Ann Rheum Dis 1992b; 51:182–185.

de Juan MD, Belmonte I, Barado J, Martinez LJ, Figueroa M, Arnaiz-Villena A, Cuadrado E: Differential associations of HLA-DR antigens with rheumatoid arthritis (RA) in Basques: high frequency of DR1 and DR10 and lack of association with HLA-DR4 or any of its subtypes. Tissue Antigens 1994; 43:320–323.

Del Puente A, Knowler WC, Pettitt DJ, Bennett PH: High incidence and prevalence of rheumatoid arthritis in Pima Indians. Am J Epidemiol 1989; 129:1170–1178.

Dobloug JH, Forre O, Kass E, Thorsby E: *HLA* antigens and rheumatoid arthritis. Association between HLA-DRw4 positivity and IgM rheumatoid factor production. Arthritis Rheum 1980; 23:309–313.

Doita M, Hirohata K, Maeda S: Association of *HLA-DR* antigens with disease severity in Japanese patients with rheumatoid arthritis. Kobe J Med Sci 1990; 36:103–114.

Dorner RW, Alexander RL Jr, Moore TL: Rheumatoid factors. Clin Chim Acta 1987; 167:1–21.

Drosos AA, Lanchbury JS, Panayi GS, Moutsopoulos HM: Rheumatoid arthritis in Greek and British patients. A comparative clinical, radiologic, and serologic study. Arthritis Rheum 1992; 35:745–748.

Drosos AA, Moutsopoulos HM: Rheumatoid arthritis in Greece: clinical, serological and genetic considerations. Clin Exp Rheumatol 1995; 13(Suppl 12):S7–12.

Eberhardt K, Fex E, Johnson U, Wollheim FA: Associations of *HLA-DRB* and *-DQB* genes with two and five year outcome in rheumatoid arthritis. Ann Rheum Dis 1996; 55:34–39.

Ebringer A, Wilson C: HLA molecules, bacteria and autoimmunity. J Med Microbiol 2000; 49:305–311.

Elliott MJ, Maini RN, Feldmann M, Kalden JR, Antoni C, Smolen JS, Leeb B, Breedveld FC, Macfarlane JD, Bijl H: Randomised double-blind comparison of chimeric monoclonal antibody to tumour necrosis factor α (cA2) versus placebo in rheumatoid arthritis. Lancet 1994; 344:1105–1110.

Engel A, Roberts J, Burch TA: Rheumatoid Arthritis in Adults. United States 1960–1962. Washington DC: US Public Health Service, 1966.

Feldmann M, Maini RN: The role of cytokines in the pathogenesis of rheumatoid arthritis. Rheumatology (Oxford) 1999; 38(Suppl 2):3–7.

Field M, Gallagher G, Eskdale J, McGarry F, Richards SD, Munro R, Oh HH, Campbell C: Tumor necrosis factor locus polymorphisms in rheumatoid arthritis. Tissue Antigens 1997; 50:303–307.

Fries JF, Hochberg MC, Medsger TA Jr, Hunder GG, Bombardier C: Criteria for rheumatic disease. Different types and different functions. The American College of Rheumatology Diagnostic and Therapeutic Criteria Committee. Arthritis Rheum 1994; 37:454–462.

Friman C, Schlaut J, Davis P: HLA-DR4 in Felty's syndrome [letter]. J Rheumatol 1985; 12:628–629.

Fugger L, Svejgaard A: The HLA-DQ7 and -DQ8 associations in DR4-positive rheumatoid arthritis patients. A combined analysis of data available in the literature. Tissue Antigens 1997; 50:494–500.

Gabriel SE: The epidemiology of rheumatoid arthritis. Rheum Dis Clin North Am 2001; 27:269–281.

Gao X, Gazit E, Livneh A, Stastny P: Rheumatoid arthritis in Israeli Jews: shared sequences in the third hypervariable region of *DRB1* alleles are associated with susceptibility. J Rheumatol 1991; 18:801–803.

Gao XJ, Olsen NJ, Pincus T, Stastny P: *HLA-DR* alleles with naturally occurring amino acid substitutions and risk for development of rheumatoid arthritis. Arthritis Rheum 1990; 33:939–946.

Gaston JS, Life PF, Bailey LC, Bacon PA: In vitro responses to a 65-kilodalton mycobacterial protein by synovial T cells from inflammatory arthritis patients. J Immunol 1989; 143:2494–2500.

Gladman DD, Anhorn KA: *HLA* and disease manifestations in rheumatoid arthritis—a Canadian experience. J Rheumatol 1986; 13:274–276.

Gonzalez A, Nicovani S, Massardo L, Aguirre V, Cervilla V, Lanchbury JS, Jacobelli S: Influence of the *HLA-DRβ* shared epitope on susceptibility to and clinical expression of rheumatoid arthritis in Chilean patients. Ann Rheum Dis 1997; 56:191–193.

Gonzalez-Gay MA, Hajeer AH, Dababneh A, Makki R, Garcia-Porrua C, Thomson W, Ollier W: Seronegative rheumatoid arthritis in elderly and polymyalgia rheumatica have similar patterns of *HLA* association. J Rheumatol 2001; 28:122–125.

Goronzy JJ, Weyand CM: Rheumatoid arthritis. A. Epidemiology, pathology, and pathogenesis. In: Klippel JH (ed). Primer on the Rheumatic Diseases. Atlanta: Arthritis Foundation, 1987:155–161.

Gough A, Faint J, Salmon M, Hassell A, Wordsworth P, Pilling D, Birley A, Emery P: Genetic typing of patients with inflammatory arthritis at presentation can be used to predict outcome. Arthritis Rheum 1994; 37:1166–1170.

Gran JT, Husby G, Thorsby E: The association between rheumatoid arthritis and the *HLA* antigen *DR4*. Ann Rheum Dis 1983; 42:292–296.

Gregersen PK: The North American Rheumatoid Arthritis Consortium—bringing genetic analysis to bear on disease susceptibility, severity, and outcome. Arthritis Care Res 1998; 11:1–2.

Gregersen PK, Silver J, Winchester RJ: The shared epitope hypothesis. An approach to understanding the molecular genetics of susceptibility to rheumatoid arthritis. Arthritis Rheum 1987; 30:1205–1213.

Hajeer AH, Lazarus M, Turner D, Mageed RA, Vencovsky J, Sinnott P, Hutchinson IV, Ollier WE: *IL-10* gene promoter polymorphisms in rheumatoid arthritis. Scand J Rheumatol 1998; 27:142–145.

Hajeer AH, Worthington J, Silman AJ, Ollier WE: Association of tumor necrosis factor microsatellite polymorphisms with *HLA-DRB1*04*-bearing haplotypes in rheumatoid arthritis patients. Arthritis Rheum 1996; 39:1109–1114.

Hameed K, Bowman S, Kondeatis E, Vaughan R, Gibson T: The association of *HLA-DRB* genes and the shared epitope with rheumatoid arthritis in Pakistan. Br J Rheumatol 1997; 36:1184–1188.

Harada S, Yamamura M, Okamoto H, Morita Y, Kawashima M, Aita T, Makino H: Production of interleukin-7 and interleukin-15 by fibroblast-like synoviocytes from patients with rheumatoid arthritis. Arthritis Rheum 1999; 42:1508–1516.

Hardwick LJ, Walsh S, Butcher S, Nicod A, Shatford J, Bell J, Lathrop M, Wordsworth BP: Genetic mapping of susceptibility loci in the genes involved in rheumatoid arthritis. J Rheumatol 1997; 24:197–198.

Harris ED Jr: Rheumatoid arthritis. Pathophysiology and implications for therapy [published erratum appears in N Engl J Med 1990; 323:996]. N Engl J Med 1990; 322:1277–1289.

Harvey J, Lotze M, Arnett FC, Bias WB, Billingsley LM, Harvey E, Hsu SH, Sutton JD, Zizic TM, Stevens MB: Rheumatoid arthritis in a Chippewa band. II. Field study with clinical serologic and *HLA-D* correlations. J Rheumatol 1983; 10:28–32.

Harvey J, Lotze M, Stevens MB, Lambert G, Jacobson D: Rheumatoid arthritis in a Chippewa band. I. Pilot screening study of disease prevalence. Arthritis Rheum 1981; 24:717–721.

Hazes JM, Dijkmans BA, Vandenbroucke JP, de Vries RR, Cats A: Pregnancy and the risk of developing rheumatoid arthritis. Arthritis Rheum 1990; 33:1770–1775.

Hazes JM, Silman AJ: Review of UK data on the rheumatic diseases—2. Rheumatoid arthritis. Br J Rheumatol 1990; 29:310–312.

Hazes JM, van Zeben D: Oral contraception and its possible protection against rheumatoid arthritis. Ann Rheum Dis 1991; 50:72–74.

Heliovaara M, Aho K, Knekt P, Impivaara O, Reunanen A, Aromaa A: Coffee consumption, rheumatoid factor, and the risk of rheumatoid arthritis. Ann Rheum Dis 2000; 59:631–635.

Hellgren L: The prevalence of rheumatoid arthritis in different geographical areas in Sweden. Acta Rheumatol Scand 1970; 16:293–303.

Hellier JP, Eliaou JF, Daures JP, Sany J, Combe B: *HLA-DRB1* genes and patients with late onset rheumatoid arthritis. Ann Rheum Dis 2001; 60:531–533.

Hillarby MC, Davies EJ, Donn RP, Grennan DM, Ollier WE: *TAP2D* is associated with HLA-B44 and DR4 and may contribute to rheumatoid arthritis and Felty's syndrome susceptibility. Clin Exp Rheumatol 1996; 14:67–70.

Holoshitz J, Klajman A, Drucker I, Lapidot Z, Yaretzky A, Frenkel A, van Eden W, Cohen IR: T lymphocytes of rheumatoid arthritis patients show augmented reactivity to a fraction of mycobacteria cross-reactive with cartilage. Lancet 1986; 2:305–309.

Holoshitz J, Koning F, Coligan JE, De Bruyn J, Strober S: Isolation of $CD4^-$ $CD8^-$ mycobacteria-reactive T lymphocyte clones from rheumatoid arthritis synovial fluid. Nature 1989; 339:226–229.

Hong GH, Park MH, Takeuchi F, Oh MD, Song YW, Nabeta H, Nakano K, Ito K, Park KS: Association of specific amino acid sequence of *HLA-DR* with rheumatoid arthritis in Koreans and its diagnostic value. J Rheumatol 1996; 23:1699–1703.

Hormell RS: Notes on the history of rheumatism and gout. N Engl J Med 1940; 223:754–760.

Hutchings CJ, Hillarby MC, McMahon MJ, Ollier WE, Grennan DM: *HLA-DPA1* and *HLA-DPB1* in rheumatoid arthritis and its subsets. Dis Markers 1993; 11:37–44.

Jain A, Nanchahal J, Troeberg I, Green P, Brennan F: Production of cytokines, vascular endothelial growth factor, matrix metalloproteinases, and tissue inhibitor of

metalloproteinases 1 by tenosynovium demonstrates its potential for tendon destruction in rheumatoid arthritis. Arthritis Rheum 2001; 44:1754–1560.
Jajic Z, Jajic I, Jajic I, Kerhin-Brkljacic V: *HLA* antigens in a Yugoslav population with rheumatoid arthritis. Clin Rheumatol 1990; 9:48–50.
Jaraquemada D, Ollier W, Awad J, Young A, Silman A, Roitt IM, Corbett M, Hay F, Cosh JA, Maini RN: *HLA* and rheumatoid arthritis: a combined analysis of 440 British patients. Ann Rheum Dis 1986; 45:627–636.
Jaraquemada D, Pachoula-Papasteriadis C, Festenstein H, Sachs JA, Roitt IM, Corbett M, Ansell B: *HLA-D* and *DR* determinants in rheumatoid arthritis. Transplant Proc 1979; 11:1306.
Jarvinen P, Aho K: Twin studies in rheumatic diseases. Semin Arthritis Rheum 1994; 24:19–28.
Jawaheer D, Seldin MF, Amos CI, Chen WV, Shigeta R, Monterio J, Kern M, Criswell LA, Albani S, Nelson JL, et al.: A genomewide screen in multiplex rheumatoid arthritis families suggests genetic overlap with other autoimmune diseases. Am J Hum Genet 2001; 68:927–936.
Jawaheer D, Thomson W, MacGregor AJ, Carthy D, Davidson J, Dyer PA, Silman AJ, Ollier WE: "Homozygosity" for the HLA-DR shared epitope contributes the highest risk for rheumatoid arthritis concordance in identical twins. Arthritis Rheum 1994; 37:681–686.
John S, Myerscough A, Marlow A, Hajeer A, Silman A, Ollier W, Worthington J: Linkage of cytokine genes to rheumatoid arthritis. Evidence of genetic heterogeneity. Ann Rheum Dis 1998; 57:361–365.
Jones MA, Silman AJ, Whiting S, Barrett EM, Symmons DP: Occurrence of rheumatoid arthritis is not increased in the first degree relatives of a population based inception cohort of inflammatory polyarthritis. Ann Rheum Dis 1996; 55:89–93.
Jonsson T, Thorsteinsson J, Valdimarsson H: Elevation of only one rheumatoid factor isotype is not associated with increased prevalence of rheumatoid arthritis—a population based study. Scand J Rheumatol 2000; 29:190–191.
Kaarela K, Alekberova Z, Lehtinen K, Puolakka K, Koskimies S, Nassonova V, Pospelov L: Seronegative rheumatoid arthritis: a clinical study with HLA typing. J Rheumatol 1990; 17:1125–1129.
Kaltenhauser S, Wagner U, Schuster E, Wassmuth R, Arnold S, Seidel W, Troltzsch M, Loeffler M, Hantzschel H: Immunogenetic markers and seropositivity predicts radiological progression in early rheumatoid arthritis independent of disease activity. J Rheumatol 2001; 28:735–744.
Karr RW, Rodey GE, Lee T, Schwartz BD: Association of *HLA-DRw4* with rheumatoid arthritis in black and white patients. Arthritis Rheum 1980; 23:1241–1245.
Kay CR, Wingrave SJ: Oral contraceptives and rheumatoid arthritis [letter]. Lancet 1983; 1:1437.
Khan MA, Khan MK: HLA studies in familial and sporadic rheumatoid arthritis. Dis Markers 1986; 4:67–76.
Kim HY, Kim TG, Park SH, Lee SH, Cho CS, Han H: Predominance of *HLA-DRB1*0405* in Korean patients with rheumatoid arthritis. Ann Rheum Dis 1995; 54:988–990.
Kim HY, Min JK, Yang HI, Park SH, Hong YS, Jee WH, Lee SH, Cho CS, Kim TG, Han H: The impact of *HLA-DRB1*0405* on disease severity in Korean patients with seropositive rheumatoid arthritis. Br J Rheumatol 1997; 36:440–443.
King RA: Rheumatoid arthritis. In: King RA, Rotter JI, Motulsky AG (eds). The Genetic Basis of Common Diseases. New York: Oxford University Press, 1992:596–624.
Klimiuk PA, Sierakowski S, Latosiewicz R, Cylwik B, Skowronski J, Chwiecko J: Serum cytokines in different histological variants of rheumatoid arthritis. J Rheumatol 2001; 28:1211–1217.
Konenkov V, Sartakova M, Kimura A: Oligonucleotide genotyping of *HLA-DRB1 04* and *HLA-DQB1 03* among Russians in west Siberia suffering from rheumatoid arthritis. Exp Clin Immunogenet 1994; 11:187–191.
Koumantaki Y, Giziaki E, Linos A, Kontomerkos A, Kaklamanis P, Vaiopoulos G, Mandas J, Kaklamani E: Family history as a risk factor for rheumatoid arthritis: a case-control study. J Rheumatol 1997; 24:1522–1526.
Kwoh CK, Venglish C, Lynn AH, Whitley DM, Young E, Chakravarti A: Age, sex, and the familial risk of rheumatoid arthritis. Am J Epidemiol 1996; 144:15–24.
Laiho K, Tuomilehto J, Tilvis R: Prevalence of rheumatoid arthritis and musculoskeletal diseases in the elderly population. Rheumatol Int 2001; 20:85–87.
Lanchbury JS, Jaeger EE, Sansom DM, Hall MA, Wordsworth P, Stedeford J, Bell JI, Panayi GS: Strong primary selection for the *Dw4* subtype of *DR4* accounts for the *HLA-DQw7* association with Felty's syndrome. Hum Immunol 1991; 32:56–64.
Lawrence JS: Heberden Oration, 1969. Rheumatoid arthritis—nature or nurture? Ann Rheum Dis 1970; 29:357–379.
Lawrence JS: Rheumatism in Populations. London: William Heinemann, 1977.
Lawrence JS, Bremner JM, Ball J, Burch TA: Rheumatoid arthritis in a subtropical population. Ann Rheum Dis 1966; 25:59–66.
Lawrence RC, Helmick CG, Arnett FC, Deyo RA, Felson DT, Giannini EH, Heyse SP, Hirsch R, Hochberg MC, Hunder GG, et al.: Estimates of the prevalence of arthritis and selected musculoskeletal disorders in the United States. Arthritis Rheum 1998; 41:778–799.
Lawrence RC, Hochberg MC, Kelsey JL, McDuffie FC, Medsger TA Jr, Felts WR, Shulman LE: Estimates of the prevalence of selected arthritic and musculoskeletal diseases in the United States. J Rheumatol 1989; 16:427–441.
Lee DM, Weinblatt ME: Rheumatoid arthritis. Lancet 2001; 358:903–911.
Legrand L, Lathrop GM, Marcelli-Barge A, Dryll A, Bardin T, Debeyre N, Poirier JC, Schmid M, Ryckewaert A, Dausset J: *HLA-DR* genotype risks in seropositive rheumatoid arthritis. Am J Hum Genet 1984; 36:690–699.
Loughran TP Jr, Starkebaum G: Large granular lymphocyte leukemia. Report of 38 cases and review of the literature. Medicine (Baltimore) 1987; 66:397–405.
MacGregor A, Ollier W, Thomson W, Jawaheer D, Silman A: *HLA-DRB1*0401/0404* genotype and rheumatoid arthritis: increased association in men, young age at onset, and disease severity. J Rheumatol 1995a; 22:1032–1036.
MacGregor AJ, Bamber S, Carthy D, Vencovsky J, Mageed RA, Ollier WE, Silman AJ: Heterogeneity of disease phenotype in monozygotic twins concordant for rheumatoid arthritis. Br J Rheumatol 1995b; 34:215–220.
MacGregor AJ, Bamber S, Silman AJ: A comparison of the performance of different methods of disease classification for rheumatoid arthritis. Results of an analysis from a nationwide twin study. J Rheumatol 1994; 21:1420–1426.
Maeda H, Juji T, Mitsui H, Sonozaki H, Okitsu K: *HLA DR4* and rheumatoid arthritis in Japanese people. Ann Rheum Dis 1981; 40:299–302.
Maini RN, Feldmann M: Rheumatoid arthritis: immmunopathogenesis of rheumatoid arthritis. In: Maddison PJ, Isenberg DA, Woo P, Glass DN (eds). Oxford Textbook of Rheumatology. Oxford: Oxford University Press, 1998:983–1004.
Marsal S, Hall MA, Panayi GS, Lanchbury JS: Association of *TAP2* polymorphism with rheumatoid arthritis is secondary to allelic association with *HLA-DRB1*. Arthritis Rheum 1994; 37:504–513.
Martell RW, Du Toit ED, Kalla AA, Meyers OL: Association of rheumatoid arthritis with HLA in three South African populations—white, blacks and a population of mixed ancestry. S Afr Med J 1989; 76:189–190.
Martel RW, Stein M, Davis P, West G, Emmanuel J, du Toit ED: The association between HLA and rheumatoid arthritis in Zimbabwean blacks. Tissue Antigens 1990; 36:125–126.
Massardo L, Jacobelli S, Rodriguez L, Rivero S, Gonzalez A, Marchetti R: Weak association between HLA-DR4 and rheumatoid arthritis in Chilean patients. Ann Rheum Dis 1990; 49:290–292.
Mattey DL, Dawes PT, Gonzalez-Gay MA, Garcia-Porrua C, Thomson W, Hajeer AH, Ollier WE: *HLA-DRB1* alleles encoding an aspartic acid at position 70 protect against rheumatoid arthritis. J Rheumatol 2001a, 28:232–239.
Mattey DL, Hassell AB, Dawes PT, Cheung NT, Poulton KV, Thomson W, Hajeer AH, Ollier WE: Independent association of rheumatoid factor and the *HLA-DRB1* shared epitope with radiographic outcome in rheumatoid arthritis. Arthritis Rheum 2001b; 44:1529–1533.
McCusker CT, Reid B, Green D, Gladman DD, Buchanan WW, Singal DP: HLA-D region antigens in patients with rheumatoid arthritis. Arthritis Rheum 1991; 34:192–197.
McDaniel DO, Alarcon GS, Pratt PW, and Reveille JD: Most African-American patients with rheumatoid arthritis do not have the rheumatoid antigenic determinant (epitope). Ann Intern Med 1995; 123:181–187.
McMahon MJ, Hillarby MC, Clarkson RW, Hollis S, Grennan DM: Major histocompatibility complex variants and articular disease severity in rheumatoid arthritis. Br J Rheumatol 1993; 32:899–902.
McMichael AJ, Sasazuki T, McDevitt HO, Payne RO: Increased frequency of *HLA-Cw3* and *HLA-Dw4* in rheumatoid arthritis. Arthritis Rheum 1977; 20:1037–1042.
Merriman TR, Cordell HJ, Evaes IA, Danoy PA, Cordaddu F, Barber R, Cucca F, Broadley S, Sawcer S, Compston A, et al.: Suggestive evidence for association of human chromosome 18q12–q21 and its orthologue on rat and mouse chromosome 18 with severe autoimmune disease. Diabetes 2001; 50:184–194.
Mijiyawa M: Epidemiology and semiology of rheumatoid arthritis in Third World countries. Rev Rhum Engl Ed 1995; 62:121–126.
Mikkelsen WM, Dodge HJ, Duff IF, Kato H: Estimates of the prevalence of rheumatic diseases in the population of Tecumseh, Michigan, 1959–60. J Chronic Dis 1967; 20:351–369.
Miossec P: Are T cells in rheumatoid synovium aggressors or bystanders? Curr Opin Rheumatol 2000; 12:181–185.
Miyazawa K, Mori A, Okudaira H: IL-6 synthesis by rheumatoid synoviocytes is autonomously upregulated at the transcriptional level. J Allergy Clin Immunol 1999; 103:S437–S444.
Mody GM, Hammond MG, Naidoo PD: HLA associations with rheumatoid arthritis in African blacks. J Rheumatol 1989; 16:1326–1328.
Molkentin J, Gregersen PK, Lin X, Zhu N, Wang Y, Wang Y, Chen S, Chen S, Baxter-Lowe LA, Silver J: Molecular analysis of HLA-DRβ and DQβ polymorphism in Chinese with rheumatoid arthritis. Ann Rheum Dis 1993; 52:610–612.
Moolenburgh JD, Valkenburg HA, Fourie PB: A population study on rheumatoid arthritis in Lesotho, southern Africa. Ann Rheum Dis 1986; 45:691–695.
Moran H, Chen SL, Muirden KD, Jiang SJ, Gu YY, Hopper J, Jiang PL, Lawler G, Bai MX: A comparison of changes seen on radiographs of rheumatoid arthritis patients in Australia and in China. Arthritis Rheum 1987; 30:1298–1302.
Moran H, Chen SL, Muirden KD, Jiang SJ, Gu YY, Hopper J, Jiang PL, Lawler G, Chen RB: A comparison of rheumatoid arthritis in Australia and China. Ann Rheum Dis 1986; 45:572–578.
Moreno I, Valenzuela A, Garcia A, Yelamos J, Sanchez B, Hernanz W: Association of the shared epitope with radiological severity of rheumatoid arthritis. J Rheumatol 1996; 23:6–9.
Mottonen TT: Prediction of erosiveness and rate of development of new erosions in early rheumatoid arthritis. Ann Rheum Dis 1988; 47:648–653.
Mulcahy B, Waldron-Lynch F, McDermott MF, Adams C, Amos CI, Zhu DK, Ward RH, Clegg DO, Shanahan F, Molloy MG, et al.: Genetic variability in the tumor necrosis factor-lymphotoxin region influences susceptibility to rheumatoid arthritis. Am J Hum Genet 1996; 59:676–683.
Myerscough A, John S, Barrett JH, Ollier WE, Worthington J: Linkage of rheumatoid arthritis to insulin-dependent diabetes mellitus loci: evidence supporting a hypothesis for the existence of common autoimmune susceptibility loci. Arthritis Rheum 2000; 43:2771–2775.
Nakai Y, Wakisaka A, Aizawa M, Itakura K, Nakai H, Ohashi A: *HLA* and rheumatoid arthritis in the Japanese. Arthritis Rheum 1981; 24:722–725.

Nelson JL, Boyer G, Templin D, Lanier A, Barrington R, Nisperos B, Smith A, Mickelson E, Hansen JA: HLA antigens in Tlingit Indians with rheumatoid arthritis. Tissue Antigens 1992; 40:57–63.

Nelson JL, Dugowson CE, Koepsell TD, Voigt LF, Branchaud AM, Barrington RA, Wener MH, Hansen JA: Rheumatoid factor, *HLA-DR4*, and allelic variants of *DRB1* in women with recent-onset rheumatoid arthritis. Arthritis Rheum 1994; 37:673–680.

Nepom BS, Nepom GT, Mickelson E, Schaller JG, Antonelli P, Hansen JA: Specific *HLA-DR4*-associated histocompatibility molecules characterize patients with seropositive juvenile rheumatoid arthritis. J Clin Invest 1984; 74:287–291.

Nepom GT: The role of the *DR4* shared epitope in selection and commitment of autoreactive T cells in rheumatoid arthritis. Rheum Dis Clin North Am 2001; 27:305–315.

Nepom GT, Byers P, Seyfried C, Healey LA, Wilske KR, Stage D, Nepom BS: *HLA* genes associated with rheumatoid arthritis. Identification of susceptibility alleles using specific oligonucleotide probes. Arthritis Rheum 1989; 32:15–21.

Nepom GT, Gersuk V, Nepom BS: Prognostic implications of *HLA* genotyping in the early assessment of patients with rheumatoid arthritis. J Rheumatol Suppl 1996; 44:5–9.

Nepom GT, Nepom BS: Prediction of susceptibility to rheumatoid arthritis by human leukocyte antigen genotyping. Rheum Dis Clin North Am 1992; 18:785–792.

Nepom GT, Seyfried CE, Holbeck SL, Wilske KR, Nepom BS: Identification of *HLA-Dw14* genes in *DR4*$^+$ rheumatoid arthritis. Lancet 1986; 2:1002–1005.

O'Brien WM, Bennett PH, Burch TA, Bunim JJ: A genetic study of rheumatoid arthritis and rheumatoid factor in Blackfeet and Pima Indians. Arthritis Rheum 1967; 10:163–179.

O'Dell JR, Nepom BS, Haire C, Gersuk VH, Gaur L, Moore GF, Drymalski W, Palmer W, Eckhoff PJ, Klassen LW, et al.: *HLA-DRB1* typing in rheumatoid arthritis: predicting response to specific treatments. Ann Rheum Dis 1998; 57:209–213.

Oen K, Postl B, Chalmers IM, Ling N, Schroeder ML, Baragar FD, Martin L, Reed M, Major P: Rheumatic diseases in an Inuit population. Arthritis Rheum 1986; 29:65–74.

Ohta N, Nishimura YK, Tanimoto K, Horiuchi Y, Abe C, Shiokawa Y, Abe T, Katagiri M, Yoshiki T, Sasazuki T: Association between HLA and Japanese patients with rheumatoid arthritis. Hum Immunol 1982; 5:123–132.

Ollier W, Venables PJ, Mumford PA, Maini RN, Awad J, Jaraquemada D, D'Amaro J, Festenstein H: HLA antigen associations with extra-articular rheumatoid arthritis. Tissue Antigens 1984; 24:279–291.

Ollier WE, Stephens C, Awad J, Carthy D, Gupta A, Perry D, Jawad A, Festenstein H: Is rheumatoid arthritis in Indians associated with HLA antigens sharing a DRβ1 epitope? Ann Rheum Dis 1991; 50:295–297.

Olsen NJ, Callahan LF, Brooks RH, Nance EP, Kaye JJ, Stastny P, Pincus T: Associations of HLA-DR4 with rheumatoid factor and radiographic severity in rheumatoid arthritis. Am J Med 1988; 84:257–264.

Panayi GS, Celinska E, Emery P, Griffin J, Welsh KI, Grahame R, Gibson T: Seronegative and seropositive rheumatoid arthritis: similar diseases. Br J Rheumatol 1987; 26:172–180.

Panayi GS, Corrigall VM, Pitzalis C: Pathogenesis of rheumatois arthritis: the role of T cells and other beasts. Rheum Dis Clin North Am 2001; 27:317–334

Panayi GS, Wooley P, Batchelor JR: Genetic basis of rheumatoid disease: HLA antigens, disease manifestations, and toxic reactions to drugs. BMJ 1978; 2:1326–1328.

Papadopoulos IA, Katsimbri P, Katsataki A, Temekonidis T, Georgiadis A, Drosos AA: Clinical course and outcome of early rheumatoid arthritis. Rheumatol Int 2001; 20:205–210.

Pawelec G, Reekers P, Brackertz D, Sansom D, Schneider EM, Blaurock M, Muller C, Rehbein A, Balko I, Wernet P: *HLA-DP* in rheumatoid arthritis. Tissue Antigens 1988; 31:83–89.

Pemberton R Osgood RB: The Medical and Orthopedic Management of Chronic Arthritis. New York: Macmillin, 1934.

Perdriger A, Semana G, Quillivic F, Chales G, Chardevel F, Legrand E, Meadeb J, Fauchet R, Pawlotsky Y: *DPB1* polymorphism in rheumatoid arthritis: evidence of an association with allele *DPB1 0401*. Tissue Antigens 1992; 39:14–18.

Pinet V, Combe B, Avinens O, Caillat-Zucman S, Sany J, Clot J, Eliaou JF: Polymorphism of the *HLA-DMA* and *DMB* genes in rheumatoid arthritis. Arthritis Rheum 1997; 40:854–858.

Plant MJ, Jones PW, Saklatvala J, Ollier WE, Dawes PT: Patterns of radiological progression in early rheumatoid arthritis: results of an 8 year prospective study. J Rheumatol 1998; 25:417–426.

Ploski R, Mellbye OJ, Ronningen KS, Forre O, Thorsby E: Seronegative and weakly seropositive rheumatoid arthritis differ from clearly seropositive rheumatoid arthritis in HLA class II associations. J Rheumatol 1994; 21:1397–1402.

Pociot F, Wilson AG, Nerup J, Duff GW: No independent association between a tumor necrosis factor-alpha promotor region polymorphism and insulin-dependent diabetes mellitus. Eur J Immunol 1993; 23:3050–3053.

Quadri SA, Taneja V, Mehra NK, Singal DP: HSP70-1 promoter region alleles and susceptibility to rheumatoid arthritis. Clin Exp Rheumatol 1996; 14:183–185.

Queiros MV, Sancho MR, Caetano JM: HLA-DR4 antigen and IgM rheumatoid factors. J Rheumatol 1982; 9:370–373.

Radstake TR, Barrera P, Albers JM, Swinkels HL, van de Putte LB, van Riel PL: Familial vs sporadic rheumatoid arthritis (RA). A prospective study in an early RA inception cohort. Rheumatology (Oxford) 2000; 39:267–273.

Radstake TR, Barrera P, Albers JM, Swinkels HL, van de Putte LB, van Riel PL: Genetic anticipation in rheumatoid arthritis in Europe. European Consortium on Rheumatoid Arthritis Families. J Rheumatol 2001; 28:962–967.

Rigby AS, Silman AJ, Voelm L, Gregory JC, Ollier WE, Khan MA, Nepom GT, Thomson G: Investigating the HLA component in rheumatoid arthritis: an additive (dominant) mode of inheritance is rejected, a recessive mode is preferred. Genet Epidemiol 1991; 8:153–175.

Ronningen KS, Spurkland A, Egeland T, Iwe T, Munthe E, Vartdal F, Thorsby E: Rheumatoid arthritis may be primarily associated with HLA-DR4 molecules sharing a particular sequence at residues 67–74. Tissue Antigens 1990; 36:235–240.

Roudier J: Association of MHC and rheumatoid arthritis. Association of RA with HLA-DR4: the role of repertoire selection. Arthritis Res 2000; 2:217–220.

Roudier J, Petersen J, Rhodes GH, Luka J, Carson DA: Susceptibility to rheumatoid arthritis maps to a T-cell epitope shared by the HLA-Dw4 DR β-1 chain and the Epstein-Barr virus glycoprotein gp110. Proc Natl Acad Sci USA 1989; 86:5104–5108.

Roudier J, Rhodes G, Petersen J, Vaughan JH, Carson DA: The Epstein-Barr virus glycoprotein gp110, a molecular link between HLA DR4, HLA DR1, and rheumatoid arthritis. Scand J Immunol 1988; 27:367–371.

Rubin LA, Voorneveld CR: High prevalence of rheumatoid arthritis (RA) among North American Native Indians (NANI): support for the New World theory of RA. Arthritis Rheum 1991; 34(Suppl): D108.

Sage DA, Evans PR, Cawley MI, Smith JL, Howell WM: *HLA DPB1* alleles and susceptibility to rheumatoid arthritis. Eur J Immunogenet 1991; 18:259–263.

Salmon M, Wordsworth P, Emery P, Tunn E, Bacon PA, Bell JI: The association of *HLA DRβ* alleles with self-limiting and persistent forms of early symmetrical polyarthritis. Br J Rheumatol 1993; 32:628–630.

Salvarani C, Macchioni PL, Mantovani W, Bragliani M, Collina E, Cremonesi T, Battistel B, Boiardi L: *HLA-DRB1* alleles associated with rheumatoid arthritis in northern Italy: correlation with disease severity. Br J Rheumatol 1998; 37:165–169.

Sanchez B, Moreno I, Magarino R, Garzon M, Gonzalez MF, Garcia A, Nunez-Roldan A: HLA-DRw10 confers the highest susceptibility to rheumatoid arthritis in a Spanish population. Tissue Antigens 1990; 36:174–176.

Sansom DM, Bidwell JL, Maddison PJ, Campion G, Klouda PT, Bradley BA: HLA *DQα* and *DQβ* restriction fragment length polymorphisms associated with Felty's syndrome and *DR4*-positive rheumatoid arthritis. Hum Immunol 1987; 19:269–278.

Sarkissian M, Lafyatis R: Integrin engagement regulates proliferation and collagenase expression of rheumatoid synovial fibroblasts. J Immunol 1999; 162:1772–1779.

Sattar MA, al Saffar M, Guindi RT, Sugathan TN, Behbehani K: Association between HLA-DR antigens and rheumatoid arthritis in Arabs. Ann Rheum Dis 1990; 49:147–149.

Scherak O, Smolen JS, Mayr WR: Rheumatoid arthritis and B lymphocyte alloantigen HLA-DRw4. J Rheumatol 1980; 7:9–12.

Schiff B, Mizrachi Y, Orgad S, Yaron M, Gazit E: Association of HLA-Aw31 and HLA-DR1 with adult rheumatoid arthritis. Ann Rheum Dis 1982; 41:403–404.

Seglias J, Li EK, Cohen MG, Wong RW, Potter PK, So AK: Linkage between rheumatoid arthritis susceptibility and the presence of *HLA-DR4* and *DRβ* allelic third hypervariable region sequences in southern Chinese persons. Arthritis Rheum 1992; 35:163–167.

Seidl C, Koch U, Brunnler G, Buhleier T, Frank R, Moller B, Markert E, Koller-Wagner G, Seifried E, Kaltwasser JP: HLA-DR/DQ/DP interactions in rheumatoid arthritis. Eur J Immunogenet 1997; 24:365–376.

Seidl C, Korbitzer J, Badenhoop K, Seifried E, Hoelzer D, Zanelli E, Kaltwasser JP: Protection against severe disease is conferred by DERAA-bearing *HLA-DRB1* alleles among *HLA-DQ3* and *HLA-DQ5* positive rheumatoid arthritis patients. Hum Immunol 2001; 62:523–529.

Seitz M, Perler M, Pichler W: Only weak association between disease severity and *HLA-DRB1* genes in a Swiss population of rheumatoid arthritis patients. Rheumatol Int 1996; 16:9–13.

Sen M, Lauterbach K, El Gabalawy H, Firestein GS, Corr M, Carson DA: Expression and function of wingless and frizzled homologs in rheumatoid arthritis. Proc Natl Acad Sci USA 2000; 97:2791–2796.

Sherritt MA, Tait B, Varney M, Kanaan C, Stockman A, Mackay IR, Muirden K, Bernard CC, Rowley MJ: Immunosusceptibility genes in rheumatoid arthritis. Hum Immunol 1996; 51:32–40.

Short CL: The antiquity of rheumatoid arthritis. Arthritis Rheum 1974; 17:1029–1032.

Shunichi S, Hayashi S, Tsukamoto Y, Yasuda N, Goko H, Kawasaki H, Wada T, Shimizu K, Takasugi K, Yanaka Y, et al.: Identification of the gene loci that predispose to rheumatoid arthritis. Arthritis Rheum 1997; 40:S329.

Silman AJ, MacGregor AJ, Thomson W, Holligan S, Carthy D, Farhan A, Ollier WE: Twin concordance rates for rheumatoid arthritis: results from a nationwide study. Br J Rheumatol 1993; 32:903–907.

Singal DP, Ye M: *HLA-DM* polymorphisms in patients with rheumatoid arthritis. J Rheumatol 1998; 25:1295–1298.

Singal DP, Ye M, Qiu X, D'Souza M: Polymorphisms in the *TAP2* gene and their association with rheumatoid arthritis. Clin Exp Rheumatol 1994; 12:29–33.

Smith MD, Slavotinek J, Au V, Weedon H, Parker A, Coleman M, Roberts-Thomson PJ, Ahern MJ: Successful treatment of rheumatoid arthritis is associated with a reduction in synovial membrane cytokines and cell adhesion molecule expression. Rheumatology (Oxford) 2001; 40:965–977.

Snijders A, Elferink DG, Geluk A, van der Zanden AL, Vos K, Schreuder GM, Breedveld FC, de Vries RR, Zanelli EH: An *HLA-DRB1*-derived peptide associated with protection against rheumatoid arthritis is naturally processed by human APC. J Immunol 2001; 166:4987–4993.

So AK, Warner CA, Sansom D, Walport MJ: *DQβ* polymorphism and genetic susceptibility to Felty's syndrome. Arthritis Rheum 1988; 31:990–994.

Solomon L, Robin G, Valkenburg HA: Rheumatoid arthritis in an urban South African Negro population. Ann Rheum Dis 1975; 34:128–135.

Sorensen K: Rheumatoid arthritis in Denmark. Two population studies. Dan Med Bull 1973; 20:86–93.

Spector TD: Rheumatoid arthritis. Rheum Dis Clin North Am 1990; 16:513–537.

Spector TD, Hochberg MC: The protective effect of the oral contraceptive pill on rheumatoid arthritis: an overview of the analytical epidemiological studies using meta-analysis. Br J Rheumatol 1989; 28(Suppl 1):11–12.

Speerstra F, Reekers P, van de Putte LB, Vandenbroucke JP, Rasker JJ, de Rooij DJ: HLA-DR antigens and proteinuria induced by aurothioglucose and D-penicillamine in patients with rheumatoid arthritis. J Rheumatol 1983; 10:948–953.

Starkebaum G, Loughran TP Jr, Gaur LK, Davis P, Nepom BS: Immunogenetic similarities between patients with Felty's syndrome and those with clonal expansions of large granular lymphocytes in rheumatoid arthritis. Arthritis Rheum 1997; 40:624–626.

Stastny P: Association of the B-cell alloantigen *DRw4* with rheumatoid arthritis. N Engl J Med 1978; 298:869–871.

Stavropoulos C, Spyropoulou M, Koumantaki Y, Kappou I, Kaklamani V, Linos A, Giziaki E, Kaklamani E: *HLA-DRB1* alleles in Greek rheumatoid arthritis patients and their association with clinical characteristics. Eur J Immunogenet 1997; 24:265–274.

Stephens HA, Sakkas LI, Vaughan RW, Teitsson I, Welsh KI, Panayi GS: *HLA-DQw7* is a disease severity marker in patients with rheumatoid arthritis. Immunogenetics 1989; 30:119–122.

Suarez-Almazor ME, Tao S, Moustarah F, Russell AS, Maksymowych W: *HLA-DR1*, *DR4*, and *DRB1* disease related subtypes in rheumatoid arthritis. Association with susceptibility but not severity in a city wide community based study. J Rheumatol 1995; 22:2027–2033.

Sutton B, Corper A, Bonagura V, Taussig M: The structure and origin of rheumatoid factors. Immunol Today 2000; 21:177–183.

Takeuchi F, Nabeta H, Kuwata S, Tanimoto K, Ito K: Association of *DMA* and *DMB* with RA in Japanese. Clin Exp Rheumatol 1997; 15:189–192.

Takeuchi F, Nakano K, Matsuta K, Nabeta H, Bannai M, Tanimoto K, Ito K: Positive and negative association of *HLA-DR* genotypes with Japanese rheumatoid arthritis. Clin Exp Rheumatol 1996; 14:17–22.

Tan PL, Farmiloe S, Roberts M, Geursen A, Skinner MA: HLA-DR4 subtypes in New Zealand Polynesians. Predominance of Dw13 in the healthy population and association of Dw15 with rheumatoid arthritis. Arthritis Rheum 1993; 36:15–19.

Taneja V, Giphart MJ, Verduijn W, Naipal A, Malaviya AN, Mehra NK: Polymorphism of *HLA-DRB*, *-DQA1*, and *-DQB1* in rheumatoid arthritis in Asian Indians: association with *DRB1*0405* and *DRB1*1001*. Hum Immunol 1996; 46:35–41.

Teller K, Budhai L, Zhang M, Haramati N, Keiser HD, Davidson A: *HLA-DRB1* and *DQB* typing of Hispanic American patients with rheumatoid arthritis: the "shared epitope" hypothesis may not apply. J Rheumatol 1996; 23:1363–1368.

Thomas R: Antigen-presenting cells in rheumatoid arthritis. Springer Semin Immunopathol 1998; 20:53–72.

Thomsen M, Morling N, Snorrason E, Svejgaard A, Sorensen SF: *HLA-Dw4* and rheumatoid arthritis. Tissue Antigens 1979; 13:56–60.

Thomson W, Pepper L, Payton A, Carthy D, Scott D, Ollier W, Silman A, Symmons D: Absence of an association between *HLA-DRB1*04* and rheumatoid arthritis in newly diagnosed cases from the community. Ann Rheum Dis 1993; 52:539–541.

Thould AK, Thould BT: Arthritis in Roman Britian. BMJ 1983; 287:1909–1911.

Tiwana H, Wilson C, Alvarez A, Abuknesha R, Bansal S, Ebringer A: Cross-reactivity between the rheumatoid arthritis-associated motif EQKRAA and structurally related sequences found in *Proteus mirabilis*. Infect Immun 1999; 67:2769–2775.

Toda Y, Minamikawa Y, Akagi S, Sugano H, Mori Y, Nishimura H, Arita S, Sugino Y, Ogawa R: Rheumatoid-susceptible alleles of *HLA-DRB1* are genetically recessive to non-susceptible alleles in the progression of bone destruction in the wrists and fingers of patients with RA. Ann Rheum Dis 1994; 53:587–592.

Udalova IA, Nedospasov SA, Webb GC, Chaplin DD, Turetskaya RL: Highly informative typing of the human TNF locus using six adjacent polymorphic markers. Genomics 1993; 16:180–186.

Ueno Y, Iwaki Y, Terasaki PI, Park MS, Barnett EV, Chia D, Nakata S: *HLA-DR4* in Negro and Mexican rheumatoid arthritis patients. J Rheumatol 1981; 8:804–807.

van Eden W, Holoshitz J, Nevo Z, Frenkel A, Klajman A, Cohen IR: Arthritis induced by a T-lymphocyte clone that responds to *Mycobacterium tuberculosis* and to cartilage proteoglycans. Proc Natl Acad Sci USA 1985; 82:5117–5120.

van Eden W, Thole JE, van der ZR, Noordzij A, van Embden JD, Hensen EJ, Cohen IR: Cloning of the mycobacterial epitope recognized by T lymphocytes in adjuvant arthritis. Nature 1988; 331:171–173.

van Zeben D, Hazes JM, Zwinderman AH, Cats A, Schreuder GM, D'Amaro J, Breedveld FC: Association of *HLA-DR4* with a more progressive disease course in patients with rheumatoid arthritis. Results of a followup study. Arthritis Rheum 1991; 34:822–830.

Vandevyver C, Geusens P, Cassiman JJ, Raus J: Peptide transporter gene (*TAP*) polymorphisms and genetic susceptibility to rheumatoid arthritis. Br J Rheumatol 1995; 34:207–214.

van der Horst-Bruinsma IE, de Vries RR, de Buck PD, van Schendel PW, Breedveld FC, Schreuder GM, Hazes JM: Influence of HLA-class II incompatibility between mother and fetus on the development and course of rheumatoid arthritis of the mother. Ann Rheum Dis 1998; 57:286–290.

Veerapen K, Mangat G, Watt I, Dieppe P: The expression of rheumatoid arthritis in Malaysian and British patients: a comparative study. Br J Rheumatol 1993; 32:541–545.

Vehe RK, Nepom GT, Wilske KR, Stage D, Begovich AB, Nepom BS: Erosive rheumatoid factor negative and positive rheumatoid arthritis are immunogenetically similar. J Rheumatol 1994; 21:194–196.

Venables P: Epstein-Barr virus infection and autoimmunity in rheumatoid arthritis. Ann Rheum Dis 1988; 47:265–269.

Vinasco J, Beraun Y, Nieto A, Fraile A, Mataran L, Pareja E, Martin J: Polymorphism at the TNF loci in rheumatoid arthritis. Tissue Antigens 1997a; 49:74–78.

Vinasco J, Beraun Y, Nieto A, Fraile A, Pareja E, Mataran L, Martin J: Heat shock protein 70 gene polymorphisms in rheumatoid arthritis. Tissue Antigens 1997b; 50:71–73.

Vinasco J, Fraile A, Nieto A, Beraun Y, Pareja E, Mataran L, Martin J: Analysis of *LMP* and *TAP* polymorphisms by polymerase chain reaction-restriction fragment length polymorphism in rheumatoid arthritis. Ann Rheum Dis 1998; 57:33–37.

Volin MV, Koch AE: Cell cycle implications in the pathogenesis of rheumatoid arthritis. Front Biosci 2000; 5:594–601.

Wagner U, Kaltenhauser S, Sauer H, Arnold S, Seidel W, Hantzschel H, Kalden JR, Wassmuth R: HLA markers and prediction of clinical course and outcome in rheumatoid arthritis. Arthritis Rheum 1997; 40:341–351.

Wakitani S, Murata N, Toda Y, Ogawa R, Kaneshige T, Nishimura Y, Ochi T: The relationship between *HLA-DRB1* alleles and disease subsets of rheumatoid arthritis in Japanese. Br J Rheumatol 1997; 36:630–636.

Wallin J, Carlsson B, Strom H, Moller E: A *DR4*-associated *DR-DQ* haplotype is significantly associated with rheumatoid arthritis. Arthritis Rheum 1988; 31:72–79.

Wallin J, Hillert J, Olerup O, Carlsson B, Strom H: Association of rheumatoid arthritis with a dominant *DR1/Dw4/Dw14* sequence motif, but not with T cell receptor beta chain gene alleles or haplotypes. Arthritis Rheum 1991; 34:1416–1424.

Westedt ML, Breedveld FC, Schreuder GM, D'Amaro J, Cats A, de Vries RR: Immunogenetic heterogeneity of rheumatoid arthritis. Ann Rheum Dis 1986; 45:534–538.

Weyand CM, Goronzy JJ: Association of MHC and rheumatoid arthritis. *HLA* polymorphisms in phenotypic variants of rheumatoid arthritis. Arthritis Res 2000; 2:212–216.

Weyand CM, Hicok KC, Conn DL, Goronzy JJ: The influence of *HLA-DRB1* genes on disease severity in rheumatoid arthritis. Ann Intern Med 1992a; 117:801–806.

Weyand CM, McCarthy TG, Goronzy JJ: Correlation between disease phenotype and genetic heterogeneity in rheumatoid arthritis. J Clin Invest 1995; 95:2120–2126.

Weyand CM, Schmidt D, Wagner U, Goronzy JJ: The influence of sex on the phenotype of rheumatoid arthritis. Arthritis Rheum 1998; 41:817–822.

Weyand CM, Xie C, Goronzy JJ: Homozygosity for the *HLA-DRB1* allele selects for extraarticular manifestations in rheumatoid arthritis. J Clin Invest 1992b; 89:2033–2039.

Wigley RD, Zhang NZ, Zeng QY, Shi CS, Hu DW, Couchman K, Duff IF, Bennett PH: Rheumatic diseases in China: ILAR-China study comparing the prevalence of rheumatic symptoms in northern and southern rural populations. J Rheumatol 1994; 21:1484–1490.

Williams RC, Jacobsson LT, Knowler WC, Del Puente A, Kostyu D, McAuley JE, Bennett PH, Pettitt DJ: Meta-analysis reveals association between most common class II haplotype in full-heritage Native Americans and rheumatoid arthritis. Hum Immunol 1995; 42:90–94.

Willkens RF, Nepom GT, Marks CR, Nettles JW, Nepom BS: Association of HLA-Dw16 with rheumatoid arthritis in Yakima Indians. Further evidence for the "shared epitope" hypothesis. Arthritis Rheum 1991; 34:43–47.

Wilson AG, de Vries N, van de Putte LB, Duff GW: A tumour necrosis factor alpha polymorphism is not associated with rheumatoid arthritis. Ann Rheum Dis 1995; 54:601–603.

Witte T, Hartung K, Sachse C, Matthias T, Fricke M, Kalden JR, Lakomek HJ, Peter HH, Schmidt RE: Rheumatoid factors in systemic lupus erythematosus: association with clinical and laboratory parameters. SLE study group. Rheumatol Int 2000; 19:107–111.

Wollheim FA: Rheumatoid arthritis: the clinical picture. In: Maddison PJ, Isenberg DA, Woo P, Glass DN (eds). Oxford Textbook of Rheumatology. Oxford: Oxford University Press. 1998:1004–1031.

Woodrow JC, Nichol FE, Zaphiropoulos G: *DR* antigens and rheumatoid arthritis: a study of two populations. BMJ 1981; 283:1287–1288.

Wooley PH, Griffin J, Panayi GS, Batchelor JR, Welsh KI, Gibson TJ: *HLA-DR* antigens and toxic reaction to sodium aurothiomalate and D-penicillamine in patients with rheumatoid arthritis. N Engl J Med 1980; 303:300–302.

Wordsworth BP, Lanchbury JS, Sakkas LI, Welsh KI, Panayi GS, Bell JI: *HLA-DR4* subtype frequencies in rheumatoid arthritis indicate that *DRB1* is the major susceptibility locus within the HLA class II region. Proc Natl Acad Sci USA 1989; 86:10049–10053.

Wordsworth P: T cell genetics and rheumatoid arthritis (RA). Clin Exp Immunol 1998; 111:469–471.

Wordsworth P, Bell J: Polygenic susceptibility in rheumatoid arthritis. Ann Rheum Dis 1991; 50:343–346.

Wordsworth P, Pile KD, Buckely JD, Lanchbury JS, Ollier B, Lathrop M, Bell JI: HLA heterozygosity contributes to susceptibility to rheumatoid arthritis. Am J Hum Genet 1992; 51:585–591.

Yelamos J, Garcia-Lozano JR, Moreno I, Aguilera I, Gonzalez MF, Garcia A, Nunez-Roldan A, Sanchez B: Association of HLA-DR4-Dw15 (DRB1*0405) and DR10 with rheumatoid arthritis in a Spanish population. Arthritis Rheum 1993; 36:811–814.

Yen JH, Chen CJ, Tsai WC, Tsai JJ, Chang JG, Liu HW: *HLA-DMA* and *DMB* genotyping in patients with rheumatoid arthritis. J Rheumatol 1997; 24:442–444.

Yen JH, Chen CJ, Tsai WC, Ou TT, Lin CH, Lin SC, Liu HW: *HLA-DQA1* genotyping in patients with rheumatoid arthritis in Taiwan. Kao Hsiung I Hsueh Ko Hsueh Tsa Chih 2001; 17:183–189.

Yen JH, Chen JR, Tsai WJ, Tsai JJ, Liu HW: *HLA-DRB1* genotyping in patients with rheumatoid arthritis in Taiwan. J Rheumatol 1995; 22:1450–1454.

Young A, Jaraquemada D, Awad J, Festenstein H, Corbett M, Hay FC, Roitt IM: Association of HLA-DR4/Dw4 and DR2/Dw2 with radiologic changes in a prospective study of patients with rheumatoid arthritis. Preferential relationship with HLA-Dw rather than HLA-DR specificities. Arthritis Rheum 1984; 27:20–25.

Zanelli E, Breedveld FC, de Vries RR: HLA class II association with rheumatoid arthritis: facts and interpretations. Hum Immunol 2000; 61:1254–1261.

Zhao Y, Dong Y, Zhu X, Qui C: *HLA-DRB1* allele genotyping in patients with rheumatoid arthritis in Chinese. Chin Med Sci J 1996; 11:232–235.

Zoschke D, Segall M: *Dw* subtypes of DR4 in rheumatoid arthritis: evidence for a preferential association with Dw4. Hum Immunol 1986; 15:118–124.

30 Seronegative Spondyloarthropathies

R. HAL SCOFIELD

More than 25 years ago, the association of ankylosing spondylitis (AS) with the class I major histocompatability complex (MHC) gene product HLA-B27 was recognized. Shortly thereafter, HLA-B27 was associated with the other spondyloarthropathies. Today, these genetic associations and the genetic linkage of AS to the MHC remain among the strongest known for a genetically complex disease. Greater than 90% of those with AS carry HLA-B27, while from 1 in 10 to 1 in 50 persons with HLA-B27 will develop a spondyloarthropathy. Despite data that HLA-B27 is directly involved in pathogenesis and a number of theories, no compelling data have come forth to demonstrate the mechanism by which HLA-B27 leads to disease.

DISEASE DEFINITION

The seronegative spondyloarthropathies are a group of related disorders of which AS is the prototype. This illness usually presents in young adulthood with persistent low back pain and stiffness. It is more commonly diagnosed in men than women. Its characteristic clinical feature is sacroiliitis, and its characteristic pathological feature is enthesopathy with new bone formation. Axial involvement gradually proceeds up the spine, with bony ankylosis occurring such that vertebrae are fused together and motion is severely limited. Oligoarticular peripheral arthritis is common in addition to the axial disease. *Seronegative* refers to the fact that, in contrast to rheumatoid arthritis, the rheumatoid factor is consistently negative in spondyloarthropathies, as are antinuclear antibodies.

Spondyloarthropathy also includes a spectrum of diseases distinct from classic AS. These subtypes include reactive arthritis, psoriatic arthritis, enteropathic arthritis, and Whipple's disease. AS and most of these other spondyloarthropathies are associated with the presence of HLA-B27 (Table 30–1). Reactive arthritis is the result of infection with several bacterial pathogens and is typically manifested by a peripheral, asymmetric oligoarthritis. Among the bacteria which can trigger reactive arthritis are salmonella, shigella, yersinia, and sexual transmitted chlamydia. Because viable bacteria cannot be recovered from involved joints, this syndrome has been considered a noninfectious sequela of these infections. However, bacterial products are present in the joints of individuals with reactive arthritis (Granfors et al., 1990; Nikkari et al., 1992; Bas et al., 1995). In addition to arthritis, reactive arthritis can be accompanied by noninfectious inflammation of the conjunctivae and urethra (Reiter, 1916; Paronen, 1948), while some patients may have arthritis alone. The term *Reiter's syndrome*, as an eponym for reactive arthritis syndrome including arthritis, urethritis, conjunctivitis, and psoriasiform rash, is best avoided for scientific reasons (Inman, 1999) as well as because of Reiter's role in medical atrocities during the Nazi regime (Wallace and Weismann, 2000, 2001; Maitra 2001).

Arthritis occurs in some patients in the course of either psoriasis or inflammatory bowel disease, such as ulcerative colitis or Crohn's disease. Axial or peripheral arthritis can predominate in this setting. Peripheral arthritis is usually asymmetric, more likely to involve the lower limb, and not associated with an increase in HLA-B27. About 50% of patients with sacroiliitis or spondylitis in the setting of psoriasis or inflammatory bowel disease have HLA-B27. In some patients, arthritis may precede the skin disease psoriasis or inflammatory bowel disease. Many patients with AS may have subclinical bowel inflammation (Mielants et al., 1985). Finally, many individuals have a spondyloarthropathy that does not fit into the well-defined clinical entities discussed above and are best described as having undifferentiated or overlap spondyloarthropathy. Such disease may be more common in those of American Indian ancestry (reviewed in Scofield, 2000).

Useful classification criteria for the spondyloarthropathies have been difficult to achieve given the similarities and differences of the clinical syndromes seen. The diseases which can be included under the umbrella of *spondyloarthropathy* and their association with HLA-B27 are shown in Table 30–1. Because of the wide variation of diseases present in spondyloarthropathy, especially the presence of undifferentiated forms, criteria for individual diseases (Willkens et al., 1981; van der Linden et al., 1984a) have been seen as too restrictive. Thus, criteria that encompass a wider spectrum of illness and serve diagnostic purposes for spondyloarthropathy in general have been proposed (Dougados et al., 1991). Of course, there is no gold standard for diagnosis, so these criteria rely on expert opinion for final determination of diagnosis. The relatively simple criteria proposed by the European Spondyloarthropathy Study Group to classify spondyloarthropathy are shown in Table 30–2.

GENERAL GENETIC AND EPIDEMIOLOGICAL EVIDENCE

Spondyloarthropathies occur throughout the world in every ethnic population that has been studied, except perhaps in West Africa (Brown et al., 1997a). AS is probably an old disease, putatively found in skeletons as ancient as 5500 years before the present (Russell, 1998). The prevalence of disease is correlated with the prevalence of HLA-B27 in the population (Tiware and Terisaki, 1985; Khan, 1995). This has been well studied in American Indians, several tribal groups having HLA-B27 in up to 50% of members compared to about 10% in most Caucasian popula-

Table 30–1. The Distinct Categories of Spondyloarthropathies and Their Relationship to the Presence of HLA-B27

Disease Entity	HLA-B27 Association
Ankylosing spondylitis	>90%
Reactive syndrome	50%–75%
Psoriatic arthropathy	50%
Enteropathic arthropathy	
Peripheral arthritis	No increase
Spondylitis/sacroiliitis	50%
Whipple's disease	No increase
Undifferentiated	60%–90%

tions. These tribes, which include the Inuit and Yupic Eskimos (Oen et al., 1986; Boyer et al., 1988, 1990, 1994) as well as the Hadia (Gofton et al., 1972) and Navajo (Muggia et al., 1971; Rate et al., 1980; Morse et al., 1980), have a very high rate of spondyloarthropathy. Norwegian Lapps also have a high rate of HLA-B27 carriage and a high prevalence of AS (Johnsen, 1992). The only population that is incongruent in this regard is the Fula in Gambia. Among over 1000 members of this west African ethnic group, including an HLA-B27-positive cohort, not a single case of AS was found, despite 6% of the Fula population carrying HLA-B27 (Brown et al., 1997a).

AS has a strong predilection for males as opposed to females; however, with other forms of spondyloarthropathy the male:female ratio is different (Kennedy et al., 1993). The gender ratio is equal in enteropathic disease and greater than that in AS in psoriatic arthritis (Kennedy et al., 1993). Some of the gender differences may not reflect an increase of disease prevalence in men but instead increased severity. Thus, men are more likely to be diagnosed than women. However, the risk of disease within a given population may also affect the sex ratio (James, 1991). Genetic linkage of disease to the X chromosome has been excluded. Thus, genes on this chromosome do not explain the sex bias (Hoyle et al., 2000). Another study has found that a CAG microsatellite repeat of exon 1 of the androgen receptor (which is related to transactivation function) is significantly shorter in AS patients compared to controls (Mori et al., 2000). This interesting observation will need further investigation at the biochemical and genetic levels. Finally, there may be an influence of sex on disease among offspring of AS patients: children of female AS patients were more likely to develop disease than children of male AS patients [odds ratio (OR) of 1.9] in a study of more than 4000 AS patients (Calin et al., 1999).

Table 30–2. European Spondyloarthropathy Study Group Criteria for the Classification of Spondyloarthropathy[a]

Criteria 1: must satisfy one of the following
- Inflammatory spinal pain: characterized by at least four of the following traits: onset before age 45, insidious onset, improved by exercise, morning stiffness, over 3 months in duration
- Synovitis: past or present, asymmetric or predominately in the lower limbs

Criteria 2: must satisfy one of the following
- Positive family history: first- or second-degree relative with ankylosing spondylitis, psoriasis, inflammatory bowel disease, or reactive arthritis
- Psoriasis: past or present, diagnosed by a physician
- Inflammatory bowel disease: past or present Crohn's disease or ulcerative colitis, diagnosed by a physician and confirmed by radiographic or endoscopic study
- Alternating buttock pain: past or present
- Enthesopathy: past or present pain or tenderness of the insertion site of the Achilles tendon or plantar fascia
- Acute diarrhea: Episode of diarrhea within 1 month before onset of arthritis
- Urethritis: non-gonococcal, within 1 month before onset of arthritis
- Sacroiliitis: Bilateral grade 2–4 or unilateral grade 3–4, where grade 0, normal; 1, possible; 2, minimal; 3, moderate; 4, ankylosis

[a]An individual must satisfy either inflammatory spinal pain or synovitis and one of the conditions from criteria 2 in order to be classified as having a spondyloarthropathy.

Family studies show that there is a markedly increased risk of AS among HLA-B27-positive individuals with an affected first-degree relative compared to HLA-B27-positive individuals with no family history of spondyloarthropathy (Møller and Berg, 1983; van der Linden et al., 1984b; Gran et al., 1985). Among HLA-B27-positive persons with an affected first-degree relative, the risk of disease may be as high as 50%. AS has been studied in the Finnish Twin Cohort (Järninen, 1995). From this nationwide twin registry, the investigators identified six pairs of monozygotic (MZ) twins and 20 pairs of dizygotic (DZ) twins. These are thought to be every twin pair in Finland where at least one of the pair has AS. Three (50%) of the MZ twin pairs were concordant, while only three of the 20 (6.7%) DZ pairs were concordant. In another study of twins, six of eight MZ pairs were concordant for AS, while only four of 15 DZ pairs were concordant (Brown et al., 1997b). The rate of concordance among DZ twins was significantly increased when both members of a pair had HLA-B27. This study estimated that 97% of the population variance was accounted for by additive genetic effects. Brown and colleagues (2000b) extended these results in a larger study of familial occurrence and assessed the genetic model that might explain the results. Recurrence in MZ twins was 13%, 8.2% in first-degree relatives, and only 1.0% in second-degree relatives. The parent–child rate was 7.9%, not significantly different from that of first-degree relatives. The genetic model best fitting the data was a five-locus one with multiplicative interaction between the loci (Brown et al., 2000a,b). Another study has shown similar familial aggregation (Liu et al., 2001). The severity of disease may also have familial aggregation that suggests a genetic basis (Hamersma et al., 2001). This study examined 384 AS patients, all of whom had at least one affected relative. Using both the Bath AS Disease Activity Index and the Bath AS Functional Index, the authors found high correlations among family members. No adoption studies have been reported to the author's knowledge, nor have twin or family studies of spondyloarthropathies other than AS been reported.

There are several diseases associated with spondyloarthropathy. As has been discussed above, spondyloarthropathy can be associated with psoriasis or inflammatory bowel disease. AS is associated with certain cardiac abnormalities, such as aortic valve disease, and conduction abnormalities leading to heart block. Complete heart block (without evidence of spondyloarthropathy) is associated with the presence of HLA-B27 (Bergfeldt, 1997).

Reactive arthritis, with or without other associated features such as urethritis and uveitis, is clearly the result of enteric or urogenital bacterial infection. In certain populations, a high incidence of triggering infection is in part responsible for a high incidence of spondyloarthropathy (Rate et al., 1980). T lymphocytes reactive with triggering bacteria are found at increased frequencies within involved joints of patients with reactive arthritis, including T cells restricted by HLA-B27 (Hermann et al., 1993; Duchmann et al., 1996). The notion that a particular bacterium might trigger AS is quite controversial. There is evidence linking AS with *Klebsiella* infection or intestinal carriage (Ebringer, 1992) as well as substantial evidence that *Klebsiella* is not related to AS (Russell and Suarez Almazor, 1992). In AS, circulating T cells reactive to *Klebsiella* were decreased compared to HLA-B27-positive controls (Hermann et al., 1995). Another study showed that immunoglobulin G (IgG), IgA, and IgM anti-*Klebsiella* antibodies were elevated in the circulation of patients with AS, while antibodies to other enteric bacteria were not elevated (Mäki-Ikola et al., 1995a,b). Also, anti-*Klebsiella* titers are associated with the presence of intestinal inflammation in those with AS (Mäki-Ikola et al., 1997a), but there is no increase in anti-*Klebsiella* antibodies in the synovium compared to the serum (Mäki-Ikola et al., 1997b).

PATHOPHYSIOLOGY: BIOLOGICAL BASIS OF GENETIC SUSCEPTIBILITY

The pathological basis of the spondyloarthropathies is not known. The illnesses are associated with HLA-B27 and linked to the MHC region. The products of the MHC gene play a pivotal role in the immune system. In association with β_2-microglobulin, the class I human leukocyte antigen (HLA) molecules *HLA-A*, *HLA-B*, and *HLA-C* present short peptides to cytotoxic (CD8-positive) T cells. The complex of class I molecule and peptide is recognized as self or foreign by these T cells via interaction with the T-cell receptor on the T-cell membrane. Thus, this knowledge, along with the known association of the diseases with certain bacterial agents, has led to several theories of pathoetiology that are related to the immune function of HLA-B27 (Benjamin and Parham, 1990). For example, the pathogenic basis of disease has been ascribed to an arthritogenic peptide. Such a peptide is proposed to be bound by HLA-B27 and to induce disease (Geczy et al., 1986). Putative arthritogenic peptides might be derived from the organisms associated with disease and mimic HLA-B27 (Schwimmbeck et al., 1987). Others have proposed that the critical peptide might come from HLA-B27 itself and be presented by MHC class II molecules (Davenport, 1995), or an arthritogenic HLA-B27-derived peptide might be presented by HLA-B27 itself (Scofield et al., 1993, 1995). Interesting immunological data on MZ twins discordant for AS once again suggest that T-cell stimulation is involved in the pathogenesis of AS (Duchmann et al., 2001).

HLA-B27 might be involved in the pathogenesis of disease by virtue of an altered or novel function. For example, a direct effect of the presence of HLA-B27 on bacterial interaction with cells has been found (Kapasi and Inman, 1992, 1994; Virala et al., 1997; Laitio et al., 1997). Alternatively, bacterial infection may have an effect on HLA-B27 (Huang et al., 1997; Wuorela et al., 1997). Further, the unusual stability of HLA-B27 may allow either binding of peptides in a manner distinct from other class I molecules or empty HLA-B27 to be present on the cell surface (Benjamin et al., 1991; Peh et al., 1998). HLA-B27 without bound peptide may have immunological properties that are involved in the pathogenesis of disease. Finally, the most recent hypothesis is that misfolding of HLA-B27 within the endoplasmic reticulum may be responsible for the disease (Mear et al., 1999; Colbert, 2000).

Direct involvement of HLA-B27 in the pathophysiology of the diseases has been studied in several animal models of spondyloarthropathy. Rats transgenic for HLA-B27 and human β_2-microglobulin develop joint, skin, and nail disease that is similar to human spondyloarthropathy (Hammer et al., 1990; Breban et al., 1993). The disease occurs only in transgenic lines with very high copy number of the HLA-B27 transgene (Taurog et al., 1993). When these animals are raised in a germ-free environment, no disease is seen. Studies have also been performed in mice, showing that disease arises in mice with transgenic HLA-B27 and β_2-microglobulin knocked out (Khare et al., 1995). Furthermore, disease occurred only upon transfer of these animals from ultraclean to regular housing. Thus, these data indicate that HLA-B27 itself, not a closely linked gene, is a direct part of pathogenesis. However, similar to the human condition, the environment, presumably exposure to particular bacteria, is critical for disease expression.

GENE IDENTIFICATION

The association of AS with HLA-B27 has been known for over 25 years (Brewerton et al., 1973). More than 95% of AS patients carry the HLA-B27 allele. Thus, the association of this marker with AS is one of the strongest MHC–disease associations known. In addition, HLA-B27 is found in excess among persons with AS in every racial and ethnic group examined (Tiware and Terisaki, 1985). Thus, the association of HLA-B27 and AS is one of only a few MHC–disease associations that crosses ethnic and racial lines (reviewed in Mignot, 1998). Subsequent to the original report of Brewerton and colleagues (1973), other disease entities that were clinically related to AS were examined for an association with HLA-B27. While a lower percentage of these patients had HLA-B27, there was still a considerable association between the presence of HLA-B27 and arthritis in the setting of inflammatory bowel disease (Asquith et al., 1974; Brewerton et al., 1974; Morris et al., 1974), reactive arthritis syndrome (Brewerton et al., 1975), and psoriatic arthritis (Brewerton et al., 1974; Metzger et al., 1975).

More recently, genetic linkage to the MHC or *HLA-B* has been demonstrated for AS. Rubin et al. (1994) studied 15 multiple-case Canadian families and found evidence of genetic linkage between AS and the MHC. The maximal OR (LOD) score was 3.48 at a recombination rate of 0.05. When the population association of HLA-B27 and AS was considered in a second analysis, the LOD score obtained was 7.5 at $\theta = 0.05$ (Rubin et al., 1994). The first screening of the entire genome was performed in 105 white British families in which at least two persons were diagnosed with AS (Brown et al., 1998a). The highest LOD score was obtained with a microsatellite marker within the MHC III region. The maximal LOD score found with a marker not located within the MHC was 2.6 for D16S422 on chromosome 16q. In total, nine markers from seven regions outside the MHC had a $p < 0.01$. Thus, this genomic screening confirms linkage of AS to the MHC and suggests other areas of the genome which might contain genes impacting on acquisition of AS. This same group has extended their work in 185 AS families containing 225 affected sibling pairs (Laval et al., 2001). Again, the MHC region showed the strongest linkage, with a LOD score of 15.6. The second most powerful effect was found for a genetic interval on chromosome 16q, with a LOD score of 4.7 (Laval et al., 2001). A separate study of chromosome 22 using an association strategy (in 617 AS patients and 402 controls) showed that homozygosity for poor metabolizer alleles of the cytochrome P-450 enzyme CYP2D6 (dibrisoquine hydroxylase) was associated with AS (Brown et al., 2000a). Using a linkage approach (in 200 affected sibling pairs), there was weak evidence of linkage between CYP2D6 and AS (Brown et al., 2000a).

Serologically identified HLA-B27 is a family of highly related alleles. A large number (>20) of HLA-B27 subtypes have been identified (reviewed in Khan, 2000). The sequence mutations distinguishing the HLA-B27 subtypes tend to be located in the peptide binding cleft and therefore affect peptide binding and T-cell activation (Galocha et al., 1996; Garcia et al., 1997, 1998). Structural and functional aspects of the differences and similarities among the HLA-B27 subtypes (Lopez de Castro, 1995; Boisgérault et al., 1996) as well as their worldwide distribution (Khan, 1995) have been reviewed. Some of these alleles, such as B*2701, B*2710, B*2708, and B*2711, have been found in only a few individuals or a single kindred. Their relationship to spondyloarthropathy is unknown. The common allele in Caucasian populations is B*2705, which along with B*2702 is associated with spondyloarthropathy (Brown et al., 1996).

The alleles B*2704, B*2706 and B*2707 are found in Asian populations, while B*2703 is found in west Africa (Khan, 1995; Gonzales-Roces et al., 1997). A study of AS in Thailand found that B*2704, but not B*2706, was associated with the disease (López-Larrea et al., 1995). A subsequent study found two Chinese AS patients with the B*2706 subtype among 22 patients examined (Gonzales-Roces et al., 1997). This same study also found three AS patients in west Africa with B*2703. Of course, if these subtypes are not related to disease, one expects to find a few individuals with AS and either B*2703 or B*2706 by chance. Thus, while suggestive of an association, these data are incomplete. Population studies of larger numbers of spondyloarthropathy patients are needed to definitively determine whether these HLA-B27 subtypes are associated with disease.

One study used the transmission disequilibrium test (TDT) to assess genetic effects for AS and found an effect of HLA-B27. However, in this study of 13 families (97 individuals with 42 affected by AS), no effect of HLA-B40 was found (Amos et al., 1997). We used a modified version of the TDT (Harley et al., 1995) to study transmission of alleles at *HLA-B* in a previously published set of families with AS (R.H. Scofield, B.R. Neas, and J.B. Harley, unpublished data). This data set contains 38 pedigrees with 83 affecteds as well as HLA data on at least one affected and both parents and complete family structures (Møller and Berg, 1983). The logistic transmission model of the TDT compares the probability of transmission to affected or unaffected offspring of each allele at a locus using stepwise logistic regression (Harley et al., 1995; Neas et al., 1997). The allele with the most prominent effect in a univariate analysis enters the model first and remains while the contribution to the model of other alleles is evaluated. Thus, no prior population association is required, nor is an assumption concerning the mode of inheritance required. For logistic transmission modeling, the paired, matched parental alleles serve as controls. HLA-B27 has the most statistically powerful effect ($\chi^2 = 31$, $p < 0.0001$, df = 7) and enters the model in step 1. Once incorporated into the model, B27 accounts for approximately 75% of the variability of transmission of the *HLA-B* alleles (OR = 5.9, Wald $\chi^2 = 24.2$, $p <$ 0.0001). Next, HLA-B40 enters in step 2, significantly improves the model, and therefore is incorporated. HLA-B12 then enters with a negative contribution in affected individuals but does not reach statistical significance and is therefore removed. When the unaffected siblings from the Møller and Berg (1983) families were examined by logistic transmission modeling, we found that only HLA-B35 had a statistically significant contribution. This allele was statistically likely to be transmitted to the unaffecteds (OR = 12.9, $\chi^2 = 6.1$, $p = 0.013$).

Over the past several years, a few reports have associated spondyloarthropathy with other *HLA-B* alleles. HLA-B7, -B40, and -B22 (the HLA-B27 cross-reactive group) have been found in excess (Arnett et al., 1977). HLA-B7 has been associated with the development of reactive arthritis after a well-characterized outbreak of salmonellosis (Inman et al., 1988). In Israel, both HLA-B7 and -B22 are found in excess among reactive arthritis syndrome patients (Ben-Chetrit et al., 1985). In a Japanese (Yamaguchi et al., 1995) and a Caucasian (Khan et al., 1978) population, HLA-B39 was found in HLA-B27-negative patients with AS. Our analyses demonstrate that HLA-B40 contributes to genetic linkage to AS, but we have not found an independent contribution of HLA-B7 or -B22. The effect of HLA-B40 in these families is large and significantly participates with HLA-B27. The risk of AS in HLA-B27/B40 heterozygotes was increased threefold over those with HLA-B27 alone, a finding similar in magnitude to previous reports (Robinson et al., 1989; Rubin et al., 1994; Brown et al., 1996).

We have also identified HLA-B35 as being negatively associated with disease. This allele was uncommonly transmitted to affected individuals and tended to be transmitted to unaffected siblings. A previous report found less HLA-B35 in AS patients compared to controls in one of four cohorts examined for population effects (Robinson et al., 1989). However, another study found the HLA-B35 cross-reactive group to be increased in HLA-B27-negative AS (Wagener et al., 1980). The effect was not due to transmission by HLA-B27/B35 parents as the HLA-B35 effect is independent of HLA-B27 in the multivariate analysis. Serological HLA-B35 is now known to identify a family of almost 20 subtypes. If confirmed, the effect of HLA-B35 may be restricted to one or a few subtypes or could be a broad effect seen with most subtypes. The finding of differential effects for HLA-B27 and HLA-B35 in AS is especially interesting given the reports of opposing effects of HLA-B27 and HLA-B35 in the progression of human immunodeficiency virus disease (McNeil et al., 1996; Tomiyama et al., 1997).

Several candidate genes within the MHC other than *HLA-B* have been studied. A 9.2 kb restriction fragment length polymorphism (RFLP) was associated with the presence of AS as well as the presence of peripheral arthritis (McDaniel et al., 1987). However, further studies have failed to confirm the association with AS (Durand and Taurog, 1988; Ahearn et al., 1989; Reveille et al., 1994). Also, polymorphisms of the tumor necrosis factor (TNF) gene located in the MHC III region have been examined. The TNF gene is a candidate in AS by virtue of evidence supporting it as a mediator of inflammation in the disease (Gratacos et al., 1994; Toussirot et al., 1994), including a spondyloarthropathy-like illness in mice expressing a *Peromyscus leucopus* TNF-α transgene (Crew et al., 1998). A study of RFLP of the TNF-α and TNF-β genes in 73 AS patients and 81 controls found no differences in frequency of the RFLPs (Verjans et al., 1991). Two subsequent studies, one analyzing a single-base polymorphism (Verjans et al., 1994) and the other examining RFLP genotypes (Fraile et al., 1998), confirmed the original findings. Another study of 311 B27-positive subjects (of whom 161 had AS) found no association of TNF polymorphisms with disease (Martinez-Borra et al., 2000). Nonetheless, some data can be interpreted to support a second, weaker, non-*HLA-B* locus within the MHC that is a risk factor for disease (Milicic et al., 2000; Ricci-Vitiani et al., 2000). Several other candidate genes distant from the MHC have been studied. A polymorphism in the interleukin-6 promoter was not associated with AS (Collado-Escobar et al., 2000). The T-cell receptor (TCR) genes have been studied in AS patients and controls as candidate genes. Neither of the two studies found polymorphisms in either the TCRα or TCRβ genes associated with AS (Durand et al., 1988; Brown et al., 1998b).

Other candidate genes investigated have a role in the processing of peptides to be bound and presented by MHC class I molecules. The low molecular weight polypeptide 2 (*LMP2*) gene encodes a subunit of the proteasome that is in part responsible for the generation of short (8–11 amino acids) peptides that will be bound by MHC class I molecules. The *LMP2* gene is located within the MHC class II region between *HLA-DR* and *HLA-DP*. Several studies have investigated its potential role in spondyloarthropathy. Using the biallelic RFLPs induced by the restriction enzyme CfoI and studying 125 AS patients, Maksymowych and colleagues (1994) found that AS complicated by iritis was associated with homozygosity for the *b* allele of *LMP2* (72.7% vs. 38.6% of AS without iritis vs. 45.2% of controls). In subsequent studies, these investigators found the *LMP2 b/b* genotype to be associated with extraspinal disease and anterior uveitis in 193 white AS patients (Maksmowych et al., 1995a; Maksmowych and Russell, 1995) and Mexican (Maksymowych et al., 1997). There was no association with disease severity in adults with AS (Maksymowych et al., 1997), but in children with juvenile rheumatoid arthritis homozygosity for *LMP2 b* was associated with an older age at onset, oligoarticular presentation, and a polyarticular course of disease (Pryhuber et al., 1996). These effects persisted when the presence or absence of HLA-B27 was taken into account in a multiple regression analysis of juvenile spondyloarthropathy (Pryhuber et al., 1996) as well as in patients with adult-onset disease (Maksmowych et al., 2000).

Three studies have examined alleles of the transporter-associated protein (*TAP*) genes. These gene products participate in the physical association of class I MHC with peptides that occurs in the endoplasmic reticulum. One study of 30 AS patients, 30 reactive arthritis patients, 35 B27-positive controls, and 93 random controls found no association of either *TAP1* or *TAP2* alleles with disease (Westman et al., 1995). A Spanish study also found no association of either *TAP1* or *TAP2* in 44 AS patients (Fraile et al., 2000). Meanwhile, a third study of *TAP1* RFLPs found no difference between 115 AS patients and 41 B27-positive controls. However, the *TAP1B* allele was found in 17% of AS patients with extraspinal disease, while only 2.9% of those with axial disease alone and 1.9% of controls had this allele (Maksymowych et al., 1995b). Thus, both *TAP* and *LMP2* lie within the MHC, have been associated with specific phenotypes of AS, and have gene products involved in the association of MHC class I with peptides.

CLINICAL APPLICATION AND RISK ASSESSMENT OF GENETICS INFORMATION

Application of the known genetic information to spondyloarthropathy in the clinical arena is limited. At present, there is no role in the screening or prevention of AS or reactive arthritis. In a screening of random blood donors, a prevalence of 1.9% for spondyloarthropathies was found; in this cohort, 19 of 140 *B27*-positive subjects had disease, while only one of 133 B27-negative subjects did (Braun et al., 1998). Thus, spondyloarthropathies are among the most common of all rheumatic illnesses, but the risk of disease is low, even among those with HLA-B27. In other words, most individuals with HLA-B27 do not become ill and most individuals with a musculoskeletal illness do not have a spondyloarthropathy. Therefore, there is no role for population screening at present, especially since there is no preventive treatment available.

Determination of HLA-B27 in first-degree relatives of AS patients could be useful. Family members without the disease and negative for HLA-B27 could be counseled that they have little chance of developing the illness. The negative predictive value of HLA-B27 for AS is greater than 99.9% in this setting (Gran and Husby, 1995). However, a positive result for HLA-B27 in this situation will not be helpful in that about 50% of HLA-B27-positive first-degree relatives will go on to have a spondyloarthropathy.

HLA-B27 status is not routinely required in the diagnosis of individual patients. The diagnosis of spondyloarthropathy is based on, and can usually be determined with, the history and physical examination along with radiographic studies. There are no data that HLA-B27 status affects or predicts the course of disease, response to treatment, or long-term outcome in AS. Occasionally, determination of HLA-B27 is helpful in an individual patient in whom the diagnosis is not clear, but in the great majority of patients such determination is not helpful. If the clinical certainty of the AS diagnosis (prior to radiographic studies) is greater than 50% but substantially lower than 95%, the finding of HLA-B27 positivity might be useful (Hawkins et al., 1981). However, because greater than 75% of patients with low back pain and stiffness do not have AS, clinical certainty rarely, if ever, is greater than 50% (Gran and Husby, 1995). In a patient with apparent AS, a negative HLA-B27 status should alert the clinician to the possibility of undetected psoriasis or inflammatory bowel disease. However, routine determination of HLA-B27 cannot be recommended in AS.

In reactive arthritis, where the presence of HLA-B27 is associated with outcome, a case can be made for routinely determining HLA-B27 status. In 63 patients with post-salmonella reactive arthritis, extra-articular manifestations, sacroiliitis, or chronic or recurrent arthritis occurred only in those with HLA-B27 (Leirisalo-Repo et al., 1997). In another study of 116 spondyloarthropathy patients, HLA-B27 was associated with sacroiliitis and higher values for inflammatory markers such as erythrocyte sedimentation rate and C-reactive protein (Saroux et al., 1995). In several long-term follow-up studies of reactive arthritis after outbreaks of enteric infections, HLA-B27 appeared to be a predictor of chronicity (Bremell et al., 1991; Yla-Kerttula et al., 1995). Thus, determination of HLA-B27 in reactive arthritis can provide clinical information as to outcome and the possibility of extra-articular complications.

REFERENCES

Ahearn JM Jr, Calomiris JJ, Wigley FM, Jabs DA, Bias WB, Hochberg MC: Characterization of the class I HLA 9.2-kb Pvu II restriction fragment length polymorphism. Linkage to HLA-A and lack of disease association. Arthritis Rheum 1989; 32:870–876.

Amos CI, Wan Y, Siminovitch KA, Rubin LA: Estimating the strength of genetic effects: a combination of maximum likelihood and transmission disequilibrium methods in the study of ankylosing spondylitis. Hum Immunol 1997; 57:44–50.

Arnett FC, Hochberg MC, Bias WB: Cross-reactive antigens in B27-negative Reiter's syndrome and sacroiliitis. John Hopkins Med J 1977; 141:193–197.

Asquith P, Mackintosh P, Stokes PL, Holmes GK, Cooke WT: Histocompatibility antigens in patients with inflammatory bowel disease. Lancet 1974; 1:113–115.

Bas S, Griffais R, Kvien TK, Glennas A, Melby K, Visher TL: Amplification of plasmid and chromosomal chlamydia DNA in synovial fluid of patients with reactive arthritis and undifferentiated seronegative oligoarthropathies. Arthritis Rheum 1995; 38:1005–1013.

Benjamin R, Parham P: Guilt by association: HLA-B27 and ankylosing spondylitis. Immunol Today 1990; 11:137–142.

Benjamin RJ, Madrigal JA, Parham P: Peptide binding to empty HLA-B27 of viable human cells. Nature 1991; 351:74–77.

Bergfeldt L: HLA-B27-associated cardiac disease. Ann Intern Med 1997; 127:621–629.

Boisgérault F, Tieng V, Stolzenberg M, Dulphy N, Khalil I, Tamouza R, Charron D, Toubert A: Differences in endogenous peptides presented by HLA-B*2705 and B*2703 allelic variants: implications for susceptibility to spondyloarthropathy. J Clin Invest 1996; 98:2764–2770.

Boyer GS, Lanier AP, Templin DW: Prevalence rates of spondyloarthropathies, rheumatoid arthritis, and other rheumatic disorders in an Alaskan Inupiat Eskimo population. J Rheumatol 1988; 15:678–683.

Boyer GS, Lanier AP, Templin DW, Bulkow L: Spondyloarthropathy and rheumatoid arthritis in Alaskan Yupik Eskimos. J Rheumatol 1990; 17:489–498.

Boyer GS, Templin DW, Cornoni-Huntley JC, Everett DF, Lawrence RC, Heyse SF, Miller MM, Goring WP: Prevalence of spondyloarthropathies in Alaskan Eskimos. J Rheumatol 1994; 21:2291–2297.

Braun J, Bollow M, Remlinger G, Eggens U, Rudwaleit M, Distler A, Sieper J: Prevalence of spondyloarthropathies in HLA-B27 positive and negative blood donors. Arthritis Rheum 1998; 41:58–67.

Breban M, Hammer RE, Richardson JA, Taurog JD: Transfer of the inflammatory disease of HLA-B27 transgenic rats by bone marrow engraftment. J Exp Med 1993; 178:1607–1616.

Bremell T, Bjelle A, Svedham A: Rheumatic symptoms following an outbreak of Campylobacter enteritis: a five year follow up. Ann Rheum Dis 1991; 50:934–938.

Brewerton DA: HL-A 27 in Reiter's disease and psoriatic arthropathy. Int J Dermatol 1975; 14:39–40.

Brewerton DA, Caffrey M, Nicholls A, Walters D, James DC: HL-A 27 and arthropathies associated with ulcerative colitis and psoriasis. Lancet 1974; 1:956–958.

Brewerton DA, Hart FD, Nicholls A, Caffrey M, James DCO, Sturock RD: Ankylosing spondylitis and HLA A27. Lancet 1973; 1:904–907.

Brown M, Pile K, Kennedy L, Calin A, Darke C, Bell J, Wordsworth B, Cornelis F: HLA class I associations of ankylosing spondylitis in the white population in the United Kingdom. Ann Rheum Dis 1996; 55:268–270.

Brown MA, Edwards S, Hoyle E, Campbell S, Laval S, Daly AK, Pile KD, Calin A, Ebringer A, Weeks DE, et al.: Polymorphisms of the CYP2D6 gene increase susceptibility to ankylsing spondylitis. Hum Mol Genet 2000a; 9:1563–1566.

Brown MA, Jepson A, Young A, Whittle HC, Greenwood BM, Wordsworth BP: Ankylosing spondylitis in west Africans-evidence for a non-HLA-B27 protective effect. Ann Rheum Dis 1997a; 56:68–70.

Brown MA, Kennedy LG, MacGregor AJ, Darke C, Duncan E, Shatford JL, Taylor A, Calin A, Wordworth P: Susceptibility to ankylosing spondylitis in twins. Arthritis Rheum 1997b; 40:1823–1828.

Brown MA, Laval SH, Brophy S, Calin A: Recurrence risk modelling of the genetic susceptibility to ankylosing spondylitis. Ann Rheum Dis 2000b; 59:883–886.

Brown MA, Pile KD, Kennedy LG, Campbell D, Andrew L, March R, Shatford JL, Weeks DE, Calin A, Wordsworth BP: A genome-wide screen for susceptibility loci in ankylosing spondylitis. Arthritis Rheum 1998a; 41:588–597.

Brown MA, Rudwalaleit M, Pile KD, Kennedy LG, Shatford J, Amos CI, Siminovitch K, Rubin L, Calin A, Wordsworth BP. The role of germline polymorphisms in the T-cell receptor in susceptibility to ankylosing spondylitis. Br J Rheumatol 1998b; 37:454–458.

Calin A, Brophy S, Blake D: Impact of sex on inheritance of ankylosing spondylitis: a cohort study. Lancet 1999; 354:1687–1690.

Colbert RA: HLA-B27 misfolding: a solution to the spondyloarthropathy conundrum? Mol Med Today 2000; 6:224–230.

Collado-Escobar MD, Nieto A, Mataran L, Raya E, Martin J: Interluekin 6 gene promoter polymorphism is not associated with ankylosing spondylitis. J Rheumatol 2000; 27:1461–1463.

Crew MD, Effros RB, Walford RL, Zeller E, Cheroutre H, Brahn E: Transgenic mice expressing a truncated *Peromyscus leucopus* TNF-α gene manifest an arthritis resembling ankylosing spondylitis. J Interferon Cytokine Res 1998; 18:219–225.

Davenport MP: The promiscuous B27 hypothesis. Lancet 1995; 346:500–501.

Dougados M, van der Linden S, Juhlin R, Huitfeldt B, Amor B, Calin A, Cats A, Dijkmans B, Olivieri I, Pasero G, et al: The European Spondyloarthropathy Study Group preliminary criteria for the classification of spondyloarthropathy. Arthritis Rheum 1991; 34:1218–1227.

Duchmann R, Lambert C, May E, Hohler T, Marker-Hermann E: CD4+ and CD8+ clonal T cell expansions indicate a role of antigens in ankylosing spondylitis; a study in HLA-B27+ monozygous twins. Clin Exp Immunol 2001; 123:315–322.

Duchmann R, May E, Ackermann B, Goergen B, Meyer zum Büschenfelde KH, Marker-Hermann E: HLA-B27-restricted cytotoxic T lymphocyte responses to arthritogenic enterobacteria or self-antigens are dominated by closely related TCRBV gene segments. A study in patients with reactive arthritis. Scand J Immunol 1996; 43:101–108.

Durand JP, el Zaatari FA, Krieg AM, Taurog JD: Restriction length polymorphism of T cell receptor alpha and beta chain genes in patients with ankylosing spondylitis. J Rheumatol 1988a; 15:1115–1118.

Durand JP, Taurog JD: Association of ankylosing spondylitis and a 9.2 kb Pvu II class I DNA restriction fragment: a reassessment. J Rheumatol 1988b; 15:1119–1122.

Ebringer A: Ankylosing spondylitis is caused by Klebsiella. Evidence from immunogenetic, microbiologic, and serologic studies. Rheum Dis Clin North Am 1992; 18:105–121.

Fraile A, Collado MD, Mataran L, Martin J, Nieto A: TAP1 And TAP2 polymorphism in Spanish patients with ankylosing spondylitis. Exp Clin Immunogenet 2000; 17:199–204.

Fraile A, Nieto A, Beraún Y, Vinasco J, Matarán L, Martín J: Tumor necrosis factor gene polymorphisms in ankylosing spondylitis. Tissue Antigens 1998; 51:386–390.

Galocha B, Lamas JR, Villadangos JA, Albar JP, López de Castro JA: Binding of peptides naturally presented by HLA-B27 to the differentially disease-associated B*2704 and B*2706 subtypes, and to mutants mimicking their polymorphism. Tissue Antigen 1996; 48:509–518.

García F, Marina A, Albar JP, López de Castro JA: HLA-B27 presents a peptide from a polymorphic region of its own molecule with homology to proteins from arthritogenic bacteria. Tissue Antigen 1997; 49:23–28.

García F, Rognan D, Lamas JR, Marina A, López de Castro JA: An HLA-B27 polymorphism (B*2710) that is critical for T-cell recognition has limited effects on peptide specificity. Tissue Antigens 1998; 51:1–9.

Geczy AF, McGuigan LE, Sullivan JS, Edmonds JP. Cytotoxic T lymphocytes against disease-associated determinant(s) in ankylosing spondylitis. J Exp Med 1986; 164:932–937.

Gofton JP, Bennett PH, Smythe HA, Decker JL. Sacroiliitis and ankylosing spondylitis in North American Indians. Ann Rheum Dis 1972; 31:474–481.

Gonzales-Roces S, Alvarez MV, Gonzales S, Dieye A, Makni H, Woodfield DG, Housan L, Konenkov V, Abbadi MC, Grunnet N, et al: HLA-B27 polymorphism and worldwide susceptibility to ankylosing spondylitis. Tissue Antigen 1997; 49:166–123.

Goto K, Ota M, Ohno S, Mizuki N, Ando H, Katsuyama Y, Maksymowych WP, Kimura M, Bahram S, Inoko H: MICA gene and ankylosing spondylitis: linkage analysis via a transmembrane-encoded triplet repeat polymorphism. Tissue Antigens 1997; 49:503–507.

Gran J, Husby G, Hordvik M. Prevalence of ankylosing spondylitis in males and females in a young middle age population in Tromso, northern Norway. Ann Rheum Dis 1985; 44:359–367.

Gran JT, Husby G: HLA-B27 and spondyloarthropathy: value for early diagnosis? J Med Genet 1995; 32:497–501.

Granfors K, Jalkanen S, Lindberg AA, Maaki-Ikola O, von Essen R, Lahesmaa-Rantala R, Isomaki H, Saario R, Arnold WJ, Toivanen A.: Salmonella lipopolysaccharide in synovial sells from patients with reactive arthritis. Lancet 1990; 33:685–686.

Gratacos J, Collado A, Filella X, Sanmarti R, Canete J, Llena J, Molina R, Ballaesta A, Muñuz-Gomez J: Serum cytokines (IL-6, TNF-alpha, IL-1 beta, and IFN-gamma) in ankylosing spondylitis: a close correlation between serum IL-6 and disease activity and severity. Br J Rheumatol 1994; 33:927–931.

Hamersma J, Cardon LR, Bradbury L, Brophy S, van der Horst-Bruinsma I, Calin A, Brown MA: Is disease activity in ankylosing spondylitis genetically determined? Arthritis Rheum 2001; 44:1396–1400.

Hammer RE, Maika SD, Simmons WA, Breban M, Taurog JD. Spontaneous inflammatory arthritis in transgenic rats expressing HLA-B27 and human β2M: an animal model of HLA-B27associated human disorders. Cell 1990; 63:1099–1112.

Harley BJ, Moser KL, Neas BR: Logistic transmission modeling of simulated data. Genet Epidemiol 1995; 12:607–612.

Hermann E, Sucké B, Droste U, Meyer zum Büschenfelde K-H: *Klebsiella pneumoniae*-reactive T cells in blood and synovial fluid of patients with ankylosing spondylitis. Comparison with HLA-27+ healthy control subjects in a limiting dilution analysis and determination of the specificity of synovial fluid T cell clones. Arthritis Rheum 1995; 38:1277–1282.

Hermann E, Yu DTY, Meyer zum Büschenfelde K-H, Fleischer B: HLA-B27 restricted CD8 T cells derived from synovial fluids of patients with reactive arthritis and ankylosing spondylitis. Lancet 1993; 342:646–650.

Hoyle E, Laval SH, Calin A, Wordsworth BP, Brown MA: The X-chromosome and susceptibility to ankylosing spondylitis. Arthritis Rheum 2000; 43:1353–1355.

Huang F, Yamaguvhi A, Tsuchiya N, Ikawa T, Tamura N, Virtala MM, Granfors K, Yasaei P, Yu DT: Induction of alternative splicing of HLA-B27 by bacterial invasion. Arthritis Rheum 1997; 40:694–703.

Inman RD: Classification criteria for reactive arthritis. J Rheumatol 1999; 26:1338–1346.

Inman RD, Johnston ME, Hodge M, Falk J, Helewa A: Postdysenteric reactive arthritis. A clinical and immunogenetic study following an outbreak of salmonellosis. Arthritis Rheum 1988; 31:1377–1383.

James WH: The sex ratio of probands and of secondary cases in conditions of multifactorial inheritance where liability varies with sex. J Med Genet 1991; 28:41–43.

Järninen P: Occurrence of ankylosing spondylitis in nationwide series of twins. Arthritis Rheum 1995; 38:381–383.

Johnson K, Gran JT, Dale K, Husby G: The prevalence of ankylosing spondylitis among Norwegian Samis (Lapps). J Rheumatol 1992; 19:1591–1594.

Kapasi K, Inman RD: HLA-B27 expression modulates invasion by gram-negative bacteria into transfected L-cells. J Immunol 1992; 148:3554–3559.

Kapasi K, Inman RD: ME1 epitope of HLA-B27 confers class I-mediated modulation of Gram-negative bacterial invasion. J Immunol 1994; 153:833–840.

Kennedy LG, Will R, Cain A: Sex ratio in the spondyloarthropathies and its relationship to phenotypic expression, mode of inheritance and age at onset. J Rheumatol 1993; 20:1900–1904.

Khan M: HLA-B27 and its subtypes in world populations. Curr Opin Rheumatol 1995; 7:263–269.

Khan MA: Update: the twenty subtypes of HLA-B27. Curr Opin Rheumatol 2000; 12:235–238.

Khan MA, Kushner J, Braun WE: B27-negative HLA-Bw16 in ankylosing spondylitis. Lancet 1978; 1:1370–1371.

Khare SD, Luthra HS, David CS: Spontaneous inflammatory arthritis in HLA-B27 transgenic mice lacking beta 2-microglobulin: a model of human spondyloarthropathy. J Exp Med 1995; 182:1153–1158.

Laitio P, Virtala M, Salmi M, Pelliniemi LJ, Yu DT, Granfors K: HLA-B27 modulates intracellular survival of *Salmonella enteritidis* in human monocytic cells. Eur J Immunol 1997; 27:1331–1338.

Laval SH, Timms A, Edwards S, Bradbury L, Brophy S, Milicic A, Rubin L, Siminovitch KA, Weeks DE, Calin A, et al: Whole genome screening in ankylosing spondylitis: evidence of non-MHC genetic susceptibility loci. Am J Hum Genet 2001; 68:918–926.

Leirisalo-Repo M, Helenius P, Hannu T, Lehtinen A, Kreula J, Taavitsainen M, Koskimies S. Long-term prognosis of reactive salmonella arthritis, Ann Rheum Dis 1997; 56:516–520.

López de Castro JA: Structural polymorphism and function of HLA-B27. Curr Opin Rheumatol 1995; 7:270–278.

López-Larrea K, Sujirachato K, Mehra NK, Chiewsilp P, Isarangkura D, Kanga U, Dominguez O, Coto E, Peña M, Setién F, et al: HLA-B27 subtypes in Asian patients with ankylosing spondylitis. Evidence for new associations. Tissue Antigens 1995; 45:169–175.

Liu Y, Li J, Chen B, Helenius H, Granfors K: Familial aggregation of ankylosing spondylitis in southern China. J Rheumatol 2001; 28:550–553.

Maitra RT: Comments regarding Hans Reiter's role in Nazi Germany. J Clin Rheumatol 2001; 7:127–129.

Mäki-Ikola O, Leirisalo-Repo M, Turunen U, Granfors K: Association of gut inflammation with increased serum IgA class klebsiella antibody concentrations in patients with axial ankylosing spondylitis (AS): implications for different aetiopathogenetic mechanisms for axial and peripheral AS? Ann Rheum Dis 1997a; 56:180–183.

Mäki-Ikola O, Nissilä M, Lehtinen K, Leirisalo-Repo M, Granfors K: IgA1 and IgA2 subclass antibodies against *Klebsiella pneumoniae* in the sera of patients with peripheral and axial types of ankylosing spondylitis. Ann Rheum Dis 1995a; 54:631–635.

Mäki-Ikola O, Nissilä M, Lehtinen K, Leirisalo-Repo M, Tovivanen P, Granfors K: Antibodies to *Klebsiella pneumoniae*, *Escherichia coli* and *Proteus mirabilis* in the sera of patients with axial and peripheral form of ankylosing spondylitis. Br J Rheumatol 1995b; 34:413–417.

Mäki-Ikola O, Penttinen M, von Essen R, Gripenberg-Lerche C, Isomaki H, Granfors K: IgM, IgG, and IgA class enterobacterial antibodies in serum and synovial fluid in patients with ankylosing spondylitis and rheumatoid arthritis. Br J Rheumatol 1997b; 36:1051–1053.

Maksymowych WP, Chou C-T, Russell AS: Matching prevalence of peripheral arthritis and acute anterior uveitis in individuals with ankylosing spondylitis. Ann Rheum Dis 1995a; 54:128–130.

Maksymowych WP, Jhangri GS, Gorodezky C, Luong M, Wong C, Burgos-Vargas R, Morenot M, Sanchez-Corona J, Ramos-Remus C Rusell AS: Ann Rheum Dis 1997; 56:488–492.

Maksymowych WP, Russell AS: Polymorphism in the LMP2 gene influences the relative risk for acute anterior uveitis in unselected patients with ankylosing spondylitis. Clin Invest Med 1995; 18:42–46.

Maksymowych WP, Suarez-Almazor M, Chou C-T, Russell AS: Polymorphism in LMP2 gene influences susceptibility to extraspinal disease in HLA-B27 positive individuals with ankylosing spondylitis. Ann Rheum Dis 1995b; 54:321–324.

Maksymowych WP, Tao S, Suarez-Almazor M, Ramos-Remus C, Russell AS: LMP2 polymorphism is associated with extraspinal disease in HLA-B27 negative Caucasian and Mexican Mestizo patients with ankylosing spondylitis. J Rheumatol 2000; 27:183–189.

Maksymowych WP, Wessler A, Schmidt-Egenolf M, Suarez-Almazor M, Ritzel G, Von Borstel RC, Pazderka F, Russel AS: Polymorphism in an HLA-linked proteasome gene influences phenotypic expression of disease in HLA-B27 individuals. J Rheumatol 1994; 21:665–669.

Martinez-Borra J, Gonzales S, Lopez-Vazquez A, Gelaz MA, Armas JB, Kanga U, Mehra NK, Lopez-Larrea C: HLA-B27 alone rather than B27-related class I haplotypes contributes to ankylosing spondylitis susceptibility. Hum Immunol 2000; 61:131–139.

McDaniel DO, Acton RT, Barger BO, Koopman WJ, Reveille JD: Association of a 9.2-kilobase PvuII class I major histocompatibility complex restriction fragment length polymorphism with ankylosing spondylitis. Arthritis Rheum 1987; 30:894–900.

McNeil AJ, Yap PL, Gore SM, Brettle RP, McColl M, Wyld R, Davidson S, Weightman R, Richardson AM, Robertson JR: Association of HLA types A1-B8-DR3 and B27 with rapid and slow progression of HIV disease. QJM 1996; 89:177–185.

Mear JP, Schreiber KL, Munz C, Zhu X, Stevanovic S, Rammensee HG, Rowland-Jones SL, Colbert RA: Misfolding of HLA-B27 as a result of its B pocket suggests a novel mechanism for its role in susceptibility to spondyloarthropathies. J Immunol 1999; 163:6665–6670.

Metzger AL, Morris RI, Bluestone R, Terasaki PI: HL-A w27 in psoriatic arthropathy. Arthritis Rheum 1975; 18:111–115.

Mielants H, Veys Em, Cuveilier C, De Vos M, Botelberghe L: HLA-B27 related arthritis and bowel inflammation. II. Ileocolonoscopy and bowel histology in patients with HLA-B27 related arthritis. J Rheumatol 1985; 12:294–298.

Mignot E: Genetics and familial aspects of narcolepsy. Neurology 1998; 50(Suppl 2):S16–S22.

Milicic A, Lindheimer F, Laval S, Rudwaleit M, Ackerman H, Wordsworth P, Hohler T, Brown MA: Interethnic studies of TNF polymorphisms confirm the likely presence of a second MHC susceptibility locus in ankylosing spondylitis. Gene Immun 2000; 1:418–422.

Møller P, Berg K: Family studies in Bechterew's syndrome (ankylosing spondylitis) III. Genetics. Clin Genet 1983; 24:73–89.

Mori K, Ushiyama T, Inoue K, Hukuda S: Polymorphic CAG repeats of the androgen receptor in Japanese male patients with ankylsoing spondylitis. Rheumatology (Oxford) 2000; 39:530–532.

Morris RI, Metzger AL, Bluestone R, Terisaki PI: HL-A-W27—a useful discriminator in the arthropathies of inflammatory bowel disease. N Engl J Med 1974; 290:1117–1119.

Morse HG, Rate RG, Bonnell MD, Kuberski T: High frequency of HLA-B27 and Reiter's syndrome in Navajo Indians. J Rheumatol 1980; 7:900–902.

Muggia AL, Bennahum DA, William RC: Navajo arthritis—an unusual, acute, self-limited disease. Arthritis Rheum 1971; 14:348–355.

Nikkari S, Merilahti-Palo R, Saario R, Soderstrom KO, Granfors K, Skurnik M, Toivanen P: Yersinia-triggered reactive arthritis. Use of polymerase chain reaction and immunocytochemical staining in the detection of bacterial components from synovial specimens. Arthritis Rheum 1992; 35:682–687.

Neas BR, Moser KL, Harley JB: Logistic transmission modeling for the simulated data of GAW10 problem 2. Genet Epidemiol 1997; 14:857–860.

Oen K, Postl B, Chalmers IM, Ling N, Schroeder ML, Baragar FD, Martin L, Reed M, Major P: Rheumatic diseases in an Inuit population. Arthritis Rheum 1986; 29:65–74.

Paronen I: Reiter's disease. A study of 344 cases observed in Finland. Acta Med Scand 1948; 212(Suppl):1–112.

Peh CA, Burrows SR, Barnden M, Khanna R, Cresswell P, Moss DJ, McCluskey J: HLA-B27-restricted antigen presentation in the absence of tapasin reveals polymorphism in mechanisms of HLA class I peptide loading. Immunity 1998; 8:531–542.

Pryhuber KG, Murray KJ, Donnelly P, Passo MH, Maksymowych WP, Glass DN, Giannini EH, Colbert RA: Polymorphisms in the LMP2 gene influence disease susceptibility and severity in HLA-B27 associated juvenile rheumatoid arthritis. J Rheumatol 1996; 23:747–752.

Rate RG, Morse HG, Donnell MD, Kurerski TT: "Navajo arthritis" reconsidered. Relationship to HLA-B27. Arthritis Rheum 1980; 23:1299–1302.

Reiter H: Uber eine bisher unerkannte Spirochäteninfektion. Dtsch Med Wochenschr 1916; 42:1535–1536.

Reveille JD, Suarez-Almazor ME, Russell AS, Go RC, Appleyard J, Barger BC, Acton RT, Koopman WJ, McDaniel DO: HLA in ankylosing spondylitis: is HLA-B27 the only MHC gene involved in disease pathogenesis. Semin Arthritis Rheum 1994; 23:295–309.

Ricci-Vitiani L, Vacca A, Potolicchio I, Scarpa R, Bitti P, Sebastiani G, Passiu G, Mathieu A, Sorrentino R: MICA gene triplet repeat polymorphism in patients with HLA-B27 positive and negative ankylosing spondylitis from Sardinia. J Rheumatol 2000; 27:2193–2197.

Robinson WP, van der Linden SM, Khan MA, Rentsch H-U, Cats A, Russell A, Thomson G: HLA-Bw60 increases susceptibility to ankylosing spondylitis in HLA-B27+ patients. Arthritis Rheum 1989; 32:1135–1141.

Rubin LA, Amos CI, Wade JA, Martin JR, Bale SJ, Little AH, Gladman DD, Bonney GE, Rubenstein JD, Siminovitch KA: Investigating the genetic basis for ankylosing spondylitis. Linkage studies with the major histocompatibility complex region. Arthritis Rheum 1994; 37:1212–1220.

Russell AS: Ankylosing spondylitis: history. In: Klippel JH, Dieppe PA (eds). Rheumatology, 2d ed. London:Mosby 1998:6.14.1–6.14.2.

Russell AS, Suarez Almazor ME: Ankylosing spondylitis is not caused by Klebsiella. Rheum Dis Clin North Am 1992; 18:94–104.

Saroux A, de Saint-Pierre V, Baron D, Valls I, Koreichi D, Youinou P, Le Goff P: The HLA-B27 antigen-spondyloarthropathy association. Impact on clinical expression. Rev Rhum Engl Ed 1995; 62:487–491.

Schwimmbeck PL, Yu DTY, Oldstone MB. Autoantibodies to HLA-B27 in the sera of patients with ankylosing spondylitis and Reiter's syndrome: molecular mimicry with Klebsiella pneumoniae as potential mechanism of autoimmune disease. J Exp Med 1987; 166:173–181.

Scofield RH. Diseases of the immune and collagen vascular systems. In: Rhoades ER (ed.) The Health of American Indians and Alaska Natives. (Baltimore:Johns Hopkins Press 2000:328–346.

Scofield RH, Kurien B, Gross T, Warren WL, Harley JB: HLA-B27 binding of peptide from its own sequence and similar peptides from bacteria: implications for spondyloarthropathies. Lancet 1995; 345:1542–1544.

Scofield RH, Warren WL, Koelsch G, Harley JB: A hypothesis for the immune dysregulation in spondyloarthropathy: contributions from enteric organisms, B27 structure, peptides bound by B27 and convergent evolution. Proc Natl Acad Sci USA 1993; 90:9330–9334.

Taurog JD, Maika SD, Simmons WA, Breban M, Hammer RE: Susceptibility to inflammatory disease in HLA-B27 transgenic rat lines correlates with level of B27 expression. J Immunol 1993; 150:4168–4178.

Tiware JL, Terasaki PL. HLA and Disease. Berlin: Springer-Verlag, 1985:32–48.

Tomiyama H, Miwa K, Shiga H, Moore YI, Oka S, Iwamoto A, Kaneko Y, Takiguchi M. Evidence of presentation of multiple HIV-1 cytotoxic T lymphocyte epitopes by HLA-B*3501 molecules that are associated with the accelerated progression of AIDS. J Immunol 1997; 158:5026–5034.

Toussirot E, Lafforgue P, Boucraut J, Despieds P, Schiano A, Bernard D, Acquaviva PC: Serum levels of interleukin 1-beta, tumor necrosis factor-alpha, soluble interleukin 2 receptor and soluble CD8 in seronegative spondyloarthropathies. Rheumatol Int 1994; 13:175–180.

van der Linden SM, Valkenburg HA, Cats A. Evaluation of diagnostic criteria for ankylosing spondylitis: a proposal for modification of the New York criteria. Arthritis Rheum 1984a; 27:361–368.

van der Linden SM, Valkenburg HA, de Jongh, Cats A: The risk of developing ankylosing spondylitis in HLA-B27 positive individuals. A comparison of relatives of spondylitis patients with the general population. Arthritis Rheum 1984b; 27:241–249.

Verjans GMGM, Brinkman BMN, van Doornik CEM, Kijlstra A, Verweij CL: Polymorphism of tumour necrosis factor-alpha (TNF-alpha) at position −308 in relation to ankylosing spondylitis. Clin Exp Immunol 1994; 97:45–47.

Verjans GMGM, van der Linden SM, van Eys GJJM, de Waal LP, Kijlstra A. Restriction fragment length polymorphism of the tumor necrosis factor region in patients with ankylosing spondylitis. Arthritis Rheum 1991; 34:486–489.

Virala M, Kirveskari J, Granfors K: HLA-B27 modulates the survival of *Salmonella enteritidis* in transfected L cell, possibly by impaired nitric oxide production. Infect Immun 1997; 65:4236–4242.

Wallace DJ, Weismann M. Should a war criminal be rewarded with eponymous distinction? The double life of Hans Reiter (1881–1969). J Clin Rheumatol 2000; 6:49–54.

Wallace DJ, Weismann M: Response to letter from Dr. Maitra. J Clin Rheumatol 2001; 7:129–130.

Wegener S, Mach J: Association of ankylosing spondylitis (Bechterew disease) and the HLA system. Zeitschrift Arzliche Fortbildung Jena 1980; 74:895–898.

Westman P, Partanen J, Leirisalo-Repo M, Koskimies S: TAP1 and TAP2 polymorphism in HLA-B27-positive subpopulations: no allelic differences in ankylosing spondylitis and reactive arthritis. Hum Immunol 1995; 44:236–242.

Willkens RF, Arnett FC, Bitter T, Calin A, Fisher L, Ford DK, Good AE, Masi AT: Reiter's syndrome: evaluation of preliminary criteria for definite disease. Arthritis Rheum 1981; 24:844–849.

Wuorela M, Jalkanen S, Kirveskari J, Laito P, Granfors K: *Yersinia enterocolitica* serotype 0:3 alters the expression of serologic HLA-B27 epitopes on human monocytes. Infect Immun 1997; 65:2060–2066.

Yamaguchi A, Naoyuki N, Mitsui H, Ahiota M, Ogawa A, Tokunaga T, Yoshinoya S, Juji T, Ito K: Association of HLA-B39 with HLA-B27-negative ankylosing spondylitis and pauciarticular juvenile rheumatoid arthritis in Japanese patients. Arthritis Rheum 1995; 38:1672–1677.

Yla-Kerttula T, Tertti R, Toivanen A: Ten-year follow up of patients from a *Yersinia pseudotuberculosis* III outbreak. Clin Exp Rheumatol 1995; 13:333–337.

31 Genetics of Systemic Lupus Erythematosus

PATRICK M. GAFFNEY, RICHARD A. KING, AND TIMOTHY W. BEHRENS

Systemic lupus erythematosus (SLE) is an autoimmune disease characterized by a loss of immunologic tolerance to a multitude of self-antigens. The immune dysfunction of SLE involves both B and T lymphocytes of the adaptive immune system. In addition, elements of the innate immune system, such as complement protein deficiencies and genetic polymorphisms in immunoglobulin Fc receptors, may contribute to disease expression. In this chapter, we review new experimental data providing clues to genetic pathways important in the pathogenesis of SLE. In addition, we discuss individual genes implicated in SLE and the ongoing genetic mapping studies in mouse and human SLE.

DISEASE DEFINITION

The primary immunologic dysfunction in SLE is the production of high titers of serum autoantibodies. These antibodies cause disease either by directly binding to cellular epitopes (e.g., antibody-mediated cytopenias and clotting associated with antiphospholipid antibodies) or by depositing in blood vessels as immune complexes (high molecular weight lattices of antibody and antigen), leading to vascular inflammation (*vasculitis*). A typical patient with SLE is a young woman in her childbearing years who presents with fatigue, joint pain and swelling, skin rash, low white blood cell count, and pleuritis. Fewer than half of lupus patients will present with more severe manifestations of the disease, which may include glomerulonephritis, compromised renal function, and/or neurologic symptoms including cerebritis, peripheral neuropathies, or stroke.

Laboratory testing is very helpful for establishing the diagnosis of SLE and for monitoring therapy. Nearly all patients with bona fide SLE have excessive titers of autoantibodies to nuclear autoantigens in serum; thus, antinuclear antibody (ANA) testing is very sensitive, though not 100% specific, at detecting individuals with the disease. Certain autoantibodies are observed essentially only in SLE, e.g., anti-double-stranded DNA (dsDNA) antibodies and anti-Smith antibodies, and have diagnostic utility. Active disease is often accompanied by high erythrocyte sedimentation rates, elevated serum levels of acute-phase reactants (e.g., C-reactive protein), and low levels of C3 and C4 complement components.

The clinical manifestations of SLE can be quite variable between individual patients, resulting in unique diagnostic challenges. Criteria for the diagnosis of SLE have been established by the American College of Rheumatology (ACR) that are both highly specific (>95%) and sensitive (>95%) (Tan et al., 1982; Hochberg, 1997) (Table 31–1). Patients fulfilling four of the 11 criteria can be considered to have the systemic form of SLE. There are also limited forms of lupus that involve only the skin and a subtype of the systemic disease caused by certain pharmaceutical agents (drug-induced lupus). For every patient who fulfills the ACR criteria for systemic lupus, there are probably three or four patients with fewer than four criteria who are classified as "probable" or "possible" SLE. Environmental factors, such as viral infections, ultraviolet light exposure, and certain toxins, potentially have a role in triggering SLE in some patients (reviewed by Mongey and Hess, 1997).

GENERAL GENETIC AND EPIDEMIOLOGICAL EVIDENCE

Clinical Epidemiology and Ethnic Differences

Prevalence

The prevalence of SLE has been documented worldwide and in multiple ethnic groups, with estimates ranging from 12 to 64/100,000 persons (Table 31–2). Three major studies have been conducted in the United States (Siegel and Lee, 1973; Fessel, 1974; Michet et al., 1985). Michet et al. (1985) estimated the prevalence of SLE in Olmstead County, Minnesota, from 1950 through 1979. Using medical record reviews and established criteria for case definition, the overall prevalence was estimated at 40/100,000 (Table 31–2). Fessel (1974) used similar case ascertainment methods and diagnostic criteria in the more racially heterogeneous population of the Kaiser Permanente Health Plan in San Francisco, California. A total of 64 cases of SLE were identified between 1967 and 1973, for an overall prevalence of 50/100,000. Of the 64 cases, 19 were African-American (16 women, 3 men), leading to an estimated prevalence in African-American women of 283/100,000 compared with 71/100,000 in Caucasian women. The accuracy of this estimate in African-Americans is uncertain, however, given the small number of cases. Siegel and Lee (1973) focused on a well-defined region of Manhattan in New York City. Cases were identified by review of records from hospitals and clinics within the sampling frame (1950–1965), positive tests for lupus at selected laboratories, and death records. A total of 193 definite cases of SLE were identified, for an overall estimated prevalence in the New York population of 14/100,000 (Table 31–2). Again, a higher prevalence was demonstrated among African-American females (56/100,000) compared to Caucasian females (17/100,000) (Table 31–3), but these estimates were considerably lower than those obtained in the more recent studies in Minnesota and California. This discrepancy may be due to an increasing awareness of SLE in the medical community and the availability of sensi-

Table 31–1. 1997 Revised American College of Rheumatology Criteria for Systemic Lupus Erythematosus (Four of the 11 Criteria Required for Diagnosis)

1. Malar rash	Fixed malar erythema, flat or raised
2. Discoid rash	Erythematous raised patches with keratotic scaling and follicular plugging
3. Photosensitivity	Skin rash as an unusual reaction to sunlight, by patient history or physician observation
4. Oral ulcers	Oral or nasopharyngeal ulcers, usually painless, observed by physician
5. Arthritis	Nonerosive arthritis involving two or more peripheral joints, characterized by tenderness, swelling, or effusion
6. Serositis	a. Pleuritis (convincing history of pleuritic pain, rub heard by physician, or evidence of pleural effusion), or b. Pericarditis (documented by electrocardiogram, or rub or evidence of pericardial effusion)
7. Renal disorder	a. Persistent proteinuria >0.5 g/day or >3+, or b. Cellular casts of any type
8. Neurologic disorder	a. Seizures (in the absence of other causes), or b. Psychosis (in the absence of other causes)
9. Hematologic disorder	a. Hemolytic anemia with reticulocytosis, or b. Leukopenia (<4000/mm^3 on two or more occasions), or c. Lymphopenia (<1500/mm^3 on two or more occasions), or d. Thrombocytopenia (<100,000/mm^3 in the absence of offending drugs)
10. Immune disorder	a. Anti-dsDNA antibody, or b. Anti-Sm antibody, or c. Antiphospholipid antibody based on: (i) abnormal serum level of IgG or IgM anticardiolipin antibodies, (ii) a positive test result for lupus anticoagulant using a standard method, or (iii) a false-positive serologic test for syphilis known to be positive for at least 6 months and confirmed by *Treponema pallidum* immobilization or fluorescent treponemal antibody absorption test
11. Antinuclear antibody	An abnormal titer by immunofluorescence or an equivalent assay at any time and in the absence of drugs known to be associated with "drug-induced lupus syndrome"

tive immunologic methods to detect the ANAs that are characteristic of it.

Using the data from the San Francisco study (Fessel, 1974), the National Arthritis Data Workgroup in 1998 (Lawrence et al., 1998) estimated the overall nationwide prevalence of suspected (fewer than four diagnostic criteria) or definite SLE in the United States at approximately 239,000 cases, affecting 4000 Caucasian males, 41,000 Caucasian females, 31,000 African-American males, and 163,000 African-American females. These estimates represent a substantial increase in the prevalence of SLE from that estimated in the 1989 workgroup report [131,000 cases nationwide (Lawrence et al., 1989)] due primarily to the inclusion of patients with "suspected" SLE in the 1998 report. The workgroup argued that patients who do not meet the criteria for SLE also consume health-care resources and may suffer from their illness as much as those who do meet the criteria.

Table 31–2. Prevalence of Systemic Lupus Erythematosus in Various Populations

Location	Reference	Year[a]	Overall[b]
North America			
Rochester, MN	Michet et al. (1985)	1979	40
San Francisco, CA	Fessel (1974)	1973	50
New York, NY	Siegel and Lee (1973)	1965	14
Europe and Atlantic			
Denmark	Voss et al. (1998)	1995	22
Northern Ireland	Gourley et al. (1997)	1993	25
England	Johnson et al. (1995)	1992	28
Curaçao	Nossent (1992)	1992	48
England	Hopkinson et al. (1993)	1990	25
England	Samanta et al. (1992)	1989	64
Sweden	Jonsson et al. (1989)	1986	42
Iceland	Gudmundsson and Steinssan (1990)	1984	36
England	Hochberg (1987b)	1982	12[c]
Sweden	Nived et al. (1985)	1982	39
Finland	Helve (1985)	1978	28
Asia and Pacific			
Malaysia	Wang et al. (1997)	1990	43
Oahu	Serdula and Rhoads (1979)	1975	15
New Zealand			
Auckland	Hart et al. (1983)	1980	18
Dunedin	Meddings and Grennan (1980)	1980	15
Range			12–64
Mean			31

[a]Corresponds to the year the study was completed.
[b]Rates per 100,000 individuals.
[c]Females only, no cases identified in males.

International studies of SLE prevalence in predominantly European Caucasian populations range from 12 to 42/100,000, which approximates the prevalence among Caucasians in the U.S. population (Helve, 1985; Nived et al., 1985; Hochberg, 1987a; Jonsson et al., 1989; Gudmundsson and Steinsson, 1990; Gourley et al., 1997; Voss et al., 1998). In studies that sampled populations of mixed ethnicity, overall prevalence estimates ranged from 15 to 64/100,000 (Serdula and Rhoads, 1979; Meddings and Grennan, 1980; Hart et al., 1983; Nossent, 1992; Samanta et al., 1992; Hopkinson et al., 1993; Johnson et al., 1995; Wang et al., 1997). In all of these international studies, non-Caucasians had higher prevalence estimates of SLE than Caucasians and females had higher prevalence estimates than males, mirroring the data from the United States.

Age and Sex

Peak incidence rates for SLE in females show significant variability between studies. Most studies report peak incidence in the 25- to 44-year age group (Serdula and Rhoads, 1979; Hart et al., 1983; Michet et al., 1985) or the 45- to 64-year age group (Nived et al., 1985; Jonsson et al., 1989; Nossent, 1992; Hopkinson et al., 1993). However, one study reported peak incidence in the 65 and older age group (Helve, 1985). Caucasian and non-Caucasian females had similar age-specific incidence rates.

Firm conclusions about the age-specific incidence rates in males are difficult given the relatively small numbers of cases reported in the literature. In studies where age-specific preva-

Table 31–3. Prevalence[a] of Systemic Lupus Erythematosus by Sex/Race: Selected Studies

Reference	Country	CM	CF	AAM	AAF	AM	AF
Siegel and Lee (1973)	United States	3	17	3	56	—	—
Fessel (1974)	United States	7	71	53	283	—	—
Johnson et al. (1995)	England	3	36	9	197	4	97
Gourley et al. (1997)	Ireland	4	47	—	—	—	—
Voss et al. (1998)	Denmark	5	38	—	—	—	—
Nossent (1992)	Curaçao	—	—	9	84	—	—
Samanta et al. (1992)	England	7	32	—	—	32	70
Mean		5	40	19	155	18	84

[a]Rates per 100,000 individuals.
CM, Caucasian males; CF, Caucasian females; AAM, African-American males; AAF, African-American females; AM, Asian males; AF, Asian females.

lence rates were also stratified by sex, SLE onset in males tended to occur later in life, with peak age-specific incidence rates (Michet et al., 1985; Nived et al., 1985; Jonsson et al., 1989) or prevalence rates (Helve, 1985; Nossent, 1992; Hopkinson et al., 1993) after age 65.

The male-to-female ratio for SLE is approximately 1:8 to 1:9 (Table 31–3). The overall predominance of women with SLE and the earlier age at disease onset are likely due in part to hormonal influences that occur during puberty and childbearing years in females.

Race

Table 31–3 summarizes the prevalence of SLE by race in selected population-based studies. It has been commonly observed that the incidence and prevalence of SLE is higher in persons of color. In the United States, Siegel (1973) and Fessel (1974) demonstrated an approximately three- to fourfold higher prevalence of SLE in African-American females compared with Caucasian females. This is comparable to a more recent study investigating the incidence of SLE in Allegheny County, Pennsylvania (McCarty et al., 1995), which identified 191 SLE cases between 1985 and 1990 and a threefold higher incidence in African-American females. A slightly higher, fivefold, excess prevalence of SLE was documented for Afro-Caribbean women compared to Caucasians in Birmingham, UK (Johnson et al., 1995).

There also appears to be a two- to threefold increase in the prevalence of SLE in Asian females compared to Caucasian females (Samanta et al., 1992; Johnson et al., 1995) (rates per 100,000: Birmingham, UK, Caucasian females 36.2, Asian females 96.5; Leicester City, UK, Caucasian females 31.7, Asian females 69.7). While no increase in SLE prevalence was noted among Chinese in San Francisco (Fessel, 1974), a prevalence as high as 1/170 was reported in Beijing, China, although there were design flaws in this study (Nai-Cheng, 1983). Studies of ethnic populations in Malaysia have demonstrated a higher prevalence of SLE in individuals of Chinese ancestry compared to native Malays or Indians (Frank, 1980; Wang et al., 1997). Among the various ethnic groups on the island of Oahu, Hawaii, the rate of SLE in the Chinese population was 4.2 times the rate in the Caucasian population (Serdula and Rhoads, 1979). Similarly, Filipino, native Hawaiian, and Japanese prevalence rates were three to four times that of Caucasians (Serdula and Rhoads, 1979). Finally, in New Zealand, SLE prevalence in the Polynesian population was 3.5 times higher than that among Caucasians (Hart et al., 1983).

SLE is also more common in certain North American Indian populations. A large survey of Indian Health Service records between 1971 and 1975 revealed a population prevalence of 1/1506 for the Sioux, based on 20 documented cases of SLE (18 female) in a population of 30,120 (Morton et al., 1976). The Crow and Arapahoe tribes also had higher SLE prevalence rates compared to other Native American groups. The Nuu-Chah-Nulth of the Pacific Northwest and Alaskan Indians of the southeast coast also have high rates of SLE (1/288 and 1/361, respectively) compared to white populations in the United States and Europe (Atkins et al., 1988; Boyer et al., 1991).

Despite variations in study design, case ascertainment methods, geographic distribution, and ethnic composition, two major conclusions about the population genetics and epidemiology of SLE can be drawn. First, there is a clear predisposition for females to develop SLE, which crosses ethnic and geographic boundaries. Second, in all studies where direct comparisons have been made, the prevalence of SLE is greater in non-Caucasian populations. These race- and sex-specific differences are likely due to a complex interaction of many factors, including race-specific differences in genetic susceptibility to SLE (highlighted by recent gene-mapping studies in humans, see below), environmental exposures, and socioeconomic conditions.

Family Epidemiology

Family Studies

An important part of assessing the genetic predisposition for a disease is establishing familial aggregation through well-designed family studies. To establish that a disease clusters in families, a comparison is made between the disease frequency in relatives of affected individuals and the disease frequency in the general population or in the relatives of an appropriately selected control group. Two excellent studies have been performed (Table 31–4). A case-control study in Baltimore, Maryland, identified 77 SLE patients and an equal number of age-, sex-, and race-matched controls (Hochberg et al., 1985; Hochberg, 1987a). From these individuals detailed family histories were obtained, and medical records of relevant individuals were reviewed. Eight cases had a first-degree relative with SLE compared to only one control [odds ratio (OR) 8, $p = 0.02$). Subgrouping by race and age at diagnosis revealed greater familial aggregation in African-Americans compared to Caucasians (OR 3.4, $p = 0.12$) and in those diagnosed at age ≤ 30 years (OR 5.7, $p = 0.08$). In the study by Lawrence et al. (1987), 74 consecutive SLE cases were identified from the diagnostic registers at two teaching hospitals in the United Kingdom. From these probands, 335 first-degree relatives were available for examination, and 10 (3.0%) met the criteria for SLE. The control group in this study comprised the first-degree relatives identified from probands with generalized

Table 31–4. Family Studies in Systemic Lupus Erythematosus (SLE)

			SLE Families			Controls		
Reference	Year	Country	Probands	First-Degree Relatives	First-Degree Relatives with SLE (%)	Probands	First-Degree Relatives	First-Degree Relatives with SLE (%)
Hochberg et al. (1985)	1985	US	77	541	8 (1.5)	77	540	1 (0.2)
Lawrence et al. (1987)	1987	UK	74	335	10 (3.0)	759	2512	7 (0.3)

osteoarthritis, psoriasis, and colitis who were age- and sex-matched to the SLE proband relatives. In this group, there were 759 probands ascertained with 2512 evaluable first-degree relatives. Seven individuals with SLE (0.3%) were identified.

Twin Studies

Comparison of concordance rates between monozygotic (MZ) and dizygotic (DZ) twins is a powerful tool for establishing the importance of genetic factors in disease transmission. Several such studies have been performed in SLE (Table 31–5). Block et al. (1975) reported on a collection of 10 sets of twins (7 MZ, 3 DZ) and reviewed the literature on 17 previously reported sets of twins. Among the MZ twins, 11/16 (69%) were concordant for SLE by the ACR criteria. By comparison, only one of four DZ twins was concordant. In the MZ twins, concordance for ANA and hypergammaglobulinemia was 71% and 87%, respectively. Reichlin and colleagues (1992) extended the serologic studies on the seven sets of MZ twins described by Block. Autoantibody titers for Ro/SS-A, La/SS-B, U1 ribonucleoprotein (RNP), and Sm were measured by enzyme-linked immunosorbent assay along with titers for ANA and anti-dsDNA antibodies. The three sets of twins concordant for SLE demonstrated similar levels of ANA and anti-dsDNA antibodies and similar anti-RNP antibody profiles. By comparison, the four sets of twins discordant for SLE demonstrated higher ANA and anti-dsDNA antibody titers in the affected twin, while the anti-RNP antibody profiles were similar for three of the four pairs. These data provide strong evidence for the importance of genetic influences in the development of autoantibodies in SLE.

A revised estimate for the concordance of SLE in MZ twins was provided by Deapen et al. (1992) who identified twins pairs with SLE from a large twin study registry in southern California. From this registry, 107 twins pairs that met criteria for SLE were identified. Of the 45 MZ twins identified, 11 (24%) were concordant for SLE while only 1 (2%) of the 61 DZ twins was concordant. In a similar study from Finland (Jarvinen et al., 1992), twins with SLE were identified from the Finnish Twin Cohort Registry and zygosity was confirmed by genetic marker analysis. One of nine sets of MZ twins was concordant for SLE by the ACR revised criteria, although two additional sets of twins had one co-twin with three of four ACR criteria consistent with probable SLE. Inclusion of these two sets of twins would have resulted in a 30% concordance rate for SLE in the MZ twins. None of the DZ twins was concordant for SLE. A small study from Australia (Grennan et al., 1997) demonstrated similar estimates of concordance for MZ twins with SLE: one of four MZ (25%) twins was concordant for SLE compared to none of six DZ twin pairs.

In summary, twin studies of SLE support an important role for genetic factors in disease expression. Concordance rates in MZ twin pairs range from 24% to 69%. When the data from these studies are combined, the overall concordance rate for MZ twin pairs is 34% vs. 3% for DZ twin pairs (Table 31–5). These rates compare favorably with MZ concordance studies in other autoimmune diseases, such as type I diabetes mellitus, multiple sclerosis, and rheumatoid arthritis (reviewed by Vyse and Todd, 1996).

Table 31–5. Twin Studies in Systemic Lupus Erythematosus (SLE)

	MZ[a]		DZ		% Concordant	
Reference	C	D	C	D	MZ	DZ
Block et al. (1975)	11	5	1	3	69	25
Deapen et al. (1992)	11	34	1	61	24	2
Jarvinen et al. (1992)	3[b]	8	0	10	27	0
Grennan et al. (1997)	1	3	0	6	25	0
Total	26	50	2	80	34	3

[a]MZ, monozygotic; DZ, dizygotic; C, concordant twin pairs; D, discordant twin pairs.
[b]One set of twin pairs meets American College of Rheumatology revised criteria; one co-twin from each of two other pairs meet three of four criteria and probably have SLE.

PATHOPHYSIOLOGY: BIOLOGIC BASIS OF GENETIC SUSCEPTIBILITY

The pathophysiologic hallmark of SLE is the production of self-reacting antibodies directed against native DNA and other cellular constituents (Rothfield, 1985). As discussed above, these pathogenic antibodies are in some instances directly responsible for disease manifestations of lupus, examples being antiphospholipid antibody–mediated thrombosis or antibody-dependent cytopenias. However, many of the clinical manifestations of SLE result from the formation of immune complexes (ICs) which deposit in vital organs and connective tissues and lead to arthritis, dermatitis, serositis, glomerulonephritis, and vasculitis. In healthy individuals, IC formation serves as a mechanism for clearance of foreign antigens. In SLE, IC formation and deposition result from immune-regulatory defects, including loss of self-tolerance, high-level autoantibody production, and impaired IC clearance mechanisms. The loss of B- and T-cell immune tolerance in SLE and the potential role for apoptosis in SLE pathogenesis have been reviewed (Utz and Anderson, 1998; Rosen and Casciola-Rosen, 1999; Levine and Koh, 1999; Ring and Lakkis, 1999). Here, we discuss how impaired handling of ICs contributes to SLE.

The formation of ICs and their subsequent propensity to promote inflammation depend on the individual characteristics of antigen and antibody, the biologic properties of the ICs themselves, and the nature of the interaction of ICs with the mononuclear phagocyte system. The factors that influence the ability of an antibody to form ICs include concentration, affinity for antigen, and immunoglobulin (Ig) subclass. Antigen excess and high affinity of the antibody tend to promote IC formation. The efficiency with which ICs fix complement, another property important in IC pathogenicity, depends in part on the Ig subclass. Anti-dsDNA antibodies, found almost exclusively in SLE, are restricted to the Ig subclasses IgG1, IgG2, and IgG3; and these isotypes fix complement more efficiently than IgG4 (Rubin et al., 1986). In health, ICs with high numbers of antigen/antibody molecules are better at fixing complement and tend to be cleared from the circulation sooner. ICs with a low number of antigen/antibody molecules activate complement poorly and tend to circulate longer, allowing more time for redistribution to tissues.

Complement-decorated ICs are cleared from the circulation by receptors that bind complement and by Fc receptors, which recognize the constant portion of antibodies. The coating of ICs by the complement protein C3b facilitates binding to circulating erythrocytes via cell surface–expressed complement receptor 1 (Pederson et al., 1980; Hebert, 1991). This attachment of ICs to erythrocytes clears ICs from the circulation and delivers them to the liver and spleen, where they are stripped from the erythrocyte surface by Fcγ receptors expressed on mononuclear phagocytes (Cornacoff et al., 1983). This process, *immune adherence*, is important for efficient removal of ICs. Once stripped of ICs, erythrocytes are released back into the circulation, where the process begins again.

IC disease results when there is inadequate clearance of ICs and they are free to then deposit in connective tissues, vital organs, and vessel walls. IC deposition leads to generation of the complement fragments C5a and C3a, which damage tissues by activating the membrane attack complex of the terminal complement cascade and by recruiting additional inflammatory cells to the region. Interaction of ICs with neutrophils and monocytes promotes degranulation and release of inflammatory cytokines and enzymes, leading to further tissue damage. In SLE, the normal equilibrium of IC formation and clearance is significantly altered. The contributing factors include B- and T-lymphocyte hyperactivity, excessive autoantibody production, hypergammaglobulinemia, macrophage dysfunction, and alterations in cellular apoptosis. Emerging data on coding region polymorphisms of Fcγ receptors and studies of patients and mice with deficiencies in early classical pathway complement components (C1q, C2, and C4) suggest that these molecules are important in the pathophysiology of SLE.

GENE IDENTIFICATION

Spontaneous Mouse Models

There are several important mouse models for SLE that exhibit disease manifestations remarkably similar to those observed in the human disease (reviewed by Vyse and Kotzin, 1998). This section introduces several of these SLE mouse models and reviews the current status of genetic studies.

(NZB × NZW)F$_1$ Mice

Female F_1 offspring of a cross between New Zealand black (NZB) and New Zealand white (NZW) mice spontaneously accumulate high serum levels of IgG antinuclear antibodies and develop severe IC-mediated glomerulonephritis (reviewed by Drake et al., 1995). The kidney disease and autoantibody profiles present in the F_1 mice differ from those found in either of the parental strains, emphasizing that contributions to the phenotype from both parental strains are required for disease. Linkage analyses in various backcrosses have identified contributions from the major histocompatibility complex (MHC) and at least 12 non-MHC chromosomal regions to nephritis, autoantibody production, and death in this model (Vyse and Kotzin, 1998). The genetic effects attributed to the MHC are dependent on heterozygosity at this locus, the $H2^{d/z}$ genotype being associated with an increased frequency of fatal lupus nephritis compared with either the $H2^{d/d}$ or the $H2^{z/z}$ genotype (Hirose et al., 1986, 1990). Other genes located in the MHC region, such as tumor necrosis factor alpha (TNF-α), may also contribute the SLE phenotype in these mice (Jacob and McDevitt, 1988). In general, the linkage intervals for the non-MHC regions are currently quite broad, and to date, no genes have been identified.

The NZM2410 (New Zealand mixed) mouse is an inbred strain derived from an intercross of the NZB and NZW strains (Rudofsky et al., 1993). F_1 parental backcross analysis initially identified four major genetic regions that contribute to SLE in this strain: the distal portion of murine chromosome 1 (*Sle1*), intervals on chromosome 4 (*Sle2*) and chromosome 7 (*Sle3*), and the MHC region on chromosome 17 (Morel et al., 1994). These genetic intervals were found to be additive in terms of their ability to induce the autoimmune phenotype and provided evidence for a genetic threshold liability in SLE (Morel et al., 1994).

Wakeland and colleagues (1996) have generated congenic mice for each of these individual regions on the "non-autoimmune" C57Bl/6 genetic background. Interestingly, a component phenotype for SLE has been observed for each of the non-MHC regions (Morel et al., 1997; reviewed by Morel et al., 1998). In initial studies, each of the congenic strains was assayed for features of SLE, including polyclonal immunoglobulin production, ANA formation, and nephritis (Morel et al., 1997). Congenic mice for *Sle1* exhibited loss of B-cell tolerance to chromatin autoantigens (Mohan et al., 1998). This effect was dependent on the age of the mouse and peaked at 7 to 9 months of age. Surprisingly, despite the vigorous autoantibody response noted in these mice, there was little or no nephritis identified. Congenic mice for *Sle2* (from mouse chromosome 4) have significant B-cell hyperactivity (Mohan et al., 1997). B cells in Sle2 mice have an activated phenotype and respond more strongly than controls to mitogenic stimuli. These mice also have an increased number of CD5-expressing peritoneal B-1 cells and elevated levels of polyreactive/polyclonal IgM. However, *Sle2* on a B6 background was insufficient for generating IgG autoantibodies or lupus nephritis. *Sle2* may accelerate immune responses in these mice by lowering the threshold of B-cell signaling (Mohan et al., 1997). *Sle3* congenic mice have dysregulated T-cell function (Mohan et al., 1999). These mice spontaneously produced low levels of autoreactive antibodies and developed lupus nephritis by 9 months of age. Furthermore, the peripheral CD4 T-cell compartment is expanded, and T cells respond excessively to exogenous antigenic challenge compared with controls. These data suggest that *Sle3* may elevate antigen-dependent T-cell responsiveness.

The dissection of lupus-like disease into component phenotypes elegantly demonstrates the polygenic nature of SLE in this model. Interestingly, none of the monocongenic strains develop a phenotype of lethal glomerulonephritis. Wakeland and his group hypothesized that it would take a combination of two or more of the susceptibility loci to reproduce fully penetrant lethal disease. To test this hypothesis, they developed double and triple congenic strains and tested all possible combinations, including breeding with the Yaa lupus accelerator locus (Murphy and Roths, 1979), for evidence of lethal glomerulonephritis. These studies demonstrated that *Sle1* is a key locus for initiating the lethal glomerulonephritis phenotype by breaking tolerance to chromatin. Without this locus, neither the combination *Sle2/Yaa*, *Sle3/Yaa*, nor *Sle2/Sle3* resulted in any excess autoimmunity over the *Sle2* or *Sle3* phenotype alone.

Fine-mapping the *Sle1* locus revealed the presence of a cluster of functionally related loci (*Sle1a*, *-b*, and *-c*) which independently mediate the loss of tolerance to nuclear antigens (Morel et al., 2001). However, the immunologic phenotypes attributed to each of these subloci appear to be distinct. *Sle1b* accounts for most of the effect of the *Sle1* locus and displays a phenotype consistent with alterations in B-cell function (increased amounts of antichromatin antibody, high levels of IgM and IgG, and increased B7-2 expression on the surface of B cells). In contrast, *Sle1a* displays features of late T-cell activation (decreased CD62L, increased CD44) with a significant reduction in T-cell numbers (both $CD4^+$ and $CD8^+$ subsets). The phenotype attributable to *Sle1c* was more subtle and did not show any significant differences in IgM or IgG production in response to antigen challenge or specificity to any chromatin component. To determine if *Sle1a*, *-b*, *-c*, or combinations thereof were sufficient to induce proliferative glomerulonephritis, congenic mice were crossed with NZW mice (Morel et al., 2001). Glomerulonephritis was seen only in NZW mice crossed to a congenic strain containing the *Sle1b* locus with an additional NZM2410-derived region extending about 5 cM telomeric. These results suggest the presence of a fourth locus (*Sle1d*) affecting end-organ susceptibility to autoimmune damage. Genetic dissection of the NZM model by Morel and co-workers together with ongoing mapping studies in other spontaneous mouse models of SLE (BXSB, MRL/lpr) is rapidly moving into the gene-identification phase.

BXSB Mice

BXSB mice develop an SLE-like disease characterized by polyclonal B-cell expansion and autoantibody production and leading to glomerulonephritis and mild lymphadenopathy. An unusual feature of this model is that males are preferentially affected. Male mice develop a severe form of SLE that leads to 50% mortality by 6 to 8 months of age compared to females with 50% mortality at 20 months. The rapid onset of disease in males is attributed to a Y chromosome gene, *Yaa* (Y-accelerator autoimmune) (Murphy and Roths, 1979), which has yet to be cloned and characterized. *Yaa* does not accelerate SLE-like disease in the absence of the BXSB background (Hudgins et al., 1985; Izui et al., 1988), indicating a role for background genes in BXSB animals. In a genome-wide linkage analysis in BXSB mice, SLE susceptibility intervals were identified on chromosomes 1, 3, 4, and 10 (Hogarth et al., 1998). Some degree of overlap was seen with the NZB/W mouse model, with three intervals on chromosome 1 and one interval on chromosome 4 mapping in the region of *Sle1* and *Sle2*, respectively. The other two intervals on chromosome 1 and the intervals on chromosomes 3 and 10 appear to be unique to the BXSB strain.

MRL-lpr/lpr Mice

MRL mice develop a mild autoimmune syndrome late in life. The spontaneous mutation *lpr* (lymphoproliferation), a mutation in the *Fas* death receptor gene, accelerates the underlying autoimmune phenotype of the MRL strain. MRL *lpr/lpr* mice exhibit marked proliferations of $CD4^-$ $CD8^-$ (double negative) T cells and nonclonal rearrangements of the T-cell receptor genes (Cohen and Eisenberg, 1991). Full expression of this lupus-like disease is dependent on contributions from other non-MHC genes. Backcross mapping experiments have demonstrated two loci, one on the proximal arm of chromosome 7 and the other on chromosome 12, that do not appear to overlap with the loci identified from linkage analysis of other murine lupus models and are probably unique to this strain (Watson et al., 1992). A more recent genome-wide linkage study of MRL-Fas^{lpr} × C57BL/6-Fas^{lpr} F2 intercross mice identified regions on chromosomes 4, 5, 7, and 10 with significant linkage to lymphadenopathy and/or splenomegaly (Vidal et al., 1998). The intervals on chromosomes 4, 5, and 7 were also linked to the production of anti-dsDNA antibodies, while the chromosome 10 interval was associated with glomerulonephritis. The role of Fas and the Fas ligand (FasL) in autoimmune disease is under intense investigation and has been the subject of recent reviews (Cohen and Eisenberg, 1991; Nagata and Golstein, 1995; Abbas, 1996; Elkon and Marshak-Rothstein, 1996). The accelerated autoimmune phenotype in Fas- or FasL-deficient mice highlights the important role for these molecules in eliminating self-reactive lymphocytes and maintaining peripheral T-cell tolerance (Herron et al., 1993; Singer and Abbas, 1994).

Collectively, the data derived from the study of murine models of SLE have advanced our appreciation for the polygenic complexity of this disease. Genetic dissection of the relative contributions from several individual susceptibility loci through the use of congenic mice promises to enhance our understanding of how these genes interact to produce the SLE phenotype. It remains to be seen how the genetic information derived from these murine models will correlate with human SLE.

Knockout and Transgenic Mouse Models

Several transgenic and knockout mouse models have identified molecular pathways that when disrupted result in a lupus-like phenotype (Table 31–6). Genes that control immune cell apoptosis (*Fas*, *FasL*, *bcl-2*) (Strasser et al., 1991; Nagata and Suda, 1995), molecules that negatively regulate antigen receptor signaling in B and T cells (SHP-1, Lyn, CD22) (Cornall et al., 1998), components of the innate immune system involved in clearance of self-antigens from the circulation (C1q, C3, C4, Dnase-1, Sap, the Fc receptors) (Botto et al., 1998; Carroll, 1998; Clynes et al., 1998; Bickerstaff et al., 1999; Ehrenstein et al., 2000; Napirei et al., 2000), and certain cytokines [interleukin-2 (IL-2)] (Horak et al., 1995) each have the potential to contribute to an SLE phenotype in the mouse.

Mice deficient in serum amyloid P-component (Sap) or Dnase-I also develop a lupus-like phenotype, perhaps by a similar mechanism (Bickerstaff et al., 1999; Napirei et al., 2000). It has been hypothesized that the binding of Sap to chromatin may prevent its recognition by antigen receptors. In the absence of Sap, immunologic responses to chromatin may result. Similarly, Dnase-I removes soluble or deposited autoantigenic nucleoprotein complexes from the circulation, and its absence results in decreased clearance of DNA from serum. Together, these mouse models demonstrate that efficient removal of potential autoantigens is critical for the maintenance of self-tolerance. In human SLE, a truncating mutation in Dnase-I has been described in two Japanese patients with early-onset disease (Yasutomo et al., 2001). These patients had higher levels of anti-dsDNA and antinucleosomal antibodies compared to other SLE patients or normal control individuals. The exact contribution to the SLE phenotype derived from the Dnase-I mutation has yet to be defined, and confirmatory studies in other SLE cohorts are needed.

Perturbation of the intricate balance by which the immune system regulates the activation of lymphocytes and the deletion of self-reactive clones is another pathway that can lead to systemic autoimmunity. For example, deficiency of any one of several molecules that attenuate lymphocyte activation, such as Lyn, SHP-1, CD22, and PD-1, leads to a lupus-like disease (Cornall et al., 1998; Nishimura et al., 1999). Conversely, a gain-of-function point mutation in CD45 (E613R) leads to an SLE phenotype via constitutive lymphocyte activation (Majeti et al., 2000). Mice exhibiting Fas/FasL deficiency, heterozygous deficiency of the phosphatase and tensin homolog (*Pten*) tumor-supressor gene, or deficiency of the cell-cycle inhibitor p21 develop SLE-like disease through the inability to remove autoreactive lymphoctyes (Fas/FasL deficiency) (Nagata and Suda, 1995) or the uncontrolled expansion and inhibition of lymphocyte apoptosis (*Pten* heterozygous deficiency and *p21* deficiency) (Di Cristofano et al., 1999; Balomenos et al., 2000). These induced mutant mice will likely provide important clues to the identity of relevant genes in humans.

Candidate Genes in Human SLE

Currently, several candidate genes in human SLE have been described (Table 31–6).

Fcγ Receptors

There are three families of Fcγ receptors, FcγRI (CD64), FcγRII (CD32), and FcγRIII (CD16), encoded by eight distinct genes clustered on chromosome 1 at cytogenetic position 1q23. These receptors differ in their affinity for IgG, their cellular distribution, and the intracellular signaling pathways engaged following receptor cross-linking. Of interest, there is functionally significant allelic variation for several of these genes (Ravetch and Kinet, 1991; Kimberly et al., 1995; Daeron, 1997).

FcγRII is the most widely expressed of the Fc receptors and binds IgG with low affinity, interacting only with IgG in immune complexes. Three isotypes of FcγRII are encoded by three distinct genes (*FcγRIIA*, *-B*, and *-C*), which differ predominantly in their cytoplasmic tails (Salmon, 1997). Of the *FcγRII* genes, the most compelling evidence for a role in SLE exists for *FcγRIIA* (*FcγRIIA* gene, FcγRIIa protein). Two co-dominantly expressed allelic forms of FcγRIIa have been identified, which change two amino acid residues in the extracellular domain of the molecule (Rascu et al., 1997). The first polymorphism is a glutamine vs. tryptophan residue at amino acid 27 in extracellular domain 1. The second polymorphism is an arginine (R) vs. histidine (H) residue at amino acid 131 in extracellular domain 2. Only the polymorphism at position 131 appears to hold significant functional consequences by altering the affinity of the receptor to bind IgG2. The H131 (wild-type) allele is the only Fc receptor that efficiently binds IgG2 in humans. FcγRIIa-expressing phagocytes with the R131 allele have a reduced ability to bind and internalize polyclonal IgG-opsonized erythrocytes (Salmon et al., 1992). This observation also predicts differential handling of IgG2-coated ICs in vivo based on the FcγRIIa genotype. In support of this hypothesis, association studies have documented that a greater proportion African-American SLE patients are heterozygous or homozygous for the low-binding FcγRIIa-R131 allele (Salmon et al., 1996). The FcγRIIa-R131 allele was observed further when the data were stratified for African-Americans with lupus nephritis. This observation may explain, at least in part, the increased incidence and severity of SLE in African-Americans. A similar enrichment for the FcγRIIa-R131 allele was described in Korean SLE patients when compared to non-SLE controls (Song et al., 1998). However, this association was not demonstrated in Caucasian, Afro-Caribbean, and Chinese SLE populations sampled in the United Kingdom (Botto et al., 1996), suggesting that the distribution of FcγRIIa alleles may be subject to significant population and ethnic variability. A more recently identified polymorphism (lysine for glu-

Table 31–6. Candidate Genes and Pathways Implicated in Systemic Lupus Erythematosus (SLE)

Proposed Mechanism	Murine SLE	Human SLE
Antigen–immune complex clearance	C1q knockout (Botto et al., 1996) C3, C4 knockout (Carroll, 1998) Sap[a] knockout (Bickerstaff et al., 1999) Dnase-1 knockout (Napirei et al., 2000) Serum IgM knockout (Ehrenstein et al., 2000) Fcγ common chain knockout (Clynes et al., 1998)	C1q (Slingsby et al., 1996) C2, C3, C4 (Arnett, 1997) Mannose binding protein (Davies et al., 1995; Ip et al., 1998; Sullivan et al., 1996) FcγRIIA (Salmon et al., 1996) FcγRIIIA (Wu et al., 1997) Dnase I (Yasutomo et al., 2001)
Lymphoid signaling	SHP-1 knockout (Cornall et al., 1998) Lyn knockout (Cornall et al., 1998) Lyn/Fyn double knockout (Yu et al., 2001) CD22 knockout (Cornall et al., 1998) BlyS transgenic (Khare et al., 2000) PD-1 knockout (Nishimura et al., 1999) IL-2 knockout (Horak et al., 1995) CD45 E613R point mutation (Majeti et al., 2000)	T-cell receptor ζ chain (Liossis et al., 1998; Vassilopoulos et al., 1995) TNF-α (Fugger et al., 1989; Sullivan et al., 1997) IL-10 (Llorente et al., 1995, 1997; Mehrian et al., 1998)
Apoptosis	Fas knockout (Nagata and Suda, 1995) Fas-L knockout (Nagata and Suda, 1995) Bcl-2 transgenic (Strasser et al., 1991) Pten[b] heterozygous deficiency (Di Cristofano et al., 1999) p21 cyclin-dependent kinase knockout (Balomenos et al., 2000)	
Epitope modification	α-Mannosidase II knockout (Chui et al., 2001)	

[a]Serum amyloid P-component.
[b]Phosphatase and tensin homolog.

tamine at position 127) of FcγRIIa has been shown to abrogate the phagocytic defect of a patient homozygous for the low-binding R131 allele (Norris et al., 1998).

The FcγRIII receptor is encoded by two highly related genes (*FcγRIIIA* and *FcγRIIIB*). The major structural difference in the proteins is that FcγRIIIa is a conventional transmembrane protein while FcγRIIIb is anchored to the external cell membrane by a glycosyl-phosphatidylinositol moiety. FcγRIIIa is expressed on the surface of macrophages and natural killer cells and interacts with members of the CD3 family of proteins (CD3γ, ζ, η) to transmit extracellular signals to the intracellular compartment (Ravetch and Kinet, 1991; Kimberly et al., 1995; Rascu et al., 1997). FcγRIIIb is the major Fc receptor expressed on the surface of neutrophils. Both FcγRIIIa and FcγRIIIb bind preferentially to IgG1 and IgG3 subclasses. Allelic polymorphisms in FcγRIIIb impart neutrophilic phagocytic defects and may predispose to renal dysfunction in patients with Wegener's granulomatosis (Wainstein et al., 1996), but to date, no associations with SLE have been demonstrated. In contrast, of the multiple polymorphisms described in FcγRIIIa, an F-to-V substitution at amino acid position 176, a portion of the molecule involved in ligand binding, may be important for the pathophysiology of SLE. Functionally, this polymorphism enhances natural killer cell activation in response to IgG1 or IgG3 ligand binding and leads to increases in intracellular calcium concentrations and a more rapid induction of apoptosis following stimulation (Wu et al., 1997). One prediction is that individuals carrying F/F or V/F genotypes might have impaired handling of IgG1- or IgG3-bearing ICs compared with F/F individuals. In support of this, an association study of 200 ethnically diverse SLE patients demonstrated a higher proportion of individuals with SLE with the FcγRIIIa-F/F176 and FcγRIII-F/V176 alleles and an underrepresentation of the V/V176 genotype in SLE patients with nephritis (Wu et al., 1997).

A persuasive example of the importance of Fcγ receptors in SLE has been demonstrated in the NZB/W model for lupus. All of the Fc receptors share a common polypeptide chain, termed the *common γ chain*, which serves a critical structural role for the molecule. NZB/W F_1 lupus-prone mice lacking the Fc common γ chain (by genetic knockout) produce ICs that deposit in tissues and activate complement similar to control NZB/W mice (Clynes et al., 1998). However, animals deficient in the Fc common γ chain were protected from the severe nephritis observed in this model, indicating a direct role for Fcγ receptors in mediating inflammation in response to IC deposition.

Complement

The complement system consists of approximately 20 plasma proteins that mediate inflammatory responses to ICs and assist in the clearance of various infectious microbes (Schur, 1997). For many years, a strong relationship has been noted between deficiencies of early classical pathway complement components (C1q, C2, and C4) and the development of SLE (reviewed by Schur, 1997; Carroll, 1998). Homozygous C1q deficiency is an extremely rare disorder, with only 32 individuals described in the literature. Of these, 30 had SLE, one had discoid lupus, and one was healthy (Topaloglu et al., 1996; Slingsby et al., 1996). C1q-deficient patients suffer from a particularly severe form of SLE with severe glomerulonephritis and skin manifestations, beginning in the first or second decade of life (Bowness et al., 1994).

Deficiencies of C2 and C4 also predispose individuals to SLE (reviewed by Schur, 1997). The genes for both of these complement proteins are located on human chromosome 6 in the MHC region. Complete C2 or C4 deficiencies are rare (1/10,000 for C2, <1/10,000 for C4) and generally associated with a mild form of lupus, often with only skin and joint involvement (Agnello, 1978; Arnett and Reveille, 1992). Documenting deficiencies in the C4 genes is complicated by the fact that there are two isotypes of C4, C4A and C4B. Each C4 isotype has numerous allelic variants, and null alleles for each have also been identified. C4A null alleles are usually transmitted as part of the extended haplotype HLA-B8, DR3 in Caucasian populations (Schur et al., 1990), and association studies suggest that C4A *null/null* individuals are predisposed to mild SLE in most, but not all, populations.

We currently do not understand how these complement deficiencies lead to SLE. However, two studies using mice deficient in various complement components appear to provide some insights. In the first study, mice deficient in C1q were generated using targeted gene disruption. Homozygous C1q-deficient ($C1q^{-/-}$) animals developed autoantibodies and glomerulonephritis on a mixed C57BL/6 and 129/Ola genetic background (Botto et al., 1998). Histologic examination of glomeruli from $C1q^{-/-}$ mice revealed increased numbers of apoptotic cells in the kidneys compared to control animals. Membrane blebs on the surface of apoptotic cells are a particularly rich source of the various autoantigens that are targeted in patients with SLE (Casciola-Rosen et al., 1994, 1996). The autoantigens within blebs are often altered by intracellular proteases (Casciola-Rosen et al., 1995) or kinases (Utz et al., 1997) in such a way that cryptic immunologic epitopes may be revealed to immune effector cells, allowing tolerance to be broken (Rosen and Casciola-Rosen, 1999). C1q binds to apoptotic cells (Casciola-Rosen et al., 1994) and may assist in the efficient removal of autoantigen-rich apoptotic cells. In the absence of C1q, the load of autoantigen from apoptotic cells may exceed the threshold needed to maintain immunologic tolerance. In a second study, mice deficient for either C4 or the CD21/35 complement receptor showed reduced evidence of central B-cell tolerance (Prodeus et al., 1998). In the setting of either genetic deficiency, B cells could not be rendered fully anergic. In addition, accelerated autoimmunity was observed in mice doubly deficient in C4 or CD21 and the apoptotic death receptor Fas compared with animals deficient in Fas alone. These provocative data do not precisely define how complement deficiencies impair immunologic tolerance of B lymphocytes, but one possibility is that complement may be important for concentrating self-antigen in the bone marrow during the development of B cells. Humans deficient in these complement components, in turn, may possess a B-cell repertoire that has not been sufficiently purged of self-reactive cells.

CD3ζ Chain

The T-cell receptor (TCR) is a multisubunit complex consisting of antigen-specific TCRα and β chains, noncovalently associated with the invariant CD3ε, γ, δ, and ζ chains. The CD3ζ protein exists either as ζ-ζ homodimers or as ζ-η or ζ-FcγR heterodimers. The intracellular domain of CD3ζ contains sequence motifs critical for signaling through the intact TCR (Weiss and Littman, 1994). Interest in the function of the TCR in lupus lymphocytes and its role in the expression of SLE arose from observations that fresh T cells from patients with SLE displayed exaggerated elevation in intracellular calcium concentrations in response to cross-linking of the TCR–CD3 complex (Vassilopoulos et al., 1995). To determine whether this reflected an intrinsic TCR signaling defect in SLE, Liossis et al. (1998) investigated the pattern of protein tyrosine phosphorylation in patients with SLE compared to patients with other autoimmune disorders and normal controls. Following TCR ligation, tyrosine phosphorylation of intracellular proteins with a molecular weight between 36 and 64 kDa was increased in SLE patients compared to controls (Liossis et al., 1998). Interestingly, in 10 of 22 SLE patients, significant levels of CD3ζ protein could not be demonstrated by Western blot. The authors postulated that increased TCR-initiated calcium responses, increased TCR-induced protein tyrosine phosphorylation, and deficient CD3ζ expression may represent intrinsic defects which modulate T-cell function in lupus. However, there is no convincing evidence for genetic defects in CD3ζ, suggesting that this is a secondary phenomenon.

HLA

The association of particular human leukocyte antigen (HLA) alleles with human SLE has been documented (Schur, 1995; Arnett, 1997). In humans, the HLA region is located on the short arm of chromosome 6 and spans approximately 4 cM of DNA (Trowsdale, 1993). It has been subdivided into three functionally distinct regions: class I, class II, and class III. HLA class I genes include the *HLA-A*, *-B*, and *-C* loci (see Chapter 29). They encode glycoprotein molecules noncovalently bound to β_2-microglobulin and are expressed on the surface of all cell types. The HLA class II region includes genes that encode for a series of structurally similar α and β heterodimers and HLA-DR, -DQ, and -DP molecules. These are expressed on the surface of antigen-presenting cells, in particular macrophages/monocytes, B lymphocytes, and activated T lymphocytes. Genes mapped to the class III region include the *TAP1* and *TAP2* transporters, the class II transporters HLA-DMA and -DMB, and the proteasome genes (*LMP2* and *LMP7*) important in the intracellular processing of antigenic peptides. The MHC class III region also contains the early complement components C4, C2, and factor B, TNF-α, and TNF-β, heat-shock protein 70, and many other genes (Arnett, 1997).

In Caucasian SLE populations, associations with the disease have most often been documented with HLA-DR2, HLA-DR3, or both; and these alleles confer an overall relative risk for SLE of 2 to 3 (Schur, 1995; Arnett, 1997). Despite the higher incidence and severity of SLE in African-Americans, HLA class II associations with SLE in African-American populations are not very convincing or consistent (reviewed by Schur, 1995; Arnett, 1997).

Class II molecules, and especially HLA-DQ alleles, are more strongly associated with autoantibodies found in SLE than with the disease itself or individual clinical manifestations. Anti-Ro and anti-La autoantibodies are associated with HLA-DR2 or HLA-DR3 (Bell and Maddison, 1980; Arnett et al., 1989; Hartung et al., 1992). This effect may derive from heterozygosity at the DQ locus, which is in strong linkage disequilibrium with DR3 and DR2 (Hamilton et al., 1988; Harley et al., 1989; Reveille et al., 1991). Sequencing of the DQ α and β chains in a cohort of 106 patients with SLE or Sjögren's syndrome demonstrated a glutamine residue at position 34 of the α chain and a leucine residue at position 26 of the β chain, suggesting that these amino acids may be important for the anti-Ro response (Reveille et al., 1991). These polymorphisms were demonstrated in both Caucasian and African-American populations (Reveille et al., 1991). This finding was confirmed in an independent cohort of SLE patients, with the anti-Ro response being most prevalent when all four DQ alleles contained these residues (Scofield and Harley, 1994).

Anti-dsDNA antibodies, found in half of all SLE patients and very specific for SLE, are associated with DR2, DR3, DR7, and three alleles of DQB1 (Griffing et al., 1980; Ahearn et al., 1982; Schur et al., 1982; Khanduja et al., 1991; Olsen et al., 1992). HLA-DQ alleles showing the strongest association with anti-dsDNA were HLA-DQB1*0201, which is in linkage disequilibrium with DR3 and DR7; DQB1*0602, which is in linkage disequilibrium with DR2 and DR3; and DQB1*0302. These alleles were found in 96% of patients with high-level anti-dsDNA antibody production but showed no correlation with the presence of glomerulonephritis in these patients (Khanduja et al., 1991).

Antispliceosome antibodies (most often anti-U1 RNP and Sm) occur frequently in patients with SLE and other autoimmune diseases, and African-Americans are more likely to express these antibodies than Caucasians (Arnett et al., 1988). In a study comparing 49 SLE patients with either anti-RNP alone or anti-Sm alone to 139 race-matched normal controls and 59 race-matched SLE patients without anti-RNP and anti-Sm antibodies, an association with HLA-DR2 and -DR4 was made (Olsen et al., 1993). In African-American patients with anti-Sm, there were increased frequencies of HLA-DQ6 alleles (DQA1*0102 and DQB1*0602, in linkage disequilibrium with certain HLA-DR2 haplotypes) compared to normal African-American controls. In African-Americans with anti-RNP alone, significant increases in HLA-DQ5 alleles, DQA1*0101 and DQB1*0501, were demonstrated in comparison to African-American SLE patients without anti-RNP or Sm antibodies. In Caucasian patients with anti-RNP alone, allelic association was demonstrated for the DQ8-associated allele DQB1*0302 compared with normal controls as well as an increased frequency of the DQ5-associated alleles DQA1*0101 and DQB1*0501 compared with lupus patients without anti-Sm or RNP (Olsen et al., 1993). Other studies have been less conclusive, showing no HLA correlations with Sm or nRNP (Bell and Maddison, 1980; Ahearn et al., 1982) or even a negative correlation with HLA-DQ1/DQ2 heterozygosity (Hamilton et al., 1988). Taken together, data examining the correlations between HLA class II alleles and anti-Ro/La, anti-dsDNA, anti-RNP and Sm antibodies suggest that the primary influence of class II genes is at the level of autoantibody formation and specificity.

Genes mapping to the MHC class III which show associations with SLE include *TNF-α* (Jacob et al., 1990; Sturfelt et al., 1996; Rudwaleit et al., 1996; D'Alfonso et al., 1996; Sullivan et al., 1997; Hajeer et al., 1997), the transporters associated with antigen processing *TAP1* and *TAP2* genes (Takeuchi et al., 1996; Ocal et al., 1996), and the heat-shock protein gene *HSP70-2* (Pablos et al., 1995; Jarjour et al., 1996). Establishing clear-cut associations with SLE for any of these candidate genes has been difficult due to extensive linkage disequilibrium across the HLA region.

TNF

TNF-α belongs to a cytokine superfamily which includes FASL. TNF-α possesses paradoxical immunomodulatory effects that both promote and protect from autoimmunity (Vassalli, 1992; reviewed by Cope, 1998). In (NZB $\times$ NZW)F_1 SLE mice, a restriction fragment length polymorphism (RFLP) of TNF-α (NZW-derived) correlates with decreased TNF-α production (Jacob and McDevitt, 1988). Exogenous TNF-α infusions into F_1 mice significantly delayed the onset of fatal nephritis in this model. In humans, decreased but inducible TNF-α production was observed in SLE patients carrying the HLA-DR2/Dqw1 haplotype (Jacob et al., 1990). An RFLP corresponding to a 5.5 kb

NcoI fragment of the *TNF-α* gene was associated with SLE in Caucasian patients (Fugger et al., 1989). This RFLP is in linkage disequilibrium with HLA-B8/DR3 haplotypes, and clear associations due to an isolated effect from TNF-α could not be distinguished. In African-American SLE patients, a biallelic polymorphism in the TNF-α promoter region was found at higher frequency, independent of HLA-DR alleles, compared to matched controls (Sullivan et al., 1997). A relationship between these polymorphisms and levels of TNF-α expression remains to be established.

Interleukin 10

IL-10 is a potent activator of B lymphocytes, inducing both proliferation and antibody production in vitro (Moore et al., 1993), an observation which has led to studies of the role of IL-10 in SLE (Eskdale et al., 1997; Llorente et al., 1997; Lazarus et al., 1997; Mehrian et al., 1998; Mok et al., 1998). At the cellular level, IL-10 may have a role in promoting B-cell hyperactivity and autoantibody production in SLE (Llorente et al., 1995). Serum IL-10 levels are higher in patients with SLE, rheumatoid arthritis, and Sjögren's sydrome compared to controls (Llorente et al., 1994); however, IL-10 levels are elevated in both affected and unaffected members of lupus-prone families (Llorente et al., 1997). Promoter polymorphisms in the IL-10 gene have been associated with SLE in some studies (Eskdale et al., 1997) but not others (Lazarus et al., 1997; Mok et al., 1998). Also, a possible interaction between the IL-10 and *bcl*-2 loci in SLE has been suggested (Mehrian et al., 1998).

Mannose Binding Protein

Mannose binding protein (MBP) is an opsinin, binding directly to the surface of bacteria and activating complement by both the alternative and classical pathways (Kiwasaki et al., 1983; Ikeda et al., 1987; Schweinle et al., 1989). Three studies in separate racial groups have shown marginally significant associations of SLE with a polymorphism of MBP, aspartic acid at amino acid position 54 (Davies et al., 1995; Sullivan et al., 1996; Ip et al., 1998). In studies of African-American, Spanish, and Chinese SLE patients, MBP alleles that result in lower serum levels were associated with a modestly increased risk for lupus (Davies et al., 1995; Sullivan et al., 1996; Ip et al., 1998).

Linkage Studies in Human SLE

Linkage studies in human SLE include a candidate interval study focused on the long arm of chromosome 1 and, more recently, genome-wide screens. The candidate interval study examined 52 affected sib pairs from 42 racially diverse families (Tsao et al., 1997b). Linkage analysis was focused on the 1q31–q42 region, initially thought to be syntenic to the *Sle1/Nba2* susceptibility locus on mouse chromosome 1 (Morel et al., 1994; Vyse et al., 1997). Seven microsatellite markers spanning approximately 27 cM were screened. Evidence for excess allele sharing ($p > 0.05$) was found for five of the markers, D1S245, D1S229, D1S213, D1S225, and D1S103, in the region of 1q41–42. Furthermore, tentative evidence for linkage to antichromatin antibody production was also shown for the five markers ($p = 0.04$–0.12). The interval studied was subsequently determined to map 5 to 10 cM telomeric to the murine syntenic interval containing Nba2 and Sle1. Tsao and colleagues (1997a) then added 25 additional sib pairs to the original cohort for a total of 77 and performed nonparametric multipoint linkage anaylsis using 15 microsatellite markers encompassing the 15 cM susceptibility region identified in the initial study. These analyses identified a peak with a LOD score of 3.3 and narrowed the region of interest to approximately 5 cM between markers D1S2860 and D1S213. Excess allele sharing was demonstrated in all racial groups (mean allele sharing 0.71 in Asian, 0.62 in Hispanic, 0.61 in African-American, and 0.60 in Caucasian SLE sib pairs). The poly(ADP-ribosyl) transferase (PARP) gene lies within this putative susceptibility interval and was initially suggested to be the relevant candidate gene in the region (Tsao et al., 1998, 1999) due to preferential transmission of one of the *PARP* alleles to affected SLE offspring by transmission-disequilibrium testing (Spielman et al., 1993) ($p = 0.0002$) (Tsao et al., 1999). *PARP*, however, is probably not the relevant SLE gene at 1q42 as significant transmission distortion of implicated *PARP* alleles has not been reproduced in other family collections (Criswell et al., 2000; Boorboor et al., 2000).

Because of the compelling evidence emerging from congenic mouse models and the candidate interval study results discussed above, the region at 1q41–42 has been the focus of intense study. Indeed, this interval has demonstrated at least some evidence for linkage in nearly all studies reported to date. A group in Oklahoma provided the initial evidence that the susceptibility locus in this region might be centromeric of *PARP*. As part of their genome-wide screen, Moser et al. (1998) described a strong effect on chromosome 1 in the 1q41 region, with a maximized LOD score of 3.50 using a dominant model for marker D1S3462. Fine-mapping of this interval with 33 additional multiplex families and nine additional markers subdivided the linkage effect in this region based on ethnicity. African-American pedigrees demonstrated the best LOD score at marker D1S3462 (LOD = 3.03), while the best evidence for linkage in European-American families was found at marker D1S229 (LOD = 1.46) approximately 15 cM centromeric to D1S3462 (Moser et al., 1999). This finding has been confirmed by a group in Minnesota who demonstrated evidence for transmission disequilibrium for both single marker alleles and short marker haplotypes from the 1q41–42 interval in their 210 SLE sib-pair family collection, 122 trio families, and the combined data set of 332 SLE families (Graham et al., 2001). In total, the data from these groups suggest that a human SLE susceptibility locus is located in a 2.3 Mb region centromeric to *PARP* near the D1S490 marker.

Genome-wide screens in SLE have been been reported by groups from Minnesota (Gaffney et al., 1998, 2000), Oklahoma (Gray-McGuire et al., 2000; Moser et al., 1998), California (Shai et al., 1999), and Sweden (Lindqvist et al., 2000). The overall designs of these studies were somewhat different and varied by ethnic composition, primary pedigree structure, and analytical approach (Table 31–7).

Using a threshold of LOD > 1.5, the Oklahoma group identified potential linkages on 1q23, 1q31, 13q32, and 20q13 in all pedigrees combined. When the data were stratified for race, additional loci at 1q41 and 11q14–23 were identified in African-American families and loci at 14q11, 4p15, 11q25, 2q32, 19q13, 6q26–27, and 12p12–11 were identified in European-American families. The highest LOD score was seen in the Fcγ receptor region at 1q23, 3.37 with 85% penetrance in females and 60% penetrance in males at $\theta = 0$ with no admixture ($\alpha = 1.0$). Allele-sharing methods were also used to investigate the effect at 1q23, and the greatest degree of sharing was found for the FcγRIIa marker ($p = 0.0003$), with the largest contribution from the African-American pedigrees. These data support the finding that the FcγRIIa molecule predisposes to lupus nephritis, especially in African-Americans (Salmon et al., 1996). The Okla-

Table 31–7. Key Characteristics of the Published Human Systemic Lupus Erythematosus (SLE) Genome Screens

Reference	Number of Families, Individuals, SLE Patients	Family Ethnicity	Primary Method of Analysis	Average Inter-marker Distance (cM)	Total No. Loci	No. Shared Loci	No. Unique Loci
Minnesota (Gaffney et al., 1998; Gaffney et al., 2000)	187 Families 656 Individuals 399 SLE Patients	148 Caucasian 17 African-American 13 Hispanic 9 Other	Non-parametric parametric multipoint linkage	8.9	18	10	8
Oklahoma (Gray-McGuire et al., 2000; Moser et al., 1998)	126 Families 744 Individuals 295 SLE Patients	40 African-American 77 Caucasian 9 Other	Model-based two-point linkage	10	16	7	9
California (Shai et al., 1999)	80 Families 434 Individuals 80 Families	43 Hispanic 37 Caucasian 188 SLE patients	Non-parametric multipoint linkage	12	11	7	4
Uppsala (Lindqvist et al., 2000)	17 Families 201 Individuals 44 SLE Patients	6 Icelandic 11 Swedish	Model-based two-point linkage	10	13	3	10

homa group described a second strong effect on chromosome 1 in the 1q41 region, with a maximized LOD score of 3.50 using a dominant model for marker D1S3462.

A more recent analysis from the Oklahoma group included 32 additional families, for a total of 126, and utilized two newly developed regression modeling approaches for sib pairs and affected relative pairs (Gray-McGuire et al., 2000). Significant evidence for linkage was found at 4p16–15.2 ($p = 0.0003$, LOD = 3.84). These results were confirmed using the same analytical approach to analyze identical markers in 187 independent pedigrees from the Minnesota collection. A locus–locus epistatic interaction was also identified between the 4p16–15.2 region and 5p15 in a subset of 77 European-American families from the Oklahoma data set. Three regions not previously identified in any published genome scan were identified (9q21–32, 12q24, and 17p11–q21), while 10 regions identified elsewhere were supported by this analysis.

In the screen from the California group, the three best intervals identified by nonparametric multipoint analyses were 1q44, 1q24, and 18q21 (Shai et al., 1999). When the data were stratified by ethnicity, the evidence for linkage at 1q44 was provided primarily from Mexican-American families, while the intervals at 1q24 and 18q21 were supported in both Mexican-American and Caucasian families. Significant scores were also obtained at 1p36, 1p21, 1q24, 6p22, 14q23, 16q13, 20p13, and 20q11.

To reduce the inherent heterogeneity present in previous genome scans, the Swedish group focused their efforts on presumably more homogeneous pedigrees from Iceland and Sweden (Lindqvist et al., 2000). Using model-based linkage methods and a nominal LOD cut-off of 2.0 and excluding two families not carrying C4 null alleles, four regions were identified in Icelandic families, 2q37 (LOD = 2.06), 4p15–13 (LOD = 3.20), 19p13 (LOD = 2.58), and 19q13 (LOD = 2.06). No evidence for linkage was found in the HLA region or on chromosome 1. In the Swedish families, one region with a LOD score greater than 2.0 was identified in the 2q37 region (LOD = 2.18) with the same marker as in the Icelandic families (D2S125). When these two data sets were combined, the evidence for linkage at marker D2S125 increased to LOD = 4.24.

The group from Minnesota used a threshold LOD score of ≥1.0 to define regions of potential interest in their genome screen and applied the criteria of Lander and Kruglyak (1995) to further define regions of significant ($Z \geq 4.1$, LOD ≥ 3.6, $p \leq 0.00002$) or suggestive ($Z \geq 3.2$, LOD ≥ 2.2, $p \leq 0.0007$) linkage. Overall, 25 of the 341 markers tested (7%) gave LOD scores >1.00. Two of these intervals contained a marker that met criteria for significant linkage: 6p11–p21, mapping near the HLA region (D6S257, LOD = 3.90), and 16q13 (D16S415, LOD = 3.64). Two other regions fulfilled criteria for suggestive linkage: 14q21–q23 (D14S276, LOD = 2.81) and 20p12 (D20S186, LOD = 2.62). Nine additional chromosomal regions were identified with LOD scores ≥1.00 at 2p15, 1p13, 1q42, 4q28, 3cent-q11, 11p15, 2q21–33, 15q26, and 1p36. Due to sample size considerations, the data were stratified by ethnic group only for the 84 Caucasian families in the overall sample of 105 families. LOD scores dropped in 10 of the top 13 potential susceptibility intervals when non-Caucasian families were eliminated from the analysis, suggesting that families of all ethnic groups contributed to the evidence for genetic linkage in these regions. In contrast, three intervals (4q28, 11p15, and 15q26) were characterized by an improvement in LOD scores when only Caucasian families were considered.

In further studies, data from a second cohort of 82 additional sib-pair families and combined analysis of the entire 187 sib-pair collection were reported by the Minnesota group (Gaffney et al., 2000). This second cohort demonstrated evidence of suggestive linkage (LOD > 2.2) on 7p22 (LOD = 2.87), 7q21 (LOD = 2.40), and 10p13 (LOD = 2.24). In the combined analysis, two intervals (6p11–p21 and 16q13) continued to meet the criteria for significant linkage (LOD >3.6). The region near HLA at 6p11–p21 (LOD = 4.19) demontrated the strongest evidence for linkage. This finding supports a large number of previous studies that have described an association between SLE and various HLA class II alleles. Dense mapping of the HLA region in the Minnesota family collection identified dominant haplotypes that show strong evidence for both linkage and association (unpublished data). The 16q13 (LOD = 3.85) region is notable because of its identification in other autoimmune diseases, including psoriasis (Nair et al., 1997), Crohn's disease (Hugot et al., 1996; Mirza et al., 1998; Curran et al., 1998; Hampe et al., 1999), Blau syndrome (Tromp et al., 1996), insulin-dependent diabetes mellitus (Davies et al., 1994), and asthma (Daniels et al., 1996). The recently identified *NOD2* gene polymorphisms in inflammatory bowel disease need to be examined in SLE (Ogura et al., 2001; Hugot et al., 2001). Nonrandom clustering of autoimmune loci has been reported for several autoimmune diseases (Becker

Table 31–8. Regions Demonstrating Significant[a] Linkage in Human Systemic Lupus Erythematosus (SLE)[b]

Locus	Minnesota	Oklahoma	USC[c]	Uppsala
1q22–23		3.45 (FcγRIIa)	1.51 (D1S484)	
1q41–44	1.92 (D1S235)	3.50 (D1S3462)	2.40 (D1S2785)	
2q37		1.53 (D2S1363)		4.24 (D2S125)
4p16	1.50 (D4S2366)	3.84 (D4S2366)		
6p11–22	4.19 (D6S426)	1.70 (D6S2439)		
16q12–13	3.85 (D16S415)			

[a]Recommended criteria for significant linkage in a genome-wide scan for a complex trait (LOD ≥ 3.3 for complex pedigrees, LOD ≥ 3.6 for sib pairs) (Lander and Kruglyak, 1995).
[b]Shown are LOD scores (marker) meeting criteria for each interval. Supporting evidence (LOD ≥ 1.5) from an independent family collection is also shown if present.
[c]Z-scores were converted to LOD scores by the equation LOD = $Z^2/2\ln 10$ (Kong and Cox, 1997).

et al., 1998), and it appears that some SLE loci overlap with intervals identified in other autoimmune diseases, suggesting shared genetic susceptibility.

Although there are significant differences between the reported mapping results in SLE, there is an encouraging level of agreement between studies. A summary of genomic intervals demonstrating significant linkage is shown in Table 31–8 and those demonstrating evidence of suggestive linkage confirmed by a second independent data set are shown in Table 31–9. The 18 intervals shown in Tables 31–8 and 31–9 appear at present to be the most promising susceptibility intervals for human SLE. The next major task will be to prioritize these intervals for further gene-identification efforts. Given the complex genetic basis of SLE, this task is not trivial and will require the efforts of multiple groups, combined family collections, and novel analytical approaches.

The first wave of gene-identification studies in human SLE support the hypothesis that multiple genes contribute to disease susceptibility. Clearly, there is no single locus operating in all families multiplex for SLE, and the degree of ethnic and genetic heterogeneity appears to be quite significant. In this respect, the genetics of SLE resembles that of many other complex genetic diseases. The list of candidate genes and pathways (Table 31–6) implicated in the pathogenesis of SLE is expanding at a rapid rate. Understanding how alterations in these genes and pathways lead to disease is the primary objective of future genetic studies in SLE.

CLINICAL APPLICATION AND RISK ASSESSMENT

As noted throughout this chapter, genetic studies of SLE are ongoing and hold the promise of improving our understanding of the pathophysiology of the autoimmune process and the genetic basis of susceptibility. Studies to date, however, have not provided specific information that can be used in the identification of susceptible individuals or the development of preventive strategies or tailored therapy. Genetic counseling can provide risk assessment based on population data and should be offered when appropriate.

Diagnosis

The diagnosis of SLE is based on the clinical and laboratory findings listed in Table 31–1. The ACR revised criteria do not include any aspect of family history and do not depend on the presence or absence of any of the genetic markers discussed in this chapter. At the present time, genetic testing for diagnostic purposes and genetic screening of potentially susceptible individuals are not indicated. Recessive inherited deficiencies of the early components of complement (C1q, C2, C4) may present as SLE-like syndromes (Schur, 1997; Carroll, 1998), and testing for the specific complement deficiency can be used to identify susceptible family members. These families are rare, however; and routine screening of relatives of a typical patient with SLE for a complement deficiency is not cost-effective and not warranted.

Table 31–9. Regions Demonstrating Suggestive[a] Linkage in Human Systemic Lupus Erythematosus (SLE)[b]

Locus	Minnesota	Oklahoma	USC[c]	Uppsala
1q31		2.04 (lamc1)		1.61 (D1S1660)
2q32–35	1.45 (D2S126)	2.09 (D2S1391)		
4p13–15	1.31 (D4S403)	2.18 (D4S403)		3.20 (D4S1627)
6q26–27		2.04 (D6S1027)		1.35 (D6S503)
9p24–21		2.08 (D9S925)		2.27 (gata62f03)
11q23		2.10 (D11S2002)		1.15 (D11S1998)
13q31–32	1.02 (D13S170)	2.50 (D13S779)		
14q11–23	2.81 (D14S276)			1.15 (D14S592)
15q26	1.07 (D15S127)			1.95 (D15S657)
19q13.1		2.05 (D19S246)		2.06 (D19S246)
20p12–13	2.62 (D20S186)		1.13 (D20S115)	
20q11–13	1.64 (D20S119)	2.49 (D20S481)		

[a]Recommended criteria for suggestive linkage in a genome-wide scan for a complex trait (LOD ≥ 1.9 for complex pedigrees, LOD ≥ 2.2 for sibpairs) (Lander and Kruglyak, 1995).
[b]Shown are LOD scores (marker) meeting criteria for each interval. Supporting evidence (LOD ≥ 1.5) from an independent family collection is also shown if present.
[c]Z-scores were converted to LOD scores by the equation LOD = $Z^2/2\ln 10$ (Kong and Cox, 1997).

Screening and Prevention

First-degree relatives (parents, sibs, children) of an individual with SLE have an increased risk of developing SLE, as shown in Tables 31–4 and 31–5, but the risk is only modest. The linkage studies described in this chapter have identified chromosomal regions that may contain the genes involved in the development and/or progression of disease; however, the individual genes have not been identified, and direct gene testing of unaffected family members is not available. Candidate genes such as TNF-α or IL-10 do not have SLE-specific changes that can be utilized for diagnosis or screening.

The association of SLE with HLA class II antigens suggests that HLA typing in appropriate families could be useful for screening susceptible relatives of an index case. As with most autoimmune diseases, however, the association between HLA and disease is not absolute and the majority of individuals with a disease-associated allele do not develop the disease. HLA typing can be very precise (particularly molecular typing), but the predictive value of the testing is not. The probable instigating environmental agent(s) is unknown, as are the modifying genes that segregate in a family. Siblings affected with SLE share HLA haplotypes more often than expected, yet finding a sibling with the same HLA type as the proband suggests only increased susceptibility and not the level of susceptibility or the course of action to prevent disease. HLA testing of family members is not used in a clinical setting, being reserved for research studies at this time.

It is not possible to develop prevention strategies for SLE. The environmental agent(s) is unknown, and the genetic control of susceptibility has not been elucidated. Identification of the genes in the chromosomal regions identified by linkage analysis and characterization of the molecular changes that produce susceptibility with each gene will be necessary before precise methods of prevention can be developed.

Counseling

First-degree relatives of an affected individual have a modest increase in risk for developing SLE. The studies detailed in Table 31–4 show an 8- to 10-fold increase in risk for family members compared to the risk in control families (Hochberg et al., 1985; Lawrence et al., 1987). The overall prevalence of SLE in Caucasian females is 40/100,000 (0.0004), as shown in Table 31–3. The risk for their first-degree relatives will be approximately 0.3% to 0.4%, or in the range of 1/25 to 1/300, with most of the risk for female relatives. This is a substantial increase in risk but the absolute risk is still low. The prevalence of SLE in African-American females is three- to fourfold higher than that of Caucasian females (Table 31–3), and the risk to first-degree relatives of African-American probands is greater than that of Caucasian probands (Hochberg et al., 1985). As a result, the risk to first-degree relatives of an African-American woman with SLE will be at least 1.3% to 1.6%, or in the range of 1/60 to 1/80, and again, this risk is greatest for female relatives. These values can be used to provide general genetic counseling when appropriate for first-degree relatives of an individual with SLE.

Pregnancy in a woman with SLE produces an increased risk of maternal and fetal complications (Mascola and Repke, 1997; Kitrodou, 1997; reviewed by Meng and Lockshin, 1999). The lupus may flare with pregnancy, although this does not occur with the majority of pregnant women. There is a 2.0- to 2.5-fold increase in the risk of fetal loss for a woman with lupus, both spontaneous abortion and intrauterine fetal death being more common (Julkunen et al., 1993; Hardy et al., 1999). Second trimester loss is common. Fetal complications include prematurity, intrauterine growth retardation, neonatal lupus, and the development of complete heart block (Watson et al., 1984; Julkunen et al., 1993). The presence of maternal antiphospholipid antibody, identified as lupus anticoagulant and anticardiolipin antibody, correlates with increased fetal loss, intrauterine growth retardation, and prematurity (Julkunen et al., 1993). Treatment of a woman during pregnancy to reduce the levels anticoagulant antibodies is controversial and not routine at this time. Plasmapheresis has been attempted in a limited number of cases, with mixed success (Kitrodou, 1997).

Neonatal lupus and fetal congenital heart block are related to the development of specific autoantibodies to ribonucleoproteins known as anti-SS-A/Ro (52 and 60 kDa) and anti-SS-B/La (48 kDa) (Brucato et al., 1995; Julkunen et al., 1995; Miyagawa et al., 1997; Buyon et al., 1998; Colombo et al., 1999; Siren et al., 1999a,b). These antibodies cross the placenta after the 16th week of gestation. Neonatal lupus is characterized by transient skin as well as hepatic and hematologic (thrombocytopenia) abnormalities, which clear without treatment. Development of complete heart block is irreversible and associated with high morbidity and mortality (Brucato et al., 1995; Buyon et al., 1998). Development of complete heart block is complex, however, and involves genetic regulation of the immune response as well as the presence of antibodies. For example, Caucasian and African-American women with lupus who have anti-Ro or anti-La antibodies are at increased risk of having a child with neonatal lupus if they are positive for HLA-B8, -DR3, and -DQ2 rather than other HLAs (Julkunen et al., 1995; Miyagawa et al., 1997; Colombo et al., 1999; Siren et al., 1999a,b). Furthermore, it is hypothesized that additional unknown factors are necessary as mothers with the antibody do not develop heart block and twins discordant for heart block have been reported (Julkunen et al., 1995; Miyagawa et al., 1997). The birth of a second child with complete heart block after the birth of the first affected child is not common (reported recurrence risk of 16% reported by Buyon et al., 1998) but does represent an important risk for the family. Prophylactic therapy of the mother to reduce antibody levels may be considered in this situation (Julkunen et al., 1995). Fetal monitoring is indicated for pregnant women known to have anti-SS-A/Ro antibody, and early delivery to facilitate fetal pacing may be indicated.

Therapy

Therapy for SLE involves the use of antiinflammatory drugs such as salicylates and non-steroidal antiinflammatory drugs, antimalarials, corticosteroids, and cytotoxic drugs. The method of treatment is dictated by the clinical presentation and course of disease, and genetic factors such as family history of SLE or presence of a particular HLA haplotype do not influence therapy. The only exception to this may be pregnant women who have had a child with complete heart block, as noted above. It is hoped that the elucidation of the genetic basis of susceptibility will provide tailored therapies, but that will await identification of the involved genes.

REFERENCES

Abbas AK: Die and let live: eliminating dangerous lymphocytes. Cell 1996; 84:655–657.

Agnello V: Complement deficiency states. Medicine (Baltimore) 1978; 57:1–23.

Ahearn JM, Provost TT, Dorsch CA, Stevens MB, Bias WB, Arnett FC: Interrelationships of HLA-DR, MB, and MT phenotypes, autoantibody expression, and clinical features in systemic lupus erythematosus. Arthritis Rheum 1982; 25:1031–1040.

Arnett FC: The genetics of human lupus. In: Wallace DJ, Hahn BH (eds). Dubois' Lupus Erythematosus. Baltimore: Williams and Wilkins, 1997:77–117.

Arnett FC, Hamilton RG, Reveille JD, Bias WB, Harley JB, Reichlin M: Genetic studies of Ro (SS-A) and La (SS-B) autoantibodies in families with systemic lupus erythematosus and primary Sjogren's syndrome. Arthritis Rheum 1989; 32:413–419.

Arnett FC, Hamilton RG, Roebber MG, Harley JB, Reichlin M: Increased frequency of Sm and nRNP autoantibodies in American blacks compared to whites with systemic lupus erythematosus. J Rheumatol 1988; 15:1773–1776.

Arnett FC, Reveille JD: Genetics of systemic lupus erythematosus. Rheum Dis Clin North Am 1992; 18:865–892.

Atkins C, Reuffel L, Roddy J, Platts M, Robinson H, Ward R: Rheumatic disease in the Nuu-Chah-Nulth native Indians of the Pacific Northwest. J Rheumatol 1988; 15:684–690.

Balomenos D, Martin-Caballero J, Garcia MI, Prieto I, Flores JM, Serrano M, Martinez AC: The cell cycle inhibitor p21 controls T-cell proliferation and sex-linked lupus development. Nat Med 2000; 6:171–176.

Becker KG, Simon RM, Bailey-Wilson JE, Freidlin B, Biddison WE, McFarland HF, Trent JM: Clustering of non-major histocompatibility complex susceptibility candidate loci in human autoimmune diseases. Proc Natl Acad Sci USA 1998; 95:9979–9984.

Bell DA, Maddison PJ: Serologic subsets in systemic lupus erythematosus: an examination of autoantibodies in relationship to clinical features of disease and HLA antigens. Arthritis Rheum 1980; 23:1268–1273.

Bickerstaff MC, Botto M, Hutchinson WL, Herbert J, Tennent GA, Bybee A, Mitchell DA, Cook HT, Butler PJ, Walport MJ, et al.: Serum amyloid P component controls chromatin degradation and prevents antinuclear autoimmunity. Nat Med 1999; 5:694–697.

Block SR, Winfield JB, Lockshin MD, D'Angelo WA, Christian CL. Studies of twins with systemic lupus erythematosus. A review of the literature and presentation of 12 additional sets. Am J Med; 59:533–552.

Boorboor P, Drescher BE, Hartung K, Sachse C, Tsao BP, Schneider PM, Kalden JR, Lakomek HJ, Peter HH, Schmidt RE, et al.: Poly(ADP-ribose) polymerase polymorphisms are not a genetic risk factor for systemic lupus erythematosus in German Caucasians. J Rheumatol 2000; 27:2061.

Botto M, Dell'Agnola C, Bygrave AE, Thompson EM, Cook HT, Petry F, Loos M, Pandolfi PP, Walport MJ: Homozygous C1q deficiency causes glomerulonephritis associated with multiple apoptotic bodies. Nat Genet 1998; 19:56–59.

Botto M, Theodoridis E, Thompson EM, Beynon HLC, Briggs D, Isenberg DA, Walport MJ, Davies KA: FcγRIIa polymorphism in systemic lupus erythematosus (SLE): no association with disease. Clin Exp Immunol 1996; 104:264–268.

Bowness P, Davies KA, Norsworthy PJ, Athanassiou P, Taylor-Wiedeman J, Borysiewicz LK, Meyer PAR, Walport MJ: Hereditary C1q deficiency and systemic lupus erythematosus. QJM 1994; 87:455–464.

Boyer GS, Templin DW, Lanier AP: Rheumatic diseases in Alaskan Indians of the southeast coast: high prevalence of rheumatoid arthritis and systemic lupus erythematosus. J Rheumatol 1991; 18:1477–1484.

Brucato A, Gasparini M, Vignati G, Riccobono S, De Juli E, Quinzanini M, Bortolon C, Coluccio E, Massari D: Isolated congenital complete heart block: longterm outcome of children and immunogenetic study. J Rheumatol 1995; 22:541–543.

Buyon JP, Hiebert R, Copel J, Craft J, Friedman D, Katholi M, Lee LA, Provost TT, Reichlin M, Rider L, et al.: Autoimmune-associated congenital heart block: demographics, mortality, morbidity and recurrence rates obtained from a national neonatal lupus registry. J Am Coll Cardiol 1998; 31:1658–1666.

Carroll MC: The role of complement and complement receptors in induction and regulation of immunity. Annu Rev Immunol 1998; 16:545–568.

Casciola-Rosen L, Rosen A, Petri M, Schlissel M: Surface blebs on apoptotic cells are sites of enhanced procoagulant activity: implications for coagulation events and antigenic spread in SLE. Proc Natl Acad Sci USA 1996; 93:1624–1629.

Casciola-Rosen LA, Anhalt G, Rosen A: Autoantigens targeted in systemic lupus erythematosus are clustered in two populations of surface structures on apoptotic keratinocytes. J Exp Med 1994; 179:1317–1330.

Casciola-Rosen LA, Anhalt G, Rosen A: DNA-dependent protein kinase is one of a subset of autoantigens specifically cleaved early during apoptosis. J Exp Med 1995; 182:1625–1634.

Chui D, Sellakumar G, Green R, Sutton-Smith M, McQuistan T, Marek K, Morris H, Dell A, Marth J: Genetic remodeling of protein glycosylation in vivo induces autoimmune disease. Proc Natl Acad Sci USA 2001; 98:1142–1147.

Clynes R, Dumitru C, Ravetch JV: Uncoupling of immune complex formation and kidney damage in autoimmune glomerulonephritis. Science 1998; 279:1052–1054.

Cohen PL, Eisenberg RA: Lpr and gld: single gene models of systemic autoimmunity and lymphoproliferative disease. Annu Rev Immunol 1991; 9:243–269.

Colombo G, Brucato A, Coluccio E, Compasso S, Luzzana C, Franceschini F, Quinzanini M, Scorza R: DNA typing of maternal HLA in congenital complete heart block: comparison with systemic lupus erythematosus and primary Sjogren's syndrome. Arthritis Rheum 1999; 42:1757–1764.

Cope AP: Regulation of autoimmunity by proinflammatory cytokines. Curr Opin Immunol 1998; 10:669–676.

Cornacoff JB, Hebert LA, Smead WL, Van Aman ME, Birmingham DJ, Waxman FJ: Primate erythrocyte-immune complex–clearing mechanism. J Clin Invest 1983; 71:236–247.

Cornall RJ, Cyster JG, Hibbs ML, Dunn AR, Otipoby KL, Clark EA, Goodnow CC: Polygenic autoimmune traits: Lyn, CD22, and SHP-1 are limiting elements of a biochemical pathway regulating BCR signaling and selection. Immunity 1998; 8:497–508.

Criswell LA, Moser KL, Gaffney PM, Inda S, Ortmann WA, Lin D, Chen JJ, Li H, Gray-McGuire C, Neas BR, et al.: PARP alleles and SLE: failure to confirm association with disease susceptibility. J Clin Invest 2000; 105:1501–1502.

Curran ME, Lau KF, Hampe J, Schreiber S, Bridger S, Macpherson AJ, Cardon LR, Sakul H, Harris TJ, Stokkers P, et al.: Genetic analysis of inflammatory bowel disease in a large European cohort supports linkage to chromosomes 12 and 16 [see comments]. Gastroenterology 1998; 115:1066–1071.

Daeron M: Fc receptor biology. Annu Rev Immunol 1997; 15:203–234.

D'Alfonso S, Colombo G, Della Bella S, Scorza R, Momigliano-Richiardi P: Association between polymorphisms in the TNF region and systemic lupus erythematosus in the Italian population. Tissue Antigens 1996; 47:551–555.

Daniels SE, Bhattacharrya S, James A, Leaves NI, Young A, Hill MR, Faux JA, Ryan GF, le Souef PN, Lathrop GM, et al.: A genome-wide search for quantitative trait loci underlying asthma. Nature 1996; 383:247–250.

Davies EJ, Snowden N, Hillarby MC, Carthy D, Grennan DM, Thomson W, Ollier WE: Mannose-binding protein gene polymorphism in systemic lupus erythematosus. Arthritis Rheum 1995; 38:110–114.

Davies JL, Kawaguchi Y, Bennett ST, Copeman JB, Cordell HJ, Pritchard LE, Reed PW, Gough SCL, Jenkins SC, Palmer SM, et al.: A genome-wide search for human type 1 diabetes susceptibility genes. Nature 1994; 371:130–136.

Deapen DM, Escalante A, Weinrib L, Horwitz DA, Mack TM: A revised estimate of twin concordance in systemic lupus erythematosus. Arthritis Rheum 1992; 35:311–318.

Di Cristofano A, Kotsi P, Peng YF, Cordon-Cardo C, Elkon KB, Pandolfi PP: Impaired Fas response and autoimmunity in Pten$^{+/-}$ mice. Science 1999; 285:2122–2125.

Drake CG, Rozzo SJ, Vyse TJ, Palmer E, Kotzin BL: Genetic contributions to lupus-like disease in (NZB × NZW)F_1 mice. Immunol Rev 1995; 144:51–74.

Ehrenstein MR, Cook HT, Neuberger MS: Deficiency in serum immunoglobulin (Ig)M predisposes to development of IgG autoantibodies. J Exp Med 2000; 191:1253–1258.

Elkon KB, Marshak-Rothstein A: B cells in systemic autoimmune disease: recent insights from Fas-deficient mice and men. Curr Opin Immunol 1996; 8:852–859.

Eskdale J, Wordsworth P, Bowman S, Field M, Gallagher G: Association between polymorphisms at the human IL-10 locus and systemic lupus erythematosus. Tissue Antigens 1997; 49:635–639.

Fessel WJ: Systemic lupus erythematosus in the community: incidence, prevalence, outcome, and first symptoms; the high prevalence in black women. Arch Intern Med 1974; 134:1027–1035.

Frank AO: Apparent predisposition to systemic lupus erythematosus in Chinese patients in West Malaysia. Ann Rheum Dis 1980; 39:266–269.

Fugger L, Morling N, Ryder LP, Georgsen J, Jakobsen BK, Svejgard A, Andersen V, Oxholm P, Pederson FK, Friis J, et al.: NcoI restriction fragment length polymorphism (RFLP) of the tumor necrosis factor (TNF-gamma) region in four autoimmune diseases. Tissue Antigens 1989; 34:17–22.

Gaffney PM, Kearns GM, Shark KB, Ortmann WA, Selby SA, Malmgren ML, Rohlf KE, Ockenden TC, Messner RP, King RA, et al.: A genome-wide search for susceptibility genes in human systemic lupus erythematosus sib-pair families. Proc Natl Acad Sci USA 1998; 95:14875–14879.

Gaffney PM, Ortmann WA, Selby SA, Shark KB, Ockenden TC, Rohlf KE, Walgrave NL, Boyum WP, Malmgren ML, Miller ME, et al.: Genome screening in human systemic lupus erythematosus: results from a second Minnesota cohort and combined analyses of 187 sib-pair families. Am J Hum Genet 2000; 66:547–556.

Gourley IS, Patterson CC, Bell AL: The prevalence of systemic lupus erythematosus in Northern Ireland. Lupus 1997; 6:399–403.

Graham RR, Langefeld CD, Gaffney PM, Ortmann WA, Selby SA, Baechler EC, Shark KB, Ockenden TC, Rohlf KE, Moser KL, et al.: Genetic linkage and transmission disequilibrium of marker haplotypes at chromosome 1q41 in human systemic lupus erythematosus. Arthritis Res; 3:299–305.

Gray-McGuire C, Moser KL, Gaffney PM, Kelly J, Yu H, Olson JM, Jedrey CM, Jacobs KB, Kimberly RP, Neas BR, et al.: Genome scan of human systemic lupus erythematosus by regression modeling: evidence of linkage and epistasis at 4p16–15.2. Am J Hum Genet 2000; 67:1460–1469.

Grennan DM, Parfitt A, Manolios N, Huang Q, Hyland V, Dunckley H, Doran T, Gatenby P, Badcock C: Family and twin studies in systemic lupus erythematosus. Dis Markers 1997; 13:93–98.

Griffing WL, Moore SB, Luthra HS, McKenna CH, Fathman CG: Associations of antibodies to native DNA with HLA-DRw3: a possible major histocompatibility linked human immune response gene. J Exp Med 1980; 152:319s-320s.

Gudmundsson S, Steinsson K: Systemic lupus erythematosus in Iceland 1975 through 1984. A nationwide epidemiological study in an unselected population. J Rheumatol 1990; 17:1162–1167.

Hajeer AH, Worthington J, Davies EJ, Hillarby MC, Poulton K, Ollier WER: TNF microsatellite a2, b3 and d2 alleles are associated with systemic lupus erythematosus. Tissue Antigens 1997; 49:222–227.

Hamilton RG, Harley JB, Bias WB, Roebber M, Reichlin M, Hochberg MC, Arnett FC: Two Ro (SS-A) autoantibody responses in systemic lupus erythematosus: correlation of HLA-DR/DQ specificities with quantitative expression of Ro (SS-A) autoantibody. Arthritis Rheum 1988; 31:496–505.

Hampe J, Schreiber S, Shaw SH, Lau KF, Bridger S, Macpherson AJ, Cardon LR, Sakul H, Harris TJ, Buckler A, et al.: A genomewide analysis provides evidence for novel linkages in inflammatory bowel disease in a large european cohort. Am J Hum Genet 1999; 64:808–816.

Hardy CJ, Palmer BP, Mortan SJ, Muir KR, Powell RJ: Pregnancy outcome and fam-

ily size in systemic lupus erythematosus: a case control study. Rheumatology (Oxf) 1999; 38:559–563.
Harley JB, Seslak AL, Willis LG, Fu SM, Hansen JA, Reichlin M: A model for disease heterogeneity in systemic lupus erythematosus. Arthritis Rheum 1989; 32:826.
Hart HH, Grigor RR, Caughey DE: Ethnic difference in the prevalence of systemic lupus erythematosus. Ann Rhuem Dis 1983; 42:529–532.
Hartung K, Ehrfeld H, Lakomek HJ, Coldewey R, Lang B, Krapf F, Muller R, Schendel D, Deicher H, Seelig HP, et al.: The genetic basis of Ro and La antibody formation in systemic lupus erythematosus. Rheumatol Int 1992; 11:243–249.
Hebert L: The clearance of immune complexes from the circulation of man and other primates. Am J Kidney Dis 1991; 17:352–361.
Helve T: Prevalence and mortality rates of systemic lupus erythematosus and caused of death in SLE patients in Finland. Scand J Rheumatol 1985; 14:43–46.
Herron LR, Eisenberg RA, Roper E, Kakkanaiah VN, Cohen PL, Kotzin BL: Selection of the T cell receptor repertoire in *lpr* mice. J Immunol 1993; 151:3450–3459.
Hirose S, Kinoshita K, Nozawa S, Nishimura H, Shirai T: Effects of major histocompatibility complex on autoimmune disease on H-2-congenic New Zealand mice. Int Immunol 1990; 2:1091–1095.
Hirose S, Ueda G, Noguchi K, Okada T, Sekigawa I, Sato H, Shirai T: Requirement of H-2 heterozygosity for autoimmunity in (NZB × NZW)F_1 hybrid mice. Eur J Immunol 1986; 16:1631–1633.
Hochberg MC: The application of genetic epidemiology to systemic lupus erythematosus. J Rheumatol 1987a; 14:867–869.
Hochberg MC: Prevalence of systemic lupus erythematosus in England and Wales, 1981–2. Ann Rheum Dis 1987b; 46:664–666.
Hochberg MC: Updating the American College of Rheumatology revised criteria for the classification of systemic lupus erythematosus. Arthritis Rheum 1997; 40:1725.
Hochberg MC, Flórsheim P, Scott J, Arnett FC: Familial aggregation of systemic lupus erythematosus [abstract]. Arthritis Rheum 1985; 28:523.
Hogarth MB, Slingsby JH, Allen PJ, Thompson EM, Chandler P, Davies KA, Simpson E, Morley BJ, Walport MJ: Multiple lupus susceptibility loci map to chromosome 1 in BXSB mice. J Immunol 1998; 161:2753–2761.
Hopkinson ND, Doherty M, Powell RJ: The prevalence and incidence of systemic lupus erythematosus in Nottingham, UK, 1989–1990. Br J Rheumatol 1993; 32:110–115.
Horak I, Lohler J, Ma A, Smith KA: Interleukin-2 deficient mice: a new model to study autoimmunity and self-tolerance. Immunol Rev 1995; 148:35–44.
Hudgins CC, Steinberg RT, Klinman DM, Reeves MJP, Steinberg AD: Studies of consomic mice bearing the Y chromosome of the BXSB mouse. J Immunol 1985; 134:3849.
Hugot J-P, Chamaillard M, Zouali H, Lesage S, Cezard J-P, Belaiche J, Almer S, Tysk C, O'Morain CA, Gassull M, et al.: Association of NOD2 leucine-rich repeat variants with susceptibility to Crohn's disease. Nature 2001; 411:599–603.
Hugot JP, Laurent PP, Gower RC, Olson JM, Lee JC, Beaugerie L, Naom I, Dupas JL, Van GA, Orholm M, et al.: Mapping of a susceptibility locus for Crohn's disease on chromosome 16. Nature 1996; 379:821–823.
Ikeda K, Sannoh T, Kawasaki N, Kawasaki T, Yamashini I: Serum lectin with known structure activates complement through the classical pathway. J Biol Chem 1987; 262:7551–7556.
Ip WK, Chan SY, Lau CS, Lau YL: Association of systemic lupus erythematosus with promoter polymorphisms of the mannose-binding lectin gene. Arthritis Rheum 1998; 41:1663–1668.
Izui S, Higaki M, Morrow D, Merino R: The Y chromosome from autoimmune BXSB/MpJ mice induces a lupus-like syndrome in (NZW × C57BL/6)F_1 male mice, but not in C57BL/6 male mice. J Immunol 1988; 18:911–915.
Jacob CO, Fronek Z, Lewis GD, Koo M, Hansen JA, McDevitt HO: Heritable major histocompatibility complex class II–associated differences in production of tumor necrosis factor α: relevance to genetic predisposition to systemic lupus erythematosus. Proc Natl Acad Sci USA 1990; 87:1233–1237.
Jacob CO, McDevitt HO: Tumour necrosis factor-α in murine autoimmune "lupus" nephritis. Nature 1988; 331:356–358.
Jarjour W, Reed AM, Gauthier J, Hunt S, Winfield JB: The 8.5-kb *PstI* allele of the stress protein gene, *Hsp70-2*: an independent risk factor for systemic lupus erythematosus in African-Americans? Hum Immunol 1996; 45:59–63.
Jarvinen P, Kaprio J, Makitalo R, Koskenvuo M, Aho K: Systemic lupus erythematosus and related systemic diseases in a nationwide twin cohort: an increased prevalence of disease in MZ twins and concordance of disease features. J Intern Med 1992; 231:67–72.
Johnson AE, Gordon C, Palmer RG, Bacon PA: The prevalence and incidence of systemic lupus erythematosus in Birmingham, England. Arthritis Rheum 1995; 38:551–558.
Jonsson H, Nived O, Sturfelt G: Outcome in systemic lupus erythematosus: a prospective study of patients from a defined population. Medicine 1989; 68:141–150.
Julkunen H, Jouhikainen T, Kaaja R, Leirisalo-Repo M, Stephansson E, Palosuo T, Teramo K, Friman C: Fetal outcome in lupus pregnancy: a retrospective case-control study of 242 pregnancies in 112 patients. Lupus 1993; 2:125–131.
Julkunen H, Siren MK, Kaaja R, Kurki P, Friman C, Koskimies S: Maternal HLA antigens and antibodies to SS-A/Ro and SS-B/La. Comparison with systemic lupus erythematosus and primary Sjogren's syndrome. Br J Rheumatol 1995; 34: 901–907.
Khanduja S, Arnett FC, Reveille JD: HLA-DQ beta genes encode an epitope for lupus specific DNA antibodies. Clin Res 1991; 38:975–980.
Khare SD, Sarosi I, Xia XZ, McCabe S, Miner K, Solovyev I, Hawkins N, Kelley M, Chang D, Van G, et al.: Severe B cell hyperplasia and autoimmune disease in TALL-1 transgenic mice. Proc Natl Acad Sci USA 2000; 97:3370–3375.
Kimberly RP, Salmon JE, Edberg JC: Receptors for immunoglobulin G: Molecular diversity and implications for disease. Arthritis Rheum 1995; 38:306–314.
Kitrodou RC: The mother in systemic lupus erythematosus. In: Wallace DJ, Hahn BH (eds). Dubois' Lupus Erythematosus. Baltimore: Williams and Wilkins, 1997:967–1002.
Kiwasaki M, Kawasaki T, Tyamashura I: Isolation and characterization of a mannose binding protein from human serum. J Biol Chem 1983; 94:937–942.
Kong A, Cox NJ: Allele-sharing models: LOD scores and accurate linkage tests. Am J Hum Genet 1997; 61:1179–1188.
Lander E, Kruglyak L: Genetic dissection of complex traits: guidelines for interpreting and reporting linkage results. Nat Genet 1995; 11:241–247.
Lawrence JS, Martins CL, Drake GL: A family survey of lupus erythematosus. 1. Heritability. J Rheumatol 1987; 14:913–921.
Lawrence RC, Helmick CG, Arnett FC, Deyo RA, Felson DT, Giannini EH, Heyse SP, Hirsch R, Hochberg MC, Hunder GG, et al.: Estimates of the prevalence of arthritis and selected musculoskeletal disorders in the United States [see comments]. Arthritis Rheum 1998; 41:778–799.
Lawrence RC, Hochberg MC, Kelsey JL, McDuffie FC, Medsger TA, Felts WR, Shulman LE: Estimates of prevalence of selected arthritis and musculoskeletal diseases in the United States. J Rheumatol 1989; 16:427–441.
Lazarus M, Hajeer AH, Turner D, Sinnott P, Worthington J, Ollier WE, Hutchison IV: Genetic variation in the interleukin 10 gene promoter and systemic lupus erythematosus. J Rheumatol 1997; 24:2314–2317.
Levine JS, Koh JS: The role of apoptosis in autoimmunity: immunogen, antigen, and accelerant. Semin Nephrol 1999; 19:34–47.
Lindqvist AK, Steinsson K, Johanneson B, Kristjansdottir H, Arnasson A, Grondal G, Jonasson I, Magnusson V, Sturfelt G, Truedsson L, et al.: A susceptibility locus for human systemic lupus erythematosus (hSLE1) on chromosome 2q. J Autoimmun 2000; 14:169–178.
Liossis SNC, Ding XZ, Dennis GJ, Tsokos GC: Altered pattern of TCR/CD3-mediated protein-tyrosyl phosphorylation in T cells from patients with systemic lupus erythematosus. J Clin Invest 1998; 101:1448–1457.
Llorente L, Richaud-Patin Y, Couderc J, Alarcon-Segovia D, Ruiz-Soto R, Alcocer-Castillejos N, Alcocer-Varela J, Granados J, Bahena S, Galanaud P, et al.: Dysregulation of interleukin-10 production in relatives of patients with systemic lupus erythematosus. Arthritis Rheum 1997; 40:1429–1435.
Llorente L, Richaud-Patin Y, Fior R, Alcocer-Varela J, Wijdenes J, Fourrier BM, Galanaud P, Emilie D: In vivo production of interleukin-10 by non-T cells in rheumatoid arthritis, Sjogren's syndrome, and systemic lupus erythematosus. Arthritis Rheum 1994; 37:1647–1655.
Llorente L, Zou W, Levy Y, Richaud-Patin Y, Wijdenes J, Alcocer-Varela J, Morel-Fourrier B, Brouet JC, Alarcon-Segovia D, Ruiz-Soto R, et al.: Role of interleukin 10 in the B lymphocyte hyperactivity and autoantibody production of human systemic lupus erythematosus. J Exp Med 1995; 181:839–844.
Majeti R, Xu Z, Parslow TG, Olson JL, Daikh DI, Killeen N, Weiss A: An inactivating point mutation in the inhibitory wedge of CD45 causes lymphoproliferation and autoimmunity. Cell 2000; 103:1059–1070.
Mascola MA, Repke JT: Obstetric management of the high-risk lupus pregnancy. Rheum Dis Clin North Am 1997; 23:119–132.
McCarty DJ, Manzi S, Medsger TA, Ramsey-Goldman R, LaPorte RE, Kwoh CK: Incidence of systemic lupus erythematosus: race and gender differences. Arthritis Rheum 1995; 38:1260–1270.
Meddings J, Grennan DM: The prevalence of systemic lupus erythematosus (SLE) in Dunedin. N Z Med J 1980; 91:205–206.
Mehrian R, Quismorio J, Strassmann G, Stimmler MM, Horwitz DA, Kitridou RC, Gauderman WJ, Morrison J, Brautbar C, Jacob CO: Synergistic effect between IL-10 and bcl-2 genotypes in determining susceptibility to systemic lupus erythematosus. Arthritis Rheum 1998; 41:596–602.
Meng C, Lockshin M: Pregnancy in lupus. Curr Opin Rheumatol 1999; 11:348–351.
Michet CJ, McKenna CH, Elveback CR, Kaslow RA, Kurland LT: Epidemiology of systemic lupus erythematosus and other connective tissue diseases in Rochester, Minnesota 1950 through 1979. Mayo Clin Proc 1985; 60:105–113.
Mirza MM, Lee J, Teare D, Hugot JP, Laurent-Puig P, Colombel JF, Hodgson SV, Thomas G, Easton DF, Lennard-Jones JE, et al.: Evidence of linkage of the inflammatory bowel disease susceptibility locus on chromosome 16 (IBD1) to ulcerative colitis. J Med Genet 1998; 35:218–221.
Miyagawa S, Shinohara K, Kidoguchi K, Fujita T, Fukumoto T, Yamashina Y, Hashimoto K, Yoshioka A, Sakurai S, Nishihara O, et al.: Neonatal lupus erythematosus: HLA-DR and -DQ distributions are different among the groups of anti-Ro/SSA-positive mothers with different neonatal outcomes. J Invest Dermatol 1997; 108:881–885.
Mohan C, Alas E, Morel L, Yang P, Wakeland EK: Genetic dissection of SLE pathogenesis: *Sle1* on murine chromosome 1 leads to a selective loss of tolerance to H2A/H2B/DNA subnucleosomes. J Clin Invest 1998; 101:1362–1372.
Mohan C, Morel L, Yang P, Wakeland EK: Genetic dissection of systemic lupus erythematosus pathogenesis: *Sle2* on murine chromosome 4 leads to B cell hyperactivity. J Immunol 1997; 159:454–465.
Mohan C, Yu Y, Morel L, Yang P, Wakeland EK: Genetic dissection of Sle pathogenesis: Sle3 on murine chromosome 7 impacts T cell activation, differentiation, and cell death. J Immunol 1999; 162:6492–6502.
Mok CC, Lanchbury JS, Chan DW, Lau CS: Interleukin-10 promoter polymorphisms in southern Chinese patients with systemic lupus erythematosus. Arthritis Rheum 1998; 41:1090–1095.
Mongey AB, Hess EV: The role of the environment in systemic lupus erythematosus and associated disorders. In: Wallace DJ, Hahn BH (eds). Dubois' Lupus Erythematosus. Baltimore: Williams and Wilkins, 1997:31–47.

Moore KW, O'Garra A, de Waal Malefyt R, Vieira P, Mosmann TR: Interluekin-10. Annu Rev Immunol 1993; 11:165–190.

Morel L, Blenman KR, Croker BP, Wakeland EK: The major murine systemic lupus erythematosus susceptibility locus, Sle1, is a cluster of functionally related genes. Proc Natl Acad Sci USA 2001; 98:1787–1792.

Morel L, Croker BP, Blenman KR, Mohan C, Huang G, Gilkeson G, Wakeland EK: Genetic reconstitution of systemic lupus erythematosus immunopathology with polycongenic murine strains. Proc Natl Acad Sci USA 2000; 97:6670–6675.

Morel L, Mohan C, Yu Y, Croker BP, Tian N, Deng A, Wakeland EK: Functional dissection of systemic lupus erythematosus using congenic mouse strains. J Immunol 1997; 158:6019–6028.

Morel L, Rudofsky UH, Longmate JA, Schiffenbauer J, Wakeland EK: Polygenic control of susceptibility to murine systemic lupus erythematosus. Immunity 1994; 1:219–229.

Morel L, Wakeland EK: Susceptibility to lupus nephritis in the NZB/W model system. Curr Opin Immunol 1998; 10:718–725.

Morel L, Yu Y, Blenman KR, Caldwell RA, Wakeland EK: Production of congenic mouse strains carrying SLE-susceptibility genes derived from the SLE-prone NZM/Aeg2410 strain. Mamm Genome 1996; 7:335–339.

Morton RO, Gershwin ME, Brady C, Steinberg AD: The incidence of systemic lupus erythematosus in North American Indians. J Rheumatol 1976; 3:186–190.

Moser KL, Gray-McGuire C, Kelly J, Asundi N, Yu H, Bruner GR, Mange M, Hogue R, Neas BR, Harley JB: Confirmation of genetic linkage between human systemic lupus erythematosus and chromosome 1q41. Arthritis Rheum 1999; 42:1902–1907.

Moser KL, Neas BR, Salmon JE, Yu H, Gray-McGuire C, Asundi N, Bruner GR, Fox J, Kelly J, Henshall S, et al.: Genome scan of human systemic lupus erythematosus: evidence for linkage on chromosome 1q in African-American pedigrees. Proc Natl Acad Sci USA 1998; 95:14869–14874.

Murphy ED, Roths JB: A Y chromosome associated factor in strain BXSB producing accelerated autoimmunity and lymphoproliferation. Arthritis Rheum 1979; 22:1188–1194.

Nagata S, Golstein P: The Fas death factor. Science 1995; 267:1449–1456.

Nagata S, Suda T: Fas and Fas ligand: lpr and gld mutations. Immunol Today 1995; 16:39–43.

Nai-Cheng C: Rheumatic diseases in China. J Rheumatol 1983; 10(Suppl 10):41–44.

Nair RP, Henseler T, Jenisch S, Stuart P, Bichakjian CK, Lenk W, Westphal E, Guo S-W, Christophers E, Voorhees JJ, et al.: Evidence for two psoriasis susceptibility loci (HLA and 17q) and two novel candidate regions (16q and 20p) by genome-wide scan. Hum Mol Genet 1997; 6:1349–1356.

Napirei M, Karsunky H, Zevnik B, Stephan H, Mannherz HG, Moroy T: Features of systemic lupus erythematosus in Dnase1-deficient mice. Nat Genet 2000; 25:177–181.

Nishimura H, Nose M, Hiai H, Minato N, Honjo T: Development of lupus-like autoimmune diseases by disruption of the *PD-1* gene encoding an ITIM motif-carrying immunoreceptor. Immunity 1999; 11:141–151.

Nived O, Sturfelt G, Wollheim F: Systemic lupus erythematosus in an adult population in southern Sweden: incidence, prevalence and validity of ARA revised classification criteria. Br J Rheumatol 1985; 24:147–154.

Norris CF, Pricop L, Millard SS, Taylor SM, Surrey S, Schwartz E, Salmon JE, McKenzie SE: A naturally occurring mutation in FcγRIIA: a Q to K127 change confers unique IgG binding properties to the R131 allelic form of the receptor. Blood 1998; 91:656–662.

Nossent JC: Systemic lupus erythematosus on the Caribbean island of Curaçao: an epidemiological investigation. Ann Rheum Dis 1992; 51:1197–1201.

Ocal L, Russell K, Beynon H, Cruickshank K, Lanchbury JS, Walport M, Isenberg D, Briggs D: Genetic analysis of *TAP2* in systemic lupus erythematosus patients from two ethnic groups. Br J Rheumatol 1996; 35:529–533.

Ogura Y, Bonen DK, Inohara N, Nicolae DL, Chen FF, Ramos R, Britton H, Moran T, Karaliuskas R, Duerr RH, et al.: A frameshift mutation in *NOD2* associated with susceptibility to Crohn's disease. Nature 2001; 411:603–606.

Olsen ML, Arnett FC, Reveille JD: Contrasting molecular patterns of MHC class II alleles associated with the anti-Sm and anti-RNP autoantibodies in systemic lupus erythematosus. Arthritis Rheum 1993; 36:94–104.

Olsen ML, Dimou GS, Papasteriades C, Moutsopoulos HM, Arnett FC: MHC class II and III genes in Greek patients with systemic lupus erythematosus. Arthritis Rheum 1992; 36:94–104.

Pablos JL, Carreira PE, Martin-Villa JM, Montalvo G, Arnaiz-Villena A, Gomez-Reino JJ: Polymorphism of the heat-shock protein gene *HSP70-2* in systemic lupus erythematosus. Br J Rheumatol 1995; 34:721–723.

Pederson SE, Taylor RP, Morley KW, Wright E: Stability of DNA/anti-DNA complexes. IV. Complement fixation. J Immunol Methods 1980; 38:269–280.

Prodeus AP, Goerg S, Shen LM, Pozdnyakova OO, Chu L, Alicot EM, Goodnow CC, Carroll MC: A critical role for complement in maintenance of self-tolerance. Immunity 1998; 9:721–731.

Rascu A, Repp R, Westerdaal NAC, Kalden JR, van de Winkel JGJ: Clinical relevance of Fcγ receptor polymorphisms. Ann N Y Acad Sci 1997; 815:282–295.

Ravetch JV, Kinet JP: Fc receptors. Annu Rev Immunol 1991; 9:457–492.

Reichlin M, Harley JB, Lockshin MD: Serologic studies of monozygotic twins with systemic lupus erythematosus. Arthritis Rheum 1992; 35:457–464.

Reveille JD, Macleod MJ, Whittington K, Arnett FC: Specific amino acid residues in the second hypervariable region of HLA-DQA1 and DQB1 chain genes promote the Ro (SS-A)/La (SS-B) autoantibody responses. J Immunol 1991; 146:3871–3876.

Ring GH, Lakkis FG: Breakdown of self-tolerance and the pathogenesis of autoimmunity. Semin Nephrol 1999; 19:25–33.

Rosen A, Casciola-Rosen L: Autoantigens as substrates for apoptotic proteases: implications for the pathogenesis of systemic autoimmune disease. Cell Death Differ 1999; 6:6–12.

Rothfield NF: Systemic lupus erythematosus: clinical aspects and treatments. In: McCarty DJ (ed). Arthritis and Allied Conditions. Philadelphia: Lea and Febiger, 1985:911–935.

Rubin RL, Tang FL, Chan EKL, Pollard KM, Tsay G, Tan EM: IgG subclasses of autoantibodies in systemic lupus erythematosus, Sjogren's syndrome and drug-induced autoimmunity. J Immunol 1986; 137:2528–2534.

Rudofsky UH, Evans BD, Balaban SL, Mottironi VD, Gabrielsen AE: Differences in expression of lupus nephritis in New Zealand mixed H-2z homozygous inbred strains of mice derived from New Zealand black and New Zealand white mice. Origins and initial characterization. Lab Invest 1993; 68:419–426.

Rudwaleit M, Tikly M, Khamashta M, Gibson K, Klinke J, Hughes G, Wordsworth P: Interethnic differences in the association of tumor necrosis factor promotor polymorphisms with systemic lupus erythematosus. J Rheumatol 1996; 23:1725–1728.

Salmon JE: Abnormalities in immune complex clearance and Fcγ receptor function. In: Wallace DJ, Hahn BH (eds). Dubois' Lupus Erythematosus. Baltimore: Williams and Wilkins, 1997:221–243.

Salmon JE, Edberg JC, Brogle NL, Kimberly RP: Allelic polymorphisms of human Fc gamma receptor IIA and Fc gamma receptor IIIB. Independent mechanisms for differences in human phagocyte function. J Clin Invest 1992; 89:1274–1281.

Salmon JE, Millard S, Schachter LA, Arnett FC, Ginzler EM, Gourley MF, Ramsey-Goldman R, Peterson MG, Kimberly RP: FcγRIIA alleles are heritable risk factors for lupus nephritis in African Americans. J Clin Invest 1996; 97:1348–1354.

Samanta A, Roy S, Feehally J, Symmons DPM: The prevalence of diagnosed systemic lupus erythematosus in whites and Indian Asian immigrants in Leicester City, UK. Br J Rheumatol 1992; 31:679–682.

Schur PH: Genetics of systemic lupus erythematosus. Lupus 1995; 4:425–437.

Schur PH: Complement and systemic lupus erythematosus. In: Wallace DJ, Hahn BH (eds). Dubois' Lupus Erythematosus. Baltimore: Williams and Wilkins, 1997:245–261.

Schur PH, Marcus-Bagley D, Awdeh Z, Yunis EJ, Alper CA: The effect of ethnicity on major histocompatibility complex complement allotypes and extended haplotypes in patients with systemic lupus erythematosus. Arthritis Rheum 1990; 33:985–992.

Schur PH, Meyer I, Garovoy M, Carpenter CB: Associations between systemic lupus erythematosus and the major histocompatibility complex: clinical and immunological considerations. Clin Immunol Immunopathol 1982; 24:263–275.

Schweinle JE, Ezekowitz RAB, Tenner AJ, Kuhlman M, Joiner KA: Human mannose-binding protein activates the alternative complement pathway and enhances serum bactericidal activity on a mannose rich isolate of *Salmonella*. J Clin Invest 1989; 84:1821–1829.

Scofield RH, Harley JB: Association of anti-Ro/SS-A autoantibodies with glutamine in position 34 of DQA1 and leucine in position 26 of DQB1. Arthritis Rheum 1994; 37:961–962.

Serdula MK, Rhoads GG: Frequency of systemic lupus erythematosus in different ethnic groups in Hawaii. Arthritis Rheum 1979; 22:328–333.

Shai R, Quismorio FP Jr, Li L, Kwon OJ, Morrison J, Wallace DJ, Neuwelt CM, Brautbar C, Gauderman WJ, Jacob CO: Genome-wide screen for systemic lupus erythematosus susceptibility genes in multiplex families. Hum Mol Genet 1999; 8:639–644.

Siegel M, Lee S: The epidemiology of systemic lupus erythematosus. Semin Arthritis Rheum 1973; 3:1–54.

Singer GG, Abbas AK: The FAS antigen is involved in the peripheral but not thymic deletion of T lymphocytes in T cell receptor transgenic mice. Immunity 1994; 1:365–372.

Siren MK, Julkunen H, Kaaja R, Ekblad H, Koskimies S: Role of HLA in congenital heart block: susceptibility alleles in children. Lupus 1999a; 8:60–67.

Siren MK, Julkunen H, Kaaja R, Kurki P, Koskimies S: Role of HLA in congenital heart block: susceptibility alleles in mothers. Lupus 1999b; 8:52–59.

Slingsby JH, Norsworthy P, Pearce G, Vaishnaw AK, Issler H, Morley BJ, Walport MJ: Homozygous hereditary C1q deficiency and systemic lupus erythematosus. Arthritis Rheum 1996; 39:663–670.

Song YW, Han CW, Kang SW, Baek HJ, Lee EB, Shin CH, Hahn BH, Tsao BP: Abnormal distribution of Fcγ receptor type IIa polymorphisms in Korean patients with systemic lupus erythematosus. Arthritis Rheum 1998; 41:421–426.

Spielman RS, McGinnis RE, Evans WJ: Transmission test for linkage disequilibrium: the insulin gene region and insulin dependent diabetes mellitus (IDDM). Am J Hum Genet 1993; 52:506–516.

Strasser A, Whittingham S, Vaux DL, Bath ML, Adams JM, Cory S, Harris AW: Enforced BCL2 expression in B-lymphoid cells prolongs antibody responses and elicits autoimmune disease. Proc Natl Acad Sci USA 1991; 88:8661–8665.

Sturfelt G, Hellmer G, Truedsson L: TNF microsatellites in systemic lupus erythematosus—a high frequency of the TNFabc 2-3-1 haplotype in multicase SLE families. Lupus 1996; 5:618–622.

Sullivan KE, Wooten C, Goldman D, Petri M: Mannose-binding protein polymorphism in black patients with systemic lupus erythematosus. Arthritis Rheum 1996; 39:2046–2051.

Sullivan KE, Wooten C, Schmeckpeper BJ, Goldman D, Petri MA: A promotor polymorphism of tumor necrosis factor α associated with systemic lupus erythematosus in African-Americans. Arthritis Rheum 1997; 40:2207–2211.

Takeuchi F, Nakano K, Nabeta H, Hong GH, Kuwata S, Ito K: Polymorphisms of the *TAP1* and *TAP2* transporter genes in Japanese SLE. Ann Rheum Dis 1996; 55:924–926.

Tan EM, Cohen AS, Fries JF, Masi AT, McShane DJ, Rothfield NF, Schaller JG, Talal N, Winchester RJ: The 1982 revised criteria for the classification of systemic lupus erythematosus. Arthritis Rheum 1982; 25:1271–1277.

Topaloglu R, Bakkaloglu A, Slingsby JH, Mihatsch MJ, Pascual M, Norsworthy P, Morley BJ, Saatci U, Schifferli JA, Walport MJ: Molecular basis of hereditary C1q deficiency associated with SLE and IgA nephropathy in a Turkish family. Kidney Int 1996; 50:635–642.

Tromp G, Kuivaniemi H, Raphael S, Ala-Kokko L, Christiano A, Considine E, Dhulipala R, Hyland J, Jokinen A, Kivirikko S, et al.: Genetic linkage of familial granulomatous inflammatory arthritis, skin rash, and uveitis to chromosome 16. Am J Hum Genet 1996; 59:1097–1107.

Trowsdale J: Genomic structure and function in the MHC. Trends Genet 1993; 9:117–122.

Tsao BP, Cantor RM, Badsha H, Grossman JM, Kalunian KC, Hartung K, Arnett FC, Wallace DJ, Hahn BH, Rotter JI: A susceptibility gene for SLE maps to a 5 cM region of chromosome 1q. Arthritis Rheum 1997a; 40:S315.

Tsao BP, Cantor RM, Grossman JM, Shen N, Teophilov NT, Wallace DJ, Arnett FC, Hartung K, Goldstein R, Kalunian KC, et al.: PARP alleles within the linked chromosomal region are associated with systemic lupus erythematosus. J Clin Invest 1999; 103:1135–1140.

Tsao BP, Cantor RM, Grossman JM, Theophilov N, Wallace DJ, Arnett FC, Hartung K, Goldstein R, Kalunian KC, Hahn BH, et al.: *ADPRT* alleles from the chromosome 1q41–1q42 linked region are associated with SLE. Arthritis Rheum 1998; 41:S80.

Tsao BP, Cantor RM, Kalunian KC, Chen CJ, Badsha H, Singh R, Wallace DJ, Kitridoou RC, Chen S, Shen N, et al.: Evidence for linkage of a candidate chromosome 1 region to human systemic lupus erythematosus. J Clin Invest 1997b; 99:725–731.

Utz PJ, Anderson P: Posttranslational protein modifications, apoptosis, and the bypass of tolerance to autoantigens. Arthritis Rheum 1998; 41:1152–1160.

Utz PJ, Hottelet M, Schur PH, Anderson P: Proteins phosphorylated during stress-induced apoptosis are common targets for autoantibody production in patients with systemic lupus erythematosus. J Exp Med 1997; 185:843–854.

Vassalli P: The pathophysiology of tumor necrosis factors. Annu Rev Immunol 1992; 10:411–452.

Vassilopoulos D, Kovacs B, Tsokos GC: TCR/CD3 complex–mediated signal transduction pathway in T cells and T cell lines from patients with systemic lupus erythematosus. J Immunol 1995; 155:2269–2281.

Vidal S, Kono DH, Theofilopoulos AN: Loci predisposing to autoimmunity in MRL-*Fas* ^{lpr} and C57BL/6-*Fas* ^{lpr} mice. J Clin Invest 1998; 101:696–702.

Voss A, Green A, Junker P: Systemic lupus erythematosus in Denmark: clinical and epidemiological characterization of a county-based cohort. Scand J Rheumatol 1998; 27:98–105.

Vyse TJ, Kotzin BL: Genetic susceptibility to systemic lupus erythematosus. Annu Rev Immunol 1998; 16:261–292.

Vyse TJ, Rozzo SJ, Drake CG, Izui S, Kotzin BL: Control of multiple autoantibodies linked with a lupus nephritis susceptibility locus in New Zealand black mice. J Immunol 1997; 158:5566–5574.

Vyse TJ, Todd JA: Genetic analysis of autoimmune disease. Cell 1996; 85:311–318.

Wainstein E, Edberg J, Csernok E, Sneller M, Hoffman G, Keystone E, Gross W, Salmon J, Kimberly R: FcγRIIIB alleles predict renal dysfunction in Wegener's granulomatosis (WG). Arthritis Rheum 1996; 39:S210.

Wang F, Wang CL, Tan CT, Manivasagar M: Systemic lupus erythematosus in Malaysia: a study of 539 patients and comparison of prevalence and disease expression in different racial and gender groups. Lupus 1997; 6:248–253.

Watson ML, Rao JK, Gilkeson GS, Ruiz P, Eicher EM, Pisetsky DS, Matsuzawa A, Rochelle JM, Seldin MF: Genetic analysis of MRL-*lpr* mice: relationship of the *Fas* apoptosis gene to disease manifestations and renal disease-modifying loci. J Exp Med 1992; 176:1645–1656.

Watson RM, Lane AT, Barnett NK, Bias WB, Arnett FC, Provost TT: Neonatal lupus erythematosus: a clinical, serological and immunogenetic study with review of the literature. Medicine 1984; 63:362–378.

Weiss A, Littman DR: Signal transduction by lymphocyte antigen receptors. Cell 1994; 76:263–274.

Wu J, Edberg JC, Redecha PB, Bansai V, Guyre PM, Coleman K, Salmon JE, Kimberly RP: A novel polymorphism of FcγRIIIa (CD16) alters receptor function and predisposes to autoimmune disease. J Clin Invest 1997; 100:1059–1070.

Yasutomo K, Horiuchi T, Kagami S, Tsukamoto H, Hashimura C, Urushihara M, Kuroda Y: Mutation of DNASE1 in people with systemic lupus erythematosus. Nat Genet 2001; 28:313–314.

Yu CC, Yen TS, Lowell CA, DeFranco AL: Lupus-like kidney disease in mice deficient in the Src family tyrosine kinases Lyn and Fyn. Curr Biol 2001; 11:34–38.

32 Genetic Basis of Primary Osteoarthritis

JOHN LOUGHLIN AND KAY CHAPMAN

Osteoarthritis (OA) was long considered an inevitable consequence of aging, with excessive mechanical stresses leading to breakdown of the articular cartilage of the joints. This simplistic view has long been challenged, with rheumatologists highlighting the nodal form of the disease, which demonstrates familial clustering, and pointing to rare families in which the disease is apparently transmitted as a Mendelian trait. Eventually, more systematic genetic epidemiological studies confirmed that the disease has a genetic component and supported the role of nongenetic factors in disease development and progression. These studies originate from the mid- to late 1990s, which means that, apart from nodal OA, only recently has the research community had the confidence to seriously attempt the process of disease gene identification. Therefore, in comparison to many other complex diseases, the genetic dissection of OA is still in its early stages. Nevertheless, a number of candidate genes have been assessed through association and linkage analyses, while at least three genome-wide linkage scans have been completed. To determine whether any of the loci so far implicated are real susceptibility genes will require large-scale association studies and extensive research collaboration.

DISEASE DEFINITION

OA is a degenerative joint disease involving focal cartilage loss. Its histology varies from minor erosion to cartilage loss that extends to the bone (Jones and Doherty, 1995; Creamer and Hochberg, 1997). There are a number of other phenotypic components of the disease which can accompany the cartilage loss, including new bone growth (osteophytes), an increase in the density of subchondral bone (sclerosis), and an inflammatory response. When an individual presents with symptomatic disease (localized joint pain, tenderness, and movement limitation), a radiograph is still the preferred means of assessing the severity of the disease. Cartilage loss is detectable as a joint-space narrowing, and the accompanying bone response of osteophytes and sclerosis can clearly be observed. A scale for measuring narrowing and bone response was developed by Kellgren and Lawrence (1963). This scale ranges from 0 to 4 with 0 representing no OA and 4 representing severe OA. This is essentially the scale used today, although adaptations have been applied (Spector et al., 1993).

Immediately before and during cartilage loss, the cellular biology of the cartilage and underlying bone changes significantly. There is upregulation of a number of genes, such as the type II collagen gene *COL2A1* (Aigner et al. 1993), and altered activity of a number of proteins, including cytokines such as tumor necrosis factor-α and the matrix metalloproteinases and their inhibitors (Goldring, 2000a,b; Pelletier et al., 2001). These changes, which represent an attempt by the joint to repair damage, can inadvertently initiate or accelerate cartilage destruction.

Subtypes

Primary

OA can exist in two main forms: primary and secondary. Primary (or idiopathic) OA is the common late-onset form of the disease, with radiographic evidence first detectable in the fifth decade. It has no obvious cause and can be localized to a particular joint group (i.e., hands, hip, knee, shoulder, or spine) or generalized with the involvement of three or more joint groups. One form of primary OA that has long been considered a separate entity is nodal generalized OA (Kellgren and Moore, 1952). This form is characterized by the presence of multiple Heberden's and/or Bouchard's nodes on the distal interphalangeal and proximal interphalangeal joints, respectively. It is often clustered in families, accompanied by OA at other joint groups, and much more prevalent in females. It was this form that first prompted rheumatologists to suggest that primary OA may have a genetic component (Stecher, 1941, 1955; Kellgren et al., 1963).

Secondary

Secondary OA, as the name implies, arises in response to a clearly identifiable factor, such as trauma, a congenital or developmental abnormality, or a biochemical abnormality (e.g., crystal deposition in the joint, chondrocalcinosis). In a small number of cases, secondary OA is associated with developmental abnormalities that are transmitted as Mendelian traits. These diseases are members of the osteochondrodysplasia class of skeletal dysplasias and the OA in these familial cases is often of early onset (third or fourth decade), precocious, and severe. Linkage and positional cloning have identified the disease genes and the causal mutations in several of the osteochondrodysplasias whose phenotypes include precocious OA (Table 32–1). These genes have tended to encode structural proteins of the cartilage extracellular matrix. All are considered potential candidates for primary OA, the assumption being that less severe mutations at these loci may predispose to disease. Chondrocalcinosis is characterized by the deposition in the joint of crystalline forms of calcium (Fam, 1992; Schumacher, 2001). This can result in a chronic OA that is occasionally transmitted as a Mendelian trait. Two pedigrees were used to map chondrocalcinosis loci to chromosomes 5p15.1–15.2 (Hughes et al., 1995) and 8q22.1–24.1 (Baldwin et al., 1995). The locus on 5p has been fine-mapped to an interval of less than 1 cM, suitable for positional cloning and candidate gene investigation (Andrew et al., 1999). A very strong candidate gene for the 5p locus, the ankylosis gene *ANK* (Ho et al., 2000; Reichenberger et al., 2001), has been identified

Table 32–1. Examples of Single-Gene Disorders That Have Osteoarthritis as a Phenotypic Component

Phenotype	Gene	Chromosome	Polypeptide	Reference
Ocular Stickler's syndrome and mild spondyloepiphyseal dysplasia	*COL2A1*	12q12–13.1	α1 chain type II collagen	Mundlos and Olsen (1997)
Multiple epiphyseal dysplasia (EDM2)	*COL9A2*	1p32.3–33	α2 chain type IX collagen	Holden et al. (1999)
Multiple epiphyseal dysplasia (EDM3)	*COL9A3*	20q13.3	α3 chain type IX collagen	Paassilta et al. (1999)
Ocular Stickler's syndrome and Marshall's syndrome	*COL11A1*	1p21	α1 chain type XI collagen	Mundlos and Olsen (1997), Griffith et al. (1998)
Nonocular Stickler's syndrome and otospondylomegaepiphyseal dysplasia	*COL11A2*	6p21.3	α2 chain type XI collagen	Mundlos and Olsen (1997)
Multiple epiphyseal dysplasia (EDM1) and pseudoachondroplasia	*COMP*	19p13.1	Cartilage oligomeric matrix protein	Loughlin et al. (1998)
Multiple epiphyseal dysplasia (EDM5)	*MATN3*	2p24–p23	Matrilin-3	Chapman et al. (2001)

and is currently being scrutinized for mutations that can cause chondrocalcinosis.

Since primary OA is the form that impacts most significantly in the population, it is the form that we will concentrate on in this chapter.

GENERAL GENETIC AND EPIDEMIOLOGICAL EVIDENCE

Population Epidemiology

The Kellgren and Lawrence (1963) scale has been used as a standard measuring tool in a number of epidemiological tests to determine the prevalence of OA in different population groups and to assess potential risk factors. These studies have tended to concentrate on gender, occupation, and ethnic origin; and the results are often conflicting. This may be the result of inadequate test design, small study numbers, or attempts to draw conclusions from essentially unrelated tests. Felson and Zhang (1998) have reviewed a number of epidemiological studies performed on knee and hip disease. This review, along with others (Maetzel et al., 1997), permits some firmer conclusions to be drawn regarding OA risk factors.

Age and Sex

The major risk factor is age, with prevalence gradually rising and reaching a peak in the eighth decade. The prevalence then appears to stabilize. By the seventh decade, up to 50% of individuals will have some radiographic evidence of the disease in at least one joint group. Before the age of 50, males have a greater risk of disease than females. However, this disparity narrows, with women having a greater risk after age 50. This increased risk in females is strongly associated with menopause, indicating that the development and/or progression of primary OA may be heavily influenced by hormonal factors.

Occupation

Occupation is a contentious risk factor. At the extreme end, occupation may cause severe damage to a joint, which will then develop OA. An example of this can be seen in some sporting injuries, where physical damage results in early-onset OA. This form belongs better in the secondary rather than the primary class of OA. Less obvious occupational factors may, however, predispose to primary OA. The population most examined in this context includes those with manual occupations, in particular farmers. From the review of Maetzel et al. (1997) it is clear that excessive, sustained manual labor predisposes to large-joint OA (hip and knee). However, the predisposition is not strong: repetitive knee bending does appear to be a risk factor for knee OA in males but less so in females, while manual labor only moderately predisposes to hip OA in males.

Ethnicity

Ethnic differences in the prevalence of OA have been reported, although again the reports are conflicting. For example, hip OA is less prevalent in Asians than in Europeans, whereas hand OA is as common in both groups. The difference in hip OA prevalence was partially ascribed to a greater frequency of dysplasia of the acetabulum (hip socket) in Europeans (Lane et al., 2000). However, some studies have contradicted this viewpoint and have found no association between acetabular dysplasia and hip OA (Yoshimura et al., 1998; Inoue et al., 2000).

Obesity

Obesity has long been recognized as a major risk factor for OA, particularly for knee OA. The initial interpretation of the increased risk was that an obese individual applyies more mechanical loading to the joints. However, there are two observations that do not support this simple interpretation: *(1)* obesity is also a risk factor for hand OA and *(2)* obesity is more strongly associated with female OA than male OA. These two observations have begged the question whether it is the weight per se that is the risk factor or whether it is the degree of adiposity (Felson and Chaisson, 1997; Toda et al., 1998). It has been suggested that adipose tissue may act as a reservoir for metabolic factors, such as hormones and growth factors, that are regulators of cartilage and/or bone homeostasis. If this is the case, then excess adipose tissue may result in an imbalance in the levels of these factors, which could promote cartilage breakdown.

Family Epidemiology

Although primary OA has long been considered an inevitable consequence of aging, with certain environmental risk factors increasing the likelihood of developing the disease, there were those who suggested that at least some individuals had a genetic predisposition. These suggestions arose from epidemiological studies that demonstrated clustering of generalized OA in families (Stecher, 1941, 1955; Kellgren et al., 1963). However, it was correctly pointed out that clustering in families could be the result of shared environmental factors and that the involvement of genes was still not demonstrated.

Twin Studies

The point at which the arthritis research community finally had the confidence to consider primary OA as a disease with a significant genetic component came in 1996 with the publication of the first large-scale twin study (Spector et al., 1996). This study was performed on 130 monozygotic and 120 dizygotic female twin pairs from the United Kingdom who were aged 48 or over. Hand and knee X-rays were taken, and the heritability of OA was calculated to vary from 39% to 65%. The concordance rate in monozygotic twin pairs was 0.64 compared to 0.38 in dizygotic pairs. This indicated a role for the environment in disease development and that there may be only a relatively small number of susceptibility genes, placing OA into the oligogenic, multifactorial class of common diseases. A similar study performed by the same group on 135 monozygotic and 277 dizygotic female twin pairs calculated a heritability value of 58% for primary hip OA (MacGregor et al., 2000). The original twin study was soon followed by a Finnish twin study, which examined both male (577 monozygotic and 1180 dizygotic) and female (836 monozygotic and 1502 dizygotic) twin pairs, with OA at any joint group being used as the criterion for disease presence (Kaprio et al., 1996). A heritability value of 44% was obtained for females, which is comparable to that in the two UK studies. However, there was no genetic component in males, with a concordance of 0.34 in monozygotic male twin pairs and 0.38 in dizygotic male twin pairs. This study therefore suggests that genes play a more significant role in female OA. A very informative review discusses the power and utility of twin studies, with particular reference to OA (MacGregor and Spector, 1999).

Sibling Risk

Chitnavis et al. (1997) estimated the sibling relative risk (λ_s) of severe OA, with patients ascertained through the need for joint replacement surgery. They examined 402 UK patients who had undergone total hip replacement (THR) or total knee replacement (TKR) for primary OA and compared the prevalence of THR or TKR in 1171 siblings and 376 spouses. The spouses acted as controls, and λ_s values of 1.9 for THR and 4.8 for TKR were calculated. The combined λ_s for joint replacement was 2.3, which translated into a heritability of severe OA of 27%.

In a second UK study, the investigators identified 392 probands who had undergone THR and compared the frequency of hip OA between 604 siblings to the probands and 1718 unrelated, matched control individuals drawn from the same population (Lanyon et al., 2000). Again, the frequency of OA was greater in the siblings than in the controls (9.4% vs. 1.1%), translating into the siblings being 9.8 times more likely to develop severe hip OA. These investigators also stratified their data by sex. The frequency of THR for female siblings was 9% and for male siblings, 10%. Both frequencies were much greater than the frequencies in stratified controls (1.3% for female controls and 0.8% for male controls). Comparison of female siblings with female controls indicated that female siblings were 7.7 times more likely to develop severe OA. Male cases were 14.4 times more likely than male controls to develop severe OA. This result, of a high risk to male siblings, does not support the results of the Finnish twin study discussed above, which reported that genetic susceptibility may play little or no role in male OA (Kaprio et al., 1996).

In a very comprehensive sibling risk study performed in Iceland, investigators identified 2713 cases who had undergone THR for hip OA (Ingvarsson et al., 2000). Siblings to these cases were found to be three times more likely to require THR than matched population controls. As well as estimating sibling risk, the investigators carried out three additional statistical tests to quantify the hip OA genetic component in Iceland: *(1)* they determined the degree of familial clustering of the 2713 hip patients, *(2)* they estimated the minimum number of founders who could account for the genealogy of these patients and compared this to the average number of founders for their controls, and *(3)* they determined the overall degree of relatedness between these patients and compared this with the relatedness between Icelandic controls. Each of these three tests demonstrated that the cases were more related to each other than would be expected if no OA-predisposing genetic component had segregated in them. The results support the existence of a significant genetic component to the familial aggregation of hip OA in Iceland.

Hirsch et al. (1998) also analyzed aggregation of OA in families, although they did not ascertain families by the presence of OA but instead determined sibling correlations for OA in a cohort of patients previously collected for an aging project (Baltimore Longitudinal Study on Aging). From this cohort, they identified 167 nuclear families with hand radiographic data, 157 with knee radiographic data, and 148 with hand and knee radiographic data. Their analysis revealed aggregation of OA, particularly in families with severe and/or polyarticular disease.

With evidence for a genetic component to OA accumulating, Felson et al. (1998) performed a segregation analysis to elucidate the nature of the transmission of the genetic component. They examined a cohort of 337 nuclear families, with each family containing both parents and at least one offspring (average age of offspring 54 years). Parent–parent, parent–offspring, and sibling–sibling correlations for primary OA were then determined by hand and knee radiography. This analysis revealed no correlation for spouse pairs but clear correlations for parent–offspring and sibling–sibling pairs, suggesting that an OA genetic component is transmitted from parents to offspring. Mothers appeared more likely to transmit OA to their offspring than fathers. For example, the mother–daughter and mother–son correlations were 0.206 and 0.158, respectively, whereas the father–daughter and father–son correlations were 0.084 and 0.007, respectively. As the investigators reported, these results may support the Kaprio et al. (1996) finding of greater female heritability for OA.

Not all epidemiological studies have confirmed a genetic component to hip and knee OA. Bijkerk et al. (1999) identified 118 Dutch probands with radiographic OA at several joint sites and 257 siblings to the probands. They compared the joint-specific frequency of OA between probands and siblings and noted a high level of correlation for hand OA (heritability 0.56) but no correlation for knee or hip OA.

PATHOPHYSIOLOGY: BIOLOGICAL BASIS OF GENETIC SUSCEPTIBILITY

There are two simplistic mechanisms that one could apply to help explain how primary OA develops. The first is that the disease simply results from excessive and/or repetitive force being applied to a joint, which over time causes loss of cartilage. Susceptible individuals are those whose cartilage is less able to withstand these forces, and susceptibility loci may therefore be genes that encode structural proteins of the cartilage extracellular matrix (i.e., the cartilage collagen and proteoglycan genes) or genes that encode proteins which are responsible for the correct alignment of the joint or of the [illegible]ies associated with the joint. The second mechanism is [illegible] results from a shift in the catabolic/anabolic balance responsible for maintaining the integrity of the cartilage and/or the underlying bone. This shift may result from a change in the activity or prevalence of nonstructural proteins, such as growth factors, cytokines, matrix metalloproteinases, or the receptors for these three classes of protein. Obviously, there is significant scope for these two mechanisms to overlap.

The idea that hormonal and/or growth factors play a role in OA development has gathered momentum over recent years. This has partially resulted from the epidemiological findings highlighted earlier, such as the increased prevalence of the disease in females, particularly after menopause. The role of estrogen has come under particular scrutiny, with hormone replacement therapy (HRT) providing an opportunity to measure the effect of estrogen on OA progression. Dennison et al. (1998) examined 413 women with primary OA of the hip and an equal number of female controls, and their results suggest that long-term HRT does reduce the risk of disease development. A mechanism that Dennison et al. (1998) proposed, through which HRT could mediate an OA-protective effect, is slowing of subchondral bone remodeling. An increase in subchondral bone density and mass (sclerosis) does precede OA in some cases, and this greater density of underlying bone may reduce the ability of the joint to transmit mechanical force, increasing the likelihood of cartilage breakdown (Lane and Nevitt, 1994; Karvonen et al., 1998). This increase in subchondral bone mass may be one of the factors that accounts for the apparent inverse relationship between OA and osteoporosis, a disease of low bone density (Sambrook and Naganathan, 1997). This inverse relationship may be particularly insightful with regard to OA genetics since a number of genes have already been identified that are associated with osteoporosis susceptibility, including the estrogen receptor gene (Kobayashi et al., 1996): different alleles at these loci may predispose to OA. This idea is so persuasive that osteoporosis susceptibility loci have been investigated as possible OA susceptibility loci in several of the genetic association tests performed on this disease (see below).

GENE IDENTIFICATION

Association Analysis

Several OA association analyses have been performed on candidate genes using case-control cohorts (Table 32–2). The candidates targeted have tended to be genes encoding structural proteins of the extracellular matrix of cartilage and bone or genes implicated in the regulation of bone density and mass.

Of the structural genes, *COL2A1* (12q12–13.1) has received the most attention. There are two principal reasons for this: *(1) COL2A1* encodes type II collagen, the most abundant protein of articular cartilage, and *(2) COL2A1* has been implicated in several osteo-chondrodysplasias (Table 32–1) and in some rare cases of familial OA (see below). In the first *COL2A1* association study, an intragenic dimorphism was associated with disease in 86 British cases with radiographic OA (Hull and Pope, 1989). Using different *COL2A1* variants from the British study, association was not detected in a Finnish cohort of 90 cases and 48 controls (Vikkula et al., 1993a) or a Belgian cohort of 75 cases and 239 controls (Aerssens et al., 1998), but association was detected in a Dutch cohort of 123 cases and 697 controls (Meulenbelt et al., 1999). Unlike the previous studies, Meulenbelt et al. (1999) constructed haplotypes for the markers they tested, thus enhancing their power to detect an association. Loughlin et al. (1995) approached the possibility of *COL2A1* encoding OA susceptibility in a different manner, by testing for a reduction in expression of the gene in OA cartilage. Their logic was that if severe mutations result in osteochondrodysplasia, then less severe mutations may account for primary OA. Knee cartilage biopsies were collected from individuals who had undergone TKR for primary OA. Twenty-seven cases (7 men and 20 women, all >47 years of age at time of surgery) were heterozygous for one or more exonic dimorphisms in the *COL2A1* gene. These dimorphisms were used to compare the allelic output of *COL2A1* mRNA extracted from the cartilage biopsies. Three of the 27 cases (two women, one man) did demonstrate differential allelic expression. All three cases were heterozygous for a *MaeII* restriction dimorphism in exon 50 of *COL2A1*, and in each case it was the rare *MaeII*(−) allele that demonstrated reduced expression. This suggested that these three cases may have inherited a common mutant allele. To test this, the frequency of the *MaeII*(−) allele was measured in a cohort of 76 British cases with hand OA and 73 controls. The *MaeII*(−) allele was at an elevated frequency in the cases ($p < 0.05$). However, Meulenbelt et al. (1999) observed no significant difference in the frequency of this allele between Dutch cases with radiographic OA and matched controls.

Of the genes implicated in regulating bone mass and density, the *vitamin D receptor* (*VDR*, 12q12–13.1) gene has received the most attention. Alleles of this gene were associated with low bone density several years ago (Morrison et al., 1994), although there is some controversy as to whether this locus does encode susceptibility for osteoporosis (Eisman, 1995; Peacock, 1995). Two groups have reported association of *VDR* with OA. Keen et al. (1997) compared the allele frequencies and genotypes of a *VDR* intragenic TaqI dimorphism between 82 women with primary radiographic knee OA and 269 female controls, all collected in the United Kingdom. An allele of the TaqI dimorphism was associated with disease in a codominant or dominant pattern. Uitterlinden et al. (1997) compared the allele, genotype, and haplotype frequencies for three intragenic dimorphisms, one of which was the TaqI dimorphism used by Keen et al. (1997), in 405 Dutch males and 441 Dutch females stratified by the presence of osteophytes, joint-space narrowing, and a high Kellgren and Lawrence score. Their analysis supported association of *VDR* with OA, particularly OA characterized by the presence of osteophytes. This association was not restricted to one sex. The TaqI allele that was associated in the Keen et al. (1997) study was on the haplotype that was associated in the Uitterlinden et al. (1997) study. Two groups, however, have failed to detect association of the *VDR* with primary OA. Geusens et al. (1997) compared the allele and genotype frequencies of a *VDR* intragenic BsmI dimorphism (one of the three dimorphisms used by Uitterlinden et al. 1997) in females with spinal OA and in females without disease, drawn from a group of 212. No significant differences were detected. Aerssens et al. (1998) compared the allele and genotype frequencies of the BsmI dimorphism between 75 female OA cases who had undergone THR for primary OA and 239 female controls, all selected from the Belgian population. Again, no significant differences were observed. The Geusens et al. (1997) and Aerssens et al. (1998) studies did not involve knee OA cases, so it is possible that the *VDR* associations detected by Keen et al. (1997) and Uitterlinden et al. (1997) are knee-specific. Loughlin et al. (2000c) examined knee OA

Table 32–2. Osteoarthritis (OA) Association Studies

Locus	Polypeptide	Chromosome	Polymorphism	OA Type	Result[a]	Reference
COL1A1	α1 chain type I collagen	17q21.3–22	Intragenic dimorphism[b]	Female hip	No association	Aerssens et al. (1998)
			Intragenic dimorphism	Female spine	No association	Geusens et al. (1997)
			Intragenic dimorphism[b]	Hip and knee (both sexes)	No association	Loughlin et al. (2000c)
COL1A2	α2 chain type I collagen	7q21.3–22	Intragenic dimorphism[c]	Female spine	No association	Geusens et al. (1997)
COL2A1	α1 chain type II collagen	12q12–13.1	Intragenic dimorphism[c]	Female hip	No association	Aerssens et al. (1998)
			Intragenic dimorphism[c] and extragenic VNTR[d]	generalized and hand	No association	Vikkula et al. (1993a)
			Four intragenic dimorphisms[c]	Female, more than one joint	Associated	Hull and Pope (1989)
			Three intragenic dimorphisms and an extragenic VNTR[d]	Knees, hips, hands, and spine (both sexes)	Associated	Meulenbelt et al. (1999)
			Intragenic dimorphism	Hand (both sexes)	Associated	Loughlin et al. (1995)
COL9A1	α1 chain type IX collagen	6q12–13	Intragenic microsatellite	Knees, hips, and hands (both sexes)	Associated (female)	van Duijn et al. (1998)
COL11A2	α2 chain type XI collagen	6p21.3	Extragenic microsatellites	Knees, hips, and hands (both sexes)	No association	van Duijn et al. (1998)
AGC1	Aggrecan	15q26	Intragenic VNTR	Hand and knee (male)	Associated (hand)	Horton et al. (1998)
CRTM	Matrillin-1	1p35	Intragenic microsatellite[e]	Hip and knee (both sexes)	Associated (male hip)	Meulenbelt et al. (1997b)
			Intragenic microsatellite[e]	Hip and knee (both sexes)	No association	Loughlin et al. (2000a)
CRTL1	Cartilage link protein	5q13–14.1	Intragenic microsatellite	Hip and knee (both sexes)	No association	Meulenbelt et al. (1997b)
VDR	Vitamin D receptor	12q12–13.1	Intragenic dimorphism[f]	Female hip	No association	Aerssens et al. (1998)
			Three intragenic dimorphisms[f]	Knee (both sexes)	Associated	Uitterlinden et al. (1997)
			Intragenic dimorphism[f]	Female knee	Associated	Keen et al. (1997)
			Intragenic dimorphism[f]	Female spine	No association	Geusens et al. (1997)
			Intragenic dimorphism[f]	Hip and knee (both sexes)	No association	Loughlin et al. (2000c)
ER	Estrogen receptor	6q22.3–23.1	Two intragenic dimorphisms[g]	Generalized nodal (female)	Associated	Ushiyama et al. (1998)
			Intragenic dimorphism[g]	Hip and knee (both sexes)	No association	Loughlin et al. (2000c)
IGF-1	Insulin-like growth factor-I	12q21.3	Intragenic microsatellite	Hand, hip, knee, and spine (both sexes)	Associated	Meulenbelt et al. (1998)
HLA	Human leukocyte antigen cluster	6p21.3	Antigenic variation	Generalized nodal (both sexes)	Associated	Pattrick et al. (1989)
TGF-β1	Transforming growth factor-β1	19q13.1–13.3	Intragenic dimorphism	Female spine	Associated	Yamada (2000)
IL-1β	Interleukin-1β	2q13	Intragenic dimorphism	Hip or knee (both sexes)	Associated	Moos et al. (2000)
IL-1RN	Interleukin-1 receptor antagonist	2q13	Intragenic VNTR	Hip or knee (both sexes)	Associated	Moos et al. (2000)

[a]Associated if $p \leq 0.05$.
[b]Aerssens et al. (1998) and Loughlin et al. (2000c) examined the same *COL1A1* dimorphism.
[c]Aerssens et al. (1998) and Vikkula et al. (1993a) examined the same *COL2A1 PvuII* dimorphism, which was not one of the four dimorphisms examined by Hull and Pope (1989).
[d]Same variable number tandem repeat marker examined in both studies, but Meulenbelt et al. (1999) detected a greater number of alleles than Vikkula et al. (1993a).
[e]Same microsatellite marker examined in both studies.
[f]The three Uitterlinden et al. (1997) *VDR* dimorphisms affect *BsmI*, *ApaI*, and *TaqI* sites. Keen et al. (1997) and Loughlin et al. (2000c) examined the *TaqI* dimorphism; Geusens et al. (1997) and Aerssens et al. (1998) examined the *BsmI* dimorphism.
[g]Ushiyama et al. (1997) and Loughlin et al. (2000c) examined the same two *ER* dimorphisms.

cases as well as hip cases in a cohort of 371 cases and 369 controls ascertained in the United Kingdom. In their female knee cases, they observed an elevation in the frequency of heterozygotes for the TaqI dimorphism, which was the pattern reported by Keen et al. (1997). However, this increase was not significant ($p > 0.05$). Since the *VDR* and *COL2A1* genes are tightly linked (<750 kb apart), associations to 12q12–13.1 could be to either locus or to both loci simultaneously (Uitterlinden et al., 2000).

COL1A1 (17q21.3–22) encodes for the α1 chain of type I collagen, which is the major collagen of bone and is responsible for conferring tensile strength to this tissue. *COL1A1* has been associated with a low bone density phenotype (Grant et al., 1996); and of the three OA case-control studies so far performed (Geusens et al., 1997; Aerssens et al., 1998; Loughlin et al., 2000c), only Loughlin et al (2000c) reported some evidence supporting association of *COL1A1* with OA. This association was restricted to female cases but was not significant ($p > 0.05$) when corrected for the multiple comparisons performed.

The positive association reported for *COL9A1* by van Duijn et al. (1998) is given credence by two mouse models that highlight the critical role of type IX collagen in cartilage integrity and demonstrate that mutations in *COL9A1* can result in an OA phenotype (Nakata et al., 1993; Fassler et al., 1994; Hagg et al., 1997). Type IX collagen is a heterotrimeric protein composed of $\alpha1$(IX), $\alpha2$(IX), and $\alpha3$(IX) polypeptide chains, which are encoded by the *COL9A1*, *COL9A2*, and *COL9A3* genes, respectively (Ayad et al., 1998). Type IX is a quantitatively minor cartilage collagen that decorates the type II collagen fibrils, and this interaction regulates the growth of the type II fibril. In the first mouse model, a truncated form of *col9a1* resulted in a mild osteochondrodysplasia with OA (Nakata et al., 1993). In the second model, a *col9a1* knockout mouse had no congenital abnormality but developed severe OA that was comparable in timing and pathology to human primary OA (Fassler et al., 1994; Hagg et al., 1997).

In more recent years, investigators have started to investigate genes that encode proteins involved in the homeostatic balance between cartilage breakdown and cartilage maintenance. These have included the catabolic cytokine interleukin (IL)-1β, its inhibitor IL-1RN, and the anabolic cytokine (transforming growth factor-β1) (Moos et al., 2000; Yamada, 2000). This change in emphasis may reflect the ambiguous data that have arisen from extensive association analyses of genes encoding structural proteins of the cartilage extracellular matrix and the realization that an imbalance in cartilage metabolism may be where a significant proportion of OA susceptibility resides (Goldring 2000a,b; Pelletier et al., 2001).

It is apparent from Table 32–2 that positive associations are not always confirmed in follow-up studies. A number of factors could account for this: *(1)* the original positive finding represents a Type I error, possibly arising because the cohort studied was too small for a reliable inference of association; *(2)* the negative follow-up study represents a Type II error, possibly arising because this cohort was too small and therefore lacked power; *(3)* there are differences in the populations being compared, such as ethnic differences and differences in the disease phenotype (i.e., comparing hip OA with knee OA or radiographic OA with end-stage OA); *(4)* the same markers were not examined when trying to confirm the positive finding. To overcome these problems, large cohorts (>1000) of well-characterized cases will have to be collected, suitable for stratification analysis by, e.g., sex and site of disease. There will have to be consistency in the markers investigated. Several markers within each candidate gene should be examined and haplotypes constructed to extract more information and facilitate the investigation of rare alleles.

Association tests in the form of case-control cohorts have been criticized for the apparent high level of Type I errors that arise from population differences between cases and controls. This can be partly alleviated by first testing for stratification and then factoring any differences in to the association test (Pritchard and Rosenberg, 1999; Pritchard et al., 2000). Alternatively, an analysis that has matched familial controls, such as the transmission disequilibrium test (TDT), can be employed. Some groups have already identified large numbers of nuclear families that have offspring with OA and are therefore suitable for conventional TDT analysis (Felson et al., 1998). However, since primary OA is a late-onset disease, parents of probands are rarely available to participate in a study. Nevertheless, robust adaptations to the TDT that use unaffected siblings as controls are being developed, and these tests could be used in the future (Spielman and Ewens, 1998).

Linkage Analysis

Parametric linkage analysis was originally performed on a small number of families in which OA segregates as a Mendelian trait. These families are rare, and the majority of them have a mild osteochondrodysplasia which predisposes to precocious disease. They are therefore examples of secondary OA. The locus that is consistently linked in these families is the type II collagen gene *COL2A1* (Knowlton et al., 1990; Ala-Kokko et al., 1990; Vikkula et al., 1993b).

There is a report of one large family with primary OA (knee, hand, and spine) in four generations, with onset in the third to fifth decades and no evidence of an osteochondrodysplasia (Meulenbelt et al., 1997a). The transmittance of OA in this family appears to be autosomal dominant, and 10 candidate genes have been excluded as the mutant locus, including *COL2A1*, the type IX collagen gene *COL9A2*, the type XI collagen genes *COL11A1* and *COL11A2*, and the cartilage oligomeric matrix protein gene *COMP*. All of these genes have previously been implicated in Mendelian osteochondrodysplasias (Table 32–1). Roby et al. (1999) also excluded several candidate genes in a pedigree of Dutch origin in which severe early-onset hip OA (associated with severe hip dysplasia) segregates as an autosomal dominant trait. The group subsequently mapped the disease to chromosome 4q35, a region that lacks any known strong candidates.

The rarity of families in which primary OA segregates as a Mendelian trait combined with the uncertainty over the absence of an osteochondrodysplasia segregating in these families has promoted the investigation of affected sibling pairs by model-free linkage analysis. Three published reports have targeted candidate genes as susceptibility loci in affected pairs. Loughlin et al. (1994) tested for linkage of the *COL2A1* gene, the cartilage link protein gene *CRTL1*, and the cartilage matrix protein gene *CRTM* in a UK cohort of 38 affected sibling pairs with generalized OA. None of the three genes was positive for linkage, but the cohort size was small and, therefore, had the power to detect only a major effect. Baldwin et al. (1998) also targeted *COL2A1* using an unspecified number of affected pairs and did not detect linkage. Mustafa et al. (2000) targeted a number of genes encoding cartilage structural proteins using a cohort of 481 affected sibling pairs ascertained by joint replacement surgery for OA (hip, knee, or hip and knee). Suggestive linkage was obtained to the *COL9A1* gene in female affected pairs who were concordant for hip OA, with a LOD score of 2.3 ($p = 0.00053$).

Choosing candidate genes for association or linkage analysis is obviously dependent on assumptions regarding the pathophysiology of the disease. These assumptions may be inaccurate or uninformative and are therefore prone to bias and error. An alternative is to make no assumptions and to carry out a scan of the whole genome using anonymous, evenly spaced markers. Three such anonymous genome scans have been performed on OA-affected sibling-pair cohorts, ascertained radiographically (Wright et al., 1996; Leppävuori et al., 1999) and through joint replacement surgery (Chapman et al., 1999). Wright et al. (1996) have so far reported their findings only for chromosome 2q. They genotyped 12 microsatellite markers in 44 generalized nodal families ascertained in the United Kingdom, which were composed of 66 affected pairs. Three of their 12 markers demonstrated linkage at $p \leq 0.05$ (D2S326, D2S126, and GCG). Leppävuori et al. (1999) performed a genome-wide scan using 302 microsatellites on 27 Finnish families, each composed of at least two affected siblings with distal interphalangeal OA. Eight regions supported linkage with parametric LOD scores >1.0 on chromosomes 2q, 4q, 7p, 8q, 9p, 9q, 10p, and 12q. The X centromeric region also supported linkage but at a lower level of significance. Typing of these regions in additional family members supported linkage to 2q, 4q, 7p, and Xcen. The Finnish 2q linkage, which maps to 2q11–q24, showed only slight overlap with the linkage reported by Wright et al. (1996), which maps to 2q23–q35. The same 481 UK families that Mustafa et al. (2000) used in their candidate screen were subjected to a genome-wide linkage scan by Chapman et al. (1999). In a first stage of 272 microsatellite markers and 297 families, 16 microsatellites supported linkage at $p \leq 0.05$ (D2S202, D3S1266, D4S231, D4S415, D6S260, D6S273, D6S286, D6S281, D7S669, D7S530, D11S907, D11S903, D11S901, D17S807, D17S789, and DXS1068). These markers were then taken through to a second stage of an additional 184 families. This two-stage approach confirmed suggestive linkage to markers on 2q (D2S202) and 11q (D11S907, D11S903, and D11S901), with maximum multipoint LOD scores (MLS) of 1.2 on 2q and 3.1 on 11q. The linkage data for 2q and 11q from this scan were subsequently stratified into six strata: *(1)* female affected pairs, *(2)* male affected pairs, *(3)* hip-only affected pairs, *(4)* knee-only affected pairs, *(5)* female affected pairs who were concordant for hip but not knee OA, and *(6)* male affected pairs who were concordant for hip but not knee OA. This stratification highlighted that the linkage to 2q was principally accounted for by affected pairs with hip OA, with an MLS of 2.2 (Loughlin et al., 2000b), while the 11q linkage was principally accounted for by female hip pairs, with an MLS of 3.0 (Chapman et al., 1999). Stratification of the remaining markers from the first stage of the UK genome scan revealed additional regions of suggestive linkage on chromosomes 4q (MLS of 3.9 in female hip pairs), 6q (MLS of 2.9 in hip pairs) and 16 (MLS of 2.1 in female hip pairs) (Loughlin et al., 1999). Intriguingly, the UK linkage on 2q overlaps with both the Wright et al. (1996) and the Leppävuori et al. (1999) linkages.

Overall, linkage analysis of primary OA families and of affected sibling pairs has so far identified regions of suggestive linkage on chromosomes 2q, 4q, 6q, 7p, 11q, 16, and X. Some of these chromosomes have given positive results in more than one study, such as 2q and 4q, and some contain known candidate genes that merit further analysis, such as *COL9A1* on 6q. Further analysis of these regions will involve the typing of additional families combined with finer linkage mapping. Confirmed regions can then be subjected to comprehensive association analysis.

CLINICAL APPLICATION AND RISK ASSESSMENT OF GENETICS INFORMATION

The genetic analysis of primary OA is still in its early stages, and no genetic breakthroughs have yet transferred to the clinic. For some of the monogenic osteochondrodysplasias, which often have severe OA as a secondary phenotypic component, identification of the mutant loci has enabled presymptomatic diagnosis (Newman et al., 2000). For complex traits like primary OA, the relationship between DNA variant and disease will not be as clear-cut. Even so, identification of causal variants may assist in risk assessment. One novel application of the secondary forms of the disease has been to assess the effectiveness of biological markers of cartilage breakdown as predictors of disease development. Investigation of biological markers, which has gathered momentum for the rheumatological diseases as a whole (Poole, 1994), can aid clinical diagnosis and be used to determine the efficacy of therapeutic interventions. Bleasel et al. (1999) collected a group of individuals with secondary OA caused by a *COL2A1* mutation and measured the serum levels of two markers of cartilage breakdown and two markers of cartilage repair. Their results point to elevated levels of the cartilage breakdown markers COMP and keratan sulfate in OA cases and highlight the potential utility of these markers as prognostic tools.

ACKNOWLEDGMENTS

This work was supported by the Arthritis Research Campaign and The Wellcome Trust.

REFERENCES

Aerssens J, Dequeker J, Peeters J, Breemans S, Boonen S: Lack of association between osteoarthritis of the hip and gene polymorphisms of *VDR*, *COL1A1* and *COL2A1* in postmenopausal women. Arthritis Rheum 1998; 41:1946–1950.

Aigner T, Bertling W, Stoss H, Weseloh G, von der Mark K: Independent expression of fibril-forming collagens I, II and III in chondrocytes of human osteoarthritic cartilage. J Clin Invest 1993; 91:829–837.

Ala-Kokko L, Baldwin CT, Moskowitz RW, Prockop DJ: Single base mutation in the type II procollagen gene (*COL2A1*) as a cause of primary osteoarthritis associated with a mild chondrodysplasia. Proc Natl Acad Sci USA 1990; 87:6565–6568.

Andrew LJ, Brancolini V, delaPena LS, Devoto M, Caeiro F, Marchegiani R, Reginato A, Gaucher A, Netter P, Gillet P, et al.: Refinement of the chromosome 5p locus for familial calcium pyrophosphate dihydrate deposition disease. Am J Hum Genet 1999; 64:136–145.

Ayad S, Boot-Handford RP, Humphries MJ, Kadler KE, Shuttleworth CA: The Extracellular Matrix Facts Book, 2nd ed. London: Academic Press, 1998.

Baldwin C, Joost O, Chaisson C, McAlindon T, Farrer L, Ordovas J, Schaefer E, Levy D, Myers R, Felson D: The type II collagen/vitamin D receptor locus and osteoarthritis: the Framingham Osteoarthritis Study. [abstract]. Am J Hum Genet 1998; 63(Suppl):1616.

Baldwin CT, Farrer LA, Adair R, Dharmavaram R, Jimenez S, Anderson L: Linkage of early-onset osteoarthritis and chondrocalcinosis to human chromosome 8q. Am J Hum Genet 1995; 56:692–697.

Bijkerk C, Houwing-Duistermaat JJ, Valkenburg HA, Meulenbelt I, Hofman A, Breedveld FC, Pols HAP, van Duijn CM, Slagboom PE: Heritabilities of radiological osteoarthritis in peripheral joints and of disc degeneration of the spine. Arthritis Rheum 1999; 42:1729–1735.

Bleasel JF, Poole AR, Heinegard D, Saxne T, Holderbaum D, Ionescu M, Jones P, Moskowitz RW: Changes in serum cartilage marker levels indicate altered cartilage metabolism in families with the osteoarthritis-related type II collagen gene *COL2A1* mutation. Arthritis Rheum 1999; 42:39–45.

Chapman K, Mustafa Z, Irven CM, Carr AJ, Clipsham K, Smith A, Chitnavis J, Sinsheimer JS, Bloomfield VA, McCartney M, et al.: Osteoarthritis-susceptibility locus on chromosome 11q, detected by linkage. Am J Hum Genet 1999; 65:167–174.

Chapman KL, Mortier GR, Chapman K, Loughlin J, Grant ME, Briggs MD: Mutations in the region encoding the von Willebrand factor A domain of matrilin-3 are associated with multiple epiphyseal dysplasia. Nat Genet 2001; 28:393–396.

Chitnavis J, Sinsheimer JS, Clipsham K, Loughlin J, Sykes B, Burge PD, Carr AJ: Genetic influences in end-stage osteoarthritis. Sibling risks of hip and knee replacement for idiopathic osteoarthritis. J Bone Joint Surg Br 1997; 79:660–664.

Creamer P, Hochberg MC: Osteoarthritis. Lancet 1997; 350:503–508.

Dennison EM, Arden NK, Kellingray S, Croft P, Coggon D, Cooper C: Hormone replacement therapy, other reproductive variables and symptomatic hip osteoarthritis in elderly white women: a case-control study. Br J Rheumatol 1998; 37:1198–1202.

Eisman JA: Vitamin D receptor gene alleles and osteoporosis: an affirmative view. J Bone Miner Res 1995; 10:1289–1293.

Fam AG: Calcium pyrophosphate crystal deposition disease and other crystal deposition diseases. Curr Opin Rheumatol 1992; 4:574–582.

Fassler R, Schnegelsberg PNJ, Dausman J, Shinya T, Muragaki Y, McCarthy MT, Olsen BR, Jaenisch R: Mice lacking α1(IX) collagen develop noninflammatory degenerative joint disease. Proc Natl Acad Sci USA 1994; 91:5070–5074.

Felson DT, Chaisson CE: Understanding the relationship between body weight and osteoarthritis. Baillieres Clin Rheumatol 1997; 11:671–681.

Felson DT, Couropmitree NN, Chaisson CE, Hannan MT, Zhang Y, McAlindon TE, LaValley M, Levy D, Myers RH: Evidence for a Mendelian gene in a segregation analysis of generalized radiographic osteoarthritis. Arthritis Rheum 1998; 41:1064–1071.

Felson DT, Zhang Y: An update on the epidemiology of knee and hip osteoarthritis with a view to prevention. Arthritis Rheum 1998; 41:1343–1355.

Geusens P, Vandevyver C, Cassiman JJ, Philippaerts L, Vanhoof J, Mertens J, Raus J: Osteoarthritis of the spine: association with bone density in the hip, not with gene polymorphism of the vitamin D receptor or collagen-1. [abstract]. J Bone Miner Res 1997; 12(Suppl):F582.

Goldring MB: Osteoarthritis and cartilage: the role of cytokines. Curr Rheumatol Rep 2000a; 2:459–465.

Goldring MB: The role of the chondrocyte in osteoarthritis. Arthritis Rheum 2000b; 43:1916–1926.

Grant SFA, Reid DM, Blake G, Herd R, Fogelman I, Ralston SH: Reduced bone density and osteoporosis associated with a polymorphic Sp1 binding site in the *collagen type I $\alpha 1$* gene. Nat Genet 1996; 14:203–205.

Griffith AJ, Sprunger LK, SirkoOsadsa DA, Tiller GE, Meisler MH, Warman ML: Marshall syndrome associated with a splicing defect at the *COL11A1* locus. Am J Hum Genet 1998; 62:816–823.

Hagg R, Hedbom E, Mollers U, Aszodi A, Fassler R, Bruckner P: Absence of the $\alpha 1$(IX) chain leads to a functional knock-out of the entire collagen IX protein in mice. J Biol Chem 1997; 272:20650–20654.

Hirsch R, Lethbridge-Cejku M, Hanson R, Scott WW, Reichle R, Plato CC, Tobin JD, Hochberg MC: Familial aggregation of osteoarthritis—data from the Baltimore Longitudinal Study on Aging. Arthritis Rheum 1998; 41:1227–1232.

Ho AM, Johnson MD, Kingsley DM: Role of the mouse *ank* gene in control of tissue calcification and arthritis. Science 2000; 289:265–270.

Holden P, Canty EG, Mortier GR, Zabel B, Spranger J, Carr A, Grant ME, Loughlin J, Briggs MD: Identification of novel pro-$\alpha 2$ (IX) collagen gene mutations in two families with distinctive oligo-epiphyseal forms of multiple epiphyseal dysplasia. Am J Hum Genet 1999; 65:31–38.

Horton WE, Lethbridge Cejku M, Hochberg MC, Balakir R, Precht P, Plato CC, Tobin JD, Meek L, Doege K: An association between an aggrecan polymorphic allele and bilateral hand osteoarthritis in elderly white men: data from the Baltimore Longitudinal Study of Aging (BLSA). Osteoarthritis Cartilage 1998; 6:245–251.

Hughes AE, McGibbon D, Woodward E, Dixey J, Doherty M: Localisation of a gene for chondrocalcinosis to chromosome 5p. Hum Mol Genet 1995; 4:1225–1228.

Hull R, Pope FM: Osteoarthritis and cartilage collagen genes. Lancet 1989; i:1337–1338.

Ingvarsson T, Stefánsson SE, Hallgrímsdóttir IB, Frigge ML, Jónsson H, Gulcher J, Jónsson H, Ragnarsson JI, Lohmander LS, Stefánsson K: The inheritance of hip osteoarthritis in Iceland. Arthritis Rheum 2000; 43:2785–2792.

Inoue K, Wicart P, Kawasaki T, Huang J, Ushiyama T, Hukuda S, Courpied J-P: Prevalence of hip osteoarthritis and acetabular dysplasia in French and Japanese adults. Rheumatology 2000; 39:745–748.

Jones A, Doherty M: ABC of rheumatology. Osteoarthritis. BMJ 1995; 310:457–460.

Kaprio J, Kujala UM, Peltonen L, Koskenvuo M: Genetic liability to osteoarthritis may be greater in women than men. BMJ 1996; 313:232.

Karvonen RL, Miller PR, Nelson DA, Granda JL, Fernandez-Madrid F: Periarticular osteoporosis in osteoarthritis of the knee. J Rheumatol 1998; 25:2187–2194.

Keen RW, Hart DJ, Lanchbury JS, Spector TD: Association of early osteoarthritis of the knee with a TaqI polymorphism of the vitamin D receptor gene. Arthritis Rheum 1997; 40:1444–1449.

Kellgren JH, Lawrence JS: The Epidemiology of Chronic Rheumatism. Oxford: Blackwell, 1963.

Kellgren JH, Lawrence JS, Bier F: Genetic factors in generalised osteo-arthrosis. Ann Rheum Dis 1963; 22:237–254.

Kellgren JH, Moore R: Generalized osteoarthritis and Heberden's nodes. Br J Med 1952; 1:181–187.

Knowlton RG, Katzenstein PL, Moskowitz RW, Weaver EJ, Malemud CJ, Pathria MN, Jimenez SA, Prockop DJ: Genetic linkage of a polymorphism in the type II procollagen gene (*COL2A1*) to primary osteoarthritis associated with mild chondrodysplasia. N Engl J Med 1990; 322:526–530.

Kobayashi S, Inoue S, Hosoi T, Ouchi Y, Shiraki M, Orimo H: Association of bone mineral density with polymorphism of the estrogen receptor gene. J Bone Miner Res 1996; 11:306–311.

Lane NE, Lin P, Christiansen L, Gore LR, Williams EN, Hochberg MC, Nevitt MC: Association of mild acetabular dysplasia with an increased risk of incident hip osteoarthritis in elderly white women. Arthritis Rheum 2000; 43:400–404.

Lane NE, Nevitt MC: Osteoarthritis and bone mass. J Rheumatol 1994; 21:1393–1396.

Lanyon P, Muir K, Doherty S, Doherty M: Assessment of a genetic contribution to osteoarthritis of the hip: sibling study. BMJ 2000; 321:1179–1183.

Leppävuori J, Kujala U, Kinnunen J, Kaprio J, Nissilä M, Heliövaara M, Klinger N, Partanen J, Terwilliger JD, Peltonen L: Genome scan for predisposing loci for distal interphalangeal joint osteoarthritis: evidence for a locus on 2q. Am J Hum Genet 1999; 65:1060–1067.

Loughlin J, Dowling B, Mustafa Z, Smith A, Sykes B, Chapman K: Analysis of the association of the matrillin-1 gene (*CRTM*) with osteoarthritis. Arthritis Rheum 2000a; 43:1423–1424.

Loughlin J, Irven C, Athanosou N, Carr A, Sykes B: Differential allelic expression of the type II collagen gene (*COL2A1*) in osteoarthritic cartilage. Am J Hum Genet 1995; 56:1186–1193.

Loughlin J, Irven C, Fergusson C, Sykes B: Sibling pair analysis shows no linkage of generalised osteoarthritis to the loci encoding type II collagen (COL2A1), cartilage link protein (CRTL1) or cartilage matrix protein (CRTM). Br J Rheumatol 1994; 33:1103–1106.

Loughlin J, Irven C, Mustafa Z, Briggs MD, Carr A, Lynch SA, Knowlton RG, Cohn DH, Sykes B: Identification of five novel mutations in the cartilage oligomeric matrix protein gene in pseudoachondroplasia and multiple epiphyseal dysplasia. Hum Mutat 1998; (Suppl 1):S10–S17.

Loughlin J, Mustafa Z, Irven C, Smith A, Carr AJ, Sykes B, Chapman K: Stratification analysis of an osteoarthritis genome screen—suggestive linkage to chromosomes 4, 6 and 16. Am J Hum Genet 1999; 65:1795–1798.

Loughlin J, Mustafa Z, Smith A, Irven C, Carr AJ, Clipsham K, Chitnavis J, Bloomfield VA, McCartney M, Cox O, et al.: Linkage analysis of chromosome 2q in osteoarthritis. Rheumatology 2000b; 39:377–381.

Loughlin J, Sinsheimer JS, Mustafa Z, Carr AJ, Clipsham K, Bloomfield VA, Chitnavis J, Bailey A, Sykes B, Chapman K: Association analysis of the vitamin D receptor gene, the type I collagen gene *COL1A1* and the estrogen receptor gene in idiopathic osteoarthritis. J Rheumatol 2000c; 27:779–784.

MacGregor AJ, Antoniades L, Matson M, Andrew T, Spector TD: The genetic contribution to radiographic hip osteoarthritis in women. Arthritis Rheum 2000; 43:2410–2416.

MacGregor AJ, Spector TD: Twins and the genetic architecture of osteoarthritis. Rheumatology 1999; 38:583–590.

Maetzel A, Makela M, Hawker G, Bombardier C: Osteoarthritis of the hip and knee and mechanical occupational exposure—a systematic overview of the evidence. J Rheumatol 1997; 24:1599–1607.

Meulenbelt I, Bijkerk C, Breedveld FC, Slagboom PE: Genetic linkage analysis of 14 candidate gene loci in a family with autosomal dominant osteoarthritis without dysplasia. J Med Genet 1997a; 34:1024–1027.

Meulenbelt I, Bijkerk C, de Wildt SCM, Miedema HS, Valkenburg HA, Breedveld FC, Pols HAP, Te Koppele JM, Sloos VFG, Hofman A, et al.: Investigation of the association of the *CRTM* and *CRTL1* genes with radiographically evident osteoarthritis in subjects from the Rotterdam study. Arthritis Rheum 1997b; 40:1760–1765.

Meulenbelt I, Bijkerk C, De Wildt SCM, Miedema HS, Breedveld FC, Pols HAP, Hofman A, Van Duijn CM, Slagboom PE: Haplotype analysis of three polymorphisms of the *COL2A1* gene and associations with generalised radiological osteoarthritis. Ann Hum Genet 1999; 63:393–400.

Meulenbelt I, Bijkerk C, Miedema HS, Breedveld FC, Hofman A, Valkenburg HA, Pols HAP, Slagboom PE, van Duijn CM: A genetic association study of the *IGF-1* gene and radiological osteoarthritis in a population-based cohort study (the Rotterdam study). Ann Rheum Dis 1998; 57:371–374.

Moos V, Rudwaleit M, Herzog V, Höhlig K, Sieper J, Müller B: Association of genotypes affecting the expression of interleukin-1β or interleukin-1 receptor antagonist with osteoarthritis. Arthritis Rheum 2000; 43:2417–2422.

Morrison NA, Qi JC, Tokita A, Kelly PJ, Crofts L, Nguyen TV, Sambrook PN, Eisman JA: Prediction of bone density from vitamin D receptor alleles. Nature 1994; 367:284–287.

Mundlos S, Olsen BR: Heritable diseases of the skeleton. Part II: Molecular insights into skeletal development—matrix components and their homeostasis. FASEB J 1997; 11:227–233.

Mustafa Z, Chapman K, Irven CM, Carr AJ, Clipsham K, Chitnavis J, Sinsheimer JS, Bloomfield VA, McCartney M, Cox O, et al.: Linkage analysis of candidate genes as susceptibility loci for osteoarthritis—suggestive linkage of *COL9A1* to female hip osteoarthritis. Rheumatology 2000; 39:299–306.

Nakata K, Ono K, Miyazaki J-I, Olsen BR, Muragaki Y, Adachi E, Yamamura K-I, Kimura T: Osteoarthritis associated with mild chondrodysplasia in transgenic mice expressing $\alpha 1$(IX) collagen chains with a central deletion. Proc Natl Acad Sci USA 1993; 90:2870–2874.

Newman B, Donnah D, Briggs MD: Molecular diagnosis is important to confirm suspected pseudoachondroplasia. J Med Genet 2000; 37:64–65.

Paassilta P, Lohiniva J, Annunen S, Bonaventure J, LeMerrer M, Pai L, AlaKokko L: *COL9A3:* a third locus for multiple epiphyseal dysplasia. Am J Hum Genet 1999; 64:1036–1044.

Pattrick M, Manhire A, Ward AM, Doherty M: HLA-A, B antigens and $\alpha 1$-antitrypsin phenotypes in nodal generalised osteoarthritis and erosive osteoarthritis. Ann Rheum Dis 1989; 48:470–475.

Peacock M: Vitamin D receptor gene alleles and osteoporosis: a contrasting view. J Bone Miner Res 1995; 10:1294–1297.

Pelletier J-P, Martel-Pelletier J, Abramson SB: Osteoarthritis, an inflammatory disease. Arthritis Rheum 2001; 44:1237–1247.

Poole AR: Immunochemical markers of joint inflammation, skeletal damage and repair: where are we now? Ann Rheum Dis 1994; 53:3–5.

Pritchard JK, Rosenberg NA: Use of unlinked genetic markers to detect population stratification in association studies. Am J Hum Genet 1999; 65:220–228.

Pritchard JK, Stephens M, Rosenberg NA, Donnelly P: Association mapping in structured populations. Am J Hum Genet 2000; 67:170–181.

Reichenberger E, Tiziani V, Watanabe S, Park L, Ueki Y, Santanna C, Baur ST, Shiang R, Grange DK, Beighton P, et al.: Autosomal dominant craniometaphyseal dysplasia is caused by mutations in the transmembrane protein ANK. Am J Hum Genet 2001; 68:1321–1326.

Roby P, Eyre S, Worthington J, Ramesar R, Cilliers H, Beighton P, Grant M, Wallis G: Autosomal dominant (Beukes) premature degenerative osteoarthropathy of the hip joint maps to an 11-cM region on chromosome 4q35. Am J Hum Genet 1999; 64:904–908.

Sambrook P, Naganathan V: What is the relationship between osteoarthritis and osteoporosis? Baillieres Clin Rheum 1997; 11:695–710.

Schumacher HR: Crystal-associated diseases. Curr Opin Rheumatol 2001; 13:219–220.
Spector TD, Cicuttini F, Baker J, Loughlin J, Hart D: Genetic influences on osteoarthritis in women: a twin study. BMJ 1996; 312:940–943.
Spector TD, Hart DJ, Byrne J, Harris PA, Dacre JE, Doyle DV: Definition of osteoarthritis of the knee for epidemiological studies. Ann Rheum Dis 1993; 52:790–794.
Spielman RS, Ewens WJ: A sibship test for linkage in the presence of association: the sib transmission/disequilibrium test. Am J Hum Genet 1998; 62:450–458.
Stecher RM: Heberden's nodes. Heredity in hypertrophic arthritis of the finger joints. Am J Med Sci 1941; 201:801.
Stecher RM: Heberden oration. Heberden's nodes: a clinical description of osteoarthritis of the finger joints. Ann Rheum Dis 1955; 14:1–10.
Toda Y, Toda T, Takemura S, Wada T, Morimoto T, Ogawa R: Change in body fat, but not body weight or metabolic correlates of obesity, is related to symptomatic relief of obese patients with knee osteoarthritis after a weight control program. J Rheumatol 1998; 25:2181–2186.
Uitterlinden AG, Burger H, Huang Q, Odding E, van Duijn CM, Hofman A, Birkenhager JC, van Leeuwen JPTM, Pols HAP: Vitamin D receptor genotype is associated with radiographic osteoarthritis at the knee. J Clin Invest 1997; 100:259–263.
Uitterlinden AG, Burger H, van Duijn CM, Huang Q, Hofman A, Birkenhäger JC, van Leeuwen JPTM, Pols HAP: Adjacent genes, for *COL2A1* and the *vitamin D receptor*, are associated with separate features of radiographic osteoarthritis of the knee. Arthritis Rheum 2000; 43:1456–1464.
Ushiyama T, Ueyama H, Inoue K, Nishioka J, Ohkubo I, Hukuda S: Estrogen receptor gene polymorphism and generalised osteoarthritis. J Rheumatol 1998; 25:134–137.
van Duijn CM, Bijkerk C, Houwing-Duistermaat JJ, Meulenbelt I, Valkenburg HA, Hofman A, Breedveld FC, Stijnen T, Pols HAP, Slagboom PE: A population-based study of the genetics of osteoarthritis. [abstract]. Am J Hum Genet 1998; 63(Suppl):1282.
Vikkula M, Nissila M, Hirvensalo E, Nuotio P, Palotie A, Aho K, Peltonen L: Multiallelic polymorphism of the cartilage collagen gene: no association with osteoarthrosis. Ann Rheum Dis 1993a; 52:762–764.
Vikkula M, Palotie A, Ritvaniemi P, Ott J, Ala-Kokko L, Sievers U, Aho K, Peltonen L: Early-onset osteoarthritis linked to the type II procollagen gene. Arthritis Rheum 1993b; 36:401–409.
Wright GD, Hughes AE, Regan M, Doherty M: Association of two loci on chromosome 2q with nodal osteoarthritis. Ann Rheum Dis 1996; 55:317–319.
Yamada Y: Association of a $Leu^{10} \rightarrow$ Pro polymorphism of the transforming growth factor-$\beta 1$ with genetic susceptibility to osteoporosis and spinal osteoarthritis. Mech Ageing Dev 2000; 116:113–123.
Yoshimura N, Cambell L, Hashimoto T, Kinoshita H, Okayasu T, Wilman C, Coggon D, Croft P, Cooper C: Acetabular dysplasia and hip osteoarthritis in Britain and Japan. Br J Rheumatol 1998; 37:1193–1197.

33 Common Disorders of Connective Tissue

REED E. PYERITZ

Virtually all somatic cells produce an extracellular matrix (ECM) of some sort. However, certain cells, such as osteoblasts, chondroblasts, and fibroblasts, produce enough matrix that it defines, in large part, the structure and function of the local environment. Examples of such tissues include bone, cartilage, ligaments, and teeth, which fall under the general class termed *connective tissue*. However, this classification unfairly emphasizes the "glue and scaffolding" functions to the detriment of an important array of other crucial functions (Table 33–1).

While the ECM is highly variable among organs, it is ubiquitous, and defects in one or another component may have effects limited or widespread in scope and effect. This results in many of the phenotypes associated with one or another ECM defect being pleiotropic. Even a brief review of the biochemistry and cell biology of the ECM is beyond the scope of this chapter, but a number of excellent general references exist (Koopman, 1997, 2000; Rimoin et al., 2002; Royce and Steinmann, 1993, 2001; Scriver et al., 2001). A wide array of macromolecules are involved, including the collagens, elastin, and fibrillins (examples of the fibrillar components), glycoproteins (e.g., fibronectin, entactin, osteopontin, and laminin), and proteoglycans (e.g., chondroitin sulfate and heparan sulfate, examples of ground substance). These components interact with each other and with receptors on cell surfaces in highly specific ways; e.g., osteopontin binds tightly to both the cell-surface receptor vitronectin and hydroxyapatite. Understanding how genetic alterations affect phenotype is complicated by several factors. Individual components may have multiple functions; e.g., fibrillin-1 is a major constituent of extracellular microfibrils, which form part of the elastic fiber, act as the ocular zonule, and serve as structural elements at the epidermal–dermal junction. Further diversity of phenotypes associated with mutations in single genes can result from alternative splicing or a single product being cleaved into molecules that have different functions.

DISEASE DEFINITION

Because the ECM is so complex, variable, and ubiquitous, it is not surprising that a great many disorders are due to primary or secondary defects of the ECM (Table 33–2). Most of the primary defects of the ECM are categorized as "heritable disorders of connective tissue," the most common of which are listed in Table 33–2. Although the prevalences of these disorders are imprecise, none is more frequent than 1/1000, so they will not be discussed in this book. Compendia of these disorders exist (Beighton, 1993; Royce and Steinmann, 1993, 2002; Rimoin et al., 2002), while some of the more prevalent are surveyed in several texts (Pyeritz 1993, 2001, 2002; Byers 2001, 2002; Pyeritz and Dietz, 2002).

A few of the more common disorders of the skeleton, including osteoarthritis and osteoporosis, have tantalizing ties to specific genes encoding components of the ECM (Dalgleish, 1997; Meulenbelt et al., 1997; Prockop et al., 1997; Riggs, 1997; Beaven et al., 1998; Bucay et al., 1998; DeVoto et al., 1998; Nelson et al., 1998; Prockop, 1998; Taboulet et al., 1998; Uitterlinden et al., 1998; Vingsbo-Lundberg et al., 1998; Lazner et al., 1999; Zmuda et al., 1999). This evidence is reviewed in this chapter and in others in this book (see Chapter 24 on osteoporosis and Chapter 32 on osteoarthritis).

Older terminology classified a group of non-Mendelian conditions as connective tissue disorders because the histopathology of affected tissues showed alterations in the ECM. However, these disorders, such as lupus erythematosis, scleroderma, and mixed connective tissue disease, are better termed *rheumatologic disorders* and are discussed in other chapters of this section.

The disorders considered in this chapter comprise a heterogenous group of skeletal problems that share only a few features. One is that their prevalences depend on the criteria used to define them, and since various criteria have been used in published studies, no consistent frequency based on a large sample size can be reported. Another common characteristic is that many of the conditions represent one end of a phenotypic continuum. Typically, the clinical problems present in many individuals in the population represent the mild end of a particular phenotype. The notion of a continuum permeates this chapter and can be reflected in the bedside examination (Rimoin et al., 1998; Pyeritz and Dietz, 2002), radiologic features (Spranger 1989), and biochemical and genetic defects (Kuivaniemi et al., 1997; Horton, 1997). A final shared feature is a clear familial predilection but no clear Mendelian pattern in any but a small percentage of cases. While some of the basic tenets of multifactorial inheritance may apply in some of the conditions, none adheres to all (see Chapter 1). However, the importance of genetic factors in the cause and pathogenesis of all of the conditions described in this chapter cannot be overestimated (Murphy and Pyeritz 1995, 2001; Pyeritz, 1999).

DEFECTS OF THE VERTEBRAL COLUMN

Scoliosis

Scoliosis is any lateral curvature of the vertebral column of greater than 10° and is diagnosed from a posteroanterior radiograph of the spine in the standing position (Scoliosis Research Society, 1976). While the primary determinant is the lateral deformity, scoliosis virtually always is associated with some anteroposterior and rotational distortion of the usual thoracic kyphosis and cervical and lumbar lordosis. Scoliosis is classified

Table 33–1. Functions of the Extracellular Matrix and Connective Tissue

Functions	Organ or Tissue
Support	Bone, cartilage, ligament
Cushioning	Cartilage, nucleus pulposis, tendon
Flexibility	Ligament, tendon
Distensibility	Elastic lamina (arteries)
Diffusion	Basement membrane (capillaries, lung, gastrointestinal tract)
Filtration	Basement membrane (kidney)
Healing	Scar
Hemostasis	Basement membrane (skin, blood vessels)
Transmission of light	Vitreous of eye
Maintenance of cell shape	Basement membrane, extracellular matrix (various organs)
Morphogenesis	Extracellular matrix (embryo)

by the number of curves (single or compound), age at onset [congenital, infantile (to age 3 years), juvenile (years 4–10), or adolescent], and cause. Infantile scoliosis comprises about 0.5% of cases of noncongenital onset, is more common in boys (Riseborough and Wynne-Davies, 1973), and typically involves a left thoracic curve. Juvenile onset comprises 10% to 15%, and adolescent scoliosis the remainder. The juvenile form is typically right thoracic. Mild adolescent scoliosis (<30°) is equally frequent between the sexes. Development of more severe curves is three- to fourfold more common in girls, but fortunately curves >30° represent only 10% of all adolescent scoliosis cases. The overall prevalence of scoliosis in adulthood is estimated variously at 2% to 3% (Rogala et al., 1978) and 5% to 6% (Cowell et al., 1972) at the high end to 0.2% (Filho and Thompson, 1971; Risebourgh and Wynne-Davies, 1973) at the low end.

Scoliosis has many causes, but in about 80% of instances, the cause is unclear (idiopathic). Congenital scoliosis usually has a definable etiology, if only in terms of a gross anatomic defect. Defects of vertebral formation or segmentation account for most cases, and these may be associated with other congenital anomalies, particularly of the appendicular skeleton and the cardiac, gastrointestinal, and genitourinary systems. The VATER (vertebral defects, imperforate anus, tracheoesophageal fistula, and radial and renal dysplasia) and VACTERL (vertebral, anal, cardiac, tracheal, esophageal, renal, limb) anomalads include vertebral defects that usually cause scoliosis. As growth occurs, the abnormal curvatures invariably worsen due to asymmetric growth around the primary defect(s). Congenital scoliosis often causes or is associated with intraspinal complications that affect nervous function, such as syringomyelia, tethered cord, or cord or root compression.

Scoliosis of infantile and juvenile onset is most often detected by the parent concerned by truncal asymmetry, school screening examinations, or the pediatrician during well-child care and may be caused by neuromuscular disorders (e.g., muscular dystrophies, cerebral palsy, poliomyelitis), heritable disorders of connective tissues (e.g., Marfan syndrome, many skeletal dysplasias), type I neurofibromatosis, and anomalies of one or more vertebrae of severity insufficient to cause congenital curvature. However, the majority of noncongenital scoliosis is classified as idiopathic. Curves of less than 10° usually escape clinical detection, and their relevance to genetic studies (given the arbitrary criterion for what constitutes scoliosis) is unclear.

Genetics

Given the wide variety of developmental defects that can cause congenital scoliosis, the role of genetic factors is complex. Most cases are sporadic. When the cause is an isolated vertebral anomaly of no apparent syndromic association, the recurrence risk in sibs is a few percent. Some familial occurrences have been reported, usually in conjunction with segmentation defects (Rimoin et al., 1968; Cantu et al., 1971; Rivera et al., 1988; Lorenz and Rupprecht, 1990; Giacoia and Say, 1991; Romeo et al., 1991; Turnpenny et al., 1991). Brewer and colleagues (1998) queried the Human Cytogenetic Database for aberrations associated with various congenital malformations. Scoliosis was reported in deletions of 2p15–p13, 6q13, and 15q12, suggesting that undetermined loci at these regions play some role in the development of the spine. A similar line of reasoning suggests that a locus or loci at 13q34 or 17p11.2 might be involved because a patient with congenital scoliosis and hemivertebrae had a reciprocal translocation with those breakpoints (Imaizumi et al., 1997).

Table 33–2. Classification of Disorders of the Extracellular Matrix

Disorder	OMIM No.[a]
Heritable disorders of connective tissue	
Marfan syndrome	*154700
Stickler syndrome (hereditary arthroophthalmopathy)	*108300, *184840
MASS phenotype	*157700
Osteogenesis imperfecta syndromes	*166200, *166210, *166220, 166230, 259420
Ehlers-Danlos syndromes	*130000, *130010, 130020, *130050, *130060, 130080, 225310, *225410, *225400, 305200
Cutis laxa	*123700, *219100, *304150
Epidermolysis bullosa syndromes	*131705, *131750, *131760, *131800, *131900, *131950, *131960, *132000, *226450, *226500, *226600, *226650, *226670, *226700, *226730, *601001
Pseudoxanthoma elasticum	*177850, *264800
Idiopathic osteoporosis (Chapter 24)	*166710, 259250
Idiopathic osteoarthritis (Chapter 32)	165720
Idiopathic abnormalities of the vertebral column	
Scoliosis	181800
Spondylosis and spondylolisthesis	184200, 184300
Secondary defects	
Inborn errors of metabolism	
Homocystinuria	*236200
Alkaptonuria	*203500
Menkes' syndrome	*309400
Hemochromatosis (Chapter 18)	*235200, *602390
Hyperuricemia and gout (Chapter 25)	138900, *308000
Vitamin deficiencies	
Scurvy	240400
Rickets	*193100, *241530, *264700, *277420, *277440, *307800, *600785
Autoimmune and rheumatologic syndromes (Chapters 28–31)	
Lupus erythematosis	*152700, *217000, *601744
Rheumatoid arthritis	180300
Scleroderma	*181750
Spondyloarthropathies	*106300
Inflammatory bowel disease–related arthritis (Chapter 15)	*191390, *266600, *601458

[a]Numbers with an asterisk indicate a phenotype with an acknowledged inheritance pattern, often with at least one defined molecular defect. Numbers beginning with *1*, *2*, or *3* indicate an autosomal dominant, autosomal recessive, or X-linked phenotype, respectively; numbers beginning with *6* indicate an autosomal phenotype defined since 1994.

Table 33–3. Candidate Genes in the Mouse for Idiopathic Scoliosis and Their Functional Classification

Intracellular Signaling	Signal Transduction	Structural Components of ECM	Metabolism of ECM
Ihh	*Hoxd*	*Crtm*	*Mmp* cluster
Ptn	*Csk*	*Col8a1*	*Timp2*
Tgfa	*Pml*	*Col9a2*	*Acp5*
Dll3	*Gli2*	*Col11a2*	*Lax*
Tgfbr2	*Nhlh1*	*Col12a1*	
Ltbp3	*Rxrb*		
Wnt3a	*Lmx1b*		
	Pax1		
	Pax3		
	Pax4		
	Pax7		
	Msx1		
	Cbx2		

ECM, extracellular matrix.
Source: Giampietro et al. (1999).

The case for genetic factors in the etiology of idiopathic scoliosis is considerably stronger, and while no specific gene has been identified, the case for a major locus has been made (Connor et al., 1987; Axenovich et al., 1999). Twin studies show higher concordance in monozygotic compared to dizygotic twin pairs but relatively high concordance (~37%) among dizygotic pairs as well (DeGeorge and Fisher, 1967; Kesling and Reinker, 1997). Families suggestive of autosomal dominant and X-linked dominant inheritance have been reported (Garland, 1934; Cowell et al., 1972; Robin and Cohen 1975). Females are much more frequently affected, as are the first-degree relatives of probands compared to second- and third-degree relatives (Wynne-Davis, 1968; Filho and Thompson, 1971; Martin et al., 1997). These latter two relationships do not hold for infantile idiopathic scoliosis, which suggests a different etiology. For juvenile- and adolescent-onset idiopathic scoliosis, the offspring of affected males (i.e., the less commonly affected sex) are not more likely to be affected, so not all characteristics of multifactorial inheritance are satisfied. Giampietro and colleagues (1999) scrutinized various databases of the mouse and human for possible animal models of human scoliosis. Of some 400 mouse mutant phenotypes involving the skeleton or neurologic and neuromuscular systems, 266 had been mapped. Focusing just on those that involved scoliosis, vertebral anomalies, and bent or kinky tails and excluding conditions with known human homologues (e.g., Marfan syndrome) left 45 mouse phenotypes. Of these, 28 were selected for further study because comparative mapping suggested plausible human candidate genes (Table 33–3). Most of the mouse mutants represented likely examples of human congenital scoliosis. The candidate genes could be loosely grouped into four classes based on function: intracellular signaling, signal transduction, structural components of the ECM, and ECM metabolism. The human homologues of these genes should be useful candidates for exploring linkages and mutations in idiopathic scoliosis. All of the biochemical distinctions found in tissue from scoliosis patients probably represent epiphenomena.

Management

When detected, scoliosis should be documented and quantified by anterior–posterior and lateral radiographs of the entire spine performed with the patient standing in bare feet. In general, curves tend to progress during periods of rapid linear growth; hence, regular follow-up is essential at least until skeletal maturity. The ultimate severity of scoliosis is determined by age at onset, severity and flexibility at diagnosis, rate of progression, and response to therapy. Severe curves are associated with back pain, leg length discrepancy, pelvic tilt, and restrictive lung problems.

Congenital scoliosis rarely responds to bracing (McMaster and Ohtsuka, 1982). Successful surgical therapy depends on the severity of the vertebral anomalies and the occurrence of additional malformations.

Idiopathic scoliosis of infantile onset may spontaneously regress or, in 10% to 30% of cases, progress. Frequent follow-up is essential to identify children in the latter group. Juvenile-onset scoliosis is much more likely than not to progress, with the pubertal growth spurt being the period of highest vulnerability (Lonstein and Carlson, 1984). Casting and bracing are tried initially for those who progress. In most instances when bracing is effective, treatment must be continued until skeletal maturity (Green, 1986; Nachemson and Peterson 1995).

Various surgical procedures to prevent worsening lateral and rotatory curvature can be used on children and adolescents who fail conservative treatment. Arthrodesis (fusion) of vertebral levels prevents further growth at those levels and, if extensive, can result in overt truncal shortening and body asymmetry. Thus, surgery should be delayed until late adolescence or a rodding procedure has been employed for stabilization followed by fusion.

Genetic Counseling

The keys to providing accurate and useful genetic counseling regarding scoliosis, as with all of the disorders in this chapter, are obtaining an accurate and detailed family history and excluding a Mendelian syndrome associated with, in this case, scoliosis. The former is time-consuming and often not completed at one sitting with the patient or the parents. Frequently, relatives need to be contacted, informed consent and medical records obtained, and radiographs retrieved and examined. Insuring that a recognized syndrome is not the cause of the vertebral column defects in the proband may require further consultation and testing, as would be the case with possible Marfan syndrome. Assuming that no syndrome is identified, if the family history reveals one or more near relatives with idiopathic scoliosis, then even the nonmedical geneticist should feel comfortable counseling the proband of the increased risk that offspring will be affected and his or her parents about the increased chance that they themselves might have unrecognized abnormal curvature and, if they were interested in having further children, that the risk of scoliosis is increased.

Anteroposterior Vertebral Curvatures

Abnormal anteroposterior vertebral curvatures have been much less studied than scoliosis. The most common deformities are reduced thoracic kyphosis (straight back syndrome) accentuated thoracic kyphosis (widow's hump), and accentuated lumbar lordosis (sway back).

Straightening or outright reversal of the usual thoracic kyphosis accompanies some connective tissue disorders [e.g., Marfan syndrome (DePaepe et al., 1996)] and congenital cardiac defects. Although no careful epidemiologic studies have been performed, the association of mitral valve prolapse with reduced thoracic kyphosis (and with pectus excavatum) suggests an underlying defect of the ECM since fibrillin-1 defects account for a percentage of such patients (Glesby and Pyeritz, 1989; Dietz and Pyeritz, 1995). Furthermore, since mitral valve prolapse is relatively common in most populations, reduced thoracic kyphosis is likely to be present in many individuals with this valvular characteristic.

Accentuated thoracic kyphosis in adulthood is very common (5%–10%), age-dependent, and most often a concomitant of osteoporosis and anterior wedging of vertebral bodies (see Chapter 24). In children, thoracic hyperkyphosis can be due to most of the specific causes of congenital and juvenile scoliosis. However, in most cases, no diagnosis other than Scheuermann's disease, a generic radiologic diagnosis, can be applied. A lateral standing radiograph should be performed in any child with accentuated forward bending of the spine. The absence of any structural defects suggests benign postural kyphosis. Scheuermann's disease requires three adjacent vertebrae to show anterior wedging of >5°. Maximal curvature usually occurs between T7 and T9. Kyphosis lower in the spine tends to occur in athletes and those performing repetitive bending functions. Most instances fall under the category osteochondritis dissecans (see below).

Accentuated lumbar lordosis has not been studied epidemiologically or in families.

Spondylosis and Spondylolisthesis

Spondylosis is a defect in the posterior inferior process (the pars interarticularis) of a vertebra. Spondylosis is classified into five types: dysplastic (often associated with spina bifida occulta), isthmic (the most common), degenerative (as in osteoarthritis), traumatic, and pathologic (due to a metastatic lesion) (Freeman, 1996). Spondylosis to some degree occurs in at least 5% of the adult population of the United States (Talwalkar and Mencio, 1999) and is more common in white males; however, accurate prevalences in different populations at distinct ages have not been determined. The majority of those affected are asymptomatic. The most frequent type, isthmic, is characterized by elongation or fracture of the pars interventricularis. Most instances are thought to be acquired, through stress fracture from physical activity. The dysplastic form results from congenital defect of the facet joints.

Spondylolisthesis refers to the displacement of one vertebra anterior to the one below it. The most commonly affected vertebra is L5 over S1, with L4 next in frequency and other vertebrae much less frequently involved. Cervical vertebrae are affected preferentially in some families. The overall prevalence by adulthood is in the range of 2% to 4%, or about one-half the frequency of spondylosis, which is the most common cause of spondylolisthesis. Subjects come to diagnosis on account of lower back pain, difficulty with forward bending, a waddling gait, radicular numbness or weakness, or a serendipitous radiograph. Follow-up studies of spondylolisthesis detected in children have shown progression likely through adolescence but rare after that. Slippage beyond 30° is uncommon if the slip is less than that observed when diagnosis is first made as long as spina bifida or other congenital vertebral defects are not present (Blackburne and Velikas, 1977). The timing and likelihood of progression may be related to the increased physical stress during adolescence, a fact that may also contribute to males being twice as likely to be affected in older studies. Now that girls are as athletically involved as boys, this sex ratio may change. Sports that require hyperlordotic movements, such as diving and gymnastics, are especially problematic. Progression of spondylosis to spondylolisthesis through repetitive stress fractures of the pars interventricularis, while unproven, seems likely (Wiltse et al., 1975).

Genetics

Family studies have demonstrated some aggregation of both spondylolisthesis and the dysplastic and isthmic forms of spondylosis (Albanese and Pizzutillo, 1982; Haukipuro et al., 1978). Shared environmental factors, such as occupations and other lifestyle attributes, might contribute more to the predisposition than genetics in some families. The Inuit are especially predisposed (Stewart, 1931). In one study of relatives of 47 probands with L5 spondylolisthesis (12 with dysplastic and 35 with isthmic spondylosis), 19% were affected (33% of relatives of probands with the dysplastic form and 15% of probands with the isthmic form, although both types occurred in most families (Wynne-Davies and Scott, 1979).

Reports of a number of families with multiple affected relatives have led to the conclusion that an autosomal dominant susceptibility exists (Amuso and Mankin, 1967; Shahriaree et al., 1979), with a 75% penetrance for spondylosis and a 33% risk of spondylolisthesis in those with a pars interventricularis defect (Haukipuro et al., 1978). Spina bifida occulta appears to predispose to slippage but occurs no more frequently than among those with spondylosis (Wynne-Davies and Scott, 1979). No reports of genetic linkage or biochemical defects have emerged.

Management

Symptoms of spondylolisthesis are related to the degree of kyphotic angulation and the percentage of slippage of the cephalad vertebra over the caudal one. Treatment for most patients can be conservative: temporary exercise reduction, physical therapy including stretching, nonsteroidal antiinflammatories, and bracing for severe cases. Surgical fusion is unlikely to be necessary unless the superior vertebra is displaced >50% over the lower one. The role of radiographic screening of near relatives, especially young ones, or probands is unproven.

DEFECTS PRIMARILY OF THE APPENDICULAR SKELETON

Benign Joint Hypermobility

Excessive passive range of motion of multiple joints is a feature of a number of heritable disorders of connective tissue, especially the Ehlers-Danlos syndromes, Marfan syndrome, osteogenesis imperfecta, familial joint instability syndrome, and some osteochondrodysplasias. The definition of joint hypermobility is largely subjective, and even rheumatologists in practice diverge considerably in their perceptions of its prevalence, importance, and relationship to specific disorders of the ECM (Grahame and Bird, 2001). Some attempts have been made to define diagnostic criteria (Beighton and Horan, 1970; Beighton et al., 1999). Obviously, the population prevalence of joint hypermobility will depend on the criteria used to define the phenotype at one end of the continuum of joint mobility (Beighton et al., 1973, 1999; Poul and Fait, 1986). However, the positive association of complaints of joint discomfort and swelling with joint hypermobility (Kirk et al., 1967; Beighton et al., 1988) and of fibromyalgia syndrome and joint hypermobility is clear (Genalia et al., 1993; Acasuso-Diaz and Collantes-Estevez, 1998). There is also a correlation among joint hypermobility, mitral valve prolapse, asthenic habitus, easy bruisability, and thin skin, which suggests a generalized disorder of the ECM in some, and perhaps many, people. Just as defining where MASS phenotype ends and Marfan syndrome begins is arbitrary (Glesby and Pyeritz, 1989), so is differentiating MASS and Ehlers-Danlos, hypermobility type (type III) from so-called benign hypermobility syndrome (DePaepe et al., 1996). Estimates of the frequency of polyarticular hypermobility are 4% to 7% in the general adult population and up to 30% in children (Murray and Woo, 2001). Estimates for adults undoubtedly include individuals who "train" their joints to be more mobile and, thus, represent phenocopies of hereditary predispositions. Of course, individuals successful at acquiring flexibility may primarily be those who are genetically susceptible. Joint hypermobility, despite its clinical difficulties, can be advantageous in some activities, such as gymnastics and performing on some musical instruments (Larsson et al., 1993).

Extrapolating from various heritable disorders of connective tissue, complaints of joint discomfort and actual degenerative joint disease are likely to be more common in adults with polyarticular hypermobility as they age (Beighton et al., 1973).

No genetic linkage or biochemical studies of people with isolated polyarticular hypermobility have been reported. However, some ethnic groups (e.g., Iraqis, sub-Saharan Africans, Asian Indians) have more joint hypermobility than other populations (Al Rawi et al., 1985; Wordsworth et al., 1987). Hypermobility segregates in some families as an autosomal dominant trait (Beighton and Horan, 1970).

Joint Instability

Some individuals are predisposed to recurrent sprains and dislocation of one or more joints. This phenotype represents another continuum, and in the main distinguishing between abnormal and everyday wear and tear, or even bad luck, is both frustrating and pointless. Thus, the prevalence of an abnormal connective tissue condition among the population experiencing one of the most common of life's occurrences is completely unclear. The phenotype is age- and experience-dependent. The older the individual, the more likely a traumatic event that exceeds the tolerance of a joint will occur. Similarly, the more physically active an individual, the more likely a joint injury and one dislocation, to the extent that the event itself damages supporting tissues, may aggravate instability and predispose to subsequent events. Individuals with dysplastic joints, including some with congenital hip dislocation, are predisposed to recurrent joint instability. Furthermore, congenital hip dislocation without hip dysplasia may be the earliest sign of an individual prone to instability of other joints (Wynne-Davies, 1970).

One Mendelian condition, familial joint instability, has been described (Horton et al., 1980). Originally, this phenotype was categorized as Ehlers-Danlos syndrome type XI, but it was reclassified in 1986 because of the absence of signs in the skin (Beighton et al., 1988). Inheritance is autosomal dominant with considerable intrafamilial variability. Shoulders, hips, and knees (patellae) are most likely to be affected. Pain even in the absence of dislocation or evidence of inflammation (such as might be present after an acute sprain) is quite common. No defect of the ECM has been identified.

Management is difficult. Conservative measures, such as physical therapy and other effects to strengthen the periarticular muscles, should always be recommended but have never been tested formally for effectiveness. Nonsteroidal antiinflammatory medications have a role as analgesics in treating the chronic joint pain. Eventually, many people with joint instability consult orthopedists. Many different surgical procedures to stabilize inherently unstable joints are available. Any surgery is less likely to be successful in a patient who has some defect of the ECM that affects healing, native strength of articular and periarticular structures, or both. When faced with a choice of therapeutic options, a more conservative selection seems more appropriate early in the course of polyarticular instability. Similarly, a positive family history of recurrent joint instability might steer the primary care physician or consultant to a more cautious course.

Osteochondritis Dissecans

The generic term *osteochondritis dissecans*, also called *osteochondrosis*, refers to any bone with part of an articular surface seemingly cut away (*dis* meaning "from" and *secare* meaning "cut off"). Many bones can be affected, and specific bones have acquired their own terms, often eponyms (Table 33–4). The general causes include trauma (often repetitive injuries), infarction (in some cases due to trauma), and likely developmental defects. That the latter cause has some genetic component is supported by several observations. "Simple" osteochondritis dissecans of the same bone has been reported in successive generations of multiple families in a pattern consistent with autosomal dominance (Online Mendelian Inheritance in Man, 2001, numbers 165800 and 259200). In a small proportion of families, osteochondritis dissecans is part of a pleiotropic disorder. Finally, in familial cases, the condition is more likely to be bilateral. Primary care physicians should be made aware of osteochondritis dissecans of any form occurring in a near relative of a child under their care. Such a child should be monitored more closely than usual by the parents for any symptoms in the joint at risk and diagnostic radiographs ordered more readily if pain, favoring one side, or a limp appear.

Osgood-Schlatter disease is perhaps the most common type and a consideration in any child who complains of recurrent and

Table 33–4. Varieties of Osteochondritis Dissecans (König Disease)

Common Name	Affected Bone	Clinical Consequence	OMIM No.[a]
Osgood-Schlatter	Tibial tubercle	Pain, tibia vara (bow legs)	188700
Legg-Calvé-Perthes	Femoral head	Pain in the hip(s)	150600
Scheuermann	Vertebrae	Pain at affected level, hyperkyphosis	181440
Thiemann	Phalanges	Stiffness, pain	165700
Köhler	Tarsal navicular	Ankle pain	
Kienböck	Carpal lunate	Wrist pain	
Larsen-Johanssen	Patella	Anterior knee pain	
Panner	Capitellum humeri	Elbow pain	
Frieberg (also called Köhler's second disease)	2nd metatarsal head	Plantar pain	

[a]OMIM, Online Mendelian Inheritance in Man (www.ncbi.nlm.nih.gov/omim).

persistent pain in the knees. The relationship with Blount disease, or osteochondrosis deformans tibiae, is unclear; however, some cases of tibia vara (considered the hallmark of Blount disease) are clearly due to osteochondritis dissecans (Tobin, 1957). Treatment is supportive and conservative, with mild analgesics and avoidance of strenuous exertion being key.

Perthes' disease is more frequent in males by a factor of 2 to 4. It has a low recurrence risk in sibs and offspring of 1% to 3%, with a gradient of decreasing risk among first-, second-, and third-degree relatives consistent with multifactorial inheritance (Gray et al., 1972; Wynne-Davies and Gormley, 1978; Hall, 1986). Probands with bilateral disease do not have a greater risk of having an affected relative than those with unilateral disease (Harper et al., 1976). Additional evidence against the polygenic model was the equivalent risk to offspring and sibs regardless of the sex of the proband (Wynne-Davies and Gormley, 1978). The role of avascular necrosis remains unsettled. Glueck and colleagues (1994) suggested that susceptibility to thrombosis predisposes to Perthes' disease and found a number of individuals with deficiency of protein S or protein C.

Scheuermann's disease causes pain in the back and accentuated anteroposterior curvature, usually hyperkyphosis. The curvature must be quite severe (>100°) to compromise pulmonary function. Symptoms improve with decreased physical activity. Bracing, if instituted early in flexible curves, coupled with modulation of traumatic activities can be extremely helpful. Surgical stabilization is necessary for progressive curves and those associated with neurologic or pulmonary sequelae.

Osteitis Deformans (Paget's Disease)

Osteitis deformans is due to dysregulated bone turnover. The prevalence increases with age and is unclear but certainly underestimated because most affected individuals are asymptomatic. Concentrations of cases in local geographic regions suggest one or more environmental influences. Western Europe, the United States, Australia, and New Zealand have higher prevalence rates than the rest of the world. In susceptible regions of the world, the prevalence is 3% to 5% between ages 50 and 70 years and 10% in those older than 80 years. The causes are unclear. Ultrastructural analysis of involved bone has suggested cytoplasmic and intranuclear inclusions characteristic of viral infection (Harvey et al., 1982). Osseous cells remote from pagetic lesions and hematopoietic cells do not show similar inclusions.

Family studies, to be accurate, must involve routine skeletal radiographs. When adequate phenotyping has been performed, autosomal dominant inheritance has been suggested. Genetic studies initially showed linkage of some families to the major histocompatibility complex region of chromosome 6 (6p21.3) (Fortino et al., 1977). More recent studies of families not linked to the major histocompatibility complex showed linkage to 18q21–q22, in the same region to which familial expansile osteolysis (Online Mendelian Inheritance in Man, 2001, number 174810) had been mapped (Van Hul et al., 1977). The first locus is termed *PDB1* and the second *PDB2*. In one pedigree with *PDB1*, Hughes and colleagues (2000) identified duplication of 26 nucleotides in *TNFRSF11A*, which segregated with the disease. Mutations in this locus, which is known to cause familial expansile osteolysis, were not found in three other families with Paget's disease that also mapped to 18q. Nance and colleagues (2000) described a large pedigree in which Paget's disease was unliked to 18q but was clinically indistinguishable to the phenotype of *PDB1*.

Paget's disease may produce considerable deformity of bone, especially of the pelvis, femur, skull, and tibia (Kaplan and Singer, 1995). Symptomatic bones are locally painful, warm, and tender. The risk of fracture at affected sites is increased. Joints may be involved through the articular surface; the hip is especially prone, and acetabular protrusion is a frequent complication. In early stages, pagetic changes are primarily osteolytic, especially of the metaphyses and diaphyses. Later, a mixed picture of osteolysis and osteosclerosis appears. The late stage shows considerable disorganization of the medullary structure. Throughout, the serum alkaline phosphatase level is increased.

Complications are primary, due to the effect of bone lesions on the skeleton, and secondary, due to nerve impingement and increased circulation through lesions (leading to cardiac failure). Occasional pagetic lesions are the locus for sarcomatous degeneration.

A short-term clinical trial of oral risedronate in 13 patients with severe Paget's disease showed a marked decrease in serum alkaline phosphatase levels (Singer et al., 1998).

THE FUTURE

In early 2001, when the rough draft of the human genome sequence was published, a number of surprises emerged. The number of human genes, estimated at 35,000, was about one-third of that expected. While the number of genes for humans is not substantially larger than for many "lower" organisms, the number and complexity of human proteins is now understood to be greater than in any other species. The diversity of the human proteome results from several mechanisms, including alternative splicing of mRNA and the mixing of peptide motifs that expand the functional scope of a given protein. Between the current edition of this text and the next, the location and function of most, if not all, of the human genes will be known. Investigating the genetic bases of common diseases, most of which will prove to be complex in the etiologic sense, will be particularly difficult. However, the human proteome will prove much more challenging. Understanding how proteins interact, both with themselves and with small molecules, will be essential to making progress in the pathogenetics of disease (Murphy and Pyeritz, 2002), in which we deduce how the normal and abnormal products of our genes and the abnormally regulated products of our genes contribute to our risks of developing common disorders. Novel therapies will unquestionably arise from this knowledge. Moreover, once an individual's specific risks of developing, say, scoliosis, can be identified, preventive measures can be prescribed that might impact for the good those risks. Additionally, more accurate genetic counseling will be available for both the proband and his or her relatives. As useful as the current edition of this book is, I can hardly wait to read the third edition.

REFERENCES

Acasuso-Diaz M, Collantes-Estevez E: Joint hypermobility in patients with fibromyalgia syndrome. Arthritis Care Res 1998; 11:39–42.

Albanese M, Pizzutillo PD: Family study of spondylolysis and spondylolisthesis. J Pediatr Orthop 1982; 2:496–499.

Al Rawi ZS, Al-Aszawi AJ, Al-Chalabi T: Joint mobility among university students in Iraq. Br J Rheumatol 1985; 24:326–331.

Amuso SJ, Mankin HJ: Hereditary spondylolithesis and spina bifida. J Bone Joint Surg Am 1967; 49:507–513.

Axenovich TI, Zaidman AM, Zorkoltseva IV, Tregubova IL, Borodin PM: Segregation analysis of idiopathic scoliosis: demonstration of a major gene effect. Am J Med Genet 1999; 86:389–394.

Beavan S, Prentice A, Dibba B, Yan L, Cooper C, Ralston SH: Polymorphism of the collagen type Iα1 gene and ethnic differences in hip-fracture rates. N Engl J Med 1998; 339:351–352.

Beighton P (ed): McKusick's Heritable Disorders of Connective Tissue, 5th ed. St. Louis: CV Mosby, 1993.

Beighton P, de Paepe A, Danks D, Finidori G, Gedde-Dahl T, Goodman R, Hall JG, Hollister DW, Horton W, McKusick VA, et al.: International nosology of heritable disorders of connective tissue—Berlin, 1986. Am J Med Genet 1988; 29:581–594.

Beighton P, Grahame R, Bird H: Hypermobility of Joints, 3rd ed. London: Springer-Verlag, 1999.

Beighton PH, Horan FT: Dominant inheritance in familial generalized articular hypermobility. J Bone Joint Surg Br 1970; 52:145–147.

Beighton PH, Solomon L, Soskolne CL: Articular mobility in an African population. Ann Rheum Dis 1973; 32:413–418.

Blackburne JS, Velikas EP: Spondylolithesis in children and adolescents. J Bone Joint Surg Br 1977; 59:490–494.

Brewer C, Holloway S, Zawalnyski P, Schinzel A, Fitzpatrick D: A chromosomal deletion map of human malformations. Am J Hum Genet 1998; 63:1153–1159.

Bucay N, Sarosi I, Dunstan CR, Morony S, Tarpley J, Capparelli C, Scully S, Tan HL, Lacey DL, Boyle WJ, et al.: Osteoproteogerin-deficient mice develop early onset osteoporosis and arterial calcification. Genes Dev 1998; 12:1260–1268.

Byers PH: Disorders of collagen biosynthesis and structure. In: Scriver CR, Beaudet AL, Sly WS, Valle D (eds). The Metabolic and Molecular Bases of Inherited Disease, 8th ed. New York: McGraw-Hill, 2001:5241–5286.

Byers PH, Schwarze U: Ehlers-Danlos syndrome. In: Rimoin DL, Connor JM, Pyeritz RE, Korf BR (eds). Principles and Practice of Medical Genetics, 4th ed. Edinburgh: Churchill Livingstone, 2002:4021–4043.

Cantu JM, Urrusti J, Rosales G, Rojas A: Evidence for autosomal recessive inheritance of costovertebral dysplasia. Clin Genet 1971; 2:149–154.

Connor JM, Conner AN, Connor RAC, Tolmie JL, Yeung B, Goudie D: Genetic aspects of early childhood scoliosis. Am J Med Genet 1987; 27:419–424.

Cowell HR, Hall JN, MacEwen GD: Genetic aspects of idiopathic scoliosis. Clin Orthop 1972; 86:121–131.

Dalgleish R: The human type I collagen mutation database. Nucleic Acids Res 1997; 25:181–187.

DeGeorge F, Fisher R: Idiopathic scoliosis: genetic and environmental aspects. J Med Genet 1967; 4:251–257.

DePaepe A, Deitz HC, Devereux RB, Hennekem R, Pyeritz RE: Revised diagnostic criteria for the Marfan syndrome. Am J Med Genet 1996; 62:417–426.

Devoto M, Shimoya K, Caminis J, Ott J, Tenenhouse A, Whyte MP, Sereda L, Hall S, Considine E, Williams CJ, et al.: First-stage autosomal genome screen in extended pedigrees suggests genes predisposing to low bone mineral density on chromosomes 1p, 2p and 4q. Eur J Hum Genet 1998; 6:151–157.

Dietz HC, Pyeritz E: Mutations in the human gene for fibrillin-1 (*FBN1*) in the Marfan syndrome and related disorders. Hum Mol Genet 1995; 4:1799–1809.

Dietz HC, Pyeritz RE: Marfan syndrome and related disorders. In: Scriver CR, Beaudet AL, Sly WS, Valle D (eds). The Metabolic and Molecular Bases of Inherited Disease, 8th ed. New York: McGraw-Hill, 2001:5287–5311.

Filho NA, Thompson MW: Genetic studies in scoliosis. J Bone Joint Surg Am 1971; 53:199.

Fortino M, Haymovits A, Falk CT: Evidence for linkage between HLA and Paget's disease. Transplant Proc 1977; 9:1867–1868.

Freeman BL III: The pediatric spine. In: Canale ST, Beaty JH (eds). Operative Pediatric Orthopaedics. St. Louis: CV Mosby, 1996:599–615.

Garland H: Hereditary scoliosis. BMJ 1934; 1:328.

Genalia A, Press J, Klein M, Buskila D: Joint hypermobility and fibromyalgia in school children. Ann Rheum Dis 1993; 52:494–496.

Giacoia GP, Say B: Spondylocostal dysplasia and neural tube defects. J Med Genet 1991; 28:51–53.

Giampietro PF, Raggio CL, Blank RD: Synteny-defined candidate genes for congenital and idiopathic scoliosis. Am J Med Genet 1999; 83:164–177.

Glesby MJ, Pyeritz RE: Association of mitral valve prolapse and systemic abnormalities of connective tissue: a phenotypic continuum. JAMA 1989; 262:523–528.

Glueck CJ, Glueck HI, Greenfield D, Freiberg R, Kahn A, Hamer T, Stroop D, Tracy T: Protein C and S deficiency, thrombophilia, and hypofibrinolysis: pathophysiologic causes of Legg-Perthes disease. Pediatr Res 1994; 35:383–388.

Grahame R, Bird H: British consultant rheumatologists' perceptions about the hypermobility syndrome: a national survey. Rheumatology 2001; 40:559–562.

Gray IM, Lowry RB, Renwick DHG: Incidence and genetics of Legg-Perthes disease (osteochondritis deformans) in British Columbia: evidence of a polygenic determination. J Med Genet 1972; 9:197–202.

Green NE: Part-time bracing of adolescent idiopathic scoliosis. J Bone Joint Surg Am 1986; 68:738–742.

Hall DJ: Genetic aspects of Perthes' disease: a critical review. Clin Orthop 1986; 209:100–114.

Harper PS, Brotherton J, Cochlin D: Genetic risks in Perthes' disease. Clin Genet 1976; 10:178–182.

Harvey L, Gray T, Beneton MNC, Douglas DL, Kanis JA, Russell RGG: Ultrastructural features of the osteoclasts from Paget's disease of bone in relation to a viral aetiology. J Clin Pathol 1982; 35:771–779.

Haukipuro K, Keranen N, Koivisto E, Lindholm R, Rorio R, Puton L: Familial occurrence of lumbar spondylolysis and spondylolisthesis. Clin Genet 1978; 13:471–476.

Horton WA: Molecular genetics of human chondrodysplasias. Growth Genet Horm 1997; 13:49–56.

Horton WA, Collins DL, DeSmet AA, Kennedy JA, Schimke RN: Familial joint instability syndrome. Am J Med Genet 1980; 6:221–228.

Hughes AE, Ralston SH, Marken J, Bell C, MacPherson H, Wallace RGH, van Hul W, Whyte MP, Nakatsuka K, Hovy L, et al.: Mutations in *TNFRSF11A*, affecting the signal peptide of RANK, cause familial expansile osteolysis. Nat Genet 2000; 24:45–48.

Imaizumi K, Masuno M, Ishii T, Kuroki Y, Okuzumi N, Nakamura Y: Congenital scoliosis (hemivertebra) associated with de novo balanced reciprocal translocation, 46,XX,t(13;17)(q34;p11.2). Am J Med Genet 1997; 73:244–246.

Kaplan FS, Singer FR: Paget's disease of bone: pathophysiology, diagnosis, and management. J Am Acad Orthop Surg 1995; 3:336–344.

Kesling KL, Reinker KA: Scoliosis in twins: a meta-analysis of the literature and report of six cases. Spine 1997; 22:2009–2015.

Kirk JA, Ansell BM, Bywaters FGL: The hypermobility syndrome: musculoskeletal complaints associated with generalized joint hypermobility. Ann Rheum Dis 1967; 26:419–425.

Koopman WJ (ed): Arthritis and Allied Conditions: A Textbook of Rheumatology, 13th ed. Baltimore: Williams and Wilkins, 1997.

Koopman WJ (ed): Arthritis and Allied Conditions: A Textbook of Rheumatology, 14th ed. Baltimore: Williams and Wilkins, 2000.

Kuivaniemi H, Tromp G, Prockop DJ: Mutations in fibrillar collagens (types I, II, III, and XI), fibril-associated collagen (type IX), and network-forming collagen (type X) cause a spectrum of diseases of bone, cartilage, and blood vessels. Hum Mutat 1997; 9:300–315.

Larsson L-G, Baum J, Mudholkar GS, Kolla GD: Benefits and disadvantages of joint hypermobility among musicians. N Engl J Med 1993; 329:1079–1082.

Lazner F, Gowen M, Pavasovic D, Kola I: Osteopetrosis and osteoporosis: two sides of the same coin. Hum Mol Genet 1999; 8:1839–1846.

Lonstein JE, Carlson JM: The prediction of curve progression in untreated idiopathic scoliosis during growth. J Bone Joint Surg Am 1984; 66:1061–1071.

Lorenz P, Rupprecht E: Spondylocostal dysostosis: dominant type. Am J Med Genet 1990; 35:219–221.

Martin MJ, Rodriguez BC, Eguren HEM, Diaz PR, de Leon GF, Pedrosa GAI: Family prevalence of idiopathic scoliosis [in Spanish]. An Esp Pediatr 1997; 46:148–150.

McMaster MJ, Ohtsuka K: The natural history of congenital scoliosis: a study of 251 patients. J Bone Joint Surg Am 1982; 64:1128–1147.

Meulenbelt I, Bijkerk C, Breedveld C, Slagboom PE: Genetic linkage analysis of 14 candidate gene loci in a family with autosomal dominant osteoarthritis without dysplasia. J Med Genet 1997; 34:1024–1027.

Murphy EA, Pyeritz RE: Genes and disease. In: Wagner HN Jr, Szabo Z, Buchanan JW (eds). Principles of Nuclear Medicine, 2nd ed. Philadelphia: WB Saunders, 1995:18–27.

Murphy EA, Pyeritz RE: Pathogenetics. In: Rimoin DL, Connor JM, Pyeritz RE, Korf BR (eds). Principles and Practice of Medical Genetics, 4th ed. Edinburgh: Churchill Livingstone, 2002:439–455.

Murray KJ, Woo P: Benign joint hypermobility in childhood. Rheumatology 2001; 40:489–491.

Nachemson AL, Peterson LE: Effectiveness of treatment with a brace in girls who have adolescent idiopathic scoliosis: a prospective, controlled study based on data from the Brace Study of the Scoliosis Research Study. J Bone Joint Surg Am 1995; 77:815–822.

Nance MA, Nuttall FQ, Econs MJ, Lyles KW, Viles KD, Vance JM, Pericak-Vance MA, Speer MC: Heterogeneity in Paget disease of the bone. Am J Med Genet 2000; 92:303–307.

Nelson F, Dahlberg L, Laverty S, Reiner A, Pidoux I, Ionescu M, Fraser GL, Brooks E, Tanzer M, Rosenberg LC, et al.: Evidence for altered synthesis of type II collagen in patients with osteoarthritis. J Clin Invest 1998; 102:2115–2125.

Online Mendelian Inheritance in Man: McKusick-Nathans Institute for Genetic Medicine, Johns Hopkins University (Baltimore, MD) and National Center for BioInformatics, National Library of Medicine (Bethesda, MD), 2001 (www.ncbi.nlm.nih.gov/omim).

Poul J, Fait M: Generalisierte Bandlaxität bei Kindern. Z Orthop 1986; 124:336–339.

Prockop DJ: The genetic trail of osteoporosis. N Engl J Med 1998; 338:1061–1062.

Prockop DJ, Ala-Kokko L, McLain DA: Can mutated genes cause common osteoarthritis? Br J Rheumatol 1997; 36:827–830.

Pyeritz RE: The Marfan syndrome and related disorders of the microfibril. In: Royce PM, Steinmann B (eds). Connective Tissue and Its Heritable Disorders: Molecular, Genetic and Medical Aspects. New York: Wiley-Liss, 1993:437–468.

Pyeritz RE: Genetic aspects of orthopaedic disorders. In: Baratz ME, Watson AD, Imbriglia JE (eds). Orthopedic Surgery: The Essentials. New York: Thieme, 1999:65–72.

Pyeritz RE: Heritable and developmental disorders of connective tissues and bone. In: Koopman WJ (ed). Arthritis and Allied Conditions: A Textbook of Rheumatology, 14th ed. Philadelphia: Williams and Wilkins, 2001:1925–1962.

Pyeritz RE: Marfan syndrome and other disorders of fibrillin. In: Rimoin DL, Connor JM, Pyeritz RE, Korf BR (eds). Principles and Practice of Medical Genetics, 4th ed. Edinburgh: Churchill Livingstone, 2002:3977–4020.

Pyeritz RE, Dietz HC: The Marfan syndrome and other fibrillinopathies. In: Royce PM, Steinmann B (eds). Connective Tissue and Its Heritable Disorders: Molecular, Genetic and Medical Aspects, 2nd ed. New York: Wiley-Liss, 2002 (in press).

Riggs BL: Vitamin D-receptor genotypes and bone density. N Engl J Med 1997; 337:125–126.

Rimoin DL, Connor JM, Pyeritz RE, Korf BR (eds): Principles and Practice of Medical Genetics, 4th ed. Edinburgh: Churchill Livingstone, 2002.

Rimoin DL, Fletcher BD, McKusick VA: Spondylocostal dysplasia: a dominantly inherited form of short-trunked dwarfism. Am J Med 1968; 45:948–953.
Rimoin DL, Francomano CA, Giedion A, Hall C, Kaitila I, Cohn D, Gorlin R, Hall J, Horton W, Krakow D, et al.: International nomenclature and classification of the osteochondysplasias (1997). Am J Med Genet 1998; 79:376–382.
Riseborough E, Wynne-Davies R: A genetic survey of idiopathic scoliosis in Boston, Massachusetts. J Bone Joint Surg Am 1973; 55:974–982.
Rivera H, Perez-Salas JM, Nazara Z, Ramirez ML: A probably distinct autosomal recessive thoraco-limb dysplasia. J Med Genet 1988; 25:619–622.
Robin GC, Cohen T: Familial scoliosis: a clinical report. J Bone Joint Surg Br 1975; 57:146–147.
Rogala E, Drummond D, Gurr J: Scoliosis incidence and natural history: a prospective epidemiological study. J Bone Joint Surg Am 1978; 60:173.
Romeo MG, Distefano G, DiBella D, Mangiagli A, Caltabiano L, Roccar S, Mollica F: Familial Jarcho-Levin syndrome. Clin Genet 1991; 39:253–259.
Royce PM, Steinmann B (eds): Connective Tissue and Its Heritable Disorders: Molecular, Genetic and Medical Aspects. New York: Wiley-Liss, 1993.
Royce PM, Steinmann B (eds): Connective Tissue and Its Heritable Disorders: Molecular, Genetic and Medical Aspects, 2nd ed. New York: Wiley-Liss, 2001.
Scoliosis Research Society: Glossary of scoliosis terms. Spine 1976; 1:57–58.
Scriver CR, Beaudet AL, Sly WS, Valle D (eds): The Metabolic and Molecular Bases of Inherited Disease, 8th ed. New York: McGraw-Hill, 2001.
Shahriaree H, Sajadi K, Rooholamini SA: A family with spondylolithesis. J Bone Joint Surg Am 1979; 61:1256–1258.
Singer FR, Clemens TL, Eusebio RA, Becker RJ: Risedronate, a highly effective oral agent in the treatment of patients with severe Paget's disease. J Clin Endocrinol Metab 1998; 83:1906–1910.
Spranger J: Radiologic nosology of bone dysplasias. Am J Med Genet 1989; 34:96–104.
Stewart TD: Incidence of separate neural arch in the lumbar vertebrae of Eskimos. Am J Phys Anthropol 1931; 16:51–62.
Taboulet J, Frenkian M, Frendo JL, Feingold N, Jullienne A, de Vernejoul MC: Calcitonin receptors polymorphism is associated with a decreased fracture risk in postmenopausal women. Hum Mol Genet 1998; 7:2129–2133.
Talwalkar VR, Mencio GA: The pediatric spine. In: Baratz ME, Watson AD, Imbriglia JE (eds). Orthopaedic Surgery: The Essentials. New York: Thieme, 1999:711–736.
Tobin WJ: Familial osteochondritis dissecans with associated tibia vara. J Bone Joint Surg Am 1957; 39:1091–1105.
Turnpenny PD, Thwaites RJ, Boulos FN: Evidence for variable gene expression in a large inbred kindred with autosomal recessive spondylocostal dysostosis. J Med Genet 1991; 28:27–33.
Uitterlinden AG, Burger H, Huang Q, Yue F, McGuigan FE, Grant FG, Hofman A, van Leeuwen JPTM, Pols HAP, Ralston SH: Relation of alleles of the collagen type Iα1 gene to bone density and the risk of osteoporotic fractures in postmenopausal women. N Engl J Med 1998; 338:1016–1021.
Van Hul W, Bollerslev J, Gram J, Van Hul E, Wuyts W, Benichou O, Vanhoenacker F, Willems PJ: Localization of a gene for autosomal dominant osteoporosis (Albers-Schönberg disease) to chromosome 1p21. Am J Hum Genet 1997; 61:363–369.
Vingsbo-Lundberg C, Nordquist N, Olofsson P, Sundvall M, Saxne T, Pettersson U, Holmdahl R: Genetic control of arthritis onset, severity and chronicity in a model for rheumatoid arthritis in rats. Nat Genet 1998; 20:401–404.
Wiltse LL, Widell EH Jr, Jackson DW: Fatigue fracture: the basic lesion in isthmic spondylolisthesis. J Bone Joint Surg Am 1975; 57:17–22.
Wordsworth P, Oglivie D, Smith R, Sykes B: Joint mobility with particular reference to racial variation and inherited connective tissue disorders. Br J Rheumatol 1987; 26:9–12.
Wynne-Davies R: Familial (idiopathic) scoliosis: a family survey. J Bone Joint Surg Br 1968; 50:24–30.
Wynne-Davies R: Acetabular dysplasia and familial joint laxity: two etiologic factors in congenital dislocation of the hip. J Bone Joint Surg Br 1970; 52:704–716.
Wynne-Davies R, Gormley J: The aeitiology of Perthes' disease: genetic, epidemiological and growth factors in 310 Edinburgh and Glasgow patients. J Bone Joint Surg Br 1978; 60:6–14.
Wynne-Davies R, Scott JHS: Inheritance and spondylolithesis: a radiographic family survey. J Bone Joint Surg Br 1979; 61:301–305.
Zmuda JM, Cauley JA, Ferrell RE: Recent progress in understanding the genetic susceptibility to osteoporosis. Genet Epidemiol 1999; 16:356–367.

Part VIII

CANCER

34 Gastrointestinal Cancer

Randall W. Burt

This chapter will examine malignancy of the esophagus, stomach, small bowel, pancreas, and colon. In terms of U.S. incidence and mortality, colon cancer stands out in importance. It is much more common and a greater cause of mortality than all other gastrointestinal malignancies combined. A large research effort has therefore been devoted to colon cancer. This has led to important advances in both basic and clinical knowledge of this malignancy. More is now known about the inheritance, biology, and clinical management of colon cancer than about any other gastrointestinal malignancy and perhaps any other cancer. Additionally, precise and effective prevention and screening strategies for colon cancer have also emerged from ongoing research. This chapter will thus address colon cancer first, followed by a review of the other gastrointestinal (GI) tumors.

COLORECTAL CANCER

Remarkable progress has been made in understanding the inherited, genetic, and environmental pathogenesis of colorectal cancer (Potter, 1999). Epidemiological studies first demonstrated wide international differences in the incidence of this malignancy that could not be accounted for by race or ethnicity alone, thus suggesting an environmental influence in cancer pathogenesis. Changing colon cancer incidence rates were then demonstrated in migrational populations, further suggesting a role for the environment. Case-control studies have now confirmed significant associations of colon cancer with specific dietary and environmental factors.

Inherited syndromes of colon polyps and cancer have also been described and, although rare, include familial adenomatous polypsis (FAP), hereditary non-polyposis colorectal cancer (HNPCC), and several conditions of hamartomatous polyposis (Guillem et al., 1999; Hampel and Pettomäki, 2000). The genetic etiology of these syndromes is now known, and genetic tests are available for clinical diagnosis. In addition to these syndromes, a significant risk of colon cancer has been demonstrated in close relatives of persons with large bowel malignancy, even when the syndromes are excluded (Burt, 2000). The genetic etiology of this more common familial risk has not yet been defined, but it is hypothesized that additional susceptibility genes play a role (Lichtenstein et al., 2000).

At the molecular level, all colon malignancies are now known to arise when relevant genes are affected by mutation. Colon cancer genes include certain tumor suppressor genes, oncogenes, and DNA repair genes (Kinzler and Vogelstein, 1996). The histopathologic parallel is the progression of normal colonic epithelial cells to hyperproliferative epithelium, small adenomatous polyps, larger polyps, and, finally, frank malignancy. The unifying hypothesis of colon cancer pathogenesis is that inheritance determines individual susceptibility, while environmental exposures determine the expression of that susceptibility.

There is already substantial clinical application of colon cancer research findings. Guidelines for diet and lifestyle have been suggested to minimize the risk of colon cancer (Potter, 1999). Colon cancer screening algorithms now incorporate family history to stratify risk, and genetic diagnosis is used for the rare syndromes (Byers et al., 1997; Terdiman et al., 1999; Burt, 2000; Hampel and Peltomäki, 2000). It is expected that molecular genetic knowledge will soon translate into even more specific screening and treatment approaches.

Disease Definition

Diagnostic Criteria

The diagnosis of colon cancer is based on appropriate histopathology, usually obtained by colonoscopic biopsy. The X-ray and colonoscopic appearance of colon cancer can be highly suggestive but not diagnostic.

Clinical Presentation

The presenting symptoms of colorectal cancer are nonspecific and include rectal bleeding, abdominal pain (usually hypogastric), change in bowel habits, weight loss, and fatigue. The presence of symptoms correlates with later-stage disease and poor prognosis. Detection of colon cancer through screening for occult GI blood in asymptomatic persons, in contrast, correlates with early-stage disease and a high rate of surgical cure. Additionally, detection and treatment of colonic adenomatous polyps through screening effectively prevents cancer from occurring (Winawer et al., 1997). The emphasis to approaching colon cancer has therefore changed in recent years from symptom evaluation to screening and early detection.

Pathology

Adenocarcinoma of the colon is histologically similar to adenocarcinoma in general, with increased nuclear size, loss of basilar polarity of the nucleus, increased nuclear to cytoplasmic ratio, more basophylic cytoplasm, loss of cytyoplasmic glycogen, loss of goblet cells, loss of regular gland formation, and invasion through the basement membrane. Colon cancer almost always arises from colonic adenomatous polyps. Histology of these premalignant lesions is similar to cancer, but less severe, and does not include invasion through the basement membrane. The progression from normal tissue through an adenomatous polyp to colon cancer is a slow process, with estimates of 15 years and longer. Approximately 25% of large intestinal malignancies occur in the rectum and 50% to 60% distal to the splenic flexure.

Table 34–1. Occurrence and Survival of Colon Cancer, by Dukes and TNM Stages

Dukes Stage[a]	TNM Stage[b]	Description	Frequency of Occurrence (%)	5-Year Survival Rate (%)
A	I	Into the muscularis propria	15	95–100
B	II	Into the serosa and may extend into the pericolic fat	31	80–85
C	III	Involvement of regional lymph nodes	23	50–70
D	IV	Distant metastasis	30	5–15

Source: Modified from Boland (1999) with permission.

[a]Dukes is a classical staging system for colon cancer with many variations. The most common is Dukes A. A: the tumor penetrates but does not go beyond the muscularis propria; B: tumor extends into the serosa; C: lymph nose metastasis present; D: distant metastasis.

[b]The TNM staging is the preferred system. Primary tumor: T_1, submucosal invasion; T_2, muscularis propria invasion; T_3, submucosa invasion; T_4, adjacent organs invaded. Regional lymph nodes: N_0, no node involvement; N_1, 1–3 nodes involved; N_2, ≥4 nodes involved; N_3, distant nodes involved. Distant metastasis: M_0, no distant metastasis; M_1, distant metastasis. The T, N, and M codes are then combined to indicate stages. Stage I: $T_1 N_0 M_0$, $T_2 N_0 M_0$. Stage II: $T_3 N_0 M_0$, $T_4 N_0 M_0$. Stage III: $T_{any} N_1 M_0$, $T_{any} N_2 M_0$, $T_{any} N_3 M_0$. Stage IV: $T_{any} N_{any} M_1$.

The Duke's staging system is traditional and has many variations, while the tumor-node-metastasis (TNM) staging system is gradually replacing this method (Boland, 1999). In the TNM system the depth of the tumor invasion is specified, together with the presence or absence of node involvement and, finally, the presence or absence of metastasis. These three considerations together specify a tumor stage that varies somewhat with each organ and cancer. Table 34–1 summarizes the Duke's and TNM staging systems as they apply to colon cancer and also gives the frequency of diagnosis and survival statistics relative to the stage.

General Genetic and Epidemiologic Evidence

Clinical Epidemiology and Ethnic Differences

It is estimated that 130,200 new cases of colon cancer occurred in the U.S. in 2000, with 56,300 deaths (Greenlee et al., 2000). The lifetime risk is 5.69% in men and 5.62% in women. Colon cancer is uncommon before age 50 years (about 7% of cases), but its incidence rises rapidly after that age. Overall there has been an increase in incidence in the past 20 years of 0.3% but a decrease in mortality of 15.5%. Five-year survival has concurrently increased from 45.6% to 61.5%. The incidence of colon cancer in the United States varies somewhat by ethnic subgroup (see Table 34–2). Both the incidence and mortality is higher in

Table 34–2. U.S. Annual Incidence and Mortality of Colorectal Cancer per 100,000, by Ethnicity

Gender	Caucasian	African American	Asian/Pacific Islander	American Indian	Hispanic
Incidence					
Male	53.8	59.4	47.2	21.9	35.6
Female	37.2	45.5	31.2	?	24.3
Combined	44.3	51.2	38.3	16.4	29.1
Mortality					
Male	21.8	28.0	13.6	10.5	13.2
Female	14.6	20.1	9.0	8.7	8.5
Combined	17.6	23.3	11.0	9.6	10.5

Source: Modified from Landis et al. (1999) with permission.

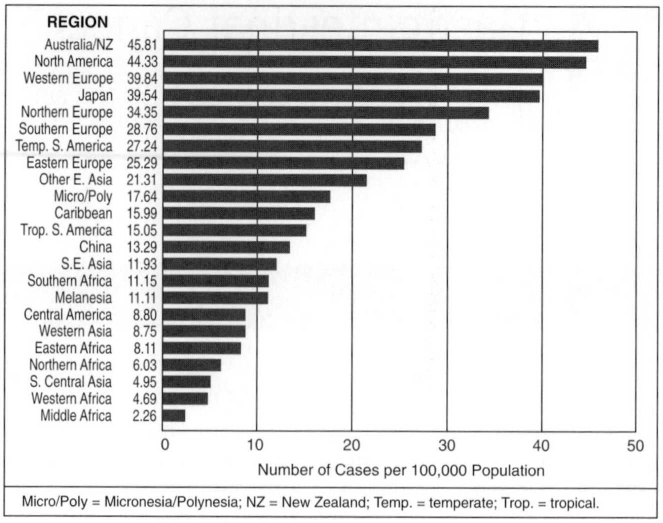

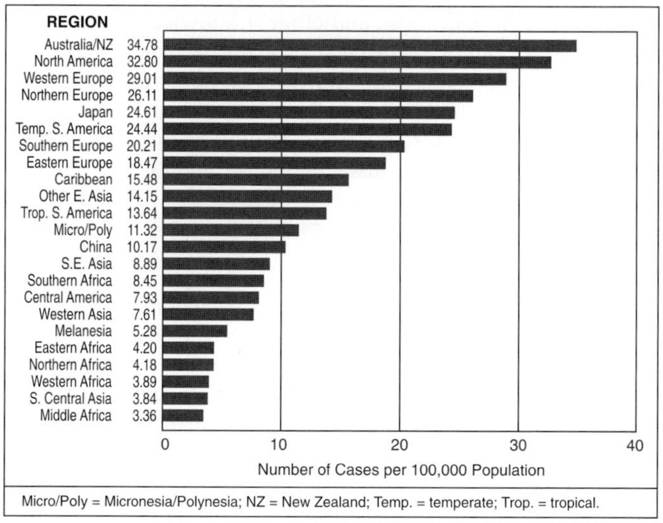

Fig. 34–1. Incidence of colorectal cancer in males (*top*) and females (*bottom*) by world region. From Parkin (1999) with permission.

African Americans than among Caucasians. It should be noted that when colon and rectal cancer are considered separately, most groups exhibit an equal or higher incidence of colon cancer in women and a higher incidence of rectal cancer in men.

International differences in colon cancer incidence are striking and have implicated environmental factors as important in pathogenesis of this malignancy (Fig. 34–1) (Parkin et al., 1999). Migration studies, particularly those of persons migrating from Japan to Hawaii, have shown a rapidly changing incidence of colon cancer in the same generation (Straszewski and Haenszel, 1965, 1971; Wynder and Hirayama, 1977; Correa and Haenszel, 1978; Weisburger et al., 1985).

Genetic Epidemiology

Colorectal cancers frequently occur in families, even when the syndromes of FAP and HNPCC are not included (Burt, 2000). Epidemiological investigations have consistently demonstrated a 2- to 3-fold increased risk of colon cancer in persons with a positive family history compared to controls (Tables 34–3, 34–4). This excess risk is not observed in spouses, suggesting that inherited rather than environmental factors account for the excess familial cases (Lovett, 1976; Jensen et al., 1980). Famil-

Table 34–3. Risk of Colorectal Cancer (CRC) in First-Degree Relatives of Person Who Died of CRC

Study Site	No. of Subjects	Control	Relative Risk	Reference
University of Utah	763	Age, gender, county of birth matched persons	3.3 ($p < .01$)	Woolf, 1958
Ohio University	145	From state cancer statistics	2.9	Macklin, 1960
St. Mark's Hospital, London	209	From national cancer statistics	3.3 ($p < .01$)	Lovett, 1976

ial risk is thus a substantial health issue, considering the already very significant lifetime risk of this disease in the general population. There also is a higher risk of colon cancer in the first-degree relatives of those persons with adenomatous polyps, and a similar higher risk of adenomas in relatives of those with colon cancer (Tables 34–4 and 34–5).

Kindred studies where both colonic adenomas and cancers have been examined indicate that this common familial risk probably arises from mildly to moderately penetrant inherited susceptibility (Cannon-Albright et al., 1988). Such studies also indicate that this type of inheritance is frequent in the population and may account for a substantial fraction of colon cancer cases. A recent twin study supports these findings and indicates that 35% of colon cancers arise from inherited susceptibility (Lichtenstein et al., 2000). The genes that give rise to this common type of inherited risk have not yet been identified, although a number of candidate genes are being investigated (see below).

The number of affected relatives and their ages at the time of cancer diagnosis can be used to stratify familial risk (Tables 34–6 and 34–7). If two or more first-degree relatives have colon cancer, the risk of large bowel malignancy for other family members is about three times the risk in the general population. A relative risk of 3-fold or greater also is observed if a first-degree relative is diagnosed with colon cancer at 50 years of age or younger. Approximately 15% of colon cancer cases fall into the high-risk group, which is defined as having two or more affected first-degree relatives or an age of diagnosis in a first-degree relative of 50 years of age. Only a small fraction of these cases has clinically diagnosed FAP or HNPCC. Although somewhat arbitrary, this definition of high risk is useful clinically to stratify screening.

If a second- or even third-degree relative has colon cancer, the risk to family members is still increased, but only by 30% to 50% above the expected risk (Slattery and Kerber, 1994) (Table 34–7). Second-degree relatives include grandparents, aunts, and uncles, while third-degree relatives are great-grandparents and first cousins. Familial risk is significant for all colonic tumor sites, including the rectum. When persons with adenomatous polyps serve as the index cases, the results are similar to colon cancer index cases (Tables 34–4 to 34–7). Refinement of these observations is needed, however, as it is known that 30% to 50% of persons will eventually develop adenomas during life. It may be that larger adenomas are more predictive of familial risk. For example, Pariente et al. (1998) found in a colonoscopy study that the odds ratio of risk for all adenomas in first-degree relatives of persons with colon cancer was 1.5 (1.0–2.4). When only high-risk adenomas (size ≥ 1 cm or villous component) were considered, the odds ratio increased to 2.6 (1.3–5.1).

Association with Other Diseases

Adenomatous Polyps. The most common associated disease is the adenomatous polyp. In fact, there is convincing evidence that most cases of colon cancer arise from adenomatous polyps. Larger and more dysplastic adenomas have a greater risk of harboring cancer, and removal of adenomas markedly lowers the incidence of colon cancer (Winawer et al., 1993). Additionally, adenomatous polyps are clonal, and the DNA mutations observed in adenomas containing cancer are identical in both the benign and malignant portions of the polyp.

Approximately 30% of adults in the United States will eventually develop adenomatous polyps. Most of these polyps reach only several millimeters in size and do not progress to cancer. A small fraction, however, progress to larger and more advanced lesions—that is, they exhibit severe dysplasia or villous change (Macrae and Young, 1999). Such adenomas are more likely to become malignant. Cross-sectional data have been used to suggest that at least 5 to 10 years are usually required for adenomatous polyps to become malignant (Winawer et al., 1997). It

Table 34–4. Frequency of Positive Family History[a] in Persons with Colorectal Cancer

		Index Case with Colon Cancer		Index Case with Adenomatous Polyp		
Study Location	Frequency in Controls (%)	Frequency (%)	Risk Compared to Controls	Frequency (%)	Risk Compared to Controls	Reference
Scotland	2.0	16	8.0			Duncan and Kyle, 1982
France	3.5	19	5.3	15	4.2	Maire et al., 1984
Australia	10.0	18	1.8			Kune et al., 1987
Italy	5.4	21	3.9	18	3.4	Ponz de Leon et al., 1987
Italy	5.1	11	2.4	14	3.2	Bonelli et al., 1988
Australia	7.5	16	2.2			St. John et al., 1993
United Kingdom	5.0	23	4.6			Stephenson et al., 1991
United States	9.9	17	1.7			Fuchs et al., 1994
United States	2.1			4.7	1.78	Winawer et al., 1996
United States	3.0			4.7	1.74	Ahsan et al., 1998

[a]Positive family history defined as one or more first-degree relatives with colon cancer.
Source: Adapted from Burt (1997) with permission.

Table 34–5. Frequency of Adenomas in First-Degree Relatives of Persons with Colorectal Cancer

Authors	Relatives (%)	Controls (%)	Study Method[a]
Gryska and Cohen, 1987	63	—	Colonoscopy
Rozen et al., 1987	8	4[b]	FOBT/FS
Cannon-Albright et al., 1988	19	12[b]	FS
Grossman and Milos, 1988	18	—	Colonoscopy
Guillem et al., 1988	14	8[b]	Colonoscopy
Baker et al., 1990	27	—	Colonoscopy
Herrera et al., 1990	12	—	FOBT/FS
McConnell et al., 1990	12	—	Colonoscopy
Orrom et al., 1990	20	—	Colonoscopy
Sauar et al., 1992	37	—	Colonoscopy
Bazzoli et al., 1995	69	36[b]	Colonosocpy
Pariente et al., 1998	23	17[b]	Colonoscopy

[a]FOBT, fecal occult blood test; FS, flexible sigmoidoscopy.
[b]Difference was statistically significant.
Source: Adapted from Burt (1997) with permission.

has recently been suggested that some "flat" cancers develop either de novo or with a much shortened benign phase. This pathway appears to be very unusual in the United States, although it may be more common in Japan where the relevant studies have been done.

As described above, adenomas exhibit a close relationship to colon cancer in terms of familial risk. Relatives of patients with adenomas have an increased risk of colon cancer. The reverse is also true (Tables 34–4 to 34–7). The epidemiology of adenomas and of adenocarcinoma of the colon is nearly identical, and the association with environmental factors is likewise similar (Potter, 1999). Finally, the pathogenesis of adenomas and cancer represents a genetic and histologic continuum. Relevant genes are affected by accumulating mutational events, and polyps become larger and more dysplastic (Kinzler and Vogelstein, 1996).

Ulcerative Colitis. Persons with ulcerative colitis exhibit a risk of colorectal cancer that parallels the duration of the illness. Excess risk of malignancy is observed after 7 to 10 years of colitis and then accumulates at about a rate of 1% per year. Persons with pancolitis and very active disease appear to have the greatest risk. If Crohn's disease involves the entire colon, the cancer risk appears to approach that of ulcerative colitis. Inflammatory bowel disease may account for as much as 1% of colon cancers. These conditions are examined in detail in other chapters of this volume.

Associated Cancers. Some, but not all, epidemiologic studies have demonstrated a high risk of colon cancer associated with the occurrence of certain other malignancies. Women who have had breast, uterine, or ovarian cancer exhibit some increased risk of colon cancer (Correa and Haenszel, 1978). Additionally, a genealogical database study found a 30% to 50% higher risk of colon cancer when first-degree relatives were affected with breast, uterine, ovarian, or prostate cancer (Slattery and Kerber, 1994).

Environmental Factors

As outlined above, international differences and changing frequencies of colon cancer in migrating populations suggest that environmental factors play a role in the etiology of this malignancy. Case-control studies have further identified specific environmental factors that associate with either an increased or a decreased risk (Sandler, 1996; Potter, 1999). These are summarized in Table 34–8. Adenomatous polyps have been associated with many of the same factors. Based on epidemiologic associations, dietary recommendations have been given to minimize colon cancer (and other cancer) risk. Interventional studies are needed to validate these recommendations. Individual risk assessment based on environmental exposure is also presently far from a reality. The difficulty lies in reliably assessing a lifetime of exposures.

Inherited Syndromes of Colon Cancer

A number of syndromes are known in which affected persons exhibit a high risk of colon cancer (Burt, 1996; Burt, 2000; Guillem et al., 1999). Each of these syndromes is a single-gene, autosomal dominantly inherited condition. All of the syndromes are rare. The syndromes that give rise to adenomatous polyps, including FAP, HNPCC, and their subtypes, have an extreme risk of colon cancer. FAP accounts for only about 0.5% of colon cancer cases and HNPCC accounts for 2% to 3% (Burt, 1996; Burt, 2000; Guillem et al., 1999). The syndromes that give rise to hamaratomatous polyps, particularly juvenile polyposis but also Peutz-Jeghers syndrome, also have a higher risk of colon cancer, although the risk is lower than it is for FAP and HNPCC. The hamartoma syndromes are less than one-tenth as common as FAP. Finally, the genetics of each of these syndromes is now known (Hampel and Peltomäki, 2000) and has interestingly led to the understanding of much of the genetics of common or sporadic colon cancers (Kinzler and Vogelstein, 1996).

Familial Adenomatous Polyposis

Clinical Characteristics. FAP is an autosomal dominantly inherited syndrome expressed as hundreds to thousands of colonic adenomatous polyps and a virtual certainty of colon cancer if the colon is not removed (Burt, 1999). The prevalence of FAP is

Table 34–6. Risk of Colon Cancer in Relatives of Persons with Large Bowel Malignancy (Odds Ratio and Confidence Interval)

Study	One Affected First-Degree Relative	Two Affected First-Degree Relatives	First-Degree Relative with Young Age at Diagnosis
St. John et al., 1993	1.8 (1.2–2.7)	5.7 (1.7–19.3)	<45 years: 3.7 (1.5–9.1)
Fuchs et al., 1994	1.72 (1.34–2.19)	2.75 (1.34–5.63	<45 years: 5.37 (1.98–14.6)
Winawer et al., 1996[a]	1.78 (1.18–2.76)	3.25 (1.92–5.52)[b]	<60 years: 2.59 (1.46–4.58)
Ahsan et al., 1998[a]	1.74 (1.24–2.45)	Not done	<50 years: 4.36 (2.24–8.51)

[a]Index cases had adenomatous polyps rather than colon cancer.
[b]A sibling had an adenomatous polyp, and a parent had colon cancer.
Source: Adapted from Burt (2000) with permission.

Table 34–7. Summary of Familial Risk of Colon Cancer

Familial Setting[a]	Lifetime Risk
General population risk in the U.S.	6%
One first-degree relative with colon cancer	2- to 3-fold increased
Two first-degree relatives with colon cancer	3- to 4-fold increased
First-degree relative with colon cancer diagnosed at ≤50 years	3- to 4-fold increased
One second- or third-degree relative with colon cancer	About 1.5-fold increased
Two second-degree relatives with colon cancer	About 2- to 3-fold increased
One first-degree relative with an	About 2-fold increased
Familial adenomatous polyposis, gene carrier adenomatous polyp	Near 100%
Hereditary nonpolyposis colorectal cancer, gene carrier	≥80%

[a]First-degree relatives include parents, siblings, and children. Second-degree relatives include grandparents, aunts, and uncles. Third-degree relatives include great-grandparents and cousins

Source: Adapted from Burt (2000) with permission.

about 1 in 10,000. Fewer than 1.0% of colon cancers arise from the disease. Polyps most often appear in the second decade of life, and the average age of colon cancer is 39 years (Burt, 1999) (Table 34–9). FAP arises from inactivating mutations of the adenomatous polyposis coli (APC) gene.

Although the extreme colon cancer risk is the central clinical focus of FAP, there are a number of extra-colonic manifestations. These include frequent fundic gland polyps of the stomach, adenomas in the duodenum, and, less frequently, adenomas of the small bowel. The gastric polyps are hamartomas with little malignancy potential. There is a 5% to 10% lifetime risk of duodenal cancer, but small bowel cancer past the duodenum is unusual. Other benign growths of FAP include osteomas, epidermoid cysts, fibromas, odontomas, supernumerary teeth, congenital hypertrophy of the retinal pigment epithelium (CHRPE), and desmoid tumors, particularly of the abdominal mesentery. Malignancies outside the gastrointestinal tract are unusual but include tumors of the central nervous system (CNS), thyroid carcinomas, hepatoblastomas, and adrenal carcinomas.

Table 34–8. Environmental Risk and Protective Factors for Colorectal Cancer

Risk Factors	Protective Factors
Strong (RR > 4.0)[a]	
Advanced age	
Country of birth (North America and Northern Europe vs. Asia and Africa)	
Long-standing ulcerative colitis	
Moderate (RR 2.1–4.0)	Moderate (RR < 0.6)
Previous adenoma or colon cancer	High physical activity
High-red-meat diet	Aspirin/selected nonsteroidal anti-inflammatory drugs
Pelvic irradiation	
Modest (RR 1.1–2.0)	Moderate (RR 0.7–1.0)
High-fat diet	High-vegetable/fruit diet
Alcohol	High-fiber diet
Cigarette smoking	High folate/methionine intake
Obesity	
Tall stature	High calcium intake
Cholecystectomy	Postmenopausal hormone replacement therapy
High sucrose consumption	

[a]RR, Relative risk.

Source: Adapted from Sandler (1996) with permission.

There are three clinical variants of FAP: Gardner syndrome (GS), Turcot syndrome (TS), and attenuated adenomatous polyposis coli (AAPC) (Table 34–9) (Burt and Ahnen, 1998). FAP families that exhibit frequent and obvious extraintestinal growths have historically been called GS. It is now known that GS also arises from mutations of the *APC* gene. The presence of CNS malignancies, together with the intestinal polyposis, is called TS. About two-thirds of TS cases also arise from *APC* mutations; the remainder are variants of HNPCC (see below) (Hamilton et al., 1995). TS associated with *APC* mutations usually exhibits medulloblastoma-type CNS malignancies. AAPC defines an attenuated form of FAP that arises from mutations of the *APC* gene but in which the average number of colonic adenomas is 30 (Spirio et al., 1993b). The appearance of both adenomas and cancer is approximately 10 years delayed compared to typical FAP.

Genetics

The *APC* Gene. The *APC* gene was localized to the long arm of chromosome 5 in 1987 (Bodmer et al., 1987; Leppert et al., 1987) and was identified and characterized in 1991 (Groden et al., 1991; Joslyn et al., 1991; Kinzler et al., 1991; Nishisho et al., 1991). Over 80% of affected FAP families have unique *APC* mutations. These are almost always nonsense mutations, giving rise to a truncated APC protein (Bisgaard et al., 1994). Very large mutations that partially or completely eliminate the APC protein coding region are also observed, but far less often. Missense mutations are found in up to 13% of *APC* genes, but they do not appear sufficient to cause FAP. Both copies of the *APC* gene must be mutated, or one copy must be mutated and the other lost (called loss of heterozygosity [LOH]) for APC function to be lost. The *APC* gene is thus a tumor suppressor gene. In FAP, one copy of the *APC* gene is inherited in a mutated form. When the remaining normal copy undergoes somatic (acquired) mutation or deletion, gene function is lost and polyps occur. It is interesting that over 80% of sporadic colon cancers also start with inactivation of the *APC* gene, but in this instance, both copies are lost by somatic events (Powell et al., 1992).

Gene Product and Function. The APC protein is approximately 300 kd with 2843 amino acids (Smith et al., 1993). The protein forms homodimers, which may be important to its function (Joslyn et al., 1993). Localization of the APC protein in normal colonic tissues by immunohistochemical staining demonstrates diffuse and variable cytoplasmic localization. It is most prominent in cells in the upper portions of the colonic epithelial crypt and has been described as exhibiting both a basolaterial (Miyashiro et al., 1995) and an apical (Sieber et al., 2000) distribution. The APC protein is found in many other tissues, and the *APC* gene is mutated in other malignancies.

The APC protein functions as a negative regulator in the Wnt growth–signaling pathway (Chung, 2000; Goss and Groden, 2000; Sieber et al., 2000; van Es et al., 2001). In the unstimulated cell, apoptosis is sustained through this pathway (Morin et al., 1996) and cellular proliferation is controlled or inhibited (Peifer, 1997). A growth signal or loss of APC gene function appears to cause a decrease of cellular apoptosis and an increase in proliferation. With APC gene function loss, these effects are constant and unregulated.

This growth regulation occurs through the interaction of the APC protein and β-catenin. The normal APC protein contains several functional domains that act as binding and degradation sites for β-catenin and thereby control its intracellular concen-

Table 34–9. Inherited Adenoma Syndromes of Colon Cancer

Syndrome[a]	Gene(s) Involved	No. of Polyps	Extra-Colonic Polyps	Other Manifestations	Clinical Genetic Testing Available	Surgery of Choice
FAP	*APC*	100s to 1000s	Gastric fundic gland polyps; duodenal and small bowel adenomas	Congenital hypertrophy of retinal pigment epithelium, desmoid tumors; increased risk for duodenal, CNS, thyroid, and adrenal cancers and for hepatoblastomas	Yes	Total colectomy with mucosal proctectomy and ileo-anal pull through
Variants of FAP				*Same as typical FAP, but also:*		
Gardner's syndrome	*APC*	100s to 1000s	Gastric fundic gland polyps; duodenal and small bowel adenomas	Osteomas, soft tissue abnormalities, dental abnormalities	Yes	Total colectomy with mucosal proctectomy and ileo-anal pull through
AAPC	*APC*	10s to >100, average of 30	Gastric fundic gland polyps; duodenal and small bowel adenomas	Possible risk of stomach and duodenal cancers	Yes	Subtotal colectomy with ileorectal anastomosis
Turcot's	*APC*	10s to >100	Gastric fundic gland polyps; duodenal and small bowel adenomas	CNS malignancy, usually medulloblastoma	Yes	Same as for FAP
HNPCC	*hMLH1, hMSH2, hMSH6, hPMS1, hPMS2*	Few	None	Gastric, biliary tract, ovarian, uterine, renal, transitional cell urinary tract, and small bowel cancers	Yes, for *hMLH1* and *hMSH2*	Subtotal colectomy
Variants of HNPCC				Same as typical HNPCC, but also:		
Muir Torre	*HMLH1, hMSH2*	Few	None	Sebaceous adenomas, epitheliomas, and carcinomas; keratocanthomas	Yes	Same as for HNPCC
Turcot's	*HMLH1, hPMS2*	Usually few	None	CNS malignancy, glioblastoma multiforme	Yes	Same as for HNPCC

Source: Modified from Burt (1998) with permission.
[a]FAP, familial adenomatous polyposis; AHPC, attenuated adenomatous polyposis coli, HNPCC, hereditary nonpolyposis colorectal cancer.

tration. A domain near the carboxyl-terminal end of APC mediates phosphorylation of β-catenin by glycogen synthase kinase 3β (GSK3b) (Rubinfeld et al., 1996). In an unstimulated cell, GSK3b promotes phosphorylation of the protein conductin/axin, which is added to the APC-GSK3b complex (Behrens et al., 1998; Willert et al., 1999). Phosphorylated axin recruits β-catenin, which, in turn, is phosphorylated and targeted for degradation through an APC-dependent ubiquitin-proteasome pathway (Aberle et al., 1997). Normal growth signaling inhibits GSK3b activity and dephosphorylates axin. β-catenin is then released from the complex (Willert et al., 1999).

In the cytoplasm, β-catenin is involved in cytoskeletal organization with binding to microtubules and in cell adhesion through interaction with E-cadherin, a membrane protein. Free β-catenin shuttles to the nucleus, where it binds to the transcription factors of the TCF/LEF family. The resulting complexes appear to activate the transcription of c-Myc (He et al., 1998), cyclin D1 (Shtutman et al., 1999; Tetsu and McCormick, 1999; Chung, 2000), and other proteins. Lack of functional APC causes unregulated intracellular accumulation of β-catenin and thus constitutive expression of c-Myc and cyclin D1).

APC protein also binds to microtubules and is believed to have a function in cell migration (Sieber et al., 2000). Two recent studies further suggest that APC has a role in chromosome segregation and that mutational inactivation in certain areas of the gene contributes to chromosomal instability by inducing ineffective kinetochore-microtubule attachment (Fodde et al., 2001; Kaplan et al., 2001). It is thereby suggested that chromosome segregation is a potential mechanism of chromosomal instability that is frequently observed in tumors with loss of APC function.

Genetic Testing. A number of highly heterogeneous DNA markers have been identified in or near the *APC* gene. Such markers can be used to identify persons who carry the mutant gene in kindreds where two or more living individuals are already clinically known to have the disease. A useful marker must be in or near the gene so as to minimize separation of the marker and gene during meiosis. At the same time, heterogeneity of a marker is important so that the marker differs between spouses, again allowing successful tracking of the mutant gene in a kindred. Markers meeting these requirements have allowed successful tracking of the mutant gene in more than 95% of FAP families, with a predicted accuracy to identify gene carriers of usually greater than 98% (Petersen et al., 1991; Spirio et al., 1993a). This approach to genetic diagnosis is called linkage testing.

In vitro protein synthesis testing (IVPS) is another approach to clinical genetic testing that has proved successful in up to 80% of FAP families (Powell et al., 1993). This testing is based on the observation that the large majority of *APC* mutations that cause FAP give rise to a shortened or truncated protein (Goss and Groden, 2000). Truncated proteins arise primarily in two ways. In the first, a nucleotide base substitution can change a base triplet from one that codes for an amino acid to one that is a "stop" codon. A stop codon is a base triplet that signals the translation of mRNA to protein to stop; it is normally found at the end of genes and defines the end of the protein. The accidental message causes a premature stop message and thus a truncated protein. The second and most common cause of accidental stop codons is the addition or deletion of a small numbers of nucleotide bases that shifts the DNA triplet reading "out of frame." Accidental stop codons always occur shortly downstream from these errors, again giving rise to truncated proteins. Both types of mutations are called *nonsense mutations* because of the complete disruption in coding. Mutations of large portions of chromosomal material sometimes cause FAP but are quite unusual.

The IVPS clinical genetic testing method takes advantage of the observation that disease-causing *APC* mutations almost always give rise to truncated APC proteins (Powell et al., 1993). The laboratory method proceeds as follows. DNA material is purified from white blood cells of a blood sample. The *APC* gene is isolated, amplified by the polymerase chain reaction (PCR), and divided into five segments for convenience of testing. DNA segments are then processed to messenger RNA and finally to protein in the test tube. This protein is then placed on an electrophoretic gel that separates by size. If both alleles (one from each parent) are of normal length, only one band is observed, as all the protein migrates at an equal speed. If there is a normal-length APC protein segment from one parent and a truncated or shortened protein segment from the FAP parent, then two bands will be observed in the electrophoretic lane, indicating the presence of a disease-causing mutation in one allele. Although the precise mutation is not defined by this method, the presence of a disease-causing mutation is clear. This method is successful in identifying the presence of mutation in about 80% of families with FAP (Hemminki et al., 1998). Once evidence of a mutation is found in an index case, however, the test is virtually 100% accurate in other members of the same family, as all affected members of the family will have the identical mutation.

An increasing number of laboratories are now directly applying sequencing to the *APC* gene to identify the specific disease-causing mutation. Often, one of several methods that narrow the area of DNA to be sequenced is first applied, such as single-stranded conformational polymorphism (SSCP) analysis and denaturing gradient gel electrophoresis (DGGE). As in IVPS, finding a specific mutation in an index case allows other family members to be tested for the presence or absence of that mutation with a high degree of accuracy.

A reasonable approach to clinical genetic testing in FAP is to first apply IVPS testing or sequencing to an index case with clinically apparent FAP. This will be successful in the majority of cases and will then allow highly accurate predictive testing in other family members. If a mutation cannot be detected by these methods, then linkage testing can be applied, providing that there are two or more known cases of FAP in the family in question. IVPS testing or sequencing can also be applied to confirm the diagnosis in questionable cases where there is no family history, although it must be kept in mind that failure to identify a mutation in this setting does not rule out FAP. Only a positive test is helpful.

It is important that both the physician and the person being tested thoroughly understand the risks, the limitations, and the interpretations of genetic tests before the tests are performed (Geller et al., 1997; Petersen et al., 1999; Wong et al., 2001). Genetic counselors can be very helpful in this regard, and consultation with centers where genetic testing for FAP is regularly performed is strongly encouraged. A recent study found that genetic testing for FAP was often done without proper patient consent or understanding and without proper counseling or advice (Giardiello, 1997). Insurance difficulties, psychological harm, and even inappropriate medical care may result from improper application of genetic testing. Genetic testing for FAP is usually not recommended before 10 to12 years of age because of the potential for emotional, psychological, and family distress at an age when the diagnosis is not clinically helpful (MacDonald and Lessick, 2000).

Genotype-Phenotype Correlations. The location of germline mutations in the *APC* gene has shown correlation with phenotype of the disease (Figure 34–2) (Chung, 2000; Sieber et al., 2000; van Es et al., 2001). The CHRPE lesion is present if mutations occur distal to exon 9 of the gene (Wallis et al., 1994). Mutations of the extreme proximal or distal end of the gene result in AAPC (Spirio et al., 1993). Profuse polyposis (>5,000

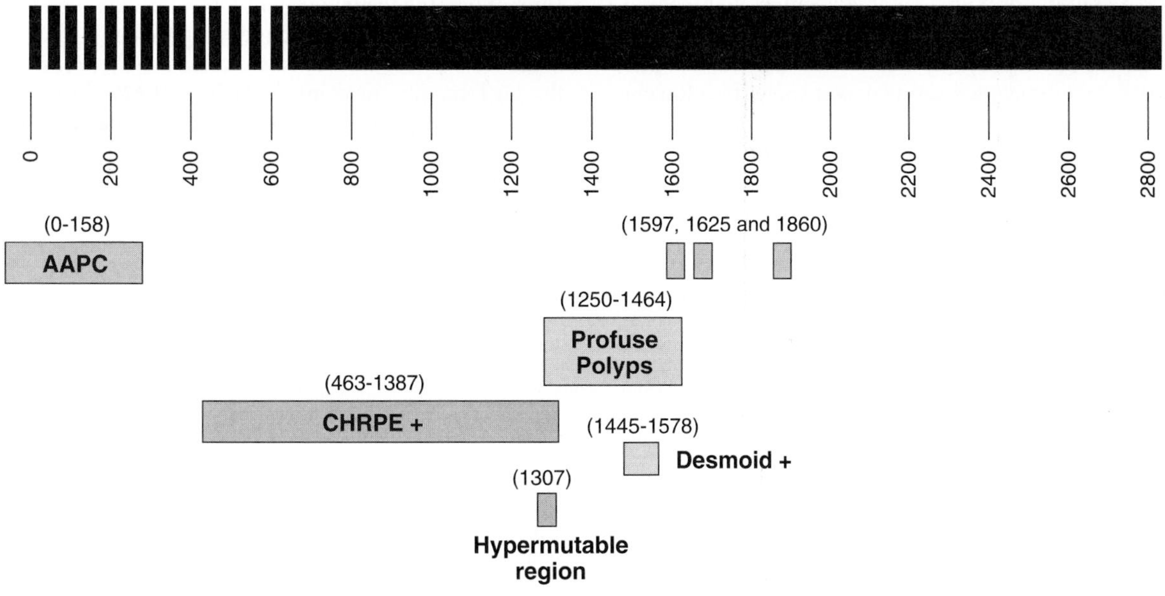

Fig. 34–2. The adenomatous polyposis coli gene with locations of mutations that correspond with extra-intestinal manifestations of the disease. From Burt (1998) with permission.

adenomas) correlates with mutation in a small region in the mid-portion of exon 15 of the gene (Nagase et al., 1992). Desmoid tumors and possibly osteomas occur more frequently when mutations occur in a region just distal to the mutations that give rise to profuse polyposis (Caspari et al., 1995). Variable colonic polyp distributions have been described in the setting of identical disease-causing mutations, suggesting modifying genetic mechanisms in some cases (Paul et al., 1993; Giardiello et al., 1994).

Clinical Application of Genetic Information. Colonic screening of persons at risk for FAP usually begins by age 10 to 12 years, as cancers have occasionally been reported by this age (King et al., 2000). Genetic testing, as described above and using peripheral blood for DNA, can also be offered at this age to direct screening (Giardiello, 2001). Biannual sigmoidoscopy is the appropriate screening in those who test positive unless the first screening is done at an older age. All family members who are at risk for FAP require sigmoidoscopy or colonoscopy screening if genetic testing is not successful in a family (King et al., 2000). Full colonoscopy should be used in families with AAPC, although screening in this condition can safely begin in the late teens. Correlations with mutation location in the *APC* gene are generally not yet sufficiently accurate to be of clinical utility but may sometimes help in favoring subtotal colectomy over proctocolectomy in persons with AAPC (Soravia et al., 2000).

Hereditary Nonpolyposis Colorectal Cancer

Clinical Characteristics. HNPCC is an autosomal dominantly inherited condition characterized by a high risk of colorectal cancer at a young age (Table 34–9) (Lynch and Lynch, 2000). Although adenomatous polyps are also the precursor of colon cancer in this disease, only one or several polyps usually form in affected individuals. Polyps, however, appear at a younger age, are larger, and exhibit more advanced histopathology than their sporadic counterparts. The average age of colon cancer diagnosis is 44 years, and the lifetime risk of this malignancy is 80% (Marra and Boland, 1995; Lynch and de la Chapelle, 1999). HNPCC accounts for 2% to 3% of colon cancer cases. Colonic cancers in HNPCC favor a proximal colonic location, and there are frequent synchronous (simultaneous) and metachronous (future) tumors. Mucinous and signet ring tumors are common, and there is an improved staged-matched survival over sporadic colon cancers.

Clinical criteria have been developed to predict HNPCC, as there is no distinct phenotype in an isolated patient (Vasen et al., 1991). These are called the Amsterdam Criteria, and include the following: (1) three relatives in a family should have colon cancer, two of them being first-degree relatives of a third; (2) cases of colon cancer must span at least two generations; and (3) one case must be diagnosed at 50 years of age or younger. When these conditions are met, 49% of families tested are found to have a mutation in one of the genes that causes HNPCC (Wijnen et al., 1997). These criteria recently have been expanded to include all of the malignancies found in HNPCC rather than just colon cancer (Vasen et al., 1999).

Uterine cancer is the most frequent extra-colonic malignancy with a lifetime risk of about 40%. There is also a 10% to 20% risk of gastric, ovarian, biliary tract, renal, and urinary tract cancer, and a small risk of small bowel cancer (Table 34–10) (Aarnio et al., 1999). Empiric guidelines for cancer screening in HNPCC are also given in Table 34–10. Muir-Torre syndrome is a variant of HNPCC with similar genetic etiology. It is characterized by benign and malignant sebaceous tumors, keratoacanthomas, and the other malignancies of HNPCC (Kolodner et al., 1994) (Table 34–9). Approximately one-third of the families with Turcot's syndrome arise from mutations of the same genes that give rise to HNPCC (Hamilton et al., 1995) (Table 34–9). In these families, the colonic adenomas are often relatively few in number, and the CNS tumors are usually glioblastoma multiform in type.

Genetics

DNA Mismatch Repair. HNPCC results from inherited mutations in one of six mismatch repair genes (Marra and Boland, 1995; Lynch and de la Chapelle, 1999). Mismatches are DNA errors that may occur during DNA transcription; the mismatch repair system normally repairs such errors. In HNPCC, one copy of one of the mismatch repair genes is inherited in a mutated form. The normal allele may later be lost or mutated, resulting in gene inactivation. DNA mismatch errors then persist into daughter cells during subsequent cell divisions. When a mismatch error occurs in a gene that is critical to cancer pathogenesis, there is progression toward adenoma and cancer.

In part, the mismatch repair (MMR) system is responsible for maintaining the integrity of DNA through repair of mismatch errors. The human mismatch repair genes now identified include *hMLH1*, *hMSH2*, *hMSH3* (also called *DUG*), *hMSH6* (also called the G–T binding protein), *hPMS1*, and *hPMS2* (Miyaki, 1997). Each of these genes was first identified in bacterial or yeast systems. The lowercase "h" preceding each gene designation indicates the human homolog of the particular gene found in a non-

Table 34–10. Cancer Risks and Screening Recommendations in Hereditary Non-polyposis Colorectal Cancer

Cancer	Cancer Risk (%)	Screening Recommendations
Colon	≥80%	Colonoscopy, every 1–2 years, beginning at age 20–25 years or 10 years younger than the earliest case in the family, whichever comes first
Endometrial	43–60	Pelvic exam, transvaginal ultrasound and/or endometrial aspirate every 1–2 years, starting at age 25–35 years
Gastric	13–19	Upper GI endoscopy every 1–2 years, starting at age 30–35 years
Urinary tract	4.0–10	Ultrasound and urinalysis (?urine cytology) every 1–2 years, starting at age 30–35 years
Biliary tract and gallbladder	2.0–18	Uncertain, possibly LFTs annually after age 30 years
Central nervous system, usually glioblastoma (Turcot's syndrome)	3.7	Uncertain, possibly annual physical examination and periodic head CT in affected families
Small bowel	1–4	Uncertain, at least small bowel X-ray if symptoms occur

Source: Modified from Burt (2000) with permission.

human DNA repair system. Over 95% of HNPCC families in which mutations are found have mutations in either *hMLH1* and *hMSH2*. Only one family has been identified with mutations of *hPMSH1*, two families with mutations of *hPMS2*, and none with mutations of *hMSH3* (Miyaki et al., 1997). Multiple families have now been found with mutations of *hMSH6*. Such families appear to have a slightly different phenotype, with later-onset colon cancer and possibly a higher risk of uterine than colon cancer (Kolodner et al., 1999; Wu et al., 1999).

The *hMSH2* gene product appears to recognize DNA mismatches (Yin et al., 1997). *hMSH2* forms heterodimers with *hMSH6* and *hMSH3*, both of which affect the specificity of error recognition (Yin et al., 1997). *hMLH1* and *hPMS2* also form a heterodimer that interacts with the *hMSH2/hMSH6* (or *hMSH2/hMSH3*) complex. Other proteins are then recruited to complete the repair process, including DNA polymerase, helicase, and ligase. The overall repair process includes recognition of the DNA mismatch error, excision of a DNA segment containing the error, re-synthesis of a new DNA segment from the parent DNA, and, finally, ligation of the new DNA strand into place. In addition to the repair of mismatches from replication, the mismatch repair system also repairs errors caused by deamination events, oxidation, adduct formation, damage to nucleotide precursors, and direct DNA damage (Marra and Borland, 1996). This system recognizes and repairs not only single base pair mismatches and mutations but also errors up to 14 bases in length.

The Mutator Phenotype. Dysfunction of the mismatch repair (MMR) system leads to the accumulation of replication errors (also called mismatches), which are usually detected in di- and trinucleotide DNA repeat regions that occur throughout the chromosome and also flank certain genes, where they are called microsatellites. Errors in these microsatellites are particularly frequent with cell division because of slippage of the DNA replication enzymes, which, in turn, leads to DNA repeat segments of different lengths. Tumors containing errors of this type are said to exhibit the mutator phenotype, or microsatellite instability (MSI). Over 90% of colon cancers in patients with HNPCC are found to exhibit MSI (Marra and Borland, 1996). About 15% of sporadic colon cancers also exhibit MSI, although the mechanism of MMR gene inactivation appears to more often involve methylation errors in the gene promotor region (Herman et al., 1998; Thibodeau et al., 1998).

Clinical Genetic Testing for HNPCC. A number of laboratory genetic approaches are used to identify persons with HNPCC. Linkage testing is possible but rarely used. IVPS is also used to look for truncating mutations, but this type of mutation is not nearly as common in HNPCC as in FAP. Thus sequencing is most commonly done of the *hMSH2* and *hMLH1* genes, as they are responsible for the large majority of disease-causing mutations. As in sequencing the *APC* gene, laboratory screening methods, such as SSCP and DGGE, are used to find the area of DNA in which the mutation occurs, followed by sequencing.

The recommended clinical approach is to use genetic testing in families that meet the Amsterdam criteria (Giardiello, 2001) and to first test the person with the youngest age of colon cancer diagnosis, thus the person least likely to have a sporadic colon cancer. If a disease-causing mutation is found, genetic testing can then be performed with high predictability in other family members. Genetic testing for HNPCC is now commercially available through a number of laboratories.

It is well recognized that some fraction of families with colon cancer from inherited MMR mutations do not meet the Amsterdam criteria (Wijnen et al., 1997). Lack of a specific phenotype for HNPCC makes its diagnosis difficult when the Amsterdam criteria are not met. Several strategies have been proposed to clinically screen colon cancer cases to detect such families. In view of cost and psychosocial issues surrounding genetic testing, it is presently unrealistic to perform genetic testing on all cases of colon cancer for this condition. Short of this, testing colon cancer tissue for MSI has been suggested as an approach, since almost all HNPCC colon cancers exhibit MSI, while only about 15% of sporadic colon cancers have this trait. Such an approach has been applied with good results in the clinical setting (Aaltonen et al., 1998; Loukola et al., 1999; Terdiman et al., 2001), especially when cases in which the tumor is to be tested for MSI are selected on the basis of having a family history of colon cancer or having a young age of diagnosis. Another approach uses extended family history with a web-based formula to determine who should have genetic testing (Wijnen et al., 1998). Finally, a simplified, single-stage approach has been suggested which appears to be both efficient and accurate in determining who should undergo DNA sequencing to detect germline MMR mutations (Syngal et al., 2000; Giardiello, 2001). With this approach, one goes directly to DNA testing if a colon cancer patient *(1)* has a family that meets the Amsterdam criteria; *(2)* has had a previous HNPCC tumor; or *(3)* has a first-degree relative with any HNPCC tumor and either the patient or the relative were diagnosed at an age less than 50 years.

Management. Colonoscopy is recommended for screening persons who are at risk in families with HNPCC (Marra and Borland, 1995; Lynch and Lynch, 2000). Screening should begin at 25 years of age, or 10 years younger than the earliest diagnosis of colon cancer in the family, whichever comes first. Screening should be repeated every one to two years because advanced cancers may occur if the intervals are longer (Burke et al., 1997; Järvinen et al., 2000; Giardiello, 2001). As in FAP, screening may be reduced or possibly even eliminated in persons who have negative genetic testing for a specific mutation already identified in a family. Periodic screening for other cancers—especially uterine—should also be performed, although the effectiveness of screening for extra-colonic tumors in persons with HNPCC is unproven (Burke et al., 1997). Nonetheless, empiric guidelines are given in Table 34–10, as a point of consideration for physicians caring for patients and families with this condition. A subtotal colectomy is the recommended treatment for colon cancer when the patient is from a family with HNPCC. Screening of the remaining rectum should then be performed every 2 years.

Syndromes of Hamartomatous Polyposis

The hamartomatous syndromes are very rare but will be included because it is now known that these syndromes exhibit a significant risk of colon and other malignancies. The genes relevant to these conditions also have now been identified, and genetic testing is available (Table 34–11) (Hampel and Peltomäki, 2000). Each of these conditions is inherited in an autosomal dominant fashion with high penetrance.

Peutz-Jeghers Syndrome. Peutz-Jeghers syndrome is characterized by melanin pigment spots on the lips, buccal mucosa, and other areas (Utsunomiya et al., 1975; Spigelman et al., 1995; McGarrity et al., 2000). Polyps are histologically characteristic and found in the small bowel and sometimes throughout the GI

Table 34–11. Function of Genes Mutated in the Inherited Syndromes of Colon Cancer

Syndrome	Gene(s)[a]	Gene Function
Familial adenomatous polyposis	*APC*	Negative regulator in a signaling pathway controlling cell proliferation and apoptosis
Hereditary nonpolyposis colorectal cancer	*MMR*	A set of genes involved in the repair of DNA errors that often arise during DNA replication
Peutz-Jeghers syndrome	*STK11*	A regulator of gene expression
Juvenile polyposis	*SMAD4/DPC4; BMPR1A; PTEN*	*SMAD4* and *BMPR1A* are modulators of the TGFβ[b] cell growth signaling pathway
Cowden syndrome	*PTEN*	A modulator in a cell growth signaling pathway

[a]APC, Adenomatous polyposis coli; MMR, Mismatch repair; STK11, Serine threonine kinase 11; SMAD4/DPC4, Sma- and Mad-related protein 4, Deleted in pancreatic carcinoma 4; BMPR1A, Bone morphogenetic protein receptor 1A; PTEN, Phosphatase and tensin homolog deleted on chromosome 10.
[b]TGFβ, Transforming growth factor β.
Source: Modified from Burt (2000) with permission.

tract. Symptoms often begin in the second decade and include bleeding, abdominal pain, and intussusception. Malignancy is the major cause of morbidity after age 40 years with a cancer risk of any site over 90% by age 65 years (Giardiello et al., 2000). Cancers of the colon, pancreas, stomach, and small bowel are all common, together with a number of extra-intestinal cancers, including breast, uterine, and ovarian. The frequencies of these malignancies, together with empiric screening guidelines, are given in Table 34–12. About 50% of Peutz-Jeghers syndrome patients are found to have a disease-causing mutation of a seronine-threonine kinase gene, *STK11*, on chromosome 19. The function of this gene appears related to DNA expression (Hemminki et al., 1998).

Juvenile Polyposis. Juvenile polypsis (JP) is defined as the presence of more than 10 juvenile polyps. About one-third of such cases inherit this condition (Jass, 1994; Desai et al., 1998; Woodford-Richens et al., 2000). The polyps are most often found in the colon but may occur throughout the small bowel and stomach. Nonspecific benign symptoms, most commonly bleeding and abdominal pain, often occur in the first decade of life. Some surveys have found a colon cancer risk approaching 50% (Desai et al., 1995). JP arises from mutations of the *SMAD4* gene on chromosome 18 (about 25% of cases) (Howe et al., 1998; Roth et al., 1999), from mutations of the *BMPRA1* gene on chromosome 10 (about 25% of cases) (Howe et al., 2001), and from mutations of the *PTEN* gene (only a few reported families) (Olschwang, 1998). The SMAD4 protein is an effector in the transforming growth factor β (TGFβ) cell growth signaling pathway (Howe et al., 1998). BMPRA1 is a serine-threonine kinase type 1 receptor of the TGFβ superfamily.

Cowden Syndrome. The hallmark of Cowden syndrome (CS) is the presence of trichilemmoma, most commonly observed over the bridge of the nose and on the gingiva and tongue (Hizawa et al., 1994; Eng, 1997, 2000). Hamartomatous polyps occur throughout the GI tract and are most often juvenile polyps, although neurofibromas, lipomas, and other hamartomatous polyps may also be seen. There is a 3% to 10% risk of thyroid cancer, a 25% to 50% risk of breast cancer, and an increased risk for ovarian and uterine cancer in Cowden syndrome. GI cancer risk has not been appreciated but will likely be observed, as juvenile polyps are common in the syndrome and are associated with colon cancer in juvenile polyposis. The syndrome is included here mainly because it must be distinguished from JP. This condition arises from mutations of the *PTEN* gene that is involved in cell growth regulation (Liaw et al., 1997). Bannayan-Ruvalcaba-Riley syndrome appears to be allelic to CS and is characterized by macrocephaly, lopomas, and pigmented macules of the glans penis, as well as other findings of CS (Gorlin et al., 1992; Marsh et al., 1997; Hampel and Peltomäki, 2000).

Table 34–12. Cancer Risks and Screening Recommendations in Peutz-Jeghers Syndrome

Type of Cancer	Cancer Risk (%)	Screening Recommendations
GI Cancers		
Colon	39	Colonoscopy, beginning with symptoms or in late teens if no symptoms occur; interval determined by number of polyps, but at least every 3 years once begun
Pancreatic	36	Endoscopic or abdominal ultrasound every 1–2 years, starting at age 30 years
Stomach	29	Upper GI endoscopy every 2 years, starting at age 10 years
Small bowel	13	Annual hemoglobin, small bowel X-ray every 2 years, both starting at age 10 years
Esophagus	0.5	None given
Non-GI Cancers		
Breast	54	Annual breast exam and mammography every 2–3 years, both starting at age 25 years
Ovarian	21	Annual pelvic exam with pap smear; annual pelvic or vaginal ultrasound and/or uterine washings, both starting at age 20 years
Uterine	9	
Adenoma malignum (cervix)	Rare	
Sex cord tumor with annular tubules (SCTAT), in almost all women	20 become malignant	
Sertoli cell tumor (males), unusual	10 to 20 become malignant	Annual testicular exam, starting at age 10 years; testicular ultrasound if feminizing features occur
Lung	15	None given

[a]Cumulative cancer risks, ages 15 to 64 years.
Source: Modified from Burt (2000) with permission.

Table 34–13. Commonly Mutated Genes in Colon Cancer and Their Function

Gene	Gene Type	Gene Function	Fraction of all Colon Cancers with Gene Mutated (%)	Condition if Gene Mutation Is Inherited
APC	Tumor suppressor gene	Normal function sustains apoptosis and regulates or decreases proliferation	80 or more	Familiae adenomatous polyposis
K-ras	Oncogene	Intracellular signal transduction of growth signals	50	Non known
p53	Tumor suppressor gene	Cell cycle arrest for mutation repair or apoptosis if repair is not possible	75	Li-Fraumeni syndrome
hMLH1 hMSH2, hMSH6, hPMS1, hPMS2	DNA mismatch repair genes	Repair of short-length DNA errors	15	Hereditary non-polyposis colorectal cancer

Colon Carcinogenesis

Colon cancer develops as relevant genes are affected by mutation (Table 34–13). The pathogenesis of this malignancy is a multistep process that occurs over years and affects the function of tumor suppressor genes, oncogenes, and DNA repair genes (Chung, 2000; Kinzler and Vogelstein, 1996). The molecular process is mirrored by the pathologic progression of normal colonic epithelium to adenomatous polyps to cancer. There appear to be two quite distinct molecular genetic pathways that lead to colon cancer. One begins with inactivation of the *APC* gene and the other with inactivation of one of the mismatch repair genes. Thus, the genetic pathogenesis of colon cancer is the same in both the inherited syndromes and the sporadic setting. The only difference is that one allele of the relevant gene is inherited in a mutated form in the syndromes and the second allele is later mutated, causing gene inactivation. In common or sporadic colon polyps and cancers, both alleles must be somatically inactivated. Additionally, only a single colonic epithelial cell is involved in the sporadic setting, while all cells begin with one mutated allele in one of the relevant genes in the inherited conditions.

APC Pathway (Chromosome Instability Pathway)

Over 80% of nonsyndromic colon cancers begin with somatic inactivation of the *APC* gene, which is a tumor suppressor gene and the same gene that gives rise to FAP (Powell et al., 1992; Chung, 2000; Sieber et al., 2000). For common colon adenomas to form, both APC alleles must be somatically mutated for gene function to be lost. Somatic, or acquired, loss of both alleles is statistically an unlikely event, so that sporadic adenomas occur much later in life and only one or several polyps are observed compared to FAP. Once *APC* is inactivated, dysplastic cells arise and progress to an adenomatous polyp through clonal expansion (Kinzler and Vogelstein, 1996). In FAP, one allele of the *APC* gene is inherited in a mutated form. Loss or mutation of the second allele is a frequent event, giving rise to the phenotype of colonic polyposis at a young age. The type of mutation carried by the inherited or germline *APC* mutation may influence the mode of inactivation of the second *APC* allele (Spirio et al., 1998).

A frequent mechanism of loss of genetic material in the APC pathway is called loss of heterozygosity (LOH) (Carethers, 1996). LOH is an important mechanism of tumorigenesis, and appears to arise, at least in part, from *APC* mutation itself (Fodde et al., 2001; Kaplan et al., 2001). With LOH, there appears to be an asymmetric distribution of chromosomal material during a flawed mitosis. This may result in loss of the entire normal allele, thereby unmasking the mutated allele of the tumor suppressor gene and causing loss of that gene's normal function. The frequent chromosomal errors in the APC pathway give rise to the term *chromosome instability (CIN) pathway*.

Once an FAP or sporadic adenoma forms, it may progress to cancer. This progression involves cumulative somatic mutations of similar genes in both settings (Kinzler and Vogelstein, 1996; Chung, 2000; Sieber et al., 2000; Terdiman, 2000) (Fig. 34–3). It is believed that the rate of somatic mutation (often by way of LOH) is increased after APC is inactivated and may be further driven by the level of luminal carcinogens. *K-ras* is an oncogene and is most frequently the next gene affected by mutation in colon tumor progression. K-ras is normally involved in growth signal transduction; it is constitutively activated when mutations occur in specific areas of one allele of the gene. The frequency of observed *K-ras* mutations increases from moderately (11%) to severely (36%) dysplastic adenomas to carcinoma (50%) (Vogelstein et al., 1988). Inactivation of a gene on chromosome 18 appears to be the next most common genetic event in the APC pathway. The deleted in colon cancer (*DCC*) gene was previously believed to be the target gene of this inactivation, although recent work suggests that this is not the case and a yet-to-be-identified gene, possibly *SMAD*, is inactivated (Vogelstein et al., 1988). *K-ras* and chromosome 18 mutations are accompanied at the histologic level by enlargement and increasing dysplasia of the adenoma (Fig. 34–3).

Inactivation of p53, a tumor suppressor gene, has been observed in 75% of invasive colon carcinomas and in over 50% of all human cancers (Vogelstein et al., 1988; Hollstein et al., 1991; Lane, 1992). The benign to malignant transformation of the adenomatous polyp appears to parallel p53 inactivation (Baker et al., 1990b). Normally, p53 is activated by the presence of mutation in any of the chromosomes. G1 cell cycle arrest is initiated, allowing time for DNA repair. If repair is not possible, apoptosis is initiated and the mutation is eliminated in this fashion. Loss of normal p53 function thus carries significant consequences to the integrity of DNA, as mutations are allowed to persist and accumulate. Loss of alleles on chromosome 18 and 22 are observed in 46% and 33% of colon cancers, respectively, although the specific genes involved on these chromosomes are still in question (Vogelstein et al., 1988).

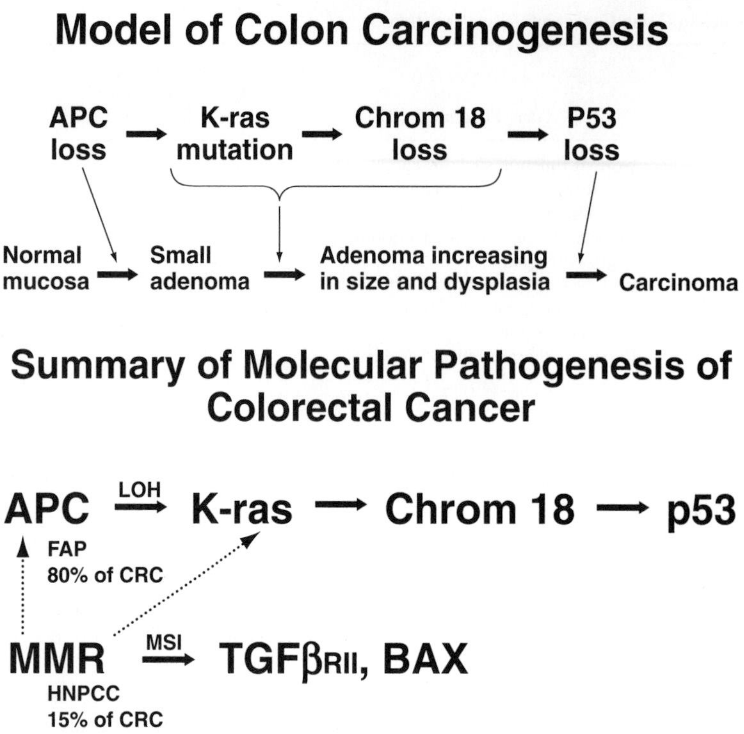

Fig. 34–3. The molecular pathogenesis of colorectal cancer: APC pathway (*top*) and APC and MMR pathway (*bottom*).

Mismatch Pathway

About 15% of sporadic colon cancers begin, or have as an early event, the inactivation of the mismatch repair process, the same process that is inactivated in HNPCC (Thibodeau et al., 1993; Loeb, 1994; Samowitz et al., 1995; Chung, 2000). In HNPCC, one of the mismatch repair genes is inherited in a mutated form. Gene inactivation occurs when the second allele is later somatically mutated. In the setting of sporadic polyps and cancer, both alleles must be mutated somatically.

Tumors beginning with mismatch repair inactivation are very different, however, than those beginning with inactivation of APC. LOH is rarely observed, and activation of K-ras or inactivation of p53 and APC are unusual (Konishi et al., 1996; Chung, 2000). Instead, MSI is observed in tumor tissues (see above, under HNPCC genetics), and different genes appear to be subsequently mutationally affected in the pathogenic process. Transforming growth factor βRII receptor (TGFβRII) and *BAX* genes, both relevant in cell growth signal transduction, have been described as affected in this pathway (Markowitz et al., 1995).

It is interesting and instructive that the initial gene inactivation of virtually all colonic adenomas and colon cancers occurs in the same genes that give rise to the inherited conditions of FAP and HNPCC. Thus, study of the rare inherited syndromes has provided the needed clues to understanding colon cancer pathogenesis in general.

Familial Occurrence of Common Colon Cancer

Clinical Characteristics

The clinical characteristics of this group of colon cancers are reviewed under "family epidemiology" above and in Tables 34–3 to 34–7. To summarize, familial risk of colon cancer outside FAP and HNPCC is very common (Lichtenstein et al., 2000) and may be stratified, to some degree, by the number of affected persons in a family and the age of cancer diagnosis (Burt, 2000).

Possible Genetic Causes

In the setting of common familial risk, it appears that inherited factors may often determine individual susceptibility to colonic neoplasm, whereas environmental factors probably determine the expression of these susceptibilities. A number of candidate genes have been suggested to explain this mild to moderate form of inherited predisposition. These include milder mutations of the genes that give rise to FAP and HNPCC, as well as certain polymorphisms of genes that are important to carcinogen or tumor promoter metabolism. Some of the likely candidate genes or mutations include the following.

APC Mutation in Ashkenazim. Laken, 1997 reported that an inherited mutation of the *APC* gene caused a mild but common colon cancer predisposition. The mutation was a substitution of lysine for isoleucine at codon 1307. It was found in 6% of the Ashkenazi Jews, in about 10% of the Ashkenazim with colon cancer, and in 28% of the Ashkenazim with colorectal cancer and a positive family history of colon malignancy. The mutation was not found outside Ashkenazim. Overall, the results suggested that the mutation was associated with about a 2-fold increased risk of colorectal cancer.

Methylenetetrahydrofolate Reductase. Dietary folate and methionine have been associated with low rates of colorectal cancer, and their deficiency with increased rates (Chen et al., 1996; Ma et al., 1997). Furthermore, both are factors in the DNA methylation process, and both hypo- and hypermethylation have been implicated in carcinogenesis. Methylenetetrahydrofolate reductase (MTFR) is an important enzyme in folate and methionine metabolism and to some extent determines the circulating levels of these nutrients. Certain polymorphisms of MTFR have been associated with decreased risk of colon cancer. Their effect is modulated by intake of alcohol, folate, and methionine (Potter, 1999).

Glutathione S-Transferases. Glutathione *S*-transferases (GSTs) are a family of phase II xenobiotic (foreign substance)-metabolizing enzymes. The gene encoding the isoenzyme, GST Mu (*GSTM1*), is polymorphic with at least four alleles. About 30% to 70% of individuals from various racial groups lack GSTM1 enzyme activity. Zhong and colleagues (1993) found a significantly increased risk of colorectal cancer in persons lacking GSTM1 activity, although other studies have not confirmed this (Chenevix-Trench et al., 1995). If *GSTM1* polymorphisms are related to colorectal cancer risk, they may be related to altered metabolism of environmental hazards, carcinogens, tumor promotors, or protective agents by this class of enzymes.

Cytochrome P450 and Acetyltransferase. The cytochrome P450 and acetyltransferase enzymes systems mediate the *N*-oxidation and *O*-acetylation of xenobiotics. Dietary heterocyclic amines are xenobiotics formed by the pyrolysis of amino acids and creatinine during cooking, particularly at high temperatures, of meats. It has been suggested that dietary heterocyclic amines are activated by certain cytochrome P450 and acetyltransferase polymorphisms to produce *N*-acetoxyarylamines, which bind to DNA to form DNA-carcinogen adducts. DNA adducts increase the risk of mutation during DNA replication. In a case-control study by Lang and colleagues (1994), case patients with rapid metabolizing phenotypes of both enzyme systems had a colon cancer prevalence that was slightly above that in the control patients. In the combined rapid phenotype, colon cancer was found in 35% of the case patients but in only 16% of the control patients (OR 2.79). Other studies, however, have not found this association (Spurr et al., 1995).

Alcohol Dehydrogenase. A high alcohol intake has been associated with increased colon cancer risk. Polymorphisms of the alcohol metabolizing enzyme, ADH, have been associated with increased oral cancer risk (Harty et al., 1997). Acetaldehyde, a metabolite of alcohol, has been shown in cell cultures to cause DNA mutations and DNA-adduct formation, to initiate cell transformation, and to inhibit DNA repair (Singh and Kahn, 1995). Suspect ADH polymorphisms have not yet been studied in colon cancer.

Vitamin D Receptor. A lower intake of calcium and vitamin D has been associated with colon cancer and adenoma risk, and supplementation with these nutrients with lower risk (Kampman et al., 1994; Baron et al., 1999; Holt, 1999). VDR may modulate vitamin D levels and therefore calcium metabolism, and one polymorphism of VDR has been associated with prostate cancer risk. VDR polymorphisms have not yet been examined in association with colon cancer risk.

Screening

Presently recommended colorectal cancer screening for the general population includes annual fecal occult blood testing and sigmoidoscopy every five years, both starting at age 50 years, or alternatively, colonoscopy every 10 years, starting at age 50 years. (Byers et al., 1997; Winawer et al., 1997) (Table 34–14). All persons with a family history of colon cancer should be encouraged to undergo standard screening, at the very least. It should probably start at age 40, however, as the colon cancer risk at age 40 when a family history is present is about the same as the risk at age 50 with no family history (Fuchs et al., 1994). If two first-degree relatives have colon cancer or a first-degree relative is diagnosed with colon cancer at 50 years of age or younger (possibly 60 years or younger), then colonoscopy is the most appropriate screening test (Burt, 2000). Colonoscopy should begin by age 40 years, or 10 years younger than the youngest case in the family, and should be repeated every five years. The American Cancer Society supports these recommendations (Byers et al., 1997), which are summarized in Table 34–14.

ESOPHAGEAL CANCER

Disease Definition

Esophageal cancer includes primarily squamous cell carcinoma and adenocarcinoma. Diagnosis is made by endoscopic biopsy, although X-ray and endoscopic appearance are usually characteristic. Dysphagia is the most common clinical presentation, and diagnosis is almost always made at late stages of the disease. There is an occasional surgical cure, but surgical and endoscopic approaches are primarily for palliation. Endoscopic ultrasound has emerged as probably the most accurate staging approach. Esophageal cancer, overall, carries a poor prognosis, with little response to chemotherapy or radiation therapy. Familial clustering of cases is unusual. Familial risk has been noted in some populations, and rare inherited syndromes have been described (see below).

Table 34–14. Suggested Colon Cancer Screening Considering Familial Risk

Setting[a]	Screening Recommendations[b]
General population	Standard screening
One first-degree relative with colon cancer	Standard screening, beginning at age 40
Two first-degree relatives with colon cancer	Colonoscopy every 5 yrs, beginning at age 40
First-degree relative with colon cancer diagnosed at ≤50 years	Colonoscopy every 5 yrs, beginning 10 years younger than earliest age of colon cancer diagnosis in family
One second- or third-degree relative with colon cancer	Standard screening, beginning at age 40
Two second-degree relatives with colon cancer	Standard screening, beginning at age 40
One first-degree relative with an adenomatous polyp	Standard screening, probably beginning at age 40
Familial adenomatous polyposis, gene carrier	Sigmoidoscopy every 2 years, beginning at age 10–12 years
Hereditary nonpolyposis colorectal cancer, gene carrier	Colonoscopy every 1–2 years, beginning at age 25 or 10 years younger than earliest age of diagnosis in family, whichever comes first

[a]First-degree relatives include parents, siblings, and children. Second-degree relatives include grandparents, aunts, and uncles. Third-degree relatives include great-grandparents and cousins.
[b]Standard screening includes annual fecal occult blood testing and sigmoidoscopy every five years, both beginning at age 50 years.

Epidemiology

There were an estimated 12,300 new cases of esophageal cancer diagnosed in the United States in 2000, and 12,100 deaths (Greenlee et al., 2000). The incidence of this malignancy in various areas of the world is shown in Figure 34–4. The incidence in the United States is slowly increasing. Men have esophageal cancer more often than women, with a ratio of 3.0:1. The mean age of diagnosis is 65 years. Squamous and adenocarcinoma are the two common types of esophageal cancer. Recent trends show an increasing fraction of cases arising in the distal one-third of the esophagus, now 48% (Devesa et al., 1998). The fraction of adenocarcinomas is also increasing and now accounts for 43% of cases; squamous cell carcinomas account for 56%. Among white males, adenocarcinoma has increased 350% in the last two decades. The fraction of all esophageal cancer cases being diagnosed in the most advanced stages is also increasing and is now 32%. There is less than a 10% five-year survival rate, with only a 20% to 25% five-year survival rate even among those operated for cure.

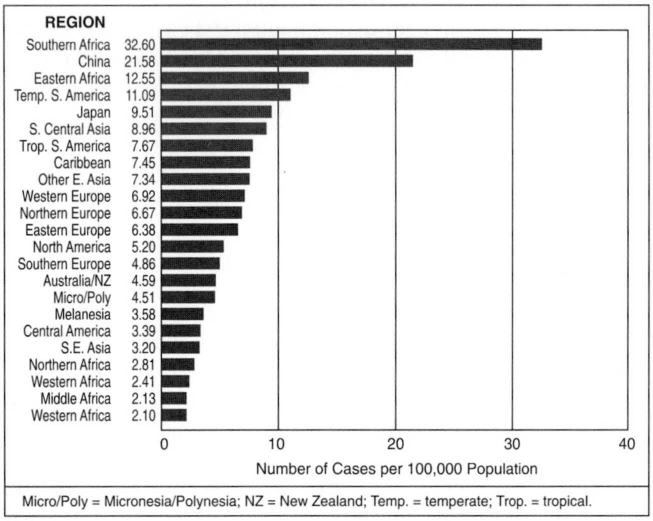

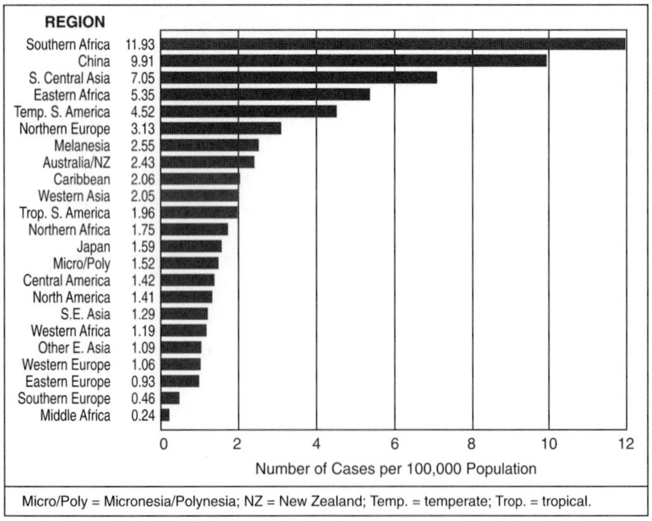

Fig. 34–4. Incidence of esophageal cancer in males (*top*) and females (*bottom*) by world region. From Parkin (1999) with permission.

Alcohol and tobacco appear to be the most important risk factors associated with squamous cell carcinoma (Rustgi, 1999). Other factors include corrosive injury; deficiencies of vitamin A, vitamin C, iron, and riboflavin; the rare inherited disease of tylosis; esophageal webs; and achalasia (Heitmiller, 2001). There are large racial differences in the incidence of esophageal squamous cell carcinoma. Black men younger than 55 years of age have a 6-fold increased risk over white men of the same age (Devesa, 1998). There are also large geographic differences of uncertain etiology and an increased risk associated with asbestos workers and rubber workers. Some countries have an especially high rate of esophageal squamous cell cancer, especially China, Iran, and South Africa (Greenlee, 2000). There is a recent suggestion that human papillomavirus may be associated with squamous cell carcinoma of the esophagus (Li, 2001).

Adenocarcinoma of the esophagus is most common in white men and is often associated with Barrett's esophagus and dysplasia (Drewitz et al., 1997). This malignancy may also arise without the presence of Barrett's esophagus, and recent evidence suggests a strong association of esophageal adenocarcinoma with gastroesophageal reflux (Lagergren et al., 1999).

Inherited Syndromes

Familial Risk in China and Iran

Esophageal cancer accounts for 64% of cancer deaths in Linxian county of the Henan province of China. Segregation analysis of 221 high-risk nuclear families from one commune in Linxian suggested autosomal recessive inheritance of predisposition to this malignancy with a predicted gene carrier frequency of 19% (Carter et al., 1992). Case-control studies from one county in the Jiangsu province demonstrated a relative risk of esophageal cancer of 2.68 ($p < .001$) when a family history of esophageal cancer was present (Li, 1982). The Turkoman population in the Caspian Littoral of northern Iran exhibits a high risk of esophageal cancer. A positive family history for esophageal cancer was reported in 47% of Turkomans with this malignancy, compared to a positive family history of 2% in non-Turkomans (Ghadirian, 1985).

Tylosis

Tylosis is an extremely rare autosomal dominant skin disease characterized by hyperkeratosis of the palms and soles. Almost one-third of the members of a London family with tylosis, spanning six generations, have been affected with esophageal cancer (Ellis et al., 1994). Linkage analysis suggests a disease locus on 17q (Risk et al., 1994). Several additional families with this condition have now also been reported in the United States and Germany.

Barrett's Esophagus

Barrett's esophagus is defined as the presence of a columnar lined distal esophagus with a distinctive histology (Morales and Sampliner, 1999). Both the cancer risk and the severity of associated gastroesophageal reflux relate to the length of the columnar lined epithelium. Overall risk for adenocarcinoma associated with Barrett's esophagus is 40 times greater than the general population, with a median incidence of 1 cancer per 100 patient-years of patient follow-up. *p53* mutations have been associated with severe dysplasia in this condition. Families with Barrett's esophagus have been reported, suggesting that this condition is at least in part familial and may be inherited in these cases.

GASTRIC CANCER

Disease Definition

Gastric cancers are primarily adenocarcinomas, with a small percentage of lymphomas and other histologic subtypes. Adenocarcinomas are most commonly of the intestinal type. These cancers are superficial and often associated with intestinal metaplasia. Diffuse gastric cancer is also an adenocarcinoma, but it is much less common than the intestinal type, often spreads submucosally and is therefore difficult to detect.

Clinical presentation of gastric cancer in general is nonspecific, with symptoms and signs including weight loss, early satiety, fatigue, nonspecific abdominal pain, and anemia. Diagnosis is by endoscopic biopsy. Screening has been discussed for several high-risk conditions (see below) but has not been agreed on because of the low overall incidence of this malignancy in the United States. Screening is advised in some high-risk countries such as Japan. Surgical cure is unusual, and the tumor responds poorly to both chemotherapy and radiation therapy. Most gastric cancer cases appear to be sporadic, although some types of gastritis that lead to gastric cancer appear to be inherited. Furthermore, the genetic marker blood group A associates with gastric cancer risk, and gastric cancer occurs as a part of several known inherited cancer syndromes.

Epidemiology

In the United States, gastric cancer was the most common cause of cancer mortality before 1930. Its rate has steadily declined since that time, so that it is now sixth in men and eighth in women as a cause of cancer mortality (Landis et al., 1999). In 2000, 21,500 new cases of gastric cancer and 13,000 deaths were estimated in the United States (Greenlee et al., 2000). This malignancy remains the second most common cancer in the world (Fig. 34–5). Its rate is declining in virtually all countries in the world, however. Gastric cancer incidence is almost double in men than in women and is almost twice as common in blacks as in whites. The five-year survival from gastric adenocarcinoma is about 17% in the United States.

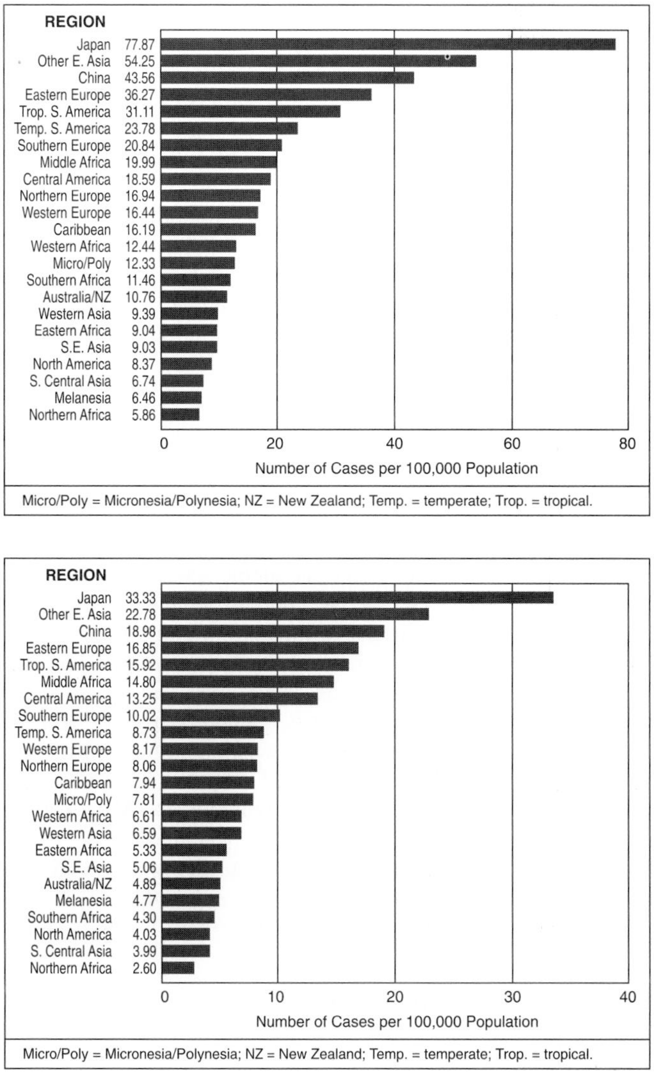

Fig. 34–5. Incidence of gastric cancer in males (*top*) and females (*bottom*) by world region. From Parkin (1999) with permission.

Gastritis and Gastric Cancer Pathogenesis

Evidence suggests a multistep process in the pathogenesis of gastric adenocarcinoma that includes both genetic and environmental risk factors. These factors affect normal gastric mucosa to sequentially produce chronic gastritis, atrophy, intestinal metaplasia, dysplasia, and finally cancer. Chronic atrophic gastritis (CAG) is found in 80% to 90% of patients with gastric cancer of the intestinal type and has several etiologies. Type A is associated with pernicious anemia and typically occurs in persons of Scandinavian and northern European descent and is considered an inherited form of gastritis.

Type B includes multifocal atrophic gastritis and *Helicobacter pylori*–associated chronic active gastritis. Multifocal atrophic gastritis exhibits foci of intestinal metaplasia and chronic inflammatory infiltrates that begin in the region of the incisura and spread with age. This type of gastritis associates with populations that have a high risk of gastric cancer and may be related to environmental factors. *H. pylori* infection is commonly found in patients with this type of atrophic gastritis and is associated with cancer risk. Unlike chronic active gastritis, however, multifocal atrophic gastritis does not regress with treatment of *H. pylori*. *H. pylori*–associated chronic active gastritis involves mainly the antrum, is the most common type found in developed countries, and does regress with the treatment of *H. pylori*.

There is a 3- to 6-fold increased risk of gastric cancer associated with *H. pylori*, but only a small fraction of persons with *H. pylori* ever develop this malignancy (McFarlane and Munro, 1997). Strains of *H. pylori* that express the CagA protein have been associated with distal gastric cancer. Treatment of *H. pylori* reverses gastritis, but not metaplasia.

H. pylori, high salt intake, and inherited gastritis all can lead to chronic atrophic gastritis. In turn, gastric atrophy then leads to a high gastric pH, allowing proliferation of bacteria in the stomach and bacterial reduction of dietary nitrates and nitrites to N-nitroso compounds. These N-nitroso compounds are carcinogenic and appear to play a part in the transition of gastritis to intestinal metaplasia and possibly dysplasia. Nitrates and nitrites are often present in meats, particularly smoke-cured meats. Compounds that inhibit this process include vitamins A and C, which are present in fresh fruits and vegetables. Salt may potentiate certain carcinogens and increase dysplastic transformation, while beta-carotene appears to inhibit this process. This proposed carcinogenic pathway is consistent with observations that fresh fruit and vegetables associate with decreased gastric cancer risk, while smoke- and salt-cured foods associate with increased risk. Societal use of refrigeration is correlated with a decreased risk of gastric cancer, probably because salt- and smoke-curing become unnecessary and fresh fruits and vegetables are available year round.

Other risk factors for gastric cancer include (1) the post-gastrectomy state, with a 2-fold increased risk after 10 to 20 years, and (2) gastric adenomas, which are rare. Hyperplastic polyps and fundic gland polyps, by themselves, appear to have no cancer potential, although hyperplastic polyps often are found in the setting of chronic gastritis. Although gastric metaplasia is a step in the carcinogenic process, it is not a good marker of malignant potential. It is so common that it simply is not a good predictor of eventual cancer development.

Other Subtypes of Gastric Cancer

The incidence of adenocarcinoma of the cardia has been increasing dramatically (see above under esophageal carcinoma), while gastric adenocarcinoma of the antrum and body has been decreasing. Prognosis for cancer of the cardia is poor, and it is believed that it may have the same risk factors as distal esophageal adenocarcinoma. Gastric lymphoma accounts for 3% to 5% of all gastric cancers but is the most common extranodal non-Hodgkin's lymphoma. Both non-Hodgkin's lymphoma and mucosa-associated lymphoid tissue lymphomas (MALTomas) are associated with *H. pylori* infection (Neubauer et al., 1997). Kaposi's sarcoma is found in homosexual men with AIDS. Benign carcinoid tumors often are induced by chronic gastrin stimulation of chronic gastritis or by Zollinger-Ellison syndrome.

Genetic Epidemiology

Familial Risk

Studies of gastric cancer have generally found a 2- to 3-fold increased risk of this malignancy in first-degree relatives of affected persons compared to controls (Macklin, 1955, 1960, 1961; Jackson et al., 1980; McConnell, 1981; Bishop and Skolnick, 1984; Zanghieri et al., 1990; La Vecchia et al., 1992). The diffuse histologic subtype is known to occur as part of the recently described syndrome of hereditary diffuse gastric cancer (see under syndromes below). It is yet to be determined, however, what fraction of familial cases is accounted for by this syndrome. The intestinal and intermediate histologic subtypes of gastric cancer are much less familial (Lehtola, 1978).

Genetic Markers

More than 70 studies from many countries have examined the relationship of gastric cancer with blood group A (Dunn, 1975). Of these, 55 have demonstrated an association with blood group A, 14 have found no difference from control, and 2 have shown a negative correlation. From the combined studies, individuals with blood group A are estimated to have a 20% increased risk over the general population for acquiring gastric carcinoma (McConnell, 1981). Although correlations of specific cancer characteristics with blood group A have been somewhat conflicting, one large study from Amsterdam demonstrated an association of antral tumors and this blood type (Haenszel et al., 1976). Another study, in a Japanese population, found blood group A to be associated only with the diffuse-type histology of gastric cancer (Haenszel et al., 1976). Finally, an excess incidence of blood group A has been found in a group of patients with pernicious anemia (Hoskins et al., 1965). It has been postulated that this association may account for the excess of blood group A in gastric cancer in general (Shearman and Finlayson, 1967), although this remains unproven. The association of blood group A with the inherited syndrome of hereditary diffuse gastric cancer must also be evaluated.

Hereditary Gastritis and Pernicious Anemia

Type A gastritis (see above), also called autoimmune gastritis (Lambert, 1972; Strickland and Mackay, 1973), appears to arise on the basis of autosomal dominant inheritance (Yardley and Hendrix, 1999). Although much less common than type B or environmental gastritis, it may affect as many as 5% of the adult population (Strickland and Mackay, 1973). This type of gastritis appears to be a precursor to pernicious anemia, although only a small fraction of persons with type A gastritis develop pernicious anemia. Of note, pernicious anemia has a number of other causes, mostly inherited, and related to the physiology of vitamin B12 absorption. Type A gastritis is the most common cause of pernicious anemia, however.

Type A gastritis involves mainly the gastric body and fundus. These areas become progressively atrophic, and the lesion eventually leads to hypochlorhydria and achlorhydria in many individuals. This gastritis is also accompanied by low levels of intrinsic factor, hypersecretion of gastrin, low levels of serum pepsinogen I, and parietal cell and intrinsic factor antibodies (McConnell, 1981). Intestinal metaplasia may also accompany type A gastritis when it is well developed. There is a strong association between this type of gastritis and gastric cancer (Siruala et al., 1966; McConnell, 1981).

Studies have shown that type A gastritis is genetically determined (Varis, 1971), with a high occurrence of the gastritis in first-degree relatives of affected patients. Furthermore, the degree of affectedness in relatives forms a bimodal distribution, suggesting monogenetic inheritance, probably autosomal dominant (Hovinen et al., 1976). It has also been found that type A gastritis is more common among relatives of patients with gastric cancer, especially the diffuse type (Kekki et al., 1975; Ihamaki et al., 1979).

In summary, type A or severe atrophic fundic gastritis appears to arise on the basis of genetic susceptibility. It exhibits immunologic features and may lead to pernicious anemia and the diffuse histologic type of gastric cancer. Much of the familial clustering observed in gastric cancer may occur on the basis of type A gastritis. Type B gastritis develops secondary to environmental factors, including *H. pylori*, as outlined above. It is prevalent in countries and populations that exhibit a high incidence of environmental gastric cancer and, as expected, is associated with the intestinal type of stomach carcinoma. Although these histologic subtypes of gastritis and gastric cancer are not always easily separated, the models have given significant insight into the underlying genesis and heterogeneity of gastric cancer.

Hereditary Syndromes with Gastric Cancer

Hereditary Diffuse Gastric Cancer Syndrome

Disease causing mutations of the E-cadherin (*CDH1*) gene have recently been demonstrated to give rise to an inherited syndrome, now called the hereditary diffuse gastric cancer (HDGC) syndrome (Guilford et al., 1998). This syndrome is now known to give rise to a young age–onset (average age 38 years) diffuse histologic type of gastric cancer with a 70% penetrance. HDGC has now been demonstrated in various populations, but it is believed to account for a minority of the familial gastric cancers (Richards et al., 1999). Because of the difficulty in making a diagnosis of gastric cancer of the diffuse type, which often presents a "linitus plastica" appearance, prophylactic gastrectomy has been recommended as a consideration for mutant gene carriers from families with known E-cadherin mutations (Chun et al., 2001; Huntsman et al., 2001).

E-cadherin is a cell–cell adhesion molecule that regulates intercellular adhesion and cell polarity in the normal gastric epithelium. Somatic mutations of the *CDH1* gene have been found in up to 80% of diffuse gastric cancers, but not in the intestinal type. Loss of E-cadherin appears related to tumor invasion and poor prognosis. The *CDH1* gene has also been found to be somatically mutated in a number of other cancers.

It remains to be determined what fraction of the familial clustering of gastric cancer overall, what fraction of diffuse histologic subtype gastric cancer, and what fraction of blood group A familial clustering of gastric cancer are accounted for by the syndrome of HDGC. It has been known for some time that the diffuse histologic type of gastric cancer is associated with a much higher frequency of a positive family history for gastric cancer than the intestinal type (Lehtola, 1978) and also that the diffuse-type gastric cancer is associated with blood group A more frequently than the intestinal type (Correa et al., 1973).

HNPCC

HNPCC outlined in detail under colon cancer, carries a near 20% lifetime risk of gastric cancer (Aarnio et al., 1999). Gastric cancers in HNPCC are of the intestinal type. It is interesting that gastric and uterine cancer were the main malignancies associated with this syndrome when it was first described in family "G." Subsequent generations of family G, however, have seen colon cancer replace gastric cancer, in parallel with the declining incidence of gastric cancer in the U.S. population.

FAP

FAP appears to exhibit an excess of gastric cancer in Asian populations, but only about a 0.5% risk of gastric cancer in non-Asian groups (Burt and Jacoby, 1999). Adenomas occasionally occur in the stomach in FAP but most often in the antrum. There have been reports of gastric cancer outside Asian populations, even arising from fundic gland polyps, leaving the possibility that there is some increased risk of gastric cancer in non-Asian FAP patients (Zwick et al., 1997; Hofgartner et al., 1999).

Peutz-Jeghers Syndrome

The occurrence of gastric cancer in Peutz-Jeghers disease has been reported to be 29% (Giardiello et al., 2000). An emperic recommendation of upper GI endoscopy screening, starting at age 10 years and repeated every 2 years, has been given.

Juvenile Polyposis

Gastric cancers have been reported in patients with juvenile polyposis, but the degree of increased risk, if any, is not known (Burt and Jacoby, 1999).

Cowden Disease

GI malignancy is unusual in Cowden disease, and it is not yet certain if the risk is even increased. There have been reports of gastric cancer in this syndrome, however (Eng, 1997; Burt and Jacoby, 1999).

Li-Fraumeni Syndrome

Li-Fraumeni syndrome arises from germline mutations of the *p53* gene and results in a marked predisposition to soft-tissue sarcomas, leukemia, brain cancer, and breast cancer, as well as gastric cancer in some families (Li et al., 1988).

SMALL BOWEL CANCER

Small bowel cancer is a rare neoplasm accounting for about 1% to 5% of gastrointestinal malignancies. There were an estimated 4700 cases in 2000, with 1200 deaths (Greenlee et al., 2000). The incidence of small bowel malignancy is equivalent for men and women. Symptoms are nonspecific and include abdominal pain, GI blood loss, and small bowel obstruction (Lance, 1999). Adenocarcinoma, lymphoma, carcinoid, and leiomyosarcoma, in that order, are the most common small bowel malignancies. Adenocarcinoma is most prevalent in the proximal small bowel, and lymphoma in the distal. Carcinoids occur more often in the distal small bowel. Predisposing conditions of small bowel cancer, all of which are now known to have a genetic etiology, include celiac sprue (both adenocarcinoma and lymphoma), Crohn's disease, HNPCC, Peutz-Jeghers disease, juvenile polyposis, and FAP (mostly duodenal). Polyp types of the small bowel include adenomas, leiomyomas, lipomas, and Peutz-Jeghers and juvenile polyps. All but the lipomas appear to have some malignancy potential. Some 50% of metastatic melanomas metastasize to the small bowel, although these lesions are often not clinically apparent.

PANCREATIC CANCER

Disease Definition

By far the most common pancreatic cancer is adenocarcinoma (Brand and Tempero, 1998; Todd et al., 1999). This malignancy is slow growing, indolent, and almost always diagnosed in late, advanced stages. Symptoms are nonspecific and include vague abdominal pain, weight loss, anorexia, depression, anemia, and fatigue. The etiology is believed to be mostly environmental, although there is some familial risk and several inherited conditions include pancreatic cancer.

Epidemiology

Adenocarcinoma of the pancreas is the fourth leading cause of cancer mortality in the United States. There were an estimated 28,300 cases, with 28,200 deaths in 2000 in the United States (Greenlee et al., 2000). This malignancy is more common in men than women (1.4 to 1), and more common in blacks than whites (1.4 to 1). There has been little change in incidence in the past 20 years. Early detection is rare, with a one-year survival rate of 18% and a five-year survival rate of 2%.

Cigarette smoking is the most significantly associated environmental factor (Boyle et al., 1996; Harnack et al., 1997), although high-fat and red-meat diets have also exhibited positive associations. Raw fruit and vegetable diets may decrease the risk of pancreatic cancer (Brand and Tempero, 1998; Todd et al., 1999). Pre-existing diabetes and chronic pancreatitis are associated with an increased risk of pancreatic cancer. The risk associated with alcohol is uncertain, and there is little, if any, evidence for an association with coffee (Harnack et al., 1997).

Syndromes and Genetic Epidemiology

Familial Risk

Several studies have demonstrated an increased risk for pancreatic cancer among relatives with this malignancy (Appel, 1974; Falk et al., 1988; Ghadirian et al., 1991; Fernandez et al., 1994). Only one of these also examined environmental factors and reported no difference in exposure between cases and controls (Ghadirian et al., 1991). A number of families have now been identified in which multiple cases of pancreatic cancer have occurred. The genetic etiology relates both to syndromes in which pancreatic cancer is sometimes observed and to families in which a specific syndrome has not been identified. These include familial atypical multiple mole-melanoma (FAMM) syndrome, breast and ovarian cancer family syndrome (BRCA1/BRCA2), hereditary pancreatitis, isolated pancreatic cancer families, FAP, and Peutz-Jeghers syndrome and, possibly, HNPCC, Li-Fraumeni syndrome, von Hippel-Lindau syndrome and ataxia-telangiectasia.

Syndromes in Which Pancreatic Cancer Has Been Observed

Familial Atypical Multiple Mole-Melanoma Syndrome. There is an increased risk of pancreatic cancer in some families with FAMM (Bergman et al., 1990). There is further evidence in some of these families that pancreatic cancer arises from mutations in the cell cycle inhibitor gene *CDKN2A/p16/INK4A* (Hussussian et al., 1994; Goldstein et al., 1995; Gruis et al., 1995; Liu et al., 1995; Whelan et al., 1995).

Breast and Ovarian Cancer Family Syndrome. Pancreatic cancer families have rarely been found to arise from disease causing mutations of *BRCA1* and *BRCA2*. These families also exhibited breast and ovarian cancers (Lal et al., 2000).

Hereditary Pancreatitis. Hereditary pancreatitis is an extremely rare condition that arises from mutations of a cationic typsinogen gene (Whitcomb et al., 1996). An international study of hereditary pancreatitis cases revealed a high incidence of pancreatic cancer (53 of 248 cases) with an estimated risk of 40% by age 70 years (Lowenfels et al., 1997).

FAP. A relative risk for pancreatic cancer of 4.46 (95% CI, 1.2–11.4) was calculated for FAP patients in a study from the Johns Hopkins registry that involved 197 kindreds (Giardiello et al., 1993).

Peutz-Jeghers Syndrome. In addition to case reports of pancreatic cancer in Peutz-Jeghers syndrome, a 36% incidence of this malignancy was noted in a large registry (Giardiello et al., 2000).

HNPCC. An increased risk of pancreatic cancer has been reported in HNPCC (Lynch et al., 1991), although the association is uncertain, as larger, more recent series have not found an excess of this malignancy (Aarnio et al., 1999).

Li-Fraumeni Syndrome. Pancreatic cancer may be related to Li-Fraumeni syndrome, as young-age cancer of the pancreas was observed in three separate families of 24 syndrome families under study (Li et al., 1988).

REFERENCES

Aaltonen LA, Salovaara R, Kristo P, Canzian F, Hemminki A, Peltomäki P, Chadwick RB, Kääriänen H, Eskelinen M, Järvinen H, et al.: Incidence of hereditary nonpolyposis colorectal cancer and the feasibility of molecular screening for the disease. N Engl J Med 1998; 338:1481–1487.

Aarnio M, Sankila R, Pukkala E, Salovaara R, Aaltonen LA, de la Chapelle A, Peltomäki P, Mecklin J-P, Järvinen HJ: Cancer risk in mutation carriers of DNA-mismatch-repair genes. Int J Cancer 1999; 81:214–218.

Aberle H, Bauer A, Stappert J, Kispert A, Kemler R: β-catenin is a target for the ubiquitin-proteasome pathway. EMBO J 1997; 16:3797–3804.

Ahsan H, Neugut AI, Garbowski GC, Jacobson JS, Forde KA, Treat MR, Waye JD: Family history of colorectal adenomatous polyps and increased risk for colorectal cancer. Ann Intern Med 1998; 128:900–905.

Appel MF: Hereditary pancreatitis. review and presentation of an additional kindred. Arch Surg 1974; 108:63–65.

Baker JW, Gathright JB Jr, Timmcke AE, Hicks TC, Ferrari BT, Ray JE: Colonoscopic screening of asymptomatic patients with a family history of colon cancer. Dis Colon Rectum 1990a; 33:926–930.

Baker SJ, Preisinger AC, Jessup JM, Paraskeva C, Markowitz S, Willson JK, Hamilton S, Vogelstein B: *p53* gene mutations occur in combination with 17p allelic deletions as late events in colorectal tumorigenesis. Cancer Res 1990b; 50:7717–7722.

Baron JA, Beach M, Mandel JS, van Stolk RU, Haile RW, Sandler RS, Rothstein R, Summers RW, Snover DC, Beck GJ, et al.: Calcium supplements for the prevention of colorectal adenomas. N Engl J Med 1999; 340:101–107.

Bazzoli F, Fossi S, Sottili S, Pozzato P, Zagari RM, Morelli MC, Taroni F, Roda E: The risk of adenomatous polyps in asymptomatic first-degree relatives of persons with colon cancer. Gastroenterology 1995; 109:783–788.

Behrens J, Jerchow BA, Wurtele M, Grimm J, Asbrand C, Wirtz R, Kuhl M, Wedlich D, Birchmeier W: Functional interaction of an axin homolog, conductin, with β-catenin, APC, and GSK3β. Science 1998; 280:596–599.

Bergman W, Watson P, de Jong J, Lynch HT, Fusaro RM: Systemic cancer and the FAMMM syndrome. Br J Cancer 1990; 61:932–936.

Bisgaard ML, Fenger K, Bulow S, Niebuhr E, Mohr J: Familial adenomatous polyposis (FAP): frequency, penetrance, and mutation rate. Hum Mutat 1994; 3:121–125.

Bishop DT, Skolnick MH: Genetic epidemiology of cancer in Utah genealogies: a prelude to the molecular genetics of common cancers. J Cell Physiol (Suppl) 1984; 3:63–77.

Bodmer WF, Bailey CJ, Bodmer J, Bussey HJ, Ellis A, Gorman P, Lucibello FC, Murday VA, Rider SH, Scambler P, et al.: Localization of the gene for familial adenomatous polyposis on chromosome 5. Nature 1987; 328:614–616.

Boland CR: Malignant tumors of the colon. In: Yamada T (ed). Textbook of Gastroenterology, 3d ed. Philadelphia: J. B. Lippincott, 1999:2023–2082.

Bonelli L, Martines H, Conio M, Bruzzi P, Aste H: Family history of colorectal cancer as a risk factor for benign and malignant tumours of the large bowel: a case-control study. Int J Cancer 1988; 41:513–517.

Boyle P, Maisonneuve P, Bueno de Mesquita B, Ghadirian P, Howe GR, Zatonski W, Baghurst P, Moerman CJ, Simard A, Miller AB, et al.: Cigarette smoking and pancreas cancer: a case control study of the search programme of the IARC. Int J Cancer 1996; 67:63–71.

Brand RE, Tempero MA: Pancreatic cancer. Curr Opin Oncol 1998; 10:362–366.

Burke W, Petersen G, Lynch P, Botkin J, Daly M, Garber J, Kahn MJ, McTiernan A, Offit K, Thomson E, Varricchio C: Recommendations for follow-up care of individuals with an inherited predisposition to cancer: I. Hereditary nonpolyposis colon cancer. JAMA 1997; 277:915–919.

Burt RW: Familial risk and colorectal cancer. Gastroenterol Clin North Am 1996; 25:793–803.

Burt RW: Screening of patients with a positive family history of colorectal cancer. Gastrointest Endosc Clin N Am 1997; 7:65–79.

Burt RW: Colon cancer screening. Gastroenterology 2000; 119:837–853.

Burt RW, Ahnen D: Genetics of colon cancer. In: Yamada T (ed). Gastroenterology Updates. Philadelphia: Lippincott Raven, 1998:1–16.

Burt RW, Jacoby R: Polyposis syndromes. In: Yamada T (ed). Textbook of Gastroenterology. Philadelphia: Lippincott Raven, 1999:1995–2022.

Byers T, Levin B, Rothenberger D, Dodd GD, Smith RA: American Cancer Society guidelines for screening and surveillance for early detection of colorectal polyps and cancer: update 1997. CA Cancer J Clin 1997; 47:154–160.

Cannon-Albright LA, Skolnick MH, Bishop DT, Lee RG, Burt RW: Common inheritance of susceptibility to colonic adenomatous polyps and associated colorectal cancers. N Engl J Med 1988; 319:533–537.

Carethers JM: The cellular and molecular pathogenesis of colorectal cancer. Gastroenterol Clin North Am 1996; 25:737–754.

Carter CL, Hu N, Wu M, Lin PZ, Murigande C, Bonney GE: Segregation analysis of esophageal cancer in 221 high-risk Chinese families. J Natl Cancer Inst 1992; 84:771–776.

Caspari R, Olschwang S, Friedl W, Mandl M, Boisson C, Boker T, Augustin A, Kadmon M, Moslein G, Thomas G, et al.: Familial adenomatous polyposis: desmoid tumours and lack of ophthalmic lesions (CHRPE) associated with *APC* mutations beyond codon 1444. Hum Mol Genet 1995; 4:337–340.

Chen J, Giovannucci E, Kelsey K, Rimm EB, Stampfer MJ, Colditz GA, Spiegelman D, Willett WC, Hunter DJ: A methylenetetrahydrofolate reductase polymorphism and the risk of colorectal cancer. Cancer Res 1996; 56:4862–4864.

Chenevix-Trench G, Young J, Coggan M, Board P: Glutathione S-transferase M1 and T1 polymorphisms: susceptibility to colon cancer and age of onset. Carcinogenesis 1995; 16:1655–1657.

Chun YS, Lindor NM, Smyrk TC, Petersen BT, Burgart LJ, Guilford PJ, Donohue JH: Germline E-cadherin gene mutations: is prophylactic total gastrectomy indicated? Cancer 2001; 92:181–187.

Chung DC: The genetic basis of colorectal cancer: insights into critical pathways of tumorigenesis. Gastroenterology 2000; 119:854–865.

Correa P, Haenszel W: The epidemiology of large-bowel cancer. Adv Cancer Res 1978; 26:1–141.

Correa P, Sasano N, Stemmermann GN, Haenszel W: Pathology of gastric carcinoma in Japanese populations: comparisons between Miyagi prefecture, Japan, and Hawaii. J Natl Cancer Inst 1973; 51:1449–1459.

Desai DC, Murday V, Phillips RKS, Neale KF, Milla P, Hodgson SV: A survey of phenotypic features in juvenile polyposis. J Med Genet 1998; 35:476–481.

Desai DC, Neale KF, Talbot IC, Hodgson SV, Phillips RK: Juvenile polyposis. Br J Surg 1995; 82:14–17.

Devesa SS, Blot WJ, Fraumeni JF Jr: Changing patterns in the incidence of esophageal and gastric carcinoma in the United States. Cancer 1998; 83:2049–2053.

Drewitz DJ, Sampliner RE, Garewal HS: The incidence of adenocarcinoma in Barrett's esophagus: a prospective study of 170 patients followed 4.8 years. Am J Gastroenterol 1997; 92:212–215.

Duncan JL, Kyle J: Family incidence of carcinoma of the colon and rectum in north-east Scotland. Gut 1982; 23:169–171.

Dunn JE: Cancer epidemiology in populations of the United States—with emphasis on Hawaii and California—and Japan. Cancer Res 1975; 35:3240–3245.

Ellis A, Field JK, Field EA, Friedmann PS, Fryer A, Howard P, Leigh IM, Risk J, Shaw JM, Whittaker J: Tylosis associated with carcinoma of the oesophagus and oral leukoplakia in a large Liverpool family: a review of six generations. Eur J Cancer Oral Oncol 1994; 2:102–112.

Eng C: Cowden syndrome. Genet Couns 1997; 6:181–192.

Eng C: Will the real Cowden syndrome please stand up: revised diagnostic criteria. J Med Genet 2000; 37:828–830.

Falk RT, Pickle LW, Fontham ET, Correa P, Fraumeni JF Jr: Life-style risk factors for pancreatic cancer in Louisiana: a case-control study. Am J Epidemiol 1988; 128:324–336.

Fernandez E, La Vecchia C, D'Avanzo B, Negri E, Franceschi S: Family history and the risk of liver, gallbladder, and pancreatic cancer. Cancer Epidemiol Biomarkers Prev 1994; 3:209–212.

Fodde R, Kuipers J, Rosenberg C, Smits R, Kielman M, Gaspar C, van Es JH, Breukel C, Wiegant J, Giles RH, Clevers H: Mutations in the *APC* tumour suppressor gene cause chromosomal instability. Nat Cell Biol 2001; 3:433–438.

Fuchs CS, Giovannucci EL, Colditz GA, Hunter DJ, Speizer FE, Willett WC: A prospective study of family history and the risk of colorectal cancer. N Engl J Med 1994; 331:1669–1674.

Geller G, Botkin JR, Green MJ, Press N, Biesecker BB, Wilfond B, Grana G, Daly MB, Schneider K, Kahn MJ: Genetic testing for susceptibility to adult-onset cancer: the process and content of informed consent. JAMA 1997; 277:1467–1474.

Ghadirian P: Familial history of esophageal cancer. Cancer 1985; 56:2112–2116.

Ghadirian P, Boyle P, Simard A, Baillargeon J, Maisonneuve P, Perret C: Reported family aggregation of pancreatic cancer within a population-based case-control study in the Francophone community in Montreal, Canada. Int J Pancreatol 1991; 10:183–196.

Giardiello FM, Brensinger JD, Tersmette AC, Goodman SN, Petersen GM, Booker SV, Cruz-Correa M, Offerhaus JA: Very high risk of cancer in familial Peutz-Jeghers syndrome. Gastroenterology 2000; 119:1447–1453.

Giardiello FM, Hamilton SR, Krush AJ, Piantadosi S, Hylind LM, Celano P, Booker SV, Robinson CR, Offerhaus GJ: Treatment of colonic and rectal adenomas with sulindac in familial adenomatous polyposis. N Engl J Med 1993; 328:1313–1316.

Giardiello FM, Krush AJ, Petersen GM, Booker SV, Kerr M, Tong LL, Hamilton SR: Phenotypic variability of familial adenomatous polyposis in 11 unrelated families with identical *APC* gene mutation. Gastroenterology 1994; 106:1542–1547.

Giardiello FM, Brensinger JD, Luce MC, Petersen GM, Cayouette MC, Krush AJ, Bacon JA, Booker SV, Bufill JA, Hamilton SR: Phenotypic expression of disease in families that have mutations in the 5′ region of the adenomatous polyposis coli gene. Ann Intern Med 1997; 126:514–519.

Giardiello FM, Brensinger JD, Petersen GM: American Gastroenterological Association Medical Position Statement: Hereditary Colorectal Cancer and Genetic Testing. Gastroenterology 2001; 121:195–197.

Giardiello FM, Brensinger JD, Petersen GM: AGA Technical Review on Hereditary Colorectal Cancer and Genetic Testing. Gastroenterology 2001; 121:198–213.

Goldstein AM, Fraser MC, Struewing JP, Hussussian CJ, Ranade K, Zametkin DP, Fontaine LS, Organic SM, Dracopoli NC, Clark WH Jr, et al.: Increased risk of pancreatic cancer in melanoma-prone kindreds with p16INK4 mutations. N Engl J Med 1995; 333:970–974.

Gorlin RJ, Cohen MM Jr, Condon LM, Burke BA: Bannayan-Riley-Ruvalcaba syndrome. Am J Med Genet 1992; 44:307–314.

Goss KH, Groden J: Biology of the adenomatous polyposis coli tumor suppressor. J Clin Oncol 2000; 18:1967–1979.

Greenlee RT, Murray T, Bolden S, Wingo PA: Cancer statistics, 2000. CA Cancer J Clin 2000; 50:7–33.

Groden J, Thliveris A, Samowitz W, Carlson M, Gelbert L, Albertsen H, Joslyn G, Stevens J, Spirio L, Robertson M, et al.: Identification and characterization of the familial adenomatous polyposis coli gene. Cell 1991; 66:589–600.

Grossman S, Milos ML: Colonoscopic screening of persons with suspected risk factors for colon cancer: I. Family history. Gastroenterology 1988; 94:395–400.

Gruis NA, van der Velden PA, Sandkuijl LA, Prins DE, Weaver-Feldhaus J, Kamb A, Bergman W, Frants RR: Homozygotes for CDKN2 (p16) germline mutation in Dutch familial melanoma kindreds. Nat Genet 1995; 10:351–353.

Gryska PV, Cohen AM: Screening asymptomatic patients at high risk for colon cancer with full colonoscopy. Dis Colon Rectum 1987; 30:18–20.

Guilford P, Hopkins J, Harraway J, McLeod M, McLeod N, Harawira P, Taite H, Scoular R, Miller A, Reeve AE: E-cadherin germline mutations in familial gastric cancer. Nature 1998; 392:402–405.

Guillem JG, Neugut AI, Forde KA, Waye JD, Treat MR: Colonic neoplasms in asymptomatic first-degree relatives of colon cancer patients. Am J Gastroenterol 1988; 83:271–273.

Guillem JG, Smith AJ, Culle J, Ruo L: Gastrointestinal polyposis syndromes. Curr Probl Surg 1999; 36:217–323.

Haenszel W, Kurihara M, Locke FB, Shimuzu K, Segi M: Stomach cancer in Japan. J Natl Cancer Inst 1976; 56:265–274.

Hamilton SR, Liu B, Parsons RE, Papadopoulos N, Jen J, Powell SM, Krush AJ, Berk T, Cohen Z, Tetu B, et al.: The molecular basis of Turcot's syndrome. N Engl J Med 1995; 332:839–847.

Hampel H, Peltomäki P: Hereditary colorectal cancer: risk assessment and management. Clin Genet 2000; 58:89–97.

Harnack LJ, Anderson KE, Zheng W, Folsom AR, Sellers TA, Kushi LH: Smoking, alcohol, coffee, and tea intake and incidence of cancer of the exocrine pancreas: the Iowa Women's Health Study. Cancer Epidemiol Biomarkers Prev 1997; 6:1081–1086.

Harty LC, Caporaso NE, Hayes RB, Winn DM, Bravo-Otero E, Blot WJ, Kleinman DV, Brown LM, Armenian HK, Fraumeni JF Jr, Shields PG: Alcohol dehydrogenase-3 genotype and risk of oral cavity and pharyngeal cancers. J Natl Cancer Inst 1997; 89:1698–1705.

He TC, Sparks AB, Rago C, Hermeking H, Zawel L, da Costa LT, Morin PJ, Vogelstein B, Kinzler KW: Identification of c-MYC as a target of the APC pathway. Science 1998; 281:1509–1512.

Heitmiller RF: Epidemiology, diagnosis, and staging of esophageal cancer. Cancer Treat Res 2001; 105:375–386.

Hemminki A, Markie D, Tomlinson I, Avizienyte E, Roth S, Loukola A, Bignell G, Warren W, Aminoff M, Hoglund P, et al.: A serine/threonine kinase gene defective in Peutz-Jeghers syndrome. Nature 1998; 391:184–187.

Herman JG, Umar A, Polyak K, Graff JR, Ahuja N, Issa JP, Markowitz S, Willson JK, Hamilton SR, Kinzler KW, et al.: Incidence and functional consequences of *hMLH1* promoter hypermethylation in colorectal carcinoma. Proc Natl Acad Sci USA 1998; 95:6870–6875.

Herrera L, Hanna S, Petrelli N, Nava H: Screening endoscopy in patients with family history positive (FH+) for colorectal neoplasia (CRN) (abstr). Gastrointest Endosc 1990; 36:211.

Hizawa K, Iida M, Matsumoto T, Kohrogi N, Suekane H, Yao T, Fujishima M: Gastrointestinal manifestations of Cowden's disease: report of four cases. J Clin Gastroenterol 1994; 18:13–18.

Hofgartner WT, Thorp M, Ramus MW, Delorefice G, Chey WY, Ryan CK, Takahashi GW, Lobitz JR: Gastric adenocarcinoma associated with fundic gland polyps in a patient with attenuated familial adenomatous polyposis. Am J Gastroenterol 1999; 94:2275–2281.

Hollstein M, Sidransky D, Vogelstein B, Harris CC: *p53* mutations in human cancers. Science 1991; 253:49–53.

Holt PR: Dairy foods and prevention of colon cancer: human studies. J Am Coll Nutr 1999; 18:379S–391S.

Hoskins LC, Loux HA, Britten A, Zamcheck N: Distribution of ABO blood groups in patients with pernicious anemia, gastric carcinoma and gastric carcinoma associated with pernicious anemia. N Engl J Med 1965; 273:633–637.

Hovinen E, Kekki M, Kuikka S: A theory to the stochastic dynamic model building for chronic progressive disease processes with an application to chronic gastritis. J Theor Biol 1976; 57:131–152.

Howe JR, Bair JL, Sayed MG, Anderson ME, Mitros FA, Petersen GM, Velculescu VE, Traverso G, Vogelstein B: Germline mutations of the gene encoding bone morphogenetic protein receptor 1A in juvenile polyposis. Nat Genet 2001; 28:184–187.

Howe JR, Roth S, Ringold JC, Summers RW, Jarvinen HJ, Sistonen P, Tomlinson IP, Houlston RS, Bevan S, Mitros FA, et al.: Mutations in the *SMAD4/DPC4* gene in juvenile polyposis. Science 1998; 280:1086–1088.

Huntsman DG, Carneiro F, Lewis FR, MacLeod PM, Hayashi A, Monaghan KG, Maung R, Seruca R, Jackson CE, Caldas C: Early gastric cancer in young, asymptomatic carriers of germ-line E-cadherin mutations. N Engl J Med 2001; 344:1904–1909.

Hussussian CJ, Struewing JP, Goldstein AM, Higgins PA, Ally DS, Sheahan MD, Clark WH Jr, Tucker MA, Dracopoli NC: Germline p16 mutations in familial melanoma. Nat Genet 1994; 8:15–21.

Ihamaki T, Varis K, Siurala M: Morphological, functional and immunological state of the gastric mucosa in gastric carcinoma families: comparison with a computer-matched family sample. Scand J Gastroenterol 1979; 14:801–812.

Jackson CE, Brownlee RW, Schuman BM, Micheloni F, Ghironzi G: Observations on gastric cancer in San Marino: I. Familial factors. Cancer 1980; 45:599–602.

Järvinen HJ, Aarnio M, Mustonen H, Aktan-Collan K, Aaltonen LA, Peltomäki P, de la Chapelle A, Mecklin J-P: Controlled 15-year trial on screening for colorectal cancer in families with hereditary nonpolyposis colorectal cancer. Gastroenterology 2000; 118:829–834.

Jass JR: Juvenile polyposis. In: Phillips RKS, Spigelman AD, Thomason JPS (eds). Familial Adenomatous Polyposis and Other Polyposis Syndromes. London: Edward Arnold, 1994:203–214.

Jensen OM, Bolander AM, Sigtryggsson P, Vercelli M, Nguyen-Dinh X, MacLennan R: Large-bowel cancer in married couples in Sweden: a follow-up study. Lancet 1980; 1:1161–1163.

Joslyn G, Carlson M, Thliveris A, Albertsen H, Gelbert L, Samowitz W, Groden J, Stevens J, Spirio L, Robertson M, et al.: Identification of deletion mutations and three new genes at the familial polyposis locus. Cell 1991; 66:601–613.

Joslyn G, Richardson DS, White R, Alber T: Dimer formation by an *N*-terminal coiled coil in the APC protein. Proc Natl Acad Sci USA 1993; 90:11109–11113.

Kampman E, Giovannucci E, van 't Veer P, Rimm E, Stampfer MJ, Colditz GA, Kok FJ, Willett WC: Calcium, vitamin D, dairy foods, and the occurrence of colorectal adenomas among men and women in two prospective studies. Am J Epidemiol 1994; 139:16–29.

Kaplan KB, Burds AA, Swedlow JR, Bekir SS, Sorger PK, Nathke IS: A role for the adenomatous polyposis coli protein in chromosome segregation. Nat Cell Biol 2001; 3:429–432.

Kekki M, Ihamaki T, Sipponen P, Hovinen E: Heterogeneity in susceptibility to chronic gastritis in relatives of gastric cancer patients with different histology of carcinoma. Scand J Gastroenterol 1975; 10:737–745.

Kervinen K, Sodervik H, Makela J, Lehtola J, Niemi M, Kairaluoma MI, Kesaniemi YA: Is the development of adenoma and carcinoma in proximal colon related to apolipoprotein E phenotype? Gastroenterology 1996; 110:1785–1790.

King JE, Dozois RR, Lindor NM, Ahlquist DA: Care of patients and their families with familial adenomatous polyposis. Mayo Clin Proc 2000; 75:57–67.

Kinzler KW, Nilbert MC, Su LK, Vogelstein B, Bryan TM, Levy DB, Smith KJ, Preisinger AC, Hedge P, McKechnie D, et al.: Identification of FAP locus genes from chromosome 5q21. Science 1991; 253:661–665.

Kinzler KW, Vogelstein B: Lessons from hereditary colorectal cancer. Cell 1996; 87:159–170.

Kolodner RD, Hall NR, Lipford J, Kane MF, Rao MR, Morrison P, Wirth L, Finan PJ, Burn J, Chapman P: Structure of the human MSH2 locus and analysis of two Muir-Torre kindreds for msh2 mutations. Genomics 1994; 24:516–526.

Kolodner RD, Tytell JD, Schmeits JL, Kane MF, Gupta RD, Weger J, Wahlberg S, Fox EA, Peel D, Ziogas A, et al.: Germ-line msh6 mutations in colorectal cancer families. Cancer Res 1999; 59:5068–5074.

Konishi M, Kikuchi-Yanoshita R, Tanaka K, Muraoka M, Onda A, Okumura Y, Kishi N, Iwama T, Mori T, Koike M, et al.: Molecular nature of colon tumors in hereditary nonpolyposis colon cancer, familial polyposis, and sporadic colon cancer. Gastroenterology 1996; 111:307–317.

Kune GA, Kune S, Watson LF: The Melbourne Colorectal Cancer Study: characterization of patients with a family history of colorectal cancer. Dis Colon Rectum 1987; 30:600–606.

Lagergren J, Bergstrom R, Lindgren A, Nyren O: Symptomatic gastroesophageal reflux as a risk factor for esophageal adenocarcinoma. N Engl J Med 1999; 340:825–831.

Laken SJ, Petersen GM, Gruber SB, Oddoux C, Ostrer H, Giardiello FM, Hamilton SR, Hampel H, Markowitz A, Klimstra D, Jhanwar S, Winawer S, Offit K, Luce MC, Kinzler KW, Vogelstein B: Familial colorectal cancer in Ashkenazim due to a hypermutable tract in APC. Nat Genet 1997; 17:79–83.

Lal G, Liu G, Schmocker B, Kaurah P, Ozcelik H, Narod SA, Redston M, Gallinger S: Inherited predisposition to pancreatic adenocarcinoma: role of family history and germ-line *p16*, *BRCA1*, and *BRCA2* mutations. Cancer Res 2000; 60:409–416.

Lambert R: Chronic gastritis: a critical study of the progressive atrophy of the gastric mucosa. Digestion 1972; 7:83–126.

Lance P: Tumors and other neoplastic diseases of the small intestine. In: Yamada T (ed). Textbook of Gastroenterology, 3d ed. Philadelphia: J. B. Lippincott, 1999:1722–1738.

Landis SH, Murray T, Bolden S, Wingo PA: Cancer statistics, 1999. CA Cancer J Clin 1999; 49:8–31.

Lane DP: Cancer: p53, guardian of the genome. Nature 1992; 358:15–16.

Lang NP, Butler MA, Massengill J, Lawson M, Stotts RC, Hauer-Jensen M, Kadlubar FF: Rapid metabolic phenotypes for acetyltransferase and cytochrome P4501A2 and putative exposure to food-borne heterocyclic amines increase the risk for colorectal cancer or polyps. Cancer Epidemiol Biomarkers Prev 1994; 3:675–682.

La Vecchia C, Negri E, Franceschi S, Gentile A: Family history and the risk of stomach and colorectal cancer. Cancer 1992; 70:50–55.

Lehtola J: Family study of gastric carcinoma; with special reference to histological types. Scand J Gastroenterol (Suppl) 1978; 13:1–54.

Leppert M, Dobbs M, Scambler P, O'Connell P, Nakamura Y, Stauffer D, Woodward S, Burt R, Hughes J, Gardner E, et al.: The gene for familial polyposis coli maps to the long arm of chromosome 5. Science 1987; 238:1411–1413.

Li FP, Fraumeni JF Jr, Mulvihill JJ, Blattner WA, Dreyfus MG, Tucker MA, Miller RW: A cancer family syndrome in twenty-four kindreds. Cancer Res 1988; 48:5358–5362.

Li JY: Epidemiology of esophageal cancer in China. Natl Cancer Inst Monogr 1982; 62:113–120.

Liaw D, Marsh DJ, Li J, Dahia PL, Wang SI, Zheng Z, Bose S, Call KM, Tsou HC, Peacocke M, et al.: Germline mutations of the *PTEN* gene in Cowden disease, an inherited breast and thyroid cancer syndrome. Nat Genet 1997; 16:64–67.

Lichtenstein P, Holm NV, Verkasalo PK, Iliadou A, Kaprio J, Koskenvuo M, Pukkala E, Skytthe A, Hemminki K: Environmental and heritable factors in the cusation of cancer. N Engl J Med 2000; 343:78–85.

Liu L, Lassam NJ, Slingerland JM, Bailey D, Cole D, Jenkins R, Hogg D: Germline p16INK4A mutation and protein dysfunction in a family with inherited melanoma. Oncogene 1995; 11:405–412.

Loeb LA: Microsatellite instability: marker of a mutator phenotype in cancer. Cancer Res 1994; 54:5059–5063.

Loukola A, de la Chapelle A, Aaltonen LA: Strategies for screening for hereditary non-polyposis colorectal cancer. J Med Genet 1999; 36:819–822.

Lovett E: Family studies in cancer of the colon and rectum. Br J Surg 1976; 63:13–18.

Lowenfels AB, Maisonneuve P, DiMagno EP, Elitsur Y, Gates LK Jr, Perrault J, Whitcomb DC: Hereditary pancreatitis and the risk of pancreatic cancer. J Natl Cancer Inst 1997; 89:442–446.

Lynch HT, de la Chapelle A: Genetic susceptibility to non-polyposis colorectal cancer. J Med Genet 1999; 36:801–818.

Lynch HT, Lanspa S, Smyrk T, Boman B, Watson P, Lynch J: Hereditary nonpolyposis colorectal cancer (Lynch syndromes I & II): genetics, pathology, natural history, and cancer control, part I. Cancer Genet Cytogenet 1991; 53:143–160.

Lynch HT, Lynch J: Lynch syndrome: genetics, natural history, genetic counseling, and prevention. J Clin Oncol 2000; 18:19s–31s.

Ma J, Stampfer MJ, Giovannucci E, Artigas C, Hunter DJ, Fuchs C, Willett WC, Selhub J, Hennekens CH, Rozen R: Methylenetetrahydrofolate reductase polymorphism, dietary interactions, and risk of colorectal cancer. Cancer Res 1997; 57:1098–1102.

MacDonald DJ, Lessick M: Hereditary cancers in children and ethical and psychosocial implications. J Pediatr Nurs 2000; 15:217–225.

Macklin MT: The role of heredity in gastrointestinal cancer. Gastroenterology 1955; 29:507–511.

Macklin MT: Inheritance of cancer of the stomach and large intestine in man. J Natl Cancer Inst 1960; 24:551–571.

Macrae FA, Young GP: Neoplastic and nonneoplastic polyps of the colon and rectum. In: Yamada T (ed). Textbook of Gastroenterology, 3d ed. Philadelphia: J. B. Lippincott, 1999:1965–1994.

Maire P, Morichau-Beauchant M, Drucker J, Barboteau MA, Barbier J, Matuchansky C: Familial occurrence of cancer of the colon and the rectum: results of a 3-year case-control survey. Gastroenterol Clin Biol 1984; 8:22–27.

Markowitz S, Wang J, Myeroff L, Parsons R, Sun L, Lutterbaugh J, Fan RS, Zborowska E, Kinzler KW, Vogelstein B, et al.: Inactivation of the type II TGF-β receptor in colon cancer cells with microsatellite instability. Science 1995; 268:1336–1338.

Marra G, Boland CR: Hereditary nonpolyposis colorectal cancer: the syndrome, the genes, and historical perspective. J Natl Cancer Inst 1995; 87:1114–1125.

Marra G, Boland CR: DNA repair and colorectal cancer. Gastroenterol Clin North Am 1996; 25:755–772.

Marsh DJ, Dahia PL, Zheng Z, Liaw D, Parsons R, Gorlin RJ, Eng C: Germline mutations in *PTEN* are present in Bannayan-Zonana syndrome. Nat Genet 1997; 16:333–334.

McConnell JC, Nizin JS, Slade MS: Colonoscopy in patients with a primary family history of colon cancer. Dis Colon Rectum 1990; 33:105–107.

McConnell RB: Genetic aspects of gut cancer. In: DeCosse JJ, Sherlock P (eds). Gastrointestinal Cancer. Boston: Martinus Nijhoff Publishers, 1981:27–62.

McFarlane GA, Munro A: *Helicobacter pylori* and gastric cancer. Br J Surg 1997; 84:1190–1199.

McGarrity TJ, Kulin HE, Zaino RJ: Peutz-Jeghers syndrome. Am J Gastroenterol 2000; 95:596–604.

Miyaki M, Konishi M, Tanaka K, Kikuchi-Yanoshita R, Muraoka M, Yasuno M, Igari T, Koike M, Chiba M, Mori T: Germline mutation of *MSH6* as the cause of hereditary nonpolyposis colorectal cancer. Nat Genet 1997; 17:271–272.

Miyashiro I, Senda T, Matsumine A, Baeg GH, Kuroda T, Shimano T, Miura S, Noda T, Kobayashi S, Monden M, et al.: Subcellular localization of the APC protein: immunoelectron microscopic study of the association of the APC protein with catenin. Oncogene 1995; 11:89–96.

Morales TG, Sampliner RE: Barrett's esophagus: update on screening, surveillance, and treatment. Arch Intern Med 1999; 159:1411–1416.

Morin PJ, Vogelstein B, Kinzler KW: Apoptosis and APC in colorectal tumorigenesis. Proc Natl Acad Sci USA 1996; 93:7950–7954.

Nagase H, Miyoshi Y, Horii A, Aoki T, Ogawa M, Utsunomiya J, Baba S, Sasazuki T, Nakamura Y: Correlation between the location of germ-line mutations in the APC gene and the number of colorectal polyps in familial adenomatous polyposis patients. Cancer Res 1992; 52:4055–4057.

Neubauer A, Thiede C, Morgner A, Alpen B, Ritter M, Neubauer B, Wundisch T, Ehninger G, Stolte M, Bayerdorffer E: Cure of *Helicobacter pylori* infection and duration of remission of low-grade gastric mucosa-associated lymphoid tissue lymphoma. J Natl Cancer Inst 1997; 89:1350–1355.

Nishisho I, Nakamura Y, Miyoshi Y, Miki Y, Ando H, Horii A, Koyama K, Utsunomiya J, Baba S, Hedge P: Mutations of chromosome 5q21 genes in FAP and colorectal cancer patients. Science 1991; 253:665–669.

Olschwang S, Serova-Sinilnikova OM, Lenoir GM, Thomas G: *PTEN* germ-line mutations in juvenile polyposis coli. Nat Genet 1998; 18:12–14.

Orrom WJ, Brzezinski WS, Wiens EW: Heredity and colorectal cancer: a prospective, community-based, endoscopic study. Dis Colon Rectum 1990; 33:490–493.

Pariente A, Milan C, Lafon J, Faivre J: Colonoscopic screening in first-degree relatives of patients with "sporadic" colorectal cancer: a case-control study. Gastroenterology 1998; 115:7–12.

Parkin DM, Pisani P, Ferlay J: Global cancer statistics. CA Cancer J Clin 1999; 49:33–64.

Paul P, Letteboer T, Gelbert L, Groden J, White R, Coppes MJ: Identical APC exon 15 mutations result in a variable phenotype in familial adenomatous polyposis. Hum Mol Genet 1993; 2:925–931.

Peifer M. β-catenin *s* oncogene: the smoking gun. Science 1997; 275:1572–1573.

Petersen GM, Brensinger JD, Johnson KA, Giardiello FM: Genetic testing and counseling for hereditary forms of colorectal cancer. Cancer 1999; 15:1720–1730.

Petersen GM, Slack J, Nakamura Y: Screening guidelines and premorbid diagnosis of familial adenomatous polyposis using linkage. Gastroenterology 1991; 100:1658–1664.

Ponz de Leon M, Antonioli A, Ascari A, Zanghieri G, Sacchetti G: Incidence and familial occurrence of colorectal cancer and polyps in a health care district of northern Italy. Cancer 1987; 60:2848–2859.

Potter JD: Colorectal cancer: molecules and populations. J Natl Cancer Inst 1999; 91:916–932.

Powell SM, Petersen GM, Krush AJ, Booker S, Jen J, Giardiello FM, Hamilton SR, Vogelstein B, Kinzler KW: Molecular diagnosis of familial adenomatous polyposis. N Engl J Med 1993; 329:1982–1987.

Powell SM, Zilz N, Beazer-Barclay Y, Bryan TM, Hamilton SR, Thibodeau SN, Vogelstein B, Kinzler KW: *APC* mutations occur early during colorectal tumorigenesis. Nature 1992; 359:235–237.

Richards FM, McKee SA, Rajpar MH, Cole TR, Evans DG, Jankowski JA, McKeown C, Sanders DS, Maher ER: Germline E-cadherin gene (*CDH1*) mutations predispose to familial gastric cancer and colorectal cancer. Hum Mol Genet 1999; 8:607–610.

Risk JM, Field EA, Field JK, Whittaker J, Fryer A, Ellis A, Shaw JM, Friedmann PS, Bishop DT, Bodmer J, et al.: Tylosis oesophageal cancer mapped. Nat Genet 1994; 8:319–321.

Roth S, Sistonen P, Salovaara R, Hemminki A, Loukola A, Johansson M, Avizienyte E, Cleary KA, Lynch P, Amos CI, et al.: *SMAD* genes in juvenile polyposis. Genes Chromosomes Cancer 1999; 26:54–61.

Rozen P, Fireman Z, Figer A, Legum C, Ron E, Lynch HT: Family history of colorectal cancer as a marker of potential malignancy within a screening program. Cancer 1987; 60:248–254.

Rubinfeld B, Albert I, Porfiri E, Fiol C, Munemitsu S, Polakis P: Binding of GSK3β to the APC-β-catenin complex and regulation of complex assembly. Science 1996; 272:1023–1026.

Rustgi AK: Esophageal neoplasms. In: Yamada T (ed). Textbook of Gastroenterology, 3d ed. Philadelphia: J. B. Lippincott, 1999:1278–1303.

Saitoh Y, Waxman I, West AB, Popnikolov NK, Gatalica Z, Watari J, Obara T, Kohgo Y, Pasricha PJ: Prevalence and distinctive biologic features of flat colorectal adenomas in a North American population. Gastroenterology 2001; 120: 1657–1665.

Samowitz WS, Slattery ML, Kerber RA: Microsatellite instability in human colonic cancer is not a useful clinical indicator of familial colorectal cancer. Gastroenterology 1995; 109:1765–1771.

Sandler RS: Epidemiology and risk factors for colorectal cancer. Gastroenterol Clin North Am 1996; 25:717–735.

Sauar J, Hausken T, Hoff G, Bjorkheim A, Foerster A, Mowinckel P: Colonoscopic screening examination of relatives of patients with colorectal cancer: I. A comparison with an endoscopically screened normal population. Scand J Gastroenterol 1992; 27:661–666.

Shearman DJ, Finlayson ND: Familial aspects of gastric carcinoma. Am J Dig Dis 1967; 12:529–534.

Shtutman M, Zhurinsky J, Simcha I, Albanese C, D'Amico M, Pestell R, Ben-Ze'ev A: The cyclin D1 gene is a target of the β-catenin/LEF-1 pathway. Proc Natl Acad Sci USA 1999; 96:5522–5527.

Sieber OM, Tomlinson IP, Lamlum H: The adenomatous polyposis coli (APC) tumour suppressor; genetics, function and disease. Mol Med Today 2000; 6:462–469.

Singh NP, Khan A: Acetaldehyde: genotoxicity and cytotoxicity in human lymphocytes. Mutat Res 1995; 337:9–17.

Siruala M, Varis K, Woljasulo M: Studies of patients with atrophic gastritis: a 10–15 year follow-up. Scand J Gastroenterol 1966; 1:40–48.

Slattery ML, Kerber RA: Family history of cancer and colon cancer risk: the Utah population database. J Natl Cancer Inst 1994; 86:1618–1626.

Smith KJ, Johnson KA, Bryan TM, Hill DE, Markowitz S, Willson JK, Paraskeva C, Petersen GM, Hamilton SR, Vogelstein B, et al.: The *APC* gene product in normal and tumor cells. Proc Natl Acad Sci USA 1993; 90:2846–2850.

Soravia C, Berk T, Cohen Z: Genetic testing and surgical decision making in hereditary colorectal cancer. Int J Colorectal Dis 2000; 15:21–28.

Spigelman AD, Arese P, Phillips RK: Polyposis: the Peutz-Jeghers syndrome. Br J Surg 1995; 82:1311–1314.

Spirio L, Nelson L, Ward K, Burt R, White R, Leppert M: A CA-repeat polymorphism close to the adenomatous polyposis coli (*APC*) gene offers improved diagnostic testing for familial APC. Am J Hum Genet 1993a; 52:286–296.

Spirio L, Olschwang S, Groden J, Robertson M, Samowitz W, Joslyn G, Gelbert L, Thliveris A, Carlson M, Otterud B: Alleles of the *APC* gene: an attenuated form of familial polyposis. Cell 1993b; 75:951–957.

Spirio L, Samowitz W, Robertson J, Robertson M, Burt R, Leppert M, White R: Alleles of *APC* modulate the frequency and classes of mutations that lead to colon polyps. Nat Genet 1998; 20:385–388.

Spurr NK, Gough AC, Chinegwundoh FI, Smith CA: Polymorphisms in drug-metabolizing enzymes as modifiers of cancer risk. Clin Chem 1995; 41:1864–1869.

Stephenson BM, Finan PJ, Gascoyne J, Garbett F, Murday VA, Bishop DT: Frequency of familial colorectal cancer. Br J Surg 1991; 78:1162–1166.

St. John DJ, McDermott FT, Hopper JL, Debney EA, Johnson WR, Hughes ES: Cancer risk in relatives of patients with common colorectal cancer. Ann Intern Med 1993; 118:785–790.

Straszewski J, Haenszel W: Cancer mortality among the Polish-born in the United States. J Natl Cancer Inst 1965; 35:291–297.

Strickland RG, Mackay IR: A reappraisal of the nature and significance of chronic atrophic gastritis. Am J Dig Dis 1973; 18:426–440.

Syngal S, Fox EA, Eng C, Kolodner RD, Garber JE: Sensitivity and specificity of clinical criteria for hereditary non-polyposis colorectal cancer associated mutations in *MSH2* and *MLH1*. J Med Genet 2000; 37:641–645.

Terdiman JP: Genomic events in the adenoma to carcinoma sequence. Semin Gastrointest Dis 2000; 11:194–206.

Terdiman JP, Conrad PG, Sleisenger MH: Genetic testing in hereditary colorectal cancer: indications and procedures. Am J Gastroenterol 1999; 94:2344–2356.

Terdiman JP, Gum JRJ, Conrad PG, Miller GA, Weinberg V, Crawley SC, Levin TR, Reeves C, Scmitt A, Hepburn M, et al.: Efficient detection of hereditary nonpolyposis colorectal cancer gene carriers by screening for tumor microsatellite instability before germline genetic testing. Gastroenterology 2001; 120:21–30.

Tetsu O, McCormick F: β-catenin regulates expression of cyclin D1 in colon carcinoma cells. Nature 1999; 398:422–426.

Thibodeau SN, Bren G, Schaid D: Microsatellite instability in cancer of the proximal colon. Science 1993; 260:816–819.

Thibodeau SN, French AJ, Cunningham JM, Tester D, Burgart LJ, Roche PC, McDonnell SK, Schaid DJ, Vockley CW, Michels VV, et al.: Microsatellite instability in colorectal cancer: different mutator phenotypes and the principal involvement of *hMLH1*. Cancer Res 1998; 58:1713–1718.

Todd KE, Gloor B, Reber HA: Pancreatic carcinomas. In: Yamada T (ed). Textbook of Gastroenterology, 3d ed. Philadelphia: J. B. Lippincott, 1999:2178–2192.

Utsunomiya J, Gocho H, Miyanaga T, Hamaguchi E, Kashimure A: Peutz-Jeghers syndrome: its natural course and management. Johns Hopkins Med J 1975; 136:71–82.

van Es JH, Giles RH, Clevers HC: The many faces of the tumor suppressor gene *APC*. Exp Cell Res 2001; 264:126–134.

Varis K: A family study of chronic gastritis: histological, immunological and functional aspects. Scand J Gastroenterol Suppl 1971; 13:1–56.

Vasen HFA, Mecklin J, Merra Khan P, Lynch HT: The International Collaborative Group on Hereditary Non-Polyposis Colorectal Cancer (ICG-HNPCC). Dis Colon Rectum 1991; 34:424–425.

Vasen HFA, Watson P, Mecklin J-P, Lynch HT, ICG-HNPCC: New clinical criteria for hereditary nonpolyposis colorectal cancer (HNPCC, Lynch syndrome) proposed by the International Collaborative Group on HNPCC. Gastroenterology 1999; 116:1453–1456.

Vogelstein B, Fearon ER, Hamilton SR, Kern SE, Preisinger AC, Leppert M, Nakamura Y, White R, Smits AM, Bos JL: Genetic alterations during colorectal-tumor development. N Engl J Med 1988; 319:525–532.

Wallis YL, Macdonald F, Hulten M, Morton JE, McKeown CM, Neoptolemos JP, Keighley M, Morton DG: Genotype–phenotype correlation between position of constitutional *APC* gene mutation and CHRPE expression in familial adenomatous polyposis. Hum Genet 1994; 94:543–548.

Weisburger JH, Reddy BS, Newell GR: Potential for personal modification of risk for developing colon cancer. Cancer Detect Prev 1985; 8:399–412.

Whelan AJ, Bartsch D, Goodfellow PJ: Brief report: a familial syndrome of pancreatic cancer and melanoma with a mutation in the *CDKN2* tumor-suppressor gene. N Engl J Med 1995; 333:975–977.

Whitcomb DC, Gorry MC, Preston RA, Furey W, Sossenheimer MJ, Ulrich CD, Martin SP, Gates LK Jr, Amann ST, Toskes PP, et al.: Hereditary pancreatitis is caused by a mutation in the cationic trypsinogen gene. Nat Genet 1996; 14:141–145.

Wijnen J, Khan P, Vasen H, van der Klift H, Mulder A, van Leeuwen-Cornelisse I, Bakker B, Losekoot M, Moller P, Fodde R: Hereditary nonpolyposis colorectal cancer families not complying with the Amsterdam criteria show extremely low frequency of mismatch-repair-gene mutations. Am J Hum Genet 1997; 61:329–335.

Wijnen J, Vasen HA, Khan M, Zwinderman A, van der Klift H, Mulder A, Tops C, Møller P, Fodde R: Clinical findings with implications for genetic testing in families with clustering of colorectal cancer. N Engl J Med 1998; 339:511–518.

Willert K, Shibamoto S, Nusse R: Wnt-induced dephosphorylation of axin releases β-catenin from the axin complex. Genes Dev 1999; 13:1768–1773.

Winawer SJ, Fletcher RH, Miller L, Godlee F, Stolar MH, Mulrow CD, Woolf SH, Glick SN, Ganiats TG, Bond JH, et al.: Colorectal cancer screening: clinical guidelines and rationale. Gastroenterology 1997; 112:594–642.

Winawer SJ, Zauber AG, Gerdes H, O'Brien MJ, Gottlieb LS, Sternberg SS, Bond JH, Waye JD, Schapiro M, Panish JF, et al.: Risk of colorectal cancer in the families of patients with adenomatous polyps. N Engl J Med 1996; 334:82–87.

Winawer SJ, Zauber AG, Ho MN, O'Brien MJ, Gottlieb LS, Sternberg SS, Waye JD, Schapiro M, Bond JH, Panish JF, et al.: Prevention of colorectal cancer by colonoscopic polypectomy. N Engl J Med 1993; 329:1977–1981.

Wong N, Lasko D, Rabelo R, Pinsky L, Gordon PH, Foulkes TW: Genetic counseling and interpretation of genetic tests in familial adenomatous polyposis and hereditary nonpolyposis colorectal cancer. Dis Colon Rectum 2001; 44:271–279.

Woodford-Richens K, Bevan S, Churchman M, Dowling B, Jones D, Norbury CG, Hodgson SV, Desai DC, Neale KF, Phillips RKS, et al.: Analysis of genetic and phenotypic and heterogeneity in juvenile polyposis. Gut 2000; 46:656–660.

Woolf CM: The incidence of cancer in spouses of stomach cancer patients. Cancer 1961; 14:199–200.

World Cancer Research Fund 1997.

Wu Y, Berends MJ, Mensink RG, Kempinga C, Sijmons RH, van Der Zee AG, Hollema H, Kleibeuker JH, Buys CH, Hofstra RM: Association of hereditary nonpolyposis colorectal cancer-related tumors displaying low microsatellite instability with *MSH6* germline mutations. Am J Hum Genet 1999; 65:1291–1298.

Wynder EL, Hirayama T: Comparative epidemiology of cancers of the United States and Japan. Prev Med 1977; 6:567–594.

Yardley JH, Hendrix TR: Gastritis, gastropathy, duodenitis, and associated ulcerative lesions. In: Yamada T (ed). Textbook of Gastroenterology, 3d ed. Philadelphia: J. B. Lippincott, 1999:1463–1499.

Yin J, Kong D, Wang S, Zou TT, Souza RF, Smolinski KN, Lynch PM, Hamilton SR, Sugimura H, Powell SM, et al.: Mutation of *hMSH3* and *hMSH6* mismatch repair genes in genetically unstable human colorectal and gastric carcinomas. Hum Mutat 1997; 10:474–478.

Zanghieri G, Di Gregorio C, Sacchetti C, Fante R, Sassatelli R, Cannizzo G, Carriero A, Ponz de Leon M: Familial occurrence of gastric cancer in the 2-year experience of a population-based registry. Cancer 1990; 66:2047–2051.

Zhong S, Wyllie AH, Barnes D, Wolf CR, Spurr NK: Relationship between the GSTM1 genetic polymorphism and susceptibility to bladder, breast and colon cancer. Carcinogenesis 1993; 14:1821–1824.

Zwick A, Munir M, Ryan CK, Gian J, Burt RW, Leppert M, Spirio L, Chey WY: Gastric adenocarcinoma and dysplasia in fundic gland polyps of a patient with attenuated adenomatous polyposis coli. Gastroenterology 1997; 113:659–663.

35 Breast Cancer

KATHERINE L. NATHANSON AND BARBARA L. WEBER

Breast cancer is the most common form of noncutaneous cancer in American women (Landis et al., 1998). In the United States alone, there are over 186,000 new cases and 46,000 deaths each year. It is estimated that 12.5% of all American women (1 in 8) will develop breast cancer and 3.4% will die from it (Ries et al., 1998). Due to breast cancer's importance as a public health problem, its usefulness as a paradigm of human cancer development, and the public interest in investigating this problem, it has been extensively studied by both clinical and basic science researchers. These efforts have begun to elucidate some of the mechanisms by which breast cancer develops from both a genetic and biochemical perspective. This work also has provided an improved understanding of why some people are more susceptible to breast cancer than others and insight into some of the important genetic and environmental factors that influence cancer susceptibility. This chapter contains (1) a review of the epidemiology of breast cancer; (2) a clinical overview of breast cancer screening and therapy; (3) a discussion of risk factors for breast cancer, with emphasis on hereditary causes; (4) a description of the breast/ovarian cancer susceptibility genes *BRCA1* and *BRCA2*, as well as other rarer cancer susceptibility syndromes that predispose to breast cancer; (5) an overview of the lower-penetrance genes thought to be involved in breast cancer susceptibility; and (6) guidelines for the clinical application of genetic information.

EPIDEMIOLOGY

The incidence of breast cancer as reported by the National Cancer Institute's Surveillance, Epidemiology, and End Results (SEER) program is 111.2 cases per 100,000 American women of all ages, averaged over the years 1992–1998 (Ries et al., 2001). On average, a woman's lifetime risk of developing breast cancer is 1 in 8. However, this overall risk is not reached until late life, and, interestingly, risk begins to decline in women who have not developed breast cancer at older ages. The overall incidence of breast cancer in all age groups increased by more than 40% from 1973 to 1998 (Howe et al., 2001). The increase in breast cancer incidence from 1992 to 1998 was most pronounced in Caucasian women aged 50 to 64 and was limited to early-stage disease. The annual rate of increase in breast cancer diagnoses was 1% from the 1940s to 1980; from 1982 to 1987 it was 4% per year, and from 1987 to 1998 it decreased to less than 1% per year (Feuer et al., 1993; Howe et al., 2001). The increase in incidence was concordant with increased utilization of mammography, which is expected to create an artificially increased incidence rate by moving diagnosis earlier in the newly screened cohort. It also is consistent with an aging of the population in the interval 1987 to 1998, but contains a true increment in incidence as well (Feuer and Wun, 1992). Since 1994, there has been an increase in the incidence of stage II lymph-node positive disease, for unknown reasons (Howe et al., 2001). Fortunately, however, the breast cancer–related mortality rate for American women of all ages declined 3.4% from 1995 to 1998 and is currently 24.5 per 100,000 (Ries et al., 2001). Of note, one-third of women diagnosed with breast cancer die of the disease, and only lung cancer supersedes breast cancer as the leading cause of cancer mortality among American women (Landis et al., 1998).

There is wide international variation in breast cancer rates. During 1983 to 1987, breast cancer incidence rates ranged more than 5-fold, from less than 6 per 100,000 women years in Japan to almost 30 in England and Wales (Brinton and Devesa, 1996). Studies showing that within two generations Japanese immigrants to the United States have a rate of breast cancer almost equal to Americans suggest certain environmental and lifestyle effects have a considerable effect on disease incidence (Parkin, 1989).

Another statistic that emphasizes population differences is the difference in incidence and mortality between American Caucasian and African American women. From 1987 to 1998 the increase in breast cancer incidence for African American women was higher than that for Caucasian women; however, while the mortality in African American women had increased by 1.3% per year between 1973 and 1991, the death rates have now stabilized and even declined among women under age 75 (Howe et al., 2001) (Fig. 35–1). While the explanation for increased breast cancer–related mortality in African American women is unclear, African American women are more frequently diagnosed with late-stage disease. This may be due to several factors, including lower use of regular mammography or socioeconomic and cultural factors that may lead to decreased access to or utilization of health care services, but could be due to underlying genetic or biological factors (Ayanian et al., 1993; Lannin et al., 1998; McCarthy et al., 1998; Yood et al., 1999). Additionally, African American women are more likely to be diagnosed with breast cancer at a younger age, and in some studies younger women have a higher breast cancer–related mortality rate (Garfinkel et al., 1994). Finally, there is some evidence that African Americans may have higher-grade tumors than Caucasian patients, with more nuclear atypia and mitoses, which may be a possible contributor to increased mortality (Chen et al., 1994; Rose and Royak-Schaler, 2001).

CLINICAL PRESENTATION

Breast cancer arises from the epithelium of the mammary gland, which includes the milk-producing lobules and the ducts that carry milk to the nipple (Fig. 35–2). Malignant transformation

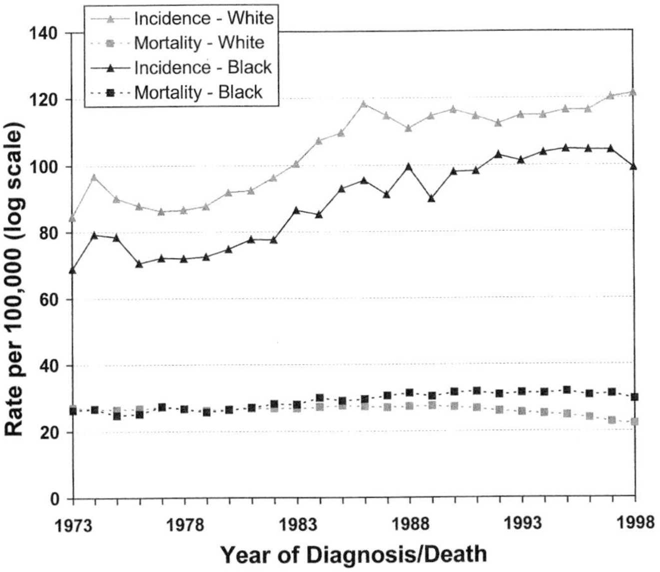

Fig. 35–1. Breast cancer incidence and mortality: White females vs. black females. Data taken from SEER (Ries et al., 2001) demonstrates the differences in breast cancer incidence and mortality between Caucasian versus African American women.

of the fatty, vascular, and stromal elements of the breast is not included in this definition and is extremely rare. Breast size is not a risk factor for breast cancer, as it is determined predominantly by fatty and stromal elements, with all women having a similar amount of breast epithelium. The transition from normal to malignant breast epithelium is not as well understood as it is for colon cancer, but it appears to progress along the same general pathway from normal tissue to hyperplasia to dysplasia and then to carcinoma in situ and invasive disease.

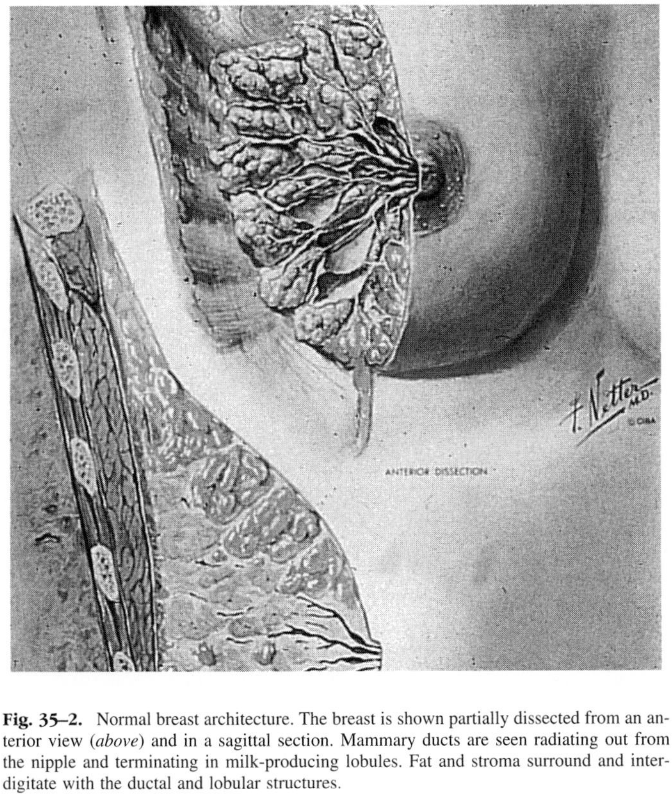

Fig. 35–2. Normal breast architecture. The breast is shown partially dissected from an anterior view (*above*) and in a sagittal section. Mammary ducts are seen radiating out from the nipple and terminating in milk-producing lobules. Fat and stroma surround and interdigitate with the ductal and lobular structures.

Ductal Carcinoma in Situ

Ductal carcinoma in situ (DCIS), also known as intraductal carcinoma, is considered a precursor lesion of invasive or infiltrating ductal carcinoma. There are two major pathological subtypes of DCIS, based on the presence or absence of comedo necrosis (Figs. 35–3, 35–4). DCIS was infrequently diagnosed before the advent of mammography, when it constituted only 1% to 5% of all breast cancer cases. Currently, DCIS is usually seen as a cluster of microcalcifications on a routine mammogram. From 1983 to 1995, the apparent incidence of DCIS rose ~250% in American women over age 50, with much of the increase a result of widespread implementation of mammographic screening (Ernster et al., 1996; Ries et al., 1998). DCIS now accounts for 50% to 60% of all breast malignancies identified by mammographically directed biopsy and 20% to 30% of all cases in women who are undergoing regular mammography (Morrow et al., 1996; Fonseca et al., 1997).

The natural history of DCIS is not well understood, because until recently the treatment of choice was mastectomy, which is almost 100% effective in preventing disease progression and death. What is known comes from patients who had a benign patriological diagnosis initially and then on re-evaluation of the original specimen were found to have DCIS. Several small series of patients show a risk of developing invasive cancer ranging from 20% to 60% within 6 to 10 years of diagnosis (Rosen et al., 1980; Eusebi et al., 1994; Page et al., 1995).

As in invasive breast cancer, breast-conserving therapy (lumpectomy followed by radiation) is emerging as the treatment of choice. Many studies have shown that lumpectomy alone is inadequate therapy, with a mean recurrence rate of 20% (range of 8%–63%), in studies with follow-up ranging from 18 to 108 months (Fonseca et al., 1997). High nuclear grade, comedo-type necrosis, tumor size, and margin width are all predictors of local recurrence (Cheng et al., 1997; Silverstein, 1997; Stallard et al., 2001). No randomized trial has specifically addressed the question of survival by comparing mastectomy and lumpectomy followed by radiation. However, studies have shown comparable survival rates for both therapies, which supports the use of breast conservation in women for whom there is no other contraindication (Fisher et al., 1993; Solin et al., 1996). Initial re-

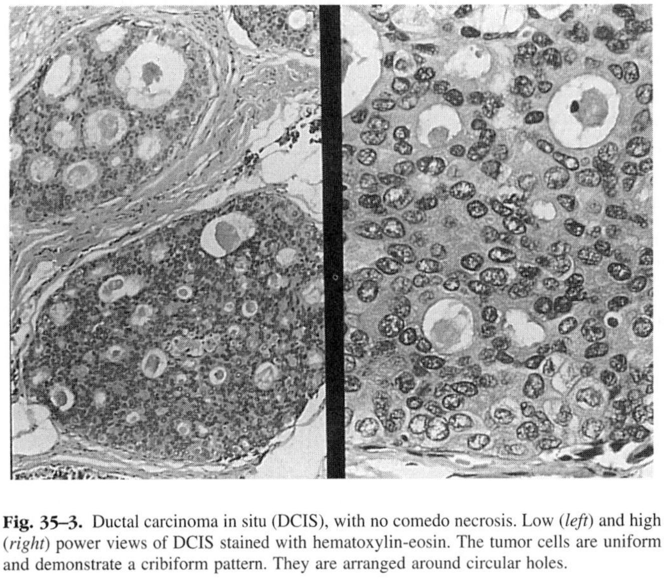

Fig. 35–3. Ductal carcinoma in situ (DCIS), with no comedo necrosis. Low (*left*) and high (*right*) power views of DCIS stained with hematoxylin-eosin. The tumor cells are uniform and demonstrate a cribiform pattern. They are arranged around circular holes.

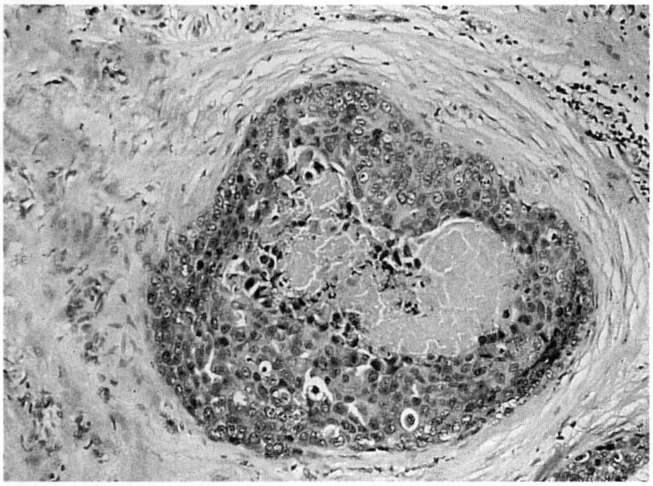

Fig. 35–4. Ductal carcinoma in situ (DCIS), with comedo necrosis. A focus of comedo-type DCIS is shown stained with hemotoxylin-eosin. The malignant cells are wholly contained within the duct and do not invade the surrounding stroma. The central region is filled with necrotic cellular debris, hence the name comdeo type.

sults from NSABP 24 suggest that tamoxifen reduces the risk of subsequent invasive cancer in women with DCIS (Fisher et al., 1999).

DCIS alone or in association with invasive cancer has been seen in almost one-half of the tumors of carriers of *BRCA1* or *BRCA2* mutations. However, the frequency of DCIS may be lower in patients with an inherited susceptibility to breast cancer than in age-matched unselected controls, and this may reflect a quicker progression through the stages of carcinogenesis than in sporadic tumors (BCL Consortium, 1997).

Lobular Carcinoma In Situ

In contrast to DCIS, lobular carcinoma in situ (LCIS) is not thought to be a preinvasive lesion but appears to be a marker of increased risk for the development of invasive cancer (Fig. 35–5). LCIS was not identified as a clinical entity until 1941 and was originally believed to be the precursor lesion of invasive lobular carcinoma. Since its original description, LCIS has been recognized as a purely histologic diagnosis. Clinical diagnosis is not possible, as LCIS does not form a palpable lesion, therefore it cannot be identified on physical examination; in addition, it is not visible on mammography. Thus, the diagnosis of LCIS always is made as an incidental finding on a breast biopsy obtained for diagnosis of an adjacent lesion. The exact incidence of LCIS in the general population is unknown, but there is general agreement that it is an uncommon finding (Morrow and Schnitt, 1996). Evidence that LCIS is a marker lesion and not a true malignant lesion comes from studies demonstrating that it is frequently multicentric or bilateral and that the risk for subsequent cancer is bilateral and is more often of ductal than lobular histology.

The risk of invasive breast cancer after a diagnosis of LCIS has been the subject of many studies; the largest series was reported by Haagenson and colleagues (1981). This series included 287 women, of whom only 2 were lost to follow-up, who were followed for a mean of 16.3 years. Some 18% of the women developed breast cancer, for a relative risk (observed/expected) of 6.9. In a similar cohort followed by Rosen and colleagues (1978) for a mean of 24 years, a relative risk of 9 for the development of breast cancer was observed; more than half of these women developed an invasive lesion at least 15 years after the initial diagnosis of LCIS. Thus a woman with LCIS has an increased risk for the development of breast cancer that is approximately 7 to 10 times that of the general population.

The treatment of LCIS presents a conundrum, because of the substantial risk of invasive carcinoma and the inability to predict where it will occur in the breasts of a woman with LCIS. Currently patients are offered a choice between frequent mammographic surveillance and bilateral mastectomies. This widely discrepant choice obviously is a difficult one and seems particularly harsh, considering the emphasis on breast conservation for the treatment of invasive disease. Tamoxifen may be considered as an alternative to these therapies. LCIS was one of the entry criteria for the recent NSABP P-1 trial; women with LCIS showed a breast cancer risk reduction of 66% when on Tamoxifen versus placebo (Fisher et al., 1998).

There has been considerable speculation on whether or not LCIS represents a histologic marker of genetic predisposition to breast cancer, particularly as it is frequently multicentric and bilateral. In the Cancer and Steroid Hormone Study (CASH) a higher familial risk was reported for LCIS than for other subtypes of breast cancer (Claus et al., 1993). Data suggest that women with LCIS and a family history of breast cancer may be more likely to develop invasive cancer than are those with LCIS alone (Haagenson et al., 1981). However, no study comparing invasive cancer risk in women with a family history with and without LCIS has been reported. Thus, the question of whether family history and LCIS represent compounding risk factors remains unanswered. While LCIS is not seen in increased frequency in *BRCA1* and *BRCA2* mutation carriers, there is evidence to suggest that LCIS is more frequent in familial breast cancer not attributable to mutations in *BRCA1* and *BRCA2* and, in fact, may be a moderately negative predictor for a *BRCA1* mutation (Lakhani et al., 2000).

Invasive Cancer

Invasive breast cancer may be ductal or lobular in histologic subtype, and while there are a few distinguishing clinical features, the natural history and treatment of the two lesions are virtually

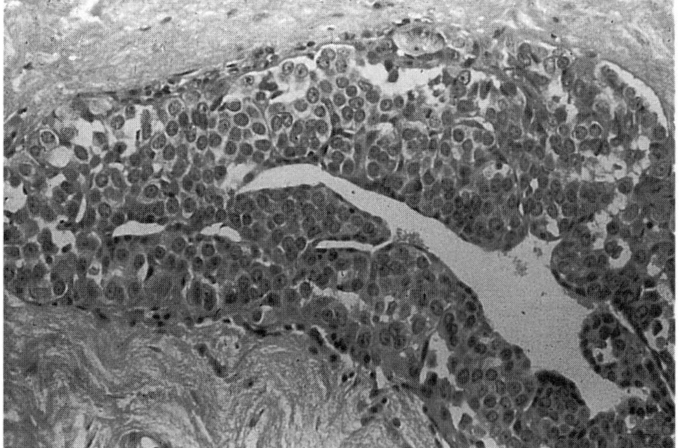

Fig. 35–5. Lobular carcinoma in situ (LCIS). This high-power section of LCIS shows clusters of tumor cells spreading along the duct. The tumor cells are characteristically uniform and round with bland nuclei.

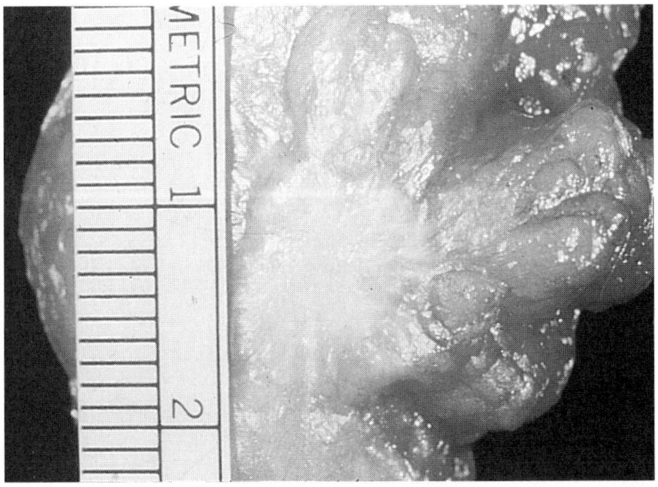

Fig. 35–6. Invasive breast cancer: gross pathology. An unfixed biopsy specimen shows the hard, white invasive cancer extending into the breast in all directions, with an ill-defined border and numerous stellate extensions.

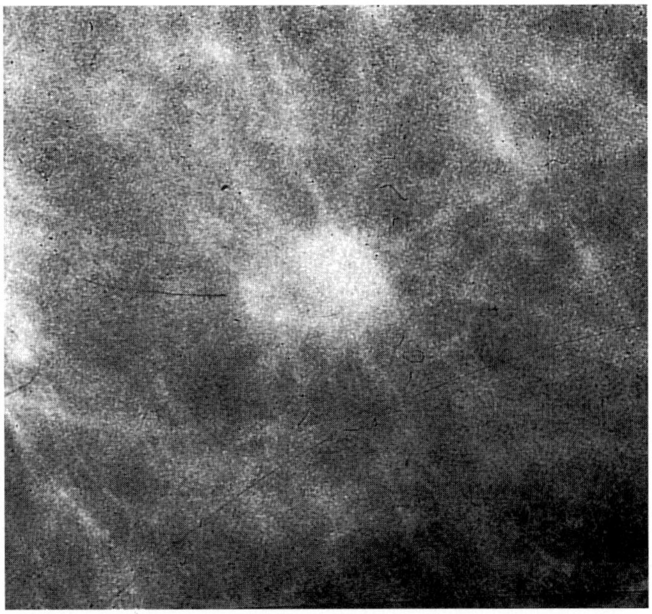

Fig. 35–8. Invasive breast cancer: X-ray. Mammogram showing a spiculated mass with poorly defined borders that is characteristic of an invasive breast cancer.

identical. About 80% of invasive breast cancers are ductal carcinomas. Infiltrating lobular carcinoma is less common, representing only 5% to 10% of breast cancers. The remainder of invasive breast cancer consists of a variety of "special types," including tubular cancer, characterized by prominent tubule formation; medullary carcinoma, a lesion that appears poorly differentiated under the microscope, but is thought to have a more favorable prognosis than other breast cancers; and mucinous (or colloid) carcinoma, characterized by the abundant accumulation of extracellular mucin, bulky tumors, and a good prognosis (Fisher et al., 1990; Harris et al., 1992). Of particular note, approximately 15% of invasive carcinomas are not detectable mammographically, particularly invasive lobular carcinomas. The clinical implication of this false negative rate is that mammography alone is not sufficient for the evaluation of a breast mass. In the presence of a palpable breast mass, a negative mammogram always should be followed by ultrasound and/or biopsy. A cystic lesion on ultrasound may be presumed benign and should be aspirated or followed. A solid or complex lesion should be

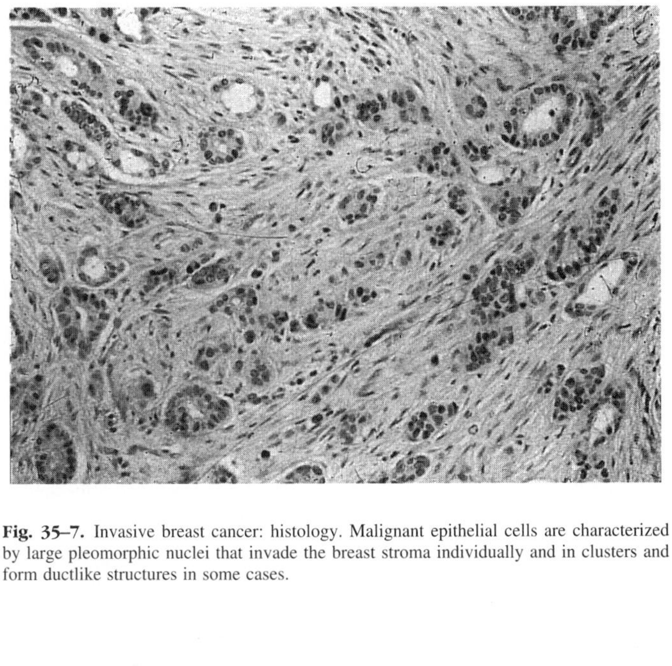

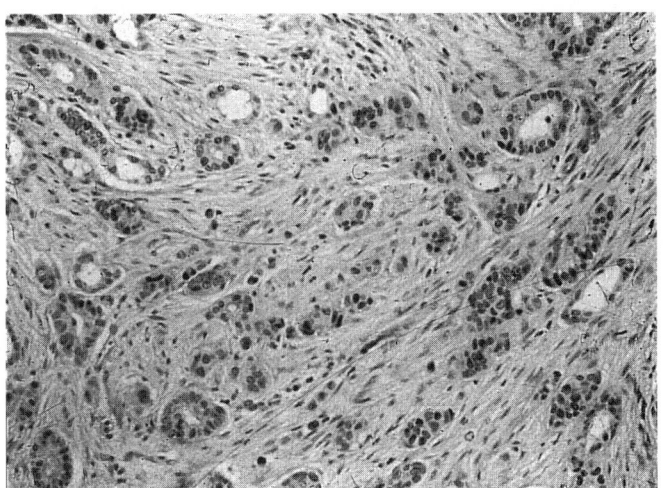

Fig. 35–7. Invasive breast cancer: histology. Malignant epithelial cells are characterized by large pleomorphic nuclei that invade the breast stroma individually and in clusters and form ductlike structures in some cases.

subjected to excisional biopsy. The mammographic and histopathologic appearance of invasive breast cancer is illustrated in Figures 35–6 and 35–7. An X-ray is shown in Figure 35–8.

Both the treatment of and prognosis for a woman with breast cancer are strongly influenced by the stage at the time of diagnosis. Multiple staging systems have been proposed, but the most commonly used system is the one adopted by both the American Joint Committee (AJC) and the International Union against Cancer (UICC) (American Joint Committee on Cancer, 1989). This staging system is a detailed TNM (tumor, nodes, metastasis) system, which is summarized as in Table 35–1. Data compiled from several studies with extensive follow-up suggest that 10-year disease-free survival rates for women with invasive breast cancer are approximately 80% for women diagnosed with stage I disease, decreasing to 55% at stage II, 40% at stage III, and 10% at stage IV, as the stage at diagnosis increases (Clark et al., 1987; Harris, 1991) (Fig. 35–9).

As breast cancer is considered a systemic disease at the time of detection, treatment is designed to achieve two distinct goals: (1) local control of the tumor in the breast and the ipsilateral axillary lymph nodes and (2) eradication of clinically occult systemic micrometastases. Local control may be obtained in most cases by mastectomy alone or by lumpectomy (removal of the tumor with histologically negative margins) followed by radiation therapy to the affected breast. Lumpectomy without radia-

Table 35–1. AJC and IUCC Staging System for Breast Cancer

Stage	Characteristics
0	Carcinoma in situ
I	Tumor ≤ 2 cm, negative axillary nodes
II	Tumor 2–5 cm and/or mobile positive axillary nodes
III	Tumor > 5 cm and/or fixed axillary nodes; inflammatory breast cancer
IV	Distant metastases beyond ipsilateral axillary nodes

Note: This table is a condensed summary of the staging system designed to provide a framework with which to interpret survival curves. A detailed schema for use in clinical practice is provided in Harris (1991).

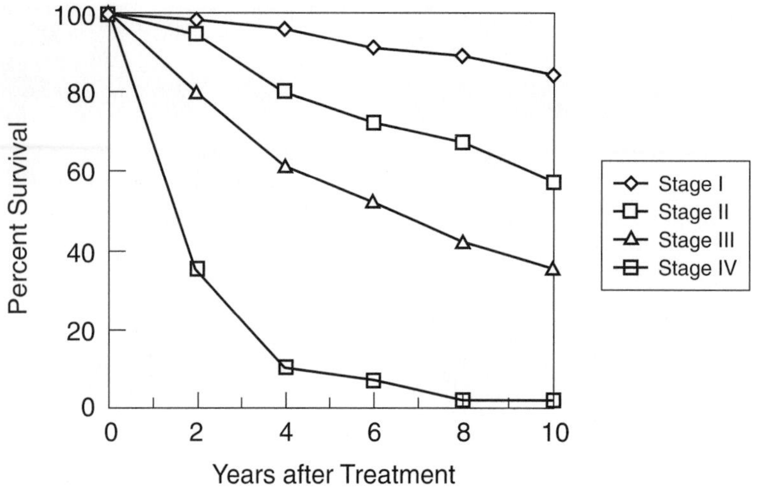

Fig. 35–9. Stage-specific survival curves for breast cancer. Survival at 2-year intervals is indicated by stage (IUCC). Adapted from Harris (1991).

tion is associated with a 35% local recurrence rate and thus is considered unacceptable and rarely used. As multiple randomized studies have shown that the breast-conserving approach of lumpectomy and radiation does not compromise survival compared to mastectomy, this therapeutic choice is often left to the individual patient. Relative contraindications to the use of breast conservation are related to the presence of a multicentric or multifocal tumor, extensive DCIS in association with an invasive tumor, or a large tumor (>5 cm). Large tumors are particularly problematic in a small breast, where the cosmetic result associated with a complete excision may be compromised by the relative amount of tissue that must be removed to obtain clear margins around the tumor. However, the choice of procedure generally is dictated only by personal preference (some patients feel more comfortable with removal of the entire breast, despite data supporting the safety of lumpectomy) and convenience (some patients choose mastectomy to avoid 6 to 7 weeks of daily radiotherapy treatments).

Once local control has been achieved by one of the two surgical options, adjuvant therapy may be used to reduce the likelihood of a systemic recurrence. Often confusing to patients, the decision to use adjuvant chemotherapy is not dictated by the choice of local therapy but by the stage of disease and the menopausal status of the patient. The adjuvant regimens most commonly used include a three- to six-month course of chemotherapy and/or a prolonged course of the partial estrogen antagonist Tamoxifen. Surgical oophorectomy (removal of both ovaries) performed after local therapy also has been shown to reduce the risk of systemic recurrence in premenopausal patients. While the needs of each patient must be addressed individually, generalizations can be made about the choice of therapy (Table 35–2). First, there is increasing evidence that women with tumors less than 1 cm in diameter, without involved axillary nodes, do not require adjuvant therapy. The 10-year survival rates for women in this category exceed 90%, and the relative benefit derived from adjuvant treatment adds little to this excellent prognosis. In contrast, numerous studies support the use of adjuvant therapy in premenopausal women with tumors greater than 1 cm in diameter, regardless of nodal status. In this setting, chemotherapy is associated with the greatest increase in overall survival, with Tamoxifen generally being added for women with tumors that appear to be hormonally responsive by virtue of expressing the estrogen receptor (ER). More controversial is the treatment of postmenopausal women, as Tamoxifen alone may be of equivalent benefit to chemotherapy, obviating the need for chemotherapy in postmenopausal women with ER-positive tumors. Postmenopausal women with ER-negative tumors, without involved axillary nodes, may receive no adjuvant therapy or a course of chemotherapy, depending on a number of variables, including the size and grade of the tumor, as well as the general health status of the patient. Postmenopausal women with involved axillary nodes may receive chemotherapy and/or Tamoxifen, depending on their ER status. Chemotherapy may be administered for three to six months, is given in the outpatient setting, and generally is well tolerated. The most commonly employed regimens include cyclophosphamide and doxorubicin or cyclophosphamide, methotrexate, and 5-fluorouracil with Taxol now being added at some centers for patients at a high risk of recurrence. Tamoxifen is self-administered orally and is taken daily for a minimum of 5 years after the diagnosis.

Metastatic Disease

Metastatic disease (stage IV) may be extremely variable in course. The 10-year survival rates are dismal at 5% to 10%, with the median survival for patients with metastatic disease being

Table 35–2. Overview of Adjuvant Treatment Options for Women with Breast Cancer

Patient Characteristics	Standard Treatment[a]
Premenopausal	
Tumor < 1 cm, node negative	None
Tumor ≥ 1 cm, node negative	Chemotherapy with Tamoxifen if ER+
Tumor ≥ 1 cm, node positive	Chemotherapy with Tamoxifen if ER+
Postmenopausal	
Tumor < 1 cm, node negative	None
Tumor ≥ 1 cm, node negative, ER+	Tamoxifen or observation
Tumor ≥ 1 cm, node negative, ER−	Chemotherapy or observation
Tumor ≥ 1 cm, node positive, ER+	Tamoxifen ± chemotherapy
Tumor ≥ 1 cm, node positive, ER−	Chemotherapy

[a]The standard treatment options (given after adequate surgical treatment) listed in this table are generalizations based on multiple studies. In clinical practice, each patient must be evaluated individually and treatment recommendations may vary with the clinical scenario.

approximately 18 months (Peters, 1995). However, while some patients with metastatic breast cancer may succumb within months of a recurrence, others, particularly those with metastases to bone as the only site of disease, may do well with minimally progressive disease for years. Time to recurrence is also extremely variable, as some patients will relapse with aggressive, drug-resistant tumors within weeks of the completion of adjuvant therapy and some patients will have disease-free intervals of up to 30 years before disease recurrence.

Treatment for metastatic disease must be individualized but may include chemotherapy, hormonal therapy, and palliative radiation therapy. Surgical resection of chest wall recurrences after mastectomy may be indicated in some cases. Unfortunately, treatment of metastatic breast cancer is uniformly considered palliative. While initial studies suggested that bone marrow transplant leads to improved survival over conventional chemotherapy, recent data (median follow-up time 37 months) have not found any significant difference in survival (Peters, 1995; Stadtmauer et al., 2000).

NONGENETIC RISK FACTORS FOR BREAST CANCER

Family history is the most significant risk factor for breast cancer and is explored in detail below. However, there are multiple nongenetic risk factors that fall into two general categories: hormonal and nonhormonal (Table 35–3). Hormonal factors can either elevate breast cancer risk due to increased exposure to estrogen or progestrone or, conversely, reduce risk by decreasing exposure to these hormones. Thus, anything that increases the number of menstrual cycles elevates breast cancer risk, such as early age at menarche (relative risk 1.2), nulliparity (relative risk 2.0), and late age at menopause (relative risk 1.5) (Trichopoulos et al., 1972; White, 1987; Kampert et al., 1988). Moderate levels of exercise can also reduce breast cancer risk, perhaps by decreasing the number of ovulatory cycles (Bernstein et al., 1994). Lactation of long duration also appears to be protective, presumably because again it results in fewer ovulatory cycles (Yuan et al., 1988). After a transient increase in breast cancer risk after childbirth, there is a long-term reduction in risk, which is directly related to age at first live birth (MacMahon et al., 1970). Women who have their first full-term pregnancy at older ages have a higher risk of breast cancer than do nulliparous women presumably because the transient increase in risk directly after childbirth outweighs the long-term reduction in risk for these women. Finally, there is an association between increased weight and breast cancer risk (Pujol et al., 1997). During the postmenopausal period, the major source of estrogen is conversion by adipose tissue of androstenedione to estrone, presumably resulting in a greater estrogen exposure.

Table 35–3. Risk Factors for Breast Cancer

Risk Factor	Relative Risk of Breast Cancer	Reference
Family history of breast cancer		
Mother dx < age 40	2.1	Colditz et al., 1993
Mother dx > age 70	1.5	Colditz et al., 1993
Two first-degree relatives	4–6	Gail et al., 1989
BRCA1/2 mutation	150	Easton et al., 1994
Hormonal factors		
Early age at menarche	1.2	Kampert et al., 1988
Nulliparity	2.0	White, 1987
Late age at menopause	1.5	Trichopoulos et al., 1972
Nonhormonal factors		
ATOMIC BOMB SURVIVORS—AGE OF DIAGNOSIS		
Breast cancer under age 35 yr	13	Tokunaga et al., 1994
Breast cancer over age 35 yr	2	
MANTLE RADIATION FOR HODGKIN DISEASE		
Treated under age 15 yr	136	Bhatia et al., 1998
Treated ages 25–29 yr	7.3	

Nonhormonal factors also contribute to breast cancer risk, particularly exposure to ionizing radiation (John and Kelsey, 1993). Young girls treated for Hodgkin's disease with radiation therapy have a greatly elevated risk of breast cancer, the exact magnitude of which appears to depend on the age at which they were treated (Bhatia et al., 1996; Wolden et al., 1998). In data from the Late Effects Study Group, the relative risk for breast cancer was 136 for those treated when they were younger than 15 years of age. This dramatic elevation in risk decreases as the age at which radiation is administered increases, to a relative risk of 7.3 for those treated when they were 25 to 29 years old (Bhatia et al., 1998). An additional weak risk factor for breast cancer is alcohol consumption, the etiology of which is unknown, but may be due to changes in estrogen metabolism (Hunter and Willett, 1996). Finally, the role of dietary factors in the etiology of breast cancer is controversial, but a high-fat diet is associated with increased risk in most studies (Wynder et al., 1997). Whether this is due to hormones stored in animal fat or other potential carcinogens is unknown.

GENETICS OF BREAST CANCER

Familial clustering of breast cancer was first recognized by physicians in ancient Rome (Lynch et al., 1976). The first documentation of familial clustering of breast cancer in the modern era was published in 1866 by Paul Broca, a French surgeon, who reported 10 cases of breast cancer in five generations in his wife's family; four other women in this family died of hepatic tumors. The literature continues to show an increased breast cancer risk among first-degree relatives of women with breast cancer (Claus et al., 1990; Colditz et al., 1993). Current estimates suggest that family history accounts for approximately 10% to 20% of breast cancer in the United States (Madigan et al., 1995). In 1984, Williams and Anderson used segregation analysis to compare various models that might explain the pattern of aggregation of breast cancer in families, and they were the first to provide evidence for an autosomal dominant breast cancer susceptibility gene with age-related penetrance.

Breast cancer is a complex disease and can aggregate in families for multiple reasons. Mutations in high-penetrance cancer-susceptibility genes, such as *BRCA1* and *BRCA2*, are inherited in an autosomal dominant fashion and confer a risk of breast cancer that is greatly above what is seen in the general population. However, they are uncommon in the population in general. There are other rare cancer susceptibility syndromes, such as Li-Fraumeni, Cowden, and Muir-Torre syndromes, among others, which are associated with a greatly elevated risk of breast cancer, as well as with other nonmalignant findings in an individual or family (Table 35–4). However, these syndromes are considerably less common than the hereditary breast and ovarian cancer syndrome due to *BRCA1* and *BRCA2* mutations.

There are probably other breast cancer susceptibility genes, as yet unidentified, in which mutations confer a slightly lower risk than *BRCA1* and *BRCA2* and are more common in the population. In addition, variants in candidate low-penetrance genes,

Table 35–4. Cancer Susceptibility Syndromes Associated with an Increased Risk of Breast Cancer

Syndrome	Susceptibility Transmission	Gene	Chromosomal Location
Hereditary breast and ovarian cancer I	Autosomal dominant	*BRCA1*	17q21
Hereditary breast and ovarian cancer II	Autosomal dominant	*BRCA2*	13q12.3
Cowden syndrome	Autosomal dominant	*PTEN/MMAC1*	10q23.3
Li-Fraumeni syndrome	Autosomal dominant	*P53*	17q13.1
Peutz-Jeughers syndrome	Autosomal dominant	*STK11/LKB1*	19q13.3
Muir-Torre syndrome	Autosomal dominant	*MSH2/MLH1*	2p22–p21 3p21.3

such as the cytochrome P450 enzymes, may confer a lower risk of breast cancer but are much more frequent in the population. Thus, variants in these low-penetrance genes may have a higher population-attributable risk of breast cancer than does the more striking susceptibility due to *BRCA1* and *BRCA2* mutations that are found in only a limited number of individuals.

In addition to the genetic factors that confer increased susceptibility, there may be other noninherited reasons that produce clustering of breast cancer in certain families. These could include (1) geographically limited environmental exposure to carcinogens that might affect an extended family living in close proximity; (2) culturally motivated behavior that alters the risk factor profile, such as age at first live birth or contraceptive choice; and (3) socioeconomic influences that, for example, might result in different dietary exposure.

High-Penetrance Genes

BRCA1: Linkage and Isolation of the Gene

In 1990, chromosome 17q21 was identified as the location of a susceptibility gene for early-onset breast cancer, now termed *BRCA1*. Linkage analysis in seven early-onset breast cancer families produced a maximum cumulative LOD score of 5.98 at a locus now known to be approximately 20 cM telomeric of *BRCA1* (Hall et al., 1990). In the study there was stratification by age of diagnosis of breast cancer, and the families with positive LOD scores were those with the earliest mean age of diagnosis. In several large kindreds, linkage between the genetic marker D17S74 on 17q21 and the appearance of either breast and ovarian cancer or ovarian cancer only was subsequently demonstrated (Narod et al., 1991). Breast cancer susceptibility in these families appeared to be inherited in an autosomal dominant fashion with high penetrance; approximately 50% of the female children of carriers developed breast and/or ovarian cancer. No information was available on the structure and function of *BRCA1* before its identification in 1994. Therefore, several groups used positional cloning in an attempt to isolate the gene. In late 1994, this effort culminated with the identification of the *BRCA1* gene by Miki and colleagues (Fig. 35–10).

BRCA1 is composed of 24 exons, 22 of which code for a protein of 1863 amino acids. The coding region begins in exon 2, and exon 4 is thought to be an artifact of the isolation method. When *BRCA1* was isolated, the majority of the gene showed no homology to any known protein. It contains a large central exon (11), which comprises 60% of the coding region, with all other exons ranging from 100 to 500 bp in size. Southern blotting of human genomic DNA detects a single band, suggesting that only one gene is present in the human genome. There have been three major *BRCA1* splice variants studied: (1) an in-frame deletion of exon 11, (2) a deletion of exon 11, 11 bp from the 5′ splice acceptor, and (3) an in-frame deletion of exon 10 (Thakur et al., 1997; Wilson et al., 1997). *BRCA1* is situated head to head and may share a bidirectional promotor sequence with 1A1.3B, a homolog of the gene encoding CA-125, an ovarian carcinoma-related serum antigen. Separating the two genes is a tandemly duplicated region of 30 kb that contains two copies of *BRCA1* exons 1 and 2, two copies of 1A1.3b exons 1 and 3, in the form of unprocessed pseudogenes, and two copies of 1A1.3B (Brown et al., 1996).

BRCA2: Linkage and Isolation of the Gene

BRCA2 was initially localized in families with early-onset female breast cancer and at least one case of male breast cancer. The 22 families in the linkage study were analyzed for linkage between breast cancer and genetic markers flanking the BRCA1 region on chromosome 17. A maximum LOD score of −16.63 was obtained, providing strong evidence against linkage to *BRCA1* in those families (Stratton et al., 1994). Shortly after the appearance of this report, a large collaborative group succeeded in identifying chromosome 13q12–13q as the candidate locus for *BRCA2* (Wooster et al., 1994).

The isolation of *BRCA2* took less time than *BRCA1* (15 months, as opposed to 4 years) partly due to the extensive physical mapping of the region (facilitated by the Human Genome Project) and large-scale sequencing of the region (provided by the Sanger Center). Importantly, a 250 kb homozygous deletion in the candidate region was found by representational difference analysis in a pancreatic cancer from a woman; this facilitated the identification process by enabling investigators to prioritize the

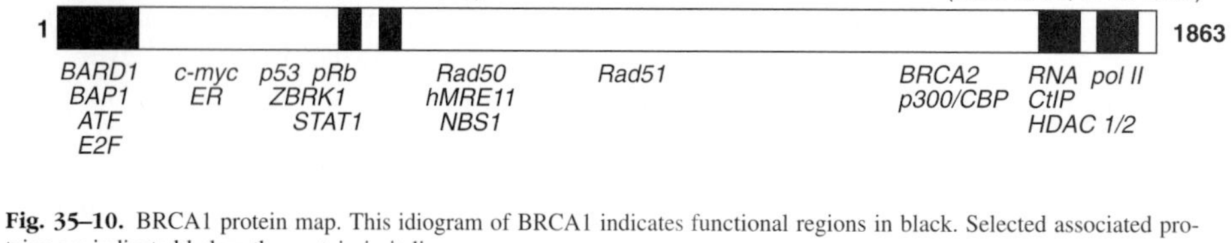

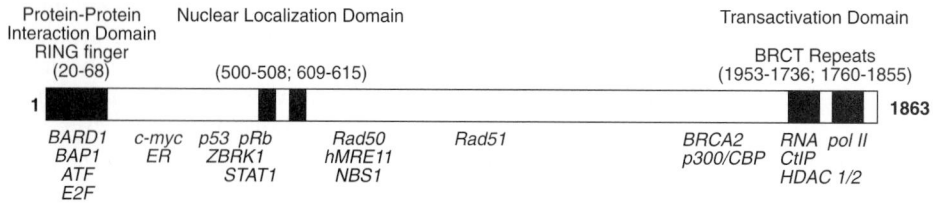

Fig. 35–10. BRCA1 protein map. This idiogram of BRCA1 indicates functional regions in black. Selected associated proteins are indicated below the protein in italics.

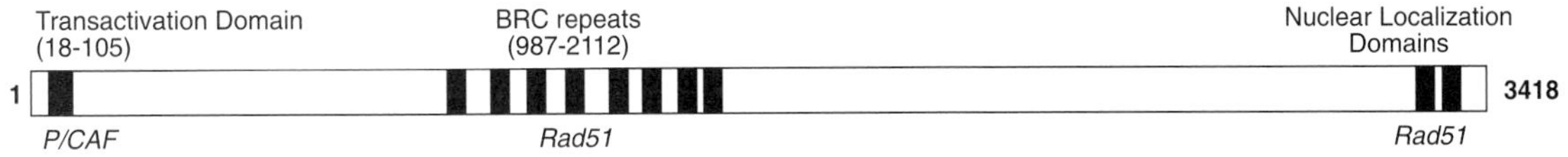

Fig. 35–11. BRCA2 protein map. This idiogram of BRCA2 indicates functional regions in black. Selected associated proteins are indicated below the protein in italics.

segment between D13S260 and D13S171 (Schutte et al., 1995). These efforts resulted in the identification of a partial sequence of the *BRCA2* gene and six germline mutations, which truncated the putative BRCA2 protein in late 1995 (Wooster et al., 1995). Shortly thereafter, the complete cDNA sequence was published by another collaborative group (Fig. 35–11) (Tavtigian et al., 1996).

The *BRCA2* cDNA is approximately 11.5 kb in length and is contained within 70 kb of genomic DNA. The coding region is 11.2 kb and is composed of 26 exons; exon 1 is not translated. The protein is 3,418 amino acids with an estimated molecular weight of 384 kDa. Like *BRCA1*, *BRCA2* has a large central exon 11 (4.8 kb). It has no strong similarity to any known protein. There are eight copies of a 30 to 80 amino acid repeat (BRC repeats) that are present in the part of the protein encoded by exon 11, which seem to be conserved between species and facilitate Rad 51 binding to BRCA2 (Bignell et al., 1997; Wong et al., 1997).

Mutational Spectrum in BRCA1 and BRCA2

A variety of mutation detection methods have been used to identify mutations in *BRCA1* and *BRCA2*, including single-strand conformational polymorphism analysis (SSCP), protein truncation test (PTT), multiplex heteroduplex analysis, conformation sensitive gel electrophoresis (CSGE), and direct DNA sequencing. A tabulated list of identified mutations in both genes and details of the detection methodology are available on the Breast Cancer Information Core (BIC) website: (*http://www.nhgri.nih.gov/Intramural_research/Lab_transfer/Bic/*). Each gene has over 850 distinct variants reported in it, with the list growing on a continuous basis.

The majority of the mutations reported in *BRCA1* are truncating mutations scattered evenly throughout the gene. These mutations presumably render *BRCA1* nonfunctional and are therefore thought to be disease associated. However, a number of the mutations reported in *BRCA1* are missense mutations. These include polymorphisms and unclassified variants, as well as true disease-associated mutations; thus, care must be taken in interpreting the clinical significance of missense mutations. Mutations within the RING finger domain (5′) and the transcriptional activation domain (3′) of *BRCA1* are thought to have functional significance, and there are four reported noncoding region defects inferred from inactivation of transcription of one allele of *BRCA1* (Miki et al., 1994; Gayther et al., 1995; Serova et al., 1996). The specific DNA alterations that result in inactivation of transcription in these families have not been determined.

Partial genomic deletions of *BRCA1* also have been found, and they are presumably caused by the high number of Alu repeats in *BRCA1* introns. Multiple studies have demonstrated that genomic rearrangements in *BRCA1* are a cause of hereditary breast and ovarian cancer. The frequency of rearrangements found in *BRCA1* has ranged from 5% to 12% in a clinic population of families with breast and ovarian cancer, tested negative from mutations in *BRCA1* and *BRCA2* (Unger et al., 2000). Two genomic rearrangements appear to have a founder effect and have been found on a recurrent basis. In the Dutch population, three large genomic deletions are estimated to account for approximately 30% of all Dutch breast cancer families (Petrij-Bosch et al., 1997). A duplication of exon 13 has been found in multiple families and is to originate from Yorkshire in England (BRCA1 Exon 13 Duplication Screening Group, 2000).

The mutational spectrum of *BRCA2* is similar to that of *BRCA1*. Mutations are spread over the entire gene; frameshift and nonsense mutations are the only mutations unequivocally classified as deleterious. More than one-half of the mutations appear only once in the BIC. Some 30% of the mutations reported are missense mutations, all of which are unclassified variants or polymorphisms. As of yet, no missense mutation in *BRCA2* has been classified as a deleterious high-penetrance mutation. However, at least one missense mutation (N372H) in *BRCA2* appears to contribute to breast cancer risk as a "low-penetrance" variant. (For further discussion, see the section on low-penetrance genes.) In addition, a nonsense mutation K3326X (10204 A → T) has been identified in multiple populations and is not thought to be associated with an increased susceptibility to breast or ovarian cancer (Mazoyer et al., 1996). While two genomic rearrangements have been described in *BRCA2*, presumably this mutation source in *BRCA2* will be less common than in *BRCA1*, as *BRCA2* is not as dense in Alu repeats as *BRCA1* (Nordling et al., 1998; Wang et al., 2001).

Founder Mutations

Several founder mutations have been identified in *BRCA1* and *BRCA2*. The most striking founder effects have been seen in the Ashkenazi Jewish population for the *BRCA1* mutations 185delAG and 5382insC and for the *BRCA2* mutation 6174delT. The carrier frequency of these mutations in the general Ashkenazi Jewish population has been determined to be 1% for 185delAG and 1.4% for 6174delT (Roa et al., 1996). The mutation 5382insC also has been seen in the Ashkenazi Jewish population, but at a lower frequency of 0.12 percent (Roa et al., 1996). The 185delAG and 6174delT mutations also have been found in the Moroccan, Iraqi, and Yemenite Jewish populations, which suggests that they arose before the Diaspora (Bar-Sade et al., 1998). Of note, the 185delAG mutation has been found in non-Ashkenazi Jewish individuals on different haplotypes, and thus it may represent a mutational "hotspot." These mutations may have arisen as there are a series of three AG dinucleotides at this locus, which may predispose to polymerase slippage (Neuhausen et al., 1996). The 5382insC mutation was initially observed in northern and eastern European families; thus a Baltic origin has been suggested (Neuhausen et al., 1996). The Icelandic population is another group with a striking founder effect, where the *BRCA2* mutation 999del5 explains nearly all of the inherited breast and ovarian cancer, and is present in 1 in 173 Icelanders (Thorlacius et al., 1996, 1997). For a review of the genetics of *BRCA1* and *BRCA2* mutations in populations, see Szabo and King (1997).

Penetrance of BRCA1/2 mutations

The original estimates of penetrance of *BRCA1* mutations were made using families from linkage analysis studies (Ford et al., 1994). The cumulative risk of breast cancer in *BRCA1* mutation carriers was estimated at 83% and of ovarian cancer at 40% to 60% by age 70 (Easton et al., 1994; Narod et al., 1995a). In this model, 20% of *BRCA1* mutation carriers would develop breast cancer by age 20: 51% by age 50; and approximately 85% by age 70. *BRCA1* mutation carriers also appeared to have an increased incidence of bilateral breast cancer, up to 65% for those who live to age 70. *BRCA2* penetrance has been estimated in the same fashion. Using linkage analysis families, *BRCA2* mutation carriers have cumulative breast cancer risk by age 70 of 84% and 27% for ovarian cancer (Ford et al., 1998). So while *BRCA1* and *BRCA2* mutations confirm a similar risk of breast cancer, the risk for ovarian cancer is substantially higher in *BRCA1* mutation carriers.

After the isolation of *BRCA1*, further studies were done to define breast cancer penetrance in populations that were not made of families highly selected for multiple early-onset breast cancer cases, thus high penetrance. The first such study, the Washington D.C. Ashkenazi Study, was undertaken looking at the founder mutations in Ashkenazi Jews; carriers of the founder mutations were identified, and cancer prevalence in the relatives of carriers was compared to that in the relatives of noncarriers (Struewing et al., 1997). The risk of breast cancer and ovarian cancer in *BRCA1* and *BRCA2* mutation carriers was estimated to be 56% and 16% by age 70, respectively. This observation of low penetrance, as compared to "high-penetrance" families selected for linkage studies, has been substantiated by four other population- and hospital-based studies, with estimates of breast cancer risk ranging from 36% at age 85 to 60% at age 70, respectively, as shown in Figure 35–12 (Fodor et al., 1998; Hopper et al., 1999; Warner et al., 1999; Antoniou et al., 2000). Interestingly, a study estimating breast cancer risk for *BRCA1* and *BRCA2* mutations in a population-based series from East Anglia found an overall higher breast cancer penetrance for *BRCA2* mutations (74%) than for *BRCA1* mutations (48%) by age 80 (TABCS Group, 2000). Genotype–phenotype correlation may account for some of the observed variability, as detailed below, but it is likely that other genetic and environmental factors act to influence penetrance as well.

Prevalence of BRCA1 and BRCA2 Mutations

There have been four types of populations studied to estimate the prevalence of *BRCA1* mutations: (1) members of high-risk families (three or more breast cancer cases usually diagnosed before age 60, and/or ovarian cancer); (2) early-onset breast cancer cases; (3) patients from "high-risk" clinics (from moderate- or high-risk families); and (4) population-based series of breast cancer cases. In studies of high-risk families, the proportion of inherited susceptibility to breast cancer attributable mutations into *BRCA1* or *BRCA2* depends on the population. For BRCA1, it ranges from 9% to 10% in Japan and Iceland to 79% in Russia. In the United States the proportion of high-risk families with mutations in *BRCA1* is estimated to be 39% (Szabo and King, 1997). For *BRCA2*, the highest prevalence is in Iceland where a founder mutation accounts for almost all of the high-risk families (Thorlacius et al., 1997). However, in general, the percentage of high-risk families accounted for by mutations *BRCA2* is fewer than *BRCA1*.

Patients who visit high-risk clinics are usually from moderate- or high-risk families. In the clinic-based cohorts described to date, the likelihood of a patient carrying a germline mutation in *BRCA1* or *BRCA2* depends on family history. A recent series looking at 615 families and predictors for mutation status in *BRCA1* and *BRCA2* found that the significant predictors were number of premenopausal women affected with breast cancer (OR 2.9, $p < .001$), number of individuals with both breast and ovarian cancer (OR 6.6, $p < .001$), presence of ovarian and/or fallopian tube cancer (OR 3.25, $p < .001$), Ashkenazi Jewish ancestry (OR 4.4, $p < .001$), and male breast cancer (OR 3.2, $p =$

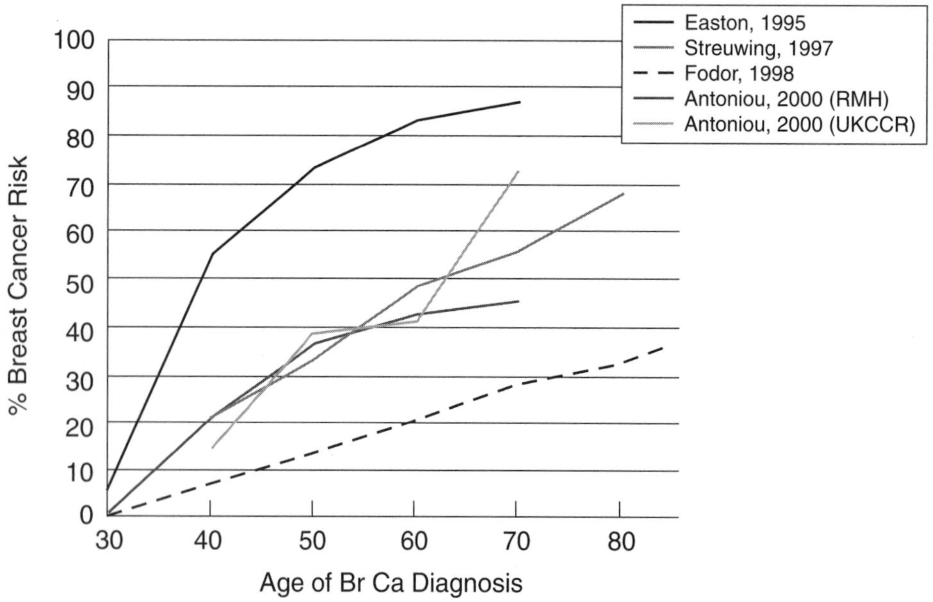

Fig. 35–12. Variable penetrance of *BRCA1* mutations. This demonstrates the different breast cancer risk estimates for *BRCA1* mutations, depending on the population of ascertainment. Easton (1994) shows the original penetrance estimates from a linkage-based series; Streuwing et al. (1997) show the estimates from an Ashkenazi Jewish population-based series; Fodor et al. (1998) show the estimates from an Ashkenazi Jewish hospital-based series.

.003) (Blackwood et al., 2001). In a large series from a referral laboratory, mutations in *BRCA1* and *BRCA2* were identified in 20% of women with breast cancer and in 34% of the women with ovarian cancer. In this moderate- to high-risk population, mutations were as prevalent in those of African ancestry as in those of European ancestry (Deffenbaugh et al., 2001).

Populations of women with early-onset breast cancer have been well studied, as it was predicted, based on age-specific penetrance, that a greater proportion would have *BRCA1* and *BRCA2* mutations than would the breast cancer population overall. In young Ashkenazi Jewish women, studies looking for the *BRCA1* common founder mutation (185delAG) describe rates of 16%, 20%, and 22% of breast cancer cases diagnosed at <50, <40, and <42 years of age, respectively (Struewing et al., 1995; FitzGerald et al., 1996; Offit et al., 1996). Studies also have been conducted in non-Ashkenazi Jewish populations that are known to have a lower rate of *BRCA1* mutations. Taking together all the studies done in young non-Ashkenazi Jewish women (diagnosed age 40 or lower), it is estimated that approximately 7% of women diagnosed with breast cancer before age 40 have mutations in *BRCA1*, irrespective of family history (FitzGerald et al., 1996; Ithier et al., 1996; Couch et al., 1997; Malone et al., 1998).

In contrast, the rate of *BRCA2* mutations in young women with breast cancer appears to be lower than that for *BRCA1*. Krainer et al. (1997) reported that 2.7% of 73 women diagnosed with breast cancer had mutations in *BRCA2*. Another study from the United Kingdom has examined *BRCA2* mutations in young women with breast cancer (755 women diagnosed under age 36; 644 women diagnosed between 36 and 45) and reported a mutation rate of 2.4% in women under age 36 and 2.2% in women ages 36 to 45 (Peto et al., 1999). This study also looks at the *BRCA1* mutation status and suggests that *BRCA1* and *BRCA2* mutations make an equivalent contribution to early-onset breast cancer in the U.K. Both this study and one from the East Anglia breast cancer study group suggest that a greater proportion of breast cancer diagnosed over age 50 is due to *BRCA2* mutations than to *BRCA1* mutations (TABES Group, 2000). The proportion of breast cancer cases in the U.K. due to *BRCA1* mutations had been previously estimated at 7.5% for women diagnosed under age 30, 5.1% for women diagnosed between 30 and 39, and 2.2% for women diagnosed between 40 and 49 (Ford et al., 1995).

Two types of population-based studies have been done to look at the prevelance of *BRCA1* mutations: the first drew on breast cancer cases diagnosed at a single institution and looked for founder mutations; the second used breast cancer cases diagnosed in a geographic region and looked for all mutations. In a consecutive series of 268 Ashkenazi Jewish breast cancer cases, unselected for family history or age of diagnosis, 6.8% had one of the three common founder mutations (*BRCA1*–185delAG, *BCRA1*–5382insC, and *BRCA2*–6174delT) (Fodor et al., 1998). In a series from North Carolina using population-based series of breast cancer cases ascertained without regard to age of onset, 3% of 120 Caucasian women and 0% of 88 African American women had mutations in *BRCA1* (Newman et al., 1998). However, because the population average for breast cancer diagnosis is approximately 62 years, this cohort was "selected" for a low rate of *BRCA1* and *BRCA2* mutations. A similar mutation rate of 1.8% was found in unselected breast cancer patients in the Finnish population (Syrjakoski et al., 2000). In the population series, family history of ovarian cancer and early age of breast cancer onset remain the strongest predictors of mutation status.

Evidence is accumulating that suggest that a large proportion of familial breast cancer risk is not accounted for by mutations in *BRCA1* and *BRCA2*. Using families with at least four cases of early-onset breast cancer (<60 yrs), Ford and colleagues (1998) found that 67% of families with four or five cases of (site-specific) breast cancer were not linked to *BRCA1* or *BRCA2*. They conclude that other more common susceptibility genes, responsible for a large fraction of familial breast cancer, remain to be identified, in which mutations confer a lower risk for breast cancer than mutations in *BRCA1* or *BRCA2*. Two population-based series of breast cancer cases have found that only 15% of the excess breast cancer risk to sisters and mothers of the cases was attributable to mutations in *BRCA1* and *BRCA2* (Peto et al., 1999; TABCS Group, 2000). Claus and colleagues (1998) have reported that family history remains a predictive factor for breast cancer risk in women who are determined to be noncarriers of *BRCA1* and *BRCA2* mutations using the Parmigiani model. The cumulative evidence from all of these studies strongly suggests that other genes contribute to familial breast cancer, in addition to *BRCA1* and *BRCA2*.

Other Cancers in BRCA1 and BRCA2 Mutation Families

In families segregating *BRCA1* and *BRCA2* mutations, there is an increased risk for cancers other than breast and ovarian. In 173 *BRCA2* families (169 with coding region mutations, 4 with LOD score >1), increased relative risks for prostate (4.65), pancreatic (3.5), stomach (2.6), gallbladder (5), melanoma (2.6), and buccal cavity/pharynx (2.4) cancers were noted (Easton and BCL, 1999). The overall cumulative risk of cancer by age 70 was estimated to be 32% in male carriers and 70% in female carriers of a *BRCA2* mutation. The overall cumulative risk of cancer by age 70 was estimated to be 32% in male carriers of a *BRCA2* mutation and 70% in female carriers. In *BRCA1* mutation carriers, there is an increased risk of prostate cancer, which has held up across studies. In the population-based study by Streuwing et. al. (1997), the risk of prostate cancer was calculated at 16% among carriers, as opposed to 3.8% among noncarriers, which is comparable to the 4-fold increased risk initially predicted by Easton and colleagues (Struewing et al., 1997). In the initial studies of BRCA1 carriers, there was a suggestion of an increased risk of colon cancer associated with BRCA1 germline mutations, but this effect was due to cancers seen in a minority of families and has not held up upon further evaluation (Easton and BCL, 1999). Taken together, these data suggest that while *BRCA2* mutations may confer a lower risk of ovarian cancer than *BRCA1* mutations do, they confer a higher risk of "other" cancers.

Nearly half of the patients with breast and another primary cancer in a series from a high-risk clinic had mutations in *BRCA1* and *BRCA2*, as opposed to 12% of patients with breast cancer and a family history of breast cancer only. *BRCA1* and *BRCA2* mutations were twice as common in women with breast cancer and a second nonovarian primary as in women with breast cancer alone (Shih et al., 2000). These data suggest that a second primary cancer is predictive of mutation status in this cohort.

Genotype–Phenotype Correlations in BRCA1 and BRCA2 Mutations

The suggestion has been made that families with mutations in the 5′ end of the *BRCA1* gene (up to exon 12) tend to have a higher proportion of ovarian cancers (OR 2) than do those with mutations in the 3′ one-third (Gayther et al., 1995; Holt et al.,

1996). In 356 families with protein truncating mutations in *BRCA1*, Easton and colleagues found that the ratio of ovarian to breast cancers was higher (OR 1.81, $p = .006$) for mutations in the central portion of the gene (nucleotides 2401–4190). The data suggest that the breast cancer risk for mutations in the central region is lower, while the ovarian cancer risk is higher in the central region than at either the 5′ or the 3′ end (DF Easton and D Thompson, unpublished data). In *BRCA2*, an ovarian cancer cluster region (OCCR) in exon 11 has been postulated, in which mutations lead to a higher relative risk (OR 2.5) of ovarian cancer than of breast cancer (Gayther et al., 1997). This study has been substantiated by the Breast Cancer Linkage Consortium using 164 families with *BRCA2* mutations (Thompson et al., 2001). There has been no difference in cancer risk observed between the two ends of the gene. However, despite the statistical significance of these observations and the potential to provide functional insight, clinical recommendations do not vary by site of mutation, as all cancer risks are much greater than those in the general population.

Potential Modifiers of Penetrance in BRCA1 and BRCA2 Mutation Carriers

Both genetic and environmental factors have been examined in preliminary studies to see how they affect the penetrance of *BRCA1* and *BRCA2* mutations. Early age of menarche and low parity, both of which increase the number of menstrual cycles a woman experiences, may be associated with an earlier age of onset of breast cancer in *BRCA1* mutation carriers, presumably through the same mechanisms by which they increase breast cancer risk in general (Narod et al., 1995b). Subsequent studies have found different effects of parity, and so, while it is clear that reproductive history has an effect on breast cancer risk in mutation carriers, the magnitude and direction of the risk has not been fully elucidated (Jernstrom et al., 1999; Modan et al., 2001). As differences in environment do not appear to completely account for the variability in cancer risk among individuals both between and within families observed in carriers of *BRCA1* and *BRCA2* mutations, it also has been hypothesized that genetic variants contribute to the variable phenotype. Therefore, a number of studies have evaluated variants in candidate genes, some examples of which are reviewed here, looking for modifiers of penetrance. In general, these studies are done using increasing age at diagnosis of breast cancer as a surrogate for decreasing penetrance.

HRAS1. The proto-oncogene HRAS1 encodes a protein involved in mitogenic signaling, the process by which an extracellular growth factor signal is transmitted to the nucleus. A microsatellite, composed of 30 to 100 units of a 28 bp repeat, is located approximately 1000 bp downstream from the HRAS coding region. Individuals with rare alleles (population frequency <5%) have an increased risk of certain types of cancer, including breast cancer (Krontiris et al., 1993). The first association study done in *BRCA1* mutation carriers suggested that in carriers of *BRCA1* mutations with 1 or 2 rare HRAS alleles, the risk for ovarian cancer was increased 2.11-fold over *BRCA1* mutation carriers that harbored only common alleles (Phelan et al., 1996).

Androgen Receptor. An association between age of breast cancer diagnosis in *BRCA1* mutation carriers and length of the CAG repeat in exon 1 of the androgen receptor (*AR*) has been recently suggested (Rebbeck et al., 1999a). The *AR*-CAG repeat was selected for study as it modulates the activity of the AR, with alleles containing longer CAG repeat lengths having a decreased ability to activate androgen-responsive genes (Szelei et al., 1997), resulting, in turn, in increased breast epithelial cell proliferation. In this series, women with *BRCA1* mutations and who had at least one *AR* allele with more than 28, 29, or 30 CAG repeats were diagnosed with breast cancer 0.8, 1.8, and 6.3 years earlier, respectively, than women who did not carry at least one such *AR* allele. These data have not been fully replicated in two further studies, but both studies were underpowered as the long repeats are very rare in the population (Kadouri et al., 2001; Menin et al., 2001). Recent data have shown that BRCA1 interacts physically with and is a co-activator of the *AR* promoter, thus providing a plausible explanation for the finding that allelic variation in *AR* affects breast cancer penetrance in *BRCA1* mutation carriers (Park et al., 2000).

AIB1. AIB1 is a member of the SRC-1 family of transcriptional co-activators that interact with steroid hormones to enhance estrogen-dependent transcription. AIB1 has been found to be amplified in 10% and overexpressed in 64% of 105 breast tumors (Anzick et al., 1997). The *AIB1* coding region contains a variable number of glutamine residues (20–29), beginning at residue 3930. In a study of 165 breast cancer cases and 139 unaffected controls, all of whom had germline *BRCA1* mutations, women with an *AIB1* allele with at least 28 polyglutamine repeats were a higher breast cancer risk than were women with shorter alleles (OR = 1.59, 95% CI, 1.03–2.47 and OR = 2.85, 95% CI, 1.64–4.96, respectively) (Rebbeck et al., 2001). Breast cancer risk increased further in association with late age at first live birth and no *AIB1* alleles with less than 28 or 29 repeats (OR = 4.62, 95% CI, 2.02–10.56 and OR = 6.97, 95% CI, 1.71–28.43, respectively). This preliminary association study suggests that expression levels of *AIB1* may vary, based on the number of glutamine repeats and, consequently, may influence breast cancer penetrance.

Variants in genes that affect penetrance in *BRCA1* and *BRCA2* mutation carriers have not been consistently associated with an increased risk of sporadic breast cancer. There are several possible explanations for this finding. First, it may be that these variants affect penetrance in *BRCA1* and *BRCA2* mutation carriers specifically and are not low-penetrance susceptibility genes in general. More likely, however, because the majority of studies evaluating hormonal risk factors in *BRCA1* and *BRCA2* mutation carriers have produced very similar results to general population studies, it may be that population-based studies have been underpowered as the associated relative risks are small. Effects on breast cancer risk in *BRCA1* and *BRCA2* mutation carriers may be more readily detected because of the much higher number of events in study cohorts at very high risk of breast cancer. In fact, this study design may be hampered by a lack of age-matched unaffected controls.

BRCA1 and BRCA2 Tumors

Somatic mutations in *BRCA1* have not been found in sporadic breast tumors and are rarely found in sporadic ovarian tumors (Futreal et al., 1994; Merajver et al., 1995). *BRCA2* is similar in that mutations are rarely found in sporadic breast and ovarian cancers (Foster et al., 1996; Lancaster et al., 1996). The reasons for this surprising finding are unclear, but it is speculated that that other mechanisms may down-regulate or inactivate BRCA1 and BRCA2 proteins in sporadic tumors. (For further explanation see section on BRCA1/2 function.)

Large studies by the Breast Cancer Linkage Consortium have been done to examine breast cancers from known *BRCA1* and *BRCA2* mutation carriers. Breast cancers from *BRCA1* mutation carriers have a higher overall grade than do sporadic cases (BCL Consortium, 1997; Jacquemier et al., 1995). Tumors of *BRCA1* mutation carriers showed more pleomorphism, a higher mitotic count, and less tubule formation than did sporadic tumors. Medullary or atypical medullary carcinoma also was more common in *BRCA1* than in *BRCA2* mutation carriers. *BRCA1* mutation carriers were less likely to have DCIS (still seen in 45% of *BRCA1* mutation carriers), but the rate in *BRCA2* mutation carriers did not differ from controls. In a second review from the same group, a higher mitotic count, continuous pushing margins, and lymphocytic infiltration were the most significant findings in *BRCA1* mutation carriers. A lower mitotic count, less tubule formation, and continuous pushing margins were features of the breast cancers in *BRCA2* mutation carriers (Lakhani et al., 1998). Breast cancers from *BRCA1* mutation carriers also have been found to be less likely to be estrogen and progestrone receptor positive than tumors from *BRCA2* mutation carriers and familial non-*BRCA1,2* cases and controls in two studies from the same group (Johannsson et al., 1997; Loman et al., 1998).

Breast cancers from non-*BRCA1/2* families also have been characterized, demonstrating a lower grade, fewer mitoses, and less nuclear pleomorphism, among other findings. Interestingly, the tumors were more likely to be of the invasive lobular type, which is consistent with earlier studies, before the identification of BRCA1/2, which suggested that hereditary tumors were more frequently lobular (Lakhani et al., 2000).

Comparative genome hybridization (CGH) has been done on breast cancers from *BRCA1* and *BRCA2* mutation carriers to determine whether the tumors have different regions of allelic imbalance than sporadic tumors (Tirkkonen et al., 1997). Interestingly, the total number of genetic changes in the tumors was twice that in the control group, and in *BRCA1* carriers, losses of 5q, 4q, 4p, 2q and 12q were significantly more common than in sporadic cases. In *BRCA2* mutation carriers, there was a higher frequency of 13q and 6q losses and gains of 17q22–4 and 20q13.

Recently data have been published on transcriptional profiling of BRCA1 and BRCA2 tumors using high-density cDNA arrays. Hedenfalk et al. (2001) measured expression in 5361 genes and compared seven *BRCA1* mutation carriers, seven *BRCA2* mutation carriers, and seven sporadic breast cancers. Although they were able to use expression profiling to differentiate the tumors associated with *BRCA1* and *BRCA2* mutations, the profiles of the *BRCA2* mutation associated tumors and mutation-negative tumors were not as distinct as those of the *BRCA1* mutation–associated tumors. While this is an important study using microarray analysis to examine the gene expression of these tumors, there were some limitations to the study; in particular, the small numbers of tumors used in the comparison were not well matched in terms of tumor grade and receptor status. Therefore, differences in gene expression could be partially due to those pathological differences rather than to germline mutation status (Lakhani et al., 2001). The data from the histological analysis, CGH studies, and expression arrays suggest that the pathway to cancer in *BRCA1* and *BRCA2* mutation carriers may be different from that in sporadic breast cancer. In particular, *BRCA1*-associated breast cancers may be more genetically unstable and thus perhaps of higher grade.

Functions of BRCA1 and BRCA2

Many functional similarities have been described for BRCA1 and BRCA2, both of which appear to be involved in the maintenance of genomic integrity and to co-localize in the nucleus with each other and Rad51 (Scully et al., 1997b; Chen et al., 1998b). While there is evidence that while BRCA2 participates directly in homologous repair (HR), BRCA1 may regulate HR as a sensor of DNA damage, either as part of the chromatin remodeling complex SWI/SNF or as a regulator of transcriptional response to DNA damage, as reviewed in Monteiro (2000) and Venkitaraman (2001). Both *BRCA1* and *BRCA2* are classic tumor-suppressor genes and demonstrate loss of the wild-type allele in tumors from mutation carriers. They are nuclear proteins with similar patterns of expression, and they co-localize during proliferation and differentiation. Mice with targeted deletions involving more than half of *Brca1* and *Brca2* die in early embryogenesis in the homozygous state and appear normal in the heterozygous state. Both appear to be important for cell proliferation during development and are up-regulated in the murine mammary gland during puberty and pregnancy. Finally, there are structural similarities as well, with the genomic organization of both genes including a large central exon containing 60% of the sequence.

BRCA1 was thought to fit the model of a classical tumor suppressor gene even before it was isolated. After linkage analysis was performed showing that 17q21 was the locus of *BRCA1*, the observation was made that in presumed mutation carriers, allele loss at this locus occurred in approximately 50% of tumors; invariably, the wild-type allele was lost (Smith et al., 1992). A similar observation—in that there was loss of the wild-type allele of 13q—was made in *BRCA2*-linked families before that gene was isolated (Collins et al., 1995). Thus it was thought that both genes would fulfill Knudson's (1971) two-hit hypothesis of inherited cancer predisposition, where the first hit is the inherited mutation and the second is somatic loss in the tumor.

However, while loss of heterozygosity has been observed on 17q and 13q in sporadic tumors, when *BRCA1* and *BRCA2* were isolated, somatic mutations were not found in either *BRCA1* or *BRCA2* in sporadic breast cancer and only rarely in sporadic ovarian cancer (Futreal et al., 1994; Merajver et al., 1995; Lancaster et al., 1996). While recently it has been demonstrated that there is reduction or loss of the BRCA1 and BRCA2 message and proteins in the majority of sporadic breast cancers, it is not yet fully understood why somatic mutations in *BRCA1* and *BRCA2* are so rare. But it has been suggested that these genes may be down-regulated in tumors by other mechanisms (Wilson et al., 1999). BRCA1 has been observed to be down-regulated by CpG methylation of a CREB (cAMP-responsive element binding) site in its promoter, which was seen in breast tumors but not in normal tissue (Mancini et al., 1998; Hedenfalk et al., 2001). Welcsh and King (2001) hypothesize that somatic loss is common in sporadic breast tumors, due to genomic rearrangement rather than mutation; however, this theory has not yet been substantiated.

As noted above, most of the *BRCA1* gene shows no homology to any previously described protein; the exceptions are two highly conserved regions: the RING finger domain and the BRCT domains. The RING finger motif at the amino terminus is 126 bp long. This domain, which has been identified in numerous transcription factors and cofactors, may be involved in mediating homo- or heterodimer formation (Brzovic et al., 1998). Two BRCT (BRCA1 carboxy terminus) domains are found in tandem at the 3′ end—motif1, aa1653–1736, and motif2, aa1760–1863. The BRCT domains, initially described in BRCA1, were retrospectively noted in many other proteins that function as cell cycle checkpoints responsive to DNA damage (Bork et al., 1997). A large superfamily of BRCT domain–containing proteins, including over 40 nonorthologous proteins from bacteria to yeast to humans, has now been described. Additional BRCA1 functional domains now have been defined, including a nuclear localization domain (aa501–507) and a Rad51 interaction domain (Thakur et al., 1997; Bertwistle and Ashworth, 1998).

BRCA2, like BRCA1, showed no homology to any known protein when it was isolated. Unlike BRCA1, it did not contain any previously defined functional domains. In the large central exon (11) there are eight copies of a 30 to 80 bp amino acid repeat (BRC repeats). These repeats are more conserved between species than the rest of exon 11 and now appear to be binding sites for Rad51, as does a C-terminal domain (Wong et al., 1997). Like BRCA1, BRCA2 appears to be a nuclear protein expressed in response to cell proliferation (Bertwistle et al., 1997).

Numerous known proteins have been described with evidence of interaction with BRCA1 (as reviewed in Scully and Livingston, 2000; Scully, 2001; Welcsh and King, 2001). Two major groups of interest are proteins involved in the DNA damage and repair pathways and in hormonal pathways. The first protein that BRCA1 was demonstrated to interact with was Rad51, suggesting that it plays a role in double-strand breast repair (DSB). hRad51, a eukaryotic equivalent of bacterial RecA, is involved in the homologous pairing of DNA strands during the process of recombination and DNA double-strand repair (Benson et al., 1994). BRCA1 co-localizes with Rad51 on unsynapsed elements of the synaptonemal complex in meiotic cells. In mitotic cells, BRCA1/Rad51/BARD1 co-localize in S phase foci. BRCA1 undergoes hyperphosphorylation and dispersal of the S phase foci in response to DNA damaging agents (Scully et al., 1997a; Thomas et al., 1997). In addition, it has been suggested that BRCA1 binds with PCNA at DNA replication forks. BRCA1 has been also shown to associate with the hRAD50/hMre11/p95 complex (Zhong et al., 1999). This complex appears to function in DSB repair as a sensor of DNA damage and may also play a role in sister chromatid exchange (Petrini, 1999). While the interaction of BRCA1 with the hRAD50/hMre11/p95 complex might suggest a role in either nonhomologous end joining (NHEJ) or HR, it is fairly clear that the BRCA genes play a role in HR and not NHEJ (Scully and Livingston, 2000). Recent data has shown that BRCA1 interacts with H2AX, a human histone that becomes phosphorylated after cells have been exposed to ionizing radiation and form foci about DSB (Paull et al., 2000). BRCA1 is recruited to the foci before Rad50 and Rad51, strongly supporting its importance in DSB repair. BRCA1 has also been shown to associate with a large complex of genes important in mismatch repair (BASC, BRCA1–associated surveillance complex) suggesting a role in sensing or signaling DNA damage (Wang et al., 2000). BRCA1 has been found to be part of the SWI/SNF complex, interacting directly with BRG1, which plays a role in chromosomal remodeling (Bochar et al., 2000).

Recent data has linked BRCA1 to hormonal pathways. BRCA1 has been shown to physically interact with the androgen receptor and enhance transcription, possibly through the effects of the p160 co-activators GRIP1, SRC-1a, and AIB1 (Park et al., 2000; Yeh et al., 2000). BRCA1 has been found to inhibit estrogen receptor activity and to interact with the estrogen receptor at its amino terminus, which is abrogated by disease-associated mutations in BRCA1 (Fan et al., 1999, 2001). As noted above, BRCA1 interacts with the chromatin remodeling complex SWI/SWF, in particular BRG1. BRG1 has been demonstrated to be required for the action of the estrogen receptor, and the association of the two proteins couples BRG1 to the estrogen-responsive promoter regions (DiRenzo et al., 2000).

BRCA1/2 Gene Expression. BRCA1 and BRCA2 have similar expression patterns in developing and adult mice, and both are co-induced in murine mammary epithelium during puberty and pregnancy, which suggests that both BRCA1 and BRCA2 are involved in cell proliferation and may be regulated by hormonal changes during pregnancy (Connor et al., 1997b; Rajan et al., 1996, 1997). In cultured breast epithelial cells, BRCA1 and BRCA2 are induced by estrogen stimulation, but this is thought to be an indirect effect linked to DNA synthesis and cell proliferation (Marquis et al., 1995; Spillman and Bowcock, 1996; Marks et al., 1997). In humans, BRCA1 and BRCA2 expression is observed in most cells, albeit at low levels, with the highest mRNA levels found in testes and thymus, consistent with their postulated role in genomic integrity, as these cells undergo multiple rounds of mitosis (Miki et al., 1994; Tavtigian et al., 1996).

Brca1/2 and Development. The murine homolog of *BRCA1* has been characterized by several groups (Abel et al., 1995; Bennett et al., 1995). The mouse cDNA sequence predicts a protein of 1812 amino acids, 51 residues shorter than the human cDNA. The human and mouse cDNAs display 58% identity and 73% similarity at the protein level with perfect conservation in the RING finger domain near the amino terminus and high homology in the BRCT domain. *Brca2* in mice contains 3329 amino acids and has 59% identity with the human sequence. Murine and human *Brca2* share higher identity in the putative transactivation domain in exon 3, a highly conserved large carboxyl region, and the BRC repeats (McAllister et al., 1997).

Brca1 and *Brca2* nullizygous mice have been created by genetic manipulation in several laboratories. *Brca1* and *Brca2* heterozygous mice do not have an evident phenotype; most notably, they do not appear to have an increased susceptibility to cancer, unlike their human counterpart (Gowen et al., 1996; Hakem et al., 1996; Liu et al., 1996; Sharan et al., 1997; Suzuki et al., 1997). In contrast to the heterozygotes, both homozygous Brca1 and Brca2$^{-/-}$ mice die between days 5.5 and 9.5 of embryogenesis. The phenotype of Brca1$^{-/-}$ mice appears to be more severe, and double Brca1$^{-/-}$: Brca2$^{-/-}$ mice display the Brca1$^{-/-}$ phenotype (Ludwig et al., 1997). A lack of cell proliferation has been suggested as the mechanism of lethality in these strains. This hypothesis is supported by several lines of evidence. First, in developing mouse embryos Brca1 and Brca2 mRNA are widely expressed and are most highly expressed in rapidly dividing tissues (Marquis et al., 1995; Rajan et al., 1997). Second, p21$^{waf1/cip1}$, a target of p53, appears to be overexpressed in these embryos (Hakem et al., 1996, Suzuki, 1997). Third, both *Brca1* and *Brca2* nullizygous embryos are partially rescued by homozygosity for null alleles of *p53* or *p21* (Hakem et al., 1997; Ludwig et al., 1997).

In addition to the nullizygous mice, mice homozygous for hypomorphic alleles of *Brca2* have been generated (Connor et al., 1997b; Patel et al., 1998). They are about one-third the size of their littermates, and have a shortened life span, and those that do live to adulthood develop thymic lymphomas. These mice display spontaneous chromosomal abnormalities and deficiency in DNA damage repair, which is discussed in more detail below. Brca1 and Brca2 appear to play critical roles in development; while their exact function is unclear, it is thought that both genes are important for cell proliferation.

BRCA1/2 and the Maintenance of Genome Integrity. Several lines of evidence point to an important role for the BRCA proteins in DNA damage response and repair. BRCA1 appears to play a role in sensing and signaling DNA damage, in regulating cell cycle checkpoint in response to DNA damage, and in modulating chromatin structure. BRCA2 complexes with Rad51 and is postulated to play a more direct role in DNA damage, complexing with Rad51 when it is not needed for DSB repair, as reviewed in Venkitaraman (2001).

Cells deficient in BRCA1 or BRCA2 are hypersensitive to ionizing radiation and undergo spontaneous chromosomal breakage (Patel et al., 1998; Deng and Scott, 2000). BRCA1 has been recently demonstrated to play an early role in the response to DSB. When DSB occurs, the histone H2AX is phosphorylated and BRCA1 along with the Rad50/MRE11/NBS1 complex is recruited to the foci around the DSB (Paull et al., 2000). These data focus on BRCA1 as one of the early proteins that assemble around DSB and are consistent with the earlier data on the interaction of BRCA1 and Rad51. As previously mentioned, BRCA1 also is part of a large complex (BASC) of proteins that are important for sensing and repair of DNA damage (Wang et al., 2000). Even though it has become clear that BRCA1 plays an important role, its exact function in the response to DNA damage has not been clearly elucidated. However, it has become clear that the BRCA proteins participate in HR and not in nonhomologous end-joining.

In addition, BRCA1 has been implicated in one of two subpathways of nucleotide excision repair—transcription coupled repair (TCR)—in which DNA damage repair occurs more rapidly in transcribed strands than in nontranscribed strands of DNA (Vrieling et al., 1998). TCR appears to depend on the presence of RNA polymerase II; when RNA polymerase II is stalled, it serves as a signal to direct repair to the transcribed strand of DNA (Leadon, 1999). BRCA1 has been demonstrated to bind to RNA polymerase II and several transcription factors, suggesting that it might be involved in TCR. Both mouse embryonic stem cells and a human breast cancer cell line (HCC1937) deficient in BRCA1 have been shown to be defective in TCR (Gowen et al., 1998; Abbott et al., 1999). Mouse embryonic stem cells deficient in BRCA1 are hypersensitive to ionizing radiation and hydrogen peroxide, due to a defect in their ability to carry out transcription-coupled repair of oxidative DNA damage, as measured by thymine glycol removal (Gowen et al., 1998). HCC1937's hypersensitivity to ionizing radiation and decreased TCR were corrected by the transfection and expression of BRCA1, demonstrating its role in TCR.

BRCA2 binds Rad51 through its BRC repeats, and cells from mouse fibroblasts from embryos (MEF) homozygous for a truncated allele of BRCA2 are unable to repair double-strand breaks that have been caused by ionizing radiation (Connor et al., 1997a; Wong et al., 1997). A pancreatic cell line (CAPAN1), which has lost one allele of BRCA2 and carries a mutation in the other allele, also is deficient in repair of double-stranded breaks due to ionizing radiation, as well as to methylmethanesulfonate and -etoposide (Abbott et al., 1998). Interestingly, the homozygous truncated BRCA2 MEFs display numerous spontaneous chromosomal breaks and the formation of triradials and quadriradials. Recently BRCA2 was found to regulate the intracellular localization of Rad51 and block the ability of Rad51 to form nucleoprotein filament, giving it a central role in the repair of DSB (Davies et al., 2001).

Similar models for the roles of BRCA1 and BRCA2 were recently proposed (Scully and Livingston, 2000; Venkitaraman, 2001). Work in prokaryotes has demonstrated an important role for sister chromatid recombination (SCR) during chromosomal replication. SCR occurs after stalling of the replication fork, a common event during replication. Roles for BRCA1 and BRCA2 in SCR at the site of the replication forks have been proposed. Rather than BRCA1 playing a primary checkpoint signaling role, it may be intrinsic to the checkpoint, and the persistent daughter strand gap (ssDNA) may lead to the activation of checkpoint signals. These models would tie in both DSB repair, which happens after the stalling of the replication fork, and SCR and TCR, which are initiated after stalling of RNA polymerase.

BRCA1/2 and Tumorigeneis. There are two postulated mechanisms by which germline mutations in BRCA1 or BRCA2 could lead to cancer. In both of the models, the cellular pathways involving *both* BRCA1 and p53 are inactivated. A high rate of *p53* mutations in both BRCA1-related breast and ovarian cancers has been demonstrated, providing suggestive evidence of the importance of the loss of the p53 pathway in BRCA1 mutation carriers (Crook et al., 1997; Rhei et al., 1998). This means that somatic mutations need to occur and result in both loss of the wild-type allele of BRCA *and* inactivation of the p53 pathway. This could occur either by a single dominant mutation or by two separate events affecting each allele. The difference between the two models is the timing with which the somatic events occur.

In the first model, put forth by Kinzler and Vogelstein (1997), the first step is loss of the wild-type allele of BRCA1 (proposed as a "caretaker gene"), leading to a defect in DNA repair. This defect in DNA repair allows mutations in "gatekeeper genes," those that regulate cell growth, in this case p53, which would allow tumor growth. The alternative view, put forth by Bertwistle and Ashworth (1998), is that loss of the p53 pathway happens first, perhaps by a dominant negative mutation in p53. Loss of the wild-type allele of BRCA1 could then happen, allowing progression to tumorigenesis. If loss of BRCA function happened first, causing genome instability, there would be checkpoint activation and ultimately apoptosis. With loss of checkpoint function, either though loss of p53 or another mechanism, genome errors would be tolerated, and eventually this would lead to tumorigenesis (Scully and Livingston, 2000). Recent data from Brca1$^{\Delta 11/\Delta 11}$ mice demonstrates that p53 loss rescues the proliferation deficiency of the Brca1 mutant but allows genomic instability, again supporting the loss of p53 as an important and perhaps a necessary step in BRCA-related tumorigenesis (Xu et al., 2001) (Fig. 35–13).

Additional Breast Cancer Susceptibility Genes

Several genomic regions have been suggested as candidate loci for additional breast cancer susceptibility genes, but none have been supported in confirmatory studies. Analysis of 56 families (three or more cases under 60) did not show evidence of linkage between breast cancer and genetic markers in the region of *PTEN* (10q23), which had been proposed because of its role in Cowden syndrome (Shugart et al., 1999). Chromosome 8p also has been proposed as a locus for a breast cancer susceptibility gene based on studies documenting allelic loss in this region in sporadic breast cancers, (Kerangueven et al., 1995; Seitz et al., 1997). The initial linkage studies evaluating 8p were performed using 11 families—1 family had a multipoint LOD score of 2.32, but only 3 of the remaining families had positive LOD scores, all less than 0.6 (Seitz et al., 1997). In a larger series of 38 site-specific breast cancer families (three or more cases under 60) no evidence of linkage was found on 8p, suggesting that if a breast cancer susceptibility gene exists at this locus, it accounts for a very small proportion of familial site-specific breast cancer (Rahman et al., 2000).

Recently, it was suggested that a breast cancer susceptibility gene may be located on 13q21(Kainu et al., 2000). Using comparative genomic hybridization (CGH) on 61 tumors from 37 families (at least three breast cancers, no germline mutations in *BRCA1* or *BRCA2*), the most common somatic alteration was

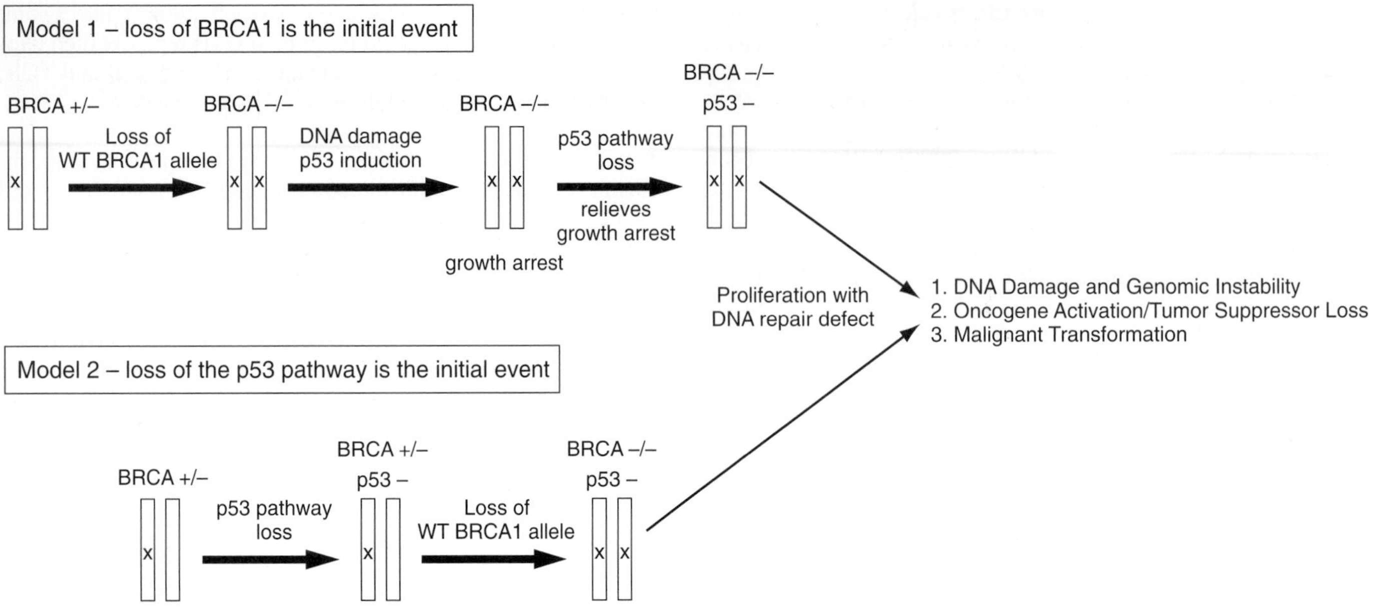

Fig. 35–13. Two models of tumor initiation in *BRCA1* mutation carriers. In both models there is loss of the wild-type allele of *BRCA1* and the *p53* pathway; however, the models differ in the timing of these events.

The initial event is loss of the wild-type *BRCA1* allele. Loss of the function of both alleles of *BRCA1* would allow for DNA damage to occur. This results in the induction of p53 and p21 leading to growth arrest. Loss of function in the p53 pathway would be required to relieve this checkpoint and allow cell division. Cell division with a defect in DNA damage and repair would lead to genomic instability, the accumulation of other mutations, and eventually malignant transformation.

Model 2: The initial event is loss of the p53 pathway. The second event is loss of the wild-type *BRCA1* allele, possibly driven by a centrosome defect caused by loss of p53 function. Again, growth with a DNA repair defect leads to malignant transformation. Modified from Bertwistle and Ashworth, with permission.

loss of 13q21–q31, which was thought to be an early event in tumorigenesis using hierarchical branching algorithms. These CGH findings were followed up with targeted linkage analysis in 77 breast cancer families, in which *BRCA1* and *BRCA2* mutations were excluded. An overall maximum 2-point LOD score of 2.76 at D13S1308 was observed, with a peak 3-point heterogeneity LOD (hLOD) of 3.46 ($\alpha = 0.65$). However markers immediately adjacent to the positive hLOD gave lower hLOD scores of 1.5. Studies from the BRCA3 Linkage Consortium using 128 families (at least three breast cancers <60, site-specific disease, no *BRCA1* or *BRCA2* mutations by both mutational and linkage analyses) do not support 13q21–q31 as a locus for a moderate- or high-penetrance breast cancer susceptibility gene (Thompson et al., 2002).

The search for BRCA3 has been difficult for several reasons. First, in the search for *BRCA1* and *BRCA2*, the associations between ovarian cancer (*BRCA1* and *BRCA2*) and male breast cancer (*BRCA2*) were recognized before either gene was isolated, allowing for targeted ascertainment of families with a high prior probability of linkage to the respective candidate regions. As no such phenotype has been associated with mutations in the putative BRCA3 gene(s), families entered into current studies are selected only for early age of breast cancer diagnosis and the absence of ovarian and male breast cancer. Additionally, BRCA3 mutations may be associated with lower breast cancer penetrance than *BRCA1* and *BRCA2*, and, if so, differentiating sporadic from hereditary cancers becomes a serious problem. Finally, multiple additional genes, each responsible for small numbers of families, may exist and limit the power of traditional linkage analyses.

Male Breast Cancer

Male breast cancer accounts for ~1% of all cancers in men. It affects 1 in 1,000 men and is therefore 100 times less common than breast cancer in women. However, the histopathology and clinical history of breast cancer in men is very similar to what is observed in women (Cutuli et al., 1995; Donegan and Redlich, 1996). The risk of breast cancer is higher in men with reduced testicular function or an increase in the estrogen : androgen ratio from conditions such as Klinefelter's syndrome (XXY), undescended testes, testicular injury, and orchitis (Donegan and Redlich, 1996). Radiation exposure and family history, particularly breast cancer in a first-degree relative, also are significant risk factors, as they are in women (Sasco et al., 1993).

The existence of a breast cancer susceptibility gene other than *BRCA1* (later shown to be *BRCA2*) was first demonstrated by showing that kindreds with both early-onset female breast cancer and male breast cancer were unlinked to *BRCA1* (Stratton et al., 1994). Linkage to a second locus (*BRCA2*) on chromosome 13 was subsequently demonstrated, and *BRCA2* was isolated as outlined above (Wooster et al., 1995). While the high relative risk for male breast cancer associated with BRCA2 germline mutations suggested that BRCA2 mutations may account for a large percentage of male breast cancer cases, several series of male breast cancers suggest that this is not the case (Couch et al., 1996; Friedman et al., 1997; Mavraki et al., 1997; Haraldsson et al., 1998). The proportion of male breast cancer cases found with germline BRCA2 mutations ranges from 7% in a series from the United Kingdom to 33% in a series from Hungary (Csokay et al., 1999). Strikingly, the majority of men with BRCA2 mutations in these unselected series did not have a family history of breast cancer. While mutations in BRCA2 were initially associated with a family history and male breast cancer, in a recent series from a large referral laboratory one-third of the germline mutations in men with breast cancer were found in BRCA1, demonstrating the importance of an evaluation of both genes in men with breast cancer (Richardson et al., 2001).

Suggesting the presence of a modifier gene for BRCA2 penetrance is the fact that within families with known BRCA2 mutations, there is clustering of male breast cancer cases. An analysis in Icelandic families has suggested that such clustering is unlikely to be due to chance and led to the hypothesis of a "male modifier gene" that segregates independently in these families and alters BRCA2 penetrance (Thorlacius et al., 1996). In one possible clue to localization of such a gene, a BRCA2 mutation family with three brothers with early-onset male breast cancer, an interstitial tandem duplication of chromosome 9p23–4 was found (Savelyeva et al., 1998). Since the initial report, other families with complex rearrangements of distal 9p have been reported (Savelyeva et al., 2001). The authors suggest that a gene(s) may be present in the region that contributes to the cancer phenotype.

Male breast cancer has been seen in a small number of families with germline mutations in the androgen receptor and partial androgen insensitivity (Wooster et al., 1992; Lobaccaro et al., 1993). However, germline mutations in the androgen receptor do not appear to contribute to male breast cancer susceptibility in a population unselected for features of androgen insensitivity (Haraldsson et al., 1998). Two male breast cancer cases with germline mutation in *PTEN* and Cowden syndrome have been reported, suggesting that Cowden syndrome may be associated with an increased risk of male breast cancer, as it is associated with an increased risk of female breast cancer.

Rare Causes of Inherited Susceptibility to Breast Cancer

Hamartomata Syndromes. Three hamartomata syndromes are associated with an increased risk of cancer. Two of the three, Peutz-Jeghers and Cowden syndromes, are associated with the development of breast cancer. The third, juvenile polyposis syndrome, is not. Peutz-Jeghers syndrome (PJS) is caused by germline mutations in *STK11/LKB1*, a serine-threonine kinase located on chromosome 19q13.3 (Hemminki et al., 1998; Jenne et al., 1998). PJS is characterized by hamartomatous polyps in the small bowel and pigmented macules of the buccal mucosa, lips, fingers, and toes. A retrospective study looking at cancer risk in Peutz-Jeghers families assigns a relative risk for breast and all gynecological tumors of 20.3 (Boardman et al., 1998). The mean age of breast cancer diagnosis in this series was 39 years. In spite of the early-onset breast cancer that can be seen in PJS patients, mutations in *STK11/LKB1* do not appear to play an important role in sporadic breast cancers (Bignell et al., 1998).

Cowden syndrome (CS) is a rare autosomal dominant phakomatosis in which patients have a predisposition to both benign and malignant neoplasms. Some 20% to 50% of affected women develop breast cancer (Eng et al., 2001). Other tumors seen in patients with CS include adenomas and follicular cell carcinomas of the thyroid gland, polyps and adenocarcinomas of the gastointestinal tract, and ovarian cysts and carcinoma (Starink et al., 1986; Hanssen and Fryns, 1995). The characteristic dermatological features include smooth facial papules (trichilemmomas and verrucae), acral and palmerplantar keratoses, and oral papillomas (Fargnoli et al., 1996). The mucocutaneous lesions are pathognomic for CS and seen in over 90% of patients (Hanssen and Fryns, 1995; Nelen et al., 1996). Some families also have Lhermitte-Duclos syndrome, a global hypertrophy or dysplastic ganglioma of the cerebellum (Eng et al., 1994).

CS is caused by germline mutations in *PTEN* (*MMAC1/TEP1*). The presence of a germline mutation in *PTEN* in clinically diagnosed CS families is associated with an increased risk of breast cancer (Marsh et al., 1998). Individuals in series of women with early-onset breast cancers (3%) and women with multiple primary cancers (5%) have been found to have germline missense mutations in *PTEN*, and thus germline mutations may be more prevalent than initially thought (FitzGerald et al., 1998; De Vivo et al., 2000). PTEN is a phosphoinositide 3-phosphatase which phosphorylates the lipid second messenger phosphatidylinositol 3,4,5-triphosphate (PIP_3) and negatively regulates survival signaling mediated by the protein kinase PKB/Akt (Maehama and Dixon, 1998; Stambolic et al., 1998). Recent data have shown that p53 is an activator of PTEN transcription and leads to a decrease in PKB/Akt phosphorylation, suggesting a role for p53 in negative regulation of cellular survival (Stambolic, 2001).

Due to the increased incidence of breast cancer among female patients with CS, there was speculation that *PTEN* would play a role in familial breast cancer (Nelen et al., 1996; Liaw et al., 1997). However, in families with a high incidence of breast cancer but without linkage to *BRCA1* or *BRCA2*, linkage has not been found to 10q (Goldgar et al., 1997). In addition, in studies of women diagnosed with breast cancer under the age of 35 without mutations in BRCA1 and of BRCA1/2 negative women with a significant family history of breast cancer, no mutations in *PTEN* have been found (Lynch et al., 1997a; Tsou et al., 1997; Carroll et al., 1999). These data strongly suggest that PTEN does not play a role in familial breast cancer apart from CS. Additionally, somatic mutations in *PTEN* have been found infrequently in sporadic breast cancer (Sakurada et al., 1997; Rhei et al., 1998). Of note, there is a common insertion polymorphism in *PTEN*, downstream of exon 4, that was associated with early age of breast cancer diagnosis in one study ($\chi^2_1 = 0.024$) in patients homozygous for the insertion. These preliminary data suggest that this variant may be a low-penetrance susceptibility allele, but additional work will be needed to confirm this observation (Carroll et al., 1999).

Li-Fraumeni Syndrome. Li-Fraumeni syndrome (LFS), now known to be associated with germline mutations in p53, was first identified as a syndrome in 1969 with a description of four kindreds in which cousins or siblings had childhood soft-tissue sarcomas and other relatives had excessive cancer occurrence (Li and Fraumeni, 1969). Subsequent epidemiological efforts resulted in the enumeration of the major component neoplasms, including breast cancer, soft-tissue sarcomas and osteosarcomas, brain tumors, leukemias, and adrenalcortical carcinomas, with several additional tumors likely to merit inclusion (Li et al., 1988; Strong et al., 1992). Segregation analysis of families identified through a family member with sarcoma confirmed the autosomal dominant pattern of transmission of cancer susceptibility, with the penetrance of mutations in *TP53* estimated to reach 90% by age 70 (Lynch et al., 1976). Unfortunately, almost 30% of the tumors in reported families occur before age 15 years (Strong et al., 1992).

The pattern of breast cancer in LFS families is remarkable. Among 24 LFS families studied in one series, 44 women were diagnosed with breast cancer, of which 77% were between 22 and 45 years old (Hisada et al., 1998). Bilateral disease was documented in 25% of these women; 11% had additional primary tumors. Although it is possible that codon 248 mutations in *TP53* are associated with an increased risk of breast cancer, the numbers are small (Eng et al., 1997). It has been suggested that males in LFS families may have later-onset tumors because they do not get breast cancer, which is so dramatic in female family members.

As noted above, in 1990, germline mutations were identified in the p53 tumor suppressor gene (*TP53*) in affected members of 6 LFS families (Malkin et al., 1990; Srivastava et al., 1990). Mutations were clustered in the conserved sequences of the gene, exons 5 through 9, known to mediate DNA binding. Additional families meeting the classical criteria for the clinical syndrome of LFS have been evaluated for the presence of germline mutations in p53, with approximately 50% of such carefully defined families carrying alterations identified in the p53 gene. In studies using direct sequencing, this number has increased to 70% suggesting that previous techniques missed some mutations (Varley et al., 1997). While *TP53* mutations in LFS patients are more frequently identified in the hotspots within conserved sequences, they have been seen throughout the gene (Law et al., 1991; Sameshima et al., 1992; Srivastava et al., 1992). *TP53* genes that are ostensibly normal by sequencing but are abnormal in a functional assay or with regard to expression also have been observed (Barnes et al., 1992). Recently germline mutations in *hCHK2* have been postulated as a cause of LFS (Bell et al., 1999). Screening of *hCHK2* is complicated as exons 10 to 14 of the gene are duplicated in several places in the genome (Sodha et al., 2000). While Haber and colleagues found mutations in screening LFS and LFS-like families, mutations in families with multiple cancers, but not typical for LFS have been more recently reported (Vahteristo et al., 2001). Interestingly, the same mutation, 1100delC, has been reported several times, suggesting it might be a low-penetrance breast cancer susceptibility gene.

The prevalence of germline p53 alterations among women diagnosed with breast cancer before age 40 has been estimated at less than 1% (Borresen et al., 1992; Sidransky et al., 1992). It is therefore a rare explanation for breast cancer in the population. Nonetheless, p53 mutation screening formed the basis for the first predisposition testing programs for breast cancer susceptibility. However, the low prevalence of TP53 mutations in the general population, and the profound psychological effect of such testing, have kept this genetic test from widespread application.

Muir-Torre Syndrome and HNPCC. Muir-Turre syndrome (MTS) is defined by a person's having had at least one sebaceous gland tumor (adenoma, epithelioma, or carcinoma) or keratocanthoma with sebaceous differentiation plus one visceral malignancy. It is inherited in an autosomal dominant fashion with high penetrance (Schwartz and Torre, 1995). About one-half of the patients have more than one malignancy. The most common malignancy is colorectal cancer, which is seen in 50% of patients. Breast cancer occurs in ~25% of women carriers, with a median age of onset of 68 years (Cohen et al., 1991). It was initially postulated that MTS and hereditary nonpolyposis colorectal cancer (HNPCC) were allelic, based on the similar pattern of malignancies, as well as the fact that patients with MTS have been found in HNPCC families (Hall et al., 1994). HNPCC is caused by germline mutations in one of the DNA mismatch repair genes (*hMSH2, hMLH1, hPMS1, hPMS2, hMSH6*) with mutations in these genes leading to the development of HNPCC through loss of the ability to repair damaged DNA, accumulation of replication errors, and genomic instability (Lynch and Lynch, 1998). In the tumors of MTS and HNPCC patients, microsatellite instability is observed. Mutational analyses in MTS kindreds have demonstrated mutations predominantly in *hMSH2* and, in two instances, in *hMLH1*, thus confirming that MTS is a variant of HNPCC (Kolodner et al., 1994). There has been a long-standing controversy about whether breast cancer is a component tumor of classic HNPCC. In a recent study looking at 96 HNPCC families, Scott et al. (2001) found an overrepresentation of breast cancer in the *hMLH1* group (SIR 14.77, 95% CI, 6.2–35) and in the mutation negative group (SIR 18.03, 95% CI, 12.2–26.7) but not in the *hMSH2* group. Previous studies, however, had not reported an increased incidence of breast cancer in HNPCC families (Watson and Lynch, 1993; Aarnio et al., 1999). A recent review of the Dutch HNPCC registry also did not reveal an increased rate of breast cancer, but Vasen and colleagues (2001) suggest that when breast cancer does develop, its progression is accelerated because of the mutations in the mismatch repair genes, and so it is diagnosed at a younger age. Further discussion of MTS and HNPCC can be seen in Chapter 34.

Low-Penetrance Genes

Low-penetrance genes are here defined as genes in which relatively common sequence variants, such as single nucleotide polymorphisms, may be associated with a small to moderate increased relative risk for breast cancer. Such variants are relatively common in the population and as such may confer a much higher population attributable risk than do the rare high-penetrance genes. Therefore, variants in low-penetrance genes could explain a greater proportion of breast cancer than the highly penetrant genes such as *BRCA1* and *BRCA2*. A hypothetical example of how a low-penetrance gene can explain more breast cancer than a high-penetrance gene is illustrated in Table 35–5. Candidate low-penetrance gene products are chosen on the basis of biological plausibility, in that alterations in the protein would affect a pathway involved in carcinogenesis. Low-penetrance candidates are found in a wide variety of pathways, ranging from the detoxification of environmental carcinogens to steroid hormone metabolism and DNA damage repair; examples of each are reviewed below and in Dunning et al. (1999). These variants are being examined to identify associations with increased breast cancer risk. However, we are just starting to learn about low-penetrance genes and the magnitude of their effect on cancer susceptibility.

Low-penetrance genes can be evaluated in two different ways. In a population-based case-control series, polymorphisms in low-penetrance genes can be evaluated for an association with an increased relative risk for cancer. Additionally, in carriers of mutations in autosomal dominant high-penetrance genes, which confer a high risk of cancer but have some variability in penetrance, the same polymorphisms in low-penetrance genes can be evaluated as modifiers by association with variable age of diagnosis or the type of cancer that develops. Many low-penetrance genes are being studied in both contexts.

Table 35–5. Example of Increased Population Attributable Risk for Low-Penetrance Genes

Gene	Risk Allele Frequency	Effect Size (RR)	Population Atttributable Risk (%)
High-penetrance	1/1,000	8.5	2
Low-penetrance	560/1,000	1.5	22

This is a theoretical example to demonstrate how a low-penetrance gene might have a higher population attributable risk than a high-penetrance gene.

P450 Enzymes

CYP1A1. *CYP1A1* encodes the enzyme aryl hydrocarbon hydroxlase (AHH), which is involved in the metabolism of polycyclic aromatic hydrocarbons (PAH) and estrogens. AHH is the primary catalyst in the conversion of estradiol (E2) to the less active hydroxylated (catechol) estrogens (Dannan et al., 1986). Decreased exposure to estrogen over a lifetime is associated with a lower risk of breast cancer: conversely, an increased exposure is associated with a higher risk of breast cancer. Therefore, changes in activity of AHH leading to differing levels of estrogen could affect breast cancer risk. AHH catalyzes the monoxygenation of PAH found in cigarette smoke to phenolic products, which may be mutagenic and carcinogenic (Nebert, 1991). PAHs do cause mammary tumors in mice and are associated with a high rate of DNA adduct formation (Liehr, 1990). At present, how the two aspects of AHH activity—decreasing active estrogens and increasing carcinogen levels—affect breast cancer risk has not been resolved. Thus polymorphisms in *CYP1A1*, which in theory change enzymatic activity, have been studied to see whether they are associated with breast cancer risk.

To date, four polymorphisms have been described in *CYP1A1*. The first (*m1*) is a T $\rightarrow$ C transition in the 3′ untranslated region at nucleotide 6235; the second (*m2*) is an A $\rightarrow$ G transition at nuceolotide 4889 (codon 462) leading to an isoleucine to valine change in the heme-binding domain of exon 7; the third (*m3*), restricted to African Americans, is another nucleotide change in the 3′ untranslated region; and the last (*m4*), is a threonine to asparagine substitution at codon 461 next to *m2*. The *m2* variant has been associated with increased enzymatic activity, but the biologic significance of the others remains to be elucidated (Crofts et al., 1994).

In an initial small study, the *m1* allele was associated with an increased risk of breast cancer in African Americans using 21 African American cases and 86 controls, demonstrating an OR of 9.7 (Taioli et al., 1995). A follow-up study using 59 African American cases did not find any association in a case-control study, nor has the *m1* allele been associated with an overall increase in breast cancer risk in Caucasian women (Bailey et al., 1998). However, one study did report a relative risk of 5 in those who carried the *m1* genotype and had commenced smoking before age 18, presumably due to AHH's role in metabolizing PAH in cigarettes to more carcinogenic products (Ishibe et al., 1998). In a study from Taiwan, the *m1* (homozygous) allele was found to be a risk factor, particularly in postmenopausal women (OR 1.98, 95% CI, 1.01–3.99) but not the *m2* allele (Huang et al., 1999b). Analysis of the *m2* allele by Ambrosone et al. (1995) demonstrated a weakly increased OR of 1.6 for breast cancer risk in postmenopausal Caucasian women using 176 cases and 228 controls. This association was most pronounced in light smokers (OR 5.2), but only 7 cases and 3 controls fell into this category, making generalization difficult (Ambrosone et al., 1995). Although this effect had not been seen in two previous studies, association with smoking was not examined (Rebbeck et al., 1994; Taioli et al., 1995). As in the previous studies, no evidence of an overall association between breast cancer and the variant *m2* allele was found in the studies by Bailey et al. (1998) using 164 matched case-controls and Ichibe et al. (1998) using 466 matched case-controls. Ichibe et al. observed an increase in breast cancer risk (RR 3.6, 95% CI, 1.1–11.7) for those who had commenced smoking prior to age 18. Krajinovic et al. (2001) observed an association of the *m2* allele with breast cancer, with an odds ratio of 3.3 (95% CI, 1.1–9.7), which was most pronounced among postmenopausal women (OR 4, 95% CI, 1.2–3.8). The *m3* and *m4* variants have not been associated with an increase in breast cancer risk (Taioli et al., 1995; Bailey et al., 1998). Taken together, these studies suggest that carriers of the *m1* and *m2* variant alleles may be associated with an increased risk of breast cancer when they are combined with exposure to cigarette smoke, which is a potentially modifiable environmental risk factor.

CYP17. The *CYP17* gene (cytochrome P450c17α enzyme), located on chromosome 10, mediates both steriod 17α hydoxylase and 17,20 lyase activities and plays a role in the intraconversion of cholesterol precursors to androgens, estrogens, or progestins, as well as mineralo- or glucocorticoids, and therefore plays an important role in determining the balance of these compounds. A polymorphism (T $\rightarrow$ C) in the 5′ untranslated region of *CYP17* (34 bp upstream from the initiation of translation) has been identified that has been shown to increase promoter activity as it creates an additional Sp-1 binding site. In a mixed population of 174 cases and 285 controls—including African American, Asian, and Latino women—an increased OR of 2.5 for having advanced breast cancer was found for the variant (C) allele. The TT genotype was associated with an older age at menarche and a lower risk of breast cancer (Feigelson et al., 1997). However, these findings were not confirmed in a case-control study of 835 cases and 591 controls in Caucasian women with a similar distribution of genotypes to the previously studied population (Dunning et al., 1998). Other studies similarly have not found an association between CC genotype and breast cancer, but they have mostly focused on postmenopausal women (Helzlsouer et al., 1998a; Weston et al., 1998; Thompson and Ambrosone, 2000). Interestingly, while Haiman et al. (1999) did not find an association with the C allele with breast cancer, they did find evidence that the protective effect of late age of menarche was only observed in carriers of the C allele, similar to the findings in initial study. Spurdle et al. (2000), focusing on pre-menopausal breast cancers, have found an association between the CC allele and breast cancer (OR 1.63, 95% CI, 1.00–2.64) and an excess of the CC allele in those with a family history of breast cancer. Thus the CC variant may be associated with an increased breast cancer risk in a subset of individuals.

Glutathione S-Transferases. The glutathione *S*-transferases (GSTs) are a family of genes that encode for enzymes that catalyze the conjugation of reactive chemical intermediates to soluble glutathione conjugates in order to facilitate clearance. GSTM1 and GSTP1 can detoxify polycyclic aromatic hydrocarbons (PAH), and GSTT1 detoxifies smaller reactive hydrocarbons. The GSTs may also have a role in the metabolism of lipids, chemotherapeutic agents, and reactive oxygen species. Interestingly, *GSTM1* and *GSTT1* are homozygously deleted at a high frequency (20%–50%) in all populations studied. *GSTP1* carries a coding region polymorphism (A313G), which changes an isoleucine to a valine, and it has been suggested that the valine allele is associated with lower enzyme activity (Helzlsouer et al., 1998b). There has been interest in determining whether homozygotes for the null alleles in *GSTT1* or *GSTM1* or the variant of *GSTP*, with consequent decrease or absence of enzyme activity, have an associated increased risk of cancer, as these enzymes regulate the ability to metabolize environmental carcinogens (Rebbeck, 1997).

The *GSTM1* null variant has been well examined in breast cancer case-control studies with variable results. Studies by

Zhong et al. (1993) and Kelsey et al. (1997) found a slight (nonsignificant) excess of the null allele in breast cancer cases. Only one study, by Helzlsouer et al. (1998b), has shown a significant OR (2.1) for developing cancer among carriers of the null allele; the association was principally seen in postmenopausal breast cancer patients (OR 2.5), and most pronounced in women with a high body mass index (OR 7), perhaps because of the additive risk factors of increased estrogen and carcinogen levels. This result is similar to that of Maugard et al. (1998), who also found more carriers of the null allele in the postmenopausal (≥55) breast cancer group (p = .006). Dunning et al. (1999) performed a meta-analysis of these studies and found an association between postmenopausal breast cancer and *GSTM1* null (OR 1.33, p = .04). In aggregate, these studies suggest that the *GSTM1* null allele may play a part in the development of postmenopausal breast cancer. However, Ambrosone et al. (1995) and Bailey et al. (1998) found no increase in the frequency of the null allele in cases, although one of these studies did suggest an increase in relative risk for breast cancer in the youngest postmenopausal women. More recent studies have not found an association between the *GSTM1* null allele and breast cancer (Krajinovic et al., 2001), although Millikan et al. (2000) did find an association in women with a family history of breast cancer (OR 2.1, 95% CI, 1.0–4.2). Therefore the role of the *GSTM1* allele continues to remain unclear; however, several studies suggest it may play a role in postmenopausal breast cancer risk.

The prevalence of the *GSTT1* variant in breast cancer cases has not been found to be significantly increased in multiple studies (Bailey et al., 1998; Helzlsouer et al., 1998b; Garcia-Closas et al., 1999; Millikan et al., 2000). In the study by Helzlsouer et al. (1998b), however, the homozygous *GSTT1* null variant in combination with a history of drinking alcohol at all increased the odds ratio to 5.3 (95% CI, 1.1–25.9). Although, the *GSTP1* variant has been less well studied than the null alleles of the other two members of the GST family, there is suggestive evidence that the hetero- or homozygosity for valine at Ile105Val is associated with an increased risk of breast cancer, consistent with the reported decrease in activity associated with this variant (Harries et al., 1997; Helzlsouer et al., 1998b). Later studies identified an Ala114Val substitution in *GSTP1* that occurs only on the 105Val allele. Maugard et al. (2001) suggest that, in fact, the presence of 114Val decreases breast cancer risk (OR for non-114Val genotype 2.18, 95% CI, 1.08–4.4); This finding has not yet been replicated.

GST null alleles also have been studied in conjugation with other variants in carcinogen-metabolizing enzyme genes in various combinations. *GSTM1* or *GSTT1* null alleles together or in combination with the *CYP1A1* variants *m2* or *m4* have not been associated with an increased risk for developing breast cancer (Ambrosone et al., 1995; Bailey et al., 1998). However, Helzlsouer et al. (1998b) did see a trend toward higher risk as the number of putative high-risk GST alleles increased. When two high-risk alleles were examined in combination, a significantly increased odds ratio for breast cancer was seen only when the *GSM1* null and the *GSTP1* valine allele were considered together. All three potentially high-risk genotypes together gave an OR of 3.77 (95% CI, 1.1–12.9), which underscores the importance of multiple genes working together to contribute to breast cancer risk.

Estrogen Metabolism and Receptor Variants

Catechol-O-Methyl Transferase. Catechol-*O*-methyltransferase (COMT) catalyzes the *O*-methylation of catechol estrogens, thus inactivating them. Some 25% of Caucasians carry a low-activity *COMT* allele (*COMT-L*), which is caused by a nucleotide transition from a G → A and results in a valine to methonine amino acid change at position 185/108 in the membrane-bound/cytosolic form of the protein. Multiple studies have looked at how this variant may be associated with breast cancer risk. Lavigne et al. (1997) used 112 matched, nested case-control subjects; in postmenopausal women, there was an increased breast cancer risk with an odds ratio of 2.2 associated with *COMT-L*. This was most pronounced in women with a high body mass index (OR 3.6), presumably because during the postmenopausal period the major source of estrogen is conversion by adipose tissue of androstenedione to estrone (Lavigne et al., 1997). Huang et al. (1999a) also found an increased risk of breast cancer associated with the *COMT-L* allele (OR 4, 95% CI, 1.12–19.08), which was more predictive of breast cancer risk than were high-risk alleles in *CYP17* or *CYP1A1*. Thompson et al. (1998) looked at 281 cases and 289 controls; they found an increased OR of 2.4 in pre-menopausal women and inverse correlation in postmenopausal women (OR 0.4), in direct contrast to Lavigne et al. (1997). In concordance with Lavigne, however, they found an even greater association of risk in heavier women carrying the variant with an OR of 5.7. Similarly, Mitrunen et al. (2001) found an inverse correlation between breast cancer and the COMT-LL allele in both pre-menopausal women (OR 0.44, 95% CI, 0.22–0.87) and postmenopausal women (OR 0.55, 95% CI, 0.31–0.98) with the COMT-LL. The effect was more pronounced in women with a low BMI. The largest study, by Millikan et al. (1998), looked at 654 cases and 642 controls and did not find an association between the COMT allele and breast cancer risk. Despite the varying results, there is the suggestion that COMT allele and BMI interact to influence breast cancer risk; the discrepancies in results may be due to different populations and other biological factors.

Estrogen and Progestrone Receptors. Estrogen and the estrogen receptor (ER) protein are believed to play a crucial role in the pathophysiology of breast cancer. The function of estrogen as a promoter of cell growth has been well documented. The ER is a critical determinant of cellular responsiveness to estrogen and therefore is thought to play an important part in the promotion of breast cancers as well (Fuqua et al., 1993). As it has such a central role in breast cancer, it is plausible that variants in the ER gene could affect breast cancer susceptibility. Therefore, several variants in the *ER* gene have been studied. Andersen et al. (1994) looked at three restriction fragment length polymorphisms in cases and controls. Only one, a XbaI site in one of the introns flanking exon 2, appeared to be associated with disease (p = .033). The same group investigated another variant (Gly160Cys), which is most likely a polymorphism, but they suggest it may be associated with increased breast cancer risk (Andersen et al., 1997). Finally, the *ER* codon 325 polymorphism (CC*C* → CC*G*) in exon 4 was initially shown to have a significant association with a family history of breast cancer. It is a small study of 34 affected women with a family history of breast cancer and 154 cases without such a history (Roodi et al., 1995). This finding was not supported by a larger study, which found no difference in association between cases and controls with the *ER* codon 325 receptor (Southey et al., 1998). In spite of the estrogen receptor's important role in breast cancer physiology as of yet, ER polymorphisms have not been shown to play a significant role in susceptibility to breast cancer.

Progesterone receptor status is also important, both for prognosis and predicting response to hormonal therapy for breast cancer (Habel and Stanford, 1993). In the progesterone receptor, there is a 306 bp Alu insertion in intron 7 termed *PROGINS*. Two transcribed isoforms of the progesterone receptor (HPR-A and HPR-B) use alternate initiation sites. The *PROGINS* variant of HPR-A isoform has been demonstrated to increase transcriptional activity and stability, and may repress estrogen receptor activation and transcriptional activity of the HPR-B isoform more effectively than the wild type does (Wang-Gohrke et al., 2000). In breast cancer case-control studies, there is evidence that carriers of *PROGINS* are at decreased risk of breast cancer, with the largest study, containing 554 cases and 559 matched controls, showing a gene dosage effect (OR 0.82, 95% CI, 0.62–1.08 for heterozygotes and OR 0.27, 95% CI, 0.10–0.74 for homozygotes) (Dunning et al., 1999; Wang-Gohrke et al., 2000).

Proto-oncogenes

Proto-oncogenes are involved in the regulation of normal growth and differentiation of the cell. Mutations or disruptions in proto-oncogenes, rendering them oncogenes, lead to disturbances in the cell cycle and can result in abnormal growth or proliferation. Somatic mutations in proto-oncogenes appear to be necessary for tumorogenesis, and many instances of such mutations have been documented in multiple types of cancers. So far, only a few instances of germline mutations in proto-oncogenes have seen which lead to cancer susceptibility, in *MET* (hereditary renal cancer, papillary type), *CDK4* (familial melanoma), and *RET* (multiple endocrine neoplasia, type 2). Germline mutations in proto-oncogenes have not been seen in syndromes that confer an increased susceptibility to breast cancer. However, in addition to mutations, which could confer a greatly increased risk of cancer, polymorphisms have been examined which would give only a modest elevation in risk.

HRAS. The proto-oncogene *HRAS1* encodes a protein involved in mitogenic signaling, the process by which an extracellular growth factor signal is transmitted to the nucleus. A microsatellite, composed of 30 to 100 units of a 28 bp repeat, is tightly linked to *HRAS1* and is located approximately 1000 bp downstream from the coding region. Rare alleles of the *HRAS1* microsatellite may be associated with an increased odds ratio for breast cancer. In one of the larger studies, Krontiris et al. (1993) evaluated 736 unselected cancer cases, of which 10% were breast cancer cases, plus 652 controls and calculated an increased relative risk of breast cancer of 2.29 (95% CI, 1.18–4.46). In the same study, a meta-analysis of all previous studies was done, which also showed an increased relative risk of 1.9 (95% CI, 1.23–2.29) associated with the rare alleles. A study looking at the rare *HRAS* alleles in both Caucasian and African American women suggested that their association with breast cancer may be strongest in African American women, as the rare alleles are more common in that population (Garrett et al., 1993). A meta-analysis made the same observation that rare HRAS alleles are associated with breast cancer and calculated a population attributable risk of 0.092 (Weston and Godbold, 1997). However, a more recent study of early-onset breast cancer (under age 40), using newly developed techniques for sizing alleles, did not show an association between breast cancer and rare HRAS alleles. The authors suggest that the association seen in other studies may need to be reexamined using newer techniques with an improved ability to discriminate between *HRAS1* common and rare alleles (Firgaira et al., 1999). While it is possible that different risk alleles contribute to early-onset versus later-onset breast cancer, the contribution of rare *HRAS1* alleles to breast cancer risk remains controversial.

DNA Damage Response Genes

The capacity of cells to repair DNA damage is, at least in part, genetically determined. Twin studies support a genetic component in DNA repair capacity, and a higher frequency of individuals with low repair capacity among relatives of patients with cancer has been described (Helzlsouer et al., 1995; Kovacs and Almendral, 1987; Pero et al., 1989). These family studies highlight the association between DNA damage response pathway defects and cancer susceptibility. Not only are multiple heritable cancer susceptibility syndromes due to germline mutations in genes involved in DNA damage response, such as hereditary non-polyposis colorectal cancer (HNPCC), breast and ovarian cancer, ataxia telangiectasia, and Nijmegen breakage syndrome, but also a reduced ability to repair DNA appears to increase cancer risk in case-control association studies. A capacity to repair DNA is associated with a higher odds ratios for cancer, ranging from 1.6 to as much as 10 (Kovacs and Almendral, 1987; Knight et al., 1993; Grossman and Wei, 1994; Scott et al., 1994; Helzlsouer et al., 1995, 1996). Cellular radiosensitivity, a measure of DNA damage response capacity, has been directly associated with breast cancer susceptibility and may be a heritable trait, with a limited number of genes contributing to the phenotype (Scott et al., 1994, 1998; Roberts et al., 1999). For genes within the multiple DNA damage response pathways, both heterozygosity for germline mutations in genes that cause autosomal recessive cancer susceptibility syndromes and common variants in genes that cause autosomal dominant cancer susceptibility syndromes may be low-penetrance risk factors for breast cancer.

Ataxia Telangiectasia. Individuals homozygous for germline mutations in *ATM* have ataxia telangiectasia (AT), an autosomal recessive disorder characterized by cerebellar ataxia, oculocutaneous telangiectasias, radiation hypersensitivity, and a high incidence of malignancy (Wright et al., 1996). AT homozygotes have cancer risks 60 to 180 times greater than the general population, including non-Hodgkins' lymphoma (nearly 100% lifetime risk) and breast and ovarian cancer (Morrell et al., 1986). Heterozygosity for germline mutations in *ATM* was initally hypothesized by Swift et al. (1986) to confer an increased breast cancer risk, a finding that could be particularly significant given that AT heterozygotes represent up to 7% of the general population and that screening mammography, a source of ionizing radiation, could theoretically increase the penetrance of such mutations. However, subsequent studies do not all support the initial claim, and the association remains controversial. Two approaches have been used to address this issue.

First, unaffected family members of AT patients consistently have a high risk of breast cancer, with relative risks ranging from 1.5 to 9 (Swift et al., 1987, 1991; Easton, 1994; Inskip et al., 1999; Janin et al., 1999). The most recent study, evaluating 609 female relatives of Nordic AT patients, found an increased breast cancer risk only in mothers of AT patients and an overall relative risk of 2.4 associated with AT heterozygosity (Olsen et al., 2001).

Second, mutational analysis has been used to define the contribution of ATM to breast cancer risk. In the first such study of 401 women under age 40 who were diagnosed with breast cancer, *ATM* mutation frequency did not differ from controls (FitzGerald et al., 1997). However, protein truncation testing (PTT) was used for mutation screening, and it may have missed some mutations. Null results also were reported by Izatt et al. (1999) in 100 breast cancer cases under the age of 40 and by Chen et al. (1998a) in 100 breast cancer patients with a family history, as well as several smaller studies (Bebb et al., 1997; Shayeghi et al., 1998; Vorechovsky et al., 1996). Finally, in a recent study of 483 unselected Norwegian breast cancer cases, 150 under age 55, screened for the Norwegian founder *ATM* mutations, no increase in prevalence over controls was found (Laake et al., 2000). However, Broeks et al. (2000) did find an increased rate of *ATM* mutations in 82 patients diagnosed with breast cancer before age 45, of whom 40% had contralateral disease and all had been exposed to low-dose radiation at a young age. The latter study suggests that exposure to even low-dose radiation at a young age may be an important component of breast cancer risk in the presence of an *ATM* mutation. Taken together, these data suggest that, in the absence of additional exposures, any increased breast cancer risk due to truncating mutations in *ATM* is likely to be minimal, with a population attributable risk of 1% to 2% (Olsen et al., 2001).

NBS. Patients with Nijmegen breakage syndrome (NBS) have an increased sensitivity to ionizing radiation and a predisposition to cancer that is similar to what patients with AT have. As such, a large case-control study of women with breast cancer diagnosed before age 51 was undertaken to determine whether the common Slavic founder mutation in nibrin, the gene associated with NBS, was associated with an increased susceptibility to breast cancer (Carlomagno et al., 1999). In this study no difference in nibrin mutation frequency was seen between cases and controls, suggesting that this variant does not predispose carriers to breast cancer.

BRCA1 and BRCA2. As deleterious germline mutations in *BRCA1* and *BRCA2* confer a greatly increased risk of breast cancer, common variants in both genes are ideal candidates for low-penetrance alleles. Several common variants in *BRCA1* have been studied, without any clear evidence for low-penetrance susceptibility alleles. The common BRCA1 haplotypes 356Q/871P/1038E/1613S (frequency 0.57) and 356Q/871L/1038G/1613G (frequency 0.32) and the variant R356Q do not significantly differ between cases and controls (Durocher et al., 1996; Dunning et al., 1999). The BRCA1 variant R841W may be associated with an increase in breast cancer susceptibility based on one study of *BRCA1* mutations in breast cancer cases; however, this variant is rare (<1% in U.S. controls) and has not been rigorously evaluated in another large case-control study (Barker et al., 1996; Petersen et al., 1998).

Recently, six variants in BRCA2 were studied for an association with breast cancer susceptibility. Of those variants (a-26g, N298H, N372H, T1915M, R2034C, K3326X), only one, N372H, appears to confer a small increased risk of breast cancer (Healey et al., 2000). N372H also is the only variant amino acid change in BRCA2 with an allele frequency greater than 6%. In a joint analysis of five series of breast cancer case-control studies (3459 cases and 2805 controls), homozygosity for the 372H allele, as compared to homozygosity for the 372N allele, was associated with an OR of 1.31 (95% CI, 1.04–1.61). Interestingly, the study also revealed that the N372H allele is not in Hardy-Weinberg equilibrium, with females having an excess of heterozygotes and a deficit of homozygotes, while the reverse is true in males. The authors suggest that there is sex-specific selection in utero, supporting a role for *BRCA2* in human development.

TP53. Given the well-described high penetrance of germline *TP53* mutations for early onset breast cancer as a component of Li-Fraumeni syndrome, sequence variants in TP53 also have been investigated as possible low-penetrance cancer susceptibility alleles (Varley et al., 1997). Three polymorphisms—IVS3 16 bp tandem repeat, IVS6 + 62 G–A, and Arg72Pro (Campbell et al., 1996; Sjalander et al., 1996; Weston et al., 1997; Mavridou et al., 1998; Wang-Gohrke et al., 1998)—all have been extensively studied. In a meta-analysis, the Arg72Pro variant (Pro carrier OR = 1.27, $p = .03$) was associated with a small increase in breast cancer risk; the other variants have not been consistently associated with high risk for breast cancer.

While candidate low-penetrance or modifier genes have been studied for their association with breast cancer risk, the question of how to find new low-penetrance genes is now being considered. As these genes cannot be easily tracked through families, as is true for the dominant high-risk genes, novel statistical and genetic methods will have to be employed to identify them and to demonstrate their importance.

Risk Assessment and Clinical Application

Molecular genetics has provided the medical profession with the capability to screen individuals for mutations in a number of cancer susceptibility genes. However, as with all new technology, it is incumbent upon us to employ such advances in a responsible manner. When an individual is tested for a mutation in a high-penetrance susceptibility gene, several questions need to be considered: Is testing the right choice for this person? Are they adequately informed about the nature and consequences of the test? Do we as health care providers understand the limitations of the test? Are there interventions that will be helpful to the person if the test is positive? What might be the psychological impact on the individual if he or she is found to be positive or negative? What are the long-term social implications for the individual? The following discussion addresses these issues for high-penetrance breast cancer susceptibility alleles; testing for low-penetrance genes is not thought to be of clinical usefulness at present and is not considered here.

Two types of risk assessment models can be used to assist patients with a family history of breast cancer. The first, exemplified by the "Claus model," predicts lifetime risk of developing breast cancer. The Claus model is based on 4730 patients with histogically proven breast cancer ages 20 to 54, and 4688 controls, which were age and frequency matched to cases (Claus et al., 1994). In this model, breast cancer risk is based on the number and relatedness of affected relatives and their ages of breast cancer diagnosis. Another such model is the "Gail model" in which risk evaluation is based on the number of first-degree relatives with breast cancer, the number of previous breast biopsies, age at menarche, and age at first childbirth (Gail et al., 1989). The Gail model is best used in Caucasian women undergoing yearly mammography and may be inaccurate in estimating risk in moderate- and high-risk breast cancer families, as it does not take into account the age of breast cancer diagnosis and paternal family history of cancer (Bondy et al., 1994). A drawback to both the Claus and Gail models is that they are entirely based on Caucasian populations, making risk assessment in non-Caucasian populations potentially inaccurate.

The second type of model is based on family history and ethnic background; it predicts the probability of finding a *BRCA1* or *BRCA2* mutation in the family. With this model, it is important to remember that the probabilities estimated are for affected individuals and must be adjusted accordingly for other individuals (e.g. half the likleihood for the daughter of an affected mother). The "Couch model" uses ethnicity, average age of onset, family history of breast or ovarian cancer, and the presence of breast and ovarian cancer in a single individual to estimate the probability of finding a mutation in *BRCA1* (Couch et al., 1997). This model was developed using a high-risk clinic population who were physician- or self-referred because of a perception of an increased risk of breast cancer. This model was recently expanded to calculate the prior probability of finding a mutation in *BRCA1* or *BRCA2* using 615 U.S. and U.K. families who were attending high-risk clinics. The mutation predictors are similar to prior studies, including the number of premenopausal women with breast cancer, the number of breast and ovarian multiple primary cancer cases, the presence of ovarian or fallopian cancer in the family, Ashkenazi Jewish ancestry, and male breast cancer (Blackwood et al., 2001). A similar model was derived from data collected on women who were undergoing commercial genetic testing (Myriad Genetics) using ethnicity, age at first diagnosis, family history of breast or ovarian cancer, and patient diagnosis (Shattuck-Eidens et al., 1997). Myriad Genetics maintains a website with mutation prevelance tables (*http://www.myriad.com/med/brac/mutptables.html*) from their moderate- to high-risk testing population.

A third type of model uses Bayesian theory in conjunction with family history of breast and ovarian cancer in first- and second-degree relatives and mutation prevalences to calculate the probability of carrying a *BRCA1* or *BRCA2* mutation (Parmigiani et al., 1998). In general, a 5% to 10% chance of finding a mutation is considered justification for testing; however, each decision must be made jointly by the individual and physician considering testing.

For those patients who decide to undergo genetic testing, informed consent is a critical part of the process (Geller et al., 1997). Despite the potential of learning more about cancer risk, there are risks involved. In addition, most patients do not have a working knowledge of genetics and the implications for their families. While educating patients, the health care provider must be aware of the limitations of the testing process. While clinical testing in the United States is done by Myriad Genetics, which employs full sequencing in both directions for *BRCA1* and *BRCA2*, there are still some drawbacks to current mutation detection systems. First, it is not possible to detect all disease-causing mutations in *BRCA1* and *BRCA2*. Current estimates based on families with linkage to *BRCA1* and *BRCA2* suggest that the sensitivity of PCR-based testing could be as low as 65% in terms of detecting mutations actually present (Ford et al., 1998). This may well be an oversimplification and underestimate of actual mutation detection sensitivity, as it is clear that not all PCR-based techniques for testing are equivalent. It also is clear that variable proportions of *BRCA1* mutation–carrying families are attributable to non-coding region mutations in different populations. First, in the Dutch population it is estimated that 30% of BRCA1 families are due to genomic deletions, whereas in other populations that does not appear to be the case. These genomic deletions are not currently detectable with commercial testing. Second, some of the mutations detected in *BRCA1* and *BRCA2* will be missense mutations. In the absence of a functional test for these mutations, one cannot always predict whether sequence variants are disease-associated. Third, up to 60% of high-risk site-specific breast cancer families are not accounted for by mutations in *BRCA1* and *BRCA2*, resulting in uncertainty transmitting anything other than a clearly positive result.

Surveillance and Prophylactic Surgery

While the ability to identify mutations in *BRCA1* and *BRCA2* has provided a significant advance in our understanding of hereditary breast cancer, what is perhaps more important is determining the optimum way in which to use the information in clinical management of mutation carriers. For breast cancer, there are several options, including surveillance, surveillance plus chemoprevention (reviewed below), and prophylactic surgery. Recent data on prophylactic mastectomy suggest that it is effective in high-risk women. In 425 women from moderate-risk families who underwent prophylactic mastectomy at the Mayo Clinic, 39 breast cancer cases were predicted using the Gail model; only 4 cases were seen ($p < .001$). In 214 women from high-risk families, using sisters as the controls, a risk reduction of over 90% for breast cancers was seen in those that had a prophylactic mastectomy (Hartmann et al., 1999). Of the 214 women in the study, 110 were screened for mutations in *BRCA1* and *BRCA2*; 12 mutations were identified, and with a median follow-up of 16 years, none had developed breast cancer (Hartmann et al., 2000). In a more recent study from the Rotterdam Family Cancer Clinic of 139 women with deleterious mutations, half of the women chose to have prophylactic surgery; none of those women developed breast cancer, however 8 of the women in the surveillance group developed breast cancer (Meijers-Heijboer et al., 2001). While there were some limitations to the study, including a short follow-up period of three years, the Rotterdam Family Cancer Clinic Study is consistent with the earlier studies, which show a significant breast cancer risk reduction for those who undergo prophylactic mastectomy. In addition, data from a larger cohort of 55 subjects and 99 controls show a breast cancer risk reduction of 80% with a mean follow-up of seven years (BL Weber and TR Rebbeck, unpublished data). While prophylactic mastectomy has been demonstrated to decrease breast cancer risk, screening for breast cancer, especially in conjunction with prophylactic oophorectomy or chemoprevention, remains a viable option and the one that many women select. Current breast cancer surveillance recommendations for *BRCA1* and *BRCA2* mutation carriers include annual mammography starting at age 25, clinic breast examination, and breast self-examination. However, increasingly, data suggest that interval cancers are a problem, and screening intervals in *BRCA1* and *BRCA2* mutation carriers may need to be decreased to every six months for optimum benefit (Armstrong et al., 2000). Breast magnetic resonance imaging remains an investigational screening method.

Unfortunately, screening for ovarian cancer is less effective than screening for breast cancer. While annual or semi-annual ovarian cancer screening is an option, using transvaginal ultrasound and serum CA-125 levels, it is clear that most women are still diagnosed with late-stage ovarian cancer disease. Thus, we currently recommend prophylactic oophorectomy when childbearing is completed, as does the American College of Obstetrics and Gynecology. In addition to reducing the risk of ovarian cancer by 97%, prophylactic oophorectomy also appears to reduce the risk of breast cancer in *BRCA1* mutation carriers by 40% (Rebbeck et al., 1999b; Eisen et al., 2000). In *BRCA1* mutation carriers, the mean familial mean age of onset of ovarian cancer (49 $\pm$ 7 years) appears to be younger than in sporadic cases (63) (Ries et al., 1998). After oophorectomy, we recommend hormone replacement therapy to age 50, and then consideration of a selective estrogen-receptor modulator (SERM). In addition, when prophylactic oophorectomy is done, hysterectomy should be considered as well, as it eliminates the risk of endometrial cancer and alleviates the need to take exogenous progesterone, which has been demonstrated to increase the risk of breast cancer over estrogen replacement therapy alone (Ross et al., 2000).

Chemoprevention

In the first large trial of chemoprevention, the National Surgical Adjuvant Breast and Bowel Project (NSABP) conducted a clinical trial of Tamoxifen vs. placebo in women at high risk of developing breast cancer (Fisher et al., 1998). Encouragingly, results of the study showed a 49% reduction in breast cancer incidence among the group treated with Tamoxifen, with an average follow-up time of 47.7 months. Patients were enrolled at or above age 60 or, using the Gail model as described above, if they were at least 35 years old and had the breast cancer risk of a 60-year-old woman. Lobular carcinoma in situ also was an entry criteria for women aged 35 or older. Tamoxifen did increase the risk of three other medical conditions: endometrial cancer, deep vein thrombosis, and pulmonary embolism. After completion of the NBASP P1 study, 288 of the 315 women who developed breast cancer were screened for mutations in *BRCA1* and *BRCA2*. Of those women, only 19 had mutations, making an analysis of the efficacy of Tamoxifen in preventing breast cancer in BRCA1 or BRCA2 mutation cancer difficult due to the small numbers (King et al., 2001).

Two European studies also looking at Tamoxifen for chemoprevention of breast cancer did not find any benefit (Powles et al., 1998; Veronesi et al., 1998). The studies had different entry criteria (using the Claus model rather than the Gail model), lower numbers of participants, and they allowed the use of concomitant hormone replacement therapy. As they used the Claus model, the participants' breast cancer risk was more likely to be due to genetic factors. Tamoxifen has been shown to reduce the risk of second breast cancer in *BRCA1* and *BRCA2* carriers by 30%, similar to the effect seen in unselected breast cancer patients (Narod et al., 2000). Further evaluation needs to be done, but Tamoxifen should be considered for prevention of breast cancer in high-risk women on an individual basis, taking into account the risks and benefits.

Exogenous Hormone Use

In *BRCA1* and *BRCA2* mutation carriers, hormone replacement therapy (HRT) is controversial. When considering use in women with mutations in *BRCA1* and *BRCA2*, it should be noted that HRT reduces exposure to estrogen as compared to the premenopausal ovary and therefore it can presumably be safely used in oophorectomized women at least until age 50 or 55. In addition, recent data suggest that estrogen use alone does not incrementally increase breast cancer risk over the risk associated with a family history of breast cancer and decreases overall mortality, suggesting that in aggregate it may be beneficial (Sellers et al., 1997; Ross et al., 2000). Oral contraceptive use in *BRCA1* mutation carriers appears to be associated with a significantly lower risk of ovarian cancer and a small increased risk of breast cancer, which is consistent with studies in the general population (Ursin et al., 1997; Narod et al., 1998). As with chemoprevention, each patient should be assessed individually, especially with respect to estrogen replacement therapy, especially as it also provides benefits in terms of cardiovascular disease and osteoporosis.

Other Issues

In addition to choosing a management plan to prevent cancer or detect cancer in at an early stage, there are other more intangible issues to consider when offering DNA-based cancer susceptibility testing. Insurance discrimination based on genetic testing has been of concern for many people. While a grave concern initially, there is no evidence that discrimination has occurred as a result of breast cancer susceptibility testing. However, those who are self-insured or have coverage as part of a small group may be at risk (Geller et al., 1995; Hall and Rich, 2000). There has been much research into the psychological ramifications of testing for BRCA1 and BRCA2 mutations. Multiple studies reinforce the importance of a genetic counseling and education program, such as the one outlined above, not only in order to allow patients to make decisions but also to help address cancer-related stress (Lerman et al., 1996; Lynch et al., 1997b). Interestingly, one study suggests that patients who decline testing and who scored high on measures of cancer-related stress had significantly higher levels of depression (Lerman et al., 1998). Most of these patients chose not to participate in the educational sessions offered. Patients who tested positive for a mutation did not have any change in their level of depression. These data suggest that the process of testing in the context of adequate counseling helps women with significant family histories deal with their cancer-related fears, or at the very least it does not adversely affect them.

SUMMARY

Breast cancer susceptibility is genetically complex. The identification of high-penetrance genes, epitomized by *BRCA1* and *BRCA2*, has led to a greater understanding of breast cancer risk in a small group of individuals. However, it is becoming increasingly clear that the mutations in the high-risk genes which have been isolated do not account for a family history of breast cancer in some, and perhaps most, individuals. Therefore mutations and polymorphisms in other genes are being examined in order to understand their contribution to breast cancer susceptibility. Candidate lower-penetrance genes, based on biological plausibility, are being examined for their association with breast cancer risk in populations, as well in carriers of mutations, in high-penetrance genes. In addition, investigators are seeking novel genes and using a variety of techniques that could be associated with all levels of breast cancer risk. Our knowledge of the genetics of breast cancer susceptibility continues to expand and open up new areas of interest and investigation.

REFERENCES

Aarnio M, Sankila R, Pukkala E, Salovaara R, Aaltonen LA, de la Chapelle A, Peltomaki P, Mecklin J-P, Jarrvinen HJ: Cancer risk in mutation carriers of DNA-mismatch-repair genes. Int J Cancer 1999; 81:214–218.

Abbott DW, Freeman ML, Holt JT: Double-strand break repair deficiency and radiation sensitivity in BRCA2 mutant cancer cells [see comments]. J Natl Cancer Inst 1998; 90:978–985.

Abbott DW, Thompson ME, Robinson-Benion C, Tomlinson G, Jensen RA, Holt JT: BRCA1 expression restores radiation resistance in BRCA1-defective cancer cells through enhancement of transcription-coupled DNA repair. J Biol Chem 1999; 274:18808–18812.

Abel KJ, Xu J, Yin GY, Lyons RH, Meisler MH, Weber BL: Mouse *Brca1*: localization sequence analysis and identification of evolutionarily conserved domains. Hum Mol Genet 1995; 4:2265–2273.

Ambrosone CB, Freudenheim JL, Graham S, Marshall JR, Vena JE, Brasure JR, Laughlin R, Nemoto T, Michalek AM, Harrington A, et al.: Cytochrome P4501A1 and glutathione S-transferase (M1) genetic polymorphisms and postmenopausal breast cancer risk. Cancer Res 1995; 55:3483–3485.

American Joint Committee on Cancer: Manual for Staging for Breast Carcinoma. Philadelphia: J. B. Lippincott, 1989.

Andersen TI, Heimdal KR, Skrede M, Tveit K, Berg K, Borresen AL: Oestrogen receptor (*ESR*) polymorphisms and breast cancer susceptibility. Hum Genet 1994; 94:665–670.

Andersen TI, Wooster R, Laake K, Collins N, Warren W, Skrede M, Elles R, Tveit KM, Johnston SR, Dowsett M, et al.: Screening for *ESR* mutations in breast and ovarian cancer patients. Hum Mutat 1997; 9:531–536.

Antoniou AC, Gayther SA, Stratton JF, Ponder BA, Easton DF: Risk models for familial ovarian and breast cancer. Genet Epidemiol 2000; 18:173–190.

Anzick SL, Kononen J, Walker RL, Azorsa DO, Tanner MM, Guan XY, Sauter G, Kallioniemi OP, Trent JM, Meltzer PS: *AIB1*, a steroid receptor coactivator amplified in breast and ovarian cancer. Science 1997; 277:965–968.

Armstrong K, Eisen A, Weber B: Assessing the risk of breast cancer. N Engl J Med 2000; 342:564–571.

Ayanian JZ, Kohler BA, Abe T, Epstein AM: The relation between health insurance coverage and clinical outcomes among women with breast cancer [see comments]. N Engl J Med 1993; 329:326–331.

Bailey LR, Roodi N, Verrier CS, Yee CJ, Dupont WD, Parl FF: Breast cancer and CYPIA1, GSTM1, and GSTT1 polymorphisms: evidence of a lack of association in Caucasians and African Americans. Cancer Res 1998; 58:65–70.

Barker DF, Almeida ER, Casey G, Fain PR, Liao SY, Masunaka I, Noble B, Kurosaki T, Anton-Culver H: BRCA1 R841W: a strong candidate for a common mutation with moderate phenotype. Genet Epidemiol 1996; 13:595–604.

Barnes DM, Hanby AM, Gillett CE, Mohammed S, Hodgson S, Bobrow LG, Leigh IM, Purkis T, MacGeoch C, Spurr NK, et al.: Abnormal expression of wild type p53 protein in normal cells of a cancer family patient. Lancet 1992; 340:259–263.

Bar-Sade RB, Kruglikova A, Modan B, Gak E, Hirsh-Yechezkel G, Theodor L, Novikov I, Gershoni-Baruch R, Risel S, Papa MZ, et al.: The 185delAG *BRCA1* mutation originated before the dispersion of Jews in the diaspora and is not limited to Ashkenazim. Hum Mol Genet 1998; 7:801–805.

BCL Consortium: Pathology of familial breast cancer: differences between breast cancers in carriers of *BRCA1* or *BRCA2* mutations and sporadic cases [see comments]. Lancet 1997; 349:1505–1510.

Bebb G, Glickman B, Gelmon K, Gatti R: "AT risk" for breast cancer [see comments]. Lancet 1997; 349:1784–1785.

Bell DW, Varley JM, Szydlo TE, Kang DH, Wahrer DC, Shannon KE, Lubratovich M, Verselis SJ, Isselbacher KJ, Fraumeni JF, et al.: Heterozygous germ line *hCHK2* mutations in Li-Fraumeni syndrome. Science 1999; 286:2528–2531.

Bennett LM, Haugen-Strano A, Cochran C, Brownlee HA, Fiedorek FT Jr, Wiseman RW: Isolation of the mouse homologue of *BRCA1* and genetic mapping to mouse chromosome 11. Genomics 1995; 29:576–581.

Benson FE, Stasiak A, West SC: Purification and characterization of the human Rad51 protein, an analogue of *E. coli* RecA. EMBO J 1994; 13:5764–5771.

Bernstein L, Henderson BE, Hanisch R, Sullivan-Halley J, Ross RK: Physical exercise and reduced risk of breast cancer in young women [see comments]. J Natl Cancer Inst 1994; 86:1403–1408.

Bertwistle D, Ashworth A: Functions of the *BRCA1* and *BRCA2* genes. Curr Opin Genet Devel 1998; 8:14–20.

Bertwistle D, Swift S, Marston NJ, Jackson LE, Crossland S, Crompton MR, Marshall CJ, Ashworth A: Nuclear location and cell cycle regulation of the BRCA2 protein. Cancer Res 1997; 57:5485–5488.

Bhatia S, Meadows AT, Robison LL: Second cancers after pediatric Hodgkin's disease [letter; comment]. J Clin Oncol 1998; 16:2570–2572.

Bhatia S, Robison LL, Oberlin O, Greenberg M, Bunin G, Fossati-Bellani F, Meadows AT: Breast cancer and other second neoplasms after childhood Hodgkin's disease [see comments]. N Engl J Med 1996; 334:745–751.

Bignell GR, Barfoot R, Seal S, Collins N, Warren W, Stratton MR: Low frequency of somatic mutations in the LKB1/Peutz-Jeghers syndrome gene in sporadic breast cancer. Cancer Res 1998; 58:1384–1386.

Bignell GR, Micklem G, Stratton MR, Ashworth A, Wooster R: The BRC repeats are conserved in mammalian BRCA2 proteins. Hum Mol Genet 1997; 6:53–58.

Blackwood MA, Yang H, Nathanson KL, Stratton MR, Easton DF, Calzone K, Stopfer J, Olopade O, Cummings SA, Ganguly A, et al.: Predicted probability of breast cancer susceptibility mutations. Paper presented at the San Antonio Breast Cancer Symposium, San Antonio 2001.

Boardman LA, Thibodeau SN, Schaid DJ, Lindor NM, McDonnell SK, Burgart LJ, Ahlquist DA, Podratz KC, Pittelkow M, Hartmann LC: Increased risk for cancer in patients with the Peutz-Jeghers syndrome. Ann Intern Med 1998; 128:896–899.

Bochar DA, Wang L, Beniya H, Kinev A, Xue Y, Lane WS, Wang W, Kashanchi F, Shiekhattar R: *BRCA1* is associated with a human *SWI/SNF*-related complex: linking chromatin remodeling to breast cancer. Cell 2000; 102:257–265.

Bondy ML, Lustbader ED, Halabi S, Ross E, Vogel VG: Validation of a breast cancer risk assessment model in women with a positive family history [see comments]. J Natl Cancer Inst 1994; 86:620–625.

Bork P, Hofmann K, Bucher P, Neuwald AF, Altschul SF, Koonin EV: A superfamily of conserved domains in DNA damage-responsive cell cycle checkpoint proteins. FASEB J 1997; 11:68–76.

Borresen AL, Andersen TI, Garber J, Barbier-Piraux N, Thorlacius S, Eyfjord J, Ottestad L, Smith-Sorensen B, Hovig E, Malkin D, et al.: Screening for germ line TP53 mutations in breast cancer patients. Cancer Res 1992; 52:3234–3236.

BRCA1 Exon 13 Duplication Screening Group: The exon 13 duplication in the *BRCA1* gene is a founder mutation present in geographically diverse populations. Am J Hum Genet 2000; 67:207–212.

Brinton L, Devesa S: Incidence, demographics, and environmental factors. In: Harris J, Lippman M, Morrow M, Hellman S (eds). Diseases of the Breast. Philadelphia: Lippincott/Raven, 1996:159–168.

Broca, P: Taite de tumerus. Asselin, 1866.

Broeks A, Urbanus JH, Floore AN, Dahler EC, Klijn JG, Rutgers EJ, Devilee P, Russell NS, van Leeuwen FE, van't Veer LJ: ATM-heterozygous germline mutations contribute to breast cancer susceptibility. Am J Hum Genet 2000; 66:494–500.

Brown MA, Xu C, Nicolai H: The 59 end of the *BRCA1* gene lies within a duplicated region of human chromosome 17q21. Cancer Res 1996; 12:2507.

Brzovic PS, Meza J, King MC, Klevit RE: The cancer-predisposing mutation C61G disrupts homodimer formation in the NH2-terminal BRCA1 RING finger domain. J Biol Chem 1998; 273:7795–7799.

Campbell IG, Eccles DM, Dunn B, Davis M, Leake V: p53 polymorphism in ovarian and breast cancer [letter; comment]. Lancet 1996; 347:393–394.

Carlomagno F, Chang-Claude J, Dunning AM, Ponder BA: Determination of the frequency of the common 657Del5 Nijmegen breakage syndrome mutation in the German population: no association with risk of breast cancer. Genes Chromosomes Cancer 1999; 25:393–395.

Carroll BT, Couch FJ, Rebbeck TR, Weber BL: Polymorphisms in *PTEN* in breast cancer families. J Med Genet 1999; 36:94–96.

Chen J, Birkholtz GG, Lindblom P, Rubio C, Lindblom A: The role of ataxia-telangiectasia heterozygotes in familial breast cancer. Cancer Res 1998a; 58:1376–1379.

Chen J, Silver DP, Walpita D, Cantor SB, Gazdar AF, Tomlinson G, Couch FJ, Weber BL, Ashley T, Livingston DM, et al.: Stable interaction between the products of the BRCA1 and BRCA2 tumor suppressor genes in mitotic and meiotic cells. Mol Cell 1998b; 2:317–328.

Chen VW, Correa P, Kurman RJ, Wu XC, Eley JW, Austin D, Muss H, Hunter CP, Redmond C, Sobhan M, et al.: Histological characteristics of breast carcinoma in blacks and whites. Cancer Epidemiol Biomarkers Prev 1994; 3:127–135.

Cheng L, Al-Kaisi NK, Gordon NH, Liu AY, Gebrail F, Shenk RR: Relationship between the size and margin status of ductal carcinoma in situ of the breast and residual disease [see comments]. J Natl Cancer Inst 1997; 89:1356–1360.

Clark GM, Sledge GW Jr, Osborne CK, McGuire WL: Survival from first recurrence: relative importance of prognostic factors in 1,015 breast cancer patients. J Clin Oncol 1987; 5:55–61.

Claus EB, Risch NJ, Thompson WD: Age at onset as an indicator of familial risk of breast cancer [see comments]. Am J Epidemiol 1990; 131:961–972.

Claus EB, Risch N, Thompson WD: Autosomal dominant inheritance of early-onset breast cancer: implications for risk prevention. Cancer 1994; 73:643–651.

Claus EB, Risch N, Thompson WD, Carter D: Relationship between breast histopathology and family history of breast cancer. Cancer 1993; 71:147–153.

Claus EB, Schildkraut J, Iversen ES Jr, Berry D, Parmigiani G: Effect of *BRCA1* and *BRCA2* on the association between breast cancer risk and family history [see comments]. J Natl Cancer Inst 1998; 90:1824–1829.

Cohen PR, Kohn SR, Kurzrock R: Association of sebaceous gland tumors and internal malignancy: the Muir-Torre syndrome. Am J Med 1991; 90:606–613.

Colditz GA, Willett WC, Hunter DJ, Stampfer MJ, Manson JE, Hennekens CH, Rosner BA: Family history, age, and risk of breast cancer: prospective data from the Nurses' Health Study [published erratum appears in JAMA 1993 Oct 6; 270(13):1548] [see comments]. JAMA 1993; 270:338–343.

Collins N, McManus R, Wooster R, Mangion J, Seal S, Lakhani SR, Ormiston W, Daly PA, Ford D, Easton DF, et al.: Consistent loss of the wild type allele in breast cancers from a family linked to the *BRCA2* gene on chromosome 13q12–13. Oncogene 1995; 10:1673–1675.

Connor F, Bertwistle D, Mee PJ, Ross GM, Swift S, Grigorieva E, Tybulewicz VL, Ashworth A: Tumorigenesis and a DNA repair defect in mice with a truncating *Brca2* mutation. Nat Genet 1997a; 17:423–430.

Connor F, Smith A, Wooster R, Stratton M, Dixon A, Campbell E, Tait TM, Freeman T, Ashworth A: Cloning, chromosomal mapping and expression pattern of the mouse *Brca2* gene. Hum Mol Genet 1997b; 6:291–300.

Couch FJ, DeShano ML, Blackwood MA, Calzone K, Stopfer J, Campeau L, Ganguly A, Rebbeck T, Weber BL: *BRCA1* mutations in women attending clinics that evaluate the risk of breast cancer [see comments]. N Engl J Med 1997; 336:1409–1415.

Couch FJ, Farid LM, DeShano ML, Tavtigian SV, Calzone K, Campeau L, Peng Y, Bogden B, Chen Q, Neuhausen S, et al.: *BRCA2* germline mutations in male breast cancer cases and breast cancer families. Nat Genet 1996; 13:123–125.

Crofts F, Taioli E, Crofts I, Taioli E, Trachman E, Cosma GN, Cumie D, Toniolo P, Garte SJ: Functional significance of different *CYP1A1* genotypes. Carcinogenesis 1994; 15:2961–2963.

Crook T, Crossland S, Crompton MR, Osin P, Gusterson BA: p53 mutations in *BRCA1*-associated familial breast cancer [letter]. Lancet 1997; 350:638–639.

Csokay B, Udvarhelyi N, Sulyok Z, Besznyak I, Ramus S, Ponder B, Olah E: High frequency of germ-line *BRCA2* mutations among Hungarian male breast cancer patients without family history. Cancer Res 1999; 59:995–998.

Cutuli B, Lacroze M, Dilhuydy JM, Velten M, De Lafontan B, Marchal C, Resbeut M, Graic Y, Campana F, Moncho-Bernier V, et al.: Male breast cancer: results of the treatments and prognostic factors in 397 cases. Eur J Cancer 1995; 31A:1960–1964.

Dannan G, Porubek D, Nelson S, Waxman D, Guengerich F: 17-estradiol and 2- and 4-hydroxylation catalyzed rat hepatic cytochrome P-450. Endocrinology 1986; 188:1952–1960.

Davies AA, Masson JY, McIlwraith MJ, Stasiak AZ, Stasiak A, Venkitaraman AR, West SC: Role of BRCA2 in control of the RAD51 recombination and DNA repair protein. Mol Cell 2001; 7:273–282.

Deffenbaugh AM, Reid JE, Hulick M, Ward BE, Lingfelter B, Gumpper KL, Scholl T, Tavitigian SV, Pruss DR, Critchfield GC, et al.: Clinical characteristics of individuals with germline mutations in *BRCA1* and *BRCA2*: analysis of 10,000 individuals. American Journal of Human Genetics, Annual Meeting Proceedings 2001; 69S:1437.

Deng CX, Scott F: Role of the tumor suppressor gene *Brca1* in genetic stability and mammary gland tumor formation. Oncogene 2000; 19:1059–1064.

De Vivo I, Gertig DM, Nagase S, Hankinson SE, O'Brien R, Speizer FE, Parsons R, Hunter DJ: Novel germline mutations in the *PTEN* tumour suppressor gene found in women with multiple cancers. J Med Genet 2000; 37:336–341.

DiRenzo J, Shang Y, Phelan M, Sif S, Myers M, Kingston R, Brown M: BRG-1 is recruited to estrogen-responsive promoters and cooperates with factors involved in histone acetylation. Mol Cell Biol 2000; 20:7541–7549.

Donegan WL, Redlich PN: Breast cancer in men. Surg Clin North Am 1996; 76:343–363.

Dunning AM, Healey CS, Pharoah PD, Foster NA, Lipscombe JM, Redman KL, Easton DF, Day NE, Ponder BA: No association between a polymorphism in the steroid metabolism gene *CYP17* and risk of breast cancer. Br J Cancer 1998; 77:2045–2047.

Dunning AM, Healey CS, Pharoah PD, Teare MD, Ponder BA, Easton DF: A systematic review of genetic polymorphisms and breast cancer risk. Cancer Epidemiol Biomarkers Prev 1999; 8:843–854.

Durocher F, Shattuck-Eidens D, McClure M, Labrie F, Skolnick MH, Goldgar DE, Simard J: Comparison of *BRCA1* polymorphisms, rare sequence variants and/or missense mutations in unaffected and breast/ovarian cancer populations. Hum Mol Genet 1996; 5:835–842.

Easton DF: Cancer risks in A–T heterozygotes. Int J Radiat Biol 1994; 66:S177–182.

Easton DF, Bishop DT, Ford D, Crockford GP, Consortium BCL: Breast and ovarian cancer incidence in *BRCA1* mutation carriers. Lancet 1994; 343:962.

Easton DF, BCLC Consortium: Cancer Risks in *BRCA2* mutation carriers. J Natl Cancer Inst 1999; 91:1310–1316.

Eisen A, Rebbeck TR, Lynch HT, Lerman C, Ghadirian P, Dube MP, Weber BL, Narod SA: Reduction in breast cancer risk after bilateral prophylactic oophorectomy in *BRCA1* and *BRCA2* mutation carriers. 2000 Annual Meeting of the American Society of Human Genetics. American Journal of Human Genetics 2000; 67S. Abstract 250.

Eng C, Hampel H, de la Chapelle A: Genetic testing for cancer predisposition. Annu Rev Med 2001; 52:371–400.

Eng C, Murday V, Seal S, Mohammed S, Hodgson SV, Chaudary MA, Fentiman IS, Ponder BA, Eeles RA: Cowden syndrome and Lhermitte-Duclos disease in a family: a single genetic syndrome with pleiotropy? J Med Genet 1994; 31:458–461.

Eng C, Schneider K, Fraumeni JF Jr, Li FP: Third international workshop on collaborative interdisciplinary studies of p53 and other predisposing genes in Li-Fraumeni syndrome. Cancer Epidemiol Biomarkers Prev 1997; 6:379–383.

Ernster VL, Barclay J, Kerlikowske K, Grady D, Henderson C: Incidence of and treatment for ductal carcinoma in situ of the breast [see comments]. JAMA 1996; 275:913–918.

Eusebi V, Feudale E, Foschini MP, Micheli A, Conti A, Riva C, Di Palma S, Rilke F: Long-term follow-up of in situ carcinoma of the breast. Semin Diagn Pathol 1994; 11:223–235.

Fan S, Ma YX, Wang C, Yuan RQ, Meng Q, Wang JA, Erdos M, Goldberg ID, Webb P, Kushner PJ, et al.: Role of direct interaction in BRCA1 inhibition of estrogen receptor activity. Oncogene 2001; 20:77–87.

Fan S, Wang J, Yuan R, Ma Y, Meng Q, Erdos MR, Pestell RG, Yuan F, Auborn KJ, Goldberg ID, et al.: BRCA1 inhibition of estrogen receptor signaling in transfected cells. Science 1999; 284:1354–1356.

Fargnoli MC, Orlow SJ, Semel-Concepcion J, Bolognia JL: Clinicopathologic findings in the Bannayan-Riley-Ruvalcaba syndrome. Arch Dermatol 1996; 132:1214–1218.

Feigelson HS, Coetzee GA, Kolonel LN, Ross RK, Henderson BE: A polymorphism in the *CYP17* gene increases the risk of breast cancer. Cancer Res 1997; 57:1063–1065.

Feuer EJ, Wun LM: How much of the recent rise in breast cancer incidence can be explained by increases in mammography utilization? A dynamic population model approach. Am J Epidemiol 1992; 136:1423–1436.

Feuer EJ, Wun LM, Boring CC, Flanders WD, Timmel MJ, Tong T: The lifetime risk of developing breast cancer [see comments]. J Natl Cancer Inst 1993; 85:892–897.

Firgaira FA, Seshadri R, McEvoy CR, Dite GS, Giles GG, McCredie MR, Southey MC, Venter DJ, Hopper JL: *HRAS1* rare minisatellite alleles and breast cancer in Australian women under age forty years. J Natl Cancer Inst 1999; 91:2107–2111.

Fisher B, Costantino J, Redmond C, Fisher E, Margolese R, Dimitrov N, Wolmark N, Wickerham DL, Deutsch M, Ore L, et al.: Lumpectomy compared with lumpectomy and radiation therapy for the treatment of intraductal breast cancer [see comments]. N Engl J Med 1993; 328:1581–1586.

Fisher B, Costantino JP, Wickerham DL, Redmond CK, Kavanah M, Cronin WM, Vogel V, Robidoux A, Dimitrov A, Atkins J, et al.: Tamoxifen for prevention of breast cancer: report of the National Surgical Adjuvant Breast and Bowel Project P-1 Study. J Natl Cancer Inst 1998; 90:1371–1388.

Fisher B, Dignam J, Wolmark N, Wickerham DL, Fisher ER, Mamounas E, Smith R, Begovic M, Dimitrov NV, Margolese RG, et al.: Tamoxifen in treatment of intraductal breast cancer: National Surgical Adjuvant Breast and Bowel Project B-24 randomised controlled trial. Lancet 1999; 353:1993–2000.

Fisher ER, Kenny JP, Sass R, Dimitrov NV, Siderits RH, Fisher B: Medullary cancer of the breast revisited. Breast Cancer Res Treat 1990; 16:215–229.

FitzGerald MG, Bean JM, Hegde SR, Unsal H, MacDonald DJ, Harkin DP, Finkelstein DM, Isselbacher KJ, Haber DA: Heterozygous ATM mutations do not contribute to early onset of breast cancer [see comments]. Nat Genet 1997; 15:307–310.

FitzGerald MG, MacDonald DJ, Krainer M, Hoover I, O'Neil E, Unsal H, Silva-Arrieto S, Finkelstein DM, Beer-Romero P, Englert C, et al.: Germ-line *BRCA1* mutations in Jewish and non-Jewish women with early-onset breast cancer [see comments]. N Engl J Med 1996; 334:143–149.

FitzGerald MG, Marsh DJ, Wahrer D, Bell D, Caron S, Shannon KE, Ishioka C, Isselbacher KJ, Garber JE, Eng C, et al.: Germline mutations in *PTEN* are an infrequent cause of genetic predisposition to breast cancer. Oncogene 1998; 17:727–731.

Fodor FH, Weston A, Bleiweiss IJ, McCurdy LD, Walsh MM, Tartter PI, Brower ST, Eng CM: Frequency and carrier risk associated with common *BRCA1* and *BRCA2* mutations in Ashkenazi Jewish breast cancer patients. Am J Hum Genet 1998; 63:45–51.

Fonseca R, Hartmann LC, Petersen IA, Donohue JH, Crotty TB, Gisvold JJ: Ductal carcinoma in situ of the breast. Ann Intern Med 1997; 127:1013–1022.

Ford D, Easton DF, Bishop DT, Narod SA, Goldgar DE: Risks of cancer in *BRCA1*-mutation carriers. Breast Cancer Linkage Consort. Lancet 1994; 343:692–695.

Ford D, Easton DF, Peto J: Estimates of the gene frequency of BRCA1 and its contribution to breast and ovarian cancer incidence. Am J Hum Genet 1995; 57:1457–1462.

Ford D, Easton DF, Stratton M, Narod S, Goldgar D, Devilee P, Bishop DT, Weber B, Lenoir G, Chang-Claude J, et al.: Genetic heterogeneity and penetrance analysis of the *BRCA1* and *BRCA2* genes in breast cancer families. Am J Hum Genet 1998; 62:676–689.

Foster KA, Harrington P, Kerr J, Russell P, DiCioccio RA, Scott IV, Jacobs I, Chenevix-Trench G, Ponder BA, Gayther SA: Somatic and germline mutations of the *BRCA2* gene in sporadic ovarian cancer. Cancer Res 1996; 56:3622–3625.

Friedman LS, Gayther SA, Kurosaki T, Gordon D, Noble B, Casey G, Ponder BA, Anton-Culver H: Mutation analysis of *BRCA1* and *BRCA2* in a male breast cancer population. Am J Hum Genet 1997; 60:313–319.

Fuqua SA, Chamness GC, McGuire WL: Estrogen receptor mutations in breast cancer. J Cell Biochem 1993; 51:135–139.

Futreal PA, Liu Q, Shattuck-Eidens D, Cochran C, Harshman K, Tavtigian S, Bennett LM, Haugen-Strano A, Swensen J, Miki Y, et al.: *BRCA1* mutations in primary breast and ovarian carcinomas. Science 1994; 266:120–122.

Gail MH, Brinton LA, Byar DP, Corle DK, Green SB, Schairer C, Mulvihill JJ: Projecting individualized probabilities of developing breast cancer for white females who are being examined annually [see comments]. J Natl Cancer Inst 1989; 81:1879–1886.

Garcia-Closas M, Kelsey KT, Hankinson SE, Spiegelman D, Springer K, Willett WC, Speizer FE, Hunter DJ: Glutathione *S*-transferase μ and θ polymorphisms and breast cancer susceptibility. J Natl Cancer Inst 1999; 91:1960–1964.

Garfinkel L, Boring CC, Heath CW Jr.: Changing trends: an overview of breast cancer incidence and mortality. Cancer 1994; 74:222–227.

Garrett PA, Hulka BS, Kim YL, Farber RA: HRAS protooncogene polymorphism and breast cancer. Cancer Epidemiol Biomarkers Prev 1993; 2:131–138.

Gayther SA, Mangion J, Russell P, Seal S, Barfoot R, Ponder BA, Stratton MR, Easton D: Variation of risks of breast and ovarian cancer associated with different germline mutations of the *BRCA2* gene. Nat Genet 1997; 15:103–105.

Gayther SA, Warren W, Mazoyer S, Russell PA, Harrington PA, Chiano M, Seal S, Hamoudi R, van Rensburg EJ, Dunning AM, et al.: Germline mutations of the *BRCA1* gene in breast and ovarian cancer families provide evidence for a genotype–phenotype correlation. Nat Genet 1995; 11:428–433.

Geller G, Bernhardt BA, Helzlsouer K, Holtzman NA, Stefanek M, Wilcox PM: Informed consent and BRCA1 testing [letter]. Nat Genet 1995; 11:364.

Geller G, Botkin JR, Green MJ, Press N, Biesecker BB, Wilfond B, Grana G, Daly MB, Schneider K, Kahn MJ: Genetic testing for susceptibility to adult-onset cancer. the process and content of informed consent [see comments]. JAMA 1997; 277:1467–1474.

Goldgar DE, Teare D, Shugart Y, Stratton M, Easton D: Candidate gene analysis and preliminary genomic search results for mapping of non-BRCA1/2 breast cancer genes. Am J Humn Genet 1997; 61:A66.

Gowen LC, Avrutskaya AV, Latour AM, Koller BH, Leadon SA: BRCA1 required for transcription-coupled repair of oxidative DNA damage. Science 1998; 281:1009–1012.

Gowen LC, Johnson BL, Latour AM, Sulik KK, Koller BH: *Brca1* deficiency results in early embryonic lethality characterized by neuroepithelial abnormalities. Nat Genet 1996; 12:191–194.

Grossman L, Wei Q: DNA repair capacity as a biomarker of human variational responses to the environment. In: Vos J (ed). DNA Repair Mechanisms. Austin, TX: Landes Co., 1994:329–347.

Haagensen C, Bodian C, Haagenson D: Lobular neoplasia (lobular carcinoma in situ): breast carcinoma, risk and detection. Philadelphia: Saunders, 1981:238.

Habel LA, Stanford JL: Hormone receptors and breast cancer. Epidemiol Rev 1993; 15:209–219.

Haiman CA, Hankinson SE, Spiegelman D, Colditz GA, Willett WC, Speizer FE, Kelsey KT, Hunter DJ: The relationship between a polymorphism in *CYP17* with plasma hormone levels and breast cancer. Cancer Res 1999; 59:1015–1020.

Hakem R, de la Pompa JL, Elia A, Potter J, Mak TW: Partial rescue of *Brca1* (5–6) early embryonic lethality by *p53* or *p21* null mutation. Nat Genet 1997; 16:298–302.

Hakem R, de la Pompa JL, Sirard C, Mo R, Woo M, Hakem A, Wakeham A, Potter J, Reitmair A, Billia F, et al.: The tumor suppressor gene *Brca1* is required for embryonic cellular proliferation in the mouse. Cell 1996; 85:1009–1023.

Hall JM, Lee MK, Newman B, Morrow JE, Anderson LA, Huey B, King MC: Linkage of early-onset familial breast cancer to chromosome 17q21. Science 1990; 250:1684–1689.

Hall MA, Rich SS: Patients' fear of genetic discrimination by health insurers: the impact of legal protections. Genetics in Medicine 2000; 2:214–221.

Hall NR, Williams MA, Murday VA, Newton JA, Bishop DT: Muir-Torre syndrome: a variant of the cancer family syndrome. J Med Genet 1994; 31:627–631.

Hanssen AM, Fryns JP: Cowden syndrome. J Med Genet 1995; 32:117–119.

Haraldsson K, Loman N, Zhang QX, Johannsson O, Olsson H, Borg A: *BRCA2* germline mutations are frequent in male breast cancer patients without a family history of the disease. Cancer Res 1998; 58:1367–1371.

Harries LW, Stubbins MJ, Forman D, Howard GC, Wolf CR: Identification of genetic polymorphisms at the glutathione *S*-transferase π locus and association with susceptibility to bladder, testicular and prostate cancer. Carcinogenesis 1997; 18:641–644.

Harris JR: Staging of breast carcioma. In: Harris JR, Hellman S, Henderson IC, Kinne DW (eds). Breast Diseases. Philadelphia: J. B. Lippincott, 1991:330.

Harris JR, Lippman ME, Veronesi U, Willett W: Breast cancer (1) [see comments]. N Engl J Med 1992; 327:319–328.

Hartmann LC, Schaid D, Sellers T, McDonnell SK, Woods J, Sitta D, Frost M, Couch FJ, Jenkins R: Bilateral prophylactic mastectomy (PM) in *BRCA1/2* mutation carriers. In: Proceedings of the 91st Annual Meeting of the American Association for Cancer Research, April 1–5, 2000. Philadelphia: American Association for Cancer Research 2000, 2000:222–223, abstract.

Hartmann LC, Schaid DJ, Woods JE, Crotty TP, Myers JL, Arnold PG, Petty PM, Sellers TA, Johnson JL, Michels VV, et al.: Efficacy of bilateral prophylactic mastectomy in women with a family history of breast cancer. N Engl J Med 1999; 340:77–84.

Healey CS, Dunning AM, Dawn Teare M, Chase D, Parker L, Burn J, Chang-Claude J, Mannermaa A, Kataja V, Huntsman DG, et al.: A common variant in BRCA2 is associated with both breast cancer risk and prenatal viability. Nat Genet 2000; 26:362–364.

Hedenfalk I, Duggan D, Chen Y, Radmacher M, Bittner M, Simon R, Meltzer P, Gusterson B, Esteller M, Kallioniemi OP, et al.: Gene-expression profiles in hereditary breast cancer. N Engl J Med 2001; 344:539–548.

Helzlsouer KJ, Harris EL, Parshad R, Fogel S, Bigbee WL, Sanford KK: Familial clustering of breast cancer: possible interaction between DNA repair proficiency and radiation exposure in the development of breast cancer. Int J Cancer 1995; 64:14–17.

Helzlsouer KJ, Harris EL, Parshad R, Perry HR, Price FM, Sanford KK: DNA repair proficiency: potential susceptiblity factor for breast cancer. J Natl Cancer Inst 1996; 88:754–755.

Helzlsouer KJ, Huang HY, Strickland PT, Hoffman S, Alberg AJ, Comstock GW, Bell DA: Association between *CYP17* polymorphisms and the development of breast cancer. Cancer Epidemiol Biomarkers Prev 1998a; 7:945–949.

Helzlsouer KJ, Selmin O, Huang HY, Strickland PT, Hoffman S, Alberg AJ, Watson M, Comstock GW, Bell D: Association between glutathione *S*-transferase M1, P1, and T1 genetic polymorphisms and development of breast cancer [see comments]. J Natl Cancer Inst 1998b; 90:512–518.

Hemminki A, Markie D, Tomlinson I, Avizienyte E, Roth S, Loukola A, Bignell G, Warren W, Aminoff M, Hoglund P, et al.: A serine/threonine kinase gene defective in Peutz-Jeghers syndrome. Nature 1998; 391:184–187.

Hisada M, Garber JE, Fung CY, Fraumeni JF Jr, Li FP: Multiple primary cancers in families with Li-Fraumeni syndrome. J Natl Cancer Inst 1998; 90:606–611.

Holt JT, Thompson ME, Szabo C, Robinson-Benion C, Arteaga CL, King MC, Jensen RA: Growth retardation and tumour inhibition by BRCA1 [see comments]. Nat Genet 1996; 12:298–302.

Hopper JL, Southey MC, Dite GS, Jolley DJ, Giles GG, McCredie MR, Easton DF, Venter DJ: Population-based estimate of the average age-specific cumulative risk of breast cancer for a defined set of protein-truncating mutations in *BRCA1* and *BRCA2*. Cancer Epidemiol Biomarkers Prev 1999; 8:741–747.

Howe HL, Wingo PA, Thun MJ, Ries LA, Rosenberg HM, Feigal EG, Edwards BK: Annual report to the nation on the status of cancer (1973 through 1998), featuring cancers with recent increasing trends. J Natl Cancer Inst 2001; 93:824–842.

Huang CS, Chern HD, Chang KJ, Cheng CW, Hsu SM, Shen CY: Breast cancer risk associated with genotype polymorphism of the estrogen-metabolizing genes *CYP17*, *CYP1A1*, and *COMT*: a multigenic study on cancer susceptibility. Cancer Res 1999a; 59:4870–4875.

Huang CS, Shen CY, Chang KJ, Hsu SM, Chern HD: Cytochrome P4501A1 polymorphism as a susceptibility factor for breast cancer in postmenopausal Chinese women in Taiwan. Br J Cancer 1999b; 80:1838–1843.

Hunter DJ, Willett WC: Dietary factors. In: Harris JR LM, Morrow M, Hellman S (eds). Diseases of the Breast. Philadelphia: Lippincott/Raven, 1996:201–212.

Inskip HM, Kinlen LJ, Taylor AM, Woods CG, Arlett CF: Risk of breast cancer and other cancers in heterozygotes for ataxia-telangiectasia. Br J Cancer 1999; 79:1304–1307.

Ishibe N, Hankinson SE, Colditz GA, Spiegelman D, Willett WC, Speizer FE, Kelsey KT, Hunter DJ: Cigarette smoking, cytochrome P450 1A1 polymorphisms, and breast cancer risk in the Nurses' Health Study. Cancer Res 1998; 58:667–671.

Ithier G, Girard M, Stoppa-Lyonnet D: Breast cancer and *BRCA1* mutations [letter]. N Engl J Med 1996; 334:1198–1199.

Izatt L, Greenman J, Hodgson S, Ellis D, Watts S, Scott G, Jacobs C, Liebmann R, Zvelebil MJ, Mathew C, et al.: Identification of germline missense mutations and rare allelic variants in the *ATM* gene in early-onset breast cancer. Genes Chromosomes Cancer 1999; 26:286–294.

Jacquemier J, Eisinger F, Birnbaum D, Sobol H: Histoprognostic grade in BRCA1-associated breast cancer [letter] [see comments]. Lancet 1995; 345:1503.

Janin N, Andrieu N, Ossian K, Lauge A, Croquette MF, Griscelli C, Debre M, Bressac-de-Paillerets B, Aurias A, Stoppa-Lyonnet D: Breast cancer risk in ataxia telangiectasia (AT) heterozygotes: haplotype study in French AT families. Br J Cancer 1999; 80:1042–1045.

Jenne DE, Reimann H, Nezu J, Friedel W, Loff S, Jeschke R, Muller O, Back W, Zimmer M: Peutz-Jeghers syndrome is caused by mutations in a novel serine threonine kinase. Nat Genet 1998; 18:38–43.

Jernstrom H, Lerman C, Ghadirian P, Lynch HT, Weber B, Garber J, Daly M, Olopade OI, Foulkes WD, Warner E, et al.: Pregnancy and risk of early breast cancer in carriers of BRCA1 and BRCA2. Lancet 1999; 354:1846–1850.

Johannsson OT, Idvall I, Anderson C, Borg A, Barkardottir RB, Egilsson V, Olsson H: Tumour biological features of BRCA1-induced breast and ovarian cancer. Eur J Cancer 1997; 33:362–371.

John EM, Kelsey JL: Radiation and other environmental exposures and breast cancer. Epidemiol Rev 1993; 15:157–162.

Kadouri L, Easton DF, Edwards S, Hubert A, Kote-Jarai Z, Glaser B, Durocher F, Abeliovich D, Peretz T, Eeles RA: CAG and GGC repeat polymorphisms in the androgen receptor gene and breast cancer susceptibility in BRCA1/2 carriers and non-carriers. Br J Cancer 2001; 85:36–40.

Kainu T, Juo SH, Desper R, Schaffer AA, Gillanders E, Rozenblum E, Freas-Lutz D, Weaver D, Stephan D, Bailey-Wilson J, et al.: Somatic deletions in hereditary breast cancers implicate 13q21 as a putative novel breast cancer susceptibility locus. PNAS 2000; 97:9603–9608.

Kampert JB, Whittemore AS, Paffenbarger RS Jr.: Combined effect of childbearing, menstrual events, and body size on age-specific breast cancer risk. Am J Epidemiol 1988; 128:962–979.

Kelsey KT, Hankinson SE, Colditz GA, Springer K, Garcia-Closas M, Spiegelman D, Manson JE, Garland M, Stampfer MJ, Willett WC, et al.: Glutathione *S*-transferase class μ deletion polymorphism and breast cancer: results from prevalent versus incident cases. Cancer Epidemiol Biomarkers Prev 1997; 6:511–515.

Kerangueven F, Essioux L, Dib A: Loss of heterozygosity and linkage analysis in breast carcinoma: indication for a putative third susceptibility gene on the short arm of chromosome 8. Oncogene 1995; 10:1023.

King MC, Wieand HS, Hale K, Walsh T, Owens KM, Lee MK, Costantino JP, Fisher B, Investigators N: Tamoxifen and breast cancer incidence among women with inherited mutations in *BRCA1* and *BRCA2*: a genomic resequencing study in the NSABP-P1 Breast Cancer Prevention Trial. Am J Hum Genet 2001; 69S:272.

Kinzler KW, Vogelstein B: Cancer-susceptibility genes: gatekeepers and caretakers [news; comment]. Nature 1997; 386:761, 763.

Knight R, Parshad R, Price F: X-ray induced chromatid damage in relation to DNA repair and cancer incidence in family members. Int J Cancer 1993; 54:589–593.

Knudson AG: Mutation and cancer: statistical study of retinoblastoma. PNAS 1971; 68:820–823.

Kolodner RD, Hall NR, Lipford J, Kane MF, Rao MR, Morrison P, Wirth L, Finan PJ, Burn J, Chapman P: Structure of the human *MSH2* locus and analysis of two Muir-Torre kindreds for *msh2* mutations [published erratum appears in Genomics 1995 Aug 10; 28(3):613]. Genomics 1994; 24:516–526.

Kovacs E, Almendral A: Reduced DNA repair synthesis in healthy women having first degree relatives with breast cancer. Eur J Cancer Clin Oncol 1987; 23:1051–1057.

Krainer M, Silva-Arrieta S, FitzGerald MG, Shimada A, Ishioka C, Kanamaru R, MacDonald DJ, Unsal H, Finkelstein DM, Bowcock A, et al.: Differential contributions of *BRCA1* and *BRCA2* to early-onset breast cancer [see comments]. N Engl J Med 1997; 336:1416–1421.

Krajinovic M, Ghadirian P, Richer C, Sinnett H, Gandini S, Perret C, Lacroix A, Labuda D, Sinnett D: Genetic susceptibility to breast cancer in French-Canadians: role of carcinogen-metabolizing enzymes and gene–environment interactions. Int J Cancer 2001; 92:220–225.

Krontiris TG, Devlin B, Karp DD, Robert NJ, Risch N: An association between the risk of cancer and mutations in the *HRAS1* minisatellite locus [see comments]. N Engl J Med 1993; 329:517–523.

Laake K, Vu P, Andersen TI, Erikstein B, Karesen R, Lonning PE, Skovlund E, Borresen-Dale AL: Screening breast cancer patients for Norwegian *ATM* mutations. Br J Cancer 2000; 83:1650–1653.

Lakhani SR, Gusterson BA, Jacquemier J, Sloane JP, Anderson TJ, van de Vijver MJ, Venter D, Freeman A, Antoniou A, McGuffog L, et al.: The pathology of familial breast cancer: histological features of cancers in families not attributable to mutations in *BRCA1* or *BRCA2*. Clin Cancer Res 2000; 6:782–789.

Lakhani SR, Jacquemier J, Sloane JP, Gusterson BA, Anderson TJ, van de Vijver MJ, Farid LM, Venter D, Antoniou A, Storfer-Isser A, et al.: Multifactorial analysis of differences between sporadic breast cancers and cancers involving *BRCA1* and *BRCA2* mutations. J Natl Cancer Inst 1998; 90:1138–1145.

Lakhani SR, O'Hare MJ, Ashworth A: Profiling familial breast cancer. Nat Med 2001; 7:408–410.

Lancaster JM, Wooster R, Mangion J, Phelan CM, Cochran C, Gumbs C, Seal S, Barfoot R, Collins N, Bignell G, et al.: *BRCA2* mutations in primary breast and ovarian cancers. Nat Genet 1996; 13:238–240.

Landis SH, Murray T, Bolden S, Wingo PA: Cancer statistics, 1998 [published erratum appears in CA Cancer J Clin 1998 May–Jun; 48(3):192]. CA Cancer J Clin 1998; 48:6–29.

Lannin DR, Mathews HF, Mitchell J, Swanson MS, Swanson FH, Edwards MS: Influence of socioeconomic and cultural factors on racial differences in late-stage presentation of breast cancer. JAMA 1998; 279:1801–1807.

Lavigne JA, Helzlsouer KJ, Huang HY, Strickland PT, Bell DA, Selmin O, Watson MA, Hoffman S, Comstock GW, Yager JD: An association between the allele coding for a low activity variant of catechol-*O*-methyltransferase and the risk for breast cancer. Cancer Res 1997; 57:5493–5497.

Law JC, Strong LC, Chidambaram A, Ferrell RE: A germ line mutation in exon 5 of the p53 gene in an extended cancer family. Cancer Res 1991; 51:6385–6387.

Leadon SA: Transcription-coupled repair of DNA damage: unanticipated players, unexpected complexities. Am J Hum Genet 1999; 64:1259–1263.

Lerman C, Hughes C, Lemon SJ, Main D, Snyder C, Durham C, Narod S, Lynch HT: What you don't know can hurt you: adverse psychologic effects in members of *BRCA1*-linked and *BRCA2*-linked families who decline genetic testing [see comments]. J Clin Oncol 1998; 16:1650–1654.

Lerman C, Narod S, Schulman K, Hughes C, Gomez-Caminero A, Bonney G, Gold

K, Trock B, Main D, Lynch J, et al.: BRCA1 testing in families with hereditary breast-ovarian cancer: a prospective study of patient decision making and outcomes [see comments]. JAMA 1996; 275:1885–1892.

Li FP, Fraumeni JF: Soft-tissue sarcomas, breast cancer, and other neoplasms: familial syndrome? Ann Intern Med 1969; 71:747.

Li FP, Fraumeni JF, Mulvihill JJ: A cancer family syndrome in 24 kindreds. Cancer Res 1988; 48:5358.

Liaw D, Marsh DJ, Li J, Dahia PL, Wang SI, Zheng Z, Bose S, Call KM, Tsou HC, Peacocke M, et al.: Germline mutations of the *PTEN* gene in Cowden disease, an inherited breast and thyroid cancer syndrome. Nat Genet 1997; 16:64–67.

Liehr JG: Genotoxic effects of estrogens. Mutat Res 1990; 238:269–276.

Liu CY, Flesken-Nikitin A, Li S, Zeng Y, Lee WH: Inactivation of the mouse *Brca1* gene leads to failure in the morphogenesis of the egg cylinder in early postimplantation development. Genes Dev 1996; 10:1835–1843.

Lobaccaro JM, Lumbroso S, Belon C, Galtier-Dereure F, Bringer J, Lesimple T, Namer M, Cutuli BF, Pujol H, Sultan C: Androgen receptor gene mutation in male breast cancer. Hum Mol Genet 1993; 2:1799–1802.

Loman N, Johannsson O, Bendahl PO, Borg A, Ferno M, Olsson H: Steroid receptors in hereditary breast carcinomas associated with *BRCA1* or *BRCA2* mutations or unknown susceptibility genes. Cancer 1998; 83:310–319.

Ludwig T, Chapman DL, Papaioannou VE, Efstratiadis A: Targeted mutations of breast cancer susceptibility gene homologs in mice: lethal phenotypes of *Brca1*, *Brca2*, *Brca1/Brca2*, *Brca1/p53*, and *Brca2/p53* nullizygous embryos. Genes Dev 1997; 11:1226–1241.

Lynch ED, Ostermeyer EA, Lee MK, Arena JF, Ji H, Dann J, Swisshelm K, Suchard D, MacLeod PM, Kvinnsland S, et al.: Inherited mutations in *PTEN* that are associated with breast cancer, Cowden disease, and juvenile polyposis. Am J Hum Genet 1997a; 61:1254–1260.

Lynch HT, Guirgis HA, Brodkey F, Lynch J, Maloney K, Rankin L, Mulcahy GM: Genetic heterogeneity and familial carcinoma of the breast. Surg Gynecol Obstet 1976; 142:693–699.

Lynch HT, Lemon SJ, Durham C, Tinley ST, Connolly C, Lynch JF, Surdam J, Orinion E, Slominski-Caster S, Watson P, et al.: A descriptive study of *BRCA1* testing and reactions to disclosure of test results [see comments]. Cancer 1997b; 79:2219–2228.

Lynch HT, Lynch JF: Genetics of colonic cancer. Digestion 1998; 59:481–492.

MacMahon B, Cole P, Lin TM, Lowe CR, Mirra AP, Ravnihar B, Salber EJ, Valaoras VG, Yuasa S: Age at first birth and breast cancer risk. Bull World Health Org 1970; 43:209–221.

Madigan MP, Ziegler RG, Benichou J, Byrne C, Hoover RN: Proportion of breast cancer cases in the United States explained by well-established risk factors. J Natl Cancer Inst 1995; 87:1681–1685.

Maehama T, Dixon JE: The tumor suppressor, *PTEN/MMAC1*, dephosphorylates the lipid second messenger, phosphatidylinositol 3,4,5-trisphosphate. J Biol Chem 1998; 273:13375–13378.

Malkin D, Li FP, Strong LC, Fraumeni JF Jr, Nelson CE, Kim DH, Kassel J, Gryka MA, Bischoff FZ, Tainsky MA, et al.: Germ line *p53* mutations in a familial syndrome of breast cancer, sarcomas, and other neoplasms [see comments]. Science 1990; 250:1233–1238.

Malone KE, Daling JR, Thompson JD, O'Brien CA, Francisco LV, Ostrander EA: *BRCA1* mutations and breast cancer in the general population: analyses in women before age 35 years and in women before age 45 years with first-degree family history [see comments]. JAMA 1998; 279:922–929.

Mancini DN, Rodenhiser DI, Ainsworth PJ, O'Malley FP, Singh SM, Xing W, Archer TK: CpG methylation within the 5′ regulatory region of the *BRCA1* gene is tumor specific and includes a putative CREB binding site. Oncogene 1998; 16:1161–1169.

Marks JR, Huper G, Vaughn JP, Davis PL, Norris J, McDonnell DP, Wiseman RW, Futreal PA, Iglehart JD: *BRCA1* expression is not directly responsive to estrogen. Oncogene 1997; 14:115–121.

Marquis ST, Rajan JV, Wynshaw-Boris A, Xu J, Yin GY, Abel KJ, Weber BL, Chodosh LA: The developmental pattern of *Brca1* expression implies a role in differentiation of the breast and other tissues. Nat Genet 1995; 11:17–26.

Marsh DJ, Coulon V, Lunetta KL, Rocca-Serra P, Dahia PL, Zheng Z, Liaw D, Caron S, Duboue B, Lin AY, et al.: Mutation spectrum and genotype–phenotype analyses in Cowden disease and Bannayan-Zonana syndrome, two hamartoma syndromes with germline *PTEN* mutation. Human Molecular Genetics 1998; 7:507–515.

Maugard CM, Charrier J, Bignon YJ: Allelic deletion at glutathione *S*-transferase M1 locus and its association with breast cancer susceptibility. Chem Biol Interact 1998; 111–112:365–375.

Maugard CM, Charrier J, Pitard A, Campion L, Akande O, Pleasants L, Ali-Osman F: Genetic polymorphism at the glutathione *S*-transferase (*GST*) *P1* locus is a breast cancer risk modifier. Int J Cancer 2001; 91:334–339.

Mavraki E, Gray IC, Bishop DT, Spurr NK: Germline *BRCA2* mutations in men with breast cancer. Br J Cancer 1997; 76:1428–1431.

Mavridou D, Gornall R, Campbell IG, Eccles DM: *TP53* intron 6 polymorphism and the risk of ovarian and breast cancer [letter]. Br J Cancer 1998; 77:676–677.

Mazoyer S, Dunning AM, Serova O, Dearden J, Puget N, Healey CS, Gayther SA, Mangion J, Stratton MR, Lynch HT, et al.: A polymorphic stop codon in *BRCA2* [letter]. Nat Genet 1996; 14:253–254.

McAllister KA, Haugen-Strano A, Hagevik S, Brownlee HA, Collins NK, Futreal PA, Bennett LM, Wiseman RW: Characterization of the rat and mouse homologues of the *BRCA2* breast cancer susceptibility gene. Cancer Res 1997; 57:3121–3125.

McCarthy EP, Burns RB, Coughlin SS, Freund KM, Rice J, Marwill SL, Ash A, Shwartz M, Moskowitz MA: Mammography use helps to explain differences in breast cancer stage at diagnosis between older black and white women [see comments]. Ann Intern Med 1998; 128:729–736.

Meijers-Heijboer H, van Geel B, van Putten WL, Henzen-Logmans SC, Seynaeve C, Menke-Pluymers MB, Bartels CC, Verhoog LC, van den Ouweland AM, Niermeijer MF, et al.: Breast cancer after prophylactic bilateral mastectomy in women with a *BRCA1* or *BRCA2* mutation. N Engl J Med 2001; 345:159–164.

Menin C, Banna GL, De Salvo G, Lazzarotto V, De Nicolo A, Agata S, Montagna M, Sordi G, Nicoletto O, Chieco-Bianchi L, et al.: Lack of association between androgen receptor CAG polymorphism and familial breast/ovarian cancer. Cancer Lett 2001; 168:31–36.

Merajver SD, Pham TM, Caduff RF, Chen M, Poy EL, Cooney KA, Weber BL, Collins FS, Johnston C, Frank TS: Somatic mutations in the *BRCA1* gene in sporadic ovarian tumours. Nat Genet 1995; 9:439–443.

Miki Y, Swensen J, Shattuck-Eidens D, Futreal PA, Harshman K, Tavtigian S, Liu Q, Cochran C, Bennett LM, Ding W, et al.: A strong candidate for the breast and ovarian cancer susceptibility gene *BRCA1*. Science 1994; 266:66–71.

Millikan RC, Pittman GS, Tse CK, Duell E, Newman B, Savitz D, Moorman PG, Boissy RJ, Bell DA: Catechol-*O*-methyltransferase and breast cancer risk. Carcinogenesis 1998; 19:1943–1947.

Millikan RC, Pittman GS, Tse CK, Savitz DA, Newman B, Bell D: Glutathione *S*-transferases *M1*, *T1*, and *P1* and breast cancer. Cancer Epidemiol Biomarkers Prev 2000; 9:567–573.

Mitrunen K, Jourenkova N, Kataja V, Eskelinen M, Kosma VM, Benhamou S, Kang D, Vainio H, Uusitupa M, Hirvonen A: Polymorphic catechol-*O*-methyltransferase gene and breast cancer risk. Cancer Epidemiol Biomarkers Prev 2001; 10:635–640.

Modan B, Hartge P, Hirsh-Yechezkel G, Chetrit A, Lubin F, Beller U, Ben-Baruch G, Fishman A, Menczer J, Ebbers SM, et al.: Parity, oral contraceptives, and the risk of ovarian cancer among carriers and noncarriers of a *BRCA1* or *BRCA2* mutation. N Engl J Med 2001; 345:235–240.

Monteiro AN: *BRCA1*: exploring the links to transcription. Trends Biochem Sci 2000; 25:469–474.

Morrell D, Cromartie E, Swift M: Mortality and cancer incidence in 263 patients with ataxia-telangiectasia. J Natl Cancer Inst 1986; 77:89–92.

Morrow M, Schnitt S: Lobular carcinoma in situ. In: Harris J, Lippman M, Morrow M, Hellman S (eds). Diseases of the Breast. Philadelphia: Lippincott/Raven, 1996:369–373.

Morrow M, Schnitt S, Harris J: Ductal carcinoma in situ. In: Harris J, Lippman M, Morrow M, Hellman S (eds). Diseases of the Breast. Philadelphia: Lippincott/Raven, 1996:355–368.

Narod SA, Brunet JS, Ghadirian P, Robson M, Heimdal K, Neuhausen SL, Stoppa-Lyonnet D, Lerman C, Pasini B, de los Rios P, et al.: Tamoxifen and risk of contralateral breast cancer in *BRCA1* and *BRCA2* mutation carriers: a case-control study. Lancet 2000; 356:1876–1881.

Narod SA, Feunteun J, Lynch HT, Watson P, Conway T, Lynch J, Lenoir GM: Familial breast-ovarian cancer locus on chromosome 17q12–q23 [see comments]. Lancet 1991; 338:82–83.

Narod SA, Ford D, Devilee P, Barkardottir RB, Lynch HT, Smith SA, Ponder BA, Weber BL, Garber JE, Birch JM, et al.: An evaluation of genetic heterogeneity in 145 breast-ovarian cancer families. Am J Hum Genet 1995a; 56:254–264.

Narod SA, Goldgar D, Cannon-Albright L, Weber B, Moslehi R, Ives E, Lenoir G, Lynch H: Risk modifiers in carriers of *BRCA1* mutations. Int J Cancer 1995b; 64:394–398.

Narod SA, Risch H, Moslehi R, Dorum A, Neuhausen S, Olsson H, Provencher D, Radice P, Evans G, Bishop S, et al.: Oral contraceptives and the risk of hereditary ovarian cancer [see comments]. N Engl J Med 1998; 339:424–428.

Nebert D: Polymorphism of human *CYP2D* genes involved in drug metabolism: possible relationship to individual cancer risk. Cancer Cells 1991; 3:93–96.

Nelen MR, Padberg GW, Peeters EA, Lin AY, van den Helm B, Frants RR, Coulon V, Goldstein AM, van Reen MM, Easton DF, et al.: Localization of the gene for Cowden disease to chromosome 10q22–23. Nat Genet 1996; 13:114–116.

Neuhausen SL, Mazoyer S, Friedman L, Stratton M, Offit K, Caligo A, Tomlinson G, Cannon-Albright L, Bishop T, Kelsell D, et al.: Haplotype and phenotype analysis of six recurrent *BRCA1* mutations in 61 families: results of an international study. Am J Hum Genet 1996; 58:271–280.

Newman B, Mu H, Butler LM, Millikan RC, Moorman PG, King MC: Frequency of breast cancer attributable to *BRCA1* in a population-based series of American women [see comments]. JAMA 1998; 279:915–921.

Nordling M, Karlsson P, Wahlstrom J, Engwall Y, Wallgren A, Martinsson T: A large deletion disrupts the exon 3 transcription activation domain of the *BRCA2* gene in a breast/ovarian cancer family. Cancer Res 1998; 58:1372–1375.

Offit K, Gilewski T, McGuire P, Schluger A, Hampel H, Brown K, Swensen J, Neuhausen S, Skolnick M, Norton L, et al.: Germline *BRCA1* 185delAG mutations in Jewish women with breast cancer [see comments]. Lancet 1996; 347:1643–1645.

Olsen JH, Hanemann JM, Borresen-Dale AL, Brondum-Neilsen K, Hammarstrom L, Kleinerman R, Kaarianen H, Lonnqvist T, Sankila R, Seersholm N, et al.: Cancer in patients with ataxia-telangiectasia and in their relatives in the Nordic countries. J Natl Cancer Inst 2001; 93.

Page DL, Dupont WD, Rogers LW, Jensen RA, Schuyler PA. Continued local recurrence of carcinoma 15–25 years after a diagnosis of low grade ductal carcinoma in situ of the breast treated only by biopsy. Cancer 1995; 76:1197–1200.

Park JJ, Irvine RA, Buchanan G, Koh SS, Park JM, Tilley WD, Stallcup MR, Press MF, Coetzee GA: Breast cancer susceptibility gene 1 (*BRCA1*) is a coactivator of the androgen receptor. Cancer Res 2000; 60:5946–5949.

Parkin DM: Cancers of the breast, endometrium and ovary: geographic correlations. Eur J Cancer Clin Oncol 1989; 25:1917–1925.

Parmigiani G, Berry D, Aguilar O: Determining carrier probabilities for breast cancer-susceptibility genes *BRCA1* and *BRCA2*. Am J Hum Genet 1998; 62:145–158.

Patel KJ, Vu VP, Lee H, Corcoran A, Thistlethwaite FC, Evans MJ, Colledge WH, Friedman LS, Ponder BA, Venkitaraman AR: Involvement of *Brca2* in DNA repair. Mol Cell 1998; 1:347–357.

Paull TT, Rogakou EP, Yamazaki V, Kirchgessner CU, Gellert M, Bonner WM: A critical role for histone H2AX in recruitment of repair factors to nuclear foci after DNA damage. Curr Biol 2000; 10:886–895.

Pero RW, Johnson DB, Markowitz M, Doyle G, Lund-Pero M, Seidegard J, Halper M, Miller DG: DNA repair synthesis in individuals with and without a family history of cancer. Carcinogenesis 1989; 10:693–697.

Peters WP: High-dose chemotherapy with autologous bone marrow transplantation for the treatment of breast cancer: yes. Important Adv Oncol 1995:215–230.

Petersen GM, Parmigiani G, Thomas D: Missense mutations in disease genes: a Bayesian approach to evaluate causality. Am J Hum Genet 1998; 62:1516–1524.

Peto J, Collins N, Barfoot R, Seal S, Warren W, Rahman N, Easton DF, Evans C, Deacon J, Stratton MR: Prevalence of *BRCA1* and *BRCA2* gene mutations in patients with early-onset breast cancer [see comments]. J Natl Cancer Inst 1999; 91:943–949.

Petrij-Bosch A, Peelen T, van Vliet M, van Eijk R, Olmer R, Drusedau M, Hogervorst FB, Hageman S, Arts PJ, Ligtenberg MJ, et al.: *BRCA1* genomic deletions are major founder mutations in Dutch breast cancer patients [published erratum appears in Nat Genet 1997 Dec; 17(4):503]. Nat Genet 1997; 17:341–345.

Petrini JH: The mammalian Mre11–Rad50–nbs1 protein complex: integration of functions in the cellular DNA-damage response. Am J Hum Genet 1999; 64:1264–1269.

Phelan CM, Rebbeck TR, Weber BL, Devilee P, Ruttledge MH, Lynch HT, Lenoir GM, Stratton MR, Easton DF, Ponder BA, et al.: Ovarian cancer risk in *BRCA1* carriers is modified by the *HRAS1* variable number of tandem repeat (VNTR) locus. Nat Genet 1996; 12:309–311.

Powles T, Eeles R, Ashley S, Easton D, Chang J, Dowsett M, Tidy A, Viggers J, Davey J: Interim analysis of the incidence of breast cancer in the Royal Marsden Hospital tamoxifen randomised chemoprevention trial [see comments]. Lancet 1998; 352:98–101.

Pujol P, Galtier-Dereure F, Bringer J: Obesity and breast cancer risk. Hum Reprod 1997; 12:116–125.

Rahman N, Teare MD, Seal S, Renard H, Mangion J, Cour C, Thompson D, Shugart Y, Eccles D, Devilee P, et al.: Absence of evidence for a familial breast cancer susceptibility gene at chromosome 8p12–p22. Oncogene 2000; 19:4170–4173.

Rajan JV, Marquis ST, Gardner HP, Chodosh LA: Developmental expression of *Brca2* colocalizes with *Brca1* and is associated with proliferation and differentiation in multiple tissues. Dev Biol 1997; 184:385–401.

Rajan JV, Wang M, Marquis ST, Chodosh LA: *Brca2* is coordinately regulated with Brca1 during proliferation and differentiation in mammary epithelial cells. Proc Natl Acad Sci USA 1996; 93:13078–13083.

Rebbeck TR: Molecular epidemiology of the human glutathione *S*-transferase genotypes *GSTM1* and *GSTT1* in cancer susceptibility. Cancer Epidemiol Biomarkers Prev 1997; 6:733–743.

Rebbeck TR, Kantoff PW, Krithivas K, Neuhausen S, Blackwood MA, Godwin AK, Daly MB, Narod SA, Garber JE, Lynch HT, et al.: Modification of *BRCA1*-associated breast cancer risk by the polymorphic androgen-receptor CAG repeat. Am J Hum Genet 1999a; 64:1371–1377.

Rebbeck TR, Levin AM, Eisen A, Snyder C, Watson P, Cannon-Albright L, Isaacs C, Olopade O, Garber JE, Godwin AK, et al.: Breast cancer risk after bilateral prophylactic oophorectomy in *BRCA1*. J Natl Cancer Inst 1999b; 91:1475–1479.

Rebbeck TR, Rosvold EA, Duggan DJ, Zhang J, Buetow KH: Genetics of *CYP1A1*: coamplification of specific alleles by polymerase chain reaction and association with breast cancer. Cancer Epidemiol Biomarkers Prev 1994; 3:511–514.

Rebbeck TR, Wang Y, Kantoff PW, Krithivas K, Neuhausen SL, Godwin AK, Daly MB, Narod SA, Brunet JS, Vesprini D, et al.: Modification of *BRCA1*- and *BRCA2*-associated breast cancer risk by *AIB1* genotype and reproductive history. Cancer Res 2001; 61:5420–5424.

Rhei E, Bogomolniy F, Federici MG, Maresco DL, Offit K, Robson ME, Saigo PE, Boyd J: Molecular genetic characterization of *BRCA1*- and *BRCA2*-linked hereditary ovarian cancers. Cancer Res 1998; 58:3193–3196.

Richardson CR, Deffenbaugh AM, Frank TS: Genetic analysis of *BRCA1* and *BRCA2* in 100 males with breast cancer. American Journal of Human Genetics, Annual Meeting Proceedings 2001; 69S: #418.

Ries LAG, Eisner MP, Kosary CL, Hankey BF, Miller BA, Clegg L, Edwards BK: SEER Cancer Statistics Review, 1973–1998. Bethesda, MD: National Cancer Institute, 2001.

Ries LAG, Kosary CL, Hankey BF, Miller BA, Edwards BK: SEER Cancer Statistics Review, 1973–1995. Bethesda, MD: National Cancer Institute, 1998.

Roa BB, Boyd AA, Volcik K, Richards CS: Ashkenazi Jewish population frequencies for common mutations in *BRCA1* and *BRCA2*. Nat Genet 1996; 14:185–187.

Roberts SA, Spreadborough AR, Bulman B, Barber JBP, Evans DGR, Scott D: Heretibility of cellular radiosensitivity: a marker of low-penetrance predisposition genes in breast cancer? Am J Hum Genet 1999; 65:784–794.

Roodi N, Bailey LR, Kao WY, Verrier CS, Yee CJ, Dupont WD, Parl FF: Estrogen receptor gene analysis in estrogen receptor-positive and receptor-negative primary breast cancer. J Natl Cancer Inst 1995; 87:446–451.

Rose DP, Royak-Schaler R: Tumor biology and prognosis in black breast cancer patients: a review. Cancer Detect Prev 2001; 25:16–31.

Rosen PP, Braun DW Jr, Kinne DE: The clinical significance of pre-invasive breast carcinoma. Cancer 1980; 46:919–925.

Rosen PP, Kosloff C, Lieberman PH, Adair F, Braun DW Jr: Lobular carcinoma in situ of the breast: detailed analysis of 99 patients with average follow-up of 24 years. Am J Surg Pathol 1978; 2:225–251.

Ross RK, Paganini-Hill A, Wan PC, Pike MC: Effect of hormone replacement therapy on breast cancer risk: estrogen versus estrogen plus progestin. J Natl Cancer Inst 2000; 92:328–332.

Sakurada A, Suzuki A, Sato M, Yamakawa H, Orikasa K, Uyeno S, Ono T, Ohuchi N, Fujimura S, Horii A: Infrequent genetic alterations of the *PTEN/MMAC1* gene in Japanese patients with primary cancers of the breast, lung, pancreas, kidney, and ovary. Jpn J Cancer Res 1997; 88:1025–1028.

Sameshima Y, Tsunematsu Y, Watanabe S, Tsukamoto T, Kawa-ha K, Hirata Y, Mizoguchi H, Sugimura T, Terada M, Yokota J: Detection of novel germ-line *p53* mutations in diverse cancer-prone families identified by selecting patients with childhood adrenocortical carcinoma. J Natl Cancer Inst 1992; 84:703–707.

Sasco AJ, Lowenfels AB, Pasker-de Jong P: Review article: epidemiology of male breast cancer: a meta-analysis of published case-control studies and discussion of selected aetiological factors. Int J Cancer 1993; 53:538–549.

Savelyeva L, Claas A, Gier S, Schlag P, Finke L, Mangion J, Stratton MR, Schwab M: An interstitial tandem duplication of 9p23–24 coexists with a mutation in the *BRCA2* gene in the germ line of three brothers with breast cancer. Cancer Res 1998; 58:863–866.

Savelyeva L, Claas A, Matzner I, Schlag P, Hofmann W, Scherneck S, Weber B, Schwab M: Constitutional genomic instability with inversions, duplications, and amplifications in 9p23–24 in *BRCA2* mutation carriers. Cancer Res 2001; 61:5179–5185.

Schutte M, da Costa LT, Hahn SA, Moskaluk C, Hoque AT, Rozenblum E, Weinstein CL, Bittner M, Meltzer PS, Trent JM, et al.: Identification by representational difference analysis of a homozygous deletion in pancreatic carcinoma that lies within the *BRCA2* region. Proc Natl Acad Sci USA 1995; 92:5950–5954.

Schwartz RA, Torre DP: The Muir-Torre syndrome: a 25-year retrospect [see comments]. J Am Acad Dermatol 1995; 33:90–104.

Scott D, Barber JB, Levine EL, Burrill W, Roberts SA: Radiation-induced micronucleus induction in lymphocytes identifies a high frequency of radiosensitive cases among breast cancer patients: a test for predisposition? Br J Cancer 1998; 77:614–620.

Scott D, Spreadborough A, Levine E, Roberts SA: Genetic predisposition in breast cancer [letter]. Lancet 1994; 344:1444.

Scott RJ, McPhillips M, Meldrum CJ, Fitzgerald PE, Adams K, Spigelman AD, du Sart D, Tucker K, Kirk J: Hereditary nonpolyposis colorectal cancer in 95 families: differences and similarities between mutation-positive and mutation-negative kindreds. Am J Hum Genet 2001; 68:118–127.

Scully R: Interactions between BRCA proteins and DNA structure. Exp Cell Res 2001; 264:67–73.

Scully R, Chen J, Ochs RL, Keegan K, Hoekstra M, Feunteun J, Livingston DM: Dynamic changes of BRCA1 subnuclear location and phosphorylation state are initiated by DNA damage. Cell 1997a; 90:425–435.

Scully R, Chen J, Plug A, Xiao Y, Weaver D, Feunteun J, Ashley T, Livingston DM: Association of *BRCA1* with Rad51 in mitotic and meiotic cells. Cell 1997b; 88:265–275.

Scully R, Livingston DM: In search of the tumour-suppressor functions of *BRCA1* and *BRCA2*. Nature 2000; 408:429–432.

Seitz S, Rohde K, Bender E, Nothnagel A, Pidde H, Ullrich O-M, El-Zehairy A, Haensch W, Jandrig B, Kolble K, et al.: Deletion mapping and linkage analysis provide strong indication for the involvement of the human chromosome region 8p12–p22 in breast carcinogenesis. Br J Cancer 1997; 76:983–991.

Sellers TA, Mink PJ, Cerhan JR, Zheng W, Anderson KE, Kushi LH, Folsom AR: The role of hormone replacement therapy in the risk for breast cancer and total mortality in women with a family history of breast cancer [see comments]. Ann Intern Med 1997; 127:973–980.

Serova O, Montagna M, Torchard D, Narod SA, Tonin P, Sylla B, Lynch HT, Feunteun J, Lenoir GM: A high incidence of *BRCA1* mutations in 20 breast-ovarian cancer families. Am J Hum Genet 1996; 58:42–51.

Sharan SK, Morimatsu M, Albrecht U, Lim DS, Regel E, Dinh C, Sands A, Eichele G, Hasty P, Bradley A: Embryonic lethality and radiation hypersensitivity mediated by Rad51 in mice lacking *Brca2* [see comments]. Nature 1997; 386:804–810.

Shattuck-Eidens D, Oliphant A, McClure M, McBride C, Gupte J, Rubano T, Pruss D, Tavtigian SV, Teng DH, Adey N, et al.: *BRCA1* sequence analysis in women at high risk for susceptibility mutations: risk factor analysis and implications for genetic testing [see comments]. JAMA 1997; 278:1242–1250.

Shayeghi M, Seal S, Regan J, Collins N, Barfoot R, Rahman N, Ashton A, Moohan M, Wooster R, Owen R, et al.: Heterozygosity for mutations in the ataxia telangiectasia gene is not a major cause of radiotherapy complications in breast cancer patients. Br J Cancer 1998; 78:922–927.

Shih HA, Nathanson KL, Seal S, Collins N, Stratton MR, Rebbeck TR, Weber BL: *BRCA1* and *BRCA2* mutations in patients with multiple primary cancers. Clin Cancer Res 2000; 11:4259–4264.

Shugart YY, Cour C, Renard H, Lenoir G, Goldgar D: Linkage analysis of 56 multiplex families excludes the Cowden disease gene *PTEN* as a major contributor to familial breast cancer. J Med Genet 1999; 36:720–721.

Sidransky D, Tokino T, Helzlsouer K, Zehnbauer B, Rausch G, Shelton B, Prestigiacomo L, Vogelstein B, Davidson N: Inherited *p53* gene mutations in breast cancer. Cancer Res 1992; 52:2984–2986.

Silverstein MJ: Ductal carcinoma in situ of the breast. Br J Surg 1997; 84:145–146.

Sjalander A, Birgander R, Hallmans G, Cajander S, Lenner P, Athlin L, Beckman G, Beckman L: *p53* polymorphisms and haplotypes in breast cancer. Carcinogenesis 1996; 17:1313–1316.

Smith SA, Easton DF, Evans DG, Ponder BA: Allele losses in the region 17q12–21 in familial breast and ovarian cancer involve the wild-type chromosome. Nat Genet 1992; 2:128–131.

Sodha N, Williams R, Mangion J, Bullock SL, Yuille MR, Eeles RA: Screening *hCHK2* for mutations. Science 2000; 289:359.

Solin LJ, Kurtz J, Fourquet A, Amalric R, Recht A, Bornstein BA, Kuske R, Taylor M, Barrett W, Fowble B, et al.: Fifteen-year results of breast-conserving surgery and definitive breast irradiation for the treatment of ductal carcinoma in situ of the breast. J Clin Oncol 1996; 14:754–763.

Southey MC, Batten LE, McCredie MR, Giles GG, Dite G, Hopper JL, Venter DJ: Estrogen receptor polymorphism at codon 325 and risk of breast cancer in women before age forty. J Natl Cancer Inst 1998; 90:532–536.

Spillman MA, Bowcock AM: BRCA1 and BRCA2 mRNA levels are coordinately elevated in human breast cancer cells in response to estrogen. Oncogene 1996; 13:1639–1645.

Spurdle AB, Hopper JL, Dite GS, Chen X, Cui J, McCredie MR, Giles GG, Southey MC, Venter DJ, Easton DF, et al.: *CYP17* promoter polymorphism and breast cancer in Australian women under age forty years. J Natl Cancer Inst 2000; 92:1674–1681.

Srivastava S, Tong YA, Devadas K, Zou ZQ, Sykes VW, Chen Y, Blattner WA, Pirollo K, Chang EH: Detection of both mutant and wild-type p53 protein in normal skin fibroblasts and demonstration of a shared "second hit" on *p53* in diverse tumors from a cancer-prone family with Li-Fraumeni syndrome. Oncogene 1992; 7:987–991.

Srivastava S, Zou ZQ, Pirollo K, Blattner W, Chang EH: Germ-line transmission of a mutated *p53* gene in a cancer-prone family with Li-Fraumeni syndrome [see comments]. Nature 1990; 348:747–749.

Stadtmauer EA, O'Neill A, Goldstein LJ, Crilley PA, Mangan KF, Ingle JN, Brodsky I, Martino S, Lazarus HM, Erban JK, et al.: Conventional-dose chemotherapy compared with high-dose chemotherapy plus autologous hematopoietic stem-cell transplantation for metastatic breast cancer. N Engl J Med 2000; 342:1069–1076.

Stallard S, Hole DA, Purushotham AD, Hiew LY, Mehanna H, Cordiner C, Dobson H, Mallon EA, George WD: Ductal carcinoma in situ of the breast—among factors predicting for recurrence, distance from the nipple is important. Eur J Surg Oncol 2001; 27:373–377.

Stambolic V, Suzuki A, de la Pompa JL, Brothers GM, Mirtsos C, Sasaki T, Ruland J, Penninger JM, Siderovski DP, Mak TW: Negative regulation of PKB/Akt-dependent cell survival by the tumor suppressor PTEN. Cell 1998; 95:29–39.

Stambolic V, Macpherson D, Sas D, Lin Y, Snow B, Jang Y: Regulation of PTEN transcription by p53. Mol Cell 2001; 8:317–325.

Starink TM, van der Veen JP, Arwert F, de Waal LP, de Lange GG, Gille JJ, Eriksson AW: The Cowden syndrome: a clinical and genetic study in 21 patients. Clin Genet 1986; 29:222–233.

Stratton MR, Ford D, Neuhasen S, Seal S, Wooster R, Friedman LS, King MC, Egilsson V, Devilee P, McManus R, et al.: Familial male breast cancer is not linked to the *BRCA1* locus on chromosome 17q. Nat Genet 1994; 7:103–107.

Strong LC, Williams WR, Tainsky MA: The Li-Fraumeni syndrome: from clinical epidemiology to molecular genetics. Am J Epidemiol 1992; 135:190–199.

Struewing JP, Abeliovich D, Peretz T, Avishai N, Kaback MM, Collins FS, Brody LC: The carrier frequency of the *BRCA1* 185delAG mutation is approximately 1 percent in Ashkenazi Jewish individuals [see comments] [published erratum appears in Nat Genet 1996; 12(1):110]. Nat Genet 1995; 11:198–200.

Struewing JP, Hartge P, Wacholder S, Baker SM, Berlin M, McAdams M, Timmerman MM, Brody LC, Tucker MA: The risk of cancer associated with specific mutations of *BRCA1* and *BRCA2* among Ashkenazi Jews [see comments]. N Engl J Med 1997; 336:1401–1408.

Suzuki A, de la Pompa JL, Hakem R, Elia A, Yoshida R, Mo R, Nishina H, Chuang T, Wakeham A, Itie A, et al.: Brca2 is required for embryonic cellular proliferation in the mouse. Genes Dev 1997; 11:1242–1252.

Swift M, Morrell D, Cromartie E, Chamberlin AR, Skolnick MH, Bishop DT: The incidence and gene frequency of ataxia-telangiectasia in the United States. Am J Hum Genet 1986; 39:573–583.

Swift M, Morrell D, Massey RB, Chase CL: Incidence of cancer in 161 families affected by ataxia-telangiectasia [see comments]. N Engl J Med 1991; 325:1831–1836.

Swift M, Reitnauer PJ, Morrell D, Chase CL: Breast and other cancers in families with ataxia-telangiectasia. N Engl J Med 1987; 316:1289–1294.

Syrjakoski K, Vahteristo P, Eerola H, Tamminen A, Kivinummi K, Sarantaus L, Holli K, Blomqvist C, Kallioniemi OP, Kainu T, et al.: Population-based study of *BRCA1* and *BRCA2* mutations in 1035 unselected Finnish breast cancer patients. J Natl Cancer Institute 2000; 92:1529–1531.

Szabo CI, King MC: Population genetics of *BRCA1* and *BRCA2* [editorial; comment]. Am J Hum Genet 1997; 60:1013–1020.

Szelei J, Jimenez J, Soto AM, Luizzi MF, Sonnenschein C: Androgen-induced inhibition of proliferation in human breast cancer MCF7 cells transfected with androgen receptor. Endocrinology 1997; 138:1406–1412.

TABCS Group: Prevalance of *BRCA1* and *BRCA2* mutations in a large population based series of breast cancer cases. Br J Cancer 2000; 83:1301–1308.

Taioli E, Trachman J, Chen X, Toniolo P, Garte SJ: A *CYP1A1* restriction fragment length polymorphism is associated with breast cancer in African-American women. Cancer Res 1995; 55:3757–3758.

Tavtigian SV, Simard J, Rommens J, Couch F, Shattuck-Eidens D, Neuhausen S, Merajver S, Thorlacius S, Offit K, Stoppa-Lyonnet D, et al.: The complete *BRCA2* gene and mutations in chromosome 13q-linked kindreds [see comments]. Nat Genet 1996; 12:333–337.

Thakur S, Zhang HB, Peng Y, Le H, Carroll B, Ward T, Yao J, Farid LM, Couch FJ, Wilson RB, et al.: Localization of *BRCA1* and a splice variant identifies the nuclear localization signal. Mol Cell Biol 1997; 17:444–452.

Thomas JE, Smith M, Tonkinson JL, Rubinfeld B, Polakis P. Induction of phosphorylation on *BRCA1* during the cell cycle and after DNA damage. Cell Growth Differ 1997; 8:801–809.

Thompson D, Easton D, Breast Cancer Linkage C: Variation in cancer risks, by mutation position, in *BRCA2* mutation carriers. Am J Hum Genet 2001; 68:410–419.

Thompson D, Szabo CI, Mangion J, Oldenburg RA, Odefrey F, Seal S, Borfoot R, Kroeze-Jansema K, Teare D, Rahman N et al.: Evaluation of linkage of breast cancer to the putative BRCA3 locus on chromosome 13q21 in 128 multiple case families from the Breast Cancer Linkage Consortium PNAS 2002; 98:827–831.

Thompson PA, Ambrosone C: Molecular epidemiology of genetic polymorphisms in estrogen metabolizing enzymes in human breast cancer. J Natl Cancer Inst Monographs 2000:125–134.

Thompson PA, Shields PG, Freudenheim JL, Stone A, Vena JE, Marshall JR, Graham S, Laughlin R, Nemoto T, Kadlubar FF, et al.: Genetic polymorphisms in catechol-*O*-methyltransferase, menopausal status, and breast cancer risk. Cancer Res 1998; 58:2107–2110.

Thorlacius S, Olafsdottir G, Tryggvadottir L, Neuhausen S, Jonasson JG, Tavtigian SV, Tulinius H, Ogmundsdottir HM, Eyfjord JE: A single *BRCA2* mutation in male and female breast cancer families from Iceland with varied cancer phenotypes [see comments]. Nat Genet 1996; 13:117–119.

Thorlacius S, Sigurdsson S, Bjarnadottir H, Olafsdottir G, Jonasson JG, Tryggvadottir L, Tulinius H, Eyfjord JE: Study of a single *BRCA2* mutation with high carrier frequency in a small population [see comments]. Am J Hum Genet 1997; 60:1079–1084.

Tirkkonen M, Johannsson O, Agnarsson BA, Olsson H, Ingvarsson S, Karhu R, Tanner M, Isola J, Barkardottir RB, Borg A, et al.: Distinct somatic genetic changes associated with tumor progression in carriers of *BRCA1* and *BRCA2* germ-line mutations. Cancer Res 1997; 57:1222–1227.

Tokunaga M, Land CE, Tokuoka S, Nishimori I, Soda M, Akiba S: Incidence of female breast cancer among atomic bomb survivors, 1950–1985. Radiation Research 1994; 138:209–223.

Trichopoulos D, MacMahon B, Cole P: Menopause and breast cancer risk. J Natl Cancer Inst 1972; 48:605–613.

Tsou HC, Teng DH, Ping XL, Brancolini V, Davis T, Hu R, Xie XX, Gruener AC, Schrager CA, Christiano AM, et al.: The role of *MMAC1* mutations in early-onset breast cancer: causative in association with Cowden syndrome and excluded in BRCA1-negative cases. Am J Hum Genet 1997; 61:1036–1043.

Unger MA, Nathanson KL, Calzone K, Antin-Ozerkis D, Shih HA, Martin AM, Lenoir GM, Mazoyer S, Weber BL: Screening for genomic rearrangements in families with breast and ovarian cancer identifies *BRCA1* mutations previously missed by conformation-sensitive gel electrophoresis or sequencing. Am J Hum Genet 2000; 67:841–850.

Ursin G, Henderson BE, Haile RW, Pike MC, Zhou N, Diep A, Bernstein L: Does oral contraceptive use increase the risk of breast cancer in women with *BRCA1/BRCA2* mutations more than in other women? Cancer Res 1997; 57:3678–3681.

Vahteristo P, Tamminen A, Karvinen P, Eerola H, Eklund C, Aaltonen LA, Blomqvist C, Aittomaki K, Nevanlinna H: *p53*, *CHK2*, and *CHK1* genes in Finnish families with Li-Fraumeni syndrome: further evidence of *CHK2* in inherited cancer predisposition. Cancer Res 2001; 61:5718–5722.

Varley JM, McGown G, Thorncroft M, Santibanez-Koref MF, Kelsey AM, Tricker KJ, Evans DG, Birch JM: Germ-line mutations of *TP53* in Li-Fraumeni families: an extended study of 39 families. Cancer Res 1997; 57:3245–3252.

Vasen HF, Morreau H, Nortier JW: Is breast cancer part of the tumor spectrum of hereditary nonpolyposis colorectal cancer? Am J Hum Genet 2001; 68:1533–1535.

Venkitaraman AR: Chromosome stability, DNA recombination and the BRCA2 tumour suppressor. Curr Opin Cell Biol 2001; 13:338–343.

Veronesi U, Maisonneuve P, Costa A, Sacchini V, Maltoni C, Robertson C, Rotmensz N, Boyle P: Prevention of breast cancer with tamoxifen: preliminary findings from the Italian randomised trial among hysterectomised women [see comments]. Lancet 1998; 352:93–97.

Vorechovsky I, Luo L, Lindblom A, Negrini M, Webster AD, Croce CM, Hammarstrom L: *ATM* mutations in cancer families. Cancer Res 1996; 56:4130–4133.

Vrieling H, van Zeeland AA, Mullenders LH: Transcription coupled repair and its impact on mutagenesis. Mutat Res 1998; 400:135–142.

Wang T, Lerer I, Gueta Z, Sagi M, Kadouri L, Peretz T, Abeliovich D: A deletion/insertion mutation in the *BRCA2* gene in a breast cancer family: a possible role of the Alu-polyA tail in the evolution of the deletion. Genes Chromosomes Cancer 2001; 31:91–95.

Wang Y, Cortez D, Yazdi P, Neff N, Elledge SJ, Qin J: BASC, a super complex of *BRCA1*-associated proteins involved in the recognition and repair of aberrant DNA structures. Genes Dev 2000; 14:927–939.

Wang-Gohrke S, Chang-Claude J, Becher H, Kieback DG, Runnebaum IB: Progesterone receptor gene polymorphism is associated with decreased risk for breast cancer by age 50. Cancer Res 2000; 60:2348–2350.

Wang-Gohrke S, Rebbeck TR, Besenfelder W, Kreienberg R, Runnebaum IB: p53 germline polymorphisms are associated with an increased risk for breast cancer in German women. Anticancer Res 1998; 18:2095–2099.

Warner E, Foulkes W, Goodwin P, Meschino W, Blondal J, Paterson C, Ozcelik H, Goss P, Allingham-Hawkins D, Hamel N, et al.: Prevalence and penetrance of *BRCA1* and *BRCA2* gene mutations in unselected Ashkenazi Jewish women with breast cancer. J Natl Cancer Inst 1999; 91:1241–1247.

Watson P, Lynch HT: Extracolonic cancer in hereditary nonpolyposis colorectal cancer. 1993; 71:677–685.

Welcsh PL, King MC: *BRCA1* and *BRCA2* and the genetics of breast and ovarian cancer. Hum Mol Genet 2001; 10:705–713.

Weston A, Godbold JH: Polymorphisms of *H-ras-1* and *p53* in breast cancer and lung cancer: a meta-analysis. Environ Health Perspect 1997; 105:919–926.

Weston A, Pan CF, Bleiweiss IJ, Ksieski HB, Roy N, Maloney N, Wolff MS: *CYP17* genotype and breast cancer risk. Cancer Epidemiol Biomarkers Prev 1998; 7:941–944.

Weston A, Pan CF, Ksieski HB, Wallenstein S, Berkowitz GS, Tartter PI, Bleiweiss IJ, Brower ST, Senie RT, Wolff MS: p53 haplotype determination in breast cancer. Cancer Epidemiol Biomarkers Prev 1997; 6:105–112.

White E: Projected changes in breast cancer incidence due to the trend toward delayed childbearing. Am J Public Health 1987; 77:495–497.

Williams WR, Anderson DE: Genetic epidemiology of breast cancer: segregation analysis of 200 Danish pedigrees. Genet Epidemiol 1984; 1:7–20.

Wilson CA, Payton MN, Elliott GS, Buaas FW, Cajulis EE, Grosshans D, Ramos L, Reese DM, Slamon DJ, Calzone FJ: Differential subcellular localization, expression and biological toxicity of BRCA1 and the splice variant BRCA1-δ11b. Oncogene 1997; 14:1–16.

Wilson CA, Ramos L, Villasenor MR, Anders KH, Press MF, Clarke K, Karlan B, Chen JJ, Scully R, Livingston D, et al.: Localization of human *BRCA1* and its loss in high-grade, non-inherited breast carcinomas. Nat Genet 1999; 21:236–240.

Wolden SL, Lamborn KR, Cleary SF, Tate DJ, Donaldson SS: Second cancers following pediatric Hodgkin's disease [see comments]. J Clin Oncol 1998; 16:536–544.

Wong AKC, Pero R, Ormonde PA, Tavtigian SV, Bartel PL: RAD51 interacts with the evolutionarily conserved BRC motifs in the human breast cancer susceptibility gene *Brca2*. J Biol Chem 1997; 272:31941–31944.

Wooster R, Bignell G, Lancaster J, Swift S, Seal S, Mangion J, Collins N, Gregory S, Gumbs C, Micklem G: Identification of the breast cancer susceptibility gene *BRCA2* [see comments] [published erratum appears in Nature 1996; 22;379(6567): 749]. Nature 1995; 378:789–792.

Wooster R, Mangion J, Eeles R, Smith S, Dowsett M, Averill D, Barrett-Lee P, Easton DF, Ponder BA, Stratton MR: A germline mutation in the androgen receptor gene in two brothers with breast cancer and Reifenstein syndrome. Nat Genet 1992; 2:132–134.

Wooster R, Neuhausen SL, Mangion J, Quirk Y, Ford D, Collins N, Nguyen K, Seal S, Tran T, Averill D, et al.: Localization of a breast cancer susceptibility gene, *BRCA2*, to chromosome 13q12–13. Science 1994; 265:2088–2090.

Wright J, Teraoka S, Onengut S, Tolun A, Gatti RA, Ochs HD, Concannon P: A high frequency of distinct *ATM* gene mutations in ataxia-telangiectasia. Am J Hum Genet 1996; 59:839–846.

Wynder EL, Cohen LA, Muscat JE, Winters B, Dwyer JT, Blackburn G: Breast cancer: weighing the evidence for a promoting role of dietary fat. J Natl Cancer Inst 1997; 89:766–775.

Xu X, Qiao W, Linke SP, Cao L, Li WM, Furth PA, Harris CC, Deng CX: Genetic interactions between tumor suppressors Brca1 and p53 in apoptosis, cell cycle and tumorigenesis. Nat Genet 2001; 28:266–271.

Yeh S, Hu YC, Rahman M, Lin HK, Hsu CL, Ting HJ, Kang HY, Chang C: Increase of androgen-induced cell death and androgen receptor transactivation by BRCA1 in prostate cancer cells. Proc Natl Acad Sci USA 2000; 97:11256–11261.

Yood MU, Johnson CC, Blount A, Abrams J, Wolman E, McCarthy BD, Raju U, Nathanson DS, Worsham M, Wolman SR: Race and differences in breast cancer survival in a managed care population. J Natl Cancer Inst 1999; 91:1487–1491.

Yuan JM, Yu MC, Ross RK, Gao YT, Henderson BE: Risk factors for breast cancer in Chinese women in Shanghai. Cancer Res 1988; 48:1949–1953.

Zhong Q, Chen CF, Li S, Chen Y, Wang CC, Xiao J, Chen PL, Sharp ZD, Lee WH: Association of BRCA1 with the hRad50–hMre11–p95 complex and the DNA damage response. Science 1999; 285:747–750.

Zhong S, Wyllie AH, Barnes D, Wolf CR, Spurr NK: Relationship between the *GSTM1* genetic polymorphism and susceptibility to bladder, breast and colon cancer. Carcinogenesis 1993; 14:1821–1824.

36 Familial and Genetic Influences on Risk of Lung Cancer

THOMAS A. SELLERS AND PING YANG

Lung cancer, a term denoting a heterogeneous group of carcinomas of the lung and bronchus, was an uncommon tumor in humans before cigarette smoking became widespread. Since 1950, lung cancer has been recognized as a major public health problem (Wynder and Graham, 1950) and has become the leading cause of all malignancies in men (Landis et al., 1998). For nearly a decade, the lung cancer mortality rate in American women has been the highest worldwide (Landis et al., 1998). It is estimated that in 1998 over 170,000 people developed lung cancer and over 160,000 people died from the disease in the United States alone. To put the problem in perspective, this is more than the total number of deaths from the next three most common cancers (breast, colon, prostate) combined (Landis et al., 1998).

The epidemic of lung cancer extends beyond the boundaries of the United States, and lung cancer continues to be the leading cause of cancer death in most countries (Kurihara et al., 1989). The average annual age-adjusted rates in some areas exceed 100/100,000, some of the highest reported for any cancer type (Parkin and Muir, 1992). Moreover, the international battle to reduce the epidemic caused by the use of tobacco products is not being won. There is clear evidence that the burden of disease is being transferred from rich to poor countries (Pandey et al., 1999). It has been projected that the tobacco-related mortality will rise from the present annual global toll of 3 million to over 10 million by the year 2025 (Mackay, 1994); 70% of these deaths will occur in developed countries.

Lung cancer has strong environmental influences. Tobacco smoke is the most obvious relevant exposure, but the list also includes radioactive ores, heavy metals, radon, and petrochemicals. Nonetheless, individuals vary widely in their response to these environmental insults. Recognizing that cigarette smoking was the principal cause of lung cancer, Goodhart (1959) noted:

> different individuals show wide variation in the type and strength of stimulus needed for a neoplastic reaction so that, although even quite light smokers run a significantly higher risk of lung cancer than nonsmokers, nine out of ten of the heaviest smokers never get it at all. Personal idiosyncrasy seems to be an important factor in carcinogenesis and this suggests the hypothesis that the population may be genetically heterogeneous for susceptibility to cancer, some individuals being more 'cancer prone' than others.

This chapter reviews the evidence to support this hypothesis.

DISEASE DEFINITION

Based on histopathology, clinical presentation, management, treatment responses, and overall prognosis, lung cancer is commonly divided into two categories: small cell lung cancer (SCLC) and non-small cell lung cancer (NSCLC). The NSCLC group includes a variety of cell types (Table 36–1), with squamous cell, adenocarcinoma, and SCLC being the three most common subtypes. Squamous cell carcinoma and SCLC are more closely associated with cigarette smoking than adenocarcinoma. Squamous cell carcinoma has been the predominant cell type in male lung cancer patients, whereas adenocarcinoma has been the predominant cell type in female patients and is more strongly associated with a positive family history of lung cancer (Satcher, 2001).

Most lung cancer cases are discovered through clinical symptoms and signs, which vary by tumor location and size (Larsson, 1973; Nesbitt et al., 1997). Typical symptoms include cough, hemoptysis, dyspnea, pneumonia, chest pain, shoulder pain, weight loss, bone pain, hoarseness, headaches, seizures, or swelling of the face or neck. A small proportion of patients are asymptomatic, and the diagnosis is an incidental finding on chest X-rays; these tumors are more likely to be small and in peripheral lung tissue (Nesbitt et al., 1997). A cough is the most common symptom, but because most patients with lung cancer are current or former smokers, many have had a cough for much of their lives. The definitive diagnosis of lung cancer always requires pathologic examination of tissue taken from biopsies, sputum, surgical resection, or autopsy. At the time of diagnosis, patients present with the disease in clinical stages ranging from stage I through stage IV. The proportion of patients in each stage at the time of diagnosis and the corresponding survival rate are given in Table 36–2. The 1-year survival rate is only 20% to 50% for advanced NSCLC (stage IIIA or above) and 25% for extensive SCLC. Five-year survival rates range from over 60% for stage IA to <3% for stage IV in NSCLC and from 10% for limited disease to 1% for extensive disease in SCLC.

GENERAL GENETIC AND EPIDEMIOLOGIC EVIDENCE

Tobacco use, especially cigarette smoking, has been recognized as a major risk factor for lung cancer for nearly 50 years throughout the world (Levin et al., 1950; Doll and Hill, 1952), and tobacco smoke is responsible for over 80% of the current lung cancer incidence (Lee and Forey, 1998). The rising prevalence of tobacco use in the United States has preceded by several decades a corresponding increase in lung cancer incidence and mortality. Searching for genetic predispositions has been motivated mainly by the paradox that fewer than 20% of long-term heavy smokers eventually develop lung cancer (Kreuzer et al., 2000; Wistuba and Gazdar, 2000).

Table 36–1. Modified World Health Organization Histologic Classification of Invasive Lung Cancer

Histologic Type	Percent
Squamous cell carcinoma	29.4
Small cell carcinoma	17.8
Pure small cell carcinoma	NA[a]
Mixed small cell and large cell carcinoma	NA
Combined small cell carcinoma	NA
Adenocarcinoma	31.5
Acinar adenocarcinoma	NA
Papillary adenocarcinoma	0.7
Bronchioloalveolar carcinoma	2.6
Solid carcinoma with mucus formation	0.1
Large cell carcinoma	9.2
Giant cell carcinoma	0.3
Clear cell carcinoma	NA
Adenosquamous carcinoma	1.4
Carcinoid tumor	1.0
Bronchial gland carcinoma	0.1
Adenoid cystic carcinoma	<0.1
Mucoepidermoid carcinoma	<0.1
Others	9.6

[a]NA, not available.
Data from World Health Organization (1981), Hirsch et al. (1988), and Travis et al. (1995).

Case Reports of Familial Aggregation of Cancer

Published case reports on the familial aggregation of lung cancer are rare. Brisman and colleagues (1967) reported a family in which four of eight siblings had lung cancer; Nagy (1968) described a family in which three of 15 siblings were affected; and Jones (1977) reported the clustering of bronchogenic carcinoma in three of five siblings. Goffman et al. (1982) studied two families with over 40% of siblings affected with lung cancer, Joishy et al. (1977) reported 58-year-old identical twins who developed alveolar cell carcinoma with nearly synchronous onset, and Paul et al. (1987) observed three siblings affected with the same histologic cell type. While dramatic case reports such as these may offer a striking clinical impression, they are insufficient evidence for the role of a genetic effect. In particular, rare familial clusters of a disease with such strong environmental influences may simply represent chance occurrence.

Table 36–2. Clinical Stage and Cumulative Survival Rate of Non-Small Cell Lung Cancer

	Cumulative Percent Survival by Years after Treatment				
Clinical Stage[a]	1	2	3	4	5
IA (n = 687)	91	79	71	67	61
IB (n = 1189)	72	54	46	41	38
IIA (n = 29)	79	49	38	34	34
IIB (n = 357)	59	41	33	26	24
IIIA (n = 511)	50	25	18	14	13
IIIB (n = 1030)	34	13	7	6	5
IV (n = 1427)	19	6	2	2	1

[a]Percentage distribution of cell types: adenocarcinoma, 47.2% (2466/5230); squamous cell carcinoma, 33.9% (1773/5230); large cell carcinoma, 3.1% (163/5230); small cell carcinoma, 11.9% (624/5230); NOS (otherwise not specified), 3.9% (204/5230).
Source: Mountain (1997) with permission.

Epidemiologic Studies of Family History and Families of Lung Cancer Patients

The question of whether or not lung cancer clusters in families has been evaluated in a number of case-control studies. The first landmark study of this type was conducted by Tokuhata and Lilienfeld (1963a,b). They showed that the occurrence of lung cancer among the parents and siblings of 270 lung cancer patients was three times greater than the frequency among relatives of the patients' spouses. This report remained uncorroborated for over 20 years, until the study by Ooi and colleagues (1986) in southern Louisiana. Studies conducted since these early reports demonstrate a wide range in the reported frequency of a family history of lung cancer (Table 36–3). However, the finding of a statistically significant excess occurrence of lung cancer among relatives of lung cancer cases is, with few exceptions (Lynch et al., 1986; Pierce et al., 1989; Wood et al., 2000), quite consistent. Similar findings have been observed when investigators considered the occurrence of cancer at all sites, although the magnitude of the risk elevation is generally lower (Samet et al., 1986; Schwartz et al., 1999). When examined on a site-specific basis, the malignancies observed to be most frequent were usually smoking-associated.

It is well known that cigarette smoking habits are familial in nature (Horn et al., 1959; Salber and MacMahon, 1961); that is, children are more likely to smoke if their parents also smoke. Therefore, when comparing the prevalence of lung cancer among relatives of lung cancer cases and controls, one must consider the distinct possibility that, unless cases and controls are matched on smoking behavior, relatives of cases would be more likely to smoke than relatives of controls. The clustering of such behaviors might well explain why lung cancer cases are more likely to have a positive family history of the disease than controls. To date, only four studies have been conducted in which smoking data on the majority of family members were collected. In the study by Tokuhata and Lilienfeld (1963a,b), the observed number of lung cancer deaths among men who smoked was twofold greater than expected (p = 0.01) and fourfold greater than expected among men who did not smoke (p = 0.02). Among nonsmoking female relatives, there was a 2.4-fold excess prevalence of lung cancer. The study by Ooi et al. (1986) in southern Louisiana found that the risk to smoking fathers of cases was increased fivefold, while the risk of lung cancer to nonsmoking female relatives of cases was elevated ninefold.

Table 36–3. Studies of Family History and Lung Cancer

	Lung Cancer		Any Cancer	
Reference	%	Odds ratio	%	Odds ratio
Ooi et al. (1986)	25.6	3.2	58.3	1.5
Samet et al. (1986)	6.9	5.3	31.3	1.6
McDuffie et al. (1988)	9.3	2.0	24.4	1.3
Shaw et al. (1991)	26.1	1.8	58.1	1.3
McDuffie et al. (1991)	2.6	2.0	13.2	1.2
Wu et al. (1996)[a]	8.9	1.3	42.2[b]	1.0
Schwartz et al. (1996, 1999)[a]	12.5	1.4	57.3	1.32[c]
Brownson et al. (1997)	13.5	1.3	61.0	1.1
Kreuzer et al. (1988)				
<45 years	10.0	2.6	33.5	1.2
55–69 years	7.0	1.4	35.5	0.9

[a]Patients were lifetime nonsmokers.
[b]Prevalence of a positive family history of cancers other than lung cancer.
[c]For the first-degree relatives who never smoked cigarettes.

The excess risk could not be explained by the distribution of age, sex, smoking status, pack-years of tobacco exposure, or a cumulative index of occupational/industrial exposures. The third study that considered specific environmental measures in family members was not restricted to patients with lung cancer. Since a number of studies had noted a greater-than-normal likelihood of cancer among relatives of lung cancer patients, Sellers and co-workers (1988) in southern Louisiana evaluated the familial risk of lung and other cancers among a randomly selected sample of cases with malignancy at any site. An excess of lung cancer was observed among relatives of lung cancer probands [odds ratio (OR) = 2.5] as well as among relatives of probands with cancers other than lung or breast (OR 1.6). This excess risk was evident even after allowing for each family member's age, sex, frequency of alcohol consumption, pack-years of tobacco consumption, and a cumulative index of occupational/industrial exposures. To more clearly delineate genetic from environmental factors that may underlie familial clusters, Schwartz et al. (1996) conducted a case-control family study of lung cancer among nonsmokers. Nonsmoking relatives of lung cancer patients were at 7.2-fold greater risk than relatives of controls among the subset of cases between the ages of 40 and 59; no excess risk was evident among nonsmoking relatives of cases aged 60 to 84 years.

In summary, studies in which specific environmental and lifestyle exposures were determined for individual family members suggest that, even after allowing for the effects of age, sex, and smoking, close relatives of lung cancer patients are still at an increased risk for the disease, especially among nonsmokers.

Studies of Family History by Histologic Cell Type

Adenocarcinoma of the lung demonstrates a weaker association with the use of tobacco products than does small cell, squamous cell, or large cell carcinomas of the lung. One might therefore expect to observe stronger evidence for familial factors in adenocarcinoma of the lung; most studies that have examined familial risk by histologic categories support this hypothesis. Wu et al. (1988) studied 336 females with adenocarcinoma of the lung and found that, after adjusting for personal smoking habits, cases were 3.9 times as likely to report a family history of lung cancer than neighborhood controls. Osann (1991) reported another study of females with lung cancer and noted a stronger association of family history of lung cancer with adenocarcinoma (OR 3.0) than with smoking-associated histologies (OR 1.4). Although Lynch et al. (1986) observed no association of histology with a family history of lung cancer, they did find that the greatest familial risk of smoking-associated cancers occurred among relatives of patients with adenocarcinoma. When Shaw et al. (1991) stratified their cases according to histology, the greatest familial risk was noted for cases with adenocarcinoma (OR 2.1) but significantly elevated risks were observed for other histologies: squamous cell (OR 1.9) and small cell (OR 1.7). In contrast to these studies is the report by Sellers et al. (1992a) of 300 lung cancer patients, which found the lowest familial risk among those with adenocarcinoma and the highest among those with small cell carcinoma. Ambrosone and colleagues (1993) examined family history of cancer at all sites in a much larger sample and observed the greatest familial risks among patients with small cell and squamous cell histologies. Carcinoid tumors of the lung have historically not been well represented in these studies, owing in part to the rarity of the disease. Investigators at the M.D. Anderson Cancer Center (Houston, TX) reviewed the medical records of 86 patients with carcinoid tumors of the lung diagnosed between 1959 and 1994. A family history of cancer was noted in 86% of the medical records and in 43% when only first-degree relatives were considered (Perkins et al., 1997). What is difficult to reconcile from these studies is the fact that cigarettes have not remained constant over time. For example, changes over time in the use of filters, the nicotine content, and the type of tobacco mean that even within a family the bronchial tissues of members may be exposed to quite different chemicals. Some studies suggest that histologic cell type presentation of lung cancer is associated with these characteristics of cigarettes (McDuffie et al., 1990)

Genetic and Environmental Models of Lung Cancer Susceptibility

Given the evidence that lung cancer clusters in families and is not accounted for by measured risk factors, it is reasonable to examine whether the pattern of disease is consistent with Mendelian transmission of a susceptibility gene. To date, few attempts to answer this question have been published.

Sellers et al. (1990) performed a complex segregation analysis on the 337 lung cancer families collected by Ooi et al. (1986) in southern Louisiana. Families included index cases (probands) and their parents, siblings, offspring, and spouses. A total of 4357 family members were studied, but because of missing values on tobacco consumption, only 3276 were included in the analysis. Excluding the probands, there were 86 families (35.6%) with at least one other family member affected with lung cancer (total $n = 106$ lung cancers). Results of the segregation analyses suggested that three hypotheses could be rejected: environmental ($p < 0.01$), no major gene ($p < 0.01$), and Mendelian recessive ($p < 0.05$). Although the Mendelian dominant hypothesis could not be rejected ($p = 0.075$), Mendelian codominant inheritance provided a significantly better fit to the data ($p > 0.90$). The estimated gene frequency, 0.052, implies that approximately 10% of the population can be expected to carry the putative gene. The model further estimates that 28% of the population, regardless of genotype, would develop lung cancer. Based on the parameters of the model, it was determined that the gene and its interaction with smoking contributed to 69%, 47%, and 22% of lung cancers through the ages of 50, 60, and 70, respectively. While these percentages are quite high, it is important to consider that only 6% of lung cancer cases are diagnosed before the age of 50 and approximately 22% before the age of 60. Therefore, based on these results, the actual number of lung cancers due to inheritance of a major susceptibility gene may be low.

Lung cancer rarely occurs in the absence of environmental exposure. The consequences of this fact on identification of inherited susceptibility are critical. In particular, if lung cancer is the result of a gene–environment interaction, then in the absence of environmental exposure (i.e., cigarette consumption), an inherited susceptibility to the disease is less likely to be expressed. Sellers et al. (1992) reasoned that in the southern Louisiana lung cancer families intergenerational differences in the prevalence of the relevant environmental exposures, particularly tobacco, may obscure the true pattern of inheritance of a genetic factor. The probands (index cases) selected for the Louisiana studies on lung cancer were ascertained over a 4-year period (1976–1979) and ranged in age at onset from 32 to 91 years. A potential complicating factor in these analyses is the temporal trend in smoking. In the United States, smoking was uncommon before World War I, after which time there was a dramatic increase in tobacco use.

Table 36–4. Penetrance Estimates of Lung Cancer Risk for Carriers and Noncarriers from Two Published Segregation Analyses

			Age in Years		
Genotype	Cigarette Smoking		50	60	70
Carrier	No	Yang et al. (1999)[a]	0.003–0.005	0.009–0.018	0.018–0.042
		Sellers et al. (1990)	0.001	0.006	0.031
	Yes	Yang et al. (1999)	0.013–0.020	0.038–0.072	0.072–0.156
		Sellers et al. (1990)[b]	0.011–0.052	0.057–0.164	0.171–0.249
Noncarrier	No	Yang et al. (1999)[c]	<0.0001	<0.0001	0.0001
		Sellers et al. (1990)	<0.0001	0.0004	0.0024
	Yes	Yang et al. (1999)	<0.0001	0.0001–0.0003	0.0003–0.0008
		Sellers et al. (1990)	0.0008–0.0044	0.0048–0.0251	0.0277–0.1060

[a]Range between female and male.
[b]Range between average and heavy smokers.
[c]Adjusted for history of passive smoking.

Because of this cohort phenomenon and the wide range in the age of the probands, there was little uniformity in the exposure of the parental generations to the use of tobacco products. Lung cancer families were partitioned into two groups: *(1)* probands older than age 60 at the time of ascertainment (born before World War I and unlikely to have parents who smoked) and *(2)* probands younger than age 60 at the time of ascertainment (higher probability of smoking among parents) (Sellers et al., 1992). Of the 337 lung cancer families studied, 106 were ascertained through a proband whose age at death was less than 60 years and 231 through a proband whose age at death was 60 years or greater. Results of the segregation analyses on the early-onset proband families (higher probability of smoking parents) suggested that the pattern of disease was consistent with autosomal dominant transmission of inherited predisposition. In contrast to the earlier publication, the proportion of the population who were susceptible increased from 28% to 60%. In the families ascertained through probands with older ages at onset, there was still evidence for a Mendelian effect, but none of the models could be distinguished as providing the best fit.

Although these findings are suggestive of a gene–environment interaction, no direct modeling of such an effect was performed. Gauderman and colleagues (1997) analyzed the same set of southern Louisiana families utilizing a Markov chain Monte Carlo approach to impute missing values on tobacco use. Evidence for a major gene effect was still determined, but the gene–environment interaction was not statistically significant.

To more fully resolve the potential confounding effect of intergenerational differences in tobacco exposure on the models of inherited susceptibility, Sellers and colleagues (1998) constructed a simulated population of lung cancer families with an underlying autosomal dominant predisposition to lung cancer. The population was constructed such that tobacco exposure varied over time in a manner consistent with the pattern observed in the United States. A total of 324 families with 380 cases of lung cancer were ascertained and analyzed. Curiously, although a dominant model of susceptibility had been simulated, both dominant and codominant hypotheses fit the data. These results underscore the potential danger of segregation analysis of complex traits in which exposure to known environmental influences may differ across generations and suggest that inherited susceptibility to lung cancer may be autosomal dominant.

Another approach to the problem of differential environmental influences is to select probands who are nonsmokers. For these individuals, the genetic susceptibility may be so high that even passive exposure to sidestream smoke could be sufficient to cause lung cancer. Yang et al. (1997a) performed a complex segregation analysis on 257 families ascertained through nonsmoking lung cancer probands. Cases were identified from the Metropolitan Detroit Cancer Surveillance System. Among the 2021 first-degree relatives, 24 males and 10 females were similarly affected. The best explanation for the family clusters was an environmental hypothesis, in apparent contrast to the results obtained from families ascertained through probands who smoke. Since previous studies have found the greatest evidence for a genetic influence on early-onset cases of lung cancer, these analyses were repeated after stratifying the families (Yang et al., 1999). The authors specifically tested the effects of a Mendelian diallelic gene, history of tobacco use, and history of selected chronic lung diseases in families with a proband diagnosed at the age of 60 years or older and in families with a younger proband. In older probands' families, no evidence of a major genetic effect was detected. A history of emphysema and tobacco-smoke exposure were found to be significant risk factors. In younger probands' families, a Mendelian codominant model with significant modifying effects of smoking and chronic bronchitis best explained the observed data (Yang et al., 1999).

As shown in Table 36–4, the results of the studies by Sellers et al. (1990) and Yang et al. (1999) are remarkably similar. This consistency lends credence to the hypothesis that familial aggregations of lung cancer may reflect an underlying single-gene predisposition. The parameters of these models may therefore be considered in efforts to localize the relevant gene or genes using model-based linkage analysis.

PATHOPHYSIOLOGY: BIOLOGIC BASIS OF GENETIC SUSCEPTIBILITY

Tobacco smoke is a complex mixture of over 4000 chemical constituents, of which at least 43 are animal carcinogens and some are known to be human carcinogens. The major categories of chemical exposures of interest include polycyclic aromatic hydrocarbons (e.g., benzo[a]pyrene), aromatic amines (e.g., 4-aminobiphenyl), tobacco-specific nitrosamines (e.g., 4-(methylnitrosamino)-1-(3-pyridyl)-1-butanone, or NNK), and free radical species. All are thought to contribute to the carcinogenic and mutagenic activity of cigarette smoke. Given our understanding of the strong environmental influences in the pathogenesis of lung cancer, the search for genetic influences has focused on interindividual variation in the metabolic activation of potentially carcinogenic chemicals and the covalent binding of the reactive carcinogen metabolites to DNA. Thus, genetic factors can be hypothesized to influence risk through the rate of mutation initiation and the efficiency of DNA repair processes. The former process is influenced by the balance of metabolic activation and detoxification of reactive electrophiles. The latter process can be assessed through measurement of DNA adducts, phenotypic measures of DNA repair capacity, or examination of genes known to be involved in the homeostasis of DNA integrity.

Chronic Pulmonary Diseases and Lung Cancer

A number of nonneoplastic lung diseases have been examined as risk factors for lung cancer and may shed some light on the underlying pathophysiology influencing risk. In a case-control study in Shanghai, risk of lung cancer was found to be increased by 50% among survivors of tuberculosis (TB) and by 100% among those diagnosed with TB within the previous 20 years (Zheng et al., 1987). The relative risk for lung cancer was higher for adenocarcinoma than squamous cell carcinoma, and the TB lesions and lung cancers were highly correlated in the anatomic site within the lung. In another study, the relative risk of lung cancer was increased significantly [OR 8.2, 95% confidence interval (CI) 1.3–54.4] in nonsmoking Hawaiian women with a previous history of TB (Hinds et al., 1982). In a study of nonsmokers with lung cancer, TB was found to be a significant risk factor in both case-control and complex segregation analyses (Schwartz et al., 1996; Yang et al., 1997a,b). A positive association of lung cancer with asthma, allergies, and pneumonia has been inconsistently reported (Vena et al., 1985; Osann, 1991; Alavanja et al., 1992; Sellers, 1996). In two population-based studies (Schwartz et al. 1996; Mayne et al. 1999), none of the latter three conditions was identified as a significant risk factor for lung cancer in never-smokers. However, in the second study, asthma was a strong risk factor (OR 4.3, 95% CI 1.2–15.2) for lung cancer among former smokers (Mayne et al., 1999).

Chronic obstructive pulmonary disease (COPD), including emphysema and chronic bronchitis, is the only group of chronic pulmonary nonmalignant diseases that has been recognized as sharing a common etiology with lung cancer with respect to both host and environmental factors (Cohen et al., 1977). Early studies suggested that both lung cancer and COPD could be due to cigarette smoking and, therefore, COPD could not be distinguished as an independent risk factor for lung cancer (Krowka, 1996). However, more recent studies on smoking and nonsmoking lung cancer cases have shown COPD to be an independent risk factor (Cohen, 1980; Samet et al., 1986; Nomura et al., 1991; Wu et al., 1995). A study from the Mayo Clinic (Skillrud et al., 1986) demonstrated that the 10-year cumulative lung cancer occurrence was four times higher in individuals with a history of COPD than in individuals without such a history. Tockman et al. (1987) also reported a significantly increased lung cancer risk among smokers with ventilatory obstruction based on a study of over 4000 individuals. Results from a large-scale genetic epidemiology study of COPD suggest that in both smokers and nonsmokers lung cancer and COPD share a familial component that is associated with pulmonary dysfunction (Cohen et al., 1977). Based on a study of 618 cases and 1402 controls, Alavanja et al. (1992) reported that 16% of lung cancer risk could be attributed to COPD after adjusting for smoking. In a study of 257 never-smoking lung cancer patients, COPD was again shown to be an independent risk factor for lung cancer (Schwartz et al., 1996; Yang et al., 1997b). These investigators found that emphysema (but not chronic bronchitis) was a significant risk factor for later-onset lung cancer (≥60 years at diagnosis) whereas chronic bronchitis (but not emphysema) was a significant risk factor for earlier-onset lung cancer (<60 years at diagnosis). COPD has also been shown to aggregate not only in families with the same diseases but also in families identified through lung cancer probands (Tokuhata and Lilienfeld, 1963a; Schwartz et al., 1996). One of the earliest studies found not only a greater than a twofold increase of lung cancer deaths in smoking and nonsmoking relatives of lung cancer cases, but also an excess of nonmalignant respiratory disease deaths in relatives of lung cancer cases (Tokuhata and Lilienfeld, 1963). Similar results were reported from a family study based on nonsmoking lung cancer probands (Schwartz et al., 1996; Yang et al., 1999). All of this evidence suggests a common genetic factor or pathologic mechanism that not only causes COPD but also confers a higher lung cancer risk.

α_1-Antitrypsin and α_1-Antitrypsin Deficiency

α_1-Antitrypsin (α_1AT), a protease inhibitor, is a secretory glycoprotein produced in the liver that neutralizes the effects of proteases in several organ systems, although predominantly in the lung (Cox, 1995). The major physiologic role of α_1AT in the lung is to bind and inhibit elastase, primarily elastase released from leukocytes in the lower respiratory tract. This release prevents the destruction of lung tissue (Paul, 1989). The level of α_1AT is a codominant trait determined by the *Pi* (protease inhibitor) locus on chromosome 14q32.1 [also referred to as the α_1AT deficiency (α_1AD) gene]. The normal range of serum or plasma α_1AT levels is 120 to 200 mg/dl by standard nephelometry (Beckman, 1994) but with marked increases due to a wide range of inflammatory conditions, infections, cancer, liver disease, or pregnancy (Crystal, 1989; Paul, 1989). Homozygotes for the deficient alleles of the α_1AD gene have serum/plasma concentrations at 0% to 60% of the normal α_1AT level, depending on the specific allele, and can develop α_1AD and its sequelae (Cox, 1995). It has been known for more than 30 years that individuals who are homozygous for α_1AD alleles can develop young age at onset and severe COPD (Cox, 1995). However, heterozygotes for the deficient alleles usually have approximately 60% of normal serum levels and normally do not have clinical diseases caused by α_1AD without additional environmental insults such as tobacco smoking.

It is believed that COPD develops in α_1AD individuals because of an imbalance between neutrophil elastase (a protease) and α_1AT levels in lung tissue. This imbalance leads to the destruction of alveolar cells by elastase and could be due to an excess of elastase and/or a lack of functional α_1AT (Fletcher and Peto, 1977). Tobacco smoke disturbs the balance between protease and protease inhibitor activity in lung tissue by stimulating neutrophils to secrete more elastase (Hunninghake and Crystal, 1983) and inactivating α_1AT (Hubbard et al., 1987). This process can lead to elastolytic destruction of lung tissue (Gadek et al., 1979). An important mechanism for the increased destruction of lung tissue in smokers appears to be oxidation. Free radicals, which are found in tobacco smoke, readily oxidize the methionine residue at position 358 of the α_1AT active site, interfering dramatically with complex formation of α_1AT with elastase (Crystal, 1989). In addition to its oxidative effects, smoking can act on neutrophils, which are increased in smokers. Neutrophils not only release oxidants and elastase but also release myeloperoxidase, which is an important inactivator of α_1AT (Kueppers, 1992).

Cigarette smoking has a major effect on both the age at onset and the course of pulmonary deterioration in individuals with α_1AT deficiency. In a study of 33 patients with emphysema and α_1AD, Janus et al. (1985) indicated a mean age at onset of dyspnea of 32 years in smokers and 51 years in nonsmokers. Measuring lung function, Evald et al. (1990) found that the decline to 50% of predicted forced expiratory volume occurred 17 years later in those who had never smoked than in smokers. The same authors also concluded that patients with severe α_1AD who smoked were at increased risk of developing emphysema at a significantly earlier age than nonsmokers (Evald et al., 1990). Cox et al. (1976) examined 163 COPD patients and reported that 17.8% carried a Z allele. Comparing patients with Pi MZ type and those with Pi MM type, the authors found that 50% of the Pi MZ patients developed emphysema before the age of 50 years vs. 13% of patients with Pi MM.

The potentially important role of proteases and protease inhibitors has been demonstrated using tumor tissue studies targeting neutrophil elastase (NE). As just mentioned, NE is the major substrate of α_1AT. Yamashita et al. (1997) measured the NE from NSCLC tumor extracts by an enzyme immunoassay and showed that it was closely involved in tumor progression. The immunoreactive NE concentration was significantly higher in patients with higher clinical stage disease (T4) with aortic invasion than in those with lower-staged disease. Similar results were observed for the free form of immunoreactive NE and for α_1AT–ir-NE complex form, i.e., 7.9 mg% to 17.4 mg% in higher-staged tumors vs. 1.2 mg% to 4.9 mg% in lower-staged tumors ($p < 0.003$). These results indicate that tumor NE is closely associated with the direct extension of NSCLC. In another study using an enzyme-linked immunosorbent assay, Sakuma et al. (1995) measured NE activity in pleural effusion and peripheral blood of lung cancer patients who underwent lobectomy. NE levels were increased significantly; however, α_1AT levels did not increase in pleural effusion, showing an imbalance between NE and α_1AT in surgically treated lung cancer patients. Both of these studies focused on NE or the counterpart of α_1AT, suggesting that α_1AT may act as a suppressor in tumor progression. From these types of study, it is hard to draw a concrete causal relationship between NE and tumor progression without knowing the NE levels before disease development. In addition, a protease inhibitor derived from soybeans, Bowman Birk inhibitor (BBI) (Kennedy et al., 1996), has been reported to significantly decrease tumor growth in SCLC and other cancer cell lines (Clark et al., 1993). BBI decreases mRNA for prohormone convertases 1 and 2 by 50%. These results suggest that inhibitors of proteases may be potent suppressors of SCLC growth at the level of genes. BBI was also shown to block the development of lung tumors in mice (Witschi and Kennedy, 1989; Ekrami et al., 1993). As a naturally produced protease inhibitor, α_1AT could possess the same tumor-suppressing property as BBI. Further research in this area is necessary.

GENE IDENTIFICATION

As reviewed above, several studies suggest that the clustering of lung cancer in families may reflect an underlying single-gene defect. Unfortunately, efforts to locate the major gene(s) predisposing to lung cancer in the human genome, by either traditional parametric or nonparametric linkage methods, have not proven fruitful. This is mainly due to the extreme difficulty in collecting multiplex families that would be informative for analysis. In particular, the high case fatality and short survival rates from lung cancer make it rare to identify families with multiple living lung cancer cases. As a result, no published studies of lod score linkage analysis can be found in the literature, although a number of investigators are actively working in this area.

An alternative strategy to identify lung cancer susceptibility genes is to conduct association studies employing case-control designs. Most of the studies conducted to date have used unrelated cases and controls to examine the association of genetic polymorphisms in candidate genes with lung cancer risk. The candidate genes that have been considered are those mentioned in the earlier section on the biologic basis of genetic susceptibility. In the following sections, we provide a more detailed description of the loci that have been evaluated along with evidence that they influence risk of lung cancer.

Genetic Variation in Metabolic Activation

The cytochrome P-450 (CYP)–dependent mono-oxygenases are the first line of defense in the human body against toxic lipophilic chemicals (Bouchardy et al., 2001). They function by adding an atom of molecular oxygen into the substrate, which leads to an increase in hydrophilicity and facilitation of further metabolic processing and excretion (Nebert, 1991). However, during this process, certain inactive carcinogens are transformed into active forms capable of causing DNA damage. This in turn can lead to additional acquired mutations and ultimately cancer development. Many of the CYP-dependent genes are genetically polymorphic in the population, and three of them, *CYP1A1*, *CYP2D6*, and *CYP2E1*, have been studied in multiple populations in relation to lung cancer risk.

The *CYP1A1* gene is involved in the metabolism of polycyclic aromatic hydrocarbons. *CYP1A1* has several polymorphisms, depending on the restriction endonuclease used. The first is the MspI restriction fragment length polymorphism, which produces an M_1 (common) and an M_2 (rare) allele. In a Japanese study, individuals who were homozygous for the M_2 allele were at sevenfold greater risk of smoking-associated lung cancer (Nakachi et al., 1991). A second MspI polymorphism in *CYP1A1* has been identified (substitution of isoleucine for valine in the heme-binding region). These polymorphisms have been associated with lung cancer risk in two Japanese populations, particularly in squamous cell carcinoma, but not in at least five Caucasian populations (Hirvonen, 1995). The frequency of the polymorphisms is higher among the Japanese than Caucasians (Hirvonen et al., 1992), but it is unlikely that the inconsistency in the literature is simply a reflection of relatively small studies in Caucasian populations. Rather, there is emerging consensus that structural variation at the *CYP1A1* locus is unrelated to lung cancer risk. In fact, since *CYP1A1* is inducible, there is considerable rationale for further studies of the aromatic hydrocarbon (Ah) receptor, which induces *CYP1A1* expression after appropriate stimulation by polycyclic aromatic hydrocarbons.

Debrisoquine hydroxylase (encoded by *CYP2D6*) is one of the most thoroughly studied human enzyme deficiencies. Impaired enzyme activity is associated with a common polymorphism that affects 5% to 10% of the Caucasian population. Debrisoquine is an adrenergic blocking agent used to control blood pressure in hypertensive patients. Metabolism of the drug varies considerably in the population (10- to 200-fold difference); poor metabolizers (homozygous recessive carriers) experience a toxic acute response to the drug. Ayesh and colleagues (1984) examined the association of phenotypic ability to metabolize debrisoquine in a case-control study of 245 lung cancer patients and 234 controls. All subjects were smokers, and study groups were comparable on age and sex distributions. Among the cases, nearly 80% were characterized as extensive metabolizers compared to only 28% of controls. These striking differences spurred numerous subsequent investigations to replicate the findings.

The *CYP2D6* polymorphism (located on chromosome 22) has been conventionally classified as either a poor metabolizer or an extensive metabolizer, determined by the input–output ratio of a test drug, debrisoquine (Hirvonen, 1995). An obvious concern is that the disease itself might influence the ability to metabolize the drug, thereby causing misclassification of genotype. The studies that have relied on phenotyping have yielded conflicting results (Shaw et al., 1998). Consequently, investigations have relied on direct genotyping. Polymerase chain reaction–based methods have been developed to characterize the five major poor metabolizer–associated alleles and a deletion allele. The three most defective alleles of *CYP2D6* in Caucasians are *CYP2D6A* (deletion of A 2637 in exon 5), *CYP2D6B* (G 1934 $\rightarrow$ A transition), and *CYP2D6D* (entire gene deletion) (Hirvonen, 1995). Given the knowledge that *CYP2D6* is capable of activating the procarcinogen NNK found in tobacco smoke (Penman et al., 1993), this gene merits consideration as having some role in lung cancer susceptibility. Unfortunately, the weight of the evidence suggests that if *CYP2D6* does influence lung cancer risk, it is a minor contribution (Wolf et al., 1992; London et al., 1997; Shaw et al., 1998).

CYP2E1 is another P-450 enzyme that is involved in the metabolic activation of chemical carcinogens, especially nitrosamines contained in tobacco smoke and other low molecular weight compounds. In addition, it reduces dioxygen to radical species, thereby contributing to lipid peroxidation and oxidative stress (Ekstrom and Ingelman-Sundberg, 1989). Polymorphisms in *CYP2E1* have been identified using DraI and RsaI restriction enzymes. Two Japanese studies (Uematsu et al., 1991; Oyama et al., 1997) initially reported that lung cancer cases had a lower frequency of the DraI variant allele than controls, especially at lower levels of tobacco exposure (Uematsu et al., 1994). The association with the DraI polymorphism was not replicated in studies conducted in Finland (Hirvonen et al., 1993), Sweden (Persson et al., 1993), and the United States (Kato et al., 1992). The DraI polymorphism was determined to be a risk factor for lung cancer in a small case-control study of minority populations in the United States (overall OR 2.4, 95% CI 1.1–5.3) (Wu et al., 1998). The risk was evident among men who had ever smoked but not among women or never-smokers. Moreover, the association was evident among Mexican Americans but not African Americans (Wu et al., 1998).

A third case-control study conducted in Japan examined the *CYP2E1* RsaI polymorphism but found no association (Watanabe et al., 1995). A case-control study of lung cancer that included Caucasians and African Americans in southern California also failed to observe an association with the RsaI polymorphism (London et al., 1996). Le Marchand and colleagues (1998) examined the DraI and RsaI polymorphisms in a large population-based case-control study of lung cancer among Caucasian, Japanese, and native Hawaiians in Hawaii. Individuals who were homozygous for the rare variants were at 10-fold lower risk of lung cancer than subjects homozygous for the wild-type allele. This association was especially evident for adenocarcinoma and small cell histologies, which is consistent with results from a smaller study conducted in Texas (el-Zein et al., 1997) that found an overall 3.5-fold greater risk for carriers of a rare PstI site polymorphism, largely a reflection of a 16-fold greater risk for adenocarcinoma. One interpretation of these results is that there exists a tobacco-specific nitrosamine association with lung cancer that is influenced by genetically mediated differences in metabolism.

Many of the aromatic hydrocarbons and aromatic amines contained in cigarette smoke may also be activated by *CYP1A2*, *CYP3A4*, *CYP3A5*, *NQO1*, epoxide, and myeloperoxidase hydrolases. The association of these genetic markers with lung cancer risk has not been adequately studied. Some of the early results are worth noting, however. Metabolism of polycyclic aromatic hydrocarbons can frequently result in the production of reactive and toxic epoxides. Epoxides can be detoxicated and activated by the polymorphic enzyme epoxide hydrolase. Two functional polymorphisms have been identified in exons 3 and 4 of the gene. A hospital-based case-control study of French Caucasian smokers found that intermediate and high activities of microsomal epoxide hydrolase were associated with 1.7- and 2.7-fold greater risk of lung cancer, respectively (Benhamou et al., 1998). The association was independent of *GSTM1* and *CYP1A1* genotypes. NQO1, also known as NAD(P)H:quinone oxidoreductase 1 (Lind et al, 1990), is a flavoprotein catalyzing carcinogenic quinoid compounds into their reduced forms. The *NQO1* gene is located on chromosome 16q22, and its C $\rightarrow$ T point mutation results in a proline to serine substitution in the amino acid sequence of the protein. In a study by Xu and coworkers (2001) on 814 lung cancer patients and 1123 controls, an interaction between *NQO1* genotype and cigarette smoking was found. Individuals with the *T/T* genotype are at greater risk of lung cancer if they are long-term smokers.

Genetic Variation in Carcinogen Detoxification

Metabolic enzymes in the glutathione (GSH) family are important candidates in lung cancer susceptibility because of their involvement in the metabolism of a wide range of carcinogens and chemotherapeutic agents (Hayes and Pulford, 1995). Polymorphisms of GSH and the related enzyme system (Fig. 36–1) have been well characterized for glutathione *S*-transferase π (GSTπ), GSTμ, GSTθ (Zhong et al., 1991). GSTμ detoxifies tobacco-related and other carcinogens (e.g., benzo[*a*]pyrene, styrene-7,8-oxide, and *trans*-stilbene oxide). The gene *GSTM1*, which encodes GSTμ (chromosome 1p13.3), has three identified alleles (a, b, and null). GSTθ (chromosome 22q11.2) detoxifies low molecular weight toxins such as ethylene oxide and methyl-halogenids, methyl bromide, epoxybutanes, and holomethanes (Hayes and Pulford, 1995; Rebbeck, 1997). The gene *GSTT1*, which encodes GSTθ, has the same allele system as *GSTM1*. GSTθ detoxifies tobacco-related carcinogens and anticancer agents. *GSTP1*, the gene encoded for GSTπ polymorphisms (Mannervik et al., 1992; Harris et al., 1998), has been associated with acquired resistance to certain anticancer drugs (Hayes and Strange, 1995). Substrate specificity could influence their capacity to metabolize different environmental carcinogens and pharmacologic agents. Therefore, absence of or deficiency in GST activity could result in retention of active carcinogens or toxic compounds (e.g., drugs) in the body, which may cause DNA damage or drug resistance, respectively.

γ-Glutamyl cysteine synthetase (γ-GCS) is the rate-limiting enzyme in GSH biosynthesis (Walsh et al., 1996). A trinucleotide (GAG) marker with multiple alleles has been identified. Three

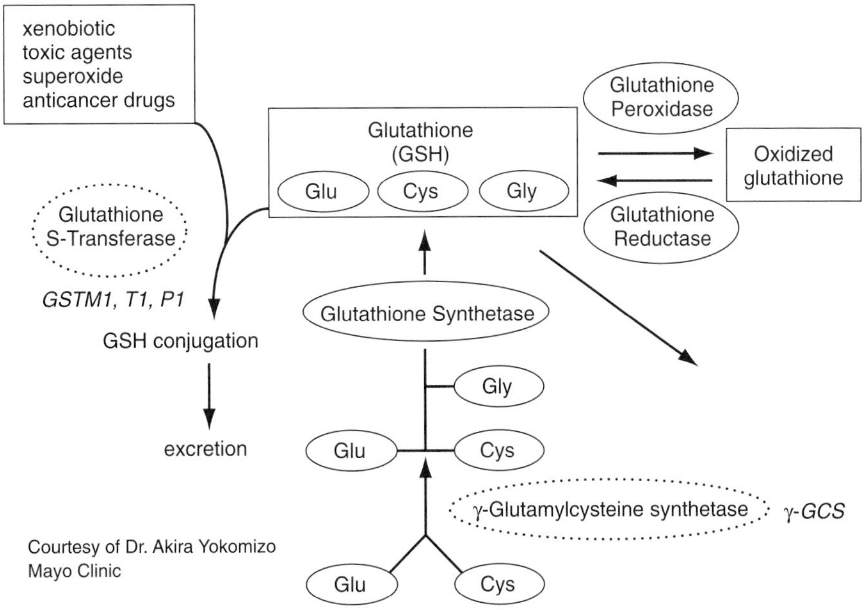

Fig. 36–1. Glutathione and its associated enzymes.

frequent alleles for this marker are labeled 7, 8, and 9 (Liu et al., 1998). The relationship of the allele types with cancer has not been reported, although GSH levels have been associated with anticancer agent sensitivity and response.

Because of the strong correlation between phenotype (enzyme activity levels) and genotype assays for *GST* genes in general (Zhong et al., 1991; Kempkes et al., 1996), it is reliable to use polymorphic genotypes to identify individuals who lack or have low activity of these enzymes. The frequency of homozygous deletion (null) genotypes in both *GSTM1* and *GSTT1* varies substantially by ethnicity (Rebbeck, 1997). For *GSTM1*, the null genotype ranges from 0.36 to 0.67 in Caucasians, from 0.33 to 0.63 in East Asians, and from 0.22 to 0.35 in Africans and African Americans. Approximately 45% of U.S. Caucasians lack a functional allele, and the null genotype is a risk factor for multiple cancers including lung (Rebbeck, 1997). For the *GSTT1* null type, the highest frequency is observed in East Asians (0.38–0.58), then Africans and African Americans (0.24–0.38), and the lowest in Caucasians. Twenty percent of U.S. Caucasians lack a functional allele, and the null genotype has been associated with a group of cancers (Zhong et al., 1991; Rebbeck, 1997). The reported frequency for lacking one allele at codon 105 of *GSTP1* is 18% to 42% (Harris et al., 1998).

McWilliams et al. (1995) conducted a review and meta-analysis of 12 case-control studies with a total of 1593 cases and 2135 controls. They concluded that the *GSTM1* null genotype confers a moderate but significant increased risk for lung cancer (OR 1.4, 95% CI 1.2–1.6). The association appears to be evident for all histologic types, and because the prevalence of *GSTM1* deficiency is high, genetic variation at this locus could account for 17% of all lung cancer cases. A more recent review that included *GSTT1* and additional studies, Rebbeck (1997) suggested that much of the published evidence comes from studies in Japan. In fact, the estimated OR among Caucasian populations is only 1.17. Subsequent studies have not clarified the picture. Three additional studies conducted in the United States have found weak associations. A study in southern California (London et al. 1995) found a modest and non-statistically significant association of homozygous null genotype and lung cancer risk among African Americans (OR 1.20, 95% CI 0.72–2.00) and Caucasians (OR 1.37, 95% CI 0.91–2.06). The association was evident among light, but not heavy, smokers. A large case-control study conducted in Boston also generated null results (Garcia-Closas et al., 1997), as did a case-control study in Texas that included African Americans and Mexican Americans (Kelsey et al., 1997). A small study conducted in Spain (To-Figueras et al., 1997) found a greater frequency of the null genotype among cases than population-based controls (OR 1.57, 95% CI 0.99–2.51). The association appeared to be most evident for small cell and adenocarcinoma histologies, light rather than heavy smokers (50 pack-years cut point), and those with onset at older ages (cut point 59 years). A Swedish study found a slightly inverse association of *GSTM1* null genotype and lung cancer risk in a sample enriched for women (74.6%) and never-smokers (48.2%) (Nyberg et al., 1998). A similar lack of association was observed in a Portuguese population (Moreira et al., 1996). In summary, the null genotype at the *GSTM1* locus appears to be a risk factor in Japanese but not in Caucasian populations.

Given that tobacco smoke is a complex mixture of chemicals, several groups of investigators have begun to examine several GSHs in combination as risk factors for lung cancer. For example, there is little evidence that either the *GSTT1* or *GSTP1* null genotype alone increases lung cancer risk (Deakin et al., 1996; Kelsey et al., 1997; Ryberg et al., 1997; To-Figueras et al., 1997; Harris et al., 1998; Saarikoski et al., 1998). However, individuals null for both *GSTM1* and *GSTT1* appear to be at elevated risk, especially for squamous cell carcinoma and with low levels of cigarette exposure (Saarikoski et al., 1998). Kelsey and colleagues (1997) found that individuals who lacked functional genes at both loci were at 2.9-fold elevated risk ($p < 0.05$). This result is similar to that of Saarikoski et al. (1998) in Finland, who observed a 2.3-fold excess risk ($p < 0.05$). Lung cancer patients in a Norwegian study who had null genotypes at the *GSTP1* and *GSTM1* loci had higher DNA adduct levels than cases with other genotype distributions (Ryberg et al., 1997), suggesting biologic plausibility for the association. However, results are not entirely consistent (Deakin et al., 1996; To-Figueras et al., 1997). Therefore, additional studies with larger sample sizes are required to clarify the issue.

N-Acetyltransferases (NATs), encoded by *NAT1* and *NAT2*, constitute another xenobiotic metabolizing enzyme system that detoxifies and/or bioactivates carcinogens found in tobacco or occupation-related exposures such as aromatic amines (Kadlubar et al., 1992). Rapid, normal, and slow acetylators have been classified in human populations by phenotypic and genotypic assays (Bell et al., 1993; Lin et al., 1993; Vineis et al., 1994). A Swedish study showed no association overall but a potential interaction between *NAT2* genotype and smoking history: slow acetylators are at higher lung cancer risk among never-smokers, whereas rapid acetylators are at a higher risk among smokers (Nyberg et al., 1998). Without adjusting for smoking status, a Spanish study (Martinez et al., 1995) observed that cases were 1.75 times more likely (95% CI 0.99–3.12) to be homozygous slow acetylators than controls. Similar observations were made by a group of Japanese investigators, who found a twofold greater risk ($p < 0.5$), primarily among patients younger than 65 years at diagnosis who had adenocarcinomas (Oyama et al., 1997). In contrast, a study from Germany found that fast acetylators were at 2.4-fold increased risk (Cascorbi et al., 1996). Adjustment for age, sex, and smoking increased the OR to 3.0 (95% CI 1.37–6.75). In addition to these conflicting findings, other studies have found no association (Bouchardy et al., 1998).

In a study of French Caucasian smokers in Switzerland (Bouchardy et al., 1998), homozygous *NAT1* rapid acetylators were found to be at the lowest cancer risk. The significant ORs were 4.0, 6.4, and 11.7 for heterozygous rapid, homozygous normal, and heterozygous slow acetylators, respectively. These results were evident after adjustment for age, sex, smoking, and occupational exposures. A small study (45 cases and 47 controls) from Texas found a 6.8-fold increased risk for rapid acetylators among subjects younger than 60 years and a 2.2-fold excess for subjects older than 60 years (Abdel-Rahman et al., 1998). If verified in other studies, these data suggest that *NAT1* polymorphisms may be some of the strongest genetic risk factors for lung cancer yet identified.

Yang et al. (1996) investigated whether clusters of various cancers in lung cancer families were associated with combined enzyme genotypes of the lung cancer probands. They found that the *mut/mut NAT2* genotype was associated with an increased cancer risk in first-degree relatives of lung cancer patients. Moreover, patients with combined *null* at *GST*μ and *mut/mut* at *NAT2* had an over threefold increased risk of having cancer-affected first-degree relatives. In a pilot study at the Mayo Clinic, Yang et al. (1998) found that *GSTM1* null and *NAT2** slow genotypes may be related to earlier age at onset of lung cancer and increased cancer risk in first-degree relatives of lung cancer probands. Interactions between *NAT2* and *GSTM1* genotypes, between *NAT2* genotype and aromatic DNA adduct level, and between *NAT2* genotype and *HPRT* reporter gene mutation frequency were examined in a Swedish case-control study (Hou et al., 2001). *NAT2* slow genotype combined with *GSTM1* null genotype may increase adduct level, mutation frequency and lung cancer risk among smokers with relatively low exposure (<24 pack-years of cigarettes).

As pointed out by Raunio et al. (1995), there are three limitations to research investigating genetic polymorphisms and risk of lung cancer: *(1)* many of the observed polymorphisms represent mutations in introns or other silent areas of DNA and, thus, any reported marker–disease association could simply reflect chance (or linkage disequilibrium); *(2)* underlying biologic mechanisms are sometimes lacking, making it difficult to understand a correlation of genotype and cancer; and *(3)* wide-range heterogeneity for background allele frequencies exists in most of the genes investigated so far.

α_1AD and Lung Cancer

It is not known whether α_1AD or carriers are associated with an increased lung cancer risk, especially after exposure to tobacco smoke. Because of the debilitating consequences (Brantly et al., 1988; Crystal et al., 1989), individuals who are known to have α_1AD usually have minimal or no tobacco smoke exposure (Alpha$_1$-Antitrypsin Deficiency Registry Study Group, 1994). These homozygous and symptomatic α_1AD individuals have a much shorter life span (<50 years) than the general population, decreasing the likelihood that lung cancer will be observed (Larsson, 1978). Although α_1AD carriers do not normally suffer from severe α_1AD-related diseases, they may be especially vulnerable to carcinogen-containing tobacco smoke, especially when their α_1AT levels are compromised under physiologic stress or from subclinical lung tissue damage. In a small study at the Mayo Clinic, Yang et al. (1997b) reported a possible association between α_1AD carriers and lung cancer compared to the expected general population carrier rate. Schwartz et al. (1998) found 15.6% and 5.8% α_1AD carrier rates for nonsmoking cases ($n = 32$) and controls ($n = 137$), respectively. After adjusting for age, gender, race, and passive smoking, there was a 13.7-fold increased risk of lung cancer in nonsmoking α_1AD carriers who were under 60 years of age. Given the biologic plausibility, it is somewhat surprising that more research in this area has not been conducted. Part of the answer may lie in the results of Harris et al. (1976). They reported that there was no difference in the α_1AT allele distribution between patients diagnosed with lung cancer and controls who were referred for sputum cytology evaluation to rule out lung cancer. Among the 196 controls in that study, however, only 53 (27.0%) had normal cytology while the remainder had regular or atypical (mild to marked) squamous metaplasia. The α_1AD carrier rate ranged from 13.2% for those with normal cytology to 27.8% for those with marked atypical squamous metaplasia; all rates were greater than the expected carrier rate in the general population. Thus, use of a control group with an unusually high carrier rate might have disguised the higher carrier rate in lung cancer patients. An investigation using appropriate control groups is clearly needed to directly test the association between α_1AD carriers and lung cancer risk.

CLINICAL APPLICATION AND RISK ASSESSMENT OF GENETICS INFORMATION

Primary Prevention

Primary prevention of lung cancer is obviously predicated upon the ability to control cigarette smoking. Tremendous effort has been expended by the Centers for Disease Control and Prevention (CDC) of the United States government and numerous non-profit agencies, clinicians, and public health professionals to reduce smoking prevalence in the U.S. population from 29% in 1987 to 15% in 2000. Based on a recent CDC report (Center for Disease Control, 1997), 50 million Americans are current smokers and each year 1.5 million become daily smokers. Each day in the United States 3000 adolescents begin smoking. In fact, 95% of all smokers become addicted before their eighteenth birthday. An appalling fact is that even if someone quits smoking today, it will still take 15 to 20 years to normalize the chance of dying from lung cancer. Over one-fourth of children under age 6 are regularly exposed to passive smoke. Passive smoking alone kills over 3000 Americans from lung cancer each year (American Cancer Society, 1998). Therefore, it could be a century-long effort to wipe out the effect of tobacco smoking on lung cancer incidence and mortality from current smokers, passive smokers, and former smokers. Meanwhile, a large number of lung cancer cases will continue to occur, with dismal chances of survival (Girard et al., 2000; Merrill, 2000). It is conceivable that knowledge of genetic susceptibility might provide additional impetus for individuals to quit smoking or to not adopt the habit in the first place.

Screening and Early Detection

Since even with the best primary prevention efforts lung cancer will continue to be a major medical problem, secondary prevention of lung cancer will be increasingly important. This implies efforts in early detection and screening. It is well known that cancers detected early have an inherently better outcome and chance for a cure. Of the four most common cancers, lung cancer is the only one for which screening is not recommended. That may be changing soon because of exciting new technological breakthroughs in spiral computed tomography (CT). Briefly, spiral CT is the newest generation of CT and lends special promise as a screening tool (Kaneko et al., 1996). Unfortunately, despite its potential, the high cost of spiral CT precludes its use in the general population as a routine screening tool. However, its value may be greatly enhanced when applied to high-risk individuals (Tockman and Mulshine, 2000; Allan et al., 2001).

Therapy

Tertiary prevention of lung cancer includes strategies to improve prognosis and minimize sequelae. Identification of factors that affect survival is vitally important for clinicians in predicting outcome and selecting the best treatment (Komaki et al., 1985). For both NSCLC and SCLC, disease staging is the most important predictor of survival (Mountain, 1997; Nesbitt et al., 1997). Many of these prognostic factors overlap with etiologic factors in lung cancer, such as gender, age, and concurrent pulmonary diseases. Several tumor markers, e.g., mutations in the *p53* and *Rb* genes and deletions on the short arm of chromosome 3, have been associated with both lung cancer development and prognosis (Testa, 1996). However, based on the myriad genetic alterations found in tumor tissues, it is difficult to distinguish those that play a role in susceptibility or early tumorigenicity from those that are important for disease progression or prognosis. It is very important to detect and compare genetic changes in biologic specimens between high-risk individuals and lung cancer patients.

Identifying genetic markers for cancer prognosis is a new and rapidly evolving field in translational research (Goto et al., 1996; Lear et al., 1997). When exposed to anticancer drugs, a critical survival trait is the maintenance of cellular homeostasis (Shen et al., 1997). Sequential and coordinated pathways are required for the conjugation and elimination of drugs and their metabolites. Drug resistance is a consequence of changes in the expression of multiple gene products. Genetic markers of this complex metabolic system, particularly those in the GSH pathway (discussed earlier), are emerging as candidate genes responsible for chemosensitivity and clinical responses and thus bear great prognostic potential (Carmichael et al., 1988). Evidence from tumor tissue and in vitro cell line studies over the past decade indicates that levels of GSH and GSH-dependent enzymes are partially responsible for anticancer drug resistance as well as for prognosis of various human cancers. For example, a number of detoxification and/or protective gene products have been shown to be overexpressed in experimental tumor cell lines with the drug-resistant phenotypes γ-GCS, GSTπ, GSTμ, and GSTθ. Two lines of evidence have demonstrated the important role of these enzymes in anticancer treatment responses and sensitivity. First, elevated GSH and/or GSH-dependent enzyme levels correlate with poorer treatment responses (Bedford et al., 1987; Ali-Osman et al., 1989). Second, inhibition or reduction of GSH and/or GSH-dependent enzymes could sensitize the treatment responses (Lutzky et al., 1989; Benathan et al., 1992). Nakanishi et al. (1997) reported that GSH derivatives inhibited GST activity in human lung cancer cell lysates, PC-9, suggesting that GSH derivatives (*S*-decyl, *S*-octyl, and *S*-hexyl GSHs) enhance doxorubicin (Adriamycin)–induced cytotoxicity. Thus, inhibition of GST may be useful as a chemosensitizer for doxorubicin treatment. Fujiwara et al. (1990) did not find a difference in mRNA expression and protein levels of GSTπ or -μ between two NSCLC cell lines, one being the wild-type line PC-9 and the other the cisplatin-resistant line PC-9/CDDP. However, the investigators did not test the expression and protein level of the more relevant gene, γ-*GCS*.

Most studies suggest that overexpression of *GSTM1*, *GSTT1*, and especially *GSTP1* or elevated levels of the corresponding enzymes is associated with poor prognosis in cancer patients. Inoue et al. (1995) tested a series of 105 NSCLC tissues and determined that 52% had elevated GSTπ expression. In the group with high GSTπ expression, all cases demonstrated a relapse when using cisplatin after a complete resection. Bai et al. (1996) studied bronchial biopsy samples from 38 NSCLC patients treated with cisplatin-based combination chemotherapy. The response rate of GSTπ-negative patients was 69% and that of GSTπ-positive patients was 12% ($p = 0.0012$). However, Campling et al. (1993) failed to find alterations in the levels of GSH and related enzymes in association with chemosensitivity in SCLC tumors. A common drawback of these studies is the lack of adjustment for disease stage or tumor histology; thus, comparability is poor.

Although these studies of altered gene expression are interesting, a more appropriate question is whether the response is a reflection of inherited variation at these loci. Only a handful of studies have examined the prognostic significance of polymorphic genes that encode drug detoxification enzymes (Chen et al., 1997; Lear et al., 1997), and only one has examined lung cancer (Goto et al., 1996). In a group of 232 patients with NSCLC, Goto et al. (1996) reported that the *GSTM1* null type was associated with the extent of regional lymph node metastasis (N factor) and the extent of distant metastasis (M factor). However, *GSTM1* null type had no effect on the 3-year survival rate. Treatment methods were not considered in their analysis, and other GSH-dependent enzyme genes were not measured. This area would appear to be both important and ripe for further investigation.

REFERENCES

Abdel-Rahman SZ, el-Zein RA, Zwischenberger JB, Au WW: Association of the NAT1*10 genotype with increased chromosome aberrations and higher lung cancer risk in cigarette smokers. Mutat Res 1998; 398:43–54.

Alavanja MCR, Brownson RC, Boice JD, Hock E: Preexisting lung disease and lung cancer among nonsmoking women. Am J Epidemiol 1992; 136:623–632.

Ali-Osman F, Caughlan J, Gray GS: Decreased DNA interstrand cross-linking and cytotoxicity induced in human brain tumor cells by 1,3-bis(2-chloroethyl)-1-nitrosourea after in vitro reaction with glutathione. Cancer Res 1989; 49:5954–5958.

Allan JM, Hardie LJ, Briggs JA, Davidson LA, Watson JP, Pearson SB, Muers MF, Wild CP: Genetic alterations in bronchial mucosa and plasma DNA from individuals at high risk of lung cancer. Int J Cancer 2001; 91:359–365.

Alpha$_1$-Antitrypsin Deficiency Registry Study Group: A registry of patients with severe deficiency of alpha$_1$-antitrypsin. Chest 1994; 106:1223–1232.

Ambrosone CB, Rao U, Michalek AM, Cummings KM, Mettlin CJ: Lung cancer histologic types and family history of cancer. Analysis of histologic subtypes of 872 patients with primary lung cancer. Cancer 1993; 72:1192–1198.

American Cancer Society: Cancer Facts and Figures—1998. Atlanta: American Cancer Society, 1998.

Ayesh R, Idle JR, Ritchie JC, Crothers MJ, Hetzel MR: Metabolic oxidation phenotypes as markers for susceptibility to lung cancer. Nature 1984; 312:169–170.

Bai F, Nakanishi Y, Kawasaki M, Takayama K, Yatsunami J, Pei XH, Tsuruta N, Wakamatsu L, Hara N: Immunohistochemical expression of glutathione *S*-transferase-π can predict chemotherapy response in patients with nonsmall cell lung carcinoma. Cancer 1996; 78:416–421.

Beckman: Instructions 015-247517-E. Brea, CA: Beckman Instruments, 1994.

Bedford P, Walker MC, Sharma HL, Perera A, McAuliffe CA, Masters JR, Hill BT: Factors influencing the sensitivity of two human bladder carcinoma cell lines to *cis*-diamminedichloroplatinum(II). Chem-Biol Interact 1987; 61:1–15.

Bell DA, Taylor JA, Butler MA, Stephens EA, Wiest J, Brubaker LH, Kadlubar FF, Lucier GW: Genotype/phenotype discordance for human arylamine *N*-acetyltransferase (*NAT2*) reveals a new slow-acetylator allele common in African-Americans. Carcinogenesis 1993; 14:1689–1692.

Benathan M, Alvero-Jackson H, Mooy AM, Scaletta C, Frenk E: Relationship between melanogenesis, glutathione levels and melphalan toxicity in human melanoma cells. Melanoma Res 1992; 2:305–314.

Benhamou S, Reinikainen M, Bouchardy C, Dayer P, Hirvonen A: Association between lung cancer and microsomal epoxide hydrolase genotypes. Cancer Res 1998; 58:5291–5293.

Bouchardy C, Benhamou S, Jourenkova N, Dayer P, Hironen A: Metabolic genetic polymorphisms and susceptibility to lung cancer. Lung Cancer 2001; 32:109–112.

Bouchardy C, Mitrunen K, Wikman H, Husgafvel-Pursiainen K, Dayer P, Benhamou S, Hirvonen A: *N*-Acetyltransferase *NAT1* and *NAT2* genotypes and lung cancer risk. Pharmacogenetics 1998; 8:291–298.

Brantly ML, Paul LD, Miller BH, Falk RT, Wu M, Crystal RG: Clinical features and natural history of the destructive lung disease with alpha-1-antitrypsin deficiency of adults with pulmonary symptoms. Am Rev Respir Dis 1988; 138:327–336.

Brisman R, Baker RR, Elkins R, Hartmann WH: Carcinoma of the lung in four siblings. Cancer 1967; 20:2048–2053.

Brownson RC, Alavanja MC, Caporaso N, Berger E, Chang JC: Family history of cancer and risk of lung cancer in lifetime non-smokers and long-term ex-smokers. Int J Epidemiol 1997; 26:256–263.

Campling BG, Baer K, Baker HM, Lam YM, Cole SP: Do glutathione and related enzymes play a role in drug resistance in small cell lung cancer cell lines? Br J Cancer 1993; 68:327–335.

Carmichael J, Forrester LM, Lewis AD, Hayes JD, Hayes PC, Wolf CR: Glutathione *S*-transferase isoenzymes and glutathione peroxidase activity in normal and tumour samples from human lung. Carcinogenesis 1988; 9:1617–1621.

Cascorbi I, Brockmoller J, Mrozikiewicz PM, Bauer S, Loddenkemper R, Roots I: Homozygous rapid arylamine *N*-acetyltransferase (*NAT2*) genotype as a susceptibility factor for lung cancer. Cancer Res 1996; 56:3961–3966.

Centers for Disease Control: Smoking-attributable mortality and years of potential life—United States, 1984. Morbidity and Mortality Weekly Report. 46(20), 1997:444–451.

Chen CL, Liu Q, Pui CH, Rivera GK, Sandlund JT, Ribeiro R, Evans WE, Relling MV: Higher frequency of glutathione *S*-transferase deletions in black children with acute lymphoblastic leukemia. Blood 1997; 89:1701–1707.

Clark DA, Day R, Seidah N, Moody TW, Cuttitta F, Davis TP: Protease inhibitors suppress in vitro growth of human small cell lung cancer. Peptides 1993; 14:1021–1028.

Cohen BH: Chronic obstructive pulmonary disease: a challenge in genetic epidemiology. Am J Epidemiol 1980; 112:274–288.

Cohen BH, Graves CG, Levy DA, Permutt S, Diamond EL, Kreiss P, Menkes HA, Quaskey S, Tockman MS: A common familial component in lung cancer and chronic obstructive pulmonary disease. Lancet 1977; 2:523–526.

Cox DW: Alpha-1 antitrypsin deficiency. In: Scriver CR, Beaudet AL, Sly WS, Valle D (eds). The Metabolic and Molecular Bases of Inherited Disease. New York: McGraw-Hill, 1995:4125–4158.

Cox DW, Hoeppner VH, Levinson H: Protease inhibitors in patients with chronic obstructive pulmonary disease: the alpha-1 antitrypsin heterozygote controversy. Am Rev Respir Dis 1976; 113:601–606.

Crystal RG: The alpha-1 antitrypsin gene and its deficiency state. Trends Genet 1989; 5:411–417.

Crystal RG, Brantly ML, Hubbard RC, Curiel DT: The alpha$_1$-antitrypsin gene and its mutations. Chest 1989; 95:196–208.

Deakin M, Elder J, Hendrickse C, Peckham D, Baldwin D, Pantin C, Wild N, Leopard P, Bell DA, Jones P, et al.: Glutathione *S*-transferase *GSTT1* genotypes and susceptibility to cancer: studies of interactions with *GSTM1* in lung, oral, gastric and colorectal cancers. Carcinogenesis 1996; 17:881–884.

Doll R, Hill AB: A study of the aetiology of carcinoma of the lung. BMJ 1952; 2:1271–1286.

Ekrami H, Kennedy AR, Witschi H, Shen WC: Cationized Bowman-Birk protease inhibitor as a targeted cancer chemopreventive agent. J Drug Target 1993; 1:41–49.

Ekstrom G, Ingelman-Sundberg M: Rat liver microsomal NADPH-supported oxidase activity and lipid peroxidation dependent on ethanol-inducible cytochrome P450 (P-450 IIE1). Biochem Pharmacol 1989; 38:1313–1319.

el-Zein RA, Zwischenberger JB, Abdel-Rahman SZ, Sankar AB, Au WW: Polymorphism of metabolizing genes and lung cancer histology: prevalence of *CYP2E1* in adenocarcinoma. Cancer Lett 1997; 112:71–78.

Evald T, Dirksen A, Keittelmann S, Viskum K, Kok-Jensen A: Decline in pulmonary function in patients with α_1-antitrypsin deficiency. Lung 1990; 168(Suppl):579–585.

Fletcher C, Peto R, Tinker C, Speizer FE: The natural history of chronic airflow obstruction. Br Med J. 1977 Jun 25; 1(6077):1645–1648.

Fujiwara Y, Sugimoto Y, Kasahara K, Bungo M, Yamakido M, Tew KD, Saijo N: Determinants of drug response in a cisplatin-resistant human lung cancer cell line. Jpn J Cancer Res 1990; 81:527–535.

Gadek JE, Fells GA, Crystal RG: Cigarette smoking induces functional antiprotease deficiency in the lower respiratory tract of humans. Science 1979; 206:1315–1316.

Garcia-Closas M, Kelsey KT, Wiencke JK, Xu X, Wain JC, Christiani DC: A case-control study of cytochrome P450 1A1, glutathione *S*-transferase M1, cigarette smoking and lung cancer susceptibility. Cancer Causes Control 1997; 8:544–553.

Gauderman WJ, Morrison JL, Carpenter CL, Thomas DC: Analysis of gene–smoking interaction in lung cancer. Genet Epidemiol 1997; 14:199–214.

Girard L, Zochbauer-Muller S, Virmani AK, Gazdar AF, Minn JD: Genome-wide allelotyping of lung cancer identifies new regions of allelic loss, differences between small cell lung cancer and non-small cell lung cancer, and loci clustering. Cancer Res 2000; 60:4894–4906.

Goffman TE, Hassinger DD, Mulvihill JJ: Familial respiratory tract cancer: opportunities for research and prevention. JAMA 1982; 247:1020–1023.

Goodhart CB: Cancer-proneness and lung cancer. Practitioner 1959; 182:578–584.

Goto I, Yoneda S, Yamamoto M, Kawajiri K: Prognostic significance of germ line polymorphisms of the *CYP1A1* and glutathione *S*-transferase genes in patients with non-small cell lung cancer. Cancer Res 1996; 56:3725–3730.

Harris CC, Cohen MH, Connor R, Primack A, Saccomanno G, Talamo RC: Serum alpha$_1$-antitrypsin in patients with lung cancer or abnormal sputum cytology. Cancer 1976; 38:1655–1657.

Harris MJ, Coggan M, Langton L, Wilson SR, Board PB: Polymorphism of the pi class glutathione *S*-transferase in normal populations and cancer patients. Pharmacogenetics 1998; 8:27–31.

Hayes JD, Pulford DJ: The glutathione *S*-transferase supergene family: regulation of GST and the contribution of the isoenzymes to cancer chemoprotection and drug resistance. Crit Rev Biochem Mol Biol 1995; 30:445–500.

Hayes JD, Strange RC: Potential contribution of the glutathione *S*-transferase supergene family to resistance to oxidative stress. Free Radic Res 1995; 22:193–207.

Hinds MW, Cohen HI, Kolonel LN: Tuberculosis and lung cancer risk in nonsmoking women. Am Rev Respir Dis 1982; 125:776–778.

Hirsch FR, Matthews MJ, Aisner S, Campobasso O, Elema JD, Gazdar AF, Mackay B, Nasiell M, Shimosato Y, Steele, RH, et al.: Histopathologic classification of small cell lung cancer: changing concepts and terminology. Cancer 1988; 62:973–977.

Hirvonen A: Genetic factors in individual responses to environmental exposures. J Occup Environ Med 1995; 37:37–43.

Hirvonen A, Husgafvel-Pursiainen K, Anttila S, Karjalainen A, Vainio H: The human *CYP2E1* gene and lung cancer: *Dra*I and *Rsa*I restriction fragment length polymorphisms in a Finnish study population. Carcinogenesis 1993; 14:85–88.

Hirvonen A, Husgafvel-Pursiainen K, Karjalainen A, Vainio H: Point-mutational *Msp*I and *Ile-Val* polymorphisms closely linked in the *CYP1A1* gene: lack of association with susceptibility to lung cancer in a Finnish study population. Cancer Epidemiol Biomarkers Prev 1992; 1(6):485–489.

Horn D, Courts FA, Taylor RM, Solomon ES: Cigarette smoking among high school students. Am J Public Health 1959; 49:1497–1511.

Hou SM, Falt S, Nyberg F, Pershagen G, Hemminki K, Lambert B: Differential interactions between *GSTM1* and *NAT2* genotypes on aromatic DNA adduct level and *HPRT* mutant frequency in lung cancer patients and population controls. Cancer Epidemiol Biomarkers Prev 2001; 10:133–140.

Hubbard RC, Ogushi F, Fells GA, Cantin AM, Courtney M, Crystal RG: Oxidants spontaneously released by alveolar macrophages of cigarette smokers can inactivate the active site of α_1-antitrypsin rendering it ineffective as an inhibitor of neutrophil elastase. J Clin Invest 1987; 80:1289–1295.

Hunninghake GW, Crystal RG: Cigarette smoking and lung destruction: accumulation of neutrophils in the lungs of cigarette smokers. Am Rev Respir Dis 1983; 128:833–838.

Inoue T, Ishida T, Sugio K, Maehara Y, Sugimachi K: Glutathione *S*-transferase pi is a powerful indicator in chemotherapy of human lung squamous-cell carcinoma. Respiration 1995; 62:223–227.

Janus ED, Philips NT, Carrell RW: Smoking, lung function, and alpha-1-antitrypsin deficiency. Lancet 1985; 1:152–154.

Joishy SK, Cooper RA, Rowley PT: Alveolar cell carcinoma in identical twins: similarity in time of onset, histochemistry and site of metastases. Ann Intern Med 1977; 87:447–450.

Jones FLJ: Bronchogenic carcinoma in three siblings. Bull Geisinger Med Center 1977; 29:23–25.

Kadlubar FR, Butler MA, Kaderlik KR: Polymorphisms for aromatic amine metabolism in humans: relevance for human carcinogenesis. Environ Health Perspect 1992; 98:69–74.

Kaneko M, Eguchi K, Ohmatsu H, Kakinuma R, Naruke T, Suemasu K, Moriyama N: Peripheral lung cancer: screening and detection with low-dose spiral CT versus radiography. Radiology 1996; 201:798–802.

Kato S, Shields PG, Caporaso NE, Hoover RN, Trump BF, Sugimura H, Weston A, Harris CC: Cytochrome P450IIE1 genetic polymorphisms, racial variation, and lung cancer risk. Cancer Res 1992; 52:6712–6715.

Kelsey KT, Spitz MR, Zuo ZF, Wiencke JK: Polymorphisms in the glutathione *S*-transferase class mu and theta genes interact and increase susceptibility to lung cancer in minority populations (Texas, United States). Cancer Causes Control 1997; 8:554–559.

Kempkes M, Wiebel FA, Golka K, Heitmann P, Bolt HM: Comparative genotyping and phenotyping of glutathione *S*-transferase *GSTT1*. Arch Toxicol 1996; 70:306–309.

Kennedy AR, Beazer-Barclay Y, Kinzler KW, Newberne PM: Suppression of carcinogenesis in the intestines of min mice by the soybean-derived Bowman-Birk inhibitor. Cancer Res 1996; 56:679–682.

Komaki R, Cox JD, Hartz AJ, Byhardt RW, Perez-Tamayo C, Clowry L, Choi H, Wilson F, Lopes da Conceicao A, Rangala N: Characteristics of long-term survivors after treatment for inoperable carcinoma of the lung. Am J Clin Oncol 1985; 8:362–370.

Kreuzer M, Kreienbrock L, Gerken M, et al.: Risk factors for lung cancer in young adults. Am J Epidemiol 1998; 147:1028–1037.

Kreuzer M, Boffetta P, Whitley E, Ahrens W, Gaborieau V, Heinrich J, Jockel KH, Kreienbrock L, Mallone S, Merletti F, et al.: Gender differences in lung cancer risk by smoking: a multicentre case-control study in Germany and Italy. Br J Cancer 2000; 82:227–233.

Krowka MJ: Recent pulmonary observations in α_1-antitrypsin deficiency, primary biliary cirrhosis, chronic hepatitis C, and other hepatic problems. Clin Chest Med 1996; 17:67–82.

Kueppers F: Chronic obstructive pulmonary disease. In: King RA, Rotter JI, Motulsky AG (eds). The Genetic Basis of Common Diseases. New York: Oxford University Press, 1992:222–239.

Kurihara M, Aoki K, Hisamichi S: Cancer Mortality Statistics in the World, 1950–1985. Nagoya: Nagoya University Press, 1989.

Landis SH, Murray T, Bolden S, Wingo PA: Cancer statistics, 1998. CA Cancer J Clin 1998; 48:6–29.

Larsson C: Natural history and life expectancy in severe alpha$_1$-antitrypsin deficiency, Pi Z. Acta Med Scand 1978; 204:345–351.

Larsson S: Pretreatment classification and staging of bronchogenic carcinoma. Scand J Thorac Cardiovasc Surg 1973; 10:1.

Lear JT, Smith AG, Heagerty AH, Bowers B, Jones PW, Gilford J, Alldersea J, Strange RC, Fryer AA: Truncal site and detoxifying enzyme polymorphisms significantly reduce time to presentation of further primary cutaneous basal cell carcinoma. Carcinogenesis 1997; 18:1499–1503.

Lee PN, Forey BA: Trends in cigarette consumption cannot fully explain trends in British lung cancer rates. J Epidemiol Community Health 1998; 52:82–92.

Le Marchand L, Sivaraman L, Pierce L, Seifried A, Lum A, Wilkens LR, Lau AF: Associations of *CYP1A1*, *GSTM1*, and *CYP2E1* polymorphisms with lung cancer suggest cell type specificities to tobacco carcinogens. Cancer Res 1998; 58:4858–4863.

Levin ML, Goldstein H, Gerhardt PR: Cancer and tobacco smoking: a preliminary report. JAMA 1950; 143:336–338.

Lin HJ, Han CY, Lin BK, Hardy S, and Lucier GW: Slow acetylator mutations in the human polymorphic *N*-acetyltransferase gene in 786 Asians, blacks, hispanics, and whites: application to metabolic epidemiology. Am J Hum Genet 1993; 52:827–834.

Lind C, Cadenas E, Hochstein P, Ernster L: DT-diaphorase: purification, properties, and function. Methods Enzymol 1990; 186:287–301.

Liu W, Smith DI, Rechtzigel KJ, Thibodeau SN, James CD: Denaturing high performance liquid chromatography (DHPLC) used in the detection of germline and somatic mutations. Nucleic Acids Res 1998; 26:1396–1400.

London SJ, Daly AK, Cooper J, Carpenter CL, Navidi WC, Ding L, Idle JR: Lung cancer risk in relation to the *CYP2E1* RsaI genetic polymorphism among African-Americans and Caucasians in Los Angeles County. Pharmacogenetics 1996; 6:151–158.

London SJ, Daly AK, Cooper J, Navidi WC, Carpenter CL, Idle JR: Polymorphism of glutathione *S*-transferase M1 and lung cancer risk among African-Americans and Caucasians in Los Angeles County, California. J Natl Cancer Inst 1995; 87:1246–1253.

London SJ, Daly AK, Leathart JB, Navidi WC, Carpenter CC, Idle JR: Genetic polymorphism of *CYP2D6* and lung cancer risk in African-Americans and Caucasians in Los Angeles County. Carcinogenesis 1997; 18:1203–1214.

Lutzky J, Astor MB, Taub RN, Baker MA, Bhalla K, Gervasoni JE Jr, Rosado M, Stewart V, Krishna S, Hindenburg AA: Role of glutathione and dependent enzymes in anthracycline-resistant HL60/AR cells. Cancer Res 1989; 49:4120–4125.

Lynch HT, Kimberling WJ, Markvicka SE, Biscone KA, Lynch JF, Whorton EJ, Mailliard J: Genetics and smoking-associated cancers. A study of 485 families. Cancer 1986; 57:1640–1646.

Mackay JL: The fight against tobacco in developing countries. Tuber Lung Dis 1994; 75:8–24.

Mannervik B, Awasthi YC, Board PG, Hayes JD, Di Ilio C, Ketterer B, Listowsky I, Morgenstern R, Muramatsu M, Pearson WR, et al.: Nomenclature for human glutathione transferases. Biochem J 1992; 282:305–306.

Martinez C, Agundez JA, Olivera M, Martin R, Ladero JM, Benitez J: Lung cancer and mutations at the polymorphic *NAT2* gene locus. Pharmacogenetics 1995; 5:207–214.

Mayne ST, Buencosejo J, Janerich DT: Previous lung disease and risk of lung cancer among men and women nonsmokers. Am J Epidemiol 1999; 149:13–20.

McDuffie HH, Klaassen DJ, Dosman JA: Cancer, genes and agriculture. Principles of Health and Safety in Agriculture. Boca Raton, FL: CRC Press. 1988:258–261.

McDuffie HH, Klaassen DJ, Dosman JA: Determinants of cell type in patients with cancer of the lungs. Chest 1990; 98:1187–1193.

McDuffie HH: Clustering of cancer in families of patients with primary lung cancer. J Clin Epidemiol 1991; 44:69–76.

McWilliams JE, Sanderson BJS, Harris EL, Richert-Boe KE, Henner WD: Glutathione *S*-transferase M1 (GSTM1) deficiency and lung cancer risk. Cancer Epidemiol Biomarkers Prev 1995; 4:589–594.

Merrill RM: Measuring the projected public health impact of lung cancer through lifetime and age-conditional risk estimates. Ann Epidemiol 2000; 10:88–96.

Moreira A, Martins G, Monteiro MJ, Alves M, Dias J, da Costa JD, Melo MJ, Matias D, Costa A, Cristovao M, et al.: Glutathione *S*-transferase mu polymorphism and susceptibility to lung cancer in the Portuguese population. Teratog Carcinog Mutagen 1996; 16:269–274.

Mountain CF: Revisions in the international system for staging lung cancer. Chest 1997; 111:1710–1717.

Nagy I: Zur Beobachtung von Bronchialkarzinomen bei drei Brudern. Prax Pneumol Vereinigt Tuberkul 1968; 22:718–723.

Nakachi K, Imai K, Hayashi S-i, Watanabe J, Kawajiri K: Genetic susceptibility of squamous cell carcinoma of the lung in relation to cigarette smoking dose. Cancer Res 1991; 51:5177–5180.

Nakanishi Y, Matsuki H, Takayama K, Yatsunami J, Kawasaki M, Abe M, Hara N: Glutathione derivatives enhance Adriamycin cytotoxicity in a human lung adenocarcinoma cell line. Anticancer Res 1997; 17:2129–2134.

Nebert DW: Role of genetics and drug metabolism in human cancer risk. Mutat Res 1991; 247:267–281.

Nesbitt JC, Lee JS, Komaki R, Roth JA: Cancer of the lung. In: Holland JF, Frei E III, Bastet RJ, et al. (eds). Cancer Medicine. Baltimore: Williams and Wilkins, 1997:1723–1803.

Nomura A, Stemmerman GN, Chyou P-H, Marcus EB, Buist AS: Prospective study of pulmonary function and lung cancer. Am Rev Respir Dis 1991; 144:307–311.

Nyberg F, Hou SM, Hemminki K, Lambert B, Pershagen G: Glutathione *S*-transferase mu1 and *N*-acetyltransferase 2 genetic polymorphisms and exposure to tobacco smoke in nonsmoking and smoking lung cancer patients and population controls. Cancer Epidemiol Biomarkers Prev 1998; 7:875–883.

Ooi WL, Elston RC, Chen VW, Bailey-Wilson JE, Rothschild H: Increased familial risk for lung cancer. J Natl Cancer Inst 1986; 76:217–222.

Osann KE: Lung cancer in women: the importance of smoking, family history of cancer, and medical history of respiratory disease. Cancer Res 1991; 51:4893–4897.

Oyama T, Kawamoto T, Mizoue T, Sugio K, Kodama Y, Mitsudomi T, Yasumoto K: Cytochrome P450 2E1 polymorphism as a risk factor for lung cancer: in relation to *p53* gene mutation. Anticancer Res 1997; 17:583–587.

Pandey M, Matthew A, Nair MK: Global perspective of tobacco habits and lung cancer: a lesson for third world countries. Eur J Cancer Prev 1999; 8:271–279.

Parkin DM, Muir CS: Cancer Incidence in Five Continents. Comparability and Quality of Data. IARC Scientific Publication 120. Lyon: IARC, 1992:45–173.

Paul LD: Alpha$_1$-antitrypsin deficiency. Pulm Crit Care Update 1989; 5:2–8.

Paul SM, Bacharach B, Goepp C: A genetic influence on alveolar cell carcinoma. J Surg Oncol 1987; 36:249–253.

Penman BW, Reece J, Smith T, Yang CS, Gelboin HV, Gonzalez FJ, Crespi CL: Characterization of a human cell line expressing high levels of cDNA-derived CYP2D6. Pharmacogenetics 1993; 3:28–39.

Perkins P, Lee JR, Kemp BL, Cox JD: Carcinoid tumors of the lung and family history of cancer. J Clin Epidemiol 1997; 50:705–709.

Persson I, Johansson I, Bergling H, Dahl M-L, Seidegard J, Rylander R, Rannug A, Hogberg J, Sundberg MI: Genetic polymorphism of cytochrome P4502E1 in a Swedish population; relationship to incidence of lung cancer. FEBS Lett 1993; 319:207–211.

Pierce RJ, Kune GA, Kune S, Watson LF, Field B, Merenstein D, Hayes A, Irving LB: Dietary and alcohol intake, smoking pattern, occupational risk, and family history in lung cancer patients: results of a case-control study in males. Nutr Cancer 1989; 12:237–248.

Raunio H, Husgafvel-Pursiainen K, Anttila S, Hietanen E, Hirvonen A, Pelkonen O: Diagnosis of polymorphisms in carcinogen-activating and inactivating enzymes and cancer susceptibility—a review. Gene 1995; 159:113–121.

Rebbeck TR: Molecular epidemiology of the human glutathione *S*-transferase genotypes *GSTM1* and *GSTT1* in cancer susceptibility. Cancer Epidemiol Biomarkers Prev 1997; 6:733–743.

Ryberg D, Skaug V, Hewer A, Phillips DH, Harries LW, Wolf CR, Ogreid D, Ulvik A, Vu P, Haugen A: Genotypes of glutathione transferase M1 and P1 and their significance for lung DNA adduct levels and cancer risk. Carcinogenesis 1997; 18:1285–1289.

Saarikoski ST, Voho A, Reinikainen M, Anttila A, Karjalainen A, Malaveille C, Vainio H, Husgafvel-Pursiainen K, Hirvonen A: Combined effect of polymorphic GST genes on individual susceptibility to lung cancer. Int J Cancer 1998; 77:516–521.

Sakuma T, Nishimura T, Usuda K, Handa M, Okaniwa G, Nakada T, Tabata T, Hoshikawa Y, Fujimura S: Neutrophil elastase in postoperative pleural effusion of patients who had undergone pulmonary resections. Nippon Kyobu Geka Gakkai Zasshi 1995; 43:153–158.

Salber EJ, MacMahon B: Cigarette smoking among high school students related to social class and parental smoking habits. Am J Public Health 1961; 51:1780–1789.

Samet JM, Humble CG, Pathak DR: Personal and family history of respiratory disease and lung cancer risk. Am Rev Respir Dis 1986; 134:466–470.

Satcher D: Women and Smoking. A Report of the Surgeon General—2001. Washington DC: US Department of Health and Human Services, Centers for Disease Control and Prevention, National Center for Chronic Disease Prevention and Health Promotion, Office on Smoking and Health, 2001:193–212.

Schwartz AG, Lassige D, Gillen-Caralli D, Shriver M: Alpha-1-antitrypsin carrier status and lung cancer risk among nonsmokers. Am J Epidemiol 1998; 147:S21.

Schwartz AG, Rothrock M, Yang P, Swanson GM: Increased cancer risk among relatives of nonsmoking lung cancer cases. Genet Epidemiol 1999; 17:1–15.

Schwartz AG, Yang P, Swanson GM: Familial risk of lung cancer among nonsmokers and their relatives. Am J Epidemiol 1996; 144:554–562.

Sellers TA: Familial predisposition to lung cancer. In: Eeles RA, Ponder BAJ, Easton DF, Horwich A (eds). Genetic Predisposition to Cancer. London: Chapman and Hall, 1996:344–353.

Sellers TA, Bailey-Wilson JE, Elston RC, Wilson AF, Elston GZ, Ooi WL, Rothschild H: Evidence for Mendelian inheritance in the pathogenesis of lung cancer. J Natl Cancer Inst 1990; 82:1272–1279.

Sellers TA, Bailey-Wilson JE, Potter JD, Rich SS, Rothschild H, Elston RC: Effect of cohort differences in smoking prevalence on models of lung cancer susceptibility. Genet Epidemiol 1992; 9:261–271.

Sellers TA, Elston RC, Atwood LD, Rothschild H: Lung cancer histologic type and family history of cancer. Cancer 1992a; 69:86–91.

Sellers TA, Elston RC, Stewart C, Rothschild H: Familial risk of cancer among randomly selected cancer probands. Genet Epidemiol 1988; 5:381–391.

Sellers TA, Potter JD, Bailey-Wilson JE, Rich SS, Rothschild H, Elston RC: Lung cancer detection and prevention: evidence for an interaction between smoking and genetic predisposition. Cancer Res 1992b; 52(Suppl):2694s–2697s.

Sellers TA, Weaver TW, Phillips B, Altmann M, Rich SS: Environmental factors can confound identification of a major gene effect: results from a segregation analysis of lung cancer in a simulated population. Genet Epidemiol 1998; 15:251–262.

Shaw GL, Falk RT, Frame JN, Weiffenbach B, Nesbitt JC, Pass HI, Caporaso NE, Moir DT, Tucker MA: Genetic polymorphism of *CYP2D6* and lung cancer risk. Cancer Epidemiol Biomarkers Prev 1998; 7:215–219.

Shaw GL, Falk RT, Pickle LW, Mason TJ, Buffler PA: Lung cancer risk associated with cancer in relatives. J Clin Epidemiol 1991; 44:429–437.

Shen H, Kauvar L, Tew KD: Importance of glutathione and associated enzymes in drug response. Oncol Res 1997; 9:295–302.

Skillrud DM, Offord KP, Miller RD: Higher risk of lung cancer in chronic obstructive pulmonary disease. Ann Intern Med 1986; 105:503–507.

Testa JR: Chromosome alterations in human lung cancer. In: Pass HI, Mitchell JB, Johnson DH, Turrisi AT, (eds). Lung Cancer: Principles and Practice. Philadelphia: Lippincott-Raven, 1996:55–71.

Tockman MS, Anthonisen NR, Wright EC, Donithan MG, The Intermittent Positive Pressure Breathing Trial Group, and the Johns Hopkins Lung Project for Early Detection of Lung Cancer: Airway obstruction and the risk for lung cancer. Ann Intern Med 1987; 106:512–518.

Tockman MS, Mulshine JL: The early detection of occult lung cancer. Chest Surg Clin N Am 2000; 10:737–749.

To-Figueras J, Gene M, Gomez-Catalan J, Galan MC, Fuentes M, Ramon JM, Rodamilans M, Huguet E, Corbella J: Glutathione *S*-transferase M1 (*GSTM1*) and T1 (*GSTT1*) polymorphisms and lung cancer risk among northwestern Mediterraneans. Carcinogenesis 1997; 18:1529–1533.

Tokuhata GK, Lilienfeld AM: Familial aggregation of lung cancer in humans. J Natl Cancer Inst 1963a; 30:289–312.

Tokuhata GK, Lilienfeld AM: Familial aggregation of lung cancer among hospital patients. Public Health Rep 1963b; 78:277–283.

Travis WD, Travis LB, Devesa SS: Lung cancer incidence and survival by histologic type. Cancer 1995; 75(1 Suppl):191–202.

Uematsu F, Ikawa S, Kikuchi H, Sagami I, Kanamaru R, Abe T, Satoh K, Motomiya M, Watanabe M: Restriction fragment length polymorphism of the human *CYP2E1* (cytochrome P450IIE1) gene and susceptibility to lung cancer: possible relevance to low smoking exposure. Pharmacogenetics 1994; 4:58–63.

Uematsu F, Kikuchi H, Motomiya M, Abe T, Sagami I, Ohmachi T, Wakui A, Kanamaru R, Watanabe M: Association between restriction fragment length polymorphism of the human cytochrome P450IIE1 gene and susceptibility to lung cancer. Jpn J Cancer Res 1991; 82:254–256.

Vena JE, Bona JR, Byers TE: Allergy-related diseases and cancer: an inverse association. Am J Epidemiol 1985; 122:66–74.

Vineis P, Bartsch H, Caporaso N, Harrington AM, Kadlubar FF, Landi MT, Malaveille C, Shields PG, Skipper P, Talaska G, et al.: Genetically based *N*-acetyltransferase metabolic polymorphism and low-level environmental exposure to carcinogens. Nature 1994; 369:154–156.

Walsh AC, Li W, Rosen DR, Lawrence DA: Genetic mapping of *GLCLC*, the human gene encoding the catalytic subunit of gamma-glutamyl-cysteine synthetase, to chromosome band 6p12 and characterization of a polymorphic trinucleotide repeat within its 5′ untranslated region. Cytogenet Cell Genet 1996; 75:14–16.

Watanabe J, Yang JP, Eguchi H, Hayashi S, Imai K, Nakachi K, Kawajiri K: An RsaI polymorphism in the *CYP2E1* gene does not affect lung cancer risk in a Japanese population. Jpn J Cancer Res 1995; 86:245–248.

Wistuba II, Gazdar AF: Molecular pathology of lung cancer. Verh Dtsch Ges Pathol 2000; 84:96–105.

Witschi H, Kennedy AR: Modulation of lung tumor development in mice with the soybean-derived Bowman-Birk protease inhibitor. Carcinogenesis 1989; 10:2275–2277.

Wolf CR, Smith CA, Gough AC, Moss JE, Vallis KA, Howard G, Carey FJ, Mills K, McNee W, Carmichael J, et al.: Relationship between the debrisoquine hydroxylase polymorphism and cancer susceptibility. Carcinogenesis 1992; 13:1035–1038.

Wood ME, Kelly K, Mullineaux LG, Bunn PA Jr: The inherited nature of lung cancer: a pilot study. Lung Cancer 2000; 30:135–144.

World Health Organization: Histologic Typing of Lung Cancer, 2d ed. Geneva: World Health Organization, 1981, pp. 1–36.

Wu X, Amos CI, Kemp BL, Shi H, Jiang H, Wan Y, Spitz MR: Cytochrome P450 2E1 DraI polymorphisms in lung cancer in minority populations. Cancer Epidemiol Biomarkers Prev 1998; 7:13–18.

Wu AH, Fontham ETH, Reynolds P, Greenberg RS, Buffler P, Liff J, Boyd P, Henderson BE, Correa P: Previous lung disease and risk of lung cancer among lifetime nonsmoking women in the United States. Am J Epidemiol 1995; 141:1023–1032.

Wu AH, Fontham ETH, Reynolds P, et al.: Family history of cancer and risk of lung cancer among lifetime nonsmoking women in the United States. Am J Epidemiol 1996; 143:535–542.

Wu AH, Yu MC, Thomas DC, Pike MC, Henderson BE: Personal and family history of lung disease as risk factors for adenocarcinoma of the lung. Cancer Res 1988; 48:7279–7284.

Wynder EL, Graham EA: Tobacco smoking as a possible etiologic factor in bronchiogenic carcinoma: a study of six hundred and eighty-four proved cases. JAMA 1950; 143:329–336.

Xu LL, Wain JC, Miller DP, Thurston SW, Su L, Lynch TJ, Christiani DC: The NAD(P)H:quinone oxidoreductase 1 gene polymorphism and lung cancer: differential susceptibility based on smoking behavior. Cancer Epidemiol 2001; 10:303–309.

Yamashita J, Ogawa M, Abe M, Hayashi N, Kurusu Y, Kawahara K, Shirakusa T: Tumor neutrophil elastase is closely associated with the direct extension of non-small cell lung cancer into the aorta. Chest 1997; 111:885–890.

Yang P, Lerdtragool S, Marks R, Lesnick T, Wentzlaff K, Swensen S, Edell E, Miller D, Jett J, Romkes M: *GSTM1* null and *NAT2** slow genotypes, age-at-diagnosis, and cancer risk in first-degree relatives of lung cancer probands. In: Proceedings from the Eighty-ninth Annual Meeting. Association for Cancer Research; March 28–April 1, 1998; New Orleans, LA: p. 182.

Yang P, Romkes M, Schwartz AG, Rittmeyer L, Adedoyin A, Landreneau R, Mauro K, Branch RA: Polymorphisms at the NAT2* locus associated with increased cancer risk in first-degree relatives of lung cancer patients. Genet Epidemiol 1996; 3:308–309.

Yang P, Schwartz AG, McAllister AE, Aston CE, Swanson GM: Genetic analysis of families with nonsmoking lung cancer probands. Genet Epidemiol 1997; 14:181–197.

Yang P, Schwartz AG, McAllister AE, Swanson GM, Aston CE: Lung cancer risk in families of nonsmoking probands: heterogeneity by age at diagnosis. Genet Epidemiol 1999; 17:253–273.

Yang P, Wentzlaff KA, Marks R, Patel A, Allen M, Edell E, Katzmann J, Lesnick T, Deschamps C, Midthun D, et al.: Higher rate of alpha-1-antitrypsin (α_1AT) deficiency carriers found in lung cancer patients. Am J Hum Genet 1997b; 61: A15.

Zheng W, Blot WJ, Liao ML, Qang ZX, Levin LI, Zhao JJ, Fraumeni JF Jr, Gao YT: Lung cancer and prior tuberculosis infection in Shanghai. Br J Cancer 1987; 56:501–504.

Zhong S, Howie AF, Ketterer B, Taylor J, Hayes JD, Beckett GJ, Wathen CG, Wolf CR, Spurr NK: Glutathione *S*-transferase μ locus: use of genotyping and phenotyping assays to assess association with lung cancer susceptibility. Carcinogenesis 1991; 12:1533–1537.

37 Reproductive Organ Cancers

MAREN T. SCHEUNER AND BETH Y. KARLAN

Reproductive organ cancers represent several different cancer types that are collectively an important cause of morbidity and mortality in both women and men. The reproductive cancers in women include cancers of the breast, uterus, cervix, ovary, fallopian tube, vulva, and vagina. In men, these cancers involve the prostate, testicle, epididymis, and penis. Both genetic and environmental factors are important in the etiology of reproductive organ cancers, and in some cases, the environment is thought to play the greatest role in cancer susceptibility [e.g., human papillomavirus (HPV) and cervical and penile cancers]. Yet even in those cases where environment predominates in determining susceptibility, genetic factors have been identified that may influence the predisposition to cancer.

Several lines of evidence support a role for genetics in the etiology of reproductive organ cancers. These include family studies, twin studies, population association studies, segregation analyses, linkage analyses, and cytogenetic and molecular studies of tumors. In some cases, a rare Mendelian disorder may feature a particular reproductive cancer type, lending further evidence that genetics may play an important role in the susceptibility to such cancers (Table 37–1). Perhaps the most conclusive evidence supporting a role for genetics in reproductive organ cancer-susceptibility is the finding of deleterious mutations in known cancer susceptibility genes, including mismatch repair genes in endometrial and ovarian cancers, as well as the *BRCA1* and *BRCA2* tumor-suppressor genes in breast and ovarian cancers.

In this chapter, we review those reproductive organ cancers for which a body of evidence exists describing genetic susceptibility, including ovarian, endometrial, cervical, and testicular cancers. Excluded are breast cancer (reviewed in Chapter 35) and prostate cancer (reviewed in Chapter 39). In addition, the clinical application of such genetic susceptibility is also addressed.

OVARIAN CANCER

Disease Definition

Most ovarian carcinomas are epithelial (80%–90%), arising from the serosal mesothelial layer of the ovaries (Scully, 1977). This epithelium may invaginate to create small cysts, which can differentiate into endometrioid, mucinous, or serous epithelium, the common histologic subtypes of epithelial ovarian cancers. Epithelial tumors may be classified as benign, borderline, or malignant. About 15% of all epithelial ovarian tumors are borderline with a more favorable prognosis (Nikrui, 1981). The prognosis of malignant epithelial ovarian cancers depends most on the degree of cellular differentiation rather than the histologic type (Aure et al., 1971). There are no specific signs or symptoms of ovarian cancer. Symptoms may include nausea, dyspepsia, lower abdominal discomfort, and bloating. At the time of diagnosis, ovarian cancer has usually spread beyond the ovary in 75% of cases and beyond the pelvis in 60% (Sall and Stone, 1973).

Stromal tumors comprise about 10% of ovarian tumors, including granulosa, theca, Sertoli, and Leydig cell tumors (Scully, 1977). Granulosa cell tumors can be associated with feminizing effects and precocious puberty. Fewer than 5% of ovarian tumors are germ cell tumors, characterized as dysgerminoma, endodermal sinus tumor, embryonal carcinoma, polyembryoma, choriocarcinoma, teratoma, and mixed forms. These tumor types occur in younger women and are associated with a better prognosis.

General Genetic and Epidemiologic Evidence

Approximately 1 in 70 women will develop ovarian cancer. In 2001, 23,400 new ovarian cancer cases and 13,900 deaths due to ovarian cancer are expected (Greenlee et al., 2001). Ovarian cancer is the leading cause of gynecologic cancer death in the United States, accounting for approximately 1% of all female deaths. Women living in industrial countries have the greatest risk, except for Japanese women, who have the lowest risk for this disease. Epithelial ovarian cancers usually occur after age 40, whereas germ cell tumors occur in children and young adults.

Hormonal factors are most important in determining ovarian cancer risk. Infertility and failure to conceive increase the risk of ovarian cancer (Whittemore et al., 1992). Use of fertility drugs and ovulation induction might also increase ovarian cancer risk, especially that of borderline tumors (Rossing et al., 1994; Shushan et al., 1996). However, these medications do not appear to be independent risk factors for ovarian cancer development (Bristow and Karlan, 1996). Conversely, increasing number of pregnancies and oral contraceptive use decrease the risk of ovarian cancer (Whittemore et al., 1992), suggesting a role for ovulation suppression in ovarian cancer risk reduction. Tubal ligation and, to a lesser extent, hysterectomy, are also associated with a decreased ovarian cancer risk (Whittemore et al., 1992; Hankinson et al., 1993).

Approximately 5% of ovarian cancer patients report a family history of ovarian cancer (Greggi et al., 1990). Because this is a relatively rare malignancy, whenever there are two or more close relatives affected with ovarian cancer, an inherited susceptibility due to a mutation in a single cancer-susceptibility gene should be suspected. Of those families with a suspected inherited susceptibility to epithelial ovarian cancer due to a mutation in a single gene, three distinct clinical genetic syndromes are recognized: hereditary site-specific ovarian cancer, hereditary breast–ovarian cancer syndrome, and hereditary nonpolyposis

Table 37–1. Mendelian Disorders That Feature Reproductive Organ Cancers

Mendelian Disorder	OMIM No.	Gene(s)	Reproductive Organ Neoplasm	Other Clinical Features
Site-specific breast cancer/breast–ovary syndrome	113705/ 600185	*BRCA1*, *BRCA2*	Ovarian, breast, and prostate cancer	Increased risk for colorectal cancer associated with *BRCA1* mutations; increased risk for pancreatic cancer, ocular melanoma, and male breast cancer associated with *BRCA2* mutations
Hereditary nonpolyposis colon cancer (HNPCC)/ Lynch syndrome I and II/Family cancer syndrome	120435/ 120436/ 114400	*MSH2*, *MLH1*, *PMS1*, *PMS2*, *MSH6*	Ovarian, endometrial, and, in some families, breast cancer	Increased risk for cancers of the colon, stomach, biliary tract, and uroepithelium; Muir-Torre variant features sebaceous adenomas and keratoacanthomas; Turcot's syndrome variant features glioblastomas.
Basal cell nevus syndrome (a.k.a. Gorlin syndrome)	109400	*PTCH*	Ovarian fibromas	Dysmorphic features, skeletal abnormalities, pits on the palms and soles, ophthalmic abnormalities, odontogenic keratocysts of the jaw, lamellar calcification of the falx cerebri, and, less commonly, cleft lip/palate, mental retardation, medulloblastoma, and cardiac fibroma
Peutz-Jeghers syndrome	175200	*STK11*	Granulosa cell tumors, Sertoli cell tumors, adenoma malignum of the endocervix, and breast cancer	Melanin spots of the lips, buccal mucosa, hands (palms), arms, feet (soles), and legs; increased risk for pancreatic cancer and other gastrointestinal tract cancers
Cowden disease	158350	*PTEN*	Breast cancer, uterine leiomyoma, ovarian cysts, and vaginal and vulvar cysts	Multiple hamartomas, especially of the skin, mucous membranes, breast, thyroid, and gastrointestinal tract; multiple facial trichilemmomas, macrocephaly, and genitourinary malformations; increased risk for thyroid cancer
Carney complex	160980	Not known	Myxoid uterine leiomyoma, testicular cancer (large-cell calcifying Sertoli cell tumor, Leydig cell tumor, or adrenocortical rest tumor)	The acronym *NAME* represents the main features of the disorder (nevi, atrial myxoma, mucinosis of the skin, endocrine overactivity or nevi, atrial myxoma, myxoid neurofibromata, ephides); ophthalmologic abnormalities include eyelid myxomas and lentigines, pigmented lesions of the caruncle or conjunctiva
Li-Fraumeni syndrome	151623	*TP53*	Breast and testicular cancer, possibly gonadal germ cell tumors and prostate cancer	Soft tissue sarcomas (usually in childhood), brain tumors, osteosarcomas, leukemia, adrenocortical carcinoma, and laryngeal and lung cancer; possibly melanoma and pancreatic cancer; early age at onset and multiple primary cancers characteristic
Von Hippel-Lindau syndrome	193300	*VHL*	Cystadenomas of the epididymis and broad ligament papillary cystadenoma	Cardinal features include angiomata of the retina and hemangioblastoma of the cerebellum. Other findings include hemangiomas of the adrenals, lungs, and liver; multiple cysts of the pancreas and kidneys; and renal cell carcinoma
Russell-Silver syndrome	180860	Not known	Testicular seminoma	Clinical findings include lateral asymmetry, low birth weight and small stature, dysmorphic features (triangular facies with frontal prominence); occasional malignancies include craniopharyngioma, hepatocellular carcinoma, and Wilms' tumor
Ataxia-telangiectasia	208900	*ATM*	Ovarian fibromas and breast cancer (in heterozygotes)	Autosomal recessive disorder characterized by cerebellar ataxia, telangiectasias, immune defects, and predisposition to malignancy (leukemias, lymphomas, medulloblastomas, and gliomas); progressive spinal muscular atrophy occurs in the 20s and 30s. ataxia-telangiectasia cells are sensitive to ionizing radiation; chromosomal instability increased
WAGR complex	194072	Contiguous gene syndrome with deletion of 11p13	Gonadoblastoma	The acronym *WAGR* has been used to describe the contiguous gene complex with Wilms' tumor; aniridia; gonadoblastoma, genitourinary abnormalities, or ambiguous genitalia; and retardation

colon cancer (HNPCC) (Houlston et al., 1992; Grover et al., 1993). Additional rare single-gene disorders that feature primarily nonepithelial ovarian tumors include Gorlin syndrome (also known as basal cell nevus syndrome) and Peutz-Jeghers syndrome (Table 37–1).

Women who report a family history of ovarian cancer have an increased risk for ovarian cancer. The risk is increased 3.6-fold and 2.9-fold in first- and second-degree relatives of an affected woman, respectively (Schildkraut and Thompson, 1988). The absolute risk for ovarian cancer associated with an affected first-degree relative is about 5% by age 70 (Amos et al., 1992). If there are two affected close relatives, the risk is increased to 30% to 40% (Kerlikowske et al., 1992). Women with a first-degree relative with breast cancer also have an increased risk for ovarian cancer of 1.7-fold (Schildkraut et al., 1989). Having a first-degree relative affected with ovarian cancer is also associated with an increased breast cancer risk of 1.6-fold compared to women without such a history (Schildkraut et al., 1989). The empiric risk for breast cancer given a first-degree relative with ovarian cancer is only modestly increased at 13.5% by age 89 (Claus et al., 1993). For women with two first-degree relatives with ovarian cancer, the empiric lifetime risk for breast cancer has been estimated to be 30.8% (Claus et al., 1993). The Iowa Women's Health Study identified a twofold increase in risk of adenocarcinoma of the lung associated with a family history of ovarian cancer (Anderson et al., 1997).

The risks for breast and ovarian cancer associated with a family history of these cancers are greater for Ashkenazi Jewish women than others (Egan et al., 1996; Steinberg et al., 1998; Moslehi et al., 2000). This is despite the fact that the frequencies of breast and ovarian cancer are not significantly increased among Ashkenazi Jewish women, suggesting more familial aggregation in Ashkenazi Jewish families. Breast cancer risk due to a family history of breast cancer is 2.28 times greater in Jewish women with breast cancer than non-Jewish women (Egan et al., 1996), and ovarian cancer risk is 2.93 times greater given a family history of ovarian cancer in Jewish compared to non-Jewish cases (Steinberg et al., 1998). The absolute risk associated with a first-degree relative affected with ovarian cancer in Ashkenazi Jewish families is 7% by age 70 (Moslehi et al., 2000) compared to 5% in the general population (Amos et al., 1992). This disproportionate familial cancer risk in Ashkenazi Jewish families is due in large part to three prevalent founder mutations in the *BRCA1* and *BRCA2* genes (Kaufman and Struewing, 1999; Moslehi et al., 2000). If the three Ashkenazi Jewish *BRCA* founder mutations are excluded in an unaffected mother or sister of a woman with ovarian cancer, her empiric ovarian cancer risk is reduced to 4% (Moslehi et al., 2000).

Gene Identification

Mutations in the *BRCA1* and *BRCA2* genes and the mismatch repair genes responsible for cancer susceptibility in HNPCC are important determinants of an inherited susceptibility to ovarian cancer. A woman from an HNPCC family who carries a mismatch repair gene mutation has about a 9% to 12% risk for ovarian cancer by age 70 (Vasen et al., 1996; Aarnio et al., 1995, 1999). However, HNPCC represents a minority of cases with an inherited susceptibility to ovarian cancer. The diagnoses of hereditary site-specific ovarian cancer and breast–ovary syndrome represent most inherited ovarian cancer susceptibility, and the *BRCA1* and *BRCA2* genes account for most of the genetic susceptibility in these clinical syndromes. The identification of these genes, their protein products, and details regarding their mutational spectrum, prevalence, and penetrance are reviewed in Chapter 35.

Cytogenetic studies of ovarian tumors reveal frequent structural abnormalities and deletions of chromosomes 1, 3, 6, and 11 (Gallion et al., 1992), suggesting candidate genes at these loci. Additionally, loss of heterozygosity (LOH) involving chromosomes 6p, 6q, 9q, 13q, 17p, and 17q has been identified in ovarian tumors (Cliby et al., 1993). The *TP53* gene on 17p and *BRCA1* on 17q are likely candidates associated with LOH of these chromosomes in ovarian cancer.

Clinical Application and Risk Assessment

Women with a family history of ovarian cancer may benefit from genetic risk assessment, counseling, and testing. If their empiric ovarian cancer risk is elevated, preventive strategies of early detection, chemoprevention and prophylactic surgery are available. If the family history is suggestive of an inherited cancer risk, genetic testing might clarify the specific genetic susceptibility. If a *BRCA* or mismatch repair gene mutation is identified, early detection and prevention of the associated spectrum of cancers should be considered. In families with HNPCC, the most important risks are for colorectal and endometrial cancers. Screening and prevention of ovarian or endometrial cancer are reviewed below. In families with *BRCA* gene mutations in addition to ovarian cancer, the most important risks are for breast, colon, and prostate cancers. Clinical management of these associated cancers is discussed in Chapters 35 and 39, respectively.

For women suspected or known to carry a *BRCA1, BRCA2,* or mismatch repair gene mutation, recommendations for early detection include annual serum CA-125 tumor marker testing and transvaginal ultrasound beginning at age 25. Unfortunately, this type of screening has a low yield of early diagnosis, and prophylactic bilateral salpingo-oophorectomy (BSO) is more effective for ovarian cancer risk reduction and should be considered when childbearing is complete (NIH Consensus Development Panel on Ovarian Cancer, 1995; Burke et al., 1997a, 1997b). In addition to BSO, prophylactic hysterectomy should be considered for women with HNPCC, especially at the time of surgery for an HNPCC-associated colorectal cancer (Moslein et al., 2000). Prophylactic BSO has been associated with a 95% reduction in the risk of ovarian cancer in women with *BRCA* gene mutations (Weber et al., 2000). However, even after prophylactic oophorectomy, a risk for peritoneal carcinomatosis remains (Tobacman et al., 1982; Piver et al., 1993). This risk is thought to be due to cancer arising in cells of similar origin in the peritoneum.

Similar to the general population, women with a genetic susceptibility for ovarian cancer may reduce their ovarian cancer risk with oral contraceptive use. Narod and co-workers (1998) describe a 70% reduction in ovarian cancer risk among *BRCA* mutation carriers who used oral contraceptives for 6 or more years. However, a population-based case-control study of ovarian cancer among Jewish women in Israel did not find a protective effect of oral contraceptive use in *BRCA* gene mutation carriers (Modan et al., 2001). This study did find that the risk of ovarian cancer among carriers of *BRCA* gene mutations decreased with each birth. There have been no studies to date assessing ovarian cancer risk reduction associated with oral contraceptive use in women with HNPCC. Additionally, at least one study suggests that women with *BRCA* mutations who take oral contraceptives may have an increased risk for breast cancer

(Ursin et al., 1997). This study found that the likelihood of being a *BRCA* mutation carrier was significantly increased among women who had breast cancer prior to age 40 who used oral contraceptives for more than 48 months prior to their first full-term pregnancy (odds ratio (OR) = 7.8, 95% confidence interval (CI) 1–55, trend $p = 0.004$).

Hormone replacement therapy is an important clinical issue for women with known or suspected *BRCA* gene mutations. Often because of prophylactic oophorectomy, these women become menopausal much before the natural age of menopause. Once menopause occurs, the decision to use hormone replacement therapy must be carefully considered because of the potential increase in risk for breast cancer (Burke et al., 1997b). A meta-analysis of five studies has shown that women with family history of breast cancer who used hormone replacement therapy had a 3.4-fold increase (95% CI 2.0–6.0) in breast cancer risk. This was more than twice the 1.5-fold increase (95% CI 1.2–1.7) in risk for women who used hormone replacement therapy and did not have a family history of breast cancer compared to control women (Steinberg et al., 1991). Another study has found that overall mortality was not increased among women using hormone replacement therapy with a family history of breast cancer compared to those without a family history (Sellers et al., 1997). However, women using hormone replacement therapy with a family history of breast cancer did have a 1.3-fold higher (95% CI 0.6–3.0) risk of death from breast cancer. This result was based on only 84 deaths and did not reach statistical significance. It is suspected that use of hormone replacement therapy might also contribute to an increased breast cancer risk in women with *BRCA* mutations, similar to that reported for women with a family history of breast cancer.

Women with *BRCA* gene mutation who undergo prophylactic BSO prior to menopause benefit from reducing not only their ovarian cancer risk but also their breast cancer risk, by as much as 50% (Rebbeck et al., 1999). This protective effect of prophylactic oophorectomy on breast cancer risk appears to be sustained in *BRCA* mutation-positive women who choose to use hormone replacement therapy (Rebbeck et al., 1999). This is probably due to an overall net reduction in exposure to hormones since the usual amount of hormone in replacement therapy is less than half of endogenous production. Thus, short-term use of hormone replacement therapy for such women appears to be appropriate.

Estrogen deficiency can increase the risk for osteoporosis and have an unfavorable effect on several cardiovascular disease risk factors. Additionally, vasomotor symptoms and problems related to urogenital atrophy associated with estrogen deficiency can be disabling for some women. Therefore, it is important that a woman with a suspected or known *BRCA* mutation review her entire medical and family history during a genetics evaluation so that appropriate preventive strategies are planned. Alternative therapies are available to protect against the medical complications of estrogen deficiency. Both raloxifene and tamoxifen have beneficial effects on bone density (Fisher et al., 1998; Cummings et al., 1999), and both are associated with favorable affects on lipids. Furthermore, tamoxifen reduces the occurrence of breast cancer by 50% in women with an increased risk (Fisher et al., 1998), and raloxifene might also be effective at reducing breast cancer incidence in women at risk (Cummings et al., 1999). However, a recent study has shown that tamoxifen is not effective at reducing breast cancer incidence in women with *BRCA1* gene mutations, although *BRCA2* gene mutation carriers had a 62% reduction in risk (King et al., 2001). This difference in response to tamoxifen might be related to a disproportionate number of estrogen and progesterone receptor-negative tumors in *BRCA1* gene mutation carriers (King et al., 2001). Prophylactic bilateral mastectomy is another approach to reducing the likelihood of breast cancer occurrence. In women with both moderate- and high-risk family histories of breast cancer, prophylactic bilateral mastectomy reduced the incidence of breast cancer by 90% (Hartmann et al., 1999). A statistically significant reduction in breast cancer risk has also been observed for women with *BRCA* mutations electing to undergo prophylactic bilateral mastectomy (Meijers-Heijboer et al., 2001). In a prospective study, after 3 years of follow-up, there were no cases of breast cancer among the 76 women who chose mastectomy vs. eight cases in the 63 women who participated in surveillance ($p = 0.003$).

ENDOMETRIAL CANCER

Disease Definition

Endometrial cancer arises from the epithelial lining of the uterine cavity, with most tumors displaying glandular differentiation. Abnormal vaginal bleeding is the usual presenting symptom in most women with endometrial cancer. A definitive diagnosis is usually made by endometrial biopsy or curretage. Two broad categories of endometrial cancer exist (Bokhman, 1983). Type I carcinomas are the most common form. They are estrogen-related cancers that develop from normal epithelium through a continuum of hyperplastic changes. These tumors tend to have endometrioid characteristics, are generally low-grade, and have a good prognosis. Type II endometrial cancers are unrelated to estrogenic stimulation, arising in atrophic rather than hyperplastic endometrium, and are aggressive in nature. These tumors are composed of cuboidal cells that grow in glandular or papillary structures, similar to serous carcinoma of the ovary.

General Genetic and Epidemiologic Evidence

Endometrial cancer is the most prevalent form of female genital tract cancer, with an estimated 38,300 new cases expected in 2001 and contributing to 6600 deaths (Greenlee et al., 2001). Most cases of endometrial cancer occur after menopause, with a median age at diagnosis of 61.1 years; only 5% occur in women under age 40 (Gallup and Stock, 1984).

Medical conditions that are associated with an increased risk of endometrial cancer include diabetes, hypertension, obesity, polycystic ovary disease, estrogen-secreting tumors of the ovary, arthritis, and hypothyroidism (MacMahon, 1974). To date, there are no known genetic associations between these conditions and endometrial cancer. Hormonal factors have been identified as important risk factors for endometrial cancer, including late menopause, nulliparity, and unopposed estrogen use.

Family history is an important risk factor; however, little is known regarding the genetic aspects of this disease. Lynch et al. (1966) found that 13% (20/154) of endometrial cancer probands had a similarly affected first-degree relative. Boltenberg et al. (1990) found similar familial aggregation, with 7 of 51 endometrial cases (14%) having either a family history of an affected mother or sister (four cases) or a family history of colon, ovarian, and/or endometrial cancer consistent with HNPCC (three additional cases). Sandles et al. (1992) found similar estimates. Among 64 endometrial cancer cases, in four families (6%), multiple first-degree relatives had endometrial, colon, and/or ovarian cancer, suggesting HNPCC. In four additional families (6%), at least one first-degree relative had endometrial cancer. Furthermore, in one of these latter four families, multiple family members in multiple generations were affected with endometrial cancer, suggesting a site-specific Mendelian form of the disease. These data suggest that at least half of familial cases, or 6% of all endometrial cancer cases, are due to an autosomal dominant disorder. Additionally, they suggest that genetic heterogeneity may exist in these hereditary forms of the disease, with the majority of cases classified as HNPCC and a minority classified as site-specific endometrial cancer.

The Cancer and Steroid Hormone (CASH) study reported the magnitude of risk associated with a family history of endometrial cancer (Gruber and Thompson, 1996). In 455 cases of endometrial cancer in women age 20 to 54 compared to 3216 controls, a family history of endometrial cancer in a first-degree relative was associated with a threefold increase in endometrial cancer risk (OR = 2.8, 95% CI 1.9–4.2). There was also an increased risk for colorectal cancer among cases (OR = 1.9, 95% CI 1.1–3.3). This increased colorectal cancer risk may be explained by occurrence of HNPCC.

HNPCC is a hereditary cancer syndrome associated with mutations in mismatch repair genes (see Chapter 39). The cancer spectrum in HNPCC includes colorectal, endometrial, ovarian, gastric, biliary tract, small bowel, urinary tract (ureter and kidney), and brain (Mecklin and Jarvinen, 1991; Lynch et al., 1993; Marra and Boland, 1995; Vasen et al., 1996; Aarnio et al., 1999). Endometrial cancer is the most frequent extraintestinal malignancy in HNPCC (Watson et al., 1994). The average age at endometrial cancer onset in HNPCC families is 48 years (Hakala et al., 1991), occurring approximately 15 years earlier than the sporadic form. By age 70, the risk of endometrial cancer for a woman in an HNPCC kindred is 20% vs. a population risk of 3% (Watson et al., 1994). If a germline mutation in the *MSH2* or *MLH1* gene can be identified, the risk can be refined further, with estimates of 20% by age 50 and 60% by age 70 (Vasen et al., 1996; Aarnio et al., 1999).

Gene Identification

Cancer-susceptibility genes have not been identified for site-specific endometrial cancer, although some of these pedigrees may have mutations in one of the mismatch repair genes associated with HNPCC. One report found that the presence of endometrial cancer in kindreds with familial clustering of colon cancer or other cancer associated with HNPCC was an independent predictor of germline mutations in the *MSH2* or *MLH1* gene (Wijnen et al., 1998).

At least five mismatch repair genes have been identified that underlie the cancer susceptibility associated with HNPCC: *MSH2*, *MLH1*, *MSH6*, *PMS1*, and *PMS2*. In the majority of families with HNPCC, the mutations affect the *MSH2* or *MLH1* gene (Peltomaki and Vasen, 1997). These genes are members of a DNA "repair crew." They orchestrate repair of DNA mismatches that occur during DNA replication. When mutated, these DNA repair enzymes typically cause a characteristic DNA pattern in malignant or premalignant tumors. This pattern is called *microsatellite instability*. Microsatellite instability has been demonstrated in 75% of endometrial cancers from HNPCC families compared to only 17% in sporadic endometrial cancers (Risinger et al., 1993).

The most consistent findings in LOH studies of endometrial cancer include loci on chromosomes 3p, 10q, 17p, and 18q (Jones et al., 1994; Fujino et al., 1994). An important candidate gene on chromosome 3p is *MLH1*.

Clinical Application and Risk Assessment

Because of the significant risk for endometrial cancer in cases with a possible inherited susceptibility, several authors support preventive strategies for endometrial cancer risk reduction in these high-risk women (Sandles et al., 1992; Watson et al., 1994; Burke et al., 1997a). These strategies might include patient education regarding abnormal vaginal discharge and bleeding, avoidance of periods of anovulation, avoidance of unopposed estrogen use, maintenance of ideal body weight, and surveillance with periodic transvaginal ultrasound examinations with endometrial biopsies. Prophylactic hysterectomy including BSO should be considered after childbearing is complete and especially at the time of surgery for an HNPCC-associated colorectal cancer (Moslein et al., 2000). Oral contraceptives might also be effective at decreasing endometrial and ovarian cancer risk associated with HNPCC.

In addition to early detection and prevention strategies for gynecologic cancers associated with HNPCC, the other cancers associated with this diagnosis must be considered (see Chapter 34).

CERVICAL CANCER

Disease Definition

Most cervical cancers arise within the transformation zone of the cervix, where the columnar epithelium of the endocervix meets the squamous epithelium of the ectocervix. Cervical cancers less commonly arise from the endocervical columnar epithelium itself (adenocarcinomas). Adenosquamous carcinomas are a mixture of malignant adenocarcinoma and squamous cell carcinoma; they are poorly differentiated and associated with decreased survival. Clear cell carcinoma, glassy cell carcinoma, adenoid cystic carcinoma, and mucoepidermoid carcinoma are rare variants that usually behave like poorly differentiated carcinoma (Hoskins et al., 1993).

Squamous cervical carcinomas progress from normal epithelium to carcinoma in a series of distinct changes. HPV infection is an early and probably initiating event in this process. Classification of preinvasive cervical carcinoma characterizes the progressive types of cervical intraepithelial neoplasia (CIN) as mild, moderate, and severe (CIN-1, CIN-2, and CIN-3, respectively). A more recent classification divides all preinvasive cervical lesions into two groups: low-grade squamous cell intraepithelial lesion, which includes HPV-related changes and CIN-1 (mild dysplasia), and high-grade squamous cell intraepithelial lesion, which includes CIN-2 and CIN-3 or moderate dysplasia, severe dysplasia, and carcinoma in situ (Richart, 1990). Preinvasive cervical lesions can regress, persist, or progress (Öster, 1993). The higher-grade lesions are most likely to progress to invasive carcinoma. However, there are no distinguishing morphologic characteristics that can predict which lesions will progress or regress.

Preinvasive cervical cancers are not associated with symptoms. Early invasive cancers can cause vaginal discharge or bleeding, usually after sexual activity. Serosanguineous or purulent discharge or bleeding might develop as the tumor becomes more invasive. Symptoms of advanced disease include pain in the pelvis, lower back, and legs associated with inflammation; tumor necrosis; and nerve root compression or involvement. Urinary frequency or urgency, hematuria, rectal tenesmus, and rectal bleeding can result from direct tumor invasion (Hoskins et al., 1993).

General Genetic and Epidemiologic Evidence

Cervical cancer is the third most common cancer of the female genital tract. In the United States, 12,900 new cervical cancer cases and 4400 deaths from cervical cancer are estimated in 2001 (Greenlee et al., 2001). The prevalence of CIN lesions ranges from 0.5% to 6.5% of the American female population. Invasive cervical cancer usually develops between 48 and 55 years, with a mean of 53.8 years and a median of 51.5 years (Cramer and Cutler, 1974). Carcinoma in situ is usually seen between the ages of 25 and 40 (Cramer and Cutler, 1974). Risk factors include low socioeconomic status, sexual intercourse at a young age, numerous sexual partners, early pregnancy, and multiparity. Conversely, nulliparity, sexual inactivity, and mutually monogamous relationships are protective (Rotkin, 1967). The incidence of cervical cancer among Hispanic women is almost twice that among non-Hispanic white women (Peters et al., 1986; Becker et al., 1992). Cervical cancer is infrequent in Jewish and Moslem women, and this may be due to circumcision of their male partners or possibly genetic factors (Terris et al., 1973; Ackerman and del Regato, 1977).

HPVs are thought to be the causative agents of most cervical carcinomas and preinvasive lesions. HPV types 6 and 11 are common in benign condylomata acuminata, and HPV types 16 and 18 are frequently identified in high-grade cervical intraepithelial neoplasms and invasive carcinomas (Bosch et al., 1995).

Familial risks for cervical cancer and in situ cervical cancer have been estimated from the Swedish Family-Cancer Database, a comprehensive database that has been collecting information on all invasive cancers since 1958 and on in situ cancers since 1970 (Hemminki and Vaittinen, 1998). The familial relative risk (FRR) associated with invasive cervical cancer between mothers and daughters was 2.0 (Weiss et al., 1996). A similar value was observed for in situ cervical cancer (FRR = 1.8, 95% CI 1.7–1.8) (Hemminki and Vaittinen, 1998). A maternal history of in situ and invasive cervical cancer was also associated with rectal and other female genital tract cancers in daughters (Hemminki and Vaittinen, 1997b, 1998). The risk of rectal cancer in sons of mothers with cervical cancer followed a similar trend, but it was not significant. Similar FRRs for in situ cancers in daughters of mothers who had invasive cervical cancer were observed. In the case of cervical cancer in situ, the FRR was 1.6 (95% CI 1.5–1.7), and for rectal cancer in situ, it was 5.5 (95% CI 1.5–14.6). The FRR for in situ cervical cancer in daughters of mothers and fathers with an invasive lung cancer was also significantly increased, 1.4 (95% CI 1.3–1.5) and 1.2 (95% CI 1.2–1.3), respectively. The FRR associated with invasive cervical cancer in daughters of mothers with in situ cervical cancer was also significant, 1.7 (95% CI 1.4–2.0). The authors of these studies suggested that the association of familial risk observed with these invasive and noninvasive cancers might be due to shared exposures to HPV or other agents. Tobacco smoke might be implicated because of the significant increase of in situ cervical cancer in daughters of parents with invasive lung cancer. Additionally, when both mothers and daughters had invasive cervical cancer as a first primary cancer, there was an excess of lung cancer occurring as a second primary cancer, providing further evidence that smoking might be a risk factor in families with aggregation of cervical cancer (Hemminki and Vaittinen, 1997a). Results from the State Health Registry of Iowa also support a role for smoking and cervical cancer risk (Anderson et al., 1997). Women with a family history of cervical cancer in a first-degree relative had a relative risk (RR) of lung cancer of 1.6 after multivariate adjustment (95% CI 0.98–2.6) compared to women without such a history. The risk was even greater among those lung cancer types associated with smoking, including squamous cell, small cell, and large cell tumors (RR = 2.0, 95% CI 1.1–3.7).

Pathophysiology: Biologic Basis of Genetic Susceptibility

The E6 and E7 proteins from high-risk HPVs can immortalize primary cells in culture and appear to play an important role in carcinogenesis (Hawley-Nelson et al., 1989). The E6 gene product of HPV types 16 and 18 interacts with and promotes degradation of p53 protein (Scheffner et al., 1990). The E7 protein of HPV16 binds to and inactivates the retinoblastoma gene protein, which acts downstream from TP53 in the growth arrest response to DNA damage (Dyson et al., 1989; Hickman et al., 1994). Thus, high-risk HPVs might indirectly contribute to cervical carcinogenesis by abolishing the cell cycle arrest seen after DNA damage, leading to genomic instability and accumulation of mutations (Kastan et al., 1991). The HPV E6 and E7 proteins probably affect other aspects of the cell cycle besides the G_1/S checkpoint, as evidenced by increased cellular levels and activity of mitotic regulatory proteins in HPV-infected keratinocytes (Steinmann et al., 1994), and other HPV proteins may play a role in cellular transformation (Straight et al., 1993).

Gene Identification

Cytogenetic studies have shown nonrandom involvement of many chromosomes, particularly chromosomes 1, 3, 5, 11, and 17; and the abnormalities detected are usually deletions (Atkin, 1997). LOH has been observed at high frequency involving chromosomes 3p, 4, 5, 6, 11p, and 17p (Kersemaekers et al., 1998). LOH of 6q, 6p, and 17p correlated marginally with HPV16 positivity. LOH of 3p was weakly correlated with high mitotic activity, while LOH of 11q, 15q, and 17p correlated with low mitotic activity. LOH of 18q was associated with poor prognosis.

A candidate tumor-suppressor gene, *FHIT* at 3p14.2, contains the fragile site FRA3B and the breakpoint of the t(3;8) translocation of familial renal cell carcinoma (Ohta et al., 1996). The *FHIT* gene contains a spontaneous HPV16 integration site (Wilke et al., 1996). When HPV16 is integrated, a short chromosomal deletion limited to the local FRA3B region is induced. In a series of 28 cervical cancers, allelic loss of *FHIT* was found in 59% of tumors and 43% of these cervical cancers showed inactivation of the *FHIT* gene in both alleles (Yoshino et al., 1998). These findings suggest that inactivation of the *FHIT* gene plays an important role in cervical carcinogenesis. The *E6* and *E7* oncogenes of HPV were expressed in 85% of the 28 cervical cancers; however, no correlation was observed between LOH at the *FHIT* locus and HPV integration or expression. The authors suggest that this might indicate that alterations of *FHIT* and HPV integration occur independently in cervical carcinogenesis. Aberrant *FHIT* transcripts have also been associated with marked reduction or loss of expression of the Fhit protein in cervical cancer, providing further evidence that *FHIT* gene alterations may be important in cervical carcinogenesis (Greenspan et al., 1997).

Cytogenetic deletion and LOH of chromosome 11p are frequent in cervical cancer (Kersemaekers et al., 1998). Two candidate genes mapping to 11p include *H19*, a gene producing an RNA that is thought to have an anticarcinogenic effect, and *IGF2*. These genes are in close proximity to one another on 11p15.5 in a region subject to LOH, and both are subject to imprinting effects; *IGF2* is expressed by the paternal allele and *H19* by the maternal allele. In a study of 29 cervical cancers, LOH of *H19* and *IGF2* was found in 48% and 45% of tumors, respectively (Douc-Rasy et al., 1996). In addition, loss of imprinting effects was observed in 17% and 50% of tumors with no evidence of LOH, respectively. Hypomethylation of *H19* was also observed in cervical tumors, suggesting disruption of the normal imprinting process. Thus, the authors suggested that both *H19* and *IGF2* might play an important role in cervical carcinogenesis.

A common amino acid polymorphism in the p53 protein exchanges a proline for an arginine at position 72. The arginine form of p53 is more susceptible to E6-mediated degredation, and one study has found a significant association of p53 arginine homozygosity with cervical cancer (Storey et al., 1998). The frequency of homozygosity for the p53 arginine allele was detected in 76% of tumors compared with 37% of controls, and proline/arginine heterozygosity was identified in 17% of tumors and 58% of controls. The authors estimated that individuals homozygous for the arginine form of p53 protein would be associated with a seven-fold increase in risk for cervical cancer. Thus, this p53 allele might represent a risk factor for HPV-associated cervical carcinogenesis.

HPV has been detected in 33% of college-aged women (Schneider, 1988). However, not all women with HPV infection will develop cervical cancer, suggesting that host factors influence cervical cancer development. In a study of 98 Hispanic women with invasive cervical cancer and 220 ethnically matched controls, human leukocyte antigen (HLA) DR-DQ haplotype associations with susceptibility and resistance were found (Apple et al., 1994). The DRB1*1501-0602 haplotype was increased among all cervical cancer cases compared to controls (OR = 2.87, 95% CI 1.25–6.65, $p = 0.005$), and it was even greater among HPV16-positive cases (OR = 4.78, 95% CI 1.90–11.83, $p = 0.00007$). No increase in risk was observed with this haplotype among other HPV-positive cases, indicating HPV16 specificity. An increase in susceptibility was also observed with the most common DR4 subtype among Hispanics. However, the OR associated with the DRB1*0407-DQB1*0302 haplotype was significant only with HPV16-positive cases (OR = 2.61, 95% CI 1.04–6.49, $p = 0.022$), and the DRB1*0405-DQB1*0302 haplotype was not increased among total cases but was increased among other HPV-positive cases (OR = 4.24, 95% CI 1.0–16.89, $p = 0.037$). Combining the risks associated with HPV16 and the DRB1*1501-DQB1*0602 haplotype resulted in an estimated 75-fold increase in risk. The risk associated with the co-occurrence of HPV16 and DRB1*1302-DQB1*0604 could not be calculated due to inadequate sample size. In studies investigating HLA alleles and non-invasive cervical cancers, the same susceptibility HLA alleles associated with invasive cervical cancer were associated with severe cervical dysplasia in a population of Mexican-American women (Apple et al., 1995), and this has been identified in Swedish and Norwegian women as well (Sanjeevi et al., 1996; Helland et al., 1998).

Protective effects were also observed with certain DR-DQ haplotypes in the study of Mexican-American women (Apple et al., 1994). Three DR13 haplotypes (DRB1*1301-DQB1*0603, DRB1*1302-DQB1*0604, and DRB1*1303-DQB1*0301) were significantly decreased among all cases. This association was found with HPV16 positive cases (OR = 0.26, 95% CI 0.07–0.77, $p = 0.009$) but not others, suggesting that the protection was HPV16-specific. The DRB1*0411-DQB1*0302 haplotype of serogroup DR14 was also associated with a protective effect. In contrast, this protective effect was significantly decreased only in cases with HPV infection other than type 16 (OR = 0.15, 95% CI 0.00–0.95, $p = 0.033$) and not with total cases or HPV16-positive cases, suggesting that the protection associated with DR14 is related to HPV types other than 16. In one study, from France, a protective effect was associated with DRB1*1301/02 alleles and HPV-positive tumors (Sastre-Garau et al., 1996). However, no association between HLA type and susceptibility to cervical cancer was observed.

In keeping with the postulated role of DRB1 amino acid position 57 in disease susceptibility (Erlich et al., 1993), the two DR4 alleles associated with cervical cancer susceptibility, DRB1*0407 and 0403/6, encode aspartic acid at position 57, while the protective DR4 allele, DRB1*0411, encodes a serine.

Clinical Application and Risk Assessment

Early detection of cervical cancer is very achievable, and when found at noninvasive or early invasive stages, it is amenable to cure. Exfoliated cervical cells can be collected, stained, and microscopically examined for abnormal cells (by Pap smear). When low-grade preinvasive lesions are detected, some physicians opt to follow patients with repeat Pap smears, whereas high-grade lesions are typically treated by excisional biopsy or some other ablative therapy, such as laser, cryotherapy, or electrocautery.

Women with a family history of invasive or in situ cervical cancer have about a twofold increase in cervical cancer risk. Because HPV and tobacco smoking are thought to underlie this increased familial risk, such women can be counseled about high-risk behaviors that might increase their cervical cancer risk. In addition, women with a family history of in situ or invasive cervical cancer might benefit from more frequent screening with Pap smears (e.g., every 6 months), and such frequent screening would continue despite consecutive normal results.

Further risk stratification in the population might be feasible with genotyping, including the p53 proline/arginine polymorphism, the molecular typing of HLA DR and DQ, as well as HPV analysis. However, the efficacy, utility, and cost-effectiveness of this strategy must be investigated to determine the appropriateness of such an approach. However, such genotyping might improve the ability to target individuals who are more likely to progress from preinvasive to invasive carcinoma and for whom more aggressive treatment would be appropriate. It might also be expected that as the pathophysiologic mechanisms of these genetic associations are more clearly defined, chemotherapeutic and chemopreventive agents targeted for specific genetic susceptibilities will be created. This might include HPV-based vaccines.

TESTICULAR CANCER

Disease Definition

In 2001, 7200 new cases of testicular cancer and 400 related deaths are expected (Greenlee et al., 2001). Testicular cancer is the most common cancer among men aged 15 to 35, and it is also seen in men over age 60. Most testicular tumors arise from germ cells. They are pluripotent and can differentiate into embryonal and extraembryonal tissue types. Germ cell tumors usually present in the testis; however, a small proportion occur in the mediastinum, retroperitoneum, and pineal gland. Histologically, they are classified as seminomas, tumors that do not differentiate, and nonseminomas, tumors that display embryonal differentiation. The different types of nonseminoma include embryonal carcinomas (embryonal differentiation), choriocarcinomas and yolk sac tumors (extraembryonal differentiation), and teratomas (somatic differentiation). Teratomas may differentiate into other mature lineages, such as cartilage, neuronal tissue, and mucinous and nonmucinous glands. Teratomas can also undergo malignant transformation, including sarcoma, carcinoma, myeloid leukemia, and neuroectodermal tumor (Murty and Chaganti, 1998). Nongerminal neoplasms account for the minority of testicular cancers and are classified as stromal tumors, gonadoblastomas, and other miscellaneous types.

Testicular cancers usually present as a painless unilateral swelling. Occasionally, a patient might complain of a dull ache in the lower abdomen or scrotum. In about 10% of patients, pain might be the presenting symptom, and rarely the presenting complaint may be related to metastatic disease. Survival of germ cell tumors is related to the stage at diagnosis, and this is often delayed in most patients. Despite this, survival of germ cell tumors has improved dramatically over the decades; with the advent of multidrug chemotherapy, the overall cure rate for all stages is higher than 90%.

General Genetic and Epidemiologic Evidence

Established risk factors involved in the development of germ cell tumors include cryptorchidism, testicular atrophy due to increased levels of gonadotropins, and family history (Forman et al., 1990). Incidence rates of testicular cancer are different among ethnic groups, with whites more often affected than Hispanics and blacks (Spitz et al., 1986). Never-married men have a greater risk of developing nonseminoma testicular cancer than their married counterparts (Forman et al., 1990).

A large, population-based prospective study from Germany and Austria described the proportion of familial testicular cancer as 1.7% of cases (Dieckmann and Pichlmeier, 1997). Of the 28 patients reporting a family history, 18 had an affected first-degree relative (nine brothers and nine fathers) and 10 had an affected second- or third-degree relative. In six of the 28 families, there were more than two affected family members. This estimate is similar to estimates of 1% to 2% derived from retrospective studies of smaller size (Dieckmann et al., 1987; Nicholson and Harland, 1995).

In a retrospective case-control study, the OR associated with a family history of testicular cancer was 4.53 (95% CI 1.23–24.9, $p = 0.018$) when all relatives were included. When only first-degree relatives were evaluated, the OR was 3.11 (95% CI 0.77–17.95, $p > 0.05$) (Dieckmann and Pichlmeier, 1997). Higher estimates of testicular cancer risk, ranging from 7.6 to 12.3 due to an affected first-degree relative, have been obtained from studies that calculated actuarial cancer risks described as standardized incidence rates derived from national cancer registries (Forman et al., 1992; Heimdal et al., 1996a; Westergaard et al., 1996). Case-control studies did not adjust for the number of relatives at risk and the years of exposure. This may explain the considerable difference in testicular cancer risk due to a family history estimated by the cancer registries (Dieckmann and Pichlmeier, 1997). In studies using cancer registry data, having a brother with testicular cancer conferred a higher risk than having a father with testicular cancer. Among the Norwegian and Swedish cancer registries, the standardized incidence rates for brothers was 10.2 (95% CI 6.2–15.7) and for fathers, 4.3 (95% CI 1.6–9.3). The cumulative risk of testicular cancer to brothers of affected cases was 2.8% (95% CI 1.2%–4.4%) at age 50 and 4.1% (95% CI 1.7%–6.6%) at age 60.

Studies provide conflicting results when age at onset of testicular cancer is compared between patients with a family history and those without. However, when father-to-son transmission has been recorded, a significantly earlier age at onset is observed in the sons vs. the fathers, suggestive of anticipation (Forman et al., 1992; Heimdal et al., 1996a). No statistically significant correlation between histologic type of testicular cancer and familial disease has been demonstrated. When the histologic groups of seminoma and nonseminoma were examined separately, there appeared to be a trend toward younger age at onset among familial cases (Dieckmann and Pichlmeier, 1997; Heimdal et al., 1996a). Familial testicular cancer cases more often have bilateral cancer compared to sporadic cases (Heimdal et al., 1996b). The well-recognized risk factor of cryptorchidism does not appear to be more prevalent among familial cases compared to nonfamilial cases of testicular cancer (Heimdal et al., 1996a).

Cancer at sites other than the testis has been studied in the families of 797 Norwegian and 178 Swedish testicular cancer cases diagnosed between 1981 and 1991 (Heimdal et al., 1996b). The total number of cancers was less than expected among the Norwegian families; fewer prostate and gastrointestinal cancer occurrences accounted for most of this discrepancy. In the Swedish cohort, the number of cancers was very close to the expected. Although there were significantly fewer prostate cancers than expected among fathers, with a standardized incidence rate of 0.51, mothers had more lung and endometrial cancers than expected, with standardized incidence rates of 2.11 and 1.73, respectively. The authors suggested that these findings support the theory of hormonal dysfunction as causing testicular cancer. Although this study did not identify an increase in breast cancer among relatives, Moss and co-workers (1986) found an increase in breast cancer among mothers of nonseminoma testicular cancer cases. Testicular cancer was not associated with several known inherited Mendelian cancer susceptibilities, including hereditary site-specific breast cancer, breast–ovary cancer, and HNPCC. However, in this study, one patient belonged to a family consistent with the Li-Fraumeni syndrome. Males and females with germ cell cancer have been reported in at least four additional families (Hartley et al., 1989; Scott et al., 1993).

A study of 194 twins from England and Wales found an increased risk of testicular cancer in monozygotic twins of men affected with testicular cancer, 76.5 (95% CI 11.2–518, $p < 0.001$), and in dizygotic twins, it was increased 35.7-fold (95% CI 5.2–244.7, $p < 0.001$) (Swerdlow et al., 1997). The difference in testicular cancer risk between monozygotic and dizygotic twins was not statistically significant ($p = 0.45$). The cumulative risk of testicular cancer by age 40 in monozygotic twins of cases was estimated to be 14% by age 40. When seminomas were analyzed separately, a 50% higher risk for testicular cancer was found in dizygotic twins compared to monozygotic twins, with an OR of 3.2 (95% CI 1.6–6.5, $p = 0.001$). There was no trend with age at onset. The authors suggested that the excess risk among dizygotic twins was due to in utero hormonal effects, possibly raised concentrations of maternal unbound estrogens in the first trimetster of pregnancy, since gonadotropin and estrogen concentrations are greater in dizygotic compared to monzygotic pregnancies (Martin et al., 1984). Page and co-workers (1998) also found an increased rate of testicular cancer among dizygotic twins compared to monozygotic twins (0.18% vs. 0.08%; OR = 2.12, $p = 0.038$). Interestingly, in their study, none of the twins carried a diagnosis of cryptorchidism.

An excess of testicular germ cell tumors has been observed in Down syndrome patients (Satge et al., 1997). In a study of testicular cancer incidence in males with Down syndrome, two invasive testicular germ cell tumors were found among 137 cases over an 8-year period. The annual incidence of malignant germ cell tumors in the population during the same period was estimated to be 3 to 5.9 per 100,000 person-years. Thus, the incidence of testicular cancer in Down syndrome patients was increased 50-fold. Correspondingly, in two series of testicular germ cell tumors, an excess of Down syndrome has been identified (Dexeus et al., 1988; Mann et al., 1989).

Gene Identification

A segregation analysis performed with family history reports from 978 Scandinavian patients with testicular cancer found that a recessive model best fit the data, with an estimated gene frequency of 3.8% (Heimdal et al., 1997). Thus, this study estimated that 7.6% of men in the population are carriers of the cancer-susceptibility allele and 0.1% are homozygous and at risk for testicular cancer with a lifetime testicular cancer risk of 43%. The authors of this study also estimated that 25% of testicular cancer cases diagnosed before age 35, 14% of cases diagnosed between ages 35 and 54, and 12% of cases diagnosed after the age of 55 could be attributed to this susceptibility. Because the incidence of testicular cancer has changed over the past generations, the authors attempted to correct for this factor in their analyses. Varying assumptions about the relative incidence of testicular cancer in parental and proband generations did not appreciably change the outcome of a recessive major gene model as most parsimonious. The family studies that demonstrated an increased RR of testicular cancer among brothers of cases compared to fathers of cases also support a recessive model of inheritance. Linkage analyses employing a genomic scan have been performed in brothers with testicular cancer (Leahy et al., 1995). A number of candidate genetic regions have been implicated, and evidence for linkage was strongest under recessive models in those regions with the highest LOD scores.

A few population association studies have identified susceptibility alleles for testicular cancer. The HLA class II allele DRB1*0410 was significantly associated with testicular cancer in Japanese cases vs. controls (5.45% vs. 1.79%, RR = 3.26, $p = 0.006$) (Ozdemir et al., 1997). The proportion of risk due to this allele was estimated to be 0.69. Within the entire population, it was estimated that 8% of Japanese patients developed testicular cancer because of this allele. DQB1*0602 was identified as a protective allele, found in 1.81% of cases compared to 6.22% of controls (RR = 0.26, $p = 0.02$). It was estimated that this allele prevented 74% of the testicular cancer cases that would have otherwise occurred among those males with this allele, and within the population, the DQB1*0602 allele would have prevented 3% of such cases. Histologic type or clinical stage of the tumors was not associated with any particular HLA allele.

Another study, from the United Kingdom, found that individuals homozygous for the *b* allele of the GSTP1 locus, involved in the inactivation of cigarette smoke carcinogens and toxins, was significantly increased among testicular cancer cases compared to controls (18.7% vs. 6.5%, OR = 3.3, 95% CI 1.5–7.7, $p = 0.002$) (Harries et al., 1997). This association was found in both teratoma and seminoma cancer cases.

Expansion of $(CAG)_n$ repeats has also been associated with testicular tumors (King et al., 1997). This was observed in 5 of 11 testicular tumor cell lines, in 1 of 11 sporadic testicular tumors, and in the germline DNA of members of testicular cancer families. The methodology used in this study revealed the presence, but not the location, of expanded CAG repeats within a given genomic DNA sample. Thus, the authors suggested that a single expanded $(CAG)_n$ tract may define a locus that resides within or near a gene important to testicular cancer development or that a form of genomic instability affecting multiple triplet repeats may be associated with testicular cancer.

Other candidate genes for testicular cancer susceptibility and progression may be discovered through identification of nonrandom cytogenetic studies (Murty and Chaganti, 1998). The most consistent nonrandom chromosomal change found in testicular tumors is isochromosome 12p. One or more copies of isochromosome 12p are found in about 80% of all subsets of tumors, including in situ tumors. A tandem duplication of 12p may be found in the remaining 20% of tumors. Although less frequent, other nonrandom chromosome abnormalities include deletion or rearrangement breakpoints at 12q12 to q24, 6q13–25, 1p31–36, and 7q. With regard to ploidy level, chromosomes that are overrepresented in testicular cancers include 8, 21, and X. Chromosomes that are underrepresented are 18, 13, 11, 5, 4, and 9. LOH has been observed frequently at 3p, 11p, 5p, and 5q, as well as three loci on chromosome 1p (1p13, 1p22, and 1p31.3–32.2) and one on 1q (1q32). LOH at 12q13.2–13.3 and 12q22 has also been observed, consistent with the cytogenetic findings, and additional studies have identified a minimal region of deletion (Murty et al., 1996). These studies suggest the presence of tumor-suppressor genes that might be implicated in a genetic susceptibility to the development or progression of testicular cancer.

Clinical Application and Risk Assessment

Delay in diagnosis of testicular cancer might be avoided if regular testicular self-exam were practiced. In addition, periodic physician testicular exams coupled with ultrasound of any suspicious lesions might improve early detection in those men with an increased risk due to history of cryptorchidism, twinning, Down syndrome, or family history (Richie et al., 1982). Ultrasound might also be useful for identification of occult testicular malignancies (Glazer et al., 1982). The serum tumor markers alpha-fetoprotein and human chorionic gonadotropin are useful in the diagnosis of germ cell testicular cancers, and they might be useful in early detection of such tumors in men at high risk. Discussion regarding cryopreservation of sperm might also be appropriate with males at increased risk for testicular cancer.

REFERENCES

Aarnio M, Mecklin J-P, Aaltonen LA, Nystrom-Lahti M, Jarvinen HJ: Life-time risk of different cancers in hereditary colorectal cancer (HNPCC) syndrome. Int J Cancer 1995; 64:430–433.

Aarnio M, Sankila R, Pukkala E, Salovaara R, Aaltonen LA, de la Chapelle A, Peltomaki P, Mecklin JP, Jarvinen HJ: Cancer risk in mutation carriers of DNA-mismatch-repair genes. Int J Cancer 1999; 81:214–218.

Ackerman LV, del Regato JA: Cancer Diagnosis, Treatment, and Prognosis. St. Louis: Mosby, 1977.

Amos CI, Shaw GL, Tucker MA, Hartge P: Age at onset for familial epithelial ovarian cancer. JAMA 1992; 268:1896–1899.

Anderson KE, Woo C, Olson JE, Sellers TA, Zheng W, Kushi LH, Folsom AR: Association of family history of cervical, ovarian, and uterine cancer with histological categories of lung cancer: the Iowa Women's Health Study. Cancer Epidemiol Biomarkers Prev 1997; 6:401–405.

Apple RJ, Becker TM, Wheeler CM, Erlich HA: Comparison of human leukocyte antigen DR-DQ disease associations found with cervical dysplasia and invasive cervical carcinoma. J Natl Cancer Inst 1995; 87:427–436.

Apple RJ, Erlich HA, Klitz W, Manos MM, Becker TM, Wheeler CM: HLA DR-DQ associations with cervical carcinoma show papillomavirus-type specificity. Nat Genet 1994; 6:157–162.

Atkin NB: Cytogenetics of carcinoma of the cervix uteri: a review. Cancer Genet Cytogenet 1997; 95:33–39.

Aure JC, Hoeg K, Kolstad P: Clinical and histologic studies of ovarian carcinoma: long-term follow-up of 900 cases. Obstet Gynecol 1971; 37:1–9.

Becker TM, Wheeler CM, Key CR, Samet SM: Cervical cancer incidence and mortality in New Mexico's Hispanics, American Indians, and non-Hispanic whites. West J Med 1992; 156:376–379.

Bokhman JV: Two pathogenetic types of endometrial carcinoma. Gynecol Oncol 1983; 15:10–517.

Boltenberg A, Furgyik S, Kullander S: Familial cancer aggregation in cases of adenocarcinoma corporis uteri. Acta Obstet Gynecol Scand 1990; 69:249–258.

Bosch FX, Manos MM, Muñoz N, Sherman M, Jansen AM, Peto J, Schiffman MH, Moreno V, Kurman R, Shah, KV: Prevalence of human papillomavirus in cervical cancer: a worldwide perspective. International Biological Study of Cervical Cancer (IBSCC) study group. J Natl Cancer Inst 1995; 87:796–802.

Bristow RE, Karlan BY: Ovulation induction, infertility, and ovarian cancer risk. Fertil Steril 1996; 66:499–507.

Burke W, Daly M, Garber J, Botkin J, Ellis Kahn MJ, Lynch P, McTiernan A, Offit K, Perlman J, Petersen G, et al.: Recommendations for follow-up care of individuals with an inherited predispostion to cancer. I Hereditary nonpolyposis colon cancer. JAMA 1997a; 277:915–919.

Burke W, Daly M, Garber J, Botkin J, Ellis Kahn MJ, Lynch P, McTiernan A, Offit K, Perlman J, Petersen G, et al.: Recommendations for follow-up care of individuals with an inherited predispostion to cancer. II *BRCA1* and *BRCA2*. JAMA 1997b; 277:997–1003.

Claus EB, Risch N, Thompson WD: The calculation of breast cancer risk for women with a first degree family history of ovarian cancer. Breast Cancer Res Treat 1993; 28:115–120.

Cliby W, Ritland S, Hartmann L, Dodson M, Halling KC, Keeney G, Podratz KC, Jenkins RB: Human epithelial ovarian cancer allelotype. Cancer Res 1993; 53(Suppl 10):2393–2398.

Cramer DW, Cutler SJ: Incidence and histopathology of malignancies of the female genital organs in the United States. Am J Obstet Gynecol 1974; 118:443–460.

Cummings SR, Eckert S, Krueger KA, Grady D, Powles TJ, Cauley JA, Norton L, Nickelsen T, Bjarnason NH, Morrow M, et al.: The effect of raloxifene on risk of breast cancer in postmenopausal women. Results of the MORE randomized trial. JAMA 1999; 281:2189–2197.

Dexeus FH, Logothetis CJ, Chong C, Sella A, Ogden S: Genetic abnormalities in men with germ cell tumors. J Urol 1988; 140:80–84.

Dieckmann K-P, Becker T, Jonas D, Bauer HW: Inheritance and testicular cancer: arguments based on a report of 3 cases and a review of the literature. Oncology 1987; 44:367–377.

Dieckmann K-P, Pichlmeier U: The prevalence of familial testicular cancer. An analysis of two patient populations and a review of the literature. Cancer 1997; 80:1954–1960.

Douc-Rasy S, Barrois M, Fogel S, Ahomadegbe JC, Stéhelin D, Coll J, Riou G: High incidence of loss of heterozygosity and abnormal imprinting of *H19* and *IGF2* genes in invasive cervical carcinomas. Uncoupling of *H19* and *IGF2* expression and biallelic hypomethylation of *H19*. Oncogene 1996; 12:423–430.

Dyson N, Howley P, Munger K, Harlow E: The human papillomavirus-16 E7 oncoprotein is able to bind to the retinoblastoma gene product. Science 1989; 243:934–937.

Egan KM, Newcomb PA, Longnecker MP, Trentham-Dietz A, Baron JA, Trichopoulos D, Stampfer MJ, Willett WC: Jewish religion and risk of breast cancer. Lancet 1996; 347:1645–1646.

Erlich HA, Zeidler A, Chang J, Shaw S, Raffel LJ, Klitz W, Beshkov Y, Costin G, Pressman S, Bugawan T: HLA class II alleles and susceptibility and resistance to insulin dependent diabetes mellitus in Mexican-American families. Nature Genetics 1993; 3:358–364.

Fisher B, Costantino JP, Wickerham DL, Redmond CK, Kavanah M, Cronin WM, Vogel V, Robidoux A, Dimitrov N, Atkins J, et al.: Tamoxifen for prevention of breast cancer: report of the National Surgical Adjuvant Breast and Bowel Project P-1 Study. J Natl Cancer Inst 1998; 90:1371–1388.

Forman D, Gallagher R, Moller H, Swerdlow TJ: Aetiology and epidemiology of testicular cancer: report of consensus group. Prog Clin Biol Res 1990; 357:245–253.

Forman D, Oliver RTD, Brett AR, Marsh SGE, Moses JH, Bodmer JG, Chilvers CE, Pike MC: Familial testicular cancer: a report of the UK family register, estimation of risk and an HLA class 1 sib-pair analysis. Br J Cancer 1992; 65:255–262.

Fujino T, Risinger JI, Collins NK, Liu F-S, Nishii H, Takahashi H, Westphal E-M, Barrett JC, Sasaki H, Kohler MF, et al.: Allelotype of endometrial carcinoma. Cancer Res 1994; 54:4294–4298.

Gallion HH, Powell DE, Smith LW, Vaugh CC, Case EA: Cytogenetic changes in human epithelial ovarian cancer. In: Sharp F, Mason WP, Creasman W (eds). Ovarian Cancer 2. London: Chapman and Hall Medical, 1992:17–22.

Gallup DG, Stock RJ: Adenocarcinoma of the endometrium in women 40 years of age or younger. Obstet Gynecol 1984; 64:417–420.

Glazer HS, Lee JKT, Melson GL, McClennan BC: Sonographic detection of occult testicular neoplasms. AJR Am J Roentgenol 1982; 138:673–675.

Greenlee RT, Hill-Harmon MB, Murray T, Thun M: Cancer statistics, 2001. CA Cancer J Clin 2001; 51:15–36.

Greenspan DL, Connolly DC, Wu R, Lei RY, Vogelstein JTC, Kim Y-T, Mok JE, Muñoz N, Bosch FX, Shah K, et al.: Loss of *FHIT* expression in cervical carcinoma cell lines and primary tumors. Cancer Res 1997; 57:4692–4698.

Greggi S, Genuardi M, Benedetti-Panici P, Cento R, Scambia G, Neri G, Mancuso S: Analysis of 138 consecutive ovarian cancer patients: incidence and characteristics of familial cases. Gynecol Oncol 1990; 39:300–304.

Grover S, Quinn MA, Weideman P: Patterns of inheritance of ovarian cancer. An analysis from an ovarian cancer screening program. Cancer 1993; 72:526–530.

Gruber SB, Thompson WD: A population-based study of endometrial cancer and familial risk in yougner women. Cancer and Steroid Hormone Study Group. Cancer Epidemiol Biomarkers Prev 1996; 5:411–417.

Hakala T, Mecklin J-P, Forss M, Jarvinen H, Lehtovirta P: Endometrial carcinoma in the cancer family syndrome. Cancer 1991; 68:1656–1659.

Hankinson SE, Hunter DJ, Colditz GA, Willett WC, Stampfer MJ, Rosner B, Hennekens CH, Speizer FE: Tubal ligation, hysterectomy, and risk of ovarian cancer. JAMA 1993; 270:2813–2816.

Harries LW, Stubbins MJ, Forman D, Howard GCW, Wolf CR: Identification of genetic polymorphisms at the glutathione *S*-transferase *Pi* locus and association with susceptibility to bladder, testicular and prostate cancer. Carcinogenesis 1997; 18:641–644.

Hartley AL, Birch JM, Kelsey AM, Marsden HB, Harris M, Teare MD: Are germ cell tumors part of the Li-Fraumeni cancer family syndrome? Cancer Genet Cytogenet 1989; 42:221–226.

Hartmann LC, Schaid DJ, Woods JE, Crotty TP, Myers JL, Arnold PG, Petty PM, Sellers TA, Johnson JL, McDonnell SK, et al.: Efficacy of bilateral prophylactic mastectomy in women with a family history of breast cancer. N Engl J Med 1999; 340:77–84.

Hawley-Nelson P, Vousden KH, Hubbert NL, Lowy DR, Schiller JT: HPV 16 E6 and E7 proteins cooperate to immortalize human foreskin keratinocytes. EMBO J 1989; 8:3905–3910.

Heimdal K, Olsson H, Tretli S, Flodgren P, Borresen A-L, Fossa SD: Familial testicular cancer in Norway and southern Sweden. Br J Cancer 1996a; 73:964–969.

Heimdal K, Olsson H, Tretli S, Flodgren P, Borresen A-L, Fossa SD: Risk of cancer in relatives of testicular cancer patients. Br J Cancer 1996b; 73:970–973.

Heimdal K, Olsson H, Tretli S, Fossa SD, Borresen A-L, Bishop DT: A segregation analysis of testicular cancer based on Norwegian and Swedish families. Br J Cancer 1997; 75:1084–1087.

Helland A, Olsen AO, Gjøen K, Akselsen HE, Sauer T, Magnus P, Børresen-Dale A-L, Rønningen KS: An increased risk of cervical intra-epithelial neoplasia grade II–III among human papillomavirus positive patients with the HLA-DQA1*0102-DQB1*0602 haplotype: a population-based case-control study of Norwegian women. Int J Cancer 1998; 76:19–24.

Hemminki K, Vaittinen P: Effect of paternal and maternal cancer on cancer in the offspring: population-based study. Cancer Epidemiol Biomarkers Prev 1997a; 6:993–997.

Hemminki K, Vaittinen P: Familial cancer in Sweden: population-based study. Int J Oncol 1997b; 11:273–280.

Hemminki K, Vaittinen P: Familial risks of in situ cancers from the Family-Cancer Database. Cancer Epidemiol Biomarkers Prev 1998; 7:865–868.

Hickman ES, Picksley SM, Vousden KH: Cells expressing HPV16 E7 continue cell cycle progression following DNA damage induced by p53 activation. Oncogene 1994; 9:2177–2818.

Hoskins WJ, Perez CA, Young RC: Gynecologic tumors. In: DeVita VT Jr, Hellman S, Rosenberg SA (eds). Cancer: Principles and Practice of Oncology, 4th ed. Philadelphia: Lippincott, 1993:1152–1225.

Houlston RS, Bourne TH, Davies A, Whitehead MI, Campbell S, Collins WP, Slack J: Use of family history in a screening clinic for familial ovarian cancer. Gynecol Oncol 1992; 47:247–252.

Jones MH, Koi S, Fujimoto I, Hasumi K, Kato K, Nakamura Y: Allelotype of uterine cancer by analysis of RFLP and microsatellite polymorphisms: frequent loss of heterozygosity on chromosome arms 3p, 9q, 10q, 17p. Genes Chromosomes Cancer 1994; 9:119–123.

Kastan MB, Onyekwere O, Sidransky D, Vogelstein B, Craig RW: Participation of p53 protein in the cellular response to DNA damage. Cancer Res 1991; 51:6304–6311.

Kaufman DJ, Struewing JP: Re: Effect of *BRCA1* and *BRCA2* on the association between breast cancer risk and family history [letter]. J Natl Cancer Inst 1999; 91:1250–1251.

Kerlikowske K, Brown JS, Grady DG: Should women with familial ovarian cancer undergo prophylactic oophorectomy? Obstet Gynecol 1992; 80:700–707.

Kersemaekers A-MF, Kenter GG, Hermans J, Fleuren GJ, van de Vijver MJ: Allelic loss and prognosis in carcinoma of the uterine cervix. Int J Cancer 1998; 79:411–417.

King BL, Peng H-Q, Goss P, Huan S, Bronson D, Kacinski BM, Hogg D: Repeat expansion detection analysis of $(CAG)_n$ tracts in tumor cell lines, testicular tumors, and testicular cancer families. Cancer Res 1997; 57:209–214.

King M-C, Wieand S, Hale K, Lee M, Walsh T, Owens K, Tait J, Ford L, Dunn BK, Costantino J, et al.: Tamoxifen and breast cancer incidence among women with inherited mutations in *BRCA1* and *BRCA2*. JAMA 2001; 286:2251–2256.

Leahy MG, Tonks S, Moses JH, Brett AR, Huddart R, Forman D, Oliver RTD, Bishop DT, Bodmer JG: Candidate regions for a testicular cancer susceptibility gene. Hum Mol Genet 1995; 4:1551–1556.

Lynch HT, Krush AL, Mangnuson CW: Endometrial carcinoma: multiple primary malignancies, constitutional factors, and heredity. Am J Med Sci 1966; 36:381–390.

Lynch HT, Smyrk TC, Watson P, Lanspa SJ, Lynch JF, Lynch PM, Cavalieri RJ, Boland CR: Genetics, natural history, tumor spectrum, and pathology of hereditary nonpolyposis colorectal cancer: an updated review. Gastroenterology 1993; 104:1535–1549.

MacMahon B: Risk factors for endometrial cancer. Gynecol Oncol 1974; 2:122–129.

Mann JR, Pearson D, Barrett A, Raafat F, Barnes JM, Wallendszus KR: Results of the United Kingdom Children's Cancer Study Group's malignant germ cell tumor studies. Cancer 1989; 63:1657–1667.

Marra G, Boland CR: Hereditary nonpolyposis colorectal cancer: the syndrome, the genes, and historical perspectives. J Natl Cancer Inst 1995; 87:1114–1125.

Martin NG, el Beaini JL, Olsen ME, Bhatnagar AS, Macourt D: Gonadotropin levels in mothers who have had two sets of DZ twins. Acta Genet Med Gemellol (Roma) 1984; 33:131–139.

Mecklin JP, Jarvinen HJ: Tumor spectrum in cancer family syndrome (hereditary nonpolyposis colorectal cancer). Cancer 1991; 68:1109–1112.

Meijers-Heijboer H, Van Geel B, Van Putten WLJ, Henzen-Logmans SC, Seynaeve C, Menke-Pluymers MBE, Bartels CCM, Verhoog LC, Van Den Ouweland AMW, Niermeijer MF, et al.: Breast cancer after prophylactic bilateral mastecomy in women with a *BRCA1* or *BRCA2* mutation. N Engl J Med 2001; 345:159–164.

Modan B, Hartge P, Hirsh-Yechezkel G, Chetrit A, Lubin F, Beller U, Ben-Baruch G, Fishman A, Menczer J, Struewing JP, et al.: Parity, oral contraceptives, and the risk of ovarian cancer among carriers and noncarriers of a *BRCA1* or *BRCA2* mutation. N Engl J Med 2001; 345:235–240.

Moslehi R, Chu W, Karlan B, Fishman D, Risch H, Fields A, Smotkin D, Ben-David Y, Rosenblatt J, Russo D, et al.: *BRCA1* and *BRCA2* mutation analysis of 208 Ashkenazi Jewish women with ovarian cancer. Am J Hum Genet 2000; 66:1259–1272.

Moslein G, Krause-Paulus R, Hegger R, Peterschulte G, Vogel T: Clinical aspects of hereditary nonpolyposis colorectal cancer. Ann NY Acad Sci 2000; 910:75–84.

Moss AR, Osmond D, Bacchetti P, Torti FM, Gurgin V: Hormonal risk factors in testicular cancer. A case-control study. Am J Epidemiol 1986; 124:39–52.

Murty VVVS, Chaganti RSK: A genetic perspective of male germ cell tumors. Semin Oncol 1998; 25:133–144.

Murty VVVS, Renault B, Falk CT, Bosl GJ, Kucherlapati R, Chaganti RS: Physical mapping of a commonly deleted region, the site of a candidate tumor suppressor gene, at 12q22 in human male germ cell tumors. Genomics 1996; 35:562–570.

Narod SA, Risch H, Moslehi R, Dorum A, Neuhausen S, Olsson H, Provencher D, Radice P, Evans G, Bishop S, et al.: Oral contraceptives and the risk of hereditary ovarian cancer. N Engl J Med 1998; 339:424–428.

Nicholson PW, Harland SJ: Inheritance and testicular cancer. Br J Cancer 1995; 71:421–426.

NIH Consensus Development Panel on Ovarian Cancer: Ovarian cancer. Screening, treatment, and follow-up. JAMA 1995; 273:491–497.

Nikrui N: Survey of clinical behavior of patients with borderline tumors of the ovary. Gynecol Oncol 1981; 12:107–119.

Ohta M, Inoue H, Cotticelli MG, Kastury K, Baffa R, Palazzo J, Siprashvili Z, Mori M, McCue P, Druck T, et al.: The *FHIT* gene, spanning the chromosome 3p14.2 fragile site and renal carcinoma-associated t(3;8) breakpoint, is abnormal in digestive tract cancers. Cell 1996; 84:587–597.

Öster AG: Natural history of cervical intraeithelial neoplasia—a critical review. Int J Gynecol Pathol 1993; 12:186–192.

Ozdemir E, Kakehi Y, Mishina M, Ogawa O, Okada Y, Ozdemir D, Yoshida O: High-resolution HLA-DRB1 and DQB1 genotyping in Japanese patients with testicular germ cell carcinoma. Br J Cancer 1997; 76:1348–1352.

Page WF, Braun MM, Caporaso NE: Twinning, cancer, and genetics. Lancet 1998; 351:910–911.

Peltomaki P, Vasen HF: Mutations predisposing to hereditary nonpolyposis colorectal cancer: database and results of a collaborative study. The International Collaborative Group on Hereditary Nonpolyposis Colorectal Cancer. Gastroenterology 1997; 113:1146–1158.

Peters RK, Thomas D, Hagan DG, Mack TM, Henderson BE: Risk factors for invasive cervical cancer among Latinas and non-Latinas in Los Angeles County. J Natl Cancer Inst 1986; 77:1063–1077.

Piver MS, Jishi MF, Tsukada Y, Nava G: Primary peritoneal carcinoma after prophylactic oophorectomy in women with a family history of ovarian cancer. Cancer 1993; 71:2751–2755.

Rebbeck TR, Levin AM, Eisen A, Snyder C, Watson P, Cannon-Albright L, Isaacs C, Olopade O, Garber JE, Godwin AK, et al.: Breast cancer risk after bilateral prophylactic oophorectomy in *BRCA1* mutation carriers. J Natl Cancer Inst 1999; 91:1475–1479.

Richart RM: A modified terminology for cervical intraepithelial neoplasia. Obstet Gynecol 1990; 75:131–133.

Richie JP, Birnholz J, Garnick MB: Ultrasonography as a diagnostic adjunct for the evaluation of masses in the scrotum. Surg Gynecol Obstet 1982; 154:695–698.

Risinger JI, Berchuck A, Kohler MF, Watson P, Lynch HT, Boyd J: Genetic instability of microsatellites in endometrial cancer. Cancer Res 1993; 53:5100–5103.

Rossing MA, Daling JR, Weiss NS, Moore DE, Self SG: Ovarian tumors in a cohort of infertile women. N Engl J Med 1994; 331:771–776.

Rotkin ID: Epidemiology of cancer of the cervix. III. Sexual characteristics of a cervical cancer population. Am J Public Health Nations Health 1967; 57:815–829.

Sall S, Stone ML: The treatment of ovarian cancer. Prog Clin Cancer 1973; 5:249–262.

Sandles LG, Shulman LP, Elias S, Photopulos GJ, Smiley LM, Posten WM, Simpson JL: Endometrial adenocarcinoma: genetic analysis suggesting heritable site-specific uterine cancer. Gynecol Oncol 1992; 47:167–171.

Sanjeevi CB, Hjelmstrom P, Hallmans G, Wiklund F, Lenner P, Angstrom T, Dillner J, Lernmark A: Different HLA-DR-DQ haplotypes are associated with cervical intraepithelial neoplasia among human papillomavirus type-16 seropositive and seronegative Swedish women. Int J Cancer 1996; 68:409–414.

Sastre-Garau X, Loste M-N, Vincent-Salomon A, Favre M, Mouret E, de la Rochefordiere A, Durand J-C, Tartour E, Lepage V, Charron D: Decreased frequency of HLA-DRB1*13 alleles in French women with HPV-positive carcinoma of the cervix. Int J Cancer 1996; 69:159–164.

Satge D, Sasco AJ, Cure H, Leduc B, Sommelet D, Vekemans MJ: An excess of testicular germ cell tumors in Down's syndrome. Cancer 1997; 80:929–935.

Scheffner M, Weness BA, Huibregste JM, Levine AJ, Howley PM: The E6 oncoprotein encoded by human papilloma virus types 16 and 18 promotes the degradation of p53. Cell 1990; 63:1129–1136.

Schildkraut JM, Risch N, Thompson WD: Evaluating genetic association among ovarian, breast, and endometrial cancer: evidence for a breast/ovarian cancer relationship. Am J Hum Genet 1989; 45:521–529.

Schildkraut JM, Thompson WD: Familial ovarian cancer: a population-based case-control study. Am J Epidemiol 1988; 128:456–466.

Schneider A: HPV infection in women and their male partners. Contemp Obstet Gynecol 1988; 32:131.

Scott RJ, Krummeernacher F, Mary JL, Weber W, Spycher M, Muller H: Hereditary p53 mutation in a patient with multiple tumors: significance for genetic counseling. Schweiz Med Wochenschr 1993; 123:1287–1292.

Scully RE: Ovarian tumors. Am J Pathol 1977; 87:686–720.

Sellers TA, Mink PJ, Cerhan JR, Zheng W, Anderson KE, Kushi LH, Folsom AR: The role of hormone replacement therapy in the risk for breast cancer and total mortality in women with a family history of breast cancer. Ann Intern Med 1997; 127:973–980.

Shushan A, Paltiel O, Isocvich J, Elchalal U, Peretz R, Schenker JG: Human menopausal gonadotropin and the risk of epithelial ovarian cancer. Fertil Steril 1996; 65:13–18.

Spitz MR, Saider JG, Pollack ES, Lynch HK, Newell GR: Incidence and descriptive features of testicular cancer among United States whites, blacks, and Hispanics, 1973–1982. Cancer 1986; 58:1785–1790.

Steinberg KK, Pernarelli JM, Marcus M, Khoury MJ, Schildkraut JM, Marchbanks PA: Increased risk for familial ovarian cancer among Jewish women: a population-based case-control study. Genet Epidemiol 1998; 15:51–59.

Steinberg KK, Thacker SB, Smith SJ, Stroup DF, Zack MM, Flanders D, Berkelman RL: A meta-analysis of the effect of estrogen replacement therapy on the risk of breast cancer. JAMA 1991; 265:1985–1990.

Steinmann KE, Pei XF, Stoppler H, Schlegel R: Elevated expression and activity of mitotic regulatory proteins in human papillomavirus-immortalized keratinocytes. Oncogene 1994; 9:387–394.

Storey A, Thomas M, Kalita A, Harwood C, Gardiol D, Mantovani F, Breuer J, Leigh IM, Matlashewski G, Banks L: Role of a p53 polymorphism in the development of human papillomavirus-associated cancer. Nature 1998; 393:229–234.

Straight SW, Hinkle PM, Jewers RJ, McCance DJ: The E5 oncoprotein of human papillomavirus type 16 transforms fibroblasts and effects the downregulation of the epidermal growth factor receptor in keratinocytes. J Virol 1993; 67:4521–4532.

Swerdlow AJ, De Stavola BL, Swanwick MA, Maconochie NES: Risks of breast and testicular cancers in young adult twins in England and Wales: evidence on prenatal and genetic aetiology. Lancet 1997; 350:1723–1728.

Terris M, Wilson F, Nelson JJ: Relation of circumcision to cancer of the cervix. Am J Obstet Gynecol 1973; 117:1056–1066.

Tobacman JK, Tucker MA, Kase R, Greene MH, Costa J, Fraumeni JF Jr: Intra-abdominal carcinomatosis after prophylactic oophorectomy in ovarian-cancer-prone families. Lancet 1982; 2:795–797.

Ursin G, Henderson BE, Haile RW, Pike MC, Zhou N, Diep A, Bernstein L: Does oral contraceptive use increase the risk of breast cancer in women with *BRCA1/ BRCA2* mutations more than in other women. Cancer Res 1997; 57:3678–3681.

Vasen HFA, Wunen JT, Menko FH, Kleibeuker JH, Taal BG, Griffioen G, Nagengast FM, Meijers-Heijboer EH, Bertario L, Varesco L, et al.: Cancer risk in families with hereditary nonpolyposis colorectal cancer diagnosed by mutation analysis. Gastroenterology 1996; 110:1020–1027.

Watson P, Vasen HFA, Mecklin JP, Jarvinen H, Lynch HT: The risk of endometrial cancer in hereditary nonpolyposis colorectal cancer. Am J Med 1994; 96:516–520.

Weber BL, Punzalan C, Eisen A, Lynch HT, Narod SA, Garber JE, Isaacs C, Daly MB, Neuhausen SL, Rebbeck TR: Ovarian cancer risk reduction after bilateral prophylactic oophorectomy (BPO) in *BRCA1* and *BRCA2* mutation carriers. Am J Hum Genet 2000; 67(Suppl 2):59.

Weiss HA, Brinton LA, Brogan D, Coates RJ, Gammon MD, Malone KE, Schoenberg JB, Swanson CA: Epidemiology of in situ and invasive breast cancer in women aged under 45. Br J Cancer 1996; 73:1298–1305.

Westergaard T, Olsen JH, Frisch M, Kroman N, Nielsen JW, Melbye M: Cancer risk in fathers and brothers of testicular cancer patients in Denmark: a population-based study. Int J Cancer 1996; 66:627–631.

Whittemore AS, Harris R, Itnyre J, and the Collaborative Ovarian Cancer Group: Characteristics relating to ovarian cancer risk: collaborative analysis of 12 U.S. case-control studies. IV. The pathogenesis of epithelial ovarian cancer. Am J Epidemiol 1992; 136:1184–1203.

Wijnen JT, Vasen HF, Khan PM, Zwinderman AH, van der Klift H, Mulder A, Tops C, Moller P, Fodde R: Clinical findings with implications for genetic testing in families with clustering of colorectal cancer. N Engl J Med 1998; 339:511–518.

Wilke CM, Hall BK, Hoge A, Paradee W, Smith DI, Glover TW: FRA3B extends over a broad region and contains a spontaneous HPV 16 integration site: direct evidence for the coincidence of viral integration sites and fragile sites. Hum Mol Genet 1996; 5:187–195.

Yoshino K, Enomoto T, Nakamura T, Nakashima R, Wada H, Saitoh J, Noda K, Murata Y: Aberrant FHIT transcripts in squamous cell carcinoma of the uterine cervix. Int J Cancer 1998; 76:176–181.

38 Skin Cancer

ALLEN E. BALE, SUZANNE J. BROWN, AND WILLIAM D. POSTEN

The majority of skin cancers are basal cell or squamous cell carcinomas, which arise from keratinocytes and have relatively benign clinical behavior. Melanomas are malignant neoplasms arising from melanocytes. Although nonmelanoma skin cancer is approximately 20 times as common as melanoma, melanoma causes three times as many deaths.

Most skin cancer occurs in fair-skinned people, and on a population basis sunlight exposure is the most important determinant of skin cancer risk. Hereditary factors, beside those influencing skin color, play a relatively minor role in predisposition to nonmelanoma skin cancer. In contrast, at least 5% of melanoma appears to be attributable to high-penetrance autosomal dominant genes. The genetics and molecular pathophysiology of melanoma and nonmelanoma skin cancer are almost entirely distinct, and they will be treated as separate entities in this chapter.

NONMELANOMA SKIN CANCER

Disease Definition

Nonmelanoma skin cancers (NMSCs) represent approximately one-half of all cancers diagnosed in the United States but cause only about 2000 deaths per year (Greenlee et al., 2000). Basal cell carcinomas (BCCs) account for 80% of NMSCs, and nearly all of the remainder are squamous cell carcinomas (SCCs) (Scotto and Fraumeni, 1982). Other rare types making up a small fraction of the total include eccrine carcinoma, apocrine and sebaceous gland carcinoma, Kaposi's sarcoma, liposarcoma, cutaneous lymphoma, leiomyosarcoma, and extramammary Paget's disease (Weinstock, 1994). Both BCCs and SCCs tend to occur in sun-exposed areas of the skin. SCCs have a predilection for the hands and forearms, while BCCs are more common on the head or neck (Marks, 1995).

There are several subtypes of basal cell carcinoma (BCC), which present with clinically diverse features. A common histopathologic classification system (Lang and Maize, 1986) divides the tumors into five main categories. The most common, nodular BCC, appears grossly as a translucent or pearly papule with telangiectasias coursing through it. Microscopically, nodular BCC is characterized by a compact mass of cells that resemble the basal layer of the epidermis but extend into the dermis. These tumors have sharp margins with a palisaded peripheral border that separates tumor from normal tissue. Micronodular BCCs are similar in gross appearance to nodular BCCs, but microscopically they are composed of many small tumor nodules rather than a single compact tumor mass. The superficial subtype consists of a flat erythematous plaque, which variably has scale; a translucent border; and areas of hypopigmentation, atrophy, or scarring. Histology shows tumor nests budding from the epidermis. Infiltrating BCCs can have many different gross appearances but are characterized histologically as irregular islands of tumor cells with jagged projections into surrounding tissue. The morpheaform subtype resembles a plaque of localized scleroderma, with indistinct borders. Microscopically, there is intense stromal proliferation and collagen production surrounding small irregular islands of tumor cells. All subtypes can contain melanin and superficially may resemble melanomas. Some tumors differentiate toward sebaceous, apocrine, or eccrine structures (Fig. 38–1).

Histopathologic subtype correlates with the risk of recurrence after surgical excision (Sexton et al., 1990). Surgical margins of nodular and superficial types are rarely positive for residual tumor, but infiltrative and morpheaform BCCs have positive margins in more than 25% of cases. Micronodular tumors have an intermediate risk of recurrence. Beside subtype, tumors occurring in men, large tumors, and tumors in unusual sites such as the ear canal or anal area are more likely to recur (Karagas, 1994).

BCCs rarely metastasize (0.0028%), but metastatic disease is almost always fatal (Paver et al., 1973). The average age of patients with metastatic BCC is 45, and the male to female ratio is 2:1. Conditions associated with metastatic disease include AIDS, systemic amyloidosis, and prior exposure to radiation (Snow et al., 1994).

Detailed histologic evaluation of BCCs suggests that many arise from hair follicles and that the cell of origin may be located in the superficial portion of the hair follicle. However, experimental data with genetically transformed interfollicular keratinocytes indicate that nonfollicular cells may also give rise to tumors with typical characteristics of BCCs (Fan et al., 1997). BCCs appear to arise de novo without a preexisting precursor lesion (Miller, 1991).

SCCs are malignant neoplasms derived from keratinocytes. Grossly they appear as indurated and often ulcerated papules, and microscopically they consist of atypical squamous cells invading the underlying dermis and producing an irregular disorganized architecture (Johnson et al., 1992). Actinic keratosis and Bowen's disease (SCC in situ) are precursor lesions on which invasive SCCs arise (Gloster and Brodland, 1996). Actinic keratoses are dysplastic keratotic, irregularly shaped, angular papules that develop on skin exposed to sun or UV light, especially in light-skinned people. Bowen's disease is intraepidermal SCC without invasion of the dermis. Typically, Bowen's disease appears as a well-circumscribed, scaling plaque without ulceration.

Like BCCs, SCCs can cause morbidity by local invasion and tissue destruction. In addition, the risk of metastasis is not insignificant (Weinstock, 1994). Risk factors for recurrence include large size, anatomic site (ear and lip greater than other sun-exposed sites), histologic factors such as thickness and depth,

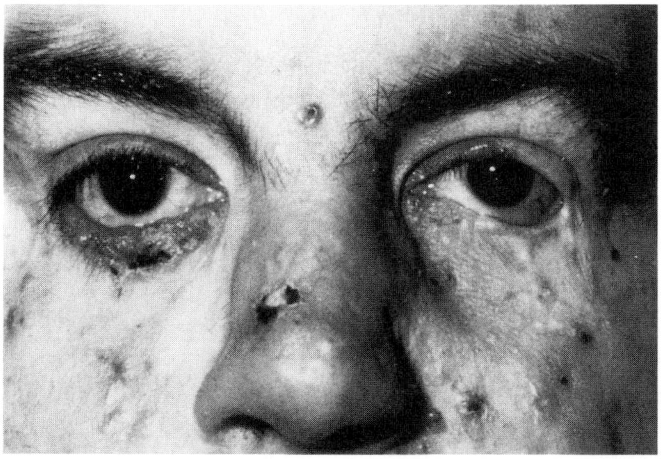

Fig. 38–1. Multiple basal cell carcinomas in a patient with hereditary skin cancer predisposition (the nevoid basal cell carcinoma syndrome). These tumors can present as pearly lesions, ulcers, or scars.

and degree of differentiation (Rowe et al., 1992). In scars, the edges of ulcers, skin damaged by ionizing radiation, and mucosal surfaces the metastatic potential is high, with a risk of 8% to 20% (Goltz, 1998). Immunosuppression is also a risk factor for metastatic disease (Haas, 1998).

General Genetic and Epidemiologic Evidence

Clinical Epidemiology and Ethnic Differences

Nonmelanoma skin cancer is not reported in most tumor registries, and few studies have accurately measured its frequency (Weinstock, 1994). Estimates from the American Cancer Society (Greenlee et al., 2000) place the incidence at more than 1 million cases per year in the United States, and the cumulative lifetime risk for developing this type of tumor is approximately one in six. The frequency of this disease is increasing 3% to 7% annually in white people in the United States, Canada, and Australia (Gloster and Brodland, 1996). SCC is responsible for most of the mortality in NMSC, resulting in death 2% of the time and accounting for three-quarters of all deaths attributable to NMSC (Gloster and Brodland, 1996).

The incidence of NMSC shows an inverse correlation with latitude. For example, the incidence of NMSC is approximately 40 per 100,000 among the Caucasian population in the United States and over 200 per 100,000 among a similar ethnic population in Australia. In a U.S. survey of six geographical sites, including Albuquerque, Atlanta, Detroit, New Orleans, Salt Lake City, San Francisco, and Seattle, NMSC incidence showed an excellent inverse correlation with latitude and positive correlation with total sunlight, with the highest rate in Albuquerque and the lowest rate in Seattle (Scotto and Fraumeni, 1982).

Skin cancer is seen almost exclusively in fair-skinned people and especially in those with blue eyes, freckles, and light hair color (Scotto and Fraumeni, 1982). Both constitutive color (the baseline level of melanin pigmentation in the absence of exogenous factors) and facultative color (which results from environmental exposures and hormonal stimuli) contribute to skin cancer risk (Marks, 1995). A sun reactivity classification scheme proposed by Fitzpatrick (1983) divides skin types into four categories believed to correlate with skin cancer risk (Table 38–1). Celtic ancestry (Scottish, Irish, Welsh) seems to be an additive risk factor in addition to skin color. NMSC is uncommon in blacks, Asians, and Hispanics. The incidence of NMSC in whites is 70 times greater than in blacks, and BCCs in blacks are much more likely to occur on non-sun-exposed skin than are BCCs in whites (Abreo and Sanusi, 1991). SCC is more common than BCC in blacks, causing more than two-thirds of their skin cancers. SCCs in blacks have a higher mortality rate (17% to 24%) than in whites presumably because SCCs in blacks more often arise in scars, burns, or ulcers, and these SCCs are inherently more aggressive (Halder and Bridgeman-Shah, 1995; Gloster and Brodland, 1996).

As with many other malignancies, elderly people are more likely to develop NMSC, with 95% of tumors occurring in people 40 to 79 years old (Scotto and Fraumeni, 1982). Depending on the geographic location, incidence of NMSC can be four times greater among 55- to 75-year-olds than that of people 20 years old or younger. NMSC is twice as frequent in men than in women (Gloster and Brodland, 1996), possibly reflecting differing occupational and recreational exposure to sunlight (Marks, 1995).

Associated Disease

The risk of NMSC is high in individuals who are immunosuppressed due to AIDS or to immunosuppressive therapy after transplantation (Marks, 1995). Nonhealing skin lesions after burns or other trauma and large scars are also associated with skin cancer, particularly squamous cell carcinoma. Chronic human papilloma virus infections may predispose to NMSC, especially (but not exclusively) in the context of epidermodysplasia verruciformis, a rare genetic disorder (Lutzner and Blanchet-Bardon, 1985).

Environmental Factors

Several lines of evidence implicate ultraviolet radiation (UV) exposure as the major environmental determinant of skin cancer risk. NMSCs occur in sun-exposed areas of skin and are far more common in light-skinned than in dark-skinned ethnic groups. Presumably, skin pigmentation acts as a screen against UV. Measurements of regional levels of UV have demonstrated strong correlation between the incidence of SCC and UVB—that is, people living in areas with greater intensity and duration of solar radiation are at higher risk for SCC than others. The correlation between UVB and BCC is weaker but still quite significant (Scotto and Fraumeni, 1982; Gloster and Brodland, 1996). On an individual basis, total cumulative sun exposure seems to be the main risk factor for SCC. Intermittent exposure to sunlight, particularly during childhood, appears to be more important than cumulative exposure in BCC risk (Kricker et al., 1995). Laboratory studies indicate that UVB light (290–320 nm) is more carcinogenic than UVA. UVB damages cells either directly, by inducing the formation of pyrimidine dimers in DNA and damaging other cellular constituents, or indirectly, by altering the immune system and host response. UVA is the major component of ultraviolet radiation in sunlight but is not directly absorbed

Table 38–1. Fitzpatrick Classification of Skin Types

Type	Characteristics
I	Always burn, never tan
II	Usually burn, tan less than average (with difficulty)
III	Sometimes mild burn, tan about average
IV	Rarely burn, tan more than average (with ease)

by DNA. Nevertheless, UVA generates free radicals and indirectly may produce single-strand breaks and other gross changes in DNA (Peak et al., 1987).

Although sunlight is the best-characterized environmental risk factor in NMSC, a smaller proportion of tumors are at least partially attributable to other environmental agents (Scotto and Fraumeni, 1982). Ionizing radiation in the context of radiotherapy or occupational exposure increases risk. Chemical carcinogens associated with NMSC include polyaromatic hydrocarbons, arsenicals, and psoralens in combination with UVA (PUVA therapy). Cigarette smoking is associated with cutaneous SCC, as well as internal malignancies (Grodstein et al., 1995).

Gene Identification

Skin Pigmentation

As with many common cancers, particularly those that are strongly associated with environmental agents, the risk of NMSC cancer attributable to strict Mendelian disease genes is small. However, hereditary traits may still play an important role in modifying host response to carcinogens. Fair skin in combination with UV exposure predisposes to the development of NMSC, and genetic studies provide strong evidence that the two components of skin color—constitutive and facultative—are both under genetic control (Harrison, 1973; Banerjee, 1984; Barsh, 1996).

Oculocutaneous albinism is an extreme form of genetically inherited fair skin that has a prevalence of at least 1 in 20,000 in the United States. Most albinism follows an autosomal recessive pattern of inheritance. Mutations in numerous genes can lead to congenital hypomelanosis in the skin, hair, and eyes, as well as to nystagmus, photophobia, and decreased visual acuity (reviewed in Oetting and King, 1994; Barsh, 1996). Complete defects in the tyrosinase gene, which catalyzes three steps in melanin biosynthesis, result in white hair, pink-white skin, and blue-gray irides, regardless of race. Tyrosinase mutations with some residual tyrosinase activity produce variable amounts of pigment in the eyes and in yellow or light brown hair, as well as variable pigment in skin, depending on racial background. Several types of tyrosinase-positive albinism have been described. A major category is caused by defects in the P gene (Rinchik et al., 1993; Durham-Pierre et al., 1994), which probably plays a role in melanosome formation and maintenance. Less common forms of albinism include Hermansky-Pudlak syndrome (Oh et al., 1996), with lysosomal storage of lipofuscin and a platelet defect, and Chediak-Higashi syndrome (Barbosa et al., 1996; Nagle et al., 1996), with intracytoplasmic granules and severe immunologic deficiency due to defective leukocytes.

Individuals with most forms of OCA are at high risk for actinic keratoses, squamous cell carcinomas, and, to a lesser extent, basal cell carcinomas (Oettle, 1963; King et al., 1980; Witkop, 1983; Kromberg et al., 1989; Aquaron, 1990; Yakubu and Mabogunje, 1993). Skin cancer is much more common in albinos living in tropical climates than those in regions farther from the equator and is often the cause of death in African albinos.

One of the genes believed to be responsible for normal variation in skin color is the melanocortin receptor (*MC1R*) gene. There are two types of melanin in skin, red phaeomelanin with little or no sun-protective effect and black eumelanin which is photoprotective. Binding of melanocyte stimulating hormone (MSH) to *MC1R* stimulates the synthesis of eumelanin. Limited data suggest that individuals with no functional copy of *MC1R* have red hair and Fitzpatrick type I skin (Frandberg et al., 1998). In British and Irish populations, heterozygotes and homozygotes for the Asp84Glu, Val92Met, Arg151Cys, Arg160Trp, and Asp294His polymorphisms of *MC1R* are reported to have an increased frequency of red hair and Fitzpatrick type I or type II skin (Valverde et al., 1995; Smith et al., 1998). The Asp294His variant has been reported to show an association with NMSC in the British population and possibly other groups (Smith et al., 1998; Bastiaens et al., 2001; Box et al., 2001). However, the role of *MC1R* in determining skin color and cancer susceptibility is somewhat controversial, and other data from Britain populations as well as other European Caucasian populations indicates this gene may have a very limited role in skin and hair color, as well as cancer susceptibility (Ichii-Jones et al., 1998; Smith et al., 1998).

Another potential candidate gene in determining skin color in humans is Agouti, a secreted protein that is a natural antagonist of *MC1R*. In mice, loss of function of Agouti results in black hair, while gain of function results in yellow hair. In humans, however, variance in the Agouti gene has not been described (Barsh, 1996).

DNA Repair Defects

Other host factors besides skin color are important in mediating the deleterious effects of sunlight. Xeroderma pigmentosum (XP), a genetically heterogeneous, rare autosomal recessive disease characterized by DNA repair deficiency, exemplifies the importance of repair of UV-induced damage (reviewed in Copeland et al., 1997). Clinical symptoms include enhanced acute sensitivity of skin to sunlight, cutaneous pigmentary abnormalities, and high incidence of cancer in sun-exposed sites. Seven complementation groups (A through G) have been defined on the basis of assays in which cells from different individuals are fused and the fusion products tested for UV sensitivity. The genes for these groups all appear to play roles in the complex process of excision repair and function as endonucleases, helicases, and DNA-binding proteins. People with the XP mutations have at least a 100-fold higher probability of developing skin tumors than do normal individuals (Suarez et al., 1989). XP heterozygotes are not uncommon in the population, but there are no data linking the heterozygous state to skin cancer predisposition.

More minor variation in DNA repair may influence skin cancer risk as well. In a study of DNA-repair capacity in peripheral blood T lymphocytes, individuals who had low repair capacity had a higher incidence of BCCs (Wei et al., 1993); a genetic basis for this variation in DNA repair has not been established, however.

Nevoid Basal Cell Carcinoma Syndrome

The nevoid basal cell carcinoma syndrome is a rare autosomal dominant disorder characterized by predisposition to BCCs but not SCCs or melanoma. In addition to BCCs, the syndrome is associated with pits in the palms and soles, keratocysts in the jaw, cleft palate, characteristic coarse facies, strabismus, dysgenesis of the corpus callosum, calcification of the falx cerebri, spina bifida occulta, bifid ribs, polydactyly, macrocephaly and generalized overgrowth (Gorlin, 1995). The frequency of NBCCS is only 1 in 50,000, but the molecular pathogenesis of this disorder has implications for both sporadic and hereditary forms of skin cancer.

The multiplicity, random distribution, and early age of onset of basal cell carcinomas in individuals with NBCCS is consistent with a two-hit model for tumorigenesis (Strong, 1977); that is, the underlying gene is a tumor suppressor and BCCs develop in precursor cells sustaining two genetic alterations. This theory is strongly supported by the demonstration that both hereditary and sporadic basal cell carcinomas show frequent loss of heterozygosity at 9q22 and that the *NBCCS* gene maps to the exact same region (Gailani et al., 1992).

The *NBCCS* gene is a human homolog of the *Drosophila* developmental gene, *patched* (Hahn et al., 1996; Johnson et al., 1996). *Drosophila patched* was originally identified as a gene important in establishing anterior–posterior relationships (segment polarity) in developing embryos. *Patched* encodes a large transmembrane protein that does not resemble any known tumor suppressor genes, although several membrane proteins involved in intercellular adhesion and signaling function as tumor suppressors. *Patched*, in a complex with *smoothened*, another transmembrane molecule, is believed to serve as the receptor for the secreted molecule hedgehog (reviewed in Bale and Yu, 2001). In the absence of hedgehog, *smoothened* and *patched* form an inactive complex. Upon hedgehog binding, *smoothened* is released from inhibitory effects of *patched* and transduces a signal (Fig. 38–2).

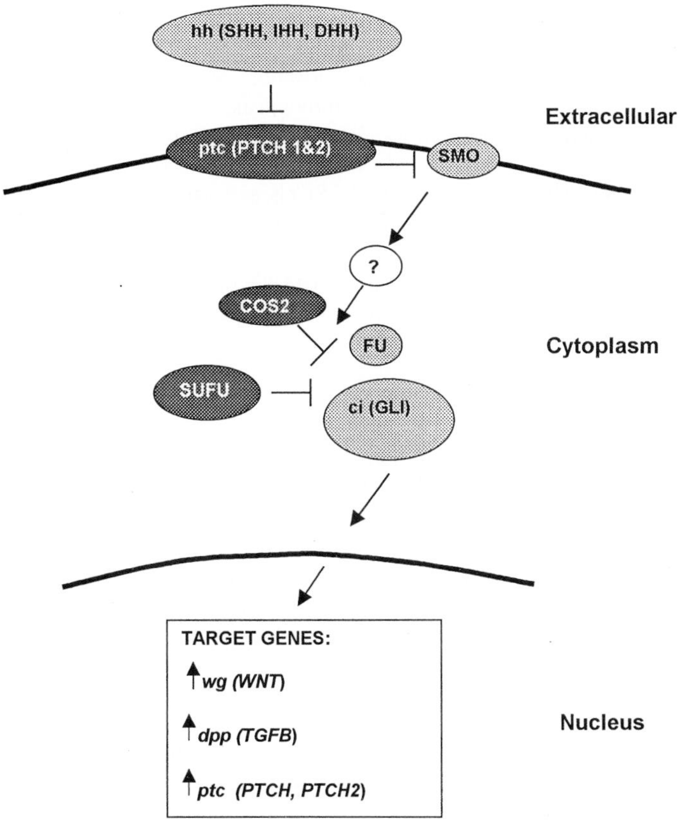

Fig. 38–2. The hedgehog pathway was originally delineated by genetic interaction studies in *Drosophila*, but subsequently biochemical interactions have been confirmed for many of the protein products of these genes. The signaling molecules intermediate between smoothened and fused are not yet known. Human homologs of most members of the *Drosophila* pathway have been isolated (*gene symbols shown in parentheses*). Either binding of hedgehog to patched or inactivating mutations of *patched* release the pathway from inhibition, resulting in activation of several downstream, growth-promoting genes. Protein symbols: hh, hedgehog; SHH, IHH, and DHH, sonic, indian, and desert hedgehog; ptc, patched; PTCH and PTCH2, two human patched homologs; SMO, *Drosophila* smoothened and human homolog; FU, fused; COS2, costal 2; ci, cubitus interruptus; GLI, human gli oncogene family; *wg*, wingless; *WNT*, human wnt oncogene family; *dpp*, decapentaplegic; *TGFB*, transforming growth factor β superfamily, including bone morphogenic proteins.

Inactivating mutations of *patched* switch on the hedgehog pathway (Gailani et al., 1996b), resulting in several molecular alterations that could be related to carcinogenesis. Inactivation of *patched* results in biochemical activation of *smoothened*. *Smoothened* has been shown to function as an oncogene when switched on in mouse skin, and, in fact, basal cell carcinomas can arise with activating mutations of *smoothened* instead of inactivating mutations of *patched* (Xie et al., 1998). GLI1, a downstream member of the hedgehog pathway that functions as a transcription factor, was originally identified as an oncogene in brain tumors, and its overexpression has been shown to cause epidermal proliferation in frogs (Dahmane et al., 1997). Activation of GLI turns on transcription of both WNT, which is known to act as an oncogene in mammary tumors in mice, and members of the TGF-α family. The latter genes have complex roles in regulating differentiation and growth of cells. It is plausible that changing the expression of these genes contributes to tumorigenesis.

Although NBCCS is rare, there is growing evidence that segmental forms of the disease, due to somatic mutations during embryonic development, may be fairly common as a cause of multiple BCCs in a limited, unilateral distribution of the body. Furthermore, it is possible that common variants of the gene contribute to skin cancer risk, although data to support this hypothesis are very limited (Chidambaram et al., 1996).

Patched and Multistep Carcinogenesis in Sporadic BCCs

Activation of the hedgehog pathway—usually through loss of *patched* function—may be a necessary if not sufficient step in basal cell carcinoma development. Mutation analysis of BCCs indicates that a high percentage have inactivating *patched* mutations (Gailani et al., 1996b). Almost all of those without *patched* mutations have activating mutations in *smoothened* (Xie et al., 1998). Combining older data from allelic loss studies and more recent direct mutation analyses, it appears that minute BCCs are as likely as large tumors to have *patched* mutations. In addition, all histological subtypes, whether primary or recurrent, have a high frequency of loss of *patched* or activation of *smoothened*. Tumors with allelic loss on chromosome 9 sometimes show additional areas of loss on other chromosomes, but no tumors have loss on other chromosomes without involvement of chromosome 9 (Gailani et al., 1992).

Patched appears to function as a "gatekeeper gene" in basal cell carcinogenesis. Inactivation of this gene (or, less commonly, loss of its effect on *smoothened* due to *smoothened* mutations) seems to be necessary before clonal expansion and accumulation of other genetic hits can lead to BCC formation (Harris, 1996; Sidransky, 1996). *Patched* mutations do not correlate with clinical subtypes of BCCs since all subtypes have mutations in this gene. Neither of two other genes (*p53* and *RAS*) known to undergo mutation in BCCs correlate with tumor size, histology, or rate of recurrence; and mutations in additional genes must confer histologic and other biologic characteristics observed clinically. Nevertheless, *p53* and *RAS* mutations no doubt contribute to the malignant characteristics of tumors.

Molecular Epidemiology of NMSC

BCCs

Epidemiological studies strongly suggest that sunlight exposure is an important etiologic agent in BCC carcinogenesis. Over 80%

of tumors occur on the head and neck, the areas of greatest sun exposure; and BCCs affect Caucasians almost exclusively, especially those who sunburn easily. However, there is a limited correlation between BCC incidence and cumulative exposure to the specific component of sunlight considered to be most carcinogenic, UVB. Furthermore, up to 33% of BCCs on the head and neck occur in areas with minimal sun exposure.

For some tumors, particular agents have been associated with specific genetic alterations; for example, aflatoxin B1 appears to lead to mutation in codon 249 of the *p53* gene in hepatocellular carcinoma (Bressac et al., 1991; Hsu et al., 1991). Ultraviolet radiation can cause several types of genetic damage, including formation of photodimers that most commonly result in a G:C to A:T transition opposite a dipyrimidine site (primarily UVB exposure), as well as single-strand breaks (primarily ultraviolet-A exposure) (Drobetsky et al., 1987; Peak et al., 1987). UVB-related point mutations have been found in the *p53* gene of 40% to 56% of BCCs (Rady et al., 1992; Ziegler et al., 1993). In addition, mutations in the ras family of proto-oncogenes are often of the type caused by UVB (Ananthaswamy and Pierceall, 1990; van der Schroeff et al, 1990).

The role of ultraviolet radiation in the pathogenesis of the genetic alterations in *patched* is less clear. The data from NBCCS patients suggests that agents other than UVB may cause somatic alterations on chromosome 9. The "first hit" in hereditary tumors is a germline point mutation or submicroscopic deletion. Any allelic loss observed in these tumors must reflect the somatic "second hit." Nearly all hereditary tumors have allelic loss, and UVB does not characteristically cause this type of gross rearrangement of genetic material. Mutations in sporadic tumors also suggest the possibility of an etiologic agent other than UVB. As in hereditary tumors, allelic loss is frequent. In one-third of tumors with allelic loss the remaining allele has a mutation characteristic of UVB, but in two-thirds the genetic alteration of the remaining allele is not a typical UVB-induced alteration (Gailani et al., 1996a,b).

The mutational spectrum in the *patched* gene is distinctly different from that in the *p53* gene, where most mutations can be linked to UVB. This discrepancy could reflect the stage at which the genetic damage occurs. Basal cell carcinomas are believed to arise from hair follicle cells. The initial "hits" that begin the process of carcinogenesis must be caused by agents that can penetrate through the superficial layer of the skin nearly into the dermis. UVB does not penetrate very deeply, and other factors such as ultraviolet A or cosmic rays may play a role in mutating *patched* in this initial stage. Chemicals such as arsenicals and polyaromatic hydrocarbons could also be involved in some cases. Once a tumor begins to grow, some of the more superficial cells might undergo *p53* mutation by UVB. These cells might derive a growth advantage, ultimately making up the bulk of the tumor. Whether this model is correct or not, the data may have clinical implications in the area of prevention because UVB sunscreen alone may not have a completely protective effect against BCCs. It remains to be seen whether sunscreens that block UVA as well will be more efficacious in preventing these tumors.

SCC

In contrast to BCC, squamous cell carcinoma of the skin shows a strong correlation with cumulative UVB exposure and a distribution on the head and neck that correlates closely with areas of greatest sun exposure. Mutations in the *p53* gene play an important role in SCCs and provide molecular evidence for the role of UVB in induction and probably promotion of early tumors. The great majority of typical SCCs occuring in sun-exposed regions of the body bear mutations in *p53*, and all of these mutations are found opposite dipyrimidine sites (Brash et al., 1991). At least 60% of actinic keratoses, the precursor lesions to SCCs, bear UVB-induced mutations in *p53*. The true frequency of mutations in these premalignant lesions may be close to 100%, but mutation detection is limited by technical problems in microdissecting actinic keratosis tissue from surrounding normal skin (Ziegler et al., 1994).

Even before the appearance of clinically recognizable actinic keratoses, normal skin in sun-exposed regions of the body bears thousands of clones with *p53* mutations (Jonason et al., 1996). These clones contain 60 to 3000 cells and typically have a conical configuration with the point of the cone at the basal layer of the skin. Presumably these clones arise from a precursor cell in the basal layer that has suffered a *p53* mutation. The mutation may increase the growth rate of the cell, but, perhaps more important, it renders the cell immune from UV-induced apoptosis. With successive exposures to sunlight, surrounding normal cells undergo apoptosis, leaving more room for the surviving mutant clone to grow and expand laterally. Hence, sunlight both initiates the clone by mutating a precursor cell and promotes clonal expansion by killing surrounding normal cells (Brash, 1997). The role of UV in promoting cancer is supported by the observation that *p53*-mutated clones in mice regress in the absence of UV exposure (Brash, 1997).

Since most of the *p53*-mutated clones in skin do not develop into actinic keratoses or SCCs, additional genetic events are almost certainly required for carcinogenesis. A small minority of SCCs have mutations in the *RAS* genes (Ananthaswamy et al., 1990; van der Schroeff et al., 1990). Allelic loss of chromosome 9q is a fairly frequent finding in SCCs as well as BCCs (Quinn et al., 1994), but the region lost is different from that in BCCs and probably does not involve the *patched* gene. *Patched* mutations have not often been found in SCCs of the skin. Mutations in other genes are almost certainly essential for progression of a normal keratinocyte to SCC.

Clinical Application and Risk Assessment

Typically, NMSC is found on sun-exposed sites in elderly, light-skinned people. Even one NMSC in a person below 40 years of age or multiple tumors at any age should raise suspicion of a genetic disorder. In a series of 63 children and teenagers with basal cell carcinomas, nearly one-half of those without an environmental cause had a predisposing genetic syndrome (Rahbari and Mehregan, 1982). NMSC in dark-skinned ethnic groups in the absence of scars, burns, or ulcers is almost always due to a hereditary condition. The differential diagnosis for early onset or multiple NMSCs includes unusual exposure to environmental carcinogens. A history of childhood exposure to X-rays or other forms of ionizing radiation, tanning salons, carcinogenic chemicals such as arsenic, and an exceptional history of trauma or burns should be sought. Childhood or a significant portion of adult life in a sunny tropical climate should also be taken into account. If no environmental risk factors are evident, both hereditary factors and other host factors, such as immunosuppression, should be considered. A careful family history should be obtained, paying close attention to relatives with a history of skin cancer and unusual skin phenotypes. A thorough physical examination for associated findings should be performed. The presence of severe actinic damage with actinic keratoses, squamous cell, and basal cell carcinomas would suggest xeroderma pigmentosum. Basal cell carcinomas without severe actinic damage or other neoplastic or preneoplastic skin lesions, especially with developmental abnormalities such as palmar pits, would suggest a diagnosis of NBCCS. In the absence of findings suggesting a known single-gene trait, the most likely cause of skin cancer predisposition is polygenic fair skin. DNA-based diagnostic tests are available for the majority of rare syndromes predisposing to NMSC. Based on current knowledge of the role of *MC1R* in NMSC predisposition, testing for common *MC1R* variants is premature and probably provides little information about risk that is independent of the risk estimate based on Fitzpatrick skin type.

Epidemiologic evidence indicates that sunlight exposure is the most important environmental risk factor for sporadic NMSC. NMSC risk in patients with albinism or XP is almost certainly mediated entirely through UV exposure, and sunlight appears to influence the risk of BCCs in individuals affected with NBCCS (Goldstein et al., 1993). Sunscreen has been shown to affect the incidence of actinic keratoses in the general population (Thompson et al., 1993), and long-term studies are in progress to evaluate the effects on sunscreen on NMSC development. Based on knowledge of the molecular mechanisms of skin cancer predisposition, it seems prudent to advise individuals with hereditary risk factors to avoid midday sunlight exposure and to use sunscreens that block both UVA and UVB. XP patients are at extreme risk of developing skin cancer and may suffer from indoor sources of UV as well. Therapeutic radiation should be avoided when possible in patients with NBCCS.

Beside avoidance of sunlight, patients with genetic disorders may benefit from chemoprophylaxis. Chemoprevention with vitamin A derivatives has shown some promise in prevention of basal cell carcinomas. Initial trials of oral isotretinoin showed clinical and histological remission in 10% of tumors in 12 patients with multiple BCCs at an oral dose of 4.5 mg/kg per day for 8 months (Peck et al., 1982). A subsequent study with doses of oral isotretinoin at 2 mg/kg per day for two years in XP patients showed a decrease in tumor frequency and size in a one-year period after treatment, compared to the two-year observational period before treatment (Kraemer et al., 1988). These positive results prompted a large prospective double-blind multicenter clinical trial by the ISO-BCC study group, which evaluated the efficacy of low-dose isotretinoin at 10 mg/day or 0.14 mg/kg per day for three years, in preventing new BCCs in patients with a history of at least two BCCs in the five years before entry into the study. In contrast to previous studies, this study showed no significant difference between drug and placebo treatment in preventing BCCs (Tangrea et al., 1992). These results may be due to a much lower dose of isotretinoin used, compared to prior studies. Unfortunately, high-dose isotretinoin treatment is associated with many adverse side effects, including mucocutaneous toxicities, hypertriglyceridemia, and vertebral abnormalities. Complications of therapy limit the long-term use of high-dose isotretinoin, but other vitamin A analogs with fewer side effects may be developed in the future.

Once NMSC has developed, surgical management is commonly employed to treat localized disease. The choice of surgical technique must be customized for each individual tumor and patient, taking into account anatomic site, tumor size, biopsy results, cosmetic concerns, and general health of the patient. Overall, the most common approach used to treat solitary SCCs and BCCs is electrodessication and curretage (Salasche, 1983). For more complicated, high-risk tumors, including recurrent tumors and those that require sparing of tissue, Mohs micrographic surgery is warranted. Mohs surgery consists of tumor debulking, followed by excision of thin slices of surrounding tissue and intraoperative, histologic "mapping" of residual tumor tissue. The surgeon removes additional regions of residual tumor based on mapping of tumor margins. This process is repeated until all the tumor is cleared (Tromovitch and Stegman, 1978). Mohs surgery leads to 5-year cure rates for primary BCCs in the range of 99%, and 94% for recurrent BCCs (Rowe et al., 1989).

Experimental studies with the teratogen cyclopamine suggest a possible application of this compound to rational medical treatment of basal cell carcinomas. Cyclopamine was discovered as an agent causing holoprosencephaly and cyclopia in sheep. The same phenotype is caused in humans by inactivating mutations of hedgehog. Cyclopamine has been shown to repress the hedgehog pathway at a point downstream from *patched*, and Taipale et al. (2000) showed that cyclopamine used at doses that do not affect normal cells result in arrest of cell growth and reversion of several malignant characteristics in cells mutant for *patched*. The findings of Taipale et al., in conjunction with the epidemiologic studies in sheep showing no ill effects of cyclopamine on adults, suggest the possibility that this agent could be used to treat basal cell carcinomas. Cyclopamine therapy of basal cell carcinomas would be predicted to suppress tumor cells but not necessarily kill them. There are few precedents in cancer therapy for the use of compounds that act in this way. However, there is some evidence that the body's natural defenses eradicate arrested tumor cells. If not, then tumors treated with cyclopamine will reappear after some brief period of latency when the drug is removed.

CUTANEOUS MELANOMA

Disease Definition

Cutaneous melanomas are malignant neoplasms arising from the melanin-producing cells of the basal layer of the epidermis. The vast majority of cutaneous pigmented lesions are benign nevi. Common nevi begin as pigmented macular lesions 1 to 2 mm in diameter, enlarge to several mm, become papular, and ultimately loose pigmentation. At all stages, benign nevi have a round or oval shape with smooth, distinct borders and even pigmentation throughout. Melanoma characteristics include asymmetry, irregular shape, indistinct borders, color variegation, elevation of some regions while other regions remain macular, and size larger than 6 mm in diameter. As cutaneous melanomas progress, their neoplastic cells penetrate from the epidermis into the subjacent dermis. A lesion may continue to expand both horizontally and vertically and become an enlarging pigmented macule with superimposed papules or nodules, a pigmented plaque, or a single nodule (Clark et al., 1969; Greene et al., 1985a). The association between nevi and melanomas is not entirely clear. It is likely that some melanomas arise from common nevi (Sagabiel, 1993). "Atypical moles" or "dysplastic" nevi (Clark et al., 1978; Piepkorn et al., 1994) may represent an intermediate precursor lesion to melanomas. Dysplastic nevi are larger than common nevi, have indistinct or irregular borders, and maintain a flat macular component as a portion of the lesion becomes papular. Histologically, they can be distinguished from melanomas in showing less aggressive behavior and more variable cytologic atypia (Fig. 38–3, 38–4).

Cutaneous melanomas tend to occur in sun-exposed areas of the body, although the association with sun-exposed sites is less striking than that for NMSC (Franceschi et al., 1996; Bulliard et

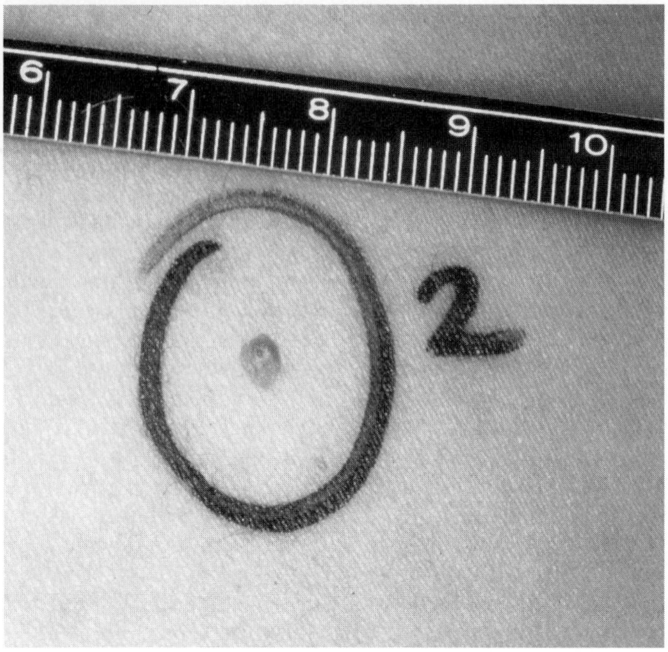

Fig. 38–3. A typical benign nevus with uniform pigmentation and clearly demarcated borders. These lesions begin as 1 to 2-mm pigmented macules; they enlarge and become papular, and ultimately they lose pigmentation. Photograph courtesy of Margaret Tucker.

al., 1997). The face is a common site in both sexes. Other areas of the head and neck are common in men, and the legs are a common site in women. The trunk is an increasingly common site, possibly related to increasing recreational sunlight exposure.

Four common subtypes are defined, based on clinical appearance and histology (Clark et al., 1969):

1. Superficial spreading melanoma presents as an asymmetric plaque with irregular borders and variegated pigmentation. Histologically, individual atypical melanocytes and small nests of cells are scattered throughout the epidermis. This subtype may be indolent with little growth or vertical invasion for years.
2. Lentigo maligna melanoma is often found in areas of sun-damaged skin in elderly, fair-skinned individuals. This lesion typically begins as a uniformly light brown macule with irregular borders and progresses to an irregularly pigmented maculo-papular melanoma. Histologically lentigo maligna is characterized by atypical epidermal melanocytes in the basal layer of the skin without abnormal cells in other layers of the epidermis.
3. Acral lentiginous melanomas are similar to lentigo maligna melanomas but arise on volar regions of hands and feet, as well as in subungual regions. They are epidemiologically distinct from lentigo maligna in that they occur with equal frequency in all races.
4. Nodular melanomas present as symmetrical, well-circumscribed nodules that are usually very dark in color and enlarge rapidly. Histologically, these tumors are composed of large masses of cells invading the dermis without a surrounding intraepidermal component.

Superficial spreading and nodular melanomas are the most common types and account for 85% of all cutaneous melanoma. Most melanomas are darkly pigmented, but any subtype may be "amelanotic" and appear reddish or skin-colored.

Important histologic features in evaluating prognosis and formulating a treatment plan include desmoplasia, neurotrophism, microscopic satellites, true vascular invasion, adequacy of surgical margins, radial or horizontal growth phase, mitotic rate, ulceration, and local invasiveness of the tumor measured as Clark level or Breslow thickness. Clark levels measure tumor invasion anatomically (Clark et al., 1969). Clark Level I is intraepidermal melanocytic atypia (i.e., melanoma in situ); Level II indicates invasion into the papillary dermis; filling and expansion of

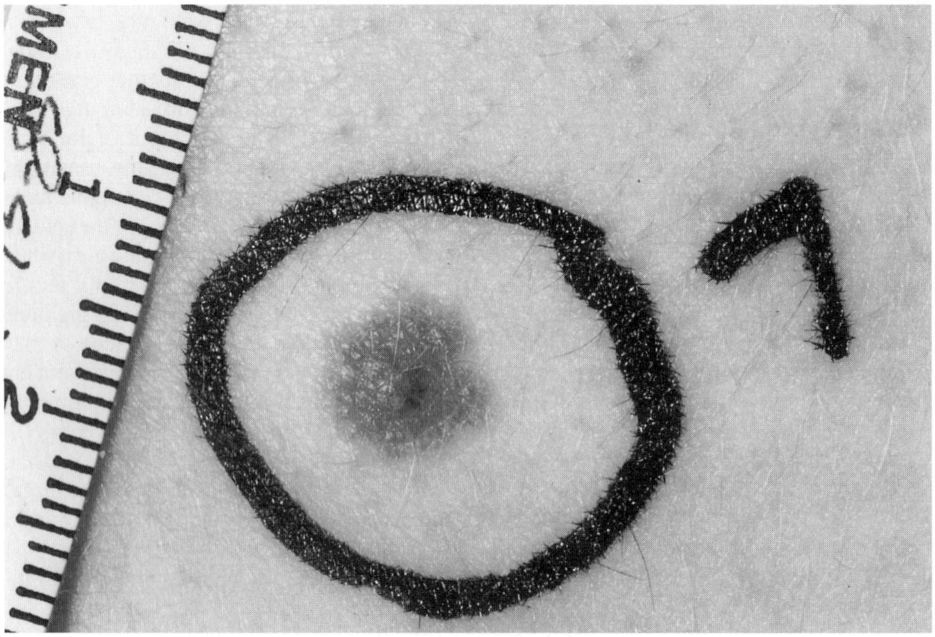

Fig. 38–4. A dysplastic nevus with irregular borders fading into surrounding skin, haphazard pigmentation, and a combination of macular and papular components. Grossly, this lesion appears similar to an early melanoma, but it could be distinguished microscopically by less aggressive histology and more varied cytologic atypia. Photograph courtesy of Margaret Tucker.

the papillary dermis defines Level III; Level IV is involvement of the reticular dermis; and Level V indicates invasion into the subcutaneous fat or deeper. Breslow depth (Breslow, 1970) measures tumor thickness in millimeters from the top of the granular layer or base of superficial ulceration to the greatest depth of tumor invasion. Prognosis is inversely related to the depth of penetration of the tumor from the epidermis into the dermis, and tumor thickness appears to be the best independent predictor of survival (Balch et al., 1978; Buzaid et al., 1997).

Genetic and Epidemiologic Evidence

Clinical Epidemiology and Ethnic Differences

Cutaneous melanoma is an increasingly common malignancy in Caucasian populations (Elwood and Koh, 1994; Armstrong and Kricker, 1994; Albino et al., 1998). In the United States the yearly incidence of invasive melanoma is 42,000 (3% of new cancers), and melanoma accounts for 1% of cancer deaths (Greenlee et al., 2000). The incidence of melanoma-in-situ, often not recorded in tumor registries, is estimated at 21,000. Melanoma incidence has been doubling every 6 to 10 years (Balch et al., 1997), and the lifetime risk of developing melanoma is projected to exceed 1% in the early twenty-first century (Rigel et al., 1996).

Melanoma is one and one-half times more common in men than women, possibly reflecting different patterns of sun exposure. In general, melanoma incidence increases with age, particularly for lentigo maligna melanoma. Superficial spreading and nodular melanoma have a median age of onset in the sixth decade but are not uncommon during the second and third decades of life (Sagabiel, 1998).

Similar to NMSC, skin color is the major determinant of melanoma risk. Melanoma is at least 10 times more common in U.S. Caucasians than in African Americans and Asian Americans. Hispanics fall between U.S. blacks and U.S. caucasians in melanoma incidence (Bergfelt et al., 1989; Cress and Holly, 1997). Among Caucasians, significant differences in risk are seen, such as decreased risk among those of southern European descent compared with those of Celtic or Scandinavian descent. Light skin color and light hair color, red hair in particular, increase melanoma risk among Caucasians when each factor is examined independently, while eye color is not an independent risk factor (Holman and Armstrong, 1984; Khlat et al., 1992). Inability to tan may be the single most important pigment-related risk factor.

Controlling for ethnic background, worldwide melanoma incidence shows an inverse correlation with latitude, with those living in more equatorial regions having a higher risk than those living in the most northern or southern regions (Lee, 1997). In the U.S. Caucasian population, there is an association between living in a more southern state and increased melanoma risk. However, the upward gradient in risk from north to south is decreasing, presumably due to increased mobility of the population. In addition to current residence, place of origin is important for the risk of melanoma among those who migrate after childhood. In a study of non-Hispanic Caucasians in Los Angeles, those migrating from a more northern latitude retained the relatively low risk associated with their place of origin rather than the higher risk associated with Los Angeles. This relative safety was unaffected by decades of life in Los Angeles (Mack and Floderus, 1991). Among Australians, those who migrated from Europe during childhood are at much greater risk for melanoma than those who migrated as adults, although duration of stay in Australia also was a risk factor (Khlat et al., 1992).

Associations with Other Diseases

Immunosuppression, either as a result of HIV infection or post-transplant therapy, is a risk factor for melanoma (Bouwes Bavinck et al., 1996; Massi et al., 1998). Benign nevi also occur to excess in immunosuppressed patients (Szepietowski et al., 1997). Melanoma has been reported to occur to excess in inflammatory bowel disease (Greenstein et al., 1992) and chronic lymphocytic leukemia (Greene et al., 1978), possibly due to alterations in immune function.

Environmental Factors

Epidemiologic evidence strongly points to sunlight exposure as the major environmental factor determining the risk of cutaneous melanoma (Armstrong and Kricker, 1993). Melanoma is far more common in fair-skinned people than in dark-skinned people, consistent with dark skin shielding melanocytes from sunlight. Melanoma tends to occur at anatomic sites that receive the greatest ultraviolet radiation, particularly sites exposed during recreational activities. Like NMSC, melanoma risk increases with decreasing latitude and increasing incident sunlight (Scotto and Fears, 1987). On an individual basis, melanoma risk is more closely associated with acute intermittent exposure and a history of sunburns, particularly during childhood, than with cumulative sunlight exposure (Elwood et al., 1985; Osterlind et al., 1988). As with NMSC, UVB is presumed to be the major carcinogenic component of sunlight associated with melanoma risk. However, UVA exposure has been shown to induce melanoma in an animal model (platyfish-swordtail hybrids), raising concerns about UVA effects as well as UVB (Setlow et al., 1993).

Occupational studies suggest that environmental factors other than sunlight exposure may have a role in melanoma risk. Exposure to PCBs, volatile photographic chemicals, and ionizing radiation appear to increase risk (Pion et al., 1995; Austin and Reynolds, 1997; Loomis et al., 1997). Non-sunlight UV exposure from fluorescent lights may be a risk factor (Walter et al., 1992). However, among all occupational studies, sunlight exposure is probably a greater risk factor than any other exposure.

Evidence for Hereditary Factors

Similar to NMSC, fair skin and the inability to tan are important risk factors for melanoma. As mentioned previously, both constitutive and facultative skin color are polygenic traits.

Melanomas do not necessarily arise from nevi, but the host factor correlating most strongly with melanoma risk is the total number of benign nevi (Holman and Armstrong, 1984). Although sun exposure itself can influence the number of nevi, twin studies indicate that most of the variance in nevi counts is attributable to genetic factors (Roudil et al., 1995).

Approximately 10% of individuals with cutaneous melanoma have at least one first-degree relative with the disorder (Reimer et al., 1978; Lynch et al., 1983; Grange et al., 1995), and a family history increases the risk of melanoma two to four times compared with the risk in the general population (Ford et al., 1995; Cutler et al., 1996). Familial forms are often associated with multiple dysplastic nevi (Clark et al., 1978; Lynch et al., 1983; Greene et al., 1985b).

The pattern of inheritance in multiplex melanoma families is autosomal dominant with the lifetime risk of melanoma in gene carriers that may approach 100% (Lynch et al., 1983). The median age of diagnosis for the first malignant lesion is 40 years, and multiple primaries are common. Dysplastic nevi and melanomas occur on sun-exposed areas, as well as on areas not exposed to the sun, such as the buttocks and female breast (Greene et al., 1985b). Compared with nonfamilial cases, patients with familial melanomas are more likely to have an early age at onset of the first tumor, multiple primaries, and superficial spreading or lentigo maligna histopathologic subtypes. Hereditary tumors tend to have a smaller diameter and are thinner at diagnosis than their sporadic counterparts, probably because patients with a family history of melanoma have increased dermatologic surveillance. NMSC is also less frequent in patients with hereditary melanoma than in sporadic controls, and this finding probably relates to a higher dose of UV for tumorigenesis in patients without hereditary predisposition to melanoma compared with familial cases (Ford et al., 1995; Grange et al., 1995; Kopf et al., 1986).

Dysplastic nevi may occur sporadically or in a familial pattern. When familial they are often but not always associated with melanoma (Kraemer et al., 1983). On a population basis, dysplastic nevi are an independent predictor of melanoma risk (Barnhill, 1991; Tucker et al., 1993).

Gene Identification

Nonsyndromic Hereditary Melanoma

A great deal of progress has been made over the past few years in delineating the molecular basis for hereditary predisposition to melanoma. Cytogenetic analysis of atypical nevi and melanomas identified deletions of chromosome 9p, suggesting that loss of a tumor suppressor gene at this location might be an early step in carcinogenesis (Cowan et al., 1988). Molecular studies showed both allelic loss and homozygous deletions of this region (Fountain et al., 1992). Strong evidence for a susceptibility locus on chromosome 9 came from a patient with early onset of multiple melanomas and a germline deletion of 9p (Cannon-Albright et al., 1992; Petty et al., 1993), and linkage studies showed cosegregation of hereditary melanoma with chromosome 9p21 markers in at least 50% of large families (Cannon-Albright et al., 1992; Nancarrow et al., 1993; MacGeoch et al., 1994; Goldstein et al., 1994).

A gene encoding a cyclin dependent kinase inhibitor (*CDKN2A*, also know as the *p16* gene) was mapped to chromosome 9p21 and shown to be deleted in melanoma cell lines, as well as a variety of other tumors (Serrano et al., 1993). *CDKN2A* mutations have been identified in many melanoma-prone kindreds, particularly those in which the disorder is linked to chromosome 9 markers (Hussussian et al., 1994; Kamb et al., 1994). In prospective studies, germline *CDKN2A* mutations increase the risk of melanoma 75-fold over the general population risk and also increase the risk of pancreatic cancer at least 10-fold (Goldstein et al., 1995; Whelan et al., 1995). *CDKN2A* encodes a 16 kD protein (p16INK4) that is an inhibitor of CDK4 and CDK6. Switching on CDK4 and CDK6 results in phosphorylation of the Rb protein and transition from the G1 to S phase of the cell cycle (reviewed in Weinberg, 1995). Mutations seen in melanoma kindreds are inactivating and contribute to malignant transformation by releasing the cell from normal cell cycle control (Ranade et al., 1995).

At the germline level most individuals with hereditary melanoma are heterozygous for *CDKN2A* mutations, but tumors lose the normal allele consistent with a two-hit mechanism for cancer susceptibility. There is compelling evidence that homozygous inactivation of *CDKN2A* is not sufficient for tumorigenesis. Germline homozygotes for inactivating *CDKN2A* mutations (Gruis et al., 1995) do not have a more severe phenotype than heterozygotes. Other alterations must be required for development of tumors, or else every melanocyte would form a tumor in these homozygous individuals.

Not all melanoma kindreds have mutations in *CDKN2A*. Of those families without *CDKN2A* mutations, a small percentage have a mutation (R24C) in cyclin-dependent kinase 4 (CDK4), which is presumed to activate the gene by releasing the gene product from negative regulation by CDKN2A (Zuo et al., 1996). Estimates of the frequency of CDKN2A and CDK4 mutations in familial melanoma vary widely from study to study. The highest rate reported was 50% (Hussussian et al., 1994), but other studies have found few families with mutations in these genes (Holland et al., 1995; Platz et al., 1997). These discrepant results may reflect differences in study populations or in the sensitivity of techniques used to detect mutations. Several reports in the late 1990s (Fitzgerald et al., 1996; Flores et al., 1997; Harland et al., 1997; Soufer et al., 1998), based on highly sensitive screening methods and similar diagnostic criteria for hereditary melanoma found *CDKN2A* mutations in 20% to 40% of families and *CDK4* mutations in few or no families. *CDKN2A* mutations are seen in 10% to 15% of individuals selected on the basis of multiple primary melanomas without regard to family history (Monzon et al., 1998; Hashemi et al., 2000) and segregate in families with the combination of pancreatic cancer and melanoma (Goldstein et al., 1995; Whelan et al., 1995).

Cytogenetic and molecular studies of melanoma tumor tissue and cell lines have identified a large number of genetic rearrangements, which may point to the locations of other melanoma susceptibility loci (Diffey et al., 1995; Thompson et al., 1995; Walker et al., 1995). Chromosome 1 rearrangements are the most frequent genetic aberrations detected in melanomas. One study linked hereditary melanoma to markers on chromosome 1p (Bale et al., 1989), but this location has been ruled out by four independent groups (van Haeringen et al., 1989; Cannon-Albright et al., 1990; Kefford et al., 1991; Nancarrow et al., 1992).

Chromosome 6 rearrangements, predominantly losses of 6q, are the second most frequent type of genetic aberrations detected in melanoma. Linkage studies have failed to detect a melanoma susceptibility locus on this chromosome (Bale et al., 1985; Walker et al., 1994; Holland et al., 1997).

Chromosome 7 duplications, and losses on chromosomes 10q, 11, 19, 22, and Y, have been described in primary and metastatic melanomas, suggesting other possible sites of melanoma susceptibility loci.

DNA Repair Defects and Albinism

Although SCCs and BCCs are more common than melanomas in xeroderma pigmentosum patients, the risk of melanoma is increased approximately 1000-fold in patients under the age of 20, compared with a normal control population (Kraemer et al., 1994; Kocabalkan et al., 1997). Some 20% of XP patients develop melanoma, and the distribution of tumors on the body resembles that in the general population. These data suggest that DNA repair plays a major role in the prevention of cutaneous melanoma and that sunlight exposure is responsible for the induction of melanoma, as well as nonmelanoma, skin cancer in patients with XP.

Albinism increases melanoma risk but probably to a lesser extent than it increases the risk of SCC or BCC (Kromberg et al., 1989; Levine et al., 1992; Ihn et al., 1993). Among African albinos, NMSC is almost universal, but melanoma is rarely reported.

Table 38–2. Association of Melanoma with Variant Alleles of the Melanocortin Receptor Gene (MC1R)

Study	Type of Subject	*N*	Percentage of Patients Bearing at Least One Allele with: Val92Met	Asp294His	Asp84Glu	Any Variant
Ichii-Jones et al., 1998	Melanoma cases	275	18.8	6.8	6.7[a]	30.6[b]
	Controls	167	17.3	7.2	3.5	26.4
Valverde et al., 1996	Melanoma cases	43	20.9	7.0	23.3	51.2[c]
	Controls	44	18.2	0.0	0.0	18.2

[a]p = .069 (not significant).
[b]Not significant.
[c]p = .0094

Common Low-Penetrance Susceptibility Loci

Glutathione *S*-transferase activity has been associated with the risk of several cancer types. In a study of 197 melanoma patients and 147 controls, a null allele at the *GSTM1* locus was significantly more frequent in melanoma patients. Based on these data, patients lacking *GSTM1* had an estimated 2-fold greater risk of developing melanoma than the rest of the population (Lafuente et al., 1995). However, another study failed to find an excess of the *GSTM1* null genotypes among melanoma patients (Shanley et al., 1995).

As with NMSC, variants of the *MC1R* locus may be associated with an increased risk of melanoma (Table 38–2). In a case-control study of 43 melanoma patients and 44 unaffected individuals in Britain, *MC1R* variants were significantly more common in melanoma patients (Valverde et al., 1996). The estimated relative risk of melanoma in *MC1R* variant carriers was nearly four times that in controls. The Asp84Glu variant, in particular, was seen only in melanoma patients. A larger study involving 190 controls and 306 melanoma cases from a similar population failed to replicate these results (Ichii-Jones et al., 1998). The Asp84Glu variant was more common in melanoma patients than in controls, but this difference did not reach statistical significance. No other variants in *MC1R* were associated with melanoma. In 101 carriers of a 19 bp deletion of *CDKN2A* in related Dutch melanoma kindreds, the Arg151Cys variant of *MC1R* was significantly overrepresented in 33 family members affected with melanoma, compared with 68 gene carriers who had not developed melanoma. These data indicate that *MC1R* modifies the risk of melanoma in people with a strong hereditary predisposition. The association was independent of Fitzpatrick skin type, suggesting that *MC1R* variants may contribute to melanoma predisposition through mechanisms other than producing fair skin (Gruis et al., 1997). With the current state of knowledge of the relationship between melanoma risk and *MC1R* variants, clinical applications of *MC1R* testing are probably premature.

Molecular Epidemiology of Melanoma

Epidemiologic evidence strongly points to sunlight exposure as the major environmental factor determining the risk of cutaneous melanoma, particularly acute intermittent exposure and a history of sunburns. Like basal cell carcinoma, melanomas do not necessarily occur on the most sun-exposed portions of the body, and melanoma risk does not show a simple correlation with cumulative UVB exposure. The mutational spectrum of *CDKN2A* in sporadic melanomas includes a high proportion of large deletions and other rearrangements probably not attributable to UVB (Fountain et al., 1992; Piccinin et al., 1997; Matsumura et al., 1998). Another common mechanism accounting for transcriptional silencing of *CDKN2A* is abnormal methylation of the 5′ CpG island of the gene (Merlo et al., 1995). Among the point mutations in primary tumors, a high percentage are typical of UVB induction (Herbst et al., 1997), and UVB-induced mutations are common in melanoma cell lines (Kamb et al., 1994; Pollock et al., 1995). The p53 gene is frequently mutated in tumors of all types, and its mutational spectrum has been analyzed in melanoma. Mutations of this gene are not as common in melanoma as in NMSC, but a high percentage are typical of UVB induction (Weiss et al., 1995; Hartmann et al., 1996). Both *p53* mutations and *CDKN2A* mutations have been identified in dysplastic nevi, and the majority have a typical UVB-induced spectrum (Lee et al., 1997). These data indicate that UVB exposure plays a part in development of some melanomas, but other factors, possibly UVA, may be more important. That PUVA therapy increases the risk of melanoma after a 15-year latency period (Stern, 2001) supports a role for UVA in pathogenesis of this tumor.

Clinical Applications

Hereditary factors underlie a significant proportion of melanoma cases, and detection of carriers of high-penetrance melanoma genes could have a major effect on mortality from this disease. Based on the characteristics of hereditary melanoma families, clues to a genetic etiology include a family history of melanoma or pancreatic cancer, multiple primary melanomas with or without a family history, early age at onset, and possibly the presence of a large number of nevi or dysplastic nevi. *CDKN2A* is the only gene currently known to cause a significant percentage of nonsyndromic hereditary melanoma predisposition. Clinic-based and population-based studies of germline *CDKN2A* mutations indicate that patients with a family history of melanoma in three or more relatives may have as high as a 50% risk of carrying *CDKN2A* mutations (Fitzgerald et al., 1996; Flores et al., 1997; Harland et al., 1997; Platz et al., 1997; Soufer et al., 1998). Some 10% to 20% of patients with multiple primary melanomas and no known family history of melanoma had germline *CDKN2A* mutations in one study (Monzon et al., 1998), indicating that this population is enriched for carriers of a melanoma-predisposition gene. Early age at onset in the absence of a family history of melanoma is less well validated as a marker of germline *CDKN2A* mutations (Tsao et al., 1998), and dysplastic nevi can occur with or without *CDKN2A* mutations (Kraemer et al., 1983).

Genetic Counseling and Testing

Hereditary melanoma is a genetically heterogeneous disorder, and the predisposition genes that are currently known probably account for fewer than 50% of melanoma kindreds. Genetic testing for hereditary melanoma in families and especially in the broader population of unselected melanoma patients has been controversial because the proportion of hereditary melanoma attributable to *CDKN2A* and *CDK4* mutations is unknown and may be low and the value of either a positive or negative test may be limited (Kamb, 1996; Goldstein and Tucker, 1997). Although early detection and treatment greatly increase survival, there is currently no effective medical intervention specific for patients with *CDKN2A* or *CDK4* mutations (e.g., a pharmaceutical compound that prevents melanomas or specifically treats melanomas in patients with germline mutations). It is not clear that a positive test for genetic predisposition would have much effect on the medical followup for melanoma patients because most of these patients, irrespective of family history, are already in a surveillance program. Another important consideration in testing for *CDKN2A* is that mutations in this gene predispose to pancreatic cancer as well as melanoma, and there is no effective early detection or treatment for this tumor type.

Nevertheless, a very high proportion of melanoma patients offered testing in a research setting express an interest, regardless of their risk factors for carrying a melanoma gene (Martin et al., 1997). If testing is to be offered, an affected family member should be tested first, and the pros and cons of testing should be discussed. Potential benefits of a positive test result include (1) greater certainty about one's risk for recurrence, which may motivate continued prevention and detection behaviors; (2) knowledge that first-degree relatives are at increased risk for carrying the mutation and for developing cancer, which may motivate them to increase prevention and detection behaviors and may affect reproductive decisions in the family; and (3) possibility of genetic testing for these individuals. One caveat is that the penetrance of melanoma genes in patients identified through population screening is unknown. It is possible that some mutations have low penetrance or that modifying genes significantly influence the effects of *CDKN2A* mutations. The risk to relatives in low-penetrance kindreds could be quite low. Potential costs of a positive test result include (1) negative psychological impact of knowing of increased risk to oneself and family members and (2) insurance or job discrimination.

Because the prevalence of *CDKN2A* and *CDK4* mutations among the total population of patients diagnosed with melanoma, even those with a family history, is low, the probability of receiving a negative test result is greater than receiving a positive test result. The potential benefit of a negative test in a proband is quite limited: reassurance that one does not carry either of the two mutations known to be associated with melanoma. Limitations of receiving a negative test result are that (1) one cannot be reassured that the melanoma was not hereditary and associated with another, yet unknown, mutation; (2) one's own risk for recurrence remains elevated, and standards for follow-up care do not change; (3) the risk of melanoma for unaffected family members remains ambiguous; (4) unaffected family members cannot be tested. Potential costs of a negative test result are (1) insurance discrimination simply because the test was performed; (2) psychological distress related to the uncertainty about one's own and family members' melanoma risk.

First-degree relatives of any melanoma patient are at 2- to 4-fold increased risk for developing melanoma, and an argument could be made for screening these family members without genetic testing. Large numbers of nevi or dysplastic nevi have some value in distinguishing gene carriers from noncarriers (Cannon-Albright et al., 1994), and those at highest risk could be evaluated by a dermatologist semiannually. Other family members might be followed less frequently. In kindreds with many affected members in which melanoma predisposition appears to follow an autosomal dominant inheritance pattern, offspring of affected family members are likely to be at 50% risk of carrying a melanoma predisposition gene. In lieu of genetic testing, it would be reasonable to follow these at-risk individuals semiannually by dermatologic screening.

Management

Management of hereditary melanoma patients involves frequent examination by a dermatologist familiar with pigmented lesions. Typically, semiannual appointments include photography of the entire body, to allow for objective determination of differences in size or appearance of moles, and excision of any suspicious lesions. Within melanoma-prone kindreds with *CDKN2A* mutations, sun exposure is a risk factor for development of melanoma (Cannon-Albright et al., 1994; Goldstein et al., 1998). Patients should be counseled regarding preventative measures, including the use of sunscreens and appropriate clothing.

With early diagnosis and surgical treatment, melanoma is often curable. Of patients with melanoma in situ, 5% to 50% will progress to primary melanoma and 10% to metastatic disease. Surgical excision is the treatment of choice, while other options include laser treatments, destructive modalities, and topical chemotherapy (Bernstein and Roenigk, 1998). Stage I/II is primarily a surgical disease and is defined as disease limited to the primary lesion without spread to regional nodes or distant sites. Treatment should include wide excision of the primary lesion. Elective lymph node dissection is controversial but may improve outcome in the 20% of patients with microscopic nodal metastases who can be detected by sentinal node biopsy. Neither adjuvant chemotherapy, limb perfusion, nor radiotherapy of this stage has shown improvement in survival (Kim and Coit, 1998). Stage III involves regional nodes, and stage IV has spread to distant sites. The outlook for both is poor, despite innovative therapies over the last 15 to 20 years. Nearly 75% of stage III and 100% of stage IV eventually succumb. Stage III should have nodal dissection and should be considered for adjuvant interferon, limb perfusion, or systemic treatment, depending on size, symptoms, and rate of tumor growth. For treatment of Stage IV, chemotherapy results in modest response rates and only rare cures. Combination chemotherapies yield no better response than single-agent therapy with dacarbazine (DTIC). IL-2 has a similar response rate to DTIC but probably a higher rate of durable remissions, and this may be combined with combination chemotherapy. Vaccines and gene therapies are in clinical trials (Sharfman 1998; Shimizu et al., 2001).

REFERENCES

Abreo F, Sanusi ID: Basal cell carcinoma in North American blacks. J Am Acad Dermatol 1991; 25(6 Pt 1):1005–1011.

Albino AP, Reed JA, Fountain JW: Molecular biology. In: Miller SJ, Maloney ME (eds). Cutaneous Oncology: Pathophysiology, Diagnosis, and Management. Malden Massachusetts: Blackwell Science, 1998, pp. 183–199.

Ananthaswamy HN, Pierceall WE: Molecular mechanisms of ultraviolet radiation carcinogenesis. Photochem Photobiol 1990; 52(6):1119–1136.

Aquaron R. Oculocutaneous albinism in Cameroon: a 15-year follow-up study. Ophthalmic Paediatr Genet 1990; 11(4):255–263.

Armstrong BK, Kricker A: How much melanoma is caused by sun exposure? Melanoma Res 1993; 3:395–401.

Armstrong BK, Kricker A: Cutaneous melanoma: trends in cancer incidence and mortality. Cancer Surv 1994; 19:219–240.
Austin DF, Reynolds P: Investigation of an excess of melanoma among employees of the Lawrence Livermore National Laboratory. Am J Epidemiol 1997; 145:524–531.
Balch CM, Murad TM, Soong SJ, Ingalls AL, Halprn NB, Maddox WA: A multifactorial analysis of melanoma: prognostic histopathological features comparing Clark's and Breslow's staging methods. Ann Surg 1978; 188:732–742.
Balch CM, Reintgen DS, Kirkwood JM, Houghton A, Peters L, Ang KK: Cutaneous melanoma. In: DeVita VT, Hellman S, Rosenberg SA (eds). Cancer: Principles and Practice of Oncology. Philadelphia: Lippincott-Raven, 1997, 1947–1994.
Bale AE, Yu KP: The hedgehog pathway and basal cell carcinomas. Hum Mol Genet 2001; 10:757–762.
Bale SJ, Dracopoli NC, Tucker MA, Clark WH Jr, Fraser MC, Stranger BZ, Green P, Doni-Keller J, Housman DE, Green MG: Mapping the gene for hereditary cutaneous malignant melanoma-dysplastic nevus to chromosome 1p. N Engl J Med 1989; 320:1367–1372.
Bale SJ, Greene MH, Murray C, Goldin LR, Johnson AH, Mann D: Hereditary malignant melanoma is not linked to the HLA complex on chromosome 6. Int J Cancer 1985; 36:439–443.
Banerjee S: The inheritance of constitutive and facultative skin color. Clin Genet 1984; 25:256–258.
Barbosa MD, Nguyen QA, Tchernev VT, Ashley JA, Detter JC, Blaydes SM, Brandt SJ, Chotai D, Hodgman C, Solari RC, et al.: Identification of the homologous beige and Chediak-Higashi syndrome genes. Nature 1996; 382:262–265.
Barnhill RL: Current status of the dysplastic melanocytic nevus. J Cutan Pathol 1991; 18:147–159.
Barsh GS: The genetics of pigmentation: from fancy genes to complex traits. Trends Genet 1996; 12:299–305.
Bastiaens MT, ter Huurne JA, Kielich C, Gruis NA, Westendorp RG, Vermeer BJ, Bavinck JN, the Leiden Skin Cancer Study Team: Melanocortin-1 receptor gene variants determine the risk of nonmelanoma skin cancer independently of fair skin and red hair. Am J Hum Genet 2001; 68:884–894.
Bergfelt L, Newell GR, Sider JC, Kripke ML: Incidence and anatomic distribution of cutaneous melanoma among United States Hispanics. J Surg Oncol 1989; 40:222–226.
Bernstein SC, Roenigk RK. Therapy of melanoma in situ (Lentigo Maligna). In: Miller SJ, Maloney ME (eds). Cutaneous Oncology: Pathophysiology, Diagnosis, and Management. Massachusetts: Malden Blackwell Science, 1998; 297–302.
Bouwes Bavinck JN, Hardie DR, Green A, Cutmore S, MacNaught A, O'Sullivan B, Siskind V, Van Der Woude FJ, Hardie IR: The risk of skin cancer in renal transplant recipients in Queensland, Australia: a follow-up study. Transplantation 1996; 61:715–721.
Box NF, Duffy DL, Irving RE, Russell A, Chen W, Griffyths LR, Parsons PG, Green AC, Sturm RA: Melanocortin-1 receptor genotype is a risk factor for basal and squamous cell carcinoma. J Invest Dermatol 2001; 116:224–229.
Brash DE: Sunlight and the onset of skin cancer. Trends Genet 1997; 13:410–414.
Brash DE, Rudolph JA, Simon JA, Lin A, McKenna GJ, Baden HP, Halperin AJ, Ponten J: A role for sunlight in skin cancer: UV-induced *p53* mutations in squamous cell carcinoma. Proc Natl Acad Sci USA 1991; 88:10124–10128.
Breslow A: Thickness, cross-sectional areas and depth of invasion in the prognosis of cutaneous melanoma. Ann Surg 1970; 172:902–908.
Bressac B, Kew M, Wands J, Ozturk M: Selective G to T mutations of *p53* gene in hepatocellular carcinoma from southern Africa. Nature 1991; 350:429–431.
Bulliard JL, Cox B, Elwood JM: Comparison of the site distribution of melanoma in New Zealand and Canada. Int J Cancer 1997; 72:231–235.
Buzaid AC, Ross MI, Balch CM, Soong S, McCarthy WH, Tinoco L, Mansfield P, Lee JE, Bedikian A, Eton O, et al.: Critical analysis of the current American joint committee on cancer staging system for cutaneous melanoma and proposal of a new staging system. J Clin Oncol 1997; 15:1039–1051.
Cannon-Albright LA, Goldgar DE, Meyer LJ, Lewis CM, Anderson DE, Fountain JW, Hegi ME, Wiseman RW, Petty EM, Bale AE, et al.: Assignment of a locus for familial melanoma, MLM, to chromosome 9p13–p22. Science 1992; 258:1148–1152.
Cannon-Albright LA, Goldgar DE, Wright EC, Turco TC, Bishop DT, Skolnick MH, Burt RW: Evidence against the reported linkage of the cutaneous malignant melanoma-dysplastic nevus syndrome locus to chromosome 1p36. Am J Hum Genet 1990; 46:912–918.
Cannon-Albright LA, Meyer LJ, Goldgar DE, Lewis CM, McWhorter WP, Jost M, Harrison D, Anderson DE, Zone JJ, Skolnick MH: Penetrance and expressivity of the chromosome 9p melanoma susceptibility locus (MLM). Cancer Res 1994; 54:6041–6044.
Chidambaram A, Goldstein AM, Gailani MR, Gerrard B, Bale SJ, Digiovanna JJ, Bale AE, Dean M: Mutations in the human homologue of the *Drosophila patched* gene in Caucasian and African-American nevoid basal cell carcinoma syndrome patients. Cancer Res 1996; 56:4599–4601.
Clark WH Jr, From L, Bernardino EA, Mihm MC: The histogenesis and biologic behavior of primary human malignant melanoma of the skin. Cancer Res 1969; 29:705–727.
Clark WH Jr, Reimer RR, Greene M, Ainsworth AM, Mastrangelo MJ: Origin of familial malignant melanomas from heritable melanocytic lesions "the B–K mole syndrome." Arch Dermatol 1978; 114:732–738.
Copeland NE, Hanke CW, Michalak JA: The molecular basis of xeroderma pigmentosum. Dermatol Surg 1997; 23:447–455.
Cowan JM, Halaban R, Francke U: Cytogenetic analysis of melanocytes from premalignant nevi and melanomas. J Natl Cancer Inst 1988; 80:1159–1164.
Cress RD, Holly EA: Incidence of cutaneous melanoma among non-Hispanic whites, Hispanics, Asians, and blacks: an analysis of California cancer registry data, 1988–1993. Cancer Causes Control 1997; 8:246–252.
Cutler C, Foulkes WD, Brunet JS, Flanders TY, Shibata H, Narod SA: Cutaneous malignant melanoma in women is uncommonly associated with a family history of melanoma in first-degree relatives: a case-contol study. Melanoma Res 1996; 6:435–440.
Dahmane N, Lee J, Robins P, Heller P, Ruiz i Altaba A: Activation of the transcription factor Gli1 and the Sonic hedgehog signalling pathway in skin tumours. Nature 1997; 389(6653):876–881.
Diffey BL, Healy E, Thody AJ, Rees JL: Melanin, melanocytes and melanoma. Lancet 1995; 346:1713.
Drobetsky EA, Grosovsky AJ, Glickman BW: The specificity of UV-induced mutations at an endogenous locus in mammalian cells. Proc Natl Acad Sci USA 1987; 84:9103–9107.
Durham-Pierre D, Gardner JM, Nakatsu Y, King RA, Francke U, Ching A, Aquaron R, del Marmol V, Brilliant MH: African origin of an intragenic deletion of the human P gene in tyrosinase positive oculocutaneous albinism. Nat Genet 1994; 7:176–179.
Elwood JB, Koh HK: Etiology, epidemiology, risk factors, and public health issues of melanoma. Curr Opin Oncol 1994; 6:179–187.
Elwood JM, Gallagher RP, Hill GB, Pearson J: Cutaneous melanoma in relation to intermittent and constant sun exposure: the Western Canada Melanoma Study. Int J Cancer 1985; 35:427–433.
Fan H, Oro AE, Scott MP, Khavari PA: Induction of basal cell carcinoma features in transgenic human skin expressing Sonic Hedgehog. Nat Med 1997; 3:788–792.
Fitzgerald MG, Harkin DP, Silva-Arrieta S, MacDonald DJ, Lucchina LC, Unsal J, O'Neill E, Koh J, Finkelstein DM, Isselbacher KJ, et al.: Prevalence of germ-line mutations in p16, p19ARF, and CDK4 in familial melanoma: analysis of a clinic-based population. Proc Natl Acad Sci USA 1996; 93:8541–8545.
Fitzpatrick TB, Pathak MA, Greiter F, Mosher DB, Parrish JA: Heritable melanin deficiency syndromes. In Fitzpatrick TB, Eisen AZ, Woff K, Freedberg IM, Austen KF (eds.). Update: Dermatology in General Medicine. New York: McGraw-Hill, 1983, pp 46–60.
Flores JF, Pollack PM, Walker GJ, Glendening JM, Lin AH, Palmer JM, Walters MK, Hayward NK, Fountain JW: Analysis of the CDKN2A, CDKN2B and CDK4 genes in 48 Australian melanoma kindreds. Oncogene 1997; 15:2999–3005.
Ford D, Bliss JM, Swerdlow AJ, Armstrong BK, Franceschi S, Green A, Holly EA, Mack T, MacKie RM, Osterlind A, et al.: Risk of cutaneous melanoma associated with a family history of the disease. Int J Cancer 1995; 62:377–381.
Fountain JW, Karayiorgou N, Graw SL, Ernstoff MS, Kirkwood JM, Vlock DR, Titus-Ernstroff L, Bouchard B, Vijayasaradhi S, Houghton AN, et al.: Homozygous deletions within human chromosome 9p band 9p21 in melanoma. Proc Natl Acad Sci USA 1992; 89:10557–10561.
Franceschi S, Levi F, Randimbison L, La Vecchia C: Site distribution of different types of skin cancer: new aetiological clues. Int J Cancer 1996; 67(1):24–28.
Frandberg PA, Doufexis M, Kapas S, Chhajlani V: Human pigmentation phenotype: a point mutation generates nonfunctional MSH receptor. Biochem Biophys Res Commun 1998; 245(2):490–492.
Gailani MR, Bale SJ, Leffell DJ, DiGiovanna JJ, Peck GL, Poliak S, Drum MA, Pastakia B, McBride OW, Kase R, et al.: Developmental defects in Gorlin syndrome related to a putative tumor suppressor gene on chromosome 9. Cell 1992; 69:111–117.
Gailani MR, Leffell DJ, Ziegler AM, Gross EG, Brash DE, Bak AE: Relationship between sunlight exposure and a key genetic alteration in basal cell carcinoma. J Natl Cancer Inst 1996a; 88:349–354.
Gailani MR, Ståhle-Bäckdahl M, Leffell DJ, Glynn M, Zaphiropoulos PG, Pressman C, Undén AB, Dean M, Brash DE, Bale AE, Toftgård R: The role of the human homologue of *Drosophila patched* in sporadic basal cell carcinomas. Nat Genet 1996b; 14:78–81.
Gloster Jr HM, Brodland DG: The epidemiology of skin cancer. Dermatol Surg 1996; 22:217–226.
Goldstein AM, Dracopoli NC, Engelstein M, Fraser MC, Clark Jr WH, Tucker MA: Linkage of cutaneous malignant melanoma/dysplastic nevi to chromosome 9p, and evidence for genetic heterogeneity. Am J Hum Genet 1994; 54:489–496.
Goldstein AM, Dracopoli NC, Ho EC, Fraser MC, Kearns KS, Bale SJ, BcBride OW, Clark WH Jr, Tucker MA: Futher evidence for the locus for cutaneous malignant melanoma-dysplastic nevus (CMM/DN) on chromosome 1p, and evidence for genetic heterogeneity. Am J Hum Genet 1993; 52:527–550.
Goldstein AM, Falk RT, Fraser MC, Dracopoli NC, Sikorski RS, Clark WH Jr, Tucker MA: Sun-related factors in melanoma-prone families with *CDKN2A* mutations. J Natl Cancer Inst 1998; 90:709–711.
Goldstein AM, Fraser MC, Struewing JP, Hussussian CJ, Ranade K, Zametkin DP, Fontaine LS, Organic SM, Dracopoli NC, Clark WH Jr, et al.: Increased risk of pancreatic cancer in melanoma-prone kindreds with p16INK4 mutations. N Engl J Med 1995; 333:970–974.
Goldstein AM, Tucker MA: Screening for *CDKN2A* mutations in hereditary melanoma. J Natl Cancer Inst 1997; 89:676–678.
Goltz RW: Clinical presentation. In: Miller SJ, Maloney ME (eds). Cutaneous Oncology. Malden, Massachusetts: Blackwell Science, 1998:468–480.
Gorlin RJ: Nevoid basal cell carcinoma syndrome. Dermatol Clin 1995; 13:113–125.
Grange F, Chompret A, Guilloud-Bataille M, Guillaume JC, Margulis A, Prade M, Demenais F, Avril MF: Comparison between familial and nonfamilial melanoma in France. Arch Dermatol 1995; 131:1154–1159.
Greene MH, Clark WH Jr, Tucker MA, Elder DE, Kraemer KH, Guerry D, Witmer WK, Thompson J, Matozzo I, Fraser MC: Acquired precursors of cutaneous ma-

lignant melanoma: the familial dysplastic nevus syndrome. N Engl J Med 1985a; 312:91–97.

Greene MH, Clark WH Jr, Tucker MA, Kraemer KH, Elder DE, Fraser MC: High risk of malignant melanoma in melanoma-prone families with dysplastic nevi. Ann Intern Med 1985b; 102:458–465.

Greene MH, Hoover RN, Fraumeni JF Jr: Subsequent cancer in patients with chronic lymphocytic leukemia: a possible immunologic mechanism. J Natl Cancer Inst 1978; 61:337–340.

Greenlee RT, Murray T, Bolden S, Wingo PA: Cancer statistics, 2000. CA Cancer J Clin 2000; 50:7–33.

Greenstein AJ, Sachar DB, Shafir M, Rosenberg IR, Lewis C, Raju T, Szporn A, Janowitz HD, Aufses AH Jr. Malignant melanoma in inflammatory bowel disease. Am J Gastroenterol 1992; 87:317–320.

Grodstein F, Speizer FE, Hunter DJ: A prospective study of incident squamous cell carcinoma of the skin in the Nurses Health Study. J Natl Cancer Inst 1995; 87:1061–1066.

Gruis NA, van der Velden PA, Sandkuijl LA, Bergman W, Frants RR: Melanocortin 1 receptor (MC1R) variant Arg151Cys is generally associated with fair skin and modifies melanoma risk in Dutch Familial Atypical Multiple Mole-Melanoma (FAMMM) syndrome families. Am J Hum Genet 1997; 61:A200.

Gruis NA, van der Velden PA, Sandkuijl LA, Prins DE, Weaver-Feldhaus J, Kamb A, Bergman W, Frants RR: Homozygotes for *CDKN2* (p16) germline mutation in Dutch familial melanoma kindreds. Nat Genet 1995; 10:351–353.

Haas AF: Features associated with metastasis. In: Miller SJ, Maloney ME (eds). Cutaneous Oncology. Malden, Massachusetts: Blackwell Science, 1998:500–505.

Hahn H, Wicking C, Zaphiropoulos PG, Gailani MR, Shanley S, Chidambaram A, Vorechovsky I, Holmberg E, Unden AB, Gillies S, et al.: Mutations of the human homolog of *Drosophila patched* in the nevoid basal cell carcinoma syndrome. Cell 1996; 85:841–851.

Halder RM, Bridgeman-Shah S: Skin cancer in African Americans. Cancer 1995; 75(suppl.):667–673.

Harland M, Meloni R, Gruis M, Pinney E, Brookes S, Spurr NK, Frischauf AM, Bataille V, Peters G, Cuzick J, et al.: Germline mutations of the *CDKN2* gene in U.K. melanoma families. Hum Mol Genet 1997; 6:2061–2067.

Harris C: Molecular epidemiology of basal cell carcinoma [editorial; comment]. J Natl Cancer Inst 1996; 88:315–317.

Harrison GA: Differences in human pigmentation: measurement, geographic variation and causes. J Invest Dermatol 1973; 60:418–426.

Hartmann A, Blaszyk H, Cunningham JS, McGovern RM, Schroeder JS, Helander SD, Pittelkow MR, Sommer SS, Kovach JS: Overexpression and mutations of *p53* in metastatic malignant melanomas. Int J Cancer 1996; 67:313–317.

Hashemi J, Platz A, Ueno T, Stierner U, Ringborg U, Hansson J: CDKN2A germline mutations in individuals with multiple cutaneous melanomas. Cancer Res 2000; 60:6864–6867.

Herbst RA, Gutzmer R, Matiaske F, Mommert S, Kapp A, Weiss J, Arden KC, Cavenee WK: Further evidence for ultraviolet light induction of *CDKN2* (p16INK4) mutation in sporadic melanoma in vivo. J Invest Dermatol 1997; 108:950.

Holland EA, Beaton SC, Becker TM, Grulet OM, Peters BA, Rizos H, Kefford RF, Mann GJ: Analysis of the p16 gene, *CDKN2*, in 17 Australian melanoma kindreds. Oncogene 1995; 11:2289–2294.

Holland EA, Beaton SC, Kefford RF, Mann GJ: Linkage analysis of familial melanoma and chromosome 6 in 14 Australian kindreds. Genes Chromosomes Cancer 1997; 19:241–249.

Holman CD, Armstrong BK: Pigmentary traits, ethnic origin, benign nevi, and family history as risk factors for cutaneous malignant melanoma. J Natl Cancer Inst 1984; 72:257–266.

Hsu IC, Metcalf RA, Sun T, Welsh JA, Wang NJ, Harris CC: Mutational hotspot in the *p53* gene in human hepatocellular carcinoma. Nature 1991; 350:427–428.

Hussussian CJ, Struewing JP, Goldstein AM, Higgins PA, Ally DS, Sheahan MD, Clark WH Jr, Tucker MA, Dracopoli NC: Germline p16 mutations in familial melanoma. Nat Genet 1994; 8:15–21.

Ichii-Jones F, Lear JT, Heagerty AH, Smith AG, Hutchinson PE, Osborne J, Bowers B, Jones PW, Davies E, Ollier WE, et al.: Susceptibility to melanoma: influence of skin type and polymorphism in the melanocyte stimulating hormone receptor gene. J Invest Dermatol 1998; 111:218–221.

Ihn H, Nakamura K, Abe M, Furue M, Takehara K, Nakagawa H, Ishibashi Y: Amelanotic metastatic in a patient with oculocutaneous albinism. J Am Acad Dermatol 1993; 28:895–900.

Johnson RL, Rothman AL, Xie J, Goodrich LV, Bare JW, Bonifas JM, Quinn AG, Myers RM, Cox DR, Epstein EH Jr, Scott MP: Human homolog of *patched*, a candidate gene for the basal cell nevus syndrome. Science 1996; 272:1668–1671.

Johnson TM, Rowe DE, Nelson BR, Swanson NA: Squamous cell carcinoma of the skin. J Am Acad Dermatol 1992; 26:467–484.

Jonason AS, Kunala S, Price GJ, Restifo RJ, Spirvelli HM, Persing JA, Leffell DJ, Tarone RE, Brash DE: Frequent clones of *p53*-mutated keratinocytes in normal human skin. Proc Natl Acad Sci USA 1996; 93:14025–14029.

Kamb A: Human melanoma genetics. J Invest Dermatol 1996; 2:177–182.

Kamb A, Gruis NA, Weaver-Feldhaus J, Liu Q, Harshman K, Tavtigian SV, Stockert E, Day RS III, Johnson BE, Skolnick MH: A cell-cycle regulator potentially involved in genesis of many tumor types. Science 1994; 264:436–440.

Karagas MR: Occurrence of cutaneous basal cell and squamous cell malignancies among those with a prior history of skin cancer. J Invest Dermatol 1994; 102(Suppl.):10S–13S.

Kefford RF, SalmonJ, Shaw HM, Donald JA, McCarthy WH: Hereditary melanoma in Australia: variable association with dysplastic nevi and absence of genetic linkage to chromosome 1p. Cancer Genet Cytogenet 1991; 51:45–55.

Khlat M, Vail A, Parkin M, Green A: Mortality from melanoma in migrants to Australia: variation by age at arrival and duration of stay. Am J Epidemiol 1992; 135:1103–1113.

Kim SH, Coit DG: Surgical treatment of stage I and II disease. In: Miller SJ, Maloney ME (eds). Cutaneous Oncology: Pathophysiology, Diagnosis, and Management. Malden: Blackwell Science, 1998:303–315.

King RA, Creel D, Cervenka J, Okoro AN, Witkop CJ: Albinism in Nigeria with delineation of new recessive oculocutaneous type. Clin Genet 1980; 17:259–270.

Kocabalkan O, Ozgur F, Erk Y, Gursu KG, Gungen Y: Malignant melanoma in xeroderma pigmentosum patients: report of five cases. Eur J Surg Oncol 1997; 23:43–47.

Kopf AW, Hellman LJ, Rogers GS, Gross DF, Rigel DS, Friedman RJ, Levenstein M, Brown J, Golomb FM, Roses DF, et al.: Familial malignant melanoma. JAMA 1986; 256:1915–1919.

Kraemer K, Greene M, Tarone R, Elder DE, Clark WH Jr, Guerry D 4th: Dysplastic naevi and cutaneous melanoma risk. Lancet 1983; 2:1076–1077.

Kraemer KH, DiGiovanna JJ, Moshell AN, Tarone RE, Peck GL: Prevention of skin cancer in xeroderma pigmentosum with the use of oral isotretinoin. N Engl J Med 1988; 318:1633–1637.

Kraemer KH, Lee MM, Andrews AD, Lambert WC: The role of sunlight and DNA repair in melanoma and non-melonoma skin cancer. Arch Dermatol 1994; 130:1018–1021.

Kricker A, Armstrong BK, English DR, Heenan PJ: Does intermittent sun exposure cause basal cell carcinoma? A case control study in Western Austrailia. Int J Cancer 1995; 60:489–494.

Kromberg JG, Castle D, Zwane EM, Jenkins T: Albinism and skin cancer in Southern Africa. Clin Genet 1989; 36:43–52.

Lafuente A, Molina R, Palou J, Castel T, Moral A, Trias M: Phenotype of glutathione *S*-transferase MU (*GSTM1*) and susceptibility to malignant melanoma. Br J Cancer 1995; 72:324–326.

Lang PG Jr, Maize JC: Histologic evolution of recurrent basal cell carcinoma and treatment implications. J Am Acad Dermatol 1986; 14:186–196.

Lee JA: Declining effect of latitude on melanoma mortality rates in the United States. Am J Epidemiol 1997; 146:413–417.

Lee JY, Dong SM, Shin MS, Kim SY, Lee SH, Kang SJ, Lee JD, Kim CS, Kim SH, Yoo NJ: Genetic alterations of *p16INK4a* and *p53* genes in sporadic dysplastic nevus. Biochem Biophys Res Commun 1997; 237:667–672.

Levine EA, Ronan SG, Shirali SS, Das Gupta TK: Malignant melanoma in a child with oculocutaneous albinism [review]. J Surg Oncol 1992; 51:138–142.

Loomis D, Browning SR, Schenck AP, Gregory E, Savitz DA: Cancer mortality among electric utility workers exposed to polychlorinated biphenyls. Occup Environ Med 1997; 54:720–728.

Lutzner MA, Blanchet-Bardon C: Epidermodysplasia verruciformis. Curr Probl Dermatol 1985; 13:164–185.

Lynch HT, Fusaro RM, Kimberling WJ, Lynch JF, Danes BS: Familial atypical multiple mole-melanoma (FAMMM) syndrome: segregation analysis. J Med Genet 1983; 20:342–344.

MacGeoch C, Bishop JA, Bataille V, Bishop DT, Frischauf AM, Meloni R, Cuzick J, Pinney E, Spurr NK: Genetic heterogeneity in familial malignant melanoma. Hum Mol Genet 1994; 3:2195–2200.

Mack TM, Floderus B: Malignant melanoma risk by nativity, place of residence at diagnosis, and age at migration. Cancer Causes Control 1991; 2:401–411.

Marks R: The epidemiology of non-melanoma skin cancer: who, why and what can we do about it. J Dermatol 1995; 22:853–857.

Martin CAD, Alvarez-Franco M, Matloff ET, Salovey P, Bale AE: Melanoma gene testing in a Connecticut Tumor Registry (CTR) population. Am J Hum Genet 1997; 61:A224.

Massi D, Borgognoni L, Reali UM, Franchi A: Malignant melanoma associated with human immunodeficiency virus infection: a case report and review of the literature. Melanoma Res 1998; 8:187–192.

Matsumura Y, Nishigori C, Yagi T, Imamura S, Takebe H: Mutations of the p16 and p15 suppressor genes and replication errors contribute independently to the pathogenesis of sporadic malignant melanoma. Arch Dermatol Res 1998; 290:175–180.

Merlo A, Herman JG, Mao L, Lee DJ, Gabrielson E, Burger PC, Baylin SB, Sidransky D: 5′ CpG island methylation is associated with transcriptional silencing of the tumor suppressor p16/CDKN2/MTSI in human cancers. Nat Med 1995; 1:686–692.

Miller SJ: Continuing medical education: biology of basal cell carcinoma (Part 1). J Am Acad Dermatol 1991; 24:1–13.

Monzon J, Liu L, Brill H, Goldstein AM, Tucker MA, From L, McLaughlin J, Hogg D, Lassam NJ: CDKN2A mutations in multiple primary melanomas. N Engl J Med 1998; 338:879–887.

Nagle DL, Karim MA, Woolf EA, Holmgren L, Bork P, Misumi DJ, McGrail SH, Dussault BJ Jr, Perou CM, Boissy RE, et al.: Identification and mutation analysis of the complete gene for Chediak-Higashi syndrome. Nat Genet 1996; 14:307–311.

Nancarrow DJ, Mann GJ, Holland EA, Walker GJ, Beaton SC, Walters MK, Luxford C, Palmer J, Donald JA, Weber JL, et al.: Confirmation of chromosome 9p linkage in familial melanoma. Am J Hum Genet 1993; 53:936–942.

Nancarrow DJ, Palmer JM, Walters MK, Kerr BM, Hofner GJ, Garske L, McLeod GR, Hayward NK: Exclusion of the familial melanoma locus (MLM) from the PND/D1S47 and MYCL1 regions of chromosome arm 1p in 7 Australian pedigrees. Genomics 1992; 12:18–25.

Oetting WS, King RA: Molecular basis of oculocutaneous albinism. J Invest Dermatol 1994; 103:131S–136S.

Oettle AG: Skin cancer in Africa. Natl Cancer Inst Monogr 1963; 10:197–214.

Oh J, Bailin T, Fukai K, Feng GH, Ho L, Mao JI, Frenk E, Tamura N, Spritz RA: Positional cloning of a gene for Hermansky-Pudlak syndrome, a disorder of cytoplasmic organelles [see comments]. Nat Genet 1996; 14:300–306.

Osterlind A, Tucker MA, Stone BJ, Jensen OM: The Danish case-control study of cutaneious malignant melanoma: II. Importance of U.V. light exposure. Int J Cancer 1988; 42:319–324.

Paver K, Royser K, Burry N: The incidence of basal cell carcinoma and their metastases in Australia and New Zealand. Australas J Dermatol 1973; 14:53.

Peak MJ, Peak JG, Carnes BA: Induction of direct and indirect single-strand breaks in human cell DNA by far and near ultraviolet radiations: action spectrums and mechanisms. Photochem Photobiol 1987; 45:381–387.

Peck GL, Gross EG, Butkus D, DiGiovanna JJ: Chemoprevention of basal cell carcinoma with isotretinoin. J Am Acad Dermatol 1982; 6:815–823.

Petty EM, Gibson LH, Fountain JW, Bolognia J, Yang-Feng TL, Housman DE, Bale AE: Molecular definition of a chromosome 9p21 germline deletion in a woman with multiple melanomas and a plexiform neurofibroma: Implications for a 9p tumor suppressor gene. Am J Hum Genet 1993; 53:96–104.

Piccinin S, Doglioni C, Maestro R, Vukosavljevic T, Gasparotto D, D'Orazi C, Boiocchi M: p16/CDKN2 and CDK4 gene mutations in sporadic melanoma development and progression. Int J Cancer 1997; 74(1):26–30.

Piepkorn MW: Genetic basis of susceptibility to melanoma. J Am Acad Dermatol 1994; 31:1022–1039.

Pion IA, Rigel DS, Garfinkel L, Silverman MK, Kopf AW: Occupation and the risk of malignant melanoma. Cancer 1995; 75(2 Suppl):637–644.

Platz A, Hansson J, Mansson-Brahme E, Lagerlof B, Linder S, Lundqvist E, Sevigny P, Inganas M, Ringborg U: Screening of germline mutations in the *CDKN2A* and *CDKN2B* genes in Swedish families with hereditary cutaneous melanoma. J Natl Cancer Inst 1997; 89:697–702.

Pollock PM, Yu F, Parsons PG, Hayward NK: Evidence for u.v. induction of *CDKN2* mutations in melanoma cell lines. Oncogene 1995; 11:663–668.

Quinn AG, Campbell C, Healy E, Rees JL: Chromosome 9 allele loss occurs in both basal and squamous cell carcinomas of the skin. J Invest Dermotol 1994; 102(3):300–303.

Rady PF, Scinicariello F, Wagner RF, Tyring SK: *p53* mutations in basal cell carcinomas. Cancer Res 1992; 52:3804–3806.

Rahbari H, Mehregan AH: Basal cell epithelioma in children and teenagers. Cancer 1982; 49:350–353.

Ranade K, Hussussian CJ, Sikorski RS, Varmus HE, Goldstein AM, Tucker MA, Serrano M, Hannon GJ, Beach D, Dracopoli NC: Mutations associated with familial melanoma impair p16/INK4 function. Nat Genet 1995; 10(1):114–116.

Reimer RR, Clark WH, Greene MH, Ainsworth AM, Fraumeni JF: Precursor lesions in familial melanoma. JAMA 1978; 239:744–746.

Rinchik EM, Bultman SJ, Horsthernke B, Lee ST, Strunk KM, Spritz RA, Avidano KM, Jong MT, Nicholls RD: A gene for the mouse pink-eyed dilution locus and for human type II oculocutaneous albinism. Nature 1993; 361:72–76.

Roudil F, Grob JJ, Gouvernet J, Richardallemand MA, Basseres N, Bonerandi JJ: Influence of sun exposure after childhood on the development of nevi: a study in monozygotic twins. Eur J Dermatol 1995; 5:477–480.

Rowe DE, Carroll RJ, Day CL: Mohs surgery is the treatment of choice for recurrent (previously treated) basal cell carcinoma. J Dermatol Surg Oncol 1989;15:424–431.

Rowe DE, Carroll RJ, Day CL: Prognostic factors for local recurrence, metastasis, and survival rates in squamous cell carcinoma. J Am Acad Dermatol 1992; 26:1–26.

Sagebiel RW: Cutaneous malignant melanoma: the party line and more, with a word on "safe sun." Compr Ther 1993; 19:225–231.

Sagabiel RW: Clinical presentation. In: Miller SJ, Maloney ME (eds). Cutaneous Oncology: Pathophysiology, Diagnosis, and Management. Malden: Blackwell Science, 1998:253–261.

Salasche SJ: Status of curettage and electrodessication in the treatment of primary basal cell carcinoma. J Am Acad Dermatol 1984; 10:285–287.

Scotto J, Fears TR: The association of solar ultraviolet and skin melanoma incidence among caucasians in the United States. Cancer Invest 1987; 5:275–283.

Scotto J, Fraumeni JFJ: Skin (other than melanoma). In: Schottenfeld D, Fraumeni JFJ (eds). Cancer Epidemiology and Prevention. Philadelphia: W. B. Saunders, 1982:996–1011.

Serrano M, Hannon GJ, Beach D: A new regulatory motif in cell-cycle control causing specific inhibition of cyclin D/CDK4. Nature 1993; 366:704–707.

Setlow RB, Grist E, Thompson K, Woodhead AD: Wavelengths effective in induction of malignant melanoma. Proc Natl Acad Sci USA 1993; 90:6666–6670.

Sexton M, Jones DB, Maloney ME: Histologic pattern analysis of basal cell carcinoma. J Am Acad Dermatol 1990; 23:1118–1126.

Shanley SM, Chenevix-Trench G, Palmer J, Hayward N: Glutathione *S*-transferase GSTM1 null genotype is not overrepresented in Australian patients with nevoid basal cell carcinoma syndrome or sporadic melanoma. Carcinogenesis 1995; 16:2003–2004.

Sharfman WH: Therapy of stage III and IV disease. In: Miller SJ, Maloney ME (eds). Cutaneous Oncology: Pathophysiology, Diagnosis, and Management. Malden: Blackwell Science, 1998:331–341.

Shimizu K, Thomas EK, Giedlin M, Mule JJ: Enhancement of tumor lysate- and peptide-pulsed dendritic cell-based vaccines by the addition of foreign helper protein. Cancer Res 2001; 61:2618–2624.

Sidransky D: Is human *patched* the gatekeeper of common skin cancers? Nat Genet 1996; 14:7–8.

Smith R, Healy E, Siddiqui S, Flanagan N, Steijlen PM, Rosdahl I, Jacques JP, Rogers S, Turner R, Jackson IJ, et al.: Melanocortin-1 receptor variants in an Irish population. J Invest Dermatol 1998; 111:119–122.

Snow SN, Sahl W, Lo JS, Mohs FE, Warner T, Dekkinga JA, Feyzi J: Metastatic basal cell carcinoma: report of five cases. Cancer 1994; 73:328–335.

Soufer N, Avril MF, Chompret A, Demenais F, Bombled J, Spatz A, Stoppa-Lyonnet D, Benard J, Bressac-de Paillerets B: Prevalence of *p16* and *CDK4* germline mutations in 48 melanoma-prone families in France. Hum Mol Genet 1998; 7:209–216.

Stern RS: The risk of melanoma in association with long-term exposure to PUVA. J Am Acad Dermatol 2001; 44:755–761.

Strong L: Genetic and environmental interactions. Cancer 1977; 40:1861–1866.

Suarez HG, Daya-Grosjean L, Schlaifer D, Nardeux P, Renault G, Bos JL, Sarasin A: Activated oncogenes in human skin tumors from a repair-deficient syndrome, xeroderma pigmentosum. Cancer Res 1989; 49:1223–1228.

Szepietowski J, Wasik F, Szepietowski T, Wlodarczyk M, Sobczak-Radwan K, Czyz W: Excess benign melanocytic naevi in renal transplant recipients. Dermatology 1997; 194:17–19.

Taipale J, Chen JK, Cooper MK, Wang B, Mann RK, Milenkovic L, Scott MP, Beachy PA: Effects of oncogenic mutations in *Smoothened* and *Patched* can be reversed by cyclopamine. Nature 2000; 406:1005–1009.

Tangrea JA, Edwards BK, Taylor PR, Hartman AM, Peck GL, Salasche SJ, Menon PA, Benson PM, Mellette JR, Guill MA: ISO-BCC Study Group: Long-term therapy with low-dose isotretinoin for prevention of basal cell carcinoma: a multicenter clinical trial. J Natl Cancer Inst 1992; 84:328–332.

Thompson FH, Emerson J, Olson S, Weinstein R, Leavitt SA, Leong SP, Emerson S, Trent JM, Nelson MA, Salmon SE: Cytogenetics in 158 patients with regional or disseminated melanoma. Cancer Genet Cytogenet 1995; 83:93–104.

Thompson SC, Jolley D, Marks R: Reduction of solar keratoses by regular sunscreen use. N Engl J Med 1993; 329:1147–1151.

Tromovitch TA, Stegman SJ: Microscopic-controlled excision of cutaneous tumors: chemosurgery, fresh tissue technique. Cancer 1978; 41:653–658.

Tsao H, Zhang X, Sober A, Haluska F: Prevalence of germline p16/CDKN2A and CDK4 mutations in patients who develop melanoma before age 40. Am J Hum Genet 1998; 63(.):A21.

Tucker MA, Crutcher WA, Hartge P, Sagebiel RW: Familial and cutaneous features of dysplastic nevi: a case-control study. J Am Acad Dermatol 1993; 28(4):558–564.

Valverde P, Healy E, Jackson I, Rees JL, Thody AJ: Variants of the melanocyte-stimulating hormone receptor gene are associated with red hair and fair skin in humans [see comments]. Nat Genet 1995; 11(3):328–330.

Valverde P, Healy E, Sikkink S, Haldane F, Thody AJ, Carothers A, Jackson IJ, Rees JL: The Asp84Glu variant of the melanocortin-1 receptor (MC1R) is associated with melanoma. Hum Mol Genet 1996; 5(10):1663–1666.

van der Schroeff JG, Evers LM, Boot AJM, Bos JL: *Ras* oncogene mutations in basal cell carcinomas and squamous cell carcinomas of human skin. J Invest Dermatol 1990; 94(4):423–425.

van der Schroeff JG, Evers LM, Boot AJM, Bos JL: *Ras* oncogene mutations in basal cell carcinomas and squamous cell carcinomas of human skin. J Invest Dermatol 1990; 94(4):423–425.

van Haeringen A, Bergman W, Nolen MR, van der Kooij-Meijs E, Hendrikse I, Wijnen JT, Khan PM, Klasen EC, Frants RR: Exclusion of the dysplastic nevus syndrome (DNS) locus from the short arm of chromosome 1 by linkage studies in Dutch families. Genomics 1989; 5:61–64.

Walker GJ, Nancarrow DJ, Walters MK, Palmer JM, Weber JL, Hayward NK: Linkage analysis in familial melanoma kindreds to markers on chromosome 6p. Int J Cancer 1994; 59(6):771–775.

Walker GJ, Palmer JM, Walters MK, Hayward NK: A genetic model of melanoma tumorigenesis based on allelic losses. Genes Chromosomes Cancer 1995; 12:134–141.

Walter SD, Marrett LD, Shannon HS, From L, Hertzman C: The association of cutaneous malignant melanoma and fluorescent light exposure. Am J Epidemiol 1992; 135(7):749–762.

Wei Q, Matanoski GM, Farmer ER, Hedayati MA, Grossman L: DNA repair and aging in basal cell carcinoma: a molecular epidemiology study. Proc Natl Acad Sci USA 1993; 90:1614–1618.

Weinberg RA: The retinoblastoma protein and cell cycle control. Cell 1995; 81:323–330.

Weinstock MA: Epidemiologic investigation of nonmelanoma skin cancer mortality: the Rhode Island follow-back study. J Invest Dermatol 1994; 102 Supplement: 6S–9S.

Weiss J, Heine M, Arden KC, Korner B, Pilch H, Herbst RA, Jung EG: Mutation and expression of TP53 in malignant melanomas. Recent Results Cancer Res 1995; 139:137–154.

Whelan AJ, Bartsch D, Goodfellow PJ. A familial syndrome of pancreatic cancer and melanoma with a mutation in the *CDKN2* tumor-suppressor gene. N Engl J Med 1995; 333:975–977.

Witkop CJ: Abnormalities of pigmentation. In: Nora, James J, Fraser, F Clarke (eds). Principles and Practice of Medical Genetics. New York: Churchill Livingstone, 1983:622–637.

Xie J, Murone M, Luoh SM, Ryan A, Gu Q, Zhang C, Bonifas JM, Lam CW, Hynes M, Goddard A, et al.: Activating *smoothened* mutations in sporadic basal-cell carcinoma. Nature 1998; 391:90–92.

Yakubu A, Mabogunje OA: Skin cancer in African albinos. Acta Oncol 1993; 32(6):621–622.

Ziegler A, Jonason AS, Leffell DJ, Simon JA, Sharma HW, Kimmelman J, Remington L, Jacks T, Brash DE: Sunburn and *p53* in the onset of skin cancer. Nature 1994; 372:773–776.

Ziegler A, Leffell DJ, Subrahmanyam K, Sharma HW, Gailani M, Simon JA, Halperin AJ, Baden HP, Shapiro PE, Bale AE, Brash DE: Mutation hotspots due to sunlight in the *p53* gene of nonmelanoma skin cancers. Proc Natl Acad Sci USA 1993; 90:4216–4220.

Zuo L, Weger J, Yang Q, Goldstein AM, Tucker MA, Walker GJ, Hayward N, Dracopoli NC: Germline mutations in the p16INK4a binding domain of CDK4 in familial melanoma. Nat Genet 1996; 12(1):97–99.

39 Prostate Cancer

WILLIAM B. ISAACS AND JIANFENG XU

In 1990, prostate cancer became the most common form of cancer (other than skin cancer) diagnosed in the U.S. male population, surpassing lung cancer. In 2001, there will be an estimated 198,000 new prostate cancer cases diagnosed, accounting for over 30% of all cancers affecting men, and over 31,000 deaths will result from this disease (Greenlee et al., 2000). The lifetime probability of a man in the U.S. developing prostate cancer is predicted to be one in six. Despite these figures, our understanding of the molecular genetics of prostate cancer is still in an embryonic stage. As research in this area gains momentum, this situation will undoubtedly change rapidly.

DIAGNOSTIC CRITERIA AND CLINICAL PRESENTATION

Prostate cancers are typically diagnosed on histological evaluation of needle biopsy samples of prostate tissue, taken because of an abnormal physical examination or an elevated serum PSA level, or both. Prostate cancers are graded based on tissue architectural patterns according to the system proposed by Gleason (1992). Due to the common morphological heterogeneity of prostate cancer, two different grades are given for the first and second most prevalent patterns, and the sum of these two grades is added to give the Gleason score. Staging is categorized using a TNM (tumor, node, metastasis) classification (Montie, 1993), with lymph nodes and bone being the most common sites of metastatic spread. Prostate cancer develops in two different regions of the gland, with most lesions (~80%) being found in the periphery, where more often than not, the disease is multifocal (see below). The remaining cancers are found in a periurethral region termed the *transition zone* (McNeal et al., 1988). Transition zone cancers are generally well differentiated and tend to have a better prognosis than tumors arising in the periphery (Greene et al., 1994). Curiously, it is the transition zone of the prostate in which the virtually ubiquitous process of benign prostatic hyperplasia (BPH) originates (McNeal, 1978). Based primarily on this regional difference in the incidence of benign and malignant growth, and the fact that stromal cell proliferation is typically a major component of BPH, these benign lesions are not thought to be the precursors of invasive adenocarcinoma in the prostate. Instead, prostatic intraepithelial neoplasia, or PIN, is the term given to characteristic foci of dysplastic ductal and acinar cells thought to be the precursor lesions of this disease (Bostwick, 1989). More recently, an interesting lesion, proliferative inflammatory atrophy, has been proposed as a precursor lesion as well (DeMarzo et al., 1999). Adenocarcinomas account for the vast majority of cancers in the prostate, although small cell carcinoma, ductal (endometroid) carcinoma, and other variants are observed (Randolph et al., 1997). Prostate cancer is commonly multifocal—that is, the prostate of a man diagnosed with prostate cancer contains an average of five apparently independent lesions (Bastacky et al., 1995); these lesions are genetically heterogeneous, both inter- and intratumorally (Sakr et al., 1994; Mirchandani et al., 1995; Qian et al., 1995); interestingly, this multifocality is independent of family history of prostate cancer (Bastacky et al., 1995).

The past dozen years or so have witnessed dramatic changes in the clinical presentation of prostate cancer. Previously, the development of symptoms—either from local disease, resulting primarily in voiding dysfunction, or from disseminated disease, commonly resulting in bone pain—has historically been an initial sign of prostatic malignancy, resulting in many men being diagnosed with advanced disease. The introduction of serum prostate specific antigen (PSA) as a screening tool, combined with digital rectal exam and transrectal ultrasound, has resulted in a much greater ability to detect prostate cancer while it is still confined to the gland. The widespread use of PSA testing is primarily responsible for the over 2-fold increase in incidence rates that were observed between 1988 and 1994 (Brawley and Kramer, 1996), as well as the substantial decline in the percentage of cases diagnosed annually with disseminated disease. There has been an equally dramatic decline in prostate cancer incidence observed since 1994, ascribed mainly to the diagnosis of prevalent cases within the population during the previous five- to six-year interval. It is unclear at present whether the incidence rates will stabilize at a rate equal to or higher than the rate observed in the pre-PSA era. The absolute mortality rates for prostate cancer declined in the United States for the first time in 1995 (SEER, 1999), quite possibly as a result of early detection due to increased disease screening, although there is debate over this issue.

The prostate gland is an androgen-dependent organ, and thus it undergoes a dramatic involution upon androgen deprivation. Similarly, prostate cancers generally respond to androgen ablation, achieved through either castration or, more commonly, interruption of the pituitary–gonadal axis with agents that block the action of luteinizing hormone. The death of prostate cancer cells triggered by androgen deprivation forms the basis for the most common therapies currently used for treatment of advanced prostate cancer. Although very effective in a palliative sense, such androgen ablation therapy is almost never curative, as the disease invariably progresses to an androgen-independent, incurable state. Early-stage prostate cancer, when thought to be localized to the prostate, is typically treated with either surgical removal or localized radiotherapy. Unfortunately, between 15% and 40% of patients thought to have localized disease in fact have disseminated disease, thus emphasizing the difficulties in staging prostate cancer accurately. Increasing serum PSA levels after prostatectomy or other treatment for prostate cancer is a very reliable indication of disease progression (Oesterling et al., 1988), and this may take years to become apparent. The tendency for prostate cancers to have a long natural history is emphasized by tumor doubling times often measured in years (Berges et al., 1995), although there are certainly exceptions. This long natural history greatly complicates the determination of the actual age of onset of disease, with the more appropriate term on identification of prostate cancer being age at diagnosis, which in numerous cases is age at first screening for prostate cancer.

PSA is a serine protease with a chymotrpysin-like substrate specificity; it is normally secreted by the prostate in large amounts into the seminal plasma (Lilja and Abrahamsson, 1988). The PSA level in the bloodstream of men is normally below 4 ng/ml, although this amount varies with age (Dalkin et al., 1993). With prostate pathology, these levels can increase—in particularly dramatic fashion in the case of carcinoma. While highly elevated PSA levels are most often associated with prostate cancer, a current focus of intense research effort is on the ability to accurately interpret slightly elevated PSA levels, which can be indicative of either benign or malignant disease (Oesterling, 1991; Carter and Pearson, 1997; Pannek and Partin, 1998). While PSA is an extremely useful tool for prostate cancer diagnosis, it is not as useful in determining prognosis. In fact, the inability to determine, at diagnosis, which prostate cancers will progress or already have progressed to disseminated disease is a major dilemma in the clinical management of this disease.

GENETIC AND EPIDEMIOLOGIAL EVIDENCE

Clinical Epidemiology and Ethnic Differences

The incidence of prostate cancer shows strong age, race, and geographical dependence. More so than any other cancer, it is primarily a disease of older men, with an incidence rate for men 65 and over being 20-fold greater than that for men under 64 years of age, reaching a peak frequency of ~1 in 9 in men aged 70–74 years (SEER Cancer Statistics Review, 1973–1997; http://seer.cancer.gov/publications/CSR1973_1997/prostate.pdf). Fewer than 1% of cases are diagnosed under the age of 40, although this may represent an underestimate as screening for disease in young men is rare. This disease is uncommon in Asian populations and high in Scandinavian countries, and the highest incidence (and mortality) rates known are in African American males, with mortality 2-fold higher than for American white males (Boring et al., 1992). Mortality rates vary significantly by country, ranging from over 32 per 100,000 in Trinidad and 23 per 100,000 for Caucasians in the United States to 4 per 100,000 in Japan.

The *initiation* of prostate cancer—the formation of a histologically identifiable lesion—is a very frequent event, occurring in nearly one-third of men over age 45 (Dhom, 1983), although the majority of such lesions do not progress to clinically detectable tumors. Interestingly, the rate of histological cancer incidence is roughly the same worldwide (Breslow et al., 1977; Yatani et al., 1982), suggesting an important role for environmental factors as potential promoting agents to explain the large regional differences observed in the incidence of clinically detectable disease and mortality rates (Carter et al., 1990). This feature of prostate cancer, as with many cancers, is emphasized by studies demonstrating large increases in risk in Japanese men when they move to the United States (Haenszel and Kurihara, 1968). Like most common cancers, the etiologic factors associated with prostate cancer are varied, encompassing both host genetic and environmental factors. Etiologic factors include aging, familial clustering, race, hormonal influences, diet (both inductive and preventive factors), and lifestyle factors (Brawley et al., 1998; Chan et al., 1998a; Haas and Sakr, 1997). Age, familial clustering, and race are clearly important, well-documented risk factors, while dietary influences such as high fat (elevated risk), antioxidants (e.g., selenium and lycopene, lowered risk), and hormone levels are less well documented but potentially critical factors as well. Recent findings of increased risk associated with increased serum levels of insulin-like growth factor 1 (IGF-1) need confirmation (Chan et al., 1998b), but they implicate nonandrogenic growth regulatory pathways as potentially important in determining prostate cancer risk.

Increasing age has long been appreciated as a powerful risk factor in prostate cancer. The exponential increases in prostate cancer incidence rates that occur in the seventh and eighth decades of life, combined with the almost ubiquitous occurrence of histologic prostate cancer in aging males, have led to the notion that the processes of aging and prostate carcinogenesis may be causally related. This relationship emphasizes the need to understand prostate cancer development in the context of aging.

Genetic Epidemiology

Family Studies

Results from multiple studies using either retrospective or cohort study designs provide evidence for aggregation of prostate cancer in families. Four major findings emerge from these studies: (1) there is an increased risk for developing prostate cancer among first- and second-degree relatives of prostate cancer patients; (2) the risk for developing prostate cancer among first- and second-degree relatives increases with an increase in the number of affected individuals in the families; (3) the risk for developing prostate cancer among first- and second-degree relatives increases with a decrease in the age at diagnosis of index prostate cancer cases; (4) having an affected brother tends to increase risk to a greater extent than does having a father with prostate cancer.

Woolf (1960) first described the association between a positive family history and increased risk for developing prostate cancer. He studied 228 prostate cases and age-matched controls and found a relative risk of 3 among first-degree relatives of prostate cancer cases. Cannon et al. (1982) demonstrated that prostate cancer showed the fourth strongest degree of familial clustering after lip, skin melanoma, and ovarian cancer, resulting in a stronger familial aggregation than both colon and breast carcinoma. Meikle and Stanish (1982) reported a 4-fold increased relative risk for development of prostate cancer in 257 brothers of 150 prostate cancer cases, compared to the brother-in-laws of the cases and males in the general population of the state of Utah. A retrospective case-control study by Steinberg et al. (1990) found that 15% of prostate cancer patients undergoing radical prostatectomy had an affected father or brother, compared to 8% of controls, and men with two or three first-degree affected relatives had a 5- and 11-fold increased risk for developing prostate cancer, respectively. Spitz et al. (1991) found 13.0% of 185 histologically confirmed prostate cancer patients had a positive family history, compared to 5.7% in race- and age-matched controls; they found a nonstatistically significant elevated risk for prostate cancer for having a second-degree relative with prostate cancer.

Keetch et al. (1995) surveyed the relatives of 1084 prostate cancer probands and the relatives of 935 controls (spouses of the probands). They found the presence of prostate cancer in the father, grandfather, or uncle of the proband significantly increased the risk of prostate cancer in brothers of the proband. Early age at onset in the proband was associated with an increased risk to the probands' brothers. Narod and colleagues (1995) collected information of family history of prostate cancer from 6390 men before they were screened for prostate cancer in Quebec City. They found a 2.6-fold higher risk in men with an affected brother than for men with no reported affected relative; this number was 1.2 for men with an affected father. Monroe et al. (1995) studied a population-based sample of blacks, whites, Japanese, and Hispanics. Independent of race, the age-adjusted relative risk for prevalent prostate cancer in subjects with affected brothers was approximately two times that in subjects with affected fathers. Hayes et al. (1995) reported similar results. In a population-based case-control study, prostate cancer risk was significantly elevated among those who reported a history of prostate cancer in first-degree relatives (odds ratio, OR = 3.2), with blacks and whites having similarly elevated risks. The ORs associated with a history of prostate cancer in fathers and brothers were 2.5 and 5.3, respectively. Risks associated with a family history of prostate cancer were consistently elevated among younger and older subjects. Whittemore et al. (1995) found a consistently increased risk for prostate cancer (OR = 2.5) among men with a positive family history across African Americans, Caucasians, and Asian Americans, despite the large difference in incidence among these ethnic groups. Lesko and colleagues (1996) performed a population-based case-control study in Massachusetts. Cases were 563 newly diagnosed prostate cancer patients, and controls were 703 age- and geographically matched nonprostate cancer subjects. Prostate cancer risk was increased among men who reported a history of this cancer in either their fathers or brothers, with an OR of 2.3. The OR was positively related with the number of relatives affected—from 2.2 for a history of prostate cancer in one relative to 3.9 for a history in two or more affected relatives. The OR was inversely related to the subject's age and to the age at diagnosis of prostate cancer in his affected relatives. Among probands younger than 60 years, the OR was 5.3; for those 60 to 64 years of age, the OR was 2.7; for those 65 years of age and older, the OR was 1.6. For prostate cancer diagnosed in a relative before age 65, the OR was 4.1; for diagnosed after age 74, the OR was 0.76. In another population-based case-control study of prostate cancer conducted in Montreal, Toronto, and Vancouver, a total of 640 newly diagnosed cases and 639 age-matched population controls were interviewed. Ghadirian et al. (1997) found 15% cases reported positive family history, compared with 5% of controls, giving a relative risk of 3.3. The results were consistent among the three centers.

There are at least two potential biases toward a significant finding in the retrospective family studies of prostate cancer. The first is a recall bias. Prostate cancer patients may be more likely to be aware of the diagnosis of prostate cancer in relatives than healthy controls. The second potential bias is detection bias. A diagnosis of prostate cancer may prompt a screening test in a case's relative, increasing the likelihood of an additional diagnosis in the family. This bias is particularly important in light of the increased sensitivity of disease testing using PSA screening. To decrease the effect of these biases, several cohort studies were performed.

Goldgar et al. (1994) reported the results of a cohort study of prostate cancer and other cancers using the Utah Population Database. The familial relative risk for prostate cancer in first-degree relatives of prostate cancer probands was 2.2. When the analyses were restricted to the cases diagnosed before age 67 years, the familial relative risk increased to 4.1. Grönberg et al. (1996) conducted another unselected population cohort study. A cohort of 5496 sons of Swedish men diagnosed with prostate cancer was followed, and all prostate cancers diagnosed in this cohort were identified through the Swedish Cancer Register. They observed 302 cases, compared with 178 expected prostate cancer cases, calculated using incidence rates obtained from the same registry. The standardized ratio (SIR) was 1.7. The SIR was 3.4 among patients aged 45 to 49 years at diagnosis, with the risk gradually decreasing to 1.4 among patients older than 80 years. In a follow-up study of 58,279 men ages 55 to 69 years, Schuurman et al. (1999) found 704 new prostate cancer cases after 6.3 years of follow-up. Having an affected father or brother increased the risk for prostate cancer to 1.4 and 5.6, respectively. The association was stronger for cases diagnosed before age 70. In a cohort study conducted in Iowa, 1557 men, ages 40 to 86 years, were followed for the occurrence of prostate cancer from 1987 to 1989 (Cerhan et al., 1999). By the year 1995, 101 new cases of prostate cancer were identified. A family history of prostate cancer in a brother or father was positively associated with prostate cancer risk after adjusting for age, with a relative risk (RR) of 3.2. Risk was greater if a brother had prostate cancer (RR = 4.5) than if a father had prostate cancer (RR = 2.3).

Both genetic components and common environmental risk factors within a family can lead to a significant finding in family studies. An estimation of gene and environmental contributions can be determined through twin studies and complex segregation analyses.

Twin Studies

The goal of twin studies is to compare the similarities (concordance rate) of a trait or disease in monozygotic (MZ) and dizygotic (DZ) twins to dissect the genetic and environmental components of a familial aggregation. Several twin studies of prostate cancer reported higher concordance rates in MZ twins than in DZ twins, thus implicating a genetic contribution for familial aggregation of prostate cancer. Grönberg et al. (1994) studied an unselected Swedish twin population. In 4840 male twin pairs, 458 prostate cancers were identified. Some 16 of the 1649 monozygotic twin pairs were concordant for prostate cancer (1.0%), compared with 6 of the 2983 dizygotic twin pair concordant for prostate cancer (0.2%). Using a cohort of 31,848 veteran twins born from 1917 to 1927, Page et al. (1997) identified 1009 prostate cancer cases. There was a significantly higher concordance rate among MZ twin pairs, 27.1%, than among DZ twin pairs, 7.1%. Most recently, in an analysis of 44,788 pairs of twins from the Swedish, Danish, and Finnish twin registries, Lichtenstein et al. (2000) found concordance rate for prostate cancer of 21% in MZ twin pairs and 6% in DZ twin pairs; they concluded that 42% (95% CI, 29%–50%) of prostate cancer risk may be accounted for by heritable factors. This is the highest rate of all cancers examined.

Complex Segregation Analysis

By testing the fit of several explicit models of inheritance (e.g., a major Mendelian gene model, an environmental model, and a polygene model) to the distribution of a disease in families, complex segregation analysis can identify the specific model that best describes the transmission of the disease in families. Four complex segregation analyses of the prostate cancer have been reported, and each is consistent with the hypothesis that there is a autosomal dominant susceptibility gene (Carter et al., 1992; Grönberg et al., 1997a; Schaid et al., 1998). The first complex segregation analysis was performed on 691 families ascertained through single prostate cancer probands undergoing radical prostatetecomy for clinically localized prostate cancer at Johns Hopkins Hospital (Carter et al., 1992). The segregation analysis revealed that the familial aggregation of prostate cancer can best be explained by autosomal dominant inheritance of a rare (disease gene frequency $q = 0.003$) high-risk allele, leading to an early onset of prostate cancer. The estimated cumulative risk of prostate cancer by age 85 years was 88% for carriers vs. 5% for noncarriers. This inherited form of prostate cancer was estimated to account for a significant proportion of early-onset disease and, overall, is responsible for ~9% of all prostate cancer occurrence. The second complex segregation analysis was performed in an unselected population-based sample of 2857 nuclear families ascertained through an affected father diagnosed with prostate cancer in Sweden during 1959 to 1963 (Grönberg et al., 1997a). The results suggested that the observed familial aggregation of prostate cancer is best explained by a high-risk allele inherited in a dominant mode, with a high population frequency and a moderate lifetime penetrance (63%). The third complex segregation analysis was performed to assess the genetic contribution to age at diagnosis and the familial aggregation of prostate cancer in a sample of 5486 men who underwent a radical prostatectomy for clinically localized prostate cancer in the Mayo Clinic during 1966 to 1995 (Schaid et al., 1998). The best-fitting model to explain the age at diagnosis and the familial aggregation proposed a rare autosomal dominant susceptibility gene, with the best fit observed when probands were diagnosed at less than 60 years. The frequency of the rare allele was estimated to be 0.006 in the population, and the penetrances were 89% by age 85 years for the carriers and 3% for the noncarriers. The last report was recently published based on 1476 men with prostate cancer diagnosed at less than 70 years of age and ascertained through population registries in Melbourne, Sydney, and Perth, Australia (Cui et al., 2001). The best-fitting models include a dominantly inherited increased risk that was greater, in multiplicative terms, at younger ages, as well as a recessively inherited or X-linked increased risk that was greater, in multiplicative terms, at older ages. More interestingly, all two-locus models gave better fits than did single-locus models, suggesting more than one major gene is involved.

GENE IDENTIFICATION

Linkage Studies

With strong evidence for a genetic component in the etiology of prostate cancer and evidence for a major susceptibility gene, mapping the gene(s) using linkage approaches is a natural next step. However, linkage analysis of prostate cancer has proved to be a difficult undertaking for the following reasons. First, as prostate cancer is a late-onset disease, individuals in the parental generation of the probands are usually deceased and individuals in the offspring generations are usually too young to manifest the phenotype, thus making many pedigrees only marginally informative for linkage analysis. Second, segregation analyses notwithstanding, there are likely multiple modes of inheritance (dominant, recessive, and X-linked) and multiple genes (i.e., genetic and allelic heterogeneity) involved in prostate cancer susceptibility, which largely decreases the power to detect the effect of any single major gene. Third, with such a high prevalence of disease, and such a strong environmental component, phenocopies (non-gene carriers with disease) are likely to be common. Fourth, incomplete and age-dependent penetrance of prostate cancer genes may decrease the power to detect linkage. In spite of these difficulties, at least four different loci have been implicated by linkage studies in the past several years.

Genome-Wide Screen

The first genome-wide screen for prostate cancer susceptibility genes was performed on 66 prostate cancer families ascertained at Johns Hopkins Hospital (Smith et al., 1996). Each of these families met an operational definition of hereditary prostate cancer: having at least three cases of prostate cancer in first-degree relatives. The average age at diagnosis in these families was 65, which is more than 5 years younger than the average age of diagnosis in the United States. A total of 341 dinucleotide repeat markers, covering the genome with ~10 cM resolution, were genotyped and analyzed in these families. Two-point parametric linkage analysis identified seven regions with LOD scores greater than 1 (Fig. 39–1). The highest LOD score observed was 2.75 at marker D1S218, which maps to the long arm of chromosome 1 (1q24–q25). The other regions were 1q33–q42, 4q26–q27, 5p12–q13, 7p21, 13q31–q33, and Xq27–q28. Recently, three other genome-wide screens were published. A second screen was published by the Fred Hutchinson group (Gibbs et al., 2000), reporting 2-point LOD scores of ≥1.5 for chromosomes 10q, 12q, and 14q, when the entire 94 families were analyzed under an autosomal dominant model of inheritance and for chromosomes 1q, 8q, 10q, and 16p when a recessive model of inheritance was considered. The third screen was performed in 504 brothers from 230 multiplex sibships; five regions with nominal evidence for linkage on 2q, 12p, 15q, 16q, and 16p were identified (Suarez et al., 2000a). The last one was based on 98 families from the United States and Canada that had three or more verified diagnoses of prostate cancer among first- and second-degree relatives (Hsieh et al., 2001). Positive linkage signals of nominal statistical significance were found in two regions (5p–q and 12p). It is worth noting that linkage at two chromosomal regions (5p and 12p) were reported multiple times.

HPC1

The region with the highest LOD score from the above-mentioned genome-wide screen from the Johns Hopkins Hospital was further studied in 25 additional hereditary prostate cancer families—13 collected at Johns Hopkins, and the remaining 12 families from Sweden. The overall 2-point LOD scores in the total 91 families was 3.65 at the recombinantion fraction (θ) of 0.18 with marker D1S2883 at 1q24–q25. Multipoint analyses using different combinations of three consecutive markers were performed and LOD scores above 4 were observed. Significant evidence for locus heterogeneity was obtained by an admixture test with an estimate of 34% of families linked to the region. The maximum multipoint LOD score under the assumption of heterogeneity was 5.43. The nonparametric analysis provided consistent results, with a peak multipoint nonparametric linkage (NPL) score of 4.71 (P = 1E-5). This locus was termed *HPC1* (Smith et al., 1996).

The results of analysis of HPC1 linkage by other research groups have been variable. Several independent studies corroborated linkage to HPC1. Cooney et al. (1997) reported a linkage

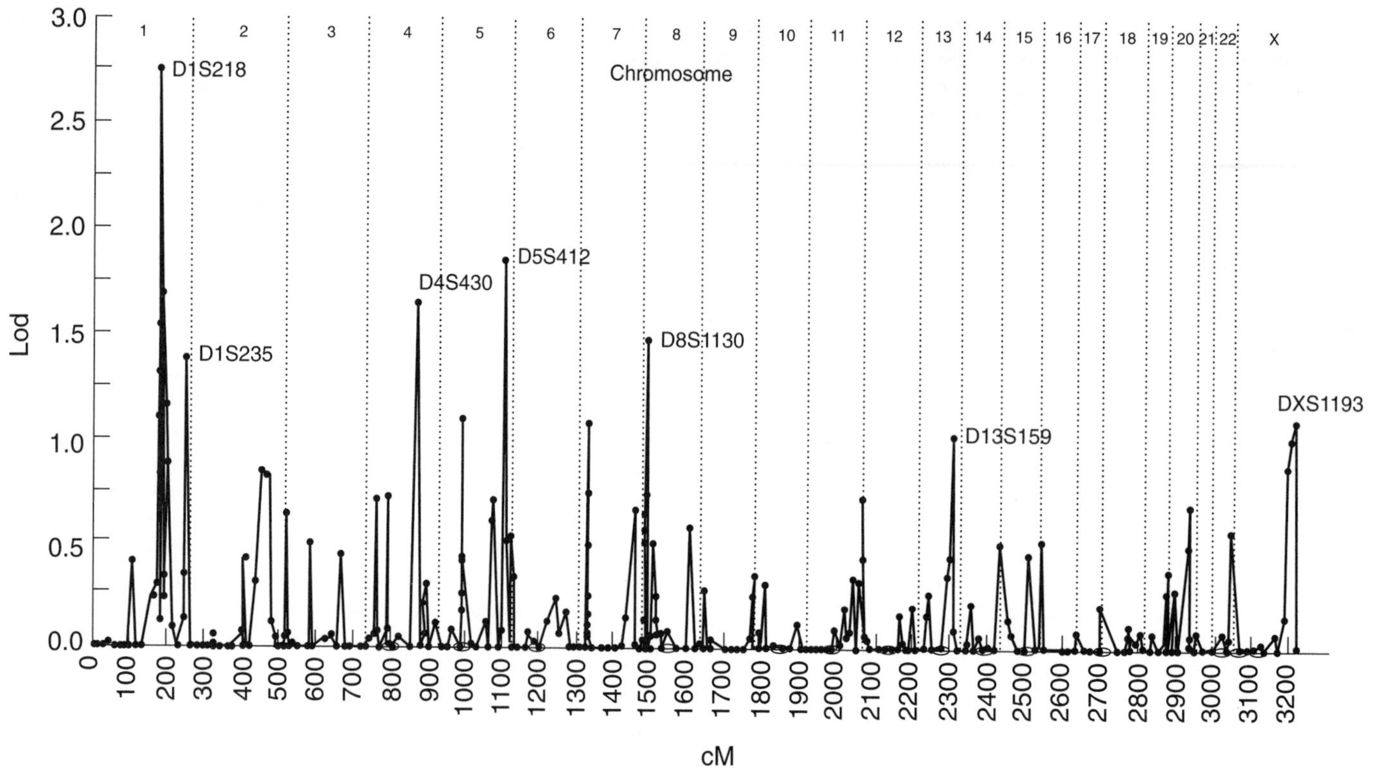

Fig. 39–1. Genome-wide screen for prostate cancer susceptibility gene. A total of 341 dinucleotide repeat markers were genotyped in 66 prostate cancer families ascertained at the Johns Hopkins Hospital (Smith et al., 1996). Maximum 2-point LOD scores were plotted. Chromosomal number is designated at the top of the plot.

study of 1q24–q25 in 59 prostate cancer families, each with two or more affected individuals. The peak NPL score was 1.58 at D1S466 (p = .057) in the total 59 families, but was 1.72 (p = .045) in the subset of 20 families that met the criteria for hereditary prostate cancer families (three or more affected individuals within one nuclear family; affected individuals in three successive generations; clustering of two or more individuals affected under 55 years old). Hsieh et al. (1997) reported further evidence to support HPC1. In 92 unrelated families having three or more affected individuals, the NPL score was 1.71 (p = .046). The evidence for linkage was stronger in the 46 families, with mean age at diagnosis less than 67. The NPL score was 2.04 (p = .023). Neuhausen et al. (1999) presented positive evidence for linkage in 41 large HPC families ascertained in Utah. The peak 2-point LOD was 1.73 (p = .005) in the total families and a 2-point LOD of 2.82 (p = .0003) in early age of onset of families. Finally, in a study of 144 HPC families collected at the Mayo Clinic, Berry et al. (2000) did not find evidence for linkage at the HPC1 region in the total sample, but found evidence for HPC1 linkage in a subset of 102 families with male-to-male disease transmission. The peak NPL score was 1.99 (p = .03) at D1S212.

Four other groups, however, reported no significant evidence for linkage of HPC1 in their study populations. McIndoe et al. (1997) reported no evidence for linkage in this region in 49 high-risk prostate cancer families, using either a parametric LOD score approach and assuming homogeneity or nonparametric analysis. There was also no evidence for linkage in the 18 families with early age at diagnosis (<65 years). Linkage analysis was further extended to 150 HPC families in this study population, and the linkage to HPC1 was strongly rejected (Goode et al., 2000). Berthon et al. (1998) reported results of a genome-wide screen and specific results from the 1q24–q25 region in 47 French and German families. For the three markers in the 1q24–q25 region, they found negative two-point LOD scores, assuming a dominant model. Eeles et al. (1998) reported a linkage study of 1q24–q25 in 136 prostate cancer families ascertained in the United Kingdom, Quebec, and Texas, 76 of which have three or more affected individuals. They found negative NPL scores in this region in the total sample, but positive NPL scores in a subset of 35 families with four or more affected members. Suarez et al. (2000a) reported no evidence for the HPC1 locus in their 230 multiplex sibships, although positive linkage results in the region were observed. The Zlr was 2.10 (p = .018) at D1S2141 in families with a positive family history and 2.72 (p = .003) at D1S1677 in families with a negative family history. Suarez et al. (2000b) reported further negative findings for HPC1 in their 45 new multiplex sibships and 4 expanded families. Interestingly, Goddard et al. (2001) reanalyzed this family collection with a total of 189 families. They reported a significant linkage at 1q24–q25 (LOD score = 3.25, p = .0001) after including the Gleason score as a covariate.

To clarify the inconsistent replication results and to test for linkage in a larger data set, a combined analysis for six markers in the 1q24–q25 regions was performed in 772 HPC families ascertained by members of the International Consortium for Prostate Cancer Genetics (ICPCG) from North America, Australia, Finland, Norway, Sweden, and the United Kingdom (Xu and ICPCG, 2000). Overall, there was some evidence for linkage, with a peak parametric multipoint LOD score assuming heterogeneity (HLOD) of 1.40 (p = .01) at D1S212. The estimated α was 6%. The evidence for linkage was stronger in families with male-to-male disease transmission. The peak HLOD was 2.56 (p = .0006) and α of 11% in the subset of 491 families with male-to-male disease transmission families, compared to HLOD of 0 in the remaining 281 families. Within the male-to-male disease transmission families, the α increased with early mean age of diagnosis (<65, α = 19%) and the number of affected family members (<5, α = 0.15%). The highest α was observed for the 48 families that met all three criteria (peak HLOD = 2.25, p = .001, α = 29%). The results from nonparametric analyses were consistent with the parametric analysis, with a peak NPL score of 1.14 at D1S212 in the total 772 HPC families. The strongest evidence for linkage at this region was observed in the 491 families with male-to-male disease transmission, with a peak NPL of 2.3 (p = .01). These results support the finding of a prostate cancer susceptibility gene linked to 1q24–q25.

HPCX

In a combined study population of 360 prostate cancer families collected at four different sites in North America, Finland, and Sweden, a linkage to Xq27–q28 was observed, which was termed HPCX (Xu et al., 1998). The peak 2-point LOD score was 4.6 at *DXS1113*, and the peak multipoint LOD score was 3.85 between *DXS1120* and *DXS297*. Significant evidence for locus heterogeneity was observed. The proportion of families linked to *HPCX* was estimated to be 16% in the combined study population and was similar in each separate family collection. The linkage of a prostate cancer gene to the X-chromosome is consistent with the results of several population-based studies, suggesting an X-linked mode of inheritance of prostate cancer (Woolf, 1960; Hayes et al., 1995; Monroe et al., 1995; Narod et al., 1995; Cerhan et al., 1999; Schuurman et al., 1999). Two subsequent studies have provided weak confirmatory evidence of linkage to Xq27–q28 (Lange et al., 1999; Peters et al., 2001). One study did not confirm the linkage (Bergthorsson et al., 2000).

PCaP

By the combination of genome-wide screening and fine mapping on a selection of 47 French and German families, Berthon et al. (1998) reported a prostate cancer susceptibility locus at 1q42–q43 (*PCaP*). The maximum 2-point LOD score was 2.7 with marker D1S2785. Multipoint parametric analysis yielded an LOD score of 2.2 assuming heterogeneity, and nonparametric analysis yielded an NPL score of 3.1. They estimated 50% of the 47 families were linked to the locus. Two replication studies did not confirm the locus (Gibbs et al., 1999; Whittemore et al., 1999), while two other studies provided some confirmation in subset of their study population (Berry et al., 2000; Xu et al., 2001b). In a linkage study of 50 markers spanned the entire chromosome 1, Xu et al. (2001b) found evidence for the linkage at this locus in 159 HPC families; however, conditional analysis revealed that evidence for linkage at 1q24–q25 and 1q42–q43 were related.

CaPB

Based on initial results of a genome-wide screen in 70 prostate cancer families and candidate-region mapping in 71 additional families, Gibbs et al. (1999) reported linkage to 1p36. Further evaluation of this data set revealed the exciting observation of an association between 1p36 linkage and the presence of brain cancer in a subset of the linked prostate cancer families. The overall 2-point LOD score was 3.22 at D1S507 for 12 families with a history of prostate cancer and a blood relative with primary brain cancer. In the younger age group (mean age at diagnosis less than 66 years), a maximum 2-point LOD of 3.65 at D1S407 was observed. However, the evidence for linkage was weaker in the multipoint analyses, with the peak multipoint LOD score assuming heterogeneity being 0.81. This linkage was rejected in both early- and late-age onset families without a history of brain cancer. Interestingly, tumors of the central nervous system were the only cancers found to be in excess in a study of other cancers in multiplex prostate cancer families reported by Isaacs et al. (1995). The group at Johns Hopkins and Wake Forest Universities investigated this linkage and provided consistent results (Xu et al., 2001b). One other study by Berry et al. (2000) did not replicate the finding. Badzioch et al. (2000) found evidence of linkage to CaPB in families with early-onset prostate cancer, although no association with other cancer was seen.

HPC20

This locus (20q13) was identified in 162 North American families with at least three members affected with prostate cancer (Berry et al., 2000). The highest 2-point LOD score was 2.69 at D20S196, and the maximum multipoint NPL score was 3.02 (p = .002) at D20S887, ~3 cM from D20S196. The evidence for linkage at this region was stronger in subsets of 46 families without male-to-male disease transmission using multipoint analyses (NPL = 3.94; p = .00007), 101 families with fewer than five family members affected with prostate cancer (NPL = 3.22; p = .0008), and 89 families with later average age of diagnosis ≥66 years (NPL = 3.40; p = .0006). The subset of 19 families with all three of these characteristics had an NPL of 3.69 (p = .0001). Two independent studies (including our collaborative group) provided confirmative evidence (Bock et al., 2001; Zheng et al., 2001).

ELAC2/HPC2

A genome-wide scan of extended high-risk pedigrees from Utah provided evidence for linkage to a locus on chromosome arm 17p (Tavtigian et al., 2001). Positional cloning and mutation screening within the defined region allowed identification of a gene, *ELAC2*, harboring mutations that segregate with prostate cancer in two pedigrees; one mutation is a frame shift and the other is a nonconservative missense change. In addition, two common missense variants in the gene have been shown to be associated with the occurrence of prostate cancer (Rebbeck et al., 2000; Tavtigian et al., 2001). This association, however, was not confirmed by two other studies (including our collaborative group) (Vesprini et al., 2001; Xu et al., 2001a). The role of ELAC2/HPC2 in affecting prostate cancer clinical characteristics and in increasing risk for other cancers remains to be investigated.

Linkage at 8p22–23

Most recently, evidence for a prostate cancer susceptibility gene at 8p22–p23 was provided by a genetic linkage analysis in 159 hereditary prostate cancer (HPC) families (Xu et al., 2001c). The prostate cancer linkage at this region was also observed in a recent genome-wide screen performed in 94 HPC families ascertained in the Seattle-based Prostate Cancer Genetic Research Study (PROGRESS) (Gibbs et al., 2000). The likelihood of a prostate cancer susceptibility gene in this region is strengthened by the accumulated evidence that 8p is the site of the most frequent loss of heterozygosity (LOH) in prostate cancer tumors (Macoska et al., 1995; Bova et al., 1996; MacGrogan et al., 1996; Vocke et al., 1996; Deubler et al., 1997; Prasad et al., 1998; Oba et al., 2001).

Association Studies

The regions identified as the potential locations of prostate cancer susceptibility genes by linkage studies tend to be broad, which causes great difficulty for fine mapping and cloning the relevant genes. The reasons for this inability of linkage analysis to provide more precise or more reliable mapping information in prostate cancer include (1) the limited number of informative recombinants is due to the small number of meioses in available family data; (2) locus heterogeneity decreases the relevant number of families useful for fine mapping; (3) the number of relevant families may be further decreased by the presence of phenocopies, resulting in negative evidence for linkage in truly linked families, and by incomplete penetrance of disease alleles; (4) with few exceptions, LOD scores for individual families are not large enough to unambiguously indicate whether a family is linked to a specific locus; (5) without a clear clinical discriminator of genetic vs. nongenetic cases, there is uncertainty whether a key recombinant in a linked family is a true recombinant or a phenocopy. To supplement fine mapping efforts in linkage studies, association studies can be taken as an alternative approach.

Association studies are generally case-control studies based on a comparison of the frequency of an allele in unrelated cases and normal controls. A significant difference in the allele frequency between cases and controls can be expected if the allele sequence itself is causal or if the allele is in linkage disequilibrium (LD) with a disease-causing mutation. Since LD can only be observed when two markers are closely linked, a significant finding of LD can pinpoint the location of the disease gene. Association studies are commonly used for testing the relevance of candidate genes as disease susceptibility genes and for testing the LD of anonymous marker allele in the regions, as implicated through linkage studies. This approach is becoming increasingly popular as more candidate genes are identified and denser maps of single nucleotide polymorphisms (SNPs) become available.

Although association studies for fine mapping have been performed successfully in many simple Mendelian diseases, this approach encounters some difficulty in complex diseases. As discussed above in relation to linkage analysis, one of the major problems is heterogeneity. Association studies are not only susceptible to etiological heterogeneity (genetic or environmental), inheritance (dominant, recessive, or X-linked), and locus heterogeneity, they are also very sensitive to allelic (same gene but different mutations) and founder (same mutation exists in different genetic background) heterogeneity. Despite these difficulties, a large number of association studies have been reported.

BRCA1 and BRCA2

As a result of various epidemiological studies over the past four decades, a link between prostate and breast cancer etiology has been suspected for many years (Thiessen, 1974; McCahy et al., 1996; Ekman et al., 1997). Anderson and Badzioch (1993) observed an increase in breast cancer risk as a function of family history of prostate cancer in families ascertained through male or female probands having breast cancer. However, as mentioned above, an examination of a large number of prostate cancer families for other cancers by Isaacs et al. (1995) found only tumors of the central nervous system to be in significant excess; the number of breast cancer cases was not significantly elevated in this study. More recent studies have demonstrated an association between *BRCA1* and *BRCA2* mutations and increased risk of prostate cancer in carriers (Ford et al., 1994; Easton et al., 1997; Sigurdsson et al., 1997; Struewing et al., 1997). The most direct evidence for a role of these genes in prostate cancer susceptibility comes from an observation of Ashkenazi men known to harbor *BRCA1* or *BRCA2* gene mutations. In this cohort, the rate of prostate cancer diagnosis by age 70 was 16%, compared to 3.8% for nonmutation carriers. Furthermore, in an extensive study of other cancers in *BRCA2* carriers from the Breast Cancer Linkage Consortium (1999), a strong association with prostate cancer was seen (estimated RR = 4.65, 95% CI, 3.48–6.22) for mutation carriers, particularly for men below 65 years of age (RR = 7.33). Other studies examining a role for these genes in prostate cancer have been less supportive of a prominent effect, although these studies have been mainly restricted to the Ashkenazi Jewish population. Lehrer et al. (1998) reported an absence of *BRCA1* and *BRCA2* founder mutations in Ashkenazi prostate cancer cases, although only a limited number of these men reported a positive family history of the disease. Langston et al. (1996) found a *BRCA1* 185delAG mutation in an affected member of a Jewish prostate cancer family, although no other family members were tested. A study of multiplex Ashkenazi Jewish prostate cancer families did not find elevated rates of common mutations in either *BRCA1* or *BRCA2* (Wilkens et al., 1999). A similar finding was reported by Nastiuk et al. (1999), who determined the rate of founder *BRCA1* and *BRCA2* mutations in early onset prostate cancer to be the same as the general Ashkenazi population. Overall, while it is clear that mutations in *BRCA1* and *BRCA2* increase the risk for prostate cancer, particularly in the case of *BRCA2* for early-onset disease, the contribution of germline mutations in these genes to familial clustering of prostate cancer in general remains to be more fully determined.

Androgen Action Pathway

It is becoming more apparent that common polymorphisms that result in quantitative or qualitative functional differences in protein products involved in normal tissue physiology may play an important role in modifying disease risk. For prostate cancer, polymorphic variants in a number of genes have been correlated with disease risk, including the androgen receptor and related 5 α-reductase gene, the vitamin D receptor, and various members of the cytochrome P450 family (Febbo et al., 1998; Murata et al., 1998; Rebbeck et al., 1998). Of these, most attention has focused on the genes involved in androgen action (Ross et al., 1998), particularly androgen receptor polymorphisms that result in variable androgen receptor activity. Specifically, there are two polymorphic triplet repeats in of exon 1 which code for polyglutamine (CAG) and polyglycine (GGN) repeats of varying lengths of between 11–31 and 10–22 residues, respectively (Edwards et al., 1992; Macke et al., 1993; Sleddens et al., 1993; Irvine et al., 1995). Although variations in the polyglycine repeat length are of unknown biological consequence, it has been demonstrated that the polyglutamine repeat length is inversely related to the ability of the androgen receptor (AR) to stimulate androgen-specific transcriptional activity (Chamberlain et al., 1994; Sobue et al., 1994; Kazemi-Esfarjani et al., 1995). This is of particular interest since the population with the shortest average glutamine repeat length observed is the African American population, which has the highest incidence and mortality rates reported for prostate cancer, whereas Asian individuals, which have low risk for prostate cancer, tend to have longer repeat lengths (Edwards et al., 1992; Irvine et al., 1995). Indeed, a number of studies have documented the correlation between shorter AR polyglutamine repeats and increased prostate cancer risk (Giovannucci et al., 1997; Stanford et al., 1997; Kantoff et al., 1998). Stanford et al. (1997) demonstrated an additional effect of shorter polyglutamine repeats, so that men with short repeat lengths for both polymorphisms (CAG < 22 and GGN ≤ 16) had a 2-fold increase in risk compared to men with two long repeats. An effect of the GGN repeat was also noted by Platz et al. (1998). Several studies have suggested that AR genes with shorter repeat lengths may increase the risk of developing more aggressive prostate cancer (Hakimi et al., 1996; Giovannucci et al., 1997). Polymorphisms in other genes involved in androgen metabolism also have been implicated in determining one's risk for prostate cancer development (e.g., 5 α-reductase, 3 β-hydroxysteroid dehydrogenase) (Reichardt et al., 1995; Devgan et al., 1997; Makridakis et al., 1997; Ross et al., 1998). Further study will be necessary to determine the overall role of these polymorphisms in determining or modifying prostate cancer risk.

Vitamin D Receptor

Although conflicting reports exist, a variety of epidemiologic data support the hypothesis that vitamin D deficiency is a risk factor for prostate cancer (Lyles et al., 1980; Schwartz and Hulka, 1990; Corder et al., 1993; Braun et al., 1995; Gann et al., 1996), and the ability of this vitamin to suppress the growth of prostate cancer cells has been documented in experimental settings (Peehl et al., 1994; Miller et al., 1995; Krill et al., 1999). The finding of polymorphisms within the 3′ untranslated region of the vitamin D receptor gene (*VDR*) which potentially affected receptor expression, led to studies examining the frequency of VDR alleles in prostate cancer cases compared to controls. Two studies found that having either one or two copies of the VDR allele containing a BsmI restriction enzyme site (i.e., allele *b*, or the putative less active variant [Morison]) was associated with an increased prostate cancer risk (Taylor et al., 1996; Ingles et al., 1997), and possibly for more advanced disease (Ingles et al., 1997). However, this result was not observed in a study by Kibel et al. (1998), which examined VDR genotpyes in a study of men who had died from prostate cancer. In this study, however, there was an interesting tendency for men with a strong family history to be homozygous for the less active allele. An extensive case-control study in the Physicians' Health Study in Boston (Ma et al., 1998) examined both serum vitamin D metabolite levels (1,25 dihydroxyvitamin D) and VDR polymorphisms in cases and controls. Although there was no increased risk associated with the allelic variants overall, in men with below median plasma levels of vitamin D, a significant reduction in risk was observed for homozygous carriers of the *B* allele. The interpretation of all these data has been complicated by recent reports indicating that the polymorphisms examined in these studies do not, as originally thought, affect receptor function, suggesting that the observed associations may reflect the influence of a different, nearby gene (Getzenberg et al., 1997; Gross et al., 1998; Durrin et al., 1999).

Regions of Loss of Heterozygosity

By analogy to other common cancers, characterization of both somatic alterations in genes and chromosomal segments in sporadic prostate cancers can be used to identify candidate prostate cancer susceptibility genes. Work from a large number of laboratories has identified a number of commonly occuring alterations in prostate cancer DNA (reviewed in Isaacs and Bova, 1999). Deletion of sequences from the short arm of chromosome 8 is perhaps the most frequent chromosomal alteration in sporadic prostate cancer, occurring at high frequency even in precursor lesions. Gain of sequences on chromosome 8q and loss of sequences on 13q are only slightly less common than 8p LOH. Gain and deletion of chromosome 7 sequences, along with deletions of chromosomes 5q, 6q, 10q, and 16q are also frequent events in the prostate cancer cell genome.

The genes driving the apparent selection of these abnormalities are largely unknown, although numerous candidates have been proposed. Methylation of a CpG island in the promoter of the gene encoding the phase II detoxification enzyme, glutathione *S*-transferase π, is the most common genomic alteration yet identified in prostate cancer, occurring in virtually every case. The common inactivation of this carcinogen-defense pathway suggests a potentially important role of environmental carcinogens during prostatic carcinogenesis. Mutations of *p53*, *PTEN*, *Rb*, *ras*, *CDKN2*, and other tumor suppressor and oncogenes have been detected at varying frequencies in prostate cancer, although no single gene has been identified as being mutated in the majority of prostate cancers. The androgen receptor gene, when either mutated or amplified, has been proposed to play a critical role in both early stages and during progression to androgen-insensitive disease. In terms of linkage analysis, no significant findings have been reported to date for genes known to undergo somatic alterations in sporadic prostate cancer, although only a handful have been analyzed (e.g., *PTEN*, *Mxi1*, *GSTP1*, *AR*).

CLINICAL APPLICATION AND RISK ASSESSMENT

To date, studies of the molecular genetics of prostate cancer have had little effect on the clinical evaluation and diagnosis of the disease. Obviously this could change dramatically when the genes identified through linkage analyses are cloned and characterized. In this regard, it is likely that much of the current study aimed at the most efficient use of genetic information for risk assessment for breast cancer and colorectal cancer will have direct relevance to prostate cancer, although prostate cancer is certain to have its unique characteristics and barriers. In the meantime, there is certainly a possibility that genotypic data for a series of polymorphisms in genes demonstrated to modulate risk (e.g., *AR*, *VDR*, *CYPs*) could be used to formulate an individual prostate cancer risk profile. DNA chip-based genotpying methodologies under development could allow such a profile to be generated rapidly and economically.

While molecular genetics may yet have a major effect on prostate cancer in the clinic, the same cannot be said for the demonstration of family history as a risk factor for prostate cancer. Family history information is now widely used in counseling individuals with respect to prostate cancer screening, and both the American Cancer Society (ACS) and the American Urological Association (AUA) recommend beginning disease screening earlier in men with a family history. Additionally, the ability to identify high-risk individuals by virtue of family history has important implications in terms of identifying appropriate participants for clinical trials to test novel chemopreventive and therapeutic strategies. Specifically, the AUA makes the following recommendations regarding regular testing for prostate cancer: all males of 50 years or more should have an annual prostate examination comprising a digital rectal examination and a PSA test; all males of 40 years or more with a family history of prostate cancer should have an annual prostate examination comprising a digital rectal examination and a PSA test. According to the ACS, beginning at age 50, an annual prostate examination, including a digital rectal examination and a PSA test, should be *offered* annually to men who have a life expectancy of at least 10 years and to younger men who are at high risk. The ACS emphasizes the benefits of beginning annual screening at age 45 in certain high-risk populations (e.g., African American men and men with two or more first-degree relatives with prostate cancer). While these guidelines are based on the idea that disease screening actually affects disease survival, this is not clear at present; certainly, the recent observation of a decline in the absolute number of deaths due to prostate cancer is encouraging in this respect. A number of clinical trials are being carried out in the United States (e.g., the National Cancer Institute's PCLO Trial) and in Europe to address the screening question, although it will be years before the results of these trials are known.

What is clear presently is that localized prostate cancer is readily curable by prostatectomy, but there is currently no effective curative therapy for disseminated disease. Thus, early detection is a critical aspect for effective prostate cancer treatment, and early detection is greatly facilitated by disease screening. It is anticipated that advances in the molecular genetics of prostate cancer will result in a more refined ability to identify which individuals will be most likely to benefit from efforts aimed at early detection. Additionally, as the molecular determinants of prostate cancer susceptibility are identified, and the pathways by which they modulate prostate cancer risk are defined, novel approaches will become available for the development of more effective prognostic, diagnostic, and therapeutic regimens for this common cancer.

REFERENCES

Anderson DE, Badzioch MD: Familial effects of prostate and other cancers on lifetime breast cancer risk. Breast Cancer Res Treat 1993; 28:107–113.

Badzioch M, Eeles R, Leblanc G, Foulkes WD, Giles G, Edwards S, Goldgar D, Hopper JL, Bishop DT, Moller P, et al.: Suggestive evidence for a site specific prostate cancer gene on chromosome 1p36. J Med Genet 2000; 37:947–949.

Bastacky SI, Wojno KJ, Walsh PC, Carmichael MJ, Epstein JI: Pathological features of hereditary prostate cancer. J Urol 1995; 153:987–992.

Berges RR, Vukanovic J, Epstein JI, CarMichel M, Cisek L, Johnson DE, Veltri RW, Walsh PC, Isaacs JT: Implication of cell kinetic changes during the progression of human prostatic cancer. Clin Cancer Res 1995; 1:473–480.

Bergthorsson JT, Johannesdottir G, Arason A, Benediktsdottir KR, Agnarsson BA, Bailey-Wilson JE, Gillanders E, Smith J, Trent J, Barkardottir RB: Analysis of HPC1, HPCX, and PCaP in Icelandic hereditary prostate cancer. Hum Genet 2000; 107(4):372–375.

Berry R, Schaid DJ, Smith JR, French AJ, Schroeder JJ, McDonnell SK, Peterson BJ, Wang ZY, Carpten JD, Roberts SG, et al.: Linkage analyses at the chromosome 1 loci 1q24–25 (HPC1), 1q42.2–43 (PCAP), and 1p36 (CAPB) in families with hereditary. Am J Hum Genet 2000; 66:539–546.

Berry R, Schroeder JJ, French AJ, McDonnell SK, Peterson BJ, Cunningham JM, Thibodeau SN, Schaid DJ: Evidence for a prostate cancer-susceptibility locus on chromosome 20. Am J Hum Genet 2000; 67:82–91.

Berthon P, Valeri A, Cohen-Akenine A, Drelon E, Paiss T, Wohr G, Latil A, Millasseau P, Mellah I, Cohen N, et al.: Predisposing gene for early-onset prostate cancer, localized on chromosome 1q42.2–43. Am J Hum Genet 1998; 62:1416–1424.

Bock CH, Cunningham JM, McDonnell SK, Schaid DJ, Peterson BJ, Pavlic RJ, Schroeder JJ, Klein J, French AJ, Marks A, et al.: Analysis of the prostate cancer-susceptibility locus HPC20 in 172 families affected by prostate cancer. Am J Hum Genet 2001; 68:795–801.

Boring CC, Squires TS, Tong T: Cancer statistics, 1992 [published erratum appears in CA Cancer J Clin 1992; 42(2):127–128]. CA Cancer J Clin 1992; 42:19–38.

Bostwick DG: Prostatic intraepithelial neoplasia (PIN). Urology 1989; 34:16–22.

Bova GS, Carter BS, Bussemakers MJ, Emi M, Fujiwara Y, Kyprianou N, Jacobs SC, Robinson JC, Epstein JI, Walsh PC, et al.: Homozygous deletion and frequent allelic loss of chromosome 8p22 loci in human prostate cancer. Cancer Res 1993; 53:3869–3873.

Braun MM, Helzlsouer KJ, Hollis BW, Comstock GW: Prostate cancer and prediagnostic levels of serum vitamin D metabolites (Maryland, United States). Cancer Causes Control 1995; 6:235–239.

Brawley OW, Knopf K, Thompson I: The epidemiology of prostate cancer, part II: The risk factors. Semin Urol Oncol 1998; 16:193–201.

Brawley OW, Kramer BS: Epidemiology of prostate cancer. In: Vogelsang NJ, Scardino PT, Shipley WU, Coffey DS (eds). Comprehensive Textbook of Genitourinary Oncology. Baltimore: Williams and Wilkins, 1996:565–572.

Breast Cancer Linkage Consortium: Cancer risks in *BRCA2* mutation carriers. 1999; 91(15):1310–1316.

Breslow N, Chan CW, Dhom G, Drury RA, Franks LM, Gellei B, Lee YS, Lundberg S, Sparke B, Sternby NH, Tulinius H: Latent carcinoma of prostate of autopsy in seven areas. Int J Cancer 1977; 20:680–688.

Cannon L, Bishop DT, Skolnick M, Hunt S, Lyon JL, Smart CR: Genetic epidemiology of prostate cancer in the Utah Mormon genealogy. Cancer Surv 1982; 1:47–69.

Carter BS, Beaty TH, Steinberg GD, Childs B, Walsh PC: Mendelian inheritance of familial prostate cancer. Proc Natl Acad Sci USA 1992; 89:3367–3371.

Carter BS, Carter HB, Isaacs JT: Epidemiologic evidence regarding predisposing factors to prostate cancer [review]. Prostate 1990; 16:187–197.

Carter HB, Pearson JD: Prostate-specific antigen velocity and repeated measures of prostate-specific antigen. Urol Clin North Am 1997; 24:333–338.

Cerhan JR, Parker AS, Putnam SD, Chiu BC, Lynch CF, Cohen MB, Torner JC, Cantor KP: Family history and prostate cancer risk in a population-based cohort of Iowa men. Cancer Epidemiol Biomarkers Prev 1999; 8:53–60.

Chamberlain NL, Driver ED, Miesfeld RL: The length and location of CAG trinucleotide repeats in the androgen receptor *N*-terminal domain affect transactivation function. Nucleic Acids Res 1994; 22:3181–3186.

Chan JM, Stampfer MJ, Giovannucci EL: What causes prostate cancer? A brief summary of the epidemiology. Semin Cancer Biol 1998a; 8:263–273.

Chan JM, Stampfer MJ, Giovannucci E, Gann PH, Ma J, Wilkinson P, Hennekens CH, Pollak M: Plasma insulin-like growth factor-I and prostate cancer risk: a prospective study [see comments]. Science 1998b; 279:563–566.

Cooney KA, McCarthy JD, Lange E, Huang L, Miesfeldt S, Montie JE, Oesterling JE, Sandler HM, Lange K: Prostate cancer susceptibility locus on chromosome 1q: a confirmatory study [see comments]. J Natl Cancer Inst 1997; 89:955–959.

Corder EH, Guess HA, Hulka BS, Friedman GD, Sadler M, Vollmer RT, Lobaugh B, Drezner MK, Vogelman JH, Orentreich N: Vitamin D and prostate cancer: a prediagnostic study with stored sera [see comments]. Cancer Epidemiol Biomarkers Prev 1993; 2:467–472.

Cui J, Staples MP, Hopper JL, English DR, McCredie MR, Giles GG: Segregation analyses of 1,476 popultaion-based Australian families affected by prostate cancer. Am J Hum Genet 2001; 68:1207–1218.

Dalkin BL, Ahmann FR, Kopp JB: Prostate specific antigen levels in men older than 50 years without clinical evidence of prostatic carcinoma. J Urol 1993; 150:1837–1839.

De Marzo AM, Marchi VL, Epstein JI, Nelson WG: Proliferative inflammatory atrophy of the prostate: implications for prostatic carcinogenesis. Am J Pathol 1999; 155(6):1985–1992.

Deubler DA, Williams BJ, Zhu XL, Steele MR, Rohr LR, Jensen JC, Stephenson RA, Changus JE, Miller GJ, Becich MJ, Brothman AR: Allelic loss detected on chromosomes 8, 10, and 17 by fluorescence in situ hybridization using single-copy P1 probes on isolated nuclei from paraffin-embedded prostate tumors. Am J Pathol 1997; 150:841–850.

Devgan SA, Henderson BE, Yu MC, Shi CY, Pike MC, Ross RK, Reichardt JK: Genetic variation of 3 β-hydroxysteroid dehydrogenase type II in three racial/ethnic groups: implications for prostate cancer risk. Prostate 1997; 33:9–12.

Dhom G: Epidemiologic aspects of latent and clinically manifest carcinoma of the prostate. J Cancer Res Clin Oncol 1983; 106:210–218.

Durrin LK, Haile RW, Ingles SA, Coetzee GA: Vitamin D receptor 3′-untranslated region polymorphisms: lack of effect on mRNA stability. Biochim Biophys Acta 1999; 1453:311–320.

Easton DF, Steele L, Fields P, Ormiston W, Averill D, Daly PA, McManus R, Neuhausen SL, Ford D, Wooster R, et al.: Cancer risks in two large breast cancer families linked to *BRCA2* on chromosome 13q12–13. Am J Hum Genet 1997; 61:120–128.

Edwards A, Hammond HA, Jin L, Caskey CT, Chakraborty R: Genetic variation at five trimeric and tetrameric tandem repeat loci in four human population groups. Genomics 1992; 12:241–253.

Eeles RA, Durocher F, Edwards S, Teare D, Badzioch M, Hamoudi R, Gill S, Biggs P, Dearnaley D, Ardern-Jones A, et al.: Linkage analysis of chromosome 1q markers in 136 prostate cancer families. Am J Hum Genet 1998; 62:653–658.

Ekman P, Pan Y, Li C, Dich J: Environmental and genetic factors: a possible link with prostate cancer. Br J Urol 1997; 79(Suppl 2):35–41.

Febbo PG, Kantoff PW, Giovannucci E, Brown M, Chang G, Hennekens CH, Stampfer M: Debrisoquine hydroxylase (CYP2D6) and prostate cancer. Cancer Epidemiol Biomarkers Prev 1998; 7:1075–1078.

Ford D, Easton DF, Bishop DT, Narod SA, Goldgar DE: Risks of cancer in *BRCA1*-mutation carriers. Lancet 1994; 343:692–695.

Gann PH, Ma J, Hennekens CH, Hollis BW, Haddad JG, Stampfer MJ: Circulating vitamin D metabolites in relation to subsequent development of prostate cancer. Cancer Epidemiol Biomarkers Prev 1996; 5:121–126.

Getzenberg RH, Light BW, Lapco PE, Konety BR, Nangia AK, Acierno JS, Dhir R, Shurin Z, Day RS, Trump DL, Johnson CS: Vitamin D inhibition of prostate adenocarcinoma growth and metastasis in the Dunning rat prostate model system. Urology 1997; 50:999–1006.

Ghadirian P, Howe GR, Hislop TG, Maisonneuve P: Family history of prostate cancer: a multi-center case-control study in Canada. Int J Cancer 1997; 70:679–681.

Gibbs M, Stanford JL, Jarvik GP, Janer M, Badzioch M, Peters MA, Goode EL, Kolb S, Chakrabarti L, Shook M, et al.: A genomic scan of families with prostate cancer identifies multiple regions of interest. Am J Hum Genet 2000; 67:100–109.

Gibbs M, Stanford JL, McIndoe RA, Jarvik GP, Kolb S, Goode EL, Chakrabarti L, Schuster EF, Buckley VA, Miller EL, et al.: Evidence for a rare prostate cancer-susceptibility locus at chromosome 1p36. Am J Hum Genet 1999; 64:776–787.

Giovannucci E, Stampfer MJ, Krithivas K, Brown M, Dahl D, Brufsky A, Talcott J, Hennekens CH, Kantoff PW: The CAG repeat within the androgen receptor gene and its relationship to prostate cancer [published erratum appears in Proc Natl Acad Sci USA 1997; 94(15):8272]. Proc Natl Acad Sci USA 1997; 94:3320–3323.

Gleason DF: Histologic grading of prostate cancer: a perspective [review]. Hum Pathol 1992; 23:273–279.

Goddard KA, Witte JS, Suarez BK, Catalona WJ, Olson JM: Model-free linkage anal-

ysis with covariates confirms linkage of prostate cancer to chromosomes 1 and 4. Am J Hum Genet 2001; 68:1197–1206.
Goldgar DE, Easton DF, Cannon-Albright LA, Skolnick MH: Systematic population-based assessment of cancer risk in first-degree relatives of cancer probands. J Natl Cancer Inst 1994; 86:1600–1608.
Goode EL, Stanford JL, Chakrabarti L, Gibbs M, Kolb S, McIndoe RA, Buckley VA, Schuster, EF, Neal CL, Miller EL, et al.: Linkage analysis of 150 high-risk prostate cancer families at 1q24–25. Genet Epidemiol 2000; 18:251–275.
Greene DR, Rogers E, Wessels EC, Wheeler TM, Taylor SR, Santucci RA, Thompson TC, Scardino PT: Some small prostate cancers are nondiploid by nuclear image analysis: correlation of deoxyribonucleic acid ploidy status and pathological features [see comments]. J Urol 1994; 151:1301–1307.
Greenlee RT, Murray T, Bolden S, Wingo PA: Cancer statistics, 2000. CA Cancer J Clin 2000; 50:7–33.
Grönberg H, Damber L, Damber JE: Studies of genetic factors in prostate cancer in a twin population. J Urol 1994; 152:1484–1487.
Grönberg H, Damber L, Damber JE: Familial prostate cancer in Sweden: a nationwide register cohort study. Cancer 1996; 77:138–143.
Grönberg H, Damber L, Damber JE, Iselius L: Segregation analysis of prostate cancer in Sweden: support for dominant inheritance. Am J Epidemiol 1997a; 146:552–557.
Gross C, Musiol IM, Eccleshall TR, Malloy PJ, Feldman D: Vitamin D receptor gene polymorphisms: analysis of ligand binding and hormone responsiveness in cultured skin fibroblasts. Biochem Biophys Res Commun 1998; 42:467–473.
Haas GP, Sakr WA: Epidemiology of prostate cancer. CA Cancer J Clin 1997; 47:273–287.
Hakimi JM, Rondinelli RH, Schoenberg MP, Barrack ER: Androgen-receptor gene structure and function in prostate cancer. World J Urol 1996; 14:329–337.
Haenszel W, Kurihara M: Studies of Japanese migrants. I. Mortality from cancer and other diseases among Japanese in the United States. J Natl Cancer Inst 1968; 40(1):43–68.
Hayes RB, Liff JM, Pottern LM, Greenberg RS, Schoenberg JB, Schwartz AG, Swanson GM, Silverman DT, Brown LM, Hoover RN: Prostate cancer risk in U.S. blacks and whites with a family history of cancer. Int J Cancer 1995; 60:361–364.
Hsieh Cl, Oakley-Girvan I, Balise RR, Halpern J, Gallagher RP, Wu AH, Kolonel LN, O'Brien LE, Lin IG, Van Den Berg DJ, et al.: A genome screen of families with multiple cases of prostate cancer: evidence of genetic heterogeneity. Am J Hum Genet 2001; 69:148–158.
Hsieh CL, Oakley-Girvan I, Gallagher RP, Wu AH, Kolonel LN, Teh CZ, Halpern J, West DW, Paffenbarger RS Jr, Whittemore AS: Re: prostate cancer susceptibility locus on chromosome 1q: a confirmatory study [letter; comment]. J Natl Cancer Inst 1997; 89:1893–1894.
Ingles SA, Ross RK, Yu MC, Irvine RA, La Pera G, Haile RW, Coetzee GA: Association of prostate cancer risk with genetic polymorphisms in vitamin D receptor and androgen receptor [see comments]. J Natl Cancer Inst 1997; 89:166–170.
Irvine RA, Yu MC, Ross RK, Coetzee GA: The CAG and GGC microsatellites of the androgen receptor gene are in linkage disequilibrium in men with prostate cancer. Cancer Res 1995; 55:1937–1940.
Isaacs SD, Kiemeney LA, Baffoe-Bonnie A, Beaty TH, Walsh PC: Risk of cancer in relatives of prostate cancer probands. J Natl Cancer Inst 1995; 87:991–996.
Isaacs WB, Bova GS: Vogelstein B, Kinzler K (eds). New York: McGraw Hill, 1999, pp. 653–660.
Kantoff P, Giovannucci E, Brown M: The androgen receptor CAG repeat polymorphism and its relationship to prostate cancer. Biochim Biophys Acta 1998; 1378:C1–C5.
Kazemi-Esfarjani P, Trifiro MA, Pinsky L: Evidence for a repressive function of the long polyglutamine tract in the human androgen receptor: possible pathogenetic relevance for the (CAG)n-expanded neuronopathies. Hum Mol Genet 1995; 4:523–527.
Keetch DW, Rice JP, Suarez BK, Catalona WJ: Familial aspects of prostate cancer: a case control study. J Urol 1995; 154:2100–2102.
Kibel AS, Isaacs SD, Isaacs WB, Bova GS: Vitamin D receptor polymorphisms and lethal prostate cancer. J Urol 1998; 160:1405–1409.
Krill D, Stoner J, Konety BR, Becich MJ, Getzenberg RH: Differential effects of vitamin D on normal human prostate epithelial and stromal cells in primary culture, Urology 1999; 54:171–177.
Lange EM, Chen H, Brierley K, Perrone EE, Bock CH, Gillanders E, Ray ME, Cooney KA: Linkage analysis of 153 prostate cancer families over a 30-cM region containing the putative susceptibility locus HPCX. Clin Cancer Res 1999; 5:4013–4020.
Langston AA, Stanford JL, Wicklund KG, Thompson JD, Blazej RG, Ostrander EA: Germ-line *BRCA1* mutations in selected men with prostate cancer [letter]. Am J Hum Genet 1996; 58:881–884.
Lehrer S, Fodor F, Stock RG, Stone NN, Eng C, Song HK, McGovern M: Absence of 185delAG mutation of the *BRCA1* gene and 6174delT mutation of the *BRCA2* gene in Ashkenazi Jewish men with prostate cancer. Br J Cancer 1998; 78:771–773.
Lesko SM, Rosenberg L, Shapiro S: Family history and prostate cancer risk. Am J Epidemiol 1996; 144:1041–1047.
Lichtenstein P, Holm NV, Verkasalo PK, Iliadou A, Kaprio J, Koskenvuo M, Pukkala E, Skytthe A, Hemminki K: Environmental and heritable factors in the causation of cancer: analyses of cohorts of twins from Sweden, Denmark, and Finland. N Engl J Med 2000; 343:78–85.
Lilja H, Abrahamsson PA: Three predominant proteins secreted by the human prostate gland. Prostate 1988; 12:29–38.
Lyles KW, Berry WR, Haussler M, Harrelson JM, Drezner MK: Hypophosphatemic osteomalacia: association with prostatic carcinoma. Ann Intern Med 1980; 93:275–278.
Ma J, Stampfer MJ, Gann PH, Hough HL, Giovannucci E, Kelsey KT, Hennekens CH, Hunter DJ: Vitamin D receptor polymorphisms, circulating vitamin D metabolites, and risk of prostate cancer in United States physicians. Cancer Epidemiol Biomarkers Prev 1998; 7:385–390.
MacGrogan D, Levy A, Bova GS, Isaacs WB, Bookstein R: Structure and methylation-associated silencing of a gene within a homozygously deleted region of human chromosome band 8p22. Genomics 1996; 35:55–65.
Macke JP, Hu N, Hu S, Bailey M, King VL, Brown T, Hamer D, Nathans J: Sequence variation in the androgen receptor gene is not a common determinant of male sexual orientation. Am J Hum Genet 1993; 53:844–852.
Macoska JA, Trybus TM, Benson PD, Sakr WA, Grignon DJ, Wojno KD, Pietruk T, Powell IJ: Evidence for three tumor suppressor gene loci on chromosome 8p in human prostate cancer. Cancer Res 1995; 15:5390–5395.
Makridakis N, Ross RK, Pike MC, Chang L, Stanczyk FZ, Kolonel LN, Shi CY, Yu MC, Henderson BE, Reichardt JK: A prevalent missense substitution that modulates activity of prostatic steroid 5α-reductase. Cancer Res 1997; 57:1020–1022.
McCahy PJ, Harris CA, Neal DE: Breast and prostate cancer in the relatives of men with prostate cancer. Br J Urol 1996; 78:552–556.
McIndoe RA, Stanford JL, Gibbs M, Jarvik GP, Brandzel S, Neal CL, Li S, Gammack JT, Gay AA, Goode EL, et al.: Linkage analysis of 49 high-risk families does not support a common familial prostate cancer-susceptibility gene at 1q24–25. Am J Hum Genet 1997; 61:347–353.
McNeal JE: Origin and evolution of benign prostatic enlargement. Invest Urol (Berl) 1978; 15:340–345.
McNeal JE, Redwine EA, Freiha FS, Stamey TA: Zonal distribution of prostatic adenocarcinoma: correlation with histologic pattern and direction of spread. Am J Surg Pathol 1988; 12:897–906.
Meikle AW, Stanish WM: Familial prostatic cancer risk and low testosterone. J Clin Endocrinol Metab 1982; 54:1104–1108.
Miller GJ, Stapleton GE, Hedlund TE, Moffat KA: Vitamin D receptor expression, 24-hydroxylase activity, and inhibition of growth by 1α,25-dihydroxyvitamin D3 in seven human prostatic carcinoma cell lines. Clin Cancer Res 1995; 1:997–1003.
Mirchandani D, Zheng J, Miller GJ, Ghosh AK, Shibata DK, Cote RJ, Roy-Burman P: Heterogeneity in intratumor distribution of *p53* mutations in human prostate cancer. Am J Pathol 1995; 147:92–101.
Monroe KR, Yu MC, Kolonel LN, Coetzee GA, Wilkens LR, Ross RK, Henderson BE: Evidence of an X-linked or recessive genetic component to prostate cancer risk [see comments]. Nat Med 1995; 1:827–829.
Montie JE: 1992 staging system for prostate cancer. [Review]. Semin Urol 1993; 11:10–13.
Murata M, Shiraishi T, Fukutome K, Watanabe M, Nagao M, Kubota Y, Ito H, Kawamura J, Yatani R: Cytochrome P4501A1 and glutathione *S*-transferase M1 genotypes as risk factors for prostate cancer in Japan. Jpn J Clin Oncol 1998; 28:657–660.
Narod SA, Dupont A, Cusan L, Diamond P, Gomez JL, Suburu R, Labrie F: The impact of family history on early detection of prostate cancer [letter]. Nat Med 1995; 1:99–101.
Nastiuk KL, Mansukhani M, Terry MB, Kularatne P, Rubin MA, Melamed J, Gammon MD, Ittmann M, Krolewski JJ: Common mutations in *BRCA1* and *BRCA2* do not contribute to early prostate cancer in jewish men. Prostate 1999; 40:172–177.
National Cancer Institute: SEER Program. 1996.
Neuhausen SL, Farnham JM, Kort E, Tavtigian SV, Skolnick MH, Cannon-Albright LA: Prostate cancer susceptibility locus HPC1 in Utah high-risk pedigrees. Hum Mol Genet 1999; 8:2437–2442.
Neuhausen SL, Skolnick MH, Cannon-Albright L: Familial prostate cancer studies in Utah. Br J Urol 1997; 79(Suppl 1):15–20.
Oba K, Matsuyama H, Yoshihiro S, Kishi F, Takahashi M, Tsukamoto M, Kinjo M, Sagiyama K, Naito K: Two putative tumor suppressor genes on chromosome arm 8p may play different roles in prostate cancer. Cancer Genet Cytogenet 2001; 124:20–26.
Oesterling JE: Prostate specific antigen: a critical assessment of the most useful tumor marker for adenocarcinoma of the prostate [review]. J Urol 1991; 145:907–923.
Oesterling JE, Chan DW, Epstein JI, Kimball AW Jr, Bruzek DJ, Rock RC, Brendler CB, Walsh PC: Prostate specific antigen in the preoperative and postoperative evaluation of localized prostatic cancer treated with radical prostatectomy. J Urol 1988; 139:766–772.
Page WF, Braun MM, Partin AW, Caporaso N, Walsh P: Heredity and prostate cancer: a study of World War II veteran twins. Prostate 1997; 33:240–245.
Pannek J, Partin AW: The role of PSA and percent free PSA for staging and prognosis prediction in clinically localized prostate cancer. Semin Urol Oncol 1998; 16:100–105.
Peehl DM, Skowronski RJ, Leung GK, Wong ST, Stamey TA, Feldman D: Antiproliferative effects of 1,25-dihydroxyvitamin D3 on primary cultures of human prostatic cells. Cancer Res 1994; 54:805–810.
Peters MA, Jarvik GP, Janer M, Chakrabarti L, Kolb S, Goode EL, Gibbs M, DuBois CC, Schuster EF, Hood L, Ostrander EA, Stanford JL: Genetic linkage analysis of prostate cancer families to Xq27–28. Hum Hered 2001; 51(1-2):107–113.
Platz EA, Giovannucci E, Dahl DM, Krithivas K, Hennekens CH, Brown M, Stampfer MJ, Kantoff PW: The androgen receptor gene GGN microsatellite and prostate cancer risk. Cancer Epidemiol Biomarkers Prev 1998; 7:379–384.
Prasad MA, Trybus TM, Wojno KJ, Macoska JA: Homozygous and frequent deletion of proximal 8p sequences in human prostate cancers: identification of a potential tumor suppressor gene site. Genes Chromosomes Cancer 1998; 23:255–262.

Qian JQ, Bostwick DG, Takahashi S, Borell TJ, Herath JF, Lieber MM, Jenkins RB: Chromosomal anomalies in prostatic intraepithelial neoplasia and carcinoma detected by fluorescence in situ hybridization. Cancer Res 1995; 55:5408–5414.

Randolph TL, Amin MB, Ro JY, Ayala AG: Histologic variants of adenocarcinoma and other carcinomas of prostate: pathologic criteria and clinical significance. Mod Pathol 1997; 10(6):612–629.

Rebbeck TR, Jaffe JM, Walker AH, Wein AJ, Malkowicz SB: Modification of clinical presentation of prostate tumors by a novel genetic variant in CYP3A4. J Natl Cancer Inst 1998; 90:1225–1229.

Rebbeck TR, Walker AH, Zeigler-Johnson C, Weisburg S, Martin AM, Nathanson KL, Wein AJ, Malkowicz SB: Association of *HPC2/ELAC2* genotypes and prostate cancer. Am J Hum Genet 2000; 67:1014–1019.

Reichardt JK, Makridakis N, Henderson BE, Yu MC, Pike MC, Ross RK: Genetic variability of the human *SRD5A2* gene: implications for prostate cancer risk. Cancer Res 1995; 55:3973–3975.

Ross RK, Pike MC, Coetzee GA, Reichardt JK, Yu MC, Feigelson H, Stanczyk FZ, Kolonel LN, Henderson BE: Androgen metabolism and prostate cancer: establishing a model of genetic susceptibility. Cancer Res 1998; 58:4497–4504.

Sakr WA, Macoska JA, Benson P, Grignon DJ, Wolman SR, Pontes JE, Crissman JD: Allelic loss in locally metastatic, multisampled prostate cancer. Cancer Res 1994; 54:3273–3277.

Schaid DJ, McDonnell SK, Blute ML, Thibodeau SN: Evidence for autosomal dominant inheritance of prostate cancer. Am J Hum Genet 1998; 62:1425–1438.

Schuurman AG, Zeegers MP, Goldbohm RA, van den Brandt PA: A case-cohort study on prostate cancer risk in relation to family history of prostate cancer. Epidemiology 1999; 10:192–195.

Schwartz GG, Hulka BS: Is vitamin D deficiency a risk factor for prostate cancer? (Hypothesis). Anticancer Res 1990; 10:1307–1311.

SEER: Cancer Statistics. www-seer ims nci nih gov/Publication/ProstMono. 1999.

Sigurdsson S, Thorlacius S, Tomasson J, Tryggvadottir L, Benediktsdottir K, Eyfjord JE, Jonsson E: *BRCA2* mutation in Icelandic prostate cancer patients. J Mol Med 1997; 75:758–761.

Sleddens HF, Oostra BA, Brinkmann AO, Trapman J: Trinucleotide (GGN) repeat polymorphism in the human androgen receptor (*AR*) gene. Hum Mol Genet 1993; 2:493.

Smith JR, Freije D, Carpten JD, Gronberg H, Xu J, Isaacs SD, Brownstein MJ, Bova GS, Guo H, Bujnovszky P, et al.: Major susceptibility locus for prostate cancer on chromosome 1 suggested by a genome-wide search [see comments]. Science 1996; 274:1371–1374.

Sobue G, Doyu M, Morishima T, Mukai E, Yasuda T, Kachi T, Mitsuma T: Aberrant androgen action and increased size of tandem CAG repeat in androgen receptor gene in X-linked recessive bulbospinal neuronopathy. J Neurol Sci 1994; 121:167–171.

Spitz MR, Currier RD, Fueger JJ, Babaian RJ, Newell GR: Familial patterns of prostate cancer: a case-control analysis. J Urol 1991; 146:1305–1307.

Stanford JL, Just JJ, Gibbs M, Wicklund KG, Neal CL, Blumenstein BA, Ostrander EA: Polymorphic repeats in the androgen receptor gene: molecular markers of prostate cancer risk. Cancer Res 1997; 57:1194–1198.

Steinberg GD, Carter BS, Beaty TH, Childs B, Walsh PC: Family history and the risk of prostate cancer. Prostate 1990; 17:337–347.

Struewing JP, Hartge P, Wacholder S, Baker SM, Berlin M, McAdams M, Timmerman MM, Brody LC, Tucker MA: The risk of cancer associated with specific mutations of *BRCA1* and *BRCA2* among Ashkenazi Jews [see comments]. N Engl J Med 1997; 336:1401–1408.

Suarez BK, Lin J, Burmester JK, Broman KW, Weber JL, Banerjee TK, Goddard KA, Witte JS, Elston RC, Catalona WJ: A genome screen of multiplex sibships with prostate cancer. Am J Hum Genet 2000a; 66:933–944.

Suarez BK, Lin J, Witte JS, Conti DV, Resnick MI, Klein EA, Burmester JK, Vaske DA, Banerjee TK, Catalona WJ: Replication linkage study for prostate cancer susceptibility genes. Prostate 2000b; 45:106–114.

Tavtigian SV, Simard J, Teng DH, Abtin V, Baumgard M, Beck A, Camp NJ, Carillo AR, Chen Y, Dayananth P, et al.: A candidate prostate cancer susceptibility gene at chromosome 17p. Nat Genet. 2001; 27:172–180.

Taylor JA, Hirvonen A, Watson M, Pittman G, Mohler JL, Bell DA: Association of prostate cancer with vitamin D receptor gene polymorphism. Cancer Res 1996; 56:4108–4110.

Thiessen EU: Concerning a familial association between breast cancer and both prostatic and uterine malignancies. Cancer 1974; 34:1102–1107.

Vesprini D, Nam RK, Trachtenberg J, Jewett MA, Tavtigian SV, Emami M, Ho M, Toi A, Narod SA: HPC2 variants and screen-detected prostate cancer. Am J Hum Genet 2001; 68(4):912–917.

Vocke CD, Pozzatti RO, Bostwick DG, Florence CD, Jennings SB, Strup SE, Duray PH, Liotta LA, Emmert-Buck MR, Linehan WM: Analysis of 99 microdissected prostate carcinomas reveals a high frequency of allelic loss on chromosome 8p12–21. Cancer Res 1996; 56:2411–2416.

Whittemore AS, Lin IG, Oakley-Girvan I, Gallagher RP, Halpern J, Kolonel LN, Wu AH, Hsieh CL: No evidence of linkage for chromosome 1q42.2–43 in prostate cancer. Am J Hum Genet 1999; 65:254–256.

Whittemore AS, Wu AH, Kolonel LN, John EM, Gallagher RP, Howe GR, West DW, Teh CZ, Stamey T: Family history and prostate cancer risk in black, white, and Asian men in the United States and Canada. Am J Epidemiol 1995; 141:732–740.

Wilkens EP, Freije D, Xu J, Nusskern DR, Suzuki H, Isaacs SD, Wiley K, Bujnovsky P, Meyers DA, Walsh PC, Isaacs WB: No evidence for a role of *BRCA1* or *BRCA2* mutations in Ashkenazi Jewish families with hereditary prostate cancer. Prostate 1999; 39:280–284.

Woolf CM: An investigation of familial aspects of carcinoma of the prostate. Cancer 1960; 13:739–744.

Xu J, International Consortium for Prostate Cancer Genetics: Combined analysis of hereditary prostate cancer linkage to 1q24–25: results from 772 hereditary prostate cancer families from the international consortium for prostate cancer genetics. Am J Hum Genet 2000; 66:945–957.

Xu J, Meyers D, Freije D, Isaacs S, Wiley K, Nusskern D, Ewing C, Wilkens E, Bujnovszky P, Bova GS, et al.: Evidence for a prostate cancer susceptibility locus on the X chromosome. Nat Genet 1998; 20:175–179.

Xu J, Zheng SL, Carpten JD, Nupponen NN, Robbins C, Mestre J, Moses T, Faith D, Kelly B, Isaacs SD, et al.: Evaluation of linkage and association of *HPC2/ELAC2* in familial and unrelated prostate cancer patients. Am J Hum Genet 2001a; 68:901–911.

Xu J, Zheng SL, Chang B, Smith JR, Carpten JD, Stine OC, Isaacs SD, Wiley K, Henning L, Ewing C, et al.: Linkage of prostate cancer susceptibility loci to chromosome 1. Hum Genet 2001b; 108:335–345.

Xu J, Zheng SL, Chang B, Isaacs SD, Wiley K, Hawkin GA, Bleecker ER, Walsh PC, Trent JM, Meyers DA, Isaacs WI: Linkage and association studies of prostate cancer susceptibility gene on 8p22–23. Am J Hum Genet 2001c; 69:341–350.

Yatani R, Chigusa I, Akazaki K, Stemmermann GN, Welsh RA, Correa P: Geographic pathology of latent prostatic carcinoma. Int J Cancer 1982; 29:611–616.

Zheng SL, Xu J, Chang B, Isaacs SD, Wiley K, Bleecker ER, Walsh PC, Trent JM, Meyers DA, Isaacs WI: Evaluation of linkage of *HPC20* in 159 hereditary prostate cancer pedigrees. Hum Genet 2001; 108:430–435.

40 Hematologic Cancer

MARSHALL HORWITZ

Unlike many diseases where anecdotal reports can be traced to Talmudic tracts or other antiquity, the discovery of leukemia and other hematopoietic malignancies could only occur after at least two major advances: the invention of the microscope and an initial understanding of cellular biology. Leukemia as such was first described independently in 1845 within a single month by Bennett and Virchow; the latter named it ("leukämie") (Freireich and Lemark, 1991). Hodgkin first reported on his eponymic disease in 1832, but the complicated nosology of the lymphoproliferative disorders took some time to be delineated (Greer et al., 1995) by Virchow, who differentiated them from leukemia in about 1865 as "lymphosarcoma" or "aleukemia," with later work by the likes of Billroth, Kundrat, and Reed and Sternberg. The first description and naming of "multiple myeloma" is credited to Rusitzky in 1873 (Sullivan, 1993). It was not until about the time of publication of Osler's milestone text, *The Principles and Practice of Medicine*, in 1892, that hematopoietic malignancy came to be generally described in reasonably modern clinical and pathological terms. Most cases of hematopoietic malignancy before then were probably clinically indistinguishable from infectious disease. These are thus illnesses in which the opportunity for genetic observations has been limited to no more than the last three or four generations. Recent years have witnessed enormous gains in understanding the molecular genetic pathology of these diseases. Until recently, the focus has been at the level of somatic mutations in sporadically occurring cases, where acquired chromosomal rearrangements have been well investigated and abundantly reviewed (Caligiuri et al., 1997; Look, 1997; Bohlander, 2000; Burmeister and Thiel, 2001). Less is known of molecular mechanisms that might be responsible for inherited predisposition, although epidemiologic evidence suggests that such factors may contribute substantially to the risk for developing hematopoietic malignancy.

DISEASE DEFINITION

Incidence of Hematopoietic Malignancy

Leukemia is the tenth most common malignancy and the seventh most frequent cause of cancer death in the United States. Lymphoma ranks fifth and sixth in cancer incidence and mortality, respectively. Multiple myeloma is the sixteenth most frequent malignancy and the twelfth leading cause of cancer death. These three major categories of hematopoietic malignancy were collectively estimated to have had an incidence of 103,200 cases for 1997 in the United States, causing 57,496 fatalities, which is equal to 2.5% of all deaths and 10.9% of all cancer-related deaths (Parker et al., 1997). Because of a relatively younger age of onset than for most solid tumors, leukemia and some lymphomas account for a relatively greater number of total years of life lost; leukemia is second only to accidents as a cause of death in the United States before the age of 15 years. Incidence figures are summarized in Table 40–1.

Diagnostic Criteria, Clinical Description, and Defined Subtypes

Leukemia

Leukemia and other hematopoietic malignancies are categorized on the basis of which cell is malignantly transformed during the course of differentiation from a single hematopoietic progenitor stem cell to the mature lineages distributed in peripheral blood and lymphoid organs.

Acute myelogenous leukemia (AML; also known as acute nonlymphocytic leukemia, ANLL) and acute lymphocytic leukemia (ALL) are classified according to the French-American-British (FAB) scheme based on morphologic appearance of bone marrow and blood leukemic blasts that was introduced in 1976 and most recently revised in 1985 (Table 40–2). Histochemical, immunocytochemical, and cytogenetic data are routinely used to corroborate FAB hematopathologic subtype.

Myelodysplasia or "myelodysplastic syndrome" (MDS) represents a heterogeneous group of disorders characterized by cytopenias that are associated with dysmorphic bone marrow. Five FAB subtypes are recognized (Table 40–3): refractory anemia (RA), refractory anemia with ringed sideroblasts (RARS), refractory anemia with excess blasts (RAEB), refractory anemia with excess blasts in transformation (RAEBT, which often evolves into AML), and chronic myelomonocytic leukemia (CMML). Myelodysplasia and AML can occur as a treatment-related side effect of chemotherapy for other malignancies. Measurements of the incidence of myelodysplasia are crude and are complicated by clinical overlap with AML, but they range from about 3.5 to 12.6 cases per 100,000 population per year (Dunbar and Nienhuis, 1995; Aul et al., 1998).

Chronic myelogenous leukemia (CML) is a "myeloproliferative syndrome," whose spectrum also consists of polycythemia vera, idiopathic myelofibrosis, and essential thrombocythemia. ("Agnogenic myeloid metaplasia" is also included within the myeloproliferative syndromes.) CML is nearly always associated with the translocation 9;22 Philadelphia chromosome first observed in 1960 by Nowell and Hungerford that results in a bcr-abl fusion oncogene (Lukens, 1993).

Table 40–1. Incidence of Hematopoietic Malignancy in the United States for 1997

Malignancy	Male	Female	Total
Leukemia	*15,900*	*12,400*	*28,300*
Acute myelogenous leukemia	4,700	4,500	9,200
Acute lymphocytic leukemia	1,600	1,400	3,000
Chronic lymphocytic leukemia	4,300	3,100	7,400
Chronic myelogenous leukemia	2,400	1,900	4,300
Other leukemia	2,900	1,500	4,400
Lymphoma	*34,200*	*26,900*	*61,100*
Hodgkin's disease	3,900	3,600	7,500
Non-Hodgkin's lymphoma	30,300	23,300	53,600
Multiple myeloma	*7,900*	*5,900*	*13,800*

Source: Parker et al. (1997) with permission.

Chronic lymphocytic leukemia (CLL) results from transformation of a mature lymphocyte, which produces a monoclonal, differentiated-appearing lymphocytosis, 90% of the time involving B-cells. CLL variants are rare and include T-cell CLL, prolymphocytic leukemia, large granular lymphocyte leukemia (LGL), hairy cell leukemia, splenic lymphoma with villous lymphocytes, and non-Hodgkin's lymphoma in leukemic phase.

Lymphoma

Hodgkin's disease (HD) is a lymph node malignancy characterized by the presence of a binucleated Reed-Sternberg (R-S) giant cell. The cellular origin of the R-S cell is uncertain, although it has some characteristics of both macrophages and lymphocytes. In contrast to almost all other tumors, the R-S cell is a minority component of the malignant lymph node, and the majority of the tumor cell population is comprised of normal inflammatory cells. There are four histologic subtypes of Hodgkin's disease, based on the number and appearance of the R-S cells, as well as the composition of the infiltrate of inflammatory cells: nodular sclerosing (NSHD), lymphocyte predominant (LPHD), mixed cellular (MCHD), and lymphocyte depleted (LDHD). Treatment decisions in Hodgkin's disease are generally based on the Ann Arbor clinical anatomic staging classification introduced in 1971 (Greer et al., 1993).

Non-Hodgkin's lymphoma (NHL) is a neoplasm involving B or T lymphocytes in lymphoid tissues. Although several pathologic classification schemes have been developed, the National Cancer Institute Working Formulation of 1982 based on clinical prognosis is most widely employed (Table 40–4). "Low-grade" lymphomas include small lymphocytic (SLL), follicular small cleaved cell (FSCL), and follicular mixed small cleaved and large cell (FML) subtypes and tend to follow an indolently progressive course. "Intermediate-grade" lymphomas include follicular large cell (FLCL), diffuse small cleaved cell (DSCL), diffuse mixed small cleaved and large cell (DML), and diffuse large cell (DLCL). "High-grade" lymphomas consists of large cell immunoblastic (IBL), lymphoblastic (LL), and small noncleaved cell (SNCL); these malignancies often appear abruptly, are fast growing, and are complicated by extranodal involvement. A miscellaneous category of lymphoma included in the Working Formulation consists of mycosis fungoides, a rare cutaneous helper T-cell lymphoma; lymphomas that are of composite histologic subtypes; and histiocytic lymphoma. Since the Working Formulation's establishment in 1982, additional peripheral T-cell lymphomas have been recognized. The majority of non-Hodgkin's lymphomas with follicular histology demonstrate a chromosome 14;18 translocation fusing BCL2 to the Ig heavy chain locus.

Multiple Myeloma

Multiple myeloma is a neoplasm arising as a monoclonal proliferation of a bone marrow plasma cell engaged in the production of IgG. The tumor frequently invades adjacent bone. Waldenstrom macroglobulinemia is similar, except that there is monoclonal proliferation of an IgM-producing cell. It clinically differs from multiple myeloma by the general absence of bone lesions and the presence of hyperviscosity of the blood, lymphadenopathy, and hepatosplenomegally. Other neoplastic plasma cell disorders include monoclonal gammopathy of undetermined significance (MGUS), osteoslcerotic myeloma (POEMS syndrome), plasma cell leukemia, nonsecretory myeloma, IgD myeloma, heavy chain disease, and primary amyloidosis.

Table 40–2. French-American-British (FAB) Classification of Acute Leukemias

Malignancy	Morphology	Typical Somatic Cytogenetic Abnormalities
Acute myelogenous leukemia (AML)		
M0, acute undifferentiated leukemia	Uniform and undifferentiated	
M1, AML with minimal differentiation	Undifferentiated with a few azurophilic granules	
M2, AML with differentiation	Granulated blasts ± Auer rods	t(8;21) producing AML1-eto fusion
M3, acute promyelocytic leukemia	Hypergranular promyelocytes	t(15;17) (or else t(11;17) or t(5;17), all involving rar-α on 17
M4, acute myelomonocytic leukemia	Both monoblasts and myeloblasts present	inv(16q22.1) involving CBFB for M4 eosinophilic type
M5, acute monocytic leukemia	Monoblasts predominate	t(9;11) producing MLL-AF9 fusion
M6, acute erythroleukemia	Erythroblasts and megaloblastic red cell precursors	
M7, acute megakaryocytic leukemia	Undifferentiated blasts, often fibrotic	
Acute lymphocytic leukemia (ALL)		
L1, ALL childhood variant	Small uniform blasts with indistinct nucleoli	
L2, ALL adult variant	Larger blasts with more irregular nucleoli	t(1;19) resulting in E2a-pbx1 fusions in pre-B cell types
L3, Burkitt-like ALL	Large blasts with basophilic cytoplasm and vacuoles	t(8;14), t(2;8), t(8;22) fusions of myc to Ig enhancers

Source: Lukens, 1993.

Table 40–3. French-American-British (FAB) Classification of Myelodysplastic (MDS) Syndrome

Subtype	Case Distribution (%)
Refractory anemia (RA)	27
Refractory anemia with ringed sideroblasts (RARS)	20
Refractory anemia with excess blasts (RAEB)	26
Refractory anemia with excess blasts in transformation (RAEBT)	13
Chronic myelomonocytic leukemia (CMML)	14

Source: Distribution of cases is taken from Dunbar and Nienhuis (1995) with permission.

GENERAL GENETIC AND EPIDEMIOLOGIC EVIDENCE

Clinical Epidemiology and Ethnic Differences

Age and Sex

Each hematopoietic malignancy has a characteristic age distribution. In general, AML incidence increases exponentially with age, beginning at about 20 years. ALL incidence logarithmically declines from early childhood and then exponentially increases from about 30 years. Myelodysplasia appears to linearly increase in frequency from about the age of 50 years, before which it is uncommon. Non-Hodgkin's lymphoma logarithmically increases with aging, while Hodgkin's disease demonstrates a bimodal age distribution, peaking in the mid-twenties and mid-sixties. For multiple myeloma, the incidence increases linearly with age, commencing from the mid-thirties, before which the disease is nearly absent. Most hematopoietic malignancy is more common among males, but the magnitude of the skewing in sex ratios depends on the particular malignancy.

Ethnic Differences

Jews. Numerous retrospectively performed studies have found an excess of leukemia among Ashkenazi (eastern European) Jews (reviewed in detail in Linet, 1985). In general, the relative risks range between 2- and 3-fold and are greatest for CLL and AML, at the expense of ALL. Russian- and Polish-born Jews are overrepresented among leukemic patients in such surveys. For example, in a study relying on the religious affiliation of the cemetery of burial for 1636 leukemics in Brooklyn, New York, between 1943 and 1952, there was a relative risk among Ashkenazim of 2.4 for CLL, 2.7 for AML, and 1.9 for CML (MacMahon and Koller, 1957). High risk occurred across both sexes and all ages. Other studies using death certificates and state registries have found similar magnitude risk elevations, although most have been confined to the East Coast of the United States and were performed in the 1950s and 1960s. A more recent study of 288 CLL patients in Jerusalem confirmed an overrepresentation of Ashkenazi Jews, compared to Sephardic (non-European) Jews and Arabs (Bartal et al., 1978). It was also noted that none of the Sephardic or Arab patients had coexisting malignancies, yet 12.5% of the Ashkenazim had a second malignancy, while 3% had, in addition to CLL, two coexisting malignancies.

Table 40–4. National Cancer Institute (NCI) Working Formulation Classification of Non-Hodgkin's Lymphoma and Immunophenotypes

Lymphoma	B cell	T cell
Low grade		
Small lymphocytic (SLL)	Yes	Rare
Follicular, small cleaved cell (FSCL)	Yes	
Follicular, mixed small cleaved and large cell (FML)	Yes	
Intermediate grade		
Follicular, large cell (FLCL)	Yes	
Diffuse, small cleaved cell (DSCL)	Yes	Occasional
Diffuse, mixed small cleaved and large cell (DML)	Yes	Yes
Diffuse, large cell (DLCL)	Yes	Yes
High grade		
Large cell immunoblastic (IBL)	Yes	Yes
Lymphoblastic (LL)		Yes
Small noncleaved cell (SNCL)	Yes	

Source: Greer et al., 1993.

These studies would seem to substantiate a role for genetic risk factors for leukemia, but note that studies ascertaining the diagnosis of leukemia at death are vulnerable to biases that reflect either a worsened survival or a relative lessening of contribution of death by other diseases. Two smaller studies found no differences in leukemia incidence between Jews and non-Jews (King et al., 1965; Cuneo,1976), although it is possible that these studies lacked the statistical power to resolve an effect. Another study of 201 children with leukemia and 117 children with lymphoma identified by death certificate in Israel between 1950–1954 and 1958–1964 found that for each of three ethnicities (European, Asian, and African), the leukemia rate was higher among foreign-born children than for native-born Israeli children (Royston and Modan, 1968); this could be taken as evidence against genetic factors and in support of environmental factors causing leukemia. A meta-analysis of several studies found a consistent risk elevation for Jews (Haenszel, 1971), and the risk was again greater for Ashkenazi Jews than for those of Sephardic ancestries. The possibility of ascertainment bias in diagnosis has been raised, but because of the presence of socialized medicine in Israel, it was assumed in one study (Bartal et al., 1978) that access to medical care was equal between Ashkenazi and Sephardic populations in Israel.

A comparison of the racial backgrounds of 339 patients with myeloproliferative disorders (excluding CML) diagnosed in northern Israel between 1975 and 1989 (Chaiter et al., 1992) found that the expected incidence in Ashkenazi Jews was 10 times greater than that for Sephardic Jews and 20 times greater than that for Arabs. A higher proportion of the patients had emigrated from Poland, the former Soviet Union, and Romania than compared to western European countries.

In a series of rare intestinal lymphoma reported from Israel, all patients were either Sephardic Jews or Arabs (Ramot and Hulu, 1969).

In a small series of 100 Israeli patients treated for multiple myeloma, nine patients developed a treatment-related myelodysplastic syndrome, and all were Ashkenazi (Mittelman et al., 1994).

Several studies have suggested that polycythemia vera occurs disproportionately commonly among Ashkenazi Jews. These studies have been criticized for having inadequate control populations and for not allowing for the possibility that this group might have better access to medical care (Modan, 1965).

Hispanics. M3 AML (acute promyelocytic leukemia) appears more commonly among Hispanic populations. Some 37.5% of 80 Hispanic AML patients treated between 1987 and 1994 at the Los Angeles County medical center had the M3 subtype, whereas M3 was the subtype in just 6.5% of 62 non-Latinos (Douer et al., 1996). The authors further surveyed a non-overlapping Los Angeles County cancer registry and found that M3 was the subtype in 24.3% of the 47 Latinos with AML compared to 8.3% among the 229 non-Hispanic AML patients. The effect was still significant even after adjustments for a younger average age among the Latino AML population. The study found no evidence for an increased risk among Hispanics for other subtypes of AML, in that the ratio of Hispanic to non-Hispanic patients for each of the non-M3 subtypes did not differ significantly from each other or from the population served by the hospital. Numerous other surveys of the frequency of M3 AML, in mostly Caucasian populations of North America and Europe, have ranged between 5% and 13% (as reviewed by (Douer, 1996). In a follow-up letter to the prior study, it was noted that M3 accounted for 23% of 104 Spanish AML patients treated between 1986 and 1994 in Madrid (Tomas and Fernandez-Ranada, 1996). This finding is somewhat difficult to reconcile in light of the extreme heterogeneity of Spanish-speaking populations. An increased frequency of M3 AML has also been reported in Italian children (Biondi et al., 1994).

Hematopoietic malignancy of all types may be more frequent in the Hispanic population. A tumor registry survey in Dade County, Florida, of cases between 1980 and 1989 found a standardized rate ratio between 10,417 Hispanic and 17,013 non-Hispanic males to be 3.29 for AML, 1.11 for CML, 1.30 for ALL, 2.27 for CLL, 2.75 for Hodgkin's disease, and 12.98 for non-Hodgkin's lymphoma (Trapido et al, 1994). It is possible that the increased risk for AML reflects an increased rate of M3 AML; however, AML subtypes were not available. It is possible that the high frequency of lymphoma reflects a higher frequency of HIV infection among Hispanic males of south Florida. Although data on HIV seropositivity was not available, the rate ratio for Kaposi sarcoma was also elevated 6-fold, and both Kaposi sarcoma and lymphoma are complications of AIDS (see later under Environmental Factors). A survey of 320 Puerto Rican–born males in the Connecticut state cancer registry was notable for what was concluded to be a statistically significant 1.77 relative risk in leukemia of all types, but no statistically significant risk elevation was seen among Hispanic females (Polednak, 1992). A review of population-based tumor registries from 28 countries found the highest incidence for all types of childhood leukemia to occur among Hispanics, with the highest rates in Costa Rica and Los Angeles, followed by Puerto Rico and Spain (Linet and Devesa, 1991). However, a smaller study of 189 Hispanic children in the New Mexico Tumor Registry found no significant differences in the incidence of leukemia or lymphoma compared to 235 non-Hispanic whites in the study (Duncan et al., 1986).

Given the heterogeneity of "Hispanic" populations in the United States, such discrepancy is not surprising. For example, among Hispanics in Florida (Wilkinson et al., 2001), primarily of Cuban and Central American origin, pediatric lymphatic leukemia and lymphoma appears 30% more frequently. While elevated frequencies of leukemia were not unexpected, no similar elevations in lymphoma had been appreciated in prior studies of Hispanic populations in Texas (Weiss et al., 1996) and California (Glazer et al., 1999), where Mexican ancestry predominates, but the frequency in Florida did match the incidence of pediatric lymphoma in Cuba.

Asians. CLL is thought to be rare in Japan and China. A review of all death certificates for Singapore from 1949 to 1958 identified just three cases of CLL but 250 cases of other types of leukemia among Chinese residents (Wells and Lau, 1960). In a review of 3925 autopsy cases of leukemia in Japan between 1958 and 1965, Nishiyama et al. (1969) found that the total leukemia mortality rate of 30.1 per million population per year was about half that in the United States. The difference was almost entirely due to a markedly decreased frequency of CLL, which was calculated to be 1/40 as common as in the United States, and confirms prior population-based surveys of a low CLL incidence in Japan in the 1950s (Hibino et al., 1958; Heyssel et al., 1960; Tomonaga, 1966). The study by Tomonaga was interpreted to suggest a role for genetic, and not environmental, factors because of an impression of continued low incidence of CLL in Japanese who have migrated to Hawaii (Finch and Linet, 1992), which is further substantiated by detailed investigations. An examination of death rates compiled by the United States National Office of Vital Statistics between 1949 and 1953 found a mortality rate for lymphatic forms of leukemia among Japanese and Chinese living in the United States to be 40% to 45% of that reported for the white population (Shimkin and Loveland, 1961). A study of Japanese immigrants to the United States determined that the percentages of leukemia deaths of persons over 55 attributable to lymphatic leukemia were 2.9% in Japan and 5.0% for Issei (first-generation) Japanese Americans but 31.5% for American whites (Haenszel et al., 1968). The authors attributed the difference between the first two figures to possible underdiagnosis of the disease in Japan (but did not seem to consider overrepresentation of other types of leukemia among Hiroshima and Nagasaki atomic bombing survivors as a factor that might depress the relative contribution of CLL—the only type of leukemia that was not high among nuclear blast survivors). A prior study of Issei in California found a reduced frequency of leukemia compared to the white population but did not separate leukemia types (Buell and Dunn, 1965). A study of CLL in Los Angeles County confirmed a markedly lower incidence of CLL among individuals of Chinese, Japanese, Filipino, and Korean ancestry; neither birthplace nor socioeconomic status accounted for this difference suggesting a role for genetic or other environmental factors in decreasing CLL risk (Gale et al., 2000). Similar low rates of CLL have also been reported in Korea (Lee et al., 1967).

A survey of international cancer registries revealed a low incidence of childhood AML among Indian children from Bombay and a high incidence among New Zealand Maoris (Linet and Devesa, 1991). CLL, however, was found to be rare among Maoris (Gunz, 1961).

American Samoans living in Hawaii were found to have an approximately 1.5- to 2-fold higher frequency of both leukemia and lymphoma than people of Hawaiian ancestry, but the rate was the same as for Samoans residing in Western Samoa (Mishra et al., 1996). The small risk elevation for hematopoietic malignancy in this study therefore seems more closely associated with ethnicity than with geographic environment.

Multiple myeloma in Shanghai, Singapore, and Osaka occurs at about half the frequency of whites in the United States (as reviewed in Bergsagel, 1995). A similar low frequency is observed among Chinese Americans in the San Francisco metropolitan area and Japanese Americans in Hawaii (Devesa, 1991), again mitigating potential environmental etiologies and substantiating a role for genetic factors.

African Americans. A lower frequency of leukemia among African Americans than white Americans has been appreciated for some time. Because there was a smaller difference in leukemia incidence in post–World War II Brooklyn than in less well racially integrated regions of the country, it was suggested that the differences could be accounted for by socioeconomic status, specifically underreporting of cases consequent to poorer access to medical care (MacMahon and Koller, 1957). More recent studies, however, continue to demonstrate similar differences in frequency; the incidence rate for ALL in all age groups was nearly 2-fold greater in white patients than in black patients in a National Cancer Institute (NCI) survey of 31,850 leukemia cases in the United States between 1973 and 1987 (Hernandez et al., 1995). Most of this appears to result from a reduced frequency of childhood ALL among African American populations in the United States (Linet and Devesa, 1991) , where the most significant differences in incidence occur between the ages of two and five years (Gurney et al., 1995). In a study of 4210 American children diagnosed with ALL between 1989 and 1991 in the Children's Cancer Group and Pediatric Oncology Group institutions, there was no significant correlation between socioeconomic status and incidence of childhood ALL (Swensen et al., 1997). More recent studies in Florida have confirmed a decreased frequency of pediatric lymphatic leukemia among African Americans, while also finding a marked reduction in frequency of pediatric lymphoma among this group, as well (Wilkinson et al., 2001).

While there is historically poorer survival of black children with ALL, no difference in survival rates using current treatment protocols was found at St. Jude Hospital in Memphis, a tertiary referral center (Pui et al., 1995). However, a small study of seven African American patients from a total of 75 patients who underwent allogeneic bone marrow transplantation for hematopoietic malignancy confirmed the authors' anecdotal impression that graft-vs.-host disease is more severe among African Americans (Easwa et al., 1996).

Several epidemiologic approaches indicate that there is an approximately 2-fold increase in the frequency of multiple myeloma among African Americans compared to whites in the United States (as reviewed in Bergsagel, 1995). Multiple myeloma is the most common hematopoietic malignancy among African Americans in the United States. Perhaps the largest study was an NCI survey of 12,237 reported myeloma cases in the Unites States between 1973 and 1986 (Hernandez et al., 1995); the incidence rate for both sexes in the black population was 7.6 to 7.8×10^{-5} and in the white population for both sexes was 3.3 to 3.4×10^{-5}. Efforts to identify environmental factors in a study of 889 patients with multiple myeloma in Dekalb and Fultan counties of Georgia, metropolitan Detroit, and New Jersey, excluded significant differences in cigarette and alcohol consumption between black and white myeloma patients (Brown et al., 1997).

The reported incidences likely reflect a true discrepancy in disease frequency between whites and blacks, as presumably the same socioeconomic conditions that might result in apparent mitigation of childhood ALL risk would not easily explain the excess incidence of myeloma.

Some older studies have suggested that polycythemia vera occurs disproportionately uncommonly among African Americans (Modan, 1965).

Family Epidemiology

Family Studies

One approach taken to determine if genetic factors account for malignancy risk is to determine whether there is an elevated frequency of disease among close relatives. Numerous such "proband studies" document a high risk for hematopoietic malignancy among family members of affected individuals. The conclusions of many of the older studies must be tempered against the fact that many clinical syndromes with familial disposition to leukemia and lymphoma (as discussed below under Associations with Other Diseases) had not yet been widely recognized.

Overall Hematopoietic Malignancy. A survey of 189 Israeli patients with all types of hematologic malignancy between 1987 and 1990 found a 3.62-fold increase in the disease among 4061 first- and second-degree relatives, compared to control populations from the same hospital (Shpilberg et al., 1994). Most of the neoplasms in the relatives were of different types than in the index case; the authors considered this as evidence of underlying inherited defects in the pluripotent hematopoietic stem cell.

Leukemia and Lymphoma. Obvious familial relationships in leukemia first became apparent with CLL. For example, in an unselected sample of 40 cases of CLL in Kansas City before 1959, there were two pairs of affected brothers (Hudson and Wilson, 1960). In 30 consecutive patients with CLL at the Johns Hopkins Hospital from 1976 to 1978, seven were found to have relatives with leukemia, four of which were CLL (Conley et al., 1980). A survey of 590 New Zealand and Australian leukemia patients questioned immediately after diagnosis between 1958 and 1961 found that 1.9% were aware of at least one first-degree relative with leukemia, compared to just 0.6% of controls (Gunz, 1963). Some 2.2% of leukemics reported at least one second-degree relative with leukemia, in contrast to 0.8% of controls. A follow-up study of what was thought to be all cases of CLL between 1962 and 1966 on the South Island of New Zealand (62 patients), found an incidence of CLL among first-degree relatives of 8.8% (Gunz and Veale, 1969); no control population was employed, but the reported CLL incidence in the studied community was 0.65%. There was no elevation in frequencies of other types of cancer among the relatives of leukemia patients.

From the pathological reporting of death on 909 patients with leukemia of all types in Sydney between 1968 and 1973 (Gunz et al., 1975), 41,807 relatives were identified and surveyed for leukemia. Some 72 patients were found to have one or more relatives with leukemia. The increase in the incidence of leukemia among first-degree relatives of a proband was found to be 2.8 to 3.0 and 2.5 to 2.8 among more distantly related individuals. Two families were found with three cases of leukemia, and one family had 10 affected individuals. The proband effect was the greatest for CLL.

A survey in eastern Nebraska between 1958 and 1966 identified 92 families whose probands had leukemia or lymphoma (Rigby et al., 1966). The occurrence of leukemia and lymphoma was 2.5 times more frequent in the family members of the identified families than in a control group. No differences were observed for environmental exposures between the leukemia and control families. One family apiece was found with three, four, five, and six affected individuals. Two of these multiplex families also had other individuals with cancer, but the two largest leukemia families demonstrated few cases of other malignancy.

A study of 20,000 cases of childhood malignancy occurring in England, Scotland, and Wales between 1953 and 1974 identified a total of 21 families with concordant sib pairs for leukemia and lymphoma (Draper et al., 1977). The authors determined relative risk for the siblings of children identified to have a particular malignancy: The relative risk for a sibling of a proband with leukemia was 2.3 for leukemia and 2.3 for lymphoma. The relative risk of a proband with lymphoma was 2.9 for leukemia and 5.4 for lymphoma. However, the relative risk for other types of cancer in a sib of a proband with leukemia or lymphoma was just 1.3 and 0.7, respectively, and, conversely, the relative risk for leukemia or lymphoma in a sib of a proband with another type of cancer was just 1.2 and 0.6, respectively. These data suggest that the risk factor for hematopoietic malignancy between siblings does not confer a risk for other types of malignancy.

A case-control study of all subtypes of AML occurring after age 15 years in Yorkshire, England, between 1979 and 1986 examined past medical history, occupational and other environmental factors, and family history (Cartwright et al., 1988a). A family history of leukemia or lymphoma was equivalent in risk effect to a prior personal history of malignancy, each conferring a 5.6-fold elevation in risk (95% CI, 1.6–24.5-fold). In this study, then, family history was of the same significance as apparent treatment-related disease. A similar study of 330 cases of CLL or related lymphomas in Yorkshire between 1979 and 1984 found a relative risk for a family history of lymphocytic forms of leukemia, myeloid leukemias, and non-Hodgkin's lymphoma of 4.3, 3.4, and 3.4, respectively, compared to a control group (Cartwright et al., 1987). Another case-control study of 130 Serbian CLL patients presenting before 1994 found an odds ratio of 5.50 for a family history of leukemia within first- through fourth-degree relatives when compared to a control population (Radovanovic et al., 1994). There was no significant increased risk for other types of cancer.

Perhaps the most comprehensive studies have been performed in Utah, where there is a state cancer registry that is linked to genealogical records maintained by the Church of Jesus Christ of Latter-day Saints ("Mormons") (Cannon-Albright et al., 1994; Goldgar et al., 1994). Detailed genealogical information is available for about one-third of all cancer patients. Among 125,000 cancer patients from 1952 to 1966, a relative risk for the same type of malignancy among first-degree relatives of probands with leukemia was 5.69 for lymphocytic types, and 2.97 for myeloid types. The relative risk for Hodgkin's and non-Hodgkin's lymphoma was just 1.27 and 1.68, respectively.

A survey of 183 patients with Hodgkin's lymphoma and 532 patients with non-Hodgkin's lymphoma in Haifa, Israel, between 1968 and 1980 identified first-degree relatives concordant for the same disease among four Hodgkin's patients and three non-Hodgkin's patients, compared to an expected number based on population incidence of 0.45 and 3.86 relative pairs, respectively (Haim et al., 1982). The authors concluded there was a relative risk of about 9 for Hodgkin's lymphoma among first-degree relatives of patients with Hodgkin's lymphoma, but no apparent increase in risk for non-Hodgkin's lymphoma. An incidence survey of Hodgkin's disease in greater Boston between 1959 and 1973 identified five affected sibling pairs, and the authors determined a relative risk of 7 for Hodgkin's disease in a sibling of an affected individual (Grufferman et al., 1977). Curiously, in this survey and in a review of the literature performed by the authors, most of the sibling cases concordant for Hodgkin's disease were also sex concordant. The authors weighed the significance of this finding and speculated that it supports relationships with environmental features that are more likely to be shared by sibs of the same sex, such as a bedroom (an alternative explanation, pseudoautosomal linkage, is offered below).

A case-control study of all cases of non-Hodgkin's lymphoma in Yorkshire, England, between 1979 and 1984 examined potential environmental and familial risk factors (Cartwright et al., 1988b). The three most significant risk factors identified among patients were being Jewish (5.1 relative risk), a history of infectious mononucleosis (5.0 relative risk), and a family history of leukemia or lymphoma (3.3 relative risk). A case-control study of 342 patients with CLL from metropolitan Baltimore diagnosed between 1969 and 1982 found a relative risk among first-degree relatives for all lymphoproliferative malignancy (Hodgkin's and non-Hodgkin's lymphoma and CLL) of 3.93 and for CLL of 6.57 (Linet et al., 1989). A total of 578 and 622 white males older than 30 years newly diagnosed with leukemia and lymphoma, respectively, from non-urban areas were identified in Iowa and Minnesota tumor registries (Pottern et al., 1991) to examine proband effects for lymphoproliferative malignancy. A parental history of lymphoproliferative malignancy was not associated with any type of leukemia or non-Hodgkin's lymphoma. However, having at least one sibling with lymphoproliferative malignancy was associated with a 2.3-fold relative risk for all types of leukemia and a 2.7-fold risk elevation for non-Hodgkin's lymphoma. A specific risk elevation for SLL or DSCL type non-Hodgkin's lymphoma of 7.3 and 5.4, respectively, was observed among subjects who had a sibling with lymphoma. The study also found a risk association between family history of solid tumors and non-Hodgkin's lymphoma, including pancreatic cancer, colorectal cancer, stomach cancer, and breast cancer.

In a small series of 29 CLL patients attended by a single hematologist in New York City (Cuttner, 1992), 10 (34%) had a first-degree relative with hematologic malignancy, which for three of the patients (10%) was also CLL. There was one pair of identical twins concordant for CLL in the study population. Seven of the ten patients with a family history of hematologic malignancy were Ashkenazi Jews. This study is also remarkable for the fact that two patients lacked a family history but had spouses with a lymphoid malignancy, although both spouses were also Ashkenazi Jewish, making it difficult to separate environmental, genetic, and—given the anecdotal nature of the study—coincidental factors. To identify potential biochemical correlates for familial CLL risk, a study examining the complement system identified abnormalities in the classic and alternative pathways among CLL patients and their healthy relatives (Schlesinger et al., 1996). A study of organophosphate and chlorinated hydrocarbon pesticide exposure in relation to non-Hodgkin's lymphoma found that exposure-related risks were greatest for those with a family history of hematopoietic cancer (Zahm et al., 1993).

An examination of the medical records of 193 patients with myelodysplasia referred to a single hospital in Wales between 1982 and 1988 found that there were five first-degree relative pairs among the register of patients (Lucas et al., 1989). The authors estimated a 15-fold risk elevation for myelodysplasia among first-degree relatives of myelodysplastic patients; these figures were conservative in that an additional three patients in whom a family history of myelodysplasia in a first-degree relative, including a member of a family with three myelodysplastic patients, were excluded, apparently, because they were not all treated at the same institution. A case-control study of 288 cases of hairy cell leukemia diagnosed in France between 1980 and 1990 found a relative odds ratio of leukemia occurring in a first-degree relative of 3.6 compared to controls (Clavel et al., 1997). Another proband study of patients with lymphoma found an elevated occurrence of gastric carcinoma among family members (Gencik et al., 1987).

Of 526 consecutive patients presenting with mycosis fungoides, 21 had first-degree relatives with hematopoietic malignancy, with other types of leukemia being the most frequently seen (Greene et al., 1982). One family was identified in this study in which one sib developed mycosis fungoides, another multiple myeloma, another Hodgkin's lymphoma, and still another non-Hodgkin's lymphoma (although other branches of the family had members with solid tumors)—a remarkable proof in principle that diverse types of hematopoietic malignancy could have a common genetic root.

Multiple Myeloma. A survey of the four northernmost counties represented in the Swedish cancer registry between 1982 and 1986 identified 239 myeloma patients (Eriksson and Hallberg, 1992). A relative risk for multiple myeloma among first-degree family members of 5.64 was reported. The relative risk for all types of hematologic malignancy was 2.36, and risk elevations were noted for solid tumors (1.21 relative risk), especially prostate cancer (3.11 relative risk) and brain tumors (6.61 relative risk). In the previously mentioned Utah registry, the relative risk for multiple myeloma among first-degree relatives of patients with the same diagnosis was 4.34 (Goldgar et al., 1994). A laboratory investigation of first-degree relatives of patients with Waldenstrom macroglobulinemia (Linet et al., 1993) identified frequent immunologic abnormalities, including some individuals with asymptomatic IgM monoclonal gammopathy. Initial, yet controversial, reports of a viral cause of multiple myeloma due to the Kaposi sarcoma–associated herpesvirus force a re-evaluation of the genetic significance of proband studies for multiple myeloma and possibly other types of hematopoietic malignancy. (See later under Environmental Factors.)

Myeloproliferative Disease. Among 652 cases registered in the International Polycythemia Vera Study Group (Brubaker et al., 1984), five patients were found to have parents who also had polycythemia vera, which is statistically greater than that expected from control populations. In a study population of 133 Italian patients with myeloproliferative syndromes from a single institution between 1978 and 1988, one pair of sisters (one with essential thrombocythemia and the other with polycythemia vera) were identified (Randi et al., 1988). The medical history of family members not treated for myeloproliferative disease during the 10-year window of time at that institution was not investigated. Although the authors interpreted this as evidence minimizing familial factors in this disease, it is perhaps all the more remarkable that a possible familial case would be detected within such a small study.

Consanguinity

Consanguinity often suggests the possibility of autosomal recessive inheritance. Consanguinity in the form of parents being second cousins was found in only one patient in a survey of 249 children with acute leukemia (Steinberg, 1960). However, in a North American Hutterite community, a significant excess of consanguinity was detected in the families of pediatric ALL patients (Martin et al., 1980). In a case-control study in Israel, a significant difference in parental consanguinity was noted among individuals with Hodgkin's disease (Abramson et al., 1978). Among 20 Japanese families with two or more cases of varying types of leukemia, consanguinity was present in 10 (50%), compared to a rate of consanguinity of just 4.5% among parents of 200 sporadic control patients with leukemia and what was interpreted as a much lower rate of consanguineous marriages in the general Japanese population (Kurita et al., 1974). Cases in which the parents were first cousins also had a younger age of onset, with the median being 6 years of age versus 27 years of age in the non-consanguineous families. A 30-fold higher than expected occurrence of pediatric ALL in a Brooklyn Syrian Jewish community was associated with consanguineous marital customs (Feldman et al., 1976). Pediatric ALL patients in the United Arab Emirates (Bener et al., 2001) were more likely to come from consanguineous families (80%) compared to the general population (where 50.5% of parents are consanguineous), although no adjustment was made to match marital customs to socioeconomic status, which, in turn, could influence reporting and environmental exposures, and which the authors had previously correlated (Bener et al., 1996).

Twin Studies

Given both the generally low frequency of leukemia and twinning, it was estimated that if the two were independent events, then a set of identical twins concordant for leukemia should appear approximately once every 150 (Anderson et al., 1955) to 200 years (Pearson et al., 1963) in the United States. There are now about 50 or so case reports, however, of monozygous twins concordant for leukemia, indicating that the risks for each individual of a twin pair are not independent events. The concordance rate for leukemia among identical twins is between 5% and 25% (Buckley et al., 1996; Miller, 1968), and declines with increasing age (Buckley et al., 1996), such that the concordance rate approaches 100% if one member of the identical twin pair develops leukemia before the age of one year (Degos, 1973) and is negligible after about age four years (Schmitt and Degos, 1978). In contrast, the concordance rate for dizygotic twins has been estimated at between 1 in 9 to 1 in 80 (Falleta et al., 1973). A possible nongenetic explanation for concordance in monozygotic twins was proposed in which the leukemic transformation happens in utero in one twin and metastasizes to the immunologically identical second fetus through the common placental circulation (Clarkson and Boyse, 1971). Strong support for this hypothesis is the finding of identical cytogenetic abnormalities and other clonal markers in concordant identical twins, including MLL rearrangements on 11q23 in four infant twin pairs with ALL (Ford et al., 1993; Gill Super et al., 1994); 15-month-old twins with ALL and a chromosome 1–derived marker chromosome (Chaganti et al., 1979), identical T-cell receptor rearrangements in a 9-year-old with non-Hodgkin's lymphoma and two years later in his twin with ALL (Ford et al., 1997); 17- and 36-month-old twin girls, both with acute undifferentiated leukemia and some blasts with trisomy 19 (Hartley and Sainsbury, 1981), 7-month-old conjoined twins separated at 42 days old, presenting simultaneously with L1 ALL with identical immunocytochemical markers and immunoglobulin heavy chain rearrangements (Pombo de Oliveira et al., 1986); and identical TEL-AML t(12p13;21q22) translocations and immunoglobulin heavy chain rearrangements in two twins with ALL diagnosed at age 3.5 and 5 years (Ford et al., 1997).

Another line of support for this interpretation comes from the observation of twins concordant for the development of ALL at ages 2 and 5 years (Wiemels et al., 1999).These twins also had in common TEL-AML translocations, the expression of the products of the resulting gene transfusion which could be detected using the reverse transcriptase-mediated polymerase chain reaction in routinely obtained neonatal blood spots, thus proving that the translocation was present at birth and had occurred in utero. Furthermore, in six of nine non-twin children with ALL manifesting this same translocation, the eldest of whom was 5 years, the fusion transcript was also detectable in neonatal blood spots, suggesting that prenatal origin of pediatric leukemia may be a common phenomenon.

There are a few reports of twin concordance that cannot all be explained by this phenomenon, however. Case reports of sets of monozygous twins concordant for Hodgkin's disease (such as Gracz et al., 1979) and non Hodgkin's lymphoma (such as Bjerrum et al., 1986) are known. In a larger twin study, 187 dizygotic and 179 monozygotic twin pairs where at least one member developed Hodgkin's disease were identified (Mack et al., 1995). None of the dizygotic twins were concordant for disease, but 10 of the monozygotic twins were concordant for disease. The majority of the twin pairs had NSHD. There was little evidence for the role of infection with Epstein-Barr virus.

Associations with Other Diseases

There are several Mendelian syndromes where an elevated risk for hematopoietic malignancy is a component feature.

DNA Repair Deficiency Syndromes

Bloom Syndrome. Bloom syndrome is an autosomal recessive illness characterized by growth retardation, characteristic facies, photosensitive telangiectatic erythema, café-au-lait skin pigmentation, and immunodeficiency with recurrent infections (German, 1997). It is most common in the Ashkenazi Jewish population. About one-fourth of patients will develop ALL, AML, lymphoma, or other malignancy. The cellular phenotype of Bloom syndrome is an increased frequency of sister chromatid exchanges, and this property was used to molecularly clone the responsible gene through a strategy selecting for spontaneous correction of the cellular deficiency (Ellis et al., 1995). The gene responsible is on chromosome 15q26.1 and encodes a putative DNA helicase, BLM, related to *E. coli* RecQ, yeast SGS1, and the gene causative of the human progeroid-like Werner syndrome. DNA damage resulting in double-strand breaks appears to induce BLM expression, where it assembles onto nuclear foci with other DNA repair enzymes (Bischof et al., 2001). While much attention has been focused on the possibility that heterozygous carriers of ataxia-telangiectasia may be predisposed to cancer (see immediately below), the possibility that Bloom syndrome carriers have high cancer frequency rates is a surprisingly neglected area of study. One wonders if this might not be one explanation for the high frequency of hematopoietic malignancy among Ashkenazim.

Ataxia-Telangiectasia. Ataxia-telangiectasia is autosomal recessive, and its clinical features include progressive cerebellar ataxia, telangiectatic skin lesions, and recurrent sinopulmonary infections as a result of the combined effects of neurologic depression and mild immunodeficiency (Taylor et al., 1996; Gatti 1998). Approximately 15% to 20% of patients develop malignancy, usually by 15 years of age, and most are of lymphoid origin, including Hodgkin's and non-Hodgkin's lymphoma and T-cell ALL (Morrell et al., 1986; Deiss, 1993; Stankovic et al., 1998). The responsible gene on chromosome 11q22–q23 codes for ATM, a phosphatidylinositol kinase homologous to yeast proteins that is involved in meiotic recombination and cell cycle control. The cellular defect is characterized by failure to heed the G1-S cell cycle transition checkpoint after DNA damage (Hartwell, 1992; Kastan and Lim, 2000), which presumably predisposes cells to accumulate somatic mutation without appropriate DNA repair. Spontaneous chromosome breaks are frequent, and sensitivity to chromosome breaks after exposure to bleomycin may offer clinically useful cytogenetic confirmation of the diagnosis. An autosomal dominant syndrome with similar clinical features to ataxia-telangiectasia has been reported in a Japanese family (Ishikawa et al., 2000).

While long suspected, it remains unclear as to whether heterozygous carriers of ATM are at elevated risk for cancer, particularly breast cancer (Gatti et al., 1999). However, some sporadic lymphatic leukemias and lymphomas display acquired ATM mutations (as reviewed in Boultwood, 2001). In particular, acquired ATM mutations are frequent in sporadic cases of T-cell prolymphocytic leukemia, B-cell CLL, and mantle cell lymphoma (Stilgenbauer et al., 1997; Vorechovsky et al., 1997; Stoppa-Lyonnet et al., 1998; Yuille et al., 1998), but not T-cell ALL (Luo et al., 1998). It has been asserted that some of the individuals who develop sporadic T-cell prolymphocytic leukemia are actually carriers of germline, heterozygous ATM mutations (Vanasse et al., 1999), but this is often difficult to verify, as there may not be non-tumor tissue (in this case, something other than blood) available from the patients. In a collection of 16 patients with this leukemia where constitutional genetic material for this leukemia was available, however, no germline ATM mutations could be identified (Stoppa-Lyonnet et al., 2000), suggesting that the ATM mutations were actually sporadic. Moreover, in a sample collection comprised largely only of tumor material, the ATM mutations tended not to occur on common ancestral haplotypes (Stankovic et al., 2001); the authors took this as support of a somatic origin of the mutations. However, it could be argued that a reduced fitness associated with potential leukemia-predisposing alleles might make founder effects, and hence common haplotypes, unlikely. Rare germline ATM mutations have also been considered as a cause of familial CLL (see below, in Familial CLL).

Nijmegen Breakage Syndrome and Berlin Breakage Syndrome. These are two autosomal recessive disorders that are clinically similar to ataxia-telangiectasia but that also include the presence of a characteristic birdlike facies with microcephaly (van der Burgt et al., 1996). Linkage evidence suggests the two syndromes to be the same. The gene responsible for Nijmegen syndrome, p95/NBS1, residing on chromosome 8q21 was cloned (Carney et al., 1998; Matsuura et al., 1998.) and appears to be a component of the MRE11/RAD50 double-strand break repair complex. This complex, in turn, is part of a large multisubunit protein complex that tracks to aberrant DNA structures and which is comprised of tumor suppressors, DNA damage sensors, and signal transducers; the complex also includes ATM; BLM; the hereditary nonpolyposis colorectal carcinoma mismatch DNA repair proteins MSH2, MSH6, and MLH1; the familial breast cancer protein BRCA1; and the RFC1-RFC2-RFC4 complex (Wang et al., 2000). An illness reported earlier with similar clinical features but an absence of chromosomal instability now appears to be one part of this syndrome, on the basis of cellular complementation studies (Jaspers et al., 1988).

Fanconi Anemia. Fanconi anemia is inherited in an autosomal recessive fashion and consists of pancytopenia with an assortment of congenital abnormalities that include short stature and skeletal dysplasia with hypoplastic thumbs, mental and sexual retardation, skin pigmentary changes, and renal malformations (Auerbach, 1995). A clinical test for Fanconi anemia involves the demonstration of chromosomal breaks after treatment with mitomycin C or diepoxybutane (Auerbach, 1993). Some 52% of Fanconi anemia patients develop myelodysplasia or AML by age 40 (Butturini et al., 1994). Fanconi anemia patients therefore have a 15,000-fold increase in relative risk for myelodysplasia and AML. The disease is genetically heterogeneous, and at least eight cellular complementation groups have been defined (Joenje et al., 1997). Mutations responsible for six complementation groups have been identified: C (Strathdee et al., 1992), encoding the *FANCC* gene on 9q22.3; A (Lo Ten Foe et al., 1996), encoding the gene *FANCA* on 16q24.3; E (de Winter et al., 2000a) encoding the gene *FANCE* on 6p22–p21; F (de Winter et al., 2000b) encoding the gene *FANCF* on 11p15; G (de Winter et al., 1998), encoding the gene *XRCC9/FANCG* on 9p13, which had previously been identified as defective in a Chinese hamster ovary cell-line-deficient DNA post-replication repair and cell cycle checkpoint control; and D2 (Timmers et al., 2001), encoding *FANCD2* on 3p25.3. Of all the identified genes, only *FANCD2* has a homolog among nonvertebrate model organisms (*Arabidopsis thaliana*, *Caenorhabditis elegans*, and *Drosophila Melanogaster*). It appears that all of the identified genes, except for *FANCD2*, encode proteins that assemble into a multiprotein nuclear complex required for the product of *FANCD2* to become monoubiquitylated, which then co-localizes with BRCA1 to subnuclear foci induced by DNA damage (Joenje and Patel, 2001). There is evidence that components of the nuclear complex are translocated from the cytoplasm.

There is evidence for modifier genes regulating the severity of Fanconi anemia. The most common FANCC allele is a splice mutation in intron 4 (IVS4 +4 A to T), which was first detected exclusively among Ashkenazi Jews, and is associated with a severe phenotype. The same mutation was recently detected in Japanese patients, where it appears by haplotype analysis to have arisen independently (Futaki et al., 2000). In the Japanese patients, however, this mutation is not associated with a severe phenotype.

Inherited Immunodeficiency Syndromes

Several heritable immunodeficiency syndromes are associated with a high frequency of hematopoietic malignancy (Table 40–5). In collectively considering the predisposition to hematopoietic malignancy with various inherited immunodeficiency syndromes, it is probable that hematopoietic malignancy results as a consequence of the immunodeficiency, rather than as a direct result of the genetic defect per se. For example, there is an increase in hematopoietic malignancy among acquired immunodeficiency syndromes, including AIDS, autoimmune disease, cancer treatment–associated immunodeficiency, and transplant-related immunosuppression (Mueller and Pizzo, 1995).

Hematopoietic Malignancy

Neurofibromatosis Type 1. Neurofibromatosis type 1 is a relatively common (1 in 3000) autosomal dominant genodermatosis characterized by café-au-lait skin lesions, intertriginous freckling, and neurofibromas. It results from mutations in the GAP family neurofibromin tumor suppressor gene on chromosome 17q11.2 that down-regulates the p21-ras proto-oncogene (Gutmann and Collins, 1995). Individuals with neurofibromatosis type 1 are at markedly increased risk for developing tumors of the central and peripheral nervous system, including gliomas, Schwannomas, and neurofibrosarcomas, and also skeletal muscle rhabdomyosarcomas. Hematopoietic malignancy is less frequent, but the risk for developing juvenile CML, usually in association with monosomy 7, is estimated at 221-fold; there is a 10-fold increase in risk for non-Hodgkin's lymphoma and a 5-fold increased risk for ALL (Stiller et al., 1994). Myelodysplasia, sometimes evolving to AML, occurs disproportionately among neurofibromatosis type 1 patients (Largaespada et al., 1996). There may be an association between the additional skin finding of xanthogranuloma and leukemia in neurofibromatosis (Zvulunov et al., 1995). Loss of heterozygosity of the neurofibromatosis type 1 locus occurs in patients with myeloid malignancy. There is evidence of sex-skewing and/or imprinting effects in that myeloproliferative disease occurs more commonly in boys with neurofibromatosis type 1 and is most often inherited maternally (Shannon et al., 1992; Stiller et al., 1994). Neurofibromatosis type 1 might also be associated with an increased risk of treatment-related AML after treatment with alkylating agents (Papageorgio et al., 1999); this finding was corroborated experimentally using a gene-targeted mouse model of neurofibromatosis (Mahgoub et al., 1999).

Li-Fraumeni Syndrome. Inherited germline mutation of the *p53* tumor suppressor/cell-cycle control gene on chromosome 17p13.1 causes the Li-Fraumeni syndrome of autosomal dominantly inherited predisposition to multiple types of malignancy, including sarcomas of muscle, bone, and soft tissue; brain tumors; melanoma; breast cancer; bronchogenic lung cancer; prostate cancer; and pancreatic carcinoma (Malkin, 1994). Leukemia and lymphoma occur in the Li-Fraumeni syndrome but are less common than sarcomas and other tumor types (Imamura et al., 1994). Lymphoma, however, is the most common malignancy in *p53* knockout mice (Donehower et al., 1992).

Germline mutations in *p53* have been excluded as the etiology of pure familial leukemia (Felix et al., 1992), pure familial lymphoma (Weintraub et al., 1996; Potzsch et al., 1999), or pure familial multiple myeloma (Willems et al., 1993).

A few rare families with the Li-Fraumeni syndrome are negative for germline mutations in p53 and have been found to have

Table 40–5. Immunodeficiency Disorders Predisposing to Hematopoietic Malignancy

Syndrome	Malignancy	Inheritance	Locus	Gene
Wiskott-Aldrich	B-cell lymphoma, ALL, AML, (Sullivan et al., 1994; Filipovich et al., 1987)	X-linked recessive	Xp11.22–p11.23	*WAS* (Derry et al., 1994)
Bruton's agammaglobulinemia	Lymphoreticular (Groopman and Broder, 1989; Frizzera et al., 1980)	X-linked recessive	Xq21.3–q22	Bruton tyrosine kinase (Vetrie et al., 1993)
X-linked lymphoproliferative syndrome (Duncan disease)	Non-Hodgkin's lymphoma (Grierson et al., 1993)	X-linked recessive	Xq25–q26	*SH2D1A* (Coffey et al., 1998)

mutations in the *hCHK2* gene (Bell et al., 1999), encoding the human homolog of the yeast Cds1 and Rad53 G2 checkpoint kinases, which, when activated by DNA damage, blocks entry into mitosis.

Congenital Cytopenias

Severe Congenital Neutropenia. Severe congenital neutropenia (SCN) also known as Kostmann syndrome or infantile agranulocytosis, is a genetically heterogeneous disorder comprised of constitutional neutropenia and promyelocytic arrest and dysgranulopoiesis in the bone marrow. About 10% of affected individuals develop myelodysplasia or AML (Freedman et al., 2000), often with acquired cytogenetic abnormalities, including monosomy 7 and trisomy 21. It was first described by Kostmann, occurring among consanguineous northern Swedes, where it appears to be transmitted through autosomal recessive inheritance. While it was once thought that mutations in the gene encoding the G-CSF receptor were the cause of some cases of SCN (Dong et al., 1995), it is now appreciated that these are acquired events of the bone marrow, sometimes accompanying neoplastic evolution (for example, Bernard et al., 1998). The majority of sporadic and multigenerational cases of SCN result from heterozygous, germline mutations in *ELA2* on 19pter (Dale et al., 2000), encoding neutrophil elastase, the target of α_1-antitrypsin and a serine protease of neutrophil and monocyte granules. Owing to its attendant lethality, the disease often occurs sporadically as a result of new germline mutations. Different mutations of *ELA2* cause cyclic neutropenia (Horwitz et al., 1999), which is an unusual disorder characterized by a 21-day cycle of nearly sinusoidal oscillations of the peripheral neutrophil count, but in which only rare cases of leukemia have been recognized. A rare X-linked form of SCN arising from mutations in WASP, allelic to the the Wiskott-Aldrich syndrome, has also been reported (Devriendt et al., 2001).

Blackfan-Diamond Anemia. The Blackfan-Diamond syndrome comprises congenital hypoplastic macrocytic anemia with growth retardation and congenital anomalies, particularly of the head and upper limbs (Halperin and Freedman, 1989). There is a high risk for AML. Both autosomal dominant and autosomal recessive inheritance have been reported. A patient with Blackfan-Diamond anemia and a X;19 translocation led to the identification of the causative gene, *RPS19* on 19q13, encoding a ribosomal protein (Draptchinskaia et al., 1999). Not all cases appear to result from mutations of *RPS19*, and other potential loci have been suggested in genomewide screens for linkage (Gazda et al., 2001).

Other Inherited Disorders Predisposing to Leukemia

Some miscellaneous inherited syndromes associated with hematopoietic malignancy are listed in Table 40–6.

Environmental Factors

Blood Transfusion

Several attempts have been made to purposefully transmit leukemia or lymphoma from an affected patient to recipients through blood transfusion, bone marrow transplant, and cross-circulation. Fortunately, none of these disturbing experiments ever succeeded. (The subjects of these experiments ranged from those with "hopelessly incurable neoplastic diseases" [Bierman et al., 1951] to "clinically well" cancer patients and syphilitics [Thiersch, 1946], one of whom had previously had his tongue resected for squamous cell carcinoma and therefore it could be imagined might have had difficulty articulating unwillingness to participate.) Follow-up studies have also been performed among individuals who accidentally received transfusion of blood from donors who were later found to have had leukemia or lymphoma (Greenwald et al., 1976); 34 transfusion recipients were identified, and no evidence of malignant transmission was observed. One conclusion of these weird studies is that viruses and other potential bloodborne factors are rare causes of leukemia.

Viruses

Numerous epidemiologic and association studies have sought evidence for viral etiologies for hematopoietic malignancy. This topic is beyond the scope of this chapter but is selectively reviewed here. In certain regions of the world, viral etiologies are significant and account for some familial clusterings of disease. Retroviruses do appear to be a significant cause of leukemia in non-human animals, however.

Human T-Cell Leukemia Virus I (HTLV-1) and Adult T-Cell Leukemia and Lymphoma. Chronic HTLV-1 infection causes a form of adult T-cell leukemia and lymphoma. There are several reported occurrences of familial adult T-cell leukemia and lymphoma caused by HTLV-1 infection, most often in areas of endemicity for the virus (southwest Japan, the Caribbean basin, and parts of Central Africa, where the virus is also the cause of the neurodegenerative disorder "tropical spastic paraparesis"). The disease has been documented in siblings who were presumably infected by the vertical transmission through an HTLV-1 positive mother (Matutes et al., 1995). Vertical transmission is thought to occur primarily through breast feeding (Fujino and Nagata, 2000), although it also may be spread by intrauterine

Table 40–6. Other Inherited Disorders Predisposing to Hematopoietic Malignancy

Syndrome	Malignancy	Inheritance	Locus
Shwachman syndrome	Myelodysplasia and AML (Woods et al., 1981; Passmore et al., 1995)	Autosomal recessive	Unknown
Pearson mitochondrial syndrome	Myelodysplastic-like changes (Casademont et al., 1994)	Mitochondrial	Mitochondrial deletions
Dubowitz syndrome	Myelodysplasia, ALL, Lymphoma (Bader-Meunier et al., 1996b)	Autosomal recessive	Unknown

transmission and saliva. Segregation analysis, performed in a large-scale genetic epidemiology investigation of familial aggregation of HTLV-1 infection in French Guiana, detected a major gene predisposing to infection (Plancoulaine et al., 2000). Under this genetic model, it was predicted that 1.5% of this population would be predisposed to HTLV-1 infection, and almost all seropositive children under the age of 10 years are likely to represent genetic cases, whereas most HTLV-1 seropositive adults likely represent sporadic cases.

Human T-Cell Leukemia Virus II (HTLV-II) and T-Cell Hairy Leukemia. There has been a single report of a patient with a rare T-cell variant of hairy cell leukemia (the disease almost always being of the B cell variety) in whom a novel retrovirus virus, HTLV-II, was isolated (Kalyanaraman, 1982), but this report apparently has not been confirmed in other patients (Saven et al., 1995). HTLV-II has also been isolated in a patient with LGL leukemia (Loughran et al., 1992).

Epstein-Barr Virus and Burkitt's Lymphoma. Endemic to equatorial Africa is a unique B cell lymphoma, typically of the jaw, first reported by Burkitt in 1958 (reviewed in Okano, 1998, and Takada, 2001). This tumor is nearly always positive for the Epstein-Barr herpesvirus genome. Sporadic forms of the disease occurring elsewhere in the world are less frequently positive for the viral genome, being present in only about 20% to 50% of cases. Malaria is considered a cofactor for the endemic form of the disease. Burkitt's lymphoma is histologically characterized by diffuse and closely packed undifferentiated cells that lack a morphologic appearance typical of either lymphocytes or histiocytes. Interspersed are large phagocytes with abundant cytoplasm, which mark the appearance of small cleared spaces that lend a "starry sky" pattern to the tumor. Burkitt's lymphoma has characteristic chromosomal abnormalities involving translocation of *c*-myc on chromosome 8 to immunoglobulin loci on chromosome 8, 14, or 22. Epstein-Barr virus–associated lymphoproliferative disorders also occur with immunodeficiency syndromes, including AIDS, ataxia-telangiectasia, and the Wiskott-Aldrich syndrome, or they occur in patients receiving immunosuppression after organ transplantation.

Epstein-Barr Virus and Hodgkin's Disease. Epidemiological studies have suggested links between Hodgkin's disease and Epstein-Barr virus (as reviewed in Klitz et al., 1994, and Dolcetti et al., 2000); EBV DNA is directly detected in tumor DNA from up to 50% of Hodgkin's disease cases. As with Burkitt's lymphoma, however, the overwhelming majority of individuals infected with this virus do not develop hematological malignancy and so other infectious co-factors or genetic predispostions are likely to be involved.

HIV and Lymphoma. Both non-Hodgkin's and Hodgkin's lymphoma may be features of AIDS (reviewed in Diebold et al., 1997, and Spina et al., 2001). A Burkitt-type lymphoma can result early in the course of evolution of HIV infection, with the majority of cases demonstrating myc rearrangements and latent Epstein-Barr virus being detectable in about 30% to 45%. Other non-Hodgkin's lymphomas, typically DLCL subtypes, occur later in AIDS when CD4 counts have become critically low. In these cases myc rearrangements are present in about 30% to 40% of cases, and about 70% are positive for Epstein-Barr virus. Hodgkin's disease can occur at any stage in HIV infection.

Kaposi's Sarcoma-Associated Herpesvirus and Multiple Myeloma. Recently, it has been claimed that the Kaposi's sarcoma–associated herpesvirus (human herpesvirus 8) can be amplified by PCR from dendritic bone marrow stromal cells in the majority of patients with multiple myeloma and among many patients with monoclonal gammopathy of undetermined significance (MGUS) (Rettig et al., 1997a). These results were initially largely unconfirmed by other investigators, however. It was further noted that there has not been serological evidence for infection with this virus among most patients with plasma cell neoplasms, nor does there appear to be an increased incidence of plasma cell neoplasia in the Mediterranean areas in which Kaposi's sarcoma and infection with this herpesvirus is endemic. (See Rettig et al., 1997b), and the associated letters to which this reference is responding.) More recently, it has been appreciated that human herpesvirus 8 DNA sequences are common in the bone marrow of healthy individuals at frequencies not markedly different from those with lymphoproliferative disorders (Azzi et al., 2001). A prospective study of healthy human herpesvirus 8–infected individuals identified among 39,000 Finnish subjects who donated serum samples from 1968 to 1972 failed to find an association with subsequent development of multiple myeloma (Tedeschi et al., 2001). The role of this virus in the development of plasma cell neoplasia therefore is difficult to substantiate at this time.

Common Variants in Enzymes of Intermediate Metabolism

An extensive number of studies have sought to associate common polymorphic variants of enzymes involved in intermediate metabolism with risk for hematopoietic malignancy (reviwed in Perentesis, 2001). Potential roles in the etiology of primary or treatment-related leukemias have been examined for glutathione *S*-transferases, NAD(P)H reductases, myeloperoxidase, *N*-acetyltransferase, P450 cytochromes, methylenetetrahydrofolate reductase (MTHFR), and cystathionine β-syntase. Notable findings include MTHFR variants associated with infant ALL or AML with MLL rearrangements and childhood ALL associated with either TEL-AML1 fusions or hyperdiploidy (Wiemels et al., 2001); low NAD(P)H:quinine oxidoreductase 1 activity at higher frequency among adult AML and ALL cases (Smith et al., 2001); and NAT2 slow acetylator, CYP1A1*2A and GSTM1 null genotypes in excess in childhood ALL (Sinnett et al., 2000). Conceivably, common variants in the enzymes could allow for individual variation in susceptibility to environmental exposures. One of the difficulties with this hypothesis, however, is that potential environmental carcinogens remain largely unidentified (see Horwitz, 2001, for review).

PATHOPHYSIOLOGY: BIOLOGIC BASIS OF GENETIC SUSCEPTIBILITY

Genetic Studies of Pathophysiology

A remarkably successful approach to the identification of genes that are causative of malignancy is to study those relatively uncommon families that demonstrate single-gene inheritance to cancer predisposition. A number of families transmit hematopoietic malignancy in a Mendelian fashion and are not associated with any other recognizable syndrome. To differentiate true familial occurrence from chance clustering of sporadic cases, the discussion here is confined to reports of three or more cases within a family, except as noted. Families where there are multiple occurrences of non-hematologic malignancy have also been excluded, since these may represent Li-Fraumeni syndrome.

Estimates of the Proportion of Cases That Are Familial

Although familial hematopoietic malignancy would appear to be exceptionally rare, there is reason to suppose it is not so uncommon.

First, the proband studies find a risk in first-degree relatives equivalent to that for breast and colorectal cancer, in which a large proportion of cases have been substantiated to result from Mendelian inheritance. For example, in the Utah cancer registry (Goldgar et al., 1994), the relative risk in first-degree relatives of patients with breast and colorectal carcinoma was 1.83 and 2.67, respectively. It is now estimated that perhaps as much as 10% of breast cancer (chapter 35, by Weber and Nathanson, in this volume) and 20% of colorectal cancer (chapter 34, by Burt, in this volume) have a Mendelian basis. Recall that the same survey found a first-degree relative risk for lymphocytic leukemia of 5.69. While the absolute risk for leukemia among family members is still small due to the relative overall rarity of the disease, the proband studies suggest that the proportion of Mendelian cases is as large, or larger, than that for breast and colorectal carcinoma.

Second, most large surveys have found a surprisingly high proportion of familial cases (two or more cases among close relatives). An early survey of 209 Danish leukemia patients found a family history in 8.1% of cases (Videbaek, 1947a, 1947b). All families of probands with leukemia and lymphoma occurring in central Nebraska between 1958 and 1963 were identified; 39 families of a total of 151 (25.8%) had familial disease (Rigby et al., 1968). Three separate surveys led by Gunz in Australia and New Zealand concluding in 1975 and incorporating a total of 1553 families in which a proband with leukemia was identified, found 69 families with two cases and three families with three or more cases occurring among first-degree relatives (as summarized in Gunz et al., 1975). An estimate by Gausch in 1954 (based on a review of literature reports of leukemia and his personal experiences with leukemia in Barcelona) showed a 4.5% incidence of familial cases. A family survey of 942 patients representing all cases of hematopoietic malignancy in Jamtland County, Sweden, from 1963 to 1984 uncovered a family history of hematopoietic malignancy in first- through third-degree relatives in 36 families (Eriksson and Bergstrom, 1987), such that the authors reported 5% of all cases of hematopoietic malignancy occurring in a family where one close relative was also affected. Cases of myelodysplasia with monosomy of chromosome 7 occurring in siblings were reviewed; a family history of this illness was detected in 7 of 27 patients, and it was concluded that one-third of childhood myelodysplasia with monosomy 7 is familial (Carroll et al., 1985). In a survey of 37 younger French adults with myelodysplasia, 5 had affected relatives, leading the authors to conclude that about one-third of all myelodysplasia in this age group is familial (Fenaux, 1993). A similar high frequency of genetic syndromes or potentially inherited disease was found in two surveys of 44 and 49 French children with myelodysplasia (Bader-Meunier et al., 1996b). A review of 68 children with myelodysplasia evaluated at the Hospital for Sick Children in Toronto between 1971 and 1991 found that 6% also had relatives with myelodysplasia and 19 (28%) of the patients had potentially heritable syndromes accompanying myelodysplasia (Passmore et al., 1995). A contrasting population-based survey of Danish children between 1980 and 1991 suggested that the proportion of familial forms of myelodysplasia is only 2% or less (Hasle et al., 1995; Hasle and Olsen, 1997). Note, however, that such a survey ignores patients who, although lacking a family history, might have clinical findings consistent with an inherited or de novo syndrome. In a meta-analysis of reports of familial Hodgkin's disease, it was estimated that 4.5% of all cases of Hodgkin's disease have a single-gene Mendelian basis (Ferraris et al., 1997). For ALL and non-Hodgkin's lymphoma, outside of case reports of rare families, there has been no evidence, however, of single-gene Mendelian transmission; no increased incidence of malignancy was found in the offspring of 382 surviving patients (Hawkins et al., 1995).

Third, it is possible that there are common yet low-penetrance alleles analogous to that been postulated for other common cancers.

Autosomal Recessive Childhood Myelodysplasia with Monosomy 7

There are at least 14 pedigrees in which multiple siblings have developed myelodysplasia, sometimes progressing to AML (Brandwein et al., 1990; Daghistani et al., 1990; Luna-Fineman et al., 1995; Horwitz, 1997). The invariant features of these families are bone marrow monosomy 7 and pediatric onset of illness. The consistent absence in other generations and a nearly equal sex ratio suggests autosomal recessive inheritance (although, there are also scattered reports of childhood monosomy 7 where a parent becomes myelodysplastic or develops AML (Luna-Fineman et al., 1995), which could be consistent with autosomal dominant transmission). There is evidence to suggest that the predisposing gene is not located on chromosome 7, however (Shannon et al., 1989); no common overlapping segment was definable among three pairs of affected sibs from different families, in contrast to the expectation that there would be a commonly deleted region if this followed a tumor suppressor gene/loss of heterozygosity model. In one sibship with two affected brothers, both were found to have constitutional inversion of chromosome 1p22–q23, possibly suggesting a locus at either breakpoint as causative (Paul et al., 1987).

Autosomal Dominant Myelodysplasia and AML

The multigenerational transmission of myelodysplasia, myelodysplasia progressing to AML, and AML without antecedent myelodysplasia have all been reported (as summarized in Horwitz, 1997). These families have a general absence of other disease and no impressive tendency toward other malignancy, and individuals are generally healthy without any premorbid phenotype until they become myelodysplastic. There appears to be just one family inheriting exclusively myelodysplasia; at least four families in which individuals inherited AML or myelodysplasia with or without progression to AML; and at least 16 families in which individuals developed nearly exclusively AML, without significant prior myelodysplasia. In one of the multigenerational families, most of the affecteds were demonstrated to have somatic monosomy for chromosome 5q (Olopade et al., 1996); a pair of adult sisters who both developed myelodysplasia also apparently had somatic monosomy 5q (Grimwade et al., 1993).

There are other reports of myelodysplasia and AML in which the affecteds are confined to a single generation. In this case, the inheritance is likely to be autosomal recessive, but in contrast to the childhood monosomy 7 syndrome, this cytogenetic abnormality is not seen and the onset can be in the adult years. It is also possible that these cases represent autosomal dominant inheritance with incomplete penetrance in the previous generations. A consanguineous family in which the parents were first cousins produced three children who had a similar syndrome of facial dysmorphism, birth defects, and myelodysplasia. Neither had monosomy 7. One of the children developed M2 AML at age 14 (Stoll et al., 1994). At least three adult sibships are known with multiple occurrences of myelodysplasia (Kaur et al., 1972; Palmer et al., 1987). In the first family, a 29-year-old sister and 26-year-old brother developed myelodysplasia six months apart and had complicated bone marrow cytogenetics without monosomy 7. In common, they both had a somatic chromosome 1 duplication (1q21–1q42). Two other large sibships with multiple children developing acute leukemia have been mentioned, but the absence of clinical details make further categorization impossible (Steinberg, 1957).

Another family (Kaur et al., 1972) has been described in which two sibs developed AML, one had myelofibrosis, and all three and an additional two individuals demonstrated a Pelger-Huet cellular anomaly with hypolobated (bisegmented) granulocytes. The two with AML had trisomy for a chromosome of group C (chromosomes 6–12). Although the affecteds were all confined to one generation, low levels of IgA were documented in individuals from three generations in this family.

Autosomal Dominant Familial Platelet Disorder and AML

In contrast to the above situation in which there is no premorbid phenotype, there are several multigenerational AML families with a constitutional platelet phenotype characterized by thrombocytopenia, platelet granule defect, and bleeding tendency (Weiss et al., 1969; Dowton et al., 1985; Gerrard et al., 1991; Ho et al., 1996). This disorder has been termed "autosomal dominant familial platelet disorder with predisposition to acute myelogenous leukemia." Other hematopoietic malignancies found in these families include lymphoid leukemia, lymphoma, and sarcoma. A genome-wide screen for linkage followed by a positional cloning strategy identified mutations in *AML1/CBFA/RUNX1* (Song et al., 1999), a gene that is among the most frequent sites of acquired chromosomal translocation in sporadic cases of luekmia. There is evidence that the molecular pathogenesis of this disorder proceeds through both haploinsufficiency (Song et al., 1999) and dominant negative action (Michaud et al., in press). Heterozygous mutations of *AML1* have also been detected at a high frequency among sporadic Japanese patients with AML and ALL (Osato et al., 1999). It was unclear from this study whether the mutations were somatic events or constitutional, thus leaving open the possibility that these could represent common, low-penetrance alleles for a gene that confers leukemia risk. Arguing against this possibility is a corroborating study that detected a similarly high frequency of heterozygous and biallelic point mutations in *AML1*, and where material was available following induction to complete remission, suggested that the mutations were acquired (Preudhomme et al., 2000).

Autosomal Dominant Erythroleukemia

In familial AML, the subtypes tend to vary among individuals within the family, but there are two exceptions. For erythroleukemia (M6 AML), there seems to be consistency of subtype among all affected family members in the five families that have been reported (Lee et al., 1987; Horwitz, 1997), with apparent multigenerational transmission of erythroleukemia or its myelodysplastic precursor ("erythremic myelosis," also known as "DiGuglielmo syndrome").

Autosomal Dominant Monocytic Leukemia

The second exception to variance of AML subtypes within a single AML family is monocytic leukemia (M5 AML). Only two families (one being sibs within a single generation and the other a multigenerational family) are reported with all affected individuals having just this subtype (Horwitz, 1997).

Familial CLL

At least 17 families with the multigenerational transmission of CLL are known (Bartal et al., 1978; Blattner et al., 1979; Cohen et al., 1979; Conley et al., 1980; LeDeist et al., 1991; Horwitz, 1997). Also included are families with just two cases of CLL confined to a parent–child pair (Horwitz, 1997; Horwitz et al., 1996), since the later age of onset of this disease may result in poorer ascertainment of such families. One of these families had a mixture of CLL, hairy cell leukemia, and lymphoma (Cohen et al., 1979). Nine families are known with multiple occurrences (three or more) within a sibship (Gunz et al., 1966; Fitzgerald et al., 1969; Potolsky et al., 1971; Schweitzer et al., 1973; LeDeist et al., 1991; Hakim et al., 1995; Horwitz, 1997). In two of these families, the type of CLL is LGL (LeDeist et al., 1991; Loughran et al., 1994).

A survey of the family history of 268 CLL patients, along with a qualitative review of the published familial cases, suggested the existence of an autosomal dominantly acting gene with pleiotrophic effects that may also predispose to other lymphoproliferative disorders (Yuille et al., 2000).

There have been two reports of a high frequency of ataxia-telangiectasia carriers among sporadic cases of B-cell CLL (Bullrich et al., 1999; Stankovic et al., 1999). It is possible, then, that at least some cases of sporadic CLL occur among individuals who carry common, but incompletely penetrant, genes (in this case, ATM heterozygotse) conferring CLL risk. However, one of the frequent alleles of ATM, C3161G, reported by Stankovic et al., also appears at somewhat similar frequencies in a control population (Vorechovsky et al., 1999), making it difficult to draw a conclusion about the association of risk for CLL among carriers for ataxia-telangiectasia. Furthermore, analysis in a collection of 24 families with CLL failed to establish genetic linkage to chromosome 11q, the region containing ATM (Bevan et al., 1999).

Familial ALL

At least eight families with the multigenerational transmission of ALL are known (Ferguson and Lynn, 1970; Kato et al., 1983; Horwitz, 1997). Eight families have multiple affected individuals within a sibship (Bertolani and Massolo, 1975; Pendergrass et al., 1975; Blattner et al., 1978; Schmitt and Degos, 1978; Kende et al., 1994; Horwitz, 1997). In two of the latter families (Johnson and Peters, 1957; Kende et al., 1994) and a third family confined to just two affected sibs (Kende et al., 1994), there is consanguinity. There is thus good evidence for both autosomal dominant and autosomal recessive forms of familial ALL. It should be noted, however, that a study of 382 offspring of survivors of childhood leukemia (usually ALL) and non-Hodgkin's lymphoma found no increased risk of malignancy (Hawkins et al., 1995), suggesting that such families are quite rare.

Familial Hairy Cell Leukemia

Hairy cell leukemia is a chronic lymphoproliferative disorder of B cells. At least four pedigrees are described with the multigenerational transmission of hairy cell leukemia (Ramseur et al., 1980; Begley et al., 1987; Gramatovici et al., 1993; Clavel et al., 1997). At least another four pedigrees occur in which there are multiple affected sibs (Cohen et al., 1979; Wylin et al., 1982; Milligan et al., 1987; Ward et al., 1990). Because of the rarity of hairy cell leukemia, reports of at least two occurrences within a family are probably significant, and some of these families have three occurrences (Cohen et al., 1979; Wylin et al., 1982; Gramatovici et al., 1993). A possible linkage or association with HLA has been investigated. In two different sibships of two (Ward et al., 1990) and three affecteds (Wylin et al., 1982), each patient within a family was HLA identical, but in the latter family one unaffected sibling also had the identical HLA haplotype. A father–son pair was also found to have identical HLA haplotypes (Ramseur et al., 1980). In another family with three individuals with lymphoproliferative disease, two brothers with CLL and hairy cell leukemia had identical HLA haplotypes, but a nephew with lymphoma did not (Cohen et al., 1979). In a family with three separate cases, there was sharing of the HLA B locus (Gramatovici et al., 1993). A viral etiology for hairy cell leukemia has been suspected (as noted above under General Genetic and Epidemiologic Evidence), but it has not been confirmed and remains uninvestigated in familial cases.

Autosomal Dominant Inheritance of Multiple Leukemia Types

There are at least 25 families with the multigenerational inheritance of multiple or unspecified types of leukemia (Weiner, 1965; Horwitz, 1997). In some of the families there is co-segregation of acute and chronic myeloid leukemia, while in other families there are mixtures of myeloid and lymphoid varieties.

Familial Myeloproliferative Syndromes

Families demonstrating genetic transmission of fairly consistent subcategories of myeloproliferative disease and families in which affected individuals develop differing subtypes of myeloproliferative disease have both been reported. Because of the rarity of myeloproliferative syndromes, some families are reviewed here that are as small as two affected members. Several pedigrees with mixtures of the myeloproliferative syndromes are known (Tatti et al., 1984; Bondare et al., 1985; Tosato et al., 1985; Perez-Encinas et al., 1994). In one family, three affected siblings were found to be identical for HLA and ABO and Rh blood groups, as were two unaffected siblings (Tatti et al., 1984). Although the categorization of relatively diverse diseases under the umbrella term "myeloproliferative syndrome" may seem somewhat arbitrary, such families would apparently confirm these entities to have a common pathogenic origin.

Polycythemia Vera

Evidence of familial polycythemia is complicated by the fact that many early reports of familial polycythemia were actually a secondary polycythemia that resulted as the consequence of a subsequently proven hemoglobinopathy (Adamson, 1975; Modan, 1965) or other disorder. Another form of apparently "benign" familial polycythemia is genetically linked to the erythropoietin receptor (de la Chapelle et al., 1993). In fact, because so many of the early reports of polycythemia vera occurred in a familial setting, it was once concluded that polycythemia vera was always an inherited disease (Owen, 1924). While this is obviously not true, there are several reports of what would appear to be the familial occurrence (both within and between generations) of genuine polycythemia vera in association with clinical or laboratory evidence of a true increase in red cell mass with a bone marrow hyperproliferative state (reviewed by Kralovics and Prchal et al., 2000, and see Nichamin, 1908; Doll, 1922; Nadler and Cohn, 1939; Efr, 1956; Manoharan et al., 1976; Kaufman et al., 1978; Ratnoff and Gress, 1980; Waddell et al., 1982; Miller et al., 1989; Gilbert, 1995), including between identical twins (Burnside et al., 1981; Fairrie et al., 1981; Friedland et al., 1981) and in association with leukemia (Lawrence and Goetsch, 1950; Longpre, 1966) or genetic deafness syndromes (Muftuoglu et al., 1975; Fairrie et al., 1981). Additional family cases have been critically evaluated with respect to their validity (Modan, 1965).

Myelofibrosis

There are scattered reports of small families, including sibling and parent–child pairs, with myelofibrosis (Decastello, 1954; Bernard et al., 1967; Patakfalvi et al., 1969; Kaufman et al., 1978; Sieff and Malleson, 1980; Gilbert, 1995).

Essential Thrombocythemia

Familial thrombocytosis, appearing to be an autosomal dominant disease with multigenerational transmission, has been reported many times (Bernard et al., 1967; Fickers and Speck, 1974; Dodsworth, 1980; Eyster et al., 1986; Randi et al., 1987; Fernandez-Robles et al., 1990; Janssen et al., 1990; Yagisawa et al., 1990; Williams and Shahidi, 1991; Schlemper et al., 1994; Gilbert, 1995; Kikuchi et al., 1995). It has only been rarely associated with malignant transformation; in one family (Slee et al., 1981) one individual developed AML and another myelofibrosis with monosomy 7 and ring chromosome 7 formation, respectively. The authors attributed the chromosomal abnormalities as a possible consequence of treatment with alkylating agents and ^{32}P, however.

In the late 1990s it was determined that splice site mutations in the gene encoding the cytokine thrombopoietin, which regulates megakaryocyte maturation, on chromosome 3q26.3–q27 are responsible for hereditary thrombocythemia in a four-generation Dutch kindred (Weistner et al., 1998). A few individuals with nonhereditary leukemia complicated by thrombocytosis were found to have acquired chromosomal abnormalities in this region of the long arm of chromosome 3 (for example, Bernstein et al., 1982; Carroll et al., 1986).

Familial CML

There are at least three reports of the multigenerational transmission of CML (Horwitz, 1997) and four pedigrees with multiple cases of CML within a sibship (Holton and Johnson, 1968; Tokuhata et al., 1968; Lardi et al., 1994). Another family has had multiple sibships related as cousins who manifest with a childhood myeloproliferative disease nearly identical to CML (Randall et al., 1965). In the latter family, the disease was lethal in some of the affected children, but apparently spontaneously remitted in others. Acquired chromosomal aneuploidy was observed.

Hodgkin's Disease

Numerous familial clusters of Hodgkin's disease (in the general absence of other cancer or non-Hodgkin's lymphoma predisposition) have been reported, both within a sibship and across generations (DeVore et al., 1957; Manigand et al., 1964; Kajii et al.,

1968; Creagan et al., 1972; Halazun et al., 1972; Maldonado et al., 1972; Thorling, 1973; Hanganu, 1976; Robertson et al., 1987; Cimino et al., 1988; Durosinmi et al., 1989). In a review of familial cases (Fraumeni, 1974) it was pointed out that onset of illness tends to occur at a younger mean age than it does with sporadic disease. Subclinical immune deficiencies have been reported in unaffected individuals from Hodgkin's disease families (Salimonu et al., 1980; Cimino et al., 1988), as well as relatives of sporadic patients (Merk et al., 1990). One unique family had a 16-year-old girl who developed Hodgkin's disease at age 20 years but was also noted to have the Gorlin syndrome of multiple nevoid basal cell carcinoma, as did her mother (Potaznik and Steinherz, 1984). The patient's maternal grandfather also had Hodgkin's disease at age 41 but was not thought to have the Gorlin syndrome. Mutations in the *PTCH* gene on 9q22.3 have now been identified as the cause of the autosomal dominant Gorlin syndrome (Wicking et al., 1997), but this pedigree remains as a unique report of the occurrence of Hodgkin's disease in this syndrome, and there are no reports linking mutations in *PTCH* in sporadic cases of Hodgkin's disease. It is presently unclear whether this occurrence represents coincidence, a rare manifestation of the Gorlin syndrome possibly resulting from a unique mutant allele, or contributions from a contiguous gene deletion syndrome.

Familial Non-Hodgkin's Lymphoma

Numerous familial aggregations of non-Hodgkin's lymphoma (typically without significant other types of cancer) have been identified. These were most recently and comprehensively reviewed in Linet and Pottern (1992), but some other cases have been reported since then (Donadieu et al., 1996); still other cases are not cited (Freeman et al., 1970; Coughlin et al., 1980), and some probably represent Li-Fraumeni syndrome (Escobar and Bixler, 1976) or other inherited cancer syndromes, such as hereditary non-polyposis colorectal carcinoma (Law et al., 1977). Two reviewers (Linet and Pottern, 1992; Lynch et al., 1992) concluded there to be three familial patterns. First, there are families where the disease appears confined to within a sibship, consistent with autosomal recessive inheritance. In these cases, there is a preponderance of males, the disease usually occurs during adolescence or preadolescence, is usually of B cell origin, and largely arises at extranodal locations, especially the gastrointestinal tract. The second category is disease that again is confined to a sibship but among adults, most typically postmenopausal women. A third category is defined by families with multigenerational transmission (consistent with autosomal dominant transmission). There tends to be an excess of other types of hematologic and non-hematologic malignancies within these families, especially colorectal carcinoma. In one family of father, son, and daughter with predominantly extranodal T-cell lymphoma, evidence for chronic infection with the Epstein-Barr virus was found in all three affected individuals (Donadieu et al., 1996).

Families with Both Hodgkin's and Non-Hodgkin's Lymphoma

There are numerous reports of both uni- and multigenerational families in which multiple individuals have developed Hodgkin's lymphoma while others have developed non-Hodgkin's lymphoma (reviewed in Linet and Pottern, 1992) and other reports (Buehler et al., 1975; Spremolla et al., 1981; Greene et al., 1982; Bjerrum et al., 1986; Donhuijsen-Ant et al., 1988; Lynch et al., 1989; Weintraub et al., 1996). This is striking evidence in support of the possibility that both Hodgkin's and non-Hodgkin's lymphoma have a common genetic foundation or environmental etiology in individuals with an inherited risk for complications of exposure to certain agents. (It should also be noted that hematopathological differentiation of Hodgkin's disease from non-Hodgkin's lymphoma is difficult, and conceivably some or all of these families represent errors in diagnosis. Ironically, it would appear that Hodgkin himself may have misdiagnosed three of his first seven cases [Dawson, 1968]). Subclinical immune deficiency has been observed in some of the nonaffected members of some of the families (Buehler et al., 1975; Lynch et al., 1989). In one family there were three brothers between the ages of 11 and 21 years old who developed Hodgkin's disease and one brother with non-Hodgkin's lymphoma in whom persistent Epstein-Barr virus infection could be demonstrated (Donhuijsen-Ant et al., 1988). Aspects of this disease are thus similar to the Duncan syndrome of X-linked lymphoproliferative syndrome, but the later age on onset of disease and the occurrence of Hodgkin's disease are contrasting features.

Familial Burkitt's Lymphoma

Burkitt's lymphoma has been reported in at least five pairs of siblings (Lynch and Schuelke, 1984; Anderson et al., 1986) residing in nonendemic areas. An additional five Tanzanian families, residing within the "lymphoma belt," have been reported with multiple cases of Burkitt's lymphoma in association with other forms of cancer (Brubaker et al., 1980).

Familial Mycosis Fungoides

There are at least six familial instances of mycosis fungoides or related cutaneous T-cell lymphoproliferative disease occurring in sibling or parent–child pairs (as reviewed in Shelley, 1980), including in identical twin women at ages 46 and 47 (Schneider et al., 1995).

Familial Multiple Myeloma

There are numerous reports of familial multiple myeloma and related plasma cell disorders. A population based survey in Sweden in 1962 sought to discover the frequency of monoclonal IgM disorders (Axelsson and Hallen, 1965). All of the adults over age 25 in one province (6995 in total) were sampled. Of these, 64 were found with apparent monoclonal IgM spikes on serum protein electrophoresis, and 7 of the identified individuals could be placed in one of three pedigrees. All of the identified family members, however, were asymptomatic, but one had plasma cell proliferation on bone marrow examination. Reports of familial occurrences of multiple myeloma and related disorders are probably too common to exhaustively reference (Nadeau et al., 1956; Manson, 1961; Thomas, 1964; Alexander and Benninghoff, 1965; Berlin et al., 1968; Grant et al., 1971; Zawadzki et al., 1977; Isobe et al., 1981; Shoenfeld et al., 1982; Horwitz et al., 1985; Bizzaro and Pasini, 1990; Crozes-Bony et al., 1995). In general, the disease has been confined to a sibship and the number of affected individuals in the family remains limited, but multigenerational reports exist. There are also at least two monozygous twin pairs concordant for multiple myeloma (Judson et al., 1985; Comotti et al., 1987). Many of these families contain individuals with subclinical monoclonal gammopathies of undetermined significance (MGUS) or various other indicators of immune disorders. A search for germline *p53* mutations in familial multiple myeloma was negative (Willems et al., 1993). There is also a report of isolated familial AL-amyloidosis among three siblings (Miliani et al., 1996) and several reports of Waldenstrom macroglobulinemia occurring across and between generations (Seligmann et al., 1963; Vannotti, 1963; Brown et al., 1967; Blattner et al., 1980; Renier et al., 1989) and including monozygotic twins (Fine et al., 1986).

Constant Somatic Mutation in Familial Disease

A notable phenomenon in familial leukemia is concordance for similar somatic and therefore acquired chromosomal abnormalities between affected family members. This is the nearly unwavering case for the autosomal recessive syndrome of pediatric myelodysplasia with monosomy 7. The monosomy 7 is not constitutional, and it appears that the predisposing gene is not located in the region of loss, but affected individuals within a family develop similar somatic cytogenetic abnormalities. Other examples of this process include two families with myelodysplasia, where both affecteds developed monosomy of 5q. One family consisted of two sisters becoming ill at age 36 and 38 years (Grimwade et al., 1993). In another family with seven cases of myelodysplasia and/or AML, four of five individuals available for bone marrow cytogenetics had acquired monosomy 5q (Olopade et al., 1996). There is, however, insignificant evidence for linkage of the familial predisposition to 5q (Gao et al., 2000). In a family with erythroleukemia (M6 AML) involving six affected individuals, two patients were available for bone marrow cytogenetic studies, and acquired monosomy 20q was observed in both. No linkage studies have been performed in this family. In a family with the multigenerational transmission of ALL, affected individuals demonstrated in vitro chromosomal instability (Kato et al., 1983), in which there was a tendency for rearrangements on chromosome 1p22 (Sasaki et al., 1980). In a unique Japanese family with an apparently autosomal dominant ataxia-telangiectasia-like disorder, multiple familiy members demonstrated tendency toward somatic 14q11.2 rearrangements (Ishikawa et al., 2000). Thus, in contrast to what might be expected based on numerous loss of heterozygosity studies in other cancer family syndromes, these nearly invariant abnormalities surprisingly do not necessarily point to the location of the predisposing gene but may, rather, represent significant secondary events required for cellular transformation.

A remarkable phenomenon has been reported for Rothmund-Thomson syndrome, an autosomal recessive disorder that results from mutations in the RECQL4 DNA helicase on 8q24.3 (Kitao et al., 1999) of skin and skeletal abnormalities associated with some characteristics of premature aging and a predisposition to malignancy, predominately osteosarcoma, but also including hematologic neoplasia (Vennos and James, 1995). Five Rothmund-Thomson patients have been karyotyped (as reported and reviewed in Lindor et al., 1996), and four are mosaic for trisomy 8. One family had karyotypically normal parents, but three of six children had the Rothmund-Thomson syndrome, two of whom were karyotyped. One had mosaic trisomy 8, and the other had mosaicism for isochromosome i(8q). Thus, individuals with Rothmund-Thomson syndrome seem predisposed to develop somatic trisomy 8, apparently as the result of mitotic, postzygotic non-disjunction. One possible mechanism is that the development of trisomy 8 somehow rescues an otherwise nonviable conception and is thus clonally selected during early embryogenesis.

Anticipation in Familial Leukemia

Anticipation refers to the observation of increasing severity or an earlier age of onset of disease occurring with each subsequent generation. It was first reported at the turn of the century for Huntington disease and myotonic dystrophy. The phenomenon was widely accepted until the 1948 publication of a paper by the influential geneticist Penrose (reviewed in Horwitz, 1997), who argued that it was a statistical artifact attributable to ascertainment bias. The subject was largely forgotten until the identification of a mutational mechanism involving expansion of DNA triplet repeats as the cause of anticipation in Huntington disease, myotonic dystrophy, and other—chiefly neurological—diseases demonstrating intergenerational worsening in concert with lengthening repeats.

We have reported that familial leukemia appears to be inherited with anticipation (Horwitz et al., 1996). We reviewed defined reports of familial leukemia and found that for 49 affected individuals in nine families transmitting AML the mean age at onset is 57 years in the grandparental generation, 32 years in the parental generation, and 13 years in the youngest generation; for 18 affected individuals in seven families inheriting CLL (limited to two-generation pedigrees), the mean age at onset in the parental generation is 66 years vs. 51 years in the youngest generation (Fig. 40–1). Support for anticipation in familial leukemia also can be extrapolated from earlier studies. Videbaek (1947a, 1947b; Busk, 1949) collectively analyzed all pedigrees with familial leukemia reported in the literature and that he observed prior to 1947. He found a mean age of onset in parents of 57.0 years, children at 33.8 years, and grandchildren at 11.7 years. Sampling biases were mitigated by the observation that there was a similar intergenerational drop in age between affected uncle–aunt and nephew–niece pairs that was not apparent when comparing the age of onset between the eldest and youngest members of a sibship. In a population-based survey that considered familial relationships for all types of hematopoietic malignancy, a mean difference between ages at death in affected par-

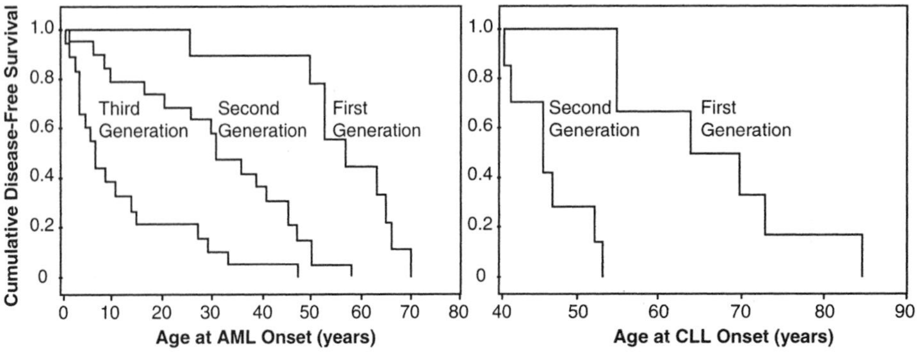

Fig. 40–1. Age of onset in familial leukemia stratified by generation.

ent–child pairs was 38 years (Rigby et al., 1968). Anticipation also appears to exist in a collection of Japanese leukemia families (Kurita and Kamei, 1969). Inspection of pedigrees transmitting multiple types of leukemia and lymphoma (Horwitz et al., 1996), including Hodgkin's disease (Shugart, 1998), also is consistent with anticipation. The statistical biases elaborated by Penrose can only be confidently overcome by a prospective study, which is virtually impossible for something as rare as familial leukemia. Nevertheless, one exceptionally large AML family with at least 16 cases of leukemia has been observed for nearly 20 years (Gunz et al., 1978; Horwitz et al., 1996). The family continues to demonstrate anticipation. The most recently observed case of AML occurred with congenital onset in an infant simultaneous with the presentation of disease in the father.

Two follow-up surveys of proprietary collections of familial CLL pedigrees confirmed anticipation with similar mean ages of onset for each generation (Yuille et al., 1998b; Goldin et al., 1999). Significant evidence for anticipation remained even after censoring the data in an attempt to control for the potential ascertainment biases noted by Penrose.

Collateral support for anticipation comes from the observations of familial hematopoietic malignancy among sibships related as first or second cousins who develop disease without a history in prior generations (Ward et al., 1952; Jelicka et al., 1958; Randall et al., 1965; Rigby et al., 1966; McPhedran et al., 1969; Machura et al., 1970; Banihashemi et al., 1973; Feldman et al., 1976; Larsen and Schimke, 1976; Chitamber et al., 1983; Kato et al., 1983; Eriksson and Bergstrom, 1987; Markkanen et al., 1987; Gramatovici et al., 1993; Kende et al., 1994) (Fig. 40–2). There are numerous other examples of affected cousin pairs identified in proband studies (for example, Kurita and Kamei, 1974; Eriksson and Bergstrom, 1987). This pattern is not easily explained by either autosomal recessive or autosomal dominant inheritance. The fact that some of the affected indi-

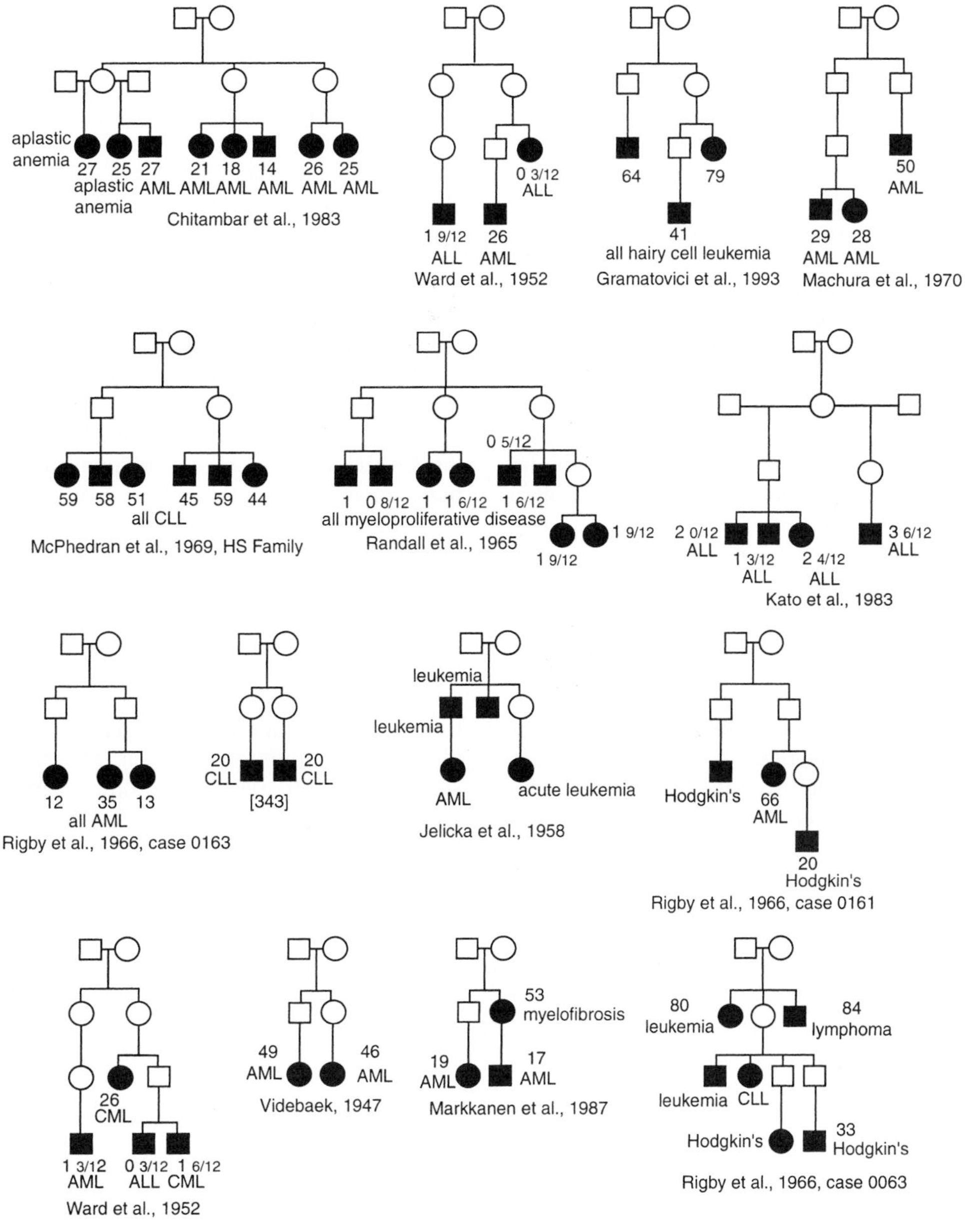

Fig. 40–2. Examples of families with hematopoietic malignancy that demonstrate the "affected cousin" pattern of inheritance. Age of onset in years or months (*n*/12) is indicated.

viduals in these families had affected children by more than one mate further removes autosomal recessive inheritance as a possible explanation. Perhaps the most plausible explanation is to suppose that there is autosomal dominant inheritance with anticipation and that the parental or grandparental generation has reduced penetrance because of a requirement for a greater age of onset in this generation. The founder mutation would then be expected to have occurred de novo in a preceding generation but, due to anticipation, not resulted in disease until one or two further generations had passed.

One explanation for anticipation in familial leukemia and lymphoma, assuming it to be a genuine phenomenon unrelated to statistical biases in ascertainment, is that the responsible gene involves an unstable repeat that is dynamically mutated. There are several arguments going against this possibility. First, thus far, trinucleotide repeats have been implicated only in syndromes in which neurodegenerative disease is a substantial component. Except for a few rare families with ataxia in conjunction with apparent autosomal recessive familial myelodysplasia with monosomy 7 (Li et al., 1981; Daghistani et al., 1990; Luna-Fineman et al., 1995), and one family with polycythemia vera and Huntington disease (Doll and Rothschild, 1922); such occurrences appear to be rare. Second, CAG repeats, at least, seem to be capable of causing only central neurodegenerative changes when expressed ubiquitously as isolated polyglutamine-encoding sequences in transgenic mice (Ordway et al., 1997). Third, using the "RED" assay, we have failed to find expanded CAG trinucleotide repeat tracts in genomic DNA from one leukemia family (Horwitz et al., 1997). Fourth, most trinucleotide repeats show preferential expansion through a particular sex. There is no expansion, for example, of the Fragile X CGG repeat through paternal meiosis; large expansions of the CAG repeat in myotonic dystrophy occur only through maternal meiosis, and expansions of the Huntington disease locus CAG repeat occur mostly through male meiosis. In contrast, we were not able to resolve sex effects in the anticipation associated with familial leukemia (Horwitz et al., 1996). The mechanism for anticipation in familial hematopoietic malignancy, should it prove to be a genuine phenomenon, remains to be determined.

It is interesting that targeted homologous recombination in mice, to knock out the telomerase gene responsible for the intergenerational maintenance of telomere length, results in, among other features, a phenotype of aneuploidy and impaired hematopoiesis that abruptly begins five generations later (Lee et al., 1998). This results from the fact that the telomeres in mice are sufficiently long so it is not until after the lapse of four generations without telomerase activity that these DNA sequences become depleted. The pattern of inheritance, then, is similar to that seen in the case of leukemia families with the affected "cousin pattern" of inheritance (Fig. 40–3). This suggests that there might be novel mechanisms responsible for anticipation that await discovery.

GENE IDENTIFICATION

Constitutional Chromosomal Abnormalities

Down Syndrome

Down syndrome of mental retardation, dysmorphism, and visceral malformations results from trisomy of chromosome 21 (as reviewed by Epstein, 1995). Down syndrome patients have an overall 10- to 18-fold relative risk for leukemia (reviewed by Taub, 2001). In the neonatal period there is a high frequency of a usually transient clonal myeloproliferative syndrome. Before age 3, M7 AML is most commonly encountered with a 400-fold risk elevation for this subtype compared to the general population. About one-third to one-half of AML in Down syndrome is preceded by myelodysplasia. As the Down syndrome individual ages, ALL predominates. In individuals constitutionally mosaic for trisomy 21, the clonal leukemoid reactions of infancy (Homans et al., 1993) or the leukemic blasts (Rowley, 1981) invariably arise from the trisomy 21 population of cells. Some attempts have been made to refine the region responsible for leukemia in Down syndrome by comparing atypical karyotypes, such as isochromosome 21 and ring chromosomes (Korenberg et al., 1994; Shen et al., 1995).

Trisomy 21 is among the most commonly observed acquired chromosomal abnormality in the bone marrow of leukemic individuals. A recent study, albeit of a single patient with erythroleukemia in which constitutional mosaicism was diligently pursued, suggests that occult trisomy 21 Down syndrome may be a mechanism for apparently sporadic cases of leukemia in which the cytogenetic abnormality is confined to the bone marrow (Minelli et al., 2001).

Most often Down syndrome results from maternal non-disjunction in meiosis I, in which the extra chromosome 21 represents that from a third grandparent. It is also possible, however, to have meiosis II non-disjunction (from either parent) or mitotic non-disjunction in the zygote or early embryo. The origin of the extra chromosome 21 has been investigated in the transient myeloproliferative syndrome of infancy in Down syndrome. In nine patients where determination of the parental ori-

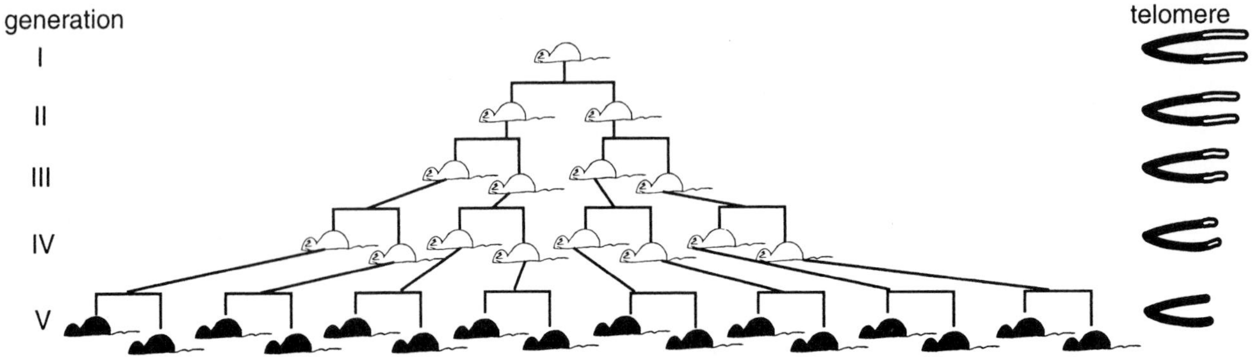

Fig. 40–3. Schematized pedigree for mouse telomerase knockout in which the phenotype abruptly appears among third cousins.

gin was possible, the extra chromosome 21 resulted from duplication of a parental chromosome, rather than meiosis I errors (Abe et al., 1989; Niikawa et al., 1991). This result was confirmed to some degree in a subsequent study (Shen et al., 1995). Thus, a theory of "disomic homozygosity" has been advanced to account for the transient myeloproliferative syndrome and possibly increased frequency of leukemia in Down syndrome (Niikawa et al., 1991; Shen et al., 1995). It holds that the hematopoietic disorders (or other phenotypic components) of Down syndrome result from two identical copies of a susceptibility allele inherited from the parent of origin of the trisomy (as a consequence of meiotic II non-disjunction or postzygotic mitotic non-disjunction). This susceptibility allele could be either a rare mutation or a common polymorphism. A supportive piece of evidence is the absence of a maternal age effect in transient myeloproliferative syndrome (Iselius and Gustavson, 1984) (although it does not appear to be true for leukemia in Down syndrome), which would be expected for mitotic, postzygotic non-disjunction. One patient with Down syndrome and transient myeloproliferative syndrome was found to have an inversion inv(21) (q11.2–q22.13) in the two copies of chromosome 21 that were maternally inherited (as a meiosis I or mitotic error) (Niikawa et al., 1991); in another five patients, analysis of cross-over sites seemed to confine the gene to between the centromere and the q21.3 segment. Additional evidence for the localization of this putative gene comes from the finding that the pericentromeric region of the long arm of chromosome 21 is the site of greatest disomic homozygosity (Shen et al., 1995). This region includes AML1, frequently somatically translocated in sporadic leukemia and heterozygous germline mutations of which are responsible for the syndrome of dominant familial platelet disorder with predisposition to acute myelogenous leukemia.

Klinefelter Syndrome

Early reports suggested that constitutional sex chromosome abnormalities may be present at higher frequency among leukemic children. Klinefelter syndrome of male hypogonadism (constitutional 47,XXY) is present in 1 in 700 males and constitutionally mosaic in 1 in 4000 cases (Jacobs et al., 1974). There is convincing evidence that Klinefelter syndrome is associated with an increased frequency of male breast cancer and germ cell tumors of the mediastinum (Robinson et al., 1997). At least 26 patients with Klinefelter syndrome and leukemia have been reported (for example, Shaw et al., 1992). In contrast to Down syndrome, in which there is general concordance of leukemia type and subtype, ALL, CLL, CML, and M1-, M2-, M4-, and M5-AML subtypes have all been reported in Klinefelter patients. Two Klinefelter patients have been reported with lymphoma, one a non-Hodgkin's germinal center (B cell type) (Becher, 1986) and the other a reticulum-cell sarcoma in a patient mosaic for XY/XXY/XXXY (MacSween, 1965).

An initial series of 5 patients with leukemia and Klinefelter syndrome from a total patient population of about 60 adult males (Geraedts et al., 1980; Muts-Homsma et al., 1981), suggested that a high frequency of males with the syndrome develop leukemia; however, a retrospective study of 1200 patients with hematological malignancy found only one Klinefelter syndrome case (Horsman et al., 1987). Two patients have been apparent constitutional mosaics: in one insufficient information is given about whether the leukemia was also mosaic for XXY (Geraedts et al., 1980; Muts-Homsma et al., 1981) and in the other (Shaw et al., 1992)—in contrast to Down syndrome—the leukemia cells had the same proportion of XXY cells as skin fibroblasts. It is therefore difficult to conclude that there is a true increased risk for leukemia in Klinefelter syndrome, and it is possible that these reports are coincidences resulting from the high background frequency for this syndrome.

Inherited Fragile Sites

A fragile site on the terminus of the short arm of chromosome 11 in the region of both ATM, causing ataxia-telangiectasia, and MLL, frequently mutated or rearranged in sporadic leukemia, has been associated with leukemia. Specifically, an 11q23 unstably inherited CGG trinucleotide repeat causing a folate-sensitive fragile site in the *CBL2* proto-oncogene (*FRA11B*) is the cause of the Jacobsen syndrome of mental retardation and dysmorphism, which results from the meiotic deletion or translocation at this chromosomal region (Jones et al., 1995). The mother of a patient with the Jacobsen syndrome, who would presumably have an expansion of this repeat, died from leukemia in her early adult years (Jacobsen et al., 1973). A 2-month-old girl who developed myelodysplasia is also reported with congenital deletion of 11q23 (Groupe Français de Cytogenetique Hematologique, 1997). A previously well 54-year-old woman with constitutional deletion of chromosome 11q23 developed M5 AML; she was additionally mosaic for trisomy X (Bigazzi et al., 1993); it is then possible that she had Jacobsen syndrome and that the deletion could have resulted from meiotic expansion of a parental fragile site. Deletions of 11q23 are frequent somatic events in sporadic CLL. A recent study indicated that deletion breakpoints cluster near CCG triplet repeats, including *FRA11B* (Auer et al., 2001). These observations remain of interest in light of the evidence of aniticipation in familial CLL, frequent somatic deletion of ATM in sporadic cases of CLL, and the suggestion that ATM heterozygotes may have a greater risk for developing CLL. One possible hypothesis is that an inherited fragile site in this region accounts for familial CLL by predisposing to somatic loss of this region; the potential for intergenerational triplet repeat expansion could then conceivably explain anticipation in familial CLL.

In contrast, a CGG repeat polymorphism is present in the BCR gene on chromosome 22, in which there is translocation with ABL on chromosome 9 to form the Philadelphia chromosome. Polymorphic expansions of this repeat, however, do not appear to be a risk factor for development of the Philadelphia chromosome and subsequent leukemia (Riggins et al., 1994).

Other Constitutional Structural Chromosomal Abnormalities

Other constitutional chromosomal abnormalities that are probable or possible risk factors for hematopoietic malignancy are listed in Table 40–7.

Linkage

Leukemia

HLA. Searches for possible HLA linkage or association were fueled by, among other factors, early studies of viral-induced leukemia in mice. Vulnerability to some murine leukemia viruses appears to map to the H-2 region of the MHC (Lilly and Pinkus, 1973; Meruelo and Bach, 1983). One obvious approach then is to test for possible HLA conservation among individuals from leukemia-prone families. These studies have been largely discouraging or inconclusive, however. In a sibship of four sisters

Table 40–7. Constitutional Chromosomal Abnormalities Associated with Hematopoietic Malignancy

Strength of Association	Chromosomal Anomaly	Malignancy
Probable	Monosomy 21	Myelodysplasia (Huret et al., 1995; Huret and Leonard, 1997)
	Trisomy 8	Myelodysplasia, AML, CML (Secker-Walker and Fitchett, 1995; Zollino et al., 1995)
Possible	Paracentric inversion of 7	AML (Stanley et al., 1997; Johnson et al., 1996)
	Christchurch chromosome (loss of short arm of acrocentric chromosome)	CLL, AML (Fitzgerald and Hamer, 1969; Gunz et al., 1962; Juberg and Jones, 1970)
	Fragile sites	
	16q22	AML (Ferro et al., 1994; Meisner et al., 1978)
	11q23	Myelodysplasia, AML (Jacobsen et al., 1973; Stanley et al., 1997)

with AML, only one affected woman was available for HLA analysis, but she was HLA identical to several siblings who had no disease (Pendergrass et al., 1975). Two brothers who developed ALL in adolescence were found to be HLA identical (Blattner et al., 1978). In another family, two first cousins with ALL (whose parents were half siblings of one another) shared a common HLA haplotype (Kato et al., 1983). Two brothers with CLL were HLA identical (Fazekas et al., 1978), as were three sisters with CLL (Hakim et al., 1995), but in another family with multiple siblings with CLL, there was no HLA conservation between affected individuals (Schweitzer et al., 1973). The largest known leukemia family, with 16 cases of AML, demonstrates no evident HLA or blood group linkage (Gunz et al., 1978). Recent genetic linkage analysis excluded HLA as a locus for familial CLL (Bevan et al., 2000).

Other studies have sought simple associations between HLA types and leukemia. These have been previously reviewed (Taylor and Birch, 1996). In general, there is only weak support for association between particular HLA types and leukemia risk. The most significant effect seems to apply to HLA-C locus alleles, where there is an approximately 2-fold association between certain alleles and risk for certain types of leukemia in some studies. Underrepresentation of some alleles has also been reported, suggesting the possibility of a protective effect.

Ha-ras Polymorphisms. The *c*-Ha-ras-1 locus on chromosome 11p15.5 contains a "hypervariable" region of repetitive DNA downstream from the coding region. An initial report found rare allelic variants in this region occurring in six of seven patients with myelodysplastic syndrome (Krontiris, et al., 1985). A subsequent study found rare alleles in 4.8% of myelodysplastic patients and 15.7% of patients with AML, but no variant alleles in normal subjects (Carter et al., 1988).

Chromosome 21q: AML1/CBFA. As noted above, heterozygous germline mutations in this gene are responsible for autosomal dominant familial platelet disorder with predisposition to acute myelogenous leukemia. This gene also resides in the critical region to which predisposition to leukemia in Down syndrome is putatively mapped.

Chromosome 16q. In two other families inheriting autosomal dominant AML and myelodysplasia without evidence of a premorbid phenotype, we excluded linkage to *AML1* on chromosome 21q22.1–q22.2, thereby demonstrating that familial AML/CBFA is a genetically heterogeneous disease (Horwitz et al., 1997; Gao et al., 2000). We tested for linkage on a candidate region basis to several loci, choosing to investigate chromosome 16q22 because of reports of two families with a fragile site in this region and multiple cases of leukemia and because it is the locus for AML1/CBFA's heterodimeric partner, CBFB. We determined a combined LOD score of 3.39 for both families at a recombination fraction $\theta = 0$, spanning a 14.9 cM (13 Mb) interval at chromosome 16q21–q22.3. Mutational analysis in this region is in progress.

Homozygosity for Mismatch Repair Genes. Recently, three families have been described in which some individuals are homozygous for mutations in the mismatch repair genes (either MLH1 (Ricciardone et al., 1999) or MSH2 (Andrew et al., 2001)) responsible for hereditary non-polyposis colorectal carcinoma (HNPCC). Several of these individuals developed the childhood onset of leukemia (the type not being described), curiously, with clinical features of neurofibromatosis 1. It may be of relevance that MSH2 "knockout" mice are susceptible to lymphoma (Reitmair et al., 1995).

Lymphoma

HLA Linkage in Hodgkin's Disease. Older case-control studies found an increased frequency of the HLA antigens A1, B5, B8, and B18 among Hodgkin's disease patients (Hors and Dausset, 1983). Potential linkage to HLA has been investigated using sib pair methods. A number of studies taken individually and analyzed in total provide support for HLA linkage for Hodgkin's disease. One study of 32 sib pairs suggested excess sharing of haplotypes at HLA; the author proposed recessive inheritance and pointed out that a low penetrance among heterozygotes might explain a large proportion of seemingly non-familial cases (Bodmer, 1986). Another study of 37 sib and cousin pairs found evidence for HLA linkage among 60% of the cases, best fitting a recessive form of inheritance with an LOD score of 3.67. An increased concordance of histological types was observed between affected relatives but was found to be independent of HLA sharing. Molecular typing of class II HLA DR-DQ loci has shown excesses and deficits of particular alleles and haplotypes among 155 consecutive Caucasian NSHD subtype patients presenting to Stanford medical center (Klitz et al., 1994). Similar results were previously reported for HLA DPB among a smaller, but more ethnically diverse, population of Hodgkin's disease patients not selected by histologic subtype (Tonks et al., 1992). These studies distinguish between an HLA association and HLA linkage in that, while certain HLA types may occur in excess among sporadic Hodgkin's disease patients, there is intrafamily, but not interfamily, HLA conservation among affected individuals in hereditary cases.

Pseudoautosomal Linkage in Hodgkin's Disease. It has been suggested that there may be a locus conferring risk for Hodgkin's disease in the pseudoautosomal region of the sex chromosomes (Horwitz and Wiernik, 1999). A unique pair of sisters was reported with both Hodgkin's disease and Leri-Weill dyschondrosteosis, a skeletal dysplasia (Gokhale et al., 1995). There was a further family history of both Hodgkin's disease and dyschondrosteosis, and the authors suggested that the two disorders might be linked. Subsequently, it was determined that Leri-Weill dyschondrosteosis results from mutations in the *SHOX* gene residing in the short-arm pseudoautosomal region of the X and Y chromosomes. (The pseudoautosomal regions, present on the termini of both arms of both sex chromosomes, represent the only regions of the X and Y chromosomes that undergo recombination during meiosis.) Diseases resulting from mutations in genes in the pseudoautosomal region should show a unique segregation pattern, in which affected sib pairs will be gender concordant (because if the gene is inherited from the father, then it must reside on either the X or Y chromosome, which is also responsible for conferring gender). Interestingly, an excess of gender-condordant sex pairs for Hodgkin's disease had been previously appreciated, but attributed to environmental factors (Grufferman et al., 1977). Review of additional reports of sib pairs concordant for Hodgkin's disease confirmed an excess of gender concordance, including a remarkable sibship with five affected males (Kajii et al., 1968). The excess of gender concordance provided significant support for a pseudoautosomal locus conferring as much as 40% of the heritability for Hodgkin's disease.

A subsequent study was performed to test for potential pseudoautosomal linkage in sibships concordant for CLL (Houlston et al., 2000). Although there was a statistically significant excess of gender-concordant sib pairs, even when allowing for the greater frequency of CLL among males, the LOD score achieved 1.51, falling short of statistical significance (although no power study was included to determine whether the sample size was capable of achieving significance).

Multiple Myeloma

PARP Polymorphisms. A polymorphism of the poly(ADP-ribose)polymerase (PARP) pseudogene on chromosome 13q33–qter has been correlated with multiple myeloma, prostate cancer, and colorectal carcinoma in African Americans. This allele was found to have a frequency of 0.35 in the general African American population, but a frequency of 0.66, 0.72, and 0.64 among African Americans with multiple myeloma, prostate cancer, and colon cancer, respectively (Lyn et al., 1993). The allele is not associated with cancer among Caucasians. The results have been extended to monoclonal gammopathy of undetermined significance (MGUS), and there appears to be increased expression of the malignancy associated allele (Cao et al., 1995). These data are interesting in light of an increased frequency of plasma cell neoplasms and prostate carcinoma among African Americans, but they require substantiation.

CLINICAL APPLICATION AND RISK ASSESSMENT

Although there is substantial genetic epidemiologic evidence for inherited risk factors for predisposition to both general and specific categories of hematopoietic malignancy, except for a few rare syndromes, the responsible genes remain uncloned and their prospective role in sporadic cases must remain uninvestigated. The field is unlikely to remain static, however, and it is probable that the coming years will witness the identification of genes responsible for the rare familial syndromes that may more broadly elucidate mechanisms for the far more common and seemingly sporadic cases. This will undoubtedly have attendant implications for new forms of treatment and diagnosis.

ACKNOWLEDGMENTS

This work was supported by grants from the National Institutes of Health (DK55820, DK58161), the Doris Duke Charitable Foundation (T98006), the Leukemia and Lymphoma Society of America (6443-00), and the American Cancer Society (RPG-99-319-01-LBC).

REFERENCES

Abe K, Kajii T, Niikawa N: Disomic homozygosity in 21-trisomic cells: a mechanism responsible for transient myeloproliferative syndrome. Hum Genet 1989; 82:313–316.

Abramson JH, Pridan H, Sacks MI, Avitzour M, Peritz E: A case-control study of Hodgkin's disease in Israel. J Natl Cancer Inst 1978; 61:307–314.

Adamson JW: Familial polycythemia. Semin Hematol 1975; 12:383–396.

Alexander LL, Benninghoff DL: Familial multiple myeloma. J Natl Med Assoc 1965; 57:471–475.

Anderson KC, Jamison DS, Peters WP, Li FP: Familial Burkitt's lymphoma: association with altered lymphocyte subsets in family members. Am J Med 1986; 81:158–162.

Anderson RC, Hermann HW: Leukemia in twin children. JAMA 1955; 158:652–654.

Andrew SE, Whiteside D, Steckley J, Booth K, Graham GE, McLeod DR: A novel homozygous mutation in the human *NSH2* gene predisposes to leukemia and multiple café-au-lait spots. Am J Hum Genet 2001; 69:A365.

Auer RL, Jones C, Mullenbach RA, Syndercombe-Court D, Milligan DW, Fegan CD, Cotter FE: Role for CCG-trinucleotide repeats in the pathogenesis of chronic lymphocytic leukemia. Blood 2001; 97:509–515.

Auerbach AD: Fanconi anemia, diagnosis and the diepoxybutane (DEB) test. Exp Hematol 1993; 21:731–733.

Auerbach AD: Fanconi anemia. In: Cohen PR, Kurzrock R (eds). Dermatologic Clinics. Genodermatoses with malignant potential Vol. 13. Philadelphia: W. B. Saunders, 1995:41–49.

Aul C, Germing U, Gattermann N, Minning H: Increasing incidence of myelodysplastic syndromes: real or fictitious? Leuk Res 1998; 22:93–100.

Axelsson U, Hallen J: Familial occurrence of pathological serum proteins of different γ-globulin groups. Lancet 1965; 2:369–370.

Azzi A, Fanci R, De Santis R, Ciappi S, Paci C: Human herpesvirus 8 DNA sequences are present in bone marrow from HIV-negative patients with lymphoproliferative disorders and from healthy donors. Br J Haematol 2001; 113:188–190.

Bader-Meunier B, Mielot F, Tchernia G, Buisine J, Delsol G, Duchayne E, Lemerle S, Leverger G, de Lumley L, Manel A-M, et al.: Myelodysplastic syndromes in childhood: report of 49 patients from a French multicentre study. Br J Haematol 1996a; 92:344–350.

Bader-Meunier B, Mielot F, Tchernia G, Lavergene JM, Leonard C, Dommergues J-P: Dubowitz syndrome: an etiology for childhood myelodysplasia. Int J Pediatr Hematol Oncol 1996b; 3:105–107.

Banihashemi A, Nasr K, Heayatee H, Mortazavee H: Familial lymphoma including a report of familial primary upper small intestinal lymphoma. Blut 1973; 26:363–368.

Bartal A, Bentwich Z, Manny N, Izak G: Ethnical and clinical aspects of chronic lymphocytic leukemia in Israel: a survey on 288 patients. Acta Haematol 1978; 60:161–171.

Becher R: Klinefelter's syndrome and malignant lymphoma. Cancer Genet Cytogenet 1986; 21:271–273.

Begley CG, Tait B, Crapper RM, Briggs PG, Brodie GN, MacKay IR: Familial hairy cell leukemia. Leuk Res 1987; 11:1027–1029.

Bell DW, Varley JM, Szydlo TE, Kang DH, Wahrer DC, Shannon KE, Lubratovich M, Verselis SJ, Isselbacher KJ, Fraumeni JF, et al.: Heterozygous germ line *hCHK2* mutations in Li-Fraumeni syndrome. Science 1999; 286:2433–2434.

Bener A, Abdulrazzaq YM, al-Gazali LI, Micallef R, al-Khayat AI, Gaber T: Consanguinity and associated socio-demographic factors in the United Arab Emirates. Hum Hered 1996; 46:256–264.

Bener A, Denic S, Al-Mazrouei M: Consanguinity and family history of cancer in children with leukemia and lymphomas. Cancer 2001; 92:1–6.

Bergsagel D: The incidence and epidemiology of plasma cell neoplasms. Stem Cells (Dayt) 1995; 13(Suppl 2):1–9.

Berlin SO, Odeberg H, Weingart L: Familial occurrence of M-components. Acta Med Scand 1968; 183:347–350.

Bernard J, Seligmann M, Loirat C, Chassigneux J, Basch A, Gueudet A: Splenomegalie myeloide familiale. Nouv Rev Fr Hematol 1967; 7:499–506.

Bernard T, Gale RE, Evans JP, Linch DC: Mutations of the granulocyte-colony stimulating factor receptor in patients with severe congenital neutropenia are not required for transformation to acute myeloid leukaemia and may be a bystander phenomenon. Br J Haematol 1998; 101:141–149.

Bernstein R, Pinto M, Behr A, Mendelow B: Chromosome 3 abnormalities in acute nonlymphocytic leukemia (ANLL) with abnormal thrombopoiesis: report of three patients with a "new" inversion anomaly and a further case of homologous translocation. Blood 1982; 60:613–617.

Bertolani MF, Massolo F: La leucemia familiare: recenti osservazioni tratte dall casistica della Clinica Pediatrica di Modena. Clin Pediat (Bologna) 1975; 57:41–51.

Bevan S, Catovsky D, Marossy A, Matutes E, Popat S, Antonovic P, Bell A, Berrebi A, Gaminara E, Quabeck K, et al.: Linkage analysis for *ATM* in familial B cell chronic lymphocytic leukaemia. Leukemia 1999; 13:1497–1500.

Bevan S, Catovsky D, Matutes E, Antunovic P, Auger MJ, Ben-Bassat I, Bell A, Berrebi A, Gaminara EJ, Junior ME, et al.: Linkage analysis for major histocompatibility complex–related genetic susceptibility in familial chronic lymphocytic leukemia. Blood 2000; 96:3982–3984.

Bierman HR, Byron RL, Kelley KH, Dod KS, Black PM: Studies on cross circulation in man: I. Methods and clinical changes. Blood 1951; 6:487–503.

Bigazzi C, Galienci P, Scarinci R, Vivarelli R, Bucalossi A, Biancolini G, Falbo R, Vessichelli F, Dispensa E, et al.: 11q- and constitutional X trisomy in a patient with M5B acute non-lymphocytic leukemia. Haematologica 1993; 78:185–186.

Biondi A, Rovelli A, Cantu-Rajnoldi A, Fenu S, Basso G, Luciano A, Rondelli R, Mandelli F, Masera G, Testi A: Acute promyelocytic leukemia in children: experience of the Italian pediatric hematology and oncology group (AIEOP). Leukemia 1994; 8:1264–1268.

Bischof O, Kim SH, Irving J, Beresten S, Ellis NA, Campisi J: Regulation and localization of the Bloom syndrome protein in response to DNA damage. J Cell Biol 2001; 153:367–380.

Bizzaro N, Pasini P: Familial occurrence of multiple myeloma and monoclonal gammopathy of undetermined significance in 5 siblings. Haematologica 1990; 75:58–63.

Bjerrum OW, Hasselbalch HC, Drivsholm A, Nissen NI: Non-Hodgkin malignant lymphomas and Hodgkin's disease in first-degree relatives. Scand J Haematol 1986; 36:398–401.

Blattner WA, Dean JH, Fraumeni JF: Familial lymphoprolfierative malignancy: clinical and laboratory follow-up. Ann Intern Med 1979; 90:943–944.

Blattner WA, Garber JE, Mann DL, McKeen EA, Henson R, McGuire DB, Fisher WB, Bauman AW, Goldin LR, Fraumeni JF: Waldenstrom's macroglobulinemia and autoimmune disease in a family. Ann Intern Med 1980; 93:830–832.

Blattner W, Naiman L, Mann D, Wimer RS, Dean JH, Fraumeni JF: Immunogenetic determinants of familial acute lymphocytic leukemia. Ann Int Med 1978; 89:173–176.

Bodmer WF: Personal communication. In OMIM Online Mendelian Inheritance in Man. MIM Number: 236000 Johns Hopkins University, Baltimore, MD. 1986: http://www.ncbi.nlm.nih.gov/omim/

Bohlander SK: Fusion genes in leukemia: an emerging network. Cytogenet Cell Genet 2000; 91:52–56.

Bondare DK, Teilane H, Resikart LB, Rotsena A, Grasmane DV: Familial myeloproliferative syndrome (study of 4 families and review of the literature). Ter Arkh 1985; 57:59–64.

Boultwood J: Ataxia telangiectasia gene mutations in leukaemia and lymphoma. J Clin Pathol 2001; 54:512–560.

Brandwein JM, Horsman DE, Eaves AC, Eaves CJ, Massing BG, Wadsworth LD, Rogers PCJ, Dalousek DK: Childhood myelodysplasia: suggested classification as myelodysplastic syndromes based on laboratory and clinical findings. Am J Pediatr Hematol Oncol 1990; 12:63–70.

Brown AK, Elves MW, Gunson HH, Pell-Ilderton R: Waldenstrom's macroglobulinaemia: a family study. Acta Haematol 1967; 38:184–192.

Brown LM, Pottern LM, Silverman DT, Schoenberg JB, Schwartz AG, Greenberg RS, Hayes RB, Liff JM, Swanson GM, Hoover R: Multiple myeloma among blacks and whites in the United States: role of cigarettes and alcoholic beverages. Cancer Causes Control 1997; 8:610–614.

Brubaker G, Levin AG, Steel CM, Creasley G, Cameron HM, Linsell CA, Smith PG: Multiple cases of Burkitt's lymphoma and other neoplasms in families in the north Mara district of Tanzania. Int J Cancer 1980; 261:165–170.

Brubaker H, Wasserman LR, Goldberg JD, Pisciotaa AV, McIntryre R, Kaplan ME, Modan B, Flannery J, Harp R: Increased prevalence of polycythemia vera in parents of patients on polycythemia vera study group protocols. Am J Hematol 1984; 16:367–373.

Buckley JD, Buckley CM, Breslow NE, Draper GJ, Roberson PK, Mack TM: Concordance for childhood cancer in twins. Med Pediatr Oncol 1996; 26:223–229.

Buehler SK, Fodor G, Marshall WH, Firme F, Fraser GR, Vaze P: Common variable immunodeficiency, Hodgkin's disease, and other malignancies in a Newfoundland family. Lancet 1975; 1:195–197.

Buell P, Dunn JE: Cancer mortality among Japanese Issei and Nisei of California. Cancer 1965; 8:656–664.

Bullrich F, Rasio D, Kitada S, Starostik P, Kipps T, Keating M, Albitar M, Reed JC, Croce CM: *ATM* mutations in B-cell chronic lymphocytic leukemia. Cancer Res 1999; 59:24–27.

Burmeister T, Thiel E: Molecular genetics in acute and chronic leukemias. J Cancer Res Clin Oncol 2001; 127:80–90.

Burnside P, Salmon DC, Humphey CA, Robertson JH, Morris TC: Polycythaemia rubra vera in monozygotic twins. Br Med J 1981; 283:560–561.

Busk T: Some observations on heredity in breast cancer and leukemia. Ann Eugenics 1949; 14:213–229.

Butturini A, Gale RP, Verlander PC, Adler-Brecher B, Gillio AP, Auerbach AD: Hematologic abnormalities in Fanconi anemia: an international Fanconi anemia registry study. Blood 1994; 84:1650–1655.

Caligiuri MA, Strout MP, Gilliland DG: Molecular biology of acute myeloid leukemia. Semin Oncol 1997; 24:32–44.

Cannon-Albright L, Thoma A, Goldgar DE, Gholami K, Rowe K, Jacobsen M, McWhorter WP, Skolnick MH: Familiarity of cancer in Utah. Cancer Res 1994; 54:2378–2385.

Cao J, Hong CH, Rosen L, Vescio RA, Smulson M, Lichenstein A, Berenson JR: Deletion of genetic material from a poly(ADP-ribose) polymerase-like gene on chromosome 13 occurs frequently in patients with monoclonal gammopathies. Cancer Epidemiol Biomarkers Prev 1995; 4:759–763.398.

Carney JP, Maser RS, Olivares H, Davis EM, Le Beau M, Yates JR, Hays L, Morgan WF, Petrini JHJ: The hMRE11/hRad50 protein complex and Nijmegen breakage syndrome: linkage of double-strand break repair to the cellular DNA damage response. Cell 1998; 93:477–486.

Carroll AJ, Poon M-C, Robinson NC, Crist WM: Sideroblastic anemia associated with thromocytosis and a chromosome 3 abnormality. Cancer Genet Cytogenet 1986; 22:183–187.

Carroll WL, Morgan R, Glader BE: Childhood bone marrow monosomy 7 syndrome: a familial disorder? J Pediatr 1985; 107:578–580.

Carter G, Worwood M, Jacobs A: The ha-ras polymorphism in myelodysplasia and acute myeloid leukaemia. Leuk Res 1988; 12:385–391.

Cartwright RA, Bernard SM, Bird CC, Darwin CM, O'Brien C, Richards ID, Roberts B, McKinney PA: Chronic lymphocytic leukaemia: case control epidemiological study in Yorkshire. Br J Cancer 1987; 56:79–82.

Cartwright RA, Darwin C, McKinney PA, Roberts B, Richards ID, Bird CC: Acute myeloid leukemia in adults: a case-control study in Yorkshire. Leukemia 1988a; 2:687–690.

Cartwright RA, McKinney PA, O'Brien C, Richard IDG, Roberts B, Lauder I, Darwin CM, Bernard SM, Bird CC: Non-Hodgkin's lymphoma: case control epidemiological study in Yorkshire. Leuk Res 1988b; 12:81–88.

Casademont J, Barrientos A, Cardellach F, Rotig A, Grau J-M, Montoya J, Beltran B, Cervantes F, Rozman C, Estivill X, et al.: Multiple deletions of mtDNA in two brothers with sideroblastic anemia and mitochondrial myopathy and in their asympotomatic mother. Hum Mol Genet 1994; 3:1945–1949.92.

Chaganti RSK, Miller DR, Meyers PA, German J: Cytogenetic evidence of the intrauterine origin of acute leukemia in monozygotic twins. N Engl J Med 1979; 300:1032–1034.

Chaiter Y, Brenner B, Aghai E, Tatarsky I: High incidence of myeloproliferative disorders in Ashkenazi Jews in northern Israel. Leuk Lymphoma 1992; 7:251–255.

Chitambar CR, Robinson WA, Glode LM: Familial leukemia and aplastic anemia associated with monosomy 7. Am J Med 1983; 75:756–762.

Cimino G, LoCoco F, Cartoni C, Gallerano T, Luciani M, Lopez M, de Rossi G: Immune deficiency in Hodgkin's disease (HD): a study of patients and healthy relatives in families with multiple cases. Eur J Cancer Clin Oncol 1988; 24:1595–1601.

Clarkson BD, Boyse EA: Possible explanation of the high concordance for acute leukaemia in monozygous twins. Lancet 1971; 1:669–701.

Clavel J, Glandrin G, Hemon D: Hairy cell leukaemia and familial history of leukaemia. Br J Haematol 1997; 97:239–241.

Coffey AJ, Brooksbank RA, Brandau O, Oohashi T, Howell GR, Bye JM, Cahn AP, Durham J, Heath P, Wray P, et al.: Host response to EBV infection in X-linked lymphoproliferative disease results from mutations in an SH2-domain encoding gene. Nat Genet 1998; 20:129–135.

Cohen HJ, Shimm D, Paris SA, Buckley CE, Kremer WB: Hairy cell leukemia–associated familial lymphoproliferative disorder: immunologic abnormalities in unaffected family members. Ann Intern Med 1979; 90:174–179.

Comotti B, Bassan R, Buzzetti M, Finazzi G, Barbui T: Multiple myeloma in a pair of twins. Br J Haematol 1987; 65:123–124.

Conley CL, Missiti J, Laster AJ: Genetic factors predisposing to chronic lymphocytic leukemia and to autoimmune disease. Medicine 1980; 59:323–334.

Consortium FABC: Positional cloning of the Fanconi anaemia group A gene. Nat Genet 1996; 14:324–328.

Coughlin C, Greenwald ES, Becker NH: Familial malignant lymphoma. N Y State J Med 1980; 80:1111–1115.

Cozzolino F, Merlini G: Familial AL-amyloidosis in three Italian siblings. Haematologica 1996; 81:105–109.

Creagan ET, Fraumeni JF: Familial Hodgkin's disease. Lancet 1972; 2:547.

Crozes-Bony P, Palazzo E, Meyer O, de Bandt M, Kahn M-F: Familial multiple myeloma: report of a case in a father and daughter—review of the literature. Rev Rhum Engl Ed 1995; 62:439–445.

Cuneo JM: Leukemia incidence and ethnicity in Nassau County, New York. Am J Public Health 1976; 66:1094–1095.

Cuttner J: Increased incidence of hematologic malignancies in first-degree relatives of patients with chronic lymphocyte leukemia. Cancer Invest 1992; 10(2):103–109.

Daghistani D, Toledano SR, Curless R: Monosomy 7 syndrome: clinical heterogeneity in children and adolescents. Cancer Genet Cytogenet 1990; 44:263–269.

Dale DC, Person RE, Bolyard AA, Aprikyan AG, Bos C, Bonilla MA, Boxer LA, Kannourakis G, Zeidler C, Welte K, et al.: Mutations in the gene encoding neutrophil elastase in congenital and cyclic neutropenia. Blood 2000; 96:2317–2322.

Dawson PJ: The original illustrations of Hodgkin's disease. Arch Intern Med 1968; 121:288–290.

Decastello A: Osteomyosclerose bei Vater und Tochter. Wien Med Wochenschr 1954; 66:655–660.

Degos L: Depidemiologie de la leucemie aigue humaine: le risque de leucemie aigue. Rev Prat 1973; 23:91–94.

Deiss A: Non-neoplastic diseases, chemical agents, and hematologic disorders that may precede hematologic neoplasms. In: Lee GR, Bithell TC, Foerster J, Athens JW, Lukens JN (eds). Wintrobe's Clinical Hematology, 9th ed. Philadelphia: Lea and Febiger, 1993:1946–1968.

de la Chapelle A, Sistonen P, Lehvaslaiho H, Ikkala E, Juvonen E: Familial erythrocytosis genetically linked to erythropoietin receptor gene. Lancet 1993; 341:82–84.

Derry JMJ, Ochs HD, Francke U: Isolation of a novel gene mutated in Wiskott-Aldrich syndrome. Cell 1994; 78:635–644.

Devesa SS: Descriptive epidemiology of multiple myeloma. In: Obrams GI, Potter M (eds). Epidemiology and Biology of Multiple Myeloma. Berlin: Springer-Verlag, 1991:3–12.

Devriendt K, Kim AS, Mathijs G, Frints SG, Schwartz M, Van Den Oord JJ, Verhoef GE, Boogaerts MA, Fryns JP, You D, et al.: Constitutively activating mutation in WASP causes X-linked severe congenital neutropenia. 2001; Nat Genet 27:313–317.

de Winter JP, Leveille F, van Berkel CG, Rooimans MA, van Der Weel L, Steltenpool J, Demuth I, Morgan NV, Alon N, Bosnoyan-Collins L, et al.: Isolation of a cDNA representing the Fanconi anemia complementation group E gene. Am J Hum Genet 2000a; 67:1306–1308.

de Winter JP, Rooimans MA, van Der Weel L, van Berkel CG, Alon N, Bosnoyan-Collins L, de Groot J, Zhi Y, Waisfisz Q, Pronk JC, et al.: The Fanconi anaemia gene *FANCF* encodes a novel protein with homology to ROM. Nat Genet 2000b; 24:15.

de Winter JP, Waisfisz Q, Rooimans MA, van Berkel CG, Bosnoyan-Collins L, Alon N, Carreau M, Bender O, Demuth I, Schindler D, et al.: The Fanconi anaemia group G gene *FANCG* is identical with *XRCC9*. Nat Genet 1998; 20:281–283.

Diebold J, Raphael M, Prevot S, Audouin J: Lymphomas associated with HIV infection. Cancer Surv 1997; 30:263–293.

Dodsworth H: Primary thrombocythaemia in monozygotic twins. Br Med J 1980; 280:1506.

Dolcetti R, Boiocchi M, Gloghini A, Carbone A: Pathogenetic and histogenetic features of HIV-associated Hodgkin's disease. Eur J Cancer 2000; 37:1276–1287.

Doll H, Rothschild K: Familiares aufreten von polycythaemia rubra in Verbendung mit chorea progressiva hereditaria Huntington. Wien Klin Wochnschr 1922; 1:2580.

Donadieu J, Canioni D, Cuenod B, Fraitag S, Bodemer C, Stephan JL, Sigaux F, Le Deist F, Schraub S, Ranfraing E, et al.: A familial T-cell lymphoma with γ-Δ phenotype and an original location: possible role of chronic Epstein-Barr virus infection. Cancer 1996; 77:1571–1577.

Donehower LA, Harvey M, Slagle BL, McArthur M, Montgomery CA, Butel JS, Bradley A: Mice deficient for p53 are developmentally normal but susceptible to spontaneous tumours. Nature 1992; 356:215–221.

Dong F, Brynes RK, Tidow N, Welte K, Lowenberg B, Touw IP: Mutations in the gene for the granulocyte colony-stimulating-factor receptor in patients with acute myeloid leukemia preceded by severe congenital neutropenia. N Engl J Med 1995; 333:487–493.

Donhuijsen-Ant R, Abken H, Bornkamm G, Donhuijsen K, Grosse-Wilde H, Neumann-Haefelin D, Westerhausen M, Wiegand H: Fatal Hodgkin and non-Hodgkin lymphoma associated with persistent Epstein-Barr virus in four brothers. Ann Intern Med 1988; 109:946–952.

Douer D, Preston-Martin S, Chang E, Nichols PW, Watkins KJ, Levine AM: High frequency of acute promyelocytic leukemia among Latinos with acute myeloid leukemia. Blood 1996; 87:308–313.

Dowton SB, Beardsley D, Jamison D, Blattner S, Li FP: Studies of a familial platelet disorder. Blood 1985; 65:557–563.

Draper GJ, Heaf MM, Kinnier Wilson LM: Occurrence of childhood cancers among sibs and estimation of familial risks. J Med Genet 1977; 14:81–90.

Draptchinskaia N, Gustavsson P, Andersson B, Pettersson M, Willig TN, Dianzani I, Ball S, Tchernia G, Klar J, Matsson H, et al.: The gene encoding ribosomal protein S19 is mutated in Diamond-Blackfan anaemia. Nat Genet 1999; 21:169–175.

Dunbar C, Nienhuis A: The myelodysplastic syndromes. In: Handin R, Lux S, Stossel T (eds). Blood, Principles and Practice of Hematology. Philadelphia: J. B. Lippincott, 1995:373–393.

Duncan MH, Wiggins CL, Samet JM, Key CR: Childhood cancer epidemiology in New Mexico's American Indians, Hispanic whites, and non-Hispanic whites, 1970–82. J Natl Cancer Inst 1986; 76:1013–1018.

Durosinmi MA, Nwosu SO, Ogunniyi JO, Dada O, Okunola MA: Hogkin's disease in siblings: a case report. Afr J Med Med Sci 1989; 18:219–222.

Easwa SJ, Lake DE, Beer M, Seiter K, Feldman EJ, Ahmed T: Graft-versus-host disease: possible higher risk for African American patients. Cancer 1996; 78:1492–1497.

Efr LA: Radioactive phosphorus in the treatment of primary polycythemia. Prog Hematol 1956; 1:153–165.

Ellis NA, Groden J, Ye T-Z, Straughen J, Lennon DJ, Ciocci S, Proytcheva M, German J: The Bloom's syndrome gene product is homologous to RecQ helicases. Cell 1995; 83:655–666.

Epstein CJ: Down syndrome (trisomy 21). In: Scriver CR, Beaudet AL, Sly WS, Valle D (eds). The Metabolic and Molecular Bases of Inherited Disease, 7th ed. New York: McGraw-Hill, 1995:749–794.

Eriksson M, Bergstrom M: Familial malignant blood disease in the county of Jamtland, Sweden. Eur J Haematol 1987; 38:241–245.

Eriksson M, Hallberg B: Familial occurrence of hematologic malignancies and other diseases in multiple myeloma: a case-control study. Cancer Causes Control 1992; 3:63–67.

Escobar V, Bixler D: Familial reticulum cell sarcoma. Birth Defects 1976; 12:151–158.

Eyster ME, Saletan SL, Rabellino EM, Karanas A, McDonald TP, Locke LA, Luderer JR: Familial essential thrombocythemia. Am J Med 1986; 80:497–502.

Fairrie G, Black AJ, McKenzie AW: Polycythaemia rubra vera and congenital deafness in monozygotic twins. Br Med J 1981; 283:192–193.

Falleta JM, Starling KA, Fernbach DJ: Leukemia in twins. Pediatrics 1973; 52:846–849.

Fazekas VT, Bach K, Toth S, Bodor F: Familiares vorkommen von chronischer lymphatischer Leukamie: HLA-antigen und zytogenetische Untersuchungen. Wien Med Wochenschr 1978; 9:262–264.

Feingold et al.: 1995.

Feldman JG, Lee SL, Seligman B: Occurrence of acute leukemia in females in a genetically isolated population. Cancer 1976; 38:2548–2550.

Felix CA, D'Amico D, Mitsudomi T, Nau MM, Li FP, Fraumeni JF Jr, Cole DE, McCalla J, Reaman GH, Whang-Peng J, et al.: Absence of hereditary *p53* mutations in 10 familial leukemia pedigrees. J Clin Invest 1992; 90:653–658.

Fenaux P: Myelodysplastic syndromes or refractory anemias. (In French.) Rev Prat 1993; 43(11):1379–1385.

Ferguson SW, Lynn TN: Familial leukemia: a report of 4 cases of acute leukemia in 4 consecutive generations. South Med J 1970; 63:1337–1340.

Fernandez-Robles E, Verymlen C, Martiat P, Ninane J, Cornu G: Familial essential thrombocythemia. Pediatr Hematol Oncol 1990; 7:373–376.

Ferraris AM, Racchi O, Rapezzi D, Gaetani GF, Boffetta P: Familial Hodgkin's disease: a disease of young adulthood? Ann Hematol 1997; 74:131–134.

Ferro MT, Garcia-Sagredo JM, Resino M, del Potro E, Villegas A, Mediavilla J, Espinos D, San Roman C: Chromosomal disorder and neoplastic diseases in a family with inherited fragile 16. Cancer Genet Cytoget 1994; 78:160–164.

Fickers M, Speck B: Thrombocythaemia: familial occurrence and transition into blastic crisis. Acta Haematol 1974; 51:257–265.

Filipovich AH, Heinitz KJ, Robison LL, Frizzera G: The immunodeficiency cancer registry: a research resource. Am J Pediatr Hematol Oncol 1987; 9:183–184.

Finch SC, Linet MS: Chronic leukaemias. Baillieres Best Pract Res Clin Haematol 1992; 5:27–56.

Fine JM, Muller JY, Rochu D, Marneux M, Gorin NC, Fine A, Lambin P: Waldenstrom's macroglobulinemia in monzygotic twins. Acta Med Scand 1986; 220:369–373.

Fitzgerald PH, Hamer JW: Third case of chronic lymphocytic leukaemia in a carrier of the inherited Ch1 chromosome. Br Med J 1969; 3:752–754.96.

Ford AM, Bennett CA, Price CM, Bruin MCA, van Wering ER, Greaves MF: Fetal origins of the TEL-AML fusion gene in identical twins with leukemia. Proc Natl Acad Sci USA 1998; 8:4584–4588.

Ford AM, Pombo de Oliveira MS, McCarthy KP, MacLean JM, Carrico KC, Vincent RF, Greaves M: Monoclonal origin of concordant T-cell malignancy in identical twins. Blood 1997b; 89:281–285.

Ford AM, Ridge SA, Cabrera ME, Mahmoud H, Steel CM, Chan LC, Greaves M: In utero rearrangements in the trithorax-related oncogene in infant leukaemias. Nature 1993:358–360.

Fraumeni JF: Family studies in Hodgkin's disease. Cancer Res 1974; 34:1164–1165.

Freedman MH, Bonilla MA, Fier C, Bolyard AA, Scarlata D, Boxer LA, Brown S, Cham B, Kannourakis G, Kinsey SE, et al.: Myelodysplasia syndrome and acute myeloid leukemia in patients with congenital neutropenia receiving G-CSF therapy. Blood 2000; 96:429–436.

Freeman AI, Sinks LF, Cohen MM: Lymphosarcoma in siblings, associated with cytogenetic abnormalities, immune deficiency, and abnormal erythropoiesis. J Pediatr 1970; 77:996–1003.

Freireich EJ, Lemark NA: Milestones in Leukemia Research and Therapy. Baltimore: Johns Hopkins University Press, 1991.

Friedland ML, Wittels EG, Robinson RJ: Polycythemia vera in identical twins. Am J Hematol 1981; 10:101–103.

Frizzera G, Rosai J, Dehner LP, Spector BD, Kersey JH: Lymphoreticular disorders in primary immunodeficiencies: new findings based on an up-to-date histologic classification of 35 cases. Cancer 1980; 46:692–699.

Fujino T, Nagata Y: HTLV-I transmission from mother to child. J Reprod Immunol 2000; 47:197–206.

Futaki M, Yamashita T, Yagasaki H, Toda T, Yabe M, Kato S, Asano S, Nakahata T: The IVS4 +4 A to T mutation of the fanconi anemia gene *FANCC* is not associated with a severe phenotype in Japanese patients. Blood 2000; 95:1493–1498.

Gale RP, Cozen W, Goodman MT, Wang FF, Bernstein L: Decreased chronic lymphocytic leukemia incidence in Asians in Los Angeles County. Leuk Res 2000; 24:665–669.

Gao Q, Horwitz M, Roulston D, Hagos F, Zhao N, Freireich EJ, Gastinaeu D, Olopade OI: Linkage of a familial acute myeloid leukemia (AML) locus to 16q22 and evidence for a secondary critical region at 5q32–33. Genes Chromosomes Cancer 2000; 28:164–172.

Gatti RA: Ataxia-telangiectasia. In: Vogelstein B and Kinzler KW (eds). The Genetic Basis of Human Cancer. New York: McGraw-Hill, 1998:275–300.

Gatti RA, Tward A, Concannon P: Cancer risk in ATM heterozygotes: a model of phenotypic and mechanistic differences between missense and truncating mutations. Mol Genet Metab 1999; 68:419–423.

Gausch J: Heredite des leucemies. Sang 1954; 25:384–421.

Gazda H, Lipton JM, Willig TN, Ball S, Niemeyer CM, Tchernia G, Mohandas N, Daly MJ, Ploszynska A, Orfali KA, et al.: Evidence for linkage of familial Diamond-Blackfan anemia to chromosome 8p23.3–p22 and for non-19q non-8p disease. Blood 2001; 97:2145–2150.

Gencik A, Buser M, Temminck B, Obrecht JP, Weber W, Muller H: High incidence of stomach cancer in relatives of patients with malignant lymphoproliferative disorders. Cancer Detect Prev Suppl 1987; 1:121–125.

Geraedts JP, Ford CE, Briet E, Hartgrink-Groeneveld CA, den Ottolander GJ: Klinefelter syndrome: a predisposition to acute non-lymphocytic leukaemia? Lancet 1980; 1:1092.

German J: Bloom's syndrome: XX. The first 100 cancers. Cancer Genet Cytogenet 1997; 93:100–106.

Gerrard JM, Israels ED, Bishop AJ, Schroeder ML, Beattle LL, McNicol A, Israels SJ, Walz D, Greenberg AH, Ray M, et al.: Inherited platelet-storage pool deficiency associated with a high incidence of acute myeloid leukaemia. Br J Haematol 1991; 79:246–255.

Gilbert HS: Familial meyloproliferative disease. In: Wasserman BB (ed). Polycythemia vera and the myeloproliferative disorders. New York: W. B. Saunders, 1995:222–225.

Gill Super HJ, Rothberg PG, Kobayashi H, Freeman A, Diaz MD, Rowley JD: Clonal, nonconstitutional rearrangements of the MLL gene in infant twins with acute lymphoblastic leukemia: in utero chromosome rearrangment of 11q23. Blood 1994; 83:641–644.

Glazer ER, Perkins CI, Young JL, Schlag RD, Campleman SL, Wright WE. Cancer among Hispanic children in California 1988–1994. Cancer 1999; 86: 1070–1079.

Gokhale DA, Evans DG, Crowther D, Woll P, Watson CJ, Dearden SP, Fergusson WD, Stevens RF, Taylor GM: Molecular genetic analysis of a family with a history of Hodgkin's disease and dyschondrosteosis. Leukemia 1995: 9:826–833.

Goldgar DE, Easton DF, Cannon-Albright LA, Skolnick MH: Systematic population-based assessment of cancer risk in first-degree relatives of cancer probands. J Natl Cancer Inst 1994; 86:1600–1608.

Goldin LR, Sgambati M, Marti GE, Fontaine L, Ishibe N, Caporaso N: Anticipation in familial chronic lymphocytic leukemia. Am J Hum Genet 1999; 65:265–269.

Gracz K, Kofman S, Economou SG: Hodgkin's disease in monozygotic twins: a case report. J Surg Oncol 1979; 12:221.

Gramatovici M, Bennett JM, Hiscock JG, Grewal KS: Three cases of familial hairy cell leukemia. Am J Hematol 1993; 42:337–339.

Grant JA, Blumenschein GR, Buckley CE: Familial paraproteinemia. Arch Intern Med 1971; 128:427–431.

Greene MH, Pinto H, Kant J, Siler K, Vonderheid E, Lamberg SI, Dalager NA: Lymphomas and leukemias in the relatives of patients with mycosis fungoides. Cancer 1982; 49:731–741.

Greenwald P, Woodard E, Nasca PC, Hempelmann L, Dayton P, Maksymowicz G, Blando P, Hanrahan R, Burnett WS: Morbidity and mortality among recipients of blood from preleukemic and prelymphomatous donors. Cancer 1976; 38:324–328.

Greer JP, Macon WR, List AF, McCurley TL: Non-Hodgkin's lymphomas. In: Lee GR, Bithell TC, Foerster J, Athens JW, Lukens JN (eds). Wintrobe's Clinical Hematology, 9th ed. Philadelphia: Lea and Febiger, 1993:2082–2142.

Grierson HL, Skare J, Church J, Silberman T, Davis JR, Kobrinsky N, McGregor R, Israels S, McCarty J, Andrews LG, et al.: Evaluation of families wherein a single male manifests a phenotype of X-linked lymphoproliferative disease (XLP). Am J Med Genet 1993; 47:458–463.

Grimwade DJ, Stephenson J, DeSilva C, Dalton RG, Mufti GJ: Familial MDS with 5q-abnormality. Br J Haematol 1993; 84:536–538.

Groopman JE, Broder S: Cancers in AIDS and other immunodeficiency states. In: DeVita VT, Hellman S, Rosenberg SA (eds). Cancer: Principles and Practice of Oncology, 3rd ed. Philadelphia: J. B. Lippincott, 1989:1953–1970.

Groupe Français de Cytogenetique Hematologique: Cytogenetic findings in leukemic cells of 56 patients with constitutional chromosome abnormalities: a cooperative study. Cancer Genet Cytogenet 1988; 35:243–252.

Groupe Français de Cytogenetique Hematologique: Forty-four cases of childhood myelodysplasia with cytogenetics, documented by the Groupe Français de Cytogenetique Hematologique. Leukemia 1997; 11:1478–1485.

Grufferman S, Cole P, Smith PG, Lukes RJ: Hodgkin's disease in siblings. N Engl J Med 1977; 296:248–250.

Gunz FW: Incidence of some aetiological factors in human leukaemia. Br Med J 1961; 1:326–327.

Gunz FW: Leukaemia in New Zealand and Australia. Path Microbiol 1963; 27:697–704.

Gunz FW, Fitzgerald PH, Adams A: An abnormal chromosome in chronic lymphocytic leukaemia. Br Med J 1962; 2:1097.

Gunz FW, Fitzgerald PH, Crossen PE, Mackenzie IS, Powles CP, Jensen GR: Multiple cases of leukemia in a sibship. Blood 1966; 27:482–489.

Gunz FW, Gunz JP, Veale AM, Chapman CJ, Houston IB: Familial leukaemia: a study of 909 families. Scand J Haematol 1975; 15:117–131.

Gunz FW, Gunz JP, Vincent PC, Bergin M, Johnson FL, Bashir H, Kirk RL: Thirteen cases of leukemia in a family. J Natl Cancer Inst 1978; 60:1243–1250.

Gunz FW, Veale AM: Leukemia in close relatives: accident or predisposition? J Natl Cancer Inst 1969; 42:517–524.

Gunz G, Dameshek W: Chronic lymphocytic leukemia in a family, including twin brothers and a son. J Am Med Assoc 1957; 164:1323–1325.

Gurney JG, Severson RK, Davis S, Robison LL: Incidence of cancer in children in the United States. Cancer 1995; 75:2186–2195.

Gutmann DH, Collins FS: von Recklinghausen Neurofibromatosis. In: Scriber CR, Beaudet AL, Sly WS, Valle D (eds). The Metabolic and Molecular Bases of Inherited Disease, 7th ed. New York: McGraw-Hill, 1995:677–696.

Haenszel W: Cancer mortality among U.S. Jews. Isr J Med Sci 1971; 7:1437–1450.

Haim N, Cohen Y, Robinson E: Malignant lymphoma in first-degree blood relatives. Cancer 1982; 49:2197–2200.

Hakim I, Amariglio N, Brok-Simoni F, Berkowitz M, Rosner E, Kneller A, Hulu N, Ramot B, Ben-Bassat I, Silverman GJ, Rechavi G: Preferred usage of specific immunoglobulin gene segments in chronic lymphocytic leukaemia cells of three HLA-identical sisters. Br J Haematol 1995; 91:915–917.

Halperin DS, Freedman MH: Diamond-Blackfan anemia: etiology, pathophysiology, and treatment. Am J Pediat Hemat Oncol 1989; 11:380–394.

Hartley SE, Sainsbury C: Acute leukaemia and the same chromosome abnormality in monozygotic twins. Hum Genet 1981; 58:408–410.

Hartwell L: Defects in a cell cycle checkpoint may be responsible for the genomic instability of cancer cells. Cell 1992; 71:543–546.

Hasle H, Kerndrup G, Jacobsen BB: Childhood myelodysplastic syndrome in Denmark: incidence and predisposing conditions. Leukemia 1995; 9:1569–1572.

Hasle H, Olsen J: Cancer in relatives of children with myelodsyplastic syndrome, acute and chronic myeloid leukemia. Br J Haematol 1997; 97:123–126.

Hawkins MM, Draper GJ, Winter DL: Cancer in the offspring of survivors of childhood leukaemia and non-Hodgkin lymphomas. Br J Cancer 1995; 71:1335–1339.

Hernandez JA, Land K, McKenna RW: Leukemias, myeloma, and other lymphoreticular neoplasm. Cancer 1995; 75:381–394.

Heyssel R, Brill B, Woodbury LA, Nishimura ET, Ghose T, Hoshino T, Yamasaki M: Leukemia in Hiroshima atomic bomb survivors. Blood 1960; 15:313–331.

Hibino S, Takikawa K, Kimura K: Incidence and treatment of leukemia in Japan, with reference to alanine nitrogen mustard. In: Proceedings of the Sixth International Congress of International Society of Hematology. New York: Grune and Stratton, 1958:172.

Ho CY, Otterud B, Legare RD, Varvil T, Saxena R, DeHart DB, Kohler SE, Aster JC, Dowton SB, Li FP, et al.: Linkage of a familial platelet disorder with a propensity to develop myeloid malignancies to human chromosome 21q22.1–22.2. Blood 1996; 87:5218–5224.

Holton CP, Johnson WW: Chronic myelocytic leukemia in infant siblings. J Pediatr 1968; 72:377–383.

Homans A, Verissimo AM, Vlacha V: Transient abnormal myelopoiesis of infancy associated with trisomy 21. Am J Pediatr Hematol Oncol 1993; 15:392–399.

Hors J, Dausset J: HLA and susceptibility to Hodgkin's disease. Immunol Rev 1983; 70:167–192.

Horsman DE, Tapio Pantzar J, Dill FJ, Kalousek DK: Klinefelter's syndrome and acute leukaemia. Cancer Genet Cytogent 1987; 26:275–276.

Horwitz LJ, Levy RN, Rosner F: Multiple myeloma in three siblings. Arch Intern Med 1985; 145:1449–1450.

Horwitz M: The genetics of familial leukemia. Leukemia 1997; 11:1347–1359.

Horwitz M: Epidemiology and genetics of acute and chronic leukemia. In: Weirnik PH (ed). Adult Leukemias. Hamilton, ON: B.C. Decker, 2001:1–18.

Horwitz M, Benson KF, Li F-Q, Wolff J, Leppert MF, Hobson L, Mangelsdorf M, Yu S, Hewett D, Richards RI, Raskind WH: Genetic heterogeneity in familial acute myelogenous leukemia: evidence for a second locus at chromosome 16q21–23.2. Am J Hum Genet 1997; 61:873–881.

Horwitz M, Benson KF, Person RE, Aprikyan AG, Dale DC: Mutations in *ELA2*, encoding neutrophil elastase, define a 21-day biological clock in cyclic haematopoiesis. Nat Genet 1999; 23:433–436.

Horwitz M, Goode EL, Jarvik GP: Anticipation in familial leukemia. Am J Hum Genet 1996; 59:990–998.

Horwitz M, Wiernik PH: Pseudoautosomal linkage of Hodgkin disease. Am J Hum Genet 1999; 65:1413–1422.

Houlston RS, Catovsky D, Yuille MR: Pseudoautosomal linkage in chronic lymphocytic leukaemia. Br J Haematol 2000; 109:899–900.

Hudson RP, Wilson SJ: Hypogammaglobulinemia and chronic lymphatic leukemia. Cancer 1960; 13:200–204.

Huret JL, Leonard C, Chery M, Philippe C, Shafei-Benaissa E, Lefaure G, Labrune B, Gilgenkrantz S: Monosomy 21q: two cases of del(21q) and review of the literature. Clin Genet 1995; 48:140–147.

Imamura J, Miyoshi I, Koeffler HP: p53 in hematologic malignancies. Blood 1994; 84:2412–2421.

Iselius L, Gustavson KH: Spatial distribution of the gene for infantile genetic agranulocytosis. Hum Hered 1984; 34:358–363.

Ishikawa S, Ishikawa M, Tokuda T, Yoshida K, Wakui K, Matsuura S, Ohara S, Sekijima Y, Hidaka E, Fukushima Y, et al.: Japanese family with an autosomal dominant chromosome instability syndrome: a new neurodegenerative disease? Am J Med Genet 2000; 94:265–270.

Isobe et al., 1981.

Jacobs PA, Melville M, Ratcliffe S: A cytogenetic survey of 11,680 newborn infants. Ann Hum Genet 1974; 37:359–376.

Jacobsen P, Hauge M, Henningsen K, Hobolth N, Mikkelsen M, Philip: An (11;21) translocation in four generations with chromosome 11 abnormalities in the offspring. Hum Hered 1973; 23:568–585.

Janssen JW, Anger BR, Drexler HG, Bartram CR, Heimpel H: Essential thrombocythemia in two sisters originating from different stem cell levels. Blood 1990; 75:1633–1636.

Jaspers NG, Gatti RA, Baan C, Linssen PC, Bootsma D: Genetic complementation analysis of ataxia telangiectasia and Nijmegen breakage syndrome: a survey of 50 patients. Cytogenet Cell Genet 1988; 49:259–263.

Jelicka VL, Hermanska Z, Smida I, Kouba A: Paramyeloblastic leukaemia appearing simultaneously in two blood cousins after simultaneous contact with gammexane (hexachlorcylohexane). Acta Med Scand 1958; 141:447–451.

Joenje H, Oostra AB, Wijker M, di Summa FM, van Berkel CG, Rooimans MA, Ebell W, van Weel M, Pronk JC, Buchwald M, Arwert F: Evidence for at least eight Fanconi anemia genes. Am J Hum Genet 1997; 61:940–944.

Joenje H, Patel KJ: The emerging genetic and molecular basis of Fanconi anemia. Nat Rev Genet 2001; 2:446–457.

Johnson EJ, Scherer SW, Osborne L, Tsui LC, Oscier D, Mould S, Cotter FE: Molecular definition of a narrow interval at 7q22.1 associated with myelodysplasia. Blood 1996; 87:3579–3586.

Johnson MJE, Peters CH: Four cases of leukemia reported in one South Dakota family. J Indiana State Med Assoc 1957; 50:206.

Jones C, Penny L, Mattina T, Yu S, Baker E, Voullaire L, Langdon WY, Sutherland GR, Richards RI, Tunnacliffe A: Association of a chromosome deletion syndrome with a fragile site within the proto-oncogene *CBL2*. Nature 1995; 376:145–149.

Juberg RC, Jones B: The Christchurch chromosome (Gp-). Mongolism, erythroleukemia and an inherited Gp- chromosome (Christchurch). N Engl J Med 1970; 282:292–297.

Judson IR, Wiltshaw E, Newland AC: Multiple myleoma in a pair of monozygotic twins: the first reported case. Br J Haematol 1985; 60:551–554.

Kajii T, Neu RL, Gardner LI: Chromosome abnormalities in lymph node cells from patient with familial lymphoma. Cancer 1968; 22:218–224.

Kalyanaraman VS, Sarngadharan MG, Robert-Guroff M, Miyoshi I, Golde D, Gallo RC: A new subtype of human T-cell leukemia virus (HTLV-II) associated with a T-cell variant of hairy cell leukemia. Science 1982; 218:571–573.

Kastan MB, Lim DS: The many substrates and functions of ATM. Nat Rev Mol Cell Biol 2000; 1:179–186.

Kato S, Tsuji K, Tsunematsu Y, Koide R, Utsumi J: Familial leukemia: HLA system and leukemia predisposition in a family. Am J Dis Child 1983; 137:641–644.

Kaufman S, Briere J, Bernard J: Syndromes myeloproliferatifs familiaux: ètude à propos de six families et revue de la litterature. Nouv Rev Fr Hematol 1978; 20:1–16.

Kaur J, Catovsky D, Valdimarsson H, Jensson O, Sjpiers ASD: Familial acute myeloid leukaemia with acquired Pelger-Huet anomaly and aneuploidy of C group. Br Med J 1972; 4:327–333.

Kende G, Toren A, Mandel M, Neumann Y, Kenet G, Brok-Simoni F, Ramot B, Ben-Bassat I, Rechavi G: Familial leukemia: description of two kindreds and a review of the genetic aspects of the disease. Acta Haematol 1994; 92:208–211.

Kikuchi M, Tayama T, Hayakawa H, Takahashi I, Hoshino H, Ohsaka A: Familial thrombocytosis. Br J Haematol 1995; 89:900–902.

King H, Diamond E, Bailar JC: Cancer mortality and religious preference: a suggested method in research. Milbank Mem Fund Q 1965; 43:349–358.

Kitao S, Shimamoto A, Goto M, Miller RW, Smithson WA, Lindor NM, Furuichi Y: Mutations in RECQL4 cause a subset of cases of Rothmund-Thomson syndrome. Nat Genet 1999; 22:82–84.

Klitz W, Aldrich CL, Fildes N, Horning SJ, Begovich AB: Localization of predisposition to Hodgkin disease in the HLA class II region. Am J Hum Genet 1994; 54:497–505.

Korenberg JR, Chen X-N, Schipper R, Sun Z, Gonsky R, Gerwehr S, Carpenter N, Daumer C, Dignan P, Disteche C, et al.: Down syndrome phenotypes: the consequences of chromosomal imbalance. Proc Natl Acad Sci USA 1994; 91:4997–5001.

Kralovics R, Prchal JT: Congenital and inherited polycythemia. Curr Opin Pediat 2000; 12:29–34.

Krontiris TG, DiMartino NA, Colb M, Parkinson DR: Unique allelic restriction fragments of the human Ha-ras locus in leukocyte and tumour DNAs of cancer patients. Nature 1985; 313:369–374.

Kurita S, Kamei Y: Genetics of familial leukemia. Jinrui Idengaku Zasshi 1969; 14:163–179. In Japanese.

Kurita S, Kamei Y, Ota K: Genetic studies on familial leukemia. Cancer 1974; 34:1098–1101.

Lardi A, Taha OM, Al-Jefri A, Ahmed MA: Familial chronic myelocytic leukaemia-like syndrome probably of congenital origin. Acta Paediatr 1994; 83:558–560.

Largaespada DA, Brannan CI, Shaughnessy JD, Jenkins NA, Copeland NG: The neurofibromatosis type 1 (NF1) tumor suppressor gene and myeloid leukemia. Curr Top Microbiol Immunol 1996; 211:233–239.

Larsen WE, Schimke RN: Familial acute myelogenous leukemia with associated C-monosomy in two affected members. Cancer 1976; 38:841–845.

Law IP, Herberman RB, Oldham RK, Bouzoukis J, Hanson SM, Rhode MC: Familial occurrence of colon and uterine carcinoma and of lymphoproliferative malignancies: clinical description. Cancer 1977; 39:1224–1228.

Lawrence JH, Goetsch AT: Familial occurrence of polycythemia and leukemia. Calif Med 1950; 73:361–364.

LeDeist F, de Saint Basile G, Coulombel L, Breton-Gorius J, Maier-Redelsperger M, Beljorde K, Bremard C, Griscelli C: A familial occurrence of natural killer cell-T-lympocyte proliferation disease in two children. Cancer 1991; 67:2610–2617.

Lee HW, Blasco MA, Gottlieb GJ, Horner JW 2nd, Greider CW, DePinho RA: Essential role of mouse telomerase in highly proliferative organs. Nature 1998; 392(6676):569–574.

Lee EJ, Schiffer CA, Misawa S, Testa JR: Clinical and cytogenetic features of familial erythroleukaemia. Br J Haematol 1987; 65:313–320.

Lee M, Lee JO, Seo HZ: Clinical and statistical observations on malignant tumors. Korean J Hematol 1967; 2:23.

Legare RD, Lu D, Gallagher M, Ho C, Tan X, Barker G, Shimizu K, Ohki M, Lenny N, Hiebert S, Gilliland DG: *CBFA2*, frequently rearranged in leukemia, is not responsible for a familial leukemia syndrome. Leukemia 1997; 11:2111–2119.

Li F, Hecht F, Kaiser-McCaw B, Baranko PV, Upp Potter N: Ataxia-pancytopenia: syndrome of cerebellar ataxia, hypoplastic anemia, monosmy 7, and acute myelogenous leukemia. Cancer Genet Cytogenet 1981; 4:189–196.

Lilly F, Pincus T: Genetic control of murine viral leukemogenesis. Adv Cancer Res 1973; 17:231–277.

Lindor NM, Devries EMG, Michels VV, Schad CR, Jalal SM, Donovan KM, Smithson WA, Kvols LK, Thibodeau SN, Dewald GW: Rothmund-Thomson syndrome in siblings: evidence for acquired in vivo mosaicism. Clin Genet 1996; 49:124–129.

Linet MS: The Leukemias: Epidemiologic Aspects. New York: Oxford University Press, 1985.

Linet MS, Devesa SS: Descriptive epidemiology of childhood leukaemia. Br J Cancer 1991; 63:424–429.

Linet MS, Humphrey RL, Mehl ES, Brown LM, Pottern LM, Bias WB, McCaffrey L: A case-control and family study of Waldenstrom's macroglobulinemia. Leukemia 1993; 7:1363–1369.

Linet MS, Pottern LM: Familial aggregation of hematopoietic malignancies and risk of non-Hodgkin's lymphoma. Cancer Res 1992; 52:5468s–5473s.

Linet MS, Van Natta ML, Brookmeyer R, Khoury MJ, McCaffrey LD, Humphrey RL, Szklo M: Familial cancer history and chronic lymphocytic leukemia. Am J Epidemiol 1989; 130:655–664.

Longpre B: Deux nouveaux cas d'erythremie familiale: association de l'erythremie et d'une hemopathie maligne. Can Med Assoc J 1966; 95:859–861.

Look AT: Oncogenic transcription factors in the human acute leukemias. Science 1997; 278:1059–1064.

Lo Ten Foe JR, Rooimans MA, Bosnoyan-Collins L, Alon N, Wijker M, Parker L, Lightfoot J, Carreau M, Callen DF, Savoia A, et al.: Expression cloning of a cDNA for the major Fanconi anaemia gene, *FAA*. Nat Genet 1996; 14:320–323.

Loughran TP, Coyle T, Sherman MP, Starkebaum G, Ehrlich GD, Ruscetti FW, Poiesz BJ: Detection of human T-cell leukemia/lymphoma virus, type II in a patient with LGL leukemia. Blood 1992; 80:1116–1119.

Loughran TP, Kidd P, Poiesz BJ: Familial occurrence of LGL leukaemia. Br J Haematol 1994; 87:199–201.

Lucas GS, West RR, Jacobs A: Familial myelodysplasia. Br Med J 1989; 299:551.

Lukens JN: Classification and differentiation of the acute leukemia. In: Lee GR, Bitnell TC, Foerster J, Athens JW, Lukens JN (eds). Wintrobe's Clinical Hematology. 9th Edition. Philadelphia: Lea and Febiger, 1993:1873–1891.

Luna-Fineman S, Shannon KM, Lange BJ: Childhood monosomy 7: epidemiology, biology, and mechanistic implications. Blood 1995; 85:1985–1999.

Luo L, Lu FM, Hart S, Foroni L, Rabbani H, Hammarstrom L, Yuille MR, Catovsky D, Webster AD, Vorechovsky I: Ataxia-telangiectasia and T-cell leukemias: no evidence for somatic *ATM* mutation in sporadic T-ALL or for hypermethylation of the ATM-NPAT/E14 bidirectional promoter in T-PLL. Cancer Res 1998; 58:2293–2297.

Lyn D, Cherney BW, Lalande M, Berenson JR, Lichenstein A, Lupold S, Bhatia KG, Smulson M: A duplicated region is responsible for the poly(ADP-ribose) polymerase polymorphism, on chromosome 13, associated with a predisposition to cancer. Am J Hum Genet 1993; 52:124–134.

Lynch HT, Marcus JN, Lynch JF: Genetics of Hodgkin's and non-Hodgkin's lymphoma: a review. Cancer Invest 1992; 10:247–256.

Lynch HT, Marcus JN, Weisenburger DD, Watson P, Fitzsimmons ML, Grierson H, Smith DM, Lynch J, Purtilo D: Genetic and immunopathological findings in a lymphoma family. Br J Cancer 1989; 59:622–626.

Lynch HT, Schuelke GS: Mendelian predisposition to lymphomagenesis. In: Purtilo DT (ed). Immune Deficiency and Cancer. New York: Plenum Medical Book Co., 1984:401–425.

Machura B, Piestrak J, Kreps Z: Przypadek rodzinnej bialaczki. Przegl Lek: A case of familial leukemia (Polish) 1970; 26:720–722.

Mack TM, Cozen W, Shibata DK, Weiss LM, Nathwani BN, Hernandez AM, Taylor CR, Hamilton AS, Deapen DM, Rappaport EB: Concordance for Hodgkin's disease in identical twins suggesting genetic susceptibility to the young-adult form of the disease. N Engl J Med 1995; 7:413–418.

MacMahon B, Koller KF: Ethnic differences in the incidence of leukemia. Blood 1957; 12:1–10.

MacSween RN: Reticulum-cell sarcoma and rheumatoid arthritis in a patient with XY/XXY/XXXY Klinefelter's syndrome and normal intelligence. Lancet 1965; 1:460–461.

Mahgoub N, Taylor BR, Le Beau MM, Gratiot M, Carlson KM, Atwater SK, Jacks T, Shannon KM: Myeloid malignancies induced by alkylating agents in Nf1 mice. Blood 1999; 93:3617–3623.

Malkin D: Germline *p53* mutations and heritable cancer. Annu Rev Genet 1994; 28:443–465.

Manoharan A, Garson OM: Familial polycythaemia vera: a study of three sisters. Scand J Haematol 1976; 17:10–16.

Manson DI: Multiple myeloma in sisters. Scott Med J 1961; 6:188.

Markkanen A, Ruutu T, Rasi V, K Franssila, Knuutila S, de la Chapelle A: Constitutional translocation t(3;6)(p14;p11) in a family with hematologic malignancies. Cancer Genet Cytogenet 1987; 25:87–95.

Martin AO, Dunn JK, Smalley B: Use of geneologically linked data base in the analysis of cancer in a human isolate. Banbury Rep 1980; 4:235–255.

Matsuura S, Tauchi H, Nakamura A, Kondo N, Sakamoto S, Endo S, Smeets D, Solder B, Belohradsky BH, Der Kaloustian VM, et al.: Positional cloning of the gene for Nijmegen breakage syndrome. Nat Genet 1998; 19:179–181.

Matutes E, Spittle MF, Smith NP, Eady RAJ, Catovsky D: The first report of familial adult T-cell leukaemia lymphoma in the United Kingdom. Br J Haematol 1995; 89:615–619.

McPhedran P, Clar WH, Lee J: Patterns of familial leukemia: ten cases of leukemia in two interrelated families. Cancer 1969; 24:403–407.

Meisner L, Gilbert E, Ris H, Haverty G: Genetic mechanisms in cancer predisposition: report of a cancer family. Cancer 1978; 43:679–689.

Merk K, Bjorkholm M, Tullgren O, Mellstedt H, Holm G: Immune deficiency in family members of patients with Hodgkin's disease. Cancer 1990; 66:1938–1943.

Meruelo D, Bach R: Genetics of resistance to virus-induced leukemias. Adv Cancer Res 1983; 40:107–188.

Michaud J, Wu F, Osato M, Cottles GM, Yanagida M, Asou N, Shigesada K, Ito Y, Benson KF, Raskind WH, et al.: In vitro analyses of known and novel *RUNX1* mutations in dominant familial platelet disorder with predisposition to acute myelogenous leukemia (FPD/AML): implications for mechanisms of pathogenesis. Blood; in press.

Miliani A, Bergesio F, Salvadori M, Amantini A, Macucci M, Arbustini E, Becucci A, Sodi A, Zuccarini S, Menicucci A, et al.: Familial AL-amyloidosis in three Italian siblings. Haematologica 1996; 81(2):105–109.

Miller RL, Purvis JD, Weick JK: Familial polycythemia vera. Cleve Clin J Med 1989; 56:813–818.
Miller RW: Deaths from childhood cancer in sibs. N Engl J Med 1968; 279(3):122–126.
Milligan DW, Stark AN, Bynoe AG: Hairy cell leukaemia in two brothers. Clin Lab Haematol 1987; 9:321–325.
Minelli A, Morerio C, Maserati E, Olivieri C, Panarello C, Bonvini L, Leszl A, Rosanda C, Lanino E, Danesino C, Pasquali F: Meiotic origin of trisomy in neoplasms: evidence in a case of erythroleukaemia. Leukemia 2001; 15:971–975.
Mishra SI, Luce-Aoelua PH, Wilkens LR: Cancer among indigenous populations: the experience of American Samoans. Cancer 1996; 78:1553–1557.
Mittelman M, Lewinski UH, Weiss H, Cohen AM, Djaldetii M, Pick AI: Secondary myelodysplastic syndrome in multiple myeloma: a study of nine patients with an attempt to detect myeloma patients at risk. Haematologia 1994; 26:67–74.
Modan B: An epidemiological study of polycythemia vera. Blood 1965; 26:657–667.
Morrell D, Cromartie E, Swift M: Mortality and cancer incidence in 263 patients with ataxia-telangiectasia. J Natl Cancer Inst 1986; 77:89–92.
Mueller BU, Pizzo PA: Cancer in children with primary or secondary immunodeficiencies. J Pediatrics 1995; 126:1–10.
Muftuoglu AU, Akman N, Savas I: Polycythemia vera associated with Usher's syndrome. Am J Ophthalmol 1975; 80:93–95.
Muts-Homsma SJM, Muller HP, Geraedst JPM: Klinefelter's syndrome and acute nonlymphocytic leukemia. Blut 1981; 44:15–20.
Nadeau LA, Magalini SI, Stefanini M: Familial multiple myeloma. Arch Path 1956; 61:101–106.
Nadler SB, Cohn I: Familial polycythemia. Am J Med Sci 1939; 198:41–48.
Nichamin SB: Ein Fall von Erythamie (*Polyglobulia splenomegalica*). Folia Haemtol 1908; 6:301.
Niikawa N, Deng H-X, Abe K, Harada N, Okada T, Tsuchiya H, Akaboshi I, Matsuda I, Fukushima Y, Kaneko Y, et al.: Possible mapping of the gene for transient myeloproliferative syndrome at 21q11.2. Hum Genet 1991; 87:561–566.
Nishiyama H, Mokuno J, Inoue T: Relative frequency and mortality rate of various types of leukemia in Japan. Jpn J Cancer Res 1969; 60:71–81.
Okano M: Epstein-Barr virus infection and its role in the expanding spectrum of human diseases. Acta Paediatr 1998; 87:11–18.
Olopade OI, Roulston D, Baker T, Narvid S, LeBeau MM, Freireich EJ, Larson RA, Golomb, HM: Familial myeloid leukemia associated with loss of the long arm of chromosome 5. Leukemia 1996; 10:669–674.
Ordway JM, Tallaksen-Greene S, Gutekunst CA, Bernstein EM, Cearley JA, Wiener HW, Dure LS, Lindsey R, Hersch SM, Jope RS, et al.: Ectopically expressed CAG repeats cause intranuclear inclusions and a progressive late onset neurological phenotype in the mouse. Cell 1997; 91:753–763.
Osato M, Asou N, Abdalla E, Hoshino K, Yamasaki H, Okubo T, Suzushima H, Takatsuki K, Kanno T, Shigesada K, Ito Y: Biallelic and heterozygous point mutations in the runt domain of the AML1/PEBP2αB gene associated with myeloblastic leukemias. Blood 1999; 93:1817–1824.
Osler W: The Principles and Practice of Medicine. New York: D. Appleton, 1892.
Owen T: A case of polycythemia vera with special reference to the familial features and treatment with phenyl-hydrazin. Bull Johns Hopkins Hosp 1924; 35:258–260.
Palmer CG, Heerema NA, Greist A, Tricot G, Hoffman R: Cytogenetic findings in siblings with a myelodysplastic syndrome. Cancer Genet Cytogenet 1987; 27:241–249.
Papageorgio C, Seiter K, Feldman EJ: Therapy-related myelodysplastic syndrome in adults with neurofibromatosis. Leuk Lymphoma 1999; 32:605–608.
Parentesis JP: Genetic predisposition and treatment-related leukemia. Med Pediatr Oncol 2001; 36:541–548.
Parker SL, Tong T, Bolden S, Wingo PA: Cancer statistics. CA Cancer J Clin 1997; 47:5–27.
Passmore SJ, Hann IM, Stiller CA, Ramani P, Swansbury GJ, Gibbons B, Reeves BR, Chessells JM: Pediatric meylodysplasia: a study of 68 children and a new prognostic scoring system. Blood 1995; 85:1742–1750.
Patakfalvi A, Csete B, Horvath T: Familial myelofibrosis. Haematologia 1969; 3214–3218.
Pendergrass TW, Stoller RG, Mann DL, Halterman RH, Fraumeni JF: Acute myelocytic leukaemia and leukaemia-associated antigens in sisters. Lancet 1975; 2:429–431.
Paul B, Reid MM, Davison EV, Abela M, Hamilton PJ: Familial myelodysplasia: progressive disease associated with emergence of monosmy 7. Br J Haematol 1987; 65:321–323.
Pearson HA, Grello FW, Cone TE: Leukemia in identical twins. N Engl J Med 1963; 268:1151–1156.
Perez-Encinas M, Bello JL, Perez-Crespo S, De Miguel R, Tome S: Familial myeloproliferative syndrome. Am J Hematol 1994; 46:225–229.
Plancoulaine S, Gessain A, Joubert M, Tortevoye P, Jeanne I, Talarmin A, de The G, Abel L: Detection of a major gene predisposing to human T lymphotropic virus type I infection in children among an endemic population of African origin. J Infect Dis 2000; 182:405–412.
Polednak A: Cancer incidence in the Puerto Rican-born population of Connecticut. Cancer 1992; 70:1172–1176.
Pombo de Oliveira MS, Awad El Seed FER, Foroni L, Matutes E, Morilla R, Luzzatoo L, Catovsky D: Lymphoblastic leukaemia in Siamese twins: evidence for identity. Lancet 1986; 2:969–970.
Potaznik D, Steinherz P: Multiple nevoid basal cell carcinoma syndrome and Hodgkin's disease. Cancer 1984; 53:2713–2715.
Potolsky A, Heath CW, Buckley CE, Rowlands DT: Lymphoreticular malignancies and immunologic abnormalities in a sibship. Am J Med 1971; 50:42–48.
Pottern M, Linet M, Blair A, Dick F, Burmeister LF, Gibson R, Schuman M, Fraumeni JF: Familial cancers associated with subtypes of leukemia and non-Hodgkin's lymphoma. Leuk Res 1991; 15:305–314.
Potzsch C, Schaefer HE, Lubbert M: Familial and metachronous malignant lymphoma: absence of constitutional *p53* mutations. Am J Hematol 1999; 62:144–149.
Preudhomme C, Warot-Loze D, Roumier C, Grardel-Duflos N, Garand R, Lai JL, Dastugue N, Macintyre E, Denis C, Bauters F, et al.: High incidence of biallelic point mutations in the Runt domain of the *AML1/PEBP2* αB gene in Mo acute myeloid leukemia and in myeloid malignancies with acquired trisomy 21. Blood 2000; 96:2862–2869.
Pui C-H, Boyett JM, Hancock ML, Pratt CB, Meyer WH, Crist WM: Outcome of treatment for childhood cancer in black as compared with white children: The St. Jude Children's Research Hospital experience 1962 through 1992. JAMA 1995; 273:633–637.
Radovanovic Z, Markovic-Denic L, Jankovic S: Cancer mortality of family members of patients with chronic lymphocytic leukemia. Eur J Epidemiol 1994; 10:211–221.
Ramot B, Hulu N: Clinical and pathological aspects of intestinal lymphoma and the relation to paraproteinemia of α chain. Harefuah 1969; 76:396–398.
Ramseur WL, Golomb HM, Vardiman JW, Oleske D, Collins JL: Hairy cell leukemia in father and son. Cancer 1980; 48:1825–1829.
Randall DL, Reiquam CW, Githen JH, Robinson A: Familial myeloproliferative disease. Am J Dis Child 1965; 110:479–500.
Randi ML, Fabris F, Vio C, Girolami A: Familial thrombocythemia and/or thrombocytosis: apparently a rare disorder. Acta Haematol 1987; 78:63.
Randi ML, Fabris F, Visentin I, Girolami A: Low incidence of familial occurrence of thrombocythaemia and/or thrombocytosis. Folia Haematol Int Mag Klin Morphol Blutforsch 1988; 115:695–699.
Ratnoff WD, Gress RE: The familial occurrence of polycythemia vera: report of a father and son, with consideration of the possible etiologic role of exposure to organic solvents, including tetrachorethylene. Blood 1980; 56:233–236.
Renier G, Ifrah N, Chevailler A, Saint-Andre JP, Boasson M, Hurez D: Four brothers with Waldenstrom's macroglobulinemia. Cancer 1989; 64:1554–1559.
Reitmair AH, Schmits R, Ewel A, Bapat B, Redston M, Mitri A, Waterhouse P, Mittrucker HW, Wakeham A, Liu B, et al.: MSH2 deficient mice are viable and susceptible to lymphoid tumours. Nat Genet 1995; 11(1):64–70.
Rettig MB, Mah HJ, Vescio RA, Pold M, Schiller G, Belson D, Savage A, Nishikubo C, Wu C, Fraser J, et al.: Kaposi's sarcoma-associated herpesvirus infection of bone marrow dendritic cells from multiple myeloma patients. Science 1997a; 276:1851–1854.
Rettig MB, Said JW, Sun R, Vescio RA, Berenson JR: Kaposi's sarcoma–associated herpesvirus infection and multiple myeloma [technical comments, response]. Science 1997b; 278:1972–1973.
Ricciardone MD, Ozcelik T, Cevher B, Ozdag H, Tuncer M, Gurgey A, Uzunalimoglu O, Cetinkaya H, Tanyeli A, Erken E, Ozturk M: Human MLH1 deficiency predisposes to hematological malignancy and neurofibromatosis type 1. Cancer Res 1999; 59(2):290–293.
Rigby PG, Pratt PT, Rosenlof RC, Lemon HM: Genetic relationships in familial leukemia and lymphoma. Arch Int Med 1968; 121:67–71.
Rigby PG, Rosenlof RC, Pratt PT, Lemon HM: Leukemia and lymphoma. JAMA 1966; 197:25–30.
Riggins GJ, Sherman SL, Philips CN, Stock W, Westbrook CA, Warren ST. CGG-repeat polymorphism of the *BCR* gene rules out predisposing alleles leading to the Philadelphia chromosome. Genes Chromosomes Cancer 1994; 9:141–144.
Robertson SJ, Lowman JT, Grufferman S, Kostyu D, van der Horst CM, Matthews TJ, Borowitz MJ, Bigner SH: Familial Hodgkin's disease. Cancer 1987; 59:1314–1319.
Robinson A, de la Chapelle A: Sex chromosome abnormalities. In: Rimoin DL, Connor JM, Pyeritz RE (eds). Emery and Rimoin's Principles and Practice of Medical Genetics, 3rd ed. New York: Churchill Livingstone, 1997:985.
Rowley JD: Down syndrome and acute leukaemia: increased risk may be due to trisomy 21. Lancet 1981; 2:1020–1022.
Royston I, Modan B: Comparative mortality of childhood leukemia and lymphoma among the immigrants and native born in Israel. Cancer 1968; 22:385–390.
Salimonu LS, Bryant DG, Buehler SK, Chandra RK, Crumley J, Marshall WH: Immunoglobulins in familial Hodgkin's disease and immunodeficiency in Newfoundland. Int Arch Allergy Appl Immunol 1980; 63:52–63.
Sasaki MS, Tsunematsu Y, Utsunomiya J, Utsumi J: Site-directed chromosome rearrangements in skin fibroblasts from persons carrying genes for hereditary neoplasms. Cancer Res 1980; 40:4796–4803.
Saven A, Piro LD: Hairy cell leukemia. In: Hoffman R, Benz EJ, Shattil SJ, Furie B, Cohen HJ, Silberstein LE (eds). Hematology: Basic Principles and Practice, 2nd ed. New York: Churchill Livingstone, 1995:1322–1331.
Schlemper RJ, van der Maas APC, Eikenboom JCJ: Familial essential thrombocythemia: clinical characteristics of 11 cases in one family. Ann Hematol 1994; 68:153–158.
Schmitt TA, Degos L: Leucemies familiales. Bull Cancer 1978; 65:83–88.
Schlesinger M, Broman I, Lugassy G: The complement system is defective in chronic lymphatic leukemia patients and in their healthy relatives. Leukemia 1996; 10(9):1509–1513.
Schneider BF, Christian M, Hess CE, Williams ME: Familial occurrence of cutaneous T cell lymphoma: a case report of monozygotic twin sisters. Leukemia 1995; 9:1979–1981.
Schweitzer M, Melief CJM, Ploem JE: Chronic lymphocytic leukemia in five siblings. Scand J Haematol 1973; 11:97–105.
Secker-Walker LM, Fitchett M: Constitutional and acquired trisomy 8. Leuk Res 1995; 19:737–740.

Seligmann M, Danon F, Fine JM: Immunological studies in familial β_2-macroglobulinaemias. Proc Soc Exp Biol Med 1963; 114:482–486.

Shannon KM, Turhan AG, Chang SSY, Bowcock AM, Rogers PCJ, Carroll WL, Cowan MJ, Glader BE, Eaves CJ, Eaves AC, Kan YW: Familial bone marrow monosomy 7: evidence that the predisposing locus is not on the long arm of chromosome 7. J Clin Invest 1989; 84:984–989.

Shannon KM, Watterson J, Johnson P, O'Connell P, Lange B, Shah N, Steinherz P, Kan YW, Priest JR: Monosomy 7 myeloproliferative disease in children with neurofibromatosis, type 1: epidemiology and molecular analysis. Blood 1992; 79:1311–1318.

Shaw MP, Eden OB, Grace E, Ellis PM: Acute lymphoblastic leukemia and Klinefelter's syndrome. Pediatr Hematol Oncol 1992; 9:81–85.

Shelley WB: Familial mycosis fungoides revisited. Arch Dermatol 1980; 116:1177–1178.

Shen JJ, Williams BJ, Zipursky A, Doyle J, Sherman SL, Jacobs PA, Shugar AL, Soukup SW, Hassold TJ: Cytogenetic and molecular studies of Down syndrome individuals with leukemia. Am J Hum Genet 1995; 56:915–925.

Shimkin MB, Loveland DB: A note on the mortality from lymphatic leukemia in Oriental populations of the United States. Blood 1961; 17:763–766.

Shoenfeld Y, Berliner S, Shaklai M, Gallant LA, Pinkhas J: Familial multiple myeloma: a review of thirty-seven families. Postgrad Med J 1982; 58:12–16.

Shpilberg O, Modan M, Modan B, Chetrit A, Fuchs Z, Ramot B: Familial aggregation of haematological neoplasms: a controlled study. Br J Haematol 1994; 87:75–80.

Shugart YY: Anticipation in familial Hodgkin lymphoma. Am J Hum Genet 1998; 63:270–272.

Sieff CA, Malleson P: Familial myelofibrosis. Arch Dis Child 1980; 55:888–893.

Sinnett D, Krajinovic M, Labuda D: Genetic susceptibility to childhood acute lymphoblastic leukemia. Leuk Lymphoma 2000; 38:447–462.

Slee PH, van Everdingen JJ, Geraedts JP, te Velde J, den Ottolander GJ: Familial myeloproliferative disease: hematological and cytogenetic studies. Acta Med Scand 1981; 210:321–327.

Smith MT, Wang Y, Kane E, Rollinson S, Wiemels JL, Roman E, Roddam P, Cartwright R, Morgan G: Low NAD(P)H:quinone oxidoreductase 1 activity is associated with increased risk of acute leukemia in adults. Blood 2001; 97:1422–1426.

Song WJ, Sullivan MG, Legare RD, Hutchings S, Tan X, Kufrin D, Ratajczak J, Resende IC, Haworth C, Hock R, et al.: Haploinsufficiency of *CBFA2* causes familial thrombocytopenia with propensity to develop acute myelogenous leukaemia. Nat Genet 1999; 23:166–175.

Spremolla G, Petrini M, Ambrogi F, Grassi B: Lymphoma in three members of the same family. Haematologica 1981; 66:228–232.

Stankovic T, Kidd AM, Sutcliffe A, McGuire GM, Robinson P, Weber P, Bedenham T, Bradwell AR, Easton DF, Lennox GG, et al.: ATM mutations and phenotypes in ataxia-telangiectasia families in the British Isles: expression of mutant ATM and the risk of leukemia, lymphoma, and breast cancer. Am J Hum Genet 1998; 62:334–345.

Stankovic T, Taylor AM, Yuille MR, Vorechovsky I: Recurrent *ATM* mutations in T-PLL on diverse haplotypes: no support for their germline origin. Blood 2001; 97:1517–1518.

Stankovic T, Weber P, Stewart G, Bedenham T, Murray J, Byrd PJ, Moss PA, Taylor AM: Inactivation of ataxia telangiectasia mutated gene in B-cell chronic lymphocytic leukaemia. Lancet 1999; 353:26–29.

Stanley WS, Burkett SS, Segel B, Quiery A, George B, Lobel J, Shah N: Constitutional inversion of chromosome 7 and hematologic cancers. Cancer Genet Cytogenet 1997; 96:46–49.

Steinberg AG: A genetic and statistical study of acute leukemia in children. In: Proceedings of the Third National Cancer Conference, 1956. Philadelphia: J. B. Lippincott, 1957:353–356.

Steinberg AG: The genetics of acute leukemia in children. Cancer 1960; 13:985–999.

Stilgenbauer S, Schaffner C, Litterst A, Liebisch P, Gilad S, Bar-Shira A, James MR, Lichter P, Dohner H: Biallelic mutations in the *ATM* gene in T-prolymphocytic leukemia. Nat Med 1997; 3:1155–1159.

Stiller CA, Chessels JM, Fitchett M: Neurofibromatosis and childhood leukaemia/lymphoma: a population-based UKCCSG study. Br J Cancer 1994; 70:969–972.

Stoll C, Alembik Y, Lutz P: A syndrome of facial dysmorphia, birth defects, myelodsyplasia and immunodeficiency in three sibs of consaguineous parents. Genet Couns 1994; 5:161–165.

Stoppa-Lyonnet D, Lauge A, Sigaux F, Stern MH: No germline *ATM* mutation in a series of 16 T-cell prolymphocytic leukemias. Blood 2000; 96:374–376.

Stoppa-Lyonnet D, Soulier J, Lauge A, Dastot H, Garand R, Sigaux F, Stern MH: Inactivation of the *ATM* gene in T-cell prolymphocytic leukemias. Blood 1998; 91:3920–3926.

Strathdee CV, Gavish H, Shannon WR, Buchwald M: Cloning of cDNAs for Fanconi's aneaemia by functional complementation. Nature 1992; 356:763–767.

Sullivan AK: Classification, pathogenesis, and etiology of neoplastic diseases of the hematopoietic system. In: Lee GR, Bithell TC, Foerster J, Athens JW, Lukens JN (eds). Wintrobe's Clinical Hematology, 9th ed. Philadelphia: Lea and Febiger, 1993:1725–1791.

Sullivan KE, Mullen CA, Blaese RM, Winkelstein JA: A multiinstitutional survey of the Wiskott-Aldrich syndrome. J Pediatr 1994; 125:876–885.

Swensen AR, Ross JA, Severson RK, Pollock BH, Robison LL: The age peak in childhood acute lymphoblastic leukemia: exploring the potential relationship with socioeconomic status. Cancer 1997; 79:2045–2051.

Takada K: Role of Epstein-Barr virus in Burkitt's lymphoma. Curr Top Microbiol Immunol 2001; 258:141–151.

Tatti V, Marfut P, Sirchia G, Pescia G, Luscieti P, Losa G: Familial myeloproliferative syndrome. Schweiz Med Wochenschr 1984; 114:196–204. In French.

Taub JW: Relationship of chromosome 21 and acute leukemia in children with Down syndrome. Am J Pediatr Hematol 2001; 23:175–178.

Taylor AMR, Metcalfe JA, Thick J, Mak Y-F: Leukemia and lymphoma in ataxia telangiectasia. Blood 1996; 87:423–438.

Taylor GM, Birch JM: The hereditary basis of human leukemia. In: Greaves MF (ed). William Dameshek and Frederick Gunz's Leukemia, 6th ed. Philadelphia: W. B. Saunders, 1996:210–245.

Tedeschi R, Kvarnung M, Knekt P, Schulz TF, Szekely L, De Paoli PD, Aromaa A, Teppo L, Dillner J: A prospective seroepidemiological study of human herpesvirus-8 infection and the risk of multiple myeloma. Br J Cancer 2001; 84:122–125.

Thiersch JB: Attempted transmission of acute leukemia from man to man by the sternal marrow route. Cancer Res 1946; 6:695–698.

Thomas TF: Multiple myeloma in siblings. N Y J Med 1964; 64:2096–2099.

Timmers C, Taniguchi T, Hejna J, Reifsteck C, Lucas L, Bruun D, Thayer M, Cox B, Olson S, D'Andrea AD, et al.: Positional cloning of a novel Fanconi anemia gene, *FANCD2*. Mol Cell 2001; 7:241–248.

Tokuhata GK, Neely CL, Williams DL: Chronic myelocytic leukemia in identical twins and a sibling. Blood 1968; 31(2):216–225.

Tomas JF, Fernandez-Ranada JM: About the increased frequency of acute promyelocytic leukemia among Latinos: the experience from a center in Spain. Blood 1996; 88:2357–2358.

Tomonaga M: Statistical investigation of leukaemia in Japan. N Z Med J Haematol (Suppl) 1966; 65:863–869.

Tonks S, Oza AM, Lister TA, Bodmer JG: Association of HLA-DPB with Hodgkin's disease. Lancet 1992; 340:968–969.

Tosato F, Pirrone S, Manzo M, Diplotti L, Sponza E: Metaplasia mieloide agnogenica e policitemia vera nella stessa famiglia. Haemtologica 1985; 70:240–241. In Italian.

Trapido EJ, Chen F, Davis K, Lewis N, MacKinnon JA: Cancer among Hispanic males in south Florida. Arch Intern Med 1994; 154:177–185.

Vanasse GJ, Concannon P, Willerford DM: Regulated genomic instability and neoplasia in the lymphoid lineage. Blood 1999; 94(12):3997–4010.

van der Burgt I, Chrzanowska KH, Smeets D, Weemaes C: Nijmegen breakage syndrome. J Med Genet 1996; 33:153–156.

Vannotti A: Etude clinique d'un cas de macrogloublinemie de Waldenstrom a caractère familial associé a des troubles endocriniens. Schweiz Med Wochenschr 1963; 93:1744–1746.

Vennos EM, James WD: Rothmund-Thomson syndrome. In: Cohen PR, Kurzrock R (eds). Dermatologic Clinics, Genodermatoses with Malignant Potential. Vol. 13. Philadelphia: W. B. Saunders, 1995:143–150.

Vetrie D, Vorechovsky I, Sideras P, Holland J, Davies A, Flinter F, Hammarstrom L, Kinnon C, Levinsky R, Bobrow M, et al.: The gene involved in X-linked agammaglobulinaemia is a member of the src family of protein-tyrosine kinases. Nature 1993; 361:226–233.

Videbaek A: Familial leukemia: a preliminary report. Acta Med Scand 1947a; 127:26–52.

Videbaek A: Heredity in Human Leukemia and Its Relation to Cancer. Copenhagen: Ejnar Munksgaard, 1947b.

Vorechovsky I, Luo L, Dyer MJ, Catovsky D, Amlot PL, Yaxley JC, Foroni L, Hammarstrom L, Webster AD, Yuille MA: Clustering of missense mutations in the ataxia-telangiectasia gene in a sporadic T-cell leukaemia. Nat Genet 1997; 17:96–99.

Vorechovsky I, Luo L, Ortmann E, Steinmann D, Dork T: Missense mutations at *ATM* gene and cancer risk. Lancet 1999; 353:1276.

Waddell C, Brown JA, Riggs SA, White MR: Polycythemia vera occurring in two brothers. South Med J 1982; 75:1010–1011.

Wang Y, Cortez D, Yazdi P, Neff N, Elledge SJ, Qin J: BASC, a super complex of BRCA1-associated proteins involved in the recognition and repair of aberrant DNA structures. Genes Dev 2000; 14:927–939.

Ward FT, Baker J, Krishnan J, Dow N, Kjobech CH: Hairy cell leukemia in two siblings: a human leukocyte antigen-linked disease? Cancer 1990; 65:319–321.

Ward JE, Galinsky I, Newton BL: Familial leukemia: a report of three cases of leukemia and one leukemoid reaction in one family. Am J Hum Genet 1952; 4:90–93.

Weiner L: A family with high incidence of leukemia and unique Ph' chromosome findings. Blood 1965; 26:871.

Weintraub M, Lin AY, Franklin J, Tucker MA, Magrath IT, Bhatia KG: Absence of germline *p53* mutations in familial lymphoma. Oncogene 1996; 12:687–691.

Weiss HJ, Chervenick PA, Zalusky R: Factor A: a familial defect in platelet function associated with impaired release of adenosine diphosphate. N Engl J Med 1969; 281:1264–1270.

Weiss NS, Katz JA, Frankel LS, Lloyd LE, McClain KL, Torges K, Thomas PJ, Bleyer WA: Incidence of childhood and adolescent cancer in Texas. Tex Med 1996; 92:54–60.

Weistner A, Schlemper RJ, van der Maas APC, Skoda RC: An activating splice donor mutation in the thrombopoietin gene causes hereditary thrombocythaemia. Nat Genet 1998; 18:49–52.

Wells R, Lau KS: Incidence of leukemia in Singapore, and rarity of chronic lymphocytic leukemia in Chinese. Br Med J 1960; 1:759–763.

Wicking C, Shanley S, Smyth I, Gillies S, Negus K, Graham S, Suthers G, Haites N, Edwards M, Wainwright B, Chenevix-Trench G: Most germ-line mutations in the nevoid basal cell carcinoma syndrome lead to a premature termination of the PATCHED protein, and no genotype–phenotype correlations are evident. Am J Hum Genet 1997; 60:21–26.

Wiemels JL, Cazzaniga G, Daniotti M, Eden OB, Addison GM, Masera G, Saha V, Biondi A, Greaves MF: Prenatal origin of acute lymphoblastic leukaemia in children. Lancet 1999; 354:1499–1503.

Wiemels JL, Smith RN, Taylor GM, Eden OB, Alexander FE, Greaves MF, United Kingdom Childhood Cancer Study investigators: Methylenetetrahydrofolate reductase (MTHFR) polymorphisms and risk of molecularly defined subtypes of childhood acute leukemia. Proc Natl Acad Sci USA 2001; 98:4004–4009.

Wilkinson JD, Fleming LE, MacKinnon J, Voti L, Wohler-Torres B, Peace S, Trapido E: Lymphoma and lymphoid leukemia incidence in Florida children: ethnic and racial distribution. Cancer 2001; 91:1402–1408.

Willems PMW, Kuypers WHM, Meijerink JPP, Holdrinet RSG, Mensink JBM: Sporadic mutations of the *p53* gene in multiple myeloma and no evidence for germline mutations in three familial multiple myeloma pedigrees. Leukemia 1993; 7:986–991.

Williams EC, Shahidi NT: Benign familial thrombocytosis. Am J Hematol 1991; 37:124–125.

Woods WG, Roloff JS, Lukens JN, Krivit W: The occurrence of leukemia in patients with the Shwachman syndrome. J Pediatr 1981; 99:425–428.

Wylin RF, Greene MH, Palutke M, Khilanani P, Tabaczka P, Swiderski G: Hairy cell leukemia in three siblings. Cancer 1982; 49:538–542.

Yagisawa M, Kamizaki K, Nagase T, Toba K, Oochi M, Fukuchi Y, Orishige J, Hino M, Miyazono K: Familial thrombocythemia in a daughter and mother. Nippon Naika Gakkai Zasshi 1990; 79:531–532. In Japanese.

Yuille MA, Coignet LJ, Abraham SM, Yaqub F, Luo L, Matutes E, Brito-Babapulle V, Vorechovsky I, Dyer MJ, Catovsky D: ATM is usually rearranged in T-cell prolymphocytic leukaemia. Oncogene 1998a; 16:789–796.

Yuille MR, Houlston RS, Catovsky D: Anticipation in familial chronic lymphocytic leukaemia. Leukemia 1998b; 12:1696–1698.

Yuille MR, Matutes E, Marossy A, Hilditch B, Catovsky D, Houlston RS: Familial chronic lymphocytic leukaemia: a survey and review of published studies. Br J Haematol 2000; 109:794–799.

Zahm SH, Weisenburger DD, Saal RC, Vaught JB, Babbitt PA, Blair A: The role of agricultural pesticide use in the development of non-Hodgkin's lymphoma in women. Arch Environ Health 1993; 48:353–358.

Zawadzki ZA, Aizawa Y, Kraj MA, Haradin AR, Fisher B: Familial immunopathies: report of nine families and survey of literature. Cancer 1977; 40:2094–2101.

Zollino M, Genuardi M, Bajer J, Tornesello A, Mastrangelo S, Zampino G, Mastrangelo R, Neri G: Constitutional trisomy 8 and myelodsyplasia: report of a case and review of the literature. Leuk Res 1995; 9:733–736.

Zvulunov A, Barak Y, Metzker A: Juvenile xanthogranuloma, neurofibromatosis, and juvenile chronic myelogenous leukemia. World statistical analysis. Arch Dermatol 1995; 131(8):904–908.

Part IX

NEUROPSYCHIATRIC DISORDERS

41 Epilepsy

MAGALI FERNANDEZ AND THOMAS D. BIRD

The familial occurrence of epilepsy has been known for centuries and is mentioned in the Talmud (Goodman, 1979). Heberden's Commentaries written in 1802 contains one of the earliest references to familial epilepsy in the English medical literature (McHenry, 1969). In 1878, Berger noted that 23 of 71 of his patients with epilepsy showed evidence of inheritance (One Hundred Years Ago, 1978). However, scientific interest in genetics and the clinical significance of Mendel's laws of inheritance did not occur until after the beginning of the twentieth century. Early in the last century, several attempts to apply genetic principles to epilepsy were confused and oversimplified. In 1911, Davenport and Weeks carefully documented the familial occurrence of epilepsy. They misunderstood the biologic and genetic relationship of epilepsy to disorders such as mental retardation, alcoholism, and economic poverty, and they strongly advocated legal measures to eliminate the reproduction of persons with epilepsy. Subsequent studies have shown increasing sophistication in both the genetic and social aspects of disorders of the nervous systems. In 1912 and 1929, human geneticists analyzing Lundborg's data on progressive myoclonic epilepsy demonstrated one of the first instances of autosomal recessive transmission of human disease (Stevenson, 1955).

DISEASE DEFINITION

The term *epilepsy* comes from a Greek word meaning to be seized by forces from without. The simplest clinical definition of epilepsy is recurrent seizures. In the nineteenth century, John Hulings Jackson deduced that a seizure was the result of an occasional excessive and disorderly discharge of nervous tissue. Paroxysmal discharges of neurons occur when the threshold for firing of the neuronal membrane is reduced beyond the capability of intrinsic membrane threshold-stabilizing mechanisms to prevent firing. The attack may be localized and remain restricted in a focal area, or it may spread to other brain regions (Glaser, 1997). Electroencephalographic (EEG) signs of seizure activity within the brain include spikes and sharp waves followed by slow waves.

The clinical manifestations of a seizure can be quite variable. A focally limited seizure discharge in the motor cortex of the brain may result in repetitive twitching of one extremity, one part of an extremity, or one side of the face. Restricted seizure activity in other parts of the brain may lead to mental confusion and repetitive stereotype movements. A generalized seizure produces loss of consciousness and is often associated with tonic or clonic movements of the extremities. Other generalized seizures may produce brief lapses in consciousness (absence attacks), myoclonic jerking of the limbs, or sudden loss of muscle tone. The earliest part of a seizure is called the *aura*. The seizure itself is referred to as the *ictus*, and the immediate period after the seizure is called *postictal*. The time between seizures is the *interictal* period.

There has been considerable controversy over the best terminology for describing seizures (Everitt and Sander, 1999). A useful advance in this field has been the adoption in 1981 of a uniform classification of epileptic seizures supported by the International League against Epilepsy (ICES) (Commission on Classification and Terminology, 1981). This classification is shown in Table 41–1. Partial seizures are those that can be determined to begin as a local cortical discharge. Such seizures were often previously called focal. Simple partial seizures usually produce only motor or sensory signs and symptoms and do not impair consciousness. Complex partial seizures impair consciousness. They were often previously called temporal lobe or psychomotor seizures, but they do not necessarily always originate in the temporal lobe. Generalized seizures are bilaterally symmetric, both clinically and electrically, and cannot be determined to have a local cortical onset. They can include convulsive action of the limbs. Generalized seizures include either absence or petit mal attacks, various kinds of myoclonic and tonic-clonic seizures, as well as atonic seizures in which there is loss of muscle tone. Not surprisingly, the third major category of epileptic seizures is "unclassified." It is important to note that the international classification of seizures in most useful in describing a single seizure and is not meant to give information about underlying causes of epilepsy or specific diagnosis. A patient with epilepsy may have a partial motor seizure one day and a generalized tonic-clonic seizure the next. Partial seizures may secondarily become generalized. A child with absence attacks may develop generalized tonic-clonic seizures at an older age. Any given seizure type in the classification may have dozens of different causes. ICES was supplemented in 1989 to include epileptic syndromes: international classification of epilepsies and epileptic syndromes (ICE) (Commission on Classification and Terminology, 1989). This classification is shown in Table 41–2. Two subdivisions continue to be used: the first separates epilepsies with generalized seizures (generalized epilepsies and syndromes) from epilepsies with partial or focal seizures (localization related, partial or focal epilepsies and syndromes). The other separates epilepsies by etiology: symptomatic (secondary) from those that are idiopathic (primary) and cryptogenic. The term *idiopathic* means that there is no underlying cause other than a possible hereditary predisposition. These are defined by age-related, clinical, and electrographic characteristics and have a presumed genetic etiology. The term *cryptogenic* refers to a disorder whose cause is hidden or occult. These are presumed to be symptomatic, but the etiology is not known. These are also age-

Table 41–1. Summary of International Classification of Epileptic Seizures

- I. Partial (focal, local) seizures
  - A. Simple partial seizures (consciousness not impaired)
    - 1. With motor signs
    - 2. With sensory symptoms
    - 3. With autonomic symptoms or signs
    - 4. With psychic symptoms
  - B. Complex partial seizures (temporal lobe or psychomotor seizures; consciousness impaired)
    - 1. Simple partial onset, followed by impairment of consciousness
      - a. With simple partial features (A.1 to A.4), followed by impaired consciousness
      - b. With automatism
    - 2. With impairment of consciousness at onset
      - a. With impairment of consciousness only
      - b. With automatism
  - C. Partial seizures, evolving to secondarily generalized seizures (tonic-clonic, tonic, or clonic)
    - 1. Simple partial seizures (A), evolving to generalized seizures
    - 2. Complex partial seizures (B), evolving to generalized seizures
    - 3. Simple partial seizures, evolving to complex partial seizures, then evolving to generalized seizures
- II. Generalized seizures (convulsive or nonconvulsive)
  - A. Absence (petit mal) seizures
  - B. Myoclonic seizures
  - C. Clonic seizures
  - D. Tonic seizures
  - E. Tonic-clonic (grand mal) seizures
  - F. Atonic seizures
- III. Unclassified epileptic seizures

Source: Commission on Classification and Terminology of the International League against Epilepsy (1981) with permission.

Table 41–2. Summary of International Classifications of Epilepsies and Epileptic Syndromes (Supplement)

- I. Localization-related (focal, local, partial) epilepsies and syndromes
  - • Temporal lobe epilepsies
  - • Frontal lobe epilepsies
  - • Parietal lobe epilepsies
  - • Occipital lobe epilepsies
  - A. Idiopathic (with age-related onset)
    - 1. Benign childhood epilepsy with centro-temporal spike
    - 2. Childhood epilepsy with occipital paroxysm
    - 3. Primary reading epilepsy
  - B. Symptomatic
    - 1. Chronic progressive epilepsia partialis continua of childhood (Kojewnikow's syndrome)
    - 2. Syndromes characterized by seizures with specific modes of precipitation
  - C. Cryptogenic
- II. Generalized epilepsies and syndromes
  - A. Idiopathic (with age-related onset, listed in order of age)
    - 1. Benign neonatal familial convulsions
    - 2. Benign neonatal convulsions
    - 3. Benign myoclonic epilepsy in infancy
    - 4. Childhood absence epilepsy (pyknolepsy)
    - 5. Juvenile absence epilepsy
    - 6. Juvenile myoclonic epilepsy (impulsive petit mal)
    - 7. Epilepsy with grand mal (GTLS) seizures on awakening
    - 8. Other generalized idiopathic epilepsies not defined above
    - 9. Epilepsies with seizures precipitated by specific modes of achration
  - B. Cryptogenic or symptomatic (in order of age)
    - 1. West syndrome (infantile spasms, Blitz-Nick-Salaam Krampfe)
    - 2. Lennox Gastaut syndrome
    - 3. Epilepsy with myoclonic-astatic seizures
    - 4. Epilepsy with myoclonic absences
  - C. Symptomatic
    - 1. Nonspecific etiology
      - a. Early myoclonic encephalopathy
      - b. Early infantile epileptic encephalopathy with suppression burst
      - c. Other symptomatic generalized epilepsies not defined above
    - 2. Specific syndromes (disease in which seizures are a presenting or predominant feature)
- III. Epilepsies and syndromes undetermined whether focal or generalized
  - A. With both generalized and focal seizure
    - 1. Neonatal seizures
    - 2. Severe myoclonic epilepsy in infancy
    - 3. Epilepsy with continuous spike waves during slow wave sleep
    - 4. Acquired epileptic aphasia (Landau-Kleffner syndrome)
    - 5. Other undetermined epilepsies not defined above
  - B. Without unequivocal generalized or focal features
- IV. Special syndromes
  - A. Situation-related seizures (Gelegenheit san falle)
    - 1. Febrile convulsions
    - 2. Isolated seizures or isolated status epilepticus
    - 3. Seizures occurring only when there is an acute metabolic or toxic event

Source: Commission on Classification and Terminology of the International League against Epilepsy (1989) with permission.

related, but often do not have well-defined electroclinical characteristics. However, it has to be recognized that patients may move from one syndrome to another during the evolution of their epileptic condition.

As a general rule, partial seizures are more likely to be the result of environmental insults such as trauma or infection, whereas generalized seizures are more apt to have an unknown cause. Genetic factors may underlie any type of seizure but seem to be more common in the generalized seizure category. Concise reviews of epilepsy for the practicing physician are the texts by Willey (1997) and Engel (1989). Because the terminology of epilepsy is complicated and has undergone many changes, definitions and synonyms for the various types of seizure disorders discussed in this chapter are listed in Table 41–3. Duchowny and Harvey (1996) have reviewed the epileptic syndromes of childhood.

GENERAL GENETIC AND EPIDEMIOLOGIC EVIDENCE

Clinical Epidemiology and Family Epidemiology

Epidemiologic studies of epilepsy have suffered from four major problems. First, terminology has been highly confused, as noted above (see Disease Definition). This was especially true before the wide application of EEG techniques and before the international classification of seizures. Second, different studies have used varying criteria for whether a patient or family member has epilepsy. For example, a single seizure such as a febrile seizure does not technically constitute epilepsy (which should imply *recurrent* seizures). However, a single seizure in a family member may represent an important clue to a subtle genetic influence. Therefore, some investigators have included single seizures in their epidemiologic net, and others have not. Third, there are large differences in investigative methodology. Some studies have used control groups; others have not. Some studies measure prevalence, others incidence, and still others cumulative risk. Fourth, interpretation of the accumulated data has been a difficult and puzzling business. One investigator may interpret results as suggesting dominant inheritance with reduced penetrance, whereas another will interpret the same figure as supporting polygenic or multifactorial inheritance. In fact, a single study may be interpreted as showing no genetic influence in epilepsy by one observer and as showing clear evidence of a genetic influence by another. These caveats must be kept in mind

Table 41–3. Definitions of Seizure Types Discussed

Seizure Type	Other Terms	Definition
Partial simple	Focal	Paroxysmal activity from cortical structures of one hemisphere *without* impairment of consciousness; may be motor, sensory, or autonomic
Partial complex	Psychomotor, temporal lobe	Partial seizure that *includes* impairment of consciousness but *without* initial diffuse bilateral cortical activity
Generalized, tonic-clonic	Grand mal	First clinical change involvement of both hemispheres with bilateral motor manifestations and impairment of consciousness (partial seizures may become secondarily generalized)
Childhood absence	Petit mal, 3 Hz spike and wave, centrencephalic pyknolepsy	Brief episodes of decreased responsiveness without preictal warning or postictal symptoms and often with automatisms, blinking, or brief changes in postural tone
Myoclonic	(Part of many syndromes)	Brief involuntary muscle contractions of one or several muscles; may be epileptic or nonepileptic, have numerous causes, and be progressive or nonprogressive
Atonic	Astatic, jackknife, salaam seizures, flexor spasms	Brief loss of postural tone from nodding of head, to sagging of body, to complete fall; multiple causes, often part of infantile spasms syndrome
Tonic		Brief contractions of all or only certain muscle groups; multiple causes
Juvenile absence epilepsy		Absences are the same as in pyknolepsy, but less frequent; association with generalized tonic clonic seizures is frequent; onset in adolescence; sex distribution is equal; EEG spike and wave discharges are often faster than 3 Hz
Juvenile benign myoclonic-seizures (Janz)	Janz's syndrome, impulsive petit mal	Juvenile or adolescent onset of nonprogressive seizure disorder that often includes grand mal seizure on awaking, sporadic myoclonic jerks, normal mentation, and diffuse 4–6 Hz EEG multi-spike-wave complexes
Primary generalized myoclonic astatic seizures	Doose's syndrome	Early childhood onset of myoclonic, atonic, tonic-clonic, or absence seizures with 3–6 Hz multi-spike-wave complexes, normal mentation, male predominance
Lennox-Gastaut syndrome		Childhood-onset seizure disorder with interictal slow and spike EEG atypical absence, myoclonic or tonic-atonic seizures, with changes, mental retardation and neurologic deficits
Infantile spasms	Salaam-seizures, jackknife seizures, flexor spasms, infantile myoclonic epilepsy	Early-onset seizure disorder frequently associated with atonic spells, diffusely slow EEG (hyperarrhythmia), mental retardation; multiple causes
Simple febrile seizures	Seizure with fever	Generalized (nonfocal) seizure of less than 15 minutes in a 3-month to 5-year old child with temperature of 30°C or higher; any seizure with fever (not simple) may be prolonged, focal, orcomplicated
Reflex epilepsy	Stimulus or sensory induced	A seizure precipitated by a specific environmental stimulus, e.g., visual, auditory, tactile, gustatory, olfactory
Rolandic epilepsy	Centrotemporal	Childhood onset of nonprogressive seizures with EEG spike focus in the central-temporal regions; often partial motor seizures of the face during sleep or waking
Benign infantile seizures	Benign neonatal seizures	Onset in first few weeks of life of generalized clonic seizures, often disappearing after a few months with normal psychomotor development
Acquired	Environmental, nongenetic, symptomatic	Seizure resulting from a previously known environmental agent or insult

in reviewing the epidemiologic data bearing on the question of genetic factors underlying epilepsy.

Epilepsy has a prevalence of approximately 0.5% to 1.0% in the general population (Glaser, 1997). It has also been found that 2.2% of the nonepileptic general population has evidence of electrical seizure activity on routine EEG studies, with the activity being more frequent in children than in adults (Zivin and Ajmone-Marsen, 1968; Cavazzuti et al., 1980). Relative incidence and prevalence of the various major types of epilepsy are shown in Table 41–4. Harvald (1954) has reviewed investigations of the inheritance of epilepsy through the first half of the twentieth century and presented a detailed study of his own. Reviews of epidemiologic studies regarding the inheritance of epilepsy are the text by Anderson et al. (1982), and the studies by Ottman et al. (1996) and Shorvon (1996).

Family Studies

Some family studies of epilepsy are presented in Table 41–5. Several studies especially in the older literature have deemphasized the importance of genetics. These include Alstrom (1950), Eisner and colleagues (1960), Beaussart and Loiseau (1969), Sorel (1969). However, most of these studies uncovered several subgroups of epilepsy in which genetic factors seemed important.

The majority of epidemiologic studies of epilepsy have found an increased frequency of epilepsy in other relatives and supported an increased recurrence risk for epilepsy in siblings and children of epileptic probands. Thom and Walker (1922) found that 7.7% of 431 offspring of epileptic parents had seizures; seizures were more common (21%) in the children of epileptic

Table 41–4. Relative Prevalence of Epilepsy by Type of Seizure

Seizure Type	Prevalence per 1,000 Population[a]	Incidence in 235 Children (0–9 years) with Seizures (%)[b]	Incidence Age Adjusted per 100,000 Person-Years[d]
Partial complex	1.7	17	16
Partial simple	1.3	16	6
Partial unclassified	1.0	—	3
Tonic-clonic only	1.3	68	10
Incompletely generalized	0.4	—	—
Absence	0.4	13[c]	3
Miscellaneous	0.2	—	2
Infantile spasms	—	8	—
Rolandic, centrotemporal	—	8	—
Myoclonic	—	—	1

[a]Modified from Hauser and Kurland, 1975.
[b]Modified from Doose and Sitepu, 1983.
[c]Includes a few myoclonic or astatic cases.
[d]Modified from Hauser et al., 1993.

mothers than in the children of epileptic fathers (15%). Stein (1933) found epilepsy in 2.2% of the children of 87 parents with epilepsy compared with 0.9% in the relatives of controls. Stein also found that 4.1% of the siblings of epileptics had a history of epilepsy compared with 0.8% of the siblings of controls. Harvald (1954) found that 4.3% of brothers and 2.1% of sisters of patients with epilepsy also had seizures. Harvald also found a history of seizures in 3.5% of close relatives and in 2.3% of distant relatives of probands with idiopathic seizures, while only 1 of 310 relatives of patients with "symptomatic" epilepsy had a history of seizures.

In the 1940s and 1950s, William Lennox (1945, 1947a, 1947b, 1951) published an important series of studies investigating genetic influences in a large number of epileptics. In 1951, he reported that a history of seizures was obtained for 3.2% of the 20,000 near relatives of 4231 epileptic patients. The incidence was 3.6% if evidence of brain damage before the patient's seizure was lacking and 1.8% if such evidence was present. These percentages were, respectively, 7 and 3.5 times the inci-

Table 41–5. Selected Family Studies in Epilepsy

References	Index Cases (*N*)	Type	Relatives Affected with Epilepsy
Thom and Walker, 1922	—	Epilepsy	7.79% of offspring 21% of offspring of affected mother 15% of offspring of affected mother
Stein, 1933	87	Epilepsy	2.2% of offspring 4.1% of offspring
		Controls	0.9% of offspring 0.8% of siblings
Harvald, 1954	—	Epilepsy	4.3% of brothers 2.1% of sisters
Lennox, 1947a, 1947b, 1951; Lennox and Gibbs, 1945	4231	Epilepsy	3.2% of relatives 7.6% of relatives if proband onset in infancy 1.5% of relatives if proband onset after age 30 years
Pederson and Krogh, 1971	109	Idiopathic or cryptogenic	42 families had a family history
Tsuboi and Endo, 1977	263	Epilepsy	2.4% of offspring 9.1% of offspring if febrile seizures included
		Idiopathic	11% of offspring
		Secondary	3.2% of offspring
		Awaking grand mal, absence, myoclonic petit mal, grand mal without aura	12–16% of offspring
Janz and Scheffner, 1980	—	Epilepsy	3.74% of offspring
Anderson et al., 1979	—	Epilepsy	6.2% of siblings if proband and mother with seizures 16.7% of siblings if proband had a single seizures and both parents had seizures 33% of siblings if proband and both parents had recurrent seizures
Beaussart and Loiseau, 1969	5200	Epilepsy (all)	2.5% with a family history
		Petit mal	10.0% with a family history
		Infantile with rolandic EEG	3.5% with a family history
		Idiopathic generalized	3.2% with a family history
Alstrom, 1950		Epilepsy	1.1–1.7% of relatives 4.1% of relatives including single attack
Sorel, 1969	2690	Epilepsy	42 families with high rate of centrencephalic 11 families with high rate of seizures
Eisner et al., 1960	669	Idiopathic major motor	7.6% of relatives by age 19 9.4% of relatives by age 39
		Controls	1.4% of relatives by age 19 2.3% of relatives by age 39
Annegers et al., 1982	196	Idiopathic	See Table 41–6
Ottman et al., 1996	1560	Idiopathic/cryptogenic	1.8% parents by age 40 3.2% siblings by age 40 6.7% offspring by age 40
Miller et al., 1999	613	Several types	Monozygotic vs dizygotic twin studies

dence of epilepsy among draftees into the U. S. Army. He also pointed out that in the group without a history of brain trauma, the incidence of epilepsy among relatives decreased progressively with a later onset of seizures—from 7.6% if onset was in infancy to 1.5% if it was after the age of 30 years. Lennox (1951) concluded that "a transmitted predisposition to seizures *and* brain damage are both important factors in the origin of a person's epilepsy. The genetic factor in epilepsy is probably no greater than it is in many other common diseases. Hence, advice regarding marriage and children must be individualized." Lennox also strongly advocated the use of the EEG in the classification of seizures and in the study of possible genetic predisposition to epilepsy in other family members.

Pederson and Krogh (1971) found that, of 109 patients with cryptogenic or idiopathic epilepsy, 42 of the families had another relative with seizures. Tsuboi and Endo (1977) studied the incidence of seizures and EEG abnormalities in 506 offspring of 263 patients with epilepsy. The total group of epileptic parents included several different classifications of seizure. The incidence of seizures among all offspring was 2.4%; it was 9.1% if febrile convulsions were included. Overall morbidity for seizures was 11% in the offspring of a parent with idiopathic epilepsy and 3.2% in the offspring of a parent with symptomatic epilepsy (known environmental cause). Incidence of seizures was 12% to 16% in the offspring of a parent with awakening grand mal, absence, or myoclonic petit mal seizures or with grand mal seizures without aura. In addition, 37% of offspring exhibited epileptic EEG abnormalities, and the ratio of epileptic EEG abnormality to clinical seizures was about 4 to 1.

Janz and Scheffner (1980) found afebrile epileptic seizures in 3.74% of 721 children who had one parent with epileptic seizures.

Annegers and colleagues (1982) evaluated the frequency of seizures in the close relatives of 196 patients with idiopathic epilepsy. These results are summarized in Table 41–6. Cumulative risks for epilepsy (recurrent seizures) for siblings, children, and the control population to age 20 years were 2.7%, 10.6%, and 1.1%, respectively. Cumulative risks for epilepsy or an isolated seizure for siblings, children, and the control population to age 20 years were 3.9%, 10.6%, and 1.4%, respectively. Cumulative risks for all seizures, including febrile seizures, for siblings, children, and the control population to age 20 years were 10.8%, 14.3%, and 4.1%, respectively. Cumulative risks for all seizures for nieces and nephews of the probands were not increased over control (4.6% vs. 4.1%).

Table 41–6. Cumulative Risk of Seizures for Relatives of 196 Probands with Idiopathic Epilepsy

To Age (Years)	Siblings (%)	Children (%)	Nieces and Nephews (%)	General Population (%)
Risk of epilepsy				
5	0.7	2.7	—	0.4
10	1.2	4.9	—	0.7
20	2.7	10.6	—	1.1
40	3.6	10.6	—	1.7
Risk of epilepsy and isolated idiopathic nonfebrile seizures				
5	1.2	2.7	—	0.5
10	1.9	4.9	—	0.9
20	3.9	10.6	—	1.4
40	4.7	—	—	2.1
Risk of all types of seizures including febrile				
5	8.1	6.7	4.1	3.1
10	9.0	8.8	4.6	3.5
20	10.8	14.3	4.6	4.1
40	11.6	—	—	5.1

Source: Modified from Annegers et al. (1982).
— = not available

Anderson and colleagues (1979) found a seizure risk in siblings of 6.2% if both the proband and the mother had seizures and 16.7% if the proband and both parents had seizures. These data were based on probands with single seizures. If the proband had recurrent seizures and both parents also had seizures, then the risk to siblings became 33.3%.

Ottman et al. (1996) evaluated genetic susceptibility to epilepsy in relatives of 1560 probands with idiopathic or cryptogenic epilepsy and 391 with symptomatic epilepsy. The risk for epilepsy for parents, siblings, and offspring to age 40 of probands with idiopathic and cryptogenic epilepsy were 1.8%, 3.2%, and 6.7%, respectively. The risk for epilepsy for parents, siblings, and offspring to age 40 of probands with postnatal symptomatic epilepsy were 1.4%, 1.3%, 1.5%; and the cumulative incidence among all relatives to age 40 was 1.5%, which is similar to the general population of 1.6%. The idiopathic/cryptogenic group, which in this study was mostly cryptogenic, included 13% with generalized onset epilepsy and 83% with partial onset, 1% with both, and 3% unclassifiable. The authors pointed out that the risk of epilepsy in relatives is defined by the proband's age at onset and found that the risk of epilepsy in parents was not associated with the proband's age of onset of idiopathic/cryptogenic epilepsy. The risk was higher in siblings of probands with onset of idiopathic/cryptogenic epilepsy between the ages 10 to 19 than in those of probands with earlier or later ages of onset. However, the risk was more than twice as high in offspring of probands with onset of idiopathic/cryptogenic epilepsy less than 10 years as in offspring of those with later ages at onset. They concluded that genetic susceptibility is likely to contribute to the risk of some forms of cryptogenic epilepsy, and it is unlikely to contribute to the risk of epilepsy associated with postnatal insults to the central nervous system (CNS). Seizure type and age at onset of epilepsy were predictors of familial risk. Among relatives of probands without identified CNS lesions, the influences on risk in offspring may differ from those in parents and siblings.

Degen and colleagues (1996) studied the presence of epileptiform activity in the EEG of relatives of patients with symptomatic generalized tonic-clonic seizures. They recorded waking and sleep EEGs in 83 siblings of 54 patients suffering symptomatic generalized tonic-clonic seizures. Epileptiform activity was recorded in at least one sibling of 27 (50%) of the 54 patients. When the 83 siblings were reviewed, epileptiform activity was found in 34 (41%). Generalized spike-wave discharges were seen in 32 cases, and two siblings showed benign sharp wave foci in the right parietal area. It was seen only in sleep in 44.1%. They also found the highest rates of epileptiform activity in the age range up to 15 years and more in female siblings (54.5%) than in male siblings (30%).

A general conclusion from these wide-ranging epidemiologic studies is that there is definite and reproducible genetic influence in large populations of index epilepsy cases. These studies are highly different in terms of methodology and definition of epilepsy. Earlier studies had serious ascertainment bias, but this is less of a problem with more recent investigations. The substantial amount of heterogeneity in the epilepsies is also a major problem for epidemiologic surveys. Nevertheless, it would appear that 2% to 10% of siblings or children of index patients with epilepsy are also likely to develop a seizure disorder. This risk increases with increasing numbers of affected individuals in the family and with less rigorous definition of a seizure disorder that includes single seizures or febrile seizures. The risk decreases with increasing genetic distance from the index case and when there is a strong history for an acquired environmental brain insult.

In their study of genetic influences in epilepsy, Ottman et al. (1998), p. 343 suggested that for "parents and siblings some susceptibility genotypes raise the risk for both generalized and localization-related epilepsies, but are more common in persons affected with generalized epilepsy. In the offspring of the probands with localization-related epilepsies, an additional influence may raise the risk for localization-related epilepsies specifically".

Of additional note in these studies is a trend for a difference between the sexes. There are small but consistent tendencies for idiopathic seizures to be more common in females, for females with epilepsy to have a high number of children with epilepsy, and for the prognosis to be somewhat worse in females with recurrent seizures. These trends have been noted in the studies by Lennox (1947), Tsuboi and Endo (1977), Janz and Scheffner (1980), Annegers et al. (1982), and Benninger et al. (1982).

There is relatively little evidence for ethnic differences in the influence of genetic factors on epilepsy. The studies reviewed here support that conclusion and include investigations from Scandinavia, Germany, France, the United States, and Japan. However, small isolated ethnic groups may have an increased frequency of a seizure disorder on a genetic basis. An example may be a genetically complex form of epilepsy occurring in an isolated tribe in the interior of Tanzania (Jilek-Aall et al., 1979; Neuman et al., 1995). There is some evidence that febrile seizures may be more common in Japan (Tsuboi, 1977). A study in New Haven, Connecticut, found that black children had a higher risk for epilepsy than white children (cumulative risks to age 15 years of about 2% and 1%, respectively; Shamansky and Glaser, 1979). The socioeconomic differences between these two groups could be of major importance (e.g., rates of infant mortality, prematurity, accidents, lead poisoning, and poor nutrition).

Twin Studies

Newmark and Penry (1979) reviewed the results of 13 separate reports describing twins with epilepsy. Rosanoff et al. (1934) reported concordance for epilepsy in 14 of 23 monozygotic twins (61%) and in 20 of 84 dizygotic twins (24%). In a study by Lennox (1947), 20 of 24 monozygotic twins (83%) without evidence of acquired brain damage were concordant for seizures. In 19 monozygotic twins with a history of brain injury there were three (15%) concordant for seizures. Of 16 dizygotic epileptic twins, only 1 pair (6%) was concordant. Inouye (1960) studied 40 twin pairs in which at least 1 individual had seizures. Of the monozygotic twins, 36% of the female pairs and 67% of the male pairs were concordant. None of the female dizygotic twins were concordant, and 14% of the dizygotic male twins were concordant. Gedda and Taterelli (1971) found concordance in 18 of 19 monozygotic twins (95%) and in 3 of 26 dizygotic twins (12%). Vercelletto and Courjon (1969) found 10 of 14 (71%) monozygotic twins concordant for epilepsy and 1 of 4 dizygotic pairs concordant. Miller et al. (1999) found concordance rates of 28% to 39% and 1% to 13% of monozygotic twins vs. dizygotic twins (ages 16–35 years) for several types of epilepsy in a large twin study from Virginia. When all published twin studies are considered, the average concordance rate for epilepsy in monozygotic twins is 57%, with a range of 30% to 95%. The average concordance rate for epilepsy in dizygotic twins is ~11%, with a range of 5% to 20%. These figures support the argument for a strong genetic influence in epilepsy but allow little more in the way of conclusions. Heterogeneity for type of seizures, sex differences, birth order, birth weight, perinatal trauma, and ascertainment are all undefined variables in most of the investigations.

Several other types of twin studies can conveniently be noted here. Identical twins concordant for photosensitive epilepsy have been reported and the various case reports summarized by Newmark and Penry (1979). Three pairs of monozygotic twins concordant for adult temporal lobe epilepsy have been described (Barslund and Danielson, 1963). A later study first identified familial temporal epilepsy in five concordant monozygotic twin pairs (Berkovic et al. 1996). Twin studies have also supported a prominent hereditary influence in the EEG patterns of normal individuals without epilepsy, including the early study of Lennox and Gibbs (1945) and a study by Lykken and colleagues (1974). A further study comparing monozygotic with dizygotic twins has documented a genetic influence in cerebral, including visual, auditory, and somatosensory (1972) evoked potentials. A more recent review article on the genetics of the EEG and evoked potentials is that by van Beijsterveldt and Boomsma (1994), who concluded that most EEG parameters are genetically determined. However, the evoked potentials studies are based on a much smaller number of studies and show genetic influences, but not as strong as for the EEG. Berkovic et al. (1998) found concordances for generalized epilepsies in monozygotic twins of 0.82 and in dizygotic twins of 0.26 that were greater than those for partial epilepsies in which the concordance for monozygotic twins was 0.36 and for dizygotic was 0.05. They concluded that genetic factors are important in the generalized epilepsies but also have a role in the partial epilepsies. The data suggested that there are syndrome-specific genetic determinants rather than a broad genetic predisposition to seizures (Berkovic et al., 1998).

Several studies have evaluated twins with febrile seizures. In 19 pairs of monozygotic twins, Lennox-Buchthal (1971) found 68% concordance for febrile seizures and 89% concordance for febrile or nocturnal convulsions. Schiottz-Christensen (1972) found 17% concordance for febrile seizures in 14 pairs of male monozygotic twins and 58% concordance in 12 pairs of female monozygotic twins. The same study showed 16% concordance for febrile seizures in 19 pairs of male dizygotic twins and 11% concordance for 18 pairs for female dizygotic twins. Tsuboi and Endo (1991) found a 69% concordance rate for febrile seizures in monozygotic twins in Japan and a 20% concordance rate in dizygotic twins. Berkovic et al. (1998) found a concordance rate for febrile seizures in monozygotic twins of 58% and 14% in dizygotic twins. Miller et al. (1999) found a concordance rate for febrile seizures of 39% to 42% in monozygotic twins and 12% to 14% in dizygotic twins, confirming the likelihood of genetic factors in this disorder.

FAMILY STUDIES OF SPECIFIC SEIZURE TYPES

Generalized Epilepsy

Childhood Absence Epilepsy

Generalized absence seizures have also been called *petit mal*, *centrencephalic* epilepsy, or pyknolepsy. The absence attack is a sudden brief episode of decreased responsiveness or altered consciousness without aura and without postictal symptoms. There may be brief motor automatisms such as lip smacking, chewing, swallowing, finger fumbling, or leg shuffling. Autonomic phenomena such as pupil dilation, flushing, or brief respiratory arrest may occur. Formed speech rarely occurs. Typically, the seizures have an onset between 5 and 10 years of age. All seizure activity ceases following puberty in 50% to 90% of patients. Some patients develop generalized major motor seizures later in life, and a small number continue to have absence attacks in adulthood (Browne and Mirsky, 1983).

An analysis by Bouma et al. (1996) to ascertain the outcome of absence epilepsy found that of patients with absence epilepsy, 78% were later seizure free. However, evolution to tonic-clonic seizures with or without coexisting freedom from absence seizures occurred in 50% of patients and of these 35% became seizure free. Wirell et al. (1996) analyzed patients with typical childhood absence epilepsy and concluded that while 65% of these children eventually have remission of their epilepsy, nearly half of those without remission will develop juvenile myoclonic epilepsy (JME). If a child develops generalized tonic-clonic or myoclonic seizures during treatment with antiepileptic drugs, remission from absence epilepsy is infrequent and development of JME is very likely (Wirrell et al., 1996).

Simple or classic petit mal epilepsy includes the typical description of the absence attack described above without other complicated phenomena and in association with a bilaterally synchronous and symmetric 3 Hz spike and wave EEG pattern (see Fig. 41–1). Lennox and coworkers (1945; Lennox, 1951) reported (1) a family history of epilepsy in 34% of patients with 3 Hz spike and wave discharges, (2) a concordance rate of 75% for absence seizures in monozygotic twins, (3) a concordance rate of 84% for 3 Hz spike and wave EEG discharges in monozygotic twins, and (4) a concordance rate of 0% for both absence seizures and 3 Hz spike wave discharges in dizygotic twins.

One of the most interesting and provocative investigations into the genetics of epilepsy was performed by Metrakos and Metrakos (1961, 1966; Metrakos et al., 1966) and involved patients with classic petit mal epilepsy with 3 Hz spike and wave EEG complexes. These studies are documented in several reports by Metrakos and Metrakos between 1961 and 1966. They presented evidence that at least one form of petit mal epilepsy is the result of a single autosomal dominant gene with low penetrance. They studied 211 probands with "typical or atypical centrencephalic epilepsy." These index patients had "a history of recurrent petit mal and/or grand mal seizures, no obvious neuropathology to account for their seizures, and a centrencephalic EEG." In addition to the author's genetic hypothesis, the studies emphasized two further important points: (1) that an individual carrying a gene for epilepsy may never have clinical seizures but may have an abnormal EEG and (2) that the penetrance of the epilepsy gene may vary with age. Thus, between ages 4.5 and 16.5 years, ~45% of the siblings of patients with petit mal epilepsy demonstrated the trait on EEG. The penetrance was low before the age of 4.5 years and decreased after adolescence. Only ~25% of those individuals inheriting the trait according to EEG criteria actually had clinical seizures. Furthermore, 35% of the offspring of patients with petit mal epilepsy demonstrated the 3 Hz spike and wave trait in the EEG, and this was uncorrected for age effect. The investigators interpreted their data as showing that at least one form of idiopathic generalized absence epilepsy is determined by a single autosomal dominant gene that has a low penetrance for clinical seizures but an al-

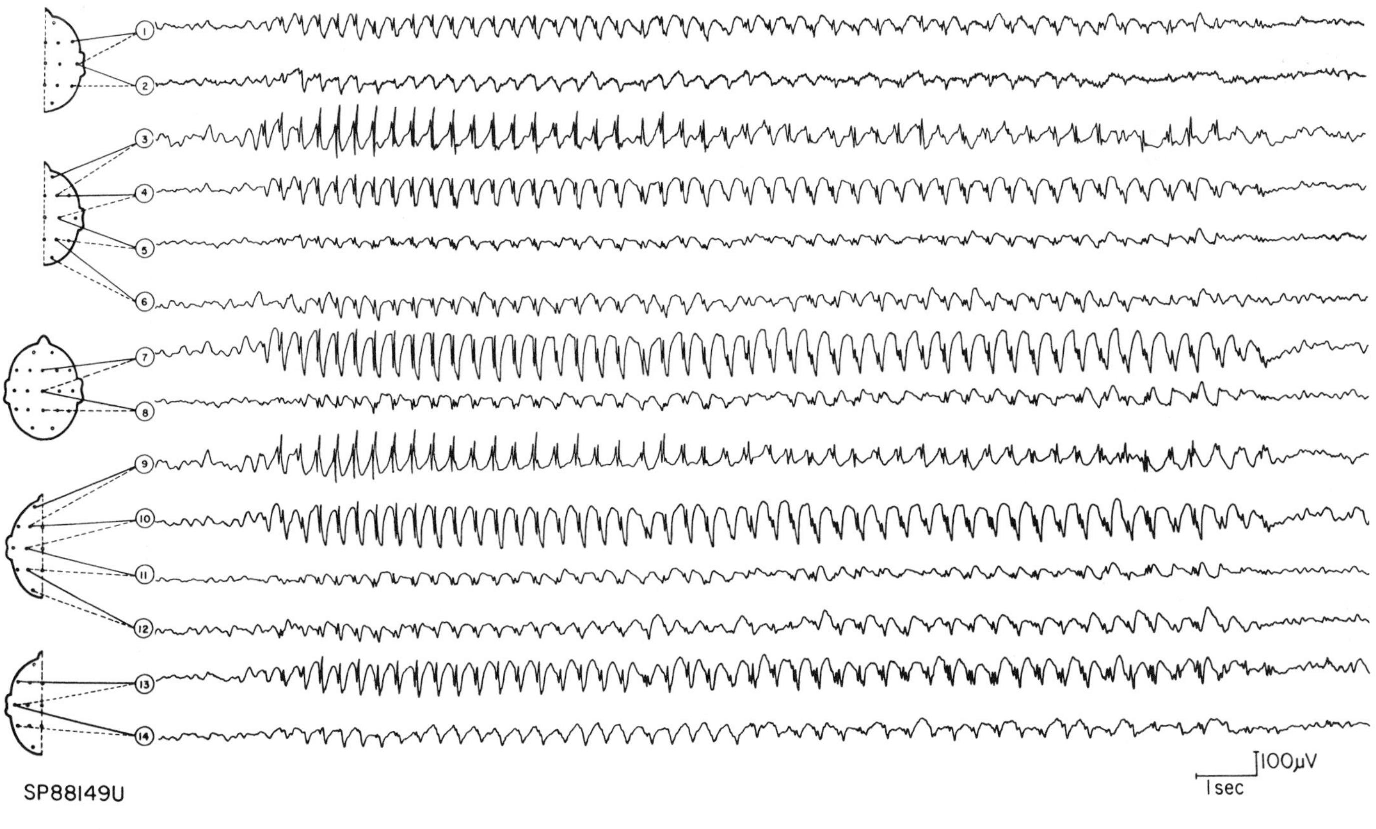

Fig. 41–1. EEG demonstrating 3 Hz per second spike and wave pattern typical of one form of generalized absence petit mal epilepsy. (Courtesy of Dr. G. Chatrian, University of Washington.)

most complete penetrance for an abnormal EEG during a restricted age period. The data suggested that genetic counseling of children or siblings of an affected person should include a 50% risk of inheriting the gene for this type of absence epilepsy, but only about a 12% risk (0.5×0.25) of actually having clinical seizures.

The findings of Metrakos and Metrakos have been criticized primarily on the basis of their criteria for an abnormal EEG and on the probable heterogeneity of their patient population. The identification of the "centrencephalic EEG abnormality" in their families included EEG changes other than the typical 3 Hz spike and wave complexes. Doose et al. (1968b, 1973) studied 252 probands with absence seizures and 3 Hz spike and wave EEG, 242 of their siblings, and 685 control patients. They reported that (1) 7.6% of siblings of probands had 3 Hz spike and wave EEG, (2) 20% of siblings of probands between the ages of 5 and 16 years had 3 Hz spike and wave EEG, and (3) 1.9% of control children had 3 Hz spike and wave EEG. They concluded that, "taken as a whole, the results suggest that epilepsies with spike and wave absences are not inherited by an autosomal gene, but that several genetic factors are responsible, some mutually independent and some either reinforcing or inhibiting the others."

Matthes and Weber (1968) found that 13.3% of patients with absence attacks and 3 Hz spike and wave EEG had a family history of convulsions and that 5.4% of parents and 11% of siblings had had a previous seizure (isolated or recurrent). Note that this latter figure of 11% is remarkably close to the 12% recurrence risk computed from the data of Metrakos and Metrakos. Fong et al. (1998) found evidence for linkage to chromosome 8q24 in a large Indian family with childhood absence seizures. Wallace et al. (2001) reported a large family with epilepsy, the main phenotypes being childhood absence epilepsy and febrile seizures. A mutation in a gene in chromosome 5, encoding a $GABA_A$ receptor subunit was identified. The mutations, as in the case of the $GABA_A$ receptor subunit gene may have an age-dependent effect on the neuronal pathways, resulting in phenotypic heterogeneity (Wallace et al. 2001).

The Commission on Classification and Terminology of the International League against Epilepsy (1989) recognizes three other epileptic syndromes with typical absences besides childhood absence epilepsy: juvenile absence epilepsy, juvenile myoclonic epilepsy, and epilepsy with myoclonic absences.

Juvenile Absence Epilepsy

In juvenile absence epilepsy (JAE), the absences are the same as in childhood absence epilepsy, but manifestation occurs in puberty (Commission on Classification and Terminology, 1989). Absences with retropulsive movements are less common. Seizure frequency is lower, with absences occurring less frequently than every day and mostly sporadically. Association with generalized tonic-clonic seizures (GTCS) is frequent, and GTCS precede the absence manifestation more often than in childhood absence epilepsy, often occurring on awakening. Patients might also have myoclonic seizures. The sex distribution is equal. The EEG spike and waves are often more than 3 Hz. The response to therapy is excellent. Sander et al. (1997) found an association of JAE with allelic variants of the GluR5 kainate receptor gene (*GRIK1*) on chromosome 21q22.1.

Juvenile Myoclonic Epilepsy

Another form of juvenile absence may be associated with myoclonic, tonic-clonic, or clonic tonic-clonic seizures and is part of the impulsive petit mal syndrome of Janz or juvenile myoclonic epilepsy (JME) (Delgado-Escueta and Enrile-Bascal, 1984). Onset of the seizures is typically between ages 10 and 20 years. Absence attacks start with 4 to 6 Hz diffuse multispike and wave complexes in the EEG instead of the well-formed 3 Hz spike and wave complexes of classic petit mal. There may be mild myoclonic jerks of neck and shoulder flexor muscles and also tonic-clonic seizures shortly after awakening. Some 37% of the patients have absence attacks. The prognosis is reported to be good with a favorable response to valproic acid. Persistence of the trait throughout life explains the high recurrence rate (90%) after withdrawal of drug treatment. Tsuboi and Christian (1973) completed a genetic study of 319 patients with sporadic myoclonic impulsive petit mal epilepsy. They concluded that 34% of female and 21% of male probands had some evidence for a genetic predisposition. The incidence of epilepsy was 4.1% in near relatives (higher among female than male relatives and higher among mothers than fathers). Of the 116 relatives found to have epilepsy, 15% had impulsive petit mal, 17% had awakening grand mal, and 14% had absence attacks. EEG examinations showed nonspecific paroxysmal abnormalities in 40% and specific abnormalities in 15% of 390 family members, which is significantly higher than those in the relatives of control subjects. Relatives of female probands had a higher frequency of paroxysmal EEG abnormalities than those of male probands (61% vs. 47%). Of 1618 near relatives, 7.3% had either epileptic seizures or specific EEG abnormalities, or both. The investigators found it difficult to distinguish between a dominant single-gene disorder with greatly reduced penetrance or a multifactorial model. However, they favored the latter explanation. The reasons for the sex differences were unexplained and, in fact, are somewhat in conflict with the multifactorial model, which would predict that the sex with the greater family history (females) should be less frequently affected among the relatives. Panayiotopoulos and Obeid (1989) found evidence for autosomal recessive inheritance in 17 families with juvenile myoclonic epilepsy.

Greenberg et al. (1988) found evidence for genetic linkage of this disorder to the HLA locus on chromosome 6. Delgado-Escueta et al. (1990) verified in 19 families that JME was present in 45% of all affected members, 55% of affected siblings, 44% of affected parents, 9% of all siblings, and 4% of all parents. Childhood absence epilepsy (CAE) was present in only 18% of affected siblings and not in affected parents. CAE plus epilepsy with GTCS was present in 22% of affected parents. Epilepsy with GTCS only was present in 23% of all affected family members. The authors concluded that "clearly, only idiopathic generalized epilepsies were present as phenotypes in family members of patients with JME" (Delgado-Escueta et al., 1990). Their linkage studies, which included an increase in the sample since their last analysis (Greenberg and Delgado-Escueta, 1988), strongly indicated that linkage to chromosome 6p existed, no matter what mode of inheritance was assumed. In 1991, Weissbecker et al. confirmed the linkage to the HLA region of chromosome 6p (EJM1) although, at a larger recombination factor. The same year, Durner et al. (1991) reported tight linkage to DNA markers in the HLA-DQ locus. In 1995, Lui et al. provided genetic linkage evidence that improved the map position of the JME locus to 35 cM below HLA in the chromosome 6p11 region. In 1996, Lui et al. further reduced the JME locus to a 7 cM region flanked by D6S272 and D6S257. Linkage analysis of JME has been confounded when families with JME have absences, when families with CAE evolve to JME, or when families with CAE with or without GTCS are mixed with families of classic JME (Minassian et al., 1996). Greenberg et al. (1996)

concluded that in families with JME mixed with absence, the JME gene is within the HLA area at chromosome 6p21.3. In their study of German JME patients, Sander et al. (1997) refined a candidate region of 10.1 cM in chromosome region 6p21. Additional genetic and physical mapping of this locus is necessary to further reduce the locus and identify the gene for JME.

The JME phenotype may have underlying genetic heterogeneity. Delgado-Escueta et al. (1990) found linkage to chromosome 1p in one large family from Mexico City and Guadalajara with a proband with CAE that evolved to JME (Minassian et al., 1996). Using nonparametric methods of linkage analysis in 10 families with 38 affected subjects, Zara et al. (1995) found evidence for involvement of a locus at chromosome 8q24. The families did not represent a particular subgroup but cluster different types of idiopathic generalized epilepsy; three families had at least one affected member with JME. In the majority of families studied, Elmslie et al. (1997) found a major susceptibility locus for JME on chromosome 15q14.

A recent article discusses the clinical heterogeneity in JME families and found only myoclonic jerks in 15 (8%) of 186 individuals with JME (Jain et al., 1997). Four of 15 persons diagnosed as having JME with only myoclonic jerks had a first-degree relative with definite JME. They proposed that individuals with only myoclonic jerks may represent a benign type of JME, that is possibly genetically distinct from classic JME (Jain et al., 1997).

Epilepsy with Generalized Tonic-Clonic Seizures upon Awakening

Epilepsy with generalized tonic clonic seizures upon awakening has an age of onset mostly in the second decade (Commission on Classification and Terminology, 1981). The seizures occur shortly after awakening. In its pure form, it has no myoclonic or absence seizures. Greenberg et al. (1995) found evidence that the pure form is linked to the EJM-1 locus.

Myoclonic Astatic Epilepsy

Primary generalized myoclonic astatic epilepsy is a rare seizure disorder with a strong genetic predisposition. It occurs between the ages of 1 and 5 in children with normal intelligence and affects boys three times more often than girls. Clinically there may be myoclonic, tonic, absence, or tonic-clonic seizures. The EEG shows bilaterally synchronous irregular 2 to 3 Hz multispike and wave complexes. Doose and colleagues (1970; Doose and Gundel, 1982) have conducted a genetic investigation of myoclonic astatic petit mal epilepsy. Their study of 50 probands showed convulsions in 13% of siblings and in 7.1% of parents. EEG studies in 72 siblings showed distinct pathologic changes in 46%, photosensitivity in 44% of children aged 6 to 10 years, and abnormal q rhythms in 43% of siblings aged 1 to 5 years. Taking the history of seizures and the EEG findings together, a total of 34 families (68%) suggested a familial convulsive susceptibility. This figure rose to 80% of families by including cases in which seizures were reported in more distant family members. Again, it was difficult to differentiate fully the autosomal dominant inheritance with reduced penetrance from a multifactorial model, although the data would seem to favor the former.

Finally, it needs to be emphasized that a major complication of genetic studies of childhood and juvenile generalized epilepsies is that the clinical syndromes are indistinct with overlapping and subjective definitions that produce groups of subjects likely to represent considerable genetic and etiologic heterogeneity (Reutens and Berkovic, 1995).

Benign Familial Neonatal Convulsions

Benign familial neonatal convulsions (BFNC) is a dominantly inherited epilepsy characterized clinically by the onset on the second and third days of life of clonic or apneic seizures. In most cases remission is seen by the age of 6 months. Interictal EEG is normal. There is normal physical examination and subsequent intellectual development. It has a benign outcome, but about 10% to 15% of the patients later develop epilepsy.

In 1989, Leppert et al. localized the gene (*EBN1*) causing BFNC to chromosome 20q. This was later confirmed by Malafosse et al. (1992), who found closed linkage of BFNC to chromosome 20q in six French pedigrees, and by Ronen et al. (1993) in one large Newfoundland kindred. Genetic heterogeneity was shown by Ryan et al. (1991) in a large pedigree from San Antonio, Texas, that failed to have linkage to the chromosome 20q locus. Also, Schiffman et al. (1991) presented a consanguineous family with BFNC. The mode of transmission in this family seems to be autosomal recessive. Linkage analysis failed to show tight linkage between this family and the locus on chromosome 20q. In 1993 Lewis et al. demonstrated that a large Mexican American kindred with BFNC was found to have linkage with chromosome 8q. None of the affected subjects in the family had seizures after 12 months of age (distinct from the chromosome 20q-linked BFNC families), suggesting that early and complete remission of BFNC is specific to the chromosome 8 locus. Steinlein et al. (1995b) also confirmed genetic heterogeneity and linkage to chromosome 8. Three individuals in their family had epileptic events after 12 months of age. For this reason, they concluded that exclusion of linkage to chromosome 20q in a BFNC family allows no prediction about the risk of subsequent seizures later in life. Both Singh et al. (1998) and Charlier et al. (1998) found that the genes responsible for BFNC are two related voltage-gated potassium channel genes that belong to a new KQT-like class of potassium channels. *KCNQ2* is the gene mutated in BFNC linked to chromosome 20q and *KCNQ3* is the gene mutated in the EBN2 locus linked to chromosome 8q.

Partial Epilepsy

Frontal Lobe Epilepsy

Nocturnal frontal lobe epilepsy was described by Scheffer et al. (1995), who saw the syndrome of autosomal dominant nocturnal frontal lobe epilepsy in five families containing 47 affected individuals. Onset of seizures varied from infancy to the sixth decade, but in 88% of cases was under age 20; the mean age was 11.7 years. Seizures occurred almost exclusively in sleep, usually as the subject dozed or before awakening. Seizures typically began with vocalization and had prominent motor manifestations of thrashing or tonic activity, and awareness was usually retained (76% of patients). Seizures occurred in clusters, with an average of eight attacks over a few hours. Individuals were of normal intellect with no neurologic abnormalities. Neuroimaging studies were normal. Seizures often persisted through adult life. The clinical features are consistent with seizure of frontal lobe origin. The interictal EEG recording lacked epileptiform activity in 84% of subjects studied. Six individuals showed epileptiform abnormalities, localized to the anterior quadrant. Seizures occurred predominantly in non-REM sleep, most commonly in stage 2. Ictal recordings were often obscured by movement artifact, but the ictal recording shows sharp and slow wave activity localized to the anterior quadrants bilaterally. Carbamazepine produced good response.

Segregation analysis strongly supported autosomal dominant inheritance with a penetrance of 69% (Scheffer et al., 1995). Phillips et al. (1995) reported the chromosomal assignment to chromosome 20q13.2 in one large Australian kindred with 27 affected individuals over six generations. Steinlein et al. (1995a) knowing that the gene for autosomal dominant frontal lobe epilepsy maps to chromosome 20q 13.2q13.3 and that neuronal nicotinic acetylcholine receptor α subunit (CHRNA4) maps to the same region of 20q, screened affected family members for mutations within CHRNA4. They found a missense mutation that replaces serine with phenylalanine at codon 248, is a strongly conserved amino acid residue in the second domain of the receptor ion channel and is likely to impair cholinergic transmission. In 1997 Steinlein et al. identified a different mutation in the same gene in a Norwegian family with a similar phenotype. A second locus for nocturnal frontal lobe epilepsy was found at 15q24 in one family (Phillips et al. 1998). Other families with typical autosomal dominant frontal lobe epilepsy are not linked to 20q13.2q13.3 or to 15q24, thus demonstrating further genetic heterogeneity for autosomal dominant nocturnal frontal lobe epilepsy. (Berkovic et al., 1995; Oldani et al., 1998; Phillips et al., 1998). A third locus for autosomal dominant nocturnal frontal lobe epilepsy was identified on chromosome 1 (Gambardella et al., 2000). De Fusco and collaborators (2000) reported a mutation in the acetylcholine receptor subunit $\beta 2$ (*CHRNB2*) gene in chromosome 1p21 as responsible for autosomal dominant nocturnal frontal lobe epilepsy. This is the second acetylcholine receptor subunit associated with autosomal dominant nocturnal frontal lobe epilepsy.

Temporal Lobe and Rolandic Epilepsy

A relatively benign epilepsy of childhood is associated with an EEG spike focus in the rolandic-centrotemporal region. The attacks are usually partial (focal) motor seizures (often of the face) that occur during sleep or waking. The seizures usually begin between ages 5 and 9 years, are controlled by anticonvulsants, and disappear after age 15 years. There is evidence that this is an autosomal dominant condition with expression limited to a short time span and occurrence of only the EEG abnormality in some affected individuals. Some 15% of siblings of index cases have had the same limited seizure disorder (Beaussart 1972; Blom et al., 1972; Heijbel and Blom, 1975; Heijbel 1980; Blom and Heijbel, 1982; Loiseau et al., 1988). The studies by Bray and Wiser (1964, 1965) showing a genetic influence in childhood temporal lobe epilepsy probably included patients with the rolandic-centrotemporal trait.

Degen and Degen in 1992 performed waking and sleep EEG studies in 69 siblings of 43 patients. Five siblings had a history of seizures (three febrile and two GTCS). Epileptiform activity was recorded in at least one sibling (51.2%) of 43 patients with 26 siblings of 69 (37.7%) having epileptiform activity recorded. Most epileptic activity was recorded in siblings aged 5 to 12 years (54.3%). Only four siblings had focal discharges. All others had generalized 3 to 4 second spike wave complexes. The finding that 54.3% of siblings ages 5 to 12 had EEG abnormalities supported an autosomal dominant genetic factor. A multifactorial mode of inheritance, however, was considered a possibility (Degen and Degen, 1992). Linkage in 22 families has been shown to chromosome 15q14 and was most consistent with an autosomal recessive model (Neubauer et al., 1998).

A syndrome related to benign rolandic epilepsy was described by Scheffer et al. in 1995. They described nine affected individuals over three generations with Rolandic epilepsy with speech dyspraxia and cognitive impairment (Scheffer et al., 1995b). Rolandic epilepsy with exercise-induced dystonia has been linked to 16p12–p11 (Guerrini et al. 1999).

Other studies show increased familial incidence of seizures in the relatives of patients with several varieties of complex partial or temporal lobe epilepsy. This includes the studies of Rodin and Gonzales (1966) and of Loiseau and Beaussart (1969). Falconer (1971) reviewed a series of patients receiving temporal lobe surgery for the treatment of complex partial seizures. About one-half of the cases had mesial temporal sclerosis on neuropathologic examination. Their seizures were characterized by early onset (usually in the first decade of life), a high incidence of prolonged febrile convulsions in infancy, and a positive family history of epilepsy. A family history of epilepsy was not found in the other patients with temporal lobe hamartomas or cerebral developmental abnormalities. Some of the patients with temporal lobe scarring and infarction did have a family history of seizures. Jensen (1975) also studied 74 patients undergoing temporal lobe surgery for drug-resistant epilepsy. Some 30% had a positive family history of epilepsy, 49% a family history of other neurologic disease, and 46% a family history of a major psychiatric disorder. Most probably genetic factors do make a contribution.

Familial temporal lobe epilepsy was initially identified through a twin study of epilepsy and is now recognized in an increasing number of families (Berkovic et al., 1996). It begins in adolescence or early adult life (median 19 years). Patients have seizures typical of mesial temporal lobe epilepsy with simple partial seizures with psychic or autonomic features, infrequent complex partial seizures, and rare secondarily generalized partial seizures. Interictal EEG abnormalities are uncommon (Berkovic and Scheffer, 1997). Electroencephalogram revealed sparse focal temporal discharges in 22% of the subjects. MRI appeared normal. The condition appears to be inherited in an autosomal dominant manner with a penetrance of approximately 60% (Berkovic et al., 1996). Cendes et al. (1998) studied 11 families with familial temporal lobe epilepsy autosomal sdominant inheritance with incomplete penetrance. They found heterogeneous clinical manifestations with some members presenting a benign course, but there was also a severe course with refractory seizures in 41% of their patients. This suggested genetic heterogeneity. Further studies are necessary to clarify this.

Ottman et al. (1995) described a family with 11 affected individuals over three generations with a partial epilepsy in which auditory hallucinations were common. The inheritance pattern was strongly suggestive of autosomal dominant inheritance with reduced penetrance. Linkage analysis provided evidence for an epilepsy susceptibility gene located within a 10 cM interval on chromosome 10 (Ottman et al., 1995). In a large family with temporal epilepsy Poza and collaborators (1999) found linkage to chromosome 10q in a 15 cM interval overlapping the previous locus reported by Ottman et al. (1995). Mutations in the LGI1 gene have been reported in this disease (Kalachikov et al., 2002).

Occipital Lobe Epilepsy: Benign Familial Infantile Convulsions

Vigevano et al. (1992) described a benign idiopathic epilepsy with onset between 3.5 and 12 months of life. It also has an autosomal dominant mode of transmission. The seizures are thought to be of the partial type because there is often an occipital-parietal EEG ictal focus. Patients display no signs of neurological abnormality and have spontaneous seizure remission and normal development. Interictal EEG shows no abnormalities. The seizure-free neonatal period distinguishes benign familial infantile convulsions (BFIC) from BFNC. Guipponi et al. in 1997 mapped the BFIC gene to chromosome 19q by linkage analysis in five Italian families. They concluded that BFNC and BFIC are not allelic, and their results indicate that BFIC is a distinct syndrome from 20q BFNC. Moreover, the existence of a founder effect in these Italian families is suggested by the common haplotype found in their pedigrees. However, larger families and more information are needed before reaching any conclusions. Guipponi et al. (1997) suggested that the ages of onset of BFNC and BFIC might indicate that their genes play a role in the maturation of regulatory processes of cerebral excitability. Szepetowski et al. (1997) reported four families from northwestern France with benign infantile convulsions inherited as an autosomal dominant trait and paroxysmal choreoathetosis. They found linkage for the disease gene in the pericentromeric region of chromosome 16 (16p12–q12) and provided evidence for a common basis of convulsive and choreoathetotic diseases. This association has been confirmed by Swoboda et al. (2000). Caraballo and collegues (2001) reported seven families with pure BFIC linked to the same region in chromosome 16p12–q12. More recently, a third locus was mapped to chromosome 2q24 (Malacarne et al., 2001).

A form of epilepsy with visual symptoms has been reported to be "familial" but requires further study. It has been referred to as "benign partial epilepsy of childhood with occipital spike-waves" (Riggio et al., 1987). Later, another occipital lobe epilepsy syndrome was described in which seizures were triggered by visual stimuli, mainly from television and computer screens (Guerrini et al., 1995). A family history was found in 30% of probands. This could also be considered a form of reflex epilepsy (see below).

Simple Partial, Acquired, and Posttraumatic Epilepsy

As noted earlier, partial or focal seizures are likely to have an identifiable environmental or acquired etiology. However, after brain trauma or infection, only a certain proportion of individuals develop epilepsy. While subsequent epilepsy clearly depends on the severity of the brain insult, there may also be subtle underlying genetic factors that predispose these individuals to seizures. Dencker (quoted by Caveness [1976]) came to this conclusion after his study of closed head injury in monozygotic twins. Evans (1962) studied 422 Korean War veterans who had sustained head injury. A family history of epilepsy was reported by 7% of the patients who had posttraumatic seizures, in contrast to only 2% of those who did not develop seizures. Giaquinto (1980) studied a small group of 41 subjects with head injury. Of the 18 who developed posttraumatic epilepsy, 28% had a family history of epilepsy, whereas there was a family history of epilepsy in only 4.3% of the 23 head injury subjects who did not have posttraumatic epilepsy. In contrast, Schaumann and colleagues (1982) found no increased familial occurrence of epilepsy in the relatives of 143 patients with posttraumatic seizures or of 50 patients with seizures related to alcoholism.

A pertinent historical anecdote is the famous case of H. M. (Corkin, 1984). This young man developed a severe and much-studied memory defect after he had bilateral temporal lobe surgery for intractable epilepsy. His seizure disorder was thought to be the result of a relatively mild head injury, yet it was noted that three paternal first cousins also had epilepsy.

Andermann (1982) reported the largest and most careful genetic study of focal (partial) epilepsy. She and her colleagues studied the families of 60 patients with focal seizures who underwent surgical treatment for epilepsy. These patients presumably included both complex partial and other forms of focal seizure disorder. There was no significant increase in seizures in first-degree or more distant relatives of focal probands, as compared to the relatives of a control population. However, there was a significant increase in EEG abnormalities in the relatives of these focal probands. Andermann (1982) reported the following empiric risk figures for purposes of genetic counseling of patients with focal epilepsy: for siblings or offspring of patients with focal epilepsy, the risk of having as epileptiform EEG abnormality is 20%, the risk of one or more isolated seizure is 7%, and the risk of chronic epilepsy is 4%. Muller and associates (1973) studied 151 children with focal seizures and found seizures in 3.2% of parents of siblings, compared with 2.1% in a control group. Abnormal EEGs were also more common in the relatives of the focal seizure probands. Treiman (1987) found some evidence for hereditary factors in adults with symptomatic partial epilepsy (28% positive history in first- and second-degree relatives).

There is additional evidence that there may be genetic susceptibility to epileptiform environmental agents. Doose and coworkers (1968a) reported an unusual study of infants having convulsions following smallpox vaccination. Of 171 children with postvaccinial convulsions, 58% had a past history of seizures, a history of seizures in a near relative, or an EEG abnormality of a "genetic type." Similar to Schaumann et al. (1982), Meyer and colleagues (1976) found no significant genetic tendency in the families of patients whose epilepsy was associated with alcohol abuse. It is of interest that Kakihana (1979) has reported differences between genetic strains of mice for susceptibility to alcohol withdrawal seizures; this remains an interesting hypothesis for humans. Women having seizures during pregnancy may demonstrate an increased family history of epilepsy, although this has not been studied in detail (MacIntosh, 1952). Children having an acquired hemiparesis or hemiplegia associated with a seizure disorder have a higher percentage of relatives with seizures than do hemiplegic children who have not had a seizure. In fact, the hemiplegic children without a seizure history had a lower family history of epilepsy than a control population had (Rimoin and Metrakos, 1972).

To summarize, genetic factors seem important in partial epilepsy. Single gene and complex (multifactorial) inheritances are the suggested inheritance for partial epilepsies. Among patients with acquired factors for epilepsy, such as head injury, not all develop epilepsy. Family studies have shown that genetic factors do make a contribution. A listing of the chromosomal location of primary epilepsy syndromes, generalized and partial, is presented in Table 41–7.

Reflex and Stimulus-Sensitive Epilepsies

Clinical seizures may sometimes be precipitated by specific environmental stimuli. Hyperventilation and photic stimulation with a flashing light have long been known to induce seizures in some individuals. Certain movements, noises, visual patterns, sudden emotional changes, or changes in body temperature have also been reported to produce seizures on rare occasions.

An individual who develops spike and wave EEG abnormalities during stimulation with a flashing light is considered to have a special kind of photosensitivity called the photoconvulsive response (PCR). Some but not all of these patients will occasionally have a clinical convulsion produced by the flashing light. This response is to be distinguished from the photo myogenic response in which the individual has only blinking or muscle twitching in response to the flash and no epileptiform EEG activity. Approximately 5% to 8% of neurologically healthy children show the PCR. Several studies have demonstrated that the

Table 41–7. Chromosomal Locations of Primary Epilepsy Syndromes

Epilepsy Syndrome[a]	Inheritance[b]	Localization	Gene	References
Generalized				
Benign familial neonatal convulsions	AD	20q 8q24	*KCNQ2* *KCNQ3*	Singh et al., 1998; Charlier et al., 1998; Biervert and Steinlein, 1999
Benign familial infantile convulsions	AD	19q 16p12–q12 2q24	—	Guiponni et al., 1997; Szepetowski et al., 1997; Caraballo et al., 2001; Malacarne et al., 2001
Febrile seizures	AD	8q 19p 2q23–q24 5q14–q15	*FEB1* *FEB2* *FEB3* *FEB4*	Wallace et al., 1996; Johnson et al., 1998; Peiffer et al., 1999; Nakayama et al., 2000
Generalized epilepsy with febrile seizures	AD	19q 2q21–q33 5q34	*SCN1B* *SCN1A* *GABRG2*	Wallace et al., 1998; Baulac et al., 1999; Moulard et al., 1999; Lopes-Cendes et al., 2000; Escayg et al., 2001; Baulac et al., 2001
Childhood absence epilepsy	AD	8q24 5q34	— *GABRG2*	Fong et al., 1998; Wallace et al., 2001
Benign myoclonic epilepsy in infancy	AR	16p13	—	Zara et al., 2000
Severe myoclonic epilepsy of infancy	sporadic	2q	*SCN1A*	Claes et al., 2001
Juvenile myoclonic epilepsy	AD, AR?	6p 15q	*EJM1* *EJM2*	Durner et al., 1991; Greenberg et al., 1995 Elmslie et al., 1997
Adult myoclonic epilepsy	AD	8q24	—	Mikami et al., 1999; Plaster et al., 1999
Baltic myoclonic epilepsy	AR	21q	Cystatin B	Pennacchio et al., 1996; Lalioti et al., 1997, 1998
Autosomal dominant cortical myoclonus and epilepsy (ADCME) with complex partial and generalized seizures	AD	2p11.2–q12.2	—	Guerrini et al., 2001
Myoclonic epilepsy with mental retardation and spasticity	XL	Xp22.3-p21.1	ARX	Stromme et al., 2002
Partial				
Nocturnal frontal lobe epilepsy	AD	20q 15q 1p21	*CHRNA4* — *CHRNB2*	Steinlein et al., 1995a; Phillips et al., 1998; De Fusco et al., 2000
Partial epilepsy with auditory features	AD	10q	—	Ottman et al., 1995
Familial temporal lobe epilepsy	AD	10q	—	Berkovic et al., 1996; Poza et al., 1999
Rolandic epilepsy	?AR	15q	—	Neubauer et al., 1998
Partial epilepsy with variable foci	AD	2q 22q11–q12	— —	Scheffer et al., 1998; Xiong et al., 1999.

[a]Complex diseases with additional neurologic characteristics such as Lafora-type epilepsy and the ceroid storage diseases are not included in this table.
[b]AD, autosomal dominant; AR, autosomal recessive; XL, x-linked.
—: not available.

PCR has a strong genetic component (Newmark and Penry, 1979; Doose, 1982, Doose and Waltz, 1993). It can be detected in up to 40% of siblings of index cases between the ages of 5 and 15 years. Females are more often affected than males. The PCR is different from the 3 Hz spike and wave EEG pattern seen in classic petit mal epilepsy, and the two disorders do not show significant overlap genetically. In one study of index cases with both epilepsy and PCR, the prevalence of clinical seizures in close relatives was 9%, 6.5%, 7%, and 1.8% for sisters, brothers, mothers, and fathers, respectively (Rabending and Klepel, 1970). This could be an example of a single dominant gene with low clinical penetrance and variability of expression, depending on both age and sex. A multifactorial explanation is also possible.

Seizures occurring during reading have been reported in more than one member of several families and may represent a dominant gene in some instances (Daly and Foster, 1975). A recent study by Radhakrishnan et al. (1995) reported a family history of seizures including reading epilepsy. Most of the reported familial cases involved idiopathic generalized epilepsy. Epilepsy sensitive to certain visual patterns has been described in siblings (Chatrian et al., 1970). Brinciotti et al. (1992) reported two families with pattern sensitive epilepsy. All affected members, except for the mother of the family, had electroclinical seizures induced by intermittent light stimulus and pattern stimulation. They suggested a common inheritance model for photo and pattern sensitivity: "Patients may exhibit only one phenotype (pattern or photosensitivity) at a given time, and this could be explained by a different age-dependent penetrance and expressivity."

Reflex seizures induced by calculation, card or board games, and spatial task have been reported in 25 individuals (Goossens et al., 1990). The activity seems to be related to a function of the parietal lobe. The clinical and electroencephalogram findings confirm the presence of a generalized epileptic abnormality. The onset is during adolescence, and myoclonus is most commonly present, along with absences with myoclonus and eventually generalized convulsions. The response to medication is generally good. In this study there was sensitivity to calculation and card games in one family. Two siblings probably had epileptic seizures induced by such stimuli.

Schubert and Cracco (1992) reported a family with rectal and other pain triggering a reaction with autonomic changes and tonic posturing. Some forms of paroxysmal choreoathetosis are thought to represent seizures induced by body movement. A controversy exists over whether this is a reflex epilepsy or a nonepileptic disorder (Cesare, 1995). Many families with various types of paroxysmal choreoathetosis have been reported, often suggesting autosomal dominant inheritance (Lance, 1977). In the late 1990s a gene locus for paroxysmal choreoathetosis and spasticity was demonstrated on chromosome 1p (Auburger et al. 1996), along with another locus on 2q for paroxysmal dystonia and choreoathetosis (Fink et al. 1997). Szepetowski et al. (1997) provided evidence for a common basis of convulsive and choreoathetotic disorders in their study of four families with benign infantile convulsions and paroxysmal choreoathetosis linked to chromosome 16.

Febrile Seizures

Controversy continues over the definition, prognosis, treatment, and pathophysiology of so-called febrile seizures. Millichap (1981) defines these as a seizure in infancy or childhood, usually occurring between 3 months and 5 years of age, associated with fever but without evidence of intracranial infection or defined cause. Seizures with fever in children who have suffered a previous nonfebrile seizure are excluded. Febrile seizures are to be distinguished from epilepsy that is characterized by recurrent nonfebrile seizures. However, children with initial febrile seizures may go on to develop epilepsy. In white populations, 2% to 5% of all children will have a febrile seizure before age 5 years (Hauser, 1981). Some 7% of Japanese children have been reported to experience febrile seizures (Tsuboi, 1977). Approximately one-third of children with a first febrile seizure will suffer another (Hirtz and Nelson, 1983). Approximately 1% to 3% of children with a febrile seizure will eventually develop nonfebrile recurrent seizures (Fishman, 1981; Hirtz and Nelson, 1983). This is more likely to happen if the child has a history of serious developmental or neurologic handicap. As association of febrile seizures in childhood with the later development of partial complex (temporal lobe) seizures has been noted (Falconer, 1971; Hirtz and Nelson, 1983; Maher and McLachlan, 1995).

A family history of febrile seizures or other convulsive disorders can be elicited in 7% to 58% of affected children. The incidence of similar febrile convulsive episodes in first-degree relatives and siblings ranges from 9% to 22% (Fukuyama et al., 1979; Hausser, 1981; Beck-Mannagetta and Janz, 1982; Hauser et al., 1982). Tsuboi (1977) reported that 17% of parents and 22% of siblings of febrile seizure probands were similarly affected, and 36% of siblings were affected if both the proband and one parent had febrile seizures. Rich et al. (1984) and Hauser et al. (1985) have reported that siblings and children of probands with a febrile seizure have a recurrence risk for a febrile seizure of about 8%, which is three to four times the normal background risk. This increases to 10 times the background risk if the proband and one parent are affected and to 25 times the background risk if the proband and both parents are affected. These studies are summarized in Table 41–8. Twin studies of febrile seizures (Table 41–8) have shown a concordance rate in monozygotic twins of between 17% and 80% (Lennox-Buchtal, 1971; Schiottz-Christensen, 1972; Tsuboi and Endo, 1991; Miller et al., 1999). Tsuboi (1987) interprets these data as indicating a multifactorial mode of inheritance (genes plus environment) for febrile convulsions, with an estimated heritability of 75%.

It is not clear if siblings of febrile seizure probands are at increased risk for epilepsy unrelated to fever. Approximately 3% to 5% of siblings of febrile convulsion probands will have a nonfebrile seizure that is slightly higher than expected in the control population. A family history of afebrile seizures may be a risk factor for developing epilepsy in a proband with an initial febrile seizure. In addition, Doose and colleagues (1983) found "genetically determined EEG probands" in 81% of children with febrile seizures, and 42% of these patients had an EEG PCR. Degen et al. (1991) recorded waking and sleeping EEG in siblings of patients with febrile seizures to study the role of genetics in these seizures. Some 67 siblings of 52 patients with febrile seizures were studied. They found in 53.8% of the patients with febrile seizures that at least one sibling had epileptic activity by EEG. Epileptic discharges were recorded in 33 (49.2%) of the 67 siblings. In 32 siblings 3 to 4 spike-wave complexes were noted, and one sibling had two independent centrotemporal sharp wave foci. A history of febrile seizure or epilepsy in other family members was noted in 25 (48.1%) of the 52 patients. Hauser and coauthors (1985) reported that the risk for epilepsy or a single unproved seizure in siblings of probands with febrile seizures is ~3.2%, which is 2.5 times the background risk.

Wallace et al. (1996) reported a linkage analysis in one family with febrile seizures and one member who later developed temporal lobe epilepsy secondary to mesial temporal sclerosis that suggested a major gene for familial febrile seizures mapping to chromosome 8q13–q21. However, linkage was only suggestive because maximizing the LOD score over different penetrance and phenocopy values can inflate the result (Wallace et al., 1996). Further studies are needed before establishing chromosome 8 as the locus of a major gene for febrile seizures. Jonhson et al. (1998) identified a linkage to chromosome 19p13.3 in a family from the midwest of the United States with autosomal dominant febrile convulsions. They called the unidentified gene *FEB2*. Peiffer and collaborators (1999) found a large Utah family linked to chromosome 2q23–q24 (*FEB3*). Nakayama and collegues (2000) recently reported a large Japanese family with linkage to chromosome 5q14q–q15 (*FEB4*).

Scheffer and Berkovic (1997) described a large family with 25 individuals with generalized epilepsy over four generations. The epilepsy phenotypes were highly heterogeneous within this one family. Febrile seizures "plus" means early febrile seizures with persistence of GTCS with fever beyond six years of age, or the later occurrence of afebrile seizures of several different types. They conceptualized this as a single genetic syndrome named "generalized epilepsy with febrile seizures plus" (GEFS+). They found strong evidence for an autosomal dominant gene segregating with the seizure disorder. They postulated that the "most likely explanation for the phenotype variability in GEFS+ is an effect of other genes." Wallace and collegues (1998) reported another large family with a similar GEFS+ phenotype which

Table 41–8. Risk of Febrile Seizures to Siblings of Affected Child (Probands)

References	Only Proband Affected	Proband and One Parent Affected	Proband and Both Parents Affected	Control Population
Tsuboi, 1977	18.5%	36.5%	~45%	6.2%
Rich et al., 1984	3.2 times control	10 times control	25 times control	3%—4%
Tsuboi et al., 1991	20%	29%	41%	9.8%

shows linkage to chromosome 19q13.1. They identified a mutation in the voltage-gated sodium channel $\beta 1$ subunit gene (*SCN1B*) in this second family. Moulard and collaborators (1999) found a new locus of GEFS+ on chromosome 2q24–q33. Lopes-Cendes et al. (2000) identified a large family with GEFS+ also linked to chromosome 2q23–q31. Mutations in the neuronal voltage-gated sodium channel $\alpha 1$ subunit gene, *SCN1A*, were described in two of these families with linkage to chromosome 2q24 (Escayg et al., 2001). A mutation in the GABAA receptor $\gamma 2$ subunit gene (*GABARG2*) on chromosome 5q34 was identified in a large French family with GEFS+ (Baulac et al., 2001). This is the same gene in which Wallace and collaborators (2001) found a mutation on a family with childhood absence epilepsy and febrile seizures.

Infantile Spasms and Lennox-Gastaut Syndrome

Infantile spasms is a poorly understood form of epilepsy, occurring in infancy or early childhood in ~1 of every 5000 children (Lombrosos, 1983). These spasms are brief, often involve the entire body (including the neck and trunk), and may be flexor or extensor in nature. Other descriptive terms have included massive jerks, salaaam seizures, jackknife convulsions, and flexor spasms. Moderate-to-severe psychomotor retardation is common, and the EEG usually shows a highly abnormal irregular spike and wave pattern referred to as hypsarrhythmia, as shown in Figure 41–2. Infantile spasm is also called West's syndrome after the first physician to describe it in the nineteenth century. The pathophysiology is not understood, and it is a heterogeneous

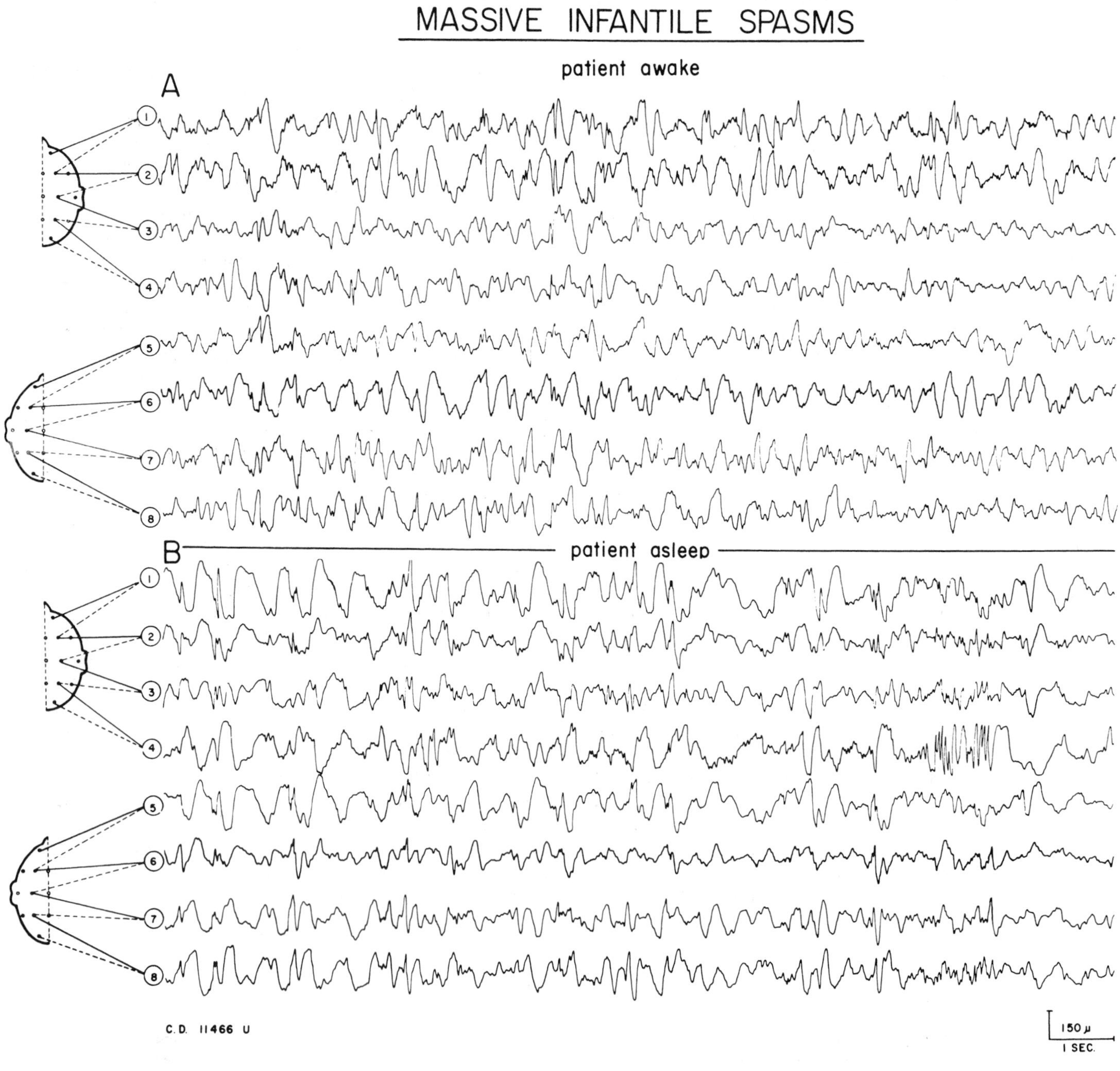

Fig. 41–2. EEG, showing severe generalized disturbance typical of the hypsarrhythmia pattern associated with infantile spasms. (Courtesy of Dr. G. Chatrian, University of Washington.)

condition with multiple causes. About one-third of patients have a history of perinatal trauma or distress. Other infants with infantile spasms may have congenital brain defects. About 5% to 17% of affected children have a family history of epilepsy, and 3% to 6% have a family history of infantile spasms.

The genetic implications of infantile spasms depend on the physician's ability to make a more specific diagnosis. A wide range of genetic disorders may occasionally be associated with this type of epilepsy. Tuberous sclerosis, the most commonly mentioned entity, occurred in 1% of the infantile spasm patients studied by Jeavons and Bower (1964) and in 13% of those studied by Charlton (1975). Another autosomal dominant disorder associated with infantile spasms is neurofibromatosis. Autosomal recessive disorders that may include infantile spasms include phenylketonuria (PKU), Sjögren-Marinesco (ataxia, cataract, mental retardation) syndrome, lipid storage disorders, pyridoxine deficiency, Leigh's syndrome, Wilson's disease. PEHO syndrome is a congenital encephalopathy with progressive encephalopathy, edema, hypsarrythmia, and optic atrophy (Somer and Sainio, 1993). The X-linked disorders that may be associated with infantile spasms include incontinentia pigmenti, Lowe's syndrome, and a disorder associated with mental retardation and spasticity having mutations in the ARX gene (Feinberg and Leahy, 1977; Stromme et al., 2002). Claes et al. (1997) demonstrated linkage in two families with X linked infantile spasms to Xp11.4–Xpter. Infantile spasms may also occur in patients with trisomy 21 (Down syndrome; Cassidy et al., 1983a).

The Lennox-Gastaut syndrome is a seizure disorder of childhood that is characterized by interictal slow and spike and wave discharge on EEG; atypical absence spells; and myoclonic, atonic, and tonic seizures—all occurring in the same patient (Erba and Browne, 1983). There is an associated encephalopathy with mental retardation and neurologic deficits. Boys are somewhat more commonly affected than girls, and at least 20% of patients have a past history of infantile spasms. Thus there is clinical overlap with the infantile spasm syndrome. The Lennox-Gastaut syndrome is also highly heterogeneous, with known causes that include neonatal anoxia, trauma, infection, and congenital brain defects. A family history of epilepsy can be found in 2.5% to 27% of patients. The causes include well-defined single-gene disorders, as noted above for infantile spasms.

RARE SYNDROME ASSOCIATIONS

Single-Gene Disorders Associated with Epilepsy

More than 100 single-gene Mendelian disorders are known to be associated with recurrent seizures in humans. A partial listing of these conditions is given in Table 41–9. Several examples of these disorders are discussed here to emphasize the importance of identifying single-gene diseases. Each disorder is followed in parentheses by its number in McKusick's catalog (McKusick, 1998) so that the reader can locate additional references.

Autosomal Recessive Disorders

A large number of autosomal recessive defects in amino acid and urea metabolism may produce neonatal and infantile recurrent seizures, but these are quite rare (see Scriver et al., 2001, for review of specific disorders). PKU, caused by phenylalanine hydroxylase deficiency (261600), is an example of a relatively common inborn error of amino acid metabolism that produces both mental retardation and seizures.

Pyridoxine-dependency seizures (266100) has been established as an autosomal recessive disorder. Affected individuals require unusually high levels of blood and tissue pyridoxine. Rapid administration of pyridoxine hydrochloride to an affected infant will stop the seizure activity, and maintenance of pyridoxine therapy may prevent repeated seizures and mental retardation. Recently, a gene for pyridoxine dependency seizures was mapped to chromosome 5q31 (Comier-Daire et al., 2000).

Progressive myoclonus and epilepsy (254800) is a heterogeneous syndrome with a confusing nomenclature. These are genetically determined, but classified by the ICE under symptomatic generalized epilepsies of specific etiologies (Commission on Classification and Terminology, 1989). Several of these are Unverricht-Lundborg disease, Lafora, neuronal ceroid lipofuscinoses, juvenile Gaucher, mitochondrial encephalomyopathy with ragged red fibers (MERRF), sialidoses types 1 and 2, and juvenile GM2 gangliosidosis (type 3) (Minassian et al., 1996).

In Finland there appears to be a high frequency of progressive myoclonic epilepsy (Norio and Koskiniemi, 1979). These kindreds are autosomal recessive and perhaps genetically related to the original families of Unverricht and Lundborg. Some of these cases have been termed Baltic myoclonic epilepsy, which is worsened by phenytoin and improved by valproic acid (Eldridge et al., 1983). The Mediterranean type formerly reported as a subgroup of Ramsey Hunt disorder is found around the western Mediterranean shores (Malafosse et al., 1992b). However, the generalized seizures respond to antiepileptic therapy (valproic acid and clonazepam) and tend to diminish at 25 to 30 years of age. Both types are closely linked to the long arm of chromosome 21, thus supporting the hypothesis that both the Mediterranean and Baltic types are due to mutations of the same gene.

Pennacchio et al. (1996) provided evidence that mutations in the gene encoding cystatin B are responsible for the disease in patients with this form of PME. Lalioti et al. (1997, 1998) described that the majority of EPM1 alleles contain large expansions of dodecamer repeats located upstream of the 5′ transcription start site of the cystatin B gene.

Lafora-type epilepsy is associated with progressive myoclonus and intellectual deterioration. This disease is distinguished by typical neuronal cytoplasmic inclusions (Lafora bodies) that may be found in other tissues, including liver and muscle. The gene (*EPM2*) has been cloned and codes for a protein tyrosine phosphatase (Serratosa 1999).

Neuronal ceroid lipofuscinoses are characterized by accumulation of ceroid and liposfusin in neurons and other cell types (Minassian et al., 1996). There are five types: CLN1 infantile maps to 1p32, and the gene encodes a palmitoyl-protein thioestherase (Vesa et al., 1995); CLN2 late infantile (Jansky-Bielschowsky disease) maps to 11p15, and the gene is a lysosomal peptidase (Sleat et al., 1997); CLN3 the juvenile form (Battens disease or Spielmeyer-Vogt-Sjogren disease) maps to 16p11.2–p12.1, and the gene encodes a 438 aminoacid protein of unknown function (International Batten Disease Consortium, 1995); CLN4 the adult type (Kuff's disease)—its chromosomal site remains unknown (Minassian et al., 1996); CLN5 Finnish variant late infantile maps to 13q21.1–q23, and the gene is a putative transmembrane protein (Savukoski et al., 1998); CLN6 late infantile maps to 15q21–q23, and the gene is still unknown (Sharp et al. 1997). CLN8 (northern epilepsy syndrome, or EPMR) is a recessive disease with epilepsy and mental retardation that is associated with a mutation in a transmembrane protein similar to that found in the motor degeneration mouse (Ranta et al. 1999).

Table 41–9. Examples of Single-Gene Disorders Associated with Seizures

Autosomal Dominant
Alopecia, psychomotor epilepsy, pyorrhea, and mental subnormality (104103)
Basal cell nevus syndrome (multiple basal cell nevi, odontogenic kepatocysts, and skeletal anomalies) (109400)
Centrencephalic (Centralopathic) epilepsy (117100)
Convulsions, benign familial neonatal (121200)
Coproporphyria (121300)
Dentatorubral-pallidoluysian atrophy (DRPLA; 125370)
Epilepsy, photogenic (132100)
Epilepsy, reading (132300)
Huntington's chorea (143100)
Myoclonic epilepsy, Hartung type (159600)
Myoclonus and ataxia (159700)
Myoclonus, cerebellar ataxia, and deafness (159800)
Myoclonus, hereditary essential (159900)
Neurofibromatosis (162200)
Photo myoclonus, diabetes mellitus, deafness, neuropathy, and cerebral dysfunction (172500)
Porphyria, acute intermittent (Swedish type of porphyria) (176000)
Porphyria, variegata (176200)
Telangiectases of brain (187200)
Tuberous sclerosis (191100)

Autosomal Recessive
Argininosuccinicaciduria (207900)
Ataxia with myoclonus epilepsy and presenile dementia (208700)
Cerebello-parenchymal disorder V (CPA V; spino dentate atrophy: dyssynergia cerebellaris myoclonica of Hunt) (213400)
Cerebro-hepato-renal syndrome (Zellweger's syndrome) (214100)
Convulsive disorder, familial, with prenatal or early onset (217200)
Corpus callosum, agenesis of, with neuropathy (Charlevoix's disease) (218000)
Deaf-mutism and familial myoclonus epilepsy (220300)
Dementia, progressive, with lipomembranous polycystic osteodysplasia (221770)
Epilepsy and yellow teeth (226750)
Epilepsy, photogenic, with spastic diplegia and mental retardation (226800)
Fructose and galactose intolerance (229500)
Fructose intolerance, hereditary (fructosemia) (229600)
Galactosemia (230400)
Gangliosidosis, generalized $GM_{(1)}$, type I (230500)
Gangliosidosis, generalized $GM_{(1)}$, type II (230600)
Gangliosidosis $GM_{(2)}$, type III (230700)
Gaucher's disease type III (juvenile and adult, cerebral) (231000)
Glycogen storage disease I (232200)
Hallervorden and Spatz, syndrome of (234200)
Homocystinuria (236200)
Hyperglycinemia, isolated (238300)
Hyperparathyroidism, neonatal familial primary (239200)
Hypoglycemia with deficiency of glycogen synthetase in the liver (240600)
Hypoglycemia, leucine induced (240800)
Krabbe's disease (globoid cell sclerosis) (245200)
Lactic acidosis, congenital infantile (245400)
Lafora myoclonus epilepsy (254780)
Leigh's necrotizing encephalopathy (256000)
Lipidosis, juvenile dystonic (246800)
Maple syrup urine disease (branched-chain ketoaciduria; 248600)
Metachromatic leukodystrophy, late infantile (metachromatic leukoencephalopathy; metachromatic form of diffuse cerebral sclerosis; sulfatide lipidosis) (250100)
Methylmalonicaciduria I (251000)
Mucolipidosis II (I-cell disease) (252500)
Myoclonic epilepsy of Unverricht and Lundberg (254800)
Neuaminidase deficiency (256550)
Neuroaxonal dystrophy, infantile (Seitelberger's disease) (256600)
Neuronal ceroid lipofuscinosis, adult type (204300)
Neuronal ceroid lipofuscinosis, EPMR (600143)
Neuronal ceroid lipofuscinosis, infantile (256731)
Neuronal ceroid lipofuscinosis, infantile Finnish type (256730)
Neuronal ceroid lipofuscinosis, juvenile type (204200)
Neuronal ceroid lipofuscinosis, late infantile (204500)
Neuronal ceroid lipofuscinosis, late infantile variant (601780)
Niemann-Pick disease (spingomyelin lipidosis) (257200)
Phenylketonuria (261600)
Pyridoxine dependency with seizures (266100)
Pyruvate carboxylase deficiency (266150)
Sandhoff disease (268800)
Sialidosis type I and Sialidosis type II (256550)
Tay-Sachs disease: GM_2 gangliosidosis, type I (272800)
Pelizaeus-Merzbacher disease (311601)

X-linked Phenotypes
Adrenoleukodystrophy (300100)
Aicardi agenesis of corpus callosum with chorioretinal abnormality (304050)
Doublecortin; DCX (300121)
Epilepsy, female restricted, with mental retardation (EFMR) (300088)
Periventricular heterotopia (300049)
X-linked lissencephaly (300067)
Corpus callosum, partial agenesis of (304100)
Hypoparathyroidism (307700)
Hypoxanthine guanine phosphoribosyltransferase deficiency (Lesch-Nyhan syndrome) (308000)
Infantile spasms (X-linked) (308350)
Menkes syndrome (kinky hair disease) (309400)
Mental deficiency (Martin-Bell, or Renpenning, type); X-linked mental retardation (309500)
Ornithine transcarbamylase deficiency (311250)
Paines syndrome (microcephaly with spastic diplegia) (311400)
Progressive myoclonus epilepsy (310370)
X-linked mental retardation with marker X chromosome (309550)
Myoclonic epilepsy, X-linked, with mental retardation and spasticity (300382)

Mitochondrial
MELAS (540000)
Mitochondrial encephalomyopathy with ragged red fibers (MERFF) (545000)

Numbers in parentheses are the numbers in McKusick's (1998) catalog.

"MERRF" designates a syndrome of myoclonus epilepsy and ragged red muscle fibers. Myoclonus, ataxia, seizures, dementia, short stature, hearing loss, optic atrophy, and neuropathy may all occur in affected persons. The abnormal mitochondria and the family pedigrees in this disorder suggest that it and similar conditions may be inherited by the maternal transmission of mitochondrial DNA (Berkovic et al., 1986; Lombes et al. 1989; Holt et al., 1989). Shoffner et al. (1990) reported a mutation in the mitochondrial DNA in MERRF: an *A8344G* nucleotide substitution in the tRNA (Lys) gene was detected. In 1996 three groups reported that a point mutation at nucleotide 3243 in tRNA (Leu) may also produce a syndrome that includes MERRF (Campos et al., 1996; Fabrizi et al., 1996; Verma et al. 1996).

Autosomal Dominant Disorders

Von Recklinghausen's neurofibromatosis (162200) occurs once in every 3000 births and is thought to have a high mutation rate. The most common clinical features are multiple café-au-lait spots, axillary freckling, and peripheral cutaneous neurofibromas. The incidence of seizures in this disorders is ~12% (Canale and Bebin, 1972; Fienman and Yakavoc, 1970). The convulsions are presumably related to the intracranial hamartomatous lesions and the heterotopias of glial and neuronal elements. The *NF-1* tumor suppressor gene (neurofibromin) is on chromosome 17 (Basu et al., 1992).

Tuberous sclerosis (191100) is less common then neurofibromatosis, having a prevalence of 1 in 3000 to 1 in 100,000 individuals. Typical clinical findings include mental retardation, facial angiofibroma, depigmented skin patches, periungual fibromas, and hamartomatous tumors in multiple organs including brain, kidney, and heart. A thorough review of tuberous sclerosis is that edited by Gomez (1979). In this series of 160 patients, 88% had seizures. Of the group with seizures, 84% of seizures were generalized, 29% were partial or focal, and 15% were both.

Infantile spasms occurred in 30% of those with seizures. There were no patients with classic petit mal epilepsy. About 60% of the entire patient population was mentally retarded, and 64% of patients with seizures were retarded. All mentally retarded patients had a history of seizures. Of those patients with average intelligence, 68% had seizures. All patients who had no history of a seizure had average intelligence. Almost all patients who had seizures in the first two years of life proved to be mentally retarded. It remains unclear whether the seizures early in childhood contributed to the development of mental retardation or whether the combination of seizures and mental retardation simply reflect the more severely affected patients.

Many "sporadic cases" have been described, but the number of such reports has been decreasing, with more vigorous attempts to identify subtle expression of the disease in one of the parents. Careful inspection of the skin, including examination with a Wood's lamp, and the advent of CT brain scans has greatly increased the diagnosis of tuberous sclerosis in mildly affected or even asymptomatic persons (Cassidy et al., 1983b). New mutations are frequent (Halley, 1996). Locus heterogeneity exists with one gene on chromosome 9q34 (*TSC1*) and the other on chromosome 16p13.3 (*TSC2*). The 16p gene is called tuberin and is a tumor suppressor gene (European Chromosome 16 Tuberous Sclerosis Consortium, 1993; Green et al., 1994). The 9q gene is called hamartin (Van Slegtenhorst et al., 1997).

X-Linked Disorders

X-linked mental retardation associated with a trinucleotide repeat expansion (309550) is recognized to be a relatively common cause of mental retardation in males. Occasional carrier females may also have mild retardation. Affected boys clearly have a high frequency of seizures, but the precise prevalence of seizures has not been determined. Review of the literature suggests that between 5% and 30% of affected males have epilepsy (Howard-Peebles et al., 1979; Jacobs et al., 1980, 1983), with 15% occurrence of seizures in a study by Neilson (1983); Wisniewski et al. (1991) reported 22% occurrence of seizures. However, the prevalence of epilepsy in patients with Fragile X syndrome varies from 9.1% to 45% in the different series (Guerrini et al., 1993). Kluger et al. (1996) suggested a possible effect of the Fragile X mental retardation-1 gene mutations on brain maturation and epileptogenesis. Ryan et al. (1997) described a family with epilepsy and mental retardation limited to females (EFMR; 300088). The disorder is transmitted by the females and by completely unaffected male carriers. This is an X-linked dominant disorder with male sparing.

Another X-linked disorder associated with seizures is periventricular heterotopia (300049). Periventricular heterotopia is a disorder that involves a cortical malformation and is frequently associated with seizures (Eksioglu et al., 1996). It is linked to chromosome Xq28. Dobyns et al. (1997) reported a new X-linked syndrome with bilateral periventricular nodular heterotopia, mental retardation, cerebellar hypoplasia, epilepsy, and syndactyly in boys; they hypothesize that it involves the same Xq28 locus as isolated bilateral periventricular heterotopia. X-linked lissencephaly (300067) and double cortex syndrome (300121) are disorders of neuronal migration that produce mental retardation and seizures. These are allelic disorders mapping to Xq22.3–Xq23. The gene encodes a protein name double cortin whose likely role is signal transduction (Gleeson et al., 1998). Another autosomal gene that causes lissencephaly is called LIS1 on chromosome 17p13 (Reiners et al., 1993). The phenotype is indistinguishable from the X-linked lissencephaly. More recently mutations have been found in the ARX gene associated with an X-linked form of myoclonic epilepsy and spasticity (Stromme et al., 2002). Additional autosomal recessive, autosomal dominant and X-linked disorders associated with seizures are listed in Table 41–9.

Chromosomal Disorders Associated with Epilepsy

The most readily diagnosed and most common known cause of mental retardation is trisomy 21 (Down syndrome). The frequency of seizures in this disorder is 1% to 9% (Paulson et al., 1969; Tangye, 1979; Pueschel et al., 1991). The prevalence of seizures seems to increase with age, being about 2% below age 20 years and 12% over age 55 years (Veal, 1974). An article by Johannsen et al. (1996) reported a prevalence study of epilepsy in patients with Down syndrome in Denmark: age groups were 14–16, 23–29, and 50–60 years, and 17% of patients had epilepsy. Infantile spasms have been reported in 4.8% of Down syndrome patients (Cassidy et al., 1983a). The prognosis for children with Down syndrome and infantile spasm appears to be better than for children with infantile spasms in the general population (Stafstrom and Konkol, 1994).

Seizures may also occur in many individuals with other autosomal chromosomal abnormalities. For example, two cases of trisomy 12p and abnormalities of chromosome 15 have been reported by Elia et al. (1998). Seizures were present in seven patients with myoclonic absence-like seizures. In all cases the EEG showed 2 to 3 Hz spike and wave discharges. Other chromosomal anomalies associated with epilepsy include trisomy 9p (Stern, 1996), inverted duplication 15 (Battaglia et al., 1997), and ring chromosome 20 (Inoue et al., 1997; Augustijn et al., 2001).

The abnormalities of sex chromosomes are generally not associated with the severe systemic morbidity that is seen with autosomal chromosome imbalance. For example, there is probably no increased frequency of epilepsy in patients with Turner's syndrome (45,XO). The prevalence of epilepsy in patients with Klinefelter syndrome (47,XXY) has been reported to be higher than in the normal population, but not higher than the background occurrence of epilepsy in other patients in the mental institution from which the Klinefelter's patients were selected (Boltshauser et al., 1978). The clinical manifestations of the 47,XXY syndrome are controversial. About 15% of patients institutionalized with this syndrome had seizures, but this incidence did not differ from the 18% incidence of seizures in the institutionalized control population (Hook, 1973).

TERATOGENIC EFFECTS OF ANTICONVULSANT DRUGS

The possible teratogenic effects of anticonvulsant medication remains a highly controversial topic. A full discussion of this field and a detailed review of the voluminous literature are clearly beyond the scope of this chapter. However, it is appropriate to briefly review some of the salient findings and issues and to provide general guidelines for clinicians dealing with epileptic patients. Excellent reviews of the larger field can be found in the publication edited by Delgado-Escueta and Janz (1992) and the paper by Lindhout and Omtzigt (1994).

Several reports in the early 1970s found an increased frequency of certain congenital malformations in the children of epileptic mothers taking anticonvulsants (Monson et al., 1973; Annegers et al., 1974). These initial findings have generally been confirmed by subsequent investigations, although exact frequencies and types of malformations have varied. The overall risk for congenital malformations in the offspring of epileptic mothers taking anticonvulsants seems to be on the order of 5% to 15%. In addition, certain types of malformations appear to have a higher frequency in this population, including cleft lip and palate, congenital heart defects, congenital urogenital malformations, and neural tube defects. Animal and human research had shown that antiepileptic drugs are teratogens predisposing to fetal malformations; however, important confounding variables in most of the large studies of teratogens and antiepileptic drugs include the potential influence of epilepsy itself, the difficulties in controlling for socioeconomic factors, possible predisposing genetic influences, blood levels of the drugs, and the importance of various drug combinations. Investigations with both human and animal models are clearly in order.

Some observers have noted a high frequency of spontaneous abortions and congenital malformations in the children of women taking trimethadione. A "trimethadione syndrome," which included mental retardation, speech difficulties, abnormal face with V-shaped eyebrows, and dental abnormalities, has been discussed (Feldman et al., 1977). Furthermore, "fetal hydantoin syndrome" has been reported in the offspring of women taking phenytoin during pregnancy (Hanson and Smith, 1975; Hanson et al., 1976; Nulman et al., 1997). This apparent syndrome includes craniofacial anomalies, nail and digital hypoplasia, prenatal onset growth deficiency, and mental retardation. It is claimed that 10% of offspring of women taking phenytoin during pregnancy may develop the entire hydantoin syndrome, and 30% may show partial mild conical manifestations (Hanson and Smith, 1975; Hanson et al., 1976). The existence of the hydantoin syndrome and the increased risk of minor anomalies among offspring of treated epileptics have been confirmed (Nulman et al., 1997). Similar anomalies were shown among offspring of nonepileptics exposed to phenytoin (DPH). Nulman et al. suggested that drugs and epilepsy have independent effects on the developing fetus. However, it has been suggested that craniofacial anomalies in children of epileptic mothers may be linked to epilepsy itself and may be genetically determined (Kelly et al., quoted in Nulman et al., 1997). There also is increasing evidence that valproic acid therapy during pregnancy may be associated with congenital defects, including neural tube abnormalities (Clayton-Smith and Donnai, 1995). Carbamazepine may be also associated with congenital defects, predominantly spina bifida and hypospadia although at a lower risk than valproic acid (Nulman et al., 1997).

The teratogenic effects of several anticonvulsants, especially phenytoin, have also been studied in mice and other laboratory animals (Paulson et al., 1979; Finnell, 1981). Several different congenital malformations have been produced, including those of the brain, heart, urogenital system, and extremities. The experimental evidence in these animal studies supports a dose–response effect of plasma phenytoin level and the importance of reactive intermediates on frequency of malformation. Studies with a mouse mutant with a genetic seizure disorder support the hypothesis that it is the serum phenytoin level and not the maternal seizure disorder that is the most important agent responsible for the congenital malformation (Finnell and Chernoff, 1982). Recommendations for epileptic women contemplating pregnancy thus become of importance (European Chromosome 16 Tuberous Sclerosis Consortium, 1993; Montouris et al., 1998) and are reviewed under Clinical Applications below. Several new anticonvulsants are now commercially available, and knowledge regarding their teratogenic effect will be forthcoming (Morrell, 1996; Leppik et al., 1999).

PATHOPHYSIOLOGY: BIOLOGIC BASIS OF GENETIC SUSCEPTIBILITY

Neurochemical and Electrophysiologic Mechanisms

It is not possible to fully document the large number of investigations into the basic mechanisms of epilepsy. The interested reader can find numerous review articles (Catterall 1984; Dichter and Ayala, 1987; Schwartzkroin 1997; Johnston, 1997; McNamara, 1999). However, a brief overview is given for proper perspective. During a seizure, the intracellular recording from a neuron reveals a sustained depolarization that triggers bursts of action potentials. This typical depolarization is called a paroxysmal depolarization shift (PDS). The PDS has been observed so frequently that it may be the final common pathway to the neuronal production of a seizure. All neurons have a calcium conductance mechanism that tends to depolarize the cell. Usually the calcium currents do not dominate neuron behavior because of large repolarizing conductances to potassium. However, any imbalance in the microcurrents through these channels could lead to self-sustained firing and epileptic activity. The balance of inhibitory and excitatory synaptic activity is also important.

Focal neuronal discharges that occur interictally are probably initiated in small units within the cerebral cortex by hyperexcitable cells that altered membrane properties. The paroxysmal activity at a cellular level consists of PDSs at the center of the focus, with a mixture of potentials that are predominantly inhibitory in the surrounding area. In the scalp EEG the activity appears as intermittent spikes. At the onset of a clinical seizure, the local paroxysmal actvity becomes more intense and spreads to other areas. The high-frequency bombardment of distant areas can be strong enough to develop self-sustained discharges in bilateral structures and at times can involve the entire cortex.

A number of chemical convulsant agents are known to have several different mechanisms of action. Strychnine competes for glycine receptors, and glycine is a potent inhibitory neurotransmitter. Picrotoxin and bicuculline are $GABA_A$ antagonists (competitive or noncompetitive), and GABA is also a potent inhibitory agent. Isoniazid may produce seizures by inhibiting glutamic acid decarboxylase, the synthetic enzyme for GABA. Aminophylline produces seizures presumably through the inhibition of phosphodiesterase and disruption of cAMP metabolism. High concentrations of penicillin block neuronal chloride conductance, and ouabain blocks ATPase-mediated potassium clearance. Major contemporary areas of research in basic mechanisms of epilepsy involve the excitatory amino acids L-glutamate and the important glutamate receptors *N*-methyl-D-aspartate (NMDA) and *d*-amino-3-hydroxy-5-methyl-4-isoxazole-propionic acid (AMPA)-kinate receptor (Johnston, 1997).

Few studies have demonstrated consistent biochemical differences between control subjects and patients with idiopathic epilepsy. The development and use of positron emission tomography (PET) have provided new information about cerebral metabolic activity during various types of seizures (Savic et al., 1997). Nuclear magnetic resonance (NMR) spectroscopy has permitted the study of pathological neurochemistry associated with epilepsy (Kuzniecky and Jackson, 1995).

Figure 41–3 presents a schematic of how one or more mutations could modulate or precipitate clinical seizures. Because the genome directly or indirectly affects all of the housekeeping activities of neurons and glial cells, the possibilities for interaction are immense. Likely areas of genetic influence include inherited enzyme deficiencies that cause blockades of important metabolic pathways. This could result in the accumulation of toxic substances (as occurs in the recessive lipid storage disorders and PKU) or in the decreased production of critical metabolic products, such as inhibitory neurotransmitters. It is interesting to note that although GABA and glycine are both inhibitory agents, and a deficiency of GABA may underlie pyridoxine dependency seizures (Lott et al., 1978), convulsions also occur in disorders associated with an *excess* of either of these amino acids (Perry et al., 1975; Jaeken et al., 1984). Genetic defects in the binding of enzymes to apoenzyme could underlie vitamin-dependency seizure disorders. Audiogenic seizures in mice are correlated with reduced calcium ATPase and serotonin receptor activity (Palayoor and Seyfried, 1984; Brennan et al., 1997). Mutations might also result in the abnormal assembly of membrane protein components that could adversely affect the structure of ionic channels, receptor sites, or the myelination of axons. Recently, two voltage-gated potassium channel genes were found responsible for benign familial neonatal convulsions (Charlier et al., 1998; Singh et al., 1998; Biervert and Steinlein, 1999), and a voltage-gated sodium channel gene is responsible for a form of febrile seizures, the GEFS+ (Wallace et al., 1998). Another potassium channel gene disease, episodic ataxia type 1 (Kv1.1), has a high frequency of partial epilepsy (Zuberi et al., 1999). Autosomal dominant frontal lobe epilepsy is caused by mutations in the neuronal nicotinic acetylcholine receptor α subunit gene (*CHRNA4*; Steinlein et al., 1995a). Thus, ion channelopathies are beginning to make a substantial genetic contribution to human epilepsies (McNamara, 1999; Ryan, 1999) The murine mutants jimpy, quaking, and shiverer are genetic models of seizures associated with deficient myelination in the central nervous system (Table 41–10). Mutations could also produce aberrations in the packaging, release, or reuptake of excitatory and inhibitory neurotransmitters. Figure 41–3 emphasizes the fact that epilepsy is not a single biochemical or genetic disease, that it will be shown to have a multitude of metabolic causes.

The strategy of positional cloning has become a major approach to identifying genes involved in epilepsy and was used in the recent discovery of the gene responsible for autosomal dominant nocturnal frontal lobe epilepsy (Steinlein et al., 1995a) and others. The general principals of mapping human epilepsy genes are reviewed by Treiman (1993) and Lowenstein (1994). The study of the genetics of epilepsy through the use of molecular genetic techniques will eventually lead to the identification of the epilepsy-related genes, their protein products, and, finally, specific biochemical treatments and preventions.

Genetic Basis of the Normal Human Electroencephalogram

The human scalp-recorded EEG reflects the summation of electrical events occurring at the neuronal level in multiple areas of the brain. Normal background EEG activity varies considerably with age and reflects the growth and maturation of the human brain (Kellaway, 1982). In 1945, Lennox and Gibbs found 85% concordance for background EEG pattern in monozygotic twins compared with 5% concordance for EEG pattern in dizygotic twins. These investigators concluded that "the brain wave pattern is an hereditary trait and, in the absence of acquired conditions which may have modified the brain wave pattern, the EEG can be used in human genetic studies and in tracing the heredity of neuropsychiatric diseases associated with cerebral dysrhythmia" (Lennox and Gibbs, 1945). The familial occurrence of the 14 and 6 Hz positive spike EEG phenomenon was noted by Rodin, 1964.

Vogel (1970, 1982) produced the greatest amount of evidence for heritability of the human EEG pattern. His studies indicate that simple autosomal dominant inheritance can explain the familial occurrence of the low-voltage EEG, fast α-variant (16–19 Hz), and monotonous α-waves. Steinlein et al. (1992) localized a gene (*EEGV1*) for human low-voltage EEG on chromosome 20q13.2–q13.3. They also presented evidence for genetic heterogeneity: only one-third (33%) of the families with low-voltage EEG showed linkage to 20q (Steinlein et al., 1992). Other types of normal EEG background activity may have genetic in-

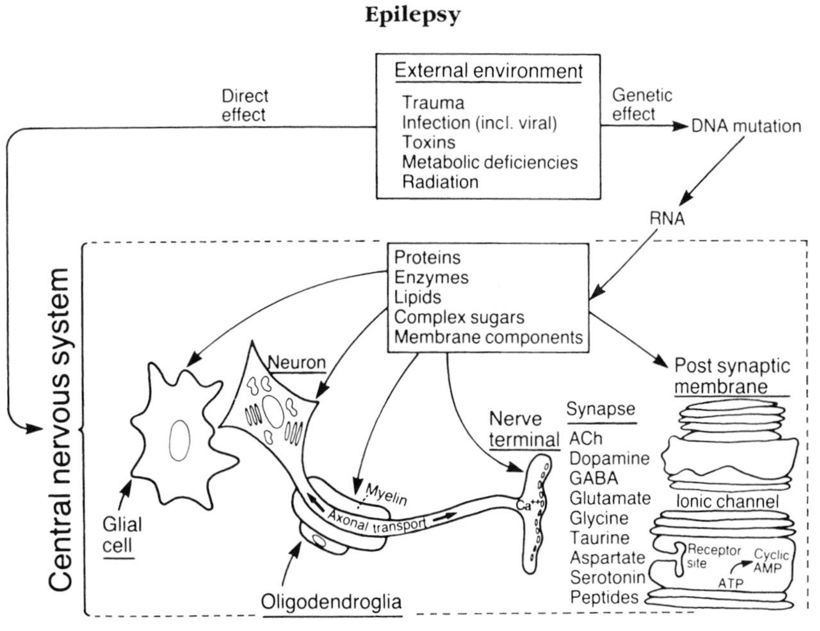

Fig. 41–3. Schematic diagram illustrating the multiple sites within the central nervous system at which genetic mutations might alter neuronal excitability and produce a lower threshold for seizures.

Table 41–10. Animal Models of Epilepsy

Animal	Genetics[a]	References
Mouse		
Audiogenic seizures	AD Juvenile onset	Seyfried et al., 1986
	AR Adult onset	Skradski et al., 2001
Quaking (gk)	AR	Guenet, 1980
Jimpy (jp)	XLR	Guenet, 1980
Shiverer (shi)	AR	Bird et al., 1978
Tottering (tr)	AR	Fletcher et al., 1996
Epileptic (El)	AD	Garey et al., 1994
Spontaneous seizures (Sps)	AR	Maxson et al., 1983
Stargazer	AR	Letts et al., 1998
Lethargic	AR	Hosford et al., 1992
Others		
Baboon *Papio papio*; photic-sensitive	Wild type (Senegal)	Naquet and Meldrum, 1972
Dog (Beagle)	AR (sex influence)	Edmonds et al., 1979
Genetic epilepsy prone rat (GERP)	AD	Buchhalter, 1993
Genetic absence epilepsy rat (GAER)	AD (variable penetrance)	Buchhalter, 1993
Rabbit; audiogenic and THC-sensitive strains	AR	Fish et al., 1983
Gerbil	Inbred strain (AR?)	Loskota et al., 1974
Fowl; photic-sensitive chicken	AR	Johnson et al., 1979
GENETIC KNOCKOUT MODELS		
Mice lacking type 1 inositol 1,4,5-triphosphate receptor	KO	Matsumoto et al., 1996
Mice lacking glutamate transporter GIT-1	KO	Tanaka et al., 1997
Sound-induced seizures in serotonin $5HT_{2c}$ receptor mutant mice	KO	Treiman, 1993
Mice lacking 65 kDa glutamic acid decarboxylase GAD65	KO	Kash et al., 1997
Mice lacking voltage-gated potassium channel α subunit Kv1.1	KO	Smart et al., 1998

[a]AR, autosomal recessive; AD, autosomal dominant; XLR, X-linked recessive; THC, tetrahydrocannabinol; KO, knockout mouse

fluences, but these have been more difficult to document. Lykken and collegues (1974), Whitton and coauthors (1985), and van Beijsterveldt et al. (1996) have supported these observations with twin studies of EEG frequency spectra. In a study of 46 monozygotic and 46 dizygotic twins, Lewis and coauthors (1972) documented a strong hereditary component in the wave characteristics of visual-, auditory-, and somatosensory-evoked responses. A good review article on the genetics of the human EEG and evoked responses is that by van Beijsterveldt and Boomsma (1994). Thus there is considerable experimental evidence for a genetic influence on the normal background human EEG pattern, but this provides little clarification of the biologic basis of epilepsy.

Genetic Animal Models of Epilepsy

Spontaneous and stimulus-induced seizures have been frequently reported in a variety of animals. Several specific genes have been identified that cause spontaneous seizures when mutated. The tottering mouse has similarities to petit mal absence seizures in humans and a mutation in the α 1A voltage-sensitive calcium channel gene has been identified in these mice (Fletcher et al., 1996). The Stargazer mouse also has seizures characteristic of absence epilesy and has a mutation in the γ subunit of the voltage-gated calcium channel (Letts et al., 1998). Knockouts of several different mouse genes have also produced epilepsy. Many other animal species with seizures have been studied from genetic, electrophysiologic, and biochemical approaches (Buchhalter, 1993). A partial listing of these animal models is given in Table 41–10. These studies have not yet explained the genetic or biochemical interactions responsible for human epilepsy and will not be further delineated in this chapter.

CLINICAL APPLICATION AND RISK ASSESSMENT OF GENETICS INFORMATION

Genetic Counseling in Epilepsy

This chapter has amply demonstrated that there is no single genetic cause of epilepsy. Genetic influences may be chromosomal, dominant or recessive, autosomal or X-linked, or multifactorial. Patients with epilepsy represent a large heterogeneous group with a vast array of etiologies. Some causes of epilepsy will be easily identifiable and others obscure. For genetic counseling of a family, the major practical questions are "What is the relative magnitude of the genetic influence for epilepsy in this particular family and what are the implications for other family members?" (Jennings and Bird, 1981).

The first and most important step in answering these questions is obtaining a specific diagnosis. Monogenic disorders can carry a recurrence risk as high as 50%, whereas environmentally induced seizures carry relatively low recurrence risks for other family members. Therefore, diagnosis is critical. The diagnosis, as always, rests on the triad of history, physical examination, and laboratory studies. The history first documents the type of seizure occurring in the index patient. This includes age at onset, clinical characteristics, and precipitating factors. The history must also include a meticulously obtained family pedigree: Who else in the family has seizures? Were the seizures single or repeated? Did they occur in infancy, childhood, or adulthood? Is there any documentation that they were produced by environmental insults such as trauma or infection, or is such documentation weak or missing? Are there other neurologic diseases in the family (e.g., mental retardation, movement disorder, dementia, muscle disease, or paralysis)?

The physical examination should search for subtle signs of a specific diagnosis. Examples would be the café-au-lait spots of neurofibromatosis, visceromegaly or macular cherry-red spots in certain lipid-storage disorders, signs of self-mutilation in Lesch-Nyhan disease, and cutaneous hyperpigmentation in adrenoleukodystrophy. Sometimes the finding of such physical characteristics will require that other family members be examined. Positive physical findings in other relatives may also identify them as carriers of a dominant gene.

Laboratory studies must be tailored to the particular clinical situation. CT scan or MRI and ophthalmologic examination may help identify family members with tuberous sclerosis. Urine amino acid analysis will be important in the diagnosis of aminoacidurias. White cell or skin fibroblast enzyme assays may be necessary for the identification of lipid-storage diseases. An EEG should always be obtained from a patient with a seizure disorder. The EEG is important in clinical classification of the seizure. It is not yet clear how useful the EEG is in identifying other family members at risk for epilepsy. In general, an EEG is not obtained from asymptomatic relatives of probands with idiopathic epilepsy except during research studies. However, it is conceivable that young siblings of probands with 3 Hz spike and wave absence seizures should have an EEG. An abnormal EEG in such children (especially one showing 3 Hz spike and wave) is likely to indicate a gene carrier and would be important for genetic counseling later in life when the EEG may have reverted to normal.

A few general statistics are given here for use as guidelines in the counseling of families with idiopathic forms of epilepsy. It is important to stress that these figures are based primarily on empiric data rather than on known Mendelian patterns of inheritance and should be presented in this context to each family. Blandfort et al. (1987) have also published useful guidelines for genetic counseling in the epilepsies.

Although neonatal seizures are usually the result of acquired causes, recall that there is a form of neonatal seizure with a good prognosis, inherited as an autosomal dominant disorder (Leppert et al., 1989; Ryan et al., 1991; Schiffmann et al., 1991; Malafosse et al., 1992a; Lewis et al., 1993; Ronen et al., 1993; Steinlein et al., 1995b). For febrile seizures it is known that ~2% to 5% of white infants have a convulsion associated with fever. Siblings of a child with febrile seizures have an increased risk for similar seizures of ~8% to 15%. The risk of developing subsequent epilepsy (recurrent seizures) in a patient with a febrile seizure is on the order of 2% to 6%.

Siblings and children of an individual with classic 3 Hz spike and wave absence epilepsy have an increased risk for a similar seizure disorder. The evidence that this is an autosomal dominant disorder has already been presented, but remains controversial. It is agreed that many more people in these families have abnormal EEGs than develop a seizure disorder. The risk for actual clinical seizures in the first-degree relatives of affected persons in on the order of 6% to 12%. At the present time, perhaps a recurrence risk of 10% is most reasonable.

It has been emphasized that infantile spasms and Lennox-Gastaut syndrome are highly heterogeneous. A careful search should be made for more specific diagnosis, especially tuberous sclerosis, which is an autosomal dominant disorder.

Each individual in the general population has a ~1% to 2% risk of developing a nonfebrile seizure by the age of 40 years (Annegers et al., 1982). The siblings or children of person with true idiopathic epilepsy without any distinguishing clinical characteristics (including EEG pattern) have a seizure risk greater than that of the general population. This risk is on the order of 2% to 14% by age 40 years. It has yet to be clarified how many variables increase or decrease these recurrence risks. Age may be one factor. Onset of seizures in the proband before age 10 years may increase the risk to siblings. Additional family members with epilepsy increase the general family risk. For example, recurrence risk for seizures in siblings was found to be 6.2% if both the proband and *both* parents had seizures. These data were based on probands with single seizures. If the proband had recurrent seizures and both parents also had seizures, then the risk to siblings became 33.3% (Anderson et al., 1979). It must also be emphasized that some of these more specific figures are based on only a few studies; the precision of these empiric risks is not well delineated, and this imprecision must be conveyed in counseling.

Finally, recurrence risk for seizures in the children or siblings of probands with partial (focal) epilepsy is little if any increase above the background rate. A risk of 1% to 3% would seem most reasonable without other confounding variables in the family. Remember, however, that the specific focal disorder of benign centrotemporal epilepsy of childhood carries a higher risk for seizures in siblings of ~15% (Heijbel et al., 1975; Heijbel, 1980).

Management of Pregnancy in a Woman with Epilepsy

Given the present incomplete information concerning the teratogenicity of anticonvulsants, what plan of management should physicians pursue with epileptic women contemplating pregnancy? The following guidelines seem most prudent (Commission on Genetics, Pregnancy, and the Child, 1993; Lindhout and Omtzigt, 1994; Montouris et al., 1998). First, determine if the patient truly requires anticonvulsant medications. Some patients are placed on anticonvulsant drugs for inappropriate or marginal indications. Some patients who have been seizure free for many years can be weaned from the drugs without high risk of seizure recurrence. Neurologic consultation would be advisable in such cases. If anticonvulsant treatment is clearly indicated, the patient must be educated about potential teratogenic risks vs. therapeutic benefits. The possible teratogenic factors should not dissuade the physician from the use of anticonvulsant medication during pregnancy when it is clearly indicated. However, it would be advisable to avoid multiple drug combinations, to attempt to limit therapy to a single anticonvulsant, and to use the lowest effective dose. Anticonvulsant blood levels should be monitored, and excessive blood levels should be avoided. Yerby (1996) has suggested careful monitoring for complications of pregnancy and childbirth in epileptic women.

Thus it is clear that there is a significant genetic component to many of the epilepsies. As genetic and physiologic studies are conducted in concert, there will be increased understanding of the etiology and improved genetic counseling and therapy for the patients affected with these many different disorders.

REFERENCES

Augustijn PB, Parra J, Wouters CH, Joosten P, Lindhout D, van Emde Boas W: Ring chromosome 20 epilepsy syndrome in children: electroclinical features. Neurology 2001; 57:1108–1111.

Alstrom CH: A study of epilepsy in its conical, social and genetic aspects. Acta Psychiatr Neurol 1950; 25(Suppl 63):1–284.

Andermann E: Multifactorial inheritance of generalized and focal epilepsy: In: Anderson VE, Hauser WA, Penry JK, King CF (eds). Genetic Basis of the Epilepsies. New York: Raven Press, 1982:355–374.

Anderson VE, Chern MM, Hauser WA, Schwanebeck E, Kouri T: Genetic heterogeneity and empirical risks in seizures. Am J Hum Genet 1979; 31:130A.

Anderson VE, Hauser WA, Penry JK, Sing CF: Genetic Basis of the Epilepsies. New York: Raven Press, 1982.

Annegers JF, Elveback LR, Hauser WA, Kurland LT: Do anticonvulsants have a teratogenetic effect? Arch Neurol 1974; 31:364–373.

Annegers JF, Hauser WA, Anderson VE: Risk of seizures among relatives of patients with epilepsy: families in a defined population. In: Anderson VE, Hauser WA, Penry JK, Sing CF (eds). Genetic Basis of the Epilepsies. New York: Raven Press, 1982:151–161

Auburger G, Ratzlaff T, Lunkes A, Nelles HW, Leube B, Binkofski F, Kugel H, Heindel W, Seitz R, Benecke R, et al.: A gene for autosomal dominant paroxysmal choreoathetosis/spasticity (CSE) maps to the vicinity of a potassium channel gene cluster on chromosome 1p, probably within 2 cM between D1S443 and D1S197. Genomics 1996; 31:90–94.

Barslund I, Danielson J: Temporal epilepsy in monozygotic twins. Epilepsia 1963; 4:138–150.

Basu TN, Gutmann DH, Fletcher JA, Glover TW, Collins FS, Downward J: Aberrant regulation of ras proteins in malignant tumour cells from type I neurofibromatosis patients. Nature 1992; 356:663–664.

Battaglia A, Guerrini F, Bertini E, Bellacosa A, Pomponi MG, Paravastou-Petsotas M, Mazza S, Neri G: The inv dup(15) symdrome: a clinically recognizable syndrome with altered behavior, mental retardation, and epilepsy. Neurology 1997; 48:1081–1086.

Baulac S, Gourfinkel-An I, Picard F, Rosenberg-Bourgin M, Prud'homme JF, Baulac M, Brice A, LeGuern E: A second locus for familial generalized epilepsy with febrile seizures plus maps to chromosome 2q21–q33. Am J Hum Genet 1999; 65:1078–1085.

Baulac S, Huberfeld G, Gourfinkel-An I, Mitropoulou G, Beranger A, Prud'homme J-F, Baulac M, Brice A, Bruzzone R, LeGuern E: First genetic evidence of $GABA_A$ receptor dysfunction in epilepsy: a mutation in the γ2-subunitgene. Nat Genet 2001; 28:46–48.

Beaussart M: Benign epilepsy of children with rolandic (centrotemporal) paroxysmal foci. Epilepsia 1972; 13:795–811.

Beaussart M, Loiseau P: Hereditary factors in a random population of 5,200 epileptics. Epilepsia 1969; 10:55–63.

Beck-Mannagetta G, Janz D: Febrile convulsions in offspring of epileptic probands. In: Anderson VE, Hauser WA, Penry JK, Sing CF (eds). Genetic Basis of the Epilepsies. New York: Raven Press, 1982:145–150.

Benninger CK, Matthis P, Scheffner D: EEG findings in children of epileptic parents. In: Anderson VE, Hauser WA, Penry JK, Sing CF (eds). Genetic Basis of the Epilepsies. New York: Raven Press, 1982:95–99.

Berkovic SF, Andermann F, Carpenter S, Wolfe LS: Progressive myoclonus epilepsies: specific causes and diagnosis. N Engl J Med 1986; 315:296–305.

Berkovic SF, Howell RA, Hay DA, Hopper JL: Epilepsies in twins: genetics of the major epilepsy syndromes. Ann Neurol 1998; 43:435–445.

Berkovic SF, McIntosh A, Howell RA, Mitchell A, Sheffield LJ, Hopper JL: Familial temporal lobe epilepsy: a common disorder identified in twins. Ann Neurol 1996; 40:227–235.

Berkovic SF, Phillips HA, Scheffer IE, Lopes-Cendes I, Bhatia KP, Fish DR, Marsden CD, Andermann F, Sutherland G, Mulley JC: Genetic heterogeneity in autosomal dominant nocturnal frontal lobe epilepsy. Epilepsia 1995; 36:147.

Berkovic SF, Scheffer IE: Genetics of human partial epilepsy. Curr Opin Neurol 1997; 10:110–114.

Biervert C, Steinlein OK: Structural and mutational analysis of *KCNQ2*, the major gene locus for benign familial neonatal convulsions. Hum Genet 1999; 104:234–240.

Bird TD, Farrell DF, Sumi SM: Brain lipid composition of the *shiverer* mouse: genetic drift in myelin development. J Neurochem 1978; 31:387–391.

Blandfort M, Tsuboi T, Vogel F: Genetic counseling in the epilepsies. Hum Genet 1987; 76:303–331.

Blom S, Heijbel J: Benign epilepsy of childhood with centrotemporal EEG: a follow-up study in adulthood of patients initially studied as children. Epilepsia 1982; 23:629–632.

Blom S, Heijbel J, Bergfars PG: Benign epilepsy of children with centrotemporal electroencephalographic foci: prevalence and follow-up study of forty patients. Epilepsia 1972; 13:609–619.

Boltshauser E, Meyer M, Deonna T: Klinefelter syndrome and neurological disease. J Neurol 1978; 219:253–259.

Bouma PAD, Wetendorp RGJ, van Dijk JG, Peters ACB, Brouwer OF: The outcome of absence epilepsy: a meta analysis. Neurology 1996; 47:802–808.

Bray PF, Wiser WC: Evidence for a genetic etiology of temporal-central abnormalities in focal epilepsy. N Engl J Med 1964; 271:926–933.

Bray PF, Wiser WC: Hereditary characteristics of familial temporal-central focal epilepsy. Pediatrics 1965; 36:206–211.

Brennan TJ, Seeley WW, Kilgard M, Schreiner CE, Tecott LH: Sound-induced seizures in serotonin 5-HT2c receptor mutant mice. Nat Genet 1997; 16:387–390.

Brinciotti M, Trasatti G, Pelliccia A, Matricardi M: Pattern-sensitive epilepsy: genetic aspects in two families. Epilepsia 1992; 33:88–92.

Browne TR, Mirsky AF: Absence (petit mal) seizures. In: Browne TR, Feldman RG (eds). Epilepsy. Boston: Little, Brown, 1983:61–74.

Buchhalter JR: Animal models of inherited epilepsy. Epilepsia 1993; 34(suppl. 3):S31–S41.

Campos Y, Martin MA, Lorenzo G, Aparicio M, Cabello A, Arenas J: Sporadic MERRF/MELAS overlap syndrome associated with the 3243 tRNA (Leu(UUR)) mutation of mitochondrial DNA. Muscle Nerve 1996; 19:187–190.

Canale DJ, Bebin J: Von Recklinghausen disease of the nervous system. In: Vinken PJ, Bruyn GW (eds). Handbook of Clinical Neurology. Amsterdam: North-Holland, 1972; 14:132–161.

Caraballo R, Pavek S, Lemainque A, Gastaldi M, Echenne B, Motte J, Genton P, Cersosimo R, Humbertclaude V, Fejerman N, et al.: Linkage of benign familial infantile convulsions to chromosome 16p12–q12 suggest allelism to the infantile convulsions and choreoathestosis syndrome. Am J Hum Genet 2001; 68:788–794.

Cassidy S, Gainey A, Holmes G, Greenstein R: Infantile spasms in Down syndrome: an unprecedented association. Am J Hum Genet 1983a; 35:82A.

Cassidy S, Pagon RA, Pepin M, Blumhagen JD: Family studies in tuberous sclerosis: evaluation of apparently unaffected parents. JAMA 1983b; 249:1302–1304.

Catterall WA: The molecular basis of neuronal excitability. Science 1984; 223:653–661.

Cavazzuti GB, Capella L, Nalin A: Longitudinal study of epileptiform EEG patterns in normal children. Epilepsia 1980; 21:43–55.

Caveness WF: Epilepsy, a product of trauma in our time. Epilepsia 1976; 17:207–215.

Cendes F, Lopes-Cendes I, Andermann E, Andermann F: Familial temporal lobe epilepsy: a clinically heterogeneous syndrome. Neurology 1998; 50:554–557.

Cesare L: Paroxysmal choreoathetosis: an epileptic or non-epileptic disorder? Ital J Neurol Sci 1995; 16:271–277.

Charlier C, Singh NA, Ryan SG, Lewis TB, Reus BE, Leach RJ, Leppert M: A pore mutation in a novel KQT-like potassium channel gene in an idiopathic epilepsy family. Nat Genet 1998; 18:53–55.

Charlton JW: Infantile spasms in myoclonic seizures. In: Charlton MW (ed). Myoclonic Seizures. Amsterdam: Excerpta Medica, 1975:111–120.

Chatrian GE, Lettich E, Miller HH, Green JR: Pattern sensitive epilepsy: I. An electrographic study of its mechanism. Epilepsia 1970; 11:125–149.

Claes L, Del-Favero J, Ceulemans B, Lagae L, VanBroeckhoven C, DeJonghe P: De novo mutations in the sodium channel gene *SCN1A* cause severe myoclonic epilepsy of infancy. Am J Hum Genet 2001; 68:1327–1332.

Claes S, Devriendt K, Lagae L, Ceulemans B, Dom L, Casaer P, Raeymaekers P, Cassiman JJ, Fryns JP: The X-linked infantile spasm syndrome (MIM308350) maps to Xp11.4–Xpter in two pedigrees. Ann Neurol 1997; 42:360–364.

Clayton-Smith J, Donnai D: Fetal valproate syndrome. J Med Genet 1995; 32:724–727.

Commission on Classification and Terminology of the International League against Epilepsy: Proposal for revised clinical and electroencephalographic classification of epileptic seizures. Epilepsia 1981; 22:489–501.

Commission on Classification and Terminology of the International League against Epilepsy: Proposal for revised classification of epilepsies and epileptic syndromes. Epilepsia 1989; 30:389–399.

Commission on Genetics, Pregnancy, and the Child, International League against Epilepsy: Guidelines for the care of women of childbearing age with epilepsy. Epilepsia 1993; 34:588–589.

Corkin S: Lasting consequences of bilateral medial temporal lobectomy: clinical course and experimental findings in H.M. Semin Neurol 1984; 4:249–259.

Cormier-Daire V, Dagoneau N, Nabbout R, Burglen L, Penet C, Soufflet C, Desguerre I, Munnich A, Dulac O: A gene for pyridoxine-dependent epilepsy maps to chromosome 5q31. Am J Hum Genet 2000; 67:991–993.

Daly FR, Foster RM: Inheritance of reading epilepsy. Neurology 1975; 25:1051–1054.

Davenport CB, Weeks DF: A first study of inheritance of epilepsy. J Nerv Ment Dis 1911; 38:641–670.

De Fusco M, Becchetti A, Patrignani A, Annesi G, Gambardella A, Quattrone A, Ballabio A, Wanke E, Casari G: The nicotinic receptor B2 subunit is mutant in nocturnal frontal lobe epilepsy. Nat Genet 2000; 26:275–276.

Degen R, Degen HE: Contribution to the genetics of rolandic epilepsy: waking and sleep EEG's in siblings. In: Degen R, Dreifuss FE (eds). Benign Localized and Generalized Epilepsies of Early Childhood. Amsterdam: Elsevier Science, 1992; 6:49–52.

Degen R, Degen HE, Ahlemeyer K: Contribution to the genetics of symptomatic generalized tonic clonic seizures: waking and sleep EEGs in siblings. Acta Neurol Scand 1996; 93:9–13.

Degen R, Degen HE, Hans K: A contribution to the genetics of febrile seizures: waking and sleep EEG in siblings. Epilepsia 1991; 32:515–522.

Delgado-Escueta AV, Enrile-Bascal F: Juvenile myoclonic epilepsy of Janz. Neurology 1984; 34:285–294.

Delgado-Escueta AV, Greenberg D, Weissbecker K, Liu A, Treiman L, Sparkes R, Park MS, Barbetti A, Terasaki PI: Gene mapping in the idiopathic generalized epilepsies. Epilepsia 1990; 31(Suppl. 3):S19–S29.

Delgado-Escueta AV, Janz D (eds): Pregnancy and teratogenesis in epilepsy. Neurology 1992; 42(suppl. 5):7–160.

Dichter M, Ayala GF: Cellular mechanisms of epilepsy: a status report. Science 1987; 237:157–164.

Dobyns WB, Guerrini R, Czapansky-Beilman DK, Pierpont ME, Breningstall G, Yock DH Jr., Bonanni P, Truwit CL: Bilateral periventricular heterotopia with mental retardation and syndactyly in boys: a new X-linked mental retardation syndrome. Neurology 1997; 49:1042–1047.

Doose H: Photosensitivity: genetics and significance in the pathogenesis of epilepsy. In: Anderson VE, Hauser WA, Penry JK, Sing CF (eds). Genetic Basis of the Epilepsies. New York: Raven Press, 1982:113–121.

Doose H, Eckel U, Volke E: Convulsion after smallpox vaccination. Z Kinderheilkd 1968a; 103:214–236.

Doose H, Gerken H, Horstmann T, Volzke E: Genetic factors in spike-wave absences. Epilepsia 1973; 14:47–75.

Doose H, Gerken H, Leonhardt R, Volzke E, Volz E, Volz C: Centrencephalic myoclonic-astatic petit mal. Neuropediatrics 1970; 2:59–78.

Doose H, Gerken H, Volzke E: Genetics of centrencephalic epilepsy in childhood. Epilepsia 1968a; 9:107–115.

Doose H, Gundel A: 4 to 7 CPR rhythms in the childhood EEG. In: Anderson VE, Hauser WA, Penry JK, Sing CF (eds). Genetic Basis of the Epilepsies. New York: Raven Press, 1982:83–94.

Doose H, Ritter K, Volzke E: EEG longitudinal studies in febrile convulsions: genetic aspects. Neuropediatrics 1983; 14:81–87.

Doose H, Sitepu B: Childhood epilepsy in a German city. Neuropediatrics 1983; 14:220–224.

Doose H, Waltz S: Photosensitivity: genetics and clinical significance. Neuropediatrics 1993; 24:249–255.

Duchovney M, Harvey AS: Pediatric epilepsy syndromes: an update and critical review. Epilepsia 1996; 37(S1):S26–S40.

Durner M, Sander T, Greenberg DA, Jonhson K, Beck-Mannagetta G, Janz D: Localization of idiopathic generalized epilepsy on chromosome 6p in families of juvenile myoclonic epilepsy patients. Neurology 1991; 41:1651–1655.

Edmonds HL, Hegreberg GA, VanGelder NM, Sylvester DM, Clemmons RM, Chatburn CG: Spontaneous convulsions in beagle dogs. Fed Proc 1979; 38:2424–2428.

Eisner V, Pauli LL, Livingston S: Epilepsy in the families of epileptics. J Pediatr 1960; 56:345–354.

Eksioglu YZ, Scheffer IE, Cardenas P, Knoll J, DiMario F, Ramsby G, Berg M, Kamuro K, Berkovik SF, Duyk GM, et al.: Periventricular heterotopia: an X-linked dominant epilepsy locus causing aberrant cerebral cortical development. Neuron 1996; 16:77–87.

Eldridge R, Iivanainen M, Stern R, Koerber T, Wilder BJ: Baltic myoclonic epilepsy: hereditary disorder of childhood made worse by phenytoin. Lancet 1983; 2:838–842.

Elia M, Guerrini R, Musumeci SA, Bonanni P, Gambardella A, Aguglia U: Myoclonic absence-like seizures and chromosome abnormality syndromes. Epilepsia. 1998;39:660–663.

Elmslie FV, Rees M, Williamson MP, Kerr M, Kjelsen MJ, Pang KA, Sundqvist A, Friis ML, Chadwick D, Richens A, et al.: Genetic mapping of a major susceptibility locus for juvenile myoclonic epilepsy on chromosome 15q. Hum Mol Genet 1997; 6:1329–1334.

Engel JL: Seizures and Epilepsy. Philadelphia: F. A. Davis, 1989.

Erba G, Browne TR: Atypical absence, myoclonic, atonic and tonic seizures, and the "Lennox-Gastaut syndrome." In: Browne RT, Feldman RG (eds). Epilepsy. Boston: Little, Brown, 1983:75–94.

Escayg A, Heils A, MacDonald BT, Haug K, Sander T, Meisler MH: A novel SCNIA mutation associated with generalized epilepsy with febrile seizures and prevalence of variants in patients with epilepsy. Am J Hum Genet 2001; 68:866–873.

European Chromosome 16 Tuberous Sclerosis Consortium: Identification and characterization of the tuberous sclerosis gene on chromosome 16. Cell 1993; 75:1305–1315.

Evans JH: Post-traumatic epilepsy. Neurology 1962; 12:665–674.

Everitt A, Sander JWAS: Classification of the epilepsies: time for a change. Eur Neurol 1999; 42:1–10.

Fabrizi GM, Cardaioli E, Grieco GS, Cavallaro T, Malandrini A, Manneschi L, Dotti MT, Federico A, Guazzi G: The A to G transition at nt 3243 of the mitochondrial tRNA Leu(UUR) may cause MERRF syndrome. J Neurol Neurosurg Psychiatry 1996; 61:47–51.

Falconer MA: Genetic and retarded aetiological factors in temporal lobe epilepsy: a review. Epilepsia 1971; 12:13–31.

Feinberg AP, Leahy WR: Infantile spasms: case report of sex-linked inheritance. Dev Med Child Neurol 1977; 19:524–526.

Feldman GL, Weaver DD, Lourien EW: The fetal trimethadione syndrome. Am J Dis Child 1977; 131:1389–1392.

Fienman NL, Yakavoc WC: Neurofibromatosis in childhood. J Pediatr 1970; 76:339–346.

Fink JK, Hedera P, Mathay JG, Albin RL: Paroxysmal dystonic choreoathetosis linked to chromosome 2q: clinical analysis and proposed pathophysiology. Neurology 1997: 49:177–183.

Finnell RH: Phenytoin-induced teratogenesis: a mouse model. Science 1981; 211:483–484.

Finnell RH, Chernoff GF: Mouse fetal hydantoin syndrome: effects of maternal seizures. Epilepsia 1982; 23:423–429.

Fish BS, Consroe P, Fox R: Convulsant-anticonvulsant properties of Δ-9-tetrahydrocannabinol in rabbits. Behav Genet 1983; 13:205–210.

Fishman MA: An approach to the management of children with febrile seizures: a child neurologist's point of view. In: Nelson KB, Ellenberg JH (eds). Febrile Seizures. New York: Raven Press, 1981:87–92.

Fletcher CF, Lutz CM, O'Sullivan TN, Shaughnessy JD Jr.: Absence epilepsy in tottering mutant mice is associated with calcium channel defects. Cell 1996; 87:607–617.

Fong GC, Shah PU, Gee MN, Serratosa JM, Castroviejo IP, Khan S, Ravat SH, Mani J, Huang Y, Zhao HZ, et al.: Childhood absence epilepsy with tonic-clonic seizures and electroencephalogram 3–4-Hz spike and multispike–slow wave complexes: linkage to chromosome 8q24. Am J Hum Genet. 1998; 63:1117–1129.

Fukuyama Y, Kagawa K, Tanaka K: A genetic study of febrile convulsions. Eur Neurol 1979; 18:166–182.

Gambardella A, Annesi G, De Fusco M, Patrignani A, Aguglia U, Annesi F, Pasqua AA, Spadafora P, Oliveri RL, Valentino P, et al.: A new locus for autosomal dominant nocturnal frontal lobe epilepsy maps to chromosome 1. Neurology 2000; 53:1467–1471.

Garey CE, Schwarzman AL, Rise ML, Seyfried TN: Ceruloplasmin gene defect associated with epilepsy in EL mice. Nat Genet 1994; 6:426–431.

Gedda L, Tatarelli R: Essential isochronic epilepsy in MZ twin pairs. Acta Genet Med 1971; 20:380–383.

Giaquinto S: Traumatic epilepsy: the value of a family study. In: Canger R, Angeleri R, Penry JK (eds). Advances in Epileptology: XIth Epilepsy Int Symp. New York: Raven Press, 1980:331–337.

Gleeson JG, Allen KM, Fox JW, Lamperti ED, Berkovik S, Scheffer I, Cooper EC, Dobyns WB, Minnerath SR, Ross ME, Walsh CA: Doublecortin, a brain specific gene mutated in human X-lissencephaly and double cortex syndrome, encodes a putative signaling protein. Cell 1998; 92:63–72.

Gomez MR (ed): Tuberous Sclerosis. New York: Raven Press, 1979.

Goodman RM: A perspective on genetic diseases among the Jewish people. In: Goodman RM, Motulsky AG (eds). Genetic Diseases among Ashkenazi Jews. New York: Raven Press, 1979:1–17.

Goossens LAZ, Andermann F, Andermann E, Remillard GM: Reflex seizures induced by calculation, card, or board games, and spatial tasks: a review of 25 patients and delineation of the epileptic syndrome. Neurology 1990; 40:1171–1176.

Green AJ, Smith M, Yates JRW: Loss of heterozygozity on chromosome 16p13.3 in hamartomas from tuberous sclerosis patients. Nat Genet 1994; 6:192–196.

Greenberg DA, Delgado-Escueta, Widelitz H, et al.: Epilepsy (juvenile myoclonic) and its associated EEG traits are linked to the HLA-BF locus. Am J Hum Genet 1988; 43(Suppl):A145.

Greenberg DA, Durner M, Resor S, Rosenbaum D, Shinnar S: The genetics of idiopathic generalized epilepsies of adolescent onset: differences between juvenile myoclonic epilepsy and epilepsy with random grand mal and with awakening grand mal. Neurology 1995; 45:942–946.

Greenberg DA, Durner M, Shinnar S, Resor S, Rosenbaum D, Klotz I, Dicker E, Keddache M, Zhou G, Yang X, Altstiel L: Association of HLA class II alleles in patients with juvenile myoclonic epilepsy compared with patients with other forms of adolescent onset generalized epilepsy. Neurology 1996; 47:750–755.

Guenet JL: Mutants of the mouse with an abnormal myelination: a review for geneticists. In: Baumann N (ed). Neurological Mutations Affecting Myelination. Amsterdam: Elsevier/North Holland, 1980:11–22.

Guerrini R, Bonanni P, Nardocci N, Parmeggiani L, Piccirilli M, De Fusco M, Aridon P, Ballabio A, Carrozzo R, Casari G: Autosomal recessive rolandic epilepsy with paroxysmal exercise-induced dystonia and writer's cramp: delineation of the syndrome and gene mapping to chromosome 16p12–11.2. Ann Neurol 1999; 45:344–352.

Guerrini R, Dravet C, Ferrari AR, Battaglia A, Mattei MG, Salvadori P, Genton P, Pfanner P: The evolution of epilepsy in the most common genetic forms with mental retardation (Down's syndrome and the fragile X syndrome). Pediatr Med Chir 1993; 15(suppl. 1):19–22.

Guerrini R, Dravet C, Genton P, Bureau M, Bonanni P, Ferrari AR, Roger J: Idiopathic photosensitive occipital lobe epilepsy. Epilepsia 1995; 36:883–891.

Guerrini R, Bonanni P, Patrignani A, Brown P, Parmeggiani L, Grosse P, Brovedani P, Moro F, Aridon P, Carrozzo R, et al.: Autosomal dominant cortical myoclonus and epilepsy (ADCME) with complex partial and generalized seizures: A newly recognized epilepsy syndrome with linkage to chromosome 2p11.1–q12.2. Brain. 2001; 124:2459–2475.

Guipponi M, Rivier F, Vigevano F, Beck C, Crespel A, Echenne B, Lucchini P, Sebastianelli R, Baldy-Moulinier M, Malafosse A: Linkage mapping of benign familial infantile convulsions (BFIC) to chromosome 19q. Hum Mol Genet 1997; 6:473–477.

Halley DJJ: Tuberous sclerosis: between genetic and physical analysis. Acta Genet Med Gemellol (Roma) 1996; 45:63–75.

Hanson JW, Myrianthopoulos NC, Harvey MAS, Smith DW: Risks to the offspring of women treated with hydantoin anticonvulsants, with emphasis of the fetal syndrome. J Pediatr 1976; 89:662–668.

Hanson JW, Smith DW: The fetal hydantoin syndrome. J Pediatr 1975; 87:285–290.

Harvald B: Heredity in Epilepsy. Copenhagen: Munksgaard, 1954.

Hauser WA: The natural history of febrile seizures. In: Nelson KB, Ellenberg JG (eds). Febrile Seizures. New York: Raven Press, 1981:5–12.

Hauser WA, Annegers JF, Anderson VE, Kurland LT: The risk of seizure disorders among relatives of children with febrile convulsions. Neurology 1985; 35:1268–1273.

Hauser WA, Annegers JF, Kurland LT: Risk of seizures among relatives of patients with febrile convulsions. Neurology 1982; 32:A185.

Hauser WA, Annegers JF, Kurland LT: Incidence of epilepsy and unprovoked seizures in Rochester, Minnesota: 1935–1984. Epilepsia 1993; 34:453–468.

Hauser WA, Kurland LT: The epidemiology of epilepsy in Rochester, Minn., 1935 through 1967. Epilepsia 1975; 16:1–10.

Heijbel J: Genetics of benign epilepsy in childhood. In: Canger R, Angeleri F, Penry JK (eds). Advances in Epileptology: XIth Epilepsy Int Symp. New York: Raven Press, 1980:319–322.

Heijbel J, Blom S, Rasmuson J: Benign epilepsy of childhood with centrotemporal EEG foci: a genetic study. Epilepsia 1975; 16:285–293.

Hirtz DG, Nelson KB: The natural history of febrile seizures. Annu Rev Med 1983; 34:453–471.

Holt IJ, Harding AE, Cooper JM, Schapira AH, Toscano A, Clark JB, Morgan-Hughes

JA: Mitochondrial myopathies: clinical and biochemical features of 30 patients with major deletions of muscle mitochondrial DNA. Ann Neurol 1989; 26:699–708.

Hook EB: Behavioral implications of the human XYZ genotype. Science 1973; 179:139–148.

Hosford DA, Clark S, Cao Z, Wilson WA Jr, Lin FH, Morrisett RA, Huin A: The role of GABAβ receptor activation in absence seizures of lethargic (lh/lh) mice. Science 1992; 257:398–401.

Howard-Peebles PN, Stoddard GR, Mims MG: Familial X-linked mental retardation, verbal disability, and marker X chromosomes. Am J Hum Genet 1979; 31:214–222.

Inouye E: Observations on forty twin index cases with chromic epilepsy and their co-twins. J Nerv Ment Dis 1960; 130:401–416.

Inoue Y, Fujiwara T, Matsuda K, Kubota H, Tanaka M, Yagi K, Yamamori K, Takahashi Y: Ring chromosome 20 and nonconvulsive status epilepticus: a new syndrome. Brain 1997; 120:939–953.

International Batten Disease Consortium: Isolation of a novel gene underlying Batten disease, *CLN3*. Cell 1995; 82:949–957.

Jacobs PA, Glover TW, Mayer M, Fox P, Gerrard JW, Dunn HG, Herbst DS: X-linked mental retardation: a study of 7 families. Am J Med Genet 1980; 7:471–489.

Jacobs PA, Mayer M, Matsuura J, Rhoads F, Yee SC: A cytogenetic study of a population of mentally retarded males with special reference to the marker X syndrome. Hum Genet 1983; 63:139–148.

Jaeken J, Casaer P, Decock P: γ-amino butyric acid-transaminase deficiency: a newly recognized inborn error of neurotransmitter metabolism. Neuropediatrics 1984; 15:165–169.

Jain S, Padma MV, Maheshwari MC: Occurrence of only myoclonic jerks in juvenile myoclonic epilepsy. Acta Neurol Scand 1997; 95:263–267.

Janz D, Scheffner D: Seizures in children of epileptic parents. In: Canger R, Angeleri F, Penry JK (eds). Advances in Epileptology: XIth Epilepsy Int Symp. New York: Raven Press, 1980:311–318.

Jeavons PM, Bower BD: Infantile spasms. Clin Dev Med 1964; 15:1–82.

Jennings MT, Bird TD: Genetic influences in the epilepsies: review of the literature with practical implications. Am J Dis Child 1981; 135:450–458.

Jenson I: Genetic factors in temporal epilepsy. Acta Neurol Scand 1975; 52:381–394.

Jilek-Aall L, Jilek W, Miller JR: Clinical and genetic aspects of seizures disorders prevalent in an isolated African population. Epilepsia 1979; 20:613–622.

Johannsen P, Christensen JE, Goldstein H, Nielsen VK, Mai J: Epilepsy in Down's syndrome: prevalence in three age groups. Seizure 1996; 5:121–125.

Johnson DD, Davis HL, Crawford RD: Pharmacological and biochemical studies in epileptic fowl. Fed Proc 1979; 38:2417–2423.

Johnson EW, Dubovsky J, Rich SS, O'Donovan CA, Orr HT, Anderson VE, Gil-Nagel A, Ahmann P, Dokken CG, Schneider DT, Weber JL: Evidence for a novel gene for familial febrile convulsions, *FEB2*, linked to chromosome 19p in an extended family from the midwest. Hum Mol Genet 1998; 7:63–67.

Johnston MV: Neurotransmitters and epilepsy. In: Willey E (ed). The Treatment of Epilepsy: Principles and Practice. Philadelphia: Lea and Febiger, 1997:111–125.

Kakihana R: Alcohol intoxication and withdrawal in inbred strains of mice. Behav Neurol Biol 1979; 26:97–105.

Kalachikov S, Evgrafov O, Ross B, Winawer M, Barker-Cummings C, Boneschi FM, Choi C, Morozov P, Das K, Teplitskaya E et al.: Mutations in LGI1 cause autosomal-dominant partial epilepsy with auditory features. Nat Genet 2002; 30:335–341.

Kash SF, Johnson RS, Tecott LH, Noebels JL, Mayfield RD, Hanahan D, Baekkeskov S: Epilepsy in mice deficient in the 65kDa isoform of glutamic acid decarboxylase. Proc Natl Acad Sci USA 1997; 94:14060–14065.

Kellaway P: Maturational and biorhythmic changes in the electroencephalogram. In: Anderson VE, Hauser JK, Penry JK, Sing CR (eds). Genetic Basis of the Epilepsies. New York: Raven Press, 1982:21–34.

Kluger G, Bohm I, Laub MC, Waldenmaier C: Epilepsy and fragile X gene mutations. Pediatr Neurol 1996; 15:358–360.

Kuzniecky RI, Jackson GD: Magnetic resonance in epilepsy. New York: Raven Press, 1995.

Lalioti MD, Scott HS, Buresi C, Rossier C, Bottani A, Morris MA, Malafosse A, Antonarakis SE: Dodecamer repeat expansionin cystatin B gene in progressive myoclonus epilepsy. Nature 1997; 386:847–851.

Lalioti MD, Scott HS, Genton P, Grid D, Ouazzani R, M'Rabet A, Ibrahim S, Gouider R, Dravet C, Chkili T, et al.: A PCR amplification method reveals instability of the dodecamer repeat in progressive myoclonus epilepsy (*EPM1*) and no correlation between size of the repeat and age at onset. Am J Hum Genet 1998; 62:842–847.

Lance JW: Familial paroxysmal dystonic choreoathetosis and its differentiation from related syndromes. Ann Neurol 1977; 2:285–293.

Lennox WG: The genetics of epilepsy. Am J Psychiatry 1947a; 103:457–462.

Lennox WG: Sixty-six twin pairs affected by seizures. Assoc Res Nerv Ment Dis Proc 1947b; 26:11–34.

Lennox WG: The heredity of epilepsy as told by relatives and twins. JAMA 1951; 146:529–536.

Lennox WG, Gibbs FA: The brain-wave pattern, an hereditary trait: evidence for 74 "normal" pairs of twins. J Hered 1945; 36:233–243.

Lennox-Buchthal M: Febrile and nocturnal convulsions in monozygotic twins. Epilepsia 1971; 12:147–156.

Leppert M, Anderson VE, Quattlebaum T, Stauffer D, O'Connell P, Nakamura Y, Lalouel JM, White R: Benign familial neonatal convulsions linked to genetic markers on chromosome 20. Nature 1989; 337:647–648.

Leppik IE, Wolff D, Purves S: Treatment of Epilepsy in women of childbearing potential, issues in management. CNS drugs 1999; 11:191–206.

Letts VA, Felix R, Biddlecome GH, Arikkath J, Mahaffey CL, Valenzuela A, Bartlett FS II, Mori Y, Campbell KP, Frankel WN: The mouse stargazer gene encodes a neuronal calcium channel γ subunit. Nat Genet 1998; 19:340–347.

Lewis EG, Dustman RE, Beck EC: Evoked response similarity in monozygotic, dizygotic and unrelated individuals. Electroencephalogy Clin Neurophysiol 1972; 23:309–316.

Lewis TB, Leach RJ, Ward K, O'Connell P, Ryan SG: Genetic heterogeneity in benign familial neonatal convulsions: identification of a new locus on chromosome 8q. Am J Hum Genet 1993; 53:670–675.

Lindhout D, Omtzigt JGC: Teratogenic effects of antiepileptic drugs: implications for the management of epilepsy in women of childbearing age. Epilepsia 1994; 35(suppl. 4):S19–S28.

Loiseau P, Beaussart M: Hereditary factors in partial epilepsy. Epilepsia 1969; 10:23–31.

Loiseau P, Duche B, Cordova S, Cohadon S: Prognosis of benign childhood epilepsy with centrotemporal spikes: a follow-up study of 168 patients. Epilepsia 1988; 29(3):229–235.

Lombes A, Mendell JR, Nakase H, Barohn RJ, Bonilla E, Zeviani M, Yates AJ, Omerza J, Gales TL, Nakahara K, et al.: Myoclonic epilepsy and ragged-red fibers with cytochrome oxide deficiency: neuropathology, biochemistry, and molecular genetics. Ann Neurol 1989; 26:20–33.

Lombrosos CT: Infantile spasms. In: Browne TR, Feldman RG (eds). Epilepsy. Boston: Little, Brown, 1983:95–109.

Lopes-Cendes I, Scheffler IE, Berkovic SF, Rousseau M, Andermann E, Rouleau GA: A new locus for generalized epilepsy with febrile seizures plus to chromosome 2. Am J Hum Genet 2000; 66(2):698–701.

Loskota WJ, Lomax P, Rich ST: The gerbil as a model for the study of the epilepsies. Epilepsia 1974; 15:109–119.

Lott IT, Coulombe T, Di Paolo RV, Richardson EP Jr, Levy H: Vitamin B6-dependent seizures: pathology and chemical findings in the brain. Neurology 1978; 28:47–54.

Lowenstein DH: Basic concepts of molecular biology for the epileptologist. Epilepsia 1994; 35(suppl. 1):S7–S19.

Lui AW, Delgado-Escueta AV, Gee MN, Serratosa JM, Zhang QW, Alonso ME, Medina MT, Cordova S, Zhao HZ, Spellman JM, et al.: Juvenile myoclonic epilepsy in chromosome 6p12–p11: locus heterogeneity and recombinations. Am J Med Genet 1996; 63:438–446.

Lui AW, Delgado-Escueta AV, Serratosa JM, Alonso ME, Medina MT, Gee MN, Cordova S, Zhao HZ, Spellman JM, Ramos Peek JR, et al.: Juvenile myoclonic epilepsy locus in chromosome 6p21.2–p11: linkage to convulsions and electroencephalography trait. Am J Hum Genet 1995; 57:368–381.

Lykken DT, Tellegen A, Thorkelson K: Genetic determination of EEG frequency spectra. Biol Psychol 1974; 1:245–259.

MacIntosh RR: The significance of fits in eclampsia. J Obstet Gynaecol Br Emp 1952; 59:197–201.

Maher J, McLachlan RS: Febrile convulsions: is seizure duration the most important predictor of temporal lobe epilepsy? Brain 1995; 118:1521–1528.

Malacarne M, Gennaro E, Madia F, Pozzi S, Vacca D, Barone B, dalla Bernardina B, Bianchi A, Bonanni P, De Marco P, et al.: Benign familial infantile convulsions: mapping of a novel locus on chromosome 2q24 and evidence of genetic heterogeneity. Am J Hum Genet 2001; 68:788–794.

Malafosse A, Leboyer M, Dulac O, Navalet Y, Plouin P, Beck C, Laklou H, Mouchnino G, Grandscene P, Vallee L, et al.: Confirmation of linkage of benign familial neonatal convulsions to *D20S19* and *D20S20*. Hum Genet 1992a; 89:54–58.

Malafosse A, Lehesjoki AE, Genton P, Labauge P, Durand G, Tassinari CA, Dravet C, Michelucci R, De La Chapelle A: Identical genetic locus for Baltic and Mediterranean myoclonus. Lancet 1992b; 339:1080–1081.

Matsumoto M, Nakagawa, Inoe T, Nagata E, Tanaka K, Tanako H, Minowa O, Kuno J, Sakakibara S, Yamada M, et al.: Ataxia and epileptic seizures in mice lacking type 1 inositol 1,4,5-triphosphate receptor. Nature 1996; 379:168–171.

Matthes A, Weber H: Clinical and electroencephalographic family studies in pyknolepsies. Dtsch Med Wochenschr 1968; 93:429–435.

Maxson SC, Fine MD, Ginsburg BE, Koniecki DL: A mutant for spontaneous seizures in C57BL/10Bg mice. Epilepsia 1983; 34:15–24.

McHenry LC: Garrison's History of Neurology. Springfield, IL: Charles C. Thomas, 1969.

McKusick VA: Mendelian Inheritance in Man. 12th ed. Baltimore: Johns Hopkins University Press, 1998.

McNamara JO: Emerging insights into the genesis of epilepsy. Nature 1999; 399(6738 Suppl):A15–22.

Metrakos JD, Metrakos K: Childhood epilepsy of subcortical (cent encephalic) origin. Clin Pediatr (Phila) 1966; 5:536–542.

Metrakos JD, Metrakos K, Polizos P, Valle F: Genetics and ontogenesis of the centrencephalic EEG. Electroencephalogr Clin Neurophysiol 1966; 21:404.

Metrakos K, Metrakos JD: Genetics of convulsive disorders: II. Genetics and electroencephalographic studies in centrencephalic epilepsy. Neurology 1961; 11:414.

Meyer JG, Holzinger H, Urban K: Epileptic seizures in alcoholic pre-delirium: clinical and electroencephalographic studies on the differentiation of genetic conditioned attack predisposition and epilepsy. Nervenarzt 1976; 47:375–379. In German.

Mikami M, Yasuda T, Terao A, Nakamura M, Ueno S, Tanabe H, Tanaka T, Onuma T, Goto Y, Kaneko S, Sano A: Localization of a gene for benign adult familial myoclonic epilepsy to chromosome 8q23.3–q24.1. Am J Hum Genet 1999; 65:745–751.

Miller LL, Pellock JM, Boggs JG, DeLorenzo RJ, Meyer JM, Corey LA: Epilepsy and seizure occurrence in a population-based sample of Virginian twins and their families. Epilepsy Res 1999; 34:135–143.

Millichap JG: The definition of febrile seizures. In: Nelson KB, Ellenberg JH (eds). Febrile Seizures. New York: Raven Press, 1981:1–4.

Minassian BA, Sainz J, Delgado-Escueta AV: Genetics of myoclonic and myoclonus epilepsies. Clin Neurosci 1996; 3:223–235.

Monson RR, Rosenberg L, Harts SC, Shapiro S, Heinonen OP, Slone D: Diphenylhydantoin and selected congenital malformations. N Engl J Med 1973; 289:1049–1052.

Montouris G, Cefalo R, Harden C, Hayashi R, Samuels P, Shah A, Yerby M: The treatment of epilepsy among women of childbearing age. Medical Tribune Suppl. May 1998; 1–18.

Morrell MJ: The new antiepileptic drugs and women: efficacy, reproductive health, pregnancy, and fetal outcome. Epilepsia 1996; 37(suppl. 6):S34–S44.

Moulard B, Guipponi M, Chaigne D, Mouthon D, Buresi C, Malafosse A: Identification of a new locus for generalized epilepsy with febrile seizures plus (GEFS+) on chromosome 2q24–q33. Am J Hum Genet 1999; 65:1396–1400.

Muller K, Arnold H, Bruhn B, Daute KH, Degen R, Kirsten G, Kulz J, Klust E, Lassker G, Munde B, et al.: Familial predisposition in focal epilepsy. Schweiz Arch Neurol Neurochir Psychiatr 1973; 113:45–55. In German.

Nakayama J, Hamono K, Iwasaki N, Nakahara S, Horigome Y, Saitoh H, Aoki T, Maki T, Kikuchi M, Migiti T, et al.: Significant evidence for linkage of febrile seizures to chromosome 5q14–15. Hum Mol Genet 2000; 9:87–91.

Naquet R, Meldrum BS: Photogenic seizures in baboon. In: Purpura DP, Penry JK, Woodbury DM, Tower DB, Walter RD (eds). Experimental Models of Epilepsy. New York: Raven Press, 1972:373–406.

Neilson KB: Diagnosis of the fragile X syndrome (Martin-Bell syndrome): clinical findings in 27 males with the fragile site at Xg28. J Ment Defic Res 1983; 27:211–226.

Neubauer BA, Fiedler B, Himmelein B, Kämpfer F, Läßker U, Schwabe G, Spanier I, Tams D, Bretscher C, Moldenhauer K, et al.: Centrotemporal spikes in families with rolandic epilepsy: linkage to chromosome 15q14. Neurology 1998; 51:1608–1612.

Neuman RJ, Kwon JM, Jilek-Aall L, Rwiza HT, Rice JP, Goodfellow PJ: Genetic analysis of Kifafa, a complex familial seizure disorder. Am J Hum Genet 1995; 57:902–910.

Neville HE, Brooke MH, Austin JH: Studies in myoclonus epilepsy (Lafora body form). Arch Neurol 1974; 30:466–474.

Newmark ME, Penry JK: Photosensitivity and Epilepsy: A Review. New York: Raven Press, 1979.

Newmark ME, Penry JK: Genetics of Epilepsy: A Review. New York: Raven Press, 1980.

Norio R, Koskiniemi M: Progressive myoclonus epilepsy: genetic and nosological aspects with special reference to 107 Finnish patients. Clin Genet 1979; 15:382–398.

Nulman I, Scolnik D, Chitayat D, Farkas LD, Koren G: Findings in children exposed in utero to phenytoin and carbamazepine monotherapy: independent effects of epilepsy and medications. Am J Med Genet 1997; 68:18–24.

Oldani A, Zucconi M, Asselta R, Modugno M, Bonati MR, Dalpra L, Malcovati M, Tenchini ML, Smirnes S, Ferini-Strambi L: Autosomal dominant nocturnal frontal epilepsy: a video-polysomnographic and genetic appraisal of 40 patients and delineation of an epileptic syndrome. Brain 1998; 121:205–223.

One hundred years ago. Br Med J 1978; 2:1456.

Ottman R, Annegars JF, Risch N, Hauser WA, Susser M: Relations of genetic and enviromental factors in the etiology of epilepsy. Ann Neurol 1996a; 39:442–449.

Ottman R, Lee JH, Hauser WA, Risch N: Are generalized and localization-related epilepsies genetically distinct? Arch Neurol 1998; 55:339–344.

Ottman R, Lee JH, Risch N, Hauser WA, Susser M: Clinical indicators of genetic susceptibility to epilepsy. Epilepsia 1996b; 37:353–361.

Ottman R, Risch N, Hauser WA, Pedley TA, Lee JH, Baker-Cummings C, Lustenberger A, Nagle KJ, Lee KS, Scheuer ML, et al.: Localization of a gene for partial epilepsy to chromosome 10q. Nat Genet 1995; 10:56–60.

Palayoor ST, Seyfried TN: Genetic association between Ca^{++} ATPase activity and audiogenic seizures in mice. J Neurochem 1984; 42:1771–1774.

Paulson GW, Son GD, Nance WE: Neurologic aspects of typical and atypical Down's syndrome. Dis Nerv Syst 1969; 30:632–636.

Paulson RB, Paulson GW, Jreissaty S: Phenytoin and carbamazepine in production of cleft palate in mice. Arch Neurol 1979; 36:832–836.

Pederson HE, Krogh E: The prognosis consequences of familial predisposition and sex in epilepsy. Acta Neurol Scand 1971; 47:105–116.

Peiffer A, Thompson J, Charlier C, Otterud B, Varvil T, Pappas C, Barnitz C, Gruenthal K, Kuhn R, Leppert M: A locus for febrile seizures (FEB3) maps to chromosome 2q23–24. Ann Neurol 1999; 46:671–678.

Pennacchio LA, Lehesjoki AE, Stone NE, Willour VL, Virtaneva K, Miao J, D'Amato E, Ramirez L, Faham M, Koskiniemi M, et al.: Mutations in the gene encoding cystatin B in progresive myoclonus epilepsy (EPM1). Science 1996; 271:1731–1734.

Perry Tl, Urquhart N, MacLean J, Evans ME, Hansen S, Davidson AGF, Applegarth DA, MacLeod PJ, Lock JE: Nonketotic hyperglycinemia: glycine accumulation due to absence of glycine clearage in the brain. N Engl J Med 1975; 292:1269–1273.

Phillips HA, Scheffer IE, Berkovic SF, Hollway GE, Sutherland GR, Mulley JC: Localization of a gene for autosomal dominant nocturnal frontal lobe epilepsy to chromosome 20q 13.2. Nat Genet 1995; 10:117–118.

Phillips HA, Scheffer IE, Crossland KM, Bhatia KP, Fish DR, Marsden CD, Howell SJ, Stephenson JB, Tolmie J, Plazzi G, et al.: Autosomal dominant nocturnal frontal-lobe epilepsy: genetic heterogeneity and evidence for a second locus at 15q24. Am J Hum Genet 1998; 63:1108–1116.

Plaster NM, Uyama E, Uchino M, Ikeda T, Flanigan KM, Kondo I, Ptacek LJ: Genetic localization of the familial adult myoclonic epilepsy (FAME) gene to chromosome 8q24. Neurology 1999; 53:1180–1183.

Poza JJ, Saenz A, Martinez-Gil A, Cheron N, Cobo AM, Urtasun M, Marti-Masso JF, Grid D, Beckmann JS, Prud'homme JF, Lopez de Munain A: Autosomal dominant lateral temporal epilepsy: clinical and genetic study of a large Basque pedigree linked to chromosome 10q. Ann Neurol 1999; 45:182–188.

Pueschel SM, Louis S, Mcknight P: Seizure disorders in Down's syndrome. Arch Neurol 1991; 48:318–320.

Rabending G, Klepel H: Photoconvulsive and photomyoclonic reactions: age dependent genetic determined variations of enhanced photosensitivity. Neuropediatrics 1970; 2:164–172.

Radhakrishnan K, Silbert PL, Klass DW: Reading epilepsy: an appraisal of 20 patients diagnosed at the Mayo Clinic, Rochester, Minnesota, between 1949 and 1989, and delineation of the epileptic syndrome. Brain 1995; 118:75–89.

Ranta S, Zhang Y, Ross B, Lonka L, Takkunen E, Messer A, Sharp J, Wheeler R, Kusumi K, Mole S, et al.: The neuronal ceroid lipofuscinoses in human *EPMR* and mnd mutant mice are associated with mutations in *CLN8*. Nat Genet 1999; 23:233–236.

Reiner O, Carrozzo R, Shen Y, Wehnert M, Faustinella F, Dobyns WB, Caskey CT, Ledbetter DH: Isolation of a Miller-Dieker lissencephaly gene containing G protein β-subunit-like repeats. Nature 1993; 364:717–721.

Reutens DC, Berkovic SF: Idiopathic generalized epilepsy of adolescence: are the syndromes clinically distinct? Neurology 1995; 45:1469–1476.

Rich SS, Hauser WA, Annegers JF, Anderson VE: Genetic analysis of febrile convulsions. Am J Hum Genet 1984; 36:179S.

Riggio S, Santiago M, Niedermeyer E: Benign occipital lobe epilepsy. Neurology 1987; 37(Suppl):106.

Rimoin DL, Metrakos JD: The genetics of convulsive disorders in the families of hemiplegic. In: Proceedings of the Second International Bureau for Epilepsy. London: 1972:11–14.

Rodin E: Familial occurrence of the 14 and 6/sec positive spike phenomenon. Electroencephalogr Clin Neurophysiol 1964; 17:566–570.

Rodin E, Gonzales S: Hereditary components in epileptic patients. JAMA 1966; 198:221–225.

Ronen GM, Rosales TO, Connolly M, Anderson VE, Leppert M: Seizure characteristics in chromosome 20 benign familial neonatal convulsions. Neurology 1993; 43:1355–1360.

Rosanoff AK, Handy LM, Rosanoff IA: Etiology of epilepsy with special reference to its occurrence in twins. Arch Neurol Psychiatr 1934; 31:1165–1193.

Ryan SG: Ion channels and the genetic contribution to epilepsy. J Child Neurol 1999; 14:58–66.

Ryan SG, Chance PF, Zou CH, Spinner NB, Golden JA, Smietana S: Epilepsy and mental retardation limited to females: an X-linked dominant disorder with male sparing. Nat Genet 1997; 17:92–95.

Ryan SG, Wiznitzer M, Hollman C, Torres MC, Szekeresova M, Schneider S: Benign familial neonataal convulsions: evidence for clinical and genetic heterogeneity. Ann Neurol 1991; 29:469–473.

Sander T, Bockenkamp B, Hildmann T, Blasczyk R, Kretz R, Wienker TF, Volz A, Schmitz B, Beck-Mannagetta G, Rieß O, et al.: Refined Mapping of the epilepsy susceptibility locus EJM1 on chromosome 6. Neurology 1997; 49:842–847.

Sander T, Hildman T, Kretz R, Furst R, Sailer U, Bauer G, Schmitz B, Beck-Mannagetta G, Wienker TF, Janz D: Allelic association of juvenile absence epilepsy with GluR5 kainate receptor gene (*GRIK1*) polymorphism. Am J Med Genet 1997; 74:416–421.

Savic I, Altshuler L, Baxter L, Engel J Jr.: Pattern of interictal hypometabolism in PET scans with fludeoxyglucose F 18 reflects prior seizure types in patients with mesial temporal lobe seizures. Arch Neurol 1997; 54:129–136.

Savukoski M, Kolkars T, Holmberg V, Santavuori P, Landers ES, Peltonen L: *CLN5*, a novel gene encoding a putative transmembrane protein mutated in Finnish variant late infantile neuronal ceroid lipofuscinosis. Nat Genet 1998; 19:286–288.

Schaumann BA, Chern MM, Johnson SB: Risk of seizure in siblings of patients with post-traumatic and alcohol related seizures. Am J Hum Genet 1982; 34:193A.

Scheffer IE, Berkovic SF: Generalized epilepsy with febrile seizures plus: a genetic disorder with heterogeneous clinical phenotypes. Brain 1997; 120:479–490.

Scheffer IE, Bhatia KP, Lopes-Cendes I, Fish DR, Marsden CD, Andermann E, Desbiens R, Keene D, Cendes F, et al.: Autosomal dominant nocturnal frontal lobe epilepsy: a distinctive clinical disorder. Brain 1995a; 118:61–73.

Scheffer IE, Jones L, Pozzebon M, Howell RA, Saling MM, Berkovic SF: Autosomal dominant rolandic epilepsy and speech dyspraxia a new syndrome with anticipation. Ann Neurol 1995b; 38:633–642.

Scheffer IE, Phillips HA, O'Brien CE, Saling MM, Wrennall JA, Wallace RH, Mulley JC, Berkovic SF: Familial partial epilepsy with variable foci: a new partial epilepsy syndrome with suggestion of linkage to chromosome 2. Ann Neurol 1998; 44:890–899.

Schiffmann R, Shapira Y, Ryan SG: An autosomal recessive form of benign familial neonatal seizures. Clin Genet 1991; 40:467–470.

Schiottz-Christensen E: Genetic factors in febrile convulsions: an investigation of 64 same sexed twin pairs. Acta Neurol Scand 1972; 48:538–546.

Schubert R, Cracco JB: Familial rectal pain: a type of reflex epilepsy. Ann Neurol 1992; 32:824–826.

Schwartzkroin PA: Basic mechanism of epileptogenesis. In: Willey E (ed). The Treatment of Epilepsy: Principles and Practice. Philadelphia: Lea and Febiger, 1997:83–98.

Scriver C, Beaudet A, Valle D, Sly W, Childs B, Kinzler K, Vogelstein B (eds): The Metabolic and Molecular Bases of Inherited Disease. 8th ed. New York: McGraw-Hill, 2001.

Serratosa JM, Gomez-Garre P, Gallardo ME, Anta B, Beltran-Valero de Bernabe D,

Lindhout D, Augustijn PB, Tassinari CA, Michelucci R, Mallafosse A, et al.: A novel protein tyrosine phosphatase gene is mutated in progressive myoclonus epilepsy of the Lafora type (EPM2). Hum Mol Genet 1999; 8(2):345–352.

Seyfried TN, Glaser GH, Yu RK, Palayoor ST: Inherited convulsive disoders in mice. In: Delgado-Escueta AV, Ward AA Jr., Woodbury DM, Porter RJ (eds). Basic Mechanisms of the Epilepsies: Molecular and Cellular Approach. New York: Raven Press, 1986:115–133.

Shamansky SL, Glaser GH: Socioeconomic characteristics of childhood seizure disorders in the New Haven area: an epidemiologic study. Epilepsia 1979; 20:457–474.

Sharp JD, Wheeler RB, Lake BD, Savukoski M, Jarvela IE, Peltonen L, Gardiner RM, Williams RE: Loci for classical and a variant late infantile neuronal ceroid lipofuscinosis map to chromosomes 11p15 and 15q21–23. Hum Mol Genet 1997; 6:591–595.

Shoffner JM, Lott MT, Lezza AM, Seibel P, Ballinger SW, Wallace DC: Myoclonic epilepsy and ragged red fiber disease (MERRF) is associated with a mitochondrial mutation DNA, tRNA (Lys) mutation. Cell 1990; 61:931–937.

Shorvon SD: The epidemiology and treatment of chronic and refractory epilepsy. Epilepsia 1996; 37(S2):S1–S3.

Singh NA, Charlier C, Stauffer D, DuPont BR, Leach RJ, Melis R, Ronen GM, Bjerre I, Quattlebaum T, Murphy JV, et al.: A novel potassium channel gene, *KCNQ2*, is mutated in an inherited epilepsy of newborns. Nat Genet 1998; 18:25–29.

Skradski SL, Clark AM, Jiang H, White HS, Fu YH, Ptacek LJ: A novel gene causing a mendelian audiogenic mouse epilepsy. Neuron 2001; 31:537–544.

Sleat DE, Donnelly RJ, Lackland H, Liu CG, Sohar I, Pullarkat RK, Lobel P: Association of mutations in a lysosomal protein with classical late-infantile neuronal ceroid lipofuscinosis. Science 1997; 277:1802–1805.

Smart SL, Lopantsev V, Zhang CL, Robbins CA, Wang H, Chiu SY, Schwartzkroin PA, Messing A, Tempel BL: Deletion of the Kv1.1 potassium channel causes epilepsy in mice. Neuron 1998; 20:809–819.

Somer M, Sainio K: Epilepsy and the electroencephalogram in progressive encephalopathy with edema, hypsarrhythmia, and optic atrophy (the PEHO syndrome). Epilepsia 1993; 34:727–731.

Sorel L: The descendants of epileptic patients. Epilepsia 1969; 10:91–96.

Stafstrom CE, Konkol RJ: Infantile spasm in children with Down syndrome. Dev Med Child Neurol 1994; 36:576–585.

Stein C: Hereditary factors in epilepsy: a comparative study of 1,000 institutionalized epileptics and 1,115 non-epileptic controls. Am J Pediatr 1933; 12:989–1037.

Steinlein O, Anokhin A, Yping M, Schalt E, Vogel F: Localization of a gene for the human low-voltage EEG on 20q and genetic heterogeneity. Genomics 1992; 12:69–73.

Steinlein O, Schuster V, Fischer C, Haussler M: Benign familial neonatal convulsions: confirmation of genetic heterogeneity and further evidence for a second locus on chromosome 8q. Hum Genet 1995b; 95:411–415.

Steinlein OK, Magnusson A, Stoodt J, Bertrand S, Weiland S, Berkovik SF, Nakken KO, Propping P, Bertrand D: An insertion mutation of the *CHRNA4* gene in a family with autosomal dominant nocturnal frontal lobe epilepsy. Hum Mol Genet 1997; 6:943–947.

Steinlein OK, Mulley JC, Propping P, Wallace RH, Phillips HA, Sutherland GR, Scheffer IE, Berkovic SF: A missense mutation in the neuronal nicotinic acetylcholine receptor $\alpha 4$ subunit is associated with autosomal dominant nocturnal frontal lobe epilepsy. Nat Genet 1995a; 11:201–203.

Stern JM: The epilepsy of trisomy 9p. Neurology 1996; 47:821–824.

Stevenson AC: Progressive familial myoclonic in three families: its clinical features and pathological basis. Brain 1955; 78:325–349.

Strømme P, Mangelsdorf ME, Shaw MA, Lower KM, Lewis SME, Bruyere H, Lütcherath V, Gedeon AK, Wallace RH, Scheffer IE et al.: Mutations in the human ortholog of Aristaless cause X-linked mental retardation and epilepsy. Nat Genet 2002; 30:441–445.

Swoboda KJ, Soong B, McKenna C, Brunt ER, Litt M, Bale JF Jr, Ashizawa T, Bennett LB, Bowcock AM, Roach ES, et al.: Paroxysmal kinesigenic dyskinesia and infantile convulsions: clinical and linkage studies. Neurology 2000; 55:224–230.

Szepetowski P, Rochette J, Berquin P, Puissan C, Lathrop GM, Monaco AP: Familial infantile convulsions and paroxysmal choreoathetosis: a new neurological syndrome linked to the pericentromeric region of human chromosome 16. Am J Hum Genet 1997; 61:889–898.

Tanaka K, Watase K, Manabe T, Yamada K, Watanabe M, Takahashi K, Iwama H, Nishikawa T, Ichihara N, Kikuchi T, et al.: Epilepsy and exacerbation of brain injury in mice lacking the glutamate transporter GLT-1. Science 1997; 276:1699–1702.

Tangye SR: The EEG and incidence of epilepsy in Down's syndrome. J Ment Defic Res 1979; 23:17–24.

Thom DA, Walker GS: Epilepsy in the offspring of epileptics. Am J Psychiatry 1922; 1:613–627.

Treiman D: Evidence for hereditary factors in adult symptomatic partial-onset epilepsy. Neurology 1987; 37(Suppl 1):140.

Treiman LJ: Genetics of epilepsy: an overview. Epilepsia 1993; 34(Suppl. 3):S1–S11.

Tsuboi T: Genetic aspects of febrile convulsions. Hum Genet 1977; 38:169–173.

Tsuboi T: Genetic analysis of febrile convulsions: twin and family studies. Hum Genet 1987; 75:7–14

Tsuboi T, Christian W: On the genetics of the primary generalized epilepsy with sporadic myoclonias of impulsive petit mal type. Humangenetik 1973; 19:155–182.

Tsuboi T, Endo S: Incidence of seizures and EEG abnormalities among offspring of epileptic patients. Hum Genet 1977; 36:173–189.

Tsuboi T, Endo S: Genetic studies of febrile convulsions: analysis of twin and family data. In: Anderson VE, Hauser WA, Leppik, JL, Noebels JL, Rich SS (eds). Genetic Strategies in Epilepsy Research. Amsterdam: Elsevier Science Publishers, 1991:119–128.

van Beijsterveldt CEM, Boomsma DI: Genetics of the human electroencephalogram (EEG) and event-related brain potentials (ERPs): a review. Hum Genet 1994; 94:319–330.

Van Beijsterveldt CEM, Molenaar PCM, deGeus EJC, Boomsma DI: Heritability of human brain functioning as assessed by electroencephalography. Am J Hum Genet 1996; 58:562–573.

Van Slegtenhorst M, de Hoogt R, Hermans C, Nellist M, Janssen B, Verhoef S, Lindhout D, van den Ouweland A, Halley D, Young J, et al.: Identification of the tuberous sclerosis gene *TSC1* on chromosome 9q34. Science 1997; 277:805–808.

Veal RM: The prevalence of epilepsy among Mongols related to age. J Ment Defic Res 1974; 18:99–106.

Vercelletto P, Courjon J: Heredity and generalized epilepsy. Epilepsia 1969; 10:7–21.

Verma A, Moraes CT, Shebert RT, Bradley WG: A MERRF?PEO overlap syndrome associated with the mitochondrial DNA 3243 mutation. Neurology 1996; 46:1334–1336.

Vesa J, Hellsten E, Verkruyse L, Camp LA, Rapola J, Santavuori P, Hofmann SL, Peltonen L: Mutations in the palmitoyl protein thioesterase gene causing infantile neuronal ceroid lipofuscinosis. Nature 1995; 376:584–588.

Vigevano F, Fusco L, Di Capua M, Ricci S, Sebastianelli R, Lucchini P: Benign infantile familial convulsions. Eur J Pediatr 1992; 151:608–612.

Vogel F: The genetic basis of the normal human EEG. Humangenetik 1970; 10:71–114.

Vogel F: Relationship between behavioral maturation measured by the Baum Test and EEG frequency: a pilot study on monozygotic and dizygotic twins. Hum Genet 1982; 62:60–65.

Wallace RH, Berkovik SF, Howell RA, Sutherland GR, Mulley JC: Suggestion of a major gene for familial febrile convulsions mapping to 8q13–21. J Med Genet 1996; 33:308–312.

Wallace RH, Schefter IE, Barnett S, Richards M, Dibbens L, Desai RR, Lerman-Sagie T: Neuronal sodium-channel α1-subunit mutations in generalized epilepsy with febrile seizures plus. Am J Hum Genet 2001; 68:859–865.

Wallace RH, Wang DW, Singh R, Scheffer IE, Geoge AL, Phillip HA, Saar K, Reis A, Johnson EW, Sutherland GR, et al.: Febrile seizures and generalized epilepsy associated with a mutation in the sodium channel β1 subunit gene *SCN1B*. Nat Genet 1998; 19:366–370.

Weissbecker KA, Durner M, Janz D, Scaramelli A, Sparkes RS, Spence MA: Confirmation of linkage between juvenile myoclonic epilepsy locus and the HLA region of chromosome 6. Am J Med Genet 1991; 38:32–36.

Whitton JL, Elgie SM, Kugel H, Moldofsky H: Genetic dependence of the electroencephalogram bispectrum. Electroencephalogr Clin Neurophysiol 1985; 60:293–298.

Willey E (ed). The Treatment of Epilepsy: Principles and Practice. Philadelphia: Lea and Febiger, 1997.

Wirrell EC, Camfield CS, Camfield PR, Gordon KE, Dooley JM: Long term prognosis of typical childhood absence epilepsy: remission or progression to juvenile myoclonic epilepsy. Neurology 1996; 47:912–918.

Wisniewski KE, Segan SM, Miezejeski CM, Sersen EA, Rudelli RD: The fra (X) syndrome: neurological, electrophysiological, and neuropathological abnormalities. Am J Med Genet 1991; 38:476–480.

Xiong L, Labuda M, Li DS, Hudson TJ, Desbiens R, Patry G, Verret S, Langevin P, Mercho S, Seni MH, et al.: Mapping of a gene determining familial partial epilepsy with variable foci to chromosome 22q11q12. Am J Hum Genet 1999; 65:1698–1710.

Yerby MS: Contraception, pregnancy and lactation in women with epilepsy. Baillieres-Clin-Neurol 1996; 5:887–908.

Zara F, Bianchi A, Avanzini G, Di Donato S, Castelloti B, Patel PI, Pandolfo M: Mapping of genes predisposing to idiopathic generalized epilepsy. Hum Mol Genet 1995; 4:1201–1207.

Zara F, Gennaro E, Stablie M, Carbone I, Marlacarne M, Majello L, Santangelo R, DeFalco FA, Bricarelli FD: Mapping of a locus for a familial autosomal recessive idiopathic myoclonis epilepsy of infancy to chromosome 16p13. Am J Hum Genet 2000; 66:1552–1557.

Zivin L, Ajmone-Marsen C: Incidence and prognostic significance of epileptiform activity in the EEG of non-epileptic subjects. Brain 1968; 91:751–775.

Zuberi SM, Eunson LH, Spauschus A, De Silva R, Tolmie J, Wood NW, McWilliam RC, Stephenson JP, Kullmann DM, Hanna MG: A novel mutation in the human voltage-gated potassium channel gene (Kv1.1) associates with episodic ataxia type 1 and sometimes with partial epilepsy. Brain 1999; 122:817–825.

42 Multiple Sclerosis

LEENA PELTONEN, JANNA SAARELA, AND SATU KUOKKANEN

TYPICAL CLINICAL FEATURES AND DIAGNOSIS

Multiple sclerosis (MS) is a chronic neurological disease of the central nervous system (CNS) and is characterized by multicentric inflammation, demyelination, and axonal damage (Allen, 1991; Trapp et al., 1998). Inflammation results in multiple patches of demyelination that leave sclerotic scars (MS plaques) during healing. Typical predilection areas are the spinal cord, optic nerves, brain stem, and cerebrum, although any part of the CNS can be involved. The classical clinical features include disturbances in sensation (paresthesiae) and mobility (pareses), ataxia, and dysfunction of bowel, bladder, and sexual functions. During the course of the disease, most patients have episodes of impaired vision caused by optic neuritis.

MS shows a high degree of individual variability in severity and clinical course, with some patients being only mildly affected. In most cases (85%), the disease follows a relapsing-remitting course, with episodes of neurological manifestations followed by complete or partial recovery. As time passes, neurological disability usually accumulates and many patients enter a chronic progressive stage. In a minority of cases (15%), the decline in neurological functions is gradual, and the disease takes a chronically progressive course that may result in severe neurological disability within a few years. The typical age of onset is between 20 and 40, and the disease is 1.5 to 2 times more common in females than in males. The etiology of MS is still unknown, and no curative treatment for the disease is available, although some recent therapeutic trials have been encouraging as to the progress of symptoms. There is clinical and neuroimaging evidence that β-interferons may delay the clinical worsening in certain patient groups. Some positive effects have also been observed in the disease progression of MS patients treated with intravenous IgG (Soelberg-Sorensen et al., 1998). The true benefits of these treatments and the duration of benefits await further follow-up clinical studies (Noseworthy, 1999).

The diagnosis of MS is still based mainly on characteristic clinical symptoms; no specific laboratory tests exist. For clinical practice, a few laboratory tests can help establish a symptom-based diagnosis. An increased cerebrospinal fluid (CSF) : serum immunoglobulin G (IgG) ratio as a sign of increased intrathecal IgG production and the presence of oligoclonal bands in CSF are both indicative of MS. However, these changes are not specific for MS but can also result from other conditions, such as neurosyphilis, sarcoidosis, and borreliosis. Magnetic resonance imaging (MRI) and spectroscopic techniques have proven most useful in viewing the patches of inflammation and demyelination in the CNS. MRI is sensitive enough for detection of both acute (inflammatory) and chronic (sclerotic) MS lesions, as well as sites of the blood–brain barrier breakage that can be an early sign of a new lesion (Miller et al., 1988; Kesserling et al., 1990). Again, the MRI findings are not specific for MS but can also be seen in the aging process, as well as in other conditions such as cerebral vasculitis and acute disseminated encephalomyelitis. However, an MRI finding with hypointense lesions using T1-weighted pulse sequences, reduced magnetization transfer ratios (MTRs), progressive cerebral and spinal atrophy, and loss of anisotrophy on diffusion MRI—all indicate axonal loss and demyelination and are highly suggestive for MS (Fazekas et al., 1988; Miller et al., 1998; Paty et al., 1988; Gass et al., 1994).

Given the high degree of variability in the clinical picture of MS, an international consensus for diagnostic criteria has been established to facilitate the consistent determination of the diagnosis especially for research purposes (Table 42–1), (Poser et al., 1983). Based on these criteria, objective or subjective evidence for neurological dysfunction having lasted more than 24 hours is regarded as an MS attack. For two attacks to be considered to be distinct episodes, they should involve different parts of the CNS, with each attack separated by a period of at least one month.

Thousands of studies have been published on the etiology and pathogenesis of MS, but the basic molecular events in the initiation and progression of the disease are still poorly understood. The acute myelin lesion of CNS in MS is characterized by the invasion of lymphocytes and macrophages and is facilitated by increased permeability of the blood–brain barrier. The disease process results in gradual loss of myelin sheath, with reactive gliosis, while axons remain relatively preserved. There is a considerable amount of evidence that MS is an inflammatory disease, and autoimmunity has become the most popular pathogenesis explanation. The target for the putative autoimmune reaction is not identified; it may be a myelin protein or a component of another CNS protein. Alternatively, autoimmunity may also develop only after the initiation of the disease as a secondary event, being relevant only for the progression of the disease. Although abnormalities of both humoral and cell-mediated immune systems have been reported in MS patients, it is difficult to judge which of these features are directly linked to molecular pathogenesis. Also the role of resident cells within the CNS—such as oligodendrocytes, astrocytes, or microglial cells in the disease process—has been difficult to define. A question remains whether if some of these cell populations are initially dysfunctional or whether inflammatory cells invading CNS interfere with the normal function of resident cells, thus contributing to myelin damage (for a review, see Noseworthy, 1999).

As in many other complex diseases in which epidemiological studies suggest a genetic component in etiology, new molecular tools produced by the Human Genome Project have been

Table 42–1. Diagnostic Criteria for MS According to Poser (1983)

Diagnostic Category	No. of Attacks	No. of Clinical Signs[a]		No. of Paraclinical Evidence[b]	CSF OB/IgG[c]
A. Clinically definitive	2	2			
(CDMS)	2	1	*and*	1	
B. Laboratory-supported	2	1	*or*	1	+
definitive (LSDMS)	1	2			+
	1	1	*and*	1	+
C. Clinically probable	2	1			
(CPMS)	1	2			
	1	1	*and*	1	
D. Laboratory-supported probable (LSPMS)	2				+

[a]Clinical signs = Signs of neurological dysfunction demonstrable by neurological examination.
[b]Paraclinical evidence = Lesions demonstrable by means of tests (evoked potential and MR imaging) but cause no signs of neurological dysfunction demonstrable by neurological examination.
[c]CSF OB/IgG = Olicoglonal banding or increased IgG in the cerebrospinal fluid.

applied to provide evidence for a genetic component and to identify predisposing genes for MS. So far, all the trials to identify specific or definitive MS genes have failed. This review can only introduce the readers to the epidemiological studies that provide initial evidence for genetic involvement in MS and describe the research strategies and partially contradictory findings produced in molecular genetic analyses of MS study samples collected from different populations.

GENETIC EPIDEMIOLOGY

Most MS cases are sporadic, and patients are typically unaware of other affected family members. However, occasional familial clustering is reported from several populations, suggesting a genetic predisposition, although the effect of a shared environment within families could also to some extent explain this finding (Compston, 1997; Sadovnick et al., 1997). Similar to most late-onset common diseases, the epidemiology of MS has been difficult to study. Early signs of MS are often ignored, and in some instances another disease is wrongly diagnosed as MS. Despite much effort and published consensus criteria for diagnosis, standardization of clinical criteria has proven to be difficult in practice and several studies reveal inconsistency in diagnostic criteria. However, if current consensus criteria are applied, MS is distributed worldwide, with ethnic factors playing a role in determining the prevalence of the disease. On a global scale, the highest incidence and prevalence rates of MS have been reported in populations of northern European descent (Kurtzke, 1983). Approximately 1 in 1000 persons of northern European origin and living in temperate climate will have MS during their lifetime. The highest prevalence has been reported in Northeast Scotland, with a prevalence of 200 in 100,000 (Poskanzer et al., 1980). In other northern European countries, the prevalence falls to between 50 and 100 per 100,000 and the incidences to between 2 and 4 per 100,000, whereas in Mediterranean countries, except in Sardinia (Rosati et al., 1987), the figures are considerably lower. The north–south gradient present in the population frequency of MS in Europe is seen also in the United States: the prevalence has been shown to vary markedly between different states, with the highest figures in the northernmost states (Kurtzke, 1983). Also, a link with Scandinavian immigration has been reported (Ebers et al., 1986), thus providing an ethnic perspective to these findings. In Australia, the high-prevalence region is related to the presence of a Caucasian population (Hammond et al., 1988), and, in general, MS is much more rare among Asians (for example, with the prevalence of 2 per 100,000 in Japan), as well as among Africans and African Americans (Kurtzke, 1983). These findings demonstrate a significant variability in the frequency of MS among human populations, as well as uneven geographical distribution.

In addition to well-established population differences, several other lines of evidence implicate genetic factors in the etiology of MS. Familial cases are reported from multiple populations, and the risk of first-degree relatives being affected is considerably increased; the recurrence in siblings has been suggested to be as high as 5%. The degree of the familial clustering of the disease can be measured by the quantity of the λ_r, which is the ratio of recurrence risk for relatives of patients vs. disease prevalence in the population. The most commonly used λ_r is the risk ratio for siblings' λ_s. In MS, the λ_s value is approximated to be between 20 and 40 (Sadovnick et al., 1988), reflecting significantly higher recurrence risks for relatives of MS patients. When compared to other complex diseases, this represents a relatively high value. The corresponding λ_s value for Type 1 diabetes is 15 (Vyse and Todd, 1996), and for rheumatoid arthritis it is 8 (Wordsworth, 1995). Comparisons between familial and sporadic MS cases have not revealed any differences in clinical features or in age of onset, which suggests that there is a similar etiological background in disease pathogenesis of familial and nonfamilial cases.

Carefully performed population-based twin studies have provided further evidence of a genetic component of MS. In a classical twin study, concordance rates for a trait are compared in MZ and DZ twins. The higher concordance rate in MZ twins implies the involvement of genetic factors in the trait. In MS, evidence for a genetic component emerges from independent twin concordance studies that demonstrate significantly higher concordance rates for MZ twins (25%–30%) than for DZ twins (2.5%–4%) (Ebers at el., 1986; Sadovnick et al., 1993; Mumford et al., 1994).

The adoption studies that facilitate the comparison of disease prevalence in nonbiological and biological relatives of an affected individual also suggest a significant genetic component in the etiology of MS. Adoption relatives share the environment with an affected individual but there is no genetic relationship, whereas biological relatives of adopted MS cases are genetically related to an affected individual even though they live in a distinct environment. Accordingly, adoption studies provide an excellent opportunity to monitor the true influence of genetic factors on the observed familial aggregation. In a population-based adoption study of MS in the Canadian population, 238 adopted MS cases had 638 nonbiological first-degree relatives (adoptive parents, adoptive siblings, and adopted children), and non-adopted MS index cases had 563 nonbiological relatives (siblings and children). From 1201 nonbiological first-degree relatives of MS index cases, only 1 had MS. This observed recurrence rate was lower than the level in the general population and significantly lower than the expected 25.4 cases based on recurrence risks for biological relatives. These findings emphasize the role of genetic factors in MS and provide no evidence for the effect of shared environmental factors. To monitor the risk in biological first-degree relatives of adopted MS cases, only a small number of such parental individuals ($n = 64$) were available in this study. However, the observed risk for the biological parents was comparable to that of first-degree relatives of MS cases, which again emphasizes that genetic factors are a major determinant for the familial clustering of MS (Ebers et al., 1995).

Additional support for a genetic component in MS has emerged from half-sib studies. An indication of operating genetic factors in a disease would present as a higher risk for full-sibs than for half-sibs. Because half-sibs often live in somewhat different environments, a study design including both half-sibs who were raised together and apart would allow the analysis of the effect of familial environmental factors on the disease occurrence. In a half-sib study performed in the Canadian population, consisting of 939 MS patients with 1395 full-sibs and 1839 half-sibs, the data demonstrated a greater age-adjusted risk for full-sibs (3.46%) than for half-sibs (1.32%), with the difference being statistically significant ($p < .001$). The age-adjusted risks for MS of half-sibs living together and in different familial environments were not significantly different; however, the age-adjusted risk for full-sibs (3.46%) living in the same familial environment was significantly greater than that for half-sibs (1.17%) who shared the familial environment. Thus, the data from the half-sib study were consistent with the results of the adoption study, indicating that familial aggregation of MS is more likely due to a genetic component than to environmental factors shared by family members (Sadovnick et al., 1996).

When evaluating the character of the genetic component of MS, the drop in risk for MS from MZ twins to first-degree relatives, and a further drop to more distant relatives, suggests an oligo- or polygenic mode of inheritance (Sadovnick et al., 1988). Both the polygenic character and the epidemiological evidence for the involvement of genetic and environmental factors in the pathogenesis of MS emphasize the complex etiological nature of this disorder. The families with multiple affected members probably demonstrate the effect of some rare, high-impact genes and thus provide an exceptional avenue to identify genes and metabolic pathways involved in the molecular pathogenesis of MS.

In summary, all of the data from genetic epidemiological studies of MS would indicate that familial clustering of the disease is mostly due to genetic factors. Also, sporadic MS cases have a genetic predisposition that may differ from that in familial cases. However, it is equally obvious that genes are not the sole determinants of MS because only 30% of monozygotic twins are concordant for the disease. The uneven regional and population distribution of MS could also be interpreted to reflect the involvement of the environmental factors in the etiology. Furthermore, reported changes in disease risk associated with immigration from a high-risk geographical area to a low-risk area or vice versa also emphasize the importance of environmental factors in the etiology (Dean and Kurtzke, 1971; Kurtzke, 1983).

ENVIRONMENTAL FACTORS: VIRUS INFECTIONS

Viruses are the most studied environmental factors in MS. Epidemiological data suggest that a transmissible agent could be the environmental trigger of MS, and the viral etiology is supported by the finding that viral infection seems to precede even 25% of relapses in MS patients (Sibley et al., 1985). A vast amount of literature reports increased antibody (IgG) titers against viruses in serum and in CSF of MS patients. Most suggested MS associations have been to viruses, which are known to be able to induce demyelinating disease in both humans and experimental animals. In humans, postinfectious encephalomyelitis is a complication of acute viral infections such as measles, chicken pox, and rubella. Tropical spastic paraparesis is an MS-like disease in the population of Africa and Caribbean, and HTLV-associated myelopathy is a similar disease in Japan, both caused by the retrovirus HTLV-1. In animals, demyelinating disease can be induced with several viruses such as corona virus in rodents and visna virus in sheep.

Several potential mechanisms explain how viruses might be involved in MS: a unique, yet undiscovered virus could cause direct tissue damage; alternatively, a common virus could produce a persistent infection in genetically susceptible individuals, or a common virus could trigger an autoimmune reaction in genetically susceptible individuals although not persisting in the body. At the molecular level, such a triggering event has been suggested to be associated with a molecular mimicry, referring to the antigenic similarity between viral proteins and human tissue components. This would result in the indirect immune-mediated injury to normal tissue in an attempt to destroy the virus particles. Since the specific tissue destruction in MS is seen in myelin, several studies have been targeted to identify molecular similarities between virus proteins and myelin components.

Based on molecular mimicry, several common viruses can potentially trigger the immune system to damage the CNS (Noseworthy, 1999). These include measles, mumps, parainfluenza, influenza C, herpes simplex, rubella, varicella zoster, and vaccinia (Adams and Imagawa 1962; Brody et al., 1971; Catalano,1972; Haire et al., 1973; Horikawa et al., 1973; Salmi et al., 1974; Miyamoto et al., 1976). The number of virus candidates suggested to be involved in MS is high and in some studies, increased antibody titers in MS patients were detected against more than one virus, each patient exhibiting a unique, fingerprint-like antibody-pattern (Salmi et al., 1983). Measles virus antibodies have been detected in the majority of studies, whereas antibodies against other viruses have been encountered less systematically. Most recent research interest has been targeted to a neurotropic human herpesvirus type 6 (HHV-6), which can establish a latent CNS infection in man (Herndon, 1996). Both DNA and protein of HHV-6 have been identified from neuroglial cells in active MS lesions in several studies, and increased HHV-6 IgM titers in MS patients would suggest recent active viral infection (Soldan et al., 1997).

Evidently, the elevated antibody titers represent only an indirect evidence for the role of viral infections in MS. More convincing evidence—direct isolation of a virus from an MS lesion—have almost systematically not been supported by replication studies. The more sensitive in situ hybridization techniques and polymerase chain reaction (PCR) have recently been applied, but the high sensitivity of these methods makes them also prone to artifacts. These methods have revealed viral genomic sequences in brain tissue and in peripheral blood mononuclear lymphocytes of MS patients. Detected viruses include retroviruses, measles, and coronaviruses. However, viral sequences isolated from MS tissues have also been found in control tissues. It should also be emphasized that MS patients have predominantly shown low-affinity antibodies against most viral pathogens, whilst patients with primary viral infections show predominantly high-affinity antibodies (Luxton et al., 1995).

Both measles and coronaviruses are among viruses which show molecular mimicry to short amino acid stretches of myelin basic protein (MBP) (Fujinami and Oldstone, 1985; Jouvenne et al., 1992). This observation has prompted a hypothesis that antigenic cross-reactivity between these viruses and a body's own molecules would initiate an autoimmune process in MS. The molecular mimicry has also been suggested for HHV-6 due to immunological cross-reactivity between HHV-6 and myelin antigens (Steinman and Oldstone, 1997). Another possible mechanism associated with molecular mimicry is that a virus displaying antigenic similarities with human proteins would escape the defense mechanisms of the immune system and produce a persistent infection. Viral persistence has also been proposed in association with the function of HLA antigens since, in MS patients, impaired HLA class II–restricted cytotoxic responses have been observed for measles and herpes simplex virus (Jacobson et al., 1985; de Silva and McFarland 1991).

In summary, the accumulated data of viral involvement in the etiology of MS, rather than evidence for any direct involvement of viruses in MS pathogenesis, can still reflect a more genetically defined sensitivity to specific viral infections or genetic variations in the immuno response, generally. Also, several environmental nonviral factors or pre-existing autoimmunity to CNS antigens could influence the disease-triggering process in MS. Suggestions have been made that, for example, an inappropriate stress response could influence the permeability of the blood–brain barrier and the expression of heat shock proteins and initiate the MS lesions analogously to viral infections (van Noort et al., 1995).

SEARCH FOR PREDISPOSING GENES

The attempts to characterize the genetic background of MS using DNA-based strategies have followed a traditional route. Typically, the first genetic studies of any complex disease aim to correlate the inheritance of specific candidate genes with disease susceptibility. In this approach, genetic markers flanking or located within genes encoding for proteins that could putatively be involved in disease pathophysiology are selected for genotyping in available study samples. These study samples representing sporadic cases are suitable for association-type statistical analyses simply comparing the allele frequencies between MS patients and controls. Study materials of affected sib-pairs or families with multiple affecteds are suitable for linkage analyses that monitor segregation and sharing of marker alleles among affected family members. Parametric linkage analyses are most powerful in relatively rare MS families with multiple affected individuals and involve determination of an inheritance model for a disease in a pedigree. On the basis of the selected model, the co-segregation of disease and marker locus is monitored and compared to by chance probability of co-segregation (linkage). Parametric linkage analyses require specification of other parameters like penetrance, disease allele frequency, and phenocopy rate, which are difficult to define for a complex disease like MS. Concordant sib-pair analysis tests whether affected siblings share alleles more frequently than would be expected from random Mendelian transmission. Discordant sib-pair analysis tests, if there is non-sharing of alleles, is more frequent than would be expected by chance. These analyses are in some sense nonparametric since they do not require a specific definition of an inheritance model (Terwilliger and Ott, 1994).

Animal models, especially the experimental autoimmune encephalomyelitis (EAE) in rodents in the case of MS, have provided an alternative resource to select rationally justified DNA regions for genetic analyses. The use of an inbred strain of rodents allows an investigator to study a genetically homogeneous population and breed the disease susceptibility in a controlled manner. In addition, a strict control over confounding environmental factors is possible in laboratory conditions. Once the disease locus is mapped in the inbred mouse strain, the genetic markers on the syntenically conserved region of the human genome can be tested in human study samples for association and linkage. Advancing or finished genome sequence projects of many species facilitate efficient synteny and homology searches, thus providing shortcuts to identify disease-associated DNA regions and all the genes in these regions across species.

The most random approach to dissect susceptibility genes underlying a complex disease like MS is by a genome-wide scan in which all chromosomes are systematically screened using evenly spaced polymorphic markers to look for genetic regions co-segregating with the disease. For a genome-scan approach, neither a priori knowledge of disease pathophysiology nor animal models is required. Genome-wide scans have proved to be efficient in detecting chromosomal locations for single-gene diseases and have also recently been performed in a number of various complex diseases (e.g., Davies et al., 1994; Moises et al., 1995; Williams et al., 1999; Brzustowicz et al., 2000). Commonly, a two-stage protocol has been employed for genome-wide scans. In the initial stage, all chromosomes are screened in the first study sample of moderate size by genotyping a relatively sparse set of some 400 multiallelic markers, providing a resolution level of 10 cM (roughly 10 Mb) along chromosomal DNA strands. Only the regions showing some evidence for co-segregation or linkage with disease in families or association in case-control studies are then selected for follow-up. In the second stage, a denser set of markers over these putative chromosomal regions is analyzed in an additional, preferably more sizeable study sample in an effort to confirm the true involvement of this particular chromosomal DNA region. The resolution of a dense marker set is typically 1 to 2 cM; however, due to many uncertainties in parameters applied (inheritance pattern, disease gene frequency, genetic heterogeneity, etc.) in statistical analyses of complex diseases, the critical DNA region can often be restricted relatively poorly, to some 5 to 25 cM region that still contains hundreds of genes.

Candidate Gene–Based Approach

Functional candidate genes tested in genetic studies of MS have been selected based on the hallmarks of tissue pathology: inflammation and demyelination. In addition to making educated guesses about involved genes, candidate genes have also been selected based on the transcripts found in affected tissues of a given disease—for example, in demyelinated lesions of MS.

Tissue findings in MS are characterized by damage to myelin and neuronal axons at multiple sites in the CNS (Allen, 1991; Trapp et al., 1998). Penetration of the blood–brain barrier by activated lymphocytes seems to be the initial step required for the process that leads to local inflammation and demyelination in the CNS. The immune reaction has been speculated to be targeted against different myelin antigens that turn on a cascade of events leading to local destruction of the myelin sheath and following destruction of axons (Steinman, 1996; Trapp et al., 1998). The histopathological picture of a typical MS lesion involves perivenular inflammation with infiltration of several inflammatory cells (T- and B-lymphocytes and macrophages), as well as accumulation of cytokines and adhesion molecules (Steinman, 1996; Archelos and Hartung, 1997). Both macrophages and proliferating resident cells of the CNS such as astrocytes and glial cells seem to be involved in myelin phagocytosis. As inflammation proceeds, production of new myelin by proliferating oligodendrocytes (remyelination) comes gradually into the effect (Raine and Wu, 1993). Occasionally, characteristic sclerotic scars replace the patches of demyelination, and the pathophysiological defect remains permanent.

The tissue destruction in MS is widely speculated to have an autoimmune background, based on the histopathological features of MS lesions and immunological abnormalities encountered in patients, including increased intrathecal production of IgG and the presence of oligoclonal bands in CSF. Furthermore, pathophysiological and histopathological findings in a rodent model of MS support an autoimmune etiology for the disease (Martin and McFarland, 1995).

Given the known characteristics of demyelination and autoimmunity, rational candidate genes to be analyzed in MS study materials have been genes that encode the multiple molecular components involved in the human immune system. Another group of potential candidate genes encodes target molecules of tissue damage, such as structural components of myelin or other putative autoantigens in the CNS. Additional candidate genes have been identified by screening transcript (cDNA) libraries constructed from mRNA obtained from the demyelinating lesions (plaques) of MS brains (Becker et al., 1997).

Multiple groups have made extensive effort to identify whether the major genes that influence MS susceptibility could be identified among functional candidate genes. Except for a repeatedly identified association between MS and both the major histocompatibility complex (MHC) and the human leukocyte antigen (HLA) on 6p21 (Vyse and Todd, 1996), most initially promising findings of candidate genes involved in myelin loss in MS have suffered from the lack of replication. This may be due to a false positive finding in the first study or, alternatively, the second data set has not been large enough to show replication. Contradictory findings expose the heterogeneity of predisposing genes between populations or even between study samples within a population. Association studies are also sensitive to study sample stratification, but this problem is sometimes difficult to identify. In this review, we try to summarize the vast literature reporting an association or a lack of association to potential candidate genes in various MS study samples. Table 42–2 summarizes the findings of studies on candidate genes that have been analyzed in several populations. The results obtained for the most popular candidate genes are described briefly in the following paragraphs.

HLA Region

The oldest and only systematic finding concerning immunological candidate genes in MS is the relationship with the HLA locus on chromosome 6p that was reported over 20 years ago. The HLA complex of about 100 genes covers about 4,000 kb and is organized to class I, class II, and class III antigens. Classical HLA antigens (class I: HLA-A, -B, -C and class II: HLA-DR, -DQ, -DP) are heterodimeric glycoproteins that present foreign and self-antigens to T cells. The HLA complex also includes genes for several complement components (class III), as well as genes that are not known to associate with the immune system. The HLA complex is the most polymorphic gene cluster known in humans, and more than 40 diseases have been associated with specific HLA haplotypes.

The role of the HLA complex in MS has been confirmed by several independent studies. As in numerous autoimmune diseases, the strongest association with MS is found to the class II antigens. Due to strong linkage disequilibrium within the HLA region, the MS-associated haplotype extends over a long interval that contains multiple genes. Centromerically the association does not extend HLA-DP or MHC class III genes, and telometrically no association is found to the peptide transporter genes *TAP1* and *TAP2* (Olerup et al., 1990; Spurkland et al., 1994). It should be emphasized that as opposed to other HLA-associated diseases, the majority of MS patients do not have common HLA haplotypes and thus a specific HLA haplotype is neither sufficient nor essential for disease susceptibility. Estimates of the contribution of HLA genes to genetic susceptibility in MS vary from 10% to 30% (Risch, 1987; Haines et al., 1998). In populations of northern European descent, the MS-associated HLA haplotype is HLA-B7, -DR15, translating to the alleles DRB1*1501 or DRB5*0101 and to DQ 6; the corresponding alleles are DQA1*0102 and DQB1*0602 (Olerup and Hillert, 1991; Tienari et al., 1993). Although this association is also seen outside northern European populations including southern European and Mediterranean populations, a trend toward a declining strength of association is apparent toward the south. A distinct exception to the DR15 haplotype associated with MS is the association between MS and the DR4 haplotype in the Sardinians (Marrosu et al., 1988).

In all earlier studies, a puzzling discrepancy existed between a failure to establish linkage between MS and the HLA locus in family studies, despite the strong association observed. If linkage was found, it was typically with the polymorphic markers at a significant genetic distance from the HLA complex. This discrepancy is probably again due to admixtures of linked and nonlinked families or to false parameters adapted in linkage analyses for the inheritance pattern of this complex disease. The first tight linkage to the DQ1DQB HLA region was reported in Finnish MS families with multiple affected individuals and a seemingly dominant inheritance pattern of MS (Tienari et al., 1993). Again, because of the tight linkage disequilibrium between the HLA class II alleles, it has been extremely hard to pinpoint which specific allele(s) of the associated haplotype is in fact responsible for disease susceptibility, even in this exceptional study sample from a genetic isolate.

Immunoglobulin Heavy Chain Region

Since the test demonstrating abnormal immunoglobulin bands in the cerebrospinal fluid of the MS patients is one of the few "diagnostic" laboratory tests for MS and since B cells have been linked to the demyelination process, the genes encoding immunoglobulin chains have been tested as candidate genes in several studies. Immunoglobulins are built from paired heavy and light chains, both composed via somatic gene rearrangement of variable, diversity, joining, and constant region genes. Suggestive associations have been reported between MS and both protein and DNA markers of constant region genes on chromosome 14q in MS (Pandey et al., 1981; Propert et al., 1982; Blanc et al., 1986; Gaiser et al., 1987). In each study, association was detected to a different area of this large gene cluster, covering about

Table 42–2. Candidate Gene Studies in MS: Classification to Positive, Suggestive, and Negative Results as Reported by the Respective Authors (Type of Study)[a]

Candidate Gene[b]	Negative Results	Suggestive Results	Positive Results
CH 45	Barcellos et al., 2001 (1)		Jacobsen et al., 2000 (2)
*HLA-DR15, DQ6, Dw2 (HLA-DRB1**1501/ *DQA1**0102/*DQB1**0602)	Kellar-Wood et al., 1995 (3)		Jersild et al., 1972 (1) Hauser et al., 1989 (1) Sheritt et al., 1992 (1) Hillert and Olerup, 1993 (1) Tienari et al., 1993 (1, 2, 3) Allen et al., 1994 (1) Kellar-Wood et al., 1995 (1) Sawcer et al., 1996 (2) Ebers et al., 1996 (2) Haines et al., 1996 (2)
HLA-DP	Begovich et al., 1990 (1) Howell et al., 1991 (1) Sherrit et al., 1992 (1)		Odum et al., 1988 (1)
TNFα/TNFβ	Fugger et al., 1990a (TNFα) (1) Roth et al., 1994 (1) Garcia-Merino et al., 1996 (1) Wingerchuk et al., 1997 (TNFα) (1)		Kirk et al., 1997 (1)
TAP1/TAP2/LMP	Liblau et al., 1993 (1) Kellar-Wood et al., 1994 (1) Spurkland et al., 1994 (TAP2) (1) Vandenbroeck et al., 1994c (TAP1/2) (1)		
IGH, constant region	Hillert, 1993 (1) Yu et al., 1993 (3)		Pandey et al., 1981 (1) Gaiser et al., 1987 (1)
IGH, variable region	Hashimoto et al., 1993 (3) Wood et al., 1995a (1)		Walter et al., 1991 (1) Hashimoto et al., 1993 (1)
Il-1ra, IL-1β	Huang et al., 1996 (Il-1ra) (1) Semana et al., 1997 (Il-1ra) (?)	Schrijver et al., 1999 (4)	Crusius et al., 1995 (Il-1ra) (1)
Il-4		Vandenbroeck et al., 1997 (4)	
ICAM-1	Luomala et al., 1999 (1)		Mycko et al., 1998 (7)
INF-γ			Vandenbroeck et al., 1998 (1)
hsp 70-2 hsp 7-*hom*	Ramachandran and Bell, 1995 (7)		
MPO			Nagra et al., 1997
Apo E	Rubinsztein et al., 1994 (1) Gervais et al., 1998 (1)		
TRCα	Lynch et al., 1992 (2) Hashimoto et al., 1992 (3) Hillert et al., 1992 (1) Vandenbroeck et al., 1994a (1) Eoli et al., 1994 (3) Droogan et al., 1996 (1)		Oksenberg et al., 1989 (1)
TCRβ	Fugger et al., 1990b (1) Hillert et al., 1991 (1) Lynch et al., 1991 (2) Vandenbroeck et al., 1994a (1) Wei et al., 1995 (1) Droogan et al., 1996 (1)	Wood et al., 1995b (3)	Seboun et al., 1989 (3) Beall et al., 1989 (1) Charmley et al., 1991 (1) Martinez-Naves et al., 1993 (1) Epplen et al., 1997 (1) Hockertz et al., 1998 (1)
MBP	Rose et al., 1993 (2) Graham et al., 1993 (1) Vandenbroeck et al., 1994b (1) Coppin et al., 2000 (1) Wood et al., 1994 (1, 3) Barcellos et al., 1997 (1) He et al., 1998 (1, 2)	Ibsen and Clausen, 1995 (1)	Boylan et al., 1990 (1) Tienari et al., 1992 (1, 2)
VDR	Niino et al., 2000 (1)		Steckley et al., 2000

[a](1), association study; (2), family study using parameter linkage analysis; (3), affected sib-pair study; (4), association with disease severity or time of onset.
[b]CD 45, protein-tyrosine phosphatase, receptor-type-C; HLA-DR, DQ, DW, *HLA-loci*; TNF, tumor necrosis factor; TAP, transporter associated with antigen processing; LMP, large multifuctional protease; IGH, immunoglobulin heavy chain; IL-1ra, interleukin-1 receptor antagonist; IL-1β, interleukin-1β; IL-4, interleukin-4; ICAM-1, intercellular adhesion molecule-1; IFN-γ, Interferon-γ; hsp 70-2 and hsp 70-*hom*, heat shock protein 70 gene family; MPO, myeloperoxidase; ApoE, apolipoprotein E; TCR, T-cell receptor; MBP, myelin basic protein; VDR, vitamin D receptor.

400 kb of genomic DNA. However, the lack of association has also been reported (Bulman et al., 1987; Hillert 1993; Wansen et al., 1997). Similarly, conflicting results have emerged in the family-based linkage studies. Although an allelic association with a gene on the IgH region was initially found in Canadian MS patients, no linkage could be detected in Canadian multiplex families. Conversely, in a large British family study, a weak evidence of linkage but no association to IgH genes was found. MS-study samples from the United States, Sweden, and Finland have failed to reveal either association or linkage to the IgH gene cluster (Hillert and Olerup, 1993; Yu et al., 1993; Wansen et al., 1997).

T-Cell Receptor Germline Genes

Based on suggestive evidence for T-cell mediated tissue destruction in MS and on the well-established association to HLA antigens which functionally interact with T-cell receptors (TCR), the *TCR* genes have been considered as good candidates genes in MS. *TCR* germline gene clusters (α, β, γ, δ) are distributed in distinct regions on chromosomes 7 and 14. *TCR* gene clusters include dozens of homologous genes distributed into gene families, which similarly to *IgH* genes, are divided into variable, diversity, joining, and constant region genes encoding respective domains of the TCR molecule. In activated T cells, *TCR* germline genes are rearranged to produce clonally restricted TCRs. TCRs are heterodimeric proteins, of which $\alpha\beta$ and $\gamma\delta$ TCRs have been identified to date.

Analogously to studies on *IgH* genes, studies on the role of *TCR* germline genes in MS have produced contradictory data. Associations with TCRα (Oksenberg et al., 1989) and *TCRβ* genes (Beall et al., 1989; Martinez-Naves et al., 1993) have been reported, but others have not been able to reproduce these findings (Hillert et al., 1991, 1992; Fugger et al., 1990b; Hashimoto et al., 1992).

Family-based linkage studies to the *TCR* genes have been equally controversial. Affected sib-pair analysis of TCRβ haplotypes produced initial evidence for linkage at the level of $p < .005$ (Seboun et al., 1989), but when more families were included, diminishing evidence for linkage was encountered (Stephen Hauser, personal communication). Others have not been able to demonstrate linkage with TCRβ (Lynch et al., 1991), with TCRα or TCRδ (Lynch et al., 1992; Hashimoto et al., 1992). Recent study of the Finnish MS families revealed no evidence of linkage or association to the TCRβ genes. Stratification of the families or cases based on the predisposing HLA haplotype, DR15DQ1 did not change this result (Wansen et al., 1997). All the genome scans have also failed to show any major involvement of the chromosomal regions containing genes for TCR components.

Myelin Basic Protein

Genes encoding components of the myelin sheet, the target of the tissue destruction, are obvious candidates to be tested in various MS study samples. The gene coding for a myelin basic protein (MBP) on chromosome 18q has been tested in numerous studies due to its direct link to the rodent model, EAE. Certain MBP-derived peptides are among the agents that trigger EAE in genetically susceptible mouse strains (Martin and McFarland, 1995). The association to the MBP gene was first identified in a Canadian case-control study (Boylan et al., 1990), and later multiplex Finnish pedigrees with unusual clustering of MS cases revealed both linkage and association to a long repeat polymorphism $(TGGA)_n$ in the 5′ end of the MBP gene (Tienari et al., 1992). This tetranucleotide repeat is located 2 kb upstream from the initiator codon of the MBP gene. The association and linkage in the Finnish study sample were detected to the large 1.27 kb allele of the long repeat polymorphism. Subsequent reports in MS study samples from other populations have failed to show either linkage or association (Graham et al., 1993; Rose et al., 1993; Vandenbroeck et al., 1994b; Wood et al., 1994; Coppin et al., 2000) except in a Danish study sample (Ibsen and Clausen, 1995). It might be of interest that the genetic marker that was analyzed in most of the "negative" studies was a short tandem repeat instead of the original long repeat polymorphism, which is more tedious to genotype because of its length.

The characterization of the MBP locus has exposed some interesting features. This gene is actually part of a larger gene complex, the golli-MBP gene (golli = gene expressed in oligodendrocyte lineage) (Pribyl et al., 1993). The sequencing of the coding and regulatory regions of the gene in a number of individuals has revealed several single nucleotide polymorphisms (SNPs). These SNPs and the long repeat polymorphism and three short tandem repeats were analyzed for association in the Finnish case-control and family data sets that originally revealed the linkage (Tienari et al., 1998). No other polymorphisms than the previously identified 1.27 kb allele of the long repeat polymorphism showed an association with MS. When the transmission of the haplotype containing the 1.27 kb allele was analyzed in MS families, an increased transmission of one specific subhaplotype of the 1.27 kb allele to MS patients was detected (Tienari et al., 1998). The extended haplotype analyses in the subset of Finnish MS families revealed that a potential "predisposing haplotype" was observed only over a 20 to 25 kb interval, between the enhancer element upstream of the long repeat polymorphism and the MBP exon 3. This suggests that the genetic variant predisposing to MS would lie within this restricted DNA region and perhaps provides further evidence to support the role of the Golli-MBP locus in MS susceptibility, although this effect might be specific to Scandinavian populations such as Finns and Danes.

Candidate Chromosomal Region Approach Based on Conserved Syntenies to Rodent Loci

Comparative mapping, an integral part of genome projects of different species, has revealed significant amount of homology between mammalian genomes, including mouse and man (Nadeau et al., 1992). Using the published genetic maps and sequences in comparative maps, it is fairly easy to look for syntenically conserved chromosomal regions between any two species. Once the equivalent regions of loci predisposing to an animal disease with phenotypic features similar to a human disease have been identified, the syntenically conserved human chromosomal regions can be analyzed. Typically, a dense set of markers providing a relatively high resolution of the region is analyzed in available study samples to see whether syntenic genomic regions are involved in the corresponding human disease.

Furthermore, while fine mapping of the susceptibility genes of complex diseases in humans is complicated due to genetic heterogeneity and poorly definable parameters in statistical analyses, possibilities for the locus restriction in animal models are excellent. It is significantly easier to fine-map and eventually identify the disease gene in a mouse strain than in humans. It is possible to create congenic mouse strains in which a specific chromosomal segment is the only genetic difference between two otherwise clonal mouse strains (Frankel, 1995). This is generated by successive backcrosses of mice with a trait of interest

Table 42–3. EAE Modifying Loci and Human Synteny Regions

EAE Locus	Chromosome No.	Human Synteny
eae1	17	6p21
eae2	15	5p13–p15, 8q22–q23
eae3	3	3q25–q27, 4q28–q33, 1p12–p31
eae4	7	11q13–q15, 15q11–q26
eae5	17	6p21–p22, 19p13
eae6	11	22q12, 7p11–p13, 2p12–p23, 16p13, 5q31–q35
eae7	11	17q11–q23
eae8	2	20q13
eae9	9	11q22–q23, 15q21–q23
eae10	3	4q21–q25, 1p25

Source: Modified from Butterfield et al. (1998) with permission.

and selection of the progeny that have inherited alleles of the genetic markers spanning the trait locus. Subsequently, it is possible to compare strains of mice that differ only at this specific chromosomal segment and to create additional backcrosses to restrict the locus to a segment of only 100 to 300 kb. The sequence variation causing the disease trait can be identified within this restricted interval by sequencing. All progeny will carry the same sequence variation and no problems of locus heterogenity and multiple DNA variants are encountered—as opposed to the problems with human study samples of complex diseases. Subsequently, the homologous gene can then become a target of extensive sequence analyses in human patients.

Experimental autoimmune encephalomyelitis (EAE) is widely regarded as a relevant animal model for MS based on clinical and histopathological (inflammation and demyelination) similarities between these two disorders (Martin and McFarland, 1995). EAE is a T-cell-mediated autoimmune disease in rodents that can be induced by immunization with CNS tissue, with myelin basic protein, or with certain peptides derived from MBP (Fritz et al., 1985; Traugott et al., 1985; Zamvil et al., 1986; Kono et al., 1988; Zamvil and Steinman, 1990). Susceptibility to EAE in rodents is influenced by the MHC complex, corresponding the HLA region in man (Fritz et al., 1985). To date, three independent genome-wide screens for non-MHC loci predisposing to murine EAE have been performed in different crosses between mouse strains that are either resistant to or susceptible to EAE (Baker et al., 1995; Sundvall et al., 1995; Encinas et al., 1996). Loci on several mouse chromosomes have been identified and are either directly linked to the susceptibility to EAE or suggested to modify the disease severity. Detection of multiple predisposing loci for EAE in these scans is consistent with the previous assertion of the polygenic nature of this rodent disease. The putative EAE modifying loci and corresponding syntenically conserved regions in man are listed in Table 42–3.

Some evidence for additional loci with gender-specific effects governing susceptibility to different disease subtypes (remitting/relapsing and monophasic remitting/nonrelapsing) has recently emerged from the studies of EAE in rodents (Butterfield et al., 1999). Such underlying genetic differences may explain the heterogeneity in disease course and prognosis, which is so characteristic of human MS. These differences may also confound the interpretation of genetic data in MS or even mask the presence of susceptibility loci. This would encourage researchers to stratify their MS study samples more stringently with respect to sex and other features of well-defined clinical phenotype. Recently reported associations between the *APOE* gene, clinical type, and progression rate could represent evidence for modifying genes.

A good example of the use of conserved syntenies is the identification of human MS loci based on the information from a genome-wide screen for non-MHC EAE-loci carried out in an experimental cross between EAE-induced resistant (RIIIS/J) and susceptible (B10.RIII) mouse strains (Sundvall et al., 1995). Although these mouse strains share the same MHC haplotype, they differ in disease susceptibility. The genome-wide scan provided evidence for the involvement of three novel loci in predisposition to EAE in this cross: *Eae2* on chromosome 15, *Eae3* on chromosome 3, and a third putative locus on mouse chromosome X. With the aid of the comparative human-mouse maps, the human chromosomal regions, which revealed conserved syntenies to the murine chromosomal regions containing the novel EAE loci, were subsequently identified. *Eae2* on mouse chromosome 15 was found to show conserved synteny to human 5p14–p12, *Eae3* on mouse chromosome 3 showed syntenies to three different regions on human chromosome 1; and a putative locus on mouse chromosome X was syntenically conserved to a human Xq13.2–q22 region.

When dense sets of microsatellite markers spanning the syntenically conserved human chromosomal regions were genotyped and linkage analyses were carried out in Finnish multiplex MS families, only markers on 5p14–p12, homologous to the *Eae 2* region in mice, yielded significant evidence for linkage (Kuokkanen et al., 1996). Markers on this chromosomal region also have revealed some evidence for linkage in a genome-wide scan performed in the Canadian family material (Ebers et al., 1996). These observations would be consistent with the hypothesis of a putative susceptibility gene for human MS in this particular chromosomal region.

Genome-wide Scans

A total of four genome-wide scans for MS loci, as well as meta-analyses of three of these scans, have been published so far. Table 42–4 compares the study materials used in the original scans. Unfortunately, direct comparison of the obtained results is somewhat complicated because the marker sets used in the different screens were only partially overlapping. Table 42–5 makes an effort to summarize the most significant findings (maximum

Table 42–4. Comparison of Study Samples in Genome Scans

Sample Type	Canada[a]	Finland[b]	United Kingdom	United States and France[d]
Stage 1				
Families	61	16	129	52
Sibling pairs	100	29	143	81
Total individuals	330	104	447	471
Total affecteds	137	50	265	129
Markers	261	328	311	443
Stage 2				
Families	114	21	98	23
Sibling pairs	122	37	108	45
Total individuals	506	191	322	172
Total affecteds	232	58	201	63
Markers	8	40	44	3

[a]Sowcer et al., 1996.
[b]Kuokkanen et al., 1997.
[c]Ebers et al., 1996.
[d]Haines et al., 1996.

Table 42–5. Highest Maximum LOD Scores Reported for Chromosomal Regions

	Maximum LOD Score Values in the Region			
Region	Canada[a]	Finland[b]	United Kingdom[c]	United States and France[d]
1p/1cen	0.95		2.2	
2p	1.24		1.4	1.71
3p	0.77		1.4	
3q	1.01	1.8		1.00
4q	0.60	1.35	1.4	0.81
5p/5cen	4.24	3.4	2.6	
5q	0.42			1.14
6p	0.72	6.43	2.8	3.57
7p	0.87		1.8	
7q	0.70			2.86
10q	0.97	0.95		1.39
11q	1.38	2.0		
17q		2.8	2.7	
18p		1.2		0.93
19q	0.73	0.9	1.7	1.47
Xp	1.85		1.8	

[a]Ebers et al., 1996
[b]Tienari et al., 1993; Kuokkanen et al., 1996, 1997
[c]Sawcer et al., 1996; Chataway et al., 1998
[d]Haines et al., 1996

LOD scores) and corresponding chromosomal regions, except in these four genome wide scans and in a few other studies. No major locus outside the HLA region influencing the genetic susceptibility to MS could be detected in any of the genome scans, and thus it is unlikely that such a major MS gene would exist. The modest (barely significant at genome-wide level) linkage results for any single locus would be in agreement with the earlier assertion of an oligo- or polygenic model for this disease. All the study samples were too small to detect multiple loci of minor significance.

The HLA complex on 6p21 is the only locus revealed by each screen, and evidence for its role in the etiology of MS is compelling (Hillert and Olerup, 1993; Tienari et al., 1993; Ebers et al., 1996; Haines et al., 1996; Sawcer et al., 1996; Kuokkanen et al., 1997). In Caucasian populations, the associated haplotype, HLA-DRB1*1501–DQA1*0102–DQB1*0602, seems to account for a small but constant portion of the overall risk. The role of other genes on the HLA region remains to be clarified, and even the actual number of predisposing genes is still open. Each of the genome-wide screens reported several provisional loci, some of which were found in more than one study and were obvious targets for further fine mapping analyses that have provided further support for loci on 5p and 17q (Table 42–5).

Failure to replicate linkage in regions of interest identified in different populations and study samples is conspicuous and somewhat expected (Dyment et al., 1997; Sawcer et al., 1997). It is in agreement with the previous assertion that genetic heterogeneity exists in MS susceptibility, but it may also reflect general difficulties in demonstrating replication (Suarez et al., 1994; Sawcer et al., 1997). None of these family data sets alone is large enough to replicate the other studies. Simulation studies have established that replication may require several hundreds of families, particularly if the effect of a given predisposing variant is small (Suarez et al., 1994). Consequently, any single locus cannot be excluded as "false positive" even if it is found in only one of the genome scans. Since one study is unlikely to be definitive, pooled analysis of the data could be advocated to achieve a sample size that overcomes statistical power limitations—although this might increase the potential for increased genetic heterogeneity if study samples from different populations, for example from Finland and Canada, are pooled. In meta-analysis of three genome scans, two regions, chromosome 17q and 6p, emerged as most interesting in nonparametric linkage analysis (Transatlantic Multiple Sclerosis Genetics Cooperative, 2001).

With regard to further investigations, clearly the regions that emerged in two or more genome scans are of first priority since the odds in favor of them to be "true MS-loci" are higher. For example, a locus on chromosome 19q13 provided some evidence for linkage in all data sets. Furthermore, haplotype analysis for association with multiple markers (D19S178, D19S574, APOE, APOC1, APOC2, and D19S219) revealed some evidence that a locus on 19q13 may confer susceptibility to MS in the American and Chinese data sets (Barcellos et al., 1997). Accordingly, the 19q13 region is an important target of further analyses.

Another putative MS locus is on 17q22–q24. This was first detected by the British genome-wide scan and then was identified with exactly the same markers in the Finnish scan (Sawcer et al., 1996; Kuokkanen et al., 1997). In the Finnish study, positive LOD scores were for the most part contributed to the families collected from the internal isolate of western Finland, revealing a high risk for MS. Such a regional subisolate should provide excellent possibilities for linkage disequilibrium mapping since one would assume only a limited number of ancestral predisposing variants to be segregating in these families. The construction of the physical map over the critical region on 17q22–q24 is warranted once the locus has been narrowed to a reasonable size. Interestingly, several candidate genes have been localized to the region of 17q22–q24—for example, genes encoding for platelet endothelial cell adhesion molecule 1, CD79B antigen (immunoglobulin-associated β), intracellular adhesion molecule-2, nerve growth factor receptor, tumor necrosis factor, and α-induced protein 1. Recent analyses targeted to this chromosomal region have supported linkage in a Scandinavian study sample (Larsen et al., 2000), whereas no support is obtained in an American-French study sample (Fontaine et al., 1999).

In addition to loci implicated in two or more genome-wide scans, the potential MS locus on chromosome 5 showing conserved synteny to mouse EAE2 is worthy of mentioning. The markers showing linkage in Finnish families are flanked by "hits" in the Canadian, UK, and American screens. Fine mapping of this region has been carried out both in English and Scandinavian study samples, both providing some supportive evidence for an MS locus on this region (Feakes et al., 1999; Oturai et al., 1999). Thus the pericentrometric region of chromosome 5 remains another interesting target of further studies.

In the English study sample, the data from the genome scan also was analyzed after conditioning the cases for the presence of HLA-DR15. The outcome suggested that depending on DR15 sharing, the linked regions were divided into two distinct groups: the evidence for linkage was mostly obtained from the DR15-sharing cohort to loci on chromosomes 1p, 17q, and X, whereas the DR15 nonsharing cohort revealed most of the evidence to linkage to 1 cen, 3p, 7p, 14q, and 22q. However, for each of these, as for most reported loci, the statistical significance remained only suggestive (Chataway et al., 1998).

Figure 42–1 provides a schematic presentation of numerous genetic loci so far reported to show some evidence of linkage or association to MS. Although, it is likely that some of these loci represent false positive findings, the busy Figure 42–1 well dem-

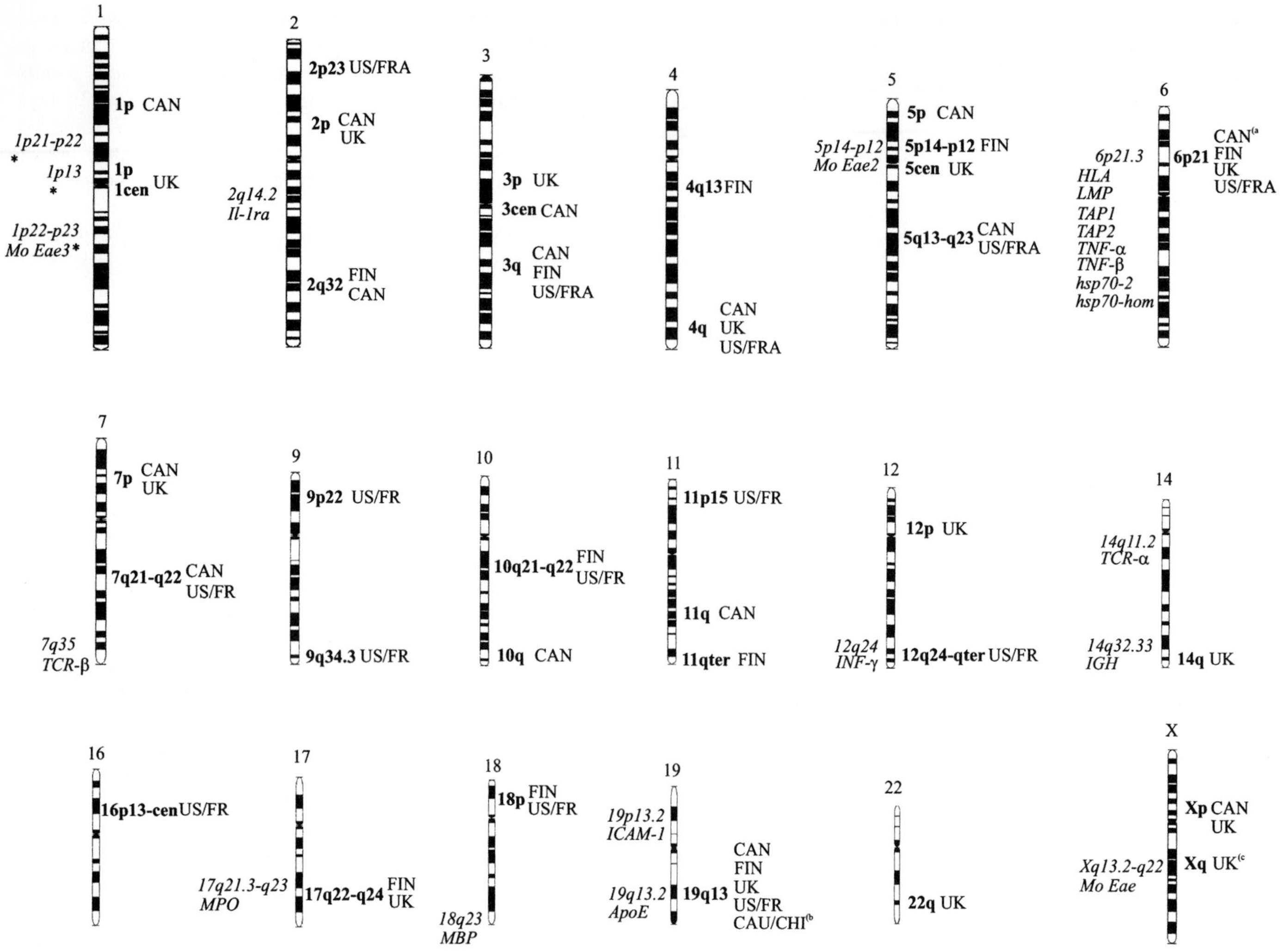

Fig. 42–1. Chromosomal loci showing evidence of linkage or association to MS. This figure depicts loci (chromosomal areas and/or candidate genes) so far reported to show some evidence of linkage or association to MS. Indicated to the left side of each chromosome are loci where individual gene associations or suggestive associations have been reported. Indicated to the right of each chromosome are areas that have been identified in genome scans. Boldface indicates; italics indicate. The population used in the genome scan are represented by the following abbreviations: CAN, Canadian; FIN, Finnish; FRA, French; US, United States; CAU, Caucasian population in the United States; CHI, Chinese.

onstrates the current complex view to the genetic background of MS. All the data from candidate gene studies, genome scans, and searches based on syntenically conserved EAE regions clearly provide evidence for the polygenic and complex genetic background of MS. In addition, predisposing genes to MS may be different in various populations. The constant findings of association to the HLA region is likely to reflect an important modifying role of this locus, as well as suggest individual immunological tolerance to MS susceptibility.

CLINICAL APPLICATIONS OF GENETIC INFORMATION

Evaluation of genetic risk for MS is still based on epidemiological studies. Siblings have 13 times increased risk, and children have 7 times increased risk, when compared with the lifetime risk for European Caucasians. Despite all the impressive research efforts and emerged evidence of potential predisposing loci, these facts still represent the best genetic information a clinician can deliver to an individual patient and his or her family. All available genetic data suggest that MS depends on independent or epistatic effects of several genes, each contributing relatively little to the phenotype. Some evidence would further hint that different clinical phenotypes would represent diseases with different genetic backgrounds. Recent results from U.K. study material would imply that the HLA type could be used to divide MS patients to different subgroups with deviating genetic backgrounds. This remains to be confirmed in other study samples. Future genetic studies, using denser marker maps, better-defined clinical study materials, and novel statistical strategies will hopefully provide conclusive evidence for some genetic loci predisposing to MS. With the human genome map at hand, these findings should rapidly result in the identification of most MS genes and DNA variants in these genes, which are found more often in MS patients than in the general population. Current data would indicate that genetic predisposition to MS consists of DNA variants in multiple genes, of which none represents "the MS mutation" or is solely responsible for the initiation or the progress of the disease. It seems obvious that novel strategies monitoring multiple loci in the same study sample must be applied to establish the definitive proof for the network of genes behind MS.

Most probably in the future, a limited number of characteristic "genetic profiles" containing different DNA variants in a limited number of genes can be identified in MS patients and genetically predisposed individuals. Hopes are high that this type of genetic profiling can be used for presymptomatic diagnosis and criteria for selection of specific treatment. After MS-associated DNA variants are identified, they will become targets of extensive investigation to clarify their functional role in the molecular pathogenesis of MS. Information from these functional studies will provide the basis for the development of novel, targeted therapies. Once the details and character of genetic component of MS are known, the character and role of environmental triggers can also be solved, hopefully resulting in protective actions that can be taken to minimize these environmental risks for individuals at high risk based on their genetic profile.

REFERENCES

Adams JM, Imagawa DT: Measles antibodies in multiple sclerosis. Proc Soc Biol Med 1962; 111:562–566.

Allen I: Pathology of Multiple Sclerosis. In: Matthew W (ed). Multiple Sclerosis. Edinburgh: Churchill Livingstone, 1991:341–378.

Allen M, Sandberg-Wolheim M, Sjögren K, Erlich HA, Petterson U, Gyllensten U: Association of susceptibility to multiple sclerosis in Sweden with HLA class II DRB1 and DQB1 alleles. Hum Immunol 1994; 39:41–48.

Archelos JJ, Hartung H: The role of adhesion molecules in multiple sclerosis: biology, pathogenesis and therapeutic implications. Mol Med Today 1997; 4:310–321.

Baker D, Rosenwasser OA, O'Neil JK, Turk JL: Genetic analysis of experimental allergic encephalomyelitis in mice. J Immunol 1995; 155:4046–4051.

Barcellos LF, Caillier S, Dragone L, Elder M, Vittinghoff E, Bucher P, Lincoln RR, Pericak-Vance M, Haines JL, Weiss A, et al.: PTPRC (CD45) is not associated with the development of multiple sclerosis in U.S. patients. Nat Genet 2001; 29:23–24.

Barcellos LF, Thomson G, Carrington M, Scafer J, Begovich AB, Lin P, Xu X-h, Min B-q, Marti D, Klitz W: Chromosome 19 single-locus and haplotype associations with multiple sclerosis. JAMA 1997; 15:1256–1261.

Beall SS, Concannon P, Charmley P, McFarland HF, Gatti RA, Hood LE, McFarlin DE, Biddison WE: The germline repertoire of T cell receptor β-chain genes in patients with chronic progressive multiple sclerosis. J Neuroimmunol 1989; 21:59–66.

Becker KG, Mattson DH, Powers JM, Gado AM, Biddison WE: Analysis of a sequenced cDNA library from multiple sclerosis lesions. J Neuroimmunol 1997; 77:27–38.

Begovich AB, Helmuth RC, Oksenberg JR, Sakai K, Tabira T, Sasazuki T, Steinman L, Erlich HA: HLA-DP β and susceptibility to multiple sclerosis: an analysis of Caucasoid and Japanese patient populations. Hum Immunol 1990; 28:365–372.

Blanc M, Clanet M, Berr C, Dugoujon JM, Ruydavet B, Ducos SJ, Rascol A, Alperovitch A, et al.: Immunoglobulin allotypes and susceptibility to multiple sclerosis. J Neurol Sci 1986; 75:1–5.

Boylan KB, Takahashi N, Paty DW, Sadovnick AD, Diamond M, Hood LE, Prusiner SB: DNA length polymorphisn 5′ to the myelin basic protein gene is associated with multiple sclerosis. Ann Neurol 1990; 27:291–297.

Brody JA, Sever JL, Heson TE: Virus antibody titers in multiple sclerosis patients, siblings and controls. JAMA 1971; 216:1441–1446.

Brzustowicz LM, Hodgkinson KA, Chow EW, Honer WG, Bassett AS: Location of a major susceptibility locus of familial schizophrenia on chromosome 1q21–q22. Science 2000; 288(5466):678–682.

Bulman DE, Pandey JP, Ebers GC: Gm allotypes in multiple sclerosis. In: Lowenthal A, Raus J (eds). Cellular and Humoral Immunological Components of Cerebrospinal Fluid in Multiple Sclerosis. Plenum Publishing, 1987:81–86.

Butterfield RJ, Blankenhorn EP, Roper RJ, Zachary JF, Doerge RW, Sudweeks J, Rose J, Teuscher C: Genetic analysis of disease subtypes and sexual dimorphisms in mouse experimental allergic encephalomyelitis (EAE): relapsing/remitting and monophasic remitting/nonrelapsing EAE are immunogenetically distinct. J Immunol 1999; 162(5):3096–3102.

Butterfield RJ, Sudweeks JD, Blankenhorn EP, Korngold R, Marini JC, Todd JA, Roper RJ, Teuscher C: New genetic loci that control susceptibility and symptoms of experimental allergic encephalomyelitis in inbred mice. J Immunol 1998; 161(4):1860–1867.

Catalano Jr LW: Herpesvirus hominis antibody in multiple sclerosis and amyotrophic later sclerosis. Neurology 1972; 22:473–478.

Charmley P, Beall SS, Concannon P, Hood L, Gatt RA: Further localization of a multiple sclerosis susceptibility gene on chromosome 7q using a new T cell receptor β-chain DNA polymorphism. J Neuroimmunol 1991; 32:231–240.

Chataway J, Freakes R, Coraddu F, Gray J, Deans J, Fraser M, Robertson N, Broadley S, Jones H, Clayton D, et al.: The genetics of multiple sclerosis: principles, background and updated results of the United Kingdom systematic genome screen. Brain 1998; 121:1869–1887.

Compston A: Genetic epidemiology of multiple sclerosis. J Neurol Neurosurg Psychiatry 1997; 62:553–562.

Coppin H, Ribouchon MT, Bausero P, Pessac B, Fontaine B, Semana G, Clanet M, Roth MP, French Multiple Sclerosis Genetics Group: No evidence for transmission disequilibrium between a new marker at the myelin basic protein locus and multiple sclerosis in French patients. Genes Immunol 2000; 1(8):478–482.

Crusius JB, Pena AS, Van Oosten BW, Bioque G, Garcia A, Dijkstra CD, Polman CH: Interleukin-1 receptor antagonist gene polymorphism and multiple sclerosis. Lancet 1995; 346:979.

Davies JL, Kawaguchi Y, Bennett ST, Copeman JB, Cordell HJ, Pritchard LE, Reed PW, Gough SCL, Jenkins SC, Palmer SM, et al.: A genome-wide search for human type 1 diabetes susceptibility genes. Nature 1994; 371:130–136.

Dean G, Kurtzke JF: On the risk of multiple sclerosis according to age at immigration to South Africa. Br Med J 1971; 3:725–729.

de Silva SM, McFarland HF: Multiple sclerosis patients have reduced HLS class II–restricted responses specific for both measles and herpes virus. J Neuroimmunol 1991; 35:219–226.

Droogan AG, Kirk CW, Hawkins SA, McMillan SA, Nevin NC, Graham CA: T-cell receptor α, β, γ, and δ chain gene microsatellites show no association with multiple sclerosis. Neurology 1996; 47:1049–1053.

Dyment DA, Sadovnick AD, Ebers GC: Genetics of multiple sclerosis. Hum Mol Genet 1997; 6(10):1693–1698.

Ebers GC, Bulman DE, Sadovnick AD, Paty DW, Warren S, Hader W, Murray TJ, Seland TP, Duquette P, Grey T, et al.: A population-based study of multiple sclerosis in twins. N Engl J Med 1986; 315:150–151.

Ebers GC, Kukay K, Bulman DE, Sadovnick AD, Rice G, Anderson C, Armstrong H, Cousin K, Bell RB, Hader W, et al.: A full genome search in multiple sclerosis. Nat Genet 1996; 13:472–476.

Ebers GC, Sadovnick AD, Risch NJ: A genetic basis for familial aggregation in multiple sclerosis. Nature 1995; 377:150–151.

Encinas JA, Lees MB, Sobel RA, Symonowicz C, Greer JM, Shovlin CL, Weiner HL, Seidman CE, Seidman JG, Kuchroo VK: Genetic analysis of susceptibility to experimental autoimmune encephalomyelitis in a cross between SJL/J and B10.S mice. J Immunol 1996; 157:2186–2192.

Eoli M, Pandolfo M, Milanese C, Gasparini P, Salmaggi A, Zeviani M: The myelin basic protein gene is not a major susceptibility locus for multiple sclerosis in Italian patients. J Neurol 1996; 241:615–619.

Eoli M, Wood NW, Kellar-Wood HF, Holmans P, Clayton D, Compston DA: No linkage between multiple sclerosis and the T cell receptor α chain locus. J Neurol Sci 1994; 124:32–37.

Epplen C, Jäckel S, Santos EJM, D'Souza M, Poehlau D, Dotzauer B, Sindern E, Haupts M, Rude K-P, Weber F, et al.: Genetic predisposition to multiple sclerosis as revealed by immunoprinting. Ann Neurol 1997; 41:341–352.

Fazekas F, Offenbacher H, Fuchs S, Schmidt R, Niederkorn K, Horner S, et al.: Criteria for increased specificity of MRI interpretation in elderly subjects with suspected multiple sclerosis. Neurology 1988; 38:1822–1825.

Feakes R, Sawcer S, Chataway J, Coraddu F, Broadley S, Gray J, Jones HB, Clayton D, Goodfellow PN, Compston A: Exploring the dense mapping of a region of potential linkage in complex disease: an example in multiple sclerosis. Genet Epidemiol 1999; 17(1):51–63.

Fontaine B, Cournu I, Arnaud I, Babron MC, Eichenbaum-Voline S, Oksenberg JR, Pericak-Vance MA, Haines JL, Semama G, Liblau R, et al.: Chromosome 17q22–q24 and multiple sclerosis genetic susceptibility. Genes Immunol 1999; 1(2):149–150.

Frankel WN: Taking stock of complex trait genetics in mice. Trends Genet 1995; 11:471–477.

Fritz RB, Skeen MJ, Chou C-HJ, Carcia M, Egorov IK: Major histocompatibility complex–linked control of the murine immune response to myelin basic protein. J Immunol 1985; 134:2328–2332.

Fugger L, Morling N, Sandberg-Wollheim M, Ryder LP, Svejgaard A: Tumor necrosis factor α gene polymorphism in multiple sclerosis and optic neuritis. J Neuroimmunol 1990a; 27:85–88.

Fugger L, Sandberg-Wollheim M, Morling N, Ryder LP, Svejgarrd A: The germline repertoire of T-cell receptor β chain genes in patients with relapsing/remitting multiple sclerosis or optic neuritis. Immunogenetics 1990b; 31:278–280.

Fujinami RS, Oldstone MBA: Amino acid homology between the encephalitogenic site of myelin basic protein and virus: mechanism for autoimmunity. Science 1985; 230:1043–1045.

Gaiser CN, Johnson MJ, de Lange G, Rassenti L, Cavalli-Sforza LL, Steinman L: Susceptibility to multiple sclerosis associated with an immunoglobulin γ 3 restriction fragment length polymorphism. J Clin Invest 1987; 79:309–313.

Garcia-Merino A, Alper CA, Usuku K, Marcus-Bagley D, Lincoln R, Awdeh Z, Yunis EJ, Eisenbarth GS, Brink SJ, Hauser SL: Tumor necrosis factor (TNF) microsatellite haplotypes in relation to extended haplotypes, susceptibility to diseases associated with the major histocompatibility complex and TNF secretion. Hum Immunol 1996; 50:11–21.

Gass A, Barker GJ, Kidd D, Thorpe JW, MacManus D, Brennan A, Tofts PS, Thompson AJ, McDonald WI, et al.: Correlation of magnetization transfer ratio with clinical disability in multiple sclerosis. Ann Neurol 1994; 36:62–67.

Gervais A, Gaillard O, Plassart E, Reboul J, Fontaine B, Schuller E: Apolipoprotein E polymorphism in multiple sclerosis. Ann Clin Biochem 1998; 35(1):135–136.

Graham CA, Kirk CW, Nevin NC, Droogan AG, Hawkins SA, McMillan SA, McNeill TA: Lack of association between myelin basic protein gene microsatellite and multiple sclerosis. Lancet 1993; 341:1596.

Haines JL, Ter-Minassian M, Bazyk A, Gusella JF, Kim DJ, Terwedow H, Pericak-Vance MA, Rimmler JB, Haynes CS, Roses AD, et al.: A complete genomic screen for multiple sclerosis underscores a role for the major histocompatibility complex. Nat Genet 1996; 13:469–471.

Haines JL, Terwedow HA, Burgess K, Pericak-Vance MA, Rimmler JB, Martin ER, Oksenberg JR, Lincoln R, Zhang DY, Banatao DR, et al.: Linkage of the MHC

to familial multiple sclerosis suggests genetic heterogeneity. Hum Mol Genet 1998; 7(8):1229–1234.
Haire M, Frazer KB, Millar JHD: Virus-specific immunoglobulins in multiple sclerosis. Clin Exp Immunol 1973; 14:409–416.
Hashimoto LL, Mark TW, Ebers GC: T cell receptor α chain polymorphisms in multiple sclerosis. J Neuroimmunol 1992; 40:41–48.
Hashimoto LL, Walter MA, Cox DW, Ebers GC: Immunoglobulin heavy chain variable region polymorphisms and multiple sclerosis susceptibility. J Neuroimmunol 1993; 44:77–83.
Hauser SL, Fleischnick E, Weiner HL, Marcus D, Awdeh Z, Yunis EJ, Alper CA: Extended major histocompatibility complex haplotypes in patients with multiple sclerosis. Neurology 1989; 39:275–277.
He B, Yang B, Lundahl J, Fredrikson S, Hillert J: The myelin basic protein gene in multiple sclerosis: identification of discrete alleles of a 1.3 kb tetranucleotide repeat sequence. Acta Neurol Scand 1998; 97:46–51.
Herndon RM: Herpesvirus in multiple sclerosis. Arch Neurol 1996; 53(2):123–124.
Hillert J: Immunoglobulin γ constant region polymorphisms in multiple sclerosis. J Neuroimmunol 1993; 43:9–14.
Hillert J, Leng C, Olerup O: No association with germline T cell receptor β-chain gene alleles or haplotypes in Swedish patients with multiple sclerosis. J Neuroimmunol 1991; 31:141–147.
Hillert J, Leng C, Olerup O: T-cell receptor α chain germline gene polymorphisms in multiple sclerosis. Neurology 1992; 42:80–84.
Hillert J, Olerup O: Multiple sclerosis is associated with genes within or close to the HLA-DR-DQ subregion on a normal DR15, DQ6, Dw2 haplotype. Neurology 1993; 43:163–168.
Hockertz MK, Paty DW, Beall SS: Susceptibility to relapsing-progressive multiple sclerosis is associated with inheritance of genes linked to the variable region of the TCR β locus: use of affected family-based controls. Am J Hum Genet 1998; 62:373–385.
Horikawa Y, Tsubaki T, Nakajima M: Rubella antibody in multiple sclerosis. Lancet 1973; I:996–997.
Howell WM, Sage DA, Evans PR, Smith JL, Francis GS, Haegert DG: No association between susceptibility to multiple sclerosis and HLA-DPB 1 alleles in the French Canadian population. Tissue Antigens 1991; 37:156–160.
Huang WX, He B, Hillert J: An interleukin-1 receptor-antagonist gene polymorphism is not associated with multiple sclerosis. J Neuroimmunol 1996; 67:143–144.
Ibsen SN, Clausen J: A repetitive DNA sequence 5′ to the human myelin basic protein gene may be linked to MS in Danes. Acta Neurol Scand 1995; 93:236–240.
Jacobsen M, Schweer D, Ziegler A, Gaber R, Schock S, Schwinzer R, Wonigeit K, Lindert R-B, Kantarci O, Schaefer-Klein J, et al.: A point mutation in PTPRC is associated with the development of multiple sclerosis. Nat Genet 2000; 26:495–499.
Jacobson S, Flerlage ML, McFarland HF: Impaired measles virus-specific cytotoxic T cell responses in multiple sclerosis. J Exp Med 1985; 162:839–850.
Jersild C, Svejgaard A, Fog T: HL-A antigens and multiple sclerosis. Lancet 1972; I:1240–1241.
Jouvenne P, Mounir S, Stewart JN, Richardson CD, Talbot PJ, et al.: Sequence analysis of human coronavirus 229E mRNAs 4 and 5; evidence for polymorphism and homology with myelin basic protein. Virus Res 1992; 22:125–141.
Kellar-Wood HF, Powis SH, Gray J, Compston DAS: MHC-encoded TAP1 and TAP2 dimorphisms in multiple sclerosis. Tissue Antigens 1994; 43:129–132.
Kellar-Wood HF, Wood NW, Holmans P, Clayton D, Robertson N, Compston DA: Multiple sclerosis and the HLA-D region: linkage and association studies. J Neuroimmunol 1995; 58(2):183–190.
Kesserling J, Miller DH, Robb SA, et al.: Acute disseminated encephalomyelitis: MRI findings and the distinction from multiple sclerosis. Brain 1990; 113:291–302.
Kirk CW, Droogan AG, Hawkins SA, McMillan SA, Nevin NC, Graham CA: Tumour necrosis factor microsatellites show association with multiple sclerosis. J Neurol Sci 1997; 147:21–25.
Kono DH, Urban JL, Horvath SJ, et al.: 2 Minor Determinants of Myelin Basic-Protein Induce Experimental Allergic Encephalomyelitis in SJL/J Mice. J Exp Med 1988; 168(1):213–227.
Kuokkanen S, Gschwend M, Rioux JD, Daly MJ, Terwilliger JD, Tienari PJ, Wikstöom J, Palo J, Stein LD, Hudson TJ, et al.: Genomewide scan of multiple sclerosis in Finnish multiplex families. Am J Hum Genet 1997; 61:1379–1387.
Kuokkanen S, Sundvall M, Terwilliger JD, Tienari PJ, Wikström J, Holmdahl R, Pettersson U, Peltonen L: A putative vulnerability locus to multiple sclerosis maps to 5p14–p12 in region syntenic to the murine locus *Eae2*. Nat Genet 1996; 13:477–480.
Kurtzke JF: Epidemiology of multiple sclerosis. In: Hallpike JF, Adams CWM, Tourtelotte WW (eds). Multiple Sclerosis. Baltimore: Williams and Wilkins, 1983:47–96.
Larsen F, Oturai A, Ryder LOP, Madsen HO, Hillert J, Fredrikson S, Sandberg-Wollheim M, Laaksonen M, Harbo HF, Sawcer S, et al.: Linkage analysis of a candidate region in Scandinavian sib pairs with multiple sclerosis reveals linkage to chromosome 17q. Genes Immunol 2000; 1(7):456–459.
Liblau R, van Endert PM, Sandberg-Wollheim M, Patel SD, Lopez MT, Land S, Fugger L, McDevitt HO: Antigen processing gene polymorphisms in HLA-DR2 multiple sclerosis. Neurology 1993; 1192–1197.
Luomala M, Elovaara I, Koivula T, Lehtimäki T: Intercellular adhesion molecule-1 K/E 469 polymorphism and multiple sclerosis. Ann Neurol 1999; 45(4):546–547.
Lynch SG, Rose JW, Petajan JH, Leppert M: Discordance of T cell receptor β-chain genes in familial multiple sclerosis. Ann Neurol 1992; 42:839–844.
Lynch SG, Rose JW, Petajan JH, Stauffer D, Kamerath C, Leppert M: Discordance of T cell receptor β-chain genes in familial multiple sclerosis. Ann Neurol 1991; 30:402–410.
Marrosu MG, Muntoni F, Murru MR, Spinicci G, Pischedda MP, Goddi F, Cosso P, Pirastu M, et al.: Sardinian multiple sclerosis is associated with HLA-DR4. Neurology 1988; 38:1749–1752.
Martell M, Marcadet A, Strominger J, et al.: Le genes α du recepteur des cellules T: une possible implication dans la susceptibilite genetique a al scerose en plaques. C R Acad Sc Paris 304, Serie III 1987; 5:105–110.
Martin R, McFarland HF: Immunological aspects of experimental allergic encephalomyelitis and multiple sclerosis. Crit Rev Clin Lab Sci 1995; 32:121–182.
Martinez-Naves E, Victoria-Gutierrez M, Uria DF, Lopez-Larrea C: The germline repertoire of T cell receptor β-chain genes in multiple sclerosis patients from Spain. J Neuroimmunol 1993: 47:9–13.
Miller DH, Grossman RI, Reingold SC, McFarland HF: The role of magnatic resonance techniques in understanding and managing multiple sclerosis. Brain 1998; 121:3–24.
Miyamoto H, Walker JE, Ginsberg AH, Burks JS, McIntosh K, Kempe CH: Antibodies to vaccinia and measles virus in multiple sclerosis patients. Arch Neurol 1976; 33:414–418.
Moises HW, Yang L, Kristbjarnarson H, Wiese C, Byerley W, Macciardi F, Arolt V, Blackwood D, Liu X, Sjögren B, et al.: An international two-stage genome-wide search for schizophrenia susceptibility gene. Nat Genet 1995; 11:321–324.
Mumford CJ, Wood NW, Kellar-Wood H, Thorpe JW, Miller DH, Compston DA: The British Isles survey of multiple sclerosis in twins. Neurology 1994; 44:11–15.
Mycko MP, Kwinkowski M, Tronczynska E, Szymanska B, Selmaj KW: Multiple sclerosis: the increased frequency of the ICAM-1 exon 6 gene point mutation genetic type K469. Ann Neurol 1998; 44(1):70–75.
Nadeau JH, Davisson MT, Doolittle DP, Grant P, Hillyard AL, Kosowsky MR, Roderick TH: Comparative map for mice and humans. Mamm Genome 1992; 3:480–536.
Nagra RM, Becher B, Tourtellotte WW, Antel JP, Gold D, Paladino T, Smith RA, Nelson JR, Reynolds WF: Immunohistochemical and genetic evidence of myeloperoxidase involvement in multiple sclerosis. J Neuroimmunol 1997; 78:97–107.
Niino M, Fukuzawa T, Yabe I, Kikuchi S, Sasaki H, Tashiro K: Vitamin D receptor gene polymorphism in multiple sclerosis and the association with HLA class II alleles. J Neurol Sci 2000; 177(1):65–71.
Noseworthy J: MS clinical trials: old and new challenges. Semin Neurol 1998; 18:377–388.
Odum N, Hyldig-Nielsen JJ, Morling N, Sandberg-Wollheim M, Platz P, Svejgaard A: HLA-DP antigens are involved in the susceptibility to multiple sclerosis. Tissue Antigens 1988; 31:235–237.
Oksenberg JR, Sherritt M, Begovich AB, Erlich HA, Bernard CC, Cavalli-Sforza LL, Steinman L: T-cell receptor Vα and Cα alleles associated with multiple sclerosis and myasthenia gravis. Proc Natl Acad Sci USA 1989; 86:988–992.
Olerup O, Hillert J: HLA class II-associated genetic susceptibility in multiple sclerosis: a critical evaluation. Tissue Antigens 1991; 38:1–15.
Olerup O, Hillert J, Fredrikson S: The HLA-D region-associated MS-susceptibility genes may be located telomeric to the HLA-DP subregion. Tissue Antigens 1990; 36(1):37–39.
Oturai A, Larsen F, Ryder LP, Madsen HO, Hillert J, Fredrikson S, Sandberg-Wollheim M, Laaksonen M, Koch-Henriksen N, Sawcer S, et al.: Linkage and association analysis of susceptibility regions ion chromosomes 5 and 6 in 106 Scandinavian sibling pair families with multiple sclerosis. Ann Neurol 1999; 46(4):612–616.
Pandey JP, Goust J-M, Salier J-P, Fundenberg HH: Immunoglobulin G heavy chain (Gm) allotypes in multiple sclerosis. J Clin Invest 1981; 67:1797–1800.
Paty DW, Oger JJ, Kastrukoff LF, Hashimoto SA, Hooge JP, Eisen AA, Eisen KA, Purves SJ, Low MD, Brandeis V, Robertson WD, Li DKB: MRI in the diagnosis of MS: a prospective study with comparison of clinical evaluation, evoked potentials, olicoclonal banding, and CT. Neurology 1988; 38:180–185.
Poser CM, Paty DW, Scheinberg L: New diagnostic criteria for multiple sclerosis: guidelines for research protocols. Ann Neurol 1983; 13:227–231.
Poskanzer DC, Prenney LB, Sheridan JL, Yon Kondy J: Multiple sclerosis in the Orkney and Shetland Islands I: epidemiology, clinical factor, methodology. J Epidemiol Common Health 1980; 34:229–239.
Pribyl TM, Campagnoni CW, Kampf K, Kashima T, Handley VW, McMahon J, Campagnoni AT: The human myelin basic protein gene is included within a 179-kilobase transcription unit: expression in the immune and central nervous systems. Proc Natl Acad Sci USA 1993; 90(22):10695–10699.
Propert DN, Bernard CCA, Simons MJ: Gm allotypes and multiple sclerosis. J Immunogenet 1982; 9:359–361.
Raine CS, Wu E: Multiple sclerosis: remyelinatin in acute lesions. J Neuropathol Exp Neurol 1993; 52:199–204.
Ramachandran S, Bell RB: Heat shock protein 70 gene polymorphisms and multiple sclerosis. Tissue Antigens 1995; 46:140–141.
Risch N: Assessing the role of HLA-linked and unlinked determinants of disease. Am J Hum Genet 1987; 40(1):1–14.
Rosati G, Aiello I, Pirastu MI, Mannu L, Demontis G, Becciu S, Sau G, Zoccheddu A: Sardinia, a high-risk area for multiple sclerosis: a prevalence and incidence study in the district of Alghero. Ann Neurol 1987; 21:190–194.
Rose J, Gerken S, Lynch S, Pisani P, Varvil T, Otterud B, Leppert M: Genetic susceptibility in familial multiple sclerosis not linked to the myelin basic protein gene. Lancet 1993; 341:1179–1181.
Roth MP, Nogueira L, Coppin H, Clanet M, Clayton J, Cambon-Thomsen A: Tumor necrosis factor polymorphism in multiple sclerosis: no additional association independent of HLA. J Neuroimmunol 1994; 51:93–99.
Rubinsztein DC, Hanlon CS, Irving RM, Goodburn S, Evans DG, Kellar-Wood H, Xuereb JH, Bandmann O, Harding AE: ApoE genotypes in multiple sclerosis,

Parkinson's disease, schwannomas and late-onset Alzheimer's disease. Mol Cell Probes 1994; 8(6):519–525.

Sadovnick AD, Armstrong H, Rice GP, Bulman D, Hashimoto L, Paty DW, Hashimoto SA, Warren S, Hader W, Murray TJ, et al.: A population-based study of multiple sclerosis in twins: update. Ann Neurol 1993; 33:281–285.

Sadovnick AD, Baird PA, Ward RH: Multiple sclerosis: updated risks for relatives. Am J Med Genet 1988; 29:533–541.

Sadovnick A, Dyment D, Ebers G: Genetic epidemiology of multiple sclerosis. Epidemiol Rev 1997; 19:99–106.

Sadovnick AD, Ebers GC, Dyment DA, Risch NJ: Evidence for genetic basis of multiple sclerosis. Lancet 1996; 347:1728–1730.

Salmi A, Leinikki P, Panelius M: Vaccinia antibodies in cerebrospinal fluid of patients with multiple sclerosis. Z Neurol 1974; 206(4):345–348.

Salmi A, Reunanen M, Ilonen J, Panelius M: Intratechal antibody synthesis to virus antigens in multiple sclerosis. Clin Exp Immunol 1983; 52:241–249.

Sawcer S, Goodfellow PN, Compston A: The genetic analysis of multiple sclerosis. Trends Genet 1997; 13:234–239.

Sawcer S, Jones HB, Feakes R, Gray J, Smaldon N, Chataway J, Robertson N, Clayton D, Goodfellow PN, Compston A: A genome screen in multiple sclerosis reveals susceptibility loci on chromosome 6p21 and 17q22. Nat Genet 1996; 13:444–468.

Schrijver HM, Crusius JBA, Uitdehaag BMJ, González G, Kostense PJ, Polman CH, Peña AS: Association of interleukin-1β and interleukin-1 receptor antagonist genes with disease severity in MS. Neurology 1999; 52(3):595–598.

Seboun E, Robinson MA, Doolittle TH, Ciulla TA, Kindt TJ, Hauser SL: A susceptibility locus for multiple sclerosis is linked to the T cell receptor β chain complex. Cell 1989; 57:1095–1100.

Semana G, Yaouanq J, Alizadeh M, Clanet M, Edan G: Interleukin-1 receptor antagonist gene in multiple sclerosis. Lancet 1997; 349:476.

Sherritt MA, Oksenberg J, de Rosbo NK, Bernard CC: Influence of HLA-DR2, HLA-DPw4, and T cell receptor α chain genes on the susceptibility to multiple sclerosis. Int Immunol 1992; 4:177–181.

Sibley WA, Bamford, CR, Clark K: Clinical viral infections and multiple sclerosis. Lancet 1985; 1:1313–1315.

Soelberg-Sorensen PS, Wanscher B, Jensen CV, Schreiber K, Blinkenberg M, Ravnborg M, Kirsmeier H, Larsen VA, Lee ML: Intravenous immunoglobulin G reduces MRI activity in relapsing multiple sclerosis. Neurology 1998; 50:1273–1281.

Soldan S, et al.: Association of human herpes virus 6 (HHV-6) with multiple sclerosis: increased IgM response to HHV-6 early antigen and detection of serum HHV-6 DNA. Nat Med 1997; 3:1394–1397.

Spurkland A, Knutsen I, Undlien DE, Vartdal F: No association of multiple sclerosis to alleles at the TAP2 locus. Hum Immunol 1994; 39:299–301.

Steckley JL, Dyment DA, Sadovnick AD, Risch N, Hayes C, Ebers GC: Genetic analysis of vitamin D related genes in Canadian multiple sclerosis patients. Neurology 2000; 54(3):729–732.

Steinman L: Multiple sclerosis: a coordinated immunological attack against myelin in the central nervous system. Cell 1996; 85:299–302.

Steinman L, Oldstone MB: More mayhem from molecular mimics. Nat Med 1997; 3(12):1321–1322.

Suarez BK, Hampe CL, Van-Eerdewegh P: In: Gershon ES, Cloninger CR (eds). Genetic Approaches to Mental Disorders. Washington DC: American Psychiatric Press, 1994:000–000.

Sundvall M, Jirholt J, Yang H-T, Jansson L, Engström Å, Pettersson U, Holmdahl R: Identification of murine loci associated with susceptibility to chronic experimental autoimmune encephalomyelitis. Nat Genet 1995; 10:313–317.

Terwilliger JD, Ott J: Handbook of Human Genetic Linkage. Baltimore and London: Johns Hopkins University Press, 1994.

Tienari PJ, Kuokkanen S, Pastinen T, Wikström J, Sajantila A, Sandberg-Wollheim M, Palo J, Peltonen L: Golli-*MBP* gene in multiple sclerosis susceptibility. J Neuroimmunol 1998; 81:158–167.

Tienari PJ, Wikström J, Koskimies S, Partanen J, Palo J, Peltonen L: Reappraisal of HLA in multiple sclerosis: close linkage in multiplex families. Eur J Hum Genet 1993; 1:257–268.

Tienari PJ, Wikström J, Sajantila A, Palo J, Peltonen L: Genetic susceptibility to multiple sclerosis linked to myelin basic protein gene. Lancet 1992; 340:987–991.

Transatlantic Multiple Sclerosis Genetics Cooperative: A meta-analysis of genomic screens in multiple sclerosis. Mult Scler 2001; 7(1):3–11.

Trapp BD, Peterson J, Ransohoff RM, Rudick R, Mörk S, Bö L: Axonal transection in the lesions of multiple sclerosis. N Engl J Med 1998; 29:278–285.

Traugott U, Raine CS, McFarlin DE: Acute experimental allergic encephalomyelitis in the mouse: immunopathology of the developing lesion. Cell Immunol 1985; 91(1):240–254.

Vandenbroeck K, Martino G, Marrosu M, Consiglio A, Zaffaroni M, Vaccargiu S, Franciotta D, Ruggeri M, Comi G, Grimaldi L: Occurrence and clinical relevance of an interleukin-4 gene polymorphism in patients with multiple sclerosis. J Neuroimmunol 1997; 76:189–192.

Vandenbroeck K, Opdenakker G, Goris A, Murru R, Billiau A, Marrosu MG: Interferon-γ gene polymorphism: associated risk for multiple sclerosis in Sardinia. Ann Neurol 1998; 44:841–842.

Vandenbroeck C, Buyse I, Philippaerts L, Ghabanbasani Z, Medaer R, Carton H, Cassiman JJ, Raus J: HLA and T-cell receptor polymorphisms in Belgian multiple sclerosis patients: no evidence for disease association with the T-cell receptor. J Neuroimmunol 1994a; 52:25–32.

Vandenbroeck C, Stinissen P, Cassiman JJ, Raus J: Myelin basic protein gene polymorphism is not associated with chronic progressive multiple sclerosis. J Neuroimmunol 1994b; 52:97–99.

Vandenbroeck C, Stinissen P, Cassiman JJ, Raus J: *TAP 1* and *TAP 2* transporter gene polymorphisms in multiple sclerosis: no evidence for disease association with TAP. J Neuroimmunol 1994c; 54:35–40.

van Noort J, van Sechel AC, van Stipdonk MJB, Bajramovic JJ: The small heat-shock protein $\alpha\beta$-crystallin as candidate autoantigen in multiple sclerosis. Nature 1995; 375:798–801.

Vyse TJ, Todd JA: Genetic analysis of autoimmune disease. Cell 1996; 85:311–318.

Walter MA, Gibson WT, Ebers GC, Cox DW: Susceptibility to multiple sclerosis is associated with the proximal immunoglobulin heavy chain variable region. J Clin Invest 1991; 87:1266–1273.

Wansen K, Pastinen T, Kuokkanen S, Wilstöm J, Palo J, Peltonen L, Tienari PJ: Immune system genes in multiple sclerosis: genetic association and linkage analyses on TCR-β, IGH, INF-γ and IL-1ra/IL-1β. J Neuroimmunol 1997; 79:29–36.

Wei S, Charmley P, Birchfield RI, Concannon P: Human T-cell receptor Vβ gene polymorphism and multiple sclerosis. Am J Hum Genet 1995; 56:963–969.

Williams NM, Rees MI, Holmans P, Norton N, Cardno AG, Jones LA, Murphy KC, Sanders RD, McCarthy G, Gray MY, et al.: A two-stage genome scan for schizophrenia susceptibility genes in 196 affected sibling pairs. Hum Mol Genet 1999; 8(9):1729–1739.

Wingerchuk D, Liu Q, Sobell J, Sommer S, Weinshenker BG: A population-based case-control study of the tumor necrosis factor α-308 polymorphism in multiple sclerosis. Neurology 1997; 49(2):626–628.

Wood NW, Holmans P, Clayton D, Robertson N, Compston DA: No linkage or association between multiple sclerosis and the myelin basic protein gene in affected sibling pairs. J Neurol Neurosurg Psychiatry 1994; 57:1191–1194.

Wood NW, Sawcer SJ, Kellar-Wood HF, Holmans P, Clayton D, Robertson N, Compston DA: Susceptibility to multiple sclerosis and the immnoglobulin heavy chain variable region. J Neurol 1995a; 242:677–682.

Wood NW, Sawcer SJ, Kellar-Wood HF, Holmans P, Clayton D, Robertson N, Compston DA: The T-cell receptor β locus and susceptibility to multiple sclerosis. Neurology 1995b; 45(10):1859–1863.

Wordsworth P: Genes and arthritis. Br Med Bull 1995; 51:249–266.

Yu JS, Pandey JP, Massacesi L, Lincoln R, Usuku K, Seboun E, Hauser SL: Segregation of immunoglobulin heavy chain constant region genes in multiple sclerosis sibling pairs. J Neuroimmunol 1993; 8:579–621.

Zamvil SS, Mitchell DJ, Moore AC, Kitamura K, Steinman L, Rothbard JB: T-cell epitope of the autoantigen myelin basic protein that induces encephalomyelitis. Nature 1986; 324(6094):258–260.

Zamvil SS, Steinman L: The T cell in experimental allergic encephalomyelitis. Annu Rev Immunol 1990; 8:579–621.

43 Alzheimer's Disease

MARGARET A. PERICAK-VANCE AND JONATHAN L. HAINES

Alzheimer's disease (AD) is characterized clinically by an insidious, progressive loss of memory, higher intellectual function, and cognitive abilities. It is the leading cause of dementia in the elderly and the most common form of dementia occurring after the age of 40. There are over four million affected individuals in the United States (Max, 1993), a number estimated to increase to 10 million in the next decade. Thus, not only is AD currently a common disease, it will become an increasing burden as the U.S. and world populations continue to age. Tremendous progress has been made in understanding the etiology of AD, particularly in dissecting the genetics of AD, over the past decade. Nonetheless, the causes of AD are only now beginning to be understood. The vast literature on the disease clearly demonstrates that it has a very complex etiologic architecture with strong genetic and environmental determinants.

DEFINITION OF ALZHEIMER'S DISEASE

Clinical Presentation and Diagnosis

The clinical diagnosis of AD is one of exclusion. Clinically, it is described as slowly progressive memory loss with alteration of higher intellectual function and cognitive abilities (Khachaturian, 1985; Growden, 1995). A confirmed diagnosis requires neuropathologic examination of brain tissue and thus can be obtained only after the patient is deceased. However, clinical diagnosis done according to standardized criteria (McKhann et al., 1984) is accurate in 85% to 90% of cases diagnosed at a tertiary care facility (Growden, 1995; Rasmusson et al., 1996; Welsh-Bohmer et al., 1997).

The clinical diagnosis of AD requires both physical and neuropsychologic examinations. A typical neurologic exam will detect the presence of gross sensory and motor disturbances that are generally not considered part of the AD phenotype, suggesting an alternate diagnosis and exclusion of AD. However, moderate disturbances, particularly those similar to Parkinson's disease (tremor, rigidity, bradykinesia), have been described in pathologically confirmed AD and, thus, do not rule out the diagnosis (Molsa et al., 1984; Mayeux et al., 1985; Chen et al., 1991). Cognitive impairment is detected through a series of neuropsychological tests, such as the Mini-Mental State Exam (Folstein et al., 1975) or the Modified Mini-Mental State Exam (Teng and Chui, 1987). These tests measure visuospatial abilities, praxis, language, and memory. Of particular importance in detecting early AD are tests of delayed recall (Knopman and Ryberg, 1989; Welsh et al., 1992).

One of the major milestones in AD research was the development of standardized criteria (the National Institute of Neurological and Communicative Disorders and Stroke-Alzheimer's Disease and Related Disorders Association (NINCDS-ADRDA) criteria) for categorizing patients (McKhann et al., 1984). These criteria divide patients into probable, possible, and definite AD. A diagnosis of *probable* AD requires that dementia be documented by clinical examination, deficits in two or more areas of cognition, progression of symptoms, no disturbance of consciousness, and absence of other acute causes, such as medication use or other inherited diseases. A diagnosis of *definite* AD requires pathologic confirmation with the finding of amyloid plaques, neurofibrillary tangles, neuronal and synaptic loss, and brain atrophy. A diagnosis of *possible* AD is given when the presentation is unusual (rapid onset, absence of a second affected area of cognition) or when another possible cause is present (e.g., another brain disorder such as stroke) but not considered to be the primary cause of the dementia.

Subtypes

The most common stratification of AD is by age at onset. Most cases occur after age 65, with fewer than 5% occurring before that age (Schoenberg, 1987; Rocca et al., 1991). Most autosomal dominantly inherited forms occur before age 60 (St George-Hyslop et al., 1990; Sherrington et al., 1995), while most sporadic cases and cases in smaller family aggregates occur after age 65 (Pericak-Vance et al., 1988). Since the distribution of age at onset is continuous, there is no obvious age at which to separate the two groups. The usual convention is to divide cases into either early- or late-onset forms using age 60 or 65 as a demarcation point.

Another aspect of AD that has been used to identify subtypes is the neuropathologic data. While most clinically diagnosed cases have only the typical pathology, several other variations have been seen. In particular, Lewy bodies in both the substantia nigra (characteristic of Parkinson's disease) and elsewhere have been observed in up to 20% of cases (Ditter and Mirra, 1987; Growden, 1995; McKeith et al., 1996). A growing body of literature suggests substantial overlap between AD, dementia with Lewy bodies, and Parkinson's disease. While some researchers consider the Lewy body variant of AD, AD with Parkinson's disease, and dementia with Lewy bodies to be separate entities, this nosology remains controversial (Perry et al., 1997; Ala et al., 1997; Brown et al., 1998; Dickson, 2001).

GENERAL GENETIC AND EPIDEMIOLOGIC EVIDENCE

Clinical Epidemiology

Many epidemiologic studies have measured the incidence and prevalence of AD. Both incidence and prevalence are age-dependent, increasing dramatically after age 60. Incidence rates for AD increase from about 0.1% in the 60 to 69 age group to approximately 2% after age 80 (Schoenberg, 1987; Newens et al., 1993; Bickel and Cooper, 1994). Prevalence rates also increase from approximately 0.3%–0.5% to 11%–15% in the respective age groups (Rocca et al., 1991; Bachman et al., 1992; Prencipe et al., 1996). There is substantial variability in these rates, however, since rates as high as 47% have been reported after age 84 (Evans et al., 1989; Polvikoski et al., 2001).

Surprisingly little has been written about the incidence and prevalence of AD in different ethnic groups. Most studies have been performed on Caucasians of northern or western European background (Schoenberg, 1987) or southern European background (Evans et al., 1989). A study including African-American patients suggested a prevalence similar to that in Caucasians (Schoenberg et al., 1981). However, incidence rates were lower in an African community compared to an African-American community (Hendrie et al., 1995, 2001). A study of a Japanese cohort gave an overall prevalence of dementia of 7% after age 65, with a prevalence of over 30% by age 90 (Ogura et al., 1995). Another study suggested that mild cognitive impairment typical of early-stage AD was higher in Caucasians than in African Americans, with Hispanics intermediate (Molgaard et al., 1990). Two studies have suggested localized geographic increases in the prevalence of AD, with some small areas of Newfoundland and of Scotland having substantially higher prevalence rates than surrounding areas (Frecker, 1991; Whalley et al., 1995). Conversely, studies of an Amish community in the midwestern United States have suggested a substantially lower prevalence of dementia (Johnson et al., 1997).

Genetic Epidemiology

Clues to the underlying genetic architecture of AD come from a number of different studies. These studies include differences in AD prevalence rates in different populations, familial aggregation and studies of risks to specific types of relative, twin studies, and segregation analyses, as described below. Taken together there are compelling data indicating that a substantial proportion of the total susceptibility to AD is inherited.

Family Studies

Familial aggregation of AD has been noted for a long time (Sjogren et al., 1952; Heyman et al., 1983; Nee et al., 1983). The simplest, but most misleading, way of estimating the genetic component in AD is simply to review all of the published pedigrees. Such a literature review in 1989 led to the obvious conclusion that AD was inherited in most cases as an autosomal dominant trait, with onset typically in the 40s to 60s (St George-Hyslop et al., 1989). While autosomal dominant inheritance is often true for early-onset families, the sample was highly biased since only the most atypical pedigrees are likely to be published and smaller pedigrees without an obvious inheritance pattern will not generally be published. Smaller pedigrees are more typical of late-onset AD. Specific studies of late-onset AD have noted familial aggregation in the much more common form (Pericak-Vance et al., 1988) and suggest a more complex genetic etiology.

Early studies reported elevated risks to first-degree relatives (generally parents, sibs, and children all lumped together) varying between approximately 4% and 14% (St George-Hyslop et al., 1989). Numerous methodologic problems, however, make these numbers dubious. Because this is a late-onset disorder, parental information is most likely obtained only through a family informant and, more rarely, from medical records. Direct examination is almost always impossible. In addition, diagnostic procedures and accuracy have changed substantially over the past 30 years, making it hard to interpret a solitary notation of "dementia" or AD in a medical record. While the data for siblings are better, younger siblings may not have moved through the risk period and older siblings may be lost to direct examination. Children have rarely entered the risk period for AD.

More recent studies have taken into account the specific family relationship, quality of the reported data, and the age dependence of the disease. Estimates for first-degree relatives still vary greatly but are substantially higher, with several studies suggesting rates as high as 50% compared to approximately 10% in the relatives of controls (Mohs et al., 1987; Breitner et al., 1988b; Huff et al., 1988; Mayeux et al., 1991). Another study suggested a rate of 24% compared to 16% in controls (Farrer et al., 1989).

Comparison of the recurrence rates in the relatives of AD patients to the general population prevalence (Risch, 1990a–c) generates a recurrence risk ratio (λ) that can be calculated for different degrees of relationship. As siblings are most readily available for study, the sibling recurrence risk ratio (λ_S) is most often reported. Estimates of λ_s calculated from various studies are surprisingly constant for AD (Breitner et al., 1988a; Sadovnick et al., 1989; Hirst et al., 1994) and range from 4 to 5. While this is substantially less than the λ_s for a Mendelian dominant disorder such as Huntington's disease ($\lambda_s = 5000$) or a recessive disorder such as cystic fibrosis ($\lambda_s = 500$), it is well within the range necessary for gene mapping (see below).

Twin Studies

Another method for identifying and quantifying the genetic component in AD is to examine the concordance rates in twins. If genes are involved in AD, the concordance rates should be higher in monozygotic (MZ) twins, who share all of their germline genes, than in dizygotic (DZ) twins, who share on average half of their genes. As with family studies, the late age at onset of AD makes twin studies difficult. Given the wide range of age at onset, a cross-sectional study will substantially underestimate concordance, particularly for MZ twins. Another limitation specific to twin studies in AD is small sample size. The largest of the twin studies to date was done in 1956 where 108 (54 MZ, 54 DZ) twins were examined. In more recent studies, sample sizes have been smaller, ranging from 10 to 40. Despite these limitations, concordance rates are generally higher in MZ twins (22%–83%) than in DZ twins (0%–50%) (Breitner et al., 1993, 1995; Bergen, 1994, 1997; Steffens et al., 2000). The overall concordance in the six studies surveyed by Bergen et al. (1994) was 0.49 for MZ twins and 0.18 for DZ twins. The fact that the MZ risk is elevated suggests a genetic component, but the fact that it is not near 100% suggests that other factors, including environmental factors, may also be important.

Segregation Analysis

Segregation analysis is a statistical method to determine the existence and mode of inheritance of a disease gene. By its very nature, segregation analysis, which attempts to estimate many different parameters, requires very large data sets to be accurate. To be representative of the general population, families must be collected (or ascertained) in a known and very rigorous fashion. In addition, the analysis requires intricate statistical calculations, which are very laborious.

Numerous segregation analyses have been performed in AD, and virtually all point toward at least one autosomal dominant gene, reduced penetrance, and a probable multifactorial (polygenic and environmental) component (Farrer et al., 1991; van Duijn et al., 1993; Rao et al., 1994). Models postulating only sporadic AD, no major genes, or only Mendelian inheritance have been rejected (Rao et al., 1996). When the families are divided into early- and late-onset subgroups, the results are somewhat clearer. Early-onset families clearly demonstrate autosomal dominant inheritance (confirmed as discussed below), while late-onset families show a more complicated inheritance, most likely a combination of genes with various modes of inheritance and nongenetic factors (Rao et al., 1994). In addition, it is likely that the mode of action of the susceptibility genes differs by sex (Rao et al., 1996) and by apolipoprotein E (*APOE*) genotype (Rao et al., 1996; Jarvik et al., 1996).

Taken together, these data overwhelmingly support a strong yet very complex genetic component to AD. Embedded in this complexity are several Mendelian genes that account for only a small proportion of disease and other genes that confer substantial susceptibility to a large proportion of the population.

Associations with Other Diseases

Clinically, AD can be very hard to distinguish from other dementias such as dementia with Lewy bodies, Pick's disease, frontal lobe degeneration, parkinsonism with dementia, vascular dementia, and hypothyroidism and vitamin B_{12} deficiency (Roses and Pericak-Vance, 1997). A confirmed diagnosis of AD requires neuropathologic examination and can then be differentiated from the other dementias. While amyloid plaques and neurofibrillary tangles can be observed in other diseases and in normal aging, the number and location of the plaques and tangles are different (Khachaturian, 1985).

Several families with apparent autosomal dominant inheritance of a specific frontotemporal dementia with parkinsonism (pallidoponto nigral-degeneration) have been described (Wijker et al., 1996; Lendon et al., 1998). One gene for this dementia was localized to chromosome 17q, in the vicinity of the neurofibromatosis type 1 gene (Wijker et al., 1996). In 1998, mutations in the gene that encodes the tau protein were described in several of these families (Clark et al., 1998), leading them to be considered tau-opathies.

AD has been strongly associated with Down syndrome (DS). Virtually all persons with DS who survive to their 30s and 40s exhibit the classical AD neuropathology (Burger and Vogel, 1973; Ellis et al., 1974; Ball and Nuttall, 1980; Wisniewski et al., 1985). However, given the extent of mental retardation in DS, it is difficult to determine with certainty that all adult DS patients exhibit clinical dementia. Several reports have suggested that the risk of developing AD is increased (two- to threefold) if there is a first-degree relative with DS (Heston et al., 1981; Heyman et al., 1984; Broe et al., 1990; van Duijn et al., 1991). This risk appears to be most prominent (fivefold) in mothers who had DS children before the age of 35 (Schupf et al., 1994).

Environmental Factors

While many putative risk factors for AD have been reported in the literature, only advanced age and family history have been consistently reported across studies (van Duijn et al., 1991; Macera et al., 1994). More typically, risk factors have been inconsistently supported. For example, early studies with small (<350) numbers of cases and controls provided conflicting evidence on whether history of head trauma increased the risk of AD. Over time, the association was more consistently detected in studies with larger sample sizes (van Duijn et al., 1991; Mayeux et al., 1993; Rasmusson et al., 1995; Plassman et al., 2000). Mayeux et al. (1995) suggested that history of head trauma interacts with the presence of the *APOE-4* allele (see below) to significantly increase the risk of AD over the risk due to either risk factor alone. However, another study suggested that lack of the *APOE-4* allele was associated with a higher risk of AD after head trauma (Guo et al., 2000).

Other risk factors with less consistent association with increased risk of AD include lower formal education (Canadian Study of Health and Aging, 1994; Macera et al., 1994; Stern et al., 1994), low linguistic ability early in life (Snowdon et al., 1996), history of depression or depressed mood (van Duijn et al., 1994a; Speck et al., 1995) manual labor occupations (Fratiglioni et al., 1993), and exposure to heavy metals, solvents, and pesticides (Canadian Study of Health and Aging, 1994; Savory et al., 1996). As well, potential protective effects of nonsteroidal anti-inflammatory drugs (NSAIDS) (Andersen et al., 1995; Breitner et al., 1995; Anthony et al., 2000) and postmenopausal estrogen replacement therapy (Brenner et al., 1994; Paganini-Hill and Henderson, 1994; Slooter et al., 1999) have been reported. A protective effect of smoking (Lee, 1994; van Duijn et al., 1995b) has been reported, but this is controversial since other studies have shown an increased risk (Ott et al., 1998; Merchant et al., 1999; Guo et al., 2000). The wide variability in associations between risk factors and AD across studies may reflect population differences in exposure, susceptibility, or both.

PATHOPHYSIOLOGY: BIOLOGIC BASIS OF GENETIC SUSCEPTIBILITY

Pathologic Definition

Pathologically, AD is characterized by neurofibrillary tangles found in the neurons of the cerebral cortex and hippocampus and deposition of amyloid within senile plaques and cerebral blood vessels (Wisniewski et al., 1993). As discussed above, a confirmed diagnosis of AD requires pathologic examination of brain tissue and, thus, can be made only after the patient is deceased. A pathologic diagnosis requires finding numerous senile plaques in the extracellular parenchyma and numerous neurofibrillary tangles in neurons. An example of plaques and tangles is shown in Figure 43–1. The primary locations for the plaques and tangles are in the cerebral cortex and the hippocampus.

There are several different sets of neuropathologic diagnostic criteria published in the literature (Khachaturian, 1985; Tierney et al., 1988; Mirra et al., 1991; Braak and Braak, 1991). The two most commonly used are the criteria published by Khachaturian (1985) and by the Consortium to Establish a Registry for Alzheimer Disease (Mirra et al., 1991). The former requires examination of three neocortical regions, and an increasing number of senile or neuritic plaques (from 2 to 15) based on the age of the patient (<50 to >75). Neurofibrillary tangles must be seen in all but the oldest age group but are not quantified. The latter uses a semiquantitative scale (sparse, moderate, or frequent) for senile plaques, with the occurrence of even sparse numbers of plaques indicating a definite diagnosis for all but the oldest patients. Such a diagnosis also requires clinical evidence of dementia. Neurofibrillary tangles are not required for diagnosis.

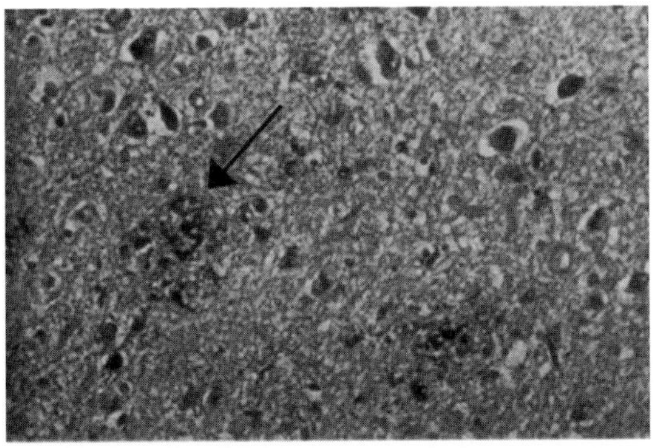

A

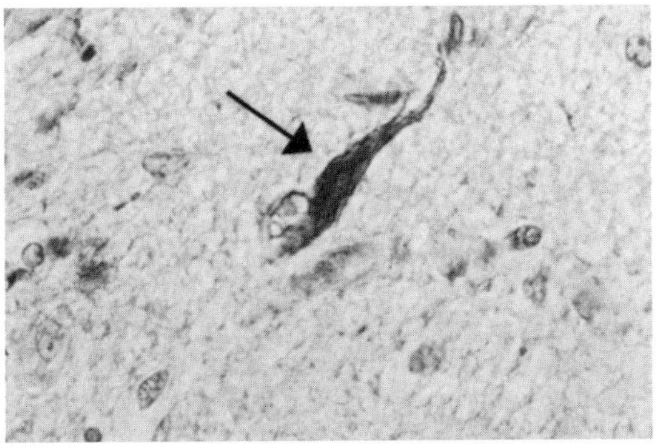

B

Fig. 43–1. Examples of senile plaques (*A*) and neurofibrillary tangles (*B*). Photo courtesy of T. Montine.

Pathophysiologic Studies

Numerous studies have been done to identify the components of the plaques and tangles characteristic of AD. Plaques consist of a central core of an amyloid protein (Mann, 1994). This protein (often referred to as β-amyloid or Aβ) is a fragment of the full protein encoded by the amyloid precursor protein (*APP*) gene on chromosome 21 (Tanzi et al., 1987a; Goldgaber et al., 1987). The gene and its role in the genetics of AD are discussed below. The central core also contains other proteins including APOE (Namba et al., 1991; Strittmatter et al., 1993), various complement factors (Eikelenboom and Stam, 1984), α_1-antichymotrypsin (Abraham et al., 1988), amyloid P (Kalaria et al., 1991), and heparan sulfate proteoglycan (Snow et al., 1990). Other cellular debris from both neurons and glial cells, along with additional Aβ, surrounds the central core (Mann, 1994). Neurofibrillary tangles are composed mainly of paired helical filaments, with a substantial component of tau protein, an interesting observation given the finding that tau mutations cause frontotemporal dementia (Clark et al., 1998).

GENE IDENTIFICATION

Almost since the first suggestions of a genetic component in AD, studies have been conducted to identify the genes involved. The two basic approaches are candidate gene studies and linkage analysis studies. In the 1960s and 1970s, a few candidate genes were examined in case-control studies, and some chromosomal regions were tested using the new methods of statistical linkage analysis. The human leukocyte antigen (HLA) region on chromosome 6 was initially rejected as a potential locus for AD (Goudsmit et al., 1981); it was later thought to possibly play some role (Weitkamp et al., 1983), but this was not confirmed in additional families (Clemenceau et al., 1986; Muller et al., 1986). One of the first studies to look at genetic linkage to a number of markers (Spence et al., 1986) found no linkage to 27 known red blood cell and serum protein polymorphisms. These early studies found no significant results but were hampered by looking at only a very small proportion ($<$5%) of the entire genome. In 1983, a lod score of 1.37 was found in one large family with immunoglobulin (*GM*) allotypes on chromosome 14 (Weitkamp et al., 1983), but this marker maps quite far away from the presenilin I (*PS1*) gene, mutations in which are now known to cause AD in this family (Sherrington et al., 1995).

With the advent of restriction fragment length polymorphisms (RFLPs) (Botstein et al., 1980) and microsatellite markers (Weber and May, 1989), the entire genome was opened for examination through linkage analysis. Thus, searching for a gene could now use a genomic screening approach. In addition, with the completion of the draft human genome sequence, virtually all genes have been identified and at least partially described (Venter et al., 2001; Lander et al., 2001), thus allowing many more candidate genes to be tested.

Methods for Testing Candidate Genes

Genes can become candidates for AD in two ways. Functional candidate genes are defined by what is known of the biology of the gene and of AD. Thus, any gene that affects (or, more commonly, could be hypothesized to affect) that biology becomes a candidate. Since AD is a central nervous system disease where the cerebral cortex and the hippocampus are affected, genes that are expressed in neurons are candidates for analysis. The strength and weakness of this approach arise from the confidence placed on the role these genes play. If the evidence is strong that a direct role is played, only one or a few such genes may need to be tested to find a true susceptibility gene. If the evidence is more circumstantial, then many genes may have an equal chance of being involved, and not much has been gained over a random genomic screen.

Locational candidate genes are defined simply by residing in a chromosomal region that is interesting for other reasons, not because of any known function the gene might have. Chromosomal regions may be of interest because an initial genomic screen has defined several "interesting" regions or a chromosomal abnormality (e.g., a duplication, deletion, or translocation) has been observed in one or more patients.

At the population level, there are several ways to test candidate genes for an effect in AD. The first, and most common, is the case-control design. This has the advantage of being able to use many, if not most, of the patients coming through the clinic. In the simplest formulation, the allele frequencies for a polymorphism within the gene are compared between the case and control groups. However, the case-control design is very sensitive to sample size, stringency of diagnosis, and particularly, appropriate matching of the control group. In addition, the case-control design cannot distinguish between a true genetic effect (either linkage disequilibrium or biologic interaction) and a marker of population admixture that is biologically irrelevant to AD.

The second approach for testing candidate genes is to use genetic linkage analysis for polymorphisms within or very near the gene in question. If significant evidence of linkage is found (using any one of several different linkage methods), then a role for that gene is supported, though not proven since the linkage could represent the effect of nearby genes. This approach has the advantage of not requiring a control group. However, it requires families with multiple affected individuals, and these can be difficult to find.

The third approach for testing candidate genes is to apply the new family-based association study designs. This combines the advantages of the case-control design (only one affected per family) with the family approach, using genetically well-matched controls (either the parents or siblings of the patient or both). This exciting approach is described in more detail below.

Candidate gene approaches have been the most widely applied to AD primarily because genomic screening is a very recent technology. Unfortunately, with the exception of the *APOE* gene, candidate gene studies have been largely unsuccessful, as described below.

Methods for Genomic Screening

The alternative to trying to understand the biology of AD before knowing the genes is to try to know the genes before understanding the biology. This can be accomplished by testing families with multiple cases of AD for linkage to polymorphic markers spread throughout the genome. The type of family to be tested varies from study to study, but the most commonly tested family type is the affected sib pair. This is the most common constellation of affected individuals in a family. Given the generally late age at onset of AD, it is often difficult to find living parents or to trace the family history to other living affected relatives, such as affected aunts, uncles, or cousins.

A good random genomic screen will cover the entire human genome using markers evenly spaced across a given genetic map. The most common spacing of markers is 10 cM, resulting in screens using between 300 and 400 markers. It does not require any knowledge of the function of any genes or even of the biology of AD. The goal in an initial genomic screen is to quickly scan through the genome and identify those regions most likely to harbor AD genes. This approach is purposely liberal in that many regions will yield false-positive results, but this allows high power in that regions that do harbor AD genes are far less likely to be missed. To eliminate the false-positive results, a second data set is usually tested only for those regions that were identified in the first data set. Once confirmed, the region is further dissected to identify candidate genes for specific study.

Known Genes in Alzheimer's Disease

As described above, early linkage analyses identifed a few mildly positive lod scores but with inconsistent results across families (Weitkamp et al., 1983; Clemenceau et al., 1986). In the past 10 years, the powerful tools of genetic analysis have been refined and have allowed the definition of approximately half of the genetic etiology of AD.

Early-Onset Alzheimer's Disease

Three of the four known AD genes [*APP* (Goate et al., 1991) and *PS1* and *PS2* (Levy-Lahad et al., 1995; Rogaev et al., 1995; Sherrington et al., 1995)] were identified using standard positional cloning methods. These initial studies used genetic linkage analysis to identify the probable location of AD genes and were greatly facilitated by well-defined autosomal dominant inheritance in families with early-onset AD.

The first of the genes in which AD-causing mutations were identified was *APP*. The gene was initially cloned in 1987 and soon localized to chromosome 21 (Goldgaber et al., 1987; Tanzi et al., 1987b). This localization was exciting because of the dual observation that DS patients almost universally develop AD and that some families with AD also have an increased rate of DS. Although a number of families initially showed linkage to chromosome 21 (St George-Hyslop et al., 1987), numerous families did not (Pericak-Vance et al., 1988; Schellenberg et al., 1987) or demonstrated recombinants with the *APP* gene (Tanzi et al., 1987b). Strong evidence for genetic heterogeneity was shown soon thereafter, suggesting that only a small subset of families actually segregated a chromosome 21 AD gene (St George-Hyslop et al., 1990). In 1991, a few families with linkage to chromosome 21 and no recombinants with *APP* were shown to have mutations in this gene (Goate et al., 1991). To date, only about 25 families carrying *APP* mutations have been described. Thus, *APP* represents a very small proportion of the overall genetic burden in AD (Table 43–1). In general, onset in these families is in the fifth decade.

Additional studies to identify the AD genes in the remaining large autosomal dominant families resulted in the finding of linkage to chromosome 14 (Schellenberg et al., 1992; St George-Hyslop et al., 1992; Van Broeckhoven et al., 1992). Mutations in the responsible *PS1* gene were identified (Sherrington et al., 1995). *PS1* was then a novel gene of unknown function. It is a transmembrane domain gene with sequence homology to the *Caenorhabditis elegans* gene *sel-12*, which facilitates signaling mechanisms in intercellular receptors. Mutations in *PS1* have been found in the majority of early-onset families. In addition, most mutations in *PS1* are unique to the family in which it is described. In general, onset in these families is in the fourth decade.

Table 43–1. Known Alzheimer's Disease Risk Loci

Chromosome	Gene	Onset Range	Proportion of Cases (%)	Inheritance	Comments
21	Amyloid precursor protein (*APP*)	40s–50s	<<1	Autosomal dominant	~25 families worldwide
1	Presenilin II (*PS2*)	40s–80s	<<1	Autosomal dominant	Mainly Volga German ancestry
14	Presenilin I (*PS1*)	30s–40s	<2	Autosomal dominant	Responsible for most early-onset families
19	Apolipoprotein E (*APOE*)	60s–90s	30–45	Susceptibility locus	Dose effect on risk and age of onset
12	?	60s–90s	<20	Susceptibility locus	
10q	?	60s–90s	?	Susceptibility locus	
9p	?	60s–90s	?	Susceptibility locus	

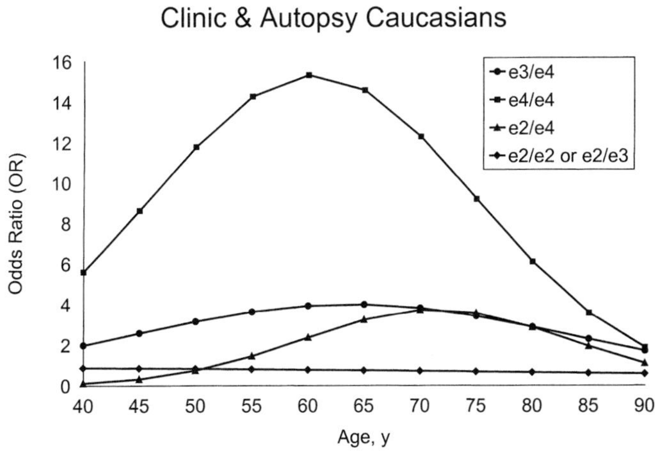

Fig. 43–2. Risk of Alzheimer's disease (*AD*) for Caucasians by age and *APOE* genotype. From Farrer et al. (1997) with permission. © 1997 American Medical Association.

A few families did not segregate either *APP* or *PS1* mutations and did not link to either chromosome 21 or 14. One such group can trace their origin to two villages in the Volga River basin of Russia, to which they migrated from Germany (Bird et al., 1988). Simultaneously with the cloning of the *PS1* gene in early-onset families, these families were shown to have genetic linkage to chromosome 1 (Levy-Lahad et al., 1995). In the cloning of the *PS1* gene, a larger, 7.5 kb, alternative polyadenylation message was also identified and found to represent another gene homologous to *PS1*. This gene mapped to chromosome 1 in the same region as the putative linkage and was quickly identified as *PS2*. Mutations in *PS2* have been described in the Volga German families and in an Italian pedigree (Levy-Lahad et al., 1995; Rogaev et al., 1995). Onset in these families is variable, ranging from the fourth to the eighth decades.

These three genes account for the majority of early-onset familial AD, but collectively they account for fewer than 2% of all AD cases (Table 43–1). While their identification represents a tremendous accomplishment and has provided new substrates for understanding the pathophysiologic process underlying AD, they represent a minor proportion of the total genetic etiology of AD.

Late-Onset Alzheimer's Disease

APOE. The vast majority of AD patients develop symptoms after age 60. However, large families with living affected individuals and late-onset AD are nearly impossible to find, in part because they are not ascertained until after most family members are deceased. Specific genetic studies in late-onset families have been done only in the past decade. The first evidence of a genetic linkage to chromosome 19q13 was published in 1991 (Pericak-Vance et al., 1991). In 1992, one of the components of the senile plaques was identified as apolipoprotein E (apo E), a plasma lipoprotein involved in lipid transport and metabolism, which also maps to 19q13. Thus, *APOE* became a candidate gene for AD by the congruence of biology (Namba et al., 1991; Wisniewski and Frangione, 1992) and genetic mapping.

The three common *APOE* alleles (2, 3, 4), when translated, result in different protein isoforms (Menzel et al., 1983; Saunders et al., 1993a). The approximate Caucasian allele frequencies are *APOE-2* (0.07), *APOE-3* (0.77), and *APOE-4* (0.16). Testing for an association between *APOE* alleles and AD resulted in the identification of an association of the *APOE-4* allele with AD in both familial late-onset and sporadic AD patients (Saunders et al., 1993b; Strittmatter et al., 1993). Simultaneously with the identification of the *APOE-4* allelic association, Corder et al. (1993) showed that the *APOE-4* allele acts in a dose-dependent manner to increase risk and decrease age at onset in both late-onset familial sporadic and early-onset sporadic AD (Corder et al., 1993; Okuizumi et al., 1994; van Duijn et al., 1994b; Roses and Pericak-Vance, 1997). The *APOE-2* allele affords protection against late-onset AD (Corder et al., 1994; Locke et al., 1995), but its effect in early-onset sporadic AD is still unclear (van Duijn et al., 1995a; Sorbi et al., 1994; Scott et al., 1997).

Over 300 studies have confirmed the association of *APOE-4* with AD (Roses and Pericak-Vance, 1997). While there are some differences between studies, overall the risk for the *APOE-3/4* genotype is about threefold, while the risk for the *APOE-4/4* genotype is about eightfold relative to the common *3/3* genotype. The risk for the *APOE-2* allele is approximately 0.5-fold. The effect of the *APOE-4* allele seems to be modified by age, sex, and ethnic origin. The *APOE-4*–related risk is greatest in the sixth decade and decreases through the seventh and eighth decades (Fig. 43–2). The effect is also modified by sex, with men showing a substantial increase in risk only for the *APOE-4/4* homozygotes and women showing a modestly increased risk for the *APOE-3/4* heterozygotes and a substantially increased risk for the *APOE-4/4* homozygotes (Fig. 43–3). The risks are also different in different ethnic groups. The highest risk occurs in the Japanese and the lowest in Hispanics (Fig. 43–4). The risk in African Americans is more variable, with some studies finding highly elevated risk and others finding relatively modest risk (Farrer et al., 1997).

The mechanism by which the specific *APOE* isoforms uniquely contribute to disease expression is still not known. Hypotheses abound, including altered levels of lipoprotein transport and interaction with both Aβ and presenilin (Roses and Pericak-Vance, 1997). *APOE* represents the fourth confirmed genetic factor and is the single most significant biologic risk factor identified for AD.

Several lines of evidence indicate that *APOE* does not account for all of the genetic variation seen in AD. While the heritability of AD has been estimated at about 80% (Bergen, 1994), more than one-third of AD cases do not have even a single

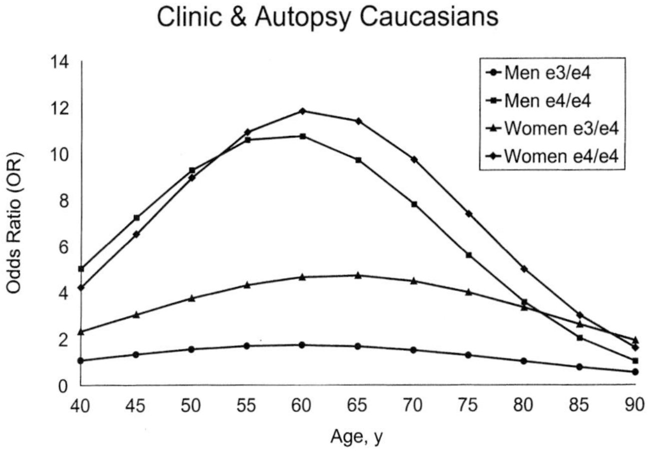

Fig. 43–3. Risk of Alzheimer's disease (*AD*) for Caucasians by age and sex. From Farrer et al. (1997) with permission. © 1997 American Medical Association.

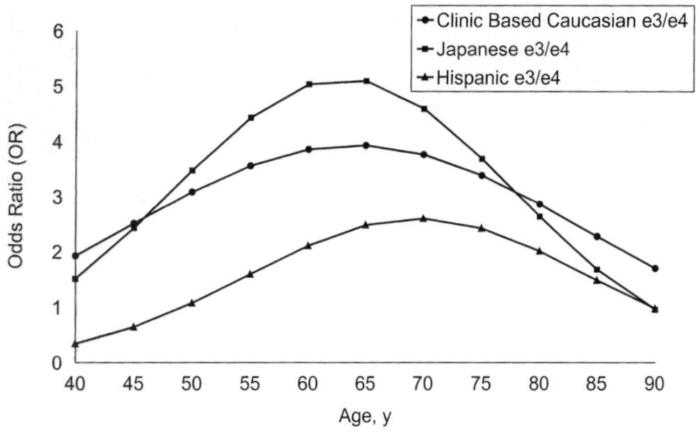

Fig. 43–4. Risk of Alzheimer's disease (*AD*) by age, sex, and ethnic group. From Farrer et al. (1997) with permission. © 1997 American Medical Association.

APOE-4 allele. In addition, studies of an Amish population (Pericak-Vance et al., 1996) show familial aggregation of AD despite a low *APOE-4* allele frequency. As well, the *APOE-4*–associated risk of AD appears to differ among ethnic groups, suggesting that ethnic background may influence the genetic risk of AD (Farrer et al., 1997; Tang et al., 1996; Maestre et al., 1995). Finally, the λ_s for the *APOE* locus has been estimated (Roses et al., 1995) to be approximately 2. Since the overall λ_s is estimated to be between 4 and 5, *APOE* is likely to account for at most 50% of the total genetic effect in AD (Roses et al., 1995; Slooter et al., 1998).

Other Genes. Genomic screening has been applied to late-onset AD (Pericak-Vance et al., 1997, 2000; Kehoe et al., 1999b), with the identification of three new loci on chromosomes 12 (Pericak-Vance et al., 1997; Rogaeva et al., 1998; Kehoe et al., 1999a), 10 q (Kehoe et al., 1999a; Myers et al., 2000; Pericak-Vance et al., 2000) and 9p (Pericak-Vance et al., 2000; Haines and Pericak-Vance, 2001). Two interesting candidate genes (A2M and LRP1) lie within the chromosome 12 candidate gene region and one (IDE; Bertram et al., 2000) in the chromosome 10 region (Table 43–2). While some elevated risk associated with the chromosome 12 genes (A2M, LRP1) has been suggested (Lendon et al., 1997; Blacker et al., 1998), it has not been confirmed (Scott et al., 1998; Rogaeva et al., 1999; Dow et al., 1999; Rudrasingham et al., 1999). Similarly the IDE locus has also not been confirmed (Abraham et al., 2001).

The chromosome 9p region is one of the most interesting new regions (Pericak-Vance et al., 2000; Haines and Pericak-

Table 43–2. Some Candidate Genes in Late-Onset Alzheimer's Disease

Gene	Gene Name	Location	Reference
A2M	α_2-Macroglobulin	12p13–12	Blacker et al. (1998)
AACT	α_1-Antichymotrypsin	14q32	Kamboh et al. (1995)
APOA4	Apolipoprotein A-IV	11q23	Csaszar et al. (1997)
APOE	Apolipoprotein E	19q13	Strittmatter et al. (1993)
APBB1	Amyloid precursor protein–binding family B	11p15	Hu et al. (1998)
APP	Amyloid precursor protein	21q21	Li et al. (1998)
BACE	β-Secretase	11q23	Murphy et al. (2001)
BCHE	Butyrylcholinesterase	3q26	Lehmann et al. (1997)
BLMH	Bleomycin hydrolase	17q11	Montoya et al. (1998)
CSEN	Calsenilin	2q11	Buxbaum et al. (2000)
CST3	Cystatin C	20p11	Finckh et al. (2000)
CTSD	Cathepsin D	1p15	Papassotiropoulos et al. (1999a)
CYP2D	Cytochrome P-450	22q13	Tanaka et al. (1998)
DCP1	Angiotensin I–converting enzyme	17q23	Kehoe et al. (1999b)
DLST	Dihydrolipoamide *S*-succinyltransferase	14q23	Nakano et al. (1997)
ESR1	Estrogen receptor 1	6q25	Brandi et al. (1999)
HFE	Hereditary hemochromatosis	6p21	Moalem et al. (2000)
HLA-A	Major histocompatibility complex A	6p21	Small et al. (1991)
HLA-B	Major histocompatibility complex B	6p21	Renvoize (1984)
HLA-DR	Major histocompatibility complex DR	6p21	Curran et al. (1997)
HTR6	5-Hydroxytryptamine receptor 6	1p36	Tsai et al. (1999)
IDE	Insulin Degrading Enzyme	10q	Bertram et al. (2000)
IL1A	Interleukin-1α	2q14	Grimaldi et al. (2000)
IL6	Interleukin-6	7p21	Papassotiropoulos et al. (1999b)
LRP1	Low-density lipoprotein receptor–related protein 1	12q13	Lendon et al. (1997)
LRPAP1	LRP-associated protein	4p	Sanchez et al. (2001)
MAPT	Microtubule-associated protein τ	17q21	Lilius et al. (1999)
Mitochondria	Mitochondrial genes	Mitochondria	Shoffner et al. (1993)
MPO	Myeloperoxidase	17q23	Reynolds et al. (1999)
MTHFR	Methylenetetrahydrofolate reductase	1p36	Nishiyama et al. (2000)
NOS3	Endothelial nitric oxide synthase	7q35	Dahiyat et al. (1999)
PNMT	Phenylethanolamine *N*-methyltransferase	17q21	Mann et al. (2001)
PS1	Presenilin 1	14q24	Wragg et al. (1996)
SLC6A4	Serotonin transporter	17q11–12	Oliveira et al. (1998)
SNCA	α-Synuclein	4q21–22	Xia et al. (1996)
Tf	Transferrin	3q21	Namekata et al. (1997)
TFCP2	Transcriptional factor CP2	12q13	Lambert et al. (2000)
TGFB	Transforming growth factor-β1	19q13	Luedecking et al. (2000)
TNFA	Tumor necrosis factor-α	6p21	Collins et al. (2000)
VLDLR	Very low-density lipoprotein receptor	9p24	Okuizumi et al. (1995)

Vance, 2001). This linkage region was recently confirmed in an independent data set comprised of inbred Arab-Israeli families (Farrer et al., 2001). The Farrer et al. linkage region completely overlaps the area of linkage reported previously (Pericak-Vance et al., 2001; Haines et al., 2001). Potential candidate genes in the region include p16 (CDKNA2)/p15 (CDKN2B) and methylthioadenosine phosphorylase (MTAP). P16 has been shown to highly colocalize with nNOS and $p21^{ras}$ in pyramidal neurons in AD (Luth et al., 2000). P15 is a closely related gene believed to be involved in growth regulation. MTAP is shown to play a major role in the salvage of adenine and methionine and polyamine metabolism (Ragione et al., 1996).

Numerous candidate gene studies have been performed over the past 10 years, testing nearly 40 different genes (Table 43–2); but with the singular exception of *APOE*, none of the results has been widely replicated. Almost universally, the approach for testing candidate genes has been the standard unmatched case-control design. There are numerous weaknesses in this approach. The three most common are small sample size, failure to correct for multiple comparisons, and poor matching of cases and controls. Many candidate gene studies are performed with sample sizes of 50 to 100 patients and similar numbers of controls. Such a sample has only modest power to detect moderate effects, and any effect seen is subject to possible random sampling variation (e.g., has a large variance). Many patient samples are tested for numerous candidate genes, but only positive results are reported. By performing multiple comparisons, the probability of a chance positive result is increased. Finally, much effort has been expended to carefully characterize the patient population using standardized criteria (McKhann et al., 1984). However, there is no standard for control populations. Many are not matched for age or sex and often are not tested or are tested minimally for cognitive ability. The variability in allele frequencies across studies is often greater for the control populations than the patient populations (Grubber et al., 1999).

To alleviate some of these problems and to control for any possible ethnic or population structure variations, family-based association methods have been developed. The most commonly applied is the transmission-disequilibrium test (TDT) (Spielman et al., 1993), which examines the frequencies of alleles transmitted and not transmitted to children. This allows the use of single affected individuals but also requires sampling their parents. The power of this simple test arises from its reliance on linkage disequilibrium, which usually exists over only very small intervals (usually <1 cM). Thus, it is complementary to standard linkage analysis, where the effect is broad (up to 30 cM), but the discriminative power over small regions is low. The TDT is best applied to the candidate genes that fall within the critical regions. Since AD is an adult late-onset disorder, most patients will not have both parents alive and available for sampling. The discordant sib pair, or sib-TDT approach (Spielman and Ewens, 1998; Boehnke and Langefeld, 1998; Horvath and Laird, 1998), and the more general extension to complete pedigrees [the Pedigree Disequilibrium Test (Martin et al., 2000)] remove the requirement of parental sampling by instead sampling and using unaffected siblings as a control group. While the power of such a test is not as strong as that of the TDT, it allows greatly increased sample sizes, overcoming any inherent loss of power. This approach was applied to the *A2M* gene on chromosome 12. Unfortunately, the initial strongly positive result (Blacker et al., 1998) was not replicated on follow-up (Rogaeva et al., 1999).

Interactions

As the number of known AD genes increases, it will be important to understand if and how each of these genes interacts with the others. This will not be limited to gene–gene interactions but will include gene–environment interactions. While tools to identify linkage and/or association exist and are being refined, tools to look for interactions between genes are still in their infancy. Initial studies have looked at potential modifying effects among the four known genes, with few positive results. In early-onset families with *APP* mutations, *APOE* genotype modifies age at onset since the presence of the *APOE-4* allele apparently decreases the age at onset of affected family members (Houlden et al., 1993; St George-Hyslop et al., 1993; Nacmias et al., 1995). Another study looking at the interaction of *APOE* and *PS1* in early-onset families found no evidence of an effect (Van Broeckhoven et al., 1994). While the effect of a single gene may be detected independently, it is important to examine any proposed susceptibility allele in relation to other known genes. Two studies have proposed such an interactive effect, the first examining the gene coding for α_1-antichymotrypsin (Kamboh et al., 1995, 1997) and the second examining the gene coding the receptor for the very low-density lipoprotein receptor (Okuizumi et al., 1995). As with the other candidate gene studies, these results have not been confirmed (Pritchard et al., 1996; Haines et al., 1996, 1997).

Fully understanding AD as a complex multifactorial disorder ultimately will require moving beyond genetic studies to include environmental factors as well. The power to identify such risk factors will be increased by controlling for as many known genetic susceptibility loci as possible. This approach is exemplified by studies on head trauma and AD (Roberts et al., 1994; Mayeux et al., 1995) where the risk from head trauma may be altered by *APOE* genotype. Possible interactions with other environmental factors, such as estrogen and NSAID use, are currently being explored.

CLINICAL APPLICATION AND RISK ASSESSMENT OF GENETICS INFORMATION

Diagnosis

The diagnosis of AD does not currently depend on obtaining genotypic information. In the few families with mutations in the *APP*, *PS1*, or *PS2* genes, a positive result could be used to confirm a clinical diagnosis. This would require a strong family history of early-onset AD and evidence of cosegregation of any mutation in multiple affected members of the family. Thus, a full family study would have to be performed.

Much controversy surrounds the use of *APOE* genotyping within a clinical diagnostic regimen for late-onset AD (Farrer et al., 1995; Mayeux et al., 1995; Roses et al., 1996; Relkin et al., 1998). While the positive predictive value of the *APOE-4* allele appears high in most studies, its sensitivity is quite variable between studies (Roses et al., 1996). Mayeux et al. (1998) indicated that the sensitivity of a clinical diagnosis of AD was 93% and the specificity was 55%. *APOE-4* carrier status (e.g., *APOE-2/4*, *-3/4*) alone had a sensitivity of 65% and a specificity of 68%. Used together, the sensitivity decreased to 61% but the specificity increased to 84%. The *APOE-4/4* genotype had a high specificity (95%) but a low sensitivity (14%) (Mayeux et al., 1998). There is consensus that *APOE* genotyping should not be used as a sole diagnostic test. However, it can be and is often used as an adjunct to other clinical tests and will provide some additional discriminatory power.

Screening

The controversy over the use and value of *APOE* genotyping for diagnosis extends to its use as a presymptomatic test. A few have advocated that any information is better than no information, but the consensus is that a presymptomatic test needs to be definitive and that the risks associated with the various *APOE* genotypes are not sufficiently strong to warrant such testing (Farrer et al., 1995; Relkin et al., 1996). Virtually all studies to date have been based on clinic populations and, thus, do not represent the risks in the general population. Studies looking at the long-term predictive value of *APOE* genotyping in community-based samples are ongoing.

Population screening for any of the known AD genes is not warranted. Mutations in *APP*, *PS1*, and *PS2* are too rare to justify the effort and expense, and the risks related to *APOE* are not sufficiently strong to be predictive of disease. In addition, there is no known cure and little effective treatment for AD. Screening symptomatic clinic populations for *APP*, *PS1*, and *PS2* mutations is also not warranted without some other suggestive findings, such as very early age at onset and extensive family history.

Prevention

There is no known effective prevention for AD.

Counseling

Patients with AD and their families need careful and thorough counseling. Patients and their caregivers will need to be guided as to the clinical course and the physical and psychological changes that can be expected. They should be provided with information about local, regional, and national support groups and any local home care, nursing home, or hospice options.

Patients in families with mutations in *APP*, *PS1*, or *PS2* must receive more specific genetic counseling. While the risk of developing AD in families segregating one of these dominant mutations is high, it is also age-dependent and, in some cases (e.g., *PS2*), penetrance may not be 100% even at very old age. Patients and families need to receive careful and thorough pre-test counseling, to be sure that they understand all of the personal, family, social, economic, and legal complications that may arise from the results of the test. As mentioned above, presymptomatic testing for *APOE* is not recommended. However, in symptomatic patients where *APOE* genotype is determined, counseling must still be done carefully as it has an impact not only on the patient but on other blood relatives as well. For example, a patient who has the *APOE-4/4* genotype must transmit at least one *APOE-4* allele to each child. Thus, without genotyping the children, knowledge that the children are at increased risk is given.

Therapy

There have been few reports of *APOE* genotypic effects related to drug regimens in AD. The most commonly tested drug is the anticholinesterase tacrine. Initial reports indicated that individuals who do not carry an *APOE-4* allele responded much better to tacrine therapy than did those who carried at least one *APOE-4* allele (Poirier et al., 1995; Farlow et al., 1996). The effect of gender on *APOE*-mediated response to tacrine is unclear, with studies reporting that either men (MacGowan et al., 1998) or women (Farlow et al., 1998) have a stronger response. *APOE* genotype is routinely obtained in most ongoing clinical trials.

REFERENCES

Abraham CR, Selkoe DJ, Potter H: Immunochemical identification of the serine protease inhibitor alpha$_1$-antichymotrypsin in the brain amyloid deposits of Alzheimer's disease. Cell 1988; 52:487–501.

Ala TA, Yang KH, Sung JH, Frey WH: Hallucinations and signs of parkinsonism help distinguish patients with dementia and cortical Lewy bodies from patients with Alzheimer's disease at presentation: a clinicopathological study. J Neurol Neurosurg Psychiatry 1997; 62:16–21.

Andersen K, Launer LJ, Ott A, Hoes AW, Breteler MM, Hofman A: Do nonsteroidal anti-inflammatory drugs decrease the risk for Alzheimer's disease? The Rotterdam Study. Neurology 1995; 45:1441–1445.

Anthony JC, Breitner JC, Zandi PP, Meyer MR, Jurasova I, Norton MC, Stone SV: Reduced prevalence of AD in users of NSAIDs and H2 receptor antagonists: the Cache County Study. Neurology 2000; 54:2066–2071.

Bachman DL, Wolf PA, Linn R, Knoefel JE, Cobb J, Belanger A, D'Agostino RB, White LR: Prevalence of dementia and probable senile dementia of the Alzheimer type in the Framingham Study. Neurology 1992; 42:115–119.

Ball MJ, Nuttall K: Neurofibrillary tangles, granulovacuolar degeneration, and neuron loss in Down syndrome: quantitative comparison with Alzheimer dementia. Ann Neurol 1980; 7:462–465.

Bergen AL: Heredity in dementia of the Alzheimer type. Clin Genet 1994; 46:144–149.

Bergen AL, Engedal K, Kringlen E: The role of heredity in late-onset Alzheimer disease and vascular dementia: a twin study. Arch Gen Psychiatry 1997; 54:264–270.

Bertram L, Blacker D, Mullin K, Keeney D, Jones J, Basu S, Yhu S, McInnis M, Go RCP, Vekrellis K, Selkoe DJ, Saunders A, Tanzi R: Evidence for genetic linkage of Alzheimer's disease to chromosome 10q. Science 2000; 290:2302–2305.

Bickel H, Cooper B: Incidence and relative risk of dementia in an urban elderly population: findings of a prospective field study. Psychol Med 1994; 24:179–192.

Bird TD, Lampe TH, Nemens EJ, Miner GW, Sumi SM, Schellenberg GD: Familial Alzheimer's disease in American descendants of the Volga Germans: probable genetic founder effect. Ann Neurol 1988; 23:25–31.

Blacker D, Wilcox MA, Laird NM, Rodes L, Horvath SM, Go RCP, Perry R, Watson B, Bassett SS, McInnis MG, et al.: Alpha-2 macroglobulin is genetically associated with Alzheimer disease. Nat Genet 1998; 19:357–360.

Boehnke M, Langefeld CD: Genetic association mapping based on discordant sib pairs: the discordant alleles test (DAT). Am J Hum Genet 1998; 62:950–961.

Botstein D, White RL, Skolnick M, Davis RW: Construction of a genetic linkage map in man using restriction fragment length polymorphisms. Am J Hum Genet 1980; 32:314–331.

Braak H, Braak E: Neuropathological stageing of Alzheimer-related changes. Acta Neuropathol (Berl) 1991; 82:239–259.

Brandi ML, Becherini L, Gennari L, Racchi M, Bianchetti A, Nacmias B, Sorbi S, Mecocci P, Senin U, Govoni S: Association of the estrogen receptor α gene polymorphisms with sporadic Alzheimer's disease. Biochem Biophys Res Commun 1999; 265:335–338.

Breitner JC, Gatz M, Christian JC, Mortimer JA, McClearn GE, Heston LL, Welsh KA, Anthony JC, Folstein MF: Use of twin cohorts for research in Alzheimer's disease. Neurology 1993; 43:261–267.

Breitner JC, Murphy EA, Silverman JM, Mohs RC, Davis KL: Age-dependent expression of familial risk in Alzheimer's disease. Am J Epidemiol 1988a; 128:536–538.

Breitner JC, Silverman JM, Mohs RC, Davis KL: Familial aggregation in Alzheimer's disease: comparison of risk among first degree relatives of early- and late-onset cases, and among male and female relatives in a successive generation. Neurology 1988b; 38:207–212.

Breitner JC, Welsh KA, Helms MJ, Gaskell PC, Gau BA, Roses AD, Pericak-Vance MA, Saunders AM: Delayed onset of Alzheimer's disease with nonsteroidal anti-inflammatory and histamine H2 blocking drugs. Neurobiol Aging 1995; 16:523–530.

Brenner DE, Kukull WA, Stergachis A, van Belle G, Bowen JD, McCormick WC, Teri L, Larson EB: Postmenopausal estrogen replacement therapy and the risk of Alzheimer's disease: a population-based case-control study. Am J Epidemiol 1994; 140:262–267.

Broe GA, Henderson AS, Creasey H, McCusker E, Korten AE, Jorm AF, Longley W, Anthony JC: A case-control study of Alzheimer's disease in Australia. Neurology 1990; 40:1698–1707.

Brown DF, Dababo MA, Bigio EH, Risser RC, Eagan KP, Hladik CL, White CLI: Neuropathologic evidence that the Lewy body variant of Alzheimer disease represents coexistence of Alzheimer disease and idiopathic Parkinson disease [see comments]. J Neuropathol Exp Neurol 1998; 57:39–46.

Burger PC, Vogel FS: The development of the pathologic changes of Alzheimer's disease and senile dementia in patients with Down's syndrome. Am J Pathol 1973; 73:457–476.

Buxbaum JD, Lilliehook C, Chan JY, Go RC, Bassett SS, Tanzi RE, Wasco W, Blacker D: Genomic structure, expression pattern, and chromosomal localization of the human calsenilin gene: no association between an exonic polymorphism and Alzheimer's disease. Neurosci Lett 2000; 294:135–138.

Canadian Study of Health and Aging: The Canadian Study of Health and Aging: risk factors for Alzheimer's disease in Canada. Neurology 1994; 44:2073–2080.

Chen JY, Stern Y, Sano M, Mayeux R: Cumulative risks of developing extrapyramidal signs, psychosis, or myoclonus in the course of Alzheimer's disease. Arch Neurol 1991; 48:1141–1143.

Clark LN, Poorkaj P, Wszolek Z, Geschwind DH, Nasreddine ZS, Miller B, Li D, Payami H, Awert F, Markopoulou K, et al.: Pathogenic implications of mutations in the *tau* gene in pallido-ponto-nigral degeneration and related neurodegenerative disorders linked to chromosome 17. Proc Natl Acad Sci USA 1998; 95:13103–13107.

Clemenceau S, Foncin JF, Muller JY, Halle L, Hauptmann G, Seger J, Salmon C: Absence of a connection between Alzheimer's disease and complement markers [in French]. C R Acad Sci III 1986; 303:149–154.

Collins JS, Perry RT, Watson B Jr, Harrell LE, Acton RT, Blacker D, Albert MS, Tanzi RE, Bassett SS, McInnis MG, et al.: Association of a haplotype for tumor necrosis factor in siblings with late-onset Alzheimer disease: the NIMH Alzheimer Disease Genetics Initiative. Am J Med Genet 2000; 96:823–830.

Corder EH, Saunders AM, Risch NJ, Strittmatter WJ, Schmechel DE, Gaskell PC Jr, Rimmler JB, Locke JL, Conneally PM, Schmader KE, et al.: Protective effect of apolipoprotein E type 2 allele for late onset Alzheimer disease. Nat Genet 1994; 7:180–184.

Corder EH, Saunders AM, Strittmatter WJ, Schmechel DE, Gaskell PC, Small GW, Roses AD, Haines JL, Pericak-Vance MA: Gene dose of apolipoprotein E type 4 allele and the risk of Alzheimer's disease in late onset families. Science 1993; 261:921–923.

Csaszar A, Kalman J, Szalai C, Janka Z, Romics L: Association of the apolipoprotein A-IV codon 360 mutation in patients with Alzheimer's disease. Neurosci Lett 1997; 230:151–154.

Curran M, Middleton D, Edwardson J, Perry R, McKeith I, Morris C, Neill D: *HLA-DR* antigens associated with major genetic risk for late-onset Alzheimer's disease. Neuroreport 1997; 8:1467–1469.

Dahiyat M, Cumming A, Harrington C, Wischik C, Xuereb J, Corrigan F, Breen G, Shaw D, St Clair D: Association between Alzheimer's disease and the *NOS3* gene. Ann Neurol 1999; 46:664–667.

Dickson DW: Neuropathology of Alzheimer's disease and other dementias. Clin Geriatr Med 2001; 17:209–228.

Ditter SM, Mirra SS: Neuropathologic and clinical features of Parkinson's disease in Alzheimer's disease patients. Neurology 1987; 37:754–760.

Dow DJ, Lindsey N, Cairns NJ, Brayne C, Robinson D, Huppert FA, Paykel ES, Xuereb J, Wilcock G, Whittaker JL, et al.: Alpha-2 macroglobulin polymorphism and Alzheimer disease risk in the UK [letter] [see comments]. Nat Genet 1999; 22:16–17.

Eikelenboom P, Stam FC: An immunohistochemical study on cerebral vascular and senile plaque amyloid in Alzheimer's dementia. Virchows Arch B Cell Pathol Mol Pathol 1984; 47:17–25.

Ellis WG, McCulloch JR, Corley CL: Presenile dementia in Down's syndrome. Ultrastructural identity with Alzheimer's disease. Neurology 1974; 24:101–106.

Evans DA, Funkenstein HH, Albert MS, Scherr PA, Cook NR, Chown MJ, Hebert LE, Hennekens CH, Taylor JO: Prevalence of Alzheimer's disease in a community population of older persons. Higher than previously reported [see comments]. JAMA 1989; 262:2551–2556.

Farlow MR, Lahiri DK, Poirier J, Davignon J, Hui S: Apolipoprotein E genotype and gender influence response to tacrine therapy. Ann NY Acad Sci 1996; 802:101–110.

Farlow MR, Lahiri DK, Poirier J, Davignon J, Schneider L, Hui SL: Treatment outcome of tacrine therapy depends on apolipoprotein genotype and gender of the subjects with Alzheimer's disease. Neurology 1998; 50:669–677.

Farrer LA, Bowirrat A, Friedland RP, Warasaka K, Adams JC, Korczyn AD, Baldwin CT: Identification of multiple loci for Alzheimer Disease in an inbred Israeli-Arab community. Am J Hum Genet 2001; 69(supp):200.

Farrer LA, Brin MF, Elsas L, Goate A, Kennedy J, Mayeux R, Myers RH, Reilly PR, Risch NJ: Statement on use of apolipoprotein E testing for Alzheimer disease. JAMA 1995; 274:1627–1628.

Farrer LA, Cupples LA, Haines JL, Hyman B, Kukull WA, Mayeux R, Myers RH, Pericak-Vance MA, Risch N, van Duijn CM, APOE and Alzheimer Disease Meta Analysis Consortium: Effects of age, sex, and ethnicity on the association between apolipoprotein E genotype and Alzheimer disease. JAMA 1997; 278:1349–1356.

Farrer LA, Myers RH, Connor L, Cupples A, Growdon JH: Segregation analysis reveals evidence of a major gene for Alzheimer disease. Am J Hum Genet 1991; 48:1026–1033.

Farrer LA, O'Sullivan DM, Cupples LA, Growden JH, Myers RH: Assessment of genetic risk for Alzheimer's disease among first-degree relatives. Ann Neurol 1989; 25:485–493.

Finckh U, von der Kammer H, Velden J, Michel T, Andresen B, Deng A, Zhang J, Muller-Thomsen T, Zuchowski K, Menzer G, et al.: Genetic association of a *cystatin C* gene polymorphism with late-onset Alzheimer disease. Arch Neurol 2000; 57:1579–1583.

Folstein MF, Folstein SE, McHugh PR: "Mini-Mental State": a practical method for grading the cognitive state of patients for the clinician. J Psychiatr Res 1975; 12:189–198.

Fratiglioni L, Ahlbom A, Viitanen M, Winblad B: Risk factors for late-onset Alzheimer's disease: a population-based, case-control study. Ann Neurol 1993; 33:258–266.

Frecker MF: Dementia in Newfoundland: identification of a geographical isolate? J Epidemiol Community Health 1991; 45:307–311.

Goate AM, Chartier-Harlin MC, Mullan MC, Brown J, Crawford F, Fidani L, Guiffra L, Haynes A, Irving N, James L, et al.: Segregation of a missense mutation in the amyloid precursor protein gene with familial Alzheimer's disease. Nature 1991; 33:53–56.

Goldgaber D, Lerman MI, McBride OW, Saffiotti U, Gajdusek DC: Characterization and chromosomal localization of a cDNA encoding brain amyloid of Alzheimer's disease. Science 1987; 235:877–880.

Goudsmit J, White BJ, Weitkamp LR, Keats BJ, Morrow CH, Gajdusek DC: Familial Alzheimer's disease in two kindreds of the same geographic and ethnic origin. A clinical and genetic study. J Neurol Sci 1981; 49:79–89.

Grimaldi LM, Casadei VM, Ferri C, Veglia F, Licastro F, Annoni G, Biunno I, De Bellis G, Sorbi S, Mariani C, et al.: Association of early-onset Alzheimer's disease with an *interleukin 1α* gene polymorphism. Ann Neurol 2000; 47:361–365.

Growden JH: Advances in the diagnosis of Alzheimer's disease. In: Iqbal K, Mortimer JA, Winblad B, Wisniewski H (eds). Research Advances in Alzheimer's Disease and Related Disorders. New York: John Wiley and Sons, 1995:139–153.

Grubber J, Saunders AM, Crane-Gatherum AR, Scott WK, Martin E, Haynes CS, Conneally PM, Small GW, Roses AD, Haines JL, et al.: Analysis of association between Alzheimer disease and the K variant of butyrylcholinesterase (BCHE-K). Neurosci Lett 1999; 269:115—119.

Guo Z, Cupples LA, Kurz A, Auerbach SH, Volicer L, Chui H, Green RC, Sadovnick AD, Duara R, DeCarli C, et al.: Head injury and the risk of AD in the MIRAGE study. Neurology 2000; 54:1316–1323.

Haines JL, Pritchard ML, Saunders AM, Schildkraut JM, Growdon JH, Gaskell PC, Farrer LA, Auerbach SA, Gusella JF, Locke PA, et al.: No genetic effect of α1-antichymotrypsin in Alzheimer disease. Genomics 1996; 33:53–56.

Haines JL, Pericak-Vance MA: A genomic search for Alzheimer's Disease genes. In: Iqbal K, Sisodia SS, Winblad B (eds) Alzheimer's Disease: Advances in Etiology, Pathogenesis and Therapeutics. John Wiley & Sons, London, 2001:33–43.

Haines JL, Scott WK, Pericak-Vance MA: Reply to "Genetic effect of α1-antichymotrypsin on the risk of Alzheimer disease" [letter]. Genomics 1997; 40:384–385.

Hendrie HC, Ogunniyi A, Hall KS, Baiyewu O, Unverzagt FW, Gureje O, Gao S, Evans RM, Ogunseyinde AO, Adeyinka AO, et al.: Incidence of dementia and Alzheimer disease in 2 communities: Yoruba residing in Ibadan, Nigeria, and African Americans residing in Indianapolis, Indiana. JAMA 2001; 285:739–747.

Hendrie HC, Osuntokun BO, Hall KS, Ogunniyi AO, Hui SL, Unverzagt FW, Gureje O, Rodenberg CA, Baiyewu O, Musick BS: Prevalence of Alzheimer's disease and dementia in two communities: Nigerian Africans and African Americans. Am J Psychiatry 1995; 152:1485–1492.

Heston LL, Mastri AR, Anderson VE, White J: Dementia of the Alzheimer type. Clinical genetics, natural history, and associated conditions. Arch Gen Psychiatry 1981; 38:1085–1090.

Heyman A, Wilkinson WE, Hurwitz BJ, Schmechel D, Sigmon AH, Weinberg T, Helms MJ, Swift M: Alzheimer's disease: genetic aspects and associated clinical disorders. Ann Neurol 1983; 14:507–515.

Heyman A, Wilkinson WE, Stafford JA, Helms MJ, Sigmon AH, Weinberg T: Alzheimer's disease: a study of epidemiological aspects. Ann Neurol 1984; 15:335–341.

Hirst C, Sadovnick AD, Yee IML: Familial risks for Alzheimer disease: data from an Alzheimer clinic population. Genet Epidemiol 1994; 11:365–374.

Horvath S, Laird NM: A discordant-sibship test for disequilibrium and linkage: no need for parental data. Am J Hum Genet 1998; 63:1886–1897.

Houlden H, Collinge J, Kennedy A, Newman S, Rossor M, Lannfelt L, Lillius L, Winbald B, Crook R, Duff K, et al.: *ApoE* genotype and Alzheimer's disease. Lancet 1993; 342:737–738.

Hu Q, Kukull WA, Bressler SL, Gray MD, Cam JA, Larson EB, Martin GM, Deeb SS: The human *FE65* gene: genomic structure and an intronic biallelic polymorphism associated with sporadic dementia of the Alzheimer type. Hum Genet 1998; 103:295–303.

Huff FJ, Auerbach J, Chakravarti A, Boller F: Risk of dementia in relatives of patients with Alzheimer disease. Neurology 1988; 38:786–790.

Jarvik G, Larson EB, Goddard K, Schellenberg GD, Wijsman EM: Influence of apolipoprotein E genotype on the transmission of Alzheimer disease in a community-based sample [published erratum appears in Am J Hum Genet 1996; 58:648]. Am J Hum Genet 1996; 58:191–200.

Johnson CC, Rybicki BA, Brown G, D'Hondt E, Herpolsheimer B, Roth D, Jackson CE: Cognitive impairment in the Amish: a four county survey. Int J Epidemiol 1997; 26:387–394.

Kalaria RN, Galloway PG, Perry G: Widespread serum amyloid P immunoreactivity in cortical amyloid deposits and the neurofibrillary pathology of Alzheimer's disease and other degenerative disorders. Neuropathol Appl Neurobiol 1991; 17:189–201.

Kamboh MI, Aston CE, Ferrell RE, DeKosky ST: Genetic effect of α1-antichymotrypsin on the risk of Alzheimer disease [letter]. Genomics 1997; 40:382–385.

Kamboh MI, Sanghera DK, Ferrell RE, DeKosky ST: APOE*4-associated Alzheimer's disease risk is modified by alpha1-antichymotrypsin polymorphism. Nat Genet 1995; 10:486–488.

Kehoe P, Wavrant-De VF, Crook R, Wu WS, Holmans P, Fenton I, Spurlock G, Norton N, Williams H, Williams N, et al.: A full genome scan for late onset Alzheimer's disease. Hum Mol Genet 1999a; 8:237–245.

Kehoe PG, Russ C, McIlory S, Williams H, Holmans P, Holmes C, Liolitsa D, Vahidassr D, Powell J, McGleenon B, et al.: Variation in DCP1, encoding ACE, is associated with susceptibility to Alzheimer disease [letter]. Nat Genet 1999b; 21:71–72.

Khachaturian Z: Diagnosis of Alzheimer's disease. Arch Neurol 1985; 42:1097–1104.

Knopman DS, Ryberg S: A verbal memory test with high predictive accuracy for dementia of the Alzheimer type. Arch Neurol 1989; 46:141–145.

Lambert JC, Goumidi L, Vrieze FW, Frigard B, Harris JM, Cummings A, Coates J, Pasquier F, Cottel D, Gaillac M, et al.: The transcriptional factor *LBP-1c/CP2/LSF* gene on chromosome 12 is a genetic determinant of Alzheimer's disease. Hum Mol Genet 2000; 9:2275–2280.

Lander ES, Linton LM, Birren B, Nusbaum C, Zody MC, Baldwin J, Devon K, Dewar K, Doyle M, FitzHugh W, et al.: Initial sequencing and analysis of the human genome. Nature 2001; 409:860–921.

Lee PN: Smoking and Alzheimer's disease: a review of the epidemiological evidence. Neuroepidemiology 1994; 13:131–144.

Lehmann DJ, Johnston C, Smith AD: Synergy between the genes for butyrylcholinesterase K variant and apolipoprotein E4 in late-onset confirmed Alzheimer's disease. Hum Mol Genet 1997; 6:1933–1936.

Lendon CL, Ashall F, Goate AM: Exploring the etiology of Alzheimer disease using molecular genetics. JAMA 1997; 277:825–831.

Lendon CL, Lynch T, Norton J, McKeel DWJ, Busfield F, Craddock N, Chakraverty S, Gopalakrishnan G, Shears SD, Grimmett W, et al.: Hereditary dysphasic disinhibition dementia: a frontotemporal dementia linked to 17q21–22 [see comments]. Neurology 1998; 50:1546–1555.

Levy-Lahad E, Wasco W, Poorkaj P, Romano DM, Oshima J, Pettingell WH, Yu CE, Jondro PD, Schmidt SD, Wang K, et al.: Candidate gene for the chromosome 1 familial Alzheimer's disease locus. Science 1995; 269:973–977.

Li L, Perry R, Wu J, Pham D, Ohman T, Harrell LE, Go RC, Fukuchi K: Polymorphic tetranucleotide repeat site within intron 7 of the beta-amyloid precursor protein gene and its lack of association with Alzheimer's disease. Hum Genet 1998; 103:86–89.

Lilius L, Froelich FS, Basun H, Forsell C, Axelman K, Mattila K, Andreadis A, Viitanen M, Winblad B, Fratiglioni L, et al.: *Tau* gene polymorphisms and apolipoprotein E epsilon4 may interact to increase risk for Alzheimer's disease. Neurosci Lett 1999; 277:29–32.

Locke P, Conneally PM, Tanzi RE, Gusella J, Haines JL: APOE and Alzheimer's disease: examination of allelic association and effect on age at-onset in both early and late-onset cases. Genet Epidemiol 1995; 12:83–92.

Luedecking EK, DeKosky ST, Mehdi H, Ganguli M, Kamboh MI: Analysis of genetic polymorphisms in the transforming growth factor-beta1 gene and the risk of Alzheimer's disease. Hum Genet 2000; 106:565–569.

Macera CA, Huang Y, Eleazer GP, Scott WK, Cornman CB: Epidemiology of Alzheimer's disease. J SC Med Assoc 1994; 90:404–406.

MacGowan SH, Wilcock GK, Scott M: Effect of gender and apolipoprotein E genotype on response to anticholinesterase therapy in Alzheimer's disease. Int J Geriatr Psychiatry 1998; 13:625–630.

Maestre G, Ottman R, Stern Y, Gurland B, Chun M, Tang MX, Shelanski M, Tycko B, Mayeux R: Apolipoprotein E and Alzheimer's disease: ethnic variation in genotypic risks. Ann Neurol 1995; 37:254–259.

Mann DM: Pathological correlates of dementia in Alzheimer's disease. Neurobiol Aging 1994; 15:357–360.

Mann MB, Wu S, Rostamkhani M, Tourtellotte W, MacMurray J, Comings DE: Phenylethanolamine *N*-methyltransferase (*PNMT*) gene and early-onset Alzheimer disease. Am J Med Genet 2001; 105:312–316.

Martin ER, Monks SA, Warren LL, Kaplan NL: A test for linkage and association in general pedigrees: the pedigree disequilibrium test. Am J Hum Genet 2000; 67:146–154.

Max W: The economic impact of Alzheimer's disease. Neurology 1993; 43:56–510.

Mayeux R, Ottman R, Maestre G, Ngai C, Tang MX, Ginsberg H, Chun M, Tycko B, Shelanski M: Synergistic effects of traumatic head injury and apolipoprotein-epsilon 4 in patients with Alzheimer's disease [see comments]. Neurology 1995; 45:555–557.

Mayeux R, Sano M, Chen J, Tatemichi T, Stern Y: Risk of dementia in first-degree relatives of patients with Alzheimer's disease and related disorders. Arch Neurol 1991; 48:269–273.

Mayeux R, Saunders AM, Shea S, Mirra S, Evans D, Roses AD, Hyman BT, Crain B, Tang MX, Phelps CH: Utility of the apolipoprotein E genotype in the diagnosis of Alzheimer's disease. Alzheimer's Disease Centers Consortium on Apolipoprotein E and Alzheimer's Disease [published erratum appears in N Engl J Med 1998; 338:1325] N Engl J Med 1998; 338:506–511.

Mayeux R, Stern Y, Ottman R, Tatemichi TK, Tang MX, Maestre G, Nagi C, Tycko B, Ginsberg H: The apolipoprotein epsilon4 allele in patients with Alzheimer's disease. Ann Neurol 1993; 34:742–754.

Mayeux R, Stern Y, Sano M: Heterogeneity and prognosis in dementia of the Alzheimer type. Bull Clin Neurosci 1985; 50:7–10.

McKeith IG, Galasko D, Kosaka K, Perry EK, Dickson DW, Hansen LA, Salmon DP, Lowe J, Mirra SS, Byrne EJ, et al.: Consensus guidelines for the clinical and pathologic diagnosis of dementia with Lewy bodies (DLB): report of the Consortium on DLB International Workshop. Neurology 1996; 47:1113–1124.

McKhann G, Drachman G, Folstein M: Clinical diagnosis of Alzheimer's disease: report of the NINCDS-ADRDA Work Group under the auspices of the Department of Health and Human Services Task Force on Alzheimer's Disease. Neurology 1984; 34:939–944.

Menzel H-J, Kladetzky RG, Asman G: Apolipoprotein E polymorphism and coronary artery disease. Arteriosclerosis 1983; 3:310–315.

Merchant C, Tang MX, Albert S, Manly J, Stern Y, Mayeux R: The influence of smoking on the risk of Alzheimer's disease. Neurology 1999; 52:1408–1412.

Mirra SS, Heyman A, McKeel D, Sumi SM, Crain BJ, Brownlee LM, Vogel FS, Hughes JP, van Belle G, Berg L: The Consortium to Establish a Registry for Alzheimer's Disease (CERAD). Part II. Standardization of the neuropathologic assessment of Alzheimer's disease. Neurology 1991; 41:479–486.

Moalem S, Percy ME, Andrews DF, Kruck TP, Wong S, Dalton AJ, Mehta P, Fedor B, Warren AC: Are hereditary hemochromatosis mutations involved in Alzheimer disease? Am J Med Genet 2000; 93:58–66.

Mohs RC, Breitner JC, Silverman JM, Davis KL: Alzheimer's dsiease: morbid risk among first degree relatives approximates 50% by age 90. Arch Gen Psychiatry 1987; 44:405–408.

Molgaard CA, Stanford EP, Morton DJ, Ryden LA, Schubert KR, Golbeck AL: Epidemiology of head trauma and neurocognitive impairment in a multi-ethnic population. Neuroepidemiology 1990; 9:233–242.

Molsa PK, Marttila RJ, Rinne UK: Extrapyramidal signs in Alzheimer's disease. Neurology 1984; 34:1114–1116.

Montoya SE, Aston CE, DeKosky ST, Kamboh MI, Lazo JS, Ferrell RE: Bleomycin hydrolase is associated with risk of sporadic Alzheimer's disease [letter] [published erratum appears in Nat Genet 1998; 19:404]. Nat Genet 1998; 18:211–212.

Muller JY, Clemenceau S, Foncin JF, Salmon D, Halle L, Castellano F, Salmon C: Absence of linkage between Alzheimer's disease and the HLA system [in French]. C R Acad Sci III 1986; 303:105–108.

Murphy T, Yip A, Brayne C, Easton D, Evans JG, Xuereb J, Cairns N, Esiri MM, Rubinsztein DC: The *BACE* gene: genomic structure and candidate gene study in late-onset Alzheimer's disease. Neuroreport 2001; 12:631–634.

Myers AJ, Goate AM, Holmans P, Williams J, Owen MJ, Crook R, Wavrant-De Vrieze F, Hardy JA: Susceptibility locus for late-onset Alzheimer's disease on chromosome 10. Presented at the World Alzheimer Congress 2000, Washington, DC, July 2000.

Nacmias B, Latorraca S, Piersanti P, Forleo P, Piacentini S, Bracco L, Amaducci L, Sorbi S: *ApoE* genotype and familial Alzheimer's disease: a possible influence on age onset in APP717 Val-Ile mutated families. Neurosci Lett 1995; 183:1–3.

Nakano K, Ohta S, Nishimaki K, Miki T, Matuda S: Alzheimer's disease and *DLST* genotype. Lancet 1997; 350:1367–1368.

Namba Y, Tamonaga M, Kawasaki H, Otomo E, Ikeda K: Apolipoprotein E immunoreactivity in cerebral amyloid deposits and neurofibrillary tangles in Alzheimer's disease and cru plaque amyloid in Creutzfeldt-Jakob disease. Brain Res 1991; 541:163–166.

Namekata K, Imagawa M, Terashi A, Ohta S, Oyama F, Ihara Y: Association of transferrin C2 allele with late-onset Alzheimer's disease. Hum Genet 1997; 101:126–129.

Nee L, Polinsky RJ, Eldridge R, Weingartner H, Smallberg S, Ebert M: A family with histologically confirmed Alzheimer's disease. Arch Neurol 1983; 40:203–208.

Newens AJ, Forster DP, Kay DW, Kirkup W, Bates D, Edwardson J: Clinically diagnosed presenile dementia of the Alzheimer type in the Northern Health Region: ascertainment, prevalence, incidence and survival. Psychol Med 1993; 23:631–644.

Nishiyama M, Kato Y, Hashimoto M, Yukawa S, Omori K: Apolipoprotein E, methylenetetrahydrofolate reductase (MTHFR) mutation and the risk of senile dementia—an epidemiological study using the polymerase chain reaction (PCR) method. J Epidemiol 2000; 10:163–172.

Ogura C, Nakamoto H, Uema T, Yamamoto K, Yonemori T, Yoshimura T: Prevalence of senile dementia in Okinawa, Japan. COSEPO Group. Study Group of Epidemiology for Psychiatry in Okinawa. Int J Epidemiol 1995; 24:373–380.

Okuizumi K, Onodera O, Namba Y, Ikeda K, Yamamoto T, Seki K, Ueki A, Nanko S, Tanaka H, Takahashi H, et al.: Genetic association of very low density lipoprotein (VLDL) receptor gene locus with sporadic Alzheimer's disease. Nat Genet 1995; 11:207–209.

Okuizumi K, Onodera O, Tanaka H, Kabayaski H, Tsuji S, Takahashi H, Oyanagi K, Seki K, Tanaja M, Naruse S: ApoE-epsilon 4 and early-onset Alzheimer's disease. Nat Genet 1994; 7:10–11.

Oliveira JR, Gallindo RM, Maia LG, Brito-Marques PR, Otto PA, Passos-Bueno MR, Morais MAJ, Zatz M: The short variant of the polymorphism within the promoter region of the serotonin transporter gene is a risk factor for late onset Alzheimer's disease. Mol Psychiatry 1998; 3:438–441.

Ott A, Slooter AJC, Hofman A, van Harskamp F, Witteman JC, Van Broeckhoven C, van Duijn CM, Breteler MM: Smoking and risk of dementia and Alzheimer's disease in a population-based cohort study: the Rotterdam Study [see comments]. Lancet 1998; 351:1840–1843.

Paganini-Hill A, Henderson VW: Estrogen deficiency and risk of Alzheimer's disease in women. Am J Epidemiol 1994; 140:256–261.

Papassotiropoulos A, Bagli M, Feder O, Jessen F, Maier W, Rao ML, Ludwig M, Schwab SG, Heun R: Genetic polymorphism of cathepsin D is strongly associated with the risk for developing sporadic Alzheimer's disease. Neurosci Lett 1999a; 262:171–174.

Papassotiropoulos A, Bagli M, Jessen F, Bayer TA, Maier W, Rao ML, Heun R: A genetic variation of the inflammatory cytokine interleukin-6 delays the initial onset and reduces the risk for sporadic Alzheimer's disease. Ann Neurol 1999b; 45:666–668.

Pericak-Vance MA, Bass MP, Yamaoka LH, Gaskell PC, Scott WK, Terwedow HA, Menold MM, Conneally PM, Small GW, Vance JM, et al.: Complete genomic screen in late-onset familial Alzheimer disease: evidence for a new locus on chromosome 12. JAMA 1997; 278:1237–1241.

Pericak-Vance MA, Bebout JL, Gaskell PC, Yamaoka LH, Hung W-Y, Alberts MJ, Walker AP, Bartlett RJ, Haynes CS, Welsh KA, et al.: Linkage studies in familial Alzheimer's disease: evidence for chromosome 19 linkage. Am J Hum Genet 1991; 48:1034–1050.

Pericak-Vance MA, Grubber J, Bailey LR, Hedges D, West S, Santoro L, Kemmerer B, Hall JL, Saunders AM, Roses AD, et al.: Identification of novel genes in late-onset Alzheimer's disease. Exp Gerontol 2000; 35:1343–1352.

Pericak-Vance MA, Johnson CC, Rimmler JB, Saunders AM, Robinson LC, D'Hondt

EG, Jackson CE, Haines JL: Alzheimer's disease and apolipoprotein E-4 allele in an Amish population. Ann Neurol 1996; 39:700–704.

Pericak-Vance MA, Yamaoka LH, Haynes CS, Speer MC, Haines JL, Gaskell PC, Hung W-Y, Clark CM, Heyman A, Trofatter J, et al.: Genetic linkage studies in Alzheimer's disease families. Exp Neurol 1988; 102:271–279.

Perry R, McKeith I, Perry E: Lewy body dementia—clinical, pathological and neurochemical interconnections. J Neural Transm 1997; 51:95–109.

Plassman BL, Havlik RJ, Steffens DC, Helms MJ, Newman TN, Drosdick D, Phillips C, Gau BA, Welsh-Bohmer KA, Burke JR, et al.: Documented head injury in early adulthood and risk of Alzheimer's disease and other dementias. Neurology 2000; 55:1158–1166.

Poirier J, Delisle MC, Quirion R, Aubert I, Farlow M, Lahiri D, Hui S, Bertrand P, Nalbantoglu J, Gilfix BM: Apolipoprotein E4 allele as a predictor of cholinergic deficits and treatment outcome in Alzheimer disease. Proc Natl Acad Sci USA 1995; 92:12260–12264.

Polvikoski T, Sulkava R, Myllykangas L, Notkola IL, Niinisto L, Verkkoniemi A, Kainulainen K, Kontula K, Perez-Tur J, Hardy J, et al.: Prevalence of Alzheimer's disease in very elderly people: a prospective neuropathological study. Neurology 2001; 56:1690–1696.

Prencipe M, Casini AR, Ferretti C, Lattanzio MT, Fiorelli M, Culasso F: Prevalence of dementia in an elderly rural population: effects of age, sex, and education. J Neurol Neurosurg Psychiatry 1996; 60:628–633.

Pritchard ML, Saunders AM, Gaskell PC, Small GW, Conneally PM, Rosi BL, Yamaoka LH, Roses AD, Haines JL, Pericak-Vance MA: No association between very low density lipoprotein receptor (VLDL-R) and Alzheimer disease in American Caucasians. Neurosci Lett 1996; 209:105–108.

Ragione FD, Takabayashi K, Mastropietro S, Mercurio C, Oliva A, Russo GL, DellaPietra V, Borriello A, Nobori T, Carson DA, Zappia V: Purification and characterization of recombinant human 5′-methylthioadenosine phosphorylase: definite identification of coding cDNA. Biochem Biophys Res Commun 1996; 223:514–519.

Rao VS, Cupples A, van Duijn CM, Kurz A, Green RC, Chui H, Duara R, Auerbach SA, Volicer L, Wells J, et al.: Evidence for major gene inheritance of Alzheimer disease in families of patients with and without apolipoprotein E epsilon 4. Am J Hum Genet 1996; 59:664–675.

Rao VS, van Duijn CM, Connor-Lacke L, Cupples LA, Growdon JH, Farrer LA: Multiple etiologies for Alzheimer disease are revealed by segregation analysis. Am J Hum Genet 1994; 55:991–1000.

Rasmusson DX, Brandt J, Martin DB, Folstein MF: Head injury as a risk factor in Alzheimer's disease. Brain Inj 1995; 9:213–219.

Rasmusson DX, Brandt J, Steele C, Hedreen JC, Troncoso JC, Folstein MF: Accuracy of clinical diagnosis of Alzheimer disease and clinical features of patients with non-Alzheimer disease neuropathology. Alzheimer Dis Assoc Disord 1996; 10:180–188.

Relkin NR, Kwon YJ, Tsai J, Gandy S: The National Institute on Aging/Alzheimer's Association recommendations on the application of apolipoprotein E genotyping to Alzheimer's disease. Ann N Y Acad Sci 1996; 802:149–176.

Relkin NR, Younga JK, Tsai J, Gandy SE: The National Institute on Aging/Alzheimer's Association recommendations on the application of apolipoprotein E genotyping to Alzheimer's disease. Ann N Y Acad Sci 1998; 802:149–171.

Renvoize EB: An HLA and family study of Alzheimer's disease. Psychol Med 1984; 14:515–520.

Reynolds WF, Rhees J, Maciejewski D, Paladino T, Sieburg H, Maki RA, Masliah E: Myeloperoxidase polymorphism is associated with gender specific risk for Alzheimer's disease. Exp Neurol 1999; 155:31–41.

Risch N: Linkage strategies for genetically complex traits I. Multilocus models. Am J Hum Genet 1990a; 46:222–228.

Risch N: Linkage strategies for genetically complex traits II. The power of affected relative pairs. Am J Hum Genet 1990b; 46:229–241.

Risch N: Linkage strategies for genetically complex traits III. The effect of marker polymorphism on analysis of affected pairs. Am J Hum Genet 1990c; 46:242–253.

Roberts GW, Gentleman SM, Lynch A: Beta-amyloid protein deposition in the brain after severe head injury. J Neurol Neurosurg Psychiatry 1994; 57:419–425.

Rocca WA, Hofman A, Brayne C, Breteler MM, Clarke M, Copeland JR, Dartigues JF, Engedal K, Hagnell O, Heeren TJ: Frequency and distribution of Alzheimer's disease in Europe: a collaborative study of 1980–1990 prevalence findings. The EURODEM-Prevalence Research Group. Ann Neurol 1991; 30:381–390.

Rogaev EI, Sherrington R, Rogaeva EA, Levesque G, Ikeda M, Liang G, Chi H, Lin C, Holman K, Tsuda T, et al.: Familial Alzheimer's disease in kindreds with missense mutations in a gene on chromosome 1 related to the Alzheimer's disease type 3 gene. Nature 1995; 376:775–778.

Rogaeva E, Premkumar S, Song Y, Sorbi S, Brindle N, Paterson A, Duara R, Levesque G, Yu G, Nishimura M, et al.: Evidence for an Alzheimer disease susceptibility locus on chromosome 12 and for further locus heterogeneity. JAMA 1998; 280:614–618.

Rogaeva EA, Premkumar S, Grubber J, Serneels L, Scott WK, Kawarai T, Song Y, Hill DL, Abou-Donia SM, Martin ER, et al.: An alpha-2-macroglobulin insertion-deletion polymorphism in Alzheimer disease [letter] [see comments]. Nat Genet 1999; 22:19–22.

Roses AD, Devlin B, Conneally PM, Small GW, Saunders AM, Pritchard M, Locke PA, Haines JL, Pericak-Vance MA, Risch N: Measuring the genetic contribution of APOE in late-onset Alzheimer disease (AD). Am J Hum Genet 1995; 57:A202.

Roses AD, Pericak-Vance MA: Alzheimer's disease and other dementias. In: Connon JM (ed). Emery and Rimoin's Principles and Practice of Medical Genetics. Edinburgh: New York: Churchill Livingstone, 1997:1807–1825.

Roses AD, Saunders AM, Corder EH, Risch NJ, Haines JL, Pericak-Vance MA, Han S-H, Einstein G, Hulette C, Schmechel DE, et al.: Apolipoprotein E and Alzheimer disease. In: Shibuya T (ed). New Drug Design for the Treatment of Neurological and Mental Disorders. Basel: Karger, 1996:187–197.

Rudrasingham V, Wavrant-DeVrieze F, Lambert JC, Chakraverty S, Kehoe P, Crook R, Amouyel P, Wu W, Rice F, Perez-Tur J, et al.: Alpha-2 macroglobulin gene and Alzheimer disease [letter] [see comments]. Nat Genet 1999; 22:17–19.

Sadovnick AD, Irwin ME, Baird PA, Beattle BL: Genetic studies on an Alzheimer clinic population. Genet Epidemiol 1989; 6:663–643.

Sanchez L, Alvarez V, Gonzalez P, Gonzalez I, Alvarez R, Coto E: Variation in the LRP-associated protein gene (*LRPAP1*) is associated with late-onset Alzheimer disease. Am J Med Genet 2001; 105:76–78.

Saunders AM, Schmader KE, Breitner JC, Benson MD, Brown WT, Goldfarb L, Goldgaber D, Manwaring MG, Szymanski MH, McCown N, et al.: Apolipoprotein E ϵ4 allele distributions in late-onset Alzheimer's disease and in other amyloid-forming diseases. Lancet 1993a; 342:710–711.

Saunders AM, Strittmatter WJ, Breitner JC, Schmechel D, St George-Hyslop PH, Pericak-Vance MA, Joo SH, Rosi BL, Gusella JF, Crapper-MacLachlan DR, et al.: Association of apolipoprotein E allele 4 with late-onset familial and sporadic Alzheimer's disease. Neurology 1993b; 43:1467–1472.

Savory J, Exley C, Forbes WF, Huang Y, Joshi JG, Kruck T, McLachlan DR, Wakayama I: Can the controversy of the role of aluminum in Alzheimer's disease be resolved? What are the suggested approaches to this controversy and methodological issues to be considered? J Toxicol Environ Health 1996; 48:615–635.

Schellenberg GD, Bird TD, Wijsman EM, Orr HT, Anderson L, Nemens E, White JA, Bonnycastle L, Weber JL, Alonso ME: Genetic linkage evidence for a familial Alzheimer's disease locus on chromosome 14. Science 1992; 258:668–671.

Schellenberg GD, Deeb SS, Boehnke M, Bryant EM, Martin GM, Lampe TH, Bird TD: Association of an apolipoprotein CII allele with familial dementia of the Alzheimer type. J Neurogenet 1987; 4:97–108.

Schoenberg BS: Environmental risk factors for Parkinson's disease: the epidemiologic evidence. Can J Neurol Sci 1987; 14:407–413.

Schoenberg BS, Anderson DW, Haerer AF: Prevalence and clinical features of dementia in a biracial population: neuroepidemiological study of a county in rural Mississippi. Trans Am Neurol Assoc 1981; 106:22–25.

Schupf N, Kapell D, Lee JH, Ottman R, Mayeux R: Increased risk of Alzheimer's disease in mothers of adults with Down's syndrome [see comments]. Lancet 1994; 344:353–356.

Scott WK, Saunders AM, Gaskell PC, Locke PA, Growdon JH, Farrer LA, Auerbach SA, Roses AD, Haines JL, Pericak-Vance MA: Apolipoprotein E ϵ2 does not increase risk of early-onset sporadic Alzheimer disease. Ann Neurol 1997; 42:376–378.

Scott WK, Yamaoka LH, Bass MP, Gaskell PC, Conneally PM, Small GW, Farrer LA, Auerbach SA, Saunders AM, Roses AD, et al.: No genetic association between the LRP receptor and sporadic or late-onset familial Alzheimer disease. Neurogenetics 1998; 1:179–183.

Sherrington R, Rogaev E, Liang Y, Rogaeva EA, Levesque G, Ikeda M, Chi H, Lin C, Li G, Holman K, et al.: Cloning of a gene bearing missense mutations in early-onset familial Alzheimer's disease. Nature 1995; 375:754–760.

Shoffner JM, Brown MD, Torroni A, Lott MT, Cabell MF, Mirra SS, Beal MF, Yang CC, Gearing M, Salvo R: Mitochondrial DNA variants observed in Alzheimer disease and Parkinson disease patients. Genomics 1993; 17:171–184.

Sjogren T, Sjogren H, Lindgren AGH: Morbus Alzheimer and morbus Pick: a genetic, clinical and patho-anatomical study. Acta Psychiatr Neurol Scand 1952; 82:1–66.

Slooter AJ, Bronzova J, Witteman JC, Van Broeckhoven C, Hofman A, van Duijn CM: Estrogen use and early onset Alzheimer's disease: a population-based study. J Neurol Neurosurg Psychiatry 1999; 67:779–781.

Slooter AJC, Cruts M, Kalmijn S, Hofman A, Breteler MM, Van Broeckhoven C, van Duijn CM: Risk estimates of dementia by apolipoprotein E genotypes from a population-based incidence study: the Rotterdam Study. Arch Neurol 1998; 55:964–968.

Small GW, Ebeling SC, Matsuyama SS, Heyman A, Reisner EG, Renvoize EB, Sulkava R: Variable association of HLA-A2 in men with early-onset Alzheimer disease. Neurobiol Aging 1991; 12:375–377.

Snow AD, Wight TN, Nochlin D, Koike Y, Kimata K, DeArmond SJ, Prusiner SB: Immunolocalization of heparan sulfate proteoglycans to the prion protein amyloid plaques of Gerstmann-Straussler syndrome, Creutzfeldt-Jakob disease and scrapie. Lab Invest 1990; 63:601–611.

Snowdon DA, Kemper SJ, Mortimer JA, Greiner LH, Wekstein DR, Markesbery WR: Linguistic ability in early life and cognitive function and Alzheimer's disease in late life. Findings from the Nun Study [see comments]. JAMA 1996; 275:528–532.

Sorbi S, Nacmias B, Forleo P, Latorraca S, Gobbini I, Bracco L, Piacentini S, Amaducci L: ApoE allele frequencies in Italian sporadic and familial Alzheimer's disease. Neurosci Lett 1994; 177:100–102.

Speck CE, Kukull WA, Brenner DE, Bowen JD, McCormick WC, Teri L, Pfanschmidt ML, Thompson JD, Larson EB: History of depression as a risk factor for Alzheimer's disease. Epidemiology 1995; 6:366–369.

Spence MA, Heyman A, Marazita ML, Sparkes RS, Weinberg T: Genetic linkage studies in Alzheimer's disease. Neurology 1986; 36:581–584.

Spielman RS, Ewens WJ: A sibship test for linkage in the presence of association: the sib transmission/disequilibrium test. Am J Hum Genet 1998; 61:450–458.

Spielman RS, McGinnis RE, Ewens WJ: Transmission test for linkage disequilibrium: the insulin gene region and insulin-dependent diabetes mellitus (IDDM). Am J Hum Genet 1993; 52:506–516.

Steffens DC, Plassman BL, Helms MJ, Welsh-Bohmer KA, Newman TT, Breitner JC: APOE and AD concordance in twin pairs as predictors of AD in first-degree relatives. Neurology 2000; 54:593–598.

Stern Y, Gurland B, Tatemichi TK, Tang MX, Wilder D, Mayeux R: Influence of education and occupation on the incidence of Alzheimer's disease. JAMA 1994; 271:1004–1010.

St George-Hyslop P, Haines JL, Rogaev E, Mortilla M, Vaula G, Pericak-Vance MA, Foncin J-F, Montesi M, Bruni A, Sorbi S: Genetic evidence for a novel familial Alzheimer's disease locus on chromosome 14. Nat Genet 1992; 2:330–334.

St George-Hyslop PH, Crapper-MacLachlan DR, Tuda T, Rogaev E: Alzheimer's disease and possible gene interaction. Science 1993; 263:537.

St George-Hyslop PH, Haines JL, Farrer LA, Polinsky RJ, Van Broeckhoven C, Goate AM, McLachlan DR, Orr H, Bruni AC, Sorbi S: Genetic linkage studies suggest that Alzheimer's disease is not a single homogenous disorder. Nature 1990; 347:194–197.

St George-Hyslop PH, Myers RH, Haines JL, Farrer LA, Tanzi RE, Abe K, James MF, Conneally PM, Polinsky RJ, Gusella JF: Familial Alzheimer's disease: progress and problems. Neurobiol Aging 1989; 10:417–425.

St George-Hyslop PH, Tanzi RE, Polinsky RJ, Haines JL, Watkins PC, Myers RH, Feldman RG, Pollen D, Drachman D: The genetic defect causing familial Alzheimer's disease maps on chromosome 21. Science 1987; 235:885–890.

Strittmatter WJ, Saunders AM, Schmechel D, Pericak-Vance MA, Enghild J, Salvesen GS, Roses AD: Apolipoprotein E: high avidity binding to beta-amyloid and increased frequency of type 4 allele in late-onset familial Alzheimer's disease. Proc Natl Acad Sci USA 1993; 90:1977–1981.

Tanaka S, Chen X, Xia Y, Kang DE, Matoh N, Sundsmo M, Thomas RG, Katzman R, Thal LJ, Trojanowski JQ, et al.: Association of CYP2D microsatellite polymorphism with Lewy body variant of Alzheimer's disease. Neurology 1998; 50:1556–1562.

Tang MX, Jacobs D, Stern Y, Marder K, Schofield P, Gurland B, Andrews H, Mayeux R: Effect of oestrogen during menopause on risk and age at onset of Alzheimer's disease [see comments]. Lancet 1996; 348:429–432.

Tanzi RE, Gusella JF, Watkins PC, Bruns GA, St George-Hyslop P, Van Keuren ML, Patterson D, Pagan S, Kurnit DM, Neve RL: Amyloid beta protein gene: cDNA, mRNA distribution, and genetic linkage near the Alzheimer locus. Science 1987a; 235:880–884.

Tanzi RE, St George-Hyslop PH, Haines JL, Polinsky RJ, Nee L, Foncin JF, Neve RL, McClatchey AI, Conneally PM, Gusella JF: The genetic defect in familial Alzheimer's disease is not tightly linked to the amyloid beta-protein gene. Nature 1987b; 329:156–157.

Teng EL, Chui HC: The Modified Mini-Mental State (3MS) examination. J Clin Psychiatry 1987; 48:314–318.

Tierney MC, Fisher RH, Lewis AJ, Zorzitto ML, Snow WG, Reid DW, Nieuwstraten P: The NINCDS-ADRDA Work Group criteria for the clinical diagnosis of probable Alzheimer's disease: a clinicopathologic study of 57 cases [see comments]. Neurology 1988; 38:359–364.

Tsai SJ, Liu HC, Liu TY, Wang YC, Hong CJ: Association analysis of the 5-HT6 receptor polymorphism C267T in Alzheimer's disease. Neurosci Lett 1999; 276:138–139.

Van Broeckhoven C, Backhovens H, Cruts M: *APOE* genotype does not modulate age of onset in families with chromosome 14 encoded Alzheimer's disease. Neurosci Lett 1994; 169:179–180.

Van Broeckhoven C, Backhovens H, Cruts M, De Winter G, Bruyland M, Cras P, Martin JJ: Mapping of a gene predisposing to early-onset Alzheimer's disease to chromosome 14q24.3. Nat Genet 1992; 2:335–339.

van Duijn CM, Clayton DG, Chandra V, Fratiglioni L, Graves AB, Heyman A, Jorm AF, Kokmen E, Kondo K, Mortimer JA, et al.: Interaction between genetic and environmental risk factors for Alzheimer's disease: a reanalysis of case-control studies. EURODEM Risk Factors Research Group. Genet Epidemiol 1994a; 11:539–551.

van Duijn CM, deKnijff P, Cruts M, Wehnert A, Havekes LM, Hofman A, Van Broeckhoven C: Apolipoprotein E4 allele in a population-based study of early-onset Alzheimer's disease. Nat Genet 1994b; 7:74–78.

van Duijn CM, Farrer LA, Cupples LA, Hofman A: Genetic transmission of Alzheimer's disease among families in a Dutch population based study. J Med Genet 1993; 30:640–646.

van Duijn CM, Farrer LA, Cupples LA, Kurz A, Zimmerman R, Muller U, Green RC, Clarke V, Shoffner J, Wallace DC: Apolipoprotein E genotype in patients with Alzheimer's disease: implications for the risk of dementia among relatives. Ann Neurol 1995a; 38:797–808.

van Duijn CM, Havekes LM, Van Broeckhoven C, de Knijff P, Hofman A: Apolipoprotein E genotype and association between smoking and early onset Alzheimer's disease. BMJ 1995b; 310:627–631.

van Duijn CM, Stijnen T, Hofman A: Risk factors for Alzheimer's disease: overview of the EURODEM collaborative re-analysis of case-control studies. Int J Epidemiol 1991; 20:S4–S11.

Venter JC, Adams MD, Myers EW, Li PW, Mural RJ, Sutton GG, Smith HO, Yandell M, Evans CA, Holt RA, et al.: The sequence of the human genome. Science 2001; 291:1304–1351.

Weber JL, May PE: Abundant class of human DNA polymorphisms which can be typed using the polymerase chain reaction. Am J Hum Genet 1989; 44:388–396.

Weitkamp LR, Nee L, Keats B, Polinsky RJ, Guttormsen S: Alzheimer disease: evidence for susceptibility loci on chromosomes 6 and 14. Am J Hum Genet 1983; 35:443–453.

Welsh KA, Butters N, Hughes JP, Mohs RC, Heyman A: Detection and staging of dementia in Alzheimer's disease: use of the neuropsychological measures developed for the Consortium to Establish a Registry for Alzheimer's Disease. Arch Neurol 1992; 49:448–452.

Welsh-Bohmer KA, Gearing M, Saunders AM, Roses AD, Mirra S: Apolipoprotein E genotypes in a neuropathological series from the Consortium to Establish a Registry for Alzheimer's Disease. Ann Neurol 1997; 42:319–325.

Whalley LJ, Thomas BM, Starr JM: Epidemiology of presenile Alzheimer's disease in Scotland (1974–88) II. Exposures to possible risk factors. Br J Psychiatry 1995; 167:732–738.

Wijker M, Wszolek ZK, Wolters EC, Rooimans MA, Pals G, Pfeiffer RF, Lynch T, Rodnitzky RL, Wilhelmsen KC, Arwert F: Localization of the gene for rapidly progressive autosomal dominant parkinsonism and dementia with pallido-ponto-nigral degeneration to chromosome 17q21. Hum Mol Genet 1996; 5:151–154.

Wisniewski KE, Dalton AJ, McLachlan C, Wen GY, Wisniewski HM: Alzheimer's disease in Down's syndrome: clinicopathologic studies. Neurology 1985; 35:957–961.

Wisniewski T, Frangione B: Apolipoprotein E: a pathological chaperone protein in patients with cerebral and systemic amyloid. Neurosci Lett 1992; 135:235–238.

Wisniewski T, Golabek A, Matsubara E, Ghiso J, Frangione B: Apolipoprotein E: binding to soluble Alzheimer beta-amyloid. Biochem Biophys Res Commun 1993; 192:359–365.

Wragg M, Hutton M, Talbot C, Alzheimer's Disease Collaborative Group: Genetic association between an intronic polymorphism in the presenilin 1 gene and late onset Alzheimer's disease. Lancet 1996; 347:509–512.

Xia Y, da Silva R, Rosi BL, Yamaoka LH, Rimmler JB, Pericak-Vance MA, Roses AD, Chen X, Masliah E, DeTeresa R, et al.: Genetic studies in Alzheimer's disease with an NACP/alpha-synuclein polymorphism. Ann Neurol 1996; 40:207–215.

44 Affective Disorders

SEVILLA D. DETERA-WADLEIGH AND LYNN R. GOLDIN

Bipolar affective disorder is a debilitating dysfunction of mood that is characterized by episodic and recurring oscillations of mania and depression. Family, twin, and adoption studies that span decades provide compelling evidence for a genetic etiology and a likely contribution of environmental factors to trigger full expression of the disease. Disentangling its biological complexity has been formidable and vexing. In fact, the past history of affective disorder genetics has been marked by uncertainty and ambivalence (Risch and Botstein, 1996). By contrast, now the field seems to be experiencing a revival because promising findings of potential susceptibility regions have begun to unfold.

Bipolar disorder and unipolar major depression have a combined prevalence rate of ~7%, indicating the pervasive reach of these diseases in the population. Global Burden of Disease (GBD) surveys conducted by the World Health Organization in recent years document the profound effect of mood disorders on families, the health care system, the economy, and society as a whole. In the GBD survey of 1999, unipolar major depression and bipolar disorder were respectively ranked as the fifth and twentieth leading causes of "disability-adjusted life years" (DALY), defined as premature mortality and years lost due to disability (Michaud et al., 2001). In the United States alone, a survey in 1996 revealed that unipolar major depression was the tenth and second leading cause of DALY, in men and women, respectively, and this is a cogent depiction of the magnitude of burden on even the most advanced economy in the world. Mortality due to unipolar disorder was estimated at 1 in 1000 (Michaud et al., 2001), highlighting the striking loss of productivity of individuals afflicted with this illness. It is stunning that unipolar major depression was projected to be the second leading cause of DALY worldwide in the year 2020 (Murray and Lopez, 1997).

The sequencing of the human genome (International Human Genome Sequencing Consortium, 2001; Venter et al., 2001) provides an unparalleled foothold for the dissection of complex disease etiology. The comprehensive cataloging of all human genes in every region of every chromosome would boost the momentum toward the identification of susceptibility genes and, in turn, hasten the development of tools for early and accurate diagnosis, investigations on function of disease-predisposing genes and gene–environment interactions, progress in formulating preventive modalities, and drug discovery and drug response prediction. Advances in these efforts may help reduce the burden attributable to mood disorders and other complex diseases.

This chapter will review data demonstrating familial aggregation of affective disorders and the current status of the search for genomic regions that contain susceptibility genes; we also discuss future strategies that need to be applied to find these genes. Several reviews on various aspects of the genetics of affective disorders have been published recently (Blackwood and Muir, 2001; Detera-Wadleigh, 2001; Evans et al., 2001; Jones and Craddock, 2001; Niculescu III and Kelsoe, 2001; Prathikanti and McMahon, 2001).

DIAGNOSTIC CRITERIA

Diagnoses of the major psychiatric disorders in the past several decades have become more precise and reliable by the widespread use of structured assessment and the application of standardized criteria (such as the Research Diagnostic Criteria [RDC]; Spitzer et al., 1978) or the *Diagnostic and Statistical Manual of Mental Disorders*, 4th ed (*DSM-IV*; American Psychiatric Association, 1994). The affective (or mood) disorders are a class of psychiatric disorders that include depression and mania. The classic affective disorder is bipolar affective disorder (manic-depressive illness), which is characterized by episodes of mania and depression. Unipolar illness (major depression) is characterized by episodes of depression only. Typically, individuals are symptom free between episodes. There are rare individuals who experience episodes of mania only, but these individuals are considered to have bipolar disorder since they respond to similar drugs as do classic bipolar patients and it is assumed that such individuals will eventually experience depressive episodes.

Tables 44–1 and 44–2 summarize the *DSM-IV* criteria for a major depressive episode and manic episode, respectively. Episodes of depression are characterized by depressed mood, loss of interest in usual activities, feelings of worthlessness, insomnia or hypersomnia, suicidal thoughts, and others. Episodes of mania are characterized by euphoric or irritable mood, grandiosity, flight of ideas, decreased need for sleep, and others. Milder forms of mood disorders, such as minor depression and hypomania, can also be diagnosed. Bipolar individuals are often divided into those who have depressive and manic episodes (bipolar I) and those who have depressive and hypomanic episodes (bipolar II). Schizoaffective disorder refers to patients who meet criteria for an affective disorder but also experience the psychotic symptoms such as hallucinations and delusions that occur in schizophrenic individuals.

GENERAL GENETIC AND EPIDEMIOLOGIC EVIDENCE

Prevalence

The lifetime prevalence of bipolar disorder ranges from 0.5% to 1.0% (Boyd and Weissman, 1981). The range for unipolar de-

Table 44–1. DSM-IV Criteria for Major Depressive Episode

Criterion	Symptom
A. Five or more of the nine symptoms have been present during the same two-week period and represent a change from previous functioning: at least one symptom is depressed mood or loss of interest.	1. Depressed mood most of the day nearly every day 2. Markedly diminished interest or pleasure in almost all activities 3. Significant weight loss or weight gain 4. Insomnia or hypersomnia nearly every day 5. Psychomotor agitation or retardation nearly every day 6. Fatigue or loss of energy nearly every day 7. Feelings of worthlessness or excessive or inappropriate guilt 8. Diminished ability to think or concentrate 9. Recurrent thoughts of death or suicide
B. Marked impairment in occupational or social functioning	
C. Symptoms not due to substance abuse, medication, or other medical conditions	
D. Symptoms not due to recent bereavement	

pression is very large and partly due to different diagnostic criteria that can be applied, such as length and severity of episode and number of episodes (Coryell et al., 1981). A study of rates in a national sample in the United States found that the lifetime prevalence of *DSM-IIIR* major depressive episode to be 17.1% (13% in men and 21% in women; Blazer et al., 1994). A recent analysis of a cross-national sample found the lifetime rates for depression to vary between 1.5% and 19% in the 10 different countries studied when the same methods were used in each location (Weissman et al, 1996); however, the rates of bipolar disorder were more consistent, varying from 0.3% to 1.5%.

Age of Onset and Sex Differences

The median age of onset for bipolar illness is in the mid-20s and for unipolar illness about 30 (Gershon et al., 1982), with onsets starting in adolescence. Childhood onset of affective disorder is rare, but these patients and their families have been studied to determine if childhood onset is associated with a higher genetic loading. This will be discussed in more detail later. The prevalence of bipolar illness has been found to be approximately equal in males and females, but the prevalence of unipolar depression is usually found to be approximately 2-fold higher in women. Data from a number of different studies are described by Weissman et al. (1993, 1996) and show that the approximately 2:1 female : male ratio was found in several different populations where both different diagnostic criteria and measurements of risk were applied. Even with the increase in rates of depression over recent decades (see below), the gender difference is still present (Leon et al., 1993).

Cohort Effect

A cohort effect has been found in mood disorders in a number of studies (both epidemiological and family) where individuals born after 1940 have significantly higher lifetime rates of affective illness and suicide than do cohorts born earlier (Solomon and Hellon, 1980; Hagnell et al., 1982; Robins et al., 1984; Klerman et al., 1985; Gershon et al., 1987; Wittchen et al., 1994). In fact, epidemiological studies show increases for every decade of birth since 1940. There is also evidence for a period effect, where more onsets of affective disorder took place during the 1960s and 1970s (Lavori et al., 1987). Recent data also show the increase in childhood onsets of affective disorder in recently born cohorts (Joyce et al., 1990; Ryan et al., 1992). This secular effect must represent some environmental influences on the susceptibility to development of affective disorders but could also be partly due to artifacts of recall or reporting. For example, one study found that, in all age groups, the reporting of the first onset of depression clustered in the 10-year period before the study (Simon and Von Korff, 1992). A different study involving reinterview of relatives several years after initial interview found no differences in recall between the two interviews for each subject (Warshaw et al., 1991). Other conditions such as drug and alcohol abuse are also more frequent in younger cohorts. However, the increase in depression is not simply due to comorbid-

Table 44–2. Summary of DSM-IV Criteria for Manic Episode

Criterion	Symptom
A. A distinct period of abnormally and persistently elevated, expansive, or irritable mood, lasting at least one week (or any duration if hospitilization required)	
B. Three or more of the symptoms must be present during the mood disturbance	1. Inflated self-esteem or grandiosity 2. Decreased need for sleep 3. More talkative 4. Flight of ideas 5. Distractibility 6. Increase in goal-directed activity 7. Excessive involvement in pleasurable activities that have a high potential for painful consequences
C. Marked impairment in occupational or social functioning	
D. Symptoms not due to substance abuse, medication, or other medical conditions	

ity with alcohol or drug abuse (Klerman et al., 1996). Whatever the explanation, the cohort effect will bias genetic studies because relatives from several cohorts will be pooled for risk estimates. Thus, segregation and linkage analyses must take the birth cohort of an individual into account.

Family Epidemiology

Family Studies

Prevalences in Relatives. The familial concentration of affective disorders is evident in several case-control and numerous other family studies (see Table 44–3). These data show the risk of affective disorder to first-degree relatives of bipolar and unipolar and control patients in studies since 1970. Earlier family studies are described by Tsuang and Faraone (1990). While the prevalences vary substantially among studies, it can be seen that first-degree relatives of bipolar probands have a several-fold higher prevalence of both bipolar and unipolar disorders than do relatives of controls. The relatives of unipolar patients have a several-fold higher risk of unipolar disorders but only a slightly higher risk of bipolar disorder than do controls. The large variation among studies in prevalence is most likely due to differences in diagnostic definitions, proband ascertainment, and other clinical methods.

Age of Onset-Related Risk. A number of studies have examined the recurrence risk in relatives as a function of the age of onset of the proband. Tsuang and Faraone (1990) tabulated 19 family studies that examined morbidity risk of early- vs. late-onset probands (generally dividing early vs. late onset at 40 years) and found that the risks were higher in early-onset probands in 17 of the 19 studies. Some studies have also found that relatives of childhood onset cases have increased risks of affective disorder, compared to relatives of normal controls (Puig-Antich et al., 1989; Todd et al., 1993). Later, Neuman et al. (1997) found that the relatives of prepubertal probands had a lifetime risk of affective disorder twice that of relatives of adult probands, even when controlling for birth cohort. This suggests that very early age of onset may identify a form of affective illness with a greater genetic loading.

Table 44–3. Lifetime Prevalence of Affective Illness in First-Degree Relatives of Patients and Controls

Study	Bipolar (%)	Unipolar (%)
A. Bipolar probands		
Goetzl et al., 1974	2.8	13.7
Helzer and Winokur, 1974	4.6	10.6
Mendlewicz and Rainer, 1974	17.7	22.4
Gershon et al., 1975	3.8	8.7
James and Chapman, 1975	6.4	13.2
Johnson and Leeman, 1977	15.5	19.8
Pettersen, 1977	3.6	7.2
Smeraldi et al., 1977	5.8	7.1
Angst et al., 1980	2.5	7.0
Taylor et al., 1980	4.8	4.2
Tsuang et al., 1980	5.3	12.4
Gershon et al., 1982	8.0	14.9
Fieve et al., 1984		
Rice et al., 1987	10.4	23.1
Sadovnick et al., 1994	3.5	5.7
B. Unipolar probands		
Gershon et al., 1975	2.1	14.2
Smeraldi et al., 1977	0.6	8.0
Angst et al., 1980	0.1	5.9
Taylor et al., 1980	4.1	8.3
Tsuang et al., 1980	3.0	15.2
Gershon et al., 1982	2.9	16.6
Weissman et al., 1984 (severe)	2.1	17.5
Rice et al., 1987	5.4	28.6
Sadovnick et al., 1994	0.65	5.5
C. Normal probands		
Gershon et al., 1975	0.2	0.7
Tsuang et al., 1980	0.3	7.5
Gershon et al., 1982	0.5	5.8
Weissman et al., 1984	1.8	5.6

Anticipation. Over the last few years, it has been shown that some neurological disorders are caused by trinucleotide repeats (reviewed in La Spada, 1997). These disorders also show anticipation where each generation in a pedigree may have earlier onset of disease or a more severe disease due to continued expansion of repeat sequences. Some studies have addressed the question of anticipation in psychiatric disorders. Two studies of anticipation in bipolar pedigrees (Nylander et al., 1994; McInnis et al., 1993) and one in unipolar disorder (Engstrom et al., 1995) found earlier age of onset in the offspring generation than in the parent generation. The study by McInnis et al. (1993) also controlled for cohort effect. One study (Grigoroiu-Serebanescu et al., 1997) looked at families of a group of bipolar probands (unselected for having family history) and found that the parental generation had a higher age of onset than the offspring generation. Despite these positive results, it is hard to conclude that anticipation is present in psychiatric disorders because of possible ascertainment bias (Hodge and Wickramaratne, 1995). The families most likely to be ascertained will have probands with early onset and parents with later onset since individuals with early onset of severe mental illness are less likely to become parents. Nonetheless, a number of studies have looked for expansion of trinucleotide repeats in bipolar disorder (see below).

Twin Studies

The clear difference between monozygotic (MZ) and dizygotic (DZ) twin concordance in numerous twin studies of affective illness over a 70-year period argues strongly for heritability of affective illness. The concordances range from 33% to 93% in MZ twins and from 0% to 24% in DZ twins (Tsuang and Faraone, 1990). The twin study by Bertelsen et al. (1977) is the most methodologically sound since the investigators used the Danish Twin Registry from which they identified affectively ill probands. Psychiatric information from twins of patients was obtained by case history and personal interviews. This study found an MZ concordance rate of 67% and a DZ concordance rate of 20%. The concordance for bipolar disorder was higher than the concordance for unipolar disorder.

More recently, twin studies have gone a step beyond simply looking at heritability of bipolar and unipolar disorder. Large samples from twin registries have been analyzed with more sophisticated models to test the importance of genetic and environmental factors in the liability to depression and related disorders (Kendler et al., 1992, 1995a, 1995b; Karkowski and Kendler, 1997). From these studies, there is some evidence that liability to depression is due to genetic factors and individual environmental factors, but not to shared environmental factors (Kendler et al., 1992, 1995a). Genetic factors also explain some of the co-morbidity between anxiety disorders and affective disorders (Kendler et al., 1995b).

Adoption Studies

Adoption studies also provide support for heritability of major affective disorders. Mendlewicz and Rainer (1977) reported on a study of bipolar adoptees. They found affective disorder in 31% of the biological parents of these probands compared with 2% in biological parents of normal adoptees. Another study (Schulsinger et al., 1979) found that biological relatives of 71 adoptees with affective disorder had a higher frequency of suicide (3.9%) than did biologic relatives of control group of adoptees (0.3%). A study in Sweden (von Knorring et al., 1983) found no increased frequency of affective illness in biological relatives of adoptees with affective disorder; however, most of the adoptees had milder depressions. Wender et al. (1986) carried out an adoption study of affective disorders in Denmark similar in design to their earlier landmark study of schizophrenia (Kety et al., 1976). They ascertained adoptees who had been hospitalized for an affective disorder and then searched for hospitalization records for biologic relatives of these adoptees and those of a matched control group. They found an increase of severe affective disorders (but not of mild affective disorders) in the biologic relatives of the affectively ill adoptees over biologic relatives of control adoptees.

Associations with Other Diseases: Affective Disorders Spectrum

It is also of interest to determine which other psychiatric disorders aggregate in families of affective disorders patients. Schizoaffective disorder has been described above and is associated with bipolar illness in families. Relatives of schizoaffective individuals have the highest prevalence of affective disorders (Gershon et al., 1982). One study divided schizoaffective into bipolar and depressed subtypes and found that the bipolar subtype had similar familial risks as do bipolar patients, but the depressed subtype was associated with more schizophrenia in relatives (Andreasen et al, 1987). There is substantial co-morbidity of affective disorders and alcoholism (Regier et al., 1990; Maier et al., 1995), but there does not appear to be an increase in alcoholism in families of affective disorders patients unless the proband has co-morbid alcoholism (Winokur et al., 1996). Recently, analyses of genome scan data was performed on the NIMH Genetics Initiative bipolar disorder families and families from the Collaborative Study of the Genetics of Alcoholism to identify regions linked to the three phenotypes of co-morbid alcoholism and depression, alcoholism or depression, and depression (Nurnberger et al., 2001). The highest ASPEX multipoint lod score was 5.12 at markers on 1p33–p22 for alcoholism or depression. When analysis was performed for the co-morbid alcoholism and depression phenotype, the strongest evidence of linkage was at D2S1371 (lod = 4.12), on 2q35. These results imply possible sharing of molecular components that underlie the risk for alcoholism and affective disorders. MacKinnon et al. (1998) evaluated the co-morbidity of panic disorder with affective disorder in a panel of families that displayed evidence of linkage on 18q. Their analysis revealed that families whose probands had panic attacks produced the strongest evidence of linkage on 18q. A number of studies have supported a genetic relationship between anorexia and affective disorders where first-degree relatives of anorexics have an increased risk of affective illness (Cantwell et al., 1977; Winokur et al., 1980; Gershon et al., 1984). However, there is no increase in anorexia in the relatives of bipolar patients, probably due to its rarity in the population.

MODELS OF GENETIC TRANSMISSION

A number of different approaches have been used to model the genetic transmission of affective disorders. Some studies have tested whether the probability of a relative being ill is related to factors such as the sex, age, and cohort of the relative and to characteristics of the proband such as sex and age of onset. Some of these factors have already been discussed. Studies have found that sex of the proband does not affect the risk to relatives (Smeraldi et al., 1981; Weissman et al., 1984). This allows us to rule out a class of models that assume different genetic liabilities for males and females. In two sets of pedigrees ascertained for linkage (i.e., multiple cases), mothers of probands were more often affected than were fathers of probands (McMahon et al., 1995; Gershon et al, 1996). It is hard to draw conclusions about a parent of origin effect since these findings were not derived from systematically ascertained families from the population. However, in a family study of systematically ascertained probands, a maternal effect was detected (Rice et al., 1984).

A number of analyses have assumed that there is an underlying continuous liability to affective disorders as a result of additive genetic and environmental factors. Some studies have found the family data to be consistent with a continuum of liability where unipolar is less severe than bipolar disorder (Gershon et al., 1982; Tsuang et al., 1985a). Other studies have found this model to be inconsistent with familial prevalences (Price et al., 1985).

A number of segregation analyses have been carried out to determine if the transmission in families could be modeled as a single major locus. Ideally, a study should test both single locus and polygenic alternatives. Most of these studies have found that a single major locus is inconsistent with the family data or that Mendelian transmission can be rejected (Bucher and Elston, 1981; Crowe et al., 1981; Goldin et al., 1983; Tsuang et al., 1985b; Rice et al., 1987; Cox et al., 1989; Sham et al., 1991). A segregation analysis of affective disorder in several extended pedigrees from the Old Order Amish reported by Pauls et al. (1995) found that a single dominant locus for bipolar I illness could be supported in a subset of families that were more closely related; however, a large number of analyses were carried out, and the findings did not hold for any other diagnostic classification or for the whole series of families. Spence et al. (1995) found that a single dominant locus was not rejected for bipolar illness, although a polygenic model could not be tested. Marazita et al. (1997) carried out segregation analysis in a sample of early-onset (less than 25 years) recurrent unipolar patients. They found evidence for a single locus when affective disorder was defined as either bipolar or unipolar; they also found significant residual parent and spouse effects.

It has been argued that single-locus and even two-locus models are not compatible with familial recurrence risks when MZ twin concordances are included (Neuman and Rice, 1992; Craddock et al., 1995). The study by Craddock et al. (1995) examined the constraints of allele frequencies and penetrances on the population prevalence and recurrence risks in relatives for bipolar disorder only. Assuming that the risks for MZ twins is .45 to .75, for siblings' parents, and offspring is .045 to .09 and that the population risk is .005 to .015, they found that single-locus and two-locus models were not compatible but multiplicative models with three or more loci were consistent with the data. Relevant to this discussion is the exchange of letters between Craddock et al. (1997) and Spence et al. (1997).

It appears that the weight of the evidence is against there being a single major locus that could account for the familial aggregation of affective disorders. Since the goal in complex disease genetics is to detect susceptibility loci, even those with relatively small effects, it is not necessary to have evidence for a single major locus from segregation analysis of a trait in order to proceed with gene searches. Risch (1990a) has developed an approach to determine what is the largest effect of any one locus that can account for population, family, and twin data. Risch defines λ_r as being the risk ratio of a relative of type r, the risk ratio being defined as the recurrence risk to relatives of type r compared to the population risk. If there is no dominance, then λ for parents will be the same as for sibs. Thus, λ_{sibs} is generally the most reliable measurement for complex traits with late onset. Given the midpoint of the prevalences shown above from Craddock et al. (1995), λ_{sibs} is about 6.7 and λ_{MZ} is about 60. For unipolar illness, the total λ_{sibs} is much lower. Based on the data of Gershon et al. (1982), shown here in Table 44–3, λ for first-degree relatives for unipolar illness is 2.6 in bipolar families and 2.9 in unipolar families. Different models can then be fitted to the values of λ_{sibs} and λ_{MZ} involving one or more genes. For example, there may be three multiplicative loci, each with a λ of 2 to account for a total λ of 6. Given the largest λ for any one locus, one can determine the number of families needed to detect linkage. Sample sizes of sib-pairs as a function of locus-specific λ have been given by Risch (1990b) and by Hauser et al. (1996) for the case of interval mapping. The advantage of this approach is that the disease can be due to a mechanism involving multiple genes, heterogeneity, and environmental factors, but one need only determine the likely locus-specific λ.

PATHOPHYSIOLOGY: BIOLOGIC BASIS OF GENETIC SUSCEPTIBILITY

One approach to unraveling the underlying biology of affective disorders is to find some biological measurement associated with illness. For many years, investigators have studied peripheral measures of enzymes of catecholamine metabolism, metabolites of neurotransmitters, neurotransmitter receptors, and others in hope of detecting biological markers that contributed to genetic vulnerability for affective disorders (see Goodwin and Jamison, 1990). Much knowledge has been obtained from studying the effects of antidepressant and antimanic drugs and also from studying the underlying biology of some of the symptoms of affective disorder, especially sleep and neuroendocrine disturbances. While these studies have contributed to understanding the biology of psychiatric disorders, they have not led to the identification of specific susceptibility genes. At this point, numerous genes have been identified that code for many interesting proteins involved in central nervous system function, including those previously studied in peripheral tissues. The emphasis has now shifted to looking for association of illness with mutations or polymorphisms of these candidate genes or studying the in vitro function of these genes. A number of genome-wide screens of affective disorder—that is, looking for genetic linkage to anonymous markers—have been reported and continue to be actively pursued by investigators on various sample collections. In addition, functional genomics is starting to be exploited in an attempt to peer into the global expression profile of an affected phenotype or models of that phenotype.

Gene Identification

Linkage studies of bipolar illness started well before the DNA era. These are reviewed by Tsuang and Faraone (1990). In the late 1980s up to the early 1990s, initial reports of strong linkage of bipolar disorder to chromosomes X and 11 could not be reproduced in follow-up studies in the original samples (Baron et al., 1987, 1993; Egeland et al., 1987; Kelsoe et al., 1989) or in independent cohorts (Detera-Wadleigh et al. 1987; Hodgkinson et al., 1987; Mendlewicz et al., 1987; Berrettini et al., 1990; Gejman et al., 1990). Early attempts to scan the genome have yielded rare, nonsignificant positive linkage signals (e.g., Coon et al., 1993; Detera-Wadleigh et al., 1994; LaBuda et al., 1996). The question then was whether any linkage for affective disorders would be detectable.

The recent advances in our knowledge of the human genome have provided powerful tools for a genetic approach to unraveling the biology of complex diseases. There is currently a very dense map of markers across the entire human genome that permits whole genome linkage analysis to any disorder. In bipolar disorder, several genome scans on independent data sets have been conducted (see below). Although some findings remain ambiguous, and in some cases possibly spurious, convincing data have begun to emerge.

A working draft of the human genome sequence is now publicly accessible (e.g., University of California Santa Cruz Genome Browser and Ensembl Genome Server of the Sanger Centre), and the imminent completion of the sequence will enable candidate gene association testing on a genome-wide scale. Chromosomes 21 and 22 are considered finished sequences, providing a complete genetic template for dissection by investigators with well-supported findings in these chromosomes (see below).

Annotations of the human genome sequence published in February 2001 (International Human Genome Sequencing Consortium, 2001; Venter et al., 2001) cataloged and predicted a total of ~30,000 genes. If this was indeed the total count, then broad linkage regions that are characteristic of complex diseases would contain fewer genes than expected, and molecular screening for genetic variants would be confined to fewer targets. But this number appears to be an underestimate. Continued evaluation and annotations on the existing human genome sequence have cast doubts on the count (Hogenesch et al., 2001) and led to the prediction of at least twice the previous estimate (Wright et al., 2001). Regardless of the actual number, researchers will be able to conduct a comprehensive screening of their regions of interest, searching primarily for variants that disrupt gene function or those that exhibit linkage disequilibrium (LD). LD could pinpoint a short stretch of DNA encoding a susceptibility gene, and central to LD detection are single nucleotide polymorphisms (SNPs) that are spaced at an average distance of ~1 kb. Millions of SNPs have been deposited in the databases, and millions more will be detected (International SNP Map Working Group, 2001).

Gene identification strategies that complement linkage and association are also being pursued. One such approach involves the detection of a cytogenetic aberration that co-segregates with affective disorders (see below). This approach restricts the search to a very narrow region because the gene disrupted at a translocation breakpoint may contain the risk variant. A new strategy stemming from the spectacular progress in human genome sequencing involves the application of functional genomics. The goal is to find a correlation of gene expression with phenotype, disease state, drug or effect disease predisposition (see below).

Some caution is required in applying these technologies to affective disorders. Two mechanisms that have been proposed to explain the genetic basis of complex diseases are (a) the common disease/common variant (CD/CV) hypothesis (Reich and Lander, 2001; Wright and Hastie, 2001) and (b) the multilocus-multiallele (ML/MA) hypothesis (Pritchard, 2001; Wright and Hastie, 2001). The CD/CV hypothesis assumes that susceptibility alleles occur at high frequencies in the population, and the ML/MA hypothesis proposes extensive allelic heterogeneity in multiple loci. Either of these two mechanisms would require large sample sizes in order to have adequate power to detect these alleles. As discussed previously, each of the risk genes most likely exert relatively small effects on the overall susceptibility to affective disorders. In addition, as for most complex diseases or traits, the definition of who is ill or well can vary, depending on where one chooses to draw the line in the range of mild to severe illness. For example, one can argue that it is worth testing linkage to only narrowly defined bipolar illness since it has the highest risk ratio in first-degree relatives. In contrast, it can be argued that unipolar illness should also be included in the spectrum, given the evidence for aggregation from family studies, even though the risk ratio is lower. Generally, investigators test more than one hypothesis about illness classification. There may also be other subsamples tested, based on age of onset or other characteristic. When multiple linkage hypotheses are tested, this can lead to an increase in type I error in linkage and association studies and must be taken into account when reporting results.

Thresholds for Statistical Significance

In terms of linkage studies, the *p*-value threshold needed for a significant statistic has been determined for a whole genome scan to be on the order of 10^{-5} (Feingold et al., 1993; Lander and Kruglyak, 1995). This stringency accounts for all of the independent tests that are required in a whole genome scan and is set in order to have a 5% false positive rate for an entire genome scan. However, Lander and Kruglyak (1995) emphasized that even if one does not obtain a "significant" finding in an initial scan, a *p* value of about 10^{-4} or less can be considered "suggestive" linkage (leading to an average of one false positive rate per genome scan) and an indication that an area should be studied further. For association studies, each marker tested is independent because association is not expected to be correlated, even at relatively small genetic distances. This is especially an issue for candidate gene studies because often only one or two genes are tested for association in a study. However, one can argue that there are actually thousands of candidate genes for psychiatric illnesses and that the known candidates are only a small subset of the possible candidates that we happen to know about because of the hypothesized biology of the disorders. Association studies generally do not account for the number of possible genes that could be tested (see Crowe, 1993). Risch and Merikangas (1996) have argued that it will soon be practical to screen the entire genome for association using single nucleotide polymorphism markers. In this case, they have determined the total possible number of statistical tests and calculate sample sizes needed given the stringent statistical threshold required (*p* value of 10^{-8}) for the approximately 1 million tests that would be required.

Genetic Linkage

The advent of dense chromosomal maps saturated with highly informative, easy-to-read markers, improvement in the quality and quantity of patient samples, and advances in methods of statistical analysis are factors that have laid the groundwork for new findings in the genetics of affective disorders, leading to the current palpable optimism in this field. Genome scan data on samples consisting of either an extended pedigree or a panel of sib-pair, nuclear, medium, and large families have been reported. Some studies have employed finer intermarker distances than others. From these studies a pattern has emerged indicating the following:

- Suggestive or significant linkage based on the criteria proposed by Lander and Kruglyak (1995)
- A convergence of linkage peaks on distinct genomic regions serving to reinforce the evidence for risk-conferring genes in these locations, albeit the apex of linkage peaks from various studies may not coincide, and the original findings are not universally supported
- Eight linkage regions with support at the level of lod ≥2 from one initial study and at least two independent replication studies
- At least eight overlapping susceptibility regions for mood disorders and schizophrenia, with support at the level of lod 22 from one initial study and at least one replication study
- Broad linkage regions, and in some chromosomal arms there are more than one linkage peaks separated by a wide genetic distance

In Table 44–4, we list 20 chromosomal regions where linkage signals at the level of ≥2 have been reported in at least one study. Most of the original studies included here obtained lod scores greater than 3, while others generated lod scores between 2 and 3. Studies that showed lod scores of less than 2 were not included, but these have been cited in reports from the Chromosome Workshops at the World Congress on Psychiatric Genetics (Barden and Morissette, 1999; Craddock and Lendon, 1999; Crowe and Vieland, 1999; Curtis, 1999; Detera-Wadleigh, 1999; Hallmayer, 1999; Kennedy et al., 1999; Nurnberger and Foroud, 1999; Paterson, 1999; Schwab and Wildenauer, 1999; Van Broeckhoven and Verheyen, 1999; Wildenauer and Schwab, 1999; DeLisi et al., 2000).

Many of the implicated regions shown in Table 44–4 have support from one or more independent studies at the level of lod 2 or higher except for chromosomes 3, 5, 8, 10p,14, 15, 16, 20, and X. The highest lod scores on chromosomes 3, 5, 6, 8, and 16 are less than 3 (Ewald et al.,1995; Ginns et al., 1996; Friddle et al., 2000; Kelsoe et al., 2001; Turecki et al., 2001). Linkage signals on chromosome 6p24 (lod score >2) were derived from a genome scan of the large Old Order Amish kindred (Ginns et al., 1996). A recent genome scan on lithium-responsive families yielded a lod score of 2.0 with D6S1050 on 6p23 under a recessive genetic model (Turecki et al., 2001). These findings overlap the schizophrenia region on 6p24–p22 that has received a lot of attention and on which several studies have reported evidence of linkage (Schwab et al., 1995, 2000; Straub et al., 1995; Wang et al., 1995; Maziade et al., 1997; Lindholm et al., 1999).

On 14q23–q31, one of the largest pedigrees in our 22 multiplex pedigrees consisting of more than 350 members available for genotyping (from here on we will refer to this sample set as the Bethesda bipolar series), yielded a parametric lod greater than 3 with D14S617 under a dominant, 85% penetrance model of transmission (Detera-Wadleigh et al., 1999). Although this could be a spurious finding, it is interesting that this was the only marker among more than 600 employed in genotyping that gen-

Table 44–4. Genomic Regions Associated with Bipolar Illness and Overlap with Schizophrenia

Genomic Region	Affective Disorder	Schizophrenia
1q25; 1q32q–q42	Turecki et al., 1995; Detera-Wadleigh et al., 1999; Blackwood et al., 2001	Hovatta et al., 1999; Brzustowicz et al., 2000; Ekelund et al., 2000, 2001; Gurling et al., 2001; Blackwood et al., 2001
3p21 and 3q27	Kelsoe et al., 2001	
4p16–p15	Blackwood et al., 1996; Ewald et al., 1998b; Detera-Wadleigh et al., 1999	
4q31–q35	Adams et al., 1998; Friddle et al., 2000	Hovatta et al., 1999; Gurling et al., 2001
6p24–p22	Ginns et al., 1996; Turecki et al., 2001	Straub et al., 1995; Wang et al., 1995; Schwab et al., 1995; Maziade et al., 1997; Lindholm et al., 1999; Schwab et al., 2000
5p15–p13	Kelsoe et al., 2001	Silverman et al., 1996
8q24	Friddle et al., 2000	
10p14–p11	Rice et al., 1997; Foroud et al., 2000	Faraone et al., 1998; Straub et al., 1998; Schwab et al., 1998a, 2000;
10q25–q26	Cichon et al., 2001; Kelsoe et al., 2001	Levinson et al., 1998; Mowry et al., 2000
12q23–q24	Craddock et al., 1994; Ewald et al., 1998a; Morissette et al., 1999	
13q14–q32	Detera-Wadleigh et al., 1999; Liu et al., 2001; Kelsoe et al., 2001; Badenhop et al., 2001	Lin et al., 1997; Blouin et al., 1998; Brzustowicz et al., 1999
14q13–q32	Detera-Wadleigh et al., 1999	Blouin et al., 1998
15q14	Turecki et al., 2001	
16p13	Ewald et al., 1995	
18pericen, 18p11.2	Berrettini et al., 1994; Stine et al., 1995; Detera-Wadleigh et al., 1999 Nothen et al., 1999	Schwab et al., 1998b; Yoshikawa et al., 2001 (association)
18q21–q23	Stine et al., 1995; De Bruyn et al., 1996; Freimer et al., 1996; McMahon et al., 1997, 2001	
20p11.2–q11.2	Radhakrishna et al., 2001	Gurling et al., 2001
21q22	Straub et al., 1994; Detera-Wadleigh et al., 1996, 1997; Smyth et al., 1997; Aita et al., 1999; Kelsoe et al., 2001	
22q11–q13	Edenberg et al., 1997; Lachman et al., 1997; Detera-Wadleigh et al., 1999; Kelsoe et al., 2001	Coon et al., 1994; Blouin et al., 1998
Xq24–q27	Pekkarinen et al., 1995	

erated this level of signal for this pedigree. Furthermore, the entire sample set generated a lod score higher than 2 at D14S1060 on 14q under a recessive, 85% penetrance model. Turecki et al. (2001) conducted a genome-wide screening of bipolar disorder on 31 families ascertained through lithium responders, and this study revealed the strongest evidence of linkage at *ACTC* on 15q14, with a lod score of 3.43, assuming recessive inheritance. In a genome survey on a large Turkish pedigree, markers on the pericentromeric region of chromosome 20 exhibited a maximum 2-point lod score greater than 4 under a dominant, fully penetrant model, suggesting the presence of a major locus for bipolar disorder (Radhakrishna et al., 2001). On the 20q12–q11 region, possibly overlapping the peak observed in the Turkish pedigree, a single pedigree gave a lod score of 2.9 under a recessive genetic model in a genome scan on a European schizophrenia family series (Gurling et al., 2001). Analysis of an extended Finnish pedigree with chromosome X markers yielded evidence of linkage with a peak lod of 3.54 at DXS994 under a single major locus model (Pekkarinen et al., 1995).

Genetic linkage studies have uncovered the exciting phenomenon that portrays overlaps of peaks for mood disorders and schizophrenia in various regions of the genome (some were reviewed in Wildenauer et al., 1999; Berrettini, 2000), although there are at least four regions that seem to be involved in risk solely to affective illness (Table 44–4). As shown, there are a minimum of eight shared regions, and findings on 1q, 4q, 10p, 13q, 18p, and 22q have been supported by one or more independent studies at the lod ≥2 level.

More than a century ago Kraepelin postulated a dichotomy between dementia praecox (schizophrenia) and manic-depressive psychosis (bipolar disorder), and this has proved beneficial in diagnosis and treatment. The nosologic distinction between these diseases implies disparate clinical course and outcome. However, clinical, epidemiologic and family studies also provide clues to some degree of relatedness between affective disorders and schizophrenia. Transitions from affective disorder to schizophrenia have been documented (Coryell et al., 1985); schizoaffective disorder, an intermediate phenotype, exists in schizophrenia and mood disorder families (Kendell and Gourlay, 1970; Taylor and Amir, 1994); and schizophrenia and affective disorders have been shown to co-occur in the same families (Gershon et al., 1988; Taylor, 1992; Maier et al., 1993). Recent data on the overlaps of susceptibility regions for mood disorders and schizophrenia may provide molecular evidence of shared genetic mechanisms for these diseases. It is conceivable that shared risk alleles may predispose to psychosis. Likewise, in a shared gene the susceptibility allele for affective disorder may be distinct from that for schizophrenia.

The most important findings are described in greater detail below.

Chromosome 1q

We conducted a whole genome screen of affective disorders on the Bethesda bipolar disorder series comprised of pedigrees with least four affected members under affection status model II (ASM II), which included bipolar I (BPI), bipolar II (BPII) with major depression, schizoaffective disorder (SA), and recurrent unipolar major depression (RUP) (Detera-Wadleigh et al., 1999). Statistical analysis was done under both ASM II and ASM I (ASM II minus RUP), using both nonparametric and parametric methods. Analysis using GENEHUNTER PLUS on nuclear families from the pedigrees displayed a maximum lod score of 2.67 between D1S1660 and D1S1678 on 1q31–q32, representing suggestive linkage. Analysis using ASPEX shifted the peak to 1q32–q41 between D1S471 and D1S237. Under a dominant, 85% penetrance mode of transmission, a lod score of 2.37 for the entire series was generated by GATA124F08 on 1q32. Consistent with this finding was a report that indicated a frequent occurrence of a fragile site on 1q32 in patients with bipolar disorder (Turecki et al., 1995).

A recent report by Blackwood and colleagues (2001) supplements evidence for the importance of 1q in affective disorder vulnerability. This group studied an extended family with a (1;11)(q42;q14.3) translocation that co-segregated with both affective disorder and schizophrenia phenotypes. When the phenotype classification was restricted to either disease, linkage analysis showed that the cytogenetic aberration was linked to affective disorders (lod score of 4.5) and schizophrenia (lod score of 3.6). A lod score of 7 was generated when schizophrenia and affective disorders were both classified as affected. Previously this group cloned *DISC1*, the disrupted gene at the translocation breakpoint (Millar et al., 2000). This work illustrates potential sharing of susceptibility components on 1q for mood disorders and schizophrenia. It is noteworthy that 15 of our 22 pedigrees had members with schizoaffective diagnosis; therefore, the genes found in regions of overlap may contribute to risk for psychosis (Detera-Wadleigh et al., 1999).

Evidence has accumulated suggesting the involvement of 1q in predisposition to schizophrenia. Genome screening of schizophrenia in an internal isolate from Finland revealed significant linkage (maximum lod score of 3.82), where the highest pairwise lod scores were observed in markers mapping to1q32–q41 (Hovatta et al., 1999). A follow-up study that combined the subisolate with families from other parts of Finland shifted the peak distally. The whole family series, exclusive of the internal isolate, generated the strongest evidence of linkage on 1q, at D1S2709, a marker within the *DISC1* gene (Ekelund et al., 2000, 2001).

So far, the strongest evidence of linkage to schizophrenia (maximum lod score of 6.5) has been found in 22 multiply affected Canadian families by Brzustowicz and colleagues (2000). The multipoint peak was broad, extending up to 50 cM and higher on both proximal and distal sides, and the apex centered at 1q21–q22. Similarly, a genome-wide scan on 13 British and Icelandic schizophrenia families produced a maximum lod score greater than 3 in several regions of the genome, including 1q23–q33 (Gurling et al., 2001). Inspection of studies on 1q indicates that the apex of the linkage peaks and the translocation breakpoint do not converge at the same restricted site. Whether there are more than one predisposing genes on 1q for affective disorders and schizophrenia remains to be determined.

Chromosome 4p

Genetic analysis of extended Scottish pedigrees generated a maximum heterogeneity lod score of 4.1, with markers on chromosome 4p16–p15 under a dominant model of inheritance, indicating significant linkage to bipolar affective disorder (Blackwood et al., 1996). Three-point analysis on a single extended pedigree produced a lod score of 4.8. Support for this finding was reported in Danish pedigrees (lod score of 2) (Ewald et al., 1998b) and in one kindred from our Bethesda series (lod score higher than 3) (Detera-Wadleigh et al., 1999).

Chromosome 4q

A maximum 3-point lod score of 3.19 between D4S408 and D4S2924 on 4q35 was found in a single Australian pedigree segregating bipolar disorder (Adams et al., 1998). In a genome scan conducted on 50 families with affective disorders, multipoint heterogeneity lod scores higher than 2 under a recessive genetic model were displayed by markers on 4q34–q35 (Friddle et al., 2000), thus increasing support for a potential linkage to mood disorders in the long arm of chromosome 4.

Two reports on schizophrenia screens seem to support a convergence schizophrenia and affective disorder loci on 4q. In an extended pedigree from a Finnish internal isolate, a maximum lod score of 2.71 was found in the 4q31 region under a dominant, 90% penetrance model (Hovatta et al., 1999). In another extended European kindred, a lod score of 3.2 was found at 4q13–q31, assuming a dominant inheritance (Gurling et al., 2001).

Chromosome 10p

A genomic survey on the NIMH Genetics Initiative Bipolar series that included 540 members in 97 families produced evidence of a potential linkage to chromosome 10p (Rice et al., 1997). A MOD (model lod) score of 3.4 was found when BPI, BPII, and SA were counted as affected. A follow-up whole-genome analysis on the same data set using GENEHUNTER PLUS revealed that the highest lod score of 2.5 was displayed by D10S1423 at 10p14–p11 (Foroud et al., 2000).

Screening of several independent schizophrenia samples has yielded support for a susceptibility locus on 10p14–p11. Faraone et al. (1998) found the highest nonparametric linkage (NPL) score, $Z = 3.4$ at D10S1423, in the European American schizophrenia families collected through the NIMH Genetics Initiative. This is the same marker that yielded the highest lod score in the genome scan of the bipolar series collected through the NIMH Genetics Initiative (see above). In a subset of 88 Irish families, the highest pairwise heterogeneity lod (HLOD) score on chromosome 10 was 3.2 with D10S674 at 10p15–p11 under a recessive mode of inheritance (Straub et al., 1998). When all 265 families were examined, the maximum Hlod of 1.95 on chromosome 10 was detected by D10S2443. Schwab et al. (1998a) analyzed chromosome 10 on a combined set of 72 families from Germany and Israel and found the highest NPL score of 3.2 with D10S1714 on 10p14–p11. A genome-wide scan on these latter pedigrees sustained support for suggestive linkage on 10p (Schwab et al., 2000). These studies suggest that the short arm of chromosome 10 is a shared predisposing region for bipolar disorder and schizophrenia.

Chromosome 10q

A 10 cM genome screen of bipolar affective disorder on 75 German and Israeli families generated the most prominent evidence of linkage (maximum NPL score >3) between D10S1483 and D10S217 on 10q25–q26 (Cichon et al., 2001). Another whole-genome scan displayed suggestive evidence in the same region, specifically at D10S1223, that yielded a lod score above 2 under an autosomal recessive, 50% penetrance model (Kelsoe et al., 2001). In the NIMH Genetics Initiative Bipolar series a MOD score over 3 was generated by D10S188, a marker mapping to 10q22–q23 (Rice et al., 1997). Suggestive evidence for an overlap with schizophrenia at the level of NPL >2 with D10S1239 and D10S168 on 10q23–q24 was observed in a screening study on 71 Australian/U.S. pedigrees (Mowry et al., 2000).

Chromosome 12q

Linkage analysis on a number of independently ascertained families has implicated the long arm of chromosome 12 in conferring risk to affective disorders. A genome survey on large, homogeneous pedigrees from the Saguenay-Lac-St. Jean area in the Quebec province of Canada revealed that the strongest evidence of linkage localized on 12q23–q24 (Morissette et al., 1999). Multipoint analysis using GENEHUNTER PLUS displayed two peaks, one at D12S82 (Z score = 3.92) and the other at D12S86 (Z score = 2.5). Significant linkage to this region at D12S1639 (2-point lod score = 3.37) was reported in Danish families under a dominant mode of inheritance (Ewald et al., 1998a). Craddock et al. (1994) studied a family that exhibited co-segregation of affective disorders with Darier's disease, an illness linked to 12q23. Despite this co-segregation, no definitive correlation between variants in the Darier's disease gene, *ATP2P2*, and affective disorders has been detected (Jacobsen et al., 1999).

Chromosome 13q

Whole-genome scans conducted on mood disorder and schizophrenia pedigrees by different groups have heightened the evidence for risk-conferring genes on the long arm of chromosome 13. The first compelling evidence for linkage to affective disorders was derived from a high-density genome scan conducted by our group on the 22 Bethesda bipolar disorder series. The strongest finding centered at 13q32 with a peak lod of 3.5 (Detera-Wadleigh et al., 1999). Multipoint analysis using GENEHUNTER PLUS on nuclear families localized the apex of the peak between D13S1271 and D13S779 under ASM I, and between D13S1252 and D13S1271 under ASM II. Also, as discussed in a previous section and will be discussed in later ones, in the entire series suggestive linkage was generated by markers that map to 1q32, 18p11.2, and 22q (Detera-Wadleigh et al., 1999). A follow-up screening on this same set of families at a finer intermarker spacing further supported the finding on 13q32 and shifted the peak a few cM distally, between D13S779 and D13S225 (Liu et al., 2001).

Confirmatory data was generated from a genome-wide scan on a 20-affective disorder family data set (Kelsoe et al., 2001). Lod scores higher than 2 were produced by markers on 13q32. In a genome screen of mood disorders on 50 families by Friddle et al. (2000), a simultaneous-search analysis revealed the highest points in the lod-plot range to be 3.4 to 3.8 at the locus pairs D8S272 and D9S264, and D9S264 and D13S151. Interestingly, D13S151 maps to 13q32. In addition, a genome survey on a single Australian pedigree produced a maximum 3-point lod score of 3 under a recessive, 90% penetrance model at a more centromeric location on 13q14, between D13S291 and D13S153.

Linkage studies have localized a schizophrenia susceptibility region on 13q32. A 5-point model free-linkage analysis on 21 English and Welsh schizophrenic families provided support for suggestive linkage (maximum lod score = 2.58) around D13S122 and D13S128, markers located on 13q32 (Lin et al., 1997). This was followed by two studies that showed significant evidence of linkage. In a genome-wide scan conducted on 54 multiplex pedigrees segregating schizophrenia, the highest evidence of linkage was on 13q32 with a peak NPL score of 4.18 detected by D13S174 (Blouin et al., 1998). The HLOD score assuming a recessive model was 3.19. Genetic analysis of chromosome 13 in 21 extended Canadian pedigrees affected with schizophrenia revealed a maximum 3-point lod score of 3.92, with a peak proximal to D13S793 on 13q32, under the assumption of homogeneity (Brzustowicz et al., 1999). Under the assumption of heterogeneity, the maximum 3-point lod score was 4.42 at the marker pair D13S793 and D13S779. These reports disclose corroborating evidence for the existence of affective disorder- and schizophrenia-predisposing genes on 13q.

A genome-wide scan conducted on panic disorder families uncovered evidence for linkage on 13q32, specifically at D13S779 (Weissman et al., 2000). Co-morbidity of panic disorder and affective disorder was previously evaluated by MacKinnon et al. (1998), with respect to bipolar disorder linkage on 18q. The strongest evidence of linkage was found in families where the proband had panic attacks. Weissman et al. (2000) reported evidence of linkage at D13S779 in panic families with bladder/kidney problems (lod score above 3), under a dominant genetic model. The lod score rose to over 4 when the phenotype classification (panic disorder plus other syndromes) was broadened. The joint findings in affective disorders, schizophrenia, and panic disorder with other medical syndromes involving the same marker is quite intriguing.

Chromosome 18p

The pericentromeric region of chromosome 18 was first implicated in risk to bipolar disorder in a study by Berrettini and colleagues (1994). Affected pedigree member five-locus analysis on the 22 Bethesda bipolar disorder series yielded $p < .0001$ and $< .0007$, under two respective weighting functions. Support for linkage on 18p was demonstrated in a panel of 28 affective disorder families by Stine et al. (1995), who also found that the excess allele sharing was attributable to the paternal families. Five data sets were submitted to the Genetic Analysis Workshop 10 (Goldin et al., 1997), two of which were already known to be positive. Overall, there was suggestive evidence for linkage in these data sets (Rice, 1997). Analysis of chromosome 18 in 57 German families generated results consistent with linkage on 18p in paternal pedigrees under a recessive genetic model (lod score of 2.54) (Nothen et al., 1999). Follow-up analysis on the Bethesda bipolar families with increased marker coverage to an average ~3 cM spacing elicited a peak lod of 2.32 between D18S1150 and D18S71, on 18p11.2 under ASM I (Detera-Wadleigh et al., 1999).

Chromosome 18p seems to be another site that shows a convergence of peaks for mood disorders and schizophrenia. A sample panel consisting of 59 German and Israeli families with schizophrenia index patients that included members diagnosed with affective illness was screened with chromosome 18 markers (Schwab et al., 1998b). The highest pairwise lod score (>2) was detected by an intragenic marker in G-olfα (GNAL) under an affected classification that included only schizophrenia and schizoaffective disorder. Broadening the affected phenotype to incorporate affective disorders generated a maximum lod score of 3.1 with D18S53, a marker physically close to G-olfα on 18p11.2. Linkage disequilibrium tests showed significant transmission distortion of the 124 bp allele of G-olfα.

Myo-inositol monophosphatase-2 (*IMPA2*) was cloned and mapped to 18p11.2 (Yoshikawa et al., 1997). This is an interesting functional candidate gene because the enzyme is inhibited by lithium. The genomic structure was determined and all exons, splice junctions, and the promoter region were screened for mutations, single nucleotide polymorphisms (SNPs) and other genetic variants (Sjoholt et al., 2000, Yoshikawa et al., 2000, 2001). Three clusters of SNPs were found, and a representative SNP from each cluster was used to test for association in Japanese affective disorder and schizophrenia patients using a case-control paradigm (Yoshikawa et al., 2001). Significant association with schizophrenia was detected but not with affective disorders. GNAL and *IMPA2* are located within 100 kb of each other (Reyes et al., in press; University of California–Santa Cruz Genome Browser), suggesting that there is a restricted region on 18p11.2 that is in linkage disequilibrium with schizophrenia.

Chromosome 18q

In contrast to the chromosomal stretch on 18p, the predisposing region on 18q has been shown to correlate solely with affective disorder vulnerability. In addition to their chromosome 18p finding, Stine and coworkers (1995) reported evidence for linkage on 18q21–q22, with the highest lod score of 3.52 at D18S41 in paternal pedigrees. This study was extended by the same group employing a new panel of 30 pedigrees and linkage signals were detectable only on 18q and not on 18p (McMahon et al., 1997). Nonparametric analysis on the combined data set (new plus original) yielded a maximum NPL score of 2.84 at D18S38. This same group further investigated the possibility of a correlation between sib-pair diagnostic subtypes and evidence of linkage (McMahon et al., in press). The study revealed that BPII-BPII sharing could account for all of the evidence of linkage on 18q, and the peak paternal lod increased to 4.67 in BPII sib-pair families (McMahon et al., 2001).

De Bruyn et al. (1996) reported evidence of linkage to 18q21 in two large families collected in Belgium. Although the lod scores were less than 2, simulations on these kindreds showed that the values fell within the range suggesting linkage. In another sample consisting of two extended Costa Rican bipolar pedigrees, a joint linkage and association analysis of chromosome 18 revealed the highest evidence at 18q22–q23, specifically with markers D18S554 (Z_{max} = 3.70) and D18S70 (Z_{max} = 4.06) (Freimer et al., 1996). Haplotype sharing among affected members was demonstrable, but it covered a wide region on 18q. The chromosome 18 genetic data reported by Nothen et al. (1999) were also consistent with linkage to 18q, with a maximum parametric lod score of 2.1 observed at D18S554 and D18S461 under a dominant, ASM I model.

Chromosome 21q

Genetic studies published so far indicate that the risk-conferring locus on 21q is unique to bipolar affective disorder. The first report of affective disorder linkage to chromosome 21q22.3 was derived from the analysis of a large, multigenerational Israeli pedigree that displayed a pairwise lod score of 3.41 with PFKL (Straub et al., 1994). Support for linkage on 21q was found in our Bethesda bipolar disorder kindreds (Detera-Wadleigh et al., 1996). Two peaks of excess allele sharing were apparent, but these were ~10 Mb and ~3 Mb proximal to *PFKL*, respectively. (Note: Mb distances cited here were taken from the Genetics Location Database; Collins et al. [1996], with recent updates on chromosomes 21 and 22.) Excess allele sharing was observed also in the NIMH Genetics Initiative Bipolar set of 97 kindreds, with a broad peak spanning ~10 Mb, between D21S1265 and D21S1255 (Detera-Wadleigh et al., 1997).

Aita and colleagues (1999) typed additional markers on the original sample (including the large Israeli kindred that showed evidence of linkage to PFKL) that was studied by Straub et al. (1994). Analysis of the whole sample of 47 families confirmed linkage to 21q with a pairwise heterogeneity lod score of 3.35 at D21S1260, indicating that the linkage peak was shifted 5 cM proximal to PFKL. Similarly, genetic data derived from extended homogeneous pedigrees from Quebec revealed a peak at D21S263, a marker ~10 Mb centromeric of D21S1260 but about 1 Mb from the more proximal peak in our prior study (Detera-Wadleigh et al., 1996), thus increasing support for a bipolar disorder locus on 21q (Morissette et al., 1999). A two-locus admixture test using PFKL/D21S171 and tyrosine hydroxylase on 23 multiply affected pedigrees generated an lod score of 3.87 (Smyth et al., 1997). Recently, Kelsoe et al. (2001) reported a lod score above 2 at PFKL under a dominant mode of transmission with 85% penetrance. These reports raise the possibility that 21q encodes more than one gene that contributes to bipolar disorder susceptibility.

Chromosome 22q

A significant percentage of patients with velo-cardio-facial syndrome (VCFS) also exhibit symptoms characteristic of either affective disorders or schizophrenia (Pulver et al. 1994). This observation suggests the existence on 22q of a locus that confers risk to mood disorders and schizophrenia, and support for this idea has been elicited by recent genetic studies. Significant evidence of linkage to bipolar disorder was detected on 22q in a genome-wide scan conducted on a panel of 20 North American pedigrees (Kelsoe et al., 2001). The highest lod score was 3.84, generated by D22S278 under an autosomal dominant, 85% penetrance model. In addition, D22S419, which is located ~10 Mb centromeric of D22S278, gave a lod score of 2.19, assuming an autosomal recessive, 50% penetrance model. A prior study on a subset of these families by Lachman et al. (1997) displayed a maximum lod score of 2.51 at D22S303, ~13 Mb proximal to D22S278. Consistent with the latter finding was the linkage data derived from the initial genome scan of the NIMH Genetics Initiative Bipolar Disorder 97 family set, where a multipoint lod score of 2.46 (ASPEX) was found at D22S533, located les than 100 kb from D22S419 (Edenberg et al., 1997). Kelsoe et al. (2001) analyzed a subset of 57 families from the NIMH Genetics Initiative bipolar families and reproduced the evidence for suggestive linkage, with the highest lod score of 2.72 at D22S419 under an autosomal recessive, 50% penetrance model. Our genome scan on the Bethesda family set provided further support for a predisposing locus on 22q with a multipoint ASPEX lod of 2.1 between D22S689 and D22S685, a peak spanning ~5 Mb and >2 Mb distal to D22S419 (Detera-Wadleigh et al., 1999). There seems to be more than one linkage peak for bipolar disorder on 22q, which parallels the observation in other chromosomes.

The degree of evidence for a schizophrenia locus on 22q does not match that for bipolar affective disorder. Lod score greater than 2 was generated in Utah schizophrenia pedigrees under a recessive genetic model (Coon et al., 1994). In their genome scan on 54 families, Blouin et al. (1998) found a maximum NPL score of 2.42 at D22S1265, on 22q. This region could be another area in the genome that encodes both bipolar disorder and schizophrenia loci.

Not presented here are many studies that were not supportive of the findings summarized in Table 44–4. This lack of universal reproducibility may be due to one or a combination of the following:

- Proposed linkage may be a false positive
- Genetic heterogeneity—i.e., interfamilial variability in the individual genetic components of the group of genes required to confer full expression of the affected phenotype

- Inadequate representation of families linked to specific regions in a sample set; therefore, low power to detect genes with weak effect
- Ascertainment and diagnostic differences between studies
- Suarez's (1994) prediction that replicating a finding requires an exponential number of families

Data derived from genome scans on independent sample sets support the hypothesis that mood disorders are caused by multiple, possibly interacting, genes that exert moderate effects. There may be some infrequent exceptions where a major effect gene acts in rare pedigrees. As shown, we included 20 different chromosomal regions that have linkage signals for affective disorders but with the obvious caveat that some of these may be false positives and do not encode a susceptibility locus. Additional caution is in order, given that each study involved multiple hypothesis tests being applied. Linkage statistics are often computed under multiple genetic models, multiple phenotypes, and sample stratification. Nonetheless, we believe that it is now reasonable to fully explore regions that have compelling evidence of linkage to expedite the discovery of risk-conferring genes.

Association/Linkage Disequilibrium

Findings that are reproduced in other data sets are consequently strengthened, increasing the likelihood that they are valid and credible. But the detection of susceptibility genes remains an imposing task. Recombinants cannot be used reliably to narrow the region of significance because of imperfect genotype–phenotype correspondence. As previously mentioned, if either CD/CV (Reich and Lander, 2001; Wright and Hastie, 2001) or ML/MA (Pritchard, 2001; Wright and Hastie, 2001) is the genetic mechanism that underlies affective disorders, very extensive analysis of both positional and functional candidate genes in large samples must be undertaken. An exhaustive screening for SNPs or other genetic variants followed by fine linkage disequilibrium (LD) mapping is a widely accepted strategy to advance toward the eventual detection of susceptibility alleles. A primary goal is to find variants that could potentially alter gene function. Informative variants that do not have obvious functional effect must be evaluated also for LD.

Linkage Disequilibrium Mapping in Susceptibility Regions

The occurrence of LD is determined by a number of factors that include population history, population size, bottlenecks and rates of mutation and recombination in diverse genomic regions. In LD mapping two critical issues need to be considered: (a) the range and extent of LD in the human population and (b) sample size. Sample size has been thoroughly discussed by Risch and Merikangas (1996). The sample size required to achieve detecting power depends on the locus relative risk, as can be gleaned from the association/LD studies on *APOE4* (Corder et al., 1993) in Alzheimer's disease and *PPARG* in Type 2 diabetes (Altshuler et al., 2000). It is important to emphasize the need to pool and collect very large sample sizes to enhance the possibility of identifying risk-conferring genes. However, the success of LD methods for fine mapping of genes for complex diseases will have limitations, given the likely high population frequency and the heterogeneity of susceptibility alleles (Terwilliger and Weiss, 1998; Jorde, 2000).

The question of how much LD exists in different human populations has been actively debated. Knowledge of the range and extent of LD in regions of interest would help guide the decision on the number of markers needed to detect disequilibrium. Fortunately, given the availability of dense markers, empirical data are actively being generated to measure levels of LD in various regions of the genome and in different populations. We picked two recent studies as examples. Abecasis et al. (2001) examined markers (SNPs, VNTRs, and microsatellites) on 2q13 (63 markers spanning 0.6 Mb), 13q13 (38 markers spanning 1.2 Mb), and 14q11 (26 markers spanning 0.8 Mb) in 575 chromosomes from individuals of British ancestry. The study revealed that LD was irregular, detectable at less than 50 kb in more than 50% of marker pairs, with occasional LD at 500 kb. Reich et al. (2001) analyzed 19 randomly selected genomic regions in families from Utah, Sweden, and Nigeria. In the populations of northern European ancestry, LD had an average size of 60 kb, although variability in range was also evident. The Nigerian sample displayed a much shorter LD than those of European ancestry. However, it is important to remember that both theoretical studies and empirical data demonstrate that LD coefficients are quite variable at small distances (Nickerson et al., 1998).

Although more empirical data are needed, these LD findings can guide us in determining the density of markers and sample size for studying bipolar disorder in outbred populations. Also, the exponential growth in SNP detection suggests that an adequate marker density can be achieved. Currently, there are millions of SNPs that have been deposited in the SNP database (International SNP Map Working Group, 2001), and the number will continue to burgeon. However, it is common knowledge that a substantial fraction of the SNPs in the database may not be polymorphic or sufficiently informative, therefore experimental validation would be necessary. We find that many of the known and predicted genes in our regions of interest have not been examined for SNPs, and therefore extensive SNP detection on these loci needs to be done. To increase the likelihood of detecting LD, it is vital to interrogate all informative SNPs and SNP haplotypes in each candidate gene.

Genotyping of SNPs is still expensive, and a number of techniques and instruments have been developed for this purpose (reviewed by Kwok, 2000). A few examples are allele-specific oligo ligation, pyrosequencing, fluorescence polarization, and mass spectrometry. Perhaps the most efficient, high-throughput genotyping technique that is currently available is matrix-assisted laser desorption ionization-time-of-flight (MALDI-TOF) mass spectrometry, but this requires a substantial capital outlay.

Association with Biologically Relevant Genes

The unveiling of all human genes via the expected completion of the human genome sequence (International Human Genome Sequencing Consortium, 2001; Venter et al., 2001) is hugely propitious for a genome-wide association strategy (Risch and Merikangas, 1996). Emergent high-throughput technologies, particularly whole-genome SNP chips, would accelerate the process tremendously. Presently, the cost is steep and the technology needs to mature so that it could be applied to most laboratory settings. So far, association studies have focused on individual genes that have potential relevance to pathophysiology. Scrutinizing genes on an individual basis is slow; besides, there are potentially thousands of brain-expressed genes that could qualify as candidates for affective disorders. Nonetheless, we believe that this type of effort will continue, particularly in small laboratories, because it is both biologically based and affordable.

Genetic association is designed to test whether a marker allele is significantly enriched in patients. The associated allele either may be the disease-predisposing variant itself or is in linkage disequilibrium with the disease-predisposing variant. Association may be conducted by using a case-control design or family-based paradigm, or both. The chief advantage of the case-control approach is that sample collection is easier and cheaper; the main disadvantage is that it is susceptible to false association due to population stratification. The family-based approach is robust to ethnic differences, but sample collection is expensive and difficult. A comparison of these two paradigms was reviewed recently (Jones and Craddock, 2001).

Inspection of association studies in affective disorders leads to the conclusion that the approach has yielded mostly negative results; while some potentially significant data exist, their reproducibility is low (Jones and Craddock, 2001). Some possible reasons include:

- Wrong gene targets
- Correct targets, but all possible gene variants or SNP haplotypes were not interrogated; a comprehensive analysis of variants is crucial because of variable intragenic LD profile and possible allelic heterogeneity
- Inadequate sample size

Genetic components of pathways involving neurotransmitters such as serotonin and dopamine and pathways perturbed by lithium, antidepressants, or other relevant therapeutic agents are plausible targets for intensive investigation. We will discuss studies on four genes for which potentially significant association has been reported, and here we present only selected key reports. A list of nonconfirmatory reports have been presented in the review by Jones and Craddock (2001), and they will not be discussed here.

The serotonin transporter is vital to the recycling of serotonin into the neurotransmitter pool in the presynaptic terminal and is an important target of tricyclic antidepressants. An example of a family-based study using intragenic marker haplotypes was reported recently (Mynett-Johnson et al., 2000). A total of 106 Irish trios were genotyped using the markers: promoter 5-HTTLPR, intron 2 VNTR, and 3′ UTR G/T. Transmission disequilibrium tests (TDT) (Spielman et al. 1993) using single polymorphism revealed modest evidence of transmission distortion only with 5–HTTLPR ($p = .022$). Construction of multimarker haplotypes revealed that the HHTPLR-3′ UTR haplotype showed an increased evidence for association ($p = .005$), suggesting that the promoter variant that supports lower transcriptional activity (5-HTTLPR) in combination with a 3′ UTR allele may either contribute to risk or is in LD with a risk allele. Modest linkage signals on 17q11–q12 (Murphy et al., 2000), the region to which serotonin transporter maps, may concur with this LD finding.

The dopamine transporter (DAT) is central to the dopamine reuptake process from the synapse into the presynatic terminal. Several studies attempting to correlate DAT variants with various psychiatric disorders have been reported. The DAT gene maps to 5p15, a region that displayed lod scores above 2 in one pedigree of the sample set subjected to a genome scan by Kelsoe et al. (2001). We chose to present the recent report by Greenwood et al. (2001) because it illustrates an approach that involved an extensive search for SNPs and the analysis of multiple haplotypes generated from these SNPs. In the presence of an adequate sample size, this type of approach could expose any detectable LD. By the use of TDT on 50 triads, a five-marker haplotype detected association with bipolar disorder (allelewise $p = .001$, genotype-wise $p = .0004$). Because none of the SNPs had any apparent deleterious functional effect, it is possible that this haplotype is in LD with a nearby risk allele.

Catecholamine-*O*-methyltransferase (COMT) catalyzes a critical metabolic step that involves the methylation of biogenic amines. The COMT gene has been mapped to 22q11, which as shown in Table 44–4 is a susceptibility region for both affective disorders and schizophrenia. Microdeletions in VCFS have been shown to occur at 22q11. Lachman and colleagues (1996) performed an association test on VCFS patients using the COMT Val158Met missense mutation and found evidence of association of the low-activity Met allele with rapid-cycling bipolar disorder in these patients. A follow-up study by the same group on bipolar disorder cases exhibited a similar finding in ultra–ultra rapid cycling (Papolos et al., 1998). Meta-analysis on 13 case-control studies that included more than 900 probands and more than 1,000 controls displayed support for association of the Met allele, raising the possibility that this variant has a minor role in bipolar disorder susceptibility (Jones and Craddock, 2001).

Monoamine oxidase A (MAOA) catalyzes the oxidative deamination of monoamine neurotransmitters, which is a key step in their degradation. The gene has been mapped to Xp11.23, and many reports have been published on association studies in bipolar affective disorder, but we will present only two studies that analyzed relatively larger number of samples. A meta-analysis was performed on several sets of samples comprising 67 males and 113 females with bipolar disorder and a similar number of matched controls using data from a microsatellite and an restriction fragment length polymorphism (RFLP) marker (Rubinsztein et al., 1996). In the pooled and females-only samples, the microsatellite detected significant association yielding $p =$ .003 and .0009, respectively. With the Fnu4H1 RFLP, which detects a silent mutation, the combined and female-only samples generated $p = .0045$ and .012, respectively. Association was not found in males with either marker. A multicenter association study in France and Switzerland was conducted on 272 bipolar disorder patients and 122 controls employing the microsatellite, RFLP and VNTR markers on MAOA (Preisig et al. 2000). This analysis recapitulated results with the microsatellite marker from the previous study of Rubinsztein et al. (1996), but association was not evident with either the RFLP or the VNTR marker. Preisig et al. (2000) subsequently performed a meta-analysis on all available data, and results paralleled those found in their initial sample set, except that in the combined sample association was detected with the RFLP marker also.

MAOA is a particularly intriguing candidate gene because it is one of 113 genes with orthologs in vertebrates and bacteria but none in lower eukaryotes that have been sequenced so far (International Human Genome Sequencing Consortium, 2001). It has been proposed that these genes may have been integrated into the human genome through horizontal transfer from bacterial infection. This integration may have provided a selective advantage favoring its preservation in evolution. If MAOA is indeed a risk gene for bipolar disorder, we believe that it could have potent ramifications for the mechanisms that underlie susceptibility to mental illness.

Expression-Based Strategies for Finding Susceptibility Genes

Expression-based strategies could be exploited to complement genetic linkage and association. It is conceivable that these strategies could quickly detect susceptibility genes for complex psychiatric disorders. Gene expression profiling is global, and either the transcriptome or the proteome can be interrogated. cDNA microarrays or oligonucleotide chips that contain a full representation of transcripts encoded by the genome could be used to evaluate altered gene expression in affecteds vs controls. Advances in protein profiling are also gaining speed. The proteome is a very attractive target for exploration because proteins act as the engine that drives the cellular machinery. Also, proteins are not as labile as mRNA. Compared to the transcriptome, the proteome is more complex because proteins undergo multiple posttranslational modifications.

To study gene differential gene expression in affective disorders, the following tissues could be used as a source of mRNA or proteins: postmortem brains, cerebrospinal fluid, hematopoietic cells, or other cellular models. When using brain tissues, it is important to target structures that have been shown to exhibit abnormal neuroanatomical patterns in bipolar affective disorder, and a review of this topic was published recently (Baumann and Bogerts, 2001). The principal disadvantage of the expression-profiling approach arises from the confounding effect of unmatched samples caused by differences in therapeutic exposure, disease states, and postmortem delay. Conceivably, these nongenetic factors are the main cause of altered gene expression; consequently, the majority of transcripts or proteins that exhibit changes in levels of expression would have no relevance to etiology. However, this global exploration at the transcript and protein level could expose differentially expressed genes that map to proposed susceptibility regions, and these genes then become priority candidates for an exhaustive mutation analysis.

So far, microarray analysis and protein profiling in bipolar disorder have not yet been reported. Another method for detecting differential gene expression referred to as serial analysis of gene expression (SAGE) was conducted in frontal cortices of bipolar disorder patients and controls (Sun et al., 2001). Altered transcript levels were found for the serotonin transporter and components of the NF-κB complex. This finding elevates the importance of serotonin transporter in bipolar disorder and tends to support the association finding described previously (see above).

In schizophrenia, two studies that employed microarray technology using postmortem brains have been reported. Many varied types of differentially expressed genes were detected (Mirnics et al., 2000; Hakak et al., 2001). Mirnics et al. (2000) reported a decrease in expression of genes involved in synaptic transmission, while Hakak et al. (2001) observed consistent altered levels of myelination-related genes.

Another approach involves the use of animal models treated with certain drugs that induce and mimic specific symptoms associated with the affective disorder phenotype, followed by assessment of differential gene expression using transcript microarrays. Niculescu et al. (2000) treated rats with metamphetamine to model manic and psychotic symptoms. RNA from brains of untreated and treated rats were used to synthesize cDNA that, in turn, was used to hybridize Affymetrix expression chips. This exploration detected many differentially expressed genes, including *GRK3*, which maps to 22q11, a region that showed a linkage peak for bipolar disorder (see above). It would be important to determine whether any of these genes contributes to disease risk.

Examining genetic components of signal transduction pathways that are perturbed by therapeutic agents for affective disorders represents another plausible strategy to hunt for susceptibility genes. To detect lithium-responsive genes, Cordeiro et al. (2000) probed cDNA microarrays with cDNA derived from nerve growth factor differentiated and undifferentiated PC12 cells. Changes in transcript levels were displayed by a total of 29 genes, 15 in differentiated cells and 8 in both differentiated and undifferentiated cells. A list of these genes—including components of lithium-responsive pathways involved in phosphoinositide, Wnt, and Akt signaling, and corresponding chromosomal locations—was published recently (Detera-Wadleigh, 2001).

Cytogenetic Abnormalities

For many years there have been anecdotal reports on individuals with chromosomal aberrations having major psychiatric disorders (Craddock and Owen, 1994). Recently, there have been reports of single families or pedigrees where a balanced translocation segregates with bipolar illness. St. Clair et al (1990) examined 282 pedigrees from the MRC Cytogenetics Registry in Edinburgh to attempt to find families with mental illness. One large pedigree was identified, where 34 individuals carried a balanced translocation between chromosomes 1 and 11. Sixteen of the 34 individuals had a diagnosed mental disorder, including schizophrenia, schizoaffective depression, and recurrent major depression. As mentioned in the previous section, the disrupted gene *DISC1*, at the 1q42 translocation breakpoint, was cloned by Millar et al. (2000), and the translocation was shown to be significantly linked to schizophrenia and affective disorders (Blackwood et al., 2001). Whether *DISC1* is the risk-conferring gene remains to be established.

Another pedigree has been reported by Baysal et al. (1998), where 11 individuals carry a balanced translocation between chromosomes 9 and 11 (although not the same part of chromosome 11 that was described above): 5 of the 11 carriers had bipolar disorder, and 1 had unipolar disorder. There were no affected individuals who were not carriers. Several years ago, it was discovered that many patients with velo-cardo-facial syndrome (VCFS), which involves a microdeletion of chromosome 22, had diagnoses of schizophrenia (Pulver et al., 1994). Later, Papolos et al. (1996) systematically assessed 25 patients with VCFS for psychiatric symptoms: 16 of 25 patients had bipolar disorder or some bipolar spectrum disorder. In addition, Lachman et al. (1997) found some evidence for linkage in bipolar families to markers in this region of chromosome 22.

Trinucleotide Repeats

As discussed earlier, one hypothesis about bipolar disorder is that some cases may be caused by an expanded trinucleotide repeat. Several studies have tried to detect expanded repeats in patients by using the repeat expansion detection (RED) method. Lindblad et al. (1995) and O'Donovan et al. (1996) found a longer average repeat length in bipolars than in controls. Oruc et al. (1997) found that increased repeat length was only found in familial bipolar patients but not in the group of bipolars as a whole. However, some studies have found no differences between bipolars and controls (Vincent et al., 1996; Guy et al., 1997). It has also been shown that 94% of the repeat sizes detected by the RED method can be accounted for by two loci, one on chromosome 18 and one on chromosome 17q (Sidransky et al., 1998). Thus, studies need to test for these specific loci to consider the possibility that size differences between groups are due to a small number of individuals who by chance carry the very long alleles. If expanded repeats were found to be a mechanism for bipolar disorder in some cases, then one would also have to demonstrate actual expansion of allele size from one generation to another in a pedigree. Five different CAG repeats containing loci in the genome were screened in lithium-responsive bipolar patients and controls, but association was not found (Serretti et al., 1998). Vincent et al. (2000) reviewed published studies on trinucleotide repeats in major psychosis and concluded that these unstable repeats may not have a major effect in risk for psychosis.

CLINICAL APPLICATION AND RISK ASSSESSMENT

Therapy

A number of drugs are available for treatment of depression and mania (Thase and Kupfer, 1996). Pharmacotherapy for depression includes tricyclic antidepressents, monoamine oxidase inhibitors, and selective serotonin reuptake inhibitors (the most well known being fluoxetine, or Prozac). Severe or refractory depression may respond to treatment with electoconvulsive therapy (ECT). For treatment of manic episodes, lithium is the first-line therapy. Interestingly, over time, the effectiveness of lithium has decreased, and now only about 40% to 50% of patients respond. Anticonvulsant drugs, such as carbamazapine, are also used to treat mania. As new etiologic mechanisms are defined from identification of underlying genes for affective disorders, it should be possible to develop more specific therapies.

Genetic Counseling

The most common questions that the psychiatric genetic counselor is asked are, "What is the chance of my child developing the same disorder that I or my spouse has?" and "What are the chances of my developing the same disorder that my relative has?" A request for counseling should also be approached as a problem in short-term psychotherapy. The first of these questions is often asked in the context, "Should I have children?" Here there are issues of self-esteem, competency, and feelings of being damaged that need to be addresssed by the clinician. There is also a tendency for psychiatric patients to minimize the burden and risk of these illnesses (Schulz et al., 1982).

Because no single-gene mode of inheritance has been established for affective disorders, empirical risk estimates should be used in counseling. As stated above, the risk of all affective disorders in first-degree relatives of affective disorders patients is 20% to 25%, with most of the risk being due to unipolar depression. When counseling siblings of patients, their age must be taken into account. These risks are for adult affective disorder. Children of parents with major affective disorder also appear to have an increased risk of childhood depression and other disorders. A long-term follow-up study of a high-risk sample was reported by Weissman et al. (1997); it showed that offspring of depressed parents are at high risk for a number of psychiatric disorders in childhood, adolescence, and early adulthood. The clinician may be asked by parents with affective disorder for interventions for children that will decrease their risk of becoming ill. There is no known intervention for preventing affective disorder, but the best hope is for early recognition and treatment of symptoms of major affective disorder if they develop. When onset of illness is in adolescence, the symptoms are often denied or mistaken for adolescent acting out, but treatment is important to avoid disruption of early adulthood.

The largest issue for women with affective disorder is how to safely manage the pregnancy and postpartum period to avoid exposure of the fetus during the first trimester to drugs such as lithium and antidepressants or exposure through breast milk, while also minimizing the risk of a severe affective episode to the mother (Packer, 1992; Llewellyn et al., 1998). There is also an increased risk for postpartum episodes of affective illness in women with affective disorder.

Several recent surveys have addressed the issue of attitudes toward genetic testing for bipolar disorder if a gene were found. One study, including both patients and normals (Smith et al., 1996), found that half of the respondents would abort a fetus if the child were certain to develop bipolar illness. The percentage favoring abortion was related to the risk of developing the disorder. A survey of bipolar patients and their spouses (Trippitelli et al., 1998) found that the majority of them would favor genetic testing because of a perceived benefit of early, preventive treatment. The majority of patients and spouses indicated that they would definitely not have an abortion if a fetus were found to have a gene for bipolar illness, but a fair percentage of them were uncertain. Because a number of loci with small effect may be identified that together cause susceptibility to bipolar disorder, these studies also indicate the need for education about the meaning of genetic risks for complex diseases.

CONCLUSIONS AND FUTURE APPROACHES

Detection of risk-conferring genes for affective disorders is a persistently challenging endeavor. There are now a number of promising regions, although findings of linkage have not been consistently supported. Based on findings from genome scans on various sample collections, it is likely that there are at least several susceptibility genes for affective disorders, each with a relatively small effect, with possible very rare exceptions where a major locus may be operational. Suarez et al. (1994) have shown that in the case of disease caused by several additive genes, it takes severalfold more families to replicate any one particular locus than to initially detect a locus. Thus, it is not surprising that some of the genomic regions identified for affective disorder have not been replicated. But the question remains: How do we distinguish nonreplication from false positive findings? As more genome scans are carried out for psychiatric disorders, techniques of meta-analyses will become important as a way to summarize the likelihood of any particular region containing a susceptibility gene. Another way to find genes with small effects is to increase the sample size. This is extremely important, particularly because affective disorders may be caused by high-frequency alleles and extensive allelic heterogeneity on multiple loci may exist. With the availability of an extensive family collection, perhaps stratifying them on the basis of specific endophenotypes may reduce the level of heterogeneity and expose higher linkage signals. There is a realization among investigators in the field of complex diseases that consortia of studies need to be organized and methods designed so that data from multiple studies can be combined.

The spectacular progress in human genome sequencing would facilitate whole-genome screening for association since genes with smaller effects can be more efficiently detected (Risch and Merikangas, 1996). The generation of millions of SNPs throughout the genome should favor this approach. In this respect, high-throughput techniques have been developed and are being improved to permit analysis of numerous SNP markers on massive numbers of samples. But, as shown by Altshuler et al. (2000), for a locus with a relative risk of 1.25, several thousands of individuals had to be analyzed to extract a definitive evidence of association. Just as importantly, this work revealed that negative findings in reality may not be so, because the study interrogated insufficient number of samples to have enough power of detecting association. This serves as a cautionary reminder that exclusion or inclusion of the contribution of a gene to genetic risk should not be done hastily.

Another approach is to conduct linkage and association studies in population isolates in the hope that they will carry fewer genes for a particular disorder; however, this is not a panacea. When susceptibility loci are common, population isolates are also expected to be segregating for multiple susceptibility loci. Population isolates may be more powerful for detecting susceptibility genes by association because they will have larger regions of linkage disequilibrium than do outbred populations.

Currently, functional genomics has started to be exploited to help dissect the complexity of mood disorders. Clearly, a combination of all of these strategies is needed to increase the chance of identifying affective disorder–predisposing genes. The comprehensive elucidation of all human genes provides an unprecedented advantage that is certain to speed up this process. Knowledge of susceptibility genes would allow investigations into their biological function and associated pathophysiology. The effect on these genes of various environmental insults can be investigated. Furthermore, the question of whether mood disorders and schizophrenia share some risk genes could be evaluated. Conceptually, a potential outcome of the susceptibility gene identification would be the development of improved diagnostic tools that could be used to molecularly classify subtypes of the affective disorder phenotypes. These varied approaches could also provide multiple potential targets for drug discovery. It is likely that by the time the third edition of this volume is published, new susceptibility genes will have been elucidated and these preceding questions will be under investigation.

REFERENCES

Abecasis GR, Noguchi E, Heinzmann A, Traherne JA, Bhattacharyya S, Leaves NI, Anderson GG, Zhang Y, Lench NJ, Carey A, et al.: Extent and distribution of linkage disequilibrium in three genomic regions. Am J Hum Genet 2001; 68:191–197.

Adams LJ, Mitchell PH, Fielder SL, Rosso A, Donald JA, Schofield PR: A susceptibility locus for bipolar affective disorder on chromosome 4q35. Am J Hum Genet 1998; 62:1084–1091.

Aita VM, Liu J, Knowles JA, Terwilliger JD, Baltazar R, Grunn A, Loth JE, Kanyas K, Lerer B, Endicott J, et al.: A comprehensive linkage analysis of chromosome 21q22 supports prior evidence for a putative bipolar affective disorder locus. Am J Hum Genet 1999; 64:210–217.

Altshuler D, Hirschhorn JN, Klannemark M, Lindgren CM, Vohl MC, Nemesh J, Lane CR, Schaffner SF, Bolk S, Brewer C, et al.: The common PPARγ Pro12Ala polymorphism is associated with decreased risk of Type 2 diabetes. Nat Genet 2000; 26:76–80.

American Psychiatric Association: Diagnostic and Statistical Manual of Mental Disorders, 4th ed. Washington, DC: American Psychiatric Association, 1994.

Andreasen NC, Rice J, Endicott J, Coryell W, Grove WM, Reich T: Familial rates of affective disorder. Arch Gen Psychiatry 1987; 44:461–469.

Angst J, Frey R, Lohmeyer B, Zerbin-Rudin E: Bipolar manic depressive psychoses: results of a genetic investigation. Hum Genet 1980; 55:237–254.

Badenhop RF, Moses MJ, Scimone A, Mitchell PB, Ewen KR, Rosso A, Donald JA, Adams LJ, Schofield PR: A genome screen of a large bipolar affective disorder pedigree supports evidence for a susceptibility locus on chromosome 13q. Mol Psychiatry 2001; 6:396–403.

Barden N, Morissette J: Chromosome 13 workshop report. Am J Med Genet 1999; 88:260–262.

Baron M, Freimer NF, Risch N, Lerer B, Alexander JR, Straub RE, Asokan S, Das K, Peterson A, Amos J, et al.: Diminished support for linkage between manic depressive illness and X-chromosome markers in three Israeli pedigrees. Nat Genet 1993; 3:49–55.

Baron M, Risch N, Hamburger R, Mandel B, Kushner S, Newman M, Drumer D, Belmaker RH: Genetic linkage between X chromosome markers and bipolar affective illness. Nature 1987; 326:289–292.

Baumann B, Bogerts B: Neuroanatomical studies on bipolar disorder. Br J Psychiatry Suppl 2001; 41:S142–147.

Baysal BE, Potkin SG, Farr JE, Higgins MJ, Korcz J, Gollin SM, James MR, Evans GA, Richard CW III: Bipolar affective disorder partially cosegregates with a balanced t(9;11)(p24:q23.1) chromosomal translocation in a small pedigree. Am J Med Genet 1998; 81:81–91.

Berrettini WH. Are schizophrenic and bipolar disorders related? A review of family and molecular studies. Biol Psychiatry 2000; 48(6):531–538.

Berrettini WH, Ferraro TN, Goldin LR, Weeks DE, Detera-Wadleigh S, Nurnberger JI Jr, Gershon ES: Chromosome 18 DNA markers and manic-depressive illness: evidence for a susceptibility gene. Proc Natl Acad Sci USA 1994; 91:5918–5921.

Berrettini WH, Goldin LR, Gelernter J, Gejman PV, Gershon Es, Detera-Wadleigh S: X-chromosome and manic depresion: rejection of linkage to Xq28 in nine bipolar pedigrees. Arch Gen Psychiatry 1990; 47:366–373.

Bertelsen A, Harvald B, Hauge MA: A Danish twin study of manic-depressive disorders. Br J Psychiatry 1977; 130:330–351.

Blackwood DH, Fordyce A, Walker MT, St Clair DM, Porteous DJ, Muir WJ: Schizophrenia and affective disorders: cosegregation with a translocation at chromosome 1q42 that directly disrupts brain-expressed genes—clinical and P300 findings in a family. Am J Hum Genet 2001; 69:428–433.

Blackwood DH, Muir W: Molecular genetics and the epidemiology of bipolar disorder. Ann Med 2001; 33:242–247.

Blackwood DH, He L, Morris SW, McLean A, Whitton C, Thomson M, Walker MT, Woodburn K, Sharp CM, Wright AF, et al.: A locus for bipolar affective disorder on chromosome 4p. Nat Genet 1996; 12:427–430.

Blazer DG, Kessler RC, McGonagle KA, Swartz MS: The prevalence and distribution of major depression in a national community sample: the National Comorbidity Survey. Am J Psychiatry 1994; 151:979–986.

Blouin JL, Dombroski BA, Nath SK, Lasseter VK, Wolyniec PS, Nestadt G, Thornquist M, Ullrich G, McGrath J, Kasch L, et al.: Schizophrenia susceptibility loci on chromosomes 13q32 and 8p21. Nat Genet 1998; 20:70–73.

Boyd JH, Weissman MM: Epidemiology of affective disorders: a reexamination and future directions. Arch Gen Psychiatry 1981; 38:1039–1046.

Brzustowicz LM, Hodgkinson KA, Chow EW, Honer WG, Bassett AS: Location of a major susceptibility locus for familial schizophrenia on chromosome 1q21–q22. Science 2000; 288:678–682.

Brzustowicz LM, Honer WG, Chow EW, Little D, Hogan J, Hodgkinson K, Bassett AS: Linkage of familial schizophrenia to chromosome 13q32. Am J Hum Genet 1999; 65:1096–1103.

Bucher KD, Elston RC: The transmission of manic depressive illness: I. Theory, description of the model and summary of results. J Psychiatr Res 1981; 16:53–63.

Cantwell DP, Struzenberger S, Burroughs J, Salkin B, Green JK: Anorexia nervosa: an affective disorder. Arch Gen Psychiatry 1977; 234:1087–1093.

Cichon S, Schmidt-Wolf G, Schumacher J, Muller DJ, Hurter M, Schulze TG, Albus M, Borrmann-Hassenbach M, Franzek E, Lanczik M, et al.: A possible susceptibility locus for bipolar affective disorder in chromosomal region 10q25–q26. Mol Psychiatry 2001; 6:342–349.

Collins A, Frezal J, Teague J, Morton NE: A metric map of humans: 23,500 loci in 850 bands. Proc Natl Acad Sci USA 1996; 93:14771–14775.

Coon H, Jensen S, Hoff M, Holik J, Plaetke R, Reimherr F, Wender P, Leppert M, Byerley W: A genome-wide search for genes predisposing to manic-depression, assuming autosomal dominant inheritance. Am J Hum Genet 1993; 52:1234–1249.

Coon H, Holik J, Hoff M, Reimherr F, Wender P, Myles-Worsley M, Waldo M, Freedman R, Byerley W: Analysis of chromosome 22 markers in nine schizophrenia pedigrees. Am J Med Genet 1994; 54:72–79.

Corder EH, Saunders AM, Strittmatter WJ, Schmechel DE, Gaskell PC, Small GW, Roses AD, Haines JL, Pericak-Vance MA: Gene dose of apolipoprotein E type 4 allele and the risk of Alzheimer's disease in late onset families. Science 1993; 261:921–923.

Cordeiro ML, Umbach JA, Gundersen CB: Lithium ions up-regulate mRNAs encoding dense-core vesicle proteins in nerve growth factor-differentiated PC12 cells. J Neurochem 2000; 75(6):2622–2625.

Coryell W, Endicott J, Keller M, Andreasen NC: Phenomenology and family history in DSM-III psychotic depression. J Affect Disord 1985; 9:13–18.

Coryell W, Winokur G, Andreasen N: Effect of case definition on affective disorder rates. Am J Psychiatry 1981; 138:1106–1109.

Cox N, Reich T, Rice J, Elston R, Schober J, Keats B: Segregation and linkage analyses of bipolar and major depressive illnesses in multigenerational pedigrees. J Psychiatr Res 1989; 23:109–123.

Craddock N, Khodel V, Van Eerdewegh P, Reich T: Mathematical limits of multilocus models: the genetic transmission of bipolar disorder. Am J Hum Genet 1995; 57:690–702.

Craddock N, Lendon C: Chromosome workshop: chromosomes 11, 14, and 15. Am J Med Genet 1999; 88:244–254.

Craddock N, Owen M: Chromosomal abberations and bipolar affective disorder. Br J Psychiatry 1994; 164:507–512.

Craddock N, Owen M, Burge S, Kurian B, Thomas P, McGuffin P: Familial cosegregation of major affective disorder and Darier's disease (keratosis follicularis). Br J Psychiatry 1994; 164:355–358.

Craddock N, Van Eerdewegh P, Reich T: Single major locus models for bipolar disorder are implausible. Am J Med Genet 1997; 74:18.

Crowe RR: Candidate genes in psychiatry: an epidemiological perspective. Am J Med Genet 1993; 48:74–77.

Crowe RR, Namboodiri KK, Ashby HB, Elston RC: Segregation and linkage analysis of a large kindred of unipolar depression. Neuropsychobiology 1981; 7:20–25.

Crowe RR, Vieland V: Report of the Chromosome 5 Workshop of the Sixth World Congress on Psychiatric Genetics. Am J Med Genet 1999; 88:229–232.

Curtis D: Chromosome 21 workshop. Am J Med Genet 1999; 88:272–275.

De Bruyn A, Souery D, Mendelbaum K, Mendlewicz J, Van Broeckhoven C: Linkage analysis of families with bipolar illness and chromosome 18 markers. Biol Psychiatry 1996; 39:679–688.

DeLisi LE, Craddock NJ, Detera-Wadleigh S, Foroud T, Gejman P, Kennedy JL,

Lendon C, Macciardi F, McKeon P, Mynett-Johnson L, et al.: Update on chromosomal locations for psychiatric disorders: report of the interim meeting of chromosome workshop chairpersons from the VIIth World Congress of Psychiatric Genetics, Monterey, California, October 14–18, 1999. Am J Med Genet 2000; 96:434–449.

Detera-Wadleigh SD: Chromosomes 12 and 16 workshop. Am J Med Genet 1999; 88:255–259.

Detera-Wadleigh SD: Lithium-related genetics of bipolar disorder. Ann Med 2001; 33:272–285.

Detera-Wadleigh SD, Badner JA, Berrettini WH, Yoshikawa T, Goldin LR, Turner G, Rollins DY, Moses T, Sanders AR, Karkera JD, et al.: A high-density genome scan detects evidence for a bipolar-disorder susceptibility locus on 13q32 and other potential loci on 1q32 and 18p11.2. Proc Natl Acad Sci USA 1999; 96:5604–5609.

Detera-Wadleigh SD, Badner JA, Goldin LR, Berrettini WH, Sanders AR, Rollins DY, Turner G, Moses T, Haerian H, Muniec D, et al.: Affected sib-pair analyses reveal support of prior evidence for a susceptibility locus for bipolar disorder on 21q. Am J Hum Genet 1996; 58:1279–1285.

Detera–Wadleigh SD, Badner JA, Yoshikawa T, Sanders AR, Goldin LR, Turner G, Rollins DY, Moses T, Guroff JJ, Kazuba D, et al.: Initial genome scan of the NIMH genetics initiative bipolar pedigrees: chromosomes 4, 7, 9, 18, 19, 20, and 21q. Am J Med Genet 1997; 74:254–262.

Detera-Wadleigh S, Berrettini WH, Goldin LR, Boorman D, Anderson S, Gershon ES: Close linkage of c-harvery-ras-1 and Insulin to affective disorder is ruled out in 3 North American pedigrees. Nature 1987; 325:806–808.

Detera-Wadleigh SD, Hseih WT, Berrettini WH, Goldin LR, Rollins DY, Muniec D, Grewal R, Guroff JJ, Turner G, Coffman D, et al.: Genetic linkage mapping for a susceptibility locus to bipolar illness: chromosomes 2, 3, 4, 7, 9, 10p, 11p, 22, and Xpter. Am J Med Genet 1994; 54:206–218.

Edenberg HJ, Foroud T, Conneally PM, Sorbel JJ, Carr K, Crose C, Willig C, Zhao J, Miller M, Bowman E, et al.: Initial genomic scan of the NIMH genetics initiative bipolar pedigrees: chromosomes 3, 5, 15, 16, 17, and 22. Am J Med Genet 1997; 74:238–246.

Egeland JA, Gerhard DS, Pauls DL, Sussex JN, Kidd KK, Allen CR, Hostetter AM, Housman DE: Bipolar affective disorders linked to DNA markers on chromosome 11. Nature 1987; 325:783–787.

Ekelund J, Hovatta I, Parker A, Paunio T, Varilo T, Martin R, Suhonen J, Ellonen P, Chan G, Sinsheimer JS, et al.: Chromosome 1 loci in Finnish schizophrenia families. Hum Mol Genet 2001; 10:1611–1617.

Ekelund J, Lichtermann D, Hovatta I, Ellonen P, Suvisaari J, Terwilliger JD, Juvonen H, Varilo T, Arajarvi R, Kokko-Sahin ML, et al.: Genome-wide scan for schizophrenia in the Finnish population: evidence for a locus on chromosome 7q22. Hum Mol Genet 2000; 9:1049–1057.

Engstrom C, Thornlund AS, Johansson EL, Langstrom M, Chotai J, Adolfsson R, Nylander PO: Anticipation in unipolar affective disorder. J Affect Disord 1995; 35:31–40.

Ensemble Gene View: http://www.ensembl.org, Dec 5, 2001.

Evans KL, Muir WJ, Blackwood DH, Porteous DJ: Nuts and bolts of psychiatric genetics: building on the Human Genome Project. Trends Genet 2001; 17:35–40.

Ewald H, Degn B, Mors O, Kruse TA: Support for the possible locus on chromosome 4p16 for bipolar affective disorder. Mol Psychiatry 1998b; 3:442–448.

Ewald H, Degn B, Mors O, Kruse TA: Significant linkage between bipolar affective disorder and chromosome 12q24. Psychiatr Genet 1998a; 8:131–140.

Ewald H, Mors O, Flint T, Koed K, Eiberg H, Kruse TA: A possible locus for manic depressive illness on chromosome 16p13. Psychiatr Genet 1995; 5:71–81.

Faraone SV, Matise T, Svrakic D, Pepple J, Malaspina D, Suarez B, Hampe C, Zambuto CT, Schmitt K, Meyer J, et al.: Genome scan of European-American schizophrenia pedigrees: results of the NIMH Genetics Initiative and Millennium Consortium. Am J Med Genet 1998; 81:290–295.

Feingold E, Brown PO, Siegmund D: Gaussian models for genetic linkage analysis using complete high resolution maps of identity by descent. Am J Hum Genet 1993; 53:234–251.

Fieve RR, Go R, Dunner DL, Elston R: Search for biological/genetic markers in a long-term epidemiological and morbid risk study of affective disorders. J Psychiatr Res 1984; 18:425–445.

Foroud T, Castelluccio PF, Koller DL, Edenberg HJ, Miller M, Bowman E, Rau NL, Smiley C, Rice JP, Goate A, et al.: Suggestive evidence of a locus on chromosome 10p using the NIMH genetics initiative bipolar affective disorder pedigrees. Am J Med Genet 2000; 96:18–23.

Freimer NB, Reus VI, Escamilla MA, McInnes LA, Spesny M, Leon P, Service SK, Smith LB, Silva S, Rojas E, et al.: Genetic mapping using haplotype, association and linkage methods suggests a locus for severe bipolar disorder (BPI) at 18q22–q23. Nat Genet 1996; 12:436–441.

Friddle C, Koskela R, Ranade K, Hebert J, Cargill M, Clark CD, McInnis M, Simpson S, McMahon F, Stine OC, et al.: Full-genome scan for linkage in 50 families segregating the bipolar affective disease phenotype. Am J Hum Genet 2000; 66(1):205–215.

Gejman P, Detera-Wadleigh S, Martinez MM, Berrettini WH, Goldin LR, Gelernter J, Hsieh WT, Gershon ES: Manic depressive illness not linked to factor IX region in an independent series of pedigrees. Genomics 1990; 8:648–655.

Gershon ES, Badner JA, Detera-Wadleigh SD, Ferraro TN, Berrettini WH: Maternal inheritance and chromosome 18 allele sharing in unilineal bipolar illness pedigrees. Am J Med Genet 1996; 67:202–207.

Gershon ES, DeLisi LE, Hamovit J, Nurnberger JI Jr, Maxwell ME, Schreiber J, Dauphinais D, Dingman CW 2nd, Guroff JJ: A controlled family study of chronic psychoses: schizophrenia and schizoaffective disorder. Arch Gen Psychiatry 1988; 45:328–336.

Gershon ES, Hamovit J, Guroff JJ, Dibble ED, Leckman J, Sceery W, Targum SD, Nurnberger JI Jr, Goldin L, Bunney WE Jr: A family study of of schizoaffective, bipolar I, bipolar II, unipolar and normal control probands. Arch Gen Psychiatry 1982; 39:1157–1167.

Gershon ES, Hamovit JH, Guroff JJ, Nurnberger JI Jr: Birth cohort changes in manic and depressive disorders in relatives of bipolar and schizoaffective patients. Arch Gen Psychiatry 1987; 44:314–319.

Gershon ES, Mark A, Cohen N, Belizon N, Baron M, Knobe KE: Transmitted factors in the morbidity of affective disorders: a controlled study. J Psychiatr Res 1975; 12:283–299.

Gershon ES, Schreiber JL, Hamovit JR, Dibble ED, Kaye W, Nurnberger JI Jr, Andersen AE, Ebert M: Clinical findings in patients with anorexia nervosa and affective illness in their relatives. Am J Psychiatry 1984; 141:1419–1422.

Ginns EI, Ott J, Egeland JA, Allen CR, Fann CSJ, Pauls DL, Weissenbach J, Carulli JP, Falls KM, Keith TP, Paul SM: A genome-wide search for chromosomal loci linked to bipolar affective disorder in the Old Order Amish. Nat Genet 1996; 12:431–435.

Goetzl V, Green R, Whybrow P, Jackson R: X-linkage revisited: a further family study of manic depressive illness. Arch Gen Psychiatry 1974; 31:665–673.

Goldin LR, Gershon ES, Berrettini WH, Stine OC, DePaulo R, McMahon F, Meyers D, Nothen M, Propping P, Cichon S, et al.: Description of the Genetic Analysis Workshop: 10 bipolar disorder linkage data sets. Genet Epidemiol 1997; 14:563–568.

Goldin LR, Gershon ES, Targum SD, Sparkes RS, McGinniss M: Segregation and linkage analysis in families of patients with bipolar, unipolar, and schizo-affective mood disorders. Am J Hum Genet 1983; 35:274–287.

Goodwin FK, Jamison KR: Manic-Depressive Illness. New York: Oxford University Press, 1990.

Greenwood TA, Alexander M, Keck PE, McElroy S, Sadovnick AD, Remick RA, Kelsoe JR: Evidence for linkage disequilibrium between the dopamine transporter and bipolar disorder. Am J Med Genet 2001; 105:145–151.

Grigoroiu-Serebanescu M, Wickramaratne P, Hodge SE, Milea S, Mihailescu R: Genetic anticipation and imprinting in bipolar I illness. Br J Psychiatry 1997; 170:162–166.

Gurling HM, Kalsi G, Brynjolfson J, Sigmundsson T, Sherrington R, Mankoo BS, Read T, Murphy P, Blaveri E, McQuillin A, et al.: Genomewide genetic linkage analysis confirms the presence of susceptibility loci for schizophrenia, on chromosomes 1q32.2, 5q33.2, and 8p21–22 and provides support for linkage to schizophrenia, on chromosomes 11q23.3–24 and 20q12.1–11.23. Am J Hum Genet 2001; 68:661–673.

Guy C, Bowen T, Daniels JK, Speight G, McKeon P, Mynett-Johnson L, Claffey E, McGuffin P, Owen MJ, Craddock N, O'Donovan MC: Exclusion of expansion of 50 CAG/CTG trinucleotide repeats in bipolar disorder. Am J Psychiatry 1997; 154:1146–1147.

Hagnell O, Lanke J, Rorsman B, Ojesjo L: Are we entering an age of melancholy? Depressive illness in a prospective epidemiological study over 25 years: the Lundby Study, Sweden. Psychol Med 1982; 12:279–289.

Hakak Y, Walker JR, Li C, Wong WH, Davis KL, Buxbaum JD, Haroutunian V, Fienberg AA: Genome-wide expression analysis reveals dysregulation of myelination-related genes in chronic schizophrenia. Proc Natl Acad Sci USA 2001; 98:4746–4751.

Hallmayer J: Chromosomes 1, 2, and 7 workshop. Am J Med Genet 1999; 88:219–223.

Hauser ER, Boehnke M, Guo SW, Risch N: Affected sib-pair interval mapping and exclusion for complex genetic traits: sampling considerations. Genet Epidemiol 1996; 13:117–137.

Helzer JE, Winokur G: A family interview study of male manic depressives. Arch Gen Psychiatry 1974; 31:73–77.

Hodge SE, Wickramaratne PJ: Statistical pitfalls in detecting age-of-onset anticipation and detecting ascertainment bias. Psychiatr Genet 1995; 5:43–47.

Hodgkinson S, Sherrington R, Gurling H, Marchbanks R, Reeders S, Mallet J, McInnis M, Petursson H, Brynjolfsson J: Molecular evidence for heterogeneity in manic depression. Nature 1987; 325:805–806.

Hogenesch JB, Ching KA, Batalov S, Su AI, Walker JR, Zhou Y, Kay SA, Schultz PG, Cooke MP: A comparison of the Celera and Ensembl predicted gene sets reveals little overlap in novel genes. Cell 2001; 106:413–415.

Hovatta I, Varilo T, Suvisaari J, Terwilliger JD, Ollikainen V, Arajarvi R, Juvonen H, Kokko-Sahin ML, Vaisanen L, Mannila H, et al.: A genomewide screen for schizophrenia genes in an isolated Finnish subpopulation, suggesting multiple susceptibility loci. Am J Hum Genet 1999; 65:1114–1124.

International Human Genome Sequencing Consortium: Initial sequencing and analysis of the human genome. Nature 2001; 409:860–921.

International SNP Map Working Group: A map of human genome sequence variation containing 1.42 million single nucleotide polymorphisms. Nature 2001; 409:928–933.

Jacobsen NJ, Lyons I, Hoogendoorn B, Burge S, Kwok PY, O'Donovan MC, Craddock N, Owen MJ: *ATP2A2* mutations in Darier's disease and their relationship to neuropsychiatric phenotypes. Hum Mol Genet 1999; 8:1631–1636.

James NM, Chapman CJ: A genetic study of bipolar affective disorder. Br J Psychiary 1975; 126:449–456.

Johnson GFS, Leeman MM: Analysis of familial factors in bipolar affective illness. Arch Gen Psychiatry 1977; 34:1074–1083.

Jones I, Craddock N: Candidate gene studies of bipolar disorder. Ann Med 2001; 33:248–256.

Jorde LB: Linkage disequilibrium and the search for complex disease genes. Genome Res 2000; 10:1435–1444.

Joyce PR, Oakley-Browne MA, Wells JE, Bushnell JA, Hornblow AR: Birth cohort

trends in major depression: increasing rates and earlier onset in New Zealand. J Affect Disord 1990; 18:83–89.
Karkowski LM, Kendler KS: An examination of the genetic relationship between bipolar and unipolar illness in an epidemiological sample. Psychiatr Genet 1997; 7:159–163.
Kelsoe JR, Ginns EI, Egeland JA, Gerhard DS, Goldstein AM, Bale SJ, Pauls DL, Long RT, Kidd KK, Conte G, et al.: Re-evaluation of the linkage relationship between chromosome 11p and the gene for bipolar affective disorder in the Old Order Amish. Nature 1989; 342:238–243.
Kelsoe JR, Spence MA, Loetscher E, Foguet M, Sadovnick AD, Remick RA, Flodman P, Khristich J, Mroczkowski-Parker Z, Brown JL, et al.: A genome survey indicates a possible susceptibility locus for bipolar disorder on chromosome 22. Proc Natl Acad Sci USA 2001; 98:585–590.
Kendell RE, Gourlay J: The clinical distinction between the affective psychoses and schizophrenia. Br J Psychiatry 1970; 117(538):261–266.
Kendler KS, Neale MC, Kessler RC, Heath AC, Eaves LJ: A population-based twin study of major depression in women: the impact of varying definitions of illness. Arch Gen Psychiatry 1992; 49:257–266.
Kendler KS, Pedersen NL, Neale MC, Mathe AA: A pilot Swedish twin study of affective illness including hospital- and population-ascertained subsamples: results of model fitting. Behav Genet 1995a; 25:217–232.
Kendler KS, Walters EE, Neale MC, Kessler RC, Heath AC, Eaves LJ: The structure of the genetic and environmental risk factors for six major psychiatric disorders in women: phobia, generalized anxiety disorder, panic disorder, bulimia, major depression, and alcoholism. Arch Gen Psychiatry 1995b; 52:374–383.
Kennedy JL, Basile VS, Macciardi FM. Chromosome 4 workshop summary: Sixth World Congress on Psychiatric Genetics, Bonn, Germany, October 6–10, 1998. Am J Med Genet 1999; 88:224–228.
Kety SS, Rosenthal D, Wender PH, Schulsinger F, Jacobsen B: Mental illness in the biological and adoptive families of adopted individuals who have become schizophrenic. Behav Genet 1976; 6:219–225.
Klerman GL, Lavori PW, Rice J, Reich T, Endicott J, Andreasen NC, Keller MB, Hirschfeld RMA: Birth cohort trends in rates of major depressive disorder among relatives of patients with affective disorder. Arch Gen Psychiatry 1985; 42:689–695.
Klerman GL, Leon AC, Wickramaratne P, Warshaw MG, Mueller TI, Weissman MM, Akiskal H: The role of drug and alcohol abuse in recent increases in depression in the United States. Psychol Med 1996; 26:343–351.
Kwok PY: High-throughput genotyping assay approaches. Pharmacogenomics 2000; 1(1):95–100.
LaBuda MC, Maldonado M, Marshall D, Otten K, Gerhard D: A follow-up report of a genome search for affective disorder predisposition loci in the Old Order Amish. Am J Hum Genet 1996; 59:1343–1362.
Lachman HM, Kelsoe JR, Remick RA, Sadovnick AD, Rapaport MH, Lin M, Pazur BA, Roe AMA, Saito T, Papolos DF: Linkage studies suggest a possible locus for bipolar disorder near the velo-cardio-facial syndrome region on chromosome 22. Am J Med Genet 1997; 74:121–128.
Lachman HM, Morrow B, Shprintzen R, Veit S, Parsia SS, Faedda G, Goldberg R, Kucherlapati R, Papolos DF. Association of codon 108/158 catechol-*O*-methyltransferase gene polymorphism with the psychiatric manifestations of velo-cardio-facial syndrome. Am J Med Genet 1996; 67:468–472.
Lander E, Kruglyak L: Genetic dissection of complex traits: guidelines for interpreting and reporting linkage results. Nat Genet 1995; 11:241–247.
La Spada AR: Trinucleotide repeat instability: genetic features and molecular mechanisms. Brain Pathol 1997; 7:943—963.
Lavori PW, Klerman GL, Keller MB, Reich T, Rice J, Endicott J: Age-period-cohort analysis of secular trends in onset of major depression: findings in siblings of patients with major affective disorder. J Psychiatr Res 1987; 21:23–35.
Leon AC, Klerman GL, Wickramaratne P: Continuing female predominance in depressive illness. Am J Public Health 1993; 83:754–757.
Levinson DF, Mahtani MM, Nancarrow DJ, Brown DM, Kruglyak L, Kirby A, Hayward NK, Crowe RR, Andreasen NC, Black DW, et al.: Genome scan of schizophrenia Am J Psychiatry 1998; 155:741–750.
Lin MW, Sham P, Hwu HG, Collier D, Murray R, Powell JF: Suggestive evidence for linkage of schizophrenia to markers on chromosome 13 in Caucasian but not Oriental populations. Hum Genet 1997; 99:417–420.
Lindblad K, Nylander PO, Debruyn A, Sourey D, Zander C, Engstrom C, Holmgren G, Hudson T, Chotai J, Mendlewicz J. et al.: Detection of expanded CAG repeats in bipolar affective disorder using the repeat expansion detection (RED) method. Neurobiol Dis 1995; 2:55–62.
Lindholm E, Ekholm B, Balciuniene J, Johansson G, Castensson A, Koisti M, Nylander PO, Pettersson U, Adolfsson R, Jazin E. Linkage analysis of a large Swedish kindred provides further support for a susceptibility locus for schizophrenia on chromosome 6p23. Am J Med Genet 1999; 88:369–377.
Liu C, Badner JA, Christian SL, Guroff JJ, Detera-Wadleigh SD, Gershon ES: Fine mapping supports previous linkage evidence for a bipolar disorder susceptibility locus on 13q32. Am J Med Genet 2001; 105:375–380.
Llewellyn A, Stowe ZN, Strader JR Jr: The use of lithium and management of women with bipolar disorder during pregnancy and lactation. J Clin Psychiatry 1998; 59(Suppl 6):57–64.
MacKinnon DF, Xu J, McMahon FJ, Simpson SG, Stine OC, McInnis MG, DePaulo JR: Bipolar disorder and panic disorder in families: an analysis of chromosome 18 data. Am J Psychiatry 1998; 155(6):829–831.
Maier W, Lichtermann D, Minges J, Delmo C, Heun R: The relationship between bipolar disorder and alcoholism: a controlled family study. Psychol Med 1995; 25:787–796.
Maier W, Lichtermann D, Minges J, Hallmayer J, Heun R, Benkert O, Levinson DF. Continuity and discontinuity of affective disorders and schizophrenia: results of a controlled family study. Arch Gen Psychiatry 1993; 50:871–883.
Marazita ML, Neiswanger K, Cooper M, Zubenko GS, Giles DE, Frank E, Kupfer DJ, Kaplan BB: Genetic segregation analysis of early-onset recurrent unipolar depression. Am J Hum Genet 1997; 61:1370–1378.
Maziade M, Bissonnette L, Rouillard E, Martinez M, Turgeon M, Charron L, Pouliot V, Boutin P, Cliche D, Dion C, et al.: 6p24–22 region and major psychoses in the Eastern Quebec population. Am J Med Genet 1997; 74:311–318.
McInnis MG, McMahon FJ, Chase GA, Simpson SG, Ross CA, DePaulo JR Jr: Anticipation in bipolar affective disorder. Am J Hum Genet 1993; 53:385–390.
McMahon FJ, Hopkins PJ, Xu J, McInnis MG, Shaw S, Cardon L, Simpson SG, MacKinnon DF, Stine OC, Sherrington R, et al.: Linkage of bipolar affective disorder to chromosome 18 markers in a new pedigree series. Am J Hum Genet 1997; 61:1397–1404.
McMahon FJ, Simpson SG, McInnis MG, Badner JA, MacKinnon DF, DePaulo JR: Linkage of bipolar disorder to chromosome 18q and the validity of bipolar II disorder. Arch Gen Psychiatry, 2001; 58:1025–1031.
McMahon FJ, Stine OC, Meyers DA, Simpson SG, DePaulo RJ Jr: Patterns of maternal transmission in bipolar affective disorder. Am J Hum Genet 1995; 56:1277–1286.
Mendlewicz J, Rainer JD: Morbidity risk and genetic transmission in manic depressive illness. Am J Hum Genet 1974; 26:692–701.
Mendlewicz J, Rainer JD: Adoption study supporting genetic transmission in manic depressive illness. Nature 1977; 268:327–329.
Mendlewicz J, Simon P, Sevy S, Charon F, Brocas H, Legrus S, Vassart G: Polymorphic DNA marker on X-chromosome and manic depressive illness. Lancet 1987; 1:1230–1232.
Michaud CM, Murray CJ, Bloom BR: Burden of disease: implications for future research. JAMA 2001; 285:535–539.
Millar JK, Wilson-Annan JC, Anderson S, Christie S, Taylor MS, Semple CA, Devon RS, Clair DM, Muir WJ, Blackwood DH, Porteous DJ: Disruption of two novel genes by a translocation co-segregating with schizophrenia. Hum Mol Genet 2000; 9:1415–1423.
Mirnics K, Middleton FA, Marquez A, Lewis DA, Levitt P: Molecular characterization of schizophrenia viewed by microarray analysis of gene expression in prefrontal cortex. Neuron 2000; 28:53–67.
Morissette J, Villeneuve A, Bordeleau L, Rochetter D, Laberge C, Gagne B, Laprise C, Bouchard G, Plante M, Gobeil L, et al.: Genome-wide search for linkage of bipolar affective disorders in a very large pedigree derived from a homogeneous population in Quebec points to a locus of major effect on chromosome 12q23–24. Am J Med Genet 1999; 88:567–587.
Mowry BJ, Ewen KR, Nancarrow DJ, Lennon DP, Nertney DA, Jones HL, O'Brien MS, Thornley CE, Walters MK, Crowe RR, et al.: Second stage of a genome scan of schizophrenia: study of five positive regions in an expanded sample. Am J Med Genet 2000; 96(6):864–869.
Murphy VE, Mynett-Johnson LA, Claffey E, Bergin P, McAuliffe M, Kealey C, McKeon P: Search for bipolar disorder susceptibility loci: the application of a modified genome scan concentrating on gene-rich regions. Am J Med Genet 2000; 96:728–732.
Murray CJL, Lopez AD. Alternative projections of mortality and disability by cause 1990–2020: global burden of disease survey. Lancet 1997; 349:1498–1504.
Mynett-Johnson L, Kealey C, Claffey E, Curtis D, Bouchier-Hayes L, Powell C, McKeon P: Multimarker haplotypes within the serotonin transporter gene suggest evidence of an association with bipolar disorder. Am J Med Genet 2000; 96(6):845–849.
Neuman RJ, Geller B, Rice JP, Todd RD: Increased prevalence and earlier onset of mood disorders among relatives of prepubertal versus adult probands. J Am Acad Child Adolesc Psychiatry 1997; 36:466–473.
Neuman RJ, Rice JP: Two-locus models of disease. Genet Epidemiol 1992; 9:347–365.
Nickerson DA, Taylor SL, Weiss KM, Clark AG, Hutchinson RG, Stengard J, Salomaa V, Vartiainen E, Boerwinkle E, Sing CF: DNA sequence diversity in a 9.7 kb region of human lipoprotein lipase gene. Nat Genet 1998;19:233–240.
Niculescu AB III, Kelsoe JR. Convergent functional genomics: application to bipolar disorder. Ann Med 2001; 33:263–271.
Niculescu AB III, Segal DS, Kuczenski R, Barrett T, Hauger RL, Kelsoe JR: Identifying a series of candidate genes for mania and psychosis: a convergent functional genomics approach. Physiol Genomics 2000; 4:83–91.
Nothen MM, Cichon S, Rohleder H, Hemmer S, Franzek E, Fritze J, Albus M, Bormann-Hassenbach M, Kreiner R, Weigelt B, et al.: Evaluation of linkage of bipolar affective disorder to chromosome 18 in a sample of 57 German families. Mol Psychiatry 1999; 4:76–84.
Nurnberger JI Jr, Foroud T. Chromosome 6 workshop report. Am J Med Genet 1999; 88:233–238.
Nurnberger JI Jr, Foroud T, Flury L, Su J, Meyer ET, Hu K, Crowe R, Edenberg H, Goate A, Bierut L, et al.: Evidence for a locus on chromosome 1 that influences vulnerability to alcoholism and affective disorder. Am J Psychiatry 2001; 158:718–724.
Nylander PO, Engstrom C, Chotai J, Wahlstrom J, Adolfsson R: Anticipation in Swedish families with bipolar affective disorder. J Med Genet 1994; 31:686–689.
O'Donovan MC, Guy C, Craddock N, Bowen T, McKeon P, Macedo A, Maier W, Wildenauer D, Aschauer HN, Sorbi S, et al.: Confirmation of association between expanded CAG/CTG repeats and both schizophrenia and bipolar disorder. Psychol Med 1996; 26:1145–1153.
Oruc L, Lindblad K, Verheyen GR, Ahlberg S, Jakovljevic M, Ivezic S, Raeymaek-

ers P, Van Broeckhoven C, Schalling M: AG repeat expansions in bipolar and unipolar disorders. Am J Hum Genet 1997; 60:730–732.

Packer S: Family planning for women with bipolar disorder. Hosp Community Psychiatry 1992; 43:479–482.

Papolos DF, Faedda GL, Veit S, Goldberg R, Morrow B, Kucherlapatic R, Shprintzen RJ: Bipolar spectrum disorders in patients diagnosed with velo-cardio-facial syndrome: does a hemizygous deletion of chromosome 22q11 result in bipolar affective disorder? Am J Psychiatry 1996; 153:1541–1547.

Papolos DF, Veit S, Faedda GL, Saito T, Lachman HM: Ultra-ultra rapid cycling bipolar disorder is associated with the low activity catecholamine-*O*-methyltransferase allele. Mol Psychiatry 1998; 3:346–349.

Paterson AD: Report of the Sixth World Congress of Psychiatric Genetics X Chromosome Workshop. Am J Med Genet 1999; 88:279–286.

Pauls DL, Bailey JN, Carter AS, Allen CR, Egeland JA: Complex segregation analyses of Old Order Amish families ascertained through bipolar I individuals. Am J Med Genet 1995; 60:290–297.

Pekkarinen P, Terwilliger J, Bredbacka PE, Lonnqvist J, Peltonen L: Evidence of a predisposing locus to bipolar disorder on Xq24–q27.1 in an extended Finnish pedigree. Genome Res 1995; 5:105–115.

Pettersen U: Manic depressive illness: a clinical, social and genetic study. Acta Psychiatr Scand Suppl 1977; 269:1–93.

Prathikanti S, McMahon FJ: Genome scans for susceptibility genes in bipolar affective disorder. Ann Med 2001; 33:257–262.

Preisig M, Bellivier F, Fenton BT, Baud P, Berney A, Courtet P, Hardy P, Golaz J, Leboyer M, Mallet J, et al.: Association between bipolar disorder and monoamine oxidase A gene polymorphisms: results of a multicenter study. Am J Psychiatry 2000; 157:948–955.

Price RA, Kidd KK, Pauls DL, Gershon ES, Prusoff BA, Weissman MM, Goldin LR: Multiple threshold models for the affective disorders: the Yale-NIMH collaborative family study. J Psychiatr Res 1985; 19:256–259.

Pritchard JK: Are rare variants responsible for susceptibility to complex diseases? Am J Hum Genet 2001; 69:124–137.

Puig–Antich J, Goetz D, Davies M, Kaplan T, Davies S, Ostrow L, Asnis L, Twomey J, Iyengar S, Ryan ND: A controlled family history study of prepubertal major depressive disorder. Arch Gen Psychiatry 1989; 46:406–418.

Pulver AE, Nestadt G, Goldberg R, Shprintzen RJ, Lamacz M, Wolyniec PS, Morrow B, Karayiorgou M, Antonarakis SE, Housman D: Psychotic illness in patients diagnosed with velo-cardio-facial syndrome and their relatives. J Nerv Ment Dis 1994; 182:476–478.

Radhakrishna U, Senol S, Herken H, Gucuyener K, Gehrig C, Blouin JL, Akarsu NA, Antonarakis SE: An apparently dominant bipolar affective disorder (BPAD) locus on chromosome 20p11.2–q11.2 in a large Turkish pedigree. Eur J Hum Genet 2001; 9:39–44.

Regier DA, Farmer ME, Rae DS, Locke BZ, Keith SJ, Judd LL, Goodwin FK: Comorbidity of mental disorders with alcohol and other drug abuse. JAMA 1990; 264:2511–2518.

Reich DE, Cargill M, Bolk S, Ireland J, Sabeti PC, Richter DJ, Lavery T, Kouyoumjian R, Farhadian SF, Ward R, Lander ES. Linkage disequilibrium in the human genome. Nature 2001; 411:199–204.

Reich DE, Lander ES: On the allelic spectrum of human disease. Trends Genet 2001; 17:502–510.

Reyes GD, Esterling LE, Corona W, Ferraren D, Rollins DY, Padigaru M, Monje VD, Detera-Wadleigh SD. Map of candidates genes and STSs on 18p11.2, a bipolar disorder and schizophrenia susceptibility region. Mol Psychiatry, in press.

Rice J: Genetic analysis of bipolar disorder: summary of GAW10. Genet Epidemiol 1997; 14:549–561.

Rice J, Goate A, Williams JT, Bierut L, Dorr D, Wu W, Shears S, Gopalakrishnan G, Edenberg HJ, Foroud T, et al.: Initial genome scan of the NIMH genetics initiative bipolar pedigrees: chromosomes 1, 6, 8, 10, and 12. Am J Med Genet 1997; 74:247–253.

Rice J, Reich T, Anderson NC, Endicott J, Van Eerdewegh M, Fishman R, Hirschfeld RMA, Klerman GL: The familial transmission of bipolar illness. Arch Gen Psychiatry 1987; 44:441–447.

Rice J, Reich T, Andreasen NC, Lavori PW, Endicott J, Clayton PJ, Keller MB, Hirschfeld RM, Klerman GL: Sex-related differences in depression: familial evidence. J Affect Disord 1984; 7:199–210.

Risch N: Linkage strategies for genetically complex traits: I. Multilocus models. Am J Hum Genet 1990a; 46:222–228.

Risch N: Linkage strategies for genetically complex traits: II. The power of affected relative pairs. Am J Hum Genet 1990b; 46:229–241.

Risch N, Botstein D: A manic depressive history. Nat Genet 1996; 12(4):351–353.

Risch N, Merikangas K: The future of genetic studies of complex human diseases. Science 1996; 273:1516–1517.

Robins LN, Helzer JE, Weissman MM, Orvaschel H, Gruenberg E, Burke JD, Regier DA: Prevalence of specific psychiatric disorders in three sites. Arch Gen Psychiatry 1984; 41:949–958.

Rubinsztein DC, Leggo J, Goodburn S, Walsh C, Jain S, Paykel ES: Genetic association between monoamine oxidase A microsatellite and RFLP alleles and bipolar affective disorder: analysis and meta-analysis. Hum Mol Genet 1996; 5:779–782.

Ryan ND, Williamson DE, Iyengar S, Orvaschel H, Reich T, Dahl RE, Puig-Antich J: A secular increase in child and adolescent onset affective disorder J Am Acad Child Adolesc Psychiatry 1992; 31:600–605.

Sadovnick AD, Remick RA, Lam R, Zis AP, Yee IML, Huggins MJ, Baird PA: Mood disorder service genetic database: morbidity risks for mood disorders in 3,942 first-degree relatives of 671 index cases with single depression, recurrent depression, bipolar I, or bipolar II. Am J Med Genet 1994; 54:132–140.

Schulsinger F, Kety SS, Rosenthal D, Wender PH: A family study of suicide. In Shou M, Stromgren E (eds). Origin, Prevention, and Treatment of Affective Disorders. London: Academic Press, 1979:277–287.

Schulz PM, Schulz SC, Dibble E, Targum SD, vanKammen DP, Gershon ES: Patient and family attitudes about schizophrenia: implications for genetic counselling. Schizophr Bull 1982; 8:504–514.

Schwab SG, Albus M, Hallmayer J, Honig S, Borrmann M, Lichtermann D, Ebstein RP, Ackenheil M, Lerer B, Risch N, et al.: Evaluation of a susceptibility gene for schizophrenia on chromosome 6p by multipoint affected sib-pair linkage analysis. Nat Genet 1995; 11:325–327.

Schwab SG, Hallmayer J, Albus M, Lerer B, Eckstein GN, Borrmann M, Segman RH, Hanses C, Freymann J, Yakir A, et al.: A genome-wide autosomal screen for schizophrenia susceptibility loci in 71 families with affected siblings: support for loci on chromosome 10p and 6. Mol Psychiatry 2000; 5:638–649.

Schwab SG, Hallmayer J, Albus M, Lerer B, Hanses C, Kanyas K, Segman R, Borrman M, Dreikorn B, Lichtermann D, et al.: Further evidence for a susceptibility locus on chromosome 10p14–p11 in 72 families with schizophrenia by nonparametric linkage analysis. Am J Med Genet 1998a; 81:302–307.

Schwab SG, Hallmayer J, Lerer B, Albus M, Borrmann M, Honig S, Strauss M, Segman R, Lichtermann D, Knapp M, et al.: Support for a chromosome 18p locus conferring susceptibility to functional psychoses in families with schizophrenia, by association and linkage analysis. Am J Hum Genet 1998b; 63:1139–1152.

Schwab SG, Wildenauer DB. Chromosome 22 workshop report. Am J Med Genet 1999; 88:276–278.

Serretti A, Macciardi F, Cusin C, Verga M, Pedrini S, Smeraldi E: Tyrosine hydroxylase gene in linkage disequilibrium with mood disorders. Mol Psychiatry 1998; 3:169–174.

Sham PC, Morton NE, Rice JP: Segregation analysis of the NIMH collaborative study family data on bipolar disorder. Psychiatr Genet 1991; 2:175–184.

Sidransky E, Burgess C, Ikeuchi T, Lindblad K, Long RT, Philibert RA, Rapoport J, Schalling M, Tsuji S, Ginns EI: A triplet repeat on 17q accounts for most expansions detected by the repeat-expansion-detection technique. Am J Hum Genet 1998; 62:1548–1551.

Silverman JM, Greenberg DA, Alstiel LD, Siever LJ, Mohs RC, Smith CJ, Zhou G, Hollander TE, Yang XP, Kedache M, et al.: Evidence of a locus for schizophrenia and related disorders on the short arm of chromosome 5 in a large pedigree. Am J Med Genet 1996; 67:162–171.

Simon Ge, VonKorff M: Reevaluation of secular trends in depression rates. Am J Epidemiol 1992; 135:1411–1422.

Sjoholt G, Gulbrandsen AK, Lovlie R, Berle JO, Molven A, Steen VM: A human myo-inositol monophosphatase gene (IMPA2) localized in a putative susceptibility region for bipolar disorder on chromosome 18p11.2: genomic structure and polymorphism screening in manic-depressive patients. Mol Psychiatry 2000; 5:172–180.

Smeraldi E, Negri R, Heimbuch RC, Kidd KK: Familial patterns and possible modes of inheritance of primary affective disorder. J Affect Disord 1981; 3:173–182.

Smeraldi E, Negri F, Melica AM: A genetic study of affective disorder. Acta Psychiatr Scand 1977; 56:382–398.

Smith LB, Sapers B, Reus VI, Freimer NB: Attitudes towards bipolar disorder and predictive genetic testing among patients and providers. J Med Genet 1996; 33:544–549.

Smyth CS, Kalsi G, Curtis D, Brynjolfsson J, O'Neill J, Rifkin L, Moloney E, Murphy P, Petursson H, Gurling H: Two locus admixture linkage analysis of bipolar and unipolar disorder supports the presence of susceptibility loci on chromosomes 11p15 and 21q22. Genomics 1997; 39:1–8.

Solomon MI, Hellon CP: Suicide and age in Alberta, Canada, 1951–1977. Arch Gen Psychiatry 1980; 37:511–513.

Spence MA, Flodman PL, Sadovnik AD, Ameli H, Bailey-Wilson JE, Remick RA: Response to Craddock et al. Am J Med Genet 1997; 74:19–20.

Spence MA, Flodman PL, Sadovnick AD, Bailey-Wilson JE, Ameli H, Remick RA: Bipolar disorder: evidence for a major locus. Am J Med Genet 1995; 60:370–376.

Spielman RS, McGinnis RE, Ewens WJ: Transmission test for linkage disequilibrium: the insulin gene region and insulin-dependent diabetes mellitus (IDDM). Am J Hum Genet 1993; 52:506–516.

Spitzer RL, Endicott J, Robins E: Research diagnostic criteria: rationale and reliability. Arch Gen Psychiatry 1978; 35:773–782.

St. Clair D, Blackwood D, Muir W, Carothers A, Walker M, Spowart G, Gosden C, Evans HJ: Association within a family of a balanced autosomal translocation with major mental illness. Lancet 1990; 336:13–16.

Stine OC, Xu J, Koskela R, McMahon FJ, Gschwend M, Friddle C, Clark CD, McInnis MG, Sinpson SG, Breschel TS, et al.: Evidence of linkage of bipolar disorder to chromosome 18 with a parent-of-origin effect. Am J Hum Genet 1995; 57:1384–1394.

Straub RE, Lehner T, Luo Y, Loth JE, Shao W, Sharpe L, Alexander JR, Das K, Simon R, Fieve RR, et al.: A possible vulnerability locus for bipolar affective disorder on chromosome 21q22.3. Nat Genet 1994; 8:291–296.

Straub RE, MacLean CJ, Martin RB, Ma Y, Myakishev MV, Harris-Kerr C, Webb BT, O'Neill FA, Walsh D, Kendler KS: A schizophrenia locus may be located in region 10p15–p11. Am J Med Genet 1998; 81:296–301.

Straub RE, MacLean CJ, O'Neill FA, Burke J, Murphy B, Duke F, Shinkwin R, Webb BT, Zhang J, Walsh D, et al.: A potential vulnerability locus for schizophrenia on chromosome 6p24–22: evidence for genetic heterogeneity. Nat Genet 1995; 11:287–293.

Suarez BK, Hampe CL, Van Eerdewegh P: Problems of replicating linkage claims in psychiatry. In: Gershon ES, Cloninger CR (eds). Genetic Approaches to Mental Disorders. Washington DC: American Psychiatric Press, 1994:23–46.

Sun Y, Zhang L, Johnston NL, Torrey EF, Yolken RH: Serial analysis of gene expression in the frontal cortex of patients with bipolar disorder. Br J Psychiatry Suppl 2001; 41:S137–141.
Taylor MA: Are schizophrenia and affective disorder related? A selective literature review. Am J Psychiatry 1992; 149:22–32.
Taylor MA, Abrams R, Hayman MA: The classification of affective disorders: a reassessment of the bipolar-unipolar dichotomy. J Affective Disord 1980; 2:95–109.
Taylor MA, Amir N: Are schizophrenia and affective disorder related? The problem of schizoaffective disorder and the discrimination of the psychoses by signs and symptoms. Compr Psychiatry 1994; 35:420–429.
Terwilliger JD, Weiss KM: Linkage disequilibrium mapping of complex disease: fantasy or reality? Curr Opin Biotechol 1998; 9:578–594.
Thase ME, Kupfer DJ: Recent developments in the pharmacotherapy of mood disorders. J Consult Clin Psychol 1996; 64:646–659.
Todd RD, Neuman R, Geller B, Fox LW, Hickok J: Genetic studies of affective disorders: should we be starting with childhood onset probands? J Am Acad Child Adolesc Psychiatry 1993; 32:1164–1171.
Trippitelli CL, Jamison KR, Folstein MF, Bartko JJ, DePaulo JR: Pilot study on patients' and spouses' attitudes toward potential genetic testing for bipolar disorder. Am J Psychiatry 1998; 155:899–904.
Tsuang MT, Bucher KD, Fleming JA, Faraone SV: Transmission of affective disorders and application of segregation analysis to blind family study data. J Psychiatr Res 1985b; 19:23–29.
Tsuang MT, Faraone SV: The Genetics of Mood Disorders. Baltimore: Johns Hopkins University Press, 1990.
Tsuang MT, Faraone SV, Fleming JA: Familial transmission of major affective disorders: is there evidence supporting the distinction between unipolar and bipolar disorders? Br J Psychiatry 1985a; 146:268–271.
Tsuang MT, Winokur G, Crowe RR: Morbidity risks of schizophrenia and affective disorders among first degree relatives of patients with schizophrenia, mania, depression and surgical conditions. Br J Psychiatry 1980; 137:497–504.
Turecki G, Grof P, Grof E, D'Souza V, Lebuis L, Marineau C, Cavazzoni P, Duffy A, Betard C, Zvolsky P, et al.: Mapping susceptibility genes for bipolar disorder: a pharmacogenetic approach based on excellent response to lithium. Mol Psychiatry 2001; 6:570–578.
Turecki G, Smith M, Mari JJ. Type I bipolar disorder associated with a fragile site on chromosome 1. Am J Med Genet 1995; 60:179–182.
University of California–Santa Cruz Genome Browser: http://genome.ucsc.edu/, August 6, 2001.
Van Broeckhoven CV, Verheyen G: Report of the chromosome 18 workshop. Am J Med Genet 1999; 88:263–270.
Venter JC, Adams MD, Myers EW, Li PW, Mural RJ, Sutton GG, Smith HO, Yandell M, Evans CA, Holt RA: The sequence of the human genome. Science 2001; 291:1304–1351.
Vincent JB, Klempan T, Parikh SS, Sasaki T, Meltzer HY, Sirugo G, Cola P, Petronis A, Kennedy JL: Frequency analysis of large CAG/CTG trinucleotide repeats in schizophrenia and bipolar affective disorder. Mol Psychiatry 1996; 1:141–148.
Vincent JB, Paterson AD, Strong E, Petronis A, Kennedy JL: The unstable trinucleotide repeat story of major psychosis. Am J Med Genet 2000; 97:77–97.
von Knorring AL, Cloninger CR, Bohman M, Sigvardsson A: An adoption study of depressive disorders and substance abuse. Arch Gen Psychiatry 1983; 40:943–950.
Wang S, Sun CE, Walczak CA, Ziegle JS, Kipps BR, Goldin LR, Diehl SR: Evidence for a susceptibility locus for schizophrenia on chromosome 6pter–p22. Nat Genet 1995; 10:41–46.
Warshaw MG, Klerman GL, Lavori PW: Are secular trends in major depression an artifact of recall? J Psychiatr Res 1991; 25:141–151.
Weissman MM, Bland RC, Canino GJ, Faravelli C, Greenwald S, Hwu HG, Joyce PR, Karam EG, Lee CK, Lellouch J, et al.: Cross-national epidemiology of major depression and bipolar disorder. JAMA 1996; 276:293–299.
Weissman MM, Bland R, Joyce PR, Newman S, Wells JE, Wittchen H: Sex differences in rates of depression: cross national perspectives. J Affect Disord 1993; 29:77–84.
Weissman MM, Fyer AJ, Haghighi F, Heiman G, Deng Z, Hen R, Hodge SE, Knowles JA: Potential panic disorder syndrome: clinical and genetic linkage evidence. Am J Med Genet 2000; 96:24–35.
Weissman MM, Gershon ES, Kidd KK, Prusoff BA, Leckman JF, Dibble E, Hamovit J, Thompson WD, Pauls DL, Guroff JJ: Psychiatric disorders in the relatives of probands with affective disorders: the Yale-NIMH collaborative family study. Arch Gen Psychiatry 1984; 41:13–21.
Weissman MM, Kidd KK, Prusoff BA: Variability in rates of affective disorders in relatives of depressed and normal probands. Arch Gen Psychiatry 1982; 39:1397–1403.
Weissman MM, Warner V, Wickramaratne P, Moreau D, Olfson M: Offspring of depressed parents: 10 years later. Arch Gen Psychiatry 1997; 54:932–940.
Wender PH, Kety SS, Rosenthal D, Schulsinger F, Ortmann J: Psychiatric disorders in the biological and adoptive families of adopted individuals with affective disorders. Arch Gen Psychiatry 1986; 43:923–929.
Wildenauer DB, Schwab SG: Chromosomes 8 and 10 workshop. Am J Med Genet 1999; 88:239–243.
Wildenauer DB, Schwab SG, Maier W, Detera-Wadleigh SD: Do schizophrenia and affective disorder share susceptibility genes? Schizophr Res 1999; 39:107–111.
Winokur G, Coryell W, Endicott J, Keller M, Akiskal H, Solomon D: Familial alcoholism in manic-depressive (bipolar) disease. Am J Med Genet 1996; 67:197–201.
Winokur A, March V, Mendels J: Primary affective disorder in relatives of patients with anorexia nervosa. Am J Psychiatry 1980; 137:695–698.
Wittchen H, Knauper B, Kessler RC. Lifetime risk of depression. Br J Psychiatry 1994; 165(suppl. 26):16–22.
Wright AF, Hastie ND: Complex genetic diseases: controversy over the Croesus code. Genome Biol 2001; 2: comment 2007.1–2007.8.
Wright FA, Lemon WJ, Zhao WD, Sears R, Zhuo D, Wang JP, Yang HY, Baer T, Stredney D, Spitzner J, et al.: A draft annotation and overview of the human genome. Genome Biol 2001; 2:25.1–25.8.
Yoshikawa T, Kikuchi M, Saito K, Watanabe A, Yamada K, Shibuya H, Nankai M, Kurumaji A, Hattori E, Ishiguro H, et al.: Evidence for association of the myo-inositol monophosphatase 2 (*IMPA2*) gene with schizophrenia in Japanese samples. Mol Psychiatry 2001; 6:202–210.
Yoshikawa T, Padigaru M, Karkera JD, Sharma M, Berrettini WH, Esterling LE, Detera-Wadleigh SD: Genomic structure and novel variants of myo-inositol monophosphatase 2 (*IMPA2*). Mol Psychiatry 2000; 5:165–171.
Yoshikawa T, Turner G, Esterling LE, Sanders AR, Detera-Wadleigh SD: A novel human myo-inositol monophosphatase gene, *IMP.18p*, maps to a susceptibility region for bipolar disorder. Mol Psychiatry 1997; 2:393–397.

45 Schizophrenia

ANN E. PULVER, GODFREY D. PEARLSON, JOHN A. McGRATH,
VIRGINIA K. LASSETER, KAREN L. SWARTZ, AND GEORGE PAPADIMITRIOU

Schizophrenia is a clinical syndrome of markedly abnormal mental experiences including hallucinations, delusions, and disorganized thoughts and behavior. Significant heterogeneity in the clinical presentation of schizophrenia has prompted researchers to propose the existence of multiple subtypes of the illness. The heterogeneity likely relates to complex interactions between multiple genes and environmental risk factors. As the underlying etiology of this illness is not known, its diagnostic classification is based on clinical symptoms.

HISTORY

Schizophrenia was first conceptualized as a unique illness by Emil Kraepelin (1856–1926) and colleagues (1919), who focused on the course of illness in differentiating dementia praecox from manic-depression. *Dementia praecox*, the earliest term for schizophrenia, highlighted the cognitive decline, or dementia, seen with the chronic course of the illness and the relatively early onset (praecox) which distinguished this condition from late-onset dementia. In his differentiation between manic-depressive illness and dementia praecox, Kraepelin focused on the contrast between the typical deterioration in functioning and chronic psychotic symptoms of schizophrenia and the episodic course with return to baseline functioning between episodes characteristic of manic-depressive illness. This dichotomous differentiation of the two major subtypes of psychotic illness continues to influence the diagnostic criteria for schizophrenia significantly. Kraepelin's diagnostic term *dementia praecox* has been universally replaced by *schizophrenia*, a termed attributed in 1911 to Eugen Bleuler (1857–1939) (Bleuler, 1950). Unlike Kraepelin, Bleuler did not see deteriorating course as a critical symptom. Instead, he focused on the disordered thinking and emotions of patients with the condition.

In contrast, Kurt Schneider (1887–1967) (1974), like Kraepelin, focused on hallucinations and delusions when enumerating his "first-rank symptoms" of schizophrenia. Mood changes were included in his "second-rank symptoms." In the current diagnostic criteria, the ideas of Kraepelin and Schneider predominate, with distinct disease categories differentiating types of psychotic illness.

DIAGNOSTIC CRITERIA

No symptoms are pathognomonic. Because diagnosis is based entirely on clinical history and symptoms, operational criteria have been developed to maximize the reliability of diagnoses, the most common being the *Diagnostic and Statistical Manual*, 4th edition (DSM-IV) developed by the American Psychiatric Association and the International Classification of Disease (ICD-10) developed by the World Health Organization (WHO) (APA, 1994). The DSM-IV diagnostic criteria require at least two of the following: delusions, hallucinations, disorganized speech, disorganized or catatonic behavior, or negative symptoms including affective flattening or avolition. Symptoms should persist for at least 6 months. Impairment in work, interpersonal relationships, or self-care is also a necessary criterion for the diagnosis. Mood symptoms or cognitive impairment should not be prominent features of the clinical presentation. The ICD-10 criteria closely match those of the DSM-IV as the two organizations worked to maximize international agreement.

CLINICAL PRESENTATION

A 20-year-old male college student began to feel uncomfortable around his fellow students and became increasingly socially isolated. Over the course of the following 4 months, he became delusional, believing that he was being controlled by a device implanted in his mouth during a previous dental visit. He experienced auditory hallucinations, hearing voices making comments about him such as "he's going across the room, he's opening the door now." He also believed that his thoughts could be heard by those around him. He could not explain why he had been singled out for this treatment and denied feeling grandiose or of particular importance. His mood was not depressed or elated, but he felt confused and distressed by his symptoms. He had very little insight into his illness, arguing with family and physicians when they told him that he had an illness.

CLINICAL SUBTYPES

Subtypes have primarily been determined by identifying symptoms that commonly co-occur. The DSM-IV classification includes five subtypes: paranoid, disorganized (hebephrenic), catatonic, undifferentiated, and residual. The stability of these subtypes has not been consistently demonstrated. A study by Kendler et al. (1985) of paranoid, hebephrenic, catatonic, and undifferentiated subtypes found the highest stability for the paranoid subtype, particularly in those with later onset (after age 30).

Other clinical subtypes have been described based on age at onset. Late-onset schizophrenia, previously termed *paraphrenia*, is seven times more common in women. Patients with late-onset schizophrenia typically have more complex hallucinations and delusions of a paranoid nature (Rabins, 1992).

GENERAL GENETIC AND EPIDEMIOLOGIC EVIDENCE

Clinical Epidemiology

Our understanding of the epidemiology of schizophrenia will face new challenges once schizophrenia susceptibility genes are identified. Epidemiologic research will then focus on detecting environmental factors that increase susceptibility to disease given specific genetic mutations, and these studies will benefit from the ascertainment of homogeneous groups of patients; clinical diagnosis will be of less importance.

For the present, the validity of the diagnosis remains problematic. No identifiable, continuous trait marker for schizophrenia exists, leaving diagnosis based on assessment of self-reported experiences (Jablensky and Eaton, 1995). Diagnosis also requires adequate longitudinal information about the onset and course of the illness. This information is frequently difficult to obtain from an affected individual and/or his relatives.

Methods of obtaining clinical information on which to base a diagnosis can vary widely across studies and further confuse the epidemiology of schizophrenia. For example, the use of lay interviewers failed to elicit a report of ever experiencing hallucinations in 36% of cases in which a psychiatrist had previously detected them; the corresponding failure rate for delusions was 14% (Pulver and Carpenter, 1983). Studies based on standardized assessments made or reviewed by psychiatrists or psychologists are therefore believed to be stronger (Kendler et al., 1996a,b).

Although inconsistent research findings may be attributed to both disease heterogeneity and differences in representation of subgroups in different study samples, the complicating effect of varying diagnostic methods on the epidemiology of schizophrenia should not be underestimated. Without accurate diagnosis, study of the distribution and determinants of the disease is difficult.

Incidence, Prevalence, and Geographic Differences

Despite these obstacles, progress has been made in incidence and prevalence methodology. Past studies often relied on first psychiatric hospitalization data to calculate incidence rates for schizophrenia. Such rates are biased because some cases are not hospitalized and not all those hospitalized receive the diagnosis of schizophrenia at the first hospitalization. When the case-finding "net" is broadened to include outpatient cases as well as those who did not have a first-admission diagnosis of schizophrenia, incidence rates increase to more accurately reflect the population. For example, Goldacre et al. (1994) found a rate of 8.7/100,000 among hospitalized males, but the actual rate was 15.1/100,000 when ascertainment was broadened as mentioned above; a similar increase was seen for females.

Even better are studies that go beyond mental health facility screening to ascertain incident cases, such as the WHO Collaborative Study on Determinants of Outcome of Severe Mental Disorders (Sartorius et al., 1986; Hafner and an der Heiden, 1997). Table 45–1 lists incidence rates derived from the WHO study (Jablensky et al., 1992), using common diagnostic criteria among the psychiatrists from each country. These rates are remarkably similar across settings, especially for the narrowly defined diagnosis of schizophrenia.

Prevalence is the product of incidence and length of illness. In a broad review of the epidemiology of schizophrenia, Eaton (1985) reported a range of prevalence rate findings for schizophrenia from 0.6 to 8.2/1000; an update by Jablensky and Eaton (1995) documented several more recent results within this range.

Incidence Trends over Time

Studies in several different countries have pointed to the possibility that the incidence of schizophrenia may have decreased in the past 15 to 25 years (Geddes et al., 1993; Munk-Jorgensen and Mortensen, 1993; Brewin et al., 1997). Future incidence studies of cross-regional and longitudinal differences will focus on the incidence of specific genetic mutations rather than symptom or syndrome clusters.

Table 45–1. Selected Incidence Rates for Schizophrenia

Study	Diagnosis	Sample	1-Year Incidence Rates (1979–1980) by Location	Incidence Rate per 100,000	
				Male	Female
Jablensky et al. (1992)	Narrowly defined schizophrenia, CATEGO[a] S+ (research diagnosis)	Community members with diagnosis at first contact with a broad spectrum of "helping" agencies (including inpatient and outpatient), ages 15–54	Aarhus, Denmark	9	5
			Chandigarh, India (rural)	13	9
			Chandigarh, India (urban)	8	11
			Honolulu, HI	10	8
			Moscow, USSR	10	14
			Nagasaki, Japan	11	9
			Nottingham, UK	17	12
	Broadly defined schizophrenia, clinical diagnosis or CATEGO S, P, or O (research diagnosis)	As above	Aarhus, Denmark	18	13
			Chandigarh, India (rural)	37	48
			Chandigarh, India (urban)	34	35
			Dublin, Ireland	23	21
			Honolulu, HI	18	14
			Moscow, USSR	25	31
			Nagasaki, Japan	23	18
			Nottingham, UK	28	15

[a]CATEGO is a computerized classification system; CATEGO class S+, first-rank (Schneiderian) symptoms of schizophrenia; CATEGO class S, schizophrenic psychoses with delusions or auditory hallucinations of specified types; class P, nonaffective paranoid psychoses; class O, other psychoses or borderline conditions.

Ethnic Differences in Incidence

A higher incidence of schizophrenia among immigrant vs. native populations in the same geographic region has been reported (Thomas et al., 1993; Selten and Sijben, 1994; Bhugra et al., 1997). Interpretation of these data is difficult due to potential selection bias and differential diagnoses in the native and immigrant populations. However, immigrants may be subject to some environmental factors that increase risk for schizophrenia. This idea is bolstered by findings of increased risk among siblings, but not parents, of affected probands and especially increased risk for second-generation relatives (born in the land to which the proband's family migrated) (Sugarman and Craufurd, 1994; Hutchinson et al., 1996).

Sex and Age at Onset

Males have an earlier age at onset (age first psychotic or age first hospitalized) of schizophrenia than females (Eaton, 1985; Hambrecht et al., 1992; Hafner et al., 1994). The distribution of male age at onset rises rapidly in the late teenage years to peak in the early to mid-20s. Female age at onset rises more gradually and peaks later, at around age 30.

Several studies have found a second, milder peak for women around menopause (see below). However, the lifetime morbidity risk for schizophrenia is believed to be the same for the two sexes. Hafner et al. (1994) calculated morbidity risks to age 60 for schizophrenia (ICD code 295): 16.4/100,000 for males and 16.6/100,000 for females.

Hafner et al. (1993, 1994) demonstrated the robustness of the sex difference in onset across four different *onset* definitions: age at first sign of illness, first psychotic symptom, first episode (peak of positive symptom accumulation), and first psychiatric hospitalization. Regardless of which onset definition was examined, males preceded females in onset by 3 to 4 years. For example, the mean age at onset for the earliest sign of illness was 24.3 years in males and 27.5 years in females. WHO researchers found that male onset significantly preceded female onset by 3.4 years (Hambrecht et al., 1992).

The Estrogen Hypothesis

Onset sex differences may be a function of the different levels of estrogen in males vs. females. Multiple studies have shown a second, albeit lower incidence peak in the female distribution of onsets, around ages 45 to 49: e.g., the Hafner ABC study (Hafner et al., 1994) and the Camberwell Psychosis Registry study (Castle et al., 1998). According to the estrogen hypothesis, the late-onset peak in women results from the waning supply of estrogen at the time of menopause and thereafter, and the general lag in age at onset for women relative to men results from the protective effects of estrogen earlier in adolescence and adulthood (Hafner et al., 1998). Some evidence exists that lower estrogen levels at points in the menstrual cycle are associated with more psychopathology in schizophrenic women (Riecher-Rossler et al., 1994). These hypotheses are intriguing but require further study before definite conclusions can be made.

Sex and Onset Effects on Symptom Profiles

Despite the sex difference in age at onset, there appear to be few differences in first-admission schizophrenia symptom profiles associated with different onsets or sexes; i.e., patients stricken with the illness at varying ages appear to be remarkably similar in the core symptoms of schizophrenia at the time of first admission (Hafner et al., 1994).

Family Epidemiology

Sex, Onset, and Familial Schizophrenia

Schizophrenia probands may be classified as either *familial* (probands have an affected relative) or *sporadic* (no other affected relative). Cases of familial schizophrenia are expected to include a higher genetic loading among earlier-onset cases and, thus, more affected relatives in families with earlier-onset cases (Childs and Scriver, 1986). Two types of study have been undertaken: the *familial/sporadic paradigm* classifies probands as familial or sporadic and then examines onset differences; the *family risk paradigm* classifies a proband by sex and onset status (early vs. late) and then ascertains the risk for schizophrenia among family members. The latter approach is preferred; calculations can be adjusted for individuals who, based on age, have not advanced through the disease risk period (Kendler et al., 1987; Maclean et al., 1990).

Familial/Sporadic Paradigm. Some studies under the familial/sporadic paradigm have reported that among familial cases the typical sex difference in age at onset is not found (Baron et al., 1982; Albus and Maier, 1995). This suggests that the genetic factors affecting age at onset may be "stronger than any sex-related hormonal and/or environmental or non-genetic effects" (DeLisi et al., 1994).

Family Risk Paradigm. These studies of sex and/or onset and familiality have produced more complex results, likely owing to heterogeneity among the samples studied. Goldstein et al. (1990) found a significantly higher morbidity risk for schizophrenia among first-degree relatives of female vs. male probands: 5.2% vs. 2.2%. Sham et al. (1994a,b), MacLean et al. (1990), and Kendler and MacLean (1990) examined the joint effects of proband sex and age at onset on familial risk using life table methods and proportional hazards modeling and did not find an effect for proband sex. However, they found that the risk declined in relatives as proband age at onset increased; e.g., among early-onset (≤20 years) male and female probands, risks were 4.75% and 5.38%, respectively, while among late-onset (≥41 years) probands, the comparable risks were 1.39% and 3.09%.

Other studies have addressed proband sex and onset effects. A higher morbidity risk of schizophrenia was found among the first-degree relatives of female vs. male probands (respective unadjusted rates were 4.1% and 2.1%) (Pulver et al., 1990; Wolyniec et al., 1992). A significant age-at-onset effect was also found but only among relatives of male probands; however, the male:female ratio was 2.7:1, and the authors noted possible sampling biases in the female proband group.

Sham et al. (1994a,b) built a systematic sample that nevertheless seems underrepresentative of female schizophrenics, with a male:female ratio of 3.4:1. They found a pattern of results similar to that of Pulver et al. (1990) and Wolyniec et al. (1992), with stronger risk for schizophrenia among relatives of female vs. male probands and among earlier-onset cases (with an extremely high risk of 31.3% among relatives of early-onset female probands). However, their sample was admittedly biased toward younger ages, and the small number of female probands ($n = 23$) may not be representative of female schizophrenics on the whole.

The bulk of the above studies support the idea that early onset among schizophrenic probands is related to increased risk for schizophrenia in relatives, although the association is mild (Kendler and MacLean, 1990). However, the above studies do not allow conclusions to be made about proband sex and familial risk. The apparent proband sex effect may be an artifact of ignoring pleiotropy (Goldstein et al., 1990). Goldstein et al. (1990) looked at the risk for a more broadly defined illness, including not only schizophrenia, schizoaffective disorder, and schizophreniform disorder but also schizotypal personality disorder, and found that the proband sex effect disappeared: the morbidity risks for this "full-spectrum" disorder were 9.4% vs. 8.7% among relatives of female vs. male probands, respectively. Also supporting the possibility that schizotypal disorder may represent pleiotropy in schizophrenia, Kendler et al. (1993a) found comparable morbid risks for schizophrenia in relatives of DSM-III-R schizophrenic vs. schizotypal disorder probands in the Roscommon Family Study. In another study based on this data set, they found a high prevalence of schizotypal personality disorder among relatives of schizophrenic probands and a higher prevalence of schizotypal or paranoid personality disorder among parents vs. siblings of schizophrenic probands (Kendler et al., 1993b). These findings are especially consistent with the interpretation of these personality disorders as part of the schizophrenia spectrum (pleiotropy): parents are at a reduced risk of schizophrenia compared to other first-degree relatives of schizophrenic probands by virtue of the reduced reproductive fitness associated with schizophrenia, but the higher rate of spectrum personality disorders among parents suggests that these may reflect alternative phenotypes of schizophrenia.

Paternal Age and Risk in Offspring

The risk of advancing paternal age and its association with schizophrenia was examined in a population-based cohort of 87,907 individuals born in Jerusalem from 1964 to 1976 (Malaspina et al., 2001). The relative risk of schizophrenia increased monotonically with each 5-year age group of paternal age, culminating in a relative risk of 2.96 [95% confidence interval (CI) 1.6–5.5] in offspring of men aged 50 or more. Malaspina et al. (2001) concluded that schizophrenia may be associated with de novo mutations from paternal germ cells. Pulver et al. (unpublished) tested a corollary of the paternal age hypothesis, that there is a decreased risk of schizophrenia in the relatives of probands born to older fathers compared to the relatives of probands born to younger fathers. There was no support for this hypothesis in the sample of 376 individuals with schizophrenia (Pulver et al., unpublished). This hypothesis should be tested in other large samples.

Family, Twin, and Adoption Studies

Family studies have established patterns of risk for schizophrenia consistent with contributing genetic factors. When compared to the approximate 1% general population risk for schizophrenia, relatives of schizophrenic patients show higher risk of illness, and this increased risk correlates with their degree of relationship.

As seen in Table 45–2, the highest risk among first-degree relationships is for children of two schizophrenic parents (47%) and the lowest is for parents of a schizophrenic child (5.6%) (Gottesman et al., 1982).

For siblings of schizophrenics, the risk can vary from 9.6% when parents are unaffected to 16.7% when one parent is affected to 46.3% when both parents are affected. Risk to second- and third-degree relatives is low and approaches the general population rate. An important study using the Danish Psychiatric Case Register of 1.75 million cases found 2669 schizophrenics, giving a relative risk of 9.31 if a mother, father, or sib has schizophrenia (Mortensen et al., 1999). The caveat of family studies is that the same risk patterns may result from genetic or environmental factors.

Table 45–2. Risks of Schizophrenia for Relatives of Schizophrenics (SZ)

Relationship	No. of Studies	Total Relatives (BZ)	Schizophrenic (Including Probable)	Morbid Risk (%)
First-degree				
Parents	14	8020	477	5.6
Siblings				
All	13	9920.7	1002	10.1
Parents not SZ	9	7264	698	9.6
One parent SZ	5	623.5	104	16.7
Children	7	1577.3	202	12.8
Children of 2 SZ	5	134	62	46.3
Second-degree				
Half-siblings	5	499.5	21	4.2
Uncles, aunts	3	2421	57	2.4
Nephews, nieces	6	3965.5	120	3.0
Grandchildren	5	739.5	27	3.7
Third-degree				
First cousins	3	1600.5	39	2.4
Genetically unrelated spouses	4	399	9	2.3

BZ, pooled sample sizes.
Source: Gottesman et al. (1982).

Studies of monozygotic (MZ) and dizygotic (DZ) twins attempt to control for environmental factors. When twin pairs are reared in the same household, MZ pairs experience the same environmental similarity as DZ pairs. Because MZ pairs are genetically identical and DZ pairs share on average half of their genes, differences in concordance rates between the two types show the relative contribution of genetics and environment to the development of schizophrenia. Table 45–3 shows concordance rates from several schizophrenia twin studies.

Higher concordance rates between MZ twins (45% probandwise concordance for MZ vs. 13% same-sex probandwise concordance for DZ) suggest a large genetic contribution to disease development, although lack of complete concordance is evidence that environmental factors are also at play. The estimated heritability of liability to schizophrenia is between 0.6 and 0.9 (Cannon et al., 1998). Cardno et al. (1999) studied 224 same-sex twin probands (106 MZ and 118 DZ) based on the Maudsley Twin Registry (1948–1993) in London, England. The twins studied included the 114 studied originally by Gottesman and Shields (1972) with 25-year follow-up on 107 of the twin pairs. Estimates of heritability from the 1999 study are 83% to 85%, with probandwise concordance of 40.8% (20/49) for MZ twin pairs and 5.3% (3/57) for DZ twin pairs.

A small sample of MZ twins discordant for schizophrenia was studied by Fischer (1971). If nonschizophrenic co-twins carry genetic liability to the disease, their children should experience the same risk as those of the genetically identical but affected twins. Fischer (1971) found that the children of the schizophrenic co-twins had a 9.6% rate of illness, not significantly different from the 12.9% rate for children of the unaffected co-twins. Risk for children of discordant and concordant pairs was the same. Thus, genetic susceptibility was transmitted despite disease status ("obligate carriers").

Adoption studies are another method of examining genetic and environmental contributions to disease development. When genes and prenatal environment are the only contributions of the biologic family, comparison studies between adopted-away children of schizophrenics, schizophrenic adoptees, and matched controls can shed light on the cultural transmission of schizophrenia from parent to offspring. Does the presence of a schizophrenic parent precipitate disease in the offspring? Several stud-

Table 45–3. Concordances in Schizophrenic Twin Series

	MZ Pairs			Same-Sex DZ Pairs		
References, Location	*Total*	Percent Pairwise Concordance	Percent Probandwise Concordance	*Total*	Percent Pairwise Concordance	Percent Probandwise Concordance
Tienari (1971), Finland	17	0–36	35	20	5–14	13
Kringlen (1976), Norway	55	25–38	45	90	4–10	15
Fischer et al. (1969), Denmark	21	24–48	56	41	10–19	27
Kendler and Robinette (1983), U.S.	164	18	31	268	3	7
Gottesman and Shields (1972), U.K.	22	40–50	58	33	9–19	12
Weighted average			38			11
Median			45			13

Source: Gottesman et al. (1982)

ies have followed the adopted-away offspring of schizophrenics (Heston, 1966; Tienari et al., 1987). Overall, these studies suggest an excess of schizophrenia in adopted-away children of schizophrenic parents.

Studies of schizophrenic adoptees by Kety et al. (1968, 1978) looked at risk to biologic and adoptive relatives and showed that biologic relatives had the highest rates of schizophrenia despite lack of contact with the proband. Also studied were biologic paternal half-siblings of ill and well adoptees. The results showed greater risk to biologic paternal half-siblings of schizophrenic adoptees than to biologic paternal half-siblings of control adoptees.

Family, twin, and adoption studies provide strong evidence for a genetic factor contributing to the familiality of schizophrenia. These studies also suggest that genes do not suffice; some other factors play a role.

Associations with Other Diseases

Rheumatoid Arthritis

Studies dating back to the 1930s have indicated that schizophrenic patients have a lower prevalence of rheumatoid arthritis (RA) than the general population. Eaton et al. (1992) analyzed the methodologic weaknesses in 14 such studies, including lack of direct assessment of RA in many cases, nonexplicit or nonstandardized diagnostic criteria for both RA and schizophrenia, limitation of controls to other psychiatric inpatient groups, and failure to include controls at all; yet 12 of the 14 studies revealed a decreased prevalence of RA in schizophrenic patients (median 0.47%) compared with an expected population prevalence of 1% to 3%. This negative association is not a mutually exclusive one; i.e., co-occurrence of RA and schizophrenia has been noted (Tsuang et al., 1983; Eaton et al., 1992). However, in the five studies reviewed by Eaton et al. (1992) that included psychiatric controls, the prevalence of RA was consistently lower in the schizophrenic patients. Thus, the negative association appears to be relatively specific to schizophrenia (Vinogradov et al., 1991). A more recent study based on discharge registry data found a normal prevalence of schizophrenia among RA patients (0.96%) but a significantly decreased prevalence (0.47%) in a group of appendicitis patient controls (Lauerma et al., 1998). However, this finding was due to an unusually high rate of schizophrenia discharge diagnoses (22.6/1000) in the 18- to 27-year-old RA group and calls for replication in a more general sample (i.e., including nonhospitalized RA cases) and use of research diagnoses rather than discharge diagnoses of schizophrenia.

RA is believed to be an autoimmune disorder, and researchers have hypothesized that, like RA, some subtype(s) of schizophrenia results from a primary or secondary autoimmune process (Vinogradov et al., 1991), with specific antibodies directed against the brain (Ganguli et al., 1993). To explore this possibility, studies have examined various human leukocyte antigen (HLA) associations, the presence of non-specific autoantibodies (e.g., antinuclear antibody), immunoglobulin M (IgM) and IgG concentrations, production of various interferons as well as interleukin-2 (IL-2) and IL-6, serum cortisol concentration, changes in the concentrations of different lymphocyte subsets, T-cell receptor rearrangements, and antihippocampal antibodies. However, results are incomplete and sometimes inconsistent (Vinogradov et al., 1991; Ganguli et al., 1993; Kirch, 1993). The present consensus is that the heterogeneity of schizophrenia includes some percentage of affected people for whom the disorder results from one or more autoimmune responses (see Gene Identification below).

Seizures / Epilepsy

Researchers have studied the relationship between schizophrenia and epilepsy because of the frequency of psychotic states occurring in epileptic patients, psychoses being either confined to the period around the seizure or occurring between periods of seizure (*interictal*) but brief. The more chronic interictal psychoses that resemble schizophrenia are of the greatest interest to schizophrenia researchers. Sachdev (1998) summarized eight epidemiologic studies of the association between epilepsy and the more chronic schizophrenia-like psychosis and found that schizophrenia-like psychosis was prevalent in 1.8% to 9.25% of epileptic patients, exceeding the 1% prevalence of schizophrenia in the general population. In the study showing the highest prevalence (9.25% among 1611 epileptic outpatients), a control group of 2167 migraine outpatients showed a prevalence of only 1.06%, very close to the general population expectation; this study had the additional strength of employing DSM-IIIR diagnoses made by a psychiatrist (Mendez et al., 1993).

Three broad explanations for the relationship between epilepsy and schizophrenia-like psychosis are that *(1)* the repeated electrical or biochemical disturbances associated with epilepsy create neurophysiologic abnormalities that lead to psychosis; *(2)* both epilepsy and schizophrenia-like psychosis result from a common neuropathology (Sachdev, 1998); and *(3)* nonspecific brain damage can lead to either or both. The fact that the mean onset of epilepsy precedes the onset of schizophrenia-like psychosis by 10 or more years (Mendez et al., 1993; Sachdev, 1998) does not necessarily contradict the common neuropathological explanation since the manifestation of schizophrenia symptoms under the neurodevelopmental hypothesis is dependent on both an initial early lesion and later cerebral maturational events (Hyde and Weinberger, 1997).

The temporal lobe has been frequently implicated in schizophrenia-like psychosis since temporal lobe epilepsy (complex partial seizure disorder) is a risk factor for schizophrenia-like psychosis (Mendez et al., 1993; Hyde and Weinberger, 1997; Sachdev, 1998). Studies have found fetal lesions or putative perinatal temporal lobe lesions (mesial temporal sclerosis) to be more common among epileptic patients with psychosis or schizophrenia-like psychosis (Roberts et al., 1990); however, the former finding was not replicated in a later study (Bruton et al., 1994). Other studies have examined schizophrenic vs. epileptic patients for similarities and differences in morphologic structures, such as ventricular enlargement and volume reduction in the temporal lobe and hippocampus. Barr et al. (1997) compared 32 first-episode schizophrenic patients with 39 temporal lobe epilepsy patients and 42 normal controls. Both the epileptic and schizophrenic patients showed significantly higher total ventricular volume than controls and reductions in left hippocampal volume compared to controls. These findings offer some insight into the association between epilepsy and schizophrenia, but, as pointed out by Sachdev (1998), both epilepsy and schizophrenia are heterogeneous disorders.

Environmental Factors

Season of Birth

One of the most consistent findings in schizophrenia is that the distribution of birth dates of individuals with schizophrenia differs from that of the general population. Schizophrenics are more likely to be born in the winter and early spring (Bradbury and Miller, 1985; Boyd et al., 1986; Torrey et al., 1997). The proportional excess of winter or early-spring births among schizophrenic subjects is estimated to range from 5% to 15%. Although the basis for the association is unknown, several explanations have been offered. One is that some seasonally varying factor, occurring sometime during intrauterine life or during the initial postnatal months, alters the central nervous system (CNS) and increases an individual's risk for the later development of schizophrenia. The seasonally varying risk has been hypothesized to be a virus, a diet low in protein, or pregnancy and birth complications (Bradbury and Miller, 1985; Boyd et al., 1986). A second explanation is that genetic susceptibility to schizophrenia may confer a protective biologic advantage against allergies or infections that may cause mortality and may be more prevalent in the winter. Thus, during the winter and spring months there may be a preferential survival of infants who are genetically susceptible to schizophrenia (Bradbury and Miller, 1985; Boyd et al., 1986). A third explanation is that parents of schizophrenic patients (those who may have a schizophrenia genotype) have an unusual pattern of conception. This hypothesis has been tested by studying the distribution of birth dates of the siblings of schizophrenic probands. Results have been conflicting (Pulver et al., 1992a,b; Torrey et al., 1997).

Many studies have been conducted to determine if season of birth is important to the etiology of an identifiable subgroup of schizophrenic patients. Although inconsistent findings have been reported regarding the association between season of birth and patients' family history of schizophrenia (Baron and Gruen, 1988; O'Callaghan et al., 1991; Pulver et al., 1992; Hettema et al., 1996; Chen WJ et al., 1996; Dassa et al., 1996), there is some support for an association between season of birth and the following variables: platelet 5-hydroxytryptamine (5-HT) concentration (Muck-Seler et al., 1999), eye-tracking dysfunction (Kinney et al., 1999), urban birth (O'Callaghan et al., 1995; Mortensen et al., 1999), deficit syndrome (Kirkpatrick et al., 1998), electroencephalogram power abnormalities (Sponheim et al., 1997), obstetric complication (Dassa et al., 1996), sex (Pulver et al., 1992a,b; O'Callaghan et al., 1995), and electrodermal activity (Ohlund et al., 1991; Schnur et al., 1995).

Viral Infections

The viral hypothesis of schizophrenia has been around for many decades (Torrey and Peterson, 1976). Rubella virus illustrates well that intrauterine viral infections can cause seasonal birth patterns and can have a devastating effect on fetal development. Furthermore, viral infections can produce effects many years after entry. A considerable number of studies have been published over the last two decades, but, in general, results of epidemiologic studies have been inconsistent. There is some consistent support for an association between the 1957 influenza epidemic and later development of schizophrenia (McGrath and Castle, 1995). However, a case-control study comparing individuals who were and were not exposed prenatally to the 1957 influenza epidemic did not find an increased rate among those who were exposed (Cannon et al., 1996). A study conducted in Denmark using the Danish computerized case register (involving over 9000 patients born between 1915 and 1970 and admitted to Danish psychiatric hospitals between 1971 and 1991) found that maternal exposure to influenza, during the later part of the second trimester, marginally increased the fetal risk for later development of schizophrenia.

Rantakallio et al. (1997) examined the association between CNS infection through age 14 and later development of schizophrenia in the 1966 birth cohort of northern Finland. Individuals who experienced a viral CNS infection during childhood were at an increased risk to develop schizophrenia [odds ratio (OR) = 4.8, 95% CI 1.6–14.0]. Sequences homologous to retroviral *pol* genes have been found in the cerebrospinal fluid (CSF) of 10 of 35 (29%) individuals with recent-onset schizophrenia or schizoaffective disorder and in neither of two control samples (22 diagnosed with neurologic disease, 30 without neurologic or psychiatric disorder; $p = 0.01$) (Karlsson et al., 2001). Retroviral sequences homologous to retroviral *pol* genes were also found in the CSF of 1 of 20 individuals with chronic schizophrenia (Karlsson et al., 2001).

Inconsistent results in studies of Borna virus associations with schizophrenia susceptibility (Sierra-Honigmann et al., 1995; Salvatore et al., 1997; Chen et al., 1999) may be due to differences in laboratory methods and/or criteria for positivity (Iwata et al., 1998).

Pregnancy and Birth Complications

Considerable attention has been paid to the potential role that pregnancy and birth complications may play in the development of schizophrenia. The results of two longitudinal studies of national cohorts provide support for the role of pregnancy and birth complications in the etiology of schizophrenia (Jones et al., 1998; Dalman et al., 1999). The study of the 1966 northern Finnish population suggested that both low birth weight and short gestation (37 weeks) were more common among individuals who developed schizophrenia (Jones et al., 1998). The study of a Swedish birth cohort of 507,516 individuals born between 1973 and 1977 suggested that pre-eclampsia, vacuum extraction, and malformations noted at birth were associated with later development of schizophrenia (Dalman et al., 1999).

PATHOPHYSIOLOGY

Neuropathology

The emerging picture of neuropathology in schizophrenia is one of subtle changes in cellular architecture and brain circuitry (Selemon and Goldman-Rakic, 1999). Grossly, the brain in schizophrenia is reduced in weight and volume by approximately 5%, with modestly enlarged ventricles. None of these changes is diagnostically specific. Neuropathologic studies provide strong evidence against a classic neurodegenerative pathogenesis of schizophrenia and moderate support for prenatal development abnormalities. Given that these brain changes may be developmental, they are likely to be risk or trait factors for the subsequent development of the disease rather than state or illness indices (Lawrie and Abukmeil, 1998). Available clinical and experimental models of late deterioration after static early brain lesions are unconvincing. However, a progressive developmental mechanism active into adult life can reconcile the neuropathologic and imaging data while being compatible with both early onset and late deterioration in schizophrenia (Woods, 1998).

Local circuit neurons in the prefrontal cortex containing the inhibitory neurotransmitter γ-aminobutyric acid (GABA) differentially regulate the activity of pyramidal cells, the principal type of excitatory output neuron. Lewis (1998), in an elegant series of experiments, showed that a subclass of prefrontal GABA axon terminals (from chandelier cells) is decreased by 40% in the prefrontal cortex of schizophrenic subjects compared with matched groups of normal controls and non-schizophrenic psychiatric subjects. Of interest, studies in nonhuman primates show that the connectivity for the prefrontal cortex is substantially refined during adolescence (Lewis, 1997).

A series of quantitative neuropathologic studies (Selemon et al., 1998; Rajkowska et al., 1998; Selemon and Goldman-Rakic, 1999) reveals several abnormalities, including a reduction in the interneuronal neuropil in the prefrontal cortex and neuronal loss in the temporal and cingulate cortex. The schizophrenic prefrontal cortex was characterized by a downward shift in neuronal sizes accompanied by a 70% to 140% per layer increase in the density of small neurons, supporting the hypothesis that neuronal degeneration in the prefrontal cortex is not a prominent feature of the neuropathology of schizophrenia.

Akbarian et al. (1993) argued that cortical connectivity is disrupted by an observed abnormal neuronal distribution, implying a developmental disturbance (such as impaired neuronal migration or an alteration in the death cycle of transitory subcortical neurons). The findings are consistent with a subplate disturbance during development, in which the normal pattern of programmed cell death is disrupted and accompanied by defective neuronal migration toward the cortical plate.

Structural Imaging

Structurally, both global and local brain changes occur in schizophrenia (Shenton et al., 1997). There is a precedent for this in other brain disorders, including developmental disorders such as Down syndrome (Pearlson et al., 1998), Rett syndrome (Subramaniam et al., 1997), and degenerative conditions such as Alzheimer's disease (Pearlson et al., 1992).

Many researchers agree that schizophrenics show widespread, if small, alterations in ventricular size and cortical gray matter. As reviewed by Pearlson and Marsh (1993) and by Shenton et al. (1997), regional volume changes on magnetic resonance imaging (MRI) occur in the following anatomic systems: mesial temporal (amygdala, hippocampus, entorhinal, and parahippocampal cortices), temporal neocortical (superior temporal gyrus, planum temporale surface area), frontal neocortical [Broca's area, dorsolateral prefrontal cortex (DLPFC)], thalamic/basal ganglia, and cerebellum.

Ventricular enlargement and decreased cerebral cortical and hippocampal volume have been confirmed by meta-analysis and are characteristics of the disease as a whole; i.e., they are not restricted to a clinical subtype and are present in first-episode, unmedicated patients (Harrison, 1999).

Results from initial MRI segmentation methods (Schlaepfer et al., 1995; Pearlson et al., 1996; Ross and Pearlson, 1996) suggested that the primary cerebral lesions in schizophrenia lie within the heteromodal association cortex (Mesulam, 1985). A reversal in the expected asymmetry of the surface area of the planum temporale (Petty et al., 1995; Barta et al., 1997) is consistent with a hypothesis of heteromodal association cortex involvement.

Recent discussions have focused on disturbed relations between different brain regions in schizophrenia (Liddle, 1996). An exploratory factor analysis of MRI brain structure measures in schizophrenia (Tien et al., 1996) concluded that several brain regions are affected, that structural relationships between groups of regions are abnormal, and that heteromodal regions seem particularly affected.

Functional Imaging

Functional imaging data with positron emission tomography (PET) of blood flow and metabolism and functional MRI activation generally suggest that the pathophysiology of schizophrenia reflects aberrant activity in, and integration of, the components of distributed circuits involving various neocortical, limbic, and subcortical structures. It is hypothesized that the neuropathologic features represent the anatomical substrate of these functional abnormalities in neural connectivity (Harrison, 1999).

Abnormalities of the language system have long been hypothesized to underlie two positive symptoms, thought disorder and auditory hallucinations. Studies using cerebral activation tasks in conjunction with functional MRI have shed some light on the functional basis for speech and language abnormalities associated with the disorder. McGuire et al. (1998) found that verbal disorganization was inversely correlated with activity in regions implicated in generating, regulating, and monitoring speech.

Curtis et al. (1998) studied frontal activation during a verbal fluency task in schizophrenic patients and matched volunteers using functional MRI. This experiment showed abnormal activation in frontal association cortical regions as well as imbalance in a cortical loop linking the frontal and parietal cortices.

Functional neuroanatomical differences between schizophrenic and control subjects characterized by Fletcher et al. (1998) highlighted similar imbalances.

Brain areas believed to be functionally abnormal in schizophrenia, e.g., DLPFC (Weinberger et al., 1986), Broca's area (McGuire et al., 1993), superior temporal gyrus (Woodruff et al., 1997), and thalamus (Silbersweig and Stern, 1996), also have significant structural abnormalities documented by either MRI or neuropathology (Barta et al., 1990; Shenton et al., 1992; Andreasen et al., 1995; Buchanan et al., 1998).

Overall, functional neuroimaging techniques illuminate normal and abnormal functions of neocortical circuits concerned with speech, language, and other self-generated mental activities. Dynamic neuroimaging studies reveal that components of these neuronal networks fail to communicate normally with one another in patients with schizophrenia. Such experiments emphasize the failure of *systems* rather than isolated brain regions.

Biochemistry

Nicotinic Cholinergic System

Patients suffering from schizophrenia may have a primary defect in the CNS nicotinic system that leads to abnormal sensory gating (Dalack et al., 1998). Cholinergic nicotinic receptors in the hippocampus were diminished in specimens of hippocampal brain tissue obtained post mortem from schizophrenic patients (Freedman et al., 1995).

Dopamine

The dopamine hypothesis of schizophrenia continues to be based mainly on pharmacologic evidence that dopamine receptor antagonists alleviate certain symptoms, such as delusions and hallucinations, whereas dopamine agonists exaggerate them (Carlsson, 1995). The dopaminergic overactivity may be due to excess dopamine itself or to overly sensitive receptors.

The efficacy of antipsychotic drugs is due to their antagonistic effects on dopamine D_2 receptors. In schizophrenic patients, D_2 receptor densities are increased postmortem, but this increase may be attributed to antipsychotic drugs (Zakzanis and Hansen, 1998). Laruelle (1998) reviewed the results of 15 brain imaging studies and concluded that schizophrenic patients possess a significant but mild elevation of D_2 receptor density. Regarding the other types of dopamine receptor, D_1 (Okubo et al., 1997), D_4, and D_3 (Gurevich et al., 1997) have been reported to be altered in schizophrenic patients, but these findings are unconfirmed or controversial (Harrison, 1999).

The origins of a neurocognitive decline in the disease may be related to a reduction in dopaminergic activity in the prefrontal cortex (Borison, 1996). The positive symptoms of schizophrenia are more likely to be associated with disturbances in the temporal lobe. However, dopamine systems in the temporal lobe are poorly explored (Joyce and Meador-Woodruff, 1997). In addition to the limitations of a simple dopamine hyperactivity theory, there is increasing evidence for abnormal interactions between the dopamine and serotonin systems.

Serotonin

Post mortem brain tissue analysis, CSF studies, and pharmacologic challenges suggest a deficit in serotonin function in the cortex of schizophrenic patients (reviewed in Abi-Dargham et al., 1997). Hypotheses to explain serotonin involvement in schizophrenia include alterations in the trophic role of serotonin in neurodevelopment, impaired 5-HT_{2A} receptor–mediated activation of the prefrontal cortex, and interactions between serotonin and dopamine (Kapur and Remington, 1996).

The serotonin system inhibits dopamine function, and serotonin antagonists release the dopamine system from this inhibition, alleviating neuroleptic-induced extrapyramidal symptoms and ameliorating negative symptoms (Kapur and Remington, 1996).

Current research interest in the role of the 5-HT_{2A} receptor is due to the high affinity that novel antipsychotics have for the receptor, and the research may ultimately explain the different therapeutic and side-effect profiles of typical vs. atypical drugs (Meltzer, 1996). Lowered 5-HT_{2A} receptor expression in the frontal cortex in schizophrenia (Harrison, 1996) and elevated numbers of cortical 5-HT_{1A} receptors (Burnet et al., 1997) have been reported. Polymorphisms of 5-HT receptor genes are reported to be a minor risk factor for schizophrenia (Williams et al., 1997) and may predict response to the atypical antipsychotic drug clozapine (Arranz et al., 1998). PET studies have not shown any change in 5-HT_{2A} receptors in younger, medication-free patients (Trichard et al., 1998).

Glutamatergic Systems

Several clinical, neurochemical, and postmortem tissue anomalies of glutamatergic neurotransmission have suggested a role for excitatory amino acid neuronal systems in the pathophysiology of schizophrenia and have driven a glutamatergic deficiency hypothesis for the disease (Moghaddam and Bolinao, 1994; Tamminga, 1998). The *N*-methyl-D-aspartate (NMDA) receptor has been implicated in processes such as synaptogenesis, learning, and memory and is the site of action of NMDA antagonists such as phencyclidine, ketamine, and related anesthetics that can reproduce in normal individuals some of the symptomatic features of schizophrenia. NMDA receptor abnormalities may be involved in the neurodevelopmental predisposition to schizophrenia or in symptom production (Catts et al., 1997; Heresco-Levy and Javitt, 1998).

Glutamatergic dysfunction may be relevant to those forms of schizophrenia in which negative symptoms, cognitive deficits, and deterioration are prominent features (Coyle, 1996). Glutamatergic function is reportedly decreased in the medial temporal lobe (Eastwood et al., 1997). A functional link may exist between glutamatergic and dopaminergic neural systems (Riederer et al., 1991).

GABA

GABA, an inhibitory neurotransmitter, may play a role in schizophrenia, and a GABA imbalance hypothesis has been proposed (Roberts and Caird, 1976). Post mortem studies have shown an increased number of GABA receptors in the brain of schizophrenic patients (reviewed in Benes, 1997). Neither biochemical nor pharmacologic studies have demonstrated a clear GABAergic disturbance in schizophrenia. Evidence for GABAergic predominance/glutamatergic deficit as a common etiologic factor in schizophrenia has been reported (Squires and Saederup, 1991).

Neurocognitive Studies

Neurocognitive studies have suggested that schizophrenia includes both general and specific cognitive problems involving memory (particularly verbal memory) and visual and auditory attention. The magnitude of the cognitive deficit in schizophrenia can be considerable and remains relatively stable despite fluctuations in other symptoms (Weinberger and Gallhofer, 1997). Compared to normal individuals, schizophrenic patients present problems in general intelligence, other aspects of memory, spatial ability, language, and interhemispheric tactile-transfer test performance (Heinrichs and Zakzanis, 1998).

Physiology/Electrophysiology

Eye-tracking deficits have long been observed in 60% to 80% of schizophrenic patients and in a proportion of their relatives. The smooth pursuit eye-movement impairment is not due to inattention and is not substantially affected by neuroleptic medication (MacAvoy and Bruce, 1995). Lipton et al. (1983) suggested that eye-tracking patterns appear to be under genetic control and that some impairment may reflect a predisposition to functional psychosis.

Studies of evoked potentials have shown that both chronic and first-episode schizophrenic patients display smaller amplitudes of the P300 cognitive event-related potential over the left temporal lobe, implicating underlying left temporal lobe dysfunction in the etiology of the disease (Salisbury et al., 1998).

Electrodermal activity measurements are abnormal and perhaps abnormally lateralized in schizophrenia. These differences may be consistent with higher left than right hemispheric activity in the presence of positive symptoms and the opposite for negative ones (Gruzelier and Raine, 1994).

Timing and Evolution of Changes

Despite its usual onset in adolescence or early adult life, there is an emerging consensus that schizophrenia may be a neurodevelopmental disorder (Jakob and Beckmann, 1986; Weinberger, 1995). Evidence for this hypothesis includes documentation of neurobehavioral abnormalities in infancy and childhood, years prior to the onset of the disorder (Weinberger, 1996; Jones, 1997). Also, epidemiologic evidence suggests that schizophrenia is associated with pregnancy, and obstetric and perinatal abnormalities (Kendell et al., 1996). Neuropathologic and neuroimaging evidence for brain abnormalities suggests a neurodevelopmental etiology, possibly involving abnormal neuronal migration. These changes occur in association with mild somatic defects, congruent with an ectodermal developmental etiology (Green et al., 1994). Structural abnormalities in patients with first-episode schizophrenia also support a neurodevelopmental hypothesis because they precede clinical manifestation of the disease (Gur et al., 1998). For example, non-ill adolescents and young adults at high risk of developing schizophrenia by virtue of their family history show enlarged ventricles and smaller medial temporal lobes (Lawrie et al., 1999; Harrison, 1999).

Some of the above evidence has been disputed (reviewed in Gur and Pearlson, 1993). The evidence for schizophrenia as a disorder of neurodevelopment is suggestive rather than conclusive. An important question is one of similarity in schizophrenia to brain changes seen in other developmental disorders, such as Down syndrome (Schmidt-Sidor et al., 1990; Raz et al., 1995).

The topic of schizophrenia as a neurodegenerative disorder has generated two major opposing views. One is that of Weinberger (1987), which views schizophrenia as a "static encephalopathy" of neurodevelopmental origin without a progressive element (over and above changes caused by normal aging). An opposing view (reviewed in DeLisi et al., 1997) is that clinical onset is followed by a continuing, active neurodegenerative process in either all patients or a significant subgroup. Several longitudinal studies have found no evidence of excessive change (Illowsky et al., 1988; Vita et al., 1988), nor have cross-sectional investigations (Lim et al., 1996). Some MRI studies (Kemali et al., 1989; Woods et al., 1990; DeLisi et al., 1995; Turetsky et al., 1995; Mathalon et al., 1997) detected small decreases in brain volume with time in schizophrenia. However, in first-episode cases, Jaskiw et al. (1994) and Vita et al. (1994) detected no such change. Elderly, institutionalized schizophrenic patients develop non-Alzheimer's disease dementia (Purohit et al., 1993).

DeLisi et al. (1997) conducted the largest study to date, on 50 schizophrenic patients followed since first clinical onset and 20 controls, with annual scans for 4+ years. They found volume changes at a greater rate in patients. Gur et al. (1998) rescanned 40 schizophrenics (half first-episode) at a mean of 30 months, reporting greater frontal lobe volume decreases than in normals. The few existing neuroimaging studies are generally unclear and contradictory, and the timing of neuro-degeneration, if present, is unknown.

A possible way out of the static/neurodevelopmental vs. continuing/neurodegenerative debate was suggested by Woods (1998), who reviewed the evidence that schizophrenia is a progressive neurodevelopmental disorder that continues into adult life. Since there is increasing evidence that myelination and pruning in the brain continue well into adult life, our view of neurodevelopmental disorders may be updated to include conditions representing continuing disturbances of these processes well into adult life. Thus, schizophrenia may turn out to be both neurodevelopmental and progressive without necessarily being degenerative.

Etiopathology

The putative gene(s) may influence cortical migration or development (Ross and Pearlson, 1996). One view, in light of data suggesting a link between hippocampal dysfunction and genetic risk for schizophrenia (Adler et al., 1998; Callicott et al., 1998), is that hippocampal function may be at fault (Weickert and Weinberger, 1998; Weinberger, 1999).

Above, we noted a developmental hypothesis of schizophrenia. Additional evidence in support of this is documentation of loss or reversal of normally occurring cerebral structural asymmetries in schizophrenia. In addition, chemical (Kitamura et al., 1998) and electrophysiologic (Reite et al., 1997) asymmetries have been documented. Crow (1989) argued that one human gene, an asymmetry or cerebral dominance factor essential to the evolution of human language and hand dominance, is abnormal in schizophrenia and "contributes substantially to the predisposition to psychosis."

Specificity within Schizophrenia (Subgroups), within Families, and vs. Other Neuropsychiatric Disorders

It is plausible that some brain changes are markers for symptom groups across disorders, i.e., within all patients who share psychotic symptoms (e.g., dopaminergic markers across psychotic illnesses). The specificity of structural brain changes identified in schizophrenia has not been clearly shown but is an important issue to resolve in view of arguments over the continuum concept of psychosis.

Brain Changes in Siblings of Schizophrenics

The high prevalence of biologic abnormalities and of schizophrenia spectrum disorders in the first-degree relatives of schizophrenia patients make it likely that a proportion of clinically unaffected first-degree relatives carry one or more pathologic genes for the disorder (Kremen et al., 1994). Consequently, use of appropriate biologic markers such as structural brain abnormalities could *(1)* allow identification and exclusion of phenocopies, *(2)* identify homogeneous subtypes, and *(3)* clarify the relationship of the genotype to the CNS phenotype as relevant disease genes are identified. Such data, which highlight genetic influences, are a useful counterpoint to discordant MZ twin studies, which emphasize environmental factors.

Supporting and Contradictory Evidence

Twin studies in normal volunteers emphasize the role of heritability of total brain and sulcal volumes (Reveley et al., 1982). Non-schizophrenic siblings of schizophrenics have ventricular volumes intermediate between those of patients and controls (Weinberger et al., 1981; DeLisi et al., 1986). In MZ twins discordant for schizophrenia, the schizophrenic twin has larger ventricles while the unaffected twin has ventricular size intermediate between those of schizophrenic patients and normal controls (Reveley et al., 1982, 1984). Shihabuddin et al. (1996) assessed lateral ventricular enlargement and frontoparietal atrophy on computed tomography (CT) in one large family containing multiple cases of schizophrenia. They hypothesized that these changes were associated with a schizophrenia-related gene and denote a susceptibility to schizophrenia-related conditions. Cannon et al. (1997) studied MRIs of schizophrenic patients and nonschizophrenic siblings: schizophrenic patients had increased CSF, especially in the frontal lobes and left hemisphere. Seidman (1997) found that nonschizophrenic sisters of schizophrenic patients had increased ventricular size and reduced volumes of gray matter and right amygdala relative to normal controls. Sharma et al. (1997) examined 16 families multiply affected with schizophrenia. MRI scans showed that ventricular volume in the patients was larger than that in first-degree relatives and controls. Most unaffected relatives resembled normals, but presumed obligate carriers showed the same abnormalities as the schizophrenic patients.

Few other anatomical regions have been explored in this context. Dauphinais et al. (1990) reported smaller temporal lobe size in nonschizophrenic sibs. Silverman et al. (1998) showed that within sibships the ventricle:brain ratios of schizophrenic patients were similar to those of their siblings with schizotypal personality disorder but different from those of family members without any schizophrenia-related disorders. The nonpsychotic siblings of schizophrenic patients have a regionally specific reduction of *N*-acetyl-aspartate measures in the hippocampal area (Callicott et al., 1998).

Twin Studies

Although anatomical changes can be detected in almost every twin with schizophrenia, they tend to be less marked in the unaffected twin (Levy et al., 1994). Evaluation of MZ twin pairs discordant for schizophrenia demonstrated decreased prefrontal physiologic cerebral blood flow activation during the Wisconsin Card Sorting Test for the affected twins, which correlated with decreased hippocampal volume determined by MRI. In schizophrenic vs. nonschizophrenic co-twins, there is more marked brain ventricular enlargement and hippocampal reduction (Stabenau and Pollin, 1993). In most MZ twin pairs discordant for schizophrenia, rostral hippocampal volume is smaller (by a mean of 10%), ventricles are larger (Suddath et al., 1990), and cortical and hippocampal sizes are smaller (Noga et al., 1996) in the affected twin. Studies of twins discordant for schizophrenia and of normal twins strongly support genetic control of eye-tracking performance (Levy et al., 1994). Concordance rates for eye tracking in MZ twins are approximately twice those found in DZ twins and are approximately 30% as high as would be expected for a trait under complete genetic control.

GENE IDENTIFICATION

Linkage and Association

One of the greatest problems in this field has been an inability to identify homogenous groups of patients. Although most investigators believe that schizophrenia is etiologically heterogeneous, few studies attempt to determine if a relationship exists between some genetic factor and a subgroup of patients and their families. Although there are some generally accepted findings, the majority of reports have been conflicting.

Earliest efforts to identify a genetic component contributing to schizophrenia liability involved blood serum measurements focusing on the blood groups and HLA (Gaekwad et al., 1972; Czechowicz and Pamnany, 1972; Eberhard et al., 1975; Ivanyi et al., 1976; Smeraldi et al., 1976). With the development of polymerase chain reaction technology, researchers were no longer limited to known trait markers and began to use restriction fragment length polymorphisms in linkage studies. By the late 1980s, several other classes of highly polymorphic DNA markers were discovered, which gave association and linkage studies higher resolution and greater scope; but in spite of these advances, results of early studies were conflicting.

The 5q region was first implicated due to partial trisomy of 5q11.2–5q13.3 in two related schizophrenics (Bassett et al., 1988). Linkage evidence for schizophrenia was reported for the genetic markers *D5S76* and *D5S39* (Sherrington et al., 1988), and these same markers were shown in 1991 to be tightly linked to the serotonin receptor, HTR1A (Melmer et al., 1991). However, evidence against linkage in this region quickly followed (Kennedy et al., 1988; Kaufmann et al., 1989; Detera-Wadleigh et al., 1989). These initial efforts were hampered by the use of very small samples in an environment in which genetic heterogeneity is likely to exist not only across families but even within families. Sufficient statistical power to detect linkage in this environment requires large and informative population samples.

Systematic/Random Markers Used in Linkage and Association Studies of Clinical Disease

Using clinical diagnosis in conjunction with polymorphic genetic markers, completed scans of the human genome for schizophrenia susceptibility loci have been reported by 19 investigators (Table 45–4). In addition, results from a nearly complete genome scan (Kendler et al., 1996b; Straub et al., 1996, 1997, 1998) are considered in Table 45–4.

The regions of greatest interest are those in which a suggestion of linkage in one sample has been explored with other samples. The criteria for a suggestion of linkage are either the most significant finding in a completed genome scan or a p value ≤ 0.01. Supporting studies in regions 1q21–q41, 5q23–q31, 6p25–21, 6q13–q26, 8p23–p21, 10p15–p13, 13q14–q32, and 22q are reviewed in Tables 45–5 through 45–12, respectively.

Chromosome 6p and HLA. Early studies by McGuffin et al. (1983), Chadda et al. (1986), and Goldin et al. (1987) using small multiplex family samples found no evidence for linkage to the HLA region or chromosome 6p. However, strong findings in 6p24–p22 by Straub et al. (1995) renewed interest in the HLA

Table 45–4. Characteristics of the Samples and Diagnostic Methods in Completed Genome Scans for Schizophrenia Susceptibility Loci

Reference	Multiplex Families No. Affected	Sample Ethnicity	Average No. Affected
Coon et al. (1994a,b)	9 (35)	European Caucasian	3.9
Barr et al. (1994a,b)	1 (31) 7 branches	Swedish	31
Moises et al. (1995)			
Stage I	5 (37)	Iceland	7.4
Stage II	65 families	Mixed	3.3
	11	Swedish kindred	5.4
	10	American (Utah)	3.6
	15	Austrian	2.1
	6	Italian	4.0
	11	Taiwanese	2.1
	6	German	3.3
	4	Scottish	5.0
	2	Canadian	2.0
Stage III	113 trios	Chinese	1.0[a]
	93 trios	Italian/German	1.0[a]
Wildenauer et al. (1996)	59 (155)	48 German 11 Sephardic	2.6
Levinson et al. (1998)	43 (126)	31 European Caucasian 9 African American 1 Hispanic 1 Aboriginal 1 Asian	2.9
Faraone et al. (1998)	43 (96)	European Caucasian	2.2
Kaufmann et al. (1998)	30 (79)	African American	2.6
Blouin et al. (1998)			
Stage I	54 (142)	European Caucasian	2.6
Stage II	51 (133)	European Caucasian	2.2
Shaw et al. (1998)	70 (171)	European Caucasian	2.4
Straub et al. (1998)	265 (577)	Irish	2.3
Williams et al. (1999)			
Stage I	85 (170)	European Caucasian	2.0
Stage II	65 (157)	European Caucasian	2.2
Rees et al. (1999)	13 (45)	11 European Caucasian 2 Japanese	3.8
Brzustowicz et al. (2000)	22 (80)	Celtic	3.6
Hovatta et al. (1999)	Stage I:1 (17) Stage II:20 (40)	Finnish	I:17 II:2
Schwab et al. (2000)	71 (171)	56 German 13 Israeli 2 Hungarian	2.4
Bailer et al. (2000)	5 (16)	Austrian	2.8
Ekelund et al. (2000)	I:52 (104) II:134 (268)	Finnish	2.3
Gurling et al. (2001)	13 (39)	5 British 8 Icelandic	4.3
Lindholm et al. (2001)	1 (39)	Swedish	39

[a]These trios may be familial or nonfamilial; i.e., some may have other relatives affected with schizophrenia.

region. Although the region identified by Straub et al. was telomeric of the HLA region in 6p21, other linkage reports suggested a locus nearer to the HLA region (Schwab et al., 1995; Moises et al., 1995). Still other linkage reports were negative (Mowry et al., 1995; Gurling et al., 1995) or equivocal (Antonarakis et al., 1995). Brzustowicz et al. (1997) reported linkage to the 6p region using a quantitative trait based on positive and negative symptoms. Arolt et al. (1996) found positive lod scores greater than 3 in linkage studies of 6p21–23 using the phenotype of eye-tracking dysfunction, but no linkage evidence was found using the schizophrenia phenotype. Schwab et al. (2000) genotyped HLA polymorphisms as part of a 10 cM genome scan in 71 multiplex schizophrenia pedigrees and reported a nonparametric lod score (NPL) of 3.3 for *HLA-DQB1* ($p = 0.001$) (Schwab et al., 2000).

Pseudoautosomal Region(s) on X and Y. Two pseudoautosomal regions on the sex chromosomes are now recognized: 2.6 Mb on Xp22:Y and a 350kb region on Xq28:Yq12. Crossing over between the X and Y chromosomes is confined to these regions, with the result that recombination rates for males are at their highest for the entire genome. Pseudoautosomal genes are not subject to X inactivation in females. Crow (1988) reviewed the evidence for a relationship between psychosis and the sex chromosomes, concluding that a pseudoautosomal locus could explain same-sex concordance in paternally inherited illness, sex differences in age at onset, and by unequal recombination rates, the high mutation rate required for the persistence of psychotic illness in the population.

A locus (*DXYS14*) unlinked to sex was tested in 83 affected European Caucasian sib pairs (Collinge et al., 1991). Affected

Table 45–5. Supportive Linkage Evidence in Region 1q21–q32

Reference	Sample	Marker in LDB[a]	Evidence
Brzustowicz et al. (2000)	21 Celtic, 1 German	D1S1679 182.3 cM (1q24.2)	m-pt HLOD 6.5 ($p < 0.00002$)
Gurling et al. (2001)	5 British, 8 Icelandic	D1S196 185.4 cM (1q24.2)	5-pt HLOD 2.8 ($p = 0.0003$)
Hovatta et al. (1999)	I: 1 large Finnish II: 20 Finnish	D1S2891 221.8 cM (1q32.2)	2-pt LOD 3.82
Ekelund et al. (2000)	52 Finnish	D1S2833 245.3 cM (1q32–q42)	2-pt LOD 2.65
Ekelund et al. (2001)	221 Finnish	D1S2709 245.6 cM (1q42)	2-pt LOD 2.71

[a]LDB, Location Database (*http://cedar.genetics.soton.ac.uk/public_html/gmap.html*); m-pt, multipoint analyses.

Table 45–6. Supportive Linkage Evidence in Region 5q23–q31

Reference	Sample	Marker in LDB[a]	Evidence
Schwab et al. (1997)	I: 14 German/Israeli II: 40 German/Israeli	IL9 142.6 cM (5q31.1) D5S399 144.9 cM (5q31.2)	2-pt HLOD 1.8 2-pt HLOD 1.3
Straub et al. (1997)	265 Irish	D5S393 142.9 cM (5q31.1) D5S804 135.7 cM (5q23.3)	2-pt HLOD 3.04 ($p = 0.0005$) m-pt HLOD 3.35 ($p = 0.0002$) n-par Z 2.84 ($p = 0.002$)
Sherrington et al. (1988)	7 British/Icelandic	D5S76 60.3 cM (5q11.2) D5S39 68.8 cM (5q12.3)	m-pt LOD 6.49
Schwab et al. (2000)	13 Israeli 56 German 2 Hungarian	D5S2066 174.5 cM (5q34)	m-pt LOD 1.36
Gurling et al. (2001)	5 British 8 Icelandic	D5S422 174.4 cM (5q34)	3-pt HLOD 3.6 ($p = .0001$)

[a]LDB, Location Database (*http://cedar.genetics.soton.ac.uk/public_html/gmap.html*); m-pt, multipoint analyses; n-par, nonparametric.

Table 45–7. Supportive Linkage Evidence in Region 6p25–21

Reference	Sample	Marker in LDB[a]	Evidence
Wildenauer et al. (1996)	59 German/Israeli	D6S260 17.8 cM (6p22.3)	2-pt LOD 2.31
Moises et al. (1995)	I : 5 Icelandic II: 65 mixed replication III: 113 Chinese trios	D6S274 17.0 cM (6p21.3)	n-par WRPC ($p = 0.005$)
Straub et al. (1995)	265 Irish	D6S296 03.1 cM (6p25.2)	2-pt LOD 3.51 ($p = 0.0002$)
Schwab et al. (1995)	44 German/Israeli	D6S274 17.0 cM (6p21.3)	2-pt LOD 2.2
Schwab et al. (2000)	13 Israeli 2 Hungarian 56 German	HLA-DQB1 37.6 cM (6p21.3)	m-pt NPL 3.3 ($p = 0.001$)
Bailer et al. (2000)	5 Austrian	D6S309 2.8 cM (6p24)	m-pt NPL 2.75 ($p = 0.005$)

[a]LDB, Location Database (*http://cedar.genetics.soton.ac.uk/public_html/gmap.html*); m-pt, multipoint analyses; n-par, nonparametric; NPL, nonparametric LOD; WRPC, Weighted Rank Pairwise Correlation.

Table 45–8. Supportive Linkage Evidence in Region 6q13–q26

Reference	Sample	Marker in LDB[a]	Evidence
Cao et al. (1997)	I: 53 (77% Caucasian, 7% Slavic, 3.5% African American, 12.4% other) II: 69 (51% Caucasian, 35% African American, 14% other)	I: D6S454 123.8 cM (6q16–q23) II: D6S424 107.8 cM (6q14)	I: m-pt LOD 3.06 ($p = 0.00018$) II: m-pt LOD 2.35 ($p = 0.00095$)
Martinez et al. (1999)	I: 53 (see above) II: 69 (see above) III: 43 (18, from Australia, 23 from U.S.)	I : D6S416 123.4 cM (6q22) II: D6S301 118.7 cM (6q22) III: D6S301 (see above) II+III: D6S301 (see above)	I: m-pt LOD 2.17 II: m-pt LOD 3.18 III: m-pt LOD 1.07 ($p = 0.013$) II+III: m-pt LOD 3.82 ($p = 0.000014$)
Bailer et al. (2000)	5 Austrian	D6S290 157.7 cM (6q21–q24)	n-par NPL 2.20 ($p = 0.02$)
Levinson et al. (2000)	8 samples and 734 pedigrees	D6S424 107.8 cM (6q14)	m-pt LOD 3.10 ($p = 0.0036$)
Lindholm et al. (2001)	1 large Swedish	D6S264 180.0 cM (6q25–q27) D6S253 173.2 cM (6q25–q27))	2-pt LOD 3.45 m-pt LOD 6.6

[a], LDB, Location Database (*http://cedar.genetics.soton.ac.uk/public html/gmap.html*); m-pt, multipoint analyses; n-par, nonparametric; NPL, nonparametric LOD.

Table 45–9. Supportive Linkage Evidence in Region 8p23–p21

Reference	Sample	Marker in LDB[a]	Evidence
Blouin et al. (1998)	54 European Caucasian	D8S1771 33.3 cM (8p21.1)	m-pt Z-ALL 3.64 (p = 0.0001)
Shaw et al. (1998)	70 European Caucasian	D8S560 26.6 cM (8p21.2)	2-pt HLOD 1.99
Kendler et al. (1996b)	Blouin et al. (1998)	D8S1715 23.9 cM (8p21.3)	2-pt HLOD 2.52
Kaufmann et al. (1998)	30 African American	D8S1819 4.4 cM (8p23.2) D8S532 48.6 cM (8p11)	m-pt Z-ALL 2.27 (p = 0.01) Z-ALL 1.88 (p = 0.03)
Moises et al. (1995)	I : 5 Icelandic II: 65 mixed replication	D8S298 28.0 cM (8p21.2)	n-par WRPC ($p < 0.05$)
Brzustowicz et al. (2000)	22 Celtic	D8S136 25.5 cM (8p21.2)	3-pt LOD 2.8
Gurling et al. (2001)	5 British 8 Icelandic	D8S503 5.7 cM (8p23–p22) D8S1771 33.3 cM (8p21)	3-pt HLOD 3.6 (p = 0.0001) 5-pt HLOD 3.2 (p = 0.0005)

[a]LDB, Location Database (*http://cedar.genetics.soton.ac.uk/public_html/gmap.html*); m-pt, multipoint analyses; n-par, nonparametric; Z-ALL, non-parametric lod score from GeneHunter; WRPC, Weighted Rank Pairwise Correlation.

Table 45–10. Supportive Linkage Evidence in Region 10p15–13

Reference	Sample	Marker in LDB[a]	Evidence
Straub et al. (1998)	265 Irish	D10S2443 4.8 cM (10p15.2)	m-pt n-par 1.88 (p = 0.03)
Schwab et al. (1998a)	72 German/Israeli	D10S1714 19.0 cM (10p13)	m-pt Z-ALL 3.2 (p = 0.0007)
Faraone et al. (1998)	43 European Caucasian	D10S1423 19.1 cM (10p13)	m-pt Z-ALL 3.4 (p = 0.0004)
Schwab et al. (2000)	13 Israeli 2 Hungarian 56 German	D10S1714 19.1 cM (10p13)	m-pt NPL 3.13 (p = 0.001)
Levinson et al. (2000)	734 pedigrees from 8 centers	D10S189–D10S1220 (10p15–10q11)	Logistic regression HLOD 3.41 (p = 0.045)
Gurling et al. (2001)	13 Israeli 2 Hungarian 56 German	D10S1714 19.1 cM (10p13)	m-pt LOD 2.1 m-pt NPL 3.13 (p = 0.0015)

[a]LDB, Location Database (*http://cedar.genetics.soton.ac.uk/public_html/gmap.html*); m-pt, multipoint analyses; n-par, nonparametric; Z-ALL, non-parameter lod score from GeneHunter; NPL, non-parametric LOD.

Table 45–11. Supportive Linkage Evidence in Region 13q21–q32

Reference	Sample	Marker in LDB[a]	Evidence
Blouin et al. (1998)	54 European Caucasian	D13S174 99.7 cM (13q32.3)	m-pt Z-ALL 4.18 (p = 0.00002)
Shaw et al. (1998)	70 European Caucasian	D13S170 85.0 cM (13q31.1) D13S1293 29.4 cM (13q12.3)	m-pt Z-ALL 1.83 (p = 0.03) m-pt Z-ALL 1.80 (p = 0.01)
Brzustowicz et al. (2000)	22 Celtic	D13S793 95.8 cM (13q32.1)	3-pt LOD 3.81
Lin et al. (1995)	9 English/Welsh	D13S144 69.4 cM (13q21.3)	2-pt HLOD 1.61
Lin et al. (1997)	9 English 1 Welsh 34 Taiwan	D13S128 96.3 cM (13q32.2)	5-pt n-par 2.58

[a]LDB, Location Database (*http://cedar.genetics.soton.ac.uk/public_html/gmap.html*); m-pt, multipoint analyses; n-par, nonparametric; Z-ALL, non-parametric lod score from GeneHunter.

Table 45–12. Supporting Linkage Evidence on Region 22q

Reference	Sample	Region
Blouin et al. (1998)	54 European Caucasian	(22q13.1)
Pulver et al. (1994a–c)	39 European Caucasian	(22q13.2)
Shaw et al. (1998)	70 European Caucasian	(22q12.1)
Gill et al. (1996)	Combined 11 studies	(22q13.2)
Coon et al. (1994a,b)	9 Utah	(22q13.2)
Lindsay et al. (1995) (22q11 deletions)	100 SZ European Caucasian	(22q11.21)
Yan et al. (1998)	Childhood-onset SZ	(22q11.21)
Gothelf et al. (1997)	15 SZ with cardiac cleft	(22q11.21)

SZ, schizophrenia.

sibs shared alleles more frequently than predicted by Mendelian inheritance ($p < 0.05$), and there was a suggestion of an excess of maternally inherited alleles ($p = 0.07$). The sample was later enlarged by 16 sibships with similar results (d'Amato et al., 1994). This work was replicated using 33 French sibships ($p < 0.05$) (d'Amato et al., 1992). Other reports subsequently found no evidence: linkage analyses in 25 multiplex families from Wales (Asherson et al., 1992); association studies in 46 Japanese schizophrenics and 146 healthy controls (Ishida et al., 1993); Barr et al. (1994a) in a large Swedish kindred; Crow et al. (1994) in linkage analysis of 85 families; and Wang et al. (1994). Kalsi et al. (1995) excluded *DXYS14* and *MIC2* in British and Icelandic kindreds, and Maier et al. (1995) excluded pseudoautosomal linkage to DXYS14 in 14 German families. A multicenter collaborative effort using 92 pedigrees selected for exhibiting a maternal inheritance pattern found evidence for linkage at Xp11(DXS7) (Dann et al., 1997). A follow-up study of 34 pedigrees unselected for mode of transmission supported a locus at MAOB (Xp11) (Dann et al., 1997). Families from an internal isolate of Finland, a population founded in the seventeenth century, supported a predisposing locus at Xp11 ($Z_{max} = 2.01$) (Hovatta et al., 1999).

DeLisi et al. (2000) comprehensively studied the X chromosome by genotyping 19 polymorphisms in a large sample of 309 multiplex schizophrenia pedigrees and reported no confirmation of linkage. Weak positive lod scores were found in the pericentromeric region in the entire sample and in the maternally inherited families. The authors suggested that other genetic mechanisms, such as abnormal patterns of imprinting of a gene or epigenetic modification, may account for the sex differences associated with schizophrenia (DeLisi et al., 2000).

Heterogeneity Analyses of Linkage Evidence. The partitioning of linkage evidence by defining groups of families based on heritable characteristics is one approach to the question of genetic heterogeneity. These studies are just beginning but will be more common as family samples increase in size. In an initial attempt to address genetic heterogeneity, striking evidence for chromosome 8p21 has been associated with the presence of schizophrenia spectrum personality disorders in non-schizophrenic first-degree relatives of schizophrenic probands (D8S1771, $p = 0.000002$) (Pulver et al., 2000). Using periodic catatonia as a distinct inherited clinical subtype of the schizophrenias, significant evidence for chromosome 15q15 ($p = 2.6 \times 10^{-5}$) was found in a genome scan of 12 pedigrees (average 4.75 affected per family) as well as suggestive evidence for 22q13 ($p = 0.0018$) (Stober et al., 2000b). The 22q13 evidence was further supported by a report of a Leu^{309}Met mutation in *WKL1*, a positional candidate gene on chromosome 22q13.33 encoding a putative nonselective cation channel expressed exclusively in brain and cosegregating with periodic catatonia in an extended pedigree (Meyer et al., 2001). Age at onset of schizophrenia has been used in quantitative trait analyses to search for susceptibility loci or modifying loci in a 20 cM genome scan of 94 affected sib pairs (Cardno et al., 2001). The mean age at onset was 24.5 years and the range, 12 to 45 years. The highest lod scores were on chromosome 17q (lod = 2.54). An additional peak on chromosome 13q (lod = 1.68) coincides with the region showing maximum evidence for linkage in the study by Blouin et al. (1998), using a narrow phenotype of categorical schizophrenia.

Clinical variability may be due to genetic heterogeneity. Pulver et al. (2000) explored the possibility that there may be clinically observable differences in the expression of the schizophrenia phenotype in a stratified analysis looking at chromosome 8p–linked families vs. other strata. There were no differences in symptom profiles. The hypothesis was also tested for regions on chromosome 5q, 6p, 8p, and 10p in the linkage evidence from an Irish study of high-density schizophrenia families ($n = 265$ pedigrees); affected individuals from families with linkage to chromosome 8p had significantly more affective deterioration, more thought disorder, fewer depressive symptoms, and poorer outcome than affected individuals from other families (Kendler et al., 2000).

Evidence for Overlap in Susceptibility Regions for Other Psychiatric Disorders. Compilation of results from both family studies and linkage scans over the last decade for schizophrenia, schizoaffective disorder, and bipolar disorder supports a consideration of overlap in epidemiologic evidence and genetic susceptibility (Berrettini, 2000; Wildenauer et al., 1999). Independent studies from families with bipolar disorder and families with schizophrenia now implicate regions on chromosomes 10p13–p12, 13q32, 18p, and 22q11–q13 (Berrettini et al., 1994; Blouin et al., 1998; Schwab et al., 1998b, 2000; Detera-Wadleigh et al., 1999; Brzustowicz et al., 2000; Foroud et al., 2000).

Systematic/Random Markers Used in Linkage and Association Studies of Physiologic Traits Associated with Disease

Definition of affected status for studies in schizophrenia may rely on an associated trait or characteristic known to be heritable. Decreased P300 or P50 auditory evoked potential inhibition, smooth pursuit eye-tracking abnormality, neurophysiologic measurements such as those obtained from PET and MRI brain scans, or electroencephalographic changes observed during mental tasks have been used in linkage and association studies.

Freedman et al. (1997) studied nine families with multiple cases of schizophrenia and found that decreased P50 inhibition occurred not only in most schizophrenics but also in many of their nonschizophrenic relatives, in a distribution consistent with inherited vulnerability for the disease. A genome-wide linkage analysis, assuming autosomal dominant transmission, showed that the deficit is linked (maximum lod = 5.3 with zero recombination) to a dinucleotide polymorphism at 15q13–q14, the site of the α7-nicotinic receptor (*CHRNA7*) gene (Freedman et al., 1997). It was considered relevant that many schizophrenics are heavy smokers.

The authors speculated that heavy use of nicotine and nicotine dependence may represent self-treatment for the defect at the α7-nicotinic receptor. Twenty multiplex families with at least three affecteds from the National Institute of Mental Health Genetics Initiative Study were used in linkage analyses between chromosome 15 markers and the schizophrenia phenotype, and excess sib pair sharing for D15S1360 ($p = 0.0024$) near *CHRNA7* was found. A sample of five Canadian multiplex families showed no evidence of linkage to *CHRNA7* (Neves-Pereira et al., 1998) using the schizophrenia phenotype.

Candidate Genes Used in Linkage and Association Studies

Because the biologic underpinnings for schizophrenia are not known with any certainty, many candidate genes can be hypothesized.

Studies of chromosomal aberrations in schizophrenic patients have identified regions (5q,11q, 18q, 19p, 22q) worthy of attention (Bassett, 1992; Bassett et al., 2000). Significant advances in molecular cytogenetic techniques, in particular fluorescence in situ hybridization, highlight the evidence for associating a cytogenetic abnormality (22q11.2 microdeletion) with schizophrenia (Pulver et al., 1994a–c; Karayiorgou et al., 1995; Bassett et al., 1998). In a large Scottish pedigree in which a balanced translocation segregates with major mental illness (1;11)(q42.1;q14.3) (St. Clair et al., 1990), two novel genes (*DISC1*, *DISC2*) have been shown to be disrupted in the chromosome 1q42 region (Millar et al., 2000), and linkage evidence in a nearby region from studies of bipolar disorder and schizophrenia make *DISC1* and *DISC2* interesting candidates for susceptibility to psychiatric disorders (Hovatta et al., 1999; Detera-Wadleigh et al., 1999; Gurling et al., 2001; Ekelund et al., 2001).

Propping (1983) described biologic disorders with apparent schizophrenia-like psychotic symptoms, another source of potential candidates. The biologic mechanism characterizing mutations in certain genes (i.e., expanded trinucleotide repeats) makes genes of that type potential candidates, particularly in candidate regions, e.g., *NOTCH4* in chromosome 6p21.3 (Wei and Hemmings, 2000) or *KCNN3* in chromosome 1q21 (Dror et al., 1999). Pharmacologic research and autoimmune, neurodevelopmental, and neuropsychologic hypotheses of disease etiology also suggest potential candidates. Comparison of genome-wide microarray expression analysis of postmortem tissues from schizophrenics and control patients may identify candidate genes with altered expression levels important in biologic processes relevant to schizophrenia, e.g., myelination-related genes (Hakak et al., 2001). The large number of potential schizophrenia susceptibility genes and the consequent low prior probability of success in association studies raise the issue of setting stringent significance levels for reporting results, to avoid misallocation of limited scientific resources (Crowe, 1993). Case-control studies and family-based studies provide a potentially powerful way to detect genes of smaller effect, which may not be detectable using linkage methods. The inhibiting factor may be ascertainment of the larger samples required (Owen et al., 1997).

Candidate Genes Used with Clinical Disease

If there is an autoimmune pathogenesis for schizophrenia, transmission of specific alleles identified in the MHC, particularly the HLA class I (*HLA-A, -B, -C*) and class II (*HLA-DR, -DQ, -DP*) alleles, are excellent candidates for testing in cases and controls. The products of the class I and class II genes are involved in the presentation of processed antigens to T cells. HLA subtypes have also been postulated to influence neuronal postsynaptic membrane sensitivity to central neurotransmitters such as dopamine.

Early reports of associations between schizophrenia and the MHC were reviewed by McGuffin (1979), McGuffin and Sturt (1986), Nimgaonkar et al. (1993, 1997), and Ganguli et al. (1994a). A meta-analysis of nine studies (McGuffin and Sturt, 1986) provided some support for strong positive associations ($p = 0.0003$) with *HLA-A9*. Luchins et al. (1980) found a significant association of *HLA-A2* with schizophrenia among African Americans; these findings were related to reverse cerebral asymmetry (Luchins et al., 1981). A study among male cases and controls in Czechoslovakia found a strong positive association for *HLA-A28* ($p < 0.001$) and *HLA-Cw4* ($p < 0.01$) (Ivanyi et al., 1978), restricted to the paranoid subtype. The incidence of the combined alleles *HLA-B38*, *-DR4*, and *-DQw3* in a haplotype was significantly elevated in patients of Ashkenazi Jewish descent experiencing agranulocytosis after treatment with clozapine (Lieberman et al., 1990). Three findings of negative associations of schizophrenia with *DQB1*0602* among African Americans, particularly among females, were reported by Nimgaonkar et al. (1993, 1995a, 1997). Straub et al. (1995) found evidence supporting linkage in the 6p region in a genome-wide scan, which once again focused attention on the HLA region. Schwab et al. (2000) reported an NPL of 3.3 for *HLA-DQB1* ($p = .0001$) in 71 German and Israeli pedigrees.

The autoimmune hypothesis also offers candidate genes from the class of protein mediators generically called *cytokines*. Neurotransmitters stimulate cytokine secretion in the CNS (Norris and Benveniste, 1993), which Muller et al. (1998) propose as a regulative mechanism affecting autoimmune disorders, susceptibility to infection, and psychiatric illness.

Ganguli et al. (1993) revealed that a subgroup of schizophrenics have several significant immunologic abnormalities, including increased prevalence of autoimmune diseases and antinuclear and anticytoplasmic antibodies, decreased lymphocyte IL-2 production (replicated in Ganguli et al., 1995), increased serum IL-2 receptor concentration, increased serum IL-6 concentration (Ganguli et al., 1994b), and an association with HLAs. Gaughran et al. (1998) showed soluble *IL-2RA* levels to be significantly higher in 27 Irish patients compared to 32 controls ($p = 0.0019$). Additional studies report elevated serum soluble IL-2 receptor levels (Rapaport et al., 1993, 1994; Barak et al., 1995). Association and linkage studies related to loci *IL2Rb* and *IL1B* have been negative (Nimgaonkar et al., 1995a,b; Tatsumi et al., 1997; Parsian et al., 1997; Laurent et al., 1997).

The dopamine hypothesis of schizophrenia (see Pathophysiology above) was initially supported by the action of typical antipsychotics on dopamine D_2 receptors. Lack of uniformity in pharmacologic response has led to association studies based on dopamine receptor polymorphisms combined with responder/nonresponder status to various medications, particularly clozapine. Similarly, association studies may examine side effects of antipsychotics (tardive dyskinesia), significant differences in homozygosity, or allele or genotype frequencies (Table 45–13).

In linkage analyses of nine families, Coon et al. (1993) examined three markers at each of five dopamine receptor sites used as candidate genes, and the results were strongly negative for the schizophrenia phenotype. Using the P50 auditory evoked potential gating deficit ratio as a phenotype, the results were even more negative.

Su et al. (1993) concluded that allelic variation of *DRD2* and five surrounding loci was not a major component of genetic susceptibility to schizophrenia in 112 Irish multiplex pedigrees. *DRD2* maps close to the breakpoint in 11q23 identified by St. Clair et al. (1990). The polymorphic gene variants identified in *DRD2* appear to have functional differences (Cravchik et al., 1996). A missense mutation (Cys^{311}) was identified by Itokawa et al. (1993) when sequencing *DRD2* in 50 Japanese schizophrenics, and Cys^{311} was associated with a positive family history of schizophrenia ($p = 0.047$). The evidence indicates that Cys^{311} is a rare variant, with some implication that homozygosity may be associated with schizophrenia. Arinami et al. (1997) reported two polymorphisms in *DRD2*: A-241G and −141C Ins/Del. Structural mutational studies were undertaken by Gejman et al. (1994), and no functionally relevant mutations were found to be associated with schizophrenia. Ebstein et al. (1997) reviewed 16 studies: five found association and another three found associations in subgroups. Dopamine receptor *DRD1* sequences were examined in 132 schizophrenics, and no functionally relevant polymorphisms were detected (Liu et al., 1995).

Table 45–13. Dopamine Association Studies

Gene	Reference	Cases	Controls	Results
DBH	Wei et al. (1998)	161	67	No association
DRD1	Cichon et al. (1994)	36 German	45 German	No association
	Kojima et al. (1999)	148 Japanese	148 Japanese	No association
DRD2	Li et al. (1998a,b)	229 Chinese 151 Caucasian	Trios	141 δC no association
	Stober et al. (1998)	260 German	290 German	141 δC no association
	Arinami et al. (1997)	260 Japanese	312 Japanese	141 δC negative association $p = 0.001$
	Itokawa et al. (1993)	142 Japanese	289 Japanese	Csy^{311} slightly more common in SZ
	Verga et al. (1997)	103 Italian	97 Italian	Cys^{311} no association
	Spurlock et al. (1998b)	EMASS: Wales 96 Austria 76 Ireland 33 Sweden 67 Italy 92 Total 359	EMASS: Wales 104 Austria 53 Ireland 85 Sweden 63 Italy 91 Total 396	Cys^{311} no association
	Chen et al. (1996a)	114 Taiwanese	88 Taiwanese	Cys^{311} no association
	Shaikh et al. (1994)	140 Caucasian (32 subgroups)	100	Cys^{311} $p = 0.017$
	Hori et al. (2001)	241 Japanese	201 Japanese	Ser^{311} Cys no association −141C Ins/Del no association
DRD3	Crocq et al. (1992)	68 European Caucasian 71 French	68 European Caucasian 73 French	BalI homozygous $p = 0.005$ BalI homozygous $p = 0.008$ Combined $p = 0.0001$
	Shaikh et al. (1996)	133 Caucasian (clozapine) 10 studies	109 Caucasian	Ser^{-9} $p = 0.004$ Meta-analysis 1-1 genotype $p = 0.01$
	Chen et al. (1997)	178 Chinese	100 Chinese	Ser^{9}Gly no assoc.
	Ebstein et al. (1997)	87 Israeli 80 Italian	136 Israeli 63 Italian	Allele 2 homozygous $p = 0.03$
	Williams et al. (1998)	30 studies: 2722 57 trios	 2629	Ser^{9}Gly meta-analysis BalI homozygous $p = 0.0009$ Homozygous $p = 0.004$
	Ishiguro et al. (2000)	153 Japanese 99 Japanese	122 Japanese 132 Japanese	−712G/C, −205A/G, and Ser^{9}Gly haplotype $p = 0.0007$ uncorrected $p = 0.00004$
DRD4	Sommer et al. (1993)	115 Caucasian	115 Caucasian	48 bp repeat 4.4 slightly more frequent
	Nakamura et al. (1995)	55 L^{+} Japanese 46 L^{-} Japanese	52	4.4 possible association in L group $p = 0.013$ L^{-}, no family history
	Serretti et al. (2001)	419	601	No association
DRD5	Sobell et al. (1995)	400 Caucasian	1914 Caucasian (Mayo)	No association
	Muir et al. (2001)	158	437	148 bp allele $p = 0.02$
DAT1 (*SLC6A3*)	Daniels et al. (1995)	92	84	No association
	Semwal et al. (2001)	179 trios		No association

Sokoloff et al. (1990) cloned *DRD3* (3q13) and showed that both typical and atypical neuroleptics upregulate *DRD3* expression in the brain. *DRD3*-deficient mice exhibit hyperactive behaviors and reduced anxiety-associated behavior in a test paradigm (Accili et al., 1996; Drago et al., 1998). Homozygosity of a polymorphism in the *DRD3* gene has been associated with schizophrenia. A large-scale meta-analysis of over 30 studies found an excess of homozygosity in the Bal1 polymorphism ($p = 0.0009$) (Dubertret et al., 1998).

Atypical neuroleptics, such as clozapine, have been shown to bind *DRD4* with a 10-fold greater affinity than either *DRD2* or *DRD3* (Griffon et al., 1995). Despite this affinity, numerous reports have shown no association between *DRD4* and schizophrenia. A slight trend toward greater prevalence among schizophrenics of homozygotes with a 48 bp tandem repeat allele was found by Sommer et al. (1993). Homozygosity of the 48 bp repeat allele in exon 3 was associated with good neuroleptic response during acute treatment ($p = 0.01$) in 42 of 80 Taiwanese schizophrenics and with a lower prevalence of negative symptoms at remission, especially in male schizophrenic patients (Hwu et al., 1998).

DRD5 was screened for mutations in 78 unrelated schizophrenics (Sobell et al., 1995). Four sequence changes with likely functional significance were identified, and none showed an association with schizophrenia. Studies of the *DRD5* region on 4p16–p15 have found no evidence of linkage or association (Ravindranathan et al., 1994; Kalsi et al., 1996; Asherson et al., 1998).

The principal enzymes for the biosynthesis and metabolism of catecholamines (dopamine, norepinephrine, epinephrine), including dopamine hydroxylase, tyrosine hydroxylase, and catechol-*O*-methyltransferase, have been investigated as candidate genes. Polymorphisms of the dopamine hydroxylase (*DBH*) gene were the subject of an association study by Wei et al. (1998), who found no associations between schizophrenia and *DBH* polymorphisms in 161 unrelated schizophrenics and 67 controls. A study of 34 Austrian multiplex families focusing on the 9q34 region of the *DBH* gene found no evidence of linkage (Meszaros et al., 1996). Nevertheless, variability of *DBH* activity and plasma homovanillic acid levels (the major metabolite of dopamine) in drug-free and drug-treated schizophrenics is one area of continued research interest in the catacholamine pathway of schizophrenia.

Tyrosine hydroxylase (TH) is involved in the conversion of phenylalanine to dopamine and is the rate-limiting enzyme in the synthesis of catecholamines. It plays a key role in the physiology of adrenergic neurons. TH is highly homologous in terms of both protein sequence and catalytic mechanism to phenylalanine hydroxylase and tryptophan hydroxylase. TH is mapped to 11p15.5, closely linked to the dopamine receptor D_4. A rare variant of a tetrarepeat polymorphism $(TCAT)_n$ was identified in five of 94 French schizophrenics and did not appear in 145 screened controls. A second study identified four variants in 44 Tunisian schizophrenics and none in the 44 screened controls (Meloni et al., 1995). However, a Swedish sample found the variant more frequently in controls (9/76) than cases (4/117) (Jonsson et al., 1998b). No association was found between a $Val^{81}Met$ polymorphism in the *TH* gene in a Japanese sample of 194 schizophrenics and 161 controls (Kunugi et al., 1998). In another study, a particular genotype (*AE*) in a variable number tandem repeat (VNTR) in the first exon of *TH* was more frequent in schizophrenics (30/176) compared to controls (9/107) ($p < 0.05$) (Wei et al., 1995).

Catechol-*O*-methyltransferase (COMT) is involved in the metabolism of catecholamine neurotransmitters, inactivating the neurotransmitters by methylation. Two alleles coding for high or low COMT activity in red blood cells are recognized. COMT is mapped to the candidate region 22q11. Floderus et al. (1981a) reviewed 10 small studies, the majority reporting no difference, and in a new study found no difference in enzyme activity between 18 schizophrenics and their 54 unaffected relatives from a large Swedish pedigree. A follow-up study included assays for erythrocyte COMT activity in a small sample of Swedish twins discordant for the schizophrenia phenotype and revealed no differences (Floderus et al. 1981b). Karayiorgou et al. (1998) used single-strand conformation polymorphism analysis to identify a polymorphism causing a missense mutation ($Val^{158}Met$) within the COMT coding region that results in the creation of an NlaIII restriction site in the low-activity allele. Although evidence suggests that the polymorphism is the genetic cause underlying the high/low activity of the COMT enzyme, it appears not to play a major role in schizophrenia in general. The presence of Met in both alleles is highly correlated with three- to fourfold variations in enzyme activity (Lotta et al., 1995; Lachman et al., 1996). Social behaviors in knockout mice have been studied by Gogos et al. (1998). Recent studies are shown in Table 45–14. Finally, Egan et al. (2001) suggested that the COMT Val allele, because it increases prefrontal dopamine catabolism, impairs prefrontal cortical function and is associated with an increased risk for schizophrenia, based on transmission disequilibrium studies in 104 schizophrenic parent/child trios and on tests of executive cognition using the Wisconsin Card Sorting Test in 175 patients with schizophrenia, 219 unaffected siblings, and 55 controls.

Serotonin (or 5-HT), another monoamine neurotransmitter, was first linked to schizophrenia because of the psychotomimetic actions of its agonists [lysergic acid diethylamide (LSD), mescaline] in healthy subjects (see Pathophysiology above). Williams et al. (1996) reported an association between a particular polymorphism in the $5\text{-}HT_{2A}$ receptor gene on the long arm of chromosome 13 and schizophrenia, but this finding has not been replicated. There is evidence that $5\text{-}HT_{2A}$ on chromosome 13 is in a region subject to maternal imprinting (Kato et al., 1996). Table 45–15 summarizes serotonin association studies.

The relationship between schizophrenia and glutamatergic neurotransmission (see Pathophysiology above) has been investigated in several candidate gene studies. Linkage studies of 9 multiplex families found no evidence of linkage to the *NMDAR1* or *GLUR5* glutamate receptor subunit genes (Pariseau et al., 1994), but Riley et al. (1997) found small positive two-point lod scores in 19 multiplex families for the 9q34 region near the *NMDAR1* central subunit gene (0.88) and in the 17q25 region near the *NMDAR2C* potentiating subunit gene (0.76). Decreased concentrations of glutamate in the CSF and in regions of the brain implicated in schizophrenia have been reported (Kim et al.,

Table 45–14. Catechol-*O*-Methyltransferase (COMT) Association Studies

Reference	Size	Sample Ethnicity	Control Sample	COMT Findings
Karayiorgou et al. (1998)	157	European Caucasian	129	Met^{158} no difference
Ohmori et al. (1998)	150	Japanese	150	Met^{108} positive $p = 0.028$
Lachman et al. (1998)	55	Caucasian	none	Homozygosity of low-activity allele associated with violence $p = 0.03$
Kunugi et al. (1997)	76 (63)	Welsh (7 families) English (13) Japanese (2)	Trios	Val^{158} (22 T vs. 13 NT) NS C256G, G256 positive $p = 0.03$
Strous et al. (1997)	54	Caucasian	87	NlaIII low-allele-positive >0.07
Li et al. (1996)	178	Chinese	Trios	Val^{108} TDT-positive $p = 0.005$
Chen et al. (1996b)	177	Chinese	99	BglI no association
Daniels et al. (1996)	78	Welsh, Irish, English	78	No differences
Li et al. (2000)	198	Chinese	Trios	Val^{158} allele TDT $p = 0.01$
Egan et al. (2001)	104	European American	Trios	Val^{108} allele TDT $p = 0.03$
Semwal et al. (2001)	179	Northern Indian	Trios	No association

T, transmitted; NT, not transmitted; TDT, Transmission Disequilibrium Test.

Table 45–15. Serotonin Association Studies

Gene	Reference	Cases	Controls	Results
HTR2A	Spurlock et al. (1998a)	63 trios	126 parents	$T^{102}C$ $p = 0.001$
	Williams et al. (1997)	15 studies: 1533	1771	$T^{102}C$ allele 2 excess $p = 0.0009$ meta-analysis
	Williams et al. (1996)	571	639	$T^{102}C$ allele 2 excess $p = 0.003$
	Inayama et al. (1996)	62	96	$T^{102}C$ allele 2 excess $p < 0.05$
	Erdmann et al. (1996)	45	46	$T^{102}C$ $p = 0.04$

$T^{102}C$, allele 2 is the C allele in the noncoding $T^{102}C$ polymorphism in the promoter region of 5-hydroxytryptamine$_{2A}$.

1980). Binding studies and messenger RNA studies reviewed by Hirsch et al. (1997) showed widespread changes in NMDA receptor function, with replicated findings of decreased NMDA receptors in the hippocampal area, increased kainate receptors in the prefrontal and orbitofrontal areas, and decreased kainate receptors in the hippocampus.

Metabolism of neuroleptic drugs is influenced by polymorphisms in the *CYP2D6* gene (mapped to 22q.13), which codes for the cytochrome P-450 enzyme debrisoquine hydroxylase. Reduced *CYP2D6* activity resulting in the "poor metabolizer" phenotype may be related to an increased risk of Parkinson's disease and has been hypothesized to influence persistent tardive dyskinesia (Kapitany et al., 1998), but *CYP2D6* does not appear to be important to schizophrenia liability (Vallada et al., 1992; Dawson et al., 1994; Daniels et al., 1995; Armstrong et al., 1997; Jonsson et al., 1998).

The neurodevelopmental hypothesis for schizophrenia has led to the consideration of brain-derived neurotrophic factor (*BDNF*) and neurotrophin 3 (*NT3*) as candidate genes. *BDNF* (mapped to chromosome 11p13) and *NT3* (mapped to 12p13) promote neuronal survival and differentiation. A Japanese study of *BDNF* genotypes in 60 unrelated schizophrenics and matched controls found no association with schizophrenia but did suggest population differences in allele frequencies compared to Caucasian data (Sasaki et al., 1997). An excess of allele 3 of *NT3* was found among Japanese schizophrenics vs. controls ($p = 0.011$) (Nanko et al., 1994) but was not replicated in a Swedish sample (Jansson et al., 1997) or in two other reports (Dawson et al., 1995; Arinami et al., 1996).

Expansion of repeating triplets of nucleotides in the genome has been connected with degenerative and developmental neuropsychiatric diseases. Many of these unstable DNA segments are $(CAG)_n$ repeats, coding for polyglutamine. The phenomenon of *anticipation*, a progressively earlier age at onset and/or worsening severity of symptoms over successive generations, may be inversely related to the extent of triplet expansion. Several groups have searched for expansions in patients with schizophrenia. Anticipation has been hypothesized, but methodologic difficulties in studies which rely on retrospective data make it impossible to draw firm conclusions. An age-at-onset cohort effect may introduce bias into anticipation studies of schizophrenia (Di Maggio et al., 2001).

Crowe et al. (1993) found significant sharing of alleles ($p = 0.003$) in male—male affected sib pairs using a $(CAG)_n$ polymorphism in the androgen receptor (*AR*) gene mapped to Xq11–q12. No associations have been found between schizophrenia and abnormally expanded repeats in any of the following: the gene coding for dentatorubral-pallidoluysian atrophy (DRPLA) protein (Lesch et al., 1994; Brando et al., 1996; Morris-Rosendahl et al., 1997), the spinocerebellar ataxia type 1 (*SCA1*) gene (Morris-Rosendahl et al., 1997; Pujana et al., 1997), the Huntington's disease (*HD*) genes (Rubinsztein et al., 1996), or the *AR* gene (Arranz et al., 1995). Searches for abnormally expanded repeats of greater than 300 trinucleotides in Canadian multiplex families exhibiting anticipation found no differences in the distribution patterns between affected and unaffected family members (Petronis et al., 1996). However, the presence of shorter repeats (30–130 nucleotides) could not be excluded as an etiologic factor. The results from other studies are not consistent. Some have shown support for the greater repeat size in schizophrenics compared to controls (Morris et al., 1995; O'-Donovan et al., 1995); others have not (Vincent et al., 1999).

Chandy et al. (1998) identified two polymorphic CAG triplet repeat sites in the human calcium-activated potassium channel gene (*KCNN3*, formerly named *hSKCa3*) and found significantly longer repeats in the second polymorphism (longer than the modal value of 19 repeats) in schizophrenics compared to controls ($p = 0.0035$). This study also suggested that *KCNN3* mapped to chromosome 22q. Further studies by Antonarakis et al. (1999), Guy et al. (1999), and Stober et al. (2000a) suggested no linkage or association and mapped the gene to chromosome 1q21. In addition, no evidence for an association was found using a sample of 97 schizophrenic triads from southwest China (Li et al., 1998b) or in a Japanese population (Ujike et al., 2001).

Pulver et al. (1994b) suggested linkage for 22q in a sample of 39 multiplex families with a heterogeneity lod score of 2.84 for 22q12–q13. Follow-up studies in 256 families found no support, with the caveat that if fewer than 25% of the families contributed to the linkage, then the follow-up sample most likely did not have the power to detect linkage in such a subset (Pulver et al., 1994a).

The 22q region became the focus of further studies when it was observed that patients exhibiting a microdeletion in 22q11 (velocardiofacial syndrome) often presented with severe psychiatric manifestations of illness as they entered late adolescence (Pulver et al., 1994a–c). Velocardiofacial syndrome, an autosomal dominant disorder, is characterized by cleft palate, cardiac defects, learning disabilities, and a typical facial appearance. In a random sample of 100 schizophrenics, two individuals were found to have the microdeletion characteristic of velocardiofacial syndrome (Karayiorgou et al., 1995). It is now suggested that schizophrenic patients with a history of delayed motor development, early onset of the disorder, history of learning disability, mental retardation, congenital cardiac anomalies, and/or hypernasal speech should be screened for the velo-cardio-facial syndrome deletion (Gothelf et al., 1999). Bassett et al. (1998) replicated the association of a 22q11 deletion syndrome with schizophrenia. Yamagishi et al. (1999) suggested that *UFD1L* haploinsufficiency contributes to the congenital heart and craniofacial defects seen in 22q11 deletion. The human *UFD1L* gene maps to the 22q11 region (Pizzuti et al., 1997) and is involved in neural crest development. In a study of 182 patients with 22q11 deletion, Yamagishi et al. (1999) found corresponding deletion of the *UFD1L* gene in all 182 patients. Embryonic expression patterns in mice showed that *Ufd1* was specifically expressed in most tissues affected in patients with 22q11 deletion syndrome, particularly the hippocampus.

CLINICAL APPLICATION AND RISK ASSESSMENT OF GENETICS INFORMATION

Our current understanding of the genetic basis of schizophrenia does not afford clinical applications, with one exception: it provides a framework for the development of empirical risks. It must be understood, however, that these risks do not apply to any one individual. Looking ahead, it is likely that a chapter on schizophrenia in the third edition of this book will characterize a number of schizophrenia susceptibility genes with certainty. Discovery and study of such genes will shed light on the problem of disease heterogeneity we have reviewed and discussed in this chapter, an issue vital for precision in pharmacologic treatment. Furthermore, identification of gene products will allow correlation between pathophysiologic studies, whether anatomical or neuroimaging, and clinical expression, delineating disease subtypes. The existence of such subtypes, validated by association between gene, gene product, pathophysiology, variation in clinical expression, and perhaps above all prognosis, has been predicted for years. Now, we are nearly there, but the number and frequency of the genes involved may complicate realization of this goal. We have presented evidence for many susceptibility loci. If we assume one or more alleles of polymorphic frequency in each of these many regions (and no doubt more to come), subtypes may overlap. We may even find that each individual has a unique form of schizophrenia. We are standing at the threshold of truly vital discoveries in schizophrenia research. These are stirring times.

ACKNOWLEDGMENTS

We thank Jamie Winshell for her steadfast editorial assistance in preparing this manuscript.

REFERENCES

Abi-Dargham A, Laruelle M, Aghajanian GK, Charney D, Krystal J: The role of serotonin in the pathophysiology and treatment of schizophrenia. J Neuropsychiatry Clin Neurosci 1997; 9:1–17.

Accili D, Fishburn CS, Drago J, Steiner H, Lachowicz JE, Park BH, Gauda EB, et al.: A targeted mutation of the D3 dopamine receptor gene is associated with hyperactivity in mice. Proc Natl Acad Sci USA 1996; 93:1945–1949.

Adler LE, Olincy A, Waldo M, Harris JG, Griffith J, Stevens K, Flach K, et al.: Schizophrenia, sensory gating, and nicotinic receptors. Schizophr Bull 1998; 24:189–202.

Akbarian S, Vinuela A, Kim JJ, Potkin SG, Bunney WE Jr, Jones EG: Distorted distribution of nicotinamide-adenine dinucleotide phosphate-diaphorase neurons in temporal lobe of schizophrenics implies anomalous cortical development. Arch Gen Psychiatry 1993; 50:178–187.

Albus M, Maier W: Lack of gender differences in age at onset in familial schizophrenia. Schizophr Res 1995; 18:51–57.

Antonarakis SE, Blouin JL, Pulver AE, Wolyniec P, Lasseter VK, Nestadt G, Kasch L, et al.: Schizophrenia susceptibility and chromosome 6p24–22. Nat Genet 1995; 11:235–236.

Antonarakis SE, Blouin JL, Lasseter VK, Gehrig C, Radhakrishna U, Nestadt G, Housman DE, et al.: Lack of linkage or association between schizophrenia and the polymorphic trinucleotide repeat within the KCNN3 gene on chromosome 1q21. Am J Med Genet 1999; 88:348–351.

APA. Diagnostic and Statistical Manual of Mental Disorders. In: Michael B. First E (ed). American Psychiatric Association, Washington, D.C., 1994.

Arinami T, Gao M, Hamaguchi H, Toru M: A functional polymorphism in the promoter region of the dopamine D2 receptor gene is associated with schizophrenia. Hum Mol Genet 1997; 6:577–582.

Arinami T, Takekoshi K, Itokawa M, Hamaguchi H, Toru M: Failure to find associations of the CA repeat polymorphism in the first intron and the Gly-63/Glu-63 polymorphism of the neurotrophin-3 gene with schizophrenia. Psychiatr Genet 1996; 6:13–15.

Armstrong M, Daly AK, Blennerhassett R, Ferrier N, Idle JR: Antipsychotic drug-induced movement disorders in schizophrenics in relation to CYP2D6 genotype. Br J Psychiatry 1997; 170:23–26.

Arranz MJ, Munro J, Sham P, Kirov G, Murray RM, Collier DA, Kerwin RW: Meta-analysis of studies on genetic variation in 5-HT_{2A} receptors and clozapine response. Schizophr Res 1998; 32:93–99.

Asherson P, Mant R, Williams N, Cardno A, Jones L, Murphy K, Collier DA, Nanko S, Craddock N, Morris S, et al.: A study of chromosome 4p markers and dopamine D_5 receptor gene in schizophrenia and bipolar disorder. Mol Psychiatry 1998; 3:310–320.

Asherson P, Parfitt E, Sargeant M, Tidmarsh S, Buckland P, Taylor C, Clements A, Gill M, McGuffin P, Owen M: No evidence for a pseudoautosomal locus for schizophrenia. Linkage analysis of multiply affected families. Br J Psychiatry 1992; 161:63–68.

Bailer U, Leisch F, Meszaros K, Lenzinger E, Willinger U, Strobl R, Gebhardt C, Gerhard E, Fuchs K, Sieghart W, et al.: Genome scan for susceptibility loci for schizophrenia. Neuropsychobiology 2000; 42:175–182.

Barak V, Barak Y, Levine J, Nisman B, Roisman I: Changes in interleukin-1beta and soluble interleukin-2 receptor levels in CSF and serum of schizophrenic patients. J Basic Clin Physiol Pharmacol 1995; 6:61–69.

Baron M, Gruen R: Risk factors in schizophrenia. Season of birth and family history [see comments]. Br J Psychiatry 1988; 152:460–465.

Baron M, Gruen R, Asnis L: Schizophrenia: a comparative study of patients with and without family history. Br J Psychiatry 1982; 140:516–517.

Barr CL, Kennedy JL, Pakstis AJ, Castiglione CM, Kidd JR, Wetterberg L, Kidd KK: Linkage study of a susceptibility locus for schizophrenia in the pseudoautosomal region. Schizophr Bull 1994a; 20:277–286.

Barr CL, Kennedy JL, Pakstis AJ, Wetterberg L, Sjogren B, Bierut L, Wadelius C, Wahlstrom J, Martinsson T, Giuffra L, et al.: Progress in a genome scan for linkage in schizophrenia in a large Swedish kindred. Am J Med Genet 1994b; 54:51–58.

Barr WB, Ashtari M, Bilder RM, Degreef G, Lieberman JA: Brain morphometric comparison of first-episode schizophrenia and temporal lobe epilepsy. Br J Psychiatry 1997; 170:515–519.

Barta PE, Pearlson GD, Brill LB 2nd, Royall R, McGilchrist IK, Pulver AE, Powers RE, Casanova MF, Tien AY, Frangou S, et al.: Planum temporale asymmetry reversal in schizophrenia: replication and relationship to gray matter abnormalities. Am J Psychiatry 1997; 154:661–667.

Barta PE, Pearlson GD, Powers RE, Richards SS, Tune LE: Auditory hallucinations and smaller superior temporal gyral volume in schizophrenia. Am J Psychiatry 1990; 147:1457–1462.

Bassett AS: Chromosomal aberrations and schizophrenia. Autosomes. Br J Psychiatry 1992; 161:323–334.

Bassett AS, Chow EW, Weksberg R: Chromosomal abnormalities and schizophrenia. Am J Med Genet 2000; 97:45–51.

Bassett AS, Hodgkinson K, Chow EW, Correia S, Scutt LE, Weksberg R: 22q11 deletion syndrome in adults with schizophrenia. Am J Med Genet 1998; 81:328–337.

Bassett AS, McGillivray BC, Jones BD, Pantzar JT: Partial trisomy chromosome 5 cosegregating with schizophrenia. Lancet 1988; 1:799–801.

Benes FM: The role of stress and dopamine–GABA interactions in the vulnerability for schizophrenia. J Psychiatr Res 1997; 31:257–275.

Berrettini WH: Susceptibility loci for bipolar disorder: overlap with inherited vulnerability to schizophrenia. Biol Psychiatry 2000; 47:245–251.

Berrettini WH, Ferraro TN, Goldin LR, Weeks DE, Detera-Wadleigh S, Nurnberger JI Jr, Gershon ES: Chromosome 18 DNA markers and manic-depressive illness: evidence for a susceptibility gene. Proc Natl Acad Sci USA 1994; 91:5918–5921.

Bhugra D, Leff J, Mallett R, Der G, Corridan B, Rudge S: Incidence and outcome of schizophrenia in whites, African-Caribbeans and Asians in London [see comments]. Psychol Med 1997; 27:791–798.

Bleuler E: Dementia Praecox of the Group of Schizophrenias (1911). New York: International Universities Press, 1950.

Blouin JL, Dombroski BA, Nath SK, Lasseter VK, Wolyniec PS, Nestadt G, Thornquist M, Ullrich G, McGrath J, Kasch L, et al.: Schizophrenia susceptibility loci on chromosomes 13q32 and 8p21. Nat Genet 1998; 20:70–73.

Borison RL: The role of cognition in the risk–benefit and safety analysis of antipsychotic medication. Acta Psychiatr Scand Suppl 1996; 389:5–11.

Boyd JH, Pulver AE, Stewart W: Season of birth: schizophrenia and bipolar disorder. Schizophr Bull 1986; 12:173–186.

Bradbury TN, Miller GA: Season of birth in schizophrenia: a review of evidence, methodology, and etiology. Psychol Bull 1985; 98:569—594.

Brando LJ, Yolken R, Herman MM, Kleinman JE, Ross CA, Torrey EF: Analysis of the DRPLA triplet repeat in brain tissue and leukocytes from schizophrenics. Psychiatr Genet 1996; 6:1–5.

Brewin J, Cantwell R, Dalkin T, Fox R, Medley I, Glazebrook C, Kwiecinski R, Har-

rison G: Incidence of schizophrenia in Nottingham. A comparison of two cohorts, 1978–80 and 1992–94. Br J Psychiatry 1997; 171:140–144.
Bruton CJ, Stevens JR, Frith CD: Epilepsy, psychosis, and schizophrenia: clinical and neuropathologic correlations. Neurology 1994; 44:34–42.
Brzustowicz LM, Hodgkinson KA, Chow EW, Honer WG, Bassett AS: Location of a major susceptibility locus for familial schizophrenia on chromosome 1q21–q22. Science 2000; 288:678–682.
Brzustowicz LM, Honer WG, Chow EW, Hogan J, Hodgkinson K, Bassett AS: Use of a quantitative trait to map a locus associated with severity of positive symptoms in familial schizophrenia to chromosome 6p. Am J Hum Genet 1997; 61:1388–1396.
Brzustowicz LM, Honer WG, Chow EW, Little D, Hogan J, Hodgkinson K, Bassett AS: Linkage of familial schizophrenia to chromosome 13q32. Am J Hum Genet 1999; 65:1096–1103.
Buchanan RW, Vladar K, Barta PE, Pearlson GD: Structural evaluation of the prefrontal cortex in schizophrenia. Am J Psychiatry 1998; 155:1049–1055.
Burnet PW, Eastwood SL, Harrison PJ: [^{3}H]WAY-100635 for 5-HT_{1A} receptor autoradiography in human brain: a comparison with [^{3}H]8-OH-DPAT and demonstration of increased binding in the frontal cortex in schizophrenia. Neurochem Int 1997; 30:565–574.
Callicott JH, Egan MF, Bertolino A, Mattay VS, Langheim FJ, Frank JA, Weinberger DR: Hippocampal *N*-acetyl aspartate in unaffected siblings of patients with schizophrenia: a possible intermediate neurobiological phenotype. Biol Psychiatry 1998; 44:941–950.
Cannon M, Cotter D, Coffey VP, Sham PC, Takei N, Larkin C, Murray RM, O'-Callaghan E: Prenatal exposure to the 1957 influenza epidemic and adult schizophrenia: a follow-up study [see comments]. Br J Psychiatry 1996; 168:368–371.
Cannon M, Jones P, Murray RM, Wadsworth ME: Childhood laterality and later risk of schizophrenia in the 1946 British birth cohort. Schizophr Res 1997; 26:117–120.
Cannon TD, Kaprio J, Lonnqvist J, Huttunen M, Koskenvuo M: The genetic epidemiology of schizophrenia in a Finnish twin cohort. A population-based modeling study. Arch Gen Psychiatry 1998; 55:67–74.
Cao Q, Martinez M, Zhang J, Sanders AR, Badner JA, Cravchik A, Markey CJ, Beshah E, Guroff JJ, Maxwell ME, et al.: Suggestive evidence for a schizophrenia susceptibility locus on chromosome 6q and a confirmation in an independent series of pedigrees. Genomics 1997; 43:1–8.
Cardno AG, Holmans PA, Rees MI, Jones LA, McCarthy GM, Hamshere ML, Williams NM, Norton N, Williams HJ, Fenton I, et al.: A genomewide linkage study of age at onset in schizophrenia. Am J Med Genet 2001; 105:439–445.
Cardno AG, Marshall EJ, Coid B, Macdonald AM, Ribchester TR, Davies NJ, Venturi P, Jones LA, Lewis SW, Sham PC, et al.: Heritability estimates for psychotic disorders: the Maudsley twin psychosis series. Arch Gen Psychiatry 1999; 56:162–168.
Carlsson A: Neurocircuitries and neurotransmitter interactions in schizophrenia. Int Clin Psychopharmacol 1995; 10(Suppl 3):21–28.
Castle D, Sham P, Murray R: Differences in distribution of ages of onset in males and females with schizophrenia. Schizophr Res 1998; 33:179–183.
Catts SV, Ward PB, Lloyd A, Huang XF, Dixon G, Chahl L, Harper C, Wakefield D: Molecular biological investigations into the role of the NMDA receptor in the pathophysiology of schizophrenia. Aust N Z J Psychiatry 1997; 31:17–26.
Chadda R, Kulhara P, Singh T, Sehgal S: HLA antigens in schizophrenia: a family study. Br J Psychiatry 1986; 149:612–615.
Chandy KG, Fantino E, Wittekindt O, Kalman K, Tong LL, Ho TH, Gutman GA, Crocq MA, Ganguli R, Nimgaonkar V, et al.: Isolation of a novel potassium channel gene *hSKCa3* containing a polymorphic CAG repeat: a candidate for schizophrenia and bipolar disorder? Mol Psychiatry 1998; 3:32–37.
Chen CH, Chien SH, Hwu HG: No association of dopamine D_2 receptor molecular variant Cys^{311} and schizophrenia in Chinese patients. Am J Med Genet 1996a; 67:418–420.
Chen CH, Chiu YL, Wei FC, Koong FJ, Liu HC, Shaw CK, Hwu HG, Hsiao KJ: High seroprevalence of Borna virus infection in schizophrenic patients, family members and mental health workers in Taiwan. Mol Psychiatry 1999; 4:33–38.
Chen CH, Lee YR, Liu MY, Wei FC, Koong FJ, Hwu HG, Hsiao KJ: Identification of a BglI polymorphism of catechol-*O*-methyltransferase (*COMT*) gene, and association study with schizophrenia. Am J Med Genet 1996b; 67:556–559.
Chen CH, Liu MY, Wei FC, Koong FJ, Hwu HG, Hsiao KJ: Further evidence of no association between Ser^9Gly polymorphism of dopamine D^3 receptor gene and schizophrenia. Am J Med Genet 1997; 74:40–43.
Chen WJ, Yeh LL, Chang CJ, Lin LC, Rin H, Hwu HG: Month of birth and schizophrenia in Taiwan: effect of gender, family history and age at onset. Schizophr Res 1996; 20:133–143.
Childs B, Scriver CR: Age at onset and causes of disease. Perspect Biol Med 1986; 29:437–460.
Cichon S, Nothen MM, Rietschel M, Korner J, Propping P: Single-strand conformation analysis (SSCA) of the dopamine D_1 receptor gene (*DRD1*) reveals no significant mutation in patients with schizophrenia and manic depression. Biol Psychiatry 1994; 36:850–853.
Collinge J, Delisi LE, Boccio A, Johnstone EC, Lane A, Larkin C, Leach M, Lofthouse R, Owen F, Poulter M, et al.: Evidence for a pseudoautosomal locus for schizophrenia using the method of affected sibling pairs. Br J Psychiatry 1991; 158:624–629.
Coon H, Byerley W, Holik J, Hoff M, Myles-Worsley M, Lannfelt L, Sokoloff P, Schwartz JC, Waldo M, Freedman R, et al.: Linkage analysis of schizophrenia with five dopamine receptor genes in nine pedigrees. Am J Hum Genet 1993; 52:327–334.
Coon H, Holik J, Hoff M, Reimherr F, Wender P, Myles-Worsley M, Waldo M, Freedman R, Byerley W: Analysis of chromosome 22 markers in nine schizophrenia pedigrees. Am J Med Genet 1994a; 54:72–79.
Coon H, Jensen S, Holik J, Hoff M, Myles-Worsley M, Reimherr F, Wender P, Waldo M, Freedman R, Leppert M, et al.: Genomic scan for genes predisposing to schizophrenia. Am J Med Genet 1994b; 54:59–71.
Coyle JT: The glutamatergic dysfunction hypothesis for schizophrenia. Harv Rev Psychiatry 1996; 3:241–253.
Cravchik A, Sibley DR, Gejman PV: Functional analysis of the human D_2 dopamine receptor missense variants. J Biol Chem 1996; 271:26013–26017.
Crocq MA, Mant R, Asherson P, Williams J, Hode Y, Mayerova A, Collier D, Lannfelt L, Sokoloff P, Schwartz JC, et al.: Association between schizophrenia and homozygosity at the dopamine D_3 receptor gene [see comments]. J Med Genet 1992; 29:858–860.
Crow T, Ball J, Bloom S, Brown R, Bruton C, Colter N, Frith C, Johnstone E, Owens D, Roberts G: Schizophrenia as an anomaly of development of cerebral asymmetry. A postmortem study and a proposal concerning the genetic basis of the disease. Arch Gen Psychiatry 1989; 46:1145–1150.
Crow TJ: Sex chromosomes and psychosis. The case for a pseudoautosomal locus [see comments]. Br J Psychiatry 1988; 153:675–683.
Crow TJ, Delisi LE, Lofthouse R, Poulter M, Lehner T, Bass N, Shah T, Walsh C, Boccio-Smith A, Shields G, et al.: An examination of linkage of schizophrenia and schizoaffective disorder to the pseudoautosomal region (Xp22.3) [see comments]. Br J Psychiatry 1994; 164:159–164.
Crow TJ, Poulter M, Lofthouse R, Chen G, Shah T, Bass N, Morganti C, Vita A, Smith C, Boccio-Smith A, et al.: Male siblings with schizophrenia share alleles at the androgen receptor above chance expectation. Am J Med Genet 1993; 48:159–160.
Crowe RR: Candidate genes in psychiatry: an epidemiological perspective [see comments]. Am J Med Genet 1993; 48:74–77.
Curtis VA, Bullmore ET, Brammer MJ, Wright IC, Williams SC, Morris RG, Sharma TS, Murray RM, McGuire PK: Attenuated frontal activation during a verbal fluency task in patients with schizophrenia. Am J Psychiatry 1998; 155:1056–1063.
Czechowicz AS, Pamnany L: ABO blood groups and the aetiology of schizophrenia. Med J Aust 1972; 1:1252–1254.
Dalack GW, Healy DJ, Meador-Woodruff JH: Nicotine dependence in schizophrenia: clinical phenomena and laboratory findings. Am J Psychiatry 1998; 155:1490–1501.
Dalman C, Allebeck P, Cullberg J, Grunewald C, Koster M: Obstetric complications and the risk of schizophrenia: a longitudinal study of a national birth cohort. Arch Gen Psychiatry 1999; 56:234–240.
d'Amato T, Campion D, Gorwood P, Jay M, Sabate O, Petit C, Abbar M, Malafosse A, Leboyer M, Hillaire D, et al.: Evidence for a pseudoautosomal locus for schizophrenia. II: Replication of a non-random segregation of alleles at the DXYS14 locus. Br J Psychiatry 1992; 161:59–62.
d'Amato T, Waksman G, Martinez M, Laurent C, Gorwood P, Campion D, Jay M, Petit C, Savoye C, Bastard C, et al.: Pseudoautosomal region in schizophrenia: linkage analysis of seven loci by sib-pair and lod-score methods. Psychiatry Res 1994; 52:135–147.
Daniels J, Williams J, Asherson P, McGuffin P, Owen M: No association between schizophrenia and polymorphisms within the genes for debrisoquine 4-hydroxylase (*CYP2D6*) and the dopamine transporter (DAT). Am J Med Genet 1995; 60:85–87.
Daniels JK, Williams NM, Williams J, Jones LA, Cardno AG, Murphy KC, Spurlock G, Riley B, Scambler P, Asherson P, et al.: No evidence for allelic association between schizophrenia and a polymorphism determining high or low catechol-*O*-methyltransferase activity. Am J Psychiatry 1996; 153:268–270.
Dann J, DeLisi LE, Devoto M, Laval S, Nancarrow DJ, Shields G, Smith A, Loftus J, Peterson P, Vita A, et al.: A linkage study of schizophrenia to markers within Xp11 near the *MAOB* gene. Psychiatry Res 1997; 70:131–143.
Dassa D, Sham PC, van Os J, Abel K, Jones P, Murray RM: Relationship of birth season to clinical features, family history, and obstetric complication in schizophrenia. Psychiatry Res 1996; 64:11–17.
Dauphinais ID, DeLisi LE, Crow TJ, Alexandropoulos K, Colter N, Tuma I, Gershon ES: Reduction in temporal lobe size in siblings with schizophrenia: a magnetic resonance imaging study. Psychiatry Res 1990; 35:137–147.
Dawson E, Powell JF, Nothen MM, Crocq MA, Lanczik M, Korner J, Rietschel M, van Os J, Wright P, Gill M: An association study of debrisoquine hydroxylase (*CYP2D6*) polymorphisms in schizophrenia. Psychiatr Genet 1994; 4:215–218.
Dawson E, Powell JF, Sham PC, Nothen M, Crocq MA, Propping P, Korner J, Rietschel M, van Os J, Wright P, et al.: An association study of a neurotrophin-3 (*NT-3*) gene polymorphism with schizophrenia. Acta Psychiatr Scand 1995; 92:425–428.
DeLisi LE, Bass N, Boccio A, Shields G, Morganti C: Age of onset in familial schizophrenia [letter]. Arch Gen Psychiatry 1994; 51:334–335.
DeLisi LE, Goldin LR, Hamovit JR, Maxwell ME, Kurtz D, Gershon ES: A family study of the association of increased ventricular size with schizophrenia. Arch Gen Psychiatry 1986; 43:148–153.
DeLisi LE, Sakuma M, Tew W, Kushner M, Hoff AL, Grimson R: Schizophrenia as a chronic active brain process: a study of progressive brain structural change subsequent to the onset of schizophrenia [see comments]. Psychiatry Res 1997; 74:129–140.
DeLisi LE, Shaw S, Sherrington R, Nanthakumar B, Shields G, Smith AB, Wellman N, Larach VW, Loftus J, Razi K, et al.: Failure to establish linkage on the X chromosome in 301 families with schizophrenia or schizoaffective disorder. Am J Med Genet 2000; 96:335–341.
DeLisi LE, Tew W, Xie S, Hoff AL, Sakuma M, Kushner M, Lee G, Shedlack K,

Smith AM, Grimson R: A prospective follow-up study of brain morphology and cognition in first-episode schizophrenic patients: preliminary findings. Biol Psychiatry 1995; 38:349–360.

Detera-Wadleigh SD, Badner JA, Berrettini WH, Yoshikawa T, Goldin LR, Turner G, Rollins DY, Moses T, Sanders AR, Karkera JD, et al.: A high-density genome scan detects evidence for a bipolar-disorder susceptibility locus on 13q32 and other potential loci on 1q32 and 18p11.2. Proc Natl Acad Sci USA 1999; 96:5604–5609.

Detera-Wadleigh SD, Goldin LR, Sherrington R, Encio I, de Miguel C, Berrettini W, Gurling H, Gershon ES: Exclusion of linkage to 5q11–13 in families with schizophrenia and other psychiatric disorders. Nature 1989; 340:391–393.

Di Maggio C, Martinez M, Menard JF, Petit M, Thibaut F: Evidence of a cohort effect for age at onset of schizophrenia. Am J Psychiatry 2001; 158:489–492.

Drago J, Padungchaichot P, Accili D, Fuchs S: Dopamine receptors and dopamine transporter in brain function and addictive behaviors: insights from targeted mouse mutants. Dev Neurosci 1998; 20:188–203.

Dror V, Shamir E, Ghanshani S, Kimhi R, Swartz M, Barak Y, Weizman R, Avivi L, Litmanovitch T, Fantino E, et al.: *hKCa3/KCNN3* potassium channel gene: association of longer CAG repeats with schizophrenia in Israeli Ashkenazi Jews, expression in human tissues and localization to chromosome 1q21. Mol Psychiatry 1999; 4:254–260.

Dubertret C, Gorwood P, Ades J, Feingold J, Schwartz JC, Sokoloff P: Meta-analysis of *DRD3* gene and schizophrenia: ethnic heterogeneity and significant association in Caucasians. Am J Med Genet 1998; 81:318–322.

Eastwood SL, Kerwin RW, Harrison PJ: Immunoautoradiographic evidence for a loss of alpha-amino-3-hydroxy-5-methyl-4-isoxazole propionate-preferring non-*N*-methyl-D-aspartate glutamate receptors within the medial temporal lobe in schizophrenia. Biol Psychiatry 1997; 41:636–643.

Eaton WW: Epidemiology of schizophrenia. Epidemiol Rev 1985; 7:105–126.

Eaton WW, Hayward C, Ram R: Schizophrenia and rheumatoid arthritis: a review. Schizophr Res 1992; 6:181–192.

Eberhard G, Franzen G, Low B: Schizophrenia susceptibility and HL-A antigen. Neuropsychobiology 1975; 1:211–217.

Ebstein RP, Macciardi F, Heresco-Levi U, Serretti A, Blaine D, Verga M, Nebamov L, Gur E, Belmaker RH, Avnon M, et al.: Evidence for an association between the dopamine D_3 receptor gene *DRD3* and schizophrenia. Hum Hered 1997; 47:6–16.

Egan MF, Goldberg TE, Kolachana BS, Callicott JH, Mazzanti CM, Straub RE, Goldman D, Weinberger DR: Effect of *COMT* $Val^{108/158}$ Met genotype on frontal lobe function and risk for schizophrenia. Proc Natl Acad Sci USA 2001; 98:6917–6922.

Ekelund J, Hovatta I, Parker A, Paunio T, Varilo T, Martin R, Suhonen J, Ellonen P, Chan G, Sinsheimer JS, et al.: Chromosome 1 loci in Finnish schizophrenia families. Hum Mol Genet 2001; 10:1611–1617.

Ekelund J, Lichtermann D, Hovatta I, Ellonen P, Suvisaari J, Terwilliger JD, Juvonen H, Varilo T, Arajarvi R, Kokko-Sahin ML, et al.: Genome-wide scan for schizophrenia in the Finnish population: evidence for a locus on chromosome 7q22. Hum Mol Genet 2000; 9:1049–1057.

Erdmann J, Shimron-Abarbanell D, Rietschel M, Albus M, Maier W, Korner J, Bondy B, Chen K, Shih JC, Knapp M, et al.: Systematic screening for mutations in the human serotonin-2A (5-HT2A) receptor gene: identification of two naturally occurring receptor variants and association analysis in schizophrenia. Hum Genet 1996; 97:614–619.

Faraone SV, Matise T, Svrakic D, Pepple J, Malaspina D, Suarez B, Hampe C, Zambuto CT, Schmitt K, Meyer J, et al.: Genome scan of European-American schizophrenia pedigrees: results of the NIMH Genetics Initiative and Millennium Consortium. Am J Med Genet 1998; 81:290–295.

Fischer M: Psychoses in the offspring of schizophrenic monozygotic twins and their normal co-twins. Br J Psychiatry 1971; 118:43–52.

Fischer M, Harvald B, Hauge M: A Danish twin study of schizophrenia. Br J Psychiatry 1969; 115:981–990.

Fletcher PC, McKenna PJ, Frith CD, Grasby PM, Friston KJ, Dolan RJ: Brain activations in schizophrenia during a graded memory task studied with functional neuroimaging. Arch Gen Psychiatry 1998; 55:1001–1008.

Floderus Y, Book JA, Wetterberg L: Erythrocyte catechol-*O*-methyltransferase activity in related families with schizophrenia. Clin Genet 1981a; 19:379–385.

Floderus Y, Eberhard G, Witterberg L: Erythrocyte catechol-*O*-methyltransferase activity in psychotic twins. Clin Genet 1981b; 19:386–389.

Foroud T, Castelluccio PF, Koller DL, Edenberg HJ, Miller M, Bowman E, Rau NL, Smiley C, Rice JP, Goate A, et al.: Suggestive evidence of a locus on chromosome 10p using the NIMH genetics initiative bipolar affective disorder pedigrees. Am J Med Genet 2000; 96:18–23.

Freedman R, Coon H, Myles-Worsley M, Orr-Urtreger A, Olincy A, Davis A, Polymeropoulos M, Holik J, Hopkins J, Hoff M, et al.: Linkage of a neurophysiological deficit in schizophrenia to a chromosome 15 locus. Proc Natl Acad Sci USA 1997; 94:587–592.

Freedman R, Hall M, Adler LE, Leonard S: Evidence in postmortem brain tissue for decreased numbers of hippocampal nicotinic receptors in schizophrenia. Biol Psychiatry 1995; 38:22–33.

Gaekwad RS, Niyogi AK, Jagtiani R: ABO blood group genes in schizophrenia and manic depressive psychosis. Indian J Med Sci 1972; 26:493–495.

Ganguli R, Brar JS, Chengappa KN, Yang ZW, Nimgaonkar VL, Rabin BS: Autoimmunity in schizophrenia: a review of recent findings. Ann Med 1993; 25:489–496.

Ganguli R, Brar JS, Chengappa KN, DeLeo M, Yang ZW, Shurin G, Rabin BS: Mitogen-stimulated interleukin-2 production in never-medicated, first-episode schizophrenic patients. The influence of age at onset and negative symptoms [see comments]. Arch Gen Psychiatry 1995; 52:668–672.

Ganguli R, Brar JS, Rabin BS: Immune abnormalities in schizophrenia: evidence for the autoimmune hypothesis. Harv Rev Psychiatry 1994a; 2:70–83.

Ganguli R, Yang Z, Shurin G, Chengappa KN, Brar JS, Gubbi AV, Rabin BS: Serum interleukin-6 concentration in schizophrenia: elevation associated with duration of illness. Psychiatry Res 1994b; 51:1–10.

Gaughran F, O'Neill E, Cole M, Collins K, Daly RJ, Shanahan F: Increased soluble interleukin 2 receptor levels in schizophrenia. Schizophr Res 1998; 29:263–267.

Geddes JR, Black RJ, Whalley LJ, Eagles JM: Persistence of the decline in the diagnosis of schizophrenia among first admissions to Scottish hospitals from 1969 to 1988 [see comments]. Br J Psychiatry 1993; 163:620–626.

Gejman PV, Ram A, Gelernter J, Friedman E, Cao Q, Pickar D, Blum K, Noble EP, Kranzler HR, O'Malley S, et al.: No structural mutation in the dopamine D_2 receptor gene in alcoholism or schizophrenia. Analysis using denaturing gradient gel electrophoresis. JAMA 1994; 271:204–208.

Gill M, Vallada H, Collier D, Sham P, Holmans P, Murray R, McGuffin P, Nanko S, Owen M, Antonarakis S, et al.: A combined analysis of D22S278 marker alleles in affected sib-pairs: support for a susceptibility locus for schizophrenia at chromosome 22q12. Schizophrenia Collaborative Linkage Group (Chromosome 22). Am J Med Genet 1996; 67:40–45.

Gogos JA, Morgan M, Luine V, Santha M, Ogawa S, Pfaff D, Karayiorgou M: Catechol-*O*-methyltransferase-deficient mice exhibit sexually dimorphic changes in catecholamine levels and behavior. Proc Natl Acad Sci USA 1998; 95:9991–9996.

Goldacre M, Shiwach R, Yeates D: Estimating incidence and prevalence of treated psychiatric disorders from routine statistics: the example of schizophrenia in Oxfordshire. J Epidemiol Community Health 1994; 48:318–322.

Goldin LR, DeLisi LE, Gershon ES: Relationship of HLA to schizophrenia in 10 nuclear families. Psychiatry Res 1987; 20:69–77.

Goldstein JM, Faraone SV, Chen WJ, Tolomiczencko GS, Tsuang MT: Sex differences in the familial transmission of schizophrenia. Br J Psychiatry 1990; 156:819–826.

Gothelf D, Frisch A, Munitz H, Rockah R, Aviram A, Mozes T, Birger M, Weizman A, Frydman M: Velocardiofacial manifestations and microdeletions in schizophrenic inpatients. Am J Med Genet 1997; 72:455–461.

Gothelf D, Frisch A, Munitz H, Rockah R, Laufer N, Mozes T, Hermesh H, Weizman A, Frydman M: Clinical characteristics of schizophrenia assoicated with velo-cardio-facial syndrome. Schizophr Res 1999; 35:105–112.

Gottesman I, Shields J: Schizophrenia and Genetics: A Twin Study Vantage Point. New York: Academic Press, 1972.

Gottesman I, Shields J, Hanson D: Schizophrenia: The Epigenetic Puzzle. New York: Cambridge University Press, 1982.

Green MF, Bracha HS, Satz P, Christenson CD: Preliminary evidence for an association between minor physical anomalies and second trimester neurodevelopment in schizophrenia. Psychiatry Res 1994; 53:119–127.

Griffon N, Sokoloff P, Diaz J, Levesque D, Sautel F, Schwartz JC, Simon P, Costentin J, Garrido F, Mann A, et al.: The dopamine D_3 receptor and schizophrenia: pharmacological, anatomical and genetic approaches. Eur Neuropsychopharmacol 1995; 5:3–9.

Gruzelier J, Raine A: Bilateral electrodermal activity and cerebral mechanisms in syndromes of schizophrenia and the schizotypal personality. Int J Psychophysiol 1994; 16:1–16.

Gur RE, Cowell P, Turetsky BI, Gallacher F, Cannon T, Bilker W, Gur RC: A follow-up magnetic resonance imaging study of schizophrenia. Relationship of neuroanatomical changes to clinical and neurobehavioral measures. Arch Gen Psychiatry 1998; 55:145–152.

Gur RE, Pearlson GD: Neuroimaging in schizophrenia research. Schizophr Bull 1993; 19:337–353.

Gurevich EV, Bordelon Y, Shapiro RM, Arnold SE, Gur RE, Joyce JN: Mesolimbic dopamine D_3 receptors and use of antipsychotics in patients with schizophrenia. A postmortem study. Arch Gen Psychiatry 1997; 54:225–232.

Gurling H, Kalsi G, Chih-Hui Chen A, Green M, Butler R, Read T, Murphy P, Curtis D, Sharma T, Hui-Sui Chen A, et al.: Schizophrenia susceptibility and chromosome 6p24–22 [letter; comment] [published erratum appears in Nat Genet 1996; 13:129]. Nat Genet 1995; 11:234–235.

Gurling HM, Kalsi G, Brynjolfson J, Sigmundsson T, Sherrington R, Mankoo BS, Read T, Murphy P, Blaveri E, McQuillin A, et al.: Genomewide genetic linkage analysis confirms the presence of susceptibility loci for schizophrenia, on chromosomes 1q32.2, 5q33.2, and 8p21–22 and provides support for linkage to schizophrenia, on chromosomes 11q23.3–24 and 20q12.1–11.23. Am J Hum Genet 2001; 68:661–673.

Guy CA, Bowen T, Williams N, Jones IR, McCandless F, McGuffin P, Owen MJ, Craddock N, O'Donovan MC: No association between a polymorphic CAG repeat in the human potassium channel gene *hKCa3* and bipolar disorder. Am J Med Genet 1999; 88:57–60.

Hafner H, an der Heiden W: Epidemiology of schizophrenia [see comments]. Can J Psychiatry 1997; 42:139–151.

Hafner H, an der Heiden W, Behrens S, Gattaz WF, Hambrecht M, Loffler W, Maurer K, Munk-Jorgensen P, Nowotny B, Riecher-Rossler A, et al.: Causes and consequences of the gender difference in age at onset of schizophrenia. Schizophr Bull 1998; 24:99–113.

Hafner H, Maurer K, Loffler W, Fatkenheuer B, an der Heiden W, Riecher-Rossler A, Behrens S, Gattaz WF: The epidemiology of early schizophrenia. Influence of age and gender on onset and early course. Br J Psychiatry Suppl 1994; 29–38.

Hafner H, Maurer K, Loffler W, Riecher-Rossler A: The influence of age and sex on the onset and early course of schizophrenia. Br J Psychiatry Suppl. 1993; 162:80–86.

Hakak Y, Walker JR, Li C, Wong WH, Davis KL, Buxbaum JD, Haroutunian V, Fienberg AA: Genome-wide expression analysis reveals dysregulation of myelination-related genes in chronic schizophrenia. Proc Natl Acad Sci USA 2001; 98:4746–4751.

Hambrecht M, Maurer K, Hafner H, Sartorius N: Transnational stability of gender differences in schizophrenia? An analysis based on the WHO study on determinants of outcome of severe mental disorders. Eur Arch Psychiatry Clin Neurosci 1992; 242:6–12.

Harrison PJ: Advances in post mortem molecular neurochemistry and neuropathology: examples from schizophrenia research. Br Med Bull 1996; 52:527–538.

Harrison PJ: The neuropathology of schizophrenia. A critical review of the data and their interpretation. Brain 1999; 122:593–624.

Heinrichs RW, Zakzanis KK: Neurocognitive deficit in schizophrenia: a quantitative review of the evidence. Neuropsychology 1998; 12:426–445.

Heresco-Levy U, Javitt DC: The role of *N*-methyl-D-aspartate (NMDA) receptor–mediated neurotransmission in the pathophysiology and therapeutics of psychiatric syndromes. Eur Neuropsychopharmacol 1998; 8:141–152.

Heston LL: Psychiatric disorders in foster home reared children of schizophrenic mothers. Br J Psychiatry 1966; 112:819–825.

Hettema JM, Walsh D, Kendler KS: Testing the effect of season of birth on familial risk for schizophrenia and related disorders. Br J Psychiatry 1996; 168:205–209.

Hirsch SR, Das I, Garey LJ, de Belleroche J: A pivotal role for glutamate in the pathogenesis of schizophrenia, and its cognitive dysfunction. Pharmacol Biochem Behav 1997; 56:797–802.

Hori H, Ohmori O, Shinkai T, Kojima H, Nakamura J: Association analysis between two functional dopamine D_2 receptor gene polymorphisms and schizophrenia. Am J Med Genet 2001; 105:176–178.

Hovatta I, Varilo T, Suvisaari J, Terwilliger JD, Ollikainen V, Arajarvi R, Juvonen H, Kokko-Sahin ML, Vaisanen L, Mannila H, et al.: A genomewide screen for schizophrenia genes in an isolated Finnish subpopulation, suggesting multiple susceptibility loci. Am J Hum Genet 1999; 65:1114–1124.

Hutchinson G, Takei N, Fahy TA, Bhugra D, Gilvarry C, Moran P, Mallett R, Sham P, Leff J, Murray RM: Morbid risk of schizophrenia in first-degree relatives of white and African-Caribbean patients with psychosis. Br J Psychiatry 1996; 169:776–780.

Hwu HG, Hong CJ, Lee YL, Lee PC, Lee SF: Dopamine D_4 receptor gene polymorphisms and neuroleptic response in schizophrenia. Biol Psychiatry 1998; 44:483–487.

Hyde TM, Weinberger DR: Seizures and schizophrenia. Schizophr Bull 1997; 23:611–622.

Illowsky B, Juliano D, Bigelow L, Weinberger D: Stability of CT scan findings in schizophrenia: results of an 8 year follow-up study. J Neurol Neurosurg Psychiatry 1988; 51:209–213.

Inayama Y, Yoneda H, Sakai T, Ishida T, Nonomura Y, Kono Y, Takahata R, Koh J, Sakai J, Takai A, et al.: Positive association between a DNA sequence variant in the serotonin 2A receptor gene and schizophrenia. Am J Med Genet 1996; 67:103–105.

Ishida T, Yoneda H, Sakai T, Nonomura Y, Inayama Y, Kono Y, Kobayashi S: Pseudoautosomal region in schizophrenia: sex concordance of the affected sibpairs and the association study with DNA markers. Am J Med Genet 1993; 48:151–155.

Ishiguro H, Okuyama Y, Toru M, Arinami T: Mutation and association analysis of the 5′ region of the dopamine D_3 receptor gene in schizophrenia patients: identification of the $Ala^{38}Thr$ polymorphism and suggested association between *DRD3* haplotypes and schizophrenia. Mol Psychiatry 2000; 5:433–438.

Itokawa M, Arinami T, Futamura N, Hamaguchi H, Toru M: A structural polymorphism of human dopamine D_2 receptor, $D_2(Ser^{311} \rightarrow Cys)$. Biochem Biophys Res Commun 1993; 196:1369–1375.

Ivanyi D, Zemek P, Ivanyi P: HLA antigens in schizophrenia. Tissue Antigens 1976; 8:217–220.

Ivanyi D, Zemek P, Ivanyi P: HLA antigens as possible markers of heterogeneity in schizophrenia. J Immunogenet 1978; 5:165–172.

Iwata Y, Takahashi K, Peng X, Fukuda K, Ohno K, Ogawa T, Gonda K, Mori N, Niwa S, Shigeta S: Detection and sequence analysis of Borna disease virus p24 RNA from peripheral blood mononuclear cells of patients with mood disorders or schizophrenia and of blood donors. J Virol 1998; 72:10044–10049.

Jablensky A, Eaton WW: Schizophrenia. Baillieres Clin Psychiatry Int Pract Res 1995; 1:283–307.

Jablensky A, Sartorius N, Ernberg G, Anker M, Korten A, Cooper JE, Day R, Bertelsen A: Schizophrenia: manifestations, incidence and course in different cultures. A World Health Organization ten-country study [published erratum appears in Psychol Med Monogr Suppl 1992; 22:1092]. Psychol Med Monogr Suppl 1992; 20:1–97.

Jakob H, Beckmann H: Prenatal developmental disturbances in the limbic allocortex in schizophrenics. J Neural Transm 1986; 65:303–326.

Jaskiw GE, Juliano DM, Goldberg TE, Hertzman M, Urow-Hamell E, Weinberger DR: Cerebral ventricular enlargement in schizophreniform disorder does not progress. A seven year follow-up study. Schizophr Res 1994; 14:23–28.

Jones P: The early origins of schizophrenia. Br Med Bull 1997; 53:135–155.

Jones PB, Rantakallio P, Hartikainen AL, Isohanni M, Sipila P: Schizophrenia as a long-term outcome of pregnancy, delivery, and perinatal complications: a 28-year follow-up of the 1966 north Finland general population birth cohort. Am J Psychiatry 1998; 155:355–364.

Jonsson EG, Dahl ML, Roh HK, Jerling M, Sedvall GC: Lack of association between debrisoquine 4-hydroxylase (*CYP2D6*) gene polymorphisms and schizophrenia. Psychiatr Genet 1998a; 8:25–28.

Jonsson EG, Geijer T, Gyllander A, Terenius L, Sedvall GC: Failure to replicate an association between a rare allele of a tyrosine hydroxylase gene microsatellite and schizophrenia. Eur Arch Psychiatry Clin Neurosci 1998b; 248:61–63.

Jonsson E, Brene S, Zhang XR, Nimgaonkar VL, Tylec A, Schalling M, Sedvall G: Schizophrenia and neurotrophin-3 alleles. Acta Psychiatr Scand 1997; 95:414–419.

Joyce JN, Meador-Woodruff JH: Linking the family of D_2 receptors to neuronal circuits in human brain: insights into schizophrenia. Neuropsychopharmacology 1997; 16:375–384.

Kalsi G, Curtis D, Brynjolfsson J, Butler R, Sharma T, Murphy P, Read T, Petursson H, Gurling HM: Investigation by linkage analysis of the XY pseudoautosomal region in the genetic susceptibility to schizophrenia. Br J Psychiatry 1995; 167:390–393.

Kalsi G, Sherrington R, Mankoo BS, Brynjolfsson J, Sigmundsson T, Curtis D, Read T, Murphy P, Butler R, Petursson H, et al.: Linkage study of the D_5 dopamine receptor gene (*DRD5*) in multiplex Icelandic and English schizophrenia pedigrees. Am J Psychiatry 1996; 153:107–109.

Kapitany T, Meszaros K, Lenzinger E, Schindler SD, Barnas C, Fuchs K, Sieghart W, Aschauer HN, Kasper S: Genetic polymorphisms for drug metabolism (*CYP2D6*) and tardive dyskinesia in schizophrenia. Schizophr Res 1998; 32:101–106.

Kapur S, Remington G: Serotonin–dopamine interaction and its relevance to schizophrenia. Am J Psychiatry 1996; 153:466–476.

Karayiorgou M, Gogos JA, Galke BL, Wolyniec PS, Nestadt G, Antonarakis SE, Kazazian HH, Housman DE, Pulver AE: Identification of sequence variants and analysis of the role of the catechol-*O*-methyl-transferase gene in schizophrenia susceptibility. Biol Psychiatry 1998; 43:425–431.

Karayiorgou M, Morris MA, Morrow B, Shprintzen RJ, Goldberg R, Borrow J, Gos A, Nestadt G, Wolyniec PS, Lasseter VK, et al.: Schizophrenia susceptibility associated with interstitial deletions of chromosome 22q11. Proc Natl Acad Sci USA 1995; 92:7612–7616.

Karlsson H, Bachmann S, Schroder J, McArthur J, Torrey EF, Yolken RH: Retroviral RNA identified in the cerebrospinal fluids and brains of individuals with schizophrenia. Proc Natl Acad Sci USA 2001; 98:4634–4639.

Kato MV, Shimizu T, Nagayoshi M, Kaneko A, Sasaki MS, Ikawa Y: Genomic imprinting of the human serotonin-receptor (*HTR2*) gene involved in development of retinoblastoma. Am J Hum Genet 1996; 59:1084–1090.

Kaufmann CA, DeLisi LE, Lehner T, Gilliam TC: Physical mapping, linkage analysis of a putative schizophrenia locus on chromosome 5q. Schizophr Bull 1989; 15:441–452.

Kaufmann CA, Suarez B, Malaspina D, Pepple J, Svrakic D, Markel PD, Meyer J, Zambuto CT, Schmitt K, Matise TC, et al.: NIMH Genetics Initiative Millenium Schizophrenia Consortium: linkage analysis of African-American pedigrees. Am J Med Genet 1998; 81:282–289.

Kemali D, Maj M, Galderisi S, Milici N, Salvati A: Ventricle-to-brain ratio in schizophrenia: a controlled follow-up study. Biol Psychiatry 1989; 26:756–759.

Kendell RE, Juszczak E, Cole SK: Obstetric complications and schizophrenia: a case control study based on standardised obstetric records [see comments]. Br J Psychiatry 1996; 168:556–561.

Kendler KS, Gallagher TJ, Abelson JM, Kessler RC: Lifetime prevalence, demographic risk factors, and diagnostic validity of nonaffective psychosis as assessed in a US community sample. The National Comorbidity Survey. Arch Gen Psychiatry 1996a; 53:1022–1031.

Kendler KS, Gruenberg AM, Tsuang MT: Subtype stability in schizophrenia. Am J Psychiatry 1985; 142:827–832.

Kendler KS, MacLean CJ: Estimating familial effects on age at onset and liability to schizophrenia. I. Results of a large sample family study. Genet Epidemiol 1990; 7:409–417.

Kendler KS, MacLean CJ, O'Neill FA, Burke J, Murphy B, Duke F, Shinkwin R, Easter SM, Webb BT, Zhang J, et al.: Evidence for a schizophrenia vulnerability locus on chromosome 8p in the Irish Study of High-Density Schizophrenia Families. Am J Psychiatry 1996b; 153:1534–1540.

Kendler KS, McGuire M, Gruenberg AM, O'Hare A, Spellman M, Walsh D: The Roscommon Family Study. I. Methods, diagnosis of probands, and risk of schizophrenia in relatives [see comments]. Arch Gen Psychiatry 1993a; 50:527–540.

Kendler KS, McGuire M, Gruenberg AM, O'Hare A, Spellman M, Walsh D: The Roscommon Family Study. III. Schizophrenia-related personality disorders in relatives. Arch Gen Psychiatry 1993b; 50:781–788.

Kendler KS, Myers JM, O'Neill FA, Martin R, Murphy B, MacLean CJ, Walsh D, Straub RE: Clinical features of schizophrenia and linkage to chromosomes 5q, 6p, 8p, and 10p in the Irish Study of High-Density Schizophrenia Families. Am J Psychiatry 2000; 157:402–408.

Kendler KS, Robinette CD: Schizophrenia in the National Academy of Sciences–National Research Council Twin Registry: a 16-year update. Am J Psychiatry 1983; 140:1551–1563.

Kendler KS, Tsuang MT, Hays P: Age at onset in schizophrenia. A familial perspective. Arch Gen Psychiatry 1987; 44:881–890.

Kennedy JL, Giuffra LA, Moises HW, Cavalli-Sforza LL, Pakstis AJ, Kidd JR, Castiglione CM, Sjogren B, Wetterberg L, Kidd KK: Evidence against linkage of schizophrenia to markers on chromosome 5 in a northern Swedish pedigree. Nature 1988; 336:167–170.

Kety S, Rosenthal D, Wender P, Schulsinger F: The types and prevalence of mental illness in the biological and adoptive families of adopted schizophrenics. In: Rosenthal D, Kety S (eds). The Transmission of Schizophrenia. Oxford: Pergamon, 1968:345–362.

Kety S, Rosenthal D, Wender P, Schulsinger F, Jacobsen B: The biological and adoptive families of adopted individuals who become schizophrenic: prevalence of mental illness and other characteristics. In: Wynne L, Cromwell R, Matthysse S (eds). The Nature of Schizophrenia: New Approaches to Research and Treatment. New York: Wiley, 1978:25–37.

Kim JS, Kornhuber HH, Schmid-Burgk W, Holzmuller B: Low cerebrospinal fluid glutamate in schizophrenic patients and a new hypothesis on schizophrenia. Neurosci Lett 1980; 20:379–382.

Kinney DK, Levy DL, Yurgelun-Todd DA, Lajonchere CM, Holzman PS: Eye-tracking dysfunction and birth-month weather in schizophrenia. J Abnorm Psychol 1999; 108:359–362.

Kirch DG: Infection and autoimmunity as etiologic factors in schizophrenia: a review and reappraisal. Schizophr Bull 1993; 19:355–370.

Kirkpatrick B, Ram R, Amador XF, Buchanan RW, McGlashan T, Tohen M, Bromet E: Summer birth and the deficit syndrome of schizophrenia. Am J Psychiatry 1998; 155:1221–1226.

Kitamura N, Nishino N, Hashimoto T, Kajimoto Y, Shirai Y, Murakami N, Yang CQ, Lin XH, Yamamoto H, Nakai T, et al.: Asymmetrical changes in the fodrin alpha subunit in the superior temporal cortices in schizophrenia. Biol Psychiatry 1998; 43:254–262.

Kojima H, Ohmori O, Shinkai T, Terao T, Suzuki T, Abe K: Dopamine D_1 receptor gene polymorphism and schizophrenia in Japan. Am J Med Genet 1999; 88:116–119.

Kraepelin E, Barclay RM, Robertson GM: Dementia Praecox and Paraphrenia. Edinburgh: Livingstone, 1919.

Kremen WS, Seidman LJ, Pepple JR, Lyons MJ, Tsuang MT, Faraone SV: Neuropsychological risk indicators for schizophrenia: a review of family studies. Schizophr Bull 1994; 20:103–119.

Kringlen E: Twins—still our best method. Schizophr Bull 1976; 2:429–433.

Kunugi H, Kawada Y, Hattori M, Ueki A, Otsuka M, Nanko S: Association study of structural mutations of the tyrosine hydroxylase gene with schizophrenia and Parkinson's disease. Am J Med Genet 1998; 81:131–133.

Kunugi H, Vallada HP, Sham PC, Hoda F, Arranz MJ, Li T, Nanko S, Murray RM, McGuffin P, Owen M, et al.: Catechol-*O*-methyltransferase polymorphisms and schizophrenia: a transmission disequilibrium study in multiply affected families. Psychiatr Genet 1997; 7:97–101.

Lachman HM, Nolan KA, Mohr P, Saito T, Volavka J: Association between catechol *O*-methyltransferase genotype and violence in schizophrenia and schizoaffective disorder. Am J Psychiatry 1998; 155:835–837.

Lachman HM, Papolos DF, Saito T, Yu YM, Szumlanski CL, Weinshilboum RM: Human catechol-*O*-methyltransferase pharmacogenetics: description of a functional polymorphism and its potential application to neuropsychiatric disorders. Pharmacogenetics 1996; 6:243–250.

Laruelle M: Imaging dopamine transmission in schizophrenia. A review and meta-analysis. Q J Nucl Med 1998; 42:211–221.

Lauerma H, Lehtinen V, Joukamaa M, Jarvelin MR, Helenius H, Isohanni M: Schizophrenia among patients treated for rheumatoid arthritis and appendicitis. Schizophr Res 1998; 29:255–261.

Laurent C, Thibaut F, Ravassard P, Campion D, Samolyk D, Lafargue C, Petit M, Martinez M, Mallet J: Detection of two new polymorphic sites in the human interleukin-1beta gene: lack of association with schizophrenia in a French population. Psychiatr Genet 1997; 7:103–105.

Lawrie SM, Abukmeil SS: Brain abnormality in schizophrenia. A systematic and quantitative review of volumetric magnetic resonance imaging studies [see comments]. Br J Psychiatry 1998; 172:110–120.

Lawrie SM, Whalley H, Kestelman JN, Abukmeil SS, Byrne M, Hodges A, Rimmington JE, Best JJ, Owens DG, Johnstone EC: Magnetic resonance imaging of brain in people at high risk of developing schizophrenia [see comments]. Lancet 1999; 353:30–33.

Lesch KP, Stober G, Balling U, Franzek E, Li SH, Ross CA, Newman M, Beckmann H, Riederer P: Triplet repeats in clinical subtypes of schizophrenia: variation at the DRPLA (B 37 CAG repeat) locus is not associated with periodic catatonia. J Neural Transm Gen Sect 1994; 98:153–157.

Levinson DF, Holmans P, Straub RE, Owen MJ, Wildenauer DB, Gejman PV, Pulver AE, Laurent C, Kendler KS, Walsh D, et al.: Multicenter linkage study of schizophrenia candidate regions on chromosomes 5q, 6q, 10p, and 13q: Schizophrenia Linkage Collaborative Group III. Am J Hum Genet 2000; 67:652–663.

Levinson DF, Mahtani MM, Nancarrow DJ, Brown DM, Kruglyak L, Kirby A, Hayward NK, Crowe RR, Andreasen NC, Black DW, et al.: Genome scan of schizophrenia. Am J Psychiatry 1998; 155:741–750.

Levy DL, Holzman PS, Matthysse S, Mendell NR: Eye tracking and schizophrenia: a selective review. Schizophr Bull 1994; 20:47–62.

Lewis DA: Development of the prefrontal cortex during adolescence: insights into vulnerable neural circuits in schizophrenia. Neuropsychopharmacology 1997; 16:385–398.

Lewis DA: Chandelier cells: shedding light on altered cortical circuitry in schizophrenia. Mol Psychiatry 1998; 3:466–471.

Li T, Arranz M, Aitchison KJ, Bryant C, Liu X, Kerwin RW, Murray R, Sham P, Collier DA: Case-control, haplotype relative risk and transmission disequilibrium analysis of a dopamine D_2 receptor functional promoter polymorphism in schizophrenia. Schizophr Res 1998a; 32:87–92.

Li T, Ball D, Zhao J, Murray RM, Liu X, Sham PC, Collier DA: Family-based linkage disequilibrium mapping using SNP marker haplotypes: application to a potential locus for schizophrenia at chromosome 22q11. Mol Psychiatry 2000; 5:77–84.

Li T, Sham PC, Vallada H, Xie T, Tang X, Murray RM, Liu X, Collier DA: Preferential transmission of the high activity allele of *COMT* in schizophrenia. Psychiatr Genet 1996; 6:131–133.

Li T, Vallada HP, Liu X, Xie T, Tang X, Zhao J, O'Donovan MC, Murray RM, Sham PC, Collier DA: Analysis of CAG/CTG repeat size in Chinese subjects with schizophrenia and bipolar affective disorder using the repeat expansion detection method. Biol Psychiatry 1998b; 44:1160–1165.

Liddle PF: Functional imaging—schizophrenia. Br Med Bull 1996; 52:486–494.

Lieberman JA, Yunis J, Egea E, Canoso RT, Kane JM, Yunis EJ: *HLA-B38, DR4, DQw3* and clozapine-induced agranulocytosis in Jewish patients with schizophrenia. Arch Gen Psychiatry 1990; 47:945–948.

Lim K, Sullivan E, Zipursky R, Pfefferbaum A: Cortical gray matter volume deficits in schizophrenia: a replication. Schizophr Res 1996; 20:157–164.

Lin MW, Curtis D, Williams N, Arranz M, Nanko S, Collier D, McGuffin P, Murray R, Owen M, Gill M, et al.: (1995) Suggestive evidence for linkage of schizophrenia to markers on chromosome 13q14.1–q32 [published erratum appears in Psychiatr Genet 1996; 6:37]. Psychiatr Genet 1995; 5:117–126.

Lin MW, Sham P, Hwu HG, Collier D, Murray R, Powell JF: Suggestive evidence for linkage of schizophrenia to markers on chromosome 13 in Caucasian but not Oriental populations. Hum Genet 1997; 99:417–420.

Lindholm E, Ekholm B, Shaw S, Jalonen P, Johansson G, Pettersson U, Sherrington R, Adolfsson R, Jazin E: A schizophrenia-susceptibility locus at 6q25, in one of the world's largest reported pedigrees. Am J Hum Genet 2001; 69:96–105.

Lindsay EA, Morris MA, Gos A, Nestadt G, Wolyniec PS, Lasseter VK, Shprintzen R, Antonarakis SE, Baldini A, Pulver AE: Schizophrenia and chromosomal deletions within 22q11.2 [letter]. Am J Hum Genet 1995; 56:1502–1503.

Lipton RB, Levy DL, Holzman PS, Levin S: Eye movement dysfunctions in psychiatric patients: a review. Schizophr Bull 1983; 9:13–32.

Liu Q, Sobell JL, Heston LL, Sommer SS: Screening the dopamine D_1 receptor gene in 131 schizophrenics and eight alcoholics: identification of polymorphisms but lack of functionally significant sequence changes. Am J Med Genet 1995; 60:165–171.

Lotta T, Vidgren J, Tilgmann C, Ulmanen I, Melen K, Julkunen I, Taskinen J: Kinetics of human soluble and membrane-bound catechol *O*-methyltransferase: a revised mechanism and description of the thermolabile variant of the enzyme. Biochemistry 1995; 34:4202–4210.

Luchins D, Torrey EF, Weinberger DR, Zalcman S, Delisi L, Johnson A, Rogentine N, Wyatt RJ: HLA antigens in schizophrenia: differences between patients with and without evidence of brain atrophy. Br J Psychiatry 1980; 136:243–248.

Luchins DJ, Weinberger DR, Torrey EF, Johnson A, Rogentine N, Wyatt RJ: *HLA-A2* antigen in schizophrenic patients with reversed cerebral asymmetry. Br J Psychiatry 1981; 138:240–243.

MacAvoy MG, Bruce CJ: Comparison of the smooth eye tracking disorder of schizophrenics with that of nonhuman primates with specific brain lesions. Int J Neurosci 1995; 80:117–151.

Maclean CJ, Neale MC, Meyer JM, Kendler KS: Estimating familial effects on age at onset and liability to schizophrenia II. Adjustment for censored data. Genet Epidemiol 1990; 7:419–426.

Maier W, Schmidt F, Schwab SG, Hallmayer J, Minges J, Ackenheil M, Lichtermann D, Wildenauer DB: Lack of linkage between schizophrenia and markers at the telomeric end of the pseudoautosomal region of the sex chromosomes. Biol Psychiatry 1995; 37:344–347.

Malaspina D, Harlap S, Fennig S, Heiman D, Nahon D, Feldman D, Susser ES: Advancing paternal age and the risk of schizophrenia. Arch Gen Psychiatry 2001; 58:361–367.

Martinez M, Goldin LR, Cao Q, Zhang J, Sanders AR, Nancarrow DJ, Taylor JM, Levinson DF, Kirby A, Crowe RR, et al.: Follow-up study on a susceptibility locus for schizophrenia on chromosome 6q. Am J Med Genet 1999; 88:337–343.

Mathalon D, Sullivan E, Lim K, Pfefferbaum A: Longitudinal analysis of MRI brain volumes in schizophrenia. Schizophr Res 1997; 24:152.

McGrath J, Castle D: Does influenza cause schizophrenia? A five year review. Aust N Z J Psychiatry 1995; 29:23–31.

McGuffin P: Is schizophrenia an HLA-associated disease? Psychol Med 9:721–728.

McGuffin P, Festenstein H, Murray R: A family study of HLA antigens and other genetic markers in schizophrenia. Psychol Med 1983; 13:31–43.

McGuffin P, Sturt E: Genetic markers in schizophrenia. Hum Hered 1986; 36:65–88.

McGuire PK, Quested DJ, Spence SA, Murray RM, Frith CD, Liddle PF: Pathophysiology of "positive" thought disorder in schizophrenia. Br J Psychiatry 1998; 173:231–235.

McGuire PK, Shah GM, Murray RM: Increased blood flow in Broca's area during auditory hallucinations in schizophrenia [see comments]. Lancet 1993; 342:703–706.

Melmer G, Sherrington R, Mankoo B, Kalsi G, Curtis D, Gurling HM: A cosmid clone for the $5HT_{1A}$ receptor (HTR_{1A}) reveals a TaqI RFLP that shows tight linkage to DNA loci D5S6, D5S39, and D5S76. Genomics 1991; 11:767–769.

Meloni R, Laurent C, Campion D, Ben Hadjali B, Thibaut F, Dollfus S, Petit M, Samolyk D, Martinez M, Poirier MF, et al.: A rare allele of a microsatellite located in the tyrosine hydroxylase gene found in schizophrenic patients. C R Acad Sci III 1995; 318:803–809.

Meltzer HY: Pre-clinical pharmacology of atypical antipsychotic drugs: a selective review. Br J Psychiatry Suppl 1996; 23–31.

Mendez MF, Grau R, Doss RC, Taylor JL: Schizophrenia in epilepsy: seizure and psychosis variables [see comments]. Neurology 1993; 43:1073–1077.

Mesulam M: Principles of Behavioral Neurology. Philadelphia: F A Davis, 1985.

Meszaros K, Lenzinger E, Fureder T, Hornik K, Willinger U, Stompe T, Heiden AM, Resinger E, Fathi N, Gerhard E, et al.: Schizophrenia and the dopamine-beta-hydroxylase gene: results of a linkage and association study. Psychiatr Genet 1996; 6:17–22.

Meyer J, Huberth A, Ortega G, Syagailo YV, Jatzke S, Mossner R, Strom TM, Ulzheimer-Teuber I, Stober G, Schmitt A, et al.: A missense mutation in a novel

gene encoding a putative cation channel is associated with catatonic schizophrenia in a large pedigree. Mol Psychiatry 2001; 6:302–306.
Millar JK, Wilson-Annan JC, Anderson S, Christie S, Taylor MS, Semple CA, Devon RS, Clair DM, Muir WJ, Blackwood DH, et al.: Disruption of two novel genes by a translocation co-segregating with schizophrenia. Hum Mol Genet 2000; 9:1415–1423.
Moghaddam B, Bolinao ML: Glutamatergic antagonists attenuate ability of dopamine uptake blockers to increase extracellular levels of dopamine: implications for tonic influence of glutamate on dopamine release. Synapse 1994; 18:337–342.
Moises HW, Yang L, Kristbjarnarson H, Wiese C, Byerley W, Macciardi F, Arolt V, Blackwood D, Liu X, Sjogren B, et al.: An international two-stage genome-wide search for schizophrenia susceptibility genes. Nat Genet 1995; 11:321–324.
Morris AG, Gaitonde E, McKenna PJ, Mollon JD, Hunt DM: CAG repeat expansions and schizophrenia: association with disease in females and with early age-at-onset. Hum Mol Genet 1995; 4:1957–1961.
Morris-Rosendahl DJ, Burgert E, Uyanik G, Mayerova A, Duval F, Macher JP, Crocq MA: Analysis of the CAG repeats in the *SCA1* and *B37* genes in schizophrenic and bipolar I disorder patients: tentative association between *B37* and schizophrenia. Am J Med Genet 1997; 74:324–330.
Mortensen PB, Pedersen CB, Westergaard T, Wohlfahrt J, Ewald H, Mors O, Andersen PK, Melbye M: Effects of family history and place and season of birth on the risk of schizophrenia [see comments]. N Engl J Med 1999; 340:603–608.
Mowry BJ, Nancarrow DJ, Lennon DP, Sandkuijl LA, Crowe RR, Silverman JM, Mohs RC, Siever LJ, Endicott J, Sharpe L, et al.: Schizophrenia susceptibility and chromosome 6p24–22 [see comments]. Nat Genet 1995; 11:233–234.
Muck-Seler D, Pivac N, Jakovljevic M: Sex differences, season of birth and platelet 5-HT levels in schizophrenic patients. J Neural Transm 1999; 106:337–347.
Muir WJ, Thomson ML, McKeon P, Mynett-Johnson L, Whitton C, Evans KL, Porteous DJ, Blackwood DH: Markers close to the dopamine D_5 receptor gene (*DRD5*) show significant association with schizophrenia but not bipolar disorder. Am J Med Genet 2001; 105:152–158.
Muller N, Ackenheil M: Psychoneuroimmunology and the cytokine action in the CNS: implications for psychiatric disorders. Prog Neuropsychopharmacol Biol Psychiatry 1998; 22:1–33.
Munk-Jorgensen P, Mortensen PB: Is schizophrenia really on the decrease? Eur Arch Psychiatry Clin Neurosci 1993; 242:244–247.
Nakamura M, Inoue A, Hemmi H, Suzuki J: Positive associations between dopamine D_4 receptor polymorphism and schizophrenia. A study on two schizophrenic groups with genetic loading and unloading. Proc Jpn Acad 1995; 71:241–243.
Nanko S, Hattori M, Kuwata S, Sasaki T, Fukuda R, Dai XY, Yamaguchi K, Shibata Y, Kazamatsuri H: Neurotrophin-3 gene polymorphism associated with schizophrenia. Acta Psychiatr Scand 1994; 89:390–392.
Neves-Pereira M, Bassett AS, Honer WG, Lang D, King NA, Kennedy JL: No evidence for linkage of the *CHRNA7* gene region in Canadian schizophrenia families. Am J Med Genet 1998; 81:361–363.
Nimgaonkar VL, Ganguli R, Rudert WA, Vavassori C, Rabin BS, Trucco M: A negative association of schizophrenia with an allele of the *HLA DQB1* gene among African-Americans. Schizophr Res 1993; 8:199–209.
Nimgaonkar VL, Rudert WA, Zhang X, Trucco M, Ganguli R: Negative association of schizophrenia with *HLA DQB1*0602*: evidence from a second African-American cohort. Schizophr Res 1997; 23:81–86.
Nimgaonkar VL, Rudert WA, Zhang XR, Tsoi WF, Trucco M, Saha N: Further evidence for an association between schizophrenia and the *HLA DQB1* gene locus. Schizophr Res 1995a; 18:43–49.
Nimgaonkar VL, Yang ZW, Zhang XR, Brar JS, Chakravarti A, Ganguli R: Association study of schizophrenia and the IL-2 receptor beta chain gene. Am J Med Genet 1995b; 60:448–451.
Noga JT, Bartley AJ, Jones DW, Torrey EF, Weinberger DR: Cortical gyral anatomy and gross brain dimensions in monozygotic twins discordant for schizophrenia. Schizophr Res 1996; 22:27–40.
Norris JG, Benveniste EN: Interleukin-6 production by astrocytes: induction by the neurotransmitter norepinephrine. J Neuroimmunol 1993; 45:137–145.
O'Callaghan E, Cotter D, Colgan K, Larkin C, Walsh D, Waddington JL: Confinement of winter birth excess in schizophrenia to the urban-born and its gender specificity. Br J Psychiatry 1995; 166:51–54.
O'Callaghan E, Gibson T, Colohan HA, Walshe D, Buckley P, Larkin C, Waddington JL: Season of birth in schizophrenia. Evidence for confinement of an excess of winter births to patients without a family history of mental disorder [see comments]. Br J Psychiatry 1991; 158:764–769.
O'Donovan MC, Guy C, Craddock N, Murphy KC, Cardno AG, Jones LA, Owen MJ, McGuffin P: Expanded CAG repeats in schizophrenia and bipolar disorder [letter]. Nat Genet 1995; 10:380–381.
Ohlund LS, Ohman A, Ost LG, Lindstrom LH, Wieselgren IM: Electrodermal orienting response, maternal age, and season of birth in schizophrenia. Psychiatry Res 1991; 36:223–232.
Ohmori O, Shinkai T, Kojima H, Terao T, Suzuki T, Mita T, Abe K: Association study of a functional catechol-O-methyltransferase gene polymorphism in Japanese schizophrenics. Neurosci Lett 1998; 243:109–112.
Okubo Y, Suhara T, Suzuki K, Kobayashi K, Inoue O, Terasaki O, Someya Y, Sassa T, Sudo Y, Matsushima E, et al.: Decreased prefrontal dopamine D_1 receptors in schizophrenia revealed by PET [see comments]. Nature 1997; 385:634–636.
Owen MJ, Holmans P, McGuffin P: Association studies in psychiatric genetics. Mol Psychiatry 1997; 2:270–273.
Pariseau C, Gregor P, Myles-Worsley M, Holik J, Hoff M, Waldo M, Freedman R, Coon H, Byerley W: Schizophrenia and glutamate receptor genes. Psychiatr Genet 1994; 4:161–165.
Parsian A, Suarez BK, Isenberg K, Hampe CL, Fisher L, Chakraverty S, Meszaros K, Lenzinger E, Willinger U, Fuchs K, et al.: No evidence for a schizophrenia susceptibility gene in the vicinity of *IL2RB* on chromosome 22. Am J Med Genet 1997; 74:361–364.
Pearlson GD, Breiter SN, Aylward EH, Warren AC, Grygorcewicz M, Frangou S, Barta PE, Pulsifer MB: MRI brain changes in subjects with Down syndrome with and without dementia. Dev Med Child Neurol 1998; 40:326–334.
Pearlson GD, Harris GJ, Powers RE, Barta PE, Camargo EE, Chase GA, Noga JT, Tune LE: Quantitative changes in mesial temporal volume, regional cerebral blood flow, and cognition in Alzheimer's disease. Arch Gen Psychiatry 1992; 49:402–408.
Pearlson GD, Marsh L: MRI in psychiatry. In: Oldham JM, Riba MB, Tasman A (eds). American Psychiatric Association Annual Review, Vol 12. Washington DC: American Psychiatric Press, 1993:347–382.
Pearlson GD, Petty RG, Ross CA, Tien AY: Schizophrenia: a disease of heteromodal association cortex? Neuropsychopharmacology 1996; 14:1–17.
Petronis A, Bassett AS, Honer WG, Vincent JB, Tatuch Y, Sasaki T, Ying DJ, Klempan TA, Kennedy JL: Search for unstable DNA in schizophrenia families with evidence for genetic anticipation. Am J Hum Genet 1996; 59:905–911.
Petty RG, Barta PE, Pearlson GD, McGilchrist IK, Lewis RW, Tien AY, Pulver A, Vaughn DD, Casanova MF, Powers RE: Reversal of asymmetry of the planum temporale in schizophrenia. Am J Psychiatry 1995; 152:715–721.
Pizzuti A, Novelli G, Ratti A, Amati F, Mari A, Calabrese G, Nicolis S, Silani V, Marino B, Scarlato G, et al.: *UFD1L*, a developmentally expressed ubiquitination gene, is deleted in CATCH 22 syndrome. Hum Mol Genet 1997; 6:259–265.
Propping P: Genetic disorders presenting as "schizophrenia." Karl Bonhoeffer's early view of the psychoses in the light of medical genetics. Hum Genet 1983; 65:1–10.
Pujana MA, Martorell L, Volpini V, Valero J, Labad A, Vilella E, Estivill X: Analysis of amino-acid and nucleotide variants in the spinocerebellar ataxia type 1 (*SCA1*) gene in schizophrenic patients. Hum Genet 1997; 99:772–775.
Pulver AE, Brown CH, Wolyniec P, McGrath J, Tam D, Adler L, Carpenter WT, Childs B: Schizophrenia: age at onset, gender and familial risk. Acta Psychiatr Scand 1990; 82:344–351.
Pulver AE, Carpenter WT Jr: Lifetime psychotic symptoms assessed with the DIS. Schizophr Bull 1983; 9:377–382.
Pulver AE, Karayiorgou M, Lasseter VK, Wolyniec P, Kasch L, Antonarakis S, Housman D, Kazazian HH, Meyers D, Nestadt G, et al.: Follow-up of a report of a potential linkage for schizophrenia on chromosome 22q12–q13.1: part 2. Am J Med Genet 1994a; 54:44–50.
Pulver AE, Karayiorgou M, Wolyniec PS, Lasseter VK, Kasch L, Nestadt G, Antonarakis S, Housman D, Kazazian HH, Meyers D, et al.: Sequential strategy to identify a susceptibility gene for schizophrenia: report of potential linkage on chromosome 22q12–q13.1: part 1. Am J Med Genet 1994b; 54:36–43.
Pulver AE, Liang KY, Brown CH, Wolyniec P, McGrath J, Adler L, Tam D, Carpenter WT, Childs B: Risk factors in schizophrenia. Season of birth, gender, and familial risk [see comments]. Br J Psychiatry 1992a; 160:65–71.
Pulver AE, Liang KY, Wolyniec PS, McGrath J, Melton BA, Adler L, Childs B: Season of birth of siblings of schizophrenic patients [see comments]. Br J Psychiatry 1992b; 160:71–75.
Pulver AE, Mulle J, Nestadt G, Swartz KL, Blouin JL, Dombroski B, Liang KY, Housman DE, Kazazian HH, Antonarakis SE, et al.: Genetic heterogeneity in schizophrenia: stratification of genome scan data using co-segregating related phenotypes. Mol Psychiatry 2000; 5:650–653.
Pulver AE, Nestadt G, Goldberg R, Shprintzen RJ, Lamacz M, Wolyniec PS, Morrow B, Karayiorgou M, Antonarakis SE, Housman D, et al.: Psychotic illness in patients diagnosed with velo-cardio-facial syndrome and their relatives. J Nerv Ment Dis 1994c; 182:476–478.
Purohit DP, Davidson M, Perl DP, Powchik P, Haroutunian VH, Bierer LM, McCrystal J, Losonczy M, Davis KL: Severe cognitive impairment in elderly schizophrenic patients: a clinicopathological study. Biol Psychiatry 1993; 33:255–260.
Rabins PV: Schizophrenia and psychotic states. In: Birren JE, Sloane RB, Cohen GD (eds). Handbook of Mental Health and Aging. San Diego: Academic Press, 1992:463–475.
Rajkowska G, Selemon LD, Goldman-Rakic PS: Neuronal and glial somal size in the prefrontal cortex: a postmortem morphometric study of schizophrenia and Huntington disease. Arch Gen Psychiatry 1998; 55:215–224.
Rantakallio P, Jones P, Moring J, Von Wendt L: Association between central nervous system infections during childhood and adult onset schizophrenia and other psychoses: a 28-year follow-up. Int J Epidemiol 1997; 26:837–843.
Rapaport MH, McAllister CG, Kim YS, Han JH, Pickar D, Nelson DL, Kirch DG, Paul SM: Increased serum soluble interleukin-2 receptors in Caucasian and Korean schizophrenic patients. Biol Psychiatry 1994; 35:767–771.
Rapaport MH, Torrey EF, McAllister CG, Nelson DL, Pickar D, Paul SM: Increased serum soluble interleukin-2 receptors in schizophrenic monozygotic twins. Eur Arch Psychiatry Clin Neurosci 1993; 243:7–10.
Ravindranathan A, Coon H, DeLisi L, Holik J, Hoff M, Brown A, Shields G, Crow T, Byerley W: Linkage analysis between schizophrenia and a microsatellite polymorphism for the D_5 dopamine receptor gene. Psychiatr Genet 1994; 4:77–80.
Raz N, Torres IJ, Briggs SD, Spencer WD, Thornton AE, Loken WJ, Gunning FM, McQuain JD, Driesen NR, Acker JD: Selective neuroanatomic abnormalities in Down's syndrome and their cognitive correlates: evidence from MRI morphometry. Neurology 1995; 45:356–366.
Rees MI, Fenton I, Williams NM, Holmans P, Norton N, Cardno A, Asherson P, Spurlock G, Roberts E, Parfitt E, et al.: Autosome search for schizophrenia susceptibility genes in multiply affected families. Mol Psychiatry 1999; 4:353–359.
Reite M, Sheeder J, Teale P, Adams M, Richardson D, Simon J, Jones RH, Rojas DC:

Magnetic source imaging evidence of sex differences in cerebral lateralization in schizophrenia. Arch Gen Psychiatry 1997; 54:433–440.
Reveley AM, Reveley MA, Clifford CA, Murray RM: Cerebral ventricular size in twins discordant for schizophrenia. Lancet 1982; 1:540–541.
Reveley AM, Reveley MA, Murray RM: Cerebral ventricular enlargement in non-genetic schizophrenia: a controlled twin study. Br J Psychiatry 1984; 144:89–93.
Riecher-Rossler A, Hafner H, Stumbaum M, Maurer K, Schmidt R: Can estradiol modulate schizophrenic symptomatology? Schizophr Bull 1994; 20:203–214.
Riederer P, Lange KW, Kornhuber J, Jellinger K: Glutamate receptor antagonism: neurotoxicity, anti-akinetic effects, and psychosis. J Neural Transm Suppl 1991; 34:203–210.
Riley BP, Tahir E, Rajagopalan S, Mogudi-Carter M, Faure S, Weissenbach J, Jenkins T, Williamson R: A linkage study of the *N*-methyl-D-aspartate receptor subunit gene loci and schizophrenia in southern African Bantu-speaking families. Psychiatr Genet 1997; 7:57–74.
Roberts GW, Done DJ, Bruton C, Crow TJ: A "mock up" of schizophrenia: temporal lobe epilepsy and schizophrenia-like psychosis. Biol Psychiatry 1990; 28:127–143.
Roberts M, Caird FI: Computerised tomography and intellectual impairment in the elderly. J Neurol Neurosurg Psychiatry 1976; 39:986–989.
Ross CA, Pearlson GD: Schizophrenia, the heteromodal association neocortex and development: potential for a neurogenetic approach [see comments]. Trends Neurosci 19:171–176.
Rubinsztein DC, Leggo J, Crow TJ, DeLisi LE, Walsh C, Jain S, Paykel ES: Analysis of polyglutamine-coding repeats in the TATA-binding protein in different human populations and in patients with schizophrenia and bipolar affective disorder. Am J Med Genet 1996; 67:495–498.
Sachdev P: Schizophrenia-like psychosis and epilepsy: the status of the association. Am J Psychiatry 1998; 155:325–336.
Salisbury DF, Shenton ME, Sherwood AR, Fischer IA, Yurgelun-Todd DA, Tohen M, McCarley RW: First-episode schizophrenic psychosis differs from first-episode affective psychosis and controls in P300 amplitude over left temporal lobe [published erratum appears in Arch Gen Psychiatry 1998; 55:413]. Arch Gen Psychiatry 1998; 55:173–180.
Salvatore M, Morzunov S, Schwemmle M, Lipkin WI: Borna disease virus in brains of North American and European people with schizophrenia and bipolar disorder. Bornavirus Study Group [see comments]. Lancet 1997; 349:1813–1814.
Sartorius N, Jablensky A, Korten A, Ernberg G, Anker M, Cooper JE, Day R: Early manifestations and first-contact incidence of schizophrenia in different cultures. A preliminary report on the initial evaluation phase of the WHO Collaborative Study on Determinants of Outcome of Severe Mental Disorders. Psychol Med 1986; 16:909–928.
Sasaki T, Dai XY, Kuwata S, Fukuda R, Kunugi H, Hattori M, Nanko S: Brain-derived neurotrophic factor gene and schizophrenia in Japanese subjects. Am J Med Genet 1997; 74:443–444.
Schlaepfer TE, Harris GJ, Tien AY, Peng L, Lee S, Pearlson GD: Structural differences in the cerebral cortex of healthy female and male subjects: a magnetic resonance imaging study. Psychiatry Res 1995; 61:129–135.
Schmidt-Sidor B, Wisniewski KE, Shepard TH, Sersen EA: Brain growth in Down syndrome subjects 15 to 22 weeks of gestational age and birth to 60 months. Clin Neuropathol 1990; 9:181–190.
Schneider K: Primary and secondary symptoms in schizophrenia. In: Hirsch SR, Shepherd M (eds). Themes and Variations in European Psychiatry. An Anthology. Charlottesville: University Press of Virginia, 1974:40–44.
Schnur DB, Bernstein AS, Yeager A, Smith S, Bernstein P: The relationship of the skin conductance and finger pulse amplitude components of the orienting response to season of birth in schizophrenia and depression. Biol Psychiatry 1995; 37:34–41.
Schwab SG, Albus M, Hallmayer J, Honig S, Borrmann M, Lichtermann D, Ebstein RP, Ackenheil M, Lerer B, Risch N, et al.: Evaluation of a susceptibility gene for schizophrenia on chromosome 6p by multipoint affected sib-pair linkage analysis. Nat Genet 1995; 11:325–327.
Schwab SG, Eckstein GN, Hallmayer J, Lerer B, Albus M, Borrmann M, Lichtermann D, Ertl MA, Maier W, Wildenauer DB: Evidence suggestive of a locus on chromosome 5q31 contributing to susceptibility for schizophrenia in German and Israeli families by multipoint affected sib-pair linkage analysis. Mol Psychiatry 1997; 2:156–160.
Schwab SG, Hallmayer J, Albus M, Lerer B, Eckstein GN, Borrmann M, Segman RH, Hanses C, Freymann J, Yakir A, et al.: A genome-wide autosomal screen for schizophrenia susceptibility loci in 71 families with affected siblings: support for loci on chromosome 10p and 6. Mol Psychiatry 2000; 5:638–649.
Schwab SG, Hallmayer J, Albus M, Lerer B, Hanses C, Kanyas K, Segman R, Borrman M, Dreikorn B, Lichtermann D, et al.: Further evidence for a susceptibility locus on chromosome 10p14–p11 in 72 families with schizophrenia by nonparametric linkage analysis. Am J Med Genet 1998a; 81:302–307.
Schwab SG, Hallmayer J, Lerer B, Albus M, Borrmann M, Honig S, Strauss M, Segman R, Lichtermann D, Knapp M, et al.: Support for a chromosome 18p locus conferring susceptibility to functional psychoses in families with schizophrenia, by association and linkage analysis. Am J Hum Genet 1998b; 63:1139–1152.
Seidman LJ: Clinical neuroscience and epidemiology in schizophrenia. Harv Rev Psychiatry 1997; 4:338–342.
Selemon LD, Goldman-Rakic PS: The reduced neuropil hypothesis: a circuit based model of schizophrenia. Biol Psychiatry 1999; 45:17–25.
Selemon LD, Rajkowska G, Goldman-Rakic PS: Elevated neuronal density in prefrontal area 46 in brains from schizophrenic patients: application of a three-dimensional, stereologic counting method. J Comp Neurol 1998; 392:402–412.
Selten JP, Sijben N: First admission rates for schizophrenia in immigrants to the Netherlands. The Dutch National Register. Soc Psychiatry Psychiatr Epidemiol 1994; 29:71–77.
Semwal P, Prasad S, Bhatia T, Deshpande SN, Wood J, Nimgaonkar VL, Thelma BK: Family-based association studies of monoaminergic gene polymorphisms among north Indians with schizophrenia. Mol Psychiatry 2001; 6:220–224.
Serretti A, Lilli R, Lorenzi C, Lattuada E, Smeraldi E: *DRD4* exon 3 variants associated with delusional symptomatology in major psychoses: a study on 2,011 affected subjects. Am J Med Genet 2001; 105:283–290.
Shaikh S, Collier D, Arranz M, Ball D, Gill M, Kerwin R: *DRD2* Ser^{311}/Cys^{311} polymorphism in schizophrenia [letter]. Lancet 1994; 343:1045–1046.
Shaikh S, Collier DA, Sham PC, Ball D, Aitchison K, Vallada H, Smith I, Gill M, Kerwin RW: Allelic association between a Ser-9-Gly polymorphism in the dopamine D_3 receptor gene and schizophrenia. Hum Genet 1996; 97:714–719.
Sham PC, Jones P, Russell A, Gilvarry K, Bebbington P, Lewis S, Toone B, Murray R: Age at onset, sex, and familial psychiatric morbidity in schizophrenia. Camberwell Collaborative Psychosis Study. Br J Psychiatry 1994a; 165:466–473.
Sham PC, MacLean CJ, Kendler KS: A typological model of schizophrenia based on age at onset, sex and familial morbidity. Acta Psychiatr Scand 1994b; 89:135–141.
Sharma T, du Boulay G, Lewis S, Sigmundsson T, Gurling H, Murray R: The Maudsley Family Study. I: Structural brain changes on magnetic resonance imaging in familial schizophrenia. Prog Neuropsychopharmacol Biol Psychiatry 1997; 21:1297–1315.
Shaw SH, Kelly M, Smith AB, Shields G, Hopkins PJ, Loftus J, Laval SH, Vita A, De Hert M, Cardon LR, et al.: A genome-wide search for schizophrenia susceptibility genes. Am J Med Genet 1998; 81:364–376.
Shenton ME, Kikinis R, Jolesz FA, Pollak SD, LeMay M, Wible CG, Hokama H, Martin J, Metcalf D, Coleman M, et al.: Abnormalities of the left temporal lobe and thought disorder in schizophrenia. A quantitative magnetic resonance imaging study. N Engl J Med 1992; 327:604–612.
Shenton ME, Wible CG, McCarley RW: A review of magnetic resonance imaging of brain abnormalities in schizophrenia. In: Brain Imaging in Clinical Psychiatry. New York: Marcel Dekker, 1997:297–380.
Sherrington R, Brynjolfsson J, Petursson H, Potter M, Dudleston K, Barraclough B, Wasmuth J, Dobbs M, Gurling H: Localization of a susceptibility locus for schizophrenia on chromosome 5. Nature 1988; 336:164–167.
Shihabuddin L, Silverman JM, Buchsbaum MS, Seiver LJ, Luu C, Germans MK, Metzger M, Mohs RC, Smith CJ, Spiegel-Cohen J, et al.: Ventricular enlargement associated with linkage marker for schizophrenia-related disorders in one pedigree. Mol Psychiatry 1996; 1:215–222.
Sierra-Honigmann AM, Carbone KM, Yolken RH: Polymerase chain reaction (PCR) search for viral nucleic acid sequences in schizophrenia. Br J Psychiatry 1995; 166:55–60.
Silbersweig D, Stern E: Functional neuroimaging of hallucinations in schizophrenia: toward an integration of bottom–up and top–down approaches. Mol Psychiatry 1996; 1:367–375.
Silverman JM, Smith CJ, Guo SL, Mohs RC, Siever LJ, Davis KL: Lateral ventricular enlargement in schizophrenic probands and their siblings with schizophrenia-related disorders. Biol Psychiatry 1998; 43:97–106.
Smeraldi E, Bellodi L, Cazzullo CL: Further studies on the major histocompatibility complex as a genetic marker for schizophrenia. Biol Psychiatry 1976; 11:655–661.
Sobell JL, Lind TJ, Sigurdson DC, Zald DH, Snitz BE, Grove WM, Heston LL, Sommer SS: The D_5 dopamine receptor gene in schizophrenia: identification of a nonsense change and multiple missense changes but lack of association with disease. Hum Mol Genet 1995; 4:507–514.
Sokoloff P, Giros B, Martres MP, Bouthenet ML, Schwartz JC: Molecular cloning and characterization of a novel dopamine receptor (D_3) as a target for neuroleptics. Nature 1990; 347:146–151.
Sommer SS, Lind TJ, Heston LL, Sobell JL: Dopamine D_4 receptor variants in unrelated schizophrenic cases and controls. Am J Med Genet 1993; 48:90–93.
Sponheim SR, Iacono WG, Clementz BA, Beiser M: Season of birth and electroencephalogram power abnormalities in schizophrenia. Biol Psychiatry 1997; 41:1020–1027.
Spurlock G, Heils A, Holmans P, Williams J, D'Souza UM, Cardno A, Murphy KC, Jones L, Buckland PR, McGuffin P, et al.: A family based association study of T102C polymorphism in $5HT_{2A}$ and schizophrenia plus identification of new polymorphisms in the promoter. Mol Psychiatry 1998a; 3:42–49.
Spurlock G, Williams J, McGuffin P, Aschauer HN, Lenzinger E, Fuchs K, Sieghart WC, Meszaros K, Fathi N, Laurent C, et al.: European Multicentre Association Study of Schizophrenia: a study of the *DRD2* $Ser^{311}Cys$ and *DRD3* $Ser^{9}Gly$ polymorphisms. Am J Med Genet 1998b; 81:24–28.
Squires RF, Saederup E: A review of evidence for GABergic predominance/glutamatergic deficit as a common etiological factor in both schizophrenia and affective psychoses: more support for a continuum hypothesis of "functional" psychosis. Neurochem Res 1991; 16:1099–1111.
Stabenau JR, Pollin W: Heredity and environment in schizophrenia, revisited. The contribution of twin and high-risk studies. J Nerv Ment Dis 1993; 181:290–297.
St Clair D, Blackwood D, Muir W, Carothers A, Walker M, Spowart G, Gosden C, Evans HJ: Association within a family of a balanced autosomal translocation with major mental illness. Lancet 1990; 336:13–16.
Stober G, Jatzke S, Heils A, Jungkunz G, Knapp M, Mossner R, Riederer P, Lesch KP: Insertion/deletion variant (−141C Ins/Del) in the 5′ regulatory region of the dopamine D_2 receptor gene: lack of association with schizophrenia and bipolar affective disorder. J Neural Transm 1998; 105:101–109.
Stober G, Meyer J, Nanda I, Wienker TF, Saar K, Jatzke S, Schmid M, Lesch KP, Beckmann H: *hKCNN3* which maps to chromosome 1q21 is not the causative gene

in periodic catatonia, a familial subtype of schizophrenia. Eur Arch Psychiatry Clin Neurosci 2000a; 250:163–168.

Stober G, Saar K, Ruschendorf F, Meyer J, Nurnberg G, Jatzke S, Franzek E, Reis A, Lesch KP, Wienker TF, et al.: Splitting schizophrenia: periodic catatonia-susceptibility locus on chromosome 15q15. Am J Hum Genet 2000b; 67:1201–1207.

Straub RE, MacLean CJ, Kendler KS: The putative schizophrenia locus on chromosome 6p: a brief overview of the linkage studies. Mol Psychiatry 1996; 1:89–92.

Straub RE, MacLean CJ, Martin RB, Ma Y, Myakishev MV, Harris-Kerr C, Webb BT, O'Neill FA, Walsh D, Kendler KS: A schizophrenia locus may be located in region 10p15–p11. Am J Med Genet 1998; 81:296–301.

Straub RE, MacLean CJ, O'Neill FA, Burke J, Murphy B, Duke F, Shinkwin R, Webb BT, Zhang J, Walsh D, et al.: A potential vulnerability locus for schizophrenia on chromosome 6p24–22: evidence for genetic heterogeneity [see comments]. Nat Genet 1995; 11:287–293.

Straub RE, MacLean CJ, O'Neill FA, Walsh D, Kendler KS: Support for a possible schizophrenia vulnerability locus in region 5q22–31 in Irish families [see comments]. Mol Psychiatry 1997; 2:148–155.

Strous RD, Bark N, Parsia SS, Volavka J, Lachman HM: Analysis of a functional catechol-*O*-methyltransferase gene polymorphism in schizophrenia: evidence for association with aggressive and antisocial behavior. Psychiatry Res 1997; 69:71–77.

Su Y, Burke J, O'Neill FA, Murphy B, Nie L, Kipps B, Bray J, Shinkwin R, Ni Nuallain M, MacLean CJ, et al.: Exclusion of linkage between schizophrenia and the D_2 dopamine receptor gene region of chromosome 11q in 112 Irish multiplex families. Arch Gen Psychiatry 1993; 50:205–211.

Subramaniam B, Naidu S, Reiss AL: Neuroanatomy in Rett syndrome: cerebral cortex and posterior fossa. Neurology 1997; 48:399–407.

Suddath RL, Christison GW, Torrey EF, Casanova MF, Weinberger DR: Anatomical abnormalities in the brains of monozygotic twins discordant for schizophrenia [published erratum appears in N Engl J Med 1990; 322:1616] [see comments]. N Engl J Med 1990; 322:789–794.

Sugarman PA, Craufurd D: Schizophrenia in the Afro-Caribbean community. Br J Psychiatry 1994; 164:474–480.

Tamminga CA: Schizophrenia and glutamatergic transmission. Crit Rev Neurobiol 1998; 12:21–36.

Tatsumi M, Sasaki T, Sakai T, Kamijima K, Fukuda R, Kunugi H, Hattori M, Nanko S: Genes for interleukin-2 receptor beta chain, interleukin-1beta, and schizophrenia: no evidence for the association or linkage. Am J Med Genet 1997; 74:338–341.

Thomas CS, Stone K, Osborn M, Thomas PF, Fisher M: Psychiatric morbidity and compulsory admission among UK-born Europeans, Afro-Caribbeans and Asians in central Manchester [see comments]. Br J Psychiatry 1993; 163:91–99.

Tien AY, Eaton WW, Schlaepfer TE, McGilchrist IK, Menon R, Powers R, Aylward E, Barta P, Strauss ME, Pearlson GD: Exploratory factor analysis of MRI brain structure measures in schizophrenia. Schizophr Res 1996; 19:93–101.

Tienari P: Schizophrenia and monozygotic twins [in Russian]. Vestn Akad Med Nauk SSSR 1971; 26:53–57.

Tienari P, Lahti I, Sorri A, Naarala M, Moring J, Wahlberg KE, Wynne LC: The Finnish adoptive family study of schizophrenia. J Psychiatr Res 1987; 21:437–445.

Torrey EF, Miller J, Rawlings R, Yolken RH: Seasonality of births in schizophrenia and bipolar disorder: a review of the literature. Schizophr Res 1997; 28:1–38.

Torrey FF, Peterson MR: The viral hypothesis of schizophrenia. Schizophr Bull 2:136–146.

Trichard C, Paillere-Martinot ML, Attar-Levy D, Blin J, Feline A, Martinot JL: No serotonin 5-HT_{2A} receptor density abnormality in the cortex of schizophrenic patients studied with PET. Schizophr Res 1998; 31:13–17.

Tsuang MT, Perkins K, Simpson JC: Physical diseases in schizophrenia and affective disorder. J Clin Psychiatry 1983; 44:42–46.

Turetsky B, Cowell PE, Gur RC, Grossman RI, Shtasel DL, Gur RE: Frontal and temporal lobe brain volumes in schizophrenia. Relationship to symptoms and clinical subtype. Arch Gen Psychiatry 1995; 52:1061–1070.

Ujike H, Yamamoto A, Tanaka Y, Takehisa Y, Takaki M, Taked T, Kodama M, Kuroda S: Association study of CAG repeats in the *KCNN3* gene in Japanese patients with schizophrenia, schizoaffective disorder and bipolar disorder. Psychiatry Res 2001; 101:203–207.

Vallada H, Collier D, Dawson E, Owen M, Nanko S, Murray R, Gill M: Debrisoquine 4-hydroxylase (*CYP2D*) locus and possible susceptibility to schizophrenia. Lancet 1992; 340:181–182.

Verga M, Macciardi F, Pedrini S, Cohen S, Smeraldi E: No association of the Ser/Cys^{311} *DRD2* molecular variant with schizophrenia using a classical case control study and the haplotype relative risk. Schizophr Res 1997; 25:117–121.

Vincent JB, Petronis A, Strong E, Parikh SV, Meltzer HY, Lieberman J, Kennedy JL: Analysis of genome-wide CAG/CTG repeats, and at SEF2–1B and ERDA1 in schizophrenia and bipolar affective disorder. Mol Psychiatry 1999; 4:229–234.

Vinogradov S, Gottesman II, Moises HW, Nicol S: Negative association between schizophrenia and rheumatoid arthritis. Schizophr Bull 1991; 17:669–678.

Vita A, Giobbio GM, Dieci M, Garbarini M, Morganti C, Comazzi M, Invernizzi G: Stability of cerebral ventricular size from the appearance of the first psychotic symptoms to the later diagnosis of schizophrenia. Biol Psychiatry 1994; 35:960–962.

Vita A, Sacchetti E, Valvassori G, Cazzullo CL: Brain morphology in schizophrenia: a 2- to 5-year CT scan follow-up study. Acta Psychiatr Scand 1988; 78:618–621.

Wang ZW, Black DW, Andreasen N, Crowe RR: No evidence of a schizophrenia locus in a second pseudoautosomal region. Arch Gen Psychiatry 1994; 51:427.

Wei J, Hemmings GP: The *NOTCH4* locus is associated with susceptibility to schizophrenia. Nat Genet 2000; 25:376–377.

Wei J, Ramchand CN, Hemmings GP: Association of polymorphic VNTR region in the first intron of the human TH gene with disturbances of the catecholamine pathway in schizophrenia. Psychiatr Genet 1995; 5:83–88.

Wei J, Ramchand CN, Hemmings GP: TaqI polymorphic sites at the human dopamine beta-hydroxylase gene possibly associated with biochemical alterations of the catecholamine pathway in schizophrenia. Psychiatr Genet 1998; 8:19–24.

Weickert CS, Weinberger DR: A candidate molecule approach to defining developmental pathology in schizophrenia. Schizophr Bull 1998; 24:303–316.

Weinberger DR: Implications of normal brain development for the pathogenesis of schizophrenia. Arch Gen Psychiatry 1987; 44:660–669.

Weinberger DR: From neuropathology to neurodevelopment. Lancet 1995; 346:552–557.

Weinberger DR: On the plausibility of "the neurodevelopmental hypothesis" of schizophrenia. Neuropsychopharmacology 1996; 14:1S–11S.

Weinberger DR: Cell biology of the hippocampal formation in schizophrenia. Biol Psychiatry 1999; 45:395–402.

Weinberger DR, Berman KF, Zec RF: Physiologic dysfunction of dorsolateral prefrontal cortex in schizophrenia. I. Regional cerebral blood flow evidence [see comments]. Arch Gen Psychiatry 1986; 43:114–124.

Weinberger DR, DeLisi LE, Neophytides AN, Wyatt RJ: Familial aspects of CT scan abnormalities in chronic schizophrenic patients. Psychiatry Res 1981; 4:65–71.

Weinberger DR, Gallhofer B: Cognitive function in schizophrenia. Int Clin Psychopharmacol 1997; 12(Suppl 4):S29–S36.

Wildenauer DB, Hallmayer J, Schwab SG, Albus M, Eckstein GN, Zill P, Honig S, Strauss M, Borrmann M, Lichtermann D, et al.: Searching for susceptibility genes in schizophrenia by genetic linkage analysis. Cold Spring Harb Symp Quant Biol 1996; 61:845–850.

Wildenauer DB, Schwab SG, Maier W, Detera-Wadleigh SD: Do schizophrenia and affective disorder share susceptibility genes? Schizophr Res 1999; 39:107–111, 160.

Williams J, McGuffin P, Nothen M, Owen MJ: Meta-analysis of association between the 5-HT_{2a} receptor $T^{102}C$ polymorphism and schizophrenia. EMASS Collaborative Group. European Multicentre Association Study of Schizophrenia. Lancet 1997; 349:1221.

Williams J, Spurlock G, Holmans P, Mant R, Murphy K, Jones L, Cardno A, Asherson P, Blackwood D, Muir W, et al.: A meta-analysis and transmission disequilibrium study of association between the dopamine D_3 receptor gene and schizophrenia. Mol Psychiatry 1998; 3:141–149.

Williams J, Spurlock G, McGuffin P, Mallet J, Nothen MM, Gill M, Aschauer H, Nylander PO, Macciardi F, Owen MJ: Association between schizophrenia and $T^{102}C$ polymorphism of the 5-hydroxytryptamine type 2a-receptor gene. European Multicentre Association Study of Schizophrenia (EMASS) Group [see comments]. Lancet 1996; 347:1294–1296.

Williams NM, Rees MI, Holmans P, Norton N, Cardno AG, Jones LA, Murphy KC, Sanders RD, McCarthy G, Gray MY, et al.: A two-stage genome scan for schizophrenia susceptibility genes in 196 affected sibling pairs. Hum Mol Genet 1999; 8:1729–1739.

Wolyniec PS, Pulver AE, McGrath JA, Tam D: Schizophrenia: gender and familial risk. J Psychiatr Res 1992; 26:17–27.

Woodruff PW, Wright IC, Bullmore ET, Brammer M, Howard RJ, Williams SC, Shapleske J, Rossell S, David AS, McGuire PK, et al.: Auditory hallucinations and the temporal cortical response to speech in schizophrenia: a functional magnetic resonance imaging study. Am J Psychiatry 1997; 154:1676–1682.

Woods B, Yurgelun-Todd D, Benes F, Frankenburg F, Pope H, McSparren J: Progressive ventricular enlargement in schizophrenia: comparison to bipolar affective disorder and correlation with clinical course. Biol Psychiatry 1990; 27:341–352.

Woods BT: Is schizophrenia a progressive neurodevelopmental disorder? Toward a unitary pathogenetic mechanism [see comments]. Am J Psychiatry 1998; 155:1661–1670.

Yamagishi H, Garg V, Matsuoka R, Thomas T, Srivastava D: A molecular pathway revealing a genetic basis for human cardiac and craniofacial defects. Science 1999; 283:1158–1161.

Yan W, Jacobsen LK, Krasnewich DM, Guan XY, Lenane MC, Paul SP, Dalwadi HN, Zhang H, Long RT, Kumra S, et al.: Chromosome 22q11.2 interstitial deletions among childhood-onset schizophrenics and "multidimensionally impaired." Am J Med Genet 1998; 81:41–43.

Zakzanis KK, Hansen KT: Dopamine D_2 densities and the schizophrenic brain. Schizophr Res 1998; 32:201–206.

46 Alcoholism

DHARAM P. AGARWAL

Both clinical and epidemiological studies have implicated the excessive use of alcohol in the risk of developing a variety of organ, neuronal, and metabolic disorders that affect almost all body functions. Recent human genetic studies clearly suggest that a predisposition to alcohol abuse or alcoholism is inherited. Pedigree analysis, linkage studies, and association studies have helped detect marker loci and candidate genes that may be useful for identifying individuals at risk. Elucidation of the molecular mechanisms that control and influence elimination and metabolism of alcohol is important in understanding the biochemical basis of alcohol toxicity and alcohol abuse–related pharmacological and addictive consequences in humans. It may be surprising that a disease with such an obvious exogenous cause—intake of alcohol—should be influenced by genetic factors; but even in countries where alcoholism imposes a tremendous public health problem, a great majority of the population are able to control their own alcohol intake. Because it has been known for a long time that alcoholism tends to run in families, the involvement of genetic factors in the form of genetic susceptibility is a priori a real possibility.

A necessary condition for the development of alcoholism is the availability of alcohol. Alcohol is known to mankind probably from prehistoric times. After the introduction of agriculture between 10,000 and 5,000 B.C., systematic alcohol production through fermentation of barley, honey, milk, and grapes became possible in various populations. At the time, alcohol was mainly used as a food because of its vitamin and mineral content. The preserving qualities of alcoholic solutions permitted long-term storage of food, which was an important property in the early stages of civilization. In addition, the euphoric potency of ethanol must have been detected early on. (Presumably, an essential motivation for using the psychotropic effects of alcohol was coping with existential fear, which must have been omnipresent in primitive societies.) This might also have been the cause for early integration of alcohol use in religious rites. Invention of the method of distillation of alcohol around A.D. 1000 made the production of concentrated alcoholic beverages possible. During the thirteenth and fourteenth centuries, this technique spread over Europe and paved the way for alcohol abuse and the development of alcoholism.

DISEASE DEFINITION

Alcoholism is an extremely complex disease for which no generally accepted definition exists. There is a complex interaction between the socioenvironmental context, the individual at risk, and the availability of alcohol. Therefore, it is obvious that the conditions facilitating the development of the disease and the criteria of its definition can hardly be generalized to different populations or societies. That alcoholism is a disease was recognized as early as 1785 (Keller, 1976). However, there has been widespread opposition to the disease concept of alcoholism (Fingarette, 1991; Heather, 1992). Alcohol consumption is so intimately entangled in cultural traditions and everyday life in many countries that there is no clearcut separation of "normal" from "abnormal" drinking. Nevertheless, alcoholism imposes such tremendous public health problems on society that the consequences of chronic alcohol intake undoubtedly have disease qualities. Furthermore, it has been known for decades that only a relatively small part of the population is responsible for most of the alcohol consumption.

For practical purposes, there is need for a definition of the "phenomenon" of alcoholism. The World Health Organization (WHO) provided a definition of the now preferred term Alcohol Dependency Syndrome as follows:

> A state, psychic and sometimes also physical, resulting from the interaction between a living organism and a drug, characterized by behavioral and other responses that always include a compulsion to take the drug on a continuous or periodic basis in order to experience its psychic effects, and sometimes to avoid the discomfort of its absence. Tolerance may or may not be present. A person may be dependent on more than one drug. (National Council on Alcoholism, 1972)

Although concise, this definition of dependency is not suitable for practical purposes or as a definition for research on alcoholism. Four different dimensions of definitions have been proposed instead (Feuerlein, 1984):

1. The quantity–frequency dimension attempts to gather information on drinking patterns. Although this scheme has great relevance to studies of drinking practices, its usefulness is limited by the difficulty in obtaining reliable information about individual alcohol intake. Physicians frequently regard an alcohol consumption of over 30 g [over 1 oz.] per day for males and 20 g [0.7 oz.] per day for females as critical for the development of alcohol dependence. However, such an estimate is based on retrospective data and applies only to injuries of the liver and not to other organs; it also does not take into account the age or body weight of an individual or the type of alcoholic beverage.
2. Occurrence of withdrawal or abstinence symptoms when an individual stops drinking alcohol is a category widely used by physicians. This dimension is restrictive, because many individuals who have serious life-impairment and medical problems have never demonstrated obvious signs of physiological withdrawal.
3. Existence of psychological dependence is based on subjective experiences; the individual feels uncomfortable

unless there is alcohol around. It is difficult, if not impossible, to quantify this approach objectively.

4. The dimension that probably has the greatest usefulness to clinicians centers on the occurrence of serious social or health problems related to alcohol, such as marital separation or divorce, loss of a job, problems with the law, or physical evidence that alcohol has harmed health.

The definition proposed by the National Council on Alcoholism and Drug Dependence (NACDD) and the American Society of Addiction Medicine (ASAM) reads as follows:

Alcoholism is a primary, chronic disease with genetic, psychosocial, and environmental factors influencing its development and manifestations. The disease is often progressive and fatal. It is characterized by continuous or periodic impaired control over drinking, preoccupation with the drug alcohol, use of alcohol despite adverse consequences, and distortions in thinking, most notably denial. (Flavin and Morse, 1990)

While the definitions of alcoholism as descibed above reflect substantial advances in our understanding of the disease of alcoholism, much remains to be learned about the development, expression, and effective treatment of alcohol dependence.

Diagnostic Criteria

For purposes of treatment or research, criteria for the diagnosis of alcoholism have been developed that take clinical, physiological, behavioral, and attitudinal aspects into account (National Council on Alcoholism, 1972). As formulated by the National Council on Alcoholism, the criteria cannot be used for ascertaining the nature of alcoholism, but they may be used to identify individuals at multiple levels of dependency, to promote early detection, and to prevent overdiagnosis. In addition, the National Council on Alcoholism has defined major criteria and

Table 46–1. Major Criteria for the Diagnosis of Alcoholism

Criteria	Level[a]
Physiologic and Clinical	
Physiologic dependency	
Evidence of a withdrawal syndrome when the intake of alcohol is interrupted or decreased without substitution of other sedation	
Gross tremor (differentiated from other causes of tremor)	1
Hallucinosis (differentiated from schizophrenic hallucinations or other psychoses)	1
Withdrawal seizures (differentiated from epilepsy and other seizure disorders)	1
Delirium tremens. Usually starts between the first and third day after withdrawal and minimally includes tremors, disorientation, and hallucinations. Remember that overuse of other sedative drugs can produce a similar withdrawal state. Evidence of tolerance to the effects of alcohol. (There may be a decrease in previously high levels of tolerance late in the course.) Although the degree of tolerance to alcohol in no way matches the degree of tolerance to other drugs, the behavioral effects of a given amount of alcohol vary greatly between alcoholic and nonalcoholic subjects.	1
A blood alcohol level of >150 mg/dl, without gross evidence of intoxication	1
The consumption of one-fifth of a gallon of whiskey or an equivalent amount of wine or beer daily, for more than 1 day, by a 180 pound individual	1
Alcoholic "blackout" periods (differentiated from purely psychologic fugue states and psychomotor seizures)	2
Clinical major alcohol-associated illnesses. Alcoholism can be assumed to exist if major alcohol-associated illnesses develop in a person who drinks regularly. In such individuals, evidence of physiologic and psychologic dependence should be sought	
Fatty degeneration in absence of other known cause	2
Alcoholic hepatitis	1
Laennec cirrhosis	2
Pancreatitis in the absence of cholelithiasis	2
Chronic gastritis	3
Hematologic disorders	
Anemia: hypochromic, normocytic, macrocytic, hemolytic with stomatocytosis, low folic acid	3
Clotting disorders: prothrombin elevation, thrombocytopenia	3
Wernicke-Korsakoff syndrome	2
Alcoholic cerebellar degeneration	1
Cerebral degeneration in absence of Alzheimer's disease or arteriosclerosis	2
Central pontine myelinolysis[b]	2
Marchiafava-Bignami disease[b]	2
Peripheral neuropathy	2
Toxic amblyopia	3
Alcohol myopathy	2
Alcoholic cardiomyopathy	2
Pellagra	3
Behavioral, Psychologic, and Attitudinal	
All chronic conditions of psychologic dependence occur in dynamic equilibrium with intrapsychic and interpersonal consequences. In alcoholism, similarly, there are varied effects on character and family. Like other chronic relapsing diseases, alcoholism produces vocational, social, and physical impairments. Therefore, the implications of these disruptions must be evaluated and related to the individual and the pattern of alcoholism. The following behavior patterns show psychologic dependence on alcohol in alcoholism:	
Drinking despite strong medical contraindication known to patient	1
Drinking despite strong, identified, social contraindication (job loss for intoxication, marriage disruption because of drinking, arrest for intoxication, driving while intoxicated)	1
Patient's subjective complaint of loss of control of alcohol consumption	2

[a]The signs of alcoholism are weighted by grouping them into three "diagnostic levels." Diagnostic level 1: A person who fits this criterion must be diagnosed as being alcoholic. Diagnostic level 2: A person who satisfies this criterion is under strong suspicion of alcoholism. Diagnostic level 3: These manifestations are common in alcoholism, but other evidence is needed for diagnosis.

[b]Diagnosis possible only after death.

Source: National Council on Alcoholism (1972) with permission.

a series of minor criteria that are weighted according to their specificity for alcoholism, as shown in Table 46–1.

In the course of time, three classification systems, DSM-III-R (American Psychiatric Association, 1987), DSM-IV (American Psychiatric Association, 1994), and ICD-10 (World Health Organization, 1994), have found wide application for the diagnosis of alcohol dependence syndrome and harmful use of alcohol. Researchers and clinicians usually diagnose alcohol problems using standardized structured instruments (interviews) such as SADS, DIS, SCID, SCID-A/D, AUDADIS, SCAN, and CIDI. In recent years, a number of rapid interview techniques for detecting alcohol abuse and alcoholism have been developed, such as MAST (Selzer, 1971), CAGE (Mayfield et al., 1974), REICH (Reich et al., 1975), MALT (Feuerlein et al., 1977), TWEAK (Chan et al., 1993), SADQ (Stockwell et al., 1994), AUDIT (Saunders et al., 1993), and SSAGA (Bucholz et al., 1994). In accordance with the alcoholism criteria already discussed, the focus of these interviews is mainly on detecting abnormal drinking behavior and alcohol-induced problems rather than on measuring the amount of alcohol consumed individually. The value of screening interviews is undoubtedly limited to those who recognize that alcohol plays a crucial role in their personal difficulties and are willing to admit this fact. Nevertheless, well-designed screening tests can identify a great majority of alcohol abusers and alcoholics (Fig. 46–1).

To arrive at more objective measures, various laboratory parameters (state markers) have been examined for their specificity and sensitivity to detect alcoholism. Although a large number of biochemical and hematologic parameters have been proposed as diagnostic tools for the objective identification of hazardous drinking, their application in the clinical situation has often been restricted due to their nonspecificity and low sensitivity. Gamma-glutamyl transpeptidase (γ-GT) and aspartate aminotransferase (ASAT) are traditionally considered to be markers of alcohol-related liver impairment. However, both tests are nonspecific for alcohol-induced hepatic damage (Conigrave et al., 1995). Measurement of carbohydrate-deficient transferrin (CDT) seems to be a more accurate indicator of alcohol abuse than any other laboratory test currently in routine use (Salaspuro, 1999). Recently, a multinational study was initiated to develop biological screening tools that can identify problem drinkers (Helander, 2001; Tabakoff et al., 2001).

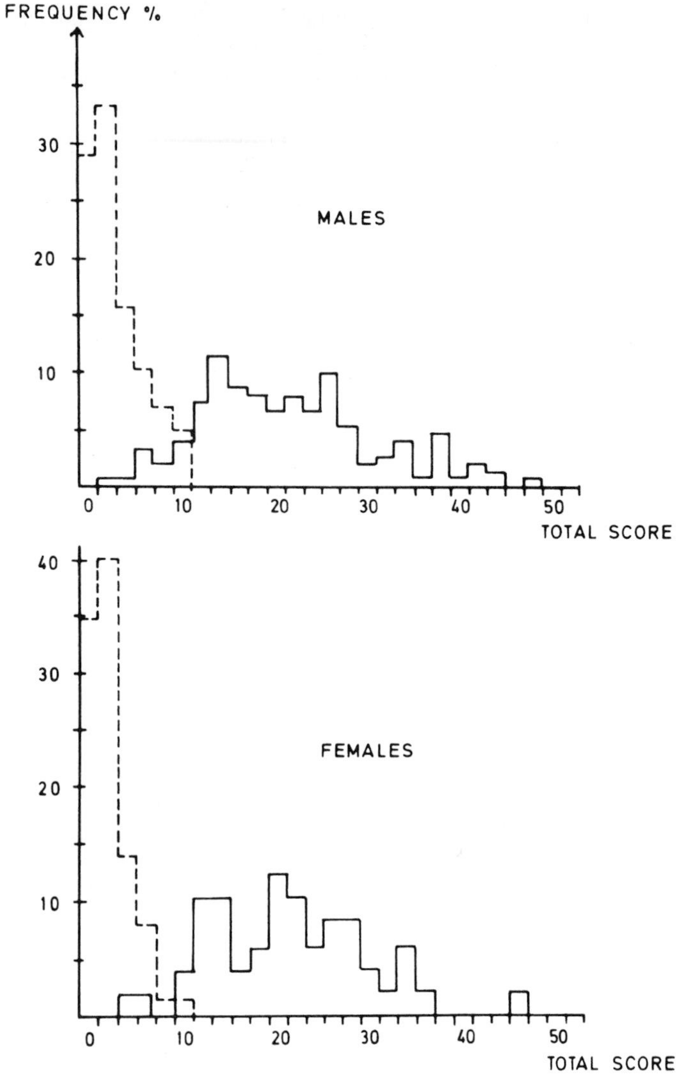

Fig. 46–1. Distribution of total scores obtained in alcoholics and controls after application of the Munich Alcoholism Test (MALT). Persons with a total score of ≥11 are regarded as alcoholics; persons with a total score of 6–10 are suspected to be alcoholics. From Feuerlein (1984) with permission.

Typology

For over a century, physicians and researchers have attempted to categorize alcoholics according to various schemes or typologies. According to Babor (1996), the history of typological thinking about alcoholics can be divided into three periods: prescientific period (1850–1940), the Jellinek era (1941–1960), and the post-Jellinek era (1961–present).

Prescientific Period

William Carpenter (1850), one of the pioneer alcohol researchers of the nineteenth century, proposed three categories of wine mania: acute, periodic, and chronic. In subsequent years many more classifications were developed. However, the early typologies were unsystematic and lacked an empirical foundation.

Jellinek Era

In the 1940s, the Canadian investigator Jellinek developed a typology of alcoholism that is still widely used. In a fruitful attempt, Jellinek (1946, 1959, 1960) hypothesized that alcoholism (a "genus") consists of different entities ("species"). He defined the types of alcoholism according to (1) etiological elements, (2) elements of the alcoholic process, and (3) damage resulting from drinking. Although this subdivision is somewhat arbitrary and to some extent overlapping, it reflects certain general tendencies observed in the population of alcoholics. Among the etiological elements, Jellinek considered psychological and physiological vulnerability and sociocultural and economic factors. He regarded psychological vulnerability to range from small deficits (such as lack of self-confidence) to neuroses and psychoses. Physiological vulnerability was only hypothetical at that time; certain biochemical lesions were claimed to play a role in the primary cause of heavy alcohol intake. Among sociocultural influences, drinking customs and particularly the degree of intoxication that is socially acceptable were regarded as important. The price of alcoholic beverages and general living conditions contributed to economic factors. The development of alcohol dependence was thought to be influenced by an increase in tissue tolerance to alcohol. However, the damage resulting from drinking did not contribute to this typology of alcoholism.

Jellinek differentiated five types of alcoholism: alpha, beta, gamma, delta, and epsilon (Table 46–2). The alpha drinker (con-

Table 46–2. Some Characteristics of the Main Types of Alcoholism

	Etiologic Elements of Various Species of Alcoholism				Elements of the Alcoholic Process				
Designation of Given Species of Alcoholism	Psychologic Vulnerability	Physiologic Vulnerability	Sociocultural Elements	Economic Elements	Acquired Increased Tissue Tolerance	Main Addictive Features	Nature of Dependence	Progressive Nature	Short Characterization, by Feuerlein (1984)
Alpha	+++ to ++++	0 to +	+ to (+++)	0 to (+++)	+ to ++	0 No loss of control but deliberate undisciplined drinking	Purely psychologic	Slight, in the sense that there are no great psychologic and social behavior changes except perhaps some guilt about drinking	Conflict drinker
Beta	+	0 to +	+++ (Culturally determined heavy weekend drinking)	0 to (+++)	+ to ++	0 No loss of control	None, unless sociocultural dependence is considered	No progression, except increase in number of arrests with incumbent social damage	Occasional drinker
Gamma	+++ to ++++	+++ to ++++	+ to (+++)	0 to (+++)	+++ to ++++	++++ With loss of control but ability to abstain entirely	First, psychologic dependence and later, marked physical dependence as manifested by the development of the main addictive features	Strongly marked progression in terms of changes in psychologic and social behavior ("phases of alcoholism"), changes caused by the addictive process, and the possible emergence of chronic alcoholic diseases	Addictive drinker
Delta	+	+++ to ++++	+++ to ++++	++ to ++++	+++ to ++++	++++ With inability to abstain even for 24 hours, but no loss of control unless in some instances as a very late development	Physical dependence, although at a late stage. Psychologic dependence could develop, too	Some progression in terms of psychologic and social behavior largely emerging after many years and in terms of the addictive process, as as well as the possible emergence of organic damage	Habitual drinker
Epsilon	Knowledge of this species or perhaps several species of true periodic alcoholism is too scant to permit rating and delimitation								

Source: Jellinek (1960), supplemented with a short characterization by Feuerlein (1984) with permission.

flict drinkers) is characterized by strong psychological vulnerability without loss of control. Dependency is exclusively psychological. Beta alcoholism (occasional drinkers) is mainly due to sociocultural causes. In gamma alcoholism (addictive drinkers), there are both strong psychological vulnerability and loss of control. Delta alcoholism (habitual drinkers) is mainly characterized by sociocultural and economic elements, whereas psychological factors are less important. Delta alcoholics are particularly common among people who produce or distribute alcoholic beverages and in certain sociocultural conditions where drinking of alcohol is part of everyday life (e.g., wine-making countries). Jellinek delineated periodic alcohol intake as epsilon alcoholism, for which he did not give further characteristics. Alpha alcoholism tends to develop to the gamma, and beta to the delta, type of alcoholism. Only the gamma and delta types have clearcut disease qualities. Alpha alcoholism cannot be regarded as a disease but as a symptom of an underlying disorder. Beta alcoholism seems to be neither a disease nor a symptom but merely a culturally determined drinking habit (Jellinek, 1960).

Jellinek's typology, although based on an empiric examination of ~2000 alcoholics (Jellinek, 1959), is essentially intuitive in origin. Nevertheless, it proved useful for scientific and practical purposes, and pharmacokinetic and pharmacodynamic findings with alcohol metabolism have substantiated such concepts as psychological and physiological vulnerability.

Post-Jellinek Era

In the post-Jellinek era, research on typologies gained momentum. For example, two or more groups of alcoholics are classified on the basis of gender, family history of alcoholism, and coexisting psychopathology and are then compared with correlates such as age of onset, rapidity of symptom development, and severity of dependence. A history of alcoholism in first-degree relatives has also been used as a typological criterion. Other studies compared alcoholics with and without coexistent psychopathologies.

Alcohol typology researchers rely on personality questionnaires to determine the category in which each alcoholic subject belongs (Ingle, 1996). Five frequently used questionnaires are the Minnesota Multiphasic Personality Inventory (MMPI), the MacAndrew Alcoholism Scale (MAC), the Eysenck Personality Questionnaire (EPQ), the Tridimensional Personality Questionnaire (TPQ), and the Connecticut Typology Questionnaire (CTQ).

Type I and Type II Alcoholism. A study of Swedish adoptees and their biological and adoptive parents resulted in the identification of two distinct alcoholism subtypes, type I and type II. Personality traits of children with varying risk for alcoholism were examined by Cloninger (1987). He distinguished type I of alcoholism (low novelty seeking, high harm avoidance, high reward dependence) from type II (male-limited) alcoholism (high novelty seeking, low harm avoidance, low reward dependence). Spontaneous alcohol-seeking behavior or inability to abstain (type II) and psychological dependence or loss of control (type I) should be associated with different personality traits.

A third type of alcoholism has been proposed by Hill (1992). Like type II alcoholism, it is significantly influenced by genetic factors but is not associated with antisocial behavior.

Type A and Type B Alcoholism. Babor and colleagues (1992) suggested another typology, type A and type B, based on the assumption that heterogeneity among alcoholics is attributable to a complex interaction among genetic, biological, psychological, and sociocultural factors. Type A alcoholics are characterized by later onset of alcoholism, fewer childhood risk factors, less severe alcohol dependence, fewer alcohol-related problems, and less psychopathology. Type B alcoholics are characterized by childhood risk factors, a family history of alcoholism, early onset of alcohol-related problems, greater severity of dependence, multiple drug use, a more chronic treatment history, greater psychopathology, and more life stress.

According to Babor and Dolinsky (1988) a useful typology would be characterized by (1) homogeneity within types, (2) stability over time, (3) inclusiveness across alcoholics, but exclusivity between subtypes, (4) multidimensionality, (5) utility—easily employed and clinically relevant, and (6) validity—demonstrable robustness across different samples. Furthermore, developing subtypes of alcoholism that clearly distinguish between individuals on the basis of relative genetic and environmental influence is essential to understanding the disease etiology, prevention, and treatment. One such typology, reported recently, distinguishes mild, severe, and dyssocial alcohol dependence across racial or ethnic groups (Johnson et al., 1998). Kendler et al. (1998) applied latent class analysis to data on the number, age at onset, and reasons for temperance board registration in all male–female twin pairs of known zygosity born in Sweden from 1902 to 1949. The two most common subtypes identified bear substantial but imperfect resemblance to previously proposed typologies.

GENERAL GENETIC AND EPIDEMIOLOGICAL EVIDENCE

Clinical Epidemiology and Ethnic Differences

The relationship between alcohol consumption and all-cause mortality is J-shaped in most industrialized countries (Rehm and Bondy, 1998). The J-shape is the result of the combination of adverse and beneficial effects of alcohol consumption. Adverse effects include several types of cancer (oropharyngeal, oesophageal, liver, laryngeal, and breast cancer), other diseases of the aerodigestive tract, diseases of the heart (alcoholic cardiomyopathy, haemorrhagic stroke, arrhythmia, hypertension), addiction-related mental disorders, and accidents and injuries. Beneficial effects are for ischaemic heart disease and ischaemic stroke. The exact shape of the all-cause mortality curve in a given region depends on the proportion of the population consuming alcohol at different levels, especially heavy consumption, and on the prevalence of the disorders named above. Thus regions with a relatively low prevalence of ischaemic cardiovascular disease show almost no benefits of consumption, along with an all-cause mortality curve that is almost exponential. Females experience a minimum mortality risk at a level of alcohol intake that is lower than that associated with the minimum risk for men. Similarly, an upturn in mortality risk occurs at lower intake levels for women than for men. However, at present, there is no satisfactory explanation for the observation that the shape of the mortality curve varies with the consumption level of the cohort under study. Heavier-drinking cohorts tend to display their minimum risk at relatively higher levels of alcohol intake than do cohorts with lower alcohol consumption (Rehm and Bondy, 1998).

Epidemiology of Alcohol Use and Abuse

A review of the literature on the epidemiology of alcohol use and abuse reveals significant variations between sexes, across various age groups, and among the several subpopulations. Immigrant populations, indigenous cultural styles, and assimilation and acculturation to the so-called Western societies have had a powerful effect on alcohol use. Thus, there is a considerable variation in the proportion of drinkers in a given population when divided by ethnicity, gender, age, religious affiliation, and socioeconomic status (Heath et al., 2001).

Several factors promote a current widespread and extremely high use of alcohol in underdeveloped countries. For example: purchasing power of alcoholic drinks over other consumer goods has increased among both urban and rural consumers; there is a strong promotion of alcoholic drinks by advertising through cinema, radio, television, newspapers, and billboards; supermarkets openly display and provide easy access to alcohol products; having a bar in private homes has become a status symbol; tourism has developed with more open recruitment to social clubs, and this has served to popularize drinking behavior; because legal punishment is extremely severe for using illicit drugs, in effect young adults are encouraged to choose alcohol.

In Europe, for instance, British and northern and eastern European societies have generally shown a stronger concern for alcoholism in the last 150 years than have central and southern European countries. The societies that admit having alcohol problems often emphasize a different nature of the problem. Finnish and Polish literature blames the social disruption associated with drinking; Germany places greater emphasis on drunk driving casualities. The French, by contrast, often focus on long-term medical problems such as liver cirrhosis.

Alcohol Drinking Pattern. Although the use of alcoholic beverages is found in virtually all societies, certain socioeconomic, cultural, and biobehavioral factors, along with ethnic and gender differences, are among the strongest determinants of drinking pattern in a society. The distribution of drinking patterns in specific racial and ethnic groups is of great interest from the public health perspective. Governing images of alcohol problems differ considerably from one society to another, and they shift over time in a particular society or culture.

Ethnicity is an important risk factor for alcohol abuse and alcohol dependence. Geneticists recognize five human races: two smaller races, the Bushmen and Australian aborigines, plus three larger races, the Caucasoids, Mongoloids, and Negroids. Each of the larger races consists of subgroups that do not always represent distinct and uniform groups; rather, they represent populations with racial mixtures that differ in geography, culture, lifestyle, and social and religious norms. In the past centuries these populations underwent severe influences of historical processes (various political, social, and economic events), migration patterns, isolation and ecological pressure, and the interactions of all of these. In addition, changing social norms, mores, and sanctions exert influences over the subgroups. While discussing interethnic differences in alcohol drinking behavior, educational level, occupational-generational differences, language, customs, and religion, attitudes toward alcohol also have to be taken into consideration. Moreover, there is a need to distinguish between important within-culture subgroups that are subsumed under the broader groups. The legacy of alcoholism among certain ethnic groups suggests that genetic factors can increase an individual's vulnerability for this disease. Alternatively, individuals within certain ethnic groups have protective genetic factors that make them sensitive to alcohol actions, thereby acting as a deterrent to alcohol abuse. A better understanding of the contribution of these variables in drinking patterns may help reduce alcohol-related problems.

A wide variety of environmental and biological factors, and the complex interactions between them, may influence the pattern and extent of alcohol consumption. Studies at the cross-cultural level have helped identify possible risk factors for alcohol abuse, thus contributing toward designing primary and secondary preventive measures. However, the reported ethnic variations in alcohol use have a meaning only in regions where alcohol is freely available without widespread religious, moral, or economic restrictions.

Per Capita Alcohol Consumption. There is no simple and reliable way of measuring yearly per capita consumption of alcohol in terms of absolute alcohol in liters in various population groups. Differences in the trends of alcohol consumption in different parts of the world may have nation-specific explanations. Considerable variation is found from one society to another in the habits and patterns of alcohol drinking, differing in terms of frequency, beverage choice, and amounts consumed, as well as in the context of drinking, including the location, social setting, and occasion. An indirect approach uses the average alcohol consumption at the population level, which has the advantage of being based on hard quantitative data. For a wide variety of populations, the distribution of the per capita consumption approximates a logarithmic normal curve: there are many persons who drink only small amounts of alcohol, and relatively few people who drink large quantities (Fig. 46–2). Thus, if the average consumption of alcohol is known, the distribution of the per capita consumption in the population can be fairly reliably estimated. This approach is suitable for estimates of drinking habits at the population level. If one makes an assumption of the average alcohol consumption of an alcoholic, it is possible to obtain a rough estimate of the alcoholism rate in a population.

Alcohol Consumption in Different Countries. Average alcohol intake per person varies remarkably among countries. Alcohol consumption is usually expressed in liters of absolute alcohol per year. To give an indication of the ethanol content of alcoholic beverages, the range of ethanol concentrations in different beverages is shown in Table 46–3. Yearly per capita consumption of alcohol in terms of absolute alcohol in liters in various countries is displayed in Table 46–4. The highest alcohol consumption is found in Europeans (Hüllinghorst, 1999). In these countries, nearly everyone drinks alcohol, usually wine, at meals,

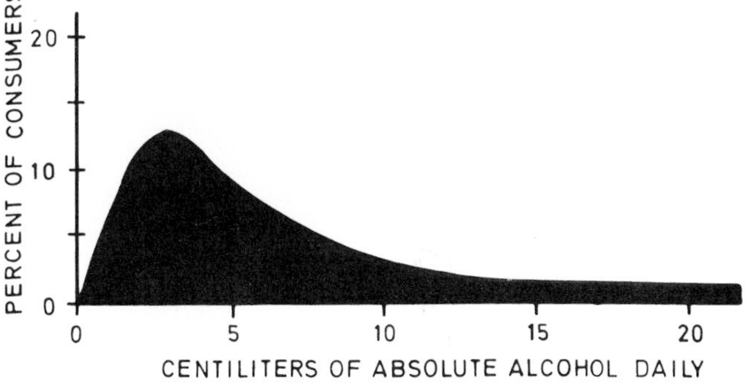

Fig. 46–2. Distribution of daily alcohol consumption in a population with an average yearly consumption of 25 liters of absolute alcohol, corresponding to 69.4 ml per day. From De Lint and Schmidt (1976) with permission.

Table 46–3. Average Alcohol Concentration in Alcoholic Beverages

	Ethanol	Concentration
Beverage	Volume %, Range (ml/100 ml)	Weight %, Mean (g/100 ml)
Beer	3.0–8.0	3.2
Wine, fruit wine	3.5–14.0	11.1
Vermouth, sherry	14.0–19.0	13.4
Liqueurs	20.0–42.0	26.0
Spirits	35.0–60.0	33.0

Source: Keup (1983) with permission.

Table 46–5. Per Capita Alcohol Consumption in Germany during the Past Century

Year	Liters of Absolute Alcohol
1900	10.1
1913	7.5
1929	5.2
1950	3.3
1960	7.8
1970	11.4
1975	12.4
1980	12.5
1985	11.8
1990	11.9
1991	12.2
1992	11.8
1993	11.3
1994	11.4
1995	11.1
1996	10.9

Source: Hüllinghorst (1999) with permission.

and the whole population is adapted to controlled drinking from childhood. In central and eastern Europe the drinking pattern is similar to that of Mediterranean populations, but alcohol ingestion with the aim of achieving a specific pharmacological effect is also known. In certain cultures, or religions, such as Islam and Hinduism, alcohol is by tradition forbidden, and consequently alcoholism has not been a public health problem in those populations. Even in countries where alcohol intake has been high for longer times, average consumption may vary remarkably over time for external reasons. In Germany, alcohol consumption was high at the beginning of this century, particularly in the lower social classes. Consumption then decreased, mainly for economic reasons; reached a minimal level during World War II; and increased after the war simultaneously with the economic improvement (Table 46–5). If people with an age of 15 years or older are considered (a realistic approach for alcoholism studies), the average annual consumption during 1980–1996 ranged between 10.9 and 12.4 liters of ethanol per person (Hüllinghorst, 1999), which is about 30 g (1 oz.) absolute alcohol per day.

Alcohol Drinking Pattern in Different Populations. The alcohol drinking pattern in different populations is usually estimated on the basis of classification by quantity, frequency, and variability. Populations are broadly divided into abstainers and drinkers. The drinking group is further divided into heavy, moderate to light, and infrequent drinkers. While it is quite difficult to classify different populations on the basis of any single criteria set for drinkers and nondrinkers, the available data do hint to a general pattern of drinking habits in these populations (Agarwal and Goedde, 1990; Agarwal et al., 1997). Whereas the number of abstainers and infrequent drinkers is significantly high in Mongoloids and Mexicans, for example, the proportion of heavy and moderate drinkers is relatively higher in Caucasians, Australian Aborigines, Chileans, Filipinos, and U.S. blacks. In most European countries, the United States, and Chile, the aggregate alcohol consumption is relatively higher than in other parts of the world except the Latin American countries. In the Scandinavian countries, particularly in Finland, the per capita alcohol consumption has grown in recent years after a long stable period due to an increase in the availability of alcohol beverages and better economic conditions (Rahkonen and Ahlström, 1989). Chinese cultural values stress moderate and infrequent drinking; intoxication is permissible only in certain social situations such as weddings, banquets, and family association meetings (Hughes et al., 1990). In contrast, drinking alcohol has spread rapidly through Japanese society during the past 20 years, as Japan achieved postwar reconstruction (Higuchi and Hayashida, 1998; Tsugane et al., 1999).

Table 46–4. Alcohol Consumption (Liter of Ethanol per Person) Between 1995 and 1997

Country	1995	1996	1997
Luxemburg	12.1	11.6	11.2
France	11.4	11.2	10.9
Germany	11.1	11.0	10.8
Portugal	11	11.2	11.3
Hungary	10	10.3	10.1
Spain	9.5	9.3	10.1
Czech Republic	10	10	10
Denmark	10	10	9.9
Austria	9.8	9.7	9.5
Switzerland	9.4	9.3	9.2
Ireland	9.2	9.2	9
Belgium	9.1	9.0	8.9
Greece	8.8	8.7	8.8
Italy	8.3	7.9	7.9
Netherlands	8	8.1	8.2
Australia	7.6	7.5	7.6
Great Britain	7.3	7.6	7.7
Japan	6.6	6.6	6.6
United States	6.5	6.6	6.6

Source: Jahrbuch Sucht 2000 (1999) with permission.

Among Asian-American groups, Koreans have the highest percentage of abstainers. But Koreans are likely to be one of the extremes, either abstainers or heavy drinkers (Chi et al., 1989). Heavy drinking among Japanese Americans and Korean Americans is as prevalent as it is among men in the general U.S. population (Kitano et al., 1988; Chi et al., 1989; Lubben et al., 1989). Data show that the drinking behavior of Filipino Americans living in Los Angeles appears more comparable to the Western pattern (Lubben et al., 1987). In the United States, a greater proportion of black men than all North Americans report lifelong abstinence, but the proportion of black men who reported to be heavy drinkers is only slightly lower than among whites (Klatsky et al., 1983). At the aggregate level, both black and white men (North Americans) appear to have similar drinking patterns. More recent epidemiological studies (Helzer et al., 1991; Bucholz, 1992) further support the notion that there are distinct ethnic differences in alcoholism prevalence, particularly among whites and nonwhites.

Gender Difference in Drinking Habits. Most research on alcoholism has focused on men, largely because men are more likely than women to drink at all and are particularly more likely to drink frequently and heavily (Wilsnack, 1996). Even if gender difference in body weight and water content are taken into account, male predominance in heavy drinking persists (Dawson and Archer, 1992; Midanik and Room, 1992). Conventionally it is believed that among women social and psychological forces are far stronger than genetics in the steps leading to alcoholism.

Alcoholism Rates

The most direct way of estimating the prevalence of alcoholism in a certain population is the application of a standardized alcoholism test (Bucholz, 1992). With this approach quantitative information can be obtained according to age, sex, social class, occupation, religion, or geographic region. Representative estimates of rates of alcoholism are possible if adequate population samples can be defined. The use of treatment prevalence or incidence, either clinical or ambulatory, usually leads to an underestimation of the rate of alcoholism, because not every alcoholic is treated. The decision for treatment is influenced by the attitude toward disease in general and alcoholism in particular in the population and by the number and quality of therapeutic institutions.

Another indirect approach proposed by Jellinek in 1942 uses the mortality caused by cirrhosis of the liver and the incidence of this disease in alcoholics as an index for estimating the prevalence of alcoholism (Brenner, 1959). This approach leads to an unreliable estimate, however, because it neglects the individual predisposition to liver cirrhosis and the varying cirrhosis-inducing potential of different alcoholic beverages.

As stated above, the frequency of alcoholism depends on the epidemiological approach and on the definition of alcoholism. In the United States, a number of national surveys on drinking problems have been conducted (Cherpital, 1999). The lifetime risk of developing alcoholism at some time varies between 4.6% and 9% for American adult men, depending on the diagnostic criteria used (Grant, 1996). According to a survey by Cahalan and Cisin (1976), a remarkable percentage of the population of the United States had some degree of one or more problems with drinking (Table 46–6).

Table 46–6. Prevalence (%) of Alcohol-Related Problems among Adults (Age 21+ Years) in the United States

	Males		Females	
Problem	Moderate	Severe	Moderate	Severe
Psychologic dependence	31	8	12	3
Frequent intoxication	3	14	1	2
Problems with current spouse or relatives	8	8	3	1
Symptomatic drinking	8	8	4	3
Belligerence	8	4	5	3
Health problems	6	6	4	4
Financial problems	6	3	2	1
Problems with friends or neighbors	5	2	3	<0.5
Job problems	3	3	2	1
Binge drinking	0	3	<0.5	<0.5
Problems with police or accidents	0	1	0	1
Combined problems score	28	15	17	4

Source: Cahalan and Cisin (1976) with permission.

Although large differences in rates of alcoholism in different cultures and countries are known, the exact knowledge about these differences is rather limited, mainly because of the tremendous methodological difficulties. The most reliable knowledge comes from North America. People of western European and Native American origin, particularly Irish and Apache, have the highest susceptibility to alcoholism, whereas Jews and Chinese are the most resistant (Murphy, 1982). The differences are obvious in terms of average alcohol consumption, death from alcoholism, rate of alcoholic psychosis and cirrhosis, alcohol-associated psychopathology, and homicide rate (Murphy, 1982). The existence of ethno-cultural differences in drinking behavior is a remarkable phenomenon of the United States. Among Catholics and liberal Protestants of most national origins there are relatively few abstainers and many heavy drinkers. Most Jewish men drink at least a little, but only a few drink heavily (Monteiro and Schuckit, 1989).

As mentioned before, in Japan, alcohol consumption was not a major problem before World War II. Since 1945, the per capita consumption has been increasing. Accordingly, the number of alcoholics has been increasing (Higuchi and Hayashida, 1998). About 5% of male Japanese over age 18 years are supposed to be habitual drinkers. Thus, under the influence of Western civilization and other changes in the society, drinking problems in Japan are approaching those of the United States and Europe.

Family Epidemiology

Family Studies

Because of a high degree of familial association, for many years, alcoholism was regarded as a distinct disease that may be transmitted from generation to generation (Dawson et al., 1992). A familial association could result from cultural factors that tend to encourage heavy drinking in family members. The family system may generate or promote the development of alcoholism in a family member. Children try to model their behavior on that of their parents, and in doing so they may also imitate their drinking habits. Alternatively, drinking may be discouraged in some families for religious, cultural, or climatic grounds, while in other families, constraints on heavy drinking may be virtually nonexistent. Moreover, interfamily and interclass differences in alcohol use may account for part of the variation in alcoholism rates among families. Therefore, "familial" does not necessarily mean "hereditary." Familial occurrences of alcoholism were already observed in the nineteenth century (Amark, 1951). A critical review of studies of the familial incidence of alcoholism summarized 39 investigations published in English that comprised family data on 6251 alcoholics and 4083 nonalcoholics (Cotton, 1979). Studies in which the target populations and methods of collecting data were inadequately described or definitions of alcoholism were insufficient or absent were excluded from this review.

The findings are summarized in Table 46–7. They clearly showed that regardless of the nature of the population of nonalcoholics studied, an alcoholic is more likely to have a mother, father, or distant relative who is an alcoholic. When lifetime prevalence of alcoholism in relatives of alcoholics were compared to that in the general population, a 4-fold increased risk in first-degree relatives and a 2-fold increased risk in second-degree relatives were observed. Higher family incidence of alcohol use and abuse does not necessarily reflect a genetic determination of alcoholism. Besides family traditions and cultural

Table 46–7. Paternal, Maternal, and Parental Alcoholism in Selected Studies of Alcoholics and Nonalcoholics

	Alcoholism		
Disease in Proband	Paternal	Maternal	Parental[a]
Alcoholism			
Studies *(N)*	32	23	23
Subjects *(N)*	4329	3500	3980
Percentage of alcoholics	27.0	4.9	30.8
Schizophrenia			
Studies *(N)*	3	2	3
Subjects *(N)*	654	553	1153
Percentage of alcoholics	9.2	0.4	7.1
Other psychiatric disease			
Studies *(N)*	5	3	3
Subjects *(N)*	1217	1082	1082
Percentage of alcoholics	9.9	1.8	12.0
No psychiatric disease			
Studies *(N)*	5	3	4
Subjects *(N)*	788	692	922
Percentage of alcoholics	5.2	1.2	4.7

[a]Parental alcoholism combines subjects who had an alcoholic mother or father, or both. Data were included from studies that reported statistics for fathers and mothers or for parents (not specifying father or mother).
Source: Cotton (1979) with permission.

habits, there are family environmental effects such as parental loss, birth order, and the sex of the immediately elder siblings that may influence an individual's alcohol drinking behavior. Heritable familial attributes, as well as similarities in the social environment of family members, also appear to play a role in familial transmission of alcoholism. Thus, family systems (family reactivity patterns, ethnic family styles, gender of the alcoholic spouse, and stages of alcoholism) are an important variable in the genesis, consequences and treatment of alcoholism.

The incidence of parental alcoholism was higher in psychiatric than in nonpsychiatric patients, but alcoholics were still much more likely than nonalcoholics to have had parents who were alcoholics. This applies to both paternal and maternal alcoholics, although the incidence figures in the parents reflect the well-known sex differences of alcoholism. Nearly one-third of the alcoholics had at least one parent who was an alcoholic. This is a considerable proportion, although not as high as the 52% reported in an earlier comprehensive review, which, in addition, included the major studies published in languages other than English (Goodwin, 1971). In one study (Guze et al., 1986), the rate of alcoholism was calculated to be significantly higher in relatives of probands (15.3%) than in nonalcoholic controls (8.7%).

The alcoholism prevalence figures given in Table 46–7 roughly approach lifetime morbidity risks because the parents of the index cases usually will have completely or nearly completely surpassed their risk period, and an age correction is therefore not necessary. Some further trends apparent from the review by Cotton (1979) should be mentioned: rates of alcoholism in siblings were consistently higher in samples of alcoholics than in all types of nonalcoholics who were studied. The incidence of alcoholism in near relatives appeared to be higher than in more distant ones. Female alcoholics were more likely than male alcoholics to come from families in which pathological drinking had been known. Although the rate of alcoholism was highest in the parents of alcoholics, it was found to be somewhat increased in the parents of patients with other psychiatric diseases (Table 46–7). This observation has two implications. First, it points to some specificity in the predisposition to alcoholism. Second, there is a certain relationship of alcoholism to other psychiatric diagnoses, particularly those with depressive and psychopathological features.

Another interesting fact emerges from the reported family studies. Alcoholics with a family history of alcoholism tend to drink early in life and have more social and personal problems than alcoholics without a family history of alcoholism (Hesselbrock, 1995). Alcoholics with a positive family history on both the paternal and maternal sides of their pedigree experience greater psychosocial and physical consequences of alcohol abuse than do other alcoholics. It is important to remember, however, that 47% to 82% of alcoholics do not come from families in which one or both parents are alcoholics (Cotton, 1979). Therefore, it is worthwhile to differentiate between alcoholics with and without family histories of alcoholism (Johnson and Pickens, 2001).

In 1966, a hypothesis was advanced that alcoholism is transmitted by an X-linked recessive gene (Cruz-Coke and Varela, 1966); however, the empirical data on alcoholism in relatives obtained in the thorough epidemiological investigation by Amark (1951) are not compatible with X-linked inheritance (Winokur, 1967; Kaij and Dock, 1975). Furthermore, it is improbable that the effect of a single gene can be defined by studying the "phenotype" of a disease that is difficult to define in patients and difficult to ascertain in families and which depends on the availability and even the price of alcohol.

Goodwin (1981) has reviewed the methodological problems of family studies on alcoholism. The information on drinking habits and alcohol abuse is usually retrospective and collected from patient records, questionnaires, or interviews. Family data are usually obtained by secondhand, even conflicting, information. Very rarely are age corrections are applied to obtain lifelong morbidity rates (Winokur et al., 1970). Another problem in the interpretation of family studies relates to assortative mating, which is known to exist for individuals with psychiatric problems and alcoholics in particular (Hall et al., 1983a, 1983b).

Twin Studies

Estimates of genetic and environmental contributions to liability are obtained from twin studies by comparing the resemblance of identical (monozygotic or MZ) and fraternal (dizygotic or DZ) twin pairs. MZ twins within a pair resemble one another because they share all of their genetic and common environmental factors, while DZ pairs share (on average) half of their segregating genes and all of their common environment. Estimates from twin studies assume that MZ and DZ pairs are equally similar in their environments relevant to the development of alcoholism. Thus, the twin study paradigm is a powerful method to study complex and heterogeneous trait disorders. Differences between identical twins would presumably reflect environmental influences, while differences between nonidentical twins may be due to either heredity or environment, or both. Therefore, if alcoholism has a hereditary basis, MZ twin pairs should tend to be more similar in their drinking behavior and alcohol-related problems than are DZ twin pairs (Pickens et al., 1991).

The use of twin studies in behavioral genetics is problematic. The special twin situation, especially in childhood and youth, may lead to certain deviations from usual development. Twins form a social group; they may show identification with one another, but role differentiation is also observed, even in identical twin pairs. Particular attention must be paid to sampling criteria, and strict epidemiological measures must be applied. The possibility that twins who are more similar to one an-

Table 46–8. Twin Studies on Alcohol Abuse and Alcoholism

References	No. of Pairs[a]	Characteristics Studied	Concordance Rates (%)[a] MZ	DZ	h^2
Kaij, 1960	48 MZ, 126 DZ males	Five degrees of alcohol abuse	55.6–71.4	20.0–32.3	
Partanen et al., 1966	172 MZ, 557 DZ males	Amount of intake, Density of drinking, Lack of control			0.36 0.39 0.14
Loehlin, 1972	850 like-sex pairs	"Had a hangover" "Never any drinking," "Used alcohol excessively" "Drink before breakfast"			0.62 0.54 0.36 0.36
Hrubec and Omenn, 1981	15,924 males	Alcoholism, including alcohol psychosis	26.3	11.9	
Gurling et al., 1981	28 MZ, 28 DZ, males and females	Alcohol dependence	21	25	
Kaprio et al., 1987	879 MZ, 1940 DZ	Frequency of beer	40.8	21.5	0.39
		Frequency of spirits	32.3	13.2	0.38
		Density of drinking	43.6	23.8	0.40
		Quantity of drinking	37.4	19.3	0.36

Some Newer Studies[b]	No. of Pairs[a]	Result
Pickens et al., 1991	50 MZ, 64 DZ male and 31 MZ, 24 DZ female same-sex twin pairs	Significant MZ/DZ differences in conconcordance in male twins for both abuse and dependence, and only dependence in female twins (h^2 = 0.35 for males, 0.24 for females)
Kendler et al., 1992	1030 pairs of female same-sex twins	Familial resemblance for alcoholism was attributable to genetic factors, with heritability of liability between 51% and 59%
Heath et al., 1997	3810 adult Australian twins	There is an important genetic influence for frequency and quantity (h^2 = 0.66 in females, 0.51–0.75 for males for frequency; 0.57 in females and 0.24–0.61 in males for quantity
Prescott and Kendler, 1999; Prescott, 2001	3049 female, 1070 male twins	Males having higher prevalence of alcohol abuse, substantial family resemblance for alcohol abuse, and alcohol problems

[a]MZ, monozygotic or identical; DZ, dizygotic or fraternal; h^2, heritability.
[b]From Johnson and Leff, 1999.

other for a particular trait under study have a higher chance of being included in an investigation has to be avoided. A number of twin studies on alcohol abuse or alcoholism have been reported (Table 46–8). These studies basically differ in methods used to identify the affected individuals.

In a thorough Finnish investigation, the twins were personally interviewed (Partanen et al., 1966). Factor analysis of the interview data produced three main factors with certain heritability: amount of alcohol intake, density of alcohol intake, and lack of control. Thus the drinking "pattern" was apparently under moderate to minimal genetic influence, but drunkenness arrests, addictive symptoms, and social complications had still lower heritabilities. Lack of control was subject to the greater genetic influence in younger twins ($h^2 = 0.54$), whereas this was not the case for the older ones ($h^2 = 0.07$). The greatest genetic influence was seen when subjects were dichotomized into drinkers and abstainers (Partanen et al., 1966).

The U.S. National Merit Twin Study was based on a self-rating questionnaire that contained 13 items related to alcohol intake and allowed the calculation of heritabilities for these items (Loehlin, 1972). Factors that might protect an individual against alcohol abuse, such as having had hangovers or having never drunk heavily, had the highest heritability, and excessive drinking or drinking before breakfast had moderate heritability. In the Swedish study, the twins were ascertained from the persons registered by the temperance board as having a drinking problem (Kaij, 1960). They were classified into five categories of alcohol abuse, and an increasing difference in concordance rates between the monozygotic (MZ) and dizygotic (DZ) pairs with increasing degree of alcohol abuse was found. Another twin study looked at genetic influence on medical consequences of alcoholism. This study, which was based on medical histories from military service records, hospital records, and questionnaires, also gave information on alcoholism (Hrubec and Omenn, 1981). The concordance rate for alcoholism, including alcoholic psychosis, was reported to be much higher in MZ twins than in DZ pairs. Reed et al. (1996) published a follow-up of this sample using medical records through 1994 and obtained similar estimates.

The British study was based on the psychiatric twin register of Maudsley Hospital (Gurling et al., 1981). A consecutive series of same sex alcoholic twin probands was established. Information on probands and their co-twins was gathered by standardized interviews and hospital records. In contrast to other studies, the concordance rates of MZ and DZ twins did not differ significantly, but more than one-third of the twins were below age 40 years when examined, suggesting that alcohol dependence may yet develop in a proportion of co-twins. Another large, population-based study from Finland confirmed a genetic influence on frequency and quantity of drinking, but did not find such an influence for passing out (Kaprio et al., 1987). One study examined a sample of 90 adult twin pairs, 37 non-twin sibling pairs, and 46 pairs of unrelated individuals reared together (Gabrielli and Plomin, 1985). The authors concluded that certain alcohol-drinking behaviors are probably genetically influenced. However, the genetic variance was found to be non-additive.

Pickens et al. (1991) reported results for same-sex twin pairs who were clinically interviewed. Twin pair similarity was high for both diagnostic definitions among males, with higher heritability estimates for alcohol abuse-dependence (AAD) and stronger evidence for family environment for AAD. A similar pattern was reported for female twins, although the magnitude of estimates was lower than those reported for males. The data reported by McGue et al. (1992b) included the earlier sample (Pickens et al., 1991) plus opposite-sex pairs and pairs whose co-twins were assessed only via questionnaire. Based on this information, MZ and DZ female pairs had similar resemblance for AAD, yielding evidence for common environmental but not genetic contributions to the familiality of alcoholism in women. Results for male twins were similar to those found previously (Pickens et al., 1991), suggesting that genetic influence may be substantial only in the etiology of early-onset male alcoholism.

Koskenvuo et al. (1984) reported results from merging Finnish psychiatric records against the national twin registry to identify twins who received alcohol-related discharge diagnoses through 1979. Substantial heritability was reported for males, but, due to very low prevalence in females, no concordant female cases were observed. A follow-up to this study published by Romanov et al. (1991) included information from hospital records through 1985 for male pairs, yielding more complete ascertainment and resulting in higher heritability estimates. Allgulander et al. (1991) used similar procedures with data from the Swedish Twin Registry to identify twins who received alcohol-related discharge diagnoses. For both male and female twin pairs, DZ pairs were nearly as similar as MZ pairs, yielding low heritability estimates and evidence for moderate common environmental effects. The prevalence of alcoholism in the sample was quite low, suggesting severe underascertainment of cases.

Genetics has been shown to be an important determinant of vulnerability to alcoholism in females (Kendler et al., 1992). The authors investigated 1080 adult pairs of female twins for their alcohol-related behavior. The study revealed that at every level of alcoholism, identical twins were significantly more likely than fraternal twins to have similar histories of alcoholism. These results support an earlier finding from a Swedish study of women who had been adopted (Cloninger et al., 1981). These authors found a pattern of genetic transmission of alcoholism from mothers to daughters. Kendler et al. (1997) reported results from merging Swedish TBR records with the Swedish twin registry for twins born between 1902 and 1949. MZ twin pairs were substantially more similar for TBR than DZ pairs, yielding moderate evidence of genetic influences plus evidence of some common environmental effects. True et al. (1996) reported results from telephone interviews with male twin pairs who are members of the Vietnam Era Twin (VET) registry. Subjects were eligible for inclusion in the registry if they were born between 1939 and 1957 and both twins served in the U.S. military. Of over 10,000 eligible twins, 79% were located and interviewed. MZ twins were significantly more similar than DZ twins, producing a heritability estimate of 0.55 with no evidence for common environmental influences.

Heath et al. (1997) reported results from a telephone interview assessment of members of the Australian National Health and Medical Research Council twin registry. Participants were eligible based on prior research participation, and 86% of those eligible were interviewed. This study found strong evidence for genetic influences on the development of alcoholism for both sexes, while the evidence for common environmental effects was negligible. Recently, a population-based sample of male twins was studied in the United States for genetic and environmental contributions to alcohol abuse and dependence (Prescott and Kendler, 1999). Results based on two definitions of treatment (inpatient or outpatient alcohol treatment, and any treatment) were compared to results from the random ascertainment method originally used in the sample. Among individuals who were diagnosed as alcoholic, males were twice as likely as females to enter alcohol treatment. This difference was not accounted for by sex differences in clinical severity or course, suggesting that there were sex-related differences in treatment entry. Among males, heritability estimates were similar across sampling methods. The treatment ascertainment methods yielded higher estimates of common environmental influences, a finding similar to the results of twin studies that employed archival and treatment-based ascertainment.

Among females, heritability estimates based on the broad definition of treatment were similar to those obtained using the random ascertainment design, but estimates based on alcoholism treatment were (nonsignificantly) lower (Prescott, 2001). These results provide partial support for the hypothesis that differences in sampling method may account for differences among studies in heritability estimates.

Twin Studies of Alcohol Consumption, Metabolism, and Sensitivity

Comparison of identical (MZ) and nonidentical (DZ) twins has provided some new insights for estimating the relative contribution of environmental and genetic factors to individual differences in alcohol consumption pattern and sensitivity to alcohol (Vesell et al., 1971; Marshall and Gurling, 1989).

Alcohol Consumption. The distribution of alcohol consumption in the Australian Twin Register study (Heath et al., 1997) showed that twin pairs were highly concordant both for teenage drinking and for early vs. late onset of drinking. Environmental influences on onset of drinking appeared to be sex-specific. Among drinkers, early vs. late onset of drinking was more strongly influenced by inherited factors in females but by shared social environment (e.g., family background or peer pressure) in males. In another large study on the Finnish Twin Cohort (Kaprio et al., 1992) significant genetic variance was found for each of the drinking measures. Co-twins in more frequent social contacts with one another reported greater similarity in their use of alcohol, but heritable variance persisted after the effects of age and social contact were removed from both mean levels and co-twin resemblance. Follow-up analyses of absolute changes in alcohol use revealed heritable influences on the disposition to change (Kaprio et al., 1992).

Alcohol Metabolism. Twin studies have clearly demonstrated that alcohol metabolism rate is under genetic control (reviewed by Martin, 1987). Four twin studies on alcohol elimination rate are compiled in Table 46–9, giving heritability estimates of 0.45

Table 46–9. Heritabilities (h^2)[a] of Alcohol Elimination (β in mg/ml $\times$ h) in Four Different Twin Studies

Applied Dose of Alcohol	No. and Zygosity of Twin Pairs	h^2	Reference
0.5 g/kg	10 MZ, 10 DZ	0.63	Lüth, 1939
1.0 ml/kg	7 MZ, 7 DZ	0.98	Vesell et al., 1971
1.2 ml/kg	19 MZ, 21 DZ	0.46	Kopun and Propping, 1977
0.75 g/kg	85 MZ, 121 DZ	0.44 m. 0.57 w.	Martin et al., 1985

[a]h^2 (heritability) was estimated with the formula $(V_{DZ} - V_{MZ})/V_{DZ}$.

to 0.60. Although studies with a large sample of twins confirmed the extensive role of ephemeral environmental influences on rates of alcohol metabolism, these studies failed to identify the nature of these environmental influences.

Psychomotor Sensitivity to Alcohol. Inherited differences in reactivity or sensitivity to a standard dose of alcohol, noted in sons of alcoholics, have been hypothesized to account for the increased propensity to alcoholism among these subjects (Schuckit and Smith, 2001a). A study of psychomotor performance and subjective intoxication, in twin pairs unselected for risk of alcoholism, after intake of alcohol (0.75g/kg body weight) has shown a significant difference in alcohol-specific reactivity such as body sway and other psychomotor performance tests (Heath et al., 1999). Multivariate genetic analysis of these studies has further helped to identify two distinct genetic factors. The first factor had high loadings on drinking history, subjective intoxication, and body sway. The second factor had high loadings on blood alcohol concentration (BAC) and on tests of psychomotor coordination, but low loading on drinking history and subjective ratings. In females only, body sway also loaded on this second, BAC-sensitive factor, as well as on the first, drinking-history sensitive factor.

Several other studies show a similarity in alcohol consumption among separated twins, eliminating the possible influence of a shared environment (Hayakawa, 1987; Kaprio et al., 1992). In addition to these studies, the general population twin studies also have demonstrated that alcohol consumption patterns are more alike in MZ than in DZ twin pairs (Kaprio et al., 1987; Heath et al., 1999). In summary, these twin studies show the important part played by genetic differences in determining how much people drink and how they are affected by alcohol.

Adoption Studies

A systematic approach to separate "nature" from "nurture" is to study individuals who were separated from their biological relatives soon after birth and raised by nonrelated foster parents and to compare them with respect to characteristics of alcohol abuse with both their biological and adoptive parents. This approach is based on the premise that the genetic trait present in the affected biological parent will still be expressed in adoptees, regardless of the genotypic status and environmental circumstances of the foster parents. In studies of intact families, the effects of genetic and common environment are not separable. Adoption studies separate these effects because adoptees receive their genetic heritage from one set of parents and their rearing environment from another set. The degree to which adoptees resemble their biological relatives is a direct measure of genetic influence, while the degree to which they resemble their adoptive relatives is a measure of the influence of family environment.

A number of studies have been published in the last decade supporting the influence of genetic susceptibility to alcoholism (Cook, 2000; Schuckit, 2000; Enoch and Goldman, 2001). Extensive adoption studies conducted in Denmark and Sweden have provided substantial evidence that alcoholism is genetically influenced, and that there are distinct patterns of alcoholism with different genetic and environmental causes (Cloninger et al., 1981; Bohman et al., 1987). Table 46–10 gives an overview on the research strategies that have been used in these adoption studies. The main adoption studies and their results are summarized in Table 46–11.

When the adopted-away sons of an alcoholic parent were compared to their siblings raised by the alcoholic biological parent, a remarkably similar rate of alcoholism was noted in both groups. Subsequent adoption studies from other countries have clearly shown that children born to alcoholic parents but adopted away during infancy were at greater risk for alcoholism than were adopted-away children born to nonalcoholic parents (Sigvardsson et al., 1996).

The first adoption study on alcoholism is the only one that failed to find a genetic influence on the development of alcoholism (Roe, 1944). This outcome might have resulted from methodological peculiarities in that the experimental and control groups of adoptees did not differ impressively in their drinking habits. Among the alcoholic parents, 7% used alcohol regularly but not necessarily heavily, 63% had occasional alcohol intake, and 30% were abstainers. The respective figures for the parents of the control adoptees were 9%, 55%, and 36%. Furthermore, adoptees had not passed the whole risk period, and the groups were not sex matched. Therefore, it is difficult to know how much credit can be given to this small study.

The extensive adoption studies carried out in Denmark using the Danish population registers substantiated the influence of genetic factors on alcoholism (Goodwin et al., 1977; Bohman et al., 1981, 1987). Four groups of subjects were interviewed: sons and daughters of alcoholics who had been raised by nonalcoholic foster parents, and sons and daughters of alcoholics who had been raised by their alcoholic biological parents. Each group was paired with a control group of adoptees. It is important to note that the interviews were conducted by Danish psychiatrists who were kept "blind" about the identity of the interviewees.

Sons of alcoholics were nearly 4 times more likely to be "alcoholic, ever" than were sons of nonalcoholics (Table 46–12). Of the adopted daughters of alcoholics, 2% were alcoholic and 2% had serious problems from drinking. In the adopted daughter control group, 4% were alcoholic. Thus, in both the female proband and control groups, a higher than expected prevalence (expected to be 0.1% to 1.0%) of alcoholism was found. The authors hypothesize that some of the biological parents of the controls had undetected alcoholism. The Danish adoption studies

Table 46–10. Research Strategies Applied in Adoption Studies on Alcoholism

Index Cases	Controls	Question Examined	References
Adopted-away offspring of alcoholic parents	Adopted-away offspring of normal parents	Is alcoholism more frequent among offspring of alcoholics than among offspring of control parents?	Roe, 1944; Goodwin et al., 1973, 1974, 1977; Bohman, 1978; Cloninger et al., 1981
Alcoholic adoptees	Normal adoptees	Is alcoholism more frequent among biologic parents than among adoptive parents?	Cadoret and Gath, 1978; Bohman et al., 1981
Alcoholics with half-siblings and an alcoholic biologic parent and raised in nonalcoholic foster homes	Half-siblings of alcoholics without biologic alcoholic parents and raised by an alcoholic foster parent	Does biologic relationship predict alcoholism with greater reliability than foster relationship?	Schuckit, 1972

Table 46–11. Main Adoption Studies on Alcoholism

Studies	Sample	Essential Results
United States		
Roe, 1944	36 adopted-away children of fathers who were "heavy drinkers" compared with 25 adoptees with normal biologic parents	At the time of follow-up (mean age, 28–31 years), there were no differences in alcohol consumption between the two groups
Schuckit, 1972	98 half-siblings of 41 alcoholic probands	Having an alcoholic biologic parent predicted alcoholism with greater reliability than being raised by an alcoholic foster parent
Cadoret and Gath, 1978	84 adoptees examined for alcoholism	Alcoholism was more frequent in those adoptees who had an alcoholic biologic parent
Denmark		
Goodwin et al., 1973	55 sons of alcoholics raised by nonalcoholic foster parents and 78 male control adoptees	Offspring of alcoholics were more likely to have alcohol problems than were offspring of controls
Goodwin et al., 1974	20 sons of alcoholics raised by nonalcoholic foster parents and 30 male siblings raised by the alcoholic biologic parents	Rates of alcoholism were increased in both groups
Goodwin et al., 1977a	49 daughters of alcoholics raised by nonalcoholic foster parents and 47 female control adoptees	Both groups of adoptees had increased rates of alcohol problems
Goodwin et al., 1977b	49 daughters of alcoholics raised by nonalcoholic foster parents and 81 female siblings raised by the alcoholic biologic parents	Adopted and nonadopted daughters of alcoholics had a higher rate of alcoholism than was the expected frequency in the general population
Sweden		
Bohman, 1978	Official registers of alcoholic adoptees and their biologic and adoptive parents	There was a significant correlation in the records between alcoholism in biologic parents and in their adopted-away sons
Bohman et al., 1981	913 female adoptees among whom 51 biologic mothers and 307 biologic fathers had abused alcohol	There was a 3-fold excess of alcohol abusers among the female adoptees of alcoholic biologic mothers; the excess was lower in adoptees of alcoholic biologic fathers
Cloninger et al., 1981	862 male adoptees among whom severity of alcohol abuse was classified	With the help of multivariate statistical procedures, two types of alcoholism were differentiated, one of which was highly heritable
Some newer studies[a]		
McGue et al., 1992	653 adopted families, with one adopted child and other siblings	Relationship between parental problem drinking, family functioning, and adolscent alcohol involvement was moderate and significant among birth offspring, not among adoptive offspring
Cadoret et al., 1996	197 adult adoptees (95 male and 102 female)	A genetic factor is present for which alcoholism is a marker
Sigvardsson et al., 1996	577 mothers and 660 female adoptees	Both type 2 and severe type 1 alcoholism were confirmed as independently heritable forms of alcoholism

[a]From: Johnson and Leff, 1999.

have been criticized because of the arbitrary nature of the drinking classification (Tolor and Tamerin, 1973). If one combines the categories of alcoholism and problem drinking, then the difference between the probands and controls disappears. Because categorization was made by the "blind" interviewers, however, interviewer bias can be eliminated.

Swedish adoption studies also point to the existence of genetic factors in the etiology of alcoholism (Cadoret and Gath, 1978; Cloninger et al., 1981; Bohman et al., 1981); however, there is no consistent trend in the genetic influences on sex differences. The conflicting results of the different adoption studies as to the two sexes probably come from the differences in the expected rates of alcoholism in men and women in the respective populations. The only recent adoption studies conducted in the United States are those by Cadoret in Iowa (Cadoret et al., 1994). These studies show significantly higher risk to adopted-away sons from alcoholic biological backgrounds than in control adoptees, which is consistent with a genetic influence on risk of alcoholism in men.

Sex Differences in the Transmission of Alcoholism

There is consistent evidence that relatives of women treated for alcoholism have higher risk for alcoholism than do relatives of treated males (Prescott and Kendler, 1999). This suggests that women in treatment tend to have higher liability than their male counterparts (McGue and Slutske, 1996; Prescott, 2001). The results for untreated female alcoholics are less clear. The evidence regarding sex-specific transmission varies across studies, providing no consensus as to whether different sets of genetic factors influence the development of alcoholism in males and females (Hill, 1995). Some evidence from molecular genetic studies supports the existence of sex-specific loci (Paterson and Petronis, 1999), and a definitive answer to this issue will probably come from molecular rather than epidemiological studies.

Taken together, the results of family, twin, and adoption studies are compatible with the existence of genetic factors in the etiology of alcohol abuse. Twin and adoption studies have established the importance of genetic influences in the etiology of alcoholism in males. The evidence for females is less consistent, but newer studies suggest a similar degree of genetic influence. Women treated for alcoholism appear to have greater liability than treated males, but it is unclear whether this is true for untreated alcoholics. Results from some, but not all, studies suggest the existence of sex-specific transmission of genetic liability for alcoholism. However, no simple mode of inheritance should be expected from such an endpoint, and none was observed. A multifactorial or multicausal system would seem most likely. Sophisticated statistical models have been applied, taking into account sex differences of psychiatric symptoms, alcoholism rates, and criminality, as well as familial transmission, but these have not reduced the degree of specific genetic factors involved. A real improvement of our understanding will ultimately depend

Table 46–12. Comparison of Drinking Problems and Patterns in Adoptees with and without Alcoholic Biologic Parents

	Probands: Alcoholic Biologic Parents (N = 55)	Controls: No Alcoholic Biologic Parents (N = 78)
Problem		
Amnesia	53	41
Delirium tremens	6	1
Drunken driving arrests	7	4
Hallucinations[a]	6	0
Hospitalized for drinking	7	0
Job trouble	7	3
Loss of control[b]	35	17
Marital trouble	18	9
Morning drinking[b]	29	11
Police trouble, other	15	8
Rum fits	2	0
Social disapproval	6	8
Treated for drinking, any[a]	9	1
Tremor	24	22
Drinking pattern		
Alcoholic, ever[b]	18	5
Heavy drinker, ever	22	36
Moderate drinker	51	45
Problem drinker, ever	9	14

[a]$P < .05$.
[b]$p < .02$.
Source: Goodwin et al. (1973) with permission.

on the integration of genetic and pathophysiological mechanisms that lead to alcoholism. In males, genetic differences are important in youth but environmental factors increasingly influence their drinking habits as they age. In females, although genetic factors determine the alcohol consumption profile, the influence of both genetic and environmental variations increases considerably with age.

Mode of Inheritance

Although adoption and twin studies have proven useful in answering the question of nature vs. nurture, the mode of inheritance of alcoholism is still an unresolved matter. None of the evidence hitherto put forward suggests that susceptibility to alcoholism is inherited via a simple Mendelian dominant, recessive, or sex-linked transmission. Even if the inheritance of certain biological factors involved in alcoholism is assumed to be Mendelian, the effect of these factors on the development of complex disorders may still not fit a simple genetic model. The observed transmission of the liability of risk for alcoholism does not indicate the involvement of a single autosomal or sex-linked gene as the first- and second-degree relatives of alcoholics are about equally at risk to become alcoholic and the sex of the proband does not influence the degree of risk in the relatives (Dinwiddie and Cloninger, 1989). Thus, a substantial degree of etiological heterogeneity in the alcoholism phenotype results in the ultimate manifestation of the disorder dependent on poorly understood gene–environment interactions.

Phenotyping Alcoholism

The family, twin, and adoption studies described above present substantial evidence suggesting a genetic contribution to alcoholism. The focus of current genetic research has therefore shifted to identifying specific symptoms of alcoholism that are more or less heritable than others. A more heritable alcoholism phenotype would facilitate discovery of specific alcoholism genes underlying the risk of alcoholism. Johnson et al. (1996) addressed this issue by identifying alcoholism symptoms that were more heritable in a sample of 113 MZ/DZ male twin pairs. They identified 7 alcoholism symptoms that were more "genetic" and 14 that were more "environmental" (nongenetic) in their etiology. A recent study (Slutske et al., 1999) has attempted to replicate and extend these findings in a much larger sample of male twin pairs. Out of 19 alcoholism symptoms assessed in both studies, 6 symptoms, classified in the original study as genetic, only 3 were classified similarly in the replication study; out of the 13 symptoms classified in the Johnson et al. study as environmental, 10 were classified as genetic and 3 as environmental in the study reported by Slutske et al. (1999). Thus the results of the original study were not replicated, probably due to limitations of the modest size of the sample in the original study. Nor was the replication study able to identify subgroups of symptoms that were clearly more genetically influenced than the others. Nevertheless, the study of Slutske et al. (1999) suggests that there may exist considerable variation in the relative magnitude of genetic influence for different alcoholism symptoms (Saccone et al., 2000; Crabbe, 2001).

Associations with Other Diseases

Conceptually, peculiarities that precede alcoholism have to be differentiated from those that are simply the consequence of alcohol abuse. Often these two possibilities are difficult to disentangle, particularly at the level of psychiatric symptomatology; depression or social pathology may exist before alcohol abuse or may be secondary to alcoholism. Nevertheless, an attempt to differentiate these factors has to be undertaken.

Psychiatric Symptoms Preceding Alcoholism

At least two of Jellinek's types of alcoholism are based on certain personality characteristics. This is not a contradiction to the failure to identify a single personality type among alcoholics. Alcoholism is more frequent than any other form of mental illness in relatives of alcoholics (Cotton, 1979). Hyperactive children are at an increased risk of developing alcoholism (Goodwin et al., 1975; Tarter and Alterman, 1984), and biological but not adoptive parents of hyperactive children have an increased incidence of alcoholism and sociopathy (Morrison and Stewart, 1973). Similarly, the three dimensions of novelty seeking, harm avoidance, and reward dependence as assessed by a semi-structured interview at ages 10 to 11 years were shown to be correlated with alcohol abuse in young adults (Cloninger et al., 1988). The two childhood variables novelty seeking and low harm avoidance distinguished the boys regarding alcohol abuse: their risk varied from 4% to 75%, depending on childhood personality type. In a prospective study of young men at high risk for alcoholism, a more disturbed school career and more frequent referrals to a school psychologist were reported, but the index and control groups did not differ with respect to alcohol consumption (Schulsinger et al., 1986; Knop et al., 1993). The probands were virtually too young to develop alcoholism. Therefore, an underlying neurophysiological abnormality could manifest itself as hyperactivity in children and as sociopathy and alcoholism in later life (Tarter and Alterman, 1984).

Alcoholism and depression are reported to occur more frequently than expected in the same individual and in members of his or her family (Swendsen and Merikangas, 2000). According to Winokur and his colleagues (1970), alcoholism and depression have common etiologies called "depressive spectrum disease." They observed that alcoholism predominated in the male relatives and depression in the female relatives of the alcoholic probands. When alcoholism and depression were considered together, the morbidity in both the sexes was approximately equal. Another study confirms that depression and alcoholism are not alternate manifestations of the same underlying disorder (Maier and Merikangas, 1996). Depressives without alcoholism did not transmit alcoholism to relatives, whereas individuals with depression and alcoholism transmitted both depression and alcoholism.

Diseases Secondary to Alcoholism

A vast number of organ diseases that are a consequence of chronic alcoholism are known (Table 46–13). Although people probably differ in their predisposition to certain diseases, only a small proportion of alcoholics develop any of these diseases. Moreover, the involvement of genetic factors is known in only in a few disorders.

Disorders without Known Genetic Predisposition. A characteristic consequence of alcoholism is the acute alcohol withdrawal syndrome (Murray, 1981). The acute withdrawal includes a broad spectrum of severity, from slight tremor, malaise, and irritability to the severe delirium tremens. Only ~1% to 15% of alcoholics develop delirium tremens (Zilker, 1999). It seems reasonable to speculate that genetically determined thresholds for withdrawal effects of alcohol exist (Schmidt and Sander, 2000).

Alcoholic Brain Damage. There is still debate as to whether alcohol per se causes brain damage. The main problem has been to identify those lesions caused by alcohol itself and those caused by other common alcohol-related factors, chiefly thiamin deficiency. Careful selection and classification of alcoholic cases into those with and without these complications, together with detailed quantitative neuropathological analyses, has provided useful data (Harper, 1998; Brooks, 2000; Wuethrich, 2001). There is brain shrinkage in uncomplicated cases of alcoholics that can largely be accounted for by the loss of white matter. Some of this damage appears to be reversible. However, alcohol-related neuronal loss has been documented in specific regions of the cerebral cortex (superior frontal association cortex), hypothalamus (supraoptic and paraventricular nuclei), and cerebellum. The data are conflicting for several regions: the hippocampus, amygdala, and locus ceruleus. No change is found in the basal ganglia, nucleus basalis, or serotonergic raphe nuclei.

Table 46–13. Main Disorders Secondary to Chronic Alcoholism

Alcoholic hepatitis
Amblyopia
Cancer of the esophagus
Cardiomyopathy
Central pontine myelinolysis
Cerebellar cortical degeneration
Cerebral degeneration
Fatty liver
Gastritis
Impairment of leukocyte mobilization
Leukopenia
Liver cirrhosis
Macrocytes
Marchiafava-Bignami disease
Pancreatitis
Pellagra
Thrombocytopenia
Wernicke-Korsakoff syndrome
Zieve's syndrome

Source: Feuerlein (1984) with permission.

Many of the regions that are normal in uncomplicated alcoholics are damaged in those with the Wernicke-Korsakoff syndrome. Dendritic and synaptic changes have been documented in uncomplicated alcoholics and these, together with receptor and transmitter changes, may explain functional changes and cognitive deficits that precede the more severe structural neuronal changes. The pattern of damage appears to be somewhat different and species-specific in animal models of alcohol toxicity. Pathological changes that have been found to correlate with alcohol intake include white matter loss and neuronal loss in the hypothalamus and cerebellum.

Alcohol and Cancer. Together with tobacco smoke, alcohol is the main cause for upper gastrointestinal tract cancer in industrialized countries. It is also a risk factor to develop liver, breast, and colorectal cancer. However, the tumor-promoting effects of alcohol intake are poorly understood, and alcohol is not carcinogenic in the animal model. There is increasing evidence, that alcohol metabolism, rather than alcohol itself, is generating carcinogenic and cell-toxic compounds. Acetaldehyde, the main metabolite of ethanol, is highly toxic and mutagenic, and it has been shown to be carcinogenic in animals. Polymorphisms and mutations in the genes coding for enzymes responsible for acetaldehyde production and degradation have been associated with an increased cancer risk in humans (Homann et al., 2000). Acetaldehyde can also be produced from ethanol by the physiological microflora. High microbial acetaldehyde levels after ethanol intake have been described in the upper gastrointestinal tact and colorectum, both sites known to represent organs susceptible for ethanol-associated carcinogenesis (Seitz et al., 1998; Jokelainen, 2001).

A great number of epidemiological data have identified chronic alcohol consumption as a significant risk factor for upper alimentary tract cancer, including cancer of the oropharynx, larynx, and esophagus, and for the liver. In contrast to these organs, the risk by which alcohol consumption increases cancer in the large intestine and in the breast is much smaller. However, although the risk may be lower, carcinogenesis can be enhanced with relatively low daily doses of ethanol. Although the exact mechanisms by which chronic alcohol ingestion stimulates carcinogenesis are not known, experimental studies in animals support the concept that ethanol is not a carcinogen, but under certain experimental conditions is a cocarcinogen or (especially in the liver) a tumor promoter (Seitz et al., 1998). The metabolism of ethanol leads to the generation of acetaldehyde and free radicals. These highly reactive compounds bind rapidly to cell constituents and possibly to DNA. Acetaldehyde decreases DNA repair mechanisms and the methylation of cytosine in DNA. It also traps glutathione, an important peptide in detoxification. Furthermore, it leads to chromosomal aberrations and seems to be associated with tissue damage and secondary compensatory hyperregeneration (Jokelainen, 2001).

More recently, the finding of considerable production of acetaldehyde by gastrointestinal bacteria was reported. Other mechanisms by which alcohol may stimulate carcinogenesis include (1) the induction of cytochrome P4502E1; (2) association with an enhanced activation of various procarcinogens present in alcoholic beverages; (3) association with tobacco smoke and specific diets, a change in the metabolism, and distribution of carcinogens; (4) alterations in cell cycle behavior such as cell cycle duration leading to hyperregeneration; (5) nutritional deficiencies such as vitamin A, folate, pyrridoxal phosphate, zinc, and selenium deficiency; (6) and alterations of the immune system, eventually resulting in an increased susceptibility to certain viral infections such as hepatitis B and hepatitis C.

In addition, localized mechanisms in the upper gastrointestinal tract and in the rectum may be of particular importance. Such mechanisms lead to tissue injury, including cirrhosis of the liver, which is a major prerequisite for hepatocellular carcinoma. All these mechanisms, functioning in concert, actively modulate carcinogenesis, leading to its stimulation. The effect of alcohol alone on the oral mucosa and its association with the development of oral cancer is difficult to establish, principally because alcohol consumption histories are difficult to verify, alter over time, both with respect to beverage type and quantity, and are frequently confounded by tobacco use. Chronic ethanol ingestion leads to an enhanced risk of upper gastrointestinal tract cancer. Although many hypotheses for the tumor-promoting effect of alcohol exist, the pathogenetic mechanisms remain unclear since alcohol in itself is not carcinogenic. Acetaldehyde, the first metabolite of ethanol, has been shown to have multiple mutagenic effects and to be carcinogenic to animals. Previous research has revealed that acetaldehyde can be formed from ethanol via microbial alcohol dehydrogenase (Homann et al., 2000). Thus, at least part of the proposed tumorigenic effect of ethanol may be linked to local production of acetaldehyde from ethanol by oral microflora (Väkeväinen et al., 2000).

Alcohol-Related Birth Defects. Prenatal exposure to alcohol can result in fetal alcohol syndrome (FAS), which is characterized by growth retardation, facial dysmorphologies, and a host of neurobehavioral impairments (Sampson et al., 1997; Prenatal Exposure to Alcohol, 2000; Streissguth, 2001). Alcohol is the most common teratogenic agent, and the birth incidence of affected children is between 1 in 400 and 1 in 1000 in western Europe and the United States. Since the identification of fetal alcohol syndrome at the end of the 1960s, substantial evidence has accumulated on a number of adverse effects that alcohol consumption during pregnancy may have on the fetus. Long-term effects on child development have also been observed. It is controversial whether there is a safe limit of alcohol intake during pregnancy. In a prospective study, it has been shown that for women drinking more than 100 g (3 to 4 oz.) of alcohol per week, the risk of delivering a baby with a birth weight below the tenth percentile is more than double than that of women drinking less than 50 g (1.5 oz.) per week (Wright et al., 1983). Although the various types of effects are well documented, less is known about threshold levels of consumption, under which there is no risk of damage. Few studies have assessed the risk associated with high episodic drinking. From a theoretical point of view, binge drinking in critical stages in organ formation may constitute a particularly high risk for adverse outcomes. The principal features are mild to moderate mental retardation, microcephaly, poor coordination, growth deficiency, and facial characteristics such as short palpebral fissures, short upturned nose, hypoplastic maxilla, thin upper lip, and micrognathia (Streissguth, 2001).

Neurobehavioral effects in FAS, and in alcohol-related neurodevelopmental disorder, include poor learning and memory, attention deficits, and motor disfunction. Many fetal alcohol effects result, at least in part, from teratogenic effects of alcohol on the hippocampus. Neurobehavioral studies show that animals exposed prenatally to alcohol are impaired in many of the same spatial learning and memory tasks that are sensitive to hippocampal damage (Berman and Hannigan, 2000). Electrophysiological studies also demonstrate changes in synaptic activity in in vitro hippocampal brain slices that were isolated from prenatal alcohol-exposed animals. Considered together, these observations demonstrate that prenatal exposure to alcohol can result in abnormal hippocampal development and function. Such studies provide a better understanding of neurological deficits associated with FAS in humans and may also contribute to the development of strategies to ameliorate the effects of prenatal alcohol exposure on behavior.

The Seattle prospective study (Sampson et al., 1997; Streissguth, 2001) shows that a pattern of neurobehavioral problems has been linked to prenatal alcohol exposure in a dose-dependent fashion. These patterns can be measured throughout the life of the child from day one through 14 years (and studies into adulthood are continuing). The documented neurobehavioral problems include attention, memory, fine and gross motor problems, language and academic problems (especially in arithmetics), and problems with speed of information processing. Furthermore, these neural problems occur against a background of behavioral problems that include impulsivity, poor comprehension, poor frustration tolerance, a rigid problem-solving approach that makes new situations difficult and behavior unpredictable.

Cirrhosis Epidemiology. Although the risk of developing alcoholic liver cirrhosis is statistically related to both average daily intake of alcohol and the duration of drinking, there is a great deal of variation in individual susceptibility to the hepatotoxic effects of alcohol (Day, 2000). Alcohol is a major cause of liver cirrhosis in the Western world and accounts for the majority of cases of liver cirrhosis seen in district general hospitals in the U.K. (Walsh and Alexander, 2000). The three most widely recognized forms of alcoholic liver disease are alcoholic fatty liver (steatosis), acute alcoholic hepatitis, and alcoholic cirrhosis. The exact pathogenesis of alcoholic liver injury is still not clear, but immune-mediated and free radical hepatic injury are thought to be important. There is increasing interest in genetic factors predisposing to hepatic injury in susceptible individuals. In the previously mentioned twin study on alcoholism and medical complications, 15,924 male pairs were ascertained and the concordance rates for liver cirrhosis were 14.6% for MZ twins and 5.4% for DZ twins (Hrubeck and Omenn, 1981), suggesting the involvement of genetic factors in the development of alcoholic cirrhosis. An early study found hypogonadism and scanty body hair to be a predisposing factor for liver cirrhosis in males (Müller, 1952).

Because immune factors are thought to influence alcoholic hepatitis and cirrhosis, the possible role of HLA antigens has been studied in alcoholics. Among Europeans, patients with alcoholic liver cirrhosis had increased frequencies of HLA-B8 (List and Gluud, 1994; Caballeria et al., 1997), but there also are studies with negative results (Llop et al., 1995). This is of interest, because HLA-B8 is well documented to be associated with a number of autoimmune diseases. Among the Japanese, an increased frequency of HLA-B40 and HLA-DRw9 was described in alcoholic liver cirrhosis, the two alleles being in linkage disequilibrium (Miyamoto et al., 1983).

Alcoholic Psychosis. Another possible outcome of chronic alcohol abuse is alcoholic psychosis. In the already mentioned twin study the concordance rate of alcoholic psychosis (delirium tremens, hallucinosis, or Korsakoff syndrome) was 21.1% in MZ twins and 6.0% in DZ twins, again pointing to the influence of genetic factors (Hrubeck and Omenn, 1981). Wernicke-Korsakoff syndrome, which is a confabulatory psychosis with a disproportionate loss of retentive memory in an otherwise clear sensorium, is related to thiamine deficiency in most cases. There is tentative evidence that people differ in their predisposition to this disorder, on the basis of a biochemical peculiarity. Thiamine deficiency, a frequent complication of alcoholism, plays an important role in the pathogenesis of the Wernicke-Korsakoff syndrome (WKS). A number of investigatons have implicated the thiamine-utilizing enzyme transketolase (Tk) as being involved mechanistically in the genetic predisposition to WKS. However, it remains to be equivocally shown whether this represents a predisposing marker.

Alcoholic Hallucinosis. Older studies have suggested a relationship between alcohol hallucinosis and schizophrenia. Relatives of index cases with alcohol hallucinosis were observed to have increased rates of schizophrenia. In some schizophrenia-like psychoses, alcohol abuse leading to a hallucinatory onset may be an antecedent of the psychosis. In recent years, little research has been focused on alcohol hallucinosis. The psychopathology of alcohol hallucinosis (vivid acoustic hallucinations, paranoid symptoms, and fear) resembles paranoid schizophrenia, but other organic mental disorders have to be excluded, too. Prognosis is usually good, but in 10% to 20% of the cases, alcohol hallucinosis tends to become chronic. Possible pathophysiological mechanisms involved in the development of the syndrome are changes in dopaminergic transmission or other neurotransmitter systems and neuronal membranes, elevated levels of β-carbolines and an impaired auditory system (Soyka, 1996). For treatment, highly potent neuroleptics (haloperidol) are the drugs of first choice. In the case of alcohol abstinence the prognosis is good, but otherwise the risk of a recurrence is high (Bowden et al., 2001).

Rare Syndrome Associations. Essential tremor is a benign autosomal dominant disorder. Small or moderate amounts of alcohol markedly reduce tremor intensity, and this improves the performance in motor skills. In a retrospective study, it was observed that patients with essential tremor have markedly elevated rates of alcohol abuse or dependence (Schroeder and Nasrallah, 1982). The authors hypothesize that the patients abused alcohol for self-medicating purposes and were therefore at a higher risk of becoming alcoholics. Koller et al. (1985) examined 100 alcoholics who had had no alcohol for more than 21 days, 100 controls, and 50 patients with essential tremor. Some 3% of the controls and 47% of the alcoholics had a postural tremor. Alcoholic tremor was never severe, and functional disability occurred in only 17% of patients. There was no relation to age or duration of drinking, and only 1% of the alcoholics had a family history of tremor, compared with 46% in those with essential tremor. Tremor frequency was significantly greater in the alcoholics than in those with essential tremor. Propranolol therapy decreased tremor more in the alcoholics than in those with essential tremor. Thus, the tremor of chronic alcoholism differs from essential tremor.

Color Blindness. Alcoholism, or the appetite for alcohol, has been linked to X-linked color blindness, particularly blue-yellow color vision defects (Cruz-Coke and Varela, 1966). However, other authors were unable to confirm the claimed higher incidence of color blindness among male alcoholics (Smith, 1972). Furthermore, the available family data on alcoholism do not favor an X-linked mode of inheritance (Winokur, 1967). Thus the color-vision defects observed in alcoholics are probably the result of alcohol abuse and the associated vitamin deficiencies (Eriksson, 1975).

Environmental Factors in Alcohol Drinking and Its Outcomes

Our knowledge of diversity in alcohol use and its outcomes in various societies has increased considerably in the past two to three decades. The influence of alcohol can be understood in terms of the interaction of the agent (alcohol), the host (the individual who ingests it), and the environment (encompassing ecological., social., and cultural variables). Different populations react to alcohol in a variety of patterns, depending on such environmental variables. If we are to understand alcohol drinking and its outcomes in any human population, environmental influences must be taken into consideration. They include moral and religious instructions; exposure to alcoholic beverages; drinking patterns of the family and peer groups; and age, gender, diet, health, lifestyle, behavior, culture, and social traditions of the individual (Cooper, 2001). As mentioned before, certain socioeconomic components such as availability of alcohol and price are among the major determinants of alcohol-seeking behavior in a society. Peer pressures and attitudes to drinking and drunkenness influence directly or indirectly the decision to drink and even to drink to excess occasionally. Moreover, drinking norms in a given society significantly influence the actual drinking behavior of an individual.

Unlike many inborn errors of metabolism, which are monogenic disorders, alcoholism is possibly a polygenic multifactorial disease with a still unknown precise mode of transmission between generations. While discussing the role of genetic factors in alcohol use and alcoholism, complex gene–environment interactions have to be taken into account. Several different genetic and environmental factors may participate in generating a heterogeneous clinical picture of the disease of alcoholism. Certain environmental factors may be playing a greater role in determining the "alcoholic phenotype" in a polygenic multifactorial disorder like alcoholism as they may modulate to a different extent the multiple gene loci involved (Vesell, 1989). Therefore, it may not be correct to separate "genes" and "environment" to elucidate their relative contribution. Rather, both genes and environment may participate simultaneously, interacting dynamically to influence the "alcoholic phenotype" (Radel and Goldman, 2001). Thus, the recognition of relative contributions of genetic and environmental factors is particularly important in the formulation of prevention and treatment strategies for alcoholism (Heath et al., 2001). One approach toward this goal, therefore, is a prospective and retrospective longitudinal study of individuals who were separated from their alcoholic biological relatives soon after birth and raised by non-alcoholic adoptive parents; another approach is the twin study of alcoholism.

The combined twin and adoption studies have clearly demonstrated an important role of genetic and environmental interactions in the development of alcoholism. What we learned from adoption studies is not that nature was important or nurture was important, but that both are important. Cross-fostering studies have shown that both genetic and environmental variables play a significant role in the development of "milieu-limited" (mild alcohol abuse) alcoholism, and the risk was increased 4-fold when both genetic and environmental factors were combined (Cloninger et al., 1981). For the moderate alcohol abuser, environmental factors played no significant role. The genetic vulnerability to alcohol use could be extensively modified by environmental factors, depending on postnatal experience. In contrast, expression of the male-limited (severe alcohol abuse) form was not significantly modified by environmental forces (Sigardsson et al., 1996).

A key role of environmental factors has also been evident in some heritable forms of alcoholism associated with antisocial personality, impulsiveness, sensation-seeking behavior, and extreme emotional volatility. Studies examining possible risk factors for the development of alcoholism have focused recently on a variety of personality factors, including those associated with risk-taking behaviors. Alcohol-seeking behavior leading to the abuse of alcohol may be associated with a variety of risk-taking behaviors that derive from certain personality traits (Limosin et al., 2000). Further, there is evidence that personality traits are transmitted across generations (Hesselbrock and Hesselbrock, 1992). This study examined the relationship of a family history of alcoholism, antisocial personality disorder (ASP), and alcohol use to several personality traits, including the Tridimensional Personality Questionnaire (TPQ) in a sample of nonalcoholic, young male volunteers. The men with ASP scored higher than the non-ASP men on the Novelty Seeking Scale of the TPQ, but not on the Harm Avoidance or Reward Dependence subscales. In addition, ASP men scored higher than non-ASP men on a measure of impulsivity and tended to score higher on measures of sensation seeking, psychopathy, and monotony avoidance. A family history of alcoholism did not differentiate the young men on any of the childhood behavior problems, personality measures, or alcohol-related variables.

To study the gene–environment interaction, particularly the effect of sociocultural influences on heritable susceptibility factors, Cloninger (1987) examined the relationship between increasing average alcohol consumption in the general population (United States and Sweden) and the risk of heavy drinking or alcohol abuse in the relatives of alcoholics. The rationale behind this study was that if there were fundamental differences between familial and nonfamilial alcoholism, then an increase in average alcohol consumption would lead to an increase in sporadic cases only and no change in the inheritance of familial alcoholism. In contrast, if the risk of alcoholism was influenced by the interaction of sociocultural influences and heritable susceptibility factors shared by biological relatives, then increasing the average alcohol consumption would lead to both an increase in sporadic cases and a marked exponential increase in the proportion of relatives who abuse alcohol. The results of this study indicate that both social and temporal trends in the use of alcohol markedly influence the inheritance profile of alcohol abuse. The study emphasized the need to distinguish between variables that influence exposure to heavy drinking and variables related to susceptibility to various social and medical outcomes of alcohol abuse in the context of various exposure patterns.

Role of a Particular Profession in Drinking. While the most important determinant of an individuals drinking problems is a positive family history of alcoholism, a particular profession or occupation may also help determine an individual's liability to alcoholism. High rates of alcoholism are usually noted among certain occupational groups, such as the military, police, firefighters, sailors, brewers, and medical practitioners.

Social, Ethnic, and Cultural Variables. Social, ethnic, and cultural factors are some of the strongest determinants of drinking patterns in a society. It has long been suspected that the influence of national and ethnic origin may account for a major part of the variance observed in comparative studies of alcoholism rates within different populations. Certain features of social structure and organization constitute environmental factors that interact with genetic and biomedical factors in shaping how, when, with whom, and for what reason people drink (Heath et al., 1997). Religions constitute environmental factors that influence individuals and groups in various ways: a religion can favor drinking, or it can preach abstinence. Education too can influence norms, attitudes, and values toward drinking at the individual or group level.

A marked difference in the extent of alcoholism and related problems among Israeli Jews of the three major ethnic communities—Ashkenazi, Sephardi, and Oriental—has been reported (Snyder, 1958; Neumark et al., 1998; Aharonovich et al., 2001). In one survey, a significantly higher percentage in the Sephardi and Oriental subgroups were found to be alcoholics than in the Ashkenazi subgroup. The differences have been explained to be due to sociological factors in terms of a historic dialectic of differentiation of Jewish minorities from the drinking norms of surrounding majorities (Aharonovich et al., 2001). Additional factors like religion and social stress also may have played an important part in the conditions that foster or thwart alcoholism (Schuckit, 2000). It was also noted that comparative freedom from alcoholism might be particularly characteristic of the more religious Orthodox Ashkenazi Jews, despite their frequent drinking (Aharonovich et al., 2001).

Effect of Acculturation. A strong correlation is alleged to exist between alcohol abuse and ethno-national origins. Genetically determined biological sensitivity to mild doses of alcohol commonly found in Asians of Mongoloid heritage has been shown to be a deterrent to alcohol abuse. This adverse response to ingestion of even small amounts of alcohol may protect sensitive individuals from developing alcoholism. However, under altered social and other environmental pressures, American Indians, who are known to be of the Mongoloid origin, still abuse alcohol despite the initial aversive reactions they might experience after drinking alcohol. Thus, the environmental factors may be quite important in some of the observed biological and behavioral concomitants in alcoholism.

Availability and Price Factors. Evidently, even an individual with a strong genetic predisposition for alcoholism would not develop the disorder in the absence of alcoholic beverages. Although limiting access to alcohol may not necessarily be an effective way to lessen alcoholism in a particular society, reducing overall consumption may be a good preventive strategy. Although some of the putative environmental factors remain obscure in their nature, there is strong evidence that there is a crucial interplay between nature and nurture, heredity and environment, and biology and culture in the development of alcoholism. Nevertheless, specific factors that interact with particular genes that predispose to alcoholism require further assessment to better comprehend the intricate interaction between predisposing genes and environmental factors in the expression, etiology, and treatment of alcoholism.

PATHOPHYSIOLOGY: BIOLOGICAL BASIS OF GENETIC SUSCEPTIBILITY

Genetic Studies of Pathophysiology

On the basis of the above review of genetic determination of alcoholism, it becomes apparent that the development of alcoholism for some individuals depends on the presence of genetically controlled predisposing factors that interact with environmentally determined precipitating factors. Thus the search for potential causative genes is rather complicated; an unknown number of genes may be involved in the development of alcoholism. For many years researchers have been looking for specific genes or genetic markers for vulnerability to alcoholism.

An association with a known hereditary trait occurring in consistently higher frequency may help identify a genetic predisposition to alcoholism. Predisposing biological markers must fulfill the following criteria:

1. Trait marker can be reliably measured in individuals and is stable over time.
2. It is genetically transmitted.
3. The abnormal trait has a low base frequency in the general population.
4. It can identify individuals at risk with high specificity and sensitivity.
5. The abnormal trait shows high prevalence in the patient population.
6. It is present during symptom remission.
7. It occurs among the first-degree relatives of the probands at a higher rate than in the general population.
8. It segregates with the illness in affected relatives of the proband.

Potential markers for genetic vulnerability to alcoholism may be divided into two broad categories: biochemical markers and electrophysiological markers.

Biochemical Vulnerability Markers

Recent molecular genetic research into the pathophysiological causes of alcoholism has drawn attention to the potential important role of alcohol and acetaldehyde metabolizing enzymes (Agarwal, 1997). Functional polymorphisms have been observed at various genes encoding these enzyme proteins, which all act to alter the rate of synthesis of the toxic metabolite acetaldehyde or to decrease its further oxidation. A positive selection of such genetic polymorphisms in some populations might act as a protective factor against alcohol abuse and alcohol-related disease outcomes (Harada et al., 2001; Yin and Agarwal, 2001). Thus, elucidation of the molecular mechanisms that control and influence elimination and metabolism of alcohol is important for understanding the biochemical basis of alcohol toxicity and alcohol abuse–related pharmacological and addictive consequences in humans.

Pharmacokinetics of Alcohol

Interplay between the kinetics of absorption, distribution, and elimination of the ingested alcohol is an important determinant of the blood alcohol concentration. Only 5% to 15% of ingested alcohol is excreted directly through the lungs, sweat, and urine; the rest is metabolized by the liver, via oxidation to carbon dioxide and water. The total alcohol eliminated by the human body per hour is usually in the range of 100 to 300 mg/liter, which is equivalent to about 6 to 9 g (0.2 to 0.3 oz.) alcohol per hour for a healthy subject with an average body weight.

Absorption, Body Distribution, and Elimination of Alcohol. Ethanol enters rapidly into the circulation by diffusion mainly across the lining or membrane of the duodenum and jejunum, and to a lesser extent from the stomach and large intestine. The absorption of ethanol is normally over in two hours and overlaps with the diffusion phase during which it is distributed throughout the body water. Variation in hormonal status—for example, stage of the menstrual cycle—affects ethanol absorption. During the absorption phase, the ethanol concentration is found to be higher in the arterial blood than in the venous blood (Jones, 2000). Historically, Widmark (1981) first introduced mathematical equations to explain the disposition and fate of ethanol in the body. Accordingly, after the absorption and distribution processes were completed, the blood alcohol concentration-time course decreased at a constant rate following a zero-order elimination kinetics. However, in the meantime, many complex pharmacokinetic models were suggested, describing alcohol concentration-time curves in blood, breath, and urine. The models varied in the number of pharmacokinetically relevant compartments, the kinetics of absorption, and the kinetics of the elimination processes of alcohol. The rate constants for absorption, distribution, and elimination of alcohol have been estimated on the one hand by experimental results and on the other by simulating whole blood curves with computers. Models involving two or more compartments have been proposed to explain differences in alcohol concentrations over time between venous and arterial blood or breath and to account for different absorption rate constants for the absorption from the stomach and the small intestine, as well as the effect of food thereupon (von Wartburg, 1989; Jones, 2000).

Various studies on the pharmacokinetics of alcohol reported in recent years indicate that a nonlinear course of ethanol elimination may best explain the observed differences in the metabolic rate of alcohol in humans. Changes in the gastrointestinal absorption rate have an influence on the so-called first-pass pharmacokinetic effect. In most pharmacokinetic models, the first-pass effect is neglected while calculating the alcohol elimination rates (Levitt and Levitt, 1998; Pastino and Conolly, 2000).

Alcohol Elimination Rate. Alcohol elimination rate (ER) is normally taken as a measure for alcohol metabolism, since only a small percentage of ingested alcohol is eliminated through breath, urine, or sweat (Jones, 2000). The slope (β) of the post-absorption pseudolinear blood curve is used to estimate alcohol elimination rate. For convenience, $\beta 60$ was introduced, which expresses the grams of alcohol eliminated per liter of blood per hour. The slope $\beta 60$ multiplied with the volume of distribution (V) yields the total elimination rate (ER) in the whole body in grams per hour. As an average, rates of 100 mg/kg/hr (range: 70–130) have been suggested. Thus maximal ER for normal human subjects would not exceed 200 to 240 g (7–8 oz.) alcohol per day for an individual with a 70 kg (155 lb.) body weight. A summary of comparative studies of ethanol metabolism in various ethnic groups is presented in Table 46–14.

Factors Affecting ER. Many factors appear to influence the course of blood alcohol concentration. As the orally ingested alcohol is absorbed in the stomach and intestine by diffusion, any change in the absorption rate will affect the ER. Factors that retard gastric emptying or that lead to dilution will cause slower absorption and thus affect the systemic availability of alcohol. Consumption of a concentrated solution of ethanol results in lower blood alcohol levels than does a dilute solution when subjects are tested in a fed state (Roine, 2000). This is probably because under fasting conditions, ingested alcohol passes rapidly from the stomach into the duodenum with minimal exposure to the gastric mucosa. High alcohol concentration can delay gastric emptying; a concentrated solution of alcohol will remain in the

Table 46–14. Summary of Comparative Studies of Ethanol Metabolism Rate in North American Indians, Whites, Chinese, and Japanese

Population	No.	$\beta(X \pm SD)^a$	Rate $(X \pm SD)^b$	References
Whites	68	0.23 ± 0.06	108 ± 31	Hanna, 1978
	30	0.26 ± 0.05	93 ± 17	Bennion and Li, 1976
	58	0.20 ± 0.13	104 ± 49	Reed et al., 1976
	17	0.016 ± 0.003	112 ± 14	Farris and Morgan-Jones, 1978
North American Indians	30	0.30 ± 0.07	92 ± 17	Bennion and Li, 1976
	24	0.43 ± 0.29	183 ± 63	Reed et al., 1976
	17	0.019 ± 0.003	123 ± 14	Farris and Morgan-Jones, 1978
Chinese/Japanese	39	0.22 ± 0.06	127 ± 33	Hanna, 1978
	10	0.21 ± 0.12	137 ± 36	Reed et al., 1976
	47	0.23 ± 0.03	134 ± 33	Hanna, 1978

[a]β (after Widmark) indicates elimination as mg/100 ml × minute except for one study (Farris and Morgan-Jones, 1978), in which the slope as percentage per hour is given.
[b]Rate of alcohol elimination as mg/kg × hour (Kalow, 1982).

stomach much longer than a dilute solution. Fasting has also been shown to decrease gastric first-pass metabolism of ethanol in humans. A swift increase in the rate of ethanol metabolism also occurs after intake of food intravenously; possibly, eating a meal increases the activity the alcohol metabolizing enzymes, and may also lead to increased blood flow through the liver post-meal (Hahn et al., 1994).

Recently, a three-compartment model for blood alcohol concentration (BAC) was applied to study the effect of sex, alcohol dose, concentration, physical exercise, and several aspects of meal consumption on BAC (Wedel et al., 1991). The ingestion of a meal before the intake of alcohol reduced both the gastric emptying rate and absorption efficiency of alcohol, increased the gastric emptying delay and reduced the rate of elimination. Ethanol elimination rate is also found to be higher in heavy drinkers when they consume higher amounts of alcohol (Keiding et al., 1983). Perhaps higher ethanol concentrations stimulate hepatic ethanol metabolism via (ADH) and also due to an increased activity of the sympathetic nerve system.

The blood alcohol concentration is roughly equal to the concentration of alcohol in the tissue fluid throughout the "lean body mass," which includes most of the body except those tissues such as fat, which do not freely exchange water with the blood. Thus, volume of distribution of alcohol is said to reflect the amount of water present in various tissues of the body. This would suggest that an obese person, with proportionately increased adipose tissue, should have a higher BAC when consuming an alcohol dose similar to that taken by a lean person. A relatively higher amount of body water, when there is less adipose tissue, would be capable of holding larger amounts of alcohol. This may explain the sex-related differences in blood alcohol concentrations: females show a higher blood alcohol concentration than males after administration of an equal dose of alcohol per kg body weight. The relatively higher body fat in females leads to a higher alcohol concentration in tissue fluids.

Alcohol Metabolizing Enzymes

The enzymatic pathways responsible for ethanol metabolism and their genetic and environmental determinants have been the focus of detailed investigations in past decades. Identification of structural gene variants and the characterization of putative alcoholism vulnerability genes may help in improving preventive and treatment approaches. In humans, more than 90% of the ingested ethanol is degraded in the liver by oxidative and nonoxidative metabolic pathways (Fig. 46–3). The major enzymes involved in the metabolism of ethanol are alcohol dehydrogenases (ADH), aldehyde dehydrogenase (ALDH) and cytochrome P450 (CYP2E1). In addition, catalase and fatty acid ethyl ester synthase (FAEES) are also involved in ethanol degradation. Some of the well-known genetically controlled biological factors that may contribute to alcoholism include alcohol elimination rate; alcohol metabolism; polymorphisms of ADH, ALDH, and CYP2E1; alcohol's biochemical effects on the central nervous system; alcohol's effects on psychophysiological performance; and alcohol's effects on electrophysiological parameters. Comparison of the blood alcohol concentration after oral ingestion vs. intravenous administration of alcohol indicates that a fraction of ingested alcohol never reaches the peripheral circulation. Recent studies have shown that, indeed, a significant fraction of ingested ethanol is metabolized in the gastrointestinal tract by the so-called first-pass metabolism (Frezza et al., 1990; Oneta et al., 1998).

Alcohol Dehydrogenases. The major enzyme responsible for ethanol oxidation in human stomach are the alcohol dehydrogenases (ADH) (Agarwal and Goedde, 1990; Edenberg and Bosron, 1997). The ADH gene family encodes enzymes that metabolize a wide variety of substrates, including ethanol, retinol, other aliphatic alcohols, hydroxysteroids, and lipid peroxidation products. Human ADH is a dimeric protein consisting of two subunits with a molecular weight of 40 kD each. At least seven different genetic loci code for human ADH arising from the association of different types of subunits. Over 20 ADH isoenzymes are known, and they vary in their pharmacokinetic properties: (1) the types of alcohols they preferentially oxidize; (2) the amount of alcohol that has to accumulate before appreciable degradation occurs; and (3) the maximal rate at which they oxidize alcohol. As presented in Table 46–15, various human ADH forms can be divided into five major classes or distinct groups (I–V) according to their subunit and isoenzyme composition, as well as their physicochemical properties.

Class I ADH. The class I ADH isoenzymes are formed by random dimeric association of any of the three types of polypeptide subunits, α, β, and γ controlled by three separate gene loci, ADH1, ADH2, and ADH3, respectively. Any one particular class I ADH isoenzyme may be composed of homodimeric subunits, consisting of two identical polypeptides (e.g., $\alpha\alpha$, $\beta\beta$, $\gamma\gamma$) coded by a specific allele at one of the loci; of heterodimeric subunits consisting of two nonidentical polypeptides (e.g., $\alpha\beta$, $\alpha\gamma$) coded

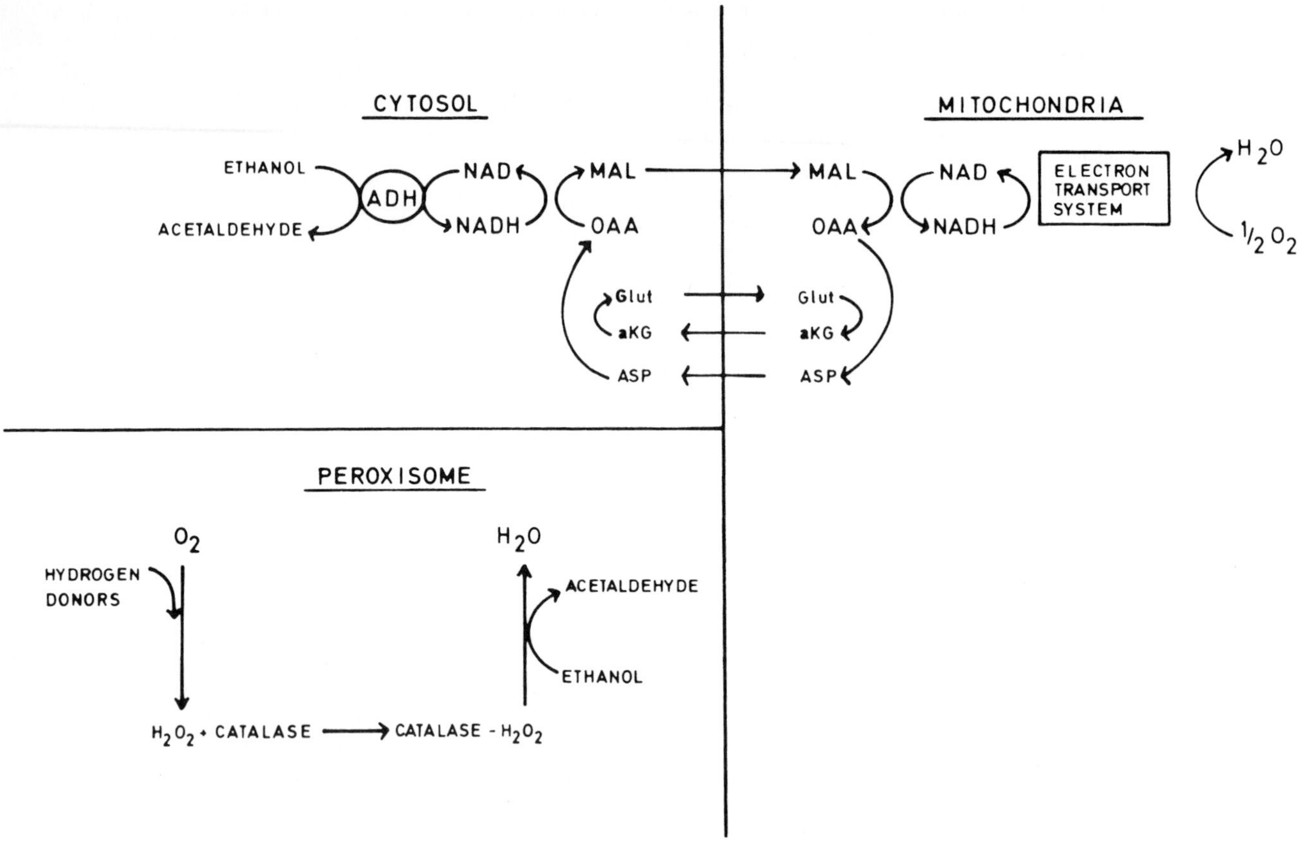

Fig. 46–3. Scheme depicting the essential pathway of hepatic ethanol metabolism. ADH, alcohol dehydrogenase; NAD, nicotinamide adenin dinucleotide; MAL, malic acid; OAA, oxalacetic acid; ASP, asparagine; Glu, glutamate; aKG, α-ketoglutaric acid.

by alleles at separate loci; or of heterodimeric subunits coded by different alleles at the same locus (e.g., $\alpha 1\alpha 2$, $\gamma 1\gamma 2$). These isoenzymes belong to the low Km forms (<4 mM) and are considered to play a major part in ethanol metabolism. The molecular characterization of the ADH2*1 allele shows that 9 exons are stretched over 15 kilobases (kb) in length. The complete nucleotide sequence of all 9 exons of an ADH2*2 allele, which encodes for the $\beta 2\beta 2$ isoenzyme, has been determined using clones from a human genomic DNA library. The nucleotide sequence data indicate that the CGC/CAC substitution, responsible for the arginine/histidine exchange, is the only nucleotide polymorphism detected between the coding regions of ADH2*1 and ADH2*2 alleles (Matsuo et al., 1989).

Class II ADH. Class II ADH, encoded by the *ADH4* gene, is composed of π subunits. It exhibits a high catalytic efficiency for oxidation of long-chain aliphatic and aromatic alcohols (Km = 18–34 mM), migrates more anodically than the class I

Table 46–15. Subunit Composition of Human ADH Genes

Class	Gene	Subunit	Dimeric Isozymes	Chromosomal Location
Class I ADH				
ADH1	*ADH1*1*	α	$\alpha\alpha$, $\alpha\beta 1$, $\alpha\beta 2$, $\alpha\gamma 1$, $\alpha\gamma 2$	4q22
ADH2	*ADH2*1*	$\beta 1$	$\beta 1\beta 1$, $\beta 1\beta 2$, $\beta 1\gamma 1$, $\beta 1\gamma 2$	4q22
	*ADH*2*	$\beta 2$	$\beta 2\beta 2$, $\beta 2\gamma 1$, $\beta 2\gamma 2$	
	*ADH2*3*	$\beta 3$	$\beta 3\beta 3$	
ADH3	*ADH3*1*	$\gamma 1$	$\gamma 1\gamma 1$	4q22
	*ADH3*2*	$\gamma 2$	$\gamma 1\gamma 2$, $\gamma 2\gamma 2$	
Class II ADH				
ADH4	*ADH4*	π	$\pi\pi$	4q21–q25
Class III ADH				
ADH5	*ADH5*	χ	$\chi\chi$	4q21–q25
Class IV ADH				
ADH7	*ADH7*	σ	$\sigma\sigma$	4q23–q24
Class V ADH				
ADH6	*ADH6*	?[a]	?[a]	4q21–q25

[a]Subunit composition not known.

isoenzymes on starch gel electrophoresis, and is far less sensitive to pyrazole inhibition. Hence it is called π (pi, pyrazole insensitive) ADH.

Class III ADH. Several ADH activity bands migrating anodically in starch gel electrophoresis and showing enzyme-specific staining activity only with medium-chain alcohols (>4 carbons) as substrate have been characterized. This class of ADH (chi or χ-ADH) is encoded by the *ADH5* gene. It has a very high Km for ethanol (>3 mM), but exhibits high activity for oxidation of long-chain alcohols. χ-ADH is a zinc-containing dimeric enzyme responsible for the oxidation of long-chain alcohols and σ-hydroxy fatty acids.

Class IV ADH. Human stomach mucosa contains an ADH isoenzyme (sigma, $\sigma\sigma$ subunits) which is moderately active with ethanol and exhibits kinetic properties, electrophoretic mobility, isoelectric point, and structural characteristics different from those previously described for other ADHs. This form is now recognized as a class IV enzyme encoded by the *ADH7* gene (Yin et al., 1997). It has nine exons and eight introns that span about 22 kb, and its intron insertion is identical to that of the other ADH genes (*ADH1* to *ADH5*). The nucleotide sequences of the exons encoding 374 amino acids are identical to the previously reported cDNA sequence of Σ-ADH. Fluorescence in situ hybridization analysis showed that ADH7 is located on human chromosome 4q23–q24, close to the ADH cluster locus (4q21–q25). These data are consistent with the view that class IV ADH is a member of the ADH family and is phylogenetically close to the other ADHs. Full-length cDNA coding for class IV ADH has been cloned and sequenced (Yokoyama et al., 1996). The deduced amino acid sequence, with 374 residues, shows about 60% to 70% identity with other human ADH classes.

Class V ADH. A recently cloned *ADH6* gene was found in liver and stomach, and an active enzyme has been expressed in *Escherichia coli* (Jörnvall and Höög, 1995). However, its expressed protein product has not yet been identified in human tissues.

Molecular Genetics of ADH. All ADH subunits consist of 374 amino acid residues and have about 10% total amino acid exchanges (Jörnvall and Höög, 1995). The β subunit differs from the α subunit at 24 amino acids, and the α subunit differs from the γ subunit at 20 residues. For class I ADH, only at three sequence positions, 143, 319 and 327, do all the three subunits differ from each other. The degrees of exchanges in the α, β, and γ subunits are very similar, thus suggesting separate but comparatively recent duplicatory diversions. Amino acid sequence data show that the "atypical" subunit (ADH2 locus) from Caucasian and Asian livers is identical, but differs from the "typical" $\beta1$ subunit by a single amino acid exchange, Arg to His at the 47th position due to a G/C to A/T base transition in exon 3. This arginine/histidine-47 mutational difference has been found to be responsible for altered catalytic and functional properties, including both a lower pH optimum and a higher turnover number of the atypical enzyme. The substitution in the $\beta3$ isoenzyme consists of a single amino acid exchange at position 369, Arg being replaced by Cys generated by C/G to T/A base transition in exon 9. Amino acid sequence analysis of the $\gamma1$ and $\gamma2$ subunits showed that both have the same sequence, Cys-Arg-Ser at their positions 46–48 but have two replacements at positions 271 (Arg/Gln) and 349 (Ile/Val).

Genetic Polymorphisms. So far, no allelic polymorphism has been reported in human populations for the α subunit of ADH1 (class I ADH), π-ADH (class II ADH), and χ-ADH (class III ADH). While about 5% to 10% of the English, 9% to 14% of the German, and 20% of the Swiss population have been found to possess an "atypical" phenotype of *ADH2* (allelic variant at the *ADH2* gene locus containing the $\beta2$ subunit), this variant form occurs in at least 85% of the Japanese, Chinese, and other Asian populations (Agarwal and Goedde, 1990). The frequency of the variant forms of the *ADH3* locus is relatively higher in Caucasians than in Asian and African populations.

Chromosome Mapping of the ADH Gene Loci. Analysis of DNA from hybrids containing fragments of human chromosome 4 has provided evidence that all classes of ADH genes are located on the long arm of human chromosome 4 between 4q21 and 4q25.

Physiological Role. The role of ADH in alcoholism and alcohol-related disorders has not been fully understood so far. Altered structures of the genes encoding for various ADH isoenzymes could potentially be the cause of observed genetic differences in alcoholics and nonalcoholics. Variants at both the *ADH2* and *ADH3* genes have been implicated in alcoholism in some populations because allele frequencies differ between alcoholics and controls (Chen et al., 1999; Osier et al., 1999; Borras et al., 2000). Specifically, controls have higher frequencies of the variants with higher V_{max} (ADH2*2 and ADH3*1). In samples of both alcoholics and controls from three Taiwanese populations (Chinese, Ami, and Atayal), Osier et al. (1999) found significant pairwise disequilibrium for all comparisons of the two functional polymorphisms and a third, presumably neutral, intronic polymorphism in *ADH2* (see below for further discussion of the role of functional polymorphisms).

Microsomal Ethanol Oxidizing System. A small but significant part of the ingested ethanol (10% or less) is metabolized by alternative pathways. The microsomal metabolism of ethanol accounts for the major non-ADH pathway of alcohol oxidation in the liver. The cytochrome P450 isoform, P4502E1 (CYP2E1), represents the major alternative system which metabolizes alcohol in the liver (Lieber, 1999). After chronic ethanol consumption, the activity of the microsomal ethanol-oxidizing system (MEOS) increases, with an associated rise in cytochrome P450, especially CYP2E1. Enhanced ethanol oxidation is associated with cross-induction of the metabolism of other drugs, resulting in drug tolerance. Furthermore, there is increased conversion of known hepatotoxic agents such as carbon tetrachloride to toxic metabolites, which may explain the enhanced susceptibility of alcoholics to the adverse effects of industrial solvents. CYP2E1 also has a high capacity to activate some commonly used drugs, such as acetaminophen, to their toxic metabolites and to promote carcinogenesis (e.g., from dimethylnitrosamine). Both ethanol-induced and constitutionally enhanced transcriptional activity of the polymorphic form of CYP2E1 (c2/c2) might play a role in the development of severe alcoholic liver disease (Tsutsumi et al., 1994; Iwahashi and Suwaki, 1998).

Polymorphic Alleles of CYP2E1. Polymorphisms in various CYP2E1 genes have been observed. A RsaI restriction fragment length polymorphism (RFLP) has been reported in the 5′-flanking region of the CYP2E1 gene. The rare mutant allele (c2 allele) that lacks the RsaI restriction site has been found to be associated with higher transcriptional activity, protein levels, and enzyme activity than is the common wild-type c1 allele. Moreover, the frequency of the RsaI c2 allele varies in different populations (Stephens et al., 1994). The highest frequency has been observed in the Taiwanese (0.28) and Japanese (0.19–0.27), while the frequency is much lower (ranging between 0.01 and 0.05) in African Americans, European Americans, and Scandinavians (Stephens et al., 1994).

Catalase. A third system with the potential to oxidize alcohols in human body is the enzyme catalase, which appears to act only at high concentrations of alcohol. However, its overall role in ethanol elimination is unclear.

Fatty Acid Ethyl Ester Synthases. Ethanol can condense with free fatty acids in a reaction catalyzed by FAEES to form abnormal compounds such as fatty acid ethyl esters. Three different synthases have been detected, designated as synthase I, II, III, and IV. Each of these enzymes has been purified and characterized, and several of them have been purified to homogeneity from the human myocardium (Beckemeier and Bora, 1998). The observation that FAEEs are synthesized at high rates in the heart and in other organs that lack oxidative ethanol metabolism provides a plausible link between the observed tissue damage, the ingestion of alcohol, and the subsequent development of alcohol-induced heart muscle disease.

Aldehyde Dehydrogenases. Acetaldehyde is the first metabolic product of enzymatic ethanol oxidation in human liver, and it is far more toxic than the parent compound ethanol. The major oxidation of acetaldehyde in the liver and other organs is catalyzed by the nicotinamide adenine dinucleotide (NAD^+)-dependent aldehyde dehydrogenase (ALDH; aldehyde : NAD^+ oxidoreductase, EC 1.2.1.3). A number of isoenzymes of ALDH coded by different gene loci have been detected in human organs and tissues; these isoenzymes differ in their electrophoretic mobility, kinetic properties, and cellular and tissue distribution. Human ALDHs are divided into nine major gene families. Members of family one are cytoplasmic ALDHs (ALDH1); members of family two are mitochondrial ALDHs (ALDH2); and members of family three are the major constitutive and inducible high Km ALDH forms (ALDH3) found in rat and mouse organs such as stomach, lung, liver, and cornea, as well as in human stomach, saliva, and hepatocarcinoma (Vasiliou et al., 1999; Agarwal, 2001).

Various ALDH isoenzymes show a broad range of substrate specificity for aliphatic and aromatic aldehydes. Whereas ALDH1 and ALDH2 both show Km values in the micromolar range with acetaldehyde and propionaldehyde, the Michaelis constants for ALDH3 and ALDH4 are in the millimolar range for these substrates. NAD^+ is the preferred coenzyme for the low Km isoenzymes (ALDH1 and ALDH2), whereas the high Km isoenzymes (ALDH3 and ALDH4) can use either NAD^+ or $NADP^+$. The major human liver ALDH1 and ALDH2 isoenzymes are homotetramers that consist of equal but isoenzyme-specific subunits with a molecular weight of about 54 kD each (Agarwal and Goedde, 1990).

Polymorphisms of ALDH Genes. Genetic polymorphisms have been reported in a number of ALDH genes. Naming of the human ALDH alleles is based on the new nomenclature (Vasiliou et al., 1999). The single genetic factor most strongly correlated with low alcohol consumption and incidence of alcoholism is a naturally occurring variant of mitochondrial aldehyde dehydrogenase (ALDH2). This variant contains a glutamate to lysine substitution at position 487 (E487K) (Yoshida et al., 1984). The E487K variant of ALDH2 is found in approximately 50% of the Asian population and is associated with a phenotypic loss of ALDH2 activity in both heterozygotes and homozygotes (Goedde et al., 1979). Functionally, a single base mutation at this position, resulting in loss of the catalytic activity, is compatible with the proximity in the primary structure between this region and the segment that contains cysteine residues. ALDH2-deficient individuals exhibit an aversive response to ethanol consumption, which is probably caused by high levels of blood acetaldehyde.

Population Distribution of ALDH2 Variants. Asian populations of Mongoloid origin widely show the presence of the inactive ALDH2 isoenzyme genotype, whereas none of the Caucasoid or Negroid populations have this isoenzyme abnormality (Goedde et al., 1992). However, this variant isoenzyme was detected in only a very small percentage of Native Americans (Table 46–16). More recent genotyping data hint to a considerable genetic heterogeneity in the distribution of the ALDH2*2 gene in American Indian and Central Asian populations (Novoradovsky et al., 1995; Santos et al., 1997; Segal, 1999).

Physiological Role of ALDH. The physiological significance of ALDH relates mainly to its role in the detoxification of acetaldehyde and other aldehydes that show a variety of toxic effects in human organs and tissues. Many biogenic amines are converted to their corresponding aldehydes via monoamine and diamine oxidase systems. Moreover, in vivo biotransformation of many drugs and xenobiotics that are not aldehydes gives rise to aldehyde metabolites. Acetaldehyde is a critical intermediate of ethanol metabolism, and its effect on the organism is thought to be important in the etiology of alcoholism (Eriksson, 2001).

Table 46–16. Frequency of ALDH2 Alleles in Different Populations

	Allele Frequency	
Population	ALDH2*1	ALDH2*2
Caucasians		
Germans	1	0
Swedes	1	0
Finns	1	0
Turks	1	0
Asian Indians	0.98	0.02
Hungarians	0.987	0.013
Asians		
Chinese	0.841	0.159
Japanese	0.764	0.236
Koreans	0.849	0.151
Fillipinos	0.994	0.006
Thais	0.950	0.050
Malayans	0.966	0.034
Africans		
Kenyans	1	0
Egyptians	1	0
American Indians		
Caboclos (Brazil)	0.826	0.174
Aboriginals		
Papua New Guineans	0.996	0.004

Source: Data from Goedde et al. (1992) with permission.

Acute Reactions to Alcohol and Its Metabolites. Alcohol is a known vasodilator, and this property is not the direct effect of alcohol on the blood vessel but is a consequence of its actions on the central nervous system. The effects of alcohol per se are influenced by its sympathomimetic activity and by its metabolites, acetaldehyde and acetate. Acetaldehyde shows stronger sympathomimetic action than alcohol and facilitates the release of catecholamines from the chromaffin cells of the adrenal medulla and from the sympathetic nerve endings. Increase of plasma catecholamines apparently leads to an elevation of heart rate, dilation of peripheral vessels accompanied with the rise of blood flow in carotid arteries and increased cardiac output (Eriksson, 2001).

In some individuals, ingestion of moderate amounts of alcohol exerts the so-called alcohol sensitivity symptoms (facial flushing, increase in heart rate, enhancement of left ventricular function, hot feeling in stomach, palpitation, tachycardia, muscle weakness, etc.). Wolff (1973) reported significant differences among the Caucasian group on one hand, with a very low percentage (5%) of subjects showing a flush response to alcohol, and the Mongoloids and American Indians on the other hand, with over 80% who showed flushing reactions. The apparent individual and racial differences in euphoric and dysphoric response to alcohol were replicated and extended in various ethnic and racial groups (Agarwal and Goedde, 1990). American Indians also are sensitive to alcohol and exhibit facial flushing associated with various subjective and objective vasomotor symptoms after drinking moderate amounts of alcohol. Wolff (1973) reported that Eastern Cree Indians who consumed no alcohol or fewer than 5 bottles of beer per week responded more intensely than those who reported drinking more than 10 bottles of beer per week or an equivalent amount of alcohol in other forms.

Mechanism of Biological Sensitivity to Alcohol. As stated above, acetaldehyde and not ethanol per se seems to be mainly responsible for most of the severe symptoms of alcohol-related cardiovascular sensitivity. Indeed, higher steady-state blood and breath acetaldehyde levels have been noted post-drink in those Japanese and Chinese subjects who show flushing after drinking mild doses of alcohol (Agarwal and Goedde, 1990). The maximum alcohol absorption takes place in the small intestine. Anatomic variations in the internal organ size may be important in this respect: Asians and American Indians have longer intestines (Hanna, 1978). Since alcohol diffuses through the lining of the stomach and the small intestine, any variation in the surface areas will lead to a more rapid absorption rate. Individual and ethnic differences in the alcohol metabolism rate (mg ethanol/kg total weight per hour) and alcohol clearence rate (mg ethanol/100 ml blood per minute) also vary considerably between and within various racial and ethnic groups (Farris and Jones, 1978; Reed et al., 1976; Reed, 1986). Thus, any genetically determined variation in the ethanol metabolism rate could also influence the steady-state blood acetaldehyde levels.

The atypical ADH, quite frequent in the Japanese, was initially thought to be responsible for a rapid oxidation of ethanol to acetaldehyde, thereby producing alcohol sensitivity symptoms. More than 90% of the Japanese and other Mongoloids possess the atypical ADH, with several times higher catalytic activity, whereas the incidence of flushing accompanied by higher blood acetaldehyde levels is only about 50%. Hence, rapid or higher than normal production of acetaldehyde via an atypical ADH alone cannot be the major cause of intense adverse reactions to alcohol (Agarwal and Goedde, 1990).

Table 46–17. Blood Acetaldehyde and Ethanol Levels in Japanese with a Normal or Deficient ALDH2 Genotype after Intake of an Acute Dose of Ethanol

	Peak Levels ($X \pm$ SD)	
ALDH2 Genotype	Acetaldehyde (μmol/liter)	Ethanol (mmol/liter)
Normal ($N = 25$)	2.1 ± 1.7	10.30 ± 1.85
Deficient ($N = 19$)	35.4 ± 12.8	10.93 ± 2.31

Source: Agarwal and Goedde (1990) with permission.

A positive correlation between alcohol sensitivity and high blood acetaldehyde level, in conjunction with ALDH2 isoenzyme abnormality, was noted in Japanese subjects who had been given an acute dose of alcohol (Harada et al., 1981). Subjects with a variant form of ALDH2 showed a significantly higher blood acetaldehyde level than did non-flushers with a normal ALDH2 isoenzyme profile, while blood ethanol concentrations were similar in both groups of subjects (Table 46–17). The subjects could be divided into three categories based on ALDH2 genotype, ALDH activity, and flushing intensity (Table 46–18). Thus, the initial vasomotor flushing after alcohol ingestion in Asians might be due to their inability to metabolize acetaldehyde quickly and effectively in the absence of the ALDH2 isoenzyme with a low Km for acetaldehyde. Apparently, slow acetaldehyde oxidation due to an ALDH2 isoenzyme abnormality leads to high blood acetaldehyde levels, resulting in catecholamine-mediated vasodilation associated with dysphoric symptoms. Indeed, a faster ethanol elimination associated with a higher blood acetaldehyde level was observed in a Japanese subject homozygous for the ALDH2*2 allele (Meier-Tackmann et al., 1990).

Functional Polymorphisms of Alcohol Metabolism Genes and Alcoholism. Comparison among racial and ethnic groups has invariably shown that (1) a larger proportion of Asians than Caucasians report no use of alcohol; (2) Caucasians report heavier alcohol use; and (3) a large proportion of Asians who drink alcohol experience facial flushing and associated sensitivity symptoms. More recent studies have focused on the putative role of functional polymorphisms of alcohol-metabolizing enzymes in alcohol elimination rate, acute reactions to alcohol, alcohol drinking habits, and alcoholism across various ethnic groups. The quantity-frequency-variability distribution indicates that the percentage of heavy and moderate drinkers is higher among Caucasians than the other ethnic groups, while the percentage of abstainers and infrequent drinkers is higher among the Chinese, Japanese, and other Asians (Agarwal and Goedde, 1990; Higuchi et al., 1995; Morimoto and Takeshita, 1996; Tanaka et al., 1997; Sun et al., 1999; Peng et al., 1999). Individuals sensitive to alcohol by virtue of their genetically controlled polymorphism of ALDH2 may be discouraged from abuse of alcohol due to initial adverse reaction (Agarwal and Goedde, 1990; Thomasson and Li, 1993; Yin and Agarwal, 2001).

Table 46–18. ALDH2 Activity and Flushing after an Acute Alcohol Dose in Asians According to *ALDH2* Genotype

Genotype	*ALDH2* Activity	Alcohol Sensitivity
ALDH2*1/ALDH2*1	Normal	Nonflusher
ALDH2*1/ALDH2*2	Intermediate	Nonflusher or light flusher
ALDH2*2/ALDH2*1	Poor or absent	Flusher

Source: Agarwal and Goedde (1990) with permission.

ALDH2 Polymorphism and Electrophysiological Response to Alcohol. Both EEG patterns and ERPs were measured in subjects homozygous or heterozygous for the functional ALDH2*1 allele (Wall et al., 1993; Wall and Ehlers, 1995; Hara et al., 2000). Homozygous subjects with the ALDH2*1 allele showed a typical EEG response, including increased θ and slow-α and decreased fast-α activity. In the heterozygous subjects, however, the slow-α EEG activity decreased significantly from that of the homozygous subjects for ALDH2*1. In the same subjects, the response to ERPs was studied. Compared with a placebo, alcohol consumption in all subjects significantly decreased the amplitude and increased the latency of the P300 wave. However, alcohol's effects on the P300 wave were significantly greater in heterozygous subjects than in the subjects homozygous for ALDH2*1. These observations support the notion that individuals heterozygous for ALDH2 experience a more intense response to alcohol than do people homozygous for the ALDH2*1 allele.

Genetic Liability to Alcohol-Related End-Organ Damage

The fact that only a small percentage of alcohol abusers develop cirrhosis and chronic pancreatitis suggests that a possible predisposing factor is involved in alcohol-related end-organ damage. Whether there are distinct genetic factors that predispose susceptibility to tissue and organ damage from alcohol (e.g., liver cirrhosis, pancreatitis, or cardiomyopathy) has been not fully elucidated. A number of biochemical and immunological mechanisms may determine susceptibility to alcohol-related organ damage.

The alcoholism rate, as well as alcohol-related end-organ damage, is found to be lower among the Japanese, Chinese, and other Asians than in Caucasian populations living in Western society (Agarwal and Goedde, 1990; Higuchi et al., 1995; Muramatsu et al., 1995; Matsumoto et al., 1996; Shen et al., 1997; Tanaka et al., 1997; Neumark et al., 1998; Chen et al., 1999; Maruyama et al., 1999). It is of interest to note the role of ADH and ALDH isoenzyme variation in the development of alcohol dependency and alcohol-related liver disease in different populations. In addition to the ALDH2*2 allele, the presence of both ADH2*2 and ADH3*1 alleles appears to be protective against the development of alcoholism among Taiwanese Han (Chen et al., 1999). A significantly fewer number of patients with alcoholism and alcoholic liver disease have been found to possess the inactive ALDH2*2 gene. Individuals heterozygous for the ALDH2 alleles are at higher risk for the development of alcoholic liver disease when they drink more than a critical level of alcohol. (Day et al., 1991; Enomoto et al., 1991; Takada et al., 1994; Yamauchi et al., 1995; Chen et al., 1999; Maruyama et al., 1999).

Taken together, the ALDH2-deficient individuals drink less, have the tendency not to become habitual drinkers, suffer less from liver disease, and are rarely alcoholics. Acetaldehyde-induced aversion to alcohol drinking may represent only one aspect of the relationship between acetaldehyde metabolism and human drinking. Thus, in future studies, the possible role of acetaldehyde and its metabolism in mediating reinforcing effects, particularly in Caucasian alcoholics, has to be elucidated.

Characterization of High-Risk and Low-Risk Individuals

In the past years, a number of investigators have tried, in prospective studies, to identify possible trait markers by studying young men and women at high risk for the future development of alcoholism based on their family history of this disorder. Having an alcoholic biological father is the best single predictor of future alcoholism in male offspring. One method of determining whether there are neuropsychological deficits before the onset of alcoholism is to study children who are at risk for becoming alcoholic (Lieberman, 2000; Schuckit and Smith, 2001a). In a typical prospective study, young men and women at high risk for the future development of alcoholism are divided into a Family History Positive (FHP) group (who report an alcoholic parent or siblings) and a Family History Negative (FHN) group (men and women who report no close alcoholic relative). The subjects are matched for demography and alcohol drinking history.

Nonspecific susceptibility factors include personality traits characterized by behavioral inhibition (e.g., novelty seeking and impulsivity). These genetically influenced traits interact with other, also genetically influenced, traits that are involved in the metabolism and pharmacodynamic effects of alcohol, and this interaction forms the basis for nominating alcoholism as a pharmacogenetic disease. Clearly, there are also many environmental factors that influence drinking behavior. Individuals have different sets of susceptibility genes and experience different kinds of environmental provocation. These factors underlie the heterogeneity and complexity of the clinical phenotype of alcoholism.

Genetic susceptibility to alcoholism may be expressed in changes in various neurobehavioral functions as alcoholism is associated with many psychiatric problems such as childhood conduct disorder, which is marked by aggression and other antisocial activities. Hyperactivity may be one aspect of the genetically mediated predisposition to alcoholism. Offspring of alcoholic parents showed higher psychiatric risk, both by the total score for psychiatric disorders and by the number of abnormalities in their psychiatric history, than the controls (Steinhausen et al., 1984). Children with alcoholic fathers tended to suffer from conduct disorders, while children with alcoholic mothers tended to suffer from emotional disorders. Factors affecting family-related environmental stress include various sex-specific drinking patterns, disorders in the maternal relationship and in the child-parent relationship, and mood and the communication patterns in families, as well as the impairment of family roles and tasks. Such factors need to be explored to explain the role of social transmission of some of the traits within a family and in the development of alcoholism in family members.

Some differences in neuropsychological deficits were observed between healthy FHP and FHN men in a large-scale study in Denmark (Drejer et al., 1985). When given a series of 12 neuropsychological tests generating 17 scores, the two groups were similar on 14 scores and differed in the remaining 3. Regarding childhood behavior, more of the FHPs had to repeat a grade, had been referred to a school psychologist, or had been placed in a special class (Knop et al., 1985). A pre-morbid assessment of the cohort clearly indicated that the FHP group is characterized by poor school career, verbal difficulties, impulsivity, abnormal EEG response after ethanol ingestion, and poor abstracting capability compared to the FHN group (Goodwin et al., 1994). Preliminary evidence suggests that a neurophysiological disorder may also characterize children who are at risk for alcoholism.

In addition, the sons of alcoholics presented a more neurotic personality profile than did the sons of nonalcoholics. Neuropsychological differences also have been found in male alcoholics who have an alcoholic first-degree relative in comparison to those who do not have any. When adolescent sons of alcoholics and nonalcoholics were compared on a battery of intellectual, neuropsychological, personality, and behavioral parameters, the former group demonstrated certain deficits in perceptual motor ability, memory, and language processing (Tarter et al., 1990). They also had auditory and visual attentional impairment in reading comprehension. In addition, the sons of alcoholics presented a more neurotic personality profile than did sons of nonalcoholics (Pihl et al., 1990). More developmental and familial problems also were noted in the offspring of alcoholics. Children with attention deficit hyperactivity disorder (ADHD) and Tourette syndrome (vocal and motor tics, learning disorder, sleep disorder, etc.) are shown to be at greater risk to develop problems with alcohol and drug abuse or dependence as adults (Comings, 1993; Ponce Alfaro et al., 2000). Both ADHD and Tourette syndrome are considered to have a genetic defect in serotonin metabolism. Individuals heterozygous for this gene can express it as alcoholism or drug addiction (Comings, 1993).

Reactions to Ethanol as a Potent Predictor of Alcoholism. Alcohol may be more positively reinforcing to sons of alcoholic fathers than to sons of nonalcoholic fathers. For example, baseline attributes of FHP and FHN individuals were measured after a beverage challenge. A decreased intensity of reaction to a challenge dose of ethanol was observed in male FHP subjects as compared to FHN controls (Schuckit and Smith, 2000, 2001b). FHPs demonstrated significantly higher levels of acetaldehyde, while similar patterns of blood alcohol concentrations were observed in FHP and FHN groups (O'Malley and Maisto, 1985). The FHP groups experienced a significantly lower level of subjective intoxication as judged by the Subjective High Assessment Scale (SHAS) and global ratings. Despite identical blood alcohol concentrations, the FHP men rated themselves as significantly less intoxicated than the FHNs (Schuckit and Smith, 2000). The FHNs reported higher scores on the overall "drug effect" scale. The FHPs demonstrated less decrement in cognitive and psychomotor performance after drinking. Moreover, the FHN subjects showed significantly greater increase in body sway after drinking an acute dose of alcohol (Schuckit and Smith, 2001b).

Trait Markers of Alcoholism

Numerous studies have been performed in the past years to identify potential markers of trait abnomarity in alcoholism (see recent reviews by Ferguson and Goldberg, 1997; Farren and Tipton, 1999). As discussed before, ADH and ALDH polymorphisms, specifically the ADH3*1, ADH2*2, and ALDH2*2 genotypes, appear to confer a protective effect against alcoholism, most notably in Asian subjects. Caucasian alcohol abusers and their first-degree relatives exhibit depressed platelet monoamine oxidase activity, the degree of which is greater in Type II than Type I alcoholics. Electrophysiological characteristics of alcoholics and those at risk for developing alcoholism also have been identified, including the reduced amplitude of the event-related brain potential and, after ethanol ingestion, characteristic EEG α-wave activity. Lower platelet adenylate cyclase activity is seen in alcoholics than in controls, presumably as a result of overexpression of an inhibitory G-protein. Markers related to other signal transduction pathways of the central nervous system—including the serotoninergic, muscarinic and dopaminergic systems—have also been studied.

In this group of markers, the putative association between the inheritance of the AI allele of the D2 dopamine receptor and the susceptibility to alcoholism provides the most dramatic illustration of the challenges that exist in this field of scientific investigation. Current limitations in the definition, diagnosis, and classification of alcoholism; the confounding influences of race and gender on association studies; and the statistical approach of linkage studies all have to be taken into consideration to uncover valid genetic markers for the risk of alcoholism. Also, linkage studies using the quantitative trait locus (QTL) mapping strategy were attempted for phenotypes relevant for alcoholism. The QTL strategy is theoretically capable of identifying determinant genes that contribute only a small portion of the variance. In human linkage studies, a genetic association was found to the DRD2 dopamine receptor. The DRD2 finding generated controversy, as a number of other groups failed to replicate it, and it focused attention on the advantages and pitfalls of the population association approach for detecting genes that influence behavior. The most promising trait markers are discussed in detail below.

Platelet Monoamine Oxidase. Monoamine oxidase (MAO) catalyzes the oxidation of monoamine neurotransmitters such as catecholamines, indolamines, and other biogenic amines that possibly play an important role in the regulation of mood and behavior. Two forms of MAO, A and B, are known; they are distributed mainly in the brain, liver, and blood platelets. In human platelets only the B form is detectable. Low platelet MAO activity associated with alcohol abuse has been thought to represent a genetic vulnerability factor for alcoholism, especially the type II form. Many earlier studies have shown the occurrence of low brain and platelet MAO activity in alcoholics with a great deal of overlap in the values (Agarwal et al., 1983; Major et al., 1985; Faraj et al., 1987).

MAO activity levels were found to be significantly low in children of a male-dominated subgroup of alcoholics with an earlier onset and severe course of alcohol-related problems (Sullivan et al., 1990; von Knorring et al., 1991). In one study, in vitro inhibition of MAO activity by ethanol was found to be significantly higher in the platelets of alcoholics than in matched controls (Tabakoff et al., 1990). The changes were long-lasting, and discriminant analysis showed that the use of values for the inhibition of MAO by ethanol correctly classified 75% of the alcoholics and 73% of the controls. Several subsequent studies have demonstrated decreased platelet MAO levels in type II alcoholics, compared with nonalcoholic controls (Anthenelli et al., 1998). However, a link between MAO activity and genetic predisposition to alcoholism remains to be unequivocally established due to an interindividual wide range of MAO activities and a great overlap between populations (Soyka et al., 2000). Also, a number of intrinsic characteristics (e.g., gender, race, comorbid psychiatric illness, metabolic factors, and personality traits) and extrinsic factors (e.g., tobacco smoking, medications, and platelet sampling differences) appear to influence MAO activity.

Adenylate Cyclase. Lymphocyte and platelet adenylate cyclase (AC) activity in alcoholic subjects were found to be less responsive to stimulation by fluoride, guanine nucleotide, or prostaglandin E (Tabakoff et al., 1990; Parsian et al., 1996; Menninger et al., 2000). A linear discriminant analysis of the distribution of fluoride-stimulated adenylate cyclase activity in the platelets of alcoholics and controls showed that by using this parameter, 75% of alcoholics and 73% of controls could be classified correctly. These abnormalities in alcoholics persisted even after weeks of abstinence, suggesting that the decreased AC activity in blood cells is a trait marker rather than a state marker. More recent work has further shown that basal and stimulated blood cell AC activity may be genetically determined (Devor et al., 1991).

Ratsma et al. (1999) studied G_s-protein stimulated AC in platelets of children of alcoholics. G_s-protein-stimulated cAMP production by NaF in platelet membranes of children of alcoholics was profoundly lower than in platelet membranes of control children. Moreover, such a reduced Gs-protein functioning was only observed in platelet membranes of children of alcoholics with a multigenerational family history of alcoholism. However, whether platelet AC activity could be used as an inherent trait marker in persons with alcoholism or as a state marker reflecting a long-term alcohol consumption of ethanol has to be further elucidated in future studies.

Serotonin Function and Uptake. Serotonin (5-HT) is an important regulator of morphogenetic activities during early central nervous system development, including cell proliferation, migration, and differentiation. The 5-HT transporter (5-HTT) plays a pivotal role in brain 5-HT homeostasis. It is also the initial target for both antidepressant drugs and drugs of abuse, some of which are potent neurotoxins. A polymorphism in the 5′-flanking regulatory region of the 5-HTT gene that results in allelic variation of 5-HTT expression is associated with anxiety-related personality traits and may influence the risk of developing affective disorders. It has been proposed that the risk for alcoholism may be associated with alterations in serotonin function related to aggression, violence, and impulsivity. The rate of serotonin uptake, a genetically influenced trait, may also mark vulnerability to alcoholism.

Rausch et al. (1991) observed that the rate of platelet serotonin uptake was higher in the high-risk individuals than in controls. Disfunction of monoamine uptake mechanisms has been implicated in the pathogenesis of alcohol dependence. A significant reduction (a mean of about 30%) in the availability of brainstem serotonin transporters was found in alcoholics, which was significantly correlated with lifetime alcohol consumption and with ratings of depression and anxiety during withdrawal. The findings support the hypothesis of serotonergic dysfunction in alcoholism and in withdrawal-emergent depressive symptoms (Heinz et al., 1998).

Transketolase. Alcohol abuse leads to lowered erythrocyte transketolase activity. A variant of transketolase having a reduced affinity for the cofactor thiamine diphosphate has been found to be associated with Wernicke-Korsakoff patients (Nixon et al., 1984; Zimtakin and Zimtakin, 1996). However, it remains to be equivocally shown whether this represents a predisposing marker.

Glutathione S-transferase. Human glutathione *S*-transferase (GST) shows at least three sets of isozymes that differ in their tissue distribution, incidence of genetic variation, susceptibility to certain inhibitors, and electrophoretic mobility. The distribution of various GST isozymes in livers and lymphocytes of patients with alcoholic and nonalcoholic liver diseases showed that the $GST1^0$ type is highly prevalent in livers of patients with acute hepatitis, alcoholic liver cirrhosis, and liver carcinoma, as compared to apparently healthy livers (Harada et al., 1987). In livers from patients with chronic hepatitis, the $GST1^2$ phenotype was found in high incidence. The null allele ($GST1^0$) was also found to be the most frequent type in the lymphocytes of alcoholics (Savolainen et al., 1996). Whether the presence of the null allele among alcoholics indicates a genetic vulnerability has yet to be established.

ABO Blood Groups. Early studies on blood groups and alcoholism revealed an association of blood group A with alcoholism. Hill et al. (1988) studied association and linkage of ABO, MNSs, Rh, Kell, Duffy, and Xg in alcoholics and their nonalcoholic first-degree relatives. Except for a higher frequency of homozygous recessive ss of the MNSs system in the nonalcoholic family members than in the alcoholics, no significant relationship between blood groups and alcoholism was noted. Subsequent studies could not establish any significant link between the MNS blood group and alcoholism (Tanna et al., 1988; Neiswanger et al., 1995).

Human Leucocyte Antigens. Significant associations between various human leucocyte antigens (HLA), including HLA-B8, HLA-B13, HLA-B40, HLA-B15, and HLA-DR3, and both alcoholic hepatitis and alcoholic cirrhosis have been observed in several studies, while in other studies no such association could be established (List and Gluud, 1994).

D2 Dopamine Receptor Gene and Alcoholism. Recently, reports suggesting an association of the D2 dopamine receptor gene, named DRD2, and alcoholism have drawn considerable attention. Restriction of DRD2 by TaqI yields polymorphic fragment lengths identifying alleles A1 and A2 that differ in average amounts of receptor sites (Blum et al., 1993). Human cadaver studies in the alcoholic group showed a significantly higher frequency of the DRD2 allele A1 than in the nonalcoholic group. This finding has been replicated in a number of subsequent studies (reviewed by Finckh, 2001). In other studies, however, no evidence of linkage of the A1 allele and increased susceptibility to alcoholism in informative families was found (Noble, 1993). More recent replication studies are highly conflicting (Sander et al., 1999; Anghelescu et al., 2001). Apparently, allele A1 confers relative susceptibility and allele A2 confers relative resistance to morbidity and mortality from chronic alcohol abuse, but the gene does not affect alcohol drinking behavior. It has been suggested that possibly the observed association of the alleles of the human D2 dopamine receptor locus may not be due to linkage with a gene for alcoholism, but could be a cause of the progression of the disease in individuals who are genetically predisposed to alcoholism (Noble, 1998).

More recent studies, nevertheless, do hint at a possible linkage of the dopamine receptor promotor region and subtypes of alcoholism (Parsian et al., 2000; Finckh, 2001). Moreover, polymorphism of the D2 dopamine receptor gene seems to be an important determinant of P300 latency (Noble et al., 1994; Nacher, 2000). P300 wave amplitude was found to be significantly longer in boys with the A1 allele than in boys carrying the A2 allele. Moreover, male and female alcoholics also differ in their visual P3 response (Hada et al., 2001; Prabhu et al., 2001).

Neurobehavioral Markers of Risk for Alcoholism

A number of studies have used psychophysiological and neurobehavioral markers for alcoholism to analyze genetic association, transmission, and linkage. These markers include the low P300 event-related potential., sensitivity to ethanol's intoxicating and euphoric effects, platelet adenylate cyclase, and neurotransmitter metabolite concentrations. Although it is highly likely that many alcoholism-associated physiologic phenotypes are secondary traits, these approaches have increased the specificity of genetic analyses and clarify their relationship to alcoholism.

Electroencephalographic Activity. Electrophysiological techniques have proven valuable in detecting subtle abnormalities in alcohol-related brain function. The human resting electroencephalogram (EEG) is a sensitive and noninvasive indicator of the central effects of drugs, particularly when combined with computational analysis. In addition, the EEG offers several advantages for the geneticist because it combines trait and state characteristics. In humans, the electroencephalogram examined under resting conditions is under strong genetic control. MZ twins have identical EEG tracings, whereas DZ twins on the average have different tracings. In addition to the average variation of the EEG pattern, certain variants of the EEG have been described, some of which follow a simple mode of inheritance (Propping, 1977).

Centrally acting drugs produce characteristic changes in the EEG according to their pharmacological classes. It is known that ethanol, when given as a single dose, increases the number of α and β waves, as well as the amplitudes of all frequency classes, a phenomenon called synchronization. In a pioneer study of 26 MZ and 26 DZ healthy adult twin pairs, it was shown that MZ twins exhibit an identical EEG response to a single dose of ethanol, whereas DZ twins on the average differ in type and extent of their response (Propping, 1977) (Figs. 46–4, 46–5). There was a considerable variation between subjects in the reaction to ethanol, depending on the type of the pre-alcohol EEG trace, and this can clearly be seen when subjects with "extreme" types of the resting EEG were exposed to alcohol (Fig. 46–6). The most pronounced synchronizing effect of alcohol was produced in the EEG with poor α activity in the pre-drug state (Figs. 46–7, 46–8). The differential response is a phenomenon at the pharmacodynamic level, because the blood alcohol concentrations do not differ among individuals with the different EEG types.

Many past studies have shown that resting-state EEGs in sober, awake alcoholics contain excess β activity and a deficiency in α, δ, and θ activity. A deficiency in α rhythm of EEG in alcoholics and their relatives was demonstrated when compared to controls (Pollock et al., 1983; Ehlers and Schuckit, 1990; Cohen et al., 1991; Enoch, 1999; Finn and Justus, 1999). Gabrielli et al. (1982) compared the male children at high risk and low risk for alcoholism. They found a faster EEG activity in the former group and concluded that this may be a potential biological marker for predisposition to alcoholism in sons of alcoholics. In a study of 115 alcoholics (78 males, 37 females) and the same number of matched controls, Propping et al. (1981) found that female alcoholics showed poorer EEG synchronization than male alcoholics or controls. The first-degree relatives who had not abused alcohol at any time also exhibited the same tendency as the corresponding index cases. The EEG with poor α wave activity may thus be regarded as a trait that increases the disposition for alcoholism, at least in females. Later studies fur-

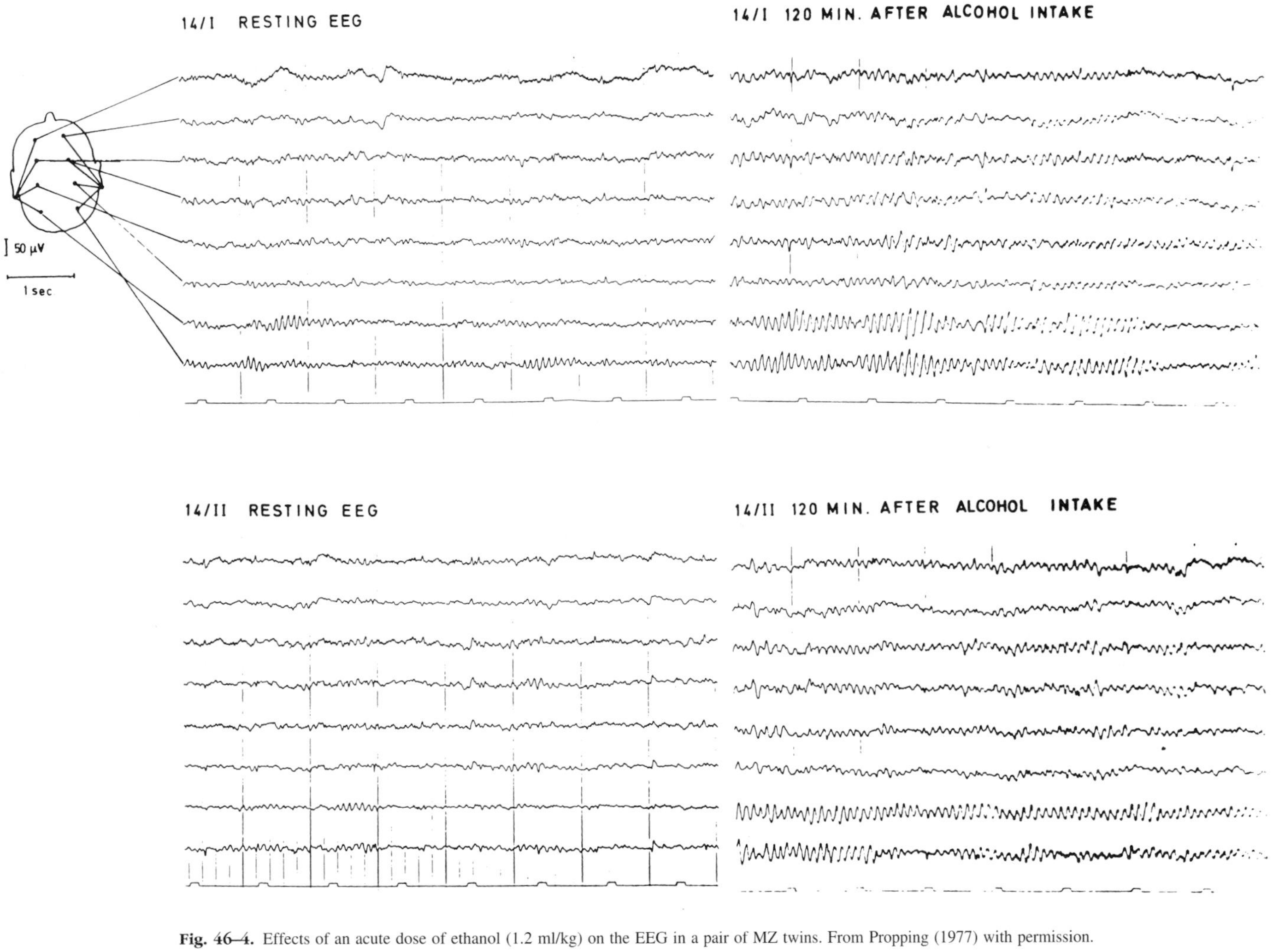

Fig. 46–4. Effects of an acute dose of ethanol (1.2 ml/kg) on the EEG in a pair of MZ twins. From Propping (1977) with permission.

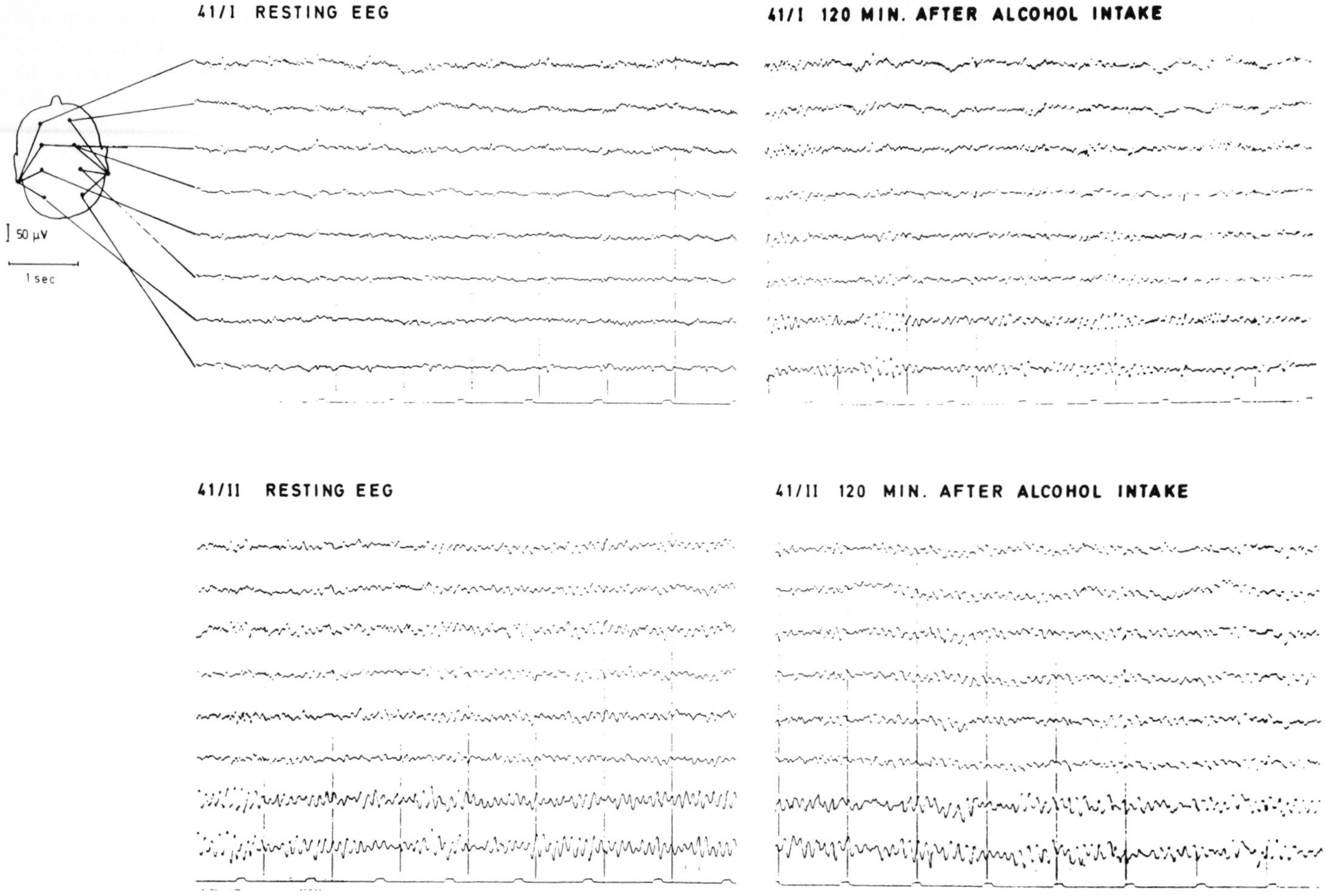

Fig. 46–5. Effects of an acute dose of ethanol (1.2 ml/kg) on the EEG in a pair of DZ twins. From Propping (1977) with permission.

ther confirmed the genetic influence on the acute adaptation of the EEG to alcohol (Christian et al., 1996; O'Connor et al., 1999). There are two possibilities, not mutually exclusive, to explain the difference between alcoholics and controls: poor EEG synchronization may be the result of alcoholic brain damage, or it may precede alcoholism and thus reflect a predisposition for development of this disease. These findings suggest that subjects at high risk for alcoholism are physiologically more sensitive to alcohol than are control subjects.

Increased fast-EEG activity can be secondary to chronic alcoholism, because this phenomenon has been described as a function of brain impairment. However, some findings favor the hypothesis that individuals with a poorly synchronized EEG are at higher risk for development of alcoholism, an idea brought forward in the early 1970s (Naitoh, 1973). Taken together, it seems reasonable to assume that a poorly synchronized EEG pattern is not specific for a certain psychiatric illness but is a basic, genetically controlled mechanism that enhances the risk of alcoholism, schizophrenia, and possibly other psychiatric diseases (Propping et al., 1981).

Event-Related Potentials. Another sensitive and noninvasive method for determining the effects of centrally-acting drugs is the determination of sensory-evoked event-related potentials (ERP). This technique consists of recording the electrical response of the brain immediately after repeated presentations of brief sensory stimuli of any modality and using signal averaging techniques to extract the precisely timed activity. ERP represents a sensitive index of brain responsivity to external visual, auditory, somatosensory, and olfactory stimuli. Differences in ERPs may also reflect differences in information processing, thus making it a useful tool for studying inherited vulnerability to alcoholism. The ERP method yields a characteristic, highly reproducible wave form, lasting between 250 and 500 msec (P300 component). Twin studies have demonstrated that the ERP pattern is under an appreciable genetic control.

In recent years great attention has focused on the P300 component of ERP, which is a wave form associated with various cognitive responses of the individual. The P300 component has been demonstrated to be significantly more similar in MZ twins than in DZ twins or control subjects, further emphasizing that ERP is under genetic control (Polich and Bloom, 1987; Rogers and Deary, 1991). Moreover, it was reported that abstinent alcoholics manifest a significantly reduced P300 component compared to matched normal control subjects (Begleiter et al., 1984; Emmerson et al., 1987; Patterson et al., 1987; Pfefferbaum et al., 1991). Subsequently, several investigators reported that sons of alcoholic fathers also exhibit a smaller P300 wave amplitude than sons of nonalcoholics in response to a visual stimulus, without exposure to alcohol (Whipple et al., 1991; Hada et al., 2001; Prabhu et al., 2001). The latency of the P300 component was found to be increased for both affected and nonaffected sibs com-

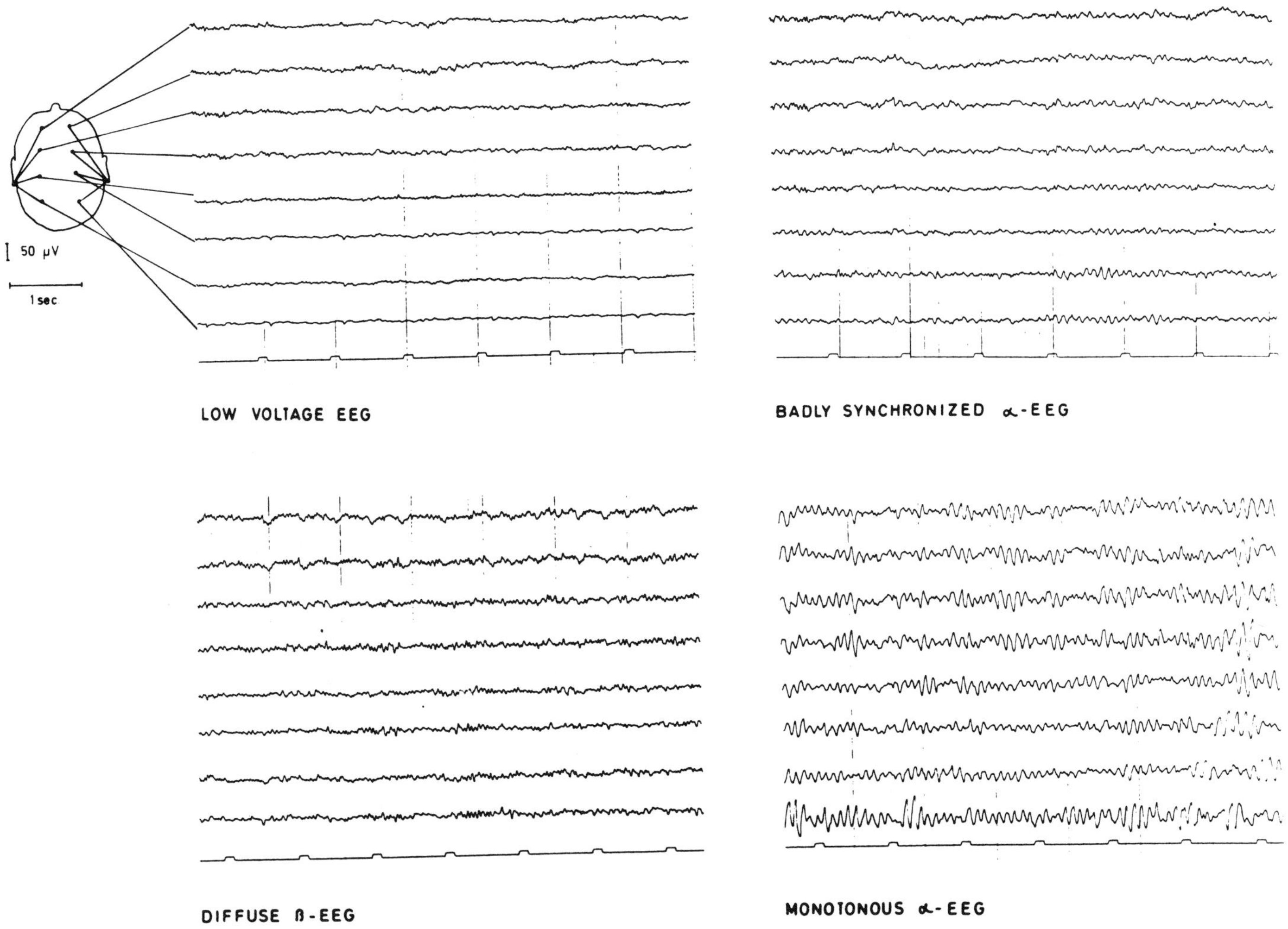

Fig. 46–6. Examples of four "extreme" types of the normal resting EEG selected by large-scale screening among healthy individuals. From Propping et al. (1980) with permission.

pared to controls, indicating a familial difference irrespective of the drinking status (Steinhauer et al., 1987). Specific neuroadaptive patterns were observed in males at high risk for alcoholism (pleasure oriented, high novelty seeking, high disinhibition, impulsivity, etc.) in contrast to those who manifest tension-reduction behavior (high harm avoidance, reduction of aversive emotional experience or stress by self-medication).

Longitudinal studies in children at high risk for developing alcohol-related disorders demonstrated that reduction in P300 amplitude is due to developmental delays in reaching age-appropriate levels in P300 ampitude (Hill et al., 1999). Systematic assessment of heritabilty of ERP in families with a history of alcoholism has further confirmed the potential of ERP as a neurophysiological marker of genetic vulnerability to alcoholism (Porjesz and Begleiter, 1998; Almasy et al., 1999; Hesselbrock et al., 2001a).

Gene Identification

Genes and Responsible Variation

Evidence for the familial transmission of alcoholism has stimulated researchers to look for specific genes that may confer vulnerability to alcoholism (Hesselbrock et al., 2001b). Existence of a variable number of possible interacting genes giving a predisposition to the diseases is likely. However, the genetic dissection has been hampered by genetic complexity, as well as by difficulties in defining the phenotypes. These include the choice of phenotype to be studied, whether narrow or broad, whether only mild or severe forms are included, and whether or not comorbidity should be excluded (Hill, 1998).

Candidate Genes

In searching for genes that contribute to alcoholism risk, several approaches may be used to identify the genetic loci that underlie alcoholism susceptibility (Kwon and Goate, 2000; Buckland, 2001). The number of mapped human genes now exceeds 30,000 of the estimated total number of 100,000 to 130,000 genes. This rapid development will facilitate gene mapping and efforts to isolate and identify the genes responsible for symptom susceptibility in many of the etiologically unclear psychiatric diseases with complex genetic origin. Genetic mapping efforts using sib pairs, twins, and individual large families have revealed preliminary or tentative evidence of susceptibility loci for alcoholism (Long et al., 1998; Reich et al., 1998; Foroud et al., 2000; Thome et al., 2000; Vadasz et al., 2000). Several candidate genes have been evaluated for their role in alcoholism; however, with the

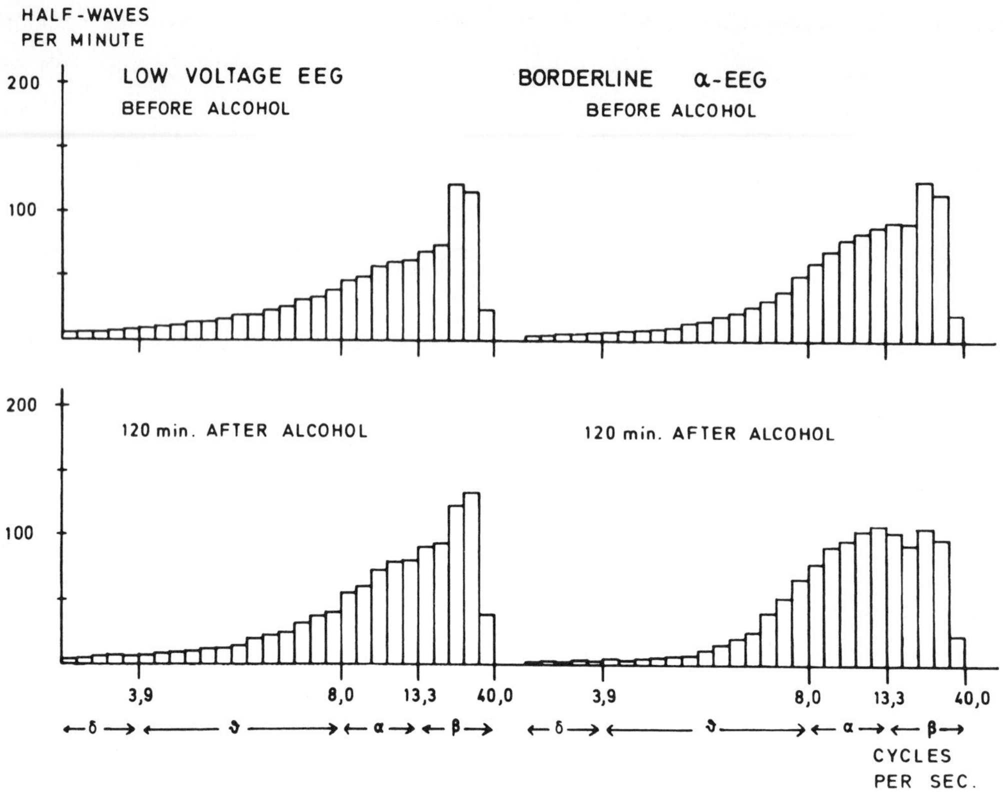

Fig. 46–7. Frequency histograms before and after intake of ethanol (1.2 ml/kg) in the low-voltage and borderline α-EEG. From Propping et al. (1980) with permission.

exception of the enzymes of alcohol metabolism, results from these studies have been inconsistent (Goldman, 1995; Chen et al., 1999; Harada et al., 2001; Li et al., 2001; Whitfield, 2001). Notably, the functional genetic variants of ADH that exhibit high alcohol oxidizing activity and the genetic variant of ALDH that exhibits low acetaldehyde oxidizing activity protect against heavy drinking and alcoholism (Agarwal, 2001).

Quantitative Trait Loci Mapping

The genetically influenced characterisrics, or traits, thought to underlie responses to alcohol (sensitivity to its effects) are called quantitative traits. Many genes influence the overall characteristics, each to a certain event. Within a population a quantitative trait differs in the degree to which individuals possess it, rather than in the kind of trait they possess. Accordingly, a small section of DNA thought to contribute to a quantitative trait is called a quantitative trait loci (QTL). Quantitative traits are said to be continuously distributed in a population because individuals exhibit them to different degrees. Locating a particular quantitative trait in the genome is called QTL mapping. Once QTL analyses have identified a chromosome region containing a gene that may affect a certain phrnotype (i.e., a candidate gene), tests can be performed to determine the magnitude of the gene's influence. However, the QTLs involved in human alcoholism remain to be characterized. Therefore, QTL mapping for alcohol-related traits is more commonly performed in animal models than in humans (Buck, 1998; Grahame, 2000). Researchers have used mouse and rat models to identify quantitative trait loci influencing alcohol preference. By studying animal models, complications imposed by environmental variations are minimized. Through the development of congenic lines and transgenic and knockout animals, candidate genes can be identified and evaluated for their role in alcohol preference. New methods for identifying chromosomal regions containing genes that affect murine responses to alcohol and drugs have been used to identify many provisional QTLs since 1991 (Crabbe et al., 1999). The syntenic (homologous) region of the human genome for these genes is often known.

For many mapped QTLs, candidate genes with relevant neurobiological function lie within the mapped region. QTLs have been confirmed for alcohol consumption and preference in regions of mouse chromosomes 1, 2, and 9 (Peirce et al., 1998; Tarantino et al., 1998). Overlapping regions of chromosomes 1 and 2 have been mapped for alcohol withdrawal (Buck et al., 1997). The ultimate goal of QTL mapping and cloning is to identify the genes contributing to alcoholism. Recently, two large studies have employed a genome screen methodology to identify novel genes contributing to the risk of alcoholism (Long et al., 1998; Reich et al., 1998; Foroud et al., 2000; Nurnberger et al., 2000; Vadasz et al., 2000). This screening has resulted in the detection of suggestive linkages on human chromosomes 1, 4, and 7, but did not identify any definitive linkage.

CLINICAL APPLICATION AND RISK ASSESSMENT

Diagnosis

Because alcohol consumption is intimately entangled in the cultural traditions of many countries and societies, an objective diagnosis of alcoholism is necessary. As stated before, several reliable interview techniques have been developed that have the

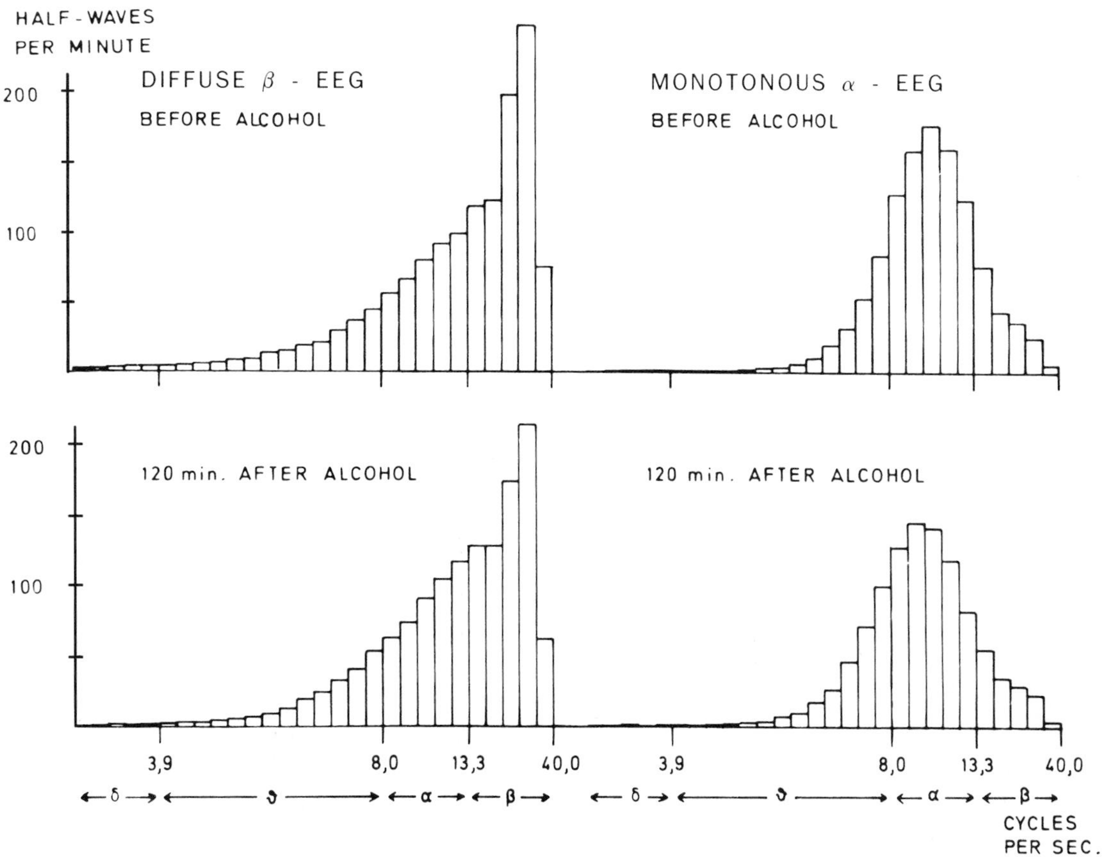

Fig. 46–8. Frequency histograms before and after intake of ethanol (1.2 ml/kg) in the EEG with diffuse β-EEG and regular α-EEG activity. From Propping et al. (1980) with permission.

advantage of being easy, inexpensive, and rapid. For clinical purposes, these tests are superior to extensive blood chemistry procedures. Alternatively, laboratory parameters, when combined with multivariate analysis, also have a high sensitivity and specificity for detection of alcoholics. In doubtful cases, familial occurrence of alcoholism can be used as an auxiliary diagnostic tool.

Screening

For screening purposes, the interview techniques can identify the great majority of alcoholics, if those being interviewed are willing to cooperate. Increased rates of alcoholism will be detected among persons with a variety of psychiatric symptoms, certain professional groups, military personnel, and, of course, offspring of alcoholics. Although some biochemical, molecular, and neurophysiological parameters such as plasma aldehyde level after acute alcohol loading, ADH and ALDH genotypes, and EEG characteristics are promising candidates for defining persons at risk for alcoholism, their practical application in screening procedures is premature. Alcoholics with certain HLA alleles presumably are at an increased risk of developing liver cirrhosis.

Prevention

Because the availability of alcohol can be drastically influenced by the price, tax policy is an important way of controlling alcohol consumption. It is problematic whether education and public warnings can be equally effective in a permissive society. Undoubtedly, the best prophylaxis against alcohol abuse has been membership in particular religious groups.

Counseling and Family Management

Alcoholism is a disease for which genetic counseling is only rarely requested. If needed, empiric recurrence risk figures can be given. Among first-degree relatives of alcoholics, it is not possible to differentiate reliably those persons at lower risk of alcoholism from those at higher risk. For such predictive purposes, more reliable knowledge from prospective studies among persons at risk is necessary.

Therapy

Providing appropriate therapy for alcoholism is one of the most difficult tasks in psychiatry and medicine. Various forms of psychotherapy are being applied. Common to all approaches is the need for patients to accept the fact that alcohol has a key role in their personal difficulties. Under certain circumstances psychotherapy might be supported by pharmacological aversion prophylaxis with disulfiram. The effect of disulfiram (antabuse) is of particular interest for the geneticist, because Asians with the deficient ALDH2 allele are physiologically in a state that can only be achieved by disulfiram in nondeficient individuals.

Thus far there is no way of applying empiric genetic knowledge to therapeutic concepts. With the advent of an improved understanding of alcohol's metabolism and action on the brain, genetic findings might prepare the way for pharmacological progress in alcoholism therapy (Brooks, 2000; Brink, 2001).

SUMMARY AND FUTURE DIRECTIONS

Some people appear greatly affected by even small doses of alcohol, while others consume large amounts without any apparent effect on their behavior or performance. The basis of this normal variation is little understood and may provide clues to the etiology of alcoholism. Scientists engaged in alcoholism research are certain that many genes are involved in determining a vulnerability to alcoholism. However, the tremendous variability shown in alcoholism has made it difficult to identify the putative "alcoholism genes" more specifically. Future research involving the genetics of predisposition to alcoholism need to take into consideration behavioral and biological assessments covering drinking and drug habits, medical history, and psychiatric problems, along with the tests of cognitive and motor skills, electrophysiological measures, and biochemical determinations. Such studies should be followed by segregation analysis to model potential mechanisms of inheritance. This will help characterize the genes that are suspected of being involved in alcohol abuse and alcoholism.

Formal linkage studies involving a large number of members from families of alcoholics should be useful for an in-depth look at candidate genes and their association with possible biological markers. Ultimately, such a study will result in capturing the full range of variation underlying alcoholism. Indeed, new technologies are now available which may enable the identification and cloning of major susceptibility genes spanning the human genome. Advances in computerized pedigree analysis and biotechnology will help in this task.

Because certain putative genetic loci that determine alcohol preference and for vulnerability to alcoholism are present in individuals at risk, prospective studies should lead to new pharmacological treatments, and to the development of tests to predict individuals at risk for alcoholism (Brooks and Lipsky, 2000). It is hoped that with the help of modern molecular biology techniques, a specific genetic profile to alcoholism will be found in the not too distant future. It might thus be possible to validate a genetic profile that associates with the future development of alcohol problems. Although much has still to be done to delineate the specific contribution of genetic and environmental factors on normal and abnormal drinking and on the development of organ damage, the discussion here clearly indicates a significant role of inherited factors in the genesis of alcoholism.

REFERENCES

Agarwal DP: Molecular genetic aspects of alcohol metabolism and alcoholism. Pharmacopsychiatry 1997; 30:79–84.

Agarwal DP: Pharmacogenetic relevance of aldehyde dehydrogenases. In: Agarwal DP, Seitz HK (eds). Alcohol in Health and Disease. New York: Marcel Dekker, 2001:49–86.

Agarwal DP, Buda B, Czeizel AE, Goedde HW: Alcohol Consumption and Alcoholism in Hungary: Ethnocultural, Epidemiological and Biomedical Aspects. Budapest: Academiai Kiado, 1997.

Agarwal DP, Goedde HW: Alcohol Metabolism, Alcohol Intolerance and Alcoholism: Biochemical and Pharmacological Approaches. Berlin, Heidelberg, New York: Springer-Verlag, 1990.

Agarwal DP, Philippu G, Milech U, Ziemsen B, Schrappe O, Goedde HW: Platelet monoamine oxidase and erythrocyte catechol-*o*-methyltransferase activity in alcoholism and controlled abstinence. Drug Alcohol Depend 1983; 12:85–91.

Aharonovich E, Hasin D, Rahav G, Meydan J, Neumark Y: Differences in drinking patterns among Ashkenazic and Sephardic Israeli adults. J Stud Alcohol 2001; 62:301–305.

Allgulander C, Nowak J, Rice JP: Psychopathology and treatment of 30,344 twins in Sweden: II. Heritability estimates of psychiatric diagnosis and treatment in 12,884 twin pairs. Acta Psychiatr Scand 1991; 83:12–15.

Almasy L, Porjesz B, Blangero J, Chorlian DV, O'Connor SJ, Kuperman S, Rohrbaugh J, Bauer LO, Reich T, Polich J, Begleiter H: Heritability of event-related brain potentials in families with a history of alcoholism. Am J Med Genet 1999; 88:383–390.

Amark C: A study in alcoholism: clinical, social-psychiatric, and genetic investigations. Acta Psychiatr Neurol Scand 1951; 70 (Suppl):1–283.

American Psychiatric Association: Diagnostic and Statistical Manual of Mental Disorders, (DSM-III-R). Washington DC: APA, 1987.

American Psychiatric Association: Diagnostic and Statistical Manual of Mental Disorders, (DSM-IV). Washington DC: APA, 1994.

Anghelescu I, Germeyer S, Muller MJ, Klawe C, Singer P, Dahmen N, Wetzel H, Himmerich H, Szegedi A: No association between the dopamine D2 receptor taqI A1 allele and earlier age of onset of alcohol dependence according to different specified criteria. Alcohol Clin Exp Res 2001; 25:805–809.

Anthenelli RM, Tipp J, Li TK, Magnes L, Schuckit MA, Rice J, Daw W, Nurnberger JI Jr: Platelet monoamine oxidase activity in subgroups of alcoholics and controls: results from the Collaborative Study on the Genetics of Alcoholism. Alcohol Clin Exp Res 1998; 22:598–604.

Babor TF: The classification of alcoholics: typology theories from the 19th century to the present. Alcohol Health Res World 1996; 20:6–14.

Babor TF, Dolinsky ZS: Alcoholic typologies: historical evolution and empirical evaluation of some common classification schemes. In: Ross RM, Barret J (eds). Alcoholism: Origins and Outcome. New York: Raven Press, 1988:245–266.

Babor TF, Hofmann M, Del Boca F, Hesselbrock V, Meyer R, Dolinsky ZS, Rounsaville B: Types of alcoholics: I. evidence for an empirically derived typology based on indicators of vulnerability and severity. Arch Gen Psychiatry 1992; 49:599–608.

Beckemeier ME, Bora PS: Fatty acid ethyl esters: potentially toxic products of myocardial ethanol metabolism. J Mol Cell Cardiol 1998; 30:2487–2494.

Begleiter H, Porjesz B, Bihari B, Kissin B: Event-related potentials in boys at risk for alcoholism. Science 1984; 225:1493–1496.

Bennion LJ, Li TK: Alcohol metabolism in American Indians and whites. N Engl J Med 1976; 294:9–13.

Berman RF, Hannigan JH: Effects of prenatal alcohol exposure on the hippocampus: spatial behavior, electrophysiology, and neuroanatomy. Hippocampus 2000; 10: 94–110.

Blum K, Noble EP, Sheridan PJ, Montgomery A, Ritchie T, Ozkaragoz T, Fitch RJ, Wood R, Finley O, Sadlack F: Genetic predisposition in alcoholism: association of the D2 dopamine receptor TaqI B1 RFLP with severe alcoholics. Alcohol 1993; 10:59–67.

Bohman M: Some genetic aspects of alcoholism and criminality. Arch Gen Psychiatry 1978; 35:269–276.

Bohman M, Cloninger CR, Sigvardsson S, von Knorring AL: The genetics of alcoholism and related disorders. J Psychiatr Res 1987; 21:447–452.

Bohman M, Sigvardsson S, Cloninger CR: Maternal inheritance of alcohol abuse: cross-fostering analysis of adopted women. Arch Gen Psychiatry 1981; 38:965–969.

Borras E, Coutelle C, Rosell A, Fernandez-Muixi F, Broch M, Crosas B, Hjelmqvist L, Lorenzo A, Gutierrez C, Santos M, et al.: Genetic polymorphism of alcohol dehydrogenase in Europeans: the ADH2*2 allele decreases the risk for alcoholism and is associated with ADH3*1. Hepatology 2000; 31:984–989.

Bowden SC, Crews FT, Bates ME, Fals-Stewart W, Ambrose ML: Neurotoxicity and neurocognitive impairments with alcohol and drug-use disorders: potential roles in addiction and recovery. Alcohol Clin Exp Res 2001; 25:317–321.

Brenner B: Estimating the prevalence of alcoholism: toward a modification of the Jellinek formula. Q J Stud Alcohol 1959; 20:255–260.

Brink S: Your brain on alcohol: a new understanding of how alcohol alters brain chemistry may transform treatment of the disease. US News World Rep 2001; 130:50–57.

Brooks PJ: Brain atrophy and neuronal loss in alcoholism: a role for DNA damage? Neurochem Int 2000; 37:403–412.

Brooks PJ, Lipsky RH: Future directions in alcoholism research: genomics and gene transfer. Alcohol Res Health 2000; 24:189–192.

Bucholz KK: Alcohol abuse and dependence from a psychiatric epidemiologic perspective. Alcohol Health Res World 1992; 16:197–208.

Bucholz KK, Cadoret R, Cloninger CR, Dinwiddie SH, Hesselbrock VM, Nurnberger JI Jr, Reich T, Schmidt I, Schuckit MA: A new, semi-structured psychiatric interview for use in genetic linkage studies: a report on the reliability of the SSAGA. J Stud Alcohol 1994; 55:149–158.

Buck KJ: Recent progress toward the identification of genes related to risk for alcoholism. Mamm Genome 1998; 9:927–928.

Buck KJ, Metten P, Belknap JK, Crabbe JC: Quantitative trait loci involved in genetic predisposition to acute alcohol withdrawal in mice. J Neurosci 1997; 17:3946–3955.

Buckland PR: Genetic association studies of alcoholism: problems with the candidate gene approach. Alcohol Alcohol 2001; 36:99–103.

Caballeria L, Pares A, Ercilla G, Montull S, Caballeria J, Rodes J: Class I and II his-

tocompatibility antigens and severity of the alcoholic liver lesion. Gastroenterol Hepatol 1997; 20:167–171.
Cadoret R, Gath A: Inheritance of alcoholism in adoptees. Br J Psychiatry 1978; 132:252–258.
Cadoret R, Troughton E, Woodworth G: Evidence of heterogeneity of genetic effect in Iowa adoption studies. Ann NY Acad Sci 1994; 708:59–71.
Cahalan D, Cisin I-H: Drinking Behavior And Drinking Problems In The United States. In: Kissin B, Begleiter H (eds). Social Aspects of Alcoholism. New York: Plenum Press, 1976:77–115.
Carpenter WB: On the Use and Abuse of Alcoholic Liquors in Health and Disease. Philadelphia; Lea and Blanchard, 1850.
Chan AW, Pristach EA, Welte JW, Russell M: Use of the TWEAK test in screening for alcoholism/heavy drinking in three populations. Alcohol Clin Exp Res 1993; 17:1188–1192.
Chen CC, Lu RB, Chen YC, Wang MF, Chang YC, Li TK, Yin SJ: Interaction between the functional polymorphisms of the alcohol-metabolism genes in protection against alcoholism. Am J Hum Genet 1999; 65:795–807.
Cherpitel CJ: Screening for alcohol problems in the U.S. general population: a comparison of the CAGE and TWEAK by gender, ethnicity, and services utilization. J Stud Alcohol 1999; 60:705–711.
Chi I, Lubben JE, Kitano HHL: Differences in drinking behaviour among three Asian-American groups. J Stud Alcohol 1989; 50:15–23.
Christian JC, Morzorati S, Norton JA Jr, Williams CJ, O'Connor S, Li TK: Genetic analysis of the resting electroencephalographic power spectrum in human twins. Psychophysiology 1996; 33:584–591.
Cloninger CR: Neurogenetic adaptive mechanisms in alcoholism. Science 1987; 236:410–416.
Cloninger CR, Bohman M, Sigvardsson S: Inheritance of alcohol abuse: cross-fostering analysis of adopted men. Arch Gen Psychiatry 1981; 38:861–868.
Cloninger CR, Sigvardsson S, Bohman M: Childhood personality predicts alcohol abuse in young adults. Alcohol Clin Exp Res 1988; 12:494–505.
Cohen HL, Porjesz B, Begleiter H: EEG characteristics in males at risk for alcoholism. Alcohol Clin Exp Res 1991; 15:858–861.
Comings DE: Serotonin and the biochemical genetics of alcoholism: lessons from studies of attention deficit hyperactivity disorder (ADHD) and Tourette syndrome. Alcohol Alcohol (Suppl) 1993; 2:237–241.
Conigrave KM, Saunders JB, Reznik RB: Predictive capacity of the AUDIT questionnaire for alcohol-related harm. Addiction 1995; 90:479–485.
Cook C: Alcohol genetics: will the promises be fullfilled? Addiction Biol 2000; 5:405–410.
Cooper B: Nature, nurture and mental disorder: old concepts in the new millennium. Br J Psychiatry (Suppl) 2001; 40:S91–S101.
Cotton NS: The familial incidence of alcoholism: a review. J Stud Alcohol 1979; 40:89–116.
Crabbe JC: Use of genetic analyses to refine phenotypes related to alcohol tolerance and dependence. Alcohol Clin Exp Res 2001; 25:288–292.
Crabbe JC, Phillips TJ, Buck KJ, Cunningham CL, Belknap JK: Identifying genes for alcohol and drug sensitivity: recent progress and future directions. Trends Neurosci 1999; 22:173–179.
Cruz-Coke R, Varela A: Inheritance of alcoholism: its association with colour-blindness. Lancet 1966; 1:1282–1284.
Dawson, DA, Archer L: Gender differences in alcohol consumption: effects of measurement. Br J Addict 1992; 87:119–123.
Dawson DA, Harford TC, Grant BF: Family history as a predictor of alcoholism. Alcohol Clin Exp Res 1992; 16:572–575.
Day CP: Who gets alcoholic liver disease: nature or nurture? J R Coll Physicians Lond 2000; 34:557–562.
Day CP, Bashir R, James OF, Bassendine MF, Crabb DW, Thomasson HR, Li TK, Edenberg HJ: Investigation of the role of polymorphisms at the alcohol and aldehyde dehydrogenase loci in genetic predisposition to alcohol-related end-organ damage. Hepatology 1991; 14:798–801.
De-Lint J, Schmidt W: Alcoholism and mortality. In: Kissin B, Begleiter H (eds). Social Aspects of Alcoholism. New York: Plenum, 1976:275–305.
Devor EJ, Cloninger CR, Hoffman PL, Tabakoff B: Adenylate cyclase activity in the families of alcoholics is controlled by a single major gene. Alcohol Alcohol (Suppl) 1991; 1:157–160.
Dinwiddie SH, Cloninger CR: Family and adoption studies of alcoholism. In: Goedde HW, Agarwal DP (eds). Alcoholism Biomedical and Genetic Aspects. New York: Pergamon, 1989:259–276.
Drejer K, Theilgaard A, Teasdale TW, Schulsinger F, Goodwin DW: A prospective study of young men at high risk for alcoholism: neuropsychological assessment. Alcohol Clin Exp Res 1985; 9:498–502.
Edenberg HJ, Bosron WF: Alcohol dehydrogenase. In: Guengerich FP (ed). Comprehensive Toxicology, vol. 3. New York: Elsevier Science, 1997:119–131.
Ehlers CL, Schuckit MA: EEG fast frequency activity in the sons of alcoholics. Biol Psychiatry 1990; 27:631–641.
Emmerson RY, Dustman RE, Shearer DE, Chamberlin HM: EEG, visually evoked and event related potentials in young abstinent alcoholics. Alcohol 1987; 4:241–248.
Enoch MA, Goldman D: The genetics of alcoholism and alcohol abuse. Curr Psychiatry Rep 2001; 3:144–151.
Enoch MA, White KV, Harris CR, Robin RW, Ross J, Rohrbaugh JW, Goldman D: Association of low-voltage α EEG with a subtype of alcohol use disorders. Alcohol Clin Exp Res 1999; 23:1312–1319.
Enomoto N, Takase S, Yashuhara M, Takada A: Acetaldehyde metabolism in different aldehyde dehydrogenase-2 genotypes. Alcohol Clin Exp Res 1991; 15:141–144.
Eriksson CJ: The role of acetaldehyde in the actions of alcohol (update 2000). Alcohol Clin Exp Res 2001; 25(5 Suppl ISBRA):15S–32S.
Eriksson K: Alcohol inhibition and behavior: a comparative genetic approach. In: Eleftheriou BE (ed). Psychopharmacogenetics. New York: Plenum, 1975:127–168.
Faraj BA, Lenton JD, Kutner M, Camp VM, Stammers TW, Lee SR, Lolies PA, Chandora D: Prevalence of low monoamine oxidase function in alcoholism. Alcohol Clin Exp Res 1987; 11:464–467.
Farren CK, Tipton KF: Trait markers for alcoholism: clinical utility. Alcohol Alcohol 1999; 34:649–665.
Farris JJ, Morgan-Jones B: Ethanol metabolism in male American Indians and whites. Alcoholism 1978; 2:77–81.
Ferguson RA, Goldberg DM: Genetic markers of alcohol abuse. Clin Chim Acta 1997; 247:199–250.
Feuerlein W: Alkoholismus-Missbrauch und Abhangigkeit. Stuttgart: Thieme, 1984: 3–9.
Feuerlein W, Ringer C, Kufner H, Antons K: Diagnose des Alkoholismus: der Münchener Alkoholismus-Test (MALT). MMW Munch Med Wochenschr 1977; 119: 1275–1282.
Finckh U: Dopamine receptor genes and alcoholism: association studies. In: Agarwal DP, Seitz HK (eds). Alcohol in Health and Disease. New York: Marcel Dekker, 2001:151–176.
Fingarette H: Alcoholism: the mythical disease. In: Pittman DJ, White HR (eds). Society, Culture, and Drinking Patterns Reexamined. Piscataway, NJ: Rutgers University Center of Alcohol Studies, 1991:417–438.
Finn PR, Justus A: Reduced EEG α power in the male and female offspring of alcoholics. Alcohol Clin Exp Res 1999; 23:256–262.
Flavin DK, Morse RM: What is alcoholism? Current definitions and diagnostic criteria and their implications for treatment. Alcohol Health Res World 1990; 20:266–271.
Foroud T, Edenberg HJ, Goate A, Rice J, Flury L, Koller DL, Bierut LJ, Conneally PM, Nurnberger JI, Bucholz KK, et al.: Alcoholism susceptibility loci: confirmation studies in a replicate sample and further mapping. Alcohol Clin Exp Res 2000; 24:933–945.
Frezza M, Di Padova C, Pozzato G, Terpin M, Baraona E, Lieber CS: High blood alcohol levels in women: the role of decreased gastric alcohol dehydrogenase activity and first-pass metabolism. N Engl J Med 1990; 322:95–99.
Gabrielli WF, Mednick SA, Volavka J, Pollock VE, Schulsinger F, Itil TM: Electroencephalograms in children of alcoholic fathers. Psychophysiology 1982; 19:404–407.
Gabrielli WF Jr, Plomin R: Drinking behavior in the Colorado adoptee and twin sample. J Stud Alcohol 1985; 46:24–31.
Goedde HW, Agarwal DP, Fritze G: Distribution of *ADH2* and *ALDH2* genotypes in different populations. Hum Genet 1992; 88:344–346.
Goedde HW, Harada S, Agarwal DP: Racial difference in alcohol sensitivity: a new hypothesis. Hum Genet 1979; 51:331–334.
Goldman D: Candidate genes in alcoholism. Clin Neurosci 1995; 3:174–181.
Goodwin DW: Is alcoholism hereditary? A review and critique. Arch Gen Psychiatry 1971; 25:545–549.
Goodwin DW: Family studies of alcoholism. J Stud Alcohol 1981; 42:156–162.
Goodwin DW, Knop J, Jensen P, Gabrielli WF Jr, Schulsinger F, Penick EC: Thirty-year follow-up of men at high risk for alcoholism. Ann NY Acad Sci 1994; 708:97–101.
Goodwin DW, Schulsinger F, Hermansen L, Guze SB, Winokur G: Alcohol problems in adoptees raised apart from alcoholic biological parents. Arch Gen Psychiatry 1973; 28:238–243.
Goodwin D, Schulsinger F, Hermansen L, Guze S, Winokur G: Alcoholism and the hyperactive child syndrome. J Nerv Ment Dis 1975; 160:349–353.
Goodwin DW, Schulsinger F, Knop J, Mednick S, Guze SB: Alcoholism and depression in adopted-out daughters of alcoholics. Arch Gen Psychiatry 1977a; 34:751–755.
Goodwin DW, Schulsinger F, Knop J, Mednick S, Guze SB: Psychopathology in adopted and nonadopted daughters of alcoholics. Arch Gen Psychiatry 1977b; 34:1005–1009.
Goodwin DW, Schulsinger F, Moller N, Hermansen L, Winokur G, Guze S: Drinking problems in adopted and nonadopted sons of alcoholics. Arch Gen Psychiatry 1974; 31:164–169.
Grahame NJ. Selected lines and inbred strains: tools in the hunt for the genes involved in alcoholism. Alcohol Res Health 2000; 24:159–163.
Grant BF: Prevalence and correlates of drug use and DSM-IV drug dependence in the United States: results of the National Longitudinal Alcohol Epidemiologic Survey. J Subst Abuse 1996; 8:195–210.
Gurling HM, Murray RM, Clifford CA: Investigations into the genetics of alcohol dependence and into its effects on brain function. Prog Clin Biol Res 1981; 69 (Pt C):77–87.
Guze SB, Cloninger CR, Martin R, Clayton PJ: Alcoholism as a medical disorder. Compr Psychiatry 1986; 27:501–510.
Hada M, Porjesz B, Chorlian DB, Begleiter H, Polich J: Auditory P3a deficits in male subjects at high risk for alcoholism. Biol Psychiatry 2001; 49:726–738.
Hahn RG, Norberg A, Gabrielsson, J, Danielsson A, Jones AW: Eating a meal increases the clearence of ethanol given by intravenous infusion. Alcohol Alcohol 1994; 29:673–678.
Hall RL, Hesselbrock VM, Stabenau JR: Familial distribution of alcohol use: I. Assortative mating in the parents of alcoholics. Behav Genet 1983a; 13:361–372.

Hall RL, Hesselbrock VM, Stabenau JR: Familial distribution of alcohol use: II. Assortative mating of alcoholic probands. Behav Genet 1983b; 13:373–382.

Hanna JM: Metabolic responses of Chinese, Japanese, and Europeans to alcohol. Alcoholism 1978; 2:89–92.

Hara K, Terasaki O, Okubo Y: Dipole estimation of α EEG during alcohol ingestion in males genotypes for *ALDH2*. Life Sci 2000; 67:1163–1173.

Harada S, Abei M, Tanaka N, Agarwal DP, Goedde HW: Liver glutathione *S*-transferase polymorphism in Japanese and its pharmacogenetic importance. Hum Genet 1987; 75:322–325.

Harada S, Agarwal DP, Goedde HW: Aldehyde dehydrogenase deficiency as cause of facial flushing reaction to alcohol in Japanese. Lancet 1981; 2:982.

Harada S, Agarwal DP, Nomura F, Higuchi S: Metabolic and ethnic determinants of alcohol drinking habits and vulnerability to alcohol-related disorder. Alcohol Clin Exp Res 2001; 25(5 Suppl ISBRA):71S–75S.

Harper C: The neuropathology of alcohol-specific brain damage, or does alcohol damage the brain? J Neuropathol Exp Neurol 1998; 57:101–110.

Hayakawa K: Smoking and drinking discordance and health condition: Japanese identical twins reared apart and together. Acta Genet Med Gemellol (Roma) 1987; 36:493–502.

Heath AC, Bucholz KK, Madden PAF, Dinwiddie SH, Slutske WS, Bierut LJ, Statham DJ, Dunne MP, Whitfield JB, Martin NG: Genetic and environmental contributions to alcohol dependence risk in a national twin sample: consistency of findings in women and men. Psychol Med 1997; 27:1381–1396.

Heath AC, Madden PAF, Bucholz KK; Dinwiddie SH, Slutske WS, Bierut LJ, Rohrbaugh JW, Statham DJ, Dunne MP, Whitfield JB, Martin NG: Genetic differences in alcohol sensitivity and the inheritance of alcoholism risk. Psychol Med 1999; 29:1069–1081.

Heath AC, Whitfield JB, Madden PA, Bucholz KK, Dinwiddie SH, Slutske WS, Bierut LJ, Statham DB, Martin NG: Towards a molecular epidemiology of alcohol dependence: analysing the interplay of genetic and environmental risk factors. Br J Psychiatry (Suppl) 2001; 40:S33–S40.

Heather N: Why alcoholism is not a disease. Med J Aust 1992; 156:212–215.

Heinz A, Ragan P, Jones DW, Hommer D, Williams W, Knable MB, Gorey JG, Doty L, Geyer C, Lee KS, et al.: Reduced central serotonin transporters in alcoholism. Am J Psychiatry 1998; 155:1544–1549.

Helander A: Biological markers of alcohol use and abuse in theory and practice. In: Agarwal DP, Seitz HK (eds). Alcohol in Health and Disease. New York: Marcel Dekker, 2001:177–206.

Helzer JE, Burnam A, McEvoy L: Alcohol abuse and dependence. In: Robins LN, Regier DA (eds). Psychiatric Disorders in America: The Epidemiologic Catchment Area Study. New York: Free Press, 1991:81–115.

Hesselbrock MN, Hesselbrock VM: Relationship of family history, antisocial personality disorder and personality traits in young men at risk for alcoholism. J Stud Alcohol 1992; 53:619–625.

Hesselbrock VM: The genetic epidemiology of alcoholism. In: Begleiter H, Kissin B (eds). Alcohol and Alcoholism, vol. 1. New York: Oxford University Press, 1995:17–39.

Hesselbrock VM, Begleiter H, Porjesz B, O'Connor S, Bauer L: P300 event-related potential amplitude as an endophenotype of alcoholism: evidence from the collaborative study on the genetics of alcoholism. J Biomed Sci 2001a; 8:77–82.

Hesselbrock VM, Foroud T, Edenberg H, Nurnberger JI Jr, Reich T, Rice J: Genetics and alcoholism: the COGA project. In: Agarwal DP, Seitz HK (eds). Alcohol in Health and Disease. New York: Marcel Dekker, 2001b:103–124.

Higuchi S, Hayashida M: Genetic and epidemiological research at the National Institute on Alcoholism, Kurihama National Hospital. Psychiatry Clin Neurosci 1998; 52(Suppl):S351–353.

Higuchi S, Matsushita S, Murayama M, Takagi S, Hayashida M: Alcohol and aldehyde dehydrogenase polymorphisms and the risk for alcoholism. Am J Psychiatry 1995; 152:1219–1221.

Hill SY: Absence of paternal sociopathy in the etiology of severe alcoholism: is there a type III alcoholism? J Stud Alcohol 1992; 53:161–169.

Hill SY: Vulnerability to alcoholism in women: genetic and cultural factors. In: Galenter M (ed). Recent Developments in Alcoholism. Vol. 12: Women and Alcoholism. New York: Plenum Press, 1995:9–28.

Hill SY: Alternative strategies for uncovering genes contributing to alcoholism risk: unpredictable findings in a genetic wonderland. Alcohol 1998; 16:53–59.

Hill SY, Aston C, Rabin B: Suggestive evidence of genetic linkage between alcoholism and the MNS blood group. Alcohol Clin Exp Res 1988; 12:811–814.

Hill SY, Yuan H, Locke J: Path analysis of P300 amplitude of individuals from families at high and low risk for developing alcoholism. Biol Psychiatry 1999; 45:346–359.

Homann N, Tillonen J, Meurman JH, Rintamaki H, Lindqvist C, Rautio M, Jousimies-Somer H, Salaspuro M: Increased salivary acetaldehyde levels in heavy drinkers and smokers: a microbiological approach to oral cavity cancer. Carcinogenesis 2000; 21:663–668.

Hrubec Z, Omenn GS: Evidence of genetic predisposition to alcoholic cirrhosis and psychosis: twin concordances for alcoholism and its biological end points by zygosity among male veterans. Alcoholism Clin Exp Res 1981; 5:207–215.

Hughes, K, Yeo PPB, Lun KC, Thai AC, Wang KW, Cheah JC: Alcohol consumption in Chinese, Malays and Indians in Singapore. Ann Acad Med Singapore 1990; 19:330–332.

Hüllinghorst R: Alkoholkonsum: Zahlen und Fakten. In: Singer MV, Teyssen S (eds). Alkohol und Alkoholfolgekrankheiten: Grundlagen, Diagnostic, Therapy. Berlin and Heidelberg: Springer-Verlag, 1999:32–39.

Ingle KG: Typology research questionnaires. Alcohol Health Res World 1996; 20:63–66.

Iwahashi K, Suwaki H: Ethanol metabolism, toxicity and genetic polymorphism. Addict Biol 1998; 3:249–259.

Jahrbuch Sucht 2000. Geesthacht: Neuland-Verlagsgesellschaft, 1999.

Jellinek EM: Phases in the drinking history of alcoholics: analysis of a survey conducted by the official organ of Alcoholics Anonymous. Q J Stud Alcohol 1946; 7:1–88.

Jellinek EM: Phases of alcohol addiction. Q J Stud Alcohol 1959; 13:673–684.

Jellinek EM: Alcoholism, a genus and some of its species. CMAJ 1960; 83:1341–1346.

Johnson EO, Pickens RW: Familial transmission of alcoholism among nonalcoholics and mild, severe, and dyssocial subtypes of alcoholism. Alcohol Clin Exp Res 2001; 25:661–666.

Johnson EO, van den Bree MBM, Gupman AE, Pickens RW: Extension of a typology of alcohol dependence based on relative genetic and environmental loading. Alcohol Clin Exp Res 1998; 22:1421–1429.

Johnson EO, van den Bree MBM, Pickens RW: Indicators of genetic and environmental influence in alcohol-dependent individuals. Alcohol Clin Exp Res 1996; 20:67–74.

Johnson JL, Leff M: Children of substance abusers: overview of research findings. Pediatrics 1999; 103:1085–1099.

Jokelainen K: Acetaldehyde and liver disease. In: Agarwal DP, Seitz HK (eds). Alcohol in Health and Disease. New York: Marcel Dekker, 2001:387–406.

Jones AW: Aspects of in vivo pharmacokinetics of ethanol. Alcohol Clin Exp Res 2000; 24:400–402.

Jörnvall H, Höög JO: Nomenclature of alcohol dehydrogenase. Alcohol Alcohol 1995; 30:153–161.

Kaij L: Alcoholism in Twins. Stockholm: Almqvist and Wiksell, 1960:17–21.

Kaij L, Dock J: Grandsons of alcoholics: a test of sex-linked transmission of alcohol abuse. Arch Gen Psychiatry 1975; 32:1379–1381.

Kalow W: Ethnic differences in drug metabolism. Clin Pharmacokinet 1982; 7:373–400.

Kaprio J, Koskenvuo M, Langinvainio H, Romanov K, Sarna S, Rose RJ: Genetic influences on use and abuse of alcohol: a study of 5,638 adult Finnish twin brothers. Alcohol Clin Exp Res 1987; 11:349–356.

Kaprio J, Viken R, Koskenvuo M, Romanov K, Rose RJ: Consistency and change in patterns of social drinking: a 6-year follow-up of the Finnish Twin Cohort. Alcohol Clin Exp Res 1992; 16:234–240.

Keiding S, Christensen NJ, Damgaard SE: Ethanol metabolism in heavy drinkers after massive and moderate alcohol intake. Biochem Pharmacol 1983; 32:3097–3120.

Keller M: The disease concept of alcoholism revisited. J Stud Alcohol 1976; 37:1694–1717.

Kendler KS, Heath AC, Neale MC, Kessler RC, Eaves LJ: A population-based twin study of alcoholism in women. JAMA 1992; 268:1877–1882.

Kendler KS, Karkowski LM, Prescott CA, Pedersen NL: Latent class analysis of Temperance Board registrations in Swedish male–female twin pairs born 1902 to 1949: searching for subtypes of alcoholism. Psychol Med 1998; 28:803–813.

Kendler KS, Prescott CA, Neale MC, Pedersen NL: Temperance board registration for alcohol abuse in a national sample of Swedish male twins born 1902–1949. Arch Gen Psychiatry 1997; 54:178–184.

Keup W: Umrechnungstabelle von Trinkmenge auf Alkoholkonsum. Suchtgefahren 1983; 29:53–54.

Kitano, HHL, Lubben JE, Chi I: Predicting Japanese American drinking behavior. Int J Addict 1988; 23:417–428.

Klatsky AL, Siegelaub AB, Landy C, Friedman GD: Racial patterns of alcoholic beverage use. Alcohol Clin Exp Res 1983; 7:372–377.

Knop J, Goodwin DW, Jensen P, Penick E, Pollock V, Gabrielli W, Teasdale TW, Mednick SA: A 30-year follow-up study of the sons of alcoholic men. Acta Psychiatr Scand Suppl 1993; 370:48–53.

Knop J, Teasdale TW, Schulsinger F, Goodwin DW: A prospective study of young men at high risk for alcoholism: school behavior and achievement. J Stud Alcohol 1985; 46:273–278.

Koller W, O'Hara R, Dorus W, Bauer J: Tremor in chronic alcoholism. Neurology 1985; 35:1660–1662.

Kopun M, Propping P: The kinetics of ethanol absorption and elimination in twins and Supplementary repetitive experiments in singleton subjects. Eur J Clin Pharmacol 1977; 11:337–344.

Koskenvuo M, Langinvainio H, Kaprio J, Lonnqvist J, Tienari P: Psychiatric hospitalization in twins. Acta Genet Med Gemellol (Roma) 1984; 33:321–332.

Kwon JM, Goate AM: The candidate gene approach. Alcohol Res Health 2000; 24:164–168.

Levitt MD, Levitt DG: Use of a two-compartment model to assess the pharmacokinetics of human ethanol metabolism. Alcohol Clin Exp Res 1998; 22:1680–1688.

Li TK, Yin SJ, Crabb DW, O'Connor S, Ramchandani VA: Genetic and environmental influences on alcohol metabolism in humans. Alcohol Clin Exp Res 2001; 25:136–144.

Lieber CS: Microsomal ethanol-oxidizing system (MEOS): the first 30 years (1968–1998)—a review. Alcohol Clin Exp Res 1999; 23:991–1007.

Lieberman DZ: Children of alcoholics: an update. Curr Opin Pediatr 2000; 12:336–340.

Limosin F, Adés J, Gorwood P: Relationships between antisocial personality and alcoholism: genetic hypotheses. Eur Psychiatry 2000; 15:123–128.

List S, Gluud C: A meta-analysis of HLA-antigen prevalences in alcoholics and alcoholic liver disease. Alcohol Alcohol 1994; 29:757–764.

Llop E, Hirsch S, de la Maza MP, Bunout D, Iturriaga H, Silva C, Ugarte G, Rothhammer F: Major histocompatibility system as a risk factor for alcoholic liver disease. Rev Med Chil 1995; 123:687–693. In Spanish.

Loehlin JC: An analysis of alcohol-related questionnaire items from the national merit twin study. Ann NY Acad Sci 1972; 197:117–120.
Long JC, Knowler WC, Hanson RL, Robin RW, Urbanek M, Moore E, Bennett PH, Goldman D: Evidence for genetic linkage to alcohol dependence on chromosomes 4 and 11 from an autosome-wide scan in an American Indian population. Am J Med Genet 1998; 8:216–221.
Lubben JE, Chi I, Kitano HHL: The relative influence of selected social factors on Korean drinking behavior in Los Angeles. Adv Alcohol Subst Abuse 1989; 8:1–17.
Lubben JE, Chi I, Kitano HHL: Exploring Filipino American drinking behavior. J Stud Alcohol 1987; 49:26–29.
Lüth KF: Untersuchungen über die Alkoholblutkonzentration nach Alkoholgaben bei 10 eineiigen und 10 zweieiigen Zwillingspaaren. Dtsch Z Ges Gerichtl Med 1939; 32:145–164.
Maier W, Merikangas K: Co-occurrence and co-transmission of affective disorders and alcoholism in families. Br J Psychiatry Suppl 1996; 30:93–100.
Major LF, Hawley RJ, Saini N, Garrick NA, Murphy DL: Brain and liver monoamine oxidase type A and type B activity in alcoholics and controls. Alcohol Clin Exp Res 1985; 9:6–9.
Martin NG: Genetic differences in drinking habits, alcohol metabolism and sensitivity in unselected samples of twins. In: Goedde HW, Agarwal DP (eds). Genetics and Alcoholism. New York: A.R. Liss, 1987:109–119.
Martin NG, Peri J, Oakeshott JG, Gibson JB, Starmer GA, Wilks AV: A twin study of ethanol metabolism. Behav Genet 1985; 15:93–109.
Marshall EJ, Gurling RM: The contribution of twin studies to alcoholism research. In: Goedde HW, Agarwal DP (eds). Alcoholism Biomedical and Genetic Aspects. New York: Pergamon, 1989:277–289.
Maruyama K, Takahashi H, Matsushita S, Nakano M, Harada H, Otsuki M, Ogawa M, Suda K, Baba T, Honma T, et al.: Genotypes of alcohol-metabolizing enzymes in relation to alcoholic chronic pancreatitis in Japan. Alcohol Clin Exp Res 1999; 23(Suppl):85S–91S.
Matsumoto M, Takahashi H, Maruyama K, Higuchi S, Matsushita S, Muramatsu T, Okuyama K, Yokoyama A, Nakano M, Ishii H: Genotypes of alcohol-metabolizing enzymes and the risk for alcoholic chronic pancreatitis in Japanese alcoholics. Alcohol Clin Exp Res 1996; 20 (Suppl): 289A–292A.
Matsuo Y, Yokoyama R, Yokoyama S: The gene for human alcohol dehydrogenase $\beta 1$ and $\beta 2$ differ by only one nucleotide. Europ J Biochem 1989; 83:317–320.
Mayfield D, McLeod G, Hall P: The CAGE questionnaire: validation of a new alcoholism screening instrument. Am J Psychiatry 1974; 131:1121–1123.
McGue M, Pickens RW, Svikis DS: Sex and age effects on the inheritance of alcohol problems: a twin study. J Abnorm Psychol 1992a; 101:3–17.
McGue M, Sharma A, Bension P: Parent and sibling influence on adolescent alcohol use and misuse: evidence from a U.S. adoption cohort. J Stud Alcohol 1992b; 57:8–18.
McGue M, Slutske WS: The inheritance of alcoholism in women. In: Howard JM, Martin SE, Mail PD, Hilton ME, Taylor ED (eds). Women and Alcohol: Issues for Prevention Research. Bethesda, MD: U.S. Department of Health and Human Services, 1996:65–91.
Meier-Tackmann D, Leonhardt RA, Agarwal DP, Goedde HW: Effect of acute ethanol drinking on alcohol metabolism in subjects with different *ADH* and *ALDH* genotypes. Alcohol 1990; 7:413–418.
Menninger JA, Baron AE, Conigrave KM, Whitfield JB, Saunders JB, Helander A, Eriksson CJ, Grant B, Hoffman PL, Tabakoff B: Platelet adenylyl cyclase activity as a trait marker of alcohol dependence. Alcohol Clin Exp Res 2000; 24:810–821.
Midanik LT, Room R: The epidemiology of alcohol consumption. Alcohol Health Res World 1992; 16:183–190.
Miyamoto K, Ishii H, Takata H, Takagi S, Shigeta Y, Sekiguchi S, Suyama K, Kohno H, Tsuchiya M: Association of HLA-B40 and DRw9 with Japanese alcoholic liver cirrhosis. Pharmacol Biochem Behav 1983; 18 (Suppl 1):467–471.
Monteiro MG, Schuckit MA: Alcohol, drug, and mental health problems among Jewish and Christian men at a university. Am J Drug Alcohol Abuse 1989; 15:403–412.
Morimoto K, Takeshita T: Low Km aldehyde dehydrogenase (ALDH2) polymorphism, alcohol-drinking behavior, and chromosome alterations in peripheral lymphocytes. Environ Health Perspect 1996; 104(Suppl 3):563–567.
Morrison J, Stewart M: The psychiatric status of the legal families of adopted hyperactive children. Arch Gen Psychiatry 1973; 28:888–891.
Müller H: Der erbkonstitutionelle Hypogenitalismus des Mannes als Dispositionsfaktor der Lebercirrhose. Med Klin 1952; 3:71–74.
Muramatsu T, Zu-Cheng W, Yi-Ru F, Kou-Bao H, Heqin Y, Yamada K, Higuchi S: Alcohol and aldehyde dehydrogenase genotypes and drinking behavior of Chinese living in Shanghai. Hum Genet 1995; 96:151–154.
Murphy HBM: Comparative Psychiatry: The International and Inter-cultural Distribution of Mental Illness. New York: Springer, 1982.
Murray TJ: Essential tremor. CMAJ 1981; 124:1559–1565.
Nacher V: Genetic association between the reduced amplitude of the P300 and the allele A1 of the gene which codifies the D2 dopamine receptor (DRD2) as possible biological markers for alcoholism. Rev Neurol 2000; 30:756–763.
Naitoh P: The value of electroencephalographv in alcoholism. Ann NY Acad Sci 1973; 215:303–320.
National Council on Alcoholism: Criteria for the diagnosis of alcoholism. Am J Psychiatry 1972; 129:127–135.
Neiswanger K, Kaplan B, Hill SY: Exclusion of linkage between alcoholism and the MNS blood group region on chromosome 4q in multiplex families. Am J Med Genet 1995; 60:72–79.
Neumark YD, Friedlander Y, Thomasson HR, Li TK: Association of the ADH2-2 allele with reduced ethanol consumption in Jewish men in Israel: a pilot study. J Stud Alcohol 1998; 59:133–139.
Nixon PF, Kaczmarek MJ, Tate J, Kerr RA, Price J: An erythrocyte transketolase isoenzyme pattern associated with the Wernicke-Korsakoff syndrome. Eur J Clin Invest 1984; 14:278–281.
Noble EP: The D2 dopamine receptor gene: a review of association studies in alcoholism. Behav Genet 1993; 23:119–129.
Noble EP: Polymorphisms of the D2 dopamine receptor gene and alcoholism and other substance use disorders. Alcohol Alcohol Suppl 1994; 2:35–43.
Noble EP: D2 dopamine receptor gene: a review of association studies in alcoholism and phenotypes. Alcohol 1998; 16:33–45.
Novoradovsky AG, Sandoval C, Guderian RH, Zimmerman PA, Nutman TB, Goldman D: Detection of aldehyde dehydrogenase deficiency in Chachi Indians, Ecuador. Alcohol 1995; 12:159–161.
Nurnberger JI Jr, Foroud T, Flury L, Su J, Meyer ET, Hu K, Crowe R, Edenberg H, Goate A, Bierut L, et al.: Evidence for a locus on chromosome 1 that influences vulnerability to alcoholism and affective disorder. Am J Psychiatry 2000; 158:718–724.
O'Connor S, Sorbel J, Morzorati S, Li TK, Christian JC: A twin study of genetic influences on the acute adaptation of the EEG to alcohol Alcohol Clin Exp Res 1999; 23:494–495.
O'Malley SS, Maisto SA: Effects of family drinking history and expectancies on responses to alcohol in men. J Stud Alcohol 1985; 46:289–297.
Oneta CM, Simanowski UA, Martinez M, Allali-Hassani A, Pares X, Homann N, Conradt C, Waldherr R, Fiehn W, Coutelle C, Seitz HK: First pass metabolism of ethanol is strikingly influenced by the speed of gastric emptying. Gut 1998; 43:612–619.
Osier M, Pakstis AJ, Kidd JR, Lee JF, Yin SJ, Ko HC, Edenberg HJ: Linkage disequilibrium at the ADH2 and ADH3 loci and risk of alcoholism. Am J Hum Genet 1999; 64:1147–1157.
Parsian A, Cloninger CR, Zhang ZH: Functional variant in the DRD2 receptor promoter region and subtypes of alcoholism. Am J Med Genet 2000; 96:407–411.
Parsian A, Todd RD, Cloninger CR, Hoffman PL, Ovchinnikova L, Ikeda H, Tabakoff B: Platelet adenylyl cyclase activity in alcoholics and subtypes of alcoholics: WHO/ISBRA Study Clinical Centers. Alcohol Clin Exp Res 1996; 20:745–751.
Partanen J, Bruun K, Markkanen T: Inheritance of Drinking Behavior: A Study on Intelligence, Personality, and Use of Alcohol of Adult Twins. Helsinki: Finnish Foundation for Alcohol Studies, 1966.
Pastino GM, Conolly RB: Application of a physiologically based pharmacokinetic model to estimate the bioavailability of ethanol in male rats: distinction between gastric and hepatic pathways of metabolic clearance. Toxicol Sci 2000; 55:256–265.
Paterson AD, Petronis A: Sex-based linkage analysis of alcoholism. Genet Epidemiol 1999; 17 (Suppl 1):S289–S294.
Patterson BW, Williams HL, McLean GA, Smith LT, Schaeffer KW: Alcoholism and family history of alcoholism: effects on visual and auditory event-related potentials. Alcohol 1987; 4:265–274.
Peirce JL, Derr R, Shendure J, Kolata T, Silver LM: A major influence of sex-specific loci on alcohol preference in C57Bl/6 and DBA/2 inbred mice. Genome 1998; 9:942–948.
Peng GS, Wang MF, Chen YC, Luu SU, Chou HC, Li TK, Yin SJ: Involvement of acetaldehyde for full protection against alcoholism by homozygosity of the variant allele of mitochondrial aldehyde dehydrogenase gene in Asians. Pharmacogenetics 1999; 9:463–476.
Pfefferbaum A, Ford JM, White PM, Marathon D: Event-related potentials in alcoholic men: P3 amplitude reflects family history but not alcohol consumption. Alcohol Clin Exp Res 1991; 15:839–850.
Pickens RW, Svikis DS, McGue M, Lykken DT, Heston LL, Clayton PJ: Heterogeneity in the inheritance of alcoholism: a study of male and female twins. Arch Gen Psychiatry 1991; 48:19–28.
Pihl RO, Peterson J, Finn P: Inherited predisposition to alcoholism: characteristics of sons of male alcoholics. J Abnorm Psychol 1990; 99:291–301.
Polich J, Bloom FE: P300 from normals and adult children of alcoholics. Alcohol 1987; 4:301–305.
Pollock VE, Volavka J, Goodwin DW. Mednick SA, Gabrielli WF, Knop J, Schulsinger F: The EEG after alcohol administration in men at risk for alcoholism. Arch Gen Psychiatry 1983; 40:857–861.
Ponce Alfaro G, Rodriguez-Jimenez Caumel R, Perez Rojo JA, Monasor Sanchez R, Rubio Valladolid G, Jimenez Arriero MA, Palomo Alvarez T: Attention-deficit hyperactivity disorder and vulnerability to the development of alcoholism: use of Wender-Utah rating scale for retrospective diagnostic of ADHD in the early ages of alcoholic patients. Actas Esp Psiquiatr 2000; 28:357–366. In Spanish.
Porjesz B, Begleiter H: Genetic basis of event-related potentials and their relationship to alcoholism and alcohol use. J Clin Neurophysiol 1998; 15:44–57.
Prabhu VR, Porjesz B, Chorlian DB, Wang K, Stimus A, Begleiter H: Visual p3 in female alcoholics. Alcohol Clin Exp Res 2001; 25:531–539.
Prenatal exposure to alcohol. Alcohol Res Health 2000; 24:32–41.
Prescott CA: The genetic epidemiology of alcoholism: sex differences and future directions. In: Agarwal DP, Seitz HK (eds). Alcohol in Health and Disease. New York: Marcel Dekker, 2001:125–150.
Prescott CA, Kendler KS: Genetic and environmental contributions to alcohol abuse and dependence in a population-based sample of male twins. Am J Psychiatry 1999; 156:34–40.
Propping P: Genetic control of ethanol action on the central nervous system: an EEG study in twins. Hum Genet 1977; 35:309–334.
Propping P, Kriiger J, Janah A: Effect of alcohol on genetically determined variants of the normal EEG. Psychiatr Res 1980; 2:85–98.

Propping P, Krüger J, Mark N: Genetic disposition to alcoholism: an EEG study in alcoholics and their relatives. Hum Genet 1981; 59:51–59.

Radel M, Goldman D: Pharmacogenetics of alcohol response and alcoholism: the interplay of genes and environmental factors in thresholds for alcoholism. Drug Metab Dispos 2001; 29:489–494.

Rahkonen O, Ahlstrom S: Trends in drinking habits among Finnish youth from 1973 to 1987. Br J Addict 1989; 84:1075–1083.

Ratsma JE, Gunning WB, Leurs R, Schoffelmeer AN: Platelet adenylyl cyclase activity as a biochemical trait marker for predisposition to alcoholism. Alcohol Clin Exp Res 1999; 23:600–604.

Rausch JL, Monteiro MG, Schuckit MA: Platelet serotonin uptake in men with family histories of alcoholism. Neuropsychopharmacology 1991; 4:83–86.

Reed TE: Between—and within—race variation in acute cardiovascular responses to alcohol: evidence for genetic determination in normal males in three races. Behav Genet 1986; 16:585–598.

Reed TE, Kalant H, Gibbins RJ, Kapur BM, Rankin JG: Alcohol and acetaldehyde metabolism in Caucasians, Chinese and Amerinds. CMAJ 1976; 115:851–855.

Reed T, Page WF, Viken RJ, Christian JC: Genetic predisposition to organ-specific endpoints of alcoholism. Alcohol Clin Exp Res 1996; 20:1528–1533.

Rehm J, Bondy S: Alcohol and all-cause mortality: an overview. Novartis Found Symp 1998; 216:223–232.

Reich T, Edenberg HJ, Goate A, Williams JT, Rice JP, Van Eerdewegh P, Foroud T, Hesselbrock V, Schuckit MA, Bucholz K, et al.: Genome-wide search for genes affecting the risk for alcoholism dependence. Am J Med Genet 1998; 81:207–215.

Reich T, Robins LN, Woodruff RA, Taibleson M, Rich C, Cunningham L: Computer-assisted derivation of a screening interview for alcoholism. Arch Gen Psychiatry 1975; 32:847–852.

Roe A: The adult adjustment of children of alcoholic parents raised in foster homes. Q J Stud Alcohol 1944; 5:378–393.

Rogers TD, Deary I: The P300 component of the auditory event-related potential in monozygotic and dizygotic twins. Acta Psychiatr Scand 1991; 83:412–416.

Roine R: Interaction of prandial state and beverage concentration on alcohol absorption. Alcohol Clin Exp Res 2000; 24:411–412.

Romanov K, Kaprio J, Rose R, Koskenvuo M: Genetics of alcoholism: effects of migration on concordance rates among male twins. Alcohol Alcohol 1991 (Suppl); 1:137–140.

Saccone NL, Kwon JM, Corbett J, Goate A, Rochberg N, Edenberg HJ, Foroud T, Li TK, Begleiter H, Reich T, Rice JP: A genome screen of maximum number of drinks as an alcoholism phenotype. Am J Med Genet 2000; 96:632–637.

Salaspuro M: Carbohydrate-deficient transferrin as compared to other markers of alcoholism: a systematic review. Alcohol 1999; 19:261–271.

Sampson PD, Streissguth AP, Bookstein FL, Little RE, Clarren SK, Dehaene P, Hanson JW, Graham M Jr: Incidence of fetal alcohol syndrome and prevalence of alcohol-related neurodevelopmental disorder. Teratology 1997; 56:317–326.

Sander T, Ladehoff M, Samochowiec J, Finckh U, Rommelspacher H, Schmidt LG: Lack of an allelic association between polymorphisms of the dopamine D2 receptor gene and alcohol dependence in the German population. Alcohol Clin Exp Res 1999; 23:578–581.

Santos BR, Monteiro MG, Thomasson HR: Allele frequency of ADH2 and ALDH2 among Brazilians of different ethnic groups. Alcohol 1997; 14:205–207.

Saunders JB, Aasland OG, Babor TF, de la Fuente JR, Grant M: Development of the Alcohol Use Disorders Identification Test (AUDIT): WHO Collaborative Project on Early Detection of Persons with Harmful Alcohol Consumption-II. Addiction 1993; 88:791–804.

Savolainen VT, Pjarinen J, Perola M, Penttila A, Karhunen PJ: Glutathione-*S*-transferase GST M1 "null" genotype and the risk of alcoholic liver disease. Alcohol Clin Exp Res 1996; 20:1340–1345.

Schmidt LG, Sander T: Genetics of alcohol withdrawal. Eur Psychiatry 2000; 15:135–139.

Schroeder D, Nasrallah HA: High alcoholism rate in patients with essential tremor. Am J Psychiatry 1982; 139:1471–1473.

Schuckit MA: Family history and half-sibling research in alcoholism. Ann NY Acad Sci 1972; 197:121–125.

Schuckit MA: Genetics of the risk for alcoholism. Am J Addict 2000; 9:103–112.

Schuckit MA, Smith TL: The relationships of a family history of alcohol dependence, a low level of response to alcohol and six domains of life functioning to the development of alcohol use disorders. J Stud Alcohol 2000; 61:827–835.

Schuckit MA, Smith TL: The clinical course of alcohol dependence associated with a low level of response to alcohol. Addiction 2001a; 96:903–910.

Schuckit MA, Smith TL: A comparison of correlates of DSM-IV alcohol abuse or dependence among more than 400 sons of alcoholics and controls. Alcohol Clin Exp Res 2001b; 25:1–8.

Schulsinger F, Knop J, Goodwin DW, Teasdale TW, Mikkelsen U: A prospective study of young men at high risk for alcoholism: social and psychological characteristics. Arch Gen Psychiatr 1986; 43:755–760.

Segal B: *ADH* and *ALDH* polymorphisms among Alaska Natives entering treatment for alcoholism. Alaska Med 1999; 41:9–12.

Seitz HK, Poschl G, Simanowski UA: Alcohol and cancer. Recent Dev Alcohol 1998; 14:67–95.

Selzer ML: The Michigan alcoholism screening test: the quest for a new diagnostic instrument. Am J Psychiatry 1971; 127:1653–1658.

Shen YC, Fan JH, Edenberg HJ, Li TK, Cui YH, Wang YF, Tian CH, Zhou CF, Zhou RL, Wang J, et al.: Polymorphism of *ADH* and *ALDH* genes among four ethnic groups in China and effects upon the risk for alcoholism. Alcohol Clin Exp Res 1997; 21:1272–1277.

Sigvardsson S, Bohman M, Cloninger CR: Replication of the Stockholm Adoption Study of alcoholism: confirmatory cross-fostering analysis. Arch Gen Psychiatry 1996; 53:681–687.

Slutske WS, True WR, Scherrer JF, Heath AC, Bucholz KK, Eisen SA, Goldberg J, Lyons MJ, Tsuang MT: Heritability of alcoholism symptoms: "indicators of genetic and environmental influence in alcohol-dependent individuals" revisited. Alcohol Clin Exp Res 1999; 23:759–769.

Smith JW: Color vision in alcoholics. Ann NY Acad Sci 1972; 197:143–147.

Snyder CR: Alcohol and the Jews: a cultural study of drinking and sobriety. New York: Free Press 1958:181.

Soyka M: Alcohol-induced hallucinosis. Clinical aspects, pathophysiology and therapy. Nervenarzt 1996; 67:891–895.

Soyka M, Bondy B, Benda E, Preuss U, Hegerl U, Moller H: Platelet monoamine oxidase activity in alcoholics with and without a family history of alcoholism. Eur Addict Res 2000; 6:57–63.

Steinhauer SR, Hill SY, Zubin J: Event-related potentials in alcoholics and their first-degree relatives. Alcohol 1987; 4:307–314.

Steinhausen HC, Gobel D, Nestler V: Psychopathology in the offspring of alcoholic parents. J Am Acad Child Psychiatry 1984; 23:465–471.

Stephens EA, Taylor JA, Kaplan N, Yang CH, Hsieh LL, Lucier GW, Bell DA: Ethnic variation in the *CYP2E1* gene: polymorphism analysis of 695 African-Americans, European-Americans and Taiwanese. Pharmacogenetics 1994; 4:185–192.

Stockwell T, Sitharthan T, McGrath D, Lang E: The measurement of alcohol dependence and impaired control in community samples. Addiction 1994; 89:167–174.

Storgaard H, Nielsen SD, Gluud C: The validity of the Michigan Alcoholism Screening Test (MAST). Alcohol Alcohol 1994; 29:493–502.

Streissguth AP: Recent advances in fetal alcohol syndrome and alcohol use in pregnancy. In: Agarwal DP, Seitz HK (eds). Alcohol in Health and Disease. New York: Marcel Dekker, 2001:303–334.

Sullivan JL, Baenziger JC, Wagner DL, Rauscher FP, Nurnberger JI Jr, Holmes JS: Platelet MAO in subtypes of alcoholism. Biol Psychiatry 1990; 27:911–922.

Sun F, Tsuritani I, Honda R, Ma ZY, Yamada Y: Association of genetic polymorphisms of alcohol-metabolizing enzymes with excessive alcohol consumption in Japanese men. Hum Genet 1999; 105:295–300.

Swendsen JD, Merikangas KR: The comorbidity of depression and substance use disorders. Clin Psychol Rev 2000; 20:173–189.

Tabakoff B, Helander A, Conigrave KM, Martinez L, Hoffman PL, Whitfield J, Degenhardt L, Saunders J, Baron A, Glanz AJ: WHO/ISBRA study on state and trait markers in alcoholism. Alcohol Clin Exp Res 2001; 25 (5 Suppl ISBRA):99S–103S.

Tabakoff B, Whelan JP, Hoffman PL: Two biological markers of alcoholism. In: Cloninger CR, Begleiter H (eds). Genetics and Biology of Alcoholism. New York: Cold Spring Harbor Laboratory Press, 1990:195–204.

Takada A, Tsutsumi M, Kobayashi Y: Genotypes of *ALDH2* related to liver and pulmonary diseases and other genetic factors related to alcoholic liver disease. Alcohol Alcohol 1994; 29:719–727.

Tanaka F, Shiratori Y, Yokosuka O: Polymorphism of alcohol-metabolizing genes affect drinking behavior and alcoholic liver disease in Japanese men. Alcohol Clin Exp Res 1997; 21:596–601.

Tanna VL, Wilson AF, Winokur G, Elston RC: Possible linkage between alcoholism and esterase-D. J Stud Alcohol 1988; 49:472–476.

Tarantino LM, McClearn GE, Rodriguez LA, Plomin R: Confirmation of quantitative traits loci for alcohol preference in mice. Alcohol Clin Exp Res 1998; 22:1099–1105.

Tarter RE, Alterman AI: Neuropsychological deficits in alcoholics: etiological considerations. J Stud Alcohol 1984; 45:1–9.

Tarter RE, Kabene M, Escallier EA, Laird SB, Jacob T: Temperament deviation and risk for alcoholism. Alcohol Clin Exp Res 1990; 14:380–382.

Thomasson HR, Li TK: How alcohol and aldehyde dehydrogenase genes modify alcohol drinking, alcohol flushing, and the risk for alcoholism. Alcohol Health Res World 1993; 17:167–172.

Thome J, Gewirtz JC, Weijers HG, Wiesbeck GA, Henn FA: Genome polymorphism and alcoholism. Pharmacogenomics 2000; 1:63–71.

Tolor A, Tamerin JS: The question of a genetic basis for alcoholism: comment on the study by Goodwin et al. Q J Stud Alcohol 1973; 34:1341–1347.

True WR, Heath AC, Bucholz K, Slutske W, Romels JC, Scherrer JF, Lin N, Eisen SA, Goldberg J, Lyons M, Tsuang MT: Models of treatment seeking for alcoholism: the role of genes and environment. Alcohol Clin Exp Res 1996; 20:1577–1581.

Tsugane S, Fahey MT, Sasaki S, Baba S: Alcohol consumption and all-cause and cancer mortality among middle-aged Japanese men: seven-year follow-up of the JPHC study Cohort I. Am J Epidemiol 1999; 150:1201–1207.

Tsutsumi M, Takada A, Wang JS, Takase S: Genetic polymorphisms of cytochrome P450IIE1 related to the development of alcoholic liver disease. Gastroenterology 1994; 107:14–30.

Vadasz C, Saito M, Gyetvai B, Mikics E, Vadasz C II: Scanning of five chromosomes for alcohol consumption loci. Alcohol 2000; 22:25–34.

Väkeväinen S, Tillonen J, Agarwal DP, Srivastava N, Salaspuro M: High salivary acetaldehyde after a moderate dose of alcohol in ALDH2-deficient subjects: strong evidence for the local carcinogenic action of acetaldehyde. Alcohol Clin Exp Res 2000; 24:873–877.

Vasiliou V, Bairoch A, Tipton KF, Nebert DW: Eukaryotic aldehyde dehydrogenase (ALDH) genes: human polymorphisms, and recommended nomenclature based on divergent evolution and chromosomal mapping. Pharmacogenetics 1999; 9:421–434.

Vesell ES: Gene–environment interactions in alcoholism. In: Goedde HW, Agarwal DP (eds). Alcoholism Biomedical and Genetic Aspects. New York: Pergamon, 1989:325–332.

Vesell ES, Page JG, Passananti GT: Genetic and environmental factors affecting ethanol metabolism in man. Clin Pharmacol Ther 1971; 12:192–201.

von Knorring AL, Hallman J, von Knorring L, Oreland L: Platelet monoamine oxidase activity in type 1 and type 2 alcoholism. Alcohol Alcohol 1991; 26:409–416.

von Wartburg JP: Pharmacokinetics of alcohol. In: Crow KE, Batt RD (eds). Human Metabolism of Alcohol. Vol. 1: Pharmacokinetics, Medicolegal Aspects, and General Interests. Boca Raton, FL: CRC Press, 1989:9–22.

Wall TL, Ehlers CL: Acute effects of alcohol on the EEG in Asians with different ALDH2 genotypes. Alcohol Clin Exp Res 1995; 19:617–622.

Wall TL, Gallen CC, Ehlers CL: Acute effects of alcohol on the EEG in Asian men with genetic variations of ALDH2. Biol Psychiatry 1993; 34:91–99.

Walsh K, Alexander G: Alcoholic liver disease. Postgrad Med J 2000; 76:280–286.

Wedel M, Pieters JE, Pikkar NA, Ockhuizen Th: Application of a three-compartment model to a study of the effects of sex, alcohol dose, and concentration, exercise and food consumption on the pharmacogenetics of ethanol in healthy volunteers. Alcohol Alcohol 1991; 26:329–336.

Whipple SC, Berman SM, Noble EP: Event-related potentials in alcoholic fathers and their sons. Alcohol 1991; 8:321–327.

Whitfield JB: Genes for alcohol metabolism and alcohol sensitivity: their role in the genetics of alcoholism. In: Agarwal DP, Seitz HK (eds). Alcohol in Health and Disease. New York: Marcel Dekker, 2001:27–48.

Widmark EMP: Kinetics of the conversion of ethyl alcohol in the organism: experimental results. In: Widmark, EMP. Principles and Applications of Medicolegal Alcohol Determination. Davis, CA: Biomedical Publications, 1981:60–84.

Wilsnack SC: Patterns and trends in women's drinking: recent findings and some implications for prevention. In: Howard JM, Martin SE, Mail PD, Hilton ME, Taylor ED. Women and Alcohol: Issues for Prevention Research. Bethesda, MD: National Institutes of Health, 1996:19–64.

Winokur G: X-borne recessive genes in alcoholism. Lancet 1967; 2:466.

Winokur G, Reich T, Rimmer J, Pitts FN Jr: Alcoholism: III. Diagnosis and familial psychiatric illness in 259 alcoholic probands. Arch Gen Psychiatry 1970; 23:104–111.

Wolff PH: Vasomotor sensitivity to alcohol in diverse Mongoloid populations. Am J Hum Genet 1973; 25:193–199.

World Health Organization: Manual of the International Statistical Classification of Disease, Injuries, and Cause of Death, 10th rev. (ICD-10). Geneva: WHO, 1994.

Wright JT, Waterson EJ, Barrison IG, Toplis PJ, Lewis IG, Gordon MG, MacRae KD, Morris NF, Murray-Lyon IM: Alcohol consumption, pregnancy, and low birth weight. Lancet 1983; 1:663–665.

Wuethrich B: Neurobiology: does alcohol damage female brains more? Science 2001; 291:2077–2079.

Yamauchi M, Maezawa Y, Mizuhara Y, Ohata M, Hirakawa J, Nakajima H, Toda G: Polymorphisms in alcohol metabolizing enzyme genes and alcoholic cirrhosis in Japanese patients: a multivariate analysis. Hepatology 1995; 22:1136–1142.

Yin SJ, Agarwal DP: Functional polymorphisms of alcohol and aldehyde dehydrogenases: alcohol metabolism, alcoholism, and alcohol-induced organ damage. In: Agarwal DP, Seitz HK (eds). Alcohol in Health and Disease. New York: Marcel Dekker, 2001:1–26.

Yin SJ, Loai CS, Wu CW, Li TT, Chen LL, Lai CL, Tsao TY: Human stomach alcohol and aldehyde dehydrogenases: comparison of expression pattern and activities in alimentary tract. Gastroenterology 1997; 112:766–775.

Yokoyama H, Baraona E, Lieber CS: Molecular cloning and chromosomal localization of the *ADH7* gene encoding human class IV (Σ) ADH. Genomics 1996; 31:243–245.

Yoshida A, Huang IY, Ikawa M: Molecular abnormality of an inactive aldehyde dehydrogenase variant commonly found in Orientals. Proc Natl Acad Sci USA 1984; 81:258–261.

Zilker T: Alcohol withdrawal syndrome and delirium tremens: diagnosis and therapy. MMW Fortschr Med 1999; 141:26–30. In German.

Zimatkin SM, Zimatkina TI: Thiamine deficiency as predisposition to, and consequence of, increased alcohol consumption. Alcohol Alcohol 1996; 31:421–427.

47 Mental Retardation

W. TED BROWN

INTRODUCTION AND DISEASE DEFINITION

Mental retardation (MR) results from a broad, heterogeneous group of disorders involving both genetic and nongenetic causes. MR is defined in terms of limitations in cognition and in daily living skills (ability to adapt to the environment) and requires an onset before adulthood. Cognitive abilities are measured by standardized psychologic tests that yield an *intelligence quotient* (IQ): mental age divided by chronologic age. The IQ score has a mean of 100 and a standard deviation (SD) of 15. Generally, individuals with an IQ below 70, −2 SD, are considered to have MR. MR has traditionally been subclassified by level of severity into mild, moderate, severe, and profound, with thresholds of 70, 50, 35, and 20, respectively. In 1992, the American Association on Mental Retardation proposed a general definition change: the IQ level defining MR was below the range of 70 to 75 and the categories were reduced from four to two, mild and severe. Further a lack of "ability to adapt to the environment" was required and defined as having limitation in at least two of the following 10 areas of adaptive behavior: communication, self-care, home living, social skills, community use, self-direction, health and safety, functional academics, leisure, and work (American Association on Mental Retardation, 1992). This definition represented a significant shift in emphasis from degree of impairment to the abilities of the individual to function in society. However, this definition has been controversial because it broadens the definition of mild MR; consolidates the moderate, severe, and profound categories into the severe group; assumes that adaptive behavior is independent of cognition; and requires more extensive psychologic testing (MacMillan et al., 1993).

GENERAL GENETIC AND EPIDEMIOLOGIC EVIDENCE

Based on the assumption of a normal distribution, the expected prevalence of MR is approximately 3%. However, the prevalence rate for MR in children varies considerably depending on study design and definition, from as low as 0.1% in children of 0 to 4 years of age to as high as 9.7% in the 10 to 14 year age range (Kiely, 1987; Murphy et al., 1998). MR most often presents during infancy or preschool years as developmental delay. The prevalence of MR peaks at ages 10 to 14 years since individuals with mild MR are identified significantly later than children with more severe MR.

Mild MR is most common as more than 85% of cases fall within the IQ range of 50 to 70. The ratio of males to females is close to 1.6:1 in mild MR but closer to 1:1 in severe MR. The recurrence risk for siblings of individuals with mild MR is high, with values typically lying between 1 in 4 and 1 in 5 (Bundey et al., 1989). There is a much higher prevalence of mild MR in lower socioeconomic classes, whereas this discrepancy is not found among severe MR cases. Therefore, it appears that some individuals with mild MR actually reflect social or cultural disadvantage and that their low IQ scores are artifactual.

The prevalence of severe MR has shown little change over the past 50 years (Kiely, 1987). This is likely to reflect the result of a balance between medical advances which can prevent the occurrence of severe MR and the emergence of new diseases or causes of MR. As examples, the morbidity and MR rates among premature infants weighing 1500 to 2500 g has decreased due to medical advances, but the survival rate of infants weighing less than 1500 g and having higher rates of morbidity and MR has increased. The decrease in prevalence of Down syndrome births because of prenatal diagnosis and reduced birth rates among older mothers and of untreated phenylketonuria because of newborn screening programs has been balanced by a rise in the prevalence of fetal alcohol syndrome, congenitally acquired immunodeficiency syndrome, and prenatal exposure to addictive drugs. Furthermore, many cases of severe MR are the result of genetic and environmental causes, which cannot be effectively anticipated or prevented.

PATHOPHYSIOLOGY: BIOLOGIC BASIC OF GENETIC SUSCEPTIBILITY

Surveys to determine the causes of MR have indicated that approximately two-thirds of severe cases, with IQ <50, are due to known (or strongly suspected) factors, with two-thirds of these due to genetic and one-third to environmental causes. Among the remaining one-third due to idiopathic causes, because of a positive family history or associated dysmorphic appearance, there is likely to be a genetic cause in at least 50%. Thus, approximately 60% of severe MR is due to known or suspected genetic causes. Among the mildly retarded group, only about 25% of cases are due to identifiable causes, of which approximately two-thirds are genetic. Improvements in cytogenetic and molecular diagnostic techniques over the last 30 years have led to a gradual reduction in the proportion of cases that remain idiopathic (Batshaw, 1993; Flint and Wilke, 1996; Raynham et al., 1996; Accardo and Capute, 1998).

GENE IDENTIFICATION

Sequencing of the human genome has indicated that there are approximately 30,000 to 40,000 human genes (Lander et al., 2001; Ventner et al., 2001). It appears that, due to alternative splicing, as many as 200,000 distinct mRNA sequences are expressed in the central nervous system, a number approximately 20-fold higher than that in specific non-neuronal tissues, such as liver or kidney (Schwartz, 2000). Thus, there exists an enormous set of genes that could be mutated and result in MR. If mutations in a significant fraction of these do result in MR, there are a large number whose identity and functions remain unknown.

Intelligence clearly has a strong genetic component. Studies of IQ correlations between relatives and between monozygotic twins reared together and apart have suggested that the genetic background component approximates 50% (McGue and Bouchard, 1998). Many milder forms of cognitive impairment compared to MR, such as developmental dyslexia, attention deficit hyperactivity disorder, specific language and reading deficits, all of which appear to have a polygenetic causation, are currently under intense scrutiny, with specific contributing loci and genes being increasingly identified (Pennington, 1997).

Pathophysiology of Disease

The underlying pathophysiology causing MR is fairly well understood for metabolic disorders associated with MR. Such defects often involve either a single enzyme or multiple enzymes in specific organelles, such as lysosomes or peroxisomes, leading to catabolic defects, accumulating substances, and neurodegeneration. Others involve defects in the synthesis or degradation of certain macromolecules that also produce a dysmorphic appearance (Clayton and Thompson, 1988). Some relatively common causes of MR involve mutations of genes related to growth or tumor suppression, such as neurofibromin in neurofibromatosis I and two different tumor-suppressor genes (*TSC1* and *TSC2*) involved in the two forms of tuberous sclerosis (North et al., 1997; Roach et al., 1998). Some mutant genes causing MR appear to involve abnormalities of transcription or translational processing, such as a small nuclear ribonucleoprotein polypeptide protein in Prader-Willi syndrome (Wevrick and Francke, 1996), a cAMP response element–binding protein in Rubinstein-Taybi syndrome (Petrij et al., 1995), and an RNA-binding protein in fragile X syndrome (Ashley et al., 1993). Some appear to involve DNA metabolic enzymes, such as the BLM protein in Bloom syndrome (Ellis et al., 1995), the ATM protein which recognizes DNA damage in ataxia-telangiectasia (Savitsky et al., 1995), or DNA repair–related enzymes in Cockayne's syndrome (Henning et al., 1995). Examples of a few specific syndromes of high prevalence and particular interest are given below.

Fragile X Syndrome

Fragile X syndrome is the leading hereditary cause of MR and second to Down syndrome as a specific genetic cause (Hagerman and Cronister, 1996). Both males and females can be affected with this genetic condition. However, the frequency of fragile X is higher in males, and they tend to be more severely affected. Current estimates are that about one male in every 2000 to 4000 will inherit the fragile X mutation and be affected. Unaffected normal males can carry the fragile X mutation in an unexpressed form. Approximately one female in every 300 inherits the fragile X premutation or mutation, of whom approximately 10% have MR. Overall, 2% to 6% of unexplained MR cases are due to this single cause (Sherman, 1996).

In comparison to some other genetic and chromosomal syndromes, males with fragile X syndrome often do not have very specific or recognizable features; hence, they are frequently quite normal in appearance and not identified as having the syndrome. Some males with fragile X syndrome show characteristic facial features that can be recognized. These may include a long and narrow face, narrow inter-eye distance, highly arched palate of the mouth, and enlarged ear size. There may be prominent thumbs, hand calluses, hyper-extensibility of the joints, and flat feet. Enlarged testicular volume, also known as macroorchidism, is commonly present and particularly noticeable after puberty. In childhood, recurrent otitis media is present in about 60% of affected boys. This often requires the insertion of one or more sets of polyethylene tubes in the tympanic membranes to correct the conductive hearing loss and resultant language and articulation deficits. Flat feet are common, which can usually be treated with orthopedic shoes. Approximately 10% of affected males develop seizures, which usually can be controlled with standard anticonvulsant therapy.

Adult males with fragile X syndrome have a variable degree of mental impairment. On IQ testing, a range of 20 to 50 is common, with an average of around 35. Some younger boys with fragile X have IQ scores that fall within the borderline to normal range (70–85), but these scores often show a decline as the boys grow older. Most boys with the syndrome have speech delay and language problems, including rapid repetitive speech, cluttering of speech, and articulation difficulties. Poor fine motor coordination, hypotonia, and gross motor delays are common. Many boys have difficulty processing sensory information and blocking out competing sensory stimulation. Behavioral problems in males with fragile X frequently include attention deficit hyperactivity disorder, impulsivity, poor eye contact, shyness, and high levels of anxiety. The anxiety of making eye contact leads to a characteristic eye gaze aversion when shaking hands, particularly with strangers. Individuals with fragile X syndrome often possess a very engaging personality and have excellent imitative skills, a good imagination, and a delightful sense of humor. Males with the syndrome often display hand-flapping and hand-biting with resulting callus formation. Some males may become aggressive, and for a few it is a daily problem. They are frequently tactilely defensive. Boys with fragile X often have difficulty adapting to changes in their routine. The majority of fragile X males have some autistic-like features, and approximately 10% have autism. Fragile X syndrome is the most common genetic syndrome associated with autism, and it may provide a clue about the nature of brain malfunction in autism. Neuroimaging studies have suggested common areas of central vermis cerebellar hypoplasia in the two conditions.

Females who are carriers of fragile X syndrome are usually perfectly normal. However, about 33% may have a mild disability in some specific area of learning or schoolwork. About 10% may have mild MR. Occasionally, an affected female will have more severe to profound MR. Physically distinct features are not commonly recognized in female carriers, but in some instances, they do resemble those seen in males with fragile X. Females who have the syndrome appear to have specific weaknesses in mathematics; motor as well as speech and language problems are also commonly seen. Females affected by fragile X syndrome tend to have behavioral problems that include shyness, social withdrawal, depression, and attention deficit hyperactivity disorder.

Fragile X syndrome is caused by a defect in the gene *FMR1* (fragile X mental retardation type 1). The common form of this syndrome is due to mutated expansion of a CGG triplet repeat in the gene. In most normal individuals, this CGG triplet is repeated approximately 10 to 59 times. In the DNA of people who are carriers of fragile X, this triplet expands to 60 to 200 repetitions (referred to as a *premutation*), and in people affected by the syndrome, the CGG triplet is usually repeated more than 200 times (referred to as a *full mutation*).

Women who carry a fragile X premutation are usually completely unaffected by the syndrome, but when they pass on their chromosome to their offspring, it usually undergoes an expansion. The risk of the premutation expanding to a full mutation is related to the premutation size, with a risk of about 30% for the size of 56 to 69 repeats, about 80% for 70 to 79 repeats, 90% for 80 to 89 repeats, and nearly 100% for 90 or more repeats. Of males who have a full fragile X mutation, 20% to 40% also have some cells that show a premutation. These males are referred to as *mosaics* and appear to be less severely affected by the syndrome. Women can also be mosaics, but fewer than 10% of women affected by the syndrome appear to be mosaic.

The fragile X gene is located near the end of the long arm of the X chromosome at band Xq27.3. When cells from an affected individual are grown under special conditions (i.e., low folic acid), the end of the chromosome appears to stretch or break; hence, the name fragile X. When the *FMR1* gene has the full mutation, it usually does not synthesize any of the fragile X protein (FMRP). It is the lack of FMRP that is the cause of the syndrome. The fragile X chromosome is inherited in an X-linked manner. If a woman is a carrier of the mutated gene, her sons are at risk of being affected by fragile X and her daughters may be carriers. With each pregnancy, there is a 50% chance that the fragile X chromosome will be passed. If a son receives the chromosome, he will have a risk of about 80% of being affected, and if a daughter receives the chromosome, she will have about a 30% risk of being affected.

Males can inherit the premutation as well. If they do, they are considered carriers and are called *nonpenetrant males*. These males do not show the fragile X chromosome in their blood; likewise, they usually do not have mental impairment or physical signs of the syndrome. They pass on their X chromosome to all of their daughters and to none of their sons. Daughters of nonpenetrant males do not inherit a full mutation. Hence, all daughters of males who are nonpenetrant are carriers and none of their sons are carriers.

DNA testing for diagnosing fragile X syndrome includes two complementary tests. The first is by polymerase chain reaction, which can accurately determine the number of triplet repeats. The second is a genomic Southern blot, which provides useful information about whether the gene is methylated and turned off or not. DNA testing can identify both carriers and affected individuals and can be used for prenatal diagnosis. Prenatal diagnosis involves either chorionic villus sampling, which is done at about 10 weeks of pregnancy, or amniocentesis, done at around 16 weeks. Cells from the fetus are obtained by either of these procedures and tested for the presence of the fragile X mutation by DNA analysis. The results of ongoing studies have shown that the prenatal DNA test is highly reliable.

Currently, no cure and no specific therapy are available for fragile X syndrome. The specific function of the missing FMRP is unknown, although it is known to be an RNA-binding protein, may regulate the translation of a limited subset of mRNAs, and appears to be important for normal brain development. Some treatments, including speech and language therapy, occupational therapy, certain medications, behavioral management techniques, educational strategies, and inclusion programs, have proven to be very beneficial and can lead to marked improvement.

Williams Syndrome

Williams syndrome (William-Beuren syndrome) is a contiguous gene syndrome due to a common recurrent deletion of a 1.5 mb segment containing some 17 genes on chromosome 7q11, with an estimated incidence of approximately 1/10,000 births (Osborne and Pober, 2001). Affected individuals typically have a characteristic facial appearance, originally described as "elf-like," with a small upturned nose, long philtrum, wide mouth, full lips, small chin, puffiness around the eyes, and a stellate iris pattern. They also commonly have supravalvular aortic stenosis or other forms of aortic narrowing, childhood hypercalcemia, and joint laxity. The associated MR is usually of a mild degree, with a mean IQ score of approximately 60. Affected individuals have a remarkable cognitive deficit profile with very deficient visual–spatial abilities but highly developed verbal abilities. Many have very well-developed vocabulary, auditory memory, social use of language, and musical abilities. They tend to be empathetic, loquacious, and sociable but very anxious, hyperactive, and bothered by increased hearing sensitivity (*hyperacusis*).

Adult Williams syndrome individuals are handicapped by their developmental disabilities and adaptive problems due in part to generalized anxiety. They commonly have cardiovascular complications, including hypertension, supravalvular aortic stenosis, aortic hypoplasia, pulmonic artery stenosis, and peripheral stenoses. Joint limitations are frequently progressive and often affect the spine. Gastrointestinal and genitourinary problems are common, and hypercalcemic symptoms are frequently present (Morris et al., 1990).

Genes within the common 1.5 mb deletion that appear to underlie aspects of the clinical phenotype include the gene for elastin (*ELN*), a protein kinase involved in brain development and possibly visual–spatial abilities (*LIMK1*), and a series of seven other genes including replication factor C subunit 2 (*RFC2*), eukaryotic initiation factor 4H (*EIF-4H*), and an RNA-binding protein (*WSCR1*) (Osborne and Pober, 2001).

Autism

Autism is a behaviorally defined syndrome of early childhood. A current definition of autism [pervasive developmental disorder (PDD) in the *Diagnostic and Statistical Manual of Mental Disorders*, 4th edition (DSM-IV, American Psychiatric Association, 1997)] divides it into five behavioral subtypes, all having impaired sociability, language, nonverbal communicative skills, and imagination together with stereotypic behaviors and preoccupations. Additional features are lack of cognitive flexibility, poor organizational skills and insight into what others may be thinking, rigidity, perseveration, and frequent heightened anxiety. The five DSM-IV subtypes are based on the presence, number, and distribution of 12 behavioral descriptors and on the age at onset. The subtypes include *(1)* classic autism, requiring at least six deficits, no fewer than two in sociability and one each in language and range of interests and activities, with a clinical onset before age 3; *(2)* Asperger's syndrome, a less severe subtype with at least tree deficits, two in sociability and one in range of interests and activities, but without delay in language development or important cognitive deficit; *(3)* disintegrative disorder, applying to children with normal early development, including speaking in sentences, who undergo a severe language, behavioral, and cognitive regression between ages 2 and 10 years, resulting in autism, and excluding those with a degenerative disease of the brain; *(4)* PDD not otherwise specified, applying to children with severe impairments in sociability, language, and range of activities who do not meet criteria for the first three disorders; and *(5)* Rett syndrome, a specific neurogenetic syndrome in girls with postnatal brain growth failure.

Autism has a strong genetic component and is significantly associated with MR (Gillberg and Coleman, 2000). Approximately 75% of autistic persons are considered to have MR (Bryson and Smith, 1998). About 20% of individuals with autism may have a currently definable biologic cause such as fragile X, tuberous sclerosis, phenylketonuria, Angelman's syndrome, or Cornelia de Lange's syndrome (Rapin, 1999). There has been an apparent increase in the prevalence of diagnosed autism over the last 20 years. Recent estimates have given a prevalence for classic autism of approximately 1/600 and of autism along with the other PDD subtypes of 1/160 (Chakrabarti and Frombonne, 2001). Twin studies show high concordance for autism in monozygotic twins (70%–90%) and a relatively small concordance in dizygotic twins (4%–7%). The recurrence risk for siblings of approximately 5% is thus significantly higher than the population risk. Genetic modeling studies have suggested that it is inherited as a complex genetic disorder and that three or four genes, or as many as 15, may act in a multiplicative manner to lead to autism (Jorde et al., 1991; Pickles et al., 1995). There is a consistent male to female ratio of about 4:1, but X-linked inheritance has been excluded while an imprinted gene on the X chromosome has not (Cook, 1998). Several genome-wide scans for autism susceptibility genes have been undertaken, and several loci on chromosomes 2, 7, 15, 16, and 17 appear to be reproducibly identified (Philippe et al., 1999; International Molecular Genetic Study of Autism Consortium, 2001). Thus, autism and PDD subtypes appear to be multifactorial, resulting from a complex genetic susceptibility of high heritability in concert with environmental or other nongenetic factors.

Clues to identifying the neuroanatomic basis of autism include cellular abnormalities in the posterioinferior cerebellar hemispheres, selective hypoplasia of the cerebellar vermis, bitemporal hypometabolism, and altered serotonin metabolism (Rapin, 1999). Various studies have reported evidence of enlarged brain size in autism (Courchesne et al., 2001), suggesting various explanations, such as a genetically determined decrease in neuronal apoptosis. Functional magnetic resonance imaging (MRI) studies of a group of high-functioning autistic subjects showed abnormal activity during face-recognition tasks, consistent with the concept that the face is processed as a nonface object, which may help to explain the profound social communication deficits seen in autism (Schultz et al., 2000).

Subtelomeric Deletions

It has long been suspected that subtle chromosomal abnormalities may account for a proportion of the unexplained cases of MR. Flint et al. (1995) and Slavotinek et al. (1999) have shown that approximately 7% of unexplained MR cases are likely due to relatively small subtelomeric deletion chromosomal abnormalities, not usually visualized by standard karyotyping. These can be detected with polymorphic subtelomeric microsatellite markers, with fluorescent in situ hybridization (FISH) probes or a multiplex amplifiable probe hybridization methodology (Sismani et al., 2001). Clinical characteristics suggesting such underlying deletions include prenatal onset of growth retardation, a positive family history of MR, and mildly dysmorphic features (De Vries et al., 2001).

Dyslexia and Learning Disabilities

In regard to milder forms of developmental disability, recent findings have provided great promise of being able to dissect the genetics of cognition. Children with developmental dyslexia have great difficulty in learning to read and spell, despite adequate educational opportunity and lack of apparent neurologic impairment. The presence of developmental dyslexia, also known as specific reading disability, is recognized in 5% to 17% of school-age children, making it the most common of the childhood learning disorders (Shaywitz, 1998). Dyslexia, first recognized over 100 years ago, is notable for the type of errors made by affected individuals, such as letter (*b* for *d*) and word (*was* for *saw*) reversals (Pennington, 1997). Multiple family and twin studies have consistently demonstrated that genetic factors are of major importance in the development of dyslexia (Grigorenko, 2001). The underlying problem appears to be due to individual differences in the accuracy and speed of single-word recognition (Perfetti, 1985). Dyslexics appear to have a deficit in phonologic coding: they have slower and less accurate single-word recognition (Rack et al., 1992). The dyslexic appears to have a deficit at the level of the phonologic ability to segment a written word into its underlying phonologic elements, which results in an inability to identify a specific word. This inability appears to be independent of other higher-order cognitive and linguistic functions involved in comprehension, such as general intelligence. Several independent studies have now generally replicated findings indicating that two major loci for developmental dyslexia are on chromosomes 6 and 15 (Fisher et al., 1999; Gayan et al., 1999; Morris et al., 2000). The specific genes have yet to be identified, but these studies suggest that genetics will be useful in the dissection of human cognition.

CLINICAL APPLICATION AND RISK ASSESSMENT OF GENETICS INFORMATION

A consensus conference dealing with recommendations for the evaluation of MR was sponsored by the American College of Medical Genetics (Curry et al., 1997). Recommendations from this conference suggested that the evaluation of MR should address the cause in order to appropriately answer questions regarding prognosis, management, recurrence risks, and future prevention. The general recommendations, as summarized below, form the basis for a rational plan for evaluation of the individual with MR.

1. The initial assessment should include a complete prenatal and perinatal history, a three-generation pedigree, and a careful physical examination, including growth parameters, physical findings, minor anomalies, neurologic abnormalities, and a behavioral phenotype.
2. If a diagnosis is not made following the initial evaluation, serial evaluations over time may lead to a diagnosis in up to 20% of individuals. Many syndromes, such as those listed in Table 47–1, have a phenotype that tends to become more recognizable over time.
3. Most individuals should have a chromosome analysis performed, with a band resolution of >500, which will im-

Table 47–1. Selected Causes of Mental Retardation in Which a Recognizable Phenotype May Evolve over Time

Angelman's syndrome
Fragile X syndrome
Hallervorden-Spatz disease
Hunter's syndrome
Hurler's syndrome
Kabuki make-up syndrome
Lesch-Nyhan syndrome
Metachromatic leukodystrophy
Neurofibromatosis I
Noonan's syndrome
Prader-Willi syndrome
Rett syndrome
Smith-Magenis syndrome
Tuberous sclerosis
Velocardiofacial syndrome
Williams syndrome

prove yields. The frequency of chromosomal abnormalities detected in various series of MR subjects has ranged from about 10% to 25%. For individuals with suggestive clinical signs, targeted FISH and molecular cytogenetic studies are recommended. Occasionally, somatic mosaicism is present, and skin fibroblast karyotyping may reveal abnormalities that are absent in the blood.

4. Molecular fragile X studies should be strongly considered in any individual being evaluated since overall 2% to 6% of unexplained MR cases are due to this single cause (Sherman, 1996).
5. Because the yield from unselected metabolic screening is extremely low, it is not recommended as part of the routine evaluation. However, if an individual presents with signs or symptom of a metabolic disease, such as those indicated in Table 47–2, then targeted testing should be undertaken.
6. Neuroimaging by MRI or computerized tomography (CT) will reveal abnormalities in a significant number of subjects (up to 60%). It is particularly useful in those with microcephaly, macrocephaly, or abnormal cranial contours. Although more costly, MRI is generally superior for revealing subtle abnormalities, while CT is better when a bone abnormality, such as a craniosynostosis, is present. Imaging studies should be considered following a thorough examination.

COUNSELING AND THERAPY

In cases of Mendelian inheritance with a specific diagnosis, the risk of recurrence can be accurately provided by a qualified health-care professional. In MR cases without a specific etiologic diagnosis, counseling is difficult and prenatal diagnosis is not available. Empiric risk figures can, however, be provided. Studies have shown that families that have a child with severe MR of unknown etiology have between a 3% and a 9% risk, depending on the specific diagnosis, of having future affected children (Costeff and Weller, 1987).

The individual with MR needs the same general medical services as any other person, including normal immunizations, normal dental care, and treatment of periodic infections. Individuals with both MR and motor difficulties, such as with cerebral palsy, are at increased risk for gastrointestinal reflux and aspiration pneumonias. Inadequate food intake can lead to insufficient weight gain. Certain disorders, such as Down syndrome, have specifically increased risks for congenital heart defects, hypothyroidism, and atlantoaxial subluxation (Palfrey et al., 1987).

Early identification and early intervention programs are important to maximize the individual's potential to stimulate cognitive, language, and motor development. Federal legislation mandates the provision of services for preschool children (Public Law 99-4570) and for school-age children (Public Law 94-142). Because of educational mainstreaming, there is a greater acceptance of young adults living in the community with MR. However, during the transition to adulthood, a number of new problems are faced by the family and the individual with MR, including appropriate employment, sexuality, and continuity of medical care. Except for profoundly retarded individuals and individuals with degenerative or certain specific disorders such as Down syndrome (Eyman et al., 1991), the expected life span of the MR adult is generally comparable to that of the nonretarded general population (Eyman et al., 1990).

Although the prospect of gene therapy for genetic disease holds great promise, actual progress in developing effective protocols has been disappointingly slow (Anderson, 1998). The problems that have yet to be completely solved include obtaining efficient delivery for the necessary viral vectors, transducing nondividing cells, sustaining long-term gene expression, and developing a cost-effective way to manufacture the vector. Treatment of disorders affecting the nervous system with its myriad of cell types and complex structures is extremely challenging but potentially possible with improvements in gene therapeutic strategies (Blömer et al., 1996). An exciting alternative strategy is the idea of brain transplants of pluripotent cells capable of differentiating into cells in the brain (Ourednik et al., 2000). Evidence indicates that there are primitive bone marrow stromal cells that can be isolated and used as vehicles for transplantation in both cell and gene therapies for a variety of diseases of the central nervous system (Azizi et al., 1998). Because they can be harvested from a patient's own tissue, they have the advantage of being able to circumvent the problems of host immunity rejection. Prospects for the future of gene therapy of the central nervous system (CNS) and some forms of MR are very promising.

Table 47–2. Selected Clinical Findings and Laboratory Abnormalities Which May Point to the Need for Metabolic Testing

Failure of appropriate growth
Recurrent unexplained illness
Seizures
Ataxia
Loss of psychomotor skill
Hypotonia
"Course" appearance
Eye abnormalities such as cataracts
Recurrent somnolence/coma
Abnormal sexual differentiation
Arachnodactyly
Hepatosplenomegaly
Metabolic/lactic acidosis
Hyperuricemia
Hyperammonemia
Low cholesterol
Structural hair abnormalities
Unexplained deafness
Bone abnormalities such as dysostosis
Skin abnormalities such as ichthyosis

REFERENCES

Accardo PJ, Capute AJ: Mental retardation. Ment Retard Dev Dis Resh Rev 1998; 4:2–5.

American Association on Mental Retardation: Mental Retardation: Definition, Classification, and Systems of Support. Washington, DC: Ninth Ed, 1992.

American Psychiatric Association: Diagnostic and Statistical Manual of Mental Disorders, 4th ed. Washington DC: American Psychiatric Association, 1997.

Anderson WF: Human gene therapy. Nature 1998; 392(Suppl):25–30.

Ashley CT, Wilkinson KD, Reines D, Warren ST: FMR1 protein: conserved RNP family domains and selective RNA binding. Science 1993; 262:563–566.

Azizi SA, Stokes D, Augelli BJ, DiGirolamo C, Prockop DJ: Engraftment and migration of human bone marrow stromal cells implanted in the brains of albino rats—similarities to astrocyte grafts. Proc Natl Acad Sci USA 1998; 95:3908–3913.

Batshaw MJ: Mental retardation. Pediatr Clin North Am 1993; 40:507–521.

Blömer U, Naldini L, Verma IM, Trono D, Gage FH: Applications of gene therapy to the CNS. Hum Mol Genet 1996; 5:1397–1404.

Bryson SE, Smith IM: Epidemiology of autism: prevalence, associated characteristics, and implications for research and service delivery. Ment Retard Dev Dis Resh Rev 1998; 4:97–103.

Bundy S, Thake A, Todd J: The recurrence risks for mild idiopathic mental retardation. J Med Genet 1989; 26:260–266.

Chakrabarti S, Frombonne E: Pervasive developmental disorders in preschool children. JAMA 2001; 285:3093–3099.

Clayton PT, Thompson E: Dysmorphic syndromes with demonstrable biochemical abnormalities. J Med Genet 1988; 25:463–472.

Cook EH: Genetics of autism. Ment Retard Dev Dis Resh Rev 1998; 4:113–120.

Costeff H, Weller L: The risk of having a second retarded child. Am J Med Genet 1987; 27:753–766.

Courchesne E, Karns CM, Davis HR, Ziccardi R, Carper RA, Tigue ZD, Chisum HJ, Moses P, Pierce K, Lord C, Lincoln AJ, Pizzo S, Schreibman L, Haas RH, Akshoomoff NA, Courchesne RY: Unusual brain growth patterns in early life in patients with autistic disorder: An MRI study. Neurology 2001; 57:245–254.

Curry CJ, Stevenson RE, Aughton D, Byrne J, Carey J, Cassidy S, Cunniff C, Graham J, Jones M, Kaback M, et al.: Evaluation of mental retardation: recommendations of a consensus conference. Am J Med Genet 1997; 72:468–477.

De Vries B, White S, Knight S, Regan R, Homfray T, Young ID, Super M, McKeown C, Splitt M, Quarrell OW, et al.: Clinical studies on submicroscopic subtelomeric rearrangements: a checklist. J Med Genet 2001; 38:145–150.

Ellis NA, Groden J, Ye T-Z, Straughen J, Lennon DJ, Ciocci S, Proytcheva M, German J: The Bloom's syndrome gene product is homologous to RecQ helicases. Cell 1995; 83:655–666.

Eyman RK, Call TL, White JF: Life expectancy of persons with Down syndrome. Am J Ment Retard 1991; 95:603–612.

Eyman RK, Grossman HJ, Chaney RH, Call TL: The life expectancy of profoundly handicapped people with mental retardation. N Engl J Med 1990; 323:584–589.

Fisher SE, Marlow AJ, Lamb J, Maestrini E, Williams DF, Richardson AJ, Weeks DE, Stein JF, Monaco AP: A quantitative-trait locus on chromosome 6p influences different aspects of developmental dyslexia. Am J Hum Genet 1999; 64:146–156.

Flint J, Wilkie AOM: The genetics of mental retardation. Br Med Bull 1996; 52:453–464.

Flint J, Wilkie AOM, Buckle VJ, Winter RM, Holland AJ, McDermid HE, et al.: The detection of subtelomeric chromosomal rearrangements in idiopathic mental retardation. Nat Genet 1995; 9:132–140.

Gayan J, Smith SD, Cherny SS, Cardon LR, Fulker DW, Browner AM, Olson RK, Pennington BF, DeFries JC: Quantitative-trait locus for specific language and reading deficits on chromosome 6p. Am J Hum Genet 1999; 64:157–164.

Gillberg C, Coleman M: The Biology of the Autistic Syndromes, 3rd ed. New York: Cambridge University Press, 2000.

Grigorenko EL: Developmental dyslexia: an update on genes, brains, and environments. J Child Psychol Psychiatry 2001; 42:91–125.

Hagerman RJ, Cronister A: Fragile X Syndrome: Diagnosis, Treatment, and Research, 2nd ed. Baltimore: Johns Hopkins University Press, 1996.

Henning KA, Li L, Iyer N, McDaniel LD, Reagan MS, Legerski R, Schultz RA, Stefanini M, Lehmann AR, Mayne LV, et al.: The Cockayne syndrome group A gene encodes a WD repeat protein that interacts with CSB protein and a subunit of RNA polymerase II TFIIH. Cell 1995; 82:555–564.

International Molecular Genetic Study of Autism Consortium: A genomewide screen for autism: strong evidence for linkage to chromosomes 2q, 7q, and 16p. Am J Hum Genet 2001; 69:570–581.

Jorde LB, Hasstedt SJ, Ritvo ER, Mason-Brothers A, Freeman BJ, Pingree C, McMahon WM, Petersen B, Jenson WR, Mo A: Complex segregation analysis of autism. Am J Hum Genet 1991; 49:932–938.

Kiely M: The prevalence of mental retardation. Epidemiol Rev 1987; 9:194–218.

Lander ES, Linton LM, Birren B, Nusbaum C, Zody MC, Baldwin J, Devon K, Dewar K, Doyle M, FitzHugh W, et al.: Initial sequencing and analysis of the human genome. Nature 2001; 860–921.

MacMillan D, Gresham F, Siperstein G: Conceptual and psychometric consensus about the 1992 AAMR definition of mental retardation. Am J Ment Retard 1993; 98:325–335.

McGue M, Bouchard TJ: Genetic and environmental influences on human behavioral differences. Annu Rev Neurosci 1998; 21:1–24.

Morris CA, Leonard CO, Dilts C, Demsey SA: Adults with Williams syndrome. Am J Med Genet 1990; (Suppl 6):102–107.

Morris DW, Robinson L, Turic D, Duke M, Webb V, Milham C, Hopkin E, Pound K, Fernando S, Easton M, et al.: Family-based association mapping provides evidence for a gene for reading disability on chr 15q. Hum Mol Genet 2000; 9:843–848.

Murphy CC, Boyle C, Schendel D, Decouflé P, Yeargin-Allsop M: Epidemiology of mental retardation in children. Ment Retard Dev Dis Resh Rev 1998; 4:6–13.

North KN, Riccard V, Samango-Sprouse C, Ferner R, Moore B, Legius E, Ratner N, Denckla M, et al.: Cognitive function and academic performance in neurofibromatosis 1: consensus statement from the NF1 Cognitive Disorder Task Force. Neurology 1997; 48:1121–1127.

Osborne L, Pober B: Genes and cognition in Williams syndrome. J Am Acad Child Adolesc Psychiatry 2001; 40:732–735.

Ourednik V, Ourednik J, Park KI, Teng YD, Aboody KA, Auguste KI, Taylor RM, Tate BA, Snyder EY: Neural stem cells are uniquely suited for cell replacement and gene therapy in the CNS. Novartis Found Symp 2000; 231:242–262.

Palfrey JS, Singer JD, Walker DK, Butler JA: Early identification of children's special needs: a study in 5 metropolitan communities. J Pediatr 1987; 111:651–659.

Pennington BF: Using genetics to dissect cognition. Am J Hum Genet 1997; 60:13–16.

Perfetti CA: Reading Ability. New York: Oxford University Press, 1985.

Petrij F, Giles RH, Dauwerse HG, Saris JJ: Rubinstein-Taybi syndrome caused by mutations in the transcriptional co-activator CBP. Nature 1995; 376:348–351.

Philippe A, Martinez M, Guillouf-Bataille M, Gillberg C, Rastam M, Sponheim E, Coleman M, Zappella M, Aschauer H, Van Maldergem L, et al.: Genome-wide scan for autism susceptibility genes. Hum Mol Genet 1999; 8:805–812.

Pickles A, Bolton P, MacDonald H: Latent-class analysis of recurrence risks for complex phenotypes with selection and measurement error: a twin and family history study of autism. Am J Hum Genet 1995; 57:717–726.

Rack JP, Snowling MJ, Olson RK: The nonword reading deficit in developmental dyslexia: a review. Read Res Q 1992; 27:28–55.

Rapin I: Autism in search of a home in the brain. Neurology 1999; 52:902–904.

Raynham H, Gibbons R, Flint J, Higgs D: The genetic basis for mental retardation. Q J Med 1996; 89:169–175.

Roach ES, Gomez MR, Northrup H: Tuberous sclerosis consensus conference: revised clinical diagnostic criteria. Child Neurol 1998; 13:624–628.

Savitsky K, Sfez S, Tagle DA, Ziv Y, Sartiel A, Collins FS, Shiloh Y, Rotman G: The complete sequence of the coding region of the *ATM* gene reveals similarity to cell cycle regulators in different species. Hum Mol Genet 1995; 4:2025–2032.

Schultz RT, Gauthier I, Klin A, Fulbright RK, Anderson AW, Volkmar F, Skudlarski P, Lacadie C, Cohen DJ, Gore JC: Abnormal ventral temporal cortical activity during face discrimination among individuals with autism and Asperger syndrome. Arch Gen Psychiatry 2000; 57:344–346.

Schwartz JH: Synthesis and trafficking of neuronal proteins. In: Kandel SR, Schwartz JH, Jessell TM (eds). Principles of Neural Science, 4th ed. New York: Elsevier, 2000; 5:88–92.

Shaywitz SE: Dyslexia. N Engl J Med 1998; 338:307–312.

Sherman S: Epidemiology of fragile X syndrome. In: Hagerman RJ, Cronister A (eds). The Fragile X Syndrome: Diagnosis, Treatment, and Research, 2nd ed. Baltimore: Johns Hopkins University Press, 1996:165–192.

Sismani C, Armour JA, Flint JA, Girgalli C, Regan R, Patsalis PC: Screening for subtelomeric chromosome abnormalities in children with idiopathic mental retardation using multiprobe telomeric FISH and the new MAPH telomeric assy. Eur J Hum Genet 2001; 9:527–532.

Slavotinek A, Rosenberg M, Knight S, Gaunt L, Fergusson W, Killoran C, Clayton-Smith J, Kingston H, Campbell RH, Flint J, et al.: Screening for submicroscopic chromosome rearrangements in children with idiopathic mental retardation using microsatellite markers for the chromosome telomeres. J Med Genet 1999; 36:405–411.

Venter JC, Adams MD, Myers EW, Li PW, Mural RJ, Sutton GG, Smith HO, Yandell M, Evans CA, Holt RA, et al.: The sequence of the human genome. Science 2001; 291:1304–1351.

Wevrick R, Francke U: Diagnostic test for the Prader-Willi syndrome by SNRPN expression in blood. Lancet 1996; 348:1068–1069.

48 Hereditary Hearing Loss

RENA ELLEN FALK AND NATHAN FISCHEL-GHODSIAN

Hearing impairment represents an important cause of pediatric and adult morbidity. While significant hearing loss affects about 2 per 1000 children under age 3 years, as many as half of the population can expect to suffer some degree of hearing loss by age 80 (Avraham, 1997). Genetic factors contribute significantly to the etiology of profound prelingual and early childhood deafness, as well as to the etiology in families with later onset, progressive hearing loss (Table 48–1). While environmental factors are thought to play a major role in acquired and sporadic hearing loss, recent evidence suggests that genetic factors provide individual susceptibilities to environmental insults. Since this book deals with the genetics of common diseases, we will focus on nonsyndromic hearing loss, unless otherwise noted.

The number of genes implicated in familial hearing impairment has been estimated to be large, based on genetic segregation studies; the number of susceptibility genes has not been estimated but is likely even larger. Nevertheless, until the past few years, nothing was known about the specific genes involved in nonsyndromic familial deafness. The emergence of powerful tools for gene mapping and identification, coupled with the recognition or development of mouse models for a number of common forms of deafness, have led to the rapid identification of over 60 chromosomal regions that are involved in hearing loss, at least 16 familial deafness genes, and 1 susceptibility gene (Hereditary Hearing Loss Homepage, 2001). Concomitantly, elucidation of the mechanism of action of some of those genes has helped to provide insight into the normal and pathogenetic mechanisms involved in hearing. Many of these findings have raised unexpected new issues, however: identical mutations may produce both syndromic and nonsyndromic hearing impairment, or no hearing impairment at all; hearing impairment transmitted in either a recessive or a dominant pattern can be caused by mutations in the same gene; the same clinical syndrome can be caused by many different genes. Hence, the explosion of molecular information regarding deafness genes serves as a microcosm of the molecular dissection of other classes of disease. The common disorder nonsyndromic hearing impairment can be caused by a great number of genes that act in a Mendelian fashion, especially in childhood and young adult life, by mitochondrial mutations, which may or may not manifest themselves even in a homoplasmic state, as well as by complex polygenic inheritance that leads to the hearing loss of older age. Detailed delineation of ear embryology and anatomy may be reviewed elsewhere (Anson et al., 1991; Sulik, 1995). For a comprehensive presentation of syndromic hearing loss, see Gorlin et al. (1995).

DISEASE DEFINITION

Deafness can be classified according to several parameters, including age of onset, severity, frequency range of sound affected at onset of hearing loss, progression versus stability, anatomic portion of the ear involved in the deficit, and presence or absence of other features. Deafness present at birth or during early infancy is considered "congenital," although diagnosis may be delayed. Congenital deafness is usually associated with an inability to acquire normal speech and may be referred to as prelingual deafness. Postlingual hearing loss may be classified as either early onset or late onset, although this subdivision is somewhat arbitrary and ill-defined. Loudness of sound is expressed by the decibel (dB). As most conversational speech occurs at 25 to 45 dB, hearing loss above this magnitude represents a significant disability. Severity of hearing loss may be expressed as mild, in the 20 to 40 dB range; moderate, at 40 to 60 dB; severe, from 60 to 80 dB; and profound, above 80 dB.

Two major subgroups are defined by the portion of the ear that is affected and, therefore, the mechanism by which the hearing loss occurs (Table 48–2). Conductive deafness results from a defect in the external or middle ear and is characterized by an abnormality in the mechanical transmission of sound. Sensorineural hearing loss (SNHL), alternatively termed perceptive or neural deafness, results from a defect involving the organ of Corti and its surrounding structures—cranial nerve VIII and/or the auditory regions of the brain. SNHL may be referred to as cochlear or retrocochlear deafness, depending on the localization of the defect. When both conductive and sensorineural components are involved, the resulting deafness is classified as a mixed loss.

Deafness may occur in individuals who have additional clinical symptoms or physical abnormalities, in which case it is referred to as *syndromic* hearing loss. In general, syndromic hearing loss is most likely to affect the outer and/or middle ear structures and is commonly associated with a conductive or mixed pattern, while the vast majority of nonsyndromic (undifferentiated) deafness is associated with cochlear pathogenesis and an SNHL. Overall, about 60% of all inherited deafness is found in individuals who are otherwise phenotypically normal. While congenital deafness largely involves the full speech range of sound frequencies, postlingual deafness is more variable. Autosomal dominant postlingual hearing loss may involve the predominantly low-frequency range (Konigsmark et al., 1971; Leon et al, 1981), mid-frequency range (Williams and Roblee, 1962; Konigsmark et al., 1970), or high frequency tones (Fraser, 1964;

Table 48–1. Etiology of Deafness

Category	Contribution (%)
Genetic	50
Nonsyndromic	70
AD	20–30
AR	70
XR	1–2
Other	?1–2
Syndromic	30
Acquired	35
Idiopathic	15–30

Table 48–3. Impact of Hearing Loss

More than 6 million deaf/hearing impaired in the United States
Worldwide, 70 million have hearing loss ≥55 dB
400,000 deaf or hearing impaired U.S. children
About 1/1,000 profoundly deaf under age 3
Hearing loss affects
4% under age 44
29% by age 65
36% over age 75
50% over age 80
At least 50% of prelingual deafness is genetic
30%–50% of adult-onset hearing loss is genetic

Huizing et al., 1966), although a broader range of tonality becomes affected with progression of the condition. Higashi (1988) further classified high-frequency SNHL into four subtypes, according to the features of the audiogram and specifically emphasized the interfamilial differences in this group.

Finally, autosomal dominant loci are identified by the nomenclature DFNA; autosomal recessive loci are termed DFNB, and X-linked loci are denoted as DFN. The various loci are then numbered roughly in the order in which they were identified.

GENERAL GENETIC AND EPIDEMIOLOGIC EVIDENCE

Clinical Epidemiology

Most epidemiologic studies (see summary, Table 48–3) have focused on the incidence, prevalence, and etiology of profound childhood hearing loss. Various modern surveys indicate an incidence in the range of 1 to 2 per 1000 for prelingual deafness in developed countries, with genetic factors accounting for at least half of the cases (Fraser, 1964; Parving, 1983; Newton, 1985). Nongenetic causes may play a more important role in developing countries (Sellars et al., 1976) where infectious etiologies are more prevalent. A recent estimate of the global impact of hearing loss suggested that 70 million people suffer from hearing loss of 55 dB or more (Wilson, 1985). The likelihood of hearing loss increases substantially with increasing age. Current estimates indicate significant hearing impairment in 4% of individuals under age 44, 29% at 65 and above, 36% over age 75 (National Center for Health Statistics, 1990), and nearly 50% above age 80 (Morton, 1991). In an earlier British survey (Davis, 1983), 25% of the population reported at least some hearing loss. There is a skewed sex ratio, with male predominance in prelingual deafness (Wilde, 1853; Reardon, 1990) as well as in adult-onset hearing loss, so that more than 50% of men over age 65 have a hearing loss substantial enough to interfere with speech comprehension (Cohen and Gorlin, 1995).

Table 48–2. Types of Hearing Loss

Type	Characteristics
Conductive	Outer and middle ear structures are involved May be associated with visible malformation Often syndromic
Sensorineural	Inner ear, auditory nerve, brain Most commonly nonsyndromic
Mixed	

While hearing impairment presents a major challenge in the areas of communication, socialization, and education (Arnos et al., 1992), there is also a significant associated socioeconomic burden. Costs upward of $30 billion per year for medical treatment, special education, and loss of productivity have been attributed to various disorders of hearing, speech, and language in the United States (Nadol, 1993).

Genetic Epidemiology

Multiple studies have evaluated the relative contribution of genetic influences and environmental factors to the occurrence of deafness (Table 48–4). As noted above, the majority have reported data for profound childhood deafness. Early series, including the seminal reports of Nance (1980), Fraser (1964), and Sellars et al. (1976) found the proportion of genetic deafness to be 30% to 85%, based on family studies in a variety of early-onset deafness populations. More recent studies confirm these findings, and most suggest a genetic etiology for greater than 50% to 60% of cases of prelingual deafness (Marazita et al., 1993; Nadol, 1993). Similarly, the very limited available studies of predominantly adult-onset populations suggest that the genetic contribution to hearing loss in this group is also in the 30% to 50% range (Sill et al., 1994). As many of these studies are based on patient response to questionnaires or on retrospective record review, ascertainment bias remains an issue. Also, the relatively large proportion of cases for whom etiology cannot be assigned (30%–50%) underscores the possibility that sporadic cases may be misclassified as nongenetic because of the absence of family history or identifying phenotypic features. Finally, ac-

Table 48–4. Genetic Contribution to Profound Prelingual Deafness

Population	Report	% Genetic
Prelingual profound hearing loss (Danes)	Lindenov, 1945	45
U.K. children in schools for the deaf	Fraser, 1964	30
Israeli families ascertained for deafness	Dar and Winter, 1969	70
U.S. children in schools for hearing impaired/deaf	Chung and Brown, 1970	70
South African white children in schools for the deaf	Sellars et al., 1976	36
U.S. children ascertained by survey (Gallaudet)	Nance, 1980	85
U.S. children with profound early-onset deafness	Marazita et al., 1993	63

quired hearing loss may occur in individuals who are genetically predisposed to the adverse affect of a specific environmental factor (see below). Thus, the genetic contribution is likely to be at the higher end of the reported ranges. Indeed, current investigators attribute up to 60% of prelingual deafness to genetic causes (Marizita et al., 1993; Nadol, 1993).

All Mendelian modes of inheritance, as well as mitochondrial and other nontraditional inheritance models (e.g., the two-locus model) have been implicated in the etiology of familial hearing loss. However, it is again useful to discriminate between profound, prelingual deafness, which is due to autosomal recessive (AR) inheritance in at least 70% to 85% of cases (Nance, 1980) and later childhood or adult-onset hearing loss, in which autosomal dominant (AD) inheritance plays a greater role (Cohen and Gorlin, 1995). Indeed, using an incidence of 1/1,000 for prelingual deafness, and attributing 50% of congenital deafness to genetic causation and 50% of that to AR inheritance, Marres and Cremers (1989) suggested that at least 1 in 4000 children are affected with prelingual AR deafness. In general, the AR loci are associated with prelingual severe to profound hearing loss. Family studies that demonstrated that most deaf by deaf matings produced hearing children yielded an early estimate of up to 36 different autosomal recessive loci (Morton, 1960). Recent estimates suggest as many as 50 loci (Zbar et al., 1998). However, although AD genes more typically are associated with postlingual onset of progressive hearing loss, 10% to 15% of prelingual deafness may be attributed to two autosomal dominant loci (see "Gene Identification").

X-linked inheritance accounts for a relatively small proportion of genetic deafness, in the range of 2% to 3% of all cases. In a striking reworking of nineteenth-century data collected by William Wilde (1853), Reardon (1990) estimated that 5% of congenital deafness in males is due to an X-linked gene. The XR deafness loci are associated with pre- or postlingual onset SNHL, except DFN3, which presents with mixed hearing loss due to stapes fixation (Nance et al., 1971).

The proportion of mitochondrial hearing loss among all people with nonsyndromic hearing impairment is not clear. While it has been argued that it may be quite common (Estivill et al., 1998b), this has not yet been confirmed in unselected populations of hearing-impaired individuals. It has also been observed that the great majority of autosomal dominant pedigrees, which could be confused with mitochondrial inheritance, do show transmission through fathers when the pedigrees are sufficiently large. The most common mitochondrial gene defect leading to nonsyndromic hearing loss is the homoplasmic A1555G mutation in the mitochondrial small ribosomal RNA gene (Fischel-Ghodsian, 1999a).

In addition to classical Mendelian inheritance, two-locus models involving nuclear genes have been suggested to explain data from an inbred Indian population (Majumder et al., 1989), as well as from a Swedish family demonstrating dominant inheritance of SNHL (Balciuniene et al., 1998). Similarly, the possibility of digenic inheritance of DFNB15 was raised in a consanguineous family, demonstrating two areas of identity by descent on a genome screen conducted with 165 polymorphic markers (Van Camp et al., 1997). An LOD score of 2.78, which was described as the maximum obtainable for this family, was demonstrated for each locus (chromosomes 3q and 19p). Interaction of a mitochondrial mutation and of as yet unidentified nuclear genes was suggested in the etiology of deafness in a large Arab-Israeli pedigree (Jaber et al., 1992; Prezant et al., 1993; Bykhovskaya et al., 1998). Subsequent data demonstrating that the specific mitochondrial mutation (A1555G) is also responsible for later onset SNHL (Estivill et al., 1998b), as well as aminoglycoside ototoxicity (Fischel-Ghodsian et al., 1993; Prezant et al., 1993) has raised a question of whether other mutations, as yet-unidentified environmental factors or both contribute to the expression of this mutation.

A different mitochondrial mutation, T7445C, implicated in the etiology of progressive postlingual SNHL (Reid et al., 1994; Fischel-Ghodsian et al., 1995), also shows decreased penetrance, again suggesting a possible interaction with other genetic or nongenetic factors. A third mitochondrial mutation, A3243G, has been associated with bilateral SNHL in a Japanese population (Oshima et al., 1996). Finally, the mitochondrial deletion most commonly associated with the Kearns-Sayre syndrome (myopathy with ragged red fibers and progressive ophthalmoplegia) has recently been described in otherwise normal Japanese adults with more than 40 dB hearing loss (Ueda et al., 1998).

Association with Other Diseases

Significant hearing loss may occur as an isolated finding or may be seen as a component of a specific syndrome. Of the roughly 35% of deafness that appears to have a genetic etiology, about 40% is syndromic. The recent edition of Gorlin's monograph on hereditary hearing loss (Gorlin et al., 1995) cites 427 conditions, of which over 400 are syndromic; these include 30 conditions with pinna anomalies; 103 involving the central nervous system or eye; 87 additional musculoskeletal disorders; 51 endocrine or metabolic conditions; 64 syndromes manifesting abnormal skin, teeth or oral structures; 12 chromosomal abnormalities; and 35 miscellaneous syndromes. Although syndromic hearing loss is heterogeneous at both the phenotypic and molecular levels, most syndromes can at least be suspected on the basis of associated findings. While a review of these conditions is beyond the scope of this chapter, specific disease categories or symptom complexes warrant further comment. In particular, the possibility of hearing loss should be considered in any individual with unilateral or bilateral malformation of the pinna, ectodermal dysplasia or other syndromes involving neural crest ectoderm derived structures, oro-motor hypotonia such as occurs in Down syndrome or various neuromuscular disorders, sclerosing bone disorders, and in a variety of connective tissue disorders including Marfan syndrome and the type II collagenopathies (Fischel-Ghodsian and Falk, 1997).

The association of diabetes and deafness is well established (Olsson et al., 1998) and should trigger a consideration of mitochondrial inheritance, as should the history of progressive hearing loss associated with encephalopathy, myopathy, ophthalmoplegia, and/or optic atrophy, lactic acidosis, or stroke episodes (Shoffner et al., 1989; Sue et al., 1998). An autosomal recessive syndrome of ovarian dysgenesis and sensorineural hearing loss (Perrault syndrome) presents as undifferentiated deafness in males and is difficult to distinguish from nonsyndromic hearing loss in affected females (Pallister and Opitz, 1979). Finally, several syndromes that are common among the deaf population may present as isolated or nonsyndromic deafness and should be considered more fully (Table 48–5).

Otosclerosis

Otosclerosis (Table 48–6) is the most common sclerosing disorder causing hearing loss in adults, with an estimated incidence of 1 in 330 in whites, 1 in 3300 in blacks, and 1 in 33,000 in Asians (Bergstrom, 1990). An autosomal dominant condition

Table 48–5. Congenital Deafness

50%–60% Mendelian
Of these, at least 70% are recessive
Most are nonsyndromic
Three common AR syndromes
3%–6% Usher syndrome
2%–5% Pendred syndrome
1% Jervell and Lange-Nielsen syndrome

with a female preponderance (Schaap and Gapany-Gapanavicius, 1978), it is characterized by markedly diminished penetrance of 25% to 40%, which has hindered gene identification efforts. However, linkage to 15q25–26 (Tomek et al., 1998) and 7q34–36 (Van den Bogaert et al., 2001) has been established in single kindreds. The typical presentation is conductive or mixed hearing loss, generally occurring in the third and fourth decades and often exacerbated by pregnancy. The pathologic lesion is progressive stapes fixation, associated with focal abnormal endochondral bone formation in the otic capsule. While surgical stapedectomy provides improved hearing in greater than 90% of patients (Bergstrom, 1990), medical benefit of fluoride treatment is less consistent. This common condition must be differentiated from DFN3 because stapedectomy in the latter condition results in profuse drainage of perilymph, increased hearing loss, and onset or worsening of vestibular dysfunction.

Alport Syndrome

Alport syndrome, the association of sensorineural hearing loss and chronic nephritis, comprises about 1% of all genetic hearing loss (Beighton and Sellars, 1982) and greater than 2% of renal transplant patients (Milliner et al., 1982). Although moderately high frequency hearing loss appears in adolescence in about 50% of cases, bilateral SNHL may occur in early childhood, thus presenting as apparently isolated SNHL. There is significant genetic heterogeneity with X-linked, AD, and AR (rare) inheritance (Hasstedt and Atkin, 1983; Atkin et al., 1988). Identification of mutations in the gene encoding the α chain of type IV collagen (*COL4A5*), which maps to Xq22 and is a constituent of glomerular basement membrane, represented the first documented molecular defect in genetic deafness (Barker et al., 1990; Hostikkia et al., 1990; Boye et al., 1991). A rare AR form of Alport syndrome has been associated with abnormalities of *COL4A3* and *COL4A4* (Mochizuki et al., 1994).

Neurofibromatosis

Unilateral or bilateral clinical hearing loss occurs in 1% to 2% of patients with neurofibromatosis (NF1, or Von Recklinghausen disease), who are generally easily identifiable based on other phenotypic findings. This common condition with incidence of about 1 in 3000 is caused by mutation in a gene-encoding neurofibromin, a GTPase activating protein with homology to the *ras* family of proto-oncogenes (Cawthon et al., 1990; Viskochil, et al., 1990; Wallace et al., 1990). Progressive SNHL, prominent tinnitus and vestibular dysfunction are typical presenting features of NF2 (central neurofibromatosis) due to the presence of bilateral vestibular schwannomas that occur in greater than 90% of affected patients (Riccardi and Eichner, 1986). NF2, which occurs with an incidence of about 1 in 40,000, is due to mutations in a tumor suppressor gene that encodes merlin (moesin-ezrin-radixin-like protein), a member of a family of cytoskeletal proteins, at 22q11.2 (Trofatter et al., 1993). It is critical to distinguish NF2 from other conditions with adult-onset progressive SNHL because the natural history and subsequent anticipatory management are quite different.

Table 48–6. Otosclerosis

AD with 25%–40% penetrance
Progressive stapes fixation
Female : male ratio about 1.8:1
Exacerbated by pregnancy
Benefit of fluoride Rx, surgical stapedectomy
Linkage established to 7q34–36 and 15q25–26

Usher Syndrome

Usher syndrome is a genetically heterogeneous phenotype constituting the most important hereditary cause of deafness with blindness (Smith et al., 1994). Usher syndrome, which comprises 3% to 5% of all profound childhood deafness (Fraser, 1964) and more than 50% of all deaf-blind adults (Boughman et al., 1983), generally presents with prelingual sensorineural hearing loss with or without vestibular dysfunction and includes later onset retinitis pigmentosa. Three phenotypes have been delineated on the basis of presence or absence of vestibular dysfunction and age of onset of the retinopathy, and molecular analysis has confirmed moderate genetic heterogeneity (Pieke-Dahl et al., 1993; Kimberling and Moller, 1995). Of note, Usher syndrome, Type 1b (*USH1B*), is due to mutations in the myosin-VIIA gene (Weil et al., 1995), which is also responsible for a form of nonsyndromic AR deafness, DFNB2 (Liu et al., 1997a; Weil et al., 1997), as well as an AD form, DFNA11 (Liu et al., 1997b). Three other nonsyndromic deafness genes—DFNB12, DFNB18, and DFNB23—have been associated with the Type 1 Usher syndrome phenotype as well (see Hereditary Hearing Loss Homepage, 2001). A recent report of Usher Type 2a families (*USH2A*) reveals that a specific deletion (2314delG) in the *USH2A* gene, which encodes an extracellular matrix protein, accounts for a major proportion of mutant alleles in British and Chinese families (Liu et al., 1999). This is a particularly important finding as USH2 accounts for more than 50% of Usher syndrome cases (Hopes et al., 1997).

Pendred Syndrome

Pendred syndrome classically presents as severe to profound SNHL, which is usually congenital but may develop in early childhood and is associated with a mild thyroid organification defect. Although moderate goiter presents in mid- to later childhood, most patients remain euthyroid. This AR condition, which accounts for 1% to 10% of hereditary deafness (Batsakis and Nishiyama, 1962; Fraser, 1965), is caused by mutations in an ion transporter gene, *PDS* (Everett et al., 1997). Although originally proposed to be a sulfate transporter on the basis of homology to a family of known sulfate transport proteins, as well as the presence of a sulfate-transporter signature domain, pendrin now appears to function as a chloride-iodide transport protein (Scott et al., 1999). Of note, mutations in this gene (also known as *SLC26A4*) can also produce apparently nonsyndromic deafness, *DFNB4* (Greinwald et al., 1998; Li et al., 1998), providing a second example of a gene that is responsible for both syndromic and nonsyndromic deafness.

Jervell and Lange-Nielsen Syndrome

Marked prolongation of the Q–T interval on EKG is a well-known cause of sudden death in children with congenital, profound SNHL (Jervell and Lange-Nielsen, 1957). This autosomal recessive condition, Jervell and Lange-Nielsen syndrome (also referred to as surdo-cardiac syndrome), accounts for up to 1% of the congenitally deaf population (Fraser et al., 1964) and is due to homozygosity for mutations in *KCNQ1* (*KVLQT1*), the common autosomal dominant long Q–T syndrome gene (Neyroud et al., 1997; Splawski et al., 1997), as well as to mutation in *KCNE1* (minK), whose gene product participates with the KCNQ1 protein in forming a K^+ channel (Schultze-Bahr et al., 1997; Tyson et al., 1997). Dysfunction of the potassium channel results in prolongation and lack of homogeneity of myocellular repolarization and to abnormal K^+ concentrations in the endolymph. Of note, another potassium channel component gene, *KCNQ4* has been implicated as the causal gene in 5 of 6 families with DFNA2, a dominant condition that maps to chromosome 1p34 (Coucke et al., 1999; Kubisch et al., 1999). The authors note that low expression of *KCNQ4* in the heart and differential expression of *KCNQ1* and *KCNQ4* in the cochlea (stria vascularis vs outer hair cells) may explain the lack of cardiac dysrhythmia in DFNA1, as well as the dominant pattern of inheritance.

Environmental Factors

While multiple physical, chemical, and infectious agents (Nadol, 1993) have been associated with hearing loss, genetic factors may increase susceptibility to the causal agent. Common causes of acquired hearing loss include meningitis, recurrent otitis media with or without mastoiditis, trauma, noise abuse, kernicterus, myxedema, and idiopathic progressive bilateral sensorineural hearing loss (IPBSNHL), which appears to be an autoimmune phenomenon (Moscicki et al., 1994). Of these, noise may be the most significant and potentially most easily controlled factor. Other immune-mediated conditions, vascular disorders, primary neoplasias and metastatic lesions may cause hearing loss. Sensitivity to various pharmaceutical agents, including aminoglycoside antibiotics, loop diuretics, quinine, salicylates, *cis*-platinum, and other agents, may have associated genetic susceptibility (see below). Prenatal infection with rubella virus (Dekaban et al., 1958; Reynolds et al., 1974) and cytomegalovirus (Hanshaw et al., 1976; Bauman et al., 1994) and exposure to ethanol (Church and Gerkin, 1988) are potent causes of teratogenic hearing loss. Of note, the findings of an increased incidence of hearing loss in close relatives of infants with rubella embryopathy suggested fetal genetic susceptibility (Anderson et al., 1970), but this interpretation may not be valid (Moroso, 1985). Prenatal exposure to thalidomide and retinoic acid have been associated with conductive hearing loss secondary to microtia, hypoplasia or atresia of the external acoustic meatus, ossicular fusion or other defects, and inner ear anomalies. Other human teratogens associated with hearing loss include quinine, trimethadione, fetal iodine deficiency, and fetal methyl mercury effects.

PATHOPHYSIOLOGY: BIOLOGIC BASIS OF GENETIC SUSCEPTIBILITY

To understand the pathophysiology of hearing loss, a short summary of the anatomy and physiology of the ear is required. Hearing begins with the capture of sound waves by the external ear or pinna, followed by concentration and transmission of the mechanical wave through the external auditory canal to the tympanic membrane, which delineates the transition from outer to middle ear. In the middle ear the vibration is amplified by an ossicular chain that terminates at the juxtaposition of the footplate of the stapes in the oval window, which separates the air-filled middle ear from the fluid filled membranous duct system of the inner ear. Vibration of the oval window produces a wave of perilymph in the cochlea, and this constitutes the auditory sensor of the inner ear. The wave deflects the basilar membrane that supports the organ of Corti, the organelle responsible for conversion of the mechanical sound wave to an electrical impulse that can be carried to the brain via the vestibulo-cochlear nerve. In addition to support cells, the organ of Corti is comprised of a single layer of inner hair cells and three rows of outer hair cells, which total only 15,000 to 17,000 cells (Bredberg, 1989). These are bathed in potassium-rich endolymph, which is secreted by the stria vascularis. Actin-containing microvilli (stereocilia) extend from the outer hair cells, articulating with each other and with the overlying, relatively acellular tectorial membrane via filamentous projections called *tip links*. Deflection of the basilar membrane initiates a process of movement of the hair cells and their stereocilia, with resulting displacement of the filamentous tip links and consequent potassium influx and cellular depolarization. This voltage-gated mechanism results in secondary activation of calcium channels, influx of calcium ions, and subsequent release of neurotransmitters (Petit, 1996).

The complexity of the inner ear provides the framework to understand the genetic data, which indicate that defects in many different genes can cause hearing impairment. Over the next few years the further elucidation of genes associated with hearing impairment will provide insights into many of the biochemical pathways and structures of the inner ear. Some of the genes already identified provide logical starting points for such efforts. For example, *GJB2* and *GJB3* encode connexin 26 and connexin 31, gap junction proteins that relate to intercellular communication in the organ of Corti with recent evidence implicating faulty gap junction assembly as a result of GJB mutations (Martin et al., 1999); *TECTA* encodes a-tectorin, which comprises a major component of the tectoral membrane and fosters the stability of that structure; *MYO VIIA* and *XV* are molecular motors, which may shed light on the function of the stereocilia and the tip links gating mechanism; *KVLQT1* (also called *KCNQ1*), *KCNE1* (minK), and *KCNQ4* are K^+ channel elements that are directly involved in the process of depolarization and the prolonged repolarization of the auditory hair cells; and *PDS* encodes a putative chloride-iodide transporter, pendrin, which presumably has a role in repolarization. For other genes, the physiological implications are not understood. Examples include *COCH*, whose product is an extracellular matrix protein, as well as *POU3F4* and *POU4F3*, which encode transcription factors. Similarly, DFNA5 encodes a novel protein whose function remains obscure (Van Laer et al., 1998). In addition to structural and motor proteins, intercellular communication channels, potassium and chloride homeostasis, and transcription factors, a recent observation in deafwaddler mice suggests that abnormal calcium homeostasis will also play a role in human deafness. Kozel et al. (1998) and Street et al. (1998) found that a mutation in the gene for Ca^{2+} ATPase, which has probable homology to human chromosomal region 3p25–26, caused the deafness phenotype in deafwaddler mice. The authors speculate that "ATP2b2 is essential for removing Ca^{2+} from specific subcellular domains of both auditory and vestibular hair cells." Mutant mice apparently cannot clear Ca^{2+} rapidly enough after the normal Ca^{2+} influx to the stereocilia. Hence, this represents a defect of calcium homeostasis in the auditory hair cells.

The pathophysiology of aminoglycoside ototoxicity due to the A1555G mutation appears to be relatively straightforward. The mutation lies exactly in the region of the gene for which the resistance mutations in yeast and *Tetrahymena* have been described, and in which aminoglycoside binding has been documented in bacteria (Li et al., 1982; Spangler and Blackburn, 1985; Gravel et al., 1987). In addition, the mutation makes the mitochondrial RNA gene in this region more similar to the bacterial ribosomal RNA gene (Prezant et al., 1993). Since aminoglycosides are concentrated within cochlear cells, and remain there for prolonged periods (Henley and Schacht, 1988), we proposed that susceptible individuals with the 1555 mutation have increased binding to aminoglycosides, leading to altered protein synthesis in the mitochondria (Prezant et al., 1993), with the tissue specificity due to preferential concentration of the drug in those cells. Subsequent binding experiments have proven that increased binding to the mitochondrial 12S ribosomal RNA occurs (Hamasaki and Rando, 1997). However, when examining lymphoblastoid cell lines of individuals with the 1555 mutation, exposure of the cell lines to high concentrations of neomycin or paromomycin led to a decreased rate of growth in glucose medium, but no mutant proteins were detected (Guan et al., 1996). Similar results of decreased protein synthesis but no mutant proteins were obtained in Japan using mitochondrial transfer from a human skin fibroblast line with the 1555 mutation to ρ_0HeLa cells exposed to very high levels of streptomycin (Inoue et al., 1996). This may indicate that the effects of aminoglycosides in these cell lines could be nonspecific and different from those in the cochlea, perhaps because of different transport of the antibiotic into the mitochondria.

For other mitochondrial mutations associated with hearing loss, it is tempting to speculate that mitochondrial mutations interfere with energy production, that the cochlea is highly dependent on sufficient energy production, and that insufficient energy production leads to degeneration of cochlear cells. However, the cochlea is not the most energy-dependent tissue in the body. In other systemic neuromuscular disorders caused by mitochondrial mutations, the extraocular muscles appear to be the most energy-sensitive cells. Also, hearing loss is neither the most prominent nor a consistent clinical sign in most of these conditions. In addition, the same mitochondrial mutation may cause severe hearing loss in some family members but not in others. This is particularly surprising since the mitochondrial mutations leading to nonsyndromic hearing loss are homoplasmic or near homoplasmic, meaning that essentially all mitochondrial chromosomes in the body harbor the mutation. It has been proposed that the differences in penetrance occur because of allelic variants in nuclear-encoded proteins involved in mitochondrial RNA processing or translation, which interact with the mitochondrial mutations (Fischel-Ghodsian, 1998). Similarly, if there are cochlea-specific splice-variants or isoenzymes of such proteins, this may explain the tissue specificity. However, at this time the pathophysiological pathways leading from the mitochondrial mutations to hearing loss remain unclear.

Mitochondrial genetics has been proposed as a paradigm for the effects of aging and associated degenerative disorders (Wallace, 1992). Acquired mitochondrial mutations may also lead to presbycusis (Seidman et al., 1996). Presbycusis is the progressive hearing loss that occurs with age in a significant proportion of individuals. Since mitochondrial DNA mutations and the resulting loss of oxidative phosphorylation activity seem to play an important role in the aging process (reviewed by Nagley et al., 1993), it is not unlikely that mitochondrial mutations in the auditory system can also lead to presbycusis. In a recent study, tissue from the spiral ganglion and membranous labyrinth from archival temporal bones of five patients with presbycusis was examined for mutations within the mitochondrially encoded cytochrome oxidase II gene (Fischel-Ghodsian et al., 1997). When compared to controls, results indicated that at least a proportion of people with presbycusis have a significant load of mitochondrial DNA mutations in auditory tissue and that there is great individual variability in both quantity and cellular location of these mutations. Similar data were obtained by Bai et al. (1997) when screening cochlear tissue from temporal bones for the presence of the 4,977 bp deletion, although the ages of the presbycusis and control groups were not well matched. Of note, a study evaluating the role of the MHC genes in several conditions associated with hearing loss found that a specific extended MHC haplotype occurred with increased frequency in patients with presbycusis, as well as in patients with several other genetic disorders of hearing, suggesting at least one of several genetic factors that may contribute to this apparently complex condition (Bernstein et al., 1996).

Gene Identification

To date, at least 29 autosomal dominant, 28 autosomal recessive, 4 X-linked, and 2 mitochondrial nonsyndromic deafness loci have been identified or reserved (see Hereditary Hearing Loss Homepage for frequent updates). For 16 of these loci, the genes have been identified. Of the DFNB loci, DFNB7 and DFNB11 map to the same region, chromosome 9q13–21 (Jain et al., 1995; Scott et al., 1996) and most likely represent the same gene (Van Camp et al., 1997). However, while DFNB8 and DFNB10 both map to chromosome 21q22, DFNB8 is associated with progressive, postlingual-onset hearing loss (Veske et al., 1996), while DFNB10 presents the typical picture of stable prelingual SNHL (Bonne-Tamir et al., 1996). Similarly, although four loci have been assigned to chromosome 11q, they appear to be distinct, with DFNB2 identified as the myosin VIIA gene (Liu et al., 1997a; Weil et al., 1997), DFNB21 identified as α-tectorin (Mustapha et al., 1999), and DFNB20 and DFNB24 apparently mapping to nonoverlapping regions (Moynihan et al., 1999; Smith, unpublished). While DFNA8, DFNA11 and DFNA12 all map to chromosome 11q12.3–q24, DFNA11 and DFNA12 involve nonoverlapping regions (Tamagawa et al., 1996; Van Camp et al., 1997) with DFNA11 now known to be caused by mutations in myosin VIIA and DFNA12 known to be caused by mutations in α-tectorin. Hence, mutations in either of these loci, as well as the important connexin 26 locus, may cause either dominant or recessive SNHL. Linkage data for DFNA8 implied overlap with both of the other loci, so that the number of loci in this region remained in doubt through the late 1990s (Van Camp et al., 1977); however, Verhoeven et al. (1998) established that DFNA8 was also caused by mutation in α-tectorin. Hence, DFNA8 and DFNA12 represent a single locus. Of note, the AD α-tectorin phenotype is one of only two DFNA loci (with DFNA3) associated with prelingual deafness.

Connexins

Despite the marked genetic heterogeneity of the autosomal deafness loci, one gene, *GJB2* (see Tables 48–7 and 48–8), which encodes the gap junction β_2 element, connexin 26, is now known to be responsible for DFNB1, which accounts for as much as half of autosomal recessive profound SNHL (Maw et al., 1995; Gasparini et al., 1997). Notably, a single base pair deletion that

Table 48–7. Connexins

Cx26 (*GJB2*) mutations cause DFNB1 and DFNA3
Cx30 (*GJB6*) also implicated in DFNA3
Cx31 (*GJB3*) mutations cause some DFNA2
Connexins are intercellular gap junction proteins that facilitate diffusion of small molecules between adjacent cells by forming intercellular channels
Mouse immunohistochemical studies reveal Cx26 expression in stria vascularis, basement membrane, limbus, and spiral prominence of the cochlea

occurs in a string of G residues, 35delG (also described as 30delG), accounts for more than 70% of the abnormal Cx26 alleles (Denoyelle et al., 1997; Zelante et al., 1997) and occurs with high frequency in both familial and sporadic cases (Estivill et al., 1998a; Lench et al., 1998) raising the possibility of effective screening (see below). The 30delG mutation has been described in populations as diverse as Italian and Spanish Mediterraneans (Estivill et al., 1998); Moroccans (Lench et al., 1998b); English, Belgians, Australians, New Zealanders, Tunisians, and Lebanese (Denoyelle et al., 1997; Lench et al., 1998a), Ashkenazi Jewish subjects (Morell et al., 1998); and others, occurring with a prevalence of approximately 1 in 30 to 1 in 40 (Estivill et al., 1998a; Green et al., 1999). This mutation appears to be responsible for 10% of all childhood hearing loss and 20% of hereditary deafness in children (Kelley et al., 1998). Another mutation, 167delT, is particularly prevalent among the Ashkenazi Jewish population, with a carrier rate of 1 in 25 in one study (Morell et al., 1998). In contrast to the 30delG mutation, which occurs on a background of different haplotypes, implying a mutational hot spot (Denoyelle et al., 1997), the 167delT mutation occurs in association with a conserved haplotype (Morell et al., 1998).

Mutations in *GJB2* and *GJB6* (connexin 30), both of which map to chromosome 13q12, have been described in an autosomal dominant form of congenital deafness, DFNA3 (Kelsell et al., 1997; Grifa et al., 1999), and mutations in *GJB3* (connexin 31) have been implicated in the etiology of DFNA2 (Xia et al., 1998). Connexin 31 is of considerable interest since some mutations in this gene are associated with variably penetrant, gender-influenced, late-onset hearing loss, while others result in a dermatologic condition, erythrokeratoderma variabilis (Richard et al., 1998). Finally, some connexin 32 mutations, which cause X-linked dominant (or intermediate) Charcot-Marie-Tooth disease (Bergoffen et al., 1993) may be associated with hearing loss as well. Hence, at least four members of the connexin family of genes have been associated with sensorineural hearing loss.

Unconventional Myosins

Myosins are divided into classes based on the structure of the motor domains and tails. Conventional muscle myosins are class

Table 48–8. Connexin 26

GJB2 (Cx26) mutations cause DFNB1 and DFNA3
GJB2 mutations are found in about half of all DFNB kindreds
Deletion 30delG accounts for 70% of mutant alleles in ethnically diverse DFNB1 kindreds and represents a deletion hot spot
Accounts for >80% of DFNB1 in Mediterraneans
GJB2 mutations found in 10% of "sporadic" cases
Most common cause of prelingual deafness
30delG carrier rate is at least 1 in 40
167delT occurs in 1 in 25 Ashkenazi Jews

Table 48–9. Unconventional Myosins

MYO7A mutations cause USH1B, DFNB2, and DFNA11
Analogous to the Shaker-1 mouse and Marine zebrafish models
An unconventional myosin that interacts with actin as a molecular "motor" to convert ATP to mechanical force
Expressed in inner and outer hair cells of organ of Corti of guinea pig and retinal pigment epithelium of adult rat
USH1B: mostly truncating or nonsense mutations
Multiple different mutations on different haplotypes
Myosin XV (MYO15) mutations are associated with DFNB3
Analogous to the Shaker-2 mouse model;
Myosin VI (MYO6) mutations cause DFNA22
Analogous to the Snell's Waltzer mouse model

2. The other 13 known myosin classes are called *unconventional myosins*. Three of these unconventional myosins have been implicated in hearing loss (Table 48–9). Mutations in myosin VIIA have been found to be responsible for DFNA11, DFNB2, and Usher syndrome type 1B (Liu et al., 1997a, 1997b; Weil et al., 1997). DFNB3 is caused by mutations in myosin XV (Wang et al., 1998). These myosins are expressed in the hair cells of the inner ear, interact with actin in these cells, and appear to affect stereocilia organization and hair cell contractility. Again note that myosin VIIA mutations have been associated with both syndromic and nonsyndromic hearing loss and with autosomal dominant and autosomal recessive transmission. Myosin VI is another candidate for human hearing loss as mutations in the mouse *MYO6* gene have been implicated as the causation of deafness in the Snell's waltzer mouse (Avraham et al., 1995). However, the human myosin VI gene has not yet been implicated as a cause of familial hearing loss.

Pou Domain Genes

The most frequent form of X-linked deafness, DFN3, comprises profound SNHL, as well as a conductive deficit, due to stapes fixation (Nance et al., 1971). DFN3 must be differentiated from other X-linked forms of deafness as affected individuals have a cochlear bony defect and increased perilymphatic pressure (Phelps et al., 1991), resulting in a persistent "gush" of perilymph during surgical stapedectomy or attempts to place cochlear implants. While moderately severe hearing loss is present congenitally, there may be delayed onset and rapid progression of hearing loss in some cases (Puissan et al., 1995).

Heterozygous females are variously affected and may present as adults with mild SNHL or with a course suggestive of classical otosclerosis. Hence, from a clinical perspective, DFN3 might best be considered an X-linked dominant disorder. As females are also at risk for a perilymphatic gusher, identification of a family history of profound male deafness should generate extreme caution in the evaluation and treatment of any woman presenting with an otosclerotic process. Using a candidate gene approach, de Kok et al. (1995) identified *Pou3F4* to be the gene responsible for DFN3. *Pou3F4* is a member of a family of highly conserved nuclear transcription factors and is expressed in the brain, neural tube, and otic vesicle of developing rat embryos. However, the exact pathogenesis of hearing loss in DFN3 is not yet understood. In addition to *Pou3F4*, another POU domain gene, *Pou4F3*, has been implicated in causation of DFNA15 (Vahava et al., 1998), in which the clinical phenotype presents the progressive nonsyndromic SNHL that is typical of autosomal dominant transmission.

Table 48–10. Pendred Syndrome

Congenital sensorineural hearing loss and goiter
Genetically homogeneous (incompletely ascertained)
Mapped to 7q22–q31.1 in 1996
Mutations in *PDS* gene at 7q31
PDS → pendrin, a chloride-iodide transporter
Pendrin expressed in adult thyroid and fetal cochlea
DFNB4 is also caused by *PDS* mutations

Mitochondrial Genes

Mutations in the mitochondrial 12S ribosomal RNA gene and the tRNAser(UCN) have been associated with maternally inherited nonsyndromic hearing loss. Three additional mitochondrial mutations in and around the tRNAser(UCN) gene, and leading to nonsyndromic hearing loss, have been identified subsequently in pedigrees from all over the world (reviewed in Fischel-Ghodsian, 1999a; Sue et al., 1999). In general, these mutations are nearly always homoplasmic in affected individuals. However, as noted earlier, hearing loss may be variable even within families transmitting the same mutation. This is particularly striking in the case of the A1555G mutation, which is sometimes associated with familial nonsyndromic hearing loss and is the major genetic predisposition to aminoglycoside-induced ototoxicity (Estivill et al., 1998b). The pathophysiological relationship between the mitochondrial mutations and hearing loss remains unclear (see above).

Pendrin

As described previously, mutations in the gene *PDS* (*SLC26A4*) can cause Pendred syndrome as well as DFNB4 (Table 48–10). While the original DFNB4 kindred was ultimately reclassified as having Pendred syndrome, a large, consanguineous DFNB4 family manifested mutations in *PDS* in association with a clinical picture of profound prelingual deafness, enlarged vestibular aqueduct, normal thyroid function, and absence of goiter (Li et al., 1998).

Other Genes

Several other genes have been identified in association with nonsyndromic hearing loss (Table 48–11). DFNB9 is associated with mutations in *OTOF*, which encodes a novel protein, otoferlin (Yasunaga et al., 1999). Otoferlin demonstrates sequence homology to a *Cunninghamella elegans* spermatogenesis factor, *FER-1*. From expression studies and observation of *FER-1* mutants, Yasunaga et al. postulate a role for otoferlin in calcium-dependent membrane function. To date, the only other DFNB gene that has been identified is *TECTA*, which is associated with DFNB21. DFNB21 was mapped to chromosome 11q23–25 by Mustapha et al. (1999), who noted mutations in the α-tectorin gene, which had been mapped to that region previously in association with DFNA8/12 (Verhoeven et al., 1998). Hence, mutations in this tectorial membrane component provide another example of a gene responsible for both AR and AD transmission of familial SNHL. Of note, evaluation of obligate heterozygotes in the DFNB21 families documented normal auditory function (Mustapha et al., 1999), providing further evidence for a dominant negative effect in the DFNA8/12 kindreds, as suggested by Verhoeven et al. (1998).

Other genes involved in DFNA include *HDIA1*, the human homolog of the *Drosophila* gene, diaphanous. Mutations in this gene, which represents the first DFNA locus for which linkage was established (Leon et al., 1992), cause an initially low frequency hearing loss that may be associated with endolymphatic hydrops (Lalwani et al., 1998). DFNA5 is caused by mutation in a novel gene for which no functional implication has been defined (Van Laer et al., 1998). A gene whose transcript is specific to the cochlea and vestibule, *COCH* (coagulation factor C homolog), is responsible for DFNA9, the only autosomal dominant nonsyndromic SNHL locus for which both cochlear and vestibular function are impaired (Robertson et al., 1998). Ob-

Table 48–11. Nonsyndromic Nuclear Deafness Genes

Locus	Gene	Function	Site
DFNB1/A3	*GJB2*	Connexin 26, gap junctions	13q12
DFNB2/A11USH1B	*MYO7A*	Myosin VIIA, molecular motor, ?structural role	11q13.5
DFNB3	*MYO15*	Myosin XV, ?maintains actin integrity	17p11.2
DFNB8/10	*TMPRSS3*	Transmembrane protease	21q22
DFNB4	*PDS*	Pendrin, chloride-iodide transporter	7q31
DFNB9	*OTOF*	Otoferlin, ?synaptic vesicle trafficking	2p22–23
DFNB12USH1D	*CDJ23*	Cadherin 23, Ca-dependent cell–cell adhesion molecule	10q21–22
DFNB23USH1F	*?PCDH15*	Proto-cadherin 15	10q11.2–21
DFNB29	*CLDN14*	Claudin 14, a cochlear tight junction component	21q22.3
DFNA1	*DIAPH1*	Formin family member, cell polarity, and cytokinesis	5q31
DFNA2	*GJB3*	Connexin 31; gap junction	1p34
DFNA2	*KCNQ4*	Potassium channel protein	1p34
DFNA3	*GJB6*	Connexin 30, gap junctions	13q12
DFNA5	*DFNA5*	Novel protein; ?function	7p15
DFNA8/12DFNB21	*TECTA*	α-tectorin, tectorial membrane element	11q22–24
DFNA9	*COCH*	Cochlear and vestibular fx, MPS deposits in temporal bones	14q12–13
DFNA10	*EYA4*	Eyes absent family transcription activator	6q22–23
DFNA13	*COL11A2*	Fibrillar ECM protein	6p21
DFNA15	*POU4F3*	A POU domain gene, DNA transcription factor; terminal neural cell differentiation	5q31
DFNA17	*MYH9*	Non-muscle myosin heavy chain.	22q11.2
DFNA22	*MYO6*	Non-muscle myosin 6, a molecular motor	6q13
DFN3	*POU3F4*	Transcription factor	Xq21.1
DFN4	*?DMD*	Dystrophin (proposed)	Xp21.2

servations of de Kok et al. (1999) and of Fransen et al. (1999) suggested a founder effect in Dutch and Belgian families. Temporal bone histopathology in DFNA9 patients demonstrates deposition of acid mucopolysaccharide material (Khetarpal et al., 1991), which would fit with the postulate that *COCH* is a vital extracellular matrix protein (Heller et al., 1998; Robertson et al., 1998). The vestibular features of DFNA9 have also suggested a relationship between *COCH* and Meniere's disease (Fransen et al., 1999). DFNA11 is due to mutation in COL11A2, which encodes the α_2 subunit of type XI collagen (Van Laer et al., 1999). Of note, mutations in this gene have been associated with some cases of several syndromic collagenopathies, including Stickler syndrome, otospondylomegaepiphyseal dysplasia, and the Weissenbacher-Zweymuller syndrome (Vikkula et al., 1995; Pihlajamaa et al., 1998). Finally, dystrophin mutations have been proposed to be responsible for DFN4, but definitive proof of this is still lacking (Pfister et al., 1999).

CLINICAL APPLICATION AND RISK ASSESSMENT

Diagnosis

The aims of diagnosing the precise cause of hearing loss include possible prevention of further hearing loss, prediction of associated clinical manifestations (particularly in syndromic hearing loss), prevention or amelioration of developmental and educational sequellae by early intervention, and provision of genetic counseling for the parents of a deaf child, as well as for interested deaf adults. To clarify the cause and severity of the hearing loss, the history, physical examination, and laboratory assessment must attempt to differentiate between acquired and inherited hearing loss and between syndromic and nonsyndromic deafness. Detailed audiometric and vestibular testing should be performed and interpreted according to standardized guidelines (American Speech–Language–Hearing Association, 1991, 1994). Temporal bone imaging is useful (Phelps, 1994), particularly in elucidating cochlear morphology, which is helpful in many situations but may be critical in identifying DFN3, which is associated with enlargement of the internal acoustic canal (de Kok et al., 1995). Imaging may also suggest molecular studies for *PDS* mutations as pendrin mutations are associated with widened acoustic canals as well (Li et al., 1998). In the absence of commercially available molecular testing for the mutations associated with the common deafness syndromes which present as isolated SNHL, electrocardiogram, urine analysis, thyroid function studies and electroretinography remain useful diagnostic tools. The latter studies should be repeated at long intervals, especially after about age 5 years. In some cases, simple pedigree analysis will suggest the likely mode of transmission, while other family histories will be confounded by multiple deaf by deaf matings, difficulty in obtaining accurate clinical information about deceased or distant family members, confounding environmental events, difficulty in communicating with the deaf patient and other factors. Hence, molecular testing for the common connexin 26 mutations, known mitochondrial mutations, and other common deafness alleles (see below) should prove valuable in documenting mode of inheritance and likely natural history and in establishing a genetic etiology in apparently sporadic cases (i.e., for connexin 26 mutations). Establishing a diagnosis of a nonsyndromic type of hearing loss will also avoid the often costly and sometimes invasive testing described above.

Screening

Despite great interest in screening for hereditary hearing loss, a number of issues must be considered before any screening program is implemented. From a clinical standpoint, the incidence of various mutations must be established for different populations. The behavior of common mutations such as those occuring in connexin 26 must be defined, particularly the degree of variability in penetrance, age of onset, rate of progression, and severity of the resulting hearing loss. Social issues to be addressed include the value of screening as measured by prevention of subsequent cases or improvement in overall outcome for affected individuals. Moreover, as many deaf individuals do not view hearing impairment as a disability, a universal screening program may be more poorly accepted than other public health initiatives.

Regardless of the aforementioned caveats, two approaches to screening hold potential for reducing the frequency of both profound childhood deafness and hearing loss in general. A systematic neonatal hearing screening program would allow the early identification of affected infants and, by extension, parents at risk to have a second affected child. In cases in which treatment or prevention of associated clinical findings might be possible, early diagnosis should decrease associated morbidity. However, universal newborn screening programs that rely on parental history and behavioral assessment may fail to detect significant hearing loss in early infancy (Robertson et al., 1994). A recent Italian survey suggested that mass screening by evaluating oto-acoustic emissions is effective in detecting cases of congenital deafness and in establishing a risk registry to identify contributing causes (Luppari and Arslan, 1996). The value of assessing transient oto-acoustic emissions was further documented in a community health setting (Bantock and Croxson, 1998), as was the usefulness of universal infant screening by automated auditory brainstem–evoked responses (Mason and Herrmann, 1998).

Despite controversy regarding universal screening, the National Institutes of Health position supported screening for children in the United States (NIH Consensus Statement, 1993). To further assess the logistics of newborn screening and the appropriate recommendations regarding access to genetic counseling and testing services, the Public Health and Clinical Practices Committees of the American College of Medical Genetics have established a subcommittee on Newborn Hearing Screening. Nevertheless, despite the absence of uniform recommendations for screening, follow-up, and treatment of affected individuals, there is a strong push for immediate implementation of universal newborn screening (see U.S. Department of Health and Human Services, 1999). Much effort must be expended before universal hearing screening is implemented in any given setting. In particular, one must account for circumstances that will prevent adequate screening, including early hospital discharge, home births, access to adequate services in small birthing units, insufficient numbers of trained personnel, and, most important, compliance with follow-up (Russ, personal communication). While work remains to be done to maximize follow-up of screen positive cases and to minimize the effect of false negative screens in children with slightly later onset of hearing loss, the overall benefits of universal newborn screening have been well delineated (Yoshinaga-Itano, 1999).

In contrast to newborn hearing screening, general population screening for common mutations has the potential of identifying at risk couples before the conception of an affected fetus. At present, the obvious candidate for screening is connexin 26 (*GJB2*), specifically the 30delG mutation that accounts for 70% of abnormal alleles, and the 167delT mutation that is prevalent in the Ashkenazi Jewish population. A strong case can be made for population screening for the mitochondrial mutation A1555G, which is the major predisposing factor to genetic aminoglycoside ototoxicity. It may also be reasonable to include the 2314delG mutation in the myosin VIIA gene, which causes Usher syndrome type 2A, in a population-based screening program. However, despite the excitement related to the high frequency of the 30delG mutation, it is unlikely that specific mutations in other genes will be found to make a similarly major contribution to the etiology of hereditary deafness (Nance et al., 1998). Hence, the usefulness of population screening, or even commercial laboratory testing of deaf patients, will be limited until mass molecular screening techniques are generally available. The development of a "deafness chip," which would identify the common mutations, as well as a large number of low-frequency mutations, would greatly improve the efficiency and cost-effectiveness of such a screening effort. However, as recently as 1998 a select group of experts underscored the inadequate knowledge base, regarding many of the "clinical, ethical, and social issues" related to genetic testing for deafness mutations, stating that "routine genetic screening for *GJB2* mutations is premature except as part of an appropriately designed clinical trial" (NIDCD Working Group, 1998). Finally, the working group stressed the importance of including "individuals with hearing impairment and individuals who are deaf as well as related organizations representing the spectrum of involved communities of deaf or hearing impaired people in the formulation and establishment of guidelines and future recommendations regarding genetic testing."

Prevention

Currently, the major areas of hearing loss prevention include education and ear protective measures to prevent noise abuse, immunization programs for rubella and *Haemophilus influenzae*, which is a major cause of otitis media in children (Berman, 1995), and health care measures to decrease the effect of predisposing conditions such as congenital cytomegalovirus, diabetes, atherosclerosis, and thyroid disease. In addition, since about 15% to 30% of patients with aminoglycoside ototoxicity have the A1555G susceptibility mutation, and a family history and genetic testing can easily prevent exposure to aminoglycosides in maternally related family members of such patients (Fischel-Ghodsian, 1999b), molecular testing would be beneficial in all patients with permanent hearing loss due to aminoglycosides. If universal newborn or population screening is implemented in the future, identification of individuals at risk for aminoglycoside ototoxicity would allow avoidance of inadvertant exposure in many cases. Identification of susceptibility genes contributing to ototoxicity of other classes of drugs might allow better anticipatory management of at-risk patients. The recent description of a mouse model for the affects of loop diuretics (Delpire et al., 1999) may provide insight to human hearing loss associated with that group of agents. Early diagnosis of patients with Jervell and Lange-Nielsen syndrome allows aggressive management and intervention to prevent sudden death associated with the long Q–T syndrome. Similarly, early identification of NF2 and otosclerosis patients provides a basis for periodic evaluations and directed therapy to prevent or retard the rate of further hearing loss. Finally, in the case of mutations associated with later-onset, progressive hearing loss, better understanding of the molecular regulation of gene expression may allow a targeted approach to delay or reverse the effect of the specific adverse allele.

Counseling

Genetic counseling for hereditary deafness poses specific problems not often encountered in other genetic counseling settings. In counseling a deaf patient, several roadblocks occur commonly, foremost among them, the difficulty in achieving direct and full communication between counselor and consultee. As the majority of deaf patients use a form of sign language to communicate, they may not be well served by a counselor who does not sign, which is the most typical scenario. Even with the availability of a skilled, nonfamily member translator to communicate with the patient, the level of communication is compromised as the geneticist or genetic counselor generally cannot evaluate the quality and accuracy of the translated historical questions and information provided both by the counselor and by the counselee. While accuracy of historical information may be improved by using a questionnaire to obtain the history (Bieber, 1981) and by review of any available medical records, the history is often confounded by family myths, which often provide incorrect, nongenetic explanations for hearing loss. Similarly, interpretation of the pedigree is further hindered by the tendency for deaf-by-deaf marriage, which may lead to complex pedigrees with several deafness genes and potentially varying modes of transmission. As some individuals with syndromic hearing loss present with subtle or late-onset clinical features, their hearing loss may be misassigned by both family members and health professionals. Finally, many deaf individuals and couples view their hearing loss as an alternate state rather than a disability. Hence, their perception of the condition and of the genetic implications are often quite different from the perceptions and evaluation of hearing family members or genetic counselors. In this regard, the very language of the genetic counselor may appear biased and insensitive to the deaf client, who values deaf culture and may prefer a deaf child (Arnos et al., 1992).

The most common scenarios encountered in the genetic counseling setting are requests for information from hearing parents of a profoundly deaf child, referral of deaf couples for preconceptional counseling, and the occasional referral of a deaf-by-hearing couple. The striking heterogeneity of hereditary hearing loss predicts the empiric data with regard to recurrence risk in these situations. As in any other medical setting, it is critical to establish a specific diagnosis if possible, particularly with regard to exclusion of a syndromic condition. While the advent of molecular testing should greatly alter the need to rely on empiric data, such testing will not establish the type of hearing loss in all affected individuals. Hence, in the absence of a well-known syndrome or a molecular diagnosis, empiric data will be necessary in many cases. While numerous studies address recurrence risk to a hearing couple with one affected child, the seminal work of Nance (1971; Nance et al., 1977) remains relevant. Overall, likelihood of hearing parents having a second affected child is in the range of 7% to 11% (Bieber and Nance, 1971; Nance, 1971; Newton, 1985), while recurrence of the hearing loss implicates an AR mode of inheritance with a 25% risk to subsequent pregnancies. The chance that a nonconsanguineous deaf-by-deaf couple will produce a child with hearing loss is about 10%, presumably reflecting both the possibility of AD inheritance in at least one parent, as well as the possibility that the partners each carry a mutation in the same DFNB. Odds tables such as those developed by Bieber and Nance may be used to predict the likelihood of deafness in subsequent children born to parents who have had both hearing and deaf children. A final situation of concern is that of the deaf individual whose hearing loss appears to be sporadic. If clinical and molecular assessment do not establish the recurrence risk, empiric data suggests a risk of about 6% (Newton, 1989).

Therapy

Targeted therapy may forestall or minimize hearing loss in such conditions as NF2 in which early institution of an anticipatory care plan provides the basis for identification of small vestibular Schwannomas, which are more amenable to ablative therapy with some preservation of hearing. Similarly, known medical problems such as the dysrhythmia associated with Jervell and Lange-Nielsen syndrome or the thyroid disease seen in Pendred patients can be treated by standard medical or surgical interventions. As noted previously, early implementation of fluoride therapy decreases the rate of progression of conductive hearing loss in some otosclerosis patients.

With regard to early intervention for profound congenital or prelingual hearing loss, there is considerable controversy regarding the benefits of an aural-oral approach versus a total communication program that combines aural amplification technology with sign language to facilitate development of communication skills. However, case-control cohort studies have established the benefits of very early intervention with regard to improved social function, emotional well-being, and academic success in addition to the more obvious gains in speech and language skills (Kuhl et al., 1992; Yoshinaga-Itano, 1999). The most exciting breakthrough in the treatment of profound congenital hearing loss is the relatively recent availability of cochlear implants in children. While the intensity and methods of rehabilitation (Waltzman et al., 1993), as well as the time from placement of the implant (Miyamoto et al., 1993; Gantz et al., 1994), influence the quality of subsequent speech and language, early implantation may be the key issue in determining ultimate speech quality. Brackett and Zara (1998) noted rapid improvement in language acquisition and intelligible speech production in children who received implants before age 5 and particular success in some parameters in children receiving implants before age 3, compared to those treated between years 3 and 5. The authors stressed the importance of "fine tuning the speech processor of the cochlear implant," as well as the importance of an intensive speech and language rehabilitation program coordinated between the school, home, and health professionals representing multiple disciplines.

A particularly exciting research area involves the concept of auditory hair cell regeneration, which occurs regularly in fish, amphibians, and, in some circumstances, in birds, but does not occur under normal circumstances in mammals (Lefebvre et al., 1993; Kelley et al., 1995). Recent implication of the Notch signaling pathway in the lateral inhibition of embryonic cochlear cells with consequent limitation of hair cell numbers (Lanford et al., 1999) may provide a novel approach to the issue of hair cell regeneration. Finally, general research in gene regulation promises the possibility of up-regulating a normal allele or down-regulating a defective one, or other genetic manipulation to compensate for the mutant gene product. However, such approaches will be limited in situations where cochlear maldevelopment or irreversible damage precludes improvement in auditory function.

CONCLUSIONS

The genetics of deafness underwent a revolution in the 1990s. At the beginning of the decade, not a single gene linked to deafness was known, while by the end of the decade, over 20 deafness genes had been identified. Nonsyndromic hearing loss in childhood and early adult life is characterized by genetic heterogeneity, with a single defect in one of at least 30 separate "deafness genes" being the causative factor in any given patient. All known modes of inheritance have been implicated, and complex models have been suggested in some forms of deafness. The mechanisms by which these genes exert their action mirror the broad range of biophysical functions. These include coding for nuclear transcription factors, structural and extracellular matrix proteins, molecular motors, ion channels, proteins involved in synaptic vesicle trafficking and gap junction formation, and a protein presumed to determine cell polarity and cytokinetic properties. Some of the identified genes defy classification at this time. Of interest and of clinical importance, molecular testing for two of these genes, connexin 26 and, possibly, the mitochondrial 12S rRNA gene, may detect more than 50% of all cases. The most common cause of hearing loss in later life, presbycusis, most likely represents a genetically complex disorder. However, despite the frequency and functional impact of this condition, almost no solid genetic information is available. The interaction between genetic and environmental factors has been demonstrated most dramatically for the mitochondrial 1555 mutation associated with aminoglycoside ototoxicity, yet noise and viral infections may exert their detrimental effect on hearing through genetically predisposing pathways as well.

What do we predict for the next decade? Most if not all of the deafness genes in man and mouse will be identified. Much of the attention will shift to a better understanding of presbycusis and to the genes that influence its age of onset and rate of progression. The major research effort will focus on the more difficult tasks of understanding the genotype–phenotype correlations and the intracellular physiological pathways that lead to hearing loss in the single-gene disorders. Progress may be slow initially but will benefit from continued improvement in genomic databases, as well as whole cell expression and protein profiling techniques. Lastly, what about prevention and treatment? Universal newborn screening programs will be implemented in most developed countries. Widespread molecular testing will allow detection of most deafness mutations at birth or even during pregnancy. The arrival of effective treatments will depend both on a much more detailed understanding of the pathological pathways and on better delivery methods and vectors. Genetics will have played a major role in providing the molecular basis for reaching this goal of effective therapeutics.

REFERENCES

American Speech-Language-Hearing Association: Guidelines for the audiologic assessment of children from birth through thirty-six months of age. Asha Suppl 1991; 5:37–43.

American Speech-Language-Hearing Association: Joint Committee on Infant Hearing 1994 Position Statement. Asha 1994; 36:38–41.
Anderson H, Bengt B, Wedenberg E: Genetic disposition: a prerequisite for maternal rubella deafness. Arch Otolaryngol 1970; 91:141–147.
Anson BJ, Davies J, Duckert LG: Embryology of the ear. In: Paparella MM, Shumrick DA, Gluckman JL, Meyerhoff WL (eds). Otolaryngology, 3d ed. Philadelphia: Saunders, 1991.
Arnos KS, Cunningham M, Israel J, Marazita ML: Innovative approach to genetic counseling services. Am J Med Genet 1992; 44:345–351.
Atkin CL, Hasstedt SJ, Menlove L, Cannon L, Kirschner N, Schwartz C, Nguyen K, Skolnick M: Mapping of Alport syndrome to the long arm of the X chromosome. Am J Hum Genet 1988; 42:249–255.
Avraham KB: Sounds from the cochlea. Nature 1997; 390:559–560.
Avraham KB, Hasson T, Steel KP, Kingsley DM, Russell LB, Mooseker MS, Copeland NG, Jenkins NA: The mouse Snell's waltzer deafness gene encodes an unconventional myosin required for the structural integrity of inner ear hair cells. Nat Genet 1995; 11:369–375.
Bai U, Seidman MD, Hinojosa R, Quirk WS: Mitochondrial DNA deletions associated with aging and possibly presbycusis: a human archival temporal bone study. Am J Otol 1997; 18:449–453.
Balciuniene J, Dahl N, Borg E, Samuelsson E, Koisti MJ, Pettersson U, Jazin EE: Evidence for digenic inheritance of nonsyndromic hereditary hearing loss in a Swedish family. Am J Hum Genet 1998; 63:786–793.
Bantock HM, Croxson S: Universal hearing screening using transient otoacoustic emissions in a community health clinic. Arch Dis Child 1998; 78:249–253.
Barker DF, Hostikka SL, Zhou J, Chow LT, Oliphant AR, Gerken SC, Gregory MC, Skolnick MH, Atkin CL, Tryggvason K: Identification of mutations in the *COL4A5* collagen gene in Alport syndrome. Science 1990; 248:1224–1227.
Batsakis JG, Nishiyama RH: Deafness with sporadic goiter: Pendred's syndrome. Arch Otolaryngol 1962; 76:401–406.
Bauman NM, Kirby-Keyser LJ, Dolan KD, Wexler D, Gantz BJ, McCabe BF, Bale JF: Mondini dysplasia and congenital cytomegalovirus infection. J Pediatr 1994; 124:71–78.
Beighton P, Sellars S: Genetics and Otology. Edinburgh: Churchill Livingstone, 1982.
Bergoffen J, Scherer SS, Wang S, Scott MO, Bone LJ, Paul DL, Chen K, Lensch MW, Chance PF, Fischbeck KH: Connexin mutations in X-linked Charcot-Marie-Tooth disease. Science 1993; 262:2039–2042.
Bergstrom LV: Otosclerosis. In Buyse ML (ed). Birth Defects Encyclopedia. Dover: Center for Birth Defects Information Services, 1990.
Berman S: Otitis media in children. N Engl J Med 1995; 332:1560–1565.
Bernstein JM, Shanahan TC, Schaffer FM: Further observations on the role of the MHC genes and certain hearing disorders. Acta Otolaryngol 1996; 116:666–671.
Bieber FR: Genetic studies of questionnaire data from a residential school for the deaf. PhD diss. Medical College of Virginia, Richmond, 1981.
Bieber FR, Nance WE: Hereditary hearing loss. In: Jackson L, Schimke N (eds). Clinical Genetics: A Course Book for Physicians. New York: Wiley, 1971:443–461.
Bonne-Tamir B, DeStefano AL, Briggs CE, Adair R, Franklyn B, Weiss S, Korostishevsky M, Frydman M, Baldwin CT, Farrer LA: Linkage of congenital recessive deafness gene (DFNB10) to chromosome 21q22.3. Am J Hum Genet 1996; 58:1254–1259.
Boughman JA, Vernon M, Shaver KA: Usher syndrome: definition and estimate of prevalance from two high-risk populations. J Chronic Dis 1983; 36:595–603.
Boye E, Vetrie D, Flinter F, Buckle B, Pihlajaniemi T, Hamalainen E-R, Myers JC, Bobrow M, Harris A: Major rearrangements in the α-5-(IV) collagen gene in three patients with Alport syndrome. Genomics 1991; 11:1125–1132.
Brackett D, Zara CV: Communication outcomes related to early implantation. Am J Otol 1998; 19:453–460.
Bredberg G: Cellular pattern and nerve supply of the human organ of Corti. Acta Otolaryngol Suppl 1989; 236:127–135.
Bykhovskaya Y, Shohat M, Ehrenman K, Johnson D, Hamon M, Cantor RM, Aouizerat B, Bu X, Rotter JI, Jaber L, Fischel-Ghodsian N: Evidence for complex nuclear inheritance in a pedigree with nonsyndromic deafness due to a homoplasmic mitochondrial mutation. Am J Med Genet 1998; 77:421–426.
Cawthon RM, Weiss R, Xu GF, Viskochil D, Culver M, Stevens J, Robertson M, Dunn D, Gesteland R, O'Connell P, White R: A major segment of the neurofibromatosis type 1 gene: cDNA sequence, genomic structure, and point mutations. Cell 1990; 62:193–201.
Chung CS, Brown KS: Family studies of early childhood deafness ascertained through the Clarke School for the deaf. Am J Hum Gen 1970; 22:630–644.
Church MW, Gerkin KP: Hearing disorders in children with fetal alcohol syndrome: findings from case reports. Pediatrics 1988; 82:147–154.
Cohen MM, Gorlin RJ: Epidemiology, etiology, and genetic patterns. In: Gorlin RJ, Toriello, HV, Cohen MM (eds). Hereditary Hearing Loss and Its Syndromes. New York: Oxford University Press, 1995:9–21.
Coucke PJ, Van Hauwe P, Kelley PM, Kunst H, Schatteman I, Van Velzen D, Meyers J, Ensink RJ, Verstreken M, Declau F, et al.: Mutations in the *KCNQ4* gene are responsible for autosomal dominant deafness in four DFNA2 families. Hum Mol Genet 1999; 8:1321–1328.
Dar H, Winter ST: A genetic study of familial deafness. Isr J Med Sci 1969; 5:1219–1226.
Davis AC: Hearing disorders in the population: first phase findings of the MRC National Study of Hearing. In: Lutman ME, Haggard MP (eds). Hearing Science and Hearing Disorders. New York: Academic Press, 1983:35.
Dekaban A, O'Rouke J, Corman T: Abnormalities in offspring related to maternal rubella during pregnancy. Neurology 1958; 8:387–392.
de Kok YJM, Bom SJH, Brunt TM, Kemperman MH, van Beusekom E, van der Velde-Visser SD, Robertson NG, Morton CC, Huygen PLM, Verhagen WIM, et al.: A Pro51Ser mutation in the *COCH* gene is associated with late onset autosomal dominant progressive sensorineural hearing loss with vestibular defects. Hum Mol Genet 1999; 8:361–366.
de Kok YJM, van der Maarel SM, Bitner-Glindzicz M, Huber I, Monaco AP, Malcolm S, Pembrey ME, Ropers H-H, Cremers FPM: Association between X-linked mixed deafness and mutations in the POU domain gene *POU3F4*. Science 1995; 267:685–688.
Delpire E, Lu J, England R, Dull C, Thorne T: Deafness and imbalance associated with inactivation of the secretory Na-K-2Cl co-transporter. Nat Genet 1999; 22:192–195.
Denoyelle F, Weil D, Maw MA, Wilcox SA, Lench NJ, Allen-Powell DR, Osborn AH, Dahl HH, Middleton A, Houseman MJ, et al.: Prelingual deafness: high prevalence of a 30delG mutation in the connexin 26 gene. Hum Mol Genet 1997; 6:2173–2177.
Estivill X, Fortina P, Surrey S, Rabionet R, Metchionda S, D'Agruma L, Mansfield E, Rappaport E, Govea N, Mila M, et al.: Connexin-26 mutations in sporadic and inherited sensorineural deafness. Lancet 1998a; 351:394–398.
Estivill X, Govea N, Barcelo A, Perello E, Badenas C, Romero E, Moral L, Scozzari R, D'Urbano L, Zeviani M, Torroni A: Familial progressive sensorineural deafness is mainly due to the mtDNA A1555G mutation and is enhanced by treatment with aminoglycosides. Am J Hum Genet 1998b; 62:27–35.
Everett LA, Glaser B, Beck JC, Idol JR, Buchs A, Heyman M, Adawi F, Hazani E, Nassir E, Baxevanis AD, et al.: Pendred syndrome is caused by mutations in a putative sulphate transporter gene (*PDS*). Nat Genet 1997; 17:411–422.
Fischel-Ghodsian N: Mitochondrial RNA processing and translation: Link between mitochondrial mutations and hearing loss? Mol Genet Metab 1998; 65:97–104.
Fischel-Ghodsian N: Mitochondrial deafness mutations reviewed. Hum Mutat 1999a; 13:261–270.
Fischel-Ghodsian N: Genetic factors in aminoglycoside ototoxicity. Ann NY Acad Sci 1999b; 884:99–109.
Fischel-Ghodsian N, Bykhovskaya Y, Taylor K, Kahen T, Cantor R, Ehrenman K, Smith R, Keithley E: Temporal bone analysis of patients with presbycusis reveals high frequency of mitochondrial mutations. Hearing Res 1997; 110:147–154.
Fischel-Ghodsian N, Falk RE: Deafness. In: Rimoin DL, Connor JM, Pyeritz R (eds). Emery and Rimoin's Principles and Practice of Medical Genetics, 3d ed. New York: Churchill Livingstone, 2001, in press.
Fischel-Ghodsian N, Prezant TR, Bu X, Oztas S: Mitochondrial ribosomal RNA gene mutation in a patient with sporadic aminoglycoside ototoxicity. Am J Otolaryngol 1993; 14:399–403.
Fischel-Ghodsian N, Prezant TR, Fournier P, Steward IA, Maw M: Mitochondrial mutation associated with nonsyndromic deafness. Am J Otolaryngol 1995; 16:403–408.
Fransen E, Verstreken M, Verhagen WIM, Wuyts FL, Huygen PLM, D'Haese P, Robertson NG, Morton CC, McGuirt WT, Smith RJH, et al.: High prevalence of symptoms of Meniere's disease in three families with a mutation in the *COCH* gene. Hum Mol Genet 1999; 8:1425–1429.
Fraser GR: Profound childhood deafness. J Med Genet 1964; 1:118–151.
Fraser GR: Association of congenital deafness with goiter (Pendred's syndrome): a study of 207 families. Ann Hum Genet 1965; 28:201–249.
Fraser GR, Groggatt P, Murphy T: Genetical aspects of the cardio-auditory syndrome of Jervell and Lange-Nielsen (congenital deafness and electrocardiographic abnormalities). Ann Hum Genet 1964; 28:133–157.
Gantz B, Tyler R, Woodworth G, TyeMurray N, Fryauf-Bertschy H: Results of multichannel cochlear implants in congenital and acquired prelinguistic deafness in children: five year followup. Am J Otol 1994; 15:1–8.
Gasparini P, Estivill X, Volpini V, Totaro A, Castellvi-Bel S, Govea N, Mila M, Della Monica M, Ventruto V, De Benedetto M, et al.: Linkage of DFNB1 to non-syndromic neurosensory autosomal-recessive deafness in Mediterranean families. Eur J Hum Genet 1997; 5:83–88.
Gorlin RJ, Toriello, HV, Cohen MM: Hereditary Hearing Loss and Its Syndromes. New York: Oxford University Press, 1995.
Gravel M, Melancon P, Brakier-Gingras L: Cross-linking of streptomycin to the 16S ribosomal RNA of *Escherichia coli*. Biochemistry 1987; 26:6227–6232.
Green GE, Scott DA, McDonald JM, Woodworth GG, Sheffield VC, Smith RJH: Carrier rates in the midwestern United States for GJB2 mutations causing inherited deafness. JAMA 1999; 281:2211–2216.
Greinwald JH, Wayne S, Chen AH, Scott DA, Zbar RIS, Kraft ML, Prasad S, Ramesh A, Coucke P, Srisailapathy CRS, et al.: Localization of a novel gene for nonsyndromic hearing loss (DFNB17) to chromosome region 7q31. Am J Med Genet 1998; 78:107–113.
Grifa A, Wagner CA, D'Ambrosio L, Melchionda S, Bernardi F, Lopez-Bigas N, Rabionet R, Arbones M, Della Monica M, Estivill X, et al.: Mutations in GJB6 cause nonsyndromic autosomal dominant deafness at DFNA3 locus. Nat Genet 1999; 23:16–17.
Guan M, Fischel-Ghodsian N, Attardi G: Biochemical evidence for nuclear gene involvement in phenotype of non-syndromic deafness associated with mitochondrial 12S rRNA mutation. Hum Mol Genet 1996; 5:963–972.
Hamasaki K, Rando RR: Specific binding of aminoglycosides to a human rRNA construct based on a DNA polymorphism which causes aminoglycoside-induced deafness. Biochemistry 1997; 36:12323–12328.
Hanshaw JB, Scheiner AP, Moxley AW, Gaev L, Abel V, Scheiner B: School failure and deafness after "silent" congenital cytomegalovirus infection. N Engl J Med 1976; 295:468–470.

Hasstedt SJ, Atkin CL: X-linked inheritance of Alport syndrome: family P revisited. Am J Hum Genet 1983; 35:1241–1251.

Heller S, Sheane CA, Javed Z, Hudspeth AJ: Molecular markers for cell types of the inner ear and candidate genes for hearing disorders. Proc Natl Acad Sci USA 1998; 95:11400–11405.

Henley CM, Schacht J: Pharmacokinetics of aminoglycoside antibiotics in blood, inner-ear fluids and tissues and their relationship to ototoxicity. Audiology 1988; 27:137–146.

Hereditary Hearing Loss Homepage: http://dnalab-www.hgins.uia.ac.be/dna/ab/hhh (2001).

Higashi K: Heterogeneity of dominant high-frequency sensorineural deafness. Clin Genet 1988; 33:424–428.

Hopes CI, Bundey S, Proops D, Fielder AR: Usher syndrome in the city of Birmingham: prevalence and clinical classification. Br J Ophthalmol 1997; 81:46–53.

Hostikka SL, Eddy RL, Byers MG, Hoyhtya M, Shows TB, Tryggvason K: Identification of a distinct type IV collagen α chain with restricted kidney distribution and assignment of its gene to the locus of X chromosome-linked Alport syndrome. Proc Natl Acad Sci USA 1990; 87:1606–1610.

Huizing EH, Van Bolhuis AH, Odenthal DW: Studies on progressive hereditary perceptive deafness in a family of 335 members: I. Genetical and general audiological results. Acta Otolaryngol 1966; 61:35–41.

Inoue K, Takai D, Soejima A, Isobe K, Yamasoba T, Oka Y, Goto Y, Hayashi J: Mutant mtDNA at 1555 A to G in the 12S rRNA gene and hypersusceptibility of mitochondrial translation to streptomycin can be co-transferred to ρ_0 Hela cells. Biochem Biophys Res Commun 1996; 223:496–501.

Jaber L, Shohat M, Bu X, Fischel-Ghodsian N, Yang H, Wang S, Rotter JI: Sensorineural deafness inherited as a tissue specific mitochondrial disorder. J Med Genet 1992; 29:86–90.

Jain PK, Fukushima K, Deshmukh D, Ramesh A, Thomas E, Kumar S, Lalwani AK, Kumar S, Ploplis B, Skarka H, et al.: A human recessive neurosensory nonsyndromic hearing impairment locus is a potential homologue of the murine deafness (nd) locus. Hum Mol Genet 1995; 4:2391–2394.

Jervell A, Lange-Nielsen F: Congenital deaf-mutism, functional heart disease with prolongation of Q–T interval and sudden death. Am Heart J 1957; 54:59–68.

Kelley MW, Talreja D, Corwin JT: Replacement of hair cells after laser microbeam irradiation in cultured organ of Corti from embryonic and neonatal mice. J Neurosci 1995; 15:3013–3026.

Kelley PM, Harris DJ, Comer BC, Askew JW, Fowler T, Smith SD, Kimberling WJ: Novel mutations in the connexin 26 gene (*GJB2*) that cause autosomal recessive (DFNB1) hearing loss. Am J Hum Genet 1998; 62:792–799.

Kelsell DP, Dunlop J, Stevens HP, Lench NJ, Liang JN, Parry G, Mueller RF, Leigh IM: Connexin 26 mutations in hereditary non-syndromic sensorineural deafness. Nature 1997; 387:80–83.

Khetarpal U, Schuknecht HF, Gacek RR, Holmes LB: Autosomal dominant sensorineural hearing loss: pedigrees, audiologic findings, and temporal bone findings in two kindreds. Arch Otolaryngol Head Neck Surg 1991; 117:1032–1042.

Kimberling WJ, Moller C: Clinical and molecular genetics of Usher syndrome. J Am Acad Audiol 1995; 6:63–72.

Konigsmark BW, Mengel MC, Berlin CI: Familial low-frequency hearing loss: report of three families. Laryngoscope 1971; 81:759–771.

Konigsmark BW, Salman S, Haskins H, Mengel MC: Dominant midfrequency hearing loss. Ann Otolaryngol 1970; 79:1–12.

Kozel PJ, Friedman RA, Erway LC, Yamoah EN, Liu LH, Riddle T, Duffy JJ, Doetschman T, Miller ML, Cardell EL, Shull GE: Balance and hearing deficits in mice with a null mutation in the gene encoding plasma membrane CA^{2+}–ATPase isoform 2. J Biol Chem 1998; 273:18693–18696.

Kubisch C, Schroeder BC, Friedrich T, Lutjohann B, El-Amraoui A, Marlin S, Petit C, Jentsch TJ: *KCNQ4*, a novel potassium channel expressed in sensory outer hair cells, is mutated in dominant deafness. Cell 1999; 96:437–446.

Kuhl PK, Williams KA, Cracerda F, Stevens KN, Lindblom B: Linguistic experience alters phonetic perception in infants by six months of age. Science 1992; 255:606–608.

Lalwani AK, Jackler RK, Sweetow RW, Lynch ED, Raventos H, Morrow J, King MC, Leon PE: Further characterization of the DFNA1 audiovestibular phenotype. Arch Otolaryngol Head Neck Surg 1998; 124:699–702.

Lanford PJ, Lan Y, Jiang R, Lindsell C, Weinmaster G, Gridley T, Kelley MW: Notch signalling pathway mediates hair cell development in mammalian cochlea. Nat Genet 1999; 21:289–292.

Lefebvre PP, Malgrange B, Staecker H, Moonen G, van de Water TR: Retinoic acid stimulates regeneration of mammalian auditory hair cells. Science 1993; 260:692–695.

Lench N, Houseman M, Newton V, Van Camp G, Mueller R: Connexin-26 mutations in sporadic non-syndromal sensorineural deafness. Lancet 1998a; 351:415.

Lench NJ, Markham AF, Mueller RF, Kelsell DP, Smith RJH, Willems PJ, Schatteman I, Capon H, Van de Heyning PJ, Van Camp G: A Moroccan family with autosomal recessive sensorineural hearing loss caused by a mutation in the gap junction protein gene connexin 26 (*GJB2*). J Med Genet 1998b; 35:151–152.

Leon PE, Bonilla JA, Sanchez JR, Vanegas R, Villalobos M, Torres L, Leon F, Howell AL, Rodriguez JA: Low frequency hereditary deafness in man with childhood onset. Am J Hum Genet 1981; 33:209–214.

Leon PE, Raventos H, Lynch E, Morrow J, King M-C: The gene for an inherited form of deafness maps to chromosome 5q31. Proc Natl Acad Sci 1992; 89:5181–5184.

Li M, Tzagaloff A, Underbrink-Lyon K, Martin NC: Identification of the paromomycin-resistance mutation in the 15S rRNA gene of yeast mitochondria. J Biol Chem 1982; 257:5921–5928.

Li XC, Everett LA, Lalwani AK, Desmukh D, Friedman TB, Green ED, Wilcox ER: A mutation in PDX causes non-syndromic recessive deafness. Nat Genet 1998; 18:215–217.

Lindenov H: The Etiology of Deaf-mutism with Special Reference to Heredity. Copenhagen: Munkgaard, 1945.

Liu X-Z, Hope C, Liang CY, Zou JM, Xu LR, Cole T, Mueller RF, Bundey S, Nance W, Steel KP, Brown SDM: A mutation (2314delG) in the Usher syndrome type IIA gene: high prevalence and phenotypic variation. Am J Hum Genet 1999; 64:1221–1225.

Liu X-Z, Walsh J, Mburu P, Kendrick-Jones J, Cope MJTV, Steel KP, Brown SDM: Mutations in the myosin VIIA gene cause non-syndromic recessive deafness. Nat Genet 1997a; 16:188–190.

Liu X-Z, Walsh J, Tamagawa Y, Kitamura K, Nishizawa M, Steel KP, Brown SD: Autosomal dominant non-syndromic deafness caused by a mutation in the myosin VIIA gene. Nat Genet 1997b; 17:268–269.

Luppari R, Arslan E: Neonatal screening: risk factors and outcome in 4400 children. Acta Otorhinolaryngol Ital 1996; 16:501–507.

Lynch ED, Lee MK, Morrow JE, Welcsh PL, Leon PE, King MC: Nonsyndromic deafness DFNA1 associated with mutation of a human homolog of the *Drosophila* gene diaphanous. Science 1997; 278:1315–1318.

MacNeill E, Shaw RF: Segregation ratios in Alport's syndrome. J Med Genet 1973; 10:23–26.

Majumder PP, Ramesh A, Chinnappan D: On the genetics of prelingual deafness. Am J Hum Gen 1989; 44:86–99.

Marazita ML, Ploughman LM, Rawlings B, Remington E, Arnos KS, Nance WE: Genetic epidemiological studies of early-onset deafness in the U.S. school-age population. Am J Med Genet 1993; 46:486–491.

Marres HAM, Cremers CWRJ: Autosomal recessive nonsyndromal profound childhood deafness in a large pedigree. Arch Otolaryngol Head Neck Surg 1989; 115:591–595.

Mason JA, Herrmann KR: Universal infant hearing screening by automated auditory brainstem response measurement. Pediatrics 1998; 101:221–228.

Maw MA, Allen-Powell DR, Goodey RJ, Stewart IA, Nancarrow DJ, Hayward NK, Gardner RJM: The contribution of the DFNB1 locus to neurosensory deafness in a Caucasian population. Am J Hum Genet 1995; 57:629–635.

Milliner, DS, Pierides AM, Holley KE: Renal transplantation in Alport's syndrome: anti-glomerular basement membrane glomerulonephritis in the allograft. Mayo Clin Proc 1982; 57:35–43.

Miyamoto RT, Osberger MJ, Robbins AM, Myres WA, Kessler K: Prelingually deafened children's performance with the Nucleus multichannel cochlear implant. Am J Otol 1993; 14:437–445.

Mochizuki T, Lemmink HH, Mariyama M, Antignac C, Gubler MC, Pirson Y, Verellen-Dumoulin C, Chan B, Schroder CH, Smeets HJ, Reeders ST: Identification of mutations in the α-3(IV) and α-4(IV) collagen genes in autosomal recessive Alport syndrome. Nat Genet 1994; 8:77–81.

Morell RJ, Kim HJ, Hood LJ, Goforth L, Friderici K, Fisher R, Van Camp G, Berlin CI, Oddoux C, Ostrer H, et al.: Mutations in the Connexin 26 gene (*GJB2*) among Ashkenazi Jews with nonsyndromic recessive deafness. N Engl J Med 1998; 339:1500–1505.

Moroso MJ: Genetic disposition to deafness in maternal rubella: fact or myth? J Otolaryngol 1985; 14:44–48.

Morton NE: The mutational load due to detrimental genes in man. Am J Hum Genet 1960; 12:348–364.

Morton NE: Genetic epidemiology of hearing impairment. Ann NY Acad Sci 1991; 630:16–31.

Moscicki RA, San Martin JE, Quintero CH, Rauch SD, Nadol JB, Bloch KJ: Serum antibody to inner ear proteins in patients with progressive hearing loss: correlation with disease activity and response to corticosteroid treatment. JAMA 1994; 272:611–616.

Moynihan L, Houseman M, Newton V, Mueller R, Lench N: DFNB20: a novel locus for autosomal recessive, non-syndromal sensorineural hearing loss maps to chromosome 11q25–qter. Eur J Hum Genet 1999; 7:243–246.

Mustapha M, Weil D, Chardenoux S, Elias EE, Beckmann JS, Loiselet J, Petit C: An α-tectorin gene defect causes a newly identified autosomal recessive form of sensorineural pre-lingual non-syndromic deafness, DFNB21. Hum Mol Genet 1999; 8:409–412.

Nadol JB: Hearing loss. N Engl J Med 1993; 329:1092–1102.

Nagley P, Zhang C, Martinus RD, Vaillant F, Linnane AW: Mitochondrial DNA mutation and human aging, molecular biology, bioenergetics, and redox therapy. In: DiMauro S, Wallace DC (eds). Mitochondrial DNA in Human Pathology. New York: Raven Press, 1993.

Nance WE: Genetic counseling for the hearing impaired. Audiology 1971; 10:222–223.

Nance WE: The genetic analysis of profound prelingual deafness. Birth Defects 1980; 16(4):263–269.

Nance WE, Pandya A, Xia XJ, Blanton SH, Oelrich K, Arnos K: Frequency of connexin 26 mutations among the deaf and in non-complementary deaf × deaf matings. Paper presented at the Third Symposium of Molecular Biology of Hearing and Deafness, Bethesda, Maryland, October 1998.

Nance WE, Rose SP, Conneally PM, Miller JZ: Opportunities for genetic counseling through institutional ascertainment of affected probands. In: Lubs HA, de la Cruz F (eds). Genetic Counseling. New York: Raven Press, 1977.

Nance WE, Setleff RC, Mcleod A, Sweeney A, Cooper C, McConnell F: X-linked mixed deafness with congenital fixation of the stapedial footplate and perilymphatic gusher. Birth Defects 1971; 7:64–69.

National Center for Health Statistics: Current Estimates from the National Health Interview Survey, 1989: Vital and Health Statistics. DHHS publication no. (PHS) 90–1504. Washington DC: Government Printing Office, 1990.

Newton VE: Aetiology of bilateral sensorineural hearing loss in young children. J Laryngol Otol Suppl 1985; 10:1–57.

Newton VE: Genetic counseling for isolated hearing loss. J Laryngol Otol 1989; 103:12–15.

Neyroud N, Tesson F, Denjoy I, Leibovici M, Donger C, Barhanin J, Faure S, Gary F, Coumel P, Petit C, et al.: A novel mutation in the potassium channel gene *KVLQT1* causes the Jervell and Lange-Nielsen cardioauditory syndrome. Nat Genet 1997; 15:186–189.

NIDCD Working Group on Early Identification of Hearing Impairment: Considerations for Developing and Implementing Genetic Diagnostic Tests for Hereditary Hearing Impairment and Other Communicative Disorders. Rockville, Md: 1998.

NIH Consensus Statement: Early Identification of Hearing Impairment in Infants and Young Children. Bethesda, MD: Office of Medical Application of Research, National Institutes of Health, 1993:1–24.

Olsson C, Zethelius B, Lagerstrom-Fermer M, Asplund J, Berne C, Landegren U: Level of heteroplasmy for the mitochondrial mutation A3243G correlates with age of onset of diabetes and deafness. Human Mutation 1998; 12:52–58.

Oshima T, Ueda N, Ikeda K, Abe K, Takasaka T: Bilateral sensorineural hearing loss associated with the point mutation in mitochondrial genome. Laryngoscope 1996; 106:43–48.

Pallister PD, Opitz JM: The Perrault syndrome: autosomal recessive ovarian dysgenesis with facultative, non-sex-limited sensorineural deafness. Am J Med Genet 1979; 4:239–246.

Parving A: Epidemiology of hearing loss and aetiological diagnosis of hearing impairment in childhood. Int J Pediatr Otorhinolaryngol 1983; 5:151–165.

Petit C: Genes responsible for human hereditary deafness: symphony of a thousand. Nat Genet 1996; 14:385–391.

Pfister MH, Apaydin F, Turan O, Bereketoglu M, Bilgen V, Braendle U, Kose S, Zenner HP, Lalwani AK: Clinical evidence for dystrophin dysfunction as a cause of hearing loss in locus DFN4. Laryngoscope 1999; 109:730–735.

Phelps PD: Imaging for congenital deformities of the ear. Clin Radiol 1994; 49:663–669.

Phelps PD, Reardon W, Pembrey M, Bellman S, Luxom L: X-linked deafness, stapes gushers and a distinctive defect of the inner ear. Neuroradiology 1991; 33:326–330.

Pieke-Dahl S, Weston MD, Kimberling WJ, Gorin MB, Shugart YY, Kenyon JB: Genetic heterogeneity of Usher syndrome type II. J Med Genet 1993; 30:843–848.

Pihlajamaa T, Prockop DJ, Faber J, Winterpacht A, Zabel B, Giedion A, Wiesbauer P, Spranger J, Ala-Kokko L: Heterozygous glycine substitution in the *COL11A2* gene in the original patient with the Weissenbacher-Zweymuller syndrome demonstrates its identity with heterozygous OSMED (nonocular Stickler syndrome). Am J Med Genet 1998; 80:115–120.

Piussan C, Hanauer A, Dahl N, Mathieu M, Kolski C, Biancalana V, Heyberger S, Strunski V: X-linked progressive mixed deafness: a new microdeletion that involves a more proximal region in Xq21. Am J Hum Genet 1995; 56:224–230.

Prezant TR, Agapian JV, Bohlman MC, Bu X, Oztas S, Qiu W, Arnos KS, Cortopassi GA, Jaber L, Rotter JI, et al.: Mitochondrial ribosomal RNA mutation associated with both antibiotic-induced and non-syndromic deafness. Nat Genet 1993; 4:289–294.

Reardon W: Sex linked deafness: Wilde revisited. J Med Genet 1990; 27:376–379.

Reid FM, Vernham GA, Jacobs HT: A novel mitochondrial point mutation in a maternal pedigree with sensorineural deafness. Hum Mutat 1994; 3:243–247.

Reynolds DW, Stagno S, Stubbs KG, Dahle AJ, Livingston MM, Saxon SS, Alford CA: Inapparent congenital cytomegalovirus infection with elevated cord IgM levels: causal relation with auditory and mental deficiency. N Engl J Med 1974; 290:291–296.

Riccardi VM, Eichner JE: Neurofibromatosis: Phenotype, Natural History and Pathogenesis. Baltimore: Johns Hopkins University Press, 1986.

Richard G, Smith LE, Bailey RA, Itin P, Hohl D, Epstein EH Jr, DiGiovanna JJ, Compton JG, Bale SJ: Mutations in the human connexin gene *GJB3* cause erythrokeratodermia variabilis. Nat Genet 1998; 20:366–369.

Robertson C, Aldridge S, Jarman F, Saunders K, Poulakis A, Oberklaid F: Late diagnosis of congenital sensorineural hearing impairment: why are detection methods failing? Arch Dis Child 1994; 72:11–15.

Robertson NG, Lu L, Heller S, Merchant SN, Eavey RD, McKenna M, Nadol JB Jr, Miyamoto RT, Linthicum FH, Neto JFL, et al.: Mutations in a novel cochlear gene cause DFNA9, a human nonsyndromic deafness with vestibular dysfunction. Nat Genet 1998; 20:299–303.

Schaap T, Gapany-Gapanavicius B: The genetics of otosclerosis. I. Distorted sex ratio. Am J Hum Genet 1978; 30:59–64.

Schulze-Bahr E, Wang Q, Wedekind H, Haverkamp W, Chen Z, Sun Y: KCNE1 mutations cause Jervell and Lange-Nielsen syndrome. Nat Genet 1997; 17:267–268.

Scott DA, Carmi R, Elbedour K, Yosefsberg S, Stone EM, Sheffield VC: An autosomal recessive nonsyndromic-hearing-loss locus identified by DNA pooling using two inbred Bedouin kindreds. Am J Hum Genet 1996; 59:385–391.

Scott DA, Wang R, Kreman TM, Sheffield VC, Karniski LP: The Pendred syndrome gene encodes a chloride-iodide transport protein. Nat Genet 1999; 21:440–443.

Seidman MD, Bai U, Khan MJ, Murphy MP, Quirk WS, Castora FJ, Hinojosa R: Association of mitochondrial DNA deletions and cochlear pathology: a molecular biologic tool. Laryngoscope 1996; 106:777–783.

Sellars S, Groeneveldt L, Beighton P: Aetiology of deafness in white children in the cape. South Afr Med J 1976; 50:1193–1197.

Shoffner JM, Lott MT, Voljavec AS, Soueidan SA, Costigan DA, Wallace DC: Spontaneous Kearns-Sayre/chronic external ophthalmoplegia plus syndrome associated with a mitochondrial DNA deletion: a slip-replication model and metabolic therapy. Proc Natl Acad Sci USA 1989; 86:7952–7956.

Sill AM, Stick MJ, Prenger VL, Phillips SL, Boughman JA, Arnos KS: Genetic epidemiologic study of hearing loss in an adult population. Am J Med Gen 1994; 54:149–153.

Smith RJH, Berlin CI, Hejtmancik JF, Keats BJB, Kimberling WJ, Lewis RA, Möller CG, Pelias MZ, Tranebjaerg L: Clinical diagnosis of the Usher syndromes. Am J Med Genet 1994; 50:32–38.

Spangler EA, Blackburn EH: The nucleotide sequence of the 17S ribosomal RNA gene of *Tetrahymena thermophila* and the identification of point mutations resulting in resistance to the antibiotics paromomycin and hygromycin. J Biol Chem 1985; 260:6334–6340.

Splawski I, Tristani-Firouzi M, Lehmann MH, Sanguinetti MC, Keating MT: Mutations in the hminK gene cause long QT syndrome and suppress Iks function. Nat Genet 1997; 17:338–340.

Street VA, McKee-Johnson JW, Fonseca RC, Tempel BL, Noben-Trauth K: Mutations in a plasma membrane CA^{2+}-ATPase gene cause deafness in deafwaddler mice. Nat Genet 1998; 19:390–394.

Sue CM, Lipsett LJ, Crimmins DS, Tsang CS, Boyages SC, Presgrave CM, Gibson WPR, Byrne E, Morris JGL: Cochlear origin of hearing loss in MELAS syndrome. Ann Neurol 1998; 43:350–359.

Sue CM, Tanji K, Hadjigeorgiou G, Andreu AL, Nishino I, Krishna S, Bruno C, Hirano M, Shanske S, Bonilla E, et al.: Maternally inherited hearing loss in a large kindred with a novel T7511C mutation in the mitochondrial DNA tRNASer(UCN) gene. Neurology 1999; 52:1905–1908.

Sulik KK: Embryology of the ear. In: Gorlin RH, Toriello HV, Cohen MM (eds). Hereditary Hearing Loss and Its Syndromes. New York: Oxford University Press, 1995:22–42.

Tamagawa Y, Kitamura K, Ishida T, Tanaka H, Tsuji S, Nishizawa M: A gene for a dominant form of non-syndromic sensorineural deafness (DFNA 11) maps within the region containing the DFNB2 recessive deafness gene. Hum Mol Genet 1996; 5:849–852.

Tomek MS, Brown MR, Mani SR, Ramesh A, Srisailapathy CR, Coucke P, Zbar RI, Bell AM, McGuirt WT, Fukushima K, et al.: Localization of a gene for otosclerosis to chromosome 15q25–q26. Hum Mol Genet 1998; 7:285–290.

Trofatter J, MacCollin M, Rutter J, Murrell J, Duyao M, Parry D, Eldridge R: A novel moesin-, ezrin-, radixin-like gene is a candidate for the neurofibromatosis 2 tumor suppressor. Cell 1993; 72:791–800.

Tyson J, Tranebjaerg L, Bellman S, Wren C, Taylor JFN, Bathen J, Aslaksen B, Sorland SJ, Lund O, Malcolm S, et al.: IsK and KvLQT1: mutation in either of the two subunits of the slow component of the delayed rectifier potassium channel can cause Jervell and Lange-Nielsen syndrome. Hum Mol Genet 1997; 6:2179–2185.

Ueda N, Oshima T, Ikeda K, Abe K, Aoki M, Takasaka T: Mitochondrial DNA deletion is a predisposing cause for sensorineural hearing loss. Laryngoscope 1998; 108:580–584.

U.S. Department of Health and Human Services: Early identification of Hearing Loss: Implementing Universal Newborn Hearing Screening Programs. Washington, DC: Government Printing Office, 1999.

Vahava O, Morell R, Lynch ED, Weiss S, Kagan ME, Ahituv N, Morrow JE, Lee MK, Skvorak AB, Morton CC, et al.: Mutation in transcription factor POU4F3 associated with inherited progressive hearing loss in humans. Science 1998; 279:1950–1954.

Van Camp G, Willems PJ, Smith RJH: Nonsyndromic hearing impairment: unparalleled heterogeneity. Am J Hum Genet 1997; 60:758–764.

Van Den Bogaert K, Govaerts PJ, Schatteman I, Brown MR, Caethoven G, Offeciers FI, Somers T, Declau P, Coucke P, Van de Heyning P, et al. A second gene for ostosclerosis, *OTSC2*, maps to chromosome 7q34-36. Am J Hum Genet 2001; 68:495–500.

Van Laer L, Huizing EH, Verstreken M, Van Zuijlen D, Wauters JG, Bossuyt PJ, Van de Heyning P, McGuirt WT, Smith RJ, Willems PJ, et al.: Nonsyndromic hearing impairment is associated with a mutation in DFNA5. Nat Genet 1998; 20:194–197.

Van Laer L, McGuirt WT, Yang T, Smith RJH, Van Camp G: Autosomal dominant nonsyndromic hearing impairment. Am J Med Genet 1999; 89:167–174.

Verhoeven K, Van Laer L, Kirschhofer K, Legan PK, Hughes DC, Schatteman I, Verstreken M, Van Hauwe P, Coucke P, Chen A, et al.: Mutations in the human α-tectorin gene cause autosomal dominant non-syndromic hearing impairment. Nat Genet 1998; 19:60–62.

Veske A, Oehlmann R, Younus F, Mohyuddin A, Muller-Myhsok B, Qasim MS, Gal A: Autosomal recessive non-syndromic deafness locus (DFNB8) maps on chromosome 21q22 in large consanguineous kindred from Pakistan. Hum Mol Genet 1996; 5:165–168.

Vikkula M, Mariman ECM, Lui VCH, Zhidkova NI, Tiller GE, Goldring MB, van Beersum SEC, de Waal-Malefijt MC, van den Hoogen FHJ, Ropers HH, et al.: Autosomal dominant and recessive osteochondrodysplasias associated with the *COL11A2* locus. Cell 1995; 80:431–437.

Viskochil D, Buchberg AM, Xu G, Cawthon RM, Stevens J, Wolff RK, Culver M, Carey JC, Copeland NG, Jenkins NA, et al.: Deletions and a translocation interrupt a cloned gene at the neurofibromatosis type 1 locus. Cell 1990; 62:187–192.

Wallace DC: Mitochondrial genetics: a paradigm for aging and degenerative diseases? Science 1992; 256:628–632.

Wallace MR, Marchuk DA, Andersen LB, Letcher R, Odeh HM, Saulino AM, Fountain JW, Brereton A, Nicholson J, Mitchell AL, et al.: Type 1 neurofibromatosis gene: identification of a large transcript disrupted in three NF1 patients. Science 1990; 249:181–186.

Waltzman SB, Cohen NL, Gomolin RH, Shapiro WH, Ozdamar SR, Hoffman RA: Long term results of early cochlear implantation in congenitally and prelingually deafened children. Am J Otol 1993; 15:9–14.

Wang A, Liang Y, Fridell RA, Probst FJ, Wilcox ER, Touchman JW, Morton CC, Morell RJ, Noben-Trauth K, Camper SA, Friedman TB: Association of unconventional myosin *MYO15* mutations with human nonsyndromic deafness DFNB3. Science 1998; 280:1147–1151.

Weil D, Blanchard S, Kaplan J, Guilford P, Gibson F, Walsh J, Mburu P: Defective myosin VIIA gene responsible for Usher syndrome type 1B. Nature 1995; 374:60–61.

Weil D, Kussel P, Blanchard S, Levy G, Levi-Acobas F, Drira M, Ayadi H, Petit C: The autosomal recessive isolated deafness, DFNB2, and the Usher 1B syndrome are allelic defects of the myosin-VIIA gene. Nat Genet 1997; 16:191–193.

Wilde WR: Practical Observations on Aural Surgery and the Nature and Diagnosis of Diseases of the Ear. London: Livingston Churchill, 1853.

Williams F, Roblee LA: Hereditary nerve deafness. Arch Otolaryngol 1962; 75:69–77.

Wilson J: Deafness in developing countries: approaches to a global program of prevention. Arch Otolaryngol 1985; 111:2–9.

Xia JH, Liu CY, Tang BS, Pan Q, Huang L, Dai HP, Zhang BR, Xie W, Hu DX, Zheng D, et al.: Mutations in the gene encoding gap junction protein β-3 associated with autosomal dominant hearing impairment. Nat Genet 1998; 20:370–373.

Yasunaga S, Grati M, Cohen-Salmon M, El-Amraoui A, Mustapha M, Salem N, El-Zir E, Loiselet J, Petit C: A mutation in *OTOF*, encoding otoferlin, a FER-1-like protein causes DFNB9, a nonsyndromic form of deafness. Nat Genet 1999; 21:363–369.

Yoshinaga-Itano C: Benefits of early intervention for children with hearing loss. Otolaryngol Clin North Am 1999; 32:1089–1102.

Zbar RIS, Ramesh A, Srisailapathy CRS, Fukushima D, Wayne S, Smith RJH: Passage to India: the search for genes causing autosomal recessive nonsyndromic hearing loss. Arch Otolaryngol Head Neck Surg 1998; 118:333–337.

Zelante L, Gasparini P, Estivill X, Melchionda S, D'Agruma L, Govea N, Mila M, Monica MD, Lutfi J, Shohat M, et al.: Connexin 26 mutations associated with the most common form of non-syndromic neurosensory autosomal recessive deafness (DFNB1) in Mediterraneans. Hum Mol Genet 1997; 6:1605–1609.

49 Migraine

AARNO PALOTIE, ROBERT BALOH, AND MAIJA WESSMAN

The familial clustering of migraine is a well-known clinical observation. However, the variable clinical features of migraine and the high frequency in the general population have made it difficult to define the pattern of genetic transmission. No specific disease-causing mutations or confirmed linked gene loci have so far been described in common forms of migraine. The best genetic evidence providing molecular insight into migraine has come from mutations in one calcium channel gene (*CACNA1A*), the same gene that causes familial hemiplegic migraine, episodic ataxia, and/or spinocerebellar ataxia type 6. Here, we discuss the heritability of migraine, rare migraine variants as models for understanding the pathophysiology of common migraine, and candidate genes that might contribute to a predisposition for common forms of migraine.

DISEASE DEFINITION

Migraine is a common neurovascular disorder characterized by recurrent, reversible focal neurological symptoms and disabling headache. It ranks seventh among reasons for outpatient visits, resulting in more than 18 million medical visits annually in the United States (Kaa et al., 1995; Gerth et al., 2001).

No laboratory or radiological findings are specific for migraine. The physical or neurological examination is usually normal and serves mostly to exclude other causes of headache. Thus, the diagnosis of migraine is based on retrospective reporting of headache characteristics and associated symptoms. A classic migraine attack has five phases: prodrome (e.g., depression, cognitive dysfunction, food craving), aura (e.g., visual, sensory, or motor phenomena preceding headache), headache (usually unilateral, throbbing), resolution (when pain wanes), and recovery (Blau, 1992). None of these phases is obligatory for the migraine diagnosis. Also, all of the phases (severity, duration, nature of prodrome or aura) vary substantially between individuals. The diagnosis of migraine thus depends on a combination of sequentially occurring symptoms in paroxysmal attacks.

The International Headache Society (IHS) has established criteria for the diagnosis and classification of migraine symptoms (Table 49–1) (Headache Classification Committee of the International Headache Society, 1988). The two most common forms of migraine are migraine without aura (MO) and migraine with aura (MA). These two forms account for more than 95% of all migraine cases. Conclusive epidemiological data are missing, but it has been estimated that MO accounts for about 70% and MA about 30% of migraine cases (Stewart et al., 1991). Some of the rare subtypes, however, provide interesting information for understanding the underlying pathophysiological mechanisms.

A set of multiple etiological factors, both genetic and environmental, is not unique to migraine but is characteristic for most complex diseases, such as epilepsy, multiple sclerosis, myocardial infarction, or diabetes. Many aspects of epilepsy are similar to migraine in that genetic factors are important; some seizure syndromes are monogenic, yet anyone can have a seizure with adequate provocation. Similarly, several inherited syndromes are associated with migraine headaches, and genetic factors are important in determining the threshold for migraine headache. However, structural lesions, such as vascular malformations and vasculopathies, can probably trigger migraine headaches in anyone.

GENERAL GENETICS AND EPIDEMIOLOGY

A number of studies have been carried out in Caucasian populations to determine the frequency of headaches and migraine (for ethnic variations, see the section Prevalence of Migraine in Ethnically Different Populations below). These studies vary widely in their prevalence estimations, most likely because of methodological and diagnostic differences. Unfortunately, many of these studies do not distinguish between the two major subclasses of migraine (MA vs. MO). Prevalence figures based on population surveys in adults range from as low as 3% to as high as 26% in the general population (females range 7.3%–24.9% and males 2%–7.8%) (Stewart et al., 1992; Henry et al., 1992; Honkasalo et al., 1993; O'Brien et al., 1994; Lavados and Tennham, 1997; Hagen et al., 2000). Corresponding figures for MA range from 5% to 13% in females and from 1% to 3% in males (Lipton et al., 1994b; Launer et al., 1999). In the prepubertal period, boys and girls are approximately equally affected; but at puberty, migraine decreases in boys and increases in girls so that a 2.5:1 female preponderance is established in adulthood (Stewart et al., 1992; O'Brien et al., 1994). The age at onset is a debated issue as migraine is likely to be underdiagnosed in children and adolescents (Sillanpää and Anttila, 1996; Lee and Olness, 1997). However, population-based studies suggest that about half of the patients had migraine before the age of 18 years (Bille, 1997; Stewart et al., 1997).

Three lines of evidence suggest that significant genetic mechanisms underlie migraine: *(1)* familial aggregation, *(2)* twin studies, and *(3)* racial distribution.

Familial Aggregation

Although familial aggregation of migraine is well-recognized and numerous studies in the past have supported this empirical observation, few of these studies would meet modern method-

Table 49–1A. Common Factors That Trigger Migraine Symptoms

Stress, emotional upset
Hormones: menstruation, oral contraceptives, pregnancy
Sleep deprivation
Food: red wines, fermented cheeses, chocolate, coffee
Eating disorders: fasting, binging

Table 49–1B. Abbreviated International Headache Society Classification of Migraine

Migraine without aura
Migraine with aura
Migraine with typical aura
Migraine with prolonged aura
Familial hemiplegic migraine
Basilar migraine
Migraine aura without headache
Migraine with acute-onset aura
Ophthalmoplegic migraine
Retinal migraine

Source: Olesen (1989).

Table 49–1C. Diagnostic Criteria for Migraine Without Aura

A. At least five attacks fulfilling B–D
B. Headache lasts 4–72 hours (untreated)
C. Headache has at least two of the following features:
1. Unilateral
2. Pulsating
3. Moderate or severe (inhibits or prohibits daily activities)
4. Aggravated by walking, stairs, or similar physical activities
D. During headache at least one of the following:
1. Nausea and vomiting
2. Photophobia and phonophobia
E. Other causes of headache have been ruled out

Source: Headache Classification Committee of the International Headache Society (1988).

ological standards. Apart from problems in collecting data (questionnaires, interviews), most studies lack rigorous diagnostic criteria like those of the IHS. Two newer population-based studies randomly selected individuals who were subsequently interviewed (Russell and Olesen, 1995; Stewart et al., 1997). Russell and Olesen (1995) selected 4000 40-year-old individuals (3000 men and 1000 women) from the Danish Central Person Registry. Based on a questionnaire, they selected those with self-reported migraine and invited them for a headache interview and a physical and neurological examination. Spouses and first-degree relatives were interviewed by phone and classified according to the IHS criteria. This resulted in 270 probands with migraine: 126 had MO, 127 had MA, and 17 had both. Interestingly, different patterns of familial risk were observed for MA and MO. Compared with the general population, the first-degree relatives of probands with MO had 1.9 times the risk of MO but only 1.4 times the risk of MA and first-degree relatives of probands with MA had nearly four times the risk of MA but no increased risk of MO. The authors concluded that MO was caused by a combination of genetic and environmental factors, whereas MA was determined largely by genetic factors.

In another population-based study, Stewart et al. (1997) collected a random sample of households in Baltimore County, Maryland, using a random digit dialing method. The survey was based on either a telephone interview or a self-administered questionnaire. Those with probable migraine were invited to the clinic for an interview and general medical and neurological examinations. This resulted in 73 migraine probands and 511 first-degree relatives. Probands were stratified into those having more disabling symptoms, missing work or school, and those who only rarely had to skip work or school due to migraine. The risk for migraine was considerably higher among relatives of probands with disabling migraine [relative risk (RR) 2.17] compared to relatives of probands with minimal disability (RR 1.20). This risk was not influenced by the type of migraine: they found an increased risk for both types of migraine in family members, independent of whether the proband had MA or MO. The authors concluded that familial factors contribute to fewer than 50% of all migraine cases.

Twin Studies

Five large population-based twin studies (Harvald and Hauge, 1956; Honkasalo et al., 1995; Larsson et al., 1995; Gervil et al., 1999; Ulrich et al., 1999) studying the concordance of migraine in monozygotic (MZ) twins have been published. Unfortunately, three of these studies were performed before the introduction of the standard IHS criteria for the diagnosis of migraine. Also, most of these studies used questionnaires in which only very few questions were dedicated to migraine. Thus, many methodological uncertainties exist. Nevertheless, all of these studies have a similar trend, suggesting concordance rates for MZ twins of 29% to 67% for migraine (Table 49–2) in many populations.

The most recent of these studies was performed in a Danish twin cohort by Ulrich et al. (1999). They focused on individuals having migraine with visual aura. Subjects who were tentative migraineurs based on questionnaires were interviewed by telephone. Thus, most of the criticisms of twin studies were addressed in this study and IHS criteria were applied. The concordance rate for MZ twins was somewhat higher than in previous studies, but the overall results were similar (Table 49–2). These twin data indicate that genetic factors are a major contributor to the pathogenesis of migraine.

Gervil et al. (2001) analyzed the RR of MO in parents and siblings of MO twins. The RR of MO was significantly higher in female first-degree relatives of concordant than of discordant MZ male and female twin pairs. An opposite trend was observed in male first-degree relatives. This suggests a genetic contribution in MO as well, although it is less clear than that in MA.

Another type of twin study takes advantage of twins raised apart. This provides an even more direct estimate of genetic influence since the effect of a shared environment is excluded. A drawback of these studies, however, is that the sample size is inevitably small. Ziegler et al. (1998) found that, in general, MZ twins had a higher concordance rate for migraine than dizygotic (DZ) twins (total of 197 twin pairs) but no statistically significant evidence that MZ twins raised apart (23 pairs) had a higher concordance rate for migraine than DZ twins raised apart (20 pairs). A small case study reported that two sets of MZ twins raised apart were concordant not only for migraine but also for the age at onset of the attacks (Juel-Nielsen, 1964).

Prevalence of Migraine in Ethnically Different Populations

The prevalence of migraine in African and Asian populations is lower than that in European and North American populations (Osuntokun et al., 1992; Tokio et al., 1993). These differences among racial groups are probably due to genetic rather than cultural or environmental factors since they persist in the United

Table 49–2. Population-Based Twin Studies of Migraine Concordance

	Monozygotic Twin Pairs			Dizygotic Twin Pairs		
Reference	Concordant	Discordant	Concordance (%)	Concordant	Discordant	Concordance (%)
Migraine with aura						
Lucas (1977)	4	20	29	0	19	0
Ulrich et al. (1999)	26	51	48	16	118	21
Migraine without aura						
Gervil et al. (1999)	38	99	43	47	211	31
Migraine unspecified						
Harvald and Hauge (1956)	12	12	67	6	54	18
Ziegler et al. (1975)	2	7	36	2	12	25
Honkasalo et al. (1995)	57	257	31	58	594	16
Larsson et al. (1995)	219	479	48	268	1,190	31

States. Stewart et al. (1996) randomly selected and interviewed (by telephone) 12,328 individuals 18 to 65 years of age living in Baltimore County, Maryland. The IHS criteria were used for the diagnosis of migraine. Migraine prevalence was significantly higher in Caucasians than in African or Asian Americans. African Americans reported a higher level of headache pain but were less likely to report nausea and vomiting with their attacks compared to Caucasians. By contrast, African Americans were less disabled by their attacks than Caucasians. Asian Americans and Caucasians did not have significant differences in associated features.

Mode of Inheritance

A number of attempts have been made to analyze the mode of inheritance of migraine. The early reports resulted in a number of conclusions, from autosomal recessive to autosomal dominant with or without incomplete penetrance. In most studies, X-linked and mitochondrial inheritance have been ruled out (Mochi et al., 1993; Ulrich et al., 1997). These two modes of inheritance have been of special interest due to the higher prevalence of migraine in females. A number of technical details, such as difference in diagnostic criteria and statistical analyses, contribute to the somewhat contradictory conclusions.

The more recent studies have been performed with up-to-date diagnostic criteria and statistical tools. Four studies published during the past 10 years have used the IHS criteria for diagnostics, and all study subjects were individually interviewed. Three (Russell et al., 1995; Kalfakis et al., 1996; Ulrich et al., 1997) of these studies suggested a multifactorial inheritance; the other suggested a recessive inheritance (Mochi et al., 1993). A multifactorial inheritance was suggested regardless of whether families were recruited from headache clinics (Mochi et al., 1993; Kalfakis et al., 1996; Ulrich et al., 1997) or from a population survey (Russell et al., 1995). Although various criticisms can be addressed to all of these studies, there is a consistency to the results that suggests a multifactorial mode of inheritance for migraine.

PATHOPHYSIOLOGY: BIOLOGICAL BASIS OF GENETIC SUSCEPTIBILITY

Background

Before considering candidate genes for MO and MA, it is useful to briefly consider the pathophysiology of migraine as we currently understand it. Probably the most characteristic of migraine symptoms is the classic visual aura. It typically begins with a small scintillating scotoma, which gradually enlarges over 20 to 30 minutes. There is convincing evidence that the visual aura is secondary to a wave of cortical depression, which begins at the occipital pole and gradually spreads across the cortex before stopping at the central sulcus (Leao, 1944; Lauritzen, 1994). Although decreased cerebral perfusion is associated with the spreading wave of depression, it is probably a secondary, rather than a primary, process. The spreading wave of cortical depression is associated with a marked accumulation of extracellular potassium, which must be cleared before neural activity can return to normal. Although the exact mechanism for the spreading wave of depression is not known, most agree that the initial event is a local build-up of potassium in the extracellular space (Lauritzen, 1994). Nearby synaptic terminals then depolarize in response to the high extracellular potassium, and both excitatory and inhibitory neurotransmitters are released. This release in turn leads to the opening of subsynaptic channels, resulting in further ionic exchange between the intracellular and extracellular fluid. During the spreading wave of depression, neurons are completely silent for approximately 1 minute and then slowly recover their predepression level of firing. The rate of movement of the spreading wave of depression across the visual cortex nicely correlates with the rate of enlargement of the scintillating scotoma observed by the patient. A spreading wave of cortical depression has been observed using positron emission tomography (PET) in a patient during a typical migraine headache without a visual aura (Woods et al., 1994; Weiller at al., 1995; Goadsby, 2001). Consistent with a basic neuronal defect, patients with migraine have cortical abnormalities not only during their attacks but also in the interictal period. Paroxysmal slowing on interictal electroencephalography (EEG) is commonly seen in migraine, and the clinical association of migraine and epilepsy is well documented (Lipton et al., 1994a). Identical paroxysmal slowing on EEG is seen in patients with episodic ataxia type 2 (EA-2). Magnetic resonance spectroscopy shows decreased interictal energy metabolism in the cortex of patients with MA or MO (Welch et al., 1989; Montagna et al., 1994). Single-photon emission computed tomography (SPECT) and other techniques for measuring cerebral blood flow have shown areas of regional hypoperfusion not only during migraine attacks but also in the interictal phase (Schlake et al., 1992). These changes were found in migraine without visual aura, with visual aura, and with episodes of hemiplegia. Acetazolamide reversed these interictal areas of hypoperfusion in all three classes of migraine patient (Schlake et al., 1992). Moskowitz (1984, 1990) proposed a mechanism to explain how the spreading wave of depression and associated increase in extracellular potassium could lead to a typical migraine headache. He introduced the concept of the trigeminal vascular system in the pathogenesis of vascular headaches. Trigeminal nerve fibers surrounding pial arteries on the ventral surface of the brain are depolarized by the high potassium concentration. This in turn leads to the release of neurotransmitters, such as substance P and calcitonin gene–related peptide by both orthodromic and antidromic conduction. The result is an increase in vascular permeability, dilatation of cerebral vessels, and a local inflammatory response that further activates pain-provoking fibers of the trigeminal vascular system. Thus, the headache of migraine could be a secondary phenomenon, the end result of a local increase in extracellular potassium concentration.

Ion Channels

Genes that code for calcium channels are intriguing candidates for migraine as mutations in one calcium channel gene (*CACNA1A*) result in familial hemiplegic migraine (FHM). FHM is a rare disorder compared to the common forms of migraine (for more details, see the section Familial Hemiplegic Migraine and Episodic Ataxia Type 2 below). Also, *CACNA1A* mutations result in the most severe phenotypes in the migraine disease spectrum (ataxias of various severity, hemiplegic episodes). The pathophysiology of the more common forms of migraine may be more complicated. However, many of the characteristic features of a migraine attack can be explained by an ion channel disorder. The growing number of disorders caused by mutations in ion channel genes further emphasizes their critical role in muscle and neuronal excitability (Tables 49–3, 49–4).

A number of mammalian models with ion channel mutations also exist (Table 49–3). The animals typically exhibit a combination of seizures and ataxia. Whether any of these animal models exhibits migraine-like symptoms is obviously impossible to determine. Long QT syndrome is of particular interest since mutations in a number of different ion channels can result in a similar phenotype, paroxysmal arrhythmia. Only a fraction of ion channel mutations have been described so far. The fact that even the nematode *Caenorhabditis elegans* genome contains close to 200 ion channel genes (Bargmann, 1998) likely reflects the diversity of specific signaling needs and the complexity of the family of these molecules. One could speculate that in a multifactorial disorder like migraine a complex combination of seemingly minor variations in ion channel genes combined with variations in other molecules of downstream signaling pathways might predispose to the migraine attack. However, studies in families with a strong inheritance pattern of migraine may reveal individual genes with major influences on the predisposition.

Serotonin

The neurotransmitter serotonin, or 5-hydroxytryptamine (5-HT), has long been implicated in the pathogenesis of migraine. For example, platelets release serotonin, and urinary excretion of 5-hydroxyindoleacetic acid, a breakdown product of 5-HT, is increased during an attack (Ferrari and Saxena, 1993). Also, changes in intracellular calcium concentrations are linked to 5-HT release. Furthermore, locus caeruleus and *nucleus raphe* are serotonergic and have been implicated as migraine generators. More than a dozen different 5-HT signal-mediating receptors have been described. Most of them belong to the metabotropic type of receptors, being composed of a single polypeptide, which transmits their action through G proteins. The only exception is the 5-HT_3 receptor type, which is an ionotropic receptor permeable to Na and K ions. This receptor is coded by one single gene on chromosome 11q22 and forms a homomeric complex composed of five copies of the same subunit, a relatively unique structure for neurotransmitter receptors.

Nyholt et al. (1996) studied the potential association of the $5\text{-}HT_{2A}$ receptor (chromosome 13q14–q21) in 96 migraine patients and 91 controls. Migraine patients were diagnosed based on the IHS criteria but not divided into MA and MO groups. No association was found between polymorphic markers on 5-HT_{2A} and migraine patients, nor was any evidence found for linkage in three large migraine families. As the sample is not very large, the results are not definitive but suggest that $5\text{-}HT_{2A}$ is not a good candidate gene for migraine.

Maassen VanDenBrink et al. (1998) studied the possible involvement of the $5\text{-}HT_{1F}$ receptor gene (chromosome 13p12) in 51 migraine patients with different responses to sumatriptan, a 5-HT_1 receptor agonist. The entire coding region of the gene was screened for nucleotide variations using single-strand conformation polymorphism (SSCP). No nucleotide alterations were detected. These investigators also studied an intragenic biallelic polymorphism in the 5-HT_{1B} receptor (Goto et al., 1990) but did not detect any differences in allelic distributions in different patient groups.

Dopamine

There is considerable laboratory/experimental evidence for a role of dopamine in the pathophysiology of certain subtypes of migraine. Moreover, many symptoms, such as nausea, vomiting, and hypotension, suggest that brain stem dopaminergic neurotransmission is involved in the migraine attack. Further support for the involvement of the dopaminergic system in migraine comes from the finding that dopamine antagonists are effective at the treatment of migraine symptoms. Dopamine blockers such as prochlorperazine and haloperidol are effective in suppressing and preventing migraine symptoms (see below).

Peroutka et al. (1997) studied the association of an intragenic polymorphism in the dopamine D_2 receptor (DRD_2) in 129 unrelated migraneurs (77 MO, 52 MA) and 121 controls. They found an excess of the *NcoI* polymorphic allele in MA individuals (69%) compared to both controls (49%) and MO individuals (52%). Lea et al. (2000) reported an association but no linkage to the dopamine *β-hydroxylase* gene in Australian migraine families. Del Zompo et al. (1998) studied 50 nuclear families from the island of Sardinia. Patients were affected by MO, divided into nondopaminergic (27 probands) and dopaminergic (23 probands) groups, and analyzed by the transmission disequilibrium test (TDT) on dopamine receptors D_2, D_3, and D_4. The subgroup of dopaminergic migraineurs was selected based on the presence of both yawning and nausea immediately before or during the pain phase of migraine. No association was detected for intragenic polymorphisms in DRD_3 or DRD_4 to MO. However, in the dopaminergic subgroup, an allelic association to DRD_2 was detected using TDT. The association vanished if the DRD_2 polymorphism was analyzed in the entire set of MO individuals. Both of these studies have their merits as well as methodological weaknesses. In the study by Peroutka et al. (1997), only scanty information was provided about patients' phenotypes and genetic background. Del Zompo et al. (1998) had an almost optimal population design, utilizing a genetic isolate and modern methodology (TDT), but subgrouping of patients resulted in quite small patient sets. Thus, it is not possible to make a definitive conclusion about the role of the DRD_2 locus based on these two

Table 49–3. Disorders Associated with Ion Channel Mutations

Disorders in Human	Ion Channel and Gene	Chromosomal Localization	References
Neuronal Diseases			
Episodic ataxia with myokymia (EA-1)	*KCNA1* (potassium voltage-gated channel, *Drosophila* shaker-related subfamily, member 1 (mouse Kv1.1 homolog), localized in terminal and juxtaparanodal regions of neuron)	12p13	Browne et al. (1994)
Episodic ataxia (EA-2)	*CACNA1A* (calcium channel, voltage-dependent, P/Q type, α1A subunit)	19p13	Ophoff et al. (1996), Yue et al. (1998), Denier et al. (1999)
Familial hemiplegic migraine	*CACNA1A*	19p13	Ophoff et al. (1996), Ducros et al. (2001)
Spinocerebellar ataxia (SCA6)	*CACNA1A*	19p13	Zhuchenko et al. (1997), Yue et al. (1997)
Benign neonatal familial convulsions			
Epilepsy, benign neonatal, type 1	*KCNQ2* (potassium voltage-gated channel, KQT-like subfamily, member 2)	20q13.3	Singh et al. (1998), Biervert et al. (1998)
Epilepsy, benign neonatal, type 2	*KCNQ3* (potassium voltage-gated channel, KQT-like subfamily, member 3)	8q24	Charlier et al. (1998)
Generalized epilepsy with febrile seizures	*SCN1B* (sodium channel, voltage-gated, type I, β polypeptide)	19q13.1	Wallace et al. (1998)
Autosomal dominant, nocturnal frontal lobe epilepsy	*CHRNA4* (cholinergic receptor, nicotinic, α polypeptide 4)	20q13.2–13.3	Steinlein et al. (1995)
Startle disease (hyperexplexia), autosomal dominant)	*GLRA1* (glycine receptor α1, stiff-man syndrome)	5q32	Shiang et al. (1993)
Jervell and Lange-Nielsen syndrome	*KCNQ1 (KVLQT1)* (potassium voltage-gated channel, KQT-like subfamily, member 1)	11p15.5	Neyroud et al. (1997), Splawski et al. (1997a)
	KCNE1 (MinK) (potassium voltage-gated channel, Isk-related family, member 1)	21q22.1–22.2	Tyson et al. (1997)
Autosomal dominant deafness	*KCNQ4*	1p34	Kubisch et al. (1999), Coucke et al. (1999)
Skeletal muscle			
Hyperkalemic periodic paralysis	*SCN4A* (sodium channel, voltage-gated, type IV, α polypeptide)	17q23–q25	Fontaine et al. (1990), Ptacek et al. (1991)
Paramyotonia congenita	*SCN4A*		Ptacek et al. (1992)
Potassium-activated myotonia	*SCN4A*		McClatchey et al. (1992)
Hypokalemic periodic paralysis	*CACNA1S (CACNL1A3)* (calcium channel, voltage-dependent, L type, α1S subunit)	1q32	Ptacek et al. (1994)
Autosomal recessive (Becker's) myotonia	*CLCN1*		Koch et al. (1992)
Autosomal dominant (Thomsen disease) myotonia	*CLCN1* (chloride channel 1, skeletal muscle)	7q32–7qter	George et al. (1993)
Malignant hyperthermia	*RYR1* (ryanodine receptor 1)	19q13.1	Quane et al. (1993)
Central core disease	*RYR1*		Zhang et al. (1993)
Congenital myasthenic syndrome	*CHRNA1* (cholinergic receptor, nicotinic, α polypeptide 1 muscle)	2q24–q32	Sine et al. (1995)

(continued)

Table 49–3. Disorders Associated with Ion Channel Mutations (*Continued*)

Disorders in Human	Ion Channel and Gene	Chromosomal Localization	References
Cardiac muscle			
Long QT syndrome 1	*KCNQ1 (KVLQT1)* (potassium voltage-gated channel, KQT-like subfamily, member 1	11p15.5	Wang et al. (1996)
Long QT syndrome 2	*KCNH2 (HERG)* (encodes a human homolog of the *Drosophila melanogaster eag* gene, a potassium channel protein. Along with five other human genes, mutations in *KCNH2* that result in loss of function or dominant negative function cause long QT syndrome)	7q35–q36	Curran et al. (1995)
Long QT syndrome 3	*SCN5A* (sodium channel, voltage-gated, type V, α polypeptide)	3p21–p23	Wang et al. (1995), Bennett et al. (1995)
Long QT syndrome 5	*KCNE1 (MinK)*	21q22.1–q22.2	Splawski et al. (1997b)
Idiopathic ventricular fibrillation	*SCN5A*	3p21–p23	Chen et al. (1998)
Jervell and Lange-Nielsen syndrome	*KCNE1 (MinK)* (potassium voltage-gated channel, Isk-related family, member 1)	21q22.1–q22.2	Schulze-Bahr et al. (1997), Tyson et al. (1997)
	KCNQ1 (KVLQT1) (potassium voltage-gated channel, KQT-like subfamily, member 1)	11p15.5	Neyroud et al. (1997), Splawski et al. (1997a)
Phenotype in mouse			
Tottering ataxia + seizures	*Cacna1a*, missense	Chr 8	Campbell and Hess (1996), Doyle et al. (1997), Burgess et al. (1997)
Leaner: ataxia + seizures	*Cacna1a*, splicing error	Chr 8	Campbell and Hess (1996), Burgess et al. (1997), Doyle et al. (1997), Fletcher et al. (2001)
Rolling Nagoya: ataxia, no seizures	*Cacna1a*, charge-neutralizing arginine to glycine substitution at position 1262	Chr 8	Mori et al. (2000)
Lethargic: ataxia + seizures	*Cacnb4*, splicing error	Chr 2	Escayg et al. (1998)
Stargazer: ataxia + seizures + vestibular dysfunction	*Cacnγ2*, early transposon insertion	Chr 15	Letts et al. (1997), Letts et al. (1998), Chen et al. (2000)

Source: Cooper and Jan (1999).

Table 49–4. Chromosomal Location for Calcium Channel Genes

Subunit	Gene	Chromosomal Location
α1A	*CACNA1A*	19p13.2–p13.1
α1B	*CACNA1B*	9q34
α1C	*CACNA1C*	12p13.3
α1D	*CACNA1D*	3p14.3
α1E	*CACNA1E*	1q25–q31
α1F	*CACNA1F*	Xp11.23
α1G	*CACNA1G*	17q22
α1H	*CACNA1H*	16p13.3
α1I	*CACNA1I*	22q13.1
α1S	*CACNA1S*	1q32
$\alpha2\delta1$	*CACNA2D1*	7q21–q22
$\alpha2\delta2$	*CACNA2D2*	3p21.3
$\alpha2\delta3$	*CACNA2D3*	3p21.1
$\gamma1$	*CACNG1*	17q24
$\gamma2$	*CACNG2*	22q13.1
$\gamma3$	*CACNG3*	16p12–p13.1
$\gamma4$	*CACNG4*	17q24
$\gamma5$	*CACNG5*	17q24
$\gamma6$	*CACNG6*	19q13.4
$\gamma7$	*CACNG7*	19q13.4
$\gamma8$	*CACNG8*	19q13.4
$\beta1$	*CACNB1*	17q21–22
$\beta2$	*CACNB2*	10p12
$\beta3$	*CACNB3*	12q13
$\beta4$	*CACNB4*	2q22–q31

Source: http://www.ncbi.nlm.nih.gov/LocusLink as of July 2001.

studies, and further work is clearly indicated. Peroutka et al. (1997) found a DRD_2 association to individuals having MA but not to individuals having MO. On the contrary, Del Zompo et al. (1998) reported an association of a subgroup of individuals having MO. The reason for this is not clear, but it might reflect the need of stratification of migraneurs to more specific clinical subgroups.

Genes on the X Chromosome

An unequal sex distribution with female dominance is a well-known finding in both MA and MO (Stewart et al., 1991; Rasmussen and Olesen, 1992). There is also evidence of a higher frequency of migraneurs in first-degree relatives of male probands (Russell and Olesen, 1993; Stewart et al., 1997). These findings have stimulated studies of a possible involvement of X-chromosomal loci in migraine etiology. Nyholt et al. (1998a, 2000) reported on a limited genome scan using 28 X-chromosomal markers. Using three large Australian migraine families, they found significant excess of allele sharing and suggestive evidence for linkage on a relatively large area on chromosome Xq. Although the clinical information was limited, families represented rather common migraine forms with both MA and MO individuals. Further studies are necessary to confirm the role of X-chromosomal loci in the genetic predisposition to migraine.

GENE IDENTIFICATION

Familial Hemiplegic Migraine and Episodic Ataxia Type 2

The only true molecular insight into migraine pathophysiology was provided by the isolation of the gene for a rare subtype of MA. This rare subtype is an autosomal dominant disease characterized by headache attacks preceded, or accompanied, by episodes of hemiplegia, sometimes lasting days (IHS). Unlike MO and MA, the prevalence rate is the same in men and women. In reported families with FHM, some affected members have interictal nystagmus, ataxia, and essential tremor (Ohta et al., 1967; Zifkin et al., 1980; Bisgärd et al., 1992; Joutel et al., 1993; Baloh et al., 1997). Also, it has been suggested that FHM is a subtype of basilar migraine (Haan et al., 1995).

Ophoff et al. (1996) reported mutations in a brain-specific P/Q-type calcium channel gene, *CACNA1A*, in four families with hemiplegic migraine. Mutations in this same gene can also cause EA-2 or spinocerebellar ataxia type 6 (SCA6). Although mutations in this gene represent only a minor fraction of all migraine cases and only about 50% of families with the FHM subtype, this finding provides the first true insight into the molecular pathogenesis of migraine. After assignment of the phenotype to chromosome 19p13 (Joutel et al., 1993), the gene was discovered through co-localization of EA-2 to the same chromosomal region and positional candidate gene strategy.

Another FHM locus has been reported, chromosome 1q21 (Ducros et al., 1997; Gardner et al., 1997). This locus is responsible for about 20% of FHM families. The FHM gene on this locus has not been identified.

Although the exact nature of the effect of the FHM mutations is not fully elucidated, it is logical that an episodic disease like FHM is caused by an ion channel disorder. There are a number of ion channel disorders, for most of which episodic symptoms are characteristic. Another characteristic feature for channel disorders is that they typically result in neural or neuromuscular disorders (Table 49–3). A general hypothesis is that a defective Ca^{2+} channel could explain the local build-up of extracellular potassium that initiates the spreading wave of depression in migraine. As Ca^{2+} enters neurons, potassium exits. Many of the well-known triggers for migraine symptoms, including stress and menstruation, could result from hormonal influences on the defective calcium channels. Finally, prophylactic drugs, such as β-blockers, calcium channel blockers, acetazolamide, and tricyclic amines, might work by stabilizing the abnormal calcium channels (see below).

Not enough mutations of *CACNA1A* have been described to provide us with a good insight into the phenotype–genotype correlation. However, expansions of the CAG repeat resulting in a polyglutamine stretch in the C-terminal end of the protein result in SCA6, a gradually progressive pancerebellar dysfunction beginning usually in the fourth or fifth decade and resulting in cerebellar and brain stem atrophy. The outcome of missense point mutations is very different, resulting in FHM mostly associated with cerebellar symptoms (Table 49–5). A handful of mutations resulting in FHM have been described (Ducros et al., 2000, 2001). It is remarkable that in a number of linked families no mutation has been detected; thus, our understanding of mutation–phenotype mechanisms in FHM is incomplete. In more than 80% of FHM families with *CACNA1A* mutations, ataxia or nystagmus or both were included in the symptoms (Terwindt et al., 1998; Ducros et al., 2001). All of the FHM-associated mutations in *CACNA1A* are missense point mutations, whereas truncating point mutations tend to result in EA-2 (Ophoff et al., 1996; Yue et al., 1997, 1998; Terwindt et al., 1998; Denier et al., 1999; Ducros et al., 2001). An additional complicating finding is that *CACNA1A* mutations are sometimes nonpenetrant, resulting in healthy gene carriers. The reason for this has not been discovered.

Functional studies of mutated calcium channel genes have been performed in vitro by cotransfecting calcium channel subunits with the mutant *CACNA1A* construct into cultured cells

Table 49–5. Phenotypes Associated with Different Mutations in *CACNA1A*

Phenotype in Human	Mutation	Age at Onset (years)	Ataxia Course
Hemiplegic migraine/basilar migraine	Missense mutation	2–30	Stable, exam often normal
Episodic ataxia type 2	Interrupts reading frame	3–30	Mildly progressive
Spinocerebellar ataxia	CAG repeats in open reading frame	>30	Moderately progressive
Episodic and progressive ataxia	Missense mutation	5–15	Severely progressive

(Kraus et al., 1998; Hans et al., 1999). Both groups studied the same four missense point mutations causing FHM. Based on multiple experiments, Hans et al. (1999) concluded that all four mutations affected both the biophysical properties of individual channels and the density of functional channels on the cell surface. Even detailed studies do not provide a simple explanation to conclude which mutations cause gain of function and which cause loss of function. For example, two of the mutations, I1811 L and V714A, result in a gain of function (increased Ca^{2+} influx) at the single-channel level, due to the higher open probability and a faster rate of recovery from inactivation, whereas they may lead to an overall loss of function (reduction of Ca^{2+} influx) at the level of the whole-cell calcium current, given that there is decreased density of functional channels. The in vivo situation might be even more complicated; the overall effect of these mutations might be different in different neurons. This is supported by the finding that even the expression studies appear to give different results in these two reports, depending on the cell type used.

One fascinating hypothesis is that *CACNA1A* mutations connected with an overall loss of function of P/Q-type Ca^{2+} channels, caused by either decreased density of functional channels or both decreased density and decreased single-channel conductance, result in an ataxic phenotype. This is further supported by findings that both the SCA6 polyglutamine expansion (Matsuyama et al., 1999) and the severe ataxic phenotype of the *leaner* mouse (Lorenzon et al., 1998) seem to result from a reduction in Ca^{2+} influx. However, the two FHM mutations where no ataxia has been reported appear to be connected with an increased Ca^{2+} influx (Hans et al., 1999). Hans et al. (1999) also found in two of the mutations that the reduction in single-channel conductance was not observed in some patches or periods of activity, suggesting that the abnormal channel may switch on and off, perhaps depending on some unknown factor, an intriguing parallel with the episodic nature of the disorder.

Relevance of Mutations in *CACNA1A* for More Common Forms of Migraine

The episodic nature of migraine attacks as well as the spreading phenomenon are features which could well suit a calcium channel disorder. To determine whether *CACNA1A* is involved in families with MA or MO, four (Hovatta et al., 1994; May et al., 1995; Nyholt et al., 1998b; Terwindt et al., 2001) linkage-based family studies have been performed. All of these studies differ in their statistical analyses, which somewhat complicates the interpretation.

Hovatta et al. (1994) studied four Finnish migraine families. In one of the families, MO was the predominant phenotype, whereas in the three other families there were both MO and MA individuals. The statistical analysis applied a modified autosomal dominant model, allowing for phenocopies and age-dependent penetrance. Using four polymorphic markers from the 19p13 region, two families provided suggestive evidence for excluding *CACNA1A* as a predisposing locus and the two other families were rather small and, thus, less informative but showed small negative lod scores. The cumulative lod scores of all four families were clearly negative both in two-point analysis (lod -2.26 to -2.49) and in multipoint analysis excluding a region of 50 cM (lod < -2). Similar negative values were achieved using an affected-only model.

A very different interpretation was made in a study by May et al. (1995), where 28 mostly German families with a total of 198 members were analyzed using a polymorphic marker adjacent to *CACNA1A*. Using affected sib–pair analysis by following the transmission of marker D19S394, they found that affected sibs shared the same marker allele more frequently than expected by chance (depending on the model $p = 0.04$–0.08). Also, linkage calculations provided slightly positive lod scores (cumulative two-point lod score 1.38); however, most of the positive information was contributed by a single family (lod 1.29), whereas the rest of the families were small and rather uninformative. Kim et al. (1998) screened nine families with migraine headache and episodic vertigo for mutation in *CACNA1A* using SSCP. Polymorphisms were found but no mutations.

Nyholt et al. (1998b) studied four large Australian families (total of 121 individuals) having MA or MO. Using both parametric and nonparametric approaches in one family, they found cosegregation of chromosome 19p13 markers adjacent to *CACNA1A*. In classical linkage analysis, a two-point lod score of 1.56 with marker D19S179 and a multipoint lod score of 2.4 were obtained in this family. The three other families were rather uninformative.

Terwindt et al. (2001) studied the involvement of *CACNA1A* markers in 189 affected siblings from 36 extended Dutch migraine families. They obtained multipoint lod score values of 1.41 and an increased RR of 1.56 attributed to the 19p13 locus.

White et al. (2001) reported that single-nucleotide polymorphisms in the insulin receptor gene (*INSR*) were associated with migraine. This gene is also located in the chromosome 19p13 area. This finding emphasizes the notion that the proximity of genes other than *CACNA1A* might contribute to the linkage and association findings on 19p13 to common forms of migraine.

In conclusion, the genetic evidence of the involvement of *CACNA1A* in common forms of migraine is quite vague, so far. None of the published studies provides strong evidence for this locus, but none excludes the 19p locus either. Thus, the role of this locus remains to be clarified. Three obvious possibilities exist: *(1)* the most conservative option is that these marginally significant linkages and associations represent Type I errors purely by chance; *(2)* another, more likely option is that they represent rare but true major predisposing loci in a small fraction of families with common forms of migraine; and *(3)* lastly, as with all complex traits, these results might reflect minor modifying loci that occasionally contribute to the predisposition.

Mouse Models for Migraine

The excitement over *CACNA1A* mutations and migraine was heightened by the discovery of two mouse models that carry mutations in the corresponding mouse gene (Burgess et al., 1997; Doyle et al., 1997). Contrary to FHM and EA-2, which are autosomal dominant traits, both of the mouse traits are recessive. Tottering mice have motor seizures and slowly progressive ataxia beginning around the third postnatal week, whereas leaner mice have absence spells (brief seizures) and are severely ataxic, often not surviving past weaning. Tottering mice have a missense mutation resulting in a nonconservative ($Pro^{600}Leu$) amino acid change near the second p-domain, a site putatively involved in channel formation. The more severe phenotype, leaner, is caused by a splice donor mutation, which results in truncation of the normal transcribed sequences and expression of multiple aberrant transcripts and a novel C-terminal sequence in the polypeptide. A knockout model of *CACNA1A* results in a similar phenotype as the leaner variant (Fletcher et al., 2001). This is analogous with the human mutations in which missense mutations have been detected in FHM and truncating mutations in the more severe phenotype, EA-2.

Both of these mutations in mice result in cerebellar symptoms and histological changes in Purkinje cells. Thus, the parallel disorders of these mouse models in humans are ataxias and some epileptic seizures. As migraine attacks are dominated by subjective symptoms (pain, prodromes, auras), it is obviously impossible to evaluate how these symptoms relate to these mouse models.

Cerebral Autosomal Dominant Arteriopathy with Subcortical Infarcts and Leucoencephalopathy

Cerebral autosomal dominant arteriopathy with subcortical infarcts and leucoencephalopathy (CADASIL, Online Mendelian Inheritance in Man number 125310) is an autosomal dominant condition characterized by recurrent subcortical ischemic strokes, occurring in the late 40s and leading to progressive dementia. In about 30% of patients, MA is a prominent feature. Verin et al. (1995) reported on a CADASIL family in which 40% of the affected members had isolated headache beginning in their teens as their first symptoms. CADASIL was linked to chromosome 19p (Joutel et al., 1996) and shown to be caused by mutations in the *Notch3* gene. The *Notch* genes are transmembrane proteins, which are involved in cell fate in many contexts throughout development (Joutel and Tournier-Lasserve, 1998; Lewis, 1998). The precise pathophysiological mechanism of how mutations in this gene result in CADASIL and MA remains to be clarified.

Mitochondrial Encephalopathy, Lactic Acidosis, and Stroke-like Episodes

The central role of mitochondria in energy metabolism as well as a predominance of maternal transmission in families have made mitochondrial DNA mutations potential candidates. A number of inherited disorders have been associated with specific mitochondrial DNA mutations. The syndrome of mitochondrial encephalopathy, lactic acidosis, and stroke-like episodes (MELAS) and that of myoclonus with epilepsy and ragged red fibers (MERFF) are caused by point mutations in mitochondrial DNA. Hallmarks of MELAS are lactic acidosis, strokes, and mitochondrial myopathy. MERRF is characterized by myoclonic epilepsy and specific histological findings in skeletal muscle (ragged red fibers). Mosewich et al. (1993) reported a family with a typical point mutation for MELAS but the major finding of migraine, only one member of which had stroke-like episodes. Sano et al. (1996) reported a Japanese family with features of both MELAS and MERRF and a mutation in nucleotide 8356 coding for a transfer RNA molecule. One of the prominent symptoms in this family was migraine. These reports highlight the issue that multiple underlying mechanisms might contribute to trigger the migraine attack; although the defect in mitochondrial function results in a phenotype affecting several organs, migraine is one symptom which reflects malfunction of neurons in the central nervous system. A connection between decreased adenosine triphosphate production in mitochondrial disorders potentially resulting in an increased Ca^{2+} influx into cells is an interesting hypothesis which could possibly underlie the migraine symptoms of MELAS patients.

CLINICAL APPLICATION AND RISK ASSESSMENT

With the exception of FHM, genetic information is not used in the diagnosis, screening, counseling, or treatment of patients with migraine. Some clinicians (Prensky and Sommer, 1979) have suggested that a positive family history should be added to the diagnostic criteria for migraine, but this probably would not be useful until the mode of inheritance is clarified.

Treatment of migraine can be divided into three major categories: *(1)* eliminating triggers, *(2)* symptomatic treatment, and *(3)* prophylactic treatment. Understanding how these treatments work may lead to a better understanding of the pathophysiology of migraine. Unfortunately, most of the drugs used in treating migraine were discovered empirically and have multiple actions. Furthermore, the fact that a drug is effective at relieving or preventing migraine symptoms does not necessarily indicate that it acts on the primary mechanism of migraine. A cascade of events occur with migraine symptoms, and many if not all of the drugs may affect the cascade downstream from the primary defect causing migraine. For example, drugs that suppress headache but not the prodromal or aura symptoms are not likely to teach us much about the primary mechanism of migraine.

Eliminating Triggers

Before embarking on drug treatment of migraine, it is important to recognize that there are many common triggers for migraine symptoms (Tables 49–1, 49–6) (Scharff et al., 1995). These triggers presumably initiate the cascade of events mentioned above. A basic neuronal abnormality such as an ion channel mutation could explain many of them. Similar triggers have been identified in known ion channel disorders, such as periodic paralysis, EA, and FHM. Hormonal factors in women might explain the apparent increased incidence of migraine in the female population compared to the male population.

Symptomatic Treatment

For patients who have infrequent migraine attacks, symptomatic therapy at the time of the attack is the best treatment strategy. Symptomatic treatment of migraine typically includes analgesics, antiemetics, and sedatives or some combination of these drugs. The goal of this treatment is to make the patient comfortable until the attack runs it course. It has long been

Table 49–6. Common Drugs for Prophylaxis of Migraine

Class	Actions	Sample Drugs
Serotonergic	$5\text{-}HT_1$ agonist	Sumatriptan, dihydroxyergotamine
	$5\text{-}HT_2$ antagonist	Methysergide, amitriptyline, fluoxetine
	5-HT reuptake inhibition	
Dopaminergic	DRD_2 antagonist	Prochlorperazine,[a] metoclopramide
β-blockers	$5\text{-}HT_2$ antagonist, ion channel stabilization	Propranolol, atenolol
Calcium channel blockers	Ion channel stabilization, neuronal protection, DRD_2 antagonist	Flunarizine, nimodipine
Nonsteroidal antiinflammatory drugs	Prostaglandin suppression, neurogenic inflammation	Aspirin, naproxen
Anticonvulsants	Ion channel stabilization, neuronal inhibition	Valproate, gabapentine
Carbonic anhydrase inhibitors	Ion channel stabilization	Acetazolamide

[a]Can be used for both symptomatic and prophylactic treatment.

known that if patients are able to get to sleep, the symptoms are often gone when they awaken. Thus, either primary sedatives or analgesics and antiemetics with sedating actions are beneficial. The antiemetics are primarily dopamine antagonists, presumably having their effect on dopamine receptors in the emetic centers of the brain stem. Metoclopramide also promotes normal gastric motility and may improve absorption of orally administered analgesics. For many patients, aspirin and rest are adequate to relieve the headache (O'Neill and Mann, 1978). The many combination preparations for symptomatic treatment of migraine contain sedatives that enhance sleep. Fiorinal (a combination containing aspirin, caffeine, and butalbital) is a common example.

Prophylactic and Abortive Treatment

A wide range of drugs has been used for the prophylactic treatment of migraine, and there is no uniform action that would tie all of them together (Table 49–6) (Goadsby, 1997). Some of the drugs can abort an attack if taken at the very onset, but most must be taken regularly for several weeks before their preventive action is apparent (Leone and Bussone, 1995).

A role for serotonin in the pathogenesis of migraine was initially suggested by the observation that drugs that affect serotonergic function can prevent migraine attacks. Another key observation suggesting a direct involvement of serotonin in the triggering process of migraine is that the compound *m*-chlorophenolproperazine (mCPP), a $5\text{-}HT_2$ agonist, triggers migraine attacks in certain subjects (Brewerton et al., 1988). Antagonists of the $5\text{-}HT_2$ receptors prevent attacks. Agonists of the $5\text{-}HT_1$ receptors, such as triptans, can abort migraine attacks if taken at the earliest signs of onset. As molecular biologists have focused their attention on the 5-HT receptors and their genes, the number of known receptors is rapidly expanding. At present, there are five subclasses of the $5\text{-}HT_1$ receptor and three subclasses of the $5\text{-}HT_2$ receptor. All of the $5\text{-}HT_1$ agonists affect multiple subclasses of that receptor. The $5\text{-}HT_2$ antagonists, such as methysergide, probably exert their effect through the $5\text{-}HT_{2B}$ and $5\text{-}HT_2C$ receptors since ketanserin, a relatively potent $5\text{-}HT_{2A}$ antagonist, is not an effective migraine prophylactic (Winther, 1985; Kalkman, 1994). The β-blocker propranolol is also a $5\text{-}HT_2$ antagonist, with greater potency for the $5\text{-}HT_{2B}$ receptor than the $5\text{-}HT_{2C}$ receptor (Forssman et al., 1983). The tricyclic amines, of which amitriptyline is most commonly used, block the reuptake of both noradrenaline and 5-HT into aminergic neurons (Couch and Hassanein, 1979). Selective serotonin reuptake inhibitors, such as fluoxetine, also prevent migraine symptoms, suggesting that the build-up of 5-HT is the mechanism of action. The $5\text{-}HT_1$ agonists, such as sumatriptan, prevent headache but not the aura, suggesting that these drugs act downstream from the primary metabolic defect in migraine.

The second recurring theme regarding the mode of action of migraine prophylactic drugs is their effect on ion channels. Propranolol, flunarizine, and valproate have membrane-stabilizing effects, presumably through actions on calcium and sodium channels (Leone et al., 1991). Flunarizine and acetazolamide prevent attacks in patients with FHM and familial EA due to mutations in the voltage-gated calcium channel gene *CACNA1A*. Calcium channels such as *CACNA1A* are exquisitely sensitive to changes in pH and the concentration of ions such as potassium (Hille, 1992). The mechanism of the pH-dependent control of channel function has been studied at the molecular level. A decrease in pH (increasing the number of free protons) strongly inhibits ion permeation through open calcium channels. The pronation site of the L-type voltage-regulated calcium channel lies within the pore (Chen et al., 1996). It is formed by a combination of conserved pore region glutamates, the amino acids shown to be key to calcium selectivity in these channels (Heinemann et al., 1992). This mechanism is a simple molecular explanation for the modulatory effect of H^+ ions on open channel flux and for the competition between H^+ ions and divalent cations. By increasing the extracellular proton concentration in the cerebellum (Bain et al., 1992), acetazolamide presumably stabilizes the mutant calcium channels that fail to properly inactivate. A family with progressive EA due to a missense mutation in the critical pore region of *CACNA1A* did not respond to acetazolamide, presumably because the mutation altered the stabilizing effect of H^+ (Yue et al., 1997). It is tempting to speculate that many of the triggers for migraine symptoms and many of the prophylactic drugs act through their effect on voltage-gated ion channels.

FUTURE PERSPECTIVES

No large genome scan strategies to randomly search for susceptibility loci in common forms of migraine have been published so far. Although the strategy is difficult in complex traits, if conducted with well-stratified patient samples, it might guide us to new loci and eventually to new susceptibility genes. The relevance of this approach is increasing with the rapidly evolving information and characterization of the human genome. In the near future, however, only genes with a major influence on migraine susceptibility will probably be identified. The identification of genes with less prominent effects and the understanding of their interplay will remain a challenge.

REFERENCES

Bain PG, O'Brien MD, Keevil SF, Porter DA: Familial periodic cerebellar ataxia: a problem of cerebellar intracellular pH homeostasis. Ann Neurol 1992; 31:147–154.

Baloh RW, Yue Q, Furman JM, Nelson SF: Familial episodic ataxia: clinical heterogeneity in four families linked to chromosome 19p. Ann Neurol 1997; 41:8–16.

Bargmann CI: Neurobiology of the *Caenorhabditis elegans* genome. Science 1998; 282:2028–2033.

Bennett PB, Yazawa K, Makita N, George AL Jr: Molecular mechanism for an inherited cardiac arrhythmia. Nature 1995; 376:683–685.

Biervert C, Schroeder BC, Kubisch C, Berkovic SF, Propping P, Jentsch TJ, Steinlein OK: A potassium channel mutation in neonatal human epilepsy. Science 1998; 279:403–406.

Bille B: A 40-year follow-up of school children with migraine. Cephalalgia 1997; 17:488–491.

Bisgärd C, Jensen TS, Dupont E, Hertz JM: Familial hemiplegic migraine associated with cerebellar ataxia. A distinct inherited disease entity? Acta Neurol Scand 1992; 85(Suppl 138):29.

Blau JN: Migraine: theories of pathogenesis. Lancet 1992; 339:1202–1207.

Brewerton TD, Murphy DL, Mueller EA, Jimerson DC: Induction of migrainelike headaches by the serotonin agonist *m*-chlorophenylpiperazine. Clin Pharmacol Ther 1988; 43:605–609.

Browne DL, Gancher ST, Nutt JG, Brunt ER, Smith EA, Kramer P, Litt M: Episodic ataxia/myokymia syndrome is associated with point mutations in the human potassium channel gene, *KCNA1*. Nat Genet 1994; 8:136–140.

Burgess DL, Jones JM, Meisler MH, Noebels JL: Mutation of the Ca^{2+} channel beta subunit gene *Cchb4* is associated with ataxia and seizures in the lethargic (lh) mouse. Cell 1997; 88:385–392.

Campbell DB, Hess EJ: Chromosomal localization of the neurological mouse mutations tottering (tg), Purkinje cell degeneration (pcd), and nervous (nr). Brain Res Mol Brain Res 1996; 37:79–84.

Charlier C, Singh NA, Ryan SG, Lewis TB, Reus BE, Leach RJ, Leppert MA: A pore mutation in a novel KQT-like potassium channel gene in an idiopathic epilepsy family. Nat Genet 1998; 18:53–55.

Chen L, Chetkovich DM, Petralia RS, Sweeney NT, Kawasaki Y, Wenthold RJ, Bredt DS, Nicoll RA: Stargazing regulates synaptic targeting of AMPA receptors by two distinct mechanisms. Nature 2000; 408:936–943.

Chen Q, Kirsch GE, Zhang D, Brugada R, Brugada J, Brugada P, Potenza D, Moya A, Borggrefe M, Breithardt G, et al.: Genetic basis and molecular mechanism for idiopathic ventricular fibrillation. Nature 1998; 392:293–295.

Chen XH, Bezprozvanny I, Tsien RW: Molecular basis of proton block of L-type Ca^{2+} channels. J Gen Physiol 1996; 108:363–374.

Cooper EC, Jan LY: Ion channel genes and human neurological disease: recent progress, prospects, and challenges. Proc Natl Acad Sci USA 1999; 96:4759–4766.

Couch JR, Hassanein RS: Amitriptyline in migraine prophylaxis. Arch Neurol 1979; (11):695–699.

Coucke PJ, Van Hauwe P, Kelley PM, Kunst H, Schatteman I, Van Velzen D, Meyers J, Ensink RJ, Verstreken M, Declau F, et al.: Mutations in the *KCNQ4* gene are responsible for autosomal dominant deafness in four DFNA2 families. Hum Mol Genet 1999; 8:1321–1328.

Curran ME, Splawski I, Timothy KW, Vincent GM, Green ED, Keating MT: A molecular basis for cardiac arrhythmia: *HERG* mutations cause long QT syndrome. Cell 1995; 80:795–803.

Del Zompo M, Cherchi A, Palmas MA, Ponti M, Bocchetta A, Gessa GL, Piccardi MP: Association between dopamine receptor genes and migraine without aura in a Sardinian sample. Neurology 1998; 51:781–786.

Denier C, Ducros A, Vahedi K, Joutel A, Thierry P, Ritz A, Castelnovo G, Deonna T, Gerard P, Devoize JL, et al.: High prevalence of *CACNA1A* truncations and broader clinical spectrum in episodic ataxia type 2. Neurology 1999; 52:1816–1821.

Doyle J, Ren X, Lennon G, Stubbs L: Mutations in the *Cacnl1a4* calcium channel gene are associated with seizures, cerebellar degeneration, and ataxia in tottering and leaner mutant mice. Mamm Genome 1997; 8:113–120.

Ducros A, Denier C, Joutel A, Cecillon M, Lescoat C, Vahedi K, Darcel F, Vicaut E, Bousser MG, Tournier-Lasserve E: The clinical spectrum of familial hemiplegic migraine associated with mutations in a neuronal calcium channel. N Engl J Med 2001; 345:17–24.

Ducros A, Denier C, Tournier-Lasserve E: Genetics of familial hemiplegic migraine. J Headache Pain 2000; 1: S129–S134.

Ducros A, Joutel A, Vahedi K, Cecillon M, Ferreira A, Bernard E, Verier A, Echenne B, Lopez de Munain A, Bousser MG, et al.: Mapping of a second locus for familial hemiplegic migraine to 1q21–q23 and evidence of further heterogeneity. Ann Neurol 1997; 42:885–890.

Escayg A, Jones JM, Kearney JA, Hitchcock PF, Meisler MH: Calcium channel beta 4 (*CACNB4*): human ortholog of the mouse epilepsy gene lethargic. Genomics 1998; 50:14–22.

Ferrari MD, Saxena PR: On serotonin and migraine: a clinical and pharmacological review. Cephalalgia 1993; 13:151–165.

Fletcher CF, Tottene A, Lennon VA, Wilson SM, Dubel SJ, Paylor R, Hosford DA, Tessarollo L, McEnery MW, Pietrobon D, et al.: Dystonia and cerebellar atrophy in *Cacna1a* null mice lacking P/Q calcium channel activity. FASEB J 2001; 15:1288–1290.

Fontaine B, Khurana TS, Hoffman EP, Bruns GA, Haines JL, Trofatter JA, Hanson MP, Rich J, McFarlane H, Yasek DM, et al.: Hyperkalemic periodic paralysis and the adult muscle sodium channel alpha-subunit gene. Science 1990; 250:1000–1002.

Forssman B, Lindblad CJ, Zbornikova V: Atenolol for migraine prophylaxis. Headache 1983; 23:188–190.

Gardner K, Barmada MM, Ptacek LJ, Hoffman EP: A new locus for hemiplegic migraine maps to chromosome 1q31. Neurology 1997; 49:1231–1238.

George AL Jr, Crackower MA, Abdalla JA, Hudson AJ, Ebers GC: Molecular basis of Thomsen's disease (autosomal dominant myotonia congenita). Nat Genet 1993; 3:305–310.

Gerth WC, Carides GW, Dasbach EJ, Visser WH, Santanello NC: The multinational impact of migraine symptoms on healthcare utilisation and work loss. Pharmacoeconomics 2001; 19:197–206.

Gervil M, Ulrich V, Kaprio J, Olesen J, Russell MB: The relative role of genetic and environmental factors in migraine without aura. Neurology 1999; 53:995–999.

Gervil M, Ulrich V, Kaprio J, Russell MB: Is the genetic liability in multifactorial disorders higher in concordant than discordant monozygotic twin pairs? A population-based family twin study of migraine without aura. Eur J Neurol 2001; 8:231–235.

Goadsby PJ: How do the currently used prophylactic agents work in migraine? Cephalalgia 1997; 17:85–92.

Goadsby PJ: Neuroimaging in headache. Microsc Res Tech 2001; 53:179–187.

Goto Y, Nonaka I, Horai S: A mutation in the *tRNA(Leu)(UUR)* gene associated with the MELAS subgroup of mitochondrial encephalomyopathies. Nature 1990; 348:651–653.

Haan J, Terwindt GM, Ophoff RA, Bos PL, Frants RR, Ferrari MD, Krommenhoek T, Lindhout DL, Sandkuyl LA, Van Eyk R: Is familial hemiplegic migraine a hereditary form of basilar migraine? Cephalalgia 1995; 15:477–481.

Hagen K, Zwart JA, Vatten L, Stovner LJ, Bovim G: Prevalence of migraine and non-migrainous headache—head-HUNT, a large population-based study. Cephalalgia 2000; 20:900–906.

Hans M, Luvisetto S, Williams ME, Spagnolo M, Urrutia A, Tottene A, Brust PF, Johnson EC, Harpold MM, Stauderman KA, et al.: Functional consequences of mutations in the human alpha1A calcium channel subunit linked to familial hemiplegic migraine. J Neurosci 1999; 19:1610–1619.

Harvald B, Hauge M: A catamnestic investigation of Danish twins. A preliminary report. Dan Med Bull 1956; 3:150–158.

Headache Classification Committee of the International Headache Society: Classification and diagnostic criteria for headache disorders, cranial neuralgias and facial pain. Cephalalgia 1988; 8(Suppl 7):1–96.

Heinemann SH, Terlau H, Stuhmer W, Imoto K, Numa S: Calcium channel characteristics conferred on the sodium channel by single mutations. Nature 1992; 356:441–443.

Henry P, Michel P, Brochet B, Dartigues JF, Tison S, Salamon R: A nationwide survey of migraine in France: prevalence and clinical features in adults. Cephalalgia 1992; 12: 229–237.

Hille B: Ionic Channels of Excitable Membranes, 2d ed. Sunderland, MA: Sinauer, 1992.

Honkasalo M-L, Kaprio J, Heikkilä K, Sillanpää M, Koskenvuo M: A population-based survey of headache and migraine in 22,809 adults. Headache 1993; 33:403–412.

Honkasalo M-L, Kaprio J, Winter T, Heikkilä K, Sillanpää M, Koskenvuo M: Migraine and concomitant symptoms among 8167 adult twin pairs. Headache 1995; 35:70–78.

Hovatta I, Kallela M, Färkkilä M, Peltonen L: Familial migraine: exclusion of the susceptibility gene from the reported locus of familial hemiplegic migraine on 19p. Genomics 1994; 23:707–709.

Joutel A, Bousser MG, Biousse V, Labauge P, Chabriat H, Nibbio A, Maciazek J, Meyer B, Bach MA, Weissenbach J, et al.: A gene for familial hemiplegic migraine maps to chromosome 19. Nat Genet 1993; 5:40–45.

Joutel A, Corpechot C, Ducros A, Vahedi K, Chabriat H, Mouton P, Alamowitch S, Domenga V, Cecillion M, Marechal E, et al.: *Notch3* mutations in CADASIL, a hereditary adult-onset condition causing stroke and dementia. Nature 1996; 383:707–710.

Joutel A, Tournier-Lasserve E: Notch signalling pathway and human diseases. Semin Cell Dev Biol 1998; 9:619–625.

Juel-Nielsen N: Individual and environmental. Acta Psychiatr Scand 1964; 40(Suppl 183):1–292.

Kaa KA, Carlson JA, Osterhaus JT: Emergency department resource use by patients with migraine and asthma in a health maintenance organization. Ann Pharmacother 1995; 29:251–256.

Kalfakis N, Panas M, Vassilopoulos D, Malliara-Loulakaki S: Migraine with aura: segregation analysis and heritability estimation. Headache 1996; 36:320–322.

Kalkman HO: Is migraine prophylactic activity caused by 5-HT2B or 5-HT2C receptor blockade? Life Sci 1994; 54:641–644.

Kim JS, Yue Q, Jen JC, Nelson SF, Baloh RW: Familial migraine with vertigo: no mutations found in *CACNA1A*. Am J Med Genet 1998; 79:148–151.

Koch MC, Steinmeyer K, Lorenz C, Ricker K, Wolf F, Otto M, Zoll B, Lehmann-Horn F, Grzeschik KH, Jentsch JT: The skeletal muscle chloride channel in dominant and recessive human myotonia. Science 1992; 257:797–800.

Kraus RL, Sinnegger MJ, Glossmann H, Hering S, Striessnig J: Familial hemiplegic migraine mutations change alpha1A Ca^{2+} channel kinetics. J Biol Chem 1998; 273:5586–5590.

Kubisch C, Schroeder BC, Friedrich T, Lutjohann B, El-Amraoui A, Marlin S, Petit C, Jentsch TJ: *KCNQ4*, a novel potassium channel expressed in sensory outer hair cells, is mutated in dominant deafness. Cell 1999; 96:437–446.

Larsson B, Bille B, Pedersen NL: Genetic influence in headaches: a Swedish twin study. Headache 1995; 35:513–519.

Launer LJ, Terwindt GM, Ferrari MD: The prevalence and characteristics of migraine in a population-based cohort: the GEM study. Neurology 1999; 53:537–542.

Lauritzen M: Pathophysiology of the migraine aura. The spreading depression. Brain 1994; 117:199–210.

Lavados PM, Tenhamm E: Epidemiology of migraine headache in Santiago, Chile: a prevalence study. Cephalalgia 1997; 17:770–777.

Lea RA, Dohy A, Jordan K, Quinland S, Brimage PJ, Griffiths LR: Evidence for allelic association of the dopamine betahydroxylase gene (*DBH*) with susceptibility to typical migraine. Neurogenetics 2000; 3:35–40.

Leao A: Spreading depression of activity in cerebral cortex. J Neurophysiol 1944; 7:359–390.

Lee LH, KN Olness: Clinical and demographic characteristics of migraine in urban children. Headache 1997; 37:269–276.

Leone M, Bussone G: Current approaches to the prophylaxis of migraine. CNS Drugs 1995; 3:165–173.

Leone M, Grazzi L, La Mantia L, Bussone G: Flunarizine in migraine: a minireview. Headache 1991; 31:388–391.

Letts VA, Felix R, Biddlecome GH, Arikkath J, Mahaffey CL, Valenzuela A, Bartlett FS 2nd, Mori Y, Campbell KP, Frankel WN: The mouse *stargazer* gene encodes a neuronal Ca^{2+}-channel gamma subunit. Nat Genet 1998; 19:340–347.

Letts VA, Valenzuela A, Kirley JP, Sweet HO, Davisson MT, Frankel WN: Genetic and physical maps of the *stargazer* locus on mouse chromosome 15. Genomics 1997; 43:62–68.

Lewis J: Notch signalling and the control of cell fate choices in vertebrates. Semin Cell Dev Biol 1998; 9:583–589.

Lipton RB, Ottman R, Ehrenberg BL, Hauser WA: Comorbidity of migraine: the connection between migraine and epilepsy. Neurology 1994a; 44:S28–S32.

Lipton RB, Silberstein SD, Stewart WF: An update on the epidemiology of migraine. Headache 1994b; 34:319–328.

Lorenzon NM, Lutz CM, Frankel WN, Beam KG: Altered calcium channel currents in Purkinje cells of the neurological mutant mouse leaner. J Neurosci 1998; 18:4482–4489.

Lucas RN: Migraine in twins. J Psychosom Res 1977; 21:147–156.

Maassen VanDenBrink A, Vergouwe MN, Ophoff RA, Naylor SL, Dauwerse HG, Saxena PR, Ferrari MD, Frants RR: Chromosomal localization of the 5-HT1F receptor gene: no evidence for involvement in response to sumatriptan in migraine patients. Am J Med Genet 1998; 77:415–420.

Matsuyama Z, Wakamori M, Mori Y, Kawakami H, Nakamura S, Imoto K: Direct alteration of the P/Q-type Ca^{2+} channel property by polyglutamine expansion in spinocerebellar ataxia 6. J Neurosci 1999; 19:RC14.

May A, Ophoff RA, Terwindt GM, Urban C, van Eijk R, Haan J, Diener HC, Lindhout D, Frants RR, Sandkuijl LA, et al.: Familial hemiplegic migraine locus on 19p13 is involved in the common forms of migraine with and without aura. Hum Genet 1995; 96:604–608.

McClatchey AI, Van den Bergh P, Pericak-Vance MA, Raskind W, Verellen C, McKenna-Yasek D, Rao K, Haines JL, Bird T, Brown RH Jr, et al.: Temperature-sensitive mutations in the III-IV cytoplasmic loop region of the skeletal muscle sodium channel gene in paramyotonia congenita. Cell 1992; 68:769–774.

Mochi M, Sangiorgi S, Cortelli P, Carelli V, Scapoli C, Crisci M, Monari L, Pierangeli G, Montagna P: Testing models for genetic determination in migraine. Cephalalgia 1993; 13:389–394.

Montagna P, Cortelli P, Barbiroli B: Magnetic resonance spectroscopy studies in migraine. Cephalalgia 1994; 14:184–193.

Mori Y, Wakamori M, Oda S, Fletcher CF, Sekiguchi N, Mori E, Copeland NG, Jenkins NA, Matsushita K, Matsuyama Z, et al.: Reduced voltage sensitivity of activation of P/Q-type Ca^{2+} channels is associated with the ataxic mouse mutation rolling Nagoya (tg(rol)). J Neurosci 2000; 20:5654–5662.

Mosewich RK, Donat JR, DiMauro S, Ciafaloni E, Shanske S, Erasmus M, George D: The syndrome of mitochondrial encephalomyopathy, lactic acidosis, and stroke-like episodes presenting without stroke. Arch Neurol 1993; 50:275–278.

Moskowitz MA: The neurobiology of vascular head pain. Ann Neurol 1984; 16:157–168.

Moskowitz MA: Basic mechanisms in vascular headache. Neurol Clin 1990; 8:801–815.

Neyroud N, Tesson F, Denjoy I, Leibovici M, Donger C, Barhanin J, Faure S, Gary F, Coumel P, Petit C, et al.: A novel mutation in the potassium channel gene *KVLQT1* causes the Jervell and Lange-Nielsen cardioauditory syndrome. Nat Genet 1997; 15:186–189.

Nyholt DR, Curtain RP, Gaffney PT, Brimage P, Goadsby PJ, Griffiths LR: Migraine association and linkage analyses of the human 5-hydroxytryptamine (5-HT2A) receptor gene. Cephalalgia 1996; 16:463–467.

Nyholt DR, Curtain RP, Griffiths LR: Familial typical migraine; significant linkage and localization of a gene to Xq24–28. Hum Genet 2000; 107:18–23.

Nyholt DR, Dawkins JL, Brimage PJ, Goadsby PJ, Nicholson GA, Griffiths LR: Evidence for an X-linked genetic component in familial typical migraine. Hum Mol Genet 1998a; 7:459–463.

Nyholt DR, Lea RA, Goadsby PJ, Brimage PJ, Griffiths LR: Familial typical migraine: linkage to chromosome 19p13 and evidence for genetic heterogeneity. Neurology 1998b; 50:1428–1432.

O'Brien B, Goeree R, Streiner D: Prevalence of migraine headache in Canada: a population-based survey. Int J Epidemiol 1994; 23:1020–1026.

Ohta M, Shukuro A, Kuriowa Y: Familial occurence of migraine with a hemiplegic syndrome and cerebellar infarctions. Neurology 1967; 17:813–817.

Olesen J: New international headache classification. Neuroepidemiology 1989; 8:53–55.

O'Neill BP, Mann JD: Aspirin prophylaxis in migraine. Lancet 1978; 2:1179–1181.

Ophoff RA, Terwindt GM, Vergouwe MN, van Eijk R, Oefner PJ, Hoffman SM, Lamerdin JE, Mohrenweiser HW, Bulman DE, Ferrari M, et al.: Familial hemiplegic migraine and episodic ataxia type-2 are caused by mutations in the Ca^{2+} channel gene *CACNL1A4*. Cell 1996; 87:543–552.

Osuntokun BO, Adeuja AO, Nottidge VA, Bademosi O, Alumide AO, Ige O, Yaria F, Schoenberg BS, Bolis CL: Prevalence of headache and migrainous headache in Nigerian Africans: a community-based study. East Afr Med J 1992; 69(4):196–199.

Peroutka SJ, Wilhoit T, Jones K: Clinical susceptibility to migraine with aura is modified by dopamine D2 receptor (DRD2) NcoI alleles. Neurology 1997; 49:201–206.

Prensky AL, Sommer D: Diagnosis and treatment of migraine in children. Neurology 1979; 29:506–514.

Ptacek LJ, George AL Jr, Barchi RL, Griggs RC, Riggs JE, Robertson M, Leppert MF: Mutations in an S4 segment of the adult skeletal muscle sodium channel cause paramyotonia congenita. Neuron 1992; 8:891–897.

Ptacek LJ, George AL Jr, Griggs RC, Tawil R, Kallen RG, Barchi RL, Robertson M, Leppert MF: Identification of a mutation in the gene causing hyperkalemic periodic paralysis. Cell 1991; 67:1021–1027.

Ptacek LJ, Tawil R, Griggs RC, Engel AG, Layzer RB, Kwiecinski H, McManis PG, Santiago L, Moore M, Fouad G, et al.: Dihydropyridine receptor mutations cause hypokalemic periodic paralysis. Cell 1994; 77:863–868.

Quane KA, Healy JM, Keating KE, Manning BM, Couch FJ, Palmucci LM, Doriguzzi C, Fagerlund TH, Berg K, Ording H, et al.: Mutations in the ryanodine receptor gene in central core disease and malignant hyperthermia. Nat Genet 1993; 5:51–55.

Rasmussen BK, Olesen J: Migraine with aura and migraine without aura: an epidemiological study. Cephalalgia 1992; 12:221–228.

Russell MB, Iselius L, Olesen J: Inheritance of migraine investigated by complex segregation analysis. Hum Genet 1995; 96:726–730.

Russell MB, Olesen J: The genetics of migraine without aura and migraine with aura. Cephalalgia 1993; 13:245–248.

Russell MB, Olesen J: Increased familial risk and evidence of genetic factor in migraine. BMJ 1995; 311:541–544.

Sano M, Ozawa M, Shiota S, Momose Y, Uchigata M, Goto Y: The T-C(8356) mitochondrial DNA mutation in a Japanese family. J Neurol 1996; 243:441–444.

Scharff L, Turk DC, Marcus DA: Triggers of headache episodes and coping responses of headache diagnostic groups. Headache 1995; 35:397–403.

Schlake HP, Bottger IG, Grotemeyer KH, Husstedt IW, Oberwittler C, Schober O: The influence of acetazolamide on cerebral low-flow regions in migraine—an interictal 99mTc-HMPAO SPECT study. Cephalalgia 1992; 12:284–288.

Schulze-Bahr E, Wang Q, Wedekind H, Haverkamp W, Chen Q, Sun Y, Rubie C, Hordt M, Towbin JA, Borggrefe M, et al.: *KCNE1* mutations cause Jervell and Lange-Nielsen syndrome. Nat Genet 1997; 17:267–268.

Shiang R, Ryan SG, Zhu YZ, Hahn AF, O'Connell P, Wasmuth JJ: Mutations in the alpha 1 subunit of the inhibitory glycine receptor cause the dominant neurologic disorder, hyperexplexia. Nat Genet 1993; 5:351–358.

Sillanpää M, Anttila P: Increasing prevalence of headache in 7-year-old schoolchildren. Headache 1996; 36:466–470.

Sine SM, Ohno K, Bouzat C, Auerbach A, Milone M, Pruitt JN, Engel AG: Mutation of the acetylcholine receptor alpha subunit causes a slow-channel myasthenic syndrome by enhancing agonist binding affinity. Neuron 1995; 15:229–239.

Singh NA, Charlier C, Stauffer D, DuPont BR, Leach RJ, Melis R, Ronen GM, Bjerre I, Quattlebaum T, Murphy JV, et al.: A novel potassium channel gene, *KCNQ2*, is mutated in an inherited epilepsy of newborns. Nat Genet 1998; 18:25–29.

Splawski I, Timothy KW, Vincent GM, Atkinson DL, Keating MT: Molecular basis of the long-QT syndrome associated with deafness. N Engl J Med 1997a; 336:1562–1567.

Splawski I, Tristani-Firouzi M, Lehmann MH, Sanguinetti MC, Keating MT: Mutations in the *hminK* gene cause long QT syndrome and suppress IKs function. Nat Genet 1997b; 17:338–340.

Steinlein OK, Mulley JC, Propping P, Wallace RH, Phillips HA, Sutherland GR, Scheffer IE, Berkovic SF: A missense mutation in the neuronal nicotinic acetylcholine receptor alpha 4 subunit is associated with autosomal dominant nocturnal frontal lobe epilepsy. Nat Genet 1995; 11:201–203.

Stewart WF, Linet MS, Celentano DD, Van Natta M, Ziegler D: Age- and sex-specific incidence rates of migraine with and without visual aura. Am J Epidemiol 1991; 134:1111–1120.

Stewart WF, Lipton RB, Celentano DD, Reed ML: Prevalence of migraine headache in the United States. Relation to age, income, race and other sociodemographic factors. JAMA 1992; 267:64–69.

Stewart WF, Lipton RB, Liberman J: Variation in migraine prevalence by race. Neurology 1996; 47:52–59.

Stewart WF, Staffa J, Lipton RB, Ottman R: Familial risk of migraine: a population-based study. Ann Neurol 1997; 41:166–172.

Terwindt GM, Ophoff RA, Haan J, Vergouwe MN, van Eijk R, Frants RR, Ferrari MD: Variable clinical expression of mutations in the P/Q-type calcium channel gene in familial hemiplegic migraine. Dutch Migraine Genetics Research Group. Neurology 1998; 50:1105–1110.

Terwindt GM, Ophoff RA, van Eijk R, Vergouwe MN, Haan J, Frants RR, Sandkuijl LA, Ferrari MD: Dutch Migraine Genetics Research Group. Involvement of the *CACNA1A* gene containing region on 19p13 in migraine with and without aura. Neurology 2001; 56:1028–1032.

Tokio S, Hisanori K, Toshiya N, Kazuro T: Prevalence of migraine in western Japan. Cephalalgia 1993; 13:10.

Tyson J, Tranebjaerg L, Bellman S, Wren C, Taylor JF, Bathen J, Aslaksen B, Sorland SJ, Lund O, Malcolm S, et al.: IsK and KvLQT1: mutation in either of the two subunits of the slow component of the delayed rectifier potassium channel can cause Jervell and Lange-Nielsen syndrome. Hum Mol Genet 1997; 6:2179–2185.

Ulrich V, Gervil M, Kyvik KO, Olesen J, Russell MB: Evidence of a genetic factor in migraine with aura: a population-based Danish twin study. Ann Neurol 1999; 45:242–246.

Ulrich V, Russell MB, Ostergaard S, Olesen J: Analysis of 31 families with an apparently autosomal-dominant transmission of migraine with aura in the nuclear family. Am J Med Genet 1997; 74:395–397.

Verin M, Rolland Y, Landgraf F, Chabriat H, Bompais B, Michel A, Vahedi K, Martinet JP, Tournier-Lasserve E, Lemaitre MH, et al.: New phenotype of the cerebral autosomal dominant arteriopathy mapped to chromosome 19: migraine as the prominent clinical feature. J Neurol Neurosurg Psychiatry 1995; 59:579–585.

Wallace RH, Wang DW, Singh R, Scheffer IE, George AL Jr, Phillips HA, Saar K, Reis A, Johnson EW, Sutherland GR, et al.: Febrile seizures and generalized epilepsy associated with a mutation in the Na^+-channel beta1 subunit gene *SCN1B*. Nat Genet 1998; 19:366–370.

Wang Q, Curran ME, Splawski I, Burn TC, Millholland JM, VanRaay TJ, Shen J, Timothy KW, Vincent GM, de Jager T, et al.: Positional cloning of a novel potassium channel gene: *KVLQT1* mutations cause cardiac arrhythmias. Nat Genet 1996; 12:17–23.

Wang Q, Shen J, Splawski I, Atkinson D, Li Z, Robinson JL, Moss AJ, Towbin JA, Keating MT: *SCN5A* mutations associated with an inherited cardiac arrhythmia, long QT syndrome. Cell 1995; 80:805–811.

Weiller C, May A, Limmroth V, Juptner M, Kaube H, Schayck RV, Coenen HH, Diener HC: Brain stem activation in spontaneous human migraine attacks. Nat Med 1995; 1:658–660.

Welch KM, Levine SR, D'Andrea G, Schultz LR, Helpern JA: Preliminary observations on brain energy metabolism in migraine studied by in vivo phosphorus ^{31}NMR spectroscopy. Neurology 1989; 39:538–541.

White NJ, Hosford DA, Humprey PP, Boyd PR, Griffits LR, Peroutka S, Roses AD, Purvis IJ, McCarthy LC: Single nucleotide polymorphism (SNP) alleles in the insulin receptor (*INSR*) gene are associated with migraine. Cephalalgia 2001; 21:280.

Winther K: Ketanserin—a seletive serotonin agonist, in relation to platelet aggregation and migraine attack rate. Cephalalgia 1985; 5:402–403.

Woods RP, Iacoboni M, Mazziotta JC: Bilateral spreading cerebral hypoperfusion during spontaneous migraine headache. N Engl J Med 1994; 331:1689–1692.

Yue Q, Jen JC, Nelson SF, Baloh RW: Progressive ataxia due to a missense mutation in a calcium-channel gene. Am J Hum Genet 1997; 61:1078–1087.

Yue Q, Jen JC, Thwe MM, Nelson SF, Baloh RW: De novo mutation in *CACNA1A* caused acetazolamide-responsive episodic ataxia. Am J Med Genet 1998; 77:298–301.

Zhang Y, Chen HS, Khanna VK, De Leon S, Phillips MS, Schappert K, Britt BA, Brownell AKW, MacLennan DHA: A mutation in the human ryanodine receptor gene associated with central core disease. Nat Genet 1993; 5:46–50.

Zhuchenko O, Bailey J, Bonnen P, Ashizawa T, Stockton DW, Amos C, Dobyns WB, Subramony SH, Zoghbi HY, Lee CC: Autosomal dominant cerebellar ataxia (SCA6) associated with small polyglutamine expansions in the alpha 1A-voltage-dependent calcium channel. Nat Genet 1997; 15:62–69.

Ziegler DK, Hur YM, Bouchard TJ Jr, Hassanein RS, Barter R: Migraine in twins raised together and apart. Headache 1998; 38:417–422.

Ziegler DK, Stephenson Hassanein R, Harris D, Stewart R: Headache in a non-clinic twin population. Headache 1975; 14:213–218.

Zifkin B, Andermann E, Andermann F, Kirkham T: An autosomal dominant syndrome of hemiplegic migraine, nystagmus, and tremor. Ann Neurol 1980; 8:329–332.

Part X

OTHER COMMON PROBLEMS

50 Common Skin Diseases

VIRGINIA P. SYBERT

The common skin disorders for which a genetic basis has been sought or which have excited interest are primarily limited to those suspected of having an autoimmune or immunoregulatory basis: atopic dermatitis (see Chapter 11), psoriasis, vitiligo, alopecia areata, and systemic lupus erythematosus (see Chapter 31). Other common dermatologic disorders, such as acne, have generated less interest in genetic research, even though they too appear to have genetic determinants. Perhaps the most common skin condition with clear-cut genetic dependence, male pattern baldness, has enjoyed the least rigorous study regarding genetic mechanisms.

There are genetic components to these common conditions, but we do not know what they are. For the most part, the disorders are relatively common in the general population, achieving the statistical status of polymorphisms. There is an increased, but poorly quantified, risk to family members. No predictive testing and no prenatal diagnosis are available.

VITILIGO

Vitiligo is an acquired progressive disorder of circumscribed depigmentation of the skin. It results from destruction of the melanocytes in the skin and mucous membranes. The melanocytes in the ear and eye may also be involved. The affected skin is white, with a well-defined border between involved and uninvolved skin. In some individuals, there can be variation of pigment loss within a lesion (trichrome or multichrome). Affected areas fluoresce brightly with Woods' lamp. There is no alteration in skin texture or skin appendages. The patches may be small or large and follow a segmental or a symmetric mirror image pattern or are isolated. Any cutaneous surface can be involved. Sites of predilection include periorificial areas, over bony prominences, and in folds. Vitiligo can spontaneously regress, remain stable, recur, or progress. The diagnosis is almost always evident clinically. Skin biopsy is rarely necessary.

Segmental vitiligo may be an entity distinct from generalized vitiligo. It is more common in children and almost never progresses to generalized disease. It may involve the melanocytes of the hair follicles more than classic vitiligo and, thus, is more likely to be stable and refractory to therapy.

General Genetic and Epidemiologic Evidence

Clinical Epidemiology and Ethnic Differences

Surveys suggest that the incidence of vitiligo is highest among natives of India and Mexico and lowest in Europeans (Table 50–1). This may reflect the more readily detectable loss of color in more darkly pigmented individuals or greater concern for the condition when it is cosmetically obvious as most surveys are of populations seeking specialized medical care and not of the general population.

There is no difference in the occurrence of vitiligo among different racial groups residing within the United States or between the sexes. Vitiligo can and does occur at any age. Onset is most common between 10 and 30 years of age.

Family Epidemiology

In a variety of studies using a variety of methods, most of them simply obtaining family history without documentation, estimates for a positive family history in probands range from 6.5% to 78.25%. Both extremes were found in populations in India (Nordlund and Ortonne, 1998 and references within).

Table 50–2 summarizes the occurrence of vitiligo among first-degree relatives and probands when evaluated by specific relationship.

In a study by Ando et al. (1993), 29 of 131 (22%) patients with nonsegmental vitiligo gave a positive family history as defined by one or more affected relatives within three generations. Those with a positive family history had a younger mean age at onset (12.7 vs. 32.6 years). There was no difference in distribution or extent of disease and no difference in sex ratio or presence of thyroid autoantibodies, positive antinuclear antibody or rheumatoid factor. Schallreuter et al. (1994) found a positive family history in 88 of 321 (27.8%) patients with vitiligo. There was a greater likelihood of a positive family history (37.6%) among patients with childhood-onset vitiligo than among those in whom the disease first presented in adult life. Further, 3 of 4 individuals with widespread vitiligo and onset in childhood gave a positive family history compared with 1 of 5 with adult onset of widespread disease.

Of 300 questionnaires mailed to members of the National Vitiligo Association (Majumder et al., 1993; Nath et al., 1994) requesting information regarding family history, 194 were returned. Of the 150 Caucasian probands who responded, 31 (20.7%) had affected first-degree relatives.

Bhatia et al. (1992) evaluated 400 patients with vitiligo presenting to a medical clinic in India, among whose 13,807 relatives 124 (0.89%) had vitiligo compared with 14 of 3937 (0.35%) relatives of controls ($p \leq 0.01$). The authors stated that they examined "most of the relatives" for confirmation. Of the patients with a positive family history, 60% had two or more affected family members.

Of 127 families with a child with vitiligo presenting to a pediatric hospital in Mexico, 18.1% had a positive family history (Carnevale et al., 1980), with 2.3% of first-degree relatives having vitiligo. The condition was present in 1.1% of second-degree relatives.

Table 50–1. Incidence of Vitiligo among Different Geographic Groups

Country	Incidence (%)
India	1.79–8.8
Japan	1.64
Europe	
Russia	0.14
England	0.15–0.42
Switzerland	0.39
France	0.6–3
Italy	0.3
Denmark	0.38–1.44
North America	
United States	0.14–3.2
Mexico	2.6–4

Source: Modified from Ortonne et al. (1983).

Twin Studies

There have been no systematic twin studies in vitiligo. Goudie et al. (1980) reported two sets of monozygotic twins concordant for anatomical patterns of vitiligo.

Adoption Studies

To my knowledge, there have been no adoption studies on vitiligo.

Associations with Other Diseases

Vitiligo occurs in conjunction with several other disorders of presumed autoimmune origin: thyroid disease, diabetes mellitus, pernicious anemia, and alopecia areata.

There are numerous reports demonstrating an increased prevalence of thyroid disease among individuals with vitiligo, ranging from asymptomatic increased levels of circulating thyroid autoantibodies to raging Hashimoto's thyroiditis. Estimates for concomitant thyroid disease range from 2% to 30% among different series of patients with vitiligo (Cunliffe et al., 1968; Schallreuter et al., 1994). Cunliffe et al. (1968) compared 56 patients with vitiligo to 56 psoriatics matched for age and sex: 30% of the former had evidence of thyroid disease compared to 13% of the psoriatics. Nordlund and Ortonne (1998) argued that the prevalence of thyroid disease in vitiligo is 7.5%, lower than the estimated 10% to 15% prevalence for thyroid disease in the U.S. population, and maintained that the association between the two disorders may be specious. Their figures were not, however, analyzed on the basis of age. As the incidence of thyroid disease increases with age and vitiligo is a disorder of the relatively young, one would do better to use an age-matched control population for comparison rather than the general U.S. population.

Diabetes mellitus has been reported with vitiligo in a number of series, with prevalence ranging from 1% to 7.1%. The number of patients in each series was small. The basis for this association is not understood (Ortonne et al., 1983 and references within).

Pernicious anemia occurs in 0% to 9.2% of patients with vitiligo, according to surveys. Vitiligo occurs in 1.6% to 10.6% of patients with pernicious anemia. There were 1398 subjects in the study reporting the 1.6% prevalence and 84 in the study reporting 10.6% (Ortonne et al., 1983 and references within). The basis for the association of the two disorders is unknown. A common autoimmune cause, with increased gastric parietal cell antibodies in patients with vitiligo, has been proposed.

Alopecia areata is reported in 0.4% to 16% of patients with vitiligo. Conversely, 1.6% to 15.6% of patients with alopecia areata have vitiligo (Cunliffe et al., 1968 and references within; Schallreuter et al., 1994).

Vitiligo also appears to be more common among patients with Addison's disease (3.1% to 20%). The converse is not true. This co-occurrence may represent a single-gene disorder, polyglandular insufficiency, rather than an association.

As there are melanocytes in the ear, the association of vitiligo with hearing loss has also been investigated. Tosti and colleagues (1987) found abnormal audiologic test results in the absence of clinical disease in 16% of 50 patients with vitiligo who were less than 40 years of age, had a negative family history for hearing loss, and had no history of environmental exposures deleterious to hearing. They found no audiologic abnormalities in a group of 40 control patients.

Despite these recognized associations, most patients with vitiligo are otherwise healthy and have no other disease.

Environmental Factors

Stress and trauma have long been implicated by the lay population as causal in vitiligo. The support for this is anecdotal and unconvincing.

Chemical exposures, e.g., to the monobenzylether of hydroquinone, can result in permanent loss of skin color. This untoward effect can be used therapeutically to depigment the normal skin in patients with widespread vitiligo in whom repigmentation is unlikely.

Pathophysiology: Biologic Basis of Genetic Susceptibility

The pathogenesis of vitiligo is unknown, but hypotheses abound.

Autoimmunity is believed to play a role for the following reasons:

1. There is an association with other autoimmune disorders.
2. Individuals with vitiligo have a higher likelihood of having autoantibodies to endocrine organs.

Table 50–2 Occurrence of Vitiligo in Relatives of Probands

Reference	Location	No.	Fathers	Mothers	Brothers	Sisters	Sons	Daughters	Ascertainment
Nath et al. (1994)	United States	160	7/155	7/149	8/157	9/152	9/106	11/108	Mailed questionnaire, National Vitiligo Association
Hafez et al. (1982)	Egypt	150	16/149	14/147	28/346	32/384			Not stated
Carnevale et al. (1980)	Mexico	127	1/128	9/127	6/155	13/156			Pediatric dermatology clinic
Bhatia et al. (1992)	India	400						Offspring 14/998	Outpatient dermatology clinic

3. In a single study, the majority of patients with vitiligo had antibodies to tyrosinase compared with none of the controls and 12% of patients with autoimmune endocrine disease (Song et al., 1994).

Other theories include autocytotoxicity caused by reaction against leakage of melanin into the cytoplasm and neural causation, in which a neurochemical mediator causes reduction in melanin production. This latter hypothesis is based on alterations in adrenergic and parasympathetic tone in depigmented skin (Ortonne et al., 1983 and references within).

Gene Identification

Linkage and Association

Among 20 individuals with vitiligo and a positive family history, 42% were positive for antigen BW46 compared with 15% of 19 nonfamilial cases. Among individuals with vitiligo and no family history, 42% were positive for human leukocyte antigens A31 and CW4 (Ando et al., 1993).

No linkage with blood groups ABO, Rh, Kell, or Duffy was found among 170 Sudanese patients with vitiligo (Wasfi et al., 1980). In the same population, an excess of the α_1-antitrypsin genotype *MZ* was seen (20% compared with 5% in the general population and 16% among blood donors).

Animal Models

There have been no candidate genes identified in vitiligo. Animal models of vitiligo are unsatisfying. Sinclair swine, which have been proposed as a potential model for vitiligo, are at high risk to develop melanoma. They depigment when their tumors regress. While halo nevi (loss of pigment surrounding pigmented nevocytic nevi) and vitiligo have been reported in patients with melanoma, most patients with vitiligo do not have pigment cell malignancy. C57BL/6mi^{vit} mi^{vit} mice are born with a piebald streak and progressively depigment with successive shedding of hair. The *mi* gene is not abnormal in humans with vitiligo (Nordlund and Ortonne, 1998 and references within). The Smyth chicken loses feather pigment with the second molt and develops uveitis and autoimmune thyroiditis due to a defect in tyrosinase. It is believed that the inherited defect stimulates an immune response to the melanocyte and leads to its destruction (Nordlund and Ortonne, 1998). This may be a good model for Vogt-Koyanagi-Harada syndrome.

Clinical Application and Risk Assessment of Genetics Information

Little work has been done to calculate the empiric risk of vitiligo for family members. Hafez et al. (1982), studying 150 probands, determined that the risk to develop vitiligo for first-degree relatives was 8.7%, that for second-degree relatives was 3.1%, and that for third-degree relatives was 1.1%. Carnevale et al. (1980) suggested a risk to second-degree relatives of 1.8%.

Beyond the recognition that individuals with earlier onset of vitiligo are more likely to have affected relatives and that the majority of relatives of individuals with vitiligo will not develop the disease, there is little practical utility to be gleaned from these results. There are no predictive markers that one can use for screening. There is no way to prevent the disorder from occurring, and treatment is the same for those with a family history and those without (Howitz et al., 1977; Roundtable 1986; Tosti et al., 1986).

ALOPECIA AREATA

Alopecia areata is an acquired condition of abrupt, nonscarring hair loss without underlying disease. It usually presents with an isolated, well-circumscribed, round or oval bald patch. The disorder may remit spontaneously, recur, persist, or spread. Scalp, beard, eyebrows, eyelashes, and body hairs can be involved. *Alopecia areata* refers to patchy loss, *alopecia totalis* to complete loss of head hair, and *alopecia universalis* to loss of all body hair. There has been an attempt to sort out subtypes of alopecia areata (e.g., common, atopic, prehypertensive), but these are not generally accepted. While there is general agreement that alopecia areata is heterogeneous, no studies of inheritance have analyzed patients using distinct subtypes.

General Genetic and Epidemiologic Evidence

Clinical Epidemiology and Ethnic Differences

Alopecia areata is a disorder with peak age at onset between 20 and 50 years, although it is not uncommon in children.

The prevalence of alopecia areata in surveys of the general population and among patients presenting to dermatologists ranges from <1% to 2.5% (Jackson, 1898 and references within). Males and females are equally likely to be affected. There may be racial predilection and geographic differences. For example, Arnold (1952) found that alopecia areata was more common among Hawaiians of Japanese descent than Hawaiians of other ethnic groups. Because alopecia areata is often a transient condition with little impact on health, differences in the rates at which individuals present for medical evaluation may reflect economic and social priorities rather than true geographic or ethnic differences in the disease.

Family Epidemiology

A positive family history has been reported in 3% to 28% of patients (Kianto et al., 1977; Messenger and Simpson, 1997 and references within).

Müller and Winkelmann (1963) identified 736 patients with alopecia areata treated at the Mayo Clinic between 1945 and 1954. They sent out questionnaires to 460 of these, of which 78% were returned. Ten percent reported a positive family history. There were 18 parent–child pairs, 21 sibling pairs, two sets of identical twins, one set of fraternal twins, and two other twin sets of unknown zygosity.

Shellow and colleagues (1992) sent 4000 questionnaires to members of the National Alopecia Areata Association, of which 800 were returned. Of these, 42% indicated a positive family history, with a total of 333 affected relatives: 144 individuals reported one affected relative, 47 had two, 22 had three, two had four, three had five, and one proband had six relatives with alopecia areata. Although numbers were given for each type of relative affected (e.g., 40 mothers, 73 siblings), no denominators were given.

van der Steen et al. (1992) reviewed 348 patients from two clinics, one in Nijmegen and one in Münster. Of these, 56 had one affected first-degree relative and five had two first-degree relatives with alopecia areata. Thirteen percent of patients with patchy alopecia areata had a positive family history compared to 18% of patients with alopecia totalis. There was no difference in age at onset between those with and without a positive family history. Twenty-five of 796 parents, 27 of 900 siblings, and 9 of 357 children were affected (3%, 3%, and 2.5%, respectively), with males and females equally likely to be affected.

Twin Studies

There have been no systematic twin studies on alopecia areata, solely isolated case reports of concordance (Turnacliff, 1931; Omens and Omens, 1946; Hendren, 1949; Weidman et al., 1956 and references within), most of which do not substantiate zygosity. Two of three sets of identical twins in one report were discordant for alopecia areata (Duvic et al., 1995).

Adoption Studies

To my knowledge, there have been no adoption studies on alopecia areata.

Association with Other Diseases

An association between alopecia areata and atopy has been suggested. The definition of atopy has differed from study to study, and the proportion of patients with both conditions has ranged from 52%, based on skin patch testing, to 1% (Messenger and Simpson, 1997 and references within). It is generally believed that the co-occurrence of atopy augurs a worse prognosis for alopecia areata and may be associated with earlier onset.

Alopecia areata appears to be more common in patients with Down syndrome (13/100, 60/1000) (Messenger and Simpson, 1997 and references within). The basis for this association is unclear. Messenger and Simpson (1997) suggest that the common link is an increased susceptibility to autoimmune disease of all types in Down syndrome.

Thyroid disease may be more common in patients with alopecia areata. In Müller and Winkelmann's (1963) series, 8% of patients with alopecia areata had thyroid disease. There was no control population for comparison and no indication of the age of the patients with thyroid disease. Some series have found an increased association of alopecia areata with frank thyroid disease or presence of thyroid autoantibodies; others have not.

An increased occurrence of Type 1 diabetes in relatives of probands with alopecia areata, but not in the probands themselves, has been noted (Messenger and Simpson, 1997 and references within).

Other autoimmune disorders, including vitiligo, pernicious anemia, and systemic lupus erythematosus, have been reported with alopecia areata. It can also be seen in association with the autoimmune polyglandular syndrome. Despite these reports, most patients with alopecia areata are entirely healthy.

Environmental Factors

Environmental factors have long enjoyed popularity as major players in alopecia areata, especially emotional and physical stress, though no association has been proven.

Pathophysiology: Biologic Basis of Genetic Susceptibility

Alopecia areata is believed to be an autoimmune disorder. This is based primarily on the histologic features of the disorder, which demonstrate a perifollicular lymphocytic infiltrate composed primarily of suppressor T cells. In addition, some studies have shown increased levels of autoantibodies to thyroid cells, gastric parietal cells, and smooth muscle cells (Mitchell and Krull, 1984 and references within; Messenger and Simpson, 1997 and references within) in patients with alopecia areata. These findings coupled with the co-occurrence of other autoimmune diseases in individuals with alopecia areata have provided support for this hypothesis. Furthermore, treatments for alopecia areata include corticosteroid use, believed to suppress the immune response, and autoeczematization (deliberately creating contact allergy to applied chemicals), believed to override the autoimmune phenomenon.

Evidence against the autoimmune hypothesis includes the absence of consistent immunofluorescent antibody findings in biopsies from patients with alopecia areata and no consistent finding of alterations in cell-mediated immunity.

The affected hair follicle in alopecia areata is believed to have a truncated anagen–telogen cycle, which results in failure to establish a long enough anagen phase for visible regrowth of hair. Where the abnormality in the hair follicle is situated is unknown. The keratinocytes of the precortical matrix may be the location of primary injury. Others have suggested that abnormalities of the dermal papilla may be the cause (Messenger and Simpson, 1997).

As pointed out by McDonagh and Messenger (1996), abnormalities in alopecia areata are not limited to the hair follicle. Any explanation for the pathogenesis of alopecia areata must also account for the nail involvement seen in the disorder.

Cork and colleagues (1995) suggested that there may be genes that control the severity of alopecia areata rather than susceptibility per se to the condition. They looked at polymorphisms in interleukin-1α (IL-1α) in 90 patients with alopecia areata, divided into patchy, totalis, and universalis groups. These were compared with 261 controls. IL-1α was chosen because its antagonist is reduced in other inflammatory skin diseases, it inhibits human hair follicle growth in organ culture, and the laboratory works on this molecule. Allele 2 (a VNTR polymorphism) was found in 41% of controls, 44% of patchy alopecia areata patients, 66% of alopecia totalis patients, and 77% of alopecia universalis patients ($p = 0.005$).

Gene Identification

Linkage and Association

Studies of human leukocyte antigen (HLA) associations and linkage have suggested an association with class 2 antigens, with relative risks ranging from 2- to 30-fold. There appear to be differences between those patients with longstanding and those with transient disease. Similarly, there may be differences in HLA association with extensive vs. limited disease (Colombe et al., 1995; Duvic et al., 1995). However, most studies of HLA associations have not stratified patients by phenotype. Table 50–3 presents the HLA associations that have been demonstrated.

Duvic and colleagues (1991) suggested that linkage to HLA, rather than association with it, might play a role. Valsecchi et al. (1984) saw no crossovers between HLA haplotype Aw32 or B18 and alopecia areata among six affected family members. The truncated pedigree provided in the report does not include any information about unaffected family members. Hordinsky and colleagues (1984) found no linkage with HLA in a family with six informative meioses. Zlotogorski et al. (1990) excluded linkage to HLA in two families.

Animal Models

The brown hooded rat is born with hairs that are lost subsequently. The histologic features are similar to alopecia areata in humans, and regrowth is stimulated by psoralen plus ultraviolet A (PUVA), cyclosporin A, and monoxidil. The C3H/HeJ mouse develops circular patches of hair loss associated strongly with those mice that are bred for inflammatory bowel disease (Mc-

Table 50–3. Association of Human Leukocyte Antigen (HLA) with Alopecia Areata

Reference	No. Patients	Country	HLA Association
McDonagh and Messenger (1996)[a]	Not stated	China	Bw62
	22	USA	DR4, DR5
	65	UK	DR4
	13	USA	DR4, DR5
Orecchia et al. (1987)	41	Denmark	DR4, DPw4
	54	UK	DR4
	127	Italy	DR5 (n.s.)[b]
Duvic et al. (1991)	98	USA	DR4, DwII (DR5)
Morling et al. (1991)	20	Denmark	DQB1*0301 (DQ7)
Valsecchi et al. (1984)	40	Italy	None
Hacham-Zadeh et al. (1981)	46	Israel (mixed Jewish)	B18
Colombe et al. (1995)	131	USA	DQ3[c]
			DQB1* 0301 (DQ7)[c]
			DRB1*1104 (DR11)[c]
Duvic et al. (1995)	86	USA	DR4
			DQW8
			DR5
	85	USA	DQB1*0301 (DQ7)
Kuntz et al. (1977)	70	Germany	None
Kianto et al. (1977)	47	Finland	B12

[a]See also references within.
[b]n.s., not significant.
[c]In patients with longstanding disease; no association with 31 newly diagnosed patients.

Donagh and Messenger, 1996). The Dundee experimental bald rat exhibits nonscarring hair loss characterized histologically by a lymphocytic perifollicular and intrafollicular infiltrate (Sundberg and King, 1996).

Clinical Application and Risk Assessment of Genetics Information

The diagnosis of alopecia areata is usually straightforward. Typically, there is a sudden onset of localized hair loss without scarring, activity at the margins (easy hair pull), presence of exclamation mark hairs (broken telogen hairs), and often pitting of the nails.

The disorder is not amenable either to screening or to prevention. The magnitude of the increased relative risk to family members is uncertain, as are predictions of severity and persistence. Atopy, an ophiasis pattern of hair loss (along the nuchal hairline), and/or loss of eyebrows and eyelashes are negative prognostic indicators, as are extensive disease at first presentation and young age at onset. In children with alopecia areata who appear otherwise healthy and to be growing normally, screening tests for thyroid dysfunction are not necessarily indicated. Decisions regarding testing for thyroid function and anemia in patients presenting with alopecia areata can be left to the practitioner's discretion.

Treatment for most patients with limited disease is reassurance. Use of topical or injected corticosteroids, topical irritants such as anthralin, topical sensitizers such as squaric acid dibutyl ester, or PUVA or monoxidil therapy may be indicated; but these are often unsuccessful (Mitchell and Krull, 1984; Roundtable 1987; Taylor et al., 1995; McDonagh and Messenger, 1996; Schuttelaar et al., 1996).

MALE PATTERN BALDNESS

Despite the intense interest in androgenetic hair loss (or common baldness, male premature alopecia), with an estimated $1.5 billion spent annually on treatment for hair loss (Fischer, 1997), its inheritance remains unclear.

If one defines androgenetic hair loss as the postpubescent replacement of the terminal follicles of the scalp hair by vellous follicles, almost 100% of Caucasian males and females will be affected. If one limits the definition to recognizable and readily visible areas of exposed scalp secondary to this process, about three-fifths of Caucasian males will have male pattern baldness by age 50. Although studies of the inheritance of balding have focused on those who do bald, perhaps it would be more fruitful initially to look for protective genes in the minority which does not.

Hamilton (1951) classified androgenetic baldness as idiopathic, premature, senile, or associated with seborrheic dermatitis. He provided a visual classification system for hair loss, subsequently modified by Norwood (1975), which is still used today. A similar grading system has been established for women. In general, men fitting into Hamilton/Norwood classifications IV through VIII would be considered balding or bald by the laity. Other definitions of androgenetic alopecia have differentiated between onset of noticeable hair loss before age 30 years and onset after age 50 years. This lack of a clear delineation between unaffected and affected states has complicated genetic analysis. The term *common baldness* excludes the androgenetic hair loss in females due to androgen excess.

General Genetic and Epidemiologic Evidence

Clinical Epidemiology and Ethnic Differences

There is considerable variation in the prevalence of baldness among racial groups. The Chinese are least affected. Africans and Japanese also have a relatively low prevalence of baldness. Caucasians enjoy the highest incidence.

Snyder and Yingling (1935) examined 3966 inmates over the age of 35 at state hospitals for the insane in Columbus, Ohio, and Moline, Illinois. Of the 2083 males, 43% were bald (compared with 40% of 200 "normal" individuals). Eight percent of the 1883 females had male pattern baldness.

Table 50–4. Proportion of Males with Male Pattern Baldness among 1000 Veterans Administration Hospital Patients

Degree of Hair Loss (Hamilton Classification)	Age					
	18–29	30–39	40–49	50–59	60–65	70–75
Grade III	6%	18%	20%	23%	15%	16%
>Grade III	6%	20%	27%	29%	50%	48%

Source: Norwood (1975).

Norwood (1975) evaluated 1000 white males, inpatients and outpatients at a Veterans Administration hospital. None had presented with primary complaint of hair loss (the results are given in Table 50–4).

Variation in the patterning of hair loss as well as in degree is seen. Simpson and Barth (1997) claimed that such differences in pattern are also genetically determined "as can be confirmed in any collection of family portraits." This observation has not been systematically confirmed.

Family Epidemiology

It is surprising to realize that rigorous family studies of this common condition are so few. As Küster and Happle (1984) stated: "Careful family studies of androgenetic alopecia thus far are lacking and we admit that we have not embarked on such studies either."

Osborn (1916) evaluated 22 families for baldness. She did not state how they were ascertained and did not stipulate the criteria used to determine bald or not bald. She concluded that the expected to observed number of bald offspring was consistent with the assumption that baldness is a simple autosomal dominant, sex-limited trait with expression in females only in the homozygote state. However, as she could not distinguish carrier women from homozygous normal or heterozygous from homozygous abnormal men, it is not clear how she arrived at her expected outcome. She assumed all females to be homozygous normal unless they had an affected male relative but did not stipulate which of the relatives she considered (e.g., maternal uncle vs. father). Šalamon (1968) evaluated 119 males with Hamilton IV or greater hair loss. He examined relatives and used photographs and patient recall to establish the presence of baldness in relatives. For 16 of these 119 males, there were no other affected males or no reliable data. Of the 103 with a family history of male pattern hair loss, two generations were affected in 65, three in 24, and four in 3 families. Ellis et al. (1998) studied 828 families comprised of 3000 individuals: 58 males between the ages of 18 and 30 years were bald, and 114 males between 50 and 70 years of age were not. He saw no clear pattern of inheritance of baldness among the relatives in either group. Data for 54 of the fathers of the 58 bald males were available: 32 had greater balding than the proband, and 22 had a similar degree of hair loss. Because so many fathers were bald, the authors claimed that an autosomal dominant single-gene disorder could not be the only explanation. They did not, however, exclude simple senescent hair loss in fathers and, thus, may have overdiagnosed male pattern baldness among them. Harris (1947) evaluated 120 bald males between 30 and 42 years of age: 56 of the fathers of 100 prematurely bald men were bald, 55 males with premature balding had at least one brother older than 30 years, 71 of 129 (55%) of these brothers were bald, 28 males with premature balding had prematurely bald fathers and one or more brothers older than 30, 39 of 59 (67%) of these brothers were bald, 24 males with one or more brothers older than 30 had fathers without baldness, and 19 of 41 (46%) of these brothers were prematurely bald. The authors felt that their data best fit with a single-gene autosomal dominant disorder. Maternal history was not taken into account.

Smith and Wells (1964) looked at 56 women with male pattern baldness and found a family history of baldness in 82% compared with 50% of 56 controls with alopecia areata and 43% of controls with no hair loss. Of the 18 women with severe hair loss, 33% had affected fathers and 39% had affected mothers. One-half of the brothers, one-third of the sisters, and 9 of 10 sons were also bald (no information was given regarding balding in the spouses of the probands). The authors did not attempt to distinguish between hair loss due to androgen excess in these women and common baldness.

Studies of male pattern baldness in families have been hampered by delay in age at onset, limited ability to verify historical information, lack of clear-cut diagnostic criteria, and the inability to definitively determine the carrier status of mothers, sisters, and daughters.

Twin Studies

Concordance for male pattern baldness was reported in three pairs of monozygotic twins and in four of eight pairs of dizygotic twins (cited in Küster and Happle, 1984).

Adoption Studies

I am aware of no adoption studies in the literature.

Association with Other Diseases

Although numerous conditions have at one time or another been associated with male pattern baldness, none, including early coronary artery disease, early aging, and increased virility, has been substantiated (Simpson and Barth, 1997 and references within). Hawk et al. (2000) suggested an association of male pattern baldness with an increased relative risk of prostate cancer (1.5, 95% confidence interval 1.12–2.00). This difference reached statistical significance only for the oldest age group, 64+ years. Other studies have not shown such a relationship.

Šalamon (1968) found a correlation for male pattern baldness with chest hairiness in 413 males. Others have not (Simpson and Barth, 1997). Šalamon (1968) found no correlation between hairiness of the lateral leg and male pattern baldness.

Environmental Factors

From time immemorial external causes of male pattern baldness have been sought. Tight hats, restriction of blood flow, cerebral congestion, seborrhea, infection, lack of proper toiletting, and unspecified toxins have been blamed (Osborn, 1916; Simpson and Barth, 1997 and references within). If one expands the definition of *environment* to include endogenous biology, then clearly testosterone and other androgens play a role in the expression of male pattern baldness. Eunuchs do not bald unless exposed to exogenous testosterone, nor do males with androgen insensitivity. Conversely, excess exogenous androgens can precipitate male pattern baldness in susceptible females.

Pathophysiology: Biologic Basis of Genetic Susceptibility

Histologic studies on male pattern alopecia show that the initial change is focal perivascular degeneration of the connective tissue sheath of anagen follicles; a perifollicular lymphohistiocytic infiltrate ensues at the level of the sebaceous duct. Multinucleated giant cells can be seen around hair fragments. Follicles become short and small and produce non-pigmented hairs of small diameter. The anagen growth phase of the hair is shortened.

No significant abnormalities in anagen or sebum production have been demonstrated in males with baldness. Different local metabolism of androgens by hair from balding vs. nonbalding scalps has been found, but it is not clear whether these changes are causal or subsequent. Several studies have found higher levels of, or differences in, androgen receptors between hair follicles from bald vs. nonbald scalps (Simpson and Barth, 1997 and references within).

Genetic Studies of Pathophysiology

A difference in the proportion of high- and low-activity variants of 17β-hydroxysteroid dehydrogenase in hair follicles appeared to correlate with a positive or negative family history of baldness, low activity being more common in the latter. This work was presented in abstract form only (Hodgins et al., 1985).

Gene Identification

No linkage studies have been attempted, presumably because of the inability to correctly identify female family members as gene carriers. Specific candidate genes have not been proposed, although, as a class, genes controlling androgen receptors have elicited interest.

Animal Models

Hamilton (1959) described the feather-molting pattern in the wattled starling, suggesting that it might function as a model for male pattern hair loss. The males of this species, and only the males, lose feathers over the crown in the breeding season. In contrast to male pattern baldness in humans, these feathers do regrow. However, this cyclical loss is prevented by castration. Stumptailed macaques, orangutans, and other primates also demonstrate male pattern hair loss. A mouse model has also been described (Simpson and Barth, 1997 and references within).

Clinical Application and Risk Assessment of Genetics Information

One's grandmother is as likely to be accurate in predicting the risk for male pattern baldness as one's geneticist. The diagnosis is straightforward, predictive screening is unavailable, and prevention is not a reality except by castration, which is unlikely to prove popular. Treatment options are extensive, time-consuming, variably effective, and ardently sought (Fischer, 1997).

Küster and Happle (1984) reviewed the evidence for a genetic basis in male pattern baldness and provided the following arguments against a simple autosomal dominant Mendelian model:

1. *The prevalence of male pattern baldness is so common it must be polygenic.* This argument does not impress. The ABO blood groups are common and determined by a single gene. Male pattern baldness may express a similar state of being, with no significant effect on fitness or function, and as easily could be determined by a single gene.
2. *The range of severity of male pattern baldness fits with the Gaussian curve of the theoretical distribution of genes for a polygenic trait.* Here, the concept of the threshold effect is confused with that of severity of expression. As severity in male pattern baldness is to a significant degree age-dependent, it is difficult to see how this can be interpreted as suggesting polygenic inheritance.
3. *There is an increased risk of baldness with an increasing number of affected relatives. The risk of brothers to be affected is greater when the father of a bald proband is also bald. This is again consistent with a polygenic trait.* The authors forget that the status of the mother is also a factor and that both brothers of probands with bald fathers and those of probands with nonbald fathers can still inherit baldness from the mother. Thus, an autosomal dominant single-gene mode of inheritance can readily explain this finding. No studies of male pattern baldness have compared the rates of baldness among first-, second-, and third-degree relatives.
4. *Baldness shows disparity between men and women. Women with baldness must carry more predisposing genes than men.* Küster and Happle (1984) cited a study showing that bald women were more likely than bald men to have bald mothers. These data, however, are consistent with an autosomal dominant trait requiring homozygosity in most affected women and heterozygosity in a minority. Furthermore, there was no attempt to distinguish between common baldness and androgenetic loss in females secondary to androgen excess.

Küster and Happle (1984) proposed "jettisoning" the single-gene model for male pattern androgenetic alopecia in favor of a polygenic one; however, they have failed to convince this author.

PSORIASIS

Psoriasis is a common, chronic, papulosquamous inflammatory skin disease affecting as much as 1% of the general population in the United States.

The hallmark lesion of psoriasis is a red, raised area (*plaque*) covered with a fine silvery scale, whose removal results in pinpoint bleeding (*Auspitz sign*). Diagnostic microscopic features include elongation and thickening of the rete ridges and dermal papillae with acanthosis of the epidermis, increased mitotic activity of the basal keratinocytes, a superficial lymphocytic or monocytic infiltrate, and focal collections of neutrophils in the stratum corneum and subcorneal layer (Munro microabscesses). The diagnosis of psoriasis can be made clinically or in combination with histopathology.

There are many clinical variants of psoriasis (Table 50–5), distinguished by appearance and distribution of lesions. Some of these distinctions may be indicative of underlying causal heterogeneity of the disorder. Others may reflect environmental influences on expression. All forms share the same histopathologic features and similar responses to therapy except in the pustular form. Most patients have a typical psoriatic plaque somewhere

Table 50–5. Variants of Psoriasis

Psoriasis vulgaris: stable plaque disease
Guttate psoriasis: multiple small plaques, common presentation in children
Pustular psoriasis: generalized or limited to palms and soles
Inverse psoriasis: folds-axillae, gluteal cleft
Scalp psoriasis: limited to scalp
Psoriatic arthritis: may or may not have active skin disease
Annular psoriasis
Circinate psoriasis
Follicular psoriasis
Geographic psoriasis
Gyrate psoriasis
Nummular psoriasis
Serpiginous psoriasis

on the body. All show the Koebner phenomenon, disease arising in areas of injury. Infection, stress, and injury can induce or exacerbate psoriasis.

General Genetic and Epidemiologic Evidence

Clinical Epidemiology of Ethnic Differences

Population surveys have shown disparate incidence rates of psoriasis among different geographic regions. The disorder is rare among Japanese, Eskimos, West Africans, and North American blacks. It is almost nonexistent in North American and South American natives. Table 50–6 summarizes the population data.

Males and females are affected with equal frequency and severity; psoriatic arthritis is twice as common in females. The average age at onset is in the 20s, although psoriasis has been reported at birth and as late as age 108 years.

Family Epidemiology

That psoriasis is a disorder with a significant genetic component is undisputed. However, the nature of the genetic susceptibility to the disorder remains uncertain, despite almost a century of family studies (Table 50–7). In addition to these large surveys, many individual pedigrees with multigenerational transmission have been reported (Abele et al., 1963 and references within; Kimberling and Dobson, 1973).

Most of the studies of familial occurrence of psoriasis have been survey- or questionnaire-based, with little or no verification of the self-report. Swanbeck and colleagues (1994) examined a subset of 101 probands with psoriasis and 183 of their relatives, culled from their larger study population of 5197 individuals evaluated by questionnaire. Seven of 152 (4.6%) relatives reported to be free of psoriasis were found to be affected. Three of the 101 (2.9%) probands did not have psoriasis. This suggests that data derived from self-report by patients must be viewed with healthy skepticism.

Table 50–6. Prevalence of Psoriasis

Location	%
Faroe Islands	2.8
Sweden	1.4–2.3
Denmark	1.7–2.9
Great Britain	1.6
Germany	1.3
USA	1–4.6
U.S. blacks	0.7–1.4
South America	0.97–3
China	0.36–1.67
India	0.5–1.5
West Africa	0.3–0.8
East Africa	0.7–2.8

Higher figures usually represent surveys of clinic populations rather than general population surveys.
Source: Farber and Nall (1991) and Hellgren (1967) and references within.

When viewed in toto, the data from family and population studies can be interpreted in several ways. There is a strong suggestion that a multifactorial model fits for the inheritance of psoriasis, with the absence of a clear-cut Mendelian pattern in most families, a rapid drop-off in risk to family members with lessening degree of relatedness, and recognized environmental risk factors. Conversely, the possibility of an autosomal dominant gene with reduced penetrance has not been refuted by data to date.

Twin Studies

Table 50–8 lists the twin studies in the literature. There are several caveats for these studies. Brandrup and colleagues (1982) identified 53 index cases of twins ascertained from the Danish Twin Registry, who self-reported psoriasis, originating from 46 pairs. Of the 53, 14 did not have psoriasis when evaluated by physical examination, for a false-positive rate of 26%. Duffy and colleagues (1993) evaluated 148 twins who reported they had no psoriasis. Seven were affected, giving false-negative results approaching 5%. Further, in 7% of cases, there was disagreement between the raters as to the diagnosis.

Association with Other Diseases

The major recognized association with psoriasis is psoriatic arthritis. This is a seronegative polyarticular condition that most often involves the distal interphalangeal joints and can lead to bony destruction. Sacroiliitis is also common. It may precede the development of psoriasis. It may occur in as many as 7% of psoriatics. In families, affected individuals may have either skin or joint disease or both (Tsuji et al., 1976; Marcusson et al., 1976a,b, 1978). Although several surveys of psoriatic individuals have suggested an increased or decreased risk for a variety of other dermatologic and systemic disorders, none has been consistently or convincingly demonstrated (Hellgren, 1967; Farber and Nall, 1974).

Environmental Factors

There are recognized environmental triggers that can induce or exacerbate psoriasis.

In children, streptococcal infection of the upper respiratory tract plays a major role in the development of psoriasis and its exacerbation (Rasmussen, 1986 and references within). Sunlight and warmth appear to ameliorate psoriasis; flares are common in cold weather (Farber and Nall, 1991). As for many chronic diseases with remissions and flares, stress, both physical and emotional, has been indicted as a provocative agent in psoriasis.

In psoriatics, lesions often develop at sites of injury to the skin. This is referred to as the Koebner phenomenon or the *isomorphic response*. Lithium may induce or exacerbate psoriasis.

Pathophysiology and Biologic Basis of Genetic Susceptibility

The biologic mechanisms that contribute to the development of psoriasis are complex and incompletely understood. A number of changes take place in psoriatic skin. Which is the initiator and what are the relative contributions of each is uncertain. Epidermal, dermal, vascular, and circulating alterations play roles.

Table 50–7. Family Studies of Psoriasis

Reference	No. Subjects	Findings	Ascertainment
Melski and Stern (1981)	1209 severe psoriatics	Fourfold increased risk to sibling if parent of proband also affected, threefold increased risk to sibling with age at onset <30 years, 40% of siblings of probands with onset <15 years affected: overall, 9.4% siblings, 4.5% offspring, 12.3% parents affected	Questionnaire mailed to patients receiving PUVA, 15 centers involved
Aschner et al. (1957)	239	17.9% probands with one or more affected family members	Consecutive patients with psoriasis at academic dermatology center
Hoede (1931)	1437	39% probands with positive family history: if one parent affected, 10.7% siblings of probands affected; if no parent affected, 4.5% siblings affected	Medical records reviewed, 539 personally examined and family history obtained
Lerner (1940)	172	42% probands with positive family history	Patients from private clinic, attempted to have all relatives examined personally or by other physicians
Romanus (1945)	768	Affected children: 8.5% overall, 13% children older than 30 years. Affected siblings: 7.6% overall, 9% siblings older than 30 years. Affected parents: 8.3%	Medical history reviewed, 595 patients from various hospitals examined
Steinberg et al. (1951)	464	If one parent affected, 9% siblings affected; if no parent affected, 2.45% siblings affected; 5.9% parents affected, 2.4% children affected	Histories obtained from consecutive patients in dermatology clinic at Mayo
Lomholt (1963)	11,000	25% risk to first-degree relatives; if no parent affected, 17% siblings; if one parent affected, 31% siblings; if both parents affected, 60%–75% siblings; 91% of probands with positive family history	Psoriatics culled from 11,000 individuals in inbred population of Faroe Islands
Watson et al. (1972) Farber et al. (1968)	698	10% affected first-degree relatives (13.9% parents, 9.1% siblings, 4.5% children), 4% affected second-degree relatives, 1.4% affected third-degree relatives; if no parent affected, 7.8% siblings (85/1089); if one parent affected, 16.4% siblings (42/256); if both parents affected, 50% siblings (6/12)	2144 surveys sent to psoriatics seen at Stanford dermatology clinic and private dermatologists elsewhere
Farber and Nall (1974)	5600	36% probands with positive family history: 15% of relatives had psoriasis (2698/17,903), 47% first-degree relatives (1672/3557), 23% second-degree relatives (542/2352), 6% third-degree relatives (183/2959)	Expansion of population represented in Watson et al. (1972) and Farber et al. (1968), questionnaire responses
Swanbeck et al. (1994)	5197	36% probands with one or both parents affected, 16% siblings affected (2040/12,742), 15.5% offspring affected (363/2346)	Questionnaires mailed to >10,000 members of psoriasis support groups in Sweden, pustular psoriasis and psoriatic arthritis excluded, 183 subjects from 101 families examined
Swanbeck et al. (1997)	3218	If one parent affected, 16% offspring; if both parents, 37% offspring	Expansion of population reported in Swanbeck et al. (1994), 22,000 surveys mailed, 3218 probands between ages of 50 and 70 and had children
Hellgren (1967)	762	7.8% affected first-degree relatives (44/559), 2.99% affected second-degree relatives (7/234), 3.14% relatives of control group (27/560)	Population survey using church registers in Sweden, total population 38,670

PUVA, psoralen plus ultraviolet A.

There is an increase in the proportion of basal keratinocytes that undergo turnover in both involved and uninvolved skin of psoriatics. There is a concomitant decrease in the cell cycle time required for replication. Keratinocyte differentiation is also altered. Blood vessels in the papillary dermis become dilated and tortuous, and there is an inflammatory response with polymorphonuclear leukocyte invasion of the epidermis and increased numbers of $CD4^+$ and $CD8^+$ T cells.

A laundry list of immunologic alterations, both cellular and humoral, in psoriasis has been generated. Which of these changes are primary and which are nonspecific features secondary to inflammation is uncertain (Jablonska and Glinski, 1991; Bhalerao and Bowcock, 1998). Some of the experimental studies of differences between psoriatic and normal skin include the following (reviewed by Bhalerao and Bowcock, 1998):

1. Hyperresponsiveness of β_1 integrin K1/K10 keratinocyte stem cells from normal skin of psoriatics to proliferation signals mediated by T-cell lymphokines.
2. One hundred-fold decrease in sensitivity to growth inhibition by 1,25-dihydroxyvitamin D_3 compared with keratinocytes from nonpsoriatics.
3. Abnormal expression of integrins $\alpha2\beta1$, $\alpha3\beta1$, $\alpha5\beta1$, and $\alpha6\beta4$ in psoriatic keratinocytes.
4. Overexpression of platelet-derived growth factor in normal and involved skin of psoriatics.
5. Overexpression of transforming growth factor-α, IL-6, IL-8, interferon-γ, and monocyte chemoattractant protein-1 in lesional skin.
6. In vitro keratinocyte proliferation is induced by psoriatic fibroblasts but not by fibroblasts from normal skin. Fi

Table 50–8. Concordance for Psoriasis in Twins

Reference	Monozygotic	Dizygotic
Lomholt (1963)	15/27	
Reviewed in Kimberling, and Dobson (1973)	18/26	4/26
Farber et al. (1968, 1974)	30/41	4/20
Brandrup et al. (1978, 1982)	18/32[a]	2/22
Duffy et al. (1993)	12/34	5/43
Farber and Nall (1974) and references within (summary of 30 reports)	23/35	6/25

[a]Six of the twin pairs were ascertained independently through each twin, giving a proband-wise concordance rate of 24/38.

broblasts from uninvolved skin of psoriatics proliferate faster in the presence of normal human serum compared with normal fibroblasts and even more so in the presence of serum from psoriatic individuals. Fibroblasts from both involved and uninvolved skin of psoriatics produce increased levels of IL-8.

7. Insulin-like growth factor-I and epidermal growth factor are expressed to a greater degree in lesions of psoriasis.

Gene Identification

HLA Association

There are numerous studies of the relationship between psoriasis and HLA. Russell et al. (1972) postulated that as a protein from group A β-hemolytic streptococcus cross-reacted with specific HLA antigens and as streptococcal disease was known to induce or exacerbate psoriasis, a specific HLA haplotype might confer a specific risk for psoriasis. The results of the many HLA studies performed (Russell et al., 1972; Marcusson et al., 1975; Karvonen et al., 1975; Krulig et al., 1975; Tsuji et al., 1976; Suarez-Almazor and Russell, 1990; Nakagawa et al., 1991; Schmitt-Egenolf et al., 1996; reviewed in Elder et al., 1994a,b; Henseler, 1997; Bhalerao and Bowcock, 1998) suggest that the strongest association is with Cw6 and DR7. B13, B27, and B57 have also been found with greater frequency in some studies. Attempts to correlate specific haplotypes with subsets of disease, e.g., psoriatic arthritis and early-onset disease, have not met with consistent success.

Non-HLA Associations

No association with ABH, Rh, MNS, Kell, Lewis, or Duffy blood groups; HpGc and C3 serum groups; or PGM_1, G-6PD, and AK red cell enzymes was found among 87 psoriatics compared with 198 nonpsoriatic controls from Västerbotten County, Sweden (Beckman et al., 1974).

Horne et al. (1986) provided limited evidence that heterozygosity for the *MZ* α_1-antitrypsin genotype increases the risk for psoriasis.

Linkage Studies

Table 50–9 lists the results of a number of linkage studies on psoriasis (Bhalerao and Bowcock, 1998 and references within; Barker, 2001 and references within). At least three chromosomal regions suggest strong linkage with psoriasis: 17q25, 4q, and 6p21.3 (Tomfohrde et al., 1994; Matthews et al., 1996; Bhalerao and Bowcock, 1998 and references within, Burden et al., 1998). Supportive of the concept of genetic heterogeneity in psoriasis is the exclusion of linkage to the same regions when disparate groups are evaluated (Matthews et al., 1995). Trembath et al. (1997) evaluated 254 British psoriatics, among whom there were 66 affected siblings in 41 families. Ninety-four percent had chronic plaque psoriasis, 3% had guttate disease, and 3% had palmoplantar disease. In this group and in a second cohort of 40 siblings, they demonstrated linkage to 6p21 within the major histocompatibility complex region ($p = 0.00015$) and excluded linkage to both 17q and 4q. Further, they implied that their data also supported linkage to chromosomes 2, 8q, 11, 14, 16, and 20, all with $p \leq 0.01$. Other chromosomal regions implicated included 1q21 (Bhalerao and Bowcock, 1998; Capon et al., 1999), 16q (Nair et al., 1997), 20p (Nair et al., 1997), 2p (Bhalerao and Bowcock, 1998), 14q31 (Bhalerao and Bowcock., 1998), 1p (Veal et al., 2001), 19p13 (Lee et al., 2000), and 3q21 (Enlund et al., 1999).

Bhalerao and Bowcock (1998) noted that in their largest pedigree with linkage to 17q25 the phenotypes of affected individuals ranged from mild to severe and included psoriatic arthritis in some, suggesting that phenotypic heterogeneity cannot be explained solely by genetic heterogeneity.

One of the difficulties in linkage studies on psoriasis is the variable age at onset of the disorder. At-risk individuals younger

Table 50–9. Summary of Linkage Analysis in Psoriasis

Region	No. Families	Model	LOD Score/NPL* Score	*p* value
6p21.3 (PSORS1)	68 nuclear	Recessive	6.5 (TNF-α)	
			5.01 (*D6S273*)	
			3.07 (HLA-C)	
	115	Recessive	2.31 (TNF-β)	
17q25 (PSORS2)	8	Dominant	5.33 (*D17S784*)	0.0056
	115 (29 extended, 86 nuclear)		2.09 (*D17S784*)	
4q (PSORS3)	6	Dominant	3.03	
1cen-q21 (PSORS4)	18[a]	Dominant	3.75 (*D15305*)	
3q21 (PSORS5)	20 + 104	Recessive	3.85 (*D351269*)	0.005
19p13 (PSORS6)	32	Recessive	4.06 (*D195916*)	0.0002
20p	68 nuclear	Recessive	2.01 (*D20S186*)	0.0012
	115	Recessive	2.62 (*D20S851*)	0.06
1p	158 nuclear		3.6* (*D15197, D15200, D15207*)	1.9×10^{-4}

Source: Modified from Bhalerao and Bowcock (1998).
[a]An additional four families showed no linkage to this region.
NPL, nonparametric linkage.

Table 50–10. Risk of Atopic Disease in Individuals

	Atopic Dermatitis (%)	Atopy (%)
No parent affected	3	6.9
One parent with atopic dermatitis	9.4	12.5
One parent with respiratory atopy	6.8	15.5
One sibling with atopic dermatitis	8.8	15.5
One sibling and one parent with atopic dermatitis	33.3	39.4
One sibling with atopic dermatitis, one parent with atopic dermatitis and respiratory atopy	38.9	50
One sibling with atopic dermatitis, one parent with respiratory atopy	5.9	25.5

Source: Modified from Küster et al. (1990).

than 50 years may develop the disorder with reasonable likelihood; thus, they should not be included in linkage analyses.

Genes and Responsible Variation

There is no shortage of candidate genes for psoriasis. Suggested by Henseler (1997) on chromosome 1 are psoriasin, migration inhibitory factor–related proteins (MRP8, MRP14), small proline-rich proteins (SPRRs), and calcyclin, all of which are overexpressed in epidermal shave biopsies of psoriatic skin. Further, genes at 1q21 (*S100A10*, trichohyalin, profilaggrin, involucrin, *SPRR3*, *SPRR1B*, *SPRR1A*, loricin, *S100A9*, *S100A8*, and *S100A6*) form the epidermal differentiation complex, any of which may play a role.

On chromosome 6, genes close to the HLA complex include the *S* gene, *tumor necrosis factor 1*, α and β and *HSP60.*

EXT1, mapped to chromosome 8q24.1, is a tumor-suppressor gene implicated in hereditary multiple extoses (HME). In a large family with HME and psoriasis, there appeared to be cosegregation of the disorders, suggesting the possibility of a contiguous gene defect (Trembath et al., 1997).

A locus for Crohn disease maps to a region on 16q, where psoriasis also appears to be linked (Nair et al., 1997). These authors suggested that the region might encode an "immunomodulatory locus" whose alteration could lead to one or both of these presumed autoimmune inflammatory disorders.

Clinical Application and Risk Assessment of Genetics Information

The diagnosis of psoriasis is clinical. To date, molecular and biochemical features do not permit predictive screening. Prevention is not possible. Family and linkage studies have provided no useful information vis à vis natural history or response to therapies. Beyond a certainty that a positive family history confers increased susceptibility, counseling for risks in psoriasis seems inherently inappropriate. As van Steensel and Steijlen (1997) emphasized: "we urge any practitioner involved in counseling prospective parents with psoriasis to think twice before starting to discuss relative risks and the like."

Table 50–11. Risk for Atopic Dermatitis in Offspring

	No.	Offspring with Atopic Dermatitis
Proband affected, spouse unaffected	164	180/321 (56%)
Proband and spouse affected	26	48/59 (81%)
Proband affected, spouse affected with respiratory atopy	80	88/149 (59%)
All	270	316/529 (59%)

Source: Uehara and Kimura (1993).

ATOPIC DERMATITIS

Atopic dermatitis is defined by a combination of clinical and historical features. The presence of a lichenified dermatitis that is itchy, with typical distribution patterns at different ages, and histologic evidence of epidermal spongiosis coupled with a positive personal history of atopy, including asthma, allergic rhinitis, or urticaria, supports a diagnosis of atopic dermatitis. Criteria for the diagnosis of atopic dermatitis have been generated (Hanifin, 1983) but are not universally applied by investigators. Although it has been suggested that increased immunoglobulin E responsiveness be used as a gold standard for the diagnosis of atopic dermatitis, such testing is not done routinely by practitioners, who know a purple cow when they see one.

Chapter 11 deals with the genetics of atopy, and the reader is referred there for detailed and complete discussion. As atopic dermatitis does not stand alone as an entity but requires the presence of other atopic disorders in the proband or in first-degree relatives, very few studies have looked at the inheritance of the dermatitis alone. I will limit the remarks here to a few studies which have.

Küster and colleagues (1990) sent questionnaires to a randomly chosen group of 265 inpatients with atopic dermatitis seen at a dermatology clinic. The diagnosis of atopic dermatitis was based on confirming clinical features in the probands (Hanifin, 1983). One hundred eighty-eight questionnaires were returned, with information regarding 156 families with a total of 2151 members.

For patients with atopic dermatitis only (approximately one-half), 19% of family members had atopic dermatitis, 19% had atopic dermatitis and respiratory atopy (asthma and/or rhinitis), and 23% had respiratory symptoms alone. For probands with atopic dermatitis and respiratory atopy, the results were 8%, 28%, and 43%, respectively.

Küster et al. (1990) calculated empiric risks for atopy in offspring, using information from 225 grandparents and 845 siblings of probands to calculate the risk for atopic dermatitis with no affected parent. Their results are given in Table 50–10.

Uehara and Kimura (1993) selected 270 adult patients from their outpatient dermatology clinic in whom the diagnosis of atopic dermatitis was made clinically. Information regarding 531 offspring older than 2 years was elicited on two occasions from each proband. The results are given in Table 50–11.

Table 50–12. Occurrence of Atopic Disease in First-Degree Relatives of Probands with Atopic Dermatitis and Controls

		Atopic Dermatitis (%)	Allergic Rhinitis (%)	Allergic Asthma (%)
Cases	Fathers	10.1	8.2	2.3
Controls	Fathers	1.6	2.7	1.6
Cases	Mothers	12.7	11.5	3.3
Controls	Mothers	3.4	5.3	1.8
Cases	Siblings	13.3	10	2.4
Controls	Siblings	2.2	8.6	1.1

Source: Modified from Diepgen and Blettner (1996).

Diepgen and Blettner (1996) collected information from 426 inpatients and outpatients with chronic relapsing atopic dermatitis and from 628 controls with no personal history of atopic dermatitis who were "from the area surrounding the hospital." All were interviewed by one of the authors regarding family history. Only information from siblings and parents was included, resulting in data for 1054 families with 5136 members. While none of the control cases had atopic dermatitis, 17.3% did have allergic rhinitis and 4.6% had allergic reactive airway disease. The results are listed in Table 50–12.

It is clear that there is significant heritability of atopic dermatitis in association with other atopic diseases and perhaps as an isolated disorder. Uehara and Kimura (1993) raised the question of whether atopic dermatitis and atopic respiratory diseases are controlled by the same genetic factors. They suggested that the lack of an increased risk for atopic dermatitis in offspring of one parent with atopic dermatitis and the other with respiratory atopy compared to those with only a single parent with atopic dermatitis supported the concept that there are distinct genetic contributors for the skin disease.

REFERENCES

Abele DC, Dobson RL, Graham JB: Heredity and psoriasis. Arch Dermatol 1963; 88:90–99.

Ando I, Chi H-I, Nakagawa H, Otsuka F: Difference in clinical features and HLA antigens between familial and non-familial vitiligo of non-segmental type. Br J Dermatol 1993; 129:408–410.

Arnold HL: Alopecia areata: prevalence in Japanese and prognosis after reassurance. AMA Arch Dermatol Syphilol 1952; 66:191–196.

Aschner B, Curth HO, Gross P: Genetic aspects of psoriasis. Acta Genet 1957; 7:197–204.

Barker JNWN: Genetic aspects of psoriasis. Clin Exp Dermatol 2001; 26:321–325.

Beckman L, Brönnestam R, Cedergren B, Lidén S: HLA-A antigens, blood groups, serum groups and red cell enzyme types in psoriasis. Hum Hered 1974; 24:496–506.

Bhalerao J, Bowcock AM: The genetics of psoriasis: a complex disorder of the skin and immune system. Hum Mol Genet 1998; 7:1537–1545.

Bhatia PS, Mohan L, Pandey ON, Singh KK, Arora SK, Mukhija RD: Genetic nature of vitiligo. J Dermatol Sci 1992; 4:180–184.

Brandrup F, Hauge M, Henningsen K, Eriksen B: Psoriasis in an unselected series of twins. Arch Dermatol 1978; 114:874–878.

Brandrup F, Holm N, Grunnet N, Henningsen K, Hansen H: Psoriasis in monozygotic twins: variations in expression in individuals with identical genetic constitution. Acta Derm Venereol 1982; 62:229–236.

Burden AD, Javed S, Bailey M, Hodgins M, Connor M, Tillman D: Genetics of psoriasis: paternal inheritance and a locus on chromosome 6p. J Invest Dermatol 1998; 110:958–960.

Capon F, Novelli G, Semprini S, Clementi M, Nudo M, Vultaggio P, Mazzanti C, Gobello T, Botta A, Fabrizi G, et al.: Searching for psoriasis susceptibility genes in Italy: genome scan and evidence for a new locus on chromosome 1. J Invest Dermatol 1999; 112:32–35.

Carnevale A, Zavala C, Del Castillo V, Maldonado RR, Tamayo L: Genetic analysis of 127 families with vitiligo. Rev Invest Clin 1980; 32:37–41.

Colombe BW, Price VH, Khoury EL, Lou CD: HLA class II alleles in long-standing alopecia totalis/alopecia universalis and long-standing patchy alopecia areata differentiate these two clinical groups. J Invest Dermatol 1995; 104:4S-5S.

Cork MJ, Tarlow JK, Clay FE, Crane A, Blakemore AIF, McDonagh AJG, Messenger AG, Duff GW, et al.: An allele of the interleukin-1 receptor antagonist as a genetic severity factor in alopecia areata. J Invest Dermatol 1995; 104:15S-16S.

Cunliffe WJ, Hall R, Newell DJ, Stevenson CJ: Vitiligo, thyroid disease and autoimmunity. Br J Dermatol 1968; 80:135–139.

Diepgen TL, Blettner M: Analysis of familial aggregation of atopic eczema and other atopic diseases by odds ratio regression models. J Invest Dermatol 1996; 106:977–981.

Duffy DL, Spelman LS, Martin NG: Psoriasis in Australian twins. J Am Acad Dermatol 1993; 29:428–434.

Duvic M, Hordinsky MK, Fiedler VC, O'Brien WR, Young R, Reveille JD: HLA-D locus associations in alopecia areata. Arch Dermatol 1991; 127:64–68.

Duvic M, Welsh EA, Jackow C, Papadopoulos E, Reveille JD, Amos C: Analysis of HLA-D locus alleles in alopecia areata patients and familieis. J Invest Dermatol 1995; 104:5S-6S.

Elder JT, Henseler T, Christophers E, Voorhees JJ, Nair RP: Of genes and antigens: the inheritance of psoriasis. J Invest Dermatol 1994a; 103:150S–153S.

Elder JT, Nair RP, Guo S-W, Henseler T, Christophers E, Voorhees JJ: The genetics of psoriasis. Arch Dermatol 1994b; 130:216–224.

Ellis JA, Stebbing M, Harrap SB: Genetic analysis of male pattern baldness and the 5α-reductase genes. J Invest Dermatol 1998; 110:849–853.

Enlund F, Samuelsson L, Enerbäck C, Inerot A, Wahlström J, Yhr M, Torinsson Å, et al.: Psoriasis susceptibility locus in chromosome region 3q21 identified in patients from southwest Sweden. Eur J Hum Genet 1999; 7:783–790.

Farber EM, Bright RD, Nall ML: Psoriasis: a questionnaire survery of 2,144 patients. Arch Dermatol 1968; 98:248–259.

Farber EM, Nall ML: The natural history of psoriasis in 5,600 patients. Dermatologica 1974; 148:1–18.

Farber EM, Nall ML: Epidemiology: natural history and genetics. In: Roenigk HH Jr, Maibach HI (eds). Psoriasis, 2d ed. New York: Marcel Dekker, 1991:209–258.

Farber EM, Nall ML, Watson W: Natural history of psoriasis in 61 twin pairs. Arch Dermatol 1974; 109:207–211.

Fischer D: The bald truth: Americans turn to weaves, rugs, plugs, and drugs to alleviate hair loss, creating a $1.5 billion industry. US News World Reports 1997 Aug 4:44.

Goudie RB, Goudie DR, Dick HM, Ferguson-Smith MA: Unstable mutations in vitiligo, organ specific autoimmune disease and multiple endocrine adenoma/peptic ulcer syndrome. Lancet 1980; 2:285–287.

Hacham-Zadeh S, Brautbar C, Cohen CA, Cohen T: HLA and alopecia areata in Jerusalem. Tissue Antigens 1981; 18:71–74.

Hafez M, Sharaf L, Abd El-Nabi SM: The genetics of vitiligo. Acta Derm Venereol 1982; 63:249–250.

Hamilton JB: Patterned loss of hair in man: types and incidence. Ann N Y Acad Sci 1951; 53:708–728.

Hamilton JB: A male pattern baldness in wattled starlings resembling the condition in man. Ann N Y Acad Sci 1959; 83:429–447.

Hanifin JM: Atopic dermatitis. Semin Dermatol 1983; 2:5–19.

Harris H: The inheritance of premature baldness in men. Ann Eugenics 1947; 13:172–181.

Hawk E, Breslow RA, Graubard BI: Male pattern baldness and clinical prostate cancer in the epidemiologic follow-up of the First National Health and Nutrition Examination Survey. Cancer Epidemiol Biomarkers Prev 2000; 9:523–527.

Hellgren L: Psoriasis. The Prevalence in Sex, Age and Occupational Groups in Total Populations in Sweden. Morphology, Inheritance and Association with Other Skin and Rheumatic Diseases. Stockholm: Almqvist and Wiksell, 1967.

Hendren OS: Identical alopecia areata in identical twins. Arch Dermatol Syphilol 1949; 60:793–795.

Henseler T: The genetics of psoriasis. J Am Acad Dermatol 1997; 37:S1–S11.

Hodgins MB, Murad S, Simpson NB: A search for variation in hair follicle androgen metabolism which might be linked to male pattern baldness [abstract]. Br J Dermatol 1985; 113:794.

Hoede K: Umwelt and Erblichkeit bei der Entstehung der Schuppenflechte. Wursb Abh Med 1931; 27:211–254.

Hordinsky MK, Hallgren H, Nelson D, Filipovich AH: Familial alopecia areata. Arch Dermatol 1984; 120:464–468.

Horne SL, Junk GJ, Cockcroft DW, Lovegrove A, Dosman JA: Pi MZ phenotype and an increased prevalence of reported psoriasis in a community survey. Hum Hered 1986; 36:266–268.

Howitz J, Brodthagen H, Schwartz M, Thomsen K: Prevalence of vitiligo. Epidemiological survey on the Isle of Bornholm, Denmark. Arch Dermatol 1977; 113:47–52.

Jablonska S, Glinski W: Overview of immunology. In: Roenigk HH Jr, Maibach HI (eds). Psoriasis, 2d ed. New York: Marcel Dekker, 1991:261–283.

Jackson GT: A Practical Treatise on the Diseases of the Hair and Scalp. New York: EB Treat, 1898:115–139.

Karvonen J, Tiilikainen A, Lassus A: HLA-A antigens in patients with persistent palmoplantar pustulosis and pustular psoriasis. Ann Clin Res 1975; 7:112–115.

Kianto U, Reunala T, Karvonen J, Lassus A, Tiilikainen A: HLA-B12 in alopecia areata. Arch Dermatol 1977; 113:1716.

Kimberling W, Dobson RL: The inheritance of psoriasis. J Invest Dermatol 1973; 60:538–540.

Krulig L, Farber EM, Grumet FC, Payne RO: Histocompatibility (HLA-A) antigens in psoriasis. Arch Dermatol 1975; 111:857–860.

Kuntz BME, Selzle D, Braun-Falco O, Scholz S, Albert ED: HLA antigens in alopecia areata. Arch Dermatol 1977; 113:1717.

Küster W, Happle R: The inheritance of common baldness: two B or not two B? J Am Acad Dermatol 1984; 11:921–926.

Küster W, Petersen M, Christophers E, Goos M, Sterry W: A family study of atopic dermatitis. Clinical and genetic characteristics of 188 patients and 2,151 family members. Arch Dermatol 1990; 282:98–102.

Lee YA, Rüschendorf F, Windemuth C, Schmitt-Egenolf M, Stadelmann A, Nürnberg G, Ständer M, Wienker TF, Reis A, Traupe H: Genomewide scan in German families reveals evidence for a novel psoriasis—susceptibility locus on chromosome 19p13. Am J Hum Genet 2000; 67:1020–1024.

Lerner C: Hereditary influences in psoriasis. J Invest Dermatol 1940; 3:347–356.

Lomholt G: Psoriasis. A Census Study on the Prevalence of Skin Diseases on the Faroe Islands. G.E.C. Gad. Dissertation. Copenhagen 1963.

Majumder PP, Nordlund JJ, Nath SK: Pattern of familial aggregation of vitiligo. Arch Dermatol 1993; 129:994–998.

Marcusson J, Elman A, Möller E, Thyresson N: Psoriasis, sacro-iliitis and peripheral arthritis occurring in patients with the same HLA haplotype. A preliminary family report and a hypothetical explanation of the interaction between MHS products. Tissue Antigens 1976b; 8:131–138.

Marcusson J, Möller E, Rosenthal L, Lindwall N, Thyresson N: Psoriasis and arthritic lesions in relation to the inheritance of HLA genotypes: a family study. Acta Derm Venereol 1978; 58:511–520.

Marcusson J, Möller E, Thyresson N: HL-A antigens (17, 27, UPS) in psoriasis with special reference to patients with arthritic lesions. Acta Derm Venereol 1975; 55:297–300.

Marcusson J, Möller E, Thyresson N: Penetration of HLA-linked psoriasis-predisposing gene(s): a family investigation. Acta Derm Venereol 1976a; 56:453–463.

Matthews D, Fry L, Powles A, Weber J, McCarthy M, Fisher E, Davies K, Williamson R: Evidence that a locus for familial psoriasis maps to chromosome 4q. Nat Genet 1996; 14:231–233.

Matthews D, Fry L, Powles A, Weissenbach J, Williamson R: Confirmation of genetic heterogeneity in familial psoriasis. J Med Genet 1995; 32:546–548.

McDonagh AJG, Messenger AG: The pathogenesis of alopecia areata. Dermatol Clin 1996; 14:661–670.

Melski JW, Stern RS: The separation of susceptibility to psoriasis from age at onset. J Invest Dermatol 1981; 77:474–477.

Messenger AG, Simpson NB: Alopecia areata. In: Dawber R (ed). Diseases of the Hair and Scalp. Malden, MA: Blackwell, 1997:338–369.

Mitchell AJ, Krull EA: Alopecia areata: pathogenesis and treatment. J Am Acad Dermatol 1984; 11:763–775.

Morling N, Frentz G, Fugger L, Georgsen J, Jakobsen B, Ødum N, Svejgaard A: DNA polymorphism of HLA class II genes in alopecia areata. Dis Markers 1991; 9:35–42.

Müller SA, Winkelmann RK: Alopecia areata. An evaluation of 736 patients. Arch Dermatol 1963; 88:290–297.

Nair RJ, Henseler T, Jenisch S, Stuart P, Bichakjian CK, Lenk W, Westphal E, Guo SW, Christophers E, Voorhees JJ, et al.: Evidence for two psoriasis susceptibility loci (HLA and 17q) and two novel candidate regions (16q and 20p) by genome-wide scan. Hum Mol Genet 1997; 6:1349–1356.

Nakagawa H, Akazaki S, Asahina A, Tokunaga A, Matsuki K, Kuwata S, Ishibashi Y, Juji T: Study of HLA class I, class II and complement genes (C2, C4A, C4B and Bf) in Japanese psoriatics and analysis of a newly found high-risk haplotype by pulsed field gel electrophoresis. Arch Dermatol Res 1991; 283:281–284.

Nath SK, Majumder PP, Nordlund JJ: Genetic epidemiology of vitiligo: multilocus recessivity cross-validated. Am J Hum Genet 1994; 55:981–990.

Nordlund JJ, Ortonne J-P: Genetic hypomelanoses: disorders characterized by acquired depigmentation. In: Nordlund JJ, Boissy RE, Hearing VJ, King RA, Ortonne J-P (eds). The Pigmentary System. New York: Oxford University Press, 1998:513–531.

Norwood OT: Male pattern baldness: classification and incidence. South Med J 1975; 68:1359–1365.

Omens DV, Omens HD: Alopecia areata in twins. Arch Dermatol Syphilol 1946; 53:193.

Orecchia G, Cuccia Belvedere M, Martinetti M, Capelli E, Rabbiosi G: Human leukocyte antigen region involvement in the genetic predisposition to alopecia areata. Dermatologica 1987; 175:10–14.

Ortonne J-P, Mosher DB, Fitzpatrick TB: Vitiligo and other hypomelanoses of hair and skin. In: Parrish JA, Fitzpatrick TB (eds). Topics in Dermatology. New York: Plenum, 1983.

Osborn D: Inheritance of baldness. J Hered 1916; 7:347–355.

Rasmussen J: Psoriasis in children. Dermatol Clin 1986; 4:99–106.

Romanus T: Psoriasis prognosis and heredity. Acta Dermatol 1945; 26(Suppl 12):1–137.

Roundtable: Management of vitiligo in children. Pediatr Dermatol 1986; 3:498–510.

Roundtable: Alopecia areata symposium. Pediatr Dermatol 1987; 4:136–158.

Russell TJ, Schultes LM, Kuban DJ: Histocompatibility (HL-A) antigens associated with psoriasis. N Engl J Med 1972; 287:738–740.

Šalamon T: Genetic factors in male pattern alopecia. In: Baccaredda-Boy A (ed). Biopathology of Pattern Alopecia. New York: Karger, 1968:39–49.

Schallreuter KU, Lemke R, Brandt O, Schwartz R, Westhofen M, Montz R, Berger J: Vitiligo and other diseases: coexistence or true association? Dermatology 1994; 188:269–275.

Schmitt-Egenolf M, Eiermann T, Boehncke W, Stander M, Sterry W: Familial juvenile onset psoriasis is associated with the human leukocyte antigen (HLA) class I side of the extended haplotype Cw6-B57-DRB1*0701-DQA1*0201-DQB1*0303: a population- and family-based study. J Invest Dermatol 1996; 106:711–714.

Schuttelaar M-LA, Hamstra JJ, Plinck EPB, Peereboom-Wynia JDR, Vuzevski VD, Mulder PGH, Oranje AP: Alopecia areata in children: treatment with diphencyprone. Br J Dermatol 1996; 135:581–585.

Shellow WVR, Edwards JE, Koo JYM: Profile of alopecia areata: a questionnaire analysis of patient and family. Int J Dermatol 1992; 31:186–189.

Simpson NB, Barth JH: Hair patterns: hirsuties and androgenetic alopecia. In: Dawber R (ed). Diseases of the Hair and Scalp. Malden, MA: Blackwell, 1997:101–122.

Smith MA, Wells RS: Male type alopecia, alopecia areata and normal hair in women. Family histories. Arch Dermatol 1964; 89:95–98.

Snyder LH, Yingling HC: Studies in human inheritance XII. The application of the gene frequency method of analysis to sex-influenced factors, with especial reference to baldness. Hum Biol 1935; 7:608–615.

Song YH, Connor E, Li Y, Zorovich B, Balducci P, Maclaren N: The role of tyrosinase in autoimmune vitiligo. Lancet 1994; 344:1049–1052.

Steinberg AG, Becker SW Jr, Fitzpatrick TB, Kierland RR: A genetic and statistical study of psoriasis. Am J Hum Genet 1951; 3:267–281.

Suarez-Almazor M, Russell A: The genetics of psoriasis. Haplotype sharing in sibs with the disease. Arch Dermatol 1990; 126:1040–1042.

Sundberg JP, King LE Jr: Mouse models for the study of human hair loss. Dermatol Clin 1996; 14:619–632.

Swanbeck G, Inerot A, Martinsson T, Enerbäck C, Enlund F, Samuelsson L, Yhr M, Wahlström J: Genetic counselling in psoriasis: empirical data on psoriasis among first-degree relatives of 3095 psoriatic probands. Br J Dermatol 1997; 137:939–942.

Swanbeck G, Inerot A, Martinsson T, Wahlström J: A population genetic study of psoriasis. Br J Dermatol 1994; 131:32–39.

Taylor CR, Hawk JLM: PUVA treatment of alopecia areata partialis, totalis and universalis: audit of 10 years' experience at St. John's Institute of Dermatology. Br J Dermatol 1995; 133:914–918.

Tomfohrde J, Silverman A, Barnes R, Fernandez-Vina MA, Young M, Lory D, Morris L, Wuepper KD, Stastny P, Menter A, et al.: Gene for familial psoriasis susceptibility mapped to the distal end of human chromosome 17q. Science 1994; 264:1141–1145.

Tosti A, Bardazzi F, De Padova MP, Veronesi S: Deafness and vitiligo in an Italian family. Dermatologica 1986; 172:178–179.

Tosti A, Bardazzi F, Tosti G, Monti L: Audiologic abnormalities in cases of vitiligo. J Am Acad Dermatol 1987; 17:230–233.

Trembath RC, Clough RL, Rosbotham JL, Jones AB, Camp RDR, Frodsham A, Browne J, Barber R, Terwilliger J, Lathrop GM, et al.: Identification of a major susceptibility locus on chromosome 6p and evidence for further disease loci revealed by a two stage genome-wide search in psoriasis. Hum Mol Genet 1997; 6:813–820.

Tsuji K, Nose Y, Ito M, Ozawa A, Matsuo I, Niizuma K, Ohkido M: HLA antigens and susceptibility to psoriasis vulgaris in a non-Caucasian population. Tissue Antigens 1976; 8:29–33.

Turnacliff DD: Alopecia areata in twins. Arch Dermatol Syphilol 1931; 24:1122.

Uehara M, Kimura C: Descendant family history of atopic dermatitis. Arch Derm Venereol 1993; 73:62–63.

Valsecchi R, Vicari O, Frigeni A, Foiadelli L, Naldi L, Cainelli T: Familial alopecia areata—genetic susceptibility or coincidence? Acta Derm Venereol 1984; 65:175–177.

van der Steen P, Traupe H, Happle R, Boezeman J, Strater R, Hamm H: The genetic risk for alopecia areata in first degree relatives of severely affected patients. Acta Derm Venereol 1992; 72:373–375.

van Steensel MAM, Steijlen PM: Genetics of psoriasis. Clin Dermatol 1997; 15:669–675.

Veal CO, Clough RL, Barber RC, Mason S, Tillman D, Ferry B, Jones AB, Ameen M, Balendran N, Powis SH, et al.: Identification of a novel psoriasis susceptibility locus at 1p and evidence of epistasis between *PSORS1* and candidate loci. J Med Genet 2001; 38:7–13.

Ward JH, Stephens FE: Inheritance of psoriasis in a Utah kindred. Arch Dermatol 1961; 84:589–592.

Wasfi AI, Saha N, El Munshid HA, El Sheikh FS, Ahmed MA: Genetic association in vitiligo: ABO, MNSs, Rhesus, Kell and Duffy blood groups. Clin Genet 1980; 17:415–417.

Watson W, Cann HM, Farber EM, Nall ML: The genetics of psoriasis. Arch Dermatol 1972; 105:197–207.

Weidman AI, Zion LS, Mamelok AE: Alopecia areata occurring simultaneously in identical twins. AMA Arch Dermatol Syphilol 1956; 74:424–426.

Zlotogorski A, Weinrauch L, Brautbar C: Familial alopecia areata: no linkage with HLA. Tissue Antigens 1990; 35:40–41.

51 Genetic Modulation of Aging and Longevity

GEORGE M. MARTIN

THE DEMOGRAPHIC IMPERATIVE

Diseases and disabilities of older people are increasingly dominating the practice of medicine. This is soon to be the case in the developing as well as the developed societies. As can be seen in Figure 51–1 (Murray and Lopez, 1996), over the 30-year period from 1990 to 2020, demographers project an approximately 130% to 140% increase in the global population of men and women aged 75 years but only about a 25% increase in 5-year-olds. Figure 51–1 does not show the results for individuals over the age of 75 years. In the United States, where this question has been of special interest to demographic gerontologists, it is clear that the current rate of growth of the "oldest old" (those 85 years and older) is unprecedented in human history. Projections of the current exponential rate of increase yield estimates of 4.3 million such U.S. residents by the year 2000, rising to 18.9 million by the year 2050 (Hobbs and Damon, 1996).

Demographers, epidemiologists, and physicians continue to debate the extent to which the growing ranks of the "oldest old" will be burdened with disabilities and disease. Vita and colleagues (1998) have championed the concept of a compression of morbidity near the end of a relatively fixed, species-specific life span, at least for the healthier subset with superior health habits. A population-based, longitudinal analysis of chronic disability in U.S. residents over the age of 65 years has indicated recent decreases in the proportion of chronically disabled subjects (Manton and Gu, 2001). As we shall see below, however, the evolutionary biological theory of aging predicts considerable life span plasticity, without a strict species-specific limitation. Also, these predictions are supported by experiments in model organisms. Moreover, some investigators do not support this view of morbidity compression in populations of older people (Schneider and Brody, 1983). These are quantitative arguments. All would agree that very old people require a disproportionate amount of the available medical services For example, there is a striking exponential increase in both the prevalence and the age-specific incidence of dementias beginning at about age 65, most of it due to dementias of the Alzheimer type (DAT). This has been shown for many human populations. While data for the population over the age of 90 are sparse, as one can see from Figure 51–2, by about the age of 90 years about 50% are so affected. The task of investigators with an interest in human and medical genetics is to discover the precise nature–nurture interactions that determine to which half of humanity our patients belong for disabilities such as DAT. There are, of course, numerous other serious and not so serious disabilities, all of which impact upon the quality of life for older people and their caregivers. Many of these are enumerated below. Collectively, they place an enormous economic burden upon society.

AGING AND LONGEVITY

Mammalian gerontologists generally utilize the terms *aging* and *senescence* (or *senescing*) interchangeably to refer to the panorama of changes in structure and function that gradually unfold after the organism attains full adult development with reproductive competence. We shall do likewise in this chapter. The "gold standard" methodology for defining rates of aging requires populations of organisms and is based on a determination of age-specific mortality rates. Until very recently, a simple log-linear Gompertz relationship was used to describe the entire population of organisms (Gompertz, 1825). Accordingly, it was thought that there was a continuous exponential function throughout the range of life spans. Surprisingly, however, when exceedingly large cohorts of genetically heterogeneous medflies (Carey et al., 1992) and genetically heterogeneous nematodes (Brooks et al., 1994) were studied, a sizeable proportion of the population achieving advanced ages exhibited a plateau and, in the case of medflies, a subsequent decline in age-specific death rates. That such findings cannot be due entirely to genetic heterogeneity is indicated by similar results for genetically homogeneous fruit flies (Curtsinger et al., 1992). A significant but much smaller proportion of human populations exhibited the same trends. This is illustrated in Figure 51–3 (Vaupel et al., 1998). There is not yet a widely accepted explanation for these departures from Gompertz kinetics. We shall return to consider some potential explanations when we discuss some challenges to the evolutionary biological theory of aging.

A most interesting aspect of these survival curves is the fact that their general configurations, indicative of a wide range of variation in age at death, are observed among genetically defined experimental organisms (e.g., nematodes, fruit flies, mice) aged under apparently identical environmental conditions. The most striking such example comes from research on *Caenorhabditis elegans*, which can be grown in suspension cultures with chemically defined media (Vanfleteren et al., 1998). This would seem to control for even microenvironmental perturbations. The inescapable conclusion is that stochastic factors play very important roles in the determination of life span in a given individual. These stochastic factors may play out during early development or after maturation (Finch and Kirkwood, 1999). For example, consider two individuals who undergo similar rates of somatic mutation as they age. One may be lucky in sustaining a large proportion of these mutations in pseudogenes, while the other may be unlucky in sustaining mutations in such important tumor-suppressor genes as *p53* and *Rb*. These considerations create great difficulty for geneticists interested in determining the genetic basis of longevity, e.g., via twin studies, family studies, or genetic association studies using centenarians, a currently pop-

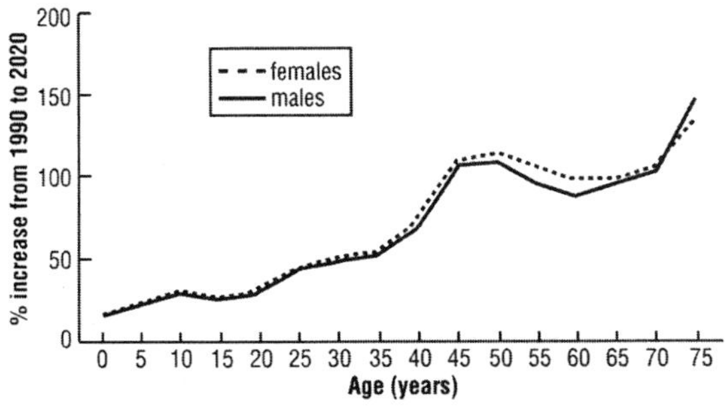

Fig. 51–1. Projections of the rates of increase in the world's population of males and females between 1990 and 2020 among cohorts of different ages. From Murray and Lopez (1996) with permission.

ular approach. There is also the considerable difficulty that the phenotype of longevity is clearly under highly polygenic controls. In the author's opinion, much more rapid progress can be made by investigations of the genetic basis of variation in rates of change in specific physiological parameters that are known to decline with age; the more specific, the better (Martin, 1998, 2000).

The late Nathan Shock devoted a large part of his career to the quantitation of rates of decline in a variety of physiological declines in human populations. The earliest studies were cross-sectional designs (reviewed in Shock et al., 1984). All of these declines were essentially linear, but the slopes varied considerably among different physiological systems. For example, the rate of decline of maximum breathing capacity was substantially greater than that of peripheral nerve conduction velocity. Later on, Shock and colleagues (1984), involved in the Baltimore Study of Aging, took care to exclude individuals with overt clinical disease and focused on longitudinal studies. The longitudinal studies uncovered considerable heterogeneity among individuals in the rate of change of specific physiological functions. For example, about one-third of their aging cohort had no detectable change in renal function (as measured by creatinine clearance) and a small number of subjects even appeared to exhibit improved function with age (Lindeman et al., 1985). Heterogeneity has also been observed with other systems. For example, while declines in cardiac output are observed in cross-sectional studies, when individuals with clinical evidence of cardiovascular disease are excluded, cardiac output is generally maintained. Such maintenance of function, however, is gained via variable degrees of compensatory alterations, such as an increase in cardiac dilatation, which results in an increased stroke volume (Lakatta, 1990, 1993). These various observations provide some partial quantification of what every physician knows on qualitative grounds, namely, that patterns of aging vary substantially among patients.

At the cellular level, it is convenient to describe age-related changes in two broad classes of cell types: those capable of proliferative replacement or expansion and those terminally differentiated and incapable of replication. An example of a biomarkers of aging for at least subsets of the latter is the accumulation of complex yellow-brownish pigments known as lipofuscins (Yin, 1996; Terman and Brunk, 1998). These accumulate in the

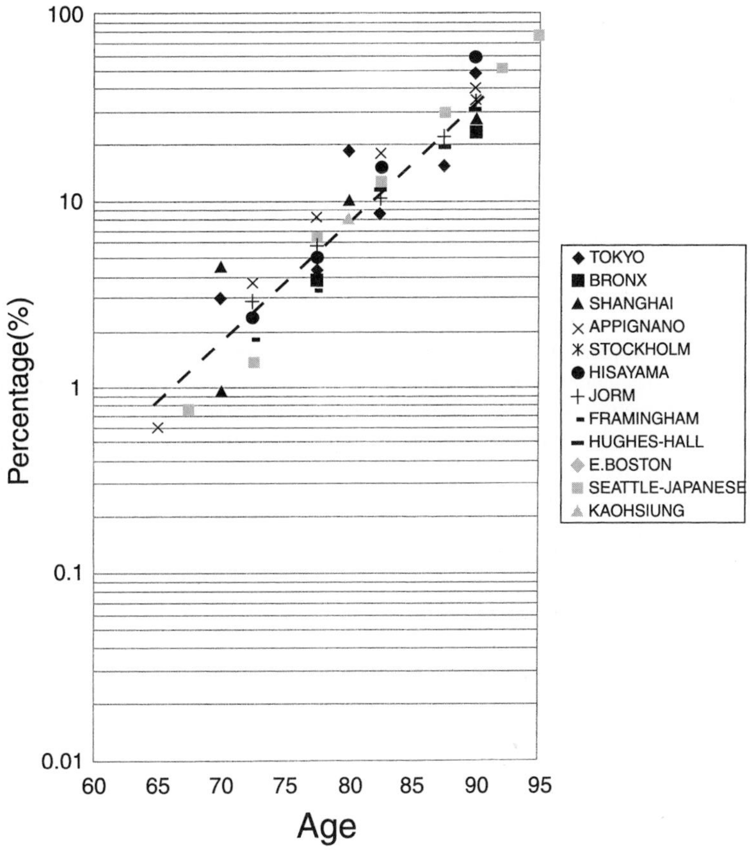

Fig. 51–2. Exponential increases in the prevalence of dementias in subjects over the age of 65 years. This pattern is found among 12 populations from around the world. From Katzman and Kawas (1998) with permission.

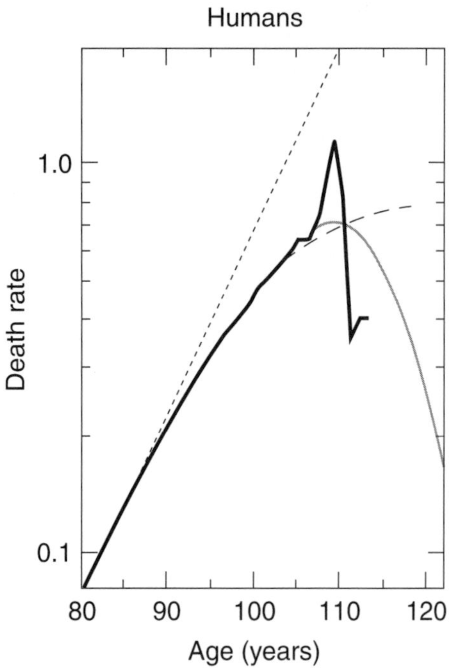

Fig. 51–3. Death rates for human females aged 80 to 122 years. The heavy solid line aggregates data from Japan and 13 Western European countries for which reliable data can be obtained over the period from 1950 to 1990 for individuals aged 80 to 109 and from 1950 to 1997 for individuals aged 110 and over. Although the data are based on 287 million person-years at risk, reliable data were available for only 82 individuals who survived beyond age 110. The best fit for an exponential (Gompertz) function at ages 80 to 84 is shown by the short dotted line. A logistic curve that best fits the entire set of data is shown with long dashes. A quadratic curve (log of death rate as a quadratic function of age), fit to data at ages 105 and higher, is shown by the light solid line. From Vaupel et al. (1998) with permission.

aging cells of an amazing variety of organisms, ranging from fungi to humans (Munkres and Rana, 1978; Fite and Bengston, 1989; Nakano and Gotoh, 1992; Wolf, 1993). Such observations have been invoked as support for the oxidative damage theory of aging because of their presumed origin via oxidative alterations of macromolecules (Terman and Brunk, 1998).

The bulk of the literature supports the contention that a large variety of mammalian somatic cell types exhibit limited replicative potentials and that these potentials decline as a function of donor age. The results of cell culture approaches to this question have been particularly convincing when employing primary and secondary cloning methodologies (Martin et al., 1983) to minimize the bias introduced by strong selection for rare cells capable of unusual replicative potential, such as occurs with mass culture methodologies; the latter methods can minimize or even obscure age-associated declines in replicative potential (Martin et al., 1970; Tesco et al., 1998; Cristofalo et al., 1998). The replicative potential of a variety of mammalian somatic cells also declines as a function of age in vivo; caloric restriction, a method leading to enhanced life span in rodents and other species (see below), conserves these replicative potentials (Wolf et al., 1995). The degree to which such limited replicative potential sets the stage for age-related aberrations remains unknown, however. It is possible that it plays a role in various tissue atrophies associated with senescence.

One of the most robust findings of age-associated changes at the molecular level is the accumulation of various posttranslational changes in proteins, particularly in long-lived proteins (Stadtman and Levine, 2000). These have been observed in organisms ranging from nematodes (Gershon and Gershon, 1970) to humans (Chen et al., 1997). Two classes of protein modification are thought to be of special significance in aging organisms, oxidative alterations [as revealed in assays for carbonyl groups (Levine et al., 2000)] and glycation [i.e., nonenzymatic glycosylation, as revealed in assays for pentosidine (Sell et al., 2000)]. Some authors emphasize the joint operation of glucose-mediated alterations of proteins with oxidative change (glycoxidation) in the pathogenesis of neurodegenerative diseases (Sayre et al., 2001) and atherosclerosis (Sakata et al., 2001).

DNA is also a target for both glycation (Lee and Cerami, 1987, 1990) and oxidation (Helbock et al., 1998). Fructose is a more efficient glycating agent than glucose and has been shown to induce DNA damage (Levi and Werman, 2001). The degree to which somatic mutation in aging organisms is due to such alterations remains to be established. It is clear, however, that somatic cells accumulate mutations in aging tissues. The rates of such accumulation in the epithelial cells of aging humans (Martin et al., 1996b) may be an order of magnitude greater than that observed for nonepithelial cells (Grist et al., 1992). This could conceivably be one of the reasons carcinomas are more prevalent than sarcomas in aging humans. Aging is also characterized by increasing degrees of chromosomal instability. A particularly striking example is the loss of X and Y chromosomes (Guttenbach et al., 1995). There is evidence that not only the inactive X but also the active X can be preferentially lost during aging, at least in peripheral blood lymphocytes (Surralles et al., 1996).

The issue of age-related DNA damage in the mitochondrial DNA of postreplicative cells such as neurons, skeletal muscle, and myocardium is currently receiving a great deal of attention (Wallace, 2001). Such lesions are even being explored as the basis for some forms of presbycusis (Fischel-Ghodian et al., 1997) and sensory neuropathology (Nagley et al., 2001). The ability to utilize polymerase chain reaction methods to amplify the entire mitochondrial genome has revealed marked increases in the number and variety of structural aberrations detectable in biopsies of skeletal muscle of aging human subjects (Melov et al., 1995). These aberrations could be associated with age-related deficiencies in the capacity to carry out oxidative phosphorylation (Pesce et al., 2001). It is likely, however, that some critical level of heteroplasmy for significant mutations is necessary to impact upon mitochondrial function within a cell. Heteroplasmy in the human brain for noncoding regions of mitochondrial DNA is much more readily detectable than lesions in coding regions (Jazin et al., 1996). It is possible that stochastic focal intracellular accumulations of mitochondrial DNA with large rearrangements and lesions in coding regions may lead to cell death. Their frequencies may therefore be underestimated. Evidence that the rate of mitochondrial mutagenesis is greater in mice than in humans supports the hypothesis that genomic instability of the mitochondrial genome may represent a general process of senescence (Wang et al., 1997) (Fig. 51–4). Some investigators believe that mitochondria are the primary targets for the oxidative damage associated with aging (Wallace, 2001).

WHY WE AGE

Although evolutionary biologists cannot tell us how we age, they are confident that they understand why we age (Rose, 1991). Simply stated, aging is thought to be inevitable in age-structured populations because of the waning of the force of natural selection with respect to the age of gene effects. Consider such an age-structured population in which aging did not occur. Given the environmental hazards of predation, starvation, drought, ac-

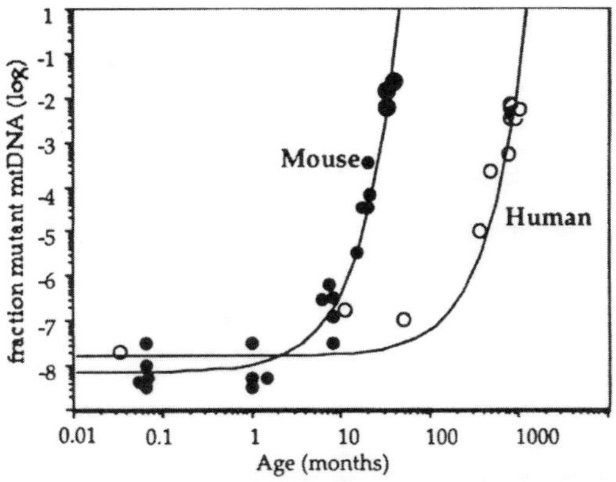

Fig. 51–4. Rates of increase in mutations in mitochondrial DNA from mouse and human myocardium. Each *open circle* (humans) and *closed circle* (mice) represents data from an individual subject. From Wang et al. (1997) with permission.

cidents, and infectious diseases under which all species have evolved, comparatively few individuals would survive to old age. Now consider those very lucky few that did exhibit exceptionally long survival. Any allele that did not reach phenotypic expression until these late ages would have virtually no representation in the gene pool of subsequent generations because it would be excessively diluted by alleles contributed by the vastly greater population of younger, reproducing individuals. By this logic, it can be seen that ecology drives life-history strategies. Given an exceptionally hazardous environment, one can anticipate strong selective pressure for alleles that contribute to very rapid sexual maturation with the production of large numbers of progeny within short periods of time. With the relaxation of such environmental hazards, there is the opportunity for selection of alleles associated with longer periods of development, longer periods of reproductive activity, and longer life spans. Such conditions can be presumed to be permissive of the evolution of genes that contribute to such phenotypes as the improved maintenance of macromolecular integrity. These theoretical ideas have received strong support from both field observations and laboratory experiments. The field experiments pursued the hypothesis that an insular species in an environment free of predators would evolve longer life spans than its mainland sibling species. Such a pair of sibling species was found among Virginia opossums living on the mainland of the southeast United States and a nearby island that had been separated from the mainland for some 4000 years. It was indeed discovered that the actuarial rate of aging of the insular species was about half that of the mainland species (Austad, 1993). Moreover, the longer-lived insular species was shown to have a lower rate of collagen cross-linking, as measured indirectly via collagen fiber breaking time. The laboratory experiments utilized both direct and indirect selection for enhanced life span, the results being in keeping with the predictions of the evolutionary theory (Luckinbill and Clare, 1987; Hutchinson and Rose, 1991; Hutchinson et al., 1991; Zwaan et al., 1995).

There are several important implications of the evolutionary biological theory of why we age. First, it is not consistent with the older idea commonly expressed in the gerontological literature that each species has a fixed maximum life span. Life span is plastic. It can be gradually modulated by selection. For model organisms with relatively short life spans, that selection can be surprisingly rapid. Second, the theory predicts that there are likely to be a large number of loci, variation at which can modulate life span and the patterns of aging. There are no genetic switches designed to "turn on" aging. Aging is thus seen to be different from development, which is subject to determinative, sequential gene action that is under strong selective pressure. By contrast, senescent phenotypes, having escaped the force of natural selection, are mere epiphenomena or by-products of gene action selected for other purposes (reproductive fitness) or the result of random mutations that accumulate in the genome but do not reach a phenotypic level of expression until late in the life course. Senescence is nonadaptive, whereas development is clearly adaptive. Given this scenario, one can anticipate a variety of mechanisms of aging, not a single mechanism. Moreover, these mechanisms are likely to be subject to stochastic variations among individuals within a species. As mentioned above, this is indeed routinely observed in life-table analyses of genetically identical individuals, such as inbred mice, inbred fruit flies, or inbred nematodes. While the theory does not falsify the hypothesis that there may be some common mechanisms of aging among different species, it suggests that there are likely to be considerable variations among species. This conclusion follows from the fact that genetic loci of importance to certain major components of fitness, such as mating behavior, are likely to differ substantially among species. Finally, there is a most interesting implication for geriatric medicine. Quantitative arguments allow one to determine the approximate age in human beings when the force of natural selection has essentially disappeared. It is earlier than one might imagine, about 45 years (Hamilton, 1966; Charlesworth, 1994). We might therefore define the sphere of geriatric medicine as beginning in middle age, not old age. There is also an important message here for geneticists interested in the genetic basis of variations in rates of decline in particular physiological domains. The time to begin a longitudinal study of such rates of change is in middle age, not old age (Martin, 1998, 2000). This has a number of advantages, including avoidance of the comorbidities that are so common in very old individuals and the potential availability of DNA from three generations.

THE EVOLUTIONARY BIOLOGICAL THEORY OF AGING

What types of gene action can escape the force of natural selection? Not surprisingly, the first insight to this question came from one of the giants of twentieth century biology, J. B. S. Haldane. Haldane (1941) wondered why an autosomal dominant mutation, e.g., that which causes Huntington's disease, was so common. [Some 40 years later, an attempt at complete ascertainment of the disorder in south Wales gave a prevalence of 7.61/100,000 individuals (Walker et al., 1981)]. Acknowledging the insights of Haldane, Medawar (1946, 1952, 1957) elaborated this idea in considerable detail. He envisioned a variety of constitutive mutations at various loci that had neutral effects early in the life span but deleterious effects in late life. Even for phenotypes that did not quite escape the force of natural selection, there would be strong selective pressure for the emergence of suppressors at other loci, which would postpone the effects of the mutation. Ultimately, however, such suppression would put the phenotype out of the reach of natural selection. The picture that emerges is that all of us have our share of such inborn mutations and suppressor alleles. The patterns likely differ among individuals, thus providing the substrate for variations in the nature–nurture and gene–gene interactions that lead to specific senescent phenotypes. The overall prevalence of any particular such constitutive mutation can be expected to vary as a function of genetic drift. Moreover, there is no necessity for such mutations (and, hence, such phenotypes) to contribute to the senescence phenotypes in all species or in all mammalian species. One can therefore refer to such genetic modulations of aging as "private" (Martin et al., 1996a; Martin, 1997).

A second class of gene action embraced by the evolutionary biological theory of aging has become known as *antagonistic pleiotropy* (Rose, 1991). It was first elucidated by Williams (1957, 1960). This idea invokes a subset of alleles that have been selected because of good effects early in the life span (leading to enhanced reproductive fitness) but with deleterious effects late in the life course, when these late phenotypic effects will have escaped the force of natural selection. The specific example cited by Williams involved loci that modulate the efficiency of incorporation of calcium into bones. One can imagine that alleles resulting in high efficiency of such incorporation would lead to improved reproductive fitness, but such alleles might, over time, result in the incorporation of calcium into arterial walls, thus resulting in a form of arteriosclerosis. Once such alleles have been selected, it seems likely that they would spread throughout the population. Moreover, it is possible that at least some such alleles would have appeared and spread within a number of independent populations, perhaps even among different species. One might therefore refer to these genetic variations as leading to "public" modulations of senescence. Polymorphisms, rather than mutations, are likely to be more relevant for our understanding of the genetic modulations of senescence associated with these pleiotropic alleles. An interesting potential molecular example involves a polymorphism coding for variable numbers of CAG repeats in the coding region of the androgen receptor gene. Individuals with relatively few such repeats are thought to have more robust responses to androgen stimulation. There appears to be a linear relationship between the length of the polyglutamine tract coded for by these repeats and the degree of inhibition of the receptors to bind androgen and to activate the transcription of downstream targets (Chamberlain et al., 1994). One can imagine that such alleles were associated with reproductive advantages in some environments of our remote ancestors. In modern societies, however, with the opportunities for long life spans, there is evidently a price to pay for being more muscular, more aggressive, and more sexually active as youngsters as these individuals have a higher risk of developing adenocarcinoma of the prostate; moreover, their prostatic cancers tend to be more aggressive (Ingles et al., 1997; Stanford et al., 1997; Giovannucci et al., 1997). Individuals with many CAG repeats are also more likely to develop their prostate cancers at a younger age (Hardy et al., 1996). A population-based case-control study has given further support for a role of these repeats in increasing the risk of developing prostate cancer (Hsing et al., 2000).

OBJECTIONS TO THE EVOLUTIONARY BIOLOGICAL THEORY OF AGING

Four arguments can be made that, at least superficially, appear to challenge the evolutionary biological theory of why we age, or at least certain implications of the theory. As indicated above, the theory predicts that there are multiple genes and multiple mechanisms contributing to senescence, but one of the most robust findings of experimental mammalian gerontology is that the simple expedient of reducing calories can postpone all of the major causes of death and greatly extend life span. For example, reducing the caloric intake of Fischer 344 rats to about 40% of that consumed by genetically identical littermates extends the maximum life span of relatively small cohorts of animals such that more than 60% of the restricted group live longer than the longest-lived member of the control group (Yu et al., 1982). The mechanism(s) of such life span extension is unknown. Hypotheses include an altered metabolic pathway of glucose fuel utilization, enhancement of protection from oxidative damage, and enhancement of the ability to cope with other stresses, perhaps via changes in neuroendocrine regulation and heat shock protein responses (Masoro, 1996; Sohal and Weindruch, 1996). These ideas were partially supported by a review of gene actions associated with genetically based enhancements of life span in organisms ranging from fungi to humans (Martin et al., 1996a). There are counterarguments that can be invoked, however. First, some may regard the ad libitum type of feeding regimen of caged rodents as being highly abnormal. Periodic caloric restriction may represent a pattern of nutrition in the wild that contributed to the evolution of rodent species. It has been suggested that the caloric restriction response evolved in these short-lived species to enhance survival during periods of unpredictable and transient food shortages (Masoro and Austad, 1996). There is no assurance that these metabolic adaptations arose in longer-lived mammalian species, such as humans, although it remains a distinct possibility. Ongoing experiments with rhesus and squirrel monkeys may provide answers to this important question (Lane and Ingram, 1998; Roth et al., 1999, 2001).

A number of simple genetic manipulations in both *C. elegans* and *Drosophila melanogaster* have led to substantial enhancements of life span. In *Drosophila*, the beneficial effects of additional superoxide dismutase expressed in motor neurons (Parkes et al., 1998) may merely reflect complementation for a "private" deficiency of the particular inbred stock of flies employed for such research. In nematodes, the single-gene mutations that have been reported to result in increased life span (Friedman and Johnson, 1988; Larsen et al., 1995; Lin et al., 1997; Tissenbaum and Ruvkun, 1998) could simply lower the metabolic rate, thus emulating the increased life span associated with lowering body temperature in poikilothermic animals. Quantitation of metabolic rates has only recently been undertaken (Van Voorhies and Ward, 1999). Nevertheless, the fact that these mutations in nematodes appear to involve alternative strategies for fuel utilization raise intriguing parallels with the caloric restriction experiments in mammals. Moreover, the key insulin-like signal-transduction pathway involved in the life span extension of nematodes has also been implicated in the life span extension of fruit flies (Clancy et al., 2001; Tatar et al., 2001; Kenyon, 2001).

As noted above, demographers have observed departures from Gompertz kinetics in old populations of animals and humans. Some have suggested that this is at variance with the evolutionary theory. Different attempts are being made by evolutionary biologists to reconcile these observations (Mueller and Rose, 1996; Charlesworth and Partridge, 1997; Pletcher and Curtsurger, 1998; Kirkwood, 1999; Wachter, 1999). There could be trivial reasons for such mortality plateaus, however. The striking limitations of motility observed in all very old animals of all species could be associated with a decreased hazard function for mortality. For fruit flies and medflies, this could occur when flight is no longer possible. For human beings, the plateaus could be associated with decreased environmental stresses resulting from such secular trends as central heating, air conditioning, and immunizations against pneumococcal and influenzal infections. Moreover, the decrease in motility could result in fewer falls and, hence, fewer hip fractures and the associated risk of fatal bronchopneumonia.

Another concern has been the intuitively appealing idea that the wisdom and nurturing of grandparents could result in enhanced reproductive fitness of grandchildren. If this were the case, there would indeed be grounds for selection for alleles expressed late in the life course. Evidence that such older humans survived in any significant numbers in the remote past is lacking, however, although some anthropologists claim to have documented such survival in extant primitive populations. While parenting skills clearly enhance the survival of anthropoid primates (Allman et al., 1998), field studies of prides of lions and of troops of olive baboons have failed to demonstrate any effect of grandparental care on survival of grandchildren (Packer et al., 1998).

Perhaps the most compelling argument comes from analyses of "time to failure" of complex structures by engineers. Wood and colleagues (1994) suggested that the absence of senescence may be an inappropriate evolutionary null model for complex metazoan animals. Animals with any degree of complexity, like complex machines (Abernathy, 1996), have some intrinsic probabilistic time to failure (Nordling, 1953).

Wood et al. (1994) argued that natural selection appears to be unnecessary to explain the origin of senescence, except indirectly, via the emergence of organismal complexity. These authors state that what we are really trying to explain with the evolutionary models is the differential delay of senescence observed among various species. Given the focus of the present chapter, one might also add that what we are really interested in, as physicians, is how evolution produced such varied patterns of senescence in our individual patients. The evolutionary theory of gene action is a satisfying framework with which to approach the origins of both interspecific and intraspecific variations in aging.

Table 51–1. A Subset of Common Geriatric Disorders*

Special senses
Ocular cataracts
Macular degeneration

Nervous system
Alzheimer's disease
Multi-infarct dementia
Frontotemporal dementia
Other dementias
Sleep disorder/insomnia
Depression
Parkinson disease
Glioma
Meningioma
Hypothermia/hyperthermia
Shingles/Herpes zoster
Trigeminal neuralgia
Peripheral neuropathy

Endocrine system
Diabetes mellitus type 2
Hypothyroidism
Hashimoto thyroiditis
Menopause

Cardiovascular system
Arteriosclerosis
Atherosclerosis/ischemic heart disease
Congestive heart failure
Calcific aortic stenosis
Cerebral amyloid angiopathy
Stroke/cerebral hemorrhage
Hypertension
Orthostatic hypotension
Giant cell arteritis
Varicose veins

Pulmonary system
Chronic obstructive pulmonary disease
Chronic interstitial pulmonary fibrosis
Pulmonary embolism
Lung cancer

Genitourinary system
Nephrosclerosis
Benign prostatic hyperplasia
Prostatic carcinoma
Renal cell carcinoma
Urinary bladder carcinoma
Ovarian carcinoma
Breast cancer

Hematopoeitic/immune systems
Iron deficiency anemia
Pernicious anemia
Aplastic anemia
Hemochromatosis
Lymphomas
Monoclonal gammopathy
Multiple myeloma
Chronic lymphocytic leukemia
Chronic myelogenous leukemia
Myelodysplastic syndrome
Atrophy of thymus
Autoimmunity
Systemic lupus erythematosus

Gastrointestinal system
Atrophic gastritis
Diverticulosis/diverticulitis
Pancreatic cancer
Gastric lymphoma
Gastric carcinoma
Polyps of the colon
Adenocarcinoma of the colon

Skin and subcutaneous tissue
Obesity
Scleroderma
Seborrheic dermatitis
Xerosis
Melanoma
Bowen disease
Basal cell carcinoma
Squamous cell carcinoma
Actinic keratosis

Miscellaneous
Amyloidosis
Osteoarthritis

*Alleles at numerous genetic loci have the potential to modulate the rates of development of these disorders, as evidenced by a large number of citations in OMIM (Online Mendelian Inheritance of Man) (http://www.ncbi.nlm.nih.gov/Omim/).

COMMON SENESCENT PHENOTYPES OF HUMANS

Table 51–1 gives a substantial, but by no means comprehensive, listing of common senescent phenotypes observed in humans. When considered collectively, there are many thousands of genetic loci with the potential to modulate the rates at which these phenotypes develop (Martin, 1978; Martin, unpublished data).

Variations at some genetic loci modulate multiple aspects of the phenotype. I have referred to these as leading to "segmental progeroid syndromes" (Martin, 1978). The classic example is Werner's syndrome (progeria of the adult) (Epstein et al., 1966). This autosomal recessive disorder is now known to result from homozygosity for a null mutation at a locus coding for a member of the *RecQ* family of DNA helicases (Yu et al., 1996). The mutation highlights the potential importance of genomic instability in the genesis of such phenotypes as atherosclerosis, Type 2 diabetes mellitus, osteoporosis, ocular cataracts, and gonadal atrophy. (A role for such genomic instability in the genesis of neoplasia, another feature of Werner's syndrome, comes as no surprise.)

Some mutations and polymorphisms appear to impact only upon a single senescent phenotype. I have referred to these as leading to "unimodal progeroid syndromes" (Martin, 1982).

Many of these segmental and unimodal progeroid mutations may represent "private" mutations. As such, there is no certainty that elucidation of their pathogenesis will inform us about the usual mechanisms for that particular phenotype in most individuals, but it may. An interesting test case, involving research in progress, is the subset of autosomal dominant mutations leading to the relatively early onset of DAT. Three such loci have been implicated to date: *APP* (coding for the β-amyloid precursor protein), *PS1* (coding for the presenilin 1 protein), and *PS2* (coding for the highly homologous presenilin 2 protein) (reviewed by Selkoe, 2001). Conventional wisdom currently ties all three mutations to the pathogenesis of DAT via altered processing of the β-amyloid precursor protein (Selkoe, 2001). Does this paradigm apply to the vastly more common late-onset sporadic forms of DAT? It is entirely possible that altered metabolism of the β-amyloid precursor protein in these cases may be a result, rather than a cause, of the pathology or, perhaps more likely, that it may be both a result and a secondary cause of additional pathology. An investigation of "public" polymorphic modulations of the disease, first initiated for a triallelic polymorphism at the apolipoprotein E locus (*APOE*) (Corder et al., 1993) and recently extended to other polymorphic loci, is indeed consistent with a unified pathogenesis. Readers should consult Blacker et al. (1998) for more details and references. There is considerable disagreement, however, regarding the validity of numerous claims of polymorphic associations for loci other than that of *APOE*. The case for the primacy of β-amyloid is by no means proven.

Charlesworth (1996) has pointed out that the three rare autosomal dominant mutations and the *APOE* polymorphism are indeed likely to constitute examples, respectively, of the Medawar notion of constitutive mutations and the Williams concept of antagonistic pleiotropic gene action. It remains for future research to uncover the putative beneficial effects, in the early life histories of our ancestors, of the $\epsilon 4$ allele of the *APOE* gene. I have suggested that endemic infectious diseases caused by lipophilic protozoa, such as *Trypanosoma brucei*, could have been the basis for such selection in human populations (Martin, 1999). The price we now pay is that the $\epsilon 4$ allele is associated with an earlier onset of DAT and atherosclerosis and a diminished probability of recovery from strokes (Basun et al., 1996).

GENETIC BASIS OF LONGEVITY IN HUMAN POPULATIONS

There has been renewed interest in discovering the genetic loci with mutations or polymorphisms that significantly impact upon human longevity. There are many ways for genes to result in decreased life span. Very few of these are likely to address fundamental mechanisms of aging as they occur in most individuals. Attention has therefore been focused on alleles that may contribute to unusually long life spans. As noted above, these are difficult studies. First, human longevity is clearly under highly polygenic control. Let us consider, e.g., only the oxidative stress theory of aging, the most popular current theory of how we age. One can quickly generate a list of hundreds of candidate genes involving such relevant processes as the rates of generation of reactive oxygen species, the degree of scavenging of such species, the structure and redundancy of macromolecular targets of oxidative damage, the repair of damage to macromolecules, the appropriate utilization of cell cycle check points to permit adequate repair, and the triggering of apoptosis as a response to unrepaired cell injury. Second, as pointed out earlier, how long we live has much to do with chance. Third, particularly for studies involving centenarians, documentation of age is often difficult and many individuals exaggerate their longevity. Fourth, variations in availability and quality of such factors as central heating, air conditioning, sanitation, nutrition, water supply, and medical care can result in large intragenerational and inter-generational effects on longevity. The same is true, of course, of exposure to accidents, tobacco smoke, and other relevant environmental agents. Despite these concerns, there is currently considerable interest on the part of many gerontologists and some geneticists in the genetic analysis of the basis of human longevity. Approaches have included twin studies, association studies, and pedigree studies.

The most recent twin studies on longevity come from the excellent Scandinavian registries, particularly those of Denmark and Sweden. Perhaps this is not surprising, given the fact that the entire field of quantitative trait analysis began with the Danish botanist Wilhelm Johannsen (the originator of the terms *gene*, *phenotype*, and *genotype*). Estimates of broadly based heritability of longevity were made in a study of all traced nonemigrant twins born in Denmark from 1870 to 1900. Inclusion criteria included a zygosity diagnosis and survival of pairs to at least age 15 years. Pairs in which one or both twins were still alive were excluded in the 1994 follow-up study, giving a total sample size of 2872 twin pairs for analysis (Herskind et al., 1996). Heritabilities were 0.26 and 0.23, respectively, for males and females. The small sex difference was thought to be the result of a greater impact of nonshared environmental factors in females. Heritability did not differ among three 10-year birth cohorts. A Swedish study determined mortality rates and within-pair similarity for age at death in a sample of 3656 identical and 6849 same-sexed fraternal twin pairs (Ljungquist et al., 1998). The authors regarded a maximum likelihood modeling of the integrated mortality risk as providing the best measure of the genetic contribution to longevity. They concluded that, over a wide age range, an upper limit of about one-third of the variance of mortality risk can be attributable to genetic factors. Almost all of the remaining variance was thought to be due to nonshared, individually unique environmental factors. They recommended further research to examine evidence that genetic factors may play a variable role as functions of age at death. An overall conclusion of these and most other such studies of twin pairs is that genetic contributions to longevity variance in human populations is substantially less than that attributable to environmental factors and intrinsic stochastic factors, if these could be considered separately from extrinsic environmental influences.

The demonstration, in populations of French centenarians, of an enrichment of the $\epsilon 2$ allele and a deficiency of the $\epsilon 4$ allele of a apolipoprotein E (Schachter, 1994) has been confirmed in Finnish populations (Louhija et al., 1994; Castro et al., 1999). This finding has prompted a number of new genetic association studies comparing centenarians with younger cohorts. Centenarians are assumed to be long-lived, in part because of their constitutional genetic makeup. These studies generally include only "healthy" centenarians, at least in terms of their ability to live relatively independently. The definition of controls is problematic. One cannot predict which members of a younger cohort would go on to achieve unusual longevity because of a robust genotype and which would not reach this potential because of chance events, such as somatic mutations involving critical loci. The degrees to which environmental cohort effects and differential migration patterns could impact upon the results would also be difficult to control. Furthermore, as noted above, it would not be surprising if one found large numbers of polymorphic alleles that characterize long-lived vs. short-lived cohorts. One might guess, moreover, that the nature–nurture interactions that led to such successful aging in one population might differ in another population. For these reasons, I believe that much more progress can be made in the elucidation of genetic mechanisms of aging by focusing on the genotypic basis of differential rates of change of highly specific physiological processes and phenotypes, rather than on age at death (Martin, 1998, 2000). Nevertheless, a number of case-control association studies are under way, using candidate loci thought to be of special relevance to the biology of aging and age-related diseases. Those being conducted by Italian investigators are the most ambitious of this type as they have segmented the Italian population into northern, southern, and central areas of Italy and have included the population of the island of Sardinia. Not surprisingly, early results suggest that statistically significant associations will be found with polymorphic alleles at many loci (De Benedictis et al., 1998a,b, 1999, 2001; Bonafe et al., 1999; Yashin et al., 1999).

An obvious question posed by genetic epidemiologists is the degree to which maternal inheritance contributes to longevity. Korpelainen (1999) estimated heritabilities, based on the pedigrees of European royal and noble families (Gavrilova et al., 1998), which led to the conclusion that the maternally inherited component in the human life span is greater than the paternal component. The extent to which specific haplotypes of mitochondrial DNA may be responsible for this putative contribution of maternal inheritance to longevity is currently being investigated among the descendents of the circa 10,000 Utah Mormon pioneers (Kerber et al., 1999).

Given the recent advances in genomics, some investigators are now conducting segregational analyses of the genetic basis of unusual longevity in pedigrees ascertained because of the occurrence of multiple centenarians and octogenarians in several generations. For at least the New England population, claims of such advanced age have been validated (Perls et al., 1999). I am not optimistic that such studies will uncover a few major polymorphic loci, but perhaps this is not out of the question for some populations that are relatively homogeneous for genetic and environmental factors.

COMMON CONSTITUTIONAL CHROMOSOMAL ANEUPLOIDIES AND THE EMERGENCE OF CERTAIN SENESCENT PHENOTYPES

Many consider Down syndrome (DS) to be a useful model of accelerated aging, at least as regards a subset of relevant phenotypes. In a 1978 review, I concluded that DS involved more relevant phenotypes than any other genetic progeroid syndrome, including Werner's syndrome (Martin, 1978). More recent literature has supported this conclusion. Examples include reports of early menopause (Schupf et al., 1997), decreased life span of erythrocytes (Bartosz and Kedziora, 1982), early onset of presbycusis (Buchanan, 1990), precocious aging of the immune system (Cossarizza et al., 1990), accelerated wrinkling of the skin (Brugge et al., 1993), altered cell membrane fluidity (Scott et al., 1994), and increased titers of thyroid autoantibodies (Karlsson et al., 1998). Molecular studies have reported defective repair of oxidative damage in mitochondrial DNA (Druzhyna et al., 1998), early glycoxidation damage in brain tissues (Odetti et al., 1998), reduction of the activity of ribosomal genes (Borsatto and Smith, 1996), and abnormal proteins thought to result from mRNA frameshifts (molecular misreading) (van Leeuwen et al., 1998a,b). The latter have also been observed in the brains of subjects with the common, late-onset, sporadic form of DAT (van Leeuwen et al., 1998a,b). The observation that virtually all subjects with DS develop the neuropathological stigmata of DAT by the fifth decade of life has received more attention than any other DS phenotype. Deposition of β-amyloid aggegates or of its precursors begins some 50 years earlier than in normal subjects (Rumble et al., 1989). This has provided important support for the β-amyloid cascade theory of the pathogenesis of DAT (Hardy and Allsop, 1991). The discovery that a proteolytic enzyme capable of initiating the β-amyloidogenic pathway of processing of the β-amyloid precursor protein is coded by a gene in the critical DS region of the long arm of chromosome 21 gives further support to the importance of DS as a model for DAT (Saunders et al., 1999). The relative importance of that protease in the β cleavage of the precursor protein compared to the protease coded for by a homologue on chromosome 11 remains to be seen (Vassar et al., 1999). The evidence (still rather sparse) that DS subjects are relatively resistant to atherogenesis (Murdoch et al., 1977; Yla-Herttuala et al., 1989) argues against an important role for that form of arteriosclerosis in the pathogenesis of DAT.

In contrast to the rather large literature on aging phenotypes in DS subjects, very little is known about the details of aging in other aneuploid syndromes, despite the fact that there are large cohorts of aging subjects with Turner's and Klinefelter's syndromes. Subjects with Turner's syndrome have insulin resistance, an increased incidence of Type 2 diabetes mellitus, elevated cholesterol levels, and hypertension (Ross et al., 1995). There is also an accelerated rate of loss of high-frequency hearing (Hultcrantz et al., 1994). They thus provide interesting models for the study of pathways of gene action leading to major age-related disorders. The loss of bone mass that has been observed in association with Klinefelter's syndrome has generally been assumed to be the result of androgen deficiency, but that lesion occurs despite adequate testosterone replacement (Wong et al., 1993). Here is then another interesting line of research of relevance to gerontology. Even less is known about the impact of autosomal aneuploidy upon aspects of aging. While full trisomies and monosomies will have severe impacts upon development and will result in short life spans, partial aneuploidies and mosaics may prove to be interesting, especially if the effects on development can be dissociated from the effects on postmaturational decline.

CLINICAL IMPLICATIONS OF RESEARCH ON THE GENETICS OF LONGEVITY AND AGING UPON DIAGNOSIS, TREATMENT, AND PREVENTION OF COMMON DISEASES OF THE ELDERLY

Like all patients, older individuals are unique, only more so. Why is this true? First, gerontologists have learned from studies of humans and nonhuman species that variance increases as a function of age for a large number of physiological measures. Longitudinal studies of human subjects have shown that rates of decline for specific parameters vary substantially among individuals (Shock et al., 1984). This behavior would be predicted by the evolutionary biological theory of aging, which invokes a large number of private and public genetic modulations and numerous gene–gene and environment–gene interactions. It should be evident that the longer one lives, the greater the collective impact of differential environmental factors. Thus, when a physician initiates some intervention in an older patient, whether medical, surgical, nutritional, or behavioral, he or she may be embarking upon an experiment that has never been done before.

A second point is the growing realization that medical geneticists can be of assistance in the evaluation of common late-onset disease. Until recently, the services of the medical geneticist have been largely confined to the pediatric population and a few relatively rare adult-dominant disorders, such as Huntington's disease. Given the anticipated impact of the new genomics with its ability to detect groups of polymorphic alleles contributing to disease susceptibility, a gradual move toward individualized prognosis, prevention, and treatment should emerge. This will especially be the case for individuals with one or a few major susceptibility alleles, but it is unlikely that physicians will be in a position to predict and influence overall life span for most subjects with any assurance, especially given the stochastic factors emphasized here. A major caveat in this conclusion of complexity in the determination of life span, however, comes from the results of the experiments on caloric restriction noted above. It is possible that the current experiments with nonhuman primates might justify clinical trials of intervention in human subjects. These are unlikely to involve strict caloric restriction, however. More likely, the trials will involve pharmacological agents that modulate the underlying mechanisms whereby caloric restriction increases life span. Should such intervention be successful, there may well be undesirable trade-offs or side effects, especially if initiated relatively early in the adult life span, when intervention is most likely to be meaningful. The major anticipated effect would be a decline in fecundity.

CONCLUSIONS

The practice of medicine is being transformed by dramatic secular changes in demography. Vast numbers of humans are living well past the peak of their reproductive activities, allowing the expression of phenotypes that were only rarely observed in the distant past because they readily escaped the force of natural selection. These phenotypes include declines in the structure and function of components of all body systems. These declines impact upon the quality of life even in the absence of clinically overt disease, including most of the major disorders of modern society, e.g., various forms of arteriosclerosis, Type 2 diabetes mellitus, carcinomas, strokes, DAT, Parkinson's disease, osteoporosis, osteoarthritis, ocular cataracts, macular degeneration, and benign prostatic hyperplasia. Two types of gene action are envisaged as modulating susceptibility to these late-life disorders: "private" constitutive mutations with neutral effects on reproductive fitness and "public" polymorphisms with positive effects on reproductive fitness but deleterious effects late in the life course. Medical geneticists have made significant progress in identifying a variety of private mutations. At least a proportion of these major genes will likely inform us as to the pathogenesis of geriatric disorders as they unfold in the general population. Much more research is required, however, to identify the public polymorphisms that serve as the polygenic substrates for susceptibility to the common disorders of older people. Such research may eventually lead to a tailoring of medical management to the needs of individual subjects. Predictions and interventions to influence longevity in most human subjects are considered unlikely for the foreseeable future, however, given the complexity of the control of rates of aging. A caveat in this conclusion comes from the strong evidence that caloric restriction can postpone disease and increase life span in a wide variety of species. Should current experiments with nonhuman primates prove to support that hypothesis, it is conceivable that pharmacological interventions may be discovered that will mimic the effects of caloric restriction and thus positively influence life span, although with anticipated decrements in fecundity.

REFERENCES

Abernathy RB (ed): The New Weibull Handbook. Houston: Gulf, 1996.

Allman J, Rosin A, Kumar R, Hasenstaub A: Parenting and survival in anthropoid primates: caretakers live longer. Proc Natl Acad Sci USA 1998; 95:6866–6869.

Austad SN: Retarded senescence in insular populations of Virginia opossums (*Didelphus virginiana*). J Zool 1993; 229:695–708.

Bartosz G, Kedziora J: Aging of the erythrocyte. XX. Decreased red cell life span in Down's syndrome. Cell Biol Int Rep 1982; 6:1119–1122.

Basun H, Corder EH, Guo Z, Lannfelt L, Corder LS, Manton KG, Winblad B, Viitanen M: Apolipoprotein E polymorphism and stroke in a population sample aged 75 years or more. Stroke 1996; 27:1310–1315.

Blacker D, Wilcox MA, Laird NM, Rodes L, Horvath SM, Go RC, Perry R, Watson B Jr, Bassett SS, McInnis MG, et al.: Alpha-2 macroglobulin is genetically associated with Alzheimer disease. Nat Genet 1998; 19:357–360.

Bonafe M, Olivieri F, Mari D, Baggio G, Mattace R, Berardelli M, Sansoni P, De Benedictis G, De Luca M, Marchegiani F, et al.: p53 codon 72 polymorphism and longevity: additional data on centenarians from continental Italy and Sardinia. Am J Hum Genet 1999; 65:1782–1785.

Borsatto B, Smith M: Reduction of the activity of ribosomal genes with age in Down's syndrome. Gerontology 1996; 42:147–154.

Brooks A, Lithgow GJ, Johnson TE: Mortality rates in a genetically heterogeneous population of *Caenorhabditis elegans*. Science 1994; 263:668–671.

Brugge KL, Grove GL, Clopton P, Grove MJ, Piacquadio DJ: Evidence for accelerated skin wrinkling among developmentally delayed individuals with Down's syndrome. Mech Ageing Dev 1993; 70:213–225.

Buchanan LH: Early onset of presbycusis in Down syndrome. Scand Audiol 1990; 19:103–110.

Carey J, Liedo P, Orozco D, Vaupel JW: Slowing of mortality rates at older ages in large medfly cohorts. Science 1992; 258:457–461.

Castro E, Ogburn CE, Hunt KE, Tilvis R, Louhija J, Penttinen R, Erkkola R, Panduro A, Riestra R, Piussan C, et al.: Polymorphisms at the Werner locus: I. Newly identified polymorphisms, ethnic variability of 1367Cy/Arg, and its stability in a population of Finnish centenarians. Am J Med Genet 1999; 82:399–403.

Chamberlain NL, Driver ED, Miesfield RL: The length and location of CAG trinucleotide repeats in the androgen receptor N-terminal domain affect transactivation function. Nucleic Acids Res 1994; 22:3181–3186.

Charlesworth B (ed): Evolution in Age Structured Populations. New York: Cambridge University Press, 1994.

Charlesworth B: Evolution of senescence: Alzheimer's disease and evolution. Curr Biol 1996; 6:20–22.

Charlesworth B, Partridge L: Ageing: leveling of the grim reaper. Curr Biol 1997; 7:R440–R442.

Chen YC, Reid GE, Simpson RJ, Truscott RJ: Molecular evidence for the involvement of alpha crystallin in the coloration/crosslinking of crystallins in age-related nuclear cataract. Exp Eye Res 1997; 65:835–840.

Clancy DJ, Gems D, Harshman LG, Oldham S, Stocker H, Hafen E, Leevers SJ, Partridge L: Extension of life-span by loss of CHICO, a *Drosophila* insulin receptor substrate protein. Science 2001; 292:104–106.

Corder EH, Saunders AM, Strittmatter WJ, Schmechel DE, Gaskell PC, Small GW, Roses AD, Haines JL, Pericek-Vance MA: Gene dose of apolipoprotein E type 4 allele and the risk of Alzheimer's disease in late onset families. Science 1993; 261:921–923.

Cossarizza A, Monti D, Montagnani G, Ortolani C, Masi M, Zannotti M, Franceschi C: Precocious aging of the immune system in Down syndrome: alteration of B lymphocytes, T-lymphocyte subsets, and cells with natural killer markers. Am J Med Genet Suppl 1990; 7:213–218.

Cristofalo VJ, Allen RG, Pignolo RJ, Martin BG, Beck JC: Relationship between donor age and the replicative lifespan of human cells in culture: a reevaluation. Proc Natl Acad Sci USA 1998; 95:10614–10619.

Curtsinger J, Fukui HH, Townsend DR, Vaupel JW: Demography of genotypes: failure of the limited life-span paradigm in *Drosophila melanogaster*. Science 1992; 258:461–463.

De Benedictis G, Carotenuto L, Cariieri G, De Luca M, Falcone E, Rose G, Cavalcanti S, Corsonello F, Feraco E, Baggio G, et al.: Gene/longevity association studies at four autosomal loci (REN, THO, PARP, SOD2). Eur J Hum Genet 1998a; 6:534–541.

De Benedictis G, Carotenuto L, Carrieri G, De Luca M, Falcone E, Rose G, Yashin AI, Bonafe M, Franceschi C: Age-related changes of the 3′APOB-VNTR genotype pool in ageing cohorts. Ann Hum Genet 1998b; 62(Pt.2):115–122.

De Benedictis G, Rose G, Carrieri G, De Luca M, Falcone E, Passarino G, Bonafe M, Monti D, Baggio G, Bertolini S, et al.: Mitochondrial DNA inherited variants are associated with successful aging and longevity in humans. FASEB J 1999; 13:1532–1536.

De Benedictis G, Tan Q, Jeune B, Christensen K, Ukraintseva SV, Bonafe M, Franceschi C, Vaupel JW, Yashin AI: Recent advances in human gene–longevity association studies. Mech Ageing Dev 2001; 122:909–920.

Druzhyna N, Nair RG, LeDoux SP, Wilson GL: Defective repair of oxidative damage in mitochondrial DNA in Down's syndrome. Mutat Res 1998; 409:81–89.

Epstein CJ, Martin GM, Schultz AL, Motulsky AG: Werner's syndrome: a review of its symptomatology, natural history, pathologic features, genetics and relationship to the natural aging process. Medicine (Baltimore) 1966; 45:177–221.

Finch CE, Kirkwood TB: Chance, Development and Aging. Oxford: Oxford University Press, 1999.

Fischel-Ghodian N, Bykhovskaya Y, Taylor K, Karen T, Cantor R, Ehrenman K, Smith R, Keithley E: Temporal bone analysis of patients with presbycusis reveals high frequency of mitochondrial mutations. Hear Res 1997; 110:147–154.

Fite KV, Bengston L: Aging and sex-related changes in the outer retina of Japanese quail. Curr Eye Res 1989; 8:1039–1048.

Friedman DB, Johnson TE: A mutation in the age-1 gene in *Caenorhabditis elegans* lengthens life and reduces hermaphrodite fertility. Genetics 1988; 118:75–86.

Gavrilova NS, Gavrilov LA, Evdokushkina GN, Semyonova VG, Gavrilova AL, Evdokushkina NN, Kushnareva YE, Kroutko VN, Andreyev A: Evolution, mutations, and human longevity: European royal and noble families. Hum Biol 1998; 70:799–804.

Gershon H, Gershon D: Detection of inactive enzyme molecules in ageing organisms. Nature 1970; 227:1214–1217.

Giovannucci E, Stampfer MJ, Krithivas K, Brown M, Dahl D, Brufsky A, Talcott J, Hennekens CH, Kantoff PW: The CAG repeat within the androgen receptor gene and its relationship to prostate cancer. Proc Natl Acad Sci USA 1997; 94:3320–3323.

Gompertz B: On the nature of the function expressive of the law of human mortality and on a new mode of determining the value of life contingencies. Philos Trans R Soc Lond 1825; 115:513–585.

Grist S, McCarron M, Kutlaca A, Turner DR, Morley AA: In vivo human somatic mutation: frequency and spectrum with age. Mutat Res 1992; 266:189–196.

Guttenbach M, Koschorz B, Bernthaler U, Grimm T, Schmid M: Sex chromosome loss and aging: in situ hybridization studies on human interphase nuclei. Am J Hum Genet 1995; 57:1143–1150.

Haldane JBS: New Paths in Genetics. London: Allen and Unwin, 1941.

Hamilton WD: The moulding of senescence by natural selection. J Theor Biol 1966; 12:12–45.

Hardy DO, Scher HI, Bogenreider T, Sabbatini P, Zhang ZF, Nanus DM, Catterall

JF: Androgen receptor CAG repeat lengths in prostate cancer: correlation with age of onset. J Clin Endocrinol Metab 1996; 81:4400–4405.
Hardy J, Allsop D: Amyloid deposition as the central event in the aetiology of Alzheimer's disease. Trends Pharmacol Sci 1991; 12:383–388.
Helbock H, Beckman KB, Shigenaga MK, Walter PB, Woodall AA, Yeo HC, Ames BN: DNA oxidation matters: the HPLC-electrochemical detection assay of 8-oxo-deoxyguanosine and 8-oxo-guanine. Proc Natl Acad Sci USA 1998; 95:288–293.
Herskind AM, McGue M, Holm NV, Sorenson TI, Harvald B, Vaupel JW: The heritability of human longevity: a population-based study of 1872 Danish twin pairs born 1870–1900. Hum Genet 1996; 97:319–323.
Hobbs FB, Damon BL: 65+ in the United States. Washington DC: US Government Printing Office, 1996.
Hsing AW, Gao YT, Wu G, Wang X, Deng J, Chen YL, Sesterhenn IA, Mostofi FK, Benichou J, Chang C: Polymorphic CAG and GGN repeat lengths in the androgen receptor gene and prostate cancer risk: a population-based case-control study in China. Cancer Res 2000; 60:5111–5116.
Hultcrantz M, Syven L, Borg E: Ear and hearing problems in 44 middle-aged women with Turner's syndrome. Hear Res 1994; 76:127–132.
Hutchinson EW, Rose MR: Quantitative genetics of postponed aging in *Drosophila melanogaster*. I. Analysis of outbred populations. Genetics 1991; 127:719–727.
Hutchinson EW, Shaw AJ, Rose MR: Quantitative genetics of postponed aging in *Drosophila melanogaster*. II. Analysis of selected lines. Genetics 1991; 127:729–737.
Ingles S, Ross RK, Yu MC, Irvine RA, La Pera G, Haile RW, Coetzee GA: Association of prostate cancer risk with genetic polymorphosis in vitamin D receptor and androgen receptor. J Natl Cancer Inst 1997; 89:166–170.
Jazin EE, Cavalier L, Eriksson I, Oreland L, Gyllensten U: Human brain contains high levels of heteroplasmy in the noncoding regions of mitochondrial DNA. Proc Natl Acad Sci USA 1996; 93:12382–12387.
Karlsson B, Gustafsoon J, Hedov G, Ivarsson SA, Anneren G: Thyroid dysfunction in Down's syndrome: relation to age and thyroid autoimmunity. Arch Dis Child 1998; 79:242–245.
Katzman R, Kawas C: Risk factors for Alzheimer's disease. Neurosci News 1998; 27–34.
Kenyon C: A conserved regulatory system for aging. Cell 2001; 105:165–168.
Kerber R, O'Brien E, Smith KR, Cawthon R: Longevity in Utah genealogies: support for both nuclear and mitchondrial genetic contributions. Gerontologist 1999; 38:6.
Kirkwood TBL: Evolution, molecular biology, and mortality plateaus. In: Bohr VA, Clark BFC, Stevnsner T (eds). Alfred Benzon Symposium 44, Molecular Biology of Aging. Copenhagen: Munksgaard, 1999:383–390.
Korpelainen H: Genetic maternal effects on human life span through the inheritance of mitochondrial DNA. Hum Hered 1999; 49:183–185.
Lakatta EG: Changes in cardiovascular function with aging. Eur Heart J 1990; 11(Suppl C):22–29.
Lakatta EG: Myocardial adaptations in advanced age. Basic Res Cardiol 1993; 88(Suppl 2):125–133.
Lane MA, Ingram DK, Roth GS: Beyond the rodent model: calorie restriction in rhesus monkeys. AGE 1998; 20:45–56.
Larsen PL, Albert PS, Riddle DL: Genes that regulate both development and longevity in *Caenorhabditis elegans*. Genetics 1995; 139:1567–1583.
Lee AT, Cerami A: Elevated glucose 6-phosphate levels are associated with plasmid mutations in vivo. Proc Natl Acad Sci USA 1987; 84:8311–8314.
Lee AT, Cerami A: In vitro and in vivo reactions of nucleic acids with reducing sugars. Mutat Res 1990; 283:185–191.
Levi B, Werman MJ: Fructose triggers DNA modification and damage in an *Escherichia coli* plasmid. J Nutr Biochem 2001; 12:235–241.
Levine RL, Wehr N, Williams JA, Stadtman ER, Shacter E: Determination of carbonyl groups in oxidized proteins. Methods Mol Biol 2000;99:15–24.
Lin K, Dorman JB, Rodan A, Kenyon C: daf-16: an HNF-3/forkhead family member that can function to double the life-span of *Caenorhabditis elegans*. Science 1997; 278:1319–1322.
Lindeman RD, Tobin J, Shock NW: Longitudinal studies on the rate of decline in renal function with age. J Am Geriatr Soc 1985; 33:278–285.
Ljungquist B, Berg S, Lanke J, McClearn GE, Pedersen NL: The effect of genetic factors for longevity: a comparison of identical and fraternal twins in the Swedish Twin Registry. J Gerontol A Biol Sci Med Sci 1998; 53:M441–M446.
Louhija J, Miettinen HE, Kontula K, Tikkanen MJ, Miettanen TA, Tilvis RS: Aging and genetic variation of plasma apolipoproteins. Relative loss of the apolipoprotein E4 phenotype in centenarians. Arterioscler Thromb 1994; 14:1084–1089.
Luckinbill L, Clare MJ: Successful selection for increased longevity in *Drosophila*: analysis of the survival data and presentation of a hypothesis on the genetic regulation of longevity. Exp Gerontol 1987; 22:221–226.
Manton KG, Gu X: Changes in the prevalence of chronic disability in the United States black and nonblack population above age 65 from 1982 to 1999. Proc Natl Acad Sci USA 2001; 98:6354–6359.
Martin GM: Genetic syndromes in man with potential relevance to the pathobiology of aging. Birth Defects 1978; 14:5–39.
Martin GM: Syndromes of accelerated aging. Natl Cancer Inst Monogr 1982; 60:241–247.
Martin GM: Genetics and the pathobiology of ageing. Philos Trans R Soc Lond B Biol Sci 1997; 352:1773–1780.
Martin GM: Towards a genetic analysis of unusually successful neural aging. In: Snyder S, Wang E (eds). Handbook of the Aging Brain. New York: Academic Press, 1998:126–134.
Martin GM: *APOE* alleles and lipophylic pathogens. Neurobiol Aging 1999; 20:441–443.
Martin GM: Some new directions for research on the biology of aging. Ann N Y Acad Sci 2000; 908:1–13.
Martin GM, Austad SN, Johnson TE: Genetic analysis of ageing: role of oxidative damage and environmental stresses. Nat Genet 1996a; 13:25–34.
Martin GM, Ogburn CE, Colgin LM, Gown AM, Edland SD, Monnat RJ Jr: Somatic mutations are frequent and increase with age in human kidney epithelial cells. Hum Mol Genet 1996b; 5:215–221.
Martin GM, Ogburn CE, Wight TN: Comparative rates of decline in the primary cloning efficiencies of smooth muscle cells from the aging thoracic aorta of two murine species of contrasting maximum life span potentials. Am J Pathol 1983; 110:236–245.
Martin GM, Sprague CA, Epstein CJ: Replicative life-span of cultivated human cells. Effects of donor's age, tissue, and genotype. Lab Invest 1970; 23:86–92.
Masoro EJ: Possible mechanisms underlying the antiaging actions of caloric restriction. Toxicol Pathol 1996; 24:738–741.
Masoro EJ, Austad SN: The evolution of the antiaging action of dietary restriction: a hypothesis. J Gerontol A Biol Sci Med Sci 1996; 51:B387–B391.
Medawar PB: Old age and natural death. Mod Q, 1946; 1:30–56.
Medawar PB: An unsolved problem in biology in The Uniqueness of the Individual London, Methuen, 1957:4–70.
Melov S, Shoffner JM, Kaufman A, Wallace DC: Marked increase in the number and variety of mitochondrial DNA rearrangements in aging human skeletal muscle. Nucleic Acids Res 1995; 23:4122–4126.
Mueller LD, Rose MR: Evolutionary theory predicts late-life mortality plateaus. Proc Natl Acad Sci USA 1996; 93:15249–15253.
Munkres KD, Rana RS: Ageing of *Neurospora crassa*. VII. Accumulation of fluorescent pigment (lipofuscin) and inhibition of the accumulation by nordihydroguairetic acid. Mech Ageing Dev 1978; 7:399–406.
Murdoch JC, Rodger JC, Rao SS, Fletcher CD, Dunnigan MG: Down's syndrome: an atheroma-free model? BMJ 1977; 2:226–228.
Murray CJL, Lopez AD (eds): The Global Burden of Disease. Boston: Harvard University School of Public Health, 1996.
Nagley P, Zhang C, Lim ML, Merhi M, Needham BE, Khalil Z: Mitochondrial DNA deletions parallel age-linked decline in rat sensory nerve function. Neurobiol Aging 2001; 22:635–643.
Nakano M, Gotoh S: Accumulation of cardiac lipofuscin depends on metabolic rate of mammals. J Gerontol 1992; 47:B126–B129.
Nordling CO: A new theory on the cancer inducing mechanism. J Cancer 1953; 7:68–72.
Odetti P, Angelini G, Dapino D, Zaccheo D, Garibaldi S, Dagna-Bricarelli F, Piombo G, Perry G, Smith M, Traverso N, et al.: Early glycoxidation damage in brains from Down's syndrome. Biochem Biophys Res Commun 1998; 243:849–851.
Packer C, Tatar M, Collins A: Reproductive cessation in female mammals. Nature 1998; 392:807–811.
Parkes TL, Elia AJ, Dickinson D, Hilliker AJ, Phillips JP, Boulianne GL: Extension of *Drosophila* lifespan by overexpression of human SOD1 in motorneurons. Nat Genet 1998; 19:171–174.
Perls TT, Bochen K, Freeman M, Alpert L, Silver MH: Validity of reported age and centenarian prevalence in New England. Age Ageing 1999; 28:193–197.
Pesce V, Cormio A, Fracasso F, Vecchiet J, Felzani G, Lezza AM, Cantatore P, Gadaleta MN: Age-related mitochondrial genotypic and phenotypic alterations in human skeletal muscle. Free Radic Biol Med 2001; 30:1223–1233.
Pletcher SD, Curtsinger JW: Mortality plateaus and the evolution of senescence: why are old-age mortality rates so low? Evolution 1998; 52:454–464.
Rose MR: The Evolutionary Biology of Aging. New York: Oxford University Press, 1991.
Ross JL, Feuillan P, Long LM, Kowal K, Kushner H, Cutler GB Jr: Lipid abnormalities in Turner syndrome. J Pediatr 1995; 126:242–245.
Roth GS, Ingram DK, Lane MA: Calorie restriction in primates: will it work and how will we know? J Am Geriatr Soc 1999; 47:896–903.
Roth GS, Lesnikov V, Lesnikov M, Ingram DK, Lane MA: Dietary caloric restriction prevents the age-related decline in plasma melatonin levels of rhesus monkeys. J Clin Endocrinol Metab 2001; 86:3292–3295.
Rumble B, Retallack R, Hilbich C, Simms G, Muthaup G, Martinis R, Hockey A, Montgomery P, Beyreuther K, Masters CL: Amyloid A4 protein and its precursor in Down's syndrome and Alzheimer's disease. N Engl J Med 1989; 320:1446–1452.
Sakata N, Uesugi N, Takebayashi S, Nagai R, Jono T, Horiuchi S, Takeya M, Itabe H, Takano T, Myint T, et al.: Glycoxidation and lipid peroxidation of low-density lipoprotein can synergistically enhance atherogenesis. Cardiovasc Res 2001; 49:466–475.
Saunders AJ, Kim T-W, Tanzi RE, Fan W, Bennett BD, Babu-Kahn S, Luo Y, Louis J-C, McCaleb M, Citron M, et al.: *BACE* maps to chromosome 11 and a *BACE* homolog, *BACE2*, reside in the obligate Down syndrome region of chromosome 21. Science 1999; 286:1255.
Sayre LM, Smith MA, Perry G: Chemistry and biochemistry of oxidative stress in neurodegenerative disease. Curr Med Chem 2001; 8:721–738.
Schachter F, Faure-Delanef L, Guenot F, Rouger H, Froguel P, Lesueur-Ginot L, Cohen D: Genetic associations with human longevity at the *APOE* and *ACE* loci. Nat Genet 1994; 6:29–32.
Schneider EL, Brody JA: Aging, natural death, and the compression of morbidity: another view. N Engl J Med 1983; 309:854–856.
Schupf N, Zigman W, Kapell D, Lee JH, Kline J, Levin B: Early menopause in women with Down's syndrome. J Intellect Disabil Res 1997; 41:264–267.
Scott RB, Collins JM, Hunt PA: Alzheimer's disease and Down syndrome: leukocyte membrane fluidity alterations. Mech Ageing Dev 1994; 75:1–10.
Selkoe DJ: Alzheimer's disease: genes, proteins, and therapy. Physiol Rev 2001; 81:741–766.
Sell DR, Kleinman NR, Monnier VM: Longitudinal determination of skin collagen

glycation and glycoxidation rates predicts early death in C57BL/6NNIA mice. FASEB J 2000; 14:145–156.

Shock NW, Greulich RC, Costa PT, Andres R, Lakatta EG, Arenberg D, Tobin JD (eds): Normal Human Aging: The Baltimore Longitudinal Study of Aging. Washington DC: US Department of Health and Human Services, 1984.

Sohal RS, Weindruch R: Oxidative stress, caloric restriction, and aging. Science 1996; 273:59–63.

Stadtman ER, Levine RL: Protein oxidation. Ann N Y Acad Sci 2000; 899:191–208.

Stanford JL, Just JJ, Gibbs M, Wicklund KG, Neal CL, Blumenstein BA, Ostrander EA: Polymorphic repeats in the androgen receptor gene: molecular markers of prostate cancer risk. Cancer Res 1997; 57:1194–1198.

Surralles J, Jeppesen P, Morrison H, Natarajan AT: Analysis of loss of inactive X chromosomes in interphase cells. Am J Hum Genet 1996; 59:1091–1096.

Tatar M, Kopelman A, Epstein D, Tu MP, Yin CM, Garofalo RS: A mutant *Drosophila* insulin receptor homolog that extends life-span and impairs neuroendocrine function. Science 2001; 292:107–110.

Terman A, Brunk UT: Lipofuscin: mechanisms of formation and increase with age. APMIS 1998; 106:265–276.

Tesco G, Vergelli M, Grassilli E, Salomoni P, Bellesia E, Sikora E, Radziszewska E, Barbieri D, Lotorraca S, Fagiolo U, et al.: Growth properties and growth factor responsiveness in skin fibroplasts from centenarians. Biochem Biophys Res Commun 1998; 244:912–916.

Tissenbaum HA, Ruvkun G: An insulin-like signaling pathway affects both longevity and reproduction in *Caenorhabditis elegans*. Genetics 1998; 148:703–717.

Vanfleteren JR, De Vreese A, Braeckman BP. Two-parameter logistic and Weibull equations provide better fits to survival data from isogenic populations of *Caenorhabditis elegans* in axenic culture than does the Gompertz model. J Gerontol A Biol Sci Med Sci 1998; 53:B393–B403.

van Leeuwen FW, Burbach JP, Hol EM: Mutations in RNA: a first example of molecular misreading in Alzheimer's disease. Trends Neurosci 1998a; 21:331–335.

van Leeuwen FW, de Kleijn DP, van den Hurk HH, Neubauer A, Sonnemans MA, Sluijs JA, Koycu S, Ramdjielal RDJ, Salehi A, Martens GJM, et al.: Frameshift mutants of beta amyloid precursor protein and ubiquitin-B in Alzheimer's and Down patients. Science 1998b; 279:242–247.

Van Voorhies WA, Ward S: Genetic and environmental conditions that increase longevity in *Caenorhabditis elegans* decrease metabolic rate. Proc Natl Acad Sci USA 1999; 96:11399–11403.

Vassar R, Bennett BD, Babu-Khan S, Kahn S, Mendia EA, Denis P, Teplow DB, Ross S, Amarante P, Loeloff R, et al.: β-Secretase cleavage of Alzheimer's amyloid precursor protein by the transmembrane aspartic protease *BACE*. Science 1999; 286:735–741.

Vaupel JW, Carey JR, Christensen K, Johnson TE, Yashin AI, Holm NV, Iachine IA, Kannisto V, Khazaeli AA, Liedo P, et al.: Biodemographic trajectories of longevity. Science 1998; 280:855–860.

Vita AJ, Terry RB, Hubert HB, Fries JF: Aging, health risks, and cumulative disability. N Engl J Med 1998; 338:1035–1041.

Wachter KW: Evolutionary demographic models for mortality plateaus. Proc Natl Acad Sci USA 1999; 96:10544–10547.

Walker D, Harper PS, Wells CE, Tyler A, Davies K, Newcombe RG: Huntington's chorea in south Wales: a genetic and epidemiological study. Clin Genet 1981; 19:213–221.

Wallace DC: A mitochondrial paradigm for degenerative diseases and ageing. Novartis Found Symp 2001;235:247–266.

Wang E, Wong A, Cortopassi G: The rate of mitochondrial mutagenesis is faster in mice than humans. Mutat Res 1997; 377:157–166.

Williams GC: Pleiotropy, natural selection, and the evolution of senescence. Evolution 1957; 11:398–411.

Williams GC: Pleiotropy, natural selection, and the evolution of senescence. In: The Biology of Aging. Washington DC: American Institute of Biological Sciences, 1960:332–337.

Wolf G: Lipofuscin, the age pigment. Nutr Rev 1993; 51:205–206.

Wolf N, Penn PE, Jiang D, Fei RG, Pendergrass WR: Caloric restriction: conservation of in vivo cellular replicative capacity accompanies life-span extension in mice. Exp Cell Res 1995; 217:317–323.

Wong FH, Pun KK, Wang C: Loss of bone mass in patients with Klinefelter's syndrome despite sufficient testosterone replacement. Osteoporos Int 1993; 3:3–7.

Wood JW, Weeks SC, Bentley GR, Weiss KM: Human population and the evolution of aging. In: Crews DE, Garruto RM (eds). Biological Anthropology and Aging. New York: Oxford University Press, 1994:332–337.

Yashin AI, DeBenedictis G, Vaupel JW, Tan Q, Andreev KF, Iachine IA, Bonafe M, De Luca M, Valensin S, Carotenuto L, et al.: Genes, demography and life span: the contribution of demographic data in genetic studies on aging and longevity. Am J Hum Genet 1999; 65:1178–1193.

Yin D: Biochemical basis of lipofuscin, ceroid, and age pigment-like fluorophores. Free Radic Biol Med 1996; 21:871–888.

Yla-Herttuala S, Luoma J, Nikkari T, Kivimaki T: Down's syndrome and atherosclerosis. Athersclerosis 1989; 76:269–272.

Yu BP, Masoro EJ, Murata I, Bertrand HA, Lynd FT: Life span of SPF Fischer 344 male rats fed ad libitum or restricted diets: longevity, growth, lean body mass and disease. J Gerontol 1982; 37:130–141.

Yu CE, Oshima J, Fu YH, Wijsman EM, Hisama F, Alisch R, Matthews S, Nakura J, Miki T, Ouais S, et al.: Positional cloning of the Werner's syndrome gene. Science 1996; 272:258–262.

Zwaan B, Bijlsmar R, Hoekstra RE: Direct selection on life span in *Drosophila melanogaster*. Evolution 1995; 49:649–659.

52 Mitochondrial Defects in Common Diseases

DOUGLAS C. WALLACE AND MARIE T. LOTT

The prevalence of mitochondrial disease has been difficult to determine. This stems from the fact that mitochondrial diseases are multifaceted in both their genetics and pathophysiology. Diseases resulting from known mitochondrial gene mutations can affect the central nervous system (CNS), heart, skeletal muscle, endocrine system, and/or kidney and result in symptoms such as deafness, blindness, diabetes, dementia, stroke, movement disorders, cardiomyopathy, and renal failure. Since these same symptoms are common medical problems, mitochondrial defects may be important in the etiology of these and related symptoms in the general population. If so, then mitochondrial diseases may not be rare but common. Indeed, the symptoms observed in mitochondrial diseases are also those of aging. If aging is a mitochondrial disease, then mitochondrial diseases are universal.

The fact that mitochondrial disease has only recently been recognized as genetic is the result of the large number of genes required for assembly of the mitochondrial bioenergetic system and the distribution of the genes between the cytoplasmic mitochondrial DNA (mtDNA) and the chromosomal nuclear DNA (nDNA). mtDNA encodes 13 components of the mitochondrial energy-generating pathway, oxidative phosphorylation (OXPHOS), and the rRNAs and tRNAs necessary for mitochondrial protein synthesis. nDNA codes for all of the remaining structural proteins for OXPHOS; the enzymes of the tricarboxylic acid (TCA) cycle and β-oxidation of fatty acids; and all of the components of the mitochondrial biosynthetic apparatus including the polymerases, ribosomal proteins, and the mitochondrial import apparatus proteins. mtDNA genes are maternally inherited and present in thousands of copies per cell, resulting in a stochastic genetics. nDNA genes are biparentally inherited and present in only two copies per cell, creating a quantized genetics. Moreover, mutations in nDNA genes can affect mtDNA maintenance, resulting in a Mendelian predisposition to mtDNA disease.

The pathophysiology of mitochondrial disease is also complex. Mitochondrial OXPHOS serves multiple functions in the cell. The central function of OXPHOS is to generate energy. This energy is stored in an electrochemical gradient across the mitochondrial inner membrane and can be used to synthesize adenosine triphosphate (ATP), take up cytosolic Ca^{2+}, and regulate the redox status of the cell. As a toxic by-product of OXPHOS, mitochondria are also the major endogenous source of cellular reactive oxygen species (ROS) or oxygen radicals. Finally, the mitochondria, through the mitochondrial permeability transition pore (mtPTP), provide one of the central signaling systems for initiating programmed cell death, or *apoptosis*. Since inhibition of OXPHOS energy production stimulates mitochondrial ROS production and can initiate opening of the mtPTP and since increased ROS production can inhibit OXPHOS, damage the mtDNA, and activate opening of the mtPTP, it is apparent that OXPHOS defects can impact on a variety of physiological processes.

Therefore, to investigate the potential role of mitochondrial defects in common disorders, it is necessary to integrate investigations on the clinical genetics of mitochondrial disease with studies on the pathophysiology of mitochondrial disease using cultured cells and mouse models. Principles of mitochondrial genetics and biochemistry that arise form these studies can then be extrapolated to common diseases to determine if they can explain the observed phenomena.

MITOCHONDRIAL GENETICS

Mammalian mtDNA (Fig. 52–1) codes for 13 key polypeptides of mitochondrial OXPHOS as well as the structural RNAs required for mitochondrial protein synthesis. The polypeptide genes include seven (*ND1-, -2, -3, -4L, -4, -5, -6*) of the roughly 43 polypeptides of OXPHOS complex I, one (cytochrome *b*, *cytb*) of the approximately 11 polypeptides of complex III, three (*COI, -II, -III*) of the 13 polypeptides of complex IV, and two (*ATP6, -8*) of the 16 polypeptides of complex V. mtDNA RNA genes include a 12S and a 16S rRNA and a complete set of the required 22 tRNAs (Fig. 52–1) (Shoffner and Wallace, 1995; Wallace et al., 1996).

Because of their endosymbiotic origin, the mitochondria and mtDNAs are semi-autonomous from the nucleus–cytosol system (Wallace, 1982b; Lang et al., 1997; Andersson et al., 1998). This has been demonstrated in cultured cells by showing that mtDNAs and associated mtDNA-encoded genetic defects can be transferred from one cell to another by enucleating the donor cell and fusing the enucleated cytoplasmic fragment (cytoplast) to a recipient cell. Transfer of the mutant cellular phenotype along with the mtDNA indicates that the phenotype is encoded by the mtDNA (Bunn et al., 1974; Wallace et al., 1975; Wallace, 1982a). This cytoplasmic hybrid, or *cybrid*, transfer technique is now standard for determining if cellular defects associated with mitochondrial disease are due to mtDNA mutations (King and Attardi, 1989; Trounce et al., 1996). The cytoplasmic inheritance of the mitochondria also means that the mtDNA is transmitted through the oocyte's cytoplasm at fertilization. Thus, mtDNA is strictly maternally inherited (Giles et al., 1980).

mtDNA has a very high mutation rate, perhaps 1 or 2 orders of magnitude greater than nDNA genes. The appearance of a new mutation in the mtDNA within a cell results in a mixture of wild-type and mutant mtDNAs, a state known as *heteroplasmy*. When such a heteroplasmic cell divides, the mutant and wild-type mtDNAs are randomly distributed into the daughter

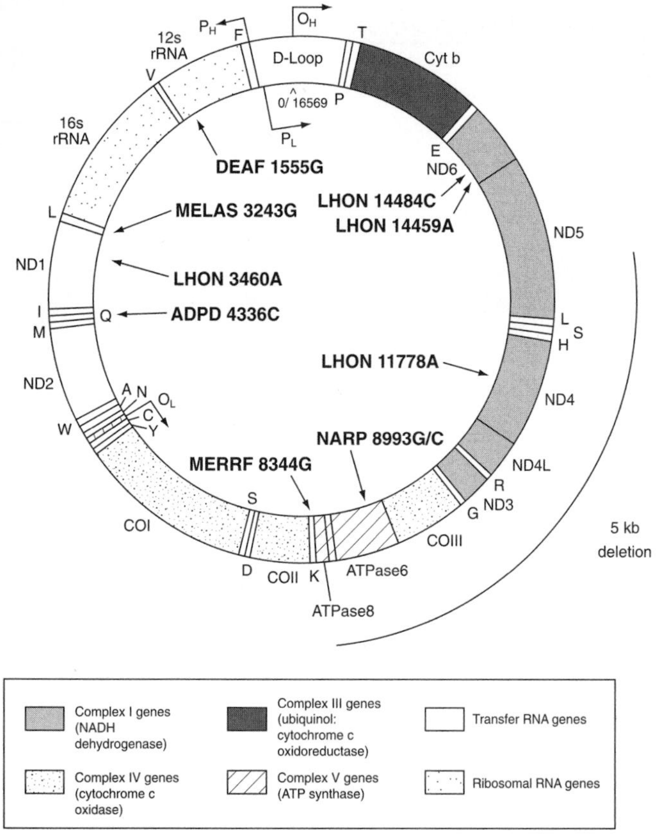

Fig. 52–1. The human mtDNA map, showing the location of selected pathogenic mutations. This genome is 16,569 nucleotide pairs and codes for seven complex I (*ND1, -2, -3, -4, -4L, -5*, and *-6*), one complex III (cytochrome *b, Cyt b*), three complex IV (*COI, -II*, and *-III*), and two complex V (*ATP6* and *-8*) genes. It also codes for the small 12S and 16S rRNA genes and 22 tRNAs, which punctuate the larger genes. The tRNAs are labeled with the letters of the cognate amino acids. The heavy (*H*)-strand origin of replication (O_H) and the H-strand and light (*L*)-strand promoters P_H and P_L are indicated in the control region (*D-loop*). The L-strand origin of replication (O_L) is located two-thirds of the way around the genome. The positions of the mentioned pathogenic base substitution mutations are shown on the inside of the circle, with the nucleotide position and disease acronym given. Each disease locus is indicated by an acronym which alludes to the clinical presentation (e.g., *DEAF* stands for sensory neural deafness and *ADPD* for late-onset Alzheimer's disease), and the nucleotide position is indicated by the mutation. Deletions associated with the disease are most commonly located in the major arc extending from O_H to O_L, although deletions have been found which encompass all regions of the mtDNA except O_H (Shoffner and Wallace, 1995; Wallace et al., 1996; Wallace and Murdock, 1999). *MELAS*, mitochondrial encephalopathy, lactic acidosis, and stroke-like episodes; *LHON*, Leber's hereditary optic neuropathy; *NARP*, neurogenic muscle weakness, ataxia, and retinitis pigmentosa; *MERRF*, myoclonic epilepsy and ragged red fibers.

cells such that, over many generations, the mtDNA genotype of a cellular lineage can drift toward predominantly mutant or wild-type mtDNAs (*homoplasmy*). This process is known as *replicative segregation*. As the percentage of mutant mtDNAs increases, the cellular energy capacity declines until it falls below the *bioenergetic threshold*, the minimum energy output necessary for a cell or tissue to function normally. Beyond this point, symptoms appear and become progressively worse (Shoffner and Wallace, 1995; Wallace et al., 1996).

MITOCHONDRIAL BIOENERGETICS

The mitochondrial OXPHOS pathway is located within the mitochondrial inner membrane and encompasses the electron transport chain (ETC), ATP synthase, and the adenine nucleotide translocator (ANT) (Fig. 52–2). The ETC oxidizes hydrogen, derived from organic acids and fatty acids and born on NAD^+, by transfer of the electrons to respiratory complex I (NADH dehydrogenase) and then to coenzyme Q_{10} (CoQ). Electrons from succinate in the TCA cycle are transmitted to complex II (succinate dehydrogenase, SDH) and to CoQ. From CoQ, the electrons pass to complex III, then to cytochrome *c*, then to complex IV (cytochrome-*c* oxidase, COX), and finally to $^1/_2$ O_2 to give H_2O. The energy released is used to pump protons (H^+) out of the mitochondrial inner membrane. This creates an electrochemical gradient ($\Delta\Psi$) across the mitochondrial inner membrane which is positive and acid on the outside and negative and alkaline on the inside. This electrochemical gradient can be depolarized by the transport of protons back into the mitochondrial matrix through the proton channel in the F0 membrane component of ATP synthase. This proton flux drives the condensation of adenosine diphosphate (ADP) + inorganic phosphate (P_i) to make ATP, which is then exported to the cytosol in exchange for the spent ADP by the ANT. Thus, oxygen consumption by the ETC is coupled to ADP phosphorylation by ATP synthase through the electrochemical gradient, $\Delta\Psi$ (Shoffner and Wallace, 1995; Wallace et al., 1996; Wallace, 1997).

While most of the electrons that enter the ETC are used to reduce atomic oxygen to water, a significant percentage can be misdirected from reduced complex I and CoQ to molecular oxygen (O_2) to give superoxide anion ($O_2^{\cdot -}$), the first of the ROS (Fig. 52–2). Blocking the electron flux through the ETC, e.g., by treatment with the complex III inhibitor antimycin A, redirects the electrons to O_2, thus maximizing the mitochondrial production of $O_2^{\cdot -}$. Mitochondrial superoxide anion is detoxified by the mitochondrial manganese superoxide dismutase (MnSOD) to give hydrogen peroxide (H_2O_2), and H_2O_2 is converted to H_2O by glutathione peroxidase (GPx). H_2O_2, in the presence of reduced transition metals, can also be converted to the highly reactive hydroxyl radical ($\cdot OH$) by the Fenton reaction. Consequently, mitochondrial OXPHOS is also the major endogenous source of ROS ($O_2^{\cdot -}$, H_2O_2, and $^{\cdot}OH$). Chronic ROS exposure can result in oxidative damage to the mitochondrial and cellular proteins, lipids, and nucleic acids, while acute ROS exposure can inactivate complex I, II, and II of the ETC aconitase of the TCA cycle (Wallace et al., 1996; Wallace, 1997). A decrease in OXPHOS appears to increase oxidative stress in patients. In patients with complex I defects, the severity of the enzymatic deficiency correlates with increased $O_2^{\cdot -}$ production and induction of MnSOD mRNA levels (Pitkanen and Robinson, 1996). In the skeletal muscle of mitochondrial myopathy patients, degenerating ragged red muscle fibers show localized increases in MnSOD protein (Ohkoshi et al., 1995).

Mitochondria are also thought to be a major site for initiating apoptosis, via opening of the mtPTP (Zoratti and Szabo, 1995; Petit et al., 1996; Green and Reed, 1998). When the mtPTP opens, the $\Delta\Psi$ collapses. The mitochondrial inner membrane space swells, apparently rupturing the outer membranes. This releases cytochrome *c*, the apoptosis initiating factor (AIF), procaspase-2, procaspase-3, procaspase-4, and a caspase-activated DNAse (CAD), which are stored in the mitochondrial intermembrane space into the cytosol (Liu et al., 1996; Mancini et al., 1998; Earnshaw, 1999; Susin et al., 1999a,b). The released cytochrome *c* activates the cytosolic Apaf-1, which activates procaspase-9 and procaspase-2. Caspases 9 and 2 activate caspases 3, 6, and 7, which destroy the cell. The AIF has a nuclear targeting sequence, is transported to the nucleus, and initiates chromatin condensation and degradation. CAD also participates in DNA degradation.

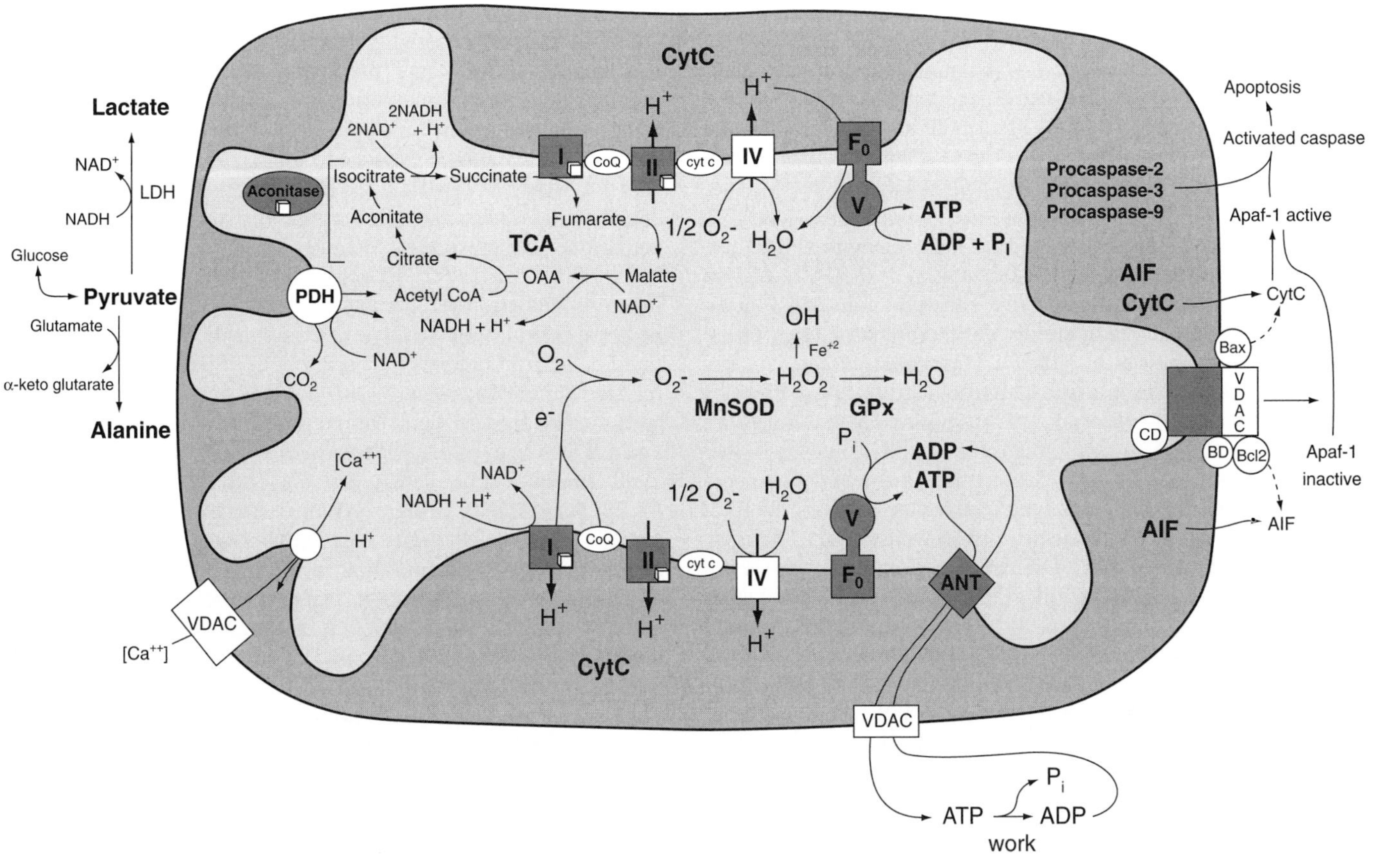

Fig. 52–2. Diagram of a mitochondrion, illustrating the relationships of mitochondrial oxidative phosphorylation to *(1)* the production of energy adenosine triphosphate, (*ATP*), *(2)* the generation of reactive oxygen species (ROS), and *(3)* the initiation of apoptosis through activation of the mitochondrial permeability transition pore (mtPTP). The enzyme complexes involved in OXPHOS, designated *I* to *V*, are complex I (NADH:ubiquinone oxidoreductase) encompassing one FMN and six Fe-S centers (designated with a *cube*); complex II (succinate:ubiquinone oxidoreductase) involving an FAD, three Fe-S centers, and a cytochrome *b*; complex III (ubiquinol:cytochrome *c* oxidoreductase) encompassing cytochromes *b* and c_1 and the Rieske Fe-S center; complex IV (cytochrome *c* oxidase) encompassing cytochromes *a* and a_3, CuA, and CuB; and complex V (H^+-translocating ATP synthase). Pyruvate from glucose enters the mitochondria via pyruvate dehydrogenase *(PDH)*, generating acetyl coenzyme A which enters the tricarboxylic acid (*acetyl CoA*), (*TCA*) cycle by combining with oxaloacetate (*OAA*). *cis*-Aconitase converts citrate to isocitrate and contains a 4Fe-4S center. Lactate dehydrogenase (*LDH*) converts excess pyruvate plus NADH to lactate (Shoffner and Wallace, 1995; Wallace et al., 1996; Wallace, 1997). Small molecules defuse through the outer membrane via the voltage-dependent anion channel (*VDAC*) or porin. The VDAC together with the adenine nucleotide translocator (*ANT*), Bax, and the cyclophilin D (*CD*) protein are thought to come together at the mitochondrial inner and outer membrane contact points to create the mtPTP. The proapoptotic Bax of the mtPTP is thought to interact with the antiapoptotic Bcl2 and the benzodiazepine receptor (*BD*). Opening of the mtPTP is associated with release of cytochrome *c* (*CytC*), apoptosis-inducing factor (AIF), and procaspases 2, 3, and 9. Cytochrome *c* interacts with and activates Apaf-1, which activates procaspases 2 and 9. Activated caspases 2 and 9 then cleave and activate procaspases 3, 6, and 7, which initiates the proteolytic degradation of cellular proteins (Liu et al., 1996; Brustovetsky and Klingenberg, 1996; Green and Reed, 1998; Marzo et al., 1998).

Opening of the pore can be initiated by the mitochondrion's excessive uptake of Ca^{2+}, increased exposure to ROS, or a decline in energetic capacity such as a drop in $\Delta\Psi$ (Liu et al., 1996; Green and Reed, 1998). Thus, defects in Ca^{2+} regulation or inhibition of OXPHOS leading to bioenergetic decline and increased ROS production could activate the mtPTP and result in cell death (Brustovetsky and Klingenberg, 1996; Green and Reed, 1998; Marzo et al., 1998).

MITOCHONDRIAL DISEASES

Mitochondrial diseases can have a variety of inheritance patterns: maternal, Mendelian, and a combination of the two. Diseases resulting from mtDNA mutations can include either base substitutions or rearrangement mutations (Mitomap, http://www.gen.emory.edu/mitomap.html). mtDNA base substitution mutations can be subdivided into missense mutations affecting the mtDNA proteins or protein synthesis mutations affecting the rRNA or tRNA genes (Shoffner and Wallace, 1995; Wallace et al., 1996).

The mtDNA mutations that cause Leber's hereditary optic neuropathy (LHON) and Leigh's disease provide good examples of the clinical variability that can accompany a missense mutation. LHON is a form of acute or subacute central vision loss leading to bilateral central scotoma, with a median age at onset around the mid-20s. Four "primary" LHON mutations have been identified, which, in order of decreasing severity, are *MTND6**LDYT14459A (Jun et al., 1994), *MTND4**LHON11778A (Wallace et al., 1988a), *MTND1**LHON3460A (Howell et al., 1991a; Huoponen et al., 1991, 1993), and *MTND6**LHON14484C (Johns et al., 1992; Mackey and Howell, 1992). The *MTND6**LDYT14459A mutation is a relatively rare cause of LHON. It is the product of a G-to-A transition that changes codon 72 of *MTND6* from a highly conserved alanine to a valine (Jun et al., 1994). This mutation results in a complex I defect and can cause either LHON or generalized dystonia as a consequence of the segregation of the heteroplasmic mutations (Novotny et al., 1986; Jun et al., 1994; Shoffner et al., 1995). The mutation also results in a complex I defect that can be transferred along with the mutant mtDNA in cybrid transfer experiments (Jun et al., 1996).

The *MTND4**LHON11778A mutation is the most common cause of LHON, accounting for 50% of European cases and the great majority of Asian cases. The mutation is a G-to-A transition in the *MTND4* gene that converts codon 340 from a highly conserved arginine to a histidine. The mutation is heteroplasmic in about 14% of cases (Wallace et al., 1988a; Newman et al., 1991; Newman, 1993). The *MTND1**LHON 3460A and *MTND6**LHON14484C mutations are moderately common causes of LHON among Europeans, each accounting for approximately 15% of cases. The *MTND1**LHON3460A mutation is a G-to-A transition in the *MTND1* gene that converts a moderately conserved alanine at codon 52 to a threonine (Howell et al., 1991a; Huoponen et al., 1991). This mutation can be heteroplasmic and results in a substantial reduction in complex I-specific activity (Howell et al., 1991b; Majander et al., 1991). The *MTND6**LHON14484C mutation is the mildest of the LHON mutations. It is a T-to-C transition in the *MTND6* gene that converts the weakly conserved methionine at codon 64 to a valine (Johns et al., 1992; Mackey and Howell, 1992). The mutation is primarily seen in LHON patients of European descent, and 80% of these patients also harbor a specific mtDNA background type, haplogroup J. Haplogroup J is defined by two missense mutations, *MTND5**LHON13708A and *MTND1**LHON4216C, of unknown etiological significance (Brown et al., 1997). Thus, LHON demonstrates that in some cases the same heteroplasmic mutation can give different phenotypes and in others different mutations can give the same phenotype. Finally, LHON has shown that in some instances more than one genetic variant may be required to give a phenotype.

Leigh's syndrome can be caused by the *MTATP6**NARP8993G mutation, a T-to-G transition that changes the conserved leucine at codon 156 in the *MTATP6* gene to an arginine (Holt et al., 1990). This mutation is invariably heteroplasmic and, when present in fewer than 75% of mtDNAs, can cause neurogenic muscle weakness, ataxia, and retinitis pigmentosa along with olivopontocerebellar atrophy and mental retardation; but when present in greater than 95% of mtDNAs, it can cause Leigh's syndrome (Shoffner et al., 1992; Tatuch et al., 1992; Ortiz et al., 1993). Leigh's syndrome is an early-onset, frequently lethal condition associated with ataxia developmental delay and subsequent regression, hypotonia, spasticity, developmental delay, optic atrophy, and ophthalmoplegia (paralysis of the extraocular eye muscles resulting in immobility of the eyeball). The end-stage disease is generally associated with degeneration of the basal ganglia (Shoffner and Wallace, 1995). The *MTATP6**NARP8993G mutation reduces mitochondrial ATP synthesis by blocking the F_0 proton channel of ATP synthase, a defect which can be transferred in cybrid experiments (Trounce et al., 1994). Thus, the varying degrees of ATP deficiency resulting from replicative segregation of the mutant mtDNA must account for the widely different clinical presentations seen in these families.

A wide variety of pathogenic base substitution mutations affecting the mtDNA protein synthesis genes have been identified. These can alter either the rRNA or tRNA genes. The tRNA mutations are frequently the most severe. Consequently, they are generally heteroplasmic and encompass CNS manifestations, including sensory neural hearing loss, epilepsy, stroke-like episodes, and progressive dementia; mitochondrial myopathy involving the proliferation of abnormal skeletal muscle mitochondria, resulting in ragged red muscle fiber pathology; cardiomyopathy; lactic acidosis; and endocrine disorders, including diabetes mellitus (Wallace et al., 1996). While these mitochondrial encephalomyopathies frequently have a number of clinical features in common, such as mitochondrial myopathy, individual mutations have a predilection to specific subsets of the clinical manifestations. Thus, the *MTTK**MERRF8344G mutation, which is an A-to-G transition in the TΨC loop of $tRNA^{Lys}$ gene, can present with myoclonic epilepsy and ragged red fibers, hence the acronym *MERRF* (Wallace et al., 1988b; Shoffner et al., 1990). The *MTTL1**MELAS3243G mutation is frequently associated with mitochondrial encephalomyopathy, lactic acidosis, and stroke-like episodes (MELAS) when the percentage of mutant mtDNA is over 85% (Goto et al., 1990) but with maternally inherited diabetes mellitus and deafness when the percentage is between 5% and 30% (Gerbitz et al., 1995; Goto, 1995). Cultured cells from patients harboring both of these mutations have reduced mitochondrial protein synthesis and complex I and IV activity, and these defects can be transferred along with the mutant mtDNA in cybrid transfer experiments (Chomyn et al., 1991, 1992; Masucci et al., 1995).

Milder mtDNA protein synthesis mutations can be homoplasmic and affect only the CNS. One example is the *MTTQ**ADPD4336C mutation in the $tRNA^{Gln}$ gene, associated with late-onset Alzheimer's disease (Shoffner et al., 1993; Hutchin and Cortopassi, 1995). A second is the pathogenic rRNA mutation *MTRNR1**DEAF1555G. This mutation alters nucleotide pair (np) 1555 of the *12S rRNA* gene, is consistently homoplasmic, and can either result in spontaneous development of sensory neural deafness or impart a predisposition to aminoglycoside-induced deafness (Fischel-Ghodsian et al., 1993; Hutchin et al., 1993; Prezant et al., 1993; Matthijs et al., 1994).

Diseases resulting from mtDNA rearrangements include chronic progressive external ophthalmoplegia (CPEO), Kearns-Sayre syndrome (KSS), maternally inherited diabetes mellitus, deafness (Ballinger et al., 1992, 1994), and the spontaneously occurring Pearson's marrow/pancreas syndrome involving pediatric pancytopenia (loss of all blood cells) and leading to death (Rotig et al., 1989). CPEO and the KSS patients present with severe mitochondrial myopathy resulting in ophthalmoplegia and ptosis (droopy eye lips), lactic acidosis, cardiac conduction defects, renal problems, diabetes mellitus, etc. Histological analysis of CPEO and KSS muscle reveals bands of COX-deficient (COX^-) and SDH-hyperreactive (SDH^+) activity along the muscle fibers. These COX^- and SDH^+ fibers generally correspond to regions of mitochondrial proliferation with ragged red fibers, high levels of mutant mtDNA, and induction of nDNA and mtDNA OXPHOS gene expression (Mita et al., 1989; Shoubridge et al., 1990; Heddi et al., 1993, 1994).

Mitochondrial diseases resulting from nDNA OXPHOS gene mutations exhibit Mendelian inheritance patterns yet share many of the clinical features of mtDNA mutations. A mutation in the complex I 18 kDa structural protein gene has been reported in a child with hypotonia, mental retardation, convulsions, and brain and basal ganglia degeneration (van den Heuvel et al., 1998). A mutation in a mitochondrial protease-like ATPase has been associated with autosomal dominant spastic paraplegia (Casari et al., 1998). Mutations in a number of nuclear genes can cause Leigh's syndrome. These include mutations in the X-linked E1α subunit of pyruvate dehydrogenase (Matthews et al., 1993), in the autosomal NDUF8 N-2 iron–sulfur center protein of complex I (Loeffen et al., 1998), in the autosomal flavoprotein subunit of complex II (Bourgeron et al., 1995), and in the autosomal *SURF-1* gene associated with complex IV defects (Tiranti et al., 1998; Zhu et al., 1998).

Mutations in nuclear genes can also exert their phenotypic effects by indirectly inactivating the OXPHOS enzymes. Friedreich's ataxia is an autosomal recessive disease that results in cerebellar ataxia, peripheral neuropathy, and hypertrophic cardiomyopathy. The mutant protein, frataxin, is targeted to the mitochondrial inner membrane and transports iron out of the mitochondrion. With loss of this protein, iron accumulates in the matrix, stimulating the conversion of H_2O_2 to $^{\cdot}OH$ by the Fenton reaction. This inactivates the mitochondrial Fe-S center enzymes (complexes I, II, and III and aconitase), reducing mitochondrial energy production (Rotig et al., 1997).

Nuclear mutations can also cause mitochondrial disease by destabilizing the mtDNA. The mitochondrial neurogastrointestinal encephalomyopathy syndrome is associated with mitochondrial myopathy with ragged red fibers and abnormal mitochondria; decreased respiratory chain activity; and multiple mtDNA deletions, mtDNA depletion, or both. This autosomal recessive disease has been linked to mutations in the thymidine phosphorylase (*TP*) gene, though the clinical symptoms are probably the result of destruction of the mtDNA. Hence, it has been hypothesized that inactivation of *TP* alters cellular thymidine pools, which are important for mtDNA maintenance (Nishino et al., 1999).

Autosomal dominant-progressive external ophthalmoplegia (AD-PEO) is a dominantly inherited nuclear mutation that predisposes patients to multiple skeletal muscle mtDNA deletions, mitochondrial myopathy, and PEO. Apparently, the nDNA mutation destabilizes the mtDNA, with the phenotypic effects being due to loss of functional mtDNA. Two different chromosomal loci have been identified for AD-PEO: one at 10q 23.3 to 24.3 and another at 3p14.2 to 21.1 (Suomalainen et al., 1995; Zeviani et al., 1995).

The mtDNA depletion syndrome involves severe reductions in the mtDNA levels of various organs (muscle, liver, or kidney), resulting in organ failure and death. This is probably the result of a nuclear mutation that disrupts regulation of the mtDNA copy number during development, leading to the chance loss of mtDNA (Moraes et al., 1991; Bodnar et al., 1993).

SOMATIC MITOCHONDRIAL DNA MUTATIONS IN AGING

Mitochondrial diseases frequently have a delayed onset and progression course. This suggests two factors in the pathogenesis of mitochondrial disease, an inherited mutation that predisposes to the disease and an age-related factor that exacerbates this defect and precipitates the onset and progression of the disease. This aging factor is now thought to be the age-related decline in mitochondrial OXPHOS enzyme activity, documented in primate skeletal muscle, liver, and brain (Trounce et al., 1989; Wallace, 1997), which is the result of the age-related accumulation of somatic mtDNA rearrangements in these same postmitotic tissues. For example, in human skeletal muscle, the activities of mitochondrial complexes I, I + II, and II + III decline with age from 20 to 80 years. Analysis of the mtDNAs of subjects under age 40, by amplification of full-length mtDNAs using the long-extension polymerase chain reaction (PCR) method, has revealed primarily full-length mtDNAs, with only an occasional mtDNA rearrangement. By contrast, the skeletal muscle mtDNAs of individuals over age 50 have been found to accumulate a wide array of mtDNA rearrangements, the nature of which is specific to each individual muscle sample (Melov et al., 1995). The skeletal muscle of elderly subjects has been found to have ragged red fibers, with each COX^- and SDH^+ fiber containing a different mtDNA mutation (Muller-Hocker et al., 1992; Wallace, 1997). This implies that each of these somatic mtDNA mutations arose de novo and was selectively amplified within the cell to create the regional respiratory defects.

Somatic mtDNA mutations also occur in the brain. Quantitation of the common 5 kb mtDNA deletion has shown that mtDNA deletions accumulate in all regions of the cortex and rise dramatically in the basal ganglia after age 75, reaching a plateau at age 80 (Corral-Debrinski et al., 1992a; Soong et al., 1992). An analogous accumulation of somatic mtDNA rearrangements also occurs in the chimpanzee (Melov et al., 1999a), mouse tissues (Melov et al., 1997), and *Caenorhabditis elegans* (Melov et al., 1999a). Thus, mtDNA rearrangements accumulate with age in multicellular animals, with the level of rearrangements being proportional to life span rather than absolute time.

The cause of the somatic mtDNA mutations is likely to be oxidative damage. Oxidative damage, quantitated using 8-hydroxydeoxyguanosine (8-OH-dG), increases in the mtDNA with age in both humans and mice (Ames et al., 1993; Mecocci et al., 1993; Wallace, 1997). Moreover, patients with chronic ischemic heart disease, which is associated with cyclic bursts of mitochondrial ROS during ischemia and repurfusion (Das et al., 1989), harbor 8- to 2000-fold more mtDNA deletions in the heart than age-matched controls (Corral-Debrinski et al., 1992b).

These observations have led to the hypothesis that somatic mtDNA mutations accumulate in postmitotic tissues with age as a result of mitochondrial ROS damage. The resulting age-related decline in OXPHOS ultimately degrades the tissue's bioenergetic capacity until it falls below expression thresholds, resulting in symptoms and senescence.

MOUSE MODELS OF MITOCHONDRIAL DISEASE

While patient studies have revealed much about the genetics of mitochondrial disease, the physiological causes of the observed symptoms have been difficult to study. This limitation is being overcome by the creation and analysis of mouse models for mitochondrial disease. Three nuclear gene mutations in the mouse have provided new insight into the pathophysiology of mitochondrial disease. These mutations affect the mitochondrial transcription factor (*Tfam*) gene, the heart/muscle ANT isoform gene (*Ant1*), and the mitochondrial *MnSOD* gene.

The *Tfam*-Deficient Mouse

Genetic inactivation of the nDNA-encoded mitochondrial transcription factor *Tfam* has provided a model for the mtDNA depletion syndrome. The *Tfam* gene was inactivated by bracketing the terminal two exons (exons 6 and 7) with loxP sites and eliminating these exons by crossing the $+/Tfam^{loxP}$ animals with animals bearing the *Cre* recombinase.

Systemic mtDNA defects were obtained by transcribing the *Cre* recombinase from a constructive β-actin promoter. The resulting heterozygous $+/Tfam^-$ animals were viable and reproductively competent, while the homozygous $Tfam^{-/-}$ animals were embryonic lethals (Larsson et al., 1998). *Tfam* heterozygous animals had a 50% reduction in *Tfam* transcripts and protein and a partial reduction in mtDNA copy number mitochondrial transcripts and cytochrome *c* oxidase polypeptide 1 (COX1) protein in heart but not liver. Homozygous $Tfam^{-/-}$ mutant animals died between embryonic day (E) 8.5 and E10.5, with a complete absence of Tfam protein and either severely reduced or completely absent mtDNA. The mitochondria in the $Tfam^{-/-}$ animals were enlarged with abnormal cristae and deficient in COX1 but not SDH (Larsson et al., 1998).

Heart- and muscle-specific mtDNA defects were obtained by combining the homozygous *Tfam*^{loxP} allele with the *Cre* recombinase gene driven by the muscle creatine kinase promoter. This resulted in selective destruction of heart and skeletal muscle *Tfam* genes. While the hearts of 18.5-day embryos had reduced levels of *Tfam*, they appeared to be otherwise morphologically and biochemically normal. By contrast, these mutant animals proved to be postnatal lethals, dying at a mean age of 20 days from dilated cardiomyopathy. The animals also developed cardiac conduction defects. This was associated with a reduction in Tfam protein and mtDNA transcript levels in heart and muscle, a reduction in heart mtDNA by three-quarters, and reductions in skeletal muscle mtDNA (40%) and respiratory complexes I and IV but not complex II. Finally, histochemical analysis of hearts revealed a mosaic staining pattern, with some of the cardiomyocytes being COX^- and SDH^+, comparable to the mosaic OXPHOS deficiencies seen in human mitochondrial myopathy (Wang et al., 1999). Hence, these animals exhibit many of the features seen in the mtDNA depletion syndrome.

The *Ant1*-Deficient Mouse

Genetic inactivation of the nDNA-encoded *Ant1* gene has provided an excellent model for demonstrating the pathophysiological effects of chronic ATP deficiency. Surprisingly, ANT1-deficient [$Ant1^{tm2Mgr(-/-)}$] animals are viable, though they developed classical mitochondrial myopathy and hypertrophic cardiomyopathy (Graham et al., 1997).

The mouse *Ant1* gene is expressed at high levels in skeletal muscle and heart and at lower levels in brain, while the other mouse isoform (*Ant2*) is expressed in all tissues but skeletal muscle (Graham et al., 1997). Consequently, mice mutant in *Ant1* have a complete deficiency of ANT in skeletal muscle, where only ANT1 is expressed; a partial deficiency in heart, where both ANT1 and ANT2 are expressed; and normal ANT levels in liver, where only ANT2 is expressed.

The skeletal muscle of $Ant1^{-/-}$ animals exhibits classic ragged red fibers and increased SDH and COX staining in the type I oxidative fibers. These elevated OXPHOS enzyme activities correlate with a massive proliferation of giant mitochondria in the skeletal muscle fibers, degeneration of the contractile fibers, and marked exercise fatigability. The hearts of ANT1-deficient mice also exhibited a striking hypertrophic cardiomyopathy, associated with a significant proliferation of cardiomyocyte mitochondria. The proliferation of mitochondria in the ANT1-deficient mouse skeletal muscle and heart is associated with the coordinate up-regulation of both nDNA and mtDNA OXPHOS genes. Upregulated transcripts identified in skeletal muscle by differential display include the nDNA complex I 18 kDa mRNA and the complex IV COXVa and COXVb mRNAs, various mtDNA transcripts, and the transcripts of several novel genes including *Mcl-1*, the muscle *Bcl-2* homologue (Murdock et al., 1999). This implies that ANT1 deficiency affects not only mitochondrial bioenergetics but also oxidative stress and possibly predisposition to mitochondrial permeability transition.

ANT1-deficient mice also had elevated serum lactate, alanine, succinate, and citrate, consistent with inhibition of the respiratory chain and TCA cycle. Inhibition of mitochondrial ADP/ATP exchange and of ADP-coupled respiration was confirmed in the skeletal muscle mitochondria of $Ant1^{-/-}$ mice by showing their complete resistance to stimulation of oxygen consumption by exogenous ADP. The heart mitochondrial respiration rate was only partially stimulated by ADP, while liver mitochondrial respiration was fully stimulated by ADP. This is consistent with the complete lack of ANT and ADP/ATP exchange in skeletal muscle mitochondria, a partial reduction in heart, and no reduction in liver. Hence, the ANT1 mouse provides direct proof that inhibition of the cell's access to mitochondrial energy production can result in the symptoms of mitochondrial myopathy and cardiomyopathy (Graham et al., 1997).

Inhibition of ADP/ATP exchange in heart and skeletal muscle would be expected to limit the availability of matrix ADP for ATP synthase, thus reducing proton flux through the ATP synthase proton channel. This would result in hyperpolarization of the mitochondrial inner membrane, $\Delta\Psi$, which would inhibit the ETC and cause the redirection of electrons from the ETC into the ROS-generating pathway.

Consistent with this expectation, the mitochondrial production rate of H_2O_2 was increased six- to eightfold in the ANT1-deficient skeletal muscle and heart mitochondria, levels comparable to those obtained for control mitochondria when the ETC was inhibited by the complex III inhibitor antimycin A. ANT1-deficient brain cortex and cerebellum mitochondria also had elevated H_2O_2 production but less than that produced in control mitochondria by antimycin A. Finally, liver mitochondrial H_2O_2 production was the same for mutant and normal animals. Thus, the increased ROS production was proportional to the reduction in mitochondrial ANT levels and associated inhibition of the respiratory chain.

The increased oxidative stress caused by the ANT1 deficiency was paralleled by an induction of the ROS-detoxifying enzymes MnSOD and GPx. In ANT1-deficient skeletal muscle, MnSOD protein was increased about 15-fold in tissue and sixfold in isolated mitochondria. GPx levels in skeletal muscle tissue and mitochondria were increased about twofold. In the ANT1-deficient heart, the MnSOD level was increased about twofold in tissue, though not in isolated mitochondria. GPx levels in heart tissue and mitochondria were also increased, about threefold. Hence, the increased oxidative stress resulting from inhibition of OXPHOS is associated with induction of the mitochondrial ROS defense systems (Esposito et al., 1999).

The increased ROS production would be expected to increase mitochondrial macromolecular damage. This was confirmed by analyses of the heart mtDNA of 16- to 20-month ANT1-deficient mice. These mutant animals had much higher levels of mtDNA rearrangements than did age-matched controls. In fact, the level of mtDNA rearrangements in the 16- to 20-month old $Ant1^{-/-}$ animals were comparable to those seen in the hearts of very old (30 month) normal mice. In skeletal muscle, the level of mtDNA rearrangements was also increased but not to the extent of heart mtDNA. Since both heart and muscle mitochondria produced maximal levels of ROS while the skeletal muscle (but not heart mitochondria) was compensated by induction of the antioxidant enzyme MnSOD, it follows that the heart would be exposed to greater residual oxidative stress than the skeletal muscle. This is reflected by the differential level of mtDNA damage. Hence, the increased ROS production does increase mitochondrial macromolecular damage, including mtDNA mutations (Esposito et al., 1999).

The MnSOD-Deficient Mouse

To better understand the origins and consequences of increased mitochondrial ROS production, mice deficient in mitochondrial MnSOD have been prepared. Two mouse lines lacking MnSOD (Sod2) have also been reported: $Sod2^{tm1Cje}$ (Li et al., 1995) and

Sod2^{tm1Leb} (Lebovitz et al., 1996). The *Sod2*^{tm1Cje} mutation was originally studied on the CD1 background and resulted in neonatal death due to dilated cardiomyopathy (Li et al., 1995). The *Sod2*^{tm1Cje} mutation was studied on the C57BL/6 background and resulted in death after about 18 days associated with degenerative injury to the large neurons, particularly in the basal ganglia and brain stem, and injury to the neuronal mitochondria (Lebovitz et al., 1996).

The *Sod2*^{tm1Cje} mutation on the CD1 background has been extensively characterized. In addition to death due to dilated cardiomyopathy at about 8 days of age (Li et al., 1995; Melov et al., 1998), histochemical analysis has revealed striking depositions of lipid in the liver and marked deficiency in SDH (complex II) in the heart (Li et al., 1995). The complex II defect was confirmed by enzymological analysis of complex II + III activity, which revealed a 65% reduction in skeletal muscle and a 76% reduction in heart. Heart complex I activity was also reduced 41%, and mitochondrial aconitase was almost entirely inactivated in heart (89%) and brain (67%–76%). Finally, urine organic acid analysis of *Sod2*$^{-/-}$ animals revealed large quantities of 3-methylglutaconic, 2-hydroxyglutaric, 3-hydroxy-3-methylglutaric, and 3-hydroxyisovaleric acids. This is characteristic of human 3-hydroxy-3-methylglutaryl coenzyme A lyase deficiency, and this enzyme was reduced 36% in the mutant mouse livers (Melov et al., 1999b).

Testing for DNA oxidation revealed that mutant hearts had large (215%–300%) increases in 8-hydroxyguanine, 8-hydroxyadenine, and 5-hydroxycytosine. The brain also had increased levels of 5-hydroxycytosine (Melov et al., 1999b).

These observations indicate that the high levels of mitochondrial superoxide anion resulting from MnSOD deficiency can cause inhibition of the ETC (complexes I and II) and the TCA cycle (aconitase), probably due to inactivation of the Fe-S centers in these enzymes. This conclusion has been confirmed by demonstrating that the cardiac defect can be rescued by treating the *Sod2*$^{-/-}$ animals with the exogenous antioxidant manganese 5,10,15,20-tetrakis (4-benzoic acid) porphyrin (MnTBAP), which catalytically converts $O_2^{\cdot -}$ to H_2O_2. Peritoneal injection of *Sod2*$^{-/-}$ mice with MnTBAP eliminated the dilated cardiomyopathy, reduced the liver lipid deposition, and extended the mean life span of the animals to about 16 days. Unfortunately, MnTBAP does not cross the blood–brain barrier, and by 12 days of age, MnTBAP-treated animals began to exhibit gait disturbances that progressed to ataxia, dystonia, repetitive movements, tremor, and immobility by 21 days of age. Histological analysis of the brains of these mice revealed a symmetrical spongiform encephalopathy together with glial fibrillary acid protein deposition in regions of the cortex and brain stem. This suggests that increased mitochondrial ROS production is extremely toxic to the brain, possibly causing neuronal cell apoptosis (Melov et al., 1998).

While the acute pathology observed in *Sod2*$^{-/-}$ animals confirms the importance of mitochondrial ROS toxicity in causing mitochondrial dysfunction, many clinical syndromes, such as Friedreich's ataxia, are associated with chronic ROS exposure. Consequently, the heterozygous +/*Sod2*$^{-}$ mouse, with a 50% reduction in MnSOD, may provide a better model for chronic mitochondrial disease. The liver mitochondria of +/*Sod2*$^{-}$ mice have a 30% reduction in mitochondrial glutathione levels, though normal levels of GPx. Mitochondrial aconitase activity was reduced 30% but could be reactivated to control levels by exposure to iron and a reducing agent, confirming the inactivation of the Fe-S centers. Mitochondrial complex I was reduced 30%, mitochondrial protein carbonyl groups (aldehydes and ketones) were increased, and the mtDNA had a 30% increase in 8-OH-dG. Respiration studies revealed a reduction in ADP-stimulated respiration, indicating partial uncoupling of the mitochondria; and the mitochondria had increased sensitivity to the calcium and oxidative stress-induced opening of the mtPTP, implying a predilection to apoptosis (Williams et al., 1998). Thus, chronic exposure to mitochondrial ROS does impair mitochondrial function, confirming that increased mitochondrial ROS production can play a significant role in the pathophysiology of mitochondrial disease.

MITOCHONDRIAL DEFECTS IN COMMON DISEASES

While individual mtDNA diseases are rare, the phenotypes associated with them are common (hearing loss, vision loss, movement disorders, dementia, diabetes, heart disease, etc.). This raises the possibility that these phenotypes might be commonly caused by mitochondrial OXPHOS defects and that they could involve defects of the mtDNA or the nDNA or an interaction of the two.

Mitochondrial Defects and Diabetes Mellitus

Diabetes mellitus is one common disease likely to have a major mitochondrial component to its etiology. Mitochondrial DNA mutations are the most common known cause of diabetes mellitus, with both tRNA mutations (Suzuki et al., 1994b; van den Ouweland et al., 1992, 1994) and rearrangement mutations (Ballinger et al., 1992, 1994) being linked to diabetes mellitus.

Diabetes mellitus patients are generally divided into two classes: insulin-dependent diabetes mellitus (IDDM), or Type 1 diabetes, and non-insulin-dependent diabetes mellitus (NIDDM) or Type 2 diabetes (Gerbitz et al., 1995; Wallace et al., 1996). Epidemiological studies have shown that a Type 2 diabetes patient's mother is more likely to be affected than the father. This bias toward female transmission of diabetes mellitus increases with the age at onset of the proband, reaching a ratio of 3:1 for a mean age of 46 years (Dorner et al., 1975, 1987; Dorner and Mohnike, 1976; Pimentel, 1979; Freinkel et al., 1986; Alcolado and Thomas, 1995).

Type 2 diabetes mellitus is a common presentation in CPEO and KSS patients harboring mtDNA rearrangements. In KSS patients harboring reciprocal duplication and deletion rearrangements, diabetes mellitus is more commonly seen with the larger deletions. These KSS patients also manifest ophthalmoplegia, ptosis, and mitochondrial myopathy (Poulton et al., 1989a,b, 1993, 1994, 1995; Dunbar et al., 1993). However, in one large African-American pedigree, maternally inherited Type 2 diabetes mellitus together with sensory neural hearing loss occurred in the absence of the other symptoms of CPEO and KSS. Moreover, molecular analysis revealed that this family harbored a trimolecular heteroplasmy including normal mtDNAs and reciprocal duplicated and deleted mtDNAs (Ballinger et al., 1992, 1994). Thus, Type 2 diabetes can be caused by mtDNA rearrangement, and it is possible that other patients with Type 2 diabetes harbor mtDNA mutations.

This has proven to be the case since it is now known that the most common cause of diabetes is the mtDNA *MTTL1**MELAS3243G mutation (van den Ouweland et al., 1992, 1994). This mutation accounts for approximately 1.4% of both Type 1 and Type 2 diabetes in surveys throughout the world

(Gerbitz et al., 1995). The mutation is invariably heteroplasmic, ranging in percentage in blood from 5% to 30% (Suzuki et al., 1994a; van den Ouweland et al., 1992, 1994). Diabetes mellitus patients with the *MTTL1**MELAS3243G mutation frequently show maternal transmission and often manifest sensory neural hearing loss (Kadowaki et al., 1994; Alcolado and Thomas, 1995). While most *MTTL1**MELAS3243G diabetes patients present as Type 2 (NIDDM), some progress to Type 1 (IDDM) and can develop islet cell autoantibodies (Oka et al., 1993, 1995). Type 2 diabetes mellitus has also been associated with the *MTTK**MERRF8344G mutation in one family (Suzuki et al., 1994b; Kadowaki et al., 1995). Clearly, additional surveys of diabetes mellitus patients for mtDNA mutations are justified.

The physiological mechanism by which mtDNA mutations induce diabetes mellitus is not understood. However, analysis of both *MTTL1**MELLAS3243G patients (Gerbitz et al., 1995) and mtDNA rearrangement patients (Ballinger et al., 1994) has revealed a defect in the response to hyperglycemia of increased blood insulin levels and decreased glucagon levels. This implies a defect in the glucose sensor system of both the alpha and beta cells of the pancreatic islets. Based on studies of maturity-onset diabetes of the young, the glucose sensor has been proposed to involve the glucokinase of the pancreatic alpha and beta cells. The K_m of pancreatic glucokinase is high such that it can only phosphorylate glucose when the blood glucose levels are high (Stoffel et al., 1992a,b, 1993; German, 1993; Gidh-Jain et al., 1993). Since glucokinase is attached to the mitochondrial outer membrane through porin and porin interacts with the ANT of the inner membrane (Malaisse-Lagae and Malaisse, 1988; Adams et al., 1991), glucose phosphorylation might be directly coupled to OXPHOS in pancreatic islet cells through this macromolecular complex. Hence, a mtDNA mutation which inhibits pancreatic OXPHOS could also inhibit the glucose sensor by limiting access to ATP (McCabe, 1994; Wallace, 1994). In addition, reduced mitochondrial ATP production could inhibit the ATP-dependent closure of the K^+ channels, inhibiting K^+ inflow into the cell and opening the voltage-activated Ca^{2+} channels. With Ca^{2+} influx inhibited, fusion of the insulin-containing vesicles to the plasma membrane could also be blocked (Gerbitz et al., 1995).

Movement Disorders

Mitochondria and Dystonia

A second common class of diseases that may have an important mitochondrial etiology are the movement disorders. A role for mtDNA mutations in movement disorders was first demonstrated by the discovery of the *MTND6**LDYT14459A mutation in a large, five-generation, Hispanic LHON and dystonia pedigree (Jun et al., 1994). Members of this pedigree with generalized dystonia had a mean age at onset of approximately 4 years and exhibited gait disturbance; rigidity of the lower extremities, which advanced with age to the upper extremities; pseudobulbar syndrome; impaired intelligence; short stature; and myopathic features (Novotny et al., 1986). Two additional families with the *MTND6**LDYT14459A mutation included an African-American mother and her daughter with LHON and a European-American singleton case of pediatric generalized dystonia with striatal necrosis (Shoffner et al., 1995).

OXPHOS enzyme analysis of skeletal muscle mitochondria from the daughter of the African-American LHON family revealed a severe respiratory complex I defect (Shoffner et al., 1995). Analysis of mitochondria from lymphoblastoid cell lines from all three families revealed an approximately 55% reduction in complex I–specific activity. This defect was encoded by the mtDNA in the cybrid transfer (Jun et al., 1996).

Other mtDNA mutations can also present as dystonia. One patient harboring the *MTND4**LHON11778A mutation lost his vision at age 37 years and later developed cerebellar–extrapyramidal tremor and left-side rigidity associated with bilateral basal ganglia degeneration at age 38 (Larsson et al., 1991). Another patient experienced visual loss at age 23 and extrapyramidal signs including spastic paraparesis, patellar and ankle clonus, diffuse muscle weakness, and a magnetic resonance image compatible with demyelinating disease (Vergani et al., 1995).

Complex I defects have also been observed in the platelet mitochondria of dystonia patients. Average complex I activity of patients with generalized or segmental dystonia was reduced 62% relative to controls, while the average activity from focal dystonia patients was reduced 37% (Benecke et al., 1992). Also, an isolated case of idiopathic dystonia, putaminal lesions, and myopathy was found to harbor a partial complex III defect (Nigro et al., 1990).

The association between mitochondrial defects and dystonia has been further supported by the discovery of homology between the nuclear genes responsible for hereditary dystonia and proteins involved in mitochondrial biogenesis. Early-onset torsion dystonia is due to mutations in the torsin A gene (*DYT1*). This is the most severe form of hereditary dystonia, inherited as an autosomal dominant, with almost all cases resulting from a 3 np deletion (GAG) that removes one glutamate codon. Torsin A was found to be homologous to the SKD3 protein, a member of the Clp/HSP104 family of proteins (Fig. 52–3) (Ozelius et al., 1997, 1998).

In analyzing the genes induced during mitochondrial proliferation in the skeletal muscle of the ANT1 knockout mouse, one of the genes identified was *SKD3*. Analysis of the cDNA revealed that the protein incorporated the Clp/HSP104 domain containing an ATP binding domain at the C-terminal end, a central domain with four ankyrin-like domains, and an amino-terminal domain with a putative mitochondria-targeting domain. The *SKD3* transcript proved to be markedly upregulated in $Ant1^{-/-}$ mouse muscle, along with other known nDNA and mtDNA OXPHOS genes. Hence, it stands to reason that *SKD3* is involved in the assembly of the mitochondrion (Murdock et al., 1999). Since *SKD3* bears homology to torsion A, it is possible that torsion A is also involved in mitochondrial biogenesis and that torsion dystonia is a mitochondrial disease (Wallace and Murdock, 1999).

The mitochondria and dystonia association has been further supported by studies on the X-linked Mohr-Tranebjaerg syndrome. The Mohr-Tranebjaerg syndrome presents in early childhood with sensory neural hearing loss that can progress to dystonia, spasticity, mental deterioration, paranoia, and cortical blindness. It is the result of mutations in the *DFN-1* gene, which encodes a 97–amino acid, 11 kDa polypeptide, designated DDP1 (Jin et al., 1996).

Concurrent studies in yeast on the mitochondrial import of nuclear-encoded inner-membrane carrier proteins like ANT has revealed a family of small polypeptides, Tim8p through Timp13p, that facilitate the import process. These proteins have a distinctive pair of $C(N)_3C$ motifs. Interestingly, the paired $C(N)_3C$ motif is also found in the Mohr-Tranebjaerg syndrome DDP1 protein (Koehler et al., 1999).

```
SKD3      CCHPLV-FLFLGSSGIGKTCLAKQTAKYKNKDAKKGFIRLDMSCFQCRHCVQKFI
torsinA   PKKPLTLSL-HGWTGTGKNFVSKIIAENIYEGGLN-------SDYVHLFVATLHF

SKD3      GSPPGYIGHCCGGQ--LTKKLKQCPNAVVLFDEVDKAHPDVLTIMLQLFDCGRLT
torsinA   PHASNITLYKDQLQLWIRGNVSACARSIFIFDEMDKMHAGLIDAIKPFLD----Y

SKD3      DGKGKTIQCKDAIFIMTSNVASDEIAQHALQLRQCALCMSRNRIACNLGDVQMSD
torsinA   YDLVDGVSYQKAMFIFLSNAGAERITDVALDFW---------RSGKQREDIKLKD

SKD3      KITISKNFKENVIRPILKAHCRRDCFLGRINCIVYFLPFCHSELIQLVNKEL
torsinA   IEHALSVSVFNNK--NSGFWHSSLIDRNLIDYFVPFLPLEYKHLKMCIRVEM
```

Fig. 52–3. Early-onset torsion dystonia gene (*DYT1*) is homologous to *SKD3*.

Moreover, comparison of the DDP1 protein to the genes that are upregulated in the skeletal muscle of the ANT mouse revealed a cDNA DD14P. The protein encoded by this cDNA had high homology with DDP1 (Fig. 52–4), again confirming that the Tim8p–Tim13p and DDP1 family of proteins are involved in mitochondrial biogenesis (Wallace and Murdock, 1999).

Therefore, three hereditary forms of dystonia have been associated with mitochondrial genetic defects: *(1)* the maternally inherited LHON plus dystonia associated with a complex I defect, *(2)* the autosomal dominant torsion dystonia possibly associated with an assembly defect, and *(3)* the X-linked recessive Mohr-Tranebjaerg syndrome associated with a carrier protein import defect. These results raise the possibility that other forms of dystonia might also have a mitochondrial basis.

Mitochondrial Defects in Parkinson's Disease

The demonstration that mtDNA mutations can cause dystonia raises the possibility that mitochondrial defects play a role in the more common movement disorder Parkinson's disease (PD). PD is clinically characterized by bradykinesia, rigidity, and tremor associated with the death of the dopaminergic neurons in the substantia nigra (Schapira, 1992, 1994b, 1995b).

The causes of PD are undoubtedly heterogeneous (Schapira, 1995a). PD can be induced in both humans and laboratory animals by 1-methyl-4-phenyl-1,2,3,6-tetrahydropyridine (MPTP), a contaminant found in illicitly synthesized meperidine (Langston et al., 1983). MPTP is oxidized by monoamine oxidase (MAO) B to its active form, MPP^+ (1-methyl-4-phenylpyridiniumoin). MPP^+ is actively taken up by the dopaminergic neurons of the substantia nigra through the dopamine transporter, is electrostatically attracted to the mitochondria (Singer et al., 1987; Schapira, 1994b; Mizuno et al., 1995), inhibits mitochondrial complex I and respiration by NADH–linked substrates (Singer et al., 1987; Schapira, 1994b; Mizuno et al., 1995), and increases mitochondrial oxidative stress (Cleeter et al., 1992; Schapira, 1994b). Thus, inhibition of complex I and increased mitochondrial oxidative stress can cause PD.

Mitochondrial OXPHOS defects may be common in PD patients. Homogenates of the substantia nigra of PD patients harbor defects in complex I (Schapira et al., 1989, 1990a; Mann et al., 1992a; Schapira, 1992, 1994a), as well as complex III in some cases (Mizuno et al., 1989; Janetzky et al., 1994). Complex I defects in PD brains have been substantiated by immunohistochemical analysis (Hattori et al., 1991). PD patients have also been reported to have complex I defects in their blood platelet mitochondria (Parker et al., 1989; Krige et al., 1992; Yoshino et al., 1992; Benecke et al., 1993) and in their skeletal muscle mitochondria (Bindoff et al., 1989; Zheng et al., 1990; Wallace et al., 1992; Blin et al., 1994), though this result has not been confirmed in a few studies (Mann et al., 1992a).

```
                      10         20         30         40         50
Tim8p     1  MGLSSIFGG- ----GAPSQQ KEAATTAKTT PNPIAKELKN QIAQELAVAN   50
hDDP1     1  MDSSS--SSS AAGLGAVD-P QLQHFIEVET QKQRFQQLVH QMT---EL--   50
mDDP1     1  MESST--SSS GSALGAVD-P QLQHFIEVET QKQRFQQLVH QMT---EL--   50
hDDP2     1         MRQ QWRLGEADEA ELQRLVAAEQ QKAQFTAQVH ---HFMEL--   50
DD14p     1         MA- --ELGEADEA ELQRLVAAEQ QKAQFTAQVH ---HFMEL--   50

                      60         70         80         90        100
Tim8p    51  ATECFEKCLT SP---YATRN DACIDQCLAK YMRSWNVISK AYISRIQNAS  100
hDDP1    51  ---CWEKCMD KPGPKLDSRA EACFVNCVER FIDTSQFILN RLEQTQKSKP  100
mDDP1    51  ---CWEKCMD KPGPKLDSRA EACFVNCVER FIDTSQFILN RLEQTQKSKP  100
hDDP2    51  ---CWDKCVE KPGNRLDSRT ENCLSSCVDR FIDTTLAITS RFAQ------  100
DD14p    51  ---CWDKCVE KPGSRLDSRT ENCLSSCVDR FIDTTLAITG RFAQ------  100

                     110        120        130        140        150
Tim8p   101  A---SGEI•• •••••••••• •••••••••• •••••••••• ••••••••••  150
hDDP1   101  VFSESLSD•• •••••••••• •••••••••• •••••••••• ••••••••••  150
mDDP1   101  VFSESLSD•• •••••••••• •••••••••• •••••••••• ••••••••••  150
hDDP2   101  -IVQKGGQ•• •••••••••• •••••••••• •••••••••• ••••••••••  150
DD14p   101  -IVQQGGQ•• •••••••••• •••••••••• •••••••••• ••••••••••  150
```

Fig. 52–4. Mohr-Tranebjaerg deafness and dystonia syndrome, a mitochondrial import disease.

Assuming that OXPHOS defects are a common feature of PD, the genetics remains unclear. A variety of germline mtDNA variants have been observed in PD mtDNA, though none has been proven to be causally related to the disease (Johns and Neufeld, 1991; Shoffner et al., 1994; Mizuno et al., 1995; Brown et al., 1996). Moreover, evidence that somatic mtDNA mutations may be increased in PD has been inconclusive (Ikebe et al., 1990; Ozawa et al., 1990; Schapira et al., 1990b; Mann et al., 1992b; Sandy et al., 1993; DiDonato et al., 1993; Shan et al., 1995).

Finally, mitochondrially generated ROS have been reported to be increased in PD pathology. The substantia nigra of PD patients showed a 33% induction of MnSOD activity, a 10-fold increase in the acutely generated hydroperoxides, and a 40% decrease in glutathione; also, reduced glutathione was decreased relative to controls (Jenner et al., 1992). Thus, PD might involve increased mitochondrially generated oxidative damage.

Mitochondria and Huntington's Disease

Huntington's disease (HD), like dystonia, shows a characteristic pathology of the basal ganglia and is associated with movement disorders as well as cognitive loss and psychiatric manifestations. The disease has an autosomal dominant mode of inheritance and is caused by a CAG repeat expansion in the *IT15* gene, located on chromosome 4p16.3. This repeat expansion causes expansion of a polyglutamine stretch within the huntington protein (Huntington's Disease Collaborative Research Group, 1993).

Treatment of rodents or primates with the complex III inhibitor 3-nitropropionic acid creates an HD-like phenotype (Beal, 1994), suggesting that OXPHOS defects may play a role in HD. Positron emission tomographic (PET) studies of striatal glucose consumption have revealed a marked reduction in all patients (Kuwert et al., 1993), and cortical glucose metabolism of HD patients is also reduced (Martin et al., 1992). HD patients also have a significant increase in lactate levels of the occipital cortex relative to controls (Jenkins et al., 1993). Thus, these results suggest a generalized energy deficit in the brains of HD patients.

Biochemical analysis of mitochondria isolated from frozen HD brains has revealed defects in complex IV in the caudate (Brennan et al., 1985). This result is supported by reports of complex II, complex III, and complex IV defects (Gu et al., 1996). Analysis of platelet mitochondria from HD patients revealed a consistent complex I defect (Parker et al., 1990a), though this was not supported in another study (Gu et al., 1996). Hence, current biochemical data support a generalized brain OXPHOS defect that progresses with the disease. However, the systemic nature of the defect remains to be proven.

A possible OXPHOS defect could increase mitochondrial ROS production and somatic mtDNA mutations. Consistent with this possibility, cortical regions of HD patients have an approximately eightfold increase in mtDNA rearrangements relative to age-matched controls. Hence, it is possible that the polyglutamine expansion in the huntington protein may in some way result in a partial OXPHOS defect.

Dementias and Alzheimer's Disease

Progressive dementia is another common manifestation of patients harboring mtDNA mutations. One patient who presented with cognitive decline, dementia, deafness, ataxia, and chorea was found to harbor a $tRNA^{Trp}$ mutation, *MTTW**DEMCHO5549A. This individual manifested mitochondrial myopathy with COX^-, ragged red fibers containing abnormal mitochondria, and a complex I defect. Autopsy histology revealed diffuse, moderate neuronal loss in the cortex and basal ganglia (Nelson et al., 1995). The prevalence of dementia in some of the more severe mtDNA diseases raises the possibility that the milder, late-onset dementias, such as Alzheimer's disease (AD), might also be associated with bioenergetic defects resulting from either inherited or acquired mtDNA mutations.

AD is an age-related, progressive dementia, associated with characteristic neuropathological findings including neurofibrillary tangles composed of highly phosphorylated forms of the microtubule-associated protein Tau and accumulation of extracellular plaques containing the amyloid β-peptide (Selkoe, 1995). Histological analysis of AD brains has revealed alterations in mitochondrial morphology in apparently normal dendrites (Saraiva et al., 1985), and metabolic and OXPHOS defects have been reported in AD patient brains and cells (Sorbi et al., 1983; Sheu et al., 1985; Sims et al., 1987; Jagust et al., 1991). A defect in OXPHOS complex IV has also been reported in blood platelets of AD patients (Parker et al., 1990b). This was reported to be associated with a heteroplasmic mtDNA mutation involving normal mtDNAs and mutant mtDNAs containing five linked mutations in the mtDNA *COI* and *COII* genes (Davis et al., 1997). However, it was subsequently revealed that the mutant mtDNAs were, in fact, nuclear DNA *COI* and *COII* pseudogenes that were being inadvertently amplified during the PCR process (Hirano et al., 1997; Wallace et al., 1997; Davis and Parker, 1998). Hence, the molecular basis of the complex IV defects remains unclear. Finally, ROS have been implicated in AD, in both damaging neurons and catalyzing the aggregation of the amyloid β-peptide (Benzi and Moretti, 1995; Mattson, 1995).

A portion of late-onset AD patients have also been associated with a T-to-C transition at np 4336 in the mtDNA $tRNA^{Gln}$ gene, *MTTQ**ADPD4336C. In European studies, this mutation has been reported in 5.2% of patients and 0.7% of controls in one study (Shoffner et al., 1993) and between 4.3% to 8.3% of patients and 0.34% and 0.63% of age-matched and total controls in a second study (Hutchin and Cortopassi, 1995; Hutchin et al., 1995). However, in a third study, the *MTTQ**ADPD4336C allele was not found at an increased frequency in AD patients (Travis, 1995). Assuming that the *MTTQ**ADPD4336C mutation is a risk factor for AD, its presence would increase the risk of the disease approximately 16-fold (Hutchin et al., 1995).

The *MTTQ**ADPD4336C variant is homoplasmic and associated with a specific European mtDNA lineage, haplogroup H. This implies that it arose in Europe as a single mutational event about 8500 to 17,000 years ago. In addition to the *MTTQ**ADPD4336C variant, several novel mtDNA variants have been observed in AD patients. These include a homoplasmic missense mutation, *MTND1**ADPD3397G, which converts a highly conserved methionine to a valine and was found to have arisen two independent times in the AD patients surveyed, one with the *MTTQ**ADPD4336C variant and one without. The other two novel variants were an insertion of five Cs between np 956 and 965 in the 12S rRNA (*MTRNR1*) and a heteroplasmic mutation in the 16S rRNA (*MTTRNR2**ADPD3197A) (Shoffner et al., 1993; Brown et al., 1996). However, the clinical significance of these later mutations remains to be determined.

If *MTTQ**ADPD4336C and *MTND1**ADPD3397G variants do contribute to AD, what might be a common underlying pathophysiological mechanism that interrelates these various mutations? One hypothesis is that these mtDNA mutations might partially inhibit mitochondrial OXPHOS, reducing ATP production and increasing ROS generation (Wallace, 1992a, b). The increase in ROS would inhibit mitochondrial function and mutate the resident mtDNAs. This would exacerbate the bioenergetic defect, ultimately activating the mtPTP, initiating apoptosis, and resulting in neuronal death (Wallace et al., 1995).

If mitochondrial function and ROS production are important factors in AD, then we might expect that ROS damage would be elevated in the mtDNAs of AD patients and that there would be a concomitant increase in somatic mtDNA mutations. Analyses of 8-OH-dG levels in AD brains has revealed a 20-fold elevation in the mtDNA over the nDNA and a significant threefold increase over controls (Mecocci et al., 1994). Moreover, this increase in oxidative damage is associated with an approximately 15-fold increase in the common 5 kb deletion levels in the cortical regions of AD patients who died prior to age 75 relative to age-matched controls and a fivefold decrease in cortical deletions in AD patients who died after age 75 (Corral-Debrinski et al., 1994). This suggests that AD patients may have an elevated ROS generation rate that increases the somatic mtDNA mutation rate. Perhaps when sufficient deleted mtDNAs accumulate in a neuron, it initiates apoptosis and the neuron self-destructs. This would account for the decline of mutant mtDNAs in older AD patients relative to controls and might contribute to the progressive dementia.

CONCLUSION

Deleterious mtDNA and nDNA mutations affecting mitochondrial bioenergetics and/or biogenesis have been associated with a wide range of clinical symptoms that encompass the major common degenerative diseases. Furthermore, somatic mtDNA mutations accumulate with age in postmitotic tissues, presumably compromising mitochondrial biogenesis and, hence, energy metabolism. Evidence continues to accumulate that inherited OXPHOS defects and age-related, acquired OXPHOS defects are cumulative, eroding the bioenergetic capacity of the mitochondria and exacerbating the disease.

Consequently, as an individual ages, mitochondrial bioenergetic capacity decreases and ROS production increases, with the result that somatic mtDNA mutations accumulate. Ultimately, these factors combine to impair bioenergetic capacity and increase oxidative stress on the mitochondria to such a degree that it opens the mtPTP, initiates apoptosis, and eliminates the cell.

If this hypothesis is valid, then it predicts that metabolic intervention of mitochondrial ROS generation should protect OXPHOS function and reduced somatic mtDNA mutations. Preservation of mtDNA integrity and mitochondrial function would in turn inhibit the onset and progression of symptoms in those diseases related to mitochondrial OXPHOS defects, thus eliminating the symptoms. Such therapies will be perfected using the various mouse models of mitochondrial disease, where genetic variability can be controlled and novel experimental drugs can be tested. The dramatic success of MnTBAP at ameliorating ROS toxicity in the MnSOD-deficient mouse indicates the power of this approach and the promise of catalytic antioxidant drugs in the treatment of degenerative diseases.

REFERENCES

Adams V, Griffin L, Towbin J, Gelb B, Worley K, McCabe ER: Porin interaction with hexokinase and glycerol kinase: metabolic microcompartmentation at the outer mitochondrial membrane. Biochem Med Metab Biol 1991; 45:271–291.

Alcolado JC, Thomas AW: Maternally inherited diabetes mellitus: the role of mitochondrial DNA defects. Diabet Med 1995; 12:102–108.

Ames BN, Shigenaga MK, Hagen TM: Oxidants, antioxidants, and the degenerative diseases of aging. Proc Natl Acad Sci USA 1993; 90:7915–7922.

Andersson SG, Zomorodipour A, Andersson JO, Sicheritz-Ponten T, Alsmark UC, Podowski RM, Naslund AK, Eriksson AS, Winkler HH, Kurland CG: The genome sequence of *Rickettsia prowazekii* and the origin of mitochondria. Nature 1998; 396:133–140.

Ballinger SW, Shoffner JM, Gebhart S, Koontz DA, Wallace DC: Mitochondrial diabetes revisited. Nat Genet 1994; 7:458–459.

Ballinger SW, Shoffner JM, Hedaya EV, Trounce I, Polack MA, Koontz DA, Wallace DC: Maternally transmitted diabetes and deafness associated with a 10.4 kb mitochondrial DNA deletion. Nat Genet 1992; 1:11–15.

Beal MF: Neurochemistry and toxin models in Huntington's disease. Curr Opin in Neurol 1994; 7:542–547.

Benecke R, Strumper P, Weiss H: Electron transfer complex I defect in idiopathic dystonia. Ann Neurol 1992; 32:683–686.

Benecke R, Strumper P, Weiss H: Electron transfer complexes I and IV of platelets are abnormal in Parkinson's disease but normal in Parkinson-plus syndromes. Brain 1993; 116:1451–1463.

Benzi G, Moretti A: Are reactive oxygen species involved in Alzheimer's disease? Neurobiol Aging 1995; 16:661–674.

Bindoff LA, Birch-Machin M, Cartlidge NEF, Parker WD Jr, Turnbull DM: Mitochondrial function in Parkinson's disease. Lancet 1989; 1:49.

Blin O, Desnuelle C, Rascol O, Borg M, Peyro Saint Paul H, Azulay JP, Bille F, Figarella D, Coulom F, Pellissier JF, et al.: Mitochondrial respiratory failure in skeletal muscle from patients with Parkinson's disease and multiple system atrophy. J Neurol Sci 1994; 125:95–101.

Bodnar AG, Cooper JM, Holt IJ, Leonard JV, Schapira AH: Nuclear complementation restores mtDNA levels in cultured cells from a patient with mtDNA depletion. Am J Hum Genet 1993; 53:663–669.

Bourgeron T, Rustin P, Chretien D, Birch-Machin M, Bourgeois M, Viegas-Pequignot E, Munnich A, Rotig A: Mutation of a nuclear succinate dehydrogenase gene results in mitochondrial respiratory chain deficiency. Nat Genet 1995; 11:144–149.

Brennan WA Jr, Bird ED, Aprille JR: Regional mitochondrial respiratory activity in Huntington's disease brain. J Neurochem 1985; 44:1948–1950.

Brown MD, Shoffner JM, Kim YL, Jun AS, Graham BH, Cabell MF, Gurley DS, Wallace DC: Mitochondrial DNA sequence analysis of four Alzheimer's and Parkinson's disease patients. Am J Hum Genet 1996; 61:283–289.

Brown MD, Sun F, Wallace DC: Clustering of Caucasian Leber hereditary optic neuropathy patients containing the 11778 or 14484 mutations on an mtDNA lineage. Am J Hum Genet 1997; 60:381–387.

Brustovetsky N, Klingenberg M: Mitochondrial ADP/ATP carrier can be reversibly converted into a large channel by Ca^{2+}. Biochemistry 1996; 35:8483–8488.

Bunn CL, Wallace DC, Eisenstadt JM: Cytoplasmic inheritance of chlormaphenicol resistance in mouse tissue culture cells. Proc Natl Acad Sci USA 1974; 71:1681–1685.

Casari G, De Fusco M, Ciarmatori S, Zeviani M, Mora M, Fernandez P, De Michele G, Filla A, Cocozza S, Marconi R, et al.: Spastic paraplegia and OXPHOS impairment caused by mutations in paraplegin, a nuclear-encoded mitochondrial metalloprotease. Cell 1998; 93:973–983.

Chomyn A, Martinuzzi A, Yoneda M, Daga A, Hurko O, Johns D, Lai ST, Nonaka I, Angelini C, Attardi G: MELAS mutation in mtDNA binding site for transcription termination factor causes defects in protein synthesis and in respiration but no change in levels of upstream and downstream mature transcripts. Proc Natl Acad Sci USA 1992; 89:4221–4225.

Chomyn A, Meola G, Bresolin N, Lai ST, Scarlato G, Attardi G: In vitro genetic transfer of protein synthesis and respiration defects to mitochondrial DNA-less cells with myopathy-patient mitochondria. Mol Cell Biol 1991; 11:2236–2244.

Cleeter MW, Cooper JM, Schapira AH: Irreversible inhibition of mitochondrial complex I by 1-methyl-4–phenylpyridinium: evidence for free radical involvement. J Neurochem 1992; 58:786–789.

Corral-Debrinski M, Horton T, Lott MT, Shoffner JM, Beal MF, Wallace DC: Mitochondrial DNA deletions in human brain: regional variability and increase with advanced age. Nat Genet 1992a; 2:324–329.

Corral-Debrinski M, Horton T, Lott MT, Shoffner JM, McKee AC, Beal MF, Graham BH, Wallace DC: Marked changes in mitochondrial DNA deletion levels in Alzheimer brains. Genomics 1994; 23:471–476.

Corral-Debrinski M, Shoffner JM, Lott MT, Wallace DC: Association of mitochondrial DNA damage with aging and coronary atherosclerotic heart disease. Mutat Res 1992b; 275:169–180.

Das DK, George A, Liu XK, Rao PS: Detection of hydroxyl radical in the mitochondria of ischemic-reperfused myocardium by trapping with salicylate. Biochem Biophys Res Commun 1989; 165:1004–1009.

Davis JN 2nd, Parker WD Jr.: Evidence that two reports of mtDNA cytochrome c oxidase "mutations" in Alzheimer's disease are based on nDNA pseudogenes of recent evolutionary origin. Biochem Biophys Res Commun 1998; 244:877–883.

Davis RE, Miller S, Herrnstadt C, Ghosh SS, Fahy E, Shinobu LA, Galasko D, Thal LJ, Beal MF, Howell N, et al.: Mutations in mitochondrial cytochrome c oxidase genes segregate with late-onset Alzheimer disease. Proc Natl Acad Sci USA 1997; 94:4526–4531.

DiDonato S, Zeviani M, Giovannini P, Savarese N, Rimoldi M, Mariotti C, Girotti F, Caraceni T: Respiratory chain and mitochondrial DNA in muscle and brain in Parkinson's disease patients. Neurology 1993; 43:2262–2268.

Dorner G, Mohnike A: Further evidence for a predominantly maternal transmission of maturity-onset type diabetes. Endokrinologie 1976; 68:121–124.

Dorner G, Mohnike A, Steindel E: On possible genetic and epigenetic modes of diabetes transmission. Endokrinologie 1975; 66:225–227.

Dorner G, Plagemann A, Reinagel H: Familial diabetes aggregation in type I diabetics: gestational diabetes an apparent risk factor for increased diabetes susceptibility in the offspring. Exp Clin Endocrinol 1987; 89:84–90.

Dunbar DR, Moonie PA, Swingler RJ, Davidson D, Roberts R, Holt IJ: Maternally transmitted partial direct tandem duplication of mitochondrial DNA associated with diabetes mellitus. Hum Mol Genet 1993; 2:1619–1624.

Earnshaw WC: Apoptosis. A cellular poison cupboard. Nature 1999; 397:387–389.

Esposito LA, Melov S, Panov A, Cottrell BA, Wallace DC: Mitochondrial disease in mouse results in increased oxidative stress. Proc Natl Acad Sci USA 1999; 96:4820–4825.

Fischel-Ghodsian N, Prezant TR, Bu X, Oztas S: Mitochondrial ribosomal RNA gene mutation in a patient with sporadic aminoglycoside ototoxicity. Am J Otolaryngol 1993; 14:399–403.

Freinkel N, Metzger BE, Phelps RL, Simpson JL, Martin AO, Radvany R, Ober C, Dooley SL, Depp RO, Belton A: Gestational diabetes mellitus: a syndrome with phenotypic and genotypic heterogeneity. Horm Metab Res 1986; 18:427–430.

Gerbitz KD, van den Ouweland JM, Maassen JA, Jaksch M: Mitochondrial diabetes mellitus: a review. Biochim Biophys Acta 1995; 1271:253–260.

German MS: Glucose sensing in pancreatic islet beta cells: the key role of glucokinase and the glycolytic intermediates. Proc Natl Acad Sci USA 1993; 90:1781–1785.

Gidh-Jain M, Takeda J, Xu LZ, Lange AJ, Vionnet N, Stoffel M, Froguel P, Velho G, Sun F, Cohen D, et al.: Glucokinase mutations associated with non-insulin-dependent (type 2) diabetes mellitus have decreased enzymatic activity: implications for structure/function relationships. Proc Natl Acad Sci USA 1993; 90:1932–1936.

Giles RE, Blanc H, Cann HM, Wallace DC: Maternal inheritance of human mitochondrial DNA. Proc Natl Acad Sci USA 1980; 77:6715–6719.

Goto Y: Clinical features of MELAS and mitochondrial DNA mutations. Muscle Nerve 1995; 3:S107–S112.

Goto Y, Nonaka I, Horai S: A mutation in the $tRNA^{Leu(UUR)}$ gene associated with the MELAS subgroup of mitochondrial encephalomyopathies [see comments]. Nature 1990; 348:651–653.

Graham B, Waymire K, Cottrell B, Trounce IA, MacGregor GR, Wallace DC: A mouse model for mitochondrial myopathy and cardiomyopathy resulting from a deficiency in the heart/skeletal muscle isoform of the adenine nucleotide translocator. Nature Genet 1997; 16:226–234.

Green DR, Reed JC: Mitochondria and apoptosis. Science 1998; 281:1309–1312.

Gu M, Gash MT, Mann VM, Javoy-Agid F, Cooper JM, Schapira AH: Mitochondrial defect in Huntington's disease caudate nucleus. Ann Neurol 1996; 39:385–389.

Hattori N, Tanaka M, Ozawa T, Mizuno Y: Immunohistochemical studies on complexes I, II, III, and IV of mitochondria in Parkinson's disease. Ann Neurol 1991; 30:563–571.

Heddi A, Lestienne P, Wallace DC, Stepien G: Mitochondrial DNA expression in mitochondrial myopathies and coordinated expression of nuclear genes involved in ATP production. J Biol Chem 1993; 268:12156–12163.

Heddi A, Lestienne P, Wallace DC, Stepien G: Steady state levels of mitochondrial and nuclear oxidative phosphorylation transcripts in Kearns-Sayre syndrome. Biochim Biophys Acta 1994; 1226:206–212.

Hirano M, Shtilbans A, Mayeux R, Davidson MM, DiMauro S, Knowles JA, Schon EA: Apparent mtDNA heteroplasmy in Alzheimer's disease patients and in normals due to PCR amplification of nucleus-embedded mtDNA pseudogenes. Proc Natl Acad Sci USA 1997; 94:14894–14899.

Holt IJ, Harding AE, Petty RK, Morgan-Hughes JA: A new mitochondrial disease associated with mitochondrial DNA heteroplasmy. Am J Hum Genet 1990; 46:428–433.

Howell N, Bindoff LA, McCullough DA, Kubacka I, Poulton J, Mackey D, Taylor L, Turnbull DM: Leber hereditary optic neuropathy: identification of the same mitochondrial ND1 mutation in six pedigrees. Am J Hum Genet 1991a; 49:939–950.

Howell N, Kubacka I, Xu M, McCullough DA: Leber hereditary optic neuropathy: involvement of the mitochondrial ND1 gene and evidence for an intragenic suppressor mutation. Am J Hum Genet 1991b; 48:935–942.

Huntington's Disease Collaborative Research Group: A novel gene containing a trinucleotide repeat that is expanded and unstable on Huntington's disease chromosomes. Cell 1993; 72:971–983.

Huoponen K, Lamminen T, Juvonen V, Aula P, Nikoskelainen E, Savontaus JL: The spectrum of mitochondrial DNA mutations in families with Leber hereditary optic neuroretinopathy. Hum Genet 1993; 92:379–384.

Huoponen K, Vilkki J, Aula P, Nikoskelainen EK, Savontaus ML: A new mtDNA mutation associated with Leber hereditary optic neuroretinopathy. Am J Hum Genet 1991; 48:1147–1153.

Hutchin T, Cortopassi G: A mitochondrial DNA clone is associated with increased risk for Alzheimer disease. Proc Natl Acad Sci USA 1995; 92:6892–6895.

Hutchin T, Haworth I, Higashi K, Fischel-Ghodsian N, Stoneking M, Saha N, Arnos C, Cortopassi G: A molecular basis for human hypersensitivity to aminoglycoside antibiotics. Nucleic Acids Res 1993; 21:4174–4179.

Hutchin T, Pericak-Vance M, Cortopassi G: Mitochondrial and ApoE genotyping and risk for Alzheimer's Disease. Abstract #1401. Am J Hum Genet 1995; 57 Suppl:A242.

Ikebe S, Tanaka M, Ohno K, Sato W, Hattori K, Kondo T, Mizuno Y, Ozawa T: Increase of deleted mitochondrial DNA in the striatum in Parkinson's disease and senescence. Biochem Biophys Res Commun 1990; 170:1044–1048.

Jagust WJ, Seab JP, Huesman RH, Valk PE, Mathis CA, Reed BR, Coxson PG, Budinger TF: Diminished glucose transport in Alzheimer's disease: dynamic PET studies. J Cereb Blood Flow Metab 1991; 11:323–330.

Janetzky B, Hauck S, Youdim MB, Riederer P, Jellinger K, Pantucek F, Zochling R, Boissl KW, Reichmann H: Unaltered aconitase activity, but decreased complex I activity in substantia nigra pars compacta of patients with Parkinson's disease. Neurosci Lett 1994; 169:126–128.

Jenkins BG, Koroshetz WJ, Beal MF, Rosen BR: Evidence for impairment of energy metabolism in vivo in Huntington's disease using localized ^{1}H NMR spectroscopy. Neurology 1993; 43:2689–2695.

Jenner P, Dexter DT, Sian J, Schapira AH, Marsden CD: Oxidative stress as a cause of nigral cell death in Parkinson's disease and incidental Lewy body disease. Ann Neurol 1992; 32(Suppl):S82–87.

Jin H, May M, Tranebjaerg L, Kendall E, Fontan G, Jackson J, Subramony SH, Arena F, Lubs H, Smith S, et al.: A novel X-linked gene, DDP, shows mutations in families with deafness (DFN-1), dystonia, mental deficiency and blindness. Nature Genet 1996; 14:177–180.

Johns DR, Neufeld MJ: Analysis of mitochondrial DNA ND-1 gene in Parkinson's disease. Mov Disord 1991; 6:271.

Johns DR, Neufeld MJ, Park RD: An ND-6 mitochondrial DNA mutation associated with Leber hereditary optic neuropathy. Biochem Biophys Res Commun 1992; 187:1551–1557.

Jun AS, Brown MD, Wallace DC: A mitochondrial DNA mutation at np 14459 of the ND6 gene associated with maternally inherited Leber's hereditary optic neuropathy and dystonia. Proc Natl Acad Sci USA 1994; 91:6206–6210.

Jun AS, Trounce IA, Brown MD, Shoffner JM, Wallace DC: Use of transmitochondrial hybrids to assign a complex I defect to the mitochondrial DNA-encoded NADH dehydrogenase subunit 6 gene mutation at nucleotide pair 14459 that causes Leber hereditary optic neuropathy and dystonia. Mol Cell Biol 1996; 16:771–777.

Kadowaki T, Kadowaki H, Mori Y, Tobe K, Sakuta R, Suzuki Y, Tanabe Y, Sakura H, Awata T, Goto Y, et al.: A subtype of diabetes mellitus associated with a mutation of mitochondrial DNA. N Engl J Med 1994; 330:962–968.

Kadowaki T, Sakura H, Otabe S, Yasuda K, Kadowaki H, Mori Y, Hagura R, Akanuma Y, Yazaki Y: A subtype of diabetes mellitus associated with a mutation in the mitochondrial gene. Muscle Nerve 1995; 3:S137–S141.

King MP, Attardi G: Human cells lacking mtDNA: repopulation with exogenous mitochondria by complementation. Science 1989; 246:500–503.

Koehler CM, Leuenberger D, Merchant S, Renold A, Junne T, Schatz G: Human deafness dystonia syndrome is a mitochondrial disease. Proc Natl Acad Sci USA 1999; 96:2141–2146.

Krige D, Carroll MT, Cooper JM, Marsden CD, Schapira AH: Platelet mitochondrial function in Parkinson's Disease. Ann Neurol 1992; 32:782–788.

Kuwert T, Lange HW, Boecker H, Titz H, Herzog H, Aulich A, Wang BC, Nayak U, Feinendegen LE: Striatal glucose consumption in chorea-free subjects at risk of Huntington's disease. J Neurol 1993; 241:31–36.

Lang BF, Burger G, O'Kelly CJ, Cedergren R, Golding GB, Lemieux C, Sankoff D, Turmel M, Gray MW: An ancestral mitochondrial DNA resembling a eubacterial genome in miniature. Nature 1997; 387:493–497.

Langston JW, Ballard P, Tetrud JW, Irwin I: Chronic parkinsonism in humans due to a product of meperidine-analog synthesis. Science 1983; 219:979–980.

Larsson NG, Andersen O, Holme E, Oldfors A, Wahlstrom J: Leber's hereditary optic neuropathy and complex I deficiency in muscle. Ann Neurol 1991; 30:701–708.

Larsson NG, Wang J, Wilhelmsson H, Oldfors A, Rustin P, Lewandoski M, Barsh GS, Clayton DA: Mitochondrial transcription factor A is necessary for mtDNA maintenance and embryogenesis in mice. Nat Genet 1998; 18:231–236.

Lebovitz RM, Zhang H, Vogel H, Cartwright J Jr, Dionne L, Lu N, Huang S, Matzuk MM: Neurodegeneration, myocardial injury, and perinatal death in mitochondrial superoxide dismutase-deficient mice. Proc Natl Acad Sci USA 1996; 93:9782–9787.

Li Y, Huang TT, Carlson EJ, Melov S, Ursell PC, Olson JL, Noble LJ, Yoshimura MP, Berger C, Chan PH, et al.: Dilated cardiomyopathy and neonatal lethality in mutant mice lacking manganese superoxide dismutase. Nat Genet 1995; 11:376–381.

Liu X, Kim CN, Yang J, Jemmerson R, Wang X: Induction of apoptotic program in cell-free extracts: requirement for dATP and cytochrome *c*. Cell 1996; 86:147–157.

Loeffen J, Smeitink J, Triepels R, Smeets R, Schuelke M, Sengers R, Trijbels F, Hamel B, Mullaart R, van den Heuvel L: The first nuclear-encoded complex I mutation in a patient with Leigh Syndrome. Am J Hum Genet 1998; 63:1598–1608.

Mackey D, Howell N: A variant of Leber hereditary optic neuropathy characterized by recovery of vision and by an unusual mitochondrial genetic etiology. Am J Hum Genet 1992; 51:1218–1228.

Majander A, Huoponen K, Savontaus ML, Nikoskelainen E, Wikstrom M: Electron transfer properties of NADH:ubiquinone reductase in the ND1/3460 and the ND4/11778 mutations of the Leber hereditary optic neuroretinopathy (LHON). FEBS Lett 1991; 292:289–292.

Malaisse-Lagae F, Malaisse WJ: Hexose metabolism in pancreatic islets: regulation of mitochondrial hexokinase binding. Biochem Med Metab Biol 1988; 39:80–89.

Mancini M, Nicholson DW, Roy S, Thornberry NA, Peterson EP, Casciola-Rosen LA, Rosen A: The caspase-3 precursor has a cytosolic and mitochondrial distribution: implications for apoptotic signaling. J Cell Biol 1998; 140:1485–1495.

Mann VM, Cooper JM, Krige D, Daniel SE, Schapira AH, Marsden CD: Brain, skeletal muscle and platelet homogenate mitochondrial function in Parkinson's disease. Brain 1992a; 115:333–342.

Mann VM, Cooper JM, Schapira AHV: Quantitation of a mitochondrial DNA deletion in Parkinson's disease. FEBS Lett 1992b; 299:218–222.

Martin WR, Clark C, Ammann W, Stoessl AJ, Shtybel W, Hayden MR: Cortical glucose metabolism in Huntington's disease. Neurology 1992; 42:223–229.

Marzo I, Brenner C, Zamzami N, Jurgensmeier JM, Susin SA, Vieira HL, Prevost MC, Xie Z, Matsuyama S, Reed JC, et al.: Bax and adenine nucleotide translocator cooperate in the mitochondrial control of apoptosis. Science 1998; 281:2027–2031.

Masucci JP, Davidson M, Koga Y, Schon EA, King MP: In vitro analysis of mutations causing myoclonus epilepsy with ragged-red fibers in the mitochondrial $tRNA^{Lys}$gene: two genotypes produce similar phenotypes. Mol Cell Biol 1995; 15:2872–2881.

Matthews PM, Marchington DR, Squier M, Land J, Brown RM, Brown GK: Molecular genetic characterization of an X-linked form of Leigh's syndrome. Ann Neurol 1993; 33:652–655.

Matthijs G, Claes S, Longo-Mbenza B, Cassiman JJ: Teenage onset non-syndromic deafness associated with a mutation and a polymorphism in the mitochondrial 12S ribosomal RNA gene in a large Zairese pedigree [abstract]. Am J Hum Genet 1994; 55 Suppl:A23.

Mattson MP: Free radicals and disruption of neuronal ion homeostasis in AD: a role for amyloid beta-peptide? Neurobiol Aging 1995; 16:679–682.

McCabe ER: Microcompartmentation of energy metabolism at the outer mitochondrial membrane: role in diabetes mellitus and other diseases. J Bioenerg Biomembr 1994; 26:317–325.

Mecocci P, MacGarvey U, Beal MF: Oxidative damage to mitochondrial DNA is increased in Alzheimer's disease. Ann Neurol 1994; 36:747–751.

Mecocci P, MacGarvey U, Kaufman AE, Koontz D, Shoffner JM, Wallace DC, Beal MF: Oxidative damage to mitochondrial DNA shows marked age-dependent increases in human brain. Ann Neurol 1993; 34:609–616.

Melov S, Coskun EP, Wallace DC: Mouse models of mitochondrial disease, oxidative stress, and senescence. Mutat Res 1999a; 434:233–242.

Melov S, Coskun P, Patel M, Tunistra R, Cottrell B, Jun AS, Zastawny TH, Dizdaroglu M, Goodman SI, Huang T, et al.: Mitochondrial disease in superoxide dismutase 2 mutant mice. Proc Natl Acad Sci USA 1999b; 96:846–851.

Melov S, Hinerfeld D, Esposito L, Wallace DC: Multi-organ characterization of mitochondrial genomic rearrangements in ad libitum and caloric restricted mice show striking somatic mitochondrial DNA rearrangements with age. Nucleic Acids Res 1997; 25:974–982.

Melov S, Schneider JA, Day BJ, Hinerfeld D, Coskun P, Mirra SS, Crapo JD, Wallace DC: A novel neurological phenotype in mice lacking mitochondrial manganese superoxide dismutase [see comments]. Nature Genet 1998; 18:159–163.

Melov S, Shoffner JM, Kaufman A, Wallace DC: Marked increase in the number and variety of mitochondrial DNA rearrangements in aging human skeletal muscle [published erratum appears in Nucleic Acids Res 1995 23:4938]. Nucleic Acids Res 1995; 23:4122–4126.

Mita S, Schmidt B, Schon EA, DiMauro S, Bonilla E: Detection of 'deleted' mitochondrial genomes in cytochrome-c oxidase-deficient muscle fibers of a patient with Kearns-Sayre syndrome. Proc Natl Acad Sci USA 1989; 86:9509–9513.

Mizuno Y, Ikebe S, Hattori N, Nakagawa-Hattori Y, Mochizuki H, Tanaka M, Ozawa T: Role of mitochondria in the etiology and pathogenesis of Parkinson's disease. Biochim Biophys Acta 1995; 1271:265–274.

Mizuno Y, Ohta S, Tanaka M, Takamiya S, Suzuki K, Sato T, Oya H, Ozawa T, Kagawa Y: Deficiencies in complex I subunits of the respiratory chain in Parkinson's disease. Biochem Biophys Res Commun 1989; 163:1450–1455.

Moraes CT, Shanske S, Tritschler HJ, Aprille JR, Andreetta F, Bonilla E, Schon EA, DiMauro S: MtDNA depletion with variable tissue expression: a novel genetic abnormality in mitochondrial diseases. Am J Hum Genet 1991; 48:492–501.

Muller-Hocker J, Schneiderbanger K, Stefani FH, Kadenbach B: Progressive loss of cytochrome c oxidase in the human extraocular muscles in ageing — a cytochemical-immunohistochemical study. Mutat Res 1992; 275:115–124.

Murdock D, Boone BE, Esposito L, Wallace DC: Up-regulation of nuclear and mitochondrial genes in the skeletal muscle of mice lacking the heart/muscle isoform of the adenine nucleotide translocator. J Biol Chem 1999; 274:14429–14433.

Nelson I, Hanna MG, Alsanjari N, Scaravilli F, Morgan-Hughes JA, Harding AE: A new mitochondrial DNA mutation associated with progressive dementia and chorea: a clinical, pathological, and molecular genetic study. Ann Neurol 1995; 37:400–403.

Newman NJ: Leber's hereditary optic neuropathy. New genetic considerations. Arch Neurol 1993; 50:540–548.

Newman NJ, Lott MT, Wallace DC: The clinical characteristics of pedigrees of Leber's hereditary optic neuropathy with the 11778 mutation. Am J Ophthalmol 1991; 111:750–762.

Nigro MA, Martens ME, Awerbuch GI, Peterson PL, Lee CP: Partial cytochrome b deficiency and generalized dystonia. Pediatr Neurol 1990; 6:407–410.

Nishino I, Spinazzola A, Hirano M: Thymidine phosphorylase gene mutations in MNGIE, a human mitochondrial disorder. Science 1999; 283:689–692.

Novotny EJ, Singh G, Wallace DC, Dorfman LJ, Louis A, Sogg RL, Steinman L: Leber's disease and dystonia: a mitochondrial disease. Neurology 1986; 36:1053–1060.

Ohkoshi N, Mizusawa H, Shiraiwa N, Shoji S, Harada K, Yoshizawa K: Superoxide dismutases of muscle in mitochondrial encephalomyopathies. Muscle Nerve 1995; 18:1265–1271.

Oka Y, Katagiri H, Ishihara H, Asano T, Kikuchi M, Kobayashi T: Mitochondrial diabetes mellitus—glucose-induced signaling defects and beta-cell loss. Muscle Nerve 1995; 3:S131–136.

Oka Y, Katagiri H, Yazaki Y, Murase T, Kobayashi T: Mitochondrial gene mutation in islet-cell-antibody-positive patients who were initially non-insulin-dependent diabetics. Lancet 1993; 342:527–528.

Ortiz RG, Newman NJ, Shoffner JM, Kaufman AE, Koontz DA, Wallace DC: Variable retinal and neurologic manifestations in patients harboring the mitochondrial DNA 8993 mutation. Arch Ophthalmol 1993; 111:1525–1530.

Ozawa T, Tanaka M, Ikebe S, Ohno K, Kondo T, Mizuno Y: Quantitative determination of deleted mitochondrial DNA relative to normal DNA in parkinsonian striatum by a kinetic PCR analysis. Biochem Biophys Res Commun 1990; 172:483–489.

Ozelius LJ, Hewett JW, Page CE, Bressman SB, Kramer PL, Shalish C, de Leon D, Brin MF, Raymond D, Corey DP, et al.: The early-onset torsion dystonia gene (DYT1) encodes an ATP-binding protein. Nat Genet 1997; 17:40–48.

Ozelius LJ, Hewett JW, Page CE, Bressman SB, Kramer PL, Shalish C, de Leon D, Brin MF, Raymond D, Jacoby D, et al.: The gene *(DYT1)* for early-onset torsion dystonia encodes a novel protein related to the Clp protease/heat shock family. Adv Neurology 1998; 78:93–105.

Parker WD, Jr., Boyson SJ, Luder AS, Parks JK: Evidence for a defect in NADH: ubiquinone oxidoreductase (complex I) in Huntington's disease. Neurology 1990a; 40:1231–1234.

Parker WD, Jr., Boyson SJ, Parks JK: Abnormalities of the electron transport chain in idiopathic Parkinson's disease. Ann Neurol 1989; 26:719–723.

Parker WD, Jr., Filley CM, Parks JK: Cytochrome oxidase deficiency in Alzheimer's disease. Neurology 1990b; 40:1302–1303.

Petit PX, Susin SA, Zamzami N, Mignotte B, Kroemer G: Mitochondria and programmed cell death: back to the future. FEBS Lett 1996; 396:7–13.

Pimentel E: Some aspects of the genetics and etiology of spontaneous diabetes mellitus. Acta Diabetol Lat 1979; 16:193–201.

Pitkanen S, Robinson BH: Mitochondrial complex I deficiency leads to increased production of superoxide radicals and induction of superoxide dismutase. J Clin Invest 1996; 98:345–351.

Poulton J, Deadman ME, Bindoff L, Morten K, Land J, Brown G: Families of mtDNA re-arrangements can be detected in patients with mtDNA deletions: duplications may be a transient intermediate form. Hum Mol Genet 1993; 2:23–30.

Poulton J, Deadman ME, Gardiner RM: Duplications of mitochondrial DNA in mitochondrial myopathy. Lancet 1989a; 1:236–240.

Poulton J, Deadman ME, Gardiner RM: Tandem direct duplications of mitochondrial DNA in mitochondrial myopathy: analysis of nucleotide sequence and tissue distribution. Nucleic Acids Res 1989b; 17:10223–10229.

Poulton J, Morten KJ, Weber K, Brown GK, Bindoff L: Are duplications of mitochondrial DNA characteristic of Kearns-Sayre syndrome? Hum Mol Genet 1994; 3:947–951.

Poulton J, O'Rahilly S, Morten KJ, Clark A: Mitochondrial DNA, diabetes and pancreatic pathology in Kearns-Sayre syndrome. Diabetologia 1995; 38:868–871.

Prezant TR, Agapian JV, Bohlman MC, Bu X, Oztas S, Qiu WQ, Arnos KS, Cortopassi GA, Jaber L, Rotter JI, et al.: Mitochondrial ribosomal RNA mutation associated with both antibiotic-induced and non-syndromic deafness. Nat Genet 1993; 4:289–294.

Rotig A, Colonna M, Bonnefont JP, Blanche S, Fischer A, Saudubray JM, Munnich A: Mitochondrial DNA deletion in Pearson's marrow-pancreas syndrome. Lancet 1989; 1:902–903.

Rotig A, de Lonlay P, Chretien D, Foury F, Koenig M, Sidi D, Munnich A, Rustin P: Aconitase and mitochondrial iron-sulphur protein deficiency in Friedreich ataxia. Nat Genet 1997; 17:215–217.

Sandy MS, Langston JW, Smith MT, DiMonte DA: PCR analysis of platelet mtDNA: lack of specific changes in Parkinson's disease. Mov Disord 1993; 8:74–82.

Saraiva AA, Borges MM, Madeira MD, Tavares MA, Paula-Barbosa MM: Mitochondrial abnormalities in cortical dendrites from patients with Alzheimer's disease. J Submicrosc Cytol 1985; 17:459–464.

Schapira AH: Nuclear and mitochondrial genetics in Parkinson's disease. J Med Genet 1995a; 32:411–414.

Schapira AH, Cooper JM, Dexter D, Clark JB, Jenner P, Marsden CD: Mitochondrial complex I deficiency in Parkinson's disease. J Neurochem 1990a; 54:823–827.

Schapira AH, Cooper JM, Dexter D, Jenner P, Clark JB, Marsden CD: Mitochondrial complex I deficiency in Parkinson's disease. Lancet 1989; 1:1269.

Schapira AH, Holt IJ, Sweeney M, Harding AE, Jenner P, Marsden CD: Mitochondrial DNA analysis in Parkinson's disease. Mov Disord 1990b; 5:294–297.

Schapira AHV: Mitochondrial abnormalities in neurodegeneration and normal aging. In: DiMauro S, Wallace DC (eds): *Mitochondrial DNA in Human Pathology*. New York: Raven Press, 1992:159–172.

Schapira AHV: Evidence for mitochondria dysfunction in Parkinson's disease—a critical appraisal. Mov Disord 1994a; 9:125–138.

Schapira AHV: Mitochondrial dysfunction in neurodegenerative disorders and aging. In: Schapira AHV, DiMauro S (eds): *Mitochondrial disorders in neurology*. Oxford: Butterworth-Heinemann Ltd, 1994b:227–244.

Schapira AHV: The role of mitochondrial dysfunction in neurodegenerative disease. In: Esser K, Martin GM (eds): *Molecular Aspects of Aging*. Chichester: John Wiley & Sons Ltd., 1995b:241–251.

Selkoe DJ: Alzheimer's disease. Missense on the membrane. Nature 1995; 375:734–735.

Shan DE, Yeh SI, Wan YC, Wei YH: Absence of 4,977–bp deletion of blood cell mitochondrial DNA in patients with young-onset Parkinson's disease. Acta Neurol Scand 1995; 91:149–152.

Sheu KF, Kim YT, Blass JP, Weksler ME: An immunochemical study of the pyruvate dehydrogenase deficit in Alzheimer's disease brain. Ann Neurol 1985; 17:444–449.

Shoffner JM, Brown M, Huoponen K, Stugard C, Koontz D, Kaufman A, Graham J, Dixon J, Wallace DC: A mitochondrial DNA (mtDNA)mutation associated with maternally inherited Parkinson's disease (PD) and deafness. Am J Hum Genet 1994; 55 Suppl:A242 (abstract 1417).

Shoffner JM, Brown MD, Stugard C, Jun AS, Pollok S, Haas RH, Kaufman A, Koontz D, Kim Y, Graham J, et al.: Leber's hereditary optic neuropathy plus dystonia is caused by a mitochondrial DNA point mutation in a complex I subunit. Ann Neurol 1995; 38:163–169.

Shoffner JM, Brown MD, Torroni A, Lott MT, Cabell MR, Mirra SS, Beal MF, Yang C, Gearing M, Salvo R, et al.: Mitochondrial DNA variants observed in Alzheimer disease and Parkinson disease patients. Genomics 1993; 17:171–184.

Shoffner JM, Fernhoff MD, Krawiecki NS, Caplan DB, Holt PJ, Koontz DA, Takei Y, Newman NJ, Ortiz RG, Polak M, et al.: Subacute necrotizing encephalopathy: oxidative phosphorylation defects and the ATPase 6 point mutation. Neurology 1992; 42:2168–2174.

Shoffner JM, Lott MT, Lezza AM, Seibel P, Ballinger SW, Wallace DC: Myoclonic epilepsy and ragged-red fiber disease (MERRF) is associated with a mitochondrial DNA $tRNA^{Lys}$ mutation. Cell 1990; 61:931–937.

Shoffner JM, Wallace DC: Oxidative phosphorylation diseases. In: Scriver CR, Beaudet AL, Sly WS, Valle D (eds): *The Metabolic and Molecular Basis of Inherited Disease*. New York: McGraw-Hill, 1995:1535–1609.

Shoubridge EA, Karpati G, Hastings KEM: Deletion mutants are functionally dominant over wild-type mitochondrial genomes in skeletal muscle fiber segments in mitochondrial disease. Cell 1990; 62:43–49.

Sims NR, Finegan JM, Blass JP, Bowen DM, Neary D: Mitochondrial function in brain tissue in primary degenerative dementia. Brain Res 1987; 436:30–38.

Singer TP, Castagnoli N Jr, Ramsay RR, Trevor AJ: Biochemical events in the development of parkinsonism induced by 1-methyl-4-phenyl-1,2,3,6-tetrahydropyridine. J Neurochem 1987; 49:1–8.

Soong NW, Hinton DR, Cortopassi G, Arnheim N: Mosaicism for a specific somatic mitochondrial DNA mutation in adult human brain. Nat Genet 1992; 2:318–323.

Sorbi S, Bird ED, Blass JP: Decreased pyruvate dehydrogenase complex activity in Huntington and Alzheimer brain. Ann Neurol 1983; 13:72–78.

Stoffel M, Bell KL, Blackburn CL, Powell KL, Seo TS, Takeda J, Vionnet N, Xiang KS, Gidh-Jain M, Pilkis SJ, et al.: Identification of glucokinase mutations in subjects with gestational diabetes mellitus. Diabetes 1993; 42:937–940.

Stoffel M, Froguel P, Takeda J, Zouali H, Vionnet N, Nishi S, Weber IT, Harrison RW, Pilkis SJ, Lesage S, et al.: Human glucokinase gene: isolation, characterization, and identification of two missense mutations linked to early-onset non-insulin-dependent (type 2) diabetes mellitus [published erratum appears in Proc Natl Acad Sci USA 1992; 89:10562]. Proc Natl Acad Sci USA 1992a; 89:7698–7702.

Stoffel M, Patel P, Lo YM, Hattersley AT, Lucassen AM, Page R, Bell JI, Bell GI, Turner RC, Wainscoat JS: Missense glucokinase mutation in maturity-onset diabetes of the young and mutation screening in late-onset diabetes. Nature Genet 1992b; 2:153–156.

Suomalainen A, Kaukonen J, Amati P, Timonen R, Haltia M, Weissenbach J, Zeviani M, Somer H, Peltonen L: An autosomal locus predisposing to deletions of mitochondrial DNA. Nat Genet 1995; 9:146–151.

Susin SA, Lorenzo HK, Zamzami N, Marzo I, Brenner C, Larochette N, Prevost MC, Alzari PM, Kroemer G: Mitochondrial release of caspase-2 and -9 during the apoptotic process. J Exp Med 1999a; 189:381–394.

Susin SA, Lorenzo HK, Zamzami N, Marzo I, Snow BE, Brothers GM, Mangion J, Jacotot E, Costantini P, Loeffler M, et al.: Molecular characterization of mitochondrial apoptosis-inducing factor. Nature 1999b; 397:441–446.

Suzuki S, Hinokio Y, Hirai S, Onoda M, Matsumoto M, Ohtomo M, Kawasaki H, Satoh Y, Akai H, Abe K, et al.: Pancreatic beta-cell secretory defect associated with mitochondrial point mutation of the $tRNA^{Leu(UUR)}$ gene: a study in seven families with mitochondrial encephalomyopathy, lactic acidosis and stroke-like episodes (MELAS). Diabetologia 1994a; 37:818–825.

Suzuki S, Hinokio Y, Hirai S, Onoda M, Matsumoto M, Ohtomo M, Kawasaki H, Satoh Y, Akai H, Abe K, et al.: Diabetes with mitochondrial gene $tRNA^{Lys}$ mutation. Diabetes Care 1994b; 17:1428–1432.

Tatuch Y, Christodoulou J, Feigenbaum A, Clarke JTR, Wherret J, Smith C, Rudd N, Petrova-Benedict R, Robinson BH: Heteroplasmic mtDNA mutation (T-G) at 8993 can cause Leigh disease when the percentage of abnormal mtDNA is high. Am J Hum Genet 1992; 50:852–858.

Tiranti V, Hoertnagel K, Carrozzo R, Galimberti C, Munaro M, Granatiero M, Zelante L, Gasparini P, Marzella R, Rocchi M, et al.: Mutations of SURF-1 in Leigh Disease associated with cytochrome c oxidase deficiency. Am J Hum Genet 1998; 63:1609–1621.

Travis J: Do brain cells run out of gas? Science News 1995; 148:84.

Trounce I, Byrne E, Marzuki S: Decline in skeletal muscle mitochondrial respiratory chain function: possible factor in ageing. Lancet 1989; 1:637–639.

Trounce I, Neill S, Wallace DC: Cytoplasmic transfer of the mtDNA nt 8993 TG (ATP6) point mutation associated with Leigh syndrome into mtDNA-less cells demonstrates cosegregation with a decrease in state III respiration and ADP/O ratio. Proc Natl Acad Sci USA 1994; 91:8334–8338.

Trounce IA, Kim YL, Jun AS, Wallace DC: Assessment of mitochondrial oxidative phosphorylation in patient muscle biopsies, lymphoblasts, and transmitochondrial cell lines. Methods Enzymol 1996; 264:484–509.

van den Heuvel L, Ruitenbeek W, Smeets R, Gelman-Kohan Z, Elpeleg O, Loeffen J, Trijbels F, Mariman E, de Bruijn D, Smeitink J: Demonstration of a new pathogenic mutation in human complex I deficiency: a 5-bp duplication in the nuclear gene encoding the 18-kD (AQDQ) subunit. Am J Hum Genet 1998; 62:262–268.

van den Ouweland JM, Lemkes HH, Trembath RC, Ross R, Velho G, Cohen D, Froguel P, Maassen JA: Maternally inherited diabetes and deafness is a distinct subtype of diabetes and associates with a single point mutation in the mitochondrial $tRNA^{Leu(UUR)}$ gene. Diabetes 1994; 43:746–751.

van den Ouweland JM, Lemkes HHP, Ruitenbeek W, Sandkjujl LA, deVijlder MF, Struyvenberg PAA, van de Kamp JJP, Maassen JA: Mutation in mitochondrial $tRNA^{Leu(UUR)}$ gene in a large pedigree with maternally transmitted type II diabetes mellitus and deafness. Nature Genet 1992; 1:368–371.

Vergani L, Martinuzzi A, Carelli V, Cortelli P, Montagna P, Schievano G, Carrozzo R, Angelini C, Lugaresi E: MtDNA mutations associated with Leber's hereditary optic neuropathy: studies on cytoplasmic hybrid (cybrid) cells. Biochem Biophys Res Commun 1995; 210:880–888.

Wallace DC: Cytoplasmic inheritance of chloramphenicol resistance in mammalian cells. In: Shay JW (ed) Techniques in Somatic Cell Genetics. New York: Plenum Press, 1982a: Volume 12:159–187.

Wallace DC: Structure and evolution of organelle genomes. Microbiol Rev 1982b; 46:208–240.

Wallace DC: Diseases of the mitochondrial DNA. Annu Rev Biochem 1992a; 61:1175–1212.

Wallace DC: Mitochondrial genetics: a paradigm for aging and degenerative diseases? Science 1992b; 256:628–632.

Wallace DC: Mitochondrial DNA mutations in diseases of energy metabolism. J Bioenerg Biomembr 1994; 26:241–250.

Wallace DC: Mitochondrial DNA mutations and bioenergetic defects in aging and degenerative diseases. In: Rosenberg RN, Prusiner SB, DiMauro S, Barchi RL (eds): The Molecular and Genetic Basis of Neurological Disease. Boston: Butterworth-Heinemann, 1997:237–269.

Wallace DC, Brown MD, Lott MT: Mitochondrial Genetics. In: Rimoin DL, Connor JM, Pyeritz RE, Emery AEH (eds): Emery and Rimoin's Principles and Practice of Medical Genetics. London: Churchill Livingstone, 1996: Volume 1:277–332.

Wallace DC, Bunn CL, Eisenstadt JM: Cytoplasmic transfer of chloramphenicol resistance in human tissue culture cells. J Cell Biol 1975; 67:174–188.

Wallace DC, Lott MT, Kogelnik AM, Brown MD, Navathe SB: MITOMAP: A Human Mitochondrial Genome Database, Center for Molecular Medicine, Emory University (Atlanta, GA). 1999.

Wallace DC, Murdock DG: Mitochondria and dystonia: the movement disorder connection? Proc Natl Acad Sci USA 1999; 96:1817–1819.

Wallace DC, Richter C, Bohr VA, Cortopassi G, Kadenbach B, Linn S, Linnane AW, Shay JW: Group Report: The Role of Bioenergetics and Mitochondrial DNA Mutations in Aging and Age-Related Diseases. In: Esser K, Martin GM (eds): Molecular Aspects of Aging. New York: John Wiley & Sons Ltd., 1995:199–225.

Wallace DC, Shoffner JM, Watts RL, Juncos JL, Torroni A: Mitochondrial oxidative phosphorylation defects in Parkinson's disease. Ann Neurol 1992; 32:113–114.

Wallace DC, Singh G, Lott MT, Hodge JA, Schurr TG, Lezza AM, Elsas LJ, Nikoskelainen EK: Mitochondrial DNA mutation associated with Leber's hereditary optic neuropathy. Science 1988a; 242:1427–1430.

Wallace DC, Stugard C, Murdock D, Schurr T, Brown MD: Ancient mtDNA sequences in the human nuclear genome: a potential source of errors in identifying pathogenic mutations. Proc Natl Acad Sci USA 1997; 94:14900–14905.

Wallace DC, Zheng X, Lott MT, Shoffner JM, Hodge JA, Kelley RI, Epstein CM, Hopkins LC: Familial mitochondrial encephalomyopathy (MERRF): Genetic, pathophysiological, and biochemical characterization of a mitochondrial DNA disease. Cell 1988b; 55:601–610.

Wang J, Wilhelmsson H, Graff C, Li H, Oldfors A, Rustin P, Bruning JC, Kahn CR, Clayton DA, Barsh GS, et al.: Dilated cardiomyopathy and atrioventricular conduction blocks induced by heart-specific inactivation of mitochondrial DNA gene expression. Nat Genet 1999; 21:133–137.

Williams MD, Van Remmen H, Conrad CC, Huang TT, Epstein CJ, Richardson A: Increased oxidative damage is correlated to altered mitochondrial function in heterozygous manganese superoxide dismutase knockout mice. J Biol Chem 1998; 273:28510–28515.

Yoshino H, Nakagawa-Hattori Y, Kondo T, Mizuno Y: Mitochondrial complex I and II activities of lymphocytes and platelets in Parkinson's disease. Journal of Neural Transmission - Parkinsons Disease & Dementia Section 1992; 2:27–34.

Zeviani M, Amati P, Comi G, Fratta G, Mariotti C, Tiranti V: Searching for genes affecting the structural integrity of the mitochondrial genome. Biochim Biophys Acta 1995; 1271:153–158.

Zheng XX, Shoffner JM, Voljavec AS, Wallace DC: Evaluation of procedures for assaying oxidative phosphorylation enzyme activities in mitochondrial myopathy muscle biopsies. Biochim Biophys Acta 1990; 1019:1–10.

Zhu Z, Yao J, Johns T, Fu K, De Bie I, Macmillan C, Cuthbert AP, Newbold RF, Wang J, Chevrette M, et al.: SURF1, encoding a factor involved in the biogenesis of cytochrome c oxidase, is mutated in Leigh syndrome. Nat Genet 1998; 20:337–343.

Zoratti M, Szabo I: The mitochondrial permeability transition. Biochim Biophys Acta 1995; 1241:139–176.

53 Constitutional Chromosome Disorders in Adults

GEORGIA L. WIESNER, DAVID B. EVERMAN, AND SUZANNE B. CASSIDY

Adulthood is not too late to think of the possibility of a constitutional chromosomal disturbance as the etiology of disease. Chromosomal imbalance is a well-recognized cause of human abnormality. Indeed, the incidence is at least 2 in 1000 for a medically significant chromosomal abnormality (Baird et al., 1988; Tawn and Earl, 1992). In many cases, this results in a recognizable pattern of developmental, structural, and functional defects that can be identified in childhood and is familiar to those physicians who provide care to children—although not often to those who care for adults. However, the most frequent of these chromosome disorders are compatible with survival well into adulthood. In addition, recent improvement in the techniques of chromosome analysis have resulted in identification of a number of chromosomal abnormalities with more subtle phenotypic consequences than was previously appreciated. In the past, the majority of chromosome studies were obtained on children with multiple congenital anomalies and developmental defects. Today, individuals without multiple physical alterations are being recognized as having chromosome disorders. This chapter is designed to describe the medical, developmental, and, in some cases, behavioral phenotype of adults with the most common disorders due to chromosomal imbalance: Down syndrome, Klinefelter syndrome, and Turner syndrome. We also review three disorders common in adults that are due to chromosomal microdeletions: velo-cardio-facial syndrome, Prader-Willi syndrome, and Williams syndrome. The intent of these descriptions is to allow recognition of these disorders and recommend appropriate guidelines for testing, health care, genetic counseling, and referral to needed community resources for patients who have them.

CHROMOSOMAL CONSTITUTION AND TYPES OF ABERRATIONS

The number of chromosomes in normal individuals is 46, or 23 pairs, one member of each pair normally being inherited from each parent. Of these, 22 pairs are autosomes and one pair consists of the sex chromosomes: two X's in females, and an X and a Y in males. Each chromosome can be distinguished on the basis of size, location of the centromere (the major constriction that divides the chromosome into a short [p] and long [q] arm), and a unique pattern of light and dark bands when stained with trypsin Giemsa. There are approximately 30,000 to 40,000 genes in the human genome, coded for by about 3×10^9 bases (3000 megabases [Mb]) of DNA. The genetic constitution of each individual is exquisitely balanced, and alterations in the amount of genetic material almost always have undesirable consequences (Therman and Susman, 1993).

Abnormalities associated with chromosomal imbalance are generally the result of abnormal gene dosage. Down syndrome (trisomy 21) and Klinefelter syndrome (47,XXY) are examples of disorders that are usually due to the presence of an entire extra chromosome. Turner syndrome is an example of a disorder most often due to loss of an entire chromosome (45,X, or monosomy X). However, altered dosage of much smaller segments of chromosomes, causing deletion (partial monosomy) or duplication (partial trisomy), can cause equally significant abnormality. Conditions with altered numbers of chromosomes arise from aberrant division of the chromosomes, a phenomenon known as nondisjunction. Older maternal age can predispose to nondisjunction of some chromosomes, particularly chromosome 21, and this is the only factor known to predispose to any type of chromosomal anomaly.

Chromosomal abnormalities can result from de novo events due to pre- or postconception errors in cell division. In that case, the likelihood of a recurrence in the family is very low. They can also be inherited from a parent who either has the same abnormality or has a structural rearrangement that involves all or part of one or more chromosomes (translocation). Translocations result from the exchange of material between two different chromosomes. If all the genetic information is present ("balanced translocation"), it is usually without phenotypic consequences in the individual but can predispose to "unbalanced" offspring. A specific type of translocation, called a Robertsonian translocation, occurs when two chromosomes in which the centromere is near the tip of the chromosome (called acrocentric chromosomes) attach to one another. Robertsonian translocation can cause Down syndrome, but does so in fewer than 5% of cases. When a parent carries a translocation, the likelihood of having an abnormal offspring is significant, in the range of 5% to 20%, depending on the sex of the parent and the type of translocation.

Post-conception errors leading to chromosome abnormalities are often present in a mosaic state in which there is an abnormal cell line and a normal (or different abnormal) cell line. This can be seen rarely in most chromosome disorders, but is relatively common in Turner syndrome (mixture of 46,XX and 45,X cells, or mixture of 47,XXX and 45,X cells) and Down syndrome (usually 46,XX and 47,XX, +21 or 46,XY and 47,XY, +21). Generally, post-conception nondisjunction carries a relatively low recurrence risk for the parents but a potentially high recurrence risk (up to 50%) for the offspring of the affected individual.

Techniques of Chromosome Analysis

Chromosomes are usually studied by putting lymphocytes, or sometimes fibroblasts or other tissues, in culture until adequate proliferation occurs, and then preparing individual metaphase cells for examination under the microscope. Development of chromosomal banding techniques in the early 1970s allowed unambiguous identification of each individual chromosome, based on patterns of banding, and allowed improved specification of the chromosomal basis of previously recognized disorders. Deletions and duplications of segments of a chromosome have been identified in increasing numbers as a result of technical advances over the past two decades. In 1976, Yunis introduced high-resolution chromosome-banding techniques, sometimes called prometaphase analysis. This is accomplished by synchronizing lymphocyte cultures to obtain a high population of cells in prophase or prometaphase rather than in metaphase, as is the case for routine chromosome analysis. High-resolution banding allows study of the chromosomes because each chromosome is much longer and has many more visible bands than when stained in the usual ways. Metaphase (standard) analysis generally involves examination of the chromosomes when a total of approximately 400 to 450 bands are visible. However, many of these bands represent two or more bands that visually appear as one. High-resolution analysis permits examination of over 500 bands and sometimes as many as 800 or more bands. This technique was introduced into clinical labs in the early 1980s and allowed testing for very small missing or extra segments of chromosomal material—so small that they were not visible or were inconsistently visible by previous techniques. It also permitted vastly improved ability to identify the origin and specific chromosomal location of deletions and duplications. Although it is labor-intensive and is not commonly used routinely, this method is extremely useful when more detailed study of a chromosome is needed to determine what material is missing or in excess.

In the early 1990s, development of a new and very powerful technique permitted recognition of chromosomal imbalances so small that they cannot normally be seen under the microscope even by using high-resolution banding techniques. Based on a combination of molecular genetics and cytogenetics, this method is called fluorescence in situ hybridization, or FISH. This technique involves attaching a fluorescent tag to a specific DNA probe complementary to a chromosomal segment of interest. When the probe hybridizes to DNA in the intact chromosome, fluorescence microscopy allows visualization of a fluorescent spot on the chromosome at the site of hybridization, indicating that the DNA segment of interest is present. Absence of a fluorescent spot indicates that the segment is missing. This technique is demonstrated in Figure 53–1. Thus, while routine chromosome analysis allows detection of deletions and duplications in the range of 5 to 10 million base pairs (megabases, Mb), and high-resolution chromosome analysis increases the sensitivity to detection of deletions or duplications in the 2 to 3 Mb range, FISH allows detection well below this level. Indeed, even abnormalities at the 30 to 100 kilobase (kb) level can be detected with sensitive probes. Thus, FISH improves sensitivity by almost two orders of magnitude over high-resolution chromosome analysis.

FISH permits detection of the abnormalities causing several disorders due to so-called microdeletions (Shapira, 1998). Three such disorders will be discussed later in this chapter. It also allows for determination of whether the correct number of chromosomes of a particular pair (for example, chromosome 21) are present in the intact cell at interphase. Using FISH probes specific to the X and the Y chromosomes, it is also possible to rapidly determine the sex chromosome complement of an intact cell. Both of these tests are used for prenatal diagnosis and are also occasionally used to make a diagnosis in an adult. Interphase analysis shortens the time needed for the analysis since the cells are studied without the necessity for prolonged culture or manipulation.

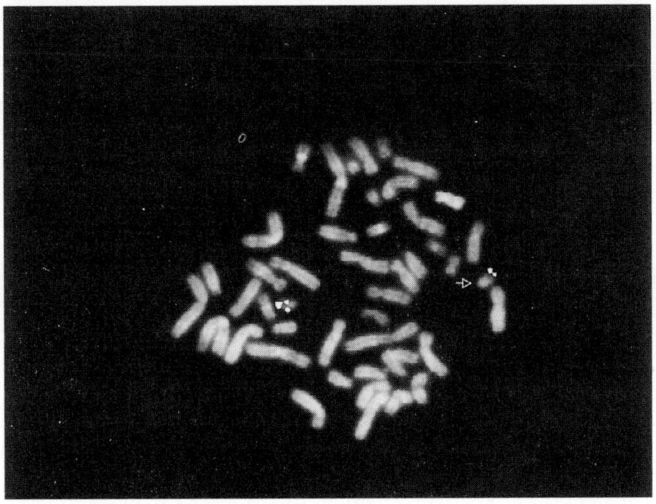

Fig. 53–1. Fluorescence in-situ hybridization (FISH). (Photo courtesy of Stuart Schwartz, PhD, University Hospitals of Cleveland and Case Western Reserve University.)

Testing for chromosomal abnormalities is now widely available in academic and commercial laboratories. Because of the necessity to culture the cells and arrest them in a phase of the cell cycle that allows optimal visualization, chromosome analysis routinely takes 10 days to 3 weeks for completion. Analysis of chromosomes from chorionic villi or amniotic fluid samples usually can be available within 10 to 14 days, and when analysis is critical for urgent diagnosis (as may be the case for a malformed infant requiring diagnosis before making critical management decisions), a preliminary reading often can be obtained in 48 to 72 hours. High-resolution analysis usually takes longer, and many labs will not perform this study unless it is specifically requested and suspected disorders or areas of the chromosome are identified by the clinician based on the patient's phenotype.

Role of the Cytogeneticist

As is true for many laboratory professionals, the cytogeneticist can be of most assistance to the clinician if clinical information is provided. Optimally, clinical cytogeneticists are certified by the American Board of Medical Genetics not only to provide technical expertise and laboratory direction but also to recognize the clinical consequences and recurrence implications of their findings. They can be excellent consultants to health-care providers requesting assistance in knowing which test to order, given the patient's clinical situation, and in how to interpret the results. They can also provide guidance concerning the genetic counseling implications of the abnormality and resources of information about detected abnormalities.

DOWN SYNDROME

Down syndrome, also known as trisomy 21, is the most widely recognized human chromosomal disorder and the most common known genetic cause of mental retardation (Gardner and Sutherland, 1989; Epstein, 2001). With an estimated incidence of 1 in

Table 53–1. Physical Findings in Down Syndrome

Area of Involvement	Manifestation
Craniofacial	Brachycephaly, flat nasal bridge
Eyes, ears, and mouth	Upslanted palpebral fissures, epicanthal folds, Brushfield spots of iris, dysplastic ears, open mouth, fissured lips, protruding/large/furrowed tongue, narrow palate
Neck, trunk, and spine	Short broad neck, flat nipples, pectus deformity, kyphosis, diastasis recti
Genitalia	Small penis and scrotum, cryptorchidism
Extremities	Broad hands, brachydactyly, single palmar crease, clinodactyly, short fifth finger with single flexion crease, wide gap between first and second toes, plantar furrow, joint hypermobility
Body habitus	Short stature, truncal obesity, sloping shoulders
Other	Hoarse voice, hypotonic gait

Source: Adapted from Gorlin et al. (1990) with permission.

650 livebirths (Gorlin et al., 1990), Down syndrome is a condition that is frequently encountered by physicians in all fields of medical practice. Although this disorder was first described by Down in 1866, almost a century elapsed before its chromosomal basis was discovered (Lejeune et al., 1959). The presence of a large amount of extra chromosome 21 material makes Down syndrome an extraordinarily complex condition featuring a wide range of physical, cognitive, and psychosocial problems. Although congenital heart disease and other medical complications once significantly limited the lifespan of individuals with Down syndrome, the majority of affected persons now live well into adulthood, with 73% surviving to age 25 and 60% reaching age 50 (Baird and Sadovnick, 1988a, 1988b, 1989). Thus, it is essential that the physicians who care for adults with Down syndrome are familiar with the many facets of this common and complex condition. For detailed discussions of the topics presented in this chapter, the reader is referred to several overviews of Down syndrome (Gorlin et al., 1990; Pueschel, 1990; Epstein, 2001), as well as a number of references regarding specific aspects of the disorder.

Diagnostic Criteria

While there are no specific clinical diagnostic criteria for Down syndrome, the disorder usually results in a distinctive pattern of findings that leads to a high degree of suspicion for this diagnosis. Ultimately, however, the diagnosis should either be made or confirmed by a blood chromosome analysis to demonstrate the presence of trisomy 21. Although the clinical manifestations of Down syndrome can vary widely, the vast majority of affected individuals are readily recognizable. In the newborn period, the disorder is usually diagnosed or suspected from the characteristic facial appearance, minor physical malformations, and hypotonia, with or without more serious cardiac or gastrointestinal malformations. Ten cardinal signs have been outlined to aid in the identification of Down syndrome at this age (Hall, 1966). Throughout childhood and into adulthood, the physical dysmorphism persists but evolves with age; mental retardation becomes evident, and growth is delayed relative to family members and peers.

While the physical phenotype of Down syndrome is relatively consistent, the nature and degree of medical, intellectual, and psychosocial problems may differ significantly among affected individuals. Most of these problems are not unique to this condition but, rather, occur with increased frequency in Down syndrome relative to the general population. Because problems can involve virtually every body system, it is easiest to consider them on a system by system basis. It should be emphasized, however, that many people with Down syndrome are in good overall health (Carr, 1994).

Clinical Findings

The phenotypic findings of adults with Down syndrome are presented in Table 53–1. The typical person with trisomy 21 has a distinctive craniofacial appearance, including brachycephaly, upslanted palpebral fissures with epicanthal folds, a flat nasal bridge, small ears, midfacial hypoplasia, and an open mouth (Figure 53–2). The hands and feet are broad, with short digits, incurved fifth fingers, transverse palmar creases, and a wide space between the first and second toes. Stature is short, with sloping

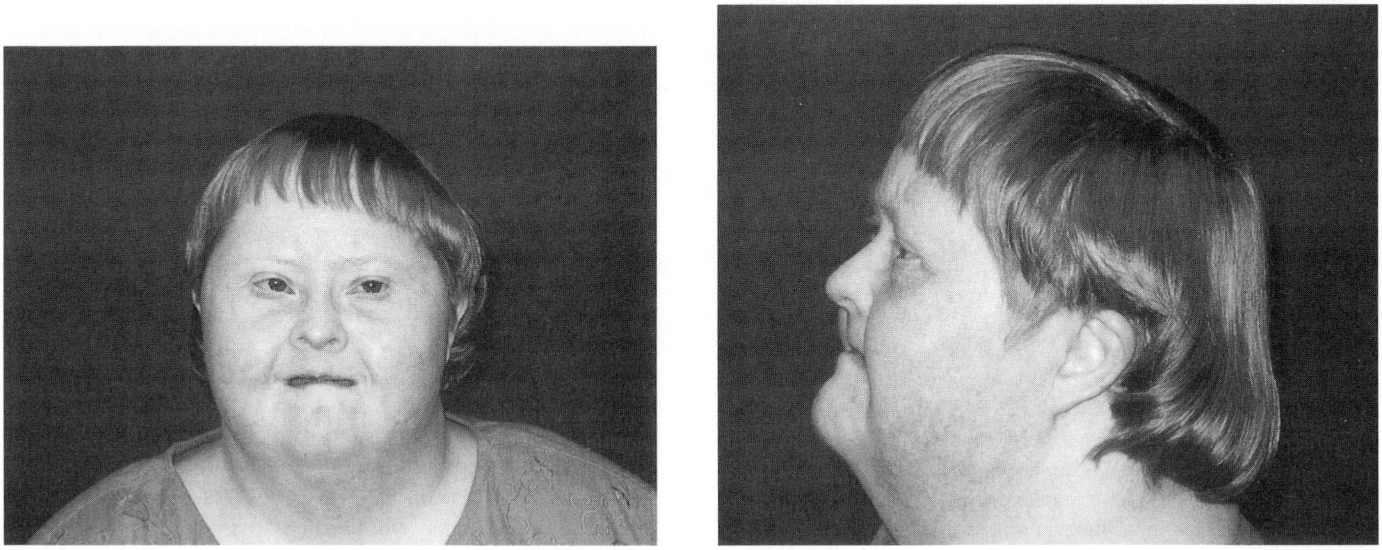

Fig. 53–2. Adult with Down syndrome.

shoulders, and obesity is often present. Any of these features may be missing in a given affected individual, and the phenotype may be subtle in patients with mosaicism. Some people with Down syndrome undergo facial plastic surgery, which may lead to difficulty in recognizing their facial phenotype. Surgical procedures may include removal of epicanthal folds, straightening of the eyelid axis, partial glossectomy, otoplasty, and implantation of silicone or cartilage in the chin, nasal bridge, and cheeks. Plastic surgery has been advocated by some as a means to improve physical appearance, speech quality, drooling, and social functioning, although they have not been conclusively demonstrated to do so in objective studies (Pueschel, 1988).

Cognitive, Neurologic, Psychiatric, and Behavioral Aspects

Mental retardation is a universal finding in Down syndrome, although the degree of cognitive impairment varies widely. On average, adults with trisomy 21 have moderate mental retardation, with a mean IQ of 45, corresponding to a mental age of 5.5 years: average IQ scores are higher in children with mosaicism, but similar data are lacking in adults (Carr, 1994). While cognitive dysfunction is usually global, selective deficits in speech/language and other specific skills have been identified (Epstein, 2001). Although there is significant variability, many adults with Down syndrome require assistance with basic activities of daily living, and the vast majority do not live independently. Participation in daytime educational programs is common, and some persons engage in work programs or paid part-time employment (Carr, 1994).

An unfortunate aspect of Down syndrome is that cognitive skills are usually lost with age. Although IQ increases early in life, intellectual abilities typically plateau and then gradually decline (Carr, 1994; Epstein, 2001). Cognitive decline is generally attributed to the premature development of neurofibrillary tangles, amyloid plaques, and other pathologic changes of Alzheimer disease within multiple areas of the brain (Oliver and Holland, 1986; Holland and Oliver, 1995), which are found in virtually all persons with Down syndrome above the age of 35 (Holland and Oliver, 1995). The pathogenesis of these changes is unknown, although overexpression of the amyloid precursor protein gene, which is located on chromosome 21, has been suggested as a possible mechanism (Holland and Oliver, 1995; Epstein, 2001). An accelerated aging process in Down syndrome has also been suggested.

Despite the consistent presence of the pathologic changes of Alzheimer disease in adults, cognitive decline is not universal (Oliver and Holland, 1986). For example, in a recent study of 75 adults with Down syndrome, aged 30 years or older, changes in personality, memory, general mental functioning, or daily living skills were found in 65% of subjects, while only 24% met criteria for a diagnosis of dementia (Holland et al., 1998). Additional studies have demonstrated rates of dementia as high as 90% in older adults (Evenhuis, 1990), while others have found a low incidence of intellectual decline when adults are followed longitudinally (Devenny et al., 1996). Despite the variability in these data, there is a clear disparity between the neuropathologic and clinical findings (Oliver and Holland, 1986).

Signs of cognitive decline in adults with Down syndrome include behavior difficulties, apathy or other mood disturbances, personality changes, daytime sleepiness, reduced social interactions, deterioration in speech and language, and loss of self-care skills (Oliver and Holland, 1986; Evenhuis, 1990; Holland et al., 1998). In a recent longitudinal study of cognitive decline in adults with Down syndrome, a sequence of declining skills was demonstrated, based on performance on specific subtests of cognitive abilities (Devenny, et al., 2000). Another recent study suggested that frontal lobe functions are the first to be affected during the development of dementia in Down syndrome (Holland et al., 2000). Seizures, muscle hypertonia, myoclonus, and gait disturbances are also commonly observed in patients with dementia (Evenhuis, 1990). Because the diagnosis of dementia is complicated by the presence of preexisting intellectual disability, specific diagnostic criteria have been proposed for use in this patient population (Aylward et al., 1997). In addition, it is important to exclude other conditions in Down syndrome that may mimic the symptoms of dementia, including hypothyroidism, hearing and visual deficits, and depression (Carr, 1994).

In light of its usefulness for patients with Alzheimer disease, the cholinergic agent donepezil hydrochloride has been suggested as a possible therapy for the cognitive and adaptive difficulties that occur in persons with Down syndrome. Use of this agent in a small pilot study of four adults ranging from 24 to 64 years of age led to improvements in communication, expressive language, attention, and mood (Kishnani et al., 1999). Randomized controlled clinical trials of donepezil in adults and children with Down syndrome are now in progress (Kishnani et al., 2001).

Seizures are more common in persons with Down syndrome than in the general population but less frequent than in other individuals with mental retardation (Stafstrom, 1993). The prevalence of seizures ranges from 1%-17%, depending upon the population studied (Romano et al., 1990; Stafstrom, 1993; Van Buggenhout et al., 1999). Seizures are most likely to begin in infancy and in the fourth and fifth decades (Stafstrom, 1993). Generalized and focal seizures of all types may occur, and they usually respond well to anticonvulsants (Romano et al., 1990; Stafstrom, 1993). The appearance of seizures in later life is correlated with the presence of the pathologic changes of Alzheimer disease and the appearance of dementia (Evenhuis, 1990; Stafstrom, 1993; Holland and Oliver, 1995).

Psychiatric disorders also occur with increased frequency in persons with Down syndrome but are less common than in other mentally handicapped populations: approximately 25% of adults have psychiatric disturbances of many different types (Myers and Pueschel, 1991; Collacott et al., 1992). Interestingly, major depression has been reported in up to 11% of adults with Down syndrome, as compared to 4% of other persons with mental retardation (Collacott et al., 1992). Depression often occurs as a reaction to the death of a family member or change in a caregiver. Signs of depression in Down syndrome include sadness, irritability, loss of interest in pleasurable activities, and disturbances in sleep, energy, and appetite, although symptoms resembling dementia or psychosis may also occur (Cohen, 1999). In addition, dementia or hypothyroidism may masquerade as depression (Collacott et al., 1992). Behavioral difficulties, including aggressive behavior and attention deficit disorder, occur in 6% to 10% of adults with Down syndrome, and repetitive or self-injurious behaviors are also relatively common; phobias, obsessive–compulsive disorder, eating disorders, Tourette syndrome, and paraphilias are less common, while schizophrenia, mania, personality disorders, and substance abuse are rare (Myers and Pueschel, 1991). When psychiatric or behavioral symptoms arise in adults with Down syndrome, care should be provided by an individual with expertise in the evaluation and management of psychiatric disorders in the mentally handicapped (Cohen, 1999).

Cardiovascular Aspects

Both congenital and acquired cardiovascular abnormalities occur in Down syndrome. Congenital heart disease is present in approximately 40% of affected individuals, most commonly as an atrioventricular canal. Patent ductus arteriosus, ventricular and atrial septal defects, Tetralogy of Fallot, and a variety of other abnormalities also occur (Gorlin et al., 1990). Since the 1970s, affected children have routinely undergone cardiac surgery, leading to significantly increased survival (Matthew et al., 1990). Adults with Down syndrome may have a variety of cardiac issues related to previous heart disease and/or surgical procedures. Interestingly, it has been suggested that adults with Down syndrome have a reduced rate of coronary atherosclerosis, although this has not been confirmed in all studies (Pueschel et al., 1992).

Adults are also at increased risk to develop valvular dysfunction, including mitral valve prolapse (MVP) with or without regurgitation, thickened mitral valve leaflets, and aortic regurgitation (Goldhaber et al., 1986, 1987, 1988; Geggel et al., 1993). These abnormalities have been hypothesized to arise from a generalized connective tissue abnormality, but their cause is unknown. Patients with valvular dysfunction are at increased risk of congestive heart failure, arrhythmias, cerebral embolism, and endocarditis, and because valve abnormalities are often asymptomatic, it is essential that adults with Down syndrome be examined routinely for suggestive clinical signs (Geggel et al., 1993). It is generally recommended that adults with Down syndrome have a baseline clinical evaluation and/or echocardiogram to screen for valvular dysfunction, especially before dental or surgical procedures (Geggel et al., 1993; Cohen, 1999). However, the natural history of cardiac dysfunction in Down syndrome is not well known, and consensus regarding routine echocardiography in adulthood is lacking. If valve dysfunction is present, endocarditis prophylaxis before dental work or other invasive procedures, regular dental care, and encouragement of good oral hygiene are indicated (Goldhaber et al., 1986, 1987, 1988; Geggel et al., 1993). If aortic regurgitation is identified, serial monitoring of valvular and ventricular function and consideration of valvular repair are warranted (Goldhaber et al., 1986, 1987).

Respiratory Aspects

Upper and lower respiratory tract problems occur with increased frequency in Down syndrome, and respiratory infections constitute the second most common cause of mortality across all ages (Baird and Sadnovnick, 1988b). The tendency to develop sinusitis, pneumonia, and other respiratory tract infections is thought to result from generalized immune dysfunction (Baird and Sadnovick, 1988b; Ugazio et al., 1990). Individuals with Down syndrome are also at increased risk to develop obstructive sleep apnea from adenotonsillar hypertrophy, obesity, and glossoptosis (Clark et al., 1980; Puseschel, 1990; Pueschel et al., 1995; Cohen, 1999). As in the general population, this condition typically presents with disrupted sleep, snoring, noisy breathing, and daytime somnolence, and it can lead to pulmonary hypertension and cor pulmonale (Pueschel et al., 1995; Cohen, 1999).

Gastrointestinal Aspects

Congenital malformations of the gastrointestinal tract occur in approximately 10% to 18% of patients and include tracheoesophageal fistula, pyloric stenosis, duodenal atresia, annular pancreas, Hirschsprung disease (colonic aganglionosis), and imperforate anus (Gorlin et al., 1990). Some adults with Down syndrome will have undergone surgery for such problems in infancy or childhood. As in other mentally handicapped and hypotonic individuals, constipation is common in Down syndrome; in many cases, a specific organic etiology of this problem cannot be identified, but hypothyroidism should be excluded (Martin, 1997). Encouragement of regular bowel habits, increased dietary fiber, and medical therapies may all be indicated in the management of this problem.

Endocrine Aspects

Thyroid dysfunction, predominantly hypothyroidism, is common in Down syndrome, affecting up to 40% of adults (Pueschel and Pezzullo, 1985; Friedman et al., 1989; Dinani and Carpenter 1990; Kennedy et al., 1992; Karlsson et al., 1998). Hypothyroidism usually results from primary thyroid dysfunction and ranges in severity with varying degrees of TSH elevation and T4 reduction. Although hypothyroidism may be congenital, it is most often acquired from childhood onward. Most cases of acquired hypothyroidism in adults with Down syndrome are thought to have an autoimmune basis, since a significant proportion of patients have antithyroid and antimicrosomal antibodies. However, many patients with these antibodies have normal thyroid function. Autoantibody production is attributed to generalized immune dysregulation (Kennedy et al., 1992). The frequency of thyroid dysfunction in adults with Down syndrome, and the fact that this problem is often asymptomatic, mandates regular thyroid screening in this population. It has been recommended that adult patients undergo measurements of TSH and T4 annually (Pueschel et al., 1995; Cohen, 1999). The signs and symptoms of hypothyroidism may also be more difficult to recognize clinically in persons with Down syndrome because of the overlap of some clinical features such as short stature, hoarse voice, coarse skin, and obesity (Pueschel and Pezzullo, 1985; Dinani and Carpenter, 1990; Kennedy et al., 1992). Furthermore, hypothyroidism can present with a variety of nonspecific symptoms and signs in Down syndrome, including cognitive decline, depression, and behavioral changes, and patients may be unable to communicate their symptoms (Friedman et al., 1989). Hence, clinicians caring for these patients should have a low threshold for obtaining thyroid function tests.

Several population-based studies have also demonstrated an increased incidence of insulin-dependent diabetes mellitus in children with Down syndrome (Van Goor et al., 1997). Obese individuals with Down syndrome are also at risk to develop adult-onset diabetes, as is true for the general population. Periodic diabetes screening for the Down syndrome population has been suggested (Martin, 1997).

Growth deficiency is the rule in Down syndrome. Height ranges between 2 and 4 standard deviations below the mean, with an average adult height of 151 cm in males and 141 cm in females (Gorlin et al., 1990). The etiology of short stature in Down syndrome is unknown. Growth hormone deficiency is not usually present, although defects in growth regulatory pathways, most notably reduced levels of insulin-like growth factor 1 (IGF-1), have been demonstrated in some cases (Epstein, 2001).

Adults with Down syndrome tend to have excessive body weight and are more often obese, as compared to both the general population and other groups of mentally handicapped individuals. Excessive weight gain often begins in childhood and continues into adulthood. Analyses of body mass index (BMI) in adults have shown that approximately 80% are overweight or obese (Bell and Bhate, 1992; Prasher, 1995). The etiology of obesity in Down syndrome is considered to be multifactorial, arising from a mixture of biologic and environmental factors such as hypotonia, hypothyroidism, short stature, reduced metabolic rate, eating behavior, and reduced physical activity (Chad et al., 1990; Prasher, 1995). Significantly greater BMIs have been shown in persons living in the community than in those in institutions, suggesting a strong environmental component (Prasher, 1995). This underscores the importance of nutritional management and physical activity in their chronic medical care.

Pubertal development is often normal in males with Down syndrome, and the majority have normal serum testosterone concentration (Hsiang et al., 1987; Pueschel, 1990). However, some men have reduced penile length and testicular volume and increased gonadotropin levels, which is consistent with partial gonadal insufficiency (Hsiang et al., 1987). There is only one documented case of reproduction by a male with complete trisomy 21, as virtually all are infertile due to abnormal spermatogenesis (Epstein, 2001). Men with mosaic trisomy 21, however, are often capable of having children, some of whom also have Down syndrome (Epstein, 2001). On average, females with Down syndrome have normal pubertal development, including onset of menarche at the same age as their unaffected peers and regular menstrual cycles (Scola and Pueschel, 1992). However, an increased rate of ovarian dysfunction—including abnormal follicular development, anovulation, and elevated gonadotropin levels—has been observed in adult women (Hsiang et al., 1987; Scola and Pueschel, 1992). Women also experience early menopause at a median age of 46 years, irrespective of hypothyroidism (Schupf et al., 1997; Seltzer et al., 2001). Although pregnancy is uncommon, women with Down syndrome may clearly be fertile, as there are over 30 documented instances of reproduction in this population; one-third of these children also had Down syndrome (Rani et al., 1990).

Given their reproductive capacity and concomitant mental retardation, women with Down syndrome are at risk to conceive unwanted children. Many persons with Down syndrome have an interest in relationships with the opposite sex, including marriage (Pueschel and Scola, 1988; Carr, 1994). Thus, it is important that they receive information about sexual activity and that contraception be provided to women who are either sexually active or who are at risk to become pregnant (Pueschel and Scola, 1988; Pueschel et al., 1995). Non-barrier contraceptive methods are often preferable in mentally handicapped persons, but decisions regarding a particular method should be individualized (Martin, 1997). Women with Down syndrome also should have regular gynecologic care, including pelvic examinations, Pap smears, and mammograms (Cohen, 1999). Recurrence risk counseling may also be appropriate for sexually active women with Down syndrome since they may have similarly affected children.

Urinary Tract Aspects

Although a variety of congenital urinary tract malformations have been described in Down syndrome, their incidence is relatively low, ranging from 2.8% to 6.7% (Lo et al., 1998). Reports of acquired renal disease are infrequent in this population, but patients may experience the range of renal disorders that is seen in the general population, and renal transplantation has been performed in some such individuals (Lo et al., 1998). In addition, autopsy studies have demonstrated an increased prevalence of glomerular microcysts in patients with Down syndrome, but this finding is of unknown significance (Ariel et al., 1991; Lo et al., 1998). Increased serum uric acid concentration and renal uric acid excretion have also been observed (Epstein, 2001).

Musculoskeletal Aspects

Ligamentous laxity is a well-recognized complication of Down syndrome, as evidenced by an increased prevalence of joint subluxations and dislocations in affected persons (Pueschel et al., 1995). This finding, along with evidence of valvular heart disease, has led to speculation that a generalized connective tissue abnormality occurs in Down syndrome (Goldhaber et al., 1987). The most significant complication of ligamentous laxity is instability of the cervical spine, occurring either between the first and second cervical vertebrae (atlantoaxial region), or, less commonly, at the craniocervical junction (atlantooccipital region) (Pueschel, 1990). Instability is generally attributed to laxity of the spinal ligaments (Pueschel and Scola, 1987; Davidson, 1988) and is present in 10% to 40% of adults with Down syndrome, depending on the radiologic criteria used for diagnosis (Alvarez and Rubin, 1986; Pueschel, 1990; Maclachlan et al., 1993). While cervical spine instability may cause neck pain, muscle weakness, hyperreflexia, gait disturbance, or other neurologic symptoms, it is most often asymptomatic (Pueschel and Scola, 1987; American Academy of Pediatrics, Committee on Sports Medicine, 1995). The presence of instability is considered a risk factor for cervical spine dislocation and catastrophic spinal cord injury in the event of head or neck trauma, although these complications are reportedly infrequent in previously asymptomatic individuals (Davidson, 1988).

Radiographic screening for cervical spine instability, beginning in early childhood, has long been considered an important aspect of the care of individuals with Down syndrome in order to identify those at risk of spinal cord injury. Lateral neck X-rays, including flexion views, have traditionally been considered the screening study of choice, but some have recommended a single lateral flexion view with the patient actively performing the flexion maneuver (O'Connor et al., 1996). Atlantoaxial instability is defined radiographically as the presence of a space 5 mm or more between the posterior portion of the anterior arch of C1 and the anterior portion of the odontoid process of C2 (Cohen, 1999), although some consider a distance 2.5 mm or higher to be abnormal in adults (Tangerud et al., 1990). The American Academy of Pediatrics, Committee on Genetics (2001) has recommended screening with a lateral neck X-ray for all children with Down syndrome between ages 3 and 5 years and when suspicious symptoms are present, and the Special Olympics requires screening X-rays on all participants. However, many consider radiologic screening to be of unproven benefit in predicting serious complications in asymptomatic patients (Davidson, 1988; American Academy of Pediatrics, Committee on Sports Medicine, 1995). Neck X-rays have also been recommended before patients undergo general anesthesia for the first time (Martin, 1997). Routine assessment for neurologic symptoms and signs referable to cervical spine instability throughout life is also warranted (Davidson, 1988; American Academy of Pediatrics, Committee on Sports Medicine, 1995; Cohen, 1999). If such symptoms or signs are detected, patients should be restricted from participating in sports or other physical activities that could lead to neck injury, and those with symptoms should be referred for surgical evaluation.

Adults with Down syndrome also are predisposed to degenerative disease at all levels of the cervical spine, including disc narrowing, osteophyte formation, deformity, subluxation, bony sclerosis, and spinal stenosis (Tangerud et al., 1990; Maclachlan et al., 1993). These problems are found in 64% of persons with

Down syndrome, as compared with 39% of the general population (Maclachlan et al., 1993). Symptoms can include reduced neck mobility, neck pain, or problems referable to encroachment on blood vessels or nerves (Maclachlan et al., 1993). Radiologic assessment and referral to a surgical specialist are indicated when symptoms are present.

Ocular Aspects

A variety of ocular problems may affect adults with Down syndrome. Congenital cataracts are an infrequent but vision-threatening complication if they are not treated early; strabismus, myopia, and astigmatism are commonly identified and may significantly impair visual acuity (Shapiro and France, 1985; Catalano, 1990; Hestnes et al., 1991). Cataracts occur in 30% to 60% of adult patients, often in the form of characteristic "flake-like" opacities, and are frequently bilateral (Catalano, 1990; Pueschel, 1990; Hestnes et al., 1991). Adults with Down syndrome also have a significantly increased rate of keratoconus, which often occurs at a younger than expected age and is more likely to be complicated by acute hydrops of the cornea (Shapiro and France, 1985; Catalano, 1990; Hestnes et al., 1991). Keratoconus is most often attributed to corneal trauma from eye-rubbing and may require surgical correction (keratoplasty) (Shapiro and France, 1985). The retinas often have an increased number of retinal vessels crossing the optic disc margin in an unusual spoke-like pattern (Catalano, 1990). Blepharitis and nystagmus also occur with increased frequency in Down syndrome (Shapiro and France, 1985). Existing visual problems and screening for keratoconus and cataracts warrant regular ophthalmologic evaluation in adults with Down syndrome. Evaluation at least every other year has been recommended (Pueschel et al., 1995; Cohen, 1999).

Hearing Aspects

Hearing loss occurs commonly in adults with Down syndrome and is more frequent in this population than in other mentally handicapped individuals; the prevalence of this problem has been reported to be as high as 90% but varies considerably with the age of the study population and the methods used to test hearing (Keiser et al., 1981; Dahle and McCollister, 1986; Evenhuis et al., 1992). Conductive hearing loss commonly develops in childhood as the consequence of middle ear pathology, including otitis media, effusion, and retracted tympanic membranes (Dahle and McCollister, 1986). In addition to conductive loss, adults are at a higher risk of developing sensorineural hearing loss, particularly involving high frequencies, with advancing age (Keiser et al., 1981; Evenhuis et al., 1992). Hearing loss may be difficult to recognize and can be mistaken for dementia in the adult population. It is recommended that adults with Down syndrome undergo regular audiologic screening, at least every other year, to facilitate early identification and treatment of reduced hearing sensitivity (Pueschel et al., 1995; Cohen, 1999).

Dental Aspects

A high frequency of periodontal disease is seen in persons with Down syndrome, particularly in institutionalized patients (Pueschel, 1990). This mandates regular dental care and judicious use of prophylactic antibiotics for those patients with valvular dysfunction to reduce the risk of bacterial endocarditis. A number of dental anomalies—including enamel hypoplasia, microdontia and macrodontia, missing teeth, and abnormal tooth alignment—have also been described in Down syndrome (Gorlin et al., 1990).

Immune System Aspects

Generalized immune dysfunction is thought to occur in Down syndrome, as suggested by an increased frequency of infectious illnesses, hematologic malignancies, and autoantibody production (Ugazio et al., 1990; Nespoli et al., 1993). In addition to being susceptible to respiratory infections, both children and adults with Down syndrome have an increased carrier rate of hepatitis B surface antigen relative to other mentally handicapped persons, irrespective of whether they are institutionalized (van Schrojenstein Lantman-deValk et al., 1996). Hence, monitoring of hepatitis B infection status and immunization with hepatitis B vaccine are warranted in this population, although the degree of immune response to the vaccine may be low (Ugazio et al., 1990; Martin, 1997).

A variety of abnormalities in immune function have been observed, including abnormal distribution of T lymphocyte subsets, abnormal antibody and cell-mediated immune responses to bacterial and viral antigens, aberrant thymic function and histology, and reduced phagocyte chemotaxis and oxygen radical production (Ugazio et al., 1990; Nespoli et al., 1993; Cuadrado and Barrena, 1996). Adults with Down syndrome tend to have a characteristic serum immunoglobulin profile, with increased levels of total IgG and IgA and reduced levels of IgM and certain IgG subclasses (Nespoli et al., 1993). IgG subclass deficiency may warrant intravenous gamma globulin therapy in some patients with recurrent infections (Cohen, 1999). Interestingly, the phagocyte dysfunction seen in Down syndrome may be related to increased levels of superoxide dismutase (SOD), an enzyme involved in degradation of oxygen free radicals required for bacterial killing (Ugazio et al., 1990). On average, persons with Down syndrome have supranormal levels of SOD activity, presumably because the SOD gene is located on chromosome 21 and is therefore present in a trisomic state. The significance and pathogenesis of many of the other immunologic abnormalities found in Down syndrome are presently unclear.

Malignancy Aspects

Leukemia occurs at a significantly increased rate in persons with Down syndrome. The risk to develop leukemia is greatest during childhood, when acute lymphocytic and non-lymphocytic leukemia are 10 to 20 times more frequent than in the general population. Adults with Down syndrome are also at a higher risk of developing leukemia, although the risk is less than that in childhood (Fong and Brodeur, 1987). Lymphomas may also be more common in Down syndrome (Satge et al., 1998). Interestingly, acquired trisomy 21 is frequently detected in the leukemic cells of patients who do not have Down syndrome, suggesting an important pathogenetic link between this karyotypic abnormality and hematopoetic dysregulation (Fong and Brodeur, 1987). Males with Down syndrome also have up to a 50-fold increased risk of testicular germ cell cancer (Satge et al., 1997; Roberge et al., 2001). Although the absolute incidence of this tumor type is low, the importance of routine testicular examination in men with Down syndrome has been emphasized (Dieckmann et al., 1997). Skin syringomas, which are benign adenomas of the sweat ducts usually involving the eyelids, are also more common in Down syndrome (Satge et al., 1998). A recent literature review of reported tumors in Down syndrome suggests that a specific tumor profile occurs in this disorder, with overrepresentation of the above tumor types and underrepresentation of others, including those derived from nervous tissue, pediatric renal tumors, and adult epithelial cancers, including those of the uterus, breast and urinary tract (Satge et al., 1998).

Life Expectancy

Survival in persons with Down syndrome is reduced at all ages relative to the general population (Baird and Sadovnick, 1989). The mortality rate in this disorder is significantly greater in the first several years of life, is relatively stable between early childhood and age 44, and increases markedly thereafter (Baird and Sadovnick, 1988a). Early mortality is principally related to congenital anomalies, especially heart disease, and respiratory problems are a significant cause of death up to age 30 (Baird and Sadovnick, 1988b). The causes of death in older adults have not been well studied.

Management

As suggested by the nature and frequency of medical, neurologic, and psychiatric complications in Down syndrome, the management of adults with this disorder is often complex. Physicians involved in the care of these individuals should be familiar with the range of health issues that are associated with Down syndrome, including their relative frequencies, presenting symptoms and signs, differential diagnosis, and methods of evaluation and management. In addition, caregivers should place special emphasis on surveillance for potential complications and refer patients for appropriate screening evaluations. Guidelines for the health care of persons with Down syndrome, including the adult population, have been published by several groups, including the International League of Societies for Persons with Mental Handicap and the Down Syndrome Medical Interest Group (Pueschel et al., 1995; Cohen, 1999). In addition, recommendations have been made by various authors in the medical literature regarding the management of specific health problems in this disorder, and a description of a multidisciplinary clinic for adults with Down syndrome has also been published (Chicoine et al., 1994). In two recent studies, the importance of continued surveillance for a variety of medical problems in middle-aged and elderly persons with Down syndrome was emphasized (van Allen et al., 1999; Van Buggenhout et al., 1999). Table 53–2 presents a summary of general management guidelines, based on these literature sources.

Table 53–2. Suggested Evaluation and Management of Health Issues in Adults with Down Syndrome

Body System	Complication	Recommended Tests	Management
Cardiovascular	Aortic and/or mitral valve dysfunction	Baseline clinical exam in early adulthood, especially prior to dental or surgical procedures; echocardiogram if symptoms or signs of valve dysfunction are present	Endocarditis prophylaxis, regular dental care and good oral hygiene, cardiac medications, consider cardiology referral
Respiratory	Upper and lower respiratory infections	None	Antibiotics, decongestants, consider ENT and/or pulmonary referral
	Sleep apnea	None; sleep study when symptoms present	ENT referral, weight management
Gastrointestinal	Constipation	None; consider hypothyroidism in differential differential diagnosis	Fiber, motility agents, enemas
Endocrine	Hypothyroidism	Annual T4 and TSH	Thyroid hormone replacement
	Diabetes mellitus	Annual plasma glucose and urine dipstick; glucose tolerance test if symptoms	Insulin, oral hypoglycemic agents, weight management
	Weight gain/obesity	Routine weight measurement; consider hypothyroidism in differential diagnosis	Nutritional management, exercise, thyroid hormone replacement if deficient
Gynecologic and reproductive	Sexual activity, pregnancy, female	If sexually active, Pap smear every 1–3 years; pelvic ultrasound every 2–3 years if bimanual exam inadequate. If not sexually active, single-finger examination with cytologic screening every 1–3 years; yearly breast exam by physician; mammogram every 1–2 years after age 40, yearly after age 50.	Contraceptives, sex and reproductive education pelvic ultrasound every
Musculoskeletal	Cervical spine instability; degenerative disease of the cervical spine	Baseline lateral C-spine X-ray (neutral, flexion, and extension views) once in adulthood; annual screening neurologic examination; C-spine imaging studies if symptoms	Limitation of physical activity, orthopedic or neurosurgical referral when symptomatic
Ocular	Cataracts; keratoconus	Ophthalmologic evaluation every 2 years	Corrective surgery
Hearing	Hearing loss	Hearing evaluation every 2 years	Hearing aids
Immune	Hepatitis B; recurrent infections	None; liver function tests and hepatitis B serology if signs of hepatitis; immunoglobulin profile if recurrent infections	Hepatitis B vaccine; immunology referral and/or IVIG if recurrent infections or IgG subclass deficiency
Malignancy	Leukemia; testicular cancer	Some suggest yearly CBC; obtain CBC if suspicious symptoms; annual testicular examination	Hematology/oncology and/or urology referral
Dental	Periodontal disease	Dental visits every 6 months	Good oral hygiene; SBE prophylaxis if valvular disease
Neurologic	Seizures	None	Anticonvulsants; neurology referral
Cognitive	Cognitive decline or dementia	None; consider hypothyroidism, hearing or vision deficits, and depression in differential diagnosis	No specific treatment
Psychiatric	Depression	None; consider hypothyroidism and dementia in differential diagnosis	Referral to mental health specialist with expertise in evaluation of patients with mental handicap

Genetics

Down syndrome occurs when an additional copy of chromosome 21 is present in an individual's cells (reviewed in Epstein, 2001). Approximately 95% of cases are attributable to trisomy of the complete chromosome 21 as a consequence of meiotic nondisjunction. The origin of the meiotic error is maternal in 90% of cases and is associated with advanced maternal age. The remaining cases of Down syndrome are roughly divided between unbalanced Robertsonian translocations involving chromosome 21 and mosaic individuals who have varying proportions of normal and trisomic cells. Although it is rare, Down syndrome may arise from partial duplications of the long (q) arm of chromosome 21.

Because the majority of cases of Down syndrome are due to random meiotic errors, the recurrence risk of this disorder is low, with usually only one affected individual within a given nuclear family (reviewed in Gardner and Sutherland, 1989). For women younger than 35 years, the empiric recurrence risk is approximately 0.5%, while for women ages 35 and older, the risk of recurrence increases with age. This risk can be significantly higher than the age related risk if a parent carries a balanced Robertsonian translocation involving chromosome 21, particularly if the mother is the carrier. If an individual of either sex carries a chromosome 21;21 translocation, all of his or her liveborn children will have trisomy 21.

Ideally, every patient with a diagnosis of Down syndrome should have a documented blood chromosome analysis to establish a definitive diagnosis and determine his or her specific chromosome constitution. This is particularly applicable to adult patients, some of whom are likely to have been diagnosed before the routine use of modern cytogenetic analysis. In caring for adults with Down syndrome, recurrence risk counseling for parents is generally not an issue, as the parents are most often well beyond their reproductive years. In cases due to Robertsonian translocations, however, parental karyotypes are indicated to determine whether the rearrangement is familial and, hence, whether other relatives are at risk of transmitting a chromosome abnormality to their children.

Many studies are in progress to investigate the causes of chromosome non-disjunction and the underlying genetic mechanisms responsible for the phenotypic features of Down syndrome. Although the pathogenesis of Down syndrome is poorly understood, some light has begun to be shed on the disorder. Abnormal patterns of chromosome recombination during meiosis have been recently recognized as a major factor associated with nondisjunction (reviewed in Hassold and Hunt, 2001). In addition, studies of individuals with partial trisomy 21 have led to the delineation of a putative Down syndrome critical region, encompassing the terminal portion of the long arm of chromosome 21 (region 21q22) (reviewed in Epstein, 2001). Trisomy of this chromosomal segment is thought to be sufficient to cause the complete Down syndrome phenotype, allowing the correlation of certain phenotypic features with specific chromosomal bands within this region (Epstein, 2001; Epstein et al., 1991). Because Down syndrome is thought to arise from increased dosage of genes on chromosome 21, there is great interest in identifying genes within the critical region and in studying the effects of their overexpression in mouse models (Hernandez and Fisher, 1996; Epstein, 2001; Reeves et al., 2001). A major advance in the study of trisomy 21 occurred in May 2000 when virtually the entire sequence of human chromosome 21 was published as part of the Human Genome Project (Hattori et al., 2000). Data from the sequence analysis indicate that this chromosome constitutes approximately 1% of the entire human genome and contains 225 known or predicted functional genes (Hattori et al., 2000). However, the relationship between specific genes and phenotypic features of Down syndrome remains unclear and is the focus of intensive investigation. Undoubtedly, future genetic research will greatly advance the understanding of this and other chromosomal disorders.

KLINEFELTER SYNDROME

Klinefelter syndrome is an important cause of male infertility that was initially described 60 years ago in a series of nine men with infertility, gynecomastia, and abnormal excretion of urinary 17-ketosteroids and follicle-stimulating hormone (FSH) (Klinefelter et al., 1942). It is now classified as one of the most common forms of hypergonadotropic hypogonadism, in which adult males have low levels of serum testosterone in the face of elevated basal levels of FSH and leutenizing hormone (LH) (Schwartz and Root, 1991). In addition to infertility caused by primary testicular failure, men with Klinefelter syndrome are at risk for other disorders, such as osteopenia, autoimmune disease, vascular abnormalities, and cancer. The chromosomal defect of 47,XXY was recognized in 1959 when cytogenetic preparations demonstrated an additional X chromosome in patients with Klinefelter syndrome (Jacobs and Strong, 1959). It occurs in all racial groups, with an estimated incidence of 1 in 500 to 1 in 1000 male births based on cytogenetic studies of consecutive prenatal, newborn, or hospitalized patients (Garson et al., 1980; Kleczkowska et al., 1988; Nielsen and Wohlert, 1991; Zhang et al., 1991; Abramsky and Chapple, 1997). Thus, Klinefelter syndrome is one of the most common chromosomal disorders in humans.

Diagnostic Criteria

While strict diagnostic criteria have not been published, Klinefelter syndrome usually refers to male patients with infertility and/or hypogonadism with a 47,XXY karyotype (Paulsen and Plymate, 1992). The diagnosis of a suspected individual with Klinefelter syndrome must include a complete cytogenetic analysis in addition to measurement of serum LH, FSH, and testosterone. Newer laboratory methods using FISH or direct DNA testing have been developed and can be used to confirm the diagnosis. Older cytogenetic methods, such as Barr body analysis of cheek swabs (Barr and Bertram, 1949; Bradbury et al., 1956), are not adequate for a genetic diagnosis because they are not always accurate and because variations in other chromosomes would be misidentified. Males with variable numbers of X and Y chromosomes have also been described, including 48,XXXY, 48,XXYY, 49,XXXXY, mosaicism for 47,XXY, and 46, XX males (Kleczkowska et al., 1988). These variant forms may result in a different prognosis and management from those for males with a 47,XXY karyotype.

Clinical Findings

The characteristic physical features of eunuchoid body habitus, sparse facial and body hair, gynecomastia, small testes, and azoospermia are found in only a small fraction of men with

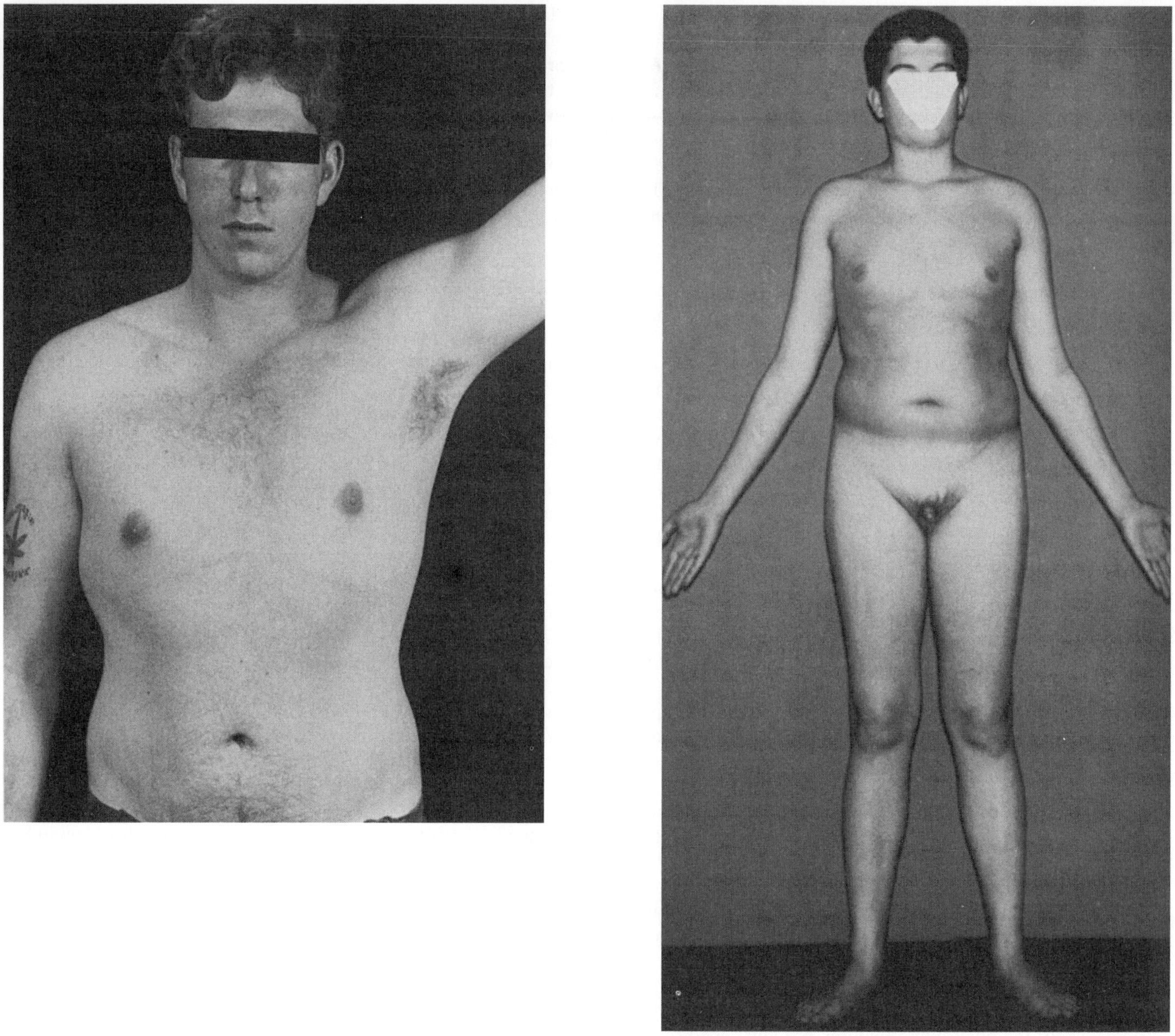

Fig. 53–3. Adults with Klinefelter syndrome.

Klinefelter syndrome. However, small firm testes are a consistent finding even when there is evidence of virilization (Garson et al.,1980; Paulsen and Plymate, 1992). Figure 53–3 shows a typical male with Klinefelter syndrome, and typical physical findings are listed in Table 53–3. Males with Klinefelter syndrome can present with variable clinical findings during all stages of life, so that a heightened clinical suspicion is necessary to make the proper diagnosis. Most males with 47,XXY will typically be identified through an evaluation for delayed puberty, infertility, or gynecomastia in adolescence or adulthood (Micic et al., 1984; Kleczkowska et al., 1988; Abramsky and Chapple, 1997; Yoshida et al., 1997b; Sher et al., 1998). In fact, cytogenetic abnormalities are commonly found in men seen in infertility clinics, in which 2% to 10% have a 47,XXY karyotype (Rivas et al., 1987; De Braekeleer and Dao, 1991; Yoshida et al., 1997b). This proportion increases to 19% of infertile males with documented azoospermia (Rivas et al., 1987). Males with Klinefelter syndrome are infrequently identified during an evaluation of developmental delay or behavioral problems in childhood or adolescence, or during prenatal amniocentesis (Kleczkowska et al., 1988; Abramsky and Chapple, 1997).

Growth and Physical Development

The body habitus of boys identified with 47, XXY karyotype is typically described as tall and thin but can be otherwise unremarkable. The mean height during childhood is at the 75th percentile, and the mean head circumference is at the 40th percentile (Robinson et al., 1990; Stewart et al., 1990). The facial features of men with Klinefelter syndrome are generally described as long and slender, with moderate mandibular prognathism. Cephalometric measurements have demonstrated differences in the size of the maxilla, mandible, and base of the cranium (Brown et al., 1993; Brkic et al., 1994; Gron et al., 1997). Taurodontism—an abnormality of tooth development with enlarged pulp chambers

Table 53–3. Physical Findings in Klinefelter Syndrome

Area of Involvement	Manifestation
Craniofacial	Long, slender face with moderate mandibular prognathism, abnormality of teeth development (taurodontism)
Genitalia	Normal to small penis, small firm testes, occasional cryptorchidism, fibrosis and hyalinization on testicular biopsy, oligospermia or aspermia leading to infertility
Extremities	Usually normal
Body habitus	Tall stature
Other	Decreased pubic and facial hair, gynecomastia

Source: Adapted from Paulsen (1992) with permission.

and apical displacement of the bifurcation or trifurcation of roots—has been identified in people with sex chromosome aneuploidy (Jaspers and Witkop, 1980) and has been reported in nearly 25% of men with Klinefelter syndrome (Komatz et al., 1978; Varrela and Alvesalo, 1988; Hillebrand et al., 1990).

Gynecomastia is a common finding in boys with Klinefelter syndrome, and the frequency increases to between 30% and 60% of adults (Ratcliffe et al., 1990; Schwartz and Root, 1991). Some experts report that up to 90% of men with Klinefelter syndrome will have gynecomastia after careful physical examination (Paulsen and Plymate, 1992). The pathogenesis of the breast enlargement is not clear but may be due to the increased rate of conversion of testosterone to estradiol (Wang et al., 1975; Stewart et al., 1990; Mandoki and Sumner, 1991). Muscle mass and hair distribution are also variable. However, muscle strength is less than in normal men, a finding also noted in boys and adolescents (Stewart et al., 1990; Paulsen and Plymate, 1992). The clinician should remember that there is wide variability in these physical features among individuals with Klinefelter syndrome.

Gonadal Function and Infertility

The primary effect of the supernumerary X chromosome is delayed sexual development after puberty. Infants and boys with a 47,XXY karyotype have normal penile and testicular size and normal levels of testosterone, FSH, and LH (Robinson et al., 1990). The onset of puberty is no different from that in the general male population and triggers a normal elevation of testosterone, which subsequently levels off to a below-normal or low–normal range in the adult (Stewart et al., 1990). Salbenblatt and colleagues (1985) prospectively followed 40 affected boys through puberty and showed that the response to gonadotropin-releasing hormone was normal at 12 years of age, but FSH and LH rose to high levels by age 14 years. Precocious puberty may also be seen, although it is rare (Bertelloni et al., 1996). Thus, by mid to late adolescence, most patients with Klinefelter syndrome will exhibit the typical hormonal profile of hypergonadotropic hypogonadism with normal to low testosterone levels and FSH and LH levels 5 to 10 times above the mean (Capell et al., 1973; Robinson et al., 1990).

Histopathologic studies of testicular tissue from men and boys with Klinefelter syndrome have shown characteristic abnormalities that explain the subsequent alteration in the hypothalamic-pituitary-gonadal axis later in life. Testicular biopsies show progressive hyalinization, fibrosis of the seminiferous tubules, and an overall decrease in Leydig cell number in pubertal boys and adults with Klinefelter syndrome (Winter, 1990; Regadera et al., 1991). The loss of functional seminiferous tubules and Sertoli cells is thought to result in a decrease in inhibin B levels (Anawalt et al., 1996; Bohring and Krause, 1999), which, in turn, regulates FSH levels, and the loss of Leydig cell function causes a decrease in serum testosterone. Immunohistochemical studies of testicular tissue show alteration in Leydig cell morphology, decrease in normal Leydig cell number, and decrease in staining for testosterone (Regadera et al., 1991). How the extra X chromosome causes the progressive testicular dysfunction is not known, but it may involve the development of antisperm antibodies (Sengul et al., 1996). However, this explanation is controversial and has not been proven. A mouse model for Klinefelter syndrome has been developed that may help answer this important question. Early studies of testicular tissue from XXY mice have shown a similar histologic pattern to men with Klinefelter syndrome with small seminiferous tubules, intraepithelial vacuolization, and absence of germ cells (Lue et al., 2001).

Small, firm testes are invariably found in men with Klinefelter syndrome, even when serum testosterone levels are within the normal range and the individual appears to be otherwise normally virilized (Paulsen and Plymate, 1992). The average testis size is less than 2 cm in length, 2 cm in width, and 4 ml in volume, which is markedly decreased from the normal 15 ml testis size (Stewart et al., 1990). Filippi (1986) reported that nearly 60% of hypogonadal Sardinian males reporting for military service had a non-mosaic 47,XXY karyotype. Sexual functioning is normal (Yoshida et al., 1997a), but the ejaculate shows either oligospermia or azoospermia, which leads to infertility in most men. One variant form of Klinefelter syndrome caused by a mosaic pattern of 46,XY/47,XXY may have a low level of sperm production, and men with this chromosome constitution have been documented to have motile spermatogonia (Bourne et al., 1997). This may explain the rare reports of fertile men with Klinefelter syndrome, although there have also been case reports of men with non-mosaic 47,XXY karyotypes who have produced children (Laron et al., 1982; Terzoli et al., 1992).

Osteoporosis

Due to relatively low levels of testosterone, adolescent and adult males with Klinefelter syndrome are at risk for osteoporosis. Foresta and colleagues (1983) studied bone density in 10 men with Klinefelter syndrome and compared them to 8 men with other forms of hypogonadism and 10 normal men. This study showed a significant loss of cortical bone when testosterone levels were below 200 ng/100 ml. Subsequently, a series of 22 men with Klinefelter syndrome documented that about 25% had measurable osteopenia (Horowitz et al., 1992). Decreased bone formation and high levels of bone resorption have been shown to cause the decrease in bone density (Luisetto et al., 1995). The loss of bone may occur early in development (Eulry et al., 1993).

Malignancy

While men with Klinefelter syndrome do not have a generalized risk for neoplasia any greater than in the normal population, those with an XXY karyotype do have an increased risk for breast cancer and germ cell tumors. Hasle et al. (1995) examined the incidence of cancer in 595 Danish men with Klinefelter syndrome and found only 39 reported neoplasms for a relative risk of 1.1 compared to the general population. There was no increase of breast cancer, lymphoma, or leukemia. However, this study did find that males with Klinefelter syndrome had a 67-fold higher relative risk for mediastinal germ cell tumors, as have other studies (Arens et al., 1988; Gohji et al., 1989). One such study showed that 5 men out of 22 patients diagnosed with a primary mediastinal germ cell tumor had Klinefelter syndrome (Nichols et al., 1987).

The first study suggesting an association between Klinefelter syndrome and breast cancer was reported in 1965, when 3 of 22 men with breast cancer were found to be positive in Barr body analysis (Jackson et al., 1965). Several subsequent studies have also suggested a 20-fold or more increase in breast cancer in males with Klinefelter syndrome (Scheike et al., 1973; Sasco et al., 1993; Hultborn et al., 1997). Hultborn et al. (1997) showed a high prevalence (7.5%) of Klinefelter syndrome cases in a retrospective FISH analysis of 93 cases of male breast cancer and suggested that men with Klinefelter syndrome may face a 50-fold increased risk in developing breast cancer. There have been numerous case reports of patients with Klinefelter syndrome with other types of tumors, including adrenal cortical cancer, leukemia, and lymphoma (Kleczkowska et al., 1988: Oguma et al., 1989). However, these types of cancers may be coincidental, due to the relatively high prevalence of Klinefelter syndrome in the general population (Muts-Homsma et al., 1982; Pascual et al., 1990; Tay et al., 1995; Humphreys et al., 1997). Men with mosaic and other variant forms of Klinefelter syndrome have been reported to have developed cancer as well (Sanchez et al., 1986; Kleczkowska et al., 1988), although no studies have been published that examine the magnitude of risk for these individuals.

Vascular Abnormalities

Men with Klinefelter syndrome have an increased incidence of venous insufficiency, leg ulceration, deep venous thrombosis, and pulmonary embolus. These conditions are more prevalent in adulthood and can be a persistent problem (Veraart et al., 1995). Campbell and Price (1981) surveyed 412 men with Klinefelter syndrome and found that 6% of cases had a history of venous leg ulceration. This survey also documented an increased incidence of deep venous thrombosis and pulmonary emboli in men over 30 years. Leg ulcerations due to underlying vascular abnormalities can be the initial finding that alerts clinicians to the diagnosis of Klinefelter syndrome (Spier et al., 1995). The underlying cause of the recurrent leg ulcers is not understood but may be due to the increased activity of plasminogen activator inhibitor 1 (PAI-1) (Veraart et al., 1994; Zollner et al., 1997), which may interfere with wound healing after minor trauma.

Other cardiovascular abnormalities have been described in Klinefelter syndrome, including mitral valve prolapse (MVP), aortic dissection, and subarachnoid hemorrhage. A single echocardiographic study of 22 men with Klinefelter syndrome showed a frequency of MVP of 55%, compared to 5% of normal males (Fricke et al., 1984). Cardiovascular events could account for the higher mortality rate of men with Klinefelter syndrome (Price et al., 1982, 1985a). Price and colleagues (1985b) examined the causes of death in 466 men with Klinefelter syndrome and found that mortality due to subarachnoid hemorrhage and aortic valve disease were elevated in this population, as were deaths from pulmonary disease and breast carcinoma.

Psychosocial Development and Adjustment

Many men with Klinefelter syndrome will complete schooling, marry, gain employment, and have productive adult lives (Kleczkowska et al., 1988). However, long-term studies of patients with Klinefelter syndrome from birth to late adolescence and early adulthood suggest that many have verbal, cognitive, and attention deficits that lead to poor school performance and other difficulties (reviewed in Mandoki et al., 1991). Robinson and colleagues (1990) followed 105 males with Klinefelter syndrome from the newborn period and reported that between 60% and 86% received special education support for dyslexia, reading comprehension, and math. Stewart et al. (1990) noted that the proportion of boys with documented cognitive and learning disabilities increased as they entered adolescence (see also Rovet et al., 1996).

There is a growing awareness that the cognitive and behavioral effects of Klinefelter syndrome are subtle and may not be completely understood (reviewed in Geschwind et al., 2000). Young men with Klinefelter syndrome may be more passive and less assertive than other men their age (Theilgaard, 1984). Many adolescents report difficulties with sports and other academic pursuits and appear to have less success in other school activities (Robinson et al., 1990). Clinical depression, bipolar disorder, and other psychiatric disorders have also been described, but most boys and young men do not have overt psychiatric problems that necessitate therapy (Everman and Stoudemire, 1994; Bender et al., 1999). Intelligence scores are lower for males with Klinefelter syndrome but may vary by the chromosomal constitution, as polysomic X males, such as 48,XXXY or 49,XXXXY, will have lower IQ scores than men with 47,XXY or mosaic 46,XY/47,XXY karyotypes (Robinson et al., 1990).

Work performance and adjustment to adult life has not been well-studied. Surveys of adult patients with Klinefelter syndrome suggest that the prevalence of slight to moderate mental retardation is 3.8% (Kleczkowska et al., 1988), and early studies of institutionalized patients showed 1.5% of men were chromatin positive (Barr et al., 1960). Subsequent studies using blood chromosome analysis show that 15% of hypogonadal institutionalized men are 47,XXY (Pecile and Filippi, 1991), although this prevalence was not compared to a control population of men with small testicular size. The older literature also suggested that men with sex chromosome anomalies, such as 47,XXY and 47,XYY, are predisposed toward criminal behavior (Witkin et al., 1976). However, this impression was most likely due to bias of ascertainment, as later studies did not support this finding for 47,XXY males (Theilgaard, 1984). As with other features of the syndrome, intellectual functioning and psychosocial adjustment are variable and are influenced by other genetic and social factors.

Other Associated Disorders

Autoimmune disorders, such as thyroid disease, systemic lupus erythematosus (SLE), rheumatoid arthritis, and Sjogren syndrome have been reported in persons with Klinefelter syndrome (Olsen and Kovacs, 1995; Kobayashi et al., 1994). No large-scale survey of this association has been published, and it is not clear whether the occurrence of these conditions may be due to the relatively high frequency of Klinefelter syndrome in the general male population. In some cases, monozygotic twins with Klinefelter syndrome have been discordant for SLE, supporting a coincidental association (Schlegelberger et al., 1984). However, testosterone treatment in two patients with Klinefelter syndrome and SLE and three patients with Sjogren syndrome resulted in a clinical remission of their disease and normalization of the abnormal T cell profile (Bizzarro et al., 1987). KoÇar and colleagues (2000) showed lower serum concentration of IgA, IgG, IgM, IL-2, and IL-4 in 26 men with Klinefelter syndrome after six months of androgen therapy. Diabetes mellitus has also been reported in men with Klinefelter syndrome (Hsueh et al., 1978), and these men can have biochemical evidence of insulin resistance (Pei et al., 1998). Seizures have also been infrequently reported in males with Klinefelter syndrome and mental retardation (Elia et al., 1995; Tatum, et al., 1998).

Management

The primary goal of treatment for Klinefelter syndrome is to correct the androgen deficiency with testosterone replacement (Paulsen and Plymate, 1992; Matsumoto, 1994; Robinson et al., 2001). As the male with Klinefelter syndrome ages, testosterone levels decline and the estradiol/testosterone ratio increases (Raboch et al., 1975; Gabrilove et al., 1979), which will continue to negatively affect muscle mass and bone strength while promoting the development of gynecomastia (Winter, 1990). Treatment with human chorionic gonadotropin (hCH) stimulates testosterone production in men with Klinefelter syndrome for a short period of time (Hirsch et al., 1984; Winter, 1990) but is not used for sustained therapy.

Case studies of testosterone injections in men with Klinefelter syndrome have shown an increase in facial and body hair, a more masculine distribution of body fat, and increased libido, as well as greater strength and higher bone mineral density (Myhre et al., 1970; Nielsen et al., 1988). A survey of 110 adult men with Klinefelter syndrome showed lower sexual activity than in normal controls (Raboch et al., 1979), and this may improve with testosterone therapy. The beneficial effects of supplemental testosterone were also supported by a double-blind, cross-over study of men with other forms of hypogonadism, who reported an improvement of fatigue, mood, and sexual activity (Skakkebaek et al., 1981). Testosterone replacement should optimally begin at 11 to 12 years when boys are entering puberty in order to enhance secondary sexual characteristics, increase bone and muscle strength, and improve behavior and social adjustment (Myhre et al., 1970; Nielsen et al., 1988; Robinson et al., 1990; Mandoki and Sumner, 1991). Supplemental testosterone should also begin at the time of diagnosis for those men who are identified later in adult life.

The goal of therapy is to maintain serum testosterone levels within age-appropriate values (Winter, 1990), and the usual route is by intramuscular injections of testosterone undecanoate, a testosterone ester. Dosages are between 100 and 200 mg every two to four weeks for the adolescent male and increase to 200 mg every two weeks for the adult male. Newer methods using scrotal and transdermal testosterone patches have been developed to provide a constant, physiologic source of testosterone that mimics the normal daily variation of physiologic testosterone (Korenman et al., 1987; Meikle et al., 1998). Hypogonadal men have reported improvement of sexual functioning while using the transdermal patch (Arver et al., 1996).

Compression fractures of the spinal column and fractures of long bones can result from osteoporosis. Thus, prevention of osteoporosis is another reason that exogenous testosterone is advocated for men with 47,XXY. However, the efficacy of this therapy on reversing osteoporosis is controversial. Studies have shown normalization of bone density of the spine in 20 subjects with Klinefelter syndrome (Choi et al., 1995), while a study of 42 males with Klinefelter syndrome showed no benefit to bone density if treatment was initiated after age 20 (Kubler et al., 1992). Similarly, Wong and colleagues (1993) showed no improvement in 14 men with Klinefelter syndrome who had been on long-term testosterone therapy. A larger study of 52 men with Klinefelter syndrome showed over half continued to have measurable deficiencies in bone mineral density after long-term androgen therapy (van den Bergh et al., 2001). A case report of an infertile man with mosaic Klinefelter syndrome showed a marked increase in bone mineral density after initiation of therapy (Yamauchi et al., 1998). These studies suggest that osteoporosis may be reversible for selected patients, but replacement therapy should at least maintain current bone density of adult patients (Leifke et al., 1998).

Unfortunately, testosterone replacement does not reverse the primary testicular failure and infertility found in the majority of men with Klinefelter syndrome. Supplemental testosterone has been shown to increase prostatic volume without a change in testicular volume in hypogonadal men (Ozata et al., 1997). Thus, adoption or artificial insemination using donor sperm have been the standard options for those men who wish to complete their families. However, newer methods using intracytoplasmic sperm injection (ICSI) are currently under investigation to assist infertile men in fathering children (Bourne et al., 1995). After sperm are collected by using testicular or epididymal sperm extraction, they are injected into the oocyte and the fertilized egg is later implanted to achieve a pregnancy (Hovatta et al., 1995; Tournaye et al., 1995; Bourne et al., 1997).

ICSI has been used successfully for many disorders that cause male infertility, including Klinefelter syndrome (reviewed in Bourne et al., 1995; Hovatta et al., 1995; Johnson, 1998). Studies of testicular biopsies and sperm extraction on men with non-mosaic forms of Klinefelter syndrome have shown viable sperm in 40 to 50% of cases (Tournaye et al., 1996; Levron et al., 2000). This technique has resulted in both viable pregnancies and liveborn children to infertile men with non-mosaic Klinefelter syndrome (Ron-El et al., 1993; Bourne et al., 1997; Hinney et al., 1997; Palermo et al., 1998; Reubinoff et al., 1998; Levron et al., 2000), and there is a suggestion that men with mosaic forms of Klinefelter syndrome will have higher success rates using this approach (Harari et al., 1995). If couples choose to use the ICSI option, chromosomes should be repeated on both parents, and prenatal or pre-implantation diagnosis should be offered to exclude the possibility of aneuploidy (Tournaye et al., 1996; Meschede and Horst, 1997; Meschede et al., 1998).

All couples who are considering advanced reproductive techniques for male infertility due to Klinefelter syndrome should receive genetic counseling and information before the procedure (Johnson, 1998). The chromosomal abnormality in Klinefelter syndrome and the potential for transmitting a similar chromosomal abnormality to the offspring should be reviewed in detail (Kim et al., 1998). For example, men with Klinefelter syndrome appear to undergo male meiosis (Cozzi et al., 1994), but an increased rate of aneuploidy has been found on examination of sperm produced by mosaic and non-mosaic men with Klinefelter syndrome (Pandiyan and Jequier, 1996; Foresta et al., 1998; Johnson, 1998; Kruse et al., 1998; Levron et al., 2000). Indeed, a fetus with a 47,XXY karyotype was reported after ICSI from a man with non-mosaic Klinefelter syndrome (Ron-El et al., 2000). Thus, Meschede et al. (1998) suggest that the chance for a subsequent fetus to have a sex chromosome anomaly is higher for men with Klinefelter syndrome than with a naturally occurring pregnancy, although no long-term studies are available. Other authors suggest that pre-implantation chromosomal diagnosis be performed as part of the ICSI protocol (Staessen et al., 1996; Kruse et al., 1998).

Genetics

The initial observation of an additional X chromosome to the normal male complement was later supported by others who showed that these individuals were phenotypically male (Ford et al., 1959; Jacobs and Strong, 1959). Subsequently, Nielsen and Wohlert (1990) documented Klinefelter syndrome in 1 of 596 male infants in a 13-year study of consecutive newborn infants. This study also confirmed other variant chromosomal forms of Klinefelter syndrome. Of the 17,872 liveborn boys, 20 had 47,XXY, 7 had 46,XX (male), and 2 had 48,XXYY karyotypes. Kleczkowska and colleagues (1988) reported the karyotypes of 569 males with Klinefelter syndrome collected over a 21-year period and found that the majority (522, or 92%) had 47,XXY, 15 patients had a mosaic pattern, and 1 case each had the 47,XXY constitution associated with autosomal rearrangements, inversions, or translocations. The most frequent mosaic pattern was 46,XX/47,XXY, and another 25 patients had a variety of X chromosome polysomies, such as 48,XXXY and 49,XXXXY. Thus, while the majority of males with Klinefelter syndrome have a 47,XXY constitutional karyotype, there are some individuals with variant karyotypes.

Chromosomal and molecular studies of samples from males with non-mosaic 47,XXY have shown that the major defect is due to non-disjunction of the X chromosome in either oogenesis or spermatogenesis. The parental origin of the additional X chromosome is paternal in approximately 50% of cases and maternal in the other 50%, and postnatal nondisjunction causes a small proportion of cases (Jacobs et al., 1988b). Harvey and colleagues (1990) studied a series of 61 newborns and 50 clinically recognized patients with Klinefelter syndrome and found 44% and 54% paternally derived X chromosomes, respectively. Of the cases in which the extra X chromosome was maternally derived, the majority (72%) resulted from an error in the first meiotic division. Other studies have confirmed the parental derivation of the additional X chromosome in patients with 47, XXY (Lorda-Sanchez et al., 1992b), as well as patients with multiple copies of the X chromosome (Lorda-Sanchez, et al., 1992a).

Differences in parental age of mothers with sons who have Klinefelter syndrome may be a factor in some cases of 47,XXY. Carothers and Filippi (1988) reviewed the parental ages of 151 males with Klinefelter syndrome and found an association with maternal but not paternal age at delivery. Of 33 cases, 19 were maternal and 14 were paternal. In addition, maternal age in the maternally derived cases was significantly older that the mothers of controls or the paternally derived cases. Other studies have also shown an association of Klinefelter syndrome with advanced maternal age due to maternal meiosis I errors but not with maternal meiosis II errors (Jacobs et al., 1988b; Harvey et al., 1990) or paternal age (Carothers et al., 1984).

These issues are of primary importance for genetic counseling of patients with 47,XXY karyotypes but have little effect on the clinical management for most males with this disorder. In general, there are no apparent differences in the clinical outcome due to the parental derivation of the additional X chromosome or the age of the parent (Harvey et al., 1990). There are reports of an increased association between Fragile-X syndrome and Klinefelter syndrome (Filippi et al., 1988). However, this seems to be due to the coincidental occurrence of a common X-linked trait and maternal nondisjunction in the affected cases (Kupke et al., 1991; Pecile and Filippi 1991), and not due to the excess of X chromosomal material (Jacobs et al., 1988a; Jenkins et al., 1994).

Variant Forms of Klinefelter Syndrome

Cytogenetic studies reveal that alternate mosaic karyotypes can occur in up to 20% of men with Klinefelter syndrome, most commonly the 46,XY/47,XXY mosaic karyotype. Individuals with this chromosomal constitution can exhibit a milder phenotype, presumably due to the presence of a normal cell line. However, there can be great variability in the clinical features of testicular size, infertility, decreased bone density, and cognitive and intellectual performance, depending on the proportion of mosaic cells (Robinson et al., 1990). Other variant forms have been identified with X chromosome polysomy, such as 48,XXXY or 49,XXXXY, that usually arise from consecutive nondisjunction events in either oogenesis or spermatogenesis. Some authors distinguish the 49,XXXXY syndrome as a separate and distinct phenotype due to X chromosome polysomy (Peet et al., 1998). It occurs in about 1 in 85,000 births (Kleczkowska et al., 1988). In addition to hypogonadism and small testes as seen in 47,XXY, these males have a small penis, microcephaly, radio-ulnar synostosis and other skeletal anomalies, and a more severe degree of mental impairment and speech delay. Males with 48,XXYY or isochromosome Xq (Arps et al., 1996) have also been identified and are generally considered to have a variant of Klinefelter syndrome (Paulsen and Plymate, 1992). These individuals can have a more severe phenotype compared to boys and men with 47,XXY karyotype. Thus, management of the variant forms of Klinefelter syndrome must be individualized based on the underlying karyotypic abnormalities.

TURNER SYNDROME

Turner (1938) first reported seven females with short stature, nuchal webbing, cubitus valgus, and sexual infantilism over 60 years ago. Since then, numerous reports have described Turner syndrome in all races worldwide, and the constellation of findings now includes gonadal dysgenesis, lymphedema, typical facial features, and short stature. The cytogenetic abnormality in Turner syndrome was identified in 1959 by Ford and colleagues, who described a female with gonadal dysgenesis and the loss of an X chromosome. Turner syndrome occurs in 1 of 2500 liveborn females based on screening of newborns (Jacobs et al., 1974; Hook and Warburton, 1983), and is caused by the loss of one of the pair of sex chromosomes (45,X), a deletion of part of all of the short arm of an X chromosome, or a mosaic complement where one cell line has lost one of the pair of sex chromosomes. This disorder is important to the practicing physician because it is common in the general population, requires lifelong management, and can escape diagnosis well into adulthood (Hall, 1992; Toth and Jogerst, 1996).

Diagnostic Criteria

While there are no standard clinical criteria for Turner syndrome, the diagnosis should be considered in any female with the combination of short stature and primary or secondary ovarian failure, with or without lymphedema. However, recent studies have detected karyotypic abnormalities of the X chromosome in a proportion of girls and women with less pronounced physical features. Most experts agree that the diagnosis should be based on a cytogenetic analysis of blood or other tissue. Relying on a buccal smear for Barr body analysis is not adequate for the diagnosis. As with other types of sex chromosome aneuploidy, patients with Turner syndrome can also have mosaic patterns, although there may be wide variability in the proportion of mosaicism (Park et al., 1999). They can also have a deletion of the short or long arm of the X chromosome, an isochromosome X (46,X,i(Xq)), or ring X pattern. In addition, a minority (5%) of females with Turner syndrome has a mosaic cell line bearing Y chromosomal material (Vlasak et al., 1999). Special molecular tests, including FISH and PCR, should be added to the standard

Table 53–4. Physical Findings in Turner Syndrome

Area of Involvement	Manifestation
Craniofacial	Triangular face, downslanting palpebral fissures, epicanthal folds, midface hypoplasia, cupped ears, high arched palate
Neck, trunk, and spine	Short neck with posterior webbing and low hairline, broad chest, hypoplastic wide-spaced nipples
Genitalia	Lack of secondary sexual characteristics, hypoplastic vaginal vault
Extremities	Edema, especially in the hands and feet, increased carrying angle of upper extremities, short fourth metacarpal, nail hypoplasia
Body habitus	Short stature, truncal obesity, short legs and spine
Other	Nevi, hearing impairment

Source: Adapted from Hall (1992) with permission.

karyotype in females with a ring chromosome or evidence of masculinization to determine whether Y material is present.

Clinical Findings

Women with Turner syndrome are classically described as having short stature with a triangular face, downslanting palpebral fissures, epicanthal folds, ptosis, high arched palate, webbed neck, broad or "shield" chest, hypoplastic nipples, and lymphedema of the hands and feet (Hall, 1992) (Table 53–4). Figure 53–4 illustrates the typical features of adult women with Turner syndrome. While most women with Turner syndrome are identified during childhood or adolescence because of poor growth, characteristic physical features, or primary amenorrhea, a small proportion are identified during adulthood. About 8% of women presenting with ovarian failure are identified as having Turner syndrome, suggesting that the diagnosis is often unrecognized by physicians (Wu et al., 1993). In addition, case reports have described the identification of women with previously unrecognized Turner syndrome during an analysis of fetal loss or pregnancy complications (Wu et al., 1993). Thus, the diagnosis should be considered in women with a less obvious or less severe presentation (Savendahl and Davenport, 2000). The following sections highlight the relevant clinical manifestations in adult women with Turner syndrome (reviewed in Elsheikh et al., 1999). Excellent review articles are available that address the clinical aspects of Turner syndrome in infants and children (American Academy of Pediatrics, Committee on Genetics, 1995; Saenger, 1993).

Growth and Physical Development

Short stature and growth failure are the cardinal physical features of Turner syndrome. The tendency to be small is evident at birth, where most newborns are in the third to tenth percentile

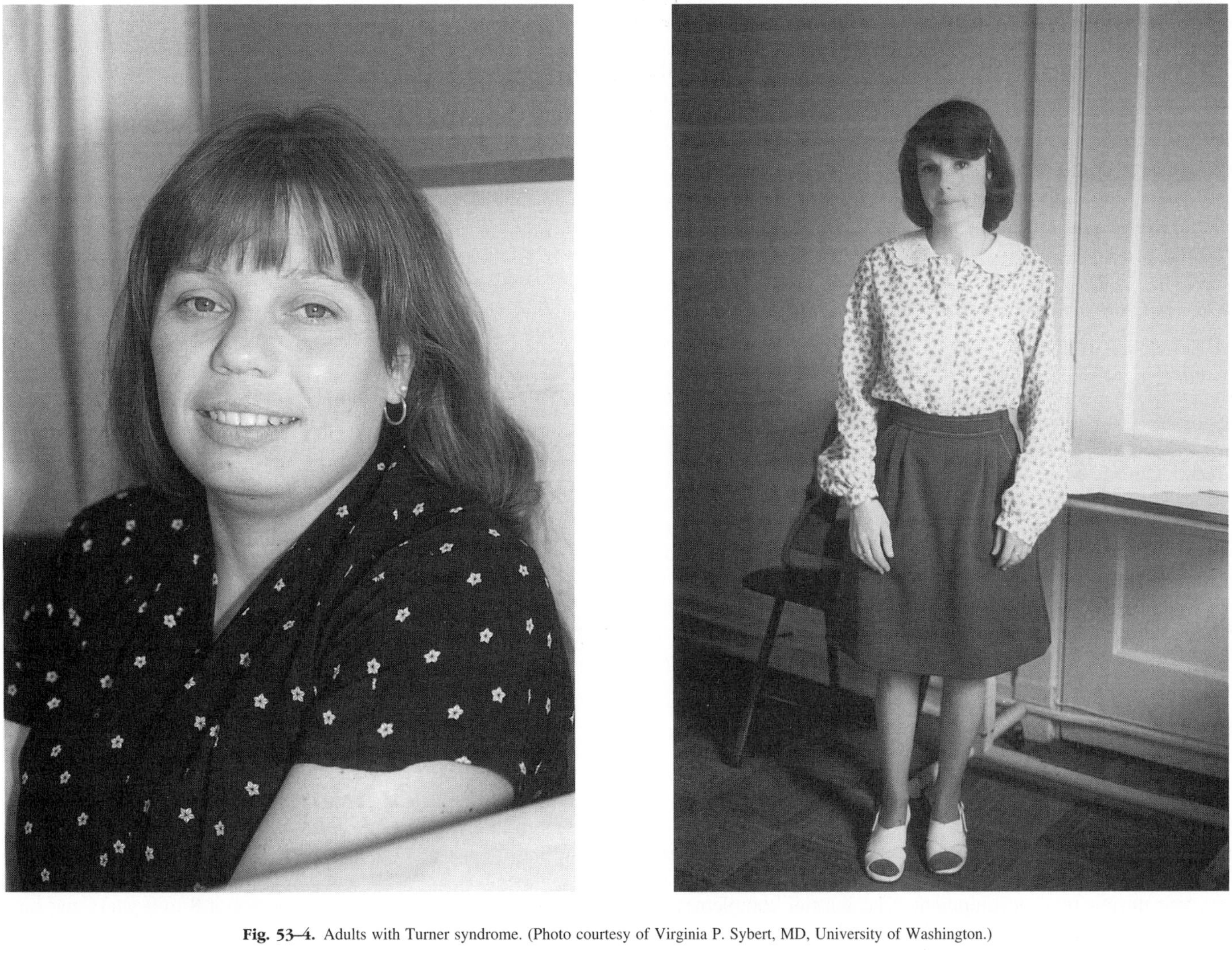

Fig. 53–4. Adults with Turner syndrome. (Photo courtesy of Virginia P. Sybert, MD, University of Washington.)

for length. As the girl with Turner syndrome develops, the rate of growth declines, and with the absence of the prepubertal growth spurt, her height will fall below the third percentile. Most girls with Turner syndrome will be 20 to 25 cm below the mean at age 12 and 30 cm below the mean at the end of the second decade (Lyon et al., 1985). Along with short stature, adult women with Turner syndrome have disproportionate skeletal features with a broad chest, large waist, and short legs. The weight/height ratio increases in childhood, and obesity can often be a continuing problem for adult women with Turner syndrome.

The short stature in Turner syndrome has been attributed to estrogen deficiency, skeletal dysplasia, and possible underlying growth hormone deficiency during development. While growth hormone production is generally normal, there are a few case reports documenting true growth hormone deficiency (Butenandt, 1980). Other studies have suggested that girls with Turner syndrome have an abnormal response to the effect of physiologic levels of growth hormone. The underlying karyotypic constitution may also influence linear growth velocity and final adult height, as mosaic females are taller than non-mosaic females (Hall, 1992).

As with the general population, final adult height is influenced by other factors, such as parental stature, nutritional status, and the presence of other endocrine abnormalities. In the future, physicians who care for adult patients need to be aware that a significant proportion of women with Turner syndrome may have been treated as girls with a regimen of growth hormone or growth hormone and anabolic steroids to increase the final adult height (Haeusler et al., 1996). However, the effectiveness of these strategies for improved linear growth have not been proven (Donaldson, 1996), as some studies showed gains (Rosenfeld et al., 1998; Chernausek et al., 2000) and others did not (Dacou-Voutetakis et al., 1998). A randomized trial of the effectiveness of growth hormone, ethinyloestradiol, and growth hormone and ethinyloestradiol therapy on the height of 58 girls with Turner syndrome showed that the greatest gain in height correlated with younger age and greater initial height deficit (Johnston et al., 2001).

Skeletal Abnormalities and Osteoporosis

The skeletal dysplasia found in girls and women with Turner syndrome is generally mild. Abnormalities are found in the bones of the hands and feet, vertebrae, long bones, pelvis, and cranium. Scoliosis is a frequent finding (10%–15%) in childhood and may be exacerbated by estrogen therapy in early adolescence (Hall, 1992). Chronic knee pain can result from patellar dislocation due to an abnormal tibial plateau. The elbow displays an increased carrying angle, which can interfere with joint mobility. Decreased bone density and osteopenia have been documented in females with Turner syndrome and are most likely due to the lack of estrogen during growth. Bone density has been shown to increase with the use of estrogens (Park, 1977) and may increase with combined growth hormone and estrogen therapy (Lanes et al., 1999; Sas et al., 2001). A longitudinal population-based study of women with Turner syndrome showed a higher risk for fractures in girls and women (Gravholt et al., 1998a); however, loss of height due to osteoporosis has not been documented.

Gonadal Dysgenesis and Infertility

Primary or secondary amenorrhea is a cardinal feature of Turner syndrome and results from ovarian failure that is histologically evident during fetal development. The normal complement of oocytes rapidly decreases in number, so that there are few remaining ova at birth. Thus, most newborns with Turner syndrome will have fibrotic "streak" gonads in place of normal ovarian tissue. In addition, these infants will have lost the normal pituitary feedback, so that FSH and LH levels may be markedly high at birth before the normal hypothalamic down-regulation that is found between the ages of 3 and 8 years (Hall, 1992).

The elevation of gonadotropins at puberty is abnormal in the majority of girls with Turner syndrome. However, approximately 10% of non-mosaic women and up to 20% of mosaic women will spontaneously initiate puberty with subsequent development of secondary sexual characteristics and the onset of menses (Pasquino et al., 1997). Breast development is usually poor, especially in young adolescents, with small or inverted nipples. Of young women who spontaneously enter puberty, most will have premature ovarian failure later in life, so that continued evaluation of hormonal status in women with Turner syndrome is warranted. Infertility or recurrent pregnancy loss should alert clinicians to the diagnosis. In one study, five (8.2%) out of 61 women with premature ovarian failure and 6 (2.9%) of 105 female partners in couples who had recurrent abortions were found to have mosaic karyotypes with abnormalities of the X chromosome, including 45,X/46,XX/47,XXX, and 45,X/46,X mosaic patterns (Wu et al., 1993).

It is estimated that only 2% of all women with Turner syndrome will spontaneously conceive (Tarani et al., 1998). Pregnancies resulting in liveborn children primarily occur in women who undergo spontaneous puberty and have ongoing menses. By the late 1980s only 13 cases of spontaneous pregnancies in apparently non-mosaic women had been reported (Kaneko et al., 1990). However, these women may have had cryptic mosaic gonadal tissue, since subsequent case reports have identified mosaicism in other tissues using newer more sensitive molecular methods (James et al., 1997; Magee et al., 1998). Follow-up of 46 pregnancies in mothers with Turner syndrome suggest a high proportion of fetal loss (48%) and chromosomal abnormalities in liveborn children (30%), including 3 cases of Down syndrome (King et al., 1978). A subsequent review of 160 pregnancies in 74 women with Turner syndrome also indicated a high rate of fetal loss and birth defects and estimated that only 38% of pregnancies would result in a normal liveborn child (Tarani et al., 1998).

Endocrine and Autoimmune Aspects

Hypothyroidism is commonly found in Turner syndrome during all stages of life and may have an autoimmune basis. Hashimoto's thyroiditis has been identified in up to 34% of cases, and leads to hypothyroidism in 10% to15% of females with Turner syndrome (Saenger, 1996). Diabetes mellitus due to insulin resistance is found in 5%, but up to 27% of females with Turner syndrome have abnormal glucose tolerance tests. The response to glucose may be aggravated by the use of estrogen replacement and by obesity. A Danish population-based study of Turner syndrome found a high incidence of both insulin-dependent diabetes mellitus and non-insulin-dependent diabetes mellitus (Gravholt et al., 1998a).

Malignancy Aspects

Females with Turner syndrome with a mosaic karyotype that includes a Y-bearing cell line face a significant risk for gonadoblastoma or other malignancy in the rudimentary gonad. Gonadoblastomas have been reported in early childhood, but it appears that the risk begins to increase at 8 to 9 years and continues to be elevated into adulthood. The link between mosaic cell lines with Y chromosomal material and the development of gonadoblastoma is supported by FISH analyses of tumors that demonstrate florescence of the Y chromosome in gonadal tumor tissue from individuals with gonadoblastoma and Turner syndrome (De Arce et al., 1992). While the likelihood of developing cancer has been estimated to be between 25% and 35% by age 30 for individuals with Y chromosomal material, a recent population-based study suggests that the rate may be on the order of 7% to 10% (Gravholt et al., 2000). In some cases, the Y chromosome material is not present using molecular analyses, leading to the rare occurrence of apparently monosomic 45,X individuals and gonadal tumors (Pierga et al., 1994). Nevertheless, prophylactic bilateral gonadectomy is usually recommended to women with Turner syndrome and documented Y chromosomal material to reduce the risk of this rare cancer.

Hasle and colleagues (1996) surveyed the risk for cancer in 597 females with Turner syndrome and found no overall increase in cancer risk compared to the general population. In addition, no instances of gonodoblastoma were identified in this cohort. Hall (1992) notes that numerous case reports have noted the occurrence of Turner syndrome and various types of cancer, including chronic myelogenous leukemia, virilizing hilus cell tumor, basal cell carcinoma, eosinophilic adenoma, thymoma, neural crest-derived tumors, bladder carcinoma, Wilms tumor, and colon cancer. Most of these cancers are coincidental and do not reflect an increased risk for malignancy. However, the risk for endometrial cancer may be high in women with Turner syndrome who receive estrogen replacement (Clement and Young, 1987).

Cardiovascular and Lymphatic Abnormalities

The majority of children and adults with Turner syndrome will have either a structural or an acquired cardiovascular abnormality that necessitates ongoing medical evaluation and treatment. Bicuspid aortic valve is the most common structural lesion and occurs in 30% to 50% of adults, depending on the population studied. Coarctation of the aorta is the most common cardiac defect identified in children and can be found in 20% of newborns. Other structural lesions have been reported, including mitral valve prolapse (MVP) and aortic aneurysms. One study reported MVP in nearly 25% of women with Turner syndrome, so that yearly echocardiograms are recommended. Lin and colleagues (1986) documented aortic root dilation in 8.8% of 57 patients with Turner syndrome and reported two patients with aortic dissection. Subsequent studies have suggested that aortic dilatation may occur in up to 42% of women with Turner syndrome (Elsheikh et al., 2001). Systemic hypertension, coarctation, and bicuspid aortic valves are risk factors for aortic aneurysms and dissection in this disorder, but they may not be found in all individuals with Turner syndrome who exhibit aortic root dilation (Bordeleau et al., 1998; Lin et al., 1998; Elsheikh et al., 2001).

Lymphedema is often a striking finding; it can cause severe hydrops and fetal demise, cystic hygroma in utero, and nuchal folds leading to neck webbing that may be identifiable at birth and later in life. Infants will often have puffy hands and feet, and this is the initial presentation in 80% of cases identified in the newborn period. Congenital hypoplasia of the lymphatics due to delay in canalization of the lymph channels is thought to be the cause of persistent lymphedema (Hall 1992). For the majority of persons with Turner syndrome, the peripheral lymphedema resolves in childhood. However, the use of estrogen replacement may aggravate this condition in a minority of adolescents and adults. Females with non-mosaic 45,X karyotype exhibit lymphedema more frequently than do those with mosaic or other cytogenetic forms of Turner syndrome.

Essential hypertension is a common problem for women with Turner syndrome and is found in about 20% of adults. The elevation in blood pressure can often be severe, with diastolic measurements over 100 mm Hg. Hypertension combined with aortic root dilatation has been shown to be a strong predictor of aortic root dissection in women with Turner syndrome (Elsheikh et al., 2001). Women with structural renal abnormalities have the highest risk for systemic hypertension, but these abnormalities may not be the underlying cause in the majority of women with Turner syndrome and high blood pressure. The hypertension may be caused by lipid abnormalities and obesity, although there is limited long-term information on adults for this (Gravholt et al., 1998b).

Psychosocial Development and Adjustment

Several studies have documented that girls with Turner syndrome have learning disabilities, although frank mental retardation is rare (reviewed by Ross et al., 2000b). Rovet (1995) compared over 200 girls with Turner syndrome to a control group of aged matched girls and found a small but statistical difference in mean IQ (94.6 vs. 103.9, respectively). School performance is usually adequate in written language, but the majority of girls with Turner syndrome have difficulties with mathematics (Rovet, 1995). Cognitive deficits have also been described in visual memory, spatial reasoning, and executive function, all of which may underlie the difficulties in math (Mazzocco, 1998). Girls may also have difficulties with fine and gross motor activities.

Most adolescents and adults with Turner syndrome are well adjusted, and there is little evidence for psychopathology. A survey of 20 adults with Turner syndrome showed one individual with hypomanic bipolar disorder. However, 50% of this group reported low self-confidence (Delooz et al., 1993). Similar feelings were expressed by a group of middle-aged woman with Turner syndrome. This group also reported negative feelings associated with infertility, which improved with the addition of hormone replacement therapy (Sylven et al., 1993). Sexual development is normal, although the initiation of sexual activity occurs at an average age of 19.5 years. Painful intercourse has been reported and may be secondary to hypoplastic vaginal vault or inadequate estrogen replacement.

Other Associated Disorders

Hearing deficits are common in adult women with Turner syndrome. Hultcrantz and colleagues (1994) found a surprisingly high frequency (90%) of sensorineural hearing loss when they tested 44 adult patients with Turner syndrome. The hearing deficit may be progressive, as 27% require hearing aids. Hearing problems are not as prevalent in childhood, although recurrent otitis media, probably due to structural craniofacial abnormalities, is a frequent problem (Gungor et al., 2000).

Genitourinary and structural renal disease are associated with Turner syndrome. Renal agenesis, horseshoe kidney, duplication of the collecting system, ureteropelvic and ureterovesicular obstruction, and aberrant renal arteries have been described, warranting renal ultrasound at the time of diagnosis. Reflux and subsequent urinary tract infections can be severe, although this is a rare complication.

Gastrointestinal problems are seen in increased frequency in all stages of life. Newborns often have gastrointestinal reflux and feeding difficulties, but this usually resolves in early infancy.

Table 53–5. Suggested Management Strategies for Adult Women with Turner Syndrome

Body System	Complication	Recommended Tests	Management
Gynecologic and reproductive	Gonadal dysgenesis, infertility, primary or secondary amenorrhea	FSH, LH prior to replacement therapy	Hormone replacement therapy with estrogen/ progesterone, fertility counseling, assisted reproduction
Cardiovascular	Hypertension, mitral valve prolapse, aortic aneurysm, undiagnosed aortic coarctation, lymphedema	Annual echocardiogram	Monitor blood pressure, endocarditis prophylaxis, regular dental care, consider cardiology referral
Endocrine	Hypothyroidism, insulin-resistant diabetes	Annual T4 and TSH, glucose	Insulin, oral hypoglycemic agents, weight management
	Obesity	Routine weight measurement; consider hypothyroidism in differential diagnosis	Nutritional management, exercise, thyroid hormone replacement if deficient
Gastrointestinal	Gastrointestinal bleeding due to vascular malformations	Colonoscopy or endoscopy if symptomatic	As indicated
Genitourinary	Structural anomalies	Renal ultrasound at diagnosis	As indicated
Hearing	Sensorineural hearing loss	Annual hearing evaluation	Hearing aids

Source: Adapted from Hall (1992) with permission.

Children and adults have been identified with vascular malformations of the gut, which lead to gastrointestinal bleeding. Telangiectases, venous malformations, and hemangiomas have all been described in the esophagus, stomach, and small and large bowel. Adults with Turner syndrome have an increased risk for inflammatory bowel disease. Four patients with either Crohn's disease or ulcerative colitis were identified in a series of 135 women with Turner syndrome (Arulanantham et al., 1980).

Management

Since the manifestations of Turner syndrome affect most major systems, women with this disorder require lifelong care and anticipatory management (Rosenfeld et al., 1994; Sybert, 2001). This section specifically reviews hormonal replacement, fertility, and endocrine management for women with Turner syndrome (Table 53–5). The strategies for children, including the use of growth hormone, are beyond the scope of this chapter, and the reader is referred to reviews by the Committee on Genetics of the American Academy of Pediatrics (1995) for a more detailed discussion of the relevant pediatric issues for Turner syndrome.

The major management issues for women with Turner syndrome are the effects of gonadal dysgenesis and subsequent ovarian failure, since it is rare for women with Turner syndrome to continue to have adequate ovarian function throughout life. Most women with Turner syndrome will require estrogen replacement therapy, which should ideally begin in adolescence and continue throughout life. For adolescent girls, the initiation of hormone replacement therapy should be adjusted by other treatment regimens for short stature, such as growth hormone. If a prepubertal girl did not receive growth hormone, some experts suggest that estrogen therapy should be delayed to 14 years of age to prolong the period of skeletal growth.

For women who are diagnosed with Turner syndrome in adulthood, estrogen treatment should be instituted immediately at the lowest effective dosage to mimic normal physiology, and estrogen should be used with progesterone to decrease the development of endometrial hyperplasia and to lower the risk for endometrial cancer. Alternatively, transdermal estrogen and estrogen vaginal creams are available, although little is known about the optimal preparation for women with Turner syndrome (Conway, 2001). A recent study of 17 young adult women with Turner syndrome directly compared low-dose to high-dose estrogen preparations, suggesting that higher doses are required to treat osteoporosis and liver function abnormalities (Guttmann et al., 2001). There are no published studies that have looked at the optimal duration of estrogen therapy, so no firm recommendations are available. Some experts have suggested that replacement be withdrawn at the time when menopause would have normally occurred (Hall, 1992), while others suggest that women with Turner syndrome be treated much as other postmenopausal women with continued hormone replacement therapy.

Infertility is the rule, and spontaneous pregnancy occurs in only about 2% of all women with Turner syndrome (Tarani et al., 1998). Newer reproductive options, such as gamete intrafallopian tube implantation (GIFT) or in vitro fertilization (IVF) have been used for a small number of women with Turner syndrome (Khastgir et al., 1997). Foudila and colleagues (1999) reported on 18 women with mosaic and non-mosaic forms of Turner syndrome who had undergone assisted reproduction with donor oocytes and reported a similar fertilization and implantation rate to women with other forms of ovarian failure. A higher rate of the viable pregnancies miscarried (40%), which was attributed to uterine and cardiovascular factors. In some mosaic women with normal FSH levels, assisted reproduction with retrieval of their own ova by ovarian biopsy is also possible (Ditkoff et al., 1996). Collection and storage of eggs for future use has been advocated for women with Turner syndrome, but there have not been any studies directly examining this option (Hovatta, 1999). In addition, pregnancy using these techniques may pose additional cardiovascular risks for women with Turner syndrome, as there have been reports of aortic dissection in two women who underwent gamete intrafallopian transfer of donor eggs (Lin et al., 1998).

Genetic counseling should be provided to patients with Turner syndrome and their families. Any woman with this disorder should learn the chromosomal basis of the disease, natural history, and management strategies at the time of diagnosis. As mentioned previously, infertility is a difficult issue for most women with Turner syndrome. However, the newer reproductive options, including in vitro fertilization, may offer a chance to bear children. At this time, the cardiovascular complications of pregnancy and the expense of such procedures should be reviewed. Women with Turner syndrome who are able to spontaneously conceive have a high rate of fetal demise as well as of liveborn children with chromosomal abnormalities. Prenatal diagnosis and genetic counseling should be offered to these individuals.

Genetics

The association between Turner syndrome and the loss of all or part of a sex chromosome from the normal female complement was first identified in 1959 by Ford and colleagues. Subsequent studies have confirmed the chromosomal basis of the disorder by examining the karyotypes of circulating lymphocytes and other tissues. The 45,X karyotype is found in about half of women with Turner syndrome, while the remainder is composed of individuals with a mosaic pattern, isochromosome Xq, or a deletion of the short or long arm of the X chromosome (Hook and Warbartun, 1983; Nielsen and Wohlert, 1990; Fernandez-Garcia et al., 2000). An isochromosome Xq, in which there is a loss of the short (p) arm and a duplication of the long (q) arm, is found in 10% to 20% of Turner syndrome cases. The presence of both a cell line with 45,X and a cell line with 46,XX is found in about 30% to 40% of females with Turner syndrome, and 2% to 5% have a combination of 45,X and 46,XY cell lines.

The loss of an intact X chromosome is the result of a pre- or postzygotic non-disjunction event of the sex chromosomes. The incidence of Turner syndrome does not increase with advancing maternal or paternal age, but between 60% and 85% of liveborn females with Turner syndrome have lost a paternally derived sex chromosome (Mathur et al., 1991; Hassold et al., 1992; Larsen et al., 1995). Cytogenetic analysis of the products of conception shows that approximately 1% of all conceptuses have Turner syndrome. In addition, the majority (98%) of these fetuses will spontaneously abort, suggesting that this sex chromosome complement is lethal in most cases. Due to the lymphatic abnormalities, some fetuses will develop hydrops or a nuchal mass that can be identified by ultrasound. Prenatal diagnosis should be considered in these circumstances for management of pregnancy, labor, and delivery.

In general, the severity of the condition is inversely related to the degree of mosaicism of the normal cell line (46,XX) (Sarkar and Marimuthu, 1983). The cardinal features of short stature and gonadal dysgenesis appear to depend on the presence of a monosomy X cell line and are not predictive of the underlying karyotypic abnormality. Other karyotype–phenotype correlations have been suggested by studies of women with nonmosaic structural X chromosome abnormalities. Terminal or interstitial deletions of the long arm of the X chromosome are found in women with short stature and either primary or secondary ovarian failure. Zinn and colleagues (1998) have identified a critical region on Xp11.2–p22.1 in a study of 22 women with interstitial Xp deletions and suggested that haploinsufficiency of genes in this region is associated with the neurocognitive phenotype (Ross et al., 2000a). However, there are case reports of women with normal stature who have deletions distal to Xq13 and of fertile women with interstitial deletions of Xq (Hall, 1992).

Mutations in the homeobox containing the SHOX gene located in the pseudoautosomal region in Xp22 may cause idiopathic short stature (Rao et al., 1997) or skeletal features seen in Turner syndrome such as Madelung deformity of the forearm (Yaegashi et al., 2000). Further, loss of both alleles of the SHOX gene is associated with prenatally diagnosed intra-uterine growth retardation in newborns with Turner syndrome (Yaegashi et al., 2000). However, the somatic effects of the loss of X chromosome material, including ovarian failure, may not be due to the presence or absence of specific genes (Hall, 1992). Recent studies suggest that the pattern of inactivation of the X chromosome may influence the outcome in females with Turner syndrome. X-chromosome inactivation occurs during normal female embryogenesis and has been found to be under the control of the XIST gene. A small proportion of females with Turner syndrome has a marker, or ring X, chromosome, that lacks the XIST gene and therefore cannot be inactivated. The more severe phenotype in these girls and women may be due to loss of the normal suppression of X chromosome material. Research correlating chromosomal regions with physical characteristics in Turner syndrome are ongoing.

It is important to note that mosaic patterns of 45,X/46,XX or 45,X/46,XY are very common and present a unique challenge to the laboratory in providing a correct diagnosis. In general, standard cytogenetic analysis of 20 cells is adequate. However, a search for a mosaic cell line by examining an additional 50 to 100 cells or analysis of cells obtained from a different tissue should be pursued if there are unexplained clinical features consistent with Turner syndrome but the standard blood chromosome study is normal, 46,XX. The presentation of a proportion of cells with Y chromosomal material deserves special consideration. The phenotypic presentation of these individuals ranges from a normal phenotypic male, to ambiguous genitalia, to a Turner syndrome phenotype (Reddy and Sulcova, 1998; Chang et al., 1990). Persons with Turner syndrome and a Y chromosome mosaic pattern are at an increased risk for gonadoblastoma so that sensitive methods using PCR or FISH have been developed to identify the presence of an occult Y chromosome. However, some studies suggest that the overall rate of cryptic Y material may be low. A study of 53 females with Turner syndrome without a karyotypically detected Y chromosome showed that only 2 (4%) had occult Y chromosomal material (Binder et al., 1995). In a recent study in which 208 patients with Turner syndrome were screened for Y chromosome sequences using PCR, occult Y chromosome sequences were identified in 12 (3%) (Vlasak et al., 1999).

MICRODELETION SYNDROMES

Microdeletion syndromes are recognizable conditions arising from deletions of small segments of DNA that are often only cytogenetically detectable by FISH. Such deletions involve a number of genes, any of which may contribute to the phenotype. Therefore, microdeletion syndromes are also referred to as contiguous gene syndromes. In many such disorders, haploinsufficiency of more than one gene is responsible for the manifestations of the disorder. Velo-cardio-facial syndrome, Prader-Willi syndrome, and Williams syndrome are among the most common microdeletion syndromes that are now being detected using FISH. Patients with each of these disorders may come to adulthood without having been diagnosed, and each is compatible with a long lifespan in a significant proportion of cases. Therefore, the clinician should be familiar with the circumstances under which these disorders should be suspected, the ways in which they can be identified in the clinical laboratory, and the medical and developmental issues that are associated with them.

Most microdeletion syndromes are now thought to share a common etiologic mechanism. Data are beginning to emerge to support the concept that these and other interstitial microdeletions arise through a common mechanism resulting from similar characteristics of the DNA at the breakpoints (Lupski, 1998). In several of the microdeletion syndromes, including the ones described below, the breakpoints have been found to be the same from person to person with the same disorder (Amos-Landgraf et al., 1999; Edelmann et al., 1999; Valero et al., 2000). Recent research suggests that the DNA at these breakpoints contains repetitive sequences. This run of repeated DNA sequences appears to predispose these spots to unequal crossing-over during meiosis, presumably resulting in looping-out and subsequent loss of the deleted segment. Therefore, the findings in individuals who have these deletions form a recognizable pattern. The following are the most common microdeletion syndromes likely to be seen in adults.

Velo-Cardio-Facial Syndrome

Velo-cardio-facial syndrome, also known as Shprintzen syndrome and previously as CATCH 22, is a highly variable multisystem disorder resulting from an interstitial microdeletion of chromosome 22q11.2. It occurs in 1 in 2000 to 1 in 4000 individuals, making it the most common microdeletion syndrome in humans (Burn and Goodship, 1996), and is compatible with a normal life span. Originally reported by Shprintzen et al. (1978, 1981), the major phenotypic findings involve the palate (velum), heart, and facial features—hence the name. Many of the affected tissues and structures are derived from the pharyngeal pouches of the developing embryo, but frequent manifestations also occur in a number of other systems, including the presence of learning disabilities and psychiatric problems in a significant percentage of affected patients. There are no obligatory or pathognomonic features.

As an indication of the frequency this disorder, one analysis of 1000 consecutive patients with clefting of the lip and/or palate showed that 5% of them had velo-cardio-facial syndrome, and 8% of the patients in the series who had cleft palate without cleft lip (including submucous cleft palate) had velo-cardio-facial syndrome (Shprintzen et al., 1985).

Diagnostic Criteria

There is no consensus on diagnostic criteria, in part because of the variability and pleiotropy of the disorder and in part because of the bias of ascertainment. However, there are some findings that are most distinctive. In two large studies, the most common findings were learning disability, cleft palate and pharyngeal hypotonia, cardiac anomalies, and slender tapering fingers (Goldberg et al., 1993; Ryan et al., 1997). Other frequent and clinically significant findings include hearing loss (mostly conductive), renal anomalies (absent, dysplastic, or multicystic kidneys; reflux; obstruction), and hypocalcemia primarily in early infancy. The latter not infrequently leads to seizures. There is considerable overlap between the features of velo-cardio-facial syndrome and the DiGeorge syndrome, which includes thymic hypoplasia, parathyroid hypoplasia leading to hypocalcemia, and outflow defects of the heart. DiGeorge syndrome is caused by the same microdeletion as velo-cardio-facial syndrome in 90% of cases, and thus the two disorders may not be distinct.

Clinical Findings

The characteristic facial appearance is subtle but distinctive (Fig. 53–5). There is a long, straight tubular nose with a somewhat bulbous tip, narrow palpebral fissures, and a somewhat small mandible. Abnormalities of the palate are very common, including cleft palate, submucous cleft palate, or just velopharyngeal insufficiency, causing a hypernasal voice (Shprintzen, 2001).

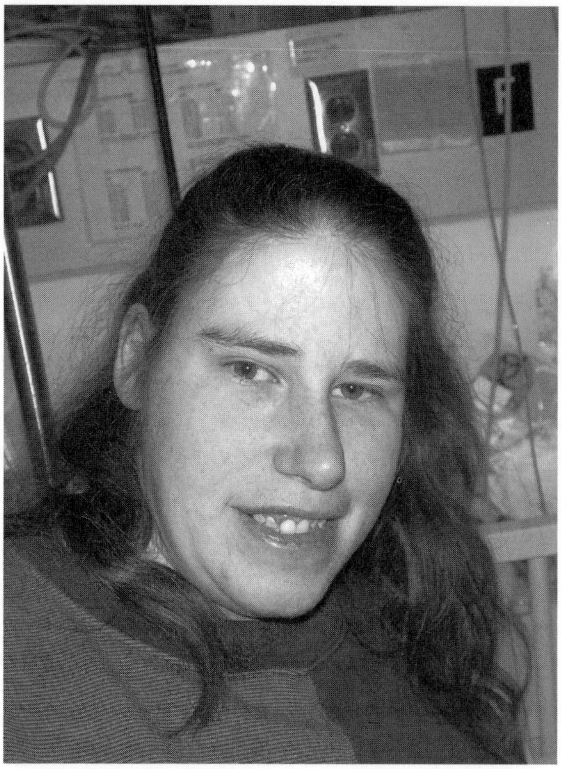

Fig. 53–5. Adult with velo-cardio-facial syndrome. (Photo courtesy of Nathaniel Robin, MD, University Hospitals of Cleveland and Case Western Reserve University.)

The congenital heart anomalies that occur most commonly in association with velo-cardio-facial syndrome are aortic arch anomalies (right-sided, double, or interrupted aortic arch type B), ventriculoseptal defects, pulmonary atresia or stenosis, tetralogy of Fallot, and truncus arteriosus. Abnormal major vessels, such as tracheal vascular rings or aberrant right or left subclavian artery, are also strong indicators of the diagnosis, especially if they occur in the absence of structural heart anomalies. Approximately 25% of affected individuals in one report had medial displacement of the internal carotid arteries (Goldberg et al., 1993). Renal anomalies are also common, and it is recommended that all affected individuals have a renal ultrasound in addition to a full cardiac evaluation at the time of diagnosis (Ryan et al., 1997).

Many of the most common anomalies in the syndrome are developmental, behavioral, and psychiatric (Arnold et al., 2001). The most frequent of such findings are mild learning disabilities, mild cognitive impairment, social immaturity, impulsivity, heightened anxiety, and phobias. In adult life, psychiatric illness is a common finding. An unusual condition, rapid cycling manic-depressive illness, is one of the more common psychiatric diagnoses, although other disorders in the manic-depressive spectrum and schizophrenia also are seen in a significant proportion of adult patients (Murphy et al., 1999). Blunt or inappropriate affect is frequently noted. Attention deficit/hyperactivity disorder is also characteristic. Paranoid and grandiose delusions were noted in two-thirds of patients in one study (Carlson et al., 1997a). In one large European collaborative study of 558 patients (Ryan et al. 1997), about 40% had abnormal cognitive development, mostly mild impairment. Some 9% of children had behavioral or psychiatric problems, and 18% of adults had psychiatric disorders. Therefore, the presence of any of these behavioral manifestations in association with hypernasal speech, cleft palate, or congenital heart disease should alert clinicians to the possible diagnosis of velo-cardio-facial syndrome.

Immune disorders resulting from lymphoid hypoplasia and T-lymphocyte dysfunction are frequently encountered in velo-cardio-facial syndrome in infancy and persist into late childhood and adulthood, leading to relatively mild chronic upper or lower respiratory infections. This is similar to what is seen in the DiGeorge sequence, where thymic hypoplasia leads to T-cell dysfunction and immunologic defects.

A total of 180 different findings have been reported in velo-cardio-facial syndrome (Shprintzen et al., 1997), so that the presence of abnormalities other than the ones mentioned above should not dissuade the clinician from suspecting this disorder.

Genetics

Although most cases of velo-cardio-facial syndrome are sporadic, it is an autosomal dominant disorder that is due to an interstitial chromosome deletion at 22q11.2 in approximately 85% of cases (Driscoll et al., 1992, 1993; Scambler et al., 1992; Kelley et al., 1993). This area is called the VCF/DiGeorge region. In approximately 15% of cases, a visible deletion can be detected on high-resolution karyotype, and in the remainder of patients FISH or other molecular techniques must be used to detect the deletion. The typical deletion that occurs in the large majority of patients encompasses approximately 3 million base pairs, with smaller deletions of several hundred thousand base pairs also being found. Therefore, the typical deletion is large enough to contain nearly 100 genes. Studies have narrowed the critical region to 250 kb (Li et al., 1994; Budarf et al., 1995). The size of the deletion has not been well correlated with the expression of the syndrome (Morrow et al., 1995; Carlson et al., 1997b). One or more genes in this region are strong candidates for involvement in the pathogenesis of velo-cardio-facial and DiGeorge syndromes (Merscher et al., 2001). Deletions at 22q11.2 have also been found in individuals with apparently isolated conotruncal heart defects and with the so-called conotruncal-anomaly face syndrome.

A few genes within the common deletion region have been identified, but to date none has been proved to be critical to causing the phenotype. Interestingly, the gene for catechol-*O*-methyltransferase (COMT) maps to the VCF/DiGeorge critical region. This gene, which is involved in the metabolism of catecholamines, including dopaminergic neurotransmitters, may well play a role in the development of the psychiatric abnormalities seen in velo-cardio-facial syndrome (Lachman et al., 1996).

Diagnostic testing for velo-cardio-facial syndrome is accomplished by FISH analysis using one or more probes within the common deletion region. The most commonly used probes are D22S75 and TUPLE I. Those cases of velo-cardio-facial and DiGeorge syndromes that do not have this deletion cannot currently be diagnosed through clinically available testing. Because of the extreme variability of manifestations related to deletion 22q11.2 and its well-documented autosomal dominant inheritance, parents and, if indicated, other family members should have diagnostic testing if a family member is found to be affected.

Prader-Willi Syndrome

Prader-Willi syndrome is a complex, multisystem mental retardation disorder that is due to a microdeletion of chromosome 15(q11–q13) in approximately 70% of cases. It is believed to represent the most common recognized genetic form of obesity. Because there are no major malformations, this disorder is compatible with survival well into adulthood, and lifespan may be normal if obesity and its complications are avoided (Greenswag, 1987; Cassidy et al., 1994).

Prader-Willi syndrome was first described in 1956 (Prader et al., 1956). Twenty-five years later, Prader-Willi syndrome captured the interest of geneticists because it was the first recognized microdeletion syndrome identified when high-resolution chromosome analysis was introduced (Ledbetter et al., 1981). It was also the first recognized human genomic imprinting disorder, and the first recognized as resulting from uniparental disomy (Nicholls et al., 1989). Prader-Willi syndrome thus occupies an important place in the contemporary history of human genetic disorders. It is also distinguished by being caused by several different genetic alterations of proximal chromosome 15q (genetic heterogeneity) and, like velo-cardio-facial syndrome, is typified by a distinctive behavioral phenotype (Dykens et al., 1992; Holm et al., 1993; Dykens and Cassidy, 1996).

It is estimated that 1 in 10,000 to 1 in 15,000 individuals are diagnosed with Prader-Willi syndrome—in both sexes and in all races. Most cases are sporadic and likely related to the associated infertility in the vast majority of patients. Despite the availability of clinical diagnostic criteria (Holm et al., 1993), many affected individuals reach adulthood without being diagnosed and present as morbidly obese and often diabetic patients with sleep disorders and severe behavior or psychiatric disorders. Making this diagnosis is important, since appropriate management can have a significant positive effect on health and quality of life and differs from that in obese patients without Prader-Willi syndrome. However, controlling the characteristic obesity and difficult behavior constitutes a major challenge, requiring cooperative input from primary care physicians, geneticists, endocrinologists, nutritionists, psychologists, psychiatrists, educators, community sources, families, and other care providers (Cassidy, 2001).

Diagnostic Criteria

Clinical diagnostic criteria were developed by consensus before completely sensitive and specific laboratory testing became available (Holm et al., 1993). These are still extremely valuable in suggesting the diagnosis and indicating the need for diagnostic testing (Table 53–6). The main features of Prader-Willi syndrome are neonatal hypotonia and failure to thrive; developmental delay and mild cognitive impairment; characteristic facial appearance; early childhood onset obesity; hypogonadism with genital hypoplasia, incomplete pubertal development, and infertility; and mild short stature. There is also a characteristic behavior disorder that usually begins in the first decade of life and becomes worse at and after adolescence. These and the more minor but often more distinctive features have been well described in a number of reviews (Cassidy, 1984, 1997; Butler, 1990; Cassidy et al., 1994). The discussion below will focus on the manifestations that are frequently present in adults.

Clinical Findings

Characteristic facial features—including narrow bifrontal diameter, almond-shaped palpebral fissures, narrow nasal bridge, and down-turned mouth with a thin upper lip—are typical (Fig. 53–6). A characteristic body habitus, including sloping shoulders, heavy mid-section, and genu valgus with straight lower leg borders, is usually present from toddlerhood (Fig. 53–6). Hypopigmentation for the family—manifested as fairer skin, hair, and eye color—occurs in about one-third of affected individu-

Table 53–6. Diagnostic Criteria for Prader-Willi Syndrome

Criterion	Manifestation
Major criteria	Characteristic facial features
	Infantile central hypotonia
	Infantile feeding problems/failure to thrive
	Rapid weight gain between 1 and 6 years
	Hypogonadism: genital hypoplasia, pubertal deficiency
	Developmental delay/mental retardation
Minor criteria	Poor fetal movement and infantile lethargy
	Typical behavior problems (temper tantrums, obsessive–compulsive behavior)
	Sleep disturbance, excessive daytime sleepiness, sleep apnea
	Short stature for the family by age 15 years
	Hypopigmentation for the family
	Small hands and feet for height age
	Narrow hands with straight ulnar border
	Esotropia, myopia
	Thick, viscous saliva
	Speech articulation defects
	Skin picking
Supportive criteria	High pain threshold
	Decreased vomiting
	Temperature control problems
	Scoliosis and/or kyphosis
	Early adrenarche
	Osteoporosis
	Unusual skill with jigsaw puzzles
	Normal neuromuscular studies (EMG, NCV, muscle biopsy)

Major criteria are worth one point, minor criteria one-half point; supportive criteria are helpful but no points. Prader-Willi syndrome should be strongly suspected in individuals above 3 years of age with 8 points (4 must be from major criteria). The original diagnostic criteria, developed before the availability of sensitive and specific genetic testing, included a major criteria of chromosome 15 deletion or other chromosome 15 anomaly.
Source: Adapted from Holm et al. (1993) with permission.

als. Strabismus is often present. Scoliosis or kyphosis is common; the former may occur at any age, and the latter develops in early adulthood.

Cognitive abnormalities are the rule in Prader-Willi syndrome, and most patients are mildly retarded (mean IQ 60s to low 70s) (Curfs and Fryns, 1992; Dykens et al., 1992). Approximately 40% have borderline retardation or low normal intelligence, and about 20% have moderate retardation. Academic performance is poor for cognitive ability. Specific patterns of cognitive strength and weakness have begun to emerge, frequently with relative strength in reading, visual-spatial skills, and long-term memory and weakness in arithmetic, sequential processing, and short-term memory (Dykens and Cassidy, 1996). Coming to the physician's office with a book of word-find puzzles can almost be considered a diagnostic sign for Prader-Willi syndrome, and unusual skill with jigsaw puzzles is common. Verbal skills are an ultimate strength in most patients, although speech is often poorly articulated, having a nasal or slurred character.

A characteristic behavior profile becomes evident in early childhood and worsens in adolescence and early adulthood, with temper tantrums, stubbornness, controlling and manipulative behavior, obsessive–compulsive characteristics, and difficulty with change in routine (Dykens et al., 1992; Dykens and Cassidy, 1996). Lying, stealing, and aggressive behavior are common. True psychosis is evident in young adulthood in approximately 5% to 10% of patients. Behavioral and psychiatric problems interfere most with quality of life in adulthood. Specific serotonin reuptake inhibitors have been of benefit in controlling behavioral and some psychiatric disturbances (Cassidy, 2001). Adults have generalized mild hypotonia. This is reflected in decreased muscle bulk and tone, as well as poor coordination and often decreased strength. One consequence of hypotonia in Prader-Willi syndrome is a decrease in lean body mass (Schoeller et al., 1988). Muscle electrophysiological and biopsy studies are usually normal or nonspecifically abnormal. The hypotonia likely contributes to a lower metabolic rate (Holland et al., 1993) and results in an inclination to inactivity. Both of these complicate the management of obesity.

Obesity is nearly always present in Prader-Willi syndrome after 6 years of age, if it is not actively avoided. The obesity is central in distribution and is the major cause of morbidity and mortality in this disorder (Greenswag, 1987; Cassidy et al., 1994). The decrease in lean body mass results in a relatively high ratio of fat-to-lean body mass even in those whose weight-to-height ratio is normal. It also is the suspected cause of decreased caloric requirement, which has been identified in Prader-Willi syndrome (Holm and Pipes, 1976). However, the major contributor to obesity is excessive eating, or hyperphagia, which characterizes the majority of affected patients. This appears to be the consequence of a hypothalamic defect resulting in lack of satiety (Holland et al., 1993), which causes the individual to constantly seek food, forage for food, and eat food that most people would consider inedible (e.g., a bag of sugar, garbage, or rotten or frozen food).

Cardiopulmonary compromise (Pickwickian syndrome) can result from uncontrolled obesity, as can Type 2 diabetes mellitus, hypertension, thrombophlebitis, and chronic leg edema. Sleep apnea occurs at increased frequency (Hertz et al., 1995).

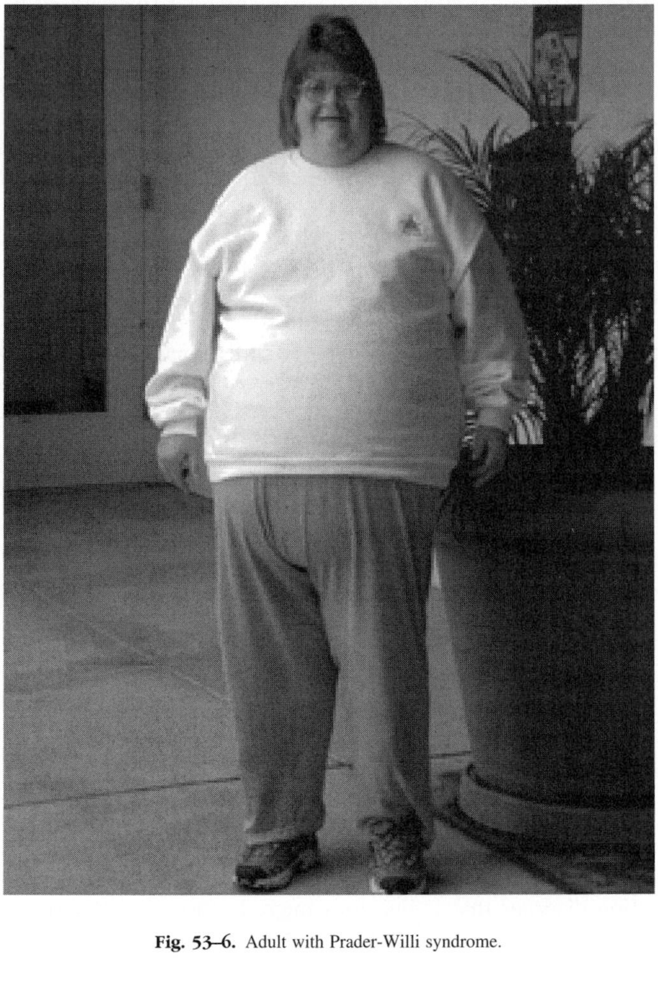

Fig. 53–6. Adult with Prader-Willi syndrome.

A low-calorie, well-balanced diet, combined with a regular exercise program and close supervision to minimize food stealing, should be instituted no later than when excessive weight gain is first noted in childhood, or whenever the diagnosis is made (Cassidy, 2001). Decreased caloric requirement should be kept in mind in planning diets, which should rarely be above 1000 to 1200 Kcal/day. Access to food should be as limited as possible, often entailing locking the kitchen or the refrigerator and pantry. Consistently enforced behavioral management programs, including firm limit setting, should be instituted simultaneously with diet. Regular exercise is also an extremely important part of weight management. Supplemental vitamins and calcium should be assured, the latter because of preliminary evidence for osteoporosis. Unfortunately, no medication or surgical procedure available at the time of writing has had long-term effectiveness in controlling appetite. There are many sources of information about weight management in Prader-Willi syndrome (Holm and Pipes, 1976; Cassidy, 1984, 2001; Greenswag and Alexander, 1995). It is unreasonable to expect that individuals with Prader-Willi syndrome will eventually learn to control their own food intake. A supportive living environment sensitive to this problem is essential.

Hypogonadism is present throughout life. It is manifested by genital hypoplasia and pubertal insufficiency in both males and females. Males are born with cryptorchidism, which in some cases has not been corrected by adulthood. Most characteristically, the scrotum is hypoplastic, often being small, hypopigmented, and poorly rugated. If the adult male has not had hormonal treatment, the penis is often small in both length and diameter. While pubic and axillary hair may develop early or normally, the remainder of pubertal development is usually delayed and incomplete. Adult males only occasionally have spontaneous voice change, male body habitus, or substantial facial or body hair. Females have hypoplasia of the labia minora and clitoris. Breast development generally begins at a normal age, but there is usually amenorrhea or oligomenorrhea. Menarche may occur as late as the 30s. In both males and females, sexual activity is rare and infertility is the rule, although two cases of successful pregnancy in affected females have appeared (Akefeldt et al., 1999). However, many affected individuals enjoy the social aspects of having a boyfriend or girlfriend.

Hypogonadism in Prader-Willi syndrome is usually due to hypothalamic insufficiency, leading to hypogonadotropic hypogonadism. Therefore, improvement in secondary sex characteristics can be accomplished by the administration of testosterone in males or estrogen in females. In males with testosterone treatment, voice can change; body hair, beard growth, and genital size can be improved; and a more masculine body habitus and increased muscle bulk and strength usually occur. Concern has been raised about the potential effect of testosterone to increase behavior problems. In females, estrogen treatment, or (preferably) cycling hormones or birth control pills, can increase breast size if desired and also results in menstrual periods. The benefits of hormone replacement therapy to the cardiovascular system and to prevention of osteoporosis in Prader-Willi syndrome have not been studied but are documented in other persons with low estrogen levels, such as those with Turner syndrome and postmenopausal women. Osteoporosis appears to be quite common in adults with Prader-Willi syndrome.

The majority of people with Prader-Willi syndrome have short stature, although the frequency is somewhat lower in blacks. Small hands and feet are also typical, although they are more normal in blacks (Hudgins et al., 1998). Without intervention, average height in Caucasians is 155 cm for males and 148 cm for females. Recent studies have shown that most patients are at least partially deficient in growth hormone, and studies documenting the benefits of growth hormone replacement in childhood have been published (Lindgren et al., 1998; Carrel et al., 1999). Improvement in muscle mass and bulk in response to growth hormone, in addition to increased height, have often resulted in improved weight management. Studies of growth hormone treatment in adults are currently ongoing.

A variety of less well understood findings are somewhat unique to this condition, including thick viscous saliva that may predispose to dental caries and contribute to articulation abnormalities, high pain threshold, skin picking, and high threshold for vomiting. Sleep disturbances, especially excessive daytime sleepiness and oxygen desaturation in REM sleep, are common, even in the absence of obesity (Hertz et al., 1995).

The Scientific Advisory Board of the Prader-Willi Syndrome Association (USA), a support and information organization, has developed Health Care Guidelines for Prader-Willi syndrome, which can be obtained by contacting them (1-800-926-4797; *www.pwsausa.org*).

Genetics

Prader-Willi syndrome is caused by the absence of normally expressed paternally-inherited genes on chromosome 15q11–q13; the maternally-inherited genes are normally not expressed due to a phenomenon called genetic imprinting by which some genes are modified differently, depending on the gender of the parent from whom they were inherited. As a result, there are three ways in which Prader-Willi syndrome can be caused. In approximately 70% to 75% of patients with Prader-Willi syndrome, there is a small deletion in the paternally-contributed chromosome 15 between bands 15q11–q13 (Ledbetter et al., 1981). In the vast majority of cases, the same breakpoints on the chromosome result in a 4 Mb deletion, although a small number of patients have a smaller or larger deletion. Most of the remaining patients with Prader-Willi syndrome have inherited two maternal chromosomes 15 but no paternal chromosome 15, a situation known as uniparental disomy (UPD) 15 (Nicholls et al., 1989). Of these two groups, approximately 2% to 5% of patients with Prader-Willi syndrome have either their deletion or their maternal UPD for the critical region as a result of a translocation or other structural abnormality involving chromosome 15. The third group of patients with Prader-Willi syndrome, which represent 1% of patients, have neither deletion nor UPD but, rather, a defect (sometimes a very small deletion or other abnormality) in the center that controls imprinting within 15q11–q13, the imprinting center (IC) (Buiting et al., 1995; Nicholls et al., 1998). All studied families in which there has been a recurrence of Prader-Willi syndrome have had an imprinting defect.

While a number of genes within 15q11–q13 have been identified and may contribute to the phenotype, the pathogenesis of the clinical findings in Prader-Willi syndrome remains unclear at this time (Nicholls, 1999; Nicholls and Knepper, 2001). Genotype–phenotype studies have indicated that individuals with Prader-Willi syndrome due to UPD have somewhat milder manifestations (Cassidy et al., 1997; Dykens et al., 1999).

Since there are three different genetic mechanisms that cause Prader-Willi syndrome, there are a number of different tests that can be used to confirm the diagnosis (American Society of Human Genetics, 1996). Inactivation of the maternal genes causing Prader-Willi syndrome is known to be caused by methylation of cytosine residues in the DNA. Methylation is the best known mechanism for genomic imprinting in general, and methylation has been demonstrated for several genes identified within the

Prader-Willi syndrome chromosome region. Unfortunately, little is known about the function of these genes or how their absence leads to the manifestations of Prader-Willi syndrome. So-called methylation analysis, originally accomplished by Southern blotting and now done by PCR, can detect all three causes of Prader-Willi syndrome since all three causes result in an exclusively maternal pattern of methylation of the genes involved in Prader-Willi syndrome (American Society of Human Genetics, 1996). This test can be done because methylated DNA is cut differently by some restriction enzymes than is unmethylated DNA, and the differences in the size of DNA fragments can be detected. Methylation analysis has been validated for both prenatal and postnatal use.

However, there are also other methods of detecting the genetic causes of Prader-Willi syndrome, and these all have a use in certain circumstances. Determining the exact cause of Prader-Willi syndrome is important primarily for genetic counseling purposes. Deletion in 15q11–q13 can be identified most accurately by doing a chromosome analysis and using the FISH probe for *SNRPN,* a candidate gene within the deletion. High-resolution chromosome analysis alone is insufficient since false positives and false negatives have occurred using this method without FISH. Uniparental disomy can be identified by using microsatellite repeat sequences on chromosome 15 in the patient and both parents; if none of the variants of those repeats present in the father are seen in the child, then all the genetic information on chromosome 15 has been derived from the mother and UPD is confirmed. This test requires DNA from both parents, as well as the child. The detection of a defect in the imprinting center is not a clinically available test but is implied from an abnormal methylation analysis in the presence of normal FISH and UPD studies. Mutations in the imprinting center can be detected in one of a few laboratories on a research basis.

Diagnostic testing for Prader-Willi syndrome has been the focus of much literature and a statement from the American Society of Human Genetics Joint Test and Technology Transfer Committee (1996).

Williams Syndrome

Also known as idiopathic hypercalcemia, Williams syndrome (or Williams-Beuren syndrome) is a recognizable pattern of abnormalities that includes a characteristic appearance, short stature, mild to moderate mental retardation, supravalvar aortic stenosis, episodic hypercalcemia, and a characteristic behavioral phenotype. As with most syndromes, not all findings must be present in a single affected individual. Williams syndrome is caused by a microdeletion of chromosome 7q11.23 (Ewart et al., 1993), which can be inherited in an autosomal dominant fashion although it is usually sporadic (Morris et al., 1993) The elastin (*ELN*) gene is present within this deletion, and FISH using the probe for *ELN* will identify 99% of individuals with the clinical phenotype of Williams syndrome (Ewart et al., 1993; Lowery et al., 1995; Mari et al., 1995; Nickerson et al., 1995). Estimates of the incidence of Williams syndrome are between 1 in 10,000 and 1 in 20,000. Most individuals survive well into adulthood.

Diagnostic Criteria

The diagnosis of Williams syndrome is based on recognizing the characteristic pattern of dysmorphic features, cardiac and other connective tissue abnormalities, short stature, cognitive impairment, and behavioral phenotype and obtaining FISH testing for confirmation. However, diagnostic scoring systems are available that may help the clinician determine if diagnostic testing is warranted (Preus, 1984; American Academy of Pediatrics, 2001). In general, individuals with cognitive impairment and supravalvar aortic stenosis deserve testing for Williams syndrome, even if the typical physical phenotype is not recognized. This is even more true in the presence of the characteristic behavior pattern of a very talkative, social, friendly person who is hyperactive. Periorbital puffiness in the context of a mildly retarded individual should also trigger testing.

Clinical Findings

The facial phenotype of Williams syndrome is distinctive but varies somewhat with age. Infants and young children generally have bitemporal narrowing, low nasal bridge with a bulbous upturned nasal tip, periorbital fullness, stellate or lacy iris pattern, malar flattening, a long philtrum with full lips and a wide mouth, full cheeks, small and widely spaced teeth, a small jaw, and prominent earlobes (Fig. 53–7). Older children and adults usually have a gaunt appearance with prominent supraorbital ridges, narrow nasal bridge of normal height, the same mouth and jaw characteristics as in earlier life, and a long neck. Dental malocclusion is common. Subcutaneous fat is often decreased.

The cognitive abilities of individuals with Williams syndrome vary from severe retardation to low average intelligence, but on average the IQ falls within the range of mild mental retardation. A characteristic cognitive profile has emerged that is typified by strengths in language and auditory memory and weak-

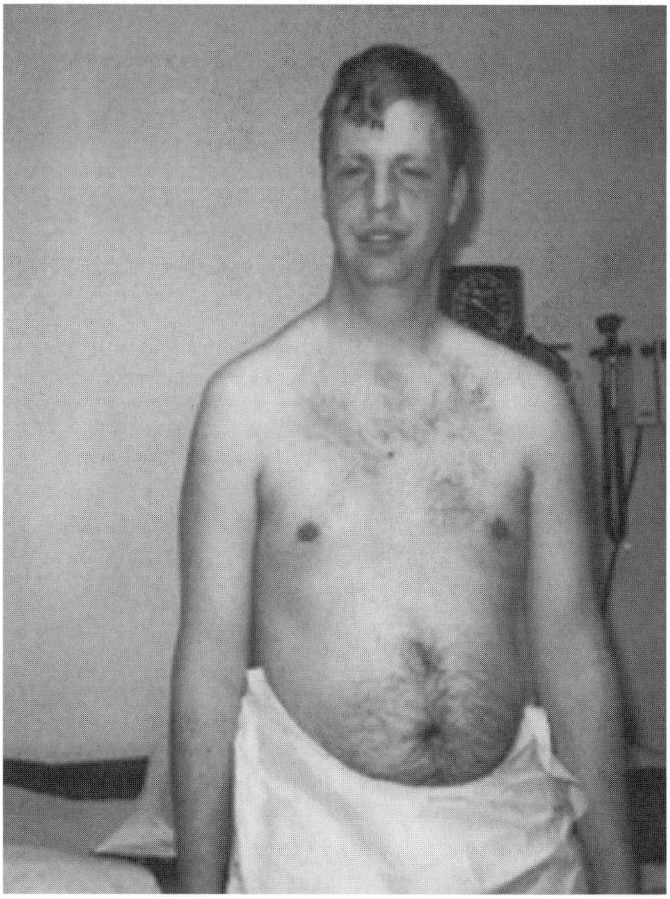

Fig. 53–7. Adult with Williams syndrome. (Photo courtesy of Nathaniel Robin, MD, University Hospitals of Cleveland and Case Western Reserve University.)

ness in visuospatial construction (Frangiskakis et al., 1996; Mervis et al., 1999; Donnai and Karmiloff-Smith, 2000). Despite mild mental retardation, 48% score in the normal range on vocabulary tests, and 65% score normal in digit recall tests (Mervis et al., 1999). Some 95% or more of affected individuals have difficulty with visual motor integration and fine motor skills. Abnormalities in depth perception lead to difficulties negotiating stairs and uneven surfaces.

The characteristic behavioral phenotype of Williams syndrome includes attention deficit disorder with or without hyperactivity in 73%, overfriendliness with strangers (97%), and generalized anxiety and preoccupations (Einfeld et al., 1997; Greer et al., 1997; Sarimski, 1997; Davies et al., 1998). There is a typical pattern of strength in interpersonal skills and weakness in daily living skills (Morris and Mervis, 1999). One study of 62 adults with Williams syndrome with a mean IQ of 61 showed an almost identical cognitive profile to that found in affected children, in whom more studies have been done (Howlin et al., 1998). Treatment with methylphenidate (Ritalin) and individual counseling have proved beneficial in some cases. Adults with Williams syndrome typically live with their parents or in group homes and work in sheltered employment (Davies et al., 1997).

Hypotonia is a common finding (80%), as is peripheral hypertonia (50%) with increased deep tendon reflexes, particularly in the lower extremities, in both children and adults. Hypersensitivity to sound occurs in 85% to 95% of affected individuals and is of unknown etiology.

Short stature for family background is seen in Williams syndrome. Most are below the third percentile in height (Morris et al., 1988, Pankau et al., 1992). Puberty often is early and is associated with a shorter than normal growth spurt (Pankau et al., 1992).

A number of connective tissue abnormalities are present, likely related to the elastin haploinsufficiency. These include a hoarse and/or deep voice, hernias, bladder and bowel diverticulae, soft and loose skin, and joint laxity or contractures, the latter being seen in 90% of adults (Morris et al., 1990). Scoliosis, kyphosis, and lordosis are common complications. The most important connective tissue problems, however, are cardiovascular. Diffuse arteriopathy is present to variable degrees, most commonly presenting as supravalvar aortic stenosis (SVAS) but also causing peripheral pulmonic stenosis (particularly in early childhood) and stenosis of virtually any blood vessel. The arterial stenosis tends to worsen over time (Ino et al., 1988). Renal artery stenosis occurs in 40% of affected individuals, and peripheral arterial stenoses are recognized in 20%. Coronary artery stenosis has been documented in some cases of sudden death (Bird et al., 1996). Hypertension occurs in 50% of people with Williams syndrome, likely as a consequence of the vascular anomalies (Kececioglu et al., 1993; Broder et al., 1999). In adults, aortic insufficiency occurs in 20% of patients and mitral valve prolapse in 15%. SVAS can lead to cardiac hypertrophy, cardiac failure, and death if untreated. About one-third of patients will ultimately require surgical correction (Kececioglu et al., 1993).

Idiopathic hypercalcemia is reported in 30% of affected individuals. Although it usually occurs in the first 18 months of life, adults may also have symptomatic hypercalcemia (Morris et al., 1990). It is recommended that the calcium : creatinine ratio be checked on a spot urine every two years; if it is above 0.22 in any individual older than 6 years, hypercalciuria is present. Despite numerous studies, the etiology of the hypercalcemia remains obscure. Nephrocalcinosis is found more frequently in persons with Williams syndrome (Pankau et al., 1996).

Structural renal anomalies occur at increased frequency. In ultrasound studies, the incidence of structural renal anomalies of a variety of types is 20% (Ingelfinger and Newburger,1991; Pober et al., 1993; Pankau et al., 1996). Bladder diverticulae and urinary tract anomalies are also common in adults (Morris et al., 1988). Therefore, it is appropriate to perform renal ultrasound and periodically check urinalysis and renal function studies.

Hypothyroidism has been reported in Williams syndrome, and diabetes mellitus occurs in 15% of affected adults. Chronic constipation occurs in 40%, rectal prolapse may occur, and diverticulosis is common (Morris et al., 1990; Morris, 2001). Chronic abdominal pain can result from hiatal hernia, gastroesophageal reflux, peptic ulcer disease, cholelithiasis, diverticulitis, ischemic bowel disease, constipation, and somatization of anxiety.

The American Academy of Pediatrics Committee on Genetics (2001) has published health care guidelines for management of Williams syndrome.

Genetics

Williams syndrome is due to an interstitial microdeletion of chromosome 7q11.23. The common deletion of Williams syndrome is 1.5 Mb, and more than 14 genes have thus far been mapped within this segment (Francke, 1999). Many of the manifestations of Williams syndrome are attributed to haploinsufficiency of the *ELN* gene. Interestingly, mutations within the *ELN* gene cause isolated autosomal dominant supravalvar aortic stenosis (Li et al., 1997). These individuals have the connective tissue findings of Williams syndrome but lack the dysmorphic features, mental retardation, and other findings. Most humans and experimental mice that are hemizygous for the *ELN* gene have a high number of lamellar units around arterial lumens, resulting in thickened arterial media and leading to obstructive vascular disease (Li et al., 1998).

LIM kinase (*LIMK1*) is also located within the usual microdeletion and has been implicated in the Williams syndrome phenotype (Frangiskakis et al., 1996). Genotype–phenotype analysis of families with smaller than normal deletions has provided evidence that the Williams syndrome cognitive profile is associated with *LIMK1* deletion, in that families that delete both *ELN* and *LIMK1* have SVAS and visuospatial constructive disability despite normal intelligence. The role of other identified genes within the usual deletion is unknown, though research is active in this area (Tassabehji et al., 1999).

REFERENCES

Abramsky L, Chapple J: 47,XXY (Klinefelter syndrome) and 47,XYY: estimated rates of and indication for postnatal diagnosis with implications for prenatal counseling. Prenat Diagn 1997; 17:363–368.

Akefeldt A, Tornhage CJ, Gillberg C: A woman with Prader-Willi syndrome gives birth to a healthy baby girl. Dev Med Child Neurol 1999; 41:789–790.

Alvarez N, Rubin L: Atlanto-axial instability in adults with Down syndrome: a clinical and radiological survey. Appl Res Ment Retard 1986; 7:67–78.

American Academy of Pediatrics, Committee on Genetics: Health supervision for children with Turner syndrome. Pediatrics 1995; 96:1166–1172.

American Academy of Pediatrics, Committee on Genetics: Healthcare supervision for children with Down syndrome. Pediatrics 2001; 107:442–449.

American Academy of Pediatrics, Committee on Genetics: Healthcare supervision for children with Williams syndrome. Pediatrics 2001; 107:1192–1204.

American Academy of Pediatrics, Committee on Sports Medicine and Fitness: Atlantoaxial instability in Down syndrome: subject review. Pediatrics 1995; 96:151–154.

American Society of Human Genetics/American College of Medical Genetics Report: Diagnostic testing for Prader-Willi and Angelman syndromes: report of the ASHG/ACMG Test and Technology Transfer committee. Am J Hum Genet 1996; 58:1085–1088.

Amos-Landgraf JM, Ji Y, Gottlieb W, Depinet T, Wandstrat AE, Cassidy SB, Driscoll DJ, Rogan PK, Schwartz S, Nicholls RD: Chromosome breakage in the Prader-Willi and Angelman syndromes involves recombination between large, transcribed repeats at proximal and distal breakpoints. Am J Hum Genet 1999; 65:370–386.

Anawalt BD, Bebb RA, Matsumoto AM, Groome NP, Illingworth PJ, McNeilly AS, Bremner WJ: Serum inhibin B levels reflect Sertoli cell function in normal men and men with testicular dysfunction. J Clin Endocrinol Metab 1996; 81:3341–3345.

Arens R, Marcus D, Engelberg S, Findler G, Goodman RM, Passwell JH: Cerebral germinomas and Klinefelter syndrome: a review. Cancer 1988; 61:1228–1231.

Ariel I, Wells TR, Landing BH, Singer DB: The urinary system in Down syndrome: a study of 124 autopsy cases. Pediatr Pathol 1991; 11:879–888.

Arnold PD, Siegel-Bartelt J, Cytrynbaum C, Teshima I, Schachar R: Velo-cardio-facial syndrome: implications of microdeletion 22q11 for schizophrenia and mood disorders. Am J Med Genet 2001; 105:354–362.

Arps S, Koske-Westphal T, Meinecke P, Meschede D, Nieschlag E, Harprecht W, Steuber E, Back E, Wolff G, Kerber S, Held KR: Isochromosome Xq in Klinefelter syndrome: report of 7 new cases. Am J Med Genet 1996; 64:580–582.

Arulanantham K, Kramer MS, Gryboski JD: The association of inflammatory bowel disease and X chromosomal abnormality. Pediatrics 1980; 66:63–67.

Arver S, Dobs AS, Meikle AW, Allen RP, Sanders SW, Mazer NA: Improvement of sexual function in testosterone deficient men treated for 1 year with a permeation enhanced testosterone transdermal system. J Urol 1996; 155:1604–1608.

Aylward EH, Burt DB, Thorpe LU, Lai F, Dalton A: Diagnosis of dementia in individuals with intellectual disability. J Intellect Disabil Res 1997; 41:152–164.

Baird PA, Anderson TW, Newcombe HB, Lowry RB: Genetic disorders in children and young adults: a population study. Am J Hum Genet 1988; 42:677–693.

Baird PA, Sadovnick AD: Causes of death to age 30 in Down syndrome. Am J Hum Genet 1988a; 43:239–248.

Baird PA, Sadovnick AD: Life expectancy in Down syndrome adults. Lancet 1988b; 2:1354–1356.

Baird PA, Sadovnick AD: Life tables for Down syndrome. Hum Genet 1989; 82:291–292.

Barr ML, Bertram EG: A morphological distinction between neurones of the male and female, and the behavior of the nucleolar satellite during accelerated nucleoprotein synthesis. Nature 1949; 163:676–677.

Barr ML, Shaver EL, Carr DH, Plunkett ER: The chromatin-positive Klinefelter syndrome among patients in mental deficiency hospitals. Resident J Ment Devic 1960; 4:89–107.

Bell AJ, Bhate MS: Prevalence of overweight and obesity in Down's syndrome and other mentally handicapped adults living in the community. J Intell Disab Res 1992; 36:359–364.

Bender BG, Harmon RJ, Linden MG, Bucher-Bartelson B, Robinson A: Psychosocial competence of unselected young adults with sex chromosome abnormalities. Am J Med Genet 1999; 88:200–206.

Bertelloni S, Baronceli G, Battini R, Saggese G: Central precocious puberty in Klinefelter syndrome: a case report with longitudinal follow-up of growth pattern. Am J Med Genet 1996; 65:52–55.

Binder G, Koch A, Wajs E, Ranke MB: Nested polymerase chain reaction study of 53 cases with Turner's syndrome: is cytogenetically undetected Y mosaicism common? J Clin Endocrinol Metab 1995; 80:3532–3536.

Bird LM, Billman GF, Lacro RV, Spicer RL, Jariwala LK, Hoyme HE, Zamora-Salinas R, Morris CA, Viskochil D, Frikke MJ, Jones MC: Sudden death in Williams syndrome: report of 10 cases. J Pediatr 1996; 129:926–931.

Bizzarro A, Valentini G, Di Martino G, DaPonte A, De Bellis A, Iacono G: Influence of testosterone therapy on clinical and immunological features of autoimmune diseases associated with Klinefelter's syndrome. Clin Endocrinol Metab 1987; 64:32–36.

Bohring C, Krause W: Serum levels of inhibin B in men with different causes of spermatogenic failure. Andrologia 1999; 31:137–141.

Bordeleau L, Cwinn A, Turek M, Barron-Klauninger K, Victor G: Aortic dissection and Turner's syndrome: case report and review of the literature. J Emerg Med 1998; 16:593–596.

Bourne H, Richings N, Harari O, Watkins W, Speirs AL, Johnston WI, Baker HW: The use of intracytoplasmic sperm injection for the treatment of severe and extreme male infertility. Reprod Fertil Dev 1995; 7:237–245.

Bourne H, Stern K, Clarke G, Pertile M, Speirs A, Baker HW: Delivery of normal twins following the intracytoplasmic injection of spermatozoa from a patient with 47,XXY Klinefelter's syndrome. Hum Reprod 1997; 12:2447–2450.

Bradbury JT, Bunge RG, Boccabella RA: Chromatin test in Klinefelter's syndrome. J Clin Endocrinol Metab 1956; 16:689.

Brkic H, Kaic Z, Poje Z, Singer Z: Shape of the craniofacial complex in patients with Klinefelter syndrome. Angle Orthod 1994; 64:371–376.

Broder K, Reinhardt E, Ahern J, Lifton R, Tamborlane W, Pober B: Elevated ambulatory blood pressure in 20 subjects with Williams syndrome. Am J Med Genet 1999; 23:356–360.

Brown T, Alvesalo L, Townsend GC: Craniofacial patterning in Klinefelter (47 XXY) adults. Eur J Orthod 1993; 15:185–194.

Budarf ML, Collins J, Gong W, Roe B, Wang Z, Sellinger B, Michaud D, Driscoll D, Emanuel BS. Cloning a balanced translocation associated with DiGeorge syndrome and identification of a disrupted candidate gene. Nat Genet 1995; 10:269–288.

Buiting K, Saitoh S, Gross S, Dittrich B, Schwartz S, Nicholls RD, Horsthemke B: Inherited microdeletions in the Angelman and Prader-Willi syndromes define an imprinting centre on human chromosome 15. Nat Genet 1995; 9:395–400.

Burn J, Goodship J: Congenital heart disease. In: Rimoin DL, Connor JM, Pyeritz RE (eds). Emery and Rimoin's Principles and Practice of Medical Genetics, 3rd ed. New York: Churchill Liviingstone, 1996:767–828.

Butenandt O: Growth hormone deficiency and growth hormone therapy in Ullrich-Turner syndrome. Klin Wochenschr 1980; 58:99–101. In German.

Butler MG: Prader-Willi syndrome: current understanding of cause and diagnosis. Am J Med Genet 1990; 35:319–332.

Campbell WA, Price WH: Venous thromboembolic disease in Klinefelter's syndrome. Clin Genet 1981; 19:275–280.

Capell PT, Paulsen CA, Derleth D, Skoglund R, Plymate S: The effect of short-term testosterone administration on serum FSH, LH and testosterone levels: evidence for selective abnormality in LH control in patients with Klinefelter syndrome. J Clin Endocrinol Metab 1973; 37:752–759.

Carlson C, Papolos D, Pandita RK, Faedda GL, Veit S, Goldberg R, Shprintzen R, Kucherlapati R, Morrow B: Molecular analysis of velo-cardio-facial syndrome patients with psychiatric disorders. Am J Hum Genet 1997a; 60:851–859.

Carlson C, Sirotkin H, Pandita R, Goldberg R, McKie J, Wadey R, Patanjali SR, Weissman SM, Anyane-Yeboa K, Warburton D, et al.: Molecular definition of 22q11 deletions in 151 velo-cardio-facial syndrome patients. Am J Hum Genet 1997b; 61:620–629.

Carothers AD, Collyer S, De Mey R, Johnstone I: An aetiological study of 290 XXY males, with special reference to the role of paternal age. Hum Genet 1984; 68:248–253.

Carothers AD, Filippi G: Klinefelter's syndrome in Sardinia and Scotland: comparative studies of parental age and other aetiological factors in 47,XXY. Hum Genet 1988; 81:71–75.

Carr J: Annotation: long term outcome for people with Down's syndrome. J Child Psychol Psychiatry 1994; 35:425–439.

Carrel AL, Myers SE, Whitman BY, Allen DB: Growth hormone improves body composition, physical strength and agility, and growth in Prader-Willi syndrome: a controlled study. J Pediatr 1999; 134:215–221.

Cassidy SB: Prader-Willi syndrome. Curr Probl Pediatr 1984; 14:1–55.

Cassidy SB: Syndrome of the month: Prader-Willi syndrome. J Med Genet 1997; 34:917–923.

Cassidy SB: Prader-Willi syndrome. In: Cassidy SB, Allanson JE (eds). Management of Genetic Syndromes. New York: Wiley, 2001:301–322.

Cassidy SB, Devi A, Mukaida C: Aging in Prader-Willi syndrome: 22 patients over age 30 years. Proc Greenwood Genet Center 1994; 13:102–103.

Cassidy SB, Forsythe M, Heeger S, Nicholls RD, Schork N, Benn P, Schwartz S: Comparison of phenotype between patients with Prader-Willi syndrome due to deletion 15q and uniparental disomy 15. Am J Med Genet 1997; 68(4):433–440.

Catalano RA" Down syndrome. Surv Ophthalmol 1990; 34:385–398.

Chad K, Jobling A, Frail H: Metabolic rate: a factor in developing obesity in children with Down syndrome? Am J Ment Retard 1990; 95:228–235.

Chang HJ, Clark RD, Bachman H: The phenotype of 45,X/46,XY mosaicism: an analysis of 92 prenatally diagnosed cases. Am J Hum Genet 1990; 46:156–167.

Chernausek SD, Attie KM, Cara JF, Rosenfeld RG, Frane J: Growth hormone therapy of Turner syndrome: the impact of age of estrogen replacement on final height. J Clin Endocrinol Metab 2000; 85:2439–2445.

Chicoine B, McGuire D, Hebein S, Gilly D: Development of a clinic for adults with Down syndrome. Ment Retard 1994; 32:100–106.

Choi HR, Lim SK, Lee MS: Site-specific effect of testosterone on bone mineral density in male hypogonadism. J Korean Med Sci 1995; 10:431–435.

Clark RW, Schmidt HS, Schuller DE: Sleep-induced ventilatory dysfunction in Down's syndrome. Arch Intern Med 1980; 140:45–50.

Clement PB, Young RH: Atypical polypoid adenomyoma of the uterus associated with Turner's syndrome: a report of three cases, including a review of "estrogen-associated" endometrial neoplasms and neoplasms associated with Turner's syndrome. Int J Gynecol Pathol 1987; 6:104–113.

Cohen WI, ed. Health care guidelines for individuals with Down syndrome: 1999 revision. Down Synd Q 1999; 4:1–16.

Collacott RA, Cooper SA, McGrother C: Differential rates of psychiatric disorders in adults with Down's syndrome compared with other mentally handicapped adults. Br J Psych 1992; 161:671–674.

Conway GS: Oestrogen replacement in young women with Turner's syndrome. Clin Endocrinol (Oxf) 2001; 54:157–158.

Cozzi J, Chevret E, Rousseaux S, Pelletier R, Benitz V, Jalbert H, Sele B: Achievement of meiosis in XXY germ cells: study of 543 sperm karyotypes from an XY/XXY mosaic patient. Hum Genet 1994; 93:32–34.

Cuadrado E, Barrena MJ: Immune dysfunction in Down's syndrome: primary immune deficiency or early senescence of the immune system? Clin Immunol Immunopathol 1996; 78:209–214.

Curfs LM, Fryns JP: Prader-Willi syndrome: a review with special attention to the cognitive and behavioral profile. Birth Defects 1992; 28:99–104.

Dacou-Voutetakis C, Karavanaki-Karanassiou K, Petrou V, Georgopoulos N, Maniati-Christidi M, Mavrou A: The growth pattern and final height of girls with Turner syndrome with and without human growth hormone treatment. Pediatrics 1998; 101(4 Pt 1):663–668.

Dahle AJ, McCollister FP: Hearing and otologic disorders in children with Down syndrome. Am J Ment Defic 1986; 90:636–642.

Davidson RG: Atlantoaxial instability in individuals with Down syndrome: a fresh look at the evidence. Pediatrics 1988; 81:857–865.

Davies M, Howlin P, Udwin O: Independence and adaptive behavior in adults with Williams syndrome. Am J Med Genet 1997; 70:188–195.

Davies M, Udwin O, Howlin P: Adults with Williams syndrome: preliminary study of social, emotional and behavioural difficulties. Br J Psych 1998; 172:273–276.

De Arce MA, Costigan C, Gosden JR, Lawler M, Humphries P: Further evidence consistent with Yqh as an indicator of risk of gonadal blastoma in Y-bearing mosaic Turner syndrome. Clin Genet 1992; 41:28–32.

De Braekeleer M, Dao TN: Cytogenetic studies in male infertility: a review. Hum Reprod 1991; 6:245–250.

Delooz J, Van den Berghe H, Swillen A, Kleczkowska A, Fryns JP: Turner syndrome patients as adults: a study of their cognitive profile, psychosocial functioning and psychopathological findings. Genet Couns 1993; 4:169–179.

Devenny DA, Krinsky-McHale SJ, Sersen G, Silverman WP: Sequence of cognitive decline in dementia in adults with Down's syndrome. J Intellect Disabil Res 2000; 44(Pt 6):654–665.

Devenny DA, Silverman WP, Hill AL, Jenkins E, Sersan EA, Wisniewski KE: Normal aging in adults with Down's syndrome: a longitudinal study. J Intellect Disabil Res 1996; 40:208–211.

Dieckmann KP, Rube C, Henke RP: Association of Down's syndrome and testicular cancer. J Urol 1997; 157:1701–1704.

Dinani S, Carpenter S: Down's syndrome and thyroid disorder. J Ment Defic Res 1990; 34:187–193.

Ditkoff EC, Vidali A, Sauer MV: Pregnancy in a woman with Turner mosaicism following ovarian stimulation and in vitro fertilization. J Assist Reprod Genet 1996; 13:447–448.

Donaldson MDC: Jury still out on growth hormone for normal short stature and Turner's syndrome. Lancet 1996; 348:3–4.

Donnai D, Karmiloff-Smith A: Williams syndrome: from genotype through to the cognitive phenotype. Am J Med Genet 2000; 97:164–171.

Down JL: Observations on an ethnic classification of idiots. Lond Hosp Rep 1866; 3:259–262.

Driscoll DA, Salvin J, Sellinger B, Budarf ML, McDonald-McGinn DM, Zackai EH, Emanuel BS: Prevalence of 22q11 microdeletions in DiGeorge and velocardiofacial syndromes: implications for genetic counselling and prenatal diagnosis. J Med Genet 1993; 30:813–817.

Driscoll DA, Spinner NB, Budarf ML, McDonald-McGinn DM, Zackai EH, Goldberg RB, Shprintzen RJ, Saal HM, Zonana J, Jones MC, et al.: Deletions and microdeletions of 22q11.2 in velo-cardio-facial syndrome. Am J Med Genet 1992; 44:261–268.

Dykens EM, Cassidy SB: Prader-Willi syndrome: genetic, behavioral and treatment issues. Child Adolesc Psychiatr Clin N Am 1996; 5:913–927.

Dykens EM, Cassidy SB, King BH: Maladaptive behavior differences in Prader-Willi syndrome due to paternal deletion versus maternal uniparental disomy. Am J Ment Retard 1999; 104:67–77.

Dykens EM, Hodapp RM, Walsh K, Nash L: Profiles, correlates and trajectories of intelligence in individuals with Prader-Willi syndrome. J Am Acad Child Adolesc Psychiatry 1992; 31:1125–1130.

Edelmann L, Pandita RK, Morrow BE: Low-copy repeats mediate the common 3-Mb deletion in patients with velo-cardio-facial syndrome. Am J Hum Genet 1999; 64:1076–1086.

Einfeld SL, Tonge BJ, Florio T: Behavioral and emotional disturbance in individuals with Williams syndrome. Am J Ment Retard 1997; 102:45–53.

Elia M, Musumeci SA, Ferri R, Scuderi C, Del Gracco S, Stefanini MC: Seizures in Klinefelter's syndrome: a clinical and EEG study of five patients. Ital J Neurol Sci 1995; 16:231–238.

Elsheikh M, Casadei B, Conway GS, Wass JA: Hypertension is a major risk factor for aortic root dilatation in women with Turner's syndrome. Clin Endocrinol (Oxf) 2001; 54:69–73.

Elsheikh M, Conway GS, Wass JA: Medical problems in adult women with Turner's syndrome. Ann Med 1999; 31:99–105.

Epstein CJ: Down syndrome (trisomy 21). In: Scriver CR, Beaudet AL, Sly WS, Valle D (eds). The Metabolic and Molecular Bases of Inherited Disease, 8th ed. New York: McGraw-Hill, 2001:1223–1256.

Epstein CJ, Korenberg JR, Anneren G, Antonarakis SE, Ayme S, Courchesne E, Epstein LB, Fowler A, Groner Y, Hurret JL, et al.: Protocols to establish genotype–phenotype correlations in Down syndrome. Am J Hum Genet 1991; 49:207–235.

Eulry F, Bauduceau B, Lechevalier D, Magnin J, Flageat J, Gautier D: Early spinal bone loss in Klinefelter syndrome: X-ray computed tomographic evaluation in 16 cases. Rev Rhum Ed Fr 1993; 60:287–291. In French.

Evenhuis HM: The natural history of dementia in Down's syndrome. Arch Neurol 1990; 47:263–267.

Evenhuis HM, van Zanten GA, Brocaar MP, Roerdinkholder WHM: Hearing loss in middle-age persons with Down syndrome. Am J Ment Retard 1992; 97:47–56.

Everman DB, Stoudemire A: Bipolar disorder associated with Klinefelter's syndrome and other chromosomal abnormalities. Psychosomatics 1994; 35:35–40.

Ewart AK, Morris CA, Atkinson D, Jin W, Sternes K, Spallone P, Stock AD, Leppert M, Keating MT: Hemizygosity at the elastin locus in a developmental disorder, Williams syndrome. Nat Genet 1993; 5:11–16.

Fernandez-Garcia R, Garcia-Doval S, Costoya S, Pasaro E: Analysis of sex chromosome aneuploidy in 41 patients with Turner syndrome: a study of "hidden" mosaicism. Clin Genet 2000; 58:201–208.

Filippi G: Klinefelter's syndrome in Sardinia: clinical report of 265 hypogonadic males detected at the time of military check-up. Clin Genet 1986; 30:276–284.

Filippi G, Pecile V, Rinaldi A, Siniscalco M: Fragile-X mutation and Klinefelter syndrome: a reappraisal. Am J Med Genet 1988; 30:99–107.

Fong C, Brodeur GM: Down's syndrome and leukemia: epidemiology, genetics, cytogenetics and mechanisms of leukemogenesis. Cancer Genet Cytogenet 1987; 28:55–76.

Ford CE, Miller O, Polani PE, de Almeida JC, Briggs JH: A sex chromosome anomaly in a case of gonadal dysgenesis (Turner's syndrome). Lancet 1959; 1:711–713.

Foresta C, Galeazzi C, Bettella A, Stella M, Scandellari C: High incidence of sperm sex chromosome aneuploidies in two patients with Klinefelter's syndrome. J Clin Endocrinol Metab 1998; 83:203–205.

Foresta C, Ruzza G, Mioni R, Meneghello A, Baccichetti C: Testosterone and bone loss in Klinefelter syndrome. Horm Metab Res 1983; 15:56–57.

Foudila T, Soderstrom-Anttila V, Hovatta O: Turner's syndrome and pregnancies after oocyte donation. Hum Reprod 1999; 14:532–535.

Francke U: Williams-Beuren syndrome: genes and mechanisms. Hum Mol Genet 1999; 8:1947–1954.

Frangiskakis JM, Ewart AK, Morris CA, Mervis CB, Bertrand J, Robinson BF, Klein BP, Ensing GJ, Everett LA, Green ED, et al.: LIM-kinase 1 hemizygosity implicated in impaired visuospatial contructive cognition. Cell 1996; 86:59–69.

Fricke GR, Mattern HJ, Schweikert HU, Schwanitz G: Klinefelter's syndrome and mitral valve prolapse, an echocardiographic study in twenty-two patients. Biomed Pharmacother 1984; 38:88–97.

Friedman DL, Kastner T, Pond WS, O'Brien DR: Thyroid dysfunction in individuals with Down syndrome. Arch Intern Med 1989; 149:1990–1993.

Gabrilove JL, Freiberg EK, Thornton JC, Nicolls GL: Effect of age on testicular function in patients with Klinefelter's syndrome. Clin Endocrinol 1979; 11:343–347.

Gardner RJM, Sutherland GR: Chromosome Abnormalities and Genetic Counseling. New York: Oxford University Press, 1989:137–143.

Garson OM, Robson MK, Weste SM, Baikie AG: Clinical findings in patients with numerical abnormalities of the X chromosome: a three-year survey of consecutive admissions to a general hospital. Med J Aust 1980; 2:33–35.

Geggel RL, O'Brien JE, Feingold M: Development of valve dysfunction in adolescents and young adults with Down syndrome and no known congenital heart disease. J Pediatr 1993; 122:821–823.

Geschwind DH, Boone KB, Miller BL, Swerdloff RS: Neurobehavioral phenotype of Klinefelter syndrome. Ment Retard Dev Disabil Res Rev 2000; 6:107–116.

Gohji K, Gogo A, Takenaka A, Arakawa S, Matumoto O, Hikosaka K, Kamidono S: Extragonadal germ cell tumor in the retrovesical region associated with Klinefelter's syndrome: a case report and review of the literature. J Urol 1989; 141:133–136.

Goldberg R, Motzkin B, Marion R, Scambler PJ, Shprintzen RJ: Velo-cardio-facial syndrome: a review of 120 patients. Am J Med Genet 1993; 45:313–319.

Goldhaber SZ, Brown WD, Robertson N, Rubin IL, St. John Sutton MG: Aortic regurgitation and mitral valve prolapse with Down's syndrome: a case-control study. J Ment Defic Res 1988; 32:333–336.

Goldhaber SZ, Brown WD, St. John Sutton MG: High frequency of mitral valve prolapse and aortic regurgitation among asymptomatic adults with Down syndrome. JAMA 1987; 258:1793–1795.

Goldhaber SZ, Rubin IL, Brown W, Robertson N, Stubblefield F, Sloss LJ: Valvular heart disease (aortic regurgitation and mitral valve prolapse) among institutionalized adults with Down's syndrome. Am J Cardiol 1986; 57:278–281.

Gorlin RJ, Cohen MM Jr, Levin LS (eds). Syndromes of the Head and Neck. New York: Oxford University Press, 1990:33–40.

Gravholt CH, Fedder J, Naeraa RW, Muller J: Occurrence of gonadoblastoma in females with Turner syndrome and Y chromosome material: a population study. J Clin Endocrinol Metab 2000; 85:3199–3202.

Gravholt CH, Juul S, Naeraa RW, Hansen J: Morbidity in Turner syndrome. J Clin Epidemiol 1998a; 51:147–158.

Gravholt CH, Naeraa RW, Nyholm B, Gerdes LU, Christiansen E, Schmitz O, Christiansen JS: Glucose metabolism, lipid metabolism, and cardiovascular risk factors in adult Turner's syndrome: the impact of sex hormone replacement. Diabetes Care 1998b; 21:1062–1070.

Greenswag LR: Adults with Prader-Willi syndrome: a survey of 232 cases. Dev Med Child Neurol 1987; 29:145–152.

Greenswag LR, Alexander RA (eds.). Management of Prader-Willi Syndrome, 2d ed. New York: Springer-Verlag, 1995.

Greer MK, Brown FR, Pai GS, Choudry SH, Lkein AJ: Cognitive, adaptive, and behavioral characteristics of Williams syndrome. Am J Med Genet 1997; 74:521–525.

Gron M, Pietila K, Alvesalo L: The craniofacial complex in 47,XYY males. Arch Oral Biol 1997; 42:579–586.

Gungor N, Boke B, Belgin E, Tuncbilek E: High frequency hearing loss in Ullrich-Turner syndrome. Eur J Pediatr 2000; 159:740–744.

Guttmann H, Weiner Z, Nikolski E, Ish-Shalom S, Itskovitz-Eldor J, Aviram M, Reisner S, Hochberg Z: Choosing an oestrogen replacement therapy in young adult women with Turner syndrome. Clin Endocrinol (Oxf) 2001; 54:159–164.

Haeusler G, Schmitt K, Blumel P, Plochl E, Waldhor T, Frisch H: Growth hormone in combination with anabolic steroids in patients with Turner syndrome: effect on bone maturation and final height. Acta Paediatr 1996; 85:1408–1414.

Hall B: Mongolism in newborn infants. Clin Pediatr 1966; 5:4–12.

Hall JG: Turner Syndrome. In: King RA, Rotter J, Motulsky AH (eds). The Genetic Basis of Common Diseases. New York: Oxford University Press, 1992:895–914.

Harari O, Bourne H, Baker G, Gronow M, Johnston I: High fertilization rate with intracytoplasmic sperm injection in mosaic Klinefelter's syndrome. Fertil Steril 1995; 63:182–184.

Harvey J, Jacobs PA, Hassold T, Pettay D: The parental origin of 47,XXY males. Birth Defects 1990; 26:289–296.

Hasle H, Mellemgaard A, Nielsen J, Hansen J: Cancer incidence in men with Klinefelter syndrome. Br J Cancer 1995; 71:416–420.

Hasle H, Olsen JH, Nielsen J, Hansen J, Friedrich U, Tommerup N: Occurrence of cancer in women with Turner syndrome. Br J Cancer 1996; 73:1156–1159.

Hassold T, Hunt P: To err (meiotically) is human: the genesis of human aneuploidy. Nat Rev Genet 2001; 2:280–291.

Hassold T, Pettay D, Robinson A, Uchida I: Molecular studies of parental origin and mosaicism in 45,X conceptuses. Hum Genet 1992; 89:647–652.
Hattori M, Fujiyama A, Taylor TD, Watanabe H, Yada T, Park HS, Toyoda A, Ishii K, Totoki Y, Choi DK, et al.: The DNA sequence of human chromosome 21. Nature 2000; 405:311–319.
Hernandez D, Fisher EMC: Down syndrome genetics: unraveling a multifactorial disorder. Hum Mol Genet 1996; 5:1411–1416.
Hertz G, Cataletto M, Feinsilver SH, Angulo M: Developmental trends of sleep-disordered breathing in Prader-Willi syndrome: the role of obesity. Am J Med Genet 1995; 56:188–190.
Hestnes A, Sand T, Fostad K: Ocular findings in Down's syndrome. J Ment Defic Res 1991; 35:194–203.
Hillebrand U, Mohr C, Plewa G: Taurodontism in patients with sex chromosome anomalies. Dtsch Z Mund Kiefer Gesichtschir 1990; 14:187–189.
Hinney B, Guttenbach M, Schmid M, Engel W, Michelmann HW: Pregnancy after intracytoplasmic sperm injection with sperm from a man with a 47,XXY Klinefelter's karyotype. Fertil Steril 1997; 68:718–720.
Hirsch M, Berezin M, Eshkol A, Goldman B, Ovadia J, Lunenfeld B: Endocrine profile in patients with Klinefelter's syndrome. Arch Androl 1984; 12:103–107.
Holland AJ, Hon J, Huppert FA, Stevens F: Incidence and course of dementia in people with Down's syndrome: findings from a population-based study. J Intellect Disabil Res 2000; 44(Pt 2):138–146.
Holland AJ, Hon J, Huppert FA, Stevens F, Watson P: Population-based study of the prevalence and presentation of dementia in adults with Down's syndrome. Br J Psych 1998; 172:493–498.
Holland AJ, Oliver C: Down's syndrome and the links with Alzheimer's disease. J Neurol Neurosurg Psychiatry 1995; 59:111–114.
Holland AJ, Treasure J, Coskeran P, Dallow J, Milton N, Hillhouse E: Measurement of excessive appetite and metabolic changes in Prader-Willi syndrome. Int J Obes 1993; 17:526–532.
Holm VA, Cassidy SB, Butler MG, Hanchett JM, Greenswag LR, Whitman BY, Greenberg F: Prader-Willi syndrome: consensus diagnostic criteria. Pediatrics 1993; 91:398–402.
Holm VA, Pipes PL: Food and children with Prader-Willi syndrome. Am J Dis Child 1976; 130:1063–1067.
Hook EB, Warburton D: The distribution of chromosomal genotypes associated with Turner's syndrome: livebirth prevalence rates and evidence for diminished fetal mortality and severity in genotypes associated with structural X abnormalities or mosaicism. Hum Genet 1983; 64:24–27.
Horowitz M, Wishart JM, O'Loughlin PD, Morris HA, Need AG, Nordin BE: Osteoporosis and Klinefelter's syndrome. Clin Endocrinol 1992; 36:113–118.
Hovatta O: Pregnancies in women with Turner's syndrome. Ann Med 1999; 31:106–110.
Hovatta O, Moilanen J, von Smitten K, Reima I: Testicular needle biopsy, open biopsy, epididymal aspiration and intracytoplasmic sperm injection in obstructive azoospermia. Hum Reprod 1995; 10:2595–2599.
Howlin P, Davies M, Udwin O: Cognitive functioning in adults with Williams syndrome. J Child Psychol Psychiatry 1998; 39:183–189.
Hsiang YH, Berkovitz GD, Bland GL, Migeon CJ, Warren AC: Gonadal function in patients with Down syndrome. Am J Med Genet 1987; 27:449–458.
Hsueh WA, Hsu TH, Federman DD: Endocrine features of Klinefelter's syndrome. Medicine 1978; 57:447–461.
Hudgins L, Geer JS, Holm VA, Cassidy SB: Phenotypic differences in African Americans with Prader-Willi syndrome. Genet Med 1998; 1:49–51.
Hultborn R, Hanson C, Kopf I, Verbiene I, Warnhammar E, Weimarck A: Prevalence of Klinefelter's syndrome in male breast cancer patients. Anticancer Res 1997; 17:4293–4297.
Hultcrantz M, Sylven L, Borg E: Ear and hearing problems in 44 middle-aged women with Turner's syndrome. Hear Res 1994; 76(1–2):127–132.
Humphreys M, Lavery P, Morris C, Nevin N: Klinefelter syndrome and non-Hodgkin lymphoma. Cancer Genet Cytogenet 1997; 97:111–113.
Ingelfinger JR, Newburger JW: Spectrum of renal anomalies in patients with Williams syndrome. J Pediatr 1991; 119:771–773.
Ino T, Nishimoto K, Iwahara M, Akimoto K, Boku H, Daneko K, Tokita A, Yabuta K, Tanaka J: Progressive vascular lesions in Williams-Beuren syndrome. Pediatr Cardiol 1988; 9:55–58.
Jackson AW, et al.: Carcinoma of male breast in association with the Klinefelter syndrome. Br Med J 1965; 1:223–225.
Jacobs PA, Bacino C, Hassold T, Morton NE, Keston M, Lee M: A cytogenetic study of 47,XXY males of known origin and their parents. Ann Hum Genet 1988a; 52:319–325.
Jacobs PA, Hassold TJ, Whittington E, Butler G, Collyer S, Keston M, Lee M: Klinefelter's syndrome: an analysis of the origin of the additional sex chromosome using molecular probes. Ann Hum Genet. 1988b; 52:93–109.
Jacobs PA, Melville M, Ratcliffe S, Deay AJ, Syme J: A cytogenetic survey of 11,680 newborn infants. Ann Hum Genet 1974; 37:359–376.
Jacobs PA, Strong JA: A case of human intersexuality having a possible XXY sex-determining mechanism. Nature 1959; 183:302–303.
James RS, Sharp AJ, Cockwell AE, Coppin B, Jacobs PA: Evidence for a cryptic 46,XX cell line in a 45,X/46,X,psu idic(Xq) patient with normal reproduction. Med Genet 1997; 34:1030–1032.
Jaspers MT, Witkop CJ Jr: Taurodontism, an isolated trait associated with syndromes and X-chromosomal aneuploidy. Am J Hum Genet 1980; 32:396–413.
Jenkins EC, Genovese M, Duncan CJ, Gu H, Stark-Houck S, Li SY, Henderson J, Morys I, Brown WT: Occurrence of aneuploidy for the X chromosome in over 1,300 unrelated specimens screened for the fragile X chromosome. Am J Med Genet 1994; 51:452–453.
Johnson MD: Genetic risks of intracytoplasmic sperm injection in the treatment of male infertility: recommendations for genetic counseling and screening. Fertil Steril 1998; 70:397–411.
Johnston DI, Betts P, Dunger D, Barnes N, Swift PG, Buckler JM, Butler GE: A multicentre trial of recombinant growth hormone and low dose oestrogen in Turner syndrome: near final height analysis. Arch Dis Child 2001; 84:76–81.
Kaneko N, Kawagoe S, Hiroi M: Turner's syndrome: review of the literature with reference to a successful pregnancy outcome. Gynecol Obstet Invest 1990; 29:81–87.
Karlsson B, Gustafsson J, Hedov G, Ivarsson SA, Anneren G: Thyroid dysfunction in Down's syndrome: relation to age and thyroid autoimmunity. Arch Dis Child 1998; 79:242–245.
Kececioglu D, Kotthoff S, Vogt J: Williams-Beuren syndrome: a 30-year follow-up of natural and postoperative course. Eur Health J 1993; 14:1458–1464.
Keiser H, Montague J, Wold D, Maune S, Pattison D: Hearing loss in Down syndrome adults. Am J Ment Defic 1981; 85:467–472.
Kelly D, Goldberg R, Wilson D, Lindsay E, Carey A, Goodship J, Burn J, Cross I, Shprintzen RJ, Scambler PJ: Velo-cardio-facial syndrome associated with haploinsufficiency of genes at chromosome 22q11. Am J Med Genet 1993; 45:308–312.
Kennedy RL, Jones TH, Cuckle HS: Down's syndrome and the thyroid. Clin Endocrinol 1992; 37:471–476.
Khastgir G, Abdalla H, Thomas A, Korea L, Latarche L, Studd J: Oocyte donation in Turner's syndrome: an analysis of the factors affecting the outcome. Hum Reprod 1997; 12:279–285.
Kim ED, Bischoff FZ, Lipshultz LI, Lamb DJ: Genetic concerns for the subfertile male in the era of ICSI. Prenat Diagn 1998; 18:1349–1365.
King CR, Magenis E, Bennett S: Pregnancy and the Turner syndrome. Obstet Gynecol 1978; 52:617–624.
Kishnani PS, Spiridigliozzi GA, Heller JH, Sullivan JA, Doraiswamy PM, Krishnan KR: Donepezil for Down's syndrome. Am J Psychiatry 2001; 158:143.
Kishnani PS, Sullivan JA, Walter BK, Spiridigliozzi GA, Doraiswamy PM, Krishnan KR: Cholinergic therapy for Down's syndrome. Lancet 1999; 353:1064–1065.
Kleczkowska A, Fryns JP, Van den Berghe H: X-chromosome polysomy in the male: the Leuven experience 1966–1987. Hum Genet 1988; 80:16–22.
Klinefelter HF Jr, Reifenstein EC Jr, Albright F: Syndrome characterized by gynecomastia, aspermatogenesis with A-Leydigism, and increased excretion of follicle-stimulating hormone. J Clin Endocrinol 1942; 2:615–627.
Kobayashi S, Yamamoto S, Tanaka M, Hashimoto H, Hirose S: Klinefelter's syndrome and rheumatoid arthritis: report of a case and review of the literature. Clin Rheumatol 1994; 13:500–503.
Koçar IH, Yesilova Z, Özata M, Turan M, Sengül A, Özdemir I: The effect of testosterone replacement treatment on immunological features of patients with Klinefelter's syndrome. Clin Exp Immunol 2000; 121:448–452.
Komatz Y, Tomoyoshi T, Yoshida O, Fujimoto A, Yoshitake K: Taurodontism and Klinefelter's syndrome. Med Genet 1978; 15:452–454.
Korenman SG, Viosca S, Garza D, Guralnik M, Place V, Campbell P, Davis SS: Androgen therapy of hypogonadal men with transscrotal testosterone systems. Am J Med 1987; 83:471–478.
Kruse R, Guttenbach M, Schartmann B, Schubert R, van der Ven H, Schmid M, Propping P: Genetic counseling in a patient with XXY/XXXY/XY mosaic Klinefelter's syndrome: estimate of sex chromosome aberrations in sperm before intracytoplasmic sperm injection. Fertil Steril 1998; 69:482–485.
Kubler A, Schulz G, Cordes U, Beyer J, Krause U: The influence of testosterone substitution on bone mineral density in patients with Klinefelter's syndrome. Exp Clin Endocrinol 1992; 100:129–132.
Kupke KG, Soreng AL, Muller U: Origin of the supernumerary X chromosome in a patient with fragile X and Klinefelter syndrome. Am J Med Genet 1991; 38:440–444.
Lachman HM, Morrow B, Shprintzen R, Veit S, Parsia SS, Faedda G, Goldberg R, Kucherlapati R, Papolos DF: Assocation of codon 108/158 catechol-*O*-methyltransferase gene polymorphism with the psychiatric manifestations of velo-cardio-facial syndrome. Am J Med Genet 1996; 7:468–472.
Lanes R, Gunczler P, Esaa S, Martinis R, Villaroel O, Weisinger JR: Decreased bone mass despite long-term estrogen replacement therapy in young women with Turner's syndrome and previously normal bone density. Fertil Steril 1999; 72:896–899.
Laron Z, Dickerman Z, Zamir R, Galatzer A: Paternity in Klinefelter's syndrome: a case report. Arch Androl 1982; 8:149–151.
Larsen T, Gravholt CH, Tillebeck A, Larsen H, Jensen MB, Nielsen J, Friedrich U: Parental origin of the X chromosome, X chromosome mosaicism and screening for "hidden" Y chromosome in 45,X Turner syndrome ascertained cytogenetically. Clin Genet 1995; 48:6–11.
Ledbetter DH, Riccardi VM, Airhart SD, Strobel RJ, Keenen SB, Crawford JD: Deletions of chromosome 15 as a cause of the Prader-Willi syndrome. N Engl J Med 1981; 304:325–329.
Leifke E, Korner HC, Link TM, Behre HM, Peters PE, Nieschlag E: Effects of testosterone replacement therapy on cortical and trabecular bone mineral density, vertebral body area and paraspinal muscle area in hypogonadal men. Eur J Endocrinol 1998; 138:51–58.
Lejeune J, Gautier M, Turpin MR: Etude des chromosomes somatiques de neuf enfants mongoliens. C R Acad Sci (Paris) 1959; 248:1721–1722.
Levron J, Aviram-Goldring A, Madgar I, Raviv G, Barkai G, Dor J: Sperm chromosome analysis and outcome of IVF in patients with non-mosaic Klinefelter's syndrome. Fertil Steril 2000; 74:925–929.
Li DY, Faury G, Taylor DG, Dais EC, Boyle WA, Mecham RP, Stenzel P, Boak B, Keating MT: Novel arterial pathology in mice and humans hemizygous for elastin. J Clin Invest 1998; 15:1783–1787.

Li DY, Toland AE, Boak BB, Atkinson D, Ensing GJ, Morris CA, Keating MT: Elastin point mutations cause an obstructive vascular disease. Hum Mol Genet 1997; 6:1021–1028.
Li M, Budarf ML, Sellainger B, Jaquez M, Matalon R, Ball S, Pagon R, Rosengren SS, Emanuel BS, Driscoll DA: Narrowing the DiGeorge region (DGCR) using DGS0VCFS associated translocation breakpoints. Am J Hum Genet 1994; 55, A10.
Lin AE, Lippe BM, Geffner ME, Gomes A, Lois JF, Barton CW, Rosenthal A, Friedman WF: Aortic dilation, dissection, and rupture in patients with Turner syndrome. Pediatrics 1986; 109:820–826.
Lin AE, Lippe B, Rosenfeld RG: Further delineation of aortic dilation, dissection, and rupture in patients with Turner syndrome. Pediatrics 1998; 102:e12.
Lindgren AC, Hagenas L, Muller J, Blichfeldt S, Rosenborg M, Brismar T, Ritzen EM: Growth hormone treatment of children with Prader-Willi syndrome affects linear growth and body composition favourably. Acta Paediatr 1998; 1:28–31.
Lo A, Brown HG, Fivush BA, Neu AM, Racusen LC: Renal disease in Down syndrome: autopsy study with emphasis on glomerular lesions. Am J Kidney Dis 1998; 31:329–335.
Lorda-Sanchez I, Binkert F, Hinkel KG, Moser H, Rosenkranz W, Maechler M, Schinzel A: Uniparental origin of sex chromosome polysomies. Hum Hered 1992a; 42:193–197.
Lorda-Sanchez I, Binkert F, Maechler M, Robinson WP, Schinzel AA: Reduced recombination and paternal age effect in Klinefelter syndrome. Hum Genet 1992b; 89:524–530.
Lowery MC, Morris CA, Ewart A, Brothman L, Zhu XL, Leonard CO, Carey JC, Keating M, Brothman AR: Strong correlations of elastin deletions, detected by FISH, with Williams syndrome: evaluation of 235 patients. Am J Hum Genet 1995; 57:49–53.
Lue Y, Rao PN, Sinha Hikim AP, Im M, Salameh WA, Yen PH, Wang C, Swerdloff RS: XXY male mice: an experimental model for Klinefelter syndrome. Endocrinology 2001; 142:1461–1470.
Luisetto G, Mastrogiacomo I, Bonanni G, Pozzan G, Botteon S, Tizian L, Galuppo P: Bone mass and mineral metabolism in Klinefelter's syndrome. Osteoporos Int 1995; 5:455–461.
Lupski JR: Genomic disorders: structural features of the genome can lead to DNA rearrangements and human disease traits. Trends Genet 1998; 14:417–422.
Lyon AJ, Preece MA, Grant DB: Growth curve for girls with Turner syndrome. Arch Dis Child 1985; 60:932–935.
Maclachlan RA, Fidler KE, Yeh H, Hodgetts PG, Pharard G, Chau M: Cervical spine abnormalities in institutionalized adults with Down syndrome. J Intellect Disabil Res 1993; 37:277–285.
Magee AC, Nevin NC, Armstrong MJ, McGibbon D, Nevin J: Ullrich-Turner syndrome: seven pregnancies in an apparent 45,X woman. Am J Med Genet 1998; 75:1–3.
Mandoki MW, Sumner GS: Klinefelter syndrome: the need for early identification and treatment. Clin Pediatr 1991; 30:161–164.
Mandoki MW, Sumner GS, Hoffman RP, Riconda DL: A review of Klinefelter's syndrome in children and adolescents. J Am Acad Child Adolesc Psychiatry 1991; 30:167–172.
Mari A, Amati F, Mingarelli R, Giannotti A, Sebastio G, Colloridi V, Novelli G, Dallapiccola B: Analysis of the elastin gene in 60 patients with clinical diagnosis of Williams syndrome. Hum Genet 1995; 96:444–448.
Martin BA: Primary care of adults with mental retardation living in the community. Am Fam Physician 1997; 56:485–494.
Mathur A, Stekol L, Schatz D, MacLaren NK, Scott ML, Lippe B: The parental origin of the single X chromosome in Turner syndrome: lack of correlation with parental age or clinical phenotype. Am J Hum Genet 1991; 48:682–686.
Matsumoto AM: Hormonal therapy of male hypogonadism. Endocrinol Metab Clin North Am 1994; 23:857–875.
Matthew P, Moodie D, Sterba R, Murphy D, Rosenkranz E, Homa A: Long-term follow-up of children with Down syndrome with cardiac lesions. Clin Pediatr 1990; 29:569–574.
Mazzocco MM: A process approach to describing mathematics difficulties in girls with Turner syndrome. Pediatrics 1998; 102:492–496.
Meikle AW, Dobs AS, Arver S, Caramelli KE, Sanders SW, Mazer NA: Androgen replacement in the treatment of Klinefelter's syndrome: efficacy and safety of a nonscrotal permeation-enhanced testosterone transdermal system. Endocr Pract 1998; 4:17–22.
Merscher S, Funke B, Epstein JA, Heyer J, Puech A, Lu MM, Xavier RJ, Demay MB, Russell RG, Factor S, et al.: TBX1 is responsible for cardiovascular defects in velo-cardio-facial/DiGeorge syndrome. Cell 2001; 104:619–629.
Mervis CB, Morris CA, Bertrand J, Robinson BF: Williams syndrome: findings from an integrated program of research. In H. Tager-Flusberg (ed). Neurodevelopmental Disorders. Cambridge, MA: MIT Press, 1999:65–110.
Meschede D, Horst J: Sex chromosomal anomalies in pregnancies conceived through intracytoplasmic sperm injection: a case for genetic counseling. Hum Reprod 1997; 12:1125–1127.
Meschede D, Lemcke B, Exeler JR, De Geyter C, Behre HM, Nieschlag E, Horst J: Chromosome abnormalities in 447 couples undergoing intracytoplasmic sperm injection: prevalence, types, sex distribution and reproductive relevance. Hum Reprod 1998; 13:576–582.
Micic M, Micic S, Diklic V: Chromosomal constitution of infertile men. Clin Genet 1984; 25:33–36.
Morris CA: Williams syndrome. In: Cassidy SB, Allanson JE (eds). Management of Genetic Syndromes. New York: Wiley, 2001:517–533.
Morris CA, Demsey SA, Leonard CO, Dilts C, Blackburn BL: Natural history of Williams syndrome: physical characteristics. J Pediatr 1988; 113(2):318–326.
Morris CA, Leonard CO, Dilts C, Dempsey SA: Adults with Williams syndrome. Am J Med Genet (Suppl) 1990; 6:102–107.
Morris CA, Mervis CB: Williams syndrome. In: Goldstein S, Reynolds C (eds). Handbook of Neurodevelopmental and Genetic Disorders in Children. New York: Guilford Press, 1999:555–590.
Morris CA, Thomas IT, Greenberg F: Williams syndrome: autosomal dominant inheritance. Am J Med Genet 1993; 47: 478–481.
Morrow B, Goldberg R, Carlson C, Gupta RD, Sirotkin H, Collins J, Dunham I, O'Donnell HO, Scambler P, Shprintzen RJ, Kucherlapati R: Molecular definition of the 22q11 deletions in velo-cardio-facial syndrome. Am J Hum Genet 1995; 56:1391–1403.
Murphy KC, Jones LA, Owen MJ: High rates of schizophrenia in adults with velo-cardio-facial syndrome. Arch Gen Psychiatry 1999; 56:940–945.
Muts-Homsma SJ, Muller HP, Geraedst JP: Klinefelter's syndrome and acute nonlymphocytic leukemia. Blut 1982; 44:15–20.
Myers BA, Pueschel SM: Psychiatric disorders in persons with Down syndrome. J Nerv Ment Dis 1991; 179:609–613.
Myhre SA, Ruvalcaba RH, Johnson HR, Thuline HC, Kelley VC: The effects of testosterone treatment in Klinefelter's syndrome. J Pediatr 1970; 76:267–276.
Nespoli L, Burgio GR, Ugazio AG, Maccario R: Immunological features of Down's syndrome: a review. J Intellect Disabil Res 1993; 37:543–551.
Nicholls RD: Incriminating gene suspects, Prader-Willi style. Nat Genet 1999; 23:132–134.
Nicholls RD, Knepper JL: Genome organization, function and imprinting in Prader-Willi and Angelman syndromes. Annu Rev Genomics Human Genet 2001; 2:153–175.
Nicholls RD, Knoll JHM, Butler MG, Karam S, Lalande M: Genetic imprinting suggested by maternal heterodisomy in non-deletion Prader-Willi syndrome. Nature 1989; 342:281–285.
Nicholls RD, Saitoh S, Horsthemke B: Imprinting in Prader-Willi and Angelman syndromes. Trends Genet 1998; 14:194–200.
Nichols CR, Heerema NA, Palmer C, Loehrer PJ Sr, Williams SD, Einhorn LH: Klinefelter's syndrome associated with mediastinal germ cell neoplasms. Clin Oncol 1987; 5:1290–1294.
Nickerson E, Greenberg F, Keating MT, McCaskill C, Shaffer LG: Deletions of the elastin gene at 7q11.23 occur in ~90% of patients with Williams syndrome. Am J Hum Genet 1995; 56:1156–1161.
Nielsen J, Pelsen B, Sorensen K: Follow-up of 30 Klinefelter males treated with testosterone. Clin Genet 1988; 33:262–269.
Nielsen J, Wohlert M: Chromosome abnormalities found among 34,910 newborn children: results from a 13-year incidence study in Arhus, Denmark. Birth Defects 1990; 26:209–223.
O'Connor JF, Cranley WR, McCarten KM, Feingold M: Commentary: atlantoaxial instability in Down syndrome: reassessment by the Committee on Sports Medicine and Fitness of the American Academy of Pediatrics. Pediatr Radiol 1996; 26:748–749.
Oguma N, Takemoto M, Oda K, Tanaka K, Shigeta C, Sakatani K, Kamada N, Kuramoto A: Chronic myelogenous leukemia and Klinefelter syndrome. Eur J Haematol 1989; 42:207–208.
Oliver C, Holland AJ: Down's syndrome and Alzheimer's disease: a review. Psychol Med 1986; 16:307–322.
Olsen NJ, Kovacs WJ: Case report: testosterone treatment of systemic lupus erythematosus in a patient with Klinefelter's syndrome. Am J Med Sci 1995; 310:158–160.
Ozata M, Bulur M, Beyhan Z, Sengul A, Saglam M, Turan M, Corakci A, Ali Gundogan M: Effects of gonadotropin and testosterone treatments on prostate volume and serum prostate specific antigen levels in male hypogonadism. Endocr J 1997; 44:719–724.
Palermo GD, Schlegel PN, Sills ES, Veeck LL, Zaninovic N, Menendez S, Rosenwaks Z: Births after intracytoplasmic injection of sperm obtained by testicular extraction from men with nonmosaic Klinefelter's syndrome. N Engl J Med 1998; 338:588–590.
Pandiyan N, Jequier AM: Mitotic chromosomal anomalies among 1210 infertile men. Hum Reprod 1996; 11:2604–2608.
Pankau R, Partsch C-J, Gosch A, Oppermann HC, Wessel A: Statural growth in Williams-Beuren syndrome. Eur J Pediatr 1992; 151:751–755.
Pankau R, Partsch C-J, Winter M, Gosch A, Wessel A: Incidence and spectrum of renal abnormalities in Williams-Beuren syndrome. Am J Med Genet 1996; 63:301–304.
Park E: Cortical bone measurements in Turner's syndrome. Am J Phys Anthropol 1977; 46:455–462.
Park JP, Brothman AR, Butler MG, Cooley LD, Dewald GW, Lundquist KF, Palmer CG, Patil SR, Rao KW, Saikevych IA, et al.: Extensive analysis of mosaicism in a case of Turner syndrome: the experience of 287 cytogenetic laboratories. Arch Pathol Lab Med 1999; 123:381–385.
Pascual J, Liano F, Garcia-Villanueva A, Salvador JL, Herrero JA, Ortuno J: Isolated primary aldosteronism in a patient with adrenal carcinoma and XY/XXY mosaic Klinefelter's syndrome. J Urol 1990; 144:1454–1456.
Pasquino AM, Passeri F, Pucarelli I, Segni M, Municchi G: Spontaneous pubertal development in Turner's syndrome. Clin Endocrinol Metab 1997; 82:1810–1813.
Paulsen CA, Plymate SR. Klinefelter's Syndrome. In: King RA, Rotter J, Motulsky AH (eds). The Genetic Basis of Common Diseases. New York: Oxford University Press, 1992:876–894.
Pecile V, Filippi G: Screening for fra(x) mutation and Klinefelter syndrome in mental institutions. Clin Genet 1991; 39:189–193.
Peet J, Weaver DD, Vance GH: 49,XXXXY: a distinct phenotype—three new cases and review. J Med Genet 1998; 35:420–424.

Pei D, Sheu WH, Jeng CY, Liao WK, Fuh MM: Insulin resistance in patients with Klinefelter's syndrome and idiopathic gonadotropin deficiency. J Formos Med Assoc 1998; 97:534–540. In Chinese.

Pierga JY, Giacchetti S, Vilain E, Extra JM, Brice P, Espie M, Maragi JA, Fellous M, Marty M: Dysgerminoma in a pure 45,X Turner syndrome: report of a case and review of the literature. Gynecol Oncol 1994; 55(3 Pt 1):459–464.

Pober BR, Lacro RV, Rice C, Mandell V, Teele RL: Renal findings in 40 individuals with Williams syndrome. Am J Med Genet 1993; 46:271–274.

Prader A, Labhart A, Willi H: Ein Syndrom von Adipositas, Kleinwuchs, Kryptochismus und Oligophrenie nach myotoniertgem Zustand im Neugeborenalter. Schweiz Med Wochenschr 1956; 86:1260–1261.

Prasher VP: Overweight and obesity amongst Down's syndrome adults. J Intellect Disabil Res 1995; 39:437–441.

Preus M: The Williams syndrome: objective definition and diagnosis. Clin Genet 1984; 25:422–428.

Price WH, Clayton JF, Collyer S, de Mey R: Mortality ratios and life expectancy in X chromatin positive males. J Epidemiol Community Health 1985a; 39:33–38.

Price WH, Clayton JF, Wilson J, Collyer S, de Mey R: Causes of death in X chromatin positive males (Klinefelter's syndrome). J Epidemiol Community Health 1985b; 39:330–336.

Price WH, Steers AJ, Wilson J: Subarachnoid hemorrhage and Klinefelter's syndrome. Lancet 1982; 2:380.

Pueschel SM: Facial plastic surgery for children with Down syndrome. Dev Med Child Neurol 1988; 30:540–543.

Pueschel SM: Clinical aspects of Down syndrome from infancy to adulthood. Am J Med Genet Suppl 1990; 7:52–56.

Pueschel SM, Anneren G, Durlach R, Flores J, Sustrova M, Verma IC: Committee report: guidelines for optimal medical care of persons with Down syndrome. Arch Pediatr 1995; 84:823–827.

Pueschel SM, Craig WY, Haddow JE: Lipids and lipoproteins in persons with Down's syndrome. J Intellect Disabil Res 1992; 36:365–369.

Pueschel SM, Pezzullo JC: Thyroid dysfunction in Down syndrome. Am J Dis Child 1985; 139:636–639.

Pueschel SM, Scola FH: Atlantoaxial instability in individuals with Down syndrome: epidemiologic, radiographic, and clinical studies. Pediatrics 1987; 80:555–560.

Pueschel SM, Scola PS: Parents' perception of social and sexual functions in adolescents with Down's syndrome. J Ment Defic Res 1988; 32:215–220.

Raboch J, Mellan J, Starka L: Klinefelter syndrome: sexual development and activity. Arch Sex Behav 1979; 8:333–339.

Raboch J, Neuwirth J, Starka L: Plasmatic testosterone values in 105 Klinefelters. Andrologia 1975; 7:77–83.

Rani AS, Jyothi A, Reddy PP, Reddy OS: Reproduction in Down's syndrome. Int J Gynecol Obstet 1990; 31:81–86.

Rao E, Weiss B, Fukami M, Rump A, Niesler B, Mertz A, Muroya K, Binder G, Kirsch S, Winkelmann M, et al.: Pseudoautosomal deletions encompassing a novel homeobox gene cause growth failure in idiopathic short stature and Turner syndrome. Nat Genet 1997; 16:54–63.

Ratcliffe SG, Butler GE, Jones M: Edinburgh study of growth and development of children with sex chromosome abnormalities. Birth Defects 1990; 26:1–44.

Reddy KS, Sulcova V: Pathogenetics of 45,X/46,XY gonadal mosaicism. Cytogenet Cell Genet 1998; 82:52–57.

Reeves RH, Baxter LL, Richtsmeier JT: Too much of a good thing: mechanisms of gene action in Down syndrome. Trends Genet 2001; 17(2):83–88.

Regadera J, Codesal J, Paniagua R, Gonzalez-Peramato P, Nistal M: Immunohistochemical and quantitative study of interstitial and intratubular Leydig cells in normal men, cryptorchidism, and Klinefelter's syndrome. J Pathol 1991; 164:299–306.

Reubinoff BE, Abeliovich D, Werner M, Schenker JG, Safran A, Lewin A: A birth in non-mosaic Klinefelter's syndrome after testicular fine needle aspiration, intracytoplasmic sperm injection and preimplantation genetic diagnosis. Hum Reprod 1998; 13:1887–1892.

Rivas F, Garcia-Esquivel L, Diaz M, Rivera H, Cantu JM: Cytogenetic evaluation of 163 azoospermics. J Genet Hum 1987; 35:291–298.

Roberge D, Souhami L, Laplante M: Testicular seminoma and Down's syndrome. Can J Urol 2001; 8:1203–1206.

Robinson A, Bender BG, Linden M: Prognosis of prenatally diagnosed children with sex chromosome aneuploidy (SCA). Am J Med Genet 1992; 44:365–368.

Robinson A, Bender BG, Linden MG: Klinefelter syndrome. In: Cassidy SB, Allanson JE (eds). Management of Genetic Syndromes. New York: Wiley 2001:195–206.

Robinson A, Bender BG, Linden MG, Salbenblatt JA: Sex chromosome aneuploidy: the Denver Prospective Study. Birth Defects 1990; 26:59–115.

Romano C, Tine A, Fazio G, Rizzo R, Colognola RM, Sorge G, Bergonzi P, Pavone L: Seizures in patients with trisomy 21. Am J Med Genet Suppl 1990; 7:298–300.

Ron-El R, Friedler S, Strassburger D, Komarovsky D, Schachter M, Raziel A: Birth of a healthy neonate following the intracytoplasmic injection of testicular spermatozoa from a patient with Klinefelter's syndrome. Osteoporos Int 1993; 3:3–7.

Ron-El R, Strassburger D, Gelman-Kohan S, Friedler S, Raziel A, Appelman Z: A 47,XXY fetus conceived after ICSI of spermatozoa from a patient with non-mosaic Klinefelter's syndrome: case report. Hum Reprod 2000; 15(8):1804–1806.

Rosenfeld RG, Attie KM, Frane J, Brasel JA, Burnstein S, Cara JF, Chernausek S, Gotlin RW, Kuntze J, Lippe BM, et al.: Growth hormone therapy of Turner syndrome: beneficial effect on adult height. J Pediatr 1998; 132:319–324.

Rosenfeld RG, Tesch L-G, Rodriguez-Rigau LJ, et al.: Recommendations for diagnosis, treatment, and management of individuals with Turner syndrome. Endocrinologist 1994; 4:351–358.

Ross J, Roeltgen D, Kushner H, Wei F, Zinn AR: The Turner syndrome–associated neurocognitive phenotype maps to distal Am J Hum Genet 2000a; 67:672–681.

Ross J, Zinn A, McCauley E: Neurodevelopmental and psychosocial aspects of Turner syndrome. Ment Retard Dev Disabil Res Rev 2000b; 6:135–141.

Rovet J: Turner syndrome. In: Rourke, BP (ed). Syndrome of Nonverbal Learning Disabilities: Neurodevelopmental Manifestations. New York: Guilford Press 1995:351–371.

Rovet J, Netley C, Keenan M, Bailey J, Stewart D: The psychoeducational profile of boys with Klinefelter syndrome. J Learn Disabil 1996; 29:180–196.

Ryan AK, Goodship JA, Wilson DI, Philip N, Levy A, Seidel H, Schuffenhauer S, Oechsler H, Belohradsky B, Prieur M, et al.: Spectrum of clinical features associated with interstitial chromosome 22q11 deletions: a European collaborative study. J Med Genet 1997; 34:798–804.

Saenger P: Clinical review 48: the current status of diagnosis and therapeutic intervention in Turner's syndrome. J Clin Endocrinol Metab 1993; 77:297–301.

Saenger, P: Turner's syndrome. New Engl J Med 1996; 335:1749–1754.

Salbenblatt JA, Bender BG, Puck MH, Robinson A, Faiman C, Winter JSD: Pituitary-gonadal function in Klinefelter syndrome before and during puberty. Pediatr Res 1985; 19:82–86.

Sanchez AG, Villanueva AG, Redondo C: Lobular carcinoma of the breast in a patient with Klinefelter's syndrome: a case with bilateral, synchronous, histologically different breast tumors. Cancer 1986; 57:1181–1183.

Sarimski K: Behavioral phenotypes and family stress in three mental retardation syndromes. Eur J Child Adolesc Psychiatry 1997; 6:26–31.

Sas TC, De Muinck Keizer-Schrama SM, Stijnen T, Van Teunenbroek A, Van Leeuwen WJ, Asarfi A, Van Rijn RR, Drop SL: Bone mineral density assessed by phalangeal radiographic absorptiometry before and during long-term growth hormone treatment in girls with Turner's syndrome participating in a randomized dose–response study. Pediatr Res 2001; 50:417–422.

Sasco AJ, Lowenfels AB, Pasker-de Jong P: Review article: epidemiology of male breast cancer—a meta-analysis of published case-control studies and discussion of selected aetiological factors. Int J Cancer 1993; 53:538–549.

Satge D, Sasco AJ, Cure H, Leduc B, Sommelet D, Vekemans MJ: An excess of testicular germ cell tumors in Down's syndrome: three case reports and a review of the literature. Cancer 1997; 80:929–935.

Satge D, Sommelet D, Geneix A, Nishi M, Malet P, Vekemans M: A tumor profile in Down syndrome. Am J Med Genet 1998; 78:207–216.

Savendahl L, Davenport ML: Delayed diagnoses of Turner's syndrome: proposed guidelines for change. J Pediatr 2000; 137:455–459.

Scambler PJ, Kelly D, Lindsay E, Williamson R, Goldberg R, Shprintzen RJ, Wilson D, Goodship J, Cross I, Burn J: Velo-cardio-facial syndrome associated with chromosome 22 deletions encompassing the DiGeorge locus. Lancet 1992; 339:1138–1139.

Scheike O, Visfeldt J, Petersen B: Male breast cancer. 3. Breast carcinoma in association with the Klinefelter syndrome. Acta Pathol Microbiol Scand 1973; 81:352–358.

Schlegelberger B, Schlegelberger T, Kekow J, Gross WL, Grote W: Monozygotic twins with Klinefelter's syndrome (concordant) and systemic lupus erythematosus (discordant). Klin Wochenschr 1984; 62:906–910.

Schoeller DA, Levitsky LL, Bandini LG, Dretz WW, Walczak A: Energy expenditure and body composition in Prader-Willi syndrome. Metabolism 1988; 39:115–120.

Schupf N, Zigman W, Kapell D, Lee JH, Kline J, Levin B: Early menopause in women with Down's syndrome. J Intellect Disabil Res 1997; 41:264–267.

Schwartz ID, Root AW: The Klinefelter syndrome of testicular dysgenesis. Endocrinol Metabol Clin N Am 1991; 20:153–163.

Scola PS, Pueschel SM: Menstrual cycles and basal body temperature curves in women with Down syndrome. Obstet Gynecol 1992; 79:91–94.

Seltzer GB, Schupf N, Wu HS: A prospective study of menopause in women with Down's syndrome. J Intellect Disabil Res 2001; 45(Pt 1):1–7.

Sengul A, Gul D, Sayli BS, Hacibektasoglu A: Antisperm antibody and Klinefelter syndrome: does autoimmunity play a role in the pathogenesis? Urol Int 1996; 57:77–79.

Shapira SK: An update on chromosome deletion and microdeletion syndromes. Curr Opin Pediatr 1998; 10:622–627.

Shapiro MB, France TD: The ocular features of Down's syndrome. Am J Ophthalmol 1985; 99:659–663.

Sher ES, Migeon CJ, Berkovitz GD: Evaluation of boys with marked breast development at puberty. Clin Pediatr (Phila) 1998; 37:367–371.

Shprintzen RJ: Velo-cardio-facial syndrome. In: Cassidy SB, Allanson JE (eds). Management of Genetic Syndromes. New York: Wiley, 2001:495–516.

Shprintzen RJ, Goldberg RB, Lewin ML, Sidoti EJ, Berkman MD, Argamaso RV, Young D: A new syndrome involving cleft palate, cardiac anomalies, typical facies, and learning disabilities: velo-cardio-facial syndrome. Cleft Palate J 1978; 15:56–62.

Shprintzen RJ, Goldberg R, Young D, Wolford L: The velo-cardio-facial syndrome: a clinical and genetic analysis. Pediatrics 1981; 67:167–172.

Shprintzen RJ, Morrow B, Kucherlapati R: Vascular anomalies may explain many of the features of velo-cardio-facial syndrome. Am J Hum Genet 1997; 61:Abstract 16, 34.

Shprintzen RJ, Siegel-Sadewitz VL, Amato J, Goldberg RB: Anomalies associated with cleft lip, cleft palate, or both. Am J Med Genet 1985; 20:585–596.

Skakkebaek NE, Bancroft J, Davidson DW, Warner P: Androgen replacement with oral testosterone undecanoate in hypogonadal men: a double blind controlled study. Clin Endocrinol 1981; 14:49–61.

Spier C, Shear NH, Lester RS: Recurrent leg ulcerations as the initial clinical manifestation of Klinefelter's syndrome. Arch Dermatol 1995; 131:230.

Staessen C, Coonen E, Van Assche E, Tournaye H, Joris H, Devroey P, Van Steirteghem AC, Liebaers I: Preimplantation diagnosis for X and Y normality in embryos from three Klinefelter patients. Hum Reprod 1996; 11:1650–1653.

Stafstrom CE: Epilepsy in Down syndrome: clinical aspects and possible mechanisms. Am J Ment Retard 1993; 98:12–26.

Stewart DA, Bailey JD, Netley CT, Park E: Growth, development, and behavioral outcome from mid-adolescence to adulthood in subjects with chromosome aneuploidy: the Toronto study. Birth Defects 1990; 26:131–188.

Sybert, VP: Turner syndrome. In: Cassidy SB, Allanson JE (eds). Management of Genetic Syndromes. New York: Wiley, 2001:459–484.

Sylven L, Magnusson C, Hagenfeldt K, von Schoultz B: Life with Turner's syndrome: a psychosocial report from 22 middle-aged women. Acta Endocrinol 1993; 129:188–194.

Tangerud A, Hestnes A, Sand T, Sunndalsfoll S: Degenerative changes in the cervical spine in Down's syndrome. J Ment Defic Res 1990; 34:179–185.

Tarani L, Lampariello S, Raguso G, Colloridi F, Pucarelli I, Pasquino AM, Bruni LA: Pregnancy in patients with Turner's syndrome: six new cases and review of literature. Gynecol Endocrinol 1998; 12:83–87.

Tassabehji M, Metcalfe K, Karmiloff-Smith A, Carette MJ, Grant J, Dennis N, Reardon W, Splitt M, Read AP, Donnai D: Williams syndrome: use of chromosomal microdeletions as a tool to dissect cognitive and physical phenotypes. Am J Hum Genet 1999; 64:118–125.

Tatum WO IVth, Passaro EA, Elia M, Guerrini R, Gieron M, Genton P: Seizures in Klinefelter's syndrome. Pediatr Neurol 1998; 19:275–278.

Tawn EJ, Earl R: The frequencies of constitutional chromosome abnormalities in an apparently normal adult population. Mutat Res 1992; 283:69–73.

Tay HP, Bidair M, Shabaik A, Gilbaugh JH III, Schmidt JD: Primary yolk sac tumor of the prostate in a patient with Klinefelter's syndrome. J Urol 1995; 153:1066–1069.

Terzoli G, Lalatta F, Lobbiani A, Simoni G, Colucci G: Fertility in a 47,XXY patient: assessment of biological paternity by deoxyribonucleic acid fingerprinting. Fertil Steril 1992; 58:821–822.

Theilgaard A: A psychological study of the personalities of XYY- and XXY-men. Acta Psychiatr Scand Suppl 1984; 315:1–133.

Therman E, Susman M: Human Chromosomes: Structure, Behavior, Effects, 3d ed. Heidelberg: Springer-Verlag, 1993.

Toth PP, Jogerst GJ: Identification of Turner's syndrome in an elderly woman: case report and review. Arch Fam Med 1996; 5:48–51

Tournaye H, Camus M, Goossens A, Liu J, Nagy P, Silber S, Van Steirteghem AC, Devroey P: Recent concepts in the management of infertility because of non-obstructive azoospermia. Hum Reprod 1995; 10:S115–119.

Tournaye H, Staessen C, Liebaers I, Van Assche E, Devroey P, Bonduelle M, Van Steirteghem A: Testicular sperm recovery in nine 47,XXY Klinefelter patients. Hum Reprod 1996; 11:1644–1649.

Turner HH: A syndrome of infantilism, congenital webbed neck, and cubitus valgus. Endocrinology 1938; 23:566–574.

Ugazio AG, Maccario R, Notarangelo LD, Burgio GR: Immunology of Down syndrome: a review. Am J Med Genet Suppl 1990; 7:204–212.

Valero MC, de Luis O, Cruces J, Perez Jurado LA: Fine-scale comparative mapping of the human 7q11.23 region and the orthologous region on mouse chromosome 5G: the low-copy repeats that flank the Williams-Beuren syndrome deletion arose at breakpoint sites of an evolutionary inversion(s). Genomics 2000; 69:1–13.

van Allen MI, Fung J, Jurenka SB: Health care concerns and guidelines for adults with Down syndrome. Am J Med Genet 1999; 89:100–110.

Van Buggenhout GJ, Trommelen JC, Schoenmaker A, De Bal C, Verbeek JJ, Smeets DF, Ropers HH, Devriendt K, Hamel BC, Fryns JP: Down syndrome in a population of elderly mentally retarded patients: genetic-diagnostic survey and implications for medical care. Am J Med Genet 1999; 85:376–384.

van den Bergh JP, Hermus AR, Spruyt AI, Sweep CG, Corstens FH, Smals AG: Bone mineral density and quantitative ultrasound parameters in patients with Klinefelter's syndrome after long-term testosterone substitution. Osteoporos Int 2001; 12:55–62.

Van Goor JC, Massa GG, Hirasing R: Increased incidence and prevalence of diabetes mellitus in Down's syndrome. Arch Dis Child 1997; 77:186.

van Schrojenstein Lantman-deValk HM, Haveman MJ, Crebolder HFJM: Comorbidity in people with Down's syndrome: a criteria-based analysis. J Intellect Disabil Res 1996; 40:385–399.

Varrela J, Alvesalo L: Taurodontism in 47,XXY males: an effect of the extra X chromosome on root development. J Dent Res 1988; 67:501–502.

Veraart JC, Hamulyak K, Neumann HA: Leg ulcers and Klinefelter's syndrome. Arch Dermatol 1995; 131:958–959.

Veraart JC, Hamulyak K, Neumann HA, Engelen J: Increased plasma activity of plasminogen activator inhibitor 1 (PAI-1) in two patients with Klinefelter's syndrome complicated by leg ulcers. Br J Dermatol 1994; 130:641–644.

Vlasak I, Plochl E, Kronberger G, Bergendi E, Rittinger O, Hagemann M, Schmitt K, Blumel P, Glatzl J, Fekete G, et al.: Screening of patients with Turner syndrome for "hidden" Y-mosaicism. Klin Padiatr 1999; 211:30–34

Wang C, Baker HW, Burger HG, De Kretser DM, Hudson B: Hormonal studies in Klinefelter's syndrome. Clin Endocrinol (Oxf) 1975; 4:399–411.

Winter JSD: Androgen therapy in Klinefelter syndrome during adolescence. Birth Defects 1990; 26:235–245.

Witkin HA, Mednick SA, Schulsinger F, Bakkestrom E, Christiansen KO, Goodenough DR, Hirschhorn K, Lundsteen C, Owen DR, Philip J, et al.: Criminality in XYY and XXY men. Science 1976; 193:547–555.

Wong FH, Pun KK, Wang C: Loss of bone mass in patients with Klinefelter's syndrome despite sufficient testosterone replacement. Osteoporos Int 1993; 3:3–7.

Wu RC, Kuo PL, Lin SJ, Liu CH, Tzeng CC: X chromosome mosaicism in patients with recurrent abortion or premature ovarian failure. J Formos Med Assoc 1993; 92:953–956.

Yaegashi N, Uehara S, Ogawa H, Hanew K, Igarashi A, Okamura K, Yajima A: Association of intrauterine growth retardation with monosomy of the terminal segment of the short arm of the X chromosome in patients with Turner's syndrome. Gynecol Obstet Invest 2000; 50:237–241.

Yamauchi M, Tadano M, Fukunaga Y, Inoue D, Minamikawa J, Koshiyama H: Low bone mineral density in a case of mosaicism Klinefelter syndrome: rapid response to testosterone therapy. Endocr J 1998; 45:601–604.

Yoshida A, Miura K, Nagao K, Hara H, Ishii N, Shirai M: Sexual function and clinical features of patients with Klinefelter's syndrome with the chief complaint of male infertility. Int J Androl 1997a; 20:80–85.

Yoshida A, Miura K, Shirai M: Cytogenetic survey of 1,007 infertile males. Urol Int 1997b; 58:166–176.

Yunis JJ: High resolution of human chromosomes. Science 1976; 191:1268–1270.

Zhang SZ, Xie T, Tang YC, Zhang SL, Xu Y: The prevalence of chromosome diseases in the general population of Sichuan, China. Clin Genet 1991; 39:81–88.

Zinn AR, Tonk VS, Chen Z, Flejter WL, Gardner HA, Guerra R, Kushner H, Schwartz S, Sybert VP, Van Dyke DL, Ross JL: Evidence for a Turner syndrome locus or loci at Xp11.2–p22.1. Am J Hum Genet 1998; 63:1757–1766.

Zollner TM, Veraart JC, Wolter M, Hesse S, Villemur B, Wenke A, Werner RJ, Boehncke WH, Jost SS, Scharrer I, Kaufmann R: Leg ulcers in Klinefelter's syndrome: further evidence for an involvement of plasminogen activator inhibitor-1. Br J Dermatol 1997; 136:341–344.

Part XI

THERAPY

54 Genetic Consequences of Modern Therapeutics: Iatrogenic Mutagenesis

JOHN J. MULVIHILL, SARAH F. WHITTON, AND PATRICK H. HORN

CLINICAL ANECDOTES

R. W. Miller has pointed out that most carcinogens and teratogens have been discovered by alert practitioners (Miller, 1978; Miller, 1981). Despite the number of patients with sporadic mutations seen by medical geneticists, clinicians do not seem to inquire about the possible environmental origins of these mutations. Over the years, one of us (JJM) has become aware of just two credible anecdotes.

Case 1: A child had unequivocal tuberous sclerosis apparently due to spontaneous mutation. To current memory, both parents had been investigated clinically, including by imaging, and were considered not to have tuberous sclerosis. The father was an air conditioning repairer and gave the intriguing history that, about three months before the conception of his affected child, a charge of Freon had exploded in his face. This highly flammable substance singed his hair and required his hospitalization (or at least emergency consultation) because of respiratory distress, perhaps from inhalation of the by-products of combustion. It seems that Freon burns to an alkylating agent, so it can be hypothesized that this transient but toxic exposure to an inhalated alkylator at a time of early sperm formation could have caused mutation in *TSC1* or *TSC2*.

Case 2: A young man survived lymphoma with multiple modality chemotherapy. He got married and experienced infertility. Through the technology of gamete in vitro transfer (GIFT), he was finally able to initiate a pregnancy, and twins were born: one was normal clinically and cytogenetically; the other had malformations, developmental delay, and a translocated chromosome. Both parents had normal karyotypes; hence, the translocation presumedly arose de novo, perhaps in association with the management of the father's lymphoma.

Perhaps it is appropriate that clinical geneticists are not reporting these anecdotes which, after all, only serve to set a hypothesis that is already valid because of other scientific considerations. Raising the suspicion that an exposure is possibly etiologic could well produce undue anxiety and further guilt in the parents of persons with "spontaneous" mutations.

That said, a major question in the mind of every person touched with disease is, "Why me? Why my child? Why my family? Why this disorder?" The central theme of this volume is providing answers to such questions, for it addresses the genetic determinants of common human disease. A large part of the clinical and research work of human and medical geneticists is the delineation of genetic variations that contribute to disease. However, "genes or changed genes" or "ecogenetics" only answers in part the question of causation. Going a step back, what has caused a gene to change?

In answering that question, the typical medical geneticist wears at least two hats. When seeing a child with achondroplasia born to normal parents, the geneticist with a *clinician's* hat explains to the parents that the new mutation in their family was a spontaneous occurrence. "Mutation just happens," says the clinical geneticist. The geneticist with a *biologist's* view knows that mutation is the building block of evolution—an essential characteristic of life itself. The very notion of "spontaneous mutation," or a mutation without an explanation, is dissatisfying and unacceptable. The genetic biologist knows that something must have caused a chromosome to be broken, a nucleotide to be changed, or a DNA sequence to be altered.

Environmental mutagenesis is the study of the extrinsic origins of sudden and permanent changes in DNA, the genetic material. The discipline is the subject of many research monographs that focus on carcinogenicity but summarize mutagenicity in detail (International Agency for Research on Cancer, 1974a, 1974b, 1975, 1976, 1977, 1978, 1979, 1980a, 1980b, 1981, 1987, 1990, 1994, 1996, 1998, 1999), and a few textbooks (Vogel and Rohrborn, 1970; Prakash et al., 1974; Hollaender and Serres, 1978; Heddle, 1982; Brusick, 1984; Grossblatt, 1989; Schottenfeld and Fraumeni, 1996; Wells, 1998). Many nations or regions have an environmental mutagen society with associated websites and journals (e.g., *http://www.ems-us.org* and *http://193.51.164.11/eems/index.htm*, for societies in the United States and Europe, respectively; *Mutation Research, Environmental and Molecular Mutagenesis*, etc.). Also, there are periodic international congresses of environmental mutagenesis.

Many clinical and research geneticists who focus on understanding the molecular and cellular pathogenesis of human hereditary disease or who care for affected persons and families may not be well versed on the possible origins of human mutation and methods for detection. Increased knowledge on their part may improve their clinical genetic counseling—for example, by providing authoritative assurance that a parental exposure to chemotherapy as a child likely did *not* result in a new sporadic genetic disease in the offspring. Recognition of the scientific challenge to understand "spontaneous mutation" may lead to insights from systematic study of the cases of new mutations that are evaluated in every genetics clinic.

Here, we review the principles of human mutagenesis, strategies for identifying environmental mutagens, and clinical counseling issues that surround possible genetic effects of human therapeutics. Finally, a note is made on a related subject: namely, the principles of human teratogenicity. The focus is on human germ cell mutagenesis, or the causes of "sporadic" genetic changes in human beings that are manifested in offspring.

PRINCIPLES OF HUMAN MUTAGENESIS

Exposures and Classes of Mutagens

Because of the chemical nature of DNA, certain classes of physical and chemical agents are more likely than others to interact with chromosomes and molecular DNA. At the same time, given the complex biostructure of chromosomes and the molecular anatomy of DNA, it is not surprising that many classes of agents can interact with chromosomes and genes.

Radiation

The subject of H. J. Müller's 1946 Nobel Prize (Müller et al., 1954) and his presidential address in the first volume of the *American Journal of Human Genetics* (Müller, 1950) was radiation, a long-studied experimental mutagen. Ionizing radiation interacts with DNA by causing ionizing events that break DNA strands and, hence, chromosomes. Likewise, X-rays cause alkylation that can permanently alter the base sequence. Ultraviolet radiation has the peculiar tendency to cause dimerization between adjacent thymidines also interrupting gene function. Both types of radiation, ionizing and ultraviolet, are known human carcinogens and thus establish the principle that a carcinogen can be a suspected mutagen.

Cancer Drugs and Other Drugs

Chemicals that produce effects similar to those of radiation are called *radiomimetic*. Their mechanism of action reflects what is known about the DNA damage by radiation. Of course, the ability to design agents that interact selectively with DNA is the foundation for much of the theory and practice of cancer chemotherapy. Again, specific classes of agents are prone to cause genetic damage.

One class is the alkylating agents that add alkyl groups to specific sites in DNA. Examples are busulfan, carboplatin, cyclophosphamide, chlorambucil, cisplatin, dacarbazine, nitrogen mustard, melphalan, and thiotepa.

Another class, the antimetabolites, interrupts the synthesis of purines and pyrimidines by blocking folate metabolism. Examples include cytarabine, uridine, and methotrexate.

A third group is the purine and pyrimidine analogs that get incorporated in place of their normal congeners in the nucleotide sequence of DNA. Examples include cladribine, pentostatin, 5-fluorouracil, 5-fluorodeoxyuridine, 6-mercaptopurine, 6-thioguanine, and cytosine arabinoside.

Finally, there are antibiotics such as mitomycin C, streptomycin, bleomycin, dactinomycin, and adriamycin hydrochloride that bind to receptor sites on a cell, enter the cell, inhibit the synthesis of RNA and DNA, and cause DNA strand breakage by reacting with or binding to the cell's DNA.

The group of cancer chemotherapeutic agents that do not act directly on DNA but on the chromosomal material is illustrated by vincristine and vinblastine. These agents paralyze the mitotic spindle and block normal cells and cancer cells from undergoing programmed mitosis. In theory, if they were mutagens, they could affect chromosome assortment and perhaps cause aneuplody, but not nucleotide substitution. It is of interest that the only epidemiologically substantiated human germ cell mutagen is of this class—trichlorfon exposure associated with the Hungarian cluster of trisomy 21 Down syndrome (see below, "*Oocyte Endpoints*").

Mechanisms

It is not sufficient to know that a chemical or physical agent interacts with DNA in vitro to declare it a mutagen. To cause human effects, the action has to take place in a complex biological system that has many other steps that could possibly increase or decrease the probability of a mutagenic effect. Such intermediary steps include the uptake of chemicals into the body by various routes and the transport of them to target sites—for example, to the lung or the liver. At the site of action, metabolic activation or inactivation of drugs can alter their mutagenic and carcinogenic potential. The transport of an active intermediate to another site by plasma proteins through cellular plasma membranes and nuclear membranes are all additional steps that could alter mutagenicity. Finally, the actual interaction with chromosomes or DNA must not be so toxic that further cellular metabolism and cell division are impossible. Hence, to be recognized as a mutagen, some other cellular genetic consequences must be observable often in daughter cells distant from the original target cell.

With all of these sources of variability, it is not surprising that there is genetic variation in the sensitivity to mutation from human drugs, an area known as pharmacogenetics.

Endpoints

Somatic Cells, Including Cancer

Many systems for detecting human mutagens hinge on nonhuman systems that detect somatic cell mutation. The prototype is the so-called Ames test based on the susceptibility of various strains of *Salmonella typhimurium* to mutagenic chemicals, first popularized by Bruce Ames, University of California at Berkeley (Ames et al., 1973a, 1973b). A huge body of literature and regulation has developed around these and other short-term test systems and their interpretation and application to human mutation, mutagenesis, and carcinogenesis. In short, the conclusion seems to be that just a few test strains are useful in predicting the mutagenicity of chemicals. However, there are important exceptions—a few known human carcinogens like benzene and diethylstilbestrol are *not* bacterial mutagens (International Commission for Protection against Environmental Mutagens and Carcinogens, 1985; Fitzgerald et al., 1989), and many *non*carcinogens are reactive in *Salmonella* (ICPEMC, 1985; Morita et al., 1989). The correlation is good, but not perfect, so there is concern that the regulatory application of the Ames test results may not be appropriate in public health and environmental regulations. Hence, many additional somatic cell mutation systems have been developed (Table 54–1). As one proceeds through the systems that include yeast, *Drosophila*, and mice, there tends to be increasing complexity and cost but also, perhaps, more relevance to human and public health.

The one test that has become a gold standard for predicting chemical carcinogens is the administration of chemicals, by various routes of exposure, depending on likely human use, followed by long-term surveillance for benign and malignant neoplasms, in the so-called rodent bioassay. The test strains are mouse strains such as the B6C3F$_1$, B6CF$_1$/An1, A, C57L, B10-A, C3H, C3H/HEN, C57B1, C57B1/6N, Sencar, SWR, and Balb/c strains, and rat strains such as the Fischer 344, Oshborne-Mendel, and Sprague-Dawley strains. Most rodent carcinogenicity assays are conducted for a two-year period of exposure.

Table 54–1. Assays for Genotoxic Effects

Effects Detected	Assays
Assays for gene mutations	
BACTERIAL ASSAYS	
Reversion of auxotrophs	*Salmonella*/mammalian microsome assay (Ames test); *E. coli* WP2 tryptophan reversion assay
Forward mutations	Arabinose resistance in *Salmonella*
FUNGAL ASSAYS	
Reversion of auxotrophs	Reversion of auxotrophs in *Neurospora* or yeast
Forward mutations and small deletions	Adenine mutants detected by colony color in *Neurospora* or yeast
MAMMALIAN CELL ASSAYS	
Forward mutations	TK mutants selected by resistance to pyrimidine analogs in Chinese hamster or human cells; HPRT mutants selected by resistance to purine analogs in Chinese human cells; HPRT mutants selected by resistance to purine analogs in Chinese hamster AS52 cells
PLANT ASSAYS	
Mutations in flowers, pollen, or seedlings	*Tradescantia* stamen hair color; corn *waxy* locus; chlorophyll mutations in various plants
DROSOPHILA ASSAYS	
Gene mutations and small deletions in germ cells	X-linked recessive lethal test
IN VIVO MAMMALIAN ASSAYS	
Gene mutations and deletions in germ cells	Mouse specific-locus test using visible markers; mouse electrophoretic specific-locus test; dominant mutations causing mouse skeletal defects or cataracts
Gene mutations in somatic cells	Mouse spot test (somatic cell specific-locus test); HPRT mutations detected by resistance to 6-thioguanine in rodent lymphocytes
Gene mutations in bacterial target genes in transgenic mice	*lacI* mutations in mice and rats; *lacZ* mutations in mice
Assays for chromosome damage	
MAMMALIAN CELL ASSAYS	
Chromosome aberrations	Metaphase analysis in Chinese hamster cells or human lymphocytes
Chromosome breakage in human lymphocytes	Cytokinesis-block micronucleus assay
PLANT ASSAYS	
Chromosome aberrations and micronuclei	Cytogenetic analysis of mitotic or meiotic cells
DROSOPHILA ASSAYS	
Chromosome aberrations	Heritable translocation assays
IN VIVO MAMMALIAN ASSAYS	
Chromosome damage in somatic cells	Metaphase analysis of rodent bone marrow or lymphocytes
Chromosome damage in germ cells	Cytogenetic analysis of oocytes, spermatogonia, or spermatocytes; micronuclei in mouse spermatids
Indirect evidence of germ cell chromosome damage	Mouse or rat dominant lethal assay
Heritable chromosome aberrations in germ cells	Mouse heritable translocation test
Assays for aneuploidy	
FUNGAL ASSAYS	
Mitotic aneuploidy	Genetic detection of chromosome loss and gain in yeast
Meiotic nondisjunction	Disomic ascospores in yeast or *Neurospora*
MAMMALIAN CELL ASSAYS	
Aberrant cell division	Disturbance of the mitotic apparatus observed by differential staining of the spindle and chromosomes
Mitotic aneuploidy	Hyperploidy detected by chromosome counts; counts for chromosome gain or loss in cells with intact cytoplasm
Centromere loss	Micronucleus assay with kinetochore labeling or FISH for centromeres
PLANT ASSAYS	Aneuploid sectors detected by pigmentation in hexaploid wheat
DROSOPHILA ASSAYS	
Sex chromosome aneuploidy	Sex chromosome loss tests
IN VIVO MAMMALIAN ASSAYS	
Mitotic aneuploidy	Hyperploidy in mouse bone marrow; mouse bone marrow micronucleus assay with kinetochore labeling or FISH for centromeres
Nondisjunction in germ cells	Hyperploidy detected by chromosome counts
Sex chromosome loss by nondisjunction or chromosome breakage	Genetic deletion of mice with a single X chromosome and no Y
Other indicators of genetic damage or mutagen exposure	
BACTERIAL ASSAYS	
Repairable DNA damage	Differential killing of repair-deficient and wild-type strains in the *Bacillus subtilis rec* assay
SOS induction	Induction of the SOS system by DNA damage in *E. coli*
FUNGAL ASSAYS	
Recombinagenicity	Mitotic crossing over and gene conversion assays in yeast

(*continued*)

Table 54–1. Assays for Genotoxic Effects (*Continued*)

Effects Detected	Assays
MAMMALIAN CELL ASSAYS	
Repairable DNA damage	Unscheduled DNA synthesis (UDS) in rat hepatocytes
DNA strand breaks	Alkaline elution, single-cell gel electrophoresis (comet assay), and pulse field gel assays
Sister chromatid exchange	SCE in human cells or Chinese hamster cells
DROSOPHILA ASSAYS	
Recombinagenicity	Mitotic recombination in eyes or wings
IN VIVO MAMMALIAN ASSAYS	
Sister chromatid exchange	SCE in rodent tissues, especially bone marrow
Repairable DNA damage	UDS in rodent hepatocytes
DNA damage in germ cells	Molecular dosimetry based on mutagen adducts; UDS in rodent germ cells; alkaline elution assays for DNA strand breaks in rodent testes

Source: Modified from Hoffmann (1996) with permission.

The results of these assays weigh heavily on predicting human carcinogenesis and are crucial in the economic decision to introduce into wide production a new or alternate chemicals, including drugs.

There have been isolated lines of evidence that suggest the mutational origins of other common diseases besides cancer, including aging (Wallace, 1994; Berdanier and Everts, 2001) and arteriosclerotic cardiovascular disease (Chung et al., 1998). Still, with regard to human endpoints, the most certain and relevant prediction from human somatic cell mutagenesis today is human carcinogenesis, justly so because of the high prevalence and severe burden of cancer.

Germ Cells, Including Reproductive Failure

Other major endpoints that have been studied over the years include mutation in human white blood cells and sperm. A now ethically inappropriate study was conducted in the United States in the 1950s (Rowley et al., 1974; Brewen and Preston, 1975). Prisoners were asked to volunteer for testicular biopsies before and after exposure to ionizing radiation. The biopsies permitted evaluation of meiotic figures as a measure of germ cell mutagenesis. The results, based on small numbers, suggested a dose–response curve for meiotic errors seen cytogenetically with increasing doses of ionizing radiation.

With regard to experimental germ cell mutagenesis, the gold standard has for many years been the seven locus murine test of the Russells at the Oak Ridge National Laboratory (Russell, 1951). In the 1960s, Udo Ehling (1965, 1966) in Munich, Germany, introduced tests of additional loci, which document mutations at a number of loci in mice by the expression of phenotypic manifestations, such as skeletal abnormalities, cataracts, coat color, hair texture, changes in eye and ear size, and limb and tail structure. Often dose–response effects are seen for various classes of chemical and physical agents, including ionizing radiation. These assays are largely done on male mice for reasons of numbers and ease of breeding. The results have become the major determinant of radiation protection standards by the World Health Organization and the U.S. National Academy of Sciences.

EVIDENCE IN HUMAN BEINGS

In human beings, the major endpoints sought as evidence for germ cell mutation are single-gene diseases, congenital malformations, spontaneous abortions, alteration in sex ratio at birth, and infertility (presumably resulting from a decreased fertilization or other impairment of the early embryo, resulting in unrecognized miscarriage). Again, surrogates for germ cell mutations have been sought in mutations in somatic cells.

Somatic Cells

Evidence for the induction of mutations in human somatic cells by drugs and other agents is beyond doubt, especially as reflected in the clinically important endpoint of carcinogenesis (Table 54–2). Several points can be gleaned from the list. Given the plethora of chemicals and drugs in use, it is somewhat reassuring that the list is as short as it is. In fact, some of the entries in Table 54–2 represent historical agents that are no longer in use, in part because of the recognition of their carcinogenicity. It is both discouraging and understandable how many of these agents are used to control an initial cancer; it seems paradoxical at first that so many antineoplastic agents are carcinogens. However, surveillance cannot be relaxed in the development of new pharmaceuticals because of the burden of human cancer. There are computer algorithms that predict carcinogenicity based on molecular structure and human cancer risk (Rosenkranz and Klopman, 1990). But, to date, regulators have insisted on the long-term rodent bioassay for cancer and relied on scrupulous reporting of the adverse effects when new pharmacologic agents are introduced.

Chromosomal breakage has largely been assayed in occupational cohorts as a sentinel for cancer, but it can be considered to be a flag for possible germ cell mutation as well. For example, in a cohort of hospital workers exposed to various agents known or suspected to induce chromosomal damage (especially ionizing radiation), 871 hospital workers and 617 controls were examined (Bonassi et al., 1997). Groups were compared by job title in their relation to the frequency of chromosomal aberrations. Compared with controls, all workers had increased aberration, but higher frequencies were seen for certain job titles, particularly for radiologists, orthopedists, anesthesiologists, other medical doctors, and nurses. The common exposure was felt to be ionizing radiation. A decrease in the amount of ionizing radiation absorbed in the medical setting in recent years and a decrease in the number of chromosomal aberrations support much other evidence that radiation promotes chromosomal breakage. An elevated frequency of chromosome aberrations has been observed in clean-up workers ("liquidators") exposed to radiation after the Chernobyl nuclear accident. They also have increases in sperm abnormalities, somatic cell chromosomal ab-

Table 54–2. Drugs That Are Carcinogenic to Humans

Drug	Human Tumors[a]	Reference[b]
Antineoplastic Drugs (proprietary name)		
Azacitidine	NAD	N, I
Azathioprine	Squamous cell cancers of the skin, non-Hodgkin's lymphoma, hepatobiliary, and mesenchymal	N, I
Bis(chloroethyl) nitrosourea (BCNU)	Acute nonlymphocytic leukemia	N, I
Bleomycins (Bleomycin hydrochloride and Bleomycin sulfate)	NAD	I
1, 4 Butanediol dimethyl sulfonate (Myleran; Busulfan)	Acute nonlymphocytic leukemia	N, I
Chlorambucil	Acute nonlymphocytic leukemia	N, I
1-(2-Chloroethyl)-3-cyclohexyl-1-nitrosourea (CCNU)	Acute nonlymphocytic leukemia	N, I
1-(2-Chloroethyl)-3-(4-methylcyclohexyl)-1-nitrosourea (Methyl-CCNU; Semustine)	Acute nonlymphocytic leukemia	N, I
Chlorozotocin	NAD	N, I
Cisplatin	NAD	N, I
Cyclophosphamide (Cytoxan)	Bladder, acute nonlymphocytic leukemia	N, I
Dacarbazine	NAD	N, I
Melphalan/Medphalan/Merphalan	Acute nonlymphocytic leukemia	N, I
8-Methoxypsoralen (Methoxsalen) with ultraviolet A therapy (PUVA)	Basal cell skin and squamous cell skin	N, I
Mitomycin C	NAD	I
MOPP and other combined chemotherapy with alkylating agents	Acute nonlymphocytic leukemia, central nervous system, lung, thyroid, gastrointestinal system	I
Mustard gas or sulfur mustard	Lung/respiratory tract	N, I
Nitrogen mustard and nitrogen mustard hydrochloride	Squamous cell carcinomas of the skin	N, I
Nitrogen mustard *N*-oxide and nitrogen mustard *N*-oxide hydrochloride	NAD	I
N-Methyl-*N*-nitrosourea (*N*-Nitroso-*N*-methylurea)	NAD	N
N, N-Bis(2-chloroethyl)-2-naphthylamine (Chlornaphazine)	Bladder	I
Procarbazine hydrochloride	Acute nonlymphocytic leukemia	N, I
Tris(1-aziridinyl)phosphine sulfide (Thiotepa)	Acute nonlymphocytic leukemia	N, I
Treosulfan	Acute nonlymphocytic leukemia	I
Uracil mustard	NAD	I
Urethane (Urethan; Ethyl carbamate)	NAD	N, I
Hormonal drugs		
ANDROGENIC (ANABOLIC) STEROIDS		
Oxymetholone	Myeloid leukemia, liver, prostate	N, I
Testosterone	Myeloid leukemia, liver, prostate	I
Testosterone enanthate	Myeloid leukemia, liver, prostate	I
Testosterone propionate	Myeloid leukemia, liver, prostate	I
ESTROGENS, STEROIDAL		
CONJUGATED ESTROGENS		
Piperazine estrone sulfate	Liver, testicular, embryonal cell, breast, endometrial	N, I
Sodium equilin sulfate	Liver, testicular, embryonal cell, breast, endometrial	N, I
Sodium estrone sulfate	Liver, testicular, embryonal cell, breast, endometrial	N, I
ESTROGENS, NOT CONJUGATED		
17β-Estradiol	Endometrial	N, I
Estriol	NAD	I
Estrone	Endometrial	N, I
Ethinylestradiol	Liver, endometrial	N, I
Mestranol	Liver, endometrial	N, I
ESTROGENS, NONSTEROIDAL		
Diethylstilbestrol and Diethylstilbestrol diproprionate	Vagina, cervix, breast, endometrial, ovary, colon-rectum	N, I
Dienestrol	NAD	I
Hexestrol	NAD	I
Estrogen replacement therapy, postmenopausal	Breast, endometrial	I
Estrogen-progestogen therapy, postmenopausal	NAD	I
Methylthiouracil	NAD	I
Oral contraceptives, combined	Endometrial, cervical, liver, pituitary	I
Oral contraceptives, sequential	Endometrial, cervical, liver, pituitary	I
PROGESTINS		
Chlormadinone acetate	NAD	I
Dimethisterone	NAD	I
Ethynodiol diacetate	NAD	I
17α-Hydroxyprogesterone caproate	NAD	I
Lynestrenal	NAD	I
Medroxyprogesterone acetate	Breast, ovary, liver, endometrium, uterus, cervix	I
Megestrol acetate	NAD	I
Norethisterone	NAD	N, I
Norethynodrel	NAD	I
Norgestrel	NAD	I

(*continued*)

Table 54–2. Drugs That Are Carcinogenic to Humans (*Continued*)

Drug	Human Tumors[a]	Reference[b]
PROGESTINS (*Continued*)		
Progesterone	NAD	N, I
Tamoxifen	Endometrial	I
Propylthiouracil	Pituitary gland, thyroid gland, leukemia	N, I
Antimicrobial drugs		
Adriamycin (Doxorubicin hydrochloride)	Bone, acute nonlymphocytic leukemia	N, I
Azaserine	NAD	I
Chloramphenicol	Acute nonlymphocytic leukemia	I
Daunomycin	NAD	I
Formaldehyde (gas)	Nasal cavity, nasopharyngeal cavity	N, I
Griseofulvin	NAD	I
Metronidazole	Lung, uterus, cervix, vagina	N, I
Niridazole	NAD	I
Streptozotocin	NAD	N, I
Other drugs		
Arsenic and arsenic compounds	Lung, respiratory tract, renal, bladder, skin, liver, colon, stomach	N, I
Cyclosporin A (Cyclosporine A; Ciclosporin)	Lymphomas, Kaposi's sarcoma, skin	N, I
Danthron (1,8-Dihydroxyanthraquinone; Chrysazin)	NAD	
Iron dextran complex	Local sarcomas at site of injection	N
Nafenopin	NAD	I
Oxazepam	NAD	I
Panfuran-S (Dihydroxymethylfuratrizine)	NAD	I
Phenacetin and analgesic mixtures with phenacetin	Urinary tract, bladder, renal pelvic, urothelial	N, I
Phenazopyridine hydrochloride	NAD	N, I
Phenobarbital	Liver, brain, lung	I
Phenoxybenzamine hydrochloride	NAD	N, I
Phenytoin	Brain, neural crest, neuroblastoma	N, I
Reserpine	Breast	N
Thorium dioxide	Liver, renal pelvis, leukemia	N, I

[a]NAD = No adequate data are available to evaluate the carcinogenicity in humans. Because this drug has been shown to promote carcinogenesis in experimental animals, it has been placed on the "*Reasonably anticipated to be a human carcinogen*" list in the National Toxicology Program's *Eighth Report on Carcinogens* and/or on the "*Probably carcinogenic to humans*" or "*Possibly carcinogenic to humans*" list in IARC monographs.
[b]N, U.S. Deptartment of Health and Human Services, Public Health Service, National Toxicology Program; I, International Agency for Research on Cancer, 1998.

normalities, carcinomas of the thyroid gland, and leukemia. De novo mutations have been claimed to occur in the progeny of the irradiated liquidators (Dubrova et al., 1996; Jeffreys, 1997; Weinberg et al., 1997, 2001)

Somatic mutagenic effects due to chemical exposure at extremely low dose levels have been detected in several occupational cohorts for ethylene oxide, which is used in hospitals for sterilization and in chemical plants to produce ethylene glycol (antifreeze), polyester fibers and films, and detergents. At ethylene oxide concentrations as low as 1 ppm, chromosomal aberrations and alterations in DNA repair have been observed as unscheduled DNA synthesis, deficits in DNA repair, and increases of sister chromatid exchanges and chromosomal aberrations, including quadriradials (Landrigan et al., 1984; Dellarco et al., 1990). These data clearly demonstrate the genetic toxicity of ethylene oxide in human somatic cells. Many cohort studies link asbestos in the industrial setting to lung cell chromosomal aberrations and lung cancer (Steenland and Stayner, 1997; Bofetta, 1998; Marczynski et al., 2000). In cohort studies involving miners, foundry workers, and ceramic workers exposed to silica, an increase in carcinomas and cellular chromosomal aberrations of the lung and stomach cells have been observed (Steenland and Stayner, 1997). Studies of workers at nickel refineries have linked nickel compounds to an increase in cellular chromosomal aberrations and cancers of the nasal cavity and lung (Anttilla et al., 1998). A century ago, an excess of bladder cancer was noted among workers exposed to the manufacture of dyestuffs (Rehn, 1895). Later studies (Meigs et al., 1986; Hemstreet et al., 2001) showed persons exposed to benzidine for more than two years had an excess of bladder cancer and chromosomal breakage in cells of the urinary tract. In short, when somatic cell mutation is looked for in occupational cancer studies, it is seen consistently.

Evidence is present but sparser in environmental carcinogens apart from occupation. Chewing betel quid accounts for the high incidence of oral cancer in India. In Hyderabad, buccal mucosa cells of chewers were compared with those of nonchewers. All participants were male vegetable market workers and most were nonsmokers. Chewers had a significant increase in the frequency of chromosomal breakage in buccal cells over nonchewers (Rupa and Eastman, 1997).

Lastly, chromosomal breakage and other measures of somatic cell mutation besides cancer have been seen by many assays in the long-term survivors of the American atomic bombs in Japan (Hakoda et al., 1988).

The few human conditions that have constitutional increases in chromosomal breakage all predispose to cancer, although highly specific cancers. For example, sister chromatid exchanges are present constitutionally at 10-fold the usual rate in persons with Bloom syndrome. These individuals have an excess of leukemia, especially acute monomyelocytic leukemia in childhood, and an excess of squamous cell carcinomas of the upper aerodigestive tract in adult life (German, 1983). Likewise, individuals with Fanconi anemia have chromosomal breakage constitutionally and in response to the mutagens diepoxybutane and mitomycin C and also have an excess risk of acute monomyelogenous leukemia, hepatic adenoma, and carcinoma, among a few other malignancies (Auerbach, 1992). Finally, the disorder ataxia-telangiectasia has excess chromosomal breakage, probably as a reflection of high rates of recombination and an excess of both leukemia and lymphoma in the homozygotes (Bridges and Harnden, 1982; Gatti and Swift, 1985).

Germ Cells

Sperm Endpoints

Beyond the observation of meiotic chromosomal abnormalities in irradiated testes, there have been exploratory studies of sperm abnormalities—for example, in occupational cohorts and in cancer patients who were exposed to large doses of chemotherapy and radiotherapy. Abnormalities in sperm number and motility, as well as direct chromosomal abnormality by the arduous human-hamster sperm chromosome assay (Martin et al., 1986, 1999) and by point mutation studies (e.g., in *HGPRT*), document the phenomenon of human sperm abnormalities in response to drugs and radiation (Hales et al., 2002).

Oocyte Endpoints

Analogous studies in oocytes are much more difficult to conduct because of the difficulty of collecting human eggs versus sperm.

Where laboratory methods have fallen short, one epidemiologic study suggested a unique episode of possible human germ cell mutagenesis in oocytes (Czeizel et al., 1993). In the rural village of Rinya, Hungary, an excess of Down syndrome over a three-year period was investigated. The epidemic correlated with the introduction of new methods for raising fish in the local water. Around the Easter religious feasts, fish were in great demand. The residents realized that the local fish farm treated the water with a pesticide trichlorfon at certain times of the year. Following such treatments, fish were often found dead or dying, floating on the top of the water—easy pickings for the Easter feast. For three years in a row after trichlorfon was introduced, there was slight excess number of births of Down syndrome that proved to be due to errors in the second division of meiosis II, in the three out of four cases that could be assayed by molecular genetic studies. The interpretation was that the new pesticide to improve yield had been taken up by the fish and ingested by the mother around the time of ovulation and conception. It may be that this agent poisoned meiotic mechanisms, leading to an epidemic of nondisjunction. Further evidence of the causal association was gained when the fish farming practices were changed and birth rates of Down syndrome returned to normal. The feasibility of even conducting this investigation is partly credited to an excellent long-term birth defects monitoring system in Hungary and its ability to recognize and mobilize on a possible change in frequency.

Offspring Studies

Gaining direct evidence of germ cell mutagenesis has been the object of studies of offspring of cohorts exposed to possible mutagens. The group studied the longest and in the greatest detail is the cohort of Japanese exposed to the American atomic bombs. The most recent update of this experience reiterated that no clear evidence of germ cell mutation was seen by eight parameters: untoward pregnancy outcomes, deaths among live-born infants (exclusive of those resulting from a malignant tumor), malignancies in the offspring, frequency of structural rearrangements of chromosomes, frequency of sex-chromosome aneuploids, frequency of mutation-altering protein charge or function, sex ratio among children of exposed mothers, and growth and development of the offspring (Satoh et al., 1996; Neel, 1998). The investigators pointed out that their observations are compatible with a doubling dose of 1.7 to 2.2 sieverts (Neel et al., 1990). This dose is in the range of the doubling effect seen in the other well-studied mammalian system, the murine multilocus systems at Oak Ridge and Munich (Neel and Lewis, 1990).

Based on several large retrospective case series (Table 54–3), some with controls, there is room for reassurance that, despite expectations, no excess of birth defects or genetic diseases has been seen in the offspring of cancer survivors who maintain fertility enough to bear or father children. In 7837 liveborns from 16 case series in the literature, the summary rate of birth defects and genetic disease is 3.7%, a rate comparable to that in the general population. The studies were not all directly comparable in how cancer survivors were identified and pregnancy outcomes were defined.

The single largest study completed, our Five Center Study, was sponsored by the National Cancer Institute and used family controls and population-expected numbers, and no excess of genetic disease was seen (Byrne et al., 1998). That study alone had a 94% power to detect a 50% increase and did not find it. Among 4256 offspring of survivors of childhood and adolescent cancer followed for over 32,000 person-years, 33 offspring had cancer; 25 of them had retinoblastoma, as did a parent of each. Except for known hereditary or familial cancer syndromes, the offspring of survivors of cancer seem to have no excess of cancer (Mulvihill et al., 1987; Hawkins et al., 1989). Preliminary results in 4,214 offspring of survivors in the new North American Childhood Cancer Survivors Study likewise showed no excess of genetic disease (3.7% in case-offspring, compared to 4.4% in offspring of sibling-controls) (Mulvihill et al., 2001). Although related more to carcinogenesis than mutagenesis, the excessive recurrence risk of cancer in siblings of children with cancer is also totally explained by known syndromes (Winther et al., 2001).

Based on just two offspring with interventricular septal defects of the heart, the question was raised of possible adverse effects on pregnancies of women who had received dactinomycin (Green et al., 1991). Special analysis of the Five Center Study data could not confirm the association (Byrne et al., 1992).

In Hungary, a study showed that offspring born to mothers after a near-lethal suicide attempt did not have higher rates of abnormalities or fetal death due to germinal mutation (Czeizel, 1996).

COUNSELING POINTS

Genetic Counseling after Mutagenic Therapy

The discussion with former cancer patients with concerns about possible mutagenicity in themselves proceeds along these lines. There are major theoretical concerns about possible somatic and germ cell mutagenesis. Cancer treatments are specifically designed to interfere with DNA, cellular metabolism, and cell division. There is good reason to suspect that cancer treatments could cause mutation and genetic disease in human beings. They do so in mice and in somatic cells of human beings (e.g., sustained chromosomal breakage or second cancers after cancer treatment). However, contrary to theoretical expectations, no environmental agent has been causally linked to human germ cell mutation, as is seen in offspring with genetic disease, with the possible exception of trichlorfon causing meiotic nondisjunction. Despite intensive study of various endpoints, an excess of ge-

Table 54–3. Large Series of Pregnancies Among Survivors of Cancer

	Exposed Parents		Completed Pregnancies			Liveborns		
Reference	Total	Females (%)	Total	Fetal Loss[a]	Elective Abortions	Total	With Defects	Defects
Li and Jaffe, 1974	46	63	107	12	3	92	2	Hirschsprung disease, asymptomatic heart murmur[c]
Ross, 1976	58[b]	100	96	18	?	78	3	Pendred syndrome, tetralogy of Fallot, hemangiomata, eczema and strabismus (1 stillborn with aplasia of the anterior abdominal wall)
Holmes and Holmes, 1978	48	60	93	19	3	83	6	Ambylopia, autism, scleroderma, rectal stenosis, absent fallopian tube and small uterus, slow learner and foot defect
Li, 1979	146	58	286	26	9	242	8	Possible trisomy 18 syndrome, Marfan syndrome, deafness, pyloric stenosis, Hirschprung disease (same as above), cardiac, brain, and multiple malformations
McKeen, 1979	66	100	87	22	12	59	6	Neurosensory deafness,[c] scoliosis and slow learner,[c] hydrocephalus,[c] cleft lip and palate,[c] hydrocephalus, tracheomalacia
Blatt, 1980	30	77	40	2	10	28	1	Congenital hip dysplasia
Horning, 1981	20	100	28	0	5	24	0	
Marradi, 1982	14	57	23	?	?	23	2	Multiple congenital anomalies with mental and growth retardation, panhypopituitarism and cerebral atrophy, gastroschisis
Bundey and Evans, 1982	24	83	48	3	0	45	1	Pyloric stenosis
Andrieu and Ochoa-Molina, 1983	22	100	30	5	4	22	1	Congenital hip dysplasia
Rustin, 1984	216[b]	100	374	54	36	275	8	Spina bifida, tetralogy of Fallot, talipes equinovares, collapsed lung, umbilical hernia, desquamative fibrosing alveolitis (2 sibs), neonatal tachycardia (plus 2 anencephalic stillbirths and 1 sudden infant death)
Goldstein, 1984	?[b]	100	222	52	6	164	5	Not specified
Li, 1987	181	65	246	53	32	190	5	Congenital hip dislocation (2), heart murmur, hypospadias, internal tibial torsion
Green, 1991	60	58	?	?	?	100	8	Ventricular septal defect, tetralogy of Fallot, hydrocele, birth marks (2), skin tags, epidermal nevus
Mulvihill, 1998	2,308	~50	?	?	?	2198	75	Rate no different from control
Mulvihill, 2001	14,054	46	?	?	?	4214	158	Rate no different from control
Total	17,293	48	>1680	>266	120	7837	289	

[a]Fetal loss is defined as elective abortion, ectopic pregnancy, spontaneous abortion (miscarriage), or stillbirth; ?, uncertain.
[b]All gestational trophoblastic neoplasia.
[c]Exposed to cancer treatment during gestation.
Source: Updated from Mulvihill (1993) with permission.

netic disease or damage has not been seen in the offspring of the survivors of the atomic bombs in Japan or in the offspring of several thousands of cancer survivors. Indicators of possible genetic damage have been birth defects, newborn death, chromosomal abnormalities, a change in protein structure or function, and growth or development of malignancies. One needs to consider the recurrence risk from genes that may have contributed to cancer in the first place.

This line of reasoning and counseling is best done as a dialogue, allowing for personalization and testing for comprehension. If the exposure was not cancer therapy, modifications are necessary to acknowledge the lack of specific relevant studies (e.g., of long-term users of noncancer drugs or substance abusers). Reference to the atomic bomb studies has the advantage of offering a familiar and intuitive frame of reference; allusion to cancer survivor studies evokes the appropriate extrapolation to a worst-case scenario: "Since untoward effects have not been seen from agents that are known carcinogens and experimental mutagens, it is not likely that your three years of alcohol and drug abuse explain why your daughter has achondroplasia."

Principles of Teratogenesis

Teratogenesis is the mechanism of fetal damage from agents that cross the placenta and harm the developing embryo and fetus directly. Human germ cell mutagenesis is different in that the damage is done to the parental germ cell and not to the developing organism. However, teratogenesis still reflects an unfavorable fetal reproductive outcome due to chemical exposure; hence, a short note on the teratogenesis by medical therapeutics merits attention. A few principles of human teratogenesis have emerged since the early embryological work on vitamin A toxicity by Warkany (1947) and the shattering epidemic of limb defects induced by thalidomide in the 1960s (Newman, 1985). Human teratogenesis is a persistent threat, as thalidomide has been reintroduced into clinical medicine for the treatment of some types of leprosy and complication of AIDS. The list of human drug teratogens (alkylators, androgen, antimetabolite, antithyroid, chlorobiphenyl, diethylstilbestrol, estrogen, heroin and methdone, hydantoin, ionizing radiation, isotretinoin, streptomycin, tetracycline, thalidomide, valproic acid, and warfarin) again is a short one. One hopes, without great confidence, that it is largely of historical interest (Shepard, 2001).

Various classes of drugs can be teratogenic and do not necessarily reflect the phenomenon of mutagenicity. The endpoints of teratogenicity may be frank malformations if the exposure is during early embryogenesis or as subtle as late behavioral consequences if the exposure is later in pregnancy, at the time of fine cerebral and cerebellar structuring. It may be that teratogens cause an excess of early fetal wastage but that endpoint is difficult to document, given the high rate of early spontaneous miscarriage.

Finally the experimental prediction of human teratogenesis is fraught with uncertainties. For example, even with the knowledge that thalidomide caused human birth defects, early systems of animal models using mice, rats, and hamsters failed to show teratogenicity, whereas it became obvious only in rabbit and monkey systems. So there is high species specificity for drug teratogenesis. This principle and the need for introducing drugs with high efficacy but with uncertain teratogenicity require scrupulous postmarketing surveillance, again largely by alert practitioners for ongoing vigilance for human teratogenicity. In practice, clinical geneticists and counselors elicit pregnancy history and possible unusual exposures; birth defect systems track the frequency of common defects; and ad hoc case control studies are launched when a suspected association is set forth. Despite great effort and cost, systematic birth defect registries have served less to suspect new teratogens than to address a proposed association with epidemiologic vigor.

REFERENCES

Ames BN, Durston WE, Yamasaki E, Lee FD: Carcinogens are mutagens: a simple test system combining liver homogenates for activation and bacteria for detection. Proc Natl Acad Sci USA 1973a; 70:2281–2285.

Ames BN, Lee FD, Durston WE: An improved bacterial test system for the detection and classification of mutagens and carcinogens. Proc Natl Acad Sci USA 1973b; 70:782–786.

Andrieu JM, Ochoa-Molina ME: Menstrual cycle, pregnancies and offspring before and after MOPP therapy for Hodgkin's disease. Cancer 1983; 52:435–438.

Anttila A, Pukkala E, Aitio A, Rantanen T, Karjalainen S: Update of cancer incidence among workers at a copper/nickel smelter and nickel refinery. Int Arch Occup Environ Health 1998; 71:245–250.

Auerbach AD: Fanconi anemia and leukemia: tracking the genes. Leukemia 1992; 6(suppl 1):1–4.

Berdanier CD, Everts HB: Mitichodrial DNA in aging and degenerative disease. Mutat Res 2001; 475:169–183.

Blatt J, Mulvihill JJ, Ziegler JL, Young RC, Poplack DG: Pregnancy outcome following chemotherapy. Am J Med 1980; 69:828–832.

Boffetta P: Health effects of asbestos exposure in humans: a quantitative assesment. Med Lav 1998; 89:471–480.

Bonassi S, Forni A, Bigatti P, Canevarollo N, De Ferrari M, Lando C, Padovani P, Bevegni M, Stella M, Vecchio D, Puntoni R: Chromosome aberrations in hospital workers: evidence from surveillance studies in Italy (1963–1993). Am J Ind Med 1997; 31:353–360.

Brewen JG, Preston RJ: Analysis of X-ray-induced chromosomal translocations in human and marmoset spermatogonial stem cells. Nature 1975; 253:468–470.

Bridges BA, Harnden DG (eds): Ataxia-Telangiectasia: A Cellular and Molecular Link between Cancer, Neuropathology, and Immune Deficiency. Chichester: Wiley, 1982.

Brusick D: Genetic toxicology. In Hayes A (ed). Principles and Methods of Toxicology. New York: Raven Press, 1984:223–272.

Bundey S, Evans K: Survivors of neuroblastoma and ganglioneuroma and their families. J Med Genet 1982; 19:16–21.

Byrne J, Nicholson HS, Mulvihill JJ: Absence of birth defects in offspring of women treated with dactinomycin. N Engl J Med 1992; 326:137.

Byrne J, Rasmussen SA, Steinhorn SC, Connelly RR, Myers MH, Lynch CF, Flannery J, Austin DF, Holmes FF, Holmes GE, et al.: Genetic disease in offspring of long-term survivors of childhood and adolescent cancer. Am J Hum Genet 1998; 62:45–52.

Chung IM, Schwartz SM, Murray CE: Clonal architecture of normal and atherosclerotic aorta: implications for atherogenesis and vascular development. Am J Pathol 1998; 152:913–923.

Czeizel AE: Human germinal mutagenic effects in relation to intentional and accidental exposure to toxic agents. Environ Health Perspect 1996; 104:615–617.

Czeizel AE, Elek C, Gundy S, Metneki J, Nemes E, Reis A, Sperling K, Timar L, Tusnady G, Viragh Z: Environmental trichlorfon and cluster of congenital abnormalities. Lancet 1993; 341:539–542.

Dellarco VL, Generoso WM, Sega GA, Fowle JR III, Jacobson-Kram D: Review of the mutagenicity of ethylene oxide. Environ Mol Mutagen 1990; 16:85–103.

Dubrova YE, Nestrov VN, Krouchinsky NG, Ostapenko VA, Neumann R, Neil DL, Jeffreys AJ: Human minisatellite mutation rate after the Chernobyl accident. Nature 1996; 380:683–686.

Ehling UH: The frequency of X-ray induced dominant mutations affecting the skeleton of mice. Genetics 1965; 51:723–732.

Ehling UH: Dominant mutations affecting the skeleton in offspring of X-irradiated male mice. Genetics 1966; 54:1381–1389.

Fitzgerald DJ, Piccoli C, Yamasaki H: Detection of non-genotoxic carcinogens in the BALB/c 3T3 cell transformation/mutation assay system. Mutagenesis 1989; 4:286–291.

Gatti RA, Swift M (eds): Ataxia-Telangiectasia: Genetics, Neuropathology and Immunology of a Degenerative Disease of Childhood. New York: Alan R. Liss, 1985.

German J: Patterns of neoplasia associated with the chrmosome-breakage syndromes. In German J (ed): Chromosome Mutation and Neoplasia. New York: Alan R. Liss, 1983:97–134.

Goldstein DP, Berkowitz RS, Bernstein MR: Reproductive performance after molar pregnancy and gestational trophoblastic tumours. Clin Obstet Gynecol 1983; 27:221–227.

Green DM, Zevon MA, Lowrie G, Seigelstein N, Hall B: Congenital anomalies in children of patients who received chemotherapy for cancer in childhood and adolescence. N Engl J Med 1991; 325:141–146.

Grossblatt N (ed): Identifying and Estimating the Genetic Impact of Chemical Environmental Mutagens. Washington, DC: National Academy Press, 1989.

Hakoda M, Akiyama M, Kyoizumi S, Awa AA, Yamakido M, Otake M: Increased somatic cell mutant frequency in atomic bomb survivors. Mutat Res 1988; 202:203–208.

Hales B, Robair B, Olshan A, Mattison D (eds): Male-Mediated Developmental Toxicity. New York: Plenum Press, 2002 (in press).

Hawkins MM, Draper GJ, Smith RA: Cancer among 1,348 offspring of survivors of childhood cancer. Int J Cancer 1989; 43:975–978.

Heddle J (ed): Mutagenicity: New Horizons in Genetic Toxicology. New York: Academic Press, 1982.

Hemstreet GP, Yin S, Ma Z, Bonner RB, Bi W, Rao JY, Zang M, Zheng Q, Bane B, Asal N, et al.: Biomarker risk assessment and bladder cancer detection in a cohort exposed to benzidine. J Natl Cancer Inst 2001; 93:427–436.

Hoffman GR: Genetic toxicology. In Klaasen CD, Amdur MO, Doull J (eds). Casarett and Doull's Toxicology: The Basic Science of Poisons, 5th ed. New York: McGraw-Hill, 1996:279–281.

Hollaender A, de Serres FJ (eds): Chemical Mutagens. New York: Plenum Press, 1978.

Holmes GE, Holmes FF: Pregnancy outcome of patients treated for Hodgkin's disease: a controlled study. Cancer 1978; 41:1317–1322.

Horning SJ, Hippe RT, Kaplan HS, Rosenburg SA: Female reproductive potential after treatment for Hodgkin's disease. N Engl J Med 1981; 304:1377–1382.

International Agency for Research on Cancer: Some Aromatic Amines, Hydrazine and Related Substances, *N*-Nitroso Compounds and Miscellaneous Alkylating Agents. IARC Monographs on the Evaluation of Carcinogenic Risks to Humans, Vol. 4. Lyon, France: IARC, 1974a:247–252.

International Agency for Research on Cancer: Some Anti-Thyroid and Related Substances, Nitrofurans and Industrial Chemicals. IARC Monographs on the Evaluation of Carcinogenic Risks to Humans, Vol. 7. Lyon, France: IARC, 1974b:53, 67–76, 95, 111.

International Agency for Research on Cancer: Some Aziridines, *N*-, *S*- and *O*-Mustards and Selenium. IARC Monographs on the Evaluation of Carcinogenic Risks to Humans, Vol. 9. Lyon, France: IARC, 1975:167–209, 235–241.

International Agency for Research on Cancer: Some Naturally Occurring Substances. IARC Monographs on the Evaluation of Carcinogenic Risks to Humans, Vol. 10. Lyon, France: IARC, 1976:43–49, 73, 145, 171.

International Agency for Research on Cancer: Some Miscellaneous Pharmaceutical Substances. IARC Monographs on the Evaluation of Carcinogenic Risks to Humans, Vol. 13. Lyon, France: IARC, 1977:113, 131–141, 157–181.

International Agency for Research on Cancer: Some *N*-Nitroso Compounds. IARC Monographs on the Evaluation of Carcinogenic Risks to Humans, Vol. 17. Lyon, France: IARC, 1978:337.

International Agency for Research on Cancer: Sex Hormones (II). IARC Monographs on the Evaluation of Carcinogenic Risks to Humans, Vol. 21. Lyon, France: IARC, 1979:95–102, 111–112, 131–362, 417–429, 519.

International Agency for Research on Cancer: Some Metals and Metallic Compounds. IARC Monographs on the Evaluation of Carcinogenic Risks to Humans, Vol. 23. Lyon, France: IARC, 1980a:39–141.

International Agency for Research on Cancer: Some Pharmaceutical Drugs. IARC Monographs on the Evaluation of Carcinogenic Risks to Humans, Vol. 24. Lyon, France: IARC, 1980b:101–124, 135–161.

International Agency for Research on Cancer: Some Antineoplastic and Immunosuppressive Agents. IARC Monographs on the Evaluation of Carcinogenic Risks to Humans, Vol. 26. Lyon, France: IARC, 1981:47–95, 97–212, 311–339.

International Agency for Research on Cancer: Genetic and Related Effects: An Updating of Selected IARC Monographs from Volumes 1 to 42. IARC Monographs on the Evaluation of Carcinogenic Risks to Humans, Supplement 6. Lyon, France: IARC, 1987a:120–125, 187, 208–209, 250–256, 293–295, 336–337, 359–360, 369–371, 421–424, 437–441, 448–450, 474–478, 558–560.

International Agency for Research on Cancer: Overall Evaluations of Carcinogenicity: An Updating of *IARC Monographs* Volumes 1 to 42. IARC Monographs on the Evaluation of Carcinogenic Risks to Humans, Supplement 7. Lyon, France: IARC, 1987b:57, 66–73, 81, 96, 100, 119, 134, 137, 144, 150, 170, 182, 184, 239, 250, 254, 259, 261, 269, 273, 280, 289, 296, 310, 313, 327, 329, 370.

International Agency for Research on Cancer: Some Pharmaceutical Drugs. IARC Monographs on the Evaluation of Carcinogenic Risks to Humans, Vol. 50. Lyon, France: IARC, 1990:47, 65, 77, 123, 169, 265.

International Agency for Research on Cancer: Some Industrial Chemicals. IARC Monographs on the Evaluation of Carcinogenic Risks to Humans, Vol. 60. Lyon, France: IARC, 1994:181.

International Agency for Research on Cancer: Some Pharmaceutical Drugs. IARC Monographs on the Evaluation of Carcinogenic Risks to Humans, Vol. 66. Lyon, France: IARC, 1996:175, 253.

International Agency for Research on Cancer: Overall Evaluations of Carcinogenicity to Humans. IARC Monographs on the Evaluation of Carcinogenic Risks to Humans. Web Site: http://www.iarc.fr/. Lyon, France: IARC, 1998.

International Agency for Research on Cancer: Hormonal Contraception and Postmenopausal Hormonal Therapy. IARC Monographs on the Evaluation of Carcinogenic Risks to Humans, Vol. 72. Lyon, France: IARC, 1999.

International Commission for Protection against Environmental Mutagens and Carcinogens: Guide to Short-Term Tests for Detecting Mutagenic and Carcinogenic Chemicals. Geneva: World Health Organization, 1985.

Jeffreys AJ: Spontaneous and induced minisatellite instability in the human genome. Clin Sci 1997; 93:383–390.

Landrigan PJ, Meinhardt TJ, Gordon J, Lipscomb JA, Burg JR, Mazzuckelli LF, Lewis TR, Lemen RA: Ethylene oxide: an overview of toxicologic and epidemiologic research. Am J Ind Med 1984; 6:103–115.

Li FP, Fine W, Jaffe N, Holmes GE, Holmes FF: Offspring of patients treated for cancer in childhood. J Natl Cancer Inst 1979; 62:1193–1197.

Li FP, Gimbere K, Gelber RD, Sallan SE, Green DM, Heyn RM, Meadows AT: Outcome of pregnancy in survivors of Wilms' tumor. JAMA 1987; 257:216–219.

Li FP, Jaffe H: Progeny of childhood-cancer survivors. Lancet 1974; 2:707–709.

Marczynski B, Rozynek P, Kraus T, Schlosser S, Raithel HJ, Baur X: Levels of 8-hydroxy-2-deoxyguanosine in DNA of white blood cells from workers highly exposed to asbestos in Germany. Mutat Res 2000; 468:195–202.

Marradi P, Schaison F, Alby N, Berger R, Jacquillat C, Boiron M: Children born of leukemic parents. Apropos of 23 children. Nouv Rev Fr Hematol 1982; 24:75–80. In French.

Martin RH, Ernst S, Rademaker A, Barclay L, Ko E, Summers N: Analysis of sperm chromosome complements before, during, and after chemotherapy. Cancer Genet Cytogenet 1999; 108:133–136.

Martin RH, Hildebrand K, Yamamota J, Rademaker A, Barnes M, Douglas G, Arthur K, Ringrose T, Brown IS: An increased frequency of human sperm chromosomal abnormalities after radiotherapy. Mutat Res 1986; 174:219–225.

McKeen EA, Mulvihill JJ, Rosner F, Zarrabi MH: Pregnancy outcome in Hodgkin's disease. Lancet 1979; 2:590.

Meigs JW, Marrett, Ulrich FU, Flannery JT: Bladder tumor incidence among workers exposed to benzidene: a thirty-year follow-up. J Natl Cancer Inst 1986; 76:1–8.

Miller RW: The discovery of human teratogens, carcinogens and mutagens: lessons for the future. In Hollaender A, de Serres FJ (eds). Chemical Mutagens: Principles and Methods for Their Detection, Vol 5. New York: Plenum Press 1978:101–126.

Miller RW: Areawide chemical contamination: lessons from case histories. JAMA 1981; 245:1548–1551.

Morita T, Iwamoto Y, Shimizi T, Masuzawa T, Yanagihara Y: Mutagenicity tests with a permeable mutant of yeast on carcinogens showing false-negative in *Salmonella* assay. Chem Pharm Bull (Tokyo) 1989; 37:407–409.

Müller HJ: Our load of mutations. Am J Hum Genet 1950; 2:111–176.

Müller HJ, Herskowitz IH, Abrahamson S, Oster II: A nonlinear relation between X-ray dose and recovered lethal mutations in drosophila. Genetics 1954; 39:741–749.

Mulvihill JJ: Genetic counseling of the cancer patient. In DeVita VT Jr, Hellman S, Rosenberg SA (eds): Cancer Principles and Practice of Oncology, 4th ed. Philadelphia: J.B. Lippincott, 1993:2529–2537.

Mulvihill JJ, Myers MH, Connelly RR, Byrne J, Austin DF, Bragg K, Cook JW, Hassinger DD, Holmes FF, Holmes GF, et al.: Cancer in offspring of long-time survivors of childhood and adolescent cancer. Lancet 1987; 2:813–817.

Mulvihill JJ, Strong LC, Robison LL: Investigators of the Childhood Cancer Survivor Study: Genetic disease in offspring of survivors of childhood and adolescent cancer. Am J Hum Genet 2001; 69:A391.

Neel JV: Reappraisal of studies concerning the genetic effects of the radiation of humans, mice, and drosophila. Environ Mol Mutagen 1998; 31:4–10.

Neel JV, Lewis SE: The comparative radiation genetics of humans and mice. Annu Rev Genet 1990; 24:327–362.

Neel JV, Schull WJ, Awa AA, Satoh C, Kato H, Otake M, Yoshimoto Y: The children of parents exposed to atomic bombs: estimates of the genetic doubling dose of radiation for humans. Am J Hum Genet 1990; 46:1053–1072.

Newman CGH: Clinical aspects of thalidomide embryopathy: a continuing preoccupation. Teratology 1985; 32:133–144.

Prakash L, Sherman F, Miller MW, Lawrence CW, Taber HW (eds): Molecular and Environmental Aspects of Mutagenesis. Springfield, IL: Charles C Thomas, 1974.

Rehn L: Blasengeschwulste bei Fuchsin-Arbeitern. Arch Klin Chir 1895; 50:588–600.

Rosenkranz HS, Klopman G: New structural concepts for predicting carcinogenesis in rodents: an artificial intelligence approach. Teratog Carcinog Mutagen 1990; 10:73–88.

Ross GT: Congenital anomalies among children born of mothers receiving chemotherapy for gestational trophoblastic neoplasms. Cancer 1976; 37:1043–1047.

Rowley MJ, Leach DR, Warner GA, Heller CG: Effect of graded doses of ionizing radiation on the human testes. Radiat Res 1974; 59:665–678.

Rupa DS, Eastmond DA: Chromosomal alterations affecting the 1cen–1q12 region in buccal mucosal cells of betel quid chewers detected using multicolor fluorescence in situ hybridization. Carcinogenesis 1997; 12:2347–2351.

Russell WL: X-ray induced mutations in mice. Cold Spring Harbor Symp Quant Biol 1951; 16:327–336.

Rustin GJ, Booth M, Dent J, Salt S, Rustin F, Bagshaw KD: Pregnancy after cytotoxic chemotherapy for gestational trophoblastic tumours. Br Med J 1984; 288:103–106.

Satoh C, Takahashi N, Asakawa J, Kodaira M, Kuick R, Hanash S, Neel J: Genetic analysis of children of atomic bomb survivors. Environ Health Perspect 1996; 104(Suppl 3):511–519.

Schottenfeld D, Fraumeni JF Jr (eds): Cancer Epidemiology and Prevention. New York: Oxford University Press, 1996.

Shepard TH: Catalog of Teratogenic Agents 10th Edition, Baltimore: Johns Hopkins, 2001.

Steenland K, Stayner L: Silica, asbestos, man-made mineral fibers, and cancer. Cancer Causes Control 1997; 8:491–503.

U.S. Department of Health and Human Services, Public Health Service, National Toxicology Program: Eighth Report on Carcinogens: Summary. Research Triangle Park, NC: National Toxicology Program, 1998.

Vogel F, Röhrborn G (eds): Chemical Mutagenesis in Mammals and Man. New York: Springer-Verlag, 1970.

Wallace DC: Mitochondrial DNA mutations in diseases of energy metabolism. J Bioenerg Biomembr 1994; 26:241–250.

Warkany J: Etiology of congenital malformations. Adv Pediatr 1947; 2:1–63.

Weinberg HS, Korol AB, Kirzhner VM, Avivi A, Fahima T, Nevo E, Shapiro S, Rennert G, Piatak O, Stepanova EI, Skvarskaja E: Very high mutation rate in offspring of Chernobyl accident liquidators. Proc R Soc Lond B Bio Sci 2001; 268:1001–1005.

Weinberg HS, Nevo E, Korol A, Fahima T, Rennert G, Shapiro S: Molecular changes in the offspring of liquidators who emigrated to Israel from the Chernobyl disaster area. Environ Health Perspect 1997; 105:1479–1481.

Wells PG: Chemical teratogenesis. In Kalant H, Roschlau WHE (eds). Principles of Medical Pharmacology. New York: Oxford University Press, 1998:873–890.

Winther J, Sankila, R, Boice J, Tulinius H, Bautz A, Barlow L, Glattre E, Langmark F, Moller T, Mulvihill JJ, et al.: Cancer in siblings of children with cancer in the Nordic countries: a population based cohort study. Lancet 2001; 358:711–717.

55 Pharmacogenetics, Ecogenetics, and Pharmacogenomics

WERNER KALOW

The main purpose of this chapter is to present the principles underlying any study of pharmacogenetics, ecogenetics, and the new field of pharmacogenomics. Examples are cited, but there is no attempt to present a comprehensive review of the pertinent data.

TERMINOLOGY AND CONCEPTS

Pharmacogenetics is a term that was coined in the 1950s (Vogel, 1959), based on a few observations of abnormal metabolism and consequent abnormal responses to a few drugs, whereby it was clear that the abnormality was inherited and thus must have had a genetic basis. Brewer (1971) coined the term *ecogenetics*, pointing out that genetic variation not only affected drug action but needed to be considered with respect to any environmental chemical or food that gets into a living creature.

In recent years, improvement in genetic methodology has allowed investigators not only to study single genes but to become interested in studies of the whole genome of different species. This broadening of interest has led also to the introduction of the term *pharmacogenomics*, as used by Marshall (1997). In practice, this term has a meaning similar to that of *pharmacogenetics* (Freeman, 2001), but it also reflects a rising interest in the genetics of common diseases, the topic of this book. The pharmaceutical industry hopes that the discovery of disease-associated genes will lead to the definition of new drug targets and thereby to the invention of new drugs (Marshall, 1997). Logically, the use of such a new drug should be restricted to patients whose genes have been tested and who carry the appropriate genetic target; this will require a radical change of attitude affecting drug therapy. In short, the term *pharmacogenomics* can be taken as forecasting genetic individualization of the choice of drugs.

In practice, use of the words *pharmaco-* and *ecogenetics* has often been restricted to monogenic variants in humans. Thus, insect resistance to insecticides, bacterial resistance to antibiotics, and multigenic variations which may affect a drug response have usually not been called *pharmacogenetics*, although they are biologically part of it. The whole field, encompassing ecogenetics and pharmacogenomics, should be looked at as part of the defenses against dangers that always lurk in the environment (Kalow, 2001a). Besides drugs and toxicants, these dangers include starvation, food incompatibilities, temperature changes, and particularly infectious diseases.

HISTORICAL ASPECTS

In 1931, the development of pharmacogenetics was foreseen by Sir Archibald Garrod in his book *Inborn Factors in Disease*, in which he suggested that individual differences in reaction to drugs and to chemicals of the environment should be anticipated. It was similar insight when J. B. S Haldane in 1949 foresaw as an implication of biochemical individuality the occurrence of unusual reactions to drugs.

Motulsky (1957) knew about the inherited atropine tolerance of some rabbits; in humans, he knew about primaquine hydrolysis, cholinesterase variation, hyperbilirubinemia, methemoglobinemia, and several other conditions. He wrote a key paper, "Drug Reactions, Enzymes, and Biochemical Genetics," which fanned interest in a new field that was called *pharmacogenetics* by Vogel (1959). Kalow (1962) was then already writing his book, quoting further examples of pharmacogenetic case histories. In the 1960s, Vesell and colleagues (e.g., Vesell and Page, 1968) investigated in twins the metabolism of various drugs and thereby established significant heritability of these processes in all cases.

In the 1970s came the double observation of the heritable lack of an important liver enzyme, the P-450 cytochrome now called CYP2D6. The defect, discovered in England, was absence of debrisoquine metabolism in some subjects (Mahgoub et al., 1977); in Germany it was the metabolic lack of sparteine (Dengler and Eichelbaum, 1977). Further studies showed that the deficiencies were the same, affected the fate of many drugs, had different frequencies in different ethnic groups, and could cause fatalities. These were major stimuli which greatly increased the medical interest in pharmacogenetics.

Changes of drug-metabolizing enzymes still represent the majority of pharmacogenetic case histories. Much less is known about pharmacogenetic alterations of drug targets. One reason is clearly the relatively long history of chemistry and its descendent biochemistry, which allowed the chemical identification of drug metabolites. By contrast, only the comparatively recent appearance of molecular biology allowed systematic studies of the variability of drug targets. Many targets are receptors, e.g., receptors serving impulse transmission in the nervous system. Only after the DNA sequence of a receptor protein is established is it possible to look for changes in the gene that is carried, e.g., by hair roots or within white bood cells. Even then, the finding of a DNA change may be biologically meaningless until its functional significance is established.

It thus remains to be established whether receptor variations are more rare than metabolic polymorphisms because of technical developments or on evolutionary grounds. The latter could be the case if a receptor mutation tends to cause a disease or other disadvantage which reduces its population frequency. Every receptor protein must be expected to fulfill a physiological function, while a drug-metabolizing enzyme may be without utility in the absence of a drug or toxicant. In any case, there are a fair number of pharmacologically important receptor mutants (Weber, 1997, 2001).

CURRENT KNOWLEDGE

Pharmacokinetics and Drug Metabolism

Pharmacokinetics is the branch of pharmacology concerned with the time course of the concentration of drugs or other chemicals in blood and tissues (Endrenyi, 1998). The determinants are rate and extent of absorption, transport within and between tissues, binding in tissues or to proteins, metabolic destruction, and excretion through kidney, bile, or gut. Every one of these factors can be subject to genetic variation. However, best studied and of greatest concern are the rates, the extent, and the pathways of metabolic destruction of drugs and other foreign chemicals; most often and most effectively investigated are the drug-metabolizing enzymes.

Drug-metabolizing enzymes (Meyer, 1996) are often divided into phase I and phase II enzymes (Riddick, 1998), phase I enzymes being those that oxidize, reduce, or split their substrates while phase II enzymes transfer and attach to them other chemical entities, e.g., methyl, acetyl sulfate, glucuronyl, or glutathione groups. There are genetic variants in each of these enzyme groups. Many drugs, perhaps most drugs, are subject to attack by more than one enzyme; the simultaneous occurrence of different enzyme variants can have devastating effects.

Table 55–1 lists genetically variable enzymes. The inclusion of glucose-6-phosphate dehydrogenase in this list could be debated because it does not directly metabolize drugs; it produces the reduced form of nicotinamide-adenine dinucleotide phosphate (NADPH) and thereby maintains a normal redox state of the cell (Kletzien et al., 1994). A particularly important group of oxidizing enzymes includes the P-450 cytochromes, which are variable (Brockmoller et al., 2000; Lin and Lu 2001; Ingelman-Sundberg, 2001) and usually located in the liver but may also be found in other tissues, e.g., gut, lungs, kidney, skin, or brain. They are heme proteins identified in print by the prefix *CYP*, followed by a system of numbers and letters. Genetically variable P-450s amount to about one-quarter of all enzymes known to be polymorphic (Kalow, 2001b), but they represented 52% of the variable enzymes studied in 12 large pharmaceutical companies (Ball and Borman, 1997).

More than 50 variants of *CYP2D6* are known (Marez et al., 1997). Variant nomenclature has been introduced by Daly et al. (1996). More than 40 drugs are substrates, but the clinical importance of deficient metabolism by *CYP2D6* varies from drug to drug (Meyer and Zanger, 1997); it depends on alternative metabolic pathways, renal excretion, and the degree of safety inherent in the drug. Some variants do not have the same order of specificity toward different substrates as the wild type (Woolhouse et al., 1985; Droll et al., 1998). For instance, a variant in Africa does not metabolize debrisoquine well but has good activity toward metoprolol (Sommers et al., 1989). A frequent variant occurring in Asia (*CYP2D6*10*) (Nishida et al., 2000) has reduced activity toward debrisoquine but apparently not to all substrates (Crespi, 1998); *CYP2D6* specificities in Asia still require more investigation. Since *CYP2D6* also occurs in the brain (Niznik et al., 1990), whether the action of perphenazine is more affected by *CYP2D6* deficiency in the brain than in the liver is under investigation; differences between side effects after *CYP2D6* inhibition appear to be greater than can be accounted for by the differences between drug levels in the blood (Ozdemir et al., 1997).

Table 55–1. Genetically Variable Drug-Metabolizing Enzymes

Esterases
Butyrylcholinesterase[a]
Paraoxonase/arylesterase[a]
Transferases
N-Acetyltransferases (Nat1)[b]
N-Acetyltransferases (Nat2)[a]
Catechol *O*-methyltransferase[c]
Histamine methyltransferase[c]
Thiol methyltransferase[c]
Thiopurine methyltransferase[c]
Platelet phenolsulfotransferase[d]
Glutathione-*S*-transferases (GSTM1)[e]
Glutathione-*S*-transferases (GSTT1)[f]
Glucuronosyltransferase (UGT1A1)[g]
Glucuronosyltransferase (UGT2B4)[h]
Glucuronosyltransferase (UGT2B7)[i]
Glucuronosyltransferase (UGT2B15)[j]
Amobarbital-glucosyltransferase[k]
Reductases
NAD(P)H:quinone oxidoreductase[l]
Glucose-6-phosphate dehydrogenase[a]
Oxidases
Alcohol dehydrogenase[a]
Aldehyde dehydrogenase[a]
Monoamine oxidase B[m]
Catalase[n]
Superoxide dismutase[o]
Trimethylamine *N*-oxidase[p]
Dihydropyrimidine dehydrogenase[q]
Cytochromes P-450
CYP1A1[r]
CYP2A6[s]
CYP2C9[t]
CYP2C19[a]
CYP2D6[a]
CYP2E1[a]
CTP3A5[u]

Sources: [a]Kalow and Bertilsson (1994). [b]Lin et al. (1998). [c]Weinshilboum et al. (1999). [d]Anderson et al. (1988). [e]Lin et al. (1994). [f]Lee et al. (1995). [g]Beutler et al. (1998). [h]Levesque et al. (1998). [i]Patel et al. (1995). [j]Levesque et al. (1997). [k]Kalow (1982a,b). [l]Kelsey et al. (1997). [m]Weyler et al. (1992). [n]Calabrese et al. (1992). [o]Canada and Calabrese (1992). [p]Mitchell et al. (1997). [q]Lu et al. (1995). [r]Cascorbi et al. (1996). [s]Fernandez-Salguero et al. (1995). [t]Inoue et al. (1997). [u]Boobis et al. (1996).
Some papers are cited because they indicate both interindividual and interethnic variations.

Genetic variation of *N*-acetyltransferase type 2 (NAT2) is one of the oldest discoveries in pharmacogenetics, initially observed as a failure of the metabolism of the then new antituberculosis drug isoniazid (Bonicke and Reif, 1953; Hughes et al., 1954). Many genetic variants of this enzyme have been identified, representing combinations of several different allelic nucleotide changes. At least 20 drugs and chemicals are affected by this polymorphism (Grant and Spielberg, 1998; Grant et al., 2000; Fretland et al., 2001). In addition, there are 11 alleles of NAT1, of which several convey functional impairment of the enzyme (Hein et al., 2000). Since the NATs are important metabolic activators of arylamine and heterocyclic amine procarcinogens, functional differences can have important toxicological consequences, affecting, e.g., the frequencies of chemically induced bladder and colon cancers (Grant et al., 1997).

Another early discovery was genetic variation of butyrylcholinesterase (Kalow, 1956). There are now numerous variants known, many without functional activity; while some are quite rare, 24% of the North American population carries at least one genetic variant allele (Lockridge and Masson, 2000). Most frequent is the K variant, with reduced activity and an allele frequency of about 20% in Caucasians (Jensen et al., 1996) and Japanese (Shibuta et al., 1994), sometimes suspected to be associated with Alzheimer's disease (Mattila et al., 2000). Of greatest clinical concern in butyrylcholinesterase failure was originally the prolonged action of the muscle relaxant succinylcholine. There is reason to suspect that severe cocaine intoxication may be a major consequence of this failure (Carmona et al., 2000; Sun et al., 2001).

Genetic deficiency of dihydropyrimidine dehydrogenase has been fatal in subjects receiving 5-fluorouracil as cancer treatment (Diasio, 1998, 2001). The attachment of glucose to amobarbital is clearly a genetically variable process, but the responsible enzyme has not been identified (Kalow et al., 1978a,b). A variant of the glucuronosyltranferase UGT2B7 showed deficiency of oxazepam glucuronidation (Patel et al., 1995). Allelic forms of UGT2B4 (Levesque et al., 1999), UGT2B15 (Levesque et al., 1997), UGT1A1, and others (Fisher et al., 2000) have been reported; however, their major clinical relevance was not obvious to Mackenzie et al. (2000).

To generalize, whenever an enzyme has been found to be genetically variable, multiple variants were found over time. Much remains to be done in studies of pharmacokinetic variation, even in the relatively well-investigated field of drug-metabolizing enzymes. Specifically required are more distinctions between genetic and environmental factors that may cause variation in enzymatic activities.

Pharmacodynamics

Pharmacodynamics describes the action of drugs or environmental chemicals and the nature of any beneficial or toxic response to an exposure (Smith, 1997). This involves identification of drug targets. It includes quantitation of the intensity of effects and thereby assessment of dose–effect relationships (Rosner and Muller, 1997; Aarons, 1999). If pharmacodynamic variation represents a difference of affinity between a drug and its target, the result may be a different target selection when there are multiple targets. There may also be differences in the number of target elements or in the transmission of messages between the target and the final response element.

The targets of numerous drugs or toxic chemicals are the internal messenger systems. These consist of not only the messengers that keep our nerves and brains responding to demands but also the regulators of growth and development, the hormones that determine much of our physiology. Genetic factors determine the chemical formation and destruction of every messenger. In addition, many of the messengers require specific transporters to reach their targets (Hafkemeyer et al., 1998) and/or to get away from them (Aszalos and Ross, 1998; Larsen et al., 2000). Genetic variation of drug transporters has become a new field of research (Kim and Wilkinson, 2001; Brinkmann and Eichelbaum, 2001).

All of the regulators, hormones, and internal messengers interact with receptors (Weber, 2001), i.e., specific proteins geared to accepting the messages. The receptors interact with G proteins and other second messengers. It is likely that every one of these substances and their function requires a gene and a genetic message. It is this multitude of genes, each one of which is potentially variable, plus environmental experiences that allows every person to differ from every other.

Let us spin out this view slightly further. While there are several types of receptor, two kinds, the nuclear (cytoplasmic) and the cell surface receptors, are particularly important (Weber, 2001). Nuclear receptors interact with relatively few but important messengers, such as steroids (Barnes, 1998), thyroxine (Apriletti et al., 1998), and retinoic acid (Folkers et al., 1998); to this categorty belongs the widely known Ah receptor, which can be activated also by smoking and several cancer-causing chemicals (Okey, 1992). The cell surface receptors are the most abundant.

There are three principal kinds of cell surface receptor. First, there are ion channels, which include the cystic fibrosis gene and the gene responsible for malignant hyperthermia. Second, there are receptors that operate with the help of a second messenger, such as G proteins. The genes that encode the G protein–linked receptors make up more than 1% of the human genome and include more than 1000 members (Weber, 2001); this is the kind of receptor that responds to rhodopsin, biogenic amines, peptides, glycoprotein hormones, and others. Considering the large number of these receptor genes, their pharmacogenetics is indeed poorly developed. Third, there are receptors that interact in a complex manner with other second-messenger systems. Among the more complex receptors are the insulin receptor (Chen et al., 1998) and growth regulators (Tarnawski and Jones, 1998).

At this time, much more receptor work is disease-related than inspired by pharmacogenetics. Nevertheless, there are some pharmacogenetic observations that are worth considering. Some specific examples follow.

Malignant hyperthermia was first described by Denborough and Lovell (1960), who reported on a patient who survived an anesthesia-induced fever and rigidity that had cost the lives of several of the patient's relatives. Kalow et al. (1970) found an unusual responsiveness of the skeletal muscle of such patients to contracture by caffeine, a diagnostically useful observation. MacLennan and Phillips (1992, 1995) identified as the cause a genetic variant of the ryanodine receptor, a calcium-release channel in skeletal muscle.

Four types of dopamine D_4 receptor variant have been identified (Van Tol, 1998). For instance, the ^{194}Val $\rightarrow$ Gly is close to the catecholamine binding site; it has lost its high affinity for dopamine and clozapine, while the low affinity for chlorpromazine is unaffected. It shows interethnic variability (Seeman and Van Tol, 1994). Another type of variant is characterized by 48 bp tandem repeats that occur between two and ten times (Van Tol et al., 1992); the number of repeats varies greatly between populations (Lichter et al., 1993). This variation does not appear to affect function very much, but it is difficult to be sure about it because the repeat sections are often not identical: 17 different repeat variants have been identified. Associations have been postulated between the repeat polymorphism and attention deficit hyperactivity (Muglia et al., 2000) as well as novelty-seeking behavior (Ronai et al., 2001). Jonsson et al. (1998) could neither confirm nor convincingly contradict this last observation.

There are a number of 5-hydroxytryptamine receptors (5-HTRs), of which several contain allelic variants (Propping and Nothen, 1995; Bunzel et al., 1998). Arranz et al. (1998a) indicated possible non-response to clozapine in the presence of both the promoter variant A1438G and the structural variant

His^{452}Tyr of the receptor subtype 5-HTR$_{2A}$. Masellis et al. (1998) reported evidence for this effect by the structural variant but indicated the absence of the effect by the promotor variant. Arranz et al. (1998b) confirmed the effect of the structural variant in a meta-analysis. Masellis et al. (2001) and Birkett et al. (2000) described several 5-HTR variants which did not seem to be associated with any different drug response.

One must conclude that there is evidence for the concurrence of pharmacogenetics and receptor variation but that knowledge in this field remains scant. A large number of gene products participate in the control of drug responses (Cicon et al., 2000), and epigenetic factors may complicate the picture (Petronis, 2000). Furthermore, any genetic observation requires an epidemiological study to assess its clinical significance.

Multifactorial Variation

The previous citations, indicating alterations of both drug-metabolizing enzymes and receptors, pertained to one or another specific protein; i.e., they presented monogenic variation. However, most person-to-person differences in drug response cannot be explained by any change of a single factor. If a drug is given to members of a population, one can usually measure an average response and the aberrations from this average in terms of a standard deviation. It is a rule that most individuals have more or less different responses to a drug, which can be pictured as a normal distribution. It therefore has become practice in pharmacology to call the dose of a drug that is sufficient for 50% of the population the ED_{50}, i.e., the effective dose for half the population. Twin studies (e.g., Vesell and Page, 1968) have shown that genetic factors are usually, at least in part, responsible for this kind of response variation. Thus, multifactorial or multigenic variations are part of pharmacogenetics.

A normal distribution of a drug response does not usually arouse much interest as long as it is a solitary event. However, this aspect changes when normal distributions differ between populations. For example, the glucuronidation of codeine shows a normally distributed variation in Swedish, Chinese, and Korean populations; the cause of this is unknown. The average rate of codeine glucuronidation differs sufficiently between Swedes and Chinese to be of clinical significance (Yue and Säwe, 1992). Furthermore, codeine glucuronidation is significantly ($p < 0.01$) faster in Chinese than in Koreans (Yue et al., 1994). Also, both glucuronidations of morphine, particularly the 3-glucuronidation, were faster in Chinese than in Caucasians (Zhou et al., 1993).

Such differences between population averages in drug response may be epidemiologically significant even if the difference is relatively small in comparison to the scatter of responses within a population (Kalow, 1992; Kalow and Bertilsson 1994). If the averages differ, the edges of the distribution curves may also differ; this means that the number of subjects close to the edges, i.e., above or below a certain critical value, may substantially differ between the populations (Fig. 55–1). If the critical value determines the absence or presence of the toxic effects of a drug, the proportion of subjects suffering toxicity may differ significantly between the populations.

It might be considered puzzling that almost nobody ever asks for the biological meaning of a mathematically presented standard deviation. In pharmacology, however, this puzzle can sometimes be solved with relative ease. A drug response, in contrast to many other measured parameters, can be repeatedly assessed within the same person. By comparing within- and between-

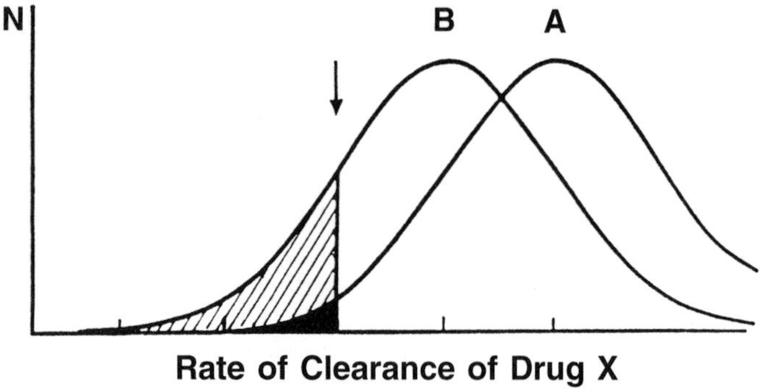

Fig. 55–1. The edge effect of different averages. Hypothetical curves *A* and *B* represent normal-frequency distributions for the elimination capacity of drug *X* in two populations; the abscissa registers the rate of drug clearance, and the ordinate indicates the number of subjects who show a particular rate of clearance. *Arrow* indicates the critical rate below which the drug causes toxicity. *Curves A* and *B* have identical standard deviations (SDs) but their means are 1 SD apart; i.e., the difference between the means is small compared to the range of variation within each population. Therefore, such differences are often neglected. *Arrow* is located 2 and 1 SD below the means of *A* and *B*, respectively. These data imply that approximately 2% of population *A* (*black area*) and 16% of population *B* (*hatched plus black area*) would suffer toxicity from the standard dose of drug *X*. The eightfold difference would grow substantially with the shift of the arrow toward lower values on the abscissa. From Kalow and Bertilsson (1994) with permission.

subject variability and using some mathematical precautions, it is possible to assess the genetic component in a series of measured standard deviations of drug responses or of rates of drug metabolism (Kalow et al., 1998).

Interethnic Differences

During the past few decades, immigration has turned many North American cities, including the city of Toronto in Canada, into ethnically mixed populations. In studies of the metabolism of amobarbital and debrisoqune among student volunteers at the University of Toronto, interethnic differences of metabolic pathways showed up as incidental observations (Kalow, 1982a,b). These observations stimulated searches for other interethnic differences in drug metabolism and response. Kalow (1984, 1992) described the term *pharmacoanthropology* as being neutral with respect to nature–nurture questions and as emphasizing science rather than politics or racism. Today, interethnic differences in drug response are well recognized (Kalow, 2001a,b; Evans et al., 2001).

As long as one had to rely on family or twin studies, it was often hard to tell whether an interethnic difference of drug response had a cultural or a genetic basis. This situation has changed with the availability of molecular techniques that revealed the operation of genetic factors (Smith and Mendoza, 1996). Therefore, the international pharmaceutical industry as well as many regulatory agencies pay increasing attention to interethnic variation in pharmacological and toxic response characteristics (Hahn, 1992; Holloway and Yam 1992; Persidis, 1998a,b; Hodgson and Marshall, 1998; Houseman and Ledley, 1998; Shi et al., 2001).

Most of the drug-metabolizing enzymes listed in Table 55–1 also show interethnic variation, at least in terms of allele frequencies. Furthermore, in most cases for which interethnic differences are not recorded, a proper search has not been made. Of the enzymes cited in Table 55–1, no interethnic differences are known for histamine and thiol methyltransferase, the three glucuronosyltransferases (UGT2B4, -7, and -15), monoamine oxidase B, and CYP3A5. Thus, of 32 polymorphic drug-metabolizing enzymes, only seven are not also known for interethnic variability; and such variability does not appear to have been studied in at least five of these.

The books edited by Kalow et al. (1986) and Lin et al. (1993) and the review articles by Kalow (1991, 2001a,b), Wood and Zhou (1991), Kudzma (1992), Kalow and Bertilsson (1994), Smith and Mendoza (1996), Wood (1998), and Bertilsson and Kalow (2001) present many examples. Johnson (1997) discusses mechanism-related ethnic differences, such as active transport, blood flow, and protein binding, besides metabolism.

In all previous sections, one or more examples of interethnic differences in drug response or metabolism have been cited. Thus, ethnicity may play a role with regard to drug-metabolizing enzymes, receptors, or multifactorial variation.

It is necessary to point out a possible complication. Since there may be ethnic differences in disease specification and different drug responses between similar diseases, an interethnic difference in drug response may be disease-related but not drug-related. For example, it has long been known that hypertensive disease is more frequent in urban blacks than in whites (Freis, 1986) on mostly genetic grounds (Winkleby et al., 1988; Seedat, 1999). The racially different therapeutic drug response may reflect differences in causative pathology (Aviv and Aladjem, 1990), perhaps related to the genetic adaptation of Africans to an environmentally enforced low-salt diet (Lifton, 1996).

CONCLUSIONS

Pharmacogenetics, ecogenetics, and pharmacogenomics are fields of science that combine genetic and various forms of medical knowledge. In spite of the accumulation of much knowledge within these fields, they deserve much more research. Particularly poorly developed at the present time is the knowledge of variability of drug targets and the influence of this variability on pharmacogenetics. In the long run, one can foresee that choice and dose of drugs will be increasingly determined by an individual's genes. Such influence of genetics on the therapeutic use of drugs will shape much of medicine, meaning that we can expect an increased, genetically based individualization of medicine.

REFERENCES

Aarons L: Pharmacokinetic and pharmacodynamic modelling in drug development. Stat Methods Med Res 1999; 8:181–182.

Anderson RJ, Jackson BL, Liebentritt DK: Human platelet thermostable phenol sulfotransferase from blacks and whites: biochemical properties and variations in thermal stability. J Lab Clin Med 1988; 112:773–783.

Apriletti JW, Ribeiro RD, Wagner RL, Feng W, Webb P, Kushner PJ, West BL, Nilsson S, Scanlan TS, Fletterick RJ, et al.: Molecular and structural biology of thyroid hormone receptors. Clin Exp Pharmacol Physiol Suppl 1998; 25:2–11.

Arranz MJ, Munro J, Owen MJ, Spurlock G, Sham PC, Zhao J, Kirov G, Collier DA, Kerwin RW: Evidence for association between polymorphisms in the promotor and coding regions of the *5-HT2A* receptor gene and response to clozapine. Mol Psychiatry 1998a; 3:61–66a.

Arranz MJ, Munro J, Sham P, Kirov G, Murray RM, Collier DA, Kerwin RW: Meta-analysis of studies on genetic variation in 5-HT2A receptors and clozapine response. Schizophr Res 1998b; 27:93–99b.

Aszalos A, Ross DD: Biochemical and clinical aspects of efflux pump relates resistance to anti-cancer drugs. Anticancer Research 1998; 18:2937–2944.

Aviv A, Aladjem M: Essential hypertension in blacks: epidemiology, characteristics, and possible roles of racial differences in sodium, potassium, and calcium regulation. Cardiovasc Drugs Ther 1990; 4(Suppl 2):335–342.

Ball S, Borman N: Pharmacogenetics and drug metabolism. Nat Biotechnol 1997; 15:925–926.

Barnes PJ: Anti-inflammatory actions of glucocorticoids: molecular mechanisms. Clin Sci (Colch) 1998; 94:557–572.

Bertilsson L, Kalow W: Interethnic differences in drug disposition and effects. In: Pacifici GM, Pelkonen O (eds). Interindividual Variability in Drug Metabolism in Man. London: Taylor and Francis, 2001:15–74.

Beutler E, Gelbart T, Demina A: Racial variability in the UDP-glucuronosyltransferase 1 (UGT1A1) promoter: a balanced polymorphism for regulation of bilirubin metabolism? Proc Natl Acad Sci USA 1998; 95:8170–8174.

Birkett JT, Arranz MJ, Munro J, Osbourn S, Kerwin RW, Collier DA: Association analysis of the *5-HT5A* gene in depression, psychosis and antipsychotic response. Neuroreport 2000; 26:2017–2020.

Bonicke R, Reif W: Enzymatische inaktivierung von isonicotinsaure-hydrazid im menschlichen und tierischen organismus. Arch Exp Path U Pharmakol Bd 1953; 220: 321–333.

Boobis AR, Edwards RJ, Adams DA, Davies DS: Dissecting the function of cytochrome P450. Br J Clin Pharmacol 1996; 42:81–89.

Brewer GJ: Annotation: Human ecology, an expanding role for the human geneticist. Am J Hum Genet 1971; 23:92–94.

Brinkmann U, Eichelbaum M: Polymorphisms in the ABC drug transporter gene *MDR1*. Pharmacogenomics J 2001; 1:59–64.

Brockmoller J, Kirchheiner J, Meisel C, Roots I: Pharmacogenetic diagnostics of cytochrome P450 polymorphisms in clinical drug development and in drug treatment. Pharmacogenomics 2000; 1:125–151.

Bunzel R, Blumcke I, Cichon S, Normann S, Schramm J, Propping J, Nothen MM: Polymorphic imprinting of the serotonin-2A (*5-HT2A*) receptor gene in human adult brain. Brain Res Mol Brain Res 1998; 15:90–92.

Calabrese EJ, Canada AT: Catalase: its role in xenobiotic detoxification. In: Kalow W (ed). Pharmacogenetics of Drug Metabolism. New York: Pergamon, 1992:397–410.

Canada AT, Calabrese EJ: Superoxide dismutase: its role in xenobiotic detoxification. In: Kalow W (ed). Pharmacogenetics of Drug Metabolism. New York: Pergamon, 1992:383–396.

Carmona GN, Jufer RA, Goldberg SR, Gorelick DA, Greig NH, Yu QS, Cone EJ, Schindler CW: Butyrylcholinesterase accelerates cocaine metabolism: in vitro and in vivo effects in nonhuman primates and humans. Drug Metab Dispos 2000; 28:367–371.

Cascorbi I, Brockmoller J, Roots I: A C4887A polymorphism in exon 7 of human *CYP1A1*: population frequency, mutation linkages, and impact on lung cancer susceptibility. Cancer Res 1996; 56:4965–4969.

Chen H, Yan GC, Gishizky ML: Identification of structural characteristics that contribute to a difference in antiapoptotic function between human insulin and insulin-like growth factor 1 receptors. Cell Growth Differ 1998; 9:939–947.

Cichon S, Nothen MM, Rietschel M, Propping P: Pharmacogenetics of schizophrenia. Am J Med Genet 2000; 97:98–106.

Crespi CL: Functional characterization of the catalytic properties of CYP2D6*10-A common CYP2D6 allele in Asians. Presented at the International Business Communications (IBC) 4th International Conference on Pharmacogenomics/Pharmacogenetics, 1998. Philadelphia, June 15–16.

Daly AK, Brockmoller J, Broly F, Eichelbaum M, Evans WE, Gonzalez FJ, Huang JD, Idle JR, Ingelman-Sundberg M, Ishizaki T, et al.: Nomenclature for human *CYP2D6* alleles. Pharmacogenetics 1996; 6:193–201.

Denborough MA, Lovell RRH: Anaesthetic deaths in a family. Lancet 1960; 2:45.

Dengler VHJ, Eichelbaum M: Polymorphismen und defekte des arzneimittelstoffwechsels als ursache toxischer reaktionen. Arzneimittelforschung 1977; 27:1836–1844.

Diasio RB: The role of dihydropyrimidine dehydrogenase (DPD) modulation in 5-FU pharmacology. Oncology (Huntingt) 1998; 12:23–27.

Diasio RB: Clinical implications of dihydropyrimindine dehydrogenase on 5-FU pharmacology. Oncology (Huntingt) 2001; 15:21–26.

Droll K, Bruce-Mensah K, Otton SV, Gaedigk A, Sellers EM, Tyndale RF: Comparison of three *CYP2D6* probe substrates and genotype in Ghanaians, Chinese and Caucasians. Pharmacogenetics 1998; 8:325–333.

Endrenyi L: Pharmacokinetics. In: Kalant H, Roschlau WHE (eds). Principles of Medical Pharmacology. New York: Oxford University Press, 1998:55–66.

Evans DAP, McLeod HL, Pritchard S, Tariq M, Mobarek A: Interethnic variability in human drug responses. Drug Metab Dispos 2001; 29:606–610.

Fernandez-Salguero P, Hoffman SMG, Cholerton S, Mohrenweiser H, Raunio H, Rautio A, Pelkonen O, Huang J, Evans WE, Idle JR, et al.: A genetic polymorphism in coumarin 7-hydroxylation: sequence of the human *CYP2A* genes and identification of variant *CYP2A6* alleles. Am J Hum Genet 1995; 57:651–660.

Fisher MB, Vandenbranden M, Findlay K, Burchell B, Thummel KE, Hall SD, Wrighton SA: Tissue distribution and interindividual variation in human UDP-glucuronosyltransferase activity: relationship between *UGT1A1* promoter genotype and variability in a liver bank. Pharmacogenetics 2000; 10:727–739.

Folkers GE, van der Burg B, van der Saag PT: Promoter architecture, cofactors, and orphan receptors contribute to cell-specific activation of the retinoic acid receptor beta2 promoter. J Biol Chem 1998; 27:32200–32212.

Freeman TR: Pharmacogenetics and pharmacogenomics: using genetic information to guide therapeutic decision making. J Am Pharm Assoc (Wash) 2001; 41:475–476.

Freis ED: Antihypertensive agents. In: Kalow W, Goedde HW, Agarwal DP (eds). Ethnic Differences in Reactions to Drugs and Xenobiotics. New York: Alan R. Liss, 1986:313–322.

Fretland AJ, Leff MA, Doll MA, Hein DW: Functional characterization of human *N*-acetyltransferase 2 (NAT2) single nucleotide polymorphisms. Pharmacogenetics 2001; 11:207–215.

Garrod AE: Inborn Factors in Disease: An Essay. New York: Oxford University Press, 1931.

Grant DM, Goodfellow GH, Sugamori K, Durette K: Pharmacogenetics of the human arylamine *N*-acetyltransferases. Pharmacology 2000; 61:204–211.

Grant DM, Hughes NC, Janezic SA, Goodfellow GH, Chen HJ, Gaedigk A, Yu VL, Grewal R: Human acetyltransferase polymorphisms. Mutat Res 1997; 376:61–70.

Grant DM, Spielberg SP: Genetic regulation of drug metabolism. In: Polin RA, Fox WW (eds). Fetal and Neonatal Physiology. Philadelphia: WB Saunders, 1998:161–169.

Hafkemeyer P, Dey S, Ambudkar SV, Hrycyna CA, Pastan I, Gottesman MM: Contribution to substrate specificity and transport of nonconserved residues in transmembrane domain 12 of human P-glycoprotein. Biochemistry 1998; 17:16400–16409.

Hahn RA: The state of federal health statistics on racial and ethnic groups. JAMA 19992; 267:268–271.

Haldane JBS: Disease and evolution. Ricerca Sci 1949; 19:68–75.

Hein DW, McQueen CA, Grant DM, Goodfellow GH, Kadlubar FF, Weber WW: Pharmacogenetics of the arylamine *N*-acetyltransferases: a symposium in honor of Wendell W. Weber. Drug Metab Dispos 2000; 28:1425–1432.

Hodgson J, Marshall A: Pharmacogenomics: will the regulators approve? Nat Biotechnol 1998; 16:243–246.

Houseman D, Ledley FD: Why pharmacogenomics? Why now? Nat Biotechnol 1998; 16:492–493.

Hughes HB, Biehl JP, Jones AP, Schmidt LH: Metabolism of isoniazid in man as related to the occurrence of peripheral neuritis. Am Rev Tuberculosis 1954; 70:266–273.

Ingelman-Sundberg M: Implications of polymorphic cytochrome P450-dependent drug metabolism for drug development. Drug Metab Dispos 2001; 29:570–573.

Inoue K, Yamazaki H, Imiya K, Akasaka S, Guengerich FP, Shimada T: Relationship between *CYP2C9* and *2C19* genotypes and tolbutamide methyl hydroxylation and *S*-mephenytoin 4′-hydroxylation activities in livers of Japanese and Caucasian populations. Pharmacogenetics 1997; 7:103–113.

Jensen FS, Nielsen LR, Schwartz M: Detection of the plasma cholinesterase K variant by PCR using an amplification-created restriction site. Hum Hered 1996; 46:26–31.

Johnson JA: Influence of race or ethnicity on pharmacokinetics of drugs. J Pharm Sci 1997; 86:1328–1333.

Jonsson EG, Nothen MM, Gustavsson JP, Neidt H, Forslund K, Mattila-Evenden M, Rylander G, Propping P, Asberg M: Lack of association between dopamine D_4 receptor gene and personality traits. Psychol Med 1998; 28:985–989.

Kalow W: Familial incidence of low pseudocholinesterase level. Lancet 1956; 2:576–577.

Kalow W: Pharmacogenetics. Heredity and the Response to Drugs. Philadelphia: WB Saunders, 1962.

Kalow W: The metabolism of xenobiotics in different populations. Can J Physiol Pharmacol 1982; 60:1–12.

Kalow W: Ethnic differences in drug metabolism. Clin Pharmacokinet 1982b; 7:373–400.

Kalow W: Pharmacoanthropology: drug metabolism. Federation Proc 1984; 43:2326–2331.

Kalow W: Interethnic variation of drug metabolism. Trends Pharmacol Sci 1991; 12: 102–107.

Kalow W: Pharmacoanthropology and the genetics of drug metabolism. In: Kalow W (ed). Pharmacogenetics of Drug Metabolism. International Encyclopedia of Pharmacology and Therapeutics, Sect 137. New York: Pergamon, 1992:865–877.

Kalow W: Interethnic differences in drug response. In: Kalow W, Meyer UA, Tyndale R (eds). Pharmacogenomics. New York: Marcel Dekker, 2001a.

Kalow W: Pharmacogenetics in perspective. Drug Metab Dispos 2001b; 29:468–470.

Kalow W, Bertilsson L: Interethnic factors affecting drug response. Adv Drug Res 1994; 25:1–59.

Kalow W, Britt BA, Terreau ME, Haist C: Metabolic error of muscle metabolism after recovery from malignant hyperthermia. Lancet 1970; 2:895–898.

Kalow W, Endrenyi L, Inaba T, Kadar D, Tang BK: Pharmacogenetic investigation of amobarbital disposition. In: Duchene-Marullaz P (ed). Advances in Pharmacology and Therapeutics. New York: Pergamon, 1978a:31–40b.

Kalow W, Goedde HW, Agarwal DP (eds). Ethnic Differences in Reactions to Drugs and Xenobiotics. New York: Alan R. Liss, 1986.

Kalow W, Tang BK, Endrenyi L: Hypothesis: comparisons of inter- and intra-individual variations can substitute for twin studies in drug research. Pharmacogenetics 1998; 8:283–289.

Kalow W, Tang BK, Kadar D, Inaba T: Distinctive patterns of amobarbital metabolites in man. Clin Pharmacol Ther 1978b; 24:576–582a.

Kelsey KT, Ross D, Traver RD, Christiani DC, Zuo ZF, Spitz MR, Wang M, Xu X, Lee BK, Schwartz BS, et al.: Ethnic variation in the prevalence of a common NAD(P)H quinone oxidoreductase polymorphism and its implications for anticancer chemotheraphy. Br J Cancer 1997; 76:852–854.

Kim RB, Wilkinson GR: Pharmacogenetics of drug transporters. In: Kalow W, Meyer UA, Tyndale RF (eds). Pharmacogenomics. New York: Marcel Dekker, 2001:81–108.

Kletzien RF, Harris PK, Foellmi LA: Glucose-6-phosphate dehydrogenase: a "housekeeping" enzyme subject to tissue-specific regulation by hormones, nutrients, and oxidant stress. FASEB J 1994; 8:174–181.

Kudzma EC: Drug response: all bodies are not created equal. Am J Nursing 1992; 92:48–50.

Larsen AK, Escargueil AE, Skladanowsi A: Resistance mechanisms associated with altered intracellular distribution of anticancer agents. Pharmacol Ther 2000; 85:217–229.

Lee EJD, Wong JYY, Yeoh PN, Gong NH: Glutathione *S*-transferase-1 (GSTT1) genetic polymorphism among Chinese, Malays and Indians in Singapore. Pharmacogenetics 1995; 5:332–334.

Levesque E, Beaulieu M, Green MD, Tephly TR, Belanger A, Hum DW: Isolation and charactertization of UGT2B15(Y85): a UDP-glucuronosyltransferase encoded by a polymorphic gene. Pharmacogenetics 1997; 7:317–325.

Levesque E, Beaulieu M, Hum DW, Belanger A: Characterization and substrate specificity of UGT2B4 (E458): a UDP-glucuronosyltransferase encoded by a polymorphic gene. Pharmacogenetics 1999; 9:207–216.

Lichter JB, Barr CL, Kennedy JL, Van Tol HH, Kidd KK, Livak KJ: A hypervariable segment in the human dopamine receptor D_4 (DRD_4) gene. Hum Mol Genet 1993; 2:767–773.

Lifton RP: Molecular genetics of human blood pressure variation. Science 1996; 272:676–680.

Lin HJ, Han CY, Bernstein DA, Hsiao W, Lin BK, Hardy S: Ethnic distribution of the glutathione transferase Mu 1-1 (*GSTM1*) null genotype in 1473 individuals and application to bladder cancer susceptibility. Carcinogenesis 1994; 15:1077–1081.

Lin HJ, Probst-Hensch NM, Hughes NC, Sakamoto GT, Louie AD, Kau IH, Lin BK, Lee DB, Lin J, Frankl HD, et al.: Variants of *N*-acetyltransferase NAT1 and a case-control study of colorectal adenomas. Pharmacogenetics 1998; 8:269–281.

Lin JH, Lu AY: Interindividual variability in inhibition and induction of cytochrome P450 enzymes. Annu Rev Pharmacol Toxicol 2001; 41:535–567.

Lin KM, Poland RE, Nakasaki G (eds): Psychopharmacology and Psychobiology of Ethnicity. Progress in Psychiatry 39. Washington DC: American Psychiatric Press, 1993.

Lockridge O, Masson P: Pesticides and susceptible populations: people with butyrylcholinesterase genetic variants may be at risk. Neurotoxicology 2000; 21:113–126.

Lu Z, Zhang R, Diasio RB: Population characteristics of hepatic dihydropyrimidine dehydrogenase activity, a key metabolic enzyme in 5-fluorouracil chemotherapy. Clin Pharmacol Ther 1995; 58:512–522.

Mackenzie PI, Miners JO, McKinnon RA: Polymorphisms in UDP glucuronosyltransferase genes: functional consequences and clinical relevance. Clin Chem Lab Med 2000; 38:889–892.

MacLennan DH, Phillips MS: Malignant hyperthermia. Science 1992; 256:789–794.

MacLennan DH, Phillips MS: The role of the skeletal muscle ryanodine receptor (*RYR1*) gene in malignant hyperthermia and central core disease. In: Society of General Physiologists (ed). Ion Channels and Genetic Diseases. New York: Rockefeller University Press, 1995:89–100.

Mahgoub A, Dring LG, Idle JR, Lancaster R, Smith RL: Polymorphic hydroxylation of debrisoquine in man. Lancet 1977; 2:584–586.

Marez D, Legrand M, Sabbagh N, Lo Guidice JM, Spire C, Lafitte JJ, Meyer UA, Broly F: Polymorphism of the cytochrome P450 *CYP2D6* gene in a European population: characterization of 48 mutations and 53 alleles, their frequencies and evolution. Pharmacogenetics 1997; 7:193–202.

Marshall A: Laying the foundations for personalized medicines. Nat Biotechnol 1997; 15:954–957.

Masellis M, Basile V, Meltzer HY, Lieberman JA, Savy S, Macciardi FM, Cola P, Howard A, Badri F, Nothen MM, et al.: Serotonin subtype 2 receptor genes and clinical response to clozapine in schizophrenia patients. Neuropsychopharmacology 1998; 19:123–132.

Masellis M, Basile VS, Meltzer HY, Lieberman JA, Sevy S, Goldman DA, Hamblin MW, Macciardi FM, Kennedy JL: Lack of association between the T $\rightarrow$ C 267 serotonin 5-HT_6 receptor gene (*HTR6*) polymorphism and prediction of response to clozapine in schizophreniza. Schizophr Res 2001; 15:49–58.

Mattila KM, Rinne JO, Roytta M, Laippala P, Pietila T, Kalimo H, Koivula T, Frey H, Lehtimaki T: Dipeptidyl carboxypeptidase 1 (*DCP1*) and butyrylcholinesterase (*BCHE*) gene interactions with the apolipoprotein E epsilon4 allele as risk factors in Alzheimer disease and in Parkinson's disease with coexisting Alzheimer pathology. J Med Genet 2000; 37:766–770.

Meyer UA: Overview of enzymes of drug metabolism. J Pharmacokinet Biopharm 1996; 24:449–459.

Meyer UA, Zanger UM: Molecular mechanisms of genetic polymorphisms of drug metabolism. Annu Rev Pharmacol Toxicol 1997; 37:269–296.

Mitchell SC, Zhang AQ, Barrett T, Ayesh R, Smith RL: Studies on the discontinuous *N*-oxidation of trimethylamine among Jordanian, Ecuadorian and New Guinean populations. Pharmacogenetics 1997; 7:45–50.

Motulsky AG: Drug reactions, enzymes, and biochemical genetics. JAMA 1957; 165:835–837.

Muglia P, Jain U, Macciardi F, Kennedy JL: Adult attention deficit hyperactivity disorder and the dopamine D_4 receptor gene. Am J Med Genet 2000; 12:273–277.

Nishida Y, Fukuda T, Yamamoto I, Azuma J: *CYP2D6* genotypes in a Japanese population: low frequencies of *CYP2D6* gene duplication but high frequency of *CYP2D6*10*. Pharmacogenetics 2000; 10:567–570.

Niznik H, Tyndale R, Sallee F, Gonzalez F, Hardwick J, Inaba T, Kalow W: The dopamine transporter and cytochrome P450IID1 (debrisoquine 4-hydroxylase) in brain: resolution and identification of two distinct [^{3}H]GBR-12935 binding proteins. Arch Biochem Biophys 1990; 276:424–432.

Okey AB: Enzyme induction in the cytochrome P-450 system. In: Kalow W (ed). Pharmacogenetics of Drug Metabolism. International Encyclopedia of Pharmacology and Therapeutics, Sect 137. New York: Pergamon, 1992:549–608.

Ozdemir V, Naranjo CA, Herrmann N, Reed K, Sellers E, Kalow W: Paroxetine potentiates the central nervous system side effects of perphenazine: contribution of cytochrome P4502D6 inhibition in vivo. Clin Pharmacol Ther 1997; 62:334–347.

Patel M, Tang BK, Grant DM, Kalow W: Interindividual variability in the glucuronidation of (*S*) oxazepam constrated with that of (*R*) oxazepam. Pharmacogenetics 1995; 5:287–297.

Persidis A: The business of pharmacogenomics. Nat Biotechnol 1998a; 16:209–210.

Persidis A: Industry trends. Biotechnology in 1998 and beyond. Nat Biotechnol 1998b; 16:1378–1379.
Petronis A: The genes for major psychosis: aberrant sequence or regulation? Neuropsychopharmacology 2000; 23:1–12.
Propping P, Nothen MM: Genetic variation of CNS receptors—a new perspective for pharmacogenetics. Pharmacogenetics 1995; 5:318–325.
Riddick DS: Drug biotransformation. In: Kalant H, Rochlau WHE (eds). Principles of Medical Pharmacology. New York: Oxford University Press, 1998:38–54.
Ronai Z, Szekely A, Nemoda Z, Lakatos K, Gervai J, Staub M, Sasvari-Szekely M: Association between novelty seeking and the −521 C/T polymorphism in the promoter region of the *DRD₄* gene. Mol Psychiatry 2001; 6:35–38.
Rosner GL, Muller P: Bayesian population pharmacokinetic and pharmacodynamic analyses using mixture models. J Pharmacokinet Biopharm 1997; 25:209–233.
Seedat YK: Hypertension in black South Africans. J Hum Hypertens 1999; 13:96–103.
Seeman P, Van Tol HHM: Dopamine receptors. Trends Pharmacol Sci 1994; 15:264–270.
Shi MM, Bleavins MR, De De La Iglesia FA: Pharmacogenetic application in drug development and clinical trials. Drug Metab Dispos 2001; 29:591–595.
Shibuta K, Abe M, Suzuki T: A new detection method for the K variant of butyrylcholinesterase based on PCR primer introduced restriction analysis (PCR-PIRA). J Med Genet 1994; 31:576–579.
Smith DA: Pharmacokinetics and pharmacodynamics in toxicology. Xenobiotica 1997; 27:513–525.
Smith MW, Mendoza RP: Ethnicity and pharmacogenetics. Mt Sinai J Med 1996; 63:285–290.
Sommers DK, Moncrieff J, Avenant J: Non-correlations between debrisoquine and metoprolol polymorphism in the Venda. Hum Toxicol 1989; 8:365–368.
Sun H, El Yazal J, Lockridge O, Schopfer LM, Brimijoin S, Pang YP: Predicted Michaelis-Menten complexes of cocaine-butyrylcholinesterase. Engineering effective butyrylcholinesterase mutants for cocaine detoxication. J Biol Chem 2001; 23:9330–9336.
Tarnawski AS, Jones MK: The role of epidermal growth factor (EGF) and its receptor in mucosal protection, adaptation to injury, and ulcer healing: involvement of EGF-R signal transduction pathways. J Clin Gastroenterol 1998; 27:12–20.
Van Tol H, Wu C, Guan HC, Ohara K, Bunzow JR, Civelli O, Kennedy J, Seeman P, Niznik HB, Jovanovic V: Multiple dopamine D_4 receptor variants in the human population. Nature 1992; 358:149–152.
Van Tol HM: Structural and functional characteristics of the dopamine D_4 receptor. Adv Pharmacol 1998; 42:486–490.
Vesell ES, Page JG: Genetic control of drug levels in man: antipyrine. Science 1968; 161:72–73.
Vogel F: Moderne Probleme der Humangenetik. Ergeb Inner Med Kinderheilkunde. 1959; 12:65–126.
Weber WW: Pharmacogenetics. New York: Oxford University Press, 1997.
Weber WW: Pharmacogenetics—receptors. In Kalow W, Meyer UA, Tyndale RF (eds). Pharmacogenomics. New York: Marcel Dekker, 2001:51–80.
Weinshilboum RM, Otterness DM, Szumlanski CL: Methylation pharmacogenetics: catechol *O*-methyltransferase, thriopurine methyltransferase, and histamine *N*-methyltransferase. Annu Rev Pharmacol Toxicol 1999; 39:19–52.
Weyler W, Hsu Y-PP, Breakefield XO: Biochemistry and genetics of monoamine oxidase. In: Kalow W (ed). Pharmacogenetics of Drug Metabolism. New York: Pergamon, 1992:333–366.
Winkleby MA, Ragland DR, Syme SL, Fisher JM: Heightened risk of hypertension among black males: the masking effects of covariables. Am J Epidemiol 1988; 128:1075–1083.
Wood AJ: Ethnic differences in drug disposition and response. Ther Drug Monit 1998; 20:525–526.
Wood AJ, Zhou HH: Ethnic differences in drug disposition and responsiveness. Clin Pharmacokinet 1991; 20:350–373.
Woolhouse NM, Eichelbaum M, Oates NS, Idle JR, Smith RL: Dissociation of coregulatory control of debrisoquin/phenformin and sparteine oxidation in Ghanaians. Clin Pharmacol Ther 1985; 37:512–521.
Yue Q, Säwe J: Interindividual and interethnic differences in codeine metabolism. In: Kalow W (ed). Pharmacogenetics of Drug Metabolism. International Encyclopedia of Pharmacology and Therapeutics, Sect 137. New York: Pergamon, 1992:721–727.
Yue QY, Svensson JO, Sawe J, Bertilsson L: Codeine metabolism in three Oriental populations: a pi Plot study in Chinese, Japanese and Koreans. Pharmacogenetics 1994; 5:173–177.
Zhou HH, Sheller JR, Nu H, Wood M, Wood AJ: Ethnic differences in response to morphine. Clin harmacol Ther 1993; 54:507–513.

INDEX

Page numbers followed by f and t indicate figures and tables, respectively.